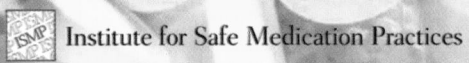

Institute for Safe Medication Practices

ISMP's List of *Error-Prone Abbreviations, Symbols,* and *Dose De...*

D0516462

Dose Designations and Other Information	Intended Meaning	Misinterpretation	Correction
Drug name and dose run together (especially problematic for drug names that end in "l" such as Inderal40 mg; Tegretol300 mg)	Inderal 40 mg Tegretol 300 mg	Mistaken as Inderal 140 mg Mistaken as Tegretol 1300 mg	
Numerical dose and unit of measure run together (e.g., 10mg, 100mL)	10 mg 100 mL	The "m" is sometimes mistaken as a zero or two zeros, risking a 10- to 100-fold overdose	Place adequate space between the dose and unit of measure
Abbreviations such as mg. or mL. with a period following the abbreviation	mg mL	The period is unnecessary and could be mistaken as the number 1 if written poorly	Use mg, mL, etc. without a terminal period
Large doses without properly placed commas (e.g., 100000 units; 1000000 units)	100,000 units 1,000,000 units	100000 has been mistaken as 10,000 or 1,000,000; 1000000 has been mistaken as 100,000	Use commas for dosing units at or above 1,000, or use words such as 100 "thousand" or 1 "million" to improve readability

Drug Name Abbreviations	Intended Meaning	Misinterpretation	Correction
ARA A	vidarabine	Mistaken as cytarabine (ARA C)	Use complete drug name
AZT	zidovudine (Retrovir)	Mistaken as azathioprine or aztreonam	Use complete drug name
CPZ	Compazine (prochlorperazine)	Mistaken as chlorpromazine	Use complete drug name
DPT	Demerol-Phenergan-Thorazine	Mistaken as diphtheria-pertussis-tetanus (vaccine)	Use complete drug name
DTO	Diluted tincture of opium, or deodorized tincture of opium (Paregoric)	Mistaken as tincture of opium	Use complete drug name
HCl	hydrochloric acid or hydrochloride	Mistaken as potassium chloride (The "H" is misinterpreted as "K")	Use complete drug name unless expressed as a salt of a drug
HCT	hydrocortisone	Mistaken as hydrochlorothiazide	Use complete drug name
HCTZ	hydrochlorothiazide	Mistaken as hydrocortisone (seen as HCT250 mg)	Use complete drug name
MgSO4**	magnesium sulfate	Mistaken as morphine sulfate	Use complete drug name
MS, MSO4**	morphine sulfate	Mistaken as magnesium sulfate	Use complete drug name
MTX	methotrexate	Mistaken as mitoxantrone	Use complete drug name
PCA	procainamide	Mistaken as patient controlled analgesia	Use complete drug name
PTU	propylthiouracil	Mistaken as mercaptopurine	Use complete drug name
T3	Tylenol with codeine No. 3	Mistaken as liothyronine	Use complete drug name
TAC	triamcinolone	Mistaken as tetracaine, Adrenalin, cocaine	Use complete drug name
TNK	TNKase	Mistaken as "TPA"	Use complete drug name
ZnSO4	zinc sulfate	Mistaken as morphine sulfate	Use complete drug name

Stemmed Drug Names	Intended Meaning	Misinterpretation	Correction
"Nitro" drip	nitroglycerin infusion	Mistaken as sodium nitroprusside infusion	Use complete drug name
"Norflox"	norfloxacin	Mistaken as Norflex	Use complete drug name
"IV Vanc"	intravenous vancomycin	Mistaken as Invanz	Use complete drug name

Symbols	Intended Meaning	Misinterpretation	Correction
ʒ	Dram	Symbol for dram mistaken as "3"	Use the metric system
℞	Minim	Symbol for minim mistaken as "mL"	
x3d	For three days	Mistaken as "3 doses"	Use "for three days"
> and <	Greater than and less than	Mistaken as opposite of intended; mistakenly use incorrect symbol; "< 10" mistaken as "40"	Use "greater than" or "less than"
/ (slash mark)	Separates two doses or indicates "per"	Mistaken as the number 1 (e.g., "25 units/10 units" misread as "25 units and 110 units)	Use "per" rather than a slash mark to separate doses
@	At	Mistaken as "2"	Use "at"
&	And	Mistaken as "2"	Use "and"
+	Plus or and	Mistaken as "4"	Use "and"
°	Hour	Mistaken as a zero (e.g., q2° seen as q 20)	Use "hr," "h," or "hour"

**These abbreviations are included on TJC's "minimum list" of dangerous abbreviations, acronyms and symbols that must be included on an organization's "Do Not Use" list, effective January 1, 2004. Visit www.jointcommission.org for more information about this TJC requirement.

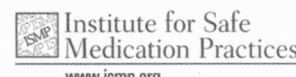

Institute for Safe Medication Practices
www.ismp.org

© ISMP 2006

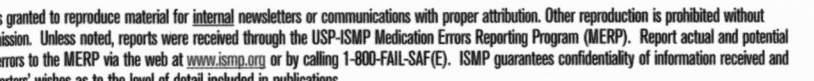

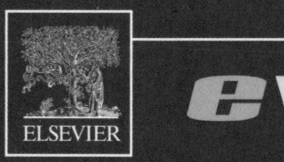

Medical-Surgical Nursing

NURSING

Clinical Management for Positive Outcomes

MEDICAL-SURGICAL
NURSING
Clinical Management for Positive Outcomes

EIGHTH EDITION

Joyce M. Black,

PhD, RN, CPSN, CWCN, FAPWCA

Associate Professor
College of Nursing
University of Nebraska Medical Center
Omaha, Nebraska

Jane Hokanson Hawks,

DNSc, RN, BC

Professor of Nursing
Midland Lutheran College
Fremont, Nebraska

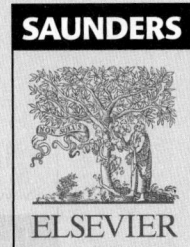

SAUNDERS

ELSEVIER

SAUNDERS
ELSEVIER

11830 Westline Industrial Drive
St. Louis, Missouri 63146

MEDICAL-SURGICAL NURSING
Clinical Management for Positive Outcomes

ISBN: 978-1-4160-3641-8 (Single Volume)
978-4160-4687-5 (Two-Volume Set)

Notice

Knowledge and best practice in this field are constantly changing. As new research and experience broaden our knowledge, changes in practice, treatment and drug therapy may become necessary or appropriate. Readers are advised to check the most current information provided (i) on procedures featured or (ii) by the manufacturer of each product to be administered, to verify the recommended dose or formula, the method and duration of administration, and contraindications. It is the responsibility of the practitioner, relying on their own experience and knowledge of the patient, to make diagnoses, to determine dosages and the best treatment for each individual patient, and to take all appropriate safety precautions. To the fullest extent of the law, neither the Publisher nor the Authors assume any liability for any injury and/or damage to persons or property arising out of or related to any use of the material contained in this book.

The Publisher

Previous editions copyrighted 2005, 2001, 1997, 1993, 1987, 1980, 1974.

Library of Congress Control Numbers: 2008922504 (Single Volume)
2008922503 (Two-Volume Set)

Executive Publisher: Tom Wilhelm
Managing Editor: Maureen Iannuzzi
Senior Developmental Editor: Jennifer Ehlers
Publishing Services Manager: Deborah L. Vogel
Design Direction: Louis Forgione

Printed in the United States of America

Last digit is the print number: 9 8 7 6 5 4 3 2 1

When I walked into the hospital, I used to see a sign that said, "Enter in to learn, go forth to serve." Therefore this book is dedicated to those patients and students who taught me the value of caring and teaching, and I hope they can serve others through my efforts here. I continue to appreciate the quiet contributions and support of my colleagues. And I thank my family—Steve, Jon, Katy, and Tricia, and my newest family members, Katie, Josh, and Elly—for their ongoing understanding of the considerable strain on my time and energy.

— J.M.B.

To the clients, nurses, students, and faculty I learned and continue to learn from; to my parents, Esther and the late Charles Hokanson, who laid the foundation for my role as a nurse, author, editor, speaker, and educator; and to my husband, Edward, and my daughter, Jennifer, whose love, support, and understanding remain constant.

— J.H.H.

About the Authors

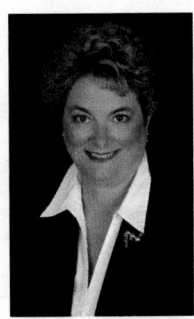

Joyce M. Black, PhD, RN, CPSN, CWCN, FAPWCA, is an Associate Professor of Nursing at the University of Nebraska Medical Center, College of Nursing, in Omaha, Nebraska. She teaches medical-surgical nursing to junior- and senior-level nursing students. Dr. Black also teaches advanced pathophysiology to graduate students. Dr. Black received her Doctor of Philosophy degree from the University of Nebraska Medical Center; her Master of Science in Nursing degree and Clinical Nurse Specialist designation from the University of Nebraska Medical Center; her Bachelor of Science in Nursing degree from Winona State University in Winona, Minnesota; and her Associate's degree in Nursing from Rochester Community College in Rochester, Minnesota.

Dr. Black has had several years of clinical experience as a medical-surgical nurse at Saint Mary's Hospital in Rochester, Minnesota, which is affiliated with the Mayo Clinic. Her clinical practice has been in orthopedics, critical care, burn care, respiratory diseases, wound care, and plastic surgery. She is certified by the Wound, Ostomy and Continence Nurses Society and the American Society of Plastic Surgical Nurses. She is also a Fellow in the American Professional Wound Care Association. Dr. Black is the immediate past president of the National Pressure Ulcer Advisory Panel. She was chairperson of the NPUAP task force to update the stages of pressure ulcers and co-chairperson of the deep tissue injury task force. Her primary research expertise is in the area of deep tissue injury, pressure ulcers, and wound healing.

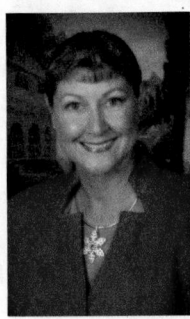

Jane Hokanson Hawks, DNSc, RN, BC, is a Professor of Nursing and Interim Nursing Department Chairperson at Midland Lutheran College in Fremont, Nebraska. She teaches students in medical-surgical nursing, advanced medical-surgical nursing, trends and issues, and nursing management. Dr. Hawks received her Doctorate in Nursing Science in collegiate nursing education from Widener University in Chester, Pennsylvania; her Master of Science in Nursing degree in medical-surgical nursing and nursing administration from the University of Nebraska Medical Center College of Nursing in Omaha, Nebraska; and her Bachelor of Science in Nursing degree from St. Olaf College in Northfield, Minnesota.

Dr. Hawks has worked in and has taught medical-surgical nursing for more than 30 years. She has practiced in a variety of areas, including critical care, renal transplantation, orthopedics, general surgery, and urology. She serves as the editor of *Urologic Nursing.* Her areas of research include empowerment, mentoring, nursing education, active teaching strategies, and alcoholism. She and her colleagues developed the NANDA nursing diagnosis Altered Family Process: Alcoholism (now known as Dysfunctional Family Processes: Alcoholism). Dr. Hawks co-authored *Mentoring for Mission: Nurturing New Faculty at Church-Related Colleges,* which was funded through a grant from the Lilly Fellows Foundation.

Section Editors

Robert G. Carroll, PhD
Professor
Department of Physiology
Brody School of Medicine
East Carolina University
Greenville, North Carolina

Susanne A. Quallich, BS, BSN, MSN, APRN, BC, NP-C, CUNP
Adjunct Faculty
University of Michigan School of Nursing
Andrology Nurse Practitioner
Division of Andrology and Microsurgery
Department of Urology
University of Michigan Medical Center
Ann Arbor, Michigan

Contributors

Donna M. Barker, MS, APRN, ANP-BC, ONC, RN-C
Pain Management Nurse Practitioner
St. Alexius Medical Center
Hoffman Estates, Illinois

Francie Bernier, PhD(c), RNC
Doctoral Candidate
University of Virginia
School of Nursing
Charlottesville, Virginia;
Principal Clinical Research Scientist
Hollister Incorporated
Libertyville, Illinois

Meg Blair, RN, MSN, CEN, PhD(c)
Associate Professor
Nebraska Methodist College of Nursing and Allied Health
Omaha, Nebraska

Lisa Bowman, MSN, RN, CRNP, CNRN
Nurse Practitioner
Division of Cerebrovascular Disease and Neurological Critical Care
Thomas Jefferson University Hospital
Philadelphia, Pennsylvania

Robert G. Carroll, PhD
Professor
Department of Physiology
Brody School of Medicine
East Carolina University
Greenville, North Carolina

Gretchen J. Carrougher, RN, MN
Research Nurse Supervisor
Department of Surgery
University of Washington Burn Center at Harborview
    Medical Center
Seattle, Washington;
Clinical Instructor
Department of Biobehavioral Nursing and Health Systems
University of Washington School of Nursing
Seattle, Washington

'Lissa D. Clark, BS, BSN, MSN, CNE
Instructor, Adult Health and Illness Department
College of Nursing
University of Nebraska Medical Center
Omaha, Nebraska

Linda Carman Copel, PhD, APRN BC, NCC, DAPA
Associate Professor
Villanova University
Villanova, Pennsylvania

Melissa Craft, RN, PhD, AOCN
Adjunct Clinical Professor
University of Oklahoma
Oklahoma City, Oklahoma;
Oncology Clinical Nurse Specialist
Breast Imaging of Oklahoma
Edmond, Oklahoma

Sherill Nones Cronin, PhD, RN, BC
MSN Program Director and Professor of Nursing
Bellarmine University
Louisville, Kentucky;
Consultant
Baptist Hospital East
Louisville, Kentucky

Beth F. Crowder, BSN, MNSc, PhD, RN, APN
Advanced Practice Nurse
Little Rock Cardiology Clinic
Little Rock, Arkansas

Susan L. Dean-Baar, RN, PhD, CRRN, FAAN
Associate Dean for Academic Affairs
University of Wisconsin–Milwaukee
Milwaukee, Wisconsin

Marie A. DeFrancesco-Loukas, MSN, CRNP
Nurse Practitioner; Clinical Manager
GoodNights Urgent Care
Hershey, Pennsylvania;
Pediatric Inpatient Nurse Practitioner
Harrisburg Hospital
Harrisburg, Pennsylvania

Jean E. DeMartinis, PhD, APRN-BC, FNP
Associate Professor and Director DNP and CNL Graduate
    Programs
School of Nursing
University of Massachusetts–Amherst
Amherst, Massachusetts

Margaret M. Ecklund, RN, MS, CCRN, APRN-BC
Clinician VI/Nurse Practitioner
Rochester General Hospital
Rochester, NY

Charlotte Eliopoulos, PhD, RNC, MPH, ND
Executive Director
American Association for Long Term Care Nursing
Glen Arm, Maryland

James A. Fain, PhD, RN, BC-ADM, FAAN
Dean and Professor, College of Nursing
University of Massachusetts-Dartmouth
North Dartmouth, Massachusetts

Kathryn Fiandt, DNS, FAANP
Professor and Associate Dean for Clinical Affairs
University of Texas Medical Branch
Galveston, Texas

Nancy J. Girard, RN, PhD, FAAN
Associate Professor and Chair
Acute Nursing Care Department
University of Texas Health Science Center-San Antonio
School of Nursing
San Antonio, Texas

Patricia E. Graham, MSN, RN, BC
Assistant Professor
Department of Nursing Education
Morningside College
Sioux City, Iowa

**Mikel Gray, PhD, FNP, PNP, CUNP, CCCN,
FAAN, FAANP**
University of Virginia
Department of Urology and School of Nursing
Charlottesville, Virginia

Sheila A. Haas, PhD, RN, FAAN
Professor
Niehoff School of Nursing
Loyola University Chicago
Chicago, Illinois

Diana P. Hackbarth, RN, PhD, FAAN
Professor
Niehoff School of Nursing
Loyola University Chicago
Chicago, Illinois

Judith S. Halpern, MS, NP, APRN, BC
Lecturer, RN Studies
School of Nursing
University of Michigan
Kalamazoo, Michigan

Allen Hanberg, RN, MSN, PhD(c)
Assistant Professor
Clinical College of Nursing
University of Utah
Salt Lake City, Utah

Karen Hanson, RN, MS, CNP
Gastroenterology Nurse Practitioner
Mayo Clinic
Rochester, Minnesota

Debra E. Heidrich, MSN, RN, ACHPN, AOCN
Palliative Care Clinical Nurse Specialist
Bethesda North Hospital, TriHealth, Inc.
Cincinnati, Ohio

Lianne F. Herbruck, MSN, RN, CNM
Health Care Consultant and Nursing Educator
Chagrin Falls, Ohio

Patricia A. Keresztes, RN, PhD, CCRN
Assistant Professor of Nursing
Saint Mary's College
Notre Dame, Indiana;
Staff Nurse, Cardiovascular Intensive Care Unit
Memorial Hospital
South Bend, Indiana

Helene J. Krouse, PhD, APRN, BC, CORLN, FAAN
Professor of Nursing
Wayne State University
Detroit, Michigan

**Judi L. Kuric, PhD, MSN, RN, APRN-BC,
CRRN-A, CNRN**
Adjunct Assistant Professor
University of Southern Indiana
Acute Care Nurse Practitioner
Tri State Neurosurgical, Inc.
Evansville, Indiana

Sharon Lanzetta, MSN, RN, C
Ambulatory Care Nurse Manager
University of Michigan Health System
Ann Arbor, Michigan

Joan M. Lappe, PhD, RN, FAAN
Criss/Beirne Endowed Chair in Nursing and Professor
  of Medicine
Creighton University
Omaha, Nebraska

Mira Lessick, PhD, RN
Associate Professor
The University of Toledo
College of Nursing
Toledo, Ohio

Patricia A. MacDonald, RN, NP
Senior Clinical Research Specialist
TAP Pharmaceutical Products, Inc.
Lake Forest, Illinois

Patricia A. Manion, RN, MS, CCRN, CEN
Trauma Program Administrator
Genesys Regional Medical Center
Grand Blanc, Michigan

Karen S. Martin, MSN, RN, FAAN
Health Care Consultant
Martin Associates
Omaha, Nebraska

Norma D. McNair, MSN, RN, CCRN, CNRN, APRN-BC
Assistant Clinical Professor
University of California-Los Angeles School of Nursing
Neuroscience Clinical Nurse Specialist
University of California-Los Angeles Medical Center
Los Angeles, California

Anita Meehan, MSN, RN, ONC, CNOR(e)
Clinical Nurse Specialist
Medical/Surgical and Gerontology
Akron General Medical Center
Akron, Ohio;
Clinical Faculty
Kent State University College of Nursing
Kent, Ohio
University of Akron College of Nursing
Akron, Ohio

Lindsay A. Middelton, BSN, CGC
Genetic Counselor and Senior Research Nurse
Urologic Oncology Branch
National Institutes of Health
National Cancer Institute
Bethesda, Maryland

Kim Miracle, MSN, RN, C
Clinical Coordinator
Quality Care and Outcomes Management Department
Jewish Hospital
Louisville, Kentucky

Anita E. Molzahn, PhD, MN, BScN
Professor
School of Nursing
University of Victoria
Victoria, British Columbia
Canada

Diana Moxness, RN, BSN, MSN
Assistant Professor
Department of Nursing
Midland Lutheran College
Fremont, Nebraska

Mark Moyad, MD, MPH
Phil F. Jenkins Director of Complementary Medicine
Urologic Oncology
Clinical Cancer Researcher/Consultant
University of Michigan
Ann Arbor, Michigan

Dawn P. Murphy, MSN, CRNP
Oncology Nurse Practitioner
Abramson Cancer Center
Hospital of The University of Pennsylvania
Philadelphia, Pennsylvania

Louise Nelson LaFramboise, RN, PhD
Director, Undergraduate Program
University of Nebraska Medical Center
Omaha, Nebraska

Susan Newton, RN, MS, AOCN, AOCNS
Oncology Advanced Practice Nurse
Project Leader, Innovex
Dayton, Ohio

Noreen Heer Nicol, MS, RN, FNP
Clinical Senior Instructor
University of Colorado
Denver, Colorado;
Affiliate Assistant Professor
University of Northern Colorado
Greeley, Colorado;
Chief Clinical Officer/Chief Nursing Officer
National Jewish Medical and Research Center
Denver, Colorado

Catherine Nosek, PhD, RN
Associate Professor
Undergraduate Nursing Education
Winona State University
Winona, Minnesota

Barbara B. Ott, RN, PhD
Associate Professor
Villanova University
Villanova, Pennsylvania

Mary Ellen Pike, RN, MSN, MA, PhD(c)
Assistant Professor
Bellarmine University
Louisville, Kentucky

Susanne A. Quallich, BS, BSN, MSN, APRN, BC, NP-C, CUNP
Adjunct Faculty
University of Michigan School of Nursing
Andrology Nurse Practitioner
Division of Andrology and Microsurgery
Department of Urology
University of Michigan Medical Center
Ann Arbor, Michigan

Sharon R. Redding, MN, RN, CNE
Associate Professor of Nursing
College of Saint Mary
Omaha, Nebraska

Dottie Roberts, MSN, MACI, RN, CMSRN, OCNS-C
Clinical Nurse Specialist
Palmetto Health Baptist
Columbia, South Carolina

Vicki M. Ross, RN, PhD
Graduate Faculty/Research Assistant Professor
University of Kansas School of Nursing
Kansas City, Kansas

Charlie Sandidge, RN, BSN, MN, CWCN
Registered Nurse, Burn Center
Harborview Medical Center
University of Washington
Seattle, Washington

Susan A. Sandstrom, MSN, RN, BC, CNE
Associate Professor in Nursing
College of Saint Mary
Omaha, Nebraska

CDR Linda M. Scott, CRNP
Nurse Practitioner
National Institute of Allergy and Infectious Diseases
Laboratory of Allergic Diseases
National Institutes of Health
Bethesda, Maryland

Clare M. Sekerak, MSN, APRN, BC, NP-C, CNRN
Nurse Practitioner
Neurosurgery
Veterans Administration Ann Arbor Healthcare System
Ann Arbor, Michigan

Nancy Christine Shoemaker, APRN-PMH, BC
Nurse Psychotherapist
University of Maryland Fayette Street Clinic;
Associate Faculty
University of Maryland School of Nursing
Baltimore, Maryland

Mary Sieggreen, MSN, APRN, BC, NP, CVN
Associate Clinical Professor
Wayne State University;
Nurse Practitioner, Vascular Surgery
Harper University Hospital
Detroit Medical Center
Detroit, Michigan

Karen A. Sikorski, MS, BSN, APN
Clinical Nurse Specialist, Pain
OSF Saint Anthony Medical Center
Rockford, Illinois

Terran Warren Sims, MSN, ACNP-C, COCN, CNN
Nurse Practitioner, ACNP-C
Genitourinary Oncology
Hematology/Oncology and Urology
University of Virginia Health System;
Course Preceptor/Lecturer
Acute Care Nurse Practitioner
Wound, Ostomy, and Continence Programs
University of Virginia School of Nursing
Charlottesville, Virginia

Sarah C. Smith, RN, MA, CRNO, COA
Medical/Surgical Nursing Division
Department of Ophthalmology
University of Iowa Hospitals & Clinics
Iowa City, Iowa

Dianne M. Smolen, PhD, CNE, RNBC, CNS
Professor
College of Nursing
The University of Toledo
Toledo, Ohio

Christina Stewart-Amidei, MSN, RN, CNRN, CCRN, CS
Instructor
University of Central Florida
Orlando, Florida

Cynthia M. Sublett, DNSc, RN
Adjunct Faculty
Xavier University
Cincinnati, Ohio

Peggy Ward-Smith, RN, PhD
Associate Professor
University of Missouri–Kansas City
School of Nursing
Kansas City, Missouri

Mary Wcisel, RN, MSN
Associate Professor of Nursing
Saint Mary's College
Notre Dame, Indiana

Carol J. Weber, RN, BSN, MSN, PhD
Professor and Chair, Online Nursing Program
Regis University
Denver, Colorado

Bernadette White, RN, MSN, APRNc, CHTP
Assistant Professor
Creighton University School of Nursing
Nurse Practitioner
Creighton University Oncology/Hematology Clinic
Omaha, Nebraska

Lynn White, MSN, CCRN, APRN, BC
Assistant Professor
Augustana College
Sioux Falls, South Dakota;
Clinical Nurse Specialist
Avera McKennan Transplant Institute
Sioux Falls, South Dakota

Connie White-Williams, RN, MSN, FAAN
Cardiothoracic Transplant Coordinator
University of Alabama at Birmingham
Birmingham, Alabama

Linda H. Yoder, RN, MBA, PhD, AOCN, FAAN
Associate Professor
Director, Nursing Systems Graduate Program
Luci Baines Johnson Fellow in Nursing
University of Texas–Austin
School of Nursing
Austin, Texas

Nancy L. York, PhD, RN
Assistant Professor of Nursing
University of Nevada-Las Vegas
Las Vegas, Nevada

Reviewers

Katrina D. Allen, RN, MSN, CCRN
Faulkner State Community College
Bay Minette, Alabama

Daria U. Amato, MSN, RN, CNE
Springfield, Virginia

Rebecca S. Appleton, RN, PhD
Marshall University
Huntington, West Virginia

Susan D. Arbogast, RN, MS
Maricopa Community College
Sun City, Arizona

Meg Blair, RN, MSN, CEN, PhD(c)
Nebraska Methodist College of Nursing and
  Allied Health
Omaha, Nebraska

Therese M. Bower, EdD, RN, MSN, CNS, CNE
Firelands Regional Medical Center School of
  Nursing
Sandusky, Ohio

Donna J. Bowles, EdD, MSN, RN, CNE
Indiana University Southeast
New Albany, Indiana

Lavoy Bray, Jr., RN, Med
Southside Regional Medical Center
  Professional Schools
Petersburg, Virginia

Patricia Louise Brown, RN, MN, PhD
Kansas Wesleyan University
Salina, Kansas

Michele Bunning, RN, MSN
Good Samaritan College of Nursing & Health
  Sciences
Cincinnati, Ohio

Catherine M. Concert, RN, MS, APRN, BC,
  FNP
Wyckoff Heights Medical Center & Long Island
  University
Brooklyn, New York

Claire Cottrell, RN, MSN
Mississippi Gulf Coast Community College
Perkinston, Mississippi

Judy A. Criner, PhD, RN
Germantown, Maryland

Mary F. Crowely, MS, RN
Regis College
Weston, Massachusetts

Sheryl L. Currie, RN, MN
Butler Community College
El Dorado, Kansas

Patricia Delmoe, RN, MN
Boswell/Mesa Nursing Education Program
Sun City, Arizona

R. Eric Doerfler, NP, MSN, AAHIVS
The Pennsylvania State University School of
  Nursing
Harrisburg, Pennsylvania

Sharon Kay Evans-Bernard, APRN-BC
The Hospital of Saint Raphael
New Haven, Connecticut

Kathleen Walsh Free, MSN, RN-C, ARNP-BC
Indiana University Southeast
New Albany, Indiana

Richard Freedberg, RN, MSN, MPA
Lansing Community College
Lansing, Michigan

Toni J. Galvan, RN, MSN, CNS, CCRN, CEN
Texas Tech University Health Sciences Center
  School of Nursing
Lubbock, Texas

Karen Heys, MN, RN
Everett Community College
Everett, Washington

Michelle N. Hough, MS, RN
Massachusetts Bay Community College
Framingham, Massachusetts

Donna Walker Hubbard, MSN, RN, CNN
University Mary Hardin-Baylor
Belton, Texas

Jaclynn A. Johnson, RNC, MSN
Otero Junior College/Arkansas Valley Regional
  Medical Center
La Junta, Colorado

Juanita F. Johnson
Oklahoma Baptist University
School of Nursing
Shawnee, Oklahoma

Leah Kelly
Jackson, New Jersey

Maria Lasater, RN, MSN, CCRN, CNRN
Texas County Technical Institute
Houston, Missouri

Gavin O'Connor, MS
Ozarks Technical Community College
Springfield, Missouri

Cynthia K. Olson, RN, MSN, C-FNP
Riverland Community College
Austin, Minnesota

Shelly Orr, RN, BS, MSN
Southside Regional Medical Center School of
  Nursing
Petersburg, Virginia

Stacey L. Rosenberg
Riverland Community College
Austin, Minnesota

Janet E. Shimek, RN, MSN, MSEd,
  CCRN, CNE
Carroll Community College
Westminster, Maryland

Fernisa Sison, MSN, RN, FNP
San Joaquin Delta College
St. Joseph's Medical Center
Lodi Hospital
Pacific Heart & Vascular
Stockton, California

In revising this textbook to keep pace with the rapidly evolving field of nursing, a perennial dilemma for us has been deciding which advancements to include in each new edition. As important new evidence-based protocols and guidelines have been issued, new legislation has taken effect, and our knowledge base has expanded in areas such as genetics, pain management, and wound healing, we've broadened our coverage to encompass each major development. Students and instructors alike have told us that even with many excellent resources available online, including those that accompany this book, they still want a reliable, comprehensive print reference. Yet as every experienced nursing instructor knows, students who are struggling to absorb the core concepts underlying this complex field can become overwhelmed by too much detail.

In this eighth edition of *Medical-Surgical Nursing: Clinical Management for Positive Outcomes*, we believe we've achieved just the right balance by offering thorough coverage in all key areas yet maintaining a constant focus on what the student needs to know. Though streamlined in design and content to approximately 2,200 pages, this eighth edition remains the most comprehensive medical-surgical nursing text in the field. It provides a solid foundation in anatomy and physiology, pathophysiology, medical management, and nursing care for the full spectrum of adult health conditions.

A key theme of this edition is evidence-based practice. Throughout the text, an integrated icon system continually highlights evidence-based content and clinical guidelines. These icons, which link in-text citations to research-based references, serve as visual reminders that clinical practice must be based on peer-reviewed research evidence and established clinical guidelines. In addition, *Translating Evidence into Practice* boxes show students that evidence-based practice is not simply an academic exercise—it's a practical way of improving measurable outcomes, such as preventing falls, ventilator-associated pneumonia, and endocarditis. To further underscore the text's evidence-based practice orientation, all Complementary and Alternative Therapy boxes report findings from research studies, many of which are randomized, controlled trials.

Another important strength of the book is its clear delineation of various healthcare professionals' roles in managing each disorder. Within each topic, nursing management is clearly identified and organized by assessment, diagnosis, desired outcome, interventions, and evaluation, allowing students to see how the nurse's actions dovetail with those of the other members of the healthcare team.

Critical thinking skills have been emphasized throughout the eighth edition, including a new chapter in Unit 1 entirely devoted to the topic. Once again, the focus is evidence based and practical. The chapter explains how sharpening their critical thinking skills can help nurses determine the significance of diagnostic findings, for example, or ensure early identification of complications ranging from dehydration to transplant rejection.

PHILOSOPHY AND APPROACH

This textbook grew out of the belief that nurses and physicians do not compete with each other but instead collaborate to reach certain outcomes in cooperation with the client and family. Nonetheless, nursing and medicine are separate disciplines and are not intermingled in this text. However, because it is often difficult for nursing students to understand one without understanding the other, we present thorough coverage of both nursing management and medical management.

With the increased emphasis on outcomes in health care, we have organized client care under the heading of Outcome Management. Several subheadings appear under this heading, including Medical Management, Nursing Management of the Medical Client, Surgical Management, and Nursing Management of the Surgical Client, as appropriate.

In this text, we use the nursing process to describe nursing management, but we do not apply the nursing process to every disorder. Instead, we have designated the nursing process for major or prototypical disorders. Within the presentation of the nursing process for those disorders, we have developed nursing diagnoses and collaborative problems, as appropriate, with their own outcomes and interventions. Collaborative problems are defined as client problems that cannot be resolved through independent nursing actions; they are complications that may develop because of a disorder, surgical procedure, or nonsurgical treatment. Collaborative problems complete the picture of nursing care and eliminate the need to force-fit every client problem into the framework of a nursing diagnosis. We have written Outcomes and Interventions sections for *each* identified nursing diagnosis and collaborative problem because we have found from our teaching experience that students cannot easily pull apart lists of diagnoses followed by lists of outcomes and interventions and then rebuild them into care plans. Each care plan is written with the problems listed in priority order and then proceeding through the trajectory of the illness. As we know from our years of teaching, setting priorities for nursing care is a skill that students struggle to master.

ORGANIZATION

This edition is organized from simple to complex and from common to uncommon disorders. The early portion of the text focuses on the care of clients usually assigned to beginning students. The book then progresses to address the care of clients with more complex disorders, which are more commonly taught in upper-division classes. Within each chapter, we begin with the most important diseases for students to grasp; this organization stems from our belief that students often trim their reading time to prioritize the most essential material. We believe that by placing the most important information first, we encourage students to read it first.

Although the text retains its familiar 18-unit format, the assessment chapters in the disorders units have been streamlined and significantly modified using simple yet innovative visual diagrams to present clinical manifestations, review-of-systems information, and standard diagnostic work-ups for many common problems, such as hematuria, anemia, and dyspnea. These concise algorithms complement the text by offering at-a-glance summaries of practical information, such as what questions to ask the client during a GI assessment and what diagnostic studies may be ordered when kidney stones are suspected. Developed in response to reviewers' suggestions, the diagrams are especially useful as study tools for today's visual learners and as quick refreshers in the clinical setting.

The first five units in the book are devoted to content that is applicable to all medical-surgical clients. The material in this first portion of the book will guide the student in learning to provide comprehensive care regardless of the specific diagnosis or problem. Concepts that span medical-surgical practice, such as health promotion, care delivery settings, physical assessment, complementary and alternative therapies, fluid and electrolyte balance, genetics, infectious diseases, pain, palliative care, perioperative care, and oncology, are found in this portion of the book. The remainder of the text, beginning with Unit 6, is divided into common

responses to health disorders. Each unit begins with a review of anatomy and physiology, followed by a chapter on health and diagnostic assessment; one or more chapters then present the nursing care of clients with specific disorders. A brief description of each unit is given below.

Unit 1 introduces the essential principles of health promotion and disease prevention (Chapter 1), such as wellness, health literacy, self-care, injury prevention, and early detection of illness. A thoroughly updated chapter on health assessment (Chapter 2) focuses on a hospital-based assessment rather than a comprehensive assessment and provides an introduction to the revised assessment format used throughout the text. A new chapter on Critical Thinking (Chapter 3; see "New Features" on p. xxii) provides a solid foundation in the increasingly important skill of thinking critically in order to provide high-level nursing care. We have approached critical thinking as a science and have provided foundational material for students to apply in the clinical setting. Chapter 4 discusses why people choose alternative therapies and considers how to discuss complementary and alternative therapies with clients.

Unit 2 presents an overview of health care delivery systems, allowing students to become oriented to care in various settings. Chapters 5 through 10 address nursing care in ambulatory care, acute care, critical care, home health care, long-term care, and rehabilitation settings.

Unit 3 explores the foundations of care for medical-surgical clients, including separate chapters on fluid and electrolyte imbalances (Chapters 11 and 12), acid-base disorders (Chapter 13), and perioperative care (Chapter 14).

Unit 4 discusses physiologic concepts basic to medical-surgical nursing care. The unit begins with a look at the field of genetics (Chapter 15) and continues with chapters related to cancer (Chapters 16 and 17), wound healing (Chapter 18), and infectious disease, including expanded information about bioterrorism (Chapter 19).

Unit 5 covers psychosocial concepts basic to medical-surgical nursing care. The unit begins with a chapter on pain management (Chapter 20) and continues with chapters on palliative care (Chapter 21), sleep and rest disorders (Chapter 22), psychosocial and mental health concerns (Chapter 23), and substance abuse (Chapter 24).

Units 6 through 17 focus on the management of clients with specific disorders. Each unit begins with an overview of the structure and function of pertinent body systems. These anatomy and physiology reviews are complemented by many new pieces of full-color artwork. Next, the unit progresses to chapters on assessment and nursing care. As mentioned earlier, the assessment chapters in the disorders units now feature concise, innovative diagrams to present clinical manifestations, review-of-systems information, and standard diagnostic work-ups for the most common problems students will encounter in daily practice. These algorithms encapsulate the assessment process and summarize critical diagnostic pathways for conditions such as neurologic pain and sensory impairments, musculoskeletal derangements, and reproductive disorders. This efficient new format puts essential information at students' fingertips for quick reference and study. In Unit 8, for example, new content related to management of chronic kidney disease has been added to Chapter 35, which concerns renal disorders. In Unit 11, author Joyce Black offers her own cutting-edge research on pressure ulcers in a chapter on managing clients with integumentary disorders (Chapter 49). In Unit 13, chronic stable heart failure is explained in Chapter 56, and STEMI versus NSTEMI is addressed in Chapter 58.

In general, the discussion of specific disorders includes section headings for Etiology, Pathophysiology, Clinical Manifestations, and Outcome Management. The etiology topics in the disorders chapters focus on health promotion, maintenance, and restoration. Within the Outcome Management sections, students are linked back to the pathophysiology of the disorder. These linkages help the student to connect the concepts of pathophysiology and the treatments used to reverse or control the pathophysiology.

Unit 18 presents the care of clients with multisystem disorders. Chapter 80 examines organ donation issues, the transplantation process, quality-of-life questions, and specific interventions for clients requiring organ transplantation. Shock and multisystem disorders are discussed in Chapter 81. Chapter 82 introduces the basic concepts of triage, ethical issues, and maintaining the chain of custody of medicolegal evidence. This chapter organizes emergency conditions according to the various nursing diagnoses identified and treated.

HALLMARK FEATURES

A completely new full-color design focuses on guiding the reader to the Evolve website, where a wealth of supplemental content resides. Each chapter opens with a list of web enhancements, which introduces the reader to that chapter's features on the Evolve website. Many of the web features—including those that begin in the text and continue on the Evolve website with interactive exercises and bonus material—contain a reference within the text and are designated with a marginal icon: *evolve*

The following is a list of the book's hallmark features, including a description and the location of the feature:

- **Anatomy and Physiology Reviews** introduce each body system unit and provide a brief review of the relevant anatomy and physiology. Many new full-color illustrations depict anatomic units, such as the cell and the genetic code, and complex physiologic processes, such as the sleep cycle and the body's response to pain.

- **Bridge to Critical Care** boxes highlight major critical care concerns, such as burn injury, defibrillation, and alarm troubleshooting. This feature appears in selected chapters in the text.

- **Bridge to Home Health Care** boxes describe specific applications and strategies for medical-surgical care in the home. Some bridges appear on the Evolve website, and others remain in the text for this edition.

- **Care Plans** use the nursing process format to highlight nursing diagnoses and collaborative problems, expected outcomes, interventions with rationales, and evaluation. These problems are presented in priority order to guide nursing care decisions anywhere along the disease trajectory. For the eighth edition, NIC and NOC designations have been incorporated into the Nursing Care Plans to demonstrate the applicability of these standardized nursing taxonomies to everyday clinical practice. Some care plans appear on the Evolve website, but most remain in the text for this edition.

- **Case Studies** present complex, in-depth client scenarios, most of which feature multiple clinical problems. Each Case Study is introduced in the text, and the body of the Case Study is continued on the Evolve website, along with discussions, multiple-choice questions, and a nursing care plan.

- **Client Education Guides** use client-centered language to help students teach clients how to collaborate in their own care. Some guides appear in the text, while others are found only on the Evolve website. All Client Education Guides in the text have been translated into Spanish and appear on the Evolve website.

- **Complementary and Alternative Therapy** boxes present nontraditional therapies used by clients and health care providers to treat various conditions. They discuss alternative and complementary therapies related to specific diseases or body systems. Some boxes are featured in the text, and others appear on the Evolve website. Each box outlines the findings of specific research studies, many of which are randomized, controlled trials.

- **Concept Maps** are full-color flowcharts linking pathophysiological processes, clinical manifestations, and medical and nursing interventions. This feature appears throughout the text, and new maps are provided for liver failure and heart failure.

- **Critical Monitoring** boxes highlight clinical manifestations that must be reported to the physician without delay and, in some cases, show how critical values are calculated. This feature appears throughout the text. New Critical Monitoring features for this edition include a consensus formula for fluid resuscitation and an explanation of arterial blood gas analysis.

- **Evolve Web Enhancement** boxes on the first page of each chapter list the supplemental features that appear on the Evolve website.
- **Genetic Links** boxes link a disease, such as breast cancer or polycystic kidney disease, with its corresponding genetics. This feature provides the student with the description, genetics, diagnosis/testing, and management of a specific disease. It appears throughout the text.
- **Integrating Pharmacology** boxes help students understand how medications can be used for disease management and examine iatrogenic complications of certain drugs by exploring common classifications of medications. This feature appears throughout the text and is designed to present material on medications for clinical consideration.
- **Management and Delegation** boxes present the primary concerns nurses need to address when delegating care activities to unlicensed assistive personnel. This feature appears in the text and includes new topics such as infection control precautions.
- **Physical Assessment Findings in the Healthy Adult** serves both to remind students of the relevant normal findings for each body system and to demonstrate how to chart those findings with clinical precision. This feature appears in the text.
- **Terrorism Alert** boxes provide cutting-edge material on bioterrorism preparedness and response. They aid the student in recognizing the clinical manifestations and diseases associated with bioterrorism. This feature appears throughout the text.
- **Thinking Critically Questions** conclude each nursing care chapter. This feature presents short, typical client scenarios and poses questions about what actions to take. Discussions of all the questions, found on the Evolve website, provide insight into the reasoning behind appropriate actions.

NEW TO THIS EDITION

In addition to the hallmark features listed in the previous section, the eighth edition includes new features that underscore the book's commitment to evidence-based practice and critical thinking.

NEW FEATURES

- **Evidence-Based Practice icons** remind students that daily clinical decision making must be based on reliable research evidence.
  - *Red lamp icons* ( ) identify primary research applicable to practice interventions, especially evidence-based recommendations that supersede

previously accepted nursing knowledge (for example, Homans' sign having been proved an unreliable indicator of DVT). Corresponding references in the bibliography are highlighted in red for easy retrieval.

- *Blue lamp icons* ( ) precede standardized guidelines, protocols, and classification systems that have evolved from evidence-based practice to govern patient care. Corresponding references in the bibliography are highlighted in blue to direct readers to print media and to the web, where they can link to online journals and to resources offered by government agencies and nonprofit health care organizations.
- **Integrating Diagnostic Testing** boxes on topics such as dyspnea and pelvic pain give students examples of the laboratory and imaging studies that may be ordered during the course of a client's illness. These boxes, accompanied by brief explanations in the text, appear in most assessment chapters and in several of the disorders chapters. They help students understand which clinical manifestations prompt specific tests and what the tests identify. However, they do not unnecessarily repeat the nursing implications of each test or the typical pre- and post-testing nursing interventions, since that information is covered in assessment courses and in diagnostic testing handbooks.
- **NIC and NOC designations** have been incorporated into the Nursing Care Plans to demonstrate how these standardized nursing taxonomies are used in everyday clinical practice.
- **Safety Alert** icons identify common hospital emergencies, National Patient Safety Goals established by The Joint Commission (TJC), and TJC sentinel events.
- **Translating Evidence into Practice** boxes present a topic in the form of a clinical question and summarize the conclusions of four to five research articles. This feature shows students that evidence-based practice occurs in the care setting, not in the ivory tower, allowing nurses to improve measurable outcomes in areas such as injury prevention, infection control, and management of chronic conditions.
- **Many new pieces of full-color art** illustrate pathologic processes such as airway obstruction and osteoarthritis, products and equipment such as a voice prosthesis and types of casts, and surgical procedures such as scleral buckling.

EXPANDED AND NEW CHAPTERS

- A **thoroughly updated chapter on Health Assessment** (Chapter 2) provides an introduction to this vital skill set and introduces the assessment format used throughout the text.

- A **new chapter on Critical Thinking** (Chapter 3) provides a solid foundation in the increasingly important skill of thinking critically in order to provide high-level nursing care. The chapter explores the necessity of applying critical thinking skills to evidence-based practice and explains how mastering the principles of critical thinking can help in setting practical priorities. Case studies are used to illustrate critical thinking skills in action in various care settings.
- An **expanded infectious-disease chapter** (Chapter 19: Perspectives on Infectious Disease and Bioterrorism) now includes vital content on bioterrorism.
- A **completely revised and newly illustrated chapter on structural cardiac disorders** (Chapter 55: Management of Clients with Structural Cardiac Disorders) provides the latest information on the expected outcomes of transplantation and the related nursing care.
- An **expanded kidney disorders chapter** (Chapter 35: Management of Clients with Renal Disorders) includes a new section on chronic kidney disease management.
- **All assessment chapters have been streamlined using simple yet innovative diagrams** to summarize clinical manifestations, review-of-systems information, and critical diagnostic pathways.

ANCILLARY PACKAGE

The ancillary package supplies both instructors and students with a variety of additional resources to enhance the utility of the book. Instructors are provided with all of the tools required for a vibrant, media-rich, successful classroom experience: Instructor's Manual, Test Bank, Image Collection, PowerPoint Presentations, and iClicker Question Suite. Students are offered content enhancements such as animations, video and audio clips, and audio pronunciations. They benefit from study and testing aids such as NCLEX® Examination Style Review Questions, Open-Book Quizzes, and Chapter Review Audio Summaries. In addition, students are given the tools to promote a successful clinical experience, such as Client Education Guides.

INSTRUCTOR RESOURCES

All Student Ancillaries, as described below, are available for instructor use. In addition, the **Instructor's Electronic Resource,** available both on **CD-ROM** and on the **Evolve Resources** website at http://evolve.elsevier.com/Black/medsurg, contains an Instructor's Manual, PowerPoint Presentations, a Test Bank, an Image Collection (including all images in the text), and an iClicker Question Suite:

- The **Instructor's Manual** consists of critical points to emphasize, to facilitate student comprehension

in both the classroom and the clinical setting. Classroom exercises include Review Activities, Class Assignments, Lectures and Discussions, suggestions for Guest Speakers, Group Activities, and Concept Map Activities (where applicable). The clinical activities include Skills Laboratories, Clinical Site Activities, and Clinical Conference Activities. For this new edition, the Chapter Objectives in the Instructor's Manual have been coordinated with those in the *Study Guide* (see below) for effective student learning.

- The **PowerPoint Presentations** include more than 2,500 slides and provide instructors with lecture aids for each chapter. Illustrations from the text as well as bonus health assessment images are included in the PowerPoint Presentations.
- The electronic **Test Bank** offers approximately 2,500 questions, including more than 300 questions in multiple-select format. Each test question includes a rationale, nursing process step, cognitive level, NCLEX category of client needs, and text reference.
- The **Image Collection** consists of more than 800 full-color images.
- **NEW!** The iClicker Question Suite contains more than 325 questions, covering topics for every chapter in the book. These questions are designed to elicit curiosity and motivate students for a dynamic classroom experience.

The **Evolve Course Management System** is an interactive learning environment that works in coordination with *Medical-Surgical Nursing: Clinical Management for Positive Outcomes,* eighth edition, to provide Internet-based course management tools you can use to reinforce and expand on the concepts you deliver in class. You can use the Evolve website to do the following:

- Publish your class syllabus, outline, and lecture notes
- Set up "virtual office hours" and e-mail communication
- Share important dates and information through the online class *Calendar*
- Encourage student participation through *Chat Rooms* and *Discussion Boards*

STUDENT RESOURCES

Student CD-ROM
The **Companion CD-ROM** for students includes the following resources:

- **Audio Pronunciations**
- **NEW! 3-D Animations** illustrating pathophysiology, drug actions, and medical treatments
- **Health Assessment Video Clips**
- **Health Assessment Audio Clips**
- **Assessment Finding Photographs**

- **Bonus Features**, including Bridges to Home Health Care; Care Plans; Case Management boxes; Clinical Pathways; discussions of Complementary and Alternative Therapy, Diversity in Health Care, and Ethical Issues; and selected tables and illustrations
- Discussions of the **Thinking Critically** questions in the text, offering students the opportunity to compare their responses to those of the authors

Student Resources on the Evolve Website

The **Evolve Resources** website, available at http://evolve. elsevier.com/Black/medsurg, contains a wealth of student assets. Students are encouraged at both the beginning and the end of each chapter to take advantage of these resources, which include all of the materials on the Companion CD-ROM in addition to the following materials:

Interactive Online Resources

- **NEW! Interactive NCLEX® Examination Style Review Questions** for every chapter, with answers and rationales
- **Interactive Open-Book Quizzes,** consisting of multiple-choice, matching, and fill-in-the-blank questions for each chapter
- **Interactive Case Studies** consisting of 12 exercise sets composed of multiple-choice quizzes and care-planning activities drawn from the Case Study feature boxes in the text
- **Interactive Concept Map Creator,** a one-of-a-kind program that allows students to create customized concept maps. Students are prompted to enter the following client data: medical diagnosis, pathophysiology, risk factors, clinical manifestations, nursing diagnoses, collaborative problems, expected outcomes, and nursing interventions. The program then generates a concept map in two formats: (1) a graphic "map" that clearly illustrates the relationships among various client data and components of the nursing process, and (2) a tabular word-processing file that students can print and use to record client responses/evaluation data, thereby completing the nursing process.

Supplemental Online Resources

- **Appendices** titled "Religious Beliefs and Practices Affecting Health Care" and "A Health History Format That Integrates the Assessment of Functional Health Patterns" supplement information in the printed text.
- **Case Management** boxes, written by a practicing case manager, present key coordination and anticipatory issues under the consistent headings of Assess, Advocate, and Prevent Readmission, thus linking nursing care with client-focused case management.
- **NEW! Chapter Review Audio Summaries** supply the major teaching points of each management chapter in downloadable MP3 files.

- **Client Education Guides,** in Spanish and English, are available for selected chapters.
- **Clinical Pathways** are excerpted from actual pathways used in specific hospitals. They are accompanied by a guide to show what should occur during specific times in the pathway and how to stay on track when caring for the client.
- **Crossword Puzzles** are supplied for each chapter.
- **Diversity in Health Care** boxes are focused discussions of health and illness related to particular populations.
- **Ethical Issues in Nursing** boxes feature an ethical dilemma in the form of a question, with the discussion immediately following.
- **Fluid and Electrolyte Tutorial** is a user-friendly module that helps students master the difficult concepts of fluid and electrolyte balance and imbalance. This self-paced program includes animations to help illustrate important concepts. Its accessible, inviting user interface helps make the program easy to navigate. The program is divided into five sections: an introduction, three sections on fluid and electrolyte balance and imbalance, and a quiz section with approximately 75 questions to test students on information learned throughout the program.
- The complete **NANDA taxonomy,** a complete listing of **NIC labels,** and a complete listing of **NOC labels** have all been updated for the new edition.
- **Spanish Assessment Phrases,** for nurses who work with Spanish-speaking clients, are supplied for selected chapters.
- **WebLinks** are provided for each chapter.

Additional Resources for Students

Other student ancillaries are available separately and include the following texts:

Study Guide for Medical-Surgical Nursing: Clinical Management for Positive Outcomes, **8th edition.** Keyed chapter-by-chapter to the text, this resource provides engaging and challenging exercises in many different formats to clarify and reinforce the textbook content. The *Study Guide* is offered in a traditional print-format text and has been completely revised for this edition, offering students the opportunity to review terminology and best practices, understand theories and trends, keep drug skills sharp, and test and apply their knowledge.

Virtual Clinical Excursions for Medical-Surgical Nursing: Clinical Management for Positive Outcomes, **8th edition.** This workbook/CD-ROM package helps students prepare for the average clinical rotation by immersing them in a realistic, yet safe, virtual hospital. The VCE workbook serves as a map, providing textbook reading assignments that correspond with the software before guiding students through the CD-ROM, where they care for patients in the virtual hospital. It presents significant real-world problems that place the student in nursing situations where they can set priorities for care, collect and analyze data, prepare and administer medications, and reach conclusions about complex and changing problems. Using multiple information sources (such as an Electronic Patient Record, Charts, a Medication Administration Record, and a Drug Guide), students make connections between what they experience in the virtual hospital and what they have learned in the text, creating a true-to-life, hands-on, multimedia learning experience.

ACKNOWLEDGMENTS

To our surprise, the preparation of this text has never become routine from one edition to the next. As medical-surgical nursing has evolved, we've only quickened our own step to see that the text keeps pace with the exciting and often momentous developments in this dynamic field. Many people have walked this path with us. Our contributing authors have led the way by lending broad clinical expertise in their respective areas of specialization. We continue to be impressed by the depth of their knowledge, the scope of their experience, and most of all, their enthusiasm for sharing it with students. Likewise, our reviewers are dedicated scholars and educators whose suggestions and comments have helped us sharpen our focus and present each topic with precision and clarity.

We would also like to thank the publishing professionals who, once again, have turned our extensively revised manuscript into a finished book. Barbara Nelson Cullen, our former Executive Publisher at Elsevier, encouraged us and gave her unflagging support to the project. Maureen Iannuzzi, Managing Editor, brought a keen eye for detail and helped us negotiate every bump in the road. Jennifer Ehlers, Senior Developmental Editor, developed the book's new features, kept the manuscript flowing in on schedule from the contributors, and handled the entire print and online ancillary package with finesse. Kathy Macciocca and Mary Ann Zimmerman, Editorial Assistants, dispatched every administrative task with an efficiency we truly appreciate. Louis Forgione, Design Director, is responsible for the bold new look that makes each page attractive and inviting. Deborah Vogel, Publishing Services Manager, and her team shepherded the manuscript through its complex production phase with an ease that could come only from experience.

Hand in hand with Elsevier, freelance editor Beth Welch overlooked nothing in copyediting the text to make it straightforward and user friendly. Melissa Kinsey and Monica Groth Farrar, of Nicholson & Stillwell Publishing Services, were thorough and responsive in developing the manuscript and the new scientific art for the book. Imagineering Media Services, of Toronto, Canada, provided contemporary, accurate medical illustration work, and Top Graphics, of St. Louis, Missouri, rendered the less complex drawings cleanly and attractively. Our thanks also go to SPi Technologies for handling the mammoth task of typesetting the manuscript.

Finally, we would like to extend our heartfelt gratitude to the educators and students nationwide who allow us to walk by their side as the practice of medical-surgical nursing is passed on to a new generation of nurses.

JOYCE M. BLACK AND JANE HOKANSON HAWKS

Contents

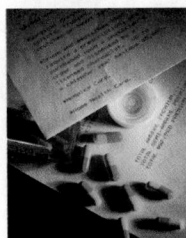

UNIT **2**
**Health Care Delivery
Systems,** 57

CHAPTER **7**

Critical Care, 84
Catherine Nosek

CHAPTER **8**

Home Health Care, 91
Karen S. Martin

CHAPTER **9**

Long-Term Care, 103
Charlotte Eliopoulos

CHAPTER **10**

Rehabilitation, 111
Susan L. Dean-Baar

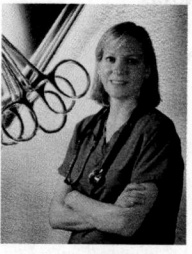

UNIT **3**
Foundations of Medical-Surgical Nursing, 119

ANATOMY AND PHYSIOLOGY REVIEW: Body Fluid Compartments and Cellular Function, 120
   Robert G. Carroll

CHAPTER **11**

Clients with Fluid Imbalances, 127
Bernadette White

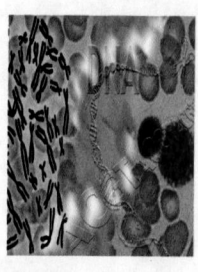

UNIT 4
Physiologic
Foundations, 229

ANATOMY AND PHYSIOLOGY REVIEW: Physiologic
Genomics, 230
  Robert G. Carroll

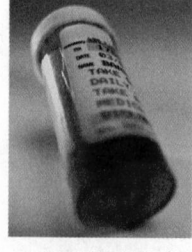

UNIT **5**

Psychosocial Foundations, 343

ANATOMY AND PHYSIOLOGY REVIEW: Arousal, Pain, and Conscious Awareness, 344

Robert G. Carroll

NEURONAL COMMUNICATION, 344

THE PHYSIOLOGY OF PAIN, 344

PAIN AS AN INTEGRATIVE EXPERIENCE, 344

Nociceptor Activation, 344

Conscious Perception of Pain, 347

Hyperalgesia, 347

CHAPTER **20**

Clients with Pain, 351

Karen A. Sikorski and Donna M. Barker

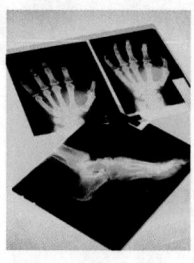

UNIT 6

Musculoskeletal Disorders, 451

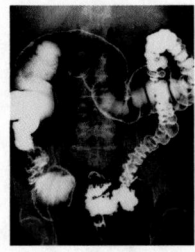

UNIT 7
Nutritional Disorders, 545

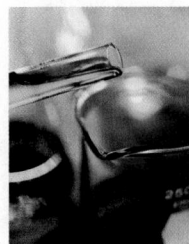

UNIT 8
Elimination Disorders, 643

CHAPTER **34**

Management of Clients with Urinary Disorders, 727
Francie Bernier and Terran Warren Sims

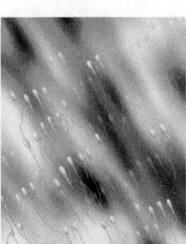

UNIT **9**

Sexuality and Reproductive Disorders, 839

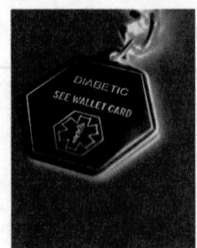

UNIT 10
Metabolic Disorders, 995

ANATOMY AND PHYSIOLOGY REVIEW: The Metabolic Systems, 996
  Robert G. Carroll

CHAPTER 42
Assessment of the Endocrine and Metabolic Systems, 1006
  Dianne M. Smolen

CHAPTER 43
Management of Clients with Thyroid and Parathyroid Disorders, 1019
  Allen Hanberg

CHAPTER **44**

Management of Clients with Adrenal and Pituitary Disorders, 1040

Allen Hanberg

CHAPTER **45**

Management of Clients with Diabetes Mellitus, 1062

James A. Fain

CHAPTER 46

Management of Clients with Exocrine Pancreatic and Biliary Disorders, 1107

Dianne M. Smolen

CHAPTER 47

Management of Clients with Hepatic Disorders, 1135

Dianne M. Smolen

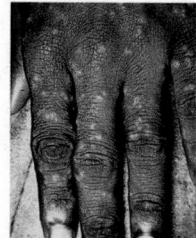

UNIT II

Integumentary Disorders, 1179

CHAPTER **50**

Management of Clients with Burn Injury, 1239

Gretchen J. Carrougher and Charles Sandidge

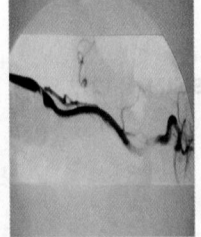

UNIT **12**

Vascular Disorders, 1271

ANATOMY AND PHYSIOLOGY REVIEW: The Vascular System, 1272

Robert G. Carroll

CHAPTER **51**

Assessment of the Vascular System, 1279

Mary Sieggreen and Susanne A. Quallich

CHAPTER **52**

Management of Clients with Hypertensive Disorders, 1290

Jean Elizabeth DeMartinis

CHAPTER **53**

Management of Clients with Vascular Disorders, 1307

Joyce M. Black

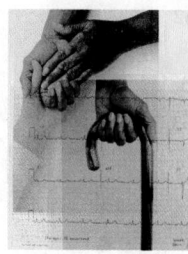

UNIT 13
Cardiac Disorders,   1341

ANATOMY AND PHYSIOLOGY REVIEW: The Heart,   1342
Robert G. Carroll

CHAPTER 54
Assessment of the Cardiac System,   1354
Beth F. Crowder

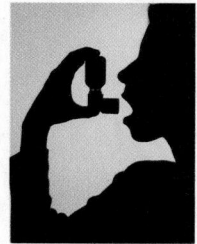

UNIT **14**

Oxygenation Disorders, 1513

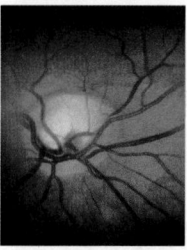

UNIT **15**
Sensory Disorders, 1667

CHAPTER **65**

Management of Clients with Visual Disorders, 1699
Sarah C. Smith

CHAPTER **66**

Management of Clients with Hearing and Balance Disorders, 1720
Helene J. Krouse

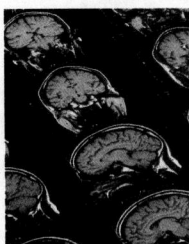

UNIT **16**

Cognitive and Perceptual Disorders, 1745

CHAPTER **67**

Assessment of the Neurologic System,   1763
Clare M. Sekerak

CHAPTER **68**

Management of Comatose or Confused Clients,   1792
Christina Stewart-Amidei

CHAPTER **69**

Management of Clients with Cerebral Disorders,   1811
Christina Stewart-Amidei

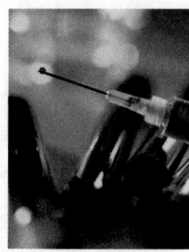

UNIT 17
Protective Disorders,   1975

CHAPTER **76**

Management of Clients with Immune Disorders, 2040

Linda M. Scott

CHAPTER **77**

Management of Clients with Rheumatic Disorders, 2053

Patricia A. MacDonald

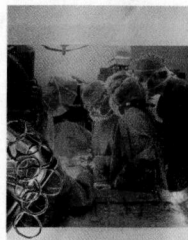

UNIT **18**
Multisystem Disorders, 2135

Special Features

GENETIC LINKS

INTEGRATING DIAGNOSTIC TESTING

INTEGRATING PHARMACOLOGY

MANAGEMENT AND DELEGATION

Physical Assessment Findings in the Healthy Adult

TERRORISM ALERT

TRANSLATING EVIDENCE INTO PRACTICE

Additional Online Content

THE FOLLOWING LEARNING TOOLS AND KEY REFERENCE CONTENT CAN BE FOUND ON THE EVOLVE WEBSITE AT

http://evolve.elsevier.com/Black/medsurg/

Audio Pronunciations for more than 250 words
Audio Clips, Animations, and Video Clips for physical examination and health assessment
Fluid & Electrolyte Module
Concept Map Creator
List of Nursing Interventions Classification (NIC) Labels
List of Nursing Outcomes Classifications (NOC) Labels
List of NANDA International Approved Nursing Diagnoses

APPENDIX A
Religious Beliefs and Practices Affecting Health Care

APPENDIX B
A Health History Format that Integrates the Assessment of Functional Health Patterns

UNIT 1

FOUNDATIONS OF PRACTICE

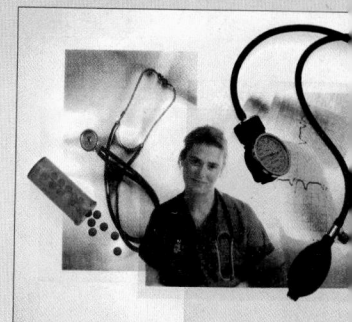

CHAPTER I

Health Promotion and Disease Prevention

KATHRYN FIANDT

It is essential that nurses be knowledgeable regarding health promotion and disease prevention. When providing holistic care, think beyond current health problems to the client's general well-being and future risks for illness or injury. As a result of the growing prevalence of chronic conditions and the related cost burden, health promotion and illness prevention are increasingly important. The emphasis of this chapter will be on health promotion and prevention of disease across the adult life span.

CONCEPT OF HEALTH AND ILLNESS

CONCEPT OF HEALTH

Nursing practice is directed and guided by an understanding of the definition of health and the factors that impact a client's health framework. The definition of health is broad and incorporates concepts of physical, mental, and social well-being. In 1947 the World Health Organization (WHO) definition of health emphasized several holistic qualities: "Health is a state of complete physical, mental, and social well-being and not merely the absence of disease or infirmity."[60] Since 1947 alternate definitions of health have been proposed. Some definitions portray health and illness on an interactive continuum, with multiple configurations ranging from depletion of health (death) to high-level wellness.[51] High-level wellness is further conceptualized as self-actualization and maximization of a person's potential. Nurses, throughout the years, have defined health in a variety of ways. Table 1-1 lists various definitions of health from nursing models. The common thread in each definition is that each person is viewed as being part of a complex, interconnected social, biologic, and environmental system.

CONCEPT OF WELLNESS

Dunn was the first to define and describe *wellness,* a term and an idea that was the precursor to the health promotion movement.[18] His now-classic definition of what he termed *high-level wellness* is "an integrated method of functioning which is oriented toward maximizing the potential of which the individual is capable within the environment where he is functioning." Dunn stressed that wellness is an ongoing process directed toward higher potential, not a static goal, and that high-level wellness is a feeling of being "alive to the tips of the fingers, with energy to burn, tingling with vitality."[18] He postulated that health professionals tend to focus on disease rather than on wellness because their training is disease focused, rather than wellness or prevention oriented. It is easier to fight against disease than to fight for a condition of greater wellness.

Travis[51] popularized the theoretical concept of wellness through development and teaching of the wellness model (Figure 1-1). The effect of this model resulted in the recognition that wellness requires attention; it does not happen automatically. The left side of the figure represents the biomedical model. The client exhibits manifestations of a disease, is treated, and is brought back to a neutral point where disease manifestations have been alleviated. In the case of chronic illness,

TABLE 1-1   Definitions of Health

Nursing Model	Definition
King's goal attainment theory	Health is a dynamic life experience. "Dynamic" implies a continuous adjustment to stressors in internal and external environments and the use of one's resources to achieve maximum potential.
Leininger's transcultural model	Health refers to "beliefs, values, and action patterns that are culturally known and used to preserve and maintain personal or group well-being, and to perform daily role activities."[23]
Levine's conservation principles	Health is defined in terms of an Anglo-Saxon word meaning "whole." Patterns of wholeness change with growth and development. Health and disease patterns reflect adaptive change.
Neuman's systems model	Health is a condition in which the parts and subparts of the whole person are in harmony.
Newman's health as expanding consciousness	Health is composed of a pattern of human-environment interaction in which the person is evolving or transforming to higher levels of consciousness characterized by new levels of understanding and decision making capacity.
Orem's self-care model	Health is a state of wholeness, including a person's parts and modes of functioning.
Pender's health promotion model	Health is a "manifestation of evolving patterns of person-environment interaction throughout the life span."[25]
Rogers' unitary person model	Health and illness are seen as expressions of the interaction of a person and the environment in the process of unfolding consciousness.
Roy's adaptation model	Health is a process or state of being and a process of becoming an integrated whole.
Watson's model of human caring	Health is more than the absence of disease. It is a harmony within the mind, body, and soul.
World Health Organization	Health is a "state of complete physical, mental, and social well-being and not merely the absence of disease or infirmity."[37]

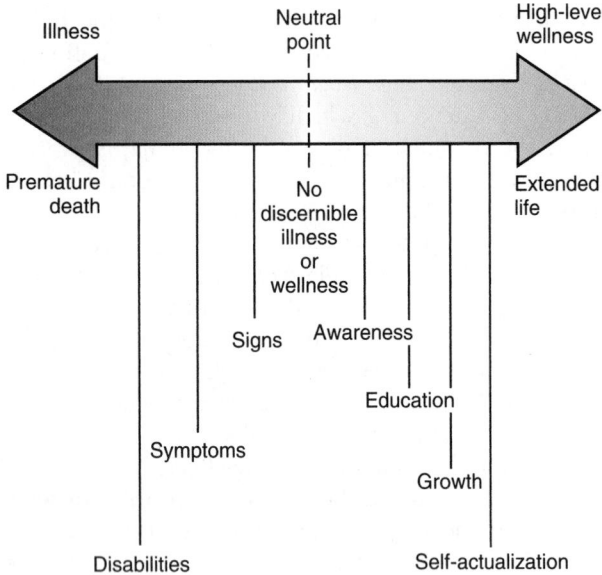

■ **FIGURE 1-1** Travis' Wellness Model.

disease manifestations are controlled and minimized. The right side represents the wellness model and the potential for high-level health and wellness. The biomedical and wellness models can work in harmony. The nurse can use the wellness model anywhere on the health-illness continuum by encouraging clients to move past the neutral point, as far toward high-level wellness as possible. For example, if clients are ill, treatment is important, but clients should not stop there. After recovery, clients should practice healthy behaviors (such as regular exercise, stress management, and eating a low-fat, balanced diet) to minimize future illnesses and progress to a higher level of wellness.

Wellness is the quality or condition of being well, even among people with chronic illness, especially of being robust, healthy, and fit. Wellness is not simply the absence of clinical manifestations; it incorporates positive mental, physical, and spiritual well-being. High-level wellness is a method of functioning oriented toward maximizing individual potential within the environment. High-level wellness involves (1) progression toward a higher level of functioning, (2) integration of the whole being, and (3) an open-ended future with the challenge of maximum potential.

CONCEPT OF DISEASE AND ILLNESS

In contrast to the concept of disease, illness has a broader meaning and includes the perception and the response of clients to the disease. Illness is a state of being with social and psychological as well as biomedical components. Illness is a disenabling response, a mismatch between a person's needs and the resources available to meet those needs; it signals that the present balance is not working.[18] A person can have a disease without feeling ill. A seemingly healthy person may have an early form of disease without clinical manifestations. For example, young adults in their teens or twenties may already have heart disease, such as atherosclerosis, without manifestations of disease. Although such people appear healthy, if they continue unhealthy habits such as smoking, eating a high-fat diet, and not exercising, the heart disease will progress until clinical manifestations appear. Similarly, injury changes the balance on the wellness continuum (see Figure 1-1). Injuries usually require treatment; after recovery or rehabilitation, people can achieve higher levels of wellness by practicing healthy behaviors.

PERCEPTION OF HEALTH

In general, today's definitions of health and wellness reflect a multidimensional, holistic, and subjective view. Individuals' personal definitions and perceptions of health must be taken into account when addressing health promotion and disease prevention. The meaning of health can be viewed in many contexts, such as historical, social, personal, scientific, philosophical, and spiritual. These meanings will always exist in the various contexts of individual human experience, are sometimes contradictory, and often overlap. Cultural ideologies and tradition also influence one's image of health.

In the nurse-client relationship, nurses respect the clients' unique psychosocial, spiritual, and cultural needs and advocate for their health choices and decisions. Nurses support client participation in the process of actualizing a defined image of health and do not negate the ability of clients to form their own image of health. They include clients' perceptions when assessing their health to understand fully the priority of their values and perceptions of these complex interactions.[33] During the course of the client's lifetime and experiences, the client's definition of health may change. Smith identified four common models of health used by our clients.[50] Because a client's model reflects the client's values, it is useful to use that perspective when working with a client in an attempt to improve health-related behavior.

Clinical Model

In this model clients consider themselves healthy if they are free from the clinical signs and symptoms of illness. Clients who function primarily in this perspective will seek out the health care system when they have a sign or symptom of a disease. Focus on improving their health status is irrelevant from their perspective but avoiding symptoms can be a motivating factor. This model is supported by the biomedical model of health and illness that is the foundation of our health care system, and it clearly fails to address many other aspects of well-being such as quality of life.

Role-Performance (Functional) Model

In this model clients consider themselves healthy if they can function well in all of their roles. Clients for whom the role-performance model is dominant will seek health care when they cannot do what they expect to be able to do. This model is common in rural communities and is typified by the farmer who seeks health care not when his knee begins to hurt, but when the pain and resultant limitations affect his ability to get up on his tractor. Clients whose dominant perspective of health is role-performance are best motivated by interventions that will improve their functional status.

Adaptive Model

Clients for whom the adaptive model is prominent define health as the ability to adapt to the expectations and challenges of the environment, both the normal day-to-day events and also the unexpected events. Challenges or changes in the environment can be physical or social; therefore adaptation can be either the biologic response to exposure to a pathogen or the social or functional response to a flat tire. More than the role-performance and clinical models of health, clients who function in the adaptive model are motivated to improve their biologic or social ability to adapt and are, therefore, motivated by interventions that will improve their health from a biologic or social perspective. For example, a harried midlife woman for whom the adaptive model is dominant and who does not take good care of herself realizes that although she feels okay and is getting through her day, she has no reserves to cope with any crisis that might develop. Building adaptive reserves might be a strong motivator for improving her lifestyle.

Eudaimonistic Model

Exuberant well-being would be one way of describing the eudaimonistic model; another would be becoming all that one is capable of becoming. The concept of high-level wellness is best seen in clients who have this perception of health. People with a eudaimonistic perception of health can also see themselves in the presence of illness and are motivated by self-actualization.

Clearly there is a great deal of interrelationship between these models. A person who generally ascribes to a eudaimonistic model of health would in all likelihood seek health care if an unusual symptom presented as would a person whose primary perception of health is adaptive. However, the models are useful in a variety of ways, perhaps most importantly to help nurses understand the values and perspectives of the clients with whom they are working. Understanding a client's perception of health helps the nurse to identify the language to use to best communicate with the client.

RELATIONSHIPS AMONG DISEASE, ILLNESS, HEALTH, AND WELLNESS

In the biomedical model, disease is identified by clinical manifestations and explained by the presence of an organic cause of a disorder. A person who has a disease has a medically defined condition similar to that suffered by others (e.g., diabetes mellitus or hepatitis). In contrast, when using a multicausal perspective to define disease, both biologic and psychological influences are important; and the interrelationship of environmental, physical, and social factors is relevant. Disease results from interacting systems at the cellular, tissue, organismal, interpersonal, and environmental levels. Disease may be defined as "the failure of a person's adaptive mechanisms to adequately counteract stimuli and stresses, resulting in functional or structural disturbances."[18]

As mentioned earlier, multicausal and biopsychosocial theories of disease causation more closely approximate reality and increase the chances of discovering factors that are amenable to intervention. See the Diversity in Health Care feature on Health and Illness Beliefs and Practices on the website.

In summary, disease, illness, health, and wellness are related concepts. Disease and health must be considered together because without disease there is no need to discuss health.[19] Disease is a state of disequilibrium, whereas health is a state of equilibrium, or balance.[18] Health and illness are dynamic patterns that change with time and social circumstances; they are not mutually exclusive. There are degrees of health and illness; clients with cancer and others with chronic diseases can achieve personal levels of wellness. Health is a resource for everyday living. High-level wellness maximizes one's potential capacity and is a component of the highest level of health.

STRATEGIES FOR PROMOTING HEALTHY BEHAVIOR

SELF-MANAGEMENT SUPPORT

Nurses tend to approach work with a client to facilitate behavior change from the perspective of health education (i.e., teaching clients and their families about health and illness). Knowledge and skills for management of health and illness are necessary but not sufficient for clients to effectively cope with their health. There is a large and evolving body of evidence that demonstrates the effectiveness of interventions a nurse can use to support a client's self-management.

One of the greatest challenges for nurses is to help their clients adopt healthy lifestyles. Although health education is foundational, there are many other effective strategies for helping clients change behaviors. These evidence-based strategies are generally called "self-management support strategies" and are based on the assumption that the client is responsible for day-to-day health-related decisions and that self-management support is aimed at helping people make the best decisions regarding their health. Although self-management support strategies have been developed based on the needs of people with chronic health problems, the same strategies can be the focus of programs to prevent a health problem. The skills needed by clients to care for themselves fall into three

categories: the first is medical or behavioral management, that is, the ability to manage the conditions of health (such as staying on a healthy diet). The second category is role management; this is the ability to make changes in life roles. An example from chronic illness would be a person with chronic lung disease who learns to move more slowly and rehabilitates to optimal function. A health promotion example would be a young woman who has recently gained 30 pounds and is now overweight; she adapts her lifestyle to include time for structured exercise and seeks more opportunities to be active. The third category of skills is affective or emotional, that is, learning to accept the illness or health challenge and to manage the emotions (such as frustration or anger) that come with the challenge.

Lorig and her colleagues have identified five self-management skills that form the core of her self-management support program. Research suggests that developing these skills can have a significant positive effect on health outcomes of people with chronic illnesses. Studies have shown that these skills are equally effective with Hispanic as well as European Americans. Nurses who understand these skills realize that knowledge of health and disease is not enough and can help clients develop the expanded skills needed to take care of themselves.[32-34]

Problem Solving

Instead of solving a problem for a client or proposing ideas for solutions, a nurse facilitating self-management support teaches a client the problem-solving process: problem identification and definition, solution options, implementation of a solution, and evaluation. The nurse who is effective in teaching this skill is not just teaching the client the concepts but is working the client through a personal problem and helping the client evaluate the outcomes. For example, when working with a client who wants to be more active, the nurse might help the client identify what the barriers to increased activity are and options for overcoming the barriers. Then the client can, with the nurse's help, develop a plan. Later the nurse will follow up with the client to evaluate the outcome and move forward.

Decision Making

When working to adopt a healthy lifestyle, clients are confronted with dozens of decisions on a daily basis. The outcome of each decision will affect their health, but more importantly, their confidence in their ability to be successful. Tools for decision making are often based on information and can include skills such as how to read a food label or how to recognize when you need to slow down in your exercise program.

Resource Utilization

There are many resources available to help the client with health-promoting lifestyle changes. These resources include social support, access to fitness facilities, and the Internet. The nurse needs to coach the client to identify possible resources and then to seek out and obtain those resources. This might be something like attending an Alcoholics Anonymous meeting, joining the local YMCA, or signing up for Weight Watchers online.

Empowered Client Role: Health Literacy

Although less common today, clients have traditionally had a great deal of respect for their health care providers and tended to defer to them without asking questions or speaking up for themselves. Even today, a client who behaves assertively is often, sadly, labeled a "difficult" client when, in fact, the client is actually empowered. The nurse can help the client learn how to be a partner in health care by strategies such as making lists of questions and reading literature about health.

Health literacy involves the ability to read, hear, comprehend, and act on health and medical information. The World Health Organization defines health literacy as ". . . the cognitive and social skills which determine the motivation and ability of individuals to gain access to, understand, and use information in ways that promote good health."[59] Low health literacy has a significant impact on clients' abilities to make effective decisions and to partner with their health care providers in their health care. Studies demonstrate that low health literacy is directly related to poorer health outcomes.[49]

Estimates of the number of people in the United States that experience some degree of health illiteracy range from one third to one half. Some groups of people are more likely to have low health literacy; these groups include people living in poverty or unemployed, older adults, and recent immigrants. Because of the prevalence of low health literacy and the significant negative impact it can have on health outcomes, nurses must devise strategies to overcome these problems. Strategies include the following: (1) use plain, lay language when talking with a client (e.g., say "high blood pressure" rather than "hypertension"); (2) limit the amount of health information provided at any one time; (3) use teach-back techniques (i.e., have the client "teach back" to you what they understood); (4) use physical diagrams whenever possible (e.g., a face on a clock for times to take medications); and (5) use written material that is at a low literacy level and visually appealing. An excellent resource for empowering a client with low health literacy is the Ask Me 3 (www.askme3.com) program. The program has downloadable brochures in English and Spanish. The program emphasizes the importance of asking 3 questions at each health encounter: (1) What is my main problem? (2) What do I need to do? (3) Why is this important?

Taking Action

All of the self-management strategies discussed thus far are the foundation for the central goal, which is to help the client take action. There are many strategies for working with clients to move to taking action; six of these strategies will be described here.

Establishing an Agenda

In a collaborative relationship, the nurse negotiates with the client to establish an agenda for an interaction based on the assumption that the client is more likely to act in response to individual values and priorities rather than those of the nurse. There are many ways to approach this. The nurse may have several ideas for an agenda and might ask the client to state which idea is most important to the client at that time, or the nurse may just ask a simple open-ended question such as, "What are you concerned about today regarding your health?"

Ask, Tell, Ask

Nurses like to teach their clients and have a great deal of information to share with them. But nurses know that cramming all the information available into an interaction is not very productive. The adult learning principle of self-directed learning is applied in the "ask, tell, ask" strategy. Using this technique, the nurse starts by asking what the client would like to learn about the topic (e.g., exercise). The client responds and the nurse can then address the information requested. The nurse would then ask if the client understood and had additional questions.

Closing the Loop

Closing the loop is a natural follow-up to the ask, tell, ask strategy and is a technique similar to "teach back." In closing the loop the client is asked to re-state the information given.

Collaborative Decision Making: Readiness to Change

Despite the logical assumption that clients are not going to change if they do not want to, nurses often do not assess a client's readiness to change as part of action planning. When working with a client to change health-related behavior, it is essential that the nurse validates that the behavior of interest is one the client truly wants to change. Readiness to change should be assessed early in the nurse-client interaction.

Transtheoretical Model of Change. The readiness to change concept comes from the Transtheoretical Model of Change (TTM).[46] The model identifies the stages of readiness to change and suggests strategies for moving clients through the change process (Table 1-2).

TABLE 1–2 Transtheoretical Model of Change

Stage	Intervention
Pre-contemplation: Client has not thought about changing behavior or has tried unsuccessfully in the past or does not want to try to change again.	Confront the client with the need to change in a personalized manner, e.g., "The shortness of breath you have is due to your smoking. You need to stop." Offer to help: "How can I help you?"
Contemplation: Client is considering change and knows that change is needed but does not know where to start; client is often anxious and lacking confidence in ability to change.	Provide encouragement and support; also acknowledge anxiety and support self-efficacy, perhaps by using an example of a change the client has made in the past.
Preparation: Client knows that change is needed but requires help with developing a plan of action.	Work with the client to develop an action plan; see Self-Management Support earlier in this chapter.
Action: Client is implementing the intended change behavior.	Provide ongoing and regular support with goal setting; see Self-Management Support earlier in this chapter.
Maintenance: Client is moving forward but remains at some risk for relapse.	Continue to support behaviors and reassure the client who relapses that this event is normal but the client needs to continue the change behavior. Support at this time is essential; the client still needs regular support or, at a minimum, occasional "booster" sessions.
Termination: New behavior has become a habit; the client has a high degree of self-confidence in maintaining the change and handling any slips or temptations.	Provide informal praise and support at encounters with the client.

From Prochaska, J.O., Norcross, J.C., & Di Clemente, C.C. (1994). *Changing for good.* New York: William Morrow and Company.

Motivational Interviewing. Another model of change based on readiness to change is Motivational Interviewing (MI).[4] Like the TTM, MI is a complex evidence-based strategy for behavior change. The basic premise of MI is that readiness to change is directly related to the importance of the change to the client and the confidence of the client in the ability to change. A nurse working with a client in health behavior change can take several key ideas from the concept of readiness to change: (1) it is essential to focus on a behavior that the client expresses an interest in changing; (2) the nurse should validate that the change being proposed is important to the client; and (3) the nurse should assess the client's level of confidence in the ability to make the change. Level of confidence can be assessed simply by asking the client, "On a scale of 1-10 with 1 = not at all and 10 = totally confident, how confident are you that you can make this change?" If clients cannot rank their confidence as 8 to 10, the nurse should ask them to consider a change that they are more confident they can make.

Collaborative Decision Making: Goal Setting

Goal setting involves the client, in negotiation with the nurse, setting a goal. The goal should be small, specific, measurable, and short term. A goal of "lose weight" is not specific and a goal of "lose 100 pounds" is not sufficiently small or short term. The goal: "I am going to walk around my block twice this week" is small, specific, measurable, and short term. After the client has set a goal the nurse should determine the client's confidence in the ability to achieve the goal (e.g., "How confident are you that you can achieve this goal this week?").

Follow-up. The final and most critical part of goal setting is follow-up. To be successful in helping a client change health behavior, the nurse must make a note of the goal and follow up with the client on a regular basis. In the case of the goal to "walk around the block 2 times this week" the nurse should call the client a week from the day the goal was set to see how the client is doing. If things went well, a new goal can be set; if the client was unable to achieve the goal, the barriers need to be discussed and the client encouraged to set a new, more achievable goal.

Helping a client change health-related behaviors is never easy but it can be much more successful if the nurse moves beyond client education and masters these simple, evidence-based self-management support strategies.

Teaching Older Adults

Because of normal developmental changes, the older clients may have difficulty with teaching strategies. The nurse should take these changes into account when planning and implementing teaching with older adults. A list of adaptive changes in client teaching that will help the nurse working with older adults is given in Box 1-1.

HEALTH PROMOTION

Health promotion involves activities that promote general well-being. These primary prevention activities are categorized as patterns of healthy eating, healthy activity, and effective coping with stress. *Healthy People 2010,*[53] the federal population-based health objectives, identified the leading indicators of health that apply to adults (Box 1-2). Nurses can assist in achieving these goals by assessing the client's lifestyle and risk status and by intervening to modify poor habits and reduce

---

BOX 1-1   Guidelines for Effectively Teaching Older Adults

VISION

1. Provide large, easy-to-read typeface.
2. Emphasize contrasting colors: black and white.
3. Avoid blues and greens.
4. Use nonglare paper.
5. Write short, simple paragraphs.
6. Make sure eyeglasses are in place and clean.

HEARING

1. Speak slowly.
2. Enunciate clearly.
3. Lower the pitch of your voice.
4. Eliminate background noise.
5. Face the learner.
6. Use nonverbal cues.
7. Make sure client's hearing aid is in place and is working properly.

ENERGY LEVEL/ATTENTION

1. Use short teaching sessions.
2. Offer liquid refreshment and bathroom breaks.
3. Promote comfort.

INFORMATION PROCESSING AND MEMORY

1. Present most important information first.
2. Clarify information with use of examples that are relevant to client.
3. Motor skills: Teach one step at a time, demonstrate, allow for return demonstration.
4. Encourage association between items.
5. Be concrete and specific.
6. Eliminate distractions.
7. Encourage verbal interactions.
8. Correct wrong answers and reinforce correct answers.
9. Offer praise and encouragement.

BOX 1-2   *Healthy People 2010* Leading Health Indicators for Young and Middle-Age Adults

1. Increase the proportion of adults who engage regularly, preferable daily, in moderate physical activity for at least 30 minutes per day.
2. Reduce the proportion of adults who are obese.
3. Reduce cigarette smoking by adults.
4. Reduce the proportion of adults using any illicit drug during the past 30 days.
5. Reduce the proportion of adults engaging in binge drinking of alcoholic beverages during the past month.
6. Increase the proportion of sexually active persons who use condoms.
7. Increase the proportion of adults with recognized depression who receive treatment.
8. Reduce deaths caused by motor vehicle accidents.
9. Reduce homicides.
10. Reduce the proportion of nonsmokers exposed to environmental tobacco smoke.
11. Increase the proportion of non-institutionalized adults who are vaccinated annually against influenza and ever vaccinated against pneumococcal disease.

Data from U.S. Department of Health and Human Services. (Jan 2000). *Healthy People 2010*. (Conference Edition, in Two Volumes). Washington, DC: Author.

---

risk. This chapter describes the components of a healthy lifestyle, including health promotion (primary prevention), risk assessment, and risk management, specifically disease prevention (*primary* prevention) and early detection (*secondary* prevention). Much of the content of the rest of the book is based on caring for people with health problems (*tertiary* prevention). Examples of client behaviors in each of the three levels of prevention are listed in Table 1-3.

HEALTHY EATING

The Institute of Medicine

Healthy eating is a cornerstone of a healthy lifestyle. The Institute of Medicine[28] suggested major revisions in the recommendations for healthy eating and activity in their 2002 report. 🥄 These recommendations were based on a comprehensive review of the research in the area of diet and exercise. The Institute of Medicine recommendations regarding a healthy diet are summarized in Box 1-3.

An important addition to dietary recommendations is that the total number of calories recommended should be based on the client's age, gender, height, weight, and one of four activity levels. The activity levels are sedentary, low active, active, and very active. Following this guideline ensures that calorie recommendations for clients take into account all the factors that determine the energy they expend, and thus their caloric needs. Too often, as will be discussed later, our clients consume more calories than needed for energy and health; this results in overweight and chronic health problems.

Nutritional Labels

To use the guidelines effectively for achieving healthy eating patterns, clients must be able to read nutrition labels. The food labeling system mandated by the U.S. Food and Drug Administration (FDA) is designed to assist consumers in making informed decisions regarding the foods they purchase. The Nutrition Facts label

TABLE 1-3 Behaviors Associated with Each Level of Prevention

Level of Prevention	Type of Behavior*
Primary	Stop smoking, or do not start smoking
	Avoid overexposure to the sun
	Support antipollution legislation
	Practice safe sex, monogamy, or abstinence
	Obtain genetic counseling for family-linked disorders
	Design and follow a regular exercise plan
	Maintain ideal body weight
	Maintain a low-cholesterol, low-fat, high-fiber nutritious diet
	Wear a seat belt and helmet
	Identify and eliminate stressors
	Limit alcohol intake, and never drink and drive
	Have regular dental care
Secondary	Obtain genetic counseling for family-linked disorders
	Undergo screening for tuberculosis
	Obtain tonometry yearly after age 40 for glaucoma screening
	Have yearly Pap smears and mammograms per recommended guidelines
	Have eye examinations every 2 years
	Practice monthly self-breast, self-testicular, self-skin, and self-oral examinations
	Undergo a physical examination yearly after age 40
	Self-monitor blood pressure for hypertension
Tertiary	Have a complete blood count before chemotherapy
	Have speech therapy after a stroke
	Participate in cardiac rehabilitation
	Have breast reconstruction
	Participate in stroke or coma rehabilitation

* Preventive behaviors identified are representative and are not intended to be inclusive.

BOX 1-3 Summary of Institute of Medicine Dietary Recommendations

1. The total recommended number of calories consumed should be based on age, gender, height, weight, and one of four activity levels. (See reference 28, Institute of Medicine, p. 5.1, for formula.)
2. Dietary Reference Intakes are recommended intakes of some nutrients (i.e., carbohydrates, fiber, fatty acids, cholesterol, protein, amino acids) for both good health and prevention of chronic disease. In addition to recommended intakes, tolerable upper intake levels of these nutrients are provided.
3. Recommended ranges of dietary sources of calories are carbohydrates 45% to 65%, protein 10% to 35%, and fat 20% to 35%. It is recommended that these be considered together to ensure that total calories per day do not exceed expenditure.
4. Fewer than 25% of total calories should be from added sugars. Added sugars are those incorporated into food and beverages during production and are distinguished from natural sugars such as those found in milk (lactose) and fruit (fructose).
5. Because saturated fat, cholesterol, and trans fatty acids serve no health benefit, it is recommended that intake be reduced to the lowest level possible needed to maintain a nutritionally adequate diet.
6. Whenever possible, monounsaturated and polyunsaturated fats should be substituted for saturated fat, cholesterol, and trans fatty acid.
7. Two polyunsaturated fats are essential and available only from food sources. These are alpha-linolenic acid (an omega-3 fatty acid) and linoleic acid (an omega-6 fatty acid).
8. The recommended intake of alpha-linolenic acid is 17 g for adult men and 12 g for adult women. Good dietary sources include vegetable oils such as safflower oil or corn oil.
9. The recommended intake of linoleic acid is 1.6 g for adult men and 1.1 g for adult women. Good dietary sources of this fat include milk and some vegetable oils, such as soybean oil and flaxseed oil.
10. Recommended daily intake of total* fiber for young and middle-aged adults is 38 g for men and 25 g for women.
11. Recommended levels of dietary protein for adults are 0.8 g per kilogram of body weight.

Data from Institute of Medicine. (2002). *Dietary reference intakes for energy, carbohydrate, fiber, fat, fatty acids, cholesterol, protein, and amino acids.* Washington, DC: National Academy Press.
* Total fiber includes both dietary fiber (the edible, nondigestible component of carbohydrates and lignin) and functional or supplemental fiber sources (such as psyllium or pectin).

(Figure 1-2) is a tool to identify both serving size and the nutritional components of the food item.

Nurses who are knowledgeable about the composition of a healthy diet and the Nutrition Facts label can assist clients to adopt healthy eating patterns. Many adults are in excellent health but may have poor eating patterns that lay the foundation for future health problems. In addition, these clients may already have health problems as a result of poor eating patterns. Health patterns of concern include obesity, cancer risk, osteoporosis, and cardiovascular disease. Obesity and cancer risks are discussed here. Chapter 26 covers osteoporosis, Chapters 54 and 56 cover heart disease, and Chapter 52 covers hypertension.

Obesity

Current estimates are that 23% of the U.S. population is obese (body mass index [BMI] >30 kg/m²). The *Healthy People 2010*[53] goals include reducing the number of obese Americans to 15%; however, in the last 20 years the percent of people who are obese has increased by 50%. In addition, the percentage of the adult U.S. population who are overweight (BMI 25 to 29.9 kg/m²) is estimated to be 55%. Both obesity and overweight pose serious health risks. Overweight people (this includes all obese people) have an increased risk for heart disease, hypertension, type 2 diabetes, degenerative joint disease, sleep apnea, and gallbladder disease.[45] When overweight

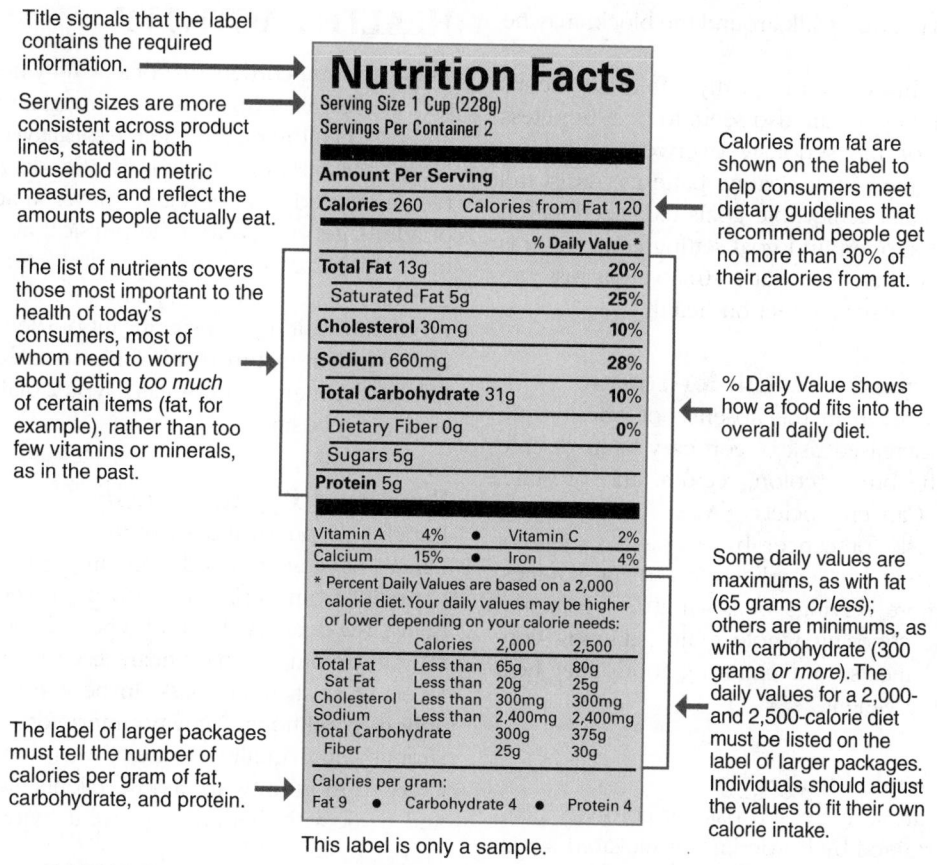

Title signals that the label contains the required information.

Serving sizes are more consistent across product lines, stated in both household and metric measures, and reflect the amounts people actually eat.

The list of nutrients covers those most important to the health of today's consumers, most of whom need to worry about getting *too much* of certain items (fat, for example), rather than too few vitamins or minerals, as in the past.

The label of larger packages must tell the number of calories per gram of fat, carbohydrate, and protein.

Calories from fat are shown on the label to help consumers meet dietary guidelines that recommend people get no more than 30% of their calories from fat.

% Daily Value shows how a food fits into the overall daily diet.

Some daily values are maximums, as with fat (65 grams *or less*); others are minimums, as with carbohydrate (300 grams *or more*). The daily values for a 2,000- and 2,500-calorie diet must be listed on the label of larger packages. Individuals should adjust the values to fit their own calorie intake.

This label is only a sample.

Nutrition Facts
Serving Size 1 Cup (228g)
Servings Per Container 2

Amount Per Serving

Calories 260   Calories from Fat 120

% Daily Value *

Total Fat 13g	**20%**
Saturated Fat 5g	**25%**
Cholesterol 30mg	**10%**
Sodium 660mg	**28%**
Total Carbohydrate 31g	**10%**
Dietary Fiber 0g	**0%**
Sugars 5g	
Protein 5g	

Vitamin A	4%	Vitamin C	2%
Calcium	15%	Iron	4%

* Percent Daily Values are based on a 2,000 calorie diet. Your daily values may be higher or lower depending on your calorie needs:

	Calories	2,000	2,500
Total Fat	Less than	65g	80g
Sat Fat	Less than	20g	25g
Cholesterol	Less than	300mg	300mg
Sodium	Less than	2,400mg	2,400mg
Total Carbohydrate		300g	375g
Fiber		25g	30g

Calories per gram:
Fat 9 • Carbohydrate 4 • Protein 4

■ **FIGURE 1–2** Guide to using a food label. *(Modified from U.S. Food and Drug Administration. [Dec 10, 1992]. The new food label. FDA Backgrounder, 1-9.)*

is associated with a high-fat diet, the risk of breast, colon, rectum, and prostate cancer increases. Take every opportunity to measure height and weight and to calculate BMI (see Chapter 28) and also to advise clients when they fall outside the range of healthy weight.

Management of the Overweight Client

The basic therapeutic approach to the overweight client is to modify eating patterns through improving the *quality* (versus *quantity*) of foods eaten. The focus is on making positive changes in eating patterns. Specific modifications include (1) decreasing portion size, (2) modifying the composition of the diet through substitution and modification of foods consumed, and (3) changing eating behaviors. The second therapeutic component of obesity management is improving activity patterns (see later discussion).

Assessment

Before recommending diet modifications, assess the client's current eating patterns. Simple dietary assessment tools include a 24-hour diet recall and use of a 3-day dietary log in which the client records all food and drink for 3 days, one of which should be a weekend day. The 24-hour diet recall is ideal for obtaining information at the time of the nurse-client encounter. The 3-day dietary log includes not only what food was eaten by the client but also when, why, and how the client ate. This tool assists both the nurse and the client in recognizing eating patterns and problematic eating behavior. Chapter 28 discusses nutritional assessment.

Intervention

Once eating patterns have been assessed, collaboratively develop a list of problems and a mutually agreeable, realistic plan for addressing these problems with the client. Interventions that focus on changing the foods eaten should include substituting foods (e.g., carrots for candy), increasing certain foods (e.g., fruits and vegetables), or decreasing other foods (e.g., fats). Interventions can also include modifying the eating circumstances, for example, adding a breakfast meal, not eating after the evening meal, setting the eating utensil down between bites, and eating only at the table.

Eating behavior has a strong emotional component. Poor eating patterns are used to cope with emotional discomfort such as depression or anger. Understanding circumstances under which the client eats helps to identify interventions specifically designed to address these problems. For example, if the client recognizes that anger or fatigue leads to eating, a more appropriate coping behavior, such as taking a walk around the block, may be identified.

Although weight loss can greatly affect a client's health and well-being, it can also seem to be a hopeless task, especially for the seriously overweight and for adults with a lifetime of poor eating patterns. Assist the client in setting small achievable goals (see sections on self-management support and goal setting earlier in this chapter). Reassure the client that a 10% weight loss can have a substantial positive effect on health.[24]

Diet and Management of Risk for Disease

Diets high in fat, even in the absence of obesity, are associated with increased risk of coronary heart disease and cancer of the breast, colon, rectum, and prostate. The American Cancer Society (ACS)[2] recommends decreasing the risk for cancer by eating a variety of healthful foods with an emphasis on plant sources, eating five or more servings of a variety of fruit and vegetables daily, choosing whole grains, limiting consumption of red meats, and choosing foods that help maintain a healthy weight.

Therapeutic Lifestyle Changes

For clients who are at increased risk for coronary heart disease, as determined by borderline or elevated serum cholesterol levels and identified risks, the National Cholesterol Education Panel recommends therapeutic lifestyle changes (TLC).[40] The TLC diet is described in Table 1-4. If the diet is not successful or is problematic for the client, a referral to a dietitian is recommended. Most recent dietary recommendations come from the American Heart Association and are listed in Box 1-2 in the section of this chapter on management of risk for heart disease.

TABLE 1–4 Nutrient Composition of the TLC Diet

Nutrient	Recommended Intake
Saturated fat*	Less than 7% of total calories
Polyunsaturated fat	Up to 10% of total calories
Monounsaturated fat	Up to 20% of total calories
Total fat	25%-35% of total calories
Carbohydrate†	50%-60% of total calories
Fiber	20-30 g/day
Protein	Approximately 15% of total calories
Cholesterol	Less than 200 mg/day
Total calories (energy)‡	Balance energy intake and expenditure to maintain desirable body weight/prevent weight gain

From *Third Report of the Expert Panel on Detection, Evaluation, and Treatment of High Blood Cholesterol in Adults (Adult Treatment Panel III)*. Retrieved Sept 2, 2002, from http://nhlbi.nih.gov/guidelines/cholesterol.
* Trans fatty acids are another LDL-raising fat that should be kept at a low intake.
† Carbohydrates should be derived predominantly from foods rich in complex carbohydrates, including grains, especially whole grains, fruits, and vegetables.
‡ Daily energy expenditure should include at least moderate physical activity (contributing approximately 200 kilocalories per day).

HEALTHY ACTIVITY

Another cornerstone of a healthy lifestyle is healthy activity. People who are active throughout life live longer and are healthier than their less active counterparts.[43] More than 60% of adults, however, do not achieve the recommended level of regular physical activity, and 40% of adults get no leisure-time physical activity.[44] Physical inactivity increases with age, and women are more inactive than men.[54] Physical inactivity is a serious, nationwide problem resulting in a significant burden of unnecessary illness and premature death. It is associated with increased risk for coronary heart disease, type 2 diabetes, hypertension, and obesity.

Benefits of Physical Activity

Benefits of physical activity include (1) weight maintenance, (2) lower blood pressure, (3) improved mood, (4) relief from depression, (5) improved sense of well-being, (6) decreased risk of type 2 diabetes, (7) reduced mortality from coronary heart disease, and (8) increased levels of peak bone mass. In people with chronic, disabling conditions, activity improves stamina, muscle strength, and quality of life. Given these benefits, take every opportunity to assess clients' activity patterns, and work with them to improve activity levels.

Management of the Inactive Client

Current activity recommendations are that every adult in the United States should accumulate an hour of moderately intense activity every day.[53] This recommendation is based on extensive research on what the average person needs to do to maintain a healthy weight. Activity can be accumulated, but it should occur in blocks of at least 8 minutes and should be perceived as moderate or high intensity.[5] In addition, people who are very fit and engage in high-intensity activity can achieve similar health benefits in 30 minutes of high-intensity activity on most days. Simple walking is an excellent initial activity that requires no special equipment and can be done anywhere. Although this level of activity is ideal, you can advise your clients that important benefits can be obtained through modest amounts of daily physical activity[43] as they begin an exercise program.

Assessment

Intervention to improve activity patterns begins with assessment of the client's current activity pattern. Two effective tools are the 24-hour recall and a 3-day activity log. In the 24-hour recall, help the client identify all forms of activity during that day. Focus on activity that was sustained for at least 8 minutes and perceived as moderate to heavy exertion. Encourage the client to be thorough by giving examples, such as time spent doing housework. Then sum the total number of minutes spent in moderate or heavy activity per day.[7] During assessment, begin developing ideas for new activity opportunities. This information will be useful later for developing an intervention plan.

Benefits outweigh the risks with the current recommendation for moderate physical activity. Before beginning an activity program, however, all clients should be screened for risks that contraindicate unsupervised activity. People with known health problems, especially those involving cardiac risk factors (including hypertension, elevated serum cholesterol level, cigarette smoking, diabetes, and a family history of early heart disease), should be evaluated by their health care provider for tolerance of increased activity before increasing physical activity levels.[42]

Intervention

Once the activity pattern has been assessed and there are no evident risks requiring further evaluation, work with the client to identify problem areas and develop a plan to increase physical activity. The Activity Pyramid is an excellent tool for beginning instruction (Figure 1-3). The Activity Pyramid is a pictorial representation of the principles of healthy activity and can be used during nurse-client encounters to provide basic information.

The Exercise Prescription. A written exercise prescription[23] specifies recommended activity. The exercise prescription has four major components:

- *Mode,* or the type of activity
- *Intensity* with which the activity is performed
- *Duration* of time
- *Frequency*

As noted earlier, the minimum goal for an exercise program is a moderate-intensity *(intensity)* physical activity performed for a total of at least 60 minutes *(duration)* most days of the week *(frequency).* Many activities that are a part of most people's daily routine can serve as the mode of a physical activity program, including walking, housework, child care, and gardening (Box 1-4).

Intensity is an essential component of an activity. The recommendations are based on moderate intensity. Instruct clients how to assess exertion level. One simple means of measuring perceived exertion is the *talk test;* clients should be able to speak only a few words at a time when engaged in the activity. If clients can carry on a normal conversation, they are not working hard enough; if they cannot talk at all, they are working too hard. Another measure of intensity is the *Borg rating* of perceived exertion.

Overcoming Barriers. Research indicates that people who successfully incorporate physical activity into their daily lives are confident in their ability to perform the

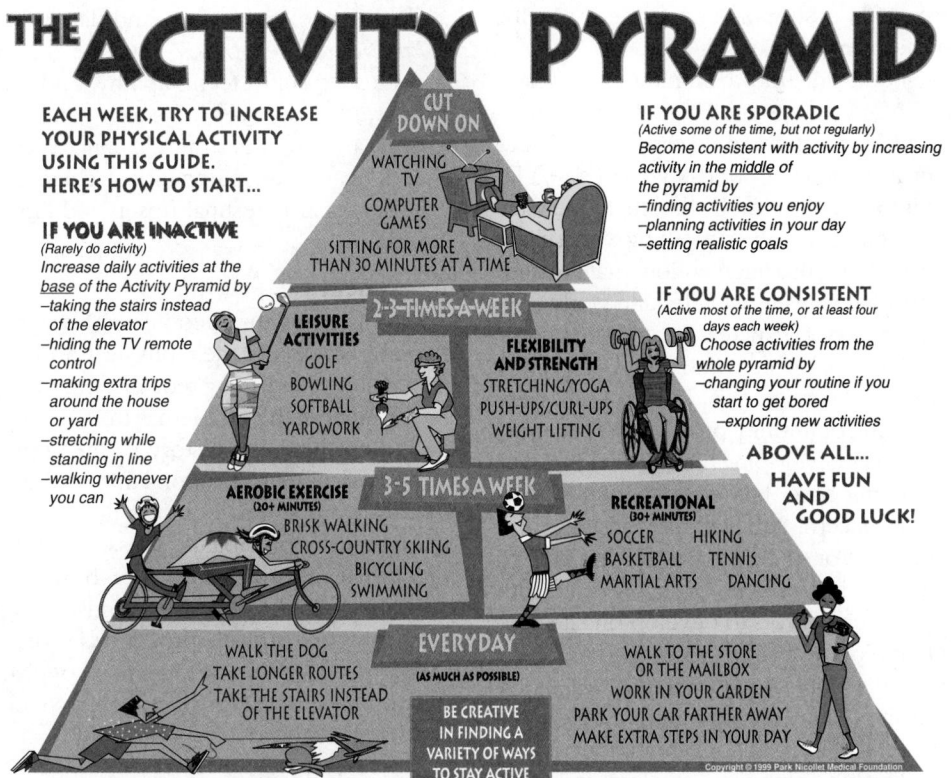

■ **FIGURE 1-3** The Activity Pyramid. *(Copyright 1999, Park Nicollet Health Source Institute for Research and Education, Minneapolis, Minn.)*

activity, find it pleasurable, and have social support.[5,7] Activities should also be convenient and realistic.

Simple strategies can increase the likelihood of success in implementing an activity program. On the basis of the assessment of the client's activity level, (1) advise the client to increase time spent in current moderate-intensity activities, (2) help the client identify pleasurable activities to incorporate into the current routine, and (3) encourage the client to identify friends or family members who can serve as a support system and, ideally, who can join in the planned activity.

Activity plans should include a monitoring method, such as a log, and a reward system. Help clients identify potential barriers and assist them in developing a plan to overcome barriers. Although the primary goal of a regular activity plan is to improve physical health, many benefits relate to feelings of well-being. When working with a client to improve activity patterns, use interventions that increase self-efficacy by choosing realistic activities and goals.

One successful strategy for increasing physical activity is to increase social support within the community as well as within the client's social circle. Use every opportunity to support community projects that promote physical activity, such as developing hiking, walking, and biking trails or opening schools for community recreation. If security is a concern, support efforts to organize a community watch unit or to develop a walking club to take advantage of safety in numbers. Occupational health nurses can encourage employers to develop on-site programs to support employee health. Nurses who regularly work with clients to develop activity programs can maintain a comprehensive listing of community resources available to support activity plans. Community nursing organizations can develop a volunteer pool to work with walking clubs in area malls, perform blood pressure screenings, and provide health education classes.

A variety of programs are available to nurses who regularly work with clients to improve their eating and activity behaviors. An excellent resource for working with overweight clients is the report of the Expert Panel on the Identification, Evaluation, and Treatment of Overweight and Obese Adults.[41] This document is a detailed guide for the treatment of overweight and obesity. Materials include information on nutrition and exercise, Weekly Food and Activity Diaries, Guides to Behavior Change and Physical Activity, and tools to help the clinician evaluate the client's risks and motivation and to set goals. The entire document is available online at www.nhlbi.nih.gov.

Stress and Stress Management

Stress, the body's response to demands, seems to be increasing in today's world. Physical demands for adaptation are compounded by the adaptive responses required by the volume of information and the decisions required for existence in today's society. Stress is usually the result of an imbalance between the demands placed on a person and one's ability to adapt. *Stress management,* the final cornerstone of a healthy lifestyle, is the ability to cope with these adaptive demands effectively.

Dysfunction in one's ability to adapt and manage stress has a negative effect on health:[14]

- *Behavioral* responses to stress include decreased ability to think clearly and function, increased tobacco and alcohol use, overeating, and disrupted sleep patterns.
- *Emotional* responses include depression, anger, decreased self-esteem, apathy, and impatience.
- *Physical* responses to stress can include tight, sore neck and shoulder muscles, increased blood pressure and heart rate, palpitations, chest discomfort, headaches, gastrointestinal upset, and fatigue.

Assessment

Today it seems that people are always "stressed," often blaming stress for their physical and mental problems. As a result, clients may request help in coping with stress. Assessment of the problem is the first step in intervention. Include a thorough history of the cognitive, emotional, and physical manifestations that lead clients to conclude that they are stressed. Assess the problems or situations that seem to precipitate stress and the behavioral and emotional responses to it (i.e., how clients feel and act when the problem is present). Also evaluate how clients currently cope with the problem (see discussion of coping in Chapter 24). Help the person recognize ineffective coping and develop a plan to cope effectively with the stress.

Intervention

Stress management has three components: stress resistance, cognitive reappraisal, and effective coping skills.

Stress Resistance

Stress resistance involves decreasing the body's response to stress; adopting healthy eating patterns, engaging in physical activity, and using relaxation techniques can help reduce the stress response. Physical activity can be a *positive* stressor; that is, activity requires an adaptive response, and, when performed properly, it results in physical changes that counter the normally negative effects of stress. Physical activity improves mental function, decreases depression, and increases physical endurance.

Healthy eating can increase resistance to stress, and unhealthy eating adds to stress. Healthy eating aids stress resistance; however, some foods are associated with effective or ineffective coping. Complex carbohydrates (e.g., breads, beans, grains) provide a sustained source of energy and have a relaxing effect, whereas fruits, vegetables, and protein provide energy and increased physiologic ability to cope. Intake of simple carbohydrates (e.g., sugar) can temporarily increase energy, but this rise is then quickly followed by weakness and lethargy as the blood glucose level drops. Overeating, an ineffective means of coping, can result in decreased energy and lowered self-esteem. The stimulant caffeine induces the fight-or-flight biologic response and when it is consumed in excess can exacerbate the physical damage that results from stress.

Sleep and rest are natural forms of relaxation that are essential for healing and repairing the physiologic consequences to stress. Inadequate rest worsens stress, especially through impaired mental functioning. Chapter 22 discusses promoting positive outcomes in clients with sleep and rest disorders. In addition to sleep and rest, people can practice techniques to facilitate physical and mental relaxation. *Progressive relaxation* is a technique of slowly focusing on each muscle group, tensing the muscles for 5 to 7 seconds, and then relaxing them. This process promotes learning how to relax the entire body and particularly benefits people with muscle tension or spasm, insomnia, and neck or back pain. Many forms of relaxation involve *breathing techniques,* such as breath awareness, deep breathing, and the purifying breath.[16]

Meditation, once considered an alternative practice, is an established form of relaxation therapy. Research has shown that physiologic changes, such as lowering blood pressure and decreasing heart disease risk, occur as a result of meditation. There are several active or passive forms of meditation, including focusing on breath awareness or a *mantra,* meditative movement such as *yoga* or *Tai Chi,* mindfulness, and prayer.

⟡ Cognitive Reappraisal

The goal of cognitive reappraisal or restructuring is to change the perception or interpretation of events as stressors. Cognitive reappraisal is based on the assumption that a major factor in stress is the individual's perception of the event or experience as a stressor.[16] Three common techniques are presented.

Thought Stopping. This technique is an ideal intervention for "worriers" (i.e., people who obsessively maintain ongoing inner dialogues of "what if" or "I can't"). Clients identify the obsessive thought and allow the self to imagine a situation involving the thought. As the obsessive dialogue begins, the person interrupts the dialogue with a loud "STOP!" and substitutes a positive thought. The goal of this process is to learn to disrupt obsessive and nonproductive thoughts automatically with a positive message.

Refuting Irrational Ideas. Like thought stopping, refuting irrational ideas involves interventions designed to disrupt obsessive, nonproductive thoughts. The intervention derives from rational emotive therapy, which is based on the belief that much stress is related to common irrational beliefs such as "I must be perfect in everything I do" and "It's absolutely necessary that I have love and approval from my peers and family at all times." To overcome these stressful beliefs, the client first identifies the irrational idea and then identifies the facts, such as "no one is perfect all the time." Clients also need to explore their emotional response to stressful thoughts. The client then substitutes rational self-talk for the previous irrational self-talk. This particular intervention is very effective for self-directed, empowered people.

Guided Imagery. Guided imagery, a form of relaxation, is an excellent method of cognitive reappraisal. Guided imagery is usually practiced under the direction of a trained therapist. The therapist assists the client to visualize a stressful event, become worried, and then to switch to a relaxing event or to rework the situation so that it is less stressful. Alternatively, the therapist may help the client into a guided dialogue with his or her inner self or may act as a guide to help with problem solving.

Effective Coping

Effective coping involves recognition of the problem causing stress and, through problem-solving skills, development and implementation of an effective strategy to cope with or solve the problem. Effective coping skills include time management, assertiveness, solution-oriented therapy, and development of a support system.[16] Clients often use ineffective coping strategies, usually designed to avoid the problem, resulting in repression of associated unpleasant emotions. Addictive behaviors, such as alcohol abuse and overeating, often begin as ineffective coping strategies.

Effective coping starts with identifying the problem. Help the client to differentiate the problem from the emotional response to the problem. Once the problem is identified, several issues must be addressed before one can work on problem-solving skills.

First, does the problem really exist, or is it imagined? People often worry about imagined problems. Help the client assess validity of the problem before working on a solution.

Second, is the problem really important or just a nuisance? If the problem is not important, use cognitive reappraisal techniques to put the problem in perspective.

Third, does the problem have feasible solutions? Some problems (an untimely death or catastrophic illness) are beyond control. In these cases, the goal is not problem resolution but acceptance that humans cannot control all aspects of life. The individual will need support to learn from the problem and to develop an ongoing support system for assistance through the crisis.

Important, controllable problems are amenable to intervention or action responses using standard problem-solving, assertiveness, and time management skills. Nurses often assist people in distress. Mastering effective coping skills can be an asset in clinical practice; however, nurses often work with people experiencing crises in which basic coping strategies are not enough. Develop a network of counseling and support resources to which clients can be referred.

DISEASE PREVENTION

The leading causes of death in young adults are motor vehicle accidents and other unintentional injuries, homicide, suicide, malignant neoplasms, and heart disease. In middle-aged adults, the risk of premature death from cancer or heart disease increases.[52] In both age groups, death from human immunodeficiency virus (HIV) infection has increased; of the more than one million persons with acquired immunodeficiency syndrome (AIDS) in the United States, most are 20 to 40 years of age.[52] The leading cause of death in older adults is cardiovascular disease, followed by cancer. However, in older adults infection from pneumonia or influenza is included in the top 10 leading causes of death; accidents are also a major cause of death in older adults.[52]

PREVENTION OF INJURY AND ILLNESS

The leading causes of injury and premature death in young and middle-aged adults include accidents, particularly motor vehicle accidents, and violence, particularly suicide and homicide.[52,53] In older adults, pneumonia and influenza, preventable infections, are also a major cause of death. Risk identification and risk management counseling can prevent illness and injury in these populations. Place particular emphasis on preventable causes of accidents, specifically the use of drugs and alcohol, and preventable causes of cancer, specifically smoking. Although chronic illnesses account for the vast majority of deaths in older adults, preventable injury is still a major cause of death.

Accidents

Because motor vehicle accidents are the leading cause of death in young adults, prevention counseling should focus on the regular use of lap and shoulder belts and refraining from drug or alcohol use while driving. Because of the significant impact of drugs, alcohol, and tobacco on health, most prevention measures are devoted to screening and intervening in alcohol, drug, and tobacco abuse. Accidents in older adults include motor vehicle accidents and accidents around the home. The following discussion focuses on screening and primary prevention measures. Chapter 24 describes secondary intervention for clients who have substance abuse problems.

Alcohol Abuse

Alcohol abuse results in specific health problems, including withdrawal syndrome; hepatitis, cirrhosis, and pancreatitis; and cancers of the liver, oropharynx (especially in smokers), and esophagus as well as an increased risk of breast cancer. In addition to diseases clearly associated with alcohol abuse, "problem drinkers" have increased mortality from all causes, beginning with four drinks per day for men and two drinks per day for women. Alcohol is associated with more than 50% of all injuries (44% of all traffic accidents), fires, drowning, homicides, and suicides.[52]

Problem drinkers are more likely to be seen in primary care clinics and hospitals. They often do not present with manifestations of dependence that would immediately result in identification of the problem. All clients, not just those with obvious problems, should be screened for problem drinking. Nurses are in a position to identify problem drinking because their role includes obtaining a comprehensive psychosocial history (see Chapter 2).

Various tools are available to screen for problem drinking, including the CAGE four-item tool. The mnemonic CAGE is a useful four item tool:[55]

C=have you ever felt you ought to **Cut** down on drinking?

A=Have people **Annoyed** you by criticizing your drinking?

G=Have you ever felt bad or **Guilty** about your drinking?

E=Have you ever had a drink first thing in the morning to steady your nerves or get rid of a hangover (**Eye-opener**)?

If problem drinking is suspected or if the client answers "yes" to any item on the CAGE, the Alcohol Use Disorders Identification Test (AUDIT) may be administered (Table 1-5). The AUDIT is a 10-item tool developed by a six-nation team in conjunction with the

TABLE 1-5 The Alcohol Use Disorders Identification Test (AUDIT) Structured Interview

	Score*				
Question	**0**	**1**	**2**	**3**	**4**
How often do you have a drink containing alcohol?	Never	Monthly or less	2-4 times/mo	2-3 times/wk	4 or more times/wk
How many drinks do you have on a typical day when you are drinking?	None	1 or 2	3 or 4	5 or 6	7-9†
How often do you have six or more drinks on one occasion?	Never	Less than monthly	Monthly	Weekly	Daily or almost daily
How often during the last year have you found that you were unable to stop drinking once you had started?	Never	Less than monthly	Monthly	Weekly	Daily or almost daily
How often last year have you failed to do what was normally expected from you because of drinking?	Never	Less than monthly	Monthly	Weekly	Daily or almost daily
How often during the last year have you needed a first drink in the morning to get yourself going after a heavy drinking session?	Never	Less than monthly	Monthly	Weekly	Daily or almost daily
How often during the last year have you had a feeling of guilt or remorse after drinking?	Never	Less than monthly	Monthly	Weekly	Daily or almost daily
How often during the last year have you been unable to remember what happened the night before because you had been drinking?	Never	Less than monthly	Monthly	Weekly	Daily or almost daily
Have you or has someone else been injured as a result of your drinking?	Never	Yes, but not in the last year (2 points)		Yes, during the last year (4 points)	
Has a relative, doctor, or other health worker been concerned about your drinking or suggested you cut down?	Never	Yes, but not in the last year (2 points)		Yes, during the last year (4 points)	

From U.S. Preventive Services Task Force. (1996). *Guide to clinical preventive services* (2nd ed.). Baltimore: Williams & Wilkins.
* Score of greater than 8 (out of 41) suggests problem drinking and indicates the need for more in-depth assessment. Cut-off of 10 points recommended by some to provide greater specificity.
† Five points if response is 10 or more drinks on a typical day.

World Health Organization (WHO). The AUDIT is highly sensitive and specific[29,48] and can easily be included in a social history format (see Chapter 2). Do not hesitate to screen for problem drinking. If you suspect that a client has a drinking problem (based on screening), briefly state so to the client. Be sure to have an established support and referral network of clinical specialists to assist the client and family with acceptance and management of problem drinking.[52] Chapter 24 also details interventions for clients who have substance abuse problems.

Alcohol abuse is not just a problem of young and midlife adults. As many as 31% of community-dwelling older adults and 18% to 49% of institutionalized older adults have serious problems related to alcohol use.[37] Both the CAGE and the AUDIT screening tools can be used with older adults.

Drug Abuse, Misuse, and Polypharmacy

🏺 Unfortunately since 1992, after years of decline in drug use, abuse of illicit and legal drugs has been on the increase. More than 5.5 million Americans are affected by drug abuse, and 50% of these people are in the criminal justice system. Drug abuse is more common among men, the unemployed, and people without a high school education. Although drug abuse is more prevalent in urban communities, rural communities are not immune. Drug abusers are at increased risk for HIV infection and other communicable diseases. Drug abuse is a significant factor in homicides, suicides, and motor vehicle accidents.[52]

Be aware of the hazards of drug abuse and of the possibility of drug abuse in clients. Several standardized tools can be used to screen for drug abuse, but none has well-established validity or reliability.[55] Take every opportunity to assess for drug abuse. Following your questions regarding tobacco and alcohol use, ask the client about drug use as a routine part of lifestyle assessment (see Chapter 2). State questions directly ("Do you currently use any other drugs such as marijuana ['pot,' 'weed'] or cocaine ['crack']?"). If the answer is "no," one can follow with "Have you ever used any other drugs?" If the client indicates current or past use of illicit drugs, further explore the patterns of use.

Advise abusing and high-risk clients (adolescents, males, people exposed to users of drugs) of the hazards of substance abuse. Advise users to stop or reduce drug use, and offer help through referral (see Chapter 24 for interventions for substance abuse problems).

It is difficult to determine the extent of prescription drug abuse by older people. Researchers contend that thousands of older Americans are "hooked" on their prescription drugs in an "inadvertent addiction."[19] In addition, it is well established drug problems in older adults include misuse of medications and the harmful effects of polypharmacy. An individual's average number of prescribed medications increases with age, with older adults filling an average of 7.5 to 17.9 prescriptions per year.[37] In addition to prescription drug use, 70% to 80% of older adults self-medicate with over-the-counter drugs without consulting a health care professional.[37]

See the Bridge to Home Health Care feature on Managing Multiple Medications.

The effects of drugs can be beneficial or harmful. A confounding factor in the effectiveness of drug therapy is related to age-related body system changes (Table 1-6). The number of adverse drug interactions increases with age and the number of drugs taken. Nearly one third of older adults report adverse reactions to medications, accounting for as many as 10% of their hospitalizations.[20]

Polypharmacy is described as the use of excessive or unnecessary medications that increase the risk of drug interactions and other adverse drug reactions. Ironically, drug reactions that mimic medical-physical complaints are often treated with another drug. Polypharmacy has many consequences, including adverse drug effects, adverse interactions with other drugs and food, duplication of therapy, decreased quality of life, and unnecessary financial and societal costs.[38] Polypharmacy is considered by *Healthy People 2010*[53] to be one of the principal drug safety problems in the United States.

SAFETY
ALERT

Nurses should screen all older adults for appropriate medication use at all health care encounters. It is useful to have older adults take all of their prescription bottles to the clinic or the hospital, and on a home visit the nurse should review all the client's prescriptions. Be sure to include over-the-counter medications, herbs, and nutritional supplements. Reviewing the medications of an older adult is an excellent time to collaborate with a pharmacist who can review all of the client's medications, herbs, and supplements for safety, contraindications, and interactions.

Smoking Cessation

 More than 25% of Americans smoke, and thousands of children begin smoking every day.[27] Smoking is directly linked to many forms of cancer, heart disease, and hypertension. It is a risk factor in health problems as diverse as osteoporosis, ulcer disease, and low birth weight in babies. Smoking accounts for one of every five deaths in the United States,[27] making tobacco the single greatest

cause of disease and premature death in the United States. All nurses should have the necessary skills both to help people who are ready to stop smoking and to help motivate people who are not ready to stop smoking.

In 2000 the *Treating Tobacco Use and Dependence Guidelines*[22] were published (Box 1-5). These guidelines were sponsored by the U.S. Public Health

🏠 BRIDGE TO HOME HEALTH CARE

Managing Multiple Medications

Clients who take several medications often need help in understanding the best administration procedure and in following instructions as closely as possible. Failure to take the right drug at the right time and in the proper way often results in relapses, rehospitalizations, or nursing home placement.

Review all prescription and nonprescription medications, and carefully explain the administration schedule to the client and family members. Tailoring the schedule to the client's lifestyle increases the likelihood that the instructions will be followed. For example, if the client goes to bed at 7:00 PM, be sure that the last dose is scheduled at that hour.

Some people need minimal help with organizing their drugs and dosages. They may benefit from any number of compliance aids that can be purchased at pharmacies, such as containers with separate compartments for each day of the week. The challenge is greater when the client has a complex medication program; reduced strength and dexterity; or a visual, hearing, cognitive, or other impairment in functional status. These clients may need to purchase an automated medication dispenser that emits visual cues, such as flashing strobe lights, or audible cues, such as beeps.

Although units vary, an automated dispenser must be simple to use. One such dispenser can be programmed easily to provide a reminder at the right time for up to four times a day for a week. This dispenser helps the client manage complex schedules, is tamper proof, and dispenses only the pills needed from a supply cassette in a removable drawer. Other automated dispensers have light-emitting diode (LED) screens on which preprogrammed messages, such as "Take with food" or "Take 30 minutes before food," serve as additional reminders.

Determine how and when the client will obtain refills. If the client has no transportation, a pharmacy may have a delivery service or a family member can obtain the prescriptions. A social service referral is needed if the client cannot pay for prescriptions.

Monitor the client for side effects. Many people stop taking essential medications because of unpleasant side effects. Sometimes the client can manage this problem effectively by changing the times of doses or by taking the medication with food.

Instruct the client on drug storage. Some drugs are sensitive to light; others must be secured to decrease the risk of overdoses. All medications must be safely kept away from any children who visit or live in the household.

Simplicity is the key to successful medication management. Regularly evaluate the client's regimen and household routines, and discuss with the client, family members, and physician any changes that would make things easier.

TABLE 1–6   Medication Effects in Older Adults[*]

Drug Dynamics	Impact on Older Person
Absorption: Movement of the drug into the circulation	Absorption is affected by age-related changes in stomach emptying, changes in gastric pH, gastrointestinal motility, and nutritional status (especially low serum albumin levels). Therefore the medication stays in the stomach or intestine longer and takes longer for effect to be obtained.
Distribution: Movement of the drug throughout the body	The adequacy of the circulatory system and the ability of the drug to enter the cell impact distribution. It is altered by reduced cardiac output, decrease in total body water, and increase of adipose tissue. These changes may result in higher than usual blood levels of water-soluble drugs and storage of lipid-soluble drugs in fatty tissue, resulting in toxicity and less drug reaching the site of action because of storage.
Metabolism: Breakdown of the drug in the body, primarily the liver	Breakdown is altered by size of liver and portal circulation; therefore the drug stays in the body longer and may show prolonged responses.
Elimination: Removal of the drug from the body, primarily the renal system	Age-related changes in renal function, renal blood flow, glomerular filtration, and tubular secretion may affect duration and intensity of drug responses in the body.
Additive effect: Two drugs with similar pharmacologic effect (e.g., $1 + 1 = 2$), which can be positive or negative	Negative additive effects can occur when a diuretic (e.g., furosemide) for a cardiovascular disorder is given with an aminoglycoside antibiotic (e.g., tobramycin) for an infection; the result can be increased damage to hearing and balance (ototoxicity) and to the kidneys (nephrotoxicity).
Synergistic effect: Two drugs whose combined effects are greater than the sum of each drug acting alone (e.g., $1 + 1 = 3$)	Positive synergistic interaction occurs when hypertension is treated with a diuretic (e.g., hydrochlorothiazide) and a beta-adrenergic blocker (e.g., atenolol). This combination lowers blood pressure than either drug alone.
Antagonistic effect: Effect of two drugs is less than the sum of the effects of the drugs acting separately, causes a diminished therapeutic effect (e.g., $2 + 2 = 3$)	Reduced anticoagulation occurs when warfarin is given with phenytoin.
Potentiation effect: One drug increases the effect of a second drug	Acetaminophen is given with codeine, with the result being increased analgesia.

Data from Gutierrez, K. (1999). *Pharmacotherapeutics: Clinical decision-making in nursing.* Philadelphia: Saunders.

[*] **Pharmacokinetics** refers to how the body handles the drug; this includes absorption, distribution, metabolism, and elimination of the drug. **Pharmacodynamics** or drug activity refers to the actual effects of the drug in the body; this includes additive, synergistic, antagonistic, and potentiation effects.

BOX 1-5   Guidelines for Tobacco Use and Dependence

1. Tobacco dependence is a chronic condition that often requires repeated intervention; however, effective treatments exist that can produce long-term or even permanent abstinence.
2. Because effective tobacco dependence treatments are available, every client who uses tobacco should be offered at least one of these treatments.
   Clients willing to try to quit tobacco use should be provided treatments identified as effective.
   Clients who are unwilling to try to quit tobacco use should be provided a brief intervention designed to increase their motivation to quit.
3. It is essential that clinicians and health care delivery systems institutionalize the consistent identification, documentation, and treatment of every tobacco user seen in a health care setting.
4. Brief tobacco dependence treatment is effective, and every client who uses tobacco should be offered at least brief treatment.
5. There is a strong dose-response relation between the intensity of tobacco dependence counseling and its

effectiveness. Treatments involving person-to-person contact are consistently effective, and their effectiveness increases with the treatment intensity (e.g., minutes of contact).
6. Three types of counseling and behavioral therapies are especially effective and should be used with all clients attempting tobacco cessation:
   a. Provision of practical counseling (problem solving/skills training)
   b. Provision of social support as a part of treatment (intratreatment social support)
   c. Help in securing social support outside of treatment (extratreatment social support)
7. Numerous effective pharmacotherapies for smoking cessation now exist. Clients attempting smoking cessation should be advised to seek pharmacologic treatment.
8. Tobacco dependence treatments are both clinically effective and cost-effective relative to other medical and disease prevention interventions. As a result, insurers and purchasers of health care should ensure that tobacco dependence treatment be a reimbursable health care service.

Modified from U.S. Public Health Service. (2000). *Treating tobacco use and dependence: Clinical Practice Guideline.* Retrieved Sept 2, 2002, from www.surgeongeneral.gov/tobacco.

Service and were the result of the collaboration of several public and private agencies to develop evidence-based guidelines on tobacco abuse. The core premise of the guidelines is that tobacco abuse is a chronic disease and as such places responsibility on the nurse, along with other health care providers, to provide ongoing counseling, support, and treatment.[3]

Intervention

Smoking cessation intervention can be seen as a stepped process. The first step is to ask all clients if they smoke. When a person who smokes is identified, the nurse then asks whether he or she is willing to quit now. The treatment algorithm then guides the nurse on means to support smoking cessation through brief support interventions or provides strategies to enhance motivation to quit. The nurse can personalize the need to stop smoking; for example, the nurse can remind parents of young children of the increased risk for ear infections and asthma in children exposed to cigarette smoke, as well as the type of role model the parent is presenting. Women should be reminded that smoking increases the risk of osteoporosis and premature aging of the skin, and asymptomatic men should be reminded of the increased risk for emphysema, heart disease, and lung cancer.

Once the client is identified as a smoker and is advised of the need to stop smoking, assessment of the motivation to change is the next step. If a client expresses any interest in changing the smoking behavior, from decreasing use to complete cessation, determine what can be done to help assure the client of the nurse's support. Success is more likely if people spend thoughtful time planning the behavior change[22] in preparation to quit. Help the client evaluate smoking patterns to personalize the plan. Suggestions include (1) cleaning the house just before stopping to rid it of tobacco odor, (2) getting rid of all cigarettes, and (3) setting up a support network. Advise the client to inform friends who smoke that he or she is trying to quit and that they should respect this by not smoking around the client or not offering cigarettes. If the client's history indicates a high degree of nicotine addiction, offer advice about or referral for nicotine replacement.

Finally, assist the client in problem-solving strategies and skills to assist in the effort. This might include addressing how the client will manage "triggers" to smoking (e.g., alcohol or anxiety-producing situations) and alternatives to smoking. When the urge to smoke strikes, advise the client to walk and to learn deep-breathing exercises to work through the urge. Box 1-6 lists suggested activities to substitute instead of smoking.

In addition to explaining smoking cessation, be aware of community resources to which clients can be referred for assistance. Provide a variety of motivational literature to clients, such as the excellent materials available from the American Cancer Society (ACS) and the American

---

BOX 1-6   Things to Do Instead of Smoking

- Take a slow, deep breath of fresh air.
- Take a walk.
- Chew on a piece of gum or a carrot or hard candy.
- Drink a glass of water.
- Think about your children.
- Brush your teeth.
- Play with worry beads.
- Pray or meditate.
- Think about the money you are saving.
- Smile.

Lung Association. Support community-based smoking cessation interventions, including a smoke-free work environment and participation in such community programs as the National Smoke-Off day.

The *Treating Tobacco Use and Dependence*[22] guidelines offer many resources to assist the nurse in smoking cessation efforts. These resources include suggestions for system-based changes as well as evidence-based strategies for increasing the likelihood of success. The guidelines are available online or can be ordered at the U.S. Public Health Service website.

Passive Smoking

Passive smoking, or exposure to second-hand smoke, also places people at increased risk for heart disease and cancer. The Atherosclerosis Risk in the Community (ARIC) study in 1994 indicated that nonsmokers who are regularly exposed to environmental tobacco smoke have a 20% increase in progression of atherosclerosis compared with nonsmokers who are not exposed to tobacco smoke.[27] Identify persons who are exposed to environmental tobacco smoke, and help them devise ways to modify their risk. Ideally, risk modification involves smoking cessation on the part of a family member; however, people are often exposed to tobacco smoke in their work environment (e.g., bars, casinos), and the client may have to make difficult decisions regarding risk management versus livelihood and family. In these cases, the nurse's role as a client advocate can be to support social efforts to limit unwanted exposure to passive smoke, such as laws to limit smoking in public places.

Safety in Older Adults

Adults older than age 65 are at increased risk for a variety of accidents not seen in younger adults. Older adults are more likely to fall and more likely to fracture bones. Thus fall prevention actions are important. As a part of discharge planning, nurses should review their older clients' home situations. The nurse should consider arranging for a home visit by a nurse or other health professional to evaluate home

safety. If clients seem frail or unstable, a physical therapy evaluation and intervention might be helpful. Vision and hearing problems can impact on safety so it is important to ensure that older clients obtain regular vision and hearing screening and appropriate treatment of any identified impairment. Falls can be prevented by some simple actions such as wearing rubber-soled shoes, using handrails, and removing throw rugs. Bathrooms can be hazardous places for older adults: use a grab bar in the tub or shower, use a rubber mat in the tub, and use rugs with rubber backing.

Driving

Physical changes associated with aging can impact the ability of an older adult to drive safely. These changes include impaired hearing and vision, slowed reaction time, and limited range of motion. Medications and medical conditions are also factors in impaired driving ability in older adults. In many communities, hospital occupational therapy departments provide comprehensive driving assessments. Driving refresher courses are available in many communities. The American Association of Retired Persons (AARP) *55 Alive/ Mature Driving Program* is a useful resource. This low-cost 8-hour course emphasizes defensive driving and helps older drivers refine their current driving skills (www.aarp.org). As an added incentive, completion of a driver refresher course often results in a discount on the cost of auto insurance.

Domestic Abuse

The Surgeon General's report in the mid-1980s identified domestic violence as a public health issue. Estimates are that from 1 million[52] to 4 million[13] women are victims of assault, robbery, or rape by a spouse, ex-spouse, or intimate partner each year. Too often, this violence escalates to murder; 50% of murders are committed by an intimate partner.[15] An estimated 35% of women are seen in emergency departments for abuse and 30% of women seen in primary care are abuse victims.[47] One study of inpatient female psychiatric clients found that 64% reported abuse as adults.[47] Although men are not immune from domestic abuse, most victims are women; therefore this discussion focuses on the abuse of women.

Nurses in all clinical settings see women who are abused; they must, therefore, be aware of the risk of violence and must be comfortable addressing abuse risk issues in client encounters. The American Nurses' Association position paper *Physical Violence Against Women*[15] supports the need to (1) increase nurses' awareness of and sensitivity to the problem of physical violence against women; (2) work to reduce injuries, psychological trauma, and costs that are a result of such violence; and (3) increase nurses' awareness of their role in assessing, intervening for, and preventing physical violence against women.[47]

Assessment

Although nurses often work with women who are victims of abuse, this text emphasizes (1) the identification of risk for abuse and (2) interventions to prevent abuse before it starts. Identification begins with recognizing characteristics common to abused women. Characteristics of women at increased risk for violence include living in households with high degrees of stress, being abused as a child, and marrying young.[47,52] Abused women often display low self-esteem and experience helplessness.[21,47] In addition, certain characteristics in the woman's partner can increase her risk, such as having been abused or observed abuse as a child, abusing drugs or alcohol, having controlling behaviors, and pathologic jealousy. In addition, men who repetitively abuse women verbally often escalate to physical violence over time, during periods of high stress, or when a woman is pregnant.[47] Remember, *any* woman can be a victim of abuse, and *any* man can be an abuser. Routine screening for a history of abuse or current abuse in all women is an appropriate component of a psychosocial history (see Chapter 2).

The Partner Violence Screen (PVS)[21] is brief, easy to use, and accurate in identifying abuse. The tool consists of three questions:

1. Have you been hit, kicked, punched, or otherwise hurt by someone within the past year? If so, by whom?
2. Do you feel safe in your current relationship?
3. Does a partner from a previous relationship make you feel unsafe now?

Intervention

Once a woman is identified as being at risk for violence either through having established risk factors or by having been abused in the past, work with her to develop an individualized plan designed to prevent future violence. The plan may include assertiveness training, participation in a woman's empowerment or support group, self-esteem work, and assistance from social services to improve her educational and economic status.[36] Additional prevention strategies include community health nurse visits to high-risk families and community-wide media campaigns to enhance public awareness of the problem.[47] Explain stress management strategies, especially effective coping (see earlier discussion), to help the client to avoid violence.

If a woman is identified as being in a currently violent relationship, intervention needs to be focused on safety. This woman is at high risk for sustaining significant injury or death. Therefore nurses who screen for domestic violence must have a clearly established protocol for ensuring that every effort has been made to protect the woman. This protocol should be developed in collaboration with local law enforcement agencies and women's safety groups (e.g., YWCAs or other agencies).[15]

Older Adult Neglect and Abuse

Unfortunately, neglect and abuse affect older adults in all settings. It is estimated that 2 million older adults are victims of abuse or neglect each year.[25] It is also estimated that only 1 out of every 14 cases of abuse or neglect comes to the attention of authorities.[17] Older adult abuse can take the form of physical or sexual abuse, emotional or psychological abuse, financial or material exploitation, abandonment, or neglect. It is not uncommon for older adults to experience several types of abuse simultaneously. Without intervention, abuse tends to escalate. Risk factors for abuse include older age, lack of access to resources, low income and/or education, social isolation, minority status, functional impairment, substance abuse by older adult or caregiver, history of family violence or psychological problems, caregiver stress, and cognitive impairment.[25] Women are at more risk for abuse than men. See the Bridge to Home Health Care feature on Detecting Elder Abuse on _evolve_ the website.

With the increasing numbers of adults living into old age, older adult abuse has emerged as a significant aspect of adult violence. It is the responsibility of the health care provider, both ethically and legally, to be aware of the obvious and subtle signs of abuse and neglect and, as a client advocate, to encourage and coordinate assistance for victims and abusers.

Assessment

Because of the prevalence of older adult abuse, the nurse should have a high index of suspicion and assess for abuse at every opportunity. Clients can be asked directly, away from their caregivers, if they feel safe where they live or if they are ever treated roughly, scolded, or threatened. They can be asked if they are ever left alone a lot or if they are afraid of anyone at home. Neglect can be assessed by asking if anyone has failed to provide care for the older adult when help was needed. Behavioral cues to possible abuse include a caregiver who will not give the nurse the opportunity to talk with the client alone or who seems indifferent or angry with the client. The nurse should suspect abuse if the caregiver exhibits aggressive behavior toward the client or if the client and caregiver have conflicting accounts of an event. Physical indicators of abuse include bruises, wounds or burns, or restraint marks on wrist or ankles. Neglect should be suspected when the client presents with dehydration or malnutrition, is inappropriately dressed, or has poor hygiene. Clients who have excoriations or pressure ulcers or fecal impaction may be suffering from neglect.[6]

Intervention

The nurse who suspects older adult abuse must address the problem from several perspectives and as part of a health care team. The safety of the client is the priority, and adult protective services and/or the police must be notified if the client is in immediate or life-threatening danger, especially if the older adult is not able to manage self-care. If the client is able and willing to accept help, the client should be advised of the options and a safety plan established. In many cases of older adult abuse the abuser is under significant caregiver stress and interventions focused on helping the caregiver can be sufficient to alleviate the abusive behavior. Finding respite care or other social support for the caregiver is important. Since caregiver stress is a major risk for abuse, the nurse should address this issue with caregivers on a regular basis as a way to prevent abuse from occurring.[6]

Infectious Diseases

With the exception of HIV disease, infectious diseases are not a major cause of illness or premature death in young or midlife adults. However, adults are not immune to problems related to infectious diseases, and as noted earlier, pneumonia and influenza are major causes of preventable death in older adults. Two activities are essential for protection from infectious diseases in adults: maintaining up-to-date immunizations and practicing safe sex.

Immunization

The U.S. Preventive Services Task Force (USPSTF)[55] recommends adults have a tetanus-diphtheria booster vaccination every 10 years and that women of childbearing age who do not have proven immunity to rubella have a rubella vaccination.

Hepatitis B. People at risk for hepatitis B should receive the hepatitis B vaccination series. These risk factors[52] include frequent occupational exposure to blood and blood products, men who have sex with men, injection drug users and their partners, people with multiple (>6 lifetime) sexual partners, people who have had a sexually transmitted disease (STD), and people who travel to countries where hepatitis B is endemic.

Meningococcal Meningitis. Recently a resurgence of concern about meningococcal meningitis in college students and discussion of the value of immunizing college students has occurred. Although the risk is low, the Centers for Disease Control and Prevention (CDC) Advisory Committee on Immunization Practices[10] (ACIP) currently recommends that clinicians inform incoming college freshman who will be living in dormitories and their families about the risk of meningococcal disease and the availability of vaccine. If the student wishes to decrease the risk, he or she should be offered the vaccine or directed to a source for vaccination. The risk for all other groups of college students is the same as that for the general population and does not justify consideration of vaccination.

Human Papillomavirus. Human papillomavirus (HPV) is sexually transmitted and the cause of genital warts. More significantly, however, several of the strains of the virus are clearly associated with the development of cervical cancer. In the last decade there has been an effort to develop a vaccine to protect women against HPV. The vaccine is now available and is currently recommended for girls and young women between age 9 and 26. This vaccination should become a part of the routine vaccinations and is recommended to be given at age 11-12 but can be given as young as 9 years of age and girls and young women under 26 should be given the vaccination as a "catch-up." The immunization schedule consists of a series of 3 doses with the second given 2 months after the first and the 3rd given 6 months after the first.[11]

Varicella (Chickenpox). The Advisory Committee on Immunization Practice (ACIP)[12] recommends varicella (chickenpox) vaccine for susceptible (i.e., nonimmune) adults in the following high-risk groups: (1) persons who live or work in environments where transmission of varicella is likely (e.g., teachers of young children, day care employees, and residents and staff members in institutional settings); (2) persons who live and work in environments where transmission can occur (e.g., college students, inmates and staff members of correctional institutions, and military personnel); (3) nonpregnant women of childbearing age; (4) adults living in households with children; and (5) international travelers.

Influenza. ACIP[13] recommendations are for all adults older than 50 to receive an annual influenza vaccination. In addition, the following high-risk individuals should receive an annual influenza vaccination: (1) persons with chronic health problems or who live in chronic care centers, (2) people working with or living with at-risk people, (3) women who will be pregnant during the influenza season, (4) health care workers and other workers who provide essential services (e.g., firefighters and police), (5) household contacts or caregivers of newborns or children up to 23 months old, and (6) students and others (e.g., military personnel) living in institutional settings such as dormitories. All high-risk people 49 years old and younger may have intranasal immunization.

Pneumococcal Vaccine. Adults older than 65 are at significant risk of severe illness or death from pneumococcal pneumonia.[9] As a result, all adults age 65 and over should have a pneumococcal vaccination. Adults younger than age 65 who are at high risk and should receive pneumococcal vaccination include those who (1) have a chronic illness, (2) are alcoholics, (3) are members of high-risk ethnic and social groups (i.e., Alaskan Natives and some Native Americans), and (4) have sickle cell anemia or have had their spleen removed. Although the pneumococcal vaccine is considered a one-time dose, if a person has the vaccination before age 65, a revaccination in 5 years is recommended.

Safe Sex

There are dozens of infectious sexually transmitted diseases (STDs). Of these, HIV infection and hepatitis B and C can result in significant morbidity and premature death; others result in permanent infection (e.g., herpes simplex) or infertility (e.g., gonorrhea). Risk factors for contracting an STD include the following:

- Having a high number of sex partners (>6 lifetime partners)
- Having sex with a person who engages in high-risk behavior (e.g., multiple partners)
- Having sex for money
- Having sex with an intravenous (IV) drug user

People who abuse drugs and alcohol are at increased risk, even if they do not abuse IV drugs, because they are more likely to engage in high-risk sexual behaviors while in an impaired state.

Do not hesitate to screen for high-risk sexual behavior, and advise clients about risks and behaviors for protection from infection. Safe sex behavior includes the following:

- Abstaining from sex
- Maintaining a mutually monogamous relationship with an uninfected partner
- Avoiding sexual contact with casual or high-risk partners
- Using male or female condoms consistently and appropriately

Present information regarding referral sources in the community to assist clients with free or low-cost screening and treatment for STDs as well as information regarding sources of low-cost condoms. If you work in an ambulatory clinic or a community-based practice, consider finding a source of low-cost condoms and making them available at little or no cost to persons at high risk. Chapters 41 and 78 cover working with clients who have STDs, including HIV/AIDS.

SCREENING FOR DISEASE

Secondary prevention includes early detection of illness. Early identification is the key to preventing premature death from many catastrophic illnesses, including coronary heart disease, cancer, and type 2 diabetes mellitus. Be aware of the risks for diseases and the current recommendations regarding screening and take every opportunity to advise clients of the need for regular screening (see Chapter 2). Facilitating early detection of disease saves lives.

Recommendations for Screening

In 1989 The U.S. Preventive Services Task Force[55] (USPSTF) issued its landmark report regarding the effectiveness of preventive services and updated its recommendations in 1996; these recommendations are now revised on a regular basis and placed on the Internet as they become available (www.ahcpr.gov/clinic/uspstf). These recommendations are the "gold standard" of screening services, and nurses should be familiar with them.

In addition to screening, the USPSTF recommends many of the counseling, immunization, and chemoprophylaxis measures discussed earlier in this chapter. The recommendations are specific to age groups (except for pregnant women) and differentiate screenings recommended for all people in the group from screenings recommended for those with high-risk characteristics.

Screening recommendations are based on several factors that apply to populations rather than to individuals. The screening test must be reasonably priced, sensitive, and specific to the problem. In addition, there is generally no value to screening for diseases for which there is no treatment or when treatment does not improve either the quality or the longevity of life. As a result, many tests do not meet requirements for an effective screening program. A summary of current USPSTF recommendations for screening, counseling, and chemoprophylaxis for adults is listed in Table 1-7.

TABLE 1–7   USPSTF Recommendations for Screening for Disease

	Frequency	Population
Screening		
Alcohol misuse	At clinic visits	All adults
Breast cancer (mammography with or without clinical breast exam)	Every 1-2 years	Women >40 years old
Cervical cancer (Pap smear)	Every 1-3 years (varies based on source of recommendation, age, and risk)	Women who have been sexually active, have a cervix, and are age 21-65 (ACS <70)
Colorectal cancer (fecal occult blood, flexible sigmoidoscopy, colonoscopy, or double-contrast barium enema)	FOBT: annual Colonoscopy: every 10 years Flexible sigmoidoscopy or barium enema: every 5 years	Adults age 50 and older
Hypertension (blood pressure)	At clinic visits	Adults age 18 and older
Lipid disorders (total cholesterol and high-density lipoprotein and cholesterol)*		Adults without risk for heart disease: men at age 35 and women at age 45 Adults with risk for heart disease: men at age 20-35 and women at age 20-45
Chlamydia infection	Not specified	Sexually active women 25 years and younger
Depression symptoms	At clinic visits[†]	All adults
Smoking behavior	At clinic visits	All adults
Obesity by BMI or circumference		
Type 2 diabetes (fasting plasma glucose [or 2-hour post-load plasma glucose or hemoglobin A_{1c}])	At least every 3 years	Adults with hypertension or hyperlipidemia
Osteoporosis (DXA scan or equivalent)	Not specified	Women age 65 and older (60 if increased risk)[‡]
Counseling		
Alcohol misuse behavior	At clinic visits	
Tobacco cessation intervention	At clinic visits	Adults who use tobacco
Behavioral intervention regarding health, diet	At clinic visits	Adults with hyperlipidemia or other cardiovascular and diet-related chronic diseases
Counseling and behavioral interventions for weight loss	At clinic visits	Obese adults
Chemoprevention		
Aspirin	Daily	Adults at increased risk for heart disease[§]

From U.S. Preventive Services Task Force. (June 2005). *The guide to preventive services 2005* (AHRQ Pub No. 05-0570). Baltimore: Williams & Wilkins.
* Diabetes, family history of early heart disease, family history of familial hyperlipidemia, tobacco use, hypertension.
† Must have systems in place to ensure accurate diagnosis, treatment, and follow-up.
‡ Body weight <70 kg.
§ Age, gender, diabetes, lipid disorders, hypertension, family history, smoking.

Cardiovascular Disease Risk

The number one cause of death in adults older than age 65 is heart disease. In adults ages 45 to 64, it is the second leading cause of death. Some risk for heart disease is unavoidable (e.g., age, gender, and family history). However, most risk is modifiable through lifestyle interventions and appropriate medical management of risks such as hypertension, type 2 diabetes, and hyperlipidemia. Healthy diet and activity were discussed earlier in this chapter, and recent American Heart Association Recommendations for Diet and Lifestyle are listed in Box 1-7. As noted in Table 1-7, the USPSTF recommends that total cholesterol and high-density lipoprotein levels be used as screening tests.

The Adult Treatment Panel III[40] recommends risk assessment with a fasting lipoprotein panel—consisting of a total cholesterol, low-density lipoprotein (LDL) cholesterol, high-density lipoprotein (HDL) cholesterol, and triglycerides—be done every 5 years on all adults age 20 and over. The ATP III panel focused their attention on the LDL cholesterol as a major cause of coronary heart disease (CHD). In addition to high LDL cholesterol, additional risk factors are considered in determining CHD risk management. These risk factors include cigarette smoking, hypertension, low HDL cholesterol (<40 mg/dl), a family history of premature CHD (CHD in a male first-degree relative <55 years or CHD in a female first-degree relative <65 years), age (men ≥45 and women ≥55), history of CHD or other atherosclerotic disease, and diabetes.

Breast Cancer

Breast cancer is the most common type of cancer among women in the United States. More than 175,000 women are diagnosed with breast cancer annually, and more than 40,000 women die of breast cancer annually. Breast cancer death can be significantly reduced by early diagnosis.

Women are screened for breast cancer in three ways: mammography, clinical breast examination, and breast self-examination. Of these, mammography is the most sensitive.[54]

The USPSTF[57] and the ACS[1] recommend that women 40 years of age and older have regular (every 1 to 2 years) mammograms. Although the USPSTF[57] states that there is insufficient evidence to support the value of clinical breast examination, the ACS[1] also recommends that women 20 to 39 years of age have clinical breast examinations every 3 years.

In addition, the USPSTF indicates that there is insufficient evidence to recommend for or against breast self-examination (BSE); however, the ACS[1] recommends that all women 20 years of age and older perform BSE on a monthly basis. Nurses can teach women how to do these self-examinations.

Women can use BSE to assess their breasts. When women perform BSE properly and regularly, they can note early changes in their breasts and seek further evaluation. A major barrier to BSE is lack of confidence. Take time when working with women to ensure that they are confident of their skill and have had all their questions addressed.

When teaching, emphasize that the examination should be done every month and at the end of menses in all menstruating women. Advise nonmenstruating women to pick one day a month (e.g., the first day of the month) to do BSE. Inform women that most breast lumps are benign but it is essential that they seek professional evaluation if they find anything that concerns them. Chapter 40 discusses physical assessment of the breast, including the clinical breast examination.

BOX 1-7 **AHA 2006 Diet and Lifestyle Recommendations for Cardiovascular Risk Reduction**

- Balance calorie intake and physical activity to achieve or maintain a healthy body weight.
- Consume a diet rich in fruits and vegetables.
- Choose whole-grain, high-fiber food.
- Consume fish, especially oily fish, at least twice a week.
- Limit your intake of saturated fat to <7% of energy, trans fat to <1% of energy, and cholesterol to <300 mg per day by:
  - Choosing lean meats and vegetable alternatives
  - Selecting fat-free (skim), 1% fat, and low-fat dairy products
  - Minimizing your intake of partially hydrogenated fats
- Minimize your intake of beverages and foods with added sugar.
- Choose and prepare food with no or little salt.
- If you consume alcohol, do so in moderation.
- When you eat food that is prepared outside the home, follow the AHA *Diet and Lifestyle Recommendations*.

Reprinted with permission. *Diet and lifestyle recommendations revision 2006: A scientific statement from the American Heart Association Committee.* © 2006, American Heart Association.

Prostate Cancer

Nearly 40,000 men die annually of prostate cancer. Men at increased risk include those who have a first-degree relative (e.g., father, brother, son) with prostate cancer and are African Americans. Despite the prevalence of the disease, neither the USPSTF[55] nor the American Academy of Family Physicians[39] recommends *routine* screening for prostate cancer because early screening and treatment have not proved beneficial in extending life expectancy or quality of life of men diagnosed with the disease. They do recommend, however, counseling clients about known risks for prostate cancer and the uncertain benefits of screening. The ACS[1] and the American Urological Association[39] suggest that men should be offered screening for prostate cancer using a prostate-specific antigen test and a digital rectal examination starting at age 50 (at age 45 for African-American men) (see Chapter 38).

When advising men about screening, keep in mind the man's prostate cancer risk factors, his general health, and his desires. Generally, prostate cancer screening should not be done in men older than 70 years of age or who have significant underlying illness that would result in a life expectancy of less than 10 years.[39]

Colorectal Cancer

Colorectal cancer is the second most common form of cancer in the United States, and it accounts for more than 55,000 deaths per year. If the disease is found while still localized, survival rates are at 91%. If the disease is found when it has spread, the survival rate is much lower.[52] Therefore early detection of the disease is essential. Uncommon risk factors include hereditary familial polyposis syndromes and ulcerative colitis of more than 10 years' duration. More common risk factors include a family history of colorectal cancer, especially in young and middle-aged adults, and possibly high-fat and low-fiber diets.[58]

Current recommendations are for annual screening of adults more than 50 years of age for colorectal cancer using fecal occult blood testing (FOBT).[58] People who are at increased risk might benefit from beginning screening at 40 years of age. FOBT is easily done at home, but the client should be instructed on dietary restrictions, specifically no raw meat, no aspirin or nonsteroidal anti-inflammatory agents, and no vitamin C in doses greater than 250 mg for 48 hours before and during specimen collection. Specimens should be kept away from heat and should be tested within 2 weeks of collection. Both the USPSTF[58] and the American Cancer Society[1] recognize the potential value of either a sigmoidoscopy every 5 years in combination with annual FOBT testing or a colonoscopy every 10 years, but there are insufficient data to support either of these options for routine screening.

Depression

More than 19 million people in the United States suffer from depression. Major depression is a significant cause of disability and accounts for two thirds of all deaths from suicide annually. In addition, depression is associated with many other medical problems, including heart disease, diabetes, and chronic obstructive pulmonary disease (COPD). Despite the significant impact of depression on the health of the population, it is estimated that fewer than 25% of people suffering from depression receive treatment. As a result, the recommendation of the USPSTF is for routine screening of adults for depression in clinical practices. A variety of depression screening tools are available (see Chapter 24). Nurses who screen for depression should have a clearly established protocol in place to ensure that the client is referred for accurate diagnosis and effective treatment.[56]

Research suggests depression occurs in approximately 10% to 15% of all community-dwelling older adults more than 65 years of age; among institutionalized older adults, the prevalence rate increases to 50% to 75%.[20] Depression is more likely to lead to cognitive impairment such as dementia or delirium in older adults. It is estimated that depression-associated cognitive disorders occur in 10% to 29% of depressed older adults.[30] Therefore differentiation between depression-related cognitive alteration and dementia may be difficult. Table 1-8 contrasts the primary clinical features of delirium, dementia, and depression.

CONCLUSIONS

Health promotion and disease prevention activities are at the core of health care. Nurses must be familiar with current recommendations regarding healthy eating and activity patterns and with strategies for coping with daily stressors. Take every opportunity to work with clients to assist them to implement healthy lifestyles. Include risk assessment, risk management, and appropriate screening for diseases when working with clients. Based on assessment results, provide education, self-management support, and appropriate referral.

TABLE 1–8 Common Mental Health Disorders in Older Adults: Clinical Features

	Delirium	Dementia	Depression
Description	A reversible, acute confusional state	A gradually progressive, irreversible cognitive decline	A reversible affective feeling associated with sadness, which may vary from mild downheartedness or a feeling of indifference to a feeling of great despair beyond hope
Onset	Rapid, acute, often at night	Slow, gradual	Gradual or sudden
Duration	Days to weeks, but usually less than 1 month	Continuous, ongoing, months to years	Varies from weeks to years
Disorientation	Present, especially for time; tendency to mistake unfamiliar for familiar persons, places	May be absent in mild states of dementia	May seem disoriented to place or time
Thinking	Slow or accelerated; may be dream-like, impoverished	Impoverished; poor abstracting ability	Slowed thinking, indecisiveness
Memory	Short-term memory impaired; long-term memory intact	Short-term memory impaired; long-term memory may be affected	May seem impaired for recent and remote events
Attention	Consistently impaired; easily distracted; fluctuates	Typically intact	Complaints or evidence of diminished ability to concentrate
Alertness	Reduced or increased, but awareness always affected	Typically normal; may be reduced	Psychomotor agitation or retardation
Perception	Invariably affected, especially at night; often have hallucinations	May be intact; usually no hallucinations	May have auditory hallucinations
Sleep	Sleep-wake cycle altered	Usually normal for age	Insomnia or hypersomnia
Course	Typically fluctuates with lucid intervals and exacerbations	Relatively stable over course of a day	Usually rapid progression
Affect	Intermittent fear, perplexity, bewilderment	Flat or indifferent	Sad, worried, anxious, hopeless; may slow agitation or apathy
Cause	Multiple potential causes (e.g., surgery, infection, drugs)	Unknown, possible environmental, hereditary, chemical	Secondary to other mental illness; related to loss, physical illness, medications, loneliness

Data from American Psychiatric Association. (2000). *Diagnostic and statistical manual of mental disorders* (4th ed.). Washington, DC: Author.

BIBLIOGRAPHY

Citations appearing in red refer to primary research.

Citations appearing in blue refer to evidence-based practice guidelines and protocols.

1. American Cancer Society. *Guidelines for the early detection of cancer.* www.cancer.org/docroot/PED.
2. American Cancer Society. Diet and Physical activity: What's the Cancer Connection? www.cancer.org/docroot/PED.
3. Anderson, J.E., et al (2002). Treating tobacco use and dependence: An evidence-based clinical practice guideline for tobacco cessation. *Chest, 121*(3), 932-941.
4. Bodenheimer, T., MacGregor, K., & Sharif, C. (2005). *Helping clients manage their chronic illnesses.* Oakland, Calif: Healthcare Foundation. Available at www.chcf.org.
5. Bonheur, B., & Young, S. (1991). Exercise as a health-promoting life-style choice. *Applied Nursing Research, 4*(1), 2-6.
6. Burke, M.M., & Laramie, J.A. (2004). *Primary care of the older adult* (2nd ed.). St. Louis: Mosby.
7. Burns, K. (1996). A new recommendation for physical activity as a means of health promotion. *Nurse Practitioner, 21*(9), 18, 21-22, 26, 27.
8. Calfas, K., et al (1996). A controlled trial of physician counseling to promote the adoption of physical activity. *Preventive Medicine, 25,* 225-233.
9. Centers for Disease Control. (April 4, 1997). Prevention of Pneumococcal Disease: Recommendations of the Advisory Committee on Immunization Practice, *Morbidity and Mortality Weekly Report, 46* (RR08), 1-24.
10. Centers for Disease Control. (June 30, 2000). Meningococcal disease and college students. *Morbidity and Mortality Weekly Report, 49*(RR07), 11-20.
11. Centers for Disease Control. (May 23, 2007). Quadrivalent Human Papilloma Vaccine: Recommendations of the Advisory Committee on Immunization Practice. *Morbidity and Mortality Weekly Report, 56* (RR02), 1-24.
12. Centers for Disease Control. (June 22, 2007). Prevention of Varicella: Recommendation of the Advisory Committee on Immunization Practice (ACIP). *Morbidity and Mortality Weekly Report, 56* (RR04), 1-40.
13. Centers for Disease Control. (July 13, 2007). Prevention and Control of Influenza. *Morbidity and Mortality Weekly Report, 56* (RR06), 1-54.
14. Chrousos, G., & Gold, P. (1992). The concepts of stress and stress system disorders. *Journal of the American Medical Association, 267*(9), 1244-1252.

15. Council of Community Health Nurses. (1991). *Physical violence against women: ANA position statement.* Kansas City, Mo: American Nurses' Association.

16. Davis, M., Eshelman, E., & McKay, M. (1995). *The relaxation and stress reduction workbook* (4th ed.). Oakland, Calif: New Harbinger Publications.

17. Dong, X. (2005). Medical implications of elder abuse and neglect. *Clinics of Geriatric Medicine, 21,* 293-313.

18. Dunn, H. (1961). *High level wellness.* Arlington, Va: R.W. Berry.

19. Edelman, C., & Mandle, C. (Eds.). (2001). *Health promotion throughout the life span* (5th ed.). St. Louis: Mosby.

20. Eliopoulos, C. (2001). *Gerontological nursing,* (5th ed.). Philadelphia: Lippincott Williams & Wilkins.

21. Feldhaus, K., et al (1997). Accuracy of three brief questions for detecting partner violence in the emergency department. *Journal of the American Medical Association, 277,* 1357-1361.

22. Fiore, M.C., et al (2000). *Treating tobacco use and dependence: Clinical practice guidelines.* Rockville, Md: U.S. Department of Health and Human Services, Public Health Service.

23. Franklin, B., Buchal, M., & Hollingsworth, V. (1991). Exercise prescription. In R. Strauss (Ed.), *Sports medicine* (2nd ed.). Philadelphia: Saunders.

24. Goldstein, D.J. (1992). Beneficial effects of modest weight loss. *International Journal of Obesity, 16,* 397-415.

25. Gorbian, M.J., & Eisenstein, A.R. (2005). Elder abuse and neglect: An Overview. *Clinics of Geriatric Medicine, 21,* 279-292.

26. Grubbs, L. (1993). The critical role of exercise in weight control. *Nurse Practitioner, 18*(4), 20, 22, 25-26, 29.

27. Howard, G., et al (1998). Cigarette smoking and progression of atherosclerosis: The Atherosclerosis Risk in Communities (ARIC) study. *Journal of the American Medical Association, 279*(2), 119-124.

28. Institute of Medicine. (2002). *Dietary reference intakes for energy, carbohydrate, fiber, fat, fatty acids, cholesterol, protein, and amino acids.* Washington, DC: National Academies Press.

29. Isaacson, J., Butler, R., & Zackarek, M. (1994). Screening with the Alcohol Use Disorders Identification Test (AUDIT) in an inner-city population. *Journal of General Internal Medicine, 9,* 550-553.

30. Kennedy-Malone, L., Flecthcer, K.R., & Plank, L.M. (2000). *Management guidelines for gerontological nurse practitioners.* Philadelphia: FA Davis.

31. Long, B.J., et al (1996). A multisite field test of the acceptability of physical counseling in primary care: Project PACE. *American Journal of Preventive Medicine, 12*(2), 73-81.

32. Lorig, K., & Holman, H.R. (2003). Self-management education: History, definition, outcomes, and mechanisms. *Annals of Behavioral Medicine, 26*(1), 1-7.

33. Lorig, K., Ritter, P., & Gonzalez, V. (2003). Hispanic chronic disease self-management: A randomized community-based outcome trial. *Nursing Research, 52*(6), 361-369.

34. Lorig, K., Ritter, P., & Jacquex, A. (2005). Outcomes of border health Spanish/English chronic disease self-management programs. *The Diabetes Educator, 31*(3), 401-409.

35. Marchione, J. (1993). *Margaret Newman: Health as expanding consciousness.* Newberry Park: Sage.

36. McWhirter, E.H. (1994). *Counseling for empowerment.* Alexandria, Va: American Counseling Association.

37. Menninger, J.A. (2002). Assessment and treatment of alcoholism and substance-related disorders in the elderly. *Bulletin of the Menninger Clinic, 66*(2), 166-183.

38. Michocki, R.J. (2001). Polypharmacy and principles of drug therapy. In A.M. Adelman, M.P. Daly. 20 Common Problems in Geriatrics. (pp. 69-81). New York: McGraw-Hill.

39. Naitoh, J., Zeiner, R.L., & Dekernion, J.B. (1998). Diagnosis and treatment of prostate cancer. *American Family Physician, 57*(7), 1531-1539.

40. *Third Report of the National Cholesterol Education Program (NCEP) Expert Panel on Detection, Evaluation, and Treatment of High Blood Cholesterol in Adults (Adult Treatment Panel III).* (2001). Bethesda, Md: U.S. Department of Health and Human Services, Public Health Service, National Institutes of Health, National Heart, Lung, and Blood Institute.

41. National Heart, Lung, and Blood Institute (NHLBI), NHLBI Obesity Education Initiative Expert Panel. (June 1998). *Clinical guidelines on the identification, evaluation, and treatment of overweight and obesity in adults: The evidence report.* Bethesda, Md: National Institutes of Health, National Heart, Lung, and Blood Institute.

42. Padden, D.L. (2002). The role of the advanced practice nurse in the promotion of exercise and physical activity. *Topics in Advanced Practice Nursing Journal, 2*(1).

43. Paffenbarger, R.S., et al (1986). Physical activity, all-cause mortality, and longevity in college alumni. *New England Journal of Medicine, 314*(10), 605-613.

44. Pate, R.R., et al (1995). Physical activity and public health. *Journal of the American Medical Association, 273*(5), 402-407.

45. Pi-Sunyer, F.X. (1993). Medical hazards of obesity. *Annals of Internal Medicine, 119*(7), 655-660.

46. Prochaska, J., Redding, C., & Evers, K. (2002). The Transtheoretical Model and stages of change. In K. Glanz, R. Rimet, & F. Lewis (Eds.), *Health behavior and health education: Theory, research and practice* (3rd ed.). San Francisco: Jossey-Bass.

47. Quillian, J.P. (1995). Domestic violence. *Journal of the American Academy of Nurse Practitioners, 7*(7), 351-358.

48. Saunders, J., et al (1993). Development of the Alcohol Use Disorders Identification Test (AUDIT): WHO collaboration project on early detection of persons with harmful alcohol consumption. II. *Addiction, 88,* 791.

49. Schillinger, D., Grumbach, K., Piette, J., et al (2002). Association of health literacy with diabetic outcomes. *Journal of the American Medical Association, 288*(4), 475-482.

50. Smith (1983). *The Idea of health.* New York: Teachers College Press.

51. Travis, J.W., & Ryan, R.S. (1988). The Wellness Workbook, 2nd ed. Berkeley, Calif: Ten Speed Press.

52. U.S. Department of Health and Human Services. (1998). *Clinician's handbook of preventive services* (3rd ed.). Washington, DC: U.S. Government Printing Office.

53. U.S. Department of Health and Human Services. (2000). *Healthy People 2010.* (Conference Edition, in Two Volumes). Washington, DC: Author.

54. U.S. Department of Health and Human Services. (1996). *Physical activity and health, S/N 017-023-00196-5.* Washington, DC: U.S. Government Printing Office.

55. U.S. Preventive Services Task Force. (1996). *Guide to clinical preventive services* (2nd ed.). Baltimore: Williams & Wilkins.

56. U.S. Preventive Services Task Force. (2002). Screening for depression: Recommendations and rationale. *Annals of Internal Medicine, 136*(10), 760-764.

57. U.S. Preventive Services Task Force. (2002). Screening for breast cancer: Recommendations and rationale. *Annals of Internal Medicine, 137*(5 pt 1), 344-346.

58. U.S. Preventive Services Task Force. (2002). Screening for colorectal cancer: Recommendations and rationale. *Annals of Internal Medicine, 137*(2), 129-131.

59. World Health Organization, Division of Health Promotion, Education and Communication, Health Education and Promotion Unit. (1998). *Health promotion glossary.* Geneva: Author.

60. World Health Organization. (1947). Constitution of the World Health Organization. *Chronicle of the World Health Organization, 1*(1-2), 29-43.

CHAPTER 2

Health Assessment

JOYCE BLACK

Assessment is the first step of the nursing process; even if you do not think you are "using the nursing process" when you talk with your clients or observe them when you enter a room, you are assessing them. This chapter will explain the importance of formal assessments in health care settings and describe how the data collected are analyzed.

There are four classic forms of physical assessment: inspection, percussion, palpation, and auscultation. You probably learned these in a health assessment course. All aspects of physical assessment begin with taking a history and then proceed to examination.

HEALTH HISTORY

Health assessment begins with the health history interview. The purpose of the interview is to collect the client's subjective data. The information contained in a health history is listed in Box 2-1. Observe the client throughout the interaction. Your observations will guide the areas to emphasize during the physical examination that follows. (A more comprehensive review of the health history process can be found on the website.)

ASPECTS OF HEALTH HISTORY

Accuracy

Collecting accurate information is the basis of the nursing process. Determine whether the client is a reliable historian, able and willing to provide information. Clients may be poor historians and cannot provide accurate data because they are (1) unconscious or disoriented and unable to cooperate; (2) willing to cooperate but hindered by circumstances, such as a language barrier or anxiety; or (3) unwilling and mistrustful about cooperating because of anger or depression. If the client

cannot provide information, seek secondary sources, such as significant others or an interpreter. However, information content and accuracy may be influenced by the perceptions and biases of the secondary sources as well as by their knowledge of the problem and recall ability.

Accuracy can also be altered by factors in the nurse. Stereotyping jeopardizes collection of accurate data. False assumptions and generalizations may alienate the client and interfere with development of trust. A mistrustful client is reluctant to divulge sensitive information, perhaps fearing rejection or ridicule, resulting in inaccurate or missed nursing diagnoses.

Generalizations, particularly those grounded in assumptions or prejudice or based on limited experience, are potentially harmful. Similarities among people can result in their being grouped according to age, gender, ethnic background, common occupation, recreational activity, health risk behavior, or type of health problem. Remember that each person is also unique. Reliable research findings concerning group characteristics or similarities may be applied to a specific client who belongs to that group. For example, the

---

BOX 2-1 Components of Health History

- Biographical and demographic information
- Current health problem (chief complaint)
- Past health history
- Family health history
- Psychosocial history
- Appraisal of the client's health maintenance and health promotion behaviors to assess health risks
- Review of systems

---

incidence of hypertension is higher in blacks than in whites, and regular blood pressure screening should be included at every health care visit.

Bias must be avoided by keeping an open mind during the physical assessment. Even physical appearance or presenting manifestations may bias perception of a client. Similar manifestations may have different origins. For example, a client with an uneven, lurching gait and garbled speech may appear to be intoxicated or under the influence of a controlled substance. In fact, the client might have residual neurologic deficits from a head injury. Initial inaccurate judgment may be costly in wasted time and effort and may result in a strained nurse-client relationship.

Computerized health history assessment is available in clinical settings, particularly ambulatory care settings. Computer programs for history taking result in accurate, legible databases when data are entered correctly. Either the client or the nurse, using interactive programs, records the data directly. Data also may be entered from a client-completed questionnaire, which is reviewed and validated by a nurse skilled in health assessment. Computerized health histories tend to be complete because pertinent assessment areas are included in the programs. Branching programs direct collection of additional data when the client responds with significant information.

Depth

Many factors influence the level of assessment. Ideally, data are collected at one time and in sufficient depth to allow problem identification; however, this may not always be practical. The interview setting may be less than ideal (for example, the scene of a motor vehicle accident). The client's reason for seeking health care may preclude in-depth interviewing (e.g., a ruptured appendix). The client's attention span, energy, and comfort level may affect the ability to participate (e.g., acute pain).

In an acute situation:

1. Collect data pertinent to the immediate problem and assess the client's present health status.
2. Tailor the health history interview to include pertinent data while striving to be thorough.
3. Update and enlarge the database as indicated by the client's condition.

Completeness

The health history model presented in this chapter is an episodic format. Refer to a health assessment text for information on the exhaustive or long format. (An example of a completed exhaustive history and physical examination is on the website.) An *episodic* health history assessment often suffices when a client presents with an uncomplicated, short-term health problem, such as an earache. Use a systematic approach to collect data significant to the problem (Box 2-2). Proficiency in all areas of health history assessment, which are discussed in this chapter, is necessary to conduct an accurate episodic assessment.

In clinical practice, many agencies provide specific health history formats. These formats are designed to meet agency purposes and may vary considerably in depth and level. Tailor the health history interview to the needs of the client and the agency. For example, you might arrange to meet several brief times with clients who have limited abilities or special needs (impaired hearing or limited intellectual capacity), or an interpreter may be required when a language barrier exists.

Components

There are many components to the health history. They are listed in Box 2-1, and are presented in priority order. When collecting information, include the date of the interview because the date and time information is gathered constitute the baseline assessment. If the client's health status changes, the health history and physical examination reflect the extent of the change over time. The baseline also provides a legal baseline, in that, in most cases, nurses are not responsible for conditions that were present at the time of admission.

Health history assessment may be organized according to a nursing theory (e.g., Orem's theory of self-care), by health behavior patterns (e.g., Gordon's functional health patterns), or by body systems (e.g., heart, lung). In this chapter, the health history format is an extended health database model (see the website). A single complete database is preferable for reference and retrieval of information.

BOX 2-2 An Episodic Health History Format

Include these elements in an episodic (short) health history:

- Client's statement of the problem (chief complaint)
- Symptom analysis
- Review the body system to which the symptom belongs
- Explore the manifestation's relationship to other body systems (include a review of associated body systems)
- Investigate the current problem's relationship to the client's past health and health maintenance and promotion practices

Biographical and Demographic Information

The extent and type of biographical and demographic information may vary, depending on agency protocol. Some computerized systems allow retrieval of this information.

History of Present Illness or Chief Complaint

The history of the present illness is a statement from the client describing the reason for seeking health care and the major presentation of the problem. Use the client's own words whenever possible. Listen closely to the client's explanation of the problem; many times the client will provide a great deal of information from which an accurate diagnosis can be made. Do not assume that you know what is wrong; allow the client to explain. At times, this section is called the chief compliant, but this phrase implies that the client "complains" and therefore is not commonly used anymore.

Determining the reason for admission to the hospital is the first question asked of clients. Many times the nurse will know the reason for admission from the admission department, the emergency department, or the operating room. If this is the case, the nurse should validate the current complaint by asking, "The ER nurse told me you came to the hospital after you fell on the ice and broke your ankle, is that right?" This statement will allow the client to validate the diagnosis and then the nurse can proceed to ask about the severity of current pain. Once the pain is controlled, the remainder of the admission can usually be conducted.

If you ask the right questions and the client is a good historian, much of the work of determining what might be wrong with the client is greatly aided. One of the most common aspects of taking a history is the recording of the client's past medical conditions and surgical interventions, along with medications and family and social history.

Symptom Analysis

Symptom analysis is a detailed description of the current health problem. In this book, the term *manifestations* is used synonymously with *signs and symptoms*. The process of symptom analysis should be used often, each time a client has a reported problem. It is especially important to fully understand the likely cause of the problem before beginning treatment. Misdiagnosis can occur, especially when inadequate data were collected. Consider this scenario: A client had a knee replacement yesterday. He asks for something for pain. The nurse brings in his oral pain medication because it was the medication he took the last time for pain. He takes the pill and then says, "I hope this helps this pain in my chest!" Except for his comment and the symptom analysis that followed, his angina could have been completely overlooked!

There are some acronyms to help you recall what questions to ask during this part of the health assessment (Table 2-1). For example, if a client reported headache, this might be the response to a symptom analysis using the acronym OLDCART:

O = Throbbing severe headache, occurring daily × 2 weeks

L = Occipital region

D = Several hours every day, starting in the morning and usually lasting until noon

C = Throbbing, constricting

A = Occasional blurred vision, accompanied by nausea at times, usually subsides as day progresses; BP 190/100 mm Hg today both arms

R = Usually subsides as day progresses without treatment; has taken Tylenol 600 mg PO with moderate relief this morning at 0900; has also used dark rooms and cold compresses

T = Recheck BP after 15 minutes; notify physician

Regardless of the process used to collect the information for symptom analysis, the same data should be collected. You may find one system works better for you and it is important to use the same process each time, so that all the data are collected.

Past Health History

The past health history may be important for determining both current and future health risk status. Past health history data include information about the client's growth and development, immunization status, past illnesses (usual childhood diseases as well as those occurring in

TABLE 2-1	Selected Acronyms for Symptom Analysis		
OLDCART	**PQRST**	**COLD SPA**	**LOCATE**
Onset	Precipitating/palliative factors	Character	Location
Location	Quality/quantity	Onset	Onset and duration
Duration	Region/radiation/related symptoms	Location	Characteristics
Characteristics	Severity	Duration	Associated symptoms
Associated manifestations	Timing	Severity	Treatments
Radiation		Pattern	Eliminates/aggravates
Treatment		Associated factors	

adulthood), presence of serious or chronic illnesses, hospitalizations, surgeries, serious injuries or accidents, obstetric history (if applicable), last visits to health care providers, allergies, and medications.

Past medical conditions are any diseases that have existed before this hospitalization. So, if the client was diagnosed with diabetes during this hospital stay, he is now a diabetic client, but diabetes would not be listed as a past medical problem. This aspect of history taking can be confusing, especially if you are collecting past medical history from a client during the hospital stay rather than on admission.

Depending upon the health care system's method of record-keeping, the nurse may or may not have to ask about previous health history. Some computerized systems detail the client's major illnesses and operations with excellent specificity (e.g., the date of diagnosis and treatment). However, it is important to confirm with the client that the list is current and correct. A second opinion may have changed the diagnosis, the disease may have been cured, or the client may have had it surgically corrected.

The list of past medical conditions can be lengthy. It is important to try to record all of the problems and what treatments are being done for them. These questions can easily be asked during this portion of the history. For example, if the client says she has asthma, the nurse can then ask what is done for the problem. If the client requires daily medication and rescue inhalers, her asthma is not as well controlled as a client who simply treats the asthma as needed with inhalers. A complete history taken in this manner will also help guide the nurse as the medications for the client are reviewed. Obviously, in the first client's situation, medications for asthma should be ordered.

Past Surgical Procedures

Recording past surgical procedures also provides a picture of the client's health. Again, it is helpful if the operation is linked to the cause. For example, recording that the client has coronary artery disease and had a coronary artery bypass graft provides more data on the seriousness of the arteriosclerosis than the two problems listed separately.

Family Health History

With the ever-increasing information about genetic profiles, the inherited risk for diseases is an important aspect of health history. The family health history helps to identify family-linked (familial) diseases that affect health status and risk for potential health problems. Health problems of interest include heart disease, hypertension, stroke, epilepsy, migraines or headaches, mental illness, Alzheimer's disease, Huntington's chorea, alcoholism, tuberculosis, asthma, allergies, diabetes mellitus, thyroid problems, eating disorders, obesity, kidney disease, arthritis, cancer (type), sickle cell anemia, anemia, hemophilia, human immunodeficiency virus infection, and developmental delay.

Health Care Maintenance

Health care maintenance includes risk factors and stressors for the age group. Depending on the age of the client, questions address use of seat belts, immunizations, and cancer screening, for example. The nurse should refer to the stages of development for ideas on typical issues as well as the usual causes of death for each age group.

Medication Use

Clients should be asked what medications they take daily and occasionally and if possible provide medication names and doses. Ask the client to include any over-the-counter medications and herbal or natural products also. This series of questions will often provide new information about diseases the client overlooked in the previous discussion. Likewise, the nurse can validate that medications are taken for the pre-existent diseases. If the client has bottles or bags of pills, they will need to be identified. Most of the time, these medications will not be administered during the hospital stay; instead, the hospital's own supply of medications will be used. Therefore these medications can be returned to the client's home with family or be secured until discharge.

Domestic Violence

Domestic violence is a more common problem than is usually recognized. Asking each client about feeling safe at home is an important first step in identifying those at risk of domestic violence. The client's safety should be the primary focus. If the batterer finds out the client revealed the abuse, the client may be in greater danger because separation is often the most dangerous time for victims. If the client admits to domestic abuse, the law requires that the nurse report these findings to the authorities.

Psychosocial History

Psychosocial assessment assists the nurse in understanding a client's response to circumstances and events, which, in turn, influences the client's ability to function. This understanding enables comprehensive and holistic care. Approximately two thirds of the disorders that nurses independently identify and treat are psychosocial. Accurate assessment of responses to health problems enables the client to return to optimal levels of both physiologic and psychological functioning.

Performing the psychosocial assessment requires sensitivity and interpersonal skills. Ability to establish a therapeutic relationship directly affects the quality of the data. Because many topics are highly personal, it is imperative to be tactful and nonjudgmental and to handle confidential information professionally. An atmosphere of trust encourages the client to divulge sensitive information. Convey interest by listening attentively, making eye contact, and using skillful interview techniques. Your personal value system may influence or bias perception of a client's behavior and experiences. Self-awareness helps one to remain nonjudgmental. Making accurate observations and sharing them allow the client opportunity to validate the nurse's perceptions and inferences.

Psychosocial Risk Factors. During the health history interview, assess factors indicating risk for or an actual psychosocial problem. Box 2-3 lists guidelines for identifying psychosocial risk factors. If risk factors are present, proceed with a detailed assessment. An interview guide for in-depth assessment of selected areas of psychosocial status appears on the website. The guide also includes questions that may be asked during a cultural assessment.

Psychological Assessment. The psychological dimension includes perceptions about mood, thoughts, feelings, motivations, stressors, personal strengths and weaknesses, values and beliefs, and spirituality. Responses and interpretations are reflected in thought processes and in what is said and done. Observe the client's appearance and behavior throughout the interview. Observations, when validated, assist in understanding psychological status. Record subjective data in the health history and objective data in the physical examination report.

General Appearance. Appearance and behavior reflect the client's mental status and comfort level with the interview. Observe the client's posture, nonverbal behavior, facial expression, manner of dress with regard to the climate and occasion, grooming and hygiene, and attitude toward the assessment interview (e.g., cooperative, hostile, withdrawn). For example, "The client is dressed in a hospital gown, is sitting erect in bed, and answers questions without hesitation."

Motor Activity. Note motor ability, gait, coordination, reaction time, and unusual body movements (e.g.,

---

BOX 2-3   Identifying Psychosocial Risk Factors

SOCIAL HISTORY

Social history includes information about the client's family members, social network, and lifestyle. Ask if others are available to provide emotional support to the client during stressful times. This support system may include pets.

PERSONAL AND FAMILY HISTORY

A personal or family history of psychosocial problems increases a client's risk of having problems. A client may fear recurrence of an emotional or mental health problem or worry that he or she has inherited a family-linked illness, such as schizophrenia.

LEVEL OF STRESS

Change and loss are two major influences that produce stress in individuals. Clients who have experienced stressful events within the past year are at risk for development of health problems. Assess the client's present stress level compared to the response to previous stressful events.

USUAL COPING PATTERN

The usual coping pattern refers to how the client copes with a serious problem or manages high levels of stress. Ask the client to describe a particularly stressful situation and how it was managed. Assess whether the client's usual coping style is adequate and appropriate for the current situation. Other coping strategies may be necessary. Psychosocial reactions to health problems are highly individual and usually occur as the client and significant others cope with the effects of illness.

CHANGES IN NEUROPHYSIOLOGIC FUNCTION

Neurophysiologic changes include physical manifestations of psychological stress. The stress response, regardless of its cause, results in altered levels of neurotransmitters, such as norepinephrine and serotonin, that then affect the sympathetic and parasympathetic nervous systems. The client's usual body functions, such as sleep and rest patterns, appetite, energy level, sexual function, and elimination patterns, can be affected.

LEVEL OF UNDERSTANDING ABOUT HEALTH PROBLEM

Explore the client's level of understanding about the health problem. The client may not comprehend what has happened or could happen as a result of a health problem. The client may have unrealistic expectations of the health care team. Determine how threatening a particular health problem is and whether the client has been able to prepare psychologically for its effects.

MENTAL STATUS

Mental status refers to the client's current emotional, intellectual, and perceptual functioning. If a dysfunction is evident, describe the problem.

PERSONALITY STYLE

Personality style is the way a client usually interacts with others. Examples include dependent, independent, controlled, relaxed, dramatic, suspicious, accepting, self-sacrificing, superior, inferior, uninvolved, involved, mixed (a combination of two predominant styles), or no predominant style.

MAJOR PSYCHOSOCIAL REACTIONS

Reactions include disruption in the ability to trust, maintain self-esteem, retain feelings of control, cope with loss and guilt, and maintain intimacy.

gestures, tics, tremors, foot tapping, hand wringing, grimacing, or other repetitive movements). For example, "The client drummed his fingers on the table before answering."

Behavior. Activities observed by others constitute behavior, and behavior is central to psychological assessment. Verbal behavior is what is said and includes voice tone; nonverbal behavior concerns observable behavior such as posture, movement, and facial expression. Observe and record both verbal and nonverbal behaviors. Accurate assessment dictates that observed behavior be described rather than interpreted. "The client is crying" is an observed behavior, whereas "The client is depressed" is a judgmental statement. Without further assessment, the nurse does not know why the client is crying. If the client states, "I feel depressed," record "States she feels depressed."

Mental Status. A mental status examination (MSE) is an assessment of a client's level of cognitive (knowledge-related) ability, appearance, emotional mood, and speech and thought patterns at the time of evaluation. It is one part of a full neurologic (nervous system) examination and includes the examiner's observations about the client's attitude and cooperativeness as well as the client's answers to specific questions. The level and depth of questioning vary, depending on individual circumstances. Assess a client who is alert and cooperative by listening and observing carefully during the interview. The client's responses provide information about orientation, mood, memory, attention span, general knowledge, language abilities, thought processes, judgment, and insight.

When assessing mental status, individualize questions to the client's circumstances. Variables affecting one's ability to respond to specific questions include the following:

- Level of education
- Cultural background
- Degree of exposure to knowledge and information
- Familiarity with the language and vocabulary
- Perceived acceptance by the nurse

For example, it may be revealing to ask a teenager the name of a current popular singer but inappropriate to ask the same question of an older person. A client who has not progressed beyond a third-grade level of education may be incapable of performing complicated arithmetic calculations. A proverb widely known in one culture may be meaningless to someone from a different cultural background. Finally, you must have access to correct answers for the questions asked, particularly those relating to personal circumstances, such as the location of the client's home, date and place of birth, and names of family members.

If a client demonstrates impaired cognitive function, perform an abbreviated mental status examination (see Chapter 23). Disturbances in mood or thought processes (such as suicidal ideation) warrant a complete, detailed mental status examination. Even though mental status data are collected during the health history, record this information with the physical examination data. The following areas are included.

Level of Consciousness. Level of consciousness is the state of awareness. The client must be alert, not just awake, for a mental status assessment (see Chapter 23). Cue the client that the questions may seem "silly" but are to be answered anyway.

Orientation to Person, Place, Time, and Circumstances. Ask the client to explain the reason for seeking health care. If the reply is unclear or if the client digresses, ask the client to state his or her name, to identify the present location, and to specify the date and time.

Mood and Affect. Mood is the subjective description of a personal emotion that is pervasive and sustained. Record whether the described mood matches the present situation. For example, "The client stated she was 'happy and going to celebrate' when informed that the results of her tests were normal."

Affect is the observable, outward demeanor that depicts the current emotional state, such as fear, anger, resentment, depression, anxiety, or elation. A flat affect is a lack of any facial expression or emotional response and is accompanied by a monotonous voice. A blunted affect is greatly reduced in intensity but still appropriate to the situation. Note whether the observed affect matches the immediate circumstances. For example, "When informed that discharge from the hospital was postponed because of an infection, the client first cried, then shouted at the nurse to leave the room." This indicates the client first was upset and then became angry that the discharge was delayed because of a complication. Both reactions are understandable, given the situation.

Speech and Communication (Language). Evaluate the physical ability to speak and communicate by focusing on how the client talks, not the topic of speech. Observe tone of voice, pitch, rate of speech, articulation, length of responses, pauses during speech, and pauses before the client replies to questions (latency).

Thought Processes and Content. Assess whether speech progresses logically and whether the stream of thought is spontaneous, natural, organized, logical, relevant, coherent, and goal-directed. What the client says should be consistent.

Other Components. Other components of the examination include attention span; immediate, recent, and remote memory; general fund of knowledge; ability to calculate; abstract reasoning and thought; perceptual distortion; judgment; and insight. Depending on the setting and the problems present, other psychological factors may be important to assess. These could include motivation, personal strengths, values and beliefs, and spirituality. Methods to collect this information are explained in health assessment textbooks and in Chapter 23.

Social History. Social history usually details the client's exposure to illness because of personal habits (e.g., alcohol, smoked and chewed tobacco, IV drugs), occupational exposure (such as exposure to second-hand smoke), life stressors (e.g., recent family events), home life (e.g., single, married), and lifestyle (e.g., homeless versus living in a private home). This area of assessment also includes information about social roles and functions, viewing the client as an individual and a member of a social network. These data provide insight into the ability of the client to return home safely, risk factors that require referral for ongoing treatment, and possible exposure to communicable diseases. The preferred method of learning is also included in this assessment.

Psychosocial Development. *Psychosocial development* refers to a person's level of growth and development, including the life developmental processes and phases of growth and maturation. Psychosocial development occurs across the life span and includes physical, emotional, psychological, social, and cognitive components. Components are not distinct from one another, and progress through life's stages and phases is neither predictable nor inflexible. An understanding of human growth and development provides a foundation from which to assess the client. Initially, consider what stage the client should be experiencing on the basis of age. Then listen to the client and as comments are made about current health status or life goals, you may gain insight into the client's current level of psychosocial development. Crises tend to send the client back to earlier levels of psychosocial development, and the nurse should listen for concerns related to trust of health care providers or need to be autonomous in doing own physical care as indications of "reworking" the earlier stages of trust versus mistrust and of autonomy versus shame and doubt, respectively. Of course, the opposite may also be true; young clients may be experiencing their integrity versus despair phase of psychosocial development as a result of fatal illnesses.

Social Network. A *social network* is the group of people that surrounds, interacts with, and sustains a person with intimacy, social integration, nurturing, reassurance, and assistance. Collect social network data by observing the client during interactions with family and visitors; ask questions about interpersonal relationships and determine whether there are certain individuals with whom the client prefers to maintain contact. Do not assume that only family members are the most important people. When planning care, include the significant others who may be experiencing stress along with the client.

Socioeconomic Status. An individual's economic position within society is referred to as *socioeconomic status*. Ask about factors that affect financial and social well-being because they have implications for planning individualized health care, such as (1) occupation, (2) current employment status, (3) work-related concerns, (4) financial concerns, (5) effect of the client's health status on the ability to work and on finances, (6) perceived effect that the client's socioeconomic status has on access to the health care system, (7) educational background, and (8) hopes and goals.

Lifestyle. Usual daily patterns of living are referred to as *lifestyle*. Lifestyle is closely associated with socioeconomic status but also includes relationships with others. Assess the following as they apply to the client's health:

- Usual roles and functions
- Work and study habits
- Leisure and relaxation activities
- Type and location of residence
- Living arrangements
- Usual manner of transportation
- Proximity of close friends
- Importance and influence of cultural beliefs on diet and health-seeking behavior or treatment
- Health habits (use of alcohol, medications, nicotine, recreational drugs)
- Stress level
- Coping methods used to relieve stress and their effectiveness
- Usual sleep pattern
- Degree of satisfaction with current status

Sexuality. *Sexuality* is the behavioral expression of one's sexual identity. It involves sexual relationships between people as well as the perception of one's maleness or femaleness (gender identification). Many aspects of sexuality affect health status and are significant to nursing care and client outcomes. Aspects include (1) physical health problems that affect sexual behavior (such as mastectomy, colostomy, skin lesions, sexually transmitted diseases, paralysis, physical deformities), (2) concerns with sexual performance (such as impotence, premature ejaculation, inability to achieve orgasm, infertility), (3) issues of sex role function (for example, homosexuality, bisexuality, sexual ambiguity, transsexual surgery), and (4) effects of environmental restrictions on sexual performance (such as residency in a long-term care facility).

Sexuality and sexual behavior are sensitive topics. Clients may want to discuss sexuality issues and may look for permission to do so. Become comfortable with sexuality issues and do not allow personal beliefs and values to interfere with professional care. Accept and interact with clients without judging them or their behavior.

Learning Preferences

The goal for most clients is to achieve independent management of chronic diseases and healing of acute diseases; therefore teaching the client and/or family to perform various treatments is cornerstone to meeting this goal. An important first step is determining how the client prefers to learn. It begins with asking the client to identify how he or she prefers to learn new material. Asking this question directly often leads to confusion; therefore ask questions such as the following: "If you needed directions, how would you like to have them presented to you? A visual map? Verbal directions? Or some other way?" The answer will identify the usual style of learning: visual, auditory, or other.

Another important component of learning is to know the client's primary language and years of formal education. Most adults can read at an eighth-grade level, so information provided in written format should be prepared with this level of language. Obviously, if the client does not speak English, translated material would *evolve* be preferred. The website has several client education documents translated into Spanish.

Cultural Assessment

Cultural assessment provides information about what shapes a client's ideas about health and illness. It may also provide insight into the client's beliefs, values, and practices that could affect health care and self-care behaviors. Components of a cultural assessment are shown in Box *evolve* 2-4. Further information about cultural assessment is available on the website, which includes Diversity in Health Care boxes on Introduction to Cultural Aspects of Health Care and on Communicating with Culturally Diverse Clients.

Health Beliefs Assessment

Factors affecting health can be understood from many angles. For example, in highly developed countries, people believe they are ill from bacterial invasion or from an imbalance in other factors such as temperature or *Yin* and *Yang*. A client's belief about the cause of the illness is important to understand.

It is important to recognize that beliefs about the significance of illness can vary greatly. Clients may not feel that diabetes is a serious disease, because "at least

---

BOX 2-4 Components of Cultural Assessment
■ Language and communication process
■ Level of ethnic identity
■ Views about the role that ethnicity plays
■ Influence of religion/spirituality on the belief system and behavior patterns
■ Views and concerns about discrimination and institutional racism
■ Importance and impact associated with physical characteristics
■ Migration experience, if applicable
■ Use of informal network and supportive institutions in the ethnic/cultural community
■ Values orientation
■ Cultural health beliefs and practices
■ Habits, customs, beliefs
■ Current socioeconomic status
■ Educational level and employment experiences
■ Self-concept and self-esteem

it isn't cancer!" Only with skilled assessment and rapport building can these health beliefs be expressed. More information on health beliefs is found in Chapter 1.

Health Promotion and Health Risk Appraisal

Biographical and demographic data provide clues about personal health risk. For example, some health risk may be ascribed to age, gender, family history, and location of residence. Various health screening procedures or recommendations are made based on age, gender, or other background data. Information on health promotion in all ages is provided in Chapter 1.

Review of Systems

The review of systems (ROS) is a head-to-toe review of the physical health history for each body system. This review provides a focus for the physical examination. Data may be collected when the client completes a checklist form that is reviewed and expanded as necessary by a health care professional. In an episodic (short-format) health history, focus on those systems pertinent to the problem. Examples of ROS data are included in the health assessment chapters in this book. A more complete listing may be found on the website.

PHYSICAL EXAMINATION

The purpose of physical examination is to differentiate normal from abnormal physical findings. A foundation of basic anatomy (structure) and physiology (function) is the key to developing skill, expertise, and an appreciation for the wide range of findings that are considered normal. Collect objective data systematically during the examination to supplement and validate subjective data. Ask about abnormal physical findings. For example, if a mass is found during palpation, ask whether the area is tender to touch. Record the client's reply in the physical examination portion of the database ("nontender") even though the data are subjective. If you palpate a lump or mass not reported initially during the history interview, ask whether the client is aware of the existence of the mass. If the client knows that the mass is present or reports related manifestations, proceed with a symptom analysis (see Symptom Analysis earlier in this chapter). Record these subjective data in the health history.

TECHNIQUES OF PHYSICAL EXAMINATION

Four primary techniques are used in physical assessment: *inspection, palpation, percussion,* and *auscultation.* These techniques enhance the data collected by observation of the ears, eyes, and senses of touch and smell, and are used during the examination of each body region (Figure 2-1).

Inspection

Inspection is the systematic, deliberate visual examination of the entire client or a body region. Inspection yields information about size, shape, color, texture, symmetry, position, and deformities. It is the first examination technique and begins at the outset of the client-nurse interaction. For example, inspect facial skin while collecting the history. Complete inspection before progressing to the hands-on techniques of palpation, percussion, and auscultation. Inspection is enhanced with special instruments such as a penlight, an oto-ophthalmoscope, and various specula (nasal and vaginal) that permit visual access to body cavities and orifices as well as with tongue blades, a marking pen, a ruler, a tape measure, skinfold calipers, a goniometer, and eye charts.

Palpation

Palpation, generally the second physical assessment technique, is the use of touch. During palpation, exert varying amounts of pressure to determine information about masses, pulsation, organ size, tenderness or pain, swelling, tissue firmness and elasticity, vibration, crepitation, temperature, texture variation, and moisture. Also use palpation to assess masses for position, size, shape, consistency, and mobility.

Technique

Use the most sensitive parts of your hands and fingers to palpate specific characteristics. For example, the *finger tips* or *pads* are the most sensitive for fine touch and are used to palpate pulses, lymph nodes, and breast tissue. Use the *dorsum,* or back of the hand and fingers, to discriminate changes in skin temperature.

Facilitate palpation by positioning the client comfortably. This minimizes muscle tension and lessens the possibility of mistaking such tension for muscle rigidity. Before palpating, ask the client to indicate tender areas. Palpate tender areas last while you observe for nonverbal signs of discomfort or pain. Examine these areas, but note that this may result in discomfort and reluctance to continue.

Percussion

Percussion is used to assess tissue density with sound produced from striking the skin. Usually the third technique in physical assessment, percussion allows examination of 3 to 5 cm of tissue depth. Evaluate the sounds and tissue vibrations that result from percussion in relation to the underlying body structures. Percussion of body structures containing air, fluid, and solids produces various sounds, depending on density.

Types of Sounds

Indirect percussion results in five characteristic sounds:

1. *Flatness,* a soft, high-pitched, short sound produced by very dense tissue such as muscle. Percussion of the thigh reproduces a characteristic flat sound.
2. *Dullness,* a soft to moderately loud sound of moderate pitch and duration. It is produced by less dense, mostly fluid-filled tissue, such as the liver and spleen, and has a thudding quality.
3. *Resonance,* a moderate to loud sound of low pitch and long duration. It results from the air-filled tissue of the normal lung and has a hollow quality.
4. *Hyperresonance,* a very loud, low-pitched sound lasting longer than resonance. It is produced by the overinflated, air-filled lungs of a person with pulmonary emphysema, or it may be heard in a child's lung because of a thin chest wall. Hyperresonance has a booming quality.
5. *Tympany,* a loud, high-pitched, moderately long sound with a drum-like, musical quality. It results from enclosed, air-containing structures, such as the stomach (gastric bubble) and bowel. It can be reproduced by percussion over a puffed cheek.

Auscultation

Auscultation is listening to internal body sounds to assess normal sounds and detect abnormal sounds. It is the final step in the physical examination. Use a stethoscope to enhance sounds. The sounds commonly assessed by auscultation include those produced by the heart, lungs, abdomen, and vascular system. Become

Inspection

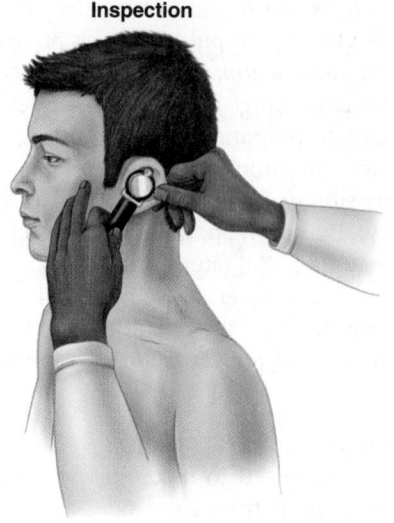

A *Inspection* is the visual examination of a patient. Instruments such as an otoscope can be used to aid inspection.

Palpation

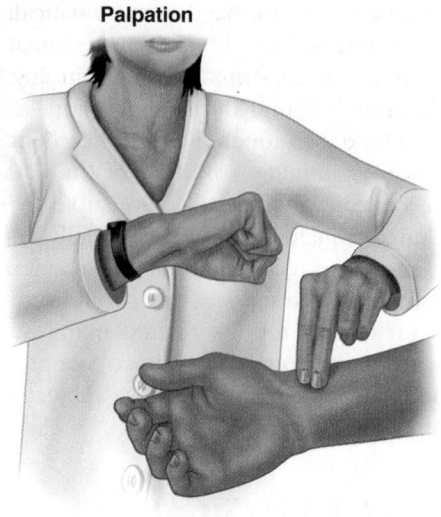

B *Light palpation* employs the lightest possible pressure to assess function or structures under the surface of the skin, such as pulses and lymph nodes.

Percussion

Direct

Indirect

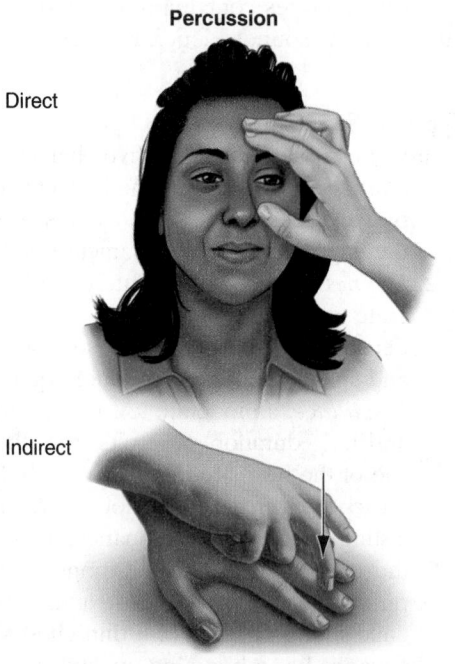

C Percussion can be direct or indirect. *Direct percussion* uses one or two fingers to percuss directly against a body surface, such as over the sinuses, to elicit tenderness. *Indirect percussion* uses the distal phalanx of the middle finger of your nondominant hand on the skin over soft tissue. Bend the middle finger of your dominant hand at its distal interphalangeal joint to create a "hammer."

Auscultation

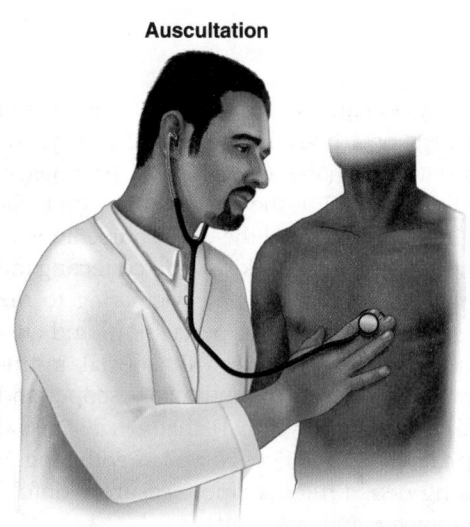

D *Auscultation* is listening to internal body sounds with a stethoscope. Hold the diaphragm of the stethoscope firmly against the skin surface.

■ **FIGURE 2–1** Components of physical assessment.

proficient at auscultation by knowing which sounds are produced by each body structure and the location at which they are most readily heard. Recognizing abnormal sounds is easier once the normal sounds have been mastered.

Technique

Hold the *diaphragm* between the index and middle fingers firmly against the skin surface; use it to hear high-pitched sounds, such as lung sounds, heart sounds, and blood pressure sounds. Place the *bell* lightly in contact with the skin to hear low-pitched sounds, such as murmurs and bruits. Place the *chestpiece* on the skin so that it is between bones and not over them, because bone does not transmit sound. Clothing and excessive chest hair interfere with sound transmission and may introduce artifacts. Snug-fitting *earpieces* occlude the external ear canal to enhance sound transmission from the chestpiece. Keep the *tubing,* no longer than 12 to 15 inches for the best sound transmission, free of contact with all surfaces to prevent extraneous noises.

Types of Sounds

There are four characteristic auscultation sounds:

1. *Pitch,* the number or frequency of sound wave cycles per second. Varying the frequency alters the pitch. For example, a high frequency results in a high-pitched sound, whereas a low frequency produces a low-pitched sound. Heart murmurs can be either high-pitched or low-pitched, depending on the structural cause. Pitch is a diagnostic clue.
2. *Intensity,* the amplitude of a sound wave. The greater the amplitude, the louder the sound; the lower the amplitude, the softer the sound.
3. *Duration,* the length of time a sound endures; it may be long, medium, or short.
4. *Quality,* a description of a sound's character, such as "gurgling," "blowing," "whistling," or "snapping."

GUIDELINES FOR PHYSICAL EXAMINATION

Physical examination proceeds in a logical, orderly fashion. The approach commonly follows a head-to-toe organization so that findings are complete (Box 2-5). This is not an absolute rule, and the nurse who is beginning to use physical assessment skills must practice and develop a system that is comfortable to use. Once a system is developed, use it routinely to avoid inadvertently omitting portions of the examination. For a successful physical assessment, you must know both the techniques and the parameters of normal findings.

Processing the Data

Skillful assessment requires careful observation and the ability to decide whether an observation is normal. Use the material you have learned in anatomy, physiology, microbiology, and sociology to recognize abnormal clinical manifestations. Always consider if the clinical manifestations you are finding are expected deviations from the normal attributable to a known disease (e.g., elevated blood glucose levels in diabetic clients), unexpected deviations (e.g., fever in a client with no other manifestations of infection), or unexpected normal findings (e.g., no pain in a client with a fracture). Psychosocial manifestations may vary much more, but again the presentation is considered in context. Depression in survivors following the death of a loved one is expected, but prolonged depression may signal mental illness. Beginning practitioners should compare their findings to textbooks and classic presentations. If an unusual presentation is seen, it is important to validate the findings with other more experienced health care providers.

Comparison of Findings

Use the client as a "control," or self-standard, for comparison during the physical examination. Compare findings from one side of the body with those from the opposite side *(bilateral comparison).* Even though both sides of the human body are not exactly identical (symmetrical), similarities in structure and appearance are individualized and unique. Comparisons are useful and valid for findings such as a joint deformity or an extremity swelling. If a part of a limb is missing (such as from an amputation), a bilateral comparison is impractical; compare findings with a known standard.

Comparison with Known Standards

Compare physical examination findings with known parameters of "normal" for age, gender, and racial background. For example, decreased skin elasticity and loss of subcutaneous adipose tissue are expected findings for an older client but not for a 30-year-old client.

BOX 2-5 Head-to-Toe Periodic Assessment Guide

1. *Vital signs:* Temperature, pulse, respirations, blood pressure
2. *Pain:* Location, type, quality, intensity
3. *Neurologic:* Orientation (person, place, time, situation), level of consciousness, gait, extremity color/movement/sensation (CMS), pupillary responses to light
4. *Pulmonary:* Respiratory pattern and effort; breath sounds; cough quality; sputum production, color, and quantity
5. *Cardiovascular:* Heart sounds and rhythm, pulses (radial, dorsalis pedis, and posterior tibial), capillary refill, edema (location and amount), skin color and temperature
6. *Gastrointestinal:* Oral assessment, abdominal appearance, bowel sounds, bowel elimination pattern
7. *Genitourinary:* Bladder distention, voiding pattern
8. *Integumentary:* Skin integrity, wounds, dressings, drainage
9. *Psychosocial:* Sociability, affect, anxiety, attitude

Note: Perform additional assessments according to the client's specific health status and needs.

Suspected Problem Areas

Examine known or suspected problem areas carefully. Include areas identified during the health history interview as well as those predicted to be at risk based on the client's history and reactions to the physical examination. For example, thoroughly assess mouth and neck structures of the client who reports difficulty swallowing. To allay anxiety, explain why a particular portion of the examination is more thorough.

Health Teaching

The physical examination process lends itself to health teaching and opportunities to provide accurate information and to correct misconceptions. Examples include reinforcing techniques for self-examination and having the client perform a return demonstration.

SPECIFIC RISK APPRAISALS

Pressure Ulcer Risk

Determining the risk of pressure ulcers at the time of admission allows the nurse to institute early preventive care to keep skin intact. The Braden pressure ulcer risk assessment is a commonly used risk assessment tool and requires that the nurse assess six areas of risk; many times these areas are fully understood on admission (nutritional status, for example). Use your best judgment to accurately identify risk. It is important to institute prevention protocols based on risk score, and an accurate score is imperative.

Fall Risk

SAFETY
ALERT

The risk of falls is usually determined at the time of admission, using various fall risk assessment tools, such as Schmid or Hendrich tools. The most common risk factors for falls are gait instability, agitated confusion, urinary incontinence/frequency, history of falls, and prescription of "culprit" drugs (especially sedative/hypnotics). When these factors or the client is identified as at risk, intercede to reduce risk of falls immediately by using interventions such as the family, bed or body alarms, or sitters. Reducing the risk of falls has been identified as a client safety goal.

DOCUMENTING FINDINGS

Document physical examination findings using accurate, descriptive terms. Avoid vague, subjective terminology, such as "normal," "slight," "moderate," "healthy," or "poor," because they are easily misinterpreted. Strive to be objective, concise, clear, and thorough. However, it is better to err on the side of verbosity than to describe a significant finding vaguely or inadequately. A detailed recording is the baseline for comparison with future physical findings.

APPLYING HEALTH ASSESSMENT TO THE NURSING PROCESS

After collecting baseline data (the results of both the health history and the physical examination), summarize the client's health problems. Assess the areas of strength and health risk profile. Formalize and prioritize nursing diagnoses. Reexamine and validate the tentative diagnoses formulated after the health history interview in light of the physical examination findings.

Determine which health problems are nursing diagnoses and which are collaborative problems. Make referrals when indicated to ensure continuity of care and either resolution or effective management of the health problems.

In health assessment, seek to gather as much data about the client as possible, both subjective and objective. Analyze the data to determine the client's needs and responses to potential and actual health problems. Consider the client's preferences when formulating nursing diagnoses that are amenable to intervention. Establishing realistic goals and outcome criteria and planning interventions follow in logical order.

ONGOING ASSESSMENTS

Clients are assessed after admission; the frequency of that assessment depends on the condition of the client. In critical care settings or during emergencies, assessments are continuous and recorded often (e.g., every 5 to 15 minutes). In acute care settings, the client is usually assessed every 4 to 12 hours, again depending upon the client's condition. There is no hard and fast rule on how often a client should be assessed, and the nurse should never hesitate to assess a client more fully than "required" in order to fully understand the situation.

Assess each of your clients at the beginning of every shift. The areas of assessment are focused on the clients' problems and usually include an abbreviated head-to-toe examination. Prioritize which clients you see first by their condition; assess the sickest patients first and then proceed to the others. Record your findings as you collect them—it is very difficult to recall all the findings hours later! This initial assessment provides a baseline for your shift. Box 2-5 provides a guide to ongoing assessment. Some of the items listed as "assessment" are conducted as you enter the room and no formal equipment is required. As you examine the client be certain that you examine all of the skin by looking under tubes and by removing stockings or anti-embolism devices. Do not assume that skin is intact simply because you cannot see it. Likewise, listen to the entire lung fields including posterior sounds. Examine the mouth closely in clients who are mouth breathers or receiving oxygen, looking for dried mucus on the soft palate and back of the throat. When bathing and bedmaking are delegated to others, the nurse remains responsible for the entire assessment.

Be certain to be complete in your assessments. Convey any unexpected abnormal findings to the physician if immediate intervention is needed. Notify the charge nurse if the problem can wait until the physician will be notified for other issues. Inform the client and family what you are doing to alleviate any problems identified. It is important that you follow up to be certain that problems identified are treated satisfactorily.

 ## CONCLUSIONS

Health assessment can range from a complete assessment of the client on admission to an ongoing and abbreviated later assessment. Health assessment includes history taking and physical examination as well as ongoing focused assessments. Completeness is crucial for analysis.

 ## BIBLIOGRAPHY

 Citations appearing in red refer to primary research.

1. Andrews, M.M., & Boyle, J.S. (Eds.). (2002). *Transcultural concepts in nursing care* (4th ed.). Philadelphia: Lippincott Williams & Wilkins.

2. Clark, C.C. (2000). *Integrating complementary health procedures into practice.* New York: Springer.
3. D'Avanzo, C.E., & Geissler, E.M. (2003). *Pocket guide to cultural assessment* (3rd ed.). St. Louis: Mosby.
4. Jarvis, C. (2004). *Physical examination and health assessment.* Philadelphia: Saunders.
5. Myers, H. (2003). Hospital fall risk assessment tools: A critique of the literature. *International Journal of Nursing Practice, 9*(4), 223-229.
6. Norred, C.L., Zamudio, S., & Palmer, S.K. (2000). Use of complementary and alternative medicines by surgical patients. *AANA Journal, 68*(1), 13-18.
7. Spector, R.E. (2000). *Cultural diversity in health and illness* (5th ed.). Upper Saddle River, NJ: Prentice-Hall.
8. Staggers, N., Thompson, C.B., & Snyder-Halpern, R. (2001). History and trends in clinical information systems in the United States. *Journal of Nursing Scholarship, 33*(1), 75-81.
9. Strub, R.L., & Black, F.W. (2000). *The mental status examination in neurology* (4th ed.). Philadelphia: F.A. Davis.

evolve *Did you remember to check out the bonus material on the Evolve website and the CD-ROM, including NCLEX®-Examination Style Review Questions, Open-Book Quizzes, and Chapter Review Audio Podcasts?*

http://evolve.elsevier.com/Black/medsurg

CHAPTER 3

Critical Thinking

JANE HOKANSON HAWKS AND JOYCE BLACK

One of the most important factors that will determine whether a nursing student or nurse will succeed or fail involves the student's or the nurse's ability to think critically. Our goal with this chapter is to focus on examples of how a nursing student will use critical thinking while preparing for a clinical experience and throughout a day of providing client care in a clinical setting. We will only summarize the literature that discusses how critical thinking is defined, measured, taught, or applied.

DEFINITIONS

Thinking is a special human characteristic that involves organization of new information and the reorganization of previously learned material into forms leading to new responses that can then be generalized to new situations. Everyone thinks; it is our nature to do so. Thinking serves as the mediator between learning and responding and uses the products of memory to synthesize new information. However, some of what we think is biased, distorted, incorrect, unclear, or even prejudicial. *Critical thinking* is a term used to describe an improved process of thinking that changes the methods of the thinking process to ensure that the conclusions are self-correctable, reasonable, informed, and precise. It is a complex process that involves purposeful[8] and informed reasoning[14] and also reflection[7] and contemplation about thinking.[11,12] It also is a cognitive process that drives problem solving and decision making.[3] *Clinical judgment, clinical decision making,* and *clinical reasoning* involve critical thinking when providing care for clients. Box 3-1 lists some of the characteristics and attitudes often found in a critical thinker. Most nursing faculty members believe that critical thinking is a skill that can be learned, and with effective communication we can learn to overcome our usual tendencies in thinking.

COGNITIVE PROCESSES USED IN CRITICAL THINKING

Many cognitive skills are involved in the process of critical thinking and were learned early in a person's education. They include the scientific process, decision making, and problem solving. In the scientific method a thinker defines a problem, collects data about the problem, formulates a hypothesis to examine the problem, tests the hypothesis, and evaluates the results of the study to determine if the hypothesis was proved or disproved. In decision making, the decision maker builds on the scientific process to identify a problem, assess all options, weigh each option, test possible options, consider the consequences of a decision, and then make the final decision. With problem solving, the problem solver identifies a problem, selects pertinent information for solution of the problem, considers the consequences of each solution, selects the best solution for problem resolution, and evaluates the solution over time to be sure the solution is still effective.

The cognitive processes discussed in the previous paragraph provide the background for the nursing process that is used when nurses provide client care. In the nursing process, the nurse assesses the client, identifies the nursing diagnosis or client problem, prioritizes the problems, establishes goals or a plan of action, provides interventions to improve the status of the client, and evaluates the client to see if the interventions were appropriate and helpful. This, similar to other cognitive processes, is a cyclical or circular process.

---

evolve **Web Enhancements**

Ethical Issues in Nursing   What Values Are Represented in the Nurse-Client Relationship?

Be sure to check out the bonus material on the Evolve website and the CD-ROM, including free self-assessment exercises. **http://evolve.elsevier.com/Black/medsurg**

BOX 3-1	Attitudes and Characteristics of a Critical Thinker		
Alert to changes	Curious	Insightful	Questioning
Analytical	Empathic	Has integrity	Realistic
Autonomous	Fair-minded	Logical	Reflective
Careful	Flexible	Open-minded	Responsible
Committed	Genuine	Patient	Sensitive
Confident	Honest	Practical	
Courageous	Humble	Proactive	
Creative	Independent	Prudent	

Modified from Alfaro-LaFevre, R. (2004). *Critical thinking and clinical judgment* (3rd ed.). St. Louis: Saunders/Elsevier; Colucciello, M. (1997). Critical thinking skills and dispositions of baccalaureate nursing students—A conceptual model for evaluation. *Journal of Professional Nursing, 13*(4), 236-245; Paul, R. (1990). *Critical thinking: What every person needs to survive in a rapidly changing world.* Rohnert Park, Calif: Center for Critical Thinking and Moral Critique; and Paul, R. (1995). *Critical thinking: How to prepare students for a rapidly changing world.* Santa Rosa, Calif: Foundation for Critical Thinking.

CRITICAL THINKING IN NURSING PRACTICE

The decisions that nurses make affect client outcomes. Making the best decisions requires the use of critical thinking and a problem-solving or decision-making process that integrates a systematic search and critical appraisal of the relevant evidence, ones' own clinical expertise, and the preferences and values of the client.[9]

Professional nurses make multiple decisions involving clients, family members, and the health care team in a variety of situations. In every clinical situation it is important for the nurse to think critically, apply knowledge, and make sound judgments so that clients receive the best care possible. To make the situation more challenging, most clients have health problems for which there are no clear textbook solutions. Each client's problem is unique and a product of many factors, including the client's physical and emotional health, lifestyle choices, cultural background, economic circumstances, religious beliefs, relationship with family and friends, and life experiences. This requires the nurse to assess, question, recall previously learned knowledge and experiences, and be self-directed in investigating various alternatives for action.

Because of the complexity of clinical care, a completely linear process of thinking can lead to erroneous conclusions. To avoid biased or erroneous conclusions, processes used in critical thinking are helpful because, once learned and called upon, the thinker is challenged to look at a problem from all aspects. Elder and Paul[6] developed Universal Intellectual Standards, often used to describe critical thinking. People who are adept at critical thinking have often assimilated these intellectual standards to augment their process of problem solving. Nurses and students providing clinical care should also use these Universal Intellectual Standards (Box 3-2).

BOX 3-2 Universal Intellectual Standards

The best examples of critical thinking in clinical settings come from thoughtful examination of all aspects of a clinical problem. Consider the standards on the left side of this box for the case presented here. Then reflect on how the questions from each standard more fully describe the problem.

Case: Mrs. Anderson enters the hospital with reported abdominal pain. She is 56 years old and has had pain "off and on" for the last week. Mrs. Anderson was just hospitalized last week for rib fractures that occurred when she was in a car accident. When her abdomen is palpated, she has severe pain for one nurse and no discomfort when another nurse examines her. She has not been eating well for the past day or two. You are going to examine her; consider how these questions could help clarify the problem.

Standard	Questions Used to Examine	Example
Clarity	Can you give me an example or elaborate further?	Can you give me an example of when your pain was at its worst? What happened just before the pain? What helped it subside?
Accuracy	How could we check on that?	Can you tell me a little more about your past health problems?
Precision	Could you be more specific?	Can you describe the severity of the pain and the nature of the pain?
Relevance	How does that relate to the problem?	How might your recent rib fractures relate to this new problem?
Depth	What are some of the complexities of this issue?	Could the abdominal pain be related to the narcotics she is taking for the rib pain?
Breadth	Do we need to consider another point of view?	Can you explain to me what has happened to you since you went home?
Significance	Is this the most important aspect to consider?	Which problem has the highest priority: her healing rib fractures or her abdominal pain?
Fairness	Am I considering everyone's interests?	What is happening at home with her family, spouse?
Completeness	Do I have all the information I need to make a decision?	Is there anything else you want to tell me about your abdominal pain?
Logic	Does this all make sense together?	Are the two problems of rib fractures and abdominal pain related? Are they potentially related, or are these two separate problems?

Modified from Elder, L., & Paul, R. (1996). *Universal intellectual standards.* Retrieved May 19, 2006, from www.criticalthinking.org/resources/articles/universal-intellectualstandards.shtml.

CRITICAL THINKING FROM NOVICE TO EXPERT

As a nursing student advances from novice or beginner to expert nurse, the use of critical thinking will undergo changes. In 1980 Dreyfus and Dreyfus introduced the Dreyfus model of skill acquisition.[4] The Dreyfus model identifies five levels of proficiency: novice, advanced beginner, competent, proficient, and expert.[4,5] These levels differ in three aspects: reliance on principles to experience, perception of the situation as component parts to perception of a whole, and detached observer to involved performer.[2] The novice must follow rules, rely on theory, and reflect upon the situation before acting. The expert is characterized by a rapid, fluid, involved kind of behavior where action precedes thought. Considerable concrete experience with real situations is what the Dreyfus model considers necessary for expertise.[4,5]

Benner[2] studied the work of nurses using the Dreyfus model of skill acquisition. In *From Novice to Expert,*[2] she shares descriptive research that identified five levels of competency in clinical nursing practice. These levels—novice, advanced beginner, competent, proficient, and expert—are adapted from the Dreyfus model and described in the words of 1200 nurses who were interviewed and observed either individually or in small groups. Box 3-3 summarizes the characteristics of the levels of competency.

BOX 3-3	Benner's Five Levels of Competency in Nurses
Novice	Has no experience in situations the nurse is expected to perform. Follows rules to guide action. Slow to act. Inflexible.
Advanced beginner	Has coped with enough real situations to note the recurring meaningful situational components. Still uses rules. Slow to act. Little flexibility.
Competent	Has been on the job or similar situations 2-3 years. Beginning to have mastery and the ability to cope with and manage many situations in clinical nursing. Not as flexible or as fast as proficient and expert nurses.
Proficient	Perceives situations as wholes rather than in terms of aspects. Perception of wholes is the result of 3-5 years of experience. No longer uses rules. Rapid recognition of subtle changes. Flexible.
Expert	Has had 5 or more years of experience in the same area. Enormous background of experience allows the nurse to intuitively grasp a situation and focus on most important aspect of a problem. No longer uses rules. Rapid recognition of subtle changes. Flexible.

Modified from Benner, P. (1984). *From novice to expert: Excellence and power in clinical nursing practice.* Menlo Park, Calif: Addison-Wesley.

An example of an expert nurse is a nurse who works in a transplant unit. She can tell when a client is beginning a kidney rejection episode often before the laboratory studies and other clinical manifestations become obvious. The nurse may notice a slight change in the quality and quantity of the urine output or that the client's color has changed somewhat. These are subtle changes that may not be observed by the novice nurse until laboratory values indicate a problem. The expert nurse notifies the physician, orders the necessary laboratory values, initiates an intravenous solution, and prepares the high-dose immunosuppressive agents. Rapid recognition is often the critical factor in determining whether the rejection episode can be successfully reversed for the client.

CRITICAL THINKING AND EVIDENCE-BASED PRACTICE

Once the problem has been identified, the interventions to provide needed care will follow. These interventions must be based on a solid foundation of all the sciences.

Critical thinking is the basis of *evidence-based practice* (EBP). Melnyk and Fineout-Overholt[10] define EPB as the use of current evidence in making decisions about client care. The University of Minnesota[15] describes *evidence-based nursing practice* (EBNP) as the process by which nurses make clinical decisions using the best available research evidence, clinical expertise, and client preferences.

Several steps are necessary for solving clinical problems encountered by nurses. The following steps are included:[9,15,16]

- Clearly identifying clinical problems in practice
- Searching the literature for relevant research and the best evidence
- Evaluating and critically appraising the literature using established criteria regarding scientific merit
- Integrating the evidence from the literature into practice with specific nursing interventions
- Evaluating the effect of the change or interventions on client outcomes

Many hospitals are rewriting their policy and procedure manuals and standards of care to incorporate evidence-based practice. Unfortunately, much of nursing care is not research based, but rather handed-down experiences. As nursing scientists continue to expand the scientific basis of nursing, some of the assessments and interventions currently used may change to reflect new evidence related to practice.

PREPARATION FOR CLINICAL EXPERIENCE

Nursing students receive an opportunity to critically think about the client and the client's health problems in clinical rotations. The critically thinking process is not exclusively used by experienced nurses; novice nurse must practice thinking in new and challenging ways to understand the client and the health problems of the client.

If the student is able to assess the client and read the chart before the clinical experience, it is important that the history and physical, doctor's orders, laboratory and other diagnostic testing results, nurses' notes, and medication records be reviewed.

Once the student has an appreciation for the reason for admission and treatments done to date, the student should introduce him/herself to the client, explain the purpose for the visit (e.g., "I will be assisting your nurse in your care tomorrow morning"). A brief head-to-toe assessment may or may not be done, depending on the expectations of the clinical faculty. During the time with the client, the student should observe equipment in the room in order to review the intravenous pump, patient-controlled analgesia (PCA) pump, or other technology as needed before the clinical experience. The introduction also allows the student to determine what cultural factors or beliefs might be important for the client.

Once the student leaves the hospital, a critical review of the information collected is performed, in order to plan for the following clinical experiences. Only if there is adequate preparation can the clinical experience provide the best education for the student and the best care for the client. Do not inadequately prepare for the clinical experience and convince yourself that it will not be obvious to your instructor or client!

Use course notes, textbooks, and other resources to gather information or review information about the client's primary diagnosis and co-morbidities (other conditions that may influence the outcome such as hypertension or diabetes mellitus). For instance, consider what is expected during the postoperative recovery for a client undergoing a total knee replacement procedure as well as how the client's diabetes may affect normal wound healing. To do this, the student should be able to explain the normal anatomy and physiology of the affected system, how a joint replacement surgery is performed, normal wound healing for a surgical client, and how diabetes mellitus may interfere with normal wound healing.

Using the standards of critical thinking, the student should consider the relevance of each of the physician's orders. Consider questions such as the following: "What usual response to this disease and/or operation is being addressed by this intervention?" For example, "What is the reason a postoperative client is prescribed iron? Did the client have an iron deficiency anemia prior to surgery? Did the client lose blood in surgery and iron is being used to rebuild blood supply?" "Why are the sequential compression devices used? Are they prescribed to reduce the risk of postoperative thrombosis? Why is this client at risk of blood clots in the legs?"

Use the principle of logic to examine diagnostic findings. Is it logical for a client with diabetes to have an elevated blood glucose level? Why might the client with sequential compressive devices also have an elevated International Normalized Ratio (INR) and prothrombin time? Could it be due to the use an anticoagulant?

Use the principle of precision and accuracy combined with logic to answer questions such as follows: "Why would this client, with no history of renal disease, have an elevated urea nitrogen level?" Consider other influences, undiagnosed disease, reactions to medications, and even error in the findings.

The student should review possible procedures that may be required while providing care for this client such as inserting a Foley catheter, scanning the bladder for residual urine, administering blood, placing the client in a continuous passive motion (CPM) machine, and injecting medications intravenously or parenterally. In addition, the student should consider unexpected events, such as deep vein thrombosis (DVT) or pulmonary embolus (PE), and the clinical manifestations and nursing interventions required to assess and treat those complications. All medications ordered for the client should be reviewed so that the student determines the following: the classification of the drug and the disorders that classification of drug may be used to treat, the action of the drug, the side effects of the drug, assessments required to determine if the medication should be held or administered, if the medication has been scheduled for administration at the correct time, and the seven rights of medication administration.

PRE-CARE CONFERENCE

Most nursing instructors and preceptors will assess the student's knowledge before the student provides client care. The student should be prepared to discuss the client's condition, pathophysiology of the primary disorder as well as the co-morbidities, expected plan of care for the day, medications, and other treatments expected. The instructor must be certain the student is adequately prepared to provide safe, supportive care for the client.

For all clients, the student should be able to recite the number of days since admission or surgery, the current activity level, the current diet, the level of pain and how it is controlled, and any relevant events scheduled for that day (e.g., MRI, surgery).

REPORT

The student providing direct client care should introduce her/himself to the nurse assigned to that client. It is the student's responsibility to tell the nurse what he or she is able to assess, medications that can be administered, skills that may be performed, and documentation that the student will complete. It is very important to determine who will

CASE STUDY

CASE I

The client is a 55-year-old man admitted for gallbladder surgery; he has a history of hypertension that is controlled with three categories of antihypertensive medications. At 0830 he asks for something for pain, and the nurse administers his postoperative pain medication. Ten minutes later, he calls the nurse again and says that his pain is not better. When assessed, it is noted that he is pale, sweating, and saying that "there is a vice on his chest."

What happened? Through faulty thinking, the nurse had a preconceived idea that any pain reported by this client would be due to the incision. This resulted in the nurse's failure to determine the true cause of the pain and delayed recognition and treatment of angina. Had the nurse clarified the source of the pain, it may have been obvious that the initial pain was not incisional. Obviously, errors like this can be costly.

CASE 2

The client is an 88-year-old woman admitted from her home with confusion. Because she is combative, she is restrained to prevent self-injury. Medical evaluation for stroke was negative and the reason for the confusion remains unclear. Her laboratory values indicate anemia (hemoglobin [Hgb] 9.2 g/dl), and her serum urea nitrogen level is elevated. The nurse assigned to her today does not spend much time with her because she is busy with her other clients. By the following morning, the client's confusion is worse.

What happened in this case? Without the data that could have been collected by adding depth to the data collection process, the nurse did not determine that this client was recently widowed and depressed and had not consumed any food or fluids for

days. Now being further deprived of food and fluids because she could not feed herself while in restraints, her situation further deteriorated.

CASE 3

The client is a 63-year-old woman with a recent fracture of her spine following a fall. She had surgery to repair the fracture using a bone graft from her left iliac crest. She also has chronic obstructive pulmonary disease (COPD) resulting from a long history of smoking. The day after surgery, her pain is very severe and she spends the majority of the day on her right side. The following day, she has significant pneumonia in the right lung.

What happened? Without considering the significance of lying on one side all day, the nurse created a new problem because of the client's immobility. While in this case the client's pain would have been a high priority, the pain should have been better controlled to prevent the complications of immobility.

CASE 4

The client is a 35-year-old homeless man with a history of diabetes mellitus. He is admitted for infected wounds on his feet. He relates that it is hard to control the disease while living and eating at the shelter. The wounds are debrided and he is sent back to the shelter.

What happened? Without examining the depth of the problem, such as access to medications and care, the problem has not been solved. It has been controlled for now, but through critical thinking other outcomes may have been achievable.

be charting intake and output records, for example. The nurse may be able to provide the student with an update on the client's status from the previous shift. The student should also communicate the assistance he or she may need as well as the skills the nursing instructor will supervise.

SETTING PRIORITIES

Setting priorities for assessment and care is sometimes very obvious . . . for example, a client who is screaming in pain needs the pain controlled before anything else is done. However, in other situations, the priority is less obvious. The case studies above are some examples of this ambiguity.

CONCLUSIONS

Critical thinking is a crucial aspect of the nurse's or student's assessment, intervention, and interaction with clients. Through critical thinking, the full understanding of the problem and potential complications can be clearly understood.

BIBLIOGRAPHY

Citations appearing in red refer to primary research.

Citations appearing in blue refer to evidence-based practice guidelines and protocols.

1. Alfaro-LaFevre, R. (2004). *Critical thinking and clinical judgment* (3rd ed.). St. Louis: Saunders.
2. Benner, P. (1984). From novice to expert: Excellence and power in clinical nursing practice. Menlo Park, Calif: Addison-Wesley.
3. Colucciello, M. (1997). Critical thinking skills and dispositions of baccalaureate nursing students—A conceptual model for evaluation. *Journal of Professional Nursing, 13*(4), 236-245.
4. Dreyfus, S., & Dreyfus, H. (1980). *A five-stage model of the mental activities involved in directed skill acquisition.* Unpublished report supported by the Air Force Office of Scientific Research, USAF (Contract F49620-79-C-0063), University of California, Berkeley.
5. Dreyfus, S., & Dreyfus, H. (1986). *Mind over machine.* New York: The Free Press.
6. Elder, L., & Paul, R. (1996). *Universal intellectual standards.* Retrieved May 19, 2006, from www.criticalthinking.org/resources/articles/universal-intellectualstandards.shtml.
7. Ennis, R., & Milman, J. (1985). *Cornell tests of critical thinking: Theory and practice.* Pacific Grove, Calif: Midwest Publications.
8. Halpern, D. (1984). *Thought and knowledge.* Hillsdale, NJ: Lawrence Erlbaum Associates.
9. Hawks, J. (2006). Why evidence-based practice? *Urologic Nursing, 26*(1), 11.
10. Melnyk, B., & Fineout-Overholt, E. (2005). *Evidence-based practice in nursing and healthcare: A guide to best practice.* Philadelphia: Lippincott Williams & Wilkins.

11. Paul, R. (1990). *Critical thinking: What every person needs to survive in a rapidly changing world*. Rohnert Park, Calif: Center for Critical Thinking and Moral Critique.

12. Paul, R. (1995). *Critical thinking: How to prepare students for a rapidly changing world*. Santa Rosa, Calif: Foundation for Critical Thinking.

13. Paul, R., & Edler, L. (2005) *Critical thinking: Concepts and tools*. Santa Rosa, Calif: Foundation for Critical Thinking.

14. Snyder, M. (1993). Critical thinking: A foundation for consumer-focused care. *The Journal of Continuing Education in Nursing, 24*(5), 206-210.

15. University of Minnesota. (2005). *Evidence-based nursing*. Retrieved Nov 10, 2005, from http://evidence.ahc.umn.edu/ebn.htm.

16. Yoder, L. (2005). Evidence-based practice: The time is now! *MEDSURG Nursing, 14*(2), 91-92.

evolve *Did you remember to check out the bonus material on the Evolve website and the CD-ROM, including NCLEX®-Examination Style Review Questions, Open-Book Quizzes, and Chapter Review Audio Podcasts?*

http://evolve.elsevier.com/Black/medsurg

CHAPTER 4

Complementary and Alternative Therapies

MARK MOYAD AND JANE HOKANSON HAWKS

Complementary and alternative medicine (CAM) has received an enormous amount of attention around the world over the past decade. Nurses need to be well informed about various CAM modalities that clients might be using because of the increased interest in CAM as well as less restrictive regulation of many products. Many clients are afraid to disclose their use of herbs and other CAM therapies. In addition, many clients who use prescription drugs concurrently with CAM therapies could face possible health risks as a result of adverse reactions. A well-informed, nonjudgmental nurse is able to instill trust and gain an accurate picture of the client's CAM use as well as provide valuable information about safety issues.

This chapter begins with an overview of CAM. The second part of the chapter discusses a few issues and regulations that could aid the health professional in understanding CAM. A list of supplements that should be avoided is also provided. A partial list of CAM therapies appears next and is followed by an explanation of the CAM boxes that appear throughout the book. CAM therapies specifically related to disorders are identified in each assessment chapter of the book.

COMPLEMENTARY, ALTERNATIVE, AND INTEGRATIVE THERAPIES

Complementary and alternative medicine is defined by the National Center for Complementary and Alternative Medicine (NCCAM) as a group of diverse medical and health care systems, practices, and products that are not presently considered part of conventional medicine.[10]

The NCCAM branch of the National Institutes of Health (NIH) was established in 1998 to ensure high-quality scientific research into CAM practices, to conduct and support basic and clinical research on CAM modalities, and to provide information about CAM to health care providers and consumers.[7,10]

According to the NCCAM,[10] complementary and alternative therapies are not the same. *Complementary* medicine is used *together with* conventional medicine. *Conventional medicine* is defined by NCCAM as medicine practiced by holders of MD (medical doctor) and DO (doctor of osteopathy) degrees and by allied health professionals, such as nurse-practitioners or advanced-practice nurses, registered nurses, physical therapists, and psychologists. Other terms for conventional medicine include allopathy; mainstream, Western, orthodox, and regular medicine; and biomedicine. Some conventional practitioners are also practitioners of CAM. An example of a complementary therapy is using aromatherapy to help lessen a client's discomfort following surgery.[7,10,13]

Alternative medicine is used *in place of* conventional medicine. An example of an alternative therapy is using a special diet to treat cancer instead of undergoing surgery, radiation, or chemotherapy that has been recommended by a practitioner of conventional medicine such as an oncologist.[7,10,13]

Integrative medicine *combines* mainstream medical therapies and CAM therapies for which there is some high-quality evidence of safety and effectiveness. Nurses often combine therapies when they use massage, touch, distraction, and relaxation techniques in addition to traditional use of analgesics for pain such as postoperative pain, cancer pain, and chronic pain control for clients.[10]

TABLE 4–1   Five Types or Classifications of CAM Therapies

Classification	Description
Alternative medical systems	Alternative medical systems are built on complete systems of theory and practice. Homeopathic medicine and naturopathic medicine are examples that have developed in Western cultures. Examples of systems that have developed in non-Western cultures include traditional Chinese medicine and ayurveda.
Mind-body interventions	Mind-body medicine uses a variety of techniques designed to enhance the mind's capacity to affect bodily function and manifestations. Some techniques that were considered CAM in the past have become mainstream (e.g., client support groups and cognitive-behavioral therapy). Other mind-body techniques are still considered CAM, including meditation, prayer, mental healing, and therapies that use creative outlets such as art, music, or dance.
Biologically based therapies	Biologically based therapies in CAM use substances found in nature, such as herbs, foods, and vitamins. Some examples include dietary supplements, herbal products, and the use of "natural" but scientifically unproved therapies such as shark cartilage to treat cancer.
Manipulative and body-based methods	Manipulative and body-based methods in CAM are based on manipulation or movement of one or more parts of the body. Some examples include chiropractic or osteopathic manipulation and massage.
Energy therapies	Energy therapies involve the use of energy fields. Biofield therapies are intended to affect energy fields that purportedly surround and penetrate the human body. The existence of such fields has not yet been scientifically proven. Some examples include qi gong, Reiki, and therapeutic touch. Bioelectromagnetic-based therapies involve the unconventional use of electromagnetic fields such as pulsed fields, magnetic fields, or alternating current or direct current fields.

Data from Hawks, J., & Moyad, M. 2003. CAM: Definition and classification overview. *Urologic Nursing, 23*(3), 221-223; and National Center for Complementary and Alternative Medicine. (2006). *What is complementary and alternative medicine (CAM)?* Retrieved 10/07/06 from http://nccam.nih.gov/health/whatiscam.

The five major categories or domains of CAM therapies are described in Table 4-1.[7,10]

WHY DO PEOPLE CHOOSE ALTERNATIVE THERAPIES?

Several factors have contributed to the increasing interest in CAM modalities.[7] High personal involvement in decision making and the hope for gaining therapeutic benefit are two main reasons why clients choose CAM therapies.[7,13] See Box 4-1 for other reasons.[7,13] All these factors contribute to the increased interest in CAM modalities.

Almost 50% of the population in the United States has used CAM at some point.[3,7] In fact, more visits to alternative medicine practitioners have occurred recently compared with total visits to all primary care providers. Internationally, widespread prevalence of these therapies has been reported. For example, in parts of Europe and Australia, more than 50% of the population have used CAM.[3,7,8] The most rapidly growing area of CAM is the use of dietary supplements (herbs, vitamins, minerals, and other compounds).[3] Currently more than 20,000 herbal and related compounds or products are being sold or used in the United States alone.[8] Sales of dietary supplements have increased substantially, from $8.8 million in 1994 to almost $16 billion in 2002.[8]

ROLE OF THE NURSE

The nurse is often the health care provider who obtains a health history from the client and has the responsibility for initiating the discussion about the use of CAM modalities.[7] As the initiator, the nurse establishes a respectful and open communication environment in which the client feels safe and welcome to speak freely. Questions related to CAM use should be asked with each interaction because the client's interest in CAM might change

BOX 4-1   Factors Affecting the Use of Alternative Therapies

- Desire for control over decision making
- Hope to gain therapeutic benefit
- Desire to avoid toxicities, invasiveness, or other qualities of conventional treatments
- Need to control undesirable side effects of conventional therapies
- Preference for natural over synthetic medications
- Dissatisfaction with attitudes and practitioners of conventional medicine
- Failure to determine diagnosis
- Failure of conventional therapy

- Chronic illnesses with poor prognosis
- Acute or chronic conditions for which conventional treatments are lacking or disappointing
- Healing system that is part of a client's cultural or identity-group heritage
- Reduced insurance coverage
- Restraints on access to health care
- Increased costs of prescriptions and services
- Increased interest in preventive strategies and holistic approaches to health such as eating a more nutritionally sound diet, maintaining fitness, and reducing stress

over time or could vary with changes in the client's health status or that of other members of the client's family or social network.[7] Box 4-2 outlines guidelines for initiating a discussion about CAM with clients.[7,9] Nurses have a responsibility to educate clients about possible adverse reactions, to provide information from the NCCAM, and to teach lifestyle-modification behaviors (such as nutritionally sound diet, weight-loss strategies, stress-reduction strategies, exercise, and fitness) that could prevent the development of acute or chronic problems.[7,9,14-16]

Issues related to regulation, quality, safety, and efficacy should be considered when discussing CAM with clients.[5,7] Many herbal products in the United States are considered dietary supplements and thus are not regulated as medicines and not required to meet the standards for drugs specified in the Federal Food, Drug, and Cosmetic Act. Quality of products from available product information should be screened and information gathered about the manufacturer, the composition and storage of the product, and its correct and safe use.[5,7,9]

Contrary to popular belief, herbal remedies and dietary supplements can pose health risks because of adverse reactions or interactions with prescribed drugs. Only a fraction of the thousands of medicinal plants used worldwide has been tested in randomized, controlled trials, many of which involved nurse researchers.[7] Further study is warranted for many commonly available products. Many of these issues are discussed in more detail in the next section.

It is important for the nurse to know that dietary supplement and herb manufacturers are not held to the same strict standards as are manufacturers of pharmaceuticals. There is poor regulation of the dietary supplement industry. Herb manufacturers are not required by law to demonstrate the safety, efficacy, or quality of their products. Therefore chemical analysis of samples labeled as the same product, but purchased from various suppliers, has revealed wide variations in quality and chemical content.[7,13] This lack of regulation is likely to continue.

As a result of the increased interest in CAM, nurses are encountering increasing numbers of clients who are using one or more of the "nontraditional" methods that constitute CAM[7] (see the box below). Clients may self-medicate with a host of CAM therapies. Some clients will not realize that these products can interfere with prescribed medication, anesthesia, or surgery. Other clients may sense "feelings of disbelief" by practitioners about the effectiveness of CAM modalities and thus not disclose their use. Because of these differing perceptions, certain issues must be considered when discussing CAM therapies with clients.

ISSUES RELATED TO DISCUSSING COMPLEMENTARY AND ALTERNATIVE THERAPIES WITH CLIENTS

1. Realize the impact of the U.S. 1994 Dietary Supplement Health and Education Act (DSHEA) and that some dietary interventions/supplements may gain U.S. Food and Drug Administration (FDA) approval to advertise a health benefit. Both Houses of Congress and President Clinton easily approved the DSHEA in 1994, and it basically allowed manufacturers to regard almost any compound as a "supplement."[8] These rules apply specifically to the labels of dietary supplements and prevent manufacturers from making

---

BOX 4-2 Methods to Facilitate Discussion of CAM Therapies

- Give permission for clients to raise the topic and ask questions.
- Ask, in every history and physical examination, "What else are you doing to care for your health?"
- Listen for nondisclosing cues or references that may represent a client's efforts to "test the waters" without making full disclosure.
- Become familiar with local patterns of use.
- Be frank about what you do not know.
- Seek more information from clients and other sources such as the NCCAM website (http://nccam.nih.gov/health).
- When asking clients about medications, ask specifically about any supplements or herbs.

Data from Hawks, J., Moyad, M. (2003). CAM: Definition and classification overview. *Urologic Nursing, 23*(3), 221-223.

COMPLEMENTARY AND ALTERNATIVE THERAPY

Internet Marketing of Herbal Products

The largest review of websites advertising and selling nutritional supplements was recently analyzed by researchers. A total of 443 websites were evaluated in this study. Interestingly, a total of 81% of the retail websites made one or more health claims, and 55% of these sites claimed to treat, prevent, diagnose, or cure specific diseases. More than 50% of the websites with a health claim omitted the standard federal disclaimer. This is a big concern because consumers may be misled by vendors' claims that herbal supplements can affect diseases, despite regulations by the government prohibiting such claims. Health professionals need to be aware of the widespread and easily accessed information. Obviously, more regulation by the government is needed.

Data from Morris, C., & Avorn, J. (2003). Internet marketing of herbal products. *Journal of the American Medical Association, 290*, 1505-1509.

unsubstantiated claims that their supplement treats, cures, mitigates, diagnoses, or prevents a disease. Therefore manufacturers can only make a general claim and no specific claims on the supplement bottle. For example, a company could state "promotes circulation health" on a vitamin E bottle, but they cannot claim something specific such as "lowers low-density lipoproteins (LDL)." Some manufacturers, however, have been guilty of outrageous claims on Internet sites or in other promotional material because the ruling applies only to bottle labels. See the Complementary and Alternative Therapy feature on Internet Marketing of Herbal Products.

The main problem with the DSHEA ruling of 1994 is that it places the actual burden of proof on the U.S. federal government.[8] Hence, even when false claims are made without any medical research or evidence, the U.S. government must prove that the claim is actually false, which is contrary to the situation for pharmaceutical manufacturers, who must prove that their product is safe and effective. Reasons why Congress should pass such an act that virtually allows free reign to one group and tight restrictions to another include the following: (1) a large proportion of Congressional men and women or their spouses used dietary supplements; (2) the large lobby group of the supplement industry has enough clout to influence the rules; and, finally, (3) Congress took a "how can it hurt" approach.[8] Regardless of the reasons, the DSHEA ruling is one of many rulings that is partially responsible for the current situation.

Interestingly, a recent large-scale survey suggests that people in the United States believe that conventional health practitioners are not well-informed about supplements and are probably biased against them.[3] Most participants surveyed, however, also favored the following: (1) increasing government regulation of supplements to determine whether claims are accurate; (2) allowing the FDA to evaluate the safety of new dietary supplements before they are marketed; and (3) increasing the overall authority of the FDA to eliminate supplements found to be unsafe.

2. Realize that the 1994 DSHEA did not apply to food manufacturers and what they may be able to claim or not claim. In the past, food manufacturers were not given as free a reign as the dietary supplement manufacturers. It was difficult to get foods passed as potential sources of health unless clinical evidence existed to support the use of the food product for health. A new ruling directed by the FDA, however, should have a profound influence on what the public will see on future food labels.[8] Food companies now can make health claims on labels if most of the scientific evidence supports a benefit. The FDA claims that the new ruling may promote better education and guidance for a public that wants to eat healthier.

Regardless, if a company exceeds the boundaries of a health claim, the FDA has a right to remove the health claim.

3. Realize that other government rulings play a role in which of the dietary supplements are available for purchase. In 2005 federal legislation expanded the steroid law that had been passed in 1990.[4] The law added more steroids to the list of substances defined as anabolic steroids and classified as Schedule III controlled substances.[4] Androstenedione (Andro), a popular supplement that was available over the counter before 2005, was one of the steroids added to the list of illegal substances.[4] The hormone precursor dehydroepiandrosterone (DHEA), another popular supplement, was added to the list of other hormonal substances excluded from the list of controlled substances.[4] Because of this exclusion and despite the fact that DHEA has caused dramatic reductions in levels of high-density lipoproteins (HDLs, or "good cholesterol") in some studies, DHEA is still available for purchase because of the passage of the 1990 Anabolic Steroid Control Act and the 2005 legislation that expanded that act. Therefore under federal law, companies are allowed to sell some types of supplements even though they may be harmful.

4. Realize the importance of the placebo effect. Randomized, controlled trials are generally considered the standard for determining causality. Some studies use a placebo group when justified. Otherwise, studies use the standard treatment as the comparison group.

A placebo is a chemically inert substance that is administered in the same manner as the chemical or substance being studied. A placebo effect suggests that the people being treated with the placebo experienced an improvement in their condition as the result of psychological or other factors rather than because of the inert substance administered. The results of drug studies that do not use placebos are always subject to doubt because the proportion of the effect that is attributable to psychological factors and the proportion that is caused by the drug cannot be determined.[6] The first article on the placebo effect was published by Pepper in 1945.[11] Ten years later Beecher proposed that about one third of clients in clinical trials experience a placebo effect.[2]

Although later studies demonstrated the placebo's dramatic effect when studying some conditions, the one-third response may be an inadequate oversimplification for research studies today. Currently many conditions have demonstrated that objective evaluations (with serum and imaging tests) demonstrate little if any placebo response. For example, drugs that use only objective evaluation (serum studies) for the assessment of benefits tend to have little to no placebo response. Statin drugs (HMG-CoA reductase inhibitors) have become the primary and standard prescription medications for the reduction of elevated cholesterol levels in men and women. Because of the increasing number of FDA-approved statins, the drugs tend to be compared with each other rather than placebo in randomized trials.

Subjective improvements or self-evaluations tend to have greater placebo responses for conditions such as depression, hair loss, benign prostatic hyperplasia, and sexual dysfunction.[2] It is not unusual to observe a 25% to 50% placebo response rate in some studies. In other words, one fourth to one half of clients taking a sugar pill claim a response that is equivalent to the drug itself, although these clients did not know they were taking a placebo. Some of the best-selling supplements in the United States today are for conditions that have enormous placebo response rates.[8]

Dietary supplements and herbal medications are enjoying an increasing amount of popularity and use, but more randomized trials are needed in this discipline before certain supplements can be recommended. With more people seeking some relief from a specific condition with a CAM, it is important for nurses to explain to clients the need for further research before the effects of many CAM modalities are known.[8]

5. Realize that at least 30% of all modern drugs are actually derived from plants. A partial list of some common drugs that are derived from plants is found on the web in the table Common Plant-Derived Conventional Medicines. Therefore the potential exists for numerous herbal medicines to have some role in our current health care system. The lack of randomized trials for most herbal products makes it difficult for health care professionals currently to recommend or not recommend many herbal products. Nurses need to emphasize this when discussing CAM modalities with clients.

6. Be careful about using the word antioxidant to describe any dietary supplement. Many people refer to dietary supplements as antioxidants; however, this is a myth because no supplement is actually a pure antioxidant.[9] Vitamins C and E and beta-carotene are redox agents. This means that in some situations (food) they are antioxidants, but in other circumstances, when given in higher doses, they can act as pro-oxidants. Pro-oxidants can produce millions if not billions of harmful free radicals and can be harmful in some situations. Antioxidant vitamins in food are balanced biochemistry. They are part of a mixture of redox agents, partly in reduced form and partly in oxidized form. In addition, these foods contain hundreds of other phytochemicals, which is why a balanced, diverse, and moderate diet of healthy foods and beverages makes the most sense unless a clinical trial suggests otherwise.[9] This important point should be discussed with clients

who believe that if they consume a vitamin C pill it might be an adequate substitute for certain fruits and vegetables high in vitamin C.

7. Realize that although numerous studies of alternative medicines have failed to demonstrate a benefit, many recent clinical trials suggest that in some qualifying people, an alternative medicine might provide a substantial benefit. Randomized, controlled trials and other studies have demonstrated that certain people should be good candidates for some dietary supplements.[8] For example, one of the best examples is derived from a randomized trial of more than 3500 people older than 60 years of age.[1] Researchers found that people diagnosed with intermediate to advanced age-related macular degeneration (AMD) who took a specific daily combination supplement (500 mg of vitamin C, 400 international units of vitamin E, 15 mg of beta-carotene, and 80 mg of zinc) for 6 years versus placebo could reduce their risk of visual impairment. This same trial revealed, however, that people with an early diagnosis of AMD did not benefit from taking the supplement.

Another, but shorter (6 month), randomized trial from Europe demonstrated that a combination B-vitamin supplement (1 mg of folic acid, 400 mcg of B_{12}, and 10 mg of B_6) could be beneficial (versus placebo) specifically for clients after coronary angioplasty.[12] Clients receiving the supplement significantly reduced their homocysteine levels, decreased the need for another revascularization procedure, and reduced the risk of early death from any cause compared with clients receiving a placebo.

Nurses should encourage a client to discuss specific supplements with their primary health care provider and realize that the final decision can be made only after an extensive medical evaluation. This method is applied when deciding on any conventional treatment for a specific medical condition. If the individual and provider agree, then a treatment or medication may be recommended. In general, CAM should not be treated any differently than conventional medicine.

8. **Realize that some supplements should be avoided under all circumstances. The FDA has developed a list of 12 supplements that should be avoided under all circumstances (Table 4-2).**

COMMON COMPLEMENTARY AND ALTERNATIVE THERAPIES ACCORDING TO NCCAM CLASSIFICATIONS

NOTE: These therapies are not necessarily advocated by the authors but are provided as a simple introduction to some of the more common CAM modalities. This is

TABLE 4–2 Twelve Supplements That Should Be Avoided (From A-Z)

Supplement	Dangers/Side Effects	Regulatory Actions Taken
Androstenedione (also known as: Andro, 4-androstene-3,17-dione, androstene)	May increase cancer risk, reduce HDL cholesterol, and increase estrogen and/or testosterone levels.	Banned in U.S. as of Jan 20, 2005. Considered a "pro-hormone" supplement. Banned by athletic associations.
Aristolochic acid (also known as: *Aristolochia*, birthwort, snakeroot, snakeweed, sangree root, sangrel, serpentary, serpentaria, asarum canadense, wild ginger); can be in Chinese herbal products labeled as fang ji, mu tong, ma dou ling, and mu xiang	Documented organ failure, and known to have cancer-causing properties. A potential human carcinogen; kidney failure (sometimes requiring transplant); deaths already reported.	FDA warning to consumers in general, and an industry and import alert in April 2001. Ingredient is banned in 7 European countries and Egypt, Japan, and Venezuela.
Bitter orange or bitter orange peel extract (also known as: *Citrus aurantium*, green orange, kijitsu, neroli oil, Seville orange, shangzhou zhiqiao, sour orange, zhi oiao, zhi xhi)	Contains a compound called "synephrine" that is similar to ephedra. Can cause high blood pressure, increased risk of heart dysrhythmias, heart attack, and stroke.	No action taken yet, and still very popular in many weight-loss supplements, especially the ones that claim that they block cortisol.
Chaparral (also known as: *Larrea divaricata*, creosote bush, greasewood, hediondilla, jarilla, larreastat)	Reported deaths, and may cause irreversible liver function or damage.	FDA first warned consumers in Dec 1992.
Comfrey (also known as: *Symphytum officinale*, ass ear, black root, blackwort, bruisewort, consolidae radix, consound, gum plant, healing herb, knitback, knitbone, salsify, slippery root, symphytum radix, wallwort)	Reported deaths, and may cause irreversible liver function or damage.	FDA advised the industry to remove it from market in July 2001.
Germander (also known as: *Teucrium chamaedrys*, wall germander, wild germander)	Reported deaths, and may cause irreversible liver function or damage.	Banned in Germany and France.
Kava (also known as: *Piper methysticum*, ava, awa, gea, gi, intoxicating pepper, kao, kavain, kawa-pfeffer, kew, long pepper, malohu, maluk, meruk, milik, rauschpfeffer, sakau, tonga, wurzelstock, yagona)	Reported deaths, and may cause irreversible liver function or damage.	FDA sent initial warning to consumers in March 2002. Banned in Canada, Germany, Singapore, South Africa, and Switzerland.
Lobelia (*Lobelia inflata*, asthma weed, bladderpod, emetic herb, gagroot, lobelia, Indian tobacco, pukeweed, vomit wort, wild tobacco)	Difficulty breathing, increased heart rate, reduced blood pressure, diarrhea, dizziness, tremors; potential deaths reported.	Banned in Bangladesh and Italy.
Organ/glandular extracts (also known as: adrenal/brain/pituitary/placenta and other gland "concentrate" or "substance")	A potential or theoretical risk of mad cow disease, especially from brain extracts.	FDA banned high-risk bovine materials from older cows in food supplements in Jan 2004. However, high-risk parts from cows under 30 months still permitted. Banned in France and Switzerland.
Pennyroyal oil (also known as: *Hedeoma pulegioides*, lurk-in-the-ditch, mosquito plant, piliolerial, pudding grass, pulegium, run-by-the-ground, squaw balm, squawmint, stinking balm, tickweed)	Liver and kidney failure, convulsions, nerve damage, abdominal pain, throat irritation, and some deaths reported.	No regulatory action yet.
Skullcap or scullcap (also known as: *Scutellaria lateriflora*, blue pimpernel, helmet flower, hoodwort, mad weed, mad-dog herb, mad-dog weed, quaker bonnet, scutellaria)	Abnormal liver function and damage.	No regulatory action yet.
Yohimbe (also known as: *Pausinystalia yohimbe*, johimbi, yohimbehe, yohimbine)	Changes in blood pressure, heart dysrhythmias, respiratory depression, heart attack, and some deaths reported.	No regulatory action yet.

only a partial list of CAM therapies. More specific clinical trials that suggest a benefit or harm with these therapies are found in boxes in many chapters of this textbook.

Table 4-3 provides examples of CAM alternative medical systems. Table 4-4 summarizes examples of CAM mind-body interventions. Table 4-5 describes examples of CAM biologically based therapies. Table 4-6 outlines examples of CAM manipulative and body-based methods. Table 4-7 provides examples of CAM energy therapies.

TABLE 4–3 Examples of CAM Alternative Medical Systems

CAM	Description
Acupuncture/traditional Chinese medicine	Practiced in China for more than 2500 years. Theory of acupuncture espouses belief that there are pathways of energy flow (qi) throughout the body that are vital for health. A trained acupuncturist can correct inadequate qi at various sites with the insertion of needles or applying heat or electrical stimulation at a number of acupuncture points.
Ayurveda (ah-yur-VAY-dah)	Practiced primarily in the Indian subcontinent for 5000 years. Includes diet, herbal remedies, and massage and emphasizes the use of body, mind, and spirit in disease prevention and treatment.
Curanderismo	This system of beliefs or folk medicine is especially popular in some Hispanic-American communities. It includes a variety of techniques such as healing rituals, spirituality, herbal medicines, and psychic healing.
Homeopathic medicine	Involves belief that "like cures like," meaning that small, highly diluted quantities of medicinal substances are given to cure manifestations, when the same substances given at higher or more concentrated doses would actually cause those manifestations.
Naturopathic medicine	Practitioners work with natural healing forces within the body with a goal of helping the body heal from disease and attain better health. Practices may include dietary modifications, massage, exercise, acupuncture, minor surgery, and various other interventions.

TABLE 4–4 Examples of CAM Mind-Body Interventions

CAM	Description
Aromatherapy	Use of fragrant compounds or essential (volatile) oils extracted from plants. They are used to improve mood and overall health. They can be inhaled or applied during massage. Some of the popular compounds include chamomile, eucalyptus, jasmine, lavender, peppermint, and rosemary.
Art, music, or dance therapy	Use of drawing or art, music, or dance to help individuals cope or express emotions.
Biofeedback	Treatment that uses monitoring devices to assist individuals to make them more aware of their physiology and to allow better self-control over such things as blood pressure, muscle tension, temperature, and bladder control.
Hypnosis	In this state of restful alertness, a practitioner makes the client more aware of his or her surroundings to change behavior or promote more healthful practices such as smoking cessation.
Imagery	In these mental exercises the client's mind and thoughts are supposed to impact or assist a certain outcome. For example, a client receiving chemotherapy has an image of the drug literally destroying cancer cells in the body. A variety of visualization techniques are used to promote mental and physical well-being.
Meditation	Uses reflection or mental concentration to create a higher sense of well-being and relaxation. The individual is supposed to eliminate extraneous and mundane thoughts with the overall goal of elevating the mind to a different level. Two broad categories of meditation exist. First, there are the techniques that place emphasis on concentration, or so-called transcendental meditation. Second are the techniques that place emphasis on mindfulness (*Vipassana*). These techniques can be acquired from experienced teachers during a series of sessions. The overall effects of meditation are derived from deep relaxation. For example, a relaxation response in the area of cardiovascular physiology may occur by reducing heart rate and blood pressure, or an endocrine response may occur by reducing the level of stress hormones.
Shamanism	This type of folk medicine uses spiritual healing and is actually performed by a shaman or an individual believed to have special religious or magical powers of healing. There is no strong scientific evidence to support a beneficial effect of shamanism, but currently it is being rigorously tested at some academic medical centers. In addition, some current uses of this therapy (imagery) may reduce stress and anxiety; however, it should not be used in place of conventional treatment.
Spiritual healing	This is the direct interaction between the healer and a client with the intention of improving the client's overall or specific condition or potentially curing the disease. The treatment itself can occur through personal contact or from a distance. Several variations of this therapy exist, including Reiki, intercessory prayer, faith healing, and therapeutic touch. Therapists of one group see themselves as separate from other groups. The primary claim of healers seems to be the promotion or facilitation of self-healing and well-being.
Tai Chi	This is actually an ancient form of martial arts that uses slow, controlled movements, meditation, and breathing to improve overall health and well-being. This form of therapy needs to be taught and should be used in addition to conventional treatment.
Yoga	This type of exercise teaches specific postures and breathing exercises. This form of therapy has been shown at least to improve quality of life for some clients by leading to relaxation and reduced stress levels. Yoga should be taught by a certified instructor because some of the postures could result in injury without proper teaching techniques.

TABLE 4–5 Examples of CAM Biologically Based Therapies

CAM	Description
Alternative diets	More than 40 alternative diets claim to prevent or treat a variety of conditions including cancer. Some examples include macrobiotic diets (based on belief that disease is caused by an imbalance of *Yin* and *Yang*) and the Gerson diet (vegan diet).
Dietary supplements (e.g., herbs, vitamins, minerals)	More than 20,000 herbal and dietary supplements are sold in the United States.

TABLE 4–6 Examples of CAM Manipulative and Body-Based Methods

CAM	Description
Chiropractic medicine	System of health care, begun in 1895 by Daniel Palmer, based on the belief that the nervous system is the most critical part of an individual's state of health. According to the theory, diseases are a result of "nerve interference," caused by spinal subluxations, which respond to manipulation of the spine. Chiropractors use spinal manipulations, mobilizations, and other types of natural medicines.
Massage	Involves rubbing, manipulation, and kneading of the body's muscle and soft tissue. It may reduce stress, anxiety, pain, and depression. Many conventional medical practitioners use or recommend massage to relieve clinical manifestations along with standard treatment. For example, the use of massage to decrease lymphedema caused by some treatments of breast and other cancers may help to reduce swelling.

TABLE 4–7 Examples of CAM Energy Therapies

CAM	Description
Cymatic therapy	Sir Peter Manners, MD, developed this non-audible sound therapy, which uses hand-held devices to transmit sound energy or waves through the skin. When the waves reach the internal body they are to restore the body's basic rhythms and boost immune function.
Magnetic therapy	Involves the use of a variety of different sizes and shapes of individual magnets on the body to reduce pain and treat disease.
Qi gong (chee-GUNG)	A component of traditional Chinese medicine that combines movement, meditation, and regulation of breathing to enhance the flow of qi (energy) in the body, improve blood circulation, and enhance immune function.
Reiki (RAY-kee)	A Japanese word representing "Universal Life Energy." Reiki is based on the belief that when spiritual energy is channeled through a Reiki practitioner, the client's spirit is healed, which in turn heals the physical body.
Therapeutic touch	Derived from an ancient technique called *laying-on of hands* and based on a premise that it is the healing force of the therapist that affects the client's recovery; healing is promoted when the body's energies are in balance; and by passing their hands over the client, healers can identify energy imbalances.

COMPLEMENTARY AND ALTERNATIVE THERAPY FEATURES THROUGHOUT THE TEXTBOOK

Effective or ineffective CAM clinical trials are included throughout this text in their appropriate setting. For example, trials of cholesterol-lowering supplements are boxed and placed in the section on cardiovascular disease. Hundreds of trials have been completed in the last decade. Many of the findings of these studies appear in boxes within specific chapters of the book to facilitate nurses who work with clients who may want to discuss CAM therapies in conjunction with conventional medical treatments.

 BIBLIOGRAPHY

Citations appearing in red refer to primary research.

1. Age-Related Eye Disease Study Research Group. (2001). A randomized, placebo-controlled, clinical trial of high-dose supplementation with vitamins C and E, beta carotene, and zinc for age-related macular degeneration and vision loss: AREDS Report No. 8. *Archives of Ophthalmology, 119*(10), 1417-1436.
2. Beecher, H.K. (1955). The powerful placebo. *Journal of the American Medical Association, 159*, 1602-1606.
3. Blendon, R.J., et al. (2001). Americans' views on the use and regulation of dietary supplements. *Archives of Internal Medicine, 161* (6), 805-810.
4. Collins, R. (2006). *Legal muscle supplements 2006.* Accessed 10/07/06 from www.steroidlaw.com/?pageID=51.
5. DeSmet, P. (2002). Herbal remedies. *The New England Journal of Medicine, 347*(25), 2046-2056.
6. Gall, M., Gall, J., & Borg, W. (2006). *Educational research: An introduction* (8th ed.). Boston: Allyn and Bacon.
7. Hawks, J., & Moyad, M. (2003). CAM: Definition and classification overview. *Urologic Nursing, 23*(3), 221-223.
8. Moyad, M.A. (2003). *The ABCs of nutrition and supplements for prostate cancer.* Ann Arbor, Mich: JW Edwards Publishing.
9. Moyad, M.A. (2006). Step-by-step lifestyle changes that can improve urologic health in men, Part II: What do I tell my patients? *Primary Care: Clinic and Office Practice, 33*, 165-185.

10. National Center for Complementary and Alternative Medicine. (2006). *What is complementary and alternative medicine (CAM)?* Retrieved 10/07/06 from http://nccam.nih.gov/health/whatiscam.

11. Pepper, O.H.P. (1945). A note on placebo. *Annals of the Journal of Pharmacology, 117,* 409-412.

12. Schnyder, G., Roffi, M., Pin, R., et al. (2001). Decreased rate of coronary restenosis after lowering of plasma homocysteine levels. *New England Journal of Medicine, 345*(22), 1593-1600.

13. Skidmore-Roth, L. (2006). *Mosby's handbook of herbs & natural supplements* (3rd ed.). St. Louis: Mosby.

14. Wender, R., & Nevin, J. (Eds.). (2002). *Primary Care: Preventive Medicine, 29*(3), 475-766.

15. Wierenga, M. (Ed.). (2002). *The Nursing Clinics of North America: Lifestyle Modification, 37*(2), 225-371.

16. Zoorob, R., & Morelli, V. (Eds.). (2002). *Primary Care: Alternative Therapies, 29*(2), 231-473.

evolve *Did you remember to check out the bonus material on the Evolve website and the CD-ROM, including NCLEX®-Examination Style Review Questions, Open-Book Quizzes, and Chapter Review Audio Podcasts?*

http://evolve.elsevier.com/Black/medsurg

UNIT 2

HEALTH CARE DELIVERY SYSTEMS

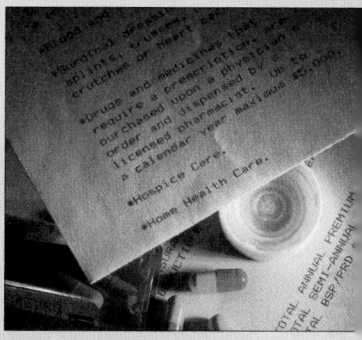

CHAPTER **5**

Ambulatory Health Care

Sheila A. Haas and Diana P. Hackbarth

In any given year, most Americans are not hospitalized, but the average person makes 3.6 ambulatory care visits per year. Infants under 1 year of age average almost seven visits, primarily for well-child care, while the older adult on Medicare averages six visits per year. These facts make ambulatory settings the major site for health care delivery in the United States. Ambulatory care visits are increasing for several reasons:

1. The length of stay in hospitals for illness, surgery, or complex treatments has decreased. More clients are seen in ambulatory settings for post-hospital visits and follow-up care.
2. As a result of new technology, ambulatory settings are increasingly common sites for people to undergo many surgical and complex procedures that previously required hospitalization.
3. Advances in the treatment of chronic health problems have made it possible to treat and monitor a client's progress in ambulatory care settings and avoid costly hospitalization. As a result, both the numbers and the acuity of people cared for in ambulatory settings have increased.

There are numerous advantages to providing health care in ambulatory settings. People prefer to receive care close to home, with providers they know and with whom they have a relationship. Clients often feel less stress because they are not separated from their family, significant others, and community. Care in the community decreases exposure to nosocomial infections and other hazards of hospitalization. Ambulatory care is often less costly than hospitalization, saving money for clients, insurance companies, employers, and the government.

Socioeconomic factors have also encouraged the growth of ambulatory care. The growth of managed care organizations has increased the demand for primary care services and ambulatory facilities. Clients who are insured through a managed care plan often must see a primary care provider before obtaining referrals to specialty or hospital care. The variety of care modalities offered in ambulatory care has escalated, and the demand for professional nurses to work in ambulatory care has never been greater. The opportunities for professional nurses to work in ambulatory care settings are expected to increase in the years to come.

DEFINITION AND CHARACTERISTICS OF AMBULATORY CARE NURSING

Nurses have worked in ambulatory care settings for many years. Ambulatory care nurses take care of people in all age groups and with all diagnoses, both those who are healthy and those with acute, chronic, or life-threatening health problems. Several characteristics of ambulatory care nursing are presented in Box 5-1.

The definition of ambulatory nursing was developed by a panel of expert ambulatory care nurses who participated in focus groups of ambulatory care nurses across the United States. Based on the characteristics listed in Box 5-1, the American Academy of Ambulatory Care Nursing (AACN) defined ambulatory care nursing as follows:

> Ambulatory care nursing includes those clinical, management, educational, and research activities provided by registered nurses for and with individuals who seek care and assistance with health maintenance, health promotion and/or health related problems. These individuals

---

evolve **Web Enhancements**

Appendix A Religious Beliefs and Practices Affecting Health Care

Be sure to check out the bonus material on the Evolve website and the CD-ROM, including free self-assessment exercises. **http://evolve.elsevier. com/Black/medsurg**

- Nursing autonomy
- Client advocacy
- Skillful, rapid assessment
- Holistic nursing care
- Client teaching
- Wellness and health promotion
- Coordination and continuity of care
- Long-term relationships with clients and families
- Telephone triage, consultation, follow-up, and surveillance
- Client and family control as major caregivers, users of the health care system, and decision makers regarding compliance with care regimen
- Collaboration with other health care providers
- Case management

engage predominantly in self-care and self-managed health activities or receive care from family and significant others outside an institutional setting.

Ambulatory care nursing takes place on an episodic basis, is less than 24 hours in duration, and occurs as a single encounter or a series of encounters over time. Ambulatory nurse-client encounters take place in health care facilities as well as in community-based settings, including but not limited to schools, workplaces, or homes. Ambulatory care nursing encounters may occur face-to-face or via phone or other communication devices. The focus of ambulatory care services encompasses use of cost-effective ways to assist clients in promoting wellness, preventing illness, and managing acute and chronic diseases to effect the most attainable positive health status over the life span.

Characteristics of ambulatory care present the following challenges for nurses:

1. Visit encounters are short, the number of client visits per day is great, and the assessment time is compressed. In contrast to the hospital nurse, who can return to a client confined to bed to retrieve data that may have been missed, the ambulatory care nurse who misses collecting data may not be able to obtain it until the next visit. Because visits are short, the ambulatory care nurse cannot perform an extensive assessment on every client but must perform a focused assessment. This change in interaction is often a difficult transition for nurses who have worked in hospital settings.
2. Control of care and treatment modalities is in the hands of the client and family, *not* the health care provider. In the hospital, the nurse administers medications, administers the treatments, or supervises others providing care to the client. In ambulatory care, however, the client chooses to schedule a visit, keep an appointment, take prescribed medications, or undergo treatments as he or she sees fit. The nurse must become a teacher, coach, and advocate as well as a treatment provider because

clients and families must follow through with the treatment plan on their own between visits.
3. In ambulatory care, many members of the health care team work together and their roles often do not have clear boundaries. Nurses must be strong communicators and collaborators, often functioning as a team leader or team facilitator.
4. In ambulatory care, contacts with the nurse are frequently maintained through *communication devices* such as the telephone and computer. Ambulatory care nurses need highly developed assessment and communication skills, as well as critical thinking and judgment, in order to interpret data and to refer the client for appropriate follow-up.
5. Finally, there is *constant pressure* to increase efficiency and effectiveness of care. Nurses are working to standardize care so that health promotion, disease prevention, and early detection and treatment of health problems become integral to the ambulatory care client encounter.

CONCEPTUAL MODELS IN AMBULATORY CARE NURSING PRACTICE

The organization of ambulatory care services in the United States is based on a complex mix of historical, philosophical, political, and economic factors. The way in which policy-makers, health care providers, and ordinary citizens conceptualize health and disease has a profound effect on how health care is delivered.

The Clinical Model

Most health policy experts agree that the current health care system is based on the clinical or medical model. In this model, health is conceptualized as the absence of the clinical manifestations of disease. It is assumed that the body is a machine and that modern medical technology can use physical and chemical interventions to "fix the machine" whenever it is broken. This has led to great emphasis on expensive, acute care with high-technology treatments and relatively little attention to prevention, public health, environmental measures, or personal responsibility for health.

Most ambulatory care services, except for certain public health programs, are outgrowths of this clinical model. Services were traditionally organized around physicians' delivery of reimbursable clinical model care to people who sought care only when they were ill. The traditional nursing role in ambulatory care supported physician control and the clinical model of care delivery. Although the clinical model has led to great advances in scientific medicine and technology, the focus on body parts rather than the whole and the lack of emphasis on prevention have been problematic.

Many nurse theorists, primary care providers, and public health advocates look at health in a *holistic* way. Nurses are educated to (1) consider the whole person, family, and environment; (2) address both actual and potential health problems; and (3) emphasize health teaching, prevention, and self-care as well as care of the sick. Newer, more holistic conceptual models are becoming increasingly important in ambulatory care. These models have been delineated by health care scholars, national and international health advocacy organizations, and ambulatory care nurses themselves.

Levels of Prevention Model

The Levels of Prevention Model, advocated by Leavell and Clark in 1965, has influenced both public health practice and ambulatory care delivery worldwide. This model suggests that the natural history of any disease exists on a continuum, with health at one end and advanced disease at the other. The model delineates three levels of the application of preventive measures that can be used to promote health and arrest the disease process at different points along the continuum. The goal is to maintain a healthy state and to prevent disease or injury.

People experiencing acute or chronic disease as well as healthy populations are all candidates for primary prevention measures. The Levels of Prevention Model is appropriate in all health care settings and in any population group. The *Healthy People 2010 Objectives for the Nation* includes two overarching goals of reducing health disparities and increasing both the length and quality of life; it also includes leading health indicators and objectives to reduce mortality and morbidity at all three levels of prevention. Most of these objectives can be implemented in ambulatory settings or through population-focused interventions in the community.

Primary Prevention

Primary prevention encompasses both health promotion and specific protection. Health promotion includes interventions such as health education, information on growth and development, nutrition, and exercise as well as the provision of adequate housing, safe working conditions, and other services. For example, an ambulatory care nurse might provide telephone consultation and teaching to a new mother concerned about well-baby care.

Specific protection interventions are targeted at specific health risks, injuries, and diseases. For example, immunizations protect against particular infectious diseases; seat belts reduce injuries in automobile crashes; smoking cessation reduces the risk of cancers and heart disease; reducing air pollution prevents exacerbations of asthma and bronchitis; a high-calcium diet with over-the-counter calcium supplements and weight-bearing exercise helps menopausal women prevent osteoporosis. Primary prevention interventions may be targeted at individual clients, families, groups, communities, or populations.

Secondary Prevention

Secondary preventive measures include early diagnosis and prompt treatment as well as disability limitation. Case finding, screening, and treatment of disease by medical or surgical interventions to arrest the disease process and prevent further complications are all part of secondary prevention. An ambulatory care nurse carrying out a multiphasic health screening for hypertension, diabetes, and hypercholesterolemia would be practicing secondary prevention. Other examples are administering chemotherapy to a client with cancer and positioning a client in the recovery room after outpatient surgery to ensure proper alignment of the extremities.

Tertiary Prevention

Tertiary prevention occurs after a disease state is present. This level of prevention is directed at measures to rehabilitate a person or group so they can maximize their remaining capacities. Cardiac rehabilitation nurses, physical and occupational therapists, and many home care nurses focus on tertiary prevention. An example of tertiary prevention in the ambulatory surgery recovery room is teaching crutch-walking to a client after foot surgery.

Primary Health Care, Primary Care, and Managed Care Models

Primary health care focuses on the universal right to basic health care. *Primary care* focuses on integrated care coordinated by one primary provider. *Managed care* approaches the use of health care services from a cost-containment perspective. *Primary prevention* is often confused with the concepts of primary health care and primary care. In addition, many managed care organizations use primary care providers, such as family practice physicians and nurse practitioners, in a "gatekeeper" function, causing further confusion. Box 5-2 compares and contrasts these conceptual models. These models, as well as the clinical model and the ambulatory care nursing conceptual framework, have influenced the organization of practice in ambulatory care settings.

AMBULATORY CARE NURSING CONCEPTUAL FRAMEWORK

The Ambulatory Care Nursing Conceptual Framework was developed by a "think tank" of experts who are also members of the AACN. The AACN member experts work in ambulatory care settings, perform research, and write

---

BOX 5-2   Health Care Models

PRIMARY HEALTH CARE

- World Health Organization (WHO) definition (1978):[45] "essential health care made universally accessible to individuals and families in the community through their full participation and at a cost the community and country can afford."
  - Assumes community involvement
  - Includes both personal health care services and population-based public health services
  - Aimed at prevention as well as treatment of disease
  - Aimed at improving health status of the population or community

PRIMARY CARE

- Institute of Medicine (IOM) definition (1994):[24] "provision of integrated accessible health care services by clinicians who are accountable for addressing a large majority of personal health care needs, developing a sustained partnership with patients, and practicing in the context of family and community."
- IOM definition (1978):[25] "personal health care services that are accessible, comprehensive, coordinated, and continuous. Care delivered by accountable providers of personal health services."
- Starfield definition (1992):[38]
  - First contact—source of care available in a timely manner
  - Longitudinal—not episodic, focused on person, not episode of disease; client sees provider as regular source of care
  - Comprehensive—includes services for common problems
  - Coordinated—provider coordinates care when client is sent elsewhere for referrals, procedures, and therapies

MANAGED CARE

- Einthoven definition (1993):[11]
  - Integrated financing and delivery systems with per capita prepayment and with providers placed at risk for cost and quality of care
  - First contact—ensure access to basic services; restrict access to specialized services through "gatekeeper" function of primary provider
- Starfield definition (1992):[38]
  - Longitudinal—not addressed
  - Comprehensive—not addressed
  - Coordinated—gatekeeper as coordinator; goal is to eliminate unnecessary and inappropriate care; may also restrict access to appropriate care
  - Reduction in cost; cost containment
  - Health status of population—not addressed; in HMO organizations, goal is to keep enrolled population healthy in order to reduce utilization cost

---

about ambulatory care nursing. A conceptual framework is a diagram or map that accomplishes the following:

- Specifies major concepts, skills, and competencies in an area of practice

- Reflects values and beliefs as well as the experiential knowledge of a practice discipline
- Delineates the relationships between major concepts and skills
- Acts as a model to help organize practice, guide the development of educational materials, create test items for certification examinations, develop orientation programs, and design ambulatory care delivery models
- Forms the basis of performance appraisal instruments for ambulatory care nurses

The conceptual framework shown in Figure 5-1 delineates the following three roles for ambulatory care nurses: (1) the clinical nursing role; (2) the organizational/systems role, and (3) the professional role. Each role has several dimensions that vary, depending on the size of the ambulatory care setting. For example, staff nurses working in large settings where there are multiple nurses and nurse managers do not need to do many of the more managerial dimensions under the organizational/systems role. In smaller settings, they would likely practice in all three roles. The Ambulatory Care Nursing Conceptual Framework was used to structure the *Core Curriculum for Ambulatory Care Nursing*, written for nurses to use in preparation for certification in ambulatory care.

As seen in Figure 5-1, client populations may be healthy, acutely ill, chronically ill, or terminally ill. Role dimensions highly valued by nurses are all included in this conceptual framework:

- Primary, secondary, and tertiary prevention
- Teaching and client advocacy
- Care management, a feature of primary care
- Evidence-based practice

AMBULATORY CARE PRACTICE SETTINGS

Historically, health services in the United States were delivered to people in their homes by itinerant physicians, midwives, barbers, nurses, and "medicine men," who learned their trade through an unregulated apprentice system. In some urban areas, freestanding dispensaries were established as charity for the poor and a place for prospective physicians to learn their trade. These dispensaries dissolved into outpatient departments once a system of voluntary hospitals was developed and nursing and medical education was upgraded and standardized in the beginning of the 20th century.

For the purposes of data collection, the National Center for Health Statistics classifies ambulatory care settings into three main groups: physicians' offices, hospital outpatient departments, and hospital emergency departments (EDs).

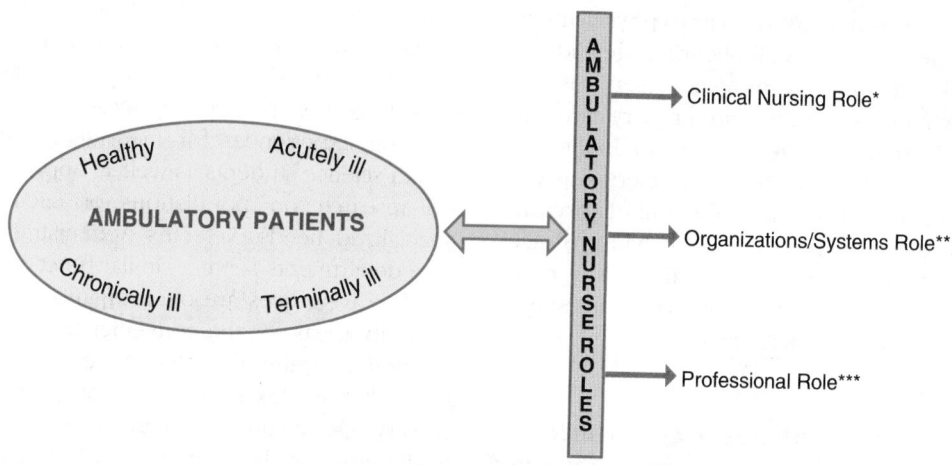

AMBULATORY PATIENTS

Healthy Acutely ill
Chronically ill Terminally ill

AMBULATORY NURSE ROLES

→ Clinical Nursing Role*

→ Organizations/Systems Role**

→ Professional Role***

*Clinical Nursing Role
Patient Education
Advocacy (compassion, caring,
    emotional support)
Care Management
Assessment, Screening, Triage
Telephone Practice
Collaboration/Resource
    Identification and Referral
Clinical Procedures,
    Independent/Interdependent/
    Dependent
Primary, Secondary, and
    Tertiary Prevention
Communication/Documentation
Outcome Management
Protocol Development/Usage

****Organizations/Systems
    Role**
Practice/Office Support
Health Care Fiscal Management
    (reimbursement and coding)
Collaboration/Conflict
    Management
Informatics
Context of Care Delivery/
    Models
Care of the Caregiver
Priority Management/
    Delegation/Supervision
Ambulatory Culture/Cross-
    Cultural Competencies
Ongoing Political/
    Entrepreneurial Skills
Structuring Customer-Focused
    Systems
Workplace Regulatory
    Compliance (EEOC, OSHA)
Advocacy (Inter-organizational
    and in Community)
Legal Issues

***Professional Role
Evidence-Based Practice
Leadership Inquiry and
    Research Utilization
Clinical Quality Improvement
Staff Development
Regulatory Compliance (Risk
    Management)
Provider Self-Care

■ **FIGURE 5–1** Ambulatory Care Nursing Conceptual Framework. *(Modified from Haas, S. [1998]. Ambulatory care nursing conceptual framework. AACN Viewpoint, 20[3], 16-17, with permission.)*

Physicians' Offices

Almost 81% of the more than 1 billion annual ambulatory care visits in the United States occur in physicians' offices. Increasingly, physicians are abandoning solo practice and aligning themselves in group practices to consolidate resources to meet the challenges of managed care and insurance contracting. About two thirds of physicians practice in a group setting, usually with two to six physicians. Some groups are specialty practices, such as cardiologists or oncologists. Larger group practices often include primary care physicians and advanced practice nurses. About 25% of physician office visits are to general and family practice physicians, and 36% of visits are to internists, pediatricians, and obstetric and gynecology physicians, all of whom are considered primary care providers. The remaining visits are to medical and surgical specialists. Nurse practitioners, nurse-midwives, and physician assistants deliver about 3% of ambulatory services in physicians' offices.

Physician group practices usually operate on a for-profit basis and seek fee-for-service payment directly from clients or through third-party payers such as insurance companies, Medicare, and Medicaid. In a *fee-for-service* system, providers get paid separately for each service they provide; the more services they provide, the more revenue they generate. In *integrated* delivery systems, hospitals align with several physician group practices to increase the hospital referral rate and provide increased coordination of care. Many physician group practices also contract with health maintenance organizations (HMOs) to provide capitated services at a prepaid, fixed rate for each person enrolled. Another way physicians get paid is by contracting with a preferred provider organization (PPO) and receive a reduced rate for each service they provide.

The predominant way of viewing health and disease in most physician group practices is the *clinical model.* However, family practice physicians may adhere to the *primary care model.* About 16% of visits to physicians are for preventive care; women of child-bearing age and children traditionally receive more preventive services than men. Nurse practitioners working with primary care physicians also ascribe to the primary care model. In the past, nurses in physicians' offices often served a clerical as well as an assistive function. The role of the ambulatory care nurse in physician group practices is evolving to meet the need for increasingly skilled technical services, especially in specialty practices such as oncology, freestanding birthing centers, and surgical centers.

Community Hospital Outpatient Departments

Community hospital clinic services began in the latter part of the 19th century and took over the functions of the freestanding dispensaries. Clinic services were consistent with the mission of the religious and ethnic groups that organized voluntary community hospitals. This mission included both a charitable function for the community and a place for local physicians to practice. Physicians were often assigned to staff hospital clinics as a duty, in return for the privilege of hospitalizing their clients. Nurses trained in diploma schools staffed both the hospitals and the clinics.

Today, nonprofit community hospitals still provide varying amounts of uncompensated care in their outpatient departments as part of their obligation to provide "community benefits" as not-for-profit corporations. However, their goal is to maximize revenues by attracting individuals or employee groups who have insurance coverage. Thus outpatient services constitute a key source of revenue for hospitals. Approximately 8.2% of all ambulatory care visits occur in hospital outpatient departments.

Both primary care and specialized care in a clinical model may be offered. Ambulatory services may be housed adjacent to the hospital or be freestanding in the community. Services may include outpatient surgery, emergency centers, cardiac rehabilitation centers, drug and alcohol treatment programs, mobile vans, women's health or breast centers, work site health promotion, oncology centers, home care, hospice, and community health promotion. Many integrated health care systems have freestanding satellite ambulatory care sites that offer primary care services for managed care enrollees. Specialized clinics and health promotion programs staffed by nurses also exist in community hospital outpatient settings. Some of these programs are organized around the ambulatory care nursing conceptual framework. Currently, 12.6% of outpatient department services are provided by nurse practitioners, midwives, or physician assistants.

Teaching Hospital Outpatient Departments

Outpatient departments of teaching hospitals were developed to fulfill the mission of academic health centers: to provide medical and other health professional education, biomedical research, and client care services. University hospital outpatient departments and most large hospitals run by local governments provide learning experiences for medical, nursing, and other health science students as well as opportunities for clinical research on populations of clients with highly specialized needs. Veterans Administration ambulatory care departments serve a similar function.

Clinical services are often organized around medical specialty areas for the convenience of providers. Some are regional referral centers, whereas others, especially those that are tax-supported, may provide a full range of services, including primary care for the poor. Most teaching hospitals maintain a nonprofit status and provide care for those with public or private insurance as well as uncompensated care for uninsured clients (whose diseases may provide good learning experiences). Many hospitals have satellite ambulatory care centers. With the growth of managed care, increased competition, and decreased reimbursement from Medicaid, Medicare, and insurance companies, teaching hospitals are increasingly concerned with maximizing revenue from insured clients and ensuring a flow of paying clients to make up for empty inpatient beds, discounted client charges, or care for the poor.

University hospital outpatient departments have traditionally espoused the clinical model and have been driven and controlled by physicians. There are, however, some nurse-managed hospital clinics that deal with specific client populations, such as clients with chronic leg ulcers or those who need monitoring of warfarin (Coumadin) therapy. Nurses play a major role in client and family teaching and as case managers for clients with catastrophic and chronic illnesses. For example, nurses case-manage the care of heart transplant clients, trauma victims, oncology clients, and high-risk mothers and infants.

Health Maintenance Organizations as Ambulatory Care Delivery Sites

HMOs began more than 50 years ago and proliferated during the 1990s in response to both federal enabling legislation and market forces. HMOs provide a defined population with a stated range of services through the prepayment of an annual or monthly capitation fee. With *capitation,* providers receive the same amount of money per client per month, no matter how many or how few services a client uses that month or year. Thus there is no incentive to provide expensive tests or treatments that the client may not need. HMOs are systems of care that integrate the insurance and payment mechanisms and the actual delivery of health care services. For example, Kaiser Permanente, the largest nonprofit HMO in the United States, operates hospitals, outpatient facilities, and large physician practices.

However, not all HMOs maintain their own ambulatory care delivery sites. The prevalence of HMOs varies in different regions of the country and about one fourth of ambulatory care visits are financed through an HMO mechanism.

HMOs began as nonprofit organizations but increasingly have been purchased by the for-profit sector. Philosophically, the concept of an HMO differs from traditional ambulatory services, in that value is placed on prevention and maintaining health in order to avoid more costly specialist or inpatient services. Care is coordinated by a primary care provider who acts as a gatekeeper. The goal is to lower costs through the provision of primary care, coordination of services, utilization management, and elimination of the "incentives" of the fee-for-service payment system.

Many HMOs employ nurse practitioners, nurse-midwives, and physician assistants as primary care providers. In addition to the clinical model, HMOs espouse wellness, health maintenance, and primary care. Nursing, with its more holistic approach to client care, can play an influential role in managed care settings.

Emergency Departments

More than 10% of ambulatory care visits in the United States are provided in emergency departments (EDs). The number of ED visits is increasing annually while the availability of EDs is decreasing in the United States. About 75% of ED visits are made by people who walk in, whereas the remaining 25% arrive by either ground or air ambulance. Triage staff in EDs classify clients in terms of the immediacy of their need to be seen in a timely manner. In 2004 ED staff classified 12.9% of visits as emergent, 37.8% as urgent, 21.8% as semi-urgent, 12.5% as not urgent, and the remaining as unclassified. The average waiting time to see a physician is 47 minutes nationally, but about one third of clients must wait an hour or more, and sometimes up to 24 hours, in some very busy, overcrowded and underfunded EDs. Low-income families, the unemployed, members of minority groups, the uninsured, and those whose health care is funded through Medicaid use disproportionately more ED services for nonurgent care than those who have private insurance. In the United States, there are 46 million uninsured and many more underinsured people who lack access to appropriate primary care services in their communities. These people often seek primary care services in EDs. However, because EDs are organized according to the clinical model and are set up to meet acute care needs, they are far from the ideal place to provide primary care services. Registered nurses play a very important client care role in EDs in that 90% of clients receive care from a nurse when they visit the ED.

Other Ambulatory Care Settings

Many other settings provide a wide array of ambulatory care services. Public health departments, federally qualified community health centers (FQCHCs), and FQCHC look-alikes provide primary health care and ambulatory services in the community. These are local, state, and federal tax-supported agencies designed to increase access to care for the poor and uninsured and serve as a safety net in many communities.

One unique type of ambulatory care organization is a nurse-managed center, nursing practice arrangement, or nursing center. These nurse-staffed community centers may provide primary health care services, home care, hospice, college health services, work site health promotion, school nursing, or wellness services. Many nursing centers were developed by schools of nursing as faculty practice sites and clinical sites for undergraduate and graduate students. Others were federally funded demonstration projects. Most nurse-managed centers employ advanced practice nurses (APNs) and are organized around a nursing or primary health care model.

Other settings in which ambulatory care nurses practice include government-funded public health clinics, migrant and community health centers, homeless shelters, school-based health centers, Native American health service clinics, and other community-based organizations that serve special population groups. These are either tax-supported or private nonprofit organizations. Many community-based organizations are organized around a primary health care or public health model. Most include population-based preventive services as well as personal health care.

CHARACTERISTICS OF AMBULATORY CARE CLIENT POPULATION

Each year in the United States, people make more than a billion ambulatory visits. Women make more visits than men, and older adults make an average 7.5 visits a year compared with about 3 visits a year for children. The overall visit rate for whites is not significantly different than that for African Americans, although African Americans are more likely to use hospital outpatient departments than whites. Figure 5-2 shows the distribution of ambulatory care visits, categorized by clients' expressed reasons for the visit. About one third of visits are for acute problems and one third are for follow-up of chronic health problems. Figure 5-3 depicts the distribution of ambulatory care visits by primary diagnosis in the United States in 2004. Respiratory problems, diseases of the nervous system, endocrine and immunity disorders, skin diseases, and mental health problems are among the most common diagnoses.

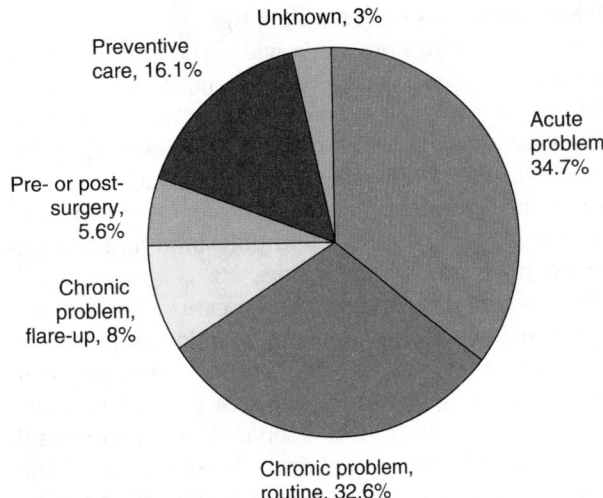

■ **FIGURE 5–2** Percent distribution of physician's office and outpatient ambulatory care visits by client's principal reason for visit: United States, 2004. *(From Hing, E., Cherry, D.K., & Woodwell, D.A. [2006]. National ambulatory medical care survey: 2004 summary. Advanced data from vital and health statistics [No. 374]. Hyattsville, Md: National Center for Health Statistics; and McCaig, L.F., & Nawar, E.W.' [2006]. National hospital ambulatory medical care survey: 2004 emergency department summary. Advance data from vital and health statistics [No. 372]. Hyattsville, Md: National Center for Health Statistics.)*

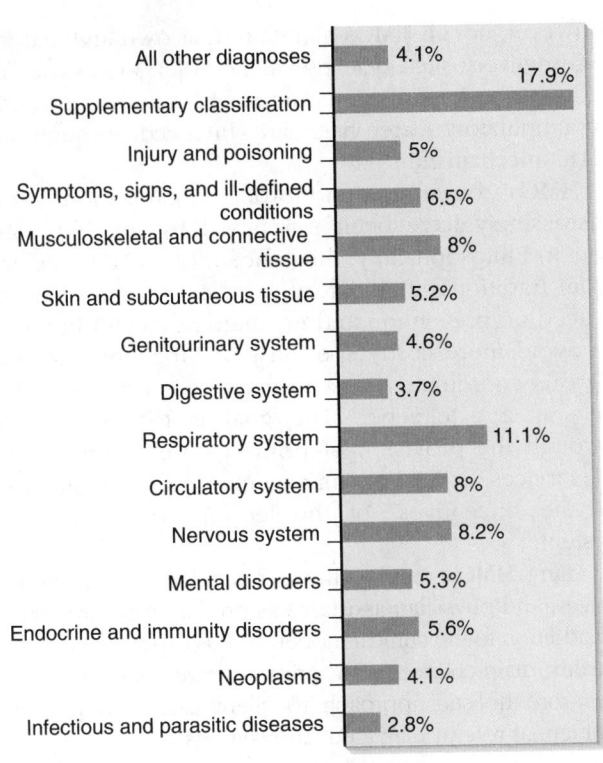

■ **FIGURE 5–3** Percent distribution of ambulatory office visits categorized by ICD-9-CM primary diagnosis categories: United States, 2004. "Supplementary classification" is used for visits not related to illness or injury, such as general medical examinations, health supervision, and normal prenatal care. *(Hing, E., Cherry, D.K., & Woodwell, D.A. [2006]. National ambulatory medical care survey: 2004 summary. Advanced data from vital and health statistics [No. 374]. Hyattsville, Md: National Center for Health Statistics; and McCaig, L.F., & Nawar, E.W. (2006). National hospital ambulatory medical care survey: 2004 emergency department summary. Advance data from vital and health statistics [No. 372]. Hyattsville, Md: National Center for Health Statistics.)*

However, many people present with signs and symptoms of ill-defined conditions.

Ambulatory clients are often classified by their *health status.* A client may be essentially healthy but acutely ill at the time of the visit, such as a client with otitis media or appendicitis. The client can be expected to return to wellness once the acute problem is cured. Another client may be chronically ill but managing the chronic illness well. A young asthmatic person with peak flow readings within normal limits is an example. A client may be chronically ill and have an acute episode, such as an older diabetic client with influenza. Finally, a client may be terminally ill with end-stage renal disease or liver failure and require supportive care.

Ambulatory clients may also be classified by a major *illness,* body system, and typical *treatment* needed. For example, teaching hospital outpatient settings often have specific clinics for people with diabetes or heart failure; some have ear, nose, and throat clinics or urology clinics for people with maladies of certain body systems. Others have programs such as a "Coumadin clinic" and "cast clinic," which classify clients according to the type of treatment to be administered. Ambulatory clients may also be classified in terms of *age,* such as pediatric, adolescent, and geriatric, or by gender, such as women's health services.

Another means of categorizing clients is by the type or source of *reimbursement* for the care provided (e.g., private insurance, Medicare, Medicaid, workers' compensation, or self-pay). Because about 16% of the U.S. population lacks health insurance, payment for care is

a problem for many individuals and families. Ambulatory care clients also may be defined by the type of *services they are seeking,* such as primary care, which includes pediatrics, obstetrics and gynecology, family practice, and internal medicine; family planning; or sports medicine.

As mentioned earlier, in ambulatory care it is the client, client's family, or significant other who initiates an encounter or visit, travels to and from the ambulatory care setting, and chooses to collaborate with the ambulatory interdisciplinary team regarding wellness behaviors and the treatment regimen. Thus the ambulatory care team must know, understand, and respect the client's culture, traditions, and perspective on health and illness. Cultural competence is essential, because the client, family, or significant other manages and provides health care during visits and during the interval between visits. The client controls health care decisions. Respectful communication facilitates the long-term relationship that clients often have with ambulatory care nurses and other providers.

RESEARCH IN AMBULATORY CARE NURSING

Although nurses have been working in ambulatory settings for many years, little research on the work and role of ambulatory care nurses has been done. Nursing research in ambulatory care is needed for many reasons:

- To help develop new models of nursing care delivery
- To delineate position descriptions for nurses working in ambulatory care
- To develop standards of client care and professional nursing practice
- To create both performance improvement programs and nursing intensity systems to determine the number and types of nursing personnel needed

One of the earliest studies, done by Hooks and colleagues in 1980, delineated barriers to ambulatory nursing practice. Verran, in 1981, developed seven areas of nursing responsibility in ambulatory care using a Delphi method and the opinion of expert ambulatory care nurses. In 1985 Tighe and associates further refined Verran's areas of responsibility by adding planning. In 1995 Hackbarth and co-workers and Haas and colleagues conducted a national survey of ambulatory care nurses working in many types of ambulatory care settings. An analysis of these data provided insight into the dimensions of the current staff nurse role and the dimensions of the future staff nurse role in ambulatory care.

In current practice, Hackbarth and co-workers found that ambulatory care nurses spent much of their time performing activities in dimensions named enabling operations and technical procedures. These activities include locating records, ordering supplies, taking vital signs, setting up rooms, assisting with procedures, and administering oral or intramuscular (IM) medications. Some of these activities could have been done by clerks or nursing assistants. Relatively less of the staff nurse's time was spent on more professional activities in the dimensions named telephone communication, advocacy, teaching, and care coordination.

When nurses surveyed by Haas and Hackbarth were asked what they would like to be doing in the future, they indicated that they would prefer to accomplish more activities in higher-level professional dimensions such as teaching, care coordination, and expert practice. They even foresaw another dimension, labeled technical procedures (Figure 5-4). The implications of this research are clear. Nurses in many ambulatory settings need to have sufficient numbers of competent assistive personnel to whom they can delegate enabling and technical procedures if they are to have sufficient time to perform activities in higher-level dimensions such as teaching, advocacy, care coordination, high-tech procedures, and expert practice.

Ambulatory care nurse researchers are involved in specifying ambulatory care nursing quality indicators and ambulatory nursing outcomes. Examples of ambulatory nursing quality indicators include appropriate services, client satisfaction, risk reduction, level of functioning, symptom severity protective factors in the client's environment, and strength of the therapeutic alliance. Seven common ambulatory care nursing outcomes are (1) vital signs' status, (2) knowledge: health promotion, (3) medication response, (4) physical aging status, (5) health-seeking behavior, (6) acceptance: health status, and (7) compliance behavior. The Nursing Outcomes Classification is

Ambulatory Professional Nurse **Current Clinical Practice** Core Role Dimensions	Ambulatory Professional Nurse **Future Clinical Practice** Core Role Dimensions
• Enabling operations • Technical procedures • Nursing process • Telephone communication • Advocacy • Teaching • Care coordination • Expert practice within setting	• Enabling operations • Technical procedures • Nursing process • Telephone communication • Advocacy • Client teaching • Care coordination • Expert practice/community outreach
Ambulatory Professional Nurse **Current Quality Improvement and Research** Core Role Dimensions	Ambulatory Professional Nurse **Future Quality Improvement and Research** Core Role Dimensions
• Quality improvement • Research • Continuing education	• Quality improvement • Research • Continuing education

■ **FIGURE 5–4** Current and future ambulatory professional nurse dimensions. *(Data from Haas, S.A., & Hackbarth, D.P. [1995]. Dimensions of the staff nurse role in ambulatory care: Part III: Using research data to design new models of nursing care delivery. Nursing Economic$, 13[4], 230–241; and Hackbarth, D.P., et al. [1995]. Dimensions of the staff nurse role in ambulatory care: Part I: Methodology and analysis of data on current staff nurse practice. Nursing Economic$, 13[2], 89-98.)*

used to define and specify each of these outcomes. Nurse staffing in ambulatory care is one of the factors that contributes to quality of care. Cusack and colleagues have developed a tool to measure client intensity in an ambulatory oncology center. Ultimately this tool can assist in development of staffing models for this setting.

DIMENSIONS UNIQUE TO NURSING PRACTICE IN AMBULATORY CARE

Telehealth Nursing Practice

One dimension of the professional nurse's role that is unique in ambulatory care settings is telephone communication, or telehealth nursing practice. Telehealth nursing is defined as "the delivery, management, and coordination of care and services provided via telecommunications technology within the domain of nursing. Telehealth nursing encompasses all types of nursing care and services delivered across distance." Criteria for telehealth nursing practice include the following:

- Using protocols, algorithms, or guidelines to assess and address client needs systematically
- Prioritizing the urgency of client needs
- Developing a collaborative plan of care with clients and their support systems; the plan of care may include wellness promotion, prevention education, care counseling, disease state management, and care coordination
- Evaluating outcomes of practice and care

Telehealth nursing practice is not new and has been described in the literature since the 1960s. Communication by telephone for health guidance is common in pediatric practices, obstetrics and gynecology practices, primary care practices, and EDs. Clients often call ambulatory care settings to report manifestations of illness and to seek advice. A 2004 document published by the AACN identifies standards that define the responsibilities of both clinical nurses and managers when providing care via the telephone.

The *Nursing Intervention Classification* (NIC) lists four telephone nursing interventions:

- Telephone consultation
- Telephone follow-up
- Telephone triage
- Telephone surveillance

Each of these interventions was proposed by Haas and Androwich in 1999:

1. With *telephone consultation,* the nurse assesses the client's need and readiness to learn, teaches clients, and provides advice based on protocols approved for use with telephone nursing practice. Assessing a client by telephone is far more difficult for the nurse than a face-to-face meeting with a client. The nurse must have expert communication skills to elicit information when no visual or physical assessment cues are available. The nurse must listen for nuances in the client's communication, such as inflection, pitch, volume, and rate of speech. The telephone encounter time is limited. There is no time to reflect or have second thoughts. Although telephone assessment has some pitfalls, there are some benefits, too.

2. *Telephone follow-up* is used for clients who have had ambulatory surgery or complex treatments. The nurse calls the client within a specified period to assess how well the client is recovering and to provide guidance for any problems. Especially when the nurse is calling the client, the nurse must protect the confidentiality of the client and should speak with family members or significant others only if the client has given permission. Many clients appreciate telephone follow-up. Follow-up denotes caring and concern on the part of the nurse and the ambulatory care organization, and it gives the client ready access to a health professional.

3. With *telephone triage,* clients are sorted by telephone encounter based on the immediacy of the need and the type of problem. In ambulatory care, a nurse talks with a client calling from home and assesses the type of problem, how the problem should be resolved, whether the client should be seen in person, and when and who should resolve the problem.

4. Nurses use *telephone surveillance* to work with data coming into a central ambulatory site from monitoring equipment used by clients at home. For example, cardiac monitoring or high-risk obstetric monitoring can be accomplished by connecting the monitoring equipment to a computer or telephone in the client's home.

Telephone triage and telephone consultation by nurses have increased with the growth of managed care health insurance plans. Nurses use commercially available protocols or protocols that have been developed by physicians and nurses in their own ambulatory care organization to assess the client over the telephone and to recommend approved interventions. Nurse telephone consultation and telephone triage have some advantages. They make nurses and expert health advice readily available, they may save a trip to the ambulatory care site, and, for many clients, they provide a knowledgeable and caring person to ask about a problem.

Professional nurses have stated strongly that telehealth nursing practice should be part of the professional nurse's role. It should not be done by licensed practical nurses (LPNs) or assistive personnel such as receptionists or schedulers. It requires critical thinking and judgment as well as assessment and evaluation skills. Nurses need to attend educational programs designed to help them develop the knowledge and skills necessary to practice these techniques effectively. Every telephone encounter should be documented on the client's medical record, including assessment data, analysis, recommendations made to the client, and the client's level of understanding of instructions (e.g., when to come in or to call back).

Expert Practice Within the Setting

Another unique dimension of the current clinical nurse's role in ambulatory care is expert practice within the setting. Ambulatory care nurses who develop expertise with specific client populations often are in charge of nurse-run clinics such as incontinence clinics, Coumadin clinics, or wound care clinics. In a nurse-run clinic, a nurse with at least a bachelor's degree in nursing, plus experience and continuing education, works with physicians to develop protocols. Nurses monitor clients during ambulatory visits and suggest interventions for common problems that clients experience.

Nurses and clients express high levels of satisfaction with nurse-run ambulatory programs. Clients can call a nurse who knows them and their problems and who has insight into their problems. The nurse often acts as their advocate in the health care system. Nurses find this type of work rewarding because they have long-term relationships with clients and families and can see the results of their teaching, advocacy, and nursing interventions.

Ambulatory Care Interdisciplinary Team

Nurses working in ambulatory settings are members of an interdisciplinary team. They work collaboratively with physicians; midlevel providers, such as nurse practitioners (NPs), nurse-midwives, and physician assistants (PAs); LPNs and licensed vocational nurses (LVN); medical assistants (MAs); nurse assistants (NAs); and clerks, receptionists, and schedulers.

The challenges in working with a large team are numerous. Roles often are blurred, especially when people have worked together in the same clinic for many years. Sometimes team members may be asked to perform beyond their legal scope of practice; at other times, nurses may do assistive or clerical work. Both situations can prevent clients from receiving care from the best prepared provider. Nurses must continually negotiate and advocate for clients within and beyond the team.

Nurses must also delegate appropriately to assistive workers. Nurses must be aware of the specifications of their state Nurse Practice Act and delegate to LPNs and LVNs only what is legally within their scope of practice. For example, MAs in some states may administer immunizations when they have the requisite training and when they are supervised by licensed professional nurses or physicians; in other states, this might be illegal.

Supervision in ambulatory care is challenging. State Nurse Practice Acts often legally define both the delegation and the supervision to be done by professional nurses.

Professional and Legal Considerations
Standards of Care

Standards are written authoritative statements developed and disseminated by a professional organizational or governmental or regulatory agency by which the quality of practice, services, research, or education can be judged. In 1987 the AACN developed *Ambulatory Care Nursing Administration and Practice Standards.* These are revised and updated periodically, most recently in 2004. There are nine standards: structure and organization of ambulatory care nursing, staffing, competency, ambulatory nursing practice, continuity of care, ethics and patient's rights, environment, research, and performance improvement. AACN also developed and published the *Telehealth Nursing Practice Administration and Practice Standards* in 1997 and the revised update *AACN Telehealth Nursing Practice Administration and Practice Standards* in 2004. The American Nurses' Association also published *Core Principles on Telehealth* in 1998.

Ambulatory care nurses are also guided by other sets of standards. To provide services, an ambulatory care setting must be in compliance with its state's department of health rules and regulations and must operate in compliance with Occupational Safety and Health Administration (OSHA) standards. Evidence-based practice guidelines are available through the Agency for Healthcare Research and Quality, which has guidelines for many common health problems such as chronic pain, incontinence care, depression, and sickle cell anemia. These are available at the website www.ahrq.gov. Professional nursing organizations, such as the American Nurses' Association and Oncology Nurses Society, also have specific client population standards.

Competence

Competence is the "demonstrated knowledge, skills, and ability to effectively carry out the requirements of a given role. Nurse competence is circumscribed by the individual nurse's education, knowledge, certification, experience and abilities." Ambulatory care nurses demonstrate competence in core clinical practice dimensions, such as client teaching. They also have competencies that reflect the unique clinical dimensions of ambulatory care nursing, such as telehealth nursing, and that correspond to the needs of the particular client populations served and the nursing interventions commonly required by such populations. For example, ambulatory oncology clients are a specific population for whom competence with chemotherapy administration is a requisite nursing intervention competence. Ambulatory care nurses who work in smaller ambulatory settings may also be required to exhibit competencies in dimensions within the leadership role, such as regulatory compliance and risk management. Any nurse who works with assistive personnel must be competent in delegation and supervision.

Certification

Holding certification in a specialty practice area such as ambulatory care nursing is a way of demonstrating competence to consumers and colleagues. To obtain certification, practicing nurses prepare for and take an examination that is developed by a panel of experts and administered by a recognized certification agency. With increasing numbers of nurses practicing in ambulatory care and the evolution of the Ambulatory Care Nursing Conceptual Framework, the AACN and the American Nurses' Credentialing Center service have developed a certification examination for nurses working in staff nursing positions in ambulatory care. The examination was administered for the first time in the fall of 1999.

To qualify for the examination, ambulatory care nurses must meet the requirement for hours of experience in ambulatory care nursing. To maintain certification, ambulatory nurses must continue to practice in the clinical area for the specified number of hours per year and accumulate a specified number of hours of sanctioned continuing education. Ambulatory care nurses are often certified in more than one area of specialty nursing practice. A nurse working with oncology clients might be certified in oncology nursing as well as ambulatory care nursing. AACN has led the development of the Core Curriculum for Ambulatory Care Nursing, and ambulatory certification. The AACN website address is www.inurse.com.

Regulatory Compliance

Ambulatory settings must be licensed in the state in which they are located; they may earn and maintain credentials, such as accreditation by a national association like The Joint Commission (TJC). Accreditation offers the opportunity for an organization to be evaluated by an external group that assesses the quality of care provided. Accreditation demonstrates compliance with a uniform set of standards; it allows comparisons with other organizations and enhances the organization's competitive edge.

All accreditation organizations use standards developed by the accreditation organization and on-site surveys done by teams of experts. Three major accreditation agencies publish standards and offer external validation of quality of care for ambulatory care organizations:

1. TJC serves hospital-affiliated ambulatory care organizations as well as freestanding ambulatory care settings.
2. The National Committee for Quality Assurance serves managed care organizations and uses the Health Plan Employer Data and Information Set report cards.

3. The Accreditation Association for Ambulatory Health Care serves freestanding ambulatory surgery centers, medical group practices, student health centers, and office-based surgeons' practices.

Regulatory agencies are very concerned about client and provider safety. TJC has just promulgated client safety goals for ambulatory care. They are as follows: improve accuracy of client identification, improve effectiveness of communication among caregivers, improve the safety of using medications, reduce the risk of health care associated infections, accurately and completely reconcile medications across the continuum of care, and reduce the risk of surgical fires.

Nursing-sensitive quality performance measures provide means by which quality of care can be judged. The National Quality Forum (NQF) has 10 priority areas for standardized performance measures in ambulatory care. These ambulatory performance areas are the following: client experience with care, coordination of care, asthma, prevention, medication management, heart disease, diabetes, hypertension, depression, and obesity. These measures are significantly different from the acute care NQF measures. Large employer groups, such as the Leapfrog Group, are also working with the health care industry to improve safety and client outcomes.

Multi-State Licensure

Multi-state licensure is an issue that has emerged because (1) there are increasing numbers of national health care systems, (2) telehealth nursing practice is more common, and (3) people are more mobile in seeking care. The legal authority for practice is a concern for any professional nurse who provides care for people located in a state in which the nurse is not licensed. Examples of nurses who must be concerned about multi-state licensure are (1) nurses working in integrated delivery systems and regional referral health care systems in which people come for care from other states, (2) flight nurses, and (3) telehealth practice nurses. If a nurse cares for a client by telephone, computer, or monitoring device and the client is located in a state where the nurse is not licensed, the nurse faces the risk of being cited for practicing without a license in the client's home state.

The *Mutual Recognition Model,* implemented through a *Nurse Licensure Compact* (NLC), has been recognized as the preferred model of nurse licensure. The National Council of State Boards of Nursing (NCSBN) has been working to educate nurses about the NLC. Information is available on their website at www.ncsbn.org. The NLC is a legal document that must be adopted by each state legislature. After adoption, nurses obtain a license in their state of residency but are able to communicate with clients in other states without violating the Nurse Practice Act in the client's home state if that state has also passed NLC legislation. The advantages of the NLC or "the one license concept" are reduced barriers to interstate practice, improved tracking for disciplinary purposes, cost-effectiveness, unduplicated counts of nurses, maintenance of a state-based system of licensure, and expanded consumer access to qualified nurses. Only a few states (19) have adopted the NLC thus far. It may be several years before all states adopt the NLC. Until all states have adopted the NLC, nurses need to be aware of the implications of practicing across state lines.

TRENDS AND DIRECTIONS FOR THE FUTURE

Demographic and socioeconomic trends in the United States are expected to continue to challenge ambulatory care nurses.

Among these challenges are (1) rapid changes in technology, (2) increased emphasis on demonstrated outcomes, (3) aging of the population as well as increasing longevity with increasing numbers of chronic diseases, (4) reduced revenue to health care organizations from state, federal, and managed care contracts, (5) the large number of uninsured people, (6) escalating concerns about safety in health care, and (7) the growing shortage of nurses. A unified system ensuring access to health care for all Americans does not seem imminent. As the electronic health record (EHR) becomes integrated into ambulatory care, ambulatory care nurses need to become expert with documentation on the EHR and the use of evidence-based practice to enhance client outcomes and safety in ambulatory care.

Many believe, however, that the nation is experiencing a fundamental shift in emphasis on the concept of health itself, with the focus changing from the old clinical model to a wellness orientation. According to Shi and Singh, health care is changing (1) from an *illness* orientation to a *wellness* orientation; (2) from an *acute* care emphasis to *primary* care; (3) from *inpatient* to *outpatient* services; (4) from *individual* health to *community* well-being; (5) from *fragmented* care to *managed* care; (6) from *independent* institutions to *integrated* systems; and (7) from service *duplication* to a *continuum* of services. If these predictions are correct, the well-educated ambulatory care nurse will be at the forefront of the health care delivery system in this new millennium.

CONCLUSIONS

Ambulatory care nursing is one of the fastest-growing areas of nursing specialty practice. Ambulatory care nurses are not only expert clinicians but also expert communicators. They play key roles in facilitating the client's successful

progress through the integrated delivery systems. Ambulatory nurses make quality health care accessible.

BIBLIOGRAPHY

 Citations appearing in red refer to primary research.

1. American Academy of Ambulatory Care Nursing. (2004). *Ambulatory care nursing administration and practice standards* (6th ed.). Pitman, NJ: Anthony J. Jannetti, Inc.
2. American Academy of Ambulatory Care Nursing. (2001). AACN Telehealth nursing practice definition. *AACN Viewpoint, 24*(4), 10.
3. American Academy of Ambulatory Care Nursing. (2004). *Telehealth nursing practice administration and practice standards* (3rd ed.). Pitman, NJ: Anthony J. Jannetti, Inc.
4. American Academy of Ambulatory Care Nursing and American Nurses' Association. (1997). *Nursing in ambulatory care: The future is here.* Washington, DC: American Nurses Publishing.
5. American Nurses' Association. (1998). *Core principles on telehealth.* Washington, DC: American Nurses Publishing.
6. Androwich, I., & Haas, S. (2006). Integrating evidence into the electronic health record. *AACN Viewpoint, 28*(5), 12-14.
7. Baker Laughlin, C. (2006). *Core curriculum for ambulatory care nursing* (2nd ed.). Pitman, NJ: Anthony J. Jannetti, Inc.
8. Bodenheimer, T., & Grumbach, K. (2004). *Understanding health policy: A clinical approach* (4th ed.). New York: Lange Medical Books/McGraw Hill.
9. Cusack, G., Jones-Wells, A., & Chisholm, L. (2004). Patient intensity in an ambulatory oncology research center: A step forward for the field of ambulatory care—Part III. *Nursing Economic$, 22*(4), 193-195.
10. Cusack, G., Jones-Wells, A., & Chisholm, L. (2004). Patient intensity in an ambulatory, oncology research center: A step forward for the field of ambulatory care. *Nursing Economic$, 22*(2), 58-63.
11. Enthoven, A. (1993). The history and principles of managed competition. *Health Affairs* (Suppl), 24-28.
12. Ginzberg, E. (1994). *The road to reform.* New York: The Free Press.
13. Haas, S. (1998). Ambulatory care nursing conceptual framework. *AACN Viewpoint, 20*(3), 16-17.
14. Haas, S., & Androwich, I. (1999). Telephone consultation. In G. Bulecheck & J. McCloskey (Eds.), *Nursing interventions: Effective nursing treatments.* Philadelphia: Saunders.
15. Haas, S., & Gold, C. (1997). Perspectives in ambulatory care: Supervision of unlicensed assistive workers in ambulatory settings. *Nursing Economic$, 15*(1), 57-59.
16. Haas, S.A., & Hackbarth, D.P. (1995). Dimensions of the staff nurse role in ambulatory care: Part III: Using research data to design new models of nursing care delivery. *Nursing Economic$, 13*(4), 230-241.
17. Haas, S.A., & Hackbarth, D.P. (1995). Dimensions of the staff nurse role in ambulatory care: Part IV: Developing nursing intensity measures, standards, clinical ladders, and QI programs. *Nursing Economic$, 13*(5), 285-294.
18. Haas, S.A., & Hackbarth, D.P. (1997). The role of the nurse manager in ambulatory care: Results of a national survey. *Nursing Economic$, 15*(4), 191-203.
19. Haas, S.A. (1995). Dimensions of the staff nurse role in ambulatory care: Part II: Comparison of role dimensions in four ambulatory settings. *Nursing Economic$, 13*(3), 152-165.
20. Hackbarth, D. (1995). Institute of Medicine revised definition of ambulatory care. *AACN Viewpoint, 17*(4), 1-4.
21. Hackbarth, D.P. (1995). Dimensions of the staff nurse role in ambulatory care: Part I: Methodology and analysis of data on current staff nurse practice. *Nursing Economic$, 13*(2), 89-98.
22. Hing, E., Cherry, D.K., & Woodwell, D.A. (2006). National ambulatory medical care survey: 2004 summary. *Advanced data from vital and health statistics* (No. 374). Hyattsville, Md: National Center for Health Statistics.
23. Hooks, M., Dewitz-Arnold, D., & Westbrook, L. (1980). The role of the professional nurse in the ambulatory care setting. *Nursing Administration Quarterly, 4*(4), 12-17.
24. Institute of Medicine. (1994). *Defining primary care: An interim report.* Committee on the future of primary care. Washington, DC: National Academy Press.

25. Institute of Medicine. (1978). Primary care medicine: A definition. In *A manpower policy for primary health care: Report of a study*. Washington, DC: National Academies Press.

26. Joint Commission on Accreditation of Healthcare Organizations. (2005). JCAHO announces 2006 patient safety goals for ambulatory care facilities. *AACN Viewpoint, 27*(4), 11-12.

27. Jones, A., Cusack, G., & Chisholm, L. (2004). Patient intensity in an ambulatory oncology research center: A step forward for the field of ambulatory care—Part II. *Nursing Economic$, 22*(3), 120-123.

28. Kovner, A.R., & Jonas, S. (2005). *Health care delivery in the United States* (8th ed.). New York: Springer.

29. Lang, N., & Kizer, K. (2005). Nursing sensitive quality performance measures: A key to health care improvement? *AACN Viewpoint, 27*(2), 1, 8-10.

30. Leavell, H.R., & Clark, E. (1965). *Preventive medicine for the doctor in his community: An epidemiologic approach*. New York: McGraw-Hill.

31. McCaig, L.F., & Nawar, E.W. (2006). National hospital ambulatory medical care survey: 2004 emergency department summary. *Advance data from vital and health statistics* (No. 372). Hyattsville, Md: National Center for Health Statistics.

32. Mastel, P. (2001). Ambulatory nursing outcomes. *AACN Viewpoint, 23*(4), 6-7.

33. Mastel, P. (2000). Report cards: Proving the value of ambulatory care nursing. *AACN Viewpoint, 22*(6), 16-22.

34. McKeown, T. (1978). Determinants of health. *Human Nature, 1*(4), 60-67.

35. Middleton, K.R., & Hing, E. (2006). National hospital ambulatory medical care survey: 2004 outpatient department summary. *Advanced data from vital and health statistics* (No. 373). Hyattsville, Md: National Center for Health Statistics.

36. Shi, L., & Singh, D.A. (2003). *Delivering health care in America: A systems approach* (3rd ed.). Gaithersburg, Md: Aspen.

37. Smith, J. (1983). *The idea of health: Implications for the nursing professional*. New York: Teachers College Press.

38. Starfield, B. (1992). *Primary care: Concept, evaluation and policy*. New York: Oxford University Press.

39. Starr, P. (1982). *The social transformation of American medicine*. Cambridge, Mass: Basic Books.

40. Swan, B.A. (2001). Ambulatory care nursing quality indicators: AACN pilot survey. *AACN Viewpoint, 23*(2), 6-10.

41. Swan, B.A. (2005). Standardizing ambulatory care performance measures: A National Quality Forum (NQF) project. *AACN Viewpoint, 27*(2), 9.

42. Tighe, M.G., (1985). A study of the oncology nurse role in ambulatory care. *Oncology Nursing Forum, 12*(6), 23-27.

43. U.S. Department of Health and Human Services. (2000). With understanding and improving health and objectives for improving health, 2 vols. In *Healthy People 2010* (2nd ed.). Washington, DC: U.S. Government Printing Office.

44. Verran, J.A. (1981). Delineation of ambulatory care nursing practice. *Journal of Ambulatory Care Management, 4*(2), 1-13.

45. World Health Organization. (1978). *Primary health care: Report of the international conference on primary health care. Alma-Ata, USSR*. Geneva: Author.

CHAPTER 6

Acute Health Care

MARY ELLEN PIKE

If you talk with a nurse who has worked in a hospital setting for the past 15 to 20 years, you are likely to hear about how drastically hospitals have changed. It is true. Today, hospitalized clients are sicker than they were years ago, in part because of advances in health care technology that have enabled them to survive disease and serious medical conditions longer. In the past, the nurse's caseload included clients who were nearly well. Today, clients who are not acutely ill are discharged from the hospital and treated in outpatient settings and by their families, significant others, or home health nurses at home. Therefore the caseload for hospital nurses today consists of seriously ill clients. This chapter discusses the many reasons for this change and addresses what it is like to work in a hospital today.

HISTORY OF HOSPITAL NURSING

At the beginning of the twentieth century, most nurses were employed by affluent clients in the client's home. Nurses worked on a fee-for-service basis and were paid by the client or the client's family. A nurse worked with only one client all day long. This early form of nursing care was called *private duty nursing*. Private duty nurses provided physical, psychological, and social care. Hospitals cared for the poor and those with communicable diseases but they were undesirable places to work. Clients were hospitalized so that society was protected from them.

During the Great Depression, even wealthy families did not have the money to pay for private duty nursing so nurses were forced to work in hospitals. Frequently they worked only for room and board rather than for a salary. The Blue Cross plan, developed in 1929, offered a form of prepaid insurance to help people pay their hospital bills. During the 1930s and 1940s, more and more people purchased such insurance to protect themselves against hospital costs. The fact that hospitals could be assured of payment put them on firmer financial footing,

and the demand for hospital-based nurses increased dramatically. World War II, wars in Korea and Vietnam, and the space program fostered advances in technology that led to the development of emergency medical services and critical care units that vastly improved client care.

Private insurance and government entitlement programs, such as Medicare and Medicaid, established in 1965, allowed clients to receive care without regard to cost. The need for nurses continued to rise and resulted in a cycle of nursing shortages every few years. The high demand for hospital care lasted until the early 1980s.

In the 1970s and 1980s, the cost of hospital care soared. Insurance companies and employers who covered health insurance premiums demanded government intervention to stem the rise in costs. In 1983 a new prospective payment system based on diagnosis-related groups (DRGs) emerged. Hospitals received monies for reimbursement based on the client's diagnosis. For example, if the client required fewer days in the hospital than the DRG allowed, the hospital made money. If the client required more days, the hospital lost money. This incentive resulted in hospitals attempting to decrease the length of stay (LOS) for every client, often to the detriment of the client. The home health care industry rapidly expanded as a result of this change in payment.

The *Balanced Budget Acts* of 1997 and 1999 emphasized cost containment and produced radical changes in hospital care. Hospitals changed from a client-driven, fee-for-service system to a payer-driven, capitated, managed

---

evolve **Web Enhancements**

Ethical Issues in Nursing Is Whistle Blowing Ever the Right Thing to Do?

Appendix A Religious Beliefs and Practices Affecting Health Care

Be sure to check out the bonus material on the Evolve website and the CD-ROM, including free self-assessment exercises. **http://evolve.elsevier.com/Black/medsurg**

care system. Physicians, subjected to utilization reviews, unhappily found third-party payers in control of hospital costs. As a consequence of cost containment, hundreds of hospitals closed. Some hospitals merged with others to form a health care "system" in efforts to reduce costs, combine services, and attract third-party payment contracts.

ACUTE CARE HOSPITALS

According to the American Hospital Association, hospitals are licensed institutions with at least six beds whose primary function is to provide diagnostic and therapeutic client services for medical conditions by an organized physician staff, and have continuous nursing services under the supervision of registered nurses. Acute care hospitals are distinguished from long-term care facilities such as nursing homes, rehabilitation centers, and psychiatric hospitals by the fact that the average client stay is less than 30 days. Such hospitals are one of several types: government, voluntary/not-for-profit, for-profit, and specialty.

TYPES OF HOSPITALS

Government-Sponsored Hospitals

Hospitals sponsored by the government receive local, state, or federal government support. Examples include the Army, Navy, Veterans Affairs, Public Health Service, and Department of Justice prison hospitals. State-supported facilities include psychiatric hospitals, state university hospitals, and state prison hospitals. Locally supported institutions include county and city hospitals. These institutions may be referred to as community hospitals. Their services are often provided at no cost or a reduced cost to the client. Many of the clients do not have health care benefits. The number of these hospitals has declined over the past 25 years.

Voluntary/Not-for-Profit Health Agencies

Voluntary health agencies are nonprofit, tax-exempt organizations designed to meet the health care needs of the general public. Despite their name, nonprofit organizations must be concerned with their financial status to meet expenses, plan for expansion, and survive economic downturns. Examples include hospitals that are church affiliated, those owned by special-interest groups, and those that treat clients with specific concerns such as cancer or other chronic disorders.

For-Profit Hospitals

For-profit (proprietary) hospitals have the same goal as businesses: to generate profit. Like nonprofit hospitals, they serve the general public. The hospitals are privately owned by large corporations, are parts of chains of hospitals, or are owned by single owners. These hospitals have stockholders. An advantage to the larger chains of hospitals is

that they can purchase medical supplies and equipment in greater volume and therefore at less cost. They may have a slight advantage when contracting for third-party payment because of their ability to reduce costs.

Specialty or Limited-Service Hospitals

Specialty hospitals are frequently owned by physician groups and are often controversial because they typically focus on lucrative services such as orthopedics or cardiac care. Physicians may refer their own clients to the institution and generally find that efficiency is improved in these hospitals. However, specialty hospitals are often accused of admitting the healthiest and wealthiest clients whose insurance has traditionally helped offset the cost of indigent care in hospitals that must provide it. Lost revenues in traditional hospitals could force cutbacks in essential programs such as behavioral health care, outpatient clinics for those with low incomes, health education, and investment in new programs and technology.

Magnet Hospitals

Hospitals may be designated a *magnet hospital*. Magnet status is an award given by the American Nurses' Credentialing Center (ANCC), an affiliate of the American Nurses Association, to hospitals where nursing delivers excellent client outcomes, nurses have a high level of job satisfaction, and there is a low staff nurse turnover rate and appropriate grievance resolution. Magnet status indicates nursing involvement in data collection and decision-making in patient care delivery, value of staff nurses, involvement in shaping research-based nursing practice, and a system that rewards nurses for advancing in nursing practice. Magnet hospitals are supposed to have open communication between nurses and other members of the health care team, and an appropriate personnel mix to attain the best patient outcomes and staff work environment. Such hospitals often provide medical services for complex problems that require a team of health care providers, which would be too expensive to replicate in multiple sites. For example, clients who require organ transplantation or care after a serious injury are commonly cared for in these institutions. The hospitals have a high staff retention rate because of their high morale and good salary and benefit programs.

CLIENT ADMISSIONS

Clients in acute care hospitals include those who are acutely ill; victims of trauma with a potential critical condition; those who need intensive monitoring, complex diagnostic studies, surgery, or complex treatments; and clients who have an exacerbation of a chronic disorder.

Clients can be admitted to a hospital in several ways (Box 6-1). Once admitted, a primary physician (also called the *attending physician*) oversees the client's

BOX 6-1 How Clients Are Admitted to a Hospital

DIRECT

A client is seen in a physician's office, and it is determined that the client needs nursing care and specialized monitoring.

EMERGENCY

A client is seen in the emergency department, and it is determined that the client needs surgery, nursing care, and/or specialized monitoring. The disease that has been diagnosed or is considered likely cannot be managed on an outpatient or self-care basis.

SCHEDULED

A client has elected to undergo surgery or special diagnostic testing that requires specialized monitoring or nursing care during recovery.

care. The clients may then be referred to one or more physician specialists to diagnose and treat problems outside the primary physician's practice area. Some hospitals are now using *hospitalists* to care for clients while they are in the acute care setting. *Hospitalists* are physicians who manage the care of only hospitalized clients, allowing primary physicians and specialists to focus on clients outside the hospital setting.

Acute care is a costly service that relies on technology and the expertise of the health care team to arrive at a diagnosis, initiate treatment, stabilize the condition, and prepare for transition to a less costly level of health care. Although nursing care is the primary reason for hospitalization, many other people are involved directly and indirectly in a client's care (Box 6-2).

BOX 6-2 Personnel and Departments in a Hospital

PROFESSIONAL SERVICES

- *Medical Staff.* Consists of private practice, group practice or academic physicians who have their own offices and use the hospital services for care of specific problems. Also made up of physicians who may work for the hospital in departments such as surgery, laboratory, radiology, and emergency.
- *Nursing Service.* Largest group of client care providers in the hospital. Nurses are employed by the nursing service department and provide client care in the hospital in areas. Nurses also work in areas where no direct client care is given (such as administration and hospital-based education programs).
- *Pharmacy.* Consists of pharmacists and technicians who dispense medications prescribed by physicians. Pharmacy staff also monitor the use of regulated medications, such as narcotics. Many pharmacists also teach clients about their medications.
- *Rehabilitation Services.* Physical therapists treat diseases and injuries by restoring, improving, or maintaining the client's functional ability or status to increase musculoskeletal strength to prevent further problems. Occupational therapists teach clients ways to overcome or reduce the problems in activities of daily living resulting from their disabilities.

SUPPORT SERVICES

- *Administration.* Hospital staff who are accountable for the operation of the entire hospital or institution. May include the hospital president, vice-presidents, and nurse-managers who supervise client care on a given nursing unit.
- *Biomedical Engineering Department.* Maintains the elaborate equipment in the hospital to ensure safe and proper functioning and adherence to government regulations.
- *Business Departments.* Several departments manage the business of the hospital based on both client income and outgoing expenses (salaries, purchasing, operation of the building). The admitting office collects information on insurance and assigns a room to the client. The business office lists all client charges, prepares the hospital bill, submits it to insurance companies, and records payments received. Payroll departments monitor hours worked, disperse salaries to the employees, and keep records. Purchasing departments disperse money for purchase of new supplies.

- *Cardiopulmonary.* Includes the specialties of respiratory therapy and cardiac diagnostics.
- *Central Service/Material Management Department.* Maintains supplies needed for client care. Provides stock supplies of routinely used items on the nursing units. Cleans and resterilizes reusable supplies.
- *Development/Community Relations.* Volunteers and professional staff who often raise funds for various hospital projects (e.g., building projects). May be combined with the marketing department.
- *Dietary.* Prepares food for client and staff daily. Dietitians assess and manage nutritional needs of hospitalized clients.
- *Environmental Services.* Clean the hospital, including client rooms.
- *Information Technology.* Computer support staff is growing in most hospitals because of the increasing use of computers. Staff members focus on design and support mechanisms for electronic data retrieval and storage.
- *Laboratory.* Conducts diagnostic tests to help identify illness. Technicians commonly work in radiology and the various laboratories. Laboratory technicians usually collect blood samples from clients; nurses often collect all other specimens and may collect blood.
- *Laundry.* Launders, sorts, and presses several hundred pounds of linen each day. New linen is delivered to each nursing unit daily. These services may be contracted out ("outsourced") to local providers.
- *Medical Records.* Stores medical records for all clients. If a client is rehospitalized, former medical records are often important in diagnosis of new problems. Also compiles data for retrieval for reimbursement, service trending, and outcomes' research.
- *Human Resources Department.* Hires new employees and concentrates on employee relations. Human resources departments may serve in public relations' roles to inform the hospital staff, clients, media, and public about the hospital and its operations. Public relations' services may also be provided by the marketing department.
- *Volunteer Services.* Operates coffee shops and gift shops, delivers mail to clients, and often raises funds for various hospital projects.

POST–ACUTE CARE

Post–acute care is one of the fastest-growing segments of health care. It is designed to fill the gap between acute care and long-term or home care and is identified by a number of terms, including telemetry, step-down, progressive, self-care, transitional, or intermediate. Not all clients require post–acute care. If clients can provide their own care at home, then discharge to home is appropriate. Even if some nursing care is still required, home health care may be employed to assist the client.

Examples of clients who benefit from post–acute care include those recovering from myocardial infarction (heart attack) or open heart surgery; those who must be weaned from a ventilator; those who need wound management after burn injury or for multiple pressure ulcers; those who require more rehabilitation after stroke or orthopedic surgery; or those who have complex medical conditions such as diabetes or digestive or renal problems.

Post–acute care units in a nursing home or rehabilitation facility include many clients who are Medicare beneficiaries, whose younger counterparts with the same level of disability would receive home care. Chronic post–acute care units manage clients with little hope of ultimate recovery and functional independence. The goal for all clients in post–acute care is to send them home or to a less expensive level of care, such as to long-term care or assisted-living centers. Communication between facilities is essential to promote continuity of care.

EFFICIENCY MEASURES

Much public attention has been focused on hospital performance. Hospitals continuously assess their outcomes and financial health by reviewing cost-benefit and clinical analysis data from their service lines. *Service lines* can be defined as care given to groups of clients with similar problems. For example, care of clients with heart disease or heart surgery would make up one service line. Many communities with two or more hospitals collaborate and then delineate service lines for each institution. For example, one hospital might provide all psychiatric services, another might have a stroke unit, and another could provide rehabilitation services. This is a cost-effective and resource-effective method of providing care because duplication is eliminated. Clinical outcomes are generally improved when the volume of cases increases because the staff members become familiar with typical responses of clients and can detect complications earlier.

As a result of the competition for clients and increased client demands for excellent care, an updated version of the service line developed: the center of excellence. Such centers are established from service lines projected to have a high potential for long-term growth and profitability. Hospitals with centers of excellence appear to increase their market share, improve the quality of client care, and increase earnings.

HOSPITALS AND DISASTER PREPAREDNESS

Hospitals have participated in disaster drills for many years, but the events of 9/11, the anthrax scare, Hurricane Katrina, and the continual threat of global terrorism resulted in disaster preparedness becoming a priority for hospitals. In 2003 the Joint Commission on Accreditation of Healthcare Organizations published, *HealthCare at the Crossroads: Strategies for Creating and Sustaining Community-wide Emergency Preparedness Systems.* It mandated that hospitals develop a cohesive, long-term strategy for disaster preparedness that includes a variety of community agencies working together.

ROLES OF NURSES IN HOSPITALS

Nursing is a service provided both to individual clients and to aggregates of people (e.g., families, groups, communities, populations). Professional nurses assume multiple roles and responsibilities. Although these roles may overlap, they are important to distinguish. Nurses in the acute care hospital setting are providers of direct care, educators, researchers, and managers.

Provider of Direct Care

Most people are familiar with nurses as providers of *direct care.* Nurses assess, care for, educate, and comfort clients and their significant others. Nurses provide direct care in all settings and along all dimensions of the health-illness continuum, from health promotion to critical care and death.

Indirect care consists of processes that support the actual bedside nursing care. Sometimes this level of care is labeled *interdependent.* The nurse interprets physicians orders, administers medication, and provides treatment for the client when performing interdependent care.

Nursing care may be provided by individuals with a variety of backgrounds. Licensed practical nurses (LPNs) and registered nurses (RNs) work together with other health care professionals as well as nurse assistants. Nurses with advanced education such as the masters of science in nursing or doctor of nursing practice may function in the role of clinical nurse leader, clinical specialist, nurse anesthetist, midwife, or nurse practitioner. Nurses holding the doctor of nursing practice degree focus on evidence-based practice to improve clinical care delivery, client outcomes, and systems' management while working with other disciplines.

Through work-redesign and skill-mix reallocation, institutions are focusing goals on achieving efficient client outcomes. *Work redesign* involves studying a job over a fixed period to discover if and how a certain job function might be made more efficient. *Skill mix* is determined by studying the ratio of RNs to LPNs and nurse assistants on a unit. The best skill mix delivers quality care while also controlling costs.

Educator

Professional nurses provide formal and informal education to their clients, individually and in groups. Informal education occurs continually; for example, clients are taught about medications while the medications are being administered or about the importance of assessment parameters when wound care is being done. The importance of informal education should not be underestimated.

Formal education is usually provided to groups of clients and their families. The nurse may use a classroom or bring videotapes, audiotapes, or a laptop computer into the client's room. Advantages of formal education are that the client is usually prepared for learning, significant others are included, and the material presented is consistent from client to client. Many hospitals have formal educators on their staff for clients with complex learning needs. Certified diabetes educators, certified lactation specialists, oncology nurse specialists, and wound ostomy and continence nurses are examples of nurses who teach clients in the hospital and often follow up with clients when they are back in the community.

Finally, some nurses specialize in education and rehabilitation. These nurses often work in cardiac and pulmonary rehabilitation and may have a subspecialty such as exercise physiology. Their role is to assist in the rehabilitation of clients after myocardial infarction, heart failure, chronic obstructive pulmonary disease, or transplantation.

Researcher

The focus on cost containment and quality improvement in hospitals has prompted clinical research to promote evidence-based practice within hospitals. Evidence-based practice is a concept used to improve care to achieve client outcomes. It uses research findings that are grounded in science along with client characteristics to guide clinical practice, thereby preventing practice that is directed by tradition or personal preference and setting the stage for quality client care.

Most nurses would not identify themselves as *researchers,* and yet they are. Most acute care hospitals have a research committee that selects topics for study. Hospital nurses can identify topics to research, help develop and implement a study, collect data, and present and utilize the study's findings. Examples may include skin care or discharge teaching protocols. A master's or doctoral prepared nurse usually directs the study.

Manager

The term *manager* in this discussion means the person who coordinates human and material resources in providing care to clients. *Human resources* include (1) the client, (2) the nurse, (3) the family or significant others, (4) professional colleagues, (5) support groups (e.g., the American Cancer Society), and (6) resource groups (e.g., Vocational Rehabilitation). *Material resources* include equipment and supplies. Time is also an important resource. Finally, outcome is an important consideration in health care management.

The first episode of client management that one encounters as a nurse is providing timely care to one client. Effective time management for one client is difficult at first because of interruptions and lack of familiarity with equipment and procedures. Even while caring for only one client, the nurse must stay on time with assessments, medications, and treatments. Most of these aspects of nursing care are scheduled more than once every 24 hours; if late, the next treatment or medication may need to be delayed. The care of multiple clients becomes more efficient with experience.

NURSING CARE DELIVERY SYSTEMS

How client care is delivered on any nursing unit is very important. Several models are in use today, and each has its advantages and disadvantages.

Functional Nursing

Functional nursing is a system of care that concentrates on duties. It can be seen as an "assembly line" of care. Functional nursing began during World War II when the demand for client care outstripped the supply of nurses. The RN coordinates care for an entire unit or team. Other nurses are assigned to pass medications and perform treatments. Personnel with less training are assigned to provide more basic care (e.g., giving baths, making beds).

An advantage of this system is that care can be provided at a lower cost. Disadvantages are that the client interacts with several people, psychosocial needs are seldom met, and the RN seldom cares directly for the client and must rely on others' assessments of the client's problems. Each member of the working group is highly dependent on the other members. Functional nursing is still commonly used in skilled nursing and long-term care facilities. When there is a shortage of nurses, functional nursing is also considered in other settings.

Team Nursing

In *team nursing,* the RN works with one or more health care personnel to provide care for four or more clients. Team nursing was developed in the 1950s. World War II drew many nurses from hospitals, creating a nursing shortage and necessitating the increased use of unlicensed assistive personnel and LPNs. Team nursing was considered one approach to using people's skills more effectively.

Advantages are that an RN is usually head of the team and generally knows the clients. In addition, the team leader can provide guidance to new or inexperienced nurses and other staff. As in functional nursing, the talents and abilities of each member of the health care team are used. Disadvantages are that (1) it is fairly expensive (because care is fragmented), (2) a lack of delegation skills by RNs may reduce efficiency, and (3) the "team" is often one RN and a nursing assistant (who may be working with more than one team).

Primary Nursing

Primary nursing is a model of care delivery that emerged during the 1980s to meet the increasingly complex needs of clients. The goal is for each client's care to be comprehensive and coordinated, from admission to discharge. Each client is assigned a primary nurse, who is an RN, and that nurse provides care for that client when he or she is working. In addition, associate nurses, who may also be RNs, provide care when the primary nurse is absent.

Advantages are obvious: (1) the client has the same nurse, (2) the client's psychosocial needs can be met, (3) communication with the physician is improved, and (4) the nurse feels autonomous. Disadvantages include (1) the increased cost in hiring a large RN staff and (2) possible role confusion between primary and associate nurses.

Case Management

Case management is a care delivery model that incorporates concepts of continuity and efficiency in addressing both long- and short-term physical, psychological, and social needs of clients. The primary goals of case management are promoting self-care, upgrading the quality of life, and using resources efficiently. Case managers are nurses who coordinate care of a group of clients, monitor the implementation of interdisciplinary care plans, and maintain communication with third-party payers and referral sources.

A key distinction in the nurse's role in the case management system is that it transcends nursing unit and physician service (e.g., cardiology) boundaries. The nurse follows the client through the entire stay in the health care system and back into the community. Case managers must have a thorough knowledge of third-party reimbursement patterns and rules, community resources, and discharge planning techniques. Many hospitals have developed plans called *clinical pathways* or case management plans to direct client care and recovery from predictable problems. Several clinical pathways are presented on the Evolve website along with a discussion of how to use them.

In reality, most acute care hospital units use a combination of nursing care delivery models to provide care to clients. For instance, an oncology unit that has repeat clients may use primary nursing, whereas a large medical-surgical unit might use a team approach; when staffing is low, functional nursing might be used to accommodate the contributions of various care providers.

MANAGEMENT AND DELEGATION

Today, in an effort to control costs, almost all hospitals have hired *unlicensed assistive personnel* (UAP) to provide care. Other than on-the-job training, these personnel receive little formal training. The use of less trained and educated personnel to perform nursing duties can pose a threat to appropriate nurse staffing in hospitals. The use of unlicensed assistive personnel remains despite the inconclusive amount of research demonstrating their effectiveness on client outcomes.

Different terms are used for *nurse extenders* (which may include unlicensed assistive personnel), such as *unit assistants, primary practice partners,* and *client care attendants.* Nurse extenders with more advanced skills might be called *clinical technicians.* Assistive personnel may help with clinical duties, nonclinical duties, or both. Some of the duties that may be delegated include giving baths, taking vital signs, serving food and collecting trays, performing unit-based laboratory tests (e.g., finger sticks for blood glucose level assessment) or 12-lead electrocardiograms (ECGs), and providing skin care.

Nurses need to learn when and how to delegate. For example, the nurse may delegate a bed bath and linen change for a client who is stable and may give the bath herself to an unstable or new client. This text offers many examples of appropriate delegation to unlicensed assistive personnel.

In planning the use of nurse extenders, nurse-managers and their staff must consider many key questions (Box 6-3). Each nurse must make reasonable efforts to determine the competence of UAP's prior to delegating tasks. Care processes that require assessment and evaluation cannot be delegated. Two issues that demand particular attention are (1) the functions that only an RN can perform and (2) the minimum level of RN staffing required to provide safe client care. Nurses may have been taught that only RNs can or should perform certain clinical duties and they may therefore have difficulty delegating them to less qualified personnel. As the pressure mounts to delegate tasks to lower-paid workers, nurses will need to develop managerial skills, especially those of leadership, delegation, and supervision. Nurses will remain professionally accountable for client outcomes whether or no

BOX 6-3   Questions to Consider Before Delegating Assessments or Tasks

- Is the assessment or task limited to a licensed RN or LPN/LVN?
- Is the UAP competent to accept the delegated assessment or task?
- Has there been proper direction and communication about what is expected?
- Is the task simple and direct?
- Can the task be performed according to exact, unchanging directions?
- Is a licensed RN or LPN/LVN available to supervise?
- If the answer is "no" to any of these questions, do not delegate the task.

BOX 6-4   The American Hospital Association (AHA) Advocacy Agenda for 2007

- Ensure that hospitals have the resources they need to provide high quality care and meet their responsibilities to their communities.
- Improve quality of care and patient safety.
- Expand health coverage to as many as possible as soon as possible.
- Make hospitals the employer of choice and prevent efforts to undermine the relationship between hospitals and their employees.
- Improve accountability for tax-exempt status.
- Ensure that a community's essential health care services are not impeded by marketplace inequity.
- Begin a national discussion on what health care should be.

the specific tasks that contribute to those outcomes have been performed by nurses or by nurse extenders. Each nurse must clearly understand what the agency defines as the roles and duties of the RN, LPN, and the various nurse extenders.

ENSURING QUALITY HEALTH CARE DELIVERY

Health care organizations are being pressured by regulatory and accrediting agencies such as the Centers for Medicaid and Medicare Services, the National Quality Forum, the Agency for Healthcare Research and Quality, and The Joint Commission (TJC) to develop quality improvement programs that demonstrate cost-effectiveness. Clients are also demanding quality improvement. Institutions that do not focus on improved standards of care and the transparency of performance and cost will jeopardize relationships with clients, government, insurers, and health care professionals.

The need for quality improvement has spawned a new industry that appraises, collects, and analyzes data on client satisfaction and quality indicators. Salaries of administrators and other employees may be connected to these results. Insurers are also aware of outcomes and pay those who perform well by referring business to them. Excellence may bring financial incentives. The American Hospital Association developed an advocacy agenda with input from hospital leaders throughout the country. It focuses on factors that can directly impact quality of care (Box 6-4).

Safety Outcomes

The Institute of Medicine's landmark document, *To Err Is Human: Building a Safer Health System* detailed safety concerns within hospitals. In addition, increased liability costs forced hospitals to examine their safety practices and to report those outcomes. This resulted in the setting of performance standards, greater transparency in reporting errors, enhanced expectations for client safety, and the goal of safe health care organizations. The passage of *The Patient Safety and Quality Improvement Act of 2005* enabled health care providers to contract voluntarily with certified client safety organizations to help identify and analyze threats to client safety without fear of reprisal.

The Clients' Rights to Quality Care

Clients have an increased awareness of the quality-of-care issue. They are demanding and receiving more information before the initiation of treatments. Increasingly, clients' requests for information about costs, risks, benefits, and alternatives to suggested therapies are being honored. No longer automatically submissive to the suggested care, the client is becoming a participant and partner in health care, with the expectation of receiving quality care from all health care professionals.

Client rights have also reached a new level of importance for the health care consumer. Regulating agencies, insurance carriers, third-party payers, and providers are responding to ensure that these fundamental rights are maintained and that clients receive quality services.

Providing Quality Client Care

Any plan for providing client care involves the following aspects: (1) strategic planning to serve as a guideline for the continued or expanded services provided by the health care agency; (2) budgeting process to assist the institution in studying, spending, and using the information to reduce costs or maintain them at the present rate; (3) performance improvement plan to show the steps taken to improve performance based on monitoring and evaluation of staff performance; (4) risk management input to identify and eliminate potential injuries to staff and clients; (5) utilization review data to explore items such as acuity levels (the degree of severity of illness that affects the amount and complexity of care the client requires), outcomes, and costs and to discover what is and is not effective care; (6) client satisfaction survey results, which gather data from clients at various stages of their stay in the agency (e.g., preprocedure, admission procedure, discharge); (7) input of all health care professionals into client care plans; and (8) census data to plot current and future trends of health care in the organization.

Changes in client population, diagnoses, programs, or staffing that would necessitate changes in the type, level, or amount of care are reviewed on an ongoing basis. Other factors contributing to quality care include the following: (1) the adherence to, monitoring of, and evaluation of care given according to professional standards; (2) The Joint Commission (TJC) and U.S. Department of Health criteria; and (3) input from other regulatory agencies. In addition, clinical pathways, clinical practice guidelines, standards of practice and care, and competence standards serve as models for professional delivery of client care. The Institutes of Health Initiative, *The 5 Million Lives Campaign*, is a national initiative focused on assisting hospitals to reduce errors by implementing research based protocols in client care.

Staffing for Quality Care

Health care institutions use a combination of methods to ensure a staff of caregivers who can deliver quality care to clients. Two methods include (1) the daily collection of census data (a count of the number of clients occupying beds on any given day) and (2) client acuity.

Staff members are assigned or reassigned to units that have the greatest need for their expertise and experience. Staffing adjustments caused by the fluctuation of census data and acuity levels are accomplished by using per diem (daily) staff and other creative measures to ensure safe client care.

Today, service-line leaders and empowered directors and managers are instrumental in adjusting strategies based on the many shifting variables that affect client care. Input from the employees who actually provide care is also helpful in redesigning and improving the quality of care. Because caregivers are directly involved with client care, they can contribute in important ways by reporting problems that can be addressed in a timely fashion. Such input, especially when acted on by management, helps staff members feel valued.

Unfortunately, adequate staffing is not always ensured. RNs remain in short supply. In an attempt to make the most effective use of available nursing staff, *cross-training* has evolved in some hospitals. Whereas in the past nurses typically were assigned to one unit, where they could become familiar with the other personnel and the unit routine, today's hospital nurses may be cross-trained to work effectively in two or more units (e.g., a surgical unit and a cardiac intensive care unit). Nurses are assigned to the unit where they are most needed and may arrive for work not knowing in advance the work assignment for that day. Nurses may also be assigned to similar areas (e.g., orthopedics) but at different hospitals within the larger system as a result of mergers and acquisitions. This new scenario is often stressful for nurses and other staff members.

Client Acuity Systems

To ensure that staffing is adequate, one must understand the acuity of illness for any given group of clients and how much nursing care they will require. Hospitalized clients are classified according to a client acuity system that identifies the needs of the client and the amount and type of nursing care needed to deliver quality care. This information may be used by nurse-managers for staffing, budgeting, and management purposes. For example, a stable comatose client might require a large amount of low-complexity care that could be provided by unlicensed assistive personnel. In contrast, a newly diagnosed diabetic teenager with several personal and family problems may require less time for care, but the care should be provided by an RN.

The type of acuity system used varies among hospitals. Many are designed by health consultants while some institutions develop their own. Examples of tools used include (1) Nursing Intervention Classification (NIC), (2) Nursing Outcomes Classification (NOC), (3) Oulu Patient Classification, and (4) Professional Assessment of Optimal Nursing Care Intensity Level (PAONCIL).

Client Satisfaction Surveys

As in business, health care providers have learned that it is easier to keep customers than to find new ones. Client satisfaction surveys are commonly given to the client on discharge or sent to the client's home shortly after discharge. Clients are often asked about their perception of medical care, nursing care, ancillary care, the environment, and follow-up care.

Sometimes client satisfaction surveys are discounted because of the fact that the client has limited knowledge of what would constitute "reasonable" care. To overcome this feeling of helplessness by the client, some hospitals inform clients of the services they can reasonably expect while hospitalized. For example, clients are told that they can reasonably expect adequate pain management. Then clients are asked to evaluate whether the outcome was met during the stay. This excellent change reminds all health care providers that the client's opinion should always be one indicator of quality of care.

REGULATORY REQUIREMENTS AND ISSUES

Regulatory agencies have the primary goal of enhancing the public's ability to secure adequate health care. Health care agencies are surveyed periodically to ensure that they comply with specific rules and regulations. A survey is an in-depth study of a health care institution (e.g., a hospital or a long-term care facility) according to specific criteria set forth by the regulating agencies involved. All aspects of the institution's services are inspected. Important performance areas include client assessment, medication administration, use of restraints, infection control practices, client and family education, staff training, information management, and organizational performance. After the survey is completed, a report of findings is compiled and the institution is notified of its status. If a criterion is not met satisfactorily, the institution is notified, given time to correct the deficiency, and reevaluated at a later date. Sometimes the reevaluation is unannounced. In extreme situations, when clients are believed to be in imminent danger by staying in the facility, the clients are transferred and the facility is closed.

Public disclosure of survey findings has begun. Hospital surveys completed after 1994 are made available to the public, media sources, insurance companies, third-party payers, clients, and competing institutions. Other health care delivery services function under the same disclosure rules for compliance with regulations of the inspecting agencies.

Regulatory Agencies and Statutes

Several regulatory agencies have statutes that must be met by hospitals. These laws govern hiring and employment, quality controls, and conditions of the work site to reduce hazards. A full description of these laws is beyond the scope of this book; we will look at only a few of them. Employment laws include the equal employment opportunity laws that ensure equal rights in the workplace for racial and ethnic minorities, women, older adults, and the handicapped.

The *Civil Rights Act* of 1964 laid the foundation for equal employment in the United States. The thrust of Title VII of the Civil Rights Act is two-fold: (1) it prohibits discrimination based on factors unrelated to job qualifications, and (2) it promotes employment based on ability and merit. The areas of discrimination specifically mentioned are race, color, religion, gender, and national origin.

In 1967 Congress enacted the *Age Discrimination and Employment Act* (ADEA). Its purpose was to promote the employment of older people based on their ability rather than on their age. In early 1978 the ADEA was amended to increase the protected age to 70 years.

Although people feared that this act would have serious consequences for labor-intensive occupations, such as nursing, many people are opting for earlier retirement and problems have not been reported.

The *Rehabilitation Act of 1973* required all employers with government contracts of more than $25,000 to take affirmative action to recruit, hire, and advance handicapped people who are qualified. In 1990 Congress passed the *Americans With Disabilities Act* to eliminate discrimination against Americans with physical or mental disabilities in the workplace and in social life. Disability is defined as "any physical or mental impairment that limits any major life activity." This includes not only all people with obvious physical disabilities but also those with cancer, diabetes, human immunodeficiency virus (HIV) infection, acquired immunodeficiency syndrome (AIDS), and recovering alcoholics and drug users. The act not only prohibits discrimination but also delineates clear, enforceable standards.

In 1970 the *Occupational Safety and Health Act* (OSHA) became law. It is broadly written legislation that requires a place of employment to be free from recognized hazards and to develop environmental safety laws for the safety of the employees. The Department of Labor enforces this act. Since the inception of OSHA, many companies have contended that the costs of meeting OSHA standards have excessively burdened American business; however, unions have asserted that the federal government has never adequately staffed or funded the Occupational Safety and Health Administration. They have charged that OSHA has been negligent in setting standards for toxic substances, carcinogens, and other disease-producing agents.

More recently, the 1996 *Health Insurance Portability and Accountability Act* (HIPAA) ushered in three major provisions: (1) promoting electronic transmission standards for claims data; (2) regulating the privacy of electronic medical records; and (3) regulating the security of medical data storage and transmission. This law has had a major impact on day to day activities within hospitals, especially in the common forms of verbal communication between health care providers.

Ethical Issues

Ethical issues commonly occur when the nurse is caught between clients, physicians, administrators, and other nurses and feels powerless to change the situation. Ethical distress can lead to negative consequences for everyone involved. Nurses are often called on to assist families in making informed decisions about client care, and they must be familiar with ethical, legal, economic, and emotional factors that affect the family's decision. Ethics committees are found in many hospitals to guide these complex decisions.

Legal Issues

Nurses have more responsibility today than in the past. Expanded roles open the doors to greater legal risk. The nurse's employer is obligated to carry malpractice insurance for employees but every nurse should consider carrying individual malpractice insurance. Nurses should also be familiar with what is covered in the policy.

Proper documentation is crucial to serve as evidence of the quality of nursing care provided. The court often assumes that if something was not noted in a chart, it was not done. Be specific, and document nursing actions taken and the client's response (e.g., pain reduction). If unusual events occur, complete an incident report. The benefit of incident reports is that they allow for analysis of adverse client events. They should not be treated as a punitive activity but rather as a method of promoting quality care and risk management. Errors are examined to determine whether or not the error was due to a system problem (e.g., a faulty electrical outlet that leads to a fire or an improperly mounted side rail that allows a client to fall).

Cultural Issues

In 2004 the Census Bureau noted that if current trends continue, by 2050 there will be no majority race in the United States. Nurses and other health professionals will interact with an increasingly multicultural American society. Such a diverse population requires that nurses be able to recognize differences and be sensitive to those differences in perceptions of health and illness, communication styles, and nontraditional approaches to health care. Culturally competent care in its broadest sense is knowing, explaining, interpreting, and predicting nursing care within the knowledge of the client's cultural and ethnic beliefs and practices, whether the client is well or sick.

The hospital workforce must also confront cultural issues in regard to staffing. *The Sullivan Commission Report* (2004) discusses the lack of diversity within the health care professions and its consequences, including major disparities in the care delivered to those of other cultures.

RISK MANAGEMENT

Risk management is a planned program of loss prevention and liability control. Its purpose is to identify, analyze, and evaluate risks followed by a plan of reducing the frequency of accidents and injuries. The program requires a team of people from all departments in the institution. The risk manager or safety committee administers the program and serves as the liaison between the hospital administration, the risk management committee, and others as well as between insurance representatives, institution attorneys, and others. Risk managers have no typical profile and can be nurses, administrators, lawyers, or former insurance representatives.

> **Nursing personnel are crucial to a successful risk management program. The areas of highest risk in the hospital are (1) medication errors, (2) complications from diagnostic or treatment procedures, (3) falls, (4) pressure ulcers, (5) client or family dissatisfaction, and (6) refusal of treatment or refusal to sign consent for treatment. Medical records and incident reports serve as documents of accountability. Incident reports are used to analyze problems within the five categories and to plan for corrective actions.**

THE FUTURE OF ACUTE CARE HOSPITAL NURSING

Acute care nursing will remain a challenging area in which to practice. Major change will continue in health care delivery and it will be essential that nurses play a primary role to help ensure that quality client care remains a priority. The following are a few of the trends that will influence the delivery of care in hospitals:

- As the acuity of clients in hospitals increases even further, the need for evidence-based research grows, and the mandate for quality with cost containment continues, the need for advanced practice nurses such as clinical nurse leaders, clinical specialists, and nurse practitioners will accelerate.
- Universal health coverage plans such as the one recently implemented in Massachusetts will offer insight into how such coverage will affect clients and hospitals.
- Mounting concern about pandemics will keep disaster preparedness as a top priority. At the same time, however, emergency departments will continue to experience overcapacity because of a lack of staffed critical care beds and inappropriate use of the emergency department to provide primary care.
- Increased technology such as improved imaging, engineered organs, designer drugs and treatments (specific to a particular client), and nanotechnology (e.g., nanobombs that can destroy cancer cells) will improve health care but increase costs.
- The 79 million baby boomers and their aging parents will present an unparalleled demand for greater hospital use and an increased complexity of care. This very likely will necessitate changes in the traditional entitlement programs in order to control costs.
- A growing number of health care workers and clients will be foreign-born. Health care professionals will need to understand how to treat and work effectively with those whose cultural background differs from theirs.

- Government and market pressure should serve as an incentive for less waste and more competitive pricing. Greater transparency in pricing will allow consumers to "shop" for the most competitive prices and highest quality care.
- Hospital systems will be involved in global health initiatives such as those of the Bill and Melinda Gates Foundation that target diseases such as malaria, AIDS, and tuberculosis.
- Public health initiatives (e.g., smoking bans) that target chronic illnesses will increase. Eighty-three percent of health care spending goes to those with chronic disease and nearly 50% of Americans suffer from at least one chronic illness.

CONCLUSIONS

Acute care hospital-based nursing has changed dramatically since its inception. Years ago, clients remained in the hospital until they were well. Today, clients spend a shortened length of stay in acute care. Professional nurses in a variety of roles are the cornerstone of high-quality care during hospitalization.

BIBLIOGRAPHY

 Citations appearing in red refer to primary research.

1. Altman, S.H., Shactman, D., & Eilat, E. (2006, Jan/Feb). Could U.S. hospitals go the way of U.S. airlines? *Health Affairs, 25*(1), 11-21.
2. American Association of Colleges of Nursing. (2004). *AACN position paper: Practice doctorates.* Washington, DC: AACN.
3. American Association of Colleges of Nursing. (2003, summer). *Working paper on the clinical nurse leader.* Washington, DC: AACN.
4. American Society for Healthcare Risk Management. (2006, July-Sept). An overview of the patient safety movement in healthcare. *Plastic Surgical Nursing, 26*(3), 116-120.
5. Boblitz, M.C., & Thompson, J.M. (2005, Oct). Assess the feasibility of developing centers of excellence. Six initial steps. *Healthcare Financial Management, 59*(1), 72-84.
6. Claudio, T.D. (2004, Oct). Questioning workload resources. *Nursing Management, 35*(10), 30-35.
7. Conn, J. (2006, Aug 7). HIPAA, 10 years after. *Modern Healthcare, 36*(31), 26-29.
8. Goals and agenda for strengthening hospitals released. (2005, March). *American Association of Operating Room Nurses Journal, 81*(3), 504.
9. Griffith, J.R., Alexander, J.A., Jelinek, R.C. (2006). Is anybody managing the store? National trends in hospital performance. *Journal of Healthcare Management, 51*(6), 392-406.
10. Guterman, S. (2006, Jan/Feb). Specialty hospitals: A problem or a symptom? *Health Affairs, 25*(1), 95-105.
11. *HealthCare at the crossroads: Strategies for creating and sustaining community-wide emergency preparedness systems.* (2003). Washington, DC: The Joint Commission on Accreditation of Healthcare Organizations.
12. *Health services for broader community put at risk by "Specialty" hospitals: Report.* (2005, Feb 16). Washington, DC: American Hospital Association.
13. Hospital care spending continues to increase. (2005, Oct). *American Association of Operating Room Nurses Journal, 82*(4), 647.
14. Kohn, L., Corrigan, J., & Donaldson, M. (1999). *To err is human: Building a safer health system.* Washington, DC: National Academy Press.
15. Mages, M.E. (2006, July/Aug). Quality-driven healthcare. *Healthcare Executive, 21*(4), 60-62.
16. Melnyk, B., & Fineout-Overholt, E. (2005). *Evidence-based practice in nursing and health care.* Philadelphia: Lippincott Williams & Wilkins.
17. New tool seeks to measure and improve patient safety. (2005, March/April). *Biomedical Instrumentation & Technology, 39*(2), 96-97.
18. Rauhala, A., & Fagerström, L. (2004). Determining optimal nursing intensity: The RAFAELA method. *Journal of Advanced Nursing, 45* (4), 351-359.
19. Saver, C. (2006, Oct). Nursing-today and beyond. *American Nurse Today, 1*(1), 18-25.
20. Scalise, D. (2006, March). Just rewards. *Hospitals & Health Networks, 80*(3), 40-46.
21. Scalise, D. (2006, Aug 7). 30 trends/innovations to watch. *Modern Healthcare*, 58-69.
22. Wall, B.M., Novak, J.C., & Wilkerson, S.A. (2005, Sept). Doctor of nursing practice program development: Reengineering health care. *Journal of Nursing Education, 44*(9), 396-403.

evolve *Did you remember to check out the bonus material on the Evolve website and the CD-ROM, including NCLEX®-Examination Style Review Questions, Open-Book Quizzes, and Chapter Review Audio Podcasts?*

http://evolve.elsevier.com/Black/medsurg

CHAPTER 7

Critical Care

CATHERINE NOSEK

Critical care (intensive care) is the practice of administering immediate and continuous care to clients experiencing actual or potentially life-threatening health disorders. More than 5 million clients are admitted annually to intensive care units in the United States. Common acute or critical disorders necessitating admission to a critical care unit include brain injuries, cardiovascular dysfunctions, pulmonary dysfunction, childbirth complications, infection/sepsis, shock, trauma, endocrine abnormalities, multisystem alterations, and complex surgical procedures (Box 7-1). According to the Society of Critical Care Medicine, the primary admitting diagnoses are, in order of frequency, respiratory failure/insufficiency, postoperative management, ischemic heart disorder, sepsis, and heart failure.

The purpose of this chapter is to provide the reader with a broad overview of concepts related to critical care as well as a description of competencies/characteristics essential for today's critical care nurses. Critical (intensive) care nursing in the 21st century will continue to be an exciting area of nursing practice.

CRITICAL CARE POPULATIONS

Although clients requiring intensive care management range throughout the life span, there are an increasing number of adults 65 years of age and older admitted to critical care. In 2004, 36.3 million older adults or 12.4% of the U.S. population was admitted to critical care. Although 36.7% of non-institutionalized older adults defined their health as very good or excellent, 80% of older adults have at least one chronic condition and 50% reported at least two. Moreover, of all adult hospital beds, more than 50% are filled with clients 65 years of age and older. Projections indicate that as the baby boomer generation ages, there will be a corresponding rise in chronic illness and hospitalizations. A predictable increase in the need for critical care will accompany these changes. Why is this important to the critical care nurse? The aging process is characterized by physiologic changes. These changes, in combination with the prevalence of chronic conditions, contribute to increased morbidity and mortality in critical care units.

CRITICAL CARE IN THE UNITED STATES

The specialties of critical care and critical care nursing have been evolving since the 1950s (Box 7-2). Historically, hospitals used monitoring technology (e.g., telemetry) to develop coronary care units. For example, coronary care units were intended to provide care to those admitted to the hospital with acute myocardial infarction. As advances in modern technology have occurred, client care has become more intense and complex. Few health care environments require as much technology as critical care. Using diagnostic technologies and information systems, the critically ill require continuous or intermittent physiologic monitoring. Information systems provide a central source of entry and storage of client history and laboratory and diagnostic testing results. Successful clinical decision making depends on the integration of data on multiple levels, as well coordinated efforts among all members of the health care team.

During the care of clients, the nurse must organize data from the medical history, physiologic monitoring, medications, and other information sources such as

evolve **Web Enhancements**

Boxes Critical Care Family Needs Inventory

Appendix A Religious Beliefs and Practices Affecting Health Care

Be sure to check out the bonus material on the Evolve website and the CD-ROM, including free self-assessment exercises. **http://evolve.elsevier. com/Black/medsurg**

BOX 7-1 Common Disorders in Intensive Care

BRAIN INJURIES
- Hemorrhage
- Stroke
- Craniotomy
- Intracranial hypertension
- Cerebral trauma/edema

PULMONARY DYSFUNCTION
- Acute respiratory failure
- Acute lung injury
- Pneumonia
- Pulmonary embolism
- Status asthmaticus
- Air leak disorders
- Thoracic surgery
- Mechanical ventilation

CARDIOVASCULAR DYSFUNCTION
- Hypotension
- Acute coronary syndromes
- Dysrhythmias
- Cardiac surgery
- Vascular surgery
- Heart failure

CHILDBIRTH COMPLICATIONS
- Premature rupture of membranes
- Hypertensive crisis
- Severe hemorrhage
- Disseminated intravascular coagulation
- Renal failure

ENDOCRINE DISORDERS
- Diabetic ketoacidosis
- Hyperglycemic/hyperosmolar state
- Diabetes insipidus
- Syndrome of inappropriate antidiuretic hormone
- Thyroid storm

MULTISYSTEM ALTERATIONS
- Shock
- Systemic inflammatory response syndrome
- Multiple organ dysfunction syndrome
- Burns
- Organ donation and transplantation
- Trauma
- Sepsis

BOX 7-2 Special Care Unit Categories

- Medical/Surgical Intensive Care
- Cardiac Intensive Care
- Neonatal Intensive Care (NICU)
- Neonatal Intermediate Care (PICU)
- Burn Care
- Other Special Care
- Other Intensive Care

mechanical ventilation, laboratory testing, and imaging. Today, fully digital client information systems are being developed. Newer intensive care information systems are integrating real-time physiologic, laboratory, and imaging results along with medications and interventions in a monitoring display at the critical care workstation. One example is eICU. An eICU facility would have the capability to link via telemedicine and computer monitors the information systems already present in the hospital critical care unit. As the technology evolves, modern eICU software allows team members to track client vital trends and intervene earlier, before complications might occur. However, regardless of the technology, an essential ingredient to successful client outcomes is coordination among the interdisciplinary critical care team members. Members of the team may include critical care nurses, physicians, intensivists, pharmacists, respiratory therapists, clergy, and social workers. Studies have shown that a 30% reduction in intensive care unit stay can be realized when care is delivered by an intensivist-lead multidisciplinary team as opposed to an attending physician. Nurses are present 24 hours per day, making the critical care nurse an integral part of the team.

So how is critical care organized institutionally in the United States? According to the American Hospital Association Annual 2005 Survey, 283 hospitals exist within the United States. The majority of critical care is provided in hospitals with 100 to 300 beds and the most common critical care unit is a combined medical-surgical specialty. The larger hospitals (>300 beds) typically organize critical care services by intensities of care, and by age or clinical condition. Examples include coronary care, neonatal, pediatric, and surgical units. Hospitals with more than 500 beds often house cardiothoracic, neurosurgical/neurologic, burn, or trauma units. In a 2005 American Hospital Association survey, 6283 hospitals were surveyed regarding service categories provided. Of the hospitals surveyed, 3250 reported 1 or more special care units, 1602 reported none, and 1431 hospitals did not respond (see Box 7-2).

CRITICAL CARE NURSING

The American Association of Critical-Care Nurses (AACN) defines critical care nursing as the specialty that deals with human responses to life-threatening problems. The critically ill client is at high risk for actual or potential life-threatening health difficulties. Entry-level nurses are prepared to function as generalists. Because critical care nurses are required to deal with complex assessment, high-intensity therapies, and interventions, they must possess a specialized body of knowledge and skills. This includes in-depth understanding of pharmacology, pathophysiology, advanced assessment, and biotechnology. Also essential for nurses to function in today's complex health care environment are advanced communication skills, problem-solving skills, and advocacy skills. These skills are essential if they are to provide holistic or humanistic care to clients and their significant others.

In general, the purpose of nursing is to meet the needs of clients and their families and to provide safe transition through the health care system during a time of crisis. Admission to critical care can be viewed as a time of crisis. Critically ill clients often experience disorientation, pain, sleep deprivation, and immobility. They may feel anxiety, isolation, and depression. Nearly everything in the environment is stress producing, including frequent interruptions, personnel and equipment noise, constant light, lack of privacy, and separation from significant others. Lack of sleep and frequent disruptions in sleep patterns further compound client illness. Research has shown that clients in critical care units may spend as much as 50% of their normal sleep time awake. Sleep deprivation may have added undesirable effects on the illness continuum. One such response is impaired immunity and healing ability. The consequence to the client is a decrease in the ability to resist and fight infection. Moreover, critical illness stimulates the stress response, or what is known as the "fight or flight" response of the sympathetic nervous system (Figure 7-1).

Beyond meeting physical needs, the nurse must identify and address the emotional, spiritual, social, and psychological needs of the client. The more compromised the client, the more severe or complex are their needs. One of the most important roles of the nurse during this crisis is that of advocate. In the advocacy role, the nurse is expected to respect and support the basic values, rights, and beliefs of the critically ill client. Box 7-3 further delineates the advocacy role of the critical care nurse. Because each client brings a unique set of characteristics to the illness experience, the nurse must be able to assess key client characteristics. The American Association of Critical-Care Nurses has identified eight such characteristics (needs) (Box 7-4). These characteristics span the health-illness continuum and are influenced by many factors. For example, educational background, resource availability, and cultural background factors influence client and family participation in care. These factors, as well as the client's capacity to make decisions and the client's level of strength during crisis, impact the client's ability to participate in decision making. Depending on the client's situation, the characteristics should be generally assessed by nurses and classified as one of three levels, for example, low, moderate, and high levels.

Families and significant others of the critically ill client also have many stressors and important needs. The impact of critical illness can generate strong emotions including shock, disbelief, denial, anger, despair, guilt, and fear of losing the client. Several studies have examined and identified the needs of family. Family members place great importance on *the need to know*. This need includes an understanding of the expected outcome, and for some family members or significant others the need to be present. The need for accurate and comprehensible information is universal, and this leaves the door open for hope. Family members want to speak with a physician regularly about the condition and prognosis. When possible, they need the same nurse to explain client care, diagnostic testing, unit activities, the equipment, and how they can be involved at the bedside. Unfortunately, research indicates that physicians and nurses tend to underestimate their role in satisfying the needs of family members, especially with respect to providing ongoing information. The Translating Evidence into Practice feature on p. 88 expands on family priorities and their implications for nursing practice.

THE CRITICAL CARE NURSE: THE CONTINUUM OF CARE

Specialized nursing care, once considered the field of critical care nurses, is now being assumed by nurses in progressive care units. Within the United States, there are an estimated 2.4 million employed registered nurses (RNs). Of these nurses, approximately 1.3 million work in hospital settings. In the 2000 RN survey, an estimated 403,000 were critical care nurses. More than 70,000 nurses work in progressive care units. According to AACN, progressive care collectively describes areas of health care including intermediate care, telemetry, transitional care, and step-down units. Many of these environments now utilize technologies and therapies that once were limited to critical care units. Progressive care is, therefore, considered part of the continuum of critical care nursing.

Continuous nursing vigilance is significant to nursing the critically ill and can make a substantial difference in client outcomes. To meet the changing needs of the client, both critical care and progressive care nurses must create an environment that promotes the best health outcomes in a caring, competent manner to ensure positive optimal outcomes for clients and families. The continuum of critical care nursing requires a specific mind-set that uses a specialized body of knowledge and skills. The AACN proposes a model for client care. This model proposes that the needs (characteristics) of clients and families influence and drive the competencies (characteristics) of the nurse (Box 7-5). According to the model, synergy results when the needs and characteristics of a client, nursing unit, or system are matched with a nurse's competencies/characteristics.

Eight essential competencies have been identified for nurses caring for the critically ill (see Box 7-4). These competencies reflect an integration of experience, skill, and knowledge of the nurse. The premise of this model is that optimal outcomes result from the *synergy*

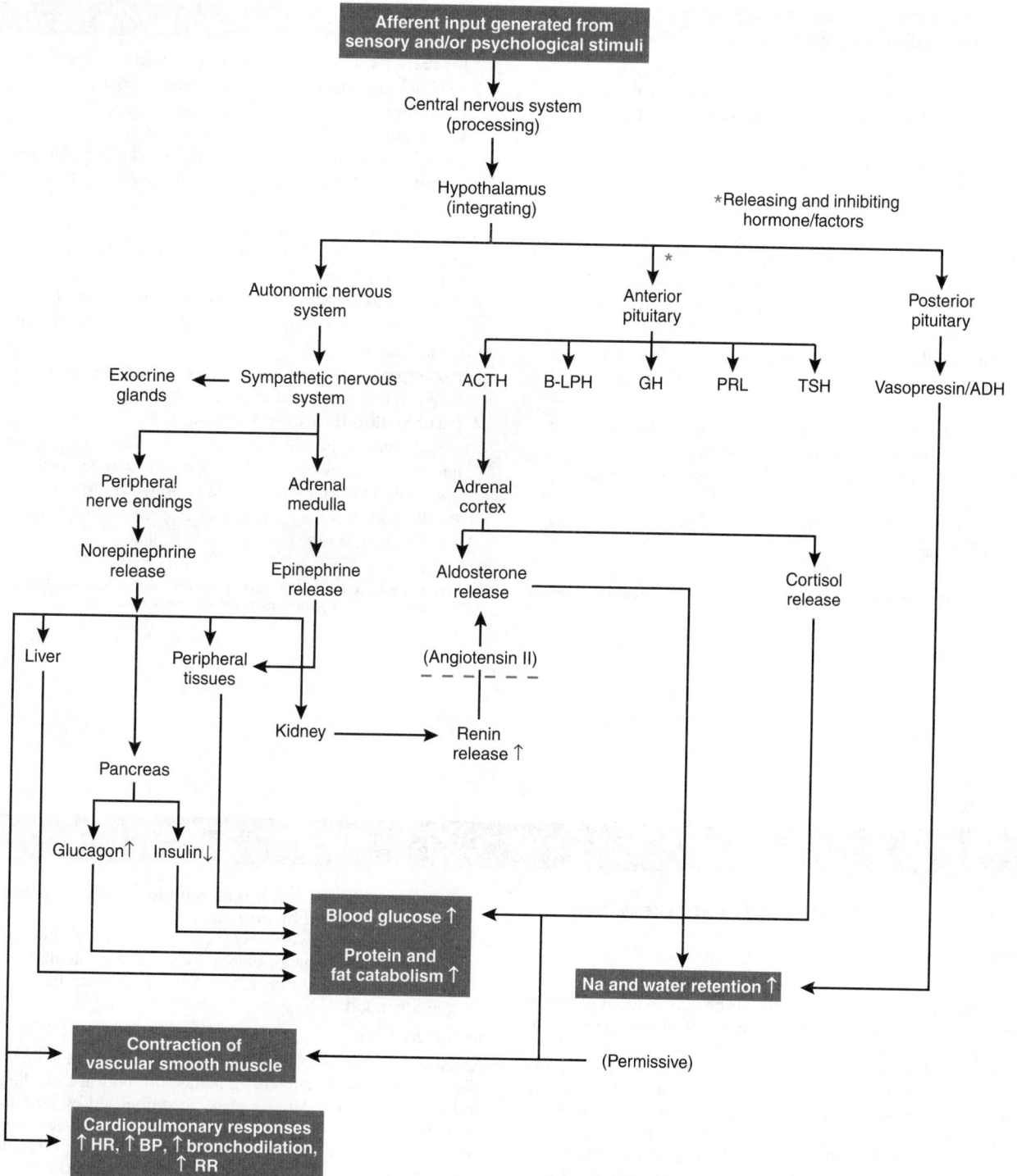

■ **FIGURE 7–1** Systems participating in the stress response. *ACTH,* Adrenocorticotropic hormone; *ADH,* antidiuretic hormone; *B-LPH,* beta-lipoprotein hormone blood pressure; *GH,* growth hormone; *HR,* heart rate; *PRL,* prolactin; *RR,* respiratory rate; *TSH,* thyroid-stimulating hormone. *(Modified from Carrieri-Kohlman, V., West, C.M., & Lindsay, A.M. [2003]. Pathophysiological phenomena in nursing [3rd ed.]. Philadelphia: Saunders.)*

of a nurse's competencies matching the needs of the clients and their families. Linking clinical practice with client outcomes is a critical component of the model. Adopted by AACN, Curley[25] has defined *outcomes* as client conditions measured along a continuum. For more information regarding outcomes refer to the AACN website (www.aacn.org).

EXPERT KNOWLEDGE, CLINICAL JUDGMENT, AND IMPROVING OUTCOMES

There is little doubt that those working with the critically ill require expert knowledge and clinical judgment.

BOX 7-3 AACN's Advocacy Statement

The critical care nurse will do the following:

1. Respect and support the right of the patient or the patient's designated surrogate to autonomous informed decision making.
2. Intervene when the best interest of the patient is in question.
3. Help the patient obtain necessary care.
4. Respect the values, beliefs, and rights of the patient.
5. Provide education and support to help the patient or the patient's designated surrogate make decisions.
6. Represent the patient in accordance with the patient's choices.
7. Support the decisions of the patient or the patient's designated surrogate, or transfer care to an equally qualified critical care nurse.
8. Intercede for patients who cannot speak for themselves in situations that require immediate action.
9. Monitor and safeguard the quality of care the patient receives.
10. Act as liaison between the patient, the patient's family, and health care professionals.

From American Association of Critical-Care Nurses. (2003). Available online at www.aacn.org.

BOX 7-4 Client Characteristics

- **Resiliency** is the client's capacity to return to a restorative level of functioning using a compensatory coping mechanism.
- **Vulnerability** is the level of susceptibility to actual or potential stressors that may adversely affect client outcomes.
- **Stability** refers to the client's ability to maintain a steady state of equilibrium.
- **Complexity** is the intricate entanglement of two or more systems (e.g., physiologic, emotional, family dynamics, environmental).
- **Resource availability** is influenced by the extent of resources brought to the situation by the client, family, and community.
- **Participation in care** is the participation by the client and family in being engaged in the delivery of care.
- **Participation in decision making** is the level of engagement of the client and family in comprehending the information provided by health care providers and acting upon this information to execute informed decisions.
- **Predictability** is the characteristic that allows one to expect a certain course of events or course of illness.

From Hardin, S.R., & Kaplow, R. (2005). *Synergy for clinical excellence: The AACN Synergy Model for patient care*. Boston: Jones & Bartlett.

TRANSLATING EVIDENCE INTO PRACTICE

Family Needs in the Intensive Care Unit

Meeting client and family needs has been a concern of nurses and managers for many years. The study of family needs in the intensive care unit (ICU) has been a research focus for many decades. Molter, a well-known critical care author and practitioner, developed a tool called the Critical Care Family Needs Inventory (CCFNI). This tool has been used by many staff nurses to ensure that nurses meet both the client's and the family's needs while their loved one is in the ICU.[4]

When the issue was first addressed, many thought that nurses' perceptions of family needs would be the same as the client's and the family's perceptions. This indeed was found to be true. In general, the three most important needs consistently identified by clients and families were proximity, assurance, and information. The top nine priorities of critical care families were as follows:[1-4]

1. To be assured that the best care was being given to their family member by caring personnel
2. To feel that there was hope
3. To know the prognosis
4. To understand how the client was being treated medically
5. To be reassured that it is all right to leave for a while
6. To feel accepted by hospital staff
7. To feel someone is concerned for the family's health
8. To feel the hospital personnel care about the client
9. To have explanations given in terms that can be understood

IMPLICATIONS

As shown by this list of priorities, nursing can do much to alleviate many of the stressors that face our critical care clients and family members. Much can be accomplished by listening to clients and their families and by taking time to meet their needs. Nurses have the knowledge base and the opportunities to address and meet almost all of the priorities listed here.

REFERENCES

1. Azoulay, E., et al. (2001). Meeting the needs of the intensive care unit patient families. *American Journal of Respiratory Critical Care Medicine, 13*(1), 135-139.
2. Bijttebier, P., et al. (2001). Needs of the relatives of critical care patients: Perceptions of relatives, physicians and nurses. *Intensive Care Medicine, 27*(1), 160-165.
3. Kosco, M., & Warren, N.A. (2000). Critical care nurses' perceptions of family needs as met. *Critical Care Nursing Quarterly, 23*(2), 60-72.
4. Molter, N.C. (1979). Needs of relatives of critically ill patients: A descriptive study. *Heart & Lung, 8*(2), 332-339.

- **Clinical judgment** is the clinical reasoning used by a health care provider in the delivery of care.
- **Advocacy** is working on another's behalf when the other is not capable of advocating for self.
- **Caring practices** are the constellation of nursing interventions that create a compassionate, supportive, and therapeutic environment for clients and staff, with the aim of promoting comfort and healing and preventing unnecessary suffering. Caring behaviors include vigilance, engagement, compassion, and responsiveness to client and family.
- **Collaboration** is the nurse working with others to promote optimal outcomes.
- **Systems thinking** comprises the tools and knowledge that the nurse uses to recognize the interconnected nature within and across the health care or non-health care system.
- **Response to diversity** is the sensitivity to recognize, appreciate, and incorporate differences into the provision of care.
- **Clinical inquiry** is the ongoing process of questioning and evaluating practice, providing informed practice, and innovating through research and experiential learning.
- **Facilitation of learning** is the promotion of learning for clients, families, nursing staff, physicians, other health care disciplines, and community through both formal and informal methods.

From Hardin, S.R., & Kaplow, R. (2005). *Synergy for clinical excellence: The AACN Synergy Model for patient care*. Jones & Bartlett.

Nurses are expected to draw on an expanding body of increasingly complex information. Today, more than ever before, nurses must know more in order to deliver safe and effective care to meet the unique needs of each client and family. Nurses may validate their knowledge of nursing of critical and progressive care clients through national certification. According to AACN, certification is the process by which a nongovernmental agency validates, based upon predetermined standards, a nurse's knowledge and qualification for practice in a defined functional or clinical area of nursing.

The AACN Certification Corporation supports critical care nurses by administering specialty certification programs. Through rigorous and comprehensive job analysis of current nursing practice, certification examinations measure what is pertinent to the care of critically ill clients today. The certification programs are based on the AACN Synergy Model for Client Care. As discussed previously, client and family needs (characteristics) drive nursing competencies. According to research, everyone in the continuum of care benefits from certified nurses, including clients, family, employers, and nurses. In addition, certification validates to clients and employers that a nurse is qualified, is competent, and has met rigorous requirements to achieve the additional certification. By helping the nurse to achieve and maintain the most up-to-date knowledge, national certification promotes continuing excellence in the nursing profession.

Improving care and improving client outcomes in critical care can also be accomplished by standardizing care through the use of practice guidelines, practice alerts, and protocols. Consistent evidence-based practice guidelines help to reduce errors and improve the quality of the care delivered. Several professional organizations have developed numerous of these resources that enable the critical care team to standardize care. These organizations also provide educational programs, professional publications, scholarship and grant money, research opportunities, Internet resources, and practitioner support. The Society of Critical Care Medicine and the American Association of Critical-Care Nurses are considered the "official" professional organizations that speak on behalf of critical care.

CONCLUSIONS

Critical care nursing occurs in a variety of settings. Health care will be pressed to provide efficient and cost-effective services. Government subsidies of health care may not be able to keep up with the demand. A growing shortage of nurses in the next several years will challenge our health care institutions. Aging nurses are retiring or leaving critical care. Young or new nurses must step up to meet the exciting challenges of critical care nursing. Despite all the challenges of the future, the center of all health care will still be the client, and the critical care nurse will be there at the client's side.

BIBLIOGRAPHY

 Citations appearing in red refer to primary research.

1. Administration of Aging. (March 2006). *A statistical profile of older Americans aged 65+, U.S.* Department of Health and Human Services. Retrieved 03/21/07 from www.aoa.gov/prof/Statistics/statistics.asp.
2. Administration of Aging. (2005). *A profile of older Americans: 2005,* U.S. Department of Health and Human Services. Retrieved 03/20/07 from www.aoa.gov/prof/Statitics/statistics.asp.
3. American Association of Critical-Care Nurses. (2007). *General information regarding certification*. AACN Certification Corp., Aliso Viejo, Calif. Retrieved 12/02/06 from www.certcorp.org/certcorp/certcorp.nsf.vwdoc/BasicCertInfo.
4. American Association of Critical-Care Nurses. (2006). *About critical care nursing*. Retrieved 12/20/06 from http://aacn.org.
5. American Association of Critical-Care Nurses. (2006). *Progressive care fact sheet*. AACN, Aliso Viejo, Calif. Retrieved 06/07/06 from www.aacn.org/AACN/pubpolcy.nsf.
6. American Association of Critical-Care Nurses. (2005). *Synergy for clinical excellence: The AACN Synergy Model for patient care*. Sudbury, Mass: Jones & Bartlett Publishers.
7. American Association of Critical-Care Nurses. (2002). *Safeguarding the patient and the profession: The value of critical care nurse certification*. AACN Certification Corp, Aliso Viejo, Calif. Retrieved 02/20/07 from www.aacn.org.
7a. American Association of Critical-Care Nurses; American College of Physicians; American Thoracic Society; Society of Critical Care Medicine. Framing options for critical care in the United States. Retrieved 03/21/07 from www.sccm.org.

8. American Hospital Association. (2007). *AHA annual survey database: Fiscal year 2005.* Chicago: Health Forum, LLC.

9. American Nurses Association. (May 1999). *Americans support rigorous standards for nursing care (press release).* Washington, DC. Retrieved 02/02/07 from www.nursingworld.org/pressrel/1999/pr0507.htm.

10. American Nurses Credentialing Center. (2007). *About the American Nurses Credentialing Center.* Retrieved 03/02/07 from http://nursingworld.org/ancc/index.htm#about.

11. Angus, D.C., Kelley, M.A., Schmitz, R.J., et al. (2000). Current and projected workforce requirements for care of the critically ill and patients with pulmonary disease. Can we meet the requirements for care of the aging population? *Journal of the American Medical Association, 284,* 2762-2770.

12. Azoulay, E., et al. (2001). Meeting the needs of the intensive care unit patient families. *American Journal of Respiratory Critical Care Medicine, 163*(1), 135-139.

13. Azoulay, E., et al. (2002). Impact of a family information leaflet on effectiveness of information provided to family members of intensive care unit patients: A multicenter, prospective, randomized, controlled trial. *American Journal of Respiratory Critical Care Medicine, 165*(4), 438-442.

14. Azoulay, E., Chevret, S., & Leleu, G. (2000). Half the families of ICU patients experience inadequate communication with physicians. *Critical Care Medicine, 28*(8), 3044-3049.

15. Benner, P., Hooper-Kyriakidis, P., & Stannard, D. (1999). *Clinical wisdom and interventions in critical care.* Philadelphia: Saunders.

16. Benner, P. (2003). Enhancing patient advocacy and social ethics. *American Journal of Critical Care, 12*(4), 374-375.

17. Bijttebier, P., et al. (2001). Needs of the relatives of critical care patients: Perceptions of relatives, physicians and nurses. *Intensive Care Medicine, 27*(1), 160-165.

18. Briggs, L.A., Brown, H., Kesten, K., et al. (2006). Certification for critical care nursing excellence. *Critical Care Nurse, 26*(6), 47-53.

19. Brunt, B. (2005). Critical thinking in nursing: An integrated review. *The Journal of Continuing Education in Nursing, 36*(2), 60-67.

20. Chant, S., Jenkinson, T., Randle, J., et al. (2002). Communication skills: Some problems in nursing education and practice. *Journal of Clinical Nursing, 11*(1), 12-21.

21. Clark, A.P., & Carter, P.A. (2002). Why do nurses see families as "trouble?" *Clinical Nurse Specialist, 16*(1), 40-41.

22. Combs, A.H., & Rainey, T.G. (2003). *Making the business case,* Critical Care Summit: ICU Quality and Cost, Society of Critical Care Medicine.

23. Committee on Quality Health Care in America, Institute of Medicine. (2001). *Crossing the quality chasm: A new health system for the 21st century.* Washington, DC: National Academy Press.

24. Culpepper, R.K. (1988). Sleep in the ICU: A description of night sleep patterns in the critical care unit. *Heart Lung, 17,* 35-42.

25. Curley, M.A.Q. (1998). Patient-nurse synergy: optimizing client's outcomes. *American Journal of Critical Care, 7*(1), 64-72.

26. Eichhorn, D.J., Meyers, T.A., Guzzetta, C.E., et al. (2001). During invasive procedures and resuscitation: Hearing the voice of the patient. *American Journal of Nursing, 101*(5), 48-55.

27. Etheridge, S.A. (2007). Learning to think like a nurse: Stories from new nurse graduates. *The Journal of Continuing Education in Nursing, 38*(1), 24-30.

28. Fontaine, D.K., Prinkey Briggs, L., & Pope-Smith, B. (2001). Designing humanistic critical care environments. *Critical Care Nursing Quarterly, 24*(3), 21-34.

29. Freedman, V.A., Martin, L.G., & Schoeni, R.F. (2002). Recent trends in disability and functioning among older adults in the United States. *Journal of the American Medical Association, 288*(24), 3137-3146.

30. Groeger, J.S., & Strosberg, M.A. (1992). Descriptive analysis of critical care units in the United States. *Critical Care Medicine, 20*(6), 846-862.

31. Groeger, J.S., Guntupalli, K.K., Strosberg, M., et al. (1993). Descriptive analysis of critical care units in the United States: Patient characteristics and intensive care unit utilization. *Critical Care Medicine, 21*(2), 279-291.

32. Haberfelde, M., & Bedecarre, D. (2005). Nurse-sensitive patient outcomes: An annotated bibliography. *Journal of Nursing Administration, 35*(6), 293-299.

33. Health Resources and Services Administration. (March 2004). *The registered nurse population. Findings from the 2004 National Sample Survey of Registered Nurses,* U.S. Department of Health and Human Services. Retrieved 01/26/07 from http://bhpr.hrsa.gov/healthworkforce/rnsurvey04.

34. Hickey, M. (1990). What are the needs of families of critically ill patients? A review of the literature since 1976. *Heart & Lung, 19,* 401-415.

35. Honkus, V.L. (2003). Sleep deprivation in critical care units. *Critical Care Nursing Quarterly, 26*(3), 179-189.

36. Joint Commission Resources. (2004). *Improving care in the ICU* (1st ed.). Oakbrook Terrace, Ill. The Joint Commission.

37. Labeau, S., Vandijck, D.M., Claes, B. et al. (2007). Critical care nurses' knowledge of evidence-based guidelines for preventing ventilator-associated pneumonia: An evaluation questionnaire. *American Journal of Critical Care, 16*(4), 371-377.

38. Lee, L.K.Y., & Lau, Y.L. (2003). Immediate needs of adult family members of adult intensive care patients in Hong Kong. *Journal of Clinical Nursing, 12,* 490-500.

39. National Commission for Certifying Agencies. (Feb 2002). *Standards for the accreditation of certification programs.* Washington, DC: National Organization for Competency Assurance.

40. Neabel, B., Fothergill-Bourbonnais, F., & Dunning, J. (2000). Family assessment tools: A review of the literature from 1978-1997. *Heart & Lung, 29,* 196-209.

41. Needleman, J., Buerhaus, P.I., Mattke, S., et al. (2002). Nurse-staffing levels and the quality of care in hospitals. *New England Journal of Medicine, 346*(22), 1715-1722.

42. Olson, D., Borel, C., Laskowitz, D., et al. (2001). Quiet time: A nursing intervention to promote sleep in neurocritical care units. *American Journal of Critical Care, 10,* 74-78.

43. Riddell, T. (2007). Critical assumptions: Thinking critically about critical thinking. *Journal of Nursing Education, 46*(3), 121-126.

44. Schmidt, L.A. (2003). Patients' perceptions of nursing care in the hospital setting. *Journal of Advanced Nursing, 44*(4), 393-399.

45. Society of Critical Care Medicine. (2007). *Surviving sepsis campaign.* Retrieved 03/20/07 from http://ssc.sccm.org.

46. Society of Critical Care Medicine. (2006). *Practicing critical medicine.* Retrieved 03/20/07 from www.sccm.org/SCCM/Press+Room/Media+Kit/PracticingCCM.htm.

47. Society of Critical Care Medicine. (2006). *Critical care statistics in the United States.* Retrieved 03/27/07 from www.sccm.org.

48. Tracy, R.F., et al. (2003). Nurses' attitudes towards the use of complementary and alternative therapies in critical care. *Heart & Lung, 32*(3), 197-209.

49. U.S. Department of Health and Human Services. (Jan 2007). *Healthy aging: preserving function and improving quality of life among older Americans,* Centers for Disease Control and Prevention.

50. Verhaeghe, S., Defloor, T., Van Zuuren, F., et al. (2005). The needs and experiences of family members of adult patients in an intensive care unit: A review of the literature. *Journal of Clinical Nursing, 14,* 507-509.

51. Visicu, Inc. (2007). *Solving the critical care crisis.* Retrieved 03/29/07 from www.visicu.com.

52. Wan, H., Sengupta, M., Velkoff, V.A., et al. (2005). *P23-209, 65+ in the United States. U.S. Census Bureau Current Population Reports.* Retrieved 03/21/07 from www.census.gov/prod/www/abs/popula.html.

53. Ward, S., & Clark, A.P. (2006). Improving patient outcomes with intensive insulin therapy. *Clinical Nurse Specialist, 20*(4), 170-174.

CHAPTER 8

Home Health Care

KAREN S. MARTIN

This chapter is designed for students and practitioners whose primary or recent clinical experiences have been in hospital, assisted living, nursing home, or other long-term care facilities as a transition to providing care in a home setting. Included is a summary of the trends, general philosophy, risks, and practice of home health care. *Home health care nursing* practice ranges from disease prevention to care of the sick in their homes and a variety of community settings; the goal is to promote and preserve the health of all.[3,27,39,42] Home health care nurses provide interventions that include teaching, guidance, and counseling; treatments and procedures; case management; and surveillance to individuals with acute, chronic, and terminal illnesses. Home health nurses also collaborate with families and designated caregivers. Nurses are usually employed by hospital-based, visiting nurse, tax-supported, and privately or corporately owned agencies. In this chapter, *community-oriented nursing* is used as a comprehensive or umbrella term. It encompasses home health care and other related services, settings, and providers such as tax-supported public health departments, nurse-managed centers, schools, wellness and occupational health programs, faith community programs, clinics, homeless centers, case management programs, and other programs.

Features called *Bridge to Home Health Care,* written by nurses and other community-oriented professionals to describe their practice, are scattered throughout this book and are included on the website. These features address environmental, psychosocial, physiological, and health-related behavior concerns experienced by clients and their families. They should help you gain insight into the roles and responsibilities of the nurse in home health care as it is practiced with clients and families every day. You can use this information as you consider and make referrals for follow-up care.

TRENDS

The need for home health care and community-oriented services has grown explosively as a result of consumer demand, the advent of Medicare reimbursement for home health services in 1965, the aging of the population, federal legislation that encouraged the expansion of home care, escalating health care costs, and the rise of managed care. Currently, more than 20,000 Medicare-certified and non-certified home health agencies provide services to nearly 8 million clients in the United States, a 1000% increase over 20 years. Between 1967 and 2003, Medicare home health expenditures grew from $50 million to $38 billion.[13,33]

These trends reflect a shift in the delivery of health care services from the hospital to the community. Ideally, this shift will decrease fragmentation and produce an improved health care system in which providers work together in the interest of their clients. The shift also has the potential to increase provider accountability and result in a more systematic delivery model that is driven by evidence-based practice and outcome data.[3,22,35,41,48,51] A *seamless health care system* is the term used to describe this model, a system that includes a wide array of services and providers who collaborate as team members.

---

evolve Web Enhancements

Bridge to Home Health Care   Finding Financial Help

Medicare and Medicaid Coverage of Home Health Services

Ethical Issues in Nursing   How Should Nurses Respond to Conflicts Between Clients and Family Members in the Home Health Care Setting?

Appendix A   Religious Beliefs and Practices Affecting Health Care

Be sure to check out the bonus material on the Evolve website and the CD-ROM, including free self-assessment exercises. **http://evolve.elsevier.com/Black/medsurg**

Although the recipients of home health care have diverse needs, circulatory disease is the most common medical diagnosis followed by neoplasms and endocrine diseases, especially diabetes. Persons 65 years of age and older constitute approximately 70% of all home health clients, and those over 85 years account for 20%.[33] These trends are likely to continue. Consider the following projections:[1,12,45]

- Cultural diversity is increasing rapidly in all subsets of the population.
- Since 1900, the percentage of people older than age 65 years has tripled; those 85 years and older increased by 34 times.
- More than 36 million people are older than age 65 years.
- People older than age 65 years account for one third of health care consumption; they may represent half of the total health care dollars spent by the year 2040.
- More than half of older adults have chronic illnesses that cause activity limitations.
- Up to 60% of older adults do not take their medications properly.
- The 4 million men and women older than age 85 years constitute the fastest-growing subset of older adults, with a growth rate nearly three times that of the overall older adult population.
- The 29 million men and women currently age 55–64 are projected to become the fastest growing segment of the adult population during the next decade.

Because the growth of home health care promises to continue, community-oriented nurses face many challenges. The number and diversity of clients and the complexity of their needs are increasing dramatically, as are the numbers and types of staff members and agency programs. At the same time, demands from consumers and payers for comprehensive, economical services are increasing, the availability of staff and reimbursement is decreasing, and regulatory demands are increasing.[21,23,24,28,35,40]

Legislation and regulations continue to modify and frequently reduce Medicare-Medicaid reimbursement to home health agencies. The stated purposes of significant regulations initiated in the late 1990s were to introduce a prospective payment system that would standardize requests for payment from all home care agencies, initiate a per-client service limit, change billing procedures, and mandate the use of the Outcome and Assessment Information Set (OASIS). Nurses and other practitioners complete versions of the OASIS when adult clients are admitted to service, at interim periods, and finally at client discharge.[13,25,26,48,52] The OASIS is an attempt by the Centers for Medicare and Medicaid Services (CMS) to quantify and track outcomes of client care nationally; agency's aggregated clinical data are released to the public. The Centers indicate that they will initiate a new program, "Pay for Performance," that will offer financial incentives to agencies when aggregate client data exceed certain outcome levels and impose financial penalties for underachievement. Regardless of what the Centers introduce, third-party payers, accreditation and certification groups, private foundations, and consumers want home health care providers to provide accurate and consistent outcome data and information.[3,34]

Nurses who practice in home health or community-oriented settings must address reimbursement (see the feature on Finding Financial Help on the website). A nurse in a hospital, nursing home, or other long-term care facility may not know the cost of service or supplies and may not need to discuss charges with clients and their families. In home health care agencies, however, it is usually nurses who collect financial data, either at intake or when providing the initial services. Data include:

- The source of payment
- Verification of eligibility for Medicare, Medicaid, or other programs providing payment
- Preauthorization approval from a managed care or other third-party payer
- Other details

Home health agencies bill third-party payers for most services; Medicare, Medicaid, and other public programs are common sources. Some clients pay for services themselves (private pay) or receive services that are paid for by private insurance, United Way, foundations, or grants. Often, reimbursement regulations are complex and require extensive paperwork for both nurses and clients.[26,48,52] Clients may ask their nurses for assistance as they try to deal with those regulations (see the feature on Medicare and Medicaid Coverage of Home Health Services on the website for a summary of eligibility, requirement, and coverage information that home health nurses must know).

PERSPECTIVES

The specialty of home health care and community-oriented nursing has a long and distinguished history in the United States, even though it received little attention from the public or the nursing profession until the 1990s. In 1877, Francis Root was employed in New York City as the first home visit nurse. In 1893, Lillian Wald and Mary Brewster established the Henry Street Settlement in the same city. Their goal was to offer public health nursing and community programs to people of all ages who were at high risk of developing health problems and to those with acute and chronic health problems. Lillian Wald had the vision to do the following:[11,15]

- Initiate programs and group activities at the settlement to meet the community's health-related, educational, social, and employment needs

- Send nurses from the settlement to make home visits and provide care to new mothers, infants, and the sick
- Forge alliances with business and political leaders to obtain support for her programs

This comprehensive approach represents a true blend of public health and home care practice. Collaboration between the Henry Street staff and the New York City Mission home visit staff followed and led to the formation of the Visiting Nurse Service of New York, the largest single provider of home health care services in the United States. Soon, organized home visit programs were established in populated areas along the East Coast. Lillian Wald's vision of preventive, curative, and social services for the entire community spread throughout New York City and the rest of the nation. By 1912, as many as 2500 nurses were employed by 900 independent visiting nurse associations.[11,15] By 1963, there were 1100 home health and home care aide organizations and hospices in the United States that employed professional registered nurses.

Agencies that provide Medicare- and Medicaid-certified services must meet minimum national standards; state standards also exist. Some agencies voluntarily participate in the Community Health Accreditation Program and The Joint Commission (formerly known as the Joint Commission on Accreditation of Healthcare Organizations or JCAHO) national accreditation programs. Nurses and other professional staff are required to meet licensure requirements but not consistent competence standards.

Accreditation and competence are becoming important concerns to administrators, practitioners, and the public because of the increased use of technology and high-risk procedures and medications in the home. To be competent, practitioners need adequate orientation, equipment, and supervision; they also need to repeat high-risk procedures with sufficient frequency that they maintain their skills.

Collaboration and communication among members of all disciplines are critical in home health care and community-oriented settings. Nurses make up the largest group of practitioners, although most home health agencies also employ or contract with home health aides, other paraprofessionals, and other professionals. Often, physical therapists, occupational therapists, social workers, and speech and language pathologists are employed. Registered dietitians, pharmacists, dentists, physicians, and clergy may be part of the team as well. Agency staff members also need to coordinate referrals and communicate about client services with various community providers.

Historically, Lillian Wald at Henry Street and other community nurses incorporated collaboration and communication skills in their practice. During the 1990s, a new type of position, that of case manager, was developed. Nurse case managers are employed by home health agencies, hospice programs, health maintenance organizations, physician group practices, private insurance companies, public health departments, school systems, and managed care organizations. Although their responsibilities vary, they attempt to coordinate the delivery and payment of services that target clients' needs.

COMMUNITY-ORIENTED PHILOSOPHY

Because home health care and other community-oriented practitioners have the opportunity to work with clients over time, they espouse a number of core values that influence their practice. Multidisciplinary collaboration and a seamless health care environment have already been mentioned. In addition, nurses provide prevention and health promotion services for topics such as immunizations; tobacco, alcohol, and drug cessation; chronic illness; exercise; healthy eating and obesity; cancer prevention and early identification; and similar concerns.[4,27,42]

Nurses in home health care and community-oriented settings refer to the individuals, families, and communities they serve as clients, patients, consumers, or customers. Regardless of the term used or whether terms are used interchangeably, nurses tend to base their practice on beliefs related to the consumer movement. Included are beliefs that people have both rights and responsibilities, must be knowledgeable about their own health care, and must be actively involved in decisions. These beliefs are linked to issues of access, cost, and quality as well as the concepts of primary health care applicable at a national and an international level. For international use, the World Health Organization[50] initially defined *health* as a state of complete physical, mental, and social well-being and not merely the absence of disease or infirmity. As the definition evolved, health was referred to as a fundamental human right and attainment of the highest possible level of health is an important worldwide social goal. Fundamental conditions and resources for health include peace, shelter, education, food, income, a stable ecosystem, sustainable resources, social justice, and equity.

The power of the client is an important core value for home health and community providers. When a practitioner enters a client's home, it is the client, not the practitioner, who is in charge. In the hospital or nursing home, the nurse gives the client medications and changes dressings. In the home, nurses assist clients in providing their own care or assist family members or informal caregivers in providing that care.[27,39,42] The family and other informal caregivers are critical members of the health care team. Their beliefs about health care practice and treatment, the extent of their skills, and their availability influence or even determine whether a client can remain at home and the outcome of the client's care.

Hospice programs provide some of the most dramatic examples of the power of clients. The agency's hospice team usually consists of nurses, home health aides, social workers, pharmacists, registered dietitians, chaplains, and volunteers. Team members also work with the client's physician and other social service agencies. The role of the team is to support end-of-life decisions made by clients and their families.

Staff members who provide services to clients, their families, and other informal caregivers in their homes are human bridges to home health care. This is true whether the staff member is a nurse, another professional, or a paraprofessional. To maximize outcomes of care, all members of the home health and community team should follow some basic principles as they practice their specialty. These principles are outlined in the Bridge to Home Health Care box below.

Risks

Home health care staff and students should consistently practice the Boy Scout motto, "Be prepared." Prepared-

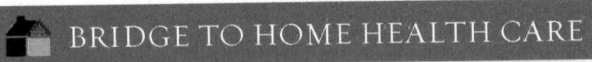

BRIDGE TO HOME HEALTH CARE

Principles of Community-Oriented Home Health Care

- You are a guest in your client's home and neighborhood. Your behavior and your manners must convey that you recognize this role.
- Respect the client's cultural, religious, and ethnic heritage. Hesitate before contradicting that heritage. Clients are more likely to follow their heritage than your advice.
- The client may not respect *your* cultural, religious, and ethnic heritage. If you are a male nurse, the client may expect, and even request, a female nurse. Develop interpersonal skills—and a tough skin.
- Almost every home health client has family members or significant others who offer advice and can serve as either your advocate or your foe. Try to enlist them as your advocate.
- The client "owns" the health-related problem that initiated your services. That problem is just one portion of the client's past, present, and future. Thus it is the client who experiences, learns to understand, and ultimately solves the problem. It is your goal to help clients and their families become independent as quickly as possible. Talk to your peers and supervisors if you sense that you may be losing that perspective.
- Enjoy the unique autonomy and challenges of providing highly complex care in the home and community setting. Home health practice requires integration of high-technology skills, teaching, case management, and monitoring. Remember the need for communication with other members of the health care team. The nurse is usually responsible for judging whether or not the client can safely remain at home, and other team members need to share the information the nurse has through oral and written means.
- Maintain your sense of humor. You will need it!

ness is essential regardless of your responsibilities, the size of your agency or organization, or its geographical location. If you work in a hospital or nursing home, colleagues, technology, supplies, and references are nearby. When you visit a home, school, clinic, or other community site, you are usually on your own. Help and information may be available via extra supplies in the trunk of your car, a cell phone, a computer, a pager, or a fax machine, but help may not be available immediately.

Always consider your safety and that of your client. Plan carefully to minimize the risks of accidents, violence, and natural or man-made disasters. Know your agency's emergency preparedness and response plan, especially since the advent of bioterrorism.[12] If an accident, violence, or disaster occurs, you must know how to intervene immediately and appropriately. For example, when selecting individuals, families, or groups for a student assignment, it is necessary to evaluate the client's needs, the student's educational and life experiences, the educator's skills and availability, where the clients are located, the timing of the visit, the availability of other sources of help, and the student's method of transportation and familiarity with the neighborhood.

It is also important to establish an excellent working relationship among the students, educators, and staff of the agencies or institutions. To enhance communication, safety, and the quality of the experience for both clients and students, strategies such as shared home visits, student learning centers, nursing centers, and homeless clinics should be used.[4,16,19,27,42] Additional strategies to link educators and students with health care providers and clients are described later in this chapter.

Resources

The home health care student and staff nurse have valuable resources that contribute to their ability to provide high-quality care: education, experience, and common sense. Use these resources consistently when making home visits.

Education

Regardless of the stage of your education or the length of time since graduation, educators and materials can provide valuable professional information. Formal and informal education beyond the professional program is important for nurses who practice in the community; many educators are increasingly interested in partnerships with practitioners and agencies.[16,27,41,49] Consider courses in first aid, cardiopulmonary resuscitation, computers, the Internet, cultural awareness, community resources, current affairs, and political, legal, financial, and ethical issues. Read relevant publications and attend relevant conferences. Remember what you learned, and keep updating your knowledge.

Experience

Your professional and life experiences contribute to your technical and interpersonal skills. Identify your strengths and take action in the areas where you need to improve.[6] Discuss your career goals and opportunities with a trusted friend. Take every opportunity to observe a colleague providing care or completing other responsibilities, such as performing complex treatments, completing documentation, or using information technology. Learn how to organize your practice and avail yourself of excellent practice pointers, including those on the web.

Common Sense

Some aspects of practice in community settings are not the same as practice in the acute care setting. Develop and use your intuition, and listen to it.[27] Expert home health care practitioners are known for their caring, flexibility, persistence, and ability to improvise. They use sound judgment to alter everything from their schedule to their interventions according to their circumstances and available resources. Expert practitioners have more than a plan A as they begin to work with a client; they can move to a plan B or plan C at a moment's notice.

PROVIDING CARE

The concepts and principles involved in home health care and other community practice settings are closely related to those of nursing practice in the hospital, outpatient departments, and long-term care. The assessment, problem identification (diagnosis), planning, intervention, and evaluation steps of the problem-solving or nursing process provide an important foundation for that practice. You may observe and use the Omaha System in home health or community care as a way to operationalize the nursing process.

The Omaha System

The Omaha System was developed and refined through three Visiting Nurse Association (VNA) of Omaha research projects funded by the Division of Nursing, U.S. Department of Health and Human Services, between 1975 and 1986. Additional reliability, validity, and usability research was completed between 1989 and 1993. Since then, more research has been conducted. Forty diverse studies have been summarized and published with their implications for practice and research.[27,36]

The Omaha System is designed to facilitate nursing practice, documentation, and information management. It is a series of cues or feedback loops that help remind the user about possible client problems and intervention options and about ways to evaluate the effect of the care provided. Structured language and codes enhance the precision of recording and ease of communication. Users

can communicate their conclusions orally, electronically, or through printed paper forms.

The Omaha System provides a data framework for agencies or programs to use with their automated or manual client records. Establishing a clinical database that is reliable and valid enables a user to generate reports that contribute to program evaluation, long-range planning, compliance with regulations required by accreditation organizations and third-party payers, and outcome statistics required by many governing board members and third-party payers. The public health nurses, managers, and administrators at Washington County Public Health and Environment, Stillwater, Minnesota, use their accurate and consistent outcomes management data for just those purposes.[30-32] Many home health and community agencies are making dramatic progress in their efforts to improve their client records and to develop integrated clinical and financial management information systems.[20,27,46-48] However, agencies and software vendors must follow the complex and lengthy regulations of the Health Insurance Portability and Accountability Act of 1996, a challenge to practitioners, administrators, third-party payers, computer vendors, educators, and students who are involved in any health care delivery.[45]

Initial users of the Omaha System were home health care, public health, and school nurses and other health care professionals in the United States. Both the number and type of users are expanding dramatically to include nurse-managed center staff, hospital-based and managed care case managers, faith community practitioners, educators and students, acute care staff, researchers, and the international community. Such expansion reflects the trends already described in this chapter and the trend among all types of health care providers to automate clinical data.[5,7,8,14,27,29,38,44] The Omaha System includes one of the vocabularies recognized and publicized by the American Nurses' Association.[2]

Figure 8-1 illustrates the concepts of the problem-solving or nursing process as they relate to the Omaha System. The circular model shown depicts the dynamic, interactive nature of the problem-solving process, the practitioner-client relationship, and the related theories of diagnostic reasoning and critical thinking, sometimes referred to as *analytic reasoning* or *expert knowledge*. The Omaha System is a research-based problem, intervention, and outcome measurement classification or taxonomy developed by nurses in community settings that incorporates evidence-based practice.[5,8,27,32] The Problem Classification Scheme, the Intervention Scheme, and the Problem Rating Scale for Outcomes are components of the system. The relationships among the problem-solving process, the Omaha System, and home health care practice are described next.

A nurse provides service to a client after the referral and intake steps are completed. During the nurse's initial visit and all other visits, the vital importance of establishing and

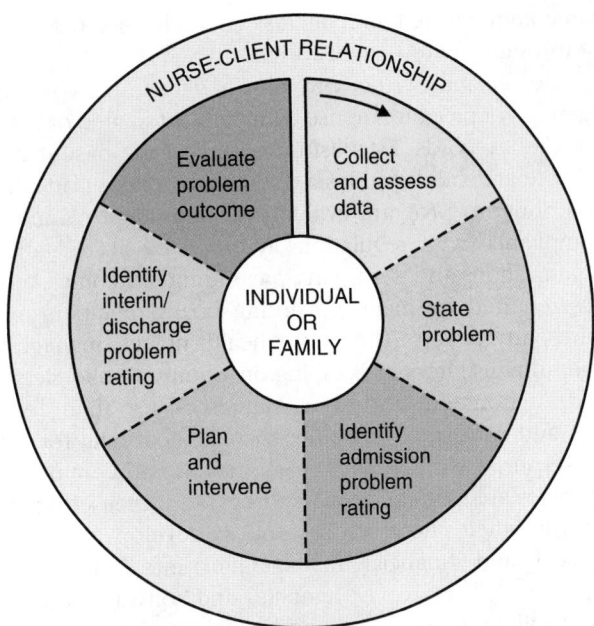

■ FIGURE 8–1 Omaha System model of the problem-solving process. *(From Martin, K.S. [2005]. The Omaha System: A key to practice, documentation, and information management [2nd ed.]. St. Louis: Mosby.)*

maintaining a positive nurse-client relationship and partnership must be recognized. Freeman and Heinrich[18] emphasized that a positive relationship is developed, not discovered. Such a relationship promotes quantity and quality of data and enhances the potential for success and client progress in relation to all components of the nursing process.

A nurse's initial activities include data collection, assessment, and analysis (i.e., Problem Classification Scheme). This process involves gathering, clustering, combining, summarizing, and validating diverse subjective and objective information about each family member, the family as an interacting unit, and the sociocultural and physical environment. A community-oriented nurse uses principles of epidemiology to enhance systematic data collection and assessment and to identify patterns within client data. The conclusion and logical end product of the data collection and assessment process is problem identification (diagnosis), which involves interpretation of the acquired data.

Planning and intervening are two of the most important concepts of the model to both a client and a nurse (i.e., Intervention Scheme). Based on client and nurse goals, assessment data, and diagnostic conclusions, the nurse and family need to collaborate to delineate alternative courses of action and choose and take action. When data about best practices are tracked over time, they become the basis of effective intervention pathways.

Identification of admission, interim, and discharge ratings quantifies the evaluation or outcomes management process (i.e., Problem Rating Scale for Outcomes). Each

rating provides a baseline for contrast with later ratings during the period of client service. The evaluation component of the Omaha System allows a nurse to compare a client's health status at different points in time to determine the degree of nursing effectiveness. The nurse uses data from the evaluation process to revise and modify plans and interventions with an individual, family, or group.[30-32]

The Problem Classification Scheme, the Intervention Scheme, and the Problem Rating Scale for Outcomes follow principles of taxonomy and consist of terms and codes arranged from general to specific. Terms are intended to be simple, clear, and concise.

The Problem Classification Scheme

The Problem Classification Scheme is a taxonomy of client problems or nursing diagnoses that has been developed from actual client data (Box 8-1). It consists of four levels, ranging from the general to specific level of abstraction:[27,36]

- *Domains* are four general areas that represent health care practice and provide organizational groupings for client problems: Environmental, Psychosocial, Physiological, and Health-Related Behaviors.
- *Problems* are 42 unique client concerns, needs, strengths, issues, foci, or conditions that affect any aspect of the client's well-being; they are nursing diagnoses stated from the client's perspective. Examples include Caretaking/parenting, Skin, and Nutrition.
- *Modifiers* are the two sets of terms (Individual, Family, Community and Health Promotion, Potential, Actual) used to identify ownership of the problem and degree of severity in relation to client strengths, concerns, risk factors, and signs and symptoms.
- *Signs and Symptoms* are more specific objective and subjective evidence of a client's problem.

The Problem Classification Scheme offers a view of the wide range of client concerns that nurses and other health care practitioners address. These include physical, emotional, social, spiritual, and economic concerns. Thus, this tool is used as a framework for assessment during a home or clinic visit and for documentation of the service provided. In that way, it constantly reminds the practitioner that the client needs to be viewed holistically and not as a "colostomy case" or a drug user, for example. The OASIS data set was not designed to be an assessment framework, but the OASIS items can be integrated into the agency's assessment form, such as a form based on the Problem Classification Scheme.[13,44,47]

Caretaking/parenting, a problem from the Psychosocial domain, is described in Box 8-2. It has 10 signs and symptoms, including difficulty providing physical care/safety as well as expectations incongruent with

BOX 8-1 Domains and Problems of the Problem Classification Scheme

Environmental Domain

Material resources and physical surroundings both inside and outside the living area, neighborhood, and broader community.

- Income
- Sanitation
- Residence
- Neighborhood/workplace safety

PSYCHOSOCIAL DOMAIN

Patterns of behavior, emotion, communication, relationships, and development.

- Communication with community resources
- Social contact
- Role change
- Interpersonal relationship
- Spirituality
- Grief
- Mental health
- Sexuality
- Caretaking/parenting
- Neglect
- Abuse
- Growth and development

Physiological Domain

Functions and processes that maintain life.

- Hearing
- Vision
- Speech and language
- Oral health
- Cognition
- Pain
- Consciousness
- Skin
- Neuro-musculo-skeletal function
- Respiration
- Circulation
- Digestion-hydration
- Bowel function
- Urinary function
- Reproductive function
- Pregnancy
- Postpartum
- Communicable/infectious condition

HEALTH-RELATED BEHAVIORS DOMAIN

Patterns of activity that maintain or promote wellness, promote recovery, and decrease the risk of disease.

- Nutrition
- Sleep and rest patterns
- Physical activity
- Personal care
- Substance use
- Family planning
- Health care supervision
- Medication regimen

From Martin, K.S. (2005). *The Omaha System: A key to practice, documentation, and information management* (2nd ed.). St. Louis: Mosby.

BOX 8-2 Problems, Modifiers, and Signs/Symptoms from the Problem Classification Scheme

Caretaking/Parenting

Health promotion
Potential
Actual

- difficulty providing physical care/safety
- difficulty providing emotional nurturance
- difficulty providing cognitive learning experiences and activities
- difficulty providing preventive and therapeutic health care
- expectations incongruent with stage of growth and development
- dissatisfaction/difficulty with responsibilities
- difficulty interpreting or responding to verbal/nonverbal communication
- neglectful
- abusive
- other

Skin

Health promotion
Potential
Actual

- lesion/pressure ulcer
- rash
- excessively dry
- excessively oily
- inflammation
- pruritus
- drainage
- bruising
- hypertrophy of nails
- delayed incisional healing
- other

From Martin, K.S. (2005). *The Omaha System: A key to practice, documentation, and information management* (2nd ed.). St. Louis: Mosby.

TABLE 8–1   Application of the Omaha System

Data	Problem Classification Scheme: Problems and Signs/Symptoms	Problem Rating Scale for Outcomes: Concepts and Ratings	Intervention Scheme: Categories	Intervention Scheme: Targets
Psychosocial Domain				
Jane Doe: 14-year-old new mother with 2-day-old infant boy. Says she is "scared." Has not cared for infants; asking how to hold and feed. Wants son to sleep at least 6 hr. No family in area.	Caretaking/parenting: actual/individual • Difficulty providing physical care/safety • Expectations incongruent with stage of growth and development	Knowledge = 2 Behavior = 3 Status = 2	Teaching, Guidance, and Counseling Case Management	Anatomy/physiology Bonding/attachment Caretaking/parenting skills Support group
Physiological Domain				
John Brown: 82-year-old just discharged after hemicolectomy. Has infected incision. Recalls some of discharge instructions.	Skin: actual/individual • Lesion/pressure ulcer • Drainage	Knowledge = 4 Behavior = 3 Status = 3	Teaching, Guidance, and Counseling Treatments and Procedures	Dressing change/wound care Signs/symptoms—physical Dressing change/wound care Signs/symptoms—physical

stage of growth and development. For example, you may visit a 14-year-old mother and her newborn to provide information about infant growth, development, and care. You record the following data that range from general to specific:

1. The problem: Caretaking/parenting.
2. Signs and Symptoms: Difficulty providing physical care/safety and expectations incongruent with stage of growth and development.
3. More specific descriptive and quantitative clinical data are recorded on the client's computerized or manual record.

Skin, a problem from the Physiological domain, also appears in Box 8-2. Skin has 11 signs and symptoms, including lesion/pressure ulcer and drainage. If you care for a client whose infected wound requires cleaning and a dressing change, you may record the following data that range from general to specific:[27]

1. The problem: Skin.
2. Signs and Symptoms: Lesion/pressure ulcer and drainage.
3. More specific descriptive and quantitative clinical data on the client's form or automated record.

Table 8-1 illustrates these two examples of documentation, which include the three components of the Omaha System. Note that it depicts only part of the documentation for two nurse-client visits, not complete record entries.

The Intervention Scheme

The Intervention Scheme is a taxonomy used to describe nurses and other practitioners' actions and activities that are intended to improve, maintain, or restore health or prevent illness (Box 8-3). The scheme consists of categories, targets, and client-specific information, ranging from the general to specific level of abstraction.

It is a research-based effort to link the effectiveness of interventions with client problems or diagnoses.[27,36]

Categories are four broad areas at the first level of the Intervention Scheme that provide a structure for describing practitioner actions or activities: Teaching, Guidance, and Counseling; Treatments and Procedures; Case Management; and Surveillance. One or more categories are used to develop a plan or document an intervention specific to a client problem.

Targets are an alphabetical listing of 75 unique objects at the second level of the Intervention Scheme. Targets are practitioner actions or activities that further describe problem-specific intervention categories. For the problem Skin and the category Treatments and Procedures, useful targets include dressing change/wound care and signs/symptoms—physical. For Caretaking/parenting and the category Teaching, Guidance, and Counseling, possible targets are anatomy/physiology, bonding/attachment, and growth/development care.

Client-specific information is at the third level of the Intervention Scheme; it is the detailed portion of a plan or intervention statement that is developed and documented by the practitioner. Client-specific information has been organized into suggested care planning guides.[27]

Table 8-1 presents the use of intervention categories, targets, and client-specific information to describe and document a plan or intervention category specific to a client problem, such as Skin or Caretaking/parenting. Again, note the definitions and diversity of community interventions. Nurses and other practitioners who provide care in the community must be generalists and must develop competence in providing "hands-on" bedside care and technical skills as well as educational, referral, monitoring, and motivational skills. Recall that the client owns the health-related problem and is the only one who ultimately solves the problem.

BOX 8-3 Intervention Scheme Categories

TEACHING, GUIDANCE, AND COUNSELING

Activities designed to provide information and materials, encourage client action and responsibility for self-care and coping, and assist the individual, family, or community to make decisions and solve problems. The overlapping concepts occur on a continuum with the variation a result of the client's self-direction capabilities.

TREATMENTS AND PROCEDURES

Technical activities such as wound care, specimen collection, resistive exercises, and medication prescriptions that are designed to prevent, decrease, or alleviate signs and symptoms for the individual, family, or community.

CASE MANAGEMENT

Activities such as coordination, advocacy, and referral that facilitate service delivery; promote assertiveness; guide the individual, family, or community toward use of appropriate resources; and improve communication among health and human service providers.

SURVEILLANCE

Activities such as detection, measurement, critical analysis, and monitoring intended to identify the status of the individual, family, or community in relation to a given condition or phenomenon.

Targets

- anatomy/physiology
- anger management
- behavior modification
- bladder care
- bonding/attachment
- bowel care
- cardiac care
- caretaking/parenting skills
- cast care
- communication
- community outreach worker services
- continuity of care
- coping skills
- day care/respite
- dietary management
- discipline
- dressing change/wound care
- durable medical equipment
- education
- employment
- end-of-life care
- environment
- exercises
- family planning care
- feeding procedures
- finances

- gait training
- genetics
- growth/development care
- home
- homemaking/housekeeping
- infection precautions
- interaction
- interpreter/translator services
- laboratory findings
- legal system
- medical/dental care
- medication action/side effects
- medication administration
- medication coordination/ordering
- medication prescription
- medication set-up
- mobility/transfers
- nursing care
- nutritionist care
- occupational therapy care
- ostomy care
- other community resources
- paraprofessional/aide care
- personal hygiene
- physical therapy care

- positioning
- recreational therapy care
- relaxation/breathing techniques
- respiratory care
- respiratory therapy care
- rest/sleep
- safety
- screening procedures
- sickness/injury care
- signs/symptoms—mental/emotional
- signs/symptoms—physical
- skin care
- social work/counseling care
- specimen collection
- speech and language pathology care
- spiritual care
- stimulation/nurturance
- stress management
- substance use cessation
- supplies
- support group
- support system
- transportation
- wellness
- other

From Martin, K.S. (2005). *The Omaha System: A key to practice, documentation, and information management* (2nd ed.). St. Louis: Mosby.

The Problem Rating Scale for Outcomes

The Problem Rating Scale for Outcomes is an outcomes management framework designed to quantify a client's problem according to three specific categories—Knowledge, Behavior, and Status. The scale is intended to measure the client's progress and provide both a guide for practice and a method of documentation. The scale was designed for use throughout the time of client service. When establishing the initial ratings for client problems, the user creates an independent data baseline, capturing the condition and circumstances of the client at a given point in time. This admission baseline is used to compare and contrast the client's condition and circumstances with those ratings completed at later intervals and at client discharge. The comparison or change in ratings over time can be used to identify the client's progress in relation to interventions and the effectiveness of the plan of care.[27,36,48]

The Problem Rating Scale for Outcomes is a five-point ordinal scale comprising three subscales, or concepts (Table 8-2). *Concepts* are three major areas that represent the basic client issues of knowing (Knowledge), doing (Behavior), and being (Status):

- *Knowledge* refers to the ability of the client to remember and interpret information.

TABLE 8–2 Problem Rating Scale for Outcomes

Concept	1	2	3	4	5
Knowledge: the ability of the client to remember and interpret information	No knowledge	Minimal knowledge	Basic knowledge	Adequate knowledge	Superior knowledge
Behavior: the observable responses, actions, or activities of the client fitting the occasion or purpose	Not appropriate behavior	Rarely appropriate behavior	Inconsistently appropriate behavior	Usually appropriate behavior	Consistently appropriate behavior
Status: the condition of the client in relation to objective and subjective defining characteristics	Extreme signs/ symptoms	Severe signs/ symptoms	Moderate signs/ symptoms	Minimal signs/ symptoms	No signs/symptoms

From Martin, K.S. (2005). *The Omaha System: A key to practice, documentation, and information management* (2nd ed.). St. Louis: Mosby.

- *Behavior* consists of the observable responses, actions, or activities of the client fitting the occasion or purpose.
- *Status* is the condition of the client in relation to objective and subjective characteristics.

The scale for each of the concepts has five categories or degrees for response. For example, for the problems Skin and Caretaking/parenting, the nurse identifies baseline Knowledge, Behavior, and Status ratings during the first home or clinic visit.

Communication and Information Technology

The presence of educators and nursing students in community settings, especially students who are just beginning their formal education, introduces numerous challenges. Unlike practice in hospitals or long-term care facilities, practice in the community usually involves educators remaining at the college or service setting while their students make independent visits and see clients at homes, clinics, schools, or other sites.[3,14,16] These educators and students, especially students in their early semesters of education, need to maintain communication while traveling and providing client care. Students may need to communicate with educators quickly and often for the safety of both clients and students. These needs can be met by using reliable and efficient cellular phones, the Internet, automated point-of-care information systems, and telehealth systems. Cellular phones are ubiquitous; community practitioners and their agencies are embracing the Internet, automation, and telehealth.[10,37,43]

Since the Internet was launched in 1992, its use has exploded nationally and internationally. Clients and their families access the Internet to become informed about medical diagnoses, providers, medications, and treatments. It is important that they are encouraged to use websites that are authenticated and accurate. It is equally important that practitioners are informed about the Internet and the sources of information that their clients are reading.

The critical need to generate, store, analyze, and distribute clinical data with the help of automated information systems exists in all health care settings. The Omaha System was described as a model for practice, documentation, and information management in the previous section. Early in the 1990s, software companies started to develop commercially available software based on the Omaha System for home health agencies, public health departments, nurse-managed centers, and colleges of nursing. The software is intended for use by practitioners at the point-of-care as a "front end" or interface terminology.[20,27,47,49] Student and educator users include associate degree, baccalaureate degree, registered nurse completion, and graduate nurse programs.[5,14,27,44] Some schools and colleges base their curriculum on the Omaha System.[27,29]

Telehealth integrates various applications such as clinical health delivery, management of health care information, education, and administrative services within a common infrastructure.[10] A system of telephones and video cameras is used to increase communication between home health care practitioners and clients. The goal is to reduce health care barriers of distance, time, and resources, not to replace visits. When nurses and clients use telehealth successfully, nurses can monitor clients' weight, oxygen saturation, glucose levels, pain, diet, symptom exacerbation, and other parameters, and provide a variety of educational interventions.[9,10,17,24,37,43,44]

CONCLUSIONS

Home health care and community-oriented settings are experiencing both unprecedented growth and financial constraints. Development of new programs, introduction of new technology, and increases in client caseloads and services, staff, and budget can be exciting. Decreased agency revenue can lead to layoffs, decreased salary and benefits, increased workloads, and a sense of insecurity. When the internal systems of agencies experience extra pressure and become overloaded, employees are more likely to become frustrated and stressed and to make errors. Quality improvement systems are critical. Practitioners, administrators, students, and educators need to use a variety of methods to monitor practice, communicate efficiently, and work together to provide effective, high-quality services.

The reference list in this chapter provides more extensive information about home care, public health, and related topics. After reading the chapter, you may discuss what community opportunities you will have as a nursing student. If you are a staff nurse, you may consider making an appointment to accompany a colleague who practices in a home care, public health, clinic, faith community, or school setting to learn more about the specialty.

BIBLIOGRAPHY

 Citations appearing in red refer to primary research.

1. Administration on Aging. (2006). *A profile of older Americans 2005: The older population and health, health care, and disability.* Available at www.aoa.dhhs.gov/.
2. American Nurses Association. (2006). *Nursing Practice Information Infrastructure's description of the 12 recognized terminologies.* Available at www.nursingworld.org/npii/terminologies.htm.
3. American Nurses Association. (in press). *Scope and standards of home health nursing practice.* Silver Spring, Md: American Nurses Association.
4. Anderson, E.T., & McFarlane, J. (2003). *Community as partner* (4th ed.). Philadelphia: Lippincott Williams & Wilkins.
5. Barton, A.J., Clark, L., & Baramee, J. (2004). Tracking outcomes in community-based care. *Home Health Care Management and Practice, 16*(3), 171-176.
6. Benner, P. (1984). *From novice to expert.* Menlo Park, Calif: Addison-Wesley.
7. Bowles, K.H. (1999). The Omaha System: Bridging hospital and home care. *On-line Journal of Nursing Informatics [On-line], 3* (1). Available at www.eaaknowledge.com/ojni/ni/dm/ojni.html.
8. Bowles, K.H. (2000). Application of the Omaha System in acute care. *Research in Nursing and Health, 23*(2), 93-105.
9. Bowles, K.H., & Baugh, A.C. (2007, Jan-Feb). Applying research evidence to optimize telehomecare. *Journal of Cardiovascular Nursing, 22*(1), 5-15.
10. Brantley, D., Laney-Cummings, K., & Spivack, R. (2004). *Innovation, demand, and investment in telehealth.* U.S. Department of Commerce, Office of Technology Policy. Available at www.technology.gov.reports/TechPolicy/Telehealth/2004/Report.pdf.
11. Buhler-Wilkerson, K. (2001). *No place like home: A history of nursing and home care in the United States.* Baltimore: Johns Hopkins University Press.
12. Centers for Disease Control and Prevention. (2006). *Public health emergency response: Guide for state, local, and tribal public health directors,* and *The burden of chronic diseases and their risk factors: National and state perspectives.* Available at www.cdc.gov/.
13. Centers for Medicare and Medicaid Services. (2006). *Medicare state operations manual: Conditions of participation* (revised 08/12/05), and *Health Insurance Portability and Accountability Act of 1996.* Available at www.cms.hhs.gov.
14. Connolly, P.M., & Novak, J.M. (2000). Teaching collaboration: A demonstration model. *Journal of the American Psychiatric Nurses Association, 6*(6), 183-190.
15. Dolan, J.A., Fitzpatrick, M.L., & Herrmann, E.K. (1983). *Nursing in society: A historical perspective* (15th ed.). Philadelphia: Saunders.
16. Donovan, N. (2002). Providing a home care clinical experience that benefits patients, students, and agencies. *Home Healthcare Nurse, 20*(7), 443-448.
17. Finkelstein, S.M., Speedie, S.M., & Potthoff, S. (2006). Home telehealth improves clinical outcomes at lower cost for home healthcare. *Telemedicine and e-Health, 12*(2), 128-136.
18. Freeman, R., & Heinrich, J. (1981). *Community health nursing practice* (2nd ed.). Philadelphia: Saunders.
19. Hamner, J.B., et al. (2002). Community-based service learning in the engaged university. *Nursing Outlook, 50*(2), 67-71.
20. Handly, M.J., et al. (2003). Essential activities for implementing a clinical information system in public health nursing. *Journal of Nursing Administration, 33*(1), 14-16.
21. Health Resources and Services Administration. (2006). *Preliminary findings: 2004 National Sample Survey of Registered Nurses.* Available at http://bhpr.hrsa.gov/healthworkforce/reports/rnpopulation/preliminaryfindings.htm.
22. Hegyvary, S.T. (2006). A call for papers on evidence-based problems. *Journal of Nursing Scholarship, 38*(1), 1-2.
23. Heineken, J., & McCoy, N. (2000). Establishing a bond with clients of different cultures. *Home Healthcare Nurse, 18*(1), 45-52.
24. Huston, C.J. (2006). *Professional issues in nursing: Challenges and opportunities.* Philadelphia: Lippincott Williams & Wilkins.
25. Madigan, E.A., Tullai-McGuiness, S., & Fortinsky, R.H. (2003). Accuracy in the Outcome and Assessment Information Set (OASIS): Results of a video simulation. *Research in Nursing and Health, 26*(4), 273-283.
26. Martin, K.S. (2000). Home health care, outcomes management, and the Land of Oz. *Outcomes Management for Nursing Practice, 4*(1), 7-12.
27. Martin, K.S. (2005). *The Omaha System: A key to practice, documentation, and information management* (2nd ed.). St. Louis: Mosby.
28. McEwen, M.M., & Slack, M.K. (2005). Factors associated with health-related behaviors in Latinos with or at risk of diabetes. *Hispanic Health Care International, 3*(3), 143-152.
29. Merrill, A.S., et al. (1998). Curriculum restructuring using the practice-based Omaha System. *Nurse Educator, 23*(3), 41-44.
30. Monsen, K.A., & Martin, K.S. (2002). Developing an outcomes management program in a public health department. *Outcomes Management, 6*(2), 62-66.
31. Monsen, K.A., & Martin, K.S. (2002). Using an outcomes management program in a public health department. *Outcomes Management, 6*(3), 120-124.
32. Monsen, K.A., et al. (2006). A public health nursing informatics data and practice quality project. *CIN: Computers, Informatics, Nursing, 24*(3), 152-158.
33. National Association for Home Care and Hospice. (2006a). *Basic statistics about home care 2004.* Available at www.nahc.org/04HC_stats.pdf.
34. National Association for Home Care and Hospice. (2006b). *Briggs National Quality Improvement/Hospitalization Reduction Study.* Available at www.nahc.org/NAHC/CaringComm/eNAHCReport/datacharts/hospredstudy.pdf.
35. Naylor, M.D., et al. (2005). Cognitively impaired older adults: From hospital to home. *American Journal of Nursing, 105*(2), 52-61.
36. Omaha System. (2006). Available at www.omahasystem.org.
37. Page, A. (Ed.). (2004). *Keeping patients safe: Transforming the work environment of nurses.* Washington, DC: National Academies Press. Available at http://nap.edu/openbook/0309090679/html/R1.html
38. Plowfield, L.A., Hayes, E.R., & Hall-Long, B. (2005). Using the Omaha System to document the wellness needs of the elderly. *Nursing Clinics of North America, 40*(4), 817-829.
39. Reif, L.J., & Martin, K.S. (1996). *Nurses and consumers: Partners in assuring quality in the home.* Washington, DC: American Nurses Publishing.
40. Schoesslet, M., & Waldo, M. (2006). The first 18 months in practice: A developmental transition model for the newly graduated nurse. *Journal for Nurses in Staff Development, 22*(2), 47-52.
41. Schumacher, K.L., & Marren, J. (2004). Home care nursing for older adults: State of the science. *Nursing Clinics of North America, 39* (3), 443-471.
42. Stanhope, M., & Lancaster, J. (Eds.). (2004). *Community and public health nursing* (6th ed.). St. Louis: Mosby.
43. Technology and Telehealth. (2004). *Home Healthcare Nurse, 22* (10), entire issue.
44. Transforming clinical data into critical outcome information: How to survive in the new data-driven world. (2004). *Home Health Care Management and Practice, 16*(3), entire issue.
45. U.S. Department of Health and Human Services, National Center for Health Statistics. (2006). *Health, United States, 2005.* Available at www.cdc.gov/nchs/hus.htm.

46. Westra, B.L., & Solomon, D.A. (1999). The Omaha System: Bridging home care and technology. *On-line Journal of Nursing Informatics [On-line]*, *3*(1). Available at www.eaaknowledge.com/ojni/ni/dm/ojni.html.

47. Westra, B.L. (2005). *National Health Information Infrastructure (NHII) and nursing: Implementing the Omaha System in community-based practice. [On-line]*. Available at www.himss.org/content/files/ImplementationNursingTerminologyCommunity.pdf and www.carefacts.com/articles.

48. Westra, B.L., Solomon, D., & Ashley, D.M. (2006). Use of the Omaha System data to validate Medicare required outcomes in home care. *Journal of Healthcare Information Management, 29* (3), 88-94.

49. Wilson, S. (2002). Development of a personal digital assistant (PDA) as point-of-care technology in nursing education. *Journal of Mobile Informatics [On-line]*. Available at www.pdacortex.com/pda_nursing_education.htm.

50. World Health Organization/UNICEF. (1978). *Primary health care: Alma-Ata Conference*. Geneva: World Health Organization.

51. Yu, F., Evans, L.K., & Sullivan-Marx, E.M. (2005). Functional outcomes for older adults with cognitive impairment in a comprehensive outpatient rehabilitation facility. *Journal of the American Geriatrics Society, 53*(9), 1599-1606.

52. Zuber, R.F. (2002). Assessing Medicare eligibility. *Home Healthcare Nurse, 20*(7), 425-430.

evolve *Did you remember to check out the bonus material on the Evolve website and the CD-ROM, including NCLEX®-Examination Style Review Questions, Open-Book Quizzes, and Chapter Review Audio Podcasts?*

http://evolve.elsevier.com/Black/medsurg

CHAPTER 9

Long-Term Care

CHARLOTTE ELIOPOULOS

Of all the types of health care settings, long-term care facilities (LTCFs) are perhaps the most misunderstood and criticized. The media gives prime coverage to the small minority of facilities that have substandard conditions while ignoring the majority that provide compassionate, competent care on a daily basis. Some professionals who have never worked in a LTCF believe that this setting is a simple, nonchallenging environment in which to work. Many families assume that nursing home staff are untrustworthy, uncaring, and lazy.

In reality, most residents of LTCFs receive competent care and enjoy a good quality of life. Despite significantly fewer resources available to them, compared with those found in hospitals and other care settings, LTCFs provide adequate care for highly dependent residents. The wide range of physical and mental conditions of residents combined with the high prevalence of individuals of advanced age make LTCF residents a complex population. Because physicians typically are not on the premises at all times, nurses must be highly competent in assessing residents, recognizing changes in status, and communicating needs to physicians. It is not unusual to find special relationships between residents and their caregivers, who often assume a family surrogate role. Why is there such a discrepancy between the reality and perception of LTCFs? Much of this is due to the lingering memories associated with some of the negative history of LTCFs. A brief review of the history of LTCFs may offer some insight into the present challenges confronting this care setting.

GROWTH OF LONG-TERM CARE FACILITIES

By the end of the seventeenth century, most European countries had created institutions to care for the mentally ill, aged, developmentally disabled, orphaned, poor,

criminals, and people with contagious diseases. It was not unusual for a single institution to house all of these various types of people together. The interest was not to provide highly specialized and individualized care but rather to segregate these people from the rest of society. Not surprisingly, low public interest and limited funds caused conditions to become inhumane in these institutions.

Until the 19th century, the United States had few institutions. People who were sick, old, or disabled were expected to receive care at home, from private help, or family. As the population grew, however, so did the number of people without the financial or family resources to provide care, and hospitals and other forms of inpatient care were needed. Hospitals, staffed by physicians who at that time were from society's elite, were less than enthusiastic about having poor people with long-term care needs remaining in their beds for extended periods. Pressure grew to create facilities that could house and care for clients over the long term. In response, communities developed institutions that were given names such as *almshouse hospital, asylum, homes for the incurable,* and *chronic disease hospital.* Most often, these institutions were located on the outskirts of town where the average citizen could avoid contact with the residents.

These early facilities relied on charities and meager public funds for their existence, and conditions were poor. A physician from that era, writing about those early institutions, described conditions such as grossly

---

evolve Web Enhancements

Appendix A Religious Beliefs and Practices Affecting Health Care

Be sure to check out the bonus material on the Evolve website and the CD-ROM, including free self-assessment exercises. **http://evolve.elsevier.com/Black/medsurg**

inadequate supplies, food so insufficient that many residents experienced recurrent incidents of scurvy, and residents forced to sleep on the floor because of overcrowding, rampant theft, open drunkenness, and sexual relations between residents and their caregivers.[8] Residents were expected to work for their keep, and recovered residents who had no family or home in the community remained in the institution and cooked, cleaned, or cared for other residents in exchange for room, board, and a small salary. In this environment, high quality of life, rehabilitation, residents' rights, and individuality were foreign concepts. With these conditions, most people did not view institutions that provided long-term care as highly desirable options.

The enactment of the Social Security Act in 1935 afforded older adults the means to purchase care privately and not rely on charitable or public institutions. An informal long-term care system began to grow as people rented rooms of their homes to older adults who needed room, board, and perhaps some basic personal care assistance. Many of these homes were operated by nurses, or women who called themselves nurses; thus the term *nursing home* began to be more widely used. Small nursing homes began to appear, often developed by religious or public agencies (e.g., Jewish homes for the aged, county rest homes) and sometimes by private individuals. At this time, the government had little involvement in nursing home operations; there were no government regulations pertaining to nursing home care and no government reimbursement for long-term care services.

In 1946 the federal government took a noticeable step in promoting nursing home growth through the Hill-Burton Hospital Survey and Construction Act. This act provided funds for hospital construction, but other institutions, such as nursing homes, could also obtain funds if they met certain conditions. Because the construction requirements were developed for hospitals, the nursing homes that obtained these funds constructed facilities that were similar to hospitals. Rather than creating an environment designed for the unique needs of chronically ill individuals who would reside in the setting for an extended length of time, nursing homes resembled acute hospitals in appearance and style of operation (e.g., white uniforms, rigid schedules, limited visitation schedules, subservient role of residents).

By the 1960s the "graying of the population" was being realized. As the numbers of older adults grew, so did their need for health services. During the Kennedy-Johnson era, federal programs proliferated to assist the disabled, aged, and other special groups. In 1965 Medicare and Medicaid were developed to ensure a minimum level of health care for the aged and poor. There was considerable interest in the existing health care system in providing nursing home reimbursement through Medicare and Medicaid. The American Medical Association

lobbied to have reimbursement for extended care facilities to ease the problems that acute hospitals were experiencing; that is, clients were staying in hospitals and often no longer needed acute care services, but remained in the hospital because they lacked the means to pay for nursing home care. The owners of LTCFs also lobbied Congress to provide government funding for care in their facilities. Congress responded by including provisions for reimbursement for nursing home care in Medicare and Medicaid.

Along with funding came regulations—the standards or conditions that facilities had to meet to qualify for funds. Initially, the regulations included requirements for 24-hour licensed nursing coverage, individualized care plans, provisions for special diets, and other good standards of practice. However, only a small minority of the existing LTCFs could meet the standards at the time and protested that it would not be possible for them to participate in the Medicare and Medicaid programs. Again, with strong lobbying efforts, these conditions were waived, and facilities were able to take advantage of government reimbursement for long-term care without having to meet what were good, basic standards. (It is interesting that there was no noticeable voice from nurses, even though these facilities were called *nursing homes*.)

With eased standards and an influx of government reimbursement, the number of nursing homes grew (Table 9-1). This rapid and unregulated growth led to problems, some of which made front page headlines. Short staffing, substandard care, and abuse were among the conditions that the media exposed and that helped to generate the negative image of LTCFs that continues to shadow this care setting. The public was outraged and demanded action. In response, the Department of Health and Human Services commissioned the Institute of Medicine (IOM) to study these facilities and recommend changes. The IOM study confirmed the widespread poor quality of care that existed in LTCFs and emphasized the need to develop stricter regulations.[6] In response, highly stringent regulations were enacted under legislation called the *Omnibus Budget*

TABLE 9–1　Growth of Nursing Homes and Nursing Home Residents

Year	Number of Nursing Homes	Residents (in Thousands)
1940	1,200	25
1960	9,582	290
1970	22,004	1,076
1980	30,111	1,396
1990	14,744	1,558
2003	16,323	1,451

From National Center for Health Statistics. (2005). *Health, United States 2005, with chartbook on trends of health of Americans* (Table 116 [2001]. Nursing homes, bed occupancy, and residents according to geographic division, United States, 1995-2003). Hyattsville, Md: USDHHS.

Reconciliation Act of 1987 (OBRA) that produced profound reforms in nursing home care. Some of the protections afforded to residents of LTCFs are described on the website of the National Citizens' Coalition for Nursing Home Reform, Fact Sheet on Residents' rights, www. nccnhr.org/public/50_156_449.cfm. Both the conditions and enforcement provisions are more stringent. Facilities that do not meet the conditions described in regulations can receive sanctions that include termination of Medicare and Medicaid reimbursement. As a result of the new regulations and strict enforcement of them, conditions in LTCFs have improved.

This history can help you understand some of the reasons for the persistent negative image of LTCFs. Furthermore, it demonstrates the importance of an active role for nursing in developing new health services and clearly defining nursing services that contribute to high-quality care. Nursing leadership was sorely lacking as nursing homes grew and as non-nurses determined nursing's function, role, and staffing requirements. The results speak for themselves.

RESIDENTS OF LONG-TERM CARE FACILITIES

Residents of LTCFs can be of any age, although most are older adults. The risk of being in an LTCF increases with each decade of life; the average age of residents is 82 years. Less than one tenth of the residents are under age 65. Women outnumber men by a ratio of 3 to 1, and 90% are single or widowed. A majority of residents are white; less than 9% are black and less than 3% Hispanic.

Most residents have conditions that impair their self-care capacity or require interventions that they cannot perform independently. About one half have a progressive cognitive impairment, such as Alzheimer's disease, arthritis, cardiovascular disease, or a combination of illnesses. About 4 of every 10 residents have impaired vision, and about one third have impaired hearing. Most residents need assistance with at least several activities of daily living (ADL). Although most residents spend the remainder of their lives in the facility, an increasing number do recover, have restored function, and return to the community. In the past, some who might have remained in the hospital during recovery are now convalescing in nursing homes as a result of changes in reimbursement policies. The quality and quantity of caregiver support, rather than the medical diagnosis, determine one's risk of being admitted to an LTCF. For every resident in a nursing home, at least two equally disabled people are living in the community, receiving care from family or paid caregivers.[7] Often it is a change in status of the caregiver that precipitates the dependent person's admission to an LTCF. This reinforces the importance

of assessing the family and assisting these caregivers in using interventions and resources that promote and maintain their health and well-being.

STAFF OF LONG-TERM CARE FACILITIES

Nearly 1 million nursing employees work in LTCFs in the United States and most of these are unlicensed personnel.[17] Regulatory standards are basic, and the only specific staffing requirements in federal regulations are the following: (1) a registered nurse (RN) must be on duty at least 8 consecutive hours per day, 7 days a week; (2) a full-time director of nursing must be on staff if the facility has more than 60 beds. The proportion of other nursing staff is not stated, although it is required that "the facility provide 24-hour nursing services which are sufficient to meet total nursing care needs."[4] The fact that most direct nursing care is provided by nursing assistants presents special challenges to nurses who must supervise these caregivers.[5]

NURSING RESPONSIBILITIES

Assessment

The Minimum Data Set (MDS) is the data collected on each resident. Depending on payment sources, the facility is required to assess residents within the first 5 days again at 14 days, then at 30, 60, 90 days and continuing quarterly. Each year, or with a significant change in condition, a full MDS assessment is required. The MDS assessment is coordinated by an RN (Figure 9-1). Problems in need of care planning are generated from the information on the MDS.

As numerous as the items are on the MDS, it is not a *comprehensive* assessment; it is a *minimum* assessment. Important pieces of information are not captured, such as the client's self-concept, spirituality, sense of power, knowledge of health condition and self-care practices, sexuality, patterns of solitude, sense of purpose, immunity, stress management, use of alternative therapies, and attitudes regarding health status and death. Because these are important areas for consideration in the long-term care of residents, you may want to supplement the MDS with these additional assessment data. Although the MDS assessment tool must be formally completed periodically, high-quality care relies on the nurse's assessment of residents with every nurse-resident contact. For example, when administering a medication, you can observe the resident's coloring and respirations, note any change in mood, and ask about the status of a previous manifestation. Often residents do not have the ability to identify and report changes in their own health status, and astute nursing assessment is thus crucial. The need to be alert to changes in status is reinforced by

Resident _____ Numeric Identifier _____

MINIMUM DATA SET (MDS) — *VERSION 2.0*
FOR NURSING HOME RESIDENT ASSESSMENT AND CARE SCREENING
FULL ASSESSMENT FORM
(Status in last 7 days, unless other time frame indicated)

SECTION A. IDENTIFICATION AND BACKGROUND INFORMATION

1. RESIDENT NAME
a. (First)   b. (Middle Initial)   c. (Last)   d. (Jr./Sr.)

2. ROOM NUMBER

3. ASSESSMENT REFERENCE DATE
a. Last day of MDS observation period
Month — Day — Year
b. Original (0) or corrected copy of form (enter number of correction)

4a. DATE OF REENTRY
Date of reentry from most recent temporary discharge to a hospital in last 90 days (or since last assessment or admission if less than 90 days)
Month — Day — Year

5. MARITAL STATUS
1. Never married   3. Widowed   5. Divorced
2. Married   4. Separated

6. MEDICAL RECORD NO.

7. CURRENT PAYMENT SOURCES FOR N.H. STAY
(Billing Office to indicate; check all that apply in last 30 days)
Medicaid per diem a.
Medicare per diem b.
Medicare ancillary part A c.
Medicare ancillary part B
CHAMPUS per diem e.
VA per diem f.
Self or family pays for full per diem g.
Medicaid resident liability or Medicare co-payment h.
Private insurance per diem (including co-payment) i.
Other per diem j.

8. REASONS FOR ASSESSMENT
[Note—If this is a discharge or reentry assessment, only a limited subset of MDS items need be completed]
a. Primary reason for assessment
1. Admission assessment (required by day 14)
2. Annual assessment
3. Significant change in status assessment
4. Significant correction of prior full assessment
5. Quarterly review assessment
6. Discharged—return not anticipated
7. Discharged—return anticipated
8. Discharged prior to completing initial assessment
9. Reentry
10. Significant correction of prior quarterly assessment
0. NONE OF ABOVE
b. Codes for assessments required for Medicare PPS or the State
1. Medicare 5 day assessment
2. Medicare 30 day assessment
3. Medicare 60 day assessment
4. Medicare 90 day assessment
5. Medicare readmission/return assessment
6. Other state required assessment
7. Medicare 14 day assessment
8. Other Medicare required assessment

9. RESPONSIBILITY/ LEGAL GUARDIAN
(Check all that apply)
Legal guardian a.
Other legal oversight b.
Durable power of attorney/health care c.
Durable power of attorney/financial d.
Family member responsible e.
Patient responsible for self f.
NONE OF ABOVE g.

10. ADVANCED DIRECTIVES
(For those items with supporting documentation in the medical record, check all that apply)
Living will a.
Do not resuscitate b.
Do not hospitalize c.
Organ donation d.
Autopsy request e.
Feeding restrictions f.
Medication restrictions g.
Other treatment restrictions h.
NONE OF ABOVE i.

SECTION B. COGNITIVE PATTERNS

1. COMATOSE
(Persistent vegetative state/no discernible consciousness)
0. No   1. Yes (If yes, skip to Section G)

2. MEMORY
(Recall of what was learned or known)
a. Short-term memory OK—seems/appears to recall after 5 minutes
0. Memory OK   1. Memory problem **2**
b. Long-term memory OK—seems/appears to recall long past
0. Memory OK   1. Memory problem **2**

▢ = When box blank, must enter number or letter.

a. = When letter in box, check if condition applies

Code "—" if information unavailable or unknown

3. MEMORY/RECALL ABILITY
(Check all that resident was **normally able to recall during** last 7 days)
Current season a.
Location of own room b.
Staff names/faces c.
That he/she is in a nursing home d.
NONE OF ABOVE are recalled e.

4. COGNITIVE SKILLS FOR DAILY DECISION-MAKING
(Made decisions regarding tasks of daily life)
0. INDEPENDENT—decisions consistent/reasonable
1. MODIFIED INDEPENDENCE—some difficulty in new situations only **2**
2. MODERATELY IMPAIRED—decisions poor; cues/ supervision required **2**
3. SEVERELY IMPAIRED—never/rarely made decisions **2, 5B**

5. INDICATORS OF DELIRIUM— PERIODIC DISORDERED THINKING/ AWARENESS
(Code for behavior in the last 7 days.) [Note: Accurate assessment requires conversations with staff and family who have direct knowledge of resident's behavior over this time.]
0. Behavior not present
1. Behavior present, not of recent onset
2. Behavior present, over last 7 days appears different from resident's usual functioning (e.g., new onset or worsening)
a. EASILY DISTRACTED—(e.g., difficulty paying attention; gets sidetracked) 2 = **1, 17***
b. PERIODS OF ALTERED PERCEPTION OR AWARENESS OF SURROUNDINGS—(e.g., moves lips or talks to someone not present; believes he/she is somewhere else; confuses night and day) 2 = **1, 17***
c. EPISODES OF DISORGANIZED SPEECH—(e.g., speech is incoherent, nonsensical, irrelevant, or rambling from subject to subject; loses train of thought) 2 = **1, 17***
d. PERIODS OF RESTLESSNESS—(e.g., fidgeting or picking at skin, clothing, napkins, etc.; frequent position changes; repetitive physical movements or calling out) 2 = **1, 17***
e. PERIODS OF LETHARGY—(e.g., sluggishness; staring into space; difficult to arouse; little body movement) 2 = **1, 17***
f. MENTAL FUNCTION VARIES OVER THE COURSE OF THE DAY—(e.g., sometimes better, sometimes worse; behaviors sometimes present, sometimes not) 2 = **1, 17***

6. CHANGE IN COGNITIVE STATUS
Resident's cognitive status, skills, or abilities have changed as compared to status of 90 days ago (or since assessment if less than 90 days)
0. No change   1. Improved   2. Deteriorated **1, 17***

SECTION C. COMMUNICATION/HEARING PATTERNS

1. HEARING
(With hearing appliance, if used)
0. HEARS ADEQUATELY—normal talk, TV, phone
1. MINIMAL DIFFICULTY when not in quiet setting **4**
2. HEARS IN SPECIAL SITUATIONS ONLY—speaker has to adjust tonal quality and speak distinctly **4**
3. HIGHLY IMPAIRED/absence of useful hearing **4**

2. COMMUNICATION DEVICES/ TECHNIQUES
(Check all that apply during last 7 days)
Hearing aid, present and used a.
Hearing aid, present and not used regularly b.
Other receptive comm. techniques used (e.g., lip reading) c.
NONE OF ABOVE d.

3. MODES OF EXPRESSION
(Check all used by resident to make needs known)
Speech a.
Writing messages to express or clarify needs b.
American sign language or Braille c.
Signs/gestures/sounds d.
Communication board e.
Other f.
NONE OF ABOVE g.

4. MAKING SELF UNDERSTOOD
(Expressing information content—however able)
0. UNDERSTOOD
1. USUALLY UNDERSTOOD—difficulty finding words or finishing thoughts **4**
2. SOMETIMES UNDERSTOOD—ability is limited to making concrete requests **4**
3. RARELY/NEVER UNDERSTOOD **4**

5. SPEECH CLARITY
(Code for speech in the last 7 days)
0. CLEAR SPEECH—distinct, intelligible words
1. UNCLEAR SPEECH—slurred, mumbled words
2. NO SPEECH—absence of spoken words

6. ABILITY TO UNDERSTAND OTHERS
(Understanding verbal information content—however able)
0. UNDERSTANDS
1. USUALLY UNDERSTANDS—may miss some part/ intent of message **2, 4**
2. SOMETIMES UNDERSTANDS—responds adequately to simple, direct communication **2, 4**
3. RARELY/NEVER UNDERSTANDS **2, 4**

7. CHANGE IN COMMUNICATION/ HEARING
Resident's ability to express, understand, or hear information has changed as compared to status of 90 days ago (or since last assessment if less than 90 days)
0. No change   1. Improved   2. Deteriorated **17***

TRIGGER LEGEND
1 - Delirium
2 - Cognitive Loss/Dementia
4 - Communication
5B - ADL Maintenance
17* - Psychotropic Drugs
(For this to trigger, O4a, b, or c must = 1-7)

Form 1728RHH   © 1997 Briggs Corporation, Des Moines, IA 50306 (800) 247-2343   PRINTED IN U.S.A.
Copyright limited to addition of trigger system.

MDS 2.0 1/30/98

■ **FIGURE 9–1** Sample section of the Minimum Data Set (MDS) assessment tool for nursing home resident assessment and care screening. Other sections would include Vision Patterns, Mood and Behavior Patterns, Psychosocial Well-Being, Physical Functioning and Structural Problems, and Continence in Last 14 Days. (© 1997, Briggs Corp., West Des Moines, Iowa.)

the reality that physicians typically do not see residents on a daily basis and must rely on nurses to detect and report manifestations.

The advanced age of the residents can create challenges in assessment. Age-related changes can cause atypical manifestations in older adults. For example, instead of high fever and coughing, clinical manifestations of pneumonia in older adults may include confusion, loss of appetite, and fatigue with activities that caused no difficulties in the past. This challenges nurses to know the norms for individual residents and to identify subtle clues of illnesses so that problems can be identified early. Timely recognition and communication of manifestations to the physician can help prevent complications.

Care Planning

Regulations require that a care plan be written for each resident within 7 days after completion of the assessment. The care plan is an *interdisciplinary* one; nurses coordinate the input offered by each discipline and ensure that the plan is written in a correct, timely manner (Box 9-1). To the extent possible, the resident and the family should actively participate in the development of the care plan.

A care plan is not merely a paperwork requirement but a working tool to guide nursing actions; it is a blueprint for nursing actions. Goals and actions that are no longer relevant need to be revised. All members of the team, particularly nursing assistants who perform most direct care activities, must be familiar with the care plan. Typically, it is the nurse's responsibility to review the care plan with unlicensed caregivers to ensure they understand the actions that must be implemented and the observations that must be reported.

Caregiving

The direct caregiving role of nurses varies from facility to facility. In some LTCFs, nurses perform selected roles, such as administering medications and treatments; in others, they may be involved in total care activities.

BOX 9-1 Characteristics of an Effective Care Plan

- Is based on needs as identified in the Minimum Data Set assessment tool
- Contains goals and actions to address current needs and to prevent new problems
- States goals that are realistic, clear, specific, and measurable
- Lists actions that are related to each goal that include discipline responsible for implementation and specific directions
- Is accessible to and used by all caregivers
- Is evaluated at least quarterly and revised as necessary, especially when a significant change in condition occurs

---

During the pre-employment interview, nurses should review the job descriptions for their specific positions to ensure that they have a realistic view of their role.

In addition to caregiving activities that might be performed in any setting (e.g., medication administration, treatments), special nursing support is required by residents and their families as they adjust to the LTCF. Few individuals have had experiences that prepared them for living in or having a loved one in a nursing home. Residents and their families face many adjustments.

Environment

Many people have lived in the same home for several decades before admission and could probably locate objects in their homes blindfolded. When moved into an LTCF, they are faced with adapting to the layout of a new setting and other new components of their environment, such as paging systems, odors, and sounds. They no longer have ready access to their own refrigerator (if they are hungry) or to a spare bedroom (where a grandchild can spend the night). Their personal space has shrunk to a bed, a few chairs, a closet, and several drawers. People can enter their space and invade their privacy at any hour of the day or night. Therefore it is extremely important to respect resident's environment as the LTCF becomes, in effect, their home.

Routines

New residents soon learn that they must adjust to facility routines and schedules. They may have to take a morning shower, although they may have taken a bedtime bath for more than 70 years. They may have a full breakfast placed before them at 8:00 AM when they seldom ate a bite of food before noon. After decades of staying awake and listening to the radio until 2:00 AM, they are told that "lights out" is 9:00 PM. Residents have rights however, and it is a challenge for LTC staff to adjust to the resident as much as it is for the resident to adjust to the LTCF.

People

After years of being on a first-name basis with neighbors, store clerks, the mail carrier, and the auto repairman, residents must learn a cast of new players. In addition to meeting other residents, they may meet at least three nurses and three nursing assistants who will care for them over a 24-hour period, the facility's medical director, administrator, social worker, housekeeper, dietitian, activities therapist, clergy, and several therapists. They must learn not only the names but also the roles of these people and how to communicate with them.

Independence

Despite a staff's best efforts to afford residents the right to make decisions, there is a loss of independence when people become residents of a nursing home. They cannot scramble an egg in the middle of the night, have a friend stay over for a few days, or paint the walls the color of their choice. They must report their whereabouts and needs to staff, and they depend on others for the basics of bringing them food and taking them to the toilet.

These adjustments also affect family members at the same time that they are facing their own changing roles and responsibilities in regard to their relationship with the resident. Both residents and their families can experience such reactions as anxiety, depression, anger, helplessness, withdrawal, grief, and inattention to self-care practices. You can protect the health of residents and their families and facilitate a positive adjustment to the LTCF by taking some of the actions described in Box 9-2.

During caregiving activities, make sure that *holistic care* is provided; such care implies that every aspect—body, mind, spirit—is being addressed. This integration of body, mind, and spirit results in more powerful and meaningful care than if each aspect was addressed separately. Some ways in which holistic nursing is demonstrated are listed in Box 9-3.

Communication

As mentioned earlier, the LTCF nurse carries significant responsibility for identifying and obtaining timely treatment of complications and new health problems. Because of their regular and close contact with residents, nursing assistants may be the first and only caregivers to detect changes in health status (e.g., a developing pressure ulcer or a change in eating pattern); therefore effective channels of communication are crucial in reporting these findings. Conducting rounds, reading what has been documented, and asking specific questions are among the measures you can use to learn about a resident's condition.

You also must make sure that physicians learn of changes in a resident's condition in a timely manner. Documenting in a resident's record is not necessarily sufficient, particularly because most attending physicians do not visit LTCF residents on a daily basis and seldom have the time to scan all notations when they do visit. You must promptly communicate any changes and relevant information (e.g., abnormal laboratory results, family complaints) to physicians.

Between their scheduled visits to the facility, physicians may generate new orders, which often are

---

BOX 9-2 Helping New Residents and Families

1. Learn about the unique characteristics of each resident.
   a. Besides determining the health conditions of residents, explore who they are as people and what kind of lives they have lived.
   b. Engage residents and families in conversations about residents' histories.
   c. Complete a Profile Poster similar to the one shown below to help staff and other residents learn about the unique backgrounds of residents and who they are as individuals.
2. Identify residents' needs, preferences, and level of physical and mental function.
   a. Assess how well residents can meet their activities of daily living and the assistance they need.
   b. Ask about their preferences in regard to food likes and dislikes, sleep and nap habits, bathing, and other activities.
   c. Incorporate findings into their plan of care.
3. Explain and educate.
   a. Orient residents and families to the layout of the facility, staff, routines, and activities.
   b. Explain procedures before doing them.
   c. Be available to discuss residents' and families' concerns and to answer questions.
4. Promote maximum independence.
   a. Encourage residents to do as much for themselves as possible.
   b. Explain to residents and families the value of residents being independent.
   c. Give residents opportunities to make decisions regarding their care and activities.
5. Make residents and families feel comfortable.
   a. Be courteous and patient; understand that the stress associated with admission can cause residents and family members to make demands, complain, ask many questions, and forget what they have been told.
   b. Provide privacy during visitation.
   c. Inform families of the location of visitor lounges, cafeteria, and vending machines.
6. Be holistic.
   a. Being holistic means that we are concerned with the whole person: body, mind, and spirit.
   b. Try to help residents meet physical, emotional, social, and spiritual needs to promote their physical, emotional, social, and spiritual health.

PROFILE POSTER

Name: *Mary Auchmeyer Luggi*   Photos of resident and
Recent home: *New York City*   family can be added
Childhood home: *Frankfurt, Germany*
Schools attended: *New York City College*
Spouse's name: *Gus Luggi (deceased)*
Occupation: *High school home economics teacher*
Children: *Son: Gus Luggi Jr, Daughter: Emily Smythe*
Grandchildren: *Tom 21, Amelia 19, Gus 15, Ginny 14, Sammie 13*
Hobbies, interests: *Quilting, baseball, singing*
Other tidbits: *Travelled on several missionary trips to India, speaks German, Italian, and French*

From Eliopoulos, C. (1997). Helping new residents and families. *Long-Term Care Educator, 8*(12), 6.

BOX 9-3   Holistic Nursing in Long-Term Care Facilities

Nurses can promote holistic care in long-term care facilities by:

- Assisting residents to achieve a higher potential of functioning
- Supporting residents in their efforts to promote health and prevent complications
- Learning about the unique life stories of residents
- Ensuring that residents receive care that is consistent with their values and beliefs and respecting cultural differences
- Aiding residents and families in discovering meaning in health status and in life and death
- Strengthening residents' abilities to live in harmony with their health condition
- Assisting residents in maintaining their connections with family, friends, and the community within and outside the facility
- Helping residents boost their natural healing abilities
- Facilitating hope and a sense of purpose in residents' lives
- Supporting residents as they respond to their spiritual identity or relate to a higher power
- Providing a nurturing and healing caregiving environment
- Offering opportunities for residents to experience joy and satisfaction
- Protecting residents from threats to their health or well-being, and promoting highest quality of life
- Adhering to accepted standards of nursing practice

From Eliopoulos, C. (2002). *Nursing administration of long-term care facilities* (6th ed.). Glen Arm, Md: Health Education Network.

communicated by telephone. Facilities may differ in regard to the personnel who can accept telephone orders; therefore it is best to check with the individual facility's policy.

The following should be done to promote safety in telephone orders:

1. **Provide the physician with complete information that can aid in medical decision-making (e.g., clinical manifestations, current and usual vital signs, prescribed medications, unusual incidents, and other relevant facts).**
2. **Avoid making a medical diagnosis. Report clinical signs and allow the physician to make a medical judgment.**
3. **Take the order directly from the prescribing physician, not through office staff.**
4. **Repeat the order; if possible, have the physician Fax a copy of the written order.**
5. **Have the order signed within 24 hours.**
6. **If there is anything that seems inappropriate about the order, question the physician. If the response from the attending physician still leaves doubt, consult with the facility's medical director and director of nursing**

Management

Nurses hold a variety of administrative and managerial positions in LTCFs, such as director of nursing, assistant director of nursing, supervisor, unit manager or head nurse, charge nurse, and staffing coordinator. Even if they do not hold these formal titles, most LTCF nurses must perform some management functions, such as the following:

- Delegating assignments
- Supervising other staff
- Evaluating performance
- Implementing disciplinary actions
- Completing reports
- Reviewing and auditing records
- Communicating needs to other departments
- Investigating, reporting, and recording incidents and accidents
- Handling complaints
- Ordering supplies
- Communicating with insurers, regulatory agencies, and other parties

To manage effectively, your knowledge and skills must exceed those used in clinical nursing activities. You must be knowledgeable of regulations, reimbursement programs, and legal aspects of nursing practice and employee-employer relations. You must also be skillful in assertiveness, coaching, counseling, accurate documentation, organization, time management, and communication.

OTHER FORMS OF LONG-TERM CARE

This chapter has focused on the role of nurses in the LTCF. However, the LTCF is only one part of the long-term care system, and other forms of long-term care are available, such as those in the following list. Other forms of long-term care and the resources to find them are presented on the website with this text:

1. *Subacute or transitional care* is for people who require ongoing care or recovery for an acute condition but do not need to receive the services on an acute hospital unit. The subacute care unit can be separate parts of a hospital or nursing home, or it can be an entire facility dedicated to this purpose.
2. *Assisted living community* is a form of housing that provides 24-hour staffing, meals, supervision of medications, and personal care assistance.
3. *Adult day care* is a daytime program for people who typically have the same level of impairments as nursing home residents but who receive care in the community, usually by family members. The client is transported to the center and receives

structured activities, meals, personal care assistance, and health care supervision.

4. *Home care* is for community-based people who are homebound and who need caregiving assistance or special treatments.

5. *Hospice* is for people who are terminally ill and in need of care. This care can be provided in the home, LTCF, or in a day hospital setting. Care of the dying is a common experience in long-term care. Caring behaviors of the staff at the time of death, allowing the family to be involved with the resident, and providing spiritual support are important and valued nursing functions.[18]

Each of these types of care has unique regulations and conditions for reimbursement.

CONCLUSIONS

The roles and responsibilities of nurses in LTCFs are varied and complex. Residents possess a wide range of physical and mental conditions that require expert assessment, interventions, and monitoring. The inability of many residents to accurately express their needs and age-related alterations in the presentation of clinical manifestations present special challenges in detecting changes in status. The absence of physicians in the facility on a daily basis places a greater responsibility on nurses to identify and seek treatment of residents' problems. The high proportion of unlicensed staff demands that nurses be effective managers. An abundance of regulatory and reimbursement requirements demand that nurses be knowledgeable of these topics.

The reality that most residents not only will receive care but also will *live* in the facility for the remainder of their lives causes nurses often to serve as surrogate family. Very few practice settings offer nurses the opportunity to fill such a wide and varied range of roles. Rather than a simple, repetitive practice setting, LTCFs challenge nurses to use a wide range of knowledge and skills as they establish meaningful long-term relationships with residents and their families. To fill the roles and responsibilities competently, LTCF nurses must be among their profession's best.

BIBLIOGRAPHY

  Citations appearing in red refer to primary research.

1. Colon-Emeric, C., Schenck, A., Gorospe, J., et al. (2006). Translating evidence-based falls prevention into clinical practice in nursing facilities: Results and lessons from a quality improvement collaborative. *Journal of the American Geriatrics Society, 54*(9), 1414-1418.

2. Eliopoulos, C. (1999). *Integrating alternative and conventional therapies: Holistic care for chronic conditions.* St. Louis: Mosby.

3. Eliopoulos, C. (2002). *Nursing administration of long-term care facilities* (6th ed.). Glen Arm, Md: Health Education Network.

4. Eliopoulos, C. (1998). *Transforming nursing homes into healing centers: A holistic model for long-term care* (p. 48). Glen Arm, Md: Health Education Network.

5. Federal Register. (1989). Rules and Regulations (Vol. 54, No. 21). Section 483.26(c) Feb 2, 1989.

6. Hall, L.M., & O'Brien-Pallas, L. (2000). Redesigning nursing work in long-term-care environments. *Nursing Economic$, 18*(2), 79-87.

7. Institute of Medicine, Committee on Implications of For-Profit Enterprise in Health Care. (1986). Profits and health care: An introduction to the issues. In B.H. Gray (Ed.), *For-profit enterprise in health care* (pp. 3-18). Washington, DC: National Academy Press.

8. Kane, R.L., & Kane, R.A. (1997). Long-term care. In C.K. Cassel, et al. (Eds.), *Geriatric medicine* (3rd ed., pp. 81-96). New York: Springer.

9. Kemper, P. (2003). Long term care research and policy. *The Gerontologist, 43*, 436-446.

10. Lawrence, C. (1905). *History of the Philadelphia almshouses and hospitals* (pp. 52, 123). Privately printed.

11. Mezey, M.D. (2006). *The encyclopedia of elder care* (2nd ed.). New York: Springer.

12. National Committee to Preserve Social Security and Medicare. (1997). *Nurse staffing in nursing homes: Viewpoint.* Legislative Agenda for the 105th Congress, April 1997.

13. Nay, R. (1998). Contradictions between perceptions and practices of caring in long-term care of elderly people. *Journal of Clinical Nursing, 7*(5), 401-408.

14. Rice, V.H. (1997). Ethical issues relative to autonomy and personal control in independent and cognitively impaired elders. *Nursing Outlook, 45*, 27-34.

15. Rosenberg, C.E. (1987). *The care of strangers: The rise of America's hospital system.* New York: Basic Books.

16. Ross, M.M., et al. (2001). Family caregiving in long-term-care facilities. *Clinical Nursing Research, 10*(4), 347-368.

17. Simmons, S.F., & Patel, A.V. (2006). Nursing home staff delivery of oral liquid nutritional supplements to residents at risk for unintentional weight loss. *Journal of the American Geriatrics Society, 54*(9), 1372-1376.

18. Strang, V.R., Koop, P.M., Duprui-Blanchard, D., et al. (2006). Family caregivers and transition to long-term care. *Clinical Nursing Research, 15*(91), 27-45.

19. Thomas, W.H. (1996). *Life worth living. How someone you love can still enjoy life in a nursing home. The Eden Alternative in action.* Acton, Mass: VanderWyk & Burnham.

20. Thurmond, J.A. (1999). Nurses' perceptions of chemical restraint use in long-term care. *Applied Nursing Research, 12*(3), 159-162.

21. U.S. Department of Commerce. (2001). Table 175: Nursing homes—Selected characteristics: 1985 to 1999. *Statistical Abstract of the United States: 2001* (121st ed., p. 116). Washington, DC: Bureau of the Census.

22. Wilson, S.A., & Daley, B.J. (1999). Family perspectives on dying in long-term-care settings. *Journal of Gerontological Nursing, 25*(11), 19-25.

23. Woods, D.L., Craven, R.F., & Whitney, J. (2005). The effect of therapeutic touch on behavioral symptoms of persons with dementia. *Alternative Therapies in Health and Medicine, 11*(1), 66-74.

evolve **Did you remember to check out the bonus material on the Evolve website and the CD-ROM, including NCLEX®-Examination Style Review Questions, Open-Book Quizzes, and Chapter Review Audio Podcasts?**

http://evolve.elsevier.com/Black/medsurg

CHAPTER 10

Rehabilitation

SUSAN L. DEAN-BAAR

Advances in science and technology are having a dramatic impact on health care as the population continues to live longer but with an increasing number of chronic conditions. Concurrent changes in health policy and the financing of health care delivery are decreasing the length of stays in acute care settings. The cumulative effect of these changes is resulting in an increasing number of clients requiring rehabilitation services after an episode of acute care. These rehabilitation services can be provided in a variety of settings. Today's nurse who is caring for clients on a medical-surgical unit needs to be familiar with the rehabilitation component of the continuum of care in order to make the appropriate referrals and prepare clients for the rehabilitation experience.

On the surface, rehabilitation settings can look much the same as acute care settings. The philosophy of these settings, however, differs significantly. In today's health care environment it is important to prepare clients and families for this change so that they can interpret provider behaviors correctly. In acute care settings clients are viewed as individuals with an illness that needs to be either cured or controlled through symptom management, and the focus is predominantly on the current episode of care. In contrast, the focus of health care providers in rehabilitation settings is to support individuals and family members in learning skills that will assist them to live with a chronic illness or disability. This difference in approach is not always easy for clients and families to see, especially when a client receives both acute care and rehabilitation care in the same hospital. When a client is transferred from one care unit to another and both units have similar physical characteristics and room layouts, it becomes critical that the client understands the differences in routines and expectations between care settings. This chapter provides an overview of important rehabilitation principles and concepts that can assist clients and their families in making a successful transition from the acute care phase of the health care continuum to the rehabilitation phase.

Rehabilitation is an interdisciplinary specialty that supports a dynamic process of helping an individual to achieve a life that is as independent and self-fulfilling as desired in the physical, emotional, psychological, social, or vocational areas of functioning. *Rehabilitation nursing* is defined as "the diagnosis and treatment of human responses of individuals and groups to actual or potential health problems relative to altered functional ability and lifestyle."[1]

WORLD HEALTH ORGANIZATION FRAMEWORK

The World Health Organization's *International Classification of Functioning, Disability, and Health (ICF)*[17] provides a framework for the description of health and health-related states that benefit from rehabilitation services. The ICF framework describes the relationship between body functions and structures, activities, participation, environmental factors, and personal factors (Figure 10-1). A review of the definitions of each of these components is important because these terms may be used differently in other areas. The ICF defines *body functions* as the physiologic functions of body systems and includes psychological functions. *Body structures* are the anatomic parts of the body, such as organs and limbs and their components. *Impairments* are problems in body function or structure that deviate significantly

---

evolve **Web Enhancements**

Appendix A   Religious Beliefs and Practices Affecting Health Care

Be sure to check out the bonus material on the Evolve website and the CD-ROM, including free self-assessment exercises. **http://evolve.elsevier. com/Black/medsurg**

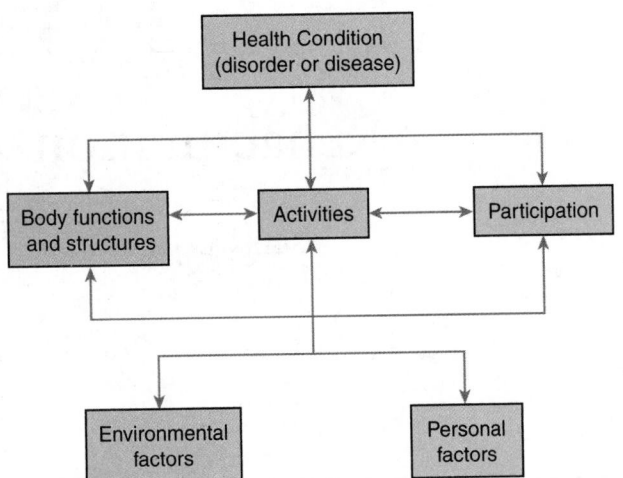

■ FIGURE 10–1 Interactions between the components of the International Classification of Functioning, Disability, and Health. *(From World Health Organization. [2001]. International classification of functioning, disability, and health [ICF]. Geneva, Switzerland: World Health Organization.)*

from the expected norm. Impairments can have different characteristics and may be slight or severe; temporary or permanent; intermittent or continuous; and progressive, regressive, or static. *Activities* are the execution of a task or action by an individual, and *participation* is involvement in a life situation. In the ICF model environmental and personal components are contextual factors that can impact an individual's health status. *Environmental factors* are the external physical, social, and attitudinal factors that can positively or negatively influence an individual's capacity to perform functions. The impacted functions may be at the body function or structure level, the individual level, or a societal level. Personal factors are the non–health condition features of an individual's life, such as gender, race, age, lifestyle habits, education, behavior, and character style.

The ICF provides a framework that shows the importance of a comprehensive assessment to determine the impact that a health condition or disease may have on an individual. A wide variation in impairment may occur as a result of changes to body function or structure. The degree to which activities and participation are affected can be influenced significantly by contextual, environmental, and personal factors. When impairments lead to a decreased ability to engage in activities and participation, the individual may benefit from rehabilitation services. The results of a comprehensive assessment would assist in determining the level of rehabilitation services required and the setting in which the services would be best provided.

REHABILITATION SETTINGS

Rehabilitation services are provided in a variety of settings, depending on the array and intensity of services that are required. Individuals with an impairment that minimally impacts functional ability may be able to receive rehabilitation services in an outpatient setting. More complex impairments may require services that can be provided in the home setting or in a day treatment program. Individuals with impairments that affect multiple functional abilities may require a period of inpatient rehabilitation services in either a subacute or an acute rehabilitation setting. Acute rehabilitation may be provided in freestanding rehabilitation hospitals or on dedicated units within hospitals. Subacute rehabilitation may be provided in long-term care facilities or on dedicated units within hospitals. Each type of setting has clear admission and discharge criteria to assist with determining the most appropriate placement for a client. As in other areas of health care, the trend has been toward shorter lengths of inpatient rehabilitation stays and the use of more community-based rehabilitation services.[2]

Current Medicare regulations require that at least 75% of clients admitted to an acute Medicare-certified rehabilitation unit have a diagnosis listed in Box 10-1. These diagnoses are the first criteria, and even if the client has one of these diagnoses, additional criteria may be required. For instance, not all clients who have had joint replacement can be admitted to an acute rehabilitation unit. A client with a joint replacement would also have to be age 85 or older, or have bilateral joint replacements, or have a body mass index of at least 50. If one of these additional criteria was not present, then the client would need to receive rehabilitation in a subacute or outpatient rehabilitation setting. Medicare revised the criteria for admission to acute inpatient rehabilitation in April 2004; the new criteria are being implemented and are expected to be fully integrated by 2008. In addition to the diagnosis requirement, Medicare requires that a

---

BOX 10-1 Conditions Suited for Admission to Medicare Facilities

- Stroke
- Spinal cord injury
- Congenital deformity
- Amputation
- Major multiple trauma
- Fracture of the femur (hip fracture)
- Brain injury
- Neurologic disorders including multiple sclerosis, motor neuron diseases, polyneuropathy, muscular dystrophy, and Parkinson's disease
- Burns
- Joint replacement
- Osteoarthritis
- Active polyarticular rheumatoid arthritis (including psoriatic arthritis and seronegative arthropathies)
- Systemic vasculitides

client be able to participate actively in at least 3 hours of therapy a day and need at least two therapeutic modalities in addition to rehabilitation nursing and medicine.

REHABILITATION GOALS

The Association of Rehabilitation Nurses defines the goal of rehabilitation nursing as "to assist the individual who has a disability and/or chronic illness in restoring, maintaining, and promoting his or her maximal health."[1] Achievement of this goal requires nurses to practice with the following foci. Rehabilitation is a client-centered approach to achieving a maximum level of functioning and self-sufficiency in all spheres of life: physical, mental, social, emotional, educational, vocational, and economic. The emphasis is on abilities and developing methods for functional substitution where appropriate. Rehabilitation is not time specific but rather an ongoing process that may include periods of intense focus. Inherent within rehabilitation is a great deal of learning or relearning of a variety of life activities to support participation in life situations. Achieving the goal of rehabilitation requires nurses to focus on an optimal level of wellness and prevention of complications, which requires early intervention in the illness stage to limit disabling effects and conditions. In all phases of health care, it is crucial to assist the client and family in understanding the health condition that has led to functional impairments and the relationship of wellness-focused interventions (e.g., nutrition, exercise, physical activity) to learning how to manage the chronic illness or disability. An additional focus important to achieving the goal of rehabilitation is a return to and successful functioning within the community. This focus must include a realistic appraisal of the client's potential functional ability and interdependence with family, the environment, and social institutions. Identifying options and alternatives available for participation in activities that are important to the individual may play a large role in returning the client to the community. A final major focus to include in determining how to fulfill the goal of rehabilitation is the need to understand what an acceptable quality of life is for each client. Each individual brings a personal perspective to defining an acceptable quality of life, and the rehabilitation process is facilitated when nurses and the health care team understand the meaning and important aspects of quality of life for a specific client.

When taken together, these goals foster an individual's ability to self-manage chronic illness or disability. The process of self-management is aimed at bringing order to the daily life of the individual. Four themes have been identified as part of the self-management process.[6] The first is the individual's ability to recognize and manage the boundaries of the illness and its impact on daily life. Learning how to recognize and manage the effects of fatigue and pain are examples of this theme. The second theme is the process of mobilizing psychological, physical, and behavioral resources in a way that maximizes wellness. The third theme focuses on managing the disruptions and shift in self-identity that occur frequently in living with a chronic illness or disability. The fourth theme is related to the ongoing efforts needed to balance, pace, plan, and prioritize numerous activities and efforts of both normal daily life and aspects of the illness. Several key principles emerge from the goal and foci of rehabilitation.

KEY PRINCIPLES IN REHABILITATION

Rehabilitation is *client centered* and de-emphasizes the medical diagnosis and the disciplines that may be involved in the treatment of the client. The client and the unique needs of the client are the focus; the rehabilitation plan is built on that focus. Health professionals provide expertise to the client and family and respect the client's ultimate right to make decisions regarding outcomes and the interventions to support achievement of outcomes. Families and significant others are an integral part of achieving client-centered care. Early assessment to identify the role family members will play in the post–acute care and rehabilitation life of the client will allow the health care team to ensure that family members are prepared with the skills and knowledge that will be needed.

Rehabilitation is also a *goal-oriented approach* to care. Individual goals are determined in conjunction with the client and the rehabilitation teams' professional expertise. Preadmission assessments are completed to ascertain the existence of reasonable goals that could be accomplished through participation in rehabilitation.

Goals are established to support the individual's improvement in *functional ability*. The rehabilitation process focuses on the functional presentation of the individual and on developing an individualized approach to maximize functional abilities by training, retraining, and the use of adaptive equipment. The focus on functional ability extends beyond physical functioning and also addresses functioning in areas such as social, emotional, and vocational issues. Assessment of functional ability and evaluation of the potential for improvement are essential components in determining an individual's potential for rehabilitation.

A common assessment tool used in clinical practice to determine an individual's level of functional ability is the Functional Independence Measures (FIM).[4] The FIM includes an assessment of 18 areas of functioning related to self-care, sphincter management, transfers, locomotion, communication, and social cognition. Each area is assessed using a seven-point scale ranging from total dependence (1) to total independence

(7). A maximum score of 126 would indicate total independence in all areas. The conceptual basis of the FIM has been incorporated into the Inpatient Rehabilitation Facility-Patient Assessment Instrument (IRF-PAI), which is the required uniform assessment tool completed for all Medicare clients admitted to acute rehabilitation settings.

Rehabilitation is provided using a *team approach*. The team comprises health care professionals who assist the client in developing and maintaining progress toward realistic goals. Box 10-2 identifies the members of the rehabilitation team. The only constant on any rehabilitation team is the client. All other members of the team vary depending on the needs of the client. The team approach to rehabilitation requires the coordination and cooperation of a variety of professionals with different areas of expertise. Teams can be described as having multidisciplinary, interdisciplinary, or transdisciplinary characteristics.[9] All three types of teams include members that are relevant to the care of the client. In a multidisciplinary team the members complete discipline-specific evaluations of and goals for the client. There is little cross-disciplinary planning, and communication between team members focuses on sharing of information about the activities of each discipline. Interdisciplinary teams include collaboration among the members on the team. The entire team sets client goals, and then each discipline develops a plan for how each will contribute to the achievement of those goals. Transdisciplinary teams identify a primary therapist who is responsible for implementing the plan of care for a client. Transdisciplinary team members show evidence of several unique attributes, including role extension, role enrichment, role expansion, and role release.[13] Other team members provide information to the primary therapist, whose role it is to provide many of the therapies that the client requires. The boundaries of specific disciplines are blurred in a transdisciplinary team. Flexibility, cross-training, and good communication are essential to the effective use of a transdisciplinary team model. This model of care can be very effective for clients who require longer-term rehabilitation and a smaller number of health care providers with whom to interact, for example, clients with significant cognitive sequelae following a traumatic brain injury.

A successful rehabilitation experience requires attention to how the client and the client's family define an acceptable *quality of life*. Quality of life is influenced by numerous personal factors that must be identified and discussed to establish a rehabilitation plan of care. This plan should facilitate the maintenance or restoration of an acceptable quality of life that recognizes the uniqueness and wholeness of each individual. Research in quality of life for individuals with chronic illness has identified numerous factors that must be taken into consideration.[14] Health and functional issues include perception of the intrusive nature of manifestations, psychological and spiritual issues, social and economic issues (e.g., emotional support, cultural life, employment, and financial factors), and family issues. These aspects of living with a chronic illness or disability must be considered when discussing quality of life with clients and families.

Rehabilitation also includes a *health promotion and wellness* focus. For many clients engaged in rehabilitation, it is not realistic to plan for a return to perfect health and an absence of illness. The focus becomes one of achieving the highest level of wellness possible. This is accomplished through maintaining, restoring, and promoting healthy lifestyles in a manner that recognizes all aspects of the client's health: physical, emotional, psychological, and spiritual. Health promotion and wellness is facilitated when interventions are included in the acute care setting to prevent and minimize complications such as pressure sores, decreased range of motion, and deconditioning.

The trajectory of many chronic illnesses and disabilities is one of continuous *change*. Coping with change is an innate characteristic of living with a chronic illness or disability. Acknowledgment of this phenomenon can be helpful to clients and families when coupled with assurance that one benefit of rehabilitation is the development of skills and knowledge that will assist with managing the many changes experienced over the trajectory of most chronic illnesses and disabilities. Most nurses and health care providers interact with clients and families at only one point of the health care delivery system. Providing care at each point in the system that acknowledges an awareness of the total trajectory and includes interventions to assist clients and their families in developing the skills needed to manage changes in their health conditions will enhance both clients' and family's abilities to cope with changes successfully.

BOX 10-2 Rehabilitation Team Members

- Client
- Family
- Registered nurse
- Physicians (physiatrists and others)
- Physical therapist
- Occupational therapist
- Speech/language pathologist
- Audiologist
- Psychologist
- Social worker
- Recreational therapist
- Vocational rehabilitation counselor
- Respiratory therapist
- Dietitian
- Chaplain
- Orthotist/prosthetist
- Insurance case manager

All people diagnosed with a chronic illness or disability will experience a psychological reaction to this change in their lives. Nurses play an important role in supporting clients and families through the *coping and adjustment* process. Each client will have a unique response that will be influenced by many personal and contextual factors. Winterhalter[16] describes the advantages of using a stage model as a theoretical base for understanding the reactions that may be observed and the interventions that are most appropriate for each stage. Mauk[8] has studied the experience of individuals who have had a stroke and has identified a six-phase process to describe the reactions and the interventions appropriate for each phase. The phases are described as agonizing, fantasizing, realizing, blending, framing, and owning. All of the staging models recognize that each client and family member will travel through an experience differently. The various responses and stages that are commonly described may or may not be present for each individual, and the intensity or length of each response can vary widely from one client to another. An individual's response may be influenced by the meaning of the event to him or her, past coping experiences, and others' reactions to the event. Common responses include denial, grieving, uncertainty, hopelessness, hopefulness, and eventual adaptation to the condition.

An understanding of the role that *culture* plays in the rehabilitation experience for clients is also needed. Cultural competence in rehabilitation nursing includes cultural awareness, cultural knowledge, cultural encounters, cultural skills, and cultural desire.[3] The provision of culturally sensitive care will enhance the ability of the rehabilitation process to achieve the predetermined rehabilitation goals. In rehabilitation settings it is important to assess the client's values regarding independence and self-care to establish an appropriate plan of care.[5]

A pivotal concept in rehabilitation is *client and family education*. In rehabilitation, this is a collaborative process among all members of the team that must be accomplished in partnership with the client and family. Several recent studies found a discrepancy in the perception of health care providers and clients and families in the effectiveness of current efforts in client education. Smith and Testani-Dufour[15] identified the need to individualize the teaching methods used to accommodate personal factors of the learner even when standardized materials have been developed. Pierce, Finn, and Steiner[11] found that families and registered nurses had very different expectations and priorities about what areas should be included in education after stroke. Paterson, Kieloch, and Gmiterek[10] report that families have limited recollection of teaching that has occurred by members of the rehabilitation team. They suggest that there are many reasons that such a discrepancy exists between what providers have documented has been taught and what

family members recall being taught. These reasons include the manner in which the content was taught, the relevance of the content to the learner, and the family's emotional state at the time the teaching occurred. These are very real constraints that providers face in today's health care systems.

To optimize the effectiveness of client and family teaching, education must be designed, delivered, and reinforced in ways that are accessible and meaningful. Education needs to be present in appropriate levels and formats at all levels of the health care system so that it is available whenever the learner is ready to learn.

REHABILITATION PROCESS

The rehabilitation process can be affected by many factors, including the attitudes of the client, the client's family, and members of the rehabilitation team; financial resources; environmental barriers; the availability of community resources; and educational and occupational barriers. The rehabilitation process involves the creative talents of various disciplines to develop a planned sequence of services designed to meet the unique needs of each client in a manner that maximizes the contributions of each member of the team.

The assessment phase of the rehabilitation process requires an initial focused assessment to determine whether a client would benefit from rehabilitation services and, if so, what would be the most appropriate setting for provision of those services. The decision about the most appropriate setting to provide rehabilitation will be determined by analyzing the client's needs and medical stability, the client's therapy needs, the services offered in that setting, the intensity and skill level of the needed nursing services, the gap between the client's current functional level and the level realistically thought to be achievable as a result of rehabilitation, and the location of the setting. Once a determination has been made that rehabilitation services are appropriate, an in-depth assessment is completed by each member of the rehabilitation team who will be involved in the provision of services for that client. The areas commonly included in this assessment are physical, functional ability, psychological, emotional, cognitive, mental status, social support, behavioral, communication, financial, previous patterns of coping, and family. Factors that may influence discharge and transition planning are identified early in the rehabilitation process.

On completion of the assessment, a set of goals and anticipated outcomes are established for the client and family and a plan is established for the achievement of those goals. Within the plan will be interventions directed at restoring lost functional abilities, promoting client and family adjustment and adaptation to the new health status and level of functioning, preventing secondary complications, and adapting the discharge environment to support the client's level of functional ability. Throughout implementation of the rehabilitation plan of care, ongoing evaluation of progress toward goals will occur. Team conferences are a standard part of comprehensive rehabilitation programs. The frequency at which team conferences occur is dictated by the setting where the client is receiving care and the requirements of the insurance or payer.

Transitions from one level of care to another can be stressful for clients and families. Without anticipatory guidance before the transfer to a rehabilitation setting, a client making the transition from an acute care setting to a rehabilitation setting might view the differences in routine in the rehabilitation setting as disturbing. Nurses and therapists often encourage the client to perform his or her own care in an effort to gain independence. This process may require that the client struggles to get the task accomplished and can lead to perception that the care being provided by the staff is not adequate, especially when compared to an acute care setting. It is important that both the client and family understand the purpose of rehabilitation is to gain independence and that independence does not happen if the client remains in a dependent role. The client or family might perceive encouragement from a nurse or a therapist in the rehabilitation setting to be independent with some aspect of daily care as poor quality of care if adequate orientation has not occurred to explain the differences in philosophy between the acute care and the rehabilitation setting.

Another stressful transition can be the discharge from the rehabilitation setting to home or other community setting. Clients and families are often not secure in their ability to use the new skills and knowledge that they have gained as a result of rehabilitation. Clients and caregivers may feel overwhelmed by the amount of information they have been given and be fearful of their ability to manage all aspects of care still needed after discharge. Anticipatory guidance regarding the stress of caregiving should also be provided to families and caregivers. Caregivers benefit from being aware that the strain and burden of caregiving can result in financial, physical, psychological, emotional, and social problems. Caregivers have identified a number of problems as they assume responsibility for care of a family member. These include difficulties associated with the level of dependence encountered even after rehabilitation, the lack of awareness by the ill family member of the level of dependence, coping with emotions in both the caregiver and the receiver, disturbances in sleep, the need to simultaneously manage other health problems, communication problems, and balancing it all.[12] It is critical for clients and families to have appropriate resources and referrals in place to ensure the most successful possible transition to the community. Lutz[7] found that the most significant factor in determining whether a client could be discharged to the community from a rehabilitation setting was how well the client's needs matched informal caregiving resources, including social support networks that were available to the family and caregivers.

CONCLUSIONS

Rehabilitation is needed by an increasing number of individuals because of the ability to live a longer, productive life with multiple chronic conditions. Nurses in acute care settings have an important role in identifying clients who will benefit from rehabilitation services. Nurses and other health care providers who understanding the rehabilitation process can help to minimize the fragmentation in care that clients sometimes feel in today's health care delivery system. Preparation for and discussion about rehabilitation and incorporation of basic rehabilitation principles in acute care will assist with a smooth transition for clients and families.

BIBLIOGRAPHY

 Citations appearing in red refer to primary research.

1. Association of Rehabilitation Nurses. (2000). *Standards and scope of rehabilitation nursing practice.* Glenview, Ill: Author.
2. Buchanan, L.C., & Neal, L.J. (2002). Community-based rehabilitation. In S. Hoeman (Ed.), *Rehabilitation nursing: Process, application, & outcomes* (3rd ed.). St. Louis: Mosby.
3. Campinha-Bacote, J. (2001). A model of practice to address cultural competence in rehabilitation nursing. *Rehabilitation Nursing, 26,* 8-11.
4. Deutsch, A., Braun, S., & Granger, C. (1997). The functional independence measure (FIM instrument). *Journal of Rehabilitation Outcomes Measurement, 1,* 67-71.
5. Galanti, G. (2005). Culturally competent rehabilitation nursing. *Rehabilitation Nursing, 30,* 123-126.
6. Kralik, D., Koch, T., Price, K., et al. (2004). Chronic illness self-management: Taking action to create order. *Journal of Clinical Nursing, 12,* 259-267.
7. Lutz, B.J. (2004). Determinants of discharge destination for stroke patients. *Rehabilitation Nursing, 29,* 154-163.
8. Mauk, K.L. (2006). Nursing interventions within the Mauk model of poststroke recovery. *Rehabilitation Nursing, 31,* 257-263.
9. Mumma, C.M., & Nelson, A. (2002). Theory and practice models for rehabilitation nursing. In S. Hoeman (Ed.), *Rehabilitation nursing: Process, application, & outcomes* (3rd ed.). St. Louis: Mosby.
10. Paterson, B., Kieloch, B., & Gmiterek, J. (2001). 'They never told us anything': Postdischarge instruction for families of persons with brain injuries. *Rehabilitation Nursing, 26,* 48-53.
11. Pierce, L.L., Finn, M.G., & Steiner, V. (2004). Families dealing with stroke desire information about self-care needs. *Rehabilitation Nursing, 29,* 14-17.
12. Pierce, L.L., Steiner, V., Hicks, B., et al. (2006). Problems of new caregivers of persons with stroke. *Rehabilitation Nursing, 31,* 166-172.
13. Reilly, C. (2001). Transdisciplinary approach: An atypical strategy for improving outcomes in rehabilitative and long-term acute care settings. *Rehabilitation Nursing, 26,* 216-220, 244.
14. Schirm, V. (2006). Quality of life. In I.M. Lubkin & P.D. Larsen (Eds.), *Chronic illness: Impact and interventions* (6th ed.). Boston: Jones & Bartlett.

15. Smith, M.S., & Testani-Dufour, L. (2002). Who's teaching whom? A study of family education in brain injury. *Rehabilitation Nursing, 27,* 209-214.

16. Winterhalter, J. (2001). Psychosocial issues for the person with chronic illness or disability. In J. Derstine & S.D. Hargrove (Eds.), *Comprehensive rehabilitation nursing.* Philadelphia: Saunders.

17. World Health Organization. (2001). *International classification of functioning, disability, and health (ICF).* Geneva, Switzerland: Author.

evolve *Did you remember to check out the bonus material on the Evolve website and the CD-ROM, including NCLEX®-Examination Style Review Questions, Open-Book Quizzes, and Chapter Review Audio Podcasts?*

http://evolve.elsevier.com/Black/medsurg

UNIT 3

FOUNDATIONS OF MEDICAL-SURGICAL NURSING

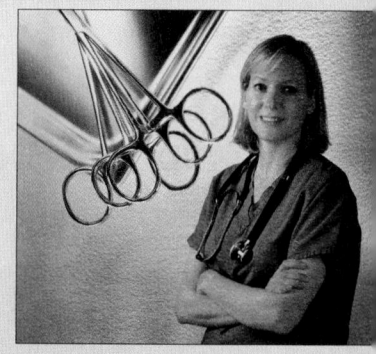

ANATOMY AND PHYSIOLOGY REVIEW:

Body Fluid Compartments and Cellular Function

Robert G. Carroll

Life requires a barrier between the organism and the environment. For animals, this barrier is the epithelium of the skin. At the microscopic level, this barrier is the cell membrane. Consequently, the anatomy and physiology review chapters focus both on (1) the external environment and the internal environment and on (2) the extracellular composition and the intracellular composition. *Anatomy* is the study of structure, including those barriers. *Physiology* is the study of movement across those barriers.

BODY FLUID COMPARTMENTS AND EXCHANGE

Water is the major body component, accounting for approximately 60% of adult body weight. The body gains water primarily from eating and drinking, and a small amount is generated from metabolism. Water is lost from the body as urine, feces, sweat, and tears, and insensibly from respiration and the skin surface. Sweat and saliva are dilute, hypotonic fluids. Most other fluids lost from the body are isotonic and have an osmolarity close to that of plasma. In all cases, water must cross an epithelial cell barrier (skin, respiratory tract, or gastrointestinal tract) to enter or exit the body.

Within the body, water is in one of two compartments. Two thirds of the body water is within the cells (intracellular fluid), and one third of body water is outside of the cells (extracellular fluid). Water can freely cross the cell membrane and move from one compartment to the other. In contrast, ions cannot easily cross the cell membrane, and intracellular ion composition is dramatically different from extracellular fluid ion composition (Table A&P3-1). Because ions cannot cross the cell membrane, they exert an osmotic pressure (or force) that determines water movement into and out of the cell. For example, if extracellular fluid osmolarity increases, water exits the cell and moves into the extracellular space to equalize each side. The most common extracellular ions are sodium, chloride, and bicarbonate.

The extracellular fluid compartment is more complex, containing interstitial and vascular fluids. Plasma is a key in the extracellular space, because compounds and fluid entering and exiting the body must first pass through the plasma before entering the cells. However, most of the extracellular fluid is in the space between the cells,

the interstitial fluid (also known as the third space). The plasma of the vascular space is also extracellular fluid. Exchange between the interstitial and plasma spaces is determined by the balance of the hydrostatic pressure and the osmotic pressure generated by the plasma proteins (see the Unit 12 Anatomy and Physiology Review for more details).

CELL STRUCTURE AND FUNCTION

The cell is the basic unit of structure and function in biologic systems. Two fundamental types of cells are recognized on the basis of composition and organization: *prokaryotic* and *eukaryotic*. Cells found in the human body and in higher plants and animals are eukaryotic, having a defined nucleus containing deoxyribonucleic acid (DNA). A less complex bacterial cell is prokaryotic, because it has DNA but lacks a nucleus. The differences between these two cell types allow clinicians to attack a prokaryotic pathogen selectively in vivo and to use drugs that do not damage eukaryotic cells. Viruses are not true cells because they cannot replicate independently. Antiviral medications are directed against the unique aspects of the viral replication process. In this chapter, the term *cell* is synonymous with eukaryotic cell.

TABLE A&P3-1 Chemical Composition of Extracellular and Intracellular Fluids

	Extracellular Fluid	Intracellular Fluid
Na^+	142 mEq/L	10 mEq/L
K^+	4 mEq/L	140 mEq/L
Ca^{2+}	2.4 mEq/L	0.0001 mEq/L
Mg^{2+}	1.2 mEq/L	58 mEq/L
Cl^-	103 mEq/L	4 mEq/L
HCO_3^-	28 mEq/L	10 mEq/L
Phosphates	4 mEq/L	75 mEq/L
SO_4^{2-}	1 mEq/L	2 mEq/L
Glucose	90 mg/dl	0 to 20 mg/dl
Amino acids	0 mg/dl	200 mg/dl ?
Cholesterol Phospholipids Neutral fat	0.5 g/dl	2-95 g/dl
Po_2	35 mm Hg	20 mm Hg ?
Pco_2	46 mm Hg	50 mm Hg ?
pH	7.4	7.0
Proteins	2 g/dl (5 mEq/L)	16 g/dl (40 mEq/L)

From Guyton, A.C., & Hall, J.E. (2006). *Textbook of medical physiology* (11th ed.). Philadelphia: Saunders.

All cells, regardless of type, have the same basic structural pattern: a cytoplasmic matrix surrounded by a plasma membrane (Figure A&P3-1). Numerous *organelles* (membrane-limited structures with a complex infrastructure and unique functions) are scattered within the cytoplasm. Their compartmentalization within the cell allows multistage metabolic and physiologic events to occur simultaneously while keeping one function separate from another.

Cells perform the basic functions of life. Cells transfer energy, take up and assimilate materials from outside the cell, synthesize macromolecules, maintain a homeostatic environment, and reproduce (Table A&P3-2).

Most of the mass of a cell is water, which aids in thermal regulation and serves as a solvent for (1) electrolytes, (2) organic molecules, and (3) chemical reactions. *Electrolytes* in the cytoplasm help maintain stable electrical and pH environments and assist with various metabolic and physiologic activities. The most prevalent intracellular electrolytes are potassium, phosphate, and magnesium. *Molecules* within the cell consist mostly of sugars, fatty acids, amino acids, and nucleotides. These are metabolized for energy or used to synthesize macromolecules (carbohydrates, lipids, proteins, nucleic acids, and their conjugates).

Cell Membrane Regulates Transport

The cell membrane is an organized layer of phospholipids and proteins (Figure A&P3-2). This dynamic structure serves a number of functions: (1) to separate the intracellular fluid from the extracellular fluid, (2) to regulate exchange and communication across the cell membrane, and (3) to provide structural support for the cell. Membranes also surround intracellular organelles, such as vacuoles, mitochondria, the Golgi apparatus, and the nucleus, where they perform an equivalent role.

Proteins in the cell membrane selectively regulate the cellular entry and exit of water-soluble materials. Movement across the membrane can be passive down a concentration gradient (from high to low concentration) or active against a gradient (from low to high concentration). Active transport processes require

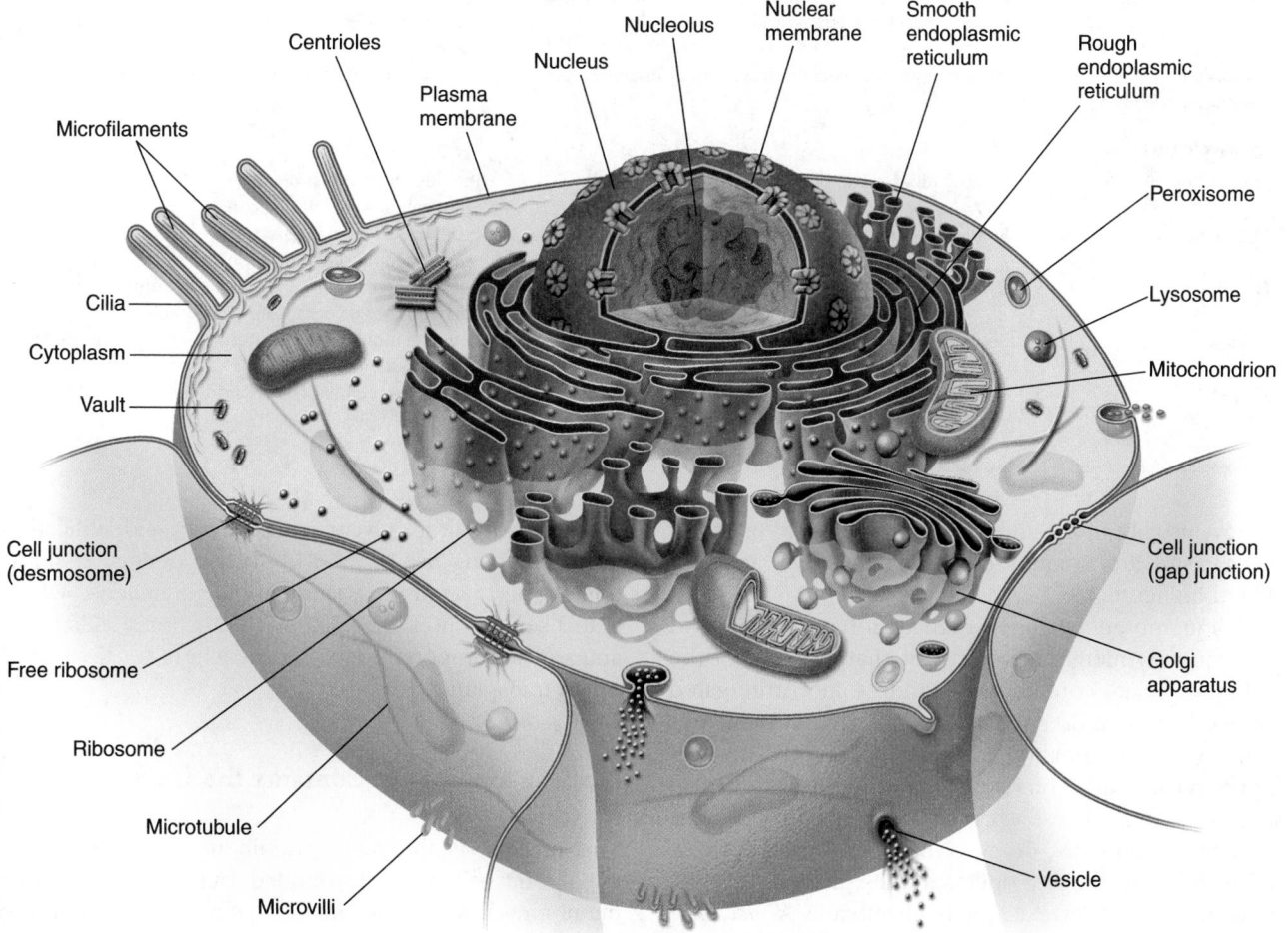

■ **FIGURE A&P3–1** A ''typical'' cell showing the internal organelles in the cytoplasm and the nucleus.

TABLE A&P3–2   Cell Structures and Their Functions

Structure	Description	Function
Cell Nucleus		
Nucleus	Large structure surrounded by double membrane; contains nucleolus and chromosomes	DNA is transcribed using RNA to make proteins
Nucleolus	Granular body; consists of RNA and protein	Ribosomal RNA synthesis; ribosome subunit assembly
Chromosomes	Complexes of DNA and protein known as chromatin become visible as rod-like structures when cell divides	Contain genes that transmit hereditary information and govern cell structure and activity
Cytoplasmic Organelles		
Cell membrane	Boundary of cell	Encloses cell contents; regulates movement of materials into and out of cell; maintains cell structure; communicates with other cells
Endoplasmic reticulum (ER)	Network of internal membranes extending throughout cytoplasm; two types: smooth and rough; smooth lacks ribosomes on outer surface; rough has ribosomes on outer surface	Site of membrane lipids and proteins; origin of intracellular transport vesicles carrying proteins to be secreted; smooth ER is used for lipid biosynthesis and drug detoxification; rough ER is site of protein manufacturing
Ribosomes	Granules composed of RNA and protein, some attached to ER, some free in cytoplasm	Synthesize polypeptides
Golgi complex	Stacks of flattened membrane sacs	Modifies proteins; packages secreted proteins; sorts other proteins to vacuoles and other organelles
Lysosomes	Membranous sacs	Contain enzymes to break down ingested materials, secretions, and waste
Vacuoles	Membranous sacs	Transport and store materials, waste, and water
Mitochondria	Sacs consisting of two membranes; inner membrane is folded to form cristae and encloses matrix	Site of most reactions of cellular respiration; transformation of energy originating from glucose or lipids into ATP
Microbodies (e.g., peroxisomes)	Membranous sacs containing variety of enzymes	Sites of many diverse metabolic reactions
Cytoskeleton		
Microtubules	Hollow tubes made of tubulin protein	Provide structural support; provide for cell movement and cell division
Microfilaments	Solid, rod-like structures consisting of actin protein	Provide structural support; provide for cell movement and cell division
Centrioles	Pairs of hollow cylinders located near center of cell	Spindles form between centrioles during mitosis; may anchor or organize microtubule formation
Cilia	Short projections extending from surface of cell, covered by plasma membrane	Regulate movement of material on surface of cell and some tissues
Flagella	Long projections made of microtubules; extend from surface of cell; covered with plasma membrane	Provide for cellular locomotion by sperm cells

ATP, Adenosine triphosphate; *DNA*, deoxyribonucleic acid; *RNA*, ribonucleic acid.

energy, usually in the form of ATP. The basic transport mechanisms are summarized in Table A&P3-3 and illustrated in Figure A&P3-3.

Cell membrane channels regulate ion movement and consequently membrane electrical charge. Some of the channels leak continuously and some are gated (opened by stimuli). A *ligand-gated* channel changes shape when a signaling molecule (e.g., peptide hormone, nitric oxide) binds to it, causing the channel to open or close. These channels are seen in cells that respond to hormones, drugs, or neurotransmitters. A *voltage-gated* channel opens or closes when there are changes in the electrical voltage across the membrane. A *mechanically gated* channel opens in response to deforming forces, such as pressure or friction.

Some cell surface glycoproteins serve as identification markers, giving rise to the ABO blood typing classification. Others act as histocompatibility antigens, which detect self and non-self in immune function. Cell surface antigens are important in tissue matching for tissue and organ transplants.

Nuclear Membrane Contains the Genetic Material

The nucleus is the most prominent organelle in the eukaryotic cell. It is surrounded by a porous double membrane, called the *nuclear envelope*. Within the nucleus are one or more nucleoli, visible among a mass of chromosomes. The nucleus contains the genetic

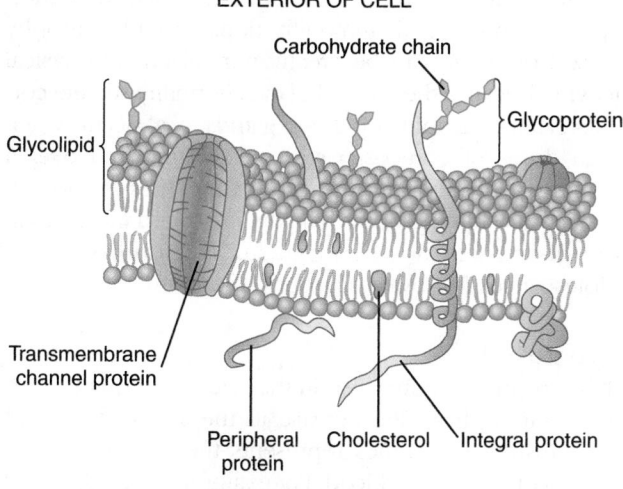

EXTERIOR OF CELL

Carbohydrate chain

Glycolipid

Glycoprotein

Transmembrane channel protein

Peripheral protein   Cholesterol   Integral protein

INTERIOR OF CELL

■ **FIGURE A&P3–2** The cell membrane is composed of a bimolecular layer of lipids, primarily phospholipid and cholesterol. Proteins can be attached or embedded in the membrane. Peripheral proteins are attached to the surface; integral proteins are embedded in the cell membrane.

TABLE A&P3–3	**Mechanisms of Membrane Transport**
Mechanism	**Common Examples**
Passive (High to Low, No ATP)	
Osmosis	Movement of water through lipid portion of membrane
Diffusion	Movement of gases and small hydrophilic molecules (oxygen, carbon dioxide, nitrogen, glycerol, urea) through lipid portion of membrane
Facilitated diffusion	Movement of glucose, some ions, and amino acids via specific carrier proteins
Active (Low to High, Uses ATP)	
Pumps	Hydrogen, sodium, and potassium ions moved by protein pumps
Endocytosis	Intake of substance by creating a vesicle
Pinocytosis	Random uptake of small amounts of extracellular fluid and solutes
Phagocytosis	Large-scale uptake of particles and cells; especially important in defense
Receptor-mediated	Specific uptake of molecules after binding to a ligand
Exocytosis	Secretion of products and wastes via secretory vesicles

ATP, Adenosine triphosphate.

material of the cell in the form of chromatin threads composed of DNA. Each cell, except the reproductive cells, contains a person's full genetic complement of DNA (46 chromosomes).

The DNA contains the blueprint for all the proteins in the body. The DNA in the nucleus is unable to pass through the nuclear envelope into the cytoplasm; products of its replication in the form of RNA are able to leave the nucleus and interact with the cytoplasmic organelles to synthesize proteins. These proteins are used for structure or control of all metabolic and physiologic activities of the cell. The processes of DNA replication and protein synthesis are described in more detail in Unit 4.

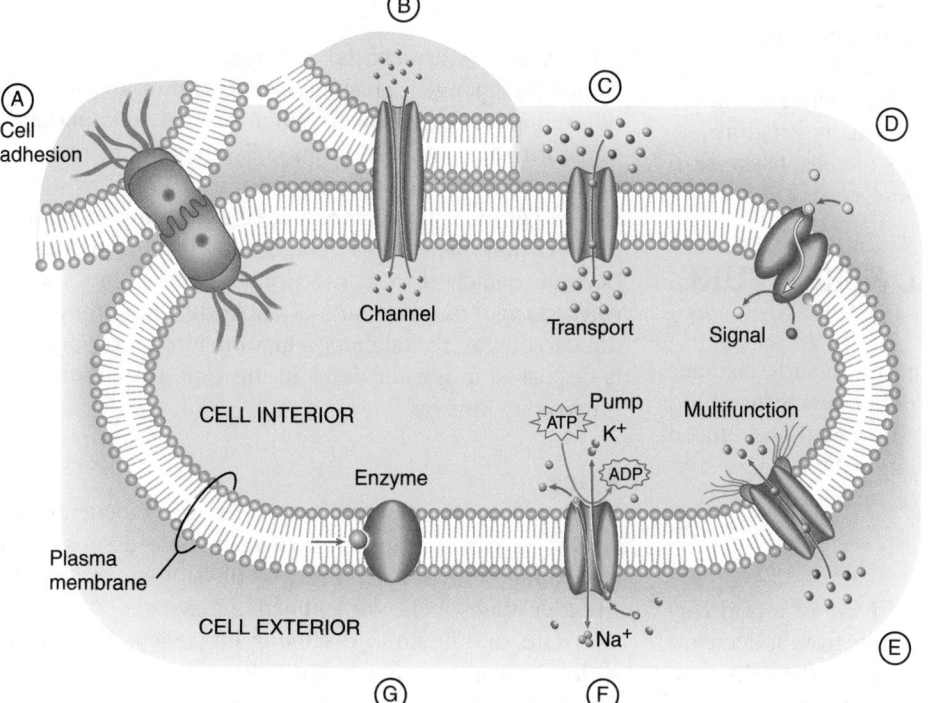

(A) Cell adhesion

(B)

(C)

(D)

Channel

Transport

Signal

CELL INTERIOR

Pump
ATP   K⁺

ADP

Multifunction

Enzyme

Plasma membrane

CELL EXTERIOR

Na⁺

(G)   (F)   (E)

■ **FIGURE A&P3–3** The cell membrane is responsible for adhesion to adjacent cells **(A)** and movement of substances in and out of the cell. Several mechanisms are required: gap junctions allow communication between neighboring cells by transfer of small molecules **(B)**; passive transport of molecules **(C)**; signal receptor proteins that bind to surface signal molecules and transfer a message to the cell interior **(D)**; use of integral proteins to transport specific molecules **(E)**; ATP-driven pumps to actively transport ions from one compartment to another **(F)**; and use of membrane-bound enzymes, which have active sites on either side of the cell membrane **(G)**. *ADP,* Adenosine diphosphate; *ATP,* adenosine triphosphate.

CELL DIFFERENTIATION

Human life begins as an undifferentiated single cell, derived from the fusion of a male gamete (sperm) with a female gamete (ovum). By about the seventh day after fertilization, the original cell (or zygote) has already undergone several cycles of replication. The progeny cells begin to develop into distinctive tissues. In the embryo and fetus, these fully differentiated cells can be distinguished on the basis of both form and function.

CELLS IN TISSUES AND ORGANS

Cells working together as a unit are called *tissues*. Tissues unite to form individual *organs*. The four major specialized types of cells that unite into larger tissue units are the following:

1. *Epithelial cells* are arranged in sheets. They cover the outside of the body (epidermis) and form the absorptive linings of the body's cavities and tubular structures (such as mucosa and glands).
2. *Nerve cells* form the highly specialized, irritable, and conductive nerve tissue.
3. *Muscle cells* allow mobility of body parts and individual cells as well as mobility of substances (such as air, blood, and waste) within the body by contracting and relaxing.
4. *Connective tissue cells* support other cells and tissues and provide the bulk mass for many organs. They include blood cells and structural cells found in bones, tendons, and ligaments. Blood cells carry oxygen to the tissues and carbon dioxide and wastes from the tissues. They also defend the body against foreign substances. Structural cells build the bony scaffolding and form the critical intercellular proteins that bind together the cells of the body. Collagen is an important extracellular connective tissue protein that provides strength to many structures.

An organ must have all four types of cells; tissues can have one or less than four cell types.

ALTERATIONS IN CELL STRUCTURE AND FUNCTION

The major causes of cellular alterations include changes in gene structure and function (either newly acquired or hereditary) and degeneration of normal tissue caused by aging, excessive use, or infiltration by foreign substances (including fat, water, glycogen, and proteins).

Atrophy

Atrophy is the wasting or decrease in size of a normally developed organ. This condition results from a decrease either in the number of cells or in the size of the cells composing it. Atrophy may follow disuse of an organ. For example, muscle atrophy may develop following denervation or prolonged immobilization. Muscular atrophy caused by aging can be greatly minimized by physical activity. Because the adrenal glands normally secrete corticosteroids, atrophy of these glands can occur when large doses of corticosteroids are administered over a prolonged period. Atrophy also accompanies the normal physiologic aging process. The thymus gland increases in size during childhood and gradually atrophies during adolescence. The ovaries atrophy after menopause.

Hypertrophy

Hypertrophy is an increase in the size of an organ or tissue resulting from an increase in the size of the cells. Hypertrophy sometimes represents the response of an organ to a greater workload. For example, when the heart is subjected to great strain, the left ventricle of the heart enlarges (hypertrophies) to handle the additional stress. Another example is the increased size of the biceps muscle in people engaged in strenuous weight training.

Hyperplasia

Hyperplasia is an increase in the number of cells. Hyperplasia can be an expected cellular response, such as increased cell regeneration in the formation of calluses. Pathologic hyperplasia can be a result of cancer. *Dysplasia* is deranged cellular growth or a form of hyperplasia. It results from genetic alterations often caused by persistent severe injury or irritation. *Metaplasia* is the transformation of one mature cell type or tissue into another. Usually, the new cell does not perform the functions of the cell it replaced. Metaplastic cells can also transform into malignant cancer cells.

Neoplastic (Cancerous) Changes

Neoplastic change is characterized by disturbances in cell differentiation and growth. When normal cells undergo transformation into cancerous cells, they fail to respond to normal regulatory forces and instead show unrestrained growth. These unregulated replicating cells *(neoplasms)* may then invade contiguous healthy tissues or become detached from the primary tumor and spread *(metastasize)* to other parts of the body where they continue to divide. This alteration in normal cell reproduction is discussed in greater detail in the Unit 4 Anatomy and Physiology Review.

Aging

In a young, healthy person, cells are biochemically active, have a high turnover rate (in some tissues), and have a high rate of metabolic and physiologic efficiency. In older adults, cells are less active, have a slower turnover rate, and begin to decline in efficiency. Aging cells shrink in size, protein synthesis slows, the Golgi apparatus shows signs of disintegration, and the mitochondria

TABLE A&P3-4   Physiologic Changes of Aging: An Overview

System	Physiologic Changes
Cardiovascular	Decreased vessel elasticity caused by calcification and connective tissue (increased pulmonary vascular resistance)
	Decreased number of heart muscle fibers, with increased size of individual fibers (hypertrophy)
	Decreased filling capacity
	Decreased stroke volume
	Decreased sensitivity of baroreceptors
	Degeneration of vein valves
Respiratory	Decreased chest wall compliance caused by calcification of costal cartilage
	Decreased alveolar ventilation
	Decreased respiratory muscle strength
	Air trapping and decreased ventilation because of degeneration of lung tissue (decreased elasticity)
Renal and urinary	Decreased glomerular filtration rate caused by nephron degeneration (decreased 33% to 50% by age 70)
	Decreased ability to concentrate urine
	Decreased ability to regulate hydrogen (H^+)
Gastrointestinal	Decreased muscular contractions
	Decreased esophageal emptying
	Decreased bowel motility
	Decreased production of hydrochloric acid (HCl), enzymes, and intrinsic factor
	Decreased hepatic enzyme production and metabolic capacity
	Thinning of stomach mucosa
Neurologic and sensory	Degeneration and atrophy of nerve cells
	Decrease of 25%-45% in neurons
	Decrease in neurotransmitters
	Decreased rate of conduction of nerve impulses
	Loss of taste buds
	Loss of auditory hair cells and sclerosis of eardrum
Musculoskeletal	Decreased muscle mass
	Bone demineralization
	Joint degeneration, erosion, and calcification
Immune	Decreased inflammatory response
	Decrease in T-cell function caused by involution of thymus gland
Integumentary	Decreased subcutaneous fat
	Decreased elastin
	Atrophy of sweat glands
	Atrophy of epidermal arterioles, causing altered temperature regulation

From Copstead-Kirkhorn, L.C., & Banasik, J. (2005). *Pathophysiology* (3rd ed.). Philadelphia: Saunders.

may undergo fragmentation. Aging affects every system of the body (Table A&P3-4).

Numerous theories exist regarding the aging process, but little is certain about how age-related changes occur. The age range of a cell is great. In the mature adult, an epithelial cell lining the intestinal tract lives only about 1½ days; a red blood cell can survive for 120 days. At the other extreme, nerve cells have a potential life expectancy of 100 years or more. Early in life, the cells with a short life span are easily replaced. One theory of aging is that unrepaired mutations accumulate on DNA, causing changes that lead to aging. For example, highly specialized cells (such as nerve cells) do not reproduce. When these cells die from injury or disease and are not replaced, the remaining cells must assume their functions. The greater workload may stress these cells, cause them to age faster, and hasten their dying.

Another hypothesis is that all people are born with a genetic clock that governs their life span. This theory is based on the observation that each cell type has a finite number of divisions. This concept is supported in part by similarities in life spans seen in various family groups.

In the immune system, immunocompetent cells appear to remain constant in numbers as people age but lose some of their interactive and regulatory properties. The resulting alteration in immune function is responsible for the increased incidence of autoimmune disease, the appearance of tumors, and the greater susceptibility to infection seen in the older population.

CONCLUSIONS

Cells are the basic units of life, and they serve many functions. The integrity and existence of the organism are dependent on the individual and collective ability of body cells to digest and assimilate substances, protect themselves by reacting to stimuli, replicate, metabolize, and produce energy. When cells lose their ability to function normally because of injury or attack by pathogens, the organism becomes distressed and disease develops.

BIBLIOGRAPHY

1. Berne, R., et al. (2004). *Physiology* (5th ed.). St. Louis: Mosby.
2. Carroll, R.G. (2007). *Elsevier's integrated physiology*. Philadelphia: Saunders.
3. Kierszenbaum, A.L. (2006). *Histology and cell biology: An introduction to pathology* (2nd ed.). St. Louis: Mosby.
4. Guyton, A., & Hall, J. (2006). *Textbook of medical physiology* (11th ed.). Philadelphia: Saunders.
5. Silverthorn, D. (2006). *Human physiology* (4th ed.). San Francisco, Calif: Pearson Benjamin Cummings.
6. Yeh, E. (1998). Life and death of the cell. *Hospital Practice*, Aug 15, 85-92.

CHAPTER 11

Clients with Fluid Imbalances

BERNADETTE WHITE

Dehydration is the most common fluid and electrolyte imbalance in the United States; more than 1 million people are admitted to the hospital yearly for dehydration. Dehydration is especially common among older adults; up to 60% of older adults have been found to have mild to moderate dehydration. This number has increased by 40% over the last decade and is expected to continue to increase as the population ages. Dehydration carries a 17% to 50% morbidity and mortality rate.

This chapter provides the basic knowledge necessary to promote positive health outcomes for clients at risk for fluid and electrolyte imbalances. Clearly, water is responsible not only for the body's structure and function but also is necessary for the maintenance of equilibrium and of life itself. The introductory chapter to this unit reviews fluid compartments and the regulation of fluid movement between compartments.

DEHYDRATION

Dehydration is loss of water from the extracellular fluid volume; loss is from the vascular and interstitial fluids. Dehydration is a common and serious fluid imbalance that leads to hypovolemia. Losses can be *mild,* with a loss of 1 to 2 L of water (2% of body weight); *moderate,* with a loss of 3 to 5 L of water (5% of body weight); or *severe,* when 5 to 10 L of water (8% of body weight) is lost. Dehydration can be called extracellular fluid volume deficit (ECFVD).

Etiology

Average daily fluid intake for adults is about 1500 to 2000 ml. In addition, about 800 ml of fluid is consumed through solid foods. Fluid balance is maintained in the body because the intake of fluids equals the excretion of fluids. This simple concept can be used to explain common causes of fluid imbalances. A lack of fluid intake, excessive fluid output, or both can lead to dehydration. Conversely, excessive fluid intake and a lack of fluid excretion can lead to overhydration. Furthermore, alteration in any of the regulators of fluid balance—thirst, hormones, lymphatic system, kidneys—increases the risk for or can cause an actual fluid imbalance (Figure 11-1).

Lack of Fluid Intake

Cognitive and physical impairments can quickly reduce water intake. For example, clients who are hospitalized, chairbound, or bedbound may not be able to reach their water or may be too confused to realize they are thirsty. Clients with dysphagia or at risk for aspiration may not be able to swallow fluids safely. Tube-fed clients who are not given adequate free water or who are fed hypertonic formulas are also at risk. Community-dwelling older adults may have decreased access to fluids because of financial or transportation barriers or debilitation. For many of these reasons, nursing home residents older than 85 years of age appear to be at greatest risk for dehydration.

Impaired thirst mechanisms can also decrease fluid intake. The thirst mechanism is usually triggered by low blood pressure or fluid volume depletion as small as 0.5%. The sensation of a dry mouth also stimulates thirst. Clients may experience dry mouth from salivary gland dysfunction, head or neck radiation, smoking, mouth breathing, oxygen therapy, hyperventilation, and anticholinergic medications (such as atropine).

---

evolve **Web Enhancements**

Appendix A Religious Beliefs and Practices Affecting Health Care

Be sure to check out the bonus material on the Evolve website and the CD-ROM, including free self-assessment exercises.

http://evolve.elsevier.com/Black/medsurg

evolve

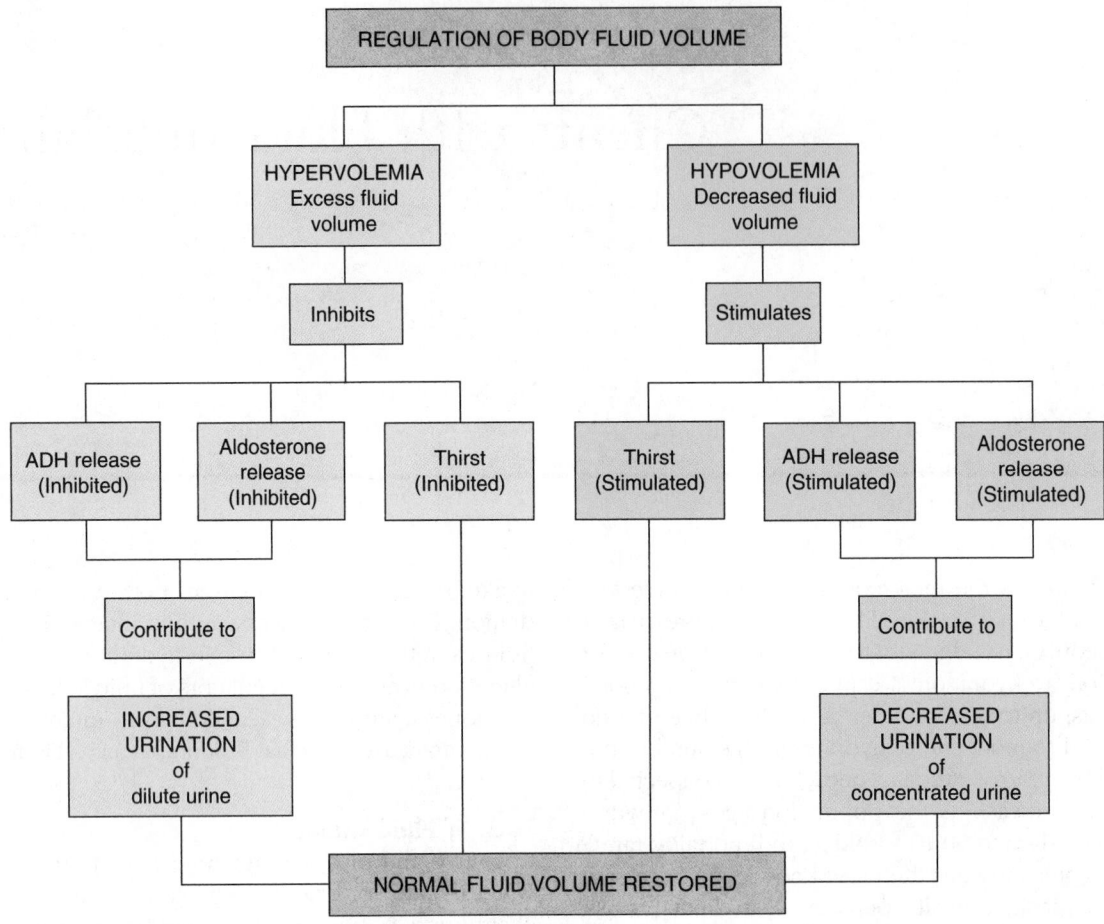

■ **FIGURE 11–1** Regulation of body fluid volume depends on antidiuretic hormone (ADH), aldosterone, and thirst and fluid dynamics. *(From White, B. [1994]. Maintaining fluid and electrolyte balance. In V.B. Bolander [Ed.], Sorensen and Luckmann's basic nursing: A psychophysiologic approach [3rd ed.]. Philadelphia: Saunders.)*

Most healthy people respond to decreased fluid levels by drinking fluids and thus maintain balance. However, the thirst mechanism is depressed in people with debilitating illnesses and in older adults, even healthy older adults. Several disorders also lead to inappropriate thirst mechanisms. Clients with excess fluids in the interstitial space but depleted fluids in the vascular space are commonly thirsty. Any stimulant that results in an increased renin-angiotensin-aldosterone response causes sodium retention that, in turn, also stimulates the thirst response. Clients with heart failure commonly experience this problem.

Osmolality also influences thirst. Hypo-osmolality inhibits the thirst response; conversely, hyperosmolality leads to thirst. It is common to find comatose and confused people with high plasma osmolality, but they are unable to recognize the urge to drink.

Excess Fluid Losses

Unmonitored use of potent diuretics (e.g., furosemide), severe vomiting, and diarrhea are common causes of dehydration. These conditions are commonly associated with changes in levels of electrolytes. Potential causes of

fluid loss include fever, diaphoresis, hyperglycemia, gastrointestinal suction, ileostomy, fistulae, burns, blood loss, hyperventilation, hyperthyroidism, decreased antidiuretic hormone (ADH) secretion, diabetes insipidus (nephrogenic and neurogenic), Addison's disease or adrenal crisis, and the diuretic phase of acute renal failure.

Again, older adults are at risk for excessive fluid losses for several reasons: (1) decreased renal concentration of urine, (2) an altered ADH response, and (3) an increase in body fat and thus a decrease in total quantity of body water in proportion to body weight. Increased drug-drug interactions and multiple chronic diseases potentiate the risk for fluid imbalances.

Thermal stressors, whether cold or relative elevations in temperature from high heat and humidity, have been reported in many studies that evaluate risks for athletes and those in the military. Recent studies have noted a 40% decline in the thirst mechanism during moderate exercise in cold temperatures.

Third-space fluid shifts (shifting of fluid from the vascular space to interstitial space where fluid cannot be easily exchanged) can result in a fluid deficit in the vascular compartment. Spaces that are susceptible to third-spacing include the peritoneal, pericardial, pleural, and joint cavities. Abdominal third-spacing is called *ascites*.

Pathophysiology

Fluids are normally found in three spaces: inside the cells (intracellular), around the cells (interstitial), and in the bloodstream (intravascular). The pathophysiology of dehydration is seen when the normal compensation for fluid loss in the bloodstream cannot be corrected by stored fluid elsewhere. When fluids are lost from the intravascular spaces because of lack of intake or excess loss, interstitial fluids move in to restore vascular volume. Because the actual volume of fluid in the interstitial space is limited, other compensation systems are initiated to restore fluid volume. ADH and aldosterone secretion increase to reabsorb water and sodium in the kidney. Fluids are also reabsorbed from the ileum and large intestine. The *baroreceptors* sense low blood pressure, and the sympathetic nervous system is stimulated to increase peripheral vasoconstriction and the heart rate. Vasoconstriction moves fluids from the periphery (legs, gastrointestinal tract) into the circulation. Increasing sodium level in the blood is also sensed by the osmoreceptors in the hypothalamus, which signals the thirst mechanism. These compensatory processes occur repeatedly in normal healthy people. When fluid loss continues or when the compensation fails to restore blood volume, the person becomes dehydrated.

If the dehydration is not corrected, fluid is shifted from the cells into the vascular system. The loss of cellular fluid is dangerous because the cells need fluid for cellular function. Less fluid is available for temperature regulation via sweating, and a lowered blood volume decreases the body's ability to transport core heat to the periphery for conductive loss. There is less cerebrospinal fluid and less fluid in the fat pads around the eyes. If cerebral cells become dehydrated, thought processes may be impaired. The cerebral vessels may be stretched and bleed or spasm. If sodium is lost, the muscle and nerve functions that depend on this electrolyte are slowed. A full discussion of sodium imbalances is provided in Chapter 12.

There are three types of extracellular fluid (ECF) volume deficits:

- *Hyperosmolar (hypertonic)* fluid volume deficit: water loss is greater than electrolyte (sodium) loss.
- *Iso-osmolar (isotonic)* fluid volume deficit: water and electrolyte (sodium) losses are equal.
- *Hypotonic* fluid volume deficit: electrolyte loss is greater than fluid loss (rare).

Clinical Manifestations
Loss of Body Weight

Fairly rapid weight loss is an early and common result of fluid loss, because water is a major portion of body weight. Mild dehydration exists when the client has lost 2% of body weight. For example, in a client who weighs 150 pounds (68 kg), a 2% loss equals 1.4 L of water. Weight is the most accurate measure of fluid status. Weight—if measured at the same time, on the same scale, and with the same clothes on the client—is less subject to errors than is measurement of intake and output.

Changes in Intake and Output

Intake and output (I&O) measurements provide another means of assessing fluid balance. These data provide insight into the cause of the imbalance (such as decreased fluid intake or increased fluid loss). These measurements are not as accurate as body weight, however, because of relative risk of errors in recording and that insensible water loss is not measured.

Thirst is an early clinical manifestation of ECFVD in a conscious person; however, thirst is diminished in older adults, so it is not an accurate indicator. Clients often request plain, cold water rather than carbonated or caffeinated beverages. This is advantageous because caffeine and glucose are diuretics and sweet fluids may not quench thirst.

Urine output usually decreases with ECFVD because of the effects of ADH and aldosterone. Urine is usually concentrated, with specific gravity greater than 1.030 and urine osmolality greater than 1000 mOsm/kg. Because of the decline in renal function in the older adult, specific gravity is not a sensitive indicator of ECFVD in this population. For many years, it was thought that the kidneys had to excrete at least 30 ml of urine per hour as a mechanism for waste removal. Currently, a urine output of 400 to 500 ml/day (16 to 20 ml/hr) is considered *oliguria* and indicates a marked compromise in kidney function. In most people (perhaps not the critically ill), urine output varies throughout the day. Normally, urine output is low and concentration is higher during the night. Thus the view that urine should flow constantly at 30 to 40 ml/hr appears to lack justification. Clients who are at risk for becoming dehydrated because they do not have the ability to concentrate urine are those who produce inadequate amounts of ADH (e.g., clients with diabetes insipidus), those who do not respond normally to ADH (e.g., older adults), and those with inability to concentrate urine (e.g., clients with kidney failure).

Changes in Vital Signs

Inadequate fluid volume also leads to a decrease in systolic blood pressure, a weak pulse, and a decrease in central venous pressure (CVP) and pulmonary capillary wedge pressure (PCWP). For every liter of fluid lost, the cardiac output decreases by 1 L/min, the heart rate increases 8 beats/min, and the core temperature increases by 0.3° C (0.6° F). Postural hypotension is one of the most sensitive indicators of decreased fluid

TABLE 11-1 Clinical Manifestations of Dehydration

Clinical Manifestations	Mild Dehydration	Moderate Dehydration	Severe Dehydration
Level of consciousness*	Alert	Lethargic	Obtunded
Capillary refill time*	2 seconds	2-4 seconds	Greater than 4 seconds, cool limbs
Mucous membranes*	Normal	Dry	Parched, cracked
Heart rate	Slight increase	Increased	Very increased
Respiratory rate	Normal	Increased	Increased and hyperpnea
Blood pressure	Normal	Normal, but orthostasis	Decreased
Pulse	Normal	Thready	Faint or impalpable
Skin turgor	Normal	Slow	Tenting
Eyes	Normal	Sunken	Very sunken
Urine output	Decreased	Oliguria	Oliguria/anuria

* Best indicators of hydration status.

volume. Postural or orthostatic hypotension is a decrease in systolic blood pressure of more than 20 mm Hg or a decrease in diastolic pressure of more than 10 mm Hg accompanied by an increase in pulse rate within 3 minutes of standing. The technique is described later in this chapter.

Sympathetic nervous system stimulation leads to vasoconstriction and increases the heart rate to compensate for the altered tissue perfusion. Without restoring fluids, vasoconstriction and tachycardia provide only a minimal and temporary compensation. If vasoconstriction continues, tissue perfusion is further compromised. Serious fluid loss can lead to systolic blood pressures less than 70 mm Hg. Low systolic pressure impairs tissue perfusion to vital organs that have high metabolic demands, such as cerebral, cardiac, and kidney tissues.

Flat jugular veins in a supine position and a prolonged peripheral venous filling time of more than 5 seconds are also noted. Because of the inability to cool the body core, an elevated temperature is common and can reach 105° F.

Other Manifestations of Dehydration

The mucous membranes of the mouth and eyes become dry even though fluid is recruited from the interstitial spaces. The lips can crack, and furrows may be seen on the tongue. Swallowing can become difficult.

Tenting of the skin (decreased turgor) occurs when the skin tissues tend to stick together because of the decreased interstitial fluid. Tenting is not diagnostic of dehydration in older adults because tenting commonly results from loss of elastin in the skin in this population. Findings of changes in mental status and decreased urine output are more common. Soft and sunken eyes may be noted. Muscle weakness from an imbalance of sodium and potassium occurs early and becomes worse as the deficit progresses. Feces become hard and decreased in number because of compensatory reabsorption of fluid from the colon.

Cerebral signs are always considered serious because it means that intracellular fluid (ICF) compartmental shifting has occurred. Early signs include apprehension,

restlessness, and headache. As the fluid deficit progresses, hallucinations, maniacal behavior, and confusion occur, followed by coma. Detection of the presentation of dehydration at various levels is presented in Table 11-1.

Diagnostic Findings

In hyperosmolar fluid deficit, more solvent (water in the plasma) is lost than solutes (cells and electrolytes in the plasma), which creates hemoconcentration. Plasma sodium concentration is also increased (*hypernatremia*). The following elevations are typical findings secondary to a hemoconcentrated state:

- Osmolality greater than 295 mOsm/kg
- Plasma sodium level greater than 145 mEq/L
- Blood urea nitrogen (BUN) level greater than 25 mg/dl (in the presence of normal creatinine)
- Plasma glucose level greater than 120 mg/dl
- Hematocrit greater than 55%
- Urine specific gravity greater than 1.030

Specific gravity is a numeric value of urine concentration using solute-solvent relationships. Very concentrated urine has a high specific gravity. High specific gravity readings indicate dehydration or increased ADH secretion. Glucose, protein, and dyes falsely elevate specific gravity. Urine specific gravity can be measured by using a urinometer or by sending a urine sample to the laboratory for testing.

Hypernatremia usually indicates hyperosmolality, and hyponatremia usually indicates hypo-osmolality. The Critical Monitoring box on p. 131 shows how to calculate plasma osmolality. Urine specific gravity may also be used as an indirect measurement of osmolality.

The seriousness of a client's manifestations and the aggressiveness of treatment are related to both the *amount* and *acuteness* of the fluid loss, and the client's state of health at the time of loss. Sudden loss of fluid does not give the compensatory mechanisms time to respond; severe loss is also often beyond the potential of compensatory mechanisms to respond, resulting in vascular collapse or shock.

How to Calculate Plasma Osmolality

To calculate plasma osmolality, you must know the plasma sodium (Na) level. Additionally, you should know the glucose level and blood urea/nitrogen (BUN) level. The first formula may be used as a rough estimate of the plasma osmolality; the second formula gives a more exact plasma osmolality value.

- $2 \times$ Plasma Na = Plasma osmolality
- $2 \times$ Plasma Na + (BUN $\div$ 3) + (Glucose $\div$ 18) = Plasma osmolality

OUTCOME MANAGEMENT

A thorough history and physical examination, including collection of such demographic variables as age, gender, culture, presence of chronic diseases, and socioeconomic status, is critical to identifying realistic and measurable outcomes. Dehydration can occur volitionally (by choice) in terminally ill clients, and for those clients treatment may be withheld to meet their desires. There is controversy in whether dehydration in the terminally ill is helpful because perception and level of consciousness are decreased by ketone and other metabolite accumulations and increased production of endorphins. Other data point to clients with increased manifestations of underlying problems and suffering from dehydration. Each client's specific wishes need to be considered in any treatment decisions.

Medical treatment of dehydration depends on the acuteness and severity of the fluid deficit. The goals of treatment are to restore normal fluid volumes by using fluids similar in composition to those lost, to replace ongoing losses, and to correct the underlying problem (such as vomiting or diarrhea).

Fluid Restoration
Oral Rehydration

If the fluid loss is mild, the thirst mechanism is intact, and the client can drink fluid, replace the fluids orally. How much is adequate? There are several standard formulas, but the one with the most positive outcomes for the older adult is based on body weight. One formula suggests providing 100 ml for the first 10 kg and 50 ml for the next 10 kg, and adding these numbers to 15 ml for the remaining number of kilograms. Another formula recommends 1.5 ml/kg of intake to meet the increased needs related to sensible losses that occur with activity and other environmental stressors. Oral glucose replacement solutions are palatable, inexpensive, and a good source of fluid, glucose, and electrolytes. For diabetic clients, who need less glucose, Pedialyte is a good alternative. These solutions are quickly absorbed even when the client has diarrhea or is vomiting. Cola drinks should be avoided because they do not contain adequate electrolyte replacement, the sugar content may lead to osmotic diuresis, and the caffeine may lead to diuresis.

Intravenous Rehydration

When the fluid loss is severe or life-threatening, intravenous (IV) fluids are used for replacement. The volume of fluid is calculated on the basis of the client's weight and the presence of any other co-morbidities, such as cardiac, renal, liver, or pulmonary disorders that would decrease the ability of the body to get rid of excess fluids. The type of solution used is based on the type of fluid lost from the body. Generally, isotonic ECFVD is treated with isotonic solutions, hypertonic ECFVD is treated with hypotonic solutions, and hypotonic ECFVD is treated with hypertonic solutions. Common IV fluids are listed in Table 11-2. Sodium solutions should be infused at a rate of 0.5 to 1 mEq/L/hr. If fluid is given too rapidly, cerebral edema may result.

Monitoring for Complications of Fluid Restoration

Fluid administration is based on the client's overall condition. A client with severe dehydration accompanied by severe heart, pulmonary, liver, or kidney disease cannot tolerate large volumes of fluid or sodium without the risk for development of heart failure. For unstable clients, monitors are used to detect increasing pressures from fluids (e.g., measurement of right atrial and pulmonary artery pressures). If the deficit has existed for more than 24 hours, it is dangerous to correct this deficit too rapidly. Urine output, body weight, and laboratory values of sodium level, osmolality, urea/nitrogen (BUN) level, and potassium level are monitored closely. However, it is important to note that BUN level may not be an accurate indicator in someone with protein deficit (lack of intake, kidney or liver disease) and BUN level can be elevated from bleeding or excessive nitrogen breakdown. Studies support that early identification and aggressive intervention of dehydration in the high-risk older adult population result in decreased complications.

Correction of the Underlying Problem

Antiemetic and antidiarrheal drugs may be prescribed to correct problems with nausea and vomiting or diarrhea. Antibiotics may be used in clients with infectious diarrhea. Antipyretic agents may be used to reduce body temperature. Clients who are taking diuretics should have a consultation regarding the benefits versus the risks of continuing the medication.

Nursing Management of the Medical Client

Assessment. At the time of admission, obtain the client's history of fluid losses. If the cause is infectious, isolation may be warranted. Determine a history of chronic illnesses that may

TABLE 11–2 Intravenous Water and Electrolyte Solutions

Solution (Abbreviation)	Contents	Uses	Comments
Hypotonic			
5% dextrose in water (D₅W)*	50 g dextrose No electrolytes	Replaces deficits of total body water Not used alone to expand ECF† volume because dilution of electrolytes can occur	Supplies 170 kcal/L and free water Distilled water cannot be given IV because it would cause hemolysis of RBCs Dextrose is metabolized on first pass through liver, leaving a solution of water but without hemolytic problems
Isotonic			
0.9% NaCl (normal saline solution, NS, 0.9% NS)	154 mEq/L Na and Cl	ECF deficits in clients with low serum levels of Na or Cl and metabolic alkalosis Before and after infusion of blood products	Not used for routine administration of IV fluids because it contains more sodium than ECF (140 mEq NaCl and 103 mEq Cl) Expands plasma and interstitial volume and does not enter cells
Lactated Ringer's solution (LR)	130 mEq/L Na 4 mEq/L K 3 mEq/L Ca 109 mEq/L Cl 28 mEq/L lactate	ECF deficits, such as fluid loss with burns and bleeding and dehydration from loss of bile or diarrhea	Solution is roughly isotonic to plasma but does not contain magnesium or phosphate Lactate is equivalent to bicarbonate, and solution can be used to treat many forms of acidosis Cannot be used in people with alkalosis; solutions of acetate Ringer's are better for these clients
Hypertonic			
Lactated Ringer's solution with 5% dextrose (D₅/LR)	50 g dextrose 130 mEq/L Na 4 mEq/L K 3 mEq/L Ca 109 mEq/L Cl 28 mEq/L lactate	ECF deficits, such as fluid loss with burns and bleeding and dehydration from loss of bile or diarrhea Provides modest calories (170 kcal)	Solution is hypertonic because it is combination of two solutions (D₅W and LR) See other comments on individual solutions
5% dextrose and normal saline (D₅/0.9 NS)	50 g dextrose 154 mEq/L Na and Cl	ECF deficits in clients with low serum levels of Na or Cl and metabolic alkalosis Before and after infusion of blood products Provides modest calories (170 kcal)	Solution is hypertonic because it is combination of two solutions (D₅W and NS) See other comments on individual solutions
5% dextrose and 0.45% normal saline (D₅/0.45 NS; D₅/½ NS)	50 g dextrose 77 mEq/L Na and Cl	Can be used as an initial fluid for hydration because it provides more water than sodium Provides modest calories (170 kcal)	Commonly used as a maintenance fluid
5% dextrose and 0.225% normal saline (D₅/0.2 NS; D₅/¼ NS)	50 g dextrose 34 mEq/L Na and Cl	Can be used as an initial fluid for hydration because it provides more water than sodium Provides modest calories (170 kcal)	Commonly used as a maintenance fluid

* Osmolarity of D₅W is 252 mOsm/L. The fluid is isotonic when in the container. After administration, the dextrose is quickly metabolized in the body, leaving only water—a hypotonic fluid.
†Ca, Calcium; Cl, chloride; ECF, extracellular fluid; IV, intravenously; K, potassium; kcal, kilocalories; Na, sodium; NS, normal saline; RBCs, red blood cells.

impair the ability to tolerate fluids at rapid speeds. Obtain any advance directives that would alter the use or course of fluid resuscitation. Examine the client completely, recording baseline data on lung and heart sounds, skin condition, vital signs, height, and weight. Ask the client for height measurement but weigh the client yourself; do not rely on the client's stated weight. Orthostatic hypotension may be present, so help the client onto the scale.

Assess the client's vital signs every 2 to 4 hours, depending on the severity of the fluid loss; compare them with baseline vital signs and report marked differences. Assess for postural (orthostatic) blood pressure and pulse changes by taking blood pressure and pulse measurements with the client lying down. Then have the client stand up; repeat the blood pressure and pulse measurements after 1 minute. Report a drop in standing systolic blood pressure of 20 mm Hg or more from the supine blood pressure measurement. Autonomic neuropathy seen in diabetes, dysrhythmias, and some medications (e.g., antihypertensive agents) can also cause postural hypotension.

Assess the peripheral vein filling time daily. Veins with normal fluid volume should fill in 3 to 5 seconds when the arm is lowered below the level of the heart.

Monitor intake, output, and daily weights accurately in high-risk clients. Be certain that all sources of intake (including liquids with meals and between meals, with medications, in IV lines, in tube-feedings, and in IV or tube flushes) and all sources of output (including urine, diarrhea, diaphoresis, and hyperventilation) are recorded accurately. If the dehydration is mild, assess urine output every 8 hours and compare daily outputs. Absence of adequate renal perfusion for several hours may result in permanent renal damage. Whenever the output decreases to less than 0.5 ml/kg/hr for 2 consecutive hours, urine output must be assessed hourly and the physician alerted about the problem. Teach unlicensed assistive personnel to report urine outputs of less than 0.5 ml/kg/hr for 2 consecutive hours or less than 240 ml for an 8-hour period. Provide other instructions as well (see the Management and Delegation feature on Care of Clients with Fluid Volume Deficit). Instruct the client to report fluids consumed in addition to the fluids on food trays and urine output not measured.

Weigh the client daily on the same scale, at the same time of day, with the client wearing clothing of similar weight. Analyze changes in daily weights. A loss of 2.2 pounds is equivalent to 1 L of fluid. Therefore an 8-pound weight loss equals about 3.5 L of fluid, or a moderate fluid volume deficit.

Care of Clients with Fluid Volume Deficit

When working with unlicensed assistive personnel in the care of clients with fluid volume deficit, remind them to do the following:
- Keep fresh water or other fluids in an easily accessible location. Remind older clients to drink fluids hourly because their thirst mechanism is diminished.
- Try to provide fluids of choice every 1 to 2 hours.
- Encourage family members to assist with fluid intake.
- Provide oral care every 2 hours to help decrease discomfort from dry mucous membranes.
- Record intake accurately. Remember, a cup of ice chips provides one-half cup of water.
- Assist clients as necessary to the bathroom, commode, or bedpan every 2 hours. If the client is wearing disposable briefs, assess for incontinence and the need for perineal care at least every 2 hours.
- Record all output accurately. Include the amount of urine, the number of episodes of incontinence, and the measured amount of any diarrhea.
- Report diarrhea, excessive sweating, or rapid breathing.
- Report urine that is dark, produced at less than 0.5 ml/kg/hr over 2 consecutive hours, or produced at more than 150 ml/hr.
- Report weight changes of 2 pounds or more from the previous day.

Assess the oral cavity between the gums and cheek for dryness of the mucous membranes and the tongue for dryness and longitudinal furrows. Use an oral assessment guide to derive a numerical rating of oral health. Another reliable method of testing for dryness of the mouth is to place your gloved finger on the mucous membranes where the gums and cheek meet. When dehydration is present, your finger will not glide easily because of dryness. Note any speech and swallowing difficulty. Assess closely for dried and adherent mucus on the soft palate.

Check skin turgor by gently pinching and lifting the skin (Figure 11-2). Usually, skin returns to a normal position within 1 or 2 seconds in people younger than 65 years of age. A slower response may indicate loss of interstitial fluids. Generalized weakness may develop because of changes in sodium levels.

Monitor plasma sodium, urea/nitrogen (BUN), glucose, and hematocrit levels to determine plasma osmolality. Assess for confusion, an early manifestation of ICF involvement.

Diagnosis, Outcomes, Interventions
Diagnosis: Deficient Fluid Volume. Deficient fluid volume is the state in which a person has vascular, interstitial, or intracellular dehydration. The nursing diagnosis is *Deficient Fluid Volume related to insufficient fluid intake, vomiting, diarrhea, hemorrhage, or third-space fluid loss such as ascites or burns*.

Outcomes. The desired outcome is return of normal levels of body fluids. The goal statement may be that the client will have restoration of normal fluid volume, improvement in fluid volume, or no further fluid losses

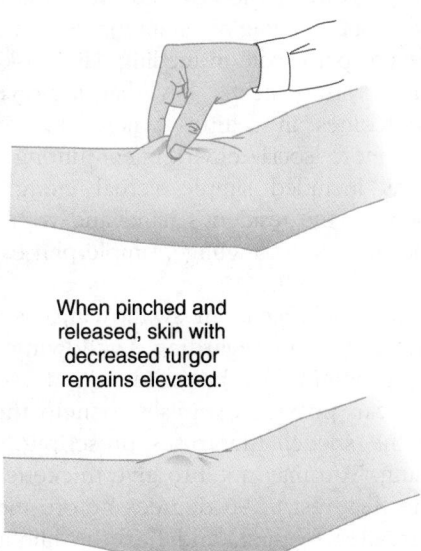

When pinched and released, skin with decreased turgor remains elevated.

■ **FIGURE 11–2** Skin turgor assessment. This assessment can be done on the forearm. Skin that does not flatten immediately after release is called "tenting," an example of fluid volume deficit in a young to middle-aged adult. Assessment for tenting is not appropriate for older adults.

depending on the clinical situation. Indicators of adequate fluid volumes include the following:

- Oral intake between 1500 and 2500 ml or more in 24 hours
- Urine output greater than 0.5 ml/kg/hr
- Stable blood pressure and pulse in the supine and standing positions
- Increasing body weight of about 0.5 to 1 pound per day
- Absence of crackles (fluid in alveoli), an indicator of pulmonary fluid overload
- Moist tongue and mucous membranes
- Mental status returned to baseline
- Urea/nitrogen (BUN), plasma sodium, hematocrit, and osmolality levels approaching normal or baseline ranges over the first 48 to 72 hours

Interventions

Restore Oral Fluid Intake. Give small amounts of fluids "of choice" hourly to older, confused, or debilitated clients and to those who require restraints. Keep fluids fresh and within reach. Use orthotic devices as appropriate for those who can assist in their own fluid intake. If a client's lips are dry, he or she may be unable to suck on a straw. Wet the lips and mouth first to facilitate sucking. When medications are given to dehydrated clients, it is helpful to give them one-at-a-time, which increases the amount of fluid consumed while taking medications. Because many dehydrated clients are also malnourished, use fluids that provide some nutrient value such as juice or oral supplements. Give antiemetics prophylactically to control nausea before drinking or taking medication that is highly emetogenic. When appropriate, begin with clear liquids, such as oral replacement fluids, broth, or gelatin. Progress to full liquids and then solid foods if tolerated without vomiting or aspiration. Encourage family members to participate in feeding. High-risk groups, such as those with dementia, have had improved fluid/nutrient outcomes in settings where the caregivers provided a more social environment during feeding. Interventions included simple verbal cuing, placing fluids/spoons in the resident's hand and with minimal guiding, positive body language, simple praises, limited distractions, and touch.

If dysphagia (difficulty in swallowing) is present, consult the physician regarding swallowing studies. Once the problem has been identified, a speech pathologist can provide exercises to help the client. Reinforce the speech therapist's prescription during each feeding. You may need to give thickened fluids, elevate the headrest to 90 degrees before meals and for 1 hour after feeding, and flex the client's head slightly forward at the start of a swallow. Decrease the risk of aspiration by placing small amounts of food on the side of the mouth that has the best sensation and muscle strength. Teaching the client to chew slowly and to swallow two or three times with each mouthful and inspecting the mouth for food pocketing can also decrease the risk of aspiration. Assessing the fit of dentures is also important. If the swallowing problem is not correctable, the client and client's family may need to consider artificial forms of feeding, such as tube-feeding.

Fluids by Intravenous Routes. Administer IV fluids cautiously to clients who are dehydrated. Ideally, a large IV gauge (e.g., 18- or 20-gauge needle) should be used; however, most clients have collapsed veins, and it is difficult to find a vein. A small IV gauge may be used initially; once fluids are reestablished, a larger catheter can be inserted if fluids or an IV access is still needed. Use an IV pump to regulate IV infusion and to decrease the risk of too rapid an infusion. Monitor IV solutions, IV sites, and client outcomes hourly.

Ensure that the rate of IV fluid via the pump is accurate; significant errors in setting IV pumps have occured.

Rapid fluid replacement often results in overflow diuresis without cellular replacement. Diuresis compounds dehydration and may result in hypernatremia. In older adults or in those with renal or cardiac disease, rapid fluid administration may also result in pulmonary overload.

Reduce the Risk of Deficient Fluid Volume. If your assessment indicates no fluid deficit but a risk of fluid deficit, the format for writing the problem statement is *Risk for Deficient Fluid Volume related to (risk factor).* The Mini Nutritional Assessment Tool is an effective tool for older adult risk assessment. Once risk is identified, interventions should focus on health promotion and maintenance strategies that decrease the likelihood of a deficit. The goal of oral fluid promotion and maintenance is to maintain the level of fluid intake at 1.5 ml/kg per 24 hours.

If the client is fed hypertonic tube-feedings, give water boluses with them. Recommended dilution is 1 ml of water per 1 kilocalorie (kcal) of feeding formula. For example, if a can of formula has 380 kcal in 240 ml of formula, give an additional 140 ml of water, for a total of 380 ml of fluid.

Control the Underlying Problems. Diarrhea has several causes. Examine the client's prescription and nonprescription (over-the-counter, herbal) medication list. If the onset of the diarrhea was at the same time as a new elixir drug with sorbitol was administered, a common cause of osmotic diarrhea, consult the pharmacist regarding pills rather than the elixir form. Consider viral infections because many infections have been known to result in lactose intolerance. If this is the cause, encourage the client to avoid milk-based products. Avoiding fatty or fried foods also decreases diarrhea and enhances digestion.

Give prescribed antiemetics for nausea, antipyretics for fever, and antibiotics for infection. Besides monitoring for positive responses to treatment, replace sensible fluid losses; for every degree of fever above 38 ° C, give an additional 500 ml of water above basal needs (approximately 1500 ml).

Monitor for Complications. When fluid balance is compromised, a person is at risk for tissue breakdown. Apply a moisturizer or skin barrier to protect the skin from the irritants, enzymes, and microorganisms found in urine and feces. Continue to assess lung sounds for manifestations of fluid overload (crackles) from overcorrection.

Diagnosis: Impaired Oral Mucous Membrane. The nursing diagnosis of *Impaired Oral Mucous Membrane related to lack of oral intake or other causes* is a common problem in clients with dehydration.

Outcomes. The desired outcome is that the mucous membranes are restored with expected outcomes of having an improvement in oral score. In addition, the client's tongue, gums, and lips should become moist and the mouth, gums, and teeth should be clean and free of accumulations of dried mucus.

Interventions. Provide oral care with a regular toothbrush or a foam toothbrush every 2 to 4 hours, and apply lip moisturizer. Rinse the client's mouth every 1 to 2 hours. Examine the client's mouth with a penlight to make sure that it remains free of debris. Avoid mouthwashes with an alcohol base, which can dry the mucous membranes. The frequency of oral care should be increased to hourly if there is no improvement. Artificial saliva can also be used for the client with a very dry and fissured mouth. Clients who have dysphagia also need oral care; a suction catheter should be used while oral care is provided to reduce the risk of aspiration.

Diagnosis: Risk for Injury. If orthostatic hypotension is present, *Risk for Injury* is another problem that needs to be addressed.

Outcomes. The desired outcome is that the client will have a reduced risk of injury as evidenced by no manifestations of falls (bruises, bumps, abrasions) or reported episodes of falls.

Interventions

Provide safety through stepped-progression position changes. Stepped-progression gives the client's body time to adapt to changes in position. First, raise the head of the bed. Next, assist the client to sit at the edge of the bed in a "dangling" position until the dizziness has subsided. Have the client stand, and assist the client to a chair. Do not progress to the next position until the client tolerates the current one (i.e., without dizziness or marked hypotension). Place alarm monitors on clients who are confused and tend to get out of bed without assistance. Sitters or restraints may be needed if all other measures to control behavior are ineffective.

Evaluation. Mild to moderate fluid deficits should be corrected in 8 to 24 hours. More severe fluid losses may take several days, especially when they occur in older adults.

Self-Care

Client teaching is one of the primary interventions for promoting and maintaining fluid balance. Teach clients with mild fluid deficit to replace fluid with clear liquids, 30 to 60 ml or more hourly, as tolerated, to decrease nausea and replace electrolytes. Teach the importance of consulting a physician if an illness lasts longer than 24 hours or if the person is older or has a chronic illness, such as diabetes mellitus or liver, kidney, or heart disease. Teach clients who take diuretics to continue to drink normally to avoid the rebound fluid retention syndrome; if the plasma volume drops too low, the renin cascade is triggered.

Health promotion teaching is critical for those who actively exercise. Teach people who exercise to do the following:

- Understand the importance of exercise and heat acclimatization over several days.
- Avoid exercise during high heat and humidity.
- Wear appropriate clothing (excess clothing decreases evaporation).
- Use more caution to prevent heat exhaustion if the client is obese, because obesity impairs the sweating mechanism.
- Drink cool water before exercise, 150 to 200 ml every 15 minutes during exercise, and after finishing exercise, and add 500 to 700 kcal of carbohydrates (for energy and sodium) if exercise is prolonged; do not wait for thirst to appear before drinking.
- Avoid rapid fluid replacement, because this fluid only overflows to the kidneys.
- Use caution when taking medications that interfere with thermoregulation, such as thyroid replacement, amphetamines, beta-blockers, haloperidol, antihistamines, anticholinergic drugs, and phenothiazines.

Encourage diabetic clients who exercise to wear or carry Medic-Alert identification, to increase their protein intake, to decrease refined sugar intake, and to reduce insulin to half the usual dosage or to an amount recommended by the physician. Teach people taking cortisone the importance of not missing doses, of carrying Medic-Alert identification, and of consulting a physician about increased dosage during physical or emotional stress to prevent adrenal crisis.

Reducing fluid intake as a way of decreasing urinary incontinence in older adults is inappropriate. Limited fluid intake increases bladder irritability, leading to uninhibited contractions, and alters the neurologic stimulus that controls normal bladder emptying. Emphasizing the importance of drinking even in the absence of thirst, teaching pelvic muscle exercises, and instituting a toilet schedule may help an older person overcome the problem of incontinence.

CELLULAR DEHYDRATION

Dehydration can become so severe that the cells become dehydrated. This condition is also called intracellular fluid volume deficit (ICFVD) and is relatively rare in a healthy adult, but it occurs often in older people and in those with conditions that result in acute water loss. Compensatory attempts to combat the fluid deficit have the same physiologic basis as in ECFVD. Thirst and oliguria are the most common compensatory signs. Cellular manifestations are due to the dysfunction in the cerebral cells and include fever and central nervous system (CNS) changes, such as confusion, and if not corrected can lead to cerebral hemorrhage and coma.

The desired outcome is restoration of fluid volume, which is initially addressed through IV replacement. Once the client becomes stable, the focus of medical management is correction or control of the underlying cause. The focus of nursing management is on prevention or early detection of complications secondary to the pathology or the treatment. Interdisciplinary communication is critical to the achievement of positive outcomes.

FLUID OVERLOAD

Fluid overload is overhydration or ECF volume excess (ECFVE). Excess fluids are in the vascular system, a problem called *hypervolemia,* or in the interstitial spaces, a problem usually called *third-spacing* (see later discussion). The water and sodium retained are in the same proportions as they exist in other ECF, and therefore this is referred to as *iso-osmolar (isotonic) fluid volume excess.*

Etiology

Fluid overload can develop from two processes: (1) simple administration of too much fluid or administering fluid too rapidly; (2) failure to excrete fluids. Fluid overload often results from an increase in the total body sodium level. Causes of fluid overload are listed in Table 11-3.

Fluid overload also results from renal disorders that impair glomerular filtration of sodium and water. As fluid volume increases, the heart attempts to compensate through tachycardia and hypertrophy. When compensatory mechanisms fail, heart failure results. Uncontrolled heart failure can lead to multiple organ failure and death from massive water retention, also known as *anasarca.*

Conditions that cause a decrease in plasma protein (mainly albumin) levels, such as liver or renal disease, burns, or protein malnutrition, result in a decreased oncotic pressure in the blood. The loss of oncotic pressure from low albumin level decreases reabsorption of water from the tissue spaces at the venous end of the capillary, which leads to peripheral edema or, if in the peritoneal cavity, ascites (Figure 11-3, *B*).

When lymphatic channels are obstructed or have been removed or damaged, tissue oncotic pressure increases and leads to edema (Figure 11-3, *C*). Edema can also develop from any condition, such as tissue trauma, that triggers the inflammatory response and thus results in increased capillary permeability (Figure 11-3, *D*).

Pathophysiology

When fluid overload is present, the hydrostatic pressure of the blood is higher than normal at the arterial end of the capillary, pushing excess fluids into the interstitial spaces. The excess fluid is not reabsorbed at the venous end of the capillary because the oncotic pressure is too low to pull the fluids back across the capillary membrane. Usually the residual fluids are removed by the

TABLE 11-3 Etiology of Extracellular Fluid Volume Excess

Etiologic Factor	Examples
Compromised regulation of fluid movement and excretion	Cirrhosis of liver Decreased plasma protein Heart failure Hypothyroidism Lymphatic or venous obstruction Renal disorders
Excessive ingestion of fluids or foods containing sodium	Excessive amounts of saline intravenous fluids Ingestion of high-sodium foods Excessive use of enemas with sodium (e.g., Fleet's) or medications with sodium (e.g., Alka-Seltzer)
Increased antidiuretic hormone (ADH) and aldosterone	Certain barbiturates and narcotics (e.g., morphine) Cushing's syndrome General anesthesia Glucocorticoid use Hyperaldosteronism Syndrome of inappropriate antidiuretic hormone (secretion)

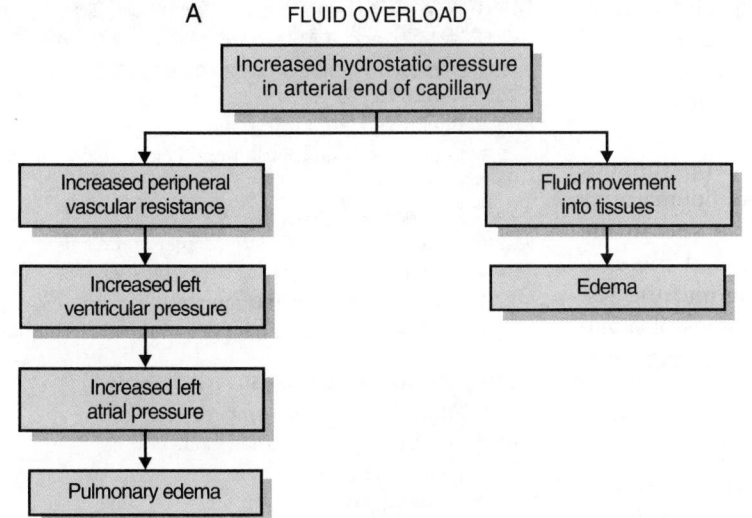

A   FLUID OVERLOAD

■ **FIGURE 11-3** Mechanisms of edema formation. **A,** Fluid overload. **B,** Decreased plasma and albumin. **C,** Altered lymphatic function. **D,** Tissue injury.

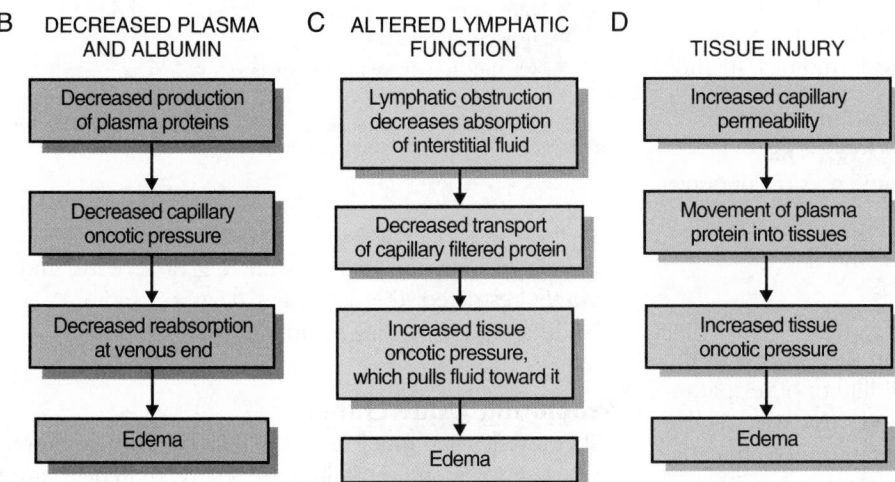

B   DECREASED PLASMA AND ALBUMIN

C   ALTERED LYMPHATIC FUNCTION

D   TISSUE INJURY

lymphatics, but in the case of edema, the fluid volume overloads the lymph system and stays in the interstitial space, leading to peripheral edema (Figure 11-3, *A*).

Edema can be progressive. As the fluid pressure increases in the interstitial area and tissues, it creates a resistance to forward blood flow and increases resistance throughout the circulatory system. This process is called *increased peripheral vascular resistance* and eventually it creates a gradient that resists left ventricular output. Blood is unable to be propelled forward and it backs up across the alveolocapillary membrane of the lungs, resulting in pulmonary fluid overload. Because the lungs are low-pressure organs, they also offer little resistance to fluid accumulation. Pulmonary edema may develop quickly in those people with an impaired left ventricle. If the right side of the heart fails, peripheral edema occurs through the same retrograde process. Left-sided heart failure may lead to right-sided failure and vice versa. Therefore pulmonary and peripheral edema may exist simultaneously.

Clinical Manifestations

Excessive fluid in the lungs leads to coughing, dyspnea, and crackles that can be auscultated over the involved lung area. The alveolar fluid accumulation also leads to impaired oxygen (O_2) and carbon dioxide (CO_2) transport between the capillaries and alveoli, resulting in pallor, cyanosis, decreased tissue oxygen levels (measured by pulse oximetry), anxiety, and increased CO_2 levels (measured in arterial blood gases). Manifestations are from increasing hydrostatic pressure in the pulmonary capillaries, which results in shifting of fluid to the alveolar sacs. If hydrostatic pressure continues to rise, fluid shifts into the pleural spaces as well; this is known as *pleural effusion.*

Cardiovascular manifestations are numerous. Delayed emptying and filling of the right ventricle leads to systemic venous engorgement, including signs of jugular venous distention, peripheral vein emptying time greater than 5 seconds, a bounding pulse and elevated blood pressure, and an increased right atrial pressure (central venous pressure [CVP]) and pulmonary capillary wedge pressure (PCWP). If the delayed ventricular filling overdistends the left ventricle, an extra heart sound (S₃) can often be auscultated with the bell of the stethoscope.

Fluid accumulates in the interstitial compartments, especially in gravity-dependent tissues. Edema may develop in the feet in ambulatory people and in the sacrum of bedridden clients. The continued increase in fluid pressure also causes fluid shifting into the visceral tissues. Thus the client may exhibit signs of organ dysfunction specific to the tissues involved (e.g., elevated liver enzymes from liver engorgement). Rapid weight gain is a classic sign of fluid overload regardless of the system responsible for the overload.

If any early changes in cerebral function develop, such as confusion and headache, suspect ICF shifting. As the fluid excess increases in the cerebral cells, lethargy occurs, followed by seizures and then coma.

With fluid overload, the excess fluid volume dilutes the concentration of solutes. Typical findings include the following:

- Plasma osmolality less than 275 mOsm/kg
- Plasma sodium level less than 135 mEq/L, depending on the type of fluid excess
- Hematocrit less than 45%
- Specific gravity less than 1.010
- BUN level less than 8 mg/dl

These results must be evaluated in the context of the client's manifestations and the possibility of other pathologic processes. For example, blood loss would also cause a decreased hematocrit; a decreased protein intake would result in decreased urea nitrogen levels. The volume of water may mask electrolyte and other solute levels. For example, the plasma sodium level may appear to be within the normal range because of excess water retention, even though the actual sodium level is increased.

OUTCOME MANAGEMENT

A thorough clinical history of contributing and causative factors, medication history, manifestations of fluid overload, and laboratory findings are essential to identifying appropriate interventions. Reduction of dietary sodium, restriction of fluids, and pharmacologic interventions are the major treatments for fluid overload.

Restriction of Sodium and Fluids

Because sodium retains water, sodium intake is commonly restricted especially in those clients with renal or heart disease. According to the usual definitions, a *mildly* restricted sodium diet contains 4 to 5 g of sodium, a

---

BOX 11-1　High-Sodium and Low-Sodium Foods

HIGH-SODIUM FOODS (APPROXIMATELY 250 MG/SERVING)

- Breads
- Cereals: most instant hot and cold cereals
- Chips
- Cheeses: all types
- Meats: sausage, luncheon, frankfurters, bacon, ham
- Convenience foods: pizza, pot pies, ravioli, soups (may have up to 5 times this amount)
- Most fast food items have 1 to 5 times this amount

LOW-SODIUM FOODS (<50 MG/SERVING)

- Fruits: fresh, frozen, canned
- Vegetables: fresh, frozen, canned
- Low-salt breads
- Unsalted pastas
- Oatmeal, cooked
- Unsalted popcorn
- Puffed rice
- Shredded wheat
- Fresh meat, chicken, fish (1 oz)

Data from Mahan, L.K., & Escott-Stump, S. (2000). *Krause's food, nutrition, and diet therapy* (10th ed.). Philadelphia: Saunders.

---

moderately restricted diet contains 2 g of sodium, and a *severely* restricted diet contains 0.5 g of sodium. Box 11-1 lists high- and low-sodium foods.

Promoting Urine Output

Mild diuretics and medications to increase cardiac output are used to promote fluid loss. Many diuretics cause potassium and magnesium to be excreted along with the sodium and water; therefore a combination of potassium-wasting and potassium-sparing diuretics may be prescribed.

Several studies have found improved myocardial contractility and decreased morbidity and mortality in clients with heart failure who have received angiotensin-converting enzyme (ACE) inhibitors, angiotensin II receptor blockers (ARBs), low-dose beta-blockers, or aldactone antagonists. Many of these clients showed such an improvement in their overall cardiac function that they did not need diuretics. When ACE inhibitors, ARBs, or aldactone antagonists are used, clients should be monitored for hyperkalemia because of the potassium-sparing effect of these drugs.

Nursing Management of the Medical Client

Assessment. Monitor the client's vital signs for a bounding pulse or elevated blood pressure, or both, every 4 to 8 hours. Assess the apical pulse if the radial pulse is irregular or if the client is taking cardiac medication. Assess breath sounds every 4 to 8 hours for crackles (especially in the bases of the lung), rhonchi, or wheezes. Assess for changes in respiratory effort with activity or rest. Note the position of comfort that the client prefers. Most dyspneic clients sit erect to ease the effort of breathing. If clients remain upright for continued periods, assess the skin of the sacrum for manifestations of edema and pressure ulcers. Use caution before lowering the client's head if a supine position worsens breathing.

Each morning, palpate the sacrum and legs for pitting edema and observe the client for hand and bilateral neck vein engorgement. Jugular vein distention at or above a 45-degree headrest and hand veins that do not flatten within 3 to 5 seconds when the hand is raised above the heart suggest fluid overload. Assess the condition of skin on the legs. Edematous skin is fragile and is at risk for injury (e.g., tearing) and decreased perfusion, which may lead to wounds.

Compare I&O every 4 to 8 hours. Weigh the client daily; do not rely on stated weights. Determine whether the client has had expected weight loss or unexpected weight gain. Edema does not usually occur until 3 L or more of excess fluid has accumulated. If edema seems pronounced in the extremities or abdomen, measure the area at the same site each shift and compare the data.

Monitor plasma osmolality, sodium level, hematocrit, and urine specific gravity. Observe for changes in level of consciousness, which may indicate the more serious complication of ICF shifting.

Diagnosis, Outcomes, Interventions

Diagnosis: Excess Fluid Volume. The diagnostic statement is written *Excess Fluid Volume* related to (specific cause, such as fluid retention secondary to heart, renal, or liver failure or excess consumption. Be certain to specify the cause in your client's case. If your client has heart failure, also consider using the nursing diagnosis *Decreased Cardiac Output.*

Outcomes. The desired outcome is return of normal levels of body fluids. Indicators of adequate fluid volumes include:

- Stable blood pressure and pulse rate
- Decreasing body weight of about 0.5 to 1 pound per day
- Absence of manifestations of ICFVE, such as confusion
- Absence of manifestations of fluid overload, such as coughing, crackles, dyspnea, jugular venous distention, peripheral edema, S_3 gallop rhythm
- Urea/nitrogen, plasma sodium, hematocrit, and osmolality levels approaching normal levels in 48 to 72 hours
- Absence of manifestations of overcorrection, such as hypotension and dry mucous membranes

Interventions

Reduce Sodium and Fluid Intake. Fluid management becomes extremely important in clients with fluid overload. Strict I&O may be crucial. Include fluids on meal trays and those given with medications as part of the total fluid intake. Collaborate with the dietitian in planning fluid restrictions. Schedule oral medications at meal times, if possible, to limit fluid intake. Use minimal amounts of water (5 to 10 ml) to dissolve crushed medications that need to be given by feeding tube. Cold fluids decrease the sensation of thirst more than warm or hot fluids. Give the client ice chips, if allowed, and provide frequent oral care to decrease the thirst sensation (1 cup of ice equals ½ cup of water). Teach clients to hold the water in the mouth for a while to rehydrate the tongue, rather than swallowing it quickly. Instruct clients about the rationale for fluid and sodium restrictions.

> **Use IV pumps to control IV fluid intake. Be cautious to set the pump correctly; adding one extra zero increases the volume ten times! Unplanned, unrestricted flow of IV fluids or medications can cause serious harm to clients. Use the devices that restrict flow on IV and PCA pumps as they are designed. Only use isotonic saline for bladder and nasogastric tube irrigations. Monitor clients who have received intraoperative irrigations with hypotonic solutions (e.g., bladder, prostate, hysteroscopic surgeries) for fluid overload and consult the physician about changing postoperative irrigations to normal saline.**

SAFETY ALERT

Sodium is a common ingredient in foods, and for many clients, the low-sodium diet is bland. Suggest alternatives for seasoning, such as lemon, garlic, or pepper, to enhance the taste of foods and increase dietary compliance. Salt substitutes are available but clients should be cautioned regarding the use of potassium salt substitutes if they are receiving ACE inhibitors or have renal disease (both cause potassium retention). Potassium salt substitutes are also "saltier" than sodium chloride, so the client should use them sparingly to avoid creating a metallic taste.

Mobilize Fluid. Instruct the client who has dependent leg edema to avoid long periods of standing and to sit with legs elevated. Bed rest alone promotes diuresis, particularly in clients with heart failure. Mobilization of edema in the supine position is probably due to decreased pooling of venous blood. When gravity no longer pulls blood to the legs, there is a rise in blood volume and usually an increase in urine output. However, some hearts cannot handle the increased fluid load. Do not elevate the legs in severe edema. Although elevation may help reduce swelling, the rapid return of pooled blood from the swollen legs can overwhelm the heart.

Reduce Complications. Elevate the head of the bed 30 to 45 degrees to decrease venous return, which decreases cardiac workload and allows for improved diaphragmatic excursion, both of which improve oxygenation. This position also promotes jugular venous drainage, which improves cerebral perfusion. If dyspnea or orthopnea is present, position the client in semi-Fowler's or Fowler's position. Consult with the physician for an order to adjust oxygen to keep oxygen saturation greater than 90%. If caring for clients undergoing hemodialysis, accurate dry weight assessments before dialysis treatments have demonstrated improvement in cardiac workload responses.

If the client is taking diuretics and digitalis, monitor plasma electrolyte levels and anticipate digitalis toxic effects resulting from hypokalemia. Report the abnormal levels of plasma electrolytes, especially potassium levels.

When peripheral tissue perfusion is altered because of edema or vascular disease, provide frequent skin care, turn the client often, control moisture, and prevent friction and shear. The heel is especially at risk for decreased capillary blood flow. Therefore it is important to keep the client's heels elevated off the mattress and to remove elastic stockings when nonblanchable erythema is noted. Lubricate the skin on the legs to prevent cracks and fissures.

Modifications for Older Clients. In general, these interventions are the same for the older client; however, response time is usually slower and the risk for side effects is higher because of poorer renal and liver function and problems with drug interactions. For instance, digitalis toxicity is much more common in older adults. Some diagnostic studies may not be as accurate in this population. For example, an older adult with protein malnutrition may have renal insufficiency but may have a normal urea/nitrogen level (BUN) because of the lack of protein. Thus it is very important to monitor creatinine levels; this provides a more precise reflection of renal function than the BUN. For persons in the high risk category for chronic kidney disease (those with diabetes, HTN, CVD, albuminuria, family history, older age, altered glomerular function for more than 3 months) a calculated glomerular filtration should be done. The Cockcroft-Gault or Levey equations are examples of formulas currently used.

Evaluation. Correcting fluid overload is a slow process, especially when it results from an organ disorder. Most clients are discharged without complete resolution of peripheral edema but with improvement in pulmonary edema and breathing. Self-care instructions are critical.

Self-Care

If the client is going home on a low-sodium diet, review allowed and restricted foods with the client and the person who prepares the meals. Many canned foods, pre-prepared foods, and seasonings are high in sodium and should be avoided; fresh and frozen foods are usually lower in sodium. Buying these items in season and freezing them for later use saves money and provides more nutrients. Encourage the food purchaser to read food labels and to avoid products with high levels of sodium or salt and food whose labels contain the word "sodium" or the symbol "Na" as a prefix. Avoid drinking or cooking with softened water, which is high in sodium. Water may need to be obtained from another source, or a water distiller may be needed.

Suggest alternatives for seasoning to enhance the taste of foods and to increase dietary compliance. Adding fresh lemon to vegetables and main dishes, condiments that come in powder form (such as garlic), or other low-sodium seasonings that can be found at food stores can improve taste. *People taking ACE inhibitors cannot use potassium salt substitutes.*

If fluids are restricted, help the client and family plan for how fluids can be spaced. Recognize the cultural variations in fluid consumption. In Western society, offering a guest something to drink is a common practice and may influence total fluid consumption.

The client should be weighed daily. Instruct the client and family to notify the physician if weight gain of more than 3 pounds per week is noted, if a marked reduction in urine output occurs, or if increased shortness of breath with exertion or especially at rest is seen. Other reasons to call the physician include new-onset headaches, confusion, seizures, or deterioration in level of consciousness.

WATER INTOXICATION

Although the cells are usually resistant to fluid shifts, certain conditions can lead to water intoxication or intracellular fluid volume excess (ICFVE). Conditions that cause acute or severe fluid volume excesses have a higher incidence of ICF overload. This is because the adaptive mechanisms may be unable to compensate for large or sudden fluid excesses.

Water intoxication results from either water excess or solute deficit, primarily sodium. In water excess, the number of solutes is normal but they are diluted by excessive water. In solute deficit, the amount of water is normal but there are too few particles per liter of water.

The most common cause of water intoxication is the administration of excessive amounts of hypo-osmolar IV fluids, such as 0.45% (half-strength) saline solution or 5% dextrose in water (D_5W). Water intoxication may occur in clients who receive continuous IV D_5W or in older clients who consume excessive amounts of tap water without adequate nutrient intake. Syndrome of inappropriate antidiuretic hormone (SIADH) also leads to ICFVE regardless of whether the SIADH is caused by CNS trauma, the stress of surgery, pain, or opioid use.

People with certain psychiatric disorders, such as schizophrenia, often drink water compulsively. Monitor intake in people with a history or current manifestations of an organic psychiatric illness.

Hypo-osmolar fluids in the vessels move by osmosis to the region of higher concentration of sodium in the cells in an attempt to maintain equilibrium. Too much fluid accumulating in the cells causes cellular edema. Cerebral cells absorb hypo-osmolar fluid more quickly than do other cells. Thus these cell changes often present the earliest warning signs of intracellular shifting.

All neurologic manifestations are secondary to the increasing intracranial pressure (ICP). Most ICP syndromes progress in a cephalocaudal order. Thus the early signs, such as changes in mental status, are seen in the brain and, as pressure increases to below the cortex, pupillary changes occur. Vital sign changes begin when the pressure is at the level of the hypothalamus and brain stem (late stages of increased ICP).

Because ICF excess is often associated with ECF excess, it is common to see a plasma sodium level of less than 125 mEq/L and a decreased hematocrit. However, there is no plasma test to reflect the cell fluid volume. Diagnostic tests, such as computed tomography and magnetic resonance imaging, are more helpful in identifying causes underlying water intoxication.

Neurologic cells are vulnerable to fluid excess or deficit. The first priority is to reduce ICP with steroids and osmotic diuretics. Equally as important is identifying and addressing the cause of the fluid volume excess. Immediate surgical intervention may be critical.

If SIADH is an impending risk, early administration of IV fluids containing some sodium chloride (NaCl) may prevent it. Saline solutions, such as $D_5/0.45\%$ NaCl, increase the osmolality of vascular fluid and prevent or help correct hypo-osmolality.

Because brain tissue has a narrow margin in which life is sustained, frequent monitoring and early intervention are critical. Perform neurologic checks, including level of consciousness, vital signs, reflexes, and pupillary responses, every hour if cranial changes are present. Cerebral perfusion is altered if systolic blood pressure drops too low or rises too high. Notify the provider if the client's neurologic response deteriorates from the baseline assessment, if systolic blood pressure is less than 100 mm Hg or greater than 160 mm Hg, or if other signs persist or worsen.

Monitor IV fluids and I&O hourly, and monitor weight daily. Polyuria is a good sign and indicates that fluid has shifted to the vascular space and to the renal tubules, where it can be excreted. Administer antiemetics prophylactically, as appropriate, to promote food and fluid ingestion and retention and to decrease the risk of vomiting, which worsens the increased ICP.

Provide safety measures when the client displays behavioral changes, such as confusion or disorientation. Keep the bed in a low position with bedside rails raised. Keep suction equipment at the bedside in anticipation of seizures. If a client has a seizure, protect the client from injury and maintain a patent airway by turning the client to one side to displace the tongue. Do not force the jaw open or attempt to insert a tongue blade. Remain at the bedside until the client is safe and document all phases of the seizure.

If the manifestations of increased ICP are improving, then the client is at less risk for complications. *Time equals brain cell survival.* The longer the manifestations of increased ICP persist and the more serious they are, the graver the prognosis.

THIRD-SPACE FLUIDS

Third-spacing is a term used to describe the accumulation of fluids in the interstitial spaces. The third-space fluid is not the fluid in the vessels or in the cells; it is the fluid around the cells and vessels. Third-space fluid is physiologically useless because it does not circulate to provide nutrients for cells. This abnormal fluid accumulation not only results from pathologic conditions but also reflects an inability of the lymphatic system to compensate. Common sites of third-spacing include the pleural cavity, peritoneal cavity, and pericardial sac.

Etiology

Fluids can move into interstitial spaces because of increased hydrostatic pressure, increased capillary permeability, decreased serum protein levels, obstruction of the venous portion of the capillary, or nonfunctional lymphatic drainage systems.

Any pathologic process that triggers the inflammatory or ischemic processes can lead to fluid shifting. For example, massive fluid shifts from the vascular to the interstitial spaces can be seen in crush injuries, major tissue trauma, major surgery, extensive burns, acid-base imbalance, bowel obstruction, and sepsis.

Decreased protein intake, production, or storage, or increased protein loss as seen in protein-calorie malnutrition and in liver and kidney disease can lead to hypoalbuminemia. Bowel disorders that reduce protein absorption can reduce serum levels. Other conditions that cause a loss of protein, such as large draining wounds or burns, also deplete protein stores. Increased protein anabolism can occur in the healing phase of fractures or wounds; increased protein catabolism can occur with fever, infection or sepsis, and malignancy.

Altered lymphatic function and venous thrombosis impair fluid return to the right atrium, thus promoting third-spacing. The decreased colloidal osmotic pressures from the impaired protein synthesis, as noted earlier, is only compounded by the portal hypertension that accompanies end-stage liver disease, leading to third-spacing in the peritoneal cavity (ascites).

Pathophysiology

Tissue injury causes the release of histamine and brady-kinin, resulting in increased capillary permeability, which allows more fluid, protein, and other solutes to move into the interstitial spaces than normal. This form of fluid shift may be time-limited. The early stages of inflammation last about 24 to 48 hours; the capillary membrane heals and the fluid returns to the venous system. It may take longer in conditions with prolonged inflammatory responses or severe tissue injury.

Protein malnutrition leads to decreased oncotic pressures because protein is not present to pull fluid back into the capillary at the venous end. This form of fluid shifting is usually long term and can be seen in children who are protein malnourished and have large protruding abdomens and pencil-thin legs.

Two phases of fluid shift are associated with tissue injury:

1. Fluid shifts from vascular to interstitial spaces, which leads to a risk for fluid volume deficit (*hypovolemia*) (see Figure 11-3, *D*). Severe hypovolemia may lead to vascular collapse and death. If cellular damage is severe, a toxic response may occur from intracellular ions, such as potassium, that leak into the vascular spaces.
2. As the capillary membrane heals, fluid shifts back from the interstitial to the vascular space, which leads to a risk for fluid volume excess (*hypervolemia*). If the hypervolemia is severe, it may lead to heart failure. Intracellular potassium ions shift back into the cell during this phase, which increases the risk for hypokalemia.

Clinical Manifestations

Clinical manifestations of a fluid shift from the vascular to the interstitial spaces are similar to the manifestations of hypovolemia because the fluid is not in the vascular system. Typical clinical manifestations include pallor, cold limbs, weak and rapid pulse, hypotension, oliguria, and decreased levels of consciousness. Body weight does not change because fluid has not been lost; it has been redistributed. Severe losses can result in hypovolemic shock.

If fluid collects and obstructs an organ, nerve, or vessel, other clinical manifestations may arise. For example, bowel sounds may change throughout the abdomen. Extremities may become pale, cool, and pulseless if fluid obstructs blood vessels or nerves. Laboratory results may indicate an elevated hematocrit, sodium level, BUN level, and urine specific gravity.

When fluid returns to the blood vessels, the clinical manifestations are similar to those of fluid overload. Signs may include a bounding pulse, crackles, engorgement of peripheral and jugular veins, and an increase in blood pressure. Laboratory results may indicate a decrease in hematocrit and BUN levels. Other abnormal findings depend on the area of the body affected.

OUTCOME MANAGEMENT

As with other types of fluid imbalances, third-spacing is only a manifestation. It is crucial that the underlying cause be identified through a thorough history and physical examination so that interventions can be targeted to the desired outcomes.

Medical treatment begins with determining the cause of the fluid volume shift. If the third-spacing of fluid has occurred around the heart (pericardial effusion), around the lung (pleural effusion), or in the peritoneal cavity (ascites), the physician removes the excess fluid by tapping the space with a large-bore needle; these procedures are known as pericardiocentesis, thoracentesis, and paracentesis, respectively.

Replace Fluids

When hypovolemia results from tissue injury, such as burns or crush injuries, a large volume of isotonic IV fluid administration is required to replace intravascular volume. When there is evidence of capillary healing (increase in urine output without additional fluids), albumin may be given to replace the protein lost from the trauma and to promote restoration of capillary oncotic pressures. Because third-spacing is a common occurrence after major surgery, maintaining IV fluid intake is essential to maintaining kidney perfusion. The amount of fluid infusion may be three times greater than urine output. Generally, fluids are titrated to maintain an adequate blood pressure, CVP, PCWP, and urine output. During the first 24 to 72 hours when there is an increase in ADH and the healing phase is beginning with fluid moving back into the vessels, the client is at risk for fluid overload if the fluid replacement is too rapid.

Stabilize Other Problems

Some etiologies of fluid shifting are life-threatening and must be treated aggressively. For example, sepsis causes major increases in capillary permeability and must be treated with IV antibiotics and, usually, vasoactive medications to maintain blood pressure. Bowel obstructions can cause major third-spacing and lead to gangrene; surgical repair is critical. Serious inflammatory disorders require massive doses of steroids to stabilize the mast cell membrane.

Nursing Management of the Medical Client

If shock-like symptoms are present, assess vital signs every hour until the blood pressure is greater than 90 mm Hg; progress up to every 8 hours as the client's condition stabilizes. If fluid loss is a result of ascites or peripheral edema, the fluid shift is slower and changes in vital signs are usually subtle.

Monitor IV Fluid Replacement Needs

If fluids are administered too rapidly, fluid overload or hypervolemia may occur. Assess for early signs of fluid overload, such as crackles, difficulty in breathing, and neck vein engorgement. Notify the physician if these signs are present. Anticipate a reduction in IV fluid needs as the third-space fluid shifts back into the plasma during the capillary repair stage.

If the third-spacing is in the abdomen, as with ascites, measure the client's abdominal girth every 8 hours. If a limb is involved, measure the circumference of the limb and assess peripheral pulses every 8 hours. Use preventive measures to prevent skin breakdown of edematous areas.

Monitor urine output every hour, and report an output of less than 0.5 ml/kg/hr if it persists for more than 2 hours. The client may need more fluids, not diuretics. Urine output is usually reduced after tissue injury because of decreased renal perfusion and a fluid shift into the injured tissue spaces. One to 3 days after tissue injury, fluid returns to the circulation and the kidneys excrete excess fluid unless renal function is impaired, the injury was massive, or the client has impaired adaptive mechanisms. Monitor plasma levels of BUN and creatinine.

SODIUM IMBALANCES

Natrium is the Latin word for sodium. Sodium deficit is known as *hyponatremia;* sodium excess is known as *hypernatremia*. Chloride is the anion that usually accompanies sodium; therefore levels of chloride usually decrease or increase along with levels of sodium. Manifestations of chloride imbalance are usually associated with the cation imbalance. Any condition that alters the renin-angiotensin-aldosterone system, kinin system, or atrial natriuretic or antidiuretic hormonal response places a person at risk for sodium imbalances.

HYPONATREMIA

Hyponatremia is defined as a plasma sodium level less than 135 mEq/L. It is one of the most common electrolyte disorders in adults, especially older adults. Hyponatremia is usually associated with changes in fluid volume status. The four types of hyponatremic states are as follows:

- Hypovolemic hyponatremia—sodium loss is greater than water loss
- Euvolemic hyponatremia—total body water (TBW) is moderately increased and sodium levels are normal
- Hypervolemic hyponatremia—there is a greater increase in TBW than in total body sodium

- Redistributive hyponatremia—there is no change in TBW or sodium but instead a shifting between intracellular and extracellular compartments

Etiology and Risk Factors

Table 11-4 lists the most common causes of hyponatremia. The most common causes of hyponatremia are conditions that lead to fluid overload. Cardiac, renal, and liver diseases increase the total body sodium levels. However, because of fluid retention the plasma sodium level may appear normal or low. Normally, when hyponatremia occurs from fluid overload, diuresis follows to promote the return of sodium and water levels to homeostasis. Renal causes of hyponatremia stem from the inability to excrete sufficiently dilute urine.

Hyponatremia can also occur in people who are considered healthy. For example, athletes, outdoor laborers, and military personnel are at risk for hyponatremia from excessive perspiration. Any person with an altered thirst mechanism or without access to fluids, or one who attempts to rehydrate too rapidly after excessive fluid loss, is at risk for hyponatremia. Older adults are at increased risk because of their relatively lower percentage of TBW. The preoperative use of laxatives, multiple pathologic conditions, spinal anesthesia, and noninfectious postoperative complications increase risk factors for death from hyponatremia in older adults after surgery. Those undergoing surgeries in which hypotonic irrigations are used have increasing risk correlated with the length of the procedure.

Hyponatremia can also develop as a side effect of medications. Hyponatremia has also been noted in clients with poor dietary intake who consume large amounts of beer and in clients after use of the recreational drug ecstasy.

TABLE 11-4 Clinical Conditions and Disorders That May Cause Hyponatremia

Type of Hyponatremia	Clinical Conditions and Disorders
Hypovolemic hyponatremia	Renal loss of sodium from diuretic use, diabetic glycosuria, aldosterone deficiency, intrinsic renal disease Extrarenal loss of sodium from vomiting, diarrhea, increased sweating, burns, high-volume ileostomy, cerebral salt wasting
Euvolemic hyponatremia	Sodium deficit resulting from SIADH* or increased secretion of ADH because of pain, emotion, medications (e.g., SSRIs); some cancers and CNS disorders
Hypervolemic hyponatremia	Edematous disorders resulting in sodium deficits: congestive heart failure, cirrhosis of liver, nephrotic syndrome, acute and chronic renal failure, psychogenic polydipsia
Redistributive hyponatremia	Pseudohyponatremia, hyperglycemia, hyperlipidemia, hyperimmunoglobinemia (as in multiple myeloma)

*ADH, Antidiuretic hormone; CNS, central nervous system; SIADH, syndrome of inappropriate (secretion of) antidiuretic hormone; SSRIs, selective serotonin reuptake inhibitors.

Pathophysiology

Recall that most of the sodium exists in the vascular fluids, and that sodium moves into the cell when the cell contracts (in exchange for potassium) or is pulled in by the negatively charged proteins in the cell. When the serum level of sodium is low, there is less sodium available to move across the excitable membrane, resulting in delayed membrane depolarization. Excitable tissues vary in their response to decreased sodium. The cells most sensitive to low serum sodium levels are the neurologic cells.

As the concentration of sodium decreases in the extracellular fluid (ECF), the fluid becomes hypo-osmolar. Water moves into the cell to the area of greater concentration to rebalance the water concentration. This osmotic shift can lead to intracellular edema. A very small increase in brain cell volume (5%) can cause brain stem herniation because of the limited space in the cerebral vault. Brain cells attempt to compensate by reducing cerebral blood flow, shifting cerebral spinal fluid, and decreasing the brain's intracellular osmolality. Intracellular osmolality is reduced through decreasing the amount of intracellular ions, such as sodium and potassium, and amino acids.

Clinical Manifestations

Clinical manifestations of hyponatremia vary with the cause, type, and rate of onset of sodium or fluid imbalance. A person with a plasma sodium level of 120 mEq/L that developed slowly may be asymptomatic. The same plasma sodium level resulting from an acute loss may be life-threatening.

When plasma sodium concentration is greater than 125 mEq/L, clinical manifestations may not be apparent. Early neurologic manifestations of headache and apprehension are from increased fluid shift into the cerebral cells. As intracranial pressure increases and plasma sodium level decreases to 115 mEq/L, severe neurologic changes such as confusion, hallucinations, behavioral changes, and seizures occur. Continued shifting of water into the intracellular compartment leads to brain herniation, resulting in coma and death.

Cardiovascular manifestations, such as a decrease in systolic and diastolic blood pressures, orthostatic hypotension, and a weak, thready pulse, are due to a decrease in vascular volume secondary to sodium and water loss. Tachycardia is a compensatory response that is the direct result of triggering of the release of sympathetic catecholamines by the baroreceptor reflex. Chemoreceptors in the aortic arch and carotid bodies also trigger sympathetic responses if the oxygen, carbon dioxide, or hydrogen levels become affected. In severe hypovolemic hyponatremia, a shock-like state occurs, with blood pressures of 60 mm Hg and below. An exception is hypervolemic hyponatremia, in which the excess volume causes elevated blood pressure and a full, rapid pulse.

Much like fluid overload, crackles in the lungs are from fluid shifting into the pulmonary alveoli secondary to increasing fluid pressures in the pulmonary capillaries. The increasing left ventricular fluid pressure leads to a retrograde increase in pressure in the left atrium and pulmonary vasculature. The changes in respiratory rate and difficulty breathing—such as tachypnea, dyspnea, orthopnea, and feeling short of breath—are from the presence of fluid in the alveoli, which alters oxygen and carbon dioxide exchange. Alterations in respiratory pattern, such as with Cheyne-Stokes respirations, neurogenic hyperventilation, apneustic breathing, or ataxic breathing, are from progressive increases in intracranial pressure.

Hyponatremia causes gastrointestinal (GI) manifestations, such as nausea, vomiting, hyperactive bowel sounds, abdominal cramping, and diarrhea, because sodium is a crucial component of normal neuromuscular activity of smooth muscle. A decrease in the level of sodium causes increased excitability of the neurons that innervate the smooth muscle.

Although not life-threatening, the dryness of the skin, tongue, and mucous membranes that results from the decreased interstitial volume caused by a sodium deficit has other, more serious implications. There is a higher risk for altered integrity of the skin and oral mucous membranes, which increases the risk of infection and results in increased health care needs and costs.

A laboratory finding of a plasma sodium level less than 135 mEq/L is diagnostic of hyponatremia. However, as noted previously, most clients are not symptomatic until levels reach 125 mEq/L or less. Because chloride is the main anion associated with sodium, a chloride level less than 98 mEq/L is a common finding. A decreased concentration of sodium is also reflected in a plasma osmolality of less than 275 mOsm/kg. The kidney attempts to compensate for the body's loss of sodium by decreasing urinary losses; thus a typical urine sodium level is less than 40 mEq/L. If the hyponatremic state and body fluid volume disorders are not corrected, potassium, calcium, chloride, and bicarbonate electrolyte imbalances may also occur.

OUTCOME MANAGEMENT

Medical Management

Medical management is determined by the cause of the hyponatremia, the type of hyponatremia, and the severity of the clinical manifestations. The more serious the manifestations, the more aggressive the treatment. The goal of medical intervention is correction of the body water osmolality, with restoration of cell volume, by raising the ratio of sodium to water in the ECF. The increased ECF osmolality draws water from the cells, thereby decreasing cellular edema.

Restore Sodium Levels

Fluids are restricted to allow the sodium to regain balance. Intake of balanced diet is usually adequate therapy for mild hyponatremia, with sodium levels of 126 to 135 mEq/L. Fluids may be restricted to a range of 1000 to 1500 ml/day.

If the plasma sodium level declines below 125 mEq/L, sodium replacement is needed. For sodium levels of 125 mEq/L or less, intravenous (IV) therapy is the treatment of choice. Dietary supplementation may still be appropriate for a client who can ingest oral fluids or food. Foods high in sodium are listed in Box 11-2. For moderate hyponatremia, with sodium levels of 125 mEq/L, IV normal saline solution (0.9% NaCl) or lactated Ringer's solution may be ordered if the client is symptomatic. When the plasma sodium level is 115 mEq/L or less, a concentrated saline solution such as 3% NaCl may be indicated until the plasma sodium concentration reaches 125 mEq/L. A diuretic such as furosemide is often given intravenously to prevent pulmonary fluid overload. Demeclocycline, an agent that antagonizes antidiuretic hormone (ADH), is the preferred agent for treatment of hyponatremia resulting from syndrome of inappropriate antidiuretic hormone (SIADH).

Rapid elevation of plasma sodium concentrations to more than 125 mEq/L increases intravascular fluid volume and may result in hypernatremia and CNS damage. Recommendations for IV replacement therapy include an infusion rate of 0.5 mEq/L/hr if the loss is chronic, not to exceed a total of 12 mEq of sodium in 48 hours, or of 1 mEq/L/hr if the loss is acute, not to exceed 25 mEq in 48 hours. To prevent fluid shifts and exacerbation of vasospasm in clients with subarachnoid hemorrhage, normal saline is usually the IV solution of choice.

Nursing Management of the Medical Client

Assessment. Take a complete history of risk factors and presenting manifestations. Collect complete and detailed information on the client's diet and medications, including over-the-counter and herbal medications. Older adults are especially susceptible to drug-drug interactions that may alter sodium balance. The client and family members should be asked about behavioral changes, headaches, increased weakness or sleepiness, dizziness, and palpitations.

Measure the client's body weight, because the stated weight may not be accurate. Compare the client's height and weight to the body mass index (BMI) chart. Assess intake and output, peripheral vein filling time, and vital signs every 4 to 8 hours. Also, monitor plasma sodium levels and estimate the plasma osmolality. It is important to remember that in hyponatremic conditions, such as hypervolemic hyponatremia, plasma sodium levels may appear to be normal to low.

Diagnosis, Outcomes, Interventions

Collaborative Problem: Risk for Hyponatremia. The collaborative problem of *Risk for Hyponatremia* can be used to label this client problem. State the problem as *Risk for Hyponatremia related to unreplaced loss or limited oral intake*. When actual hyponatremia is present, the collaborative problem is stated as *Hyponatremia related to* (e.g., *vomiting, diarrhea, gastric suctioning, burns, SIADH, surgery, or fluid overload*). The cause needs to be clear because it guides the interventions.

Outcomes. When writing an outcome statement for a collaborative problem, the role of the nurse changes. Because the nurse does not have direct responsibility for the outcome, the role of the nurse changes to monitoring. An outcome may be written as follows: The nurse will monitor laboratory sodium and chloride levels and will continue to monitor for clinical manifestations of hyponatremia. The nurse will also have a high index of suspicion for high-risk clients and will monitor clients who have had fluid losses or limited fluid intake for manifestations of hyponatremia. When assessment indicates an actual sodium deficit, restoration is the primary goal.

Interventions

Reduce Sodium Loss in High-Risk Clients. If plasma sodium levels are greater than 125 mEq/L, encourage intake of 30 to 60 ml of clear liquids or more per hour as tolerated. If the client is on a low-sodium diet, do not be concerned about sodium restriction until the vomiting or diarrhea subsides and the client is taking whole foods.

To prevent sodium loss, irrigate nasogastric tubes and wounds with isotonic saline and give only minimal ice chips, even if ordered, when a nasogastric tube is connected to suction. Never give more than three tap water or soap suds enemas in succession without consulting the physician about converting the enema solution to normal saline. Treat nausea with prophylactic antiemetics. Consult the physician if (1) the sodium level is less than 125 mEq/L or sooner if the client is symptomatic or (2) the client is receiving nothing by mouth (NPO status) and has no intake of electrolytes or has an increased loss of electrolytes.

Restore Sodium Balance. Encourage the intake of a well-balanced diet. Give nutrient-dense supplements between meals. If the client is receiving nutrition only through tube feedings, it is sometimes necessary to add extra salt to the feeding to achieve the desired sodium level. If the hyponatremia is secondary to hypervolemia, consult with the physician and dietitian to coordinate therapeutic fluid restriction. Strict behavioral modification or psychiatric consultation may be necessary for a client who drinks water compulsively.

To decrease the thirst that accompanies fluid restriction, offer ice chips, cold fluids, and frequent oral care. Some clients feel less thirsty if they hold the fluids in their mouth first to fully moisten the oral mucous membranes before swallowing. Restricting fluids is contraindicated in clients with subarachnoid hemorrhage because it increases the risk of cerebral vasospasm and central pontine myelinolysis.

When plasma sodium levels are 125 mEq/L or less and the client is symptomatic, notify the physician immediately. Administration of hypertonic IV saline (3% saline) is the most commonly prescribed therapy.

SAFETY ALERT

Caution: Hypertonic saline must be given very slowly in a large vein, using an IV pump, to decrease the risk of hypernatremia, pulmonary overload, and phlebitis. If the client is confused or agitated, also initiate safety and seizure precautions.

Evaluation. Mild to moderate deficits are usually corrected in 8 to 24 hours. More severe deficits may take several days, especially in older adults. Evaluate the client's and family members' understanding of positive health behaviors that prevent further occurrences of sodium deficit.

Self-Care

Teach the client to consult the physician if vomiting or diarrhea persists for more than 48 hours, or sooner if extreme weakness, dizziness, palpitations, irregular pulse of new onset, cough or dyspnea, or CNS changes (such as headache, confusion, or seizures) develop. Anyone who has a chronic disease—such as renal, liver, or heart disease or diabetes mellitus—should consult a physician if any manifestations persist for more than 24 hours.

Teach clients to consult a physician before taking over-the-counter or herbal medications. Review the exercise precautions discussed earlier. Refer people with eating disorders to counseling and community support groups.

HYPERNATREMIA

Hypernatremia is defined as a plasma sodium level greater than 145 mEq/L. It occurs in about 1% of hospitalized clients and carries a high mortality rate, whether it has an acute or a chronic onset. Hypernatremia is usually associated with water loss or sodium gain. It can occur with increased, decreased, or normal total body sodium levels and decreased or increased TBW levels. The underlying cause of hypernatremia is a TBW deficit relative to the total body sodium content, which results in hyperosmolality.

Etiology and Risk Factors

Body fluid loss resulting in hypernatremia may be from renal or extrarenal causes, such as GI or skin problems. Hypernatremia can be classified as one of three types:

- Hypovolemic hypernatremia—TBW is greatly decreased relative to sodium (loss of hypotonic fluid)
- Euvolemic hypernatremia—TBW is decreased relative to the normal total body sodium
- Hypervolemic hypernatremia—TBW is increased but the sodium gain exceeds the water gain

Hypervolemic hypernatremia is the least common type of hypernatremia. Table 11-5 presents clinical conditions and disorders that may contribute to the development of hypernatremia. Older adults and debilitated people are at highest risk for development of hypernatremia. Major risk factors include inadequate water intake in conjunction with decreased thirst (hypodipsia), lack of access to drinkable water, physical or chemical restraint, mental confusion, and NPO status. Excessive water loss and insufficient fluid replacement associated with fever, vomiting, diarrhea, excess drainage, polyuria, tube-feeding, or prolonged hyperventilation are also major risk factors.

Other factors that increase the risk for hypernatremia include increased sodium intake, such as with IV administration of hypertonic saline or hypertonic tube feedings. Retention of sodium occurs in heart, renal, or liver disease; Cushing's syndrome; hyperaldosteronism; corticosteroid therapy; and uncontrolled diabetes mellitus or diabetes insipidus. Uncontrolled diabetes mellitus results in polyuria, leading to dehydration and secondary hypernatremia. Hypernatremia from untreated diabetes insipidus tends to be mild. Although the ADH

TABLE 11–5   Clinical Conditions and Disorders That May Contribute to Hypernatremia

Type of Hypernatremia	Clinical Conditions and Disorders
Hypovolemic hypernatremia	Renal losses, osmotic diuresis, diuretics, severe hyperglycemia Extrarenal losses: profuse diaphoresis, decreased thirst, diarrhea occurring with inadequate volume replacement or fluid replacement with hyperosmolar solutions, burns
Euvolemic hypernatremia	Excess fluid losses from skin and lungs Hypodipsia in older adults and infants
Hypervolemic hypernatremia	Diabetes insipidus Administration of concentrated saline solutions; hypertonic feedings; excess mineralocorticoids Accidental or intentional salt ingestion; commercially prepared soups and canned vegetables

mechanism is altered, the thirst mechanism is intact and stimulates the client to drink water and fluids, which helps balance water losses and hypernatremia.

Pathophysiology

When sodium levels increase, water moves to maintain balance. However, the osmotic shift of water from the cells to the ECF in an attempt to dilute the hyperosmolar state only creates another problem: cellular dehydration. If the hypernatremia evolves slowly or is chronic, the brain develops its own osmotic particles, called *idiogenic osmoles,* to prevent fluid shifts into and out of the brain cells.

The heart is sensitive to the increasing sodium levels. Calcium must move through the calcium channels for cardiac muscle contraction to occur. However, in hypernatremia, sodium molecules compete with calcium in the slow calcium channels of the heart, resulting in decreased myocardial contractility. Myocardial depolarization, however, occurs more easily with the increased sodium levels.

Generally, the body responds to increased sodium levels by suppressing the effects of aldosterone and ADH. These two substances normally act to increase renal blood flow and cause excretion of sodium and water. In hypernatremia, the magnitude of the problem overwhelms the ability of these adaptive mechanisms to compensate.

Clinical Manifestations

In the early stages of hypernatremia, clinical manifestations are nonspecific because two thirds of body water is intracellular; primary water losses tend to cause only modest effects on circulating blood volume. Early manifestations include polyuria followed by oliguria, anorexia, nausea, vomiting, weakness, and restlessness. The anorexia, nausea, and vomiting are related to increased fluid retention in the gastric cells. Early neurologic manifestations of restlessness, agitation, irritability, and muscle weakness are related to the sensitivity of brain cells to fluid shifting.

The response of the kidneys varies with the type of hypernatremia. In a hypervolemic state, the kidneys excrete some of the excess water. In a hypovolemic state, oliguria is the method of renal compensation. As fluid levels decrease in the interstitial compartments, the skin becomes dry and flushed, the mucous membranes become dry and sticky, and tongue furrows develop. The person experiences increasing thirst and fever. Temperature elevation is from the dehydration in the hypothalamic cells from the fluid shifting out of these cells to the more hypertonic extracellular spaces.

Cardiovascular manifestations are related to the type of hypernatremia. In hypovolemic hypernatremia, orthostatic hypotension with compensatory tachycardia occurs. In hypervolemic hypernatremia, a hypertensive blood pressure, jugular venous distention, prolonged peripheral vein emptying, S_3 gallop, and generalized weight gain and edema are often present.

Dysrhythmia can result from the competition of sodium ions with calcium ions in the slow channels of the heart cells. Pulmonary manifestations, such as crackles, dyspnea, and pleural effusion, are also a result of the increasing hydrostatic pressure seen in hypervolemic hypernatremia.

When sodium levels reach 155 mEq/L or more, cells (especially brain cells) shrink because of the increased ECF osmolality. More severe neurologic changes occur, manifested as confusion, seizures, or coma, in some cases with irreversible brain damage. Altered neuromuscular contractility and irritability lead to muscle twitching, tremor, hyperreflexia, and seizures. The development of rigid paralysis is a grave sign.

The diagnosis of hypernatremia is validated when plasma sodium levels are greater than 145 mEq/L and plasma osmolality is more than 295 mOsm/kg. Because chloride is the major ECF ion that balances sodium, it is common to find a plasma chloride level greater than 106 mEq/L. Unless the sodium elevation is an acute change, many clients are not symptomatic until plasma sodium concentration reaches 155 mEq/L or more.

OUTCOME MANAGEMENT

Again, a thorough history and physical examination, including laboratory studies, is necessary for accurate diagnosis of hypernatremia. Awareness of demographic variables is essential for choosing the appropriate interventions for restoring sodium balance.

Medical Management

Medical management is determined by the type of hypernatremia. The goal of medical intervention is correction of the body water osmolality, with restoration of cell volume, by decreasing the ratio of sodium to water in the ECF.

For a client experiencing minor manifestations from hypovolemia or euvolemic hypernatremia, the focus is on correcting the underlying disorder and giving oral fluid replacement. However, clients with cardiovascular, pulmonary, or neurologic manifestations from severe hypernatremia usually require hospitalization and the more aggressive approach of IV hypotonic saline.

To decrease total body sodium and replace fluid loss, either a hypo-osmolar electrolyte solution (0.2% or 0.45% NaCl) or 5% dextrose in water (D_5W) is administered. These solutions do not cause a considerable dilution of body sodium; instead, the plasma sodium level gradually decreases as excess sodium is excreted. When administered continuously, D_5W is considered to be a hypo-osmolar solution because the dextrose is metabolized quickly and only water remains. If the plasma sodium level is lowered too rapidly, fluid shifts from the vascular fluid into the cerebral cells, causing cerebral edema. Slow administration of IV fluids with a goal of reducing plasma sodium levels, at a rate of not more than 2 mEq/L/hr for the first 48 hours, decreases this risk.

Hypernatremia caused by sodium excess may be treated with administration of D₅W and a diuretic, such as furosemide. When hypernatremia results from diabetes insipidus, desmopressin acetate, in the form of a nasal spray, is commonly ordered to slow the rate of diuresis.

Although dietary sodium restriction is useful in preventing hypernatremia in high-risk clients, it cannot bring a high sodium level down to normal. People with renal disease may need sodium intake restricted to 500 to 2000 mg/day (see Box 11-1). In hypervolemic hypernatremia, fluids must also be restricted. Clients with diabetes insipidus who are receiving antidiuretic medications must be taught to avoid excessive water intake. Drinking excess water defeats the purpose of the medication.

Nursing Management of the Medical Client

Assessment. Assess for the usual clinical manifestations, especially in head-injured and other high-risk clients. Obtain a thorough diet and medication history, including the use of corticosteroids and over-the-counter medications, such as cough medicine, herbals, food flavorings, and spices (salt).

Depending on the client's condition, assess vital signs and peripheral vein filling time every 4 to 8 hours, measure intake and output every 8 hours, and monitor body weight daily. Use oral membrane and skin assessment tools to guide your interventions. Monitor for changes in plasma sodium level and plasma osmolality (by estimated values). Report early signs of altered mental status, such as agitation, irritability, or confusion that may indicate progression of hypernatremia or hyponatremia. Monitor lung sounds every 2 to 4 hours, and notify the physician of increasing pulmonary overload.

Diagnosis, Outcomes, Interventions
Collaborative Problem: Hypernatremia. Use a collaborative problem, such as *Hypernatremia related to* (e.g., *decreased thirst, excessive administration of salt solutions,* or *impaired excretion of sodium and water*). The cause needs to be identified specifically, because it guides the choice of interventions.

Outcomes. The nurse will maintain a high index of suspicion for high-risk clients and will monitor plasma sodium and chloride levels and clinical manifestations of hypernatremia.

Interventions. Monitor the client for response to IV fluid replacement of hypo-osmolar electrolyte solutions,

absence of clinical manifestations of hypernatremia, and return to normal sodium levels. Prevent osmotic diuresis from D₅W by maintaining the prescribed rate.

Use IV pumps in high-risk clients. Initiate safety and seizure precautions if the client manifests weakness or cerebral changes.

Offer water and fluids hourly to clients with hypovolemic or euvolemic hypernatremia. Consult with the dietitian and the physician concerning the need for fluid and sodium restriction in those with hypervolemic hypernatremia. Teach the client and family members the food items that should be restricted as well as the rationale for these restrictions.

Give 1 ml of fluid per kilocalorie (kcal) of hypertonic feeding solution. Initiate new gastric feedings slowly. Increase the rate if the client tolerates the feeding, as evidenced by no diarrhea, with residuals less than half the amount of the feeding per hour, or up to 100 ml.

Consult the physician for manifestations that indicate worsening of the hypernatremia or fluid overload, such as increasing weight gain or pulmonary, cardiovascular, or neurologic manifestations.

Diagnosis: Impaired Oral Mucous Membrane. The problem statement *Impaired Oral Mucous Membrane related to lack of body water secondary to hypernatremia* can be used.

Outcomes. There are several options for outcome statements, depending upon the condition of the mouth initially. If the oral membranes are simply dry, but not open or cracked, an outcome of maintaining moist oral mucous membranes is appropriate. If the oral mucous membranes are cracked or open, the outcome should state that no further deterioration will occur and that the mouth will be moist. Additional nursing diagnoses for pain from oral ulcerations or inadequate nutrition related to mouth pain should be considered.

Interventions. Provide oral care every 2 hours with a nonalcoholic mouthwash. Dilute saline and nonalcoholic rinses have been found to be effective. Use a soft toothbrush to prevent injury to the mucosa. Moisten the client's lips every 1 to 2 hours. Offer cool, nonacidic fluids such as apple juice. Low-acid juices provide fluid while decreasing pain and irritation. Limited ice chips may also decrease the discomfort from dry mucous membranes. Teach the client to hold the fluids in the mouth for a time to hydrate the mucous membranes.

Caregivers often feel uncomfortable about giving oral care, and often the client's mouth is simply rinsed or lightly "brushed" with foam toothbrushes. This "light touch" oral care is appropriate when clients are in pain from mouth ulcers. However, lack of thorough oral care also leads to mouth ulcers, dental decay, and malnutrition. Mucus can accumulate on the roof of the mouth and impair swallowing or even breathing. Assess the mouth before and after mouth care, and be aggressive in cleaning the mouth.

Evaluation. Even if the desired outcome of sodium maintenance has been met, continue to monitor clients at high risk. The key to evaluating health promotion strategies is not only determining whether the client and family members understand the health promotion activities but also, more importantly, asking whether they have incorporated the necessary changes into their lifestyle. If change has not occurred, investigate the barriers and recommend alternatives or resources.

If the desired outcome of sodium restoration has been met or partially met, the manifestations of excess should be absent or at least lessened. Mild to moderate excesses are usually corrected in 8 to 24 hours. If the excesses are more severe or occur in very young or older clients, intervention must be more cautious, and 48 hours or more may be needed before positive outcomes are noticeable. Evaluate the client with altered oral mucous membranes every 8 to 12 hours. If improvement is not seen within a few hours, increase the frequency of oral care.

Self-Care

Teach clients the importance of taking hourly fluids—30 to 60 ml of clear liquids or more as tolerated—and avoiding excessive caffeinated beverages. Fluid intake should reach 600 ml in 24 hours. Impress upon family members the importance of keeping fresh foods and a variety of fluids on hand, especially for the client who lives alone. Encourage the use of community resources, such as Meals on Wheels. Instruct the client on how to read food labels and to avoid foods with high "Na" (sodium) content and over-the-counter medications or herbals unless physician-approved.

Teach the client to consult the physician if vomiting or diarrhea persists for more than 48 hours or sooner if extreme weakness, dizziness, palpitations, changes in mental state, new onset of cough, or increasing restlessness occurs. Clients with a concurrent chronic disease (such as diabetes mellitus or disease of the liver, heart, or kidneys) should consult a physician if any of these manifestations persist for longer than 24 hours. Explain the importance of reporting weight gains of more than 3 pounds in 1 week. Some clients are managed at home with IV fluids. Home health care nurses see their clients often (see the Bridge to Home Health Care feature on Managing Intravenous Therapy on the website).

CONCLUSIONS

Fluid imbalances are common problems, especially in high-risk populations, such as older adults and clients with acute illnesses or multiple pathologic processes. Many health care

disciplines work collaboratively toward maintaining or restoring fluid balance. The role of nursing in this collaborative effort is focused on health promotion activities, including teaching positive health behaviors, promoting health maintenance activities (including early detection and consultation with other disciplines), and preventing and early detection of complications from the underlying diseases, coexisting conditions, or treatment. Through these interventions, the nurse plays a critical role in assisting clients and their families achieve positive health outcomes.

THINKING CRITICALLY

1. A 59-year-old woman with a history of 2 days of vomiting and diarrhea and a temperature of 103° F secondary to suspected influenza virus is being admitted to the hospital. The client has a medical history of hypertension and heart failure. Home prescriptions include digoxin, 0.125 mg/day; furosemide (Lasix), 40 mg bid; and potassium chloride, 40 mEq/day. The client has also been advised to consume a low-sodium diet. An IV line of D_5/NS with 30 mEq of potassium chloride was started.

Factors to Consider. What is the priority risk/problem for this client? What are the desired outcomes? What are the critical assessments? What medical management and nursing strategies do you anticipate?

2. A middle-aged client is admitted to your unit with shock-like symptoms from a massive burn wound. He has pale skin, cold limbs, hypotension, and a weak, rapid pulse. Urine output via the indwelling catheter is decreased. His level of consciousness varies from an adequate response to little or no response to external stimuli.

Factors to Consider. What is the priority risk or problem for this client? What are the desired outcomes? What are the critical assessments? What medical management and nursing strategies do you anticipate during this phase of fluid shifting from the vascular spaces to the interstitial spaces? How will they change when the fluid shifts back into the vascular spaces?

Discussions for these questions can be found on the website.

BIBLIOGRAPHY

 Citations appearing in red refer to primary research.

Citations appearing in blue refer to evidence-based practice guidelines and protocols.

1. Amella, E.J. (2004). Feeding and hydration issues for older adults with dementia. *Nursing Clinics of North America, 39,* 607-623.
2. Arieff, A.I. (1999). Fatal postoperative pulmonary edema: Pathogenesis and literature review. *Chest, 115*(5), 1371-1377.
3. Asele, S.M. (2005). Restoring electrolyte balance. *RN, 68*(5), 34-40.
4. Ayus, J.C., Levine, R., & Arieff, A.I. (2003). Fatal dysnatraemia caused by elective colonoscopy. *British Medical Journal, 326,* 382-384.
5. Bartok, C., et al. (2004). The effect of dehydration on wrestling minimum weight assessment. *Medicine & Science in Sports & Exercise, 36*(1), 160-167.
6. Bartok, C., et al. (2004). Hydration testing in collegiate wrestlers undergoing hypertonic dehydration. *Medicine & Science in Sports & Exercise, 36*(3), 510-517.

7. Beloosesky, Y., et al. (2003). Electrolyte disorders following oral sodium phosphate administration for bowel cleansing in elderly patients. *ARCH Internal Medicine, 163*, 803-808.

8. Bennett, J. (2000). Dehydration: Hazards and benefits. *Geriatric Nursing, 21*(2), 84-88.

9. Bennett, J., Thomas, V., & Riegel, B. (2004). Unrecognized chronic dehydration in older adults. *Journal of Gerontological Nursing, 30*(11), 22-53.

10. Brewster, U.C., & Hayslett, J.P. (2005). Diabetes insipidus in the third trimester of pregnancy. *Obstetrics and Gynecology, 105*, 1173-1176.

11. Brown, O.A. (2004). Understanding postoperative hyponatremia. *Urologic Nursing, 24*(3), 197-201.

12. Cacchione, P.Z., et al. (2003). Clinical profile of acute confusion in the long-term care setting. *Clinical Nursing Research, 12*(2), 45-58.

13. Casa, D.J. (1999). Exercise in heat: I. Fundamentals of thermal physiology, performance implications, and dehydration. *Journal of Athletic Training, 34*(3), 246-252.

14. Cooper, A., & Moore, M. (1999). IV fluid therapy. *Australian Nursing Journal, 7*(5), 2-4.

15. Churchill, M., Grimm, S., & Reding, M. (2004). Risks of diuretic usage following stroke. *Neurorehabilitation and Neural Repair, 18*(3), 161-165.

16. Culp, K., Mentes, J., & Wakefield, B. (2003). Hydration and acute confusion in long-term care residents. *Western Journal of Nursing Research, 25*(3), 251-266.

17. Doorenbos, C.J., & Vermeij, C.G. (2006). Danger of salt substitutes that contain potassium in patients with renal failure. *British Medical Journal, 326*, 35-36.

18. Edwards, S. (2001). Regulation of water, sodium and potassium: Implications for practice. *Nursing Standard, 15*(22), 36-42.

19. Elgart, H.N. (2004). Assessment of fluids and electrolytes. *AACN Clinical Issues, 15*(4), 607-621.

20. Estes, C.M., & Mayne, J.P. (2003). Severe intraoperative hyponatremia in patient scheduled for elective hysteroscopy: A case report. *AANA Journal, 71*(3), 203-205.

21. Ferry, M. (2005). Strategies for ensuring good hydration in the elderly. *Nutrition Reviews, 63*(6), S22-S29.

22. Galloway, S.D. (1999). Dehydration, rehydration, and exercise in the heat: Rehydration strategies for the athletic competition. *Canadian Journal of Applied Physiology, 24*(2), 188-200.

23. Godek, S.F., Godek, J.J., & Bartolozzi, A.R. (2005). Hydration status in college football players during consecutive days of twice-a-day preseason practices. *The American Journal of Sports Medicine, 33*(6), 843-851.

24. Grandjean, A.C., Reimers, K.J., & Buyckx, M.E. (2003). Hydration: Issues for the 21st century. *Nutrition Reviews, 61*(8), 261-271.

25. Guthrie, D., & Yucha, C. (2004). Urinary concentration and dilution. *Nephrology Nursing Journal, 31*(3), 297-301.

26. Guyton, A., & Hall, J. (2001). *Textbook of medical physiology* (10th ed.). Philadelphia: Saunders.

27. Hamilton, S. (2001). Detecting dehydration malnutrition in the elderly. *Nursing, 31*(12), 56-57.

28. Hodgkinson, B., et al. (2003). Maintaining oral hydration in older adults: A systemic review. *International Journal of Nursing Practice, 9*(3), 519-528.

29. Huether, S., & McCance, K. (2004). *Understanding pathophysiology* (3rd ed.). St. Louis: Mosby.

30. Iggulden, H. (1999). Dehydration and electrolyte disturbance. *Elderly Care, 11*(3), 17-23.

31. Innis, J. (2002). Treating nephrogenic diabetes insipidus. *Dimensions of Critical Care Nursing, 21*(3), 98-99.

32. Karch, A.M. (2004). On the rebound: Maintaining normal fluid intake is critical while on diuretics. *American Journal of Nursing, 104*(10), 73-74.

33. Karlsson, A.K., & Krassioukov, A.V. (2004). Hyponatremia-induced transient visual disturbances in acute spinal cord injury. *Spinal Cord, 42*, 204-207.

34. Kenefick, R.W., et al. (2004). Thirst sensations and AVP responses at rest and during exercise-cold exposure. *Medicine & Science in Sports & Exercise, 36*(9), 1528-1534.

35. Larson, K. (2003). Fluid balance in the elderly: Assessment and intervention-important role in community health and home care nursing. *Geriatric Nursing, 24*(5), 306-309.

36. Maughan, R.J. (1999). Exercise in the heat: Limitations to performance and the impact of fluid replacement strategies. *Canadian Journal of Applied Physiology, 24*(2), 149-151.

37. May, D.L. (1998). The relationship between self-induced water intoxication and severity of psychiatric symptoms. *Archives of Psychiatric Nursing, 12*(6), 335-343.

38. McAulay, D. (2001). Dehydration in the terminally ill patient. *Nursing Standard, 16*(4), 33-37.

39. McSwan, K.L., Gontkovsky, S.T., & Splinter, M.Y. (2003). Acute changes in mental status secondary to selective serotonin reuptake inhibitor-induced hyponatremia. *Rehabilitation Psychology, 48*(3), 202-206.

40. Mentes, J. (2000). Hydration management protocol. *Journal of Gerontological Nursing, 26*(10), 6-15.

41. Mentes, J.C., & Culp, K. (2003). Reducing hydration-linked events in nursing home residents. *Clinical Nursing Research, 12*(3), 210-228.

42. Mentes, J.C. (2006). A typology of oral hydration. *Journal of Gerontological Nursing, 32*(1), 13-21.

43. Mitchell, M. (2003). *Nutrition across the lifespan* (2nd ed.). Philadelphia: Saunders.

44. Mower-Wade, D., Bartley, M., & Chiari-Allwein, J. (2001). How to respond to shock. *Dimensions of Critical Care Nursing, 20*(2), 22-27.

45. Oh, H., et al. (2005). Effects of nasogastric tube feeding on serum sodium, potassium, and glucose levels. *Journal of Nursing Scholarship, 37*(2), 141-147.

46. Purcell, W., et al. (2004). Accurate dry weight assessment: Reducing the incidence of hypertension and cardiac disease in patients on hemodialysis. *Nephrology Nursing Journal, 31*(6), 631-636.

47. Reynolds, S.A., et al. (2004). Identifying at risk nursing home residents using a polydipsia screening tool. *Archives of Psychiatric Nursing, 18*(2), 60-67.

48. Schmidt, T. (2000). Assessing a sodium and fluid imbalance. *Nursing, 30*(1), 18.

49. Sheehy, C.M., et al. (2001). Dehydration: Biological considerations, age-related changes, and risk factors in older adults. *Biological Research in Nursing, 1*(1), 30-37.

50. Sherman, F.T. (2005). Three "hypo's" of hospitalization. *Geriatrics, 60*(5), 9-10.

51. Smith, S., & Andrews, M. (2000). Artificial nutrition and hydration at the end of life. *Medical Surgical Nursing, 9*(5), 233-247.

52. Smith, J.C., Siddique, H., & Corrall, R.J.M. (2004). Misinterpretation of serum cortisol in a patient with hyponatremia. *British Medical Journal, 328*, 215-216.

53. Stookey, J.D. (2005). High prevalence of plasma hypertonicity among community-dwelling older adults: Results from NHANES III. *Journal of the American Dietetic Association, 105*(8), 1231-1242.

54. Turchin, A., Seifter, J.L., & Seely, E.W. (2003). Mind the gap. *New England Journal of Medicine, 349*(15), 1465-1469.

55. Uphold, C.R., & Graham, M.V. (2003). *Clinical guidelines in family practice* (4th ed.). Gainesville, Fla: Barmarrae Books.

56. Vacca, V.M. (2005). Cerebral salt wasting syndrome. *Nursing, 35*(10), 88.

57. Vilches, A., & Suman, A. (2004). Awareness of over-the-counter drug use by elderly patients. A hospital-based questionnaire survey. *Age Aging, 33*(2), 205-206.

58. Walsh, N.P., et al. (2004). Saliva parameters as potential indices of hydration status during acute dehydration. *Medicine & Science in Sports & Medicine, 36*(9), 1535-1542.

59. Xiao, H., Barber, J., & Campbell, E.S. (2004). Economic burden of dehydration among hospitalized elderly patients. *American Journal of Health-System Pharmacy, 61*(23), 2534-2540.

60. Zembrzuski, C. (2000). Nutrition and hydration. *Journal of Gerontological Nursing, 26*(12), 6-7.

CHAPTER 12

Clients with Electrolyte Imbalances

BERNADETTE WHITE

ELECTROLYTE IMBALANCES

Electrolytes are substances that become ions in solution and have the capacity to carry positive or negative electrical charges. Electrolytes maintain voltages across cell membranes, and cells use electrolytes to conduct electrical impulses (nerve impulses, muscle contractions) to other cells. The kidneys work to keep the electrolyte concentrations in the blood constant despite changes in the body. For example, when a person exercises heavily, electrolytes are lost in the sweat, particularly sodium and potassium. These electrolytes must be replaced to keep the electrolyte concentrations of body fluids constant.

An electrolyte imbalance is present whenever there is an excess or deficit in the plasma level of a specific ion. Terms used to describe the imbalance contain the prefix *hyper-* for increased or *hypo-* for decreased, followed by the name of the electrolyte (in its Latin form for sodium and potassium) and then the suffix *-emia* to indicate presence in the blood, as measured in the plasma. For example, *hyponatremia* means low plasma sodium, and *hyperkalemia* means elevated plasma potassium. *Hypercalcemia* and *hypermagnesemia* indicate elevated calcium and magnesium levels, respectively.

Using a "Collaborative Problem" Format

Currently there are no NANDA diagnoses for electrolyte imbalances. The Iowa Interventions Project approached these disorders as collaborative problems and developed a research-based list of critical and supporting activities for management of 15 fluid and electrolyte disorders. Because the nursing role primarily involves collaborating with the physician, the goal statements are also phrased differently. Note that each expected outcome is preceded by the phrase "The nurse will monitor the client for:" hyponatremia or hypernatremia (discussed in Chapter 11), hypokalemia or hyperkalemia, hypocalcemia or hypercalcemia, hypomagnesemia or hypermagnesemia, and

hypophosphatemia or hyperphosphatemia. Nursing diagnoses that may apply to clients with electrolyte imbalances include *Risk for Injury, Risk for Activity Intolerance, Risk for Decreased Cardiac Output, Impaired Oral Mucous Membranes,* and *Risk for Impaired Skin Integrity.* The Critical Monitoring box below lists clinical manifestations that may indicate the onset of a fluid or electrolyte imbalance secondary to another condition.

CRITICAL MONITORING

A fluid or electrolyte imbalance may cause these symptoms:
- New onset of dysrhythmia
- Worsening of dysrhythmia, such as occurrence of premature ventricular contractions at a rate greater than 6/min, bradycardia with heart rate less than 50 beats/min, tachycardia with heart rate greater than 120 beats/min
- Sudden change in level of consciousness, including sudden restlessness, lethargy, and seizures
- Tetany, laryngeal spasm, or stridor
- Postural systolic blood pressure decrease greater than 20 mm Hg, or diastolic decrease of greater than 10 mm Hg with a pulse increase
- Rapid weight loss
- Severe dryness of oral mucous membranes with tongue furrowing
- Hemorrhage
- Urine output less than 0.5 ml/kg/hr for 2 consecutive hours
- Rapid weight gain, especially with pulmonary signs of sudden onset such as crackles, dyspnea, S_3 gallop

---

evolve Web Enhancements

Bridge to Home Health Care Managing Intravenous Therapy

Appendix A Religious Beliefs and Practices Affecting Health Care

Be sure to check out the bonus material on the Evolve website and the CD-ROM, including free self-assessment exercises. **http://evolve.elsevier.com/Black/medsurg**

POTASSIUM IMBALANCES

HYPOKALEMIA

Hypokalemia is defined as a plasma potassium level less than 3.5 mEq/L. It is a common electrolyte disorder, especially in the older adult population.

Etiology and Risk Factors

The body does not conserve potassium efficiently; thus potassium deficit commonly results from inadequate potassium intake. Fortunately, potassium is found in most foods and fluids. People at high risk for hypokalemia include those who are debilitated, confused, restrained, or lacking access to dietary sources for financial or other reasons, or who are malnourished, anorexic, or bulimic. Clients on potassium-restricted diets or some weight reduction diets, or those receiving potassium-free IV solutions are also at risk.

Potassium levels can also decrease when the excretion or loss of potassium exceeds intake. People at high risk for loss include those with vomiting or diarrhea, nasogastric suctioning, intestinal fistulae, or ileostomy. Often, hypokalemia develops in surgical clients as a result of the increased cortisol levels during the stress adaptation period and from the effects of general or spinal anesthesia. Some studies suggest that hypokalemia in alcoholic clients, as well as hypocalcemia, hypophosphatemia, and hypomagnesemia, is secondary to alcohol-induced nephrotoxicity. Alcohol abstinence often results in electrolyte levels returning to normal.

Medications that commonly cause hypokalemia include the potassium-wasting diuretics (thiazide, loop, and osmotic diuretics), cathartics, steroids, aminoglycosides, amphotericin B, digitalis preparations, beta-adrenergic drugs, cisplatin, ibuprofen, and bicarbonate. Use of furosemide is the most common cause of hypokalemia, and a potassium supplement is often provided when the medication is given.

Several conditions cause redistribution of potassium. An increased level of sodium intake promotes potassium loss. Increased levels of insulin promote the movement of not only glucose but also potassium into the cell. In alkalosis, potassium exchanges with hydrogen across the cell wall, thus increasing the level of hydrogen but decreasing the level of potassium in the plasma. Clients who are in the healing phase after a severe crush injury or burn also experience hypokalemia as a result of the shifting of potassium back into the cell. An increase in catecholamines also promotes cellular uptake of potassium.

Other factors associated with an increased risk of hypokalemia include Cushing's syndrome, the diuretic phase of renal failure, hyperaldosteronism, liver disease, cancer, wounds, and Bartter syndrome, a chronic electrolyte-wasting syndrome. Other less common, but life-threatening etiologies of hypokalemia include excessive consumption of cola products, hyperthyroidism, and excessive natural licorice ingestion. The most common causes of potassium loss are presented in Box 12-1.

Pathophysiology

Decreased potassium levels in the extracellular space will require a greater than normal stimulus for depolarization of the membrane in order to initiate an action potential. Almost all of the manifestations that occur with hypokalemia result from the slowed neuronal excitability and its consequent effect on muscle function.

Clinical Manifestations

The clinical manifestations of hypokalemia include abnormal findings on the electrocardiogram (ECG) and gastrointestinal (GI), cardiac, renal, respiratory, neurologic, and musculoskeletal disturbances. Abnormalities may not be apparent with mild hypokalemia (3.3 to 3.4 mEq/L), especially if the decrease in the potassium concentration is gradual. Slowed smooth muscle contraction leads to early GI manifestations, which include anorexia, abdominal distention, and constipation. Slowed skeletal muscle contraction leads to muscle weakness and leg cramps. Decreased conduction of nerve impulses secondary to an increase in the transmembrane potential leads to the neurologic manifestations of fatigue, paresthesias, hyporeflexia, and irritability.

BOX 12-1   Etiologies of Hypokalemia

- Inadequate intake
- NPO
- IV fluids without KCl
- Renal losses
- Renal tubular acidosis
- Hyperaldosteronism
- Magnesium depletion
- Leukemia (mechanism uncertain)
- GI losses
- Vomiting or nasogastric suctioning
- Diarrhea
- Enemas or laxative use
- Medication effects
- Diuretics (thiazide, loop, osmotic; most common cause)
- Beta-adrenergic agonists
- Steroids
- Theophylline
- Aminoglycosides
- Transcellular shift
- Insulin
- Alkalosis
- Malnutrition or decreased dietary intake, parenteral nutrition

Data from Mahan, L.K., & Escott-Stump, S. (2004). *Krause's food, nutrition, and diet therapy* (11th ed.). Philadelphia: Saunders.

With severe hypokalemia, ECG changes may occur (Figure 12-1). The depressed and prolonged ST segment, depressed and inverted T wave, and prominent U wave are due to the prolongation of myocardial repolarization. Dysrhythmias are common because of increased cellular excitability. Hypokalemia also leads to a decrease in myocardial contraction, which is manifested as hypotension and a slow, weakened pulse. Potassium levels less than 2.5 mEq/L increase the risk for ventricular fibrillation and cardiac arrest. Pulmonary manifestations of shallow respirations, shortness of breath, and apnea, culminating in respiratory arrest, are also from progressive deterioration of respiratory muscular contraction.

The progressive neurologic consequences of slowed nerve conduction are manifested as dysphasia, confusion, depression, convulsions, areflexia, and coma. Extreme smooth muscle slowing leads to vomiting and an ileus as well as urinary retention. Skeletal muscle weakness may progress to paralysis. Hypokalemia also inhibits the ability of the kidney to concentrate urine, which leads to polyuria, nocturia, and a decreased plasma osmolality.

Although plasma potassium levels less than 3.5 mEq/L are diagnostic for hypokalemia, the ECG is the most reliable tool for identifying abnormalities in intracellular potassium level.

OUTCOME MANAGEMENT

A thorough history and physical examination in conjunction with appropriate diagnostic studies are essential for an accurate diagnosis and management of hypokalemia.

Medical Management

Medical management is focused on identifying and correcting the cause of the imbalance. The aggressiveness of the therapy is determined by the potassium level and the clinical manifestations. Extreme hypokalemia necessitates cardiac monitoring.

Restore Potassium Levels

Maintenance doses for clients not taking any source of potassium are 40 to 60 mEq/day in IV solution. Larger amounts are needed when there are coexisting potassium losses.

For clients with minor potassium deficits or for those who have potassium-wasting conditions, administering foods high in potassium helps correct the deficit and offsets losses. The adult recommended allowance for potassium is 1875 to 5625 mg/day. Box 12-2 includes examples of foods that are high and low in potassium.

Mild to moderate hypokalemia is treated by correcting or controlling the cause of the loss or by supplementing potassium intake through the diet or with medication. Oral potassium replacement therapy is usually prescribed for mild hypokalemia (plasma potassium level 3.3 to 3.5 mEq/L) or for potassium-wasting conditions.

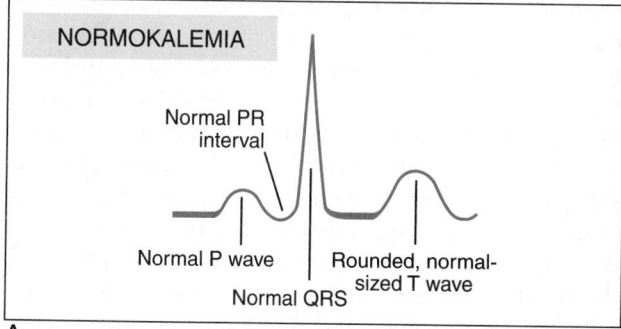

A

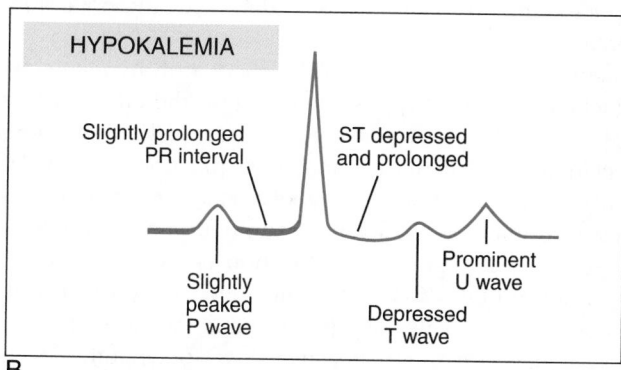

B

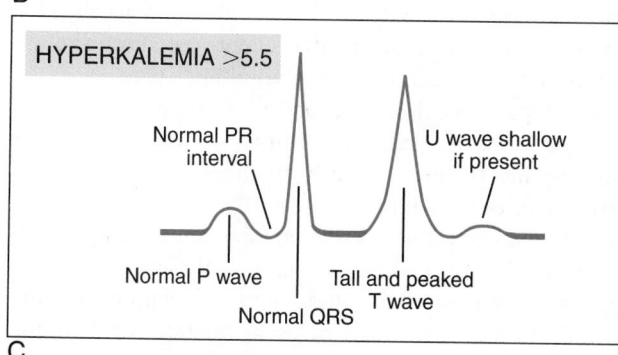

C

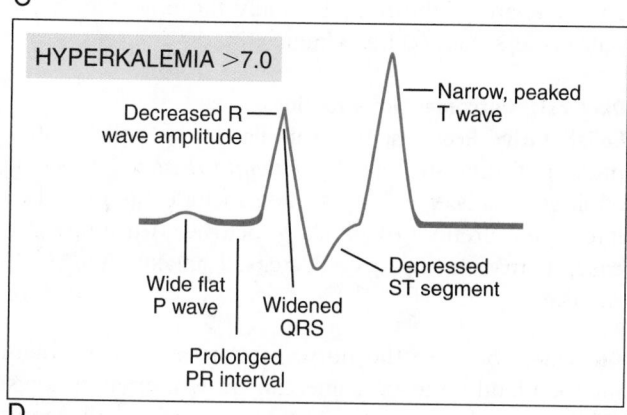

D

■ **FIGURE 12–1 A-D** Electrocardiographic changes seen in potassium imbalances.

BOX 12-2   High-Potassium and Low-Potassium Foods

HIGH-POTASSIUM FOODS (APPROXIMATELY 7 mEq/SERVING)

- Fish (not shellfish)
- Whole grains, nuts
- Vegetables: artichokes, broccoli, brussels sprouts, cabbage, carrots, celery, collards, cucumbers, mushrooms, potatoes with skins, spinach, tomatoes
- Fruits: apricots, bananas, cantaloupe, guava, honeydew melons, nectarines, oranges, prunes, strawberries, tangerines, watermelon
- Beverages: brewed coffee, tomato juice, fruit juices

LOW-POTASSIUM FOODS (APPROXIMATELY 3 mEq/SERVING)

- Vegetables: corn, sweet potatoes, lima beans, french-fried potatoes
- Fruit: apples, applesauce, apple juice, blueberries, cranberries
- Beverages: instant coffee, cola, cranberry juice, ginger ale, noncarbonated drinks, root beer, lemon-lime soda

Data from Mahan, L.K., & Escott-Stump, S. (2000). *Krause's food, nutrition, and diet therapy* (10th ed.). Philadelphia: Saunders.

Oral potassium (chloride or gluconate) is extremely irritating to the gastric mucosa and must be taken with a glass of water or juice or with meals.

Severe hypokalemia requires IV intervention. A client with a plasma potassium level between 3 and 3.4 mEq/L needs approximately 100 to 200 mEq of IV potassium for the potassium level to increase 1 mEq/L. If the plasma potassium level is less than 3 mEq/L, it takes approximately 200 to 400 mEq of IV potassium to increase the level 1 mEq/L.

SAFETY ALERT

Potassium given intravenously must always be diluted in IV fluids. The usual concentration of IV potassium is 20 to 40 mEq/L. Potassium is *not* given intramuscularly and is *never* given as a bolus (IV push) injection. Giving potassium by IV push creates sudden, severe hyperkalemia, which may result in cardiac arrest.

For severe potassium deficits, 10 to 20 mEq of potassium can be given every hour if *diluted* in IV fluids; a cardiac monitor must be used to ensure safety. Use of saline as a diluent is recommended; avoid dextrose as a diluent, because it increases intracellular potassium shifting. Because potassium is irritating to the veins, concentrations greater than 20 to 40 mEq/L increase the risk of phlebitis, and large veins should be used for administration.

If hypokalemia is refractory to the usual treatments, assess for manifestations of hypomagnesemia. Many clients who are hypokalemic are also hypomagnesemic. Hypokalemia that does not respond to treatment is frequently associated with hypomagnesemia. Magnesium is necessary for the kidney to conserve potassium.

Nursing Management of the Medical Client

Assessment. Assessment focuses on identifying risk factors for hypokalemia through history-taking and a thorough physical examination. Obtain a history that focuses on dietary intake, conditions promoting potassium loss, and use of diuretics, cortisone, over-the-counter medications, and herbals. Review laboratory reports of potassium levels. Report even borderline plasma potassium levels to the physician, especially in high-risk clients, particularly those about to undergo surgery. General anesthesia not only promotes potassium loss but also, in combination with lower plasma potassium levels, synergistically increases the risk of cardiac dysrhythmias. Consult the physician about the need for potassium supplementation in any client who has been NPO or who has an obvious cause of potassium loss or marked decrease in potassium intake.

Ongoing assessments of the client with hypokalemia include all the body systems, because the effect of low potassium level is widespread. Assess cardiac function, including apical pulses, and renal function every hour in the client with severe hypokalemia, and progress to every 8 hours as the client's condition improves. Assess neuromuscular and bowel function every 4 to 8 hours. A urine output of 0.5 ml/kg/hr is necessary to prevent rebound hyperkalemia. Hypokalemia increases the risk of digitalis toxicity because low potassium levels increase the sensitivity of the myocardium to digitalis-induced dysrhythmia. If the client receives digitalis, monitor for nausea, anorexia, vomiting, diarrhea, headache, weakness, blurring or visual halos, or marked change in cardiac rate or rhythm. Nausea and anorexia are the most common early manifestations of digitalis toxicity in older adults.

If the apical pulse is irregular, assess for pulse deficits. Because this procedure is impractical for self-monitoring, at least ensure that the client or a family member is able to assess a radial pulse accurately for 1 minute and is aware of the need to notify the physician if the pulse is less than 60 beats/min.

Diagnosis, Outcomes, Interventions

Collaborative Problem: Hypokalemia. Use a collaborative problem format such as *Hypokalemia related to* (specific etiology). Causative factors often include prolonged or intensive diuretic use, vomiting, diarrhea, Cushing's disease, cortisone therapy, decreased intake, and NPO status.

Outcomes. Because the nurse cannot treat the problem independently, the outcome can be written as follows: "The nurse will monitor potassium levels and report abnormal potassium levels or manifestations of potassium imbalance to the physician."

Interventions

Give oral or IV potassium as prescribed, ensuring that it is *diluted in IV fluids; it cannot be given as an IV push.*

Always *agitate* IV bags containing potassium before hanging them up to prevent giving a loading dose, which can cause cardiac arrest. Monitor IV sites hourly for phlebitis and infiltration, and confirm the rate of infusion. Change IV sites every 72 hours or sooner if the vein becomes tender to palpation. Tenderness indicates damage to the intima of the vein; this is an early sign of phlebitis.

Use the smallest IV catheter possible to allow maximum blood flow around the site at which the potassium enters the vein. This blood flow dilutes the potassium, thereby decreasing the risk of phlebitis. If an IV solution containing potassium infiltrates surrounding tissue, consult the pharmacist or physician for advice. Potassium infiltration can cause tissue sloughing. Give IV fluids with potassium chloride by a controlled infusion pump to ensure the correct flow rate and respond to alarms quickly.

Notify the physician if signs of hypokalemia persist or worsen, such as dysrhythmia of increasing severity, or if signs of overcorrection occur, such as manifestations of hyperkalemia. During the administration of IV potassium, consult the physician if the client's urine output is less than 0.5 ml/kg/hr for 2 consecutive hours, if the pulse deficit is greater than 20 beats/min, or if signs of impaired peripheral tissue perfusion are present. Anticipate the need for additional potassium with increased IV glucose, such as in total parenteral nutrition (TPN); increased insulin levels result in shifting of potassium into the cell.

Use of a computerized alert for clients with low potassium levels has been a very effective way of preventing severe complications related to hypokalemia in high-risk populations.

Diagnosis: Risk for Injury. Because potassium is needed for normal nerve conduction and muscle function, low plasma potassium levels often lead to weakness and can lead to falls or seizures. The nursing diagnosis is stated as *Risk for Injury or Risk for Falls related to muscle weakness and hypotension or seizures secondary to hypokalemia.*

Outcomes. The client will be at reduced risk of injury or falls, as evidenced by an absence of falls, near falls, bruises, contusions, and seizures.

Interventions

Employ safety and seizure precautions to reduce the risk of injury. Keep the bed in a low position with padded side rails up. Before the client walks, clear the path of obstacles and place nonslippery shoes and a gait belt on the client.

Use restraints only after all other alternatives to prevent inadvertent harm to self or others have been tried.

It is imperative that health care providers comply with the client's rights and follow the defined protocols for use of restraints. Side rails are considered restraints; thus the rationale for use and reevaluation of need must follow your agency's policy and be thoroughly documented.

Diagnosis: Imbalanced Nutrition: Less than Body Requirements. If the main cause of the client's hypokalemia is inadequate consumption of foods rich in potassium, then use the nursing diagnosis *Imbalanced Nutrition: Less than Body Requirements related to insufficient intake of foods rich in potassium.* However, this diagnosis can be used *only* if the client can eat and drink.

Outcomes. The client will demonstrate improved nutrition, as evidenced by consumption of adequate amounts of food and fluid to maintain a normal potassium level.

Interventions. Instruct the client to choose and consume foods rich in potassium (see Box 12-2). Instruct the client to take potassium supplements with a glass or more of water or juice and food to decrease GI irritation.

Evaluation. If the desired outcome of potassium maintenance has been met, continue to monitor high-risk clients for evidence of deficit. Continue to reinforce strategies for prevention. If the outcome of potassium restoration has been met or partially met, the manifestations of deficit should be absent or at least lessened in severity. Mild to moderate deficits are usually corrected in 8 to 24 hours. Correction of more severe deficits may take several days, especially in the older adult. Continue to evaluate the client's and family members' understanding of positive health behaviors, and assess for barriers to achieving those behaviors.

Self-Care

Teaching is essential to the promotion and maintenance of potassium balance. Provide a list of foods containing potassium, and emphasize the importance of eating a well-balanced diet. Review alternative cooking methods, reinforcing that prolonged cooking or microwaving of vegetables may result in wasting of essential nutrients. Suggest steaming or, when possible, eating raw vegetables as methods to increase nutrient retention.

Teach the basic principles of sick care. These principles include hourly ingestion of 30 to 60 ml of fluids with electrolytes; for example, carbohydrate/electrolyte solutions contain potassium as well as other electrolytes. Pedialyte is an alternative for those that have to control glucose intake. Sick care also involves teaching clients when to consult a physician. People with chronic diseases, such as heart, liver, or kidney disease or diabetes mellitus, should consult a physician for any illness that interferes with food ingestion or causes loss of nutrients and persists for more than 24 hours. Anyone who becomes symptomatic—who develops weakness of sudden onset, irregular heartbeat, or change in mental status—should consult a physician.

Teach the importance of not taking over-the-counter medicine or herbals, especially laxatives, without physician approval. Encourage clients who are lactose-intolerant to avoid milk products or to take lactase. Reinforce the label instruction that potassium products should be taken with food to avoid GI irritation.

Encourage use of support services—first, the family or extended family and then the religious community as well as respite services, Meals on Wheels, food stamps, Alcoholics Anonymous, or other community services.

HYPERKALEMIA

Hyperkalemia is defined as an elevation of the potassium level greater than 5 mEq/L. Hyperkalemia is rare in clients with normal kidney function but affects more than half of people with acute and chronic renal failure.

Etiology and Risk Factors

The three major causes of hyperkalemia are as follows:

- Retention of potassium by the body because of decreased or inadequate urine output
- Excessive release of potassium from the cells during the first 24 to 72 hours after traumatic injury or burns, or from cell lysis or acidosis
- Excessive infusion of IV solutions that contain potassium or excessive oral intake, especially in a person who has renal disease

All three potential causes of hyperkalemia limit the ability of the kidneys to excrete the excess potassium. Because the kidneys are responsible for 80% to 90% of potassium excretion, the underlying cause of hyperkalemia is often related to decreased kidney function. People with as little as 5% glomerular function can maintain normal plasma potassium levels if urine output is at least 1 L/day. Shock states compound the problem because of a low volume of circulating vascular fluids and diminished kidney function. The GI tract and skin cannot excrete enough potassium to compensate for an acute state of hyperkalemia.

Most potassium is inside the cell. Therefore conditions that destroy cells release potassium into the circulation. People with fast-growing cancers, such as non-Hodgkin's lymphoma, acute leukemia, small cell carcinomas, and some metastatic cancers, are at risk for *tumor lysis syndrome* (TLS). TLS is the consequence of rapid destruction of tumor cells by chemotherapy or irradiation and the intracellular contents are released into the blood. The

cell's destruction results in hyperkalemia, hyperphosphatemia, hypocalcemia, and hyperuricemia. Hyperkalemia can also result from burns, crush injuries, or severe infections involving extensive cell destruction. Potassium levels can also increase after the use of stored blood, and after open-heart surgery or other surgical procedures in which a perfusion pump is used.

Therapy with potassium-sparing diuretics or concurrent use of potassium supplements with angiotensin-converting enzyme (ACE) inhibitor, or angiotensin II receptor antagonists, or aldosterone antagonists may cause hyperkalemia. Each of these promotes potassium retention through inhibition of aldosterone. Other medications that have been reported to cause hyperkalemia include cyclosporine, sulfa combinations, succinylcholine, and heparin. Disorders that decrease or inhibit secretion of aldosterone, such as adrenal insufficiency, may also cause hyperkalemia. Acidosis also increases hyperkalemia owing to the compensatory shifting of potassium out of the cell in exchange for hydrogen; the exception is diabetic acidosis in which glucose-related osmotic diuresis promotes potassium wasting.

Pathophysiology

Increased levels of serum potassium result in depolarization of the membrane potentials of cells. This depolarization opens some voltage-gated sodium channels, but not enough to generate an action potential. After a short while, the open sodium channels inactivate and become refractory, increasing the threshold to generate an action potential. This leads to the impairment of neuromuscular, cardiac, and gastrointestinal organ systems. Of most concern is the impairment of cardiac conduction, which can result in ventricular fibrillation or asystole.

Clinical Manifestations

Acute hyperkalemia may cause manifestations when the plasma level is only moderately elevated to 6 mEq/L. However, if the condition developed slowly, manifestations may not be present until the plasma level reaches 7 mEq/L. Clinical manifestations can involve many body systems, including GI, cardiac, renal, neurologic, and musculoskeletal systems. Mild to moderate hyperkalemia (a plasma level near 6 mEq/L) causes nerve and muscle irritability, resulting in paresthesia (numbness, tingling), tachycardia, and intestinal colic and diarrhea.

As the plasma potassium level approaches 7 mEq/L, sodium channels become progressively inactivated, which causes disturbances in nerve and muscle function. Impaired cardiac conduction and ventricular contraction, hypotension, cardiac arrest, convulsions, and severe neuromuscular weakness progressing to flaccid paralysis and respiratory muscle paralysis can develop. There have been reported cases of pseudo-infarction in which ECG changes were consistent with an acute myocardial infarction. Other ECG findings indicated missed pacemaker capturing (approximately 50% of the time). These ECG changes resolved once the potassium levels were normalized.

The acidosis that occurs with hyperkalemia has a synergistic effect on the progressive impairment of depolarization. The renal abnormalities oliguria and anuria are commonly precursors to hyperkalemia rather than consequences of the imbalance.

As noted previously, the key to the level of severity is the amount of time the body has had to adapt to the imbalance. Although a plasma potassium level greater than 5 mEq/L is diagnostic for hyperkalemia, the ECG is the most reliable tool for identifying an imbalance (see Figure 12-1). Blood studies may yield false-positive results when hemolysis of blood specimens has occurred, when tourniquets are applied too tightly, when multiple attempts are made to obtain a sample from the same site, or when excess force is used to transfer blood into tubes or to aspirate blood into a syringe. Under these conditions, the cell ruptures and releases potassium into the sample of blood.

Other useful laboratory studies include determination of blood urea nitrogen (BUN), plasma creatinine, and carbon dioxide levels. Elevated plasma BUN and creatinine levels, which reflect decreased renal function, are important predictors of hyperkalemia. If the total carbon dioxide level in the venous blood is low, an arterial blood gas study should be done to rule out metabolic or respiratory acidosis as a possible cause of hyperkalemia.

OUTCOME MANAGEMENT

Medical Management

The goals of medical management are to correct the potassium level as quickly as possible to prevent life-threatening consequences. Although a thorough history and physical examination is desirable, if the client is critically ill, intervention may pre-empt a thorough assessment.

⬥ Restore Potassium Balance

If the plasma potassium level is less than 5.5 mEq/L, dietary restriction of potassium may be all that is needed (see Box 12-2).

If the level is higher or if the client is symptomatic, pharmacologic intervention is usually necessary. The onset of symptoms and the need for aggressive intervention are usually related to the suddenness of the development of hyperkalemia. Improving urine output by forcing fluids, giving IV saline, or giving potassium-wasting diuretics usually corrects mild hyperkalemia.

When hyperkalemia is severe, immediate action is needed to avoid lethal cardiac disturbances. Temporary corrective measures may include the following: infusion of IV calcium gluconate to decrease the antagonistic effect of the potassium excess on the myocardium; infusion of insulin and glucose or sodium bicarbonate (recommended if metabolic acidosis is present) to promote potassium uptake into the cells; and use of the beta-agonist albuterol (0.5 mg IV), which results in a decrease in plasma potassium level within 30 minutes, lasting for 6 hours. These are only temporary methods for decreasing plasma potassium level; repeating these methods may not be effective.

As hyperkalemia persists or increases, a cation-exchange resin such as sodium polystyrene sulfonate may be given orally or rectally as a retention enema. When this medication is given, the potassium ion is exchanged for the sodium ion in the intestinal tract; the potassium ion is then excreted in the stool. To prevent the constipating effect of this drug, it is usually combined with sorbitol, and diarrhea often results. In marked renal failure, peritoneal dialysis or hemodialysis may be needed.

Prevention is central to the management of TLS. Adequate hydration is the key: 3000 ml of IV fluid is given 24 hours before therapy, during therapy, and for 48 hours after therapy. Diuretics (to decrease the risk of pulmonary overload) and a uric acid blocker (to inhibit the precursors of uric acid) decrease uric acid crystallization and thus the risk of renal failure.

If hyperkalemia is secondary to respiratory acidosis, enhancing pulmonary function is the primary focus. If it is from metabolic acidosis, the immediate risks associated with the acidosis and hyperkalemia are addressed first, and then interventions are targeted at the system in which the acidosis originated.

Nursing Management of the Medical Client

Assessment. Assessment focuses on identifying risk factors for hyperkalemia through history-taking and a thorough physical examination.

> **Review laboratory reports of potassium levels. Report even borderline plasma potassium levels to the physician, especially in high-risk clients, such as those who have cancer with high tumor burdens or high mitotic rates and are undergoing chemotherapy.**

SAFETY ALERT

Ongoing assessments include checking vital signs, bowel function, urine output, lung sounds (crackles), and peripheral edema every 4 to 8 hours. Monitor plasma levels of potassium and creatinine and urea nitrogen. In severe hyperkalemia, perform hourly checks of vital signs, including apical pulses. ECG changes should be monitored continuously. In the absence of ECG monitoring, apical pulses constitute the next most valuable indicator of abnormality in intracellular potassium concentration. Monitor urine output hourly if severe hyperkalemia or a history of renal insufficiency exists or if the urine output drops to less than 0.5 ml/kg/hr for 2 consecutive hours.

Monitor not only for a therapeutic response to treatment (improvement) but also for signs of overcorrection. Rapid correction places a client at risk for hypokalemia and metabolic alkalosis. In a client taking digitalis, the occurrence of hypokalemia is associated with a digitalis toxic response.

Diagnosis, Outcomes, Interventions

Collaborative Problem: Hyperkalemia Use the following collaborative problem statement: *Hyperkalemia related to* (specify etiology). Consider the contribution of renal dysfunction, shock from traumatic injuries, or burns (tissue destruction).

Outcomes. Because nurses cannot treat the problem independently, the outcome can specify the following: "The nurse will monitor potassium levels and report abnormal findings or manifestations of hyperkalemia to the physician."

 Interventions. Administer fluids as ordered to promote renal excretion of potassium. Report manifestations indicating the development of hypokalemia and urine outputs of less than 0.5 ml/kg/hr for 2 consecutive hours, or less than 720 ml/day.

If the client is to receive a blood transfusion and is at risk for hyperkalemia, notify the blood bank so that "old" blood (more than 2 weeks old) is not supplied. Use a 19-gauge needle or 20-gauge catheter to deliver the packed cells, to prevent red blood cell (RBC) rupture with release of intracellular potassium. When obtaining blood specimens, use vacuum tubes when possible to avoid false-positive results for hyperkalemia.

High potassium levels have the potential to induce life-threatening dysrhythmias. Treat them according to protocol, and report ECG changes that indicate worsening hyperkalemia or overcorrection resulting in hypokalemia. Use a cardiac monitor to ensure safe administration of potassium to any client with renal insufficiency. Set cardiac monitor alarms with narrow limits to ensure early detection of lethal dysrhythmias. *Remember, a machine cannot replace your bedside assessment.* Cardiopulmonary resuscitation may be required, but it is seldom successful in cases of severe hyperkalemia because the heart muscle cannot respond to medications or countershock. Consult the physician for any serious change, including progression of altered tissue perfusion, especially in the heart, lungs, brain, or kidneys.

Evaluation. Evaluate the client's responses to therapy every hour if severe hyperkalemia is present or every 8 hours if mild hyperkalemia exists. Hyperkalemia must be corrected quickly because of the risk of dysrhythmia.

Self-Care

Teaching still remains one of the primary interventions to promote and maintain normal potassium balance for those at high risk for hyperkalemia. Explain the significance of potassium restriction. Crucial elements of teaching include understanding dietary potassium sources and the importance of reading labels, avoiding salt substitutes, which are usually made from a potassium salt, and avoiding over-the-counter medications not approved by a physician. Clients must also understand the importance of consulting a physician if renal function worsens or if an acute illness lasts more than 24 hours. Occasionally, a person with renal insufficiency is in a state of hypokalemia caused by an acute loss.

CALCIUM IMBALANCES

HYPOCALCEMIA

Hypocalcemia is defined as a plasma calcium level less than 4.5 mEq/L, or 9 mg/dl. Calcium levels are often reciprocal with phosphorus levels (discussed later in this chapter). It is important to remember that about 99% of the calcium is found in the bone. Of the remaining 1%, 40% is albumin bound, 45% is ionized (the active form that affects muscles and nerves), and 15% is in other anion complexes.

Low calcium levels are common in older adults because of inadequate intake. Hypocalcemia can also develop from an inadequate intake of vitamin D as a result of intentional changes in the diet, or it can result from diseases that impair calcium absorption. Diets can be deficient in vitamin D in people with lactose intolerance, GI disease, liver disease, alcoholism, anorexia, and bulimia. Decreased intake for several days, such as with NPO status, or for longer periods, as in high-protein and other weight-reduction diets, has also been linked to hypocalcemia.

Parathyroid disease decreases plasma calcium levels (Figure 12-2). A deficiency of parathyroid hormone (PTH) results in a decrease in plasma calcium levels because of decreased bone resorption, decreased GI absorption, and increased urinary excretion of calcium. Unplanned removal of the parathyroid gland can occur when the thyroid gland is removed.

Vitamin D is critical for calcium absorption and must be activated by exposure to the sun. Therefore hypocalcemia can develop in people who experience prolonged institutionalization. However, only a few minutes of sun exposure each week on the arms and face is enough to change previously ingested vitamin D to its active form. People with darkly pigmented skin require 3 to 6 times more sun exposure for the same effect.

Hypocalcemia can develop in people with pancreatitis owing to a release of lipases into soft tissue spaces, with subsequent binding of free fatty acids to calcium. Open wounds are associated with increased loss of calcium. Excess sodium, as seen in Cushing's disease, promotes the excretion of calcium. Overcorrection of

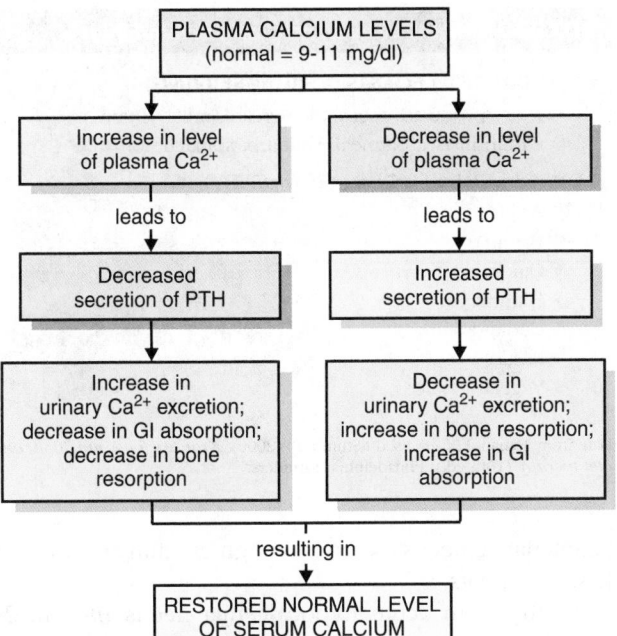

■ **FIGURE 12–2** Parathyroid hormone (PTH) regulation of plasma calcium level. *GI,* Gastrointestinal.

acidosis may also lead to hypocalcemia, because alkalosis causes decreased calcium ionization, leading to more calcium-protein binding. Clients receiving multiple transfusions of stored blood are at increased risk because of the binding of the preservative citrate with the calcium.

Several medications have been linked with hypocalcemia:

- Magnesium sulfate, colchicine, and neomycin inhibit PTH secretion.
- Aspirin, anticonvulsants (need 2 to 5 times the recommended vitamin D), and estrogen alter vitamin D metabolism.
- Phosphate preparations impair reabsorption of calcium.
- Bisphosphonates inhibit osteoclast activity.
- Steroids increase calcium mobilization.
- Loop diuretics reduce calcium reabsorption.
- Antacids and laxatives decrease calcium absorption from the intestine.

Decreased level of calcium causes a partial depolarization of nerves and muscles because of a decrease in threshold potential. Therefore a smaller stimulus initiates the action potential. The manifestations expressed by the neuromuscular system and the cardiac dysrhythmias all are due to the increased neuronal excitability and irritability in the motor and sensory nerves. The lack of calcium in the myocardium leads to weakened myocardial contraction, a prolongation of the QT interval on the

ECG, and decreased cardiac output, manifested as hypotension and a weak pulse.

The decreased calcium absorption in the intestine results in irritability of the smooth muscle in intestinal walls, resulting in increased peristalsis and diarrhea. A low calcium level impairs the intrinsic pathway and thus affects every phase of blood coagulation, leading to prolonged bleeding times and eventual hemorrhage. The bone tries to compensate for the plasma deficiency of calcium by increasing bone resorption, but the increased loss of calcium from the bone only makes the bone more brittle and results in pathologic fractures.

Clinical Manifestations

Most of the clinical manifestations of hypocalcemia are related to neuromuscular hyperexcitability. Numbness and tingling of the hands, toes, and lips and emotional lability (e.g., irritability and anxiety) are manifestations of mild hypocalcemia. In the person with hypoparathyroidism, early signs of hypocalcemia resulting from overingestion of phosphate products or protein, or both, are cardiac palpitations and restlessness. Both phosphate and protein increase calcium binding. Findings in severe hypocalcemia are cardiac insufficiency, hypotension, dysrhythmias, a prolonged QT interval, Trousseau's and Chvostek's signs (Figure 12-3), and prolonged bleeding times. These abnormalities progress to seizures, laryngeal stridor, tetany, hemorrhage, cardiac collapse, and eventual death.

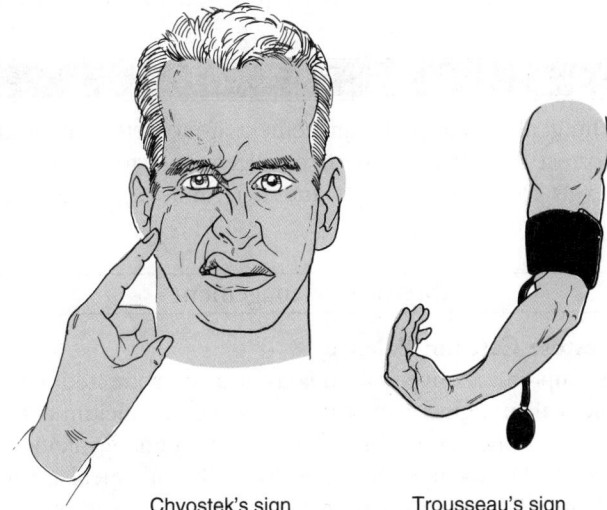

Chvostek's sign   Trousseau's sign

■ **FIGURE 12–3** Chvostek's and Trousseau's signs. A calcium deficit (hypocalcemia) or magnesium deficit (hypomagnesemia) increases the resting potential of nerves. This increase allows nerve stimulation and firing with less stimulus. Touching the facial nerve adjacent to the ear produces twitching of the client's upper lip (Chvostek's sign). The hand and fingers can also go into spasm (Trousseau's sign or carpal spasm). These spasms can occur spontaneously or when blood flow is decreased (e.g., during blood pressure cuff inflation).

With prolonged hypocalcemia, cataracts may develop because of increased uptake of sodium and water by the lens. Trophic changes, such as dry, sparse hair and rough skin, may also be noted. Spontaneous fractures can occur when the bone is depleted of calcium.

A plasma calcium level less than 4.5 mEq/L, or 9 mg/dl, is considered diagnostic for hypocalcemia. When reviewing serum calcium levels, use the ionized calcium level, because it is the true level of free (active, ionized) calcium. A level less than 1.18 mEq/L (<2.36 mg/dl) indicates hypocalcemia.

Also, abnormal plasma albumin and pH levels influence the interpretation of plasma calcium levels because of the effect on calcium binding. For example, when the albumin level is low, there is less calcium bound to the albumin, resulting in higher ionized calcium. Conversely, when plasma albumin level is high, more calcium is bound; thus the functional ionized calcium level is actually lower than the plasma level reveals. When albumin levels are low, the total plasma calcium level can be corrected by using the following formula: (4.0 − serum albumin level) × 0.8 = X; X + current calcium level = corrected calcium. Corrected calcium levels are not recommended for the critically ill. An alkaline pH causes an increase in calcium binding. The plasma level may appear normal, but the functional ionized calcium level is actually lower. The opposite is true with an acidic pH. The ionized calcium (iCa) assay is the safest way to monitor calcium level in those that are critically ill, those with marginal calcium imbalances, or those with an abnormal albumin level or acid-base imbalance. A person with true hypocalcemia has an ionized calcium level less than 1.18 mEq/L (normal equals 1.18 to 1.30 mEq/L).

OUTCOME MANAGEMENT

The goals of medical management are to determine and correct the cause of the hypocalcemia, restore calcium levels to normal values, and determine a method to reduce recurrence.

Medical Management

Restore Calcium Balance

Asymptomatic hypocalcemia is usually corrected with oral calcium gluconate, calcium lactate, or calcium chloride. For increased absorption, the calcium supplement should be given with a glass of milk with meals. The vitamin D in the milk promotes calcium absorption.

Chronic or mild hypocalcemia can be treated in part by having the client consume a diet high in calcium (Box 12-3). If hypocalcemia is secondary to parathyroid deficiency, the client must avoid high-phosphate foods, such as milk products and carbonated beverages, and excess protein. Protein binds with available calcium and only exacerbates the manifestations of hypocalcemia.

BOX 12-3 High-Calcium and Low-Calcium Foods

HIGH-CALCIUM FOODS (>100 mg/SERVING)
- Dairy products: cheese, ice cream, milk, yogurt
- Other: instant oatmeal, rhubarb, spinach, tofu

LOW-CALCIUM FOODS (<25 mg/SERVING)
- Apples
- Bananas
- Chicken
- Hamburger
- Cooked oatmeal
- Pasta
- Vegetable juices

Data from Mahan, L.K., & Escott-Stump, S. (2000). *Krause's food, nutrition, and diet therapy* (10th ed.). Philadelphia: Saunders.

Maintenance needs are met through calcium and vitamin D supplements.

Tetany from acute hypocalcemia needs *immediate* attention. IV calcium chloride or calcium gluconate must be given slowly to avoid hypotension and bradycardia and other dysrhythmias. Use D_5W solutions when dilution is necessary; avoid saline solutions, because they promote calcium loss.

> **Calcium solutions, especially calcium chloride, can extravasate and lead to severe tissue damage. Infuse calcium slowly through a small IV catheter in a large vein to quickly dilute the solution. If any blanching or pain is noted at the site of injection, stop *immediately*. Withdraw the remaining fluid from the needle and follow agency protocol for extravasation.**

Nursing Management of the Medical Client

A thorough history of the client's current and chronic illnesses, diet intake, and medications, including over-the-counter medications and herbals, assists in identifying risks for calcium deficit and guides interventions for health promotion and maintenance. If digitalis and calcium are among the medications identified, assess for digitalis toxicity as well, because hypocalcemia increases the risk of this problem.

Check for Trousseau's and Chvostek's signs in high-risk clients (see Figure 12-3). *Trousseau's sign* is the occurrence of carpal spasm, or contraction of the fingers and hand, when a blood pressure cuff is kept inflated on the upper arm for 5 minutes at diastolic pressure. *Chvostek's sign* is occurrence of spasm of the muscles innervated by the facial nerve when the client's face is tapped lightly below the temple. Spasm of the face, lip, or nose is also evidence of tetany. In addition, assess for paresthesias (finger, toes, circumoral).

Assess the client's cardiac status by monitoring the ECG and vital signs, especially the apical heart rate and rhythm. Frequency of assessment varies from 1 to 4 hours, depending on the client's condition. Assess color, warmth, motion, and sensation (CWMS) and peripheral pulses to provide data for evaluation of cardiac output.

Monitor also for bleeding in the gums and petechiae or ecchymosis in the skin. Assess for changes in the clarity of urine, because microscopic bleeding causes clear urine to become cloudy before frank bleeding is apparent. Also, note black or blood-streaked stool, which may indicate occult GI bleeding. Be suspicious of an intracerebral hemorrhage when a client reports a new onset of headache. Monitor plasma calcium levels for improvement or worsening.

Monitor IV sites for infiltration or phlebitis when IV calcium is being infused. Calcium chloride is extremely irritating to the subcutaneous tissue. Notify the physician if the client's manifestations do not resolve or if signs of overcorrection (hypercalcemia) occur. When possible, use fresh blood for transfusions. Avoid giving calcium and bicarbonate in the same IV solution, because a precipitate will form. Use filters with TPN solutions.

To prevent pathologic fractures, use caution by obtaining adequate help to turn or move the client. Use gait belts and or extra personnel to walk or transfer the client to and from bed.

Instruct the client about foods that are rich in calcium, such as milk, cheese, yogurt, and green, leafy vegetables. Encourage taking calcium supplements with meals and vitamin D milk for better absorption. *Exception:* For people with hypocalcemia resulting from hypoparathyroidism, phosphorus intake should be decreased by *omitting* milk, milk products, and other high-phosphorus foods (e.g., carbonated beverages). Calcium and vitamin D supplements are prescribed for this population as well. Several types of vitamin D are available. Therefore clients with hypoparathyroidism must be advised not to take over-the-counter forms without first consulting with a physician to ensure that the right supplement is taken. These clients should also be advised to ingest protein only in amounts recommended by the American Dietetic Association (ADA). Increased intake of protein leads only to further binding of available calcium.

Self-Care

Reinforce intake of a well-balanced diet, avoiding high-protein diets or other nonprescribed weight-loss diets, and encourage weight-bearing exercises to prevent bone resorption. Consult the physician about the need for mineral and vitamin supplements for clients who consume less than half of their meals (e.g., the older adult population). Calcium carbonate is often recommended as an inexpensive supplement.

Older clients may have difficulty incorporating large amounts of food and fluids containing calcium into the diet. Part of the difficulty is in changing long-established eating habits. Many older adults drink very little milk because of habits formed in childhood. Suggest other forms of calcium that may be more appealing, such as yogurt, cheese, milkshakes made with ice milk, or green, leafy vegetables.

HYPERCALCEMIA

Hypercalcemia is defined as a plasma calcium level greater than 5.5 mEq/L, or 11 mg/dl. Hypercalcemia can occur in any age group. It is a common electrolyte disorder that can have serious physical complications.

Etiology and Risk Factors

The three most common causes of hypercalcemia are (1) metastatic malignancy, (2) hyperparathyroidism, and (3) thiazide diuretic therapy. The most common cancers that cause hypercalcemia are malignancies of the lung, breast, ovary, prostate, bladder, bone (multiple myeloma, leukemia), kidney, head and neck, and lymph tissues. Malignancy-induced hypercalcemia is the result of either bone destruction or an increased secretion of ectopic PTH.

Other causes of hypercalcemia include an excessive intake of calcium supplements with vitamin D or of calcium-containing antacids, prolonged immobilization, metabolic acidosis, and hypophosphatemia. Prolonged immobilization causes resorption of calcium from the bone. Recall that bone density is maintained by weight-bearing stress on bone. Metabolic acidosis promotes hypercalcemia by two mechanisms: decreased binding of calcium, which increases the plasma ionized calcium levels, and inhibition of calcium excretion from the kidney. Hypophosphatemia inhibits the ability of the kidney to excrete excess calcium.

Pathophysiology

Destruction of bone tissue increases the release of calcium into the vascular spaces. Excessive PTH production promotes calcium retention, which leads to hypophosphatemia. Hypophosphatemia compounds the problem by promoting more calcium retention.

When excess calcium is present, the cell membrane threshold potential becomes more positive, which results in membranes that are refractory to depolarization. This decreased cell membrane excitability requires a stronger stimulus for a response to occur. As a result, cardiac and smooth muscle activity is decreased. Excess calcium in the bloodstream also impairs renal function and precipitates as a salt, which often forms renal stones.

Clinical Manifestations

The clinical manifestations of hypercalcemia, which are generally nonspecific, are determined by the plasma calcium level. Mild hypercalcemia, with calcium levels at or slightly above 5.5 mEq/L, or 11 mg/dl, is usually asymptomatic. In mild cases, the plasma calcium level may increase momentarily when the client consumes calcium-containing antacids, or a large dose of an oral calcium supplement, and the kidneys are initially unable to eliminate the excess.

In moderate hypercalcemia, with calcium levels of 6.2 mEq/L, or 13 mg/dl, manifestations usually include anorexia, nausea, vomiting, polyuria, muscle weakness, fatigue, lethargy, dehydration, and constipation. Increased calcium stimulates the release of hydrochloric acid, gastrin, and pancreatic enzymes and slows bowel transit time, which leads to the anorexia, nausea, vomiting, abdominal distention, and constipation. The weakness, fatigue, depression, and difficulty concentrating are due to neurologic depression. Hypercalcemia also causes osmotic diuresis; the polyuria leads to dehydration and thirst and further exacerbates the constipation.

Calcium precipitates tend to form ureteral or kidney stones, which result in urinary blockage and severe colicky pain. Excess calcium also impairs glomerular blood flow, which can lead to renal failure. Bone pain is often associated with cancer of the bone and is due to the pressure on nerve endings from the tumor cells. Pathologic fractures are due to the decalcification of the bony matrix and can occur with cancer of the bone or with any condition that causes resorption of calcium. Calcium deposits can also occur on the skin.

Progressive neurologic depression from increasing hypercalcemia is manifested as extreme lethargy, a depressed sensorium, confusion, and eventually coma. Severe hypercalcemia may result in hypercalcemic crisis, which carries a 30% to 50% mortality rate. A hypercalcemic crisis occurs when calcium levels reach 7.1 mEq/L, or 15 mg/dl. The resultant increased conduction transmission, shortened repolarization (shortened QT interval, widened T wave), and severe cardiac depression can cause cardiac dysrhythmias, ECG changes, and cardiac arrest. Hypokalemia may occur as the body eliminates potassium rather than calcium.

OUTCOME MANAGEMENT

Medical Management

The goals of medical management are to determine and correct the cause of the hypercalcemia, restore calcium levels to normal values, and determine a method to reduce recurrence. Prevention and early detection of complications such as renal stones and fractures are also important. Benefits of treatment are evaluated against risk.

Restore Calcium Balance

Immediate correction of moderate and severe hypercalcemia is essential. IV normal saline, given rapidly with furosemide to prevent fluid overload, promotes urinary calcium excretion. Antitumor antibiotics may be given that inhibit the action of PTH on osteoclasts in bone tissue, in order to reduce decalcification and the plasma calcium level.

Calcitonin decreases the plasma calcium level by inhibiting the effects of PTH on the osteoclasts and increasing urinary calcium excretion. Corticosteroid drugs decrease calcium levels by competing with vitamin D, resulting in decreased intestinal absorption of calcium, and by inhibiting prostaglandins, resulting in decreased bone resorption. IV phosphate decreases plasma calcium levels; however, it is used as a last resort because it may result in severe calcification of various tissues.

Thiazide diuretics should be changed to furosemide or to another diuretic that does not cause retention of calcium. If the cause of the hypercalcemia is excessive use of calcium or vitamin D supplements or calcium-containing antacids, these agents should be either avoided or used in a reduced dosage. If the client is not nauseated, encourage oral liquids. These actions are designed to lower the calcium level in 36 to 48 hours. Etidronate disodium reduces plasma calcium level by inhibiting precursors to calcium mineralization and, secondarily, by reducing bone formation. The client needs to be hydrated with large volumes of normal saline before etidronate administration and must be given loop diuretics to enhance urine output and calcium excretion following drug administration.

Gallium nitrate has been effective in inhibiting bone resorption and in decreasing osteoclastic activity. The drug should be stopped if the urine output is less than 2 L/day or if the plasma creatinine level is greater than 2.5 mg/dl.

Bisphosphonates (zoledronate, pamidronate) are considered the first-line therapy for hypercalcemia secondary to cancer. Second-line therapy includes glucocorticoids, mithramycin, calcitonin, and gallium nitrate.

For client teaching, review high-calcium foods that should be restricted (see Box 12-3). Instruct the client that forcing fluids helps to lower plasma levels by flushing excess calcium through the kidney. If manifestations of renal calculi (stones) are present, teach that consumption of foods and fluids that increase urine acidity helps decrease stone formation. These include meat, eggs, whole grains, cranberry juice, and prune juice.

Nursing Management of the Medical Client

Because plasma calcium levels are not routinely assessed, it is essential that the nurse identify high-risk clients. Screening assessment includes obtaining a thorough history, focusing on risk factors, medications (including over-the-counter calcium supplements or antacids), and diet history. Assess vital signs, apical pulses, and ECG every 1 to 8 hours, depending on the severity of the client's manifestations. Bowel sounds, renal function, and hydration status should be assessed every 8 hours. Also, recall that it is important to monitor for fluid volume depletion secondary to hypercalcemia.

Early treatment may prevent a hypercalcemic crisis. Unless fluids are contraindicated (as in clients with heart failure), increase fluid intake. If flank pain or renal colic is present, strain all urine to capture renal calculi for analysis. Report urine output of less than 0.5 ml/kg/hr for 2 consecutive hours. Report any manifestations that indicate worsening of the clinical status, such as an increase in severity of dysrhythmias, a decrease in sensorium, or manifestations of overcorrection (hypocalcemia).

Once the crisis is controlled, prevention of complications through teaching and safety interventions becomes the primary focus of health maintenance. Instruct the client to avoid calcium supplements. Sodium intake is increased, unless contraindicated, to promote calcium loss through the kidneys. Consumption of high-fiber foods and fluids should be increased to prevent constipation, and an acid-ash diet may be recommended to decrease the risk of stone formation. The client should also be taught to report clinical manifestations of renal calculi, such as flank pain, hematuria, or cardiac dysfunction (such as an irregular pulse or palpitations).

If the client has confusion, lethargy, or coma, institute safety precautions, including a low bed position. To prevent injury, turn and move the client with extreme caution and with adequate assistance. Gait belts, back braces, tripod canes, and walkers may be used to facilitate safer ambulation.

Assist with resistive range-of-motion and weight-bearing activities to decrease calcium loss from the bone. Report clinical manifestations of fractures immediately, such as bone pain, deformity of limbs, or ecchymosis.

Surgical Management

Surgery may be used to remove an ectopic PTH-secreting tumor. Noninvasive or invasive lithotripsy or endoscopic removal of renal or ureteral calculi may be necessary.

PHOSPHATE IMBALANCES

HYPOPHOSPHATEMIA

Hypophosphatemia is defined as plasma phosphorus level less than 1.2 mEq/L. The major risk for hypophosphatemia is loss or long-term lack of intake, increased growth or tissue repair, and recovery from malnourished states. Failure to meet these increased needs results in a state of phosphorus depletion.

Phosphorus depletion can occur as a result of prolonged and excessive intake of antacids. Administration of high levels of glucose via tube-feeding or IV line causes phosphorus to enter the cell for glucose phosphorylation;

this is known as the refeeding syndrome. The increased sodium found in Cushing's syndrome, the increased calcium found in hyperparathyroidism, and the decreased arterial partial pressure of carbon dioxide ($Paco_2$) in chronic respiratory alkalosis also cause phosphorus to move into the cell. Lead poisoning leads to a decreased availability of phosphate. Phosphate loss occurs in burns, and a mild renal loss occurs with metabolic alkalosis. Some paraneoplastic syndromes have been associated with hypophosphatemia.

Pathophysiologic changes that occur with hypophosphatemia can affect every organ system because of the effect of hypophosphatemia on optimal adenosine triphosphate (ATP) and oxygen supply. Phosphate depletion impairs the conversion of glucose and many other intermediate substances to ATP. The ultimate result is a disruption in the sole mechanism responsible for regeneration of ATP.

The plasma level, whether normal or low, does not always reflect the total body phosphate content. Careful review of a client's history, laboratory data, medications, and clinical manifestations, with emphasis on nutritional health in people at high risk, increases the likelihood of identifying phosphate deficiencies. The primary manifestations of hypophosphatemia are decreased cardiac and respiratory function, muscle weakness, fatigue, brittle bones, bone pain, confusion, and seizures.

Mild hypophosphatemia can be treated with diet and dietary supplementation. Teach the client the components of a well-balanced diet and help the client and family gain access to resources. Clients who have a serious phosphate imbalance are often deficient in many other nutrients. TPN is usually the intervention of choice until the plasma levels become stable.

HYPERPHOSPHATEMIA

Hyperphosphatemia, a plasma phosphate level greater than 3 mEq/L, is rare but serious. The most common causes are excessive intake of high-phosphate foods, excess vitamin D (especially with renal insufficiency), impaired colonic motility that causes increased absorption, hypoparathyroidism, and Addison's disease. Clinical manifestations are related to the degree of hyperphosphatemia or to secondary hypocalcemia. Tachycardia, palpitations, and restlessness are among the earliest manifestations. Anorexia, nausea, vomiting, hyperreflexia, tetany, and more serious dysrhythmias may follow if the imbalance worsens.

In certain conditions, an increased intake or decreased excretion of phosphate or an increase in cell lysis results in high levels of phosphorus. In renal failure, the kidney is less able to excrete phosphate; the excess phosphate impairs calcium reabsorption. TLS results in a state of hyperphosphatemia from tumor cell rupture. Women are at risk after menopause owing to a slight increase in phosphate secondary to a deficiency of estrogen. Hyperphosphatemia leading to death has been associated with administration of phospho-soda enemas in the presence of altered renal or bowel function. Follow manufacturer recommendations when giving phospho-soda enemas.

In mild or asymptomatic hyperphosphatemia, treatment focuses on limiting high-phosphate foods, especially milk, ice cream, cheeses, large amounts of meat and fish, and carbonated beverages, or giving calcium or aluminum products that promote the binding and excretion of phosphate. Dialysis is the primary treatment for renal failure that is refractory to conservative approaches.

MAGNESIUM IMBALANCES

HYPOMAGNESEMIA

Hypomagnesemia is defined as a plasma magnesium level less than 1.5 mEq/L, or 1.8 mg/dl. Magnesium deficits are being identified more often as a result of increased knowledge about this ion. Of the clients with calcium, phosphate, sodium, and potassium imbalances, 22% to 42% have been found to have a coexisting magnesium imbalance. However, it is a rare imbalance in people who consume a well-balanced diet. As with other intracellular ions, plasma levels may be normal in the presence of intracellular depletion. Also, hypomagnesemia is often overlooked, because tests for plasma magnesium levels are not routinely ordered until a severe deficit has occurred. Plasma levels may be helpful in severe or acute changes, but a 24-hour urinalysis after an IV magnesium challenge, ion-selective imaging scan, or nuclear magnetic resonance imaging scan (to determine soft tissue levels) is more predictive of total body magnesium levels, but these studies are rarely done because they are expensive.

Hypomagnesemia is becoming recognized as a common cause of refractory (not responsive to treatment) hypokalemia and hypocalcemia. The hypomagnesemic state inhibits potassium reabsorption; therefore the hypomagnesemia needs to be corrected before potassium and calcium imbalances respond to treatment.

Magnesium deficits are often seen in critically ill clients, alcoholic clients, in pregnancy and pregnancy-related conditions, and in clients with diabetes mellitus, infectious diseases, or ischemic heart disease. Alcoholism decreases intestinal absorption as a result of a decrease in enzymes that are normally produced by the liver. Alcoholism also promotes magnesium wasting as a result of nephrotoxicity and leads to malnutrition. Other causes of hypomagnesemia are severe or chronic malnutrition; malabsorption syndromes, such as Crohn's or celiac disease or pancreatitis; and GI losses from vomiting, GI suction, diarrhea, high-volume ileostomies, fistulae, laxative abuse, or radiation enteritis. Mechanisms for renal losses include the diuretic phase of acute renal failure and hyperphosphatemia.

Prolonged IV or TPN therapy without magnesium replacement also increases the risk for hypomagnesemia. Excess calcium (as in hyperparathyroidism) and excess sodium (as in Cushing's syndrome or hyperaldosteronism) inhibit magnesium reabsorption. The hyperglycemia seen with diabetic acidosis causes osmotic diuresis and loss of magnesium. Alkalosis is also associated with hypomagnesemia.

Excessive amounts of phosphorus in the intestine (as from overuse of antacids) inhibit the uptake of magnesium from the intestinal villi. Some medications interfere with renal handling of magnesium as either a primary action or a side effect. These include diuretics (loop, osmotic, thiazide), antibiotics (such as aminoglycoside antibiotics), carbenicillin, amphotericin B, cisplatin, corticosteroids, and digitalis. Cocaine abuse has also been linked to hypomagnesemia.

The myocardial irritability that occurs with hypomagnesemia seems to be a result of changes in the resting membrane potential caused by alterations of both potassium and magnesium ions, which stimulates beta$_2$-adrenergic cells. It is often associated with digitalis use. Magnesium depletion and digitalis both promote potassium loss from myocardial cells. Digitalis uptake also seems to be increased in hypomagnesemia. GI changes from decreased contractility, such as anorexia, nausea, and abdominal distention, can occur. Psychological disorders, such as depression, psychosis, and confusion, may also develop.

Severe hypomagnesemia causes neuromuscular manifestations such as Chvostek's and Trousseau's signs, tetany, convulsions, and vasospasm leading to stroke. Although magnesium is neuroprotective, peripheral intravenous delivery has not been shown to increase bioavailability in the brain enough to positively affect those suffering from acute ischemic strokes or subarachnoid hemorrhages.

Cardiac abnormalities include premature ventricular contractions, atrial or ventricular fibrillation, and ECG changes (prolonged QT intervals, widened QRS complexes, and broadening of T waves). Other ECG changes are related to the concomitant low levels of potassium. Low magnesium levels have been linked with an increased incidence of ventricular dysrhythmias and decreased 1-year survival rates in clients with heart failure as well as with lethal dysrhythmias in clients who have had myocardial infarctions. 🪔 Studies also suggest a link between estrogen therapy in postmenopausal women and increased coagulation risk; estrogen promotes tissue uptake of magnesium and hence hypomagnesemia.

Management

Treatment of hypomagnesemia includes oral magnesium replacement in the form of magnesium-containing antacids or parenteral magnesium sulfate. Increasing dietary intake of magnesium also helps ensure balance and stability.

IV magnesium reduces the tendency of the small airways to spasm and has been found useful in treating acute asthma that has been refractory to other therapy. The positive inotropic, negative chronotropic, and vaso-dilatory effects of magnesium have also been found to increase cardiac output and decrease oxygen consumption in people with shock and sepsis. Magnesium has also been successfully used as a mood stabilizer in clients with bipolar disease.

Nursing management includes monitoring vital signs every 4 to 8 hours and reviewing ECG readings hourly.

Initiate safety and seizure precautions for clients who are extremely confused or at risk for seizures. Monitor plasma magnesium, potassium, and calcium levels.

Also, many experts recommend assessing the client's deep tendon reflexes because normal reflexes suggest normal cellular magnesium levels. This assessment is a more sensitive indicator of the early cellular levels of this ion.

Consult a physician about the need for magnesium maintenance or replacement if the client has severe malnutrition, is on NPO status for more than 3 days (especially in the presence of coexisting losses), or has manifestations of hypokalemia or hypocalcemia even after treatment. TPN may be necessary to correct coexistent nutrient imbalances, which is common. Maintaining glucose control in people with diabetes mellitus decreases the risk of magnesium loss from the glucose-related osmotic diuresis. Rapid infusion of undiluted magnesium sulfate can cause a hot or flushed feeling and phlebitis. Avoid giving magnesium in saline solutions.

Instructing clients and family members about foods rich in magnesium provides information that may be essential in preventing magnesium deficiency or in correcting a mild deficit (Box 12-4). Caution clients about taking mineral supplements without the advice of a dietitian or pharmacist. The calcium-to-magnesium ratio should be maintained at 4:1; a higher ratio can lead to deposition of calcium in the soft tissues and vessels. Taking magnesium without potassium causes shifting of potassium into the cell. In a client with alcoholism, magnesium should be given with thiamine to promote nerve regeneration.

HYPERMAGNESEMIA

Hypermagnesemia, a plasma magnesium level greater than 2.5 mEq/L, or 3 mg/dl, is a rare disorder. Hypermagnesemia may occur with renal insufficiency, excessive use of magnesium-containing antacids or laxatives, or administration of potassium-sparing diuretics. Many potassium-sparing diuretics conserve magnesium. Hypermagnesemia is also seen with severe dehydration from ketoacidosis, with decreased synthesis of aldosterone (such as in Addison's disease or after adrenalectomy), and with overuse of IV magnesium sulfate for controlling premature labor or pre-eclampsia.

BOX 12-4   High-Magnesium and Low-Magnesium Foods

HIGH-MAGNESIUM FOODS (>75 mg/SERVING)
- Cashews
- Chili
- Halibut
- Swiss chard
- Tofu
- Wheat germ

LOW-MAGNESIUM FOODS (<25 mg/SERVING)
- Chicken
- Eggs
- Fruits
- Green peas
- Hamburger
- White bread

Data from Mahan, L.K., & Escott-Stump, S. (2000). *Krause's food, nutrition, and diet therapy* (10th ed.). Philadelphia: Saunders.

Clinical manifestations are related to the blocked release of acetylcholine from the myoneural junction, which results in a decrease in muscle cell activity. With mild hypermagnesemia, peripheral vessels dilate, causing hypotension. ECG changes include prolonged PR and QT intervals. In extreme hypermagnesemia, profound sedative effects on the neuromuscular system lead to severe muscle weakness, lethargy, drowsiness, loss of deep tendon reflexes, respiratory paralysis, and loss of consciousness. Cardiac signs include delayed myocardial conduction manifested on the ECG as wide QRS complexes, elevated T wave, heart block, and premature ventricular contractions.

Management

Management of hypermagnesemia includes decreasing the use of magnesium sulfate. Saline infusions with a diuretic increases renal elimination of magnesium. However, a side effect of the treatment is a loss of calcium. Hypocalcemia may intensify the hypermagnesemia. IV calcium may be used to antagonize the effects of hypermagnesemia. Albuterol has also been used to reduce magnesium levels. The presence of severe respiratory distress requires ventilatory assistance. If renal failure is present, hemodialysis may be necessary.

Nursing management focuses assessment on vital signs, respiratory function, ECG recordings, urine output, and the level of sensorium; these should be checked every 1 to 4 hours, depending on the client's condition.

Safety and seizure precautions should be initiated when confusion or seizure risk is present. Changes in deep tendon reflexes should be reported. Keep IV calcium salts in the code cart for emergency reversal of severe hypermagnesemia. SAFETY ⚠ ALERT

Teach clients to avoid constant use of laxatives and antacids containing magnesium, especially if urine output is decreased. Encourage eating foods that contain fiber and drinking adequate fluids to promote fecal elimination.

 CONCLUSIONS

Electrolyte imbalances are found in all age groups in every type of health care setting. It is rare for a person to have only one electrolyte imbalance; more commonly, multiple electrolyte and fluid imbalances are present, especially in high-risk populations such as the very young, older adults, and people with chronic illnesses.

Nurses play an essential role in health promotion, health maintenance, and health restoration for clients at risk for or experiencing fluid and electrolyte imbalances. Nursing management includes the following pivotal roles:

- *Teaching* clients and their families about positive health behaviors, about the importance of nutrient intake (even during nonacute illnesses), and about manifestations of fluid and electrolyte imbalance that necessitate physician consultation
- *Promoting* nutritional maintenance and replacement in clients who are at high risk for or who are experiencing fluid or electrolyte imbalance
- *Assisting* the physician in early detection of imbalances and of poor response to treatment or signs of overcorrection
- *Promoting* balanced nutrition in rehabilitation or extended care settings through family support, early physician referrals for supplements, dietary consultation, or management of imbalances

 THINKING CRITICALLY

1. An older, tube-fed resident from a nursing home is admitted with recent changes in level of consciousness. Her skin and mouth are very dry, and her urine is scant and dark yellow. Laboratory assessment reveals the following: sodium, 150 mEq/dl; chloride, 106 mEq/dl; BUN, 52 mg/dl; and creatinine, 1.2 mg/dl. Her family calls and wants to know "if she will make it." How would you respond?

Factors to Consider. What do these assessment findings suggest? What interventions would you expect to be prescribed? What precautions will be needed to prevent further fluid and electrolyte shifts?

2. A 45-year-old woman was admitted with a rapid heart rate. Her past medical history is negative for cardiac disease. One week ago, she began a new weight-loss program that included furosemide. Could her heart rate become potentially life-threatening?

Factors to Consider. Why would a client take furosemide in a weight-loss program? What side effects may be occurring? What laboratory studies do you anticipate being ordered? Which electrolytes do you think will be abnormal?

evolve *Discussions for these questions can be found on the website.*

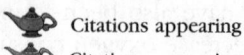 BIBLIOGRAPHY

Citations appearing in red refer to primary research.

Citations appearing in blue refer to evidence-based practice guidelines and protocols.

1. Ali, F.E., et al. (2004). Loss of seizure control due to anticonvulsant-induced hypocalcemia. *The Annals of Pharmacotherapy*, 38, 1002-1005.
2. Asele, S.M. (2005). Restoring electrolyte balance. *RN*, 68(5), 34-40.
3. Bilezikian, J.P., & Silverberg, S.J. (2004). Asymptomatic primary hyperparathyroidism. *New England Journal of Medicine*, 350(17), 1746-1751.
4. Boccalandro, C., et al. (2003). Electrocardiographic changes in thyrotoxic periodic paralysis. *The American Journal of Cardiology*, 91, 775-777.
5. Burger, C.M. (2004). Hyperkalemia. *American Journal of Nursing*, 104(10), 66-70.
6. Burger, C.M. (2004). Hypokalemia. *American Journal of Nursing*, 104(11), 61-65.
7. Cacchione, P.Z., et al. (2003). Clinical profile of acute confusion in the long-term care setting. *Clinical Nursing Research*, 12(2), 45-58.
8. Cantril, C., & Haylock, P. (2004). Tumor lysis syndrome: Prevention and early detection are crucial in caring for patients with cancer. *American Journal of Nursing*, 104(4), 49-52.
9. Champallou, C., et al. (2003). Hypocalcemia following pamidronate administration for bone metastases of solid tumor: Three clinical case reports. *Journal of Pain and Symptom Management*, 25(2), 185-190.
10. Chia-Chao, W., et al. (2003). An unrecognized cause of paralysis in ED: Thyrotoxic normokalemic periodic paralysis. *American Journal of Emergency Medicine*, 21(1), 71-73.
11. Cook, L.K. (2005). An acute myocardial infarction. *American Journal of Critical Care*, 14(4), 313-315.
12. Doorenbos, C.J., & Vermeij, C.G. (2006). Danger of salt substitutes that contain potassium in patients with renal failure. *British Medical Journal*, 326, 35-36.
13. Dyer, B.T., et al. (2004). Hypokalemia in ibuprofen and codeine phosphate abuse. *International Journal of Clinical Practice*, 58(11), 1061-1062.
14. Edwards, S. (2001). Regulation of water, sodium and potassium: Implications for practice. *Nursing Standard*, 15(22), 36-42.
15. Elinav, E., & Chajek-Shaul, T. (2003). Licorice consumption causing severe hypokalemic paralysis. *Mayo Clinic Proceedings*, 78(6), 767-768.
16. Elgart, H.N. (2004). Assessment of fluids and electrolytes. *AACN Clinical Issues*, 15(4), 607-621.
17. Gennari, F.J. (2002). Disorders of potassium homeostasis. Hypokalemia and hyperkalemia. *Critical Care Clinics*, 18(2), 273-288.
18. Gunduz, H., et al. (2004). Hypokalemia and ST elevation induced by angiotensin II type 1 receptor blocker and thiazide diuretic combination. *The Journal of Applied Research*, 4(3), 476-480.
19. Guyton, A., & Hall, J. (2001). *Textbook of medical physiology* (10th ed.). Philadelphia: Saunders.
20. Higgins, K.M. (2006). The role of intraoperative rapid parathyroid hormone monitoring for predicting thyroidectomy-related hypocalcemia. *ARCH Otolaryngology Head Neck Surgery*, 130, 63-67.
21. Hoye, A., & Clark, A. (2003). Iatrogenic hyperkalemia. *The Lancet*, 361, 2124.
22. Huether, S., & McCance, K. (2004). *Understanding pathophysiology* (3rd ed.). St. Louis: Mosby.
23. Huggins, R.M., et al. (2003). Cardiac arrest from succinylcholine-induced hyperkalemia. *American Journal of Health System Pharmacy*, 60(7), 694-697.
24. Innerarity, S. (2000). Hypomagnesemia in acute and chronic illness. *Critical Care Nursing Quarterly*, 23(2), 1-17.
25. Innis, J. (2002). Treating nephrogenic diabetes insipidus. *Dimensions of Critical Care Nursing*, 21(3), 98-99.
26. Jan de Beur, S.M. (2005). Tumor-induced osteomalacia. *JAMA*, 294(10), 1260-1267.
27. Jolobe, O.M.P. (2003). Hyperkalemic paralysis. *Age and Aging*, 3(5), 556-557.

28. Juurlink, D.N., et al. (2004). Rates of hyperkalemia after publication of the randomized aldactone evaluation study. *New England Journal of Medicine, 351*(6), 543-551.

29. Kearney, K. (2000). Hyperkalemia. *American Journal of Nursing, 100*(1), 55-56.

30. Koontz, S.L., Friedman, S.A., & Schwartz, M.L. (2004). Symptomatic hypocalcemia after tocolytic therapy with magnesium sulfate and nifedipine. *American Journal of Obstetrics and Gynecology, 190,* 1773-1776.

31. Lam, Y.W. (2003). SSRIs related to syndrome of inappropriate secretion of antidiuretic hormone. *Geriatric Psychopharmacology, 7*(12), 1, 7.

32. Lin, H.A., et al. (2003). A simple and rapid approach to hypokalemic paralysis. *American Journal of Emergency Medicine, 21*(6), 487-491.

33. Lyman, D. (2005). Undiagnosed vitamin D deficiency in the hospitalized patient. *American Family Physician, 71*(2), 299-304.

34. Marinella, M.A. (2003). The refeeding syndrome and hypophosphatemia. *Nutrition Reviews, 61*(9), 320-323.

35. McKee, J.A., et al. (2005). Analysis of the brain bioavailability of peripherally administered magnesium sulfate: A study in humans with acute brain injury undergoing prolonged induced hypermagnesemia. *Critical Care Medicine, 33*(3), 661-666.

36. Mehler, P.S. (2003). Bulimia nervosa. *The New England Journal of Medicine, 349,* 875-881.

37. Mitchell, M. (2003). *Nutrition across the lifespan* (2nd ed.). Philadelphia: Saunders.

38. Mower-Wade, D., Bartley, M., & Chiari-Allwein, J. (2001). How to respond to shock. *Dimensions of Critical Care Nursing, 20*(2), 22-27.

39. Mudge, D.W., & Johnson, D.W. (2004). Cola-Cola and kangaroos. *The Lancet, 364,* 1190.

40. Muensterer, O.J. (2003). Hyperkalemic paralysis. *Age and Aging, 32,* 114-115.

41. Norris, W., et al. (2004). Potassium supplementation, diet vs pills: A randomized trial in postoperative cardiac patients. *Chest, 125,* 404-409.

42. Oh, H., et al. (2005). Effects of nasogastric tube feeding on serum sodium, potassium, and glucose levels. *Journal of Nursing Scholarship, 37*(2), 141-147.

43. Picolos, M.K., et al. (2004). Milk-alkali syndrome in pregnancy. *Obstetrics & Gynecology, 104*(5), 1201-1204.

44. Paltiel, O., et al. (2003). Effect of a computerized alert on the management of hypokalemia in hospitalized patients. *ARCH Internal Medicine, 163,* 200-204.

45. Peter, R., Mishra, V., & Fraser, W.D. (2006). Severe hypocalcemia after being given intravenous bisphosphonate. *British Medical Journal, 328,* 335-336.

46. Sayarlioglu, H., et al. (2005). Hyperkalemia occurring in a patient with psoriatic arthritis following indomethacin use. *The Journal of Applied Research, 5*(2), 295-298.

47. Schmidt, T. (2000). How to recognize hypokalemia. *Nursing, 30*(2), 22.

48. Sellares, V.L., & Ramirez, A.T. (2004). Management of hyperphosphatemia in dialysis patients. *Drugs Aging, 21*(3), 153-165.

49. Sherman, F.T. (2005). Three "hypo's" of hospitalization. *Geriatrics, 60*(5), 9-10.

50. Shuey, K.M. (2004). Hypercalcemia of malignancy: Part I. *Clinical Journal of Oncology Nursing, 8*(2), 209-210.

51. Shuey, K.M., & Brant, J.M. (2004). Hypercalcemia of malignancy: Part II. *Clinical Journal of Oncology Nursing, 8*(3), 321-323.

52. Slomp, J., et al. (2003). Albumin-adjusted calcium is not suitable for diagnosis of hyper- and hypocalcemia in the critically ill. *Critical Care Medicine, 31*(5), 1389-1393.

53. Smith, S., & Andrews, M. (2000). Artificial nutrition and hydration at the end of life. *Medsurg Nursing, 9*(5), 233-247.

54. Stalnikowicz, R. (2003). The significance of routine serum magnesium determination in ED. *American Journal of Emergency Medicine, 21*(5), 444-446.

55. Stewart, A.F. (2005). Hypercalcemia associated with cancer. *New England Journal of Medicine, 352*(4), 373-379.

56. Sugimoto, T., et al. (2003). Central pontine myelinolysis associated with hypokalemia in anorexia nervosa. *Journal of Neurosurgical Psychiatry, 74,* 353-355.

57. Svensson, M., et al. (2003). Hyperkalemia and impaired renal function in patients taking spironolactone for congestive heart failure: Retrospective study. *British Medical Journal, 327,* 1141-1142.

58. Tanvetyanon, T., & Choudhury, A.M. (2004). Hypocalcemia and azotemia associated with zoledronic acid and interferon alfa. *The Annals of Pharmacotherapy, 38,* 418-421.

59. Turchin, A., Seifter, J.L., & Seely, E.W. (2003). Mind the gap. *New England Journal of Medicine, 349*(15), 1465-1469.

60. Uphold, C.R., & Graham, M.V. (2003). *Clinical guidelines in family practice* (4th ed.). Gainesville, Fla: Barmarrae Books.

61. Vereckei, A. (2003). Inferior wall pseudoinfarction pattern due to hyperkalemia. *Pacing Clinical Electrophysiology, 26,* 2181-2184.

62. Vilches, A., & Suman, A. (2004). Awareness of over-the-counter drug use by elderly patients. A hospital-based questionnaire survey. *Age Aging, 33*(2), 205-206.

63. Vivien, B., et al. (2005). Early hypocalcemia in severe trauma. *Critical Care Medicine, 33*(9), 1946-1952.

64. Vuckovic, K. (2004). Bradycardia induced by hyperkalemia. *AAOHN Journal, 52*(5), 186-187.

65. Wilbanks, B.A., et al. (2005). Hyperkalemia-induced residual neuromuscular blockade: A case report. *AANA Journal, 73*(6).

66. Woodman, A.M., Douglas, J.F., & Jefferson, J.A. (2004). Recurrent hyperkalemia cured by amputation. *The Lancet, 364,* 908.

67. Yamamoto, L., & Texas, V. (2004). Guillain-Barré syndrome vs electrolyte imbalances. *Topics in Emergency Medicine, 26*(3), 186-200.

68. .Yucha, C., & Guthrie, D. (2003). Renal homeostasis and calcium. *Nephrology Nursing Journal, 30*(6), 621-628.

69. Zembrzuski, C. (2000). Nutrition and hydration. *Journal of Gerontological Nursing, 26*(12), 6-7.

70. Zimmers, T., & Patel, H. (2003). Cases in electrocardiography. *American Journal of Emergency Medicine, 21*(6), 503-505.

evolve **Did you remember to check out the bonus material on the Evolve website and the CD-ROM, including NCLEX®-Examination Style Review Questions, Open-Book Quizzes, and Chapter Review Audio Podcasts?**

http://evolve.elsevier.com/Black/medsurg

CHAPTER 13

Acid-Base Balance

SUSAN A. SANDSTROM

Normal function of body cells depends on regulation of the hydrogen ion (H^+) concentration within very narrow limits. If H^+ levels exceed these normal limits, acid-base imbalances result and are recognized clinically as abnormalities of serum pH. Acid-base imbalances may be caused by disorders of any body system and are seen in the increasing numbers of acutely ill clients in clinical settings. They are frequently diagnosed with arterial blood gas results along with other diagnostic tests and the clinical manifestations of the client's illness. Nurses and other health care professionals are responsible for preventing, detecting, and intervening in acid-base imbalances.

REGULATION OF ACID-BASE BALANCE

The symbol *pH* refers to the negative logarithm of the H^+ concentration. It is used to express the acidity or alkalinity of a solution. A pH of 7.0 is *neutral,* having an equal number of acids and bases. An *acidic* solution has a pH less than 7.0, and an *alkaline* solution has a pH greater than 7.0. Because pH is a *negative* log (indicating a reciprocal relationship), a rise in pH reflects a drop in H^+. Conversely, a decline in pH indicates an increase in H^+. Normal serum pH is 7.35 to 7.45. The function of cellular proteins is seriously impaired when pH falls to 7.2 or less or rises to 7.55 or higher. Rapid rates of change in pH are especially detrimental.

Three physiologic systems act interdependently to maintain a normal serum pH:

Chemical buffering of excess acid or base by buffer systems in the blood plasma and in cells

Excretion of acid by the lungs

Excretion of acid or regeneration of base by the kidneys

MODULATION OF SERUM pH BY BUFFER SYSTEMS

A buffer system consists of a weak acid (one that does not readily release H^+ into solution) and a salt of a base. For example, carbonic acid (H_2CO_3), a weak acid, and sodium bicarbonate ($NaHCO_3$), the salt of a base with which H^+ can combine, make up the clinically important bicarbonate buffer in the blood. The organic acids formed during cellular energy metabolism are strong acids; that is, they readily contribute free H^+ to body fluids, potentially producing large alterations in pH. The pH of buffered solutions tends to remain fairly stable despite the addition of strong acids or bases because buffer system components combine with added acids or bases to convert them to weaker forms. Because only free H^+ contributes to pH, changes in pH are minimized. Examples of buffering reactions are presented next.

Strong acid buffered:

$$HCl + (H_2CO_3/NaHCO_3) \rightarrow H_2CO_3 + NaCl$$

where HCl is hydrochloric acid and NaCl is sodium chloride.

Strong base buffered:

$$NaOH + (H_2CO_3/NaHCO_3) \rightarrow NaHCO_3 + H_2O$$
$$\text{where NaOH is sodium hydroxide}$$

Several buffer systems are present in the blood, both within red blood cells (RBCs) and in the plasma. The numerous negative charges on proteins permit the

evolve **Web Enhancements**

Appendix A Religious Beliefs and Practices Affecting Health Care

Be sure to check out the bonus material on the Evolve website and the CD-ROM, including free self-assessment exercises. **http://evolve.elsevier. com/Black/medsurg**

binding of large quantities of H^+ cations. Accordingly, proteins such as hemoglobin in RBCs and albumin in the plasma are quantitatively (judged according to amount) the most important blood buffers. Negatively charged ions, such as phosphate within body cells and carbonate within bones, are important intracellular buffers.

In clinical settings, however, the bicarbonate buffer is monitored because of its accessibility within the plasma as well as its physiologic importance as an *open* buffer system. In an open buffer system, the end products of acid-buffering reactions are continuously eliminated from the body by the lungs and kidneys, allowing these reactions to continue without being slowed by the accumulation of end products. When bases must be buffered, the carbon dioxide (CO_2) consumed by carbonic acid formation is readily replenished by normal metabolism. Furthermore, the *dissociation constant* (pK_a) of this system is ideal for buffering fluids such as plasma, in which the addition of acids is more prevalent than the addition of bases. The dissociation constant (pK_a) of a buffer is the pH at which half its components are in the acid form and half are in the base form. At normal serum pH, the bicarbonate buffer has about 90% of its components in base form.

Because all intracellular and extracellular buffer systems operate interdependently, the status of the bicarbonate buffer is representative of acid-base homeostasis within the body as a whole. Buffer systems act instantly to minimize the impact of adding strong acids or bases to body fluids; thus these systems are the body's first line of defense against acid-base imbalance. Unlike the lungs and kidneys, however, buffers do not actually eliminate acid or base from the body.

REGULATION OF VOLATILE ACIDS BY THE LUNGS

Volatile acids are acids that can be converted to gases. During normal ventilation (breathing), the lungs exhale large quantities of "potential" acid in the form of CO_2 gas. CO_2 is continuously produced by body cells as an end product of complete oxidative metabolism of nutrients for energy. CO_2 diffuses from body cells into the blood, where it may combine with water to form H_2CO_3, which then dissociates, or separates, into its component ions: H^+ and HCO_3^- (bicarbonate). This *hydrolysis reaction*, which is reversible, is shown as follows:

$$H_2O + CO_2 \leftrightarrow H_2CO_3 \leftrightarrow HCO_3^- + H^+$$

It is apparent from this equation that CO_2 and H_2CO_3 are directly related. As serum CO_2 levels rise, H^+ production increases and pH falls, indicating increased acidity. Conversely, lower CO_2 levels are consistent with higher (more alkaline) pH values. The hydrolysis reaction

further demonstrates that some of the CO_2 entering the blood forms the base HCO_3^-. Although some hydrolysis occurs in the plasma, most takes place in the cytoplasm of RBCs, where the enzyme carbonic anhydrase (CA) catalyzes the reaction at much more rapid rates than in the plasma. The presence of CA in other cells, notably the renal tubular cells, is also important to acid-base homeostasis (discussed later in this chapter).

Figure 13-1, *A*, demonstrates the hydrolysis reaction at the tissue level. The *law of mass action* states that the rate of a chemical reaction is directly proportional to the molecular concentrations of the reacting substances. Consistent with this law, the rate and direction of the hydrolysis reaction are determined by (1) the addition of substrate or (2) the removal of end product. In the tissues, the addition of CO_2 to the blood by metabolizing cells drives hydrolysis in the forward direction, forming H^+ and HCO_3^-, mostly in the RBCs. The H^+ formed by hydrolysis is buffered by hemoglobin, thereby minimizing changes in the pH of the RBC cytoplasm. The HCO_3^- formed in RBCs diffuses out into the plasma, while the chloride anion (Cl^-) moves in to maintain electroneutrality. This anion countertransport is known as the *chloride shift*. HCO_3^- formed in this way accounts for the major portion (80%) of CO_2 transported in the blood. Small amounts are transported while dissolved in plasma (8%) or are combined with hemoglobin (as carbaminohemoglobin) or other proteins (12%). The amount of carbonic acid in the blood at any time is negligible (0.0006%).

In the lungs, CO_2 diffuses along its concentration gradient from the plasma to the alveoli, from which it is exhaled. Removal of CO_2 drives the hydrolysis reaction in reverse, as shown in Figure 13-1, *B*. In a reversal of the chloride shift, HCO_3^- reenters the RBCs, and Cl^- exits. HCO_3^- combines with H^+, which has been released from its buffers, regenerating CO_2 and H_2O.

REGULATION OF FIXED ACIDS AND BICARBONATE BY THE KIDNEYS

Acids that cannot be converted to gases must be eliminated in the urine. These *fixed acids* include the following:

- Sulfuric, phosphoric, and other acids produced by protein metabolism
- Ketones produced by lipid metabolism and potentially accumulating with accelerated lipid metabolism, as in diabetic ketoacidosis
- Lactic acid produced by carbohydrate metabolism and potentially accumulating with increased metabolic rates and with accelerated anaerobic glycolysis, as in shock and hypoxemia
- Occasionally, ingested toxins, such as salicylate (aspirin), drugs, and methanol

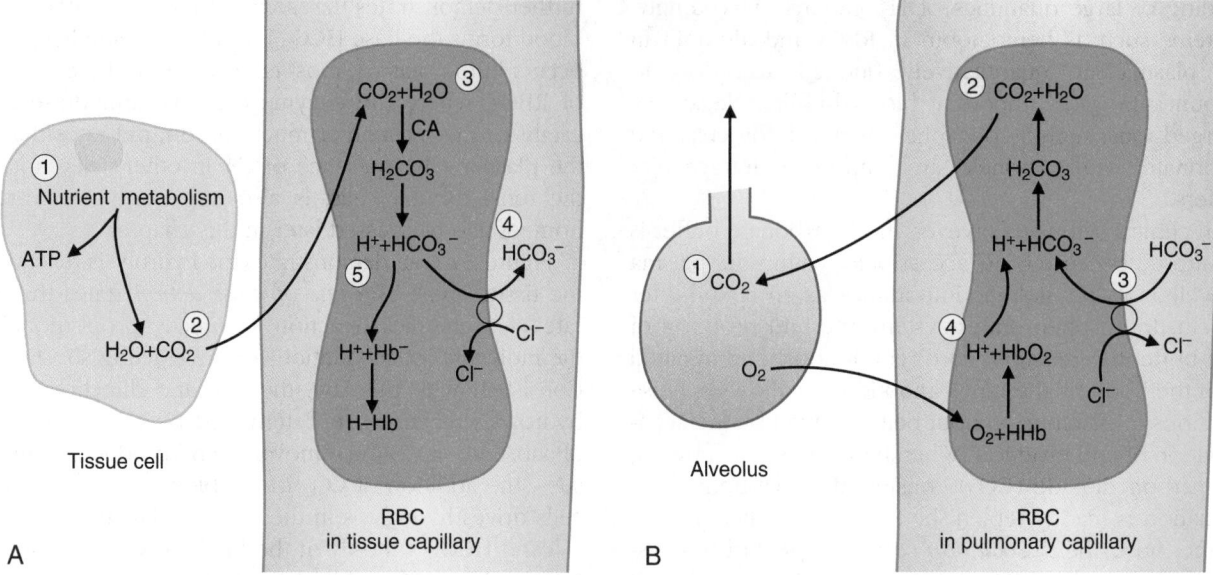

■ **FIGURE 13-1** Buffering volatile acids. **A,** Tissue level hydrolysis. *1,* Carbon dioxide (CO_2) is formed during cellular energy metabolism. *2,* CO_2 diffuses into plasma, and then into red blood cells. *3,* CO_2 enters hydrolysis catalyzed by carbonic anhydrase (CA), yielding hydrogen ion (H^+) and bicarbonate (HCO_3^-). *4,* HCO_3^- diffuses into plasma in exchange for Cl^- (chloride shift). *5,* H^+ is buffered by hemoglobin (Hb) and other intracellular buffers. *ATP,* Adenosine triphosphate; *RBC,* red blood cell. **B,** Reversal of hydrolysis in the lung. *1,* Carbon dioxide (CO_2) is exhaled, creating a gradient for diffusion of CO_2 from the blood to the alveolus. *2,* Removal of CO_2 drives reverse hydrolysis in the red blood cell (RBC). *3,* Bicarbonate (HCO_3^-) reenters the RBC in exchange for Cl^- (reverse chloride shift). *4,* Oxygen binding to hemoglobin (Hb) promotes H^+ release (reverse Haldane effect). *HHb,* Combined hydrogen/hemoglobin.

The kidneys regulate serum pH by secreting H^+ into the urine and by regenerating HCO_3^- for reabsorption into the blood. At the glomerulus, HCO_3^- is filtered from the blood into the proximal convoluted tubule. Because HCO_3^- is a large, charged particle, it is poorly reabsorbed. Any HCO_3^- filtered in excess of H^+ is excreted in the urine. H^+ is actively secreted into the renal tubules, primarily by proximal tubular cells, but also in the distal tubule and collecting duct. This system operates only until tubular pH falls to about 4.5. At lower pH values, significant amounts of H^+ leak from the tubular lumen back into the blood. Secretion of large amounts of H^+ into the renal tubules would result in a rapid fall in tubular pH and would inhibit further H^+ secretion if not for the presence of *urinary buffer systems.* These systems permit the tubular fluid to accept large quantities of H^+ while limiting how much the urinary pH decreases.

Urinary Buffer Systems

The three principal buffer systems in renal tubules are the bicarbonate, ammonia, and phosphate (titratable acid) systems.

In the *bicarbonate buffer* (Figure 13-2, *A*), H^+ is secreted into the tubular lumen by tubular cells in countertransport with sodium (Na^+). The combination of H^+ with filtered bicarbonate regenerates CO_2 in a reversal of the hydrolysis reaction. This CO_2 is reabsorbed into tubular cells, where hydrolysis proceeds efficiently

because of the presence of CA. The HCO_3^- formed is reabsorbed with sodium into the blood. Thus for every molecule of H^+ secreted, a molecule of HCO_3^- is returned to the blood to restore components of the plasma bicarbonate buffer system.

The *ammonia buffer* depends on the generation of ammonia (NH_3) from amino acids, such as glutamine, in renal tubular cells (Figure 13-2, *B*). NH_3 diffuses into the tubular lumen, where it may combine with secreted H^+ to form ammonium (NH_4^+), a large, charged particle that cannot be reabsorbed. H^+ in this form is thus trapped in the tubule. NH_4^+ is excreted in the urine in combination with Cl^- from NaCl. Na^+ is actively reabsorbed, along with tubular HCO_3^-.

The *phosphate buffer* operates similarly (Figure 13-2, *C*), resulting in the formation of weak acids that are excreted in the urine. Sodium and bicarbonate are reabsorbed.

Effects of Other Electrolytes

Although H^+ and HCO_3^- are critical determinants of acid-base balance, they are also electrolytes, subject to the *principle of electroneutrality,* which holds that total cations must equal total anions in any fluid compartment. Renal regulation of serum pH is greatly influenced by the concentrations of other electrolytes, particularly potassium (K^+), sodium (Na^+), calcium (Ca^{2+}), magnesium (Mg^{2+}), chloride (Cl^-), lactate, and protein (Pr^-).

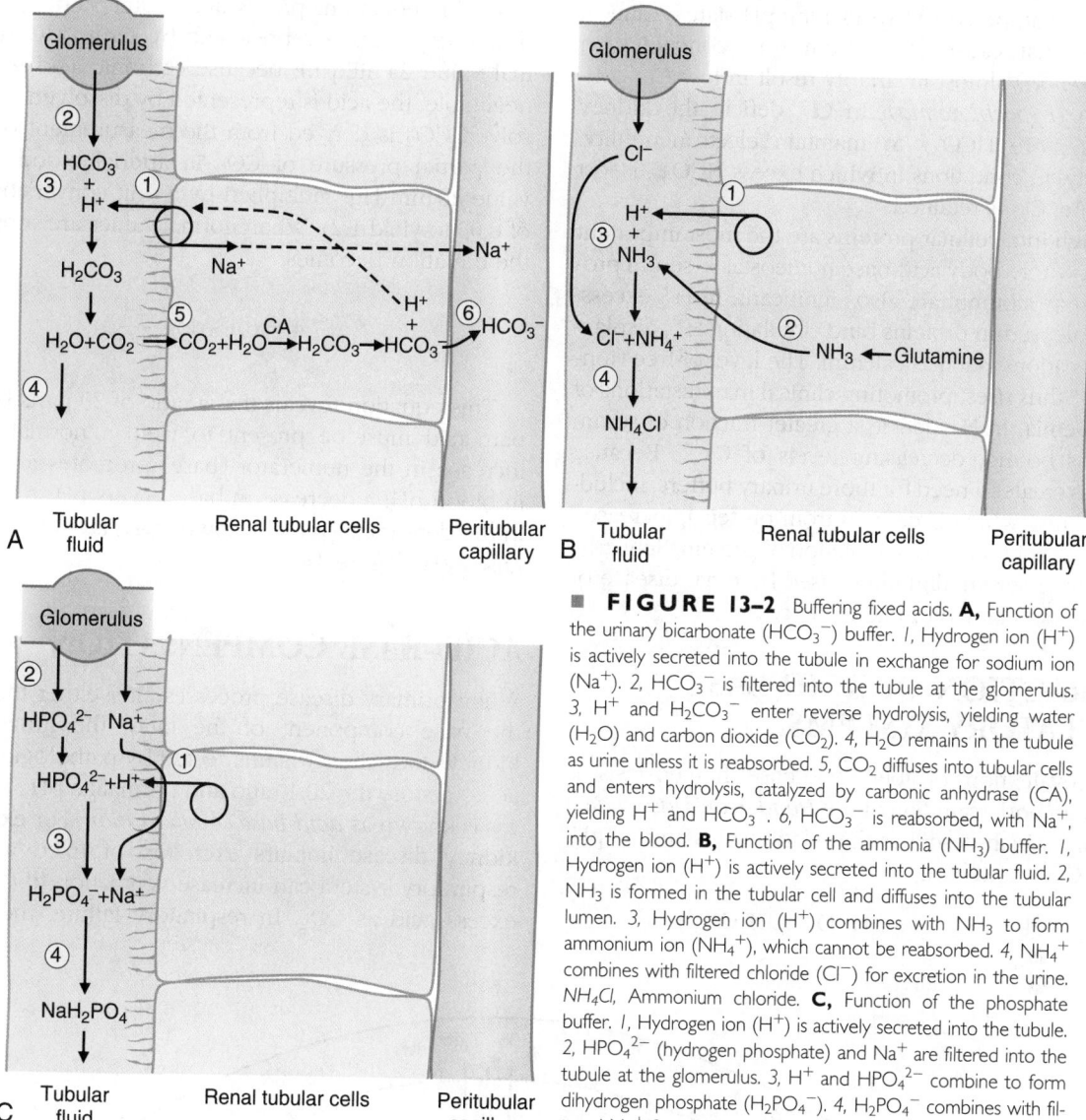

■ **FIGURE 13–2** Buffering fixed acids. **A,** Function of the urinary bicarbonate (HCO_3^-) buffer. 1, Hydrogen ion (H^+) is actively secreted into the tubule in exchange for sodium ion (Na^+). 2, HCO_3^- is filtered into the tubule at the glomerulus. 3, H^+ and $H_2CO_3^-$ enter reverse hydrolysis, yielding water (H_2O) and carbon dioxide (CO_2). 4, H_2O remains in the tubule as urine unless it is reabsorbed. 5, CO_2 diffuses into tubular cells and enters hydrolysis, catalyzed by carbonic anhydrase (CA), yielding H^+ and HCO_3^-. 6, HCO_3^- is reabsorbed, with Na^+, into the blood. **B,** Function of the ammonia (NH_3) buffer. 1, Hydrogen ion (H^+) is actively secreted into the tubular fluid. 2, NH_3 is formed in the tubular cell and diffuses into the tubular lumen. 3, Hydrogen ion (H^+) combines with NH_3 to form ammonium ion (NH_4^+), which cannot be reabsorbed. 4, NH_4^+ combines with filtered chloride (Cl^-) for excretion in the urine. *NH_4Cl,* Ammonium chloride. **C,** Function of the phosphate buffer. 1, Hydrogen ion (H^+) is actively secreted into the tubule. 2, HPO_4^{2-} (hydrogen phosphate) and Na^+ are filtered into the tubule at the glomerulus. 3, H^+ and HPO_4^{2-} combine to form dihydrogen phosphate ($H_2PO_4^-$). 4, $H_2PO_4^-$ combines with filtered Na^+ for excretion in the urine.

When serum potassium level is elevated (*hyperkalemia*), renal tubular cells secrete more K^+ but retain H^+ for electroneutrality. The opposite occurs in *hypokalemia,* which promotes renal secretion of H^+. Similarly, H^+ imbalance influences both renal regulation and cellular shifts in potassium. In cases of serum H^+ excess, renal tubular cells secrete more H^+, but K^+ is retained, promoting hyperkalemia. At the tissue level, H^+ moves into cells to be buffered by intracellular proteins, and K^+ moves out into the blood to maintain electroneutrality. This shift does not represent true K^+ excess but does contribute to clinical manifestations of hyperkalemia, which include potentially lethal cardiac dysrhythmias. Treatment of the H^+ excess causes a shift in the opposite direction, promoting hypokalemia. In response to a deficit in serum H^+, renal cells retain H^+ and secrete more K^+, and cellular proteins release H^+ to the extracellular fluid while K^+ shifts intracellularly.

Na^+ and Cl^- are of particular importance in maintaining fluid balance, and the kidney is the principal site of their regulation. Active reabsorption of Na^+ from the renal tubules creates gradients that drive the secretion of H^+ and the reabsorption of anions such as Cl^- and HCO_3^-.

The juxtaglomerular cells of the renal glomeruli sense a low extracellular volume, triggering the renin-angiotensin-aldosterone system. Release of the mineralocorticoid hormone aldosterone from the adrenal cortex stimulates renal reabsorption of Na^+ from the distal tubule and proximal collecting duct. Maintenance of electroneutrality requires concurrent increases in the secretion of H^+ and K^+ as well as reabsorption of HCO_3^-. The kidney's priority in such cases is to restore volume balance, but this happens at the cost of worsening pH status. Clinical conditions that cause low serum Na^+ concentration *(hyponatremia)* almost invariably result in low Cl^- concentration *(hypochloremia)*. In Cl^- deficit, the kidney reabsorbs more HCO_3^- to maintain electroneutrality. Conversely, in conditions in which excess HCO_3^- is lost in the urine, Cl^- is retained.

Although intracellular proteins are the most important buffers in whole-body acid-base homeostasis, serum proteins such as albumin are also significant. In H^+ excess, for example, serum proteins bind circulating H^+, displacing other cations, such as calcium. The level of free (ionized) Ca^{2+} thus rises, promoting clinical manifestations of hypercalcemia. In H^+ deficit, a greater fraction of serum calcium is bound, decreasing levels of Ca^{2+}. Because H^+ excess creates a need for more urinary buffers, including ammonia (which is derived from protein), increased buffering of acid promotes depletion of protein. Similarly, deficiency of serum albumin caused by renal disease or other disorders may promote H^+ excess.

INTERACTION OF ACID-BASE REGULATORY SYSTEMS

Clinical evaluation of total acid-base homeostasis is aided by an understanding of the *Henderson-Hasselbalch equation,*[3] which describes the relationships among pH, acid (H_2CO_3), and base (HCO_3^-):

$$pH = pK_a + \log([HCO_3^-]/[H_2CO_3])$$

In this equation, pK_a is a constant value (6.1). The base component is represented by serum HCO_3^- (normal value 24 mEq/L); because carbonic acid levels are negligible, the acid is represented by dissolved CO_2. Dissolved CO_2 is derived from the measurement of $Paco_2$, the partial pressure of CO_2 in arterial blood (normal value 40 mm Hg, multiplied by a unit conversion factor of 0.03 to yield 1.2). When normal values are substituted, the equation becomes:

$$7.4 = 6.1 + \log \frac{24}{1.2}$$

This equation reveals that a ratio of 20 parts base to 1 part acid must be present to yield a normal pH. An increase in the numerator (base) promotes an increase in blood pH; a decrease in base lowers pH. An increase in the denominator (acid) lowers pH; a decrease in acid raises pH (Figure 13-3).

ACID-BASE COMPENSATION

When primary disease processes alter either the acid or the base component of the ratio, the lungs or the kidneys (whichever is unaffected by pathologic change) act to restore the 20:1 ratio and normalize pH. This process is known as *acid-base compensation*. For example, if kidney disease impairs excretion of fixed acids, the respiratory system can increase ventilation to "blow off" excess acid as CO_2. In respiratory failure, the kidneys

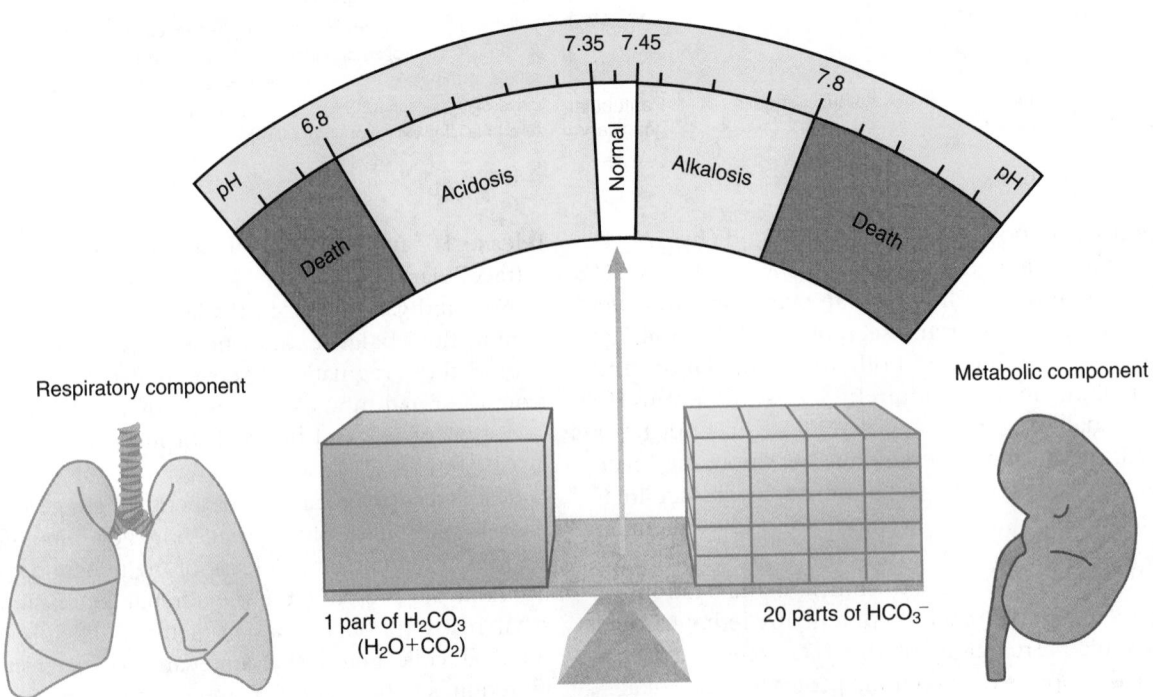

HENDERSON–HASSELBALCH RELATIONSHIP

■ **FIGURE 13-3** Regulation of acid-base balance. *CO_2*, Carbon dioxide; *HCO_3^-*, bicarbonate; *H_2CO_3*, carbonic acid; *H_2O*, water.

can compensate for retention of acid (CO_2) by secreting H^+ and regenerating HCO_3^-.

As stated, blood buffers act to modulate pH changes but do not eliminate acid or base from the body. The lungs or kidneys alter the actual amounts of acid and base, but regulation by these systems is not as fast. The lungs respond within minutes, but maximal compensation takes up to 24 hours. The kidneys may require up to 72 hours to achieve optimal compensation.

Except in mild, chronic respiratory alkalosis (see later discussion), compensation does not fully restore normal pH. Respiratory compensation is limited because reducing ventilation to compensate for a renal deficit of H^+ would eventually result in hypoxemia. Because hypoxemia is a respiratory stimulant, ventilation would again increase. Similarly, renal compensation for ventilatory disorders is potentially limited by many factors, including renal blood flow, tubular flow rates, and saturability of tubular transport processes.

ACID-BASE CORRECTION

Although compensatory responses for primary acid-base disorders may nearly restore the 20:1 ratio of base to acid, the actual amounts of acid and base remain abnormal. Thus compensation must be differentiated from *correction,* in which the ratio is restored and the absolute quantities of dissolved CO_2 (as derived from $Paco_2$) and HCO_3^- are returned to normal range. Correction occurs only with resolution of the underlying disorder.

ANALYSIS OF ARTERIAL BLOOD GASES

Arterial blood gases (ABGs) are obtained to determine oxygenation status and acid-base status. The partial pressure of oxygen (Pao_2), the percentage of hemoglobin saturated with oxygen or the oxygen saturation (Sao_2), and the partial pressure of CO_2 ($Paco_2$) directly monitor the oxygenation status. The parameters reported to monitor acid-base homeostasis are pH, $Paco_2$, and HCO_3^- concentration. The $Paco_2$ is the measure of carbon dioxide in the blood and is referred to as the respiratory component of ABGs. The HCO_3^- concentration is referred to as the metabolic or renal component of ABGs.

Current studies are comparing the accuracy of central venous blood gases and arterial blood gases.[14,15] The similarity between end-tidal partial pressure of carbon dioxide measured by capnography and arterial blood gas results is also being studied.[7] There are many systems used to interpret ABG results.[2,17,18,22,23] One method, shown in the Critical Monitoring box at right, illustrates how these values may be used to (1) determine the presence and type of acid-base imbalance and (2) evaluate the level of compensation.

CRITICAL MONITORING

Analysis of Arterial Blood Gases

STEP 1: CLASSIFY THE pH
- Normal: 7.35-7.45
- Acidemia: <7.35
- Alkalemia: >7.45

STEP 2: ASSESS $Paco_2$
- Normal: 35-45 mm Hg
- Respiratory acidosis: >45 mm Hg
- Respiratory alkalosis: <35 mm Hg

STEP 3: ASSESS HCO_3^-*
- Normal: 22-26 mEq/L
- Metabolic acidosis: <22 mEq/L
- Metabolic alkalosis: >26 mEq/L

STEP 4: DETERMINE PRESENCE OF COMPENSATION
- Compensation present: $Paco_2$ and HCO_3^- are abnormal (or nearly so) in opposite directions; that is, one is acidotic and the other alkalotic.[†]
- Compensation absent: One component ($Paco_2$ or HCO_3^-) is abnormal, the other normal. The problem is likely acute.

STEP 5: IDENTIFY PRIMARY DISORDER, IF POSSIBLE
- If pH is clearly abnormal: The acid-base component most consistent with the pH disturbance is the primary disorder.
- If pH is normal or near-normal: The more deviant component is probably primary.[‡] Also, note whether pH is on acidotic or alkalotic side of 7.4. The more deviant component should be consistent with this pH.

STEP 6: CLASSIFY DEGREE OF COMPENSATION, IF PRESENT
The limits of complete compensation are as follows:
- *Metabolic acidosis:* The decrease in $Paco_2$ is approximately equal to the last two digits of the pH.
- *Metabolic alkalosis:* The $Paco_2$ is approximately equal to 0.6 times the increase in HCO_3^- level.
- *Respiratory acidosis:* For every 10 mm Hg increase in $Paco_2$, the HCO_3^- level is increased by 1 mEq/L (in acute acidosis) or 4 mEq/L (in chronic acidosis).
- *Respiratory alkalosis:* For every 10 mm Hg decrease in $Paco_2$, the HCO_3^- level is decreased by 2 mEq/L (in acute alkalosis) or 5 mEq/L (in chronic alkalosis).

"Compensation" beyond these limits suggests the presence of a complex disorder.

*Base excess (BE) is also reported with arterial blood gas (ABG) values and is a second index of metabolic status. Normal BE is −2 to +2. Because fluctuation in BE parallels that of bicarbonate concentration, it is not usually necessary to classify both.
†It is possible, but less likely, that two or more opposing primary imbalances (i.e., a complex disorder) are present, resulting in the appearance of compensation. The detection of complex disorders is facilitated by the use of an acid-base map (see Figure 13-4) and by the use of the "formulas" described in step 6, but a complex disorder cannot always be differentiated from compensation on the basis of laboratory values.
‡It is unlikely that the more deviant component represents compensation, because except in rare cases the body does not overcompensate for imbalance. When pH approaches the normal range, compensatory mechanisms are no longer triggered.

DISORDERS OF ACID-BASE BALANCE

The four general classes of acid-base imbalance are (1) respiratory acidosis, (2) respiratory alkalosis, (3) metabolic acidosis, and (4) metabolic alkalosis. These disorders are not clinical diagnoses or diseases in themselves; rather, they are clinical syndromes associated with a wide variety of diseases.

Acidosis refers to any pathologic process that causes a relative excess of acid (volatile or fixed) in the body. *Acidemia* is excess acid in the blood. The presence of acidemia does not necessarily confirm an underlying pathologic process; technically, it is merely a laboratory finding.

The same distinction may be made between the terms alkalosis and alkalemia. *Alkalosis* indicates a primary condition resulting in excess base in the body, and *alkalemia* refers more narrowly to elevation of serum pH. Care must be taken not to confuse these terms conceptually, and they must not be used interchangeably in clinical practice.

RESPIRATORY ALKALOSIS

Respiratory alkalosis is a state of relative excess of base in body fluids resulting from increased respiratory elimination of CO_2. *Acute* respiratory alkalosis lasts for 24 hours or less; *chronic* respiratory alkalosis persists longer.

Etiology and Risk Factors

Respiratory alkalosis is caused by alveolar hyperventilation, in which excess CO_2 is eliminated. The most common cause of respiratory alkalosis is hypoxemia from such pulmonary disorders as pneumonia, pulmonary embolism, asthma, adult respiratory distress syndrome (ARDS), pulmonary edema, and cystic fibrosis—all which lead to shortness of breath. Transient respiratory alkalosis may also occur secondary to acute anxiety or pain or as a response to respiratory stimulant drugs such as epinephrine and salicylates. Neural disorders, such as stroke and intracranial lesions, may stimulate the central respiratory drive.

The most common causes of mild, chronic respiratory alkalosis are residence in high altitudes and pregnancy. Pulmonary fibrosis and other disorders that limit ventilatory volume result in an increased ventilatory rate, with a possible net excess of CO_2 elimination.

Pathophysiology

A low partial pressure of oxygen in arterial blood (Pa_{O_2}) is sensed by peripheral chemoreceptors in the carotid bodies and aortic arch. The rate of firing by these receptors then increases, stimulating the respiratory center in the medulla, which increases the rate and depth of ventilation. Peripheral chemoreceptors are also stimulated in states of low blood flow, such as shock.

Conditions that physically impede expansion of the lungs (such as pulmonary fibrosis) stimulate activation of the respiratory center via the Hering-Breuer, or stretch reflex. The J receptors, located in the alveolar-capillary membrane, are thought to stimulate increased ventilation in disorders such as ARDS, which causes thickening of this membrane.

The central chemoreceptors and respiratory center may be stimulated excessively by chemicals or toxins. In the case of salicylate overdose, it is interesting that adults usually exhibit respiratory alkalosis and that children more often have metabolic acidosis from the acid ingestion. The reason for this difference between children and adults is unknown. In severe alkalemia, changes in the ionization of structural and regulatory proteins result in widespread organ dysfunction. Cellular shifts and increased binding of Ca^{2+} to serum proteins induce electrolyte imbalance.

The buffering response in acute respiratory alkalosis results from (1) shifting of acid from intracellular fluid into the blood and (2) movement of HCO_3^- into cells in exchange for Cl^-. An adaptive increase in lactic acid production occurs secondary to stimulation of glycolysis. Renal compensation in chronic respiratory alkalosis involves decreased H^+ secretion as well as excretion of excess filtered HCO_3^-.

Clinical Manifestations

Manifestations of respiratory alkalosis in a client's ABG analysis include a high pH and a low Pa_{CO_2}. HCO_3^- levels fall with compensation in chronic respiratory alkalosis, and serum lactate dehydrogenase levels are often elevated. Compensated chronic respiratory alkalosis is the only acid-base imbalance in which serum pH may be returned to within normal limits despite persistence of the initiating cause. Hyperventilation, the underlying cause, is clinically apparent.

Central nervous system manifestations of altered blood flow and neurotransmission are usually predominant. They include paresthesias, lightheadedness, and confusion. Musculoskeletal and cardiac manifestations of hypokalemia and hypocalcemia (such as dysrhythmias and muscle weakness) may be present. Chest pain may occur secondarily to coronary artery spasm but is more often noncardiac in origin. Acute, but not chronic, respiratory alkalosis may cause gastrointestinal manifestations such as nausea, vomiting, and diarrhea attributable to sympathetic nervous system effects. Rarely seizures may occur if the alkalosis is severe or untreated.

Treatment of the Underlying Disorder

Treatment of mild, chronic respiratory alkalosis is usually not warranted because it produces little risk and few symptoms. Aggressive treatment of the underlying causes of hypoxemia is essential in cases of severe respiratory alkalosis. Electrolyte imbalances usually resolve with treatment of the underlying cause.

Respiratory Support

Oxygen therapy may be used to correct underlying hypoxemia. Rebreathing of CO_2 (as from breathing into a paper bag or other closed system) provides prompt but short-term relief in anxiety-related respiratory alkalosis.

RESPIRATORY ACIDOSIS

Respiratory acidosis is a state of relative excess of acid in body fluids resulting from retention or excessive production of CO_2. *Acute* respiratory acidosis develops and resolves within 3 days or less; *chronic* respiratory acidosis persists over a longer period.

Etiology and Risk Factors

Respiratory acidosis nearly always results from hypoventilation. Chronic respiratory acidosis is most commonly caused by chronic obstructive pulmonary disease (COPD). In end-stage COPD, pathologic changes lead to airway collapse, air trapping, and disturbance of ventilation-perfusion (V/Q) relationships. Acute respiratory acidosis also occurs when respiratory tract infection or concurrent cardiac disease increases the work of breathing. Hypoventilation with resulting respiratory acidosis is seen in diseases of the neuromuscular junction in which diaphragmatic movement is impaired (such as Guillain-Barré syndrome) and in depression of the medullary respiratory center by drugs or lesions of the central nervous system. Obesity hypoventilation syndrome, excessive fatigue or weakness, or severe deformities of the spine and rib cage muscles may also lead to respiratory acidosis.

Respiratory acidosis may occur iatrogenically (as a result of treatment) from inadequate mechanical ventilation or from excessive oxygen administration to clients with chronic CO_2 retention (as in COPD). In the latter case, hypoventilation results from the following:

- **Depression of the medullary respiratory center with removal of the hypoxemic stimulus**
- **Worsening of V/Q relationships secondary to replacement of airway nitrogen (which helps keep airways open) with oxygen**

Normally, the most important stimulus for ventilation is an increase in the acidity of cerebrospinal fluid (CSF) resulting from diffusion of CO_2 into the CSF from the blood; however, the higher level of HCO_3^- resulting from renal compensation for chronic respiratory acidosis minimizes the effect of increasing Pa_{CO_2} in these clients. Oxygen therapy may worsen V/Q relationships because it displaces nitrogen, a much less soluble gas, in alveoli. As oxygen is absorbed, alveoli may collapse, contributing to hypoventilation.

The second, much less common cause of respiratory acidosis is excessive CO_2 production from hypermetabolism or from excessive metabolism of carbohydrate fuels for energy. Clinical use of enteral feedings or parenteral nutrition formulas that are disproportionately high in carbohydrate may contribute to elevated Pa_{CO_2} levels, particularly in clients who also have impaired ventilation.

Pathophysiology

CO_2 accumulates in the blood and diffuses readily into all body compartments. This *hypercapnia* drives the hydrolysis reaction forward, generating carbonic acid that dissociates into H^+ and HCO_3^-. Immediate buffering by non-bicarbonate buffers occurs. Renal compensation proceeds over 3 to 5 days, with greater secretion of H^+ and regeneration of bicarbonate. Renal ammonia production increases, enhancing the function of the ammonia urinary buffer but depleting protein stores. As serum HCO_3^- levels rise with compensation, Cl^- is excreted in greater amounts, potentially inducing hypochloremia in chronic respiratory acidosis. Renal retention of K^+ and cellular cation shifts may lead to hyperkalemia. Displacement of Ca^{2+} from albumin may result in hypercalcemia.

In acute respiratory acidosis, the rapid rise in Pa_{CO_2} results in hypoxemia in clients who are breathing room air because retained CO_2 displaces oxygen in alveoli. Hypoxemia poses a more serious threat to life than either acidemia or hypercapnia in severe acute respiratory acidosis. Acidemia alters the ionization of structural and regulatory proteins (enzymes, for example), resulting in widespread manifestations of organ dysfunction.

Clinical Manifestations

An arterial blood sample that has a low pH signifies that the client has acidemia, and a high Pa_{CO_2} signifies hypercapnia. The client probably exhibits hypoventilation, the usual underlying cause of respiratory acidosis; manifestations of hypoxemia (confusion, irritability, or lethargy) may be present in severe cases. HCO_3^- levels are normal or, if renal compensation is occurring, elevated. Compensation is present to a greater extent in chronic respiratory acidosis than in acute respiratory acidosis.

Clinical manifestations of organ system dysfunction from acidemia include hypotension and cardiac dysrhythmias caused by decreased vascular tone, decreased myocardial contractility, and manifestations of electrolyte imbalance. Altered cerebral blood flow and depressed neurotransmission in acute respiratory acidosis may manifest as tremors, seizures, lethargy, stupor, and ultimately coma (hypercapnic encephalopathy). Because of compensation, clients with chronic hypercapnia have fewer dramatic manifestations and little alteration of cerebral blood flow.

OUTCOME MANAGEMENT

Treatment of the Underlying Disorder

Treatment of respiratory acidosis is focused primarily on resolving the underlying disorder. For example, an antibiotic may be given to treat pneumonia, an opioid antagonist to treat a drug overdose, or dialysis to clear toxins from the blood. Electrolyte imbalances usually resolve with such treatment; however, life-threatening hyperkalemia may require emergency treatment with dialysis or cation-exchange resins.

Respiratory Support

Mechanical ventilation and supplemental oxygen are often employed in conditions that cause respiratory acidosis. Currently, the trend is to use ventilation at lower tidal volumes than would be required to restore $Paco_2$ completely to the normal range. This *permissive hypercapnia* results in fewer airway injuries but comparable clinical outcomes; however, because the client's own ventilatory drive exceeds that provided by the ventilator, sedation is usually required. Oxygen therapy must be administered cautiously (at low flow rates or low percentages) to the client with chronic CO_2 retention to minimize the risk of worsening the client's respiratory status via nitrogen washout and blunting of the ventilatory drive. Noninvasive ventilatory support versus invasive mechanical ventilation is being studied. Some advantages have been seen in the treatment of chronic obstructive pulmonary disease clients with acute respiratory failure.[19]

Administration of Exogenous Alkali

If the client has adequate renal function, administration of base (typically, sodium bicarbonate) to correct the pH partially is not warranted. Such treatment may actually worsen the client's condition because bicarbonate further raises CO_2 levels by driving reverse hydrolysis. An exception may be made if the client has severe bronchospasm because alkalinization may restore the responsiveness of the airways to beta-agonist drugs.

METABOLIC ALKALOSIS

Metabolic alkalosis is a state of relative excess of base (or H^+ deficit) in body fluids resulting from a gain of bicarbonate or a loss of fixed acids.

Etiology and Risk Factors

Metabolic alkalosis develops through a two-phase mechanism. In the *generation phase,* the imbalance is first created by (1) loss of acid (as with HCl loss during vomiting or long-term gastric suctioning) or gain of base (as with administration of $NaHCO_3$) or (2) loss of fluids containing more Cl^- than HCO_3^- (as with overuse of loop or thiazide diuretics). Metabolic alkalosis associated with fluid volume loss is referred to as *contraction alkalosis.* Another common type, *posthypercapnic metabolic alkalosis,* results from too-rapid correction of chronic respiratory acidosis, in which case a compensatory increase in HCO_3^- then persists as a primary disorder.

In the *maintenance phase,* alkalosis persists because renal excretion of HCO_3^-, which would otherwise correct the disorder, is impaired. This impairment may result from hypovolemia in contraction alkalosis or, much less commonly, from aldosterone excess. In hypovolemia, greater Na^+ reabsorption by the distal tubule (stimulated by the renin-angiotensin-aldosterone system) increases both H^+ secretion and HCO_3^- regeneration. In primary aldosteronism (or with prolonged or high-dose corticosteroid administration, in which aldosterone-like effects also arise), the hormone stimulates increased Na^+ reabsorption by the same distal tubular transport mechanism.

Metabolic alkalosis from fluid loss is referred to as *saline sensitive* because restoration of volume with fluid containing NaCl permits the kidneys to restore acid-base homeostasis. Alkalosis in cases of aldosterone excess is not correctable with administration of a saline solution and so is termed *saline resistant.*

Overcorrection of acidosis with $NaHCO_3$ may cause alkalosis, as can massive transfusion of whole blood. The citrate anticoagulant used for storing blood is metabolized to bicarbonate. Packed RBCs contain much less citrate; thus their use in multiple transfusion is preferred.

Loss of gastric fluid via nasogastric suction or vomiting further contributes to metabolic alkalosis because of loss of HCl. Additional HCl must be produced by gastric cells via the hydrolysis reaction. H^+ is secreted into the stomach with Cl^-; the HCO_3^- produced during the reaction is reabsorbed into the blood.

Pathophysiology

Respiratory compensation for metabolic alkalosis is limited by the hypoxemia that quickly develops with hypoventilation. Most buffering occurs in the extracellular fluid, where the buffers are much less effective for base loads than for acid loads. Severe alkalemia leads to widespread organ dysfunction because of altered ionization of body proteins as well as enhanced Ca^{2+} binding to serum proteins. Neurologic and cardiovascular systems are primarily affected. Hypokalemia, which occurs from cellular shifts and renal or intestinal losses, is more prominent in metabolic alkalosis than in respiratory alkalosis.

Clinical Manifestations

Metabolic alkalosis is manifested in ABG values by a high pH and a high HCO_3^- level. $Paco_2$ rises with compensation. Adaptive hypoventilation may be apparent and may induce some hypoxemia. Manifestations of volume deficit are often present in association with the underlying disorder. Hypokalemia and hypomagnesemia may manifest as cardiac dysrhythmias. Central nervous system manifestations include lethargy, confusion, and seizures.

OUTCOME MANAGEMENT

Treatment of the Underlying Disorder

Prompt treatment of the underlying disease process is the primary approach. Replacement of lost fluids and electrolytes (potassium and magnesium) and support of renal function (possibly with dialysis against a high-chloride, low-bicarbonate dialysate) are often the mainstays of therapy.

Administration of Acetazolamide

Acetazolamide (Diamox) is a diuretic that inhibits CA and promotes loss of bicarbonate in the urine. Losses of potassium and phosphate are also greater with the use of acetazolamide, however, and may lead to manifestations of electrolyte imbalance.

Administration of Exogenous Acid

In severe alkalemia, the intravenous administration of acid (HCl) or HCl precursors (ammonium chloride or arginine monohydrochloride) may be warranted to enhance physiologic compensation. Risks of acid infusion are substantial, however; they include local tissue injury (sclerosis of veins or extravasation), hypervolemia, hyperosmolar imbalance (with HCl precursors), increased ammonia levels (with ammonium chloride), and hyperkalemia (with arginine monohydrochloride).

METABOLIC ACIDOSIS

Metabolic acidosis is a state of relative acid excess (or base deficit) in body fluids resulting from a gain of fixed acids or a loss of bicarbonate.

Etiology and Risk Factors

Metabolic acidosis may result from either of two mechanisms: accumulation of fixed acid or loss of base. These mechanisms often can be differentiated clinically by the presence or absence of a high *anion gap*. Normally, the anion gap is 12 ± 4 mEq/L.[16] It is calculated by subtracting the sum of the serum concentrations of the major anions, bicarbonate and chloride, from the serum concentration of sodium. The difference, or "gap," represents anions in the serum other than HCO_3^- and Cl^-, such as lactate, phosphate, sulfates, organic ions, and proteins.

When acidosis results from addition of organic acid (as in lactic acidosis), bicarbonate is consumed in buffering but is not lost from the body. When the bicarbonate level decreases, the anion gap increases, and as the level of albumin increases to buffer most of the acid load, the anion gap also increases. Common causes of *high anion gap acidosis* include the following:

- Lactic acidosis, a consequence of an increase in anaerobic carbohydrate metabolism
- Diabetic ketoacidosis, in which ketone bodies accumulate because of accelerated lipid metabolism in the absence of insulin
- Azotemic renal failure, in which acid end products of protein metabolism (phosphate, sulfates etc.) cannot be effectively excreted because of impaired glomerular filtration
- Ingestion of toxins with acid metabolites (less common)

Non–anion gap acidosis caused by loss of base is also called *hyperchloremic metabolic acidosis*. In this case, the kidneys retain chloride when excess bicarbonate is lost from the body, and the anion gap remains normal. Excess bicarbonate may be lost through either the kidneys or the intestinal tract. In renal tubular acidosis, the renal tubular cells cannot reabsorb bicarbonate, which therefore is lost in the urine. Intestinal secretions, high in bicarbonate, may be lost through enteric drainage tubes (such as an ileostomy tube) or diarrhea. Drugs that inhibit CA, such as acetazolamide, interfere with bicarbonate regeneration during urinary buffering. Critically ill clients who receive very aggressive fluid volume replacement with normal saline or other bicarbonate-free solution may develop a relative bicarbonate deficiency caused by dilution of extracellular fluids. In non–anion gap acidosis caused by a gain of mineral acid (such as HCl), chloride is ingested with the acid, and bicarbonate is excreted proportionately.

Pathophysiology

Metabolic acidosis is accompanied by a compensatory increase in ventilation. Severe acidemia induces insulin resistance and depresses glycolytic enzymes, resulting in impairment of energy metabolism. The function of regulatory and structural proteins is impaired by altered ionization, leading to widespread organ dysfunction. Increased protein catabolism also occurs. Hyperkalemia occurs because K^+ shifts out of cells as excess H^+ enters. Insulin deficiency in diabetic ketoacidosis may worsen hyperkalemia because insulin normally promotes cellular uptake of K^+ along with glucose. Uptake of lactic acid by the liver is reduced, whereas hepatic lactate production is increased.

In metabolic acidosis caused by a gain of organic acids, buffering rapidly depletes bicarbonate stores. If renal function is not impaired, renal regeneration of HCO_3^- occurs with excretion of H^+; however, this response takes several days.

Clinical Manifestations

 Metabolic acidosis is apparent in ABG values as a low pH and a low HCO_3^- level. $Paco_2$ drops as respiratory compensation occurs. Systemic manifestations of acidemia resulting from altered protein function and electrolyte imbalance are similar to those of respiratory acidosis except that compensatory hyperventilation is present. Inability to correct metabolic acidosis with hyperventilation is related to an increased occurrence of respiratory failure and the need for mechanical ventilation.[8]

OUTCOME MANAGEMENT

Treatment of the Underlying Disorder

Aggressive intervention aimed at resolving the underlying disorder is the primary form of treatment and usually involves restoration of normal tissue oxygenation and perfusion. Electrolyte imbalance is treated only if it is life-threatening because it normally resolves with correction of the underlying disorder.

Respiratory Support

Assisted mechanical ventilation may be indicated for clients whose ability to hyperventilate in compensation is limited.

Administration of Exogenous Alkali

There is controversy related to the use of exogenous alkali to treat metabolic acidosis. In metabolic acidosis associated with hyperkalemia or with toxin ingestion, administration of intravenous sodium bicarbonate or other alkalinizing substances may be warranted to minimize the detrimental effects of the acidosis until the underlying disorder is resolved or until physiologic compensation is effective. In the more common types, lactic acidosis and ketoacidosis, no evidence exists that alkali administration is beneficial. Fluid overload, hyperosmolar imbalance, and alkalosis attributable to excessive treatment are risks of this approach. As previously mentioned, administration of sodium bicarbonate results in increased CO_2 levels, which may be detrimental in clients with respiratory disease or advanced cardiac failure. Alternative alkalinizing agents, such as tromethamine (THAM), produce less CO_2 but have not proved more effective than $NaHCO_3$ for the treatment of severe acidemia.

COMPLEX ACID-BASE DISORDERS

Mixed acid-base disorders, in which two primary acid-base imbalances coexist, are common, especially in those clients in critical care units. In cardiac arrest, for example, lactic acid quickly accumulates as a result of anaerobic metabolism; the carbonic acid level is elevated because of respiratory arrest. In COPD, underlying respiratory acidosis may be complicated by metabolic alkalosis secondary to diuretic or steroid therapy.

A *triple acid-base disorder* is present when metabolic acidosis and metabolic alkalosis coexist with either respiratory acidosis or respiratory alkalosis. (The two respiratory imbalances cannot coexist because they have opposite effects on ventilation.) As an example of a triple disorder, imbalances caused by ingestion of methanol (an exogenous toxin that produces metabolic acidosis), vomiting (which produces metabolic alkalosis), and respiratory arrest from aspiration (which produces respiratory acidosis) may occur simultaneously.

A complex acid-base disorder should be suspected when a client's $Paco_2$ value and HCO_3^- level do not correlate with pH or when ABG evidence of compensation exceeds predicted levels (see the Critical Monitoring box on p. 179). Use of an acid-base map may also facilitate detection (Figure 13-4). If the plotted ABG values converge at a point outside the usual range for a primary imbalance, a complex disorder is likely.

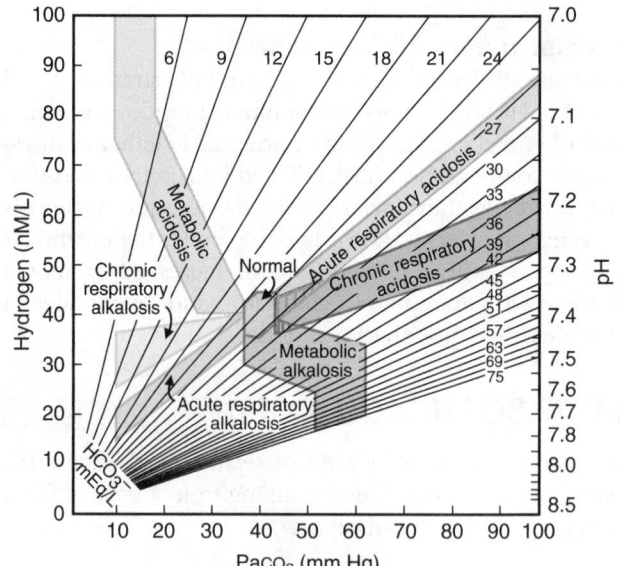

■ **FIGURE 13-4** An acid-base map. To use the acid-base map, plot the pH on the vertical axis and the partial pressure of arterial carbon dioxide ($Paco_2$) on the horizontal axis. Note the point at which the values intersect. If the result falls outside the normal area or the 95% confidence bands for the major primary disorders, the client probably has a complex acid-base imbalance; however, a point falling within one of the bands does not rule out a complex disorder. HCO_3^-, Bicarbonate.

CRITICAL MONITORING

Acid-Base Imbalances

	Respiratory Acidosis	Metabolic Acidosis	Respiratory Alkalosis	Metabolic Alkalosis
Defining Signs	Hypoventilation	Hyperventilation (Kussmaul's respirations, or air hunger)	Hyperventilation	Increasing HCO_3^- value
	Increasing $Paco_2$	Decreasing HCO_3^- value	Decreasing $Paco_2$	Increasing pH
	Decreasing pH	Decreasing pH	Increasing pH	Hypoventilation
Commonly Seen	Dyspnea	Hyperkalemia	Confusion	Confusion
	Hypercalcemia	Increasing serum Cl^- level and anion gap	Hypocalcemia	Decreasing level of consciousness
	Hyperkalemia	Stress response followed by lethargy	Hypokalemia	Hypocalcemia
	Hypochloremia	Dyspnea	Lightheadedness	Hypochloremia
	Hypernatremia			Hypokalemia
	Anxiety			Hypomagnesemia
	Confusion			Hypovolemia
				Numbness and tingling of limbs
Signs of Severe Imbalance	Hypotension	Bradycardia or other dysrhythmia	Dysrhythmias	Dysrhythmias
	Papilledema	Decreased cardiac output	Numbness and tingling of limbs and around mouth	Decreased cardiac output
	Seizures	Gastrointestinal distention	Muscle weakness	Hypotension
	Dysrhythmias	Hypotension	Chest pain	Hypoxemia
	Muscle tremors	Nausea and vomiting	Nausea, vomiting, diarrhea	Muscle cramping or tetany
	Lethargy			Muscle tremors
	Coma			Seizures
	Hypoxemia			

Nursing Management of the Medical Client

Assessment. The nurse must be alert for manifestations of acid-base imbalance in high-risk clients. These clients include those who:

- Have a known disease of the pulmonary, cardiovascular, or renal system
- Are in a hypermetabolic state, such as with fever, sepsis, or burns
- Are receiving total parenteral nutrition or enteral tube feedings high in carbohydrate
- Are receiving mechanical ventilation
- Have diabetes
- Are vomiting, have diarrhea, or have enteric drainage
- Are an older adult

Age-related decreases in respiratory and renal function may limit the client's ability to compensate for acid-base disturbances. The normal aging process results in decreased ventilatory capacity as well as loss of alveolar surface area for gas exchange; thus older adults are susceptible to respiratory acidosis from hypoventilation and to respiratory alkalosis from hypoxemia. Older adults commonly take multiple medications for hypertension or cardiovascular disease; these drugs may contribute to hypokalemia and metabolic alkalosis. Respiratory compensation in this condition is compromised because of the structural and functional changes mentioned. Decreased cardiac output in the aging person diminishes renal perfusion and glomerular filtration. Aldosterone is less effective in older people, as is ammonia buffering. These changes limit renal compensation for respiratory imbalances and may put an older client at higher risk for metabolic imbalance.

To assess for acid-base imbalances, document the findings of a comprehensive physical assessment of ventilatory status, cardiovascular function, and fluid-electrolyte balance, as described in the Critical Monitoring box above. Carefully analyze the trends in ABGs. Consider laboratory values, including ABG results and electrolyte, blood urea nitrogen, creatinine, and serum lactate dehydrogenase values.

Interpret Acid-Base Homeostasis. Knowledgeable interpretation of ABG values is critical for timely, appropriate intervention in acid-base disturbances. Often the nurse is the first to see a client's ABG results and becomes the communication link between respiratory therapists and physicians about potential changes in a client's status or treatment. In critical care units, many nurses are using bedside ABG analyzers to obtain these results. Systems for continuous in vivo monitoring of blood gases have recently been developed. Although ABG interpretation is essential to diagnosis and treatment of acid-base imbalance, ABG findings are helpful only when they are considered as part of the total clinical picture.

Protect the Client. Preventing client injury during diagnostic procedures is one of the nurse's important responsibilities.

SAFETY ALERT

To prevent injury to the hand from trauma to the radial or ulnar arteries during ABG assessments, perform Allen's test to ensure adequate circulation to the hand before an arterial puncture.

Perform Allen's test as follows:
1. With the hand over the client's head, have the client tightly close the intended test hand into a fist.
2. Apply pressure over the pulse points for both radial and ulnar arteries.
3. Ask the client to lower the hand and open the fist; the palm has a blanched look from a lack of blood.
4. Release pressure on the ulnar artery. If the artery has adequate circulation, the client's palm reddens within 7 to 15 seconds; it is safe to use the radial artery to obtain a blood specimen. This is a positive Allen's test.

Failure to assess collateral circulation may result in severe ischemic injury to the client's hand if the ulnar artery is compromised and the radial artery is injured by the puncture. Arterial blood gas specimens may be drawn from any artery with a strong pulse. Usually the radial or brachial artery is used. The femoral artery may be used as a last resort because this site is more likely to develop infections and hematomas. Critically ill clients commonly have femoral or radial arterial catheter systems from which blood specimens are drawn. Frequent sampling can result in significant blood loss when an open system is used. Nursing research recommends the minimum discard amount to avoid nosocomial anemia. Closed systems allow reinstillation of initially aspirated heparinized solution and blood. Nursing responsibilities for the procedure of obtaining ABG specimens and for clients with arterial lines are discussed in Chapter 59. The most common complications from drawing blood for ABGs are pain, vasospasm, hematoma formation, infection, hemorrhage, and neurovascular compromise.[5]

Nurses are responsible for minimizing errors in ABG analysis caused by faulty specimen collection and handling. Potential sampling errors and their consequences as well as nursing implications are summarized in Table 13-1.

Despite quality control procedures, erroneous blood gas data are sometimes reported. A sampling error or transcription error should be suspected when the reported values lack internal consistency or external congruity. *Internal consistency* means that the values make sense when considered as a whole. An alkalotic pH, for example, is inconsistent with excess $Paco_2$ and deficient HCO_3^-. *External congruity* means that the ABG findings are consistent with other laboratory data

TABLE 13–1   Arterial Blood Gas Sampling Errors

Sampling Error	Effect	Nursing Implications
Air bubbles in syringe	↑ Pao_2*	Expel all air bubbles immediately.
	↓ $Paco_2$	Do not agitate syringe.
	↑ pH	Do not use any sample that appears frothy.
Inadvertent venous sample or venous contamination of arterial sample	↓ Pao_2	Avoid use of femoral artery.
	↑ $Paco_2$	Use short-beveled needle.
	↓ pH	Do not overshoot artery and then withdraw to "catch" it. Watch for autofilling of syringe with arterial puncture. Verify questionable results with new sample.
Anticoagulant effects	↓ pH	Use lithium heparin, if possible.
Altered pH		Use 1:1000 units/ml concentration. Use minimum 2-ml discard sample with arterial line aspiration.
Dilution of sample	↑ pH	Use syringe with minimal dead space.
	↓ all other values	Use dried heparin if available. Use at least 3-ml sample.
Effects of metabolism of white blood cells in sample	↓ Pao_2	Place sample in ice water immediately.
	↑ $Paco_2$	Have sample analyzed within 20 min.
	↓ pH	Cool sample to 5° C if it cannot be analyzed quickly. Have sample analyzed immediately if client has leukocytosis.

* $Paco_2$, Partial pressure of carbon dioxide in arterial blood; Pao_2, partial pressure of oxygen in arterial blood; ↑, increase in; ↓, decrease in.
Data from Malley, W.J. (2005). *Clinical blood gases: Application and noninvasive alternatives.* Philadelphia: W.B. Saunders; and Williams, A.J. (1998). ABC of oxygen: Assessing and interpreting arterial blood gases and acid-base balance. *British Medical Journal, 317*(7167), 1213-1216.

and with clinical assessment findings. For example, a client with a pH of 7.10 should appear profoundly ill.

Diagnosis, Outcomes, Interventions

Nursing Diagnoses. Several nursing diagnoses may apply to the management of underlying causes and clinical manifestations of acid-base disturbances. For example, *Impaired Gas Exchange, Ineffective Breathing Pattern, Ineffective Tissue Perfusion, Acute Confusion,* or *Risk for Injury* may be appropriate. Acid-base imbalances are perhaps best conceptualized as collaborative problems, however, because the interventions of several health care professionals, including nurses, respiratory therapists, physicians, and pharmacists, are required for effective treatment.

Outcomes. When acid-base imbalances are approached as collaborative problems, the expected outcomes reflect timely resolution of underlying disorders and minimization of the detrimental effects of acidemia or alkalemia. The nurse's role in promoting these outcomes includes implementing medical management and watching for clinical manifestations of the imbalances and the response to treatment.

Interventions. Corrective interventions address the underlying causes of acid-base imbalances and are the mainstay of treatment in such disorders. Compensatory imbalances are not treated but instead resolve spontaneously as the primary disorder is reversed. You should optimize the client's respiratory and renal function through positioning, pulmonary hygiene, and hydration. Also, help clients cope with the anxiety that often accompanies—and may contribute to—acid-base imbalance. Collaborate in the administration of drug therapy, fluid and electrolyte replacement, oxygen therapy, and mechanical ventilation when indicated. For a detailed discussion of appropriate nursing interventions for specific disorders contributing to acid-base imbalances, consult the appropriate chapters of this book.

Provide Respiratory Support. Altered ventilation is a component of all significant acid-base imbalances, whether as a contributing cause or as a result of compensation. You can help to promote optimal ventilation through such measures as repositioning, airway management, hydration, and implementation of oxygen therapy and mechanical ventilation.

Administer Exogenous Acid or Alkali. In extreme circumstances that require intravenous administration of acid or base, these medications must be given following standard precautions to avoid injury to the vein. Nurses must be knowledgeable about the potential risks of this therapy, and must carefully monitor administration rates and therapeutic response.

Evaluation. Acid-base disorders can be acute and corrected quickly, with control of the underlying disorder, or they may be chronic and managed with compensation. Clients with chronic forms of acid-base imbalance must be assessed closely because they may decompensate quickly.

CONCLUSIONS

In collaboration with other health care professionals, you may reduce the client's risk for adverse outcomes resulting from acid-base imbalances. Because of the narrow homeostatic range of serum pH, the client at risk must be carefully monitored to detect imbalance as early as possible. Nursing interventions that promote optional respiratory and renal function are particularly important in prevention and treatment of acid-base imbalances.

THINKING CRITICALLY

1. The client is a 65-year-old widow with a long history of type 2 diabetes mellitus. She was a heavy smoker for 40 years but has not smoked in the last 5 years. She is admitted to the general medical unit because of a 1-week history of profuse diarrhea, attributed to food poisoning. She appears to be in respiratory distress. Her admission ABG values are pH, 7.26; $Paco_2$, 13 mm Hg; HCO_3^-, 5 mEq/L. What acid-base imbalance does she have? Should you encourage her to breathe more slowly? Other than ABGs, what laboratory values should you monitor closely in this case? Why?

Factors to Consider. What acids or bases are lost through diarrhea? Why might a respiratory change have developed if the client's primary problem is gastrointestinal (e.g., metabolic)?

2. A 19-year-old college student is brought to the emergency department at 4:30 AM by his friends. While studying for final examinations, he grew increasingly anxious during his "cram session," frequently voicing doubts about passing a particularly difficult course. His breathing became increasingly labored, and he seemed dazed and confused. He says his "face feels numb." His pulse is rapid (165 beats/min) and he is diaphoretic. He was seen with bleeding duodenal ulcers 2 years ago. ABG analysis of blood samples drawn in the emergency department reveals pH, 7.58; $Paco_2$, 21 mm Hg; HCO_3^-, 20 mEq/L. What acid-base imbalance does the client have? What caused it? What bedside assessments should you perform and why? What interventions should you consider that might prevent future episodes?

Factors to Consider. Can rapid breathing alone alter the excretion of components needed for acid-base balance?

3. A 72-year-old retired college professor has a 55-pack-year history of cigarette smoking and advanced emphysema. He had an acute myocardial infarction 5 years ago, from which he recovered uneventfully. He sees his physician in the clinic, complaining of a

"cold" that he "just cannot get rid of" and "soreness" in his chest. His blood pressure is 165/90 mm Hg, and he has inspiratory crackles in both lung bases. His ankles are edematous. ABG analysis of blood samples drawn during the visit revealed pH, 7.34; $Paco_2$, 65 mm Hg; HCO_3^-, 34 mEq/L. What acid-base imbalance does he have? What is the probable cause? What additional information would be helpful in planning his care? What variables should you consider in determining priorities of care?

Factors to Consider. Consider that the client has developed heart failure. When the lungs fill with fluid, what happens to O_2/CO_2 exchange and, thereby, acid-base balance?

Discussions for these questions can be found on the website.

BIBLIOGRAPHY

Citations appearing in red refer to primary research.

1. Adrogue, H.J. (2006). Mixed acid-base disturbances. *Journal of Nephrology,19*(Suppl 9), S97-S103.
2. Allen, K. (2005). Four-step method of interpreting arterial blood gas analysis. *Nursing Times, 101*(1), 42-45.
3. Bodinot, S. (2005). *Drug pathways and chemical concepts: 8a. The Henderson-Hasselbalch equation: A practical application.* Retrieved 08/07/06 from Kennesaw State University website: www.chemcases.com/pheno/pheno08a.htm. Funded by National Science Foundation.
4. Buchanon, I.B., Campbell, B.T., Peck, M.D., et al. (2005). Chest wall necrosis and death secondary to hydrochloric acid infusion for metabolic alkalosis. *The Southern Medical Journal, 98*(8), 822-824.
5. Bucher, L. (2005). Arterial puncture. In D.J. Lynn-McHale Wiegand & K.K. Carlson (Eds.), *AACN procedure manual for critical care* (5th ed., pp. 630-637). Philadelphia: Saunders.
6. Cariou, A., Vinsonneau, C., & Dhainaut, J.F. (2004). Adjunctive therapies in sepsis: An evidence-based review. *Critical Care Medicine, 32*(11 Suppl), S562-S570.
7. Corbo, J., Bijur, P., Lahn, M., et al. (2005). Concordance between capnography and arterial blood gas measurements of carbon dioxide in acute asthma. *Annals of Emergency Medicine, 46*(4), 323-327.
8. Daniel, S.R., Morita, S.Y., Yu, M., et al. (2004). Uncompensated metabolic acidosis: An under-recognized risk factor for subsequent intubation requirement. *Journal of Trauma, 57*(5), 993-997.
9. Frangiosa, A., DeSanto, L.S., Anastasio, P., et al. (2006). Acid-base balance in heart failure. *Journal of Nephrology, 19*(Suppl 9), S115-S120.
10. Funk, G.C., Doberer, D., Heinze, G., et al. (2004). Changes of serum chloride and metabolic acid-base state in critical illness. *Anaesthesia, 59*(11), 1111-1115.
11. Gunen, H., Hacievliyagil, S.S., Kosar, F., et al. (2006). The role of arterial blood gases, exercise testing and cardiac examination in asthma. *Allergy Asthma Proceedings: The Official Journal of Regional and State Asthma Societies, 27*(1), 45-52.
12. Guyton, A.C., & Hall, J.E. (2006). *Textbook of medical physiology* (11th ed.). St. Louis: Saunders,
13. Kraut, J.A., & Kurtz, I. (2006). Use of base in the treatment of acute severe organic acidosis by nephrologists and critical care physicians: Results of an online survey. *Clinical and Experimental Nephrology, 10*(2), 111-117.
14. Malinoski, D.J., Todd, S.R., Slone, S., et al. (2005). Correlation of central venous and arterial blood gas measurements in mechanically ventilated trauma patients. *Archives of Surgery, 140*(11), 1122-1125.
15. Middleton, P, Kelly, A.M., Brown, J., et al. (2006). Agreement between arterial and central venous values for pH, bicarbonate, base excess, and lactate. *Emergency Medicine Journal, 23*(8), 622-624.
16. Pagana, K.D., & Pagana, T.J. (2006). *Mosby's manual of diagnostic and laboratory tests* (3rd ed.). St. Louis: Mosby.
17. Pruitt, W.C., & Jacobs, M. (2004). Interpreting arterial blood gases: Easy as ABC. *Nursing, 34*(8), 50-53.
18. Simpson, H. (2004). Interpretation of arterial blood gases: A clinical guide for nurses. *British Journal of Nursing, 13*(9), 522-528.
19. Squadrone, E., Frigerio, P., Fogliati, C., et al. (2004). Noninvasive vs. invasive ventilation in COPD patients with severe acute respiratory failure deemed to require ventilatory assistance. *Intensive Care Medicine, 30*(7), 1303-1310. Epub 06/12/04.
20. Tasker, R.C., Lutman, D., & Peters, M.J. (2005). Hyperventilation in severe diabetic ketoacidosis. *Pediatric Critical Care Medicine, 6*(4), 405-411.
21. Tsai, W.S., Wu, C.P., Hsu, Y.J., et al. (2004). Life-threatening hypokalemia in an asthmatic patient treated with high-dose hydrocortisone. *The American Journal of the Medical Sciences, 327*(3), 152-155.
22. Woodrow, P. (2004). Arterial blood gas analysis. *Nursing Standard, 18*(21), 45-52.
23. Woodruff, D.W. (2006). Deciphering diagnostics: Take these 6 easy steps to ABG analysis. *Nursing Made Incredibly Easy, 4*(1), 4-8.

evolve **Did you remember to check out the bonus material on the Evolve website and the CD-ROM, including NCLEX®-Examination Style Review Questions, Open-Book Quizzes, and Chapter Review Audio Podcasts?**

http://evolve.elsevier.com/Black/medsurg

CHAPTER 14

Clients Having Surgery: Promoting Positive Outcomes

NANCY J. GIRARD

Having surgery is a major event in any person's life. Clients faced with surgery want to know that someone is there with them and will protect them during a time when they may have no control or any self-care abilities. Surgical clients are most likely to expect support and encouragement from the perioperative nurse.

More and more surgery today is done in ambulatory surgery centers, radiology departments, gastrointestinal laboratories, physicians' offices, and sites other than the traditional hospital setting. Much of the nursing care traditionally performed for these clients has been modified because of the short time nurses now spend with the client and family. Team work in preparing the client is essential in order to complete all assessments and interventions that promote a successful and safe procedure. The team can consist of anyone working with the client. Thus one of the most important activities a nurse can perform is coordination of care and accurate and timely communication among all concerned.

PERIOPERATIVE NURSING

The total surgical episode is called the *perioperative period*. This period in the health care continuum includes the time before surgery, or preoperative period; the time spent during the actual surgical procedure, or intraoperative period; and the period after the surgery is completed, or postoperative period. In the broadest definition of perioperative nursing practice, care can range from home, through surgery and recovery, and back to home again. A *perioperative nurse* is a registered nurse who uses the nursing process to design, plan, and deliver care to meet the identified needs of a client whose protective reflexes or self-care abilities are potentially compromised because of the operative procedures to be performed. Surgery is performed in a multitude of settings, and the nurse's role as a surgical team member is partially defined by the practice setting. Thus perioperative nursing is client-centered rather than task-oriented. The perioperative nurse must possess and apply knowledge of anatomy, physiology, psychology, and sociocultural and spiritual beliefs and practices, in addition to knowledge of all aspects of the surgical procedure to be performed. The perioperative nurse must be a good communicator, delegator, and supervisor to ensure that the needs of the client are being met throughout the surgical experience.

BASIC CONCEPTS OF PERIOPERATIVE NURSING

Nursing care of the perioperative client takes place immediately before, during, and immediately after a surgical procedure. In each of these periods, specific assessments and interventions are performed by nurses acting both as independent clinicians and as members of the health care team. The goals of perioperative nursing practice are to assist clients and their significant others through the surgical episode, to help promote positive outcomes, and to help clients achieve their optimal level of function and wellness after surgery. The management of clients' needs, both unique and predictable, may be through direct or indirect interventions. These interventions are planned to assist the client in meeting the projected outcomes in an efficient

---

evolve Web Enhancements

Case Management   The Elective Surgery Client

Ethical Issues in Nursing   Should Clients Who Have a "Do Not Resuscitate" Order Undergo Surgery?

Is It Your Job to Protect the Client's Dignity?

Appendix A   Religious Beliefs and Practices Affecting Health Care

Be sure to check out the bonus material on the Evolve website and the CD-ROM, including free self-assessment exercises. **http://evolve.elsevier. com/Black/medsurg**

and appropriate manner. Perioperative nursing care is implemented by registered nurses who strive to assist the client by functioning in various roles. Perioperative nursing strives to use a terminology data set similar to and concurrent with nursing diagnoses. It is called the Perioperative Nursing Data Set (PNDS) and was developed as a common language to promote understanding among professionals and to contribute to consistent, safe care of surgical clients.

PREOPERATIVE PERIOD

PREOPERATIVE ASSESSMENT

Each client responds differently to surgery. Therefore for each client having surgery, a care plan based on the nursing process is developed. It is vital to identify potential risks and complications that may arise during the perioperative period. In addition, a care plan can also identify the need for supportive services at home or in the hospital after surgery.

Assessment is the first step in the nursing process and is designed to provide information that enables the nurse and the client to plan for optimal postoperative outcomes. When clients are admitted on the same day as the planned operation, there is limited time for interaction with the client, so the perioperative nurse must be able to quickly and effectively complete a meaningful preoperative evaluation of the client's physical, mental, and emotional status. Preoperative assessment can take place in many different settings, including the physician's office before admission to a health care facility, at home during the days before the surgery, the night before surgery if the client is in the hospital, or on admission the day of surgery.

SAFETY

⚠

ALERT

Electronic client record systems allow easy transfer of the client's record between caregivers, contain all essential information, save time (because information does not have to be re-entered), and help ensure safe and quality care.

In the case of emergency surgery, time often does not permit complete preoperative assessment, care planning, and teaching. Nevertheless, preparation must be as thorough as possible.

Preoperative assessment includes the medical/health history, the psychosocial history, physical examination, cognitive assessment, and diagnostic testing. When surgery must be performed following a traumatic event (e.g., gunshot wound, stab wound, serious accident, or severe fall), a preoperative assessment must include details of the traumatic event described as precisely as possible. If the client was injured in a fall or a motor vehicle accident, information on injury-related factors such as the position in which the injury occurred, or whether the accident appeared to cause the victim to lose consciousness, may help to assess surgical risk or to identify underlying conditions related to the injurious event. Traumatically injured clients are usually admitted to the operating room from an emergency department. Emergency department staff provide a detailed report upon transfer.

PREOPERATIVE HEALTH HISTORY

Medical History

Obtaining a health history allows clients to explain their understanding of impending surgery and to establish rapport with the nurse conducting the interview. Reassurance by the nurse through this process may reduce anxiety in the client and family members or significant others. In most instances, the past medical history (PMH) has been previously recorded and is found in the medical record.

A complete PMH is critical, and the nurse reviews it to ensure that it is thorough, completing any missing pieces and validating information with the client. The purpose of reviewing the medical history is to determine operative risk.

The past medical history should include, but is not limited to, the following.

Previous Surgery and Experience with Anesthesia

Any untoward reactions to anesthesia (e.g., high fever, intraoperative death of family members, known malignant hyperthermia, prolonged nausea and vomiting) by the client or anyone in the family must be reported to anesthesia personnel. These problems do not preclude surgery but often require a change in the type of anesthetics used.

Serious Illness or Trauma

This information should cover anything that might influence the surgery and recovery. An ABCDE mnemonic is often used to ascertain information:

A—allergy to medications, chemicals, and other environmental products such as latex.

- All allergies are reported to anesthesia and surgical personnel before the beginning of surgery. If allergies exist, an allergy band must be placed on the client's arm and in the medical record immediately.
- *B*—bleeding tendencies or the use of medications that deter clotting, such as aspirin or products containing aspirin, heparin, or warfarin sodium. Herbal medications may also increase bleeding times or mask potential blood-related problems.
- *C*—cortisone or steroid use. The stress of the operation may require higher doses of steroids during early recovery. In addition, long-term steroid use impairs wound healing.
- *D*—diabetes mellitus, a condition that not only requires strict control of blood glucose levels but also is known to delay wound healing and is associated with increased risk of infection.

■ *E*—emboli; previous embolic events (such as lower leg blood clots) may recur because of prolonged immobility.

Alcohol, Recreational Drug, or Nicotine Use

The use of illicit drugs signals potential problems with the administration of anesthesia or analgesia and risk for withdrawal complications. 🪔

Clients who use alcohol or drugs may experience withdrawal manifestations because the drugs are not ingested during the postoperative course. In addition, clients addicted to alcohol often have malnutrition or unpredictable reactions to anesthetic agents. As little as two drinks per day can lead to withdrawal manifestations that may require dosage alterations in anesthesia and analgesia.

Smokers may be more susceptible to thrombus (clot) formation because of the hypercoagulability secondary to nicotine use. Smokers are also much more likely to have damage to lung tissue and experience atelectasis.

Clients are instructed to abstain from any nicotine product for at least 1 week before surgery. Nicotine is a potent vasoconstrictor, and the flow of blood to surgical sites is an important aspect of healing. The use of nicotine patches and nicotine gum is also inappropriate preoperatively because the client continues to receive nicotine into the bloodstream.

Current Discomforts

Clients with pre-existing painful conditions may require alternate methods of pain relief while they are receiving nothing by mouth (NPO). Clients who drink a considerable amount of caffeinated beverages such as coffee often develop headaches related to their NPO status, when their caffeine intake ceases abruptly. Without appropriate preoperative assessment, the headache may be misinterpreted as a surgical problem.

Chronic Illnesses

Arthritis of the neck or back is considered in positioning the client during surgery or in extending the neck during intubation.

Advanced Age

Older clients have specific perioperative needs that should be identified preoperatively and considered in developing and maintaining a plan of care.

Medication History

Many clients take prescription and over-the-counter (OTC) drugs that may increase operative risks.

Ask if the client is taking any medications and if these have been brought to the hospital. Dosage and administration schedules for all medications should be noted on the chart. The use of herbal and natural substances should also be noted. This topic is explored in the Complementary and Alternative Therapy feature below.

Psychological History

Knowledge of cultural beliefs and practices is a very important component of holistic nursing care. Some cultures practice traditional health care as well as alternative and complementary practices that may include use of candles, rituals, and herbs. Certain rituals are very important to the client and should be respected by all members of the health care team. For example, in some cultures, the family may make decisions regarding health care as a unit. In other cultures, the oldest woman makes all medical decisions. The nurse must be accepting of each individual's beliefs and should play an active advocate role by supporting the client in any manner possible.

Ability to Tolerate Perioperative Stress

Physiologic stressors in the perioperative client include pain, tissue damage, blood loss, anesthesia, fever, and immobilization. The stressful stimuli imposed by surgery promote the physiologic stress response by combining both psychological factors (such as anxiety and fear of the unknown) and physiologic factors (including tissue trauma, blood loss, anesthesia, pain, and immobility). The sympathetic nervous system is activated by any stressor. A person's age, physical condition, and duration of the stress determine the success of the stress response in maintaining homeostatic balance. The ability to tolerate the stress of surgery and anesthesia is decreased significantly in older and debilitated people. All body systems are affected by the stress response; therefore this

---

COMPLEMENTARY AND ALTERNATIVE THERAPY

Supplements That Should Not Be Taken During the Time of Surgery

A review of a variety of supplements has found that many of them may interact with anesthetics or may affect coagulation parameters. Some of the potential supplements include echinacea, ephedra, garlic, ginkgo, ginseng, kava, St. John's wort, and valerian. This list is expected to grow as more research is completed. Therefore, to be safe, clinicians should advise clients to eliminate all dietary supplements at least 2 to 3 weeks before any surgical procedure. When a client has recovered from surgery, an in-depth conversation with a health professional should be conducted to determine which supplements can be restarted.

REFERENCE

Ang-Lee, M., Moss, J., & Yuan, C.-S. (2001). Herbal medicines and perioperative care. *Journal of the American Medical Association, 286,* 208-216.

assessment is crucial throughout the perioperative experience. The nurse must be able to assess stress and to plan and implement appropriate interventions to effectively reduce or treat complications related to stress.

Lifestyle Habits

Sedentary lifestyles can complicate the surgical course via poor muscle tone, limited cardiac and respiratory reserves, and decreased stress response. On the other hand, an overly active lifestyle may present postoperative compliance problems.

Social History

An important component of a social history on a preoperative client is the support system. Identification of client occupation and physical and mental requirements for job performance also provides important information that may prove useful for care planning.

PREOPERATIVE PHYSICAL EXAMINATION

A physical examination is performed on all clients undergoing surgery to identify the present health status and to have baseline information for comparisons during and after surgery. These data are used to determine nursing diagnoses or to identify problems and develop pertinent outcome goals. Perform a complete physical examination whenever possible. When perioperative time is brief, such as with same-day surgery admission or trauma cases, you may be required to complete the assessment in minutes. This assessment is of the utmost importance and must be accurate. Report any abnormal findings to the surgical team members immediately, as this information may affect the initiation of the surgery.

Review preoperative laboratory and diagnostic study results, and post them on the client's chart (Table 14-1). Missing laboratory data constitute a common problem in ambulatory surgery settings, especially if the client's tests were ordered days before the scheduled procedure or in a preadmission clinic. Missing laboratory reports could lead to cancellation of the surgery.

First, examine the part of the body that will be operated on, noting any unusual findings such as skin lesions or weak or absent pulses. Next, complete a general systems assessment. Systems to be assessed include cardiovascular, pulmonary, renal, musculoskeletal, skin, and neurologic. Ask the client whether there are any particularly troublesome manifestations, and include this information in the written assessment for further investigation. Again, document all unusual findings, and communicate them to the surgical team.

The best way to organize a brief assessment in the immediate preoperative period is to develop a personal

TABLE 14–1	**Common Preoperative Screening Tests**		
Test	**Age**	**Procedure Type**	**Disease or Condition**
ECG	Males older than 40 years	Cardiovascular	Cardiovascular disease
	Females older than 50 years		Hypertension
			Diabetes
Chest x-ray	Clients older than 60 years	Any surgery requiring general anesthesia	Respiratory disease
			Cardiovascular disease
			Smoker
Hemoglobin	Any	Procedure in which >500 ml of blood loss is anticipated	Cardiovascular disease
			Renal disease
			Malignancy
			Diabetes
			Aspirin or NSAID use
			Full-dose anticoagulant use
Creatinine	Older than 50 years	Procedure with high risk for renal failure	Use of drugs with renal excretion
			Renal disease
			Cardiovascular disease
			Hypertension
			Diabetes
			NSAID use
Glucose	Older than 45 years	Any	Diabetes
	Younger clients with risk factors		Steroid use
Urinalysis	Any	Genitourinary	Use of drugs with renal excretion
		Use of bladder catheter or other infection risk, orthopedic implants or valve replacements	Renal disease
			Cardiovascular disease
			Hypertension
			Diabetes
Pregnancy (HCG)	Female of childbearing age	Any	Women of childbearing age for whom pregnancy status is uncertain
Coagulation	All	Any	Bleeding risk by history
			Plan for full-dose anticoagulation

system for conducting the examination and use it consistently. Although each person will devise a particular method for gathering data, a head-to-toe examination is a common method (Box 14-1). Assess cognition throughout the examination by noting the client's demeanor and responses to directed questioning. For example, you can assess orientation to time, place, and person in "casual" conversation with the client during the physical assessment. If possible, watch the client walk and move when he or she enters the preparation area. Include this information in the ambulatory status section of the examination.

SPECIFIC BODY SYSTEM ASSESSMENTS

Cardiovascular Assessment

Pathologic cardiac conditions or events that increase operative risk include angina pectoris, myocardial infarction within the last 6 months, uncontrolled hypertension, heart failure, and peripheral vascular disease. Clients who have drug-eluting stents must continue taking anti–platelet aggregate medications, and often cannot have elective surgery for 6 months unless the operation can be done while taking these agents. Some clients with congenital or valvular heart disease are at increased risk of developing bacterial endocarditis and receive antibiotics before undergoing oral surgery or surgery on the respiratory, gastrointestinal, or genitourinary tract. All cardiac conditions can lead to decreased tissue perfusion with impairment of surgical wound healing.

In addition to the portion of the cardiovascular assessment completed as part of the head-to-toe assessment, note specific findings that warrant further work-up. Document shortness of breath on minor exertion, hypertension, heart murmurs or S_3 gallops, and chest pain. These manifestations may be present if the client is scheduled for heart or vascular surgery, but they may make the ability to tolerate anesthesia and blood loss questionable. Laboratory studies to measure the function of the cardiovascular system include an electrocardiogram (ECG), especially for those clients older than age 40, and measurements of levels of hemoglobin, hematocrit, and serum electrolytes.

A recent study has shown that clients with and without cardiac disease have reduced mortality after surgery when they are prescribed beta-blocker therapy.

BOX 14-1 Preoperative Head-to-Toe Assessment

- Assess cognition throughout the examination by noting the client's demeanor and responses to directed questioning. For example, you can check the client's orientation to time, place, and person in the course of eliciting information during the physical assessment. This is particularly important in the older adult. The effects of the operation and of associated medications often cause temporary cognitive deficits that can be erroneously identified as a permanent condition by the health care team. Temporary deficits in memory and recall are normal and are seen in most clients, but these manifestations can persist in the older adult.
- Assess muscle strength and coordination, gait, and balance by watching the client walk and move while entering the preparation area. (This may not be possible with all clients.)
- Take a full set of vital sign measurements. Note the ease of respiration.
- Look at the client's eyes and nose, and assess the mobility of the neck.
- Listen to the heart and the lungs. Listen to the rate and rhythm of the heart. Note the character of the lung sounds, listening for any diminution of intensity or the absence of breath sounds. Shortness of breath on minor exertion should also be noted. Dyspnea, wheezing, clubbed fingers, chest pain, cyanosis, and coughing with expectoration of copious or purulent mucus should be reported to anesthesia personnel. Question the client carefully about smoking habits and recent illness with a cold or influenza. Obtain a history of respiratory allergies and infections.

- Assess range of motion of the shoulders and the strength of the arms and hand grip.
- Ask about the ability to urinate and whether the client has diabetes.
- Assess the ability to flex the spine (this is important if the client is scheduled to have spinal anesthesia).
- Examine the extremities for edema, coldness to the touch, and cyanosis.
- Palpate the presence of peripheral pulses and neurovascular function (numbness, dorsiflexion, plantiflexion).
- Assess the range of motion and strength of the legs and feet.
- Note equal movement of the face and shoulders on both sides of the body if a crude estimate of cranial nerve function is needed. Complete neurologic testing includes assessment of cranial nerve function, reflex response of the upper and lower extremities, and sensory reflexes, as well as cognitive assessment. This level of testing is performed before neurologic surgery.
- During the examination, observe the condition of the skin. Note and document lesions, pressure ulcers, necrotic tissue, skin turgor, erythema or other discoloration of the skin, and the presence of external devices. Record the approximate size, color, and location of any lesions for later comparison.
- Review the chart for results of laboratory and diagnostic tests. Tests commonly ordered for the client undergoing heart surgery include chest x-ray, electrocardiogram, hemoglobin, hematocrit, serum electrolytes, and urinalysis.
- During the physical examination, pay attention to the client's verbal and nonverbal communication. Does the client complain of any pain unrelated to the impending surgical procedure?

Respiratory Assessment

Chronic lung conditions, such as emphysema, asthma, and bronchitis, increase operative risk because these disorders impair gas exchange in the alveoli, predisposing the client to postoperative pulmonary complications. Assessment of pulmonary conditions includes examining for the presence of shortness of breath, wheezing, clubbed fingers, chest pain, cyanosis, and coughing with expectoration of copious or purulent mucus. Question the client carefully about smoking habits, especially if the smell of smoke is obvious. Obtain a complete history of respiratory allergies and infections. If a client demonstrates any respiratory distress at the time of the assessment, notify the surgeon before administration of anesthesia. Abnormal breath sounds may indicate the need for respiratory therapy both before and after surgery. Clients with severe respiratory disease are usually managed preoperatively with aerosol therapy, postural drainage, and antibiotics. Clients who smoke are strongly encouraged to stop smoking as early as possible before surgery. Nicotine patches are usually not an appropriate alternative because of vasoconstriction caused by the nicotine.

Laboratory studies performed before surgery to diagnose respiratory conditions include chest radiography and pulse oximetry. Chest radiography (or x-rays) detects abnormalities, if present, in the lungs, such as infections, collapsed alveoli or segments of the lung, tumors, fractures of the ribs, and size of the heart. The pulse oximeter is used to determine gross levels of tissue oxygenation. Explain the operation and purpose of the oximeter to the client and why it is important to monitor oxygenation throughout the surgical experience. The definitive laboratory test for blood oxygenation is arterial blood gas (ABG) analysis. Although routine ABG analyses are not ordered preoperatively, a physician may order the test if the client has been determined to be at high risk for surgical complications. Additional pulmonary function tests may be ordered in specific situations (see Chapter 59).

Assess the presence of sleep apnea. If present, alert the surgery team and document. Determine if the client uses an apnea assistance respiratory device (e.g., continuous positive airway pressure [CPAP] mask) at home and if it will be continued postoperatively during hospitalization.

Musculoskeletal Assessment

A history of arthritis, fractures, contractures, joint injury, or musculoskeletal impairment is an important factor in surgical positioning and postoperative support. The physical examination should reveal any problems with joint mobility or deformities that may interfere with operative positioning as well as with the postoperative course. For example, if the preoperative assessment identifies arthritis of the neck and shoulder, the circulating nurse can incorporate this information into the care plan. Hyperextension of the arthritic neck during intubation for general anesthesia can cause postoperative pain and discomfort unrelated to the surgery. The musculoskeletal system can be assessed through passive and active range of motion and a history provided by the client or family member, or the medical record. Documentation of impairment before the surgical procedure assists in the investigation of any impairment postoperatively.

Gastrointestinal Assessment

Gastrointestinal conditions associated with poor surgical outcomes include severe malnutrition and prolonged nausea and vomiting. The client's gastrointestinal system should be assessed if the planned operation is in the abdominal area or if the general physical examination reveals any abnormal data. Because narcotic analgesics increase constipation, obtain information about normal bowel patterns so that postoperative expectations for return of function are appropriate. A client with a long history of constipation may have more difficulty postoperatively regaining usual bowel function.

Skin Integrity Assessment

Skin integrity must be assessed and documented preoperatively to establish a baseline for comparison postoperatively. The operative site must be clear of any rashes, blisters, or infectious processes. Document and report lesions, pressure ulcers, necrotic skin or tissue, skin turgor, erythema or discoloration of the skin, and the presence of external devices. Note the size, color, and location of the skin impairment to determine whether the impaired skin remains stable or worsens during and after the surgical procedure. Padding and positioning equipment should be used to maintain skin integrity and to prevent pressure ulcers.

> **Any alterations in skin integrity that can occur intraoperatively and are not related to the actual surgical procedure are preventable by the nurse and other members of the surgical team with adequate padding and repositioning as needed during very long procedures.**

Renal Assessment

Adequate renal function is necessary to eliminate metabolic wastes, to preserve fluid and electrolyte balance, and to remove anesthetic agents. Important renal and related disorders include advanced renal insufficiency, acute nephritis, and benign prostatic hypertrophy (BPH). If renal deficiency exists, the surgical team must be made aware of the problem. To assess renal status, ask about voiding patterns such as frequency and dysuria. Also, observe the appearance of urine if a sample is collected or if an indwelling catheter is in place. Document and report abnormal urine characteristics. Monitor fluid balance by recording intake and output before and during surgery.

The most common preoperative tests to assess renal function are determination of blood urea nitrogen (BUN) and serum creatinine levels and urinalysis. BUN and serum creatinine levels indicate the ability of the kidney to excrete urea and protein wastes. Elevated levels may reflect dehydration, impaired cardiac output, or renal failure. Elevated creatinine level is associated with renal disease. Serious renal disease and urinary tract infections must be treated, if possible, before surgery. Urinalysis results may indicate urinary tract infection, diabetes, malnutrition, renal disease, or dehydration.

Liver Function Assessment

Chronic liver disease, such as cirrhosis, increases a client's surgical risk because an impaired liver cannot detoxify medications and anesthetic agents. Coagulation may also be altered. The client may also be unable to metabolize carbohydrates, fats, and amino acids. Liver disease may be manifested by decreased albumin levels, which predispose the client to fluid shifts and surgical wound infection. Faulty coagulation, noted as elevated prothrombin (PT) levels, increases the risk of bleeding. Clients with a history of alcoholism or other substance abuse require a careful assessment of liver function before surgery. If evidence of risk factors for liver disease is uncovered during the immediate preoperative assessment, information must be shared immediately with other members of the surgical team. Because a client with liver disease is often malnourished and debilitated and may have clotting disorders, the surgeon generally orders a high-calorie diet or hyperalimentation during the preoperative and postoperative periods. Clients may also experience acute alcohol withdrawal following surgery.

Cognitive and Neurologic Assessment

Serious neurologic conditions, such as uncontrolled epilepsy or severe Parkinson's disease, increase surgical risk. Important preoperative neurologic abnormalities include severe headache, frequent dizziness, lightheadedness, ringing in the ears, unsteady gait, unequal pupils, and a history of seizures. Assessment of the client's orientation to time, place, and person can be accomplished by simple questioning. To determine baseline neurologic function, include testing of cranial nerves, reflex responses of the upper and lower extremities, sensory reflexes, and cerebral responses (see Chapter 67).

Assess cognition preoperatively to determine postoperative effects of surgery. This is particularly important in an older adult. The effects of the operation and of associated medications frequently lead to temporary cognitive deficiencies that can be erroneously identified as a permanent condition. Temporary deficits in memory and recall are considered normal and are seen in the majority of clients, but the older adult can experience these symptoms for a longer time.

Endocrine Assessment

Diabetes mellitus is the most common pre-existing endocrine pathophysiologic disorder. In some ethnic groups, especially Hispanic populations, diabetes is rampant. Diabetes mellitus predisposes the affected client to poor wound healing and increased risk of surgical wound infection. Corresponding cardiovascular, peripheral vascular, neurologic, visual, and renal complications may be present as well. These factors can greatly increase the surgical risk for a client with diabetes. A client who has well-controlled diabetes (i.e., blood glucose levels are consistently monitored and kept within a normal range during the perioperative period) is less susceptible to infection. Chapter 45 describes the care of clients with diabetes mellitus.

Thyroid functioning may also need to be assessed preoperatively. Thyroid hormone replacement is usually continued throughout the perioperative period.

> **Stopping thyroid medications may precipitate a thyroid storm or crisis, with manifestations of hypertension, tachycardia, and hyperthermia.**

 SAFETY ALERT

This event can be devastating if it occurs during surgery or immediately postoperatively. In addition, the presence of hypothyroidism increases the risk of hypotension and cardiac arrest during anesthetic administration.

> **Adrenal insufficiency may develop in clients who have taken more than 5 mg of prednisone per day for more than 2 weeks in the past year.**

 SAFETY ALERT

These clients may require supplementation of steroids when their ability to muster an adrenal response to the stress of surgery is likely impaired.

Hematologic Assessment

Clients with blood coagulation disorders are at risk for hemorrhage and hypovolemic shock during and after surgery. Five factors that should be assessed preoperatively to identify potential hematologic problems are the following:

- A history of bleeding or a diagnosis of a pathologic condition such as hemophilia or sickle cell anemia
- Manifestations such as easy bruising, excessive bleeding following dental extractions and razor nicks, and severe nosebleeds
- Hepatic or renal disease
- Use of anticoagulants, aspirin, or other nonsteroidal anti-inflammatory drugs (NSAIDs)
- Abnormal bleeding time, prothrombin time, or platelet count

> **Remember that many clients take herbs, aspirin, or other OTC medications that may increase the risk of bleeding.**

SAFETY ALERT

The client may not consider nonprescription medications important and often may not include them in a medication history. Ask specific questions regarding all prescription and nonprescription medications. Specifically ask about the use of herbal preparations. Ginkgo biloba, garlic, ginger, and ginseng may prevent blood clot formation and may lead to excess blood loss in surgery. Two other popular herbs—St. John's wort (an antidepressant) and kava-kava (a relaxant)—may prolong the sedative effect of anesthesia. Advise clients to stop taking herbal products at least 2 weeks before elective surgery. Ask how often the client takes the OTC medications and when the last dose of any of those drugs was taken.

For a variety of reasons, blood transfusions are used less frequently than in past years. Many clients fear the transmission of human immunodeficiency virus (HIV) and hepatitis B. If possible, clients are encouraged to donate their own blood for use during or after surgery (autologous transfusion). Blood substitutes or fluid volume expanders can also be used in some cases to replace lost blood until the body can produce new blood cells. Blood transfusions are discussed in Chapter 75.

ADDITIONAL ASSESSMENTS

Other factors that may be considered during the planning of surgical intervention include (1) age, (2) pain, (3) nutrition, (4) fluid and electrolyte balance, and (5) infection.

Age

Normal physiologic changes that occur with aging, along with the increased presence of disease, may adversely affect surgical outcomes. Chronic conditions commonly found in the older client that may increase surgical risk include malnutrition, anemia, dehydration, atherosclerosis, chronic obstructive pulmonary disease (COPD), diabetes mellitus, cerebrovascular changes, and peripheral vascular disease.

Pain

Pain is an important physiologic indicator that must be carefully monitored (see Chapter 20). During the preoperative nursing assessment, ask if the client is experiencing any pain. If pain is present, obtain a full assessment of the pain. Determine whether the pain is chronic and unrelated to the pathologic condition necessitating surgery or is acute and attributable to the surgical procedure. Be aware that although most operations increase pain, older adults who have undergone joint replacement surgery often state that the postoperative pain is minor compared with the chronic pain of a disintegrating joint.

Nutritional Status

Nutritional status (positive nitrogen balance) is directly related to intraoperative success and postoperative recovery. The client who is well nourished preoperatively is better prepared to handle surgical stress and to return to optimal health after surgery. Improving nutrition is usually attended to in a clinic or physician's office weeks before surgery. However, if the operation is performed on an emergency basis or has not been planned, nutritional status may be a risk factor through the perioperative period. In addition, some operations are completed to improve nutrition. For example, a client who is to undergo placement of a permanent feeding tube would be expected to have evidence of malnutrition. Likewise, a client who is to have an intestinal bypass for obesity is also malnourished (in terms of excess intake).

Assessment of nutritional status preoperatively includes obtaining a diet history, observing the general appearance of the client, performing laboratory diagnostic testing, and comparing current weight with ideal body weight. Laboratory tests that can assist in the assessment of nutritional status include determinations of serum albumin, serum prealbumin, hemoglobin and hematocrit, BUN, and creatinine clearance.

Nutritional abnormalities include deficiencies and excesses. Nutritional deficiencies primarily affect clients with chronic illnesses, cancer, gastrointestinal disorders, and advanced age. Malnutrition is directly linked to delayed healing and infection.

Nursing interventions for clients who are malnourished preoperatively include encouraging high carbohydrate intake to increase energy and high protein intake to assist in wound healing, and supplementing the diet with vitamins to encourage healing. Vitamin C is beneficial in wound healing, whereas vitamin K will increase blood clotting times. Total parenteral nutrition (TPN) can be used preoperatively to bolster the client's nutritional status.

TPN and lipids (fats) supply total nutritional replacement including vitamin and mineral supplements. Tube-feeding (enteral nutrition) can be administered via a tube placed in the stomach or small intestine. The tube is placed through the nose or directly into the stomach through a skin incision. Both enteral and parenteral feeding can improve a client's nutritional status; either may be continued postoperatively until satisfactory swallowing or gastrointestinal functioning returns (see Chapter 29).

Treatment of obesity before surgery includes consuming a reduced-calorie diet, participating in mild exercise, if possible, and assessing for and controlling conditions such as hypertension and diabetes mellitus. Obese clients should not begin a weight-reduction diet while they are healing after surgery. Wound healing is delayed when protein intake is inadequate.

Obesity is also associated with poorer surgical outcomes. Adipose (fatty) tissue increases the technical difficulty of surgery. Fatty tissue is less vascular and more prone to postoperative infection, incisional hernias, and wound dehiscence or evisceration (see Figure 14-13 on p. 224). The surgeon may use an alternative closure method for a client with excess adipose tissue at or around the incision.

Obese clients frequently suffer from hypertension, heart failure, obstructive sleep apnea, and metabolic problems. An obese client is more susceptible to postoperative pulmonary complications. Obesity decreases the efficiency of coughing and deep breathing. The pressure of the abdominal contents on the diaphragm and lungs decreases expansion, which may lead to hypoventilation. An obese client is more prone to postoperative immobility. Immobility increases the risk of venous stasis and deep vein thrombosis or pulmonary embolism.

Thorough preoperative teaching that describes turning, coughing, deep breathing, and moving after surgery is essential. Most complications related to obesity can be prevented, or the risk of their occurrence reduced, with appropriate interventions.

Fluid and Electrolyte Balance

Fluid volume deficits (dehydration/hypovolemia or fluid volume excess/hypervolemia) predispose a client to complications during and after surgery. Actual or potential fluid imbalance can be assessed by evaluation of skin turgor. A coated or fissured tongue can also be a manifestation of fluid volume deficit. A decrease in urine output or urine specific gravity is also diagnostic of decreased fluid volume. If dehydration is severe, irritability or confusion can be apparent. Dehydration results from limited fluid intake, prolonged vomiting, diarrhea, or bleeding. Fluids can be administered by the IV route if dehydration is identified.

Electrolyte imbalances also increase operative risk. Preoperative laboratory results should be checked to see whether serum sodium, potassium, calcium, and magnesium concentrations are within the normal range. In-depth assessment and management of fluid and electrolyte imbalances are discussed in Chapters 11 and 12, respectively.

Infection and Immunity

Any pre-existing infection can adversely affect surgical outcomes because bacteria may be released into the bloodstream during surgery. Their release may lead to infection elsewhere in the body. When the surgical site is near a lymph node or lymphatic vessel that is draining infectious material, the likelihood of surgical infection increases.

During the preoperative assessment, documentation of any possible exposure to communicable diseases, presence of skin lesions, or manifestations of an infection (such as coughing, sore throat, or elevated body temperature) is vital.

SAFETY

ALERT

An elevated white blood cell (WBC) count also suggests an infection and should be communicated immediately to the surgical team. Because infection greatly increases surgical risk, it may be necessary to reschedule elective surgery.

A low WBC count is also a danger sign and may indicate that the client is at risk for infection. A low WBC count may be a manifestation of immunosuppression. People with diabetes mellitus, malnutrition, those who are undergoing radiation therapy or chemotherapy, and those with chronic medical conditions are at high risk of immunosuppression. Steroid use also decreases the client's ability to fight infection; therefore the client taking steroids should be assessed and monitored for immunosuppression.

ESTIMATING MEDICAL RISK FOR SURGERY

Using the information about each client's individual risk and risks associated with the planned operation, each surgeon determines the relative risk versus benefit from the operation for the specific client. In addition, the outcomes for many surgical procedures have been researched, and these figures can be presented to the client and family. The natural history of the condition requiring surgery (that is, the outcome if it remains untreated) is also presented. This information can then be considered by the client and family members before consenting to surgery. The surgeon presents a frank but optimistic discussion of risks of the procedure. Well-intentioned friends and family may wish to shield the client from unpleasant facts. Although medical facts may be unpleasant, it is imperative that the client have full and complete information before consenting. Some clients (such as those with malnutrition or anemia) benefit from waiting for elective surgery.

TABLE 14–2	Categories of Surgical Procedures	
Category	**Purpose**	**Example**
Aesthetic	Improvement of physical features that are within the "normal" range	Breast augmentation
Constructive	Repair of a congenitally defective body part	Cleft palate and cleft lip repair
Curative	Removal or repair of damaged or diseased tissue or organs	Hysterectomy
Diagnostic	Discovery or confirmation of a diagnosis	Breast biopsy
Exploratory	Estimation of extent of disease or confirmation of a diagnosis	Exploratory laparotomy
Emergent	Life-saving	Repair of traumatic punctured lung
Palliative	Relief of symptoms but without cure of underlying disease	Colostomy
Reconstructive	Partial or complete restoration of a body part	Total joint replacement
Urgent	Performed as soon as client is stable and infection is under control	Appendectomy

The type of surgery to be performed also has some inherent risk. The types of operations by category are presented in Table 14-2.

PREOPERATIVE ANESTHESIA EVALUATION

The anesthesia care provider visits the client before surgery to perform a complete respiratory, cardiovascular, and neurologic examination. The client's general surgical risk (the ability of the client to withstand the surgery) is expressed according to the American Society of Anesthesia (ASA) grading system (Box 14-2). Generally, the topics discussed with the client during this examination include the type of anesthesia planned and the sensations the client may experience when undergoing anesthesia. Fears the client has concerning anesthesia are also addressed. The client's risk of side effects and complications is assessed at this time.

The pharmacologic preparation for anesthesia is based on many variables, including the client's age and physical and psychological condition, the type of surgery, and the type of anesthesia to be used. Common preoperative and anesthetic medications are discussed later in the chapter.

PREOPERATIVE EDUCATIONAL ASSESSMENT

The client's experience with previous surgery and the level of anxiety are noted. The client's education level, sensory impairments (e.g., vision loss), expectations regarding the operation, and availability of support systems should guide plans for teaching. In general, clients who have undergone multiple operations need less educational preparation. However, do not assume that such clients need no reinforcement of preoperative and postoperative assessments and interventions.

BOX 14-2   American Society of Anesthesiologists (ASA) Physical Status Classification System

- P1 A normal healthy client
- P2 A client with mild systemic disease
- P3 A client with severe systemic disease
- P4 A client with severe systemic disease that is a constant threat to life
- P5 A moribund client who is not expected to survive without the operation
- P6 A declared brain-dead client whose organs are being removed for donor purposes

Excerpted from ASA Relative Value Guide, 2007, of the American Society of Anesthesiologists. A copy of the full text can be obtained from ASA, 520 N. Northwest Highway, Park Ridge, IL, 60068-2573.

The client undergoing elective surgery and planning to go home the same day requires some additional planning (see the Case Management feature on The Elective Surgery Client on the website).

PREOPERATIVE NURSING DIAGNOSES

Common psychosocial nursing diagnoses during the preoperative period include *Deficient Knowledge related to unfamiliar surgical experience* and *Anxiety and Fear related to pain, death, disfigurement, or the unknown.* The outcomes for these problems must be achievable in a short preoperative time frame.

PREOPERATIVE TEACHING

Preoperative teaching is very important to ensure a positive surgical experience for the client. Numerous research studies have supported the value of preoperative instructions in reducing both the incidence of postoperative complications and the length of stay in the hospital. The client's learning needs, level of anxiety, and fears about surgery are assessed individually so that an individualized teaching plan can be formulated.

The timing of preoperative teaching is highly individualized. Ideally, there would be enough time for the client to be given instructions and time to answer questions. If teaching is done too far in advance, the client may forget important components of the education. On the other hand, a client who is taught immediately before surgery may be too anxious to comprehend what is being taught. In many cases, the client is admitted on the day of surgery. It is imperative that the client has received written or oral instructions before this time, so that the nurse can simply reinforce these instructions and answer individual questions from the client and family members. Many ambulatory surgery or "same-day surgery" centers conduct telephone interviews before admission to educate and allow the client to ask questions.

Being aware of the effects of surgery on cognition, determine learning needs preoperatively and teach both client and family before surgery if at all possible. Only essential activities should be taught in the immediate preoperative period because the client's concentration is likely focused on surviving the surgery. Assess the client's ability to see, hear, and understand verbal communication. Glasses and hearing aids can be worn until the actual surgical procedure to promote learning of necessary information and to reduce apprehension and fear. As the client moves into the operating room, these important items must be carefully stored or given to an accompanying adult. To ensure retrieval after surgery, clearly document on the client record the location of items such as hearing aids and glasses. If any items are lost, the institution is responsible for replacing them.

The client should understand what the preoperative, intraoperative, and postoperative course entails. Before speaking to the client about specific or technical details, consult with the physician to ensure you understand and can clarify this information. Explain all nursing care and any possible discomfort that may result as a consequence of nursing interventions. Tell the client what you will do to minimize any discomfort. If the client is scheduled to go to the surgical intensive care unit (SICU) after the operation, ask what the client and family members already know or have heard about intensive care. Take time to address any misconceptions or incorrect information.

PREOPERATIVE ANXIETY AND FEAR

All people are anxious and fearful of surgery. The extent to which a client fears surgery depends on many factors, such as (1) the seriousness of the operation, (2) individual coping abilities, (3) cultural expectations, and (4) experiences with previous surgery. Well-meaning family members and friends often contribute to the fear level unintentionally. Fear of the unknown is one of the most prevalent causes of preoperative anxiety. During the preoperative phase, clients also fear postoperative pain, the discovery of cancer, the loss of an organ or limb, anesthesia, vulnerability while unconscious, the threat of loss of job or financial security, loss of social and familial roles, disruption of lifestyle, separation from significant others, and death.

Clients respond differently to fear. Some respond by becoming silent and withdrawn, childish, belligerent, evasive, tearful, or clinging. Most clients feel helpless to some extent when admitted to a health care facility. Although surgery may be commonplace for the health care professional, it is a frightening experience for clients and their families. Report extreme anxiety and fear to the anesthesia personnel so that a sedative can be administered. A surgical procedure can be canceled if fear is overwhelming.

Allow the client to take the lead in asking questions concerning surgery and the postoperative period. Provide only as much additional information as the client wants to know. Emphasize that a nurse will be with the client throughout the total surgical experience. Stand close to the client when taking him or her into the operating room. If touch is culturally appropriate, use touch to reassure the client.

If the surgical procedure to be performed has potential long-term effects, support groups may be contacted to offer support preoperatively. Cancer organizations, amputation support groups, and enterostomal therapist associations are examples of large national organizations that offer peer support for clients.

COMPONENTS OF PREOPERATIVE TEACHING

Information provided to the client before surgery should be geared to individual needs. This information can be (1) sensory, (2) psychosocial, or (3) procedural.

Sensory information addresses the sights, sounds, and "feel" of the operating room. Instruct the client that the operating room and skin preparation fluids will be cold but that warm blankets are available. Many surgery suites are now incorporating music into their preoperative and intraoperative areas. Clients may be given headphones and can choose from a variety of music types to help them relax and to reduce external noxious sounds in the operating room environment. If the client wears a hearing aid and music is used, check with the anesthesia personnel to determine whether the hearing aid can remain in place during surgery.

Psychosocial information involves coping abilities and worries about family and similar concerns. Typical questions the client may have are the following: "What if I die?" "Who is going to care for the children?" "What if I become an invalid?" "Who is going to earn enough money to care for my family?" You can provide answers if this information is available, or you can arrange for others, such as a social worker or a member of the clergy, to talk to the client.

Procedural information details activities during the preoperative period and postoperative care. It includes information that the client needs to know and wants to know about what is going to happen. For example, you can state as appropriate: "Your family can be in the presurgical area before you are taken into the operating room," or "There will always be a nurse with you during this time, and I will remain by your side throughout the entire operation." Provide explanations and printed information about health care facility routines, visiting hours, mealtimes, and the locations of the chapel and waiting room, for example. If you find that the client is unclear about what the operation entails, the physician must be notified. You can elaborate or clarify information regarding surgery.

The client's role in postoperative care is taught before surgery. The nurse provides instructions on (1) deep breathing, (2) coughing, (3) turning, (4) ambulating, and (5) pain control, and the client's understanding of some of these procedures is validated by return demonstration.

Deep-Breathing Exercises

To help prevent postoperative surgical complications, careful preoperative instructions and practice in deep-breathing and coughing exercises should be completed and reinforced.

Breathing and coughing exercises help to expand collapsed alveoli in the lungs and to prevent postoperative pneumonia and atelectasis. They also promote faster clearance of inhalation agents from the body. Demonstration of correct deep breathing can be done by inhaling slowly through the nose, distending the abdomen, and exhaling slowly through pursed lips. After demonstrating this method, ask the client to provide a return demonstration to ensure understanding (Figure 14-1). The client is instructed to use this breathing method as often as possible, preferably 5 to 10 times every hour during the postoperative period of immobilization.

Coughing Exercises

Coughing removes retained secretions from the bronchi and larger airways. Coughing may be painful, and analgesia may be required.

For coughing exercise, the client may remain in a sitting or supine position. Teach the client how to splint the surgical incision, to minimize pressure, and to control pain during coughing. Splinting is accomplished by lacing the fingers and holding them tightly across the incision before coughing. A small pillow or folded towel held over the incision also facilitates splinting. For example, some institutions may provide a stuffed pillow such as a heart, and teach the client to "hug the pillow" when coughing. The client is instructed to take three deep breaths, exhaling through the mouth, before coughing from deep in the lungs. Encouragement to perform deep-breathing exercises before coughing is important because the deep breathing assists in stimulating the cough reflex and mobilizing retained secretions. Many clients simply clear their throats when coughing hurts. Encourage true coughing, and use aggressive measures to control pain, with reteaching of the procedure as needed.

Breathing devices, such as incentive spirometers, are often used to promote expansion of the alveoli postoperatively by guiding the client to reach a predetermined level of lung inflation. Use of these devices also strengthens respiratory muscles that were weakened during anesthesia administration. Clients should have the opportunity to practice use of the breathing aids before surgery so that they can use it appropriately afterwards. Most facilities teach clients to use them 5 to 10 times an hour after surgery. If the client has a television in the room, a good way to help the client remember to do breathing exercises is to instruct the client to do the exercises every time there is a commercial.

Turning Exercises

Preoperative clients also need to practice turning from side to side, using the bedside rails to assist movements. Turning helps to prevent venous stasis, thrombophlebitis, pressure ulcer formation, and respiratory complications. The client should be instructed to turn and reposition in bed every 1 to 2 hours during the postoperative period.

Extremity Exercise

Postoperative extremity exercise helps to prevent circulatory problems, such as thrombophlebitis, by facilitating venous return to the heart. The client is taught to flex and extend each joint, particularly the hip, knee, and ankle joints, while lying supine; the lower back is kept flat as the leg is lowered and straightened. The feet can be moved in circular motions while the client is lying down or sitting. The client should be encouraged to practice these exercises before surgery to gain familiarity with the appropriate exercises to be used postoperatively.

Anti-embolism stockings or sequential compression devices may be used on the lower extremities after surgery and can be applied preoperatively or in the

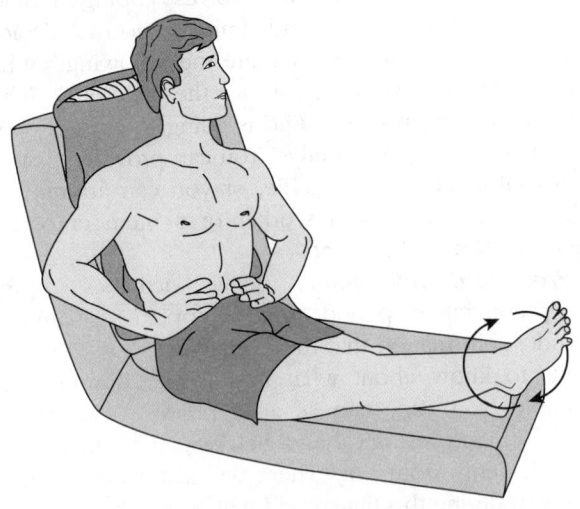

1. Have the client sit upright at the side of the bed or supported in the bed in semi-Fowler's position.
2. Instruct the client to place his or her hands on the abdomen to feel whether the chest rises to indicate that the lungs are expanding.
3. Have the client inhale through the nose until the abdomen distends.
4. Instruct the client to exhale through pursed lips while contracting the abdominal muscles.
5. Instruct the client to wiggle the toes and turn the feet in circles. The client should also try to push the knee down into the mattress or lift the leg if possible.
6. Have the client repeat this exercise every hour during the first postoperative day.

■ **FIGURE 14-1** Exercises after surgery: deep (diaphragmatic) breathing and leg exercises.

operating room. The stockings use a low compression gradient to encourage venous blood flow. Sequential pressure stockings use compression that is applied sequentially up and down the lower extremities to massage the legs rhythmically, for even more effective prevention of clot formation.

Ambulation

Early ambulation should be encouraged whenever appropriate, as it helps to prevent many postoperative complications. Clients are taught the expected ambulation schedule preoperatively so that they have an idea of when they are allowed to get out of bed after surgery. Teaching of proper methods of rising from bed to prevent pain and to minimize orthostatic hypotension is important. With abdominal surgery, one way to minimize pain upon movement is to have the client turn to the side before sitting up in bed. He or she can then push to a sitting position with their arm, which minimizes strain on the abdominal area. The client is instructed to sit up slowly and pause before attempting to stand. Teach the client to use the same splinting method for providing support to the incision that is used during coughing and deep-breathing exercises in order to decrease pain on arising and sitting.

Pain Control

Not having pain controlled after surgery is a common concern among preoperative clients. It is important to reassure clients that their pain will and can be controlled after surgery. Undertreatment of postoperative pain is unacceptable (see Chapter 20). Fears of addiction are unfounded, and clients have suffered needlessly. Preoperatively, teach clients how to communicate their level of pain to the caregiver. For example, they can rate the pain intensity on a scale from 1 to 10, with 1 being no pain to 10 being the most severe possible. Explain the type of pain relief that will be used postoperatively. For example, some surgeons inject the surgical site with a long-acting local anesthetic before closing the wound so that the client will not feel any pain in the site until the medication wears off. Clients who have ambulatory surgery will likely be home when the local anesthetic wears off. Because the stress of surgery or side effects of anesthesia can affect memory temporarily, give instructions on taking the postoperative pain medication before surgery to both the client and accompanying family members.

If the client is to be hospitalized after surgery, explain the type of pain medication used. During the immediate postoperative period, clients can receive medications by an intravenous (IV), intramuscular, or epidural route. Clients on a demand schedule should be taught to ask for pain medications when they are beginning to feel uncomfortable. Clients frequently believe that they should be stoic, and they may hesitate to ask for relief. All clients need to be assured that they will not get addicted to pain medications in the short time for which the pain medication is required. In addition, anticipate pain when the client will be moving for the first time, when breathing or ambulation exercises are performed, or when the analgesia has worn off. At such times, pain medication should be offered. If the client is to have a patient-controlled analgesia (PCA) pump after surgery, demonstrate how the machine operates, and emphasize that safety features on the equipment prevent overdosing. Explain how they can administer their own pain medication when they feel the need, rather than wait for the nurse to assist them. However, without preoperative teaching about these procedures, postoperatively the client will be groggy and sore and may not understand how to control the pain.

Pain can also be controlled through continuous infusion of analgesic agents through an epidural or IV route. Explain the method of planned pain control and how adjustments can be made for comfort.

Equipment

Whenever possible, explain about the equipment that will be used during the perioperative period. Depending on the type of surgery to be performed, various tubes, drains, and IV lines may be used. Discussion should focus on the purpose of specific pieces of equipment and how their use is related to the surgery.

Tubes

The most common type of tube used during the intraoperative period is an indwelling urinary catheter. Another tube commonly used is a nasogastric (NG) tube, which is used to decompress the stomach and upper bowel or to drain the stomach contents. These tubes are often inserted in the operating room and often remain in place until the client is able to move about and eat.

Drains

Drains are inserted to promote evacuation of fluid from the dead space (tissue planes created during the operation) in the operative site. Many different types of drains are used. Drains are frequently attached to mild suction. Hemovac and Jackson-Pratt drains are commonly used low-suction devices.

Intravenous Infusion Devices

IV infusions are usually started before surgery. The purpose of the infusion is to administer medication, fluids, and nutrition solutions. The surgeon may request IV access for use in case of emergency even if the client is not expected to need IV medications.

PREOPERATIVE TEACHING FOR OLDER ADULTS

Older clients usually desire the same basic operative information as that provided for younger clients. You must attend to this need in a sensitive and effective way. Preoperative teaching for older clients should include consideration of possible decreased sensory ability. Sit close to the client when teaching. Speak slowly and use a lower tone of voice. High-pitched sounds are frequently hard for older people to discern. Glare from lights may bother the older client's eyes. Avoid bright lights while preparing the client preoperatively. Because the older client is more prone to hypothermia, apply blankets in the preoperative area if it is the client's desire, and plan an appropriate method of warming in the operating room, where temperatures are usually cool.

IMMEDIATE PREOPERATIVE CARE

PHYSICAL CARE

Prepare the Skin

Explain shower and bathing protocols for the night before a planned surgical procedure. Usually the operative area is cleaned the night before surgery with soap and water or an antimicrobial solution to reduce the number of microbes on the skin. Allergies to chemicals (e.g., iodine) necessitate use of other cleansing agents. Piercings of the skin must be removed to reduce infection or injury. If the skin assessment has identified fragile and delicate skin in an older client, nursing care must involve a gentle method for cleansing skin and hair and for any needed hair removal. Additional considerations may include use of padding over pressure points and tape that will not irritate or rip the skin, as well as lifting—rather than pulling or sliding—the client from bed to bed, to prevent traumatizing the skin.

Prepare the Gastrointestinal Tract

The gastrointestinal tract needs special preparation on the evening before surgery to (1) reduce the possibility of vomiting and aspiration, (2) reduce the risk of possible bowel obstruction, (3) allow visualization of the intestine during bowel surgery, and (4) prevent contamination from fecal material in the intestinal tract during bowel or abdominal surgery.

NPO Status.

SAFETY ALERT

If a client undergoing surgery is to receive a general anesthetic, foods and fluids are restricted for 8 to 10 hours before the operation. This also includes tube feeding. This restriction significantly reduces the possibility of aspiration of gastric contents, which may lead to pneumonia.

Because solid food must be withheld for 8 to 10 hours before surgery, clients who are to undergo anesthetic procedures must be instructed not to eat or drink anything after midnight. Therefore clients are assigned NPO status after midnight the night before surgery is scheduled. If a client scheduled for surgery has eaten or had something to drink after midnight, the surgery may be delayed or postponed. Preoperative care for hospitalized clients also includes the restriction of food and water if anesthesia is to be used.

When a client is on NPO status, perform the following:

- Explain the reason for the fluid and food restriction.
- Remove food and water from the bedside at midnight.
- Place "NPO" signs on the door and on the bed.
- Mark the care plan or Kardex with "NPO."
- Inform the diet and nutrition department about the client's NPO status.
- Inform other caretakers and family members that the client is on NPO status.

If the client has been instructed to take important medications orally before surgery, small sips of water are permitted. For example, a client with cardiovascular disease may need to take heart medications such as digoxin on the morning of surgery. However, the client may have heard preoperative instructions not to eat or drink anything. Make sure that the medication is taken with a sip of water and inform the client that this exception is permissible. Record this medication and the amount of fluid taken on the client care record (Box 14-3).

BOX 14-3   Medications Administered Before Surgery

These medications are often given before surgery. Ask for specific instructions regarding if the client should take these medications.

- Beta-blockers
- Antidysrhythmics
- Antihypertensives
- Inhaled or nebulized bronchodilators
- Anticonvulsants

The following medications are usually not given before surgery. Ask for specific instructions to be certain.

- Oral hypoglycemics—expect that insulin will be used for blood glucose control
- Anticoagulants
- Herbals
- Vitamin supplements
- Lipid-lowering agents

When confirming the fact that a client has maintained NPO status, it is best to ask "When is the last time you had something to eat or drink?" rather than saying "You have not eaten or drank anything since midnight, right?" Some clients will be reluctant to report that they "Had a little coffee before coming in to the hospital"; therefore asking a more general question will usually elicit an accurate response.

Bowel Preparation. Enemas are not routinely ordered during the preoperative period except for surgical procedures involving the gastrointestinal tract, perianal or perineal areas, and the pelvic cavity. The client may perform the enema at home, or the nurse may complete it at the hospital. Some clients may require further bowel cleansing on the morning of surgery. Clients who are to be admitted for same-day surgery are instructed before the surgical date about the need for enemas and whether they will be self-administered. If bowel cleansing is done by the client, ensure that directions are completely understood. Gastrointestinal tubes are usually inserted during surgery for drainage. This procedure is usually performed for clients undergoing major abdominal or intestinal tract surgery.

619271 (CH Rev. 7-96)

I, _____, hereby consent to the procedures outlined below, to be performed by

_____, and his/her associates, assistants, and appropriate hospital personnel.

The procedure proposed is _____

_____

_____

for diagnosis/treatment of _____ .

This procedure has been explained in terms understandable to me, which include the following:

1. The nature and extent of the procedure to be performed and risks involved, including those which, even though unlikely to occur, involve serious consequences.
2. Alternative procedures and methods of treatment.
3. The dangers and probable consequences of such alternatives (including no procedures or treatment).
4. The estimated period of hospitalization and/or incapacity and the estimated period of convalescence (assuming there are no complications).
5. The expected consequences of the procedure upon my future health.
6. I understand that there are other risks, such as the risks of infection and other serious complications, in the preoperative and postoperative stages of my care, which can result in serious consequences such as loss of the use of parts of my body and life.
7. I have asked all of the questions that I thought were important in deciding whether or not to undergo treatment or diagnosis. Those questions have been answered to my satisfaction.
8. I understand that no assurance can be given that the procedure will be successful, and no guarantee or warranty of success or cure has been given to me.
9. I have been advised that I may have anesthesia, which in rare instances has serious and even fatal complications.
10. I further authorize and request my physician and his/her associates, assistants, and appropriate hospital personnel to perform such additional procedures that in their judgment are incidentally necessary or appropriate to carry out my diagnosis/treatment.
11. I have been afforded the opportunity to consult with other physicians to my complete satisfaction before signing this form, and I understand that I have the right to refuse any medical and surgical procedures and treatment.
12. I authorize the hospital to dispose of or use for research any tissue or body parts that may be necessary to remove in a manner consistent with state and federal regulations for such disposal.

I certify that I have read and fully understand the above consent statement, that the explanations are understood by me, that all blanks or statements requiring insertion or completion were filled in prior to the time of my signature, and that this consent was given freely, voluntarily, and without reservation.

Patient's Signature:	Date:	Time:

In the event patient is a minor, unconscious, or otherwise not competent to give consent: I, _____ the (relationship to patient) _____ , of _____ hereby give consent on his/her behalf.		
Witness to Signature:	Date:	Time:

■ **FIGURE 14–2** Consent form for surgery or diagnostic/therapeutic procedures. *(Courtesy Nebraska Medical Center, Omaha, Neb.)*

INFORMED CONSENT

Anyone undergoing any invasive procedure must give informed consent for that procedure to be performed. A *consent form* is the legal document that signifies that the client has been told about and understands all aspects of a specific invasive procedure (Figure 14-2). This document guards the client against unwanted invasive procedures. It also protects the health care facility and health care professionals when a client denies understanding the procedure that was, or is planned to be, performed. Once the operative permit—indicating the client's *informed consent*—is signed, it becomes a permanent part of the client's record. This document accompanies the record to the operating room.

Formal consent is necessary for each invasive procedure. The client or the client's legal surrogate must receive a full explanation of the operation before giving verbal and written consent. Pictures and diagrams may be necessary for a complete understanding of the surgical procedure. Moreover, the client or the surrogate must be told about who will perform the surgery; anesthesia and anesthetic choices; potential risks, complications, and risk of disfigurement or death; and whether organs or body parts may be removed. The client or the surrogate is also informed about alternative treatments. The surgeon must explain the procedure in terms and language the client or the surrogate readily understands. You are responsible for ensuring that the client or the surrogate receives an honest, accurate, and fair statement of what to expect during and after surgery and that the client understands it before informed consent is given. If the client requires consent in a language other than that printed in the form and the person obtaining consent is not fluid in his or her language, an interpreter must be used. The presence of an interpreter during consent must be documented.

The procedure for obtaining an informed consent varies from state to state and according to the individual policy for each health care facility. Generally, the surgeon explains the surgical procedure, the possible risks and complications, and the alternatives. The nurse may obtain and witness the client's signature on the consent form and may help to reinforce what the client has been told by the surgeon. It is not appropriate for the nurse to explain the surgical procedure, risks, complications, and alternatives unless this is done for reinforcement or clarification. The consent must be signed before the client receives any medication that may alter consciousness.

Adults sign their own operative permit unless they are medicated with drugs that could impair their ability to comprehend, unconscious or mentally incompetent. In such cases a surrogate, such as a relative or a legal guardian, is responsible for consent. If the relative or the guardian is out of state, consent can be secured via the telephone in the presence of one or two witnesses. If no relative or guardian can be found, one can be appointed by court order.

Children under legal age who are not emancipated minors must have consent given by the child's parent or legal guardian. Emancipated minors are considered to be those who are under the legal age of emancipation but because of marriage or other circumstances are independent of the parents. If the child's parent or guardian cannot be present to sign the permit, consent can be obtained from an appropriate person by telephone, Fax, or letter. When a minor's relatives cannot be located, the state in which the surgery is to be performed provides written procedures to follow in order to obtain consent via a court order.

PREPARING THE CLIENT ON THE DAY OF SURGERY

Many clients are admitted into the hospital or surgical center the morning of surgery. These clients can be admitted to the hospital after the procedure if their condition requires specialized observation or nursing care. For so-called ambulatory surgery or same-day surgery, clients come to the hospital or surgery suite the morning of surgery but go home the same day to the care of family members or significant others. The ambulatory surgery approach presents a dilemma in providing preoperative instruction to the client, because time is very limited during the admission period before the actual surgical event. Often, the nurse will telephone the night before the procedure to remind the client of any preoperative instructions. Instructions are reinforced about evening showers or baths, starting NPO status after midnight, wearing washable clothing that is easily removed and put back on, wearing flat shoes, not wearing pantyhose, and securing a ride home after the procedure. The nurse conducting the telephone educational session should convey a positive attitude about the planned surgical procedure and assist in allaying doubts or fears related to the surgery.

PREOPERATIVE PREPARATION IMMEDIATELY BEFORE SURGERY

Final preoperative preparation begins 1 to 2 hours before surgery for clients in the hospital or upon admission for same-day admission clients. Ask the client whether there are any unanswered questions or concerns. Make sure that the client understands the operative procedure to be performed, and continue to assess for manifestations of anxiety. Delays in performing the surgery should be communicated to the client and family.

To prevent omissions in preoperative nursing interventions, most facilities supply nurses with a preoperative checklist.

As each intervention on the list is completed, initial it on the form. An example of a preoperative checklist is provided in Box 14-4. Individual surgical centers may include various other actions on this form. You may need to give medications ordered preoperatively to the client before going to the operating room. You must know the approximate time when the surgical procedure is scheduled and must begin the preoperative activities early enough to have them completed when the operating room is ready.

The surgeon often examines the client before transportation into the operating suites. The surgical site is confirmed with the client. The surgeon then initials the surgical site so that when the client arrives in the operating room there is no confusion about which body area is to have surgery; this helps prevent wrong-site surgery.

PREOPERATIVE MEDICATIONS

An IV is started and fluids are provided to reduce any dehydration from being NPO. Preoperative medications are given IV to allay anxiety, to reduce side effects of anesthetic agents, and to induce amnesia. Specific drug choices are based on individual client variables, the goals of sedation, and the potential for undesirable side effects.

Preoperative medications may be given in the preoperative holding area or on the nursing unit.

Safety precautions must be taken when administering preoperative medications.

SAFETY ALERT

Before administering preoperative medications, ensure that the operative permit is correctly signed because legal consent cannot be given by a medicated adult. Have the client void before medication administration so the client will not have to get out of bed again. After administering preoperative medication, place the bed in the lowest position and raise the side rails of the bed to reduce the risk of falls. Instruct the client not to get up without assistance because the medications are likely to cause drowsiness or dizziness. Document all actions and reactions of the client during this time. Once the client is calm and drowsy, disruptions should take place only when necessary and then be brief. Observe the client for side effects (e.g., hypotension and respiratory distress).

TRANSPORTING THE CLIENT TO SURGERY

When surgical personnel call for the client, the client is gently transferred to a stretcher. Adequate assistance for transfer must be obtained to reduce the possibility of injury to the client and staff. Appropriate covering is provided for the client, and side rails are raised. The medical record accompanies the client to the operating room. The trip to surgery should be as smooth as possible so that the sedated client does not experience nausea and dizziness.

BOX 14-4   Immediate Preoperative Activities

Before the client enters the operating room, ensure that the following activities have been completed:

- The identification band is present and correct.
- All known allergies are recorded and an allergy wristband is present if indicated.
- Vital signs are checked and recorded. Report marked differences from baseline to the surgeon or anesthesia personnel.
- The consent form is signed and the surgical procedure is listed correctly.
- Skin preparation is completed if ordered preoperatively.
- Any special orders, such as administering enemas or starting an intravenous line, are completed.
- The client has not eaten or had fluids by mouth for the last 8 hours.
- The client has just voided; measure and record the amount of urine (if indicated).
- Oral hygiene or other physical care is completed.
- Dentures are removed and stored carefully.

- The presence of dental bridgework, loose teeth or other prostheses is noted, and the anesthesia personnel know about it.
- The perioperative nurse is notified about the presence of a hearing aid. Leave it in place so that operating room personnel can communicate with the client.
- Storage is arranged and documented for valuables according to health care facility policy, or valuables are given to family members.
- The client has removed jewelry and any piercings. (Many facilities allow the client to wear the wedding band as long as it is secured with a Band-Aid.) If jewelry is removed, it should be stored according to policy or given to the family. Assist with the removal of hairpins or wigs, for example.
- The client is wearing a hospital gown and protective cap. Elastic bandaging or anti-embolic hose has been applied, if ordered.
- Make-up is removed so skin color can be observed.

PREPARING THE CLIENT'S ROOM FOR POSTOPERATIVE CARE

For those clients that are 23-hour admit, or hospital clients, the client's room should be prepared so that the initial care of the client on return from surgery can be orderly. Furniture should be arranged so that the stretcher can easily be brought to the bedside. The bed should be placed in high position and made with clean linen in an open position. Bed rails should be down on the receiving side and up on the other side. An emesis basin should be located close to the bed. Blood pressure monitoring equipment, IV setup, suction, and oxygen should be nearby. All equipment should be tested to ensure it is in working condition before the client arrives.

CARING FOR SIGNIFICANT OTHERS

A designated waiting area is usually provided for family members during surgery. If family members plan on leaving the facility during the procedure, ensure that there is a way to contact them and supply them with a phone number to the nurses' station and client's room. Some institutions issue pagers to those waiting, so they can feel free to go to the cafeteria and still remain in touch.

When discussing the surgical procedure with the client's significant others, be sure that you are located in a private area and provide answers congruent with the information that the surgeon has already provided. Family members should also be prepared for any equipment that may accompany the client postoperatively. A preoperative explanation will assist the family in understanding what equipment is attached to their loved one, and why. Significant others need to be informed when surgery is completed or if there are any delays. The surgeon should speak with family members as soon as possible after completion of the procedure.

INTRAOPERATIVE PERIOD

Nursing care during the intraoperative phase focuses on the client's emotional well-being as well as on physical factors such as safety, positioning, maintaining asepsis, and controlling the surgical environment. The preoperative assessment assists the nurse in planning appropriate interventions for this phase of the surgical experience. The nurse remains the client's advocate during this period, anticipating and guarding against potential complications. Whereas the surgeon concentrates on performing the surgical procedure and the anesthesia provider concentrates on the client's breathing and on maintenance of the client's physiologic stability, the circulating nurse is responsible for all other activities that take place in the operating room.

MEMBERS OF THE SURGICAL TEAM

The surgical team is a group of highly trained and educated professionals who coordinate their efforts to ensure the welfare and safety of the client. Although the specifics of each type of surgical procedure may vary, certain key players must always be present, such as the surgeon, an anesthesia provider, the circulating nurse, and scrub personnel.

The surgeon heads the surgical team and makes decisions concerning the surgical procedure. Depending on the surgical procedure to be performed, a second surgeon or a registered nurse with additional education and training may serve as a first assistant (RNFA). The anesthesiologist or certified registered nurse anesthetist (CRNA) provides anesthesia, alleviates pain, and promotes relaxation with medications. The anesthesia provider maintains the airway, ensures adequate gas exchange, monitors circulation and respiration, estimates blood and fluid loss, infuses blood and fluids, administers medications to maintain hemodynamic stability, and alerts the surgeon immediately to any complications. The circulating nurse is a registered nurse and a core member of the surgical team. Other roles for RNs in surgery are discussed in Box 14-5.

> **The circulating nursing and the scrub person count together all materials that are used, such as needles, instruments, and sponges. Counts must be correct before closing any body cavity and the surgical wound.**

Depending on the specific surgical procedure, the surgical team may include other members—for instance, a pathologist may be called in to identify tissue, an x-ray technician may be needed to perform various radiologic procedures, or a perfusionist may be required when cardiac bypass is necessary.

ANESTHESIA

Anesthesia is an artificially induced state of partial or total loss of sensation with or without loss of consciousness. Anesthetic agents can produce muscle relaxation, block transmission of pain nerve impulses, and suppress reflexes. Anesthesia can also temporarily decrease memory retrieval and recall. The depth and effects of anesthesia are monitored by observing changes in respiration, oxygen saturation and end-tidal carbon dioxide (CO_2) levels, heart rate, urine output, and blood pressure.

BOX 14-5   Roles of the Perioperative Nurse

Perioperative nursing is performed preoperatively, intraoperatively, and postoperatively. Each of these periods is characterized by specific actions required by nurses, who participate both independently and as part of a health care team. Some of the more common roles for RNs are discussed below.

CIRCULATING NURSE

The circulating role is a major one for perioperative nurses. A nurse functioning as a circulator should be a registered nurse (RN). The circulator assesses the client preoperatively, plans for optimal care during the surgical intervention, coordinates all personnel within the operating room, monitors unlicensed personnel, and monitors responsible cost compliance associated with operating room procedures. The circulator does not wear sterile clothing and can go in and out of the operating room. In addition to caring directly for the client, the circulator has very defined activities during surgery. These include the following:

- Ensuring all equipment is working properly
- Guaranteeing sterility of instruments and supplies
- Assisting with positioning
- Performing surgical skin preparation
- Monitoring the room and team members for breaks in sterile technique
- Assisting anesthesia personnel with induction and physiologic monitoring
- Handling specimens
- Coordinating activities with other departments, such as radiology and pathology
- Documenting care provided
- Minimizing conversation and traffic within the operating room suite

SCRUB NURSE

An RN or surgical technician (ST) can perform the role of scrub person. The duties include gathering all equipment for the procedure, preparing all supplies and instruments using sterile technique, maintaining sterility within the sterile field during surgery, handling instruments and supplies during surgery, and cleaning up after the case. During surgery, the scrub person maintains an accurate count of sponges, sharps, and instruments on the sterile field and counts the same materials with the circulating nurse before and after the surgery.

REGISTERED NURSE FIRST ASSISTANT

The RNFA is an experienced perioperative nurse who has had additional specialized education. The RNFA works with the primary surgeon during the surgery. This is a role separate from that of the scrub person. Some of the activities of an RNFA include providing exposure of the surgical area, using instruments to hold and cut, retracting and handling tissue, providing hemostasis, and suturing. RNFAs must work with a surgeon and are not independent practitioners.

CERTIFIED REGISTERED NURSE ANESTHETIST

The CRNA is a nurse specializing in the administration of anesthetics. Entry into a CRNA program usually requires a bachelor of science degree in nursing or other appropriate field plus 1 to 2 years of acute or intensive care nursing experience. These nurses work under the direction of an anesthesiologist.

MANAGER/DIRECTOR

The manager of the operating room has extensive experience and has additional education in management. It can be any RN, but hospitals today prefer candidates with a bachelor of science in nursing (BSN). Many large hospitals now require a master's of science in nursing (MSN) degree with a major in acute care or management.

EDUCATOR

Educators are responsible for staff continuing education, orientation of new staff, and working with staff to learn how to be preceptors to students. Educators can be any RN, but usually nurses with a BSN or MSN who are experienced perioperative nurses are best qualified. These nurses may also fulfill the role of circulator or clinical nurse specialist outside their teaching responsibilities.

CASE MANAGER

The perioperative case manager coordinates the care of the perioperative client. The position requires extensive experience, an ability to communicate, and a knowledge of the total surgical episode from home before surgery to home care needs after surgery.

ADVANCED PRACTICE NURSE CLINICAL NURSE SPECIALIST

The APN is an RN with an advanced degree and skills. This nurse must hold a minimum of a master's degree in nursing, and be certified as a clinical nurse specialist or a nurse practitioner (NP). The APN is a clinical expert who practices in hospitals, ambulatory surgery centers, or surgical physician groups. APNs most often have a surgical specialty (e.g., orthopedics, cardiovascular). Their roles include consultation, education, direct client care, management, translating research to practice, and using evidence to define best practice. A perioperative APN may not always be in the operating room, but may interact with clients in offices, homes, hospital units, or other sites as needed.

Most clients are anxious about the anesthesia. Some are concerned about the adequacy of the pain-blocking effects, whereas others are concerned about being "put to sleep" with a drug. Some clients wonder whether they will talk during anesthesia or will experience nausea and vomiting postoperatively. Nurses must respond to these concerns by providing reassurance about the capability of the anesthesia provider and about the availability of other drugs to reduce any unpleasant side effects of the anesthesia.

The client needs frequent reminders to let the nurse or the physician know immediately about any side effects experienced from the anesthesia, and the nurse must remain diligent in assessing for any possible complications. Alert the anesthesia provider immediately of any side effects.

The decision about the type of anesthesia to be used is made by the anesthesia provider in consultation with the surgeon and the client. The choice of anesthetic agent for a surgical procedure depends on many variables. The two major techniques in anesthesia are general and regional.

Agents for *general anesthesia* block the pain stimulus at the cerebral cortex and induce depression of the central nervous system (CNS) that is reversed either by metabolic change and elimination from the body or by pharmacologic means. General anesthetic agents produce analgesia, amnesia, unconsciousness, and loss of reflexes and muscle tone. The neurologic, respiratory, and cardiovascular systems are affected by these agents. General anesthesia is best suited for surgery on the head, neck, upper torso, and back; for prolonged surgical procedures; or for use in clients who are unable to lie quietly for a long period of time. General anesthetic agents affect all tissues in the body to some degree.

In *regional anesthesia,* drugs are given to block the pain stimulus at its origin, along afferent neurons, or along the spinal cord. Unlike general anesthesia, regional anesthesia produces a loss of sensation and position in only one region of the body and does not result in unconsciousness. Regional anesthesia includes spinal anesthesia, epidural anesthesia, and peripheral nerve blocks. In addition to the regional anesthetic agent, the client also may receive sedative agents that produce drowsiness.

Monitored Anesthesia Care

When anesthesia providers participate in the sedation of clients having surgery, the procedure is termed monitored anesthesia care. A wide range of depths of sedation are seen, ranging from minimal sedation to brief episodes of complete unconsciousness. Monitored anesthesia is used during an operation in which the surgeon infiltrates the surgical site with a local anesthetic and the anesthesia provider supplements the local anesthetic with IV drugs to provide sedation and systemic analgesia. The anesthesia care provider monitors the client's blood pressure, heart rate, and respiration while the local anesthetic and IV support are being provided. *Local standby* and *anesthesia standby* also refer to monitored anesthesia.

Conscious Sedation

When anesthesia providers do not provide sedation, the process is generally called conscious sedation. Under conscious sedation, the client is moderately sedated with morphine or fentanyl and midazolam (Versed). The client can respond purposefully to verbal or tactile stimulation, maintains airway patency, has adequate spontaneous respirations, and maintains his or her own cardiovascular function. There is a narrow range between minimal sedation, which would be inadequate for surgery, and deep sedation, which may result in airway compromise, respiratory depression, and cardiovascular depression. Because of the risks associated with conscious sedation, clients are closely monitored by trained personnel and emergency resuscitation equipment is readily available. RNs are frequently prepared to administer conscious sedation. If so, adequate additional education and training must be provided for the nurse. Many institutions require competency testing for this skill.

General Anesthesia
Stages of Anesthesia

When clients were anesthetized with ether and chloroform many years ago, they progressed slowly from an awake state to unconsciousness. Clients would spend several minutes in a stage of excitement and agitation. Four stages of anesthesia were identified, and specific care was required at each stage. Today the stages are indistinguishable because the new anesthetic agents promote sedation and analgesia so quickly that the stages are difficult to impossible to visually determine. However, even though the stages of anesthesia are not readily apparent, they still occur.

The last sense to be depressed during induction is hearing; remember to maintain a quiet atmosphere during this time. The client can hear and may remember conversations upon awakening. The nurse, always remaining the client's advocate, ensures that all conversation during induction and throughout the case is appropriate. Clients emerge into consciousness backward through all three stages of anesthesia after the anesthetic agents are discontinued. Therefore hearing is the first sense to return.

Administration of General Anesthesia

General anesthesia can be administered in a variety of ways. The most common method of administering anesthesia is to use a combination of agents based on the client's need with consideration of the type of surgery to be performed. Anesthesia is typically achieved with a combination of an inhalation agent, oxygen, a narcotic, and a neuromuscular blocking agent. As discussed in the Integrating Pharmacology feature on p. 203, inhalation and the IV route are the most common routes of administration during surgery.

Medications Used in Surgery

Several medications are typically given to a client before, during, and even after surgery. These medications, most of them anesthetics, are given with the goal of having the client unconscious and with no memory of the event and no pain. In addition, reflexes that would impair the operation need to be suppressed. In the past 40 years tremendous advances have occurred in anesthesia. Today, medications are short acting and monitors are very sophisticated, making anesthesia for surgery a safe experience for almost all clients.

While the client is in the preoperative holding area, tranquilizers such as diazepam or midazolam are given to reduce anxiety and calm the client. Most clients will have no memory of events after they are given midazolam (Versed). However, they do remain awake and able to maintain their own airway.

Once the client is in the operating room, inhalation anesthetics are the main form of anesthesia. Nitrous oxide is the most common drug given and it produces unconsciousness and pain relief. Most clients are given nitrous oxide for induction. Depending on the type of surgery, it may or may not be given during the case. Other inhalation anesthetics, such as isoflurane, are given to maintain the anesthesia along with oxygen.

Anesthesia can also be given with intravenous medications. Thiopental is one of the most common agents used. It produces rapid unconsciousness, so it is commonly used for induction. Other agents given intravenously include propofol; this drug is commonly used for outpatient operations.

Opioids are also given to clients having surgery. Medications such as morphine or fentanyl are commonly used, and they provide analgesia and allow less of the other anesthetics to be used while maintaining an anesthetic state. Opioids can produce respiratory depression, so if they are given to clients who are not intubated, the client must be observed closely for hypoxemia.

Neuromuscular blocking agents are used for two purposes. At the beginning of the case, succinylcholine is used for intubation. It is a short-acting medication, but does have some serious potential side effects. They include triggering malignant hyperthermia in high-risk clients and muscle twitching that may cause muscle pain after surgery. Later, if the operation requires that muscles relax to gain exposure, nondepolarizing medications are used, such as vecuronium and pancuronium. Because the response to these longer-acting blocking agents is not predictable, the medications are reversed at the end of the case and the adequacy of the reversal is assessed.

If the client has a history of nausea and vomiting, medications, such as ondansetron can be given before the case is finished. Clients with reflux disease may be given medications to block production of stomach acid.

Types of General Anesthesia

Intravenous Anesthesia

When general anesthesia is administered intravenously the client experiences an extremely rapid loss of consciousness, generally 30 seconds after the medication is administered. This process promotes a rapid transition from the conscious stage to the surgical anesthesia stage. It also prepares the client for a smooth transition to the surgical stage of anesthesia, as the IV anesthetic can act as a calming agent. IV anesthesia is sufficiently potent to be used alone in such minor procedures as dental extractions and pelvic examinations. Examples of IV anesthetics are thiopental sodium and ketamine.

Inhalation Anesthesia

For inhalation anesthesia, a mixture of volatile liquids or gas and oxygen is used. The word "volatile" means that these medications are exhaled through the lungs. These are usually used to maintain the client's anesthesia following induction. The mixture is given through a mask or through an endotracheal tube (Figure 14-3).

When inhalation anesthetic agents are administered by mask, the gases generally flow into the mask via a finely calibrated vaporizer that is controlled by a machine. When an endotracheal tube is used to give the anesthetic, the gases flow directly into the client's tracheobronchial tree, resulting in a very quick response. Many different liquids and gases are used in inhalation anesthesia. A commonly used gas anesthetic is nitrous oxide, and isoflurane is a typical liquid anesthetic.

Steps in Typical General Anesthesia

Sedation

For clients who have not received an oral sedative, intravenous sedation is usually provided while still in the preoperative holding area. Common agents used include midazolam or diazepam. When the client is moved to the operating

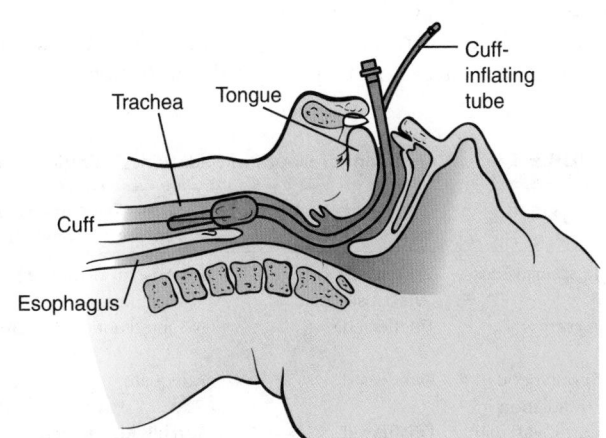

■ **FIGURE 14–3** Correct placement of the endotracheal tube for anesthesia administration.

room, they are asked to breathe oxygen through a face mask while the monitoring devices are applied. The face mask provides a reservoir of oxygen should induction or intubation be prolonged. Intubation may be prolonged in clients who are obese because of their typically thickened neck and in clients with arthritis of the neck or a neck fracture.

Induction

Induction is an important aspect of anesthesia. During induction the client is given very short-acting medications (e.g., thiopental) to produce unconsciousness and a neuromuscular blocking agent, such as succinylcholine, to cause paralysis. During induction, the client's airway is intubated.

Maintenance

Once the airway is intubated, the client can be positioned, prepped, and draped for the operation. Various medications, such as opioids, hypnotics, nitrous oxide, and anesthetics, are given to keep the client anesthetized during the various stages of the operation. For example, during skin cleansing, use of anesthetics is minimal. In contrast, when the surgeon incises and retracts the skin, stronger anesthetic agents are used to produce deep anesthesia. The depths of anesthesia are shown in Table 14-3.

Emergence

As the operation concludes, the anesthetics are stopped and reversed so that the client can emerge from anesthesia. Extubation is completed when the client can follow commands and spontaneously breathe.

Regional Anesthesia

Regional anesthetics are useful in many clinical situations. Local anesthetic agents, which are used to obtain local anesthesia, can also be administered to function as a central, peripheral, IV, regional, retrobulbar, or transbronchial nerve block. These anesthetic agents block the conduction of impulses in the nerve fibers without depolarizing the cell membrane.

Epinephrine can be added to many of the local anesthetics in an effort to prolong the anesthetic effect.

Epinephrine also causes local blood vessels to constrict, thus delaying absorption of the anesthetic agent. This vasoconstriction can also reduce bleeding. Epinephrine should be used with caution in older adults with cardiovascular or liver disease. Traditionally, epinephrine was not used in hand or foot surgery because of the small blood vessels in the area. However, as discussed in the Integrating Pharmacology feature below, the use of epinephrine in hand and foot surgery has recently been reevaluated.

INTEGRATING PHARMACOLOGY

Local Anesthetics

Local anesthetics are an important aspect of many operations and are used commonly in procedures done at the bedside or in diagnostic and treatment laboratories. The mechanism of action is dose-dependent; that is, the more anesthetic that is given, the more numbness will be created. However, it is crucial to be aware of the risk of toxicity with these agents.

Local anesthetics exist in two classes: the aminoesters and the aminoamides (often called esters and amides). The most common local anesthetics, lidocaine and bupivacaine, are amides. Lidocaine has an onset of 10 to 20 minutes and lasts up to 180 minutes. Bupivacaine's onset is slower at 15 to 30 minutes, but has twice the duration, up to 360 minutes. As common as these medications are in clinical practice, they are usually not effective in acidotic, inflamed tissues because they are in a form that cannot penetrate nerves.

When using local anesthetics, the priority is to prevent toxicity. When used for regional anesthesia, toxicity depends on the location and the speed of absorption. The main clinical manifestations of toxicity are cardiac and neurologic. The earliest signs of toxicity are numbness and tingling of the tongue, a metallic taste, lightheadedness, tinnitus, or visual problems. Toxicity can progress to slurred speech, disorientation, and seizures. Coma and respiratory arrest can ensue. It is important to talk with the client during procedures that involve local anesthesia, so that patterns of speech can be heard.

Methods to reduce risk include aspirating any syringe of local anesthetic to avoid injecting directly into blood vessels. The use of epinephrine along with local anesthetics will delay absorption by causing vasoconstriction. Toxicity is treated with oxygen and support of the airway and respirations.

	Minimal Sedation (Anxiolysis)	Moderate Sedation/Analgesia ("Conscious Sedation")	Deep Sedation/Analgesia	General Anesthesia
Responsiveness	Normal response to verbal stimulation	Purposeful response to verbal or tactile stimulation	Purposeful response following repeated or painful stimulation	Unarousable even with painful stimulus
Airway	Unaffected	No intervention required	Intervention may be required	Intervention often required
Spontaneous ventilation	Unaffected	Adequate	May be inadequate	Frequently inadequate
Cardiovascular function	Unaffected	Usually maintained	Usually maintained	May be impaired

TABLE 14-3 Continuum of Depth of Sedation, Definition of General Anesthesia, and Levels of Sedation/Analgesia

Excerpted from Continuum of Depth of Sedation, Definition of General Anesthesia, and Levels of Sedation/Analgesia, 2004, of the American Society of Anesthesiologists. A copy of the full text can be obtained from ASA, 520 N. Northwest Highway, Park Ridge, IL, 60068–2573.

Types of Regional Anesthesia

Regional anesthesia can be administered in a variety of different ways: spinal, epidural, caudal, topical, local infiltration, field block, peripheral nerve block, and IV regional block.

Spinal Anesthesia

Spinal anesthesia offers many advantages for clients undergoing surgical procedures involving the lower half of the body. It is often the anesthetic technique of choice for older adults because of its overall favorable profile. Benefits of spinal anesthesia include its relative safety, excellent lower body muscle relaxation, and absence of effect on consciousness; furthermore, its use does not require an empty stomach. Spinal anesthesia is achieved by injecting local anesthetics into the subarachnoid space (Figure 14-4).

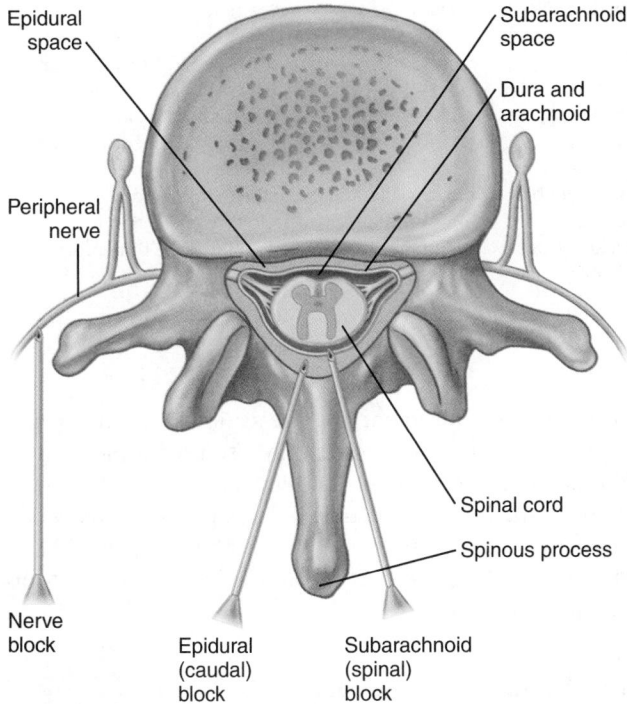

FIGURE 14–4 Cross-section of a lumbar vertebra showing injection sites for anesthesia.

Autonomic nerve fibers are affected first and are also the last to recover. After blockade of the autonomic nervous system, spinal anesthesia blocks the following fibers in this order: (1) touch, (2) pain, (3) motor, (4) pressure, and (5) proprioceptive fibers—these fibers alert the brain of physical orientation. Recovery is in the reverse order.

Spinal anesthesia can be used for almost any type of major procedure performed below the level of the diaphragm, such as a hysterectomy or appendectomy. Figure 14-5 illustrates proper positioning for injection of drugs for spinal anesthesia. Within minutes of administration the client experiences a loss of sensation and paralysis of the toes, feet, legs, and then abdomen. Most clients exhibit a slight hypotension initially because of the vasodilation that occurs with administration of the spinal anesthetic.

The complications of spinal anesthesia are listed and described in Table 14-4, along with prevention and intervention suggestions for nurses.

> **As with any anesthesia, the client who has undergone spinal anesthesia is at risk for neurologic, respiratory, or cardiovascular complications.**

SAFETY ALERT

However, usually the risk with spinal anesthesia is no greater than that with general anesthesia.

Epidural Anesthesia

An epidural block is achieved by introduction of an anesthetic agent into the epidural space (see Figure 14-4). The epidural space is generally entered by a needle at a thoracic, lumbar, sacral, or caudal interspace. The needle is carefully positioned in the epidural space without penetrating the dura and without entering the subarachnoid space. When the needle is properly positioned, the cerebrospinal fluid (CSF) cannot be aspirated. An epidural block, like spinal anesthesia, produces a blockade of the autonomic nerves and hypotension can result. If the level of the block is too high and the respiratory muscles are affected, then respiratory depression or paralysis may occur.

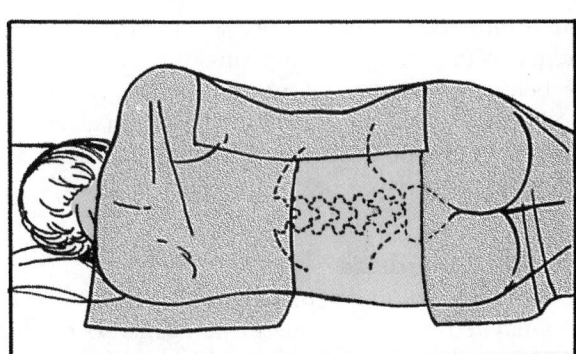
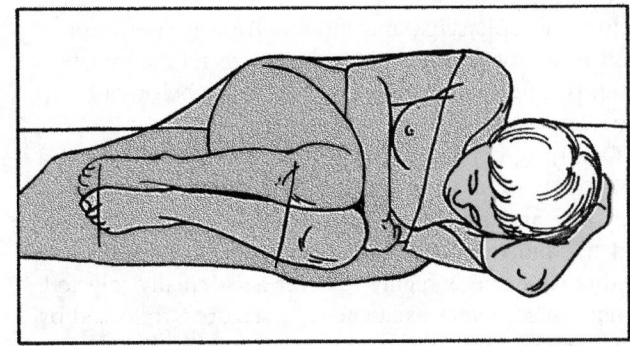

FIGURE 14–5 Proper positioning for spinal anesthesia administration flexes the client's torso to expand the space between the lumbar vertebrae.

TABLE 14-4 Complications and Discomforts of Spinal Anesthesia

Complications and Discomforts	Causes	Intervention	Prevention
Hypotension	Paralysis of vasomotor nerves; usually occurs shortly after induction of anesthesia	Administer oxygen by inhalation Administer vasoactive drugs Position in Trendelenburg's if level of anesthesia is fixed, 10-20 min after induction	In clients not prone to heart failure, 500-800 ml of IV fluids, administered rapidly before block
Nausea and vomiting	Occurs mainly from abdominal surgery because of traction placed on various structures within abdomen or from hypotension	Administer ephedrine, antiemetics, oxygen, or fluids	
Headache (can be extremely painful, may last a week)	Cerebrospinal fluid (which cushions brain) is lost through dural hole; leakage of fluid with loss of cushioning effect increased by (1) use of a large spinal needle or (2) poor hydration	Apply tight abdominal binder Provide fluids Administer analgesics In severe cases, inject 10 ml of client's blood to plug hole (blood patch)	Use of very small spinal needle reduces incidence of spinal headache to 0.9% Administer IV and oral fluids before and after induction of spinal anesthesia Keep client flat and quiet 6-8 hr postoperatively
Respiratory paralysis	Occurs if drug reaches upper thoracic and cervical spinal levels in large amounts or in heavy concentrations	Provide artificial respiration	Avoid extreme Trendelenburg's position before level of spinal anesthesia set, i.e., 10-20 min after induction
Neurologic complications (e.g., paraplegia, severe muscle weakness in legs)	Paralysis postoperatively may be due to (1) unsterile needles, syringes, and anesthetic medications; (2) pre-existing diseases of CNS (e.g., multiple sclerosis and spinal cord tumors), which cause paralysis, rather than spinal anesthesia itself; (3) transient response to anesthetics; (4) position during surgery	Provide supportive care for transient forms related to medication Provide antibiotics and steroids for infectious causes Permanent paralysis will require rehabilitation	Use strict sterile technique Use heat-sterilized medications and instruments Perform careful preoperative neurologic examination to ascertain presence of neurologic disease

CNS, Central nervous system; IV, intravenous.

Caudal Anesthesia

Caudal anesthesia, also called saddle anesthesia or block, is produced by injection of the local anesthetic into the caudal or sacral canal. Caudal anesthesia is a variation of epidural anesthesia. This method is commonly used with obstetric clients.

Topical Anesthesia

Topical anesthetic agents may be directly applied onto the area to be desensitized. The anesthetic may be a solution, an ointment, a gel, a cream, or a powder. This short-acting form of anesthesia can block peripheral nerve endings in the mucous membranes of the vagina, rectum, nasopharynx, and mouth. Topical anesthesia is used in minor procedures such as a rectal examination when painful hemorrhoids are present or before a bronchoscopy to desensitize the bronchi.

One drug commonly used for topical anesthesia is a 4% to 10% solution of cocaine. This agent is for topical use only and is primarily used to anesthetize the eye and the mucous membranes of the nose, mouth, and urethra. Cocaine is highly toxic. If accidentally injected, it may cause severe excitement or seizures, followed by shock, respiratory failure, and cardiac arrest. Emergency resuscitation equipment must be available when cocaine is used. Other agents commonly used for topical anesthesia include tetracaine, procaine, mepivacaine, bupivacaine, and lidocaine. To avoid anaphylactic reactions from previous sensitization to anesthetic agents, check the client's drug allergies before application of any topical anesthetic agent.

Local Infiltration Anesthesia

Local infiltration anesthesia involves injection of an anesthetic agent such as lidocaine (Xylocaine) into the skin and subcutaneous tissue of the area to be anesthetized. Local anesthesia blocks only the peripheral nerves around the area of the incision. When local anesthetic is administered, the person injecting the drug must aspirate before injection to ensure the needle is not in a blood vessel. If a local anesthetic agent is inadvertently injected into the bloodstream, it becomes systemic, and cardiovascular collapse or convulsions could result.

Field Block Anesthesia

The area proximal to a planned incision can be injected and infiltrated with local anesthetic agents to produce what is known as a *field block*. This block forms a barrier between the incision and the nervous system. This procedure differs from simple injection of a local anesthetic, in which only the area of the incision is injected. A field block actually barricades the area around the incision and prevents transmission of sensory impulses to the brain from that area. The anesthesia provider must take precautions when performing a field block to avoid injection of the agent into a blood vessel.

Peripheral Nerve Block Anesthesia

A *nerve block* anesthetizes individual nerves or nerve plexuses rather than all the local nerves anesthetized by a field block. Nerve blocks can be obtained in a finger (digital nerve block), the entire upper arm (brachial plexus nerve block), or the chest or abdominal wall (intercostal nerve block). Nerves most commonly blocked are those within the brachial plexus and the intercostal, sciatic, and femoral nerves. Drugs commonly used as nerve block agents are lidocaine, bupivacaine, and mepivacaine. The anesthesia provider injects the anesthetic along the nerve rather than into the nerve in an effort to decrease the risk of nerve damage. Once the drug has been injected, it takes several minutes for onset of the anesthesia.

Nerve blocks, like local infiltration blocks, can produce severe systemic response if the drug is accidentally injected into a blood vessel. Because epinephrine causes vasoconstriction, particularly in the extremities, anesthetic procedures for surgery performed below the wrist or ankle typically use agents that do not contain epinephrine.

Intravenous Regional Extremity Block Anesthesia (Bier Block)

Regional anesthesia of a limb can be achieved with an agent such as lidocaine when it is injected into a vein of the limb to be anesthetized. A pneumatic dual-cuff tourniquet applied to the anesthetized area prevents the lidocaine from circulating beyond the area undergoing the procedure. This type of anesthesia is used most commonly for procedures of the extremities that are of short duration. The tourniquet can be inflated only for 2-hour increments.

Other Methods of Anesthesia and Analgesia
Acupuncture

Acupuncture is an ancient Chinese pain-killing technique that works by the insertion of long, thin needles into specific acupuncture points located on lines called *meridians* that connect anatomic sites on the body. Practitioners of acupuncture have named and numbered approximately 1000 acupuncture points, each about 0.25 cm in diameter. When performing major surgery, Chinese doctors use acupuncture as a form of anesthesia. Some advantages of acupuncture include (1) decreased anesthesia-related side effects during or after surgery, (2) less blood loss during surgery, and (3) reduced need for postoperative analgesia, because acupuncture's pain-killing effects persist for several hours.

There are several Western hypotheses to explain why acupuncture works. One hypothesis is based on the outdated gate control theory of pain control and contends that the technique stimulates the larger sensory nerve fibers that carry non–pain impulses. Another theory suggests that acupuncture triggers the release of endorphins—endogenous polypeptides with analgesic properties. Some Western physicians remain skeptical about the technique's pain-killing capabilities.

Cryothermia

Cryothermia is the use of cold to induce anesthesia. Because a very low surface temperature reduces pain, the surgical site is treated with ice preoperatively. Although there are many acceptable alternatives to cryothermia, this technique can be used in extreme conditions that threaten life and when the client cannot tolerate conventional forms of anesthesia.

INTRAOPERATIVE NURSING ASSESSMENT

Intraoperative nursing care is the second portion of the perioperative period. It is often called "operating room nursing." Intraoperative nurses see the client immediately before surgery, either in a holding area or in an admission unit. An initial, brief assessment is completed by the intraoperative nurse. The care plans that were developed and planned preoperatively along with the findings on the extensive admission examination are used in this phase. The goals of intraoperative nursing care consider the individual needs of each client to maintain safety and prevent injury, monitor the client, and control operative resources.

INTRAOPERATIVE NURSING CARE

The nurse serves as the client's advocate during the operation by monitoring several aspects of the client's care. The nurse implements care individually designed for each client, including using proper positioning, maintaining surgical asepsis, monitoring the physiologic status, considering potential emergencies, and controlling equipment and supplies.

Identify the Client

It is imperative the each client be identified before the beginning of any portion of the surgical case. The arm band identifying the client is compared to the medical record, closely checking the name, date of birth, and medical record number. The surgical site which was marked and initialed by the surgeon is also compared to the planned operation.

SAFETY ALERT

Position the Client

Procedures vary among institutions, but after admission to the operating room the client is identified and then moved to the operating room bed. At this time, the client is anesthetized and positioned, and the skin is prepared along with any other procedures that must be completed (such as catheterization or hair removal) before draping and creating the sterile field. The perioperative nurse understands the various operative positions as well as the physiologic changes that occur when a client is placed in a specific position. Table 14-5 reviews these positions and the changes that may occur. Essential factors to consider in positioning a client on the operating table are (1) the site of the operation, (2) the age and size of the client, (3) the type of anesthetic used, and (4) pain normally experienced by the client on movement, such as that resulting from arthritis. The position must not hinder respiration or circulation, must not apply excessive pressure to skin surfaces, and must not limit surgical exposure. Common surgical positions are shown in Figure 14-6. Many other positions can be used, depending on the type of surgery and the visualization of the site required by the surgeon. Laser techniques, endoscopy, or biopsy all may require different client positioning. Interventions may include gathering special supplies that can accommodate an obese client, arranging for an appropriate operating table to withstand excess weight, and providing extra padding to assist in skin integrity maintenance. Additional padding is applied to the operating table for the very thin client or the client with kyphosis.

Whatever the client's position on the operating table, there are general guidelines to promote safety. Most clients feel stiff and sore after a long surgical procedure and may actually complain of the effects of positioning.

Safety

Almost everything in the operating room can be a source of injury if careful control is not exercised. Many procedures are in place to prevent accidents and injury.

Preventing Wrong-Site Surgery

Today an additional check to ensure safety is "time out" before the first incision in the skin. The nurse or surgeon usually calls the "time out," and all members of the team stop what they are doing and check that the client is correct, the body part to be operated upon is correct (for example, left leg), and all details are correct. If so, the surgery proceeds. Guidelines for avoiding wrong-site surgery are given in the Translating Evidence into Practice feature on p. 210.

All plugs and wires are inspected for correct attachment; all equipment is checked to ensure that it is in working order; and measures are taken to prevent electrical burns to the client. An *electrosurgical unit* (ESU) is used to sear the ends of capillaries and blood vessels to control bleeding during surgery. When unipolar cautery is used, place a grounding pad on a large body surface area (thigh or back) to "ground" the client and to prevent sparking and burns. Grounding pads must be placed over intact skin, away from any bony prominences, and not over scars or fragile tissue. Many ESUs have a safety feature that does not allow the unit to work if the grounding pad is placed inappropriately. Bipolar cautery does not require a grounding pad.

TABLE 14–5 Guidelines for Positioning the Client During Surgery

Nursing Action	Rationale
Explain to client, in simple, understandable terms, why positions and restraints are necessary.	Some clients feel that restraining straps are punitive. Some positions can be difficult or embarrassing.
Preserve client's dignity and avoid undue exposure.	Promotes a positive feeling that will encourage healing.
Place restraining straps 2 inches above knees.	This is most secure position on operating bed. Avoids pressure injury from strap on bony prominences.
Nerves, muscles, pressure points, and bony prominences are padded.	Prevents nerve and tissue damage; decreases pressure that will impair or slow circulation; prevents pressure sores during long surgical procedures.
Position client to obtain or maintain adequate respiratory exchange and vascular circulation.	Ensures tissue perfusion and oxygenation, and minimizes pooling of blood. Slow blood flow predisposes to thrombus formation.
Avoid pressure on chest and on body parts such as female breasts and male genitalia.	Prevents injury and minimizes discomfort after surgery.
Do not allow client's extremities to dangle over sides of table.	Hands or feet can be inadvertently compressed against operating room bed by surgery team personnel as they lean over client's body. Impairment of circulation or nerve and muscle damage may result.
When using an arm board, do not abduct upper extremity more than 90 degrees.	Hyperextension can result in permanent nerve damage caused by stretching or crushing the brachial plexus between first rib and scapula.
Avoid excessive strain on client's muscles.	Postoperative strain and discomfort may result.
Be certain client's ankles are not crossed when in prone position.	Circulation may be occluded.
Always move both lower extremities at same time when putting them up in stirrups and when lowering.	Hip joint could be dislocated or muscles strained when extremities are positioned one at a time.
Monitor total position throughout surgery.	Remember, client may remain in one position for hours.

Safety procedures also include counting surgical supplies and equipment that could inadvertently be left inside the body, such as needles, sponges, and instruments. Counts are performed by two people, usually the circulating nurse and the scrub person, at three different times: (1) before the initial incision, (2) during the surgery, and (3) immediately before the incision is closed. A final correct count is announced to the surgeon and charted on the intraoperative chart.

Research has shown that the most typical situations that lead to retained sponges, instruments, and needles are when the operation is an emergency, when there is a change in the planned surgery, or when the client is obese.

Maintain Surgical Asepsis

The perioperative nurse ensures the sterility of supplies and equipment.

All members of the health care team use sterile technique to minimize postoperative infections. If a suspected or actual break in the sterile field occurs, the contaminated instruments and clothing are removed and replaced with new, sterile items.

Members of the surgical team who are in the "sterile area" are those actively performing or assisting in the surgical procedure. They include the surgeon and the assistants and the scrub personnel. The circulating nurse is not sterile and monitors the sterile field to maintain sterility of supplies and personnel.

Surgical asepsis may be broken but must be immediately rectified. The nurse is the advocate of the client in maintaining a sterile surgical environment.

Monitor Body Temperature

Hypothermia occurs frequently in the operating room, either intentional or nonintentional. The operating room temperature is maintained at a standard cool level of 60° to 75° F. Humidity is regulated at 50% to 60%. Temperature control is set to allow optimal performance of the surgical team members, who must wear layers of clothing, and to inhibit bacterial growth.

The client can become cold in the operating room if appropriate covering is not provided. Heat is lost from the skin and from the area open for surgery. When tissues that are not covered with skin are exposed to the air, heat loss is greater than normal. The client should be kept as warm as possible to minimize heat loss without causing vasodilation, which may cause more bleeding.

Most operating rooms have a cabinet that warms blankets, and unless the surgical procedure requires cooling, the nurse should offer the client a blanket immediately upon transfer to the operating room bed.

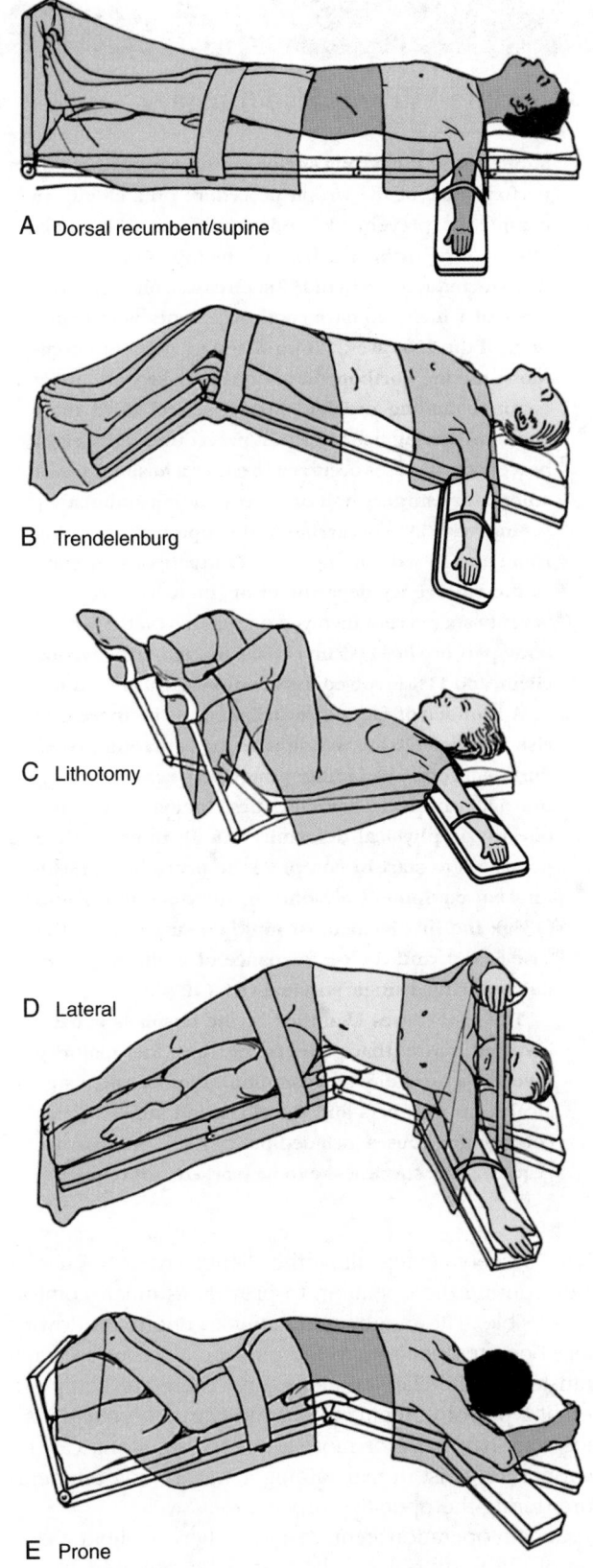

A Dorsal recumbent/supine

B Trendelenburg

C Lithotomy

D Lateral

E Prone

■ **FIGURE 14–6** Five surgical positions and their indications. **A,** Dorsal recumbent (supine): chest, cardiac, breast, and abdominal surgery. **B,** Trendelenburg: lower abdomen or pelvic surgery. **C,** Lithotomy: perineal, vaginal, and rectal surgery. **D,** Lateral: kidney, chest, or hip surgery. **E,** Prone: back surgery.

TRANSLATING EVIDENCE INTO PRACTICE

Avoiding Wrong-Site Surgery

SAFETY

⚠

ALERT

Surgeries on the wrong site or on the wrong client or performance of the wrong procedure on a client are completely preventable and should never happen. The error reporting database of The Joint Commission (TJC) includes more than 150 such cases collected since 1996, of which 126 have root cause analysis information. Of the 126 cases, wrong-site surgery is most common among orthopedic surgeries, second most common among urologic surgeries, and third most common among neurosurgical procedures. Fifty-eight percent of the cases occurred in either a hospital-based ambulatory surgery unit or a freestanding ambulatory setting, with 29% occurring in the inpatient operating room and 13% occurring in other inpatient sites such as the emergency department or intensive care unit. Seventy-six percent involved operations on the wrong body part or site, 13% involved surgery on the wrong client, and 11% involved the wrong surgical procedure.

A number of factors contributed to the increased risk for wrong-site, wrong-person, or wrong-procedure surgery, including emergency cases (19%); unusual physical characteristics, including morbid obesity or physical deformity (16%); unusual time pressures to start or complete the procedure (13%); unusual equipment or setup in the operating room (13%); the involvement of multiple surgeons in the case (13%); and the performance of multiple procedures during a single surgical visit (10%).[2]

The root causes identified by the hospitals usually involved more than one factor, but the majority involved a breakdown in communication between surgical team members and the client and family. Other contributing causes included policy issues such as not requiring the surgical site to be marked, not requiring verification in the operating room or a verification checklist, and incomplete client assessment, including an incomplete preoperative assessment. Staffing issues, distraction factors, availability of pertinent information in the operating room, and organizational cultural issues were also cited as contributing risk factors.[3]

The following activities are recommended:

- Ask the client to mark the surgical site with a permanent marker.[1]
- Ask the surgeon to sign the marked site and then actually operate through or next to the initials.[1a]
- Orally verify the surgery. Just before starting the operation in the operating room, each member of the surgical team should confirm the correct person, the correct surgical site, and the correct procedure.[4]
- Take a "time out" in the operating room. This gives the surgical team one last chance to double check among themselves about the impending procedure, to check charts, and to corroborate information with the client using active, not passive, communication techniques.[4]
- Create and use a verification checklist, including appropriate documents such as medical records, x-rays, or imaging studies, in the operating room to verify the correct client, procedure, and site.

REFERENCES

1. AORN. (2004). *Position statement: Universal protocol for preventing wrong site, wrong procedure, wrong person surgery time out.* Denver, Colo: AORN.
1a. DiGiovanni, C.W., et al. (2003). Patient compliance in avoiding wrong-site surgery. *Journal of Bone and Joint Surgery, 85A*, 815-819.
2. Joint Commission on Accreditation of Healthcare Organizations. (2001). A follow-up review of wrong-site surgery. *Sentinel Event Alert,* (24) at www.jcaho.org.
3. Saufl, N.M. (2002). Sentinel event: Wrong-site surgery. *Journal of Perianesthesia Nursing, 17*(6), 420-422.
4. Scheidt, R.C. (2002). Ensuring correct site surgery. *AORN Journal, 76*(15), 770-777.

Some surgery centers allow the client to wear booties or socks during the operation to provide as much comfort as possible. The intraoperative nurse reports the lowest core body temperature to the postoperative nurse when transferring the client after surgery. There are many different types of equipment that can warm the clients. All hospitals have one or more types. IV solutions can be warmed to assist in maintaining a warm body temperature during the operative procedure as well.

Certain operations require a hypothermic client. Cooling of the body reduces the metabolic rate, which protects the brain and other organs during the surgical procedures. Constant monitoring of the core body temperature is needed, and the nurse assists the anesthesia provider in this activity.

At other times a warm operating room is needed. A warm room is preferred for surgery for large body burns, for replantation, or for surgery in infants. Because of immature internal temperature controls, the infant's body temperature quickly equilibrates with the temperature of the room. Thus room temperatures can be in the 90° range. Hyperthermia can be a problem for the surgical team member who has adapted to the cool temperatures over time. If weakness, faintness, or nausea develops, the team member must leave the room at once.

Monitor for Emergencies

The perioperative nurse must be alert for potential emergencies. When these occur, knowledge, instant decision making, and critical thinking are essential, as is speed in performing needed skills. Although almost any imaginable emergency can occur during an operation, the most common are malignant hyperthermia, cardiac or respiratory arrest, uncontrollable hemorrhage, drug or allergic reactions and fire.

Malignant Hyperthermia. Malignant hyperthermia is a genetic disorder characterized by uncontrolled skeletal muscle contraction leading to potentially fatal hyperthermia. It occurs in predisposed clients when they receive a combination of succinylcholine and inhalation agents (especially halothane).

> **Malignant hyperthermia can occur within 30 minutes of anesthesia induction or several hours after surgery. Unless the triggering event is stopped and the body is cooled, death can result.**

The initial manifestation is increased end-tidal carbon dioxide volume, masseter (jaw) muscle rigidity, cardiac dysrhythmias, and a hypermetabolic state. The client's temperature can rise to as high as 109° F (43° C).

Everyone in the operating room must know the protocol for treatment of malignant hyperthermia. Medications for the emergency treatment of malignant hyperthermia must be on a cart near or in the operating room suite. Nurses must know where the cart is and the procedure to follow if this event occurs. Dantrolene, a skeletal muscle relaxant, is used to decrease skeletal muscle rigidity. The nurse must know how to reconstitute this drug, supplied as a powder, and must be capable of assisting the surgeon or anesthesia personnel with its administration and with any other treatments needed to save the client's life.

There is a screening test for malignant hyperthermia. A muscle biopsy specimen must be taken from the vastus lateralis or abdominal rectus muscle and sent to a malignant hyperthermia laboratory for testing. This test is very expensive and painful. A diagnosis of malignant hyperthermia can be made if there is any personal or family history of anesthesia problems. High-risk clients or those with a history of malignant hyperthermia can successfully undergo surgery if the condition is known. The triggering drugs and conditions are carefully removed from the client care plan, and all members of the surgical team are made aware of the potential problem.

Cardiac and Respiratory Arrest. Although rare, cardiac or respiratory arrest can occur in the operating room, and the same emergency procedures should be carried out as elsewhere. A code blue status may not be called when a client is in the operating room because the key people (physician, anesthetist, nurse) are already present. The emergency "crash cart" should be in the operating room suite, and everyone should know where it is kept. The nurse manager and any key people need to be notified immediately if cardiac or respiratory arrest occurs. In the case of death in the operating room, it is the surgeon's duty to talk to the family.

Uncontrollable Hemorrhage. At times blood loss exceeds the expected bleeding for which blood was prepared in advance. Emergency supplies of blood, using type O negative, may be required. The nurses role during hemorrhage is to supply the surgeon with needed sponges to absorb blood, suture to tie off bleeding vessels or other supplies. Usually the nurse does not retrieve blood, but sends another person, in order to remain in the operating room. Blood loss is always estimated at the end of each operation and further blood transfusions may be needed following surgery.

Allergic Reactions

> **Ideally, allergic reactions should not occur if an adequate history is taken. However, some clients do not recall an allergy; in other cases, the allergy is identified only with the occurrence of a second exposure to an allergen during surgery.**   SAFETY ⚠ ALERT

For example, latex allergies are becoming more frequent, and every client should be asked about latex sensitivity or allergy. Clients who are allergic to latex can successfully undergo surgery with latex-free equipment. The Translating Evidence into Practice feature on p. 212 takes a closer look at latex allergy.

Surgical Fire

> **Fire can occur from many of the instruments and procedures in the operating room.**   SAFETY ⚠ ALERT

When a laser is used, the laser light can ignite drapes or clothing. Laser light can bounce off of shiny instruments, leading to fires. In addition, alcohol found in hair gels and prep solutions is flammable. Of course, oxygen supports combustion. In addition to the laser, other pieces of surgical equipment will support combustion including the electrosurgical unit (cautery) and fiberoptic light sources.

Operating staff must take precautions before the case to ensure that measures are taken to reduce the risk of fire and that water or fire extinguishers are nearby if a fire occurs.

Completion of the Case
Assist with Wound Closure

After final counts are completed, the nurse anticipates the type of wound closure needed and obtains the supplies for the surgical team. The surgical wound may be closed with sutures, staples, or other materials or may be left open to heal by secondary intention. Common skin closures are illustrated in Figure 14-7. If a drain is needed, it is placed in a separate small incision parallel to the operative incisions to drain blood or serum from the operative site. The use of a surgical drain promotes wound healing and decreases

TRANSLATING EVIDENCE INTO PRACTICE

Latex Allergy in the Operating Room

Latex allergy is an abnormally high sensitivity to a protein in rubber that causes a physical reaction. This thin, highly stretchy rubber is found in gloves, tubes, and drains, which are common sources of latex allergy. Thin latex gloves are often coated with cornstarch or talc powder to make it easier to get the gloves on and off. When the gloves are removed, rubber particles that attach to the powder may become airborne, causing an allergic reaction in those who have a latex sensitivity.

Anyone can develop a latex allergy, but people who undergo frequent surgeries have cumulatively prolonged exposure to latex. The prevalence of latex allergy may be greater than 60% in people who have had repeated surgeries, particularly early in life—especially those with myelomeningocele (spina bifida) or urogenital abnormalities. Individuals who are allergic to latex products may experience allergic reactions resulting from cross-reactivity from avocado, banana, celery, chestnut, kiwi, melons, papaya, and tomato. Finally, people who have contact with latex in their employment, such as dental hygienists, nurses, and laboratory technicians, are at increased risk.

A latex allergy can be life-threatening. There are three types of allergic reactions to latex products. The first type is nonimmune irritant contact dermatitis, which is most commonly associated with chronic glove use. This response has a gradual onset and often appears as chapped hands, sometimes with cracking and scaling of the skin. The second type is allergic contact dermatitis; this is a type IV delayed hypersensitivity response. The onset is 6 to 48 hours after

contact. The exposed skin develops erythema, pruritus, blisters, vesicles, papules, and crusting. The most serious form of hypersensitivity reaction is a type I response, or immediate hypersensitivity. The onset is immediate, seldom longer than 2 hours after exposure. The client has localized and generalized urticaria, runny eyes and nose, feelings of faintness, feelings of impending doom, angioedema, nausea, vomiting, and abdominal cramps. Bronchospasm and anaphylactic shock can develop.

Reducing exposure to latex is important. Products containing latex are labeled. Latex exposure should be avoided whenever possible in those who show signs of latex allergy, because exposure is cumulative. Non-latex gloves are available, and powder-free surgical gloves are used to reduce airborne exposure. Admission questions are used to determine high-risk clients. Clients who are known to be allergic to latex are treated only with latex-free products.

REFERENCES

1. American Academy of Dermatology. (1998). American Academy of Dermatology's position paper on latex allergy. *Journal of American Academy of Dermatology, 39*(1), 98-106.
2. AORN. (2006). AORN latex guidelines. *AORN standards, recommended practices and guidelines* (pp. 199-214). Denver: AORN.
3. Elliott, B.A. (2002). Latex allergy: The perspective from the surgical suite. *Journal of Allergy and Clinical Immunology, 110*(2 Suppl), S117-S120.
4. Hourihane, H., et al. (2002). Impact of reported surgical procedures on the incidence and prevalence of latex allergy: A prospective study of 1263 children. *Journal of Pediatrics, 140*(4), 479-482.
5. Tesiorowski, C. (2003). Latex allergies in the healthcare worker. *Journal of Perianesthesia Nursing, 18*(1), 18-31.

the potential for infection. There are many types of surgical drains. The drain is chosen by surgeon preference and is based on the size of the wound and the type of drainage expected. Drains may be free-draining, attached to high-suction apparatus, or self-contained with low suction. The intraoperative nurse and the postoperative nurse are responsible for assessing that the drainage is flowing freely through the system. When the client is transferred out of the operative area, the responsible nurse continues to monitor the patency of the drain and the characteristics of the drainage.

Documentation of Intraoperative Care

The intraoperative nurse documents every event and action in the operating room. Information concerning any drains, tubes, or other devices remaining in the client on completion of the surgical procedure, as well as the type of closure and dressing used, is given to the postoperative care nurse upon transfer.

Moving and Transporting the Client

On completion of the operation, a member of the surgical team wipes off any excess blood, skin preparation,

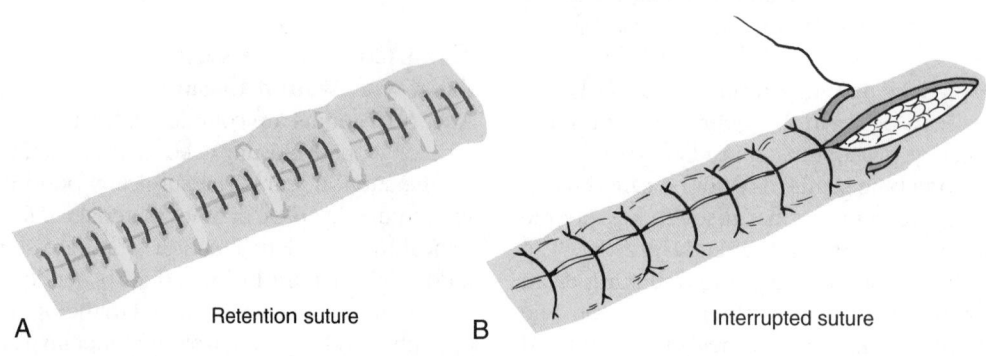

A   Retention suture   B   Interrupted suture

■ **FIGURE 14-7** Skin closures.

and debris from the client's skin and puts a clean gown and blanket on the client.

Transport presents several safety hazards for the patient.

There should always be enough personnel for moving or transferring a client postoperatively to prevent injuries to both the client and the staff. Avoid rapid movements when changing the client's position because it can predispose the development of hypotension. During emergence (revival) from anesthesia, the client is prone to nausea, confusion, and hypotension. Care must be taken not to catch, kink, or dislodge IV or catheter tubing, drains, or other equipment during the transfer. During transfer to the bed or stretcher, the client's modesty must be maintained. Avoid rough handling, which may damage fragile skin.

After being placed on the stretcher, the client is covered with warm blankets and secured with a safety belt. Make sure that the side rails of the stretcher are up to ensure the client's safety in case the client becomes agitated during transport from the operating room.

The anesthesia care provider and also another member of the operating room professional staff, and sometimes the surgeon or the assistant, accompany the client to the postoperative care unit.

In some hospitals, certain clients are transferred directly from the operating room to the intensive care unit (ICU) for continued specialized care and constant nursing supervision. The following are possible candidates for immediate transfer to intensive care:

- Clients at risk of severe complications who remain unstable for a long time after completion of the procedure and who will probably have a complicated postoperative course
- Clients who have undergone major surgery (e.g., resection of aortic aneurysm, open heart surgery, kidney transplantation)
- Clients who have suffered a cardiac or respiratory arrest during or immediately following surgery
- Clients who came to surgery from the intensive care unit and will return there

Family members should always be notified of the client's status and where the client will be immediately after surgery. The surgeon usually discusses the surgical procedure, outcomes, and postoperative course with family members.

POSTOPERATIVE PERIOD

The postoperative period is the third and final stage of the perioperative period. Nursing care continues to be a critical element in returning the client to an optimal level of functioning. The postoperative period can be divided into three phases.

- The initial period of recovery from anesthesia, during which the client is monitored closely by post-anesthesia nurses
- The time from discharge from the post-anesthesia care unit (PACU) to the first day or two after surgery, during which the client is recovering from the effects of the surgery and is beginning to eat and ambulate
- The postoperative phase, the time of healing, which may last for weeks, months, or even years after surgery

There is certainly an overlap of these phases, but in the following discussion they are dealt with separately.

POST-ANESTHESIA CARE UNIT NURSING

The goal of post-anesthesia nursing is to assist a non-complicated return to safe physiologic function after an anesthetic procedure by providing safe, knowledgeable, individualized nursing care for clients and their family members in the immediate post-anesthesia phase. The immediate post-anesthesia period is a critical time for the client. Close and constant observation is essential. The client's vital physiologic functions must be supported until the effects of the anesthetic agents abate. Until then, the client is dependent and drowsy and may be unable to call for assistance. Equipment commonly used in PACU nursing care is listed in Box 14-6.

BOX 14-6   Equipment Used in the Post-Anesthesia Care Unit (PACU)

The PACU nurse prepares and checks the function of the following equipment:

- Sphygmomanometer or automatic blood pressure monitor
- Pulse oximeter—a noninvasive device that measures oxygen saturation of arterial blood and the pulse rate; provides warning of hypoxemia
- Stethoscope—to auscultate breath sounds and blood pressure
- Cardiac monitor and electrodes
- Intravenous equipment (e.g., insertion equipment, fluids, tubing, infusion pumps)
- Suction equipment (e.g., catheters, sterile saline, sterile gloves)
- Supplies to support respiration (e.g., artificial airways, oxygen, tongue depressors, oxygen tubing with masks and cannulas, intubation equipment, and anesthesia machine)
- Medications (e.g., narcotics, narcotic antagonists, hypnotics, antihypertensives, neuromuscular blocking agents)
- Emesis basin, mouth wipes, urinals, bedpans
- Thermometers—oral, rectal, and tympanic membrane types
- Warmed blankets or electric warming units to maintain body temperature
- Emergency cart containing appropriate equipment and medications—drugs including cardiotonics, vasotonics, and respiratory agents; a tracheostomy tray; endotracheal tubes; a defibrillator; a cutdown tray; a ventilator; gastric suction equipment; and chest tube insertion equipment

The client is received in the PACU on a bed or a stretcher, where he or she remains, or is transferred to another bed or to a recovery chair. Proper positioning of a sedated, unconscious, or semiconscious client must ensure airway patency. For an unconscious adult client, extend the neck and thrust the jaw forward (Figure 14-8). The position may depend on the surgery performed. For clients without devices to protect the airway in place, the preferred position is the lateral Sims position, because the side-lying position allows the client's tongue to fall forward and mucus or vomitus to drain from the mouth. Regardless of the position used, carefully monitor the client's respiratory status. Suction equipment must be ready to suction vomit or oral secretions.

After the client has been positioned safely and has been determined to be stable, the nurse receives a verbal, detailed report of events from members of the operating room team (Box 14-7). The PACU nurse reviews the client's record with the anesthesia provider present, noting specifically:

1. The anesthesia record for IV medications and blood received during surgery
2. Any unanticipated complications
3. Significant preoperative findings
4. Presence of tubes or drains and types of wound closure
5. The length of time the client was in surgery

Ideally, a preoperative nursing assessment and nursing history are available in the record for comparison with the postoperative assessment.

Immediate Assessments in the Post-Anesthesia Care Unit

After the transfer report from the operating room, the PACU nurse performs an assessment. The ABCs (airway, breathing, and circulation) are critical and must be assessed first. Included in the assessment are the following:

Airway: Patency; presence of tubes and respiratory assistance devices.

Breathing: Respiration rate and depth; presence of bilateral breath sounds, stridor, wheezes, hoarseness, or decreased breath sounds. Stay at the bedside until the client's gag reflex returns.

Circulation: Pulse rate and strength, blood pressure measurement, skin color, pulse oximeter measurement, ECG tracing if attached, wound status, and dressings (this may include checking underneath the client's body for oozing or frank bleeding). A slight increase in a client's heart rate after surgery, resulting from the stress response, may be normal. A cardiac monitor is also recommended for postoperative clients who have been under general anesthesia so that dysrhythmias can be diagnosed and treatment can be

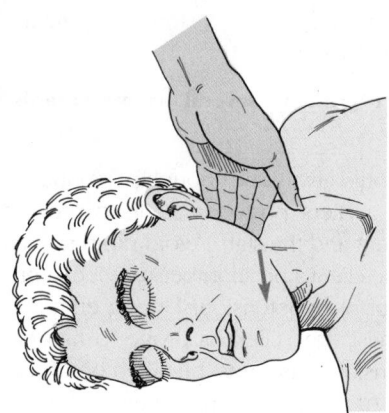

■ **FIGURE 14–8** So that the jaw can be moved forward after anesthesia, the operator's fingers are placed behind the angle of the jaw. As the jaw is moved, the tongue comes forward, opening the airway.

started immediately. Causes of postoperative cardiac dysrhythmias include hypovolemia, pain, electrolyte imbalances, hypoxemia, and acidosis. When dysrhythmias develop, the PACU nurse follows facility protocols if the disturbances are life-threatening and monitors the client's blood pressure, oxygen saturation, and ventilation.

Other: Level of consciousness, muscle strength, ability to follow commands, IV infusions, dressings, drains, special equipment, tubes and drains that must be immediately attached to containers or suction, reddened or bruised areas on skin unrelated to surgery (inspect pressure points and tape and skin preparation sites; look for signs of cautery or thermal burns), temperature (assist client to regain normal core body temperature or anticipate complications).

After receiving the admission report and reviewing the client's record, the PACU nurse documents all observations. Most PACUs use a flow-type method of charting, which includes a numerical rating scale measuring clients' respirations, level of consciousness, ability to move, body temperature or skin color, and blood pressure (Figure 14-9). As the client recovers from the anesthesia, the rating improves to a top score of 10.

BOX 14-7 Information Given to the Post-Anesthesia Care Unit Nurse by the Perioperative Team

- Operative procedure performed
- Medical diagnosis, pertinent medical history, and daily medications
- Vital signs
- Blood loss, fluid replacements
- Urine output and presence of indwelling urinary catheters
- Any events or complications that occurred during surgery
- Anesthetic agents, narcotics, neuromuscular blocking agents, or antibiotics
- Drains inserted and their locations and purpose
- Physician orders to be carried out immediately

NHS NEBRASKA HEALTH SYSTEM
CLARKSON HOSPITAL • UNIVERSITY HOSPITAL
A Partner with University of Nebraska Medical Center

NURSING NOTES:

Patient Identification (Stamp)

NAME

REG. NO.

LOCATION

DATE

Nurse Signatures	Nurse Initials

ALDRETE SCORE▲	Baseline		Post Recovery
Time			
ACTIVITY			
Able to move four extremities voluntarily or on command. 2			
Able to move two extremities voluntarily or on command. 1			
Unable to move extremities voluntarily or on command. 0			
RESPIRATION			
Able to deep breathe and cough freely. 2			
Dyspnea or limited breathing. 1			
Apneic 0			
CIRCULATION			
Baseline BP			
Systolic BP +/- 20% of preanesthetic level. 2			
Systolic BP +/- 20-49% of preanesthetic level. 1			
Systolic BP +/- 50% of preanesthetic level. 0			
CONSCIOUSNESS			
Fully awake. 2			
Arousable on calling. 1			
Unresponsive. 0			
OXYGENATION			
Able to maintain O2 saturation > 92% on room air. 2			
Needs O2 inhalation to maintain saturation > 90%. 1			
O2 saturation < 90% even with O2 supplement. 0			
TOTAL			

▲Aldrete, J.A. & Kroulik, D.J., *Clinical Anesthesia*, Vol. 7, Feb. 1995 and *Anesthesia & Analgesia*, Vol. 49, No. 6, 1970

Potential alteration in fluid volume and/or urinary elimination
Expected outcome: Maintains fluid levels

INTAKE

				On	Off
IV					
Oral			Sequential Stockings		
			Support hose		
TOTAL:			Ice		

OUTPUT

Urine	
Drain	
TOTAL:	

☐ See extended Outpatient Flowsheet

IV DC'd at _____
CATHETER TIP INTACT?   ☐ YES   ☐ NO

Narcotic Waste____ mgs of _____ #1 _____ #2 _____

Potential for Knowledge Deficit: Expected Outcome: Patient or Significant Other will Verbalize Understanding of Instructions.

DISCHARGE CRITERIA	**N/A**
☐ RX GIVEN AND EXPLAINED.	☐
☐ VITAL SIGNS STABLE_____	☐
☐ NAUSEA, VOMITING, DIZZINESS MINIMAL	☐
☐ POST ANESTHESIA RECOVERY SCORE 9-10	☐
☐ SWALLOW, COUGH AND GAG REFLEX PRESENT	☐
☐ ABSENCE OF RESPIRATORY DISTRESS	☐
☐ DRESSING CHECKED C̄ MINIMAL DRAINAGE	☐
☐ RESPONSIBLE ADULT PRESENT TO ESCORT HOME	☐
☐ ALERT AND ORIENTED	☐
☐ PAIN CONTROLLED	☐

Time discharged _____ per _____

Accompanied by _____

NHS-914 (6/99)

Postoperative Phone Call:

Phone Number: _____   Date: _____ Time: _____

	Yes	No	☐ message left
Drsg dry/intact	☐	☐	Unsuccessful Attempts: _____
Nausea/Vomiting	☐	☐	Spoke With: _____
Pain	☐	☐	
Swelling	☐	☐	
Fever	☐	☐	
Voiding easily	☐	☐	☐ Unable to reach, chart
Surgeon/Anes. Contacted	☐	☐	returned to MR

Completed by _____ RN

OUTPATIENT PACU FLOWSHEET   PROCEDURES TAB

■ **FIGURE 14–9** Post-anesthesia care unit (PACU) documentation. *(Courtesy Nebraska Medical Center, Omaha, Neb.)*

Nursing Diagnoses

Nursing diagnoses most common during this period of care are *Risk for Injury, Hypothermia, Risk for Aspiration, Acute Pain,* and *Disturbed Thought Processes.* Most common potential complications are respiratory problems, hypovolemia or hypervolemia, hemorrhage, and cardiac problems.

Nursing Care in the Post-Anesthesia Care Unit
Protect the Airway

SAFETY

⚠️

ALERT

One major complication that occurs in the PACU is airway obstruction or hypoventilation.

The primary nursing intervention to protect the airway is to position the head of a minimally responsive client to the side with the chin extended forward to prevent respiratory obstruction. The client who is unable to clear mucus or vomitus from the throat requires suctioning of secretions immediately.

An oral or nasal airway may be in place to help maintain patency and control the tongue. The airway is a hollow rubber or plastic tube. It is inserted through the nose or mouth and passes over the base of the tongue to keep the tongue from falling back into the throat and obstructing the anatomic airway (Figure 14-10). Airways should not be taped in place. When clients awaken and the gag reflex returns, they may spit out the airway. The PACU nurse may also remove the airway for the responsive client who is unable to remove it unassisted. Left in place too long, it can irritate the tissue, stimulate vomiting, or cause laryngospasm.

When the client is extubated, observe for the development of crowing respirations. The client may be experiencing laryngospasm. If this problem develops, the client could progress to respiratory arrest. Immediately try to ventilate the client using a face mask oxygen delivery system, securing a tight fit over the mouth and nose. The use of positive pressure sometimes alleviates the laryngospasm. If the spasm does not abate, anesthesia providers should be immediately notified; succinylcholine is often given to temporarily paralyze the voluntary muscles, including the muscles that control respiration. Respiration must then be supported by mechanical means (i.e., a ventilator) when muscle relaxants are used. Respiration in clients who have received muscle relaxants must be closely monitored for at least 1 hour after the relaxants appear to have worn off because of the possibility of paralysis reoccurrence. Some clients remain intubated and ventilated, such as those who have undergone open heart surgery. They require close monitoring and intermittent suctioning of secretions.

The nurse also consults with the surgeon and the anesthesia provider and administers prescribed medications as needed. Interventions may also include the continued administration of oxygen, positive-pressure airway support, and use of reversal medications. Reversal agents such as naloxone (Narcan) are administered to reverse

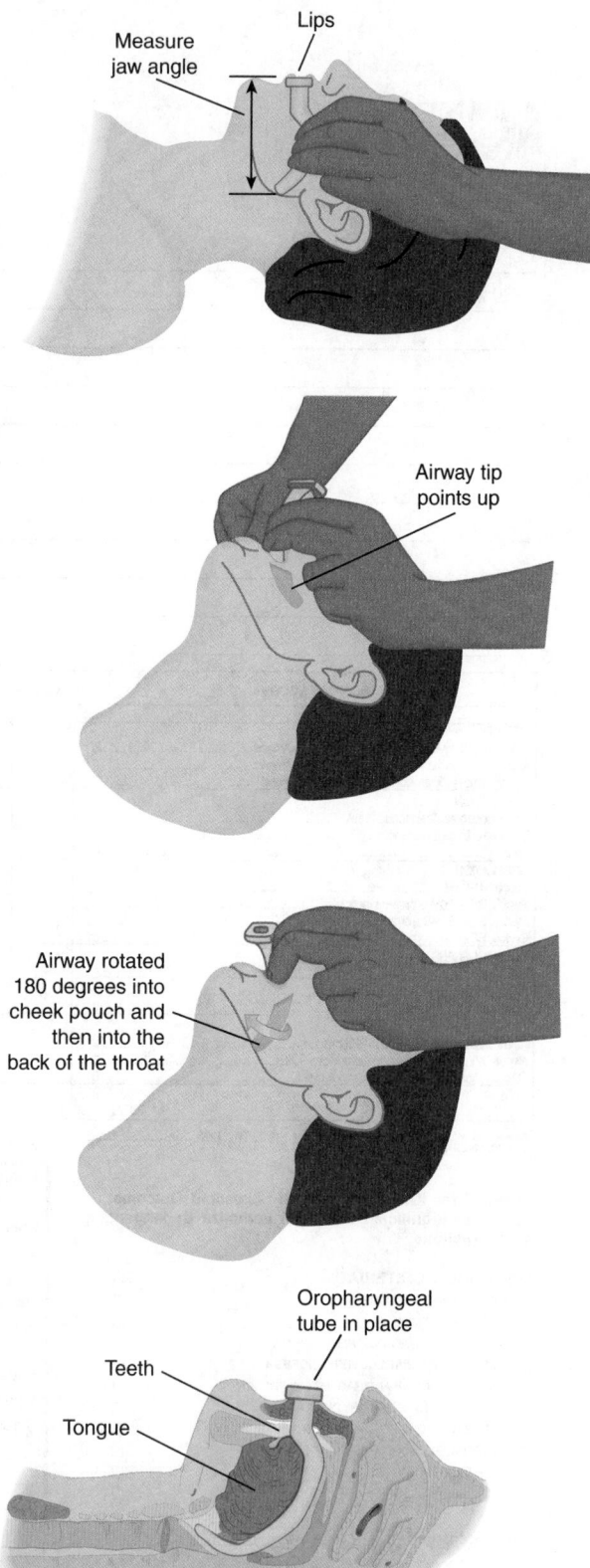

■ **FIGURE 14–10** Insertion of an artificial airway. The flattened, hollow tube prevents the tongue from falling back and occluding the natural airway.

the respiratory depression from anesthetic agents and narcotics. Neostigmine with glycopyrrolate (Robinul) is given to reverse the effect of some neuromuscular blocking agents. Most clients receive oxygen. An oximeter will usually remain on the client to monitor tissue oxygenation. The flow rate of oxygen should be closely checked against physician orders. This may be administered by a respiratory therapist, but the nurse is responsible for assessment and monitoring of treatment. Oxygen levels will vary, depending on the method of delivery, such as nasal cannula, simple face masks, or more controlled methods. Flow rates vary from 2 to 15 L/min with a positive pressure mask. Clients with COPD receive no more than 20%/2 L.

Maintain Normal Blood Pressure

Postoperative hypotension can have numerous causes, including inadequate ventilation; side effects of anesthetic agents or preoperative medications; a rapid change in position; pain, fluid, or blood loss; and peripheral pooling of blood after regional anesthesia. A drop in blood pressure slightly below a client's preoperative baseline reading is common after surgery. However, a significant drop in blood pressure, accompanied by an increased heart rate, may indicate hemorrhage, circulatory failure, or fluid shifts. Do not diagnose impending hypovolemic shock on the basis of one low blood pressure reading. If you are concerned about a dropping blood pressure (BP), measure BP every 5 minutes for 15 minutes to determine the variability. Decreased blood pressure can also mean that the anesthesia is wearing off or that the client is experiencing severe pain.

In addition to hypotension, manifestations of shock include tachycardia, restlessness and apprehension, and cold, moist, pale, or cyanotic skin. When a client appears to be going into shock, the PACU nurse intervenes as follows:

1. Administers oxygen or increases its rate of delivery
2. Raises the client's legs above the level of the heart
3. Increases the rate of IV fluids (unless contraindicated because of fluid excretion problems)
4. Notifies the anesthesia provider and the surgeon
5. Provides medications as ordered
6. Continues to assess the client and the client's response to interventions

Hypertension may also develop. Older adults with a history of hypertension may exhibit hypertensive episodes after the stress of surgery. If the blood pressure rises above the baseline, the PACU nurse should consult with the anesthesia provider or the surgeon and administer antihypertensive medication as ordered.

Monitor for Return of Consciousness

The PACU nurse monitors the level of consciousness. Orientation to person is the first cognitive response to return after anesthesia, assessed by noting whether the client responds to his or her name. Be certain that a client who normally wears a hearing aid has it in place and turned on before you attempt to talk to the client. Orientation to place is also an important indication of postoperative return of cognitive function. Because of confusion from anesthesia and analgesia medications, the client is usually not oriented to time until after the nurse provides this information. Assessment of returning cognitive functioning includes the ability to remember facts after being told. Older adults and clients with liver or kidney impairment may take longer to regain orientation. Postoperative delirium may occur with some procedures, such as open heart surgery; therefore do not assume that aberrations are a result of age-related "senility." Rather, check the present cognitive status against that noted in the preoperative assessment to gain a truer picture of the client's level of consciousness and cognition.

Assess for Return of Sensation and Motion

In the PACU, the client is monitored carefully for return of sensation as the anesthetic agent wears off. Check return of motion to the extremities by asking clients to wiggle their toes. However, the ability to move the toes will be delayed if client had spinal anesthesia. In such cases, the toe movement signifies that the motor blockade is wearing off, but blockade of the autonomic nervous system may still be present. Clients who are still experiencing autonomic blockade are prone to hypotension despite their ability to move their toes and extremities.

Assess for Normothermia

The client in the PACU is monitored for temperature and vital signs every 15 minutes until vital signs are stable, or more often if they are unstable. The frequency of monitoring and length of time over which monitoring must be done are dictated by facility PACU policy. Clients are monitored until they are discharged from the PACU. This is usually at least 1 hour. Clients must have a minimum temperature of greater than 96.8°F (36°C) before they are discharged from the PACU. The heat loss that occurs in the operating room can continue in the PACU if the client is not warmed sufficiently. Warming requires the maintenance of temperature without overwarming and causing excessive vasodilation, which can cause fluid shifts and a decrease in blood pressure. The PACU nurse must also realize that malignant hyperthermia can also occur in the PACU and should repeatedly assess for manifestations of this condition.

Assess Perfusion

Assessment of skin color, warmth, and turgor provides evidence of tissue perfusion. Verify skin color in clients with dark or brown skin with another nurse to avoid making incorrect assumptions. Dusky, pale, cold, moist skin is an important assessment finding that may be a manifestation of shock. Because it is not possible to detect systemic conditions by skin color alone, assessment should include other pertinent data. For example, when impending shock is suspected, check the client's blood pressure measurement, and inspect the lips and nails as well as the skin to detect pallor or cyanosis. Consider these findings in relation to oxygen saturation and hemoglobin level before assuming a diagnosis of shock.

Assess the Surgical Site

Check the dressing over the surgical incision frequently. If it is saturated with blood, note the color, type, and amount of drainage. Reinforce the dressing, but do not change it or open it without a physician's order. If seepage is noted, draw an outline of the fluid on the dressing and note the date and time. If oozing continues, the estimation of the amount can be more easily determined by areas outside the previously marked borders. Sometimes bleeding is present but not visible on dressings. If bleeding is suspected, look for blood that may have leaked downward out of sight, under the operated extremity, or under the back.

Promote Fluid and Electrolyte Balance

Assess intake and output hourly. Monitor all parenteral fluids to ensure that the proper amount and type of fluids are being infused. Intake can include solutions of IV fluids, medications, blood products, nutritional support, and colloid infusions. Check the amount of solution in the IV bottle on admission of the client to the PACU along with the rate of infusion. All types of delivery systems and lines must be considered: pumps, infusion machines, monitoring machines, IV lines, central venous lines, and arterial lines. Check the insertion sites for redness, soreness, and swelling, as these may be indications of infiltration. Note medications that have been added to solutions, so that when the next dose is ready to be infused a new bag of dilution fluid is present. This procedure ensures that there is no lapse in administration of ordered fluids or medications.

Changes in renal function and fluid and electrolyte balance may develop soon after surgery. The stress response to surgery stimulates the secretion of antidiuretic hormone (ADH) and aldosterone, which cause fluid retention. Until the stress subsides, urine volume decreases regardless of fluid intake. Avoid fluid overload while maintaining the client's blood pressure, cardiac output, and urinary output. If an indwelling bladder catheter is present, document the amount of output and compare it with the amount of input via IV fluids.

Manage Drainage Systems

Drainage tubes, such as a T-tube, gastric tube, urinary catheter, or wound drains, must be constantly monitored. For example, urinary catheters and T-tubes are unclamped and attached to gravity drainage systems. Gastric, chest, and intestinal tubes are attached to wall suction. Wound drainage systems are attached to self-contained suction devices. The PACU nurse must ensure that tubes are patent and draining freely. Check that there are no kinks in the tubes and that they are not occluded. Document the amount and character of drainage on a regular schedule. Compare the type and amount of drainage with those expected for the surgical procedure.

Promote Comfort

Pain is an expected outcome postoperatively, yet one of the most frequent postoperative problems is inadequate analgesic administration. You must carefully and regularly assess the client's level of pain. Pain may be caused by a factor unrelated to the surgical procedure, such as positioning that occurred during surgery. The discomfort of a full bladder can imitate abdominal pain even when appropriate doses of pain medication have been administered. Provide appropriate pain relief while not overmedicating. If there is any problem in making the postoperative client comfortable, call the anesthesia provider or surgeon to minimize the time the client is in pain.

Maintain Safety

Continue to be the client's advocate, and protect the client from injury that may be caused by equipment, medication, and postoperative risks. Side rails must remain in the up position to protect the client from falling out of the bed or off of the cart. Proper body alignment and frequent repositioning assist in maintaining circulation and relieve skin pressure. Postoperative equipment is checked to ensure that it is working properly before the client is received in the PACU. Place equipment in a safe location and electrical cords or lines out of the way so that they do not present a danger to the client or staff members.

Discharge from the Post-Anesthesia Care Unit

Common criteria for evaluating the client's readiness for discharge from the PACU are based on a general scoring system. The criteria that are scored include activity, respiration, circulation, consciousness, and skin color. A typical scoring system is shown in Figure 14-9 on p. 215.

When the client is considered ready for discharge from the PACU, a report (via telephone or verbal) must be relayed to the receiving unit. The report must include the client's condition along with a summary of details of the operative procedure and events that may affect client care. Thorough documentation of the client's progress in the PACU is included in the client's permanent medical record and is an important source of information for use in providing appropriate care. If for some reason the client is to have an extended stay in the PACU, notify the family immediately, and explain the reasons for the prolonged stay.

"Same-day surgery" clients cannot be discharged until they are able to tolerate fluids by mouth, can ambulate with a steady gait and no orthostatic hypotension, and have voided. Pain must be controllable with oral analgesia. A responsible adult must accompany the client being discharged from the ambulatory care center. Taxi cabs are not an appropriate means of transportation after a surgical procedure. Discharge instructions include written and oral information. It is best if this information is reviewed both preoperatively and postoperatively. The instructions usually include information about medications, how to care for the surgical wound, the amount and type of activity that is appropriate, when and how to seek help for any problems that may arise, and when and where follow-up appointments are scheduled. The client who has undergone a same-day procedure is telephoned by a registered nurse the day after surgery to ensure that there are no complications or further questions.

POSTOPERATIVE NURSING CARE

After the client has been released from the PACU and transferred to an inpatient nursing unit, the nursing assessments and interventions are similar to those performed in the PACU. The most common immediate postoperative complications are those related to spinal anesthesia and those affecting the respiratory, cardiovascular, and renal systems and fluid and electrolyte balance.

Establishment of Postoperative Goals

At this point, the postoperative care plan is expanded and revised. The plan should include an assessment of the client's needs and goals as well as nursing interventions. Nursing diagnoses are used to specify and define postoperative problems and to guide the plan of nursing care. Findings on the preoperative assessment constitute a very important body of information at this time because the findings can be used as baseline values for comparison with those obtained in postoperative assessments. A general nursing care plan is prepared. Specific assessment and care measures are often based upon the surgical procedure performed and the preoperative condition of the client.

ASSESSMENT OF THE POSTOPERATIVE CLIENT

Assess Respiratory Status

Assess for a patent airway. Observe the client and assess the breathing pattern at rest. Listen to sounds; breath

respirations should be unlabored and quiet. As a result of effects of general anesthetic agents and narcotics, respiratory drive and depth may be reduced, leading to hypoxia. Clinical manifestations of hypoxia include confusion, restlessness, pale skin, pulse oximetry readings below 90%, and cool skin temperature. Although restlessness is an early sign of hypoxia, there may be other causes, such as pain. Cyanosis and finally respiratory arrest are very late manifestations of hypoxia.

Major complications following surgery are decreased lung expansion, atelectasis (collapse of alveolar sacs), or aspiration of retained secretions. Lung assessment should include auscultation in all lobes as well as assessment of the rate and rhythm of respirations. Incentive spirometry, that was demonstrated and practiced preoperatively, should be used to increase lung expansion and keep alveoli open (Figure 14-11). A body temperature of greater than 100° F (37.7° C) in the first 24 hours after surgery is frequently a result of atelectasis.

Obese clients often have difficulty with airway patency. They have large chests and abdomens that put pressure on the neck and airway when the client is flat in bed. Position the client with the head of the bed elevated to reduce some of the pressure on the neck. Use continuous positive airway pressure (CPAP) masks if they were used before surgery.

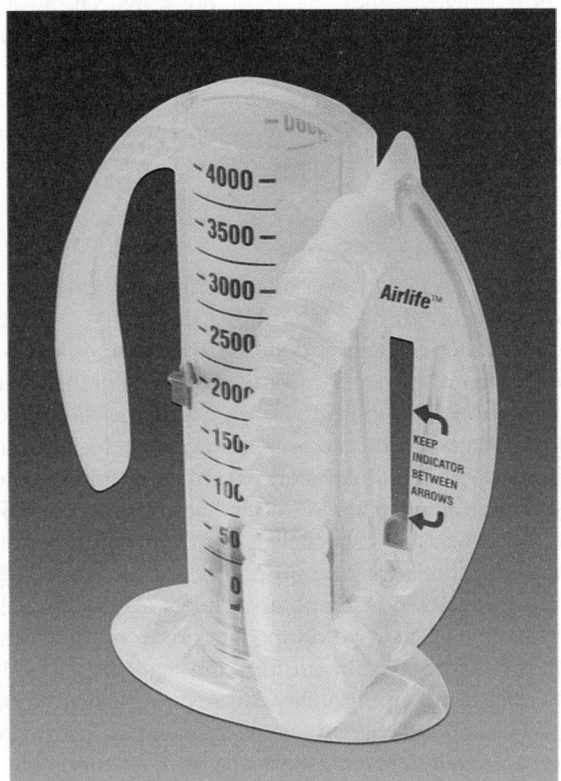

■ **FIGURE 14-11** Use of an incentive deep-breathing exerciser promotes alveolar inflation, restores and maintains lung capacity, and strengthens the respiratory muscles. (*Courtesy Cardinal Health, Dublin, Oh. All rights reserved.*)

Assess Circulation

Assess vital signs, skin color, and temperature according to facility protocols. Vital signs are assessed frequently (e.g., every 30 minutes). Reassure the client that this pattern of assessment is a matter of routine and does not indicate anything is wrong. Because the client has been immobile during the operation and may have experienced pressure on body parts that diminished circulation, extremities must be evaluated for weakness, circulation, and numbness. Bony prominences should be assessed for stage I pressure ulcers and deep tissue injury (see Chapter 49). Although all clients must be encouraged to get out of bed and walk as soon as possible after surgery to prevent the formation of thrombus and devastating emboli, early ambulation is especially important after surgery of the abdominal area. The aorta and femoral arteries may have been manipulated during the procedure. In addition, the client may find that the dorsal recumbent position (as in a recliner chair) is most comfortable because it reduces strain on the incision. However, this position slows venous return in the pelvis and can foster thrombus formation.

A thrombus can form in any blood vessel, and you should be especially alert to any complaints of extremity pain, unilateral edema, or warmth in the calf. If the thrombus dislodges and travels via the bloodstream, it can move to the lung, creating a pulmonary embolus. Walking can nullify much of the threat of thrombus formation. However, most clients do not want to move after surgery. Leg exercises should have been taught preoperatively, and you should emphasize their importance in the prevention of thrombus formation to promote an optimal outcome. Sequential compression devices are also used to enhance venous return.

Assess Neurologic Status

Assess the client for level of consciousness, orientation, and lingering effects of anesthesia in the first 24 hours. In older adults, cognitive deficits may remain for days or even weeks after surgery. Compare present mental status with preoperative ability to clearly define the client's neurologic status. Medications are slower to clear through aging kidneys, and hypothermia and pain can also affect cognition. Clients need to know that impaired cognition is to be expected—especially older clients, in whom the fear of dementia may be present. If they are not aware that the condition is temporary, clients may believe that they have had a stroke during surgery from which they will never recover. This in turn can lead to depression with decreased coping ability. Nurses can facilitate recovery by promoting cognitive activity, repeating instructions often if needed, having patience with clients slow to recover, and fostering hope. Document changes every shift. If a decrease in cognition appears, notify the physician immediately. Most clients make slow, steady progress and return to preoperative status.

Obese clients also have a delayed return of consciousness after anesthetic procedures. Greater amounts of anesthetic agents are required for these clients. Intravenous anesthetic agents are fat-soluble, and much of the drug dose is deposited from the blood into fatty tissue. In obesity, therefore, excretion of these anesthetic agents is slower because of the increased amounts of drug retained. It is not uncommon to see the obese client fall asleep mid-sentence. This is due to anesthetics being released from their storage in fat cells and usually occurs for the first 24 hours after surgery.

Postoperative Monitoring
Monitor the Wound

Assess the dressing and the amount and character of any drainage that is present. Be alert to the method of care that the surgeon prefers. Most surgeons prefer to do the first dressing change. Some surgeons leave the original surgical dressing intact for 24 to 48 hours. Others request that the dressing be changed as it becomes soiled. If the wound is closed and left to heal by first intention, dressings on the wound may be minimal, and the client may be allowed to shower after 24 hours. If the wound healing is to be by second or third intention, then it is left open to heal from the fascia to the skin, and special wound handling must occur. Measures can include wound packing, dressings, drains, and ostomy bags, depending on wound size and location and drainage from the wound. Measure and record the amount of drainage every shift for comparison with earlier assessments to guide potential care plan changes (see Chapter 18).

Each client must have an individualized care plan to facilitate the most effective healing. Document the wound's appearance and drainage and also the client's reports of discomfort at least every shift. If you are unsure how to describe the wound, it is suggested that two nurses compare observations at each change of shift.

Although it is commonplace for nurses to look at wounds, the appearance of the surgical wound is frightening to many clients. It sometimes takes days before a client can even look at the wound. Assess the client's willingness to look at the wound. Do not force the client to look at the wound until he or she is ready. Look for subtle cues—for example, the client may continue to look away from the wound while dressings are being changed. Body image is altered in response to surgery, even surgery on internal organs. Body image reintegration or restoration requires weeks or months to occur. Show acceptance of the client's appearance, and assist the client in verbalizing feelings about the postoperative appearance and the reaction of others.

Clients must learn to care for any dressing before discharge, so education must be a written intervention in the care plan on admission to the nursing unit. Training should proceed daily until the client or a family member feels comfortable with the wound care skills necessary to promote healing.

As explained in the Management and Delegation feature below, routine care of drains and dressings can be delegated to trained unlicensed assistive personnel.

Monitor Intravenous Lines

All IV lines must be checked for patency, type of fluid to be infused, and rate of infusion. For any client with an IV line, intake and output monitoring must be completed. This is a nursing decision; although there may be a

---

MANAGEMENT AND DELEGATION

Postoperative Care

The postoperative client requires special consideration with regard to delegation. Following your initial postoperative assessment you may determine that it is appropriate to delegate the measurement and recording of vital signs, urine output, drain or tube output, and the observation of surgical dressings to an unlicensed assistant. In so doing, reassure the client that the frequency of observation and measurement by the unlicensed assistant is within normal parameters for the client's condition.

Instruct your assistant as to the frequency with which the vital signs should be measured and observations are to occur. Review the vital sign measurements necessitating immediate notification to you. Reinforce the importance of timely measurement, recording, and notification with your assistant.

Instruct your assistant as to the location of any dressings and drains. Ensure the drains are appropriately secured and labeled and that the labels correlate with the output record or flow sheet before delegation of monitoring and recording drain output. Note the presence of any drainage on a new surgical dressing. Outlining the drainage with a waterproof marker at the time of your assessment establishes a baseline for comparison and progressive monitoring. The presence of drainage on a previously clean dressing is immediately reportable to you and bears further assessment and intervention. Ascertaining whether drainage may be expected is helpful information for you to have at the outset of the postoperative period.

Your knowledge of the type of surgical closure and the presence of a drain or packing below the dressing will allow you to anticipate whether drainage is expected. Your assessment should include a description of the quantity and quality of drain output or drainage on the surgical dressing. You may then delegate the continued observation of the drain or dressing to your assistant with explicit instructions that the assistant alert you to any changes in the color, amount, or other characteristics of the drainage. Additionally, any sign of redness, swelling, tenderness, warmth, pain, bleeding, discharge, or separation of wound edges is reportable. The finding of new drainage or blood on a postoperative dressing is immediately reportable to you.

Specify the frequency with which the drain is to be emptied for the assistive personnel. A frequency of every 4 hours or once per shift may be delegated, whereas you may choose to perform more frequent measurement and recording of drainage as appropriate. For example, you might best perform hourly drain emptying with subsequent IV fluid replacement of the volume measured, which requires an hourly adjustment in the IV infusion rate. Perform the assessment for air leak in chest tubes at intervals throughout your shift. Chest tube drainage may be measured and recorded by assistive personnel.

Urine output is closely monitored for 24 to 72 hours after surgery. The quantity and color of your client's urine are important indicators of fluid and hydration status. In clients with normal renal function, an average of 0.5 ml/kg/hr is desirable. Instruct the assistant as to the frequency with which urine output is to be measured and recorded. Discuss your baseline assessment of urine color, quantity, and clarity. Instruct your noncatheterized clients to collect their urine each time they void to allow measurement and observation. The assistant is to notify you of any changes from your baseline findings or a decrease in expected urine quantity.

Comfort and relief from pain are important considerations for your postoperative client. Your institution will have specific guidelines for the assessment and management of postsurgical pain. Unlicensed assistants may help in surveillance for adequacy of pain relief or reduction. Instruct your assistant to incorporate questions about pain at the time other vital signs are measured. The assistant can then relay this information to you so that you can provide further assessment and intervene to ensure that the client is achieving adequate pain relief or reduction. Your assistant may also provide comfort measures for the client such as a back rub or turning and positioning to further promote pain relief or reduction.

Coughing, deep breathing, incisional splinting, and incentive spirometry are essential to minimize respiratory complications in the postoperative period. Following your respiratory assessment and initial client instruction in the proper use of the incentive spirometer with incisional splinting, your assistant may provide encouragement and reinforce proper use of the incentive spirometer with the client. Unlicensed assistants may not provide client teaching; that remains your responsibility. Assistants may reinforce instruction and provide functional assistance to your client in this situation. Instruct your assistant to note the client's effort and frequency of spirometer use on the daily record or flow sheet. The client's responses to spirometer use (i.e., cough, sputum production, color, and consistency) should be recorded. Variations from the client's baseline performance are immediately reportable to you. This includes a client's report or appearance of difficulty breathing, increased sputum production, discolored or bloody sputum, and inability to perform incentive spirometry as previously instructed or complaints of increased pain.

The unlicensed assistant is a vital extension of your eyes and ears in providing ongoing monitoring for the stable postoperative client. As a client's postoperative condition improves, the frequency of observation may be reduced. In the event a postoperative client's condition deteriorates or becomes unstable, you will assume responsibility to assess and monitor the client's condition personally, no longer delegating these tasks to your assistant. The frequency of your assessment and intervention increases and the role of the assistant becomes more supportive of your actions and less engaged in monitoring the client directly.

physician's routine order, none is required to monitor the client. If there have been no complications during surgery, the client is drinking without nausea, and the IV line is not needed for medication delivery, the line is often capped, which allows infusions of IV medications without additional IV fluids. The locked or capped IV is usually maintained for potential emergency access until the client is considered stable. The capped IV not only is more comfortable than an IV port attached to an infusion line but also costs less and allows the client to ambulate much more easily. Assess the insertion site for any signs of redness, swelling, or pain. If any problems are noted, the catheter may have to be removed from the vein; replacement may or may not be indicated. Application of mild heat to an insertion site that has been infiltrated with IV solution may help to decrease local pain.

Monitor Drainage Tubes

Assess drainage tubes (e.g., NG tube), and check the client's postoperative physician's instructions to determine whether to attach the tubes to suction or to use gravity drainage. Note the amount, color, and consistency of drainage, and document the findings. If the client has a low-suction NG tube, it must remain patent. Irrigate the tube with normal saline according to the surgeon's orders; some tubes cannot be irrigated because of increased risk of injuring internal sutures. Make sure the tube is connected to suction if ordered.

SAFETY

⚠️

ALERT

If the tube has a dual lumen and if one side is for air, do not insert medication through the air vent. Medication can easily occlude this port. If the port gurgles, do not plug the port to quiet the system. By plugging up the air vent, the suction system becomes a closed system, thereby increasing the suction on the wall of the stomach, which can cause trauma and bleeding.

NG tubes inserted for decompression and removal of intestinal secretions remain in place until peristalsis begins. The removal of an NG tube requires an order by the surgeon. Assess for return of hunger, bowel sounds, and passage of flatus as signs of peristalsis as long as the tube is in place. When peristalsis returns, the physician will probably order the NG tube to be clamped initially and then removed if the clamping was tolerated without nausea or vomiting.

Monitor Comfort/Pain Level

All clients who have just had surgery will experience pain. Pain medication should be given when needed and before the pain becomes severe. When the "demand approach" (medicate as needed) is used for analgesia, it is crucial to medicate the client at the onset of the pain. When pain becomes too severe, more medication and a longer time are needed for the medication to take

effect. Clients may return to the surgical unit with a patient-controlled analgesia (PCA) device for pain medication administration (Figure 14-12). Repeat instructions on how to use the device, and assure the client that a "lock-out" function prevents inadvertent overdosing. Basal dosing is helpful to control pain while the client is asleep.

Document the date and time of medication administration, the amount given, and the route of administration. Also include a description of the pain the client is experiencing and the effectiveness of the pain medication in controlling it. Consider the time to onset of medication effect in determining when evaluation of pain control should be assessed. For example, reassess the client 30 minutes after oral pain medication is administered. IV medications should control pain within 5 to 10 minutes. It is usually the nurse who determines whether the client is obtaining a sufficient dose of medication, whether pain

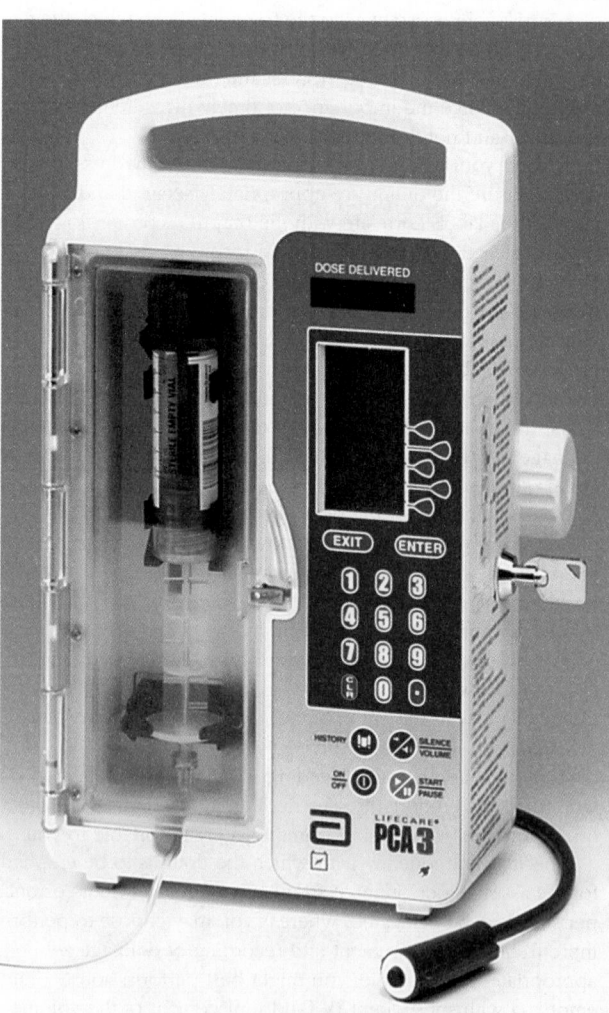

■ **FIGURE 14-12** A patient-controlled analgesia (PCA) device allows clients to control their own pain relief or pain reduction postoperatively. The printout allows the nurse to assess and record the amount of opioid analgesia. *(Courtesy Abbott Laboratories, Hospital Products Division, North Chicago, Ill.)*

is being controlled, or whether it is causing side effects such as nausea and vomiting. Communicating these details to the physician allows for a change to best suit the client's needs, leading to a positive outcome for pain relief. It is vital that pain be managed if the client is to comply with instructions for coughing, deep breathing, and ambulation. Chapter 20 addresses pain and pain management.

Monitor for Nausea and Vomiting

Postoperative nausea and vomiting (PONV) do not occur frequently; however, the surgical experience for those clients with PONV will remain uniquely unpleasant. Vomiting is a reflex, and the reflex is stimulated in many ways. Stimuli can arise from gastrointestinal tract distention on irritation, vagal stimulation, stimulation of centers in the cerebrum or the chemoreceptor trigger zone (CTZ) located in the floor of the brain's fourth ventricle, rotation or disequilibrium of the vestibular labyrinths of the ear, increased intracranial pressure, pain, or sensory perceptions (such as the sight of blood or an odor or a taste). Several medications stimulate the CTZ, including morphine, meperidine, cardiac glycosides, and amphetamines.

Risk factors are shown in Box 14-8. PONV can be prevented by reducing movement, controlling pain, and intervening early with antiemetics. Several categories of medications are used to control PONV, including the following: (1) anticholinergics and histamine type 1 (H_1) receptor antagonists, which reduce excitability of the labyrinth receptors; (2) antidopaminergic drugs, which depress the CTZ; and (3) gastrointestinal antispasmodics, which promote forward peristaltic movement. PONV has also been controlled with acupuncture.

BOX 14-8   Risk Factors for Postoperative Nausea and Vomiting

CLIENT FACTORS
- Ambulation
- Bowel obstruction/ileus
- Female gender
- History of motion sickness
- History of vomiting with previous anesthetic procedure
- Hypoglycemia
- Hypotension
- Obesity
- Swallowed blood
- Uncontrolled pain
- Young age

TYPE OF SURGERY
- Eye
- Intra-abdominal
- Intracranial
- Laparoscopic
- Middle ear
- Testicular

MEDICATIONS
- Anticholinesterases
- Etomidate
- Isoflurane
- Nitrous oxide?
- Pentothal
- Propofol
- Regional anesthetics above T5 spinal level

Suture/Staple Removal

Sutures and staples may be removed before the client is discharged. Some surgeons write standing orders to remove wound closure materials on a certain day after surgery; others write specific orders to do so. When removing suture, cut the suture at the skin and then pull on the knot to remove it. Try to avoid dragging exposed suture through the skin by cutting close to the skin. To remove staples, insert the device under the staple and push to bend the staple. Both suture and staple removal can be uncomfortable, but few clients require pain medications for the procedure. If the wound edges do not remain approximated after the suture or staples are removed, strips of paper tape (e.g., Steri-Strips) should be applied. Expect small amounts of bleeding from the suture marks, so cover the wound with sterile dressings.

SURGICAL COMPLICATIONS

Despite the best technical operation, surgical complications occur for a variety of reasons. Some complications are due to the preoperative condition of the client, such as severe heart or pulmonary disease that could not be controlled before surgery. Other complications are due to the progressive nature of the very disease for which the operation was done, such as advanced cancer. Technical errors also occur during surgery.

Wound Complications

Surgical incisions can develop collections of liquefied fat, serum, and lymphatic fluid, called a seroma. Seromas appear as swollen or tight tissue around or under the incision. They can be palpated and are usually movable. Ballottement is present. Seromas are commonly drained and sometimes require wound packing.

Hematomas, collections of blood, can also occur. Hematomas are more worrisome than seromas because they can become infected. Hematomas can be painful and also create a poor cosmetic result. Hematomas appear as a purple or bruised area of swollen skin at the surgical site. They are hard and have no ballottement. If there is no drain in the area, bloody drainage may be seeping from the hematoma. Hematomas can be large and obstruct airways or blood vessels, or they can collect in the abdomen or retroperitoneal space. Almost all hematomas are opened and drained.

If wound infection develops, the clinical manifestations appear in the wound 3 to 4 days postoperatively. Clinical manifestations include redness beyond the incision line, edema that remains after the initial swelling, increasing pain, and increased drainage. Sometimes drainage becomes purulent or foul-smelling. The client may also have fever, malaise, anorexia, and leukocytosis (increased WBC count with increased numbers of band WBCs). Notify the surgeon of any suspected wound infection. Wound cultures may be ordered to verify that organisms in the wound are sensitive to the antibiotics taken.

If collagen fibers are not mature enough to hold the incision closed without suture, the wound may open. An opening of a skin wound is called *dehiscence*. Wounds in which dehiscence has occurred are treated as open wounds—that is, they are kept clean, with application of packing or dressings, and allowed to heal by secondary or tertiary intention (see Chapter 18).

If abdominal wounds become infected and the abdominal incision opens, the fascia or internal organs may be visible (Figure 14-13). This condition is called *evisceration* and constitutes an emergency. Return the client to bed. Do not attempt to replace the organs. Cover the wound with sterile dressings moistened with normal saline. Monitor the client's vital signs, keep the client as calm as possible, and notify the surgeon immediately for emergency surgery. In many clients, evisceration is preceded by a gush of serosanguineous drainage about 48 hours earlier. Notify the surgeon of this sudden increase in drainage, and apply an abdominal binder for support.

Postoperative Fever

Persistent fever following surgery can develop from infectious or noninfectious causes (Table 14-6). Slight postoperative fever is very common and was traditionally thought to be from atelectasis, but recent evidence suggests that cytokines released from damaged and injured tissue are the more likely cause. In either case, slight fever for 72 hours following surgery is usually treated with coughing and deep-breathing exercises and

TABLE 14–6	Causes of Postoperative Fever
Infectious	**Noninfectious**
Abscess	Acute hepatic failure
Acalculous cholecystitis	Adrenal insufficiency
Bacteremia	Allergic reaction
Device-related infections	Atelectasis
Decubitus (pressure) ulcers	Dehydration
Empyema	Drug reaction
Fungal sepsis	Head injury
Hepatitis	Hepatoma
Meningitis	Hypothyroidism
Osteomyelitis	Lymphoma
Parotiditis	Pancreatitis
Perineal infection	Pheochromocytoma
Peritonitis	Pulmonary embolism
Pharyngitis	Retroperitoneal hematoma
Pneumonia	Subarachnoid hemorrhage
Pseudomembranous colitis	Systemic inflammatory response syndrome
Retained foreign body	Thrombophlebitis
Sinusitis	Transfusion reaction
Tracheobronchitis	Withdrawal syndrome
Urinary tract infection	
Wound infection	

From Townsend, C., Beauchamp, R.D., Evers, B., et al. (2004). *Sabiston textbook of surgery* (17th ed.). Philadelphia: Saunders.

fluid administration. When fever persists for 5 to 8 days, it is investigated. The most common causes of fever are called the five Ws: wind (the lungs), water (the urinary tract), wound, walking (clots in the lower legs), and waste (bowel). Some versions include wonder drugs as the sixth "W" because many medications can lead to fever.

There are many postoperative complications and they are presented in Table 14-7; the full discussion of these conditions is within this book.

Nursing Management of Clients Experiencing Postoperative Complications

A nursing diagnosis for clients who are not recovering from their operation as expected is *Delayed Surgical Recovery*. This nursing diagnosis is used when clients have extended hospital stays in order to initiate and perform activities that maintain life, health, and well-being. The diagnosis would be written as *Delayed Surgical Recovery related to severe blood loss (or other specific etiology)*. Of course, the specific issues being addressed would be included in other nursing diagnoses, such as *Impaired Gas Exchange*.

The goal for the client would be to enhance surgical recovery as evidenced by improvement in the specific problem being addressed. In some clients, the complications are so severe or life-threatening that recovery is not expected, and at that point they may be aided by hospice. In these cases, the focus of nursing care also changes.

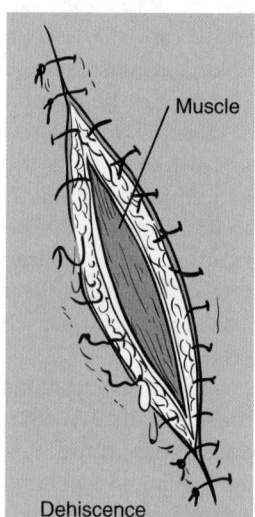
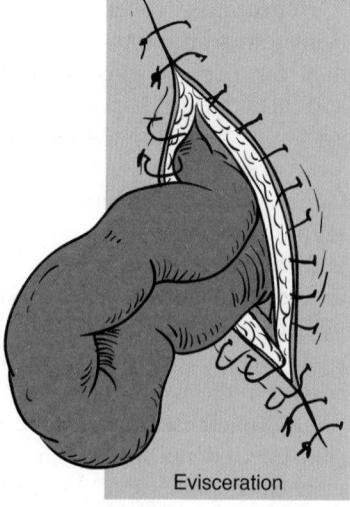

■ **FIGURE 14–13** Clients with wound dehiscence and evisceration after surgery require immediate attention (see text).

TABLE 14-7 **Postoperative Complications**

Body System	Complications
Respiratory	Atelectasis
	Pneumonia
	Aspiration pneumonitis
	Pulmonary edema
	Acute respiratory distress syndrome
	Pulmonary embolism
Cardiac	Hypertension
	Myocardial ischemia and infarction
	Cardiogenic shock
	Dysrhythmias
	Heart failure
Renal and urinary	Acute renal failure
Metabolic	Adrenal insufficiency
	Hyperthyroidism
	Hypothyroidism
	Syndrome of inappropriate antidiuretic hormone secretion (SIADH)
Gastrointestinal	Ileus and obstruction
	Abdominal compartment syndrome
	GI bleeding
	Stomal complications
	Pseudomonas colitis
	Anastomosis leak
	Fistula
Hepatobiliary	Bile duct injury
Neurologic	Delirium, dementia, psychosis
	Seizure
	Stroke
Ear, nose, and throat	Epistaxis
	Acute hearing loss
	Parotiditis
	Sinusitis

Interventions are designed to address the specific issues. For the client with severe blood loss, transfusion may be used to restore blood volume. Today, many clients donate their own blood before elective surgery, so the transfusion of autologous blood is without risk of blood-borne infection. Blood banks can provide blood quickly for clients who have been "typed and crossmatched," so that the most similar units of blood can be transfused. (See Chapter 75 for more information on blood transfusion.)

Other interventions to promote recovery might include ambulation and exercise with physical therapists to gain strength and endurance and recover energy. Ambulation also reduces the risk of thrombus. Occupational therapists may be able to assist the client in regaining some self-care abilities, by helping the client to independently dress, toilet, and eat.

It is not uncommon to find clients depressed about delays in surgical recovery. Sometimes the complications were unpredictable and clients and their families had no intention of being in the hospital or rehabilitation center for weeks to months. Find time to allow them to vent this frustration, depression, or anxiety about their outcome. Be certain that they have heard and comprehended what has been told to them by the physicians. Many times these clients have multiple teams of physicians caring for them and they lose track of "who is who." Encourage them to write questions on paper so they remember to ask. Rounds can be just a few minutes each day, and clients, oftentimes not ready to assert themselves, can be left confused or with questions. The nurse's role can be extremely valuable to help clarify and amplify the messages.

DISCHARGE INSTRUCTIONS AND CARE

Regardless of the length of stay in the hospital or surgical center, when the client is ready to go home ensure that the client and a family member (as appropriate) have the information and skills needed to continue a successful recovery.

SAFETY

ALERT

Teach skills over a period of days, with ample time for questions and "hands-on" practice. Give all information in writing to the client or family members. Consider videotaping procedures performed on the client so that the client and family can follow them at home. Most institutions provide a printed form filled out with specific postoperative information, such as instructions on medications and wound care, an appointment for a postoperative clinic visit, and names and telephone numbers in case there are further questions or an emergency arises. Drug prescriptions are also provided if medications are to be continued at home.

If the client has further health care needs after discharge, collaborate with other health care workers such as those in social services, home nursing (Bridge to Home Health Care feature Recovering from Surgery), or rehabilitation services. Many resources are available in the community for clients, and most institutions have a list for the local area. Determine the resources available in your community for the clients under your care, ascertain what each resource provides, and know how they are contacted. A partial listing of the most common resources follows:

- Child Protection Services
- Emergency social services or hospital social services
- Emergency legal assistance
- Hospice
- Local chapters of organizations offering help (e.g., American Cancer Society, American Heart Association, American Diabetes Association)
- Local mastectomy, laryngectomy, or colostomy support groups
- Local senior citizens' assistance program
- Medic Alert Foundation
- Local sexual assault center (by law, suspected sexual abuse of minors must be reported)
- Malignant Hyperthermia Hotline
- Substance abuse treatment programs or groups
- Visiting Nurse Association or home health care services

CONCLUSIONS

The nurse plays a critical role in the perioperative care of the client. Today, surgery ranges from outpatient procedures to complex inpatient procedures. No matter what type of surgery is performed, however, the client needs expert nursing care. The quality of nursing care can determine whether the client has a successful perioperative experience.

THINKING CRITICALLY

1. A young adult client in the emergency department has acute appendicitis. Surgery is scheduled in 30 minutes. What teaching should be completed before the client has the surgery? What interventions must be completed before the client is taken to the operating area?

Factors to Consider. What important client teaching is completed before any surgery in which general anesthesia is used? Are possible complications discussed at the time? What measures usually appear on a preoperative checklist?

2. An older adult client has undergone major abdominal surgery under general anesthesia. At age 80 years, she is in relatively good health following a cerebrovascular accident about 8 years ago. Her only medication is a 325-mg aspirin tablet taken once a day. What complications are most likely in an 80-year-old client? How can these complications be prevented? How is pain tolerated by the older client?

Factors to Consider. What complications are associated with general anesthesia? How do a thorough history and assessment help you in your plan to prevent complications after surgery? What age-related considerations must be made? Does the use of aspirin increase the risk of any complications?

 Discussions for these questions can be found on the website.

BIBLIOGRAPHY

 Citations appearing in red refer to primary research.

1. Allen, G. (2006). Evidence for practice. Unplanned admission after ambulatory surgery. *AORN Journal, 84*(3), 498.
2. Anonymous. (2005). New genetic test promising for malignant hyperthermia. *OR Manager, 21*(8), 7.
3. Anonymous. (2004). NICE to advise on CJD surgery risk. *Nursing Times, 100*(41), 7.
4. Anonymous. (2006). Preventing spread of 'super bugs' in the ambulatory surgery setting. *OR Manager, 22*(12), 1-26.
5. Anonymous. (2006). Ambulatory surgery leaders to identify quality measures. *OR Manager, 22*(10), 31.
6. Australian hospital warns of possible CJD exposure: More than 1,000 patients contacted. (2004). *Hospital Infection Control, 31*(10), 130-132.
7. Benefits of using the perioperative nursing data set (2002). Reprinted with permission from S.C. Beyea (Ed.), *Perioperative nursing data set* (2nd ed.). Denver: AORN. *AORN Journal, 83*(6), 1338.
8. Benson, M.K.D., Bourne, R., Hanley, E., et al. (2005). Ethics in orthopaedic surgery. *Journal of Bone and Joint Surgery, 87B*, 1449-1451.
9. Bhattacharyya, T., & Yeon, H. (2005). "Doctor, was this surgery done wrong?" Ethical issues in providing second opinions. *Journal of Bone and Joint Surgery, 87A*(1), 223-225.
10. Blanchard, J. (2005). Clinical issues. Waterborne infections; cotton swabs; patient safety goals; vancomycin; vaginal prep; battery-operated electrocautery hand pieces. *AORN Journal, 82*(3), 481.
11. Brandão, M.A. (2006). Nursing diagnosis strategies: Students' considerations. *International Journal of Nursing Terminologies & Classifications, 17*(1), 20.
12. Burden, N. (2006). Outcomes measurement in ambulatory surgery. *Journal of PeriAnesthesia Nursing, 21*(5), 342-345.
13. Burger, I., Sugarman, J., & Goodman, S. (2006). Ethical issues in evidence-based surgery. *Surgical Clinics of North America, 86*(1), 151-168.
14. Carr, A.J. (2006). Which research is to be believed? *Journal of Bone and Joint Surgery, 87B*, 1452-1453.
15. Chalfine, A., Cauet, D., Lin, W., et al. (2006). Highly sensitive and efficient computer-assisted system for routine surveillance for surgical site infection. *Infection Control & Hospital Epidemiology, 27* (8), 794-801.
16. Coleman, T., Culkin, C., & Sierka, D. (2006). Kidney transplants in HIV patients? Yes! *RN, 69*(1), 33-39.
17. Cullum, N., McInnes, E., Bell-Syer, S., et al. (2004). Support surfaces for pressure ulcer prevention. *Cochrane Library*, Issue.
18. Curtin, L. (2005). Ethics in management. Refusal of treatment. *Journal of Clinical Systems Management, 7*(5-6), 17-18.
19. Doraiswamy, N.V., Baig, H., Hammett, S., et al. (2004). Which tissue adhesive for wounds? *Injury, 35*(6), 637-638.
20. Doyle, M. (2006). Home study program. Promoting standardized nursing language using an electronic medical record system. *AORN Journal, 83*(6), 1335.
21. Dunn, D. (2006). Age-smart care: Preventing perioperative complications in older adults. *Nursing Made Incredibly Easy, 4*(3), 30.
22. Dunn, K. (2004). Music and the reduction of post-operative pain. *Nursing Standard, 18*(36), 33-39.
23. Ead, H. (2006). From Aldrete to PADSS: Reviewing discharge criteria after ambulatory surgery... Post Anesthetic Discharge Scoring System. *Journal of PeriAnesthesia Nursing, 21*(4), 259-267.
24. Elston, D. (2006). More MRSA infections are headed your way. *Clinical Advisor for Nurse Practitioners, 9*(7), 67-69.
25. Elton, G. (2004). Review: Elastic compression stockings prevent post-thrombotic syndrome in patients with deep venous thrombosis. *Evidence-Based Nursing, 7*(3), 86.
26. Fawley, W., Parnell, P., Hall, J., et al. (2006). Surveillance for mupirocin resistance following introduction of routine peri-operative prophylaxis with nasal mupirocin. *Journal of Hospital Infection, 62*(3), 327-332.
27. Gawande, A., Studdert, D., et al. (2003). Risk factors for retained instruments and sponges after surgery. *New England Journal of Medicine, 348*, 229-235.
28. Gordon, M., Gottschlich, M., Helvig, E., et al. (2004). Review of evidenced-based practice for the prevention of pressure sores in burn patients. *Journal of Burn Care & Rehabilitation, 25*(5), 388-410.
29. Gordon, H., & Mick, J. (2006). Don't be confused! Assessment of elderly surgical patients' mental status can prevent adverse events and improve outcomes. *Oncology Nursing Forum, 33*(2), 431.
30. Gurkan, I., & Wenz, J. (2006). Perioperative infection control: An update for patient safety in orthopedic surgery. *Orthopedics, 29* (4), 329-341.
31. Hickman, A., Bell, D., & Preston, J. (2005). Update for nurse anesthetists: Acupressure and postoperative nausea and vomiting. *AANA Journal, 73*(5), 379-385.
32. Hommertzheim, R., & Steinke, E. (2007). Home study program. Malignant hyperthermia—The perioperative nurse's role. *AORN Journal, 83*(1), 149.
33. Ibrahim, S.A. (2005). Racial/ethnic differences in surgical outcomes in veterans following knee or hip arthroplasty. *Arthritis & Rheumatism, 52*(10), 3143-3151.
34. Ipswich, M.A., & Rosenberg, H. (2004). A review of the malignant hyperthermia syndrome. *Current Reviews for Nurse Anesthetists, 27*(7), 75-84.

35. JCAHO issues 2007 patient safety goals. (2006). *OR Manager, 22* (7), 9.

36. Kleinbeck, S., & Dopp, A. (2006). Home study program. The Perioperative Nursing Data Set—A new language for documenting care... reprinted with permission from the American Health Information Management Association (AHIMA). *AORN Journal, 82*(1), 50.

37. Lee, M. (2006). Evidence-based surgery: Creating the culture. *Surgical Clinics of North America, 86*(1), 91-100.

38. Lee, J., Chan, A., & Phillips, D. (2006). Diagnostic practice in nursing: A critical review of the literature. *Nursing & Health Sciences, 8*(1), 57-65.

39. Leung, J., Sands, L., Mullen, E., et al. (2005). Are preoperative depressive symptoms associated with postoperative delirium in geriatric surgical clients? *Journals of Gerontology, Series A: Biological Sciences & Medical Sciences, 60A*(12), 1563-1568.

40. Lindenauer, P., Pekow, P., Wang, K., et al. (2005). Perioperative beta-blocker therapy and mortality after noncardiac surgery. *New England Journal of Medicine, 353,* 349-361.

41. Lorenz, R., Lorenz, R., & Codd, J. (2005). Home study program: Perioperative blood glucose control during adult coronary artery bypass surgery. *AORN Journal, 81*(1), 126.

42. Mathus-Vliegen, E. (2004). Old age, malnutrition, and pressure sores: An ill-fated alliance. *Journals of Gerontology, Series A: Biological Sciences & Medical Sciences, 59A*(4), 355-360.

43. McGarry, S., Engemann, J., Schmader, K., et al. (2004). Surgical-site infection due to *Staphylococcus aureus* among elderly patients: Mortality, duration of hospitalization, and cost. *Infection Control & Hospital Epidemiology, 25*(6), 461-467.

44. Rathmell, J., Wu, C., Sinatra, R., et al. (2005). Acute post-surgical pain management: A critical appraisal of current practice. *The Pain Management Summit,* Dec 2-4, 2005, Fort Lauderdale, Fla. *Regional Anesthesia & Pain Medicine [serial online], 31*(4), 1-42

45. Regez, R., Kleipool, A., Speekenbrink, R., et al. (2005). The risk of needle stick accidents during surgical procedures: HIV-1 viral load in blood and bone marrow. *International Journal of STD & AIDS, 16*(10), 671-672.

46. Render, M., Brungs, S., Kotagal, U., et al. (2006). Evidence-based practice to reduce central line infections. *Joint Commission Journal on Quality & Patient Safety, 32*(5), 253-260.

47. Sauaia, A., Min, S., Leber, C., et al. (2005). Postoperative pain management in elderly patients: Correlation between adherence to treatment guidelines and patient satisfaction. *Journal of the American Geriatrics Society, 53*(2), 274-282.

48. Schoenwald, A., & Clark, C. (2006). Acute pain in surgical patients. *Contemporary Nurse: A Journal for the Australian Nursing Profession, 22*(1), 97-108.

49. Scott, E., & Buckland, R. (2006). A systematic review of intraoperative warming to prevent postoperative complications. *AORN Journal, 83*(5), 1090.

50. Sessler, D. (2006). Non-pharmacologic prevention of surgical wound infection. *Anesthesiology Clinics of North America, 24*(2), 279-297.

51. Sigsby, L., Selzer, J., & Wilson, T. (2006). A successful nursing student practicum in an ambulatory surgery center. *AORN Journal, 84*(2), 219.

52. Sorta-Bilajac, I., Juretic, M., Muzur, A., et al. (2006). Bioethics of appearance and the quality of life issue: Who makes the decision? *Head & Neck Surgery, 134*(2), 351-352.

53. Tracy, S., Dufault, M., Kogut, S., et al. (2006). Translating best practices in nondrug postoperative pain management. *Nursing Research, 55*(2 Suppl), S57-S67.

54. Van Dorsten, B. (2006). Psychological considerations in preparing patients for implantation procedures. *Pain Medicine, 7*(Suppl 1), S47-S57.

55. Wadlund, D. (2006). Prevention, recognition, and management of nursing complications in the intraoperative and postoperative surgical patient. *Nursing Clinics of North America, 41*(2), 151-171.

56. Wagner, V. (2006). Patient safety first. Unplanned perioperative hypothermia. *AORN Journal, 3*(2), 470.

57. Woodley, K. (2004). Improving ambulatory surgical pain management. *Joint Commission Journal on Quality & Safety, 30*(1), 36-41.

58. Yellen, E.A. (2005). The effect of a preadmission videotape on patient satisfaction. *AORN Journal, 81*(4), 831-840, 842, 845.

evolve *Did you remember to check out the bonus material on the Evolve website and the CD-ROM, including NCLEX®-Examination Style Review Questions, Open-Book Quizzes, and Chapter Review Audio Podcasts?*

http://evolve.elsevier.com/Black/medsurg

UNIT 4

PHYSIOLOGIC FOUNDATIONS

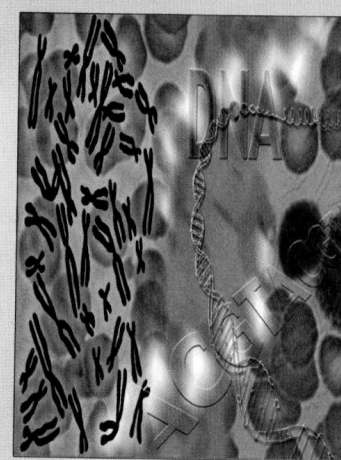

ANATOMY AND PHYSIOLOGY REVIEW:

Physiologic Genomics

Robert G. Carroll

Cellular function, and therefore body function, is governed by proteins, and proteins are governed by genes. The central tenet of molecular medicine is that the instructions for protein synthesis are encoded in the genes contained in DNA. Variations in DNA underlie the uniqueness of each individual, with significant health implications. The final health status results from the interactions of the genetic potential and the environment.

Genes do not act alone; rather, they are influenced by the genetic background of an individual and by the external or internal environment. A person's genetic constitution, or genome, is referred to as the *genotype*. How these genes express themselves (as in height, hair color, and body chemistry, for example) is referred to as the *phenotype*. With this background to the structure and function of normal genes, it is possible to consider molecular pathology and to determine how these errors relate to human disease.

In April 2003 scientists announced completion of the sequencing of the human genome, identifying the approximately 6 billion nucleotides (DNA building blocks) that make up the estimated 30,000 to 35,000 genes found in humans. This accomplishment will benefit medicine and health care by increasing knowledge about human growth and development and understanding of the role of genes in both health and disease.

Areas of clinical practice affected by the genetics revolution include the potential application of pharmacogenomics to predict individual responsiveness to drugs, prenatal diagnosis, carrier screening for select genetic disorders, diagnostic genetic testing for adult-onset disorders, presymptomatic genetic testing, and predisposition testing for complex trait disorders. Importantly, manipulation of the human genome could allow correction of diseases at the genetic level and will likely emerge as an important therapeutic adjunct to improve the care of clients. These advancements in genetic knowledge and technology also carry significant ethical, legal, and social implications that affect all levels of health care delivery.

DNA

Arranged from smallest to largest, genetic material includes the four nucleotides (bases) adenine (A), thymine (T), guanine (G), or cytosine (C); groups of three nucleotides (codon); a collection of codons (gene); a collection of genes (chromosome); and a collection of chromosomes (genotype). DNA is arranged in a double helix, with each side of the helix being a complementary mirror image, and the nucleotides arranged as base pairs joined by hydrogen bonds (Figure A&P4-1). In the base pairing, the nucleotides A and T are always joined as one base pair, and G bonds to C in the other base pair. The hydrogen bonds keep the helix joined in much the same way the teeth of a zipper interact.

The double-stranded helical arrangement plays a key role in the two major functions of DNA: protein synthesis and cellular replication. In both processes, the bonds between the complementary nucleotides are broken, exposing the interior of the DNA to allow copying. In replication, the entire complement of DNA is copied, creating a duplicate DNA. In protein synthesis, only a small portion of the DNA is copied onto a single strand of messenger RNA.

PROTEIN SYNTHESIS

The central dogma of protein synthesis is that DNA is transcribed to messenger RNA (mRNA), and mRNA is translated to protein. Only about 2% of the DNA is transcribed into the mRNA. About 98% of the DNA is not transcribed, and the function of these regions is not yet fully established. Both transcription and translation involve a complex sequence of steps (Figure A&P4-2).

Transcription

Transcription is the making of an mRNA copy from a specific segment of DNA. The initial event is the "unzipping" of a region of the DNA and creation of a single strand of mRNA. The enzyme RNA polymerase "unzips" a region of the DNA, and one side of the DNA serves as a template for the creation of mRNA. The mRNA is a mirror image of the DNA nucleotide sequence, with the exception that uracil (U) is used as the nucleotide base instead of thymine. After the mRNA is transcribed, the DNA is re-zipped, and available for future use.

The segment of mRNA that codes for the protein is called an *exon*. Most mRNAs are composed of many exons that are interrupted by noncoding sequences termed *introns*. The introns are then spliced out of the mRNA and only the exons are used for translation into proteins. The mRNA, now consisting only of exons,

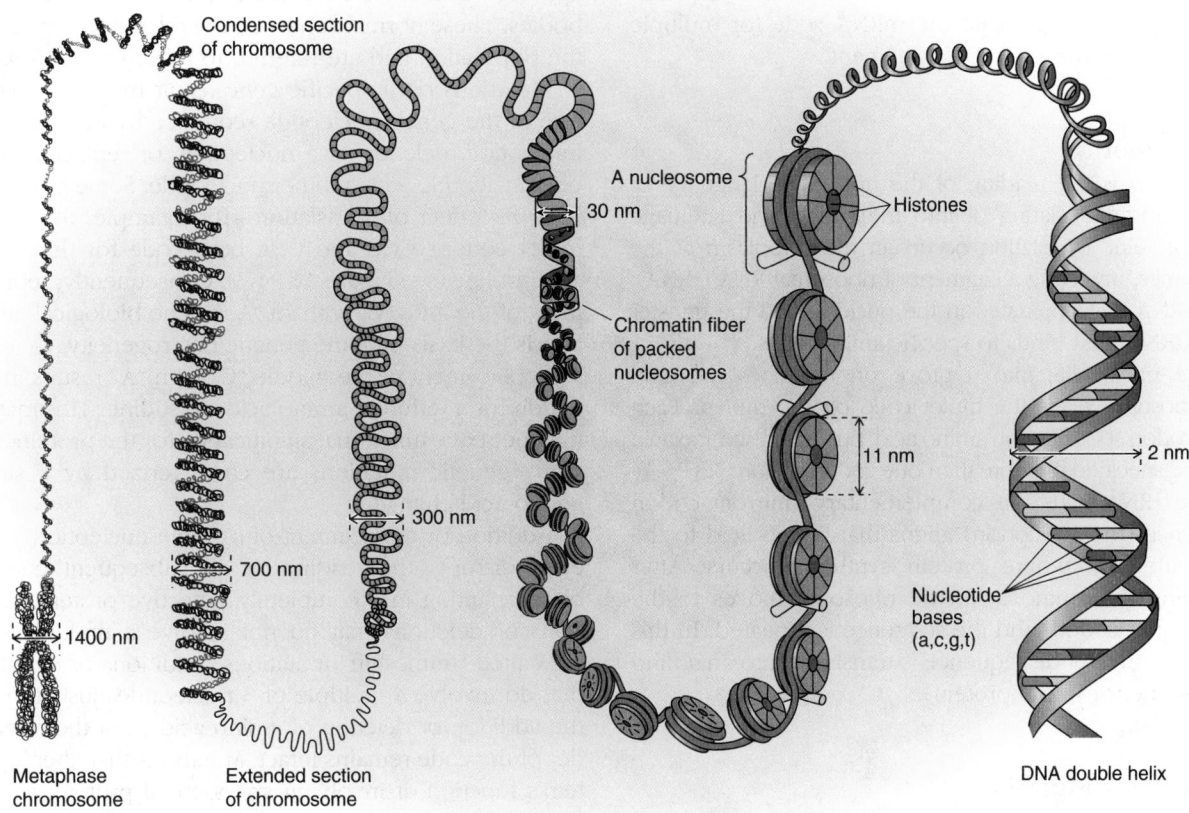

Condensed section of chromosome

A nucleosome

30 nm

Histones

Chromatin fiber of packed nucleosomes

11 nm

2 nm

300 nm

700 nm

1400 nm

Nucleotide bases (a,c,g,t)

Metaphase chromosome

Extended section of chromosome

DNA double helix

■ **FIGURE A&P4–1** From cell nucleus to DNA base pairs. *(From Lea, D. [2000]. A clinician's primer in human genetics: What nurses need to know. Nursing Clinics of North America, 35[3], 583-614.)*

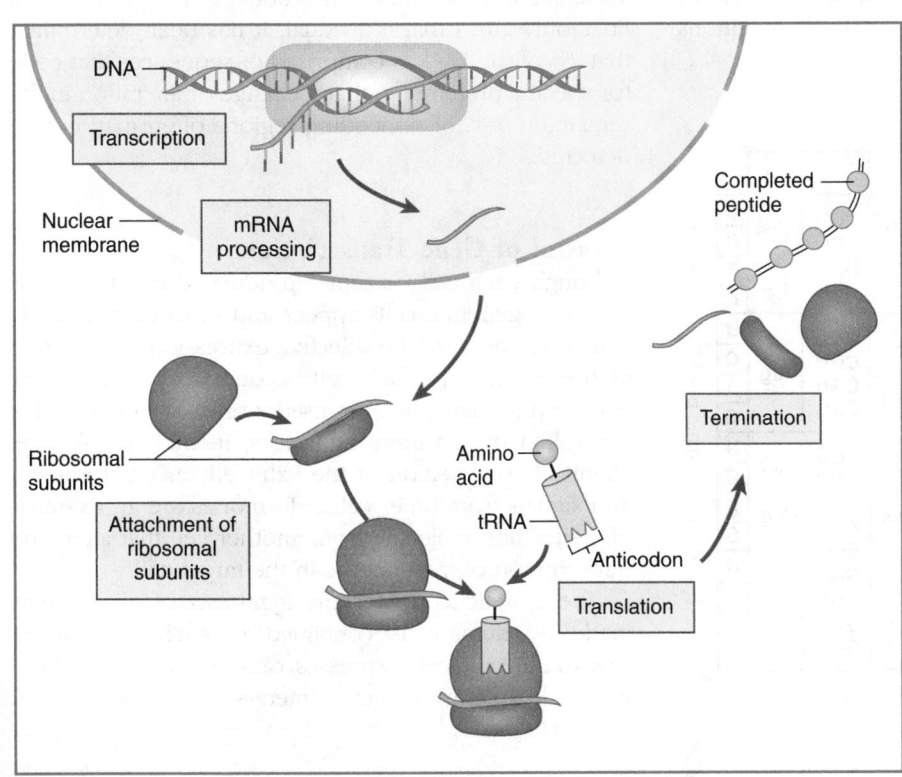

DNA

Transcription

Nuclear membrane

mRNA processing

Completed peptide

Ribosomal subunits

Attachment of ribosomal subunits

Amino acid

tRNA

Termination

Anticodon

Translation

■ **FIGURE A&P4–2** Protein synthesis requires creation of a copy of messenger RNA from the DNA template (transcription), attachment of the messenger RNA to the cytoplasmic ribosomes, and reading of the mRNA codons by the ribosome to create a specific amino acid sequence on a protein (translation).

exits the nucleus. Often, one segment of DNA encodes instructions for a variety of proteins. In these cases, alternative splicing can create the mRNA code for multiple proteins from the same DNA segment.

Translation

Translation is the reading of the nucleotide language of mRNA and "translating" it into the amino acid language of a protein. Translation occurs in the cytoplasm at the ribosomes, involving a segment of ribosomal RNA (rRNA), the mRNA that originated in the nucleus, and the transfer RNA (tRNA) that binds to specific amino acids.

The mRNA fits into a grove on the ribosome, and the ribosome reads the triplet code on the mRNA. Each RNA codon specifies one amino acid, but a single amino acid may be specified by more than one codon (Figure A&P4-3).

The tRNA with the complementary (mirror) codon sequence (the anticodon) aligns that amino acid to the ribosome site, where protein synthesis occurs. After attaching the amino acid, the ribosome moves to the next triplet codon, and the sequence is repeated. In this way, the nucleotide sequence is translated into an amino acid sequence in the protein.

DNA Point Mutations

In general, genes are generally stable and are passed from one generation to the next without change or alteration. However, genes occasionally change, referred to as *mutation*. Between the structural genes are long segments of noncoding DNA, the function of which is not completely understood. Within this DNA are mutations

or variations in nucleotide sequence, which have no apparent impact on the structure and function of human bodies. These normal variations are relatively frequent in the population and are referred to as *polymorphisms*.

Mutations on a specific gene result from the disruption of the gene's nucleotide sequence by insertion of a nucleotide, deletion of a nucleotide, or replacement of one nucleotide with another nucleotide. Some mutations have no effect on translation—for example, the mRNA triplet codons CCC and CCA both code for the amino acid proline (see Figure A&P4-3). Consequently, replacement of the third "C" with an "A" has no biological effect, and is the basis of some genetic heterogeneity.

Replacement of the middle "C" with "A" results in the codon for a different amino acid—histidine. This may or may not have functional significance for the protein, and many genetic mutations are characterized by a single amino acid change.

Addition or replacement of a single nucleotide, however, disrupts the reading of all subsequent codons, often resulting in a completely defective protein. Additions or deletions that do not involve a multiple of 3 are called "frameshift" mutations. Additions or deletions that do involve a multiple of 3 nucleotides just result in the addition or deletion of amino acids, but the remainder of the code remains intact. Mutations that alter a protein's function, if involving an essential protein, can be fatal.

Mutations can occur in the germ line (sperm and egg) cells or may occur in the somatic (body) cells after fertilization. Mutations in the germ cell line are passed to subsequent generations; mutations in the somatic cell lines only affect that individual. It has been determined that 2% of the DNA is comprised of sequences that code for specific proteins, so that a change or alteration in the remaining 98% of noncoding regions often may not be detected.

Control of Gene Transcription

Although each cell (except reproductive cells) contains the same genome, cells appear and function differently from one another. The selective expression of only part of the genome in each cell accounts for these differences. In humans, gene transcription is complex and is controlled by a variety of factors, including cell type, chemical composition of the extracellular environment, and signals from other cells. Hormones are an example of a signaling molecule from another cell that alters the transcription of the genome in the target cell.

The genetic code for the synthesis of all proteins made by humans is contained in each cell's DNA. However, each cell expresses only a fraction of these genes. Regulatory proteins interact with specific DNA

Second base

		U	C	A	G	
	U	UUU ⎤ Phe UUC ⎦ UUA ⎤ Leu UUG ⎦	UCU ⎤ UCC ⎪ Ser UCA ⎪ UCG ⎦	UAU ⎤ Tyr UAC ⎦ UAA UAG	UGU ⎤ Cys UGC ⎦ UGA UGG Trp	U C A G
First base	C	CUU ⎤ CUC ⎪ Leu CUA ⎪ CUG ⎦	CCU ⎤ CCC ⎪ Pro CCA ⎪ CCG ⎦	CAU ⎤ His CAC ⎦ CAA ⎤ Gln CAG ⎦	CGU ⎤ CGC ⎪ Arg CGA ⎪ CGG ⎦	U C A G	Third base
	A	AUU ⎤ AUC ⎪ Ile AUA ⎦ AUG Met	ACU ⎤ ACC ⎪ Thr ACA ⎪ ACG ⎦	AAU ⎤ Asp AAC ⎦ AAA ⎤ Lys AAG ⎦	AGU ⎤ Ser AGC ⎦ AGA ⎤ Arg AGG ⎦	U C A G
	G	GUU ⎤ GUC ⎪ Val GUA ⎪ GUG ⎦	GCU ⎤ GCC ⎪ Ala GCA ⎪ GCG ⎦	GAU ⎤ Asp GAC ⎦ GAA ⎤ Glu GAG ⎦	GGU ⎤ GGC ⎪ Gly GGA ⎪ GGG ⎦	U C A G

■ **FIGURE A&P4–3** Genetic code.

sequences called *response elements* to alter gene expression and to determine which genes are transcribed. These regulatory proteins are called *transcription factors,* which can increase or decrease the transcription of specific genes. Examples of regulatory elements are promoters, which enhance gene expression, and repressors, which downregulate or slow gene expression.

Control of Translation

Protein synthesis involves the creation both of the protein structure and of some additional amino acids that direct the protein folding and transport to specific intracellular locations. Post-translational modification allows enzymes to modify individual amino acids, or further alter the protein structure by folding and cross-linking to other proteins.

CELLULAR REPLICATION

Most cells in the body replicate by mitosis, although at varying rates. During replication, an exact copy of the DNA is synthesized using one half of the original material as a template. Consequently, daughter cells contain duplicate copies of all 46 chromosomes, half from the parent cell and half synthesized during mitosis. In contrast, gametes replicate by meiosis. In meiosis, the DNA is duplicated, but 4 daughter cells are formed, each with 23 chromosomes, half of the normal number. The process of fertilization, where the sperm and ovum combine, results in a return to the normal 46 chromosome count, with half of the chromosomes from the paternal sperm and half of the chromosomes from the maternal ovum.

Chromosomes

DNA in the nucleus is normally in long strands. During cellular replication, the DNA coils into chromosomes, which can be seen using a light microscope (see Figure A&P4-1). Human chromosomes consist of a short arm and a long arm separated by an area of constriction known as the *centromere*. The short arm of the chromosome is referred to as the p-arm and the long arm of the chromosome is referred to as the q-arm. For example, the designation 8q refers to the long arm of the eighth chromosome. Chromosomes are stained to reveal alternating light and dark horizontal bands. Because the banding patterns are unique to each chromosome, the bands assist in the identification of individual chromosomes and serve as geographical landmarks for localization of genetic markers and genes. In the cytogenetics laboratory, the chromosomes are stained and analyzed for number, structure, and missing (deleted) or additional (duplicated) genetic material. By convention, the

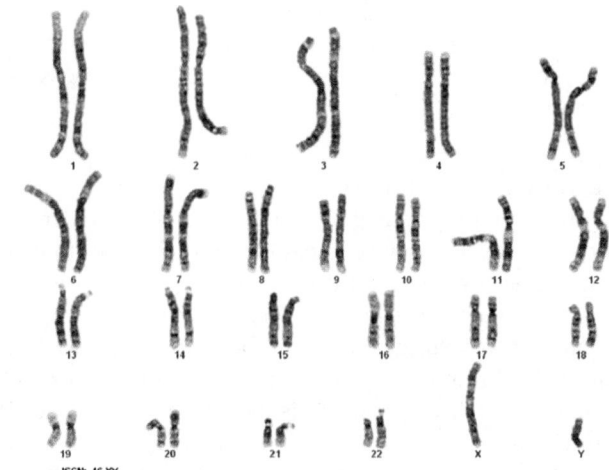

■ FIGURE A&P4–4 Normal male chromosome karyotype. *(Courtesy The Clinical Section, Laboratory of Pathology, National Cancer Institute, National Institutes of Health, Bethesda, Md.)*

chromosomes are arranged in descending order of size, and oriented such that the short arm is on top and the long arm is on the bottom.

As demonstrated in Figure A&P4-4, chromosomes are arranged in a karyotype and designated by number according to their size and shape. Chromosome pairs 1 to 22 are called *autosomes,* which are present in both males and females, and the 23rd pair consists of the sex chromosomes. Females have two X chromosomes and males have an X and a Y chromosome.

Just as there are maternal and paternal copies of each chromosome, there are also maternal and paternal copies of each gene. The nucleotide sequence, or *spelling,* of the maternal and paternal gene pair may be identical (homozygous) or different (heterozygous). For example, an individual with blood type AB inherited the type A allele (gene copy) from one parent and the type B allele from the other parent, and thus is considered to be heterozygous for the gene pair.

DIFFERENTIATION

Stem cells are undifferentiated cells, such as those of a fertilized ovum. Normally, stem cells replicate, producing identical daughter stem cells. Under specific conditions, stem cells will differentiate into specific types of tissue. Consequently, stem cells are valuable potential building blocks for tissue repair and regeneration. During fetal development, most cells of the body undergo terminal differentiation, and cannot return to the stem cell status. Certain stem cell populations persist through fetal development and possibly into adulthood.

One characteristic of differentiated cells is that they show selective gene expression. This accounts for why a liver hepatocyte and a cardiac myocyte have such different appearance and function. Despite these differences, both the hepatocyte and the myocyte still possess the same genes.

Chromosomal Mutations

During meiosis, there is crossing over of genes from one chromosome to its companion chromosome. In this case, gene(s) of paternal origin will now reside on the original maternal origin chromosome, and the complementary maternal gene(s) will be transferred to the paternal chromosome. This process contributes to genetic variability, as meiosis is the process of germ cell production.

Mutations can result during crossing over, involving a fragment of a chromosome. Deletions involve the removal of a fragment of a chromosome, and all of the genes contained in that fragment. Duplications involve a fragment attaching to the companion chromosome in addition to the complementary fragment still in place. Inversion occurs when the fragment is attached to the correct companion chromosome, but is inverted so that the code is no longer read in correct sequence. Translocation occurs when the fragment is attached to a chromosome other than the companion chromosome.

The "segregation" of chromosomes during anaphase also creates a potential for chromosome mutations. Nondisjunction is an error in chromosome distribution, leading to gametes with an abnormal chromosome count (aneuploidy, too many or to few chromosomes). Trisomy 21 is an example of an aneuploid condition that results in Down syndrome.

Regulation of Cellular Replication

Normally, cell growth and replication are regulated by a series of "checkpoint" genes. These checkpoints reduce or arrest cell division in response to cell density or to chemicals produced in the microenvironment. Consequently, most organs have a defined size and structure.

There are more than 100 genes (*proto-oncogenes*) that are a normal part of the human genome that, when activated by mutation, can participate in cancerous growth. Most of these genes interfere with key steps in cell growth or differentiation. These genes are not intrinsically active, but can become activated by a variety of chemical, viral, or environmental insults. If changes in expression of this gene result in cancer, the gene is then called an *oncogene*. The growth-stimulating proteins produced by oncogenes are not subject to normal regulation.

In general, cancers are an imbalance between normal growth repression and stimulation. At the genetic level, this is caused by underexpression of genes that inhibit growth (the tumor suppressor genes), overexpression of genes that enhance growth (tumor growth factors), or some combination of the two. Most cancers require both a genetic susceptibility and an environmental trigger to occur.

Cancer is abnormal replication of cells, in which the normal controls over cell cycling and programmed cell death have been disrupted. One characteristic of cancerous cells is an alteration in the cell membrane and the ability to adhere to both other cells and the extracellular glycoprotein matrix. Consequently, cancerous cells are likely to break free from their original location and spread through the lymphatics and circulatory system to other parts of the body (metastasize).

Cancerous cells show partial loss of differentiation (dedifferentiation) and can synthesize proteins not normally produced by that tissue. For example, 5% of clients with oat cell carcinoma of the lung have manifestations of adrenocorticotropic hormone (ACTH) excess. In this type of cancer, the gene encoding ACTH production is inappropriately transcribed and is not subject to the normal ACTH negative-feedback regulation

APOPTOSIS

Part of the genome encodes for proteins that mediate a programmed cell death, or apoptosis. This is a normal part of the aging of cells. These genes are normally suppressed and not translated. Cellular damage, however, can remove the suppressor factors, and allow synthesis of the apoptotic proteins. This mechanism allows destruction of nonfunctional cells, and allows their replacement. Some forms of cancer are linked to defects in apoptotic proteins. Figure A&P4-5 depicts apoptosis.

PHYSIOLOGIC GENOMICS

Physiologic genomics is a field of research that links gene expression to biological function. This field studies topics such as cell replication, development, metabolic function, tissue and organ function, and whole organism function. This field examines processes in which appropriate control allows growth and repair, but disordered control is the basis for cancer. Importantly, manipulation of the human genome could allow correction of diseases at the genetic level and will likely emerge as an important therapeutic adjunct to improve the care of clients.

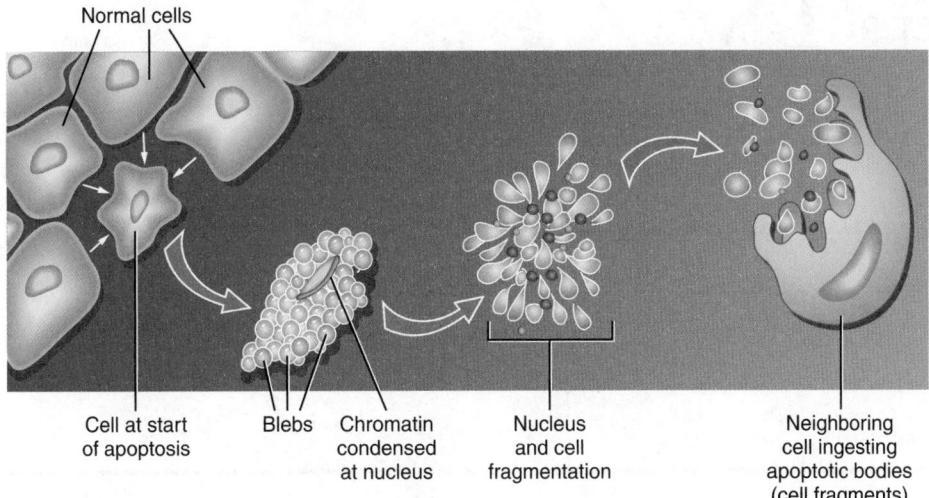

Normal cells

Cell at start
of apoptosis

Blebs

Chromatin
condensed
at nucleus

Nucleus
and cell
fragmentation

Neighboring
cell ingesting
apoptotic bodies
(cell fragments)

■ **FIGURE A&P4–5** Programmed cell death resulting from apoptosis. With apoptosis (cell suicide), the cell shrinks and pulls away from surrounding cells. Blebs appear on the surface of the cell. Chromatin condenses on the edge of the nucleus. The nucleus and then the cell itself break up. Cell fragments are ingested by other cells. *(From Duke, R.C., Ojcius, D.M., & Young, J.D. [1996]. Cell suicide in health and disease. Scientific American, 275[6], 81.)*

 BIBLIOGRAPHY

1. Berne, R., et al.. (2004). *Physiology* (5th ed.). St. Louis: Mosby.
2. Kierszenbaum, A.L. (2006). *Histology and cell biology: An introduction to pathology* (2nd ed.). St. Louis: Mosby.
3. Guyton, A., & Hall, J. (2006). *Textbook of medical physiology* (11th ed.). Philadelphia: Saunders.
4. Silverthorn, D. (2006). *Human physiology* (4th ed.). San Francisco, Calif: Pearson Benjamin Cummings.
5. Starr, C., & Taggart, R. (2004). *Biology: The unity and diversity of life* (10th ed.). Stamford, Conn: Thompson Brooks/Cole Australia.

CHAPTER 15

Perspectives in Genetics

LINDSAY ANN MIDDELTON AND MIRA LESSICK

There is a substantial body of knowledge about genetics in nursing literature written by nurse researchers, clinicians, policy-makers, and national nursing organizations. Nurses are among the few professions contributing knowledge about how clients and families are using genetic technology to improve health and quality of life.

THE GENETICS REVOLUTION AND NURSING

Revolutionary discoveries in molecular genetics that occurred through the Human Genome Project (HGP) are greatly influencing health care and the practice of nursing. These discoveries are presenting new ways of thinking about the concepts of health and disease and new approaches to the assessment, diagnosis, treatment, management, and prevention of illness. In 2001 a consortium of more than 100 organizations involved in health care developed genetic core competencies essential for all health care providers to incorporate into their practice. Nurses in all health care settings must become genetically literate if they are to effectively incorporate this burgeoning knowledge into client care. Not only are advances in genetics significantly impacting nursing practice, but widespread integration of genetics into nursing education and research is also currently underway.

The HGP began in 1990 as an international effort to analyze the structure of human DNA and determine the location of all human genes on chromosomes. In April 2003 scientists announced completion of the sequencing of the human genome, which is comprised of approximately 3 billion base pairs (DNA building blocks) that make up the estimated 30,000 to 35,000 genes of the human genome. The products of the HGP will benefit medicine and health care by increasing knowledge about human growth and development, and the role of genes in both health and disease.

Areas of clinical practice affected by the genetics revolution include the potential application of pharmacogenomics to predict individual responsiveness to drugs, carrier screening for select genetic disorders, prenatal diagnosis, diagnostic genetic testing for adult-onset disorders, presymptomatic genetic testing, and predisposition testing for complex trait disorders. In addition, genetic-based therapeutics and gene therapy hold promise for the future treatment of many conditions, including inherited and noninherited disorders. These advancements in genetic knowledge and technology also carry significant ethical, legal, and social implications that affect all levels of practice.

See the Anatomy and Physiology Review at the beginning of Unit 4 for a review of basic concepts of genes, chromosomes, and DNA. Box 15-1 lists a glossary of genetic terms.

PRIMARY CATEGORIES OF GENETIC CONDITIONS

The three primary categories of genetic conditions are chromosomal, single gene (mendelian), and multifactorial (complex trait). Disorders categorized as chromosome abnormalities involve an entire chromosome or a significant portion of a chromosome, which consists of many genes. Conditions that are categorized as "single

---

evolve Web Enhancements

Appendix A Religious Beliefs and Practices Affecting Health Care

Be sure to check out the bonus material on the Evolve website and the CD-ROM, including free self-assessment exercises. **http://evolve.elsevier. com/Black/medsurg**

BOX 15-1 Glossary of Genetic Terms

allele An alternate form of a gene or DNA segment. Of a gene pair, one allele is inherited from the father and the other allele from the mother. Sometimes the maternal and paternal alleles are identical (homozygous); other times they are different forms of the same gene (heterozygous).

aneuploidy An abnormal number of chromosomes in a cell; a number other than 46 chromosomes in somatic (body) cells or other than 23 chromosomes in germ cells (eggs and sperm).

autosome A single chromosome from any of 1 to 22 pairs of the chromosomes not involved in gender determination (XX or XY). A disease caused by mutation in an autosomal gene or gene pair shows *autosomal* inheritance.

chromosome Gene-containing structures found in the nucleus of the cell. Chromosomes occur in pairs, and a normal human cell contains 46 chromosomes, 22 pairs of autosomes, and 2 sex chromosomes.

codon Group of 3 base pairs that form the "words" identifying specific amino acids.

consanguinity Related by descent from a common ancestor, usually in the preceding few generations; blood relatives.

consultand The person referred for genetic counseling.

DNA sequencing Determining the exact order of the base pairs in a segment of DNA.

dominant A genetic trait expressed when a person has a gene mutation on one of a pair of chromosomes and the wild-type form of the gene on the other chromosome. A person who has a dominant gene usually expresses the trait.

familial Any trait that is more common in relatives of an affected individual than in the general population, whether the cause is genetic or environmental, or both.

first-degree relatives Parents, siblings, children.

gene A functional unit of inheritance consisting of DNA.

gene mapping Assignment of genes to specific sites on specific chromosomes.

genetic condition Variations, disorders, birth defects, or diseases that are caused or influenced by genes that may or may not be transmitted from parent to offspring.

genetic counseling A communication process that deals with the human problems associated with the occurrence, or risk of occurrence, of a genetic condition in a family. Genetic professionals help the individual or family to (1) comprehend the medical facts, (2) appreciate the way heredity contributes to the condition and appreciate the risk of recurrence in specified family members, (3) understand the alternatives for dealing with the risk of recurrence, (4) choose the course of action that is appropriate for them, and (5) make the best possible adjustment to the condition.

genetics The study of inherited variation.

genome The totality of the DNA of an organism.

genomics Translation of the sequence of the human genome into health benefits. Molecular analysis of the functioning organisms in health and disease.

heterozygote A person who has different alleles at a given location on a specific chromosome.

homozygote A person in whom the two alleles at a given location on a chromosome are the same.

Human Genome Project An international research project to map each human gene and to completely sequence human DNA.

multifactorial Describes traits or diseases that are due to the interaction of multiple genes and environmental factors.

mutation Any change in DNA that alters a gene; changes can produce deformity or disease or can have a neutral or beneficial effect. Mutations occur spontaneously during cell division or may be caused by environmental influences, such as radiation or chemicals.

nucleotide One of the building blocks of DNA and RNA. A nucleotide consists of a nitrogenous base (one of four chemicals: adenine, guanine, cytosine, thymine) as well as one molecule of carbohydrate and one molecule of phosphoric acid.

pedigree Also referred to as a *family tree;* a pictorial family history diagram that traces genetic characteristics and health conditions in a family.

polymorphism A genetic variation of two or more alleles that is found in 1% or more of a population.

predisposition Having increased susceptibility to a health condition (e.g., cancer) as determined by genetic analysis.

proband The affected family member through whom the family is ascertained.

recessive A genetic trait that is expressed only when a person has two copies of a mutant autosomal gene or a single copy of a mutant X-linked gene in the absence of another X chromosome.

second-degree relatives Grandparents, aunts, and uncles.

syndrome A characteristic pattern of anomalies, presumed to be causally related.

transcription The process by which complementary messenger RNA (mRNA) is synthesized from a DNA template.

translation The synthesis of amino acids, which then become proteins, from the mRNA template.

translocation Transfer of all or part of a chromosome to another chromosome.

wild-type The common allele of the gene; considered to be the "normal" allele.

X-linked Genes located on the X chromosome. One altered gene on an X chromosome in a male can produce disease, such as hemophilia.

An extensive glossary of genetic terms has been developed by the National Human Genome Research Institute and is available at the website www.genome.gov/glossary.cfm.

gene" are caused by a mutation or alteration in a single gene. This category is also referred to as mendelian, named after the Austrian monk and founding father of modern genetics Gregor Mendel. Finally, conditions categorized as multifactorial are due to the inheritance of one or more mutant genes interacting with the environment, other genes, or other factors to produce the trait or disease.

Chromosomal Disorders

The field of cytogenetics pertains to the study of chromosomes, the analysis of how chromosomes are transmitted from parents to offspring, and the mechanisms by which chromosomal aberrations occur. The two main classes of chromosome anomalies are abnormal chromosome number (aneuploidy) and structural rearrangements. The usual process by which an individual possesses an abnormal chromosome number in every cell (aneuploidy) is typically due to an error occurring during meiosis. Meiotic cell division is the process by which the sperm and egg receive one half of the genetic material, or 23 chromosomes. At conception, the sperm and egg fuse to produce a fertilized egg with the restored number of 46 chromosomes.

Aneuploidy results from errors in meiotic cell division, creating a sperm or egg with too many or too few chromosomes. This abnormal chromosome number is passed on to the child at conception. One of the most common chromosome disorders in live-born infants is Down syndrome (or trisomy 21). Most individuals with Down syndrome have three copies of chromosome 21. This syndrome is characterized by typical physical features, mild to severe mental retardation, and an increased risk for other health problems including congenital heart disease and thyroid dysfunction.

The risk of having a child with chromosomal aneuploidy increases with maternal age. Women older than 35 years are offered prenatal diagnosis by amniocentesis or chorionic villus sampling to detect changes in chromosome number. For couples who have a child with a chromosomal aneuploidy, the chance of having another child with an abnormal number of chromosomes is slightly higher (0.5% to 1%) than would be expected based on the mother's age. The risk of recurrence associated with chromosomal aneuploidy is much lower than the risks associated with single gene disorders.

The second category of chromosomal errors is the structural rearrangement of one or more chromosomes. Several types of structural abnormalities are observed, but the most common abnormality involves the breaking and rearrangement of two or more chromosomes. In these situations, usually two chromosomes break horizontally somewhere along their length and the free chromosome pieces exchange places. This is referred to as a *reciprocal translocation* (Figure 15-1). If the chromosomal break occurs in a section of the DNA that does not contain a structural gene, and there is no gain or loss of chromosomal material (balanced translocation), most likely there will be no impact on the health of the individual. However, when carriers of balanced translocations conceive, the embryo may receive an unbalanced amount of chromosomal material, resulting in an increased risk of miscarriage or a child with physical or mental abnormalities.

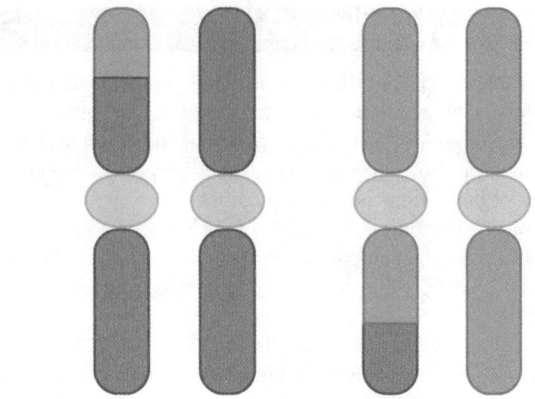

■ **FIGURE 15–1** Reciprocal translocation.

Single Gene Disorders and Patterns of Inheritance

Conditions that are categorized as "single gene" are those caused by a mutation or alteration in a single gene, transmitting in a mendelian pattern of inheritance. More than 8500 conditions are caused by a single gene that does not function at all or does not function as well as it should. Typically, single gene disorders are rare, occurring in 1 in 5000 to 100,000 live births. There are three primary single gene or mendelian inheritance patterns: autosomal recessive, autosomal dominant, and X-linked recessive. The term *autosomal* refers to conditions that are caused by mutated or altered genes on one of the chromosome pairs 1 to 22 (autosomes). Genetic conditions that follow an X-linked recessive pattern of inheritance are caused by gene alterations located on the X chromosome.

Autosomal Recessive Inheritance

Cystic fibrosis (CF) is an example of a common autosomal recessive genetic disorder in the Caucasian population. The lungs and pancreas are the primary organs affected in CF. Chronic pulmonary infection resulting from thickened secretions leads to obstructive lung disease. Thick secretions in the pancreatic ducts prevent enzymes from reaching the gastrointestinal tract, thereby interrupting proper digestion.

CF is caused by the inheritance of two copies of an altered or nonfunctioning CF gene. Parents of children with cystic fibrosis are heterozygous carriers for the CF gene, meaning they have one copy of the gene mutation and one copy of the wild-type (normal) gene. Carriers of the altered gene are usually asymptomatic, with no increased risk for other health problems. With each pregnancy, however, carriers may either transmit the mutated CF gene or transmit the wild-type gene.

Each child of heterozygous parents who are carriers of an autosomal recessive condition, such as CF, has a 25% chance of inheriting two copies of the mutated gene and therefore being affected, a 50% chance of being a carrier and unaffected, and a 25% chance of neither having the disorder nor being a carrier. These risks are independent of the gender of the child; that is, males and females can be equally affected by autosomal recessive conditions. Figure 15-2 demonstrates a pedigree that is characteristic of an autosomal recessive condition in which a horizontal pattern of inheritance involving affected siblings is observed.

When considering whether an individual is affected with an autosomal recessive condition, it is often helpful to know the ethnic background of the individual's parental ancestors. The carrier frequency of a few childhood-onset recessive disorders is known for particular ethnic groups. For example, approximately 7% of individuals of Ashkenazi Jewish ancestry are carriers of Tay-Sachs disease; 5% to 7% of African Americans are carriers of sickle cell disease; and 1 in 25 Caucasians of Northern European ancestry are carriers of CF. The carrier frequency of these and other conditions provides the basis for offering carrier screening of adults in their childbearing years.

It is also helpful to know whether the parents are biologically related (consanguineous). In general, parents who are biologically related share a proportion of genes in common, and therefore have a higher chance of carrying a copy of the same recessive gene than two unrelated individuals. For example, parents who are first cousins have a 1 in 8 chance of carrying the same genes, which increases the chance of their carrying the same mutated gene, and thus places them at increased risk for having a child with an autosomal recessive condition. However, a couple need not be related nor of a certain ethnic/racial background to have a child affected with an autosomal recessive condition.

Autosomal Dominant Inheritance

In contrast to autosomal recessive inheritance, an individual with an autosomal dominant condition needs only to have one mutated gene to be affected. The one mutated gene of the pair dominates the other parental allele. As shown in Figure 15-3, each child of an individual who has an autosomal dominant condition has a 50% chance of inheriting the gene mutation and being affected and a 50% chance of inheriting the wild-type gene and being unaffected. Similar to autosomal recessive inheritance, gender has no bearing on

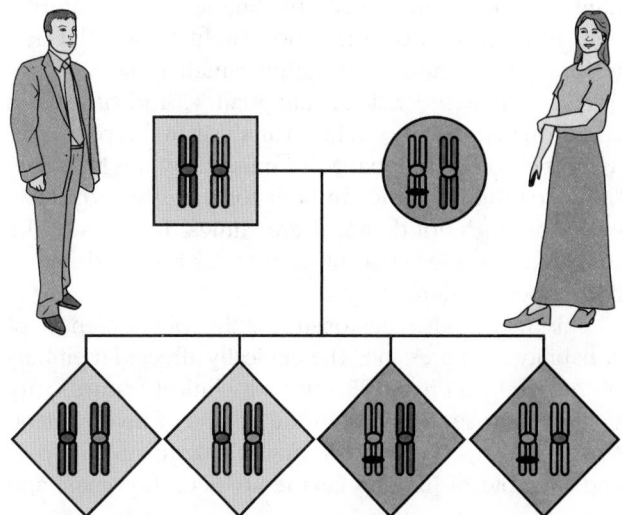

■ **FIGURE 15–3** Autosomal dominant mating outcomes. The four possible combinations of parental chromosomes in a mating between a mother with a dominant genetic condition (highlighted symbol) and a father who has two functional copies of the dominant gene. The genetic mutation is noted by a horizontal black symbol on the affected chromosome. Gender of the offspring is not specified because either gender can be affected. *(Courtesy Betty Wolf.)*

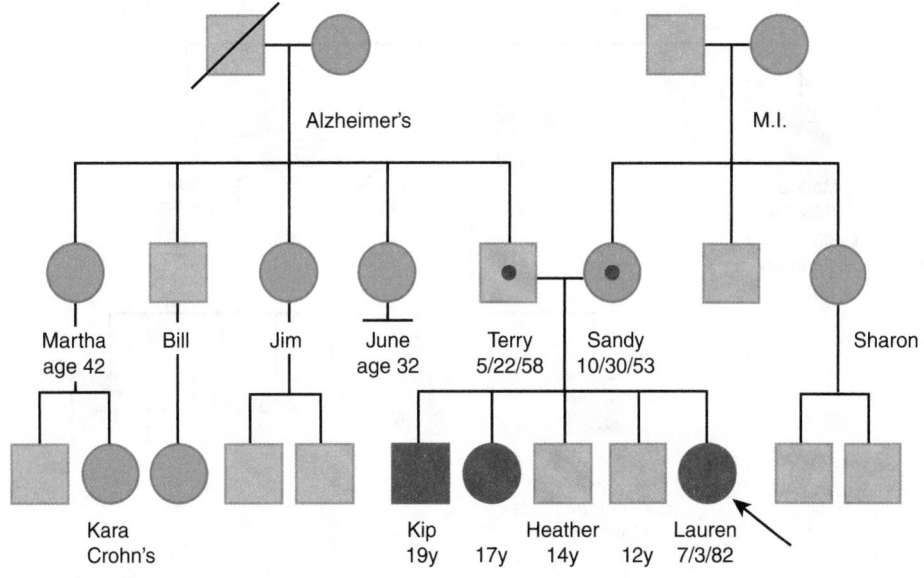

■ **FIGURE 15–2** Autosomal recessive pedigree. (Refer to Figure 15-7 on p. 245 for key to symbols).

whether an offspring is affected by an autosomal dominant condition; that is, males and females are equally affected.

Variable expressivity and incomplete penetrance are features observed frequently in autosomal dominant conditions. An altered or mutated gene may not always be expressed (incomplete penetrance) or, if expressed, may vary widely in different individuals who carry the same mutation (variable expressivity). An example of the application of these concepts is depicted in the pedigree of a family with neurofibromatosis (NF) (Figure 15-4). NF is an autosomal dominant disorder characterized by cutaneous and internal neurofibromas, café-au-lait spots (light brown, flat skin lesions), Lisch nodules (benign, small tumors of the iris), an increased risk of malignancy, and other less common manifestations. From analysis of this pedigree, it can be postulated that Mary must carry the NF gene, because both her father and her son are affected. However, she does not demonstrate clinical features of the disorder. Therefore neurofibromatosis is considered to be nonpenetrant in Mary.

This family also demonstrates the phenomenon of variability of expression. The clinically affected members of this family all have NF, but their clinical features vary both in their severity and in the organs of involvement. Mary's father, Chuck, has multiple café-au-lait spots and multiple disfiguring cutaneous neurofibromas, and

had abdominal surgery because of invasion of a large neurofibroma within the peritoneal cavity. Mary's sister, Marlene, has 15 café-au-lait spots and 1 Lisch nodule. Randy, Mary's son, has clinical manifestations consisting of multiple café-au-lait spots, an optic glioma, and a lower leg deformity (a less common manifestation of NF).

X-Linked Inheritance

In some cases, the gender of an individual does have relevance as to whether an individual will be affected with a particular genetic condition. For example, Duchenne's muscular dystrophy (DMD) is an X-linked recessive condition with onset in early childhood and is characterized by progressive muscular weakness until death, typically in the teens. DMD preferentially affects males, because it is caused by an alteration of a gene carried on the X chromosome.

Whereas males and females have two copies of autosomes (chromosomes 1 to 22), they differ in their sex chromosomes. Females have two X chromosomes, whereas males have one X chromosome and one Y chromosome. Thus males have only one copy of each of the genes carried on the X chromosome, whereas females have two copies. A deleterious mutation in a recessive gene on the X chromosome is always expressed in males because they do not have a functional copy of the gene

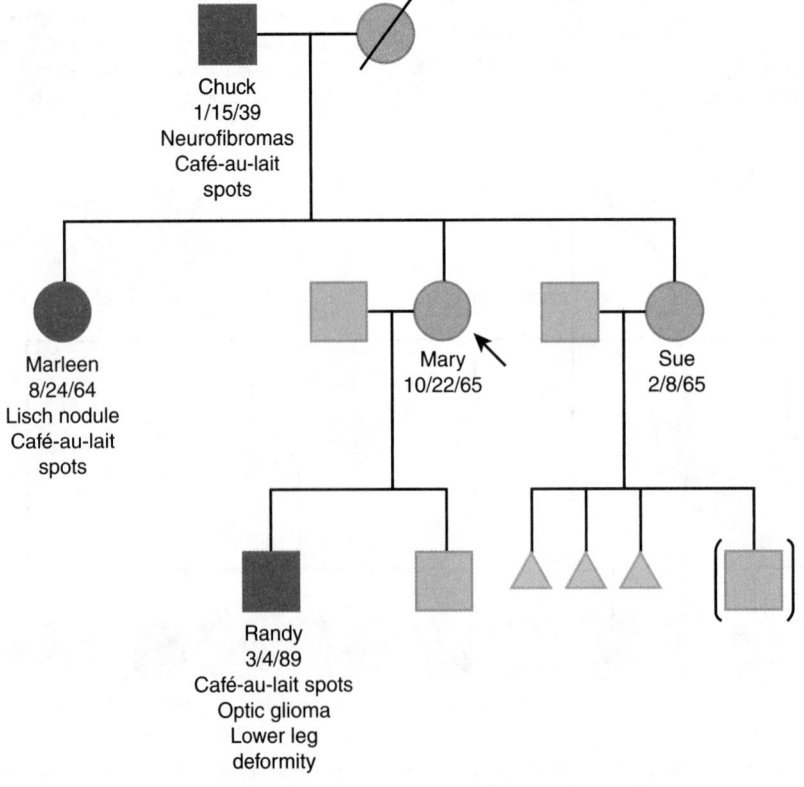

■ **FIGURE 15-4** Neurofibromatosis pedigree. (Refer to Figure 15-7 on p. 245 for key to symbols.)

on a second X chromosome. An alteration in a gene on one of the two X chromosomes in a female generally produces no manifestations, because the wild-type gene on the second X chromosome produces sufficient protein product to prevent clinical disease.

The mother of a boy affected with an X-linked recessive condition may be a carrier of the condition or the son may be affected as a result of a new mutation that occurred during the periconceptional period. A male child inherits his X chromosome only from his mother and his Y chromosome only from his father. With each pregnancy, women who are carriers of a deleterious mutation on one of their two X chromosomes face the following possible mating outcomes: each son of a woman who is a carrier of an X-linked condition has a 50% chance of inheriting the X chromosome with the gene mutation and being affected, and a 50% chance of inheriting the X chromosome with the wild-type (functional) gene and thus being free of the disease. Each daughter of a carrier female has a 50% chance of inheriting the X chromosome with the gene mutation and being an unaffected carrier, and a 50% chance of inheriting the X chromosome with the wild-type gene and being neither a carrier nor affected or at risk for having an affected son. Figure 15-5 demonstrates a pedigree that is characteristic of an X-linked recessive condition.

Because a man passes his X chromosome to his daughters, all daughters of a man affected with an X-linked genetic condition are carriers of the condition, but generally are unaffected. Sons who receive their father's Y chromosome are neither carriers of nor clinically affected with the condition. An affected father can never pass an X-linked recessive condition to his sons.

Multifactorial (Complex Trait) Inheritance

The third category of genetic conditions is one in which disorders are attributed to an interaction between one or more genes (polygenic) or between one or more genes and environmental influences. Genes do not function in isolation, but rather in concert with other genes, and they are influenced by the surrounding environment. Most human traits, including disease, are determined by the interaction of many genes and environmental influences rather than the function of a single gene. When environmental factors and gene-gene interactions are known to influence the expression of a genetic trait or disease, the term *multifactorial* or *complex inheritance* is used.

Complex inheritance is believed to be the basis for most, if not all, common diseases such as diabetes mellitus, essential hypertension, multiple sclerosis, coronary artery disease, and cancer, as well as some of the common isolated birth defects of childhood including cleft lip and cleft palate, congenital heart disease, and neural tube defects. These conditions occasionally occur in more than one member of an extended pedigree, but they do not follow clear mendelian inheritance patterns.

Every individual has genes that predispose or increase susceptibility to particular traits or disease. The presence

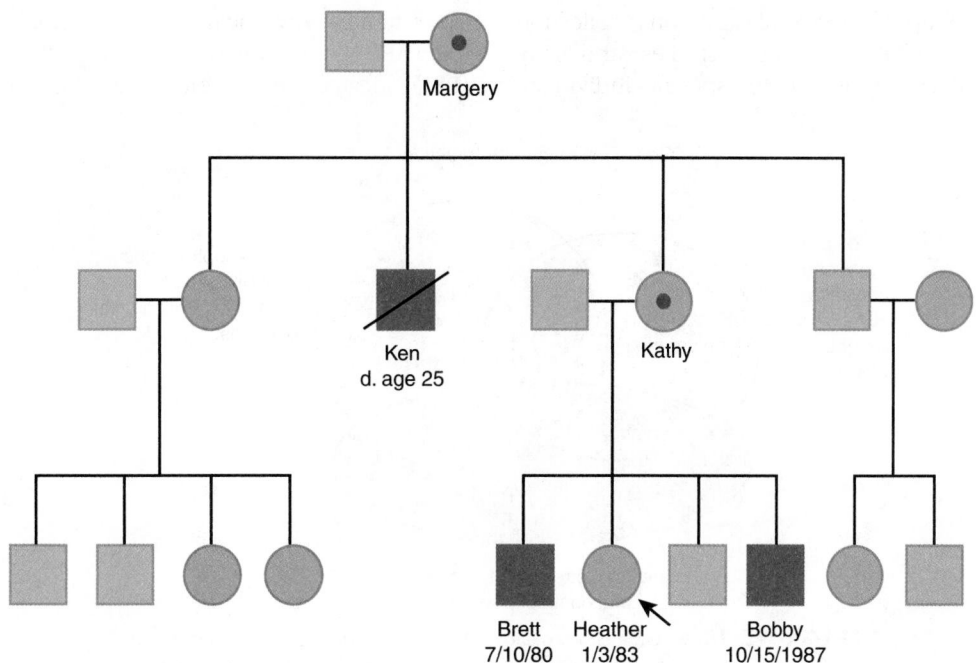

■ **FIGURE 15–5** X-linked recessive pedigree. (Refer to Figure 15-7 on p. 245 for key to symbols.)

of a predisposing gene alone may not result in the trait or disease, but confers susceptibility to that particular characteristic. The likelihood of developing a disease or having a trait increases when a person who possesses a predisposing gene also carries other genes that influence the function of that gene or provides added predisposition to that particular trait or disease. This risk is further amplified when specific environmental influences are present.

An example of the interplay between genes and environment is presented in Figure 15-6, which illustrates the multiple factors involved in coronary artery disease. An individual who carries the polygenic (multiple genes) traits of hypertension, obesity, or elevated cholesterol/triglyceride as individual conditions may not be destined to develop coronary artery disease. However, if that person possesses a major gene mutation for defective cholesterol metabolism and leads an unhealthy lifestyle, the risk of coronary artery disease is substantially increased because of this combination of factors. Alternatively, if an individual carries a major predisposing gene to coronary artery disease but is lean, normotensive, and a nonsmoker, the predisposing genetic mutation in cholesterol metabolism may not impact the health of that individual. An understanding of the genetic and environmental contributions to the pathophysiology of a particular disease may lead to more effective prevention, earlier detection, and targeted treatment modalities of the disease.

Risks to other family members often can be provided with confidence in single gene inheritance; however, it is more difficult to assess the risk in multifactorial conditions. Empirical risks are generally provided for conditions that are derived from complex inheritance (multifactorial). Empirical risks are based on a collection of large-population epidemiologic studies and may or may not reflect the risks for a specific individual.

A discussion of three examples of the role of genetics in common diseases follows.

Alzheimer's Disease

Alzheimer's disease (AD) is a chronic neurodegenerative disorder characterized by adult-onset, slowly progressive dementia involving personality changes, memory loss, deterioration of cognitive functions with neuronal cell loss, deposition of amyloid neuritic plaques, and intraneuronal neurofibrillary tangles in the cerebral cortex. AD is the most common cause of dementia in late life; it is most commonly inherited in a multifactorial manner. The disorder can be categorized as either familial or sporadic. *Familial* AD accounts for about 25% of all cases of AD and is associated with a positive family history (multiple affected family members) and early- or late-onset disease. The *sporadic* form of AD accounts for the majority (approximately 75%) of all cases of AD, and is usually associated with a negative family history and onset of disease at any time in adulthood. Sporadic AD is considered a multifactorial condition and is thought to result from a combination of aging, genetic predisposition, and exposure to environmental agents (e.g., head trauma, viruses, toxins).

Much progress has been made during the past decade in determining the role of genetics in AD. The strongest evidence for a genetic contribution to AD is found in autosomal dominant early-onset Alzheimer's disease (ADEOAD). This category comprises less than 5% of all cases of AD and refers to families in which multiple cases of AD occur with age of onset usually in the 40s or 50s (mean age of onset before age 65 years). Three gene mutations have been identified as a cause of early-onset familial AD, including the amyloid precursor protein (APP) gene located on chromosome 21, presenilin-1 (PS1) located on chromosome 14, and presenilin-2

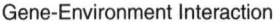

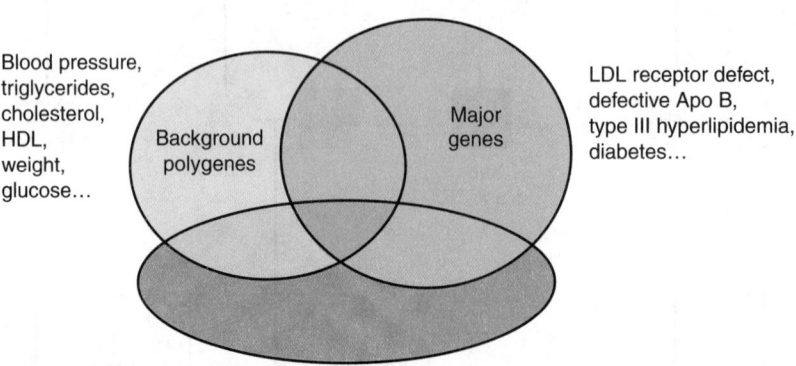

Gene-Environment Interaction

Blood pressure, triglycerides, cholesterol, HDL, weight, glucose...

Background polygenes

Major genes

LDL receptor defect, defective Apo B, type III hyperlipidemia, diabetes...

Smoking, stress, diet, inactivity, oral contraceptives...

■ **FIGURE 15–6** Gene-environment schematic for model of gene-environment interactions. *(From McCance, K.L., & Huether, S.E. [2006]. Pathophysiology: The biologic basis for disease in adults and children. St. Louis: Mosby.)*

(PS2) located on chromosome 1. Early-onset familial AD displays autosomal dominant transmission.

Genetic research has also supported the concept that late-onset familial AD is a complex disorder that may involve multiple susceptibility genes. The diagnosis of this type of AD is typically made in families with multiple affected AD members, most of whom have onset of dementia after the age of 60 or 65 years. There is a well-documented association of familial AD with the e4 allele of apolipoprotein E (APOE) located on chromosome 19. The e4 allele, by unknown mechanisms, appears to shift the age of onset curve toward an earlier age. It has been estimated that the e4 allele of APOE is a susceptibility gene for as many as one half of the cases of AD in the general population.

Diabetes Mellitus

Progress is being made in understanding the molecular and genetic basis of diabetes mellitus. Diabetes mellitus has two major clinical subtypes: type 1, or insulin-dependent diabetes mellitus (IDDM), and type 2, or non–insulin-dependent diabetes mellitus (NIDDM). Both types of diabetes mellitus demonstrate multifactorial inheritance in that both genetic and environmental factors are necessary for expression.

Type 1 diabetes mellitus tends to run in families: the risk to siblings of an affected individual with type 1 diabetes mellitus or to the offspring of a diabetic father is more than 10 times the population risk. In addition, twin studies show a concordance rate of 30% to 50% in monozygotic (identical) twins with lower rates in dizygotic (fraternal) twins. Two chromosomal locations have a well-established association with type 1 diabetes mellitus. These are the HLA region, which is the major histocompatibility complex in humans located on chromosome 6, and the insulin gene located on chromosome 11. The HLA system is estimated to contribute about 40% of the familial clustering of type 1 diabetes mellitus, and inherited genetic variations in the insulin gene region contribute about 10% of the familial clustering.

Type 2 diabetes mellitus accounts for most cases (over 90%) of diabetes. Two major risk factors for this condition are positive family history and obesity; the latter increases insulin resistance, which is a feature of type 2 diabetes mellitus. In contrast to type 1 diabetes mellitus, there is no HLA association and monozygotic twin concordance rates are substantially higher (often exceeding 90%) than in type 1 diabetes mellitus. A subset of type 2 diabetes mellitus, called maturity-onset diabetes of the young (MODY), can be inherited as an autosomal dominant trait. MODY accounts for approximately 2% to 5% of clients with type 2 diabetes mellitus and typically occurs before age 25 years. Studies have shown that about one half of cases of MODY are due to mutations in the glucokinase gene located on chromosome 7.

Cancer

Cancer is a common disease that occurs as a sporadic event in most cases. All cancer can be thought of as a genetic disease, because most cancers result from an accumulation of random mutations that occur over time in somatic (body) cells. In sporadic cancers, the cancer typically develops in a single cell. The cell progresses from a normal to a malignant cell through a series or sequence of mutations. Each of these mutations promotes uncontrolled cellular growth, which is the hallmark of cancer development.

Occasionally, pedigrees demonstrate the presence of one or more cancers in a family, suggesting familial tendency. Familial cancer clustering can occur as a result of multiple genetic effects, shared environmental factors, culturally transmitted risk factors (e.g., ethnicity, diet), or coincidence. However, in 5% to 10% of cases, the cancer may occur as a result of inheriting, from a parent, a major gene predisposing to cancer. Inheriting a major cancer-causing gene generally does not confer a 100% risk that cancer will develop, but it may confer a significant risk that at some point in a person's lifetime, a particular cancer may develop. Having this information allows for implementation of a rigorous surveillance program that will identify cancer early, which may decrease morbidity and mortality.

Nurses should become familiar with the several clinical hallmarks associated with an inherited susceptibility to cancer as listed in the Genetic Links box below. For example, inherited cancers often occur at a younger age than sporadic cancers, and they are often bilateral in paired organs (e.g., breasts, kidneys) and multifocal (multiple sites within a single organ). In addition, relatives in multiple generations are generally affected, revealing an autosomal dominant pattern of transmission. The nurse should look for the presence of these "red flags" to identify and refer clients and their families to a cancer genetic clinic for evaluation, diagnosis, and counseling.

GENETIC LINKS

Clinical "Red Flags" Suggestive of Inherited Susceptibility to Cancer

- Early age of onset (<50 years)
- Bilateral cancer in paired organs
- Multifocality—the presence of multiple distinct tumors in one organ
- Evidence of autosomal dominant inheritance
- Cancer in two or more first- or second-degree relatives
- Multiple primary cancers in one individual
- Constellation of cancers in a client or family recognized as part of an identified cancer genetic syndrome

ROLE OF NURSING IN CLINICAL GENETIC CARE

The role of the nurse in providing genetic health care varies and is dependent upon several factors, including the client's health concerns, the client's needs, and the nurse's education, expertise, role, and job description. In all roles, nurses practice within an ethical framework providing care that supports truth-telling, disclosure, privacy, nondiscrimination, and confidentiality. The nurse provides care that preserves and protects client autonomy, dignity, and rights (Box 15-2).

The nurse is often the first health professional to assess the client's medical history. Obtaining a personal and family health history is an essential component to a nursing health assessment. A thorough family history is often the first clue that a familial disorder is present or it may identify health problems to which the client may be multifactorially predisposed. Nurses should be able to provide a basic assessment of the client and family, construct a pedigree, identify potential genetic concerns, and provide basic genetic education. The nurse should also assess psychosocial aspects, including coping and adaptation styles, the client's support system, and the client's health beliefs and practices.

When the reproductive, family, or health histories in individuals suggest indications for referral to genetic professionals, the nurse makes appropriate referrals. The nurse ensures client comprehension of the health care plan, supports client autonomous decision making, and provides emotional support for the client and family. Nurses practicing at the advanced practice level in genetic health care are involved in a variety of responsibilities. Advanced practice nurses in genetics perform physical examinations and provide genetic counseling, including pedigree interpretation, risk assessment, and communication of genetic test results. Some nurses provide case management, refer clients to appropriate health care providers or community resources, collaborate with other health professionals, or manage home care and therapy. Advanced practice nurses in genetics administer state genetic screening programs, conduct genetic research, and serve as integral staff members in genetic testing laboratories (Box 15-3).

GENETIC DISEASE AND FAMILY ASSESSMENT

An expanded three-generation family medical history, in a pedigree format, is an invaluable tool for health care providers concerned not only about the identification of health risks for individual clients but also about the health status of the entire family. The pedigree is a pictorial description of the family structure that uses standardized symbols to present the family medical history in a manner that can be quickly accessed by all health care providers throughout the care of a client and a client's family. In addition to identifying familial health concerns, the process of pedigree development provides an opportunity to build or enhance rapport with clients. By carefully listening to a client's response to questions about the medical history of family members, a nurse can assess the social relationships between family members and the client's health practices.

BOX 15-2   Statement on the Scope and Standards of Genetics Clinical Nursing Practice

The International Society of Nurses in Genetics (ISONG) is responsible for defining and establishing the scope of professional nursing practice in genetics and identifying the characteristics of this unique specialty area. These characteristics pertain to standards of clinical care and standards of professional performance.

Genetic conditions are defined as variations, disorders, birth defects, or diseases that are caused or influenced by genes; these conditions may or may not be transmitted from parent to offspring.

Genetic nursing focuses on providing nursing care to clients who have, or are at risk for, known genetic conditions.

The scope of genetic nursing practice has two levels: basic and advanced. These levels of practice are distinguished by educational preparation, professional experience, practice focus, specific roles and functions, and credential status.

BOX 15-3   Advanced Practice Nurse in Genetics (APNG) and Genetics Clinical Nurse (GCN) Credentials

The ISONG-awarded APNG and GCN credentials demonstrate evidence of competence and clinical expertise based on the *Scope and Standards of Genetics Clinical Nursing Practice*. It provides recognition to professional colleagues of the nurse's ability to provide genetic health care. It provides the nurse with a sense of pride in accomplishment of advanced practice knowledge and skills in genetic health care or generalist practice knowledge and skills that every qualified nurse can attain.

The APNG and GCN credentials are awarded upon successful completion of a professional portfolio that is scientifically evaluated using carefully designed rating scales based on criteria defined in the ISONG *Scope and Standards of Genetics Clinical Nursing Practice*.

Requirements include the following:

■ Clinical practice experience in a genetic health setting
■ Education:

  ■ APNG requires a master's in nursing or equivalent; GCN requires a baccalaureate in nursing or equivalent.
  ■ Basic, advanced, or continuing education in genetics

■ Teaching of clients, families, communities, health professionals, and the public

An expanded family history usually consists of health information about the client, the client's children, and the client's siblings, parents, aunts, uncles, and grandparents. Documented information should include diagnosis, age at diagnosis, and age at death, if applicable. As shown in Figure 15-7, circles in the diagram represent females, squares represent males, and diamonds represent individuals for which the gender is unknown. An arrow identifies the client who is commonly referred to as the *consultand*. An arrow may also designate the proband—the affected family member through whom the family is ascertained. Information such as name, date of birth, medical history, and other medical problems about the various family members is noted below each symbol. A diagonal line through a symbol signifies that the represented person is deceased. A single horizontal line between two symbols represents a mating relationship. A vertical line attached to the mating line at the top and the horizontal sibship line at the bottom represents the line of descent. Symbols attached to the sibship line with an individual vertical line represent the offspring of the couple. A shaded or solid symbol represents an affected individual. To condense a pedigree, nonbiologically related individuals are often not displayed. There are several purposes for constructing a pedigree that go beyond determining health risks. The construction of a pedigree assists with determining the following:

- Statistical probability of developing a disease
- Degree of relationship among family members
- Pattern of transmission of diseases in the family
- Likelihood of a hereditary versus nonhereditary component of disease causation
- Increased risk of disease for different family members

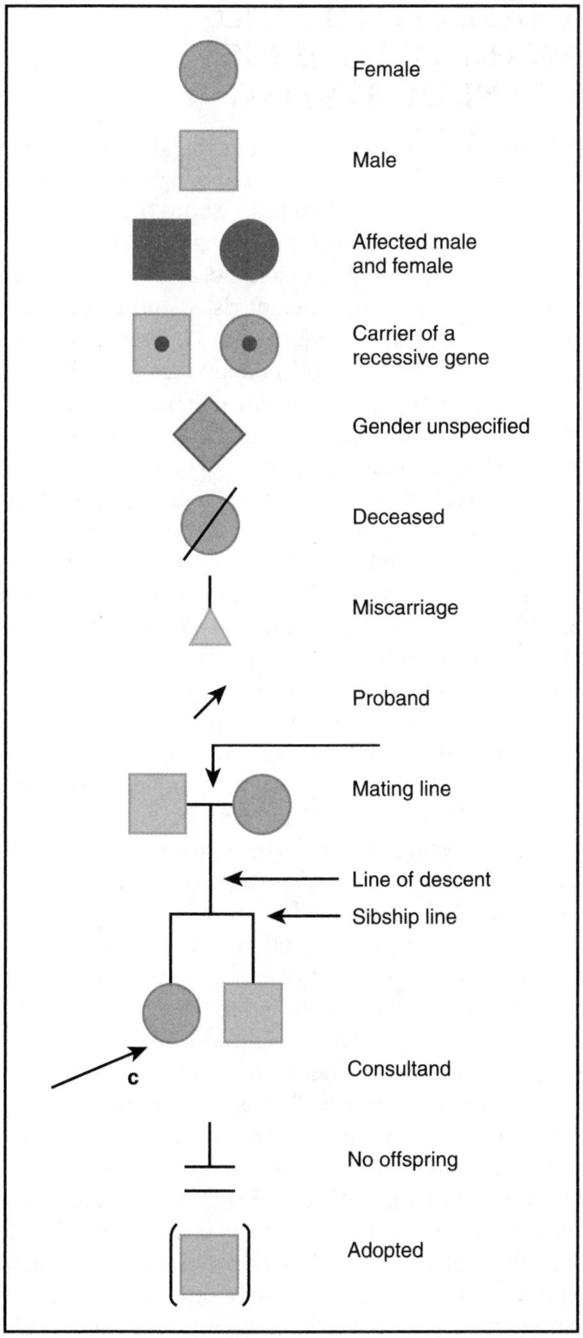

GENETIC TESTING

Advances in genetic science and technology have dramatically increased the numbers of available genetic tests. In every health care setting, nurses encounter genetic issues among their clients and are increasingly called upon to understand and effectively respond to concerns surrounding genetic testing for families. Accordingly, nurses have a responsibility to become knowledgeable about the basics of genetic testing and the accompanying ethical and psychosocial implications.

Genetic testing refers to the analysis of a person's DNA, chromosomes, proteins, or certain metabolites obtained from a sample of blood or other body tissue in order to detect changes that indicate the presence or absence of a genetic condition or a predisposition to develop one. Genetic tests are performed to (1) confirm or rule out a present condition, (2) determine whether an individual is a carrier of a genetic condition, (3) detect fetal abnormalities, and (4) predict diseases in asymptomatic individuals through presymptomatic or predisposition testing.

Screening for Carriers of Genetic Disease

The main purpose of carrier screening is the identification of individuals who are themselves healthy but carry a disease-causing gene and thus are at risk for transmitting a particular genetic condition to future offspring. Carrier screening is generally performed for autosomal recessive and X-linked recessive conditions. Examples of disorders in which carrier testing is available are

■ **FIGURE 15–7** Commonly used pedigree symbols.

Tay-Sachs disease, sickle cell disease, cystic fibrosis, thalassemia, and fragile X syndrome. Carrier testing is voluntary and focuses on individuals with a positive family history of a disorder and those who identify themselves as being members of a particular high-risk ethnic group (e.g., Tay-Sachs disease in the Ashkenazi Jewish population and sickle cell disease in the African-American population). Knowing one's carrier status may provide (1) relief from fear of the unknown and (2) information that could be useful in making life and family planning decisions.

Presymptomatic and Predisposition Testing

Both presymptomatic and predisposition (or susceptibility) tests are forms of predictive testing. In presymptomatic testing, individuals known to be at high risk for a genetic disorder because of family history can be tested to determine whether they have inherited a disease-causing genetic mutation before they develop clinical manifestations of the disorder. A classic example of presymptomatic testing is detection of the gene for Huntington's disease (HD), a progressive adult-onset neurologic disorder. Because the HD gene shows complete penetrance, a person who tests positive for the mutation has essentially a 100% chance of developing the disorder at some age.

Genetic discoveries are also making it possible to test for the presence of a genetic component that contributes to the predisposition of many common diseases such as diabetes mellitus, heart disease, and cancer. Predisposition (or susceptibility) testing is used to identify a genetic mutation that makes a person more likely, but not definitely certain, to develop a disorder. For example, gene mutations for some hereditary cancers such as hereditary breast cancer, associated with two susceptibility genes called BRCA1 and BRCA2, are detected in this manner. These two genes together account for 5% to 10% of all breast cancers. Women who carry a germ line mutation in the BRCA1 or BRCA2 gene have a 60% to 90% lifetime risk of developing breast cancer as well as a 20% to 60% risk for ovarian cancer.

Currently, both presymptomatic testing and predisposition testing are generally limited to testing in adults. However, genetic testing of minors is indicated in certain genetic disorders in which medical benefits to the minor have been established. Genetic testing can assist individuals in making informed decisions about their health care and can provide reassurance to those who learn that they do not carry a disease-causing gene. Individuals who are found to have a disease-causing gene can pursue strategies aimed at prevention and early detection.

Prenatal Diagnosis and Screening

Prenatal diagnosis and screening are an integral component of routine obstetric practice because of the availability of relatively safe tests that are cost-effective for hundreds of genetic disorders. The primary goal of prenatal genetic testing is to provide at-risk families with information to use in making informed choices during pregnancy. The methods used for prenatal diagnosis and screening are both invasive and noninvasive. Invasive techniques include amniocentesis, chorionic villus sampling, fetal blood and tissue sampling, and preimplantation genetic diagnosis. Noninvasive testing includes maternal serum screening, ultrasonography, and analysis of fetal cells in the maternal circulation.

ETHICAL, LEGAL, AND PSYCHOSOCIAL ISSUES IN GENETIC TESTING

Perhaps more so than other types of health care information, genetic information can have profound implications for individuals, families, and society. Genetic information is unique in that it relates to one's genetic identity, provides highly personal data about an individual, predicts one's future health risks, and is relevant to other family members. Issues that challenge nurses in the context of genetics and genetic testing include privacy and confidentiality, informed consent, stigmatization, potential for discrimination, and disruption of family and social relationships.

Nurses have a critical role in assuring privacy and confidentiality of genetic information obtained from such sources as family history assessments, genetic tests, and other interventions. The inadvertent loss of privacy and confidentiality with regard to genetic information can result in potential harm to clients. For example, disclosure of genetic test information to third parties, such as insurance companies or employers, may result in higher insurance rates, cancellation or denial of insurance policies, or loss of job opportunities. Because of the potential for misuse of information, it is imperative that genetic testing centers have policies and procedures in place that protect the rights of privacy and confidentiality for clients. Clients need to know that test results will not be shared with anyone other than the person being tested, unless the person gives explicit consent to disclose such information. Both federal and state legislation aimed at providing protection against discrimination has been, and continues to be, developed.

The process of informed consent is a critical component of pretest counseling, and many nurses are expected to actively participate in this process (Box 15-4). The decision to undergo a genetic test should be an autonomous decision, made on the basis of the client's consideration of the physical, psychological, or social risks and benefits, and the client's values and beliefs. Individuals should be aware that they have a right to accept or decline testing. Nursing actions in the informed consent process may

BOX 15-4 Components of Informed Consent for Genetic Testing

- Purpose of the test
- What can be learned from both a positive and a negative test result, including information on health risks associated with test results
- Possibility that test results will be ambiguous or noninformative
- Options for risk assessment without genetic testing
- Risk of transmitting a mutation to offspring
- Options for medical follow-up based on test results
- Technical accuracy of the test
- Risks of psychological distress, family disruption, and genetic discrimination following disclosure of test results
- Discussion of rules of disclosure of test results to others (e.g., family members, third parties)
- Confidentiality standards
- Risks that nonrelatedness may be discovered and policy for disclosure
- Fees associated with the genetic test as well as preventive procedures

include ensuring that written consent is obtained before testing, serving as a client advocate, assisting in providing education about testing, and ensuring that the client's autonomy is protected in making testing decisions.

The possibility of stigmatization is another ethical issue associated with genetic testing. Impairment of one's self-esteem is a potential harm that may occur with testing. Little is known about the effects of genetic information upon one's view of oneself and the emotional burden of knowing about one's own genetic makeup.

Genetic testing also carries the risk of producing psychological harm. Individuals with positive genetic test results may experience a wide range of emotions, including anger, anxiety, depression, or psychological distress. In addition, familial relationships may be negatively impacted when some family members discover they are carriers of a genetic condition while others learn they are not carriers of the condition. Family members may also have guilt feelings regardless of their genetic status. Guilt feelings for transmitting a disorder such as HD may be experienced by individuals who carry the HD gene mutation. On the other hand, individuals who have not inherited a disease-causing genetic mutation may experience feelings of survivor guilt.

Families may also develop patterns for managing disease risk in mutation carriers. An example is the pressuring of a female relative found to have a BRCA1 mutation to undergo prophylactic mastectomy. Another potential consequence of genetic testing is the discovery of misidentified paternity. This occurs when test results of both parents are inconsistent with paternity. Discussion about this possibility is an important component of the informed consent process.

FUTURE DIRECTIONS

The Genomic Era

The genomic era continues to unfold upon completion of a comprehensive sequence of the human genome. The future holds many exciting challenges for scientists to translate genome-based knowledge into health benefits. Although the genome is characterized chemically, its function is not well understood. The next phase of genomics is to catalogue and comprehend the functional elements, such as the protein-coding sequences, and to understand how genes interrelate to one another through pathways. Moreover, the genome holds much variation, and how these variations impact health and illness is yet to be understood. With enhanced knowledge of genes and their pathways, development of genome-based approaches to prediction of disease susceptibility and drug response, early detection of illness, and development of powerful new therapeutic approaches to disease are currently a reality.

Gene Therapy

Because of the influx of information from molecular genetic technology and the HGP, both the scientific and the public communities anticipate that gene therapy will revolutionize disease treatment modalities. At the onset of the new millennium, approximately 500 clinical gene therapy trials have been conducted with approximately 3000 enrolled clients. Ninety percent of the studies relate to human immunodeficiency virus or cancer and the remainder involve rare recessive disorders. To date, only a small handful of clients have benefited from gene therapy.

Many questions need to be answered before gene therapy becomes a viable option in the treatment of disease, such as the following: Will gene transfer result in adequate protein production at the correct sites? Will the transferred gene relate to or have an association with its regulatory genes or will random insertion of a transferred gene upset or negatively impact the activities of other proteins? Many scientific obstacles need to be overcome before gene therapy becomes a practical modality for treatment of disease.

Pharmacogenomics

Perhaps the most immediate and significant impact of the molecular knowledge gained in the recent past is in the field of pharmacogenomics. It has long been recognized that drugs that are safe in one individual may cause harm in another. Pharmacogenomics is the concept of individualized and rational drug selection based on the genotype of a particular client that will optimize safety and increase drug effectiveness. The science is based on genotype variations (polymorphisms) that influence an individual's response to a drug. The outcome will be customized drug therapy, that is, prescribing the right drug at the correct dose for the individual client.

A small number of metabolic pathways degrade the vast majority of drugs by means of enzymes in the liver and small intestine, and it is the family of P450 enzymes that may be responsible for degradation of a significant number of drugs. The functional differences between variants of these enzymes may, in large part, be due to genetic polymorphisms inherited as genetic traits. The allelic differences may abolish, alter, or enhance drug metabolism.

One P450 enzyme, CYP2D6, is essential in the metabolism of antidepressants and neuroleptics. The CYP2D6 genotype may be predictive of expected side effects. Individuals who lack functional CYP2D6 genes may not be able to clear drugs well and may demonstrate adverse effects resulting from increased drug plasma levels.

Another example is CYP2C9, a member of the P450 family whose genotype may be considered for optimal warfarin therapy. The clearance of warfarin in individuals who inherit two copies of the CYP2C9 allele has been shown to be reduced by 90% compared to individuals who have the wild-type allele. The differences in these two genotypes may have significant implications in the dose and schedule of warfarin treatment.

Nurses are likely to have a significant role in the application of pharmacogenomics in client care. Nurses may need to explain to clients why certain medications are being prescribed to some but not to others with the same disease. In addition, nurses will need to educate clients about the potential benefits and limitations of genotyping and the implications for therapy.

CONCLUSIONS

It is essential that nurses have a basic understanding of molecular genetics and principles of human genetics to function effectively in the modern health care arena. This knowledge is relevant in helping nurses understand the mechanisms and treatment of disease, assess genetic risk for disease, provide a scientific foundation for nursing care, and promote, retain, and restore health and wellness among clients and families.

THINKING CRITICALLY

1. *Cancer Genetic Clinical Situation:* A 46-year-old woman is informed that she carries a mutation in the dominant familial adenomatous polyposis (FAP) gene that is responsible for her colon cancer. Her physicians ordered the gene test without pretest genetic counseling. Individuals who inherit the FAP gene mutation are predisposed to development of hundreds of colon polyps with almost 100% risk of cancer. Onset of polyps may occur in adolescence. She inquires about genetic testing of her 17-year-old son and 10-year-old daughter.

Factors to Consider. Is genetic testing of the children appropriate? Who should make the decision to be tested? What is the nurse's role in this situation? Identify several psychosocial issues the family might consider before deciding to have children tested. What options are available relative to the parents' concern?

2. *Huntington Disease Clinical Situation:* A 33-year-old woman inquires about the possibility of genetic testing for Huntington's disease (HD). Her father is in advanced stages of HD, and the genetic mutation is known. HD is a chronic, progressive, neurodegenerative disease of the central nervous system with onset typically between 30 and 50 years of age. Both the client and her fiancé believe knowledge of her genotype would be helpful in their family planning.

Factors to Consider. What are some of the personal issues that may be considered by the client? What are potential ramifications to the couple's future relationship? What are the concerns if the client and her fiancé think differently about genetic testing? Is there external family pressure for the client to be tested? What is the implication to their potential offspring?

3. *Diabetes Mellitus Clinical Situation:* The client is a 24-year-old woman who has a 12-year history of type 1 diabetes mellitus. It has been difficult for her to manage her diabetes, and she has been hospitalized several times over the years for diabetic ketoacidosis. It has not been easy to maintain ideal blood glucose levels, and her insulin requirement has gradually changed. She did not adhere to dietary restrictions during her adolescent years. Having recently married, she and her husband are thinking about starting a family.

Factors to Consider. What are the risks of having a child with diabetes? Is genetic testing available? What concerns during pregnancy should be considered for this client?

Discussions for these questions can be found on the website.

BIBLIOGRAPHY

Citations appearing in red refer to primary research.

Citations appearing in blue refer to evidence-based practice guidelines and protocols.

1. Annas, G.J. (2001). Reforming informed consent to genetic research. *Journal of the American Medical Association, 286,* 2326-2328.
2. Baum, C., Kustikova, O., Modlich, U., et al. (2006). Mutagenesis and oncogenesis by chromosomal insertion of gene transfer vectors. *Human Gene Therapy, 17,* 253-263.
3. Bennett, R.L., et al. (1995). Recommendations for standardized human pedigree nomenclature. *American Journal of Human Genetics, 56,* 745-752.
4. Calzone, K.A., & Masny, A. (2004). Genetics and oncology nursing. *Seminars in Oncology Nursing, 20*(3), 178-185.
5. Collins, F.S., et al. (2003). A vision for the future of genomics research: A blueprint for the genomic era. *Nature, 422*(6934), 835-847.
6. Cuthbert, A.L. (2002). Disease genes: Flattery and deception. *Trends in Pharmacologic Sciences, 23,* 504-509.

7. Emilien, G., et al. (2000). Impact of genomics on drug discovery and clinical medicine. *Quarterly Journal of Medicine, 93*, 391-423.

8. Fischer, A., Hacien, B.A., & Cavazzana-Calvo, M. (2006). Gene therapy of metabolic diseases. *Journal of Metabolic Disease, 29*, 409-412.

9. Friedman, T. (2003). Gene therapy's new era: A balance of unequivocal benefit and unequivocal harm. *Molecular Therapy*, 8(1), 5-7.

10. Giarelli, E., & Jacobs, L.A. (2005). Modifying cancer risk factors: The gene-environment interaction. *Seminars in Oncology Nursing, 21*(4), 271-277.

11. Guttmacher, A.E., & Collins, F.S. (2002). Genomic medicine: A primer. *New England Journal of Medicine, 347*, 1512-1520.

12. Guttmacher, A.E., & Collins, F.S. (2003). Welcome to the genomic era. *New England Journal of Medicine, 349*, 996-998.

13. Guttmacher, A.E., & Collins, F. (2005). Realizing the promise of genomics in biomedical research. *Journal of the American Medical Association, 294*(11), 1399-1402.

14. Huang, Y. (2006). Apolipoprotein E and Alzheimer disease. *Neurology, 66*(2), S79-S85.

15. Human Genome Program, U.S. Department of Energy. (2001). *Genetics and its impact on society: A 2001 primer.* Available at www.ornl.gov/hgmis/publicat/primer.

16. International Society of Nurses in Genetics. (1998). *Statement on the scope and standards of genetics clinical nursing practice.* Washington, DC: American Nurses' Association.

17. International Human Genome Sequencing Consortium. (2001). Initial sequencing and analysis of the human genome. *Nature, 409*, 860-921.

18. Jenkins, J., et al. (2001). Recommendations of core competencies in genetics essential for all health professionals. *Genetics in Medicine, 3*(2), 155-159.

19. Jenkins, J., Grady, P.A., & Collins, F.S. (2005). Nurses and the genomic revolution. *Journal of Nursing Scholarship, 37*(2), 98-101.

20. Jones, K.L. (2006). *Recognizable patterns of human malformation* (6th ed.). Philadelphia: Saunders.

21. Jorde, L.B., et al. (2006). *Medical genetics* (3rd ed). St. Louis: Mosby.

22. Kwitkowski, V.E., & Daub, J.R. (2004). Clinical applications of genetics in sporadic cancers. *Seminars in Oncology Nursing, 20* (3), 155-163.

23. Lashley, F.R. (2005). *Clinical genetics in nursing practice* (3rd ed.). New York: Springer.

24. Lea, D.L., Feetham, S.L., & Monsen, R.B. (2002). A genomic-based health care in nursing: A bidirectional approach to bringing genetics into nursing's body of knowledge. *Journal of Professional Nursing, 18*(3), 120-129.

25. Lessick, M., et al. (2001). Advances in genetic testing for cancer risk. *MEDSURG Nursing, 10*(3), 123-127.

26. Loescher, L.J., & Merkel, C.J. (2005). The interface of genomic technologies and nursing. *Journal of Nursing Scholarship, 37*(2), 111-119.

27. McKusick, V.A. (2006). *Mendelian inheritance in man: A catalog of human genes and genetic disorders (OMIM).* Available at www.ncbi.nlm.nih.gov/entrez/query.fcgi?db=OMIN&itool=toolbar.

28. Middelton, L., & Lessick, M. (2003). Inherited urologic malignant disorders: Nursing implications. *Urologic Nursing, 23*(1), 15-30.

29. Miola, J. (2006). The need for informed consent: Lessons from the ancient Greeks. *Cambridge Quarterly of Healthcare Ethics, 15*, 152-160.

30. Nussbaum, R.L., McInnes, R.R., & Willard, H.F. (2006). *Thompson & Thompson genetics in medicine* (6th ed.). Philadelphia: Saunders.

31. O'Neil, O. (2003). Some limits of informed consent. *Journal of Medical Ethics, 29*, 4-7.

32. Phillips, K.A., et al. (2001). Potential role of pharmacogenomics in reducing adverse drug reactions: A systematic review. *Journal of the American Medical Association, 286*, 2270-2279.

33. Prows, C.A., & Prows, D.R. (2004). Medication selection by genotype: How genetics is changing drug prescribing and efficacy. *American Journal of Nursing, 104*(5), 60-70.

34. Raux, G., et al. (2005). Molecular diagnosis of autosomal dominant early onset Alzheimer's disease: An update. *Journal of Medical Genetics, 42*, 793-795.

35. Rushnak, J.M., et al. (2001). Pharmacogenomics: A clinician's primer on emerging technologies for improved patient care. *Mayo Clinical Proceedings, 76*, 299-309.

36. Sadelain, M. (2004). Insertional oncogenesis in gene therapy: How much of a risk? *Gene Therapy, 11*(7), 569-573.

37. Sundberg, M.I., Oscarson, M., & McLellan, R.A. (1999). Polymorphic human cytochrome P450 enzymes: An opportunity for individualized drug treatment. *Trends in Pharmaceutical Science, 20*, 342-349.

38. Williams, J., & Lessick, M. (2001). Historical evolution of nursing in genetics. *MEDSURG Nursing, 10*(6), 301-307.

evolve **Did you remember to check out the bonus material on the Evolve website and the CD-ROM, including NCLEX®-Examination Style Review Questions, Open-Book Quizzes, and Chapter Review Audio Podcasts?**

http://evolve.elsevier.com/Black/medsurg

CHAPTER 16

Perspectives in Oncology

Peggy Ward-Smith

The face of health care, including scientific knowledge and care delivery systems, is ever changing. Likewise, the experience of cancer is changing for our clients and families. Today, a person confronted with a new cancer diagnosis often knows someone who has survived cancer; yet cancer remains a frightening unknown for many. Some clients, especially older ones, still associate the word with death. Cancer nursing requires a clinical knowledge of the disease and its treatment as well as the skills to care for and support clients and their families. The pathophysiology and scientific advances discussed in this chapter provide a foundation for promoting positive outcomes for clients with cancer, discussed in the next chapter.

Approximately 1.4 million new cancers are expected to be diagnosed in the United States in 2007. Survival rates and quality of life for people living with the disease have improved. Yet this year about 564,000 Americans are expected to die of cancer. Cancer remains the second leading cause of death in the United States, exceeded only by heart disease.[2,15] See the Evolve website for the Estimated New Cancer Cases and Deaths by Sex for All Sites in the United States, 2007.

The National Cancer Institute (NCI) estimates that approximately 10.1 million Americans alive in January 2002 have a history of cancer. This number includes disease-free survivors who are considered "cured," people living with cancer as a chronic disease, and those currently receiving treatment. Sixty-five percent of clients with cancer diagnosed this year are expected to be alive 5 years after the diagnosis. This statistic is based on clients diagnosed and treated 5 years ago. It does not take into account an estimation of survival resulting from evolving detection methods and newer treatment modalities.[2]

TERMINOLOGY

The terms *cancer, neoplasm, malignant neoplasm,* and *tumor* are often used interchangeably by both professionals and the lay public. Strictly speaking, these words are not interchangeable. Although generally used as a synonym for cancer, the word *tumor* simply refers to a lump, mass, or swelling. That swelling can be a neoplastic mass, or it may be an accumulation of fluid.

The word *neoplasm* (derived from the Greek *neos,* "new," and *plasis,* "molding") is defined as an abnormal mass of tissue that serves no useful purpose and may harm the host organism. A neoplasm can be either *benign* or *malignant.* A benign neoplasm is *usually* a harmless growth that does not spread or invade other tissues. A benign tumor does occupy space. Consequently, if it is located near a vital tube or organ, it can be fatal, as with a benign brain tumor. A malignant neoplasm is a harmful mass, capable of invasion of other tissues and *metastasis* ("spread") to distant organs.

The term *cancer* is used to refer to malignant neoplasms. Cancer is a disease of the cell in which the normal mechanisms for control of growth and proliferation have been altered. It is invasive, spreading directly to surrounding tissue as well as to new sites in the body.

The term *oncology* refers to the medical specialty that deals with the diagnosis, treatment, and study of cancer. An *oncologist* is a physician who specializes in cancer therapy. There are surgical, radiation, and medical oncologists. A *medical oncologist* is a physician with expertise in treating cancer with chemotherapy or biotherapy and in handling general medical problems related to the disease or side effects of cancer treatment. Box 16-1 lists other important terms.

EPIDEMIOLOGY

Epidemiology is the study of the distribution and determinants of diseases and health problems in specified populations. The goal of epidemiologic study is the prevention or control of the health problem. Although the causes of many cancers remain unknown, epidemiologic studies have helped to identify factors that underlie theories of causation. Nurses can use their knowledge of the factors associated with cancer causation in promoting positive outcomes for their clients through nursing assessment and interventions.

The NCI established the Surveillance, Epidemiology, and End Results (SEER) program in 1973 as a way to report population-based data in site-specific incidences of cancer, mortality, and survival rates (see SEER WebLink). This report is based on a sample of 14% of the U.S. population from 11 registries. Currently these include six metropolitan areas (Atlanta, Detroit, San Francisco/ Oakland, Seattle/Puget Sound, Los Angeles, and San Jose-Monterey). It also contains data from five states (Connecticut, Hawaii, Iowa, New Mexico, and Utah) and the Commonwealth of Puerto Rico. With the addition of supplemental and expansion registries such as the Alaska Native Tumor Registry, 26% of the population are included in SEER data. The SEER reporting areas reasonably represent the subsets of the population. Data are gathered from hospital medical records. Therefore the accuracy of the data recorded in clients' medical records by physicians, nurses, and others can affect the accuracy of the SEER data. This ongoing project provides a great deal of information about cancer incidence, prevalence, and mortality for different geographic areas and ethnic groups.[23]

Incidence and Prevalence

The *incidence* rate for cancer reflects the number of new cases occurring in a specified population during a year, expressed as the number of cancer diagnoses per 100,000 people. For the year 2007, about 1,445,000 new diagnoses of cancer are expected.[2] See the Evolve website for the Estimated New Cancer Cases and Deaths by Sex for All Sites, United States, 2007. The incidence gives perspective on the current magnitude of the problem and provides a source for establishing future priorities in cancer control programs. The *prevalence* of cancer is

BOX 16-1 Cancer Terminology	
Terms	**Definitions**
Adenocarcinoma	Cancer that arises from glandular tissues. Examples include cancers of the breast, lung, thyroid, colon, and pancreas.
Anaplastic	Tumor cells that are completely undifferentiated and bear no resemblance to the cells in the tissue of origin.
Aneuploid	Tumor cells that do not have the normal 46 chromosomes in a human cell. Aneuploid tumors often have a worse prognosis.
Antigens	Substances that cause activation of the immune system.
Carcinoma	A form of cancer that is composed of epithelial cells; develops in tissues covering or lining the organs of the body, such as the skin, uterus, or breast.
Carcinoma in situ	The earliest stage of cancer in which the tumor is still confined to the local area, before it has grown to a significant size or has spread.
Cytokine	A substance secreted by immune system cells, usually to send messages to other immune cells.
Differentiation	The process of maturation of a cell line of cancer cells. When they are fully differentiated or well differentiated, they more closely resemble the normal cells in the tissue of origin.
Dysplasia	An alteration in the size, shape, and organization of differentiated cells. Cells lose their regularity and show variability in size and shape, usually in response to an irritant. Cells may revert to normal when the irritant is removed but may transform to a neoplasia.
Hyperplasia	An increase in the number of normal cells in a normal arrangement in a tissue or organ; usually leads to an increase in the size of the part and an increase in functional activity.
Metaplasia	The replacement of one type of fully differentiated cell by another fully differentiated cell that is not normal for that part of the body.
Oncogenes	Specific segments of cellular deoxyribonucleic acid (DNA) that, when inappropriately activated, contribute to the transformation of normal cells into malignant cells.
Sarcoma	A cancer of supporting or connective tissue such as cartilage, bone, muscle, or fat.
Tumor markers	Chemicals in the blood that are produced by certain cancers.

the total number of people alive today whose cancer has been diagnosed in the current year (incidence) and those whose cancer has been diagnosed previously. The 10.1 million Americans living with a history of cancer (prevalence) include the 1,445,000 people who will be diagnosed with cancer in 2007 (incidence).

The reported incidence of cancer appears to have increased since 1900 for several reasons. First, diagnostic methods have become more precise. Utilization of diagnostic tests, such as mammograms for breast cancer and the prostate-specific antigen (PSA) blood test for prostate cancer, has led to earlier detection than previously.

Second, data collection and analysis of cancer statistics have become more sophisticated over the years. Therefore reported rates of incidence and mortality resulting from cancer are more accurate. Both can result in an increase in the *reported* incidence of cancer but not a true increased incidence of cancer.

Third, Americans are living longer and most cancers take many years to develop. More people now live long enough to develop cancer. Therefore the apparent rise in cancer rates can be somewhat misleading, because more precise diagnostic and statistical methods combined with the trend toward a longer life span impact rates of cancer.

Mortality

The mortality rate is the number of deaths caused by cancer that occur in the specified population in a given year, expressed as the number of deaths that are due to cancer per 100,000 people. Figures from the American Cancer Society (ACS) show changes in the mortality rates for lung cancer for both males and females.[2] See the figures illustrating Age-Adjusted Cancer Death Rates by site in males and females on the website. Lung cancer deaths for males have declined from a high of 102.0 per 100,000 in 1984 to 77.8 in 2002, which is reflective of the decline in smoking by American men. For women, the rate of lung cancer has been stable since 1998. Since 1987 more women have died of lung cancer than of breast cancer.[5]

Increased use of mammography has resulted in breast cancer incidence rates rising rapidly in the 1980s. An estimated 178,480 new cases are expected to occur among women in 2007. Death rates from breast cancer have declined by an average of 2.3% per year from 1990 to 2002, with larger decreases seen in younger (<50 years) women. This decrease is thought to be a result of earlier detection through screening, increased awareness, and improved treatment. Assessing the genetic risk factors (BRCA1 and BRCA2) is recommended only for those with a strong inherited susceptibility for breast or ovarian cancer. Recent evidence suggests that prophylactic removal of the breasts or ovaries decreases the risk substantially.

Trends

From 1998 to 2002, the median age at diagnosis for cancer of all sites was 67 years. During this same time frame, the median age at death for cancer of all sites was 72 years. Incidence rates in males were stable between 1995 and 2002. Incidence rates among females increased 0.3% annually from 1987 to 2002.[2,15] Mortality rates for males and females with all cancers decreased by 1.1% annually between 1999 and 2002.

Factors that may explain this decline include the decrease in tobacco use, better cancer research and treatment, and earlier cancer detection and prevention.

For males, incidence rates increased for melanoma of the skin and cancers of the prostate, kidney and renal pelvis, and esophagus, while rates decreased for cancers of the lungs and bronchus, colon and rectum, oral cavity and pharynx, and stomach and larynx. For females, cancer rates increased for leukemia, non-Hodgkin's lymphoma, melanoma, and cancers of the breast, thyroid, urinary bladder, and kidney. Incidence rates decreased in females for cancers of the colon and rectum, ovary, cervix uteri, oral cavity, and stomach.

Racial and ethnic disparity in cancer incidence and deaths persists, particularly among black men (Figures 16-1 and 16-2). Cancer incidence rates for all sites combined are 25% higher in black men, when compared to white men, and 50% higher for myeloma and cancers of the prostate, lung, stomach, liver, esophagus, and larynx. Cancer death rates for all sites combined are 43% higher for black men when compared to white men. Death rates for myeloma and cancer of the prostate and stomach were more than 200% higher; rates for cancers of the esophagus and oral cavity were more than 75% higher.

Cancer incidence and death rates for Asian American and Pacific Islander (API), American Indian and Alaska Native (AI/AN), and Hispanic/Latino (H/L) populations are much lower than those among blacks and white populations. However, cancers of the stomach

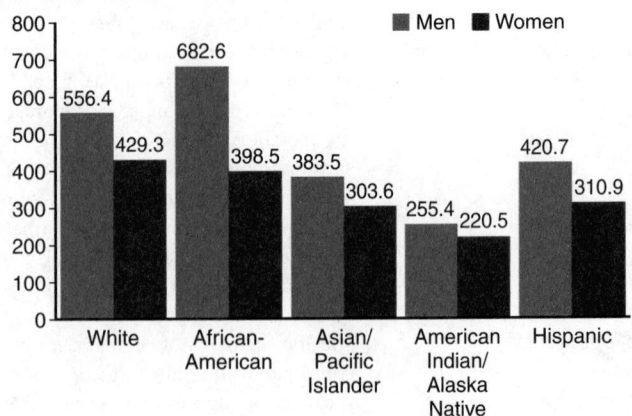

■ **FIGURE 16-1** Cancer incidence rates by race and ethnicity, 1997-2001.

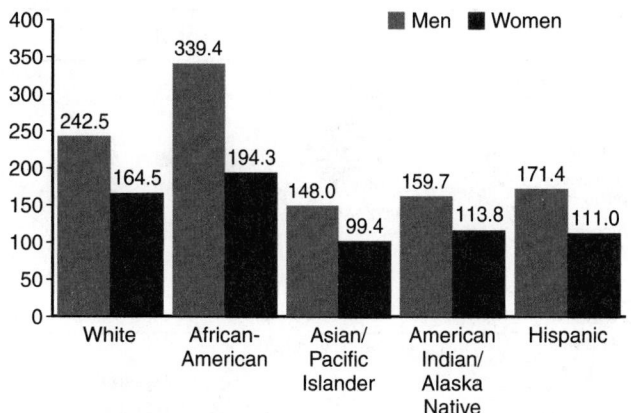

■ **FIGURE 16–2** Cancer death rates by race and ethnicity, 1997-2001.

and liver are disproportionately represented in these populations. APIs have the highest rates of stomach and liver cancers, although stomach cancer deaths are highest among black men. Women of H/L descent experience the highest rates of cancers of the cervix uteri. The incidence of gallbladder cancer was highest among women of H/L and AI/AN descent.

Most cancers are associated with controllable factors. Tobacco use is the number one cause of cancer and the number one cause of preventable death in the world. If the current trend continues, 650 million people alive today will die of tobacco-related diseases, including cancers of the lung, esophagus, and bladder.[18] In developed countries, poor diet, inadequate physical activity, and obesity are second only to tobacco as causes of cancer. These lifestyle choices are becoming apparent in all parts of the world, resulting in an increased diagnosis of cancers of the colon, breast, and prostate. Cancers linked to infectious agents (cervix, stomach, and liver) remain a threat that could be eliminated through the use of programs aimed at prevention, early diagnosis, and early, effective treatment.

PATHOPHYSIOLOGY

Knowledge about the pathophysiology of cancer will help you better understand the significance of clinical observations and the importance of planning interventions, including client teaching, for outcome management. A common misconception is that cancer is *one* disease. Cancer is many diseases.

Cancers comprise all diseases involving cells that are altered or transformed in some way but are able to multiply, grow, and spread. Cancer development begins at the molecular level and may begin with mutations or damage of one or more genomes. Cancerous cells differ from normal cells in appearance, growth, and function. The change from normal to neoplastic cells is a process, not a single event or a single alteration in cells. The

development of a cancer is a series of events that generally occur over many years. Clinical manifestations are only the final stages in the natural history of a cancer. Figure 16-3 describes the stages of cancer development.

Carcinogens

Carcinogens (factors associated with cancer causation) may be (1) radiation, (2) chemicals, (3) viruses, or (4) other physical agents.[36] In addition, hormones play a significant role in the development of many cancers.[12] The correlation between carcinogenic exposure, hormones, or genetics and the development of cancer remains under investigation. The present paradigm is that each plays a role, with the presence of one, two, or all three indicative of a cancer risk, not a cancer certainty.[3]

Radiation

More than 80% of exposure to radiation is from natural sources,[30,34] including ionizing radiation from cosmic rays and radioactive minerals, such as radon gas, radium, and uranium. Sunlight and tanning beds are two sources of ultraviolet radiation.

About 15% of radiation exposure comes from diagnostic or therapeutic procedures, including radiographs, radiation therapy, and radioisotopes used in diagnostic imaging. Individual doses vary widely with the numbers and types of procedures done.[36] The levels of radiation emitted by equipment for a given procedure have been falling significantly since the 1980s. About 5% of all secondary cancers are clearly linked to radiation therapy for a previous cancer.[34]

Chemicals

Tobacco, a chemical carcinogen, remains the most important known cause of cancer in the United States. Cole and Ralu state that *"smoking causes more cancer in the USA than do all other known causes combined."*[6] A clear linear relationship exists between the amount and number of years of smoking and cancer risk. This is documented in the medical record by the number of pack-years a client has smoked. (A *pack-year* refers to the number of packs of cigarettes smoked per day times the number of years the client has smoked.) Smokeless tobacco (chewing tobacco, snuff) is linked to oral cancers. Cancer risks associated with smokeless tobacco products may be decreasing because the suspected carcinogens, naturally occurring tobacco-specific nitrosamines, have been removed.[6]

In addition to lifestyle exposure to the chemicals in tobacco products, people can be exposed to chemicals in the workplace. Occupational exposure causes 2% to 8% of all human cancers. The risk estimates are much higher among the subpopulation of people actually

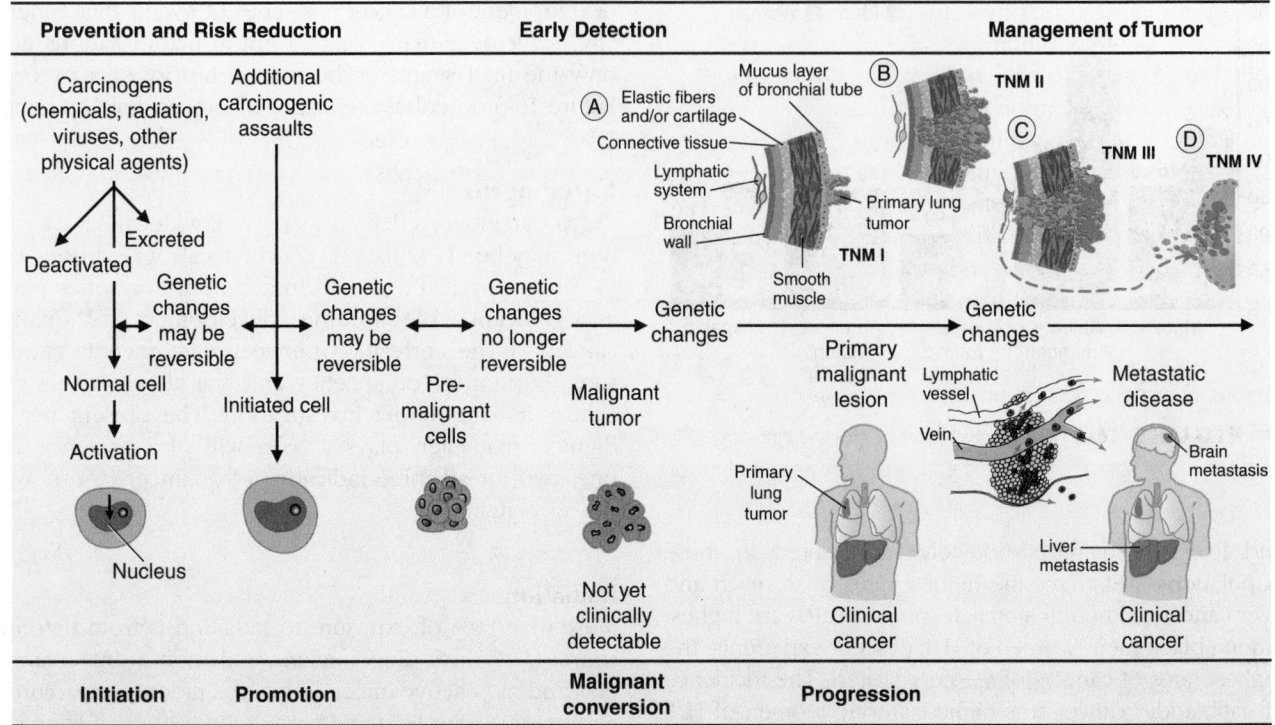

| Prevention and Risk Reduction | Early Detection | Management of Tumor |

■ FIGURE 16–3 Multistage model of carcinogenesis. The stages of cancer in the progression stage follow the T (tumor), N (node), and M (metastasis) system. **A,** Primary malignant lesion illustrates where the cancer is confined to lung tissue or the mucosa of the bronchial tube (TNM I). **B,** The cancer extends into bronchial muscle, serosa, and connective tissue (TNM II). **C,** The cancer penetrates the bronchial tube and tissue and adheres to or invades adjacent organs; or the lymphatic nodes are positive for cancer. **D,** Cancer metastasizes to distant organs such as the brain from the original lung tumor.

exposed to carcinogens in the workplace. These occupationally occurring cancers are, for the most part, preventable.[24]

SAFETY ALERT

Health care workers wear radiation badges to ensure that they do not receive unsafe levels of exposure. Most chemotherapeutic agents bind directly to genetic material or affect cellular protein synthesis.[7,24,31] The Occupational Safety and Health Administration (OSHA) outlines appropriate policies for mixing and administering chemotherapy agents. Today, chemotherapeutic agents are mixed under laminar-flow hoods that redirect air containing aerosolized drugs to prevent breathing of the chemicals. Gowns and gloves must be worn when administering chemotherapy, and spills are cleaned using special procedures that prevent absorption of the chemicals through the skin or mucous membranes. Personal protective equipment (PPE) is being used when mixing chemotherapeutic agents, but there is limited use of PPE when administering chemotherapy.[24,31] This is a potential health concern.

Viruses

Some viruses are strongly associated with cancer. Today, nine biologic agents are known to be associated with cancer causation. Of these, the hepatitis B and C viruses, the human papilloma viruses (HPV), and

Helicobacter pylori are considered public health problems in the United States.[6] In the 1970s and early 1980s, many thought cancer was contagious. Even today, a client or family member can express this fear. Even when there is a viral link, the cancer is not contagious. Rather, a virus at some point infected the cell, causing genetic damage to the cell's deoxyribonucleic acid (DNA), thus leading to the development of cancer.

Age, Gender, Genetics, Ethnicity

Host characteristics that influence cancer susceptibility include age, gender, genetic predisposition, and ethnicity or race. Age is a factor because it increases the years of potential exposure to carcinogens. Females have a generally lower risk of cancer incidence. Hormonal status is associated with an increased risk of neoplasia in tissues that are responsive to hormones, including breast, endometrium, prostate, ovary, thyroid, bone, and testes. In addition to biologic or genetic differences, cultural and socioeconomic factors may place an ethnic or racial group at increased or decreased risk of a specific cancer.[3]

For people who do not smoke, dietary patterns and physical activities become the most important cancer risk factors that they can modify. The ACS estimates that one third of cancer deaths in the United States are related to diet and physical activity.[3] Research into the relationship of diet and cancer is ongoing.[30] Changes in the ACS guidelines to decrease cancer risk include an emphasis on physical activity and weight control as well as the addition of a physical activity recommendation for youth.[2] A balanced, healthy diet that includes a high proportion of plant foods (fruits, vegetables, grains, and beans), limited intake of high-fat foods, a balance of caloric intake and physical activity, and limited consumption of alcoholic beverages can reduce cancer risks and maintain a healthy weight throughout life.[2,20]

The role of genes has been linked to between 5% and 10% of all cancers. Individuals who have had at least two blood relatives develop the same cancer, and these have occurred before the age of 65, may wish to consider genetic testing.[33] Additional information on the role of genetics in the development of cancer can be located elsewhere in this chapter and in Chapter 15.

Carcinogenesis: Transformation of Normal Cells into Cancer Cells

The process through which normal cells are transformed into malignant or cancer cells is called *carcinogenesis*. Four broadly identified stages of this process include the following:

1. *Initiation* occurs when a carcinogen damages DNA. Carcinogens cause changes in the structure and function of the cell at the genetic or molecular level. This damage may be reversible or may lead to genetic mutations if not repaired; however, the mutations may not lead immediately to cancer.
2. *Promotion* occurs with additional assaults to the cells, resulting in further genetic damage.
3. At some point, these genetic events result in a *malignant conversion.*
4. With *progression,* the cells are increasingly malignant in appearance and behavior and develop into an invasive cancer with metastases to distant body parts.

Clinical application of this process can be used to develop health promotion programs. Smoking cessation classes aim to decrease lung cancer through prevention. Health maintenance activities should include regular Papanicolaou (Pap) smears, because this procedure provides early detection of cervical dysplasia, a precancerous lesion. Precancerous colon polyps can be removed by colonoscopy before they progress to malignancy. Monitoring moles for early changes can allow a potentially lethal melanoma to be removed while it is still a localized, surgically curable disease.

Increased knowledge of the underlying biology of the process of carcinogenesis has exploded in the last decade. The identification of oncogenes, which occurred in the 1980s, has resulted in the recognition that cancer may be a genetic disease. Research shifted from carcinogenesis and mutagens to oncogenes and tumor suppressor genes. Oncogenes are genes that when mutated or expressed at abnormally high levels contribute to converting a normal cell into a cancer cell. A proto-oncogene is a gene whose protein product has the capacity to undergo cellular transformation if it sustains an insult. An oncogene is a gene that has sustained some genetic damage and thus produces a protein capable of cellular transformation. Proto-oncogenes have been classified into many different groups, and have been identified at all stages of cell growth. The list of proto-oncogenes currently identified is lengthy, and these cells have been acknowledged as critically important mechanisms that control cell growth and division, regulate embryologic development, and cause disease.[32] With this knowledge, scientists are developing better treatments. Powerful new chemotherapy drugs and new ways of delivering these drugs are becoming available. *Biotherapy* is now recognized as a fourth treatment modality in addition to surgery, radiation therapy, and chemotherapy. Biotherapy is moving from research to standard treatment.[21,22]

The process of carcinogenesis transforms normal cells into cancer cells. Anatomy and physiology of normal cells is presented in Units 3 and 4 Anatomy and Physiology Reviews. Changes that occur in the neoplastic transformation of cells are (1) alterations in the cell cycle, (2) altered differentiation, (3) altered growth characteristics, and (4) metastasis.

The Cell Cycle

The concept of the cell cycle has increased researchers' understanding of how both normal and neoplastic cells replicate. To review the cell cycle, please refer to Unit 3 Anatomy and Physiology Review. In the normal mature organ, cell cycling is carefully controlled so that the organ maintains its function. Cells that die are replaced, but no extra cells are produced. Researchers are investigating the mechanisms of this control, which are not fully understood.

Altered Cell Differentiation

Cells that were genetically identical in the embryo eventually assume varying structures and functions. In normal growth, cells become more specialized or committed to a particular cell line as they mature. This process of development is called *differentiation*. Most cells contain the entire genome. Transformation of a normal cell to a cancer cell can occur at any point in the process of differentiation. Changes in the appearance of the cell, the presence of tumor-specific antigens that are suppressed on the normal cell, and the loss of normal function can result from altered differentiation.

Appearance. The appearance of a cancer cell is obviously different from normal cells. Normal cells have well-organized cellular components, while cancer cells have variable sizes and shapes. In the cancer cell, nuclei may be disproportionately large, or there may be multiple nuclei. A variety of abnormal mitotic features may be present. There may be an abnormal number of chromosomes (*aneuploidy*) or an abnormal arrangement of chromosomes.[25] The detection of aneuploidy in a pathology report is an unfavorable prognostic factor.

The pathology report will describe the grade of the cancer cells. Cells that are well differentiated, or low grade, are more mature in appearance and more like the normal cells from which they have arisen than poorly differentiated cancer cells. Anaplastic (undifferentiated) cells appear so disorganized under the microscope that they have no resemblance to the tissue of origin. Poorly differentiated and anaplastic cancers tend to be more aggressive—an unfavorable prognostic factor. During the natural history of many malignant neoplasms, as the cancer cells grow and divide, they often lose more and more of their mature characteristics. As a result, a malignant neoplasm can be heterogeneous with more than one variation of the malignant cell line. This heterogeneity is caused by random mutations during tumor progression.[32]

At times, a neoplasm initially responds to therapy. You may read in a radiology report that the tumor has shrunk, with a partial remission (PR) or a complete remission (CR) of all radiologic evidence of the neoplasm; then the neoplasm may come back and grow aggressively. A likely explanation is that the treatment successfully eliminated one variant of the cancer cells, causing those cells to die and the overall size of the tumor to shrink. Then other variants of the cancer cells, which were resistant to the treatment, grew and multiplied, so that the tumor increased in size.

Biochemical studies may reflect differences resulting from altered cell metabolism. The cell's surface membrane is the interface between the cell and extracellular components. Cell membrane changes may result in the production of enzymes that aid in cancer spread. (A loss of glycoproteins results in a loss of cell-to-cell adhesion.) Loss of antigens that identify the cell as "self" or production of tumor-specific antigens can alter the immune system's ability to mount a response.[25]

Tumor cell membranes have a greater fluidity than normal cell membranes. This may be due to changes in the lipid composition of the membrane of tumor cells. Scientists are trying to take advantage of this difference. Some chemotherapy drugs are now being delivered in *liposomes* (spheres with an outer lipid layer and internal core of drug). The tumor cells take in more of the liposomal drug than is taken in by the normal cells. The result is a better treatment effect with fewer harmful effects on the normal cells.

Tumor-Specific Antigens. Cell surfaces express antigens. Some tumors express more of an antigen than is expressed by normal cells. These tumor-specific antigens can be used as a diagnostic tool in the detection of cancer or in monitoring the effectiveness of cancer treatment. One example is the PSA test. Normally, a man's blood level of PSA is low (i.e., 0 to 2 ng/ml). In the presence of prostate cancer, this antigen can be elevated. The PSA blood test is now being used as one early detection tool, along with the digital rectal examination, to detect prostate cancer in men who are still asymptomatic.[2] During treatment, a decline in the PSA level is an indicator of the effectiveness of the treatment. During follow-up after treatment ends, a rise in the PSA level can be an early indicator that the cancer has recurred.

Function. Unlike normal cells, cancer cells typically serve no useful purpose. The result of neoplastic growth is an abnormal tissue mass that does not contribute in any way to the well-being of the host. The mass occupies space and draws nutrition and sustenance from the host. If the cancer cells function at all, they often do not function normally and may even act in a way that causes damage to the host. For example, a functional tumor of the thyroid gland produces excess amounts of thyroid hormone, leading to a hypermetabolic state.

Altered Growth Characteristics

Another obvious difference from normal cells is the uncontrolled growth of cancer cells. Because of changes in their cell surfaces, neoplastic cells differ from normal cells in growth patterns and mobility. Cancer cells lose the contact inhibition of normal cells, can establish metastasis, avoid normal regulation by hormones, and avoid being recognized by the immune system as altered.

Cancer cells do not go through the cell cycle at a faster rate than normal cells; rather, the abnormality is that they do not stop replicating. Cancer cells are almost continuously in the process of cell division. This appears to be due to (1) lack of responses to signals to stop replicating and (2) lack of responses to cell death (*apoptosis*) signals.[26] (Apoptosis is discussed later in this chapter.)

Contact Inhibition and Doubling Time. This continuous growth results in a phenomenon referred to as *doubling time*. The doubling time of a human malignant tumor can vary from weeks to months. As depicted in Figure 16-4, it may take 10 years for a tumor to reach 1 cm in size. In only another year, that same tumor may grow to 8 cm. The smallest clinically detectable mass weighs about 1 g, or 1 cm^3 in size. A *tumor burden* (amount) of 1 kg, which requires only about 10 more doublings, is potentially lethal.[25]

Clients sometimes ask whether exposing the tumor to air during surgery can cause it to grow more rapidly. More likely, if the surgeon did not see evidence of tumor in other areas, it had already spread, but the size of the

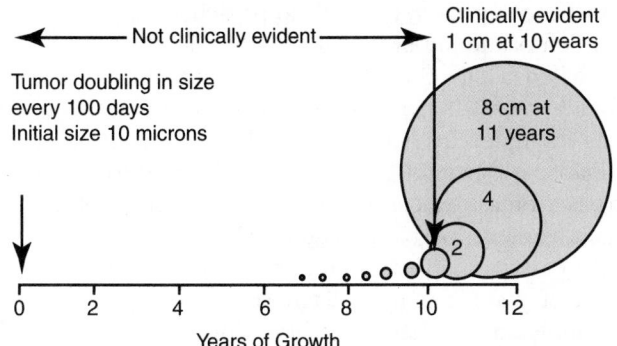

■ FIGURE 16–4 Depiction of tumor growth showing doubling time related to tumor size.

tumor mass was still too small to be seen or felt. Then in a few more doubling times, without effective treatment, it became evident and proceeded to enlarge.

Metastasis

Normal cells are adherent to the other normal cells from which they have arisen. Normal breast tissue cells, for example, are never found anywhere in the body except in the breast. Malignant or cancer cells are less adherent and more mobile than normal cells. They have the ability to spread from the original site of the tumor to distant organs. This phenomenon is called *metastasis* (from the Greek *meta,* beyond, and *stasis,* standing).

The capacity of a neoplastic tumor to metastasize to other sites is a major characteristic of malignancy and the most frequent reason why cancer treatment fails. It is the characteristic that distinguishes malignant from benign growths. Neoplastic cells must progress through a sequence of complex stages to overcome multiple barriers and successfully spread to other sites. Failure to complete any stage in the metastatic cascade disrupts formation of metastases.[32]

No single gene product is solely responsible for the highly complex processes in the metastatic cascade. Progressive alterations in cellular oncogenes and inactivation of tumor suppressor genes result in uncontrolled growth and development of metastatic potential. For the purposes of this discussion, the metastatic cascade is divided into three stages (see Figure 16-3).

Stage 1. The progressive alteration of malignant cells with additional genetic changes results in a heterogeneous population of malignant cells with varying degrees of metastatic potential. Increasing tumor size, leading to tissue pressure and mechanical expansion, may cause neoplastic invasion; however, the size of the primary tumor is not the sole predictor of metastasis. Tumors with identical size and histologic cell type can vary markedly in metastatic spread. As the malignant tumor grows, the cells at the center become hypoxic, and it begins to seek its own blood supply. Neoplastic

cells from the primary tumor invade surrounding tissue and penetrate blood or lymph vessels. Vascularization *(angiogenesis)* of the tumor dramatically increases its metastatic potential.[25,32]

Loss of tumor cell cohesiveness with increasing motility is an important factor in the metastatic cascade. These cells can detach from the primary tumor and create defects in the basement membranes with resulting stromal invasion and spread into the circulation. Tumors, even when very small, shed cells. As many as 10^7 to 10^9 cells per day may be found circulating in the bloodstream of clients with cancer.[25,32] Although surgery, for example, can cure most early breast cancers, some eventually recur because of these shed cells. Adjuvant chemotherapy or hormonal therapy, given when no visible tumor remains, may therefore be considered for clients with early-stage breast cancer to decrease the risk of recurrence. Yet fewer than 1% of circulating cancer cells successfully metastasize.[32] Emerging scientific knowledge may allow oncologists to identify the client with early-stage breast cancer who would benefit from adjuvant chemotherapy. This would allow most women for whom surgery alone was curative to avoid the adverse effects of chemotherapy.

Benign neoplasms and cancer in situ do not cause destruction of the host stroma (the supporting tissues of an organ). With progression to invasive disease, the neoplasm penetrates the epithelial basement membrane and invades the interstitial stroma at multiple stages in the metastatic cascade.[28] A client's pathology report often indicates whether there was invasion of the neoplasm into surrounding tissue or into lymphatic, perineural, or vascular tissues. Such invasion may be an indication of occult (as yet undetected) metastatic disease.

Cancer cells that successfully metastasize represent a subpopulation of the primary tumor's cells. Not all cells in the primary mass share the unique genetic and biologic properties necessary for metastasis.[25]

Stage 2. Cancer cells migrate via the lymph or blood circulation or by direct extension. The lymphatic system provides the most common pathway for the initial spread of malignant cancer cells. There may be spread to the lymph nodes draining the region of the primary tumor site. Lymph node involvement is seen in about 50% of all fatal cancers. The blood vessels (both veins and arteries) carry cancer cells from the primary tumor to the capillary beds of the lungs, liver, and bones. Metastatic spread to distant organs and tissues is almost always the result of cells moving through the bloodstream.

Direct extension of tumors to adjacent tissues also occurs. For example, a breast cancer may spread directly to the chest wall. In body cavities, cells may spread by gravity, resulting in new growths on other serosal surfaces. Cells shed by cancers of the ovary are often found to have fallen onto and "seeded" the entire peritoneal cavity with metastatic sites of the tumor.

To complete this stage in the metastatic cascade, tumor cells must survive a variety of hemodynamic and immunologic challenges.

Stage 3. Cancer cells are established at the secondary site. This may result from entrapment caused by the size of the tumor clump, from adherence to cells at the new site through specific interactions, or by binding to exposed basement membrane. Continued growth and proliferation at the metastatic site are also dependent on the development of its own blood supply (*angiogenesis*) and ability to evade eradication by immune responses. Cells from the metastatic site may then proceed to disseminate to form additional metastatic lesions.[32]

Researchers have observed that certain tumor cells have, for unknown reasons, an affinity for certain sites. Although the exact mechanism of metastasis is unclear, the metastatic sites of many cancers are fairly predictable. The predilection of certain malignant neoplasms for particular sites may be due to the ability of the tumor to live within only certain tissues or to some other unknown factor. The most common site of metastasis is lymphatic tissues; the next most common sites are the liver, lungs, bones, and brain.[25]

Angiogenesis. The metastatic cascade begins and ends with *angiogenesis*. A tumor cannot grow more than 0.5 mm without a blood supply to transport nutrients to the tumor. Very tiny tumors can receive oxygen and nutrients by diffusion. Proliferation beyond 0.5 mm requires a vasculature blood supply. Angiogenesis is the ability of cancer cells to secrete substances that stimulate blood vessel growth.[6,10] The angiogenic process involves a series of sequential steps that result in a shift in the balance between stimulators and inhibitors of angiogenesis. When the number of pro-angiogenic molecules exceeds the number of anti-angiogenic molecules, new blood vessels are formed. Scientists are studying various anti-angiogenesis strategies.[25,32] Arresting the development of new blood supplies could halt the growth of a tumor. The destruction of a single tumor capillary may be able to kill many cancer cells that rely on that vessel for nutrition. Benign tumors are sparsely vascularized and grow slowly, whereas malignant tumors are highly vascular and grow rapidly. If angiogenesis is inhibited, cancer progression may be halted or slowed by preventing metastasis. Several types of anti-angiogenic agents are currently under investigation.[11,29,34]

The growth of metastatic tumors puts severe stress on the affected person, both physiologically and psychologically. As the *tumor burden* (the amount of tumor in the body) increases, fewer metabolic resources are available for normal cells. As mentioned earlier, when the total

burden of tumor in the body approaches 1 kg, the sheer burden of the tumor is potentially lethal.

When a client's cancer metastasizes, the client and family members may erroneously believe that the client has multiple cancers; it is one cancer spread to other organs. For example, cells that have spread to the bone from a breast cancer are breast cancer cells, not malignant variants of bone tissue cells; however, a client may have two different cancers at one time. In the process of making a new diagnosis of colon cancer, for example, a clinician may also discover a previously undetected prostate cancer.

Knowing the natural history and the most likely pattern of proliferation can be very helpful to the clinician. If the cancer is likely to spread to the liver, bone, or brain, the clinician will want to rule out evidence of such distribution in making treatment decisions and in monitoring for recurrence following treatment.

Inability of the Immune System to Recognize Cancer Cells

The immune system usually defends against bacterial or viral invaders and plays a key role in controlling the growth of cancer cells. There are two critical components of the immune response: (1) the ability to recognize a pathogen as foreign and (2) the ability to mount a response to eliminate the pathogen.[21,28] The Unit 17 Anatomy and Physiology Review section discusses the immune system; this section addresses the role of the immune system in preventing carcinogenesis.

Role in Preventing Carcinogenesis

Cancer cells arise continually as a result of somatic (non–reproductive cell) mutations. The immune system—specifically the T-cell lymphocytes, macrophages, and antigens—recognizes these cells as non-self and destroys them. Immune surveillance theory, as yet unproved, proposes that immune responses, particularly cell-mediated responses, provide a defense against cancer cells by recognizing the antigens on the surface of some neoplastic cells as foreign. These cells are killed by cytotoxic T cells that have receptors for specific tumor antigens and by interferon-activated natural killer (NK) lymphocytes and macrophages.[21]

Macrophages, the important first line of defense, phagocytize the pathogen and present it as antigen to T and B lymphocytes. T-cell recognition of antigen stimulates proliferation of T and B cells, with B-cell production of antibodies against the pathogen and T-cell secretion of cytokines. Cytokines, hormone-like peptides or glycopeptides, regulate activation of the immune system against cancer cells. Cytokines both enhance and suppress complex immune interactions.

Antigens on cancer cells can take various forms, resulting in T-cell recognition of the cells as abnormal.

The cancer cells may express antigens that are not present on normal cells. Cancer cells may have antigens that are "unmasked" and thus visible to the immune system. These same antigens when present on normal cells are masked and thus are not recognized by the immune system. Cancer cells may also express antigens that are only present during oncofetal or embryonic development of normal cells. Cytotoxic T cells that have receptors for specific tumor antigens and interferon-activated NK lymphocytes and macrophages can then destroy these cancer cells.

Failure of Immune Defenses

Unfortunately, the immune defenses are not always effective. The immune system may be unable to recognize cancer cells as foreign or to mount an immune response for several reasons.

An immature, old, or weak immune system may contribute to this. People who are malnourished or chronically ill may also be immunocompromised. The tumor burden (number of cancer cells) may be too small to stimulate an immune response. Alternatively, the tumor burden may be so great as to overwhelm the immune system.

Some cancer cells escape detection because they resemble normal cells. Other cancer cells produce substances that shield them from recognition. Cancer cells may also escape detection by becoming coated with fibrin. Tumor invasion of the bone marrow can result in decreased production of lymphocytes needed to destroy the tumor mass.

The incidence of malignancy increases with the use of immunosuppressive drugs after organ transplantation to counteract rejection. Chemotherapeutics or radiation used to treat cancer can also induce suppression of the immune response.[21,25]

Apoptosis

With the development of molecular biology in the 1980s, scientists began to understand another important step in the process of carcinogenesis: the failure of cells to die.[1,10,13,35,37] In normal physiology, a damaged cell sacrifices itself for the greater good. There are two pathways to cell death:

1. *Necrosis* is cell death resulting from injury. The dead cells swell, lyse, and release their cellular contents into the intercellular spaces, causing the inflammatory response.
2. In *apoptosis* (from the Greek word for "falling off"), cellular "suicide" results in cells rapidly shrinking with loss of their intercellular contents.[25] They are quickly phagocytized and digested by macrophages and other cells in the vicinity. Inflammation is not triggered. See Figure A&P4-5 on p. 235, which depicts apoptosis. The morphologic changes of apoptosis can be completed in less than an hour.[9,13]

Most, if not all, cells manufacture a set of proteins that serve as weapons of self-destruction. As long as a cell is useful to the body, it restrains its death machinery. If the cell becomes infected or malignant or otherwise threatens the health of the organism, however, the lethal proteins are unleashed.[9]

Increasingly, scientists view cancer as a disease of both excessive cell growth and a lack of normal cell death. In the process of carcinogenesis, cells accumulate enough damage to genes that control cell growth and survival that the mutation seems irreparable. The affected cell usually kills itself rather than risk becoming deranged and potentially dangerous. If the cell does not die, it or its daughter cells may live long enough to accumulate mutations that make it possible to divide uncontrollably and to metastasize to distant sites.

When a death signal, such as tumor necrosis factor (TNF), is initiated, a survival signal is also initiated. The balance between cell survival and cell death signals determines cell fate.[37] Apoptosis may not be induced in response to a cancer cell because there has also been damage to a tumor suppressor gene. In many cancers, genetic damage apparently fails to induce apoptosis because there has been damage to the gene that codes for the p53 protein. The p53 protein is a suppressor gene that can prompt activation of cell suicide. It is estimated that as many as half of solid cancers, including lung, colon, and breast cancers, have damage to the p53 protein.[9]

Still other apoptotic triggers can lead to programmed death of cancerous cells. Normal cells also tend to self-destruct when deprived of their usual growth factors or contact with other like cells. This is probably a built-in defense mechanism against metastasis. Part of the reason some cancers are resistant to the effects of radiation therapy or chemotherapy may be due to the lack of cell death through apoptosis even after cancer treatment. Researchers are investigating genetic therapies that might overcome this resistance to apoptosis.

GENETICS AND CANCER

Medical genetics has rapidly evolved into a full-fledged scientific field, and oncology is at the forefront in utilizing these scientific strides. The Human Genome Project's goal is locating, mapping, and sequencing the genes of a human's genetic composition. Scientists have mapped the estimated 30,000 to 40,000 genes on the human chromosome and are now working to apply this knowledge to prevent or treat disease.[16,20,28] A powerful new technology combining biology with computers is emerging. This gene chip analysis technology will make possible the screening of vast numbers of genes. The potential payoff is great.[17]

Cancer may be a genetic disease. On the molecular level, cancer may result from different combinations of a few similar gene mutations.[19] Two neoplasms that are morphologically indistinguishable can have different gene profiles. In clinical practice, two women can have breast cancers with the same histology, grade, and stage and receive the same therapy and yet have different outcomes. Gene profiling provides the ability to recognize areas of genetic abnormalities on the chromosome. Different combinations of genetic mutations and environmental influences can cause a normal cell to become malignant. On the other hand, genetic mutation, such as damage to the p53 suppressor gene, can be seen in the profiles of clinically very different cancers.[14] Another person whose genetic profile carries this same abnormality may develop cancer or may never develop cancer but might pass the abnormality on to offspring.

Up to 30% of rare childhood cancers result from genetic predisposition. In adults, about 34% of cancers have a *familial* basis; only 5% to 10% of adult cancers are *hereditary*. Hereditary cancers result from a single inherited gene disorder. Patterns of occurrence are clearly predictable. These cancers usually occur at an early age, in unusual sites, and in paired organs (both breasts, for example). There also may be multiple primary (versus metastatic) sites. Hereditary cancers include some breast, colorectal, melanoma, ovarian, and renal cell cancers as well as retinoblastoma and Wilms' tumor.[21] Other cancers have no predictable pattern of inheritance because these cancers may not be linked to a single gene disorder. Cancers that may have a potential familial link include breast, ovarian, colorectal, prostate, melanoma, uterine, leukemia, sarcomas, and primary brain tumors.

At present oncologists recommend treatments and provide clients with a statistical prognosis based on research data outlining the response to treatment from groups of clients with similar type, grade, and stage of cancer. Over the coming decade, medical genetics will be able to provide scientists new tools to answer more specifically questions about cancer causation and response to treatment.[17,28] As we identify how treatments work at the genetic level, oncologists will be able to customize a treatment plan to the specific areas of genetic damage resulting in a client's cancer. New biologic agents being developed have an additive effect when combined with chemotherapy and radiation therapy.[14]

Genetic discoveries, together with the identification of oncogenes and pro-oncogenes, will impact nursing practice and change the traditional perspective on screening, identifying, preventing, and treating cancer.[4] Most nurses are already performing some genetics-related activities. Do you know the recommendation to use sunscreens has a genetic basis? Has a client ever expressed concern about familial experience of cancer? Has a client ever asked you about a vaccine for melanoma or pancreatic cancer? As clients become more aware of the role that genetics has in cancer causation, nurses will need to be able to provide client teaching or referrals to professionals who can address these concerns.[17] Precise identification of cancer-causing genetic abnormalities will significantly improve the accuracy of cancer prediction and thus the capacity to target preventive interventions to at-risk populations.[28] As a result, the perspective of nursing will shift from symptomatic clients with cancer to counseling asymptomatic clients. CA125, an identified tumor marker, is useful in monitoring the response of ovarian cancer to therapy; however, it has not been sufficiently sensitive for detecting early-stage disease. Higher levels of a new biomarker, osteopontin, may be a valuable early detection tool for ovarian cancer. Likewise, molecular profiling of prostate cancer has led to the identification of new biomarkers that may have value in analysis of prostate biopsy specimens.[29] Counseling and support are vital for any client considering genetic testing.

Issues of confidentiality and discrimination, as well as the dilemma of predicting as yet incurable illnesses, may have an enormous negative effect on the client's and family's quality of life and psychological state. Learning one's genetic test results may cause distress, sadness, depression, anxiety, or anger and may affect one's relationship with other family members. Clients considering genetic testing need to be informed of state and federal laws protecting them from insurance and job discrimination and the limitations of these laws.[11,12]

Knowledge of genetics is rapidly becoming fundamental to oncology nursing practice. Nurses will need this knowledge to help their clients understand cancer causation and their customized treatments, to recognize risk factors, and to promote effective prevention/early detection strategies. The diffusion of our evolving science of cancer genetics will be dependent on health professionals, including nurses, applying that knowledge in our clinical practices.[4]

CLASSIFICATION OF NEOPLASMS

Benign Versus Malignant

As stated, neoplastic tumors can be either benign or malignant. Benign tumors generally have a good prognosis because they do not infiltrate or metastasize. They may be fatal if located near a vital tube or organ. Malignant neoplasms represent a serious threat to the life and well-being of the host. Table 16-1 compares benign and malignant neoplasms.

Tissue of Origin

In addition to being classified as benign or malignant, neoplasms are also classified according to the tissue from which they arise. The suffix is usually attached to a term for the parent tissue of the neoplasm. When more than

TABLE 16–1   Comparison of the Characteristics of Benign and Malignant Neoplasms

Characteristic	Benign Neoplasm	Malignant Neoplasm
Speed of growth	Grows slowly	Usually grows rapidly
	Usually continues to grow throughout life unless surgically removed	Tends to grow relentlessly throughout life
	May have periods of remission	Rarely, neoplasm may regress spontaneously
Mode of growth	Grows by enlarging and expanding	Grows by infiltrating surrounding tissues
	Always remains localized; never infiltrates surrounding tissues	May remain localized (in situ), but usually infiltrates other tissues
Capsule	Almost always contained within a fibrous capsule	Never contained within a capsule
	Capsule does not prevent expansion of neoplasm but does prevent growth by infiltration	Absence of capsule allows neoplastic cells to invade surrounding tissues
	Capsule advantageous because encapsulated tumor can be removed surgically	Surgical removal of tumor difficult
Cell characteristics	Usually well differentiated	Usually poorly differentiated
	Mitotic figures absent or scanty	Large numbers of normal and abnormal mitotic figures present
	Mature cells	
	Anaplastic cells absent	Cells tend to be anaplastic (i.e., young, embryonic type)
	Cells function poorly in comparison with normal cells from which they arise	Cells too abnormal to perform any physiologic functions
	If neoplasm arises in glandular tissue, cells may secrete hormones	Occasionally a malignant tumor arising in glandular tissue secretes hormones
Recurrence	Recurrence extremely unusual when surgically removed	Recurrence common following surgery because tumor cells spread into surrounding tissues
Metastasis	Metastases never occur	Metastases very common
Effect of neoplasm	Not harmful to host unless located in area where it compresses tissues or obstructs vital organs	Always harmful to host
		Causes death unless removed surgically or destroyed by radiation or chemotherapy
	Does not produce cachexia (weight loss, debilitation, anemia, weakness, wasting)	Causes disfigurement, disrupted organ function, nutritional imbalances
		May result in ulcerations, sepsis, perforations, hemorrhage, tissue slough
		Almost always produces cachexia, which leaves person prone to pneumonia, anemia, and other conditions
Prognosis	Very good	Depends on cell type and speed of diagnosis
	Tumor generally removed surgically	Poor prognosis if cells are poorly differentiated and evidence of metastatic spread exists
		Good prognosis indicated if cells still resemble normal cells and there is no evidence of metastasis

one parent tissue enters into the formation of a neoplasm, the names of the tumors are even more descriptive.

Because epithelial tissues vary greatly, benign tumors of epithelial origin are classified according to either their *microscopic* appearance (e.g., adenoma) or their *macroscopic* appearance (e.g., polyp, from the Greek *polys* for "many" plus *pous* for "foot").

There are three common benign neoplasms. *Fibromas* may grow anywhere in the body, but they frequently make their home in the uterus. Fibromas are generally small but occasionally grow to great size. These encapsulated, relatively harmless neoplasms cause no manifestations unless, because of their location, they press on a bone or nerve. Fibromas are easily removed surgically. *Lipomas* arise in adipose tissue. Lipomas rarely cause manifestations, but they are poorly encapsulated and may exert pressure on surrounding tissues as they expand. *Leiomyomas* are benign neoplasms of smooth muscle origin and the most common benign tumor in women. Leiomyomas may develop anywhere in the body,

but most often they grow in the uterus. Rarely (approximately 1% of cases), these neoplasms become malignant.

Malignant neoplasms are also categorized by tissue origin. A malignant neoplasm that arises from epithelial tissue is called a *carcinoma;* a malignant neoplasm that arises from mesenchymal origins (i.e., blood vessels, lymphatic tissue, nerve tissue) is called a *sarcoma* (from Greek *sarx,* or flesh). Table 16-2 provides the classification of neoplasms by their tissue of origin.

Defining the Stage

In addition, cancer is staged using the TNM system. T stands for the size of the tumor, N for the degree of spread to the lymph nodes, and M for the presence of metastasis. Then a number is added to each of these letters to indicate the size and spread. This method identifies the "extent" of the tumor and its degree of spread. It provides an estimate of prognosis, since cure chances decrease as the tumor becomes more advanced or

TABLE 16–2 Classification of Neoplasms by Tissue of Origin

Tissue of Origin	Benign	Malignant
Connective tissue		Sarcoma
Embryonic fibrous tissue	Myxoma	Myxosarcoma
Fibrous tissue	Fibroma	Fibrosarcoma
Adipose tissue	Lipoma	Liposarcoma
Cartilage	Chondroma	Chondrosarcoma
Bone	Osteoma	Osteogenic sarcoma
Epithelium		Carcinoma
Skin and mucous membrane	Papilloma	Squamous cell carcinoma
Glands		Basal cell carcinoma
		Transitional cell carcinoma
	Adenoma	Adenocarcinoma
	Cystadenoma	Cystadenocarcinoma
Pigmented cells (melanocytes)	Nevus	Malignant melanoma
Endothelium		Endothelioma
Blood vessels	Hemangioma	Hemangioendothelioma
		Hemangiosarcoma
		Kaposi's sarcoma
Lymph vessels	Lymphangioma	Lymphangiosarcoma
		Lymphangioendothelioma
Bone marrow		Multiple myeloma
		Ewing's sarcoma
		Leukemia
Lymphoid tissue		Malignant lymphoma
		Lymphosarcoma
		Reticulum cell sarcoma
Muscle tissue		
Smooth muscle	Leiomyoma	Leiomyosarcoma
Striated muscle	Rhabdomyoma	Rhabdomyosarcoma
Nerve tissue		
Nerve fibers and sheaths	Neuroma	Neurogenic sarcoma
	Neurinoma	
	Neurilemoma	
	Neurofibroma	Neurofibrosarcoma
Ganglion cells	Ganglioneuroma	Neuroblastoma
Glial cells	Glioma	Glioblastoma
Meninges	Meningioma	Malignant meningioma
Gonads	Dermoid cyst	Embryonal carcinoma
		Embryonal sarcoma
		Teratocarcinoma

extensive. The staging of the tumor becomes most important when deciding on appropriate treatment and is discussed in more detail in Chapter 17.[8]

CONCLUSIONS

Effective nursing care and client teaching to achieve outcome goals require that you understand the pathophysiology of the cancer. You should know the natural history of the disease, such as the normal course of disease progression, likely sites of metastasis, potential for effective treatment, and side effects and complications of both the disease and the treatments. With a basic understanding of cancer, you can build on that knowledge base by listening to the client's history, reviewing the information provided in the medical record, and consulting with colleagues, including nursing peers, nursing leaders, physicians, and oncology nurses, both locally and nationally.

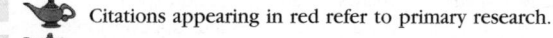

BIBLIOGRAPHY

Citations appearing in red refer to primary research.

Citations appearing in blue refer to evidence-based practice guidelines and protocols.

1. Ameisen, J.C. (1996). The origin of programmed cell death. *Science, 272,* 1278-1279.
2. American Cancer Society. (2007). *Cancer facts and figures—2007.* Atlanta: Author.
3. Calvo, K.R., Petricoin, E.F., & Liotta, L.A. (2005). Genomics and proteomics. In V.T. DeVita, S. Hellman, & S.A. Rosenberg (Eds.), *Cancer: Principles and practice of oncology* (7th ed., pp. 51-72). Philadelphia: Lippincott Williams & Wilkins.
4. Calzone, K.A., & Tranin, A.S. (2003). The scope of cancer genetics nursing practice. In A.M. Tranin & J. Jenkins (Eds.), *Genetics in oncology practice: Cancer risk assessment* (pp. 13-22). Pittsburgh: Oncology Nursing Society.
5. Chapman, D.D. (2005). Breast cancer. In C.H. Yarbro, M.H. Frogge, & M. Goodman (Eds.), *Cancer nursing: Principles and practice* (6th ed., pp 1022-1057). Boston: Jones & Bartlett.
6. Cole, P., & Ralu, B. (2001). Analytic epidemiology: Cancer causes. In V.T. DeVita, S. Hellman, & S.A. Rosenberg (Eds.), *Cancer: Principles and practices of oncology* (6th ed., pp. 241-252). Philadelphia: Lippincott Williams & Wilkins.
7. Connor, T.H., et al. (1999). Surface contamination with antineoplastics in six cancer treatment centers in Canada and the United States. *ASHP, 56,* 1427-1432.
8. DeVita, V.T., Hellman, S., & Rosenberg, S.A. (Eds.) (2005). *Cancer: Principles and practices of oncology* (7th ed.). Philadelphia: Lippincott Williams & Wilkins.
9. Duke, R.C., Ojcius, D.M., & Young, J.D. (1996). Cell suicide in health and disease. *Scientific American, 275*(6), 80-87.
10. Fidler, I.J., Langley, R.R., Kerbel, R.S., et al. (2005). Angiogenesis. In V.T. DeVita, S. Hellman, & S. Rosenberg (Eds.), *Cancer: Principles and practice of oncology* (7th ed., pp. 129-137). Philadelphia: Lippincott Williams & Wilkins.
11. Greco, K. (2003). How to provide genetic counseling and education. In A.M. Tranin & J. Jenkins (Eds.), *Genetics in oncology practice: Cancer risk assessment* (pp. 189-224). Pittsburgh: Oncology Nursing Society.
12. Groopman, J. (1998, Feb 9). Decoding destiny. *The New Yorker,* pp 42-47.
13. Hetts, S.W. (1998). To die or not to die. *Journal of the American Medical Association, 279*(4), 300-307.
14. Ishii, H., et al. (2001). Potential cancer therapy with the fragile histidine triad gene. *Journal of the American Medical Association, 286*(19), 2441-2449.
15. Jemal, A., et al. (2005). Cancer statistics, 2005, *CA: A Cancer Journal for Clinicians, 55*(1), 5-31.
16. Jenkins, J., & Masny, A. (2003). Why should oncology nurses be interested in genetics? In A.M. Tranin & J. Jenkins (Eds.), *Genetics in oncology practice: Cancer risk assessment* (pp. 1-12). Pittsburgh: Oncology Nursing Society.
17. King, H.C., & Sinha, A.A. (2001). Gene expression profile analysis by DNA microarrays: Promise and pitfalls. *Journal of the American Medical Association, 286*(18), 2280-2288.
18. Knop, C.S. (2005). Lung cancer. In C.H. Yarbro, M.H. Frogge, & M. Goodman (Eds.), *Cancer nursing: Principles and practice* (6th ed., pp. 1379-1414). Boston: Jones & Bartlett.
19. Loescher, L.J., & Whitesell, L. (2003). The biology of cancer. In A.M. Tranin & J. Jenkins (Eds.), *Genetics in oncology practice: Cancer risk assessment* (pp. 23-56). Pittsburgh: Oncology Nursing Society.
20. McKusick, V.A. (2001). The anatomy of the human genome: A neovesalian basis for medicine in the 21st century. *Journal of the American Medical Association, 28*(18), 2289-2295.

21. Merkle, C.J., & Loesher, L.J. (2005). Biology of cancer. In C.H. Yarbro, M.H. Frogge, & M. Goodman (Eds.), *Cancer nursing: Principles and practice* (6th ed., pp. 4-26). Boston: Jones & Bartlett.
22. Miaskowski, C. (1999). *Oncology nursing: An essential guide for patient care.* Philadelphia: Saunders.
23. National Cancer Institute Surveillance, Epidemiology and End Results. (2006). *About SEER.* Retrieved 04/12/06 from http://seer.cancer.gov/about.
24. Occupational Safety and Health Administration (OSHA). (2006). *Hazardous drugs: Hazards and solutions.* Retrieved 04/11/06 from www.osha.gov/SLTC/hazardousdrugs/recognition.html.
25. Omerod, K.F. (2005). Diagnosis, classification and staging. In C.H. Yarbro, M.H. Frogge, & M. Goodman (Eds.), *Cancer nursing: Principles and practice* (6th ed., pp. 153-181). Boston: Jones & Bartlett.
26. Reed, S.I. (2005). Cell cycle. In V.T. DeVita, S. Hellman, & S.A. Rosenberg (Eds.), *Cancer: Principles and practice of oncology* (7th ed., pp. 83-95). Philadelphia: Lippincott Williams & Wilkins.
27. Rieger, P.T. (2003). The impact of genetic information in the management of cancer. In A.M. Tranin & J. Jenkins (Eds.), *Genetics in oncology practice: Cancer risk assessment* (pp. 139-188). Pittsburgh: Oncology Nursing Society.
28. Rieger, P.T., & Much, J.K. (2005). Genetic risk for cancer. In C.H. Yarbro, M.H. Frogge, & M. Goodman (Eds.), *Cancer nursing: Principles and practice* (6th ed., pp. 127-153). Boston: Jones & Bartlett.
29. Rubin, M.A., et al. (2002). Methylacyl coenzyme A racemase as a tissue biomarker for prostate cancer. *Journal of the American Medical Association, 287*(13), 1662-1670.
30. Schulmeister, L. (2001). Epidemiology. In S. Otto (Ed.), *Oncology nursing* (4th ed., pp. 42-52). St. Louis: Mosby.
31. Sessink, P.J., & Bos, R.P. (1999). Drugs hazardous to healthcare workers. *Drug Safety, 20*(4), 347-357.
32. Stetler-Stevenson, W.G. (2005). Invasion and metastases. In V.T. DeVita, S. Hellman, & S.A. Rosenberg (Eds.), *Cancer: Principles and practice of oncology* (7th ed., pp. 113-128). Philadelphia: Lippincott Williams & Wilkins.
33. Tranin, A.M., Masny, A., & Jenkins, J. (Eds.) (2003). *Genetics in oncology practice: Cancer risk assessment.* Pittsburgh: Oncology Nursing Society.
34. Ullrich, R.L. (2005). Etiology of cancer: Physical factors. In V.T. DeVita, S. Hellman, & S.A. Rosenberg (Eds.), *Cancer: Principles and practice of oncology* (7th ed., pp. 193-200). Philadelphia: Lippincott Williams & Wilkins.
35. Yarbo, C.H., Frogge, M.H., & Goodman, M. (Eds.), *Cancer nursing: Principles and practice* (6th ed.). Boston: Jones & Bartlett.
36. Yuspa, S.H., & Shields, P.G. (2005). Etiology of cancer: Chemical factors. In V.T. DeVita, S. Hellman, & S. Rosenberg (Eds.), *Cancer: Principles and practice of oncology* (7th ed., pp. 185-192). Philadelphia: Lippincott Williams & Wilkins.
37. Zinkel, S.S., & Korsmeyer, S.J. (2005). Apoptosis. In V.T. DeVita, S. Hellman, & S.A. Rosenberg (Eds.), *Cancer: Principles and practice of oncology* (7th ed., pp. 95-104). Philadelphia: Lippincott Williams & Wilkins.

evolve *Did you remember to check out the bonus material on the Evolve website and the CD-ROM, including NCLEX®-Examination Style Review Questions, Open-Book Quizzes, and Chapter Review Audio Podcasts?*

http://evolve.elsevier.com/Black/medsurg

CHAPTER 17

Clients with Cancer

PEGGY WARD-SMITH

The continuum of disease progression begins with the precancerous and cellular level changes discussed in the previous chapter on the pathophysiology of malignant neoplasms. The goal of health promotion is to prevent cancer or to detect it early, in its most treatable stage. After a new diagnosis of cancer, the client may experience remission, stable disease, recurrence, progressive disease, end-stage or terminal disease, or long-term survivorship. Treatment modalities depend on the type and extent of the cancer but often include some combination of surgery, radiation therapy (XRT), chemotherapy, and biotherapy. Bone marrow transplantation (BMT) may be part of the treatment plan. Clinical trials offer the hope of new treatments for clients.

Complementary approaches are being used in combination with other cancer treatments. The disease process and the effects of treatment on normal tissue present common complications or oncologic emergencies that require effective nursing management to achieve desired outcomes. Cancer care is not just about the disease and treatment, but includes the impact cancer has on people's lives. Therefore an important role of the nurse in managing outcomes is to recognize, intervene, and provide support for the human responses to living with cancer.

HEALTH PROMOTION AND MAINTENANCE

Cancer Prevention and Control

The incidence and mortality of all cancers have changed substantially over time. The downward trend in the rates of cancer deaths in the United States is due in part to the prevention and detection of early-stage cancers. The identification of prostate-specific antigen (PSA) testing and a decrease in smoking prevalence between 1973

and 1997 resulted in a decrease in cancer deaths for men.[2] An increase in the rates of lung and breast cancer among women reflects the greater numbers of women who smoke and changes in reproductive trends (delayed childbearing)[69] and increased use of mammography.[19] Recognizing the role of health professionals in motivating clients to alter lifestyle behaviors, the National Cancer Institute (NCI) set an objective to have at least 75% of primary care providers routinely counsel clients about cessation of tobacco use, modifications of diet and exercise, and guidelines for screening.[62] These goals have been difficult to achieve from the outset, given that (1) 20% to 30% of Americans smoke; (2) 90% do not eat enough fruits, vegetables, and grains while

---

evolve Web Enhancements

Bridge to Home Health Care   Dealing with Grief Related to a New Cancer Diagnosis

Case Management   The Client with Cancer

Client Education Guide   Skin Care Within the Treatment Field (Spanish Translation)

Complementary and Alternative Therapy   Low-Residue Diet for Reducing the Complications of Pelvic Radiotherapy for Cancer

Ethical Issues in Nursing   Who Should Decide to Continue or End Cancer Treatment?

Who Should Be Screened for Cancer, and What Tests Should Be Used?

Boxes   Side Effects of Antineoplastic Drugs

Cancer-Related Resources

Classification of Chemotherapeutic Agents

Tables   Cancer Problems by Ethnic Groups

Performance Status Scales

Appendix A   Religious Beliefs and Practices Affecting Health Care

Be sure to check out the bonus material on the Evolve website and the CD-ROM, including free self-assessment exercises. **http://evolve.elsevier. com/Black/medsurg**

consuming too much fat; and (3) more than half have sedentary lifestyles.

Prevention, Screening, and Early Detection

The three interrelated activities involved in cancer prevention and control are prevention, screening, and early detection. Primary prevention involves measures to avoid or reduce exposure to carcinogens. Screening programs help to identify high-risk populations and individuals. Early detection involves diagnosing a precancerous lesion or a cancer at its earliest, most treatable stage.

Primary prevention activities are aimed at intervention before pathologic change has begun.[62] They help to reduce cancer risk through alteration of lifestyle behaviors that eliminate or reduce exposure to carcinogens. Many cancers are associated with smoking, poor dietary habits, and alcohol consumption.[58] All the cancers caused by tobacco and alcohol consumption could be avoided. Following a more healthful diet (see the Complementary and Alternative Therapy box at right), adapting to a more physically active lifestyle, limiting exposure to sun and other sources of ultraviolet radiation, modifying sexual practices, and decreasing exposure to environmental and occupational carcinogens would lead to further reduction in cancer incidence. Exposure to carcinogens can vary widely among population segments. In lower socioeconomic, medically underserved, and nonwhite segments of the population, the incidence of cancer is increased, and cancer is usually diagnosed at more advanced stages (see the website table Cancer Problems by Ethnic Groups).[60]

Secondary prevention,[62] also referred to as early detection, provides the opportunity to diagnose precancerous lesions or early-stage cancers before manifestations become readily apparent and provides for prompt treatment. Screening efforts facilitate early detection. Methods of early detection are (1) inspection, (2) palpation, and (3) the use of tests or procedures. Inspection is useful in identifying lesions of the skin, lip, mouth, larynx, external genitalia, and cervix. Lumps or nodules in the breast, mouth, salivary glands, thyroid, subcutaneous tissue, anus, rectum, prostate, testes, ovaries, and uterus as well as enlarged lymph nodes can be detected through palpation. Mammograms, Papanicolaou (Pap) smears, occult blood testing of feces, endoscopy, and radiologic imaging procedures are some of the tests or procedures that can be used. As a result of early detection, (1) premalignant lesions may be arrested, removed, or reversed; or (2) cancer treatment can be started earlier, often while the cancer is in a stage more amenable to treatment.

Screening identifies high-risk groups of people more likely to have cancer or precancerous lesions. (For current American Cancer Society [ACS][2,62] recommendations for screening, see the ACS WebLink on the website.) It is

---

COMPLEMENTARY AND ALTERNATIVE THERAPY

Mediterranean Diet and Cancer

Serra-Majem, Roman, and Estruch evaluated 43 articles that corresponded to 35 different experimental studies to determine if there was relationship between longevity of life/quality of life and the consumption of a Mediterranean diet. A Mediterranean diet is traditionally high in fruits and vegetables, legumes, nuts, cereal grains, and olive oil (monounsaturated fat); includes moderate amounts of fish, dairy (mostly cheese and yogurt), and alcohol; and is low in saturated fat. They reported that there was decreased cancer incidence among individuals who followed a Mediterranean diet, especially among those that were also considered obese. Favorable effects were also noted in lipoprotein levels, insulin resistance, and myocardial and cardiovascular mortality. Adherence to a traditional Mediterranean diet has been associated with a significant increase in longevity of life and quality of life.

This review supports the earlier findings of Trichopoulou and colleagues who reported that a traditional Mediterranean diet may reduce the risk of dying from cardiovascular disease and cancer. In this study, researchers evaluated 22,000 individuals 22 to 86 years of age in Greece. Participants were rated on how closely they followed a Mediterranean diet. After 4 years of study, the researchers found that the more closely individuals adhered to the diet, the lower their risk of death, including death from cardiovascular disease and cancer (about a 25% decrease for every 2-point increase on the scale). Thus a greater adherence to the traditional Mediterranean diet was associated with a significant reduction in total mortality.

REFERENCES

1. Serra-Majem, L., Roman, B., & Estruch, R. (2006). Scientific evidence of interventions using the Mediterranean Diet: A systematic review. *Nutrition Reviews*, S27-S47.
2. Trichopoulou, A., et al. (2003). Adherence to a Mediterranean diet and survival in a Greek population. *New England Journal of Medicine, 348,* 2599-2608.

---

estimated that 75% of all cancers in the United States could be cured if all available screening tests and self-examination methods were practiced routinely. Criteria for screening focus on the following:

- The population to be screened has a high incidence of the disease.
- The disease is detectable in its presymptomatic stage.
- Prognosis is poor if diagnosis is delayed until manifestations appear.
- An effective treatment is available for disease that is diagnosed early.
- There is an effective test for screening.
- The potential benefits of screening outweigh its potential risks and costs.

Approaches to Cancer Prevention

Three main approaches to cancer prevention are (1) education, (2) regulation, and (3) host modification.[62] A client's health beliefs can be vital determinants of learning readiness when information is made available.

The beliefs that influence the effectiveness of education consist of the client's perception of susceptibility to developing cancer, beliefs about the harmful or beneficial consequences of lifestyle behaviors, and perceptions about the benefits of prevention and early detection.

Methods of regulation used in the United States include prohibiting the sale of tobacco and alcohol to minors, limiting smoking in public places, imposing excise taxes, regulating the use of manufactured carcinogens such as asbestos, and prohibiting carcinogens in foods.

Host modification aims to alter the body's internal environment to decrease the risk of cancer or to reverse a carcinogenic process. Clinical trials of possible vaccines to immunize against some cancers, including melanoma, kidney cancer, colon cancer, cervical cancer, and pancreatic cancer, have begun. Yet another avenue for host modification being studied in clinical trials is chemoprevention. This process involves the use of non-cytotoxic (non–cell-destroying) nutrients, pharmacologic agents, or both to prevent or reverse carcinogenesis. Individuals who use chemopreventive agents or who participate in studies of potential chemopreventive agents must be willing to accept the side effects and adverse risks of the agents.[25]

Prevention and Early Detection of Common Cancers

Breast Cancer

Breast cancer is the most commonly diagnosed cancer in American women, second only to lung cancer for cancer mortality. Risk factors (early menarche, late menopause, or being either nulliparous or older than 30 years at the birth of a first child) relate to their effect on circulating hormones. Incidence increases with age; more than 77% of women diagnosed with breast cancer are older than 50 years of age at diagnosis. Onset and progression of breast cancer appear to be intimately, but not exclusively, tied to genetic alterations.[22] While significant progress has been made in the identification of inherited defects in the somatic genes responsible for hereditary and familiar breast cancer syndromes, in aggregate, it is estimated that 5% to 10% of breast cancer cases occur in families with significant inherited risk. The "two-hit" hypothesis—genetic alteration and mutation—has been used to explain this phenomenon. Many women diagnosed with breast cancer have no known risk factors.

Breast cancer mortality could be reduced by 30% through early detection using routine screening mammography alone or together with an annual clinical breast examination by a primary health care provider beginning between 40 and 50 years of age. The ACS also recommends that women perform monthly breast self-examination (BSE) beginning at 20 years of age. There are insufficient data to determine the role of BSE in decreasing mortality; however, clients who perform BSE generally present with smaller tumors.[2,62] Previous studies have shown tamoxifen to be an effective chemopreventive for breast cancer. STAR (Study of Tamoxifen and Raloxifene), a national study conducted by the National Surgical Adjuvant Breast and Bowel Project (NSABP) and supported by the NCI, is currently being conducted for postmenopausal women at high risk for breast cancer. The study is comparing the effectiveness of the osteoporosis drug raloxifene with tamoxifen as a chemopreventive.

Lung Cancer

One in two Americans who continue to smoke will ultimately die as a result of their cigarette addiction.[2] Lung cancer is the most commonly occurring cancer and the leading cause of cancer deaths worldwide.[2] The global rise in lung cancer, together with the fact that the overall 5-year survival is less than 15%, describes the magnitude of this disease. More than 80% of lung cancers are directly attributed to tobacco abuse. Other risk factors are tuberculosis (scar tumor), asbestos exposure, exposure to radiation, and air pollution. The American Society of Clinical Oncology has published steps to curb global tobacco use. These include counseling clients not to smoke, which will have the greatest effect on decreasing the rate of lung cancer. A healthy diet with at least five servings of fruits and vegetables is an added preventive step.[3] Previous clinical trials have not found chemopreventives effective in preventing lung cancer. Spiral computed tomography (CT) scanning is being investigated for use in mass screening for lung cancer in high-risk groups. The National Lung Screening Trial, initiated in 2002, will enroll 50,000 current or former smokers.[62]

Colorectal Cancer

Colorectal cancer accounts for nearly 11% of cancer mortality in the United States, with the incidence slightly higher in men. Age impacts the incidence of colorectal cancer more than any other demographic, with incidence rates dramatically increasing above the age of 50 years.[37] Risk factors include familial polyposis, familial nonpolyposis syndromes, cancer family syndrome, hereditary site-specific colon cancer, and ulcerative colitis. The incidence of colorectal cancer increases with age after 50 years. Alcohol consumption, smoking, and a sedentary lifestyle are also contributing risk factors. A weaker risk factor associated with colorectal cancer may be a high-fat, low-fiber diet. There is no known prevention, although a healthy diet (high fiber, low fat, vitamins C and E, calcium, and folic acid) and a physically active lifestyle may be of benefit. Research suggests that some pharmaceutical agents such as cyclooxygenase-2 (COX-2) inhibitors and aspirin may provide some protection.[36] Emerging technologies such as CT "virtual colonoscopies" and immunochemical fecal occult blood testing are being investigated. To date evidence is insufficient to recommend such technologies for routine screening.

Early detection through routine screening is the key to decreasing mortality. In fact, the increased use of colonoscopy with polypectomy is the prime reason for the 20% improved survival rate since 1985.[33] The ACS recommends that people with an average risk for colon cancer be screened annually with digital rectal examinations and fecal occult blood tests beginning at 40 years of age, and with sigmoidoscopy every 3 to 5 years beginning at 50 years of age. For people with a high risk for colon cancer, the ACS recommends discussing the frequency of monitoring with their physician.[38]

Prostate Cancer

Age is the greatest risk factor for prostate cancer with the median age at diagnosis currently 70 years. The incidence of being diagnosed with prostate cancer increases with each decade of life, beginning at age 50. African-American men have the highest incidence of prostate cancer in the world. Another risk factor is family history, with almost 25% of men with prostate cancer also having two first-degree relatives with the disease. An occupationally related risk factor is exposure to cadmium. Prevention strategies include limiting exposure of workers handling cadmium batteries and keeping the intake of dietary fat low.

The ACS recommends that men at age 50 years and high-risk clients at age 40 years begin receiving a digital rectal examination as part of their annual physical examination in addition to a prostate-specific antigen (PSA) blood test. The role of PSA findings in early detection is still being debated. Early-stage prostate cancer is more amenable to treatment; however, the controversy centers on whether the PSA result leads to the diagnosis and treatment of prostate cancers that would never progress if not detected. The ACS has updated their guidelines on prostate screening to recommend men be informed of the benefits and limitations of screening.[2] A clinical trial sponsored by the NCI is currently investigating the benefits of selenium or vitamin E supplements as chemoprotection for prostate cancer.[44] In 2004 a docetaxel-based chemotherapy program was shown to prolong the lives of prostate cancer clients whose disease had progressed while receiving hormonal therapy.[57]

Cervical Cancer

Among women between the ages of 20 and 39 years, cervical cancer is the second leading cause of cancer in the United States and the leading cause of cancer deaths among women in medically underserved countries.[23] Risk factors for cervical cancer are closely linked to sexual behavior and sexually transmitted infections. First intercourse at an early age, multiple sexual partners, or a sexual partner who has had multiple sexual partners put a woman at increased risk. The human papillomavirus and acquired immunodeficiency syndrome (AIDS) are also risk factors, as are low socioeconomic status and cigarette smoking. Changing sexual behavior, avoiding tobacco use, and undergoing routine screening are actions the client can take to avoid cervical cancer.

There is a correlation between the presence of the human papillomavirus (HPV) and invasive carcinoma of the cervix. Gardasil, a vaccine that works by building immunity against the sexually transmitted human papillomavirus (HPV) strains 16 and 18, which cause 70% of all cervical cancers, was approved by the FDA in June 2006. The development and availability of additional vaccines to prevent this disease and provide immunity to additional strains of HPV are underway.[20]

The Pap smear detects cancer in a premalignant stage, when it is very amenable to treatment. With adequate screening, cervical cancer should not exist; however, cultural and social barriers to prevention and early detection of this disease persist.[2] The ACS has updated their guidelines for the early detection of cervical cancer. They now recommend that cervical cancer screening begin 3 years after the onset of vaginal intercourse but no later than age 21. The harm in beginning screening earlier is from inappropriate interventions because of overdiagnosis of cervical lesions that would have regressed spontaneously. After the age of 30, women who have had two normal tests can be screened every 2 to 3 years.[56]

Head and Neck Cancer

Approximately 66% of all new cases of head and neck cancer occur in men, with the median age at diagnosis 40 years.[40] A synergistic effect of alcohol and tobacco use increases the risk for cancer of the head and neck. Poor oral hygiene, long-term sun exposure, and occupational exposures (asbestos, tar, nickel, textile, wood or leather work, and machine tool operation) are additional risk factors. Individuals from Southern China are also at greater risk. All clients who smoke or combine smoking with drinking alcohol should be counseled to stop these behaviors. Retinoids have been used as a chemopreventive. The evidence does not support the value of routine screening programs, although early detection by dentists and dental hygienists can identify precancerous lesions.[2] The management of the primary site of the cancer determines the treatment plan. Clients in poor nutritional states may require a feeding gastrostomy before initiating any therapy.

Skin Cancer

While one in five Americans will develop skin cancer during their lifetime, more than 97% of these lesions will be non-melanoma skin cancer (NMSC). NMSC has a low mortality, yet is occurring in epidemic proportions. The rising incidence of NMSC is thought to be due to an increase in outdoor activities, changes in clothing styles, increased longevity, and ozone depletion. Health care costs associated with NMSC are estimated at 600 million dollars annually.[21]

The incidence of the most serious form of skin cancer, melanoma, has been increasing by about 4% each year since 1973. Individuals with a fair complexion, a family history, multiple or atypical nevi (moles), and occupational exposure to coal tar, pitch, creosote, arsenic, or radium are at greater risk. Prevention involves avoiding ultraviolet radiation as well as limiting midday sun exposure, wearing a hat or clothing to protect the skin, using sunscreen with a sun protective factor (SPF) of 15 or higher, and avoiding severe sunburns, especially in childhood.

Early detection, especially for melanomas, is critical. Annually about 38,000 melanomas are detected at a curable in situ stage. Screening programs should include teaching clients how to inspect their own skin. Moles can be mapped as a baseline for future inspections. Basal and squamous cell skin cancer frequently appears as a pale, wax-like, pearly nodule or a red, scaly patch. Note should be made of any changes, such as new moles or a sore that repeatedly scabs over but fails to heal. Moles that are asymmetrical, that have irregular borders or uneven variations in color, or that change in diameter or height should be checked by a physician. A change in the color, surface appearance, or sensation of a mole should also be reported. Clients should be taught the importance of regular self-inspection and of seeking medical attention.[2]

HEALTH RESTORATION

Maintaining Wellness During Treatment

For the client diagnosed with cancer, tertiary prevention consists of limitation of disability and rehabilitation. For the client undergoing any cancer treatment, maintaining optimum wellness is important for both treatment outcome and quality of life. The nurse's role in caring for clients undergoing cancer treatment to maintain optimum wellness is addressed in the later discussion of outcome management during cancer treatments.

Rehabilitation

In addition to disease treatment, rehabilitation therapy is often important to the client's quality of life. Rehabilitation may consist of reconstructive surgery after breast cancer or surgery to reverse a temporary colostomy after colon cancer treatment. An important opportunity for rehabilitation may be an exercise program to help a client counteract chemotherapy-related fatigue.

A client whose treatment has resulted in lymphedema may experience an improved quality of life after a rehabilitation referral for lymphedema management. Clinicians often think of lymphedema management as benefiting only clients with breast cancer; however, professionals may overlook the possible secondary effect of lower-extremity lymphedema after treatment for prostate cancer. Treatment for other cancers that affect the lymph nodes, such as surgery for melanoma or metastatic colon cancer, may also result in lymphedema. Additional rehabilitation strategies, such as speech therapy and prosthetic devices, are described in various chapters of this book in the discussions of specific disorders.

OUTCOME MANAGEMENT

Diagnosis of Cancer

Accurate diagnosis is paramount to effective cancer treatment. The first step in the diagnostic process is obtaining a complete history and physical examination. These data, together with diagnostic tests, can be highly predictive of a cancer diagnosis. Careful attention to a client's history and physical status will result in accurate nursing diagnoses and interventions.

Obtain History

Because some cancers are known to be linked with certain genetic and environmental factors, the health history should include the presence of cancer among the client's blood relatives, the client's work history, and environmental factors associated with cancer causation. (See Chapter 2 for a discussion of health history and physical assessment. Genetic history taking is discussed in Chapter 15.) You should also determine if the client has previous life experiences with cancer—whether it was the experience of a blood relative, the client's own history, or a friend's experience. This information will be useful in assessing the client's previous knowledge, the client's perceptions about cancer, and the readiness for teaching.

Assess Clinical Manifestations

When cancer is in its early stages, clinical manifestations are few. Clinical manifestations usually appear once the cancer has grown sufficiently large to cause one or more of the following problems:

- Pressure on surrounding organs or nerves
- Distortion of surrounding tissue
- Obstruction of the lumina of vessels, intestines, and/or ureters
- Interference with the blood supply of surrounding tissues
- Interference with organ function
- Disturbance of body metabolism
- Parasitic use of the body's nutritional supplies
- Mobilization of the body's defensive response

A localized tumor usually produces manifestations related to increased pressure or obstruction in a single region. Metastatic disease and extensive tumors of major organs may display a variety of local and systemic manifestations.

Common clinical manifestations associated with cancer include weight loss, weakness or fatigue, central nervous system (CNS) alterations, pain, and hematologic and metabolic alterations. Anorexia, weight loss, weakness, and fatigue are related to the body's inability to consume and use nutrients appropriately. Mechanical interference by tumors, malabsorption, paraneoplastic endocrine secretions (such as excessive secretion of thyroid hormones), and a tumor's use of nutrients may all contribute to a process that must be interrupted to avoid general physical debility. The client who has difficulty with vision, speech, coordination, or memory may be experiencing primary or metastatic CNS disease. Increased intracranial pressure caused by tumor growth may cause headache, lethargy, nausea, and vomiting.

Although pain is not a common manifestation of early-stage cancer, it may occur during the course of the disease as a result of obstruction or destruction of a vital organ, pressure on sensitive tissues or bone, or involvement of nerves. Pain that is not adequately treated may become chronic and increasingly severe. Bone cancer is particularly painful because the rigidity of bone allows little or no expansion as the tumor cells proliferate. This pain worsens when pathologic fractures produce instability and muscle spasms. Even though pain is usually a late manifestation in cancer, it may be the manifestation that brings the client to a health care provider.

Complete Diagnostic Evaluation

In addition to the history and physical assessment, laboratory and imaging studies are useful in the detection of cancer, as explained in the Integrating Diagnostic Studies box above, right. Many diagnostic laboratory and imaging studies used to detect other diseases are used to detect cancer.

INTEGRATING DIAGNOSTIC TESTING

Laboratory and Imaging Studies Used to Diagnose Cancer

A variety of blood tests can help diagnose cancer. Some of the more routine tests, such as the complete blood count (CBC) and differential count, do not test specifically for cancer but indicate the presence of nonspecific problems. These tests are also used to monitor the treatment side effects. Other blood tests, such as tumor marker measurements and biochemical tests, identify the extent of a particular type of cancer. Tumor markers such as PSA can be indicators of cancer, and tumor markers are often used as "barometers" detecting the effectiveness of treatment. Unexplained anemia often indicates a malignancy.

Hematologic changes include leukopenia, leukocytosis, and bleeding disorders, which in some cancers may occur before local manifestations. Metabolic manifestations, such as Cushing's syndrome, hypercalcemia, syndrome of inappropriate antidiuretic hormone (SIADH) secretion, and carcinoid syndrome, also increase the possibility of cancer.

Basic x-rays, computerized tomography (CT), magnetic resonance imaging (MRI), positron emission tomography (PET), ultrasound, and other imaging studies are used in the diagnosis of cancer. When measurable amounts of tumor remain after surgery, imaging studies are repeated at regular intervals and used to evaluate the effectiveness of chemotherapy or radiation therapy.

Grading and Staging of Cancer

Microscopic evidence of malignant cells from the tumor tissue is the only definitive evidence of cancer. When a neoplastic growth is definitely diagnosed, it must be further defined in terms of its degree of malignancy (grade) and extent (stage). After tissue has been obtained through a biopsy or the surgical removal of tumor, it is sent to the pathologist for microscopic examination. The pathologist prepares a section of the tissue to examine the specimen. The tumor grade is an evaluation of the extent to which tumor cells differ from their normal precursors. In low numerical grades, grades 1 and 2, the cells are well differentiated and deviate minimally from normal cells. High grades, grades 3 and 4, refer to cells that are poorly differentiated and the most aberrant compared with normal cells. Tumor grading involves a histologic and anatomic description of the cancer. The pathologist also evaluates the biopsy specimen for other characteristics that help identify the cell type of the malignancy or provide important indicators of prognosis.

Once the diagnosis has been made and the microscopic cell type and grade of the tumor have been determined, the extent of spread (staging) of the tumor also needs to be identified. Cancer staging determines the extent of disease and is used in treatment decision making. Staging involves a systematic search for the characteristics of the primary tumor (T), involvement of lymph nodes (N), and evidence of metastasis (M), on the basis of knowledge of the natural history of the disease. The TNM system is the primary accepted system for cancer staging today (Table 17-1).

Clinical staging is based on evidence acquired before treatment and is obtained by physical examination, imaging, endoscopy, biopsy, laboratory tests, surgical exploration, and other diagnostic tests. Pathologic staging is based on the microscopic evidence acquired before treatment, which is supplemented or modified by information obtained at surgery and from the pathologic examination of resected specimens, including the primary tumor, regional lymph nodes, and metastatic nodules.

Using the TNM classification, cancers can be grouped into one of four stages (I to IV) or indicated as stage 0 for carcinoma in situ (without spread). Higher stages signify more extensive disease, with stage IV representative of distant metastasis and the worst prognosis.

Other established classifications may be used for particular malignancies, such as Clark's classification for malignant melanomas and Dukes' classification for colorectal cancer. Clark's classification considers the level of invasion of melanomas, and Dukes' system refers to the depth of invasion of colorectal cancer.

Identifying Treatment Goals

The major objective of cancer therapy is to treat the client effectively with appropriate therapy for a sufficient duration so that a cure (or control) of the cancer results with minimal functional and structural impairment. Cure is a controversial word because of the chronic nature of most cancers; for this reason, many health care providers prefer the term control. If a cure is not possible, the following are important alternative goals:

- Control of the cancer by slowing disease progression
- Palliation, or alleviation of manifestations
- Rehabilitation to maintain quality of life

Decisions made at the time of first diagnosis are crucial because early aggressive intervention usually offers the best hope of cure. Even when cure is not possible, many clients with cancer have benefited from an extended life span with a good quality of life as a result of cancer treatment.

Determining Treatment Modalities

Methods of treating clients with cancer are surgery, radiation therapy, chemotherapy, biotherapy, and bone marrow transplantation (BMT). The treatment method depends on the type of tumor, the extent of disease, the client's co-morbid conditions (such as cardiac disease), performance status, and treatment desires.

Performance status is a way of evaluating a client's overall health status and ability to tolerate treatment. A performance scale will provide quantitative data and may be used to monitor a client's response to treatment. See the table Performance Status Scales on the website for a description of two common status scales. In most cases, cancer treatment combines a variety of methods rather than a single therapy. This approach is called combined modality or multimodal therapy. Combined modality therapy is more effective in destroying cancerous cells.

TREATMENT MODALITIES

Surgery

Surgery has a major role in the diagnosis, staging, and treatment of cancer. It is also an integral part of the rehabilitation and palliation for clients with cancer. Surgery is used less frequently as a method of cancer prevention.

Although many aspects of surgical care of the client with cancer are similar to those for all clients undergoing surgery for any reason (see Chapter 14), some differences do exist. In addition to providing expert physical care, it is important that, preoperatively, you evaluate the client's understanding of the proposed procedure and the physical change that will occur. The emotional impact of the diagnosis may affect the client's expectations, coping, and ability to learn. Preoperatively, clients with cancer may be nutritionally compromised and may require nutritional therapy. Those who have undergone adjuvant (treatment after removal of all detected cancer) or palliative (comfort care) chemotherapy or radiation therapy may have low red blood cell (RBC) or white blood cell (WBC) counts, which need to be corrected before surgery.

TABLE 17-1	TNM Staging System
Stage	**Characteristics**
	Primary Tumor (T)
TX	No primary tumor can be assessed
T0	No evidence of primary tumor
Tis	Carcinoma in situ
T1, T2, T3, T4	Increasing size and extent of primary tumor
	Regional Lymph Nodes (N)
NX	Cannot be assessed
N0	No regional lymph node involvement
N1, N2, N3	Increasing involvement of regional lymph nodes
	Distant Metastasis (M)
MX	Presence of metastasis cannot be assessed
M0	No distant metastasis
M1	Distant metastasis

From Sloan, J., et al. (2005). Mapping the journey of cancer patients through the health care system. Part 3: An approach to staging. *Canadian Oncology Nursing Journal, 15*(1), 4-8.

Diagnostic Surgery

While the diagnosis of cancer is established only by microscopic identification of malignant cells from tumor tissue, a variety of surgical procedures are used to obtain tissue. The biology of the tumor, its size and location, and the proposed method of treatment determine which surgical method should be used.

Cytologic specimen collection and needle biopsy are relatively simple procedures. A negative biopsy result does not prove the absence of cancer but rather might indicate inadequate or misplaced tissue sampling. Negative needle biopsy results generally must be followed by additional specimen collections to obtain an accurate diagnosis.

Cytologic Specimens. Cytologic specimens can be obtained from tumors that tend to shed cells from their surface. Tumor cells can often be obtained from cytologic examination of fluids aspirated from effusions or ascitic fluid. Cytologic brushings or tissue biopsy specimens may be collected while using an endoscope to examine a questionable area. An endoscopy involves direct visualization of the gastrointestinal (GI) tract, bronchoscopy of the lungs, laryngoscopy of the larynx, colposcopy of the cervix and vagina, cystoscopy of the bladder, or laparoscopy of the pelvic or abdominal cavity. During these tests, areas of concern can be examined, tissue samples and aspirates taken for biopsy, the extent of the disease staged, and pathologic processes excised.

Needle Biopsy. Needle biopsy is a simple method of obtaining tissue samples. In a fine-needle aspiration, tumor cells are withdrawn from the tumor with a needle and syringe. A core-needle biopsy is essentially the same procedure; however, the needle is larger, and a core or barrel of tissue is obtained. Core-needle biopsy allows the pathologist to examine the cells with their spatial relationships intact, whereas fine-needle aspiration provides individual cells or clumps of cells for review.

Excisional Biopsy and Incisional Biopsy. The size of the tumor and the purpose of the biopsy determine if an excisional or incisional biopsy is performed. If the suspected tumor is small, the entire tumor is excised for examination; this is called a total or excisional type of biopsy. It is used for small tumors (2 to 3 cm) for which the biopsy also may serve as the treatment if the tissue margins contain no tumor cells. If tumor cells remain, a wider excision is required.

If the tumor is large, only a part of the neoplasm is excised. This procedure is termed a subtotal or incisional type of biopsy. Stereotactic breast biopsy is a radiography-guided method for localizing and sampling small, nonpalpable breast lesions that are discovered on mammography when malignancy is suspected.

Surgery as Treatment

Surgery is performed in 55% of clients with cancer. Of the clients with cancer who undergo surgery, 40% are treated with surgery alone. Cancers that are localized to the organ of origin and the regional lymph nodes are potentially curable by surgery, although multimodal treatment is more likely to be used to control any submicroscopic spread.

Historically, the generally accepted concept of tumor growth was an orderly sequence of growth from the organ of origin to adjacent tissue, regional lymph nodes, and eventually distant sites in a systematic fashion. The logical surgical approach to this type of growth was the widest excision possible of the tumor, surrounding tissue, and regional lymph nodes. Thus radical surgery became the standard for cancer treatment. Analysis of treatment results, however, demonstrated that, despite radical excisions, tumors recurred. Current concepts of tumor biology hold that tumors probably shed cells into the systemic circulation throughout their growth and therefore local therapies (surgery and radiation) generally must be combined with systemic therapies (biotherapy and chemotherapy) to improve client survival.

When surgery is performed with curative intent, the type of tumor determines the extent of the excision. For slow-growing tumors, such as squamous cell carcinoma and adenocarcinoma of the skin, a wide local excision may be sufficient. Tumors of the colon and breast that spread to the regional lymph nodes are removed with an en bloc excision of the tumor and regional lymph nodes. Sentinel node mapping for breast cancer is discussed in Chapter 40 (the procedure is also used for melanoma). Large tumors, such as sarcomas, which tend to spread locally without metastasis, are removed with radical excisions, such as amputations. In all surgical procedures, various operative techniques, such as glove changing, instrument cleaning, and wound irrigation with cytotoxic agents, are used to prevent dissemination of tumor cells into and beyond the operative field.

Surgery for Recurrence and Metastasis

Cancer that recurs locally can be resected, resulting in occasional cure, remission, or both. Local recurrences of sarcomas as well as colon, breast, and skin cancers have been successfully excised. Solitary metastatic lesions that appear in the lungs, liver, or brain can sometimes be removed and obtain surgical cure. Excision of metastatic lesions is considered if (1) no other evidence of disease exists and (2) the metastatic lesion has appeared after a relatively long disease-free interval. The metastatic lesion must exhibit some stability and must be refractory (unresponsive) to chemotherapy and XRT. Metastatic renal cell carcinomas, sarcomas, melanomas, and colon carcinomas have been removed in selected clients, resulting in cures or prolonged survival intervals.

Palliative Surgery

Because surgical procedures carry an inherent potential for morbidity, the use of surgery in palliative care is carefully considered and used only if the risk-benefit ratio is favorable. Palliative surgery that benefits the client with cancer and improves quality of life includes procedures that (1) reduce pain by such means as interrupting nerve pathways or implanting pain-control pumps, (2) relieve airway obstructions, (3) relieve obstructions in the GI and urinary tracts, (4) relieve pressure on the brain or spinal cord, (5) prevent hemorrhage, (6) remove infected and ulcerating tumors, and (7) drain abscesses.

Reconstructive Surgery

Advances in reconstructive surgery offer a different perspective on rehabilitation to the client who has experienced curative surgery. Restoration of form and function is possible to varying degrees, depending on the site and extent of surgery. Reconstructive surgery may be performed concurrently with the radical procedure, or it may be delayed. The major goal of reconstructive surgery is to improve the client's quality of life by restoring maximal function and appearance.

Preventive Surgery

The client at unusually high risk for cancer may elect to undergo a preventive (prophylactic) surgical intervention. Certain conditions or diseases increase the risk of cancer occurrence so significantly that removal of the target organ is justified to prevent cancer development. Clients with familial polyposis, for example, have a 50% risk of having colon cancer by age 40 years. By the time they are 70 years old, all clients with this inherited trait have colon cancer. Clients with ulcerative colitis also have a greater risk for colon cancer. Prophylactic subtotal colectomies may be indicated for these individuals.

Clients with multiple high-risk factors may consider preventive surgery. Prophylactic mastectomy (breast removal) and oophorectomy (ovary removal) are controversial preventive therapies. The advent of genetic testing has added further complexity to the controversy. The decision to have genetic testing can have far-reaching psychological implications for the client and other family members. Women with BRCA1 and BRCA2 mutations need to be counseled on the strengths and limitations of risk assessment in predicting their own likelihood of developing breast cancer.[55]

Nursing Management of the Surgical Client

Surgery for cancer tends to be more complex than similar procedures for benign conditions. This results in the potential for more complications. While most of the postoperative care (such as wound care and prevention of infection) is similar among all clients having the same surgical procedure, the difference for the cancer client lies in what follows. With a benign condition, although there is certainly a period of healing and perhaps rehabilitation, the surgery usually concludes the active treatment.

With cancer surgery, however, the client often has begun only one phase of multimodal treatment. Surgery is not always the first phase of treatment because many treatment protocols begin with chemotherapy or XRT to shrink the tumor mass and decrease the likelihood of micrometastasis. In the midst of the emotional impact of the diagnosis, the client and family are confronted with an often overwhelming amount of information about the diagnosis, necessary tests, treatment alternatives, and decisions to be made. The client will probably be seen or treated in multiple health care settings by many different health professionals. To help the client manage outcomes effectively, the nurse must not only provide excellent care during the hospitalization but also proactively assist the client with continuing care. The value of home nursing care for cancer clients is well documented. Hughes and colleagues found that home care nurses use a variety of interventions, especially teaching, to respond to complex problems for older postsurgical cancer clients.[32]

Assess Discharge Needs

Questions you can ask as a guide to discharge planning are as follows:

- What does the client need to know and what does the client need to be able to do?
- Does the client know how to get to the medical oncologist's office or clinic?
- Will the client need assistance with transportation, such as an ACS "Road to Recovery" volunteer driver?
- Would the client benefit from initial information about chemotherapy or from talking with someone who has "been there"?
- Would the client benefit from a referral for home health nursing?
- If the client or family members have questions you cannot answer, is there a social worker, oncology nursing colleague, or chaplain who can provide assistance?

See the Case Management feature on The Client with Cancer on the website. No one person or profession can meet all the needs of the client with cancer and his or her family. Managing outcomes effectively requires teamwork involving the client, the family, the nurse, and other health professionals.

Radiation Therapy

More than 60% of all clients with cancer receive XRT at some point during the course of their disease. XRT may be used as a primary, an adjuvant, or a palliative treatment. When XRT is used as a primary modality, it is the only treatment used and aims to achieve local cure of the cancer (e.g., early-stage Hodgkin's disease, skin cancer, prostate cancer, carcinoma of the cervix). For clients with laryngeal cancer, the potential for cure with XRT is equal to the cure rate with surgery, eliminating the need to remove the client's larynx.

As an adjuvant treatment, XRT is used either preoperatively or postoperatively to aid in the destruction of cancer cells (e.g., colorectal cancer, early breast cancer). In addition, XRT can be used in conjunction with chemotherapy to treat disease in sites not readily accessible to systemic chemotherapy, such as the brain. In some situations, chemotherapy is used as a radiosensitizer. It is combined with XRT and is administered before XRT in an attempt to enhance the effects of XRT.

As a palliative treatment, XRT can be used to reduce pain associated with obstruction, pathologic fractures, spinal cord compression, and metastasis. When the cancer is widespread, XRT is not appropriate, for too much normal tissue would be harmed. XRT may be used to destroy tumor in a localized area to relieve a distressing manifestation. A few radiation treatments can be quite effective in relieving pain from a metastatic bone lesion.

How Radiation Therapy Works

Radiosensitivity, or the relative susceptibility of tissues to radiation, depends on the individual cells and the characteristics of the tissue itself. A highly radiosensitive tumor is greatly affected by radiation because it divides rapidly, is well vascularized, and has high oxygen content.

Radiation therapy is the use of high-energy ionizing radiation to treat a variety of cancers. Ionizing radiation destroys a cell's ability to reproduce by damaging its DNA, delaying mitosis to repair DNA, or inducing apoptosis. Rapidly dividing cells are more vulnerable to radiation than more slowly dividing cells. Normal cells have a greater ability than cancer cells to repair sublethal DNA damage from radiation. Therefore the radiation oncologist may deliver a sufficient dose of radiation to kill the cancer cells while sparing normal cells from excessive cell death.

In addition to the DNA effects, a complex chain of chemical reactions occurs in the extracellular fluid, resulting in the formation of free radicals. Well-oxygenated tumors show a much greater response to radiation than poorly oxygenated tumors. Oxygen free radicals formed during ionization interact readily with nearby molecules, causing cellular damage. A well-vascularized tumor may therefore be more responsive to XRT than the same type of tumor if it is larger and, as a result, more poorly vascularized.

Types of Radiation Therapy

Radiation therapy can be administered by a variety of methods. The XRT may be delivered as external-beam therapy or via a radiation source placed close to the surface of the body or inside the body. Advances in radiation therapy include (1) increased knowledge of radiation physics, (2) the use of computers making three-dimensional treatment planning possible, (3) enhancements of treatment machines to allow more precise conformal therapy of the tumor with less effect on adjacent normal tissue, and (4) the use of stereotactic radioneurosurgery.

External-Beam Radiation Therapy. External-beam XRT, or teletherapy, is the delivery of radiation from a source placed at some distance from the target site. It is administered in the XRT department by high-energy x-ray or gamma-ray machines (e.g., linear accelerator, cobalt, betatron, or a machine containing a radioisotope). The major advantage of high-energy radiation is its skin-sparing effect; that is, the maximum effect of radiation occurs at tumor depth in the body and not on the skin surface. Neutron-beam therapy delivered from a cyclotron particle accelerator is currently used to treat many types of cancers, including salivary gland tumors, sarcomas, and tumors of the prostate and lung. Therapists do not remain in the room with the client during the treatment; rather, they monitor the client via closed-circuit television and remain in voice contact via an intercom.

Internal Radiation Therapy. Internal XRT involves placement of specifically prepared radioisotopes (radioactive isotopes) directly into or near the tumor itself (brachytherapy) or into the systemic circulation. The two major types of internal XRT are (1) sealed-source XRT, in which the radioactive material is enclosed in a sealed container; and (2) unsealed-source XRT, in which the radioactive material is administered systemically, such as by injection or orally.

Sealed-Source Radiation Therapy. Sealed-source XRT is used for both intracavity and interstitial therapy. In intracavity therapy, the radioisotope, usually cesium-137 or radium-226, is put in an applicator, which is then placed in the body cavity for a carefully calculated time, generally 24 to 72 hours. Intracavity XRT is used to treat cancers of the uterus and cervix.

In interstitial therapy, the radioisotope of choice (e.g., iridium-192, iodine-125, cesium-137, gold-198, or radon-222) is placed in needles, beads, seeds, ribbons, or catheters, which are then implanted directly into the tumor. Clients with prostate or breast cancer may receive implanted seeds as therapy. These implants may be left in the tumor either temporarily (when ribbons, needles, or catheters are used) or permanently (when prostatic seeds are used), depending on the half-life of the isotope.

With sealed sources of internal radiation, the radioisotope is completely enclosed by nonradioactive material. Thus the radioisotope cannot circulate through the client's body, nor can it contaminate the client's urine, sweat, blood, or vomitus. Consequently, the client's excretions are not radioactive. Radiation exposure can result from direct contact with the sealed radioisotope, however, such as touching the container with bare hands or from lengthy exposure to the sealed radioisotope.

Afterloading devices have been developed in which a hollow applicator (the product that holds the radiation source) is placed during an operative procedure, and the radioactive source is not loaded until the client returns to the hospital room or the radiation treatment department. The technique of remote afterloading may be used to deliver frequent, short-term, high doses of radiation directly to a selected tumor. The radioactive source is inserted into the applicator and left in place for a specific time afterward. After treatment, the radioactive source is removed, but the applicator is left in place if more than one treatment is planned. The client is returned to the hospital room until the next treatment. When brachytherapy is used in the hospital room, the radioactive source can be returned to the brachytherapy device while you are in the client's room providing care. Thus the use of afterloading devices has helped to decrease radiation exposure for staff but lengthens the total time needed to deliver the dose for the client.

Unsealed-Source Radiation Therapy. Unsealed sources of internal radiation are used in systemic therapy. Unsealed sources used for internal XRT are colloid suspensions that come into direct contact with body tissues. The radioisotopes can be administered intravenously, orally, or by instillation directly into a body cavity. Iodine-131 is given orally in very low doses to treat Graves' disease (see Chapter 43) or in high doses to treat thyroid cancer. Strontium chloride 89 (Metastron) is administered intravenously for relief of painful bony metastases.

SAFETY ALERT

With unsealed sources of internal radiation, the radioisotope circulates through the client's body. Therefore the client's urine, sweat, blood, and vomitus contain the radioactive isotope.

Radiation Safety Standards

Three key principles you should follow to protect yourself and others from excessive radiation exposure are (1) distance, (2) time, and (3) shielding.

The greater the distance from the radiation source, the less the exposure dose of ionizing rays. Distance and radiation exposure are inversely related. Thus the intensity of radiation decreases inversely with the square of the distance from the source. For example, if you stand 4 feet from a source of radiation, you are exposed to about one fourth the amount of radiation you would

receive at 2 feet (Figure 17-1). When providing care to a client with a uterine implant, you will receive less radiation exposure if you stand at the head of the client's bed rather than directly beside the client.

You should aim to minimize the amount of time you are exposed to the radiation source, although you must still meet the client's care needs.

Your exposure time should generally be limited to 30 minutes of direct care per 8-hour shift. You need to plan your time in the client's room so you can spend it efficiently while providing care to the client. Time required to organize supplies should be spent outside the room. Care for the client should be rotated among available nursing staff to limit exposure for each employee. Pregnant nurses should not be assigned to care for clients receiving XRT. SAFETY ALERT

The use of shielding devices whenever possible reduces radiation exposure. The dose of x-rays and gamma-rays is reduced as the thickness of the lead shield is increased. In practice, nurses have found that working with lead shielding is cumbersome. When shielding is not feasible, you should maintain maximum distance from the radioactive source and limit the duration of exposure.

With sealed-source internal radioactive implants, clients require a private room and bath because of the risk of implant dislodgment and consequent exposure of other people to the radiation. Rooms at the ends of halls or stairwells may be designated for use by such clients because their location lessens the chance that others will be exposed to the radiation. Institutions with a high volume of radiation implants may have specially designed rooms with lead-shielded walls. Shields, a lead container called a pig, and a pair of long-handled forceps should always be present in the client's room.

If the radiation source becomes dislodged, forceps are used to pick it up and place it immediately in the pig. Generally, the radiation therapist and the radiation safety officer are notified immediately of the situation. They retrieve and secure the radiation source. SAFETY

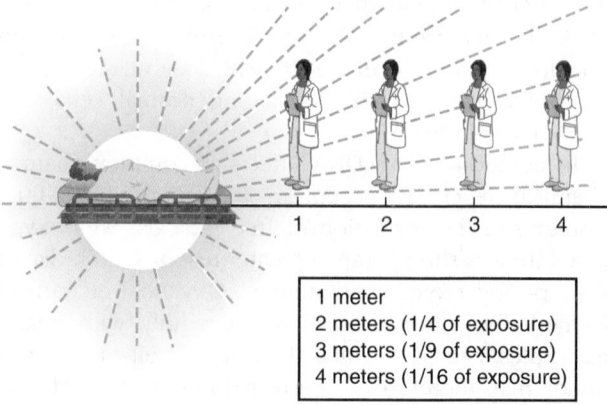

1 meter
2 meters (1/4 of exposure)
3 meters (1/9 of exposure)
4 meters (1/16 of exposure)

■ **FIGURE 17-1** Inverse relationship of distance and radiation exposure.

The staff members caring for clients with radioactive implants are rotated to limit the amount of exposure of each employee. Staff members must wear their own film badges or dosimeters while in the client's room. Because the visiting policy is restricted, the client may experience feelings of isolation. To maintain contact while keeping distance from radiation exposure, talk with the client from the doorway of the room. Encourage family and friends to telephone. Prepare the client ahead of time for limited employee contact. Before the radiation source is inserted, the client should be provided with ways to pass the time, such as reading, television, and videogames. Such clients usually feel well but safety measures dictate that they are isolated and confined to their beds.

The client receiving internal XRT with an unsealed source also needs to have a private room and bath. Further precautions must be taken because all body secretions are radioactive. All surfaces, including the floor on which the client will walk, are covered with protective covering. Foods are served on disposable plates with disposable utensils. Trash and linens are kept in the client's room and are not removed until after the client is discharged. To further decrease the risk of radiation exposure to caregivers, bed linens are generally not changed unless they are grossly soiled. The client is instructed to flush the toilet several times after each use.

Visitor and staff contact is limited, and anyone entering the room wears a new pair of booties each time to avoid tracking the radioactive isotope out into the hallway. Gloves are worn to avoid exposure when handling body fluids. Any emesis (vomiting), especially that occurring shortly after the client has ingested an oral isotope, should be covered with absorbent pads, and the radiation safety officer should be called immediately. Additional precautions may be necessary, depending on the radioisotope used and the policies and procedures of the individual practice setting.

Before being discharged, instruct the client about any precautions that should be continued at home. The radiation safety officer will scan the client to ensure that the radiation has decreased to a safe level. All precautions for the room should be continued even after the client has been discharged, until the radiation safety officer has lifted restrictions.

The U.S. Nuclear Regulatory Commission requires that radiation exposure be kept as low as reasonably achievable. All institutions using radioactive materials must have written policies concerning radiation protection. In addition, a radiation safety officer licensed by the U.S. Atomic Energy Commission to work with radioactive material must be available at all institutions that use radioactive materials.

The law also requires monitoring devices, such as film badges, for health care workers exposed to radiation and record-keeping of each worker's exposure. Do not share your film badge with anyone. The film badge provides a measure of whole-body exposure. The general precautions—distance, time, and shielding—apply for all forms of external and internal XRT. Sealed and unsealed sources of internal XRT require additional precautionary measures for their safe use.

Treatment Considerations for Radiation Therapy

The goal of XRT is to destroy the cancer while keeping dosages within the normal tissue tolerance to avoid harming surrounding normal tissues. Several factors determine treatment effects and side effects of XRT:

1. Tumor location in relation to surrounding normal tissue affects both treatment effects and side effects. Certain normal tissues are more sensitive to radiation and may incur permanent damage as a result of radiation. The spinal cord and the GI, integumentary, and myeloproliferative systems are at greatest risk for damage. If the spinal cord lies in the treatment field, the maximum safe dose of XRT is lower than if the XRT can be delivered from directions (ports) that avoid the spinal cord. Additionally, customized shielding "blocks" may be created to protect normal tissues from ionizing rays. Multileaf collimators and computer-controlled treatment machines allow the treatment field to be molded precisely to the shape of the tumor and the treatment dose to be delivered through multiple ports.

2. The size of the treatment field affects the dose of XRT. If a small area is treated, the client can tolerate a higher dose of radiation than if a larger area is treated. XRT is a regional treatment; thus when widespread or metastatic disease probably extends beyond the treatment field, XRT is not likely to be an effective treatment modality.

3. The client's overall health or performance status affects the ability to tolerate XRT. For example, a client who already has severe chronic obstructive pulmonary disease is less able to tolerate XRT to the lung.

4. The therapeutic ratio of the treatment effects on the tumor to the side effects on normal tissue is an important cost-benefit determinant in decision making about XRT.

5. The side effects a client may experience are related to the total dose of radiation. Radiation dose is prescribed in units called gray (Gy). This term has replaced the unit of dose known as the rad (radiation absorbed dose): 1 Gy equals 100 rad; 1 cGy (centigray) equals 1 rad. The XRT dose is higher when the goal is curative eradication of the cancer than when the goal is pain control or palliation. A client receiving 5000 cGy for cure experiences more side

effects than a client receiving 2000 cGy to the same body area for palliation.

6. In general, only the area in the treatment field is affected by the radiation. For example, hair loss occurs only in the area being treated with radiation. Therefore a client receiving XRT to the chest experiences hair loss on the chest but usually not on the scalp.

7. Administering the radiation in divided (fractionated) rather than single doses minimizes the side effects by allowing the normal cells time to recover. Fractionation refers to dividing the total radiation dose into small, frequent doses. A common dosage schedule for external XRT is 150 to 200 cGy, 5 days per week, for a total of 4 to 5 weeks. Fractionation also increases the probability that tumor cells will be in a vulnerable phase of the cell cycle when treated; cells are more sensitive to XRT during the late G_2 and early M phases. Fractionation allows normal cells time to repair themselves. At times, an XRT dose is hyperfractionated (divided into smaller doses given two or three times daily rather than once a day).

Some complementary therapies are also used during XRT, as described in the Complementary and Alternative Therapy box at right. (On the website, see the Complementary and Alternative Therapy feature on Low-Residue Diet for Reducing the Complications of Pelvic Radiotherapy for Cancer.)

Nursing Management of the Client Receiving Radiation Therapy

The staff of most XRT departments includes a nurse to meet the learning and manifestation management needs of the client. Yet nurses in the chemotherapy clinic, inpatient unit, or home care setting may be faced with concerns or questions from clients and family members about the side effects of XRT.

Provide Education

In addition to the emotional impact of the cancer diagnosis, XRT can be a source of fear and misunderstanding. Clients may experience fears of being burned or becoming radioactive. Because XRT cannot be seen or felt during treatment, the client may fear that the treatment is not effective. Education can dispel such common fears and misconceptions.

Comparing XRT with the effects of the sun can be helpful. One generally does not notice the full effect of the sun immediately after coming indoors; so many manifestations of XRT do not develop until about 10 to 14 days of treatment, and some do not subside until several weeks after treatment. If the cancer was not causing physical manifestations, the client may not have

---

COMPLEMENTARY AND ALTERNATIVE THERAPY

Oral Glutamine Supplements versus Placebo for the Prevention of Acute Diarrhea in Clients Receiving Pelvic Radiation Therapy

A total of 129 clients were enrolled from 14 institutions for this study. Clients received 4 g of glutamine or placebo, twice a day, beginning with the first or second day of radiation treatment and continuing for 2 weeks after radiation treatment. The median age of the clients was 69 years (range, 34 to 86 years). Quality of life scores and the average number of problems reported on the bowel function questionnaire were similar for both treatment groups. The incidence of grade 3 or higher diarrhea was 20% for the glutamine group and 19% for the placebo group. The maximum number of stools per day was 5.1 for the glutamine group and 5.2 for the placebo group. Thus no evidence of any beneficial effect of glutamine at 8 g/day was found compared with placebo during pelvic radiation therapy for cancer. Clients in this study had to be at least 18 years of age or older and have histologically confirmed adenocarcinoma or squamous cell carcinoma. Other trials are needed that use higher doses of glutamine.

REFERENCE

Kozelsky, T., et al. (2003). Phase III double-blind study of glutamine versus placebo for the prevention of acute diarrhea in patients receiving pelvic radiation therapy. *Journal of Clinical Oncology, 21*, 1669-1674.

---

evidence (like seeing a suntan) of the treatment's effect. If, however, the tumor was obstructing air flow, the client may realize a few weeks into the XRT that breathing is easier or coughing is diminished—even before imaging studies are performed to verify tumor shrinkage. Likewise, if XRT is being delivered for painful bone metastases, the client will probably note a decrease in pain or diminished need for pain medications after 1 to 2 weeks of XRT.

Minimize Side Effects

In general, skin reactions and fatigue may occur with XRT to any site, whereas other side effects occur only when specific areas are involved in the treatment field. The response of normal skin to XRT varies from mild erythema to moist desquamation similar in appearance to a second-degree burn. The term *burn* should not be used to describe these skin reactions, however, because doing so may frighten the client unnecessarily. Because megavoltage and cobalt deliver the maximum dose beneath the skin, skin reactions have become less significant than in years past. Advice for clients on caring for skin within the treatment field is given in the Client Education Guide below.

Site-specific manifestations of XRT include mucositis, xerostomia (dry mouth), radiation caries, esophagitis, dysphagia (difficulty swallowing), nausea and vomiting, diarrhea, tenesmus (straining at stool or in urination), cystitis, urethritis, alopecia (hair loss), and bone marrow suppression. These may be the result of acute changes associated with inflammation or chronic changes associated with fibrosis. During XRT, a CBC is usually performed weekly. The degree of myelosuppression varies with the amount of bone marrow within the treatment field. Areas at greatest risk are the pelvic region, sacrum, skull, lumbar and thoracic spine, ribs, shoulder region, and sternum.

In women of childbearing age, XRT may cause prolonged or permanent infertility.

In prostate brachytherapy, when radioactive seeds have been permanently implanted, there is a low, weakly penetrating radiation exposure for others. Therefore the client should use a condom for sexual intercourse in the first weeks after the procedure. Also, the client should avoid close (<6 feet) contact with pregnant women and young children (younger than 3 years) for more than 5 minutes a day during the first 2 months after implantation.[27]

Many of the manifestation management strategies for side effects of XRT are similar to those for the side effects of chemotherapy, described later in this chapter. Information on nursing management of the general side

effects of radiation therapy (RT) is included in the Oncology Nursing Society's *Manual for Radiation Oncology Nursing Practice*.[13] The NCI offers a free client education booklet titled *Radiation Therapy and You: A Guide to Self-Help*.[43] A nurse or therapist in the XRT department is a readily accessible source of information. Furthermore, you can alert the XRT staff about the client's concern and thus help the client manage outcomes of the XRT side effects.

Chemotherapy

As with surgery and XRT, the goals of chemotherapy can be cure, control, or palliation.

Chemotherapy is a systemic intervention and is appropriate in the following circumstances:

- The disease is widespread.
- The risk of undetectable disease is high.
- The tumor cannot be resected and is resistant to XRT.

The client who is at high risk for recurrence but shows no evidence of current disease may be a candidate for adjuvant chemotherapy. In this type of therapy, after initial treatment with either surgery or XRT, chemotherapeutic drugs are used to eliminate any remaining submicroscopic cancer cells that are suspected to be still present. Adjuvant therapy is now well established in the treatment of breast cancer.

Neoadjuvant chemotherapy refers to the preoperative use of chemotherapy to reduce the bulk and lower the stage of a tumor, making it amenable to surgery or possibly even cured with subsequent local therapy.

The objective of chemotherapy is to destroy malignant tumor cells without excessive destruction of normal cells. Several types of cancer are now considered curable with chemotherapy, even in advanced stages. Unfortunately, these tumors account for only about 10% of all cancers.

How Chemotherapy Works

The phases of the cell cycle are common to all cells (see the Unit 3 Anatomy and Physiology review for a description of the phases of the cell cycle). Normally, cells respond to the body's need for growth, repair, or regeneration in an orderly manner and cease production by entering a resting phase or slowing growth when the need is met. At any given time, normal cells are found in all phases of growth. Cancer cells reproduce in the same manner as normal cells; however, growth occurs in an uncontrollable manner and may not enter the resting phase. In general, cells that are actively dividing are the most sensitive to chemotherapy.

Chemotherapy directly or indirectly disrupts reproduction of cells by altering essential biochemical processes. The desired outcome is control or eradication

---

CLIENT EDUCATION GUIDE

Skin Care Within the Treatment Field

- Keep your skin dry.
- Do not wash the treatment area until you are instructed to do so. When permitted, wash the treated skin gently with mild soap, rinse well, and pat dry. Use warm or cool water, *not* hot water.
- Do not remove the lines or ink marks placed on your skin.
- Avoid using powders, lotions, creams, alcohol, and deodorants on the treated skin.
- Wear loose-fitting clothing to avoid friction over the treatment field.
- Do not apply tape to the treatment site if dressings are applied.
- Shave with an electric razor. Do not use pre-shave or after-shave lotions.
- Protect your skin from exposure to direct sunlight, chlorinated swimming pools, and temperature extremes (e.g., hot water bottles, heating pads, ice packs).
- Consult your radiation therapist or nurse about specific measures for individual skin reactions.

of all malignant cells. Experiments and clinical experience suggest that most types of chemotherapy do not kill all cancer cells during one exposure. According to the cell kill hypothesis, only a percentage of cancer cells are killed with each course of chemotherapy. Repeated doses—or cycles—of chemotherapy must therefore be used.

The use of drugs in combination, known as combination chemotherapy, has consistently been far superior to single-agent therapy. Drugs selected to be used in combination must each be effective against the type of cancer being treated. When combined, chemotherapeutic agents destroy more malignant cells and produce fewer side effects because each drug strikes the cancer cells at a different point in the cell cycle. Combination chemotherapy is now the standard in most situations. The regimens are complex, cyclic, and individualized for the client and the type of cancer.

Classification of Chemotherapeutic Agents

Chemotherapeutic agents generally are classified according to their pharmacologic actions and effects on the cell generation cycle; however, the method by which cancer cells are inhibited or destroyed is not always known. A classification of common chemotherapeutic agents is shown in Classification of Chemotherapeutic Agents on the website. This classification is also outlined in the Integrating Pharmacology box below.

INTEGRATING PHARMACOLOGY

Chemotherapy Agents

Chemotherapy agents used for the treatment of cancer are classified as cell-cycle-specific and cell-cycle-nonspecific. For a detailed list, see the Classification of Chemotherapeutic Agents on the website.

Cell-cycle-specific drugs are active on cells undergoing division in the cell cycle. These drugs are most effective against actively growing tumors that have a greater proportion of cells cycling through the phase in which the drug attacks the cancer cell. Cell-cycle-specific drugs are usually given in minimal concentration via continuous dosing methods. Examples of these types of drugs include antimetabolites, vinca plant alkaloids, and taxanes.

Cell-cycle-nonspecific drugs are active on cells in either a dividing or a resting state. These agents are active in all phases of the cell cycle and may be effective in large tumors that have few active cells dividing at the time of administration. Drugs of this nature are often given as single bolus injections. Examples include alkylating agents, antitumor antibiotics, and hormonal and steroid drugs.

Nursing Management of the Client Receiving Chemotherapy

Chemotherapy agents should be administered only by adequately prepared registered professional nurses who are skilled in the administration. At a minimum, the nurse should have completed chemotherapy administration classes. Ideally, nurses providing oncology care are also oncology-certified nurses (OCNs) who have the specialized knowledge and skills to manage potential outcomes of cancer and its treatment. It is important that the bedside nurse be aware of the potential adverse effects of the agent being administered. Nurses who have not received education in chemotherapy administration may incorrectly believe that one will need only a chemotherapy-trained nurse present long enough to initiate administration of the chemotherapeutic agent; however, careful monitoring for potential adverse reactions and side effects is required during and even after completion of the infusion. When the bedside nurse does not have the requisite knowledge, the institutional policies can ensure that a nurse with expertise in cancer care is responsible for supervising care and guiding the bedside nurse in the assessment and administration issues to provide safe, effective care to the client. Recommendations for nursing practice can be found in the Oncology Nursing Society's *Cancer Chemotherapy Guidelines.*[12]

Assessment

A thorough client assessment is necessary before cytotoxic drugs are administered. A review of the client's medical history will identify potential risk factors for chemotherapy toxicity, such as a history of impaired cardiac, pulmonary, or renal function. Carefully assess the severity and duration of previous side effects. Abnormal laboratory values may indicate organ-specific toxicities of chemotherapeutic agents. Before administering subsequent courses of chemotherapy, a CBC with differential count will ensure adequate bone marrow recovery has occurred since the previous treatment. The differential count is used to calculate the absolute neutrophil count (ANC) (see later discussion), a means of determining the percentage of mature white cells. Drug doses may have to be modified or delayed on the basis of these results.

The client's medical record should contain either a copy of the formal drug protocol or a written summary of the planned chemotherapy regimen. Chemotherapy doses are usually based on body surface area in square meters (m²), which is determined by the client's height and weight. Clear and complete chemotherapy prescriptions consist of (1) the name of the drug, (2) dose/m² and total dose, (3) route of administration, (4) administration rate for intravenous (IV) infusions, and (5) frequency of administration. Plans for antiemetic therapy, hydration, diuresis, and electrolyte supplementation are frequently included as well. Clients need to know what side effects to watch for and what to do when side effects arise. See the Care Plan on pp. 280-281 for help in managing the side effects of clients undergoing chemotherapy.

Most serious side effects of chemotherapy treatment do not occur during or immediately after administration.

Knowing the expected side effects of cancer treatment and appropriate interventions increases your ability to give prompt, effective care. You should be able to recognize variations from normal, perform a complete assessment of the client's status, and then report that information in a timely manner to the client's oncology caregivers.

You can therefore communicate pertinent data to the oncology professional as a basis for a medical or nursing diagnosis. Nurses in all practice settings must work together, sharing information and knowledge, to ensure continuity of care for the client who is undergoing chemotherapy for cancer.

Administration of Chemotherapy

Before administering antineoplastic agents, consult with the pharmacist and review chemotherapy drug handbooks and investigational drug protocols for detailed information regarding drug actions, dosages, administration guidelines, and potential side effects.

A National Patient Safety Goal issued by The Joint Commission (TJC) is to improve the safety of using medications. A critical step in the administration of chemotherapeutics is verification of the drug, route, dose, and schedule.[12,14] Chemotherapy calculations and drugs should be checked by two nurses against the written orders. Errors in chemotherapy orders may result from such factors as the misplacement of a decimal point or the dispensing of the wrong drug. An overdose of an antineoplastic agent could result in profound toxicity and death. In addition, the administration of intravenous chemotherapy must be completed with the use of an intravenous pump to control the rates of chemotherapy.

Another National Patient Safety Goal identified by TJC is to encourage clients' active involvement in their own care as a client safety strategy. This includes efforts to define and communicate the means for clients and their families to report concerns about safety and encourage them to do so.

Educating the client and the client's family about chemotherapy and the identification, prevention, and management of side effects is primarily a nursing function. As mentioned, the Care Plan in this chapter offers an example of a plan for managing side effects of chemotherapy. The NCI provides an excellent booklet, *Chemotherapy and You: A Guide to Self-help during Cancer Treatment,* free of charge for client teaching.[41] Hypersensitivity reaction and extravasation, discussed later in this chapter, can occur during the administration of chemotherapy. Potentially life-threatening side effects, such as infection during neutropenia (see later discussion), are more likely to occur after the client has left the health care facility, when no health professionals are available.

Routes of Administration

Two routes are discussed: intravenous (IV) and regional. Other routes of administration of chemotherapeutic agents include oral, subcutaneous, and intramuscular. As new chemotherapeutic agents become available in oral form, increasing numbers of clients are self-administering these drugs at home. An in-depth discussion of safe administration of oral chemotherapeutics can be found elsewhere.[10]

Intravenous Chemotherapy. Most chemotherapeutic agents are administered intravenously. Extravasation (escape from the vein) of some chemotherapeutic agents can result in significant harm to the surrounding tissue. Therefore you must always know before administering a drug whether it is a vesicant (an agent capable of causing tissue damage).

Great care should be taken in vein selection and venipuncture technique. Large veins in the fleshy part of the forearm are the preferred peripheral access sites. Avoid areas of impaired lymphatic drainage, phlebitis, invading neoplasm, hematoma, inflammation, sclerosis, impaired venous circulation, the lower extremities, and sites distal to a recent venipuncture site. Also avoid veins that are on the dorsal aspect of the hand or over an area of flexion, such as the wrist or elbow. When administering a vesicant drug, you must be prepared to deal with a potential extravasation to limit tissue damage. Preparation includes having immediate availability of an antidote, if there is one.[12]

In the past, vascular access devices (VADs) were placed as a last resort in clients with poor venous access. Today, because chemotherapy regimens are complex and supportive care is extensive, VADs are being used during the initial treatment of clients requiring continuous chemotherapy, multiple access, parenteral fluids, antibiotics, and frequent blood testing. Chemotherapy clients are generally satisfied with their VADs and find that they improve the quality of their lives.

Implanted and external vascular access catheters are usually inserted into one of the major veins of the upper chest. Centrally implanted VADs are placed by a surgeon, generally during a brief outpatient procedure. The brachial or cephalic vein in the forearm is used for peripherally inserted central catheters (PICCs), which are often placed by specially trained nurses. The distal catheter tip is advanced to the level of the superior vena cava at or above the junction of

C A R E   P L A N   *evolve*

Side Effect Management for the Client Receiving Chemotherapy

Nursing Diagnosis: Risk for Injury (NANDA) related to side effects secondary to chemotherapy.

Outcomes: Risk Control, Medication Response, Knowledge: Medication (NOC). Client will experience minimal side effects of chemotherapy, will demonstrate knowledge of rationale for chemotherapy and treatment plan, and will demonstrate knowledge about potential side effects of drugs and related self-management strategies.

Interventions	(NIC)	Rationales
1. Monitor client for side effects of chemotherapy during administration and reinforce client education.	Medication Administration	Side effects such as drug extravasation and nausea and vomiting may occur immediately.
2. Monitor client for side effects of chemotherapy after administration, such as leukopenia, diarrhea, constipation, stomatitis, hair loss.	Medication Teaching: Prescribed Medications	Side effects may also occur once drug is administered and client is home. Early intervention may minimize adverse side effects.
3. Provide individualized education related to chemotherapy regimen, expected side effects, administration schedule, knowledge of each drug used, and possible treatments to minimize side effects.	Teaching: Prescribed Medications	Written and verbal education may improve the client's willingness to participate in treatment and result in better treatment outcomes.

Evaluation: Chemotherapy will be administered without the occurrence of adverse events. Client will tolerate expected side effects of treatment and understand their presence. Side effects will be treated as indicated and potential serious effects will be identified early, with immediate treatment initiated. Client will rebound quickly from side effects of chemotherapy and resume prechemotherapy activities. Client will understand treatment plan, identify emergent problems, and be able to tolerate expected effects of treatment.

Nursing Diagnosis: Risk for Infection (NANDA) related to leukopenia secondary to chemotherapy.

Outcomes: Infection Severity, Immune Status (NOC). Client will remain free of infection as evidenced by temperature remaining within normal limits. Client will verbalize interventions that prevent infection.

Interventions	(NIC)	Rationales
1. Monitor for infection by checking vital signs.	Infection Protection	An elevated temperature is frequently the initial clinical manifestation.
2. Practice good hand-washing and use aseptic technique when providing care.	Infection Protection	Hand-washing is the most effective intervention to decrease the risk of infection. Aseptic technique minimizes risk of nosocomial infection.
3. Keep neutropenic clients separate from others.	Infection Protection	Neutropenic clients are at greatest risk for infection.
4. Monitor laboratory results, especially complete blood count, white blood cell count (WBC), differential, and absolute neutrophils.	Infection Control	Abnormal results provide data that provide a basis for early detection of infection.
5. Monitor respiratory, urinary, mucosal, and skin systems.	Infection Protection	Changes in these systems are often a basis for early detection of infection.
6. Administer Neupogen as ordered.	Infection Protection	Neupogen decreases infection risk by increasing WBCs in clients receiving chemotherapy who develop neutropenia.
7. Teach manifestations of infection and those to report immediately.	Infection Protection	Infection in the neutropenic client is life-threatening.
8. Teach measures for prevention of infection, such as avoiding crowds and not cleaning fish tanks or litter boxes.	Infection Control	These are high-risk sources of infection.

Evaluation: The client will remain free of infection or seek treatment promptly if manifestations of infection appear. The client will verbalize methods that minimize this condition from occurring.

Nursing Diagnosis: Imbalanced Nutrition: Less Than Body Requirements (NANDA) related to disease process and treatment.

Outcomes: Appetite, Nutritional Status, Weight: Body Mass (NOC). Client will identify measures to prevent nutritional deficits and will maintain adequate nutritional status, as evidenced by body weight within present parameters.

Interventions	(NIC)	Rationales
1. Weigh daily.	Nutrition Management Nutritional Monitoring	Monitors weight gain or loss. Weight loss over time is an indicator of malnutrition.

2. Monitor nutritional intake.	Nutritional Monitoring	Teaching the importance of maintaining nutrition during treatment may motivate the client to try in spite of the loss of appetite and taste alterations.
3. Discuss methods to promote good nutrition.	Nutrition Therapy	
4. Monitor hemoglobin, hematocrit, albumin, and total protein values.	Nutritional Monitoring	Monitors intake of nutrients, presence of anemia and fatigue, and colloidal osmotic pressure and edema.
5. Monitor oral cavity.	Oral Health Maintenance	Pain and taste alterations may impair nutritional intake.
6. Arrange for assistance in obtaining and preparing food.	Nutrition Management	Increases intake and provides culturally appropriate food.

Evaluation: Client will demonstrate knowledge of methods to maintain weight and body mass. Client will identify measures to prevent nutritional deficits and minimize fatigue and edema.

Nursing Diagnosis: Fatigue (NANDA) related to cancer treatment.

Outcomes: Activity Tolerance, Endurance, Energy Conservation, Nutritional Status: Energy (NOC). Client will use energy conservation techniques to maintain quality of life.

Interventions	(NIC)	Rationales
1. Assess for fatigue.	Energy Management	The first step is to identify the problem.
2. Review laboratory (RBC) or other clinical data (oxygen saturation) for physiologic manifestations of fatigue.	Energy Management	These data will identify and determine the cause of the fatigue. Fatigue is often not recognized.
3. Administer erythropoietin or blood transfusion as ordered.	Medication and Blood Product Administration	Erythropoietin stimulates RBC synthesis to prevent or treat anemia, and blood transfusion replaces RBCs.
4. Provide interventions that prevent or minimize dehydration and electrolyte imbalances.	Fluid/Electrolyte Management	Dehydration and electrolyte imbalance contribute to fatigue and weakness.
5. Promote sleep and rest. Teach relaxation and distraction techniques.	Energy Management	Sleep and rest help minimize effects of cancer-related fatigue.
6. Use community resources to minimize activities that require energy (physical therapy, home health services, transportation services, meal services).	Activity Therapy Management Energy Management Environmental	These services allow the client to conserve energy. Physical therapists can prescribe exercises to improve endurance.

Evaluation: Client will alternate rest and activity to minimize fatigue or will not experience fatigue if erythropoietin administration prevents anemia from developing. Client will demonstrate knowledge about methods that may prevent transient states of tiredness that result from treatment.

Nursing Diagnosis: Ineffective Coping (NANDA) related to cancer diagnosis.

Outcomes: Acceptance: Health Status, Coping, Decision-Making, Psychosocial Adjustment: Life Change (NOC). Client will begin to cope with the diagnosis of cancer and be aware of resources available for assistance if psychological function decreases.

Interventions	(NIC)	Rationales
1. Develop rapport; use active listening skills. Provide consistent, empathetic, and positive regard.	Coping Enhancement Emotional Support Active Listening	Client will know that you are concerned about them.
2. Ask the client directly how he or she is coping. Support client's expression of feelings.	Emotional Support Coping Enhancement	When asked, client may share fears and concerns.
3. Guide the client to community resources and refer to professional providers for emotional support.	Support Group Spiritual Support Emotional Support	These resources and referrals provide ongoing support during all phases of cancer treatment.
4. Help the client identify problem-solving and coping skills that have worked for the client in the past.	Decision-Making Support Emotional Support	The client may not recognize skills that he or she has used and could transfer these skills to make decisions and cope with the cancer diagnosis.
5. Suggest keeping a journal to identify feelings.	Emotional Support	Keeping a journal can help the client identify concerns; solutions may then be identified.
6. Emphasize the importance of social network and community resources for dealing with concerns.	Support Group Coping Enhancement Emotional Support	A social network counteracts feelings of isolation and promotes effective coping.

Evaluation: The client will cope with cancer diagnosis by maintaining interpersonal relationships and activities, participate in a social network, and use or be familiar with resources that can be of assistance if coping with the diagnosis becomes overwhelming.

the right atrium. Proper catheter tip placement of both central and peripheral VADs is confirmed by fluoroscopy or radiography. Various types of VADs are depicted in Figure 17-2.

In addition to VADs, arterial, peritoneal, and intraventricular access devices permit regional delivery of chemotherapy to the liver or peritoneal cavity or into the cerebrospinal fluid of the brain.[34] Each type of device has advantages and disadvantages, including factors such as maintenance requirements, ease of use, cost, ease of insertion, longevity, and effect on body image.

SAFETY ALERT

The most commonly reported complications are infection and catheter occlusion.[68] The prevention of VAD infection centers on catheter care, daily assessment for manifestations of infection, and client education. Intraluminal occlusion may occur secondary to a blood clot or precipitate. Prevention strategies include proper flushing, vigilance for drug incompatibilities, and adherence to proper drug dilutions. Other complications can also occur with VADs. Nurses need to be aware that the potential for extravasation is not eliminated by using a VAD rather than a peripheral IV site. When administering a vesicant agent, diligent observation is still required to ensure early intervention if an extravasation occurs.

Procedures for the care and maintenance of VADs vary with each clinical setting and type of device.

Nursing management strategies for VADs are extensively described elsewhere.[15,68]

When the procedure for accessing a VAD is performed according to institutional policy and goes as expected, use of a VAD is relatively easy.

Major, even life-threatening, problems can arise, however, if the VAD is not accessed correctly or the nurse does not know how to recognize a problem and the corrective action. Nurses who access VADs infrequently should review their institution's procedure before attempting VAD access.[68] If the procedure in any way varies from the expected, obtain the advice of a nurse who is more experienced in VADs before proceeding.

Regional Chemotherapy. Regional chemotherapy via alternative routes allows high concentrations of drugs to be directed to localized tumors. Methods are (1) topical, (2) intra-arterial, (3) intracavitary, (4) intraperitoneal, and (5) intrathecal.

Topical. Fluorouracil cream can be applied to the skin to treat actinic keratoses (sun keratoses). Squamous cell carcinoma can arise from these precancerous lesions if they are left untreated.

Intra-Arterial. Intra-arterial infusions involve some risk but enable major organs or tumor sites to receive

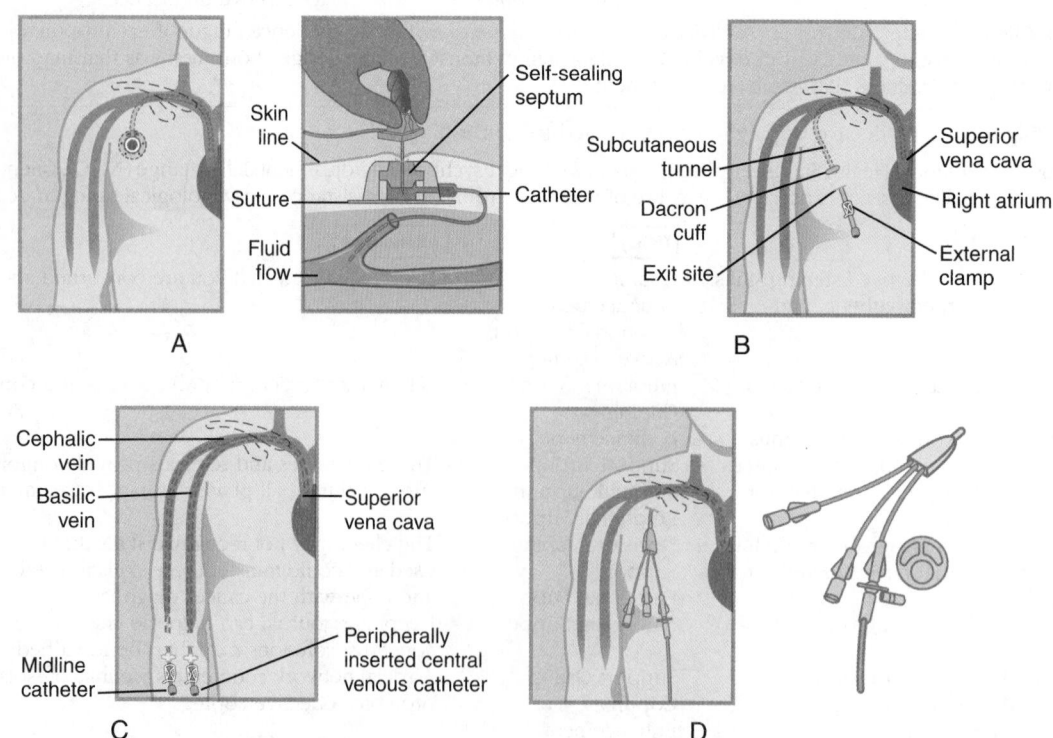

■ **FIGURE 17-2** Catheters for administration of antineoplastic medications. **A,** Implanted venous access device or port. **B,** Tunneled external venous access device (Groshong). These can be single-, double-, or triple-lumen catheters. **C,** Peripherally inserted central catheter (PICC). **D,** Subclavian catheter. These can be single-, double-, or triple-lumen catheters.

maximal exposure with limited serum levels of medications. As a result, systemic side effects are lessened.

Intracavitary. Intracavitary therapy instills the medication directly into an area such as the abdomen, bladder, or pleural space.

Intraperitoneal. Intraperitoneal chemotherapy is an option for cancer involving the intra-abdominal area, such as ovarian cancer. With this method, a high concentration of a chemotherapeutic agent is delivered to the actual tumor site with minimal exposure of healthy tissues, thereby decreasing toxic side effects.

Intrathecal. Most medications given systemically are not effective against CNS tumors because they cannot cross the blood-brain barrier. The physician may instill chemotherapeutic agents into the CNS through an implanted reservoir (an Ommaya reservoir) placed in the ventricle (Figure 17-3) or via a lumbar puncture. Kosier and Minkler[34] provide an excellent review of the nursing management of clients with an implanted Ommaya reservoir.

Adverse Reactions

Two potentially serious adverse reactions, the seriousness of which depends on the chemotherapeutic agents, may occur during administration: hypersensitivity reactions and extravasation.

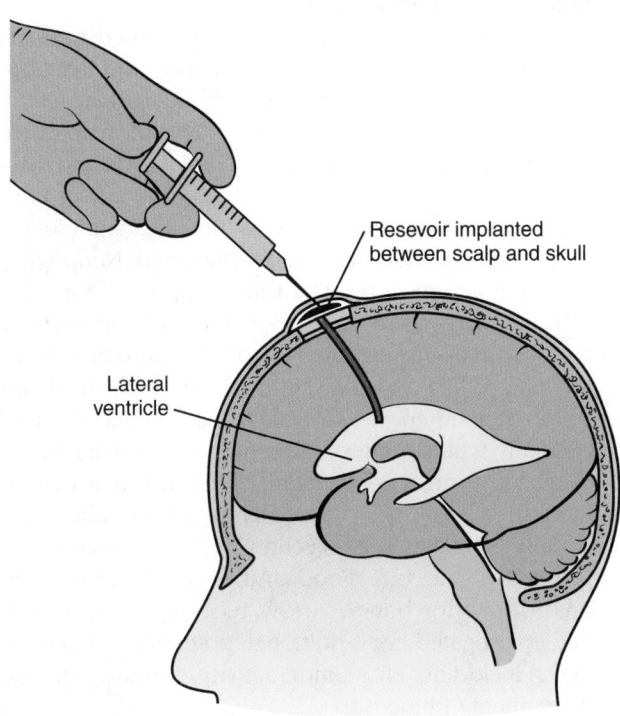

Resevoir implanted between scalp and skull

Lateral ventricle

■ **FIGURE 17-3** Ommaya reservoir. An Ommaya reservoir should only be accessed with a small-gauge non-coring or butterfly needle.

Hypersensitivity Reaction. Hypersensitivity reaction (an exaggerated immune response to a foreign substance) to chemotherapy, although uncommon, can be serious and life-threatening.[1] The antineoplastic agents most commonly implicated in the development of hypersensitivity reactions are L-asparaginase (Elspar), carboplatin (Paraplatin), cisplatin (Platinol-AQ), paclitaxel (Taxol), bleomycin (Blenoxane), rituximab (Rituxan), and teniposide (Vumon).[12]

When administering a drug with anaphylactic potential (i.e., the potential to cause a possibly fatal hypersensitivity reaction), take the following precautions to ensure client safety:

- **Obtain an allergy history.**
- **Obtain baseline vital signs.**
- **Have emergency equipment and drugs readily available.**
- **Administer a test dose if ordered by the physician.**
- **Stay with the client the entire time the drug is being administered.**
- **Establish a free-flowing IV line for the administration of fluids and emergency drugs in case they are needed.**

The manifestations of an immediate hypersensitivity reaction are (1) dyspnea, (2) chest tightness or pain, (3) pruritus (itching), (4) urticaria (wheals), (5) tachycardia, (6) dizziness, (7) anxiety, (8) agitation, (9) inability to speak, (10) abdominal pain, (11) nausea, (12) hypotension, (13) cloudy mental status, (14) flushed appearance, and (15) cyanosis. If an anaphylactic reaction is suspected, take the following actions:

- **Immediately stop drug administration.**
- **Maintain the airway.**
- **Maintain IV access with 0.9% saline.**
- **Place the client in a supine position with the feet elevated, unless contraindicated.**
- **Notify the physician.**
- **Monitor the client's vital signs every 2 minutes until stable.**
- **Administer epinephrine, aminophylline, diphenhydramine (Benadryl), and corticosteroids according to the physician's orders.**

Extravasation

Before administering a chemotherapeutic drug, note its vesicant potential and its antidote if there is one, when reviewing the drug. Careful assessment of the IV site is required during and after the infusion of antineoplastic agents because some agents cause tissue damage if extravasated (infiltrated).

Nonvesicant agents have no significant soft tissue toxicities. Vesicant chemotherapeutic agents can cause a blister to form, which results in tissue destruction. Commonly used vesicant drugs are doxorubicin (Adriamycin) and vincristine (Oncovin). Cisplatin (Platinol-AQ) and paclitaxel (Taxol) are also vesicant drugs. Because they are commonly mixed in large volumes of fluid, the extravasation can be detected more easily before serious tissue damage occurs. Irritant drugs can produce venous pain at the site and along the vein, with or without an inflammatory reaction. Pain, erythema, swelling, and lack of a blood return indicate an extravasation.[1]

Procedures for management of extravasation are controversial and unique to each clinical setting. Institutionally approved guidelines for the management of extravasation should be readily available. Guidelines for the management of extravasation are included in the Oncology Nursing Society's *Cancer Chemotherapy Guidelines*.[12] The following are general recommendations:

- Stop the administration of the drug.
- Leave the needle in place; attempt to aspirate any residual drug from the tubing, needle, and site.
- Administer an antidote, if appropriate; then remove the needle.
- Do not apply direct manual pressure to the site.
- Apply warm (for vinca alkaloid) or cold compresses as indicated.
- Observe the site regularly for pain, erythema, swelling, induration, and necrosis.
- Document the appearance of the site before and after chemotherapy.

Safe Preparation, Handling, and Disposal

The safe administration and disposal of chemotherapeutic agents decreases the risk of undue exposure to health care professionals. Most chemotherapeutic agents bind directly to genetic material in the cell nucleus or affect cellular protein synthesis. The toxic potential of significantly high workplace exposure to these agents varies and is difficult to assess. Potential risks include genotoxicity, carcinogenicity, teratogenicity, and serious organ damage. Undue exposure to antineoplastic drugs can occur from three major routes:

- Respiratory inhalation
- Skin absorption
- Oral ingestion

Several organizations, including the Occupational Safety and Health Administration (OSHA), the National Study Commission on Cytotoxic Exposure, and the Oncology Nursing Society, have prepared guidelines for the safe preparation, handling, and disposal of antineoplastics.[12,49] These guidelines call for (1) the wearing of gloves and gowns during preparation and administration and (2) the use of a biologic safety or laminar-flow cabinet for preparation. Antineoplastic agents and their metabolites are found in the excreta and body fluids of clients undergoing chemotherapy. For this reason, you should wear gloves and disposable gowns when handling body secretions of clients who have received chemotherapy within the previous 48 hours.

Biotherapy

Biotherapy is the use of agents to affect a biologic response. Efforts to understand and manipulate the human immune system have been underway for decades. Interactions between the immune system and malignant cells, such as spontaneous tumor remissions, provide a framework to isolate and identify effective biologic agents. Immune response remains the core of biotherapy. Biotherapy now also includes agents that change the relationship between the tumor and the host by altering the host's response to the tumor or by minimizing or preventing pancytopenia (neutropenia, anemia, and thrombocytopenia), which may delay scheduled chemotherapy or other therapies planned for treatment of the cancer. See the Classification of Biologic Agents on the website. In the last decade, four major technological advances have assisted scientists in their search:[5,55]

- A greater understanding of the complex cellular nature of the immune system
- Progress in genetic engineering, enabling the development of recombinant biologic agents
- Advances in molecular biology
- Refined and improved laboratory equipment and computer systems

Hematopoietic Growth Factors

Hematopoietic growth factors are glycosylated proteins that mediate hematopoiesis (the formation and development of blood cells). They stimulate bone marrow recovery after chemotherapy. Generally, they are named for the major cell lineage they mediate. Granulocyte and macrophage colony-stimulating factor (GM-CSF) affects both the granulocyte and macrophage lineage; granulocyte colony-stimulating factor (G-CSF) (filgrastim, Neupogen) affects only granulocytes. GM-CSF is approved for myeloid (bone marrow) reconstitution after autologous BMT and for use in clients experiencing BMT failure or engraftment delay. G-CSF and GM-CSF are approved for the treatment of chemotherapy-associated neutropenia. GM-CSF is generally well tolerated. Filgrastim is now available in a pegylated form, pegfilgrastim (Neulasta), that can be administered once per chemotherapy cycle rather than as a daily subcutaneous injection.[8] GM-CSF is currently approved by the U.S. Food and Drug Administration (FDA) for use for bone marrow recovery in BMT. It is being investigated for additional potential therapeutic benefits including anti-tumor activity, wound healing, and treatment of mucositis.

Side effects of these growth factors are (1) mild to moderate flu-like manifestations, such as fever, myalgia (muscular pain), bone pain, fatigue, and headache; (2) rash; (3) a transient increase in liver enzymes; and (4) thrombocytopenia (reduced platelets). The most commonly reported side effect of G-CSF is bone pain. Clients report pain in bone areas that have large marrow reserves, such as the pelvis, sternum, and long bones. This pain may be the result of the marrow expansion that occurs from the rapid increase in the neutrophil pool that G-CSF causes.

Erythropoietin, another hematopoietic growth factor, is approved by the FDA for use in treating anemia secondary to end-stage renal failure and associated with cancer chemotherapy (epoetin alfa [Procrit, Epogen]). Clients with serum erythropoietin levels greater than 200 milliunits/ml are unlikely to show a response to chemotherapy. It is important to maintain adequate levels of iron, folic acid, and vitamin B_{12} because these components are essential for the development of RBCs. The most commonly reported side effect is transient flu-like manifestations, such as arthralgias (joint pain) and myalgias.

Oprelvekin (Neumega) is a hematopoietic growth factor for chemotherapy-induced thrombocytopenia. Its most common side effects are edema, dyspnea, tachycardia, and conjunctival redness. Oprelvekin reduces the need for platelet transfusions and allows clients to receive the desired doses of chemotherapy as scheduled.

Biologic Response Modifiers

Biologic response modifiers (BRMs), which either are derived from biologic sources or affect biologic responses, are another form of biotherapy. BRMs change the relationship between the tumor and the host by altering the host's biologic response to the tumor. Many of these naturally occurring substances are hormone-like proteins or glycoproteins (proteins with a glucose molecule attached). BRMs have multiple biologic actions, including production of immunologic or other biologic effects. They may augment, modulate, or restore the immune response; they may have direct cytotoxic effects; or they may produce other biologic effects, such as maturation of cells and interference with a tumor's ability to metastasize. In addition to hematopoietic growth factors, BRM agents include interferons, interleukins, monoclonal antibodies, immunomodulators, and tumor necrosis factor.[54]

Some biologic agents have received FDA approval and are being used as standard therapy. Many others are under investigation in clinical trials. Rituximab (Rituxan) has been approved since 2001 for treatment of non-Hodgkin's lymphoma. Ongoing studies will determine if combining rituximab with chemotherapy or interferon will result in a significantly longer time before disease progression than when rituximab is used in single-agent therapy. Trastuzumab (Herceptin) is being used in combination with paclitaxel (Taxol) for treatment of HER2-positive breast cancer. Trastuzumab is being investigated as a treatment option in other solid tumors (ovarian, pancreatic, prostate) that overexpress the HER2 protein. Tositumomab (Bexxar) and ibritumomab tiuxetan (IDEC-Y2B8), two agents currently being investigated, combine a radioisotope with a monoclonal antibody (MoAb).[63]

Interferons

Interferons (IFNs) are small proteins that have cellular activity in three areas: antiviral, immunomodulatory, and antiproliferative. Interferon-alpha received FDA approval for use in hairy cell leukemia in 1986. The drug's clinical indications have been broadened to include AIDS-associated Kaposi's sarcoma. Clinical trials are being conducted to investigate its use in other hematologic malignancies, including chronic leukemias, multiple myeloma, cutaneous T-cell lymphoma, and low-grade non-Hodgkin's lymphoma.

Toxicities appear to be dose related, with lower doses of IFN associated with few side effects and high doses resulting in side effects that may require therapy to be interrupted or stopped. A flu-like syndrome, a common side effect of IFN therapy, may consist of fever, chills, tachycardia, muscle aches, malaise, fatigue, and headaches. Continued use of IFN produces a tachyphylactic response (rapidly decreasing response after administration of a few doses) such that these manifestations decrease in intensity over time. Premedication with acetaminophen (Tylenol) and diphenhydramine (Benadryl) is helpful in reducing the client's discomfort.

Interleukins

Most interleukins (proteins that serve as regulators of the immune system) are capable of inducing multiple biologic activities. A number of interleukins have been identified. Thus far, only interleukin-2 (IL-2) has received FDA approval. It is derived from T cells, augments various T-cell activities, and enhances the function of natural killer cells. It has been successfully used in clients with renal cell carcinoma and melanoma. Other areas of interest for its use are hematologic malignancies and BMT.

Major toxic responses with IL-2 therapy are due to increased capillary permeability, which may produce hypotension, ascites, pulmonary edema, fatigue, and generalized weight gain. In addition, integumentary changes occur and may include generalized redness, rash, pruritus, and occasionally skin desquamation. Toxicity resulting from IL-2 varies greatly with the dose of drug administered; higher doses produce greater toxicity, necessitating astute clinical management.

Monoclonal Antibodies

Monoclonal antibodies are specific antibodies directed against single antigenic determinants on the cell surface.[5] MoAbs provide high specificity lacking in other types of treatment modalities. They can be used either diagnostically or therapeutically. Diagnostic uses of these agents include the early detection of cancer by identification of surface markers on tumor cells and as a delivery agent of radioisotopes to the tumor site to aid in tumor visualization. Therapeutically, MoAbs may be used to deliver immunotoxins, such as ricin, chemotherapeutic agents, and radioisotopes, directly to the tumor site. To date, MoAbs have demonstrated limited success as a therapeutic option, and clinical trials continue for a variety of cancers.

Vaccines

The use of vaccines to treat cancer was first proposed more than 100 years ago. With a better understanding of the mechanisms of the immune response, new vaccine approaches are being investigated that are targeted toward specific antigens. Whereas the aim of vaccines for other diseases is to prevent contracting the disease, the goal of cancer vaccines is also to bolster the body's immune system to destroy cancer cells. Through clinical trials, vaccines are being investigated for several cancers, including B-cell lymphomas, multiple myeloma, melanoma, and renal, breast, colon, cervical, ovarian, prostate, and head and neck cancers.[63]

Anti-Angiogenesis Agents

As discussed in Chapter 16, tumors are dependent on angiogenesis (development of blood vessels) for continued growth and metastasis. Thalidomide (Thalomid) is being used to treat relapsed and refractory multiple myeloma. Thalidomide was first marketed in the 1960s in Canada and Europe as a sedative. It was removed from the market after being associated with phocomelia birth defects (absence of limbs) of children born to women who had used the drug. The anti-angiogenesis effect of the drug, which limited the normal growth of limbs in the neonate, is now being exploited to limit tumor growth and metastasis. Clinical trials using thalidomide in the treatment of other solid tumors are likely to yield other therapeutic applications of this agent. Many other anti-angiogenesis agents are also being investigated.[65]

Emerging Targeted Therapies

New approaches in cancer therapies are based on the recognition of the abnormality in the malignant cell and developing a treatment that targets the agent.

Imatinib mesylate (Gleevec) is an orally administered gene-directed therapy approved by the FDA for the treatment of chronic myelogenous leukemia (CML). It selectively blocks the abnormal *BCR-ABL* fusion gene (Philadelphia chromosome) that is vital to the survival and proliferation of CNL cells.[55]

Bone Marrow Transplantation

Bone marrow transplantation is discussed in Chapter 79. Although this is used as a primary treatment modality in leukemia, BMT may be used to counter the toxic effects of chemotherapy or XRT in the treatment of breast cancer, lymphoma, and other cancers. BMT allows the client to receive lethal and potentially more effective doses of chemotherapy and XRT without regard to hematopoietic toxicity. BMT replaces the marrow of damaged bone with healthy marrow.

The client's own marrow can be harvested before treatment (autologous BMT). An allogeneic BMT involves the use of marrow from a matching donor. If the client's own marrow was harvested, the marrow may or may not have been chemically treated to destroy any cancer cells. It is then stored (frozen) to be reinfused after the chemotherapy or XRT to "rescue" the bone marrow from the lethal effects of the treatment.

Clinical Trials

A clinical trial is a study conducted to evaluate a new treatment. The process of clinical trials allows scientific discoveries to be translated into safe, effective new therapies.[45] New drugs or treatment modalities are first evaluated through basic research studies in the laboratory and with animals. The most promising of these treatment approaches are then further assessed in clinical trials with human subjects. There are four phases of clinical trials:

- Phase 1: A small number of clients participate in phase 1 clinical trials. The purpose of these trials is to determine the maximum tolerated dose of a drug or treatment. The researchers also watch for harmful side effects. Treatments in phase 1 trials have been tested in the laboratory and in animals; it is not yet known how humans will respond. No direct benefit in terms of disease remission can be guaranteed. Because phase 1 studies involve significant risk without any promise of benefit, participation is offered only to people with advanced disease and for whom there are no other known treatment options. Safety, comfort, and ethical considerations are primary nursing concerns during phase 1 clinical trials.
- Phase 2: Phase 2 studies are developed using information obtained from the phase 1 study. The treatment is now offered to people with types of cancer

that responded in the phase 1 study. The purpose of a phase 2 study is to determine the effectiveness of the treatment against those cancers while continuing to learn more about the harmful effects of the treatment. As with phase 1 studies, participation in phase 2 studies is offered only to people for whom there are no known treatment alternatives.

- Phase 3: In a phase 3 study, a promising new treatment is compared with a standard treatment. On the basis of scientific evidence, the researchers believe that the new treatment is likely to be as good as or better than the current standard treatment. Clients who participate in phase 3 clinical trials are the first people to benefit from new, more effective treatment modalities.
- Phase 4: In phase 4 post-marketing surveillance studies, newly introduced drugs are monitored for adverse effects. Such studies may also compare two standard treatments. For example, surgery and XRT may be compared to determine whether the survival rate following XRT is similar to that after surgical treatment. Clinical trials are carried out on a nationwide basis with the pooled results used to determine and validate the effectiveness of treatment regimens.

Nurses have a major role to play in these research trials. The following are nursing responsibilities associated with caring for a client who is participating in a clinical trial:

- Client education
- Documentation of treatment benefits and side effects
- Anticipation of adverse reactions and early recognition of toxicity
- Management of side effects

Research nurses have even greater responsibilities for monitoring of clients, recruitment of participants, and dissemination of data.

Once the physician or a clinical trial nurse has identified a potential candidate, the client is invited to participate. A process to ensure informed consent could include a letter of invitation, informed consent education, and follow-up contact information for additional questions.[58] Written informed consents for participation in a clinical trial are often lengthy and can be overwhelming. In most settings, nurses are responsible for reviewing the written consent and the physician's verbal teaching with the client. You can often help by highlighting key information in the consent form, such as the purpose of the study, the treatments being compared, and whom to contact for more information. An NCI pamphlet[45] describes important questions a client should ask when considering participation in a clinical trial.

Self-Care

Complementary and Alternative Approaches

Public use of complementary and alternative medicine (CAM) therapies is growing.[30] Estimates suggest that up to 82% of clients have used CAM therapies sometime in their lives. Complementary approaches often combine one or more elements, such as (1) spiritual, psychological, nutritional, physical, pharmacologic, herbal, electromagnetic, or psychic approaches; (2) traditional medicines; (3) unconventional uses of conventional therapies; (4) unconventional instruments; and (5) humane approaches.

The Complementary and Alternative Therapy features below and on p. 288 describe two CAM therapies that may help prevent or treat cancer.

In research, prayer has been found to be a coping mechanism that correlates with perceptions of well-being.[60] Spirituality is a primary coping strategy for many people, as explained in the Translating Evidence into Practice box on p. 288. Although Sparber et al.[64] had not anticipated the high degree of importance of spirituality for clients, they concluded that there is a growing demand for integration of spirituality into health care. They also found that the use of CAM therapies increased clients' sense of control and well-being.

COMPLEMENTARY AND ALTERNATIVE THERAPY

Green Tea Supplements and Cancer

Using questionnaires, the prevalence, clinical characteristics, and pattern of use of green tea were evaluated among 102 clients with advanced malignancies who were receiving a phase 1 chemotherapy trial. Green tea was used most frequently by these clients. Other complementary treatments were also reported by the participants, including prayer, spiritual practices, and chiropractic treatment. While the use of complementary treatments among those enrolled in clinical trials is known to health care professionals, green tea may interact with investigational agents and affect adverse effects or efficacy. An earlier study by Pisters et al. found there were no major responses to green tea supplements in a small study of 49 clients with a variety of cancers (mostly non–small-cell lung cancer). The 49 clients consumed large doses of green tea supplements, equal to consuming 21 to 24 cups of green tea per day for 6 months.

REFERENCES

1. Dy, G., et al. (2004). Complementary and alternative medicine use by patients enrolled into phase 1 clinical trials. *Journal of Clinical Oncology, 22*(23), 4758-4763.
2. Pisters, K., et al. (2001). Phase 1 trial of oral green tea extract in adult patients with solid tumors. *Journal of Clinical Oncology, 19*(6), 1830-1838.

COMPLEMENTARY AND ALTERNATIVE THERAPY

Vitamin E Supplements and Cisplatin Chemotherapy for Cancer

A small study may have provided some insight into the possible benefits of certain supplements to reduce the risk of side effects from some chemotherapeutic drugs. Researchers recruited 47 clients who were randomly allocated to receive 300 mg/day of vitamin E supplements during cisplatin chemotherapy for cancer, or clients received cisplatin chemotherapy alone. Most of these clients were being treated for lung cancer, but some clients were being treated for ovarian, rhinopharynx, urethral, gastric, testicular, esophageal, ethmoidal, or tongue cancer. A total of 27 clients completed the cisplatin therapy (13 clients in the vitamin E group and 14 clients in the non–vitamin E group). The incidence of neurotoxicity (a side effect of cisplatin) was significantly reduced in the vitamin E group (30.7%) compared with the non–vitamin E group (85.7%, $p > .01$). The severity of neurotoxicity was also significantly reduced in the vitamin E group versus non–vitamin E group. Animal studies using a human tumor cell line also suggested that this combination does not inhibit treatment with cisplatin, but more clinical studies are needed. In addition, a placebo in combination with cisplatin would have been a better study. Regardless, it could be that vitamin E supplements reduce the risk of peripheral neurotoxicity associated with cisplatin chemotherapy for prostate cancer.

REFERENCE

Pace, A., et al. (2003). Neuroprotective effect of vitamin E supplementation in patients treated with cisplatin chemotherapy. *Journal of Clinical Oncology, 21*, 927-931.

TRANSLATING EVIDENCE INTO PRACTICE

Cancer Coping Strategies

Spirituality, hope, positive attitude, and support are factors reported in research studies to affect a person's ability to cope with cancer.[1-7] A research review determined that spiritual coping strategies and relationships with others and an ultimate other/God or nature were found to help individuals cope with ailments.[1] Following a review of nursing research from 1987 to 1999, Holt concluded the factors supporting hope for clients and families were social and professional support, cognitive strategies, spiritual or religious activities, reliance on inner resources, and establishment of goals.[5] Ferrell determined spirituality as the main coping mechanism of women survivors of ovarian cancer.[3] The major coping strategies for young adults with cancer were social support, belief in recovery, and returning to a normal life as soon as possible.[6] The family was the most important source of emotional support.[6] Gaining knowledge about cancer and its treatment was also a good coping strategy.[6] Moreover, a positive life attitude, belief in one's own resources, belief in God, earlier life experiences, and a willingness to fight against the disease were resources for coping with cancer.[6] Variables of self-esteem, social support, and helpfulness of religious beliefs were significant in determining levels of hope in women during breast cancer treatment.[2] A positive attitude was defined as being optimistic in the present and getting through everyday events by taking control rather than focusing on the future. Factors that affected clients' positive attitude were having good relationships with their specialists, having people around them that were positive and supportive, and having a pleasant environment at home and at the treatment center.[7]

Specific nursing interventions improved clients' perceptions of hope.[4,5] Nurses used interventions to support clients and families, assist with goal setting and distraction, affirm client worth, and provide symptom relief.[5] A quasi-experimental study sought to determine whether a specific nursing intervention program designed to enhance hope would positively influence levels of hope and quality of life in a convenience sample of 115 people with a first recurrence of cancer. The treatment group differed significantly (positively) from the control group with regard to level of hope and quality of life (QOL) immediately after intervention and across time.[4]

IMPLICATIONS

Whether a believer or nonbeliever, the onset of illness may cause an individual to realize the lack of control over his or her life. The use of spiritual coping strategies may enhance self-empowerment, leading to finding meaning and purpose in illness.[1-3] Clients with cancer must be positive for the present rather than the future. Nurses need to inspire and support client's positivity and hope while undergoing treatment for cancer.[7] Nurses should continue current practices to nurture hope in their clients. In addition, nurses need to provide spiritual care as an intervention that supports hope. Further research on nursing interventions is needed to stimulate hope as is research to understand the differences and relationships among hope, hopelessness, coping, courage, well-being, and spirituality across cultures.[5] Knowledge about the effectiveness of specific interventions designed to enhance hope is vital if nurses are to influence significantly those in their care.[4]

REFERENCES

1. Baldacchino, D., & Draper, P. (2001). Spiritual coping strategies: A review of the nursing research literature. *Journal of Advanced Nursing, 34*(6), 833-841.
2. Ebright, P., & Lyon, B. (2002). Understanding hope and factors that enhance hope in women with breast cancer. *Oncology Nursing Forum, 29*(3), 561-568.
3. Ferrell, B., et al. (2003). Meaning of illness and spirituality in ovarian cancer survivors. *Oncology Nursing Forum, 30*(2), 249-257.
4. Herth, K. (2000). Enhancing hope in people with a first recurrence of cancer. *Journal of Advanced Nursing, 32*(6), 1431-1441.
5. Holt, J. (2001). A systematic review of the congruence between people's needs and nurses' interventions for supporting hope. *Online Journal of Knowledge Synthesis Nursing, 8*(1), 10-20.
6. Kyngs, H., et al. (2001). Coping with the onset of cancer: Coping strategies and resources of young people with cancer. *European Journal of Cancer Care, 10*(1), 6-11.
7. Wilkes, L., et al. (2003). Positive attitude in cancer: Patient's perspectives. *Oncology Nursing Forum, 30*(3), 412-416.

Psychological approaches that are widely recognized yet underutilized include support groups, psychotherapy, imagery, biofeedback, and hypnosis. When used with antiemetic drugs, music can be an effective diversional therapy to decrease the frequency of nausea and vomiting. Guided imagery also can help control nausea and vomiting, create a relaxation response, and control pain. Art therapy can be used to help an adult with cancer gain insight into his or her situation.[60] See Chapter 4 for an overview of other complementary therapies and the NIH classifications.

Home Management of Side Effects

Aggressive, complex, and sophisticated cancer therapies are now being delivered in the ambulatory, office, and home care settings. This shift in care setting presents additional challenges for clients, family members, and health care providers. A high level of commitment is required from the client and family caregivers for the successful management of care in the outpatient setting. Clients and family members require education regarding complex treatment regimens. They must know how to recognize manifestations of side effects or adverse events, how to prevent side effects, and what they can do to treat the manifestations. Most important, they must know when to report manifestations and how to reach the physician—especially after office hours. When chemotherapy is administered in the home setting, provisions must be made for the safe handling and disposal of cytotoxic drugs to minimize client, family, and nurse exposure.[12]

Financial Concerns

Cancer can place a financial burden on the client and family. Direct costs include insurance deductibles and co-insurance. Unless the client has a prescription card, some medications, such as the serotonin (5-HT$_3$ [5-hydroxytryptamine]) antagonist antiemetics or oral chemotherapeutics, can cost more than the client can afford.

In addition, cancer treatment often produces many hidden costs. These costs may include transportation to appointments, meals while receiving treatment, new clothing to accommodate weight loss or gain, medical supplies, special foods or nutritional supplements, long-distance telephone calls, and loss of income for the client and/or family caregiver. Ten percent, or $104 billion, of the $1 trillion spent on health care annually is used for cancer care; of this amount, $35 billion is used for direct medical care, $12 billion for lost productivity, and $57 billion for mortality costs.[35]

EVALUATION OF TREATMENT RESPONSE

During and after treatment, each client is monitored for tumor response. These data are obtained by listening carefully to the client's history and the physical examination. If the client's cancer was symptomatic, the client may be able to predict that the treatment is working because the pain has lessened, breathing requires less effort, or other manifestations are subsiding.

When known disease remained after surgical intervention or diagnostic studies, repeating the imaging studies that were performed at the time of the diagnosis can be used to determine treatment effectiveness. Imaging studies are generally repeated after every two to three cycles of chemotherapy. If the tumor was associated with an elevated tumor marker at the time of diagnosis, testing for the marker again can be both a guide to the effectiveness of the chemotherapy and, later, a means of early detection of recurrence of the cancer. With ovarian cancer, a "second-look" surgical procedure may be performed after completion of the chemotherapy to verify that no detectable disease remains.

After treatment is completed, the client continues to be monitored for manifestations of disease recurrence and for delayed or long-term repercussions of the treatment. Depending on the type of cancer, follow-up appointments may initially be at 3-month intervals, eventually extending to 6-month and then 1-year intervals.

Nursing Management of Oncologic Treatment and Emergencies

Comprehensive and successful management of cancer-related manifestations—whether they are from the cancer itself or are side effects of treatment—is essential for achieving high-quality outcomes. For some clinical manifestations, urgent intervention is required to prevent undue morbidity or even mortality.

SAFETY ALERT

Three National Patient Safety Goals identified by TJC are (1) to comply with the current Centers for Disease Control and Prevention (CDC) hand hygiene guidelines to prevent infection (2) to manage all identified cases of unanticipated death or major permanent loss of function associated with health care associated infection as sentinel events, and (3) to recognize and report all changes in the client's health status. Infection, a potentially life-threatening complication in the client with neutropenia, is an oncologic emergency. When a person has few white blood cells, infection can progress quickly to septicemia and death unless aggressive intervention is instituted immediately. Failure to recognize, diagnose, and intervene for new-onset back pain can result in paralysis if the pain is secondary to spinal cord compression. Uncontrolled pain, discussed in Chapter 20, is often considered an oncologic emergency because it interferes with the client's relationships and activities of daily living.

Both antineoplastic medications and XRT can damage and destroy not only cancer cells but also normal cells.

See the website box titled Side Effects of Antineoplastic Drugs. Side effects to normal cells are evaluated or graded according to the degree of severity. Mild to moderate side effects generally do not warrant discontinuing or decreasing treatment. More severe or unexpected toxicities require careful evaluation, dose reduction, or treatment interruption.

Side effects associated with chemotherapy may be acute or delayed. Acute toxicities (1) tend to occur in tissues composed of rapidly dividing cells (bone marrow, hair, mucosa), (2) are frequently intermittent, and (3) generally resolve with complete recovery. In contrast, delayed or late effects can produce lifelong problems. Such effects include organ-specific treatment toxicities resulting in cardiac, renal, pulmonary, hepatic, reproductive, and neurologic dysfunction.

SAFETY ALERT

Because many of these problems appear after the client has returned home, the client and the client's caregiver must know how to recognize, monitor, and report side effects. When taking a telephone call from a client, you must be prepared to anticipate the potential complications related to the concern that led to the call. Telephone triage is a particularly challenging aspect of ambulatory care because you depend entirely on a verbal report to formulate an accurate picture of the client's situation and its urgency.

Myelosuppression

Myelosuppression may involve neutropenia, thrombocytopenia, or anemia. When all three side effects occur together, the condition is also known as pancytopenia.

Neutropenia

Infection and bleeding, often the result of diminished production of WBCs and platelets (thrombocytopenia) secondary to treatment, are common causes of death in clients with cancer. The time after chemotherapy administration when the WBC or platelet count is at the lowest point is referred to as the nadir. For most chemotherapeutic agents, the nadir occurs 7 to 14 days after drug administration. Knowledge of the blood count nadirs helps the health professional predict when the client is at greatest risk for infection and bleeding. Monitoring the CBC and differential count can identify when the nadir occurs and whether the client has adequate numbers of blood cells; it can also demonstrate evidence of impending bone marrow recovery.

The etiology of infections associated with cancer is multifactorial. Some cancers cause specific defects in the immune response. Side effects of treatment can result in myelosuppression (decreased RBCs, WBCs, and platelets). An impaired integumentary system increases vulnerability to infection. Corticosteroids, which are used in many treatment protocols, suppress immune functions. Neutropenia predisposes the client

to infection, especially infection by opportunistic endogenous (normally resident in the client's body or surroundings) organisms. More than half of the infections in clients with neutropenia are associated with organisms from the local environment. Major sources are food (raw fruits and vegetables), water, inhaled organisms, and organisms passed through direct contact. The client with neutropenia can quickly become septic, and the mortality rate from septicemia ranges from 30% to 80%.[66] For this reason, a CBC with differential count must be performed before administration of myelosuppressive (most chemotherapeutic) drugs and repeated periodically between treatments.

The two major types of WBCs are granulocytes (which include neutrophils) and agranulocytes. Neutrophils are the first and most numerous type of cell to arrive at any area of disease or tissue injury. When the number of neutrophils is substantially reduced, one of the body's prime defenses against infection is impaired. Therefore it is important to know what proportion of WBCs are neutrophils. The absolute neutrophil count (ANC) is calculated by multiplying the WBC count by the percentage of segmented and banded neutrophils in the CBC differential count:

$$ANC = WBC \times Neutrophils\ (\%)$$

In a CBC laboratory report, the neutrophils are often listed as segs (for segmented neutrophils) and as bands (banded neutrophils); the percentages of these two cells are added together to obtain the total percentage of neutrophils. For example, if the WBC count is 1200/mm^3 and the percentage of neutrophils (sum of the percentages of segmented and banded neutrophils) is 34%, the ANC is 408 ($1200 \times 0.34 = 408$).

Neutropenia is commonly defined as an ANC of less than 1000/mm^3. The frequency of infection increases (1) as the ANC decreases below 500/mm^3 and (2) with duration of the neutropenia. In the client with neutropenia, the usual manifestations of infection can be absent because of the lack of neutrophils to produce an adequate inflammatory response to the infection. Therefore a fever is the cardinal, and often the only, manifestation of infection. Three oral temperature readings exceeding 38° C (100° F) in 24 hours or one temperature reading exceeding 38.5° C (101.3° F) is considered diagnostic of a fever.

Because infections are associated with greater morbidity and mortality, the development of fever in a client with neutropenia should be treated as an oncologic emergency that mandates prompt assessment, diagnosis, and intervention. Prompt initiation of antibiotic therapy for a client with neutropenic fever will increase the likelihood of a positive outcome.[66] Measures to be taken generally consist of (1) cultures, chest x-ray, and physical evaluation to attempt to identify the source; (2) broad-spectrum antibiotic therapy; and (3) monitoring of vital signs. G-CSF or

GM-CSF may be prescribed to reduce the duration and severity of neutropenia. Nursing management of outcomes begins with teaching clients the measures to protect against infection and reinforcement of such teachings as WBC counts reach their nadir. These measures are the following:[6,48]

- Practice good personal hygiene, especially handwashing.
- Perform oral care daily and frequently rinse the mouth with an alcohol-free mouthwash, such as water or saline, four to six times per day.
- Maintain adequate nutrition and fluid intake.
- Do not share eating utensils with anyone.
- Avoid raw or uncooked foods during the nadir period. (There are few published studies on dietary restrictions to prevent infections.[61])
- Avoid crowds, people with infections, and children who have recently received any vaccinations.
- Avoid contact with animal excrement (e.g., bird, cat, or dog feces).
- Either avoid cut flowers or change the water of fresh flowers daily, adding 1 teaspoon of chlorine bleach to the new water.
- Get adequate rest and exercise.
- Avoid indiscriminate use of antipyretics (e.g., acetaminophen, aspirin) because they can mask fever.

Clients should also be taught that, even with the best precautions, infections cannot always be prevented. The importance of immediately reporting any manifestations of infection must be stressed; these manifestations include the following: (1) temperature reading greater than 38° C (100.4° F), (2) cough, (3) sore throat, (4) chills or sweating, and (5) frequent or painful urination. Prompt initiation of antibiotic therapy will increase the likelihood of a positive outcome.[6]

Thrombocytopenia

Thrombocytopenia resulting from chemotherapy can cause subtle to life-threatening bleeding. A high risk of hemorrhage exists with platelet counts less than $20,000/mm^3$. In the client with a solid (versus a hematologic) tumor, a platelet count greater than $10,000/mm^3$ puts the incidence of bleeding at less than 12%; however, fatal CNS hemorrhage or massive GI hemorrhage can occur. The platelet count usually recovers within 2 to 6 weeks after the recovery of the WBC count following chemotherapy. Chemotherapy is usually withheld until the platelet count rises to $100,000/mm$.

Nursing measures to manage outcomes are used to prevent bleeding or detect early clinical manifestations of bleeding. Instruct the client to do the following:

- Avoid injury by being cautious with sharp objects and using an electric razor rather than a blade razor.
- Use lotions to prevent dryness and cracking of the skin.
- Use lubrication (women) during sexual intercourse (if sexual activity is permitted during treatment).
- Maintain good oral hygiene; use a soft toothbrush, sponge, or oral swabs if the platelet count is very low; and report excessive bleeding of gums.
- Avoid constipation; use stool softeners if needed.
- Avoid enemas or rectal suppositories, and report any rectal bleeding.
- Avoid aspirin or nonsteroidal anti-inflammatory drugs (NSAIDs) if not prescribed.
- If nosebleeds or other external bleeding occurs, apply pressure on the source of bleeding for 10 to 15 minutes.
- Avoid taking temperatures rectally. If there is oral soreness or bleeding, take tympanic temperatures.
- Avoid intramuscular or subcutaneous injections; central lines can be used for parenteral medications.
- Notify the nurse or physician of manifestations of bleeding: petechiae (small red spots) or increased bruising, tarry stools, hypermenorrhea (heavy uterine bleeding), blood in urine or vomit, visual changes, and changes in level of consciousness (an early indication of intracranial hemorrhage).

Most oncologists use transfusions to keep a client's platelet count above $20,000/mm^3$ unless the client is known to have a platelet antibody. As previously mentioned, the thrombopoietic growth factor oprelvekin (Neumega) is available to prevent severe thrombocytopenia following myelosuppressive chemotherapy in clients with nonmyeloid malignancies.

Anemia

Anemia is experienced by half of all clients with cancer and can have multiple causes. There may be blood loss secondary to the disease. Abnormal destruction of RBCs is commonly a secondary disorder, arising from such causes as liver or spleen disease, BMT, nephrotoxic therapies, or myelosuppressive effects of chemotherapy and XRT. The most common cause of anemia in the client with cancer is inadequate production of RBCs, which can result from infiltration of the bone marrow by tumor or suppression of bone marrow production of RBCs by cancer therapy. Anemia leads to an impairment of oxygen delivery that is a common and predictable sequela of many cancer therapies. It can cause fatigue, headache, dizziness, fainting, pallor, dyspnea, palpitations, and tachycardia.

Anemia is an important component of cancer-related fatigue, which is one of the most common and distressing manifestations experienced by the client. Fatigue is poorly understood; no one definition describes all experiences. Research on cancer-related fatigue is inconclusive. It is difficult to predict with certainty which interventions will have therapeutic benefit for which clients. In addition to fatigue, anemic clients often experience decreased motivation and depression that interfere with normal activities. More clients identify fatigue as having more of a negative impact on their lives than cancer-related pain.[7,60] As advances are made in the scientific understanding of cancer-related fatigue, recommendations for interventions will very likely be altered.

Careful evaluation of exacerbating and relieving factors, the effect of fatigue on daily life, and personal and cultural influences as well as review of laboratory data add depth to the assessment of a client's fatigue and guide interventions.[7] Transfusions of packed RBCs can be used to relieve anemia that is producing manifestations. Erythropoietin may be prescribed to elevate or maintain the erythrocyte level and decrease the need for transfusions. Adequate levels of vitamin B_{12}, folic acid, and iron are also essential for erythropoiesis.[7] Other interventions can be grouped into three categories: (1) education, (2) exercise, and (3) attention-restoring activities. Clients who are taught that fatigue is expected report less fatigue than those who do not receive this information. Clients who balance exercise (such as walking) with rest report less fatigue. Engaging in activities that are interesting to the client may restore attention and the ability to think clearly.

Gastrointestinal Effects
Nausea and Vomiting
Gastrointestinal effects of chemotherapy include nausea and vomiting, anorexia, alteration in taste, weight loss, oral mucositis, diarrhea, and constipation. The vomiting center in the medulla can be stimulated by any of five different afferent pathways or by arousal of the chemoreceptor trigger zone located in the fourth ventricle of the brain. The emetic potential of a particular chemotherapeutic regimen depends on the drugs given, the dose, the route of administration, and the client's susceptibility to emesis. XRT to the chest, abdomen, or back can stimulate afferent pathways. Radiation-related emesis directly relates to the area, size, and dose delivered to the treatment field.

Adequate control of nausea and vomiting is an essential factor in a client's compliance with treatment. Uncontrolled nausea and vomiting, among the most feared treatment-related side effects, are experienced by as many as 60% of people receiving chemotherapy and can result in anorexia, malnutrition, dehydration, metabolic imbalances, psychological depression, and decreased immunity.

Three types of nausea and vomiting have been described. After the client has experienced nausea and vomiting, anticipatory nausea and vomiting may occur before the administration of further therapy. Acute post-therapy nausea and vomiting occur within minutes of the first 24 hours following therapy. Delayed nausea and vomiting consist of manifestations that persist or develop 24 hours after chemotherapy.

Management of nausea and vomiting has greatly improved because of heightened interest and research. The addition of serotonin receptor antagonists (5-HT$_3$) (e.g., ondansetron [Zofran], granisetron [Kytril], dolasetron [Anzemet]) to the drug armamentarium has improved the control of acute nausea caused by moderately to highly emetogenic (causing nausea and vomiting) chemotherapeutic agents. (For a discussion of the oral complications of cancer treatment, see the Translating Evidence into Practice box on p. 293.) These 5-HT$_3$ antagonists are particularly useful for acute nausea and vomiting during the first 24 hours. They control afferent pathway stimulation from the effects of the chemotherapy on the GI tract. Ongoing evaluation is essential to find the most effective dose, schedule, and combination of these drugs.[4]

Nonpharmacologic interventions for nausea and vomiting related to chemotherapy include adjustment of oral and fluid intake, relaxation, exercise, hypnosis, biofeedback, guided imagery, and systemic desensitization. The client and caregivers should avoid offensive odors and provide food in small, frequent meals.

Anorexia
Anorexia and weight loss occur as a result of the disease process and treatment. The client with cancer is at risk for protein-calorie malnutrition, which can lead to potentially severe consequences, including (1) diminished activity tolerance, (2) lowered survival rate, and (3) diminished quality of life. Many variables, in addition to the effects of chemotherapy, can alter the client's ability to ingest food via the oral route. Common problems are anorexia, nausea and vomiting, early satiety, alterations in taste, dry mouth, stomatitis, esophagitis, viscous saliva, lactose intolerance, pain, diarrhea, and constipation.

Nursing management to prevent a compromised nutritional state is based on assessment. Weight loss of 5% or more of body weight in a 1-month period is considered significant. When assessing the client, begin by identifying appropriate potential interventions. If indicated, a referral can be made to a dietitian for a more comprehensive assessment. When medically appropriate, oral nutrition can be enhanced by relaxing dietary restrictions and emphasizing the need for a high-protein, high-calorie diet with fortification from natural food sources or commercial supplements. An excellent source of helpful tips and recipes for nutritious foods can be found in the booklet *Eating Hints,* which can be obtained free of charge from the NCI.[42] Enteral and parenteral feedings for the client with protein-calorie malnutrition are discussed in Chapter 29.

Oral Complications of Cancer Treatment

In the past, nausea and vomiting and neutropenia were the most common dose-limiting toxicities of cancer therapy. The advent of serotonin receptor antagonists (ondansetron [Zofran], granisetron [Kytril], dolasetron [Anzemet]) and hematopoietic growth factors (G-CSF [Neupogen] and erythropoietin [Procrit]) has allowed for improved control of these treatment-related side effects. Mucositis is now the principal dose-limiting toxicity of cancer treatments.[5,8]

Mucositis is inflammation with erythema or ulceration of the mucous membrane resulting from cancer therapy. It often involves not only the oral cavity but also the mucous membrane of the entire GI tract. Pain and infection often accompany mucosal injury. The prevalence of mucositis varies widely with the multiple treatment protocols that use different chemotherapeutic agents or types of ionizing radiation. Of clients receiving chemotherapy, 30% to 40% experience oral complications. Up to 75% of clients receiving the agent 5-fluorouracil (5-FU) and 80% of clients undergoing hematopoietic stem cell transplant experience mucositis. Oral complications of head and neck radiation are often more severe than the complications of chemotherapy and can lead to permanent tissue changes.*

Oral complications can greatly affect morbidity and mortality and increase health care costs. Oral complications often necessitate dose reductions or treatment delays, which affects treatment outcomes, and prognosis. Along with the impact on the client's overall health and quality of life, this is a strong impetus for aggressive efforts to prevent or treat oral complications.[1,5,8,9,11] Because of pain and difficulty swallowing, nutritional intake can be impaired, resulting in dehydration and weight loss or cachexia. Mucositis may be further complicated by infection or bleeding. Mucosal atrophy of salivary glands secondary to radiation therapy can cause xerostomia. Oral pain, which can be severe, interferes with one's ability to talk, smile, or kiss a loved one.[2,5,8]

Recommendations gleaned from the current literature address the importance of an oral care standard. Systematic oral care is more important than any specific agent. This begins with identifying clients at risk and doing regular oral assessments.[5,6,8,11,13] Ideally, involvement of a dentist beginning before treatment may reduce the risks of oral complications.[12] The importance of hand-washing before beginning oral assessment or care is understood. Use of a tool such as the "Oral Assessment Guide" by Eilers and colleagues is helpful in ensuring a comprehensive oral assessment.[4,11] (see Fig. 28-3). A soft toothbrush has been found to be better than foam brushes and preferred by clients. A foam brush soaked in chlorhexidine can effectively remove plaque.[11] Electric toothbrushes may result in improved mouth care but may harm tender gums and cause bleeding.[10,12] Clients should also avoid whitening toothpastes.[5] Research dating back to the 1960s showed lemon-glycerin swabs do more harm than good because they decalcify the teeth, make the pH of the mouth more acidic, and dry mucous membranes. Yet it has taken decades to eliminate this nursing practice gradually.[3,5,10,11]

Dilute hydrogen peroxide was once routinely used as an oral rinse; however, studies have shown that it can harm new tissue,

interfere with healing, and promote fungal overgrowth. It should be used only for short periods as a cleansing agent.[11,12] Sodium bicarbonate or saline is often recommended as a mouthwash agent. Saline aids in the formation of granulation tissue. Sodium bicarbonate, however, creates an alkaline environment that can allow bacteria to multiply.[3,10,11] Chlorhexidine mouthwashes have the best antibacterial, antifungal effect, but they have an unpleasant taste and cause burning and stinging.[10,11] Fluoride rinses may be particularly beneficial for head and neck RT clients by preventing dental caries.[8] Clients should avoid most commercial mouthwashes because they contain 6% to 27% alcohol, which can dry the mucous membranes.[5,10,12] Frequent rinsing, however, is more important than the agent used. If clients do not like the taste of these agents, rinsing with plain water would be better than infrequent rinsing.[5] Recommendations for frequency of rinsing the mouth range from every 2 to 6 hours. Benefits of rinsing are diminished if the intervals are longer than 6 hours.[11-13]

Studies have shown conflicting findings on flossing. Flossing aids in the control of dental plaque; however, some cancer centers recommend not brushing or flossing if the platelet count falls below 30,000/mm.[3,12] Artificial salivas, often prescribed for clients with xerostomia, have short-lived action. Based on clinical experience, some clinicians recommend sugar-free gum, ice lollies, or sipping on water.[11] Pain associated with oral complications often is mild to moderate, but can be severe. It is most often described as tender, sore, burning, dull, aching, or irritating. Systemic analgesics may be necessary when topical agents such as viscous lidocaine are not sufficient for pain reduction. Clients may not experience oral pain until the mucositis or stomatitis is quite severe.[6,7,12] Teaching the client to do his or her own oral assessments and reinforcing the importance of regular mouth care are important because most cancer treatment is provided in the outpatient setting.[1,11]

IMPLICATIONS

Effective oral care must be a priority component of nursing care of the client receiving cancer treatment. Goals of oral care include cleanliness, comfort, and prevention of infection. Most research to date has focused on specific agents such as saline or other mouthwashes. Results have generally shown little difference and conflicting findings. Research and the experience of oncology professionals lend credibility to their recommendations.[9-11]

With our improved understanding of the biology of tissue injury, the potential for research is at a pivotal point. In addition to traditional agents, researchers are now looking at the potential for growth factors to reduce incidence of mucositis. Outcomes that could be studied include the extent or severity of tissue injury, pain, or infection; impairment of nutritional status; impact on health care costs or hospital length of stays; and quality of life. As new research is reported, nurses who want to provide great care must update their knowledge and adapt their caregiving to incorporate the latest scientific knowledge.[1,2,8]

REFERENCES

1. Coleman, E.A., et al. (2002). Symptom management and successful outpatient transplantation for patients with multiple myeloma. *Cancer Nursing, 25*(6), 452-460.
2. Dodd, M.J., et al. (2000). Factors influencing oral mucositis in patients receiving chemotherapy. *Cancer Practice, 8*(6), 291-297.

* References 2, 3, 5, 7, 8, 12.

(Continued)

TRANSLATING EVIDENCE INTO PRACTICE

Oral Complications of Cancer Treatment—Cont'd

3. Dose, A.M. (1995). The symptom experience of mucositis, stomatitis and xerostomia. *Seminars in Oncology Nursing, 11*(4), 248-255.
4. Eilers, J., Berger, A., & Peterson, M. (1998). Development, testing, and application of the oral assessment guide. *Oncology Nursing Forum, 15*, 325-330.
5. Eilers, J. (2003). When the mouth tells us more than it says—The impact of mucositis on quality of life. *Oncology Supportive Care, 1*(4), 31-43.
6. Ganley, B.J. (1996). Mouth care for the patient undergoing head and neck radiation therapy: A survey of radiation oncology nurses. *Oncology Nursing Forum, 23*(10), 1619-1623.
7. McGuire, D.B., et al. (1998). Acute oral pain and mucositis in bone marrow transplant and leukemia patients: Data from a pilot study. *Cancer Nursing, 21*(16), 385-393.
8. McGuire, D.B. (2002). Mucosal tissue injury in cancer therapy. More than mucositis and mouthwash. *Cancer Practice, 10*(4), 179-191.
9. Madeya, M.L. (1996). Oral complications from cancer therapy: Part 1—Pathophysiology and secondary complications. *Oncology Nursing Forum, 23*(5), 801-807.
10. Madeya, M.L. (1996). Oral complications from cancer therapy: Part 2—Nursing implications for assessment and treatment. *Oncology Nursing Forum, 23*(5), 808-819.
11. Miller, M., & Kearney, N. (2001). Oral care for patients with cancer: A review of the literature. *Cancer Nursing, 24*(4), 241-254.
12. National Cancer Institute. (2003). *Oral complications of chemotherapy and head/neck radiation*. Retrieved Aug 2003 from www.cancerinfo/pdg/supportivecare/oralcomplications/professionals.
13. Yeager, K.A., et al. (2000). Implementation of an oral care standard for leukemia and transplantation patients. *Cancer Nursing, 23*(1), 40-48.

Stomatitis

Stomatitis, or oral mucositis, is the term used to describe inflammation and ulceration of the mucosal lining of the mouth. The inflammation seen in the mouth is also present throughout the GI tract of a client receiving cancer treatment. The severity of the stomatitis can affect the client's quality of life. Consequences of stomatitis include pain, decreased nutritional and fluid intake, infections, malabsorption, diarrhea, and delay in chemotherapy and XRT treatments. *Candida* or other fungi that ordinarily live in the GI tract are generally harmless to individuals with healthy immune systems, but can become pathogenic to immunocompromised clients. *Candida* species are associated with mortality as well as significant morbidity and debility.

Nursing assessment of the oral cavity is discussed in Chapter 28, and interventions are discussed in Chapter 30. An oral hygiene program should start before therapy and should continue throughout treatment. Such a program consists of the following:

- A dental examination and completion of any treatment before beginning therapy
- Thorough and gentle dental cleaning to avoid further trauma
- Moisturization if saliva is scanty or absent
- Avoidance of alcohol and smoking
- Culture analysis and antimicrobial therapy for infections
- Topical anesthetics and analgesics for pain or discomfort

Dietary modifications include (1) avoiding extremely hot or cold foods, spices, and citrus fruits and juices; (2) eating soft foods; and (3) taking nutritional supplements.

Diarrhea and Constipation

Diarrhea is defined as an increase in stool liquid or frequency. It can result from GI mucosal damage secondary to XRT or chemotherapy. A low-residue or liquid diet is usually advised. Electrolyte levels and intake and output should be carefully monitored. Scrupulous perineal hygiene is encouraged, especially in the client with neutropenia. Antidiarrheal agents may be prescribed.

Constipation is frequently described as hard, dry stool with straining; a decrease in the number of defecations; or both. Causes include (1) a decrease in either fluid and fiber intake or mobility of clients; (2) changes in usual bowel routines; (3) mechanical changes, such as tumor pressure on the bowel; and (4) metabolic changes, such as hypokalemia or hypercalcemia. The vinca alkaloid chemotherapeutic agents (vinblastine, vincristine) can slow bowel peristalsis. Other causes of constipation are opioid use, tumor invasion of the GI tract, and depression. Preventive measures may be taken for constipation, such as increasing fluid and bulk intake, using stool softeners prophylactically, increasing physical activity, and using laxatives when necessary.

Integumentary Effects
Alopecia

Alopecia is a common side effect of many antineoplastic agents. The extent of hair loss depends on the specific drug, dosage, and method of administration. Alopecia tends to begin 2 to 3 weeks after the first treatment and is temporary. New hair growth tends to begin 4 to 6 weeks after the completion of chemotherapy and 8 to 9 weeks after XRT. Hair color and texture may change, but the hair usually returns to its former condition within a year. There can also be loss of body hair, including eyelashes, eyebrows, and pubic hair.

To help the client manage this side effect, which can be a traumatic change in body image and a constant reminder of the cancer, prepare the client for its occurrence. Begin by allowing the client to grieve for the hair loss. Having information available about where to obtain attractive wigs or turbans is helpful. Many ACS units offer a program called "Look Good, Feel Better," which involves the assistance of a volunteer beautician. Hair loss bothers men more than they acknowledge. Wigs are available for both men and women. Alternatively, many men choose to wear baseball caps to conceal the hair loss and to provide warmth.

Skin Reactions

The type of skin reactions that may occur in the client receiving chemotherapy depends on the drug administered. Red patches (erythema) or hives (urticaria) may appear at the drug injection site or on other body parts. These reactions generally disappear within several hours.

Darkening of the skin (hyperpigmentation) in the nail beds and mouth, on gums or teeth, and along the veins used for IV chemotherapy usually occurs within 2 to 3 weeks after administration of chemotherapy and continues for 10 to 12 weeks after the end of therapy. Sensitivity to sunlight (photosensitivity) may result in an acute sunburn after just a short exposure to the sun. The sensitivity disappears once treatment stops. The client should use sunscreen or protective clothing if sun exposure is anticipated.

A skin reaction called radiation recall may occur in clients who received XRT before the administration of chemotherapy. When chemotherapy is given several weeks or months later, a recall reaction occurs in the previously irradiated skin area. XRT skin effects range from redness, shedding, or peeling to blisters and oozing. After the skin heals, it is permanently darkened. It is important to maintain meticulous hygiene to avoid a superimposed infection in the area of radiation recall. Antibiotic therapy should be initiated at the first manifestation of infection.

Effects on the Reproductive System

Surgery, XRT, and chemotherapy each can have effects on sexual health and sexual self-image. Up to 25% of women undergoing modified radical mastectomy for breast cancer report problems with sexual functioning. Surgery can affect sexual functioning through impairment of the vascular supply, removal of organs, or reduction of circulating hormone levels. Among women treated with XRT for cervical cancer, 55% to 78% report sexual impairments. Body image, sexual functioning, and fertility can be affected by chemotherapy.[59] Not all clients experience these effects to the same degree. Preliminary studies suggest that the effects of chemotherapy on gonadal function vary with respect to the client's age at the time of therapy, the drugs administered, and the total drug dosage.

Administration of antineoplastic agents during the first trimester of pregnancy increases the risk of spontaneous abortion and fetal malformations. Second- and third-trimester chemotherapy exposures may result in low birth weight or prematurity. A pregnancy begun after cytotoxic

chemotherapy has about the same chance of a successful outcome as a normal pregnancy.[59] The genetic effects of chemotherapy may not be evident for several generations of offspring. You should discuss the unpredictability of occurrence, degree, and duration of genetic damage with the client and the client's significant other.

Although you may not be comfortable talking about sexuality issues, you can still be an important source of support by giving the client permission to express concerns about this aspect of cancer therapy. Begin simply by asking open-ended questions about how the cancer experience has changed the client's relationships. Beyond providing information yourself, offer to seek further information or to consult with a colleague who may have additional information or suggestions to alleviate or at least ease the concern.

The PLISSIT (permission, limited information, specific suggestions, intensive therapy) model for evaluation of sexual function can be used for assessment purposes.[59] See Chapter 41 for further discussion of the PLISSIT model. Pretreatment sperm banking offers the possibility of retaining reproductive capacity for some clients. Use of vaginal lubricants, methods of dilating the vagina after XRT for cervical cancer (see Chapter 39), and penile prostheses (see Chapter 38) are topics you can discuss. Counseling with a sexual therapist may be indicated.

Oncologic Emergencies

Infection, pain, spinal cord compression, hypercalcemia, syndrome of inappropriate antidiuretic hormone (SIADH), cardiac tamponade, superior vena cava syndrome, tumor lysis syndrome, and disseminated intravascular coagulation (DIC) are oncologic emergencies. If not identified early and treated, oncologic emergencies can result in severe morbidity and death. Each oncologic emergency is discussed only briefly here. **A TJC National Patient Safety Goal emphasizes the role of the nurse in assessing and urgently reporting sometimes subtle manifestations to ensure the best possible outcome for the client.**

SAFETY

ALERT

Consult other cancer nursing texts for further information on oncologic emergencies.

Oncologic emergencies can be grouped as follows:

- Metabolic (infection and pain, hypercalcemia, tumor lysis syndrome, SIADH, DIC)
- Structural (spinal cord compression, superior vena cava syndrome, cardiac tamponade)

Infection and Pain

Infection, which can quickly progress to a life-threatening emergency in the client with neutropenia, was previously discussed. Although pain does not usually arise suddenly or unexpectedly, it is often regarded as an oncologic emergency because it is such a pervasive problem. 🏮 As many as one third of clients in active treatment and 60% to 90% clients with advanced cancer have pain.[2,35,46] Pain interferes with the ability to enjoy activities and relationships that are meaningful. For nursing management of pain, see Chapter 20.

Hypercalcemia

Second to infection, hypercalcemia is the most commonly occurring oncologic emergency, and it can be a potentially fatal condition. Hypercalcemia is due to bone resorption (demineralization) of calcium and is defined as a serum calcium level greater than 11 mg/dl. 🏮 If the client also has a decreased level of serum albumin, a common finding with cancer, a corrected serum calcium value should be used. Of cases of cancer-related hypercalcemia, 80% occur with solid tumors, including breast, lung, head, neck, and renal cancers. The remaining 20% of cases occur in hematologic cancers, such as multiple myeloma, leukemia, and lymphoma.

If the serum calcium level rises slowly, the client may be asymptomatic for a time. When it rises swiftly, renal failure, coma, cardiac arrest, and death can result. Early manifestations may be difficult to distinguish from other cancer- or treatment-related manifestations, such as anorexia, fatigue, nausea and vomiting, constipation, excessive thirst, polyuria, poor skin turgor, and dry mucous membranes. Late manifestations include severe muscle weakness, diminished deep tendon reflexes, paralytic ileus, and electrocardiographic (ECG) changes.

Nursing management begins with the recognition of clients at risk for hypercalcemia, including clients with (1) cancer of the breast, lung, head, neck, or kidney; (2) multiple myeloma; (3) leukemia; (4) lymphoma; and (5) potential or actual bone metastases. Maintaining adequate hydration and mobility is an important preventive measure for the at-risk client. Limiting dietary intake of calcium has little or no effect. Clients and caregivers should be instructed on which manifestations should be reported.

Medical management of hypercalcemia is aimed at controlling the growth of the tumor causing the hypercalcemia and administering drugs to lower serum calcium levels, such as calcitonin (Miacalcin) and oral glucocorticoids. For the client with advanced disease, for whom other interventions are no longer effective, treatment is aimed at comfort care.

Tumor Lysis Syndrome

Tumor lysis syndrome is a potentially fatal metabolic emergency that develops as a tumor responds to treatment. When a large, bulky tumor is responsive to treatment, especially chemotherapy, the destruction of a large number of malignant cells may rapidly release intracellular potassium, phosphorus, and uric acid into the circulation. Electrolyte imbalances and acute renal failure

usually begin 1 to 2 days after treatment starts and cease within a week after completion of therapy. Clients with malignancies that are very responsive to treatment are at highest risk, especially if they have a large tumor burden. Such malignancies include aggressive lymphomas, acute leukemias, or other bulky chemosensitive solid tumors such as small-cell carcinoma of the lung. Clients with pre-existing renal compromise are also at greater risk.[11]

Medical management focuses on prevention in high-risk clients. Aggressive IV hydration is initiated before treatment and continues until after treatment ends. Allopurinol (Zyloprim) is administered to decrease uric acid concentration. Sodium bicarbonate may be given in conjunction with IV hydration to promote fecal excretion of excess phosphate.

Despite preventive measures, tumor lysis syndrome may occur. If so, the goal is to remove potassium from the extracellular fluid with medications, retention enemas, or IV 50% dextrose, all of which act to increase plasma insulin level and thereby force potassium back into the intracellular fluid. When preventive and maintenance measures are not effective, renal dialysis may be required.

The most important nursing management responsibility is to recognize and report manifestations of tumor lysis syndrome immediately. Nursing management focuses on maintaining fluid and electrolyte balance by carrying out medical orders, including IV hydration, monitoring weight daily, and maintaining a record of intake and output. Clinical manifestations to observe and report are (1) weakness, (2) nausea, (3) diarrhea, (4) flaccid paralysis, (5) ECG changes, (6) muscle cramps or twitching, (7) oliguria (diminished urine output), (8) hypotension, (9) edema, and (10) altered mental status. Especially when treatment is provided in the outpatient ambulatory setting, the client and family must be taught about which manifestations to report immediately.

Syndrome of Inappropriate Antidiuretic Hormone

Syndrome of inappropriate antidiuretic hormone (SIADH) results from the abnormal production of antidiuretic hormone (ADH). The incidence of SIADH is relatively low, occurring in only about 1% to 2% of clients with cancer. Of clients with cancer-related SIADH, 80% have an underlying diagnosis of small-cell lung cancer. Other causes of SIADH are infection, pulmonary disorders, emotional stress, CNS disorders, and some drugs, including such antineoplastic agents as cyclophosphamide (Cytoxan), vincristine (Oncovin), vinblastine (Velban), and cisplatin (Platinol-AQ). Manifestations, which are related to the rates of onset of the decrease in sodium level and the increase in water retention, include (1) confusion, (2) irritability, (3) headache, (4) muscle weakness, (5) lethargy, (6) decreased urine output, (7) edema, (8) nausea and vomiting, and (9) anorexia.

Syndrome of inappropriate antidiuretic hormone is not a preventable complication. It is a medical emergency only when the hyponatremia is severe (<120 mEq/L) and the client experiences manifestations. Mild SIADH is treated conservatively with fluid restriction (<500 to 1000 ml/day). The body should be able to normalize the serum sodium concentration and osmolality in approximately 7 to 10 days. An IV infusion of hypertonic saline (3% to 5%) is given in severe cases to prevent pulmonary edema. Pharmacologic agents for treatment of SIADH include demeclocycline (Declomycin), lithium (Lithane), and urea. Beyond symptomatic treatment, the goal of medical management is to treat the underlying disease causing the SIADH.

Disseminated Intravascular Coagulation

Disseminated intravascular coagulation (DIC) involves the development of extensive, abnormal clots throughout small blood vessels. The widespread clotting consumes all circulating clotting factors and platelets, leading to excessive bleeding from several sites. The bleeding can be minimal or life-threatening. Also, clots that are blocking blood vessels decrease blood flow to major organs, which can cause pain, stroke-like manifestations, dyspnea, tachycardia, and oliguria and bowel necrosis. The mortality rate is near 70% despite appropriate treatment.

In clients with cancer, DIC is often caused by gram-negative infection or sepsis, release of thrombin or thromboplastin (clotting factors) from cancer cells, or blood transfusions. DIC is most commonly associated with leukemia and adenocarcinomas of the lung, pancreas, stomach, and prostate. Management involves treating the cancer and other measures as discussed in Chapter 75.

Spinal Cord Compression

Even for the terminally ill client in a hospice setting, early detection and intervention in spinal cord compression are vital. Failure to intervene in this emergency can leave the client with permanent neurologic disabilities. Spinal cord compression is caused by direct pressure on the cord or by compromise of the vascular supply to the spinal cord. Back pain is often the only early presenting clinical manifestation, occurring in 95% of clients. Other early manifestations are motor weakness and decreased sensation. Depending on the rate of tumor growth, it may take only hours or days for the spinal cord compression to progress to irreversible neurologic damage with paralysis and loss of bowel and bladder control. Late manifestations are motor loss, additional sensory loss, constipation, and urinary hesitancy.[39]

In a client with known cancer, new-onset back pain is a "red flag" signaling immediate evaluation. Pain localized over the involved area of the spine or radicular (belt-like) pain is present in more than 90% of clients with spinal cord compression. Carefully assess new-onset back pain; have the client point to the location of the pain and show you the areas in which the pain is distributed. Also carefully assess for any other clinical manifestations of neurologic deficit, such as numbness, tingling, constipation, and voiding hesitancy.

Data from the medical record can be helpful in determining whether the client has known bone metastasis. Provide a complete assessment to the physician, including a description of the location and characteristics. These data will provide the physician with the information needed to consider spinal cord compression in the differential diagnosis.

Treatment is usually with XRT unless the tumor is resistant to XRT or the client has already received the maximum XRT dose in the involved area. A laminectomy for spinal cord decompression is an alternative. For the client in a hospice setting whose life expectancy is limited to days or weeks, administration of steroids to lessen the inflammation and swelling around the spinal cord can be a less aggressive but effective short-term alternative.

Superior Vena Cava Syndrome

Distressing but rarely life-threatening, superior vena cava (SVC) syndrome is a disorder that results from internal or external obstruction of the SVC. The obstruction reduces venous blood return to the heart and compromises cardiac output. SVC syndrome should be evaluated as an emergency because of concern for respiratory compromise. The onset of manifestations is usually gradual; however, if SVC syndrome was the presenting manifestation of cancer, time should be taken to diagnose accurately the underlying disease before treatment is initiated.

Typically, SVC syndrome is secondary to lung cancer, usually small-cell carcinoma (65%) or lymphoma (8%). The classical presenting manifestations are dyspnea (63%) and facial swelling (50%) with jugular vein distention. The client is often sitting up and leaning forward to breathe. Other manifestations are swelling of the arms, pain in the chest, and dysphagia.

The goals of medical management are to provide rapid palliation of the distressing manifestations and to treat the underlying cancer. External-beam XRT continues to be the standard of care for palliation; however, clients with small-cell carcinoma of the lung or lymphoma may be palliated with the appropriate curative chemotherapy regimen with or without the addition of XRT.

Cardiac Tamponade

Early detection and proper management of cardiac tamponade (acute compression of the heart) are critical to preventing cardiovascular collapse and death. When fluid collects in the pericardial sac (pericardial effusion), it affects the heart's ability to function properly and leads to cardiac tamponade. Normally the pericardium contains 15 to 50 ml of fluid; the pericardial sac may contain as much as 200 to 1800 ml of fluid before the heart begins to decompensate. The fluid prevents the heart from filling and contracting normally.

The onset of this condition may be insidious. The most common manifestations are tachycardia, severe dyspnea, cough, chest pain, edema, and hypotension. You may notice a narrowing of the pulse pressure (the difference between systolic and diastolic readings) or pulsus paradoxus (decreased or absent amplitude of the pulse with inspiration). Heart sounds may be muffled by the fluid. Jugular venous distention may be prominent. A chest x-ray is a cost-effective screening tool, although it cannot always visualize cardiac tamponade. An ECG will show a number of changes that could indicate tamponade.

Medical management of cardiac tamponade is individualized for the client. A pericardiocentesis (insertion of an 18-gauge needle into the chest to draw off the fluid) may be performed. Because the fluid can accumulate again, a pericardiotomy may be performed; this surgical procedure creates a window or opening in the pericardial sac for subsequent drainage of fluid. Even then, the pericardial fluid can accumulate again. Nursing management consists of carefully assessing clinical manifestations and teaching the client and family caregiver to watch for manifestations that may herald impending cardiac tamponade.

PSYCHOSOCIAL ASPECTS OF CANCER CARE

When cancer becomes a part of life's journey, it is hard work. (See the Bridge to Home Health Care feature on Dealing with Grief Related to a New Cancer Diagnosis on the website.) The diagnosis of cancer affects not only the individual but also the client's family. Because cancer is not just a physical disease, it compels the clients—and health care professionals—to face the meaning of their lives and their relationships. Just as life experiences affect the perceptions a client brings to the cancer experience, so do your life experiences affect the perceptions you bring to the client's care. It is therefore valuable for you to reflect on your beliefs and values about life and death and their meaning.

Providing Support for Clients

The most valuable intervention you can offer a client with cancer is your presence as a caring person. The dimensions of your presence consist of verbal expressions of empathy, positive regard, and availability of practical support.[60] Fellow clients can have a significant impact on clients with cancer. One practical source of support is taking this into consideration when making inpatient room assignments.

Hearing the stories of colleagues, clients and their families, and survivors can be a vehicle for a novice nurse to learn the art of cancer nursing. Storytelling is becoming recognized for its value.[17] A story can be a means of providing comfort by offering social comparisons (helping clients know how others have coped and felt in a similar situation) or lessons from others' experiences.

There is great variability in the distress, changes, and other effects of cancer in the lives of clients and their families. Responses to cancer depend on the following:

- The disease, the disabilities, and disfigurements it may cause
- Any pre-existing medical conditions that limit treatment options
- The client's psychological make-up and spiritual well-being
- The client's family and social community
- The availability of medical and financial resources

Providing Support for the Family

The diagnosis of cancer has an effect on the client's entire family. Daily life is changed. Other family members may need to assume the role or responsibilities of the client or serve as a caregiver. Nursing often views the family as the context of caring for the client with cancer; the family needs to be the unit of care. A family's resources, perceptions of the cancer, functioning patterns, coping strategies, and stressors are factors affecting their ability to respond to the crisis of cancer.[35,60] Much of the distress for the client and the family can be lessened with minimal assistance from the health care team. Without these services, even highly functioning families struggle.

Promoting Positive Self-Concept

Cancer affects all levels of functioning. Physical and psychological distress, medications, or the disease itself can cloud the client's intellectual function. The client's self-concept is affected by physical, role, or function changes. A breadwinner may become dependent on others and become a consumer of family savings and resources. The young adult, striving for independence, may need to revert to an earlier level of dependency.

Body image also changes for most clients. Weight loss, hair loss, and skin changes can result from treatment. Radical surgical procedures can make devastating and permanent changes in appearance and function. Procedures such as laryngectomy, glossectomy, mastectomy, and prostatectomy may result in physical changes that humiliate and overwhelm the client.

Promoting Coping Throughout the Cancer Continuum

Although each cancer experience is unique, people with cancer have some common problems. Strategies for outcome management to help clients cope with the disease and its treatment are addressed for each phase of the cancer continuum: diagnosis and treatment, survivorship, recurrent disease and progression, and terminal illness.

Diagnosis and Treatment

Clients reach the point of cancer diagnosis in many ways. A client may have had vague manifestations, such as weight loss and fatigue, that may have been ignored or a cause of some anxiety for weeks or months. Another client may have manifestations, such as pain or abdominal bloating, that evaded diagnosis. Many times, cancer is found incidentally during a routine examination. Often the client suspects cancer, but many people are shocked when the diagnosis is made. The diagnostic period may be long and extremely stressful. This period is filled with anxiety about each test result, especially when staging procedures are performed. More than 70% of clients consider the time of diagnosis and treatment as the most stressful in the cancer experience.[70]

Most clients fear death during the first few months of the cancer experience. Whether clients can express their fears or not, it is an underlying cause of distress. During diagnosis the magnitude of the client's problems becomes apparent. The client may speculate on the following questions: Is my disease curable? Will my disabilities be temporary or permanent? What types of physical impairment will occur? What will be the side effects of treatment? Will my manifestations be relieved? Will I be able to return to work? What adjustments have to be made in family life or work? Will finances be adequate? What plans need to be abandoned? Which changes in lifestyle will be temporary and which permanent?

Clients must deal with health-related problems and with the emotional distress that occurs at this time. They may feel angry and frustrated because their lives have been changed; they may feel isolated or may worry about being abandoned by family and friends. They may be shocked and unbelieving that they are the ones with cancer. They may also feel guilty if they believe they have contributed to their disease through behavior, such as by smoking, drinking, or putting themselves at risk for sexually transmitted diseases.

Clients' reactions vary greatly. The initial response to the diagnosis of cancer may be profoundly influenced by previous life experiences with the disease. When the disease is advanced at the time of diagnosis, the client and family are likely to experience more psychological distress as they are confronted with the dual stressors of a cancer diagnosis and a terminal illness.[70] Some have minimal distress, whereas others may be overwhelmed and devastated. You may sometimes feel, on the basis of your own personality and experience, that a client is responding inappropriately to a cancer diagnosis. It is crucial, however, to acknowledge every client's response as acceptable and unique for that client.

Weisman[70] identified coping styles used by many clients with cancer (Box 17-1). Denial, which is a part of coping, allows a client to "repudiate what cannot be avoided, by substituting a more favorable or agreeable idea."[53] Denial can be useful as a healthy coping mechanism in the diagnostic phase, when the number of problems may be overwhelming. Denial is harmful when it prevents the client from seeking appropriate treatment.

Clients who are good problem-solvers or who cope effectively tend to confront reality, avoid excessive denial, remain flexible, accept support, and stay hopeful and optimistic. Clients who cope poorly use avoidance and excessive denial; they are pessimistic and feel hopeless. Every client uses a variety of strategies.

Families also should be assessed for their coping abilities. Use of a specific family assessment tool may not be possible, but you may be able to identify "high-risk" families from your interaction. Unresolved past problems may affect a family's ability to cope. Families who use excessive denial, exhibit strong anger and guilt, or are unreasonably demanding may be at increased risk for dysfunction. When the client is the pivotal person in

---

BOX 17-1   General Coping Strategies

- Seek more information (rational inquiry).
- Share concern and talk with others (mutuality).
- Laugh it off; make light of the situation (affect reversal).
- Try to forget; put it out of your mind (suppression).
- Do other things for distraction (displacement, redirection).
- Take firm action on the basis of present understanding (confrontation).
- Accept but find something favorable (redefinition, revision).
- Submit to the inevitable (fatalism, passive acceptance).
- Do something—anything—however reckless or impractical (impulsivity).
- Consider or negotiate a feasible alternative (if *x*, then *y*).
- Reduce tension with excessive drink, drugs, danger (life threats).
- Withdraw into isolation; get away (disengagement).
- Blame someone or something (externalization, projection).
- Seek direction; do what you are told (cooperative compliance).
- Blame yourself; sacrifice or atone (moral masochism).

Modified from Weisman, A. 1979. *Coping with cancer.* New York: McGraw-Hill.

the family or when the family has had a previous experience of cancer with a negative outcome, their need for ongoing psychosocial support systems may be increased.

Actively listen for remarks that describe the meaning and effect of cancer as experienced by the client. Often, time limitations do not permit you to provide support separate from physical caregiving. Consequently, while giving care, take the opportunity to initiate social interactions, such as chatting about family, sharing stories, or greeting visitors. Consider these actions a professional intervention. What did you learn about the client's perceptions of cancer? What coping mechanisms did the client or significant others use with past lifestyle changes? How will the client's and the family's lives be affected? What needs for teaching or community resources did you note? Would referrals to other members of the health care team, such as the chaplain and social worker, be helpful?

Providing social support and improving the client's sense of control help to reduce anxiety. Stress reduction or relaxation techniques can be taught. Speaking with cancer survivors encourages many clients. Support groups and one-to-one visitation programs such as Reach to Recovery or CanSurmount (ACS) provide this opportunity. Internet support groups offer the same opportunity for clients who are uncomfortable with the face-to-face interactions of a traditional support group.

Informational needs of the client and family are great during the diagnostic and treatment periods. Tests, procedures, and treatments, which are often technical and complicated, must be explained. Present consistent, accurate information in as much detail as the client wants. Be sure that all health care providers are telling the client the same thing. When clients from a cancer clinic were surveyed, information and support from family, friends, and caregivers were identified as high-priority needs (Box 17-2).

Address specific problems by (1) helping the client identify them, (2) providing information when necessary, and (3) referring the client to appropriate resources. Both the NCI and the ACS provide useful written materials to reinforce teaching. Site-specific information can be obtained from the NCI via the Internet (www.nci.nih.gov or www.cancer.gov), by Fax (301-402-5874), or via telephone (1-800-4-CANCER). Other key Internet websites may be bookmarked on a computer in the clinical area or in a client library.

Survivorship

Clients who have completed successful treatment enter an indeterminate period of long-term survivorship. Survivorship has been divided into a time of acute survival followed by a period of extended survival. Transition between these periods is not precise but evolves as time passes and the cancer does not recur.

> ### BOX 17-2 Needs of Clients with Cancer
>
> The following are needs identified by those with cancer. While nurses should always treat clients as they wish to be treated, the following suggestions may make this difficult time easier.
> 1. Accept the person unconditionally.
> 2. Make plans for the future.
> 3. Keep communication open, but let the person with cancer set the pace.
> 4. Be sincere when providing support and reassurance.
> 5. Assist and encourage referrals to community services.
> 6. Be a good listener, and try to feel comfortable with silence.
> 7. Visit; if words fail, a loving look or touch can say a lot.
> 8. Ask the patient with cancer what you can do to help, and then follow-through.
> 9. Do not share privileged communication with others without permission.

Modified from *Listen with your heart: Talking with the person who has cancer.* American Cancer Society, 2002.

Depending on the extent of treatment, the period of extended survival may still be one of physical fatigue and limitation. Physical rehabilitation to improve functioning may dominate the client's energy in this early period. Efforts focus on restoring the client's previous level of functioning.

The long-term physical effects of cancer treatment are now becoming apparent as data accumulate, especially from clients with pediatric cancer.[53] The physical effects may range from minimal restriction to life-threatening complications. The effects can be organ-specific, such as cardiomyopathy or pulmonary fibrosis, or general, such as fatigue.

The potential for development of a second malignancy as a result of primary treatment is always a possibility. Although this possibility is usually rare, some studies have reported up to a 20% occurrence of another cancer after treatment of Hodgkin's disease and other cancers with alkylating agents.

Psychologically, the period of extended survival is one in which clients must assume previous roles or adjust and reorganize their lives. The possibility of recurrence may dominate their lives. Plans may be suspended. Decisions about changing jobs, buying a house, starting a family, or beginning retirement may be difficult in the face of the uncertainty of recurrence or concerns about insurance coverage.

Making sure the client adheres to routine follow-up and long-term health care with attention to prevention and early detection (health promotion) will provide early detection of recurrent cancer and second primary sites as well as early intervention for late effects of treatment. Follow-up appointments and events such as National Cancer Survivors Day celebrations (which are held in many communities each June) are opportunities to obtain emotional support, alleviate fears of recurrence, and let clients know that they are not alone in their feelings and concerns.

Employment discrimination has been problematic for cancer survivors. Despite the fact that clients with a cancer history are dependable and productive, studies show that as many as 84% of blue-collar workers and 38% of white-collar workers with cancer experience some type of discrimination in employment. Over the years, these issues have been partially rectified by state laws protecting the rights of the disabled.

Obtaining insurance coverage with a history of cancer has also been difficult, ruinously expensive, and sometimes impossible. Legislative efforts have corrected some of these problems. Insurance discrimination can be legally appealed. Federal programs such as the Consolidated Omnibus Budget Reconciliation Act (COBRA) protect the insurance coverage of an employee for 18 months after termination of employment but at an increased monthly premium. A client, spouse, or parent may be trapped in an unrewarding job to maintain the employer-funded group insurance. Direct clients who have difficulty with insurance coverage to contact the National Coalition for Cancer Survivorship, the ACS, their state department of human rights, or their state insurance department. The NCI booklet *Facing Forward* provides detailed information about resources.[66]

With time, these problems usually recede and clients move into a period of extended survival. The experience of cancer is nonetheless indelibly imprinted on their lives. Amazingly, most clients cope well and face the difficulties in their lives with courage. For many clients the experience triggers a reappraisal of goals and values, making life richer and more meaningful.

Recurrent Disease and Progression

Most clients with cancer live with the threat or reality of recurrent disease. Weisman[70] describes the effect that this phase has on the client as "the hope for a cure" becoming the "struggle for existence." With recurrent cancer, therapy may once again be used to eradicate or stabilize the disease process.

Although subsequent recurrent disease may occur, it is usually the first recurrence that causes surprise, shock, and disbelief in the client. Physical impairment may be greater, and quality of life may be limited because of disease or treatment. The client who previously projected an optimistic outlook may now express a more guarded attitude. Maintain open communication and be sensitive to the informational and support needs of the client and family.

Clients at this stage in the cancer continuum are usually not in imminent danger of dying. They are generally aware of the likely eventuality of death. Often they still want to continue treatment. Surgery, XRT, or chemotherapy may still be of value for palliation of manifestations regardless of whether the treatment extends life. Surgery, XRT, or chemotherapy may be used to palliate complications caused by persistent tumor growth. For example, surgery may be used to manage a malignant obstruction, or XRT may be used to prevent paralysis from spinal cord compression. Palliative treatment is not curative but is aimed at improving the quality of the remainder of the client's life, however long or short.

Although clients at this stage may not qualify for traditional hospice care, they could benefit from the supportive services and management of manifestations offered by hospice programs. Increasingly, hospitals are developing supportive care programs or palliative care teams to meet these needs. Palliative care is the provision of management of manifestations and psychosocial support, best offered by a multidisciplinary health care team. Palliative care can be added gradually as the cancer and its manifestations progress. Clients can participate in evaluating when the side effects of treatment modalities such as chemotherapy outweigh the benefits of palliating cancer manifestations. Increasingly today, professionals are recognizing the value of incorporating quality-of-life outcomes for clients throughout the course of their illness. Palliative care programs combine the medical model's goal to prolong life with hospice goals to relieve manifestations and improve the quality of clients' remaining time.[16,24,35] See Chapter 21 for further discussion of palliative care.

Terminal Illness

About 50% of clients with cancer will die of their disease. The time from diagnosis to death ranges from weeks to years. Not all clients with cancer become terminally ill. Some clients die during the initial treatment; others die of complications of treatment. Many, however, reach an end-point at which their cancer no longer responds to treatment and progression of the disease cannot be controlled. Then the goal of treatment is directed toward providing supportive care and minimizing distress until death occurs. See Chapter 21 for an overview of hospice and palliative care.

CONCLUSIONS

Cancer therapy is progressing rapidly at the beginning of the 21st century. Many cancers once considered incurable are now controlled with a variety of combination therapies. Even when cancer is not cured, length of life may be extended and the quality of this life has greatly improved. Professionals have greater knowledge of and skills in controlling pain and managing nausea and vomiting resulting from chemotherapy, and more options are available for helping clients cope with hair loss.

The hospice movement has demonstrated that there is still much that can be done for a client with cancer, even when cure is no longer possible. The survivorship movement has made visible the hopeful side of cancer as well as become a resource to clients in dealing with insurance, workplace, and other issues.

New treatment modalities are showing promise in clinical trials, with some already becoming standard care. The nurse for the 21st century needs to stay abreast of new developments in this rapidly expanding field.

THINKING CRITICALLY

1. You are a nurse working in a health clinic that focuses on prevention of disease. This month, the featured goal is cancer prevention. How will you assess each client for cancer risk factors?

Factors to Consider. How would you develop an assessment tool for the clinic nurses to use? How would you adapt teaching strategies to the cultural group being served? What teaching can help clients to avoid factors that increase their risk of cancer?

2. The client is a 22-year-old man who comes to the neighborhood health clinic with concern that his companion, who has pain and a lump in the right testicle, may have testicular cancer. The companion is at home. What teaching should be completed during this visit? What psychosocial concerns would the client and the companion have?

Factors to Consider. What diagnostic studies should you anticipate? What care should be given to the client awaiting diagnosis after cancer testing?

3. C.H. is a 54-year-old engineer responsible for grading, paving, and asphalting of county road surfaces. He is admitted for evaluation of chest pain and increasing shortness of breath. Because of a history of quadruple bypass surgery when he was 44, he assumes that he has additional coronary artery blockage. He has continued to smoke despite his cardiac history. Several members of his mother's family and his father died of cancer. He has lung cancer that has metastasized to the brain. He will be treated with chemotherapy and radiation therapy. What risk factors does C.H. have for lung cancer? What teaching should the nurse plan for him? What long-term plans should the nurse consider for him?

Factors to Consider. How will this client's cardiac history affect his chemotherapy regimen? What oncologic emergencies does C.H. face? Why is he not a surgical candidate?

 Discussions for these questions can be found on the website.

BIBLIOGRAPHY

Citations appearing in red refer to primary research.

Citations appearing in blue refer to evidence-based practice guidelines and protocols.

1. Albanell, J., & Baselga, J. (2000). Systemic therapy emergencies. *Seminars in Oncology, 27*(3), 347-361.
2. American Cancer Society. (2007). *Cancer facts and figures—2007.* Atlanta: Author.
3. American Society of Clinical Oncology. (2005). Policy statement update: Tobacco control—reducing cancer incidence and saving lives. *Journal of Clinical Oncology, 21,* 2777.
4. Anastasia, P.J. (2000). Effectiveness of oral 5-HT3 receptor antagonists for emetogenic chemotherapy. *Oncology Nursing Forum, 27* (3), 483-493.
5. Appel, C. (2001). Biotherapy. In S. Otto (Ed.), *Oncology nursing* (4th ed., pp. 684-730). St. Louis: Mosby.
6. Baltic, T., Schlosser, E., & Bedell, M. (2002). Neutropenic fever: One institution's quality improvement project to decrease time from client arrival to initiation of antibiotic therapy. *Clinical Journal of Oncology Nursing, 6*(6), 337-346.
7. Barnett, M. (2001). Fatigue. In S. Otto (Ed.), *Oncology nursing* (4th ed., pp. 787-801). St. Louis: Mosby.
8. Bendell, C. (2003). Pegfilgrastim for chemotherapy-induced neutropenia. *Clinical Journal of Oncology Nursing, 7*(1), 55-56, 63-64.
9. Berlin, J. (2002). Targeting vascular endothelial growth factor in colorectal cancer. *Oncology, 16*(8, Suppl 7), 13-15.
10. Birner, A. (2003). Safe administration of oral chemotherapy. *Clinical Journal of Oncology Nursing, 7*(2), 158-162, 170-172.
11. Brant, J.M. (2002). Rasburicase: An innovative new treatment for hyperuricemia associated with tumor lysis syndrome. *Clinical Journal of Oncology Nursing, 6*(1), 12.
12. Brown, K.A., et al. (2001). *Chemotherapy and biotherapy: Guidelines and recommendations for practice.* Pittsburgh, Pa: ONS Publishing Division.
13. Bruner, D.W. (2001). *Outcomes in radiation therapy: Multidisciplinary management.* Sudbury, Mass: Jones & Bartlett.
14. Burke, M.B., et al. (Eds.) (2001). *Cancer chemotherapy: A nursing process approach* (3rd ed.). Sudbury, Mass: Jones & Bartlett.
15. Camp-Sorrell, D. (2004). *Access device guidelines: Recommendations for nursing practice and education* (2nd ed.). Pittsburgh, Pa: Oncology Nursing Press.
16. Carson, M.G. (2000). Measuring patient outcomes in palliative care: A reliability and validity study of the support team assessment schedule. *Palliative Medicine, 14,* 25-36.
17. Chelf, J., et al. (2000). Storytelling: A strategy for living and coping with cancer. *Cancer Nursing, 23*(1), 1-6.
18. Chernecky, C. (2001). Satisfaction vs. dissatisfaction with venous access devices in outpatient oncology: A pilot study. *Oncology Nursing Forum, 28*(10), 1613-1616.
19. Chu, K., Tarone, R., & Kessler L.G. (1996). Recent trends in US breast cancer incidence, survival and mortality rates. *Journal of the National Cancer Institute, 88,* 1571-1577.
20. Cohen, J. (2005). Public health. High hopes and dilemmas for a cervical cancer vaccine. *Science, 308,* 618-621.
21. Cook, J., & Zitelli, J.A. (2001). Mohs micrographic surgery: A cost analysis. *Journal of the American Academy of Dermatology, 39,* 698-711.
22. Dickson, R.B., Pestell, R.G., & Lippman, M.E. (2005). Cancer of the breast. In V.T. Devita, S. Hellman, & S.A. Rosenberg (Eds.), *Cancer: Principles and practice of oncology* (7th ed., pp. 1399-1488). Philadelphia: Lippincott Williams & Wilkins.
23. Eifel, P.A., Berek, J.S., & Markman, M.A. (2005). Gynecologic cancers. In V.T. Devita, S. Hellman, & S.A. Rosenberg (Eds.), *Cancer: Principles and practice of oncology* (7th ed., pp. 1295-1498). Philadelphia: Lippincott Williams & Wilkins.
24. Esper, P., et al. (1999). A new concept in cancer care: The supportive care program. *American Journal of Hospice & Palliative Care, 16*(6), 713-722.
25. Foltz, A.T., & Mahon, S.M. (2000). Application of carcinogenesis theory to primary prevention. *Oncology Nursing Forum, 27*(9), 5-11.
26. Giarell, D. (2002). To screen or not to screen: Using spiral computerized tomography in the early detection of lung cancer. *Clinical Journal of Oncology Nursing, 6*(4), 223-227.
27. Gray, M. (2002). A prostate cancer primer. *Urologic Nursing, 22*(3), 151-169.
28. Greco, F.A. (Ed.) (1996). *Handbook of commonly used chemotherapy regimens.* Chicago: Precept Press.
29. Greene, F. (Ed.) (2002). *AJCC cancer staging manual* (6th ed.). New York: Springer-Verlag.

30. Hawks, J., & Moyad, M. (2003). CAM: Definition and classification overview. *Urologic Nursing, 23*(3), 221-223.

31. Houshamand, S., et al. (2000). Prophylactic mastectomy and genetic testing: An update. *Oncology Nursing Forum, 27*(10), 1537-1547.

32. Hughes, L.C., et al. (2002). Describing an episode of home nursing care for elderly post-surgical cancer patients. *Nursing Research, 51* (2), 110-118.

33. Jennings-Dozier, K., & Mahon, S.M. (2000). Cancer prevention and early detection—From thought to revolution. *Oncology Nursing Forum, 27*(9), 3-4.

34. Kosier, M.B., & Minkler, P. (1999). Nursing management of patients with an implanted Ommaya reservoir. *Clinical Journal of Oncology Nursing, 3*(2), 63-67.

35. Kuebler, K., Berry, P., & Heidrich, D. (2002). *End-of-life care: Clinical practice guidelines.* Philadelphia: Saunders.

36. Levin, B., et al. (2003). Emerging technologies in screening for colorectal cancer: CT colonography, immunochemical fecal occult blood tests, and stool screening. *Cancer Nursing, 23*(2), 117-121.

37. Libutti, S.K., Saltz, L.B., Rustgi, A.K., et al. (2005). Cancer of the colon. In V.T. Devita, S. Hellman, & S.A. Rosenberg (Eds.), *Cancer: Principles and practice of oncology* (7th ed., pp. 1061-1109). Philadelphia: Lippincott Williams & Wilkins.

38. Mahon, S.M. (2002). Cancer prevention and early detection. *Clinical Journal of Oncology Nursing, 5*(3), 105–107.

39. Marrs, J.A. (2006). Oncology nursing 101. Nurse, my back hurts: Understanding malignant spinal cord compression. *Clinical Journal of Oncology Nursing, 10*(1), 114–116.

40. Mendenhall, W.M., Riggs, C.E., & Cassisi, N.J. (2005). Treatment of head and neck cancers. In V.T. Devita, S. Hellman, & S.A. Rosenberg (Eds.), *Cancer: Principles and practice of oncology* (7th ed., pp. 662-732). Philadelphia: Lippincott Williams & Wilkins.

41. National Cancer Institute. (1999, Reprinted 2002). *Chemotherapy and you: A guide to self-help during cancer treatment* (NIH Pub. No. 99-1136). Washington, DC: U.S. Government Printing Office.

42. National Cancer Institute. (Revised 1998, Reprinted 2004). *Eating hints for cancer patients* (NIH Pub. No. 98-2079). Washington, DC: U.S. Government Printing Office.

43. National Cancer Institute. (Revised 1999, Reprinted 2002). *Radiation therapy and you: A guide to self-help during cancer treatment* (NIH Pub. No. 99-2227). Washington, DC: U.S. Government Printing Office.

44. National Cancer Institute. (2001). *SELECT: Selenium and vitamin E cancer prevention trial* (NIH Pub. No. D1-4978). Washington, DC: U.S. Government Printing Office.

45. National Cancer Institute. (1998). *Taking part in clinical trials: What cancer patients need to know* (NIH Pub. No. 97-4250). Washington, DC: U.S. Government Printing Office.

46. National Cancer Institute. (1997, Reprinted 2003). *Taking time: Support for people with cancer and the people who care about them* (NIH Pub. No. 97-2059). Washington, DC: U.S. Government Printing Office.

47. Nelson, R.L., Persky, V., & Turyk, M. (1999). Determination of factors responsible for the declining incidence of colorectal cancer. *Diseases of the Colon and Rectum, 42*, 741.

48. Nunez, A.M., & Liebman, M.C. (1999). Febrile neutropenia. *American Journal of Nursing*, April Suppl, 9-12.

49. Occupational Safety and Health Administration (OSHA). (1998). *Work-place guidelines for personnel dealing with cytotoxic (antineoplastic) drugs* (OSHA Instruction CPL 2-2.20B Section VI, CH 2). Washington, DC: U.S. Government Printing Office.

50. Oncology Nursing Society. (1992). *Cancer chemotherapy guidelines: Recommendations for the management of vesicant extravasation, hypersensitivity and anaphylaxis.* Pittsburgh, Pa: Author.

51. Otto, S. (2001). Protective mechanisms. In S. Otto (Ed.), *Oncology nursing* (4th ed., pp. 917-947). St. Louis: Mosby.

52. Otto, S., & Johnston, L. (2001). Home care, alternative care settings, and cancer resources. In S. Otto (Ed.), *Oncology nursing* (4th ed., pp. 802-842). St. Louis: Mosby.

53. Prouty, D., Ward-Smith, P., & Hutto, C.J. (2006). The lived experience of adult survivors of childhood cancer. *Journal of Pediatric Oncology Nursing, 23*, 143-151.

54. Rieger, P. (2001). Biotherapy: The fourth modality. In M.B. Burke, et al. (Eds.), *Cancer chemotherapy: A nursing process approach* (3rd ed., pp. 43-73). Sudbury, Mass: Jones & Bartlett.

55. Rieger, P. (2003). The impact of genetic information in the management of cancer. In A. Tranin, A. Masny, & J. Jenkins (Eds.), *Genetics in oncology practice: Cancer risk assessment* (pp. 139-187). Pittsburgh, Pa: Oncology Nursing Society.

56. Saslow, D., et al. (2002). American Cancer Society guidelines for the early detection of cervical neoplasia and cancer. *CA: A Cancer Journal for Clinicians, 52*(6), 342-362.

57. Scher, H.I., Leibel, S.A., Fuks, Z., et al. (2005). Cancer of the prostate. In V.T. Devita, S. Hellman, & S.A. Rosenberg (Eds.), *Cancer: Principles and practice of oncology* (7th ed., pp. 1192-1260). Philadelphia: Lippincott Williams & Wilkins.

58. Schulmeister, L. (2001). Epidemiology. In S. Otto (Ed.), *Oncology nursing* (4th ed., pp. 42-52). St. Louis: Mosby.

59. Shell, J. (2001). Impact of cancer on sexuality. In S. Otto (Ed.), *Oncology nursing* (4th ed., pp. 973-999). St. Louis: Mosby.

60. Shell, J., & Kirsch, S. (2001). Psychosocial issues, outcomes, and quality of life. In S. Otto (Ed.), *Oncology nursing* (4th ed., pp. 948-972). St. Louis: Mosby.

61. Smith, L.H., & Besser, S.G. (2000). Dietary restrictions for patients with neutropenia: A survey of institutional practices. *Oncology Nursing Forum, 27*(3), 515-531.

62. Smith, R., Cokkiniles, V., & Eyre, H.J. (2003). American Cancer Society guidelines for the early detection of cancer, 2003. *CA: A Cancer Journal for Clinicians, 53*(1), 27-43.

63. Sorokin, P. (2002). New agents and future directions in biotherapy. *Clinical Journal of Oncology Nursing, 6*(1), 19-24.

64. Sparber, A., et al. (2000). Using complementary medicine by adult patients participating in cancer clinical trials. *Oncology Nursing Forum, 27*(4), 623-630.

65. Tariman, J. (2003). Thalidomide: Current therapeutic uses and management of its toxicities. *Clinical Journal of Oncology Nursing, 7*(2), 143-147.

65a. The Joint Commission (2007). *2008 National Patient Safety Goals Hospital Program.* www.jointcommission.org/PatientSafety/NationalPatientSafetyGoals.

66. U.S. Department of Health and Human Services. (2002). *Facing forward: Life after cancer treatment* (NIH Pub. No. 96-2424). Washington, DC: National Cancer Institute.

67. Vanderhoof, D.D., & Brant, J.M. (1999). Alopecia: The forgotten side effect? *American Journal of Nursing*, April Suppl, 17-19.

68. Viale, P. (2003). Complications associated with implantable vascular access devices in the patient with cancer. *Journal of Infusion Nursing, 26*(2), 97-103.

69. Wier, H.R., Thun, M.J., & Hankey, B.F. (2003). Annual report to the nation of the state of cancer 1975-2000 featuring the uses of surveillance data for cancer prevention and control. *Journal of the National Cancer Institute, 95*, 1276-1289.

70. Weisman, A. (1979). *Coping with cancer.* New York: McGraw-Hill.

CHAPTER 18

Clients with Wounds

JOYCE M. BLACK

Healing is a fundamental property of living tissue. If healing did not occur, all species would eventually become extinct. Unfortunately, many health care practices seem to lack respect for this critical attribute of healing and accept the process as passive, inevitable, and unimprovable. Popular literature assumes that if people survive, they heal, and if people are healthy, they heal.

Healing activities have always formed the basis of nursing practice. Florence Nightingale defined the nursing role as preparing the client for the most favorable conditions for healing. Nurses today still serve as a crucial link in the process of wound healing. They educate clients about disease management and wound care and support them through the physical and psychological processes of healing.

Wound healing is most apparent on the skin but occurs in all areas of the body. Bones, tendons, organs, and tissues all heal by regenerating cells to restore function. The most favorable outcome of healing is the complete return to normal structure and function. Such an outcome is possible if tissue damage is minor, no complications occur, and the destroyed tissues can regenerate. Body tissues have varying capabilities for regeneration. For example, mucous membrane is completely regenerated. Full-thickness injury of the skin regenerates with a scar, which restores only a barrier. It has been thought that the central nervous system (CNS) cannot regenerate its damaged cells. Although new information is challenging that belief, today the knowledge does not exist to promote CNS tissue regeneration.

This chapter focuses on tissue injury and repair. Tissue injury is common and is seen in clients who sustain trauma as well as in those who have undergone surgery. Because tissue injury is common, the body is well equipped with mechanisms of defense and healing.

NORMAL WOUND HEALING

Wound healing has been defined as "a complex and dynamic process that results in the restoration of anatomic continuity and function."[13] Wound healing has been seen as analogous to building a house. Adequate supplies must be available to build a house, which is analogous to adequate nutrition, blood flow, and oxygen for wound healing. Cells come together, like the electrician, plumber, and painter, to do a specific task. Building the house requires a blueprint; in the body the communication must go on chemically. The work of the cells is organized and coordinated by growth factors, or cytokines, that communicate to provide an orderly sequence to the work.

Healed wounds constitute a spectrum of repair. An *ideally healed* wound is one that has returned to normal anatomic structure, function, and appearance. In humans, this degree of healing can occur only in epidermal tissue, mucous membrane, and bone. Once there is injury through the dermis, normal appearance cannot return because scar tissue replaces missing dermis and epidermis. On the other end of the spectrum, a *minimally healed* wound has anatomic continuity (the wound has closed), but it does not have sustained functional result. Hence the wound can recur. Between these two extremes of healing, an *acceptably healed* wound is characterized by restoration of sustained function and anatomic continuity.

---

evolve **Web Enhancements**

Appendix A Religious Beliefs and Practices Affecting Health Care

Be sure to check out the bonus material on the Evolve website and the CD-ROM, including free self-assessment exercises. **http://evolve.elsevier.com/Black/medsurg**

The type of injury has considerable influence on the form of repair. Clean, approximated incisions heal with minimal synthesis of new tissue and barely test a client's resources. In sharp contrast, major burn wounds require complete regeneration of tissue and stimulate massive responses from all body systems to sustain life. The location of the wound also influences healing. Perineal wounds are likely to become infected, wounds over joints are subject to motion and therefore increased scarring, and wounds in peripheral areas or those that do not receive adequate blood supply heal slowly, if at all.

Phases of Wound Healing

Regardless of the cause of the wound, healing follows a predictable course, and many actions occur simultaneously. Events can be described in four phases (Figure 18-1):

- Vascular response
- Inflammation
- Proliferation or resolution
- Maturation or reconstruction

Vascular Response Phase

Within seconds after an injury, regardless of the type, blood vessels constrict to stop bleeding and reduce exposure to bacteria. The clotting process begins. Platelets form a clot and stop bleeding. At the same time, the plasma protein system begins to form a fibrous meshwork. When the platelets come in contact with the fibrin meshwork across the open vessel wall, they become sticky and adhere (aggregate) to the fibers, forming a plug. This meshwork of clotted blood and serum covers the wound while it heals and prevents further loss of blood and plasma. Platelets also release various proteins and growth factors to stimulate healing (see later discussion).

Capillaries dilate 10 to 30 minutes after injury and remain dilated for some time because of serotonin released by the platelets. Plasma is able to flow into the wounded area to dilute toxins secreted by the organisms, transport oxygen and nutrients necessary for tissue repair, and carry phagocytes into the area. The wounded area becomes warm and red; these changes are considered classic manifestations of inflammation, and the wound begins the inflammatory phase of healing.

Inflammation Phase

Inflammation, the second phase of wound healing, is essential. Inflammation occurs whenever the cells have been injured. Cellular injury can occur from trauma, oxygen or nutrient deprivation, chemical agents, microorganism invasion, temperature extremes, or ionizing radiation. Inflammation also occurs when dead cells are present. Inflammation begins at the moment of injury and may continue for 4 to 6 days, depending on the extent of the injury. The inflammatory response is so necessary to healing that it is commonly said, "no inflammation, no healing."

The purpose of inflammation is to limit the effects of harmful bacteria or injury by destroying or neutralizing the organism and by limiting its spread throughout the body. The inflammatory response thereby sets up proper conditions to promote tissue repair, as illustrated in the Concept Map on p. 306. Unlike the *immune response,* which uses specific antibodies for a slow and deliberate response, the effects of inflammation are immediate. Unfortunately, health care terminology uses the word *inflamed* to describe a wound that is not healing normally. Do not be confused between the normal process of inflammation and the term *inflamed,* which means exaggerated inflammation and possible infection.

"Walling-Off" Effect. A walling-off effect occurs in the damaged area to prevent the spread of injurious agents to other body tissues. Fibrinogen clots block the lymphatic channels and spaces in the tissues so that fluid barely flows through the area. The process of walling off the area depends partly on the invading agent. For example, staphylococci invade and destroy nearby tissues quickly, and therefore the process of walling off also develops quickly to control the spread. In contrast, streptococci can digest the walls, allowing the streptococci to multiply and spread. As a result, streptococcal infections have a much greater tendency to invade other organs (e.g., heart valves) and are associated with a higher mortality rate.

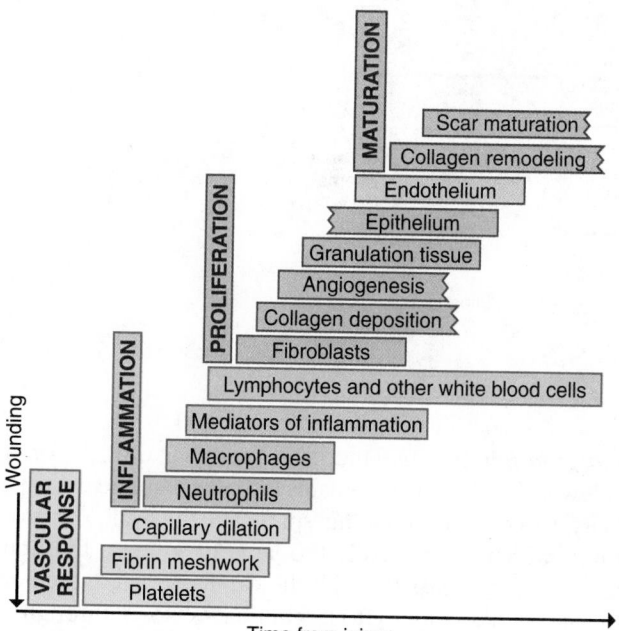

■ **FIGURE 18-1** Normal wound healing. Wound healing proceeds through four phases: (1) the vascular response, (2) inflammation, (3) proliferation of cells to heal the wound, and (4) maturation of the wound. Each step has many components. The jagged edge depicts an ongoing process. *(Modified from Cohen, I., et al. [Eds.] [1992]. Wound healing. Philadelphia: Saunders.)*

CONCEPT MAP

Understanding Inflammation and Its Treatment

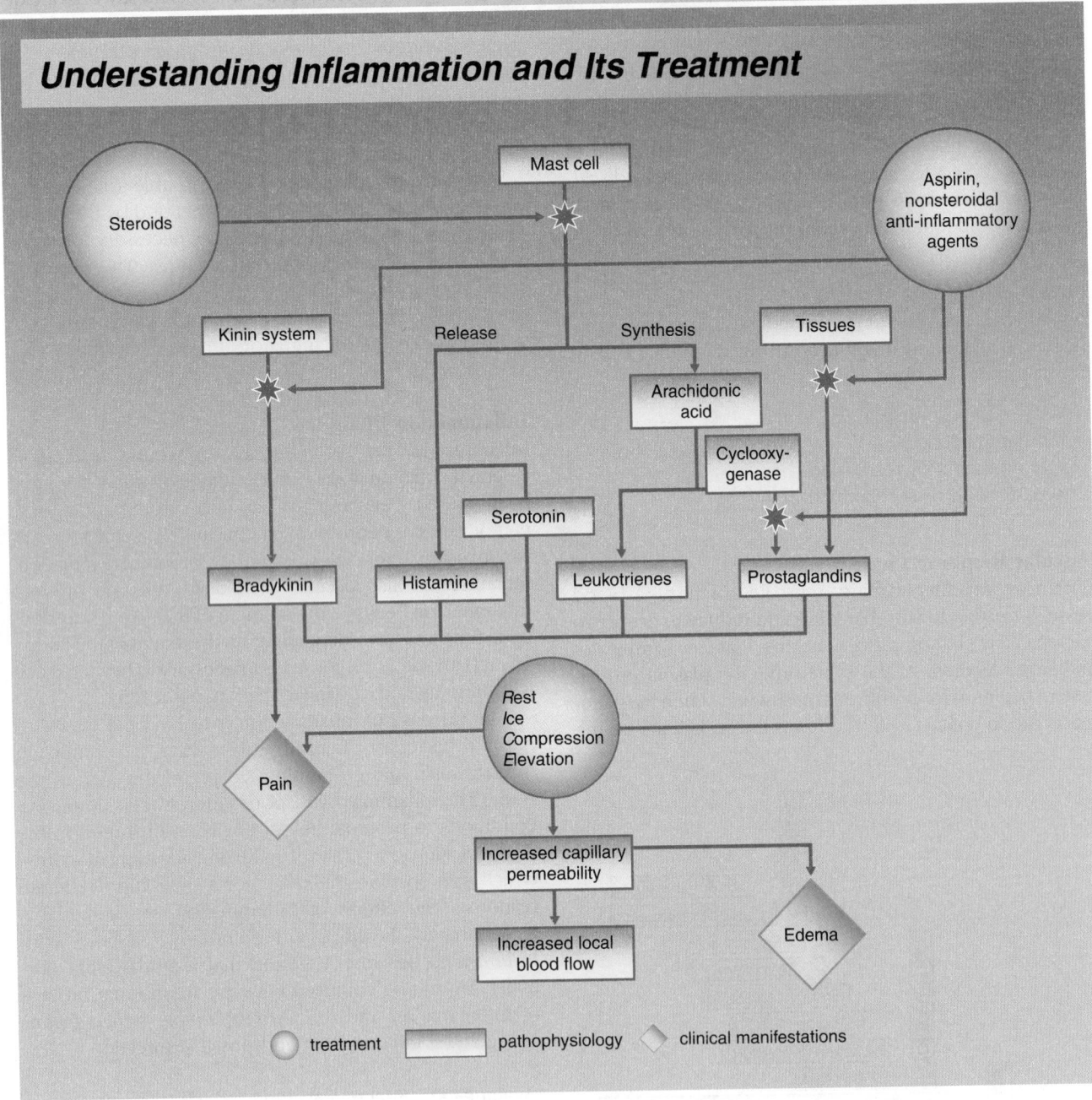

White Blood Cell Activity. During the inflammation phase, the white blood cells (WBCs) become active to clean up the wound and initiate further healing processes.

Neutrophils. Neutrophils are vital defense organisms because they are both the first and the most numerous cell types to arrive at any area of disease or injury. The slowed flow of blood allows the neutrophil to leave the center of the bloodstream and line the walls of the capillaries, a process called *pavementing,* or *marginating,* because the cells line up like bricks on a sidewalk. Histamine stimulates the cells that line the capillary to constrict, creating spaces in the wall. Neutrophils, which are normally too large to squeeze through the lining, can pass through the capillary wall and enter the site of tissue injury to begin phagocytosis, through a process called *diapedesis* (Figure 18-2). Neutrophils phagocytose bacteria, dead cells, and cellular debris. These cells are short lived, but they are effective in clearing a wound of debris if bacteria are not excessive (i.e., >100,000 per gram of tissue).

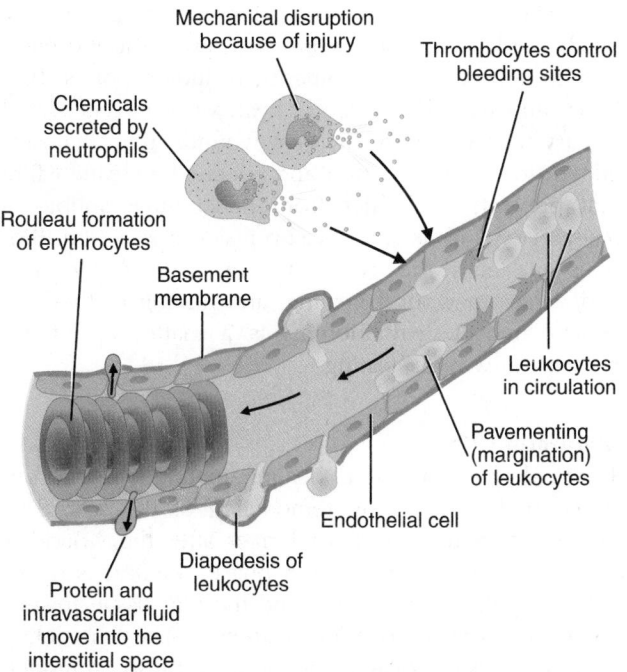

Mechanical disruption because of injury

Thrombocytes control bleeding sites

Chemicals secreted by neutrophils

Rouleau formation of erythrocytes

Basement membrane

Leukocytes in circulation

Pavementing (margination) of leukocytes

Endothelial cell

Diapedesis of leukocytes

Protein and intravascular fluid move into the interstitial space

■ **FIGURE 18–2** Several changes occur in a capillary after injury. Neutrophils are attracted to the site of injury by chemotactic factors at the site. The neutrophil leaves the blood vessel by sliding through holes in the vessel wall *(diapedesis)*. The leukocytes also line the vessel wall, and the erythrocytes stack like coins *(rouleau formation)* to slow blood flow.

Neutrophils are sometimes called *polymorphonuclear neutrophils* (PMNs), or polys, because of their irregularly shaped nuclei. Neutrophils compose about 60% of the circulating WBCs. Mature neutrophils appear segmented and are called *segs*. Immature cells are "banded" and called *bands*. Bands are not effective in phagocytosis. The presence of an increase in segmented WBCs indicates a bacterial invasion. The presence of increased band neutrophils indicates more severe infection because the bone marrow has released immature cells. Leukocytes are also the major producers of interferon.

The amount of oxygen in the wound influences the effectiveness of phagocytic cells. Both macrophages and neutrophils can function in an anaerobic environment, but their ability to digest bacteria effectively is slowed. Macrophages are inactivated when tissue levels of oxygen are below 30 mm Hg. (Normal tissue oxygen levels are not the same as levels of oxygen bound to hemoglobin or dissolved oxygen. Tissue oxygen levels are normal at or above 30 mm Hg.)

Other White Blood Cells. Eosinophils and basophils may also migrate to the injured area. Eosinophils help to control the inflammatory response by secreting antihistamine. Basophils secrete histamine. Lymphocytes help the macrophages to become more effective at the site of local injury through a number of processes. Lymphocytes are controlled by the adrenocortical hormones.

Therefore clients receiving steroid therapy have reduced numbers of lymphocytes. This change places the steroid-dependent client at increased risk for infection and delayed healing.

Mediators of the Inflammation Phase

Mast Cells. The mast cell is an important cell in inflammation. When the mast cell is stimulated, it releases histamine and serotonin, which cause capillary dilation. The mast cell can be stimulated by many factors, such as physical injury (e.g., wounds, burns, x-ray exposure), chemical injury (e.g., toxins, snake and bee venom), or immunologic means (e.g., hypersensitivity reactions seen in allergies).

Mast cells also synthesize leukotrienes and prostaglandins. These two chemicals cause the same responses as histamine, but the response lasts longer. Prostaglandins also cause pain and tend to appear in the later stages of inflammation. Aspirin and other nonsteroidal anti-inflammatory drugs (NSAIDs) block the production of prostaglandins and can assist in reducing inflammation and pain.

Kinins. Kinins are plasma proteins involved in inflammation. Early in injury, kinins increase vascular permeability and allow the leukocytes to enter the tissue. Later in the inflammatory process, kinins act with prostaglandins to cause pain and smooth-muscle contraction and to increase leukocyte chemotaxis. Kinins increase vascular permeability, fluid in the wound, and the number of leukocytes available to assist with phagocytosis. The primary kinin is bradykinin.

Cytokines. Cytokines regulate the mobility, differentiation, and growth of leukocytes. Among the best understood cytokines are interleukins and interferons. *Interleukins* promote the growth and function of several cells. Interleukin can account for many of the clinical manifestations of both acute and chronic inflammation, such as fever, anorexia, cachexia, and movement of PMNs to the site of injury. Interferons augment immunity through several processes, especially the promotion of B-cell maturation and the moderation of suppressor T-cell function.

The Complement System. The complement system is composed of a group of plasma proteins that normally lie dormant in the blood, interstitial fluid, and mucosal surfaces. Microorganisms (or antigen-antibody complexes) activate the complement system. Complement activation promotes inflammation and induces movement of leukocytes into the area of injury. The final aspect of complement activation is the coating of microbes to make them vulnerable to phagocytosis. Many bacteria have an outer capsule that resists phagocytosis. (Complement is fully discussed in the Unit 17 Anatomy and Physiology Review.)

Proliferative Phase

The third phase of wound healing, the proliferative or resolution phase, contains overlapping processes of collagen deposition, angiogenesis (formation of new blood vessels), granulation tissue development, and wound contraction. This phase ends about 2 weeks after injury, but the processes of healing are not complete and continue for 1 to 2 years.

The fibroblast is the most important cell in this phase. Fibroblasts synthesize collagen and granulation tissue. Tissue macrophages continue to patrol the wounded tissue for foreign material. The macrophage also secretes *angiogenesis factor* (AGF), which stimulates the formation of new blood vessels at the end of injured vessels. The macrophage also secretes other cytokines such as platelet-derived growth factor (PDGF), transforming growth factor (TGF), interleukin-1 (IL-1), and basic fibroblast growth factor (bFGF). This cell has a major role in wound healing. Wounds can heal without leukocytes, but wound healing is significantly impaired without macrophages.

Myofibroblasts in the wound cause the wound to contract. Wound contraction is crucial for survival. If a wound from an acute injury did not contract, infections would be lethal complications in all acute injuries. Contraction is undesirable in some wounds because of the cosmetic deformities that result. Contracture of the scar can produce profound deformities; contracture of a scar at the neck can pull the chin onto the chest. Wounds over joints can also contract severely. Contracture also occurs in internal organs, such as the intestine, breast, and liver.

Epithelialization. *Epithelialization* is the migration of epithelial cells from the edges of the wound of hair follicles within the wound. When epithelium covers a wound, the wound is considered to be closed, or healed. Large wounds or full-thickness wounds may require skin grafting because epidermal migration is normally limited to about 3 cm. Epithelialization can be hastened if a wound is kept moist.

Mediators of the Proliferative Phase

Growth Factors. Growth factors communicate between cells in the wound bed. Dozens of growth factors and cytokines govern wound healing. They can prime other cells to enter a growth phase, or they can move a cell from a growth phase to a DNA production phase. Wounds that fail to heal may be lacking growth factors, and clinical research is ongoing to determine which factors could be topically applied to stimulate wound healing.

Matrix Metalloproteases. Matrix metalloproteases (MMPs) are a group of enzymes that degrade the wound bed. Normally, a balance of wound repair and wound destruction goes on as a wound heals. Chronic wounds that are not healing have a greater amount of MMPs than wounds that are healing in a timely manner.

Biofilms. Biofilms are a collection of bacteria that exist on the surface of open wounds. They are found naturally in almost all environments, including ponds. Biofilms can cause dental decay, heart valve infection, and urinary tract infection. In open wounds, the organisms adhere to the wound bed and eventually create a film that prevents antibiotics from penetrating; antibiotic-resistant organisms can develop inside the biofilm. Biofilms are likely the cause of many wound infections and delays in wound healing, and finding methods to control and destroy biofilms is a matter of intense research in wound healing.

Maturation Phase

The final phase of wound healing, maturation or reconstruction, is marked by remodeling of the scar. This phase occurs for a year or longer after the wound is closed. During the maturation phase, the scar is remodeled, capillaries disappear, and the scar tissue regains about two thirds of its original strength. The remodeling is the process of collagen synthesis and lysis. Remodeling provides tensile strength to the wound.

Scar tissue is never as strong or as durable as normal tissue. Tensile strength never reaches more than 80% in scar tissue. During the 12 months after injury, the scar becomes mature and appears thin and white instead of the red, raised appearance seen with granulation tissue. Scarring is a normal part of wound healing. Some scars are barely visible, whereas others remain quite visible throughout the client's lifetime.

Wound Healing Intention

Wound healing intention refers to the probable process of healing for any wound. Wounds can heal by (1) primary, (2) secondary, or (3) tertiary (delayed primary) intention (Figure 18-3).

Primary Intention

Primary intention is the use of suture (stitches) or other wound closures to *approximate* (place close together) the edges of an incision or clean laceration. Healing is primarily through collagen synthesis, and little scarring or contraction is needed. The risk of infection and tissue defects is minimal. The eventual scar is usually thin and flat.

Secondary Intention

Wounds healing by secondary intention are left open rather than closed with sutures and heal by the generation of tissue. Pressure ulcers or abrasions are common examples of wounds that heal by secondary intention. Open wounds require the regeneration of much more tissue than does the wound healing by primary intention, and the risk of infection also increases. Wounds

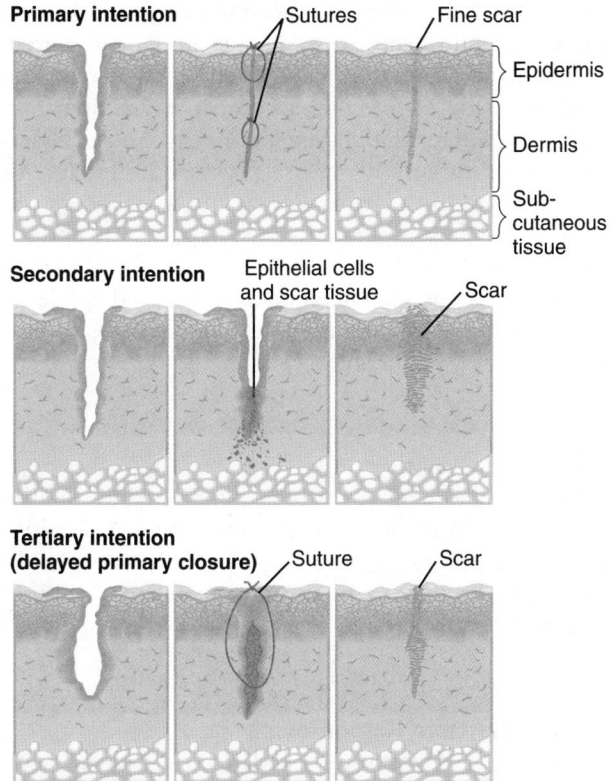

Primary intention — Sutures, Fine scar, Epidermis, Dermis, Sub-cutaneous tissue

Secondary intention — Epithelial cells and scar tissue, Scar

Tertiary intention (delayed primary closure) — Suture, Scar

■ **FIGURE 18–3** Wound healing by primary, secondary, and tertiary intention (delayed primary closure).

healing by secondary intention have a prolonged phase of inflammation because more time is required for phagocytosis of necrotic tissue. The ability of epithelial cells to migrate is limited, and epithelialization may not heal the wound. Therefore the wound is characterized by longer phases of proliferation and maturation, leading to healing by contraction and the formation of scar tissue. Sometimes healing is hastened by the application of skin grafts or musculocutaneous (myocutaneous) flaps (see Chapter 49).

Tertiary Intention

Certain wounds may be contaminated, and although they can be closed by primary intention, they are not. Because of the increased risk of infection, these wounds are closed later, when they are free of debris. This type of wound closure is called *healing by tertiary intention,* or *delayed primary closure.*

Intrinsic and Extrinsic Factors in Wound Healing

Factors in the wound itself *(intrinsic)* and within the client *(extrinsic)* can have a profound effect on how quickly a wound heals. These factors are described in Table 18-1.

TABLE 18–1   Intrinsic and Extrinsic Factors in Wound Healing

Factors	Effect on Wound Healing	Treatment
Intrinsic Factors: Local Factors in Wound Itself That Can Alter Healing		
Infection	Prolongs inflammatory response Wounds will not heal until infection is controlled	Diagnosed with wound cultures; wounds considered infected when >100,000 bacteria are present in 1 g of tissue Systemic or topical antibiotics, debridement
Foreign bodies	Increase risk of wound infection	Removal of foreign body if infected
Inadequate blood supply	Reduced fibroblast function, increased risk of infection Wounds cannot heal without adequate arterial flow	Restore blood flow with surgery or improve blood flow with medications Protect ischemic skin from injury
Smoking	Reduces arterial flow because nicotine is vasoconstrictor Carbon monoxide in cigarette smoke reduces tissue oxygen level	Abstinence from tobacco Use of smoking cessation programs, but not nicotine patches, to control urge to smoke
Neuropathy	Unintentional injury of wounded or previously healed wounds Unregulated blood flow to injured tissues	Protection from injury Daily inspection to detect wounds in early stages
Extrinsic Factors: Characteristics of Client That Have an Effect on Wound Healing		
Protein malnutrition	Reduces collagen deposition and white blood cell function	Supplements to diet Tube-feeding or hyperalimentation if acceptable to client/family
Carbohydrate malnutrition	All wound healing phases slowed; protein is used for energy	Same as above
Lack of vitamin C intake	Impaired collagen synthesis	Vitamin C supplementation
Diabetes	Increased risk of infection when blood glucose level not controlled Accelerated atherosclerosis, which impairs blood supply	Monitor and regulate blood glucose level to <200 mg/dl Monitor for methicillin-resistant *Staphylococcus aureus* (MRSA) infections
Glucocorticoid steroids	Impair all aspects of wound healing, especially inflammatory phase; also impair contraction and epithelialization	Protect paper-thin skin from injury Limit use of topical steroids on incisions Vitamin A can reverse some of effects

CLIENTS WITH ACUTE INFLAMMATION

Inflammation occurs in all clients who have sustained any form of tissue trauma. Because the response to inflammation is the same regardless of the cause, the manifestations of inflammation are relatively consistent.

Fever, leukocytosis (an increase in the number of WBCs), increased plasma proteins (e.g., fibrinogen, C-reactive protein), and malaise are the systemic reactions to inflammation: Fever is caused by a *pyrogen* (a fever-causing chemical) released from leukocytes, macrophages, and tumor necrosis factor (TNF). Prostaglandins also act on the hypothalamus to reset the internal thermostat. Fever is usually adaptive because bacterial reproduction is sensitive to even slight increases in temperature. WBC and plasma protein levels increase as the body responds to the invasion. Plasma proteins are collectively called *acute phase reactants*. They provide components of coagulation, transportation, and complement production. The *erythrocyte sedimentation rate* (ESR, or "sed rate"), the rate at which cells settle to the bottom of a glass test tube, also rises with inflammation. Increased levels of fibrinogen cause the red blood cells to stack (like coins) and therefore settle more quickly.

OUTCOME MANAGEMENT

Medical Management

Goals of medical management of a client with acute inflammation include (1) minimizing complications of the edema accompanying inflammation, (2) reducing the inflammatory response, and (3) monitoring systemic responses. Because the inflammatory response is a desired response to promote wound healing, the client with inflammation often requires only supportive care.

Control the Effects of Edema

*R*est, *I*ce, *C*ompression, and *E*levation (RICE) is a mnemonic that can be used to guide care to reduce the effect of edema. If an extremity is inflamed, it is elevated and wrapped to reduce edema. Ice is used to control the inflammatory response in the extremities, especially when edema and pain are present. Ice is usually prescribed for 24 to 72 hours to control inflammation and then apply heat is sometimes used after 72 hours to remove the accumulated waste products. When ice is ordered, be certain that the cold reaches the wound and that it is not rendered ineffective by bulky dressings. To prevent tissue injury, do not apply ice directly to unprotected skin.

If edema is causing a detrimental alteration of tissue perfusion, anti-inflammatory agents may be required. In certain areas of the body, such as the brain and extremities, the edema that accompanies inflammation can be detrimental to tissue perfusion. These clients may require surgery to release pressure in the area or restore blood flow. Fasciotomy and burr holes are examples of these operations (see Chapters 29 and 75, respectively).

The degree of inflammation is monitored to determine whether it is leading to healing. Analgesics may be required for pain control.

Reduce Inflammation

Anti-inflammatory agents may be prescribed to stabilize the mast cell and reduce edema in the area. Medications in this category range from NSAIDs to corticosteroids. Foreign bodies may be removed to reduce the cause of the inflammation.

Monitor Systemic Responses

Temperature is monitored, and fever is treated with antipyretics (e.g., acetaminophen) when temperature reaches detrimental levels (i.e., >38.3° C or 101° F). Low-grade fever should not be treated with antipyretics because the high temperature retards bacterial growth; however, fever can be detrimental if it is extreme or prolonged. Therefore the client's temperature is monitored closely to prevent harm. The client with a fever may also experience malaise, nausea, anorexia, weight loss, tachypnea, and tachycardia. The diet of the client with inflammation should be high in vitamin C, protein, calories, and fluids. Vitamin C supports WBC function, production of collagen, and angiogenesis. Protein aids in the formation of blood cells and tissue. Carbohydrates supply needed energy for fuel for healing. Additional fluids are needed to remove metabolic waste and rehydrate the client, especially if the client has been febrile. If the inflammation is in response to a probable invasion by organisms, antibiotics may be prescribed.

Leukocytosis is due to the increase in the number of leukocytes in circulation to combat infection. Sometimes, in an effort to combat infection, the bone marrow releases immature leukocytes (banded neutrophils or bands). When the number of immature neutrophils is high, the client is said to have a "left shift." At times, the release of immature cells means that the body is having difficulty combating the infection with mature cells. Interpretation of the WBC differential is shown in Table 18-2.

TABLE 18–2 Interpretation of Differential Counts Within a Complete Blood Cell Count

Cell Type	Function	Normal Value	Significance of Change
Segmented neutrophils (segs)*	Mature neutrophils act as phagocytes	50%	Elevated with infection; "left shift" means that many band (immature) cells are present as body fights infection; "right shift" is presence of more mature cells, as seen with liver disease and pernicious anemia
Banded neutrophils	Immature neutrophils	3%	Elevated in acute stages of infection
Lymphocytes	Produced by lymphoid tissue; participate in humoral response	25%	Elevated in infectious mononucleosis, cytomegalovirus infection, and infectious hepatitis; decreased in acquired immunodeficiency syndrome (AIDS), Cushing's syndrome, chronic uremia, and following trauma (e.g., burn injury)
Monocytes	Second line of defense; increase in chronic infections	2%	Elevated in chronic bacterial infection, viral disease, Hodgkin's disease, multiple myeloma, and some forms of leukemia
Eosinophils	Phagocytic; destroy antigen-antibody complexes before they can harm body	1%	Elevated in allergic disorders and parasitic infections; decreased in infectious mononucleosis, congestive heart failure, pernicious anemia, and during use of steroids, epinephrine, and thyroxine

*To calculate the absolute neutrophil count (also called an absolute granulocyte count):

$$\text{Absolute neutrophil count} = \frac{\text{Total \% of neutrophils (segs + bands)} \times \text{WBC count (cells/mm}^3)}{100}$$

When the absolute neutrophil count falls below 1000/mm^3, the client is said to be "neutropenic," and precautions must be taken to prevent infection.

Nursing Assessment of the Medical Client

Assessment. The clinical manifestations of inflammation in acute wounds include redness, swelling, heat, pain, and loss of function. Tissues are red, warm, painful, and swollen and have limited mobility. In addition, an inflammatory exudate is formed. The exudate dilutes the toxins released by bacteria, transports certain nutrients to the wound, and carries phagocytes for defense. Various types of exudate are present, depending on the stage of inflammation and its cause.

Serous exudate is seen in early inflammation and is composed of water with a small amount of colloids, ions, and phagocytic cells. A *blister* is a common example of serous exudate. Hemorrhagic or sanguineous exudate is composed of blood. Drainage is bright red or dark red. Serosanguineous exudate is drainage composed of both serous fluid and blood. It is pink and usually fairly thin. Purulent exudate is filled with more leukocytes *(pus)* and is common in chronic inflammation from walled-off lesions.

The type of drainage present in the wound is indicative of the phase of healing. For example, a surgical wound initially presents with sanguineous drainage. As hemostasis progresses, the drainage becomes serosanguineous and finally advances to serous drainage (Table 18-3).

Monitor the level of WBCs, differential counts, and fever as indicators of infection. Expect the WBC level to rise in clients with known infections and after acute injury, such as a surgical incision. Monitor also older clients, who often have infection but not necessarily elevated WBC counts.

Diagnosis, Outcomes, Interventions

Diagnosis: Ineffective Tissue Perfusion. Edema from the inflammatory response may restrict blood vessels and entrap nerves in the traumatized area. The nursing diagnosis *Ineffective Peripheral Tissue Perfusion related to edema* is an appropriate diagnosis.

Outcomes. The client will have adequate tissue perfusion as evidenced by the usual skin color, the presence of pulses in areas distal to the edema, skin warmth, lack of paresthesias, and lack of escalating pain.

TABLE 18–3 Inflammatory Exudates

Type	Appearance	Significance
Hemorrhagic, sanguineous	Bright red or bloody	Small amounts expected after surgery or trauma; large amounts may indicate hemorrhage; sudden large amounts of dark-red blood may indicate draining hematoma
Serosanguineous	Blood-tinged yellow or pink	Expected for 48-72 hr after injury or trauma; sudden increase may precede wound dehiscence
Serous	Thin, clear, yellow	Expected for up to 1 week after trauma or surgery; sudden increase may indicate draining seroma
Purulent	Thin, cloudy, foul-smelling; may be thick if filled with dead cells	Usually indicates infection; may drain suddenly from abscess (boil)
Catarrhal	Thin, clear mucus	Seen with upper respiratory tract infection

Interventions. Assess clients with visible injury causing inflammation for resolution of bleeding in the area, adequate blood flow, and nerve conduction distal to the affected site. Frequent assessments (every 2 hours) of the edematous area are needed. Measurement of the circumference of the area also enables the examiner to determine whether the area is becoming markedly edematous. To measure the same site, mark the area on the client with a pen to ensure appropriate location of serial measurements.

In addition to assessing the circumference, assess pulses, skin temperature, capillary refill, sensation, and movement in areas distal to the inflammation. Compare the involved side to the other side, using the client's uninvolved side as a baseline. Dressings or casts over the affected area can also form a constriction. This response can be called *compartment syndrome*. Clients who have been injured or had orthopedic surgery are at highest risk for compartment syndrome (see also Chapter 27).

Objects that may become entrapped in edematous tissues, such as rings, should be removed because they can cause serious damage. The inflamed area should be elevated. Application of cold compresses causes vasoconstriction and decreases the amount of edema. Prolonged use of cold compresses can lead to rebound vasodilation and increase the risk of tissue injury. Vasoconstriction can also decrease the inflow of new blood and thereby slow the removal of toxins and waste from the site of injury.

If the extremity is edematous, it should be elevated. Distal circulation and sensation should be assessed often for the first 48 hours after injury or surgery. Edematous skin is more likely to break down. Keep the skin lubricated and protected from injury. Factors that impede venous flow should be controlled. For example, rolled stockings that constrict venous return should not be worn. Compression bandages may be used to reduce edema by promoting lymphatic and venous drainage. Explain the appropriate way to apply these bandages (from distal to proximal) and when to rewrap them to maintain compression.

Evaluation. The outcome of the inflammatory response is usually time dependent. Most edema subsides over 72 hours with appropriate RICE measures. If the edema has not subsided in that time frame, consider another cause of the edematous process, such as infection.

Self-Care

Clients who are capable of caring for a wound or area that is likely to become inflamed need instructions on how to elevate the extremity, how to use heat or ice, how to follow the medication regimen, and how to change dressings. Clinical manifestations of edema and infection must be reported, such as changes in color, pulse, and pain. For clients going home, creative problem solving is needed to find a mechanism to elevate arms or legs while sleeping or sitting in a chair. The edematous extremity must remain higher than the heart to reduce edema, and this degree of elevation is hard to achieve at home and even more so while asleep.

CLIENTS WITH CHRONIC INFLAMMATION

Chronic inflammation is differentiated from acute inflammation by its duration and the cells that mediate the response. If the invading organisms were not controlled or eliminated during the acute stage of inflammation, the body attempts to protect surrounding tissues from further invasion by building a wall around the infected site called a *granuloma*. Some forms of infection, such as fungi, parasites, and perhaps antibody-antigen reactions (autoimmune disease), result in granuloma formation. Tuberculosis is a good example. When tuberculosis develops, a thick wall forms around the mycobacteria. The bacteria continue to live in the walled-off area, and it is soon filled with dead tissue. As the tissue dies, the cellular enzymes are released and the fluid leaves the granuloma. The empty sac remains.

Unlike an acutely inflamed wound, the appearance of a chronically inflamed wound often does not appear red, warm, and tender. The tissue often appears pale and odorous if infected and fails to heal.[5]

OUTCOME MANAGEMENT

The chronically inflamed wound has purulent drainage *(suppuration)* and does not heal completely. A common example of chronic inflammation is seen when foreign objects are not removed from tissues (e.g., splinter, glass, dirt). Chronic inflammation can also occur when certain forms of bacteria cannot be killed by phagocytes. For example, the organisms that cause tuberculosis, syphilis, and leprosy have cell walls with a very high lipid and wax content, which makes them impermeable to the phagocyte.

Care of the client with chronic infection is focused on determining the source of the problem. Wounds may be *debrided* (cleaned and freed of dead tissue), and the client may be given antibiotics or anti-inflammatory agents.

CLIENTS WITH INCISIONS

OUTCOME MANAGEMENT

Wounds made intentionally with a scalpel and closed with sutures, staples, glue, or strips of tape are called *incisions*. Incisions are the most common example of wounds healing by primary intention. An incision should be assessed every 8 hours. If the incision is not visible, check the dressings for drainage and odor. The incision normally appears somewhat pink and swollen; small areas of induration around the suture marks are common. Erythema should not extend beyond one-half inch from the incision. If the wound was closed primarily, you should be able to palpate the presence of newly synthesized collagen just under an intact suture line. This internal scar is known as a *healing ridge*. When this ridge is not present 5 to 7 days after suturing, suspect slowed collagen synthesis. The client may need additional protection of the nonhealing area to prevent infection.

A wound that is healing by primary intention should be protected from further trauma, including external pressure. Keep the wound free of pulling forces that stretch the sutured skin. Keep the wound clean, but do not wash the suture line because water carries microorganisms into the wound along the sutures. Protect it from the external environment and drainage with dressings.

Apply dressings using an aseptic or sterile technique. Sterile gloves are usually not required. Hold the outer side of the dressing that will not touch the client's incision by the clean or gloved hands, and tape it in place. The type of dressing used changes as the wound responds to treatment. Use dressings that best suit the wound. Gauze dressings are used most often on a wound that is healing by primary intention. Dressings for open wounds are discussed in the following section.

Wound drainage tubes can be placed in the dead space created during exposure of the operative area. Drainage of a wound is indicated when actual or potential fluid accumulation threatens the healing process. The drain facilitates removal of blood from the wound. Assess the volume and type of fluid hourly immediately after surgery. If a reservoir is attached to the drain, measure the volume of drainage by markings on the reservoir. If the drainage is emptied from the reservoir, follow standard precautions for its disposal. In addition, if the drainage is caustic (e.g., bile), the skin around the site must be protected with skin barriers.

Teach the client how to care for the incision, how to recognize the clinical manifestations of wound infection, how to care for and empty the drain reservoir, and when to return for suture removal. Sutures in areas where scarring must be controlled (e.g., on the face) are usually removed in 4 to 7 days; in other areas, sutures are usually removed in 7 to 10 days. Sutures in the hand and foot are removed in 1 to 2 weeks or longer.

CLIENTS WITH OPEN WOUNDS

OUTCOME MANAGEMENT

Medical Management

The goal of medical management of an open wound is to prepare the client and the wound for the quickest and most durable form of healing. The treatment of a wound includes the removal of its cause, the correction of underlying problems that are delaying healing, and the initiation of topical (or systemic) treatments to facilitate healing.

Control the Cause of the Wound

Open wounds are common in clients with diseases that impair blood flow to the legs (arteriosclerosis, venous insufficiency, diabetes) or that reduce sensation (paralysis, diabetes). If wound healing is delayed because of lack of venous return, the extremity requires compression and elevation. If the cause of the wound is lack of arterial flow, the extremity should be positioned flat. If pressure is a causative or contributing factor, repositioning and proper support surfaces must be considered.

Protein-calorie malnutrition may be present, which delays healing of all wounds because the protein needed to manufacture new cells is not available. The client's diet should be high in carbohydrates, protein, iron, and vitamins. In addition, the client may remain at risk of further skin breakdown, such as pressure ulcers.

Remove Devitalized Tissue from the Wound: Debridement

Wound healing is optimized and the risk of infection is reduced when all necrotic (dead) tissue, exudate, and metabolic wastes are removed from the wound. Moist, devitalized tissue supports bacterial growth. Various forms of debridement are used to remove these tissues (see later discussion). Systemic and topical antibiotics alone seldom stop infection because they cannot penetrate the avascular tissues.

Before a wound can heal, necrotic tissues must be removed. Debridement can be accomplished by means of a variety of techniques: (1) surgical or sharp, (2) mechanical, (3) enzymatic, and (4) autolytic (these last three are described later). Timely debridement is necessary to remove the devitalized tissue and reduce the risk of infection and the physical obstacles dead tissue places on the process of granulation. In addition, the true size and stage of the wound cannot be known until the necrotic tissue is removed.

Surgical or Sharp Debridement

Wounds covered with dead tissue, called *eschar* (pronounced *ES-car*) or *slough* (pronounced *sluff*), need to be cleaned to promote healing and reduce infection (Figure 18-4, *A*). *Sharp debridement* is performed by physicians or trained nurses and is the quickest method. This procedure is used for large wounds, a wound that involves a thick eschar that would not be permeated by any topical agent, and a wound that is acutely infected. The only wounds that contain eschar that should not be debrided are pressure ulcers on the heels with stable eschar and dry gangrene. These wounds are often lacking the arterial

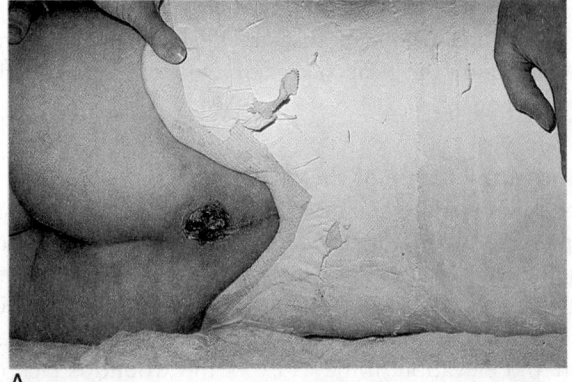

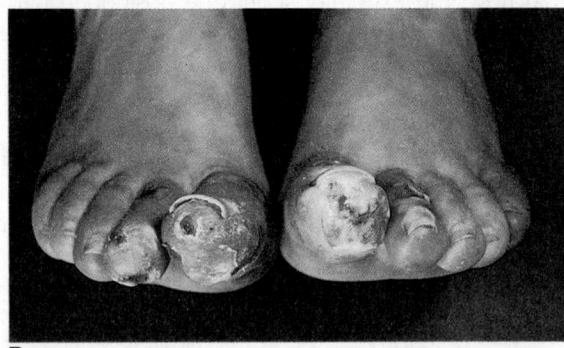

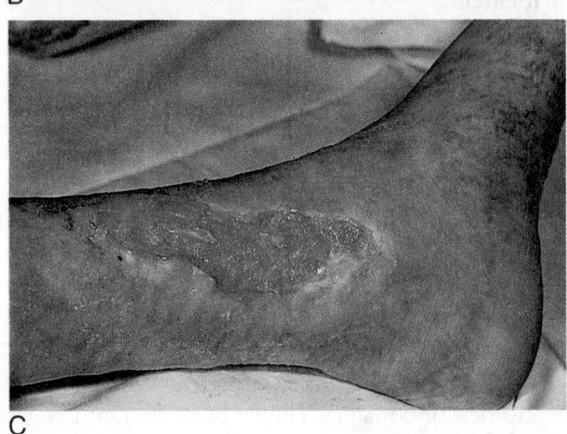

■ **FIGURE 18–4 A,** A wound on the sacrum with eschar that needs debridement, usually sharp. **B,** Diabetic foot ulcers are an example of a wound with yellow, soft slough that needs debridement, usually enzymatic. **C,** Healing venous stasis ulcers have a clean wound filled with granulation tissue that needs to be dressed with a moisture-retentive dressing.

inflow to support healing. The eschar or slough is removed to the level of bleeding tissues. The wound size, depth of the wound, contamination, and the client's status influence whether the client is in satisfactory condition to tolerate sharp debridement, which may call for general anesthesia or sedation. Pain medications should be used for clients undergoing sharp debridement.

Sharp debridement is carried out under sterile conditions, usually in an operating room, a treatment room, or an outpatient surgical setting. Risks associated with general anesthesia, blood loss, and infections are a major concern.

After sharp debridement, the client is monitored for manifestations of bleeding and bacteremia (sepsis). Sepsis is suspected if unexplained fever, tachycardia, hypotension, or deterioration in mental status develops. The physician should be notified of these changes. Sepsis can be fatal if it is not recognized early and treated aggressively (see septic shock in Chapter 81).

Once the wound is clean, surgery may be used to speed healing and to reduce the risk of infection and contracture. Skin grafts are commonly used to replace the epidermis. The partial-thickness burn wound is the best example of a wound that could heal by secondary intention but is often grafted to speed healing and reduce infection and scarring. Cutaneous or musculocutaneous flaps can also be used to close a large wound (see Chapter 49).

Nursing Management of the Medical Client

Assessment. The client's history must be taken, including a history of the wound itself. The wound history includes causative intrinsic and extrinsic factors, duration of the wound, and current and previous methods of treatment and their corresponding success. Sometimes wound treatments have been used that actually impair healing, such as hydrogen peroxide or Dakin's solution. This information is important when one is obtaining a complete wound history. Assessments should be thorough and should focus on the whole client, not just the wound.

Psychosocial assessment should include the client's age, occupation, living situation, financial status, health care benefits, roles and responsibilities, cultural and spiritual beliefs, body image and self-esteem, and ability to learn self-care and comply with the treatment plan. Also note compliance with treatment of underlying disorders, such as diabetes and collagen diseases.

A complete physical assessment should be performed. It is important to recognize that the entire client is examined, not just the wound. Focus the data collection on height and weight; degree of range of motion; muscle wasting and level of activity; circulation, such as peripheral pulses, color, edema, and the temperature of extremities; lung sounds; and level of pain. A complete wound assessment is needed (Box 18-1). Clearly document wound assessments to allow for an objective evaluation at a later date. Describe the actual size of the wound by measuring its length, width, and depth. If the wound is a pressure ulcer, use the staging system to further describe it (see Chapter 49). Describe the color, type of drainage, presence of undermining, and condition of periwound skin in the assessment data for later comparison. A photograph is an excellent means of documentation and determination of the progress in healing. Obtain consent before photographs are taken.

BOX 18-1 Wound Assessment

When assessing an open wound, obtain the following information:

1. Is the wound painful?
2. What is the size of the wound? Use objective measures to indicate the length and width (such as centimeters or millimeters). Avoid terms such as "the size of a grape." Use a sterile gloved finger or cotton swab to measure depth. Consider using photographs to provide a baseline and serial evaluations.
3. Where is the wound located anatomically?
4. What is the color of the wound? Estimate the percentage of each color when more than one color is noted.
5. Is there granulation tissue or epithelial tissue? Granulation tissue is red, shiny, and bumpy; epithelial tissue looks like pale skin.
6. Are there sinus tracts, or are the edges undermined? Use a gloved hand or swab to measure the extent. Indicate the location and direction of tunneling.
7. Are there signs of infection in the wound? Look for erythema extending beyond the edges of the wound as well as warmth, edema, odor, and purulent exudate. (Also consider systemic signs.)
8. Is there any drainage? Note the color, odor, consistency, and approximate amount by the number of dressings saturated.
9. What is the condition of the surrounding skin? Is it intact, red, indurated, or macerated?

Photographs should be taken with a consistent method that includes reproducible distance, color, and grid film or a ruler in the photo so that size can be determined.

Examine laboratory values for hemoglobin, hematocrit, albumin, prealbumin, and WBCs, specifically lymphocytes. These values indicate the degree of nutritional impairment that might contribute to the wound's lack of healing. Generally, the risk of delayed healing correlates with low serum albumin levels; however, albumin levels are a slow-to-change indicator of nutritional state. A pre-albumin level is more indicative of current nutritional status.

Diagnosis, Planning, Interventions

Diagnosis: Impaired Skin Integrity. The nursing diagnosis should be used to indicate an actual loss of skin The actual statement might be phrased *Impaired Skin Integrity related to delayed wound healing secondary to impaired circulation, to infection, or to malnutrition.*

Outcomes. The client will experience improved skin integrity, as evidenced by a cleaner wound within 1 week, less drainage from the wound, no odor from the wound, and no manifestations of infection in the wound. A long-term goal might be a smaller wound in 3 weeks.

Interventions. Many agencies have wound care nurses who should be contacted for up-to-date information and for assistance with complex wounds. Every nurse,

however, must properly identify basic concepts of wound assessment and treatment.

Keep the Wound Moist. Wound healing is optimized when the wound is kept moist. A moist environment promotes collagen synthesis, granulation tissue formation, and epithelial cell migration. This moist environment, however, can create a medium conducive to infection, and a clean technique must be used for wound care. Heat lamps or treatments that dry the wound must be avoided.

Wet-to-moist or continuously moist dressings are used in clean and granulating wounds. Open gauze dressings so that they can be inserted into the wound or placed on all surfaces of the wound while they are moist, making certain to protect normal intact skin. Remove the dressings while they are still moist to avoid disrupting the granular bed. Bleeding should not occur when the dressing is removed. If the dressing is too dry to pull off, moisten it with sterile normal saline before attempting to remove it. Foam, hydrogel and hydrocolloid dressings can also be used to keep a clean wound moist. The wound bed should be gently cleansed with normal saline to remove debris before replacing the dressings.

Prevent Injury to Healing Tissues. Normal saline or wound cleansers should be used for wound cleansing. Normal saline is physiologic, does not harm tissues, and adequately cleans most wounds. Avoid applying solutions on and in the clean wound that may impair healing. For example, full-strength iodine, hydrogen peroxide, and Dakin's solution were once commonly used for wound care; however, these solutions damage the wound (Table 18-4). If they are used for infected wounds, it is important to limit their use to the shortest time possible.

Protect the Periwound Skin. Moisture on normal, intact skin makes the skin more prone to breakdown. The cardinal rule is to keep the wound bed moist and surrounding skin dry.

Select Dressings. Dressings can protect a healing wound, absorb exudate, or debride a necrotic wound. Dressings are chosen based on the appearance of the wound bed (see Figure 18-4). Gauze still remains the most commonly used dressing. Gauze is used as a dry cover for surgical wounds or for wounds that heal by primary intention (Table 18-5). Only mesh gauze should be used in a wound because cotton dressings are likely to leave fibers behind. Use cotton-filled gauze as an outer dressing. If the wound edges are friable or if the wound will be injured when the dressing is removed, a nonadherent dressing can be used to avoid injury to the wound or periwound skin. If gauze is used to pack the wound, hydrocolloid dressings can be placed like a window frame around the wound. The tape can be applied to the window rather than the skin.

TABLE 18–4 Topical Agents Used in Treatment of Open Wounds

Agent	Indications	Impact on Wound Healing
Antiseptic Solutions		
Normal saline	Used to moisten dry wound beds; keeps clean wound healing by secondary intention	Speeds healing because solution is iso-osmolar, and it keeps wound bed moist
Hydrogen peroxide	Used to dissolve clotted blood in a wound	Retards healing; do not use as a dressing on an open wound
Povidone-iodine (Betadine)	Used for preparation of intact skin; may be used to clean very contaminated wounds	Retards healing; does not penetrate eschar
Dakin's solution	Used ½ to ¼ strength to clean contaminated wounds	Retards wound healing
Acetic acid	Used to treat wounds contaminated with *Pseudomonas*	Retards wound healing slightly
Antibiotic Solutions and Ointments		
Neomycin-bacitracin-polymyxin B (Neosporin)	Used to clean wounds contaminated with gram-negative and gram-positive bacteria	Increases epidermal healing but may sensitize tissues; high incidence of allergy
Polymyxin B-bacitracin (Polysporin)	Treatment of gram-negative bacteria	None known
Silver sulfadiazine	Used in wounds with eschar (e.g., burns); effective against gram-negative and gram-positive organisms	Enhances separation of necrotic tissue; penetrates eschar
Gentamicin	Most effective against gram-negative organisms	None known
Bacitracin	Effective against gram-positive and gram-negative organisms	May enhance epidermal healing

TABLE 18–5 Wound Dressings

Type	Product	Indications for Use	Nursing Implications
Nonadhering, nonimpregnated	Telfa	Shallow, open wounds	Second dressing or tape needed; it is nonadhesive; can lead to maceration
Impregnated	Adaptic gauze, Vaseline gauze, Xeroform	Moist wounds	Nonabsorbent, occlusive, not traumatic to remove
Gauze	Adaptic gauze, Kling gauze, NuGauze, Primapore	Wet-to-dry debridement, wound packing	Moderately absorbent; can be used as wound packing for shallow wounds; use long strips of gauze to pack deep wounds; gauze does not provide a bacterial barrier; if allowed to dry on a wound, it may remove viable tissue when removed
Transparent films	Bio-occlusive, OpSite, Tegaderm	Coverage of shallow clean wounds, intravenous sites, blisters, abrasions	Adhesive; therefore no secondary dressing is needed; retain moisture, semipermeable, water-resistant; facilitate autolytic debridement
Hydrocolloids	Comfeel, Duoderm, Intrasite, Restore, Tegasorb, Intact	Shallow clean ulcers, donor sites, partial-thickness burns; do not use on infected wounds	Retain moisture, occlusive or semipermeable, water-resistant, adhesive; require replacement because dressing melts; reduce pain
Hydrogels	Elastogel, wound gel, Spenco, Vigilon	Clean pressure ulcers, dermal ulcers, partial-thickness burns, abrasions, blisters	Have a cooling effect; maintain moist environment, relieve pain, permit autolytic debridement; easily removed unless they dry out
Exudate absorbers	Bard absorption dressing, Envisan	Deep wounds with eschar	Retain moisture, absorbent, promote autolytic debridement
Calcium alginates	Sorbsan, Kaltostat, Algiderm	Clean wounds with profuse drainage	Retain moisture, absorbent, left intact for several days
Foams	Reston, Flexan, Lyofoam, Polymen, Tielle	Full-thickness wounds with moderate to heavy drainage, skin tears	Moisture, absorbent, nonadherent, left intact for several days

Clean, granulating wounds do not require daily dressing changes (see Figure 18-4, *C*). Granulating wounds should be dressed with occlusive, moisture-retaining dressings, such as foam, moist gauze, hydrocolloid, or hydrogel. If the wound is shallow, a thin layer of antibiotic ointment and nonadhering dressing (or synthetic dressing) may be used to cover it. If the wound is deep, saline-moistened gauze can be used to pack the wound, but the dressing should not be allowed to dry out before it is changed. When a dressing adheres to a wound bed, granulation tissue and new epithelium are also removed when the dressing is changed. Continue to observe for infection. If purulent drainage develops, do not apply occlusive dressings. Allow the wound to drain by using gauze or alginates. Debriding dressings, like wet-to-dry dressings, should not be used on granulating wounds. Debridement removes new tissues, leads to bleeding, and slows healing.

Excessive exudate can delay healing. If the wound produces exudate, several absorptive dressings can be used. Absorptive dressings, calcium alginates, and hypertonic saline dressings are appropriate choices for moderate or highly exudative wounds. Foams can also be used for absorption and autolytic debridement. Table 18-5 describes the actions, indications, and nursing implications for various categories of wound dressings.

Necrotic wounds cannot be covered with occlusive dressings. Microorganisms cannot drain from the wound bed and become invasive, quickly leading to sepsis.

The selection of dressing type changes as the wound responds to treatment. Careful assessment and reassessment will indicate progress, or lack of progress, in wound healing. As the wound changes, variations in the dressing materials are made so that healing is maximized. No single dressing provides the optimal atmosphere required during all healing stages of the wound.

Fill Dead Space. *Dead space* is empty space within a wound. In an ulcer, it is the space between the base of the ulcer and the underside of the dressing around its perimeter. If this space is closed, empty pockets may develop anaerobic infection. Long-acting normal saline gel and alginate wound packing are good media to fill a clean wound and the pockets of empty space before a topical dressing is applied.

Deep wounds with tunnels or undermining are at high risk of infection. These wounds can also heal with "false floors," which trap bacteria and lead to further infection. It is important that an open wound heal from the inside out. Deep wounds are often packed with gauze strips soaked in saline or an antibiotic solution to debride the wound or prevent abnormal healing. Strips of gauze must be used to avoid having soiled single dressings lost in the wound.

The gauze is packed into the wound with enough force to hold the edges of the wound open, but not so much force that the wound is under tension. Tightly packed dressings can restrict blood flow and delay healing. The outer edge of the dressing is covered with dry dressings. Packing is usually changed every 4 to 6 hours. Some gel packing strips are changed less often. Skin surrounding the wound should be assessed for breakdown from frequent tape removal, and dressings should be secured with other methods if needed (e.g., Montgomery straps).

Remove Necrotic Tissue. Debridement is needed to remove nonviable tissue in the wound. Ulcers cannot heal with necrotic tissue present. Necrotic tissue becomes a breeding ground for microorganisms and increases the risk of septicemia, osteomyelitis, limb amputation, and death. Yellow or tan adherent material in the wound base is called *slough* (see Figure 18-4, *B*). Black, leathery material in the wound base is called *eschar*. This necrotic tissue must be removed for the wound to heal. (The only exception is dry eschar on the heel and dry gangrene, which should not be routinely removed.) The risk of infection rises in proportion to the amount of necrotic tissue present.

Several techniques can be used to debride necrotic tissue: sharp debridement (discussed earlier), mechanical debridement with irrigation and dressings, enzymatic debridement, and autolytic debridement.

Irrigation. Irrigation between 4 and 15 pounds per square inch (psi) removes debris, bacteria, and necrotic tissue without damaging tissues; 8 psi is the most pressure that should be used on a wound. High-pressure devices, such as a Waterpik, create excessive force and trauma and may cause bacteria to be driven into the wound. Wound irrigation is safe and effective small syringes of saline, or outer plastic tubing from an intravenous (IV) needle. Hydrotherapy by use of a whirlpool is also an option for wound cleaning.

When irrigating around a wound, use barrier precautions with masks or goggles, gowns, and gloves because you may be sprayed by contaminated solutions. The client may also need protection with a pad or container to collect the contaminated irrigation solution.

Wet-to-Dry Dressings. An all-gauze dressing is moistened with the prescribed solution and squeezed until the dressing is just moist. The moist dressing should be gently packed into all crevices in the wound and left long enough to begin to dry (4 to 6 hours) (Figure 18-5). As the dressing dries, debris, necrotic tissue, exudate, and drainage adhere to it. The wound is debrided as the dressing is gently removed. The dressings are not remoistened to make removal easier because this practice defeats the purpose of the dressing, which is to debride the wound. The process is often painful, and clients should have adequate analgesia before the dressing is changed. Topical skin protectant can be used to protect surrounding intact skin from exposure to moisture. Wet-to-dry dressings are a nonselective form of debridement and can inadvertently remove new granulation tissue as well as necrotic tissue, creating an environment that retards healing. Therefore they are used only until the wound is clean and granulating.

Enzymatic Debridement. Proteolytic enzymes can be applied to necrotic tissue to digest them. Enzymatic

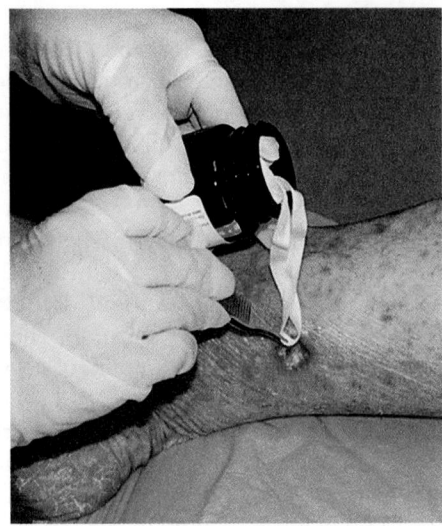

■ **FIGURE 18–5** Wet-to-dry dressings are placed into a wound with the use of strip gauze.

debridement should be considered when the client cannot tolerate surgical excision; has soft, stringy slough; or is at home or in long-term care. Enzymatic debridement is relatively slow and should not be used on wounds that appear infected. Medicate clients before the use of enzymatic agents, which cause burning. Apply the enzymatic ointment to only about 2 to 4 square inches of necrotic tissue at one time. Enzymes work best in a moist environment; use moist gauze and cover the wound with dry gauze. Enzymatic agents should not be placed on viable tissue because they cause tissue necrosis. Enzymes are inactivated by metals used in dressings, such as silver. Enzymes also cannot be used on wounds communicating with major body cavities, wounds with exposed nerves, or neoplastic ulcers. They must be used with caution around the eyes.

Autolytic Debridement. Autolytic debridement is the use of the body's own digestive enzymes to break down necrotic tissue. With this method, an occlusive dressing is placed over the ulcer and the eschar or devitalized tissue is allowed to self-digest. This is a slow process; however, autolytic debridement may be appropriate for clients who cannot tolerate other methods and are not susceptible to infection. Autolytic debridement is contraindicated for infected wounds.

Provide Nutritional Support. In addition to local wound care, the client must be provided with a diet that is high in protein, fat, carbohydrates, vitamins, and minerals to facilitate healing. Regardless of the client's actual body weight (e.g., obesity), healing a wound is not the time to begin a weight-loss diet. The wound must be healed first. Review the nutritionist's recommendations for caloric, protein, and fluid intake. Determine whether the client is receiving the needed nutrients. If the client can eat, offer supplements or adjust the diet so that the meal is more palatable. If the client cannot or will not eat, the use of tube-feeding or hyperalimentation should be considered. Many clients report that they do not have an appetite and therefore do not feel like eating. Clients and family should be encouraged to eat anyway; an appetite is not needed to consume food.

Reduce Interface Pressure. If the client has pressure ulcers, pressure redistribution is key to management and prevention. Turning and repositioning constitute the oldest form of redistributing pressure on body surfaces. Clients should be turned and repositioned every 2 hours if they do not move spontaneously. If the client cannot be moved or refuses to turn, consider changing the surface of the bed to one that creates less interface pressure. Chair cushions must also be used to reduce pressure on the ischia when sitting. Four inches of foam is adequate for most clients. Over time, however, foam develops a "memory," which reduces its effectiveness. If an imprint of the client's buttocks remains in the foam after rising from the chair, the foam needs to be replaced. Other seat cushions are also available. All clients who sit in chairs need to be repositioned hourly regardless of the surface on which they sit.

Evaluation. In hospital settings, wounds should be assessed with each dressing change. Wounds at risk of infection should be assessed every 24 hours. Clean, granulating wounds can be evaluated every 3 to 5 days, provided the dressings remain intact and clean. If the dressings appear stained or surrounding skin is red, swollen, or painful, the dressings should be removed and the wound closely assessed for infection. If the wound shows no signs of healing after 2 weeks, a 2-week trial of topical antibiotics is recommended, including quantitative bacterial cultures and a bone scan to assess for osteomyelitis.

Self-Care

The client with open wounds often requires long-term care or community resources for safe self-care. Planning for discharge should begin several days before the client is released so that the home situation can be appraised and the necessary support, supplies, and equipment obtained. Appropriate referral to the home health agency or wound-healing clinic should be made before discharge. Social services, home health care, or a discharge planner should be involved in the plan of care. The client's financial status, home environment, and support systems must be evaluated. Third-party reimbursement may cover supplies, equipment, and nursing care.

Several areas of client education are needed. The client or family should demonstrate dressing removal, wound cleaning, and dressing application before discharge. Detailed written instructions on wound care should be provided to the client, family, and home health care nurse. Videotaping the dressing change may be helpful once the client is home. Explain what changes should be expected and what changes should be reported to the health care provider. Fever, a change in drainage, or the development of an odorous drainage should be instructed as being a reportable change.

The average cost of skilled nursing services for treating wounds in the home is $1600 per healed wound. Some cost-cutting measures for saline and gloves have been designed, and it is now possible to make normal saline for home use on wounds. Use 1 gallon of distilled water or 1 gallon of tap water boiled for 5 minutes; do not use well water or seawater. Add 8 teaspoons of table salt. Mix the solution well and cool to room temperature before use. This solution can be stored for up to 1 week.

In the home, rather than purchasing gloves for dressing changes, soiled dressings can be removed using a plastic sandwich bag (Figure 18-6). The inside of the bag is used as a glove to remove the dressing, and the dressing is disposed of in the same bag. Methods of obtaining needed wound care supplies should also be discussed with the client and the client's family.

A balanced diet with frequent high-protein snacks should continue until the wound and contributing factors have been resolved. A vitamin and mineral supplement should be taken as directed. The client is often required to incorporate lifestyle changes into activities of daily living (ADL) in an effort to promote healing.

DISORDERS OF WOUND HEALING

DELAYED WOUND HEALING

Not all wounds heal in a timely manner or stay healed. Both intrinsic and extrinsic factors delay wound healing. When assessing wounds and clients with wounds, be aware of the factors that can delay healing. Some factors are controllable and some are not. The factors mentioned here are just a few of the conditions that can impede wound healing. Recent research indicates that wounds that do not heal have high levels of protein-degrading enzymes (matrix protease) in the wound bed and low levels of growth factors.

WOUND INFECTION

Wound infection is a serious consequence and a common cause of delayed wound healing. Infection is often due to lack of blood supply, lack of oxygen, autocontamination, or exposure to environmental pathogens. Clinical manifestations of wound infection include increased or more bloody drainage, purulent drainage, odor from the wound or drainage, erythema around the entire wound (not just the edges), increasing pain, fever, leukocytosis, and general malaise. The infected wound is slow to heal and may open (see later discussion on evisceration and dehiscence).

Cultures can be used in the diagnosis of wound infection. A swab culture of wound drainage can be obtained. When obtaining a swab culture, remove the excess visible drainage first, and then swab the wound bed. The value of a swab culture is limited, because all open wounds are contaminated. Therefore a swab culture does not reveal the true offending organisms within the wound; rather, it discloses only organisms growing on the wound's surface. Swab cultures can show the presence of methicillin-resistant *Staphylococcus aureus* (MRSA) or vancomycin-resistant *Enterococcus* (VRE). A quantitative culture (an actual sample of tissue) is usually needed to identify invasive infection.

A precise technique for wound care is needed to reduce the risk of cross-contamination.

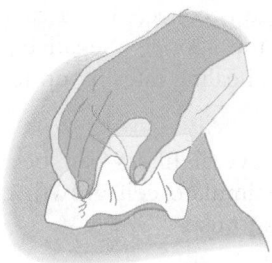

Place a small, clean bag over your hand like a mitten. Carefully lift the dressing off the sore.

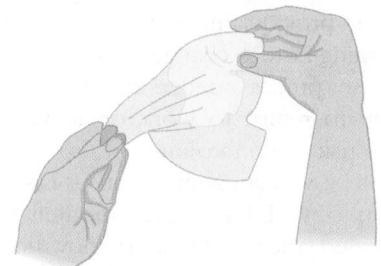

Turn the bag inside out to enclose the dressing. Seal the bag before throwing it away.

■ **FIGURE 18–6** Plastic bags used as gloves to remove a dressing in the home. *(Modified from Agency for Health Care Policy and Research. [1994]. Treating pressure sores [AHCPR Pub. No. 95-B0654]. Bethesda, Md: U.S. Department of Health and Human Services.)*

SAFETY

ALERT

OUTCOME MANAGEMENT

Topical antimicrobial agents can be used as the primary treatment. The ideal antimicrobial is a broad-spectrum agent and preserves regenerating tissues. All antimicrobials compromise wound healing to some degree by having low efficacy against a particular organism or by interfering with healing. A variety of topical agents can be used either to clean or to disinfect the wound (see Table 18-4).

Hydrogen peroxide (H_2O_2) breaks down into water and oxygen. When hydrogen peroxide is used in a wound, H_2O_2 must be rinsed off the wound bed with normal saline to remove any trapped oxygen before the tissues can absorb it. Povidone-iodine, acetic acid, and sodium hypochlorite are used only in debris-contaminated, infected, and malodorous wounds. These agents are cytotoxic and inhibit granular tissue growth and damage endothelial cells and fibroblasts. Therefore their use is usually short term only.

Medical Management

The goal of medical management of clients with wound infection is to eradicate the infection. The extrinsic and intrinsic factors that lead to nonhealing are examined. Not all of these factors can be eliminated, however. Clients cannot be made younger, and some clients refuse to stop smoking, even though their nonhealing is due to inadequate circulation. At times, bypass surgery may be required to restore adequate blood flow. Cultured epithelial grafts, wound fillers, and hyperbaric oxygen are relatively new treatments in the care of nonhealing wounds. Most chronic nonhealing wounds are managed by a team of health care providers that may include a wound care physician, vascular or orthopedic surgeons, a wound care nurse, a nutritionist, a physical therapist, hyperbaric medicine specialists, and social workers and psychologists. Even for these teams, chronic nonhealing wounds are a challenge.

Adjunctive Wound-Healing Treatments

Electrical Stimulation. Pulsed galvanic stimulation (Diapulse) is a form of electricity applied to the skin's surface. The electrical currents stimulate DNA synthesis, increase blood flow, enhance fibroblast proliferation, and promote cell migration across the wound. This modality appears to be effective in promoting healing in wounds that have been refractory to other forms of treatment. Clients who are considering the use of electrotherapy should seek centers that have proper equipment and trained personnel.

Growth Factors. The same growth factors that are found in the wound bed naturally can be grown in a laboratory and applied to the wound bed. Research is ongoing to determine the biologic activity and the potential benefits of topical application of these growth factors. Determining the timing and proper combinations of the growth factors is a subject of research. Becaplermin (Regranex), a platelet-derived growth factor, for use in diabetic foot ulcers, has gained approval by the Food and Drug Administration.

Hyperbaric Oxygen Therapy. Hyperbaric oxygen (HBO) is the administration of oxygen at greater than atmospheric pressure. When oxygen is inhaled under pressure, the level of tissue oxygen is greatly increased. The high levels of oxygen promote the action of phagocytes and encourage healing of the wound by increasing the action of fibroblasts. HBO is effective in clients with complex wounds, especially clients with osteomyelitis and other types of infection. HBO is becoming more available in the United States. As with electrical stimulation, a properly trained staff is critical. Clients who have inner ear problems and claustrophobia require pretreatment care.

Negative-Pressure Wound Therapy. The application of controlled negative pressure in a clean wound bed can assist and accelerate wound healing. A sterile, reticulated foam sponge is placed in the wound bed. A connecting evacuation tube is attached to external suction and removes excess fluid in the wound and peripheral edema. The foam and tube are secured with transparent adhesive dressing. A small electrical unit controls pressure, and drainage is collected in a canister attached to the unit and to the sponge. Negative-pressure wound therapy increases healing rates by up to 40%.[2]

Wound Fillers. Several fillers can be inserted into a wound bed to stimulate cell growth or to provide a scaffold for cells to use.

Nursing Management of the Medical Client

The nurse's role in the care of the client with a nonhealing wound is to provide ample information for self-care, including learning how to change dressings, understanding the disease process underlying the wound, and knowing how to return to work or activities without increasing the risk of nonhealing.

For example, a woman with venous stasis ulcers may need to return to work but can do so safely only when the ulcer is healed. She also needs to know how to apply bandages, how long to elevate her legs while at work, and how to move her legs while working (e.g., walking rather than standing). Nurses serve a vital role in determining whether these requirements are feasible for the client and employer.

PALLIATIVE CARE OF FRAIL CLIENTS WITH NONHEALING WOUNDS

For frail clients with little hope of recovery, wounds may never heal. Defining care for these clients is the subject of intense debate, including a change in approaches to the wound that support the client's and family's goals and promote comfort rather than aggressively promote wound healing. Palliative care that addresses pain control, odor management, drainage control, and quality of life should be the main concerns. The wound should be protected to prevent deterioration and infection.

The client's health should also be maintained so that the risk of infection or spread of infection or sepsis is minimized.

WOUND DISRUPTION

Dehiscence is the interruption of a previously intact suture line (see Chapter 14). A sharp pain in the suture line or a cough and increased serosanguineous drainage from the wound frequently will precede dehiscence. *Evisceration* is the opening of a wound with exposure of internal organs. It is obviously more serious than dehiscence. If a client experiences evisceration, cover the exposed organs with sterile wet dressings, notify the physician, and prepare the client for surgery. Also notify the physician about dehiscence, although it is not an emergency.

ALTERED COLLAGEN SYNTHESIS

Hypertrophic scars are scars that are raised above the suture line. They may be painful and itch. In general, hypertrophic scars tend to regress over time. *Keloids* are scars that extend well beyond the suture line (Figure 18-7). These scars tend to occur in African Americans and clients of Mediterranean descent. The scars can be excised from a wound but unfortunately tend to recur. Newer treatments include the use of topical forms of heat.

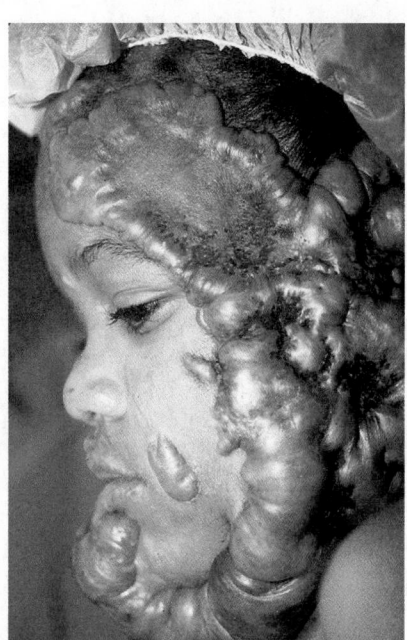

■ **FIGURE 18–7** Keloid formation. Keloids are overgrowths of scar tissue above and beyond the normal boundaries of the scar. They are fairly resistant to treatment.

THINKING CRITICALLY

1. You are caring for a man with large venous stasis ulcers on his lower legs. When he was admitted, the ulcers were covered with soft, yellow, devitalized tissue. He has been treated with wet-to-dry dressings for the past 7 days. Today you notice that the ulcers are red and wet with a lumpy appearance. What should be done?

Factors to Consider. Is the appearance of red and lumpy tissue in a wound good or bad? What might be happening? What type of dressing is best used on this red and lumpy tissue?

2. You are caring for an older homeless man after he has undergone emergency abdominal surgery. A nasogastric tube has been in place for 3 days for ileus, and he is receiving 1 L of IV fluids of 5% dextrose with 0.45% normal saline with 20 mEq of potassium every 8 hours. Before surgery, his serum albumin level was 3.2 g/dl, hemoglobin level 9.6 g/dl, and WBC count 17,000/mm^3. His weight was 104 pounds and height 5 feet 5 inches. What are this client's chances of recovery? What interventions should be considered?

Factors to Consider. Does this client have evidence of malnutrition? If so, what effect does malnutrition have on wound healing? What short-term and long-term interventions may need to be initiated? Does this client have a risk of fluid or electrolyte imbalance? If so, which ones, and what can be done (or is being done) to reduce the risk?

CONCLUSIONS

Wound healing is a complex process but often continues with little effort on the part of the client. Only when the wound does not heal or pressure ulcers develop are the many steps in wound healing evident. Wound care follows some basic principles: debride the wound of nonviable tissues, keep the clean wound bed moist, protect the surrounding skin, apply the proper dressings, use safe topical agents, fill dead space, and provide adequate protein and calories for healing.

Discussions for these questions can be found on the website.

BIBLIOGRAPHY

Citations appearing in red refer to primary research.

Citations appearing in blue refer to evidence-based practice guidelines and protocols.

1. Alvarez, O., et al. (2002). Chronic wounds: Palliative management for the frail population. *Wounds: A Compendium of Clinical Research and Practice, 14*(8 Suppl), 5S-27S.
2. Argenta, L., Morykwas, M., Marks, M., et al. (2006). Vacuum-assisted closure: State of clinic art. Wound healing: An overview. *Plastic and Reconstructive Surgery, 117* (7 Suppl), 127S-142S.
3. Boughton, G., Janis, J., & Attinger, C. (2006). Wound healing: An overview. *Plastic and Reconstructive Surgery, 117*(7 Suppl), 1eS-32eS.
4. Childress, B.B., & Stechniller, J. (2002). Role of nitric oxide in wound healing. *Biological Nursing Research, 4*(1), 5-15.
5. Collins, N. (2003). Obesity and wound healing. *Advances in Skin and Wound Care, 16*(1), 45-47.
6. Cuzzell, J. (2002). Wound healing: Translating theory into clinical practice. *Dermatology Nursing, 14*(4), 257-261.
7. Doughty, D., & Sparks-Defriese, B. (2006). Wound healing physiology. In R. Bryant & D. Nix (Eds.), *Acute and chronic wounds* (3rd ed., pp. 56-81). St. Louis: Mosby.
8. Gardner, S., et al. (2001). The validity of clinical signs and symptoms used to identify localized chronic wound infection. *Wound Repair and Regeneration, 9*(3), 178-186.
9. Greenhalgh, D.G. (2003). Wound healing and diabetes mellitus. *Clinics in Plastic Surgery, 30*(1), 37-45.
10. Hart, J. (2002). Inflammation: Its role in the healing of acute wounds. *Journal of Wound Care, 11*(6), 205-209.
11. Hunt, T.K., Hopf, H., & Hussain, Z. (2000). Physiology of wound healing. *Advances in Skin and Wound Care, 13*(2 Suppl), 6-11.
12. Kloth, L.C. (2002). How to use electrical stimulation for wound healing. *Nursing, 32*(12), 17.
13. Lazarus, G., et al. (1994). Definitions and guidelines for assessment of wounds and evaluating healing. *Archives of Dermatology, 130,* 489-493.
14. Monaco, J., & Lawrence, W. (2003). Acute wound healing: An overview. *Clinics in Plastic Surgery, 30*(1), 1-12.
15. Morykwas, M., Simpson, J., Punger, K., et al. (2006). Vacuum assisted wound closure: Stage of basic research and physiologic foundation. Wound healing: An overview. *Plastic and Reconstructive Surgery, 117*(7 Suppl), 121S-126S.
16. Nix, D. (2006). Patient assessment and evaluation of healing. In R. Bryant & D. Nix (Eds.), *Acute and chronic wounds* (3rd ed., pp. 130-148). St. Louis: Mosby.
17. Wood, Z. (2002). Hyperbaric oxygen in the management of chronic wounds. *British Journal of Nursing, 11*(16 Suppl), S16, 18-19, 22-24.

evolve *Did you remember to check out the bonus material on the Evolve website and the CD-ROM, including NCLEX®-Examination Style Review Questions, Open-Book Quizzes, and Chapter Review Audio Podcasts?*

http://evolve.elsevier.com/Black/medsurg

CHAPTER 19

Perspectives on Infectious Disease and Bioterrorism

CAROL J. WEBER

For one brief moment in human history (circa 1950 to 1980), management of infectious disease did not dominate health care practice. By the close of that era, sickness and death caused by infectious diseases had plummeted as a result of multifaceted social, public health, and medical control efforts. Environmental sanitation had curbed such killers as yellow fever, cholera, typhus, malaria, typhoid fever, and plague.

International vaccination programs had eradicated smallpox. Organized efforts to vaccinate all children lowered the occurrence of vaccine-preventable diseases, particularly measles, mumps, rubella, diphtheria, tetanus, and poliomyelitis. Improved living conditions and personal hygiene had diminished parasitic diseases and gastrointestinal (GI) infections. The widespread availability of antibiotics quelled the fear of deadly tuberculosis, syphilis, gonorrhea, bacterial meningitis, scarlet fever, and rheumatic fever. Nosocomial (hospital-acquired) infections, which had already responded to medical asepsis, responded further to antibiotics, and medical technology continued to produce anti-infective agents to match the newly developing antibiotic-resistant organisms. As a result, health professionals could focus on the prevention and management of chronic disease.

This brief moment in history did not last. The 1980s and 1990s brought new infectious agents, such as *Legionella,* the human immunodeficiency virus (HIV), and the Ebola virus (which actually first appeared in 1976), all reminders of human vulnerability to infectious disease. In 2001 the threat of bioterrorism took center stage with governments preparing for possible terrorist attacks with biologic agents such as anthrax and smallpox. In 2003 a previously unknown organism—a coronavirus—caused a worldwide outbreak of severe acute respiratory syndrome (SARS). In 2005 the World Health Organization alerted the world to prepare for a possible pandemic caused by an avian (bird) flu virus, the influenza A H5N1 virus, which had crossed the species barrier to infect humans (Box 19-1).

Meanwhile, hepatitis, tuberculosis, sexually transmitted diseases, and many vaccine-preventable diseases persist, spread, and continue to kill. Nonpathogenic organisms continue to create devastating disease in immunocompromised people and in those with chronic diseases or malnutrition. Antibiotic-resistant organisms have developed with chronic misuse and improper prescription of antibiotics. In addition, many of the major killers of the past, such as cholera and yellow fever, continue to cause death and destruction in parts of the world where poor sanitation, poor hygiene, and poverty are endemic.

All people, particularly health care professionals, must maintain vigilance to infectious diseases—to prevention rather than simply treatment. Prevention requires an understanding of the infectious process and the control measures needed. This chapter describes the process of infection, selected aspects of prevention and control, and bioterrorism. Other chapters explain the nursing care of clients with specific infectious diseases.

THE PROCESS OF INFECTION

Infection is a process by which an organism establishes a parasitic relationship with its host. The process begins with transmission of an infectious organism. Infection may end in infectious disease, a condition that depends on the response of the host to the invader. The entire process and its outcome hinge on a complex interaction of (1) the *infectious agent,* (2) an *environment* conducive

---

evolve **Web Enhancements**

Bridge to Home Health Care   Infection Control

Be sure to check out the bonus material on the Evolve website and the CD-ROM, including free self-assessment exercises. **http://evolve.elsevier. com/Black/medsurg**

BOX 19-1   Avian Influenza Pandemic Threat

Since late 2003 the world has experienced conditions that favor another pandemic. A pandemic threat exists in the form of the H5N1 virus, a highly pathogenic strain of bird flu. H5N1 has been causing outbreaks in poultry, and is now spreading in migratory and domestic fowl throughout Asia and Europe. Bird flu viruses occur mainly in birds and do not usually infect humans, but the H5N1 virus has crossed the species barrier. As of July 2007 the virus had infected 318 people, and more than half of them died.[49] H5N1 infection in people causes severe respiratory illness with rapid deterioration and high fatality commonly attributable to viral pneumonia and multi-organ failure. The virus is not yet capable of spreading from person to person, but if the virus mutates to a strain that spreads easily among humans, all prerequisites will be met to trigger a pandemic capable of killing millions. Since human-to-human transmission will most likely occur by coughing or sneezing, it is expected that the virus will spread rapidly and infect virtually all countries. Air travel will promote the distribution, especially since infected travelers can be asymptomatic but still contagious. Once international spreading begins, experts consider a pandemic unstoppable.

No one knows if the pandemic can be prevented. The best approach would be to eliminate the virus from birds, but experts are doubtful that this can be achieved within the near future. An influenza vaccine against the H5N1 virus would protect people, but there is no vaccine currently available. Vaccine development efforts are underway, but large-scale production of vaccine cannot occur until the new virus strain has emerged and the pandemic begun. Since the vaccine must closely match the pandemic virus, the new vaccine cannot be developed until the virus strain has been identified. This means that a vaccine will not be widely available until several months after a pandemic has been declared. Even then, experts predict that global production of vaccine will not be able to keep up with expected demand.

In August 2005 the World Health Organization (WHO) urged all countries to prepare for the possibility of an avian influenza pandemic. If containing or delaying the spread of a new human influenza strain is possible, it will take rapid, massive coordinated global and national actions. The primary response strategy will be to implement public health measures that reduce person-to-person transmission. When the first people are infected with a pandemic virus, the goal is to contain or delay spread of the virus. Containment measures could include a ban on large public gatherings, isolation of infected people, prophylaxis of the entire community with antiviral drugs, and possibly a large-scale quarantine.

Assuming these infection-control measures could contain the virus, many countries do not have the resources either to prepare for a pandemic or to purchase a stockpile of antiviral drugs. Furthermore, the infrastructure and skills required for surveillance and reporting are weak in several of the risk-prone countries, particularly in rural areas where most cases have occurred. Yet interventions aimed at minimizing the spread of infection depend on early detection and rapid reporting of an outbreak that occurs anywhere in the world. To mitigate some of these problems, WHO has assembled teams of experts to be deployed to provide rapid, on-site investigative support, and has

set up the infrastructure necessary to ship samples outside affected countries to certified laboratories. WHO is also establishing an international stockpile of antiviral drugs for use near the start of a pandemic, and is working with the international community to find ways to make vaccines and antiviral drugs affordable and accessible to all countries.

The United States is working closely with the World Health Organization and other international partners on surveillance, containment, and response activities. In November 2005 the Department of Health and Human Services released the *HHS Pandemic Influenza Plan* describing how the United States will prepare and respond to an influenza pandemic. The plan coordinates efforts at the federal, state, and local government levels with those of the private sector and tribal authorities. There are four major components of the plan:

1. Intensify surveillance and containment measures, both domestic and international.
2. Stockpile vaccines and antiviral medications, and work with industry to expand production capacity.
3. Create a seamless network of federal, state, and local preparedness.
4. Develop education and communication to keep the public informed.

The plan calls for purchasing enough H5N1 influenza vaccine for 20 million people and enough influenza antiviral drugs for another 20 million people. To speed the process of developing vaccines, research and development cooperating agreements have been signed by public and private agencies to produce and test multiple vaccines against H5N1 and other potential pandemic flu strains.

It is very difficult to prepare for a pandemic. While experts cannot predict the severity of the next pandemic, they predict that 15% to 35% of the U.S. population could be affected. In the absence of vaccination or drugs, it is estimated that in the United States, a pandemic could cause 89,000 to 207,000 deaths, 314,000 to 734,000 hospitalizations, 18 to 42 million outpatient visits, and another 20 to 47 million people being sick. We know that large numbers of people seeking medical treatment will overwhelm health services, and the numbers of health care workers available to work will be reduced. Other essential personnel such as law enforcement, transportation, and communications will also be affected. Compared to other public health emergencies, a pandemic will last much longer because a second wave of global spread can be expected within 3 to 12 months after the first wave.

While previous pandemics have taken the world by surprise, the present situation has given the world advanced warning and a rare opportunity to prepare for the next pandemic. WHO urges all countries to take action now to assess their level of preparedness, identify priority needs, and develop a national influenza preparedness plan. If containing or delaying the spread of a new human influenza strain is possible, it will take rapid, massive coordinated global and national actions. The success of these actions will depend on the preparations that have made in advance by each member of the international community.

Data from Weber, C.J. (2006). Infectious disease: Update on influenza pandemic threat. *Urologic Nursing, 26*(1), 67-68; Weber, C.J. (2006). Infectious disease: Update on preparing for the next influenza pandemic. *Urologic Nursing, 26*(2), 145-147; World Health Organization (2007). *Cumulative number of confirmed human cases of avian influenza A/(H5n1) reported to WHO.* Retrieved July 24, 2007 from http://www.who.int/csr/disease/avian_influenza/country/cases_table_2007_07_11/en/index.html.

to transmission of the organism, and (3) a susceptible *host*. The agent, the host, and their environmental interactions are prerequisites to infectious disease.

Agent

Humans coexist with many microorganisms in complex, mutually beneficial relationships. Many organisms establish residence on or in the host and usually cause no harm. Other organisms are parasitic, maintaining themselves at the expense of their host. Some parasites arouse a pathologic response in the host and are called *pathogens* or *pathogenic agents*. In one sense, pathogens are ineffective parasites because they stimulate an inflammatory response, leading to a disease that may harm the host and eventually kill the pathogen.

All microorganisms can be distinguished by certain intrinsic properties. These properties provide the basis for identifying and classifying bacteria, viruses, fungi, and helminths. An organism's properties include its shape, size, structure, chemical composition, antigenic make-up, growth requirements, viability under adverse environmental conditions, and ability to produce toxins. Viability is a particularly important property to health care professionals because it determines the pathogen's ability to survive outside its host. Organisms that can survive drying, sunlight, heat, or other adverse environmental conditions require more aggressive tactics to prevent transmission.

Environment

Transmission of an infectious agent from a source to a susceptible host occurs within an environment. Organisms live and multiply in a *reservoir*, which can be a person, animal, plant, soil, food, or other organic substance or combination of substances. The reservoir provides what the organism needs for survival at specific stages in its life cycle. Infected people are the reservoirs for most bacteria and viruses that affect humans.

Both human and animal reservoirs may be infected and, therefore, may also be hosts. An infected host may be asymptomatic—a *carrier* of the pathogen. A carrier maintains an environment that promotes growth, multiplication, and shedding of the parasite without exhibiting manifestations of disease.

Organisms can have one or more than one *route of transmission* from the reservoir to a new host. In fact, transmission can occur through five mechanisms:

1. *Contact transmission:* Through *direct* transmission, an organism moves from an infected person (or *carrier*) to an uninfected person via direct contact between their body surfaces. Through *indirect* transmission, an uninfected person picks up an infectious organism from an intermediate object, such as contaminated gloves, a used needle, or a dirty dressing.
2. *Droplet transmission:* An uninfected person picks up an infectious organism when an infected person coughs, sneezes, or talks. These activities propel droplets a short distance through the air, and they may land on an uninfected person's conjunctivae, nasal mucosa, or oral mucosa. Certain procedures, such as suctioning and bronchoscopy, can generate droplets as well.
3. *Airborne transmission:* Droplets can evaporate into airborne nuclei, or microbes can become attached to floating dust particles. Unlike droplets, dry nuclei and dust particles can float a long way in the air. Relatively few organisms remain viable as airborne nuclei, but those that do can be transmitted in the air and breathed into the lungs.
4. *Common vehicle transmission:* Many uninfected people can pick up an infectious organism from the same contaminated source, such as food, water, a medication, or a device.
5. *Vector transmission:* An infected creature, such as a mosquito, fly, rat, or flea, transmits an infectious organism by biting an uninfected host (Box 19-2).

BOX 19-2   West Nile Virus

West Nile virus has been commonly found in humans and birds and other vertebrates in Africa, Eastern Europe, West Asia, and the Middle East, but it was not documented in the United States until 1999. The virus can infect humans, birds, mosquitoes, horses, and some other animals.

The principal route of human infection with West Nile virus is through the bite of an infected mosquito. Mosquitoes become infected when they feed on infected birds. When the virus is injected into humans by a mosquito, it can multiply and possibly cause illness. Most people who become infected with the virus will not have any type of illness. Those who develop West Nile fever will have flu-like manifestations, lasting only a few days and without any long-term health effects. It is estimated that 1 in 150 people infected with West Nile virus will develop encephalitis or meningitis, a more severe form of the disease. Even in areas where the virus is circulating, however, very few mosquitoes are infected with the virus. The chances of becoming severely ill from any one mosquito bite are extremely small.

One cannot get West Nile virus from casual contact such as touching or kissing a person who has the disease. However, in a small number of cases, the virus has been transmitted through blood transfusion, organ transplantation, breast-feeding, and pregnancy (from mother to fetus).

You can reduce your risk of becoming infected with West Nile virus by applying insect repellent to exposed skin. Choose an insect repellant that contains diethyltoluamide (DEET) and one that provides protection for the amount of time you will be outdoors. Also spray your clothing because mosquitoes can bite through thin clothing. Wearing long-sleeved shirts, long pants, and socks while outdoors can also reduce your risk. Take special precautions from April to October, the months when mosquitoes are most active.

Data from Centers for Disease Control and Prevention. (2005). *West Nile virus: What you need to know.* Retrieved 03/10/06 from www.cdc.gov/ncidod/dvbid/westnile/wnv_factsheet.htm.

The *portal of exit* is the place where the parasite escapes the reservoir. Generally, this site corresponds to the *portal of entry* into the next host. For example, the portal of exit for GI parasites is generally the feces and the portal of entry into a new host is the mouth. As is the case with other links in the transmission chain, variability exists. Hookworm eggs, for example, are shed in the feces, but hookworm larvae enter through the skin of a person walking barefoot in soil containing hatched eggs. Common portals of exit include secretions and fluids (respiratory and vaginal secretions, blood, tears, semen, and breast milk), excretions (urine and feces), open lesions, and exudates. Some organisms, such as HIV, have more than one portal of exit. Knowledge of the portal of exit is essential for preventing transmission of a pathogen.

A pathogen may enter a new host by ingestion, inhalation, contact with mucous membranes, percutaneously, or transplacentally. Infectious diseases vary as to the number of organisms and the duration of the exposure required to start the infectious process in a new host.

Host

Some humans are more susceptible to infectious disease than others. A susceptible host has characteristics and behaviors that increase the probability of infectious disease. Factors such as age, gender, ethnicity, heredity, altitude, and temperature influence the likelihood of infection. For example, the ethnic custom of eating raw fish may increase the risk of exposure to pathogens. General health and nutritional status, hormonal balance, and the presence of concurrent disease also play a role. Living conditions and personal behaviors—such as drug use, diet, hygiene, and sexual practices—also influence the risk of exposure to pathogens and resistance once exposure has occurred. Susceptibility is also influenced by anatomic and physiologic defenses, sometimes called *lines of defense*. Even though an infectious disease is said to be caused by an etiologic (causal) agent, infection results from interactions among a variety of factors related to agent, host, and environment (Table 19-1).

The host's first-line defenses are external and act to bar invasion by pathogens. These defenses are nonspecific in that they act against any invading pathogen. First-line defenses include (1) *physical* and *chemical barriers* and (2) the body's own natural flora. Physical barriers include intact skin and mucous membranes; oil and perspiration on skin; cilia in respiratory passages; gag and cough reflexes; peristalsis in the GI tract; and the flushing action of tears, saliva, and mucus. All act to remove organisms before they have an opportunity to infect. The chemical composition of body secretions such as tears and sweat, together with the pH of saliva, vaginal secretions, urine, and digestive juices, further

prevents or inhibits the growth of organisms. Compromise of any of these natural defenses increases host susceptibility to pathogen invasion.

Another important first-line defense is the *normal flora* of microorganisms that inhabit the skin and mucous membranes of the oral cavity, GI tract, and vagina. These microorganisms are indigenous to (occur naturally in) specific tissue. They typically coexist with their host in a mutually beneficial relationship as long as they do not migrate from the specific site. Through a mechanism called *microbial antagonism,* they control the replication of potential pathogens. The importance of this mechanism is evident when the mechanism is disturbed. An example of disturbance is the overgrowth of *Candida albicans* (thrush) that results from extensive antibiotic therapy that destroys normal flora in the GI tract or vagina.

Some normal flora can become pathogenic under specific conditions, such as immunosuppression or displacement of the pathogen to another area of the body. The opportunistic infections experienced by clients with symptomatic HIV infection are an example of immunosuppression. Displacement is seen when *Escherichia coli,* normally found in the GI tract, invades the urogenital tract and becomes pathogenic. Displacement of normal flora is a common cause of nosocomial infections. Invasive procedures increase the risk of displacing these organisms. For this reason, it is essential to maintain meticulous hand-washing and asepsis.

The *second line of defense* (the inflammatory process) and the *third line* (the immune response) share several physiologic components. These include the lymphatic system, leukocytes, and a multitude of proteins and enzymes.

Even after successful transmission of a pathogen, there may be more than one possible outcome. The pathogen may merely contaminate the body surface. The process ends there if the host's first-line defenses, such as intact skin or mucous membranes, block the pathogen from further invasion. Successful invasion with replication of a pathogen that does not lead to clinical manifestations or a detectable immune response is referred to as *colonization*.

When microorganisms in or on the host cause an immune response, an infection is said to be present. The period during which the pathogen is replicating but before it is shed from the host is called the *latent period*. During latency, host inflammatory and immune responses may ward off the organism or its by-products, thus preventing tissue damage, or the pathogen or its products may begin to destroy undefended or poorly defended tissue, producing infectious disease. Disease manifestations herald the end of the *incubation period,* which is defined as the time from invasion of the disease to the appearance of manifestations. By definition, *infectious disease* is the pathophysiologic response of a host

TABLE 19–1 Agents and Sites of Selected Infectious Diseases

Disease	Infectious Agent	Site of Infection	Reservoir	Mode of Transmission
Bacteria				
Cholera	*Vibrio cholerae*	Gastrointestinal tract	Humans	Ingestion of water contaminated with feces
Diarrhea	*Escherichia coli*	Gastrointestinal tract	Humans	Ingestion of contaminated food or water
Giardiasis	*Giardia lamblia*	Gastrointestinal tract	Water, humans, wild animals	Ingestion of cysts in fecally contaminated water and food
Gonorrhea	*Neisseria gonorrhoeae*	Genitourinary tract	Humans	Sexual contact
Lyme disease	*Borrelia burgdorferi*	Skin, joints, systemic	Wild rodents and deer	Tick bite
Malaria	*Plasmodium* spp.	Red blood cells, liver	Mosquito	Bite from infected mosquito
Meningitis	*Neisseria meningitidis*	Meninges	Humans	Direct contact with droplets from respiratory passages
Pneumonia	*Streptococcus pyogenes*	Lung	Humans	Inhalation; aspiration of gastric contents
Rocky Mountain spotted fever	*Rickettsia rickettsii*	Vascular endothelium	Ticks	Tick bite
Toxoplasmosis	*Toxoplasma gondii*	Eye, lung, brain	Cats	Ingestion of cysts on fecally contaminated fingers or in food; transplacental
Tuberculosis	*Mycobacterium tuberculosis*	Lung	Humans	Inhalation of droplet nuclei
Wound infection	*Staphylococcus aureus*	Connective tissue	Humans	Contaminated hands, surgical instruments
Fungi				
Candidiasis	*Candida albicans*	Skin, mucous membranes, genital tract	Humans	Overgrowth associated with damaged skin or mucous membranes or use of antibiotics
Histoplasmosis	*Histoplasma capsulatum*	Lung	Bat or bird feces	Inhalation of spores
Helminths				
Trichinosis	*Trichinella spiralis*	Gastrointestinal tract, muscle	Animals	Ingestion of raw or undercooked meat
Viruses				
Acquired immunodeficiency syndrome (AIDS)	Human immunodeficiency virus	Helper T lymphocyte	Humans	Contaminated needles, blood transfusions, sexual contact, transplacental
Hepatitis B	Hepatitis B virus	Liver	Humans	Contaminated needles, blood transfusions, sexual contact, perinatal
Influenza A	Influenza A virus	Respiratory tract	Humans	Direct contact by aerosol droplets; airborne spread
Measles (rubeola)	Paramyxoviridae	Skin, respiratory tract, systemic	Humans	Direct contact with nasal or throat secretions; airborne spread
Rabies	*Lyssavirus*	Systemic	Dogs, wild animals	Animal bite
Severe acute respiratory syndrome (SARS)	SARS-associated coronavirus (SARS-CoV)	Respiratory tract	Under investigation: possibly first transmitted from wild animals used for food to humans, then by humans	Under investigation: probably direct contact with droplets from respiratory passages; possibly airborne spread

to the destructive action of the pathogen, to its toxic products, or to the host immune responses to fight the pathogen. This pathophysiologic response is generally symptomatic. An asymptomatic pathologic response is called a *subclinical infection*.

An important point is that an asymptomatic host can still transmit a pathogen. The host may harbor the pathogen in sufficient quantities to shed it at any time after latency and toward the end of the incubation period. The time during which an organism can be shed is called the *period of communicability*. It usually precedes manifestations and coincides with part or all of the clinical disease, sometimes extending to convalescence. The communicable period, like the incubation period, varies with the pathogen and the disease.

RISKS OF HOSPITALIZATION

Every year in the United States, close to 2 million clients contract infections in hospitals and about 90,000 of these clients die as a result of their infection.[17] Infections that are acquired in a hospital or other health care facility are referred to as *nosocomial infections*. Infections present or incubating at the time of admission to the hospital are referred to as *community-acquired infections*. Occupationally acquired infections among the staff of a hospital are also considered nosocomial.

SAFETY ALERT

Because clients are at risk of acquiring infections in hospitals, one of The Joint Commission's (TJC) National Patient Safety Goals requires health care institutions to reduce the risk of health care associated infections. Achieving this goal includes following CDC hand hygiene guidelines, reporting fatal infections, and administering flu and pneumococcus vaccines to unvaccinated clients before admission.

The source of nosocomial pathogens in health care facilities varies, but both health care workers and clients are reservoirs in most instances. For example, *Staphylococcus aureus* is often carried on the skin and in the nasopharynx. Respiratory tract secretions, feces, urine, and blood are reservoirs for some nosocomial organisms. Liquids and inanimate objects in the hospital environment may also serve as sources of nosocomial infections. The most important means of transmission is via the hands of health care workers. Hand-washing, combined with principles of asepsis and proper use of gloves, is the best method of preventing nosocomial infections.

The most common sites of nosocomial infections in clients are the urinary tract, lower respiratory tract, surgical wounds, and the bloodstream.[17,33,48] Various pathogens can cause nosocomial infections in multiple sites. For example, *Pseudomonas aeruginosa* is the organism that causes most cases of nosocomial pneumonia, but it also causes urinary tract and surgical site infections. *S. aureus* is a common cause of surgical site infection, pneumonia, and bloodstream infection. Table 19-2 lists common nosocomial pathogens.

Urinary Tract Infections

Urinary tract infections (UTIs) are the most common nosocomial infections in both acute and long-term health care facilities, and more than 80% stem from urethral catheterization.[17,48] Major risk factors for catheter-

TABLE 19–2 Most Common Causes of Nosocomial Infection*

Site of Infection	Pathogen
Bloodstream	Coagulase-negative staphylococci
	Enterococcus spp.
	Staphylococcus aureus
	Candida albicans
	Enterobacter spp.
Lung	*Staphylococcus aureus*
	Pseudomonas aeruginosa
	Enterobacter spp.
	Klebsiella pneumoniae
	Haemophilus influenzae
Surgical site	*Staphylococcus aureus*
	Coagulase-negative staphylococci
	Enterococcus spp.
	Escherichia coli
	Pseudomonas aeruginosa
Urinary tract	*Escherichia coli*
	Candida albicans
	Enterococcus spp.
	Pseudomonas aeruginosa
	Klebsiella pneumoniae

Data from Wenzel, R.P. (Ed.) (2003). *Prevention and control of nosocomial infections* (4th ed.). Philadelphia: Lippincott Williams & Wilkins.

related UTIs include female gender, old age, increased duration of catheterization, and breaks in the closed catheter system.[48]

In most catheter-related infections in women, bacteria enter the bladder by the periurethral route.[48] Organisms originating primarily from the fecal flora and found at the meatal and perineal areas may be introduced into the bladder during insertion of the catheter, or they may migrate along the external surface of the catheter into the bladder. In men, catheter-related infections usually result from *cross-infection* (transmission between clients), with bacteria introduced into the collection system at the junction of the catheter and drainage tube or at the outflow spigot; they then migrate to the bladder in 24 to 48 hours.[33] Most nosocomial UTIs are easily managed but can lead to bacteremia and death.[33]

Pneumonia

Pneumonia is the second most common nosocomial infection and is associated with more deaths than any other nosocomial infection.[17,48] Nosocomial pneumonia is defined as pneumonia that occurs 48 hours or longer after admission to the hospital. Most nosocomial pneumonias are caused by gram-negative bacteria. Aspiration of oropharyngeal or stomach organisms is the predominant mechanism by which nosocomial pneumonia develops.[33] Airborne transmission is usually not the cause.

Stasis (lack of movement) of respiratory secretions caused by immobility and a decreased cough also contributes to nosocomial pneumonia. Postoperative clients, particularly those who have had thoracic and upper abdominal surgery, and clients who require ventilatory support are at high risk of aspiration. Clients with diminished consciousness, impaired gag reflex, intubation, or tracheostomy are also at increased risk for aspiration of oral secretions. Other risk factors include old age, decreased mobility, and severe disease, such as chronic lung disease, cardiovascular disease, renal insufficiency, and malignancies.

Nosocomial pneumonia is difficult to prevent because in most cases the microorganisms are derived from the client's own flora. Soon after hospitalization, the oropharynx of many clients becomes colonized with gram-negative bacteria that may be aspirated into the lungs.[48] The use of histamine (H_2) blockers, antimicrobial therapy, and enteral nutritional therapy have been found to promote colonization of the oropharynx with gram-negative bacteria.[33,48] Contaminated respiratory therapy equipment can serve as a source of pathogens as well.

Surgical Site Infections

Surgical site infections are a major source of hospital morbidity and mortality for clients undergoing operative procedures.[17,48] These infections usually result from *endogenous* (inside the host) or *exogenous* (outside the host) microorganisms that enter the site at the time of an operation. The most common source of infecting bacteria is the client's own flora.[48] Although the physical environment of the operating room is an uncommon source of infection, operating room personnel may shed bacteria-laden skin particles that travel through the air to the open wound.

Factors that influence the development of surgical site infections include the number and types of organisms present in the wound, the type of operation, the surgeon's technique, and the duration of the operation.[48] Old age, diabetes mellitus, obesity, malnutrition, and underlying immunocompromise are client-related factors that increase the risk of surgical site infection.

The risk of surgical site infection also increases with the length of the client's preoperative hospital stay. Shortening the preoperative stay tends to reduce the risk of infection by decreasing the opportunity for colonization with nosocomial bacteria.[48] Proper preparation of the surgical site is also important. Shaving the operative site—once a common practice—is now known to damage the epithelium, impair the skin's defense mechanism, and raise the risk of infection.

Bloodstream Infections

Rates of nosocomial infection of the bloodstream are increasing, particularly in ICUs, where there is a concentrated population of seriously ill clients.[17,48] The increase is due partly to the increased use of intravascular devices in these settings. Intravascular devices may include intravenous lines; intra-arterial infusion lines; and devices used for diagnostic, therapeutic, and hemodynamic monitoring. Catheter-related bloodstream infections are associated with increased morbidity and mortality rates, prolonged hospitalization, and increased medical costs.[33] The risk of infection is influenced by factors related to the device itself, the site of insertion, the technique used to place the device, and the duration of catheterization. Short peripheral catheters inserted into the veins of the hand or forearm have rarely been associated with bloodstream infections. Central venous catheters account for up to 90% of all catheter-related bloodstream infections.[48] Partially implantable catheters and totally implanted injection ports are associated with lower infection rates.[33]

Catheter-related infections and bacteremias are usually caused by microorganisms found on the client's skin or on the hands of health care workers.[48] These microorganisms invade disrupted tissue and migrate around the site of insertion and along the device into the intravascular space. The use of semipermeable membrane dressings over the insertion site facilitates the growth of skin flora.[33] Dressing changes following institution-specific protocols must be done at regularly scheduled intervals under aseptic conditions. Colonization of skin flora can also occur around the hub of the device, the tubing-device junction, or other connectors attached to the system. Although liquids given through the device may become contaminated, infusion-related infection is relatively uncommon.

Client factors that contribute to the risk of device-related infections include age, type and severity of underlying illness, skin condition, and immunosuppressive therapy. Bacteremia is especially common in clients with chronic diseases, malnutrition, and cancer.[33]

Other Nosocomial Infections

Effective screening and processing of donated blood and blood products have greatly reduced the risk of HIV transmission to clients in health care settings. The risk of provider-to-client transmission of HIV is remote, although the matter has created much public anxiety. The risk of occupational exposure to HIV in the health care setting has been associated primarily with parenteral exposures to blood from clients infected with HIV.[33] Infection after exposure of mucous membranes to infected blood is much less common.

Nosocomial infection with *hepatitis B virus* (HBV) is another concern in hospitals because the source of a typical nosocomial HBV infection is never identified.[33] Provider-to-client transmission of HBV does not occur with routine client contact. Client-to-provider transmission is a much larger problem and is why health care workers must be vaccinated against HBV.

A resurgence of *tuberculosis* occurred in the mid 1980s and early 1990s because of delays in diagnosing and treating people with infectious TB disease, poor compliance with therapeutic drug regimens, lapses in infection control practices, and the emergence of drug-resistant strains of *Mycobacterium tuberculosis*.[16] Since then, TB control programs in the community and strict implementation of infection control measures in health care settings have substantially reduced the risk of transmission of health care associated *M. tuberculosis*. Transmission is still a risk for clients and providers, but current TB infection-control programs include prompt detection, rapid implementation of airborne precautions, and treatment of people who have suspected or confirmed TB disease.

Acute GI infections can be caused by a variety of agents, including bacteria, viruses, and protozoa, but nosocomial transmission of agents such as *Clostridium difficile* and rotavirus is on the rise.[33]

Nosocomial infections tend to occur more frequently and with more severity in ill, debilitated, malnourished, immunocompromised, and older clients (Box 19-3).

Susceptibility to infection increases when invasive procedures and indwelling devices are used. With the expanding use of invasive devices, more exposure to antimicrobial therapy, and more severely ill hospitalized clients, the risk of nosocomial infections will probably increase. Furthermore, the emergence of resistant organisms is likely to continue, resulting in infections that are more difficult to treat. Although resistance to infection is enhanced by vaccines and immune globulin, manipulation of the physical environment must be used as a supplementary measure to reduce the risk. This means that nurses must be ever more vigilant in administering care and in supervising those providing care.

Antibiotic-Resistant Microorganisms

Among researchers and health care professionals, concern is increasing over the frequent, widespread use of antimicrobial drugs in hospitals and long-term care facilities (LTCFs).

Studies in hospitals have demonstrated that 23% to 37.8% of clients receive antibiotics, of which half are used inappropriately.[34] For example, antimicrobial drugs are used routinely as prophylaxis for invasive and even noninvasive surgical procedures. Although prophylaxis may be helpful when applied wisely, many drugs are used inappropriately. In the ICU, 80% of clients receive antimicrobials.[29]

In LTCFs, antimicrobials are among the most frequently prescribed medications. Studies have shown that antibiotics account for nearly 40% of all systemic drugs used in LTCFs.[50] Nursing home studies have revealed frequent orders for antibiotics, often without adequate evidence of underlying infection. Worse, many of these drugs were prescribed for infections not responsive to antibiotic therapy, such as viral respiratory tract infections.

The most important factor in the development of antimicrobial resistance is antimicrobial use.[27,40]

BOX 19-3   Infectious Disease in Older Adults

More than any other population, older clients are at risk for infection. Infection often leads to hospitalization for nursing home residents, and it is one of the top 10 causes of death in older adults. Many common infectious diseases, such as pneumonia, urinary tract infection (UTI), sepsis, skin and soft tissue infection, tuberculosis, and herpes zoster, become more common with advancing age.

Older adults have an increased risk of infection, partly as a normal consequence of growing older. With aging, mechanical barriers—such as skin and mucous membranes—undergo structural and functional decline. The physiologic reserve capacity of organ systems dwindles, and the immune system falters. When these defense mechanisms are compromised, infection can progress locally and even spread systemically.

Many older adults have chronic diseases that further jeopardize their host defenses. Conditions associated with aging, such as diabetes mellitus and malnutrition, probably exert more influence on immunity than age itself.

Older people not only contract more infections but also tend to experience more complications of those infections. For example, an older client with pneumonia or a UTI is more likely to develop bacteremia than a younger client with the same infection.

To make matters worse, infection can be more difficult to detect and diagnose in the older client. Older people often do not manifest typical clinical manifestations of infectious diseases. Instead, they may have worsening cognition, an abnormal mental status, lethargy, agitation, loss of appetite, incontinence, or an increased tendency to fall.

Fever—the cardinal clinical manifestation of infection—may be absent in infected older clients, even those who have bacteremia or pneumonia. Many older people have a low baseline temperature. Suspect infection in any older client with an oral temperature of 99° F or higher or an increase in baseline temperature of 2° F or more. Coexisting diseases may mask clinical manifestations of infection even further.

Even drugs used to treat infections are less successful when given to older clients. The drugs produce a slower or delayed response in the older person's body while producing even more adverse reactions. Age-related changes in gastrointestinal, cardiac, and renal function alter the way in which antimicrobial agents are absorbed, distributed, and excreted.

Researchers are looking for better ways to detect and better drugs to treat infections in older adults. While these agents are being investigated in the older population, you can help already infected clients by encouraging individualized dosage regimens and monitoring these clients carefully.

Data from Yoshikawa, T.T., & Norman, D.C. (Eds.) (2001). *Infectious disease in the aging: A clinical handbook*. Totowa, NJ: Humana Press.

Areas within the hospital that have the highest rates of antimicrobial resistance also have the highest rates of antimicrobial use. In ICUs, where clients are usually undergoing intensive antibiotic therapy, the rates of antimicrobial resistance are significantly higher than in other areas of the hospital,[27] and the transfer of infected or colonized clients from hospital to LTCF is believed to be the primary way resistant bacteria have been introduced into LTCFs.[50] Once endemic to a hospital or LTCF, the antibiotic resistance genes can be transferred from one client to another and from one bacterial species to another.

Resistance to an antibiotic by a pathogen develops by spontaneous genetic mutation or genetic transfer of plasmids or chromosomal DNA. This genetic information allows bacteria to develop resistance by producing an enzyme that inactivates or destroys the antibiotic, either by altering the antibiotic target site to evade action of the antibiotic or by preventing antibiotic access to the target site.[40] Some resistance can be acquired by a single genetic change; others require a series of changes.[40] Unfortunately, resistance tends to occur to multiple antibiotics. In other words, once an organism is resistant to one antibiotic in a class, it usually is resistant to all antibiotics in that class.

S. aureus, one of the pathogens most frequently reported to cause nosocomial infections, has a remarkable ability to develop resistance to antibiotics. Before the advent of penicillin in the early 1940s, the fatality rate for bacteremia caused by *S. aureus* was about 90%.[32] The use of penicillin dramatically reduced that rate, but within a few years resistant strains of *S. aureus* evolved that produced a penicillin inactivator. New antibiotics, such as methicillin, were effective in the 1960s, but they provided only a temporary solution to the problem. In the 1980s epidemics of infections with methicillin-resistant *S. aureus* (commonly called MRSA) forced operating rooms and ICUs to close. In recent years, MRSA has accounted for approximately 80% of all *S. aureus* isolates reported to the National Nosocomial Infections Surveillance System.[8]

MRSA is the etiologic agent in many cases of conjunctivitis, skin and soft-tissue infections, pneumonia, infected pressure ulcers, and catheter-associated urinary tract infections. Once introduced into a hospital or LTCF, MRSA is difficult to eliminate because it acquires resistance to multiple antimicrobial agents.[32] The most important reservoirs of MRSA are infected or colonized clients, and the main mode of transmission of MRSA is via the hands of health care workers.[8]

With the emergence of MRSA, vancomycin became the only drug available to treat MRSA infections; however, widespread use of vancomycin has now contributed to the emergence of vancomycin-resistant organisms, including vancomycin-intermediate-sensitive *S. aureus* (VISA) and vancomycin-resistant enterococci (VRE). The first case of VISA occurred in 1997,[8] indicating the development of a strain of *S. aureus* with reduced susceptibility to vancomycin. In June 2002 the first case of an infection with vancomycin-resistant *S. aureus* (VRSA) was reported after VRSA was isolated from a swab obtained from a client's catheter exit site.[11] When MRSA began showing resistance to vancomycin, two new agents became available to treat MRSA: the combination of quinupristin and dalfopristin (Synercid) in 1999 and linezolid (Zyvox) in 2000.[29] It will only be a matter of time before resistant strains of pathogens emerge for these new drugs.

Enterococci are now the second most common pathogen in nosocomial infections.[50] Their emergence in the past two decades can be attributable to their resistance to many commonly used antimicrobial agents (aminoglycosides, aztreonam, cephalosporins, clindamycin, ampicillin, nafcillin, oxacillin, and trimethoprim-sulfamethoxazole). Strains of VRE began appearing in 1986, most likely as the result of the use of orally administered vancomycin for treating antibiotic-associated diarrhea in hospitals.[39] Enterococci are normal inhabitants of the GI tract and cause nosocomial urinary tract, bloodstream, wound, and intra-abdominal infections.[34] Treatment of VRE infections poses a major challenge because these organisms are resistant to a wide variety of antimicrobials. Synercid and Zyvox are the only drugs currently available for treatment of VRE, and for some strains there are no longer any effective antimicrobial agents.[29]

 Environmental cultures in hospital rooms have identified VRE-contaminated client gowns, bed rails, floors, door handles, blood pressure cuffs, stethoscopes, glucose meters, and telephones. It appears that VRE is transmitted directly by client-to-client contact and indirectly by the hands of health care workers, contaminated environmental surfaces, and client care equipment. Residents in LTCFs are a major reservoir for VRE, which can be transmitted to other residents, and when these clients are admitted to a hospital, to other clients.[26]

SAFETY ALERT

Streptococcus pneumoniae is a gram-positive bacterium that colonizes the nasopharynx and oropharynx and causes respiratory tract infections, otitis media, sinusitis, bloodstream infections, and meningitis.[34] Pneumonia caused by *S. pneumoniae* is one of the most frequent causes of lower respiratory tract infections. Penicillin has been the drug of choice for treating infections with *S. pneumoniae,* but penicillin-resistant pneumococci (PRP) have now emerged.[50] What is worrisome is that PRP are also resistant to erythromycin, tetracycline, and other antibiotics.

Widespread use of trimethoprim-sulfamethoxazole for UTIs, upper respiratory tract infections, and GI infections has resulted in the emergence of resistance. Major organisms resistant to this combination of antibiotics include *S. pneumoniae, Haemophilus influenzae,* and many enteric gram-negative bacilli (*Escherichia coli, Klebsiella* spp.).[50]

Other strains of bacteria have developed resistance to third-generation cephalosporins, fluoroquinolones, and imipenem. Although 90% of nosocomial infections are caused by bacteria, the fungus *Candida albicans* is the seventh most common pathogen associated with nosocomial infection in ICU clients.[34] Recent data suggest that *C. albicans* is developing resistance to some of the few antifungal agents available for treatment.[27]

Tuberculosis is an example of a resistance problem that has spread globally. Resistant *Mycobacterium* has been identified in 35 countries and regions.[2] Some *M. tuberculosis* strains are resistant to one drug, but other strains have become multi-drug–resistant. For tuberculosis, as well as many other infections, multi-drug resistance can result in treatment failure and death.

These are just a few of the increasing problems associated with antibiotic resistance. In fact, nearly all organisms have acquired resistance to some therapeutic agents.[2]

SAFETY
ALERT

Misuse of antimicrobial drugs can alter a client's normal flora and encourage resistance of pathogenic organisms. To help avoid growing resistance to antimicrobial drugs, obtain appropriate specimens for culture before starting antibiotic therapy. In addition, check sensitivity reports to ensure that the client receives an appropriate antibiotic.

Controlling the spread of antimicrobial resistance is difficult and requires appropriate selection and administration of antimicrobials, use of antibiotic combinations, and strict asepsis and infection control efforts. Finally, although infection control practices, such as hand-washing, aseptic techniques, and barrier precautions, do not directly limit the emergence of resistant strains, they do prevent transmission of resistant organisms from one client to another.

PREVENTING AND CONTROLLING INFECTION

To be effective, strategies to prevent and control infection must be based on knowledge of agent-host-environment interactions. The goal in developing and implementing interventions is to prevent the spread of an infectious agent from its reservoir or source to susceptible hosts.

Methods for controlling the transmission of infectious disease vary with the characteristics of the organism, its reservoirs, the type of pathologic response it produces, and technology available for control. In general, the aim is to intervene at the point where the greatest number of people can be protected while using the least amount of resources.

SAFETY
ALERT

The simplest and most effective way to prevent transmission is meticulous *hand-washing and the use of alcohol-based hand rubs*.[10] The hygienic hand rub is a technique that involves rubbing a fast-acting antiseptic preparation onto the hands until they are

dry. **Hand hygiene is an absolute necessity, even when gloves are worn. Wash your hands with soap and water or use an alcohol-based hand rub before donning gloves and after removing them, and before and after each client contact. Teach this procedure to all personnel and continually monitor for compliance. One of TJC's National Patient Safety Goals is to reduce the risk of health care associated infections. These simple, inexpensive techniques, used appropriately, are potent weapons against the spread of infection.**

Another method to prevent and control infectious disease involves environmental measures. Some pathogens, such as *S. aureus,* can be controlled by disinfection, sterilization, or anti-infective drugs. Other pathogens can be controlled best by eradicating their non-human reservoirs via environmental sanitation measures, such as water treatment, food safety programs, and control of animals, vectors, sewage, and solid wastes.

Transmission from the portal of exit can often be prevented by detecting and treating clients who are shedding pathogens, such as gonococci. Antimicrobials are among the drugs most frequently prescribed in the United States to treat infections, although the use of antibiotics is not without problems. Another example of prevention is the use of prophylactic antitubercular medications for clients who are exposed to tuberculosis and whose skin test result is positive.[13]

Immunization Programs

Several infectious diseases have been dramatically reduced by maximizing host defenses through active and passive vaccinations that stimulate the immune system to counteract the infectious agent:

Active vaccination refers to the deliberate administration of a modified infecting agent, called a *vaccine,* or a modified toxin, called a *toxoid,* to stimulate an immune response. Protection is not immediate: some time is needed to achieve protective antibody levels; however, induced active immunity usually results in long-lived protection against disease.

Passive vaccination refers to the administration of antibodies to a nonimmune person to provide temporary protection against a pathogenic agent or toxin. Passive immunity provides immediate but short-lived protection that lasts a few weeks.

Vaccination programs in the United States have resulted in a significant reduction in childhood infectious diseases. A major resurgence of measles occurred from 1989 to 1991, however, signaling a major problem with childhood vaccination programs.[24] Baseline data from 1989 indicated that the immunization level of preschool children was approximately 70% to 80%, with some segments of the population having levels below 50%.[43] Urban minority populations, particularly African-American and Hispanic-American children, had much lower immunization levels than those in the general population.[24] The goal of the Department of Health and Human Services is to vaccinate at least 90% of all children in the United States by age 2 years.[43,44] Entry requirements for school and day care have been one of the most effective interventions in increasing vaccination rates.[44]

An entire population does not have to be immune for prevention of a disease epidemic. When a large proportion of individual members of a community becomes immune to a disease, the chance of contact between susceptible people and infected people decreases. This type of immunity is called *herd immunity*. For example, epidemics of measles are less likely to occur when herd immunity increases and the number of susceptible people in the community decreases.

Schedules and recommendations are established by the Advisory Committee on Immunization Practices (ACIP) of the Centers for Disease Control and Prevention (CDC). ACIP recommends that all children by 2 years of age be vaccinated against measles, mumps, rubella, diphtheria, pertussis, tetanus, poliomyelitis, *Haemophilus influenzae* type b, hepatitis A, hepatitis B, pneumococcal, varicella virus, and influenza.[23] In 2007, rotavirus vaccine was added to the childhood immunization schedule.[23]

Vaccinations are as important for adolescents and adults as they are for children. Infections seen primarily in children are now occurring in adolescents and adults who never developed active immunity. Adolescents and adults who escaped natural infection or who were not immunized as children are at risk for childhood diseases and their complications. ACIP recommends a routine vaccination visit to a health care provider for adolescents 11 to 12 years old to review their vaccination status and to administer needed vaccines.[21] In 2005 pertussis was added to the adolescent (11 to 18 years old) immunization schedule to be given with the booster vaccines against diphtheria and tetanus.[21] In 2007, routine vaccination with human papillomavirus vaccine was recommended for females aged 11 to 12 years old.[23] In addition, ACIP recommends that all children should receive the meningococcal vaccine at the 11- to 12-year-old visit.[23] Unvaccinated adolescents at high school entry (15 years of age) and all college freshmen living in dormitories should also be vaccinated against meningococcal disease.[23]

Adults (people ages 19 and older) should complete a primary series of diphtheria and tetanus toxoids if they did not receive them as children.[22] A tetanus and diphtheria booster is recommended every 10 years, with a one-time booster that includes acellular pertusis.[22] Adults born during or after 1957 should receive the measles-mumps-rubella vaccine. Adults born before 1957 are likely to have been infected naturally with measles, mumps, and rubella and are generally considered immune to these diseases.[22] People who have a reliable history of varicella are considered immune; others can be tested to determine their immune status or can be vaccinated without testing.[9] Vaccination against human papillomavirus is recommended for women 19 to 26 years old who have not completed the vaccine series.[22] Vaccination for other diseases, such as influenza, pneumococcal pneumonia, hepatitis A, and hepatitis B, is recommended for people in certain age groups; for some occupational, environmental, and lifestyle groups; and for those with special health problems.

The older adult population and people with chronic diseases are at particular risk for infectious diseases because of a decline in their immune system. An important TJC National Patient Safety Goal is to reduce the risk of influenza and pneumococcal disease in older adults. More than 90% of all deaths from influenza A and B viruses occur in people 65 years and older.[19] The most effective way to reduce the impact of influenza is to vaccinate people at high risk each year before the influenza season. The ACIP recommends that influenza vaccine be administered annually to people at high risk and to all people age 50 and older.[19] For people living in nursing homes and other chronic care facilities, annual vaccination can reduce the risk of influenza outbreaks by inducing herd immunity. Health care workers and household contacts who have frequent contact with people at high risk should also be vaccinated. Annual vaccination with the current vaccine is necessary because new variants of influenza continue to occur; vaccination against one strain may not confer immunity to another.

Pneumococcal pneumonia, caused by *Streptococcus pneumoniae*, is an important cause of morbidity and mortality in the very young, in older adults, and in others with certain high-risk or chronic conditions. The ACIP recommends that these people receive a single dose of pneumococcal polysaccharide vaccine.[6]

Nurses can be instrumental in ensuring that all children, adolescents, and adults are properly immunized. (Infant, adolescent, and adult vaccine and immunization schedules can be accessed at www.cdc.gov/nip/menus/vaccines.htm#Schedules.) Every visit to a health care provider should be an opportunity to obtain a history of vaccination status and to provide vaccinations as needed. In addition, you and other health care providers should be concerned about improving your own resistance to infectious diseases. One important approach is to maintain your immunization status by being vaccinated against hepatitis B infection, measles, mumps, rubella, tetanus, diphtheria, pertussis, varicella, and influenza.

For all health care providers, hepatitis B infection is a major occupational hazard because of the likelihood of contact with blood and blood-contaminated body fluids from infected clients. The Occupational Safety and Health Administration (OSHA) has developed regulations that require employers to offer at-risk employees the hepatitis B vaccine at the employers' expense. Influenza vaccination is recommended yearly for health care providers in hospital, chronic care, and outpatient settings to reduce the risk of illness and to reduce the possibility of transmitting the virus to clients. The vaccinations you receive protect not only you but also your clients.

Infection Control in Hospitals

SAFETY ALERT

Many nosocomial infections can be prevented if health care personnel adhere to infection control practices. The CDC and TJC issue guidelines and establish standards for control of hospital infection. The CDC develops and updates guidelines related to the control and prevention of nosocomial infections, and TJC requires hospitals to establish infection control programs that meet accreditation standards. TJC standards require hospital infection control committees to establish surveillance programs, implement infection control policies and procedures, and conduct continuing education for all hospital employees regarding infection control.[33] Most hospitals employ an infection control nurse or infection control practitioner who is responsible for the coordination of a hospital-wide infection control program.

Infection control programs in hospitals address two major areas related to nosocomial infection: (1) surveillance and reporting and (2) control and prevention. The purpose of surveillance is to establish and maintain a database to track the rates of nosocomial infections. Surveillance activities include early detection of infections in clients and personnel and reporting of relevant data to designated people for appropriate action. Surveillance systems to detect both organisms and diseases are necessary components of prevention and control strategies. National data on nosocomial infections are obtained from selected hospitals in the United States by the CDC and are used to estimate rates and trends.[17]

The focus of infection control strategies is on barrier precautions to reduce infection risk for all clients and personnel and on occupational health practices to protect health care staff from infection.

Barrier Precautions

Barriers are intended to prevent the transfer of an infective organism to a susceptible host. By placing a clean layer of plastic or fabric between a susceptible site and a potential source of pathogenic organisms, the likelihood of transmitting an infection can be reduced. The prevented transmission can be from client to caregiver or from caregiver to client. The risk for clients increases when caregivers have contact with clients' mucous membranes and nonintact skin. The risk for caregivers increases whenever they have contact with clients' moist body substances. Protective barriers include gloves, gowns, masks, and protective eyewear.

None of the protective barriers is intended to replace hand-washing. *The most important means of preventing the spread of microorganisms is hand-washing.* **Hands become soiled during client care, particularly after contact with moist body sites and substances. Soiled hands have played a major role in transferring organisms to new client hosts. Unfortunately, gloves provide a false sense of security because hands can become contaminated even when gloves are used. The use of gloves is not a substitute for hand-washing.**

In the past, most barrier precautions were instituted after a client's infection was diagnosed. When an infection was suspected or recognized, a system of barrier precautions, referred to as *isolation procedures,* was instituted to prevent transmission of pathogens among hospitalized clients, health care personnel, and visitors. Depending on the diagnosis, one of several isolation strategies was used. Precautions varied, depending on the methods needed to interrupt transmission of the infection. For the isolation strategy to be effective, the diagnosis of infection had to be made or suspected early; however, most infections are communicable for some period when manifestations are absent and the infection is undetected.

In the early 1980s, unrecognized cases of HBV and HIV infection were identified as important sources of disease. Health care workers could potentially become infected through needle-sticks and body fluids contaminated with clients' blood. In response to this problem, the CDC recommended "universal precautions" as a means of preventing transmission of HIV, HBV, and other blood-borne pathogens.[3] Universal precautions focused on preventing transmission of blood-borne pathogens from infected or potentially infected clients to susceptible caregivers. Universal precautions required the use of protective barriers with all clients regardless of their presumed infection status. These precautions emphasized (1) the use of gloves and gowns to reduce contamination of skin and clothing; (2) the use of masks and goggles to reduce contamination of the mucous membranes of the mouth, nose, and eyes; and (3) prevention of needle-stick injuries. Used needles were not to be recapped by hand, and puncture-resistant containers were to be used for disposal of sharps.

In 1987 the practice of *body substance isolation* (BSI) was proposed as a system to isolate all moist and potentially infectious body substances from all clients, regardless of their presumed infection status.[30] Personnel used clean gloves during contact with nonintact skin and mucous membranes and when anticipating contact with blood, feces, urine, sputum, saliva, wound drainage, and other body fluids. BSI was based on the assumption that the blood and body substances of all clients might contain potentially infectious, transmissible organisms.

In 1996 the Hospital Infection Control Practices Advisory Committee (HICPAC) of the CDC combined the various isolation systems into one new set of guidelines.[28] The new guidelines recommend two tiers of isolation strategies: (1) standard precautions and (2) transmission-based precautions.

Standard precautions are the more important tier and are designed for the care of all clients in hospitals regardless of their diagnosis or presumed infection status. These precautions include the major components of universal precautions and BSI. Standard precautions apply to nonintact skin, mucous membranes, blood, and all body fluids, secretions, and excretions except sweat.

Transmission-based precautions form the second tier and are designed only for the care of clients who have known or suspected infections or have been colonized with transmissible pathogens. These are *additional* precautions needed to interrupt transmission of a nosocomial infection and are used with standard precautions. The three types of transmission-based precautions can be combined for infections that have more than one route of transmission:

1. *Contact precautions* are designed to reduce direct and indirect contact transmission of microorganisms.
2. *Droplet precautions* are for infections transmitted by large-particle droplets such as those generated during coughing, sneezing, speaking, or suctioning.
3. *Airborne precautions* are designed to reduce the transmission of pathogens on airborne droplet nuclei.

In many cases, the risk of transmitting a nosocomial infection is highest before a diagnosis can be made. Certain clinical syndromes and conditions warrant the addition of transmission-based precautions while the definitive diagnosis is anticipated. For example, contact precautions should be implemented for incontinent or diapered clients who have acute diarrhea with a likely infectious cause such as HAV infection. Clients with infected draining skin lesions or wounds that cannot be covered warrant contact precautions because the wound may be infected with *S. aureus*. Droplet precautions should be implemented for clients with meningitis until infection with *Neisseria meningitidis* is ruled out.

Other examples include clients admitted with rashes or respiratory tract infections with possible etiologic agents that require additional precautions beyond standard precautions. Additional precautions should also be taken with clients who have a history of infection or colonization with multi-drug–resistant organisms or who had a recent hospital or nursing home stay in a facility where multi-drug–resistant organisms were prevalent.

Control of the spread of nosocomial infections depends on meticulous attention to infection control practices. The CDC has provided excellent institutional infection control guidelines that can be tailored to meet the needs of specific situations or environments. In addition to standard and transmission-based precautions, the CDC has issued special guidelines for preventing nosocomial transmission of tuberculosis,[16] VRSA,[5] and VRE[4] in health care facilities. Some important infection control guidelines are outlined in the Management and Delegation box below.

MANAGEMENT AND DELEGATION

Infection Control Precautions

Regulatory agencies have developed specific and complete guidelines for infection control to protect clients and staff from the transmission of infectious diseases. All health care providers must receive training and education on their role in maintaining infection control practices, including standard precautions. Your role in providing and delegating care of clients in isolation for known or suspected organisms includes assessment of clients and their environment. Note the level of precaution required according to your institution's system. Ensure that strict attention to isolation techniques is maintained by all who interact with the client. For the newly isolated client, you are responsible for client and family assessment and education regarding infection control measures. Unlicensed assistive personnel may then reinforce your teachings.

Some components of infection control practice may be delegated to unlicensed assistive personnel, such as room setup and maintenance of supplies and equipment. Consider delegating the following tasks:

- Stocking of gloves, gowns, and masks
- Stocking of client-specific equipment, such as thermometers, stethoscopes, and sphygmomanometers
- Cleaning of equipment after use, such as oxygen saturation machines and wheelchairs
- Removal of linen and unused equipment from the client's room

Delegation to unlicensed assistive personnel of direct care provision for clients in isolation should include reinforcement of the outlined precautions. *Note:* Care of a client in isolation does not change the practice parameters for what unlicensed assistive personnel may provide to the client or what you can delegate. Emphasize the ways in which the isolation status might affect delivery of care. For example, a client isolated because of methicillin-resistant *Staphylococcus aureus* (MRSA) is routinely cared for with gown, gloves, and mask. If that client is actively incontinent, you may need to give unlicensed assistive personnel additional instruction to change gloves between tasks.

Instruct unlicensed assistive personnel about findings that are immediately reportable. Such findings may include a disruption of isolation technique or any difficulty the unlicensed assistive personnel experience while providing care.

Occupational Health Practices

The second major component of an infection prevention and control program is to protect health care workers from infection. Occupational health practices include evaluating personnel for existing infections, administering vaccinations, keeping records, managing exposures, educating employees, and developing and enforcing infection control procedures.

When it was recognized that health care workers who had contact with clients' blood were at increased risk for infection by blood-borne pathogens, infection control efforts focused on preventing employee exposure to blood. By 1989 most hospitals had implemented the universal precautions guidelines to protect employees at risk of transmission of HIV and HBV. In addition, efforts focused on HBV vaccination of employees at risk for blood exposure. New employees are screened for susceptibility to tuberculosis, HBV, measles, mumps, rubella, and chickenpox. Annual influenza vaccinations are strongly encouraged, and periodic tuberculin skin testing is recommended for employees at risk for exposure to tuberculosis.

In 1991 OSHA published guidelines—the *blood-borne pathogens standard*—to protect employees exposed to blood and other potentially infectious materials.[35] One of the most important components of the guidelines is the requirement that all health care employees at risk for exposure to blood and body fluids be offered an HBV vaccination free of charge. In addition, OSHA requires all care providers to wear protective attire when they are likely to have contact with blood and other moist body substances that may contain pathogens. Because one third of occupational exposures to HIV result from recapping needles after use, OSHA standards urged the use of needle-less or recessed needle systems. Injuries from contaminated needles and other sharps are also associated with hepatitis B and hepatitis C viruses.[37] The OSHA blood-borne pathogens standard incorporates most elements of universal precautions plus barrier precautions and sharps disposal systems that must be available at the point of use. Since publication of the standard, a wide variety of medical devices have been developed to reduce the risk of needle-sticks and other sharps injuries. In response to growing concern about employee protection, Congress passed the Needlestick Safety and Prevention Act in 2000 requiring OSHA to revise the standards to mandate the use of new, safer medical devices.

Another major area of concern has been the role and selection of respiratory protection equipment to prevent transmission of tuberculosis in hospitals.[36] OSHA has proposed standards for respiratory protection programs to protect hospital personnel from pathogens spread by the airborne route. In particular, surgical masks have not been effective in preventing inhalation of droplet nuclei, and the use of fit-tested disposable particulate respirators has been recommended instead.

Infection Control in Long-Term Care Facilities

Nosocomial infections are common among residents of LTCFs and are a major source of morbidity and mortality. UTIs, respiratory tract infections (influenza, pneumonia), infected pressure ulcers, gastroenteritis, and conjunctivitis are the most common infections found in long-term care facilities.[41] Many LTCFs are becoming reservoirs for antimicrobial-resistant organisms, including MRSA and VRE.[48,50]

Many hospital-oriented infection control guidelines are relevant to LTCFs, but they must be adapted, depending on the acuity of residents, facility size, resources, and other factors. The LTCF is a home to residents, one in which they usually reside for months or years. Strict barrier approaches used in hospitals can have a negative effect on the residents and the facility's social and rehabilitative goals. Infection control programs must be designed to balance the medical and social needs of long-term care residents. The Association for Practitioners in Infection Control (APIC) has addressed this problem in its guidelines for infection control programs in long-term care facilities.[41]

Infection Control in Community-Based Settings

Today health care is provided to clients in their homes, in physicians' offices, in ambulatory care centers, and in outpatient specialty clinics. Intravenous infusions, hemodialysis, and mechanical ventilation are provided in the home, and nearly half of all surgical procedures are performed in outpatient settings.[48] Venipuncture, wound care, suturing, skin biopsy, bone marrow aspiration and biopsy, plastic and reconstructive surgery, and other minor surgical procedures are commonly performed in physicians' offices. Same-day surgery centers accommodate both minor and major ambulatory surgeries and procedures. Outpatient specialty clinics are available to provide hemodialysis and peritoneal dialysis.

Infections arise during the provision of care in home and outpatient settings, but identifying a break in infection control practices can be difficult. Infection control surveillance programs in community-based settings have been limited, and specific data about infections occurring in homes and outpatient settings are not readily available.[31] Infection control guidelines from the usual resources, such as the CDC, have been written primarily for hospitals. Until setting-specific guidelines are published, commonsense adaptations of hospital infection control practices are recommended.[38,48] As the shift to managed care continues, it can be expected that infection surveillance and control issues will become more important as a basis for measuring the quality of care and as a requirement for agency certification.

Home care has grown to encompass services provided by family members, partners, and friends as well as health care professionals. Lay caregivers must be given simple guidelines for infection control in the home. Hand-washing, use of gloves, and appropriate methods for disposal of contaminated sharps and other waste products are examples of infection control practices that must be taught by the home care provider. Clients and their caregivers should be taught about safe food handling, health concerns about pets, and sanitation issues. See the Bridge to Home Health Care feature on Infection Control on the website.

Protecting the health care worker is a critical component of infection control in any health care setting, and the employee health plan should be similar to that used in hospitals. You should not assume that health care workers who are employed in outpatient settings are at lower risk for infectious diseases than those employed by hospitals. Policies should be developed that meet the requirements of OSHA and other regulating agencies and that acknowledge the unique requirements of the health care setting.

BIOTERRORISM*

The recent terrorist events in the United States have heightened awareness of the need to prepare for acts of bioterrorism. Bioterrorism—the intentional use of viruses, bacteria, and other germs as weapons—is not new.[1,15] One of the earliest uses of biologic weapons occurred in the 6th century BC when the Assyrians used rye ergot to poison the wells of their enemies. In the 14th century, a Tartan army catapulted plague-ridden bodies over the city walls of Kaffa in the Crimea. In 1763 in Pennsylvania, a Commander of British forces deliberately offered Native Americans blankets previously used by smallpox victims. Supporters of Pancho Villa may have used botulism against Mexican Federales in 1910, as there are stories about digging up buried pork and green beans to contaminate food and sharp instruments used as weapons. During the Civil War, Union soldiers were purposely sold clothing infected with smallpox and yellow fever. And more recently in 2001, letters containing anthrax spores were intentionally sent through the U.S. postal system.

The development of nationally sponsored biowarfare research programs for the purpose of gaining military advantage began in the 20th century.[1,15] In the 1930s Japan conducted experiments with disease-causing agents on allied prisoners of war and innocent civilians in nearby villages. During World War II, with fears about Japanese and German biologic weapons, the U.S. and Great Britain began their own biowarfare research programs. In 1942 British scientists exploded anthrax bombs near sheep at Gruinard Island off the coast of Scotland to test methods of dispersion. (Results showed that anthrax was effectively dispersed and remained viable in the soil for decades. The island is safe now, but it was declared off limits until it was decontaminated in the 1980s.)

The United States began research into the offensive use of biologic weapons in 1942. Harmless organisms were released to test different dispersal methods. For example, *Bacillus subtilis* was released into the subway system of New York City in 1966.[1] Results showed that release in only one station could infect the entire subway system via spread by trains. In 1969 President Nixon renounced the use of deadly biologic weapons and stopped all offensive biologic and toxin weapon research and production. By this date, the United States had weaponized seven incapacitating or lethal human agents. By executive order, all stockpiles of biologic agents and munitions from the U.S. program were destroyed. The United States continues a bioweapons program, but the focus is now on medical defense. The Terrorism Alert box below outlines the public health response to the threat of bioterrorism.

TERRORISM ALERT

Bioterrorism Preparedness and Response

The threat of bioterrorism has forever changed the role and scope of public health. The Centers for Disease Control and Prevention and the Agency for Toxic Substances and Disease Registry (CDC/ATSDR) have outlined a *National Public Health Strategy for Terrorism Preparedness and Response.*[14] The plan focuses on improving the public health system to prepare for and respond to terror-related public health emergencies, including biologic, chemical, radiologic/nuclear, and mass-trauma terrorist emergencies. The public health response to bioterrorism depends on rapid detection of the disease-producing agent and integrated response activities at the federal, state, and local levels. To achieve this complex task, the CDC/ATSDR plan calls for enhanced surveillance and epidemiology, increased laboratory capacity, coordinated communications' technology, and a national stockpile of appropriate vaccines, antidotes, and materials. In addition, an increase in the number and type of professionals that compose a preparedness and response work force must be recruited and trained, and their personal safety assured.

---

*Bioterrorism reprinted from *Urologic Nursing* (2004) *24*(5), 417-419. Reprinted with permission of the publisher, Society of Urologic Nurses and Associates, Inc. (SUNA), East Holly Avenue, Box 56, Pitman, NJ 08071-0056; Telephone: (856)256-2300; Fax: (856)589-7463; E-mail: uronsg@ajj.com; website: www.suna.org.

Biologic Warfare Agents

Since no one can predict when, where, or what agents might be used in the next terrorist attack, the most significant challenge to the terrorism preparedness and response program is planning to respond to the unknown. The CDC has identified the biologic warfare agents most likely to be involved in a terrorist attack and has grouped them into three categories.[12] Category A agents have the greatest potential for mass casualties and require broad-based public health preparedness efforts. These agents are easily disseminated and include anthrax, botulism, plague, smallpox, tularemia, and viral hemorrhagic fevers. Category A agents are being given the highest priority for preparedness, including improved surveillance and laboratory diagnosis, and stockpiling of specific medications. Category B agents have some potential for large-scale dissemination but generally cause less illness and death. These agents would require fewer special public health preparedness efforts than those in category A. Examples include Q fever, brucellosis, glanders, ricin toxin, epsilon toxin, and *Staphylococcus* enterotoxin B. Several biologic agents of concern for food and water safety are also included in this category. Category C agents do not currently present a high bioterrorism risk to public health but could emerge as future threats. Specific chapters of the book also include Terrorism Alert boxes that provide additional information on smallpox (Chapter 51), pneumonic plague (Chapter 62), botulism (Chapter 72), hemorrhagic fever viruses (Chapter 75), and sarin (Chapter 82).

The following six category A agents are high-priority agents because they pose the greatest risk to national security. Some of these enter the skin through cuts, abrasions, or mucus membranes. Others enter the gastrointestinal tract through contaminated food and water. And others enter the respiratory system via inhalation of spores, droplets, and aerosols.

Anthrax

Anthrax is at the top of the threat list for terrorism.[42] The October 2001 anthrax attacks were conducted by sending five envelopes containing *Bacillus anthracis* through the U.S. postal system. Twenty-two cases of anthrax resulted: 11 inhalational and 11 cutaneous. Five people died from inhalational anthrax. Several countries, including the United States, developed anthrax as part of a biologic weapons program in the 20th century. Anthrax released from an aircraft could create a lethal cloud of anthrax spores that are invisible and odorless. The first sign of a bioterrorist attack would most likely be clients presenting with manifestations of inhalation anthrax. Clinical manifestations would occur as soon as 2 days after exposure or as late as 6 to 8 weeks following exposure. Early manifestations of anthrax disease resemble a fever or cough, making it exceedingly difficult to diagnose. If appropriate antibiotics are not started before development of clinical manifestations, the mortality rate

is estimated to be 90%. An anthrax vaccine exists but it is only recommended for high-risk populations such as military personnel. Studies are underway to determine if the vaccine can be administered with fewer side effects and whether protection can be achieved with less than the currently recommended six inoculations.

Smallpox

Smallpox was once worldwide, and before vaccination almost everyone eventually contracted the disease. In 1980 the World Health Assembly announced that smallpox had been eradicated and recommended that all countries cease vaccination.[42] This great public health triumph has now opened the door for the smallpox virus to be used as a weapon. In fact, smallpox now represents one of the most serious bioterrorist threats. An aerosol release of smallpox virus would easily disseminate, and only a small dose is needed to be infectious. Smallpox has been universally feared as a devastating infectious disease because it is communicable from person to person, is physically disfiguring, and has a 30% case-fatality rate. Smallpox spreads primarily by droplet nuclei expelled from the mouth of the infected person or by aerosol. Infection occurs following implantation of the virus on the oral or respiratory mucosa. Contaminated clothing or bed linen could also spread the virus. A smallpox outbreak is difficult to control because an interval of as much as 2 weeks can occur between the time of an aerosol release of smallpox and diagnosis. Unless clients and close contacts are isolated, the virus can continue to spread. At this time, there is no treatment for smallpox. However, in the event of a smallpox outbreak, enough vaccine has been produced to vaccinate every person in the United States.

Plague

Plague spreads easily, kills quickly, and generates widespread fear.[42] In the 1930s and 1940s Japan used plague as a warfare weapon.[15] Bombs loaded with fleas infected with the bacteria *Yersinia pestis* were dropped over China, with devastating results. The United States tried to develop plague as a weapon, but there were problems maintaining virulence when grown in large quantities, and aerosol dissemination was difficult to control. Plague is a concern because the disease-causing agent is found in nature and in numerous biologic supply houses throughout the world.

A modern attack would most probably occur via aerosol dissemination of *Y. pestis,* causing a highly lethal pneumonic plague.[42] Clinical manifestations would appear in 1 to 2 days following an aerosol cloud exposure, with many people dying quickly after clinical manifestations appear. A vaccine that protects against inhalationally acquired pneumonic plague is under research and development. Pneumonic plague can be treated with antibiotics, and national and state public

PERSPECTIVES ON INFECTIOUS DISEASE AND BIOTERRORISM **CHAPTER 19** **339**

health officials have large supplies of drugs needed in the event of a bioterrorism attack.

Botulism

Botulinum toxin comes from the bacteria *Clostridium botulinum,* which grows in soil. It is the most lethal substance known to man.[42] During World War II, Germans developed botulism as a weapon.[15] The United States developed a weapon with botulinum toxins, but its usefulness for dissemination over large areas was inferior to that of other agents such as anthrax, and interest waned. However, botulism appears to have been Saddam Hussein's favorite weapon.[15] Iraq produced liquid botulinum toxins that were loaded into bombs. The bacterial culture to develop the weapon was obtained from a supply house in the United States! Botulinum toxin is not a great open-air biologic warfare weapon because it has a limited range, but it could be used in enclosed areas or to contaminate food supplies. Botulism results from the absorption of botulinum toxin into the circulation from a mucosal surface (gastrointestinal, lung) or a wound. The toxin prevents the release of the neurotransmitter acetylcholine, leading to muscle paralysis, and in severe cases, the need for mechanical respiration. Clinical manifestations for food-borne botulism occur from 2 hours to 8 days after ingestion. Antitoxin can reduce the severity of botulism, but it must be treated early. Licensed antitoxin is available from the CDC via state and local health departments, although supplies are limited. A human antibody against the botulinum toxin could be developed, but sufficient resources would be required to initiate the process.

Viral Hemorrhagic Fevers

Ebola and yellow fever are two of several deadly hemorrhagic fever viruses (HFVs) that can be used against mankind.[42] HFVs cause internal and external bleeding in people who get infected. None occur naturally in the United States, but risk factors for these diseases include traveling to certain geographic areas (places in Africa, Asia, the Middle East, and South America), handling of infected animals, and being bitten by an infected insect. Some of these viruses are also transmissible from person-to-person. Given the lack of readily available therapy and vaccines, a terrorist attack using aerosol dissemination of any of these viruses could cause mass illness and many deaths. Following an aerosol dissemination of an HFV, clinical manifestations would likely appear 2 to 21 days following exposure. Currently, there is no approved antiviral medication for treating any of these diseases. A vaccine exists for only one of these viruses: yellow fever. The vaccine protects travelers to areas where yellow fever is endemic, but it would not be useful following a bioterrorist attack because yellow fever has a very short incubation period.

Tularemia

In 1911 tularemia was discovered in infected ground squirrels in California.[15] *Francisella tularensis,* the organism that causes tularemia, is one of the most infectious pathogenic bacteria known.[42] Tularemia was stockpiled by the U.S. military in the late 1960s, but all of it was destroyed by 1973. Infection can occur through a variety of mechanisms such as being bit by infected deer ticks or fleas; handling meat and skin of infected animals; ingesting contaminated water, food, or soil; and inhaling infective aerosols. It is not spread person-to-person. As a weapon, tularemia bacteria can be mixed into food and water supplies, or sprayed into the air. *F. tularensis* is a hardy organism that is capable of surviving for weeks at low temperatures in water, moist soil, hay, straw, or decaying animal carcasses. Illness from tularemia would last for several weeks, with relapses occurring over several months. Clinical manifestations of pneumonia, pleuritis, and lymph node disease would occur within 3 to 5 days after exposure, and can lead to respiratory failure, shock, or death. Tularemia is found in nature and can be purchased from commercial sources for legitimate reasons. Access to these bacteria is under tight control in the United States, but not in all countries. In the United States, a live-attenuated vaccine has been used to protect laboratory personnel who routinely work with the organism, but the vaccine is not currently available for general use. Treatment with antibiotics has been successful in reducing the mortality rate.

Knowledge and preparation are the best defense against a biologic attack. By understanding the epidemiology of biologic warfare agents and diseases, strategies can be planned to decrease the morbidity and mortality associated with them. There is an urgent need for development of rapid diagnostic tests, effective vaccines, and drug therapy to defend against biologic weapon attacks. The CDC, along with other agencies and partners, is defining how the public health system is to prepare for and respond to public health threats posed by terrorism. The American Nurses' Association is working closely with the U.S. Department of Health and Human Services to establish teams of nurses, National Nurse Response Teams, who would be trained in disaster response and be ready to deploy in the event that administration of vaccines or prophylactic antibiotics is required.[25]

CONCLUSIONS

Infectious diseases have been killers of humans throughout recorded history. For most of this time, conquering infection has been the focus of health care. The nurse's role in preventing, detecting, and treating infectious disease is a vital one. And as the single largest health care professional group, nurses will be an important link in a fully developed bioterrorism response system.

BIBLIOGRAPHY

Citations appearing in blue refer to evidence-based practice guidelines and protocols.

1. Arizona Department of Health Services. (2001). *History of biowarfare and bioterrorism*. Retrieved 07/24/04 from www.hs.state.az.us/phs/edc/edrp/es/bthistor2.htm.

2. Benin, A.L., & Dowell, S.F. (2001). Antibiotic resistance and implications for the appropriate use of antimicrobial agents. In A.G. Mainous III & C. Pomeroy (Eds.), *Management of antimicrobials in infectious diseases: Impact of antibiotic resistance*. Totowa, NJ: Humana.

3. Centers for Disease Control. (1988). Update: Universal precautions for prevention of transmission of human immunodeficiency virus, hepatitis B virus, and other bloodborne pathogens in health-care settings. *Morbidity and Mortality Weekly Report, 37* (24), 377-387.

4. Centers for Disease Control and Prevention. (1995). Recommendations for preventing the spread of vancomycin resistance: Recommendations of the Hospital Infection Control Practices Advisory Committee (HICPAC). *Morbidity and Mortality Weekly Report, 44* (RR-12), 1-13.

5. Centers for Disease Control and Prevention. (1997). Interim guidelines for prevention and control of staphylococcal infection associated with reduced susceptibility to vancomycin. *Morbidity and Mortality Weekly Report, 46*(27), 626-628, 635.

6. Centers for Disease Control and Prevention. (1997). Prevention of pneumococcal disease: Recommendations of the Advisory Committee on Immunization Practices (ACIP). *Morbidity and Mortality Weekly Report, 46*(RR-8), 1-24.

7. Centers for Disease Control and Prevention. (1998). Guideline for infection control in health care personnel, 1998. *American Journal of Infection Control, 26,* 289-354.

8. Centers for Disease Control and Prevention. (1999). Antimicrobial resistance: MRSA—Methicillin resistant *Staphylococcus aureus. Issues in Healthcare Settings,* CDC online at www.cdc.gov/ncidod/hip/Aresist/mrsahcw.htm.

9. Centers for Disease Control and Prevention. (1999). Prevention of varicella. Update recommendations of the Advisory Committee on Immunization Practices (ACIP). *Morbidity and Mortality Weekly Report, 48*(RR-6), 1-5.

10. Centers for Disease Control and Prevention. (2002). Guideline for hand hygiene in healthcare settings: Recommendations of the Healthcare Infection Control Practices Advisory Committee and the HICPAC/SHEA/APIC/IDSA Hand Hygiene Task Force. *Morbidity and Mortality Weekly Report, 51*(RR 16), 1-44.

11. Centers for Disease Control and Prevention. (2002). *Staphylococcus aureus* resistant to vancomycin—United States, 2002. *Morbidity and Mortality Weekly Report, 51,* 565-567.

12. Centers for Disease Control and Prevention. (2003). *Emergency preparedness and response: Bioterrorism agents/diseases*. Retrieved 07/27/04 from www.bt.cdc.gov/agent/agentlistcategory.asp.

13. Centers for Disease Control and Prevention. (2003). *Treatment of tuberculosis*. Retrieved 03/19/06 from www.cdc.gov/mmwr/preview/mmwrhtml/rr5211a1.htm#fig2.

14. Centers for Disease Control and Prevention. (2004). *Emergency preparedness and response: CDC terrorism preparedness and response strategy*. Retrieved 07/24/04 from www.bt.cdc.gov/planning/tprstrategy/index.asp.

15. Centers for Disease Control and Prevention. (2004). *Emergency preparedness and response: The history of bioterrorism*. Retrieved 07/24/04 from www.bt.cdc.gov/training/historyofbt/index.asp.

16. Centers for Disease Control and Prevention. (2005). *Guidelines for preventing the transmission of Mycobacterium tuberculosis in health-care settings*. Retrieved 03/18/06 from www.cdc.gov/mmwr/PDF/rr/rr5417.pdf.

17. Centers for Disease Control and Prevention. (2005). *National Nosocomial Infections Surveillance System (NNIS)*. Retrieved 03/20/06 from www.cdc.gov/ncidod/dhqp/nnis.html.

18. Centers for Disease Control and Prevention. (2005). *Press release: CDC Advisory Committee offers guidance to states on developing systems for public reporting of healthcare-associated infections*. Retrieved 03/20/06 from www.cdc.gov/od/oc/media/pressrel/r050228.htm.

19. Centers for Disease Control and Prevention. (2005). *Prevention and control of influenza: Recommendations of the Advisory Committee on Immunization Practices (ACIP)*. Retrieved 03/19/06 from www.cdc.gov/mmwr/preview/mmwrhtml/rr54e713a1.htm.

20. Centers for Disease Control and Prevention. (2005). *West Nile virus: What you need to know*. Retrieved 03/10/06 from www.cdc.gov/ncidod/dvbid/westnile/wnv_factsheet.htm.

21. Centers for Disease Control and Prevention. (2006). *Preventing tetanus, diphtheria, and pertussis among adolescents: Use of tetanus toxoid, reduced diphtheria toxoid and acellular pertussis vaccines: Recommendations of the Advisory Committee on Immunization Practices (ACIP)*. Retrieved 03/19/06 from www.cdc.gov/mmwr/preview/mmwrhtml/rr55e223a1.htm.

22. Centers for Disease Control and Prevention. (2006). *Recommended adult immunization schedule– United States, October 2006—September 2007*. Retrieved 07/23/07 from http://www.cdc.gov/vaccines/recs/schedules/downloads/adult/06-07/adult-schedule.pdf.

23. Centers for Disease Control and Prevention. (2007). *Recommended immunization schedules for persons aged 0-18 years—United States, 2007*. Retrieved 07/23/07 from http://www.cdc.gov/mmwr/pdf/wk/mm5551-Immunization.pdf.

24. Cochi, S.L., et al. (1994). Meeting the challenges of vaccine-preventable diseases in child day care. *Pediatrics, 94*(6, Part 2), 1021-1023.

25. Couig, M.P. (2002). Remarks by Rear Admiral Mary Pat Couig, MPH, RN, FAAN, Chief Nurse Officer, U.S. Public Health Service, ANA Convention Opening Session, June 30, 2002. Retrieved 01/23/03 from http://nursingworld.org/conventn/2002/news/couig.htm.

26. Elizaga, M.L., Weinstein, R.A., & Hayden, M.K. (2002). Patients in long-term care facilities: A reservoir for vancomycin-resistant enterococci. *Clinical Infectious Diseases, 34,* 441-446.

27. Fridkin, S.C., & Gaynes, R.P. (1999). Antimicrobial resistance in intensive care units. *Clinics in Chest Medicine, 20,* 303-316.

28. Garner, J.S., & Hospital Infection Control Practices Advisory Committee. (1996). Guideline for isolation precautions in hospitals. *Infection Control and Hospital Epidemiology, 17,* 54-80.

29. Hamilton, D.C., & Ludlam, H. (2001). New anti-Gram-positive agents. *Current Opinion in Critical Care, 7,* 232-237.

30. Jackson, M.M., & Lynch, P. (1991). An attempt to make an issue less murky: A comparison of four systems for infection precautions. *Infection Control and Hospital Epidemiology, 12,* 448-450.

31. Jarvis, W.R. (2001). Infection control and changing health-care delivery systems. *Emerging Infectious Diseases, 7,* 170-173.

32. Maranan, M.C., et al. (1997). Antimicrobial resistance in staphylococci: Epidemiology, molecular mechanisms, and clinical relevance. *Infectious Disease Clinics of North America, 11*(4), 813-849.

33. Mayhall, C.G. (Ed.) (2004). *Hospital epidemiology and infection control* (3rd ed.). Philadelphia: Lippincott Williams & Wilkins.

34. Nelson, K.E., Williams, C.M., & Graham, N.M.H. (2001). *Infectious disease epidemiology: Theory and practice*. Gaithersburg, Md: Aspen.

35. Occupational Safety and Health Administration. (1991). Occupational exposure to bloodborne pathogens: Final rule. *Federal Register, 56,* 64003-64182.

36. Occupational Safety and Health Administration. (1997). Occupational exposure to tuberculosis: Proposed rule. *Federal Register, 62*(201), 54159-54209.

37. Occupational Safety and Health Administration. (2001). Occupational exposure to bloodborne pathogens: Needlestick and other sharps injuries; Final rule (2001, Jan 18). *Federal Register, 66,* 5317-5325.

38. Rhinehart, R. (2001). Infection control in home care. *Emerging Infectious Diseases, 7,* 208-211.

39. Rice, L.B. (2001). Emergence of vancomycin-resistant enterococci. *Emerging Infectious Diseases, 7,* 183-187.

40. Shlaes, D.M., et al. (1997). Society for Healthcare Epidemiology of America and Infectious Diseases Society of America Joint Committee on the Prevention of Antimicrobial Resistance: Guidelines for

the prevention of antimicrobial resistance in hospitals. *Infection Control and Hospital Epidemiology, 18,* 275-291.

41. Smith, P.W., & Rusnak, P.G. (1997). SHEA/APIC position paper: Infection prevention and control in the long-term-care facility. *Infection Control and Hospital Epidemiology, 18*(12), 831-849.

41a. The Joint Commission. (2007). *2008 National Patient Safety Goals Hospital Program.* www.jointcommission.org/PatientSafety/NationalPatientSafetyGoals.

42. University of Pittsburgh Medical Center. (2004). *Center for biosecurity: BW agents.* Retrieved from www.upmc-biosecurity.org/.

43. U.S. Department of Health and Human Services. (1990). *Healthy People 2000.* Washington, DC: U.S. Government Printing Office.

44. U.S. Department of Health and Human Services. (2000). *Healthy People 2010: Understanding and improving health* (2nd ed.). Washington, DC: U.S. Government Printing Office.

45. Weber, C.J. (2004). Infectious disease: Update on bioterrorism preparedness. *Urologic Nursing, 24*(5), 417-419.

46. Weber, C.J. (2006). Infectious disease: Update on influenza pandemic threat. *Urologic Nursing, 26*(1), 67-68.

47. Weber, C.J. (2006). Infectious disease: Update on preparing for the next influenza pandemic. *Urologic Nursing, 26*(2), 145-147.

48. Wenzel, R.P. (Ed.) (2003). *Prevention and control of nosocomial infections* (4th ed.). Philadelphia: Lippincott Williams & Wilkins.

49. World Health Organization (2007). *Cumulative number of confirmed human cases of avian influenza A/(H5n1) reported to WHO.* Retrieved July 24, 2007 from http://www.who.int/csr/disease/avian_influenza/country/cases_table_2007_07_11/en/index.html

50. Yoshikawa, T.T., & Norman, D.C. (Eds.) (2001). *Infectious disease in the aging: A clinical handbook.* Totowa, NJ: Humana.

evolve   *Did you remember to check out the bonus material on the Evolve website and the CD-ROM, including NCLEX®- Examination Style Review Questions, Open-Book Quizzes, and Chapter Review Audio Podcasts?*

http://evolve.elsevier.com/Black/medsurg

UNIT **5**

PSYCHOSOCIAL FOUNDATIONS

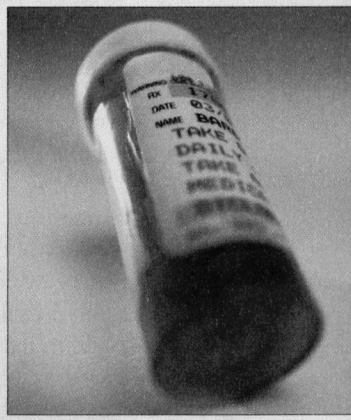

ANATOMY AND PHYSIOLOGY REVIEW:

Arousal, Pain, and Conscious Awareness

Robert G. Carroll

Awareness and response to dangerous settings are key to the survival of an organism. Humans have a variety of distinct senses (smell, sight, hearing) that can be used to identify potentially dangerous situations and allow an individual to avoid them. If avoidance fails and damage occurs, pain results.

Pain is a conscious perception that results from environmental stress. *Nociceptors,* often called *pain receptors,* are free nerve endings activated by stimuli that can cause (or already have caused) tissue damage. Neuronal transmission of nociceptors is redundant and is subject to only minor filtering before reaching the somatosensory cortex.

The reticular activating system (RAS) controls the degree of filtering of afferent sensory inputs (including pain) and therefore helps determine conscious perception. The activity of the cortex is superimposed on a normal sleep-wake cycle and can interact with this cycle.

This section uses the perception of pain to introduce the concepts of neuronal transmission, the processing of information, arousal, and conscious awareness. Unit 16 provides additional details about neuron action potential, synaptic transmission, and other somatosensory modalities.

To understand the mechanisms by which one can facilitate pain reduction, one must understand the neurologic contributions to pain perception. Pain is a perceptual interpretation of nerve activity that reaches consciousness. It depends on activation of neurons that transmit the noxious information to the central nervous system. Pain perception is initiated by activation of neurons along a pathway that eventually terminates in a sensory cortex in the brain. The pathway involves both peripheral and central nervous system components and can be activated at any point along its trajectory.

NEURONAL COMMUNICATION

At the single neuron level, action potentials generally arrive at the dendrites or cell body and initiate an action potential at the beginning of the axon; then an action potential travels along the axon to the next synapse in the sequence. Neurons in sensory pathways rarely make a 1:1 synaptic connection. The diversity of synaptic connections allows sensory information to be coded and processed before arriving at the cerebral cortex. Neuronal interconnections generally fall into a diverging or a converging pattern.

Divergence occurs when an action potential from one axon activates synapses with multiple other neurons. This arrangement allows a single stimulus to have multiple effects. One advantage of this arrangement is that the information becomes redundant, meaning that one synaptic failure will not result in loss of the message.

Convergence occurs when one neuron receives afferent connections from multiple other axons. This is important because activity at a synapse from one neuron is not sufficient to generate an action potential in the post-synaptic neuron. Convergence also increases sensitivity and the perception of the stimuli. Convergence occurs because the generation of an action potential in the post-synaptic neuron requires simultaneous activity at a number of synapses *(spatial summation)* or repetitive activation of a single synapse *(temporal summation).*

The flexibility of neuronal interconnections is enhanced by having some neurons exciting the post-synaptic neuron and other neurons inhibiting the post-synaptic neuron. Excitation or inhibition is determined by the type of post-synaptic receptor, the neurotransmitter released from the pre-synaptic neuron, and the receptor specificity of the post-synaptic neuron.

THE PHYSIOLOGY OF PAIN

PAIN AS AN INTEGRATIVE EXPERIENCE

Nociceptor Activation

Nociceptors are free nerve endings that are widely distributed throughout the body. Nociceptors can be found in the periphery in skin, fascia, bone periosteum, skeletal muscle, ligaments, and mucous membranes. In the viscera, nociceptors are found in the capsules of most organs. Chemically mediated activation of nociceptors can be initiated by (1) cell wall destruction as a result of events such as tissue injury, ulceration, tumor invasion, and cell necrosis; (2) inflammation; (3) infection; (4) nerve injury; and (5) extravasation of plasma from the circulatory system associated with edema, ischemia, or occlusion of vasculature. Mechanically mediated activation of nociceptors is accomplished by noxious stretch or pressure caused by (1) distention of viscera, fascia or periosteum; (2) occlusion of gastrointestinal or genitourinary structures; or (3) obstruction of ducts.

Chemicals that mediate nociception in the periphery include bradykinin, prostaglandins, substance P, histamine, serotonin, leukotrienes, and nerve growth factor. Bradykinin is the most potent pain-producing chemical. It is released into tissues when cell walls are destroyed and when plasma leaks from the vasculature. Bradykinin initiates a pain signal by increasing the ability of Na^+ to flow across the membrane of nociceptors.

Prostaglandins result from cell wall destruction and are derived from arachidonic acid. They most likely contribute to the pain experience by sensitizing receptors, making them more responsive to other chemical, thermal, and mechanical stimuli. They are also potent vasodilators, resulting in an increase of bradykinin release into the tissues. The resulting edema may also contribute by stimulating pressure receptors. Prostaglandins depolarize these receptors, making them responsive to the relatively weak stimulus provided by the swelling of edema.

Substance P is released into peripheral tissues when nociceptive neurons are activated. This chemical facilitates the release of plasma by increasing vascular permeability, resulting in bradykinin availability. Substance P further enhances pain responses by contributing to prostaglandin release.

Histamine is released from mast cells when inflammation is a component of the pain-producing event. In the periphery, histamine increases vascular permeability, contributing to bradykinin activity and edema. Substance P facilitates the release of histamine from mast cells.

Serotonin is released in the periphery by platelets and mast cells. Therefore any event that results in the presence of blood products in tissues or inflammation contributes to serotonin release. Serotonin causes pain directly by altering Na^+ flow in the receptive neuron membrane, causing the neuron to fire. Receptors are indirectly facilitated by serotonin as the chemical also sensitizes receptors to the effect of bradykinin.

Leukotrienes are produced by cell-wall destruction during the same process that produces prostaglandins, and also have arachidonic acid as their precursor. They contribute to pain perception by attracting neutrophils to an area of injury. Cell-wall destruction is a component of neutrophil activity to combat infection resulting in bradykinin release. Thermal and mechanical receptors have also been shown to be sensitized by leukotrienes.

Hydrogen ions are released as a result of ischemia and hypoxia. They cause Na^+ channels to open, resulting in activation of neurons in the pain pathway. Hydrogen ions cause vasodilation and also facilitate Ca^{2+} channel opening, enhancing neurotransmitter release.

Nerve growth factor (NGF) is released when neurons are injured. It is similar to bradykinin in activating nociceptive neurons. It causes injured nerves to sprout new axons and dendrites in greater numbers than existed before the injury. As a result, the area responsive to nociceptive activation is increased in the periphery, which plays a major role in chronic pain. Substance P production is also increased by NGF increasing the nociceptive effect of the neurotransmitter. In addition, the numbers of Na^+ and K^+ channels are increased, making it easier to generate an ion flow that will cause the neuron to "fire." Pain is complex and many chemical mediators are eventually involved and often synergistic.

Pain may follow the direct activation of free nerve endings, or they may become sensitized, rendering them more susceptible to nociceptive activation and causing pain to develop more quickly. Sensitizing chemicals are released into tissues as a result of cell-wall destruction and the release of plasma from the circulatory system, as seen with edema, inflammation, ischemia, and infection. Cells may be damaged by trauma and by the events that accompany inflammation and infection, including mast cell destruction during the release of histamine in inflammation and the effect of neutrophil activity in the presence of infection. Chemicals that sensitize receptors and nerve fiber membranes rendering events that do not typically produce pain sensations now are capable of initiating pain-producing signals. For example, sunburned areas produce a burning sensation when one showers with water that normally produces a pleasant warm sensation. Areas of injury are painful in response to touch and mild pressure that would not normally be painful. Normal peristalsis of the gut, which is typically undetectable, produces painful abdominal cramping in the presence of inflammation within the abdominal cavity.

The complexity of pain perception is illustrated by examination of the response to touching a hot stove with your hand. The extreme heat activates the nociceptors and generates action potentials in two different types of neurons, resulting in the perception of fast pain and slow pain.

Fast pain is carried by small *myelinated* nerves (A-delta fibers) (Figure A&P5-1). These neurons make multiple synaptic connections in the spinal cord. One connection activates the motor neurons that initiate a withdrawal reflex. This spinal reflex serves to remove the hand from the damaging environment, even before there is any cortical awareness of the injury. Other synaptic connections activate neuron sequences passing through the thalamus and terminating in the sensory cortex, the limbic system, and the hypothalamus, providing the sensation of pain. Fast pain is generally described as sharp and well localized and is generally associated with damage to the skin and muscles. A-delta fiber activity typically results in activation of the sympathetic nervous system to prepare the individual to engage in "fight-or-flight" behaviors that will allow the person to react to the pain-producing event. As a result, heart rate, respiratory rate, and blood pressure may be increased. These sympathetic reactions are not always observable in people with pain because they are relatively rapidly adapting, often short-lived responses.

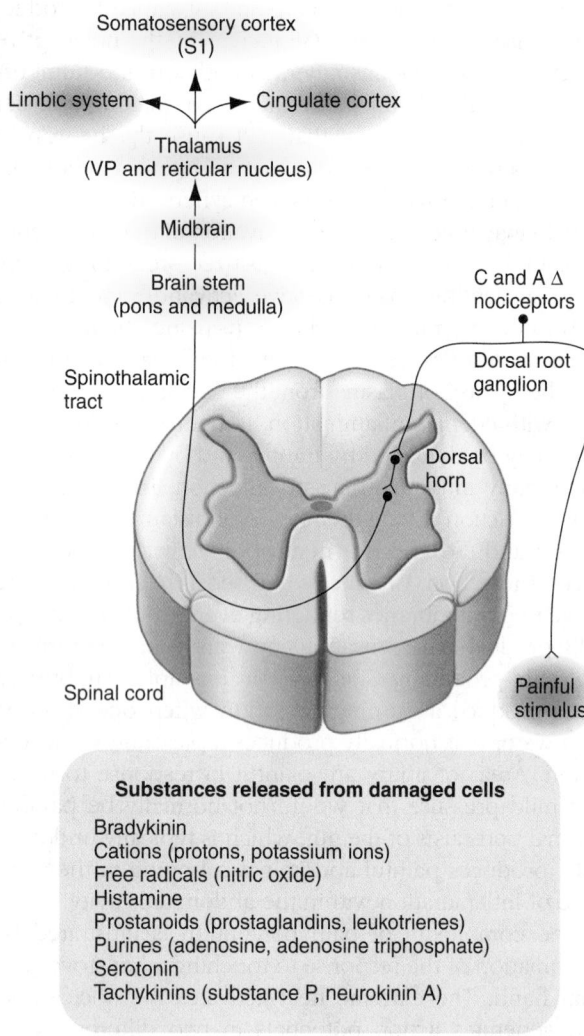

Substances released from damaged cells

Bradykinin
Cations (protons, potassium ions)
Free radicals (nitric oxide)
Histamine
Prostanoids (prostaglandins, leukotrienes)
Purines (adenosine, adenosine triphosphate)
Serotonin
Tachykinins (substance P, neurokinin A)

■ **FIGURE A&P5–1** The pathway for pain perception and response.

In contrast, *slow pain* is carried by small, *unmyelinated* nerves (C fibers). These neurons also make multiple connections in the spinal cord, and ascending information goes to the midbrain and the reticular formation and contributes to the emotional, cognitive, and situational components of pain. Slow pain is characteristic of damage to the skin, muscles, and internal organs and is characterized by dull, burning sensations. The poorly localized aspect of slow pain leads to the observation that pain originating in internal organs is perceived in areas with related dermatomes; for example, the specific cause of stomach ache is difficult to diagnose.

Spinal Cord

The dorsal horn of the spinal cord is the first synaptic relay of the nociceptor-pain pathway. The two types of pain fibers enter different layers of the dorsal horn. A-delta fibers enter the posterior marginalis and the nucleus proprius. These fibers cross to the opposite side

of the spinal cord and ascend in the spinothalamic tract and carry the pain signal to the thalamus. The C fibers enter the substantia gelatinosa and synapse on interneurons that carry the signal to the brain. Interneurons that synapse in the spinal cord use substance P and glutamate as neurotransmitters. Electrical activity resulting in pain perception can be modified at the synapse by manipulating the release of neurotransmitters. An event that inhibits neurotransmitter release decreases the potential for transmission of the nociceptive signal. The inhibition may occur to an extent that extinguishes the pain-producing signal, resulting in total pain reduction. Conversely any event that facilitates release of the neurotransmitter will enhance the transmission of the signal. For example, an event that prohibits the opening of the Ca^{2+} channels inhibits the pain response.

The signal is transmitted from the thalamus to the sensory cortex, where the pain is perceived as a sensation. The thalamus determines the location and intensity of the pain-producing event. Secondary responses to the signal are initiated throughout the brain, including the limbic system, where the emotional response to pain is generated. Signals transmitted to brain stem structures contribute to the response the individual has to the pain experience and to endogenous (naturally occurring) pain modulation systems (Figure A&P5-2).

Brain

Nociceptive sensory information is transmitted to the brain by multiple ascending pathways. Sensory information is carried through the spinothalamic tract and the spinoreticular tract to the thalamus and the RAS system, respectively. Neurons from the thalamus project to the cerebral cortex (for the conscious perception of pain) and also the limbic system (controlling the emotional response to pain). The amygdala receives nociceptive stimulation via the spinomesencephalic tract and

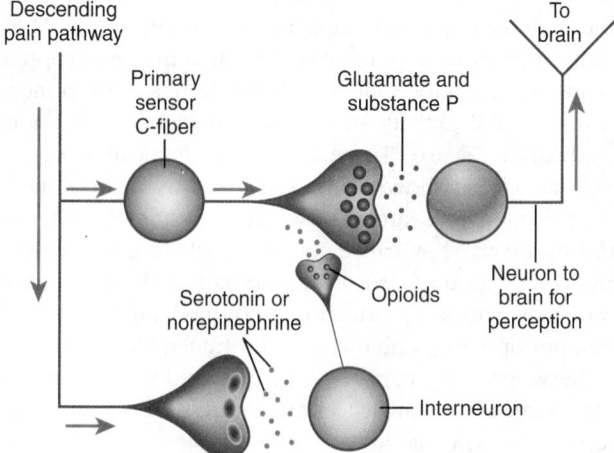

■ **FIGURE A&P5–2** Endogenous inhibition in a synapse in the spinal cord. As the pain impulse enters the dorsal horn, it has the potential of being modified by interneurons in the synapse containing endogenous opioids.

integrates feelings of fear among other basic emotions. Finally, pain elicits an autonomic response, directly via the spinohypothalamic tract and also indirectly through activity of the thalamus and cerebral cortex.

Conscious Perception of Pain

The diversity of target sites for ascending nociceptive tracts indicates the complexity of the pain perception. Fast pain is a somatosensory sensation, with the origin of the involved nociceptors being precisely localized on the somatic map of the body. In contrast, localization of slow pain is much less precise. Pain localization may actually be referred from C fibers of the same dermatome (as when myocardial ischemia is "sensed" as pain radiating down the left arm). Nociceptive afferents also synapse in the RAS, where they can regulate conscious awareness and attention. Pain elicits a sympathetic autonomic nervous system response (the "flight-or-fight response"), including an increase in pulse and respiratory rates. Finally there is a significant emotional aspect of pain, mediated through the limbic system and insular cortex.

Hyperalgesia

Hyperalgesia is an enhancement of the perception of pain. This event can be mediated both at the tissue level and at the spinal cord. Stimuli that do not originally activate nociceptors may do so after repeated application of noxious stimuli, a process called *sensitization*. Substances released from damaged cells act to decrease the threshold for nociceptors. At the spinal cord level, repetitive afferent input from C fibers causes the dorsal horn cells to become more easily excitable, a process thought to underlie the phenomenon of "phantom limb pain." Chronic phantom limb pain likely involves central nervous system reorganization and consequently can change over time.

PAIN SUPPRESSION APPROACHES

Pain is the conscious interpretation of stimuli associated with nociceptor activity. Pain management remains one of the most significant challenges in nursing. A variety of approaches are currently used to diminish the suffering from pain.

Nociceptor

Diminished stimulation of the free nerve endings will reduce the perception of pain. One approach is to use ice to cool the injured area, which diminishes the activity of the nociceptors. A second approach uses a local anesthetic (Novocain, Xylocaine) injected at the site of injury or along the motor and/or sensory nerve pathway to completely but reversibly block action potential transmission. Depending on which nerve is injected, sensory

and/or motor neuron activity can be blocked. In extreme cases, the sensory nerves can be severed to block permanently nociceptor action potential transmission.

Synaptic Interruption

The dorsal horn cell in the spinal cord is the first of the multiple synapses involved in nociceptive transmission. Glutamate, acting on α-amino-3-hydroxy-5-methylisoxazole-4-propionic acid (AMPA)-type glutamate receptors, is the major neurotransmitter. The response of the postsynaptic cell, however, is enhanced by substance P and a variety of neuropeptides released from the nociceptor axons. Blocking the *N*-methyl-D-aspartate (NMDA) receptor both diminishes nociceptor afferent transmission and also prevents the hypersensitivity caused by repetitive activity of nociceptors.

Gate Theory of Pain

Nociceptor transmission can be regulated by neurons not directly involved in the afferent pain transmission pathways (Figure A&P5-3). Non-nociceptive afferents diminish the sensitivity of dorsal horn neurons involved in nociception. The non-nociceptive afferents include sensory neurons that encode vibration. This mechanism is used to explain why rubbing a sore area reduces pain and how transcutaneous electrical nerve stimulation (TENS) is effective in modulating the sensation of pain. In addition to inhibition from sensory afferents, descending inhibitory pathways can diminish the effectiveness of the pain transmission pathways at the spinal cord and thalamic levels.

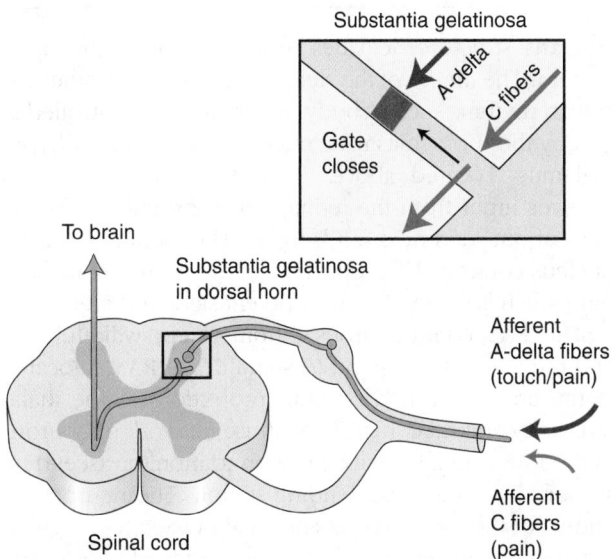

■ **FIGURE A&P5–3** The gate-control theory is a self-regulating system of pain management. Pain signals travel up the A-delta and C nerves in response to injury or inflammation. The descending nerve impulses generated by the brain close the gate, stopping pain transmission. Failure of these control mechanisms can lead to chronic pain, which persists after removal of the cause or after completion of the healing process.

Brain Chemicals and Analgesics

The importance of pain reduction led to early identification of morphine (opium) and codeine as significant analgesics. Injection of morphine into the brain inhibits the activity of the spinal cord dorsal horn cells, indicating that morphine activates descending inhibitory pathways. The localization of opiate receptors in the brain and spinal cord led to the identification of endogenous compounds that bind those receptors. Three major classes of peptides—enkephalins, endorphins, and dynorphins—are produced by the body and activate the opiate receptors, and consequently have significant analgesic actions.

The four groups of non-opioid analgesics are salicylates, acetaminophen, nonsteroidal anti-inflammatory drugs (NSAIDs), and "others." These drugs generally have both local and central analgesic effects that are tied to the inhibition of prostaglandin synthesis. For example, aspirin and NSAIDs inhibit local prostaglandin production at areas of inflammation, diminishing the sensitization of the nociceptors.

FACTORS AFFECTING PAIN

The perception of pain is shaped by emotional state and past experiences. A variety of factors cause pain perception to be a subjective experience. The person-to-person variability in the perception of pain contributes to the challenges in clinical management of pain.

THE PHYSIOLOGY OF SLEEP AND AROUSAL

Humans structure activities around a daily (circadian) rhythm. The timing of the sleep-wake cycle and other circadian rhythms such as body temperature is controlled in part by the suprachiasmatic nucleus in the anterior hypothalamus. Located above the optic chiasm, this area receives input from the retina, which provides information about darkness and light. The suprachiasmatic nucleus controls the production of the hormone melatonin, which is believed to be a potent sleep inducer.

The RAS controls arousal from sleep, wakefulness, and the ability to respond to stimuli. The RAS is located in the brain stem and contains projections to the thalamus and cerebral cortex. The diffuse network of neurons in the RAS is in a strategic position to monitor ascending sensory inputs and descending stimuli. The neurotransmitters of the RAS serve as chemical messengers regulating the sleep-wake cycle and the stages of sleep. The onset of sleep and of each subsequent sleep stage is an active process involving delicate shifts in the balance of several of these neurotransmitters.

The transition from the awake state to a non-rapid eye movement (NREM) sleep is marked by regional decreases in the concentrations of serotonin, norepinephrine, and acetylcholine. The later transition to rapid eye movement (REM) sleep is marked by a dramatic increase in acetylcholine concentration and further decreases in serotonin and norepinephrine levels. As REM sleep continues, the concentrations of serotonin and norepinephrine increase, eventually stopping REM sleep. The release of acetylcholine seems to reestablish REM sleep. The continuous interaction of these two systems produces the normal alterations between NREM and REM sleep. Other neurotransmitters such as gamma-aminobutyric acid (GABA) and dopamine contribute to the reciprocal processes involved in shift in sleep state (Figure A&P5-4).

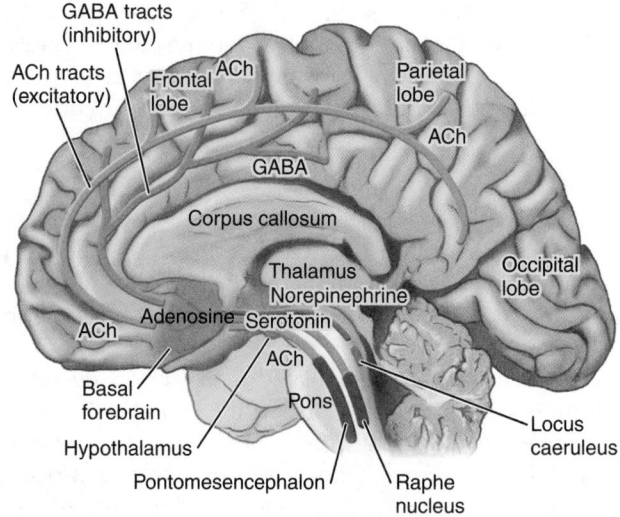

■ **FIGURE A&P5–4** The neurotransmitters of the RAS—acetylcholine, gamma-aminobutyric acid (GABA), and dopamine—are the chemical messengers regulating the sleep-wake cycle and the stages of sleep. The continuous interaction of these chemicals produces the normal alterations between NREM and REM sleep. Acetylcholine seems to reestablish REM sleep. GABA and dopamine produce the reciprocal processes involved in moving through the stages of sleep.

All of these neurotransmitters are also actively involved in the waking process. For example, neurons that produce serotonin and norepinephrine play a role in the modulation of sensory input, mood, energy, and information processing, including attention, learning, and memory. Imbalances in these neurotransmitters, such as occurs with depression, induce sleep pattern disturbances. Medications or diseases may reciprocally affect not only sleep but also aspects of sensory processing, mood, and cognition.

THE NEED FOR SLEEP

The structure of the sleep cycle is well studied and offers clues about the need for sleep. Sleep is known to have a restorative and protective function. During sleep, sympathetic activity decreases while parasympathetic activity may increase. Hormonal shifts facilitate anabolic processes. Rapid eye movement sleep may be especially important for maintaining mental activities, such as learning, reasoning, and emotional adjustment. Sleep also appears to serve as an energy-conserving measure for most of the body except for the brain.

SLEEP STAGES

Sleep can be defined behaviorally, functionally, and electrophysiologically. Electrophysiologic monitoring of sleep is called *polysomnography* and includes at least three parameters: (1) brain-wave activity, (2) eye movements, and (3) muscle tone. Polysomnography shows that sleep can be divided into REM and NREM stages. NREM sleep can further be divided into stages 1 through 4. The stages vary in depth but are characterized by slow, rolling eye movements, low-level and fragmented cognitive activity, maintenance of moderate muscle tone, and slower but generally rhythmic respiration and pulse rates. As a person progresses from stage 1 to stage 4 sleep, the wave forms recorded by electroencephalography (EEG) become more synchronized, slower, and higher in amplitude.

The stages of sleep are characterized as follows:

- *Stage 1* is very light. Respirations begin to slow, and muscles relax. At sleep onset, some erratic breathing may occur as well as sudden myoclonic jerks (sleep starts) as the body shifts from an awake to a sleep state. Stage 1 is such a light stage of sleep that people awakened from it often claim that they were not asleep at all.
- *Stage 2* is still light sleep. The brain waves are frequently mixed and low voltage in pattern, with bursts of electrical activity called *sleep spindles* and large-amplitude waves called *K complexes*. More than 50% of sleep occurs as stages 1 and 2.
- *Stages 3 and 4* are slow-wave sleep, named for the characteristic high-voltage, low-frequency delta

waves. Respirations become slow and even. The pulse rate and blood pressure fall. Oxygen consumption by muscle tissues and urine formation decrease. Dreams that occurred during the NREM stage of sleep are generally thought-like ruminations about recent events and current concerns with little story line.

REM sleep is characterized by low-voltage, random fast waves, as in stage 1 NREM. People in REM sleep have characteristic rapid eye movements, erratic respirations, changes in heart rate, and very low muscle tone. During REM sleep, ventilation depends primarily on the movements of the diaphragm because intracostal and accessory muscle tone is markedly diminished and all postural and nonrespiratory muscles are essentially paralyzed. The ventilatory response to hypoxia and hypercapnia is decreased, and thermoregulation is significantly reduced. Dreams in REM sleep are vivid, story-like, emotional, and bizarre.

Most people move through an orderly progression of NREM sleep from stages 1 to 4 and back through stages 3 to 2 before initiating a period of REM sleep (Figure A&P5-5). Although this is the typical progression, it is not essential or always seen. Atypical progressions are characteristic of some sleep disorders, such as narcolepsy, in which REM sleep is entered almost immediately after sleep onset.

In adults each sleep cycle through the stages lasts about 90 minutes. During the first few cycles, more time is spent in slow-wave sleep. The percentage of REM sleep increases later in the sleep period.

Wide variations in sleep patterns exist among individuals. By explaining the range of these variations, the nurse can help clients seek a pattern that leaves them feeling reasonably refreshed and alert. Eight hours of undisturbed sleep at night with no daytime naps has become the assumed ideal pattern in North American society. Some adults, however, do well with 6 hours or less, and other normal adults require 10 hours or more of nighttime sleep. Even young adults often awaken once or twice at night, and with aging such awakenings are more frequent. Humans may be physiologically inclined to have a long and short sleep period every 24-hour day, such as is common in warmer climates, where the siesta is a normal part of the day's schedule.

CHANGES IN SLEEP PATTERNS IN OLDER ADULTS

Older people take longer to fall asleep (called sleep latency), have increased nocturnal wakefulness, require more time to get back to sleep after arousal, and experience more sleepiness during the day than do younger adults. With aging the percentage of stage 4 decreases considerably and REM sleep decreases somewhat, with more time spent in stage 1. REM sleep is more evenly

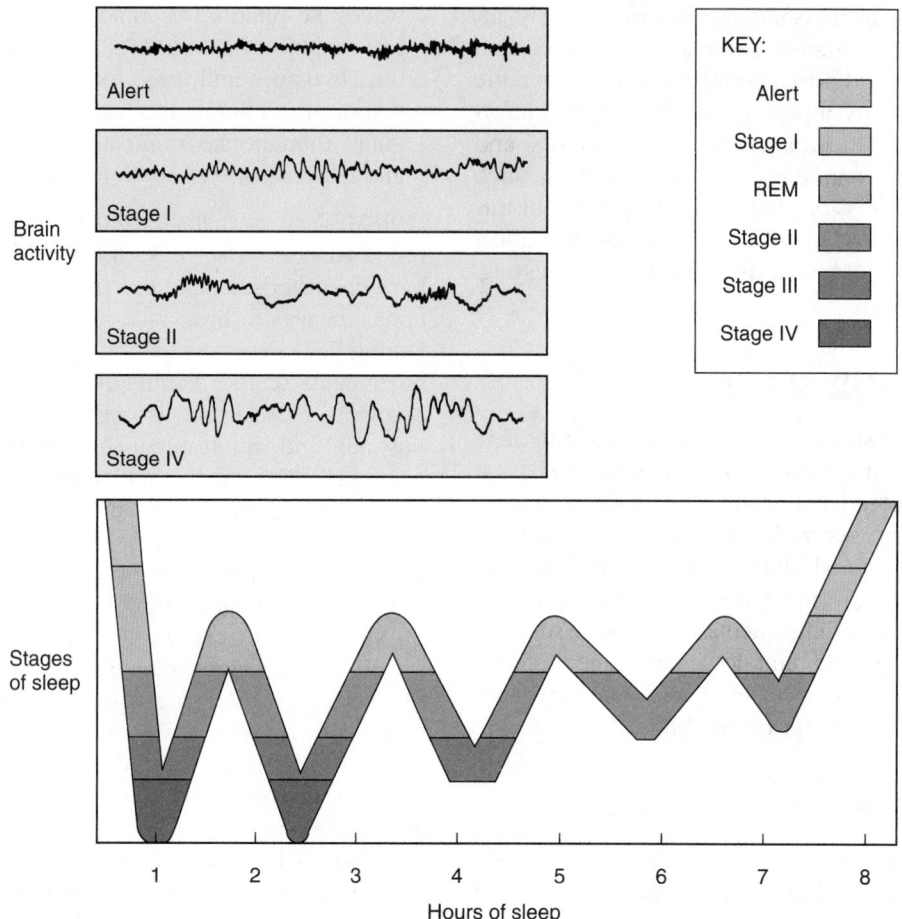

■ **FIGURE A&P5–5**   The electrical activity of the brain during various stages of sleep can be shown on electroencephalograms. During the night, people go through three to five 90-minute sleep cycles. Each cycle includes a sequence of sleep stages. *REM,* Rapid eye movement. *(From Solomon, E.P., Schmidt, R.R., & Adranga, P.J. [1990]. Human anatomy and physiology [2nd ed.]. Philadelphia: Saunders.)*

distributed through the night. Age-related respiratory dysfunction may be responsible for sleep fragmentation. Many medical problems are a common reason that elderly have difficult sleeping, such as pain, the need to void, pain from arthritis, and depression.

Hospitalization affects the quality of nocturnal and other sleep time, especially for older adults. The hospital environment often lacks light and dark cues. Confinement curtails activity or exercise that normally causes fatigue. In addition, unfamiliar sights and sounds and frequent awakenings for the assessment of vital signs and other interventions can disturb sleep. Institutionalization in a long-term care facility may perpetuate the environmental impact of noise, caregiver interruptions, inactivity, and lack of day-night cues.

CONCLUSIONS

Awareness is a neural construct based on activity of the cerebral cortex. Afferent sensory information provides a framework for constructing this awareness. The perception of pain is an example of the complexity of neuronal transmission and modulation that is applied to sensory information as it travels toward the cerebral cortex. Sleep is another example of the range of awareness experienced during the course of the day.

BIBLIOGRAPHY

1. Berne, R., et al. (2004). *Physiology* (5th ed.). St. Louis: Mosby.
2. Carroll, R.G. (2007). *Elsevier's integrated physiology.* Philadelphia: Saunders.
3. Guyton, A.C., & Hall, J.E. (2006). *Textbook of medical physiology* (11th ed.). Philadelphia: Saunders.
4. Kandel, E.R., Schwartz, J.H., & Jessel, T.M. (2000). *Principles of neural science* (4th ed.). New York: McGraw-Hill.
5. Kierzenbaum, A.L. (2007). *Histology and cell biology: An introduction to pathology* (2nd ed.). St. Louis: Mosby.
6. Silverthorn, D. (2006). *Human physiology* (4th ed.). San Francisco, Calif: Pearson Benjamin Cummings.
7. Thibodeau, G., & Patton, K. (2007). *Anatomy and physiology* (6th ed.). St. Louis: Mosby.

Pain serves as a mechanism to warn us about the potential for physical harm. Thus pain is the body's protective mechanism to prevent further damage by providing the impetus to withdraw from the pain-producing situation. The discomfort and distress associated with pain often last far beyond the tissue-damaging experience. Pain is the primary reason people seek health care and is associated with increased length of hospital stay, longer recovery time, and poorer client outcomes.[1,15] Pain is typically undertreated.[6] In the early 1970s researchers reported that pain was seriously undertreated after surgery.[23] Sadly today, this situation has changed little, even though there have been immense advances in knowledge of the causes of pain and the mechanisms that contribute to pain reduction or relief. New medications and the recognition of complementary pain management strategies have contributed to the improved ability to manage pain and to provide satisfactory pain reduction or relief. If the existing knowledge and resources were used to manage pain, 90% of people with pain would receive satisfactory reduction or relief.[24]

DEFINITION OF PAIN

How would you define *pain*? Does your definition include feelings of agony, distress, or suffering? Or is pain defined in a structural, physiologic manner only? Does your definition include individual perception of the painful stimulus? How do you include cultural and ethnic backgrounds, gender, or age?

Pain is a multidimensional phenomenon and is thus difficult to define. It is a personal and subjective experience, and no two people experience pain in exactly the same manner. Pain has been defined in many ways. It is generally related to some type of tissue damage, which serves as a warning signal, but the pain experience is much more. The International Association for the Study of Pain (IASP) offers the accepted medical definition of pain as "an unpleasant sensory and emotional experience associated with actual or potential tissue damage, or described in terms of such damage."[15]

Margo McCaffery, one of nursing's pain pioneers, defined pain as "whatever the experiencing person says it is and existing whenever the person says it does."[24] This definition makes each person the expert about his or her own pain. Because pain is subjective, the only people who can accurately define their own pain are those who are experiencing that pain. Despite its subjective nature, the nurse is charged with accurately assessing and helping to reduce or relieve pain, and McCaffery's definition helps nurses achieve this goal. All pain is real even if the cause cannot be ascertained. The nurse is not to presume to judge the presence of pain.

PAIN MECHANISMS

Scientifically, pain (a subjective experience) is separate and distinct from nociception. Nociception is a measurable physiologic event. Nociception is the system that carries

---

evolve Web Enhancements

Bridge to Home Health Care   Controlling Pain
Diversity in Health Care   Cultural Perspectives on Pain
Ethical Issues in Nursing   Pain: Who Is the Expert?
Is It Ethical to Give a Client a Placebo?
What Should the Nurse Do About an Incompetent Colleague?
Appendix A   Religious Beliefs and Practices Affecting Health Care
Be sure to check out the bonus material on the Evolve website and the CD-ROM, including free self-assessment exercises. **http://evolve.elsevier.com/Black/medsurg**

information about inflammation, damage, or near-damage in tissue to the spinal cord and brain. Nociception frequently occurs without pain being felt and is below the level of consciousness. Despite it triggering pain and suffering, nociception is a critical component of the body's defense system. The causes of nociceptive pain from stimuli are shown in Table 20-1. See the Anatomy and Physiology review on pain (pp. 344-350) for more information.

PATTERNS OF PAIN

Acute Pain

Acute pain is caused by activation of nociceptors, is usually of short duration (less than 6 months), and has an immediate onset, such as incisional pain after surgery. It is also regarded as having a limited and often predictable duration, such as postoperative pain, which usually disappears as the wound heals. Clients use words such as "sharp," "stabbing," and "shooting" to describe acute pain. Acute pain can be seen as useful, in that it indicates injury and motivates the person to seek relief by treatment of the cause. Acute pain is usually reversible or controllable with adequate treatment. People suffering from acute pain often come to terms with it because of the meaning or the limited nature of the pain, as in the pain of childbirth. When the pain is relieved, the person returns to the pre-pain state.

Acute pain may be accompanied by observable physical responses, including (1) increased or decreased blood pressure, (2) tachycardia, (3) diaphoresis, (4) tachypnea, (5) focusing on the pain, and (6) guarding the painful body area. The cardiovascular and respiratory responses are due to stimulation of the sympathetic nervous system as part of the *fight or flight response*. These responses are often interpreted as positive evidence of a person's pain. Such interpretation is not reliable, however, because these sympathetic responses are temporary and may not be present in clients with continuing acute pain. Unrelieved acute pain leads to chronic pain states.

Chronic Pain

Chronic pain is usually considered to be pain that lasts more than 6 months (or 1 month beyond the normal end of the condition causing the pain) and has no foreseeable end unless it is associated with very slow healing, as with burns. Chronic pain may have started as an acute pain or its origin may have been so obscure that the person does not know when it first developed. The course of chronic pain includes months and years of pain, not minutes or hours.

Clients with chronic pain may have localized or widespread pain and tenderness, some with tender points in predictable spots, but with few other physical findings. They often complain of fatigue, sleep disturbance, and limited function. They may have evidence of depressive mood, and exhibit behaviors of chronically ill people. They often search for a single cause of the problem and become frustrated with the medical profession when tests do not reveal a cause and multiple treatment approaches fail to give relief. As time passes and the manifestations continue, the condition becomes more complex, and other factors influence the manifestations, attitudes, and symptoms, the chronic pain client can often be noted to adopt features and behaviors that are referred to as "pain behaviors"—the client may adopt the sick role and become more limited than one would expect from the client's physical findings and functional tests. The approach of medical investigation and treatment, the attitude of family and supporters, and the practices of such organizations as workers' compensation and social agencies may become important factors by providing "rewards" for remaining unwell, and accentuating the illness behavior. The person may be quite unconscious of this, but it can be a process that worsens the condition even though the aim of these processes was to help the person.

Types of Chronic Pain

Chronic Persistent Pain

Persistent pain is a complex mix of physical and psychological manifestations. It is ideally treated with both physical and psychological interventions. Family and personal relationships, finances, work, past pain experiences, and personality are important aspects of the pain experience. The physical component of the pain

TABLE 20–1	Sources of Noxious Stimuli for Clients with Cancer
Source of Stimuli	**Cause**
Cell destruction	Chemotherapy
	Cell necrosis
	Ulceration
	Tumor invasion
	Tissue injury
Inflammation	Products of cell destruction
Infection	Bacterial invasion
Nerve injury	Direct injury through incising nerve structures
	Tumor invasion of peripheral nerves, plexuses, spinal cord, brain
	Chemotherapy/radiation injury
Ischemia/ hypoxia	Edema
	Hematoma
	Occlusion of vessels by tumor
Noxious stretch or pressure	Distention of thoracic and abdominal viscera, fascia, periosteum
	Occlusion of gastrointestinal and genitourinary structures
	Obstruction of ducts and viscus

is often a nociceptive or neuropathic problem. Common etiologies of persistent pain are a missed diagnosis, inadequate rehabilitation, a rest-reinjury cycle, complex regional pain syndrome, myofascial pain syndrome, and depression with somatization.

Chronic Intermittent Pain

Intermittent pain refers to exacerbation or recurrence of the chronic condition. The pain occurs only at specific periods; at other times, the client is free from pain. Typical conditions include migraine and cluster headache, sickle cell crisis, and the intermittent abdominal pain associated with chronic gastrointestinal disorders, such as irritable bowel syndrome and Crohn's disease. Pain management is directed toward reduction or relief of pain in much the same manner as that for individual acute pain episodes. However, chronic recurrences render the condition more difficult to control. The client anticipates continual exacerbation of the situation and is intensely influenced by psychosocial factors that are difficult to manage.

Chronic Malignant (cancer-related) Pain

Malignant pain is considered to have qualities of both acute and chronic pain. This category encompasses neuropathic, deep visceral, and bone pain, among others. Each type of pain is best managed by strategies specific to it. Therefore the nurse needs to carefully assess each type of pain and treat it appropriately. A diagnosis of cancer adds an additional psychological component associated with potential physical deformity and the possibility of impending death, preceded by agonizing suffering. The mental anguish may intensify the perception of pain.

SOURCES OF PAIN

There are several methods to classify pain; one is to classify it by its etiology, which is either nociceptive or neuropathic pain. Nociceptive pain is caused by the ongoing activation of the pain receptors in either the surface or deep tissues of the body. There are three sources of this pain. The person's pain experience depends, in part, on the source of the noxious stimulation. Therefore it is helpful to understand the typical characteristics of each pain source (Table 20-2). Neuropathic pain is due to damage to nerve cells or changes in the processing of pain information through the spinal cord.

Cutaneous (Superficial) Pain

Cutaneous pain may be characterized by an abrupt onset and a sharp or stinging quality or by a slower onset and a burning quality, depending upon the type of nerve fiber involved. Cutaneous pain receptors terminate just below the skin and, because of the high concentration of nerve endings, produce a well-defined, localized pain of short duration. Therefore cutaneous pain tends to be easily localized. For example, a client with a cut on the finger can point to the exact location of the injury.

Somatic Pain

Somatic pain originates from ligaments, tendons, bones, blood vessels, and nerves. It is detected with somatic nociceptors, but these receptors are sparse, so the pain is dull and poorly localized. For example, the pain of a sprained ankle is felt in the entire ankle, even though the injury may be only on one side. Deep somatic pain is poorly localized, may produce nausea, and may be associated with sweating and blood pressure changes. Pain from deep structures frequently radiates from the primary site (e.g., pain from a lumbar disk is felt along the sciatic nerve).

Inflammation is an important component of somatic pain. Inflammation accompanies all injuries and produces pain by the production of histamine, substance P, bradykinin, prostaglandins, and leukokinins. The inflammatory process produces vasodilation (redness, swelling, and heat). The edematous tissue distends

---

TABLE 20-2 Comparison of Cutaneous, Deep, and Visceral Pain

Characteristic	Cutaneous Pain	Deep Pain	Visceral Pain
Onset			
Location	Tends to be precise	Often diffuse and inaccurate; seems to originate in a fairly broad area	Poorly localized and cramping if hollow organ When not hollow organ, pain may be pressure-like, deep, and stabbing
Duration	Typically short	Often fairly long	Can be prolonged, especially if GI pain
Characteristics	Sharp, bright sensation or burning; felt superficially	Primarily dull and aching; may be described as boring, crushing, throbbing, or cramping; if less intense, described as soreness	Sickening pain found only when deep structures are involved, as in renal and intestinal colic, gallstones, and angina
Associated manifestations	May be hyperalgesia, paresthesia, tickling, burning, or itching	Muscle contraction and tenderness often present	Autonomic responses, including pallor, sweating, nausea, vomiting, bradycardia (at times), hypotension, syncope, faintness

stretch-sensitive tissue (periosteum, pleura), further increasing pain.

Visceral Pain

Visceral originates from body's viscera, or organs. Visceral nociceptors are located within body organs and internal cavities. The even greater scarcity of nociceptors in these areas produces pain that is usually more aching and of a longer duration than somatic pain. Visceral pain is extremely difficult to localize, and several injuries to visceral tissue exhibit "referred" pain, where the sensation is localized to an area completely unrelated to the site of injury. Myocardial ischemia or angina is possibly the best known example of referred pain; the sensation can occur in the upper chest as a restricted feeling, or as an ache in the left shoulder, arm, or even hand. Referred pain can be explained by the findings that pain receptors in the viscera also excite spinal cord neurons that are excited by cutaneous tissue. Because the brain normally associates firing of these spinal cord neurons with stimulation of somatic tissues in skin or muscle, pain signals arising from the viscera are interpreted by the brain as originating from the skin.

Visceral pain typically includes acute appendicitis, cholecystitis, and inflammation of the biliary and pancreatic tracts as well as gastroduodenal disease, cardiovascular disease, pleurisy, and renal and ureteral colic. Often visceral pain is manifested as sweating, restlessness, nausea, emesis, pallor, and agitation.

Most viscera are not sensitive to stimuli that cause pain in somatic structures (e.g., cutting, burning, or pressure). This is understandable, because viscera are not normally exposed to such traumas, and the body thus does not "need" a response system. Although these types of stimuli do not produce pain in most viscera, other stimuli may cause severe pain, for example, violent or abnormal contractions of hollow viscera, such as the ureters and alimentary tract.

In the chest, the parietal pleura are richly supplied with pain endings through the intercostal nerves and through the phrenic nerve, on the surface of the diaphragm. The visceral pleurae in the chest, however, are insensitive to pain. The bronchi, on the other hand, are sensitive to pain. Elsewhere and throughout its serous surfaces, the visceral pericardium is insensitive to pain, except for the lower portion of the fibrous pericardium, which appears to have pain fibers from the phrenic nerve.

Pain in the gastrointestinal tract is common. It appears to arise mainly from the tract's muscular and serous lining. Gastrointestinal pain seems to occur when intestinal mucosa is inflamed, ulcerated, or otherwise abnormal or when the visceral muscles contract strongly or develop spasm. Even though the wall of the intestine is not sensitive to cutting, burning, or crushing, it does produce pain under other conditions, such as widespread ischemia and distention. Abdominal pain may also occur when body organs are perforated and their contents drain into the peritoneal cavity.

Referred Pain

Referred pain is a form of visceral pain and is felt in an area distant from the site of the stimulus. It occurs when nerve fibers serving an area of the body distant from the site of the stimulus pass in close proximity to the stimulus. The referred pain sensation may be intense, and there may be little or no pain at the point of noxious stimuli. For example, myocardial ischemia typically is not felt as pain in the heart but most often as left arm, shoulder, or jaw pain. The fibers innervating these areas are close to those innervating the myocardium, resulting in the referred pain.

Referred pain is often baffling, warranting careful assessment. Examples of common patterns include pleural pain from the diaphragm referred to the shoulder and the pain of cholecystitis referred to the back and in the angle of the scapula. Figure 20-1 illustrates common sites of referred pain. It is very important to understand the locations of referred pain to avoid mistaking serious forms of pain for other problems. For example, a client with jaw pain could be treated for dental disease if the concept of referred angina was not appreciated.

Neuropathic Pain

Neuropathic pain is caused by damage or injury to nerve fibers in the periphery or by damage to the CNS. It is not attributable to nociceptor activation from injury. Noxious electrical impulses are generated at the site of the injury. Therefore the pain is felt as numbness, burning, stabbing, "needles," and electric shock. Clients may experience allodynia, "pain due to a stimulus that does not normally provoke pain."[5] The pain is perceived to occur in the area served by the nerve. For example, an injury to a nerve that serves the hand would be perceived as pain in the hand even though the injury may be at the spinal cord level. Such pain is particularly problematic for the individual, because there is no obvious pathologic process corresponding to the pain sensation (e.g., the hand). Therefore the person may not be believed. Neuropathic pain is difficult to manage because it responds poorly to typical pain medications; gabapentin and tricyclic antidepressants are commonly used.[31]

Centrally generated neuropathic pain is due to injury in the peripheral nervous system, such as phantom limb pain. It can also be due to dysfunction of the autonomic nervous system; reflex sympathetic dystrophy or complex regional pain syndromes are due to this problem.

Peripherally generated pain is felt along the distribution of the nerve. When several nerves are involved it is called a polyneuropathy. Diabetic neuropathy, alcohol

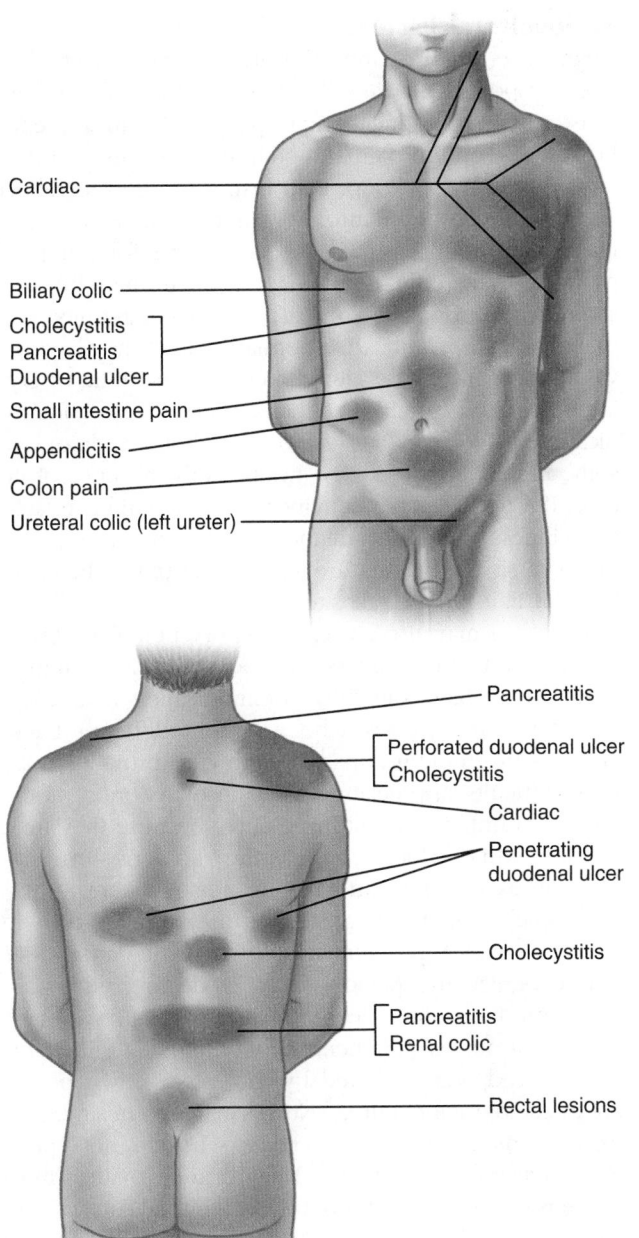

Cardiac

Biliary colic

Cholecystitis
Pancreatitis
Duodenal ulcer

Small intestine pain

Appendicitis

Colon pain

Ureteral colic (left ureter)

Pancreatitis

Perforated duodenal ulcer
Cholecystitis

Cardiac

Penetrating
duodenal ulcer

Cholecystitis

Pancreatitis
Renal colic

Rectal lesions

■ **FIGURE 20–1** Areas of referred pain.

except during physical therapy sessions, which cause a flare-up of pain. Administering short-acting medication preemptively may avoid the flare-ups and allow the client to participate more fully in therapy. Incident pain can occur with movement, coughing, and increased activity. Some clients will avoid these activities to avoid the pain. Knowing they have options to treat these flare-ups can improve functioning. Breakthrough pain can also be idiopathic, or spontaneous. It can occur randomly and unpredictably with little or no warning, and can be unrelated to activity level or adequacy of the persistent pain treatment. The intensity of breakthrough pain is generally moderate to severe. Onset tends to be rapid, with an onset of a few minutes.

Phantom Limb Sensation

Following amputation of a body part (e.g., limb, breast), a person may continue to experience sensations in the part amputated as if that part were still present or attached. The nerve fibers that served the part continue to extend to the periphery, ending at the incision site. The nerves have been injured by the surgery. As the cut nerve endings attempt to regenerate, they may form small neuromas at the incision site. When nerve fibers are stimulated as a result of injury or neuroma, they continue to mediate the sensations associated with their original location. As a result, neuropathic sensations may be generated. These abnormal sensations may be perceived as presence of the limb, paresthesia, or pain.

Sensations associated with paresthesia may consist of itching, pressure, tingling, numbness, or "pins and needles." Painful sensations include throbbing, burning, stabbing, boring, and vise-like sensations experienced in the amputated area. Phantom pain also may be experienced as cramped, twisted, and abnormal posturing of a phantom limb. As a result of the nerve injury associated with the surgery, a formerly painless phantom area may gradually become painful. For some clients, however, the abnormal sensations may persist over the long term and may never go away. Fatigue, excitement, sickness, weather changes, emotional stress, or other stimuli may exacerbate the condition.

Psychogenic Pain

Psychogenic pain is not caused by nociception, but by psychological factors. Some mental or emotional problems can cause, increase, or prolong pain. A client with psychogenic pain will report pain that does not match the underlying disorder. Headaches, muscle pain, back pain, and stomach pain are some of the most common types of psychogenic pain. Psychogenic pain is diagnosed when the other causes of pain are ruled out. Today, this problem is most often referred to as pain with psychological factors. The pain is real and saying

or nutritional neuropathies, and Guillain-Barré syndrome are polyneuropathies. Mononeuropathies are felt in one damaged nerve; spinal nerve root compression and trigeminal neuralgia are examples.

Breakthrough Pain

Breakthrough pain is defined as a transient increase in pain of moderate-to-severe intensity that occurs against a background of persistent pain of mild-to-moderate intensity that has been controlled. True breakthrough pain is either incident or idiopathic. Incident pain is predictable and occurs quickly, within minutes. A client who has just had a total knee replacement may be stable

that the client's pain is "all in their head" will not help. It is treated with psychotherapy, antidepressants, and non-narcotic analgesics.

FACTORS AFFECTING PAIN

A client's reaction to pain is intensely personal and accounts for the great variability in pain experiences from person to person.

Perception of Pain

Pain *perception,* or *interpretation,* is an important component of the pain experience. Because we perceive and interpret pain based on our own individual experience, pain is different for each person. Pain perception does not depend solely on the degree of physical damage. Both physical stimuli and psychosocial factors can influence our experience of pain. Although few agree about the specific effects of these factors, *anxiety, experience, attention, expectation,* and the *meaning of the situation* in which injury occurs affect pain perception. Cognitive functions, such as distraction, may also affect the severity and quality of the pain experience.

Pain perception is influenced by one's tolerance for pain. To understand tolerance, one must differentiate between *pain threshold* and *pain tolerance.* The pain threshold is defined as the lowest intensity of a painful stimulus that is perceived by a person as pain. The pain threshold may vary according to physiologic factors (such as inflammation or injury near pain receptors), but essentially it is similar for all people if the central nervous system (CNS) and peripheral nervous systems are intact.

Tolerance is the duration or intensity of pain that the person is willing to endure. Tolerance of pain differs by person and by experience. For example, a woman in labor can endure pain in anticipation of a new baby, but it is unlikely the woman would endure that same amount of pain again after an operation without requesting pain medication. Some people have a high tolerance; that is, they can tolerate a lot of pain without distress, whereas others have a very low tolerance. Other factors can affect tolerance of pain, such as nausea, fatigue, coping ability, sensory input, and genetic makeup.

Another aspect that can alter one's perception of pain is past experience with pain. Expectations regarding the new pain experience may be based on previous pain episodes. For example, when a person has had a bad experience with pain, the anticipation that future pain may be as bad can make subsequent pain episodes worse. If the person has had a good experience with pain management, future pain episodes may be more positively experienced. Therefore it is important for nurses to facilitate adequate pain reduction or relief that will result in positive client outcomes.

Sociocultural Factors

Race, culture, and ethnicity are critical factors in one's response to pain.[8,18,20] These factors influence all sensory responses, including responses to pain. We learn how to respond to pain and other experiences from our family and ethnic group. Pain responses tend to reflect the mores of our culture. Within this framework, we learn what is appropriate and acceptable for our peer group. For example, verbally voicing pain may be considered appropriate within the Italian community and unacceptable within the German community, which values stoicism. In the Mexican culture, moaning or crying is used to help alleviate the pain rather than communicating a need for intervention.[18] Cultural traditions of some Hispanic groups view health as the absence of illness. If a person is not convinced that the pain is related to an illness, the person might refuse treatment for it. See the Diversity in Health Care feature on Cultural Perspectives on Pain on the website.

Problems may also arise because of a person's view of health care team members. Members of various cultural groups may have difficulty communicating feelings to physicians and nurses who are from different backgrounds or ethnic groups.[13] Health care providers may have difficulty appreciating the pain experiences of clients from unfamiliar cultural groups, because they tend to adopt white, middle-class cultural traditions surrounding pain expectations and avenues for treatment.

People from different cultures may handle pain in various ways. A problem arises when the nurse does not recognize the person's way of dealing with pain or when the nurse does not accept it. Researchers found that nurses' judgments about the pain their clients experienced were affected by the nurses' own beliefs and those of their culture.[13] Nurses may also misinterpret expressions of pain from clients who do not speak English as a first language.[20] Health care providers must be sensitive to the contribution of cultural factors and language barriers in order to facilitate adequate pain management.

Age

Age may change perception and expression of pain. There are some variations in pain threshold associated with chronologic age, but no clear trends have been established. Adults may not report pain for fear that it indicates a poor diagnosis. Pain may also mean weakness, failure, or loss of control for the adult.

There is controversy regarding pain perception in the older adults. There is no reason to assume that pain perception is altered in older adults unless some damage has occurred in the CNS. The transmission and perception may be slowed with aging, but intensity of the pain is not diminished. Health care providers may underestimate the pain of older people as a result of impaired ability to express pain. Physical factors, such as paralysis and aphasia, may interfere with the ability to communicate. Confused older adults may be unable to articulate their pain experience. Altered expression does not mean absence of pain.

Age is considered an important factor in dosing of medications. Metabolic changes in older adults affect their response to opioid analgesics. Drugs are metabolized and excreted more slowly in older people. In addition, older adults frequently take combinations of medications for a variety of ailments, making them more susceptible to drug interactions.

Older people may assign different meanings to their pain. Pain may be considered a natural manifestation of aging. This may be interpreted in two ways. First, older people may think pain is simply something to be endured as a normal part of the aging process. Second, it may be seen as a sign of aging and, therefore, something to be denied because it means they are getting old. Many older people are hesitant to express pain for fear of being labeled as "complaining." These misconceptions serve to cause these people to experience pain unnecessarily. Careful assessment of the older person's pain is essential to prevent unnecessary suffering. See later discussion on modifications in older clients.

Gender

Gender can be a significant factor in the pain response, with men reporting less pain than women regardless of ethnicity. In some cultures in the United States, boys and men are expected to express pain less than women. This does not mean that men feel pain less, only that they are assumed to show it less. Yet health care providers who value bearing pain without complaint may view women as "complainers" and may ignore or devalue their pain expressions. Both men and women may experience pain unnecessarily if the nurse is not aware of personal gender biases in pain expression.

Meaning of Pain

The meaning of a person's pain influences the person's response to the pain. If the cause of pain is known, the person may be better able to interpret meaning and to deal with the experience. If the cause is unknown, more negative psychological factors (e.g., fear and anxiety) may be evoked, intensifying the degree of pain perceived. If the meaning of the experience is negative, then the pain may be perceived more intensely than pain perceived in situations with positive outcomes. For example, pain that is associated with a threat to body image may be much worse than pain that is not associated in this way. If the meaning of pain is not considered, you may make inappropriate assessments of the client's pain experience, resulting in inadequate pain control.

Anxiety

The degree of anxiety experienced by the client may also influence the response to pain. Anxiety intensifies pain perception. Anxiety is often related to the meaning of the pain. If the cause is unknown, anxiety is likely to be higher and the pain worse.

Past Experience with Pain

Past experience with pain affects the way current pain is perceived. People who had negative experiences with pain as children can have difficulty managing pain. The impact of past experiences, however, is not predictable. The person with a miserable experience in the past may perceive the next episode more intensely even though the medical conditions may be similar. Conversely, a person may view the next experience more positively because it is not as bad as the previous one. However, it is *not* true that the more pain we experience, the more accustomed we become to it. One might expect that the more pain we have experienced, the less anxious and more tolerant we may be. In actuality, we may be more anxious and desire rapid pain relief to avert a familiar and unpleasant painful experience.

Earlier pain experience allows one to adopt coping mechanisms that may or may not be used with subsequent episodes with pain. Discuss the client's past experiences with pain, including how the client managed the pain. In addition to methods that provided pain reduction or relief in the past, assess which measures did not have a positive outcome. Allow the client to use familiar positive intervention when possible.

Expectation and the Placebo Effect

Client expectations influence the perception of pain and the effectiveness of interventions for pain reduction or relief.[32] The severity of pain experienced, in addition to the emotional and cognitive overtones generated by the experience, is influenced by the client's expectations. Positive expectations engender positive outcomes; negative expectations lead to negative outcomes. Similarly, one's belief in the ability of an intervention to be effective affects the degree of pain reduction or relief attained. For example, it is not uncommon for a client to proclaim that the pain reliever Motrin is effective while Advil is not, even though the two medications are pharmaceutically identical.

The messages you deliver regarding pain and pain management strategies can affect the client's expectations. The confidence that you display regarding potential effectiveness of intervention strategies will have a significant effect on the client's ability to obtain positive pain reduction or relief outcomes. Clients must be assured that pain can be effectively treated.

Placebos have been administered when health care providers doubted that clients were truly in pain. Placebos are pills that look like medications but that have no medicinal properties. When clients are given placebos, they are told that the pills contain pain medication. It was not uncommon for these clients to obtain pain reduction or relief. It has been reported that 30% to 70% of people receiving placebos report short-lived pain reduction or relief, which in some research studies has been reversed by naloxone (Narcan).[32] The most likely explanation for the effect of placebos is the initiation of the body's endogenous opiate systems activated by the expectation of relief.[1] The response tends to be temporary, because the endogenous response is brief. A placebo response does not indicate absence of real pain; it indicates a person's ability to produce a positive outcome of pain reduction or relief internally via a real physiologic mechanism. A placebo response also indicates that the client believes that the pill will "work" and has responded to the positive attitude portrayed by the nurse administering the pill.

Health care providers have incorrectly concluded that positive responses to placebos indicate that clients did not have real pain. The client's response to placebos provides no data about the nature or severity of pain. *Placebo use is deceitful and unethical. It compromises the nurse-client relationship and the confidence the client has in the nurse's ability and desire to help with pain reduction or relief.*

SAFETY **ALERT** **Clients receiving placebos may be reluctant to report continued pain or to ask for additional pain medication, leaving them at risk for the negative physical effects of unrelieved pain.**

OUTCOME MANAGEMENT

Medical Management

Many organizations have developed guidelines or standards to aid the practitioner in pain management. The Agency for Health Care Policy and Research (AHCPR) (today the Agency for Healthcare Research and Quality [AHRQ]),[1] the American Pain Society,[4] American Pain Foundation,[3] American Society of Pain Management Nurses,[5] the Joint Commission on Accreditation of Healthcare Organizations[17] (today The Joint Commission [TJC]), and the American Geriatrics Society[2] have all published guidelines or standards for pain assessment and management. Common aspects of all of these documents include the following:

- Reducing the severity of pain by proactive management of pain
- Encouraging clients to communicate unrelieved pain so that they can receive prompt evaluation and effective treatment
- Working with all disciplines to prescribe and administer analgesics in an individualized, timely, and safe manner
- Understanding that narcotics produce dependence, and seldom addiction

- Educating clients, residents, laypersons, and their families about pain management as appropriate

History and Physical Examination

For clients with new or untreated pain, a complete medical history and physical examination (H&P) focuses on basic questions about physical, behavioral, and psychological factors (Box 20-1). This H&P helps

---

BOX 20-1   Subjective and Objective Assessment Data

HISTORY
- Age
- State of consciousness
- Medications currently taken/medication for allergies
- Physical state (fatigue, debility, lack of sleep, and prolonged suffering reduce a client's ability to tolerate pain)
- Emotional state (worry, fear, and anxiety reduce a person's ability to tolerate pain)
- Pain expectancy (the anticipation of pain)
- Pain acceptance (willingness to experience pain)
- Pain apprehension (generalized desire to avoid pain)
- Pain anxiety (the anxiety pain provokes because of its associated mystery, loneliness, helplessness, threat)
- Effects on activities and quality of life
- Methods of pain relief
- What do you do to relieve the pain?
- What has *not* worked to relieve your pain?

PHYSICAL EXAMINATION
Sympathetic Responses
- Pallor
- Increased blood pressure
- Increased pulse rate
- Increased respiration
- Skeletal muscle tension
- Dilated pupils
- Diaphoresis

Parasympathetic Responses
- Decreased blood pressure
- Decreased pulse rate
- Nausea, vomiting
- Weakness
- Pallor
- Loss of consciousness

Behavioral Characteristics
- Assumes a posture that minimizes pain (e.g., lying rigidly, guarding, drawing up the legs, or assuming the fetal position)
- Moans, sighs, grimaces, clenches the jaws or fist, becomes quiet, or withdraws from others
- Blinks rapidly
- Crying, appears frightened, exhibits restlessness
- Has a drawn facial expression
- Has twitching muscles
- Withdraws when touched
- Holds or protects affected area or remains motionless

the health care team to understand the unique pain experience of the client and to formulate a plan to resolve the pain. The H&P also provides baseline data to allow assessment of the client's progression through a pain experience. Previous medications and practitioners seen for the treatment of pain should be recorded.

Data collection by use of well-tested measurement tools is essential in assessing pain for appropriate management interventions.[50] Multidimensional assessment tools (e.g., McGill-Melzack Pain Questionnaire shown in Figure 20-2) are useful to obtain the initial H&P data and to provide information regarding the multifaceted nature of the pain experience.

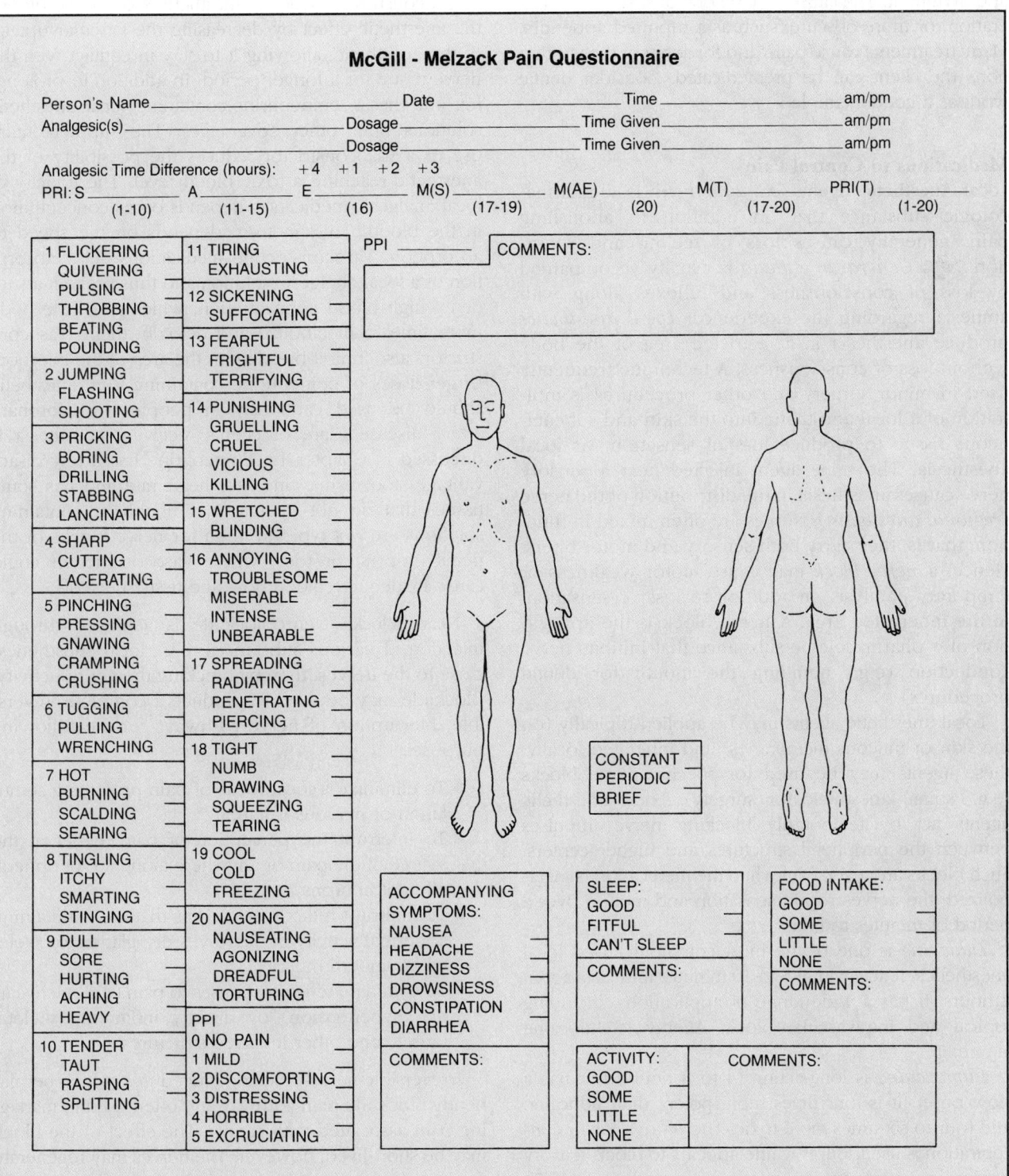

McGill - Melzack Pain Questionnaire

Person's Name_____ Date_____ Time_____ am/pm
Analgesic(s)_____ Dosage_____ Time Given_____ am/pm
_____ Dosage_____ Time Given_____ am/pm

Analgesic Time Difference (hours): +4 +1 +2 +3
PRI: S_____ A_____ E_____ M(S)_____ M(AE)_____ M(T)_____ PRI(T)_____
(1-10) (11-15) (16) (17-19) (20) (17-20) (1-20)

PPI_____ COMMENTS:

1 FLICKERING QUIVERING PULSING THROBBING BEATING POUNDING	11 TIRING EXHAUSTING
	12 SICKENING SUFFOCATING
	13 FEARFUL FRIGHTFUL TERRIFYING
2 JUMPING FLASHING SHOOTING	
3 PRICKING BORING DRILLING STABBING LANCINATING	14 PUNISHING GRUELLING CRUEL VICIOUS KILLING
	15 WRETCHED BLINDING
4 SHARP CUTTING LACERATING	16 ANNOYING TROUBLESOME MISERABLE INTENSE UNBEARABLE
5 PINCHING PRESSING GNAWING CRAMPING CRUSHING	
	17 SPREADING RADIATING PENETRATING PIERCING
6 TUGGING PULLING WRENCHING	
	18 TIGHT NUMB DRAWING SQUEEZING TEARING
7 HOT BURNING SCALDING SEARING	
8 TINGLING ITCHY SMARTING STINGING	19 COOL COLD FREEZING
9 DULL SORE HURTING ACHING HEAVY	20 NAGGING NAUSEATING AGONIZING DREADFUL TORTURING
10 TENDER TAUT RASPING SPLITTING	PPI 0 NO PAIN 1 MILD 2 DISCOMFORTING 3 DISTRESSING 4 HORRIBLE 5 EXCRUCIATING

CONSTANT
PERIODIC
BRIEF

ACCOMPANYING SYMPTOMS:
NAUSEA
HEADACHE
DIZZINESS
DROWSINESS
CONSTIPATION
DIARRHEA

COMMENTS:

SLEEP:
GOOD
FITFUL
CAN'T SLEEP
COMMENTS:

FOOD INTAKE:
GOOD
SOME
LITTLE
NONE
COMMENTS:

ACTIVITY:
GOOD
SOME
LITTLE
NONE

COMMENTS:

■ **FIGURE 20–2** The McGill-Melzack Pain Questionnaire, adapted for the study of opioid drugs. The descriptors listed at left comprise four groups: 1 to 10, sensory; 11 to 15, affective; 16, evaluative; 17 to 20, miscellaneous. The rank value for each descriptor is based on its position in the list of words. Total rank values comprise the pain-rating index (PRI). The present pain intensity (PPI) is based on a scale from 0 to 5. The drawings are used to designate the site of pain. *(From Melzack, R. (1975). The McGill Pain Questionnaire, Pain, p. 191. Copyright © R. Melzack, 1970, 1975. Reprinted with permission.)*

Goals for the medical management of pain include (1) diagnosis of the painful condition, (2) reduction of the severity and intensity of pain to tolerable levels, and (3) observation of the psychological consequences of pain. Because pain is the most common reason for seeking health care, the entire health care team will be focused on identifying the cause of the pain and treating it. The cause may be obvious, such as a laceration, or more obscure, such as a ruptured appendix. Many treatments cause pain, and for some of these situations the client can be premedicated. Consider dental work as a good example.

Medications to Control Pain

Local Anesthetic Agents. An *anesthetic* is a pharmacologic substance that, in addition to abolishing pain, generally causes loss of feeling and sensation. *General anesthesia* is usually accompanied by loss of consciousness and reflexes along with amnesia regarding the experience. *Local anesthetics* produce anesthesia in a restricted area of the body without loss of consciousness. A technique frequently used in minor surgery and other procedures is infiltration of a local anesthetic into the skin and subcutaneous tissue to produce loss of sensation, or local anesthesia. The same agent injected near a sensory nerve causes anesthesia in the distribution of the nerve *(regional anesthesia)*. Nerves are often mixed in function; that is, they carry both sensory and motor fibers. Hence, a *nerve block* may cause motor weakness or temporary paralysis, in addition to loss of sensation, in the innervated area. A nerve block is the application of a pharmacologic substance that inhibits nerve conduction (e.g., numbing the mouth for dental procedures).

Local anesthetic agents may be applied topically (on the skin or mucous membranes) and infiltrated locally; these agents may be used for specific nerve blocks (e.g., spinal anesthetic for surgery). Local anesthetic agents act by temporarily blocking nerve impulses between the peripheral structures and higher centers. Such blocks are reversible; when the medication is metabolized, the nerves regain sensation and motion over a period of minutes to hours.

Lidocaine is one of the most commonly used local anesthetics. It acts within 5 to 10 minutes and lasts about 2 hours. It has a wide range of applications, including topical and intravascular block. Allergy to lidocaine is rare.

Bupivacaine is long-acting (4 to 8 hours) but has a slow onset. It is four times more potent than lidocaine and four to six times more toxic. Therefore a lower concentration is used. Bupivacaine appears to block sensory nerves in preference to motor nerves when used in low concentration. Thus effective analgesia may result

without accompanying motor weakness. Bupivacaine is sometimes injected or infused into incisions following surgery for pain control.

Local anesthetics are usually vasodilators, increasing blood flow into the area in which they are injected. Thus they shorten the duration of their own action by enhancing their own vascular absorption. Adding epinephrine, a vasoconstrictor, to local anesthetic solutions prolongs the anesthetic effect by decreasing the vascular uptake of the anesthetic, allowing it to stay in contact with the nerve tissue for a longer period. In addition to prolonging anesthesia, epinephrine-containing local anesthetic solutions offer other advantages. The supplementary use of a vasoconstrictor reduces the possibility of the anesthetic reaching a toxic blood level. The toxicity of local analgesic medication depends on its concentration in the blood. This, in turn, depends on the speed of absorption. Vasoconstricting medications delay absorption of a local analgesic solution and thus prevent a suddenly high blood concentration, which gives the body more time to metabolize and detoxify them. Vasoconstrictors also inhibit bleeding in the area of the injection. Larger doses of epinephrine containing local anesthetic should be used cautiously in people with coronary artery disease. Care of clients receiving anesthesia is discussed in Chapter 14. Epinephrine has a few disadvantages too: it may increase heart rate and has some tissues that do not tolerate it. Epinephrine-containing solutions are *not* typically used for nerve blocks of the penis, fingers, or toes, where vasoconstriction could cause inadequate blood flow and tissue necrosis.

Nerve Blocks. Neuroblockade is achieved through injection of various substances (e.g., local anesthetics) close to the nerves, thereby blocking their conductivity. Blockade may be used to produce a complete, reversible interruption of nerve pathways for the following purposes:

- To eliminate a local focus of pain-producing stimulation or nervous irritation
- To interrupt the perception of pain, either at the source of the pain or anywhere along the peripheral afferent neurons
- To interrupt reflex mechanisms that are maintaining abnormal activity in blood vessels, glands, or skeletal or smooth muscle
- To eliminate reflex responses to pain (e.g., tachycardia, hypertension) by directly infiltrating skeletal muscle and other involved structures

Irreversible nerve-blocking procedures, which permanently block the pain pathway, are often used in managing pain associated with cancer. The effect of the block may be short-lived, however. The nerves may regenerate to some extent, with an associated return of sensory and motor functions.

Nerve blocks given for pain relief are called *analgesic blocks*. The analgesia is generally produced by injection of a local anesthetic agent. The anesthetic agent relieves pain and thus allows treatment that might otherwise be extremely uncomfortable, such as manipulation of a painful joint or wound debridement. Sometimes, by interrupting reflexes that are causing sustained pain, analgesic blocks can produce a beneficial effect that is prolonged beyond the effective duration of the agent injected.

Analgesic blocks are useful in various acute and chronic disorders. They often reduce the amounts of analgesic medication that might otherwise be needed. Injecting local anesthetics into tender points of muscle or skin *(trigger point injection)* causes a type of analgesic block that may modify pain and break the pain cycle, allowing manipulation and stretching of a joint. However, the pain may not be permanently eliminated unless the primary afferent impulses are either chemically or surgically terminated or until the underlying pathologic condition causing the pain is corrected.

Neurolytic agents (e.g., phenol, alcohol) produce prolonged nerve blocks by destroying the nerves. Neurolytic blocks may not be truly permanent because nerve fibers regrow after several months. However, the growth is often disorganized. Hence, the sensation from these nerve fibers is often abnormal or painful. Consequently, neurolytic blocks are generally used only in terminally ill clients with a short life expectancy, such as those with cancer-related pain.

Topical Local Anesthesia. Dilute solutions of local anesthetics may be applied topically in the form of pastes, sprays, or other preparations. They may reduce the severe pain of burns, abrasions, and necrosis of the mucous membranes and skin.

Remember, once an area is anesthetized, it does not transmit painful sensation and the area is thus at greater risk for injury. If topical anesthetic agents are applied to burned or abraded skin or mucous membranes, absorption of the medication is almost as rapid as that following IV administration.

EMLA cream is a mixture of lidocaine and prilocaine. It is useful in preventing pain from venipuncture, injections, heel sticks, and minor plastic surgery. It must be applied in advance to the area (45 minutes to 1 hour) and covered with an occlusive dressing. EMLA cream is an excellent strategy for eliminating the pain associated with penetration of the skin and should be encouraged.

Analgesics. Various factors are considered in selecting the most effective analgesic for a specific client. These factors include the cause, quality, intensity, duration, and distribution of the pain. The World Health Organization (WHO)[36] has suggested that decisions regarding pain medications may be aided by use of a "pain ladder" (Figure 20-3). The ladder was originally designed to guide the care of clients with cancer pain, but its use has been extended to apply to acute pain. Non-opioids, such as acetaminophen and nonsteroidal anti-inflammatory drugs (NSAIDs), are suggested by the first step. If the pain persists or increases, step 2 suggests mild opioids (such as codeine) plus non-opioid analgesics. If the pain continues to persist or increases, step 3 suggests strong opioids (such as morphine) with or without non-opioids. Adjuvant medications may be added at any step in the ladder.

Systemic analgesic medications are the most frequently used means of pain control. Analgesics are the most commonly prescribed, and thus widely used, medications. They are also purchased extensively over the counter. This is not unexpected, because pain is usually the first manifestation of injury, and most diseases begin with or include pain at some time during their course.

Types of Analgesics. Analgesics are medications developed to provide pain relief. The discussion is organized according to the WHO analgesic ladder, which is based on the notion that pain medication decisions are based in part on the intensity and controllability of the pain.[35] The three steps reflect mild, moderate, and severe degrees of pain intensity.

Non-Opioid Analgesics. Non-opioid analgesics fall into four primary categories:[4] aspirin, salicylate salts, acetaminophen, and NSAIDs. As a group, these drugs have a ceiling effect but do not cause physical

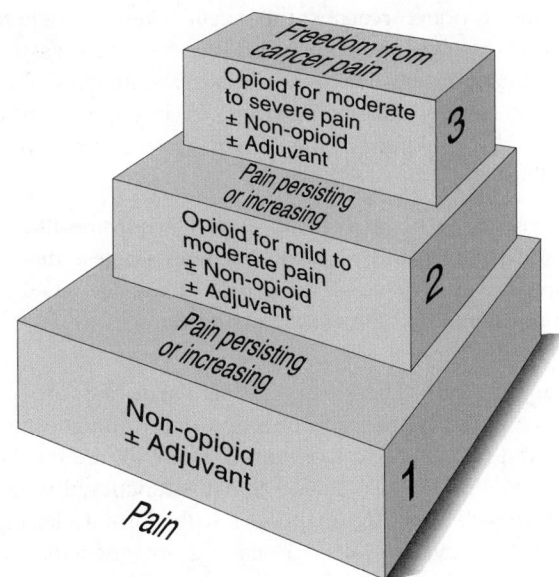

■ **FIGURE 20–3** World Health Organization (WHO) analgesic ladder describes the steps in treating cancer pain.

dependence or tolerance. Their site of action is primarily in the periphery at the receptor site, where they serve an anti-inflammatory function and prevent the production of prostaglandins. They may have a central role in pain relief, in that prostaglandins inhibit the production or the release of serotonin, removing the pain reduction or relief effect of the neurotransmitter. Preventing prostaglandin production would maintain the inhibitory effect of serotonin in the dorsal horn. An exception is acetaminophen, which produces pain reduction or relief but is not an anti-inflammatory agent and does not appear to affect prostaglandins. The physical manner by which acetaminophen produces pain relief is not known.[4]

The American Pain Society recommends that a non-opioid medication be included with any analgesic regimen, even when opioids are prescribed.[4] Opioids act centrally, within the brain and spinal cord. Non-opioids add peripherally mediated pain reduction or relief to the central effects of opioids when they are given in combination. Parenteral and rectal forms of non-opioids have been developed for individuals who cannot take oral medications. Refer to a pharmacology text for dosing information for non-opioid medications.

Aspirin. Historically, aspirin (acetylsalicylic acid, ASA) has been the primary non-opioid medication for pain. It is one of the most effective non-opioid medications available. Aspirin is available in many forms, including tablets (plain, chewable, enteric-coated, sustained-release), capsules, rectal suppositories, and topical creams. As with most nonsteroidal analgesics, aspirin has an antiplatelet effect and is a gastric irritant. Enteric-coated tablets reduce the gastric reactions because the coating remains intact until the product reaches the small intestine, where the tablet dissolves and is absorbed. Because of the association of aspirin with Reye's syndrome, a potentially fatal condition seen primarily in young children, aspirin is not used in children younger than age 12 years with viral illnesses.

SAFETY

ALERT

Recent cases of adults with Reye's syndrome–like manifestations and negative outcomes suggest that aspirin may pose a risk for people of any age when administered to those with viral infections.

Salicylate Salts. These salts are similar to aspirin but produce fewer gastric side effects. Choline magnesium trisalicylate (Trilisate) and diflunisal (Dolobid) are typical examples. Platelet aggregation remains functional when salicylate salts are used in people with normal clotting abilities. Salicylate salts containing magnesium or sodium should be avoided in clients in whom excessive amounts of these electrolytes might be harmful, such as clients with heart failure.

Acetaminophen. Acetaminophen is similar to aspirin in its ability to provide pain reduction or relief, but it does not affect the gastric mucosa. It has no effect on platelet aggregation and does not affect bleeding time. Its anti-inflammatory effect is much less than that of other non-opioids. It is tolerated well by most people of any age, and it is the drug of choice when given for pain to clients with viral infections.

Acetaminophen is metabolized by the liver, and to avoid liver injury the total dose must not exceed 4 grams in 24 hours.

NSAIDs. NSAIDs are drugs other than aspirin and acetaminophen. NSAIDs are present in numerous preparations, providing alternative medications. If one form is ineffective, another can be tried. NSAIDs were originally developed to treat arthritis, but they are also effective for mild to moderate pain of nonarthritic origin. NSAIDs act to decrease inflammation, but it is their ability to block prostaglandin synthesis that is credited for most of their pain-relieving properties.[9] NSAIDs are particularly helpful for clients with cancer or postoperative pain, because a major contributing factor to pain in these clients is cell destruction.

NSAIDs potentiate the effects of opiates and are often given in combination preparations that incorporate oxycodone or hydrocodone. NSAIDs are particularly effective for bone pain, including bone metastases of malignancy and fractures, because damaged bone produces prostaglandins. Ketoprofen and ketorolac (Toradol) also block production of leukotrienes. These agents must be used cautiously in clients with impaired renal function.

The most common side effects associated with NSAIDs are gastrointestinal upset and bleeding.

These agents also inhibit platelet aggregation, increasing the risk of hemorrhage. Clients taking NSAIDs must be monitored closely for the development of peptic ulcers.

In clients who are taking high doses for long periods (as for arthritis), a histamine H_2-receptor antagonist or proton pump inhibitor may be used.

Cyclooxygenase 2 (COX-2) inhibitors were developed in response to the negative gastrointestinal side effects of aspirin and NSAIDs. Celecoxib (Celebrex) and valdecoxib (Bextra) disrupt the synthesis of prostaglandins by interfering with the cyclooxygenase portion of the arachidonic acid cascade. Two types of cyclooxygenases predominate. COX-1 is found primarily in the stomach and has a protective function. COX-2 is usually assumed to be associated with pain initiated by inflammation. It was therefore assumed that development of an NSAID that spares the gastric protection function of COX-1 but disrupts COX-2 activity would provide pain reduction or relief while preventing the negative gastric consequences associated with existing NSAIDs.[19]

However, the COX-2 medications have been linked to increased risk of stroke and myocardial infarction (MI), attributable to clot formation. The benefit-risk profile must be individualized.

Opioid Analgesics. Opioid analgesics are derived from natural opium alkaloids and their synthetic derivatives. They tend to be grouped as opioids because their effects resemble those of opium. Opioids are typically categorized from weak to strong to aid health care providers in selecting the correct medication (see Figure 20-3). Opioids are added to the medication regimen when pain is moderate to severe and non-opioids are insufficient to manage pain effectively. Tolerance and physical dependence seen in long-term administration are not associated with short-term opioid treatment (Box 20-2).

Opioids bind with receptors that can be engaged by endogenous opioids, including mu (μ), kappa (κ), and delta (δ) receptor types. Binding with receptors in the spinal cord renders the presynaptic membrane of nociceptor fibers incapable of opening Ca^{++} channels, inhibiting nociceptive neurotransmitter release. Opiate binding with the postsynaptic membrane hyperpolarizes the membrane by altering the ability of K ions to flow across the membrane. Opiate receptors are found in the periaqueductal gray (PAG) matter and the periventricular gray (PVG) matter in the midbrain. Activation of these receptors by opioids initiates the descending effect of serotonin and norepinephrine.

All opioids produce side effects to some degree. The side effects are determined, in part, by the receptor type engaged by the medication and by the location of the receptor. The three receptor types have very different distributions and locations with the CNS. Side effects may be managed by discontinuing one form of opiate medication with untoward side effects and replacing it with another that binds to a different receptor type.

Opioid Agonists. Opioid agonists are opiate derivatives that bring about pain relief by producing the maximum degree of receptor binding. Agonists bind fully to their corresponding receptor type and do not affect the ability of other opioid preparations to engage their specific receptor. They are typically associated with mu receptors and have no ceiling effect. Opioid agonists are morphine-like medications that differ from morphine in rate of onset, duration of action, route of administration, adverse side effects, and chemical configuration. The mechanisms by which they produce pain reduction or relief are similar.

Opioid Antagonists. These agents reverse the side effects and analgesia of opioids. They have no agonist effects and thus produce no analgesia. They are used to counteract a negative effect of an opioid, typically respiratory depression. Naloxone is the most common example.

Opioid Agonist-Antagonists. These medications engage one receptor type while inhibiting receptor binding of another. When they are given following use of the opioid they inhibit, they precipitously reverse the medication's effects and can precipitate acute withdrawal. When the combination agents are given alone, they produce analgesia and the positive effects of opioids with fewer side effects. Respiratory depression is a less likely effect, although psychomimetic effects are more probable.

Methadone. A potent, long-acting opioid analgesic, methadone gained popularity in the management of cancer pain before the development of the long-acting forms of morphine. Unlike most morphine preparations, methadone has a long plasma half-life. This long plasma half-life, when repeated doses are given, may account for methadone's longer duration of analgesic action, but it also poses certain problems. This medication is not recommended for older clients and clients with compromised hepatic and renal function. The long plasma half-life necessitates close monitoring of any client receiving repeated doses because cumulative effects develop over 1 to 2 weeks. If the client becomes oversedated, the dosage should be reduced or the intervals between administrations lengthened.

BOX 20-2   Dependence, Addiction, and Tolerance

DEPENDENCE

Psychological dependence, also known as addiction, is a pattern of continual craving for opioid drugs when not experiencing pain. The pattern of drug seeking is compulsive and without control. There is continued use despite physical, social, or financial harm. The client also seeks the drug without concern for the consequences of continued use.

Physical dependence is seen when a client abruptly stops taking opioids. The client has anxiety, chills alternating with hot flashes, irritability, vomiting, abdominal cramps, and insomnia. These same manifestations are seen when the client is given opioid antagonists.

TOLERANCE

Tolerance to opioids develops when the liver becomes efficient at metabolizing the medications and higher doses are required to achieve the same level of pain control or comfort. The development of tolerance for opioids in clients who have received these medications for weeks does not mean that the client is addicted or psychologically dependent upon them.

Adverse Effects of Opioid Analgesics. Some side effects of opioid analgesics—constipation in particular—last as long as the medication is administered. Others, such as nausea and vomiting and drowsiness, decrease as the administration is continued. Other side effects (e.g., respiratory depression) are rare, and the incidence decreases precipitously with longer administration.

Constipation. Constipation is the most common side effect seen with opioid use and results from increased smooth muscle tone and decreased motility of the gastrointestinal tract. Opioids diminish the propulsive peristaltic contractions in the small and large intestine and delay the passage of gastric contents through the duodenum. Tolerance does not develop to constipation as it does to the other side effects of opioids. Clients taking opioid analgesics need to follow a bowel regimen to prevent constipation. A diet high in fiber with plenty of fluids and stool-softening or senna-based medications are used as prophylactic treatment. Constipation is treatable and is not a side effect mandating that opioid medications be discontinued. Some clients may need to discontinue opiates because of constipation.

Nausea and Vomiting. Opioids may precipitate nausea and vomiting because of their action on the brain stem centers. Morphine-like medications also affect the vestibular system, which can produce these manifestations. Changing the type of opioid used may eliminate the side effect. Antiemetic agents may also be administered. This side effect decreases with analgesic use. Clients should not be denied pain relief because of this effect. Instead, they should receive treatment for the nausea and vomiting until it subsides.

Respiratory Depression. Respiratory depression is caused by diminished sensitivity of the respiratory center to carbon dioxide. All opioids have the potential to produce respiratory depression, which can be rapidly reversed with an opioid antagonist, typically naloxone. The reaction is relatively rare, occurring primarily following the initial doses of opioid among those who never received the medication or whose last dose was a long time ago. It rarely occurs in awake individuals; however, obese clients with sleep apnea may develop respiratory depression fairly quickly.[4]

This potential for respiratory depression should not discourage the proper use of opioids to reduce or relieve pain in people of all ages. The development of respiratory depression is not necessarily dose-related. Most clients do not respond with depressed respiratory rates regardless of dose. Another person may react with decreased respiration to relatively small doses. Rather than limit the use of opioid analgesics, carefully assess and reassess each client after giving the medication for the occurrence of respiratory depression. Because sedation precedes respiratory depression, sedation scales should be used to assess and reassess clients.

Deaths that occurred secondary to opioid overdose are usually a result of respiratory depression and usually occur in people who have not received opioids in the past. With morphine, maximal respiratory depression usually occurs within 15 minutes of intravenous (IV) administration, within 30 minutes of intramuscular (IM) administration, within 90 minutes of subcutaneous administration, and within 4 to 12 hours of epidural administration. Remember these time ranges when assessing the respiratory status following administration of opioids. For an overdose to occur, however, doses well above the therapeutic level would have to be given. Accumulated doses, especially in clients with liver or renal failure and in older clients, can cause an overdose.

It is also important to clearly diagnose respiratory depression. The presence of pain may result in increased respiratory rates among clients taking frequent, shallow breaths. Providing an opioid may relieve the pain, allowing the client's respiratory pattern to return to a more normal breathing pattern. A respiratory rate of 30 breaths/min may be reduced to 15 breaths/min. Such a decrease has been interpreted as medication-caused respiratory depression, and the pain reduction or relief achieved has been reversed by naloxone administration. Assess respiratory depression in conjunction with normal functioning rather than the decrease in breaths per minute. Is the resulting respiratory rate life-threatening?

As explained in Box 20-3 and in the Critical Monitoring box on p. 365, treatment of respiratory depression includes arousing the client, establishing a patent airway, administering an opioid antagonist such as naloxone, and providing artificial ventilation as necessary. If the client stops breathing, provide rescue breathes with an Ambu bag. Oxygen is helpful, but only if the client is breathing. It does no good for a client who is apneic!

Circulatory Depression

In some clients, circulatory depression may produce hypotension. In a supine client, therapeutic dosages of morphine or synthetic opioids have little effect on blood pressure and cardiac rate or rhythm. However, some people experience orthostatic hypotension when moving from a supine position to a head-up or standing position. This hypotension is secondary to a direct dilating action on the peripheral blood vessels, caused by the opioids, that reduces the capacity of the cardiovascular system to respond to positional changes. Advise the client to avoid abrupt body position changes. For this reason, opioids are used cautiously in people with reduced blood volume, because the effect is more pronounced. Increasing fluid volume decreases the orthostatic changes.

CRITICAL MONITORING

Opioid-Induced Respiratory Depression

In the typical scenario, the nurse, summoned to the client's room because of falling oxygen saturations, finds a very somnolent client. The respiratory rate is often less than 8 breaths/minute, blood pressure is low, and pupils are pinpoint. When the client cannot be aroused to awaken, consider opioid overdose.

Opioid overdose can occur in clients receiving continuous or intermittent opioids.

Your actions need to be organized and rapid to avoid injury to the CNS. Call for help and open the client's airway using a jaw thrust. Perform rescue breathing if needed. Stop any infusion of opioids, leaving the IV line open for medications. If you do not have the keys to open the pump, remove the IV tubing at the needle and reinsert the fluids' line into the IV needle.

Dilute and inject naloxone over 10 minutes (0.1 to 0.4 mg IV every 1 to 2 minutes); do not rapidly push the drug. The client should start breathing with an improved depth and frequency. The client may awaken but need not be fully reversed to the point of experiencing severe pain to be reversed. (If the client does not improve with naloxone, the client did not overdose; consider other problems, such as carbon dioxide retention and stroke.) If the client ingested oral opiates, activated charcoal is the method of choice. Because of slowed peristalsis from narcotics, even if some time has passed since taking oral medications, the drug may still be in the stomach. Because the half-life of naloxone is shorter than those of many opioids, continue to assess the client's respiratory patterns and level of consciousness for 24 hours.

Opiate overdose is not common, but when it occurs, nurses must act promptly and skillfully. The airway must be opened and breathing established or confirmed. Be certain that all clients receiving continuously infused opiates be placed on pulse oximetry and oxygen by nasal cannula.

BOX 20-3   Naloxone Administration

1. Review end-of-life goals; naloxone administration is not indicated for clients receiving opioids who are dying, because all dying clients will at some point have altered mentation and respiratory changes. It may be necessary to have specific orders not to administer naloxone.
2. Clients should meet all of the following criteria before naloxone is administered:
   - Depressed mental status: difficult to arouse or unarousable. (If the client wakes to voice or light shake, the diagnosis is sleeping, not opioid overdose.)
   - Shallow respirations or rate <8 breaths/min associated with evidence of inadequate ventilation (e.g., low oxygen saturation, hypotension). *Note:* Some clients' respiratory rates are 6-8 breaths/min when they sleep, yet they are well ventilated.
3. Stop opioid administration.
4. Dilute 0.4 mg of naloxone (1 ampule) with normal saline to a total volume of 10 ml (1 ml = 0.04 mg).
5. Remind the client to breathe. Sometimes narcotized clients report hearing concerned staff but being unable to open their eyes or respond. Reminders to "take a deep breath" are often followed.
6. Administer 1 ml of the dilute naloxone solution (0.04 mg) intravenously every 1 minute until the client is responsive. A typical response is noted after 2-4 ml with deeper breathing and greater level of arousal. Gradual naloxone administration should prevent acute opioid withdrawal. If naloxone is given too fast, it can precipitate severe pain, which is difficult to control. The intense pain can stimulate the sympathetic nervous system, leading to tachycardia and hypertension.
7. If the client does not respond to a total of 0.8 mg of naloxone (2 ampules), consider other causes of sedation and respiratory depression (e.g., benzodiazepines, stroke).
8. The duration of action of naloxone is considerably shorter than the duration of action of most short-acting opioids. A repeat dose of naloxone, or even a continuous naloxone infusion, may be needed. Keep another syringe at the bedside for later administration.
9. Wait until there is sustained improvement in consciousness before restarting opioids at a lower dose. Provide a non-opioid for pain relief if needed.
10. Resume opioid administration at one half the original dose when the client is easily aroused and respiratory rate is >9 breaths/min.

Cutaneous Effects. Opioid medications may facilitate histamine release, resulting in pruritus, flushing, and sweating. The client becomes tolerant to this effect with repeated administration of the opioid. Clinical manifestations may be alleviated by administration of antihistamines until the client becomes tolerant.

Urinary Retention. Urinary retention may occur as the result of the increase in smooth muscle tone of the detrusor muscle of the bladder and the bladder sphincter.[25] The hypertoned muscle fibers resist opening and prevent adequate bladder emptying. Urinary retention and urgency may result, necessitating catheterization.

Adjuvant Medications. Adjuvants are medications developed for other conditions but they also have pain-reducing properties. Adjuvant medications may be used in combination with analgesics or may be used alone. A wide variety of medications can be classified as adjuvant analgesics.[4] Tricyclic antidepressants (TCAs), such as amitriptyline (Elavil), are effective for neuropathic pain. They can be given daily at bedtime so that the drowsiness associated with them promotes sleep. Other effective medications for neuropathic pain are phenytoin (Dilantin), carbamazepine (Tegretol), pregabalin (Lyrica), and gabapentin (Neurontin). Nerve compression and bone pain may respond to dexamethasone (Decadron). Muscle relaxants, such as baclofen (Lioresal) and diazepam (Valium), are used to treat muscle spasm associated with pain.

Phenothiazines are not appropriate for pain relief. They are good antiemetics, but, when given for pain, phenothiazines simply increase sedation, hypotension, and respiratory depression. A phenothiazine such as promethazine (Phenergan) should never be used for pain relief. Promethazine actually *increases* the perception of pain.

Antidepressants. TCAs contribute to pain relief via the descending pain inhibitory system by blocking cellular re-uptake of serotonin and epinephrine. They may also potentiate the effect of opiates at synapses and increase their plasma bioavailability. The analgesic effect occurs with doses lower than needed to produce an antidepressant effect. TCAs are used to enhance pain reduction or relief regardless of a depression diagnosis. However, relief of depression in clinically depressed clients with pain is a positive outcome. TCAs can be given as a single daily dose at bedtime or in divided doses. Analgesic effects usually begin within 1 week of initiation of the TCA.[31]

Anti-Anxiety Agents. Anxiety increases the pain sensation and pain increases anxiety. The treatment of anxiety along with pain is a very beneficial program. Diazepam and chlordiazepoxide (Librium) are believed to mediate pain by contributing to chloride (Cl^-) channel opening. Movement of Cl^- ions hyperpolarizes the postsynaptic membrane, making it less receptive to incoming nociceptive stimuli. Diazepam is particularly effective for relief of painful muscle spasm.

Anticonvulsants. Anticonvulsant agents are used in situations associated with nerve injury. Nerve fibers may generate electrical activity at the site of injury, causing the nerve membrane to fire with a pain-producing signal that leads to lancing pain. Agents such as phenytoin (Dilantin), gabapentin (Neurontin), pregabalin (Lyrica), duloxetine (Cymbalta), topiramate (Topamax), tiagabine (Gabitril), and zonisamide (Zonegran) stabilize the neuronal membrane.

Corticosteroids. In the periphery, steroids reduce edema and inflammation, reducing the compression caused by swelling and the availability of chemical mediators of nociception. They may also inhibit the production of prostaglandins and leukotrienes. In the CNS, they function similarly to anti-anxiety agents by modifying the flow of Cl^- ions. Corticosteroids provide pain reduction or relief from bony metastasis of cancer.

Miscellaneous Agents. *Baclofen,* a gamma-aminobutyric acid (GABA) antagonist, is used as an analgesic for lancinating or paroxysmal neuropathic pain. *Capsaicin* is a topical medication that depletes peptides (such as substance P) in small primary afferent neurons that mediate nociceptive transmission. It appears useful for postherpetic neuralgia and for postmastectomy pain in some clients.

Factors Influencing the Effectiveness of Analgesics

Relative Analgesic Potency. Relative analgesic potency refers to the ratio of the doses of two analgesics required to produce the same effect. Analgesics are compared with therapeutic doses of morphine. Estimates of relative analgesic potency provide a basis for prescribing the dose when the client is being switched from one analgesic to another or from one route of administration to another. The route used to provide pain reduction or relief affects the potency of the medication.

The availability of the analgesic is determined in part by the events encountered before the drug enters the circulatory system. Orally administered medications must be dissolved in stomach contents and absorbed by the gut and passed through the liver, before the agent can contribute to pain reduction or relief. Using the IM or subcutaneous routes necessitates that the medication be absorbed from muscle or subcutaneous tissues before it becomes available. IV medications enter the circulatory system directly. Oral and subcutaneous doses must be higher than IV doses. Doses are equally effective when equianalgesic dosing is used.

Duration of Action. The duration of action of an analgesic agent is the result of factors such as pain intensity, dose size, and the client's ability to absorb, biotransform, and eliminate the medication. The time of peak effect and the duration of action of a particular opioid vary with the route of administration. For instance, the peak analgesic effect of IV morphine occurs between 15 minutes and 40 minutes after administration. The peak analgesic effect of orally administered morphine occurs from 2 to 12 hours after administration. The duration of action of orally administered opioids is usually somewhat longer than that of IM analgesics. *Duration* of analgesia may not be the same as the *effect* of analgesia. Learn about peak and duration of analgesic effect so that activities that might produce pain can be planned to coincide with peak periods of medication action. For example, if a client is scheduled for physical therapy at 10:00 AM, give pain medication that will reach its peak effect around 10:00 AM.

Several new forms of morphine have been developed. An oral liquid can be given for more rapid but short-acting effects. A controlled-release form is also available. With long-acting morphine, the onset is somewhat slower but the duration ranges from 8 to 12 hours. Fentanyl, which is available as a patch for transdermal delivery of medication, is effective for 48 to 72 hours. Fentanyl is also available for transmucosal delivery. Oral transmucosal fentanyl citrate is available in "lollipop" form. The medication is delivered systemically directly through the transmucosal route and partially by the amount of the medication that is swallowed.

Oral Potency. As opioids are absorbed from the intestine and pass through the liver and into the systemic circulation, they differ in the degree to which they are active. Preparations with lower bioavailability require higher doses per pill. More recently developed forms of morphine have greater bioavailability, and therefore the dosages of these are lower than those of the older oral form. Opioids are available in various forms, with varying onset, peak effect, duration, and half-lives; become aware of these variations. The different equianalgesic doses are based on a single dose of IV morphine (Table 20-3). An equianalgesic dose is expected to provide the same degree of pain reduction or relief as the single IV morphine dose. Dose requirements may decrease after the client has received a loading dose. Failure of health care providers to recognize differences in the oral and intramuscular potencies of opioids and the concept of equianalgesic doses can lead to undertreatment of a person's pain.

Ceiling Effect. Some analgesics have a *ceiling effect,* which occurs when medications have a maximum effective dose; increasing the dose cannot increase pain relief but may increase side effects. Medications with a ceiling effect may be combined with other analgesics when additional pain relief is needed. Pure opiates have no ceiling dosage.

Tolerance. Tolerance, a physiologic phenomenon, occurs when larger doses of medications are needed to provide the same amount of pain relief as the previous smaller dose. It may occur in people who require long-term pain management with opioids. The person becomes tolerant to these medications because the opiate receptors become less sensitive to them. Tolerance may be managed either by continuing the dose of the opioid and adding a non-opioid analgesic or adjuvant medication or by switching to an alternate drug.

Tolerance should not be confused with *addiction,* which is rare (see Box 20-2 on p. 363). Concern about addiction in cases of tolerance has led health care providers to modify opioid prescriptions by ordering smaller doses over longer periods of time. Client response to the modification may lead one to conclude that addiction was the underlying problem, because these clients may be forced to display behaviors often associated with psychological addiction.[4] This is called *pseudoaddiction.* The client no longer receives adequate pain relief and may attempt to manipulate the provider into providing adequate medication. Such behavior is understandable but is often viewed as "medication-seeking," a classic definition of one psychologically addicted. Clients may "act out" their pain in the belief that if they look as if they have severe pain, their need for medication will be recognized by the health care provider. The client does not receive adequate pain relief in response to these behaviors and rationalizes that health care providers are no longer dependable. The health care provider concludes that the client's behavior is inappropriate and no longer values or believes the client. This atmosphere of mistrust creates a situation in which adequate pain relief for the client becomes increasingly unlikely. Addiction is discussed in Chapter 24.

Dependence. Physical dependence commonly occurs when medications are taken over a long term. Physical manifestations associated with sudden termination of the medication include anxiety, irritability, chills alternating with hot flashes, salivation, lacrimation, rhinorrhea, diaphoresis, piloerection, nausea and vomiting, abdominal cramps, and insomnia.[4] Physical dependence is not a problem unless opioids are to be discontinued. The effects of withdrawal can be avoided by weaning the client from the medication slowly. It is essential that health care providers, clients, and their significant others realize that physical dependence is not synonymous with psychological addiction. Client and family education regarding this matter is an expected nursing function.

TABLE 20–3 Equianalgesic Doses of Selected Opioid Analgesics*

Opioid	Equianalgesic Oral	Dose (mg) Parenteral
Fentanyl	—	0.1 (100 mcg)
Hydrocodone	30	—
Hydromorphone	7.5	1.5
Meperidine	300	75
Methadone	20 acute	10 acute
	2-4 chronic	2-4 chronic
Morphine	30	10
Oxycodone	20	—
OxyContin	20	—

* This chart is an estimate of drugs and their doses for pain control equal to that of 30 mg of oral morphine. Each client must be monitored for individual response.

Production of Metabolites. Meperidine (Demerol) is a popular analgesic medication but has many limitations.

SAFETY
ALERT

Meperidine should not be used on a prolonged basis, no longer than 48 hours or more than 600 mg in 24 hours, because of the potentially toxic metabolite by-product normeperidine, which is produced during its biotransformation.

Meperidine does not provide effective pain reduction or relief with repeated doses and causes untenable CNS side effects.

The metabolic by-product is toxic to the CNS and can lead to anxiety, tremors, myoclonus, and seizure activity. Nerve injury from diffusion of medication can also occur. Meperidine should not be used in clients with altered renal function or in older adults. Propoxyphene (Darvon) also has a toxic metabolite, norpropoxyphene, that accumulates and causes confusion, depression, and cardiac dysrhythmias.

Nursing Management of the Client in Pain

Misconceptions and Myths

Many misunderstandings exist about pain (Table 20-4). Examine these myths and the facts; they will become important parts of your work. If nurses continue to believe these myths, adequate pain assessment and relief are hampered. For example, many health care providers believe that it is possible to predict the amount of pain people should have, based on their medical condition. However, the diagnosis or type of surgery is *not* an effective fundamental basis for determining the amount of pain the person should be experiencing or the analgesic required to relieve that pain. The fact that clients do not visibly exhibit physiologic or behavioral signs of pain often leads to the belief by the health care provider that they do not have pain. A more likely explanation is that the client has adapted to the pain. Adaptive psychological responses include the following:

- Shifting away from the pain or guarding of the painful area
- Reporting pain only if asked directly
- Exhibiting sleepiness (which may also be due to insomnia secondary to the pain or may be used as a coping mechanism)
- Exhibiting decreased physical activity
- Showing a blank facial expression

These manifestations do not mean that the person is not experiencing pain but that the person is exhibiting adaptive responses to pain that continues to be present.

Assessment. All clients should be screened for pain, and if pain is present, a comprehensive pain assessment should be completed. The primary goals of pain assessment are to identify the cause of the pain, to understand the client's perception of the pain, to measure the characteristics of the pain, to determine the level of pain that the client can continue to participate in activities of daily living (ADL), and to implement pain management techniques. To assess a client's initial report of pain, the

TABLE 20–4 Common Misconceptions About Pain	
Myth or Misconception	**Fact**
Addiction occurs with prolonged use of morphine or morphine derivatives.	The incidence of addiction is less than 0.1%.
The nurse or physician is the best judge of a client's pain.	Only the client can judge the level and distress of the pain; pain management should be a team approach that includes the client.
Pain is a result, not a cause.	Unrelieved pain can create other problems such as anger, anxiety, immobility, respiratory problems, and delay in healing.
It is better to wait until a client has pain before giving medication.	Playing "catch-up" is not an effective way to manage pain; it is better to routinely administer analgesia, thus maintaining a low pain level.
Real pain has an identifiable cause.	There is always a cause of pain, but it may be very obscure and must be assessed carefully. Pain of a psychological origin is just as real as pain of physiologic origin.
The same physical stimulus produces the same pain intensity, duration, and distress in different people.	Intensity, duration, and distress vary with each individual.
Some clients lie about the existence or severity of their pain.	Very few people lie about pain.
Very young or very old people do not have as much pain.	All clients with an intact neurologic system experience pain; age is not a determinant of pain, but it may influence expression of pain.
Pain is a part of aging.	Pain does not accompany aging unless a disease process or ailment is present.
If a person is asleep, they are not in pain.	People in pain become exhausted and may truly be asleep or merely trying to sleep. Some people sleep as an escape mechanism.
If the pain is relieved by nonpharmaceutical pain relief techniques, the pain was not real anyway.	Nonpharmaceutical pain relief methods can be effective. A client's method of relief should be acknowledged as long as it does not harm.
Nurses should rely on their own definitions of pain and cultural beliefs about pain.	It is a mistake to impose one's own definitions, cultural beliefs, and values to another person's pain. Let the client tell you what the pain means.

nurse collects a pain history, a daily account of the current pain history (which includes pain-aggravating and pain-alleviating factors), and a collection of subjective and objective data through use of measurement tools. The client's pain goal or tolerable level of pain should be determined. Perform the assessment in an unbiased, caring manner.

For clients with expected or known and treated pain, such as postoperative pain, assessment is a constant and ongoing task, which may occur every 15 minutes for the acute, postoperative client. These clients need not be asked about the history of pain, but rather what they are experiencing now. Current pain levels should be assessed every 2 hours for the first 48 hours after surgery or trauma and every 4 hours thereafter as a standard routine, and more often if indicated. In addition, reassessment should occur within 20 to 30 minutes after administration of any medication given for pain reduction or relief and 5 to 15 minutes after intravenous (IV) medication administration at the time of the drug's peak effect.[3] However, it is important to know that the pain being treated is the same or expected pain. Ensure that the client is reporting incisional pain and not a new form of pain. New locations or characteristics of pain need a complete assessment.

Single-item assessment tools include the Visual Analog Scale (VAS), numerical scales (0-10), and visual descriptor scales. These scales can be used to measure both physical pain intensity and psychological distress (Figures 20-4 and 20-5). The tools are easy to use and provide the client and nurse with a simple means to quantify pain. The response can also be compared to the initial score, so that the degree of pain control can be maintained. The use of these scales does require the ability to think abstractly. Pictorial scales measure pain in small children, such as the widely used Faces Pain Rating Scale developed by Wong and Baker[34] (Figure 20-6). Clients with impaired cognitive ability may be better able to report their pain with the use of pictorial scales.[22] Do not assume nonverbal clients are not in pain. Watch for expressions of pain and attempt to treat pain with mild medications if you are uncertain about their pain. Table 20-5 has examples of nonverbal presentations of pain.

Ongoing Assessments. Clients may experience several types of pain during one medical episode. After surgery, a client may experience pain caused by poor body position, incisional pain, and deep visceral pain. The client may also have a condition that produces chronic pain, such as arthritis, that continues to be painful, or a secondary complication may be developing, such as pain resulting from myocardial infarction or pulmonary emboli. When planning interventions, learn to distinguish among the causes of pain. Each assessment for acute pain includes location, intensity, quality, and duration to aid in making intervention decisions. In addition, assessment for chronic pain includes sleep, appetite, function, concentration, and relationships.

Intensity. The single most important indicator of pain intensity is the client's self-report of the pain. You can obtain the client's self-report of pain intensity by asking clients to rate pain on a scale that they must mentally visualize or by showing the scale to the client. People in pain may have trouble concentrating on mental tasks and may find it particularly difficult to respond to a scale they must visualize. In some hospitals, it has been

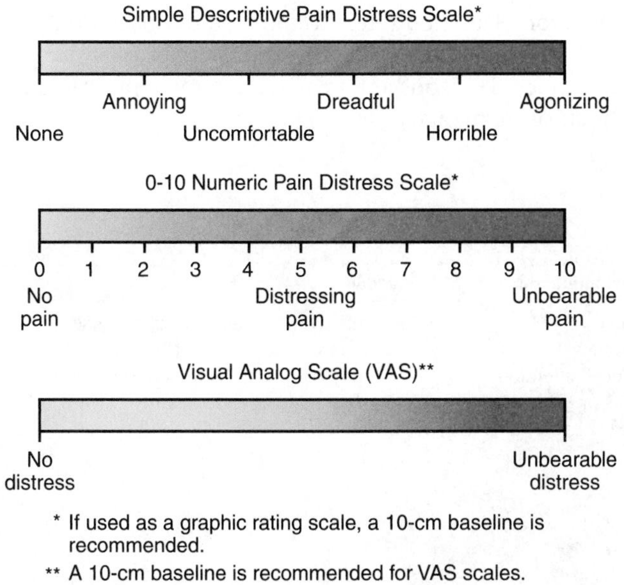

Simple Descriptive Pain Distress Scale*

| None | Annoying | Uncomfortable | Dreadful | Horrible | Agonizing |

0-10 Numeric Pain Distress Scale*

0 1 2 3 4 5 6 7 8 9 10
No pain — Distressing pain — Unbearable pain

Visual Analog Scale (VAS)**

No distress — Unbearable distress

* If used as a graphic rating scale, a 10-cm baseline is recommended.
** A 10-cm baseline is recommended for VAS scales.

■ **FIGURE 20–4** Pain distress scales.

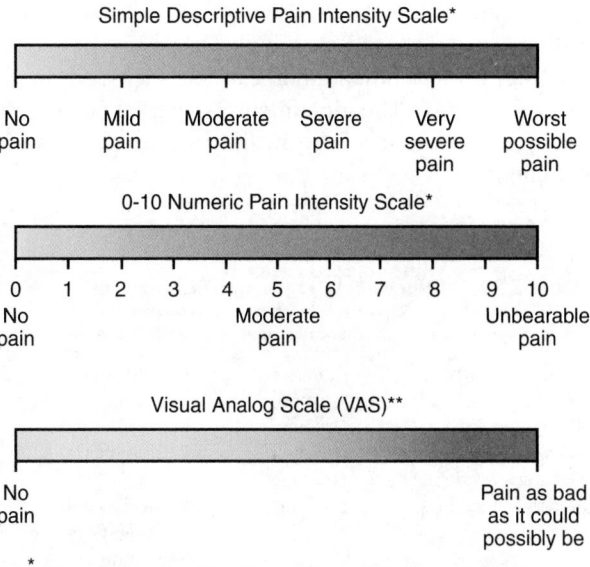

Simple Descriptive Pain Intensity Scale*

No pain | Mild pain | Moderate pain | Severe pain | Very severe pain | Worst possible pain

0-10 Numeric Pain Intensity Scale*

0 1 2 3 4 5 6 7 8 9 10
No pain — Moderate pain — Unbearable pain

Visual Analog Scale (VAS)**

No pain — Pain as bad as it could possibly be

* If used as a graphic rating scale, a 10-cm baseline is recommended.
** A 10-cm baseline is recommended for VAS scales.

■ **FIGURE 20–5** Pain intensity scales.

PAIN INTENSITY MEASURES

Faces:

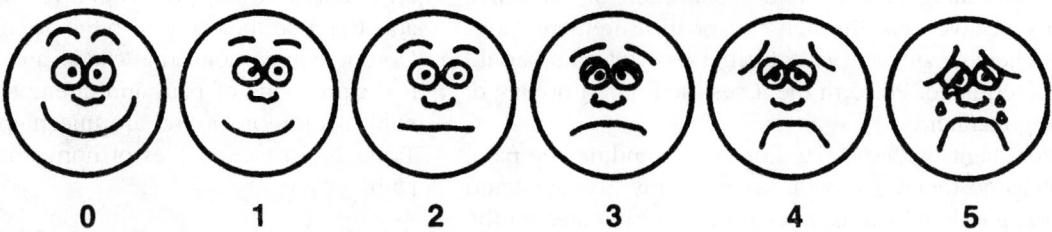

0   1   2   3   4   5

When using the Faces, explain to the person that each face is for a person who feels happy because he has no pain (hurt for young children) or sad because he has some or a lot of pain. Face 0 is very happy because he doesn't hurt at all. Face 1 hurts just a little bit. Face 2 hurts a little more. Face 3 hurts even more. Face 4 hurts a whole lot. Face 5 hurts as much as you can imagine, <u>although you don't have to be crying to feel this bad.</u>

Word:

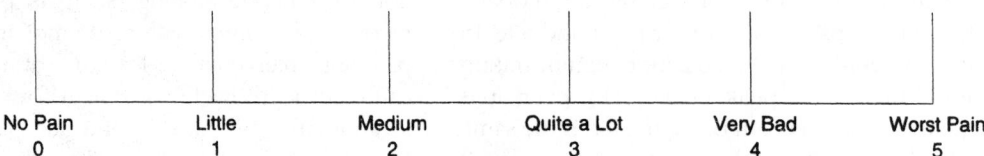

| No Pain | Little | Medium | Quite a Lot | Very Bad | Worst Pain |
| 0 | 1 | 2 | 3 | 4 | 5 |

■ **FIGURE 20–6** Faces Pain Rating Scale. Explain to the person that each face is for a person who feels happy because he or she has no pain (hurt) or sad because he or she has some or a lot of pain. Face 0 is very happy because he or she does not hurt at all. Face 1 hurts just a little bit. Face 2 hurts a little more. Face 3 hurts even more. Face 4 hurts a whole lot. Face 5 hurts as much as you can imagine, although you do not have to be crying to feel this bad. Ask the person to choose the face that best describes how he or she is feeling. This rating scale is recommended for clients age 3 years and older. *(From Wong, D.L., et al. [2001]. Wong's essentials of pediatric nursing [6th ed.]. St. Louis: Mosby. Copyrighted by Mosby.)*

beneficial to provide a copy of the intensity scale in plain view of each client, typically taped to the bedside wall.

Location. Location of pain may be ascertained by verbal description or by marking the location on a drawing of the body. Use of body drawings provides an opportunity for the client to report multiple sites of pain using a self-report document that can be included in the medical record. The document is then available for use by any member of the health care team caring for that client.

Quality. Quality of the pain is typically indicated by descriptive adjectives such as "stabbing like a knife" or "throbbing" (Box 20-4). Some clients may have difficulty describing the quality of painful sensations, or they may have problems using the term "pain" to indicate their discomfort. Showing clients a list of words to describe pain may facilitate their ability to report pain quality.

Duration. Duration refers to the time of onset, duration, and intervals of the pain. Terms used to classify the pattern include "constant, steady, intermittent, periodic, brief, or momentary."

TABLE 20–5   Nonverbal Behaviors Indicating Pain

Facial Expressions	Vocalizations	Body Movement	Social Interaction	Mood	Sleep
Clenched teeth	Crying	Restlessness	Silence	Combative	Increased, because of
Wrinkled forehead	Moaning	Guarding	Withdrawal	Confused	exhaustion
Biting lips	Gasping	Muscle tension	Reduced attention span	Cranky	Decreased, because of
Scowling	Groaning	Immobility	Focus on pain relief	Sad	frequent wakening
Closing eyes tightly	Grunting	Pacing	measures	Irritable	
Widely opened eyes	Screaming	Wringing hands			
or mouth		Rocking, fidgeting			
		Squirming			
		Resistance to			
		repositioning			
		Stiff joints			

BOX 20-4 Descriptive Terms for Pain	
Descriptive Word	**How Pain Makes Person Feel**
Sharp	Horrible
Piercing	Annoyed
Shooting	Miserable
Crushing	Frightened
Tender	Suffocated
Hurting	Tortured
Aching	Overwhelmed
Dull	Depressed
Sore	Defeated
Cramping	Anxious
Prickly	Victimized

TABLE 20–6   Pain-Related Nursing Diagnoses

Diagnosis	Etiology
Activity Intolerance	Related to unrelieved pain
Ineffective Coping	Related to lack of knowledge of possible methods of coping
Powerlessness	Related to lack of participation in decision-making process
Anxiety	Related to past experiences of poor pain control
Disturbed Sleep	Related to unrelieved pain at night pattern
Deficient Knowledge	Related to lack of exposure to informational resources
Fear	Related to anticipation of a pain experience

Aggravating and Alleviating Factors. Fatigue, muscle spasms, and anxiety can all aggravate pain. If the client has been treating the pain at home, ask "What makes the pain worse?" and "What makes the pain better?" The information obtained can be very helpful to appreciate the cause of the pain. For example, if the client says that spicy food and an empty stomach make his epigastric pain worse and food and antacids make it better, the nurse can be fairly certain that the pain is gastric and not cardiac in origin.

Distress. The psychological reactions to pain contribute to the overall pain experience. The emotional component may serve to intensify or diminish pain perception. Pain management strategies may need to be directed toward modifying the distress aspect of a pain episode.

Diagnosis, Outcomes, Interventions

Diagnosis: Acute Pain. The primary nursing diagnosis is *Acute Pain related to tissue injury from an incision, ischemia, or tumor encroachment in organs or bone.* Nurses have an impact on pain, discomfort, or suffering, no matter what the cause. In some situations, the client may be experiencing unrelieved pain or breakthrough pain. Unrelieved pain may be related to the following factors:

- Inadequate assessment of pain
- Failure to readdress uncontrolled pain
- Underadministration of ordered medication doses
- Administration of medications in inappropriate time frames
- Failure to provide stronger medications when indicated
- Failure to provide combinations of medications when indicated
- Inadequate use of nonpharmaceutical interventions

Pain may contribute to additional diagnoses as clients respond to the pain episode. Examples of such nursing diagnoses are presented in Table 20-6.

Outcomes. Outcomes and goals should be determined as a team consisting of the client, physicians, nurses, and often the extended family. A realistic outcome should be established to control or maintain the client at desired levels of pain and functioning. Desirable outcomes are that the client will (1) report acceptable pain levels, (2) request analgesia, (3) perform daily activities without limitation related to pain, and, in some cases, (4) have an improved quality of life or peaceful death.

A widely used method of providing effective care is through use of clinical care plans or clinical pathways. Care plans and pathways provide nurses with aids to diagnose the problem, plan for expected outcomes, implement interventions, state the rationale for the interventions, and evaluate the outcome. Many health care facilities provide standard care plans or clinical pathways that are part of the department protocol. Standard plans provide the beginning basis for client care. They are then individualized for the client depending on what modalities controlled or alleviated the pain.

Interventions. Effective pain reduction or relief is best achieved through the combination of both pharmaceutical and nonpharmaceutical therapies. Historically, pharmaceutical management has been the primary means of providing relief from pain, particularly acute pain. Although medications continue to serve as a major component of pain management, nonpharmaceutical techniques are being increasingly used to provide pain reduction or relief. Nonpharmacologic interventions are particularly useful (1) as adjuncts to pain reduction or relief, (2) while the client is waiting for medications to take effect, or (3) when side effects or client concerns make use of medications problematic.

Developing a Therapeutic Relationship. Therapeutic interaction with someone experiencing pain may include facilitating the client's expression of feelings about the pain, which imparts a sense of being cared for; providing support, reassurance, and understanding, which allow the client to develop confidence in the nurse; and teaching the client self-management strategies to reduce or relieve pain. Pain management strategies, including medications, are more effective when clients believe they are in control of the situation. A nurse who actively involves the client in the planning, intervention, and assessment of pain management strategies provides the client with enhanced potential to obtain satisfactory pain reduction or relief.

Administration of Pain-Relieving Medication. Numerous medications are used for pain reduction or relief. They are administered in a variety of ways: by inhalation, by subcutaneous or intramuscular injection, or orally, rectally, topically, sublingually, or intravenously. Injection is the least effective and most painful route and should be avoided. Too often nurses view the administration of pain-relieving medications as all they need to do for pain management. However, medication may be more effective when combined with other pain reduction or relief techniques such as music, massage, and biofeedback. When administering medication and repositioning the client, give a back rub or simply interact with a client; the effectiveness of the drug may be increased. Simply providing an intervention or a pill does not replace thoughtful, comprehensive pain management. A plan for pain management should be developed with the client. For clients who receive oral analgesics, the nurse should instruct the client to call when the pain is returning, and not wait until it is unbearable. Intense pain is difficult to control; it is much easier to control pain "by staying on top of it."

Managing Chronic Intractable Pain. Chronic intractable pain (pain that cannot be satisfactorily relieved by typical pharmaceutical means) causes additional difficulties for those experiencing it. Clients may require a combination of nursing interventions (cognitive, behavioral, physical, and pharmaceutical). Nursing and medical therapeutic regimens must be coordinated and consistent to ensure a unified approach. Use of balanced or preemptive analgesia is necessary.[28] Complete pain relief may be unrealistic, however, and should not be promised.

Managing Progressive Pain. People with progressive pain, such as that seen in malignancies, may require pain-relieving medications routinely as a preventive measure, in the same way that vasodilators are regularly taken by people with ischemic heart disease. As the disease progresses, clients may require increasingly stronger drug doses. Persistent intense pain can be best managed with long-acting medications. Some people hesitate to take pain-relieving medications routinely for fear of addiction. They may believe that they must avoid increasing dosages because they are afraid that they will "use up" the medication's pain relief potential and will not be able to obtain adequate medication in the future. Education of the unlimited ceiling dosage of morphine is necessary. Clients may also be concerned that they will be labeled as "drug users" if they take opioids over the long term. The analgesics at each step of the ladder are presented in Table 20-7.

Managing Breakthrough Pain. Breakthrough pain should be treated with both pharmacologic and nonpharmacologic methods. The intensity of the pain should drive the choice of medications. Short-acting medications should be used to control intense breakthrough pain. For a client whose breakthrough pain develops gradually and lasts 45 minutes to an hour,

TABLE 20–7   Analgesic Step Pain Ladder

Step One		Step Two	Step Three
NSAIDs and Others		**Opioid-Agonist Drug**	**Agonist Drugs**
Acetaminophen	Carbamazepine	Codeine	Morphine sulfate
Acetylsalicylic acid	Celecoxib	Oxycodone (with aspirin and	Methadone
(aspirin)	Meloxicam	with acetaminophen)	Hydromorphone
Ibuprofen	Phenytoin	Hydrocodone	Oxymorphone
Choline magnesium	Amitriptyline	Meperidine	Levorphanol
trisalicylate	Doxepin	Propoxyphene hydrochloride	Fentanyl
Diflunisal	Imipramine	Propoxyphene napsylate (with	
Ketoprofen	Trazodone	aspirin and with acetaminophen)	**Agonist-Antagonist Drugs**
Naproxen	Hydroxyzine		
Ketorolac tromethamine	Lidocaine	**Agonist-Antagonist Drugs**	Butorphanol
Piroxicam	Mexiletine	Pentazocine hydrochloride	Nalbuphine
Sulindac	Tocainide		Dezocine
Indomethacin	Dexamethasone		
	Dextroamphetamine		**Partial Agonist Drugs**
	Methylphenidate		Buprenorphine

From the World Health Organization. (1996). *Cancer pain relief* (2nd ed.). Geneva: Author.

conventional, shorter-acting opioids (such as oxycodone, hydrocodone, morphine, or hydromorphone) may be fine. If a client is taking sustained-release oxycodone for persistent pain and the characteristics of the break-through pain episodes match the pharmacologic profile of shorter-acting oxycodone, then that would be a clinically feasible combination.

Self-Care

Many conditions associated with pain are managed at home. The treatment of acute postoperative, chronic, and malignant pain is often performed by clients and family members. In reality, people experiencing pain attributable to widespread cancer require routine pain-relieving medications in order to function. Help is needed for clients and their significant others to understand the need for regular, often strong medications. Clients should be reassured that adequate pain reduction or relief will be possible in the future and that routine use of the medications means only that the condition warrants it, much like the routine use of medication for hypertension. See the Bridge to Home Health Care on Controlling Pain on the website.

ADMINISTRATION OF ANALGESICS

Principles of administration of analgesics are listed in Box 20-5. The goal of analgesic administration is to

provide pain reduction or relief while maintaining the ability of the client to be in control of the environment, participate in care, and reduce side effects. Assessment of the client before and after analgesic administration is necessary to ensure safe and adequate pain reduction or relief. Assess the following factors before analgesic administration:

- Medication allergies or sensitivities
- Time of last dose and response to it
- Previous response to analgesics
- Other medications being taken
- Body weight
- Individual pain experience
- Age, general state of health, mental status
- Cardiac, respiratory, renal, hepatic, and CNS status

Allergies or Sensitivities to Medications
Before administering an analgesic such as morphine, ensure that the client does not have a history of untoward reactions to the medication. When possible, ask the client or significant others, and review the chart or other documentation for such information. Allergies to opioids are rare and clients often consider side effects to be allergies.

Time of Last Dose and Client Response
Analgesics are ordered to be taken as needed by the client, such as every 3 to 4 hours. The nurse should note

BOX 20-5 Principles of Pharmaceutical Pain Management

- Provide medications in adequate doses.
- Utilize a preventive approach to pain relief. Predictable and chronic pain is managed more effectively if the client maintains a therapeutic blood level of analgesics. Use around-the-clock dosing with rescue medication available.
- Closely assess clients, with particular diligence with first doses or when the medication dose or the type is changed.
- Medication doses are specific as to type and route. For example, the dose for an oral preparation is higher than that for an intravenous dose of the same medication.
- Combinations of analgesics may be more effective than those given singularly.
- Additions of adjuvant medications enhance pain relief produced by analgesics and are not intended to replace analgesics.
- Understand and be prepared to treat side effects of medications.
- Do not consider avoidance of non–life-threatening side effects (such as constipation, nausea, pruritus) more important than providing pain relief. These concomitant conditions are easily treated.
- Recognize that respiratory depression is a rare occurrence, occurring most commonly among clients who are sedated.

Respiratory depression rarely occurs after the first few doses of an opioid.
- Asking for pain medication reflects the need for pain relief in 99.9% of people with pain and does not reflect an addictive personality.
- Do not use placebos for pain. The placebo response usually indicates that the responder has an effective endogenous opiate system and had obtained opiate-mediated pain relief.
- Believe the client's report of pain.
- Maintain a therapeutic relationship that facilitates mutual trust. Your attitudes and beliefs do affect the client's ability to respond to pain management strategies.
- Incorporate the goal of total pain relief into the pain management regimen for most clients.
- Operate as a team to provide the most effective pain relief outcomes. Include the client and significant others in pain interventions, allowing the client to maintain an adequate degree of personal control in the experience.
- *Only the client, and no one else, can determine the amount of pain experienced. There is no objective indicator of pain that can be observed by another.*

the time of the last dose, and the response to it. For example, was the last dose just 20 minutes ago? If so, the medication has not had time to take effect and another form of pain control should be used. If the dose was 30 minutes to 1 hour ago, it should have taken effect and the client may need more analgesia for pain relief. If the dose was more than 4 hours ago, the dose would appear to be working, but it would be necessary to confirm that conclusion with the client. Perhaps, the client was counting the minutes until another dose could be taken.

Concomitant Medications

Clients taking monoamine oxidase (MAO) inhibitor antidepressants should not receive meperidine. Medications that cause sedation, constipation, or orthostatic hypotension must also be considered when the client is receiving opioids. Be certain that stool softeners and fiber are being used by clients receiving opioids.

Body Weight

The standard morphine dose is 10 mg parenterally. This dose produces satisfactory analgesia in approximately 70% of people with moderate to severe postoperative pain. The analgesic effect is dose-related. Analgesics tend to be prescribed according to a standard protocol applied to all clients with similar disease, however, rather than being based on physical characteristics, including body weight. Therefore the standard dose may be too high for small adults and too low for obese adults. One cannot assume that the standard dose will produce adequate pain relief in all adults. Routinely assess degree of pain relief to ensure that adequate doses are being delivered.

Individual Differences

Given the multitude of factors that contribute to any one person's pain experience, the characteristics of one client's pain may differ from those of another client. It is not possible to design a pain management regimen that will be equally effective for all people with similar pathologic processes. For example, a person's age determines, to some extent, the length of time during which an analgesic will be effective. Age may influence the amount of relief obtained from medications. While there is most likely little difference in the ability of the CNS of an older adult to respond to stimuli, decreases in muscle mass, increases in gastric pathology, and changes in circulatory characteristics may result in a decreased ability to absorb and utilize analgesics. An older person tends to receive pain reduction or relief from an opioid for a longer time compared with a younger person. This difference in duration of action may relate to the speed

with which an opioid is cleared from the body. Opioid clearance is faster in younger people than in older people.

People with debilitating diseases, regardless of age, also have a heightened sensitivity to the effects of opioids. Because of individual differences in responses to pain medications, you must be diligent in assessing the client's responses to the medications.

Body System Assessment

Because all analgesics have the potential to produce mild to severe side effects, it is important to assess a client's cardiac, respiratory, renal, and CNS status before administering analgesics. Hepatic function is also assessed because of the important role of the liver in detoxifying analgesics. The presence of increased intracranial pressure is cause for concern. The physician typically conducts a body system assessment before ordering a specific medication regimen.

> **You must report changes in physical status that may place the client at risk if given the analgesic. The physician may then determine that an alternative regimen is needed.**

Methods of Administration

Nurse-Administered (Demand) Analgesia

The traditional method of treating pain is by nurse-administered pain medication on a schedule, or on a *prn* (as-needed) basis. This method allows the nurse to assess the pain and evaluate effectiveness of the medication, to detect or avoid untoward reactions or side effects, and to adjust the dose.

However, pain is often significantly undertreated with the as-needed system. Undertreatment may occur because (1) nurses assume authority for pain management, including determination of the amount of pain experienced by the client, and (2) the nurse, client, or significant others are overly concerned about possible opioid side effects and fear inducing opioid addiction. This concern about negative effects of pain medications often results in medications being ordered in inadequate doses for overly long intervals. When given a range of doses over a range of times, nurses tend to give the smallest dose over the longest time.

Studies have shown that nurses routinely underestimate the amount of pain being experienced. Because there is no objective indicator of pain, the only one who can determine pain medication needs is the client. Nurses who have been taught to treat medication-seeking behavior as a sign of addiction may be uncomfortable with this situation. The problem is particularly severe when medications are ordered on an as-needed basis. This order has typically been interpreted as "when the client asks for medication." When the client does ask, fears about addictive personalities surface and the client is seen as medication-seeking and may be labeled as a potential addict. The situation is especially severe when the client is young or belongs to a social or ethnic group devalued by the nurse.

The as-needed system also deprives the client of the ability to fully control the situation. Lack of control over pain experiences increases the pain endured during the episode. The pain may be worsened by anxiety about whether the next dose will be given in time to prevent the return of severe pain.

Intermittent dosing, such as occurs with as-needed medication orders, causes wide swings in the client's blood levels of the analgesic, which may result in sedation following one dose and unacceptable pain levels preceding the next dose. The as-needed dosing leads to a "hill and valley" pattern of pain relief. Clients receive a dose of medication sufficient to produce adequate pain relief. They are then expected to wait until the pain is again intense before asking for the subsequent dose.

Patient-Controlled Analgesia

Patient-controlled analgesia (PCA) entails use of an IV or subcutaneous infusion pump that contains the analgesic and that is controlled by the client. A bolus dose may be given at the onset of PCA use to provide immediate pain relief. The client can then self-administer subsequent doses by pressing a button that releases a preset dose delivered intravenously. The pumps are programmed to deliver preset demand doses of analgesic until a maximum dose is reached. Then there is a minimal interval during which no further analgesic can be administered (i.e., a lock-out period). With this system, clients control the administration of their own pain medication within the limits prescribed by the physician.

There are many advantages to PCA:

- The client usually reports good pain control.
- PCA helps to relieve the client's anxiety about waiting for the nurse to administer the medication, thereby lowering the dose needed to reduce or relieve pain.
- PCA promotes the client's independence and control over the situation.
- Clients administer lower doses of opioids compared with traditional as-needed formats.
- Clients can adjust their analgesic doses to a near-constant blood concentration.
- Clients report superior analgesia with a lower incidence of side effects compared with the traditional nurse-administered method.
- As the pain lessens, clients adjust to lower doses and eventually stop taking the analgesic.

Some problems are associated with PCA. Some clients complain of inadequate analgesia at night, requiring frequent wakening to redose themselves. At some institutions, a basal rate is added for continuous delivery at a low but constant dose through the PCA pump to avoid this situation. The device must be kept near the client and the client must understand how to use the "button." Frequent assessment by the nurse is necessary for the success of PCA. The success of this method depends on how well the client is taught to use it. Failure can often be traced to a poor understanding on the part of the client, the nurse, or both.

Oral Route

Oral (PO) dosing is usually preferred. It is noninvasive, convenient, and cost-effective and allows for the greatest flexibility in medication choices. Oral preparations may be in tablet, capsule, liquid, or sublingual forms. Some tablet preparations can be crushed and added to suspensions (e.g., to applesauce) that are more easily swallowed. Oral opioids are available in immediate and sustained-release forms. Sustained-release medications are designed to be metabolized slowly in the gastrointestinal system and must not be crushed or modified. The entire dose is released at one time if the integrity of the tablet is compromised. The peak effect of oral medications is 1½ to 2 hours for immediate-release preparations. Availability of the medication is delayed until the tablet is degraded and the medication is absorbed, passed through the liver, and made available to the circulatory system.

Intramuscular Route

IM dosing provides fairly rapid pain control, but is becoming less commonly used. Peak effects occur within 30 to 60 minutes and are accompanied by a rapid "fall-off" of effectiveness. IM injections are painful, and some people find the injections so painful to receive that they are reluctant to seek relief for their pain if the medications are to be administered this way. Additional disadvantages include wide variability and unreliable absorption from muscle and subcutaneous tissues.

Additional side effects of IM injections include trauma-induced fibrosis of muscle and soft tissues, nerve damage from chemical injury, and development of sterile abscesses. SAFETY ALERT

Intravenous Route

IV dosing provides the most rapid pain reduction or relief. Medications may be provided in bolus doses or by continuous infusions. Bolus doses are given in one administration and provide the most rapid onset of pain reduction or relief. Bolus hydromorphone reaches peak effect in 5 to 15 minutes, and morphine in 15 to 20 minutes. Continuous infusion provides a steady delivery of IV pain medication. It is usually preferred because plasma levels of the medication are maintained and the occurrence of side effects is lessened. Bolus doses may be needed if pain relief falls below acceptable levels with continuous infusion. The infusion dose may then need to be increased to maintain adequate relief.

Rectal Route

Rectal suppositories provide an alternative route to parenteral administration for people unable to take oral medications. They are provided in doses similar to those of oral preparations. Medications appropriate for the rectal route include morphine, hydromorphone (Dilaudid), oxycodone, and methadone.

Transdermal Route

Transdermal analgesia is provided by means of a skin patch. The most common opioid administered transdermally is fentanyl, which is potent. It is available in a variable-dosing transdermal application system that the client or family member can apply independently. The patch delivers specified amounts of medication over 48 to 72 hours. This system provides an easy means of maintaining independence and avoids the inconveniences of frequent dosing.

Analgesia from the first application may take up to 24 hours to reach an adequate blood level. During this period, supplemental analgesia is maintained. The patch is typically applied to clean, dry skin on the chest or upper back. These areas are less vulnerable than other areas to dislodgment of the patch. The patch may be applied to any convenient location with intact skin as long as the client can protect it. Excessive hair should be carefully clipped, not shaved, before application. The patch should not be applied over irritated or broken skin. The patch is left in place for up to 72 hours, and then is removed. A new patch is applied at a different site to prevent skin irritation. Be certain to remove the old patch when replacing it.

Transmucosal Analgesia

Transmucosal analgesia is achieved either sublingually (methadone and buprenorphine [Buprenex]) or (Fentanyl) orally by means of a lozenge (Oralet) or a lollipop (Actiq). The transmucosal route is particularly effective for breakthrough pain in clients with scheduled opioid medications around the clock. Up to two thirds of clients with chronic or malignant pain who are treated around the clock with opioids have episodes of breakthrough pain.[21,36]

Continuous Subcutaneous Analgesia

Pain reduction or relief is achieved through an infusion setup using a pump device. A 25- or 27-gauge needle is used, or a special subcutaneous needle device can be implanted. The client wears a medication reservoir that can be refilled. The needle site is rotated every 3 to 7 days according to the type and volume of medication administered. The volume delivered ranges from 2 to 4 ml/hour.

Observe the site for redness, excessive swelling, leakage of fluid around the infusion site, or edema. If an extremity is used, carefully assess it for the presence of edema, which interferes with absorption of the medication. Closely monitor the client for adequacy of the analgesic effect. If the medication is ineffective and sufficient medication is available in the reservoir, a higher concentration may be required.

Intraspinal and Epidural Analgesia

Opioids are injected intrathecally or epidurally. The epidural space is outside the dura mater of the spinal cord and brain; the intrathecal (spinal) space is inside the dura mater and contains the spinal fluid. The dorsal horns of the spinal cord contain receptors for endogenous opioid substances. By means of the intraspinal analgesia route, medication is delivered directly into the areas with the intended receptor sites. These receptors bind opioids and provide excellent pain reduction or relief of long duration (8 to 24 hours) without causing sympathetic and motor nerve blockade. Relatively small doses provide high opioid concentrations in the spinal fluid that bathes the dorsal columns. These concentrations are far higher than those in the spinal fluid after similar doses given by standard parenteral routes. Local anesthetics can be combined with opioids, thus using multiple pain pathways. Possible side effects include pruritus, urinary retention, and delayed respiratory depression occurring 6 to 12 hours after a dose. Low doses of naloxone may reverse these side effects without reducing analgesia. Clients need to have assessments of neurologic status every 4 hours initially and every 4 hours after dose increases. Pulse oximetry should be used to assess for respiratory depression. The use of low molecular weight heparins has been linked to spinal hematoma in clients with epidurals. Other forms of anticoagulation should be used.

Repeated bolus doses, PCA, or a constant infusion via an implanted refillable infusion pump of the opioid may be given through a small catheter placed in the epidural or intrathecal space. Catheters have been left in place for days to months without adverse effects.[12]

Modifications for Older Clients

Unrelieved pain is so common among older adults that it is accepted as inevitable and cynically described as "better than the alternative" (death). Financial constraints add to the problems of pain in older adults. Even when newer, sustained-release non-opioid and adjuvant drugs are prescribed, older adults may not be able to afford them. In addition, pharmacies often limit the number of doses of opioids they will dispense per prescription, a policy that increases the cost to sufferers. In many states, Medicaid, the managed health care program for the poor, will not pay for more effective, but more costly, analgesics. Comprehensive Medicare prescription drug coverage began in 2006, and its effect on pain management in older adults is still to be seen.

Fears of addiction and the side effects of analgesics, especially opioids, keep many older adults from taking medications sufficient to relieve their pain. As a result, they take smaller doses than are prescribed or wait until pain is unbearable before they "give in" and take an analgesic.

This sorry picture of pain management in older adults can be changed. With educational programs for older adults, their caregivers, and especially health care professionals, such needless suffering can be reduced.

Communicating with Older Adults

Older adults often have difficulty hearing, speaking, and seeing. These sensory and cognitive deficits may be due to common disorders of aging such as cataracts or cerebrovascular accidents and dementia. Some older adults may not be fluent in English. Because of these difficulties, these seniors need time to gather their thoughts and express their needs. Nurses need to listen carefully, speaking slowly and distinctly—and loudly enough to be heard and understood. Nurses may need to seek the assistance of a family member or caregiver to communicate more effectively with the senior. Nurses must also learn the body language of pain, as described in Table 20-5.

As medical science has overcome one physical ailment after another, life expectancy has increased, resulting in an ever-enlarging population of people more than 85 years old, the so-called old-old. Though physical stamina varies widely, many of these individuals are frail, are cared for in various institutions, and are at risk for both drug undertreatment and drug overtreatment. Age-related pharmacokinetics (absorption, excretion, and actions of drugs) vary greatly between individuals.

Assessing Pain in Older Adults

Pain assessment in older adults and people with cognitive and mental disorders includes all the same factors as in adults and children, but with some special considerations. Few assessment instruments have been tested in the geriatric population, and visual, auditory, and motor impairments, common among older adults, make typical assessment tools difficult to use.[1] The Faces Pain Rating Scale can be used in older adults, even those with mild dementia.[22] Nonverbal clues of pain can be useful in this population (see Table 20-5 on p. 370). Pain may be indicated by lack of appetite, sleeping disorders, tearing of the eyes, moaning, or splinting of a body part. Pain in older adults may result in increased falls and social isolation.

Location. Because older adults suffer many chronic conditions, they may feel pain in more than one area of the body at the same time. To gather accurate data, nurses need to inquire about specific locations of pain. They may find it useful to ask the client to touch the place that hurts. Some facilities provide line drawings of the body, front and back, on which nurses can mark the areas where the client feels pain.

Intensity. Regardless of the pain scale that is used, individuals need to understand what is asked of them. When a nurse breezes into a client's room and demands, "What is your pain number?" the older adult may not understand what is being asked. The nurse must be specific, for example, "On a scale of 0 to 10, with 0 no pain and 10 severe pain in your right hip, what number would you give it now?" Remember, older adults often feel pain in many places at once; therefore it is important to identify the exact site in question.

Quality and Pattern. Older adults often have their own terms to describe the quality of their pain. They may call throbbing pain "jumping" or sharp pain "stabbing or poking." Nurses may find it helpful to ask the client to compare the pain to a familiar experience, such as the vibration of an electric motor or the pricking of a needle.

Precipitating and Alleviating Factors. Most adults remember what they were doing when they first felt acute pain, such as "I must have tripped as I was walking down the front steps." However, chronic pain creeps up on older adults and they may not remember when or how it began. To alleviate pain, clients may first try home remedies, then experiment with over-the-counter (OTC) medicines, and, finally, seek medical intervention. For this reason it is useful to ask what remedies they have tried to ease their pain and what was most helpful.

Associated Symptoms. It is particularly important to learn what other-than-pain symptoms older adults are experiencing (e.g., dizziness, blurred vision, urinary incontinence, retention, diarrhea, constipation). These symptoms may be due to prescribed drugs, home remedies, drug interactions, or other conditions. All such symptoms should be documented, reported, and investigated.

Intervening to Relieve Pain in Older Adults

All of the pharmacologic and nonpharmacologic interventions discussed in this chapter can be used for older adults. However, adverse effects of analgesic drugs are of special concern because of age-related changes in the body systems. In older adults, these adverse effects may occur with markedly different dosages than they do in younger people. Of special concern are changes in the renal and hepatic functioning, metabolism, and clearance of analgesics such as meperidine, methadone, and acetaminophen.

When evaluating the effectiveness of medications, consider both the intended effects and the adverse effects. Intended effects are the relief of pain and the reduction of anxiety. Adverse effects include respiratory depression, mental confusion, and constipation. Adverse effects must be anticipated and steps taken to prevent them. Confusion and delirium can develop quickly after only a few doses of opioids, and when present, oral opioids or other non-opioid medications should be used for pain control.[33] Constipation is a common problem and should be managed prophylactically with fiber and stool softeners.

CLIENTS WITH ADDICTIVE DISEASE

Clients with addictive disease or who are in recovery often receive less than optimal pain relief, attributable in part to the value judgments by health professionals.[19] These clients may be involved in more acute pain episodes because of increased traumatic events, such as injuries. Clients with addictive disease are often challenging to staff who are struggling to advocate for pain relief. However, clients with addictive disease have the right to be treated with respect and to receive the same quality of pain management as all other clients. "Nurses are in an ideal position to advocate and intervene for these clients across all treatment settings."[6] Methadone has traditionally been used for clients with addictive disease to reduce withdrawal manifestations and psychological craving for the opiates. A new medication, Suboxone, is being used more often in place of methadone. Box 20-6 lists recommendations for all clients with addictive disease and recommendations for clients in recovery.

BOX 20-6 Recommendations for All Patients with Addictive Disease

- Identify and use resources available to assist with the diagnosis and treatment of both addiction and pain.
- Encourage the patient to use support systems (e.g., family, significant others, or rehabilitation sponsor); offer additional resources (e.g., addictions counselor).
- Involve the patient in pain management planning and, with the patient's consent, include family and significant others.
- Provide the patient with verbal and written information about the pain management plan, including what the patient can expect from caregivers and what the patient's responsibilities are.
- Ensure consistency in the implementation of the pain management plan.
- Educate the patient, family, and significant others about the differences between addiction, physical dependence, and tolerance.
- Help the patient make informed choices about medications by educating the patient, family, and significant others about medication options.
- Select and titrate analgesics based on pain assessment, side effects, and function, as well as sleep and mood.
- Be prepared to titrate opioid analgesics and benzodiazepines to doses higher than usual. The patient may have developed tolerance to some medications, or drug use may have caused increased sensitivity to pain.
- Benzodiazepines, phenothiazines, or other sedating medications that do not relieve pain should not be used as substitutes for analgesics.
- If pain is present most of the time, provide analgesics around-the-clock (ATC).
- Use the oral route and long acting analgesics when possible.
- Consider the use of IV or epidural patient-controlled analgesia (PCA) for acute pain management.
- Record and discuss with the patient any behavior suggestive of inappropriate medication use, especially of controlled substances.
- When opioids, benzodiazepines, or other medications with a potential for physical dependence are no longer needed, taper them very slowly to minimize the emergence of withdrawal symptoms.
- Consider nonpharmacological methods of treatment for pain but do not use them in place of appropriate pharmacological approaches.

Reprinted with permission of the American Society of Pain Management Nurses, 7794 Grow Drive, Pensacola, FL 32514. Copyright 2002. American Society of Pain Management Nurses.

NONPHARMACEUTICAL INTERVENTIONS

Although there are a myriad of drugs to relieve pain, all have some risk and cost. Fortunately, there are many nonpharmacologic interventions to provide pain relief, especially when used in conjunction with pharmacologic measures. Described as physical and cognitive-behavioral interventions, many of these approaches are noninvasive, low-risk, inexpensive, easily performed and taught, and within the scope of nursing practice. Physical interventions give comfort, increase mobility, and alter physiologic responses. Cognitive-behavioral interventions alter the perception of pain, reduce fear, and give clients a greater sense of control. The therapies are thought to cause physiologic changes. For example, peripheral blood vessels may be dilated, muscle tension is decreased, the immune system is strengthened, and brain chemicals are activated or modified. Techniques such as these can be used to manage pain and to promote healthy living. It may be possible to teach clients a combination of these techniques to maximize their opportunities for self-control over manifestations of pain.

🪔 PHYSICAL INTERVENTIONS

Comfort Measures

Clean, smooth sheets; soft, supportive pillows; warm blankets; and a soothing environment have been used by nurses throughout history to relieve pain and suffering. These measures may be difficult to provide in the noisy, mechanized health care facilities of today. Nonetheless, they are important to the mental and physical health of clients. Position change and movement are well-known pain-relieving interventions. Moving the body, even a small amount, relieves muscle spasm and provides a degree of pain relief.

Cutaneous Stimulation

Cutaneous stimulation activates the large-diameter (A-beta) fibers, which stimulate inhibitory neurons in the spinal cord and engage the descending analgesic system. Pain reduction or relief is achieved by endogenous opiate activity. Cutaneous stimulation can decrease the intensity of pain the client perceives and, in some instances, may eliminate it.[25] It also can help in changing the sensation in a painful or noxious area to a more pleasant sensation, such as warmth. This process may also be seen as a form of distraction because the client may focus on the sensation being created rather than the pain.

Massage

A back rub is a good method of providing cutaneous stimulation. It is particularly relaxing at bedtime and may block pain so as to promote more comfortable sleep. However, you should be knowledgeable in massage techniques so as not to increase discomfort; for example, too deep or rough massaging may actually increase a client's pain. Review massage techniques in a fundamentals of nursing text. Foot massage is particularly helpful and cost-effective. The feet are easily accessible, and the intervention can be applied to people in any body position.

Heat and Cold Applications

Cold and warmth receptors activate A-beta fibers when their temperature is within 4° to 5° C of body temperature. The receptors are rapid adapting, requiring that the temperature be readjusted at frequent intervals ranging from 5 to 15 minutes.

Heat is an excellent means of pain reduction or relief that is amenable to nursing autonomy.[14] Warm applications may be achieved by warming devices (e.g., heating pads, warming towels). In the clinical setting, warm applications may be achieved by warming damp disposable bed pads in the microwave. Incontinence pads can be cut to desired sizes, are inexpensive, and are disposable. Take care to avoid heat temperatures that will burn. Remember, painful areas may be hypersensitive to skin stimuli. Heat temperatures that are typically perceived as nonpainful may become painful when applied to the sensitive area.

Cold application also brings pain reduction or relief, and nurses can consider this treatment.[14] *Ice* may also be used to provide pain reduction or relief and to prevent or reduce edema and inflammation. The effectiveness of ice applications does not depend on A-beta fiber stimulation; however, ice decreases the conduction velocity of nociceptive nerve fibers, rendering the fiber incapable of transmitting the pain signal to the spinal cord. The client perceives the application area as numb. In the home setting, frozen vegetables placed in another plastic bag, rather than ice cubes, work as well as ice bags.

Transcutaneous Electrical Nerve Stimulation

Transcutaneous electrical nerve stimulation (TENS) delivers electrical bursts through the skin to superficial and deep nerves. TENS is used most often for clients with chronic pain, such as muscle pain from arthritis. TENS has been shown to reduce or relieve pain effectively in many people.[10] The client needs to learn to adjust placement of the surface electrodes and the intensity and timing of the stimuli to maximize pain reduction or relief. Electrode placement depends on the site of the pain. Positive and negative poles are usually placed within several inches of each other. Voltage and pulsation are controlled by the person wearing the device.

Acupuncture

Acupuncture has been practiced in Asian cultures for centuries for pain reduction or relief. Very thin metal needles are skillfully inserted into the body at designated locations and at various depths and angles. Approximately 1000 known acupuncture points are widely distributed over the surface of the body in patterns known as *meridians*. Each meridian contains its own group of acupuncture points and is associated with a specific visceral organ. Meridians run bilaterally just beneath the surface of the skin and begin or terminate at the tips of the fingers or toes. "Vital energy" is believed to flow through these meridians. The acupuncture points on the surface of the body provide external access to this vital energy. Through needle insertion at specific points, various physiologic processes can be influenced or controlled and are determined by the specific pathologic condition and the desired physiologic effect.

Acupressure

Acupressure is a noninvasive method of pain reduction or relief based on the principles of acupuncture. Pressure, massage, or other cutaneous stimulation, such as heat or cold, is applied over acupuncture points.

Cognitive or Biobehavioral Interventions
Deep Breathing

Deep breathing for relaxation is easy to learn and contributes to pain relief or reduction by reducing muscle tension and anxiety. First, the client clenches the fists while taking a deep breath. After holding the breath for a moment, the client exhales while letting the body "go limp." The cycle is followed by a slow, deep breath mimicking a yawn.

Progressive Relaxation

Progressive relaxation training teaches the client to gradually tighten and then deeply relax various muscle groups, proceeding systematically from one area of the body to the next. The deep relaxation produced by this method can decrease anxiety and excessive muscle contraction and can promote the onset of sleep. Instruction in this technique is available on audiotape cassettes.

Rhythmic Breathing

Rhythmic breathing is both relaxation and distraction. It may also provide effective pain reduction or relief by stimulating baroreceptors in the atria and carotid sinuses. Stimulation of these receptors initiates activity in a neuropathway that sends projections to the periaqueductal and periventricular gray matter, resulting in opioid-mediated pain inhibition. This method can be combined with rhythms such as music, a ticking clock, or a metronome. Little concentration is necessary because once the individual begins the process, it takes on an automatic quality. This method focuses attention away from the pain and on the breathing and the rhythm. The Lamaze method of childbirth is a good example of a pain control method that incorporates this technique.

Music

People in pain may find music to be relaxing. The exact physiologic mechanisms have not been determined; however, several possible theories include distraction, release of endogenous opioids, or disassociation. All three mechanisms are probably involved. Music clearly provides distraction and disassociation by focusing on the characteristics of the musical selection.[11] The auditory pathway interacts with endogenous opiate systems at several foci within the brain, including the hypothalamus and the limbic system. These areas are known to project to PAG/PVG, providing a mechanism to contribute to pain reduction or relief through both cerebral activity and spinal cord responses mediated by descending fibers from the nucleus raphe and locus ceruleus. Pain reduction or relief may also be achieved through physiologic responses to relaxation. The relaxation response is mediated through the hypothalamus.

When using music for pain reduction or relief, allow clients to choose the type of music most suited to them. Some people find the use of a radio, cassette, MP3 player, or compact disc player with headphones a quiet way to listen to music without bothering others. This allows the client to increase the music volume or to play it softly. Encourage family members to bring in the client's favorite selections. This also gives the family a sense of doing something to help.

Guided Imagery

Guided imagery helps a client visualize a pleasant experience. The client is coached to visualize a scene (e.g., relaxing on a beach). The coach instructs the client to imagine the sensory aspects of the scene: the sounds, sights, and emotions expressed. The more vivid the image, the more effective the intervention. Visualization may be combined with soft, lyrical, relaxing music. Audiotapes for guided imagery are available.

Imagery relieves pain through several mechanisms. It is a way to help people distract themselves from their pain, which may increase their pain tolerance. Imagery may also produce a relaxation response, thus relieving pain. Last, the image can be a healing one, designed not only to relieve the pain but possibly also to diminish the source of the pain (e.g., a tension headache may be alleviated).

Imagery is often combined with relaxation and biofeedback to produce a multifocal technique for pain reduction or relief. The image used in this technique can be a complex scene that requires the person to think of each detail. This image would increase distraction. The image might be a relaxing scene, such as a beach or meadow, that would help with the relaxation response, or the image might consist of visualizing the pain being worn away until it is so small that it can be "blown away." When introducing an image setting, determine which setting the client finds relaxing. Avoid using an image that may provoke anxiety, such as using a beach for someone who is afraid of water or a meadow for someone with severe allergies to pollen.

Biofeedback

Biofeedback refers to a wide variety of techniques that provide a client with information about changes in body functions of which the client is usually unaware, such as blood pressure. Biofeedback equipment provides immediate, continuous information. Some people learn to use this information to control previously involuntary functions. The purpose of biofeedback in pain management is to teach self-control over physiologic variables that relate to the pain, such as muscle contraction and blood flow.

Information used to reduce muscle contraction is obtained by an electromyogram (EMG) recorded from body surface electrodes. (Needle EMG electrodes are not used.) Changes in blood flow are produced by monitoring skin temperature, which increases with increased blood flow. Depending on the equipment used, clients can self-monitor their changes through auditory displays (decreases in muscle contractions are heard as decreases in the pitch of a tone) or visual displays (increases in skin temperature are seen as increases on a dial). The client tries to change the display of information in the desired direction, such as to reduce muscle contraction (relax muscle tension) and reduce blood flow. The continuous, precise information received shows the effectiveness of the effort and often helps the client learn physiologic control of these functions. Biofeedback can be performed at home with purchased or rented equipment under the guidance of a suitably prepared health care worker. Alternatively, it may be performed in an office or clinic setting with a biofeedback therapist or other specialist, such as a nurse trained in biofeedback. The equipment is expensive.

Distraction

Attention is directed away from the painful sensation or the negative emotional arousal associated with the pain episode. The primary theoretical explanation is that a person is able to focus attention on a limited number of foci. Actively focusing attention on a cognitive task is thought to limit one's ability to attend to the noxious sensation. To be effective, the distraction task requires considerable cognitive effort. Distraction exercises that are too easy rapidly become automatic or engage monotonous repetitive responses and are likely to be ineffective.

Interventions may be administered by a multitude of modalities that require the client to engage in highly focused interesting mental exercises. Typical techniques used in hospital settings include videotapes of favorite movies, audiotapes of favorite music, craft activities, and interacting with others. The distraction technique may be more effective if it involves action on the client's part. For example, listening to music and tapping one's fingers to the rhythm may be more effective than passive listening alone. Cognitive strategies need to be tailored to the client's personal preferences. Techniques used should be self-selected. People may want to bring their own tapes, videos, books, or craft items. If the items are supplied by an agency, a library of materials is needed to allow clients to select what is pleasing to them.

Therapeutic Touch

Therapeutic Touch has been used for disorders such as tension headaches. It is a derivative of the "laying on" of hands. The human body is believed to have energy fields that express aberrant patterns when body systems are insulted. Therapeutic Touch is thought to realign aberrant fields. Education and practice are required on the part of the nurse.

Therapeutic Touch involves three steps:
1. Become centered or focused in a meditative state. This helps you become aware of the vibrations in the surrounding energy fields.
2. Assess the client's energy field. Pass your hands over the client's body at a distance of 2 to 6 inches to sense changes in the field.
3. During the treatment step, use your hands to rearrange the client's energy field and return it to normal.

Meditation

Meditation focuses one's attention away from pain. It also provides energy and peace to the person who is meditating. The client simply sits comfortably and quietly with focused attention. The focus may vary. Examples include flow of the breath, a mantra, and a picture or mental image of a great spiritual being or peaceful place. Sometimes the person who is meditating communicates with a spiritual being. There are many meditation techniques, some with a spiritual base, such as Siddha meditation. Meditation is easily practiced anywhere, and no special equipment is required. The positive experiences available through meditation are available to anyone, including people in pain.

Hypnosis

A person's reaction to pain can be significantly altered by hypnosis. Hypnosis is based on suggestion, dissociation, and the process of focusing attention. Various procedures may be used to reduce pain following induction of a hypnotic state, including the following:

- Suggestion to alter the character of the pain or one's attitude toward it
- Body disorientation and dissociation
- Anesthesia and analgesia for superficial and deep sensation

In situations of chronic pain, a posthypnotic suggestion may be used in combination with self-hypnosis to provide prolonged relief. Many hypnotic subjects successfully learn to use deliberate spontaneous trance induction or self-hypnosis. Although hypnosis cannot change organic lesions that are producing pain, it can often reduce discomfort. The procedure itself is fairly simple and innocuous compared with the administration of many anesthetic and analgesic medications; however, take care not to probe any fears or unpleasant memories. A hypnotherapist must be skilled and informed and the client carefully selected to avoid negative effects. Increasingly, nurses are being certified to provide clinical hypnotic therapies in the United States.

Humor

It has been postulated that humor elevates endogenous opioids or endorphins. Research has revealed that humor actually increases the number of NK (natural killer) cells of the immune system. This is particularly important for implementation in clients with cancer. Regardless of the physiologic advantages, use of humor simply makes people feel better, more relaxed, and in less pain. Clients may find some degree of pain reduction or relief by watching comedic videotapes, listening to audiotapes and compact discs they find funny, or reading humorous books. The nurse might suggest that hospitalized clients bring humorous materials with them to use during their inpatient experience.[11]

Magnets

Magnets have been used to relieve a variety of painful disorders.[26] It is speculated that the pull of the magnet increases blood flow to the region, opening the Na^+ and Cl^- channels in the cells. Magnet therapy has been a mainstay in pain management in Eastern Asian countries and is gaining popularity in Western medicine. (See the Complementary and Alternative Therapy feature on Magnet Therapy for Plantar Heel Pain on p. 542.)

EVALUATION AND DOCUMENTATION

Evaluation

Evaluation is an important aspect of the nursing process because it tells the nurse if the goal was met. If the expected outcome is pain reduction, evaluation tells us if the intervention did, in fact, reduce pain.

The best source of information about pain and pain control, of course, is the client. The next best source would be the family or caregivers who watch the client over time. All aspects of the pain that were noted before the intervention, including the location, intensity, quality, and duration of the pain, must be reported for full evaluation of pain control, reduction, or relief. In addition, nurses gather data about adverse effects of an intervention, such as an allergic reaction, hypotension, or respiratory depression.

Timing of evaluation is based on the expected time frame for the interventions to work. If the client is in intense pain (10 or higher on a numerical scale), the evaluation should be within minutes after giving IV medications, because the nurse would not leave a client in that level of pain. If oral medications were used to treat the pain, the evaluation should be about 30 minutes later, when the medication is starting to work. Follow-up within an hour should also occur to be certain that pain was controlled to a tolerable level.

If the client's pain was not controlled by the interventions chosen, the nurse considers several options. Is the pain from another source and therefore not responsive to the therapy chosen? For example, angina would be best controlled with nitroglycerin, not acetaminophen. If the same pain is present, are there more potent medications that can be given? Could a nonpharmacologic measure be used to reduce anxiety, muscle tension, or fear? Does the physician need to be notified for orders for more potent medications? Never is the client "just left alone" to handle the pain; other interventions are attempted to control pain.

Barriers to pain management are present in health care professionals, clients, and even in the health care system (Box 20-7). The use of pain management flow

---

BOX 20-7 Barriers to Pain Management

PROBLEMS RELATED TO HEALTH CARE PROFESSIONALS
- Inadequate knowledge of pain management
- Poor assessment of pain
- Concern about regulation of controlled substances
- Fear of pain
- Fear of client addiction
- Concern about side effects of analgesics
- Concern about clients becoming tolerant to analgesics
- Continuing myths regarding pain

PROBLEMS RELATED TO CLIENTS
- Reluctance to report pain
- Concern about distracting physicians from treatment of underlying disease
- Fear that pain means disease is worse
- Concern about not being a "good" client
- Reluctance to take pain medications
- Fear of addiction or of being thought of as an addict
- Worries about unmanageable side effects
- Concern about becoming tolerant to pain medications

PROBLEMS RELATED TO THE HEALTH CARE SYSTEM
- Low priority given to cancer pain treatment
- Inadequate reimbursement (the most appropriate treatment may not be reimbursed or may be too costly for clients and families)
- Restrictive regulation of controlled substances
- Problems of availability of treatment or access to it

Modified from Jacox, A., et al. (1994). *Management of cancer pain. Clinical practice guidelines No. 9* (AHCPR Pub. No. 94-1592). Rockville, Md: Agency for Health Care Policy and Research, U.S. Department of Health and Human Services, U.S. Public Health Service.

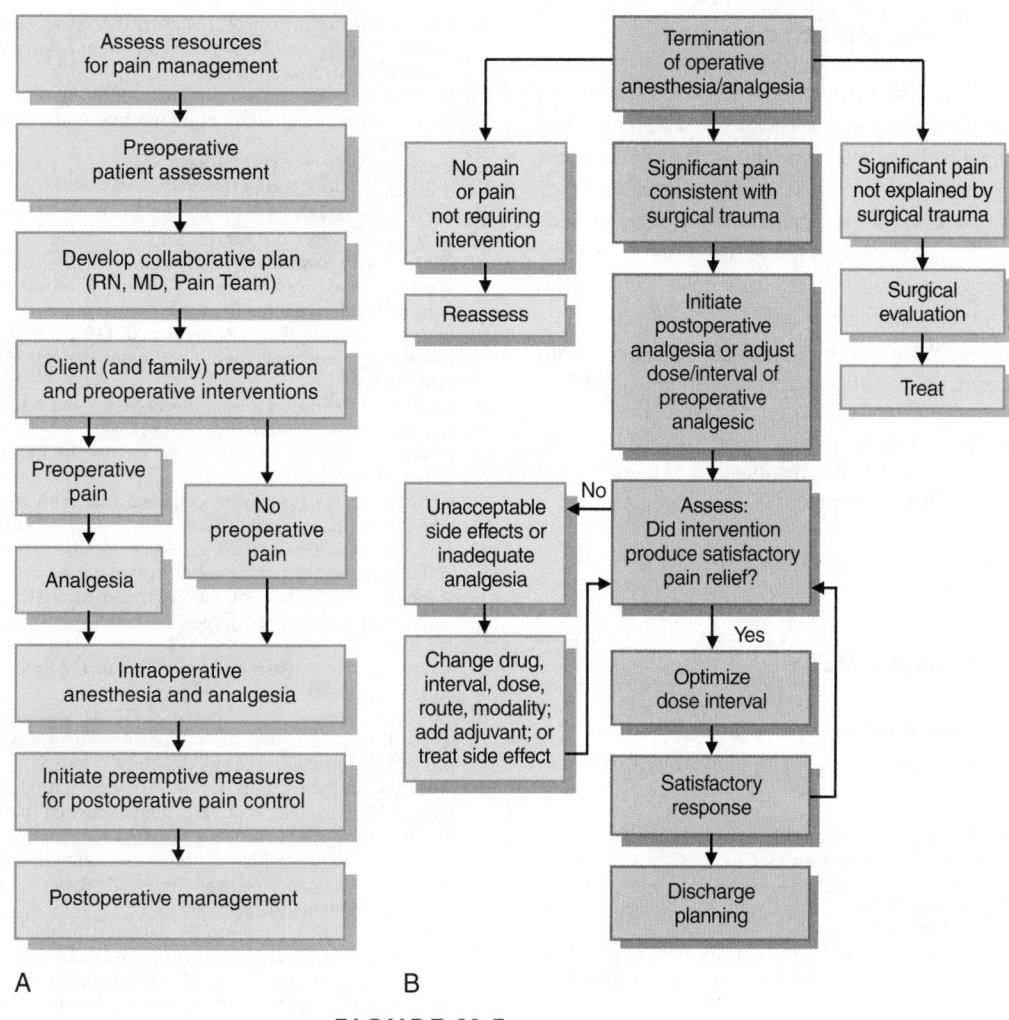

■ **FIGURE 20–7** Pain treatment flow chart.

charts will guide the health care system to monitor the effectiveness of pain management for the clients in the health care system (Figure 20-7). Your role in pain control begins with yourself and your own clients. You may have an opportunity to influence the management of pain in your agency; if so, take advantage of the willingness of a system to change.

Communication and Documentation

Communication about pain and the response of clients to interventions is facilitated by accurate and thorough documentation. This communication needs to be conveyed from nurse to nurse, from shift to shift, and from nurse to other responsible health care providers. Various tools have been devised to facilitate this communication, including pain flow sheets, running diaries, and bedside computer charting (known as "point-of-care" charting). When communicating information about pain, it is important to accurately describe the time and exact nature of an intervention, including the analgesic and dosage administered, the level of pain before and after the intervention, and adverse effects, such as respiratory depression.

CONCLUSIONS

The most effective pain management program may depend on use of a combination of medications and nonpharmaceutical interventions. Clients may benefit from the incorporation of several nonpharmaceutical interventions used simultaneously. Research has supported the efficacy of numerous nonpharmaceutical techniques. These findings plus the wide variability in the strengths and types of medications make it possible (1) to design a pain program that can be individualized and (2) to modify a pain management protocol if a component of the program is ineffective. One ineffective strategy can be replaced by another strategy until a successful combination of treatments is determined.

THINKING CRITICALLY

1. An 80-year-old client, Mrs. Parker, is terminally ill with cancer. An opiate analgesic has been prescribed for her pain. She is being cared for at home by family members who are concerned about pain control for their loved one. What should the client and family be taught about complications associated with use of opiate analgesia? Who would be the ideal person to assess and coordinate the client's response to dosing of a particular opiate or combination of opiate and non-opiate medications?

Factors to Consider. What complications are associated with the use of opiate analgesia? What factors contribute to the dosing schedule of a client with cancer-related pain? How much control over analgesia is given to the client? How should the caregiver and family monitor the response of the individual to the prescribed medication regimen?

Discussions for these questions can be found on the website.

BIBLIOGRAPHY

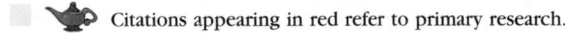

Citations appearing in red refer to primary research.

Citations appearing in blue refer to evidence-based practice guidelines and protocols.

1. Acute Pain Management Guideline Panel. (1992). *Acute pain management in adults: Operative procedures. Quick reference guide for clinicians* (AHCPR Pub. No. 92-0019). Rockville, Md: Agency for Health Care Policy and Research, U.S. Public Health Service, U.S. Department of Health and Human Services.
2. American Geriatrics Society. (2002). The management of persistent pain in older persons. *Journal of the American Geriatrics Society, 50*(6), S205-S224.
3. American Pain Foundation. (2007). Available at www.painfoundation.org.
4. American Pain Society. (2003). *Principles of analgesic use in the treatment of acute pain and cancer pain* (5th ed.). Glenview, Ill: Author.
5. American Society of Pain Management Nurses. (2002). *ASPMN Position statement: Pain management in patients with addictive disease*. Pensacola, Fla: Author.
6. American Society of Pain Management Nurses. (2002). In B. St. Marie (Ed.), *Core curriculum for pain management nursing*. Philadelphia: Saunders.
7. American Society of Pain Management Nurses. (1996). *ASPMN Position statement: Use of placebos for pain management*. Pensacola, Fla: Author.
8. Berkley, K.J., & Holdcroft, A. (1999). Sex and gender differences in pain. In P.D. Wall & R. Melzack (Eds.), *Textbook of pain* (4th ed., pp. 951-965). Edinburgh: Churchill Livingstone.
9. Brune, K., & Zeilhoffer, H.U. (1999). Antipyretic (non-narcotic) analgesics. In P.D. Wall & R. Melzack (Eds.), *Textbook of pain* (4th ed., pp. 1139-1153). Edinburgh: Churchill Livingstone.
10. Carroll, D., Moore, R.A., McQuay, H.J., et al. (2006). Transcutaneous electrical nerve stimulation for chronic pain. *Cochrane Database of Systematic Reviews, 4* (CD003222).
11. Cepedem, M.S., Carr, D.B., et al. (2006). Music for pain relief. *Cochrane Database of Systematic Reviews, 2* (CD004843).
12. Choi, P.T., Bhandari, M., et al. (2006). Epidural analgesia for pain relief following hip or knee replacement. *Cochrane Database of Systematic Reviews, 4* (CD003071).
13. Cleeland, C.S., et al. (1997). Pain and treatment of pain in minority patients with cancer: The Eastern Cooperative Oncology Group minority outpatient pain study. *Annals of Internal Medicine, 127*, 813-816.

14. French, S.D., Cameron, W., Walker, B.F., et al. (2006). Superficial heat or cold for low back pain. *Cochrane Database of Systematic Reviews, 1* (CD004750).
15. International Association for the Study of Pain. (1986). Pain terms: A current list with definitions and notes on usage. *Pain, 3*, S216-S221.
16. Jacox, A., et al. (1994). *Management of cancer pain. Clinical practice guidelines No. 9* (AHCPR Pub. No. 94-1592). Rockville, Md: Agency for Health Care Policy and Research.
17. Joint Commission on Accreditation of Healthcare Organizations. (2000). *Pain assessment and management: An organizational approach*. Oakbrook Terrace, Ill: Joint Commission on Accreditation of Healthcare Organizations.
18. Juarez, G., Ferrell, B., & Borneman, T. (1998). Influence of culture on cancer pain management in Hispanic patients. *Cancer Practice, 6*(5), 262-269.
19. Lander, J. (1990). Fallacies and phobias about addiction and pain. *British Journal of Addiction, 85*, 803-809.
20. Linton, S.J. (1999). Psychological factors. In I.K. Crombie, et al. (Eds.), *The epidemiology of pain* (pp. 25-42). Seattle: IASP Press.
21. Loitman, J.E. (2006). Enhanced analgesia with opioid antagonist administration. *Journal of Palliative Medicine, 9*(6), 1250-1253.
22. Manz, B., et al. (2000). Pain assessment in the cognitively impaired and unimpaired elderly. *Pain Management Nursing, 1*(4), 106-115.
23. Marks, R.M., & Scaher, E.J. (1973). Undertreatment of medical inpatients with narcotic analgesics. *Annals of Internal Medicine, 78*, 173-181.
24. McCaffery, M., & Pasero, C. (1999). *Pain: Clinical manual* (2nd ed.). St. Louis: Mosby.
25. Mobily, P., Herr, K., & Nicholson, A. (1994). Validation of cutaneous stimulation interventions for pain management. *International Journal of Nursing Studies, 31*, 533-544.
26. Moore, R., & Brodsgaard, I. (1999). Cross-cultural investigations of pain. In I.K. Crombie, et al. (Eds.), *Epidemiology of pain* (pp. 53-80). Seattle: IASP Press.
27. Papi, F., et al. (1995). Exposure to oscillating magnetic field influences sensitivity to electrical stimuli: II. Experiments on humans. *Bioelectromagnets, 16*, 295-300.
28. Pasero, C. (2003). Multimodal balanced analgesia in the PACU. *Journal of PeriAnesthesia Nursing, 18*(4), 265-268.
29. Payne, R., & Janjan, N. (1998). Management of metastatic bone pain. In R. Payne, et al. (Eds.), *Assessment and treatment of cancer pain: Progress in pain research and management* (Vol. 12, pp. 269-273). Seattle: IASP Press.
30. Prowse, M. (2007). Postoperative pain in older people: A review of the literature. *Journal of Clinical Nursing, 16*, 84-97.
31. Vadalouca, A., Siafaka, I., et al. (2006). Therapeutic management of chronic neuropathic pain: An examination of pharmacologic treatment. *Annals of New York Academic Science, 1088*, 164-186.
32. Wall, P. (1999). Placebos. In P.D. Wall & R. Melzack (Eds.), *Textbook of pain* (4th ed., pp. 1419-1430). Edinburgh: Churchill Livingstone.
33. Wang, Y., Sands, L.P., Mullen, E.A., et al. (2007). The effects of postoperative pain and its management on postoperative cognitive dysfunction. *American Journal of Geriatric Psychiatry, 15*(1), 50-59.
34. Wong, D., & Baker, C. (1988). Pain in children: Comparison of assessment scales. *Pediatric Nursing, 14*(1), 9-17.
35. World Health Organization (WHO). (1990). Cancer pain relief and palliative care. *Report of a WHO expert committee. Technical report series 804*. Geneva: Author.
36. Zeppetella, G., & Ribeiro, M. (2006). Opioids for the management of breakthrough (episodic) pain in cancer patients. *Cochrane Database of Systematic Reviews, 1* (CD004311).

evolve *Did you remember to check out the bonus material on the Evolve website and the CD-ROM, including NCLEX®-Examination Style Review Questions, Open-Book Quizzes, and Chapter Review Audio Podcasts?*

http://evolve.elsevier.com/Black/medsurg

CHAPTER 21

Perspectives in Palliative Care

Cynthia M. Sublett and Debra E. Heidrich

AMERICAN PERSPECTIVES ON DYING

"Passed on," "gone home," "laid to rest," "succumbed," and "passed away" are but some of the euphemisms that Carr (2006) suggests are phrases that help Americans acknowledge death. The words may or may not be a denial of death, but the truth is that Americans have lived for many years in a death-denying society. Perhaps it is the youth-oriented nature of American society that has caused this phenomenon. Scientific research that has enabled Americans to live longer has also encouraged a focus away from dying and death as a final stage of life.[14] Even the site of death has shifted from comforting the dying client at home to an aggressive cardiac and pulmonary resuscitation model in acute care institutions.[36] As a society, much community focus is and has been given to prominent individuals and celebrities who die, where grief and mourning are very public events. Yet, Americans have depersonalized death for themselves in contrast to the significance of the death of those who are celebrities and heroes.[14]

The sentinel work of Elisabeth Kübler-Ross and her phases of dying (Table 21-1)[52,53] in the 1960s, Dame Cicely Saunders and the hospice movement in England and subsequently in the United States,[6,40,72,106] the recognition that too many people were dying uncomfortable if not unnecessarily painful deaths from the SUPPORT study,[30,110] the Medicare Hospice Benefit in the 1980s,[30,67] and such programs as Last Acts[57] of the Robert Wood Johnson Foundation have brought dying and death to the forefront of American society. This surge of activity since the 1960s, summarized in the timeline presented in Table 21-2, indicates not only the increased focus on dying and death but also the fact that Americans may be acknowledging and talking about how they want to die more than in previous years. More families want to be present when their family members are dying. Although the denial of death may still have some prevalence in society, the acceptance of death as the final stage of life is increasing as well as the attitude of openness toward dying and death in families.[36,40,72]

The use of hospice care has steadily expanded since its inception in the 1960s. In 1985 about 160,000 clients were served, while in 2004 more than 1,000,000 individuals received hospice care, statistics that represent all hospice care and not just Medicare hospice.[81] Based on the preliminary data of the 2004 National Center for Health Statistics, of the 2,398,343 who died in the United States in 2004, approximately 40% of those individuals received hospice care,[80] up from 29% in 1999.[30,83]

PALLIATIVE CARE

Concept and Definitions

Palliative care, by definition of its derivative to palliate, and *palliare,* is a type of health care that focuses on alleviation of a client's symptoms, not on a cure.[36,118] The National Hospice and Palliative Care Organization (NHPCO) states that the goals of palliative care include improvement of the quality of life of those who are seriously ill and helping the family during and after any treatment they receive. Through an interdisciplinary team approach, palliative care provides support and care for individuals with life-limiting illnesses across all care settings and addresses the needs of the family as well as the client. That the client has choice is a major focus in the concept of palliative care.[82]

---

evolve **Web Enhancements**

Bridge to Home Health Care Providing Hospice Care

Diversity in Health Care Cultural Aspects of Death and Dying

Be sure to check out the bonus material on the Evolve website and the CD-ROM, including free self-assessment exercises. **http://evolve.elsevier. com/Black/medsurg**

TABLE 21–1 Stages of Dying According to Kübler-Ross

Stage	Clinical Manifestations
Denial	"This can't be true." "I'll be just fine after surgery (or radiation or chemotherapy)." Client and family may search for health care providers who will give more favorable opinion or may seek alternative therapies.
Anger	"Why me?" Client and family have feelings of resentment, envy, or anger directed at client, family, health care providers, God, and others.
Bargaining	"I just want to see my daughter's graduation, then I'll be ready . . ." Client (or family) asks for more time to reach an important life event and may make promises to God.
Depression	"I just don't know how my wife will get along after I'm gone." Family and client may grieve and mourn for impending losses.
Acceptance	"I have no regrets—I've done everything I've wanted to in my life and am proud of what I've accomplished." Client and family are neither angry nor depressed.

From Kübler-Ross, E. (1969). *On death and dying.* New York: Macmillan.

TABLE 21–2 Historical Timeline of the Evolution of Palliative and Hospice Care

1964	Elisabeth Kübler-Ross wrote *On death and dying: Acknowledging the fear of suffering and loneliness in death,* and encouraged planning of hospice movement.
1967	St. Christopher's Hospice, the first modern hospice, was opened in London by Dame Cicely Saunders.
1969	Dame Cicely Saunders came to United States at invitation of Dean Florence Wald of Yale University School of Nursing.
1972	Kübler-Ross testified before U.S. Senate Special Committee on Aging, advocating home care for dying.
1974	First home care hospice opened in United States at New Haven, Connecticut, supported by NCI funding.
1975	St. Luke's Hospital Center in New York established a second hospice within a medical center.
1978	National Hospice Organization was established, changed to National Hospice and Palliative Care Organization in 2000.
1978	U.S. Department of HEW established task force that would support hospice care for those with terminal illnesses as a viable alternative to acute curative care.
1978	National Cancer Institute (NCI) grant supports additional hospice projects, including incentive to open more hospices.
1979	Health Care Financing Administration (HCFA) supports hospice concept.
1980	44-bed inpatient unit opened at Connecticut Hospice funded by HCFA.
1982	Medicare Hospice Benefit passed by Congress.
1988	American Academy of Hospice and Palliative Medicine formed.
1989	Oncology Nursing Society developed guidelines for submission of nursing research studies for receipt of federal grants.
1989-	Phases 1 and 2 of Study to Understand Prognoses and Preferences for Outcomes and
1994	Risks of Treatment (SUPPORT): both descriptive and clinical trial research of nearly 10,000 clients that examined end-of-life care across country and found that it did not support quality end-of-life care.
1993	National Board for Certification of Hospice and Palliative Nurses (NBCHPN) to encourage certification and a higher quality of care.
1995	NHPCO established guidelines for noncancer diagnoses appropriate for palliative care.
2000	NHPCO awards Distinguished Research Award yearly to an individual who has made substantial contributions to hospice and palliative care.
2000	Center to Advance Palliative Care developed as part of Robert Wood Johnson Foundation (RWJF).
2000	Joint Commission for Accreditation of Healthcare Organizations (JCAHO) evaluates palliative care units in U.S. hospitals.
2002	Medicare Act established admission criteria for clients, including terminal illness, desiring hospice care, and doctor willing to provide records indicating terminal illness as well as a willingness to consult.
2004	End-of-Life Nursing Education Consortium (ELNEC) curriculum begun by American Association of Colleges of Nursing (AACN), RWJF, and City of Hope National Medical Center.

Modified from Goldberg, L. (2004). A survey of hospice and palliative care part I: Introduction and concepts. *Hospital Physician, 12,* 23-31; Hoffman, R. (2005). The evolution of hospice in America: Nursing's role in the movement. *Journal of Gerontological Nursing, 31*(7), 26-34; Meghani, S. (2004). A concept analysis of palliative care in the United States. *Journal of Advanced Nursing, 46*(2), 152-161.

While palliative care is a broad concept of care that focuses on the comfort of the client, one of the most well-known models of palliative care is hospice or end-of-life care that may be chosen when no further possibility of cure exists.[36] Even more typically, hospice and palliative care have been thought of specifically for cancer clients.[72] This was due, in part, if not fully, to the Medicare Hospice Benefit limitation that a client had to be diagnosed as having no more than 6 months to live. Although palliative care, hospice care, and end-of-life care may be heard in conversation interchangeably, as palliative care continues to emerge as a strong health care specialty, its broad nature becomes clearer and less confusing to health care providers as well as to the general public.[36,40,72]

Palliative care seeks to address the needs of all individuals with serious and other end-stage illnesses such as heart disease, cancer, stroke, chronic obstructive pulmonary disease, and diabetes mellitus. Many of these illnesses can cause protracted illness such that the symptoms are particularly burdensome and uncomfortable. Often, though this is changing, individuals with chronic illness other than cancer have not been treated in hospice or palliative care.[82,95] It is the hope of NHPCO and others that this fact will continue to change. In 2004 cancer diagnoses represented 46% of hospice admissions. Noncancer diagnoses such as end-stage heart disease, dementia, debility, lung disease, and end-stage kidney disease now account for the majority of the remaining admissions.[30,81]

The World Health Organization (WHO) recently expanded the definition of palliative care to include earlier integration of its precepts into the course of illness and provided the following definition:[30,122]

> Palliative care is an approach that improves the quality of life of clients and their families facing the problems associated with life-threatening illness, through the prevention and relief of suffering by means of early identification and impeccable assessment and treatment of pain and other problems that are physical, psychosocial and spiritual.

Like hospice care, palliative care recognizes that dying is a normal process that should be neither hastened nor postponed. The provision of symptom management that includes emotional and spiritual support for clients and their families is considered when developing the plan of care to promote an optimal dying experience followed by family bereavement.[9,64,68,110]

While the focus of this chapter will be primarily on palliative care at the end of life and the care models that serve that purpose, concepts that relate to palliative care before discussions of end-of-life care will also be addressed. (NOTE: in this chapter the word *symptom* is used instead of *clinical manifestations*, the term used elsewhere in the text. Common symptoms associated with comfort and the dying process differ from clinical manifestations that accompany specific medical problems. Symptom management is the preferred term often used in the care of clients with advanced illness and is the primary focus within the specialty of palliative care.)

Role of Nurses

Nurses caring for clients with advanced diseases will ultimately witness not only the symptoms that accompany the advanced diseases but also the final stage of life that is the process of dying. The dying process is usually accompanied by a myriad of psychological, spiritual, and physical needs about which nurses must be knowledgeable and able to address. Control of related symptoms, particularly pain, and working within the interdisciplinary team to provide optimal support and symptom management for dying clients and their families are major aspects of the role nurses have in palliative care.[40]

"Nurses spend more time with clients and their families than do any other health professionals and are in the most immediate position to provide care, comfort, and counsel at the end-of-life, when critical decisions must be reached and compassionate and highly specialized care provided."[63] Desirably, a less abrupt shift to palliative care decision occurs early in the client's care such that the client has the opportunity to receive the benefit of comfort measures throughout care and especially at the end of life.[36,37] Nurses are in a position not only to provide the care but also to identify clients who may be candidates for the comfort care that a hospice or palliative care unit provides.

Focus on Quality of Life

Palliative care is offered when a progressive illness is symptomatic and interferes with the quality of life. Many variables go into defining quality of life, including (1) socioeconomic status, (2) physical health, (3) relationships with friends and family, and (4) satisfaction with self.[48,93] Quality of life is defined as "a personal statement of the positivity or negativity of attributes that characterize life."[48] Olson (2001) asserts that comfort affects quality of life because of similar characteristics that exist for both. Additionally, quality of life is individually defined by clients by the closeness of client expectations and the reality of a situation. If the gap between these two concepts is large, the client may view their quality of life as less than those who have been able to achieve a new balance of body and mind in coping with progressive illness.[84] The American Geriatrics Society issued principles of quality end-of-life care and stated that clients should have quality of life in spite of declining physical health.[113]

A person's quality of life is often linked to the experience of symptom distress and the meanings that the person assigns to these physical sensations.[48,84,93] Nurses caring for clients who are experiencing distressing symptoms, such as pain, fatigue, constipation, and nausea, should understand that each client responds differently. The effect of a symptom on life routines varies from client to client, depending on overall functional status, coping abilities, and social supports. A palliative plan of care must be based not only on symptom management but also on the effect of the symptom and the burden of the intervention on the client's overall quality of living as well as the expectations.[113]

Hospice Care as a Model of Palliative Care

Goldberg[36] notes that "Hospice care is a particular model for the delivery of excellent palliative care." He further states that differing from palliative care, the hospice philosophy is clear in its acknowledgment of the eventual death. No attempt to avoid the death by furthering treatment is made.[36,49] As the historical information (see Table 21-2) supports, hospice care was initiated on the basis of a quality-oriented alternative to the traditional biomedical model of health care with the intent to ensure that clients and their families could have appropriate care at the end of life.* The genesis for hospice initially was in protest against the aggressive use of science to battle disease and choose instead the "quality-of-life alternative" offered by hospice.[42] Hospice care was enacted in part to a change in climate that rejected aggressive biotechnical interventions at the end of life, and allowed clients to die at home with quality care from a skilled interdisciplinary team.[27,41,42]

The National Hospice and Palliative Care Organization (NHPCO) stated that there are 3650 total hospice programs nationwide as of 2004. In January 2006 Medicare identified 2884 hospice organizations. For 2 decades, the Medicare Hospice Benefit has provided full coverage for terminally ill older Americans. Nearly, 65% of hospice clients are over the age of 75 years, a figure that has been steadily increasing. Although many Americans still die in hospital or nursing home beds rather than in their own homes, NHPCO reports that more than 40% of individuals who died in 2004 used hospice care services.[30,57,81] While the use of hospice care in the United States is still limited, more Americans are aware of the care that hospice can provide to improve their quality of end-of-life care and to help them avoid unnecessary suffering.[30] Although some believe there is continued lack of use possibly because of the difficulty physicians have in determining prognoses in terms of 6 months or less,[83] other leaders in this health care field are encouraged about the increase in use of hospice and palliative care services.[30,83] (See the Bridge to Home Health Care feature on Providing Hospice Care on the website.)

The concept of a "good death" is one that is noted more frequently in the literature when quality end-of-life care is considered.[7,23] Other terms that describe this phenomenon include peaceful death, natural death, healthy death, and dignified death. Numerous definitions exist to describe a good death, most of which reference being comfortable, being with family, dying with dignity, and having control over the situation such that needs and wishes are met.[7,39]

Other cultures, particularly the Asian culture, believe that providing a good death for a loved one means that the family did what they should for their family member. Western cultures focus primarily on providing the good death for the client and do not acknowledge its importance for caregivers as frequently as Asian cultures do.[39] American professional caregivers have an increased sense of self-worth if they have helped a dying person to have a good and peaceful death. In the intensive care environment where heroic attempts to save lives occur, professional caregivers have begun to examine a good death for these clients once a determination has been made that the advanced care is no longer able to provide a cure.[7]

*References 8, 9, 10, 30, 36, 40, 42, 72.

DISEASE TRAJECTORY

The leading causes of death in the United States include heart disease, cancer, stroke, chronic obstructive pulmonary disease, and dementia.[114] All of these diseases have a relatively predictable course. The disease trajectory is identified from the onset of a life-limited diagnosis until death. Some terminal diagnoses have a long disease trajectory with a gradual decline in functional status over time; others have a very short trajectory with a sharp decline; still others have variable trajectories with periods of remission and exacerbation.[66,96] The vast majority of Americans, however, who die each year are older adults with a median age of 77 years, and they typically suffer from a slow, progressive chronic disease.[80,81] Women will average about 3 years at the end of life with progressively debilitating illness, whereas men will often have 2 years with a serious progressive disability, all of whom could benefit from palliative care.[45]

Establishing specific interventions to improve each client's quality of life is determined largely by the client's position on the disease trajectory. A comprehensive assessment is essential when determining the client's disease trajectory to guide identification of appropriate palliative interventions. This assessment comprises the following actions:

1. Define the nature of the clinical findings and symptoms.
2. Perform a thorough history and physical examination, review current and previous medications, and evaluate a minimal set of diagnostic procedures to differentiate underlying pathophysiologic disorders from a reversible symptom.
3. Evaluate the problem within the context of the client's situation and allow for prioritization. For example, the priority assigned a urinary tract infection (UTI) in a cognitively impaired, dehydrated, and bedridden client will be different from that given to a UTI in a cognitively intact client with good symptom control.
4. Define the "cost" of diagnostic and therapeutic interventions and the varying differences between clients (for example, what may be considered appropriate therapy for one client may be inappropriate for another) when evaluating the risk versus benefit of treatment and the financial burden of unnecessary interventions.
5. Discuss the various care options with the client and the family and encourage informed decision making.[64]

SYMPTOMS AT THE END OF LIFE

Scientific palliative care is assessment driven and evidence based to promote the integration of rational decision making and treatment in the management of common symptoms.[24] Palliative care leaders recognize that symptom control throughout the trajectory of illness is essential.[96] Clients with advanced diseases experience multiple symptoms, some of which are more severe than others,[96,110] and each client must be assessed to determine the cause of each symptom and base the appropriate interventions on the underlying cause.[96] In one study, pain was found to be the most prevalent symptom among clients with advanced cancer (89% of respondents). In 87% of clients with pain, the severity of the pain was rated as moderate to severe. In addition to pain, the symptoms of weakness, anorexia, dyspnea, constipation, early satiety, fatigue, and dry mouth were experienced by more than 40% of clients.[91,96,110] Increasingly, the symptoms are being discussed under the concept of suffering that threatens the psychosocial and spiritual aspects of self when physical and emotional symptoms are present. It can be noted that it is rare for only one symptom to be the cause of suffering, but it can sustain the suffering.[86,108]

Symptoms vary not only in frequency and intensity but also in the distress experienced by clients. Although pain may be prevalent, it is not always identified as the most distressing symptom. Some studies have found that dyspnea, asthenia (lethargy, generalized weakness, and fatigue), dry mouth, anorexia, depression, and insomnia may actually be more distressing than pain for clients with terminal illnesses.[8,12,110] The management of symptoms includes nonpharmacologic and pharmacologic interventions. When using medications, care should always be given to titration of the dose to effect. Oftentimes, complex palliative care clients encounter polypharmacy with the idea of "one symptom, one drug," whereas the ideal is to use one medication that palliates multiple symptoms.[24,110] On occasion, pain and suffering become refractory. When this occurs, medication changes must occur along with a multidimensional assessment of physical and emotional suffering.[108] See the Case Study "Cancer of the Prostate at the End of Life," p. 896, in Chapter 38, for application of many concepts that follow.

Pain

Pain is a multidimensional phenomenon. Not only is a person's pain experience a physical response to an underlying disorder or disease state, but various emotional, intellectual, behavioral, sensory, and cultural dimensions also influence the pain experience.[29,92] When a client is nonresponsive and unable to report pain, the nurse should observe for the behavioral indicators of pain (Table 21-3). Both excellent assessment of the client and communication within the entire health care team are essential for optimal pain management.[86,103,108] Chapter 20 describes types of pain, subjective and objective assessment of pain, and pain management strategies.

TABLE 21-3 Behavioral Indicators of Pain in the Nonresponsive Client

Restlessness	Agitation
Vocalizations	Moaning
Muscle tension	Tense muscles
Facial expression	Frowning
Physiologic indicators	Fast heart rate

Data from Kuebler, K., & Ogle, K. (1998). Psychometric evaluation of an objective assessment instrument to measure pain, dyspnea, and restlessness (Abstract). *Journal of Palliative Care, 14,* 125; Sherman, D., Matzo, M., Paice, J., et al. (2004). Learning pain assessment and management: A goal of the end-of-life nursing education consortium. *The Journal of Continuing Education in Nursing, 35*(3), 107-120.

Opioid Analgesics

Opioids are the mainstay of treatment for moderate to severe pain.[2,108,122,125] These medications bind with opiate receptors in the central nervous system (CNS) and block the transmission of pain impulses to the higher brain centers. Most opioid medications bind to the mu receptor and are called mu agonists. Morphine (MS Contin), hydromorphone (Dilaudid), fentanyl (Duragesic), and oxycodone (OxyContin) are examples of mu-agonist opioids frequently used in the treatment of pain.[1,24,91] There is no ceiling to the analgesic effect of mu-agonist opioids.[17,112] See Chapter 20 for further discussion of opioid therapy.

In addition to modulating the transmission and perception of the pain impulse, opioids may bind with receptors in other tissues, leading to the potential for side effects. For example, opioid receptors are present in the gastrointestinal tract. When opioids bind with these receptors, intestinal motility is decreased and gastric emptying is delayed, leading to constipation. Prophylactic treatment of constipation with both a stool softener and a stimulant is essential and should be initiated along with the first opioid dose. The clinician should not wait for the client to complain of constipation before beginning treatment. Constipation is the only side effect of opioids to which a person does not develop tolerance. A bowel protocol must be continued for the duration of treatment with opioids.[2,96]

Other potential side effects of opioids are respiratory depression, nausea and vomiting, and sedation. Clinically significant respiratory depression is rare during treatment of pain if the opioid dose is increased slowly and decreased if sedation is noted. In addition, some clients develop tolerance to the respiratory-depressive side effects of opioids after the first several days of treatment. The client who has taken the same dose of an opioid for several weeks is not at risk for a clinically significant opioid-induced respiratory depression.[92,112]

Although nausea and vomiting may not be problems for all clients, many clients do experience these problems as a side effect of opioids. Nausea and vomiting occur when the chemoreceptor trigger zone of the brain is stimulated by these medications. A client is less likely to experience nausea when opioids are administered orally than when they are administered parenterally. As with respiratory depression, tolerance to this side effect of opioids develops over time. Clients who experience nausea and vomiting should be treated with antiemetics for the first 2 to 3 days after the opioid is initiated until tolerance develops. A small number of clients experience persistent nausea from the opioids. These clients may benefit from either changing to a different opioid or continuing to use antiemetics.[17]

A client who has been in pain and receives an initial dose of an opioid may experience some degree of sedation, in part as a result of the direct effect of opioids on the brain. In addition to the sedative side effect of the opioid, however, the client is probably exhausted from not sleeping well while in pain. The nurse should teach the client that some sleepiness is expected and that it is probably not due entirely to the new medication. As with the other side effects of opioids, tolerance to the sedation develops after the first 2 to 3 days. If, however, the client is difficult to arouse or the sedation lasts more than 2 to 3 days, the opioid dose may be too high for the intensity of the pain.[69,86]

Clients who are sedated by an opioid and still are experiencing pain probably have pain syndromes that are not completely responsive to opioids. These clients require the addition of adjuvant medications to achieve comfort. Recognize that there is no ceiling to the amount of opioid analgesic required for each client to achieve a satisfactory level of analgesia. Hence, clients may require very high doses of opioids to achieve pain reduction. Occasionally, opioid analgesics will need to be changed for varying reasons, such as an increase of morphine metabolites contributing to agitation. When this occurs, the dosage of a different drug must be equianalgesic to ensure the same or higher level of pain control and not a decrease in pain control[86,103] (see Table 20-3).

Adjuvant Analgesics

Adjuvant medications have a primary action other than pain reduction but also can serve as analgesics for some painful conditions.[17,65] They are often used in combination with other analgesic medications. At each step of the WHO analgesic ladder (see Chapter 20), adjuvant medications may be added, depending on the type of pain experienced. Several classes of medications are essential to optimal management of pain (Table 21-4). Nonsteroidal anti-inflammatory drugs (NSAIDs) can be helpful when the inflammatory process is involved and is initiating the pain impulse, such as in bone or soft-tissue damage. Clients with metastatic bone disease often require the combination of an opioid and an NSAID for comfort.

Tricyclic antidepressants (TCAs) and anticonvulsants can be effective analgesics in the management of pain syndromes that have a neurologic component.[17,86,91] TCAs appear to be most helpful for pain described as burning or aching; anticonvulsants are useful in the treatment of shooting and shock-like neurologic pains. The effective analgesic dose of a TCA is much lower than the dose required for an antidepressant effect.[2,17,86,91] Some clients are aware that these medications are used to treat depression and may be suspicious that the clinician "thinks the pain is in my head." It is important to explain to clients that these medications are used to manage pain at low doses. Because it takes 5 to 7 days for TCAs to reach the desired plasma level, inform the client that it may take several days for this new medication to be effective.

Clients who report "colicky" pain may be experiencing the discomfort of smooth muscle spasm or have pain from bowel obstruction. This type of pain is best treated with an anticholinergic medication or somatostatin analog, such as octreotide, and corticosteroids.[65]

Anxiety is a complex symptom that is caused by physical, emotional, and spiritual concerns. Clients who

---

TABLE 21-4 Adjuvant Analgesics

Pain Source	Pain Character	Medication Class	Examples
Bone or soft tissue	Tenderness over bone or joint Pain on movement	Nonsteroidal anti-inflammatory drugs	Ibuprofen Naproxen Indomethacin
Nerve damage/neuropathic	Burning, shooting, shock-like, or aching pain	Tricyclic antidepressants	Amitriptyline Doxepin
		Anticonvulsants	Carbamazepine Phenytoin Valproic acid Gabapentin
Smooth muscle spasms	Cramping or grabbing pains (intermittent)	Anticholinergics	Scopolamine Hyoscyamine Oxybutynin Dicyclomine
Anxiety	Generalized restlessness and discomfort	Benzodiazepines	Lorazepam Diazepam
		Butyrophenones	Haloperidol

are in pain often experience some anxiety, and it may be helpful to treat the anxiety to achieve comfort.[85,86,90,91] Benzodiazepine medications are frequently used for anxiety in the palliative care setting. Haloperidol, a butyrophenone, may also be used. Management of anxiety is covered in Chapter 23.

Analgesic Dosing

The initial analgesic dose is determined based on the type and intensity of pain as well as the response to current analgesics. Medication doses are titrated up or down to achieve effectiveness, both at the beginning of therapy and during the course of treatment. For example, a client receiving morphine for bone pain may find that a lower dose of morphine is possible when a NSAID is added to the regimen. Gradual escalation of the dose is required if pain reduction is inadequate. For unrelieved opioid-responsive pain problems, the opioid dose can be safely increased by 25% to 50% for mild to moderate pain (rating of 1 to 3 on a 0 to 10 scale); by 50% to 100% for moderate pain (rating of 4 to 7 on a 0 to 10 scale); and by up to 100% for severe pain (rating of 8 to 10 on a 0 to 10 scale).[69,103] The goal is to use the smallest dose that reduces the pain so that it causes the fewest side effects.

Therapeutic levels of analgesics must be maintained at all times for clients with persistent or chronic pain to manage the pain. Therefore an around-the-clock (ATC) schedule (see next section) is most appropriate.[2,86,91] The frequency of doses to maintain therapeutic levels is determined by the route of administration and the duration of action of the medication. Immediate-release (short-acting) oral morphine requires dosing every 4 hours; oral hydromorphone (Dilaudid) may need to be given every 3 hours. Controlled-release medications offer the benefit of more convenient dosing schedules (every 8, 12, or 24 hours). When a client has experienced pain relief for 24 to 48 hours, the 24-hour dose can be converted to an extended-release medication, particularly if the client has continuous pain.[103]

Rescue Dosing

The goal of ATC dosing is to keep the level of the analgesic in a range high enough to manage the pain but below the point at which the client experiences avoidable or unmanageable side effects. Unfortunately, pain does not stay at the same intensity 24 hours a day. Many clients experience pain above the normal baseline pain; this pain is often labeled breakthrough pain. The pain may spike above (break through) the therapeutic blood level of analgesia, and additional medications are required to manage such episodes. A short-acting (or immediate-release) dose of an opioid should be administered to "cover" the spike in the client's pain.[2,86,91]

For clients taking oral opioids, the recommended rescue dose is in the range of 5% to 15% of the total 24-hour ATC dose of opioid.[2,28,103] The rescue dose may be repeated hourly for oral administration, in 30 minutes for subcutaneous administration, and in 15 minutes for IV administration. For parenteral infusions, the breakthrough dose can be calculated at 50% to 100% of the hourly rate of the infusion. The client who experiences end-of-dose failure because of the development of pain before the next dose needs reevaluation of the ATC medication regimen.[103] As a rule, a client who requires more than four rescue doses during a 24-hour period or is awakened from sleep experiencing pain should have the pain experience reevaluated.[19] An increase in the ATC dose is often appropriate under these circumstances.

Dyspnea

Dyspnea is a subjective experience described as difficult breathing or an "uncomfortable awareness" of breathing that accounts for a high proportion of the client's inability to carry out activities of daily living (ADL) and gravely affects the perceived quality of life.[15,25,61,119] Dyspnea occurs in as many as 50% to 70% of clients at the end of life.[1,119] Clients also mention labored breathing, shortness of breath, and feelings of suffocation.[55] The continuous exhaustion that accompanies breathlessness can be one of the most devastating symptoms for both the client and the observing family members.[55,119]

Disease processes commonly associated with dyspnea include (1) acute and chronic pulmonary disorders, (2) heart failure, and (3) neuromuscular disorders. In the terminally ill population, anemia and generalized weakness also can contribute to dyspnea. In addition, emotions play a major role. The fear associated with the inability to "catch one's breath" can lead to panic and worsen the sensation of dyspnea.[15,24,25,55,119] As it progresses, clients experience depression, panic, anxiety, and insomnia.[1]

Assessment

Assessment of clients with dyspnea includes subjective and observational data. Clients should be asked to rate dyspnea on a scale. The scale must make sense to the client, and all people caring for that client must use the same scale. A visual analog scale such as the Borg scale[47]—with "not at all breathless" at the low end of the scale and "severely breathless" at the high end—may be helpful for quantifying this symptom.[54] This information can help determine the severity of the symptom and provides a baseline to evaluate the effectiveness of interventions.[102] Clients' evaluations of their own functional status and the effect of dyspnea on ADL provide helpful information about both the physical and the emotional responses to dyspnea.[5,119]

An objective assessment of the client provides additional information about dyspnea.[54] The nurse should observe for an increased respiratory rate, use of accessory muscles, gasping or labored breathing, restlessness, and diaphoresis.

Management

The underlying cause of dyspnea should be treated as appropriate for the client's position in the disease trajectory. For example, pneumonia in a client who is alert and oriented and has a good quality of life (as determined by the client) should be treated. It may be appropriate, however, not to treat pneumonia in a client who is clearly near the end of the disease trajectory if treatment of the pneumonia will not improve the quality of life. All treatment options should be reviewed with the client and family, including the option of no treatment.[15,54,119]

Although it may not be possible to treat the underlying cause of dyspnea at the end of life, many effective interventions can be used to manage the distress and uncomfortable sensations associated with dyspnea.[15,54,119] Interdisciplinary team support is essential in the management of dyspnea. The psychosocial and existential issues that contribute to the symptom of dyspnea require the support of professionals trained in these areas.

Opioids. Morphine is widely used for the relief of dyspnea.[15,47,116,118] There is strong evidence from a systematic review[47] that oral and parenteral opioids are effective in the treatment of breathlessness in chronic obstructive pulmonary disease (COPD) clients.[47] Exactly why opioids alleviate dyspnea is not known, but they are believed to blunt the perceptual response to dyspnea, to reduce the respiratory drive, or possibly to decrease oxygen consumption at rest and during exercise.[15,25,47,61] There is no standard optimal dose of morphine for the treatment of dyspnea, but the following recommendations are based on clinical experience:

- For the client who is already taking morphine for pain and who is dyspneic, the morphine dose should be increased by 50%.
- The dyspneic client who has not been receiving morphine should be started on 5 to 6 mg of morphine every 4 hours as needed.[61]

It may be appropriate to consider ATC dosing of morphine if the client is requiring frequent "as needed" doses. Sustained-release preparations may be more convenient and effective in this situation.[25,61]

Anti-anxiety Agents. Both benzodiazepines and phenothiazines have been effective in the management of dyspnea. Each class of drugs has the potential to depress hypoxic or ventilator responses and to alter the emotional responses to dyspnea.[25,93] Both classes of medications have the potential for side effects, but given the prevalence of anxiety associated with the experience of breathlessness, it is considered good palliative care to try anxiolytic therapy on an individual basis.[25,93]

Bronchodilators. Bronchodilators help to decrease the effort of breathing, and several studies cite their effects on breathlessness. The significant decrease in dyspnea after theophylline use is believed to result from an improvement in the length-tension relationship in the diaphragm.[24,119]

Corticosteroids. Corticosteroids are commonly used in the palliative care setting to treat dyspnea. These medications are believed to influence the symptom of dyspnea by decreasing inflammation in the pulmonary tissue and increasing bronchodilation.[15,24,119] Corticosteroid therapy is indicated when bronchodilators have been ineffective. A trial of corticosteroids is justified in almost all clients with problematic chronic airway disease, pointing out that the dose of steroid should be high enough to work efficiently but low enough not to cause potential gastric irritation or fluid retention.[25]

Oxygen Therapy. Palliative care literature does not support the use of oxygen therapy for the relief of dyspnea. Oxygen (O_2) therapy should be used only for clients who are hypoxic or who tend to have pulmonary hypertension. If O_2 saturation is less than 90% with room air, the clinician may want to (1) consider O_2 by nasal cannula at 1 to 3 L per minute, (2) recheck the client's O_2 saturation in 20 to 30 minutes, and (3) titrate the O_2 therapy up to 6 L per minute by nasal cannula if necessary.[15,25,55,119]

Nonpharmacologic Interventions. Nurses are frequently the care providers who introduce nonpharmacologic interventions to clients and families and ensure, through education and support, that the interventions are being used to maximal effectiveness. Some interventions that nurses can initiate that will contribute to the comfort of clients experiencing dyspnea are (1) pursed-lip breathing, (2) breathing exercises, (3) positioning, (4) having a fan blowing in the room, (5) coping techniques, (6) a calming presence, (7) relaxation therapy, (8) massage, (9) acupuncture, (10) hypnosis, and (11) visualization.[15,25,55,119]

Delirium

Incidence

Delirium is one of the most common complications seen in clients with advanced illness. Studies show a wide range of occurrence rates, likely resulting from nonstandardized diagnostic criteria, heterogeneous study populations, and varying study settings.[58] Two prospective studies showed that 20% to 42% of clients with advanced cancer admitted to acute palliative care units had delirium on admission and that delirium developed in 33% to 45% of the other clients over the course of their care in the palliative care unit. Additionally, these studies showed that 50% of the episodes of delirium were reversible.[31,59] Data support that early detection and appropriate intervention improve behavioral and cognitive symptoms, promote a better clinical outcome, and decrease health care costs.[31,62,75] Delirium in the last 24 to 48 hours of life, sometimes referred to as "terminal restlessness," is likely due to irreversible processes such as multiple organ failure and is often not reversible.[34]

Various terms have been used to describe delirium, such as acute brain failure, acute confusional state, acute secondary psychosis, exogenous psychosis, sundown syndrome, and organic brain syndrome.[11,20] According to the criteria of the American Psychiatric Association's *Diagnostic and Statistical Manual of Mental Disorders (DSM-IV-TR)*,[3] delirium is defined as "an etiologically non-specific, global, cerebral dysfunction characterized by concurrent disturbances of level of consciousness, attention, thinking, perception, memory, psychomotor behavior, emotion, and the sleep-wake cycle." It is often identified as a sudden and significant decline in a previous level of functioning and is conceptualized as a reversible process. Delirium can also affect sleep, psychomotor activity, and emotions.[20,44,56,111]

DSM-IV-TR criteria for delirium are as follows:[3]

1. Disturbance of consciousness with reduced ability to focus, sustain, or shift attention
2. A change in cognition (such as memory deficit, disorientation, language disturbance) or the development of a perceptual disturbance that is not better accounted for by pre-existing, established, or evolving dementia
3. Development of the disturbance over a short time (usually hours to days) and a tendency to fluctuate over the course of the day

Assessment

The diagnosis of delirium is based on careful observation and awareness of its key features. Because the clinical manifestations are nonspecific, the clinician must (1) look for manifestations of a disturbance in consciousness and a change in cognition, (2) identify the rapidity of onset, and (3) assess for associated medical and environmental risks that lead to a definitive diagnosis. Delirium is often unrecognized by clinicians and may be misdiagnosed, commonly as dementia or depression.[20,44,97]

Integrating a screening assessment tool into usual care can facilitate the early recognition and treatment of delirium.[32] The most commonly used assessment instrument for identifying cognitive impairment is the Mini-Mental State Examination (MMSE). This instrument evaluates orientation, attention, recall, and language.[20,44] While it is not specific for delirium, it does not require specialized training to administer and can be used to identify those clients that should have additional screening. The Nursing Delirium Screening Scale (Nu-DESC), a five-item tool based on the *DMS-IV* criteria for delirium, is a recently developed accurate and sensitive 24-hour screening instrument for use by nurses.[32,33]

Management

The prognosis for the client experiencing delirium is often poor. Delirium shortens the survival of cancer clients, makes the assessment of pain and symptoms difficult, and is a main cause of distress among clients, family, and health care providers.[24] This fact, however, should not deter the clinician from looking for an underlying cause because a significant number of cases are reversible. The first-line approach to the treatment of delirium is to identify and treat any reversible causes, such as (1) medications (e.g., opioids, sedatives, anticholinergics, and steroids), (2) hypoxia, (3) dehydration (see the Translating Evidence into Practice box on p. 394), (4) metabolic causes (e.g., hypercalcemia, hyponatremia), (5) sepsis, (6) polypharmacy, and (7) intracranial pressure from metastatic disease.[20,44,111] Interventions that may be helpful to reverse or lessen the symptoms of delirium are listed in Table 21-5.

Haloperidol (Haldol) is the drug of choice for managing hallucinations and agitation in the medically ill client except when alcohol or benzodiazepine withdrawal is suspected. A benzodiazepine can be added to the regimen if haloperidol alone is not effective. Caution should be considered when using benzodiazepines that have a long half-life, such as diazepam (Valium), because the active metabolites can accumulate in the dehydrated and dying client and create agitation. Lorazepam (Ativan) may be considered to reduce episodes of severe distress and anxiety. Transdermal clonidine (Catapres), an alpha-adrenergic agonist, may be useful for clients suffering from autonomic symptoms such as anxiety and tachycardia. If the agitation does not respond to these pharmacologic agents, sedation may be achieved with chlorpromazine (Thorazine) or midazolam (Versed).[20,44,85]

TRANSLATING EVIDENCE INTO PRACTICE

Dehydration

Historically the standard care in the management of dehydration is replacing fluids or hydrating the client. Traditional hospice models, however, have discouraged artificial hydration, as patients may experience less edema, dyspnea, nausea, and urinary incontinence with the "natural dehydration" of dying. Evidence can be found to support both approaches.[1-5] Near the end of life, it is important for the nurse to recognize that dehydration may actually exacerbate symptoms and create suffering.[6] Renal failure can cause the accumulation of active drug metabolites, leading to symptoms such as confusion and delirium. As an example, drug accumulation from opioid therapies can create nausea, confusion, restlessness, delirium, and myoclonus and possibly lead to hyperalgesia. As a result, clients may be less able to communicate with their families. Some hydration in this case might be helpful. Dehydration can also be helpful in avoiding the pulmonary edema that may occur because the body cannot make use of fluids during the dying process.[6] There is a fine line between hydration and dehydration in the terminally ill client, and the emphasis should be placed on comfort measures and the reduction of symptoms.[1,6] Clients and families need to make informed choices about hydration, recognizing that it can help or hinder the dying process.[6]

The nurse should not confuse edema and thirst as indicators of over-hydration or dehydration. Edema can be the result of underlying pathophysiology, for example, advanced cancer. Edema in this client is more likely a result of tumor blockage accompanied by impaired venous or lymphatic drainage, not fluid overload. Thirst or dry mouth may also be the result of specific medications frequently used in palliative care (e.g., anticholinergic medications, opioids, tricyclic antidepressants) and not necessarily a sign of a fluid deficit.

IMPLICATIONS

When making the decision to hydrate the client, the health care provider considers the various options that are available based on the client's setting. Clients able to take fluids by mouth should be encouraged to do so because oral consumption is considered the preferred route. Clients who are unable to maintain adequate fluid intake by mouth should be considered for parenteral fluid replacement. Clients in the acute care setting usually have intravenous (IV) lines inserted, which allow for replacement of fluids. Several studies have demonstrated that if the client cannot tolerate an IV or resides in the home care setting, the preferred route for hydration is a subcutaneous route, also known as hypodermoclysis or clysis.[1-5]

Hypodermoclysis is easily accomplished by inserting a 25-gauge butterfly needle subcutaneously; the site can be used for up to 7 days.[2-5] Rehydration is accomplished with the infusion of normal saline at 70 to 100 ml/hour via continuous infusion.

Hypodermoclysis is also used when providing fluid maintenance or augmentation with infusions of $^2/_3$ dextrose and $^1/_3$ normal saline via a continuous infusion of 40 to 80 ml/hour. Other rates can include 1000 ml by gravity overnight or a 500-ml bolus twice a day infused over 1 hour.

REFERENCES

1. Bruera, E., & Sweeny, B. (2001). Hydrate or dehydrate. *Supportive Care Cancer, 9*(3), 177-186.
2. Cerchietti, L., et al. (2000). Hypodermoclysis for control of dehydration in terminal stage cancer. *International Journal of Palliative Nursing, 6*(8), 370-374.
3. Frisoli, J., et al. (2000). Subcutaneous hydration by hypodermoclysis. A practical and low cost treatment for elderly patients. *Drugs and Aging, 16*(4), 313-319.
4. Lanuke, K., Fainsinger, R., & Demoissac, D. (2004). Hydrations management at the end of life. *Journal of Palliative Medicine, 7*(2):257-263.
5. Moriarty, D., & Hudson, E. (2001). Hypodermoclysis for rehydration in the community. *British Journal of Community Nursing, 6*(9), 437-443.
6. Zerwekh, J. (2003). End-of-life hydration: Benefit or burden? Teach your patient the pros and cons so they can make informed decisions. *Nursing 2003, 33*(2), 1-3.

TABLE 21–5 Reversible Causes of Delirium

Cause	Intervention
1. Medications	
a. Opioid metabolites may accumulate, especially in presence of renal insufficiency	a. Consider switching to an equianalgesic dose of a different opioid.
b. Benzodiazepine metabolites may accumulate in presence of hepatic disease	b. Hydration may be helpful to assist in eliminating these metabolites. If anti-anxiety medications are needed, consider switching client to a butyrophenone.
2. Hypoxia	2. Intervene to improve oxygenation with bronchodilators, mucolytics, and breathing techniques. Consider oxygen therapy if O_2 saturation is <90%.
3. Dehydration	3. Consider oral or parenteral hydration.
4. Metabolic	
a. Hypercalcemia	a. Evaluate benefits of hydration and use of bisphosphonates.
b. Hyponatremia	b. Encourage moderate alcohol intake before meals and encourage sodium intake.
5. Sepsis	5. Consider anti-infective therapy.
6. Polypharmacy	6. Eliminate unnecessary medications. Use medications that have more than one action to treat symptoms (e.g., Haldol to decrease delirium and nausea).
7. Increased intracranial pressure from metastatic disease	7. Use corticosteroids to decrease cerebral edema.

Depression

The prevalence of depression in clients with cancer ranges anywhere from 10% to 25%. The prevalence appears to increase in the presence of functional losses, advancing illness, and unmanaged symptoms.[85] It is believed that many cases of depression in the terminally ill go unrecognized by clinicians because many of the clinical manifestations of depression (e.g., fatigue, anorexia or weight loss, insomnia) can be attributed to the disease process itself. Key indicators of clinical depression in the terminally ill are (1) alterations in mood; (2) feelings of hopelessness, worthlessness, or excessive guilt; and (3) recurrent death wishes, including thoughts of suicide.[85] The *DSM-IV-TR* defines a major depressive syndrome when five of the following symptoms have been present for 2 weeks or longer: depressed mood, anhedonia, weight loss or gain, insomnia or hypersomnia, agitation or motor retardation, fatigue or loss of energy, depreciation or guilt feelings, concentration difficulties, or thoughts of death or suicide.[3]

Etiology

A terminal diagnosis potentiates both anxiety and depression. A client with a family or personal history of previous depressive episodes is at even higher risk for depression than the general population. Interestingly, some cancer diagnoses, such as pancreatic cancer, have been associated more strongly with depression. It is not clear whether psychological or physiologic factors are involved in this higher risk.[3,11,13]

Depression is thought to be a direct result of abnormal serotonin (5-hydroxytryptamine [5-HT]) neurotransmission in the CNS. This abnormal secretion may be genetic, or it may be induced by some unknown mechanism. Other neurotransmitters, such as gamma-aminobutyric acid (GABA) and norepinephrine, have also been closely linked in anxiety and may be associated with depression.[85]

Assessment

Nurses play a pivotal role in identifying clients with depression. A simple, valid, and reliable screening question for depression is simply to ask, "Are you depressed?"[18] Although feeling sad and anxious at times is a normal response to a terminal diagnosis, severe or prolonged depressive symptoms are not. People exhibiting signs of clinical depression should be referred to skilled health care professionals for evaluation and treatment.

Management

Optimal therapy is achieved with the combination of supportive psychotherapy, cognitive-behavioral techniques, and pharmaceutical management. This approach requires coordination of the interdisciplinary team, including a psychiatrist, psychologist, or psychiatric clinical nurse specialist. Cognitive-behavioral techniques aim to clarify misconceptions and negative patterns of thinking that lead to self-condemnation, hopelessness, and self-pity.[87] Examples of cognitive-behavioral interventions include educating clients about their terminal illness, symptoms, and depression to clarify their causes and treatments; reinforcing clients' strengths; setting realistic goals; and encouraging clients to participate in decision making.

Antidepressant medications can be effective in treating depression. There are several classes of antidepressants. The newer selective serotonin re-uptake inhibitors (SSRIs) cause fewer side effects and are at least as effective as the tricyclic antidepressants.[85] A trial of antidepressant therapy is warranted in the terminally ill client because it may greatly enhance the quality of life. Antidepressants typically take 4 to 6 weeks or longer to achieve the maximal therapeutic response. Psychostimulants (e.g., methylphenidate [Ritalin]) are sometimes used as an adjunct or an alternative to traditional antidepressants in the terminally ill. They are particularly useful when depression is accompanied by apathy, decreased energy, and poor concentration.[88] Clients may improve within the first 2 days of treatment, but these benefits must be balanced with the potential for adverse effects such as nervousness, insomnia, and anorexia.

Fatigue and Weakness

Fatigue is among the most prevalent symptoms of clients with advanced illnesses and is universally associated with advanced malignancy. It is a distressing, subjective experience that impedes functioning and impairs quality of life. Clients describe fatigue as tiredness, exhaustion, generalized weakness, diminished energy, increased need to rest or sleep, diminished motivation, diminished capacity to pay attention, or a disturbed mood.[4,74,89,109]

Etiology

Although the etiology of fatigue is not clearly understood, many physiologic, psychoemotional, and spiritual factors are recognized as contributing to the phenomenon of fatigue.[4,74,89,109] Fatigue may result from any one or combination of the following problems:

- Disease/treatment-related: Disease process, disease treatments (surgery, radiation therapy, chemotherapy, biologic therapy), infection, anemia, malnutrition or cachexia, chronic hypoxia, metabolic or electrolyte disorders, endocrine disorders, neuromuscular disorders, medication side effects (e.g., excessive sedation from opioids)

- Physiologic: Overexertion, immobility or lack of exercise, poor sleep, pain, or other discomfort
- Psychoemotional: Stress, anxiety, grief, depression
- Spiritual: Fear, distress

Assessment

Because of the multidimensional nature of fatigue and the potential for several contributing factors to be present at any one time, a comprehensive assessment is required. It is important to identify and treat reversible causes of fatigue. All medications should be reviewed and any unnecessary centrally acting drugs eliminated. If the clinician suspects that opioids are contributing to fatigue, reduction of the opioid dose by 25% should be considered, followed by evaluation of the client's cognition if pain is still controlled and fatigue is lessened.[74] If pain returns with the reduction in dose, the opioid dose should be returned to the previous level. *Note:* The client who is in pain but is sedated from opioids likely has an opioid-resistant pain syndrome; an adjuvant medication will be required (see Adjuvant Analgesics earlier in this chapter). Stress, fear, and spiritual distress are best addressed through counseling.

Management

If anemia is contributing to fatigue, transfusion with packed red blood cells may be appropriate. It appears there is no threshold hemoglobin level below which clients universally experience fatigue.[74] Because so many factors contribute to fatigue, clients with low hemoglobin levels who receive transfusions may still feel fatigued. One retrospective study showed that anemia is not one of the major contributing factors to fatigue.[77] In end-of-life care, a transfusion is not appropriate if the client's quality of life does not improve. Some clients with advanced diseases may have significant anemia but have few clinical manifestations.[35,71] These clients also would not receive a transfusion. Erythropoietin is helpful in treating the fatigue associated with chemotherapy-induced anemia,[78] but there is little research to show its effectiveness in clients with advanced diseases.

Nurses can initiate many interventions to help clients cope with fatigue. Strategies to manage stress include counseling, education, relaxation, and massage. One small study showed a combined modality treatment of aromatherapy, footsoak, and reflexology alleviates fatigue in terminally ill cancer clients.[51] Instituting a regular exercise program can be effective in lessening fatigue in clients undergoing chemotherapy. Although no studies on the effect of an exercise program on fatigue in the palliative care setting have been published, this strategy should be considered for clients who are able to participate in some form of exercise. In addition, for clients who can eat and take in fluids, you can encourage adequate nutrition and hydration.[35,74,109]

Although no studies have been reported on the effects of energy-conservation techniques for clients with fatigue,[78] modifications of activity and rest patterns are often included as intervention strategies. The nurse encourages clients to (1) incorporate rest times into their daily schedules, (2) plan their most strenuous activities for the time of day when energy levels are highest, and (3) capitalize on saving energy by accepting the assistance of others, delegating tasks, and using equipment such as a bedside commode or a portable telephone.

Medications may be helpful in treating fatigue in some clients. Corticosteroids are sometimes used to treat fatigue in clients with advanced cancer. The mechanism of action is not clear. Inhibition of tumor and tumor-induced substances that contribute to the fatigue and a central euphoric effect of these medications are two postulated mechanisms of action. If anorexia or cachexia is a contributing factor in fatigue, the appetite-stimulating effect of corticosteroids may be helpful.[109]

Psychostimulants have also been used to treat clients with fatigue (see Chapter 22). The most experience in clients with cancer has been with methylphenidate (Ritalin); dextroamphetamine (Dexedrine), pemoline (Cylert), and the wake-promoting agent modafinil (Provigil) have also been used.[12,74,76,109]

Sleep Disturbances
Etiology

Impaired sleep is a common, and often overlooked, problem in clients with advanced illnesses. Insomnia occurs in up to 59% of clients with advanced cancer. Many times a disturbance in sleep is accepted as "part of being sick"; however, it is important to recognize the importance of sleep. Sleep is associated with tissue restoration; sleep deprivation alters immune function. Although clients with a terminal illness are not going to "recuperate" from their underlying disease, they can benefit from the healing and protective functions of sleep when dealing with tissue injury and infection. Excessive sleepiness is also emotionally disabling, resulting in an inability to participate in treatment, comprehend information, and share in social interactions. Furthermore, impairment of sleep may lead to depression, irritability, and withdrawal.[60,98]

Assessment

Evaluation of the amount and quality of sleep is an important component of the overall assessment of a client in the palliative care setting.[60,98] The evaluation includes the following:

- Usual bedtime
- How long it takes to fall asleep
- Any wakefulness during the night
- Usual waking time

- Subjective feeling of being "refreshed" in the morning
- Frequency and length of daytime naps
- Use of sleep medications
- The cause of any sleep problems as identified by the client

There are many potential causes of sleep disturbances. Physiologic factors contributing to impaired sleep include pain, nausea and vomiting, itching, respiratory problems, medications (e.g., corticosteroids, bronchodilators, antihypertensives, psychostimulants), metabolic disturbances, and delirium. Sometimes medication dosing schedules interrupt sleep. Controlled-release medications provide the advantage of not needing to be awakened during the night for dose administration.

Psychoemotional factors, such as depression and anxiety, also interfere with sleep. The client's environment definitely influences the amount and quality of sleep; unfamiliar surroundings, frequent interruptions, noise, bright lighting, and unpleasant odors can all lead to a disturbance in sleep. In addition, lack of exercise, inactivity, and boredom may lead to excessive napping during the day, resulting in poor sleep at night.

Management

Treatable causes of sleep disturbance must be addressed with appropriate interventions and discontinuation of medications that interfere with sleep when possible. General sleep hygiene strategies include the following:[60,98]

- Establishing a regular sleep schedule
- Staying out of bed during the day
- Napping only when necessary
- Keeping active (mentally or physically) during the day
- Minimizing nighttime disruptions
- Avoiding stimulants at night (caffeine, nicotine)

Clients who have difficulty falling asleep may benefit from establishing a relaxing bedtime routine. Depending on individual preferences, this relaxation routine may consist of massage, progressive muscle relaxation, imagery, music, and warm milk or herbal tea.

When other interventions are not effective in promoting or maintaining sleep, sedative medications may be appropriate. Benzodiazepines are the main group of medications used to promote sleep. Some controversy remains about the long-term effectiveness of the benzodiazepines, and most are recommended for short-term use. Thus the need for sleep medications must be reevaluated on a regular basis. In general, benzodiazepines are used intermittently, at the lowest effective dose, and are never discontinued abruptly.[118] The non-benzodiazepine sedative-hypnotics (e.g., eszopiclone [Lunesta], zaleplon [Sonata], and zolpidem [Ambien]) are another option for treating insomnia. Eszopiclone and zaleplon are approved for use in treating chronic insomnia.

Knowing the half-lives of these medications may help in determining the appropriate hypnotic for an individual:

- Short half-life (1 to 4 hours): Triazolam (Halcion), zaleplon (Sonata), zolpidem (Ambien). Because of their quick onset of action, these medications are helpful for clients who have difficulty falling asleep. They do not, however, benefit clients with sleep maintenance problems. Rebound insomnia is common if the medication is abruptly stopped. Zolpidem is available in a controlled-release formulation to promote a full-night's sleep.
- Intermediate half-life (6 to 15 hours): Lorazepam (Ativan), oxazepam (Serax), temazepam (Restoril), eszopiclone (Lunesta). These medications are helpful for promoting sleep onset and maintenance. Clients who experience daytime sleepiness after using one of these medications may need to switch to one with a shorter half-life. Older adults or those with impaired hepatic or renal function may eliminate these drugs more slowly than healthy young adults.
- Long half-life (29 to 100 hours): Flurazepam (Dalmane), quazepam (Doral). Although these agents help to promote sleep onset and maintenance, daytime sedation is common because of their long half-lives. Drug accumulation may occur in older adults and those with hepatic or renal insufficiency. (See Chapter 22 on sleep management.)

Cachexia
Incidence

Cachexia is a complex syndrome associated with metabolic changes, fat and muscle wasting, loss of appetite, and involuntary weight loss. The term is derived from the Greek words *kakos* and *hexis,* meaning "poor condition." Cachexia is often associated with the symptoms of debility, chronic nausea, and constipation.[38] It is estimated that cachexia occurs in about 80% of clients with advanced cancer, 33% of clients with acquired immunodeficiency syndrome (AIDS), 20% of those with congestive heart failure, and up to 50% of clients with chronic hypoxemia associated with chronic lung disease.[6,16,22,100,117]

Etiology

Several studies have identified that numerous cytokines, including tumor necrosis factor alpha, interleukin-1, interleukin-6, and interferon, contribute to cachexia. These substances are postulated to cause anorexia, increase the metabolic rate, interfere with fat storage, and contribute to muscle protein loss.* Dietary supplementation does not reverse this process. Thus the cachexia syndrome may be viewed as a chronic inflammatory condition rather than a nutritional aberration.[70] Other contributing factors in cachexia syndrome are presented in Box 21-1.

---

*References 21, 43, 46, 70, 107, 120.

BOX 21-1 Factors Contributing to Cachexia-Anorexia Syndrome

- Tumor involvement of gastrointestinal tract
- Antitumor therapy
- Infections
- Taste change
- Medications
- Food aversions
- Pain
- Psychological factors
- Changes in metabolism
- Hormonal changes
- Fatigue, weakness
- Increased metabolic rate; altered fat, protein, or carbohydrate metabolism; fluid-electrolyte abnormalities; hormonal changes
- Malabsorption
- Tumor metabolism

Management

Interventions are as varied as the contributing factors. Supportive interventions include ensuring good mouth care, maintaining pleasant surroundings, and encouraging small, frequent meals with more emphasis on comfort (client likes and requests) than nutritional value. It is not clear if dietary supplementation can prevent cachexia, but once weight loss begins, dietary supplements do not appear to change the course of this syndrome.

Family members often worry that their loved one is "starving to death" and focus on trying to get the client to take supplements or eat big meals. It may be helpful to differentiate cachexia from starvation. The complex metabolic changes associated with cachexia cause an increase in energy expenditures that is unaffected by caloric intake. In comparison, starvation leads to energy conservation and is reversed by caloric intake. Thus cachexia is not synonymous with starvation and eating will not make their loved one well.

Some clients are distressed by their decrease appetite and want to eat more. Progestational agents (e.g., megestrol acetate [Megace]) may be trialed in an attempt to improve the client's appetite to induce weight gain.[24] Other medications to manage cachexia include dexamethasone to stimulate appetite, prokinetic agents such as metoclopramide (Reglan) to improve gastric emptying and decrease nausea, and cannabinoids (e.g., dronabinol [Marinol]) to stimulate appetite and decrease nausea. If fatigue is contributing to anorexia, a psychostimulant (e.g., methylphenidate) may be helpful.

INDICATORS OF IMMINENT DEATH

Certain physical, cognitive, and behavioral changes occur as a person enters the active dying process. Family members must be informed about the changes to expect so that they feel as prepared as possible and can recognize when death is approaching.[115] The following are common nursing diagnoses that may be observed when death is imminent:

- Impaired urinary elimination due to renal failure or decreased perfusion of the kidneys.
- Total urinary incontinence caused by changes in perception or lack of muscular control.
- Urinary retention due to medications or sensory changes causing inability to relax urinary sphincter.
- Ineffective tissue perfusion: peripheral resulting from shunting of circulation to vital organ systems, leading to tachycardia, mottling, and peripheral cyanosis.
- Impaired gas exchange and ineffective breathing pattern due to pulmonary compromise or compensation for metabolic alterations, leading to tachypnea, dyspnea, apnea, or Cheyne-Stokes respirations.
- Ineffective airway clearance resulting from weakness, leading to congested breathing (sometimes referred to as "death rattle").
- Impaired physical mobility due to generalized weakness.
- Impaired swallowing resulting from weakness and loss of gag reflex.
- Disturbed sensory perception due to altered perfusion to the brain *itself* and metabolic alterations; may progress to coma. Hearing is believed to remain intact throughout the dying process.
- Acute confusion from delirium or decreased circulation to the brain.
- Disturbed thought processes resulting from biochemical alterations.
- Anxiety, death anxiety, or fear due to physical discomfort (e.g., pain, dyspnea), unfinished business, or spiritual concerns.

Table 21-6 summarizes the indicators of impending death.

TABLE 21-6 Common Objective Body System Indicators of Imminent Death

Cognition/ orientation	Not always nonresponsive, may be agitated or restless, cannot subjectively respond to verbal stimuli
Cardiovascular	Tachycardia, irregular heart rate, lowered blood pressure or significant widening between systolic and diastolic pressures, dehydration
Pulmonary	Tachypnea, dyspnea, use of accessory muscles, acetone breath, Cheyne-Stokes breathing, pooling of secretions or noisy respirations
Gastrointestinal	Diminished appetite, smaller amounts of feces; incontinence
Renal	Diminished urine output, incontinence, concentrated urine
Mobility	Limited mobility, bedbound, requires frequent position changes

COMMUNICATION ISSUES

The dying process can be a time of emotional crisis for many clients and their families. Nurses play a critical role in supporting clients and families throughout the dying process. An open and caring discussion of what to anticipate in the dying process reduces the incidence of fear and apprehension. It is important to develop a level of comfort when communicating with dying clients and their families. Self-examination and articulation of personal feelings about death and dying are essential to providing emotional support and guidance to the dying. Uncomfortable emotions expressed by a nurse can impede the ability of clients and families to finish important issues and accomplish healthy closure.

Clients and families facing the last days of life should be given the opportunity to express any and all concerns about issues that matter the most to them. The nurse can serve as a listener, a friend, and an advocate for the client. Being available in a nonjudgmental and nonthreatening manner allows the client and family to trust the nurse. Once trust is established and the client believes that the nurse will effectively manage his or her symptoms, the client may begin to open up emotionally and discuss concerns about the illness and death.[99] Each individual is unique, and so are the conversations that occur between nurse, client, and family. The nurse can provide the therapeutic use of self through the following interventions:[104,105]

- Use active listening to encourage the client and family to tell their "story."
- Encourage a mutual participatory relationship that is not dominated by controlling conversations.
- Use less directive skills such as silence, paraphrases, reflections, and sincerity.
- Offer structure to the conversation and yet empower the client and family to express their needs.
- Promote opportunities for discussion and demonstrate a willingness to listen to difficult and painful concerns.

Communicating with dying clients and their families takes into account the multidimensional nature of people. See the Diversity in Health Care feature on Cultural Aspects of Death and Dying on the website. Sensitivity and knowledge surrounding culture, spirituality, lifestyle, and emotional connections are essential when supporting clients and their families at the end of life.

One of the most important tasks of the bedside nurse is to empower clients and families to participate in the final act of living. Through ongoing assessment, communication, and skilled physical care, you can communicate reassurance, confidence, and support for the vulnerable client and family. The seasoned hand of a skilled professional supporting and guiding the client can change the journey through dying and death from a frightening process to one of peace and comfort.

CARE FOR CAREGIVERS

The families of terminally ill clients commonly serve as primary caregivers in the home care environment and are often highly involved in providing care in other palliative care settings (e.g., extended care facility, acute care setting). This "intensive caring" is physically and emotionally exhausting. To provide and maintain this level of care, these caregivers need education and support from all members of the interdisciplinary health care team. Coping tasks for families caring for a loved one who is dying and suggested interventions are described in Table 21-7.

Even though this intensive caring is difficult, most family caregivers are able to provide appropriate levels of care for their loved ones. Despite the physical, financial, and emotional tolls of providing this care, the experience is extremely rewarding and many view it as a final act of love. Nurses play a pivotal role in assessing the educational and support needs of family members, providing information and support, and referring caregivers to other team members and community agencies to address their needs. If the physical or emotional burdens of caregiving become overwhelming, the nurse should discuss other options for care. These may include hiring additional caregivers (when financially feasible), transfer to a long-term care setting or residential hospice setting, and use of hospice continuous home care or hospice acute medical care (when medically justified).

SUPPORT OF THE GRIEVING FAMILY

Bereavement care is an important component of any palliative care program.[79] Providing bereavement care requires an understanding of the normal grieving process and the tasks of grief work. Grief is a normal and expected reaction to a loss. Family members will grieve the loss of their loved ones. One role of the health care team is to reinforce the understanding that grieving is healthy; it is a necessary process that the family must go through to be able to move on in their lives. Nurses need to validate as normal the manifestations that the bereaved may be experiencing (Table 21-8).

In addition to knowing the normal responses to grief, it is helpful for those working with the bereaved to understand the tasks of the grieving process. Four tasks of mourning that must be accomplished for the bereavement to reach a satisfactory conclusion are the following:

1. Accepting the reality of the loss
2. Experiencing the pain of the loss

3. Adjusting to the environment in which the deceased is missing
4. Finding a way to remember the deceased while moving forward with life[121]

Most people adapt to bereavement successfully, and it can even be associated with improved coping, personal growth, and a new appreciation for life.[26] However, for some, bereavement can be complicated. If any of the "normal" responses to grief are extremely intense or protracted, it may indicate a psychiatric disorder such as clinical depression, anxiety disorder, alcohol or other substance abuse, psychotic disorder, or post-traumatic stress disorder.[50]

Health care providers play a pivotal role in assisting families throughout the grieving process. Table 21-9 identifies strategies helpful to people experiencing grief.

TABLE 21–7   Family Coping Tasks in Terminal Illness

Coping Task	Support or Interventions
1. Promote acceptance versus denial.	1. Provide realistic information about illness and treatment options. Encourage open and honest communication among family members.
2. Establish a relationship with health care team.	2. Explain the roles of all interdisciplinary team members. Establish trust and maintain open lines of communication.
3. Meet the needs of the dying person: a. Physical needs	a. Provide information about pain and symptom management, use of equipment, skin care/position, rest and nutrition, infection control, and safety. Reassure caregivers that they are doing a good job. Assess need for assistance, such as home health aide. Assess need for transfer to a different care setting.
b. Emotional needs	b. Encourage caregivers to take time to sit and listen to their loved one and to share each other's feelings and concerns. Assess need for additional support/counseling from interdisciplinary team.
4. Maintain functional equilibrium (i.e., the family must maintain some sense of normalcy to continue to function as a family unit).	4. Assist family to identify and prioritize activities that must be continued (e.g., going to work or school, doing laundry, buying groceries). Assist family to identify support people to help with these tasks. Encourage caregivers to use respite care services to care for themselves and to attend family events outside of direct caregiving.
5. Regulate family affect.	5. Allow caregivers opportunity to express their feelings. Give them permission to have whatever feelings they have (i.e., "feelings just are—there's no right or wrong"). Acknowledge that normally joyful times, such as holidays, may not feel as joyful. Encourage formal counseling, if needed. Encourage caregivers to address their own needs and to care for themselves, too.
6. Negotiate relationships outside the family.	6. Give permission to take time to maintain friendships. Discuss options for maintaining jobs while caring for a dying loved one.
7. Cope with the post-death phase (healthy grieving).	7. Support family while they accept the finality of their loss. Discuss functioning of the family unit without the loved one. Encourage using available bereavement supports/counseling.

TABLE 21–8   Manifestations of Normal Grief

Behaviors	Cognitions	Feelings	Physical Sensations
1. Sleep disturbances	1. Disbelief	1. Sadness	1. Hollowness in stomach
2. Appetite disturbances	2. Confusion	2. Anger	2. Chest and throat tightness
3. Absent-minded behavior	3. Preoccupation/obsessiveness	3. Guilt	3. Oversensitivity to noise
4. Social withdrawal	4. Visual and auditory hallucinations	4. Anxiety	4. Sense of unreality
5. Dreams of deceased	5. Sense that loved one is nearby	5. Loneliness	5. Feeling short of breath
6. Avoiding reminders of deceased		6. Fatigue	6. Muscle weakness
7. Searching and calling out		7. Helplessness	7. Lack of energy
8. Restless overactivity		8. Yearning	8. Dry mouth
9. Sighing		9. Emancipation	
10. Crying		10. Relief	
11. Carrying objects as reminders		11. Numbness	
12. Visiting places as reminders			

Data from Roberts, K.F., & Berry, P.H. (2002). Grief and bereavement. In K.K. Kuebler, P.H. Berry, & D.E. Heidrich (Eds.), *End-of-life care: Clinical practice guidelines* (pp. 53-63). Philadelphia: Saunders.

TABLE 21–9 Interventions for Grieving People

Task	Interventions
Accept the reality of the loss.	Listen actively.
	Encourage gentle exploration of what future may look like without person who has died.
	Assess and encourage development of a support system.
	Encourage time with the body of the deceased at time of death.
	Offer opportunities to repeat the story of the death.
	Normalize feelings through personal contacts and written materials about grief and loss.
	Avoid use of platitudes.
	Attend funeral or visitation if possible; send a personal card to family.
	Respect survivors' feelings without judgment.
Experience the pain of the loss.	Assist in identifying feelings or behaviors and normalize them.
	Assist the survivor in placing meaning on the death.
Adjust to the environment in which deceased is missing.	Assist the survivor in further identifying the meaning of loss in practical terms (e.g., role changes).
	Provide practical assistance with developing needed skills.
	Advise survivors to minimize change and to grieve where things are familiar; discourage moving or any similar large life change.
Remember the deceased while moving forward with life.	Listen actively without judgment.
	Validate and normalize feeling.
	Encourage attendance at grief and loss support or educational groups.

Data from Roberts, K.F., & Berry, P.H. (2002). Grief and bereavement. In K.K. Kuebler, P.H. Berry, & D.E. Heidrich (Eds.). *End-of-life care: Clinical practice guidelines* (pp. 53-63). Philadelphia: Saunders.

CONCLUSIONS

It is vital for nurses to offer compassion to clients and family members facing advanced progressive illnesses, assess the multitude of symptoms associated with advanced stages of diseases, and participate with the interdisciplinary team to address the care needs of these clients and families as they experience the final phase of life. Skilled and knowledgeable nurses help the client and family attempt to make sense of life's greatest mystery—death, and promote a healthy and positive dying experience for all involved.

THINKING CRITICALLY

1. T.S., a 57-year-old man, has stage IV squamous cell carcinoma of the right lung with metastatic bony involvement. You find that he is in excruciating pain and is so sedated that he is unable to rate his pain subjectively. He is nauseated, has not had a bowel movement in 6 days, and is anorexic and dehydrated. His current medications include sustained-release morphine 60 mg every 6 hours, fentanyl 75 mcg/hr transdermal, and immediate-release morphine 20 mg every 2 hours, which have not provided relief. What can you do to make this client more comfortable?

Factors to Consider. Besides poor pain control, what other problems need attention? Consider the addition of an adjuvant analgesic, the dosing of the opioids, and the client's hydration status.

2. F.T., a 43-year-old man, entered the emergency department with complaints of severe dyspnea. The chest x-ray revealed pleural effusion of the right lung. The results of the thoracentesis, which drained 1500 ml of fluid, were positive for adenocarcinoma. After several diagnostic studies were performed, no primary site for the tumor was identified. He was referred to an oncologist for palliative chemotherapy. You are asked to make a home visit to change the dressing on his chest tube. Your first assessment reveals a very cachectic, dehydrated, constipated, dyspneic client whose pain is well managed. The chest tube drainage totals 450 ml daily. The client and his wife are questioning the relevance of the chemotherapy, given the poor prognosis as well as his continued weight loss, loss of appetite, and weakness. F.T. informs you that he does not want to be hospitalized and would like to remain at home and comfortable. After learning about this client's status and wishes, what actions should you take?

Factors to Consider. What actions should be taken to facilitate the client's request? Is 24-hour care needed now or in the future? What additional needs might the client or his wife have?

3. J.K. is a 38-year-old, unmarried teacher who has diabetes mellitus and polycystic kidney disease (PKD). Her most recent kidney-pancreas transplant has been rejected, and she is undergoing hemodialysis again. She has not been compliant with her diet and fluid restrictions, and multiple dialysis access sites have become infected. She states that she does not want to continue dialysis. What should you do next? Should her parents be told of her request?

Factors to Consider. How can you be certain that the client understands the ramifications of ending the hemodialysis? What can you do to keep her comfortable once dialysis is discontinued?

Discussions for these questions can be found on the website. **evolve**

▓ BIBLIOGRAPHY

🪔 Citations appearing in red refer to primary research.

🪔 Citations appearing in blue refer to evidence-based practice guidelines and protocols.

1. Abernethy, A., Currow, D., Frith, P., et al. (2003). Randomised, double blind, placebo controlled crossover trial of sustained release morphine for the management of refractory dyspnoea. *British Medical Journal, 327*(7414), 523. Retrieved 05/17/06 from http://proquest.umi.com/pqdweb?did=421119071&sid=2&Fmt=4&clientid=21158&RQT=309&VName=PQD.

2. Agency for Health Care Policy and Research. (1994). *Managing cancer pain.* Washington, DC: Department of Health and Human Services.

3. American Psychiatric Association. (2000). *Diagnostic and statistical manual of mental disorders (DSM-IV-TR)* (4th ed., text revision). Washington, DC: American Psychiatric Association.

4. Anderson, P.R., & Dean, G.E. (2006). Fatigue. In B.R. Ferrell & N. Coyle (Eds.), *Textbook of palliative nursing* (2nd ed., pp. 155-168). New York: Oxford University Press.

5. Andrewes, T. (2002). The management of breathlessness in palliative care. *Nursing Standard, 17*(5), 43-52.

6. Anker, S.D., Ponikowski, P., Varney, S., et al. (1997). Wasting as independent risk factor for mortality in chronic heart failure. *Lancet, 349*(9058), 1050-1053.

7. Beckstrand, R., Callister, L., & Kirchhoff, K. (2006). Providing a "good death": Critical care nurses' suggestions for improving end-life-care. *American Journal of Critical Care, 15*(1), 38-45.

8. Billings, A., Gardner, M., & Putnam, A. (2002). A one-day, hospital-wide survey of dying inpatients. *Journal of Palliative Medicine, 5*(3), 363-374.

9. Blacksher, E., & Christopher, M. (2002). On the road to reform: Advocacy and activism in end-of-life care. *Journal of Palliative Medicine, 5*(1), 13-22.

10. Block, S. (2002). Medical education in end-of-life care: The status of reform. *Journal of Palliative Medicine, 5*(2), 243-248.

11. Brietbart, W., Chochinov, H., & Passik, S. (2003). Psychiatric symptoms in palliative care. In D. Doyle, G. Hanks, N. Cherny, et al. (Eds.), *Oxford textbook of palliative medicine* (3rd ed., pp. 746-774). Oxford: Oxford University Press.

12. Bruera, E., Driver, L., Barnes, E.A., et al. (2003). Patient-controlled methylphenidate for the management of fatigue in patients with advanced cancer: A preliminary report. *Journal of Clinical Oncology, 21*(23), 4439-4443.

13. Carney, C.P., Jones, L., Woolson, R.F., et al. (2002). Relationship between depression and pancreatic cancer in the general population. *Psychosomatic Medicine, 65*(5), 884-888.

14. Carr, T. (2006). *Introducing death and dying: Readings and exercises.* Upper Saddle River, NJ: Prentice Hall.

15. Carrieri-Kohlman, V., & Stalbarg, M. (2003). Dyspnea. In V. Carrieri-Kohlman, A. Lindsay, & C. West (Eds.), *Pathophysiological phenomena in nursing* (3rd ed., pp. 177-207). Philadelphia: Saunders.

16. Castillo-Martinez, L., Orea-Tejeda, A., Rosales, M.T., et al. (2005). Anthropometric variables and physical activity as predictors of cardiac cachexia. *International Journal of Cardiology, 99*(2), 239-245.

17. Cherny, N., & Portenoy, R.K. (1999). Practical issues in the management of cancer pain. In P.D. Wall & P. Melzack (Eds.), *Textbook of pain* (4th ed., pp. 1479-1522). New York: Churchill Livingstone.

18. Chochoinov, H.M., Wilson, K.G., Enns, M., et al. (1998). Depression, hopelessness, and suicidal ideation in the terminally ill. *Psychosomatics, 39*(4), 366-370.

19. Coyle, N., & Layman-Goldstein, M. (2001). Pain assessment and management in palliative care. In M. Matzo & D. Sherman (Eds.), *Palliative care nursing: Quality care to the end of life* (pp. 362-486). New York: Springer.

20. Culp, K. (2003). Acute confusion. In V. Carrieri-Kohlman, A. Lindsay, & C. West (Eds.), *Pathophysiological phenomena in nursing* (3rd ed., pp. 155-171). Philadelphia: Saunders.

21. Davis, M.P. (2002). New drugs for the anorexia-cachexia syndrome. *Current Oncology Reports, 4*(3), 264-274.

22. Davis, M.P., & Dickerson, D. (2000). Cachexia and anorexia: Cancer's covert killer. *Supportive Care in Cancer, 8*(3), 180-187.

23. Deutsch, N. (2006). Film shows the importance of a good death. *Nursing Spectrum, 7*(2), 22.

24. Driver, L., & Bruera, E. (2002). *The M.D. Anderson palliative care handbook.* Houston, Tex: Department of Symptom Control and Palliative Care, The University of Texas M.D. Anderson Cancer Center.

25. Dudgeon, D. (2002). Managing dyspnea and cough. *Hematology Oncology Clinics of North America, 16*(3), 557-577.

26. Dutton, Y.D., & Zisook, S. (2005). Adaptation to bereavement. *Death Studies, 29*(10), 877-903.

27. Ferrell, B., & Coyle, N. (2002). An overview of palliative nursing care. *American Journal of Nursing, 102*(5), 26-33.

28. Fink, R., & Gates, R. (2001). Pain assessment. In B.R. Ferrell & N. Coyle (Eds.), *Textbook of palliative nursing* (pp. 53-75). New York: Oxford University Press.

29. Finn-Paradis, L. (1985). *The development of hospice in America: The hospice handbook.* Rockville, Md: Aspen.

30. Foley, K. (2005). The past and future of palliative care. *The Hastings Center Report, 35*(6), S42-46. Retrieved 05/24/06 from http://proquest.umi.com/pqdweb?dud=937445781&sid=3&Fmt=3&clientid=21158&RQT=309&VName+PQD.

31. Gagnon, P., Allard, P., Masse, B., et al. (2000). Delirium in terminal cancer: A prospective study using daily screening, early diagnosis, and continuous monitoring. *Journal of Pain and Symptom Management, 19*(6), 412-426.

32. Gaudreau, J.D., Gagnon, P., Harel, F., et al. (2005a). Impact on delirium detection of using a sensitive instrument integrated into clinical practice. *General Hospital Psychiatry, 27*(3), 194-199.

33. Gaudreau, J.D., Gagnon, P., Harel, F., et al. (2005b). Fast, systematic, and continuous delirium assessment in hospitalized patients: The Nursing Delirium Screening Scale. *Journal of Pain and Symptom Management, 29*(4), 368-375.

34. Gibson, C.A., Lichtenthal, W., Berg, A., et al. (2006). Psychologic issues in palliative care. *Anesthesiology Clinics of North America, 24*(1), 61-80.

35. Given, B., et al. (2002). Pain and fatigue management: Results of a nursing randomized clinical trial. *Oncology Nursing Forum, 29*(6), 949-956.

36. Goldberg, L. (2004). A survey of hospice and palliative care part I: Introduction and concepts. *Hospital Physician, 12*, 23-31.

37. Gordon, J. (2004). *Hospice offer patients expert, compassionate care. Hospice Choices.* Accessed 05/12/06 at www.hospiceschoices.com/cm/news/9530.

38. Grant, M., & Dean, G. (2003). Anorexia. In V. Carrieri-Kohlman, A. Lindsay, & C. West (Eds.), *Pathophysiological phenomena in nursing* (3rd ed., pp. 35-47). Philadelphia: Saunders.

39. Hattori, K., McCubbin, M., & Ishida, D. (2006). Concept analysis of good death in the Japanese community. *Journal of Nursing Scholarship, 38*(2), 165-170.

40. Hoffman, R. (2005). The evolution of hospice in America: Nursing's role in the movement. *Journal of Gerontological Nursing, 31*(7), 26-34.

41. Homant, S. (2002). Hospice care. In K. Kuebler & P. Esper (Eds.), *Palliative practices from A-Z for the bedside clinician* (pp. 147-150). Pittsburgh, Pa: Oncology Nursing Press.

42. Hoyer, T. (2002). Hospice and future of end-of-life care: Approaches and funding ideas. *Journal of Palliative Medicine, 5*(2), 259-270.

43. Illman, J., Corringham, R., Robinson, D., Jr., et al. (2005). Are inflammatory cytokines the common link between cancer-associated cachexia and depression? *Journal of Supportive Oncology, 3*(1), 37-50.

44. Ingham, J., & Caraceni, A. (2002). Delirium. In A. Berger, R. Portenoy, & D. Weissman (Eds.), *Principles and practice of supportive oncology* (2nd ed., pp. 555-576). Philadelphia: Lippincott Williams & Wilkins.

45. Introcaso, D., & Lynn, J. (2002). Systems of care: Future reform. *Journal of Palliative Medicine, 5*(2), 255-262.

46. Inui, A. (2002). Cancer anorexia-cachexia syndrome: Current issues in research and management. *CA: A Cancer Journal for Clinicians, 52*(2), 72-91.

47. Jennings, A., Davies, A., Higgins, J., et al. (2006). Opioids for the palliation of breathlessness in terminal illness. *The Cochrane Database of Systematic Reviews 2001,* (2), CD002066.

48. Kassa, S., & Loge, J. (2003). Quality of life in palliative medicine. In D. Doyle, G. Hanks, N. Cherny, et al. (Eds.), *Oxford textbook of palliative medicine* (3rd ed., pp. 195-206). Oxford: Oxford University Press.

49. Kinzbrunner, B. (1998). Hospice: 15 years and beyond in the care of the dying. *Journal of Palliative Medicine, 1*, 127-137.

50. Kissane, D.W. (2003). Bereavement. In D. Doyle, G. Hanks, N. Cherny, et al. (Eds.), *Oxford textbook of palliative medicine* (3rd ed., pp. 1137-1151). New York: Oxford University Press.

51. Kohara, H., Miyauchi, T., Suehiro, Y., et al. (2004). Combined modality treatment of aromatherapy, footsoak, and reflexology relieves fatigue in patients with cancer. *Journal of Palliative Medicine, 7*(6), 791-796.

52. Kübler-Ross, E. (1969). *On death and dying.* New York: Macmillan.

53. Kübler-Ross, E. (1995). *Death is of vital importance: On life, death and life after death.* New York: Station Press.

54. Kuebler, K. (1996). *Hospice and palliative care practice protocol: Dyspnea.* Pittsburgh, Pa: Hospice Nurses Association.

55. Kuebler, K. (2002). Dyspnea. In K. Kuebler, P. Berry, & D. Heidrich (Eds.), *End of life care: Clinical practice guidelines* (pp. 301-315). Philadelphia: Saunders.

56. Kuebler, K., Heidrich, D., Vena, C., et al. (2006). Delirium, confusion, and agitation. In B.R. Ferrell & N. Coyle (Eds.), *Textbook of palliative nursing* (2nd ed., pp. 401-420). New York: Oxford University Press.

57. Last Acts. (2002). *Means to a better end: A report on dying in America today.* Washington, DC: Last Acts.

58. Lawlor, P.G., Fainsinger, R.L., & Bruera, E.D. (2000). Delirium at the end of life: Critical issues in clinical practice and research. *Journal of the American Medical Association, 284*(19), 2427-2429.

59. Lawlor, P.G., Gagnon, B., Manncini, I.L., et al. (2000). Occurrence, causes, and outcomes of delirium in patients with advanced cancer: A prospective study. *Archives of Internal Medicine, 160*(6), 786-794.

60. Lee, K. (2003). Impaired sleep. In V. Carrieri-Kohlman, A. Lindsay, & C. West (Eds.), *Pathophysiological phenomena in nursing* (3rd ed., pp. 363-385). Philadelphia: Saunders.

61. LeGrand, S., et al. (2003). Opioids, respiratory function, and dyspnea. *American Journal of Hospice and Palliative Care, 20*(1), 57-61.

62. Leslie, D.L., Zhang, Y., Bogardus, S.T., et al. (2005). Consequences of preventing delirium in hospitalized older adults on nursing home costs. *Journal of the American Geriatrics Society, 53*(3), 405-409.

63. Lindell, A. (2000). Personal quote. *Journal of the American Medical Association, 284*(19), 2442.

64. Lo, B. (1995). End-of-life care after termination of SUPPORT. *Hastings Center Report Special Supplement, 25*, S6-S8.

65. Lussier, D., Huskey, A., & Portenoy, R. (2004). Adjuvant analgesics in cancer pain management. *The Oncologist, 9*(5), 571-591.

66. Lynn, J. (2000). Learning to care for people with chronic illness facing the end of life. *Journal of the American Medical Association, 284*(9), 2508-2511.

67. Mahoney, J. (1998). The Medicare hospice benefit—15 years of success. *Journal of Palliative Medicine, 1*, 139-146.

68. Marshall, P. (1995). The SUPPORT Study: Who's talking? *Hastings Center Report Special Supplement 25*, S9-S11.

69. McCaffery, M., & Pasero, C. (1999). *Pain: Clinical manual* (2nd ed.). St. Louis: Mosby.

70. McCarthy, D.O. (2003). Rethinking nutritional support for persons with cancer cachexia. *Biological Research for Nursing, 5*(1), 3-17.

71. McHale, H. (2002). Palliative care. In K. Kuebler & P. Esper (Eds.), *Palliative practices from A-Z for the bedside clinician* (pp. 193-195). Pittsburgh, Pa: Oncology Nursing Press.

72. Meghani, S. (2004). A concept analysis of palliative care in the United States. *Journal of Advanced Nursing, 46*(2), 152-161.

73. Melvin, T. (2001). The primary care physician and palliative care. *Primary Care, 28*(2), 239-248.

74. Miaskowski, C., & Portenoy, R. (2002). Assessment and management of cancer-related fatigue. In A. Berger, R. Portenoy, & D. Weissman (Eds.), *Principles and practice of supportive oncology* (2nd ed., pp. 141-153). Philadelphia: Lippincott Williams & Wilkins.

75. Morita, T., Tei, Y., Tsunoda K., et al. (2001). Underlying pathologies and their associations with clinical features in terminal delirium of cancer patients. *Journal of Pain and Symptom Management 22*(6), 997-1006.

76. Morrow, G.R., Shelke, A.R., Roscoe, J.A., et al. (2005). Management of cancer-related fatigue. *Cancer Investigation, 23*(3), 229-239.

77. Munch, T.N., Zhang, T., Willey, J., et al. (2005). The association between anemia and fatigue in patients with advanced cancer receiving palliative care. *Journal of Palliative Medicine, 8*(6), 1144-1149.

78. Nail, L. (2002). Fatigue in patients with cancer. *Oncology Nursing Forum, 29*, 537-544.

79. National Consensus Project for Quality Palliative Care. (2004). *Clinical practice guidelines for quality palliative care.* Brooklyn, NY: National Consensus Project for Quality Palliative Care.

80. National Center for Health Statistics. (2006). *Incidence and death rates.* Retrieved from www.cdc.gov/nchs/data/hestat/preliminary-deaths04_tables.pdf#.

81. National Hospice and Palliative Care Organization. (2006). *NHPCO facts and figures.* NHPCO, www.nhpco.org.

82. National Hospice and Palliative Care Organization. (2006). *What is palliative care? Caring connections.* Accessed 05/16/06 from www.caringinfo.org/i4a/pages/index.cfm?pageid=3469.

83. Ogle, K., Mavis, B., & Wyatt, G. (2002). Physicians and hospice care: Attitudes, knowledge and referrals. *Journal of Palliative Medicine, 5*(1), 85-92.

84. Olson, M. (2001). *Healing the dying* (2nd ed.). Australia: Delmar.

85. Paice, J. (2002). Managing psychological conditions in palliative care. *American Journal of Nursing, 102*(11), 36-43.

86. Panke, J. (2003). Difficulties in managing pain at the end of life. *Journal of Hospice and Palliative Nursing, 5*(2), 83-90.

87. Pasacreta, J.V., Minarik, P.A., & Nield-Anderson, L. (2006). Anxiety and depression. In B.R. Ferrell & N. Coyle (Eds.), *Textbook of palliative nursing* (2nd ed., pp. 375-399). New York: Oxford University Press.

88. Pereira, J., & Bruera, E. (2001). Depression with psychomotor retardation: Diagnostic challenges and the use of psychostimulants. *Journal of Palliative Medicine, 4*(1), 15-21.

89. Piper, B. (2003). Fatigue. In V. Carrieri-Kohlman, A. Lindsay, & C. West (Eds.), *Pathophysiological phenomena in nursing* (3rd ed., pp. 209-234). Philadelphia: Saunders.

90. Pollack, M. (1999). New treatments for panic disorders, psychiatric illness in primary care. *Clinician Reviews, 9*(3), 4-9.

91. Portenoy, R. (2001). *Contemporary diagnosis and management of pain in oncologic and AIDS patient* (3rd ed.). Newton, Pa: Handbooks in Health Care.

92. Puntillo, K., Miaskowski, C., & Summer, G. (2003). Pain. In V. Carrieri-Kohlman, A. Lindsay, & C. West (Eds.), *Pathophysiological phenomena in nursing* (3rd ed., pp. 235-254). Philadelphia: Saunders.

93. Rhodes, V., & McDaniel, R. (1998). The symptom experience and its impact on quality of life. In C. Yarbo, M. Frogge, & M. Goodman (Eds.), *Cancer symptom management* (2nd ed., pp. 3-8). Sudbury, Mass: Jones & Bartlett.

94. Robert Wood Johnson Foundation. (2002). *First state-by-state 'report card' on care for the dying finds mediocre care nationwide.* Washington, DC: Robert Wood Johnson Foundation.

95. Roscoe, L., & Schonwetter, R.S. (2006). Improving access to hospice and palliative care for patients near the end of life: Present status and future direction. *Journal of Palliative Care, 22*(1), 46-52. Retrieved 05/26/06 from http://proquest.umi.com/pqdweb?did=1032926111&sid=1&Fmt=3&clientid=21158&RQT=309&VName=PQD.

96. Ross, D., & Alexander, C. (2001). Management of common symptoms in terminally ill patients: Part II. *American Family Physician, 64*(6), 1019-1026.

97. Samuels, S.C., & Evers, M.M. (2002). Delirium: Pragmatic guidance for managing a common, confounding, and sometimes lethal condition. *Geriatrics, 57*(6), 33-38.

98. Sateia, M., & Santulli, R. (2003). Sleep. In D. Doyle, G. Hanks, N. Cherny, et al. (Eds.), *Oxford textbook of palliative medicine* (3rd ed., pp. 731-745). Oxford: Oxford University Press.

99. Scanlon, C. (2003). Ethical concerns in end-of-life care. *American Journal of Nursing, 103*(1), 48-56.

100. Schols, A.M., Soeters, P.B., Dingemans, A.M., et al. (1993). Prevalence and characteristics of nutritional depletion in patients with stable COPD eligible for pulmonary rehabilitation. *American Review of Respiratory Disease, 147*(5), 1151-1156.

101. Sepulveda, C., et al. (2002). Palliative care: The World Health Organization's global perspective. *Journal of Pain and Symptom Management, 24*(2), 91-96.

102. Shepherd, S., & Geraci, S. (1999). The differential diagnosis of dyspnea: A pathophysiological approach. *Clinician Reviews, 9*(3), 52-71.

103. Sherman, D., Matzo, M., Paice, J., et al. (2004). Learning pain assessment and management: A goal of the end-of-life nursing education consortium. *The Journal of Continuing Education in Nursing, 35*(3), 107-120.

104. Stanley, K. (2000). Silence is not golden: Conversations with the dying. *Clinical Journal of Oncology Nursing, 4*, 34-40.

105. Stanley, K. (2002). Communication. In K. Kuebler & P. Esper (Eds.), *Palliative practices from A-Z for the bedside clinician* (pp. 47-50). Pittsburgh, Pa: Oncology Nursing Press.

106. Stirling, Rev. D. (2003). Cicely Saunders, founder of the hospice movement, selected letters 1959-1999. *Journal of Palliative Care, 19*(4), 284-285.

107. Strasser, F. (2003). Eating-related disorders in patients with advanced cancer. *Supportive Care in Cancer, 11*(1), 11-20.

108. Strasser, F., Walker, P., & Bruera, E. (2005). Palliative pain management: When both pain and suffering hurt. *Journal of Palliative Care, 21*(2), 69-79.

109. Sweeney, C., Neuenschwander, H., & Bruera, E. (2003). Fatigue and asthenia. In D. Doyle, G. Hanks, N. Cherny, et al. (Eds.), *Oxford textbook of palliative medicine* (3rd ed., pp. 560-567). Oxford: Oxford University Press.

110. The SUPPORT Principal Investigators. (1995). A controlled trial to improve care for seriously ill hospitalized patients: The Study to Understand Prognoses and Preferences for Outcomes and Risks of Treatments (SUPPORT). *Journal of the American Medical Association, 274*, 1591-1598.

111. Trzepacz, P., et al. (1999). American Psychiatric Association Guidelines: Practice guidelines for the treatment of patients with delirium. *American Journal of Psychiatry, 156*, S1-S20.

112. Twycross, R.G. (1999). Opioids. In P.D. Wall & P. Melzack (Eds.), *Textbook of pain* (4th ed., pp. 1187-1214). New York: Churchill Livingstone.

113. Virani, R., & Sofer, D. (2003). Improving the quality of end-of-life care: Making changes at every level. *American Journal of Nursing, 103*(5), 52-60.

114. von Gunten, C., et al. (2002). Recommendations to improve end-of-life care through regulatory change in U.S. health care financing. *Journal of Palliative Medicine, 5*(1), 35-41.

115. Waller, A., & Caroline, N. (2000). *Handbook of palliative care in cancer* (2nd ed.). Boston: Butterworth Heinemann.

116. Walsh, D. (1998). The Medicare hospice benefit: A critique from palliative medicine. *Journal of Palliative Medicine, 1*, 147-149.

117. Wanke, C.A. (2000). Weight loss and wasting remain common complications in individuals infected with human immunodeficiency virus in the era of highly active antiretroviral therapy. *Clinical Infectious Diseases, 31*(3), 803-805.

118. *Webster's New World Dictionary* (4th ed.). (2005). Cleveland: Wiley.

119. Wickam, R. (2002). Dyspnea: Recognizing and managing an invisible problem. *Oncology Nursing Forum, 29*(6), 925-933.

120. Winter, S.M. (2002). Terminal nutrition: Framing the debate for withdrawal of nutritional support in terminally ill patients. *American Journal of Medicine, 109*(9), 723-726.

121. Worden, J.W. (1991). *Grief counseling and grief therapy: A handbook for the mental health practitioner* (2nd ed.). New York: Springer.

122. World Health Organization (WHO). (2002). *National cancer control programmes: Policies and managerial guidelines* (2nd ed.). Geneva: World Health Organization.

123. World Health Organization (WHO). (1986, 1990, 1996). *Cancer pain relief and palliative care. Report of a WHO Expert Committed* (WHO Technical Support Series, No. 804). Geneva: World Health Organization.

evolve *Did you remember to check out the bonus material on the Evolve website and the CD-ROM, including NCLEX®-Examination Style Review Questions, Open-Book Quizzes, and Chapter Review Audio Podcasts?*

http://evolve.elsevier.com/Black/medsurg

CHAPTER 22

Clients with Sleep and Rest Disorders and Fatigue

'Lissa D. Clark*

Most of us experience occasional sleep difficulties such as interrupted sleep, daytime drowsiness, or fatigue without serious health consequences. As a nurse you will frequently be involved with clients for whom these disturbances interfere with their health, healing, and activities of daily living. Many factors may contribute to these difficulties, including lifestyle, environment, circadian rhythm disturbances, and changes associated with acute or chronic illness (Box 22-1). Nurses play an important role in promoting health and healing by assessing clients for potential or real sleep difficulties, educating clients in positive sleep habits, and modifying the health care environment to promote sleep.

SLEEP AND SLEEP PATTERN DISORDERS

Sleep is a normal state of altered consciousness during which the body rests. It is characterized by decreased responsiveness to the environment; but a person can be aroused from sleep by external stimuli, whereas comatose people cannot be aroused. Sleep occurs in cycles and includes periods of dreaming and periods of physical rest. See the Anatomy and Physiology review in this section for a summary of the sleep cycle.

It has been estimated that almost one third of the general population has some difficulty with sleep during any given year. These disturbances may be secondary to situational, environmental, or developmental stressors, or they may be associated with illness or with pre-existing disorders. This relationship is often reciprocal in that the disorder often affects sleep and the altered sleep affects the disorder. Poor quality of sleep or sleep deprivation have been associated with risk for diabetes, insulin resistance, and metabolic syndrome.

Sleep pattern disorders also contribute to sensory disorders, such as sensory deprivation and sensory overload. Insomnia is a nursing diagnosis that is defined as a disruption of sleep time that causes discomfort or interferes with a desired lifestyle. Insomnia may be related to one of the more than 80 sleep disorders identified in the International Classification of Sleep Disorders. Intermittent sleep-related problems are also of concern for nursing diagnosis and intervention.

SLEEP DISORDERS

Sleep disorders are commonly divided into two categories: dyssomnias and parasomnias.

Dyssomnias

The dyssomnias include sleep disorders characterized by difficulty initiating or maintaining sleep (insomnia) or by excessive sleepiness (narcolepsy). These disorders may arise predominantly from three sources: from within the body (intrinsic), from external sources (extrinsic), or from circadian rhythm disruptions.

Intrinsic Sleep Disorders

Insomnia. Many people experience transitory periods during which they have difficulty initiating or maintaining sleep. The onset or exacerbation of illness, with or

---

* The author would like to thank Marlene Reimer for her contributions to the chapter in earlier editions.

---

evolve **Web Enhancements**

Client Education Guide Living with Obstructive Sleep Apnea Syndrome (English Version and Spanish Translation)

Appendix A Religious Beliefs and Practices Affecting Health Care

Be sure to check out the bonus material on the Evolve website and the CD-ROM, including free self-assessment exercises. **http://evolve.elsevier.com/Black/medsurg**

BOX 22-1 Chronobiology

Chronobiology refers to the study of physiologic changes as they occur in relation to time of day. Knowledge of chronobiology as it relates to sleep is important to nurses in planning client care and teaching.

Circadian rhythms follow an approximate 24-hour cycle through a complex process linked to light and dark. The *sleep-wake cycle* is one of the circadian rhythms of the body. The effects of illness and hospitalization may disrupt these rhythms, particularly in older adults, who are especially vulnerable to such changes. Nurses can minimize this effect by encouraging a regular schedule with appropriate environmental cues.

Ultradian cycles are circadian rhythms of less than 24 hours. The succession of sleep through identifiable stages, repeating approximately every 90 minutes in adults, is an example. Understanding this cycle, nurses can collaborate with other members of the health care team to cluster cares to avoid waking clients more often than absolutely necessary. As another example of ultradian cycles, serum levels of various hormones are secreted in higher levels according to time of day.

Chronopharmacology refers to the study of how time of day affects the absorption, metabolism, and excretion of drugs *(pharmacokinetics)*. For example, the serum level achieved by a continuous infusion of heparin varies throughout the day, with the risk of clotting greater in the morning and the risk of bleeding greater in the evening. The therapeutic effect of anticancer drugs varies according to the time of administration. Further, steroids should be administered in the morning to approximate most closely the body's natural elevation in cortisol levels.

---

without hospitalization, may precipitate such difficulty. These sleep pattern disturbances are most often associated with disrupted or inconsistent sleep habits *(inadequate sleep hygiene)* or environmental disruptions. These disorders do not constitute insomnia, but they do predispose individuals to insomnia. Up to 10% of the population has developed chronic difficulty in initiating or maintaining sleep. For them, the difficulty does not respond readily to improved sleep hygiene or removal of precipitating factors. This is considered insomnia. Insomnia is further categorized as *primary* or *secondary*. Primary insomnia is not related to other health problems. Secondary insomnia is environmental, emotional, or physiologic in origin.

Psychophysiologic insomnia is a primary insomnia characterized by learned or conditioned sleep-preventing associations and heightened physiologic responses to stress. This perceived difficulty in sleeping can be confirmed by polysomnographic recording, which usually shows the same pattern of long sleep latency or fragmentation that the client describes. Polysomnography is a comprehensive recording of the biophysiologic changes that occur during sleep. Polysomnography is usually performed at night during sleep. This diagnostic test monitors many body functions including brain

(electroencephalography [EEG]), eye movements (electro-oculography [EOG]), muscle activity or skeletal muscle activation (electromyography [EMG]), heart rhythm (electrocardiography [ECG]), and breathing function or respiratory effort during sleep.

In this form of insomnia, the total sleep time is often within normal range but is perceived as inadequate, thus becoming a focus of concern for the client. These clients often find that they can fall asleep unintentionally in low-stimulus situations, such as watching television, but feel increased wakefulness when they go to bed. They may also find it easier to fall asleep in places other than their usual bedroom, having become conditioned to their bedroom as a place of sleeplessness. They are often described as "trying too hard" to sleep.

Management of insomnia is complex, but there is increasing evidence to support both behavioral and pharmacologic interventions. Clients often feel they have already tried the usual interventions to promote sleep. A sleep diary may provide insight into cues and triggers. Sleep habits can become increasingly erratic if the client tries to nap during the day to compensate for sleeplessness at night. Cognitive behavioral therapy (CBT) has become an established approach for treating people with psychophysiologic insomnia. By combining sleep hygiene education, stimulus control, sleep restriction, and cognitive restructuring of beliefs about sleep over a 6- to 8-week series of individual or group sessions, clients will take less time to fall asleep and will have fewer awakenings.

Sleep hygiene is the practice of controlling environment, habits, and activities to promote restorative sleep (Box 22-2). Sleep should be consolidated or restricted by curtailing time in bed to the minimum

---

BOX 22-2 Sleep Hygiene

Sleep hygiene is a variety of habits that help promote quality sleep. The following are some suggestions you can make to your clients experiencing sleep disturbance:

- Maintain a regular sleep-wake pattern throughout the week, even on weekends.
- Avoid daytime naps.
- Avoid stimulants such as caffeine, nicotine, and alcohol close to bedtime.
- Avoid vigorous exercise within 3 hours of bedtime.
- Avoid large meals within 3 hours of bedtime.
- Ensure adequate exposure to natural light.
- Establish a regular bedtime routine with actions associated with preparing for sleep: reading, brushing teeth, listening to music.
- Associate your bed with sleep only, not TV or work.
- Ensure a quality sleep environment: comfortable bedding, clothing, temperature, light levels.

Modified from National Sleep Foundation: *Sleep Hygiene*. Available at www.sleepfoundation.org.

believed necessary, and rising time should be consistent. Relaxation exercises can be helpful, but initially they should be practiced at times other than bedtime. In this way, by the time these exercises are introduced at bedtime, they are effective. Referral to a sleep specialist or mental health professional who can work with the client over a period of time could be considered. Behavioral therapy has been found to be beneficial to some.

Narcolepsy. Narcolepsy is one of the disorders characterized by excessive daytime sleepiness. Narcolepsy is thought to be linked to malfunctioning of the mechanism controlling rapid eye movement (REM) sleep. The REM sleep that occurs appears typical, but it takes place out of sequence of the normal sleep cycle. Impaired release of neurotransmitters such as dopamine may be a factor in both narcolepsy and the associated depression. Narcolepsy is a genetically related condition with autosomal dominance in some cases. The prevalence is about 1 in 1000 people in the United States. Evidence exists for multifactorial genetic transmission. Environmental factors may also play a role.

Manifestations of narcolepsy include disturbed nocturnal sleep and repeated episodes of almost irresistible daytime drowsiness followed by brief periods of sleep at inappropriate times, such as during conversation or while driving or eating. Many narcoleptic clients also experience *cataplexy,* a sudden loss of muscle tone at times of unexpected emotion, such as fright. Upon awakening, the client may experience *sleep paralysis* for several minutes, during which time the client cannot move. Some clients may experience sleep paralysis or one of the other associated manifestations without true narcolepsy. Another REM-like manifestation of narcolepsy is *hypnagogic hallucinations,* which occur at sleep onset or awakening. Automatic behaviors during which there is a lapse of awareness are also frequent, such as the client arriving at work without remembering how she/he got there. When these symptoms are seen together with excessive sleepiness, however, they constitute the classic supporting manifestations of narcolepsy.

On polysomnography, the most characteristic finding is sleep-onset REM periods, rather than the normally occurring non–rapid eye movement (NREM) stage 1. Occurrence of REM periods at sleep onset at least twice during the test period is another criterion for the diagnosis. Multiple sleep latency tests, which measure how long it takes to fall asleep during normal waking hours, show a sleep latency of less than 5 minutes over four or five testing periods.

OUTCOME MANAGEMENT

Medical management of narcolepsy usually consists of low doses of stimulants such as modafinil (Provigil) or methylphenidate (Ritalin) to improve alertness along with tricyclic antidepressants to control cataplexy. 🪔

When counseling narcoleptic clients, emphasis should be placed on good sleep hygiene. It is important to maintain a regular schedule with adequate nighttime sleep. Regular naps at times when clients are prone to increased sleepiness should be recommended. Clients may need assistance coping with the disruptive effects of narcolepsy on family, work, and social roles.

> **Client safety is an important consideration. The effects of this disorder on lifestyle are significant, with 60% to 80% of clients reporting episodes of having fallen asleep at work, while driving, or both. The associated disruption of social and occupational roles and self-esteem may be a major factor contributing to the depression and decreased quality of life frequently reported in clients with narcolepsy.**

SAFETY
⚠
ALERT

Sleep-Disordered Breathing

Sleep apnea. Sleep apnea is characterized by cessation of breathing for 10 seconds or longer occurring at least five times per hour. Sleep apnea can be classified as obstructive, central, or mixed. More recently, other syndromes of upper airway resistance (UARS) and obesity hypoventilation syndrome have been added to the cluster of conditions known as sleep-disordered breathing. Sleep-disordered breathing with the associated recurrent hypoxia has been associated with many health problems, including memory and cognitive deficits, depression, stroke, erectile dysfunction, and decreased quality of life.

Obstructive Sleep Apnea Syndrome (OSAS). Obstructive sleep apnea is a disorder in which complete or partial obstruction of the airway during sleep causes loud snoring, oxyhemoglobin desaturations, and frequent arousals. Obstructive sleep apnea syndrome affects 2% to 4% of the adult population. Prevalence is much higher among obese adults and people older than age 65. Women are less likely than men to develop OSAS, particularly before menopause.

In OSAS, respiratory efforts of the diaphragm and intercostal muscles are apparent but ineffective against a collapsed or obstructed upper airway (Figure 22-1). Snoring indicates partial obstruction. Escalating snoring

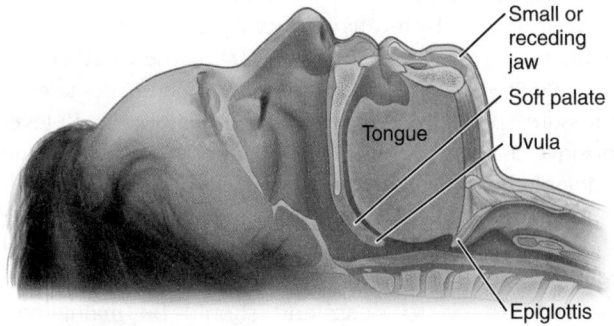

Small or receding jaw
Soft palate
Tongue
Uvula
Epiglottis

■ **FIGURE 22–1** The airway can become obstructed by the tongue, leading to apnea.

followed by a silent pause that ends with a gasp or snort may indicate complete airway obstruction. As hypoxia ensues, the person eventually awakens to breathe. These frequent awakenings interrupt the normal sleep cycle. With sleep, the muscles of the upper airway tend to relax and may occlude an airway that is already narrowed by enlarged soft tissue structures, jaw structure, or obesity. Partial obstruction may result in UARS with or without snoring. This may lead to excessive daytime sleepiness in most clients. A few clients, particularly older adults, may present with insomnia.

OUTCOME MANAGEMENT

Definitive treatment should be considered even in mild OSAS. Strong associations have been demonstrated between OSAS and elevated blood pressure, risk for stroke and heart attack, and psychological disorders. Behavioral change is an integral part of treatment for OSAS, and in milder cases of OSAS may be all that is necessary. Overweight clients may benefit from just a 10% weight loss. Clients with OSAS should avoid the use of alcohol, tobacco and sleeping pills, which make the airway more likely to collapse during sleep and prolong the apneic periods. In some clients with mild sleep apnea, apneic periods occur only when they sleep on their backs. In such cases, positioning with pillows to promote a side-lying position for sleeping has been helpful. Consider referral to a sleep disorders center for clients observed to have 15 to 20 periods of apnea lasting longer than 10 seconds, regardless of whether or not these periods are associated with snoring. Because OSAS is particularly common among men who are obese with short, thick necks who are heavy snorers, these clients should be observed during sleep for apneic periods.

SAFETY ⚠ ALERT **During assessment, question clients regarding their degree of daytime sleepiness, sudden nighttime awakening, and headache upon awakening with particular concern about safety in relation to driving and occupational activities. Clients with OSAS are involved in three times more automobile accidents than clients without OSAS.**

The application of continuous positive airway pressure (CPAP) by means of a face mask covering the nose is the treatment of choice (Figure 22-2). The CPAP device provides room air under increased pressure, providing a pressure splint to keep the upper airway open. Bi-level positive airway pressure (BiPAP) operates by the same principle but uses lower pressure during expiration.

The CPAP mask should be applied securely over the nose and held in place by the head gear (see Figure 22-2). It should be turned on whenever the client is ready to go to sleep and should be maintained throughout the sleep period. Additional humidification may be necessary, particularly in dry climates.

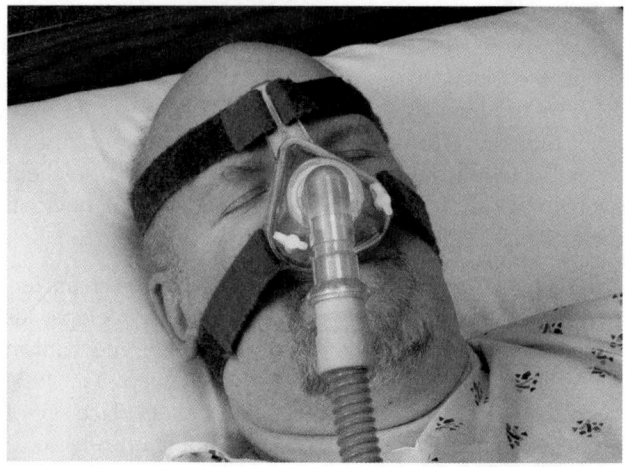

■ **FIGURE 22–2** Continuous positive airway pressure masks are used for clients with obstructive sleep apnea to help keep the airway open during sleep.

Clients may experience nasal congestion, air leaks, pressure marks on the face, or pressure intolerance. Such problems are not uncommon and may lead to discontinuation of the therapy if they are not effectively managed. It is therefore important that nurses have a working knowledge of the therapy, the importance of regularity in its use, and sources available for technical assistance (e.g., sleep disorders center, respiratory equipment supplier).

CPAP units are portable and have features such as battery operation and voltage conversion to accommodate travel requirements. Oral or dental appliances are being used increasingly as another treatment for sleep apnea. These appliances act by keeping the jaw forward and the upper airway open. Studies have found these are less effective than CPAP, but have greater compliance rates because they are less invasive and more comfortable.

Clients who regularly use CPAP should bring their units to the hospital with them. These clients must be closely monitored when recovering from anesthesia and when receiving opioids because they are at risk for ineffective breathing patterns. It should be noted on the health record at the time of admission if a client has OSAS. If the client is scheduled for surgery, the anesthetist and recovery room staff must be alerted. The CPAP unit may be requested to accompany the client to the recovery room.

Orders for benzodiazepines or other hypnotic drugs for clients with OSAS, chronic obstructive pulmonary disease (COPD), or loud snoring should be reviewed because of the risk for possible respiratory depression. Clients with such conditions should be informed that alcohol may also worsen their symptoms because of its selective effect in relaxing the muscles of the upper airway and depression of arousal (see Client Education Guide on Living with Obstructive Sleep Apnea Syndrome on the website).

Uvulopalatopharyngoplasty (UPPP) is a common surgical procedure for reducing snoring. Resecting the uvula, the posterior portion of the soft palate, tonsils, and any excessive pharyngeal tissue can reduce the propensity to obstruction in selected clients. However, concern has arisen that reducing or eliminating snoring may place clients at unknown risk for OSAS. Therefore preoperative assessment, including respiratory pattern during sleep, is recommended before UPPP or the laser-assisted UPPP procedure, which is done in stages in a physician's office. Somnoplasty is another surgical procedure for removal of excessive tissue through the use of high radiofrequencies that spare the mucosa. Tracheostomy may be required in severe OSAS.

Central Sleep Apnea Syndrome. Central sleep apnea is characterized by apneic periods during which no apparent respiratory effort occurs. It may be seen with central nervous system (CNS) lesions, such as in stroke or brain stem trauma, but it is most commonly mixed with obstructive sleep apnea. Cheyne-Stokes respirations are common with this syndrome, and CPAP is the usual treatment. As with obstructive sleep apnea, sedative-hypnotic drugs should be avoided. In severe cases with CNS involvement, the use of a diaphragmatic pacemaker or mechanical ventilation may be required.

Periodic Limb Movement Disorder. Periodic limb movement disorder is characterized by periodic episodes of repetitive, stereotypic leg (or arm) movements that occur during sleep, causing partial arousals and subsequent interruptions of the normal sleep cycle. It may also contribute to daytime sleepiness and frequent nocturnal awakenings. Periodic limb movement disorder is common in the older population.

The diagnosis can be confirmed during polysomnography with surface electromyography (EMG) of the anterior tibial muscles. Several medications can be used to treat the problem, including skeletal muscle relaxants to diminish the magnitude of the movement and the frequency of arousals. The anti-parkinsonian drug carbidopa-levodopa (Sinemet) and the tricyclic antidepressant imipramine seem to act more directly and almost eliminate the movements. Most of the other tricyclic antidepressants aggravate the condition. Anticonvulsant medications such as carbamazepine and valproic acid have brought relief for some clients. Iron and magnesium supplements may be beneficial if deficiencies are suspected.

Restless Legs Syndrome. Restless legs syndrome (RLS) involves annoying "crawling," itching, or tingling sensations of the legs while at rest and causes an almost irresistible urge to move the legs. The syndrome is most severe before sleep onset and interferes with sleep latency. Clients almost always have periodic limb movements during sleep. Treatment is similar to that for periodic limb movements.

Extrinsic Sleep Disorders

The extrinsic sleep disorders have a wide range of causes, from environmental to chemical. Some environmental factors that are present temporarily during hospitalization are discussed under Hospital-Acquired Sleep Disturbances later in this chapter.

Circadian Rhythm Sleep Disorders. In the general population the circadian rhythm sleep disorders such as *time-zone-change syndrome* and *shift-work sleep disorder* are common. In taking a nursing history, be alert to a history of long-time shift work because these clients may have developed altered sleep schedules.

Older and chronically ill clients living alone may be vulnerable to *irregular sleep-wake patterns*. In this disorder, prolonged ignoring or the absence of external cues to time, such as regular mealtimes, work periods, and daylight, leads to erratic periods of sleeping and wakefulness. Internal circadian cues may also be suppressed as a result of aging or diffuse brain disease.

Management strategies for circadian rhythm disorders include maintenance of a regular schedule and exposure to natural sunlight. For example, clients who regularly work the night shift are encouraged to maintain the same sleep schedule on their nights off. Light therapy is being used with some positive results to facilitate adjustments in circadian rhythms as well as in the treatment of seasonal affective disorder (SAD). SAD refers to the onset of a major depressive episode corresponding to a particular period of the year, usually late fall and early winter. Some seasonal variation in mood, activity level, and appetite is common in latitudes where climate and length of daylight change markedly.

Administration of bright light in the early morning is most effective in treating SAD or resetting habitual wakening to an earlier hour. Exposure to bright sunlight at those times can also be effective, but conventional indoor lighting is inadequate. The necessary level of illumination and wavelength requires special light boxes, a variety of which are now available. The combination of light box therapy and administration of melatonin has shown promising results.

Light therapy should begin only under the guidance of a clinician experienced in its use. Teaching should include appropriate positioning of the head in relation to the light source. The most common side effects are eyestrain and headache. Too much light may contribute to irritability and insomnia. The long-term risk of exposure of the eyes to bright light therapy is under investigation. Until more is known, the presence of retinopathy, glaucoma, or cataract is generally considered a contraindication.

Alternative therapies, such as melatonin and L-tryptophan, have received mixed results. The use of melatonin supplements for jet lag is considered in the Complementary and Alternative Therapy feature on p. 410.

Oral Melatonin Supplements for Jet Lag

An analysis of past studies of melatonin for jet lag was conducted, and in this analysis a total of 10 trials met the inclusion criteria. All trials compared the use of oral melatonin versus a placebo. Participants took the melatonin either at the same time after arrival at the destination or close to bedtime at the destination. All trials evaluated treatment for more than 2 days.

A meta-analysis demonstrated a reduction in jet lag with oral melatonin. Daily doses between 0.5 and 5 mg/day were similar in effectiveness, but participants who took the higher doses fell asleep more quickly. Doses greater than 5 mg were not more effective than doses of 5 mg or less. Slow-release melatonin was less effective than fast-release pills. Adverse effects were minimal but were not generally or adequately measured. Clients with epilepsy, clients taking oral anticoagulants, or clients who develop a rash are not good candidates for melatonin. Whether melatonin was better or worse than prescription agents for sleep was not tested.

REFERENCE

Herxheimer, A., & Petrie, K. (2001). Melatonin for preventing and treating jet lag. *Cochrane Database of Systematic Reviews*, 1 (CD001520)

Parasomnias

The parasomnias are disorders that occur during sleep but usually do not produce insomnia or excessive sleepiness. The underlying pathologic mechanism may involve partial arousal or abnormalities in sleep-wake transition.

Arousal Disorders

Partial arousals typically occur during slow-wave sleep. *Sleep walking,* also known as *somnambulism,* may include semi-purposeful behavior, such as dressing. The behavior may be lacking in coordination and appropriateness, however, such as voiding in the closet. Sleepwalking is primarily a pediatric problem; the occurrence of sleepwalking in adults is often associated with anxiety. *Sleep terrors* are sudden arousals from slow-wave sleep accompanied by screaming, tachycardia, tachypnea, diaphoresis, and other manifestations of intense fear. If awakened, the person is often disoriented and has little recall of the nature of the dream image. Sleep terrors typically occur in young children but may develop in adults. *Confusional arousals* manifest themselves when the client awakens, but is momentarily disoriented, has inappropriate behaviors, responds poorly to questions, and has memory impairment. For example, in response to awakening to the phone ringing, the client picks up the remote control. These symptoms most often occur when the client is awakened from deep sleep in the first third of the night. Risk for confusional arousals is increased with sleep deprivation and shift work, as well as some medication.

Sleep-Wake Transition Disorders

Sleep-wake transition disorders are common in the general population, but rarely cause enough disruption to be legitimately called disorders. *Sleep starts* refer to the sudden jerking movement of the legs that often occurs at sleep onset. Some clients may also report a feeling of falling. Nocturnal leg cramps are also common. The frequency and intensity may be greater with high caffeine intake, stress, or intense physical activity before going to bed. *Sleep talking* may occur in all stages of sleep and may also occur more frequently during times of stress.

Parasomnias Associated with Rapid Eye Movement Sleep

Like the other parasomnias, those associated with REM sleep may be distressing but are seldom serious. *Nightmares* are frightening dreams that arise in REM sleep and are often vividly recalled on awakening. In contrast, night terrors occur in slow-wave sleep, and there is little recall. *Sleep paralysis* is one of the classic manifestations of narcolepsy but can occur in isolation. At sleep onset or on awakening, people experience episodes of 1 to several minutes during which they are unable to move. This effect may be an extension of the normal state of low muscle tone during REM sleep.

Other Parasomnias

Other parasomnias are not specifically associated with a particular sleep stage. *Sleep bruxism* refers to grinding of the teeth during sleep, which may lead to dental damage. *Sleep enuresis,* or bed-wetting, may occur in adults in association with other disorders, such as OSAS, but is seen primarily in children. *Primary snoring* is distinguished from OSAS by its rhythmic nature without episodes of apnea or hypoventilation.

Sleep Patterns of Older Adults

With aging, the proportion of stage 4 sleep decreases considerably. REM sleep decreases somewhat, and more time is spent in stage 1. This change results in more frequent nighttime awakenings and less restorative sleep. *Sleep latency,* the time it takes to get to sleep, increases, as does the average length of time it takes to get back to sleep after arousal. Age-related respiratory and cardiac disease, pain, the need to void, and nocturnal dyspnea may also fragment and decrease effective sleep.

Hospitalization affects the quality of nighttime and other sleep time for all clients, but particularly for older adults as these age-related changes heighten the risk for fragmented sleep. The hospital environment often lacks light and dark cues. Anxiety increases sleep latency, and immobility limits activity and exercise. In addition, there are unfamiliar sights and sounds and frequent awakenings for assessment of vital signs and other interventions that disturb sleep.

Institutionalization in a long-term care facility may perpetuate the environmental impact of noise, caregiver interruptions, inactivity, and lack of day-night cues.

Sleep Disorders Associated with Medical and Psychological Disorders

Secondary sleep disorders are of particular relevance in considering problems common to medical-surgical clients. Whereas some clients have a pre-existing sleep dyssomnia or parasomnia, others develop a sleep disorder secondary to their disease or its symptoms. By remaining aware of the physiology of normal sleep, you can anticipate the risk of sleep pattern disturbances.

Neurotransmitter Imbalances

Neurotransmitter imbalances predispose clients to sleep pattern disturbances. These imbalances may be disease related or drug induced. More than 76% of clients being treated for Parkinson's disease report sleep pattern disturbances. Parkinson's disease is from a deficiency of the neurotransmitter dopamine. Insomnia is the most frequent initial concern, followed by sleep fragmentation, disturbances in the sleep-wake schedule, nocturnal enuresis, and visual hallucinations. Dopamine plays an important role in sleep-wake transitions.

At least 90% of people who suffer from *depression* also suffer from sleep disturbances. Milder forms of depression and those that occur in young people are often associated with sleep-onset insomnia; more severe depressions are characterized by broken sleep and early morning wakening. Some relationship appears to exist between the pathogenesis of depression and REM sleep mechanisms in that depressed people who are deprived of REM sleep often show improved mood. The action of tricyclic antidepressants in suppressing REM sleep has been proposed as the primary mechanism underlying their effectiveness in treating depression.

Neurotransmitter imbalances may also contribute to the sleep disturbances frequently seen with Alzheimer's disease and other dementias. The most typical pattern with dementias is frequent awakenings, with agitation progressing to loss of sleep-wake consolidation. Assessing sleep patterns, minimizing caregiver-initiated awakenings (e.g., for toileting), and ensuring a regular bedtime routine may help to reduce nocturnal and daytime agitation. The sleep-wake cycle may be reversed in a client with Alzheimer's disease. The client may nap during the day and be awake at night, restless, agitated, and wandering. The incidence of sleep apnea is higher in people with Alzheimer's disease, possibly as a result of associated neuronal degeneration in the brain stem. Therefore the nocturnal respiratory patterns of these clients should be carefully assessed, with referral to a sleep disorders center if apnea is suspected.

Brain Injury

All degrees of brain injury severity can affect sleep patterns. The appearance of differentiated sleep stages on EEG in comatose clients with severe brain injuries is a favorable prognostic indicator because they indicate connections between the brain stem, diencephalon, and telencephalon. Even after mild brain injury, however, some degree of sleep disturbance may persist for several months. Teaching clients and their families that this unsettled sleep is a typical sequela of *post-concussion syndrome* can allay anxiety and hasten functional recovery.

For clients in the confused, agitated stage of recovery that follows more severe brain injury, use of environmental cues such as light and darkness, regularity of daily schedule, and appropriate daytime exercise and activity can help to restore the sleep-wake cycle.

Hormonal Imbalances

Hormonal imbalances also contribute to sleep pattern disturbance. Clients with *hyperthyroidism* tend to have fragmented, short sleep periods with an excess of slow-wave sleep. *Hypothyroidism* is characterized by excessive sleepiness, with polysomnographic recordings showing a reduction in the proportion of slow-wave sleep.

Clients with *diabetes mellitus,* particularly type 1, may experience hypoglycemia during the night. Besides the usual clinical manifestations of sweating, palpitations, hunger, and anxiety, which the client may recognize as a hypoglycemic reaction, you should be alert to complaints of nightmares and early morning headaches. If these manifestations are present, check blood glucose levels at regular intervals during the night. Insulin dosage or timing may need adjusting. Diabetic clients with autonomic neuropathy have a higher prevalence of breathing abnormalities during sleep because of the associated dysfunction of autonomic respiratory control; thus their nocturnal breathing patterns should be assessed.

Sleep patterns normally vary across the menstrual cycle in response to estrogen and progesterone levels. During the latter part of the cycle, when progesterone levels are higher, the first REM sleep period occurs earlier, and some studies have shown sleep disturbances to be more frequent. Women with *premenstrual syndrome* tend to have less slow-wave sleep throughout the menstrual cycle than their asymptomatic peers. With *menopause,* many women experience poorer sleep quality that may result in mood changes. Estrogen replacement therapy may help to reduce these manifestations, but care should be taken to weigh benefits versus risks of embolic disease and cancer. *Postmenopausal* women are also at higher risk for snoring and obstructive sleep apnea.

Respiratory Disorders

Nocturnal asthma attacks contribute to frequent awakenings in up to 70% of people with asthma. Bronchial resistance and sensitivity to histamine increase during the early morning hours, even in healthy people, thus making clients with asthma more prone to difficulty breathing at night.

Chronic airway limitations, such as asthma and emphysema, contribute to difficulty initiating sleep, frequent arousals with shortness of breath or cough, and chronic fatigue. Oxygen saturation may fall, particularly during REM sleep, when ventilation depends on the diaphragm, which is often flattened and inefficient in clients with advanced chronic air flow limitation. In addition, ventilation and perfusion are altered. Dysrhythmias are common during sleep in clients with advanced respiratory disease, especially when oxygen saturation falls below 60%. Pulmonary artery pressure increases as a result of the pulmonary vascular constriction induced by the low oxygen saturation and the destructive processes of the underlying disease.

Ventilatory responses to hypoxia and hypercapnia are decreased during sleep, even in people with normal respiratory functioning. Clients with advanced respiratory disease are even more vulnerable; thus hypnotics and other CNS depressants that lessen arousal should be given with caution. Bronchodilators should be used before sleep. If the client is anxious and dyspneic, provide a calm, secure, and relaxed environment. Stimulants such as caffeine should be avoided.

The recumbent posture for sleeping is problematic for many people with respiratory disorders. Encourage clients to use several pillows or to elevate the head of the bed; during acute episodes they may find it more comfortable to sleep in a reclining chair.

Cardiovascular Disorders

It has been found that up to 25% of people with hypertension also have OSAS. An association between snoring and hypertension has also been documented. Thus it is important to assess clients with hypertension or who snore while having repeated apneic periods during sleep. In clients with severe heart failure, periodic Cheyne-Stokes breathing may occur. This pattern may result in significant hypoxemia, frequent arousals, increased stage 1 sleep, and reduced total sleep time.

The variability of heart and respiratory rates during REM sleep may be a factor in nocturnal angina. Clients recovering from myocardial infarction are often deprived of sleep during their stay in a critical care unit and may experience REM rebound on transfer to a step-down or standard unit. The greater cardiac demands during REM sleep may put some additional strain on the recovering heart, which makes continued nursing surveillance during this period particularly important.

Gastrointestinal Disorders

Gastric acid secretion normally decreases during sleep, but people with duodenal ulcers have higher than average levels of secretion. Recurrent awakenings with epigastric pain are common, especially in the first 4 hours after sleep onset. Administration of antacids or histamine antagonists may be required.

Gastroesophageal reflux disease (GERD) can be more serious when it occurs during sleep because the longer exposure of the esophagus to gastric acid can lead to esophagitis. Hypnotics should be used cautiously with such clients because the suppression of arousal makes them more vulnerable to esophagitis and pulmonary aspiration. These clients should avoid eating within 3 hours of bedtime, use antacids or histamine antagonists, and raise the head of the bed (reverse Trendelenburg position) to decrease the likelihood of reflux and subsequent aspiration.

Fibromyalgia

Fibromyalgia is a rheumatic condition characterized by unrefreshing sleep, chronic fatigue, and diffuse musculoskeletal pain. Fibromyalgia may also be associated with irritable bowel syndrome, headache, dysmenorrhea, numbness or tingling of the extremities, restless legs syndrome, and cognitive/memory difficulties. The clinical manifestations tend to be vague, and clients are often discouraged with the inability of health care professionals to diagnose and treat this condition. The nurse may be in a position to encourage referral to a sleep disorders center. The majority of clients with fibromyalgia are women. Treatment should involve a multidimensional approach of client education, stress reduction, exercise, and medication. Aerobic exercise has been shown to reduce muscle pain, as well as heat, massage, and muscle relaxants. Antidepressant medications improve mood and sleep quality.

Sleep research shows clients with fibromyalgia are lacking in stage 4 NREM sleep, the most physically restorative stage of sleep. Some suggest sleep disturbance may be an etiology rather than a symptom. Over 50% of clients diagnosed with fibromyalgia also meet the diagnostic criteria for chronic fatigue syndrome. Nurses can educate the fibromyalgia client in proper sleep hygiene. Treatment of fibromyalgia can include muscle relaxants and antidepressants to improve sleep.

Other Disorders

Numerous other disorders seem to have an effect on or an association with sleep. Any condition that results in pain, discomfort, or impaired mobility has the potential to disrupt sleep. Various skin conditions, such as atopic eczema, are associated with decreased REM sleep. Clients with multiple sclerosis experience extreme fatigue that may be related to an altered sleep cycle.

The effect of sleep or sleep deprivation on some disorders can be useful for diagnostic purposes. For example, the typical occurrence of erections in healthy men during REM sleep is used as a diagnostic measure in differentiating sources of impotence. REM-associated erections are also the reason the nurse must be careful when securing an indwelling urinary catheter in a male client to allow a sufficient amount of slack in the tubing to accommodate an erection.

Sleep deprivation and erratic sleep patterns reduce the seizure threshold, which should be considered in assessment and teaching of clients with seizure disorders. Seizure activity may also be a cause of sleep disturbance. Partial and focal seizures can arise in all phases of sleep, including REM; generalized tonic-clonic seizures are more likely to occur during slow-wave sleep than during REM. The tendency of sleep deprivation to trigger seizure activity is used diagnostically in that clients may be required to stay awake all night before they undergo a sleep-deprivation EEG. Some treatment regimens for clients susceptible to nocturnal seizures involve selective medication-induced suppression of sleep stages in which the client's seizures most frequently occur.

💡 HOSPITAL-ACQUIRED SLEEP DISTURBANCES

Clients in the hospital may report difficulty with sleep onset, latency, awakening frequently with difficulty getting back to sleep, and early morning awakening. The causes and interventions range with the type of difficulty.

Sleep Onset Difficulty

Sleep onset difficulty is a common problem in hospitals because of the strange environment and the anxieties associated with illness and hospitalization. A sleep latency time of 20 to 30 minutes is within normal range for most adults. Mimicking the usual sleep activities is helpful, such as watching TV or reading. Environmental controls, such as reduction of noise and interruptions, and conservative relaxation measures, such as a back rub, should be tried before resorting to a pharmacologic intervention. The rapid-acting hypnotics, such as zolpidem (Ambien), are most effective with this type of insomnia.

If a hypnotic is given, monitor the client's safety in getting up at night. Most hypnotics cause some degree of antegrade amnesia, meaning that otherwise cognitively intact clients may become disoriented and forget where they are. 💡 The longer-acting hypnotics also result in some "hangover" effect. An increased risk of hip fractures from falls has been documented in people who are taking long-acting benzodiazepines.

Sleep Maintenance Disturbance

Sleep maintenance disturbance may be associated with sustained use of or withdrawal from a variety of medications and related substances. Alcohol hastens sleep onset but leads to awakening later in the night. In acute intoxication, REM sleep is suppressed. Abrupt withdrawal, as occurs with hospitalization, may trigger massive REM rebound. In chronic alcoholics, sleep architecture remains disturbed even several years after abstinence. Sustained use of or withdrawal from antidepressants, monoamine oxidase inhibitors, propranolol, and phenytoin can also contribute to insomnia.

Other factors that contribute to sleep fragmentation include stimuli that tend to awaken people in the middle of the night. Internal stimuli, such as pain, discomfort, and the urge to void, are frequent causes of disturbed sleep. Sleep disorders, such as sleep apnea and periodic limb movement, are more frequently associated with excessive somnolence, but they do trigger awakenings, after which some people have difficulty getting back to sleep. Hospitalization provides an opportunity for nursing surveillance, which may be instrumental in detecting these disorders as distinct from disturbances triggered by natural or transitory stimuli.

External stimuli include environmental factors, such as light, noise, and temperature, as well as disruptions by others.

> **Nocturnal stimuli can be reduced by darkening the client's room, dimming lights, except for a small night light for safety purposes, and closing curtains. Reduce as much noise as possible by avoiding unnecessary conversation among staff and clients, minimizing equipment noise, and closing the client's door, if possible. You can adjust the temperature by providing bed coverings according to the client's preference and modifying room temperature by adjusting the thermostat or closing doors. Remove disturbing and unnecessary objects, such as equipment associated with painful procedures, to create a pleasant, uncluttered environment.**

SAFETY ALERT

You can also reduce nocturnal stimuli by spacing necessary caregiving activities such as repositioning and assessments to allow periods of 90 minutes or more of undisturbed sleep in order for clients to complete a sleep cycle. When possible, synchronize these activities with periods during which the client is already awake. Finally, coordinate the nature and timing of interruptions by other caregivers such as laboratory or respiratory therapy to preserve periods of undisturbed sleep.

Early Morning Awakening

Early morning awakening occurs frequently among older clients. Sensitivity to environmental disturbances increases toward morning in people of all ages but even more so in older adults. Clients who are disturbed by early morning awakening should be screened for depression.

Sleeplessness and agitation may be associated with an acute confusional state or delirium. This transient cognitive disorder may be associated with acute illness, infection, or admission to the hospital, particularly among older adults. Unlike that of dementia, onset is rapid and is associated with a fluctuating level of consciousness.

Thinking is disorganized and fragmented, memory is impaired, and delusions and hallucinations are common. Sleep is grossly disturbed with frightening dreams, disorientation, and restlessness. Delirium is usually precipitated by a treatable systemic illness such as dehydration, infection, drug toxicity, or renal failure. It is important to identify delirium and pursue treatment possibilities. When the cause is removed, recovery is rapid.

Sleep Deprivation

Sleep deprivation is of particular concern for clients in critical care units. Multiple factors contribute to sleep deprivation, including noise level, 24-hour lighting, and frequency of caregiver interruptions. The manifestations differ depending on the type of sleep that is deprived.

SAFETY
ALERT

Interrupted or decreased NREM sleep results in fatigue, impaired immunity, ptosis, and poor judgment. Clients experiencing a lack of REM sleep display agitation, confusion, paranoia, and hallucinations. Surgical clients are also at risk for sleep pattern disturbance because of disruptions in circadian rhythms. The cause is unclear, but the disruptions may also be related to the length and type of anesthesia, postoperative analgesia, or mechanisms associated with the procedure itself. REM sleep and slow-wave sleep are suppressed.

It may take 4 to 6 weeks for the client's sleep patterns to return to normal after open heart surgery with cardiopulmonary bypass. Specific assessment of sleep quality and quantity should be incorporated into the care of all surgical clients. Studies have shown noise levels in general surgical wards to be above the World Health Organization's guidelines for both day and night shifts.

Health problems caused or exacerbated by lack of sleep are discussed in the Complementary and Alternative Health feature below.

COMPLEMENTARY AND ALTERNATIVE THERAPY

Lack of Sleep and Health Problems

A small study may have provided some insight into the unhealthy behavior of getting too little sleep. A total of 11 healthy young men (ages 18 to 27 years) were allowed to sleep only 4 hours a night for 6 nights. They then were allowed to sleep up to 12 hours/day for another 6 nights. When the men were deprived of sleep, they experienced major imbalances in carbohydrate metabolism and hormone levels. These changes were similar to those observed in older men. These negative changes were reversed when the participants were allowed to sleep more. The researchers concluded that lack of sleep has an effect similar to an accelerated aging process.

REFERENCE
Leproult, R., Spiegel, K., dVan Cauter, E., (1999). Impact on sleep debt on metabolic and endocrine function. *Lancet, 354,* 1435-1439.

REM Rebound

REM sleep occurs later in the sleep cycle and therefore can be missed when sleep time is reduced or interrupted. In order to compensate for missing sleep, a greater proportion of REM-deprived clients' sleep will be REM. This REM rebound can last for several nights as REM sleep is recouped. Withdrawal of medications that suppress REM sleep can lead to an REM rebound effect that is accompanied by nightmares. Normal physiologic occurrences during REM sleep, such as irregular, elevated heart rate and elevated blood pressure, may place the REM rebound client at higher risk because of the longer amount of time spent in REM.

DIAGNOSTIC ASSESSMENT

The primary diagnostic test for sleep disorders is polysomnography. Clients may be referred to a sleep disorders center for overnight EEG, electro-oculography (EOG), and submental EMG with surface electrodes. Clients may also have continuous recording of arterial oxygen saturation by ear or finger oximeter, air flow as detected by monitoring expired carbon dioxide level, respiratory movements by means of transducers placed around the chest and abdomen, and an electrocardiogram (ECG) and heart rate determination with standard limb leads. Ambulatory monitoring systems are also available to facilitate studies in the natural home environment.

A multiple sleep latency test (MSLT) may also be performed to assess impairment of daytime alertness. The MSLT is performed the day after a standard overnight polysomnograph. The time required for clients to fall asleep when in a relaxed state is evaluated at 2-hour intervals, with each nap limited to 20 minutes. The type of sleep is also assessed, making the test particularly useful in diagnosing narcolepsy, a condition in which clients typically have sleep-onset REM periods.

Nursing Management of Insomnia

Assessment

Include a brief assessment of the client's usual sleep habits and recent sleep quality as part of the initial nursing history. On the care plan, note the usual bedtime and rising times as well as any preferences or rituals that may enhance sleep quality. For example, clients with ineffective breathing patterns associated with conditions such as COPD and hiatal hernia may be accustomed to sleeping with several pillows or with the head of the bed elevated.

If sleep quality is reported to be poor, explore the nature of the disturbance by noting the following:

- Usual activities in the hour before retiring
- Sleep latency
- Number and perceived cause of awakenings

- Regularity of sleep pattern (e.g., shift work)
- Consistency of rising time
- Frequency and duration of naps
- Events associated with initial onset of sleep disturbance
- Ease of falling asleep in places other than the usual bedroom
- Situations in which client fights sleepiness
- Daily caffeine intake
- Use of alcohol, sleeping pills, and other medications
- Incidence of morning headache
- Frequency of snoring, apparent pauses in breathing (apneas), and kicking movements; this last information is best obtained from the sleeping partner or from your observation while the client is in the hospital

Objective data may include visible signs of fatigue and lack of sleep, such as circles under the eyes, lack of coordination, drowsiness, diminished problem-solving ability, poor memory, and irritability.

Diagnosis, Outcomes, Interventions
Diagnosis: Sleep deprivation. Sleep deprivation is a common nursing diagnosis (e.g., *Sleep deprivation related to changes in routine secondary to hospitalization and pain*). It may be related to change in sleeping environment, shift work schedule, recurrent pain, or many other possibilities. Other nursing diagnoses may also be applicable (e.g., *Risk for Injury related to excessive daytime sleepiness*).

Outcomes. The client will have improved sleep patterns within 3 nights as evidenced by sleeping for 6 to 8 hours at one time, stated feeling of lessened fatigue, and decreased irritability.

Interventions. The client's usual bedtime routine should be followed as closely as possible. For example, if the client usually watches television before sleeping, attempt to make this possible. Schedule nursing assessments and interventions in blocks of time to allow 90 to 120 minutes of uninterrupted sleep. The environment should mimic nighttime, with lights dimmed and quiet maintained. Offer extra blankets for external warmth. Provide a light complex carbohydrate snack, such as whole wheat crackers, if the client's condition allows.

Other techniques used to promote sleep include back massage, relaxing music, and progressive relaxation techniques. Medications to promote sleep should be used judiciously because they can alter the architecture of sleep, often reducing the REM sleep and eventually leading to REM rebound. If the client is in pain, analgesics rather than sleeping medications should be given. Clients in pain do not sleep restfully.

Sleep medications may be useful during short periods of sleep disturbance (e.g., hospitalization, bereavement, relocation). These medications are usually given at bedtime, and administration may be repeated once if they are not effective. Consider the drug's half-life and the time of night before repeating administration. To avoid prolonged drowsiness, do not repeat sleeping medications after 3:00 AM. Try other measures to promote sleep, such as offering milk, analgesia, music, or back massage.

The client should be awakened with the least obtrusive stimulus possible, such as a soft touch or a soft voice. Startling the client may make it difficult for the client to go back to sleep. Many assessments and interventions can be performed without the client being completely awake.

Diagnosis: Insomnia. Insomnia is a disruption in the amount and quality of sleep that impairs functioning. This diagnosis would be fairly common in home care and long-term care settings. Specify in the diagnostic statement the specific type of problem, such as sleep latency.

Outcomes. The client will report less insomnia within a week as evidenced by feelings of refreshing sleep, less (specify clinical manifestation), and sleeping for increasing numbers of hours.

Interventions. The interventions used for insomnia depend upon the problem that led to an inability to sleep. The disease or condition that is impairing sleep should be addressed first. Instruction in sleep hygiene and behavioral therapy may be necessary. Medications for sleep must be used cautiously, as discussed in the Integrating Pharmacology feature on p. 416.

Evaluation
Some sleep disturbances are temporary and related to the stress of hospitalization. Clients with sleep disturbances may need follow-up care with repeated assessments to determine whether the problem was corrected. Clients with long-term sleep disorders may need ongoing support to maintain the effectiveness of treatment. Client report of perceived refreshing sleep or maintained sleep should be considered.

CHRONIC FATIGUE

Fatigue is a manifestation commonly associated with most acute and chronic illnesses but also experienced with normal, healthy functioning and everyday life. It can be defined as "an overwhelming sustained sense of exhaustion and decreased capacity for physical and mental work at the usual level." Fatigue can be defined as a subjective state in which a client experiences a sustained sense of exhaustion and diminished capacity for physical and mental work that is not relieved by rest. It is often the first indication of an abnormal process and may become a chronic and debilitating condition. Fatigue differs from tiredness or sleepiness in that

INTEGRATING PHARMACOLOGY

Medications for Insomnia

There are currently 10 sedative-hypnotic medications approved by the FDA for the treatment of primary insomnia; they fall into the following categories:

- Benzodiazepines such as triazolam and temazepam; non-benzodiazepines and benzodiazepine receptor agonists such as zolpidem and zaleplon
  - These medications work through similar pathways to decrease sleep latency, improve sleep maintenance, and increase total sleep time. There is little evidence for development of tolerance. Effects on daytime function and performance, anterograde amnesia, falls, and daytime sedation appear to be directly related to dosage levels, administration times, and serum concentrations. Effects of these medications on fall, injury, and cognition cannot be differentiated from similar effects from the insomnia itself. The non-benzodiazepines are becoming the preferred prescriptive treatment related to their lessened residual effects and dosage choices. Rebound insomnia after withdrawal from these medications is mostly related to higher dosing and can be lessened or eliminated by tapering dosages.
- Melatonin receptor agonists such as ramelteon
  - This medication has been found to be significantly effective for insomnia related to sleep onset difficulties. Melatonin is involved in many physiologic functions, including regulation of sleep and circadian rhythms. No studies have found reason to worry about abuse, dependence, or rebound insomnia. Interactions with some medications should be noted by the prescriber.

Other medications prescribed for insomnia but not approved by the FDA for primary insomnia include the following categories:

- Sedating antidepressants such as trazadone and amitriptyline
  - These medications have known sedative effects and are associated with more serious side effects such as leukopenia, thrombocytopenia, orthostatic hypotension, dizziness, and nausea. The residual sedation noted with these medications is thought to be related to their relatively longer half-lives. These medications are prescribed for insomnia more often than the benzodiazepines or

non-benzodiazepine agonists. It is thought this is because many prescribers are treating insomnia as secondary to depression. Recent thought on this category of medications is that there are insufficient data to justify the use of sedating antidepressants for primary insomnia, and it is not recommended.
- Antihistamines such as diphenhydramine and hydroxyzine
  - Use of these medications shows improved sleep latency and maintenance, but clients can develop tolerance in a short amount of time.
- Antipsychotics such as quetiapine and olanzepine
  - There is little research supporting the use of these medications for insomnia. These medications do possess sedative properties, but have long half-lives, resulting in residual sedation. Undesirable side effects such as drug/drug interactions and enzyme interactions are also documented.
- Alcohol
  - Alcohol is the most frequently used substance for insomnia by clients who are self-medicating. It does cause a more rapid sleep onset, but results in later nighttime sleep fragmentation. Alcohol also has been found to have an exacerbative effect on other sleep disorders such as obstructive sleep apnea and restless legs syndrome.
- Melatonin
  - Melatonin has not been evaluated by the FDA as a hypnotic. It has been found in some studies to produce a mild sleep-promoting effect, usually not considered significant. Use in blind clients, who lack the light-dark cues necessary for circadian events, has shown positive sleep effects. Long-term risks and effects are unclear.
- L-Tryptophan
  - The amino acid L-tryptophan has not been tested by the FDA in relation to sleep. Studies show supplemental L-tryptophan has been related to serious side effects such as eosinophilia-myalgia syndrome. Purity and strength of the extracts have also been found to be problematic. The effects of dietary L-tryptophan have not been studied.
- Valerian
  - The herbal supplement valerian has been shown to produce limited sedative effects. Conflicting results of its effects on REM and sleep latency exist. Valerian has been shown to produce withdrawal symptoms and to interfere with the metabolism of some medications.

Modified from Curry, D., Eisenstein, R., & Walsh, J. (2006). Pharmacologic management of insomnia: Past, present, and future. *Psychiatric Clinics of North America, 29,* 871–893.

sleepiness is a temporary state that results from lack of sleep, sleep disorders, improper nutrition, sedentary lifestyle, or a temporary increase in work or social responsibilities. Fatigue, like pain, must be understood as multidimensional, with physiologic, psychologic, social, and spiritual components. Physiologic fatigue has been associated with sleep disturbances, infection, fever, pregnancy, anemia, acquired immunodeficiency syndrome (AIDS), hyperthyroidism or hypothyroidism,

menopause, stroke, multiple sclerosis, cancer and its treatments, and hepatitis. Psychologic fatigue has been described as a state of weariness related to diminished motivation and can be associated with stress, depression, and anxiety.

Chronic fatigue has no recognized function and often has no apparent relation to activity or exertion. The affected person perceives it as being abnormal, unusual, or excessive. It typically has an insidious onset, persists over time, and is not generally relieved by usual restorative techniques.

Chronic fatigue syndrome (CFS) refers to a medical diagnosis of profound fatigue lasting at least 6 months and causing a 50% or greater reduction in physical activities not explainable by other causes. Impaired concentration and generalized aching are commonly associated. It is closely related to fibromyalgia, with about 75% of people with CFS exhibiting the same characteristic tender points as fibromyalgia. They also frequently report sleep disturbances. Coexistence of treatable sleep disorders is not uncommon, and improved sleep hygiene may reduce this overwhelming sense of fatigue.

OUTCOME MANAGEMENT

Many CFS clients are sensitive to medications, particularly sedating medications. Therapeutic benefits can often be achieved at lower than normal dosages. For instance, tricyclic antidepressants not only may improve mood but also may help with sleep and pain. Nutritional supplements and vitamins are frequently used by clients with CFS for symptom relief. While there have been few clinical trials and many CFS clients report symptom relief with supplements, these products are unregulated, and information on potency and side effects is frequently unknown. Herbal remedies such as comfrey, ephedra, kava, germander, chaparral, bitter orange, licorice root, and yohimbe should be avoided. Alternative therapies such as acupuncture, aquatic therapy, gentle massage, meditation, deep breathing, biofeedback, yoga, tai chi, and massage therapy have been helpful for some clients.

Nursing Management of Chronic Fatigue

Assessment
The major defining characteristics of chronic fatigue syndrome are listed in Box 22-3. As with any client reporting manifestations of chronic fatigue, take a detailed sleep history. Chronic fatigue has a major effect on one's activities of daily living and quality of life. Fatigue can be measured with the Revised Piper Fatigue Scale (R-PFS).

Diagnosis, Outcomes, Interventions
Diagnosis: Fatigue. The nursing diagnosis may be written as *Fatigue related to altered body chemistry secondary to chemotherapy*. Because of the complexity of chronic fatigue, a clear etiology may not be evident; in those cases, an etiology of unknown cause is used.

Outcomes. The client will experience less fatigue as evidenced by reporting quality of sleep, reduced pain, and feelings of control of his or her life. This diagnosis will require long-term goals, such as the client reporting a moderate reduction in fatigue within 3 weeks.

BOX 22-3 Manifestations of Chronic Fatigue Syndrome

The major defining characteristic of CFS is self-reported, persistent fatigue lasting 6 months or longer that is not the result of ongoing exertion, is not substantially relieved by rest, and causes a marked reduction in daily activities. Specific manifestations include the following:

- Postexertional malaise (relapse of symptoms after physical or mental exertion); unrefreshing sleep
- Substantial impairment in memory/concentration; muscle pain
- Pain in multiple joints
- Headaches of a new type, pattern, or severity
- Sore throat
- Tender neck or axillary lymph nodes

Interventions. Nurses have an important role in helping fatigued clients manage and cope effectively, whether they are in the hospital or in their own home. Understanding the debilitating effects of fatigue on individuals is an important component of effective nursing care.

Much of the management of fatigue is based on relief of manifestations, with an emphasis on the whole person, mind, and body. An excellent approach to understanding the fatigue is to have the client keep a diary of his or her fatigue. If a pattern is evident, plans can be made to perform routine activities when energy levels are high or to "save" or "bank" energy to use for more complex activities.

A prudent, well-balanced diet is the foundation of good health. Some people with CFS report varying degrees of intolerance to refined sugar, caffeine, alcohol, and tobacco, all of which should be minimized to promote optimal health.

The manifestations of CFS tend to worsen with physical or mental activity, and a prolonged relapse can be triggered by overexertion. Clients are best advised to balance gentle activity with frequent rest periods. Discourage excess rest and social withdrawal. Recommended activities include stretching, light calisthenics, light weights (1 to 2 pounds), walking, bicycling, or swimming. Most clients will need to start with 2- or 3-minute periods of exercise with frequent rest periods. The exercise should not make the individual tired. Careful planning of duration and distance allows the client to stop the activity before becoming tired. The exercise duration is then increased slowly over time but might have to be reduced or withheld temporarily during periods of relapse.

A supportive counselor can help clients cope with the prospects of long-term illness as well as family issues, anxiety, depression, grief, anger, and guilt, which frequently accompany any chronic illness. Cognitive behavioral therapists are specifically trained to provide both the guidance and the support that is helpful in

CFS and other chronic illnesses, focusing on establishing realistic goals, managing symptoms, and strengthening coping mechanisms.

The pain of CFS may be deep pain in the muscles or arthralgias in the joints. Clients may also complain of pressure headaches and allodynia, which is generalized hyperalgesia or soreness of the skin to touch. Although it is advisable to avoid opioids whenever possible, therapy should begin with simple analgesics such as acetaminophen, aspirin, or NSAIDs. Low doses of tricyclic antidepressants can also be helpful in tempering muscle pain. Clients with severe chronic pain should be advised to seek counseling about adjunctive pain management techniques, such as meditation, deep breathing, biofeedback, gentle massage, physical therapy, and others.

As a result of the loss of functional abilities and changes in brain chemistry, depression is a common manifestation in clients with CFS and should be treated when present. You can support clients in understanding the causes of their fatigue and offer support in identifying energy patterns and the need for scheduling activities. An understanding of the effects of conflict and stress on energy levels can help the client learn new fatigue coping skills. Allowing the expression of feelings regarding the effects of fatigue on one's life is therapeutic. Monitor for factors contributing to fatigue on a daily basis, and intervene in a timely manner. Intervention may include carefully planning activities of daily living and daily exercise schedules with appropriate rest periods. Assistance with self-care activities should be offered when needed, and attempts should be made to minimize sensory overload or sensory deprivation.

Evaluation

Fatigue may not resolve completely, depending on underlying factors. Thus evaluation of outcomes and revisions to interventions should be based on mutual planning with the client and family to reduce manifestations and to improve management and quality of life. Balance is needed so that strategies to reduce fatigue, such as avoidance of stress, do not preclude activities that are important to the client.

CONCLUSIONS

The adequacy of sleep and rest is important to consider in caring for clients with acute or chronic illness. Disorders of sleep and fatigue have been discussed with consideration of the reciprocity among these processes, illness, and hospitalization. The nurse can play a pivotal role in environmental modification and client teaching to minimize the impact of sleep, fatigue, and sensory disturbances.

THINKING CRITICALLY

1. The client has just been given a prescription for zolpidem (Ambien) to treat insomnia. She confides to you that she has been using a product from a health food store, recommended by a friend. Now she asks you whether it is safe to continue taking the herbal remedy as well as her new prescription.

Factors to Consider. What is zolpidem? Can it interact with other medications? Are there any worrisome side effects? How could you find more information about the herbal medication the client is taking?

2. A late-middle-age client who had a stroke and is unable to move or speak is placed in a room at the end of the hall, away from the nurses' station. This client was assigned a window bed. He has few visitors. His roommate is a young man recovering from a mild head injury. The roommate has many visitors and uses the radio and television loudly and frequently. Which client is more likely to develop sensory deprivation? Sensory overload? What nursing assessments and interventions would help prevent sensory disturbances?

Factors to Consider. What factors (age, environmental, physical, psychological) affect sensory functioning? How do clients receive and interpret incoming stimuli? Does the room assignment contribute to the development of sensory disturbance in either client?

3. A young adult comes to the neighborhood health clinic. She is unkempt, has circles under her eyes, and yawns frequently. She gives a history of being unable to sleep for any length of time since she gave birth recently to twin sons. She took a variety of prescription "sleeping pills" before she became pregnant and wants a new prescription to help her sleep. What might be causing her sleeplessness? What sleep assessments should be completed? What impact might lack of sleep have?

Factors to Consider. What measures might help this young mother sleep naturally? How would her lack of sleep affect the health of her children? How normal is it for a young adult to experience difficulty with sleep and to take medications to assist with sleep?

Discussions for these questions can be found on the website.

BIBLIOGRAPHY

Citations appearing in red refer to primary research.

Citations appearing in blue refer to evidence-based practice guidelines and protocols.

1. Aaronson, L.S., et al. (1999). Defining and measuring fatigue. *Image: Journal of Nursing Scholarship, 31*(1), 45-50.
2. Alessi, C.A., & Schnelle, J.F. (2000). Approach to sleep disorders in the nursing home setting. *Sleep Medicine Reviews, 4*(1), 45-56.
3. American Academy of Sleep Medicine (AASM). (2001). *International classification of sleep disorders, revised: Diagnostic and coding manual.* Chicago: Ill: American Academy of Sleep Medicine.
4. Armitage, R. (2000). The effects of antidepressants on sleep in patients with depression. *Canadian Journal of Psychiatry, 45,* 803-809.

5. Baldwin, C.M., & Quan, S.F. (2002). Sleep disordered breathing. *Nursing Clinics of North America, 37*, 633-654.

6. Berger, A., Parker, K., Young-McCaughan, S., et al. (2005). Sleep wake disturbances in people with cancer and their caregivers: State of the science. *Oncology Nursing Forum, 32*(6), E98-E126.

7. Carpenito, L.J. (2007). *Handbook of nursing diagnosis* (9th ed.). Philadelphia: Lippincott.

8. Castriotta, R. (2001). Sleep disorders associated with traumatic brain injury. *Archives of Physical Medicine & Rehabilitation, 82*(10), 1403-1406.

9. Christensen, M. (2002). The physiological effects of noise: Considerations for intensive care. *Nursing in Critical Care, 7*, 300-305.

10. Christensen, M. (2005). Noise levels in a general surgical ward: A descriptive study. *Journal of Clinical Nursing, 14*, 156-164.

11. Chowdhuri, S., Crook, E.D., Taylor, H.A., et al. (2007). Cardiovascular complications of respiratory disease. *American Journal of Medical Science, 334*(5), 361-380.

12. Cole, C., & Richards, K. (2006). Sleep in persons with dementia: Increasing quality of life by managing sleep disorders. *Journal of Gerontological Nursing, 32*(3), 48-53.

13. Curry, D., Eisenstein, R., & Walsh, J. (2006). Pharmacologic management of insomnia: Past, present, and future. *Psychiatric Clinics of North America, 29*, 871-893.

14. Dobbin, R. (2006). Wake up to the risks of sleep apnea. *Nursing 2006, 36*(11), 1-4.

15. Dines-Kalinowski, C. (2002). Nature's nurse: Promoting sleep in the ICU. *Dimensions of Critical Care Nursing, 21*(1), 32-34.

16. Ferguson, K., Cartwright, R., Rogers, R., et al. (2006). Oral appliances for snoring and obstructive sleep apnea: A review. *Sleep, 29*(2), 244-262.

17. Floyd, J. (2002). Sleep and aging. *Nursing Clinics of North America, 37*, 719-731.

18. Gordon, M. (2006). *Manual of nursing diagnoses* (11th ed.). St. Louis: Mosby.

19. Gupta, R.M., et al. (2001). Postoperative complications in patients with obstructive sleep apnea syndrome undergoing hip or knee replacement: A case control study. *Mayo Clinic Proceedings, 76*, 897-905.

20. Gottlieb, D., Punjabi, N., Newman, A., et al. (2005). The association of sleep time with diabetes mellitus and impaired glucose tolerance. *Archives of Internal Medicine, 165*, 863-867.

21. Guilleminault, C., & Abad, V. (2004). Obstructive sleep apnea syndromes. *Medical Clinics of North America, 88*(3), 611-630.

22. Inanici, F., & Yunus, M. (2001). Fibromyalgia syndrome: Diagnosis and management. *Journal of Clinical Outcomes Management, 8*(4), 55-67.

23. Ingles, J.L., Eskes, G.A., & Phillips, S.J. (1999). Fatigue after stroke. *Archives of Physical Medicine and Rehabilitation, 80*, 173-178.

24. Knutson, K., Ryden, A., Mander, B., et al. (2006). The role of sleep duration and quality in the risk and severity of type 2 diabetes mellitus. *Archives of Internal Medicine, 166*, 1768-1774.

25. Kulisevsky, J. (2004). Hallucinations and sleep disturbances in Parkinson's disease. *Neurology, 63*(8, Suppl 3), S28-30.

26. Kushida, C., Morgenthaler, T., Littner, M., et al. (2006). Practice parameters for the treatment of snoring and obstructive sleep apnea with oral appliances: An update for 2005. *Sleep, 29*(2), 240-243.

27. Labyak, S. (2002). Sleep and circadian schedule disorders. *Nursing Clinics of North America, 37*, 599-610.

28. Lash, A., Ehrlich-Jones, L., & McCoy, D. (2003). Fibromyalgia: Evolving concepts and management in primary care settings. *MEDSURG Nursing, 12*(3), 145-159.

29. Lee, K. (2003). Impaired sleep. In V. Carrieri-Kohlman, A.M. Lindsey, & C.M. West (Eds.), *Pathophysiological phenomena in nursing* (3rd ed., pp. 363-385). St. Louis: Saunders.

30. Lurie, S. (2006). Seasonal affective disorder. *American Family Physician, 74*(9), 1521-1524.

31. Mahowald, M.W. (2000). Sleep in traumatic brain injury and other acquired CNS conditions. In A. Culebras (Ed.), *Sleep disorders and neurological disorders* (pp. 365-385). New York: Marcel Dekker.

32. McCloskey, J., & Bulechek, G. (2000). *Nursing interventions classification* (3rd ed.). Philadelphia: Mosby.

33. Miller, A. (2005). Epidemiology, etiology, and natural treatment of seasonal affective disorder. *Alternative Medicine Review, 10*(1), 5-13.

34. North American Nursing Diagnosis Association (NANDA). (2007). *Nursing diagnoses: Definitions and classification 2007-2008*. Philadelphia: Author.

35. O'Rourke, D.J., Klaasen, K.S., & Sloan, J.A. (2001). Redesigning nighttime for personal care residents care. *Journal of Gerontological Nursing, 27*(7), 30-37.

36. Pack, A. (2006). Advances in sleep-disordered breathing. *American Journal of Respiratory and Critical Care Medicine, 173*, 7-15.

37. Piper, B., Dibble, S., Dodd, M., et al. (1998). The revised Piper fatigue scale: Psychometric evaluation in women with breast cancer. *Oncology Nursing Forum, 25*, 677-682.

38. Piper, B.F. (2003). Fatigue. In V. Carrieri-Kohlman, A.M. Lindsey, & C.M. West (Eds.), *Pathophysiological phenomena in nursing* (3rd ed., pp. 209-234). St. Louis: Saunders.

39. Revell, V., Burgess, J., Gazda, C., et al. (2006). Advancing human circadian rhythms with afternoon melatonin and morning intermittent bright light. *Journal of Clinical Endocrinology & Metabolism, 91*(1), 54-59.

40. Rogers, A.E., & Dreher, H.M. (2002). Narcolepsy. *Neurology Clinics of North America, 37*(4), 675-692.

41. Shaver, J. (2002). Women and sleep. *Nursing Clinics of North America, 37*, 707-718.

42. Smith, M., & Perlis, M. (2006). Who is a candidate for cognitive behavioral therapy for insomnia? *Health Psychology, 25*(1), 15-29.

43. Soares, C., & Murray, B. (2006). Sleep disorders in women: Clinical evidence and treatment strategies. *Psychiatric Clinics of North America, 29*(4).

44. Sleasny, K., et al. (2002). Clinical symptomatology and treatment of restless legs syndrome and periodic limb movement disorder. *Sleep Medical Review, 6*(4), 253-265.

45. Stansbury, T.T. (2001). Narcolepsy: Unveiling a mystery. *American Journal of Nursing, 101*(8), 50-53.

46. Tamburri, L., DiBrienza, R., Zoaula, R., et al. (2004). Nocturnal care interactions with patients in critical care units. *American Journal of Critical Care, 13*(2), 102-112.

47. Turkoski, B. (2006). Managing insomnia. *Orthopaedic Nursing, 25*(5), 339-347.

48. Worthington, A. (2006). Rehabilitation is compromised by arousal and sleep disorders: Results of a survey of rehabilitation centres. *Brain Injury, 20*(3), 327-332.

49. Yaggi, H., Concato, J., Kernan, W., et al. (2005). Obstructive sleep apnea as a risk factor for stroke and death. *New England Journal of Medicine, 353*(19), 2034-2041.

CHAPTER 23

Clients with Psychosocial and Mental Health Concerns

Nancy Christine Shoemaker

A sound knowledge base for responding to psychosocial and mental health concerns of clients and their families is vital in all settings where medical-surgical nursing is practiced. Psychosocial components are defined as the psychological and social aspects of the client's health status. Psychological factors include thinking, feelings, motivation, and personal strengths and weaknesses. Social issues are related to patterns of interaction with others. For all clients seeking health care for a physical problem, there is a potential for alteration in their mental or emotional status because of the stress of illness and navigating the health care system. The North American Nursing Diagnosis Association (NANDA) currently lists 188 approved nursing diagnoses; approximately 35% are related to psychosocial functioning (see the box on NANDA International 2007-2008 Nursing Diagnoses Related to Adult Psychosocial Concerns on the website). To promote successful health outcomes, the nurse must address the psychosocial and mental health concerns of each client.

Some clients have a pre-existing mental disorder that may complicate or adversely affect the outcome of their medical treatment. Within a 12-month period, approximately 40 million people suffer from anxiety disorders, approximately 20.9 million more are affected by mood disorders (depressive disorders and bipolar disorder), and approximately 2.4 million are afflicted with schizophrenia.[17] For these clients, nursing attention to psychosocial needs makes the difference between compliance with treatment and noncompliance with resulting complications.

This chapter focuses on the psychosocial concerns of clients and families who require nursing care across various treatment settings. Basic principles regarding communication are outlined, and nursing interventions to reduce anxiety are presented. Concepts of anxiety, stress, coping mechanisms, and self-esteem are reviewed. Three clients with concurrent medical disorders and serious mental illness are discussed to illustrate the challenge that these individuals present for holistic nursing care. In each case, the role of the medical-surgical nurse is presented along with a suggested nursing care plan. Finally, the dimensions of culture and spirituality are addressed (see the boxes on Psychosocial Dimensions: Spirituality and Mental Illness, Culture and Mental Illness, and Sexuality and Mental Illness on the website).

---

evolve **Web Enhancements**

Care Plan The Client with Degenerative Joint Disease and Concurrent Panic Disorder: Mrs. James

The Client with Hiatal Hernia and Concurrent Schizophrenia: Mr. Barnes

The Client with Diabetic Ketoacidosis and Concurrent Depression: Mrs. Conners

Diversity in Health Care The Significance of Cultural Assessment

Complementary and Alternative Therapy Box Exercise versus a Prescription Medication for Major Depressive Disorder

Boxes NANDA International 2007–2008 Nursing Diagnoses Related to Adult Psychosocial Concerns

Psychosocial Dimension: Spirituality and Mental Illness

Psychosocial Dimension: Culture and Mental Illness

Psychosocial Dimension: Sexuality and Mental Illness

Emotional, Physical, and Spiritual Manifestations of Anxiety

Medications for Anxiety Disorders

Selected Standardized Tools for Assessment of Psychiatric Disorders

Medications for Schizophrenia

Medications for Mood Disorders

Tables Characteristics of People with High and Low Self-Esteem

Levels of Psychiatric Treatment Services

Appendix A Religious Beliefs and Practices Affecting Health Care

Be sure to check out the bonus material on the Evolve website and the CD-ROM, including free self-assessment exercises. **http://evolve.elsevier.com/Black/medsurg**

CLIENT SCENARIOS

Picture yourself as the nurse responsible for the clients in the following scenarios. The following scenarios help illustrate the later discussion of psychosocial and mental health issues and their application in nursing care across a variety of clinical settings:

- You work the 3 to 11 PM shift in the emergency department (ED). You are assigned to Mrs. Barbara James, a 51-year-old black woman admitted several hours ago with acute chest pain and respiratory distress. Although diagnostic tests rule out myocardial infarction, she is crying and afraid to go home.
- While on duty in a busy university medical clinic, you see a client with a recently diagnosed hiatal hernia. Gregory Barnes is a 32-year-old, slightly obese black man who smiles pleasantly as you introduce yourself, and shakes your hand. He tells you that he has a problem with the elves who live in his basement and who take all his food.
- You are a staff nurse on a medical acute care unit and are assigned to Mrs. Mary Conners, a 59-year-old West Indian woman admitted the previous day with diabetic ketoacidosis. Entering her room, you notice that the lights are off, and she does not look up when she responds to your greeting.

UNIVERSAL ISSUES

Universal psychosocial concepts include anxiety, stress, coping mechanisms, and self-esteem. Additional factors that influence reactions to stress are cultural and family background, exposure to similar stressors, and repeated exposure to stressors.

Anxiety

Before addressing the psychosocial concerns of clients with concurrent mental disorders, the nurse must first develop skills to manage the anxiety that is common to all clients. *Anxiety* is a universal human phenomenon, defined as a strong feeling of fear or dread with an unknown cause. All clients (and their loved ones) are vulnerable to feeling anxiety as they seek care for medical problems. Everyone may feel anxiety at times, especially when facing an unknown situation (changing schools, starting a new job). Under normal conditions, this discomfort is short-lived and may be helpful for problem solving (see the box on Emotional, Physical, and Spiritual Manifestations of Anxiety on the website). **evolve**

Stress

Anxiety is part of the human reaction to stress. *Stress* is defined as "a particular relationship between the person and the environment that is appraised by the person as taxing and/or exceeding his or her resources and endangering his or her well-being."[12] Resources can include one's coping skills. In the case of potential physical danger, one is mobilized for self-protection with the fight-or-flight response. Most people would experience strong reactions in the face of crisis situations such as an imminent car accident or a tornado. In addition to external stressful events, people may define stress in different ways because it is the perception of the event, not the event itself, that stimulates the response. For example, one student may feel extreme stage fright when giving a speech, whereas another may feel only mild tension. Table 23-1 describes the levels of anxiety, with implications for client teaching.

Coping Mechanisms

Most people respond to anxiety by using *coping skills* that are learned external behaviors or internal thought processes consciously used to decrease discomfort. Coping behavior can be classified as follows:[25]

- *Emotion-focused* behaviors to alter one's response to the stressor, such as thinking, saying, or doing something to make oneself feel better (crying, sharing feelings with someone)
- *Problem-focused* behaviors to directly alter the stressor, such as seeking facts about a problem or making a plan to overcome the obstacle (family member asking multiple questions over and over)

TABLE 23–1 **Manifestations of Four Levels of Anxiety**

Anxiety Level	Physical Manifestations	Emotional Manifestations	Cognitive Manifestations
Mild	Increased pulse rate and blood pressure measurement	Positive affect	Alert, can solve a problem, prepared to learn new information
Moderate	Elevated vital signs, tense muscles, diaphoresis	Tense, fearful	Attention focused on one concern, may be able to concentrate with direction
Severe	Fight-or-flight response, dry mouth, numb extremities	Distressed	Decreased sensory perception, can focus only on details, unable to learn new information
Panic	Continued as in severe level	Totally overwhelmed	Ignores external cues, focused only on internal stimuli, unable to learn

Another common response to anxiety is the use of *ego defense mechanisms,* originally defined by Freud.[21] These thought processes are not deliberate or voluntary, like coping mechanisms. Instead, they exist at an unconscious level to disguise the real threat, protecting the person from feeling anxious about the real issue. One defense mechanism frequently seen in clients with serious illness is *denial.* Box 23-1 gives definitions and examples of selected defense mechanisms.

Assess the level of anxiety in all clients, and intervene as early as possible to reduce the anxiety to a manageable level. To achieve compliance with treatment, the client or family must be calm enough to understand the teaching. You can use several simple communication techniques to decrease anxiety in clients; these interventions are outlined in Box 23-2.

You must also be able to recognize positive coping efforts by clients and their families. As noted previously, these behaviors may be emotion focused or problem focused, but they function to decrease anxiety. Failure to understand these behaviors may lead to nontherapeutic staff reactions that impede recovery.

Self-Esteem

Another universal concern that affects the client's reaction to the stress of illness is self-esteem. *Self-esteem* is defined as "the individual's personal judgment of his or her own worth."[9] The client's pre-existing level of self-esteem influences the adjustment to illness. A person with high self-esteem has positive expectations even in stressful situations. In contrast, a person with low self-esteem consistently demonstrates pessimism (see the table on Characteristics of People with High and Low Self-Esteem on the website for characteristics of self-esteem with implications for nursing care).

ADDITIONAL NEEDS OF CLIENTS WITH CONCURRENT MENTAL ILLNESS

After recognizing the psychosocial concerns of clients in general, you should become aware of additional needs

---

BOX 23-1 Selected Defense Mechanisms: Definitions and Examples

Definition	Example
Denial—avoiding a problem by ignoring it or refusing to recognize it	A client with a cardiac condition tells his family that he has a "little problem" after the physician explains his diagnosis of heart attack.
Displacement—transferring feelings for a threatening topic or person to another more neutral topic or person	After a client is told that he cannot be discharged today as planned, he spends the whole shift complaining that his breakfast was cold.
Intellectualization—showing excessive thinking and logic to avoid uncomfortable feelings	After a leg amputation, a client shows great interest in the details of the surgery and even requests a textbook to identify the muscles and bones, but he does not watch while the nurse changes the dressing.
Projection—assigning one's own uncomfortable feelings or motivation to another person	A client tells the nurse, "Please explain about the operation again to my wife; she is so afraid that I won't wake up."
Rationalization—giving an apparently logical and acceptable explanation to cover up a feeling or motive that may not be socially acceptable	The nurse finds a client eating breakfast when he is on NPO status (nothing by mouth) for a diagnostic test. The nurse specifically told him about the procedure yesterday. When asked what happened, the client states, "Well, the aide brought me this tray so I thought it was okay."
Regression—demonstrating behavior characteristics of an earlier stage of development	An adult client insists on keeping multiple stuffed animals on her bed and bursts into tears when the nurse moves one to check her arm for IV access.

BOX 23-2 Nursing Interventions to Decrease Client Anxiety

Nonverbal Interventions	Verbal Interventions
Listen with full attention, looking at the client with unbroken eye contact.	Answer questions honestly.
Maintain a calm, unhurried approach.	Explain all procedures in simple terms.
Speak slowly in a clear, firm voice (not loud).	Give reassurance based on the data.
Offer or use touch (e.g., hold a hand or give a back rub).	Give information about tests, medicines, and treatments as requested.
If possible, decrease the noise and bright light.	Explain the reasons for limitations on activity or other restrictions.
	Acknowledge the client's anxiety, and encourage the client to explore the reasons.
	Include family members in discussions unless the client requests otherwise.
	If necessary, repeat directions patiently.

for successful care of clients with concurrent mental illness. These needs consist of (1) comprehensive nursing assessment, (2) self-awareness regarding communication, (3) basic mental health teaching for the client and family, and (4) referral for specialized services.

Comprehensive Nursing Assessment

As soon as you realize that the client is presenting with an altered mood or thought process, review the nursing database to ensure that it is complete. In many admission situations, limited data are obtained before treatment is initiated. Make sure that you gather a complete psychosocial history. Table 23-2 lists definitions of commonly used terms to describe abnormal findings.

Psychosocial risk factors, such as a history of self-destructive, aggressive, or socially inappropriate behavior, must also be identified. Secondary sources, such as family and medical records, are often helpful. A complete medication history also provides data about concurrent mental illness if the client names psychotropic medications.

Awareness of Communication

The second requirement in caring for psychiatric clients is to pay extra attention to all communication with them. Under ordinary circumstances, communication with clients seems fairly routine and predictable: the nurse provides necessary physical care and teaching, which the client accepts or rejects.

Human communication is complex and built upon many assumptions and unspoken rules inherent in a given culture. Communication between two participants involves all of the verbal and nonverbal behavior that they perceive in each other.[23] In addition to using selected words, we send involuntary nonverbal signals. Nonverbal communication includes tone and volume of voice, eye contact, facial expression, body posture, and other body language. We expect to find congruence between the words and nonverbal cues; the words match the feeling and tone of the body (see the Diversity in Health Care feature on The Significance of Cultural Assessment on the website).

When the words and the nonverbal signs from a sender do not match, the receiving person must pause to analyze the situation. Psychiatric clients consistently have difficulty with communicating their needs. It is generally agreed that when verbal communication and nonverbal communication are incongruent, the nonverbal communication reflects the person's true feelings.

When communicating with clients who have concurrent psychiatric problems, pay attention to the communication process. Collect thorough data to determine the nursing diagnoses and to communicate with the treatment team. Monitor your own nonverbal behavior to prevent sending negative nonverbal messages to the client. Mental illness in our society still carries a

considerable stigma: clients and their families feel ashamed because of an emotional problem; staff may have biases based on personal experience.[15]

Client and Family Teaching

The third important requirement for all clients with concurrent psychiatric disorders is basic client and family teaching. Basic teaching for all clients includes a definition of the illness, medications and treatment options, and relapse prevention.[19] This information is readily available in written teaching materials, which can be kept on file along with medical-surgical teaching guides.

TABLE 23–2 Commonly Used Terms to Describe Abnormal Mental Status Findings

Term	Mental Status Findings
Mood	
Depressed	Feeling sad, decreased energy and interest in usual activities
Elated	Feeling euphoric, overly optimistic, and energetic
Labile	Rapidly changing from one state to another (e.g., happy to sad or irritable)
Affect	
Blunted	Overall decrease in emotional tone compared with a normal reaction to a situation
Flat	No expression of feelings, regardless of variation in topics
Inappropriate	Nonverbal signs of feelings do not match the verbal report of the person (e.g., person smiles when reporting a sad event)
Motor Activity	
Agitation	Physically restless, unable to sit still
Psychomotor retardation	Physically slowed down, including all movements and speech
Perception	
Hallucination	Sensory perception originating from within the brain but attributed to external sources (e.g., hearing voices)
Illusion	Incorrect interpretation of external sensory input (e.g., seeing a shadow in the closet and thinking it is a person)
Speech	
Loose association	Speech pattern in which listener cannot follow connections between speaker's ideas, seems illogical to listener
Pressured speech	Rapid flow of speech with intense undercurrent of feeling, may refuse to be interrupted
Thought Process	
Delusion	A fixed, false belief that is strongly defended by the individual (e.g., may be paranoid [suspicious] or grandiose [unrealistically wonderful])
Psychosis	Severe impairment in reality testing, with distortion in perception and analysis of external and internal stimuli

Whenever possible, include a family member in the instruction because he or she has a significant role in caring for the client (see the WebLinks on the website for resources to educate and support clients and their families).

Specialized Referrals

The fourth important requirement to consider when caring for clients with concurrent mental disorders is the need for specialized referrals. If manifestations are severe or risk factors are significant, additional evaluation is necessary and you are in a key position to advocate for appropriate services. In the hospital or institutional environment, consulting psychiatric staff can be called for an in-depth assessment and disposition. Likewise, in the community setting, referrals can be made to specialized outpatient services.

Summary

The medical-surgical nurse has a clear role to play with clients who have concurrent psychiatric disorders. The four steps just outlined do not require training beyond that of a generalist. They do require a professional commitment to provide holistic care to all clients and to fully use the multidisciplinary team available in the health care setting. In the sections that follow, the three psychiatric clients introduced in this section are revisited in more detail. An overview of their psychiatric disorders is presented along with specific nursing care plans for management in the medical-surgical setting.

ETIOLOGY OF MENTAL DISORDERS

The causes of psychiatric disorders are not yet fully understood. Ongoing brain research has identified biologic alterations, and psychological theories have been used as a framework for treatment.

Biologic

Biologic evidence shows a genetic influence for the mental disorders: first-degree relatives have an increased risk for the same manifestations. Studies with medications and diagnostic imaging techniques have shown abnormalities in brain structures and neurotransmitters. For example, the ventricles are enlarged and brain volume is decreased in the frontal and temporal lobes in clients with schizophrenia. With mood disorders, the limbic system is altered. For anxiety disorders, frontal and temporal lobes and the brain stem are affected. Dysregulation in the following neurotransmitter systems is the target of the psychotropic medications: dopamine, serotonin, norepinephrine, gamma-aminobutyric acid (GABA), and glutamate.[8,11,24]

Psychological

Psychological approaches relate mental disorders to unconscious processes, faulty thinking, or learning.[7] Psychoanalytic theory proposes that anxiety results from inability to control painful impulses, thoughts, or memories. Cognitive theory suggests that a person consistently distorts reality to see the world in a negative way. Behavioral theory explains abnormal behavior as a learned response to specific reinforcement in the environment.

ANXIETY

Mrs. James presents with a classic case of panic attack. The acute manifestations can create severe physical distress: palpitations, chest pain, elevated vital signs, dizziness, nausea, and distinct fear that one is dying. The cardiac work-up does not reveal abnormal cardiac enzymes or any electrocardiogram (ECG) anomalies, and the manifestations subside spontaneously. After additional diagnostic testing to rule out other medical disorders, panic disorder can be identified.

Panic disorder is one of the eight subtypes of anxiety disorders identified by the *Diagnostic and Statistical Manual of Mental Disorders,* fourth edition, text revision (*DSM-IV-TR*).[1] Anxiety disorders as a group are the most common psychiatric disorders in the United States and affect 18.1% of American adults in a given year.[17] Box 23-3 describes each diagnosis.

BOX 23-3   Key Features of Anxiety Disorders

- *Panic Disorder*—recurrent panic attacks followed by a change in behavior to try and avoid another attack; persists more than 1 month
- *Generalized Anxiety Disorder* (GAD)—excessive anxiety for 6 or more months that is uncontrollable, often focused on health or money concern
- *Phobia*—severe, persistent fear of an object or situation that the person recognizes as irrational but cannot overcome
- *Obsessive-Compulsive Disorder* (OCD)—preoccupation with disturbing thoughts (obsessions) or repetitive actions (compulsions) that interferes with normal activities of daily living
- *Post-Traumatic Stress Disorder* (PTSD)—reexperiencing a real, horrifying event in nightmares or flashbacks, with a duration of manifestations more than 1 month; may be an immediate or a delayed reaction
- *Acute Stress Disorder*—similar to PTSD except that manifestations occur within 1 month of the event and last only for approximately 1 month
- *Anxiety Disorder due to General Medical Condition*—severe anxiety in the presence of clear physical findings of a somatic disorder (e.g., hypoglycemia)
- *Anxiety Disorder Not Otherwise Specified*—showing some anxiety or phobic manifestations, but not severe enough to warrant a specific diagnosis

Manifestations may range from mild to severe. Many of these clients avoid seeking treatment because of their feelings of shame. 🪔 The most recent National Comorbidity Survey Replication disclosed that there was a delay of 9 to 23 years from the onset of anxiety manifestations until the first treatment contact.[14]

OUTCOME MANAGEMENT

All of the anxiety disorders can be effectively treated through a combination of medication and psychotherapy. Several different classes of drugs that alter levels of neurotransmitters can be helpful (see the box Medications for Anxiety Disorders on the website for a list of commonly prescribed anti-anxiety medications).[18] These medicines may be prescribed for short-term or long-term use but usually are not needed permanently. Medication may offer some immediate benefit to reduce the discomfort of anxiety, but some form of psychotherapy (individual, group, or family) is necessary to achieve lasting positive outcomes. Clients have often adopted negative patterns of thinking or avoidance behaviors that are not easily given up.

Intervention

Returning to Mrs. James, the ED nurse needs to quickly devise a care plan with a discharge plan (see the Care Plan feature on The Client with Degenerative Joint Disease and Concurrent Panic Disorder on the website).[10]

Comprehensive Assessment

As the nurse explores the client's current psychological and social functioning, Mrs. James reports that she has had four episodes of respiratory distress in the past 6 months. She cannot relate the attack to any particular stressor but has started to avoid all places where she feels anxious. She also describes difficulty sleeping, increased appetite, crying spells, and decreased sexual interest.

When asked about her past level of functioning, Mrs. James states that, until 1 year ago, she was working as a nurse's aide and was independent. She drove, helped to care for her mother, and enjoyed going out with friends to church and social events. After a fall resulting in a knee injury, she never recovered full ambulation and recently applied for disability. In relation to her family history for emotional problems, Mrs. James explains that her mother is an alcoholic and her daughter takes an antidepressant, but she has always been "too strong for that kind of problem."

Communication Awareness

Throughout the interview, the nurse provides a private, supportive atmosphere. Initially, the nurse closes the curtain and moves the chair so that there is continuous eye contact. It is explained that they may have only 15 minutes before an interruption, but the nurse wants to learn as much as possible about Mrs. James. As the client talks, the nurse encourages her with nonverbal cues such as nodding her head. When the client becomes tearful at times, the nurse calmly pauses and offers her a tissue. The nurse shows no surprise or disapproval when Mrs. James mentions mental illness in her family. At the end of the assessment, the nurse explains that the discharge plan must be developed with the physician and she advises Mrs. James to call a family member to pick her up.

Client and Family Teaching

The nurse reports the findings on Mrs. James' anxiety and mood to the attending physician and recommends that the psychiatric consultant for the ED be called. The physician agrees, noting that all laboratory findings are normal. The probable diagnosis is panic disorder. As the physician goes to speak with the client, the nurse obtains material on panic attack and coping skills for families. The nurse gives these pamphlets to Mrs. James and her daughter, telling them that anxiety is a common, treatable problem. The nurse also explains the role of the psychiatric consultant and asks them to wait to talk with her. Mrs. James is uncertain, but the daughter encourages her to agree.

Specialized Referrals

In choosing the appropriate referral for discharge planning for Mrs. James, the nurse is aware that the medical center offers several levels of psychiatric care (see the table on the Levels of Psychiatric Treatment Services on the website). Because the client is not at immediate **evolve** risk to harm herself or others, referral to the inpatient unit is not indicated. If an appointment is given to the outpatient clinic for next week, she may not follow up. Thus the nurse selects the resource person who can make an immediate, specialized assessment and disposition, namely, the ED consultant.

The psychiatric consultant (social worker, advanced practice nurse, or psychologist) performs a full, diagnostic interview, including appropriate standardized tests for anxiety and depression (see the box on Selected Standardized Tools for Assessment of Psychiatric Disorders on the website for a list of commonly used rating scales for **evolve** mental health assessment). The ED nurse shares the nursing database with the consultant.

After meeting with the client and her daughter, the psychiatric consultant recommends referral to the Partial Hospital Program on the following day because of the severity of manifestations. The nurse communicates this recommendation to the physician and strongly supports this treatment in the discharge instructions to Mrs. James and her daughter.

SCHIZOPHRENIA

Mr. Barnes demonstrates clear manifestations of *schizophrenia* with fixed delusions and hallucinations. He represents a generation of young, chronically mentally ill people who have been cared for primarily in the community instead of being institutionalized. Schizophrenia is a persistent, severe mental illness that affects 1.1% of the American adult population in a given year. The onset of the disorder is usually during late teens or early twenties, and men and women are equally affected.[17] *DSM-IV-TR* lists five subtypes (Box 23-4).

In all cases, a person's thinking and communication skills are profoundly affected. Manifestations are generally classified as positive or negative.[4] *Positive* manifestations include the most obvious signs of psychosis (auditory or visual hallucinations, delusions, disorganized thinking and speech). *Negative* manifestations refer to the lack of usual emotional or social responses (blunted affect, avoidance of social contact, lack of energy and motivation).

OUTCOME MANAGEMENT

The positive manifestations of schizophrenia can be controlled by antipsychotic medication, but the negative manifestations and severe social impairment require supportive psychotherapy. Antipsychotic medicines have been used since the 1950s, and several classes of drugs have evolved over time in an effort to reduce unpleasant side effects (see the box on Medications for Schizophrenia on the website).[20] These medications usually must be taken for a lifetime to control the

manifestations. With medication, some clients report a total absence of hallucinations, but for others, internal voices become a permanent experience.

A major concern for most clients is the presence of side effects related to sedation and abnormal movements.[20] Because typical antipsychotics affect all dopamine receptors, including those for movement, muscle side effects known as *extrapyramidal symptoms* (EPS) are extremely common. Manifestations of EPS may include stiffness or tremor in arms and legs, extreme restlessness with subjective discomfort, drooling, and acute muscle spasms of the tongue, neck, or face. These side effects are usually short term and treatable with an anticholinergic agent such as benztropine or trihexyphenidyl. However, a long-term side effect of typical antipsychotics, called *tardive dyskinesia* (TD), occurs in approximately one third of clients and is usually irreversible. Common manifestations of TD are obvious, involuntary movements of the tongue, face, hands, or legs. The main benefit of the newer, atypical antipsychotics is the lower incidence of EPS and TD because the drugs are more selective in affecting neurotransmitters.

One final side effect of antipsychotics should be noted.

Neuroleptic malignant syndrome is a rare but serious condition that may appear suddenly with extreme muscle rigidity, high fever, sweating, and fluctuations in consciousness. The client requires emergency hospitalization with supportive treatment to prevent seizures, coma, or even death.

Treatment of impaired social functioning involves long-term supportive therapy and psychosocial rehabilitation. Social withdrawal and lack of interest in school or work often signal the onset of the illness and may persist throughout treatment. To develop and maintain maximal level of functioning, schizophrenic clients need individual counseling and support, psychoeducation, organized rehabilitation services, and family psychoeducation.[16]

As with any chronic illness, the client experiences episodes of remission and exacerbation. Medication noncompliance, denial of illness, and stressful events may lead to multiple, short-term hospitalizations over a lifetime. With the consistent support of family and community resources, however, many clients can progress toward higher levels of independence.

Intervention

Returning to the case of Mr. Barnes, the nurse immediately recognizes that the client has abnormal thinking (see the Care Plan feature on The Client with Hiatal Hernia and Concurrent Schizophrenia on the website). The nurse notes that he is well groomed and shows appropriate social skills for the clinic environment. Uncertain about his reliability as a historian, the nurse asks Mr. Barnes to include his mother in the interview.

BOX 23-4	Types of Schizophrenia and Manifestations
Type	**Manifestations**
Paranoid	Presence of hallucinations and delusional thinking; fairly organized in speech and behavior; may show some range in affect
Disorganized	Dominant manifestations of disorganized speech and behavior, with flat or inappropriate affect; may also have hallucinations and delusions
Catatonic	Presence of bizarre motor activity, either excessive and purposeless or immobilized as if in stupor; may be mute or show incoherent speech
Undifferentiated	Presence of two or more of the following manifestations, but without a dominant feature as in the above three types: hallucinations, delusions, disorganized speech or behavior, and flat affect
Residual	Behavior does not show obvious hallucinations, delusions, or disorganization, but alterations persist in range of affect and thinking patterns

Comprehensive Assessment

While completing the nursing assessment, the nurse evaluates the client's knowledge of his medical illness, his psychosocial functioning, and his current level of compliance with psychiatric care. Despite his bizarre speech, Mr. Barnes offers accurate dates and descriptions of his medical manifestations. He firmly repeats his belief in the elves in the basement that talk to him at night and cause him to feel hungry all the time.

His mother adds that Mr. Barnes' mental illness was first diagnosed in his last year of high school. Before that, she had not noticed any problems. He has been hospitalized 10 times for severe paranoia and hostile threats toward his family. The most recent stay was 6 months ago, and he is more compliant with his medication since his doctor switched to a long-acting intramuscular form.

Exploration of daily activities reveals that Mr. Barnes is constantly supervised by his mother. He stays at home watching television, reading, and doing chores. He has no contact with peers and never worked. He states, "My brother and his friends don't like me anymore. My schizophrenia makes me stupid."

Communication Awareness

Throughout the interview, the nurse takes care to include Mr. Barnes in the conversation, even though his mother tends to dominate. The nurse maintains a calm facial expression when the client discusses his delusions and respectfully records his answers. No attempt is made to challenge the reality of his remarks, but the nurse does not agree with his distortions. The nurse is also careful not to invade the client's personal space without asking for permission.

Client and Family Teaching

Although the client and his mother seem to be familiar with the term *schizophrenia,* it is not clear how much teaching they have received. Before giving them material about hiatal hernia, the nurse asks whether they would like to learn more about schizophrenia. They both are interested. The nurse explains that schizophrenia is a chronic illness that can be controlled and praises the client for his knowledge of his medication and medical care.

Specialized Referrals

Before setting up the next clinic appointment, the nurse considers whether any other mental health resource is indicated. Mr. Barnes' condition is stable at this time, with monthly psychiatrist appointments; however, he feels stigmatized and he is totally dependent on his mother. To promote the best overall health outcomes for Mr. Barnes, the nurse must consider *tertiary prevention* with regard to his mental illness. The nurse believes that additional professional support could improve his level of community functioning.

The nurse recommends a referral to the psychiatric clinical specialist in the outpatient clinic at the medical center to explore community resources. The nurse offers to introduce them to the psychiatric nurse at their next clinic visit. The nurse calls the clinical specialist, who explains several referrals could be made for Mr. Barnes: to a young adult supportive therapy group, a psychosocial rehabilitation program, or a mental health support group for clients and families. The clinical specialist will also call the attending psychiatrist to coordinate the treatment plan.

MOOD DISORDERS

Mrs. Conners shows the most common manifestations of a serious mood disorder. Mood disorders are classified into three major categories: (1) depressive disorders, (2) bipolar disorder (formerly called manic-depressive illness), and (3) mood disorder resulting from general medical condition or substance use.[1] Manifestations of all depressions include a sad mood, which may be accompanied by crying spells; persistent negative thinking with hopelessness; possible suicidal thinking; decreased energy and motivation; and changes in sleep, appetite, and sexual interest.

In clients with bipolar disorder, mood can fluctuate from depression to the other extreme, mania. *Manic manifestations* include excessive cheerfulness or irritability; an unrealistic, optimistic attitude toward one's accomplishments; overabundance of energy; and decreased sleep with increased physical appetite. Box 23-5 describes mood states.

BOX 23-5 Manifestations of Mood Disorders

DEPRESSION (MAJOR OR BIPOLAR)
- Sad mood, but may be irritable
- Crying spells
- Negative thinking, continuously pessimistic
- Feelings of guilt and hopelessness
- Preoccupation with usually minor somatic complaints
- Loss of pleasure in usual activities and decreased socialization
- Decreased ability to concentrate and remember current events
- Decreased energy level
- Change in sleep, increased or decreased
- Change in appetite, increased or decreased
- Decreased libido and sexual activity
- May feel suicidal
- May develop psychosis with delusions about a negative future (e.g., fatal illness)

MANIA
- Elated mood, not attributable to a reality event
- Denial of having an emotional problem
- Impulsive acts that may be dangerous or socially inappropriate (e.g., promiscuity)
- Increased energy level
- Increased socialization to the point of becoming intrusive
- Excessive, rapid speech
- Change in appetite, increased or decreased
- Decreased need for sleep
- Increased libido

The key element in mood disorders is that the person cannot control the severity of the feeling. There may or may not be a clear precipitant for the reaction. Unlike a healthy person with transient mood changes, a depressed person cannot "just get over it" and the client with mania does not wish to give up the euphoria that characterizes this mood.

 In a given year, about 9.5% of American adults suffer from mood disorders, with a median age of onset of 30 years old.[17] Adolescent and adult women are two times more likely to have depression than their male counterparts. Mood disorders frequently co-occur with other psychiatric or medical illnesses. Clients may show depression with substance abuse, an anxiety disorder, or an eating disorder. Medical problems often associated with depression include cardiovascular, endocrine, neurologic, and autoimmune disorders, as well as certain cancers. Whenever depressive manifestations are mixed with physical complaints, close collaboration between a psychiatrist and primary care provider is necessary for appropriate treatment.

SAFETY

⚠

ALERT

The most serious adverse outcome for mood disorders is suicide. In 2002, 31,655 Americans died by suicide; it is also known that 90% of people who kill themselves meet criteria for a psychiatric disorder at the time of their death.[17] Take all verbal expressions of suicide intent or threat seriously and act accordingly (see later in this chapter). There are known risk factors and protective factors associated with suicide in the United States (Box 23-6).[2] Older adults and adolescents are at special risk.

 OUTCOME MANAGEMENT

Mood disorders can almost always be managed effectively through a combination of medication and psychotherapy. In some cases, electroconvulsive therapy (ECT) is indicated. Antidepressant medication is used for up to 1 year or for a lifetime, depending on the client's potential for relapse. Particularly for bipolar disorder, mood stabilizers may be needed for long-term treatment. Several classes of antidepressant drugs affect neurotransmitters in different ways. On the website, see the boxes Medications for Mood Disorders and Exercise versus a Prescription Medication for Major Depressive Disorder.[5,6,22] The Complementary and Alternative Therapy boxes on p. 429 discuss the use of St. John's wort for major depression. Finally, the Complementary and Alternative Therapy feature on p. 429 considers how nature can ease depression.

If a client does not respond to one medication after a fair trial, the physician may switch to another class or try a combination. Unlike anti-anxiety medications, antidepressants and mood stabilizers do not produce immediate effects. Thus the depressed client often suffers for 3 to 6 more weeks after starting treatment. Hopelessness about treatment, especially if the first medication is ineffective, compounds the risk for suicide.

Several types of psychotherapy may be helpful for mood disorders. In all cases, client education is important to explain the course of the illness and the benefits of treatment, despite the delay in improvement. Often, short-term therapy is beneficial with a focus on learning to manage current stressors and relationships. Marital therapy may be indicated because a mood disorder frequently causes marital discord, and conflict with loved ones often precipitates a depressive episode.

ECT is a viable treatment alternative for some clients with depression and may be provided in an inpatient or outpatient setting. An electrical shock is administered to a specific region of the brain to induce a seizure. General anesthesia is required, and the client does not remember the experience. The mechanism of action is not entirely understood but its effect on the neurotransmitter receptors may be similar to that of the tricyclic antidepressants. The client experiences short-term memory loss, but improvement is faster than with medication treatment.[3]

BOX 23-6   Risk Factors and Protective Factors for Suicide

RISK FACTORS
- Depressed mood with suicidal intent
- History of childhood abuse
- Hopelessness
- Serious medical disorder
- Substance abuse
- Recent lack of social support (isolation)
- Unemployment
- Family history of suicide
- Recent stressful life event
- Panic attacks
- Feeling of shame or humiliation
- Impulsivity or aggressiveness
- Loss of cognitive function
- Access to firearms
- Previous attempted suicide

PROTECTIVE FACTORS
- Sense of responsibility to family
- Pregnancy
- Religious beliefs
- Satisfaction with life
- Positive social support
- Effective coping skills
- Effective problem-solving skills
- Intact reality testing

COMPLEMENTARY AND ALTERNATIVE THERAPY

St. John's Wort for Major Depression

Previous randomized studies have found that St. John's wort may reduce the manifestations of mild to moderate depression. However, its effect on major depression had not been tested until recently. A randomized, blinded, and placebo-controlled trial was conducted at 11 academic centers in the United States. A total of 200 physically healthy outpatients 18 years of age or older with major depression and without psychotic features were recruited (mean age 42.4 years, 64% women). Clients received either St. John's wort (one 300-mg tablet 3 times daily, $n = 98$) or placebo ($n = 102$) for 8 weeks. The dose was increased to 4 tablets (1200 mg) daily for individuals who did not sufficiently improve by week 4 of the study. Interestingly, both groups significantly improved over time ($p < 0.001$), but the groups did not differ significantly from each other. More clients responded to St. John's wort, but the difference was not statistically different from the placebo. This study would have been better if a standard treatment arm had been included. Regardless, this initial study demonstrated minimal to no benefit of this herb over the placebo for the reduction of major depression.

REFERENCE

Shelton, R., et al. (2001). Effectiveness of St. John's wort in major depression: A randomized controlled trial. *Journal of the American Medical Association, 285,* 1978-1986.

COMPLEMENTARY AND ALTERNATIVE THERAPY

St. John's Wort and Drug Metabolism

St. John's wort is one of the most popular antidepressant supplements sold around the world. However, this supplement has a profound effect on inducing the activity of cytochrome P450 3A4 in the liver. This observation suggests that long-term administration of this supplement could result in a decreased effectiveness or an increased dosage requirement for all drugs affected by this pathway. The biggest concern about this supplement is that at least 50% of all marketed medications are affected by this liver pathway. Therefore the ability of this supplement to affect numerous medications should be a major concern to health professionals.

REFERENCE

Markowitz, J., et al. (2003). Effect of St. John's wort on drug metabolism by induction of cytochrome P450 3A4 enzyme. *Journal of the American Medical Association, 290,* 1500-1504.

Intervention

After meeting Mrs. Conners (diagnosed with diabetic ketoacidosis), the nurse is concerned about two major problems. First, the client's mental status appears altered and she is in distress. Second, the average length of stay for this medical diagnosis is only 1 more day, and much

COMPLEMENTARY AND ALTERNATIVE THERAPY

The Effect of Nature on Depression

A study in the United Kingdom noted the therapeutic effects of water therapy and dolphin therapy on depressed clients. The researchers used the therapeutic approach of ecotherapy, intended to help people find balance, connection, and healing through interaction with the natural environment. Thirty participants with mild or moderate depression were randomly assigned to either water therapy or water therapy with dolphins for 2 weeks. The severity of depression was measured with the Hamilton Depression Rating Scale and all clients had to be free of medication for at least 4 weeks. The water therapy control group participated in an outdoor nature program at the same time as the animal care therapy group played with and cared for dolphins. The results showed that both groups improved with lower scores on the rating scale, but the dolphin group showed significantly better scores. A follow-up evaluation 3 months later showed lasting improvement in 13 participants, 10 from dolphin therapy and 3 from water therapy.

REFERENCE

Spittler, K.L. (2006). A look at "biophilia"—How does nature impact physical and mental health? *Neuropsychiatry Reviews, 7*(1), 10-11.

teaching must be done before discharge. Returning to the nursing database, the nurse notes that the psychosocial section is incomplete. It is documented that the client is a native West Indian, lives with her daughter, and has a history of depression. She has been hospitalized three times in the past year, twice on the psychiatric unit and once for ketoacidosis. (On the website, see the Care Plan feature The Client with Diabetic Ketoacidosis and Concurrent Depression.)

Comprehensive Assessment

The nurse decides to complete the psychosocial history, even though Mrs. Conners may not seem cooperative. Mrs. Conners speaks in a soft voice, with just a few words at a time. The client says that she has had diabetes for 2 years and depression for 35 years. She has been going to the same psychiatrist for 20 years and asks the nurse to notify him. When asked about her medication, Mrs. Conners knows the name and dosage of her antidepressant and admits that she occasionally misses a dose. The nurse specifically asks about suicidal thoughts.

The Joint Commission (TJC) created a new National Patient Safety Goal for 2008 that states that the organization identifies safety risks inherent in its client population; included in a subheading of this goal is that the organization identifies clients at risk for suicide. Box 23-7 presents questions to assess suicidal risk.

SAFETY

⚠

ALERT

BOX 23-7 Screening Assessment of Suicidal Risk

INTERVIEW QUESTIONS

1. Have you been thinking about death or hurting yourself?
2. If yes, do you have a plan?
3. Have you ever tried to hurt yourself before?
4. If yes, what did you do?
5. What would stop you from hurting yourself now?
6. Can you sign a written contract with me that you will not harm yourself for the next _____ (time period until next evaluation)?

ADDITIONAL INDICATIONS OF HIGHER RISK FOR SUICIDE

1. Has a specific plan that is available and dangerous (e.g., hanging, shooting, or jumping from a high location)
2. History of previous attempts
3. Cannot identify person or religious belief that would prevent action
4. Refusal to sign a safety contract
5. Living alone or estranged from loved ones
6. Use of alcohol or drugs
7. Presence of psychosis with command hallucinations to harm self (cannot safely contract)

RESULTS OF SCREENING

1. If the client shows no positive risk factors, no action is necessary except continued monitoring of behavior.
2. If the client shows positive risk factors but agrees to a written contract not to harm self, the nurse:
   a. Co-signs the contract, defining the time period from now until the next visit.
   b. Notifies the attending physician (e.g., by telephone) in front of the client to report the assessment and to request a psychiatric nurse evaluation; if the physician orders other actions, these are shared with the client.
   c. Strongly seeks the client's permission to share the contract with a family member, if available.
   d. Contacts the psychiatric nurse to give a report and schedule a visit for the following day.
3. If the client shows positive risk factors but refuses to sign a "no harm contract," the nurse must take emergency action. The nurse:
   a. Instructs the client, and family if available, that this condition is a mental health emergency and requires immediate evaluation by a physician in an emergency department.
   b. Calls 911 for assistance, explaining that there is a psychiatric emergency.
   c. Provides brief information to the police and emergency medical team upon arrival, with a follow-up telephone report to the appropriate emergency department.
   d. Notifies the attending physician of the emergency actions.

The client describes her mood as sad and becomes tearful. She denies current suicidal ideation but admits to one overdose in the past. She expresses guilt about the overdose because of her religion. Then she says that she is too tired to talk. The nurse returns at lunch time and finds Mrs. Conners dressed in a long gown and wearing a colorful turban wrapped around her hair. Her daughter is coaxing her to eat some homemade soup. The daughter states that her mother has a pattern of medication noncompliance followed by diet noncompliance, which results in rehospitalization.

Communication Awareness

During the interview, the nurse is careful to respect Mrs. Conners' low energy level. The nurse uses questions that require only short answers and speaks clearly and softly. When the client talks about feeling sad, the nurse does not try to cheer her up but reminds her that her depression has been successfully treated in the past.

After the input from the daughter, the nurse realizes how important the client's cultural background is for the care plan. In the West Indian culture, an older person may be uncomfortable around authority figures and strangers. Respect and good manners are important; people expect to be greeted with "Good morning" or "Good afternoon" and are always addressed by the last name. Personal issues are discussed only with family members who comprise the main support system. Religious beliefs are important and folk foods are considered medicinal.[13]

Client and Family Teaching

Although the client and her daughter openly discuss the diagnosis of depression, the nurse emphasizes that this is a medical illness that can be treated just like the diabetes. Reassurance may be needed about a possible change in medication or dosage. The nurse collects information on depression, the medications, and community support groups. This information is given to the client and her daughter to review and determine whether they have any questions.

Specialized Referrals

As soon as the nurse observes that the mood disorder is complicating the client's medical condition, the discharge planner is contacted along with the attending physician. Discharge planning for Mrs. Conners requires a coordinated effort between medical and psychiatric clinicians The attending physician asks the discharge planner to arrange for a consultation with the treating psychiatrist.

When the discharge planner calls the psychiatrist, he states that he can visit the client later that day. He adds that he may need to transfer her to the psychiatric unit because of her suicidal history. The nurse introduces the discharge planner to the client and her daughter and tells them to expect the psychiatrist that evening.

CONCLUSIONS

The medical-surgical nurse has a vital role in caring for the psychosocial needs of all clients. Sensitivity to client and family anxiety improves the nurse's communication skills and increases the probability that clients will achieve the desired outcomes. For clients who have concurrent mental illness, the nurse must consider several additional needs in order to provide comprehensive nursing care:

- Increased attention to completing the comprehensive nursing assessment
- Heightened awareness of verbal and nonverbal communication
- Basic teaching about illness and treatment options
- Referral to appropriate specialized resources available in the health care system

Providing holistic care to clients with concurrent mental illness does not require specialized training beyond the generalist level. However, nurses must learn about the range of multidisciplinary services available at their health care facility in a particular community. The nurse is in a prime position in the health care team to advocate for appropriate mental health services for clients. Recognition of mental health needs supports the accomplishment of general health outcomes while reducing the pain and suffering of preventable adverse events.

BIBLIOGRAPHY

Citations appearing in red refer to primary research.

Citations appearing in blue refer to evidence-based practice guidelines and protocols.

1. American Psychiatric Association. (2000). *Diagnostic and statistical manual of mental disorders (DMS-IV-TR)* (4th ed., text revision). Washington, DC: Author.
2. American Psychiatric Association. (2003). Practice guideline for the assessment and treatment of patients with suicidal behaviors. *American Journal of Psychiatry, 160*(11 Suppl), 12.
3. American Psychiatric Association. (2003). Practice guideline for the assessment and treatment of patients with suicidal behaviors. *American Journal of Psychiatry, 160*(11 Suppl), 40.
4. Brady, N., et al. (2005). Living with schizophrenia: A family perspective. *Online Journal of Issues in Nursing, 10*(1), 2. Retrieved 07/10/05 from www.medscape.com/viewarticle/499269.
5. Brown, A. (2005). New psychiatric medications in development—2005. *NARSAD Research Newsletter, 17*(2), 22-26.
6. Buckley, P.F. (2005). The bipolar spectrum: Critical diagnoses. Psychopharmacology: Beyond Conventional Wisdom CME. *Clinical Psychiatry News Supplement*, June 2005, 3-5.
7. Carson, V.B. (2006). Relevant theories and therapies for nursing practice. In E.M. Varcarolis, V.B. Carson, & N.C. Shoemaker (Eds.), *Foundations of psychiatric mental health nursing* (5th ed., pp. 25-30). St. Louis: Saunders.
8. Current Opinions in Psychiatry. (2005). Recent developments in research and treatment for social phobia (social anxiety disorder). *Current Opinions in Psychiatry, 18*(1), 51-54. Retrieved 03/05/05 from www.medscape.com/viewarticle/497225.
9. Fuhrmann, J.S. (2000). Shared attributes of every traveler. In V.B. Carson (Ed.), *Mental health nursing: the nurse-patient journey* (2nd ed., p. 167). Philadelphia: Saunders.
10. Jensen, L. (2003). Managing acute psychotic disorders in an ED. *Nursing Clinics of North America, 38*(1), 45-54.
11. Keltner, N.L. (2005). Genomic influences on schizophrenia-related neurotransmitter systems. *Journal of Nursing Scholarship, 37*(4), 322-328.
12. Lazarus, R., & Folkman, S. (1984). *Stress, appraisal and coping.* New York: Springer.
13. Leininger, M.M. (2006). Selected culture care findings of diverse cultures using culture care theory and ethnomethods. In M.M. Leininger & M.R. McFarland (Eds.), *Culture care diversity and universality* (2nd ed., pp. 281-306). Sudbury: Jones & Bartlett.
14. Mahoney, D. (2005). Mental illness prevalence high, despite advances. *Clinical Psychiatry News, 33*(7), 8.
15. Medscape Psychiatry & Mental Health. (2004). How stigma interferes with mental healthcare: An expert interview with Patrick W. Corrigan. *Medscape Psychiatry & Mental Health, 9*(2).Retrieved 01/02/05 from www.medscape.com/viewarticle/494548.
16. Mueser, K.T., et al. (2002). Illness management and recovery: A review of the research. *Psychiatric Services, 53*(10), 1272-1284.
17. National Institute of Mental Health. (2006). *The numbers count: Mental disorders in America.* Retrieved 03/30/06 from www.nimh.nih.gov/publicat/numbers.cfm.
18. Starcevic, V. (2006). Anxiety states: A review of conceptual and treatment issues. *Current Opinions in Psychiatry, 19*(1), 79-83. Retrieved 02/12/06 from www.medscape.com/viewarticle/519711.
18a. The Joint Commission. (2007). *2008 National Patient Safety Goals Hospital Program.* Retrieved 12/7/06 from www.jointcommission.org/PatientSafety/NationalPatientSafetyGoals.
19. United States Department of Health and Human Services—Substance Abuse and Mental Health Services Administration. (2003). *Evidence-based practices: Shaping mental health services toward recovery—Illness management and recovery.* Retrieved 04/09/06 from www.mentalhealth.samhsa.gov/media/ken/pdf/toolkits/illness/06.IMR_Practition.pdf.
20. Varcarolis, E.M. (2006). The schizophrenias. In E.M. Varcarolis, V.B. Carson, & N.C. Shoemaker (Eds.), *Foundations of psychiatric mental health nursing* (5th ed., pp. 404-412). St. Louis: Saunders.
21. Varcarolis, E.M. (2006). Understanding anxiety and anxiety defenses. In E.M. Varcarolis, V.B. Carson, & N.C. Shoemaker (Eds.), *Foundations of psychiatric mental health nursing* (5th ed., pp. 220-221). St. Louis: Saunders.
22. Waknine, Y. (2006). FDA approvals: Rituxan and Emsam. *Medscape Medical News.* Retrieved 04/08/06 from www.medscape.com/viewarticle/524747.
23. Watzlawick, P., Beavin, J.H., & Jackson, D.D. (1967). *Pragmatics of human communication.* New York: W.W. Norton.
24. Westanmo, A.D., Gayken, J., & Haight, R. (2005). Duloxetine: A balanced and selective norepinephrine and serotonin-reuptake inhibitor. *American Journal of Health-System Pharmacists, 62* (23), 2481-2490. Retrieved 01/08/06 from www.medscape.com/viewarticle/518683.
25. Williams, L.D., and Boyd, M.A. (2005). Stress, crisis, and disaster management. In M.A. Boyd (Ed.), *Psychiatric nursing contemporary practice* (3rd ed., p. 781). Philadelphia: Lippincott Williams & Wilkins.

evolve *Did you remember to check out the bonus material on the Evolve website and the CD-ROM, including NCLEX®-Examination Style Review Questions, Open-Book Quizzes, and Chapter Review Audio Podcasts?*

http://evolve.elsevier.com/Black/medsurg

CHAPTER 24

Clients with Substance Abuse Disorders

LINDA CARMAN COPEL

As the client passed through the hospital door, it was the beginning—the first step of many on the journey back from the world of drugs and alcohol. No longer did this person need to be entangled in the cycle of pain, ineffective coping with addictive substances, more pain, and more drugs. The client, struggling to think clearly, had the following thoughts: "I must be dying. My body hurts. Where am I? What is going on here? How did this happen? I can't stand it. What are they doing to me? They can't help me. I can't help me. No one can help me. My life has always been a mess. There is nothing I can do."

Clients with psychoactive substance abuse disorders struggle with an inability to solve problems. They are unable to use adaptive behaviors to handle life stresses, traumas, and demands. *Ineffective Coping, Defensive Coping, Ineffective Denial, Imbalanced Nutrition: Less than Body Requirements, Risk for Injury,* and *Risk for Infection* are a few of the nursing diagnoses specific to the assessment data obtained from these clients. Nurses are challenged by the myriad of physical and emotional health problems faced by clients with addiction. Their health histories and at-risk behaviors culminate in problems ranging from liver and cardiovascular disease to depression and human immunodeficiency virus (HIV) infection. The client's physical condition is further compromised by nutritional deficits and fluid and electrolyte imbalances. In addition, many clients suffer from injuries, either self-inflicted trauma or violence at the hands of others. Often, multiple injuries in various stages of healing are evident upon examination.

Underlying the physical problems are the emotional wounds from both past and present life situations. Without effective coping skills, clients tend to continuously repeat their self-destructive pattern of behavior. The inability to perceive reality accurately and to develop and maintain supportive relationships hinders successful lifestyle changes. Accelerating bouts of depression and feelings of powerlessness continue, perpetuating a sense of incompetence. A pervasive sense of failure may be overwhelming.

Studies consistently show that substance-abusing clients need both medical and psychiatric nursing care to achieve their highest level of functioning and to maintain sobriety. Nurses have the challenge of dealing not only with the addicted client's many physiologic problems but also with the effects and withdrawal symptoms of the drugs involved. Even as you seek to assess and diagnose the physiologic effects of abused substances, clients typically offer defensiveness and may remain in denial. These clients lack responsibility for their personal behavior. Constant blaming and manipulation of others is typical behavior that requires your attention and intervention along with the physiologic issues. As much as any client population, this one challenges the entire health care team to provide holistic treatment for physical, emotional, and spiritual needs.

FRAMEWORKS FOR EXPLAINING ADDICTIVE BEHAVIORS

Over the past 100 years, clinicians and researchers have attempted to develop and refine the knowledge base on substance-abusing people. Early studies of alcoholism

---

evolve Web Enhancements

Bridge to Home Health Care   Addressing Substance Abuse

Ethical Issues in Nursing   What Considerations Should Be Made for Substance Abusers Who Are Being Treated for Other Medical Problems?

What Ethical Issues Surround Your Relationship to an Impaired Nurse?

Appendix A   Religious Beliefs and Practices Affecting Health Care

Be sure to check out the bonus material on the Evolve website and the CD-ROM, including free self-assessment exercises. **http://evolve.elsevier. com/Black/medsurg**

noted generational patterns of alcoholism in families. On the basis of this observation, it was suggested that alcoholism might have a genetic component. However, there is no evidence to support this supposition with other commonly abused drugs.[12,27,28,33]

Various explanations of the causes of substance abuse have focused on three conceptual frameworks:

- Biologic
- Psychological
- Sociocultural

However, there is no one identifiable cause of substance use. Rather, a combination of factors typically coalesces to produce drug use patterns. A person may be at risk for substance abuse because of a complex combination of biologic, psychological, and sociocultural variables. All aspects of the client's background must be considered when treatment is initiated. In addition to what the client brings to the treatment setting, the theoretical approach used by the team to view the underlying dynamics of substance abuse influences the process of recovery.

Biologic Framework

The biologic theory, or disease concept, of substance abuse views addiction as a physiologic condition that can be identified and treated. The emphasis is on a physiologic cause, such as genetic predisposition, defects in metabolism, neurobiologic abnormalities, and abnormal levels of chemicals in the body.[30] Historically, studies attempting to link genetic transmission of alcoholism have been unable to identify a target gene.

Present research focuses on examining the inherited biochemical abnormalities that may predispose an individual to alcoholism.[6,24] It is believed that alcohol dependence is a combination of interwoven social and psychological variables in people who are physiologically vulnerable.[29] For example, people of East Asian ancestry tend to experience a physical reaction to alcohol characterized by tachycardia, a sensation of warmth and flushing, and generalized discomfort. The response is believed to be related to the lack of activation of the enzyme aldehyde dehydrogenase, resulting in the accumulation of acetaldehyde, a toxic product of alcohol metabolism.[6,29] This physiologic process may be the reason that Asian Americans tend to have the lowest rate of alcohol consumption and associated substance use problems compared with other racial groups.[21] Hence, an examination of biologic differences associated with the use of alcohol warrants continued investigation.

Psychological Framework

Psychological theories attempt to explain the variables that may predispose someone to substance use. According to the psychoanalytic model, the person is viewed as being fixated at the oral stage of development, seeking gratification of needs through behaviors such as drinking. With the psychodynamic approach, a person experiences both interpersonal and intrapersonal difficulties that provide the foundation for the addiction.

Behavioral theories regard addiction as a learned behavior that can be unlearned in a manner similar to that of changing negative habits or dysfunctional behaviors. A *family systems approach* emphasizes that relationships, roles, and unhealthy communication patterns among family members contribute to addictive behaviors; this dysfunctional lifestyle is transmitted to future generations.[8]

For years, researchers and clinicians have sought, without success, to discover an addictive personality type. Some common characteristics noted in clients who abuse substances are low self-esteem, low frustration tolerance, inability to cope with physical and emotional pain, depression, lack of healthy relationships, and involvement in high-risk behaviors. Proponents of the psychological theories believe that people engage in substance use in an attempt to feel better about themselves and to meet their emotional needs. Thus the use of a psychoactive substance becomes reinforced and eventually evolves into an addiction.

Sociocultural Framework

With the sociocultural theories, substance use is viewed from the perspective of cultural and social norms within various groups in society. The issues of whether to use drugs, what type of drugs to use, and how and when to use them are determined by factors in a person's background. Such factors may include values, belief systems, spiritual orientation, ethnicity, gender, family standards, or the contemporary social environment. The relationships between these variables can contribute to a person's susceptibility to drug use and potential for addiction treatment and ongoing recovery.

DEFINITIONS AND TERMINOLOGY

According to the *Diagnostic and Statistical Manual of Mental Disorders,* fourth edition, text revision *(DSM-IV-TR)*,[2] the substance-related disorders comprise the range of substance use from taking a drug of abuse, to the adverse effects of any medication, to exposure to toxic substances. *DSM-IV-TR* lists 11 types of substances commonly abused: alcohol, amphetamines, caffeine, cannabis, cocaine, hallucinogens, inhalants, nicotine, opioids, phencyclidine (PCP), and the group "sedatives, hypnotics, or anxiolytics."[2] Polysubstance dependence and other substance-related disorders, particularly toxins or prescribed and over-the-counter medications, are also included.[2]

To understand and assess substance abuse, you must learn the associated terminology (Box 24-1). In working with clients who are actively using substances, you must also know the types of drugs commonly used, the major

BOX 24-1	Substance Abuse Terms and Definitions
Psychoactive substance	A substance that affects a person's mood or behavior
Substance abuse	Continued use of a psychoactive substance despite the occurrence of physical, psychological, social, or occupational problems
Substance dependence	A range of physiologic, behavioral, and cognitive symptoms indicating that a person persists in using the substance, ignoring serious substance-related problems
Physiologic dependence	The body's physical adaptation to a drug, whereby withdrawal symptoms occur if the drug is not used
Psychological dependence	The emotional need or craving for a drug either for its effect or to prevent the occurrence of withdrawal symptoms
Addiction	A compulsion, loss of control, and progressive pattern of drug use; characterized by behavioral changes, impaired thinking, unkept promises to stop usage, obsession with the drug, neglect of personal needs, decreased tolerance, and physiologic deterioration
Polysubstance abuse	Concurrent use of multiple drugs
Intoxication	An altered physiologic state resulting from the use of a psychoactive drug
Overdose	Accidental or deliberate consumption of a drug in a dose larger than is ordinarily used, resulting in a serious toxic reaction or death
Tolerance	A state resulting from metabolic changes in cell functions, whereby the tissue reaction to a drug declines and the person needs to take increasing amounts to achieve the same effect
Cross-tolerance	A state whereby the effect of a drug is decreased and greater amounts are required to achieve the desired effect because the person has become tolerant to a similar drug
Predisposition	Any factor that increases the likelihood of an event occurring
Potentiation	The ability of one drug to increase the activity of another drug when taken at the same time
Drug misuse	Any use of a drug that deviates from medical or socially acceptable use
Dual diagnosis	The coexistence of a major psychiatric illness and a psychoactive substance abuse disorder
Blackout	An acute situation in which a person experiences a period of memory loss for actions as a direct result of using drugs or alcohol
Withdrawal	Discontinuation of a substance by a person who is dependent on it
Detoxification	The process of withdrawing a person from an addictive substance in a safe manner
Toxic dose	The amount of a drug that produces a poisonous effect
Recidivism	The tendency to relapse into a former pattern of substance use and associated behaviors
Recovery	The return to a normal state of health, whereby the person does not engage in problematic behavior and continues to meet life's challenges and personal goals
Sobriety	Complete abstinence from drugs while developing a satisfactory lifestyle
Abstinence	Voluntarily refraining from activities or the use of substances that cause problems in the physiologic, psychological, social, intellectual, and spiritual arenas of a person's life
Flashback	The reoccurring sensory or emotional experiences that happen independently of the original event

routes of administration, and the side effects (Table 24-1). The order and severity of manifestations are influenced by the size of the dose and the length of time the drug has been used.

🏮 GENERAL ASSESSMENT

The purposes of a drug and alcohol assessment are to do the following:

- Determine whether substance abuse exists.
- Evaluate the relationship between substance abuse and other health care problems.
- Implement effective health promotion and health restoration interventions.

All clients must be assessed for the use and misuse of chemical substances. Clients who struggle with addiction are found at all stages of life and therefore in all clinical specialties. It is common for a client who abuses drugs to be hospitalized for an injury, illness, or surgical procedure. The nurse-generalist must identify clients with actual or potential substance problems and institute a collaborative team approach to provide health care (see Bridge to Home Health Care on Addressing Substance Abuse on the website).

The ability of nurses to provide care is influenced by the personal thoughts and feelings about substance abuse and the people who become addicts. Self-awareness about substance use and abuse is essential if the nurse is to establish a therapeutic relationship and provide treatment. The Seaman-Mannello Scale, a Likert-type scale that assesses nurses' attitudes toward alcohol and alcoholism, and the National Council on Alcoholism and Drug Dependence Scale can provide insight about personal values and beliefs regarding substance use.[31]

TABLE 24-1 Characteristic Effects of Abuse of Major Substances

Drug Classification and Street Names (Route of Administration)	Effects*	Drug Classification and Street Names (Route of Administration)	Effects*
Alcohol (Oral)	Relaxation and sedation	"Buttons"	Palpitations
"Booze"	Decreased inhibition	"Shrooms"	Blurred vision
"Brew"	Lack of coordination		Dizziness, weakness, and tremors
"Brewskis"	Unsteady gait		Altered perceptions (flashbacks)
"Moonshine"	Slurred speech		Impaired judgment and bizarre behavior
"Shots"	Nausea and vomiting		Mood swings and psychosis-like symptoms
	Transient visual, tactile, or auditory hallucinations	Inhalants (Inhaled)	Euphoria and giddiness
		Spray can propellants	Headache
	Anxiety	Paint	Dizziness, fatigue, or drowsiness
	Psychomotor agitation	Paint thinner	Nystagmus (involuntary rapid eye movements)
	High risk of permanent liver or brain damage		
Amphetamines (Oral, injected, smoked)	Grandiosity	Glue	Unsteady gait or tremors
		Gasoline	Slurred speech
Dexedrine	Hypervigilance	Cleaning fluid	Blurred vision or diplopia (double vision)
Methamphetamine	Hypertension or hypotension	"Laughing gas"	Damage to major organs: lungs, liver, and kidneys
"Ice"	Tachycardia or bradycardia		
"Uppers"	Mydriasis (dilated pupils)	"Poppers"	Cardiac arrest
"Crank"	Euphoria	"Snappers"	
"Speed"	Appetite suppression	"Whippets"	
"Black beauties"	Personality changes	Nicotine (Inhaled, oral)	Tachycardia
"Truck drivers"	Antisocial behavior		
	Psychosis similar to paranoid schizophrenia	Cigarettes	Vasoconstriction
Caffeine (Oral)	Stimulation of senses	Cigars	Irritation of oral mucosa
Energy drinks	Alertness and enhanced performance	"Spit"	Persistent cough
		"Chew"	Damaged alveoli and bronchioli
Coffee	Anxiety and restlessness	"Snuff"	Emphysema
"Jolt"	Flushed face		High risk of oral, laryngeal, or lung cancer
"Red Bull"	Talkativeness	Opioids (Oral, injected, inhaled)	Immediate euphoria followed by dysphoria
"Monster energy"	Tremors or muscle twitching		
"Adrenaline rush"	Tachycardia or cardiac dysrhythmias	Morphine	Psychomotor retardation or agitation
"Lipovitan D"	Insomnia	Codeine	Slurred speech
	Irritation of the stomach	Methadone	Impaired judgment and memory
Cannabis (Smoked, oral)	Mild intoxication	Hydromorphone (Dilaudid)	Sedation and respiratory depression
Marijuana	Increased appetite	Heroin	Constricted pupils
"Grass"	Dry mouth	"Smack"	Decreased sexual and aggressive drives
"Pot"	Lack of coordination	"Horse"	
"Hash"	Impaired judgment and memory	"Fine China"	
"Weed"	Sexual arousal	"Monkey"	
"Mary Jane"	Tachycardia	"Dope"	
"Reefer"	Visual hallucinations	"Skag"	
Cocaine (Oral, injected, inhaled)	Talkativeness	Phencyclidine (PCP) (Oral, injected, inhaled)	Grandiosity and illusions of strength
"Coke"	Grandiosity		
"Crack"	Hypervigilance	"Angel dust"	Impulsiveness
"Snow"	Anxiety	"Hog"	Psychomotor agitation
"Blow"	Impaired judgment	"Love boat"	Assaultive behavior
"Lady"	Tachycardia or bradycardia	"Peace pill"	Decreased sensory awareness
"Powder"	Hypertension or hypotension		Hypertension and tachycardia
"Candy"	Mydriasis		Unsteady gait and lack of coordination
"Toot"	Muscle twitching		Nystagmus
	Respiratory depression		Mood swings and paranoia
	Hallucinations, paranoid delusions, or paranoia	Sedatives, Hypnotics, and Anxiolytics (Oral, injected)	Incoordination and unsteady gait
	Formication (sensation of insects crawling on the skin)		
	Personality changes	Benzodiazepine (e.g., diazepam [Valium], alprazolam [Xanax], chlordiazepoxide [Librium])	Slurred speech
	Antisocial behavior		
	Euphoria followed by depression and feeling let down		
Hallucinogens (Oral, inhaled)	Intensified perceptions and feelings	Secobarbital (Seconal)	Nystagmus
Lysergic acid diethylamide (LSD)	Synesthesia (seeing sounds or hearing colors)	Pentobarbital (Nembutal)	Sedation
"Acid"	Visual, auditory, or tactile hallucinations	Methaqualone (Quaalude)	Inappropriate sexual behavior and aggressive drives
Peyote	Fear of losing one's mind		Impaired judgment
Psilocybin	Mydriasis		Mood swings
Mescaline	Tachycardia		

*Drug effects are arranged in order of severity of effect, with prolonged use or a high dose of the drug associated with appearance of the later effects.
From Copel, L.C. (2006). *Psychiatric and mental health nursing.* Torrance, Calif: Homestead Schools Publishing.

Nurses can also examine their attitudes and their own use of drugs and alcohol by considering the questions of how, when, where, and under what conditions they use them.

Individual beliefs about drug and alcohol use come from the nurse's family background and previous knowledge about and experience with addicted people. This information allows nurses to anticipate their response patterns toward this group of clients. If nurses know their feelings and beliefs, they can recognize a judgmental attitude, rejecting behaviors, or enabling behaviors. This knowledge can prevent the nurse from being drawn into power struggles regarding the client's manipulative behavior.

In addition to self-assessment measures for nurses, some instruments allow the nurse to gain information about the client's drug and alcohol use (Box 24-2). To use a tool as part of the assessment process, the nurse must know how to score the instrument and how to correctly interpret the findings. The CAGE and Alcohol Use Disorders Identification Test (AUDIT) screen for problem drinking; they are described in Chapter 1.

Interviewing the substance abuse client presents a challenge because of the client's tendency to deny or minimize the problem. A comprehensive assessment includes the client's history and physical examination. The previously mentioned screening tools can be helpful. Laboratory studies address cardiac, liver, kidney, and respiratory functioning as well as urine toxicology. A thorough mental status assessment is a requisite part of the examination. The major components of this assessment are listed in Box 24-3.

Attention is paid to the psychosocial evaluation, especially the components that address difficulties in family, occupational, social, or leisure functioning. Some clinicians recommend that after the history and physical examination are completed, the health care provider should take a specific drug and alcohol history that asks

about drug usage for the 11 major psychoactive substances in addition to other prescription and over-the-counter substances.[7] Components of a drug and alcohol history are listed in Box 24-4.

Although all clients need to be assessed for substance abuse, of special concern are those who by virtue of lifestyle or social conditions may be at increased risk. Adolescents, women (particularly pregnant women), racial and ethnic minorities, homosexual women and men, clients with mental health problems, clients with HIV infection or acquired immunodeficiency syndrome (AIDS), homeless people, older adults, and health care

---

BOX 24-2 Examples of Substance Use Screening Tools

FOR USE WITH ADULTS
- Michigan Alcoholism Screening Test (MAST)[33]
- Short Michigan Alcoholism Screening Test (SMAST)[34]
- Addiction Severity Index[23]
- CAGE Questions[11]
- T-ACE (a modified version of the CAGE used with pregnant women)[36]
- Alcohol Use Disorders Identification Test (AUDIT)[28]
- Alcohol Dependence Scale[35]
- Self-Administered Alcoholism Screening Test (SAAST)[39]
- Alcohol Use Inventory[17]

FOR USE WITH ADOLESCENTS
- Guide's Rational Adolescent Substance Abuse Profile (GRASP)[1]
- Problem Severity Scales for Assessment of Alcohol and Drug Abuse[16]

BOX 24-3 Components of the Mental Status Assessment

GENERAL APPEARANCE
- Appearance versus stated age
- Grooming and hygiene
- Posture, gait, and station
- Interaction during the interview
- Facial expressions
- Orientation or level of consciousness

MOTOR BEHAVIOR
- Restlessness
- Agitation
- Lethargy
- Tremors

SPEECH
- Clarity and coherence of speech
- Rate of speech
- Volume and intonation
- Barriers to communication, such as confusion or delusions
- Vocabulary appropriate to socioeconomic background

AFFECT
- Flat or labile

MOOD
- Euphoric, anxious, fearful

THOUGHT PROCESSES
- Thoughts presented as normal, concrete, scattered, or illogical
- Delusions—a false belief that is firmly maintained despite evidence to the contrary

PERCEPTION
- Awareness of self and environment
- Illusions—misinterpretation of external stimuli
- Hallucinations—sensory experiences with no external stimuli present

MEMORY
- Memory for remote, recent, and immediate past
- General knowledge level
- Ability to calculate
- Ability to think abstractly
- Insight
- Judgment or problem-solving ability

- How often the drug was used (past and recent use)
- Age at first use
- Duration of use
- Age at last use
- Method of use
- Quantity used
- Initial and current reactions to the drug
- How the drug was obtained or how use of the drug was supported
- Actions taken to reduce drug use
- Client's perception of use of the drug as a problem
- Use of drug related to any health problems

professionals are identified as populations requiring special prevention, treatment, and education about substance abuse.[5,23] Extra attention must be given to clients with chronic physical or mental illnesses.

Self-medication can occur in vulnerable populations as a coping strategy to relieve physical and emotional pain associated with a chronic illness. After obtaining a comprehensive assessment, you may discover that a client struggles with polysubstance abuse. Examples of polysubstance abuse can include cocaine and alcohol, alcohol and sedatives, hypnotics and anxiolytics, and nicotine and alcohol. Such clients require specialized care during the withdrawal process according to the combination of drugs used.

ASSESSMENT AND MANAGEMENT OF SUBSTANCE-ABUSING CLIENTS

The immediate result of overconsumption of any psychoactive substance is acute intoxication. Nurses in an emergency department or a medical-surgical setting may care for clients suffering from trauma as a direct result of acute intoxication. In addition to treating the client's injuries, the nursing care of intoxication consists of monitoring vital signs, especially respiratory status, because respiratory depression or arrest can occur. Be vigilant for manifestations of shock, cardiac dysrhythmias, electrolyte imbalances, or subdural hematomas. Typically, intravenous (IV) fluids are given to prevent dehydration. Some people become intoxicated but do not seek medical intervention because no injuries or emergencies bring them to health care facilities.

When a person sharply reduces or stops use of a psychoactive substance, the process of *withdrawal* occurs. Depending on the drug, withdrawal may begin within 8 to 12 hours or be delayed for 1 to 3 days.

Prompt recognition of withdrawal symptoms can promote client safety and prevent complications. Factors that influence the withdrawal process include (1) the specific drug used, (2) the dose taken, (3) the method of intake, (4) the time of last use, and (5) the length of time during which the drug has been used. You must also consider the client's overall health, particularly the functioning of the kidneys, lungs, and liver—the principal organs that metabolize and excrete drugs. Box 24-5 lists an overview of common withdrawal symptoms for alcohol and other substances.

Alcohol

Ethyl alcohol (ethanol), a central nervous system (CNS) depressant, is found in alcoholic beverages. The ingested alcohol is absorbed directly into the bloodstream from the stomach and proximal part of the small intestine. Because alcohol is water-soluble, it circulates easily throughout the body and readily passes through the blood-brain barrier. Approximately 95% of alcohol is metabolized in the liver, with the remaining 5% being excreted through the lungs, kidneys, and skin.[29] The body's mechanism for oxidizing alcohol is accomplished through the liver enzyme alcohol dehydrogenase. This process breaks down the alcohol to acetaldehyde, which is further broken down to acetic acid. Acetic acid then goes through the citric acid cycle to become carbon dioxide and water. From this chemical process, it is evident that alcohol can affect every aspect of the body. A growing number of young people may be using alcohol to enhance a drug's effect.

A blood alcohol content (BAC) test is used to measure the concentration of alcohol in the blood. The purpose of the test is to detect and estimate the level of alcohol in the brain. The legal intoxication level varies in different countries throughout the world, ranging from zero tolerance to 100 mg/dl (0.10%). In the United States each state determines its own blood alcohol concentration limit. Today the BAC in most states is 80 mg/dl (0.08%) with several states still allowing 0.10%. The U.S. legal limit for airplane pilots and people with commercial drivers' licenses is 40 mg/dl (0.04%). For drivers under the age of 21 years, the BAC limit is 0.01% to 0.02%, also known as zero tolerance.

Although some studies suggest that small amounts of alcohol can be harmless or even healthful, moderate amounts can produce a predictable series of deleterious effects.[19] After drinking one or two alcoholic beverages, a person experiences a depression of the inhibitory regions of the brain that manage judgment, self-control, speech, and motor coordination.[16,25] Alcohol is classified as a CNS depressant that affects all levels of the brain, starting with the reticular activating system and the cerebral cortex. Alcohol suppresses the inhibitory neurotransmitter gamma-aminobutyric acid (GABA). When the release of GABA is decreased, the initial results are an excitement or euphoric response.

With acute alcohol intoxication, alcohol continues to accumulate in the brain, resulting in depression of the cerebral cortex, cerebellum, and midbrain. In severe brain depression, disruption of the spinal reflexes, respiratory system, cardiac functioning, or temperature regulation

BOX 24-5 Common Withdrawal Symptoms Associated with Psychoactive Drugs

Drug Classification	Major Withdrawal Symptoms	Drug Classification	Major Withdrawal Symptoms
Alcohol	Nausea and vomiting Tremors and weakness Sweating Tachycardia Hypertension Delusions Agitated behavior Hallucinations and nocturnal illusions	Inhalants	Symptoms appear over varying time periods following withdrawal Central nervous system damage (cerebral atrophy or peripheral neuropathies) Acute or chronic renal failure Bone marrow depression Cardiac dysrhythmias Respiratory damage (lung or sinus damage, pneumonitis, emphysema, respiratory depression) Liver disease (hepatitis, cirrhosis)
Amphetamines	Dysphoria Disorientation Fatigue and depression with suicidal potential Disturbed sleep and unpleasant dreams Hallucinations or delusions	Nicotine	Irritability and nervousness Headache Inability to concentrate Craving for cigarettes Fatigue and dizziness Tremors and palpitations
Caffeine	Irritability and nervousness Inability to concentrate Headache Tremors Lethargy	Opioids	Dysphoria Anxiety Insomnia Increased respirations and yawning Sweating Lacrimation and rhinorrhea (nasal discharge) Tremors and muscle twitching Mydriasis (dilated pupils) Piloerection (erection of the hair) Nausea, abdominal cramps, and vomiting
Cannabis	No acute withdrawal symptoms; other symptoms appear over varying time periods following withdrawal Amotivational syndrome (inability to concentrate or complete tasks) Chronic respiratory problems Memory and learning difficulty Suppressed prolactin and testosterone levels	Phencyclidine (PCP)	Symptoms may appear over varying time periods following withdrawal Anxiety Withdrawn, catatonic state Hypertension Seizures Bizarre behavior and speech associated with temporary psychosis
Cocaine	Severe craving for drug Severe depression ("post-coke blues") Fatigue Psychomotor agitation or retardation Anxiety Insomnia or hypersomnia Increased appetite	Sedatives, hypnotics, and anxiolytics	Anxiety Sweating Tachycardia Tremors Nausea and vomiting Insomnia and disturbing dreams Transient visual, auditory, or tactile hallucinations Seizures
Hallucinogens	Symptoms appear over varying time periods following withdrawal Apprehension, fear, or panic Hyperactivity Sweating Tachycardia Altered perceptions (flashbacks) Perceptual distortions, especially hallucinations		

From Copel, L.C. (2006). *Psychiatric and mental health nursing*. Torrance, Calif: Homestead Schools Publishing.
See WebLinks for links to resources.

occurs. At this point, the intoxicated person may become unconscious, and, without treatment, death may occur.

Early clinical manifestations of alcohol withdrawal (e.g., tremors, anorexia, anxiety, restlessness, insomnia) tend to occur within 6 to 8 hours after the last drink is ingested. During the next 2 to 3 days, the client may further experience disorientation, nightmares, abdominal pain, nausea, diaphoresis, and elevations in temperature, pulse, and blood pressure along with visual and auditory hallucinations. *Delirium tremens* (DTs) is a manifestation of severe alcohol withdrawal or its life-threatening complications. The client with DTs is at risk for cardiac dysrhythmias, hypertension, increased respirations, profuse sweating, delusions, and hallucinations.

Many clients are given medications to decrease the incidence of withdrawal manifestations and to prevent DTs. The benzodiazepines are commonly used because they cause less respiratory depression and hypertension compared with other drugs. Typically, the physician orders either a long-acting benzodiazepine (diazepam [Valium] or chlordiazepoxide [Librium]) or a short-acting benzodiazepine (lorazepam [Ativan] or oxazepam [Serax]). The long-acting benzodiazepines are often used to facilitate the withdrawal process; the short-acting benzodiazepines are used for clients with severe liver dysfunction or a high degree of cognitive impairment.

Since 1995 the drug naltrexone hydrochloride (ReVia) has been approved for the treatment of alcoholism. It has been successful in decreasing the craving for alcohol and, together with the client's participation in a recovery program, facilitates client compliance with treatment. The drug was originally intended to treat clients undergoing opioid detoxification. According to the manufacturer, the mechanisms of action for naltrexone in alcoholism are not completely known. However, because the drug is an opioid receptor antagonist, it blocks the effects of opioid drugs by its competitive site binding. The relatively few side effects of the drug are nausea, fatigue, dizziness, headache, anxiety, and insomnia. Contraindications include hepatitis, liver disease, and liver failure.[12,17]

Treatment with naltrexone is controversial because taking the drug conflicts with the Alcoholics Anonymous (AA) model of total abstinence from alcohol and being "drug-free." The use of any drug is seen as a "crutch" or a substitution for the alcohol. For philosophical and political reasons, some clients taking naltrexone are excluded from receiving support and the other benefits of participating in AA.

There are also nonpharmacologic approaches to treating withdrawal. The *social model,* or the nonmedicinal treatment model, incorporates the use of an extensive physical examination, followed by close medical supervision during therapy. Several studies have shown that approximately 75% of the clients enrolled in these programs improve.[14,30]

The major nursing interventions for a client experiencing withdrawal focus on the continuous monitoring of manifestations and promoting a safe, calm, and comfortable environment. During the withdrawal period, clients need reassurance and support because they may feel that they will not survive the ordeal of detoxification. In the immediate period after the withdrawal syndrome has ceased, you can refer the client for further assessment and treatment of addiction or its complications. At this time, especially after what the client has been through, address with the client the relationship between drug use and the concomitant acute or chronic physical health problems. Common medical consequences of alcohol abuse are identified in Box 24-6.

Amphetamines

Amphetamines have been used to treat *narcolepsy* (sudden sleep) and *attention deficit hyperactivity disorder* (ADHD). People often use amphetamines illegally to remain awake and alert, to increase their ability to perform physical tasks, to lose weight, or to produce a state of euphoria (a "high"). The abuse of amphetamines, according to the National Institute on Drug Abuse, is most common in the 18- to 34-year-old age group.[23] The pattern of abuse tends to be one of daily chronic use or periodic binges that end with the user being overwhelmed by exhaustion ("crashing").

Amphetamines stimulate the CNS and accelerate heart and brain activity. Amphetamines block the reuptake of

BOX 24-6	Medical Consequences of Alcohol Abuse
Body System	**Consequences**
Cardiac	Dysrhythmias
	Hypertension
	Cardiomyopathy
	Heart failure
	Beriberi heart disease
Gastrointestinal	Gastritis
	Gastric or duodenal ulcers
	Perforated gastrointestinal ulcers
	Esophageal varices
	Pancreatitis
	Interference with absorption of vitamin B_{12}, thiamine, and folic acid
	Malabsorption syndrome
	Alteration in nutrition, with potential for malnutrition
	Wernicke-Korsakoff syndrome
	Enlarged or fatty liver
	Liver enzyme changes
	Cirrhosis
	Alcoholic hepatitis
	Portal hypertension
	Ascites
	Hepatic encephalopathy
Hematologic	Anemia
	Thrombocytopenia
	Leukopenia
	Capillary fragility
	Spider nevi
	Palmar erythema
Neurologic	Peripheral neuropathy
	Brain atrophy
Musculoskeletal	Myopathy
	Decreased bone density with risk of fracture
	Fractured bones related to trauma
Immune	Depressed immune system
	Increased susceptibility to infections
Respiratory	Altered respirations
	Chronic obstructive pulmonary disease
	Pneumonia
	Tuberculosis
Endocrine	Testicular atrophy
	Gynecomastia
	Irregular menses
	Decreased libido
	Hypoglycemia
	Alcoholic ketoacidosis

dopamine and norepinephrine by interfering with the transport protein, ultimately causing accumulation of dopamine and norepinephrine at the synapses.[19,45] Amphetamines are metabolized by the liver enzymes and excreted in the urine. In some cases, after continual drug use, half of the drug may be excreted from the body unchanged.[5]

With amphetamine intoxication, the clinical findings may include cardiac dysrhythmias, hypertension, fever, labile emotions, paranoia, delusions, panic reactions, and psychosis. For client management, perform frequent assessment of vital signs and basic body functioning and provide safe, supportive care. Closely monitor the client for changes in cardiac or neurologic status, because myocardial infarction and cerebral hemorrhage have occurred after amphetamine use. Antipsychotic agents may be used to decrease CNS stimulation, or sedatives may be given. IV amino acids may be given to accelerate the detoxification process of stimulant drugs.[36]

Amphetamines commonly cause psychological dependence, often with craving behavior. Abrupt cessation of the drug can precipitate anxiety, agitation, severe depression, hyperphagia, and hypersomnolence. An amphetamine psychosis may occur after continuous high doses. Nursing care focuses on (1) providing rest, (2) orienting the client as necessary, (3) monitoring for both physical and emotional changes, and (4) intervening to prevent complications of adverse effects or withdrawal symptoms.[44]

Caffeine

In the United States, caffeine—a CNS stimulant—is the most commonly used psychoactive substance. Products containing caffeine include coffee, tea, chocolate, cola beverages, energy drinks, and prescription and nonprescription medications. People rely on caffeine to promote wakefulness, elevate their sense of well-being, decrease fatigue, and facilitate motor activity.

The mode of action within the body is stimulation of the CNS, thereby exciting the respiratory system and increasing body metabolism.[23] Caffeine is absorbed from the gastrointestinal tract, broken down in the liver, and excreted in the urine. The intake of a large quantity of caffeine can cause intoxication, manifested by cardiac dysrhythmias, sleep disturbances, mood changes, increased production of urine, gastrointestinal discomfort, and anxiety, especially panic attacks. Caffeinism and caffeine withdrawal syndrome are seen only with long-term use of caffeine, usually a documented intake of more than 500 mg/day.[12] Lack of caffeine can lead to severe headache. This problem can be seen in clients placed on NPO (nothing by mouth) status (e.g., before surgery or major diagnostic studies).

Nursing care begins with recognition of the clinical manifestations of excessive caffeine use and withdrawal. Monitoring the manifestations and observing for additional problems (such as whether the caffeine is exacerbating known health problems) are appropriate. When clients are NPO and cannot consume their usual quantities of caffeine, severe headache may develop.

Cannabis

Marijuana, a cannabis derivative, is the most widely used illegal drug in the United States, with more than 55% of young adults reporting personal use.[12] The mode of action of marijuana is not clearly understood, and researchers continue to try to identify the mechanism that accounts for its effects on the CNS and cardiovascular system.[5]

Tetrahydrocannabinol (THC) is the active ingredient in marijuana and the agent responsible for the psychological effects. The amount of marijuana that crosses the blood-brain barrier depends on the method of intake used. THC is absorbed in fatty tissues, primarily the brain and testes, and is slowly released back into the bloodstream, where it is eventually excreted in urine and feces.[12]

Clients who use marijuana experience manifestations of intoxication, such as euphoria, mood changes, memory impairment, tremors, decreased body temperature, dry mouth, lack of coordination, elevated blood pressure and heart rate, and injected conjunctivae (bloodshot eyes). The CNS and cardiac, immune, and reproductive systems are affected. Long-term use also influences respiratory functioning. Marijuana residues in the lungs are considered more carcinogenic than tobacco residues.

Withdrawal from marijuana is typically an uncomfortable but not a life-threatening process. Nursing care includes monitoring the client's physical and emotional responses to the drug. It is often helpful for a nurse, family member, or friend to stay with the client, provide reassurance, and talk the client through the anxiety. Usually the client is not hospitalized unless pre-existing medical conditions or the coexistence of another psychoactive substance complicates the withdrawal process. For most clients, the initial effects of the drug dissipate within 4 to 6 hours; however, the effects of drug intoxication may last as long as 5 days.[12]

Cocaine

Cocaine is an opioid obtained from the leaves of the coca plant; it was originally used by the Indians of the Andes to alleviate feelings of hunger and fatigue and to promote endurance. Today cocaine is readily available on the illicit market in the form of cocaine hydrochloride, which is soluble in water and used intravenously, inhaled (snorted), or smoked as "crack," a form of concentrated (freebase) cocaine.

Cocaine stimulates the CNS and blocks the conduction of peripheral nerve impulses. Continued use of cocaine increases the amount of dopamine in the synapses of nerve cells by preventing dopamine reuptake. Cocaine also decreases the breakdown of dopamine and other catecholamines, thereby increasing the level of catecholamine activity at the nerve cell synapses.

Cocaine is metabolized in the liver and excreted in the urine. Evidence of cocaine use can be extracted from a urine sample for up to 72 hours after use.

In assessing for the effects of cocaine, remember that cocaine stimulates the CNS and the cardiovascular system. Cocaine abuse has led to myocardial infarctions in young, presumably healthy individuals. An overdose causes tremors, seizures, and delirium. Death can also result from cardiac or respiratory failure. Intervention is based on treating these identified problems and acting to prevent cardiac and respiratory complications. Cocaine intoxication may not be common in medical-surgical settings, because the half-life of cocaine is approximately 60 minutes.[35] Nursing management of a cocaine overdose focuses on preventing or handling cardiovascular collapse, respiratory distress, delirium, and hyperthermia.

Withdrawal from chronic use of cocaine ("bingeing") results in an exhausted state known as crashing. Clients experience a profound sense of depression, have memories of the cocaine-induced feelings of euphoria, and have cravings for the drug. Often, clients are hospitalized if there is severe depression with suicidal risk, if coexisting medical problems necessitate intense monitoring or treatment, or if there are medical problems directly related to complications of IV use. Besides providing the physical care required for the cocaine-dependent client, the nurse helps the client become aware of the need to develop effective coping skills.

Hallucinogens

Hallucinogens, also known as *psychedelic drugs,* are both natural and synthetic substances that produce illusions, delusions, hallucinations, and alterations in thoughts, perceptions, and feelings. The effects of hallucinogens differ among individuals and are therefore unpredictable. An individual's personality may influence the reaction that occurs after hallucinogen use. Characteristic of lysergic acid diethylamide (also called LSD) and other psychedelic drugs are a subjective sensation of heightened awareness, an ability to look inward, and a feeling of oneness with the universe.

The mechanism of action is unknown. Hallucinogens are usually ingested and then absorbed from the gastrointestinal tract, metabolized in the liver, and excreted in the bile and feces.[4] The length of action is usually between 6 and 12 hours.[36]

The effects of hallucinogens are similar to those of other stimulants. The user experiences euphoria, dilated pupils, anxiety, and increased respirations, blood pressure, and heart rate. Panic attacks occur while the user is in a state of intoxication, accompanied by feelings of paranoia, confusion, hallucinations, possible dissociation, and loss of contact with reality. The resulting inability to perceive the environment accurately, impaired judgment, and the feeling of having special powers make the person susceptible to dangerous activities.

Suicide, homicide, and other acts of violence have been reported in people under the influence of hallucinogenic drugs. SAFETY ALERT

Some users also experience flashbacks. During a period of intoxication, or because of a flashback experience or the reliving of a "bad trip," a person may be brought to a health care setting.

Carefully assess the client for both physiologic and psychological problems.

Nursing care focuses on attending to the panic that the client is experiencing as well as providing for client safety and creating a nonstimulating environment. Someone should stay with the client until the side effects have worn off. In the case of a severe overdose, be prepared to intervene for possible seizures, extremely high temperatures, and cardiac distress.[8] Because withdrawal symptoms may occur over a period of time, be vigilant for possible neurologic abnormalities and psychiatric manifestations. SAFETY ALERT

Inhalants

Inhalants are chemicals that emit fumes or vapors that readily pass through the blood-brain barrier to produce an alteration in consciousness. Commonly used inhalants are (1) solvents (glue, gasoline, nail polish remover, lighter fluid, paint thinner), (2) aerosols (hair spray, insecticides), and (3) anesthetic agents used for recreational purposes (nitrous oxide, chloroform, ether).

The probable mechanism of action is that these volatile substances alter the biologic membranes of the cells of the CNS and affect the metabolism of neurotransmitters in the brain.[19] Inhalants are metabolized in the liver and kidneys. Low doses of inhalants cause initial CNS excitement within minutes of use. Immediately after inhaling a volatile substance through the nose or mouth ("huffing"), the user experiences a "high," accompanied by feelings of giddiness and euphoria. There is a decrease in inhibitions and a slowing of the heart rate, respiratory rate, and overall mental activity. With inhalant intoxication, physical manifestations include delirium, cardiac dysrhythmias, irritation of the mucous membranes of the nose and mouth, cough, and depression of brain waves. Depending on the substance inhaled, the effects may last from a few minutes to several hours.[19]

Continuous use of volatile substances results in brain, lung, liver, kidney, and bone marrow damage. Withdrawal symptoms associated with inhalants vary with the specific substance used. Sudden sniffing death (SSD) related to the use of inhalants can occur from life-threatening dysrhythmias and hypoxia.

Nursing care concentrates on prompt intervention in emergency situations (seizures, loss of consciousness, respiratory arrest). Effective management of the client's acute and chronic physiologic problems remains your primary goal.

Nicotine

Nicotine is an alkaloid substance present in tobacco leaves. Using nicotine in the form of cigarettes, cigars, or chewing or pipe tobacco is an addictive habit practiced throughout the world. It is the leading cause of preventable death in the United States. Nicotine is absorbed through the lungs and within seconds crosses the blood-brain barrier and acts to stimulate the CNS. It is metabolized in the liver and excreted in the urine. Nicotine adversely affects the cardiovascular, respiratory, and gastrointestinal systems. The use of nicotine with prescribed psychotropic medications can significantly affect the metabolism of these drugs, and this concern must be incorporated into the decision-making process related to drug dosage and desired clinical response.[34]

An overdose of nicotine is not a common occurrence. If intoxication develops, administration of oxygen and the treatment of symptoms are the nurse's priorities. Nicotine withdrawal occurs within 24 hours of smoking cessation. The withdrawal symptoms are uncomfortable, and the nurse can support the client through this process and assist with developing effective strategies for dealing with the manifestations.

Opioids

Opioids comprise drugs produced from opium along with manufactured or semisynthetic narcotics. The human body also produces natural opiates, which facilitate feelings of well-being. Chemicals known as *endorphins* are neurotransmitters that connect with opiate receptors in the brain. When a person uses opiates or other narcotics, an interference is created in the natural opioid system and the functions of the neurotransmitters in the brain are disrupted.[8] Opioids are metabolized in the liver and excreted in the bile and urine.

An opioid overdose constitutes a life-threatening situation as a result of seizures, shock, respiratory depression, or cardiac dysrhythmias. The client is usually in an unconscious or lethargic state and may die without appropriate medical treatment. The nurse assesses and intervenes with the health care team to provide the required emergency care. Establishing an airway, monitoring cardiac functioning and treating dysrhythmias, maintaining hydration, and administering an opioid antagonist such as naloxone (Narcan) are the nursing care priorities. The client should be hospitalized, with close monitoring of all body systems, for at least 24 hours.

For the client experiencing opioid withdrawal, focus on assessing and intervening for a variety of physiologic, psychological, and behavioral symptoms; these tend to occur within 72 hours of last drug use. Nursing care consists of constantly monitoring withdrawal symptoms along with providing rest, nutrition, and a comfortable environment. The administration of topiramate (Topamax) or other anticonvulsant medication is also used to facilitate safe opioid withdrawal for the client.[47]

The once popular initiation of a methadone maintenance program as an approach for treating opioid addiction is now being questioned. It has been recognized that methadone maintenance programs have become a lifelong commitment for the opiate user and these clients are often maintained on these programs 20 or 30 years after the initial detoxification period occurred. There are some addiction specialists who believe that the methadone programs switch a legal addiction (methadone) for an illegal addiction (heroin). Becoming detoxified from methadone is viewed as more difficult than being detoxified from heroin. For a safe opioid detoxification, the use of the drugs buprenorphine hydrochloride (Subutex) and buprenorphine hydrochloride plus naloxone dehydrate (Suboxone) is approved for the treatment of opiate dependence. The discontinuation of Subutex and Suboxone is done after a period of stabilization and in conjunction with the success of the overall treatment plan. Clients often are referred to residential treatment programs to learn how to develop new, drug-free lifestyles.[13]

Phencyclidine

PCP is a synthetic drug with stimulant, depressant, and hallucinogenic properties.[5,12] PCP not only increases the production of dopamine but also blocks its reuptake, thus causing increased blood pressure, heartbeat, and respiratory rates. PCP also increases acetylcholine in the CNS, thereby generating cholinergic effects manifested as diaphoresis, drooling, and pupillary constriction. Serotonin is also believed to be altered by the presence of PCP, resulting in a lack of coordination, slurred speech, and nystagmus.[22] PCP is metabolized in the liver and excreted in the urine.

Intoxication from PCP lasts up to 6 hours, and the effects of the drug are unpredictable. A person may experience euphoria, disorientation, or the racing or slowing of thoughts. In emergency departments, the client may be confused, hostile, violent, paranoid, or panicked. Nursing assessment of PCP intoxication often reveals severe cardiac or respiratory distress, which can lead to cardiac arrest. Clients under the influence of PCP can be in a psychosis-like state and can have nystagmus, abnormal muscle movements, and severe hypertension.

Nursing care concentrates on the assessment of subtle changes in vital signs and level of consciousness, gastric lavage if PCP has been ingested within the past hour, and acidification of the urine.[11] In PCP withdrawal, you may see variable presentations of manifestations, particularly abnormal muscle movements. Carefully monitor the client's physical and mental condition to minimize health problems.

Sedatives, Hypnotics, and Anxiolytics

Sedative, hypnotic, and anxiolytic agents are considered to be CNS depressants. These medications are directly absorbed from the gastrointestinal tract into the bloodstream, where they enter the brain, are metabolized in the liver, and are eliminated via the kidneys. In cases of overdose, clients experience decreased CNS functioning along with the slowing of the cardiac and respiratory systems. Monitor vital signs and initiate emergency procedures based on the clinical manifestations presented. An overdose of any of these depressant drugs constitutes a medical emergency, with some clients requiring hospitalization in an intensive care unit (ICU).

Nursing care focuses on maintenance of adequate respiratory and cardiovascular status, hydration, and possible use of gastric lavage.[5] In some emergency settings, gastric lavage is used in the following circumstances: if treatment is obtained within 1 hour after ingestion of the toxic substance, the substance slows gastric motility, the substance is a sustained-released medication, or the substance was taken in a quantity that is considered life threatening. For clients undergoing withdrawal, promote safety and rest while treating both physical and emotional manifestations. Nursing care priorities are awareness of the possibility of delirium, seizures, fever, and changes in cardiac and respiratory status as well as the interaction between adverse effects of the drug and pre-existing medical problems. Table 24-2 (pp. 444-445) summarizes common health problems observed in clients who abuse drugs other than alcohol.

Nursing Management of Substance-Abusing Clients

The nurse plays a vital role in the care of clients experiencing intoxication and withdrawal. Nurses also meet basic needs, develop a therapeutic relationship, and teach both the client and family about addiction and its effect on the entire family. Nursing strategies for meeting actual or potential health problems are implemented for nursing diagnoses generated from assessment data. Nursing diagnoses commonly applied to the substance abuse population are listed in Box 24-7.

Education is an essential component of care to help the client understand the need for lifestyle changes. The main components of a drug education plan for clients and families are outlined in Box 24-8. Sometimes clients who abuse alcohol are referred for various treatment options and given disulfiram (Antabuse) or acamprosate (Campral) to deter drinking. Clients receiving disulfiram must be carefully instructed about the drug. Clients take acamprosate to assist them in maintaining alcohol abstinence while they are establishing a sober

---

BOX 24-7   Common Nursing Diagnoses for Clients Who Abuse Substances

- Acute Confusion
- Anxiety
- Impaired Verbal Communication
- Ineffective Denial
- Dysfunctional Family Processes
- Fatigue
- Fear
- Complicated Grieving
- Hopelessness
- Ineffective Coping
- Risk for Infection
- Risk for Injury
- Deficient Knowledge (specify)
- Noncompliance (specify)
- Imbalanced Nutrition: Less than Body Requirements
- Pain
- Impaired Parenting
- Disturbed Personal Identity
- Risk for Poisoning
- Powerlessness
- Ineffective Role Performance
- Chronic Low Self-Esteem
- Disturbed Sensory Perception (Specify: visual, auditory kinesthetic, gustatory, tactile, olfactory)
- Ineffective Sexuality Patterns
- Risk for Impaired Skin Integrity
- Disturbed Sleep Pattern
- Impaired Social Interaction
- Social Isolation
- Spiritual Distress
- Disturbed Thought Processes
- Risk for Trauma
- Risk for Self-Directed Violence, Risk for Other-Directed Violence

---

BOX 24-8   Components of a Client and Family Education Plan

- Concept of addiction
- Physical health problems associated with addiction
- Nutritional status
- Feelings and behaviors of all family members associated with addiction
- Areas of life affected by substance use: family, social, spiritual, sexual, occupational, financial, legal, and leisure
- Roles family members play in addiction
- Treatment options and treatment process
- Aftercare and self-help support groups or 12-Step programs
- Community resources
- Skill building in the areas of communication, expression of feelings, socialization, and coping strategies
- Impact of both addiction and the recovery process on the roles and responsibilities of all family members
- Client confidentiality and right to privacy protected under the 1975 Federal Drug and Alcohol Abuse Act and the Health Insurance Portability and Privacy Act (HIPPA)

TABLE 24–2   Health Consequences of Commonly Abused Drugs

	Amphetamines	Caffeine	Cannabis	Cocaine	Hallucinogens	Inhalants	Nicotine	Opioids	Phencyclidine (PCP)	Sedatives, hypnotics, and anxiolytics
Abrupt withdrawal symptoms (similar to alcohol withdrawal)										X
Agitation										
Angina		X								
Acquired immunodeficiency syndrome (AIDS)				X				X		
Anemia								X		
Atelectasis								X		
Arthritis								X		
Aspiration				X						
Bone marrow depression						X				
Brain damage				X		X				
Bronchitis							X			
Cancer (laryngeal)							X			
Cancer (lung)							X			
Cancer (oral cavity)							X			
Cerebrovascular accident (stroke)				X						
Confusion									X	
Dysrhythmias	X	X		X		X	X	X		
Emphysema							X			
Endocarditis (bacterial)				X				X		
Excoriations (from scratching nonexistent bugs)	X									
Flashbacks					X					
Gastrointestinal distress/ulcers							X			
Hallucinations				X		X			X	
Hepatitis (bacterial, viral)						X		X		
Hypergammaglobulinemia								X		

Hypertension

Immune dysfunctions

Insomnia

Judgment, impaired

Lung abscess

Lung irritation

Lymphadenopathy

Mental slowness

Motor function, impaired

Muscle weakness

Myocardial infarction

Myositis ossificans (drug user's elbow)

Nasal septal damage

Nephritis

Neuropathy (peripheral)

Osteomyelitis

Paranoid psychosis

Peptic ulcers

Pharyngitis (chronic)

Phlebitis

Pneumonia

Pulmonary emboli

Pulmonary fibrosis

Renal failure

Respiratory arrest/failure

Seizures

Skin ulcers or abscesses

Sinusitis (chronic)

Splenomegaly

Testosterone (lowered levels)

Tremors

Tuberculosis

Visual loss (from adulterants in street drugs)

lifestyle. Acamprosate does not produce a reaction like disulfiram does if alcohol is ingested while taking the drug. Information to include in a teaching plan is provided in Box 24-9.

Substance abuse has a major impact on family members. The family often tries to deal with a substance-abusing member by altering his or her behavior and compensating for the addict's unfilled responsibilities. Often the family inadvertently isolates itself from others as it focuses most of its energy on the addict. Personal needs of the caregiver, other adults, and children go unmet. Family members are strongly affected by the addiction and must be involved in the recovery process. A caring, supportive, and educative response from the nurse conveys that the family's concerns are understood and will be included in the treatment program. A major role of the nurse is education of client and family. The educative response is detailed in Box 24-8.

Drug and Alcohol Intervention
Confrontation About Drug Abuse

In medical-surgical settings, nurses and other members of the health care team may receive a request for assistance from family members who believe that the client needs to obtain drug and alcohol treatment. To confront the client about drug abuse, a carefully orchestrated format (a *therapeutic intervention*) can be implemented to force the client to participate in treatment.[7,11] The intervention must be planned in advance and executed under the guidance of a health care provider with a drug and alcohol counseling background. To prepare for the intervention, all participants compose a list of situations in which they have personal knowledge about the client's drug and alcohol behaviors.

During the therapeutic intervention, a group of family and friends gather together and bring the client face to face with the addiction problem. In an objective and

---

BOX 24-9 Information to Include in a Teaching Plan About Disulfiram (Antabuse) and Acamprosate (Campral)

- Inform the client that disulfiram is not a cure for alcoholism; it only discourages drinking.
- Before initiating disulfiram therapy, ask whether the client has had any allergic reactions to substances such as sulfites, preservatives, or dyes.
- Ask whether the client has a history of seizures; severe mental illness, particularly psychosis; serious cardiac disease; kidney disease; diabetes mellitus; hypothyroidism; or skin allergies.
- Ask whether the client is taking anticoagulants or phenytoin (Dilantin), which can increase the drug effects, and isoniazid (INH) or metronidazole (Flagyl), which can precipitate psychosis.
- Instruct the client not to ingest any alcohol or use any products containing alcohol within 12 hours before taking disulfiram, while taking disulfiram, and for at least 14 days after discontinuing disulfiram.
- Explain to the client that it is necessary to read the labels on all products because alcohol is found in many foods, medicines, and personal hygiene products (e.g., sauces, vinegars, cough syrups, tonics, elixirs, mouthwash, colognes, after-shave lotions).
- Tell the client not to inhale chemicals that may contain alcohol (e.g., paints, varnish, shellac).
- Encourage the client not to use alcohol-containing products that are applied topically. Alcohol absorbed through the skin can cause redness, itching, headache, and nausea.
- Identify common side effects (e.g., headache, fatigue, a metallic or garlic-like aftertaste, skin rash) that may be experienced during the first 2 weeks of taking disulfiram. Inform the client that these manifestations resolve as the body adjusts to the medication.
- If the client ingests alcohol while taking disulfiram, blurred vision, chest pain, confusion, dizziness or fainting, palpitations, flushing, diaphoresis, nauseas, vomiting,

headache, and dyspnea may occur. These symptoms last as long as alcohol is in the body. If the client drinks a large amount of alcohol, seizures, myocardial infarction, unconsciousness, or death may result.
- Instruct the client to carry a card that specifies that he or she is taking disulfiram, lists the side effects of alcohol use, and states whom to contact in an emergency.
- Inform the client that acamprosate is not a cure for alcoholism; it is used to assist people to quit drinking alcohol.
- Before initiating acamprosate therapy, ascertain that the client is free from kidney disease or any renal impairment.
- Inform the client that acamprosate is used as a part of drug and alcohol treatment that includes counseling and participation in support groups.
- Instruct the client not to ingest any alcohol or use any products containing alcohol. If the client uses alcohol, it is acceptable to continue taking acamprosate. However, any relapse must be reported to the health care team.
- Tell the client that acamprosate can cause impairment in judgment and psychomotor skills. Caution the client against operating hazardous machinery, including motor vehicles.
- Identify common side effects (e.g., headache, tremor, anxiety, stomach pain, increased appetite, diarrhea, amnesia, disturbed vision, lack of taste, or decreased libido) that may be experienced during the initiation of the therapy. Inform the client that these manifestations resolve as the body adjusts to the medication.
- If the client experiences any severe side effects (symptoms of an allergic reaction, irregular pulse, hypotension, hypertension, abnormal bleeding or bruising), stop the medication and seek emergency medical treatment.
- Instruct the client to carry a card that specifies that he or she is taking acamprosate, a list of the side effects of the drug, and information on whom to contact in an emergency.

nonjudgmental manner, the group states its concerns about the client, its observations about the client's substance abuse behavior, and its overall caring about the client's well-being. A plan for obtaining help from these significant people is presented to the client. This plan includes treatment recommendations and may contain a reservation for a particular treatment facility. It is believed that this loving and open confrontation can break through the abuser's denial and defensiveness. The client's family and friends must also state the consequences that will immediately ensue if help is refused.

Treatment Options

After completing a comprehensive health history and providing care for the client, you are in an optimal position to recommend a treatment modality that corresponds to the needs of the client and family members. Activities that you are involved in range from primary prevention (education), to secondary prevention (outpatient services), to tertiary prevention (inpatient or outpatient detoxification and rehabilitation). The common interventions for all three levels of care are listed in Table 24-3. A list of community resources that can provide education and support to substance-abusing clients and their families appears on the website.

Prevention of Relapse

Clients in the recovery process may be at risk for relapse or a return to substance abuse. Anticipate the possibility of *relapse* (slipping back into substance use after a period of abstinence) and prepare clients with strategies to prevent it. This regression can occur any time and may be defined as one-time use, brief intermittent use, or daily long-term use. Relapse should be viewed as a potential

part of the illness process, much like the potential course of any other chronic illness. Seeing relapse as client failure sets the client up for defeat instead of recovery.

Physiologic, emotional, and social variables all contribute to relapse. Clients must be taught ways to assess their strengths and to identify situations that can distract them from their recovery. Peer pressure, stress, and negative feelings may trigger a relapse. Some relapse-prevention strategies to include in educational programs are listed in Box 24-10.

Surgery and Substance Abuse

Clients who abuse substances often experience accidents, injuries, or illnesses that require surgical intervention. In fact, many injuries seen by nurses in emergency departments are directly related to drug and alcohol use. Become skillful in observing for subtle changes, and perform frequent assessments to intervene immediately and prevent the escalation of manifestations.[3,37,42] Traumatized clients usually require immediate surgery; hence, a thorough drug and alcohol assessment may not be done. It is a challenge for the nurse to distinguish medical problems, psychiatric disorders, and substance abuse disorders in a timely manner.

Alcoholic clients who are admitted for a surgical procedure require special attention. They are told not to drink for several days before surgery, but in reality they may have been drinking up to the night before. Postoperatively, the client begins to develop withdrawal and may become combative and must be actively restrained. The challenges facing the nursing staff caring for a postoperative client with DTs are great. Client safety is a serious matter, as are wound healing and adequate nutrition. The client may be treated to reduce

SAFETY

ALERT

TABLE 24–3 **Levels of Treatment Strategies**

Level of Prevention	Activities	Resources
Primary prevention	Education to prevent substance abuse Risk factor identification Lifestyle guidance	School programs Community programs Health promotion activities
Secondary prevention (outpatient)	Assessment and intervention of early physical and emotional issues and problems Educational interventions Pharmacologic interventions Self-management strategies Support and self-help groups Psychotherapy	Medical facilities as appropriate Individual, family, or group therapy Psychoeducational groups Self-help groups (e.g., AA, NA, CA, Al-Anon, Alateen, Naranon, ACOA)*
Tertiary prevention (inpatient or outpatient)	Interventions to monitor withdrawal and prevent or treat complications Focus on relapse prevention Determine plan for aftercare and methods of obtaining support Individual, family, or group therapy	Medical services, such as detoxification Aftercare, such as partial programs, supervised living, or halfway house Individual, family, or group therapy Psychoeducational groups Self-help groups (e.g., AA, NA, CA, Al-Anon, Alateen, Naranon, ACOA)*

AA, Alcoholics Anonymous; *ACOA*, Adult Children of Alcoholics; *CA*, Cocaine Anonymous; *NA*, Narcotics Anonymous.
* See WebLinks for links to resources.

BOX 24-10   Strategies to Prevent Relapse

- Assess and build on the client's coping skills.
- Take opportunities, such as role-playing, that help the client practice coping methods.
- Assist the client in identifying personal risks of relapse.
- Identify people, places, and things that can interfere with maintaining sobriety, and encourage the client to minimize contact with these obstacles and develop ways to handle them.
- Change environmental variables when possible.
- Discuss the concept of craving, how to identify it, what may trigger it, and how to handle it.
- Focus on the client's physiologic feelings and sensations, and develop methods to handle them.
- Teach strategies that promote a healthy lifestyle, such as exercise, nutrition, stress management, and relaxation techniques.
- Encourage participation in support groups or self-help groups.
- Recommend group or individual therapy if the client has problems with the family of origin, struggles with daily functioning, or mental illness.

symptoms. In other cases, the client may be simply left to detoxify "cold turkey," a method that stops the substance abruptly. Your role as a client advocate is imperative for these clients.

If a client is addicted to CNS depressant drugs, a larger amount of an anesthetic may be needed to produce the desired effects. This situation occurs because the client has a higher tolerance to the anesthetic drug. For clients with liver impairment and overall poor health, anesthetics cannot be properly metabolized and the effect of sedation is prolonged. While undergoing surgery, the addicted client is at risk for cardiac dysrhythmias, respiratory depression, hemorrhage, and depletion of catecholamines.

In the postoperative period, these clients are susceptible to cardiac, respiratory, urinary, hemorrhagic, and wound complications. The experience of pain may be intensified because the clients often have tolerance to the pain medication. Carefully assess whether the client requires increased doses of medication for pain reduction and needs to be slowly weaned from the medication during recovery. Some addicted clients may experience drug withdrawal postoperatively because withdrawal has been delayed by the use of anesthetics.

THE IMPAIRED HEALTH CARE PROFESSIONAL

Just like other people, health care professionals can become addicted to drugs and alcohol. Research on the prevalence of substance abuse among nurses has revealed no difference between nurses and other health professionals. Furthermore, the prevalence of substance abuse among health professionals overall does not differ from that in the general population.[8,40] Many addicted health care professionals first start using drugs and alcohol in response to physical illness and pain, emotional difficulties, or work pressures.

The requirements of the professional nurse's role make nursing a stressful occupation. On a daily basis, the nurse is responsible for coordinating and directly providing care for clients who are in pain and crisis. The pressure of handling resources, making decisions, interfacing with medical and other personnel, working long hours, often with inadequate staff, and being responsible for the daily operation of the medical-surgical unit can be overwhelming. In addition, nurses have access to opioids and operate on the premise that medications are a useful vehicle for relieving or reducing pain and altering states of feelings. Specialized knowledge about drugs and experience with administering them and watching their efficacy may lead health care providers to view drugs as a "pharmacologic coping method."[15,30] It is a method that can ultimately backfire.

The signs of a chemically impaired colleague are subtle and easily overlooked by peers and supervisors. Even other health care professionals may deny and avoid the problem rather than confront the person suspected of being chemically dependent. It is essential that nurses be aware of the manifestations of chemical dependence in peers (Box 24-11). Document questionable or problematic incidents, and be willing to participate in an intervention if deemed appropriate. Remember, a peer who suffers from addiction cannot meet the requirements of your state nurse practice act. Some states have a law that mandates reporting of an impaired colleague.

As with clients, steps must be taken to assist an impaired nurse to obtain treatment. The use of an employee assistance program (EAP) and peer support or assistance groups from the state nurses' association can facilitate referrals

BOX 24-11   Signs of a Chemically Impaired Colleague

- Alcohol on breath
- Mood changes or confusion
- Difficulty making judgments and impaired memory
- Red eyes with flushed face
- Unsteady gait
- Tremors or impaired hand-eye coordination
- Irritability or hyperactivity
- Lethargy or dozing on breaks
- Disheveled appearance
- Wearing long sleeves or a sweater constantly, even in hot weather
- Incorrect drug counts
- Accidents, spillages, or drugs frequently being wasted
- Frequently found in the bathroom, nurses' lounge, or off the unit
- Recurrent unfinished assignments or client care mistakes

to treatment and can assist with recovery. Although peer assistance programs vary from state to state, most programs offer support, referral services, monitoring during recovery, and educational programs targeted to the health care professional.

CONCLUSIONS

Substance abuse remains a major health issue, affecting clients, families, and communities. Even so, many clients with substance abuse disorders are not identified and, therefore, do not obtain treatment. A lack of knowledge about addiction can perpetuate stigmatization of the client. Your challenge is to become informed about both the effects of drugs and appropriate strategies for treatment. Keen assessment skills, decision-making skills, and compassion are the prerequisites for comprehensive nursing care of the myriad physiologic and psychological needs presented by these clients.

Nurses play a vital role in developing and implementing drug and alcohol prevention strategies. Teaching how to use effective coping strategies, how to handle crises, and how to develop support systems are the primary steps that must be incorporated into the care. For you, as a nurse, it is important to spend time cultivating relationships and to allow yourself to engage in leisure activities that decrease feelings of frustration, hopelessness, and burnout.

THINKING CRITICALLY

1. A group of young college students celebrated the end of the semester with a week-long party. Alcoholic beverages were plentiful; food was not a priority. A young couple brought their friend to the emergency department. They report their suspicions that she might have a drinking problem (e.g., erratic behavior, presence of alcoholic beverages in the dormitory room, smell of alcohol on her breath). They were unable to awaken her for any length of time and are worried that she drank too much. She has not had a drink for about 6 hours. What assessment is required? What nursing actions are appropriate?

Factors to Consider. How likely is it for the client to experience DTs? How will the client be treated?

2. You are a registered nurse in the local "Driving Under the Influence of Alcohol" teaching program. Your topic is "Alcohol and the Human Body." The audience is made up of clients mandated by the court to attend. After the presentation, which focuses on the complications associated with long-term drinking, the clients ask, "If alcoholism is a disease, why are we treated as criminals?" "I didn't drink so much, why did they pull me over?" What might these questions indicate?

Factors to Consider. Is alcoholism a disease of addiction? What psychological factor is evident in such questions?

Discussions for these questions can be found on the website.

BIBLIOGRAPHY

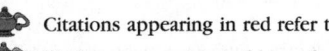 Citations appearing in red refer to primary research.

Citations appearing in blue refer to evidence-based practice guidelines and protocols.

1. Addiction Research Corporation. (1986). *GRASP: Guide's rational adolescent substance abuse profile*. Piscataway, NJ: Rutgers University Center of Alcohol Studies.
2. American Psychiatric Association. (2000). *Diagnostic and statistical manual of mental disorders DSM-IV-TR* (4th ed., text revision). Washington, DC: Author.
3. Babor, T.F., Higgins-Biddle, J., Dauser, D., et al. (2005). Alcohol screening and brief intervention in primary care settings: Implementation models and predictors. *Journal of Studies on Alcohol, 66*(3), 361-368.
4. Bond, G.R. (2002). The role of activated charcoal and gastric emptying in gastrointestinal decontamination: A state-of-the-art review. *Annals of Emergency Medicine, 39*(3):273-286.
5. Burns, E.M., Thompson, A., & Ciccone, J.K. (1993). *An addictions curriculum for nurses and other helping professionals* (Vol. 2). New York: Springer-Verlag.
6. Cook, T.A.R., Luczak, S.E., Shea, S.H., et al. (2005). Associations of ALDH2 and ADH1B genotypes with response to alcohol in Asian Americans. *Journal of Studies on Alcohol, 66*(2), 194-205.
7. Copel, L.C. (2006). *Psychiatric and mental health nursing*. Torrance, Calif: Homestead Schools Publishing.
8. Donovan, D.M., & Marlatt, G.A. (Eds.) (2005). *Assessment of addictive behaviors*. New York: Guilford Press.
9. Dunn, D. (2005). Home study program: Substance abuse among nurses—Defining the issue, first article in a two part series. *American Association of Operating Room Nurses, 82*(4), 572-575, 577-582, 585-588.
10. Ewing, J.A. (1984). CAGE. *Journal of the American Medical Association, 252*(14), 1906.
11. Finfgeld-Connett, D. (2005). Alcohol brief interventions. *Annual Review of Nursing Research, 23*, 363-389.
12. Frances, R.J., Miller, S.I., & Mack, A.H. (Eds.), *Clinical textbook of addictive disorders* (3rd ed.). New York: Guilford Press.
13. Fudala, P.J., & Woody, G.W. (2004). Recent advances in the treatment of opiate addiction. *Current Psychiatry Reports, 6*, 339-346.
14. Galanter, M., & Kleber, H.D. (2004). *Textbook of substance abuse treatment* (3rd ed.). Washington, DC: American Psychiatric Press.
15. Green, C.A. (2006). Gender and substance abuse treatment services. *Alcohol, Research, and Health, 29*(1), 55-62.
16. Handley, S.M., & Ward-Smith, P. (2005). Alcohol misuse, abuse, and addiction in young and middle adulthood. *Annual Review of Nursing Research, 23*, 213-244.
17. Hernandez, C.A., Song, C., Kuo, L., et al. (2006). Targeted versus daily naltrexone: Secondary analysis of effects on average daily drinking. *Alcoholism: Clinical and Experimental Research, 30*(5), 860-865.
18. Horn, J.L. (1984). *Alcohol use questionnaire (AUQ)*. Toronto, Canada: Addiction Research Foundation.
19. Karch, S.B. (2002). *Karch's pathology of drug abuse*. Boca Raton, Fla: CRC Press.
20. Klatsky, A.L., Gunderson, E.P., Kipp, H., et al. (2006). Higher prevalence of systemic hypertension among moderate alcohol drinkers: An exploration of the role of underreporting. *Journal of Studies on Alcohol, 67*(3), 416-420.
21. Koob, G.F., & LeMoal, M. (2006). *Neurobiology of addiction*. Philadelphia: Academic Press.
22. Laraia, M.T., & Jefferson, L.V. (2005). Chemically mediated responses and substance-related disorders. In G.W. Stuart & M. Laraia (Eds.), *Principles and practices of psychiatric nursing* (8th ed., pp. 473-516). St. Louis: Mosby.
23. Lowinson, J., Millman, R.B., Langrod, J.G., & Ruiz, P. (Eds.) (2004). *Substance abuse: A comprehensive textbook* (4th ed.). Baltimore, Md: Lippincott Williams & Wilkins.
24. Luczak, S.E., Shea, S.H., Hsueh, A.C., et al. (2006). ALDH2 is associated with a decreased likelihood of alcohol-induced blackouts in Asian American college students. *Journal of Studies on Alcohol, 67* (3), 349-353.

25. McCarthy, D.M., Pedersen, S.L., & Leuty, M.E. (2005). Negative consequences and cognitions about drinking and driving. *Journal of Studies on Alcohol, 66*(4), 567-570.

26. McLellan, A.T. (1992). The fifth edition of the addiction severity index. *Journal of Substance Abuse Treatment, 9*(3), 199-213.

27. Miller, W.R., & Carroll, K.M. (2006). *Rethinking substance abuse.* New York: Guilford Press.

28. Mulligan, M.K., Ponomarev, I., Hitzemann, R.J., et al. (2006). Toward understanding the genetics of alcohol drinking through transcriptome meta-analysis. *Proceedings of the National Academy of Sciences, 103*(16), 6368-6373.

29. Nace, E.P. (2005). Alcohol. In R.J. Frances, S.I. Miller, & A.H. Mack (Eds.), *Clinical textbook of addictive disorders* (3rd ed., pp. 91-119). New York: Guilford Press.

30. Naegle, M.A. (2006). Substance abuse and addiction in registered professional nurses. In J.J. Fitzpatrick & M. Wallace (Eds.), *The Encyclopedia for Nursing Research.* New York: Springer.

31. National Institute on Alcohol Abuse and Alcoholism. (1984). *Alcohol abuse curriculum guide for nurse practitioner faculty* (DHHS Pub. No. ADM 84-1313, Vol. 3). Rockville, Md: Health Professions Education Curriculum Resources Series.

32. National Institute on Alcohol Abuse and Alcoholism. (1990). *Seventh special report to the U.S. Congress on alcohol and health: From the Secretary of Health and Human Services* (DHHS Pub. No. ADM 90-1656). Rockville, Md: Author.

33. Peterson, K. (2004). Biomarkers for alcohol use and abuse. *Alcohol, Research, and Health, 28*(1), 30-37.

34. Pinninti, N.R., Mao, R., & de Leon, J. (2005). Coffee, cigarettes, and meds: What are the metabolic effects? *Psychiatric Times, 22*(6), 164-171.

35. Pokorney, A.D., Miller, B.A., & Kaplan, H.B. (1992). The brief MAST: A shortened version of the Michigan Alcoholism Screening Test. *American Journal of Psychiatry, 129*, 342-348.

36. Rastegar, D.A., & Fingerhood, M.I. (2005). *Addiction medicine: An evidence based handbook.* Philadelphia: Lippincott Williams & Wilkins.

37. Russell, M. (2005). Screening in general health care. *Alcohol, Research, and Health, 28*(1), 17-22.

38. Selzer, M.L. (1971). The Michigan Alcoholism Screening test: The quest for a new diagnostic instrument. *American Journal of Psychiatry, 127*, 1653-1658.

39. Selzer, M., Vinokur, A., & van Roojan, L. (1975). A self-administered short alcohol screening test (SMAST). *Journal of Studies on Alcoholism, 36*(1), 86.

40. Skinner, H.A., & Horn, J.L. (1984). *Alcohol Dependence Scale (ADS): User's guide.* Toronto, Canada: Addiction Research Foundation.

41. Shulamith, L.A.S. (Ed.) (2006). *Clinical work with substance abusing clients* (2nd ed.). New York: Guilford Press.

42. Society of Trauma Nurses. (2006). Position statement on screening for alcohol use in adult primary care. *Journal of Trauma Nursing, 13*(1), 4-5.

43. Sokol, R.J., Martier, S.S., & Ager, J.W. (1989). The T-ACE questions: Practical prenatal detection of risk-drinking. *American Journal of Obstetrics and Gynecology, 160*, 863-870.

44. Sullivan, E. (1995). *Nursing care of clients with substance abuse.* St. Louis: Mosby.

45. Sulzer, D. (2005). Mechanisms of neurotransmitter release by amphetamines: A review. *Progressive Neurobiology, 75*(6), 406-433.

46. Swenson, W., & Morse, R. (1973). The use of self-administered alcoholism screening test (SAAST) in a medical center. *Mayo Clinic Proceedings, 50*, 204-208.

47. Zullino, D.F., Krenz, S., Zimmerman, G., et al. (2005). Topiramate in opiate withdrawal—Comparison with clonidine and with carbamazepine/mianserin. *Substance Abuse, 25*(4), 27-33.

evolve *Did you remember to check out the bonus material on the Evolve website and the CD-ROM, including NCLEX®-Examination Style Review Questions, Open-Book Quizzes, and Chapter Review Audio Podcasts?*

http://evolve.elsevier.com/Black/medsurg

UNIT 6

MUSCULOSKELETAL DISORDERS

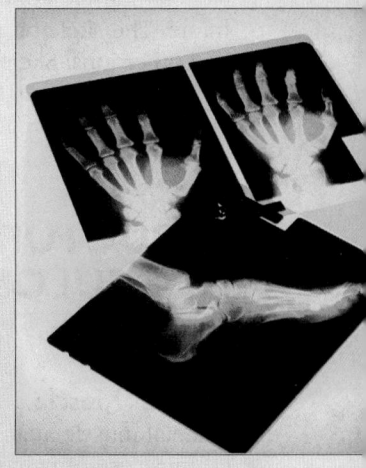

ANATOMY AND PHYSIOLOGY REVIEW:

The Musculoskeletal System

Robert G. Carroll

The musculoskeletal system consists of the bony skeleton and three types of muscles: (1) skeletal, (2) cardiac, and (3) smooth. The muscle types are distinguished based on the presence of striations, the source of innervation, and the mechanism of contraction.

Physiologically, the musculoskeletal system enables changes in movement and position. The bony skeleton provides support, protection, and a movable frame. Skeletal muscle contraction generates movement of this frame. The skeleton provides a storage pool for calcium and other ions. Skeletal muscle, which accounts for 40% to 50% of body weight, plays a major role in metabolism and temperature regulation.

STRUCTURE OF THE MUSCULOSKELETAL SYSTEM

MUSCLE

Skeletal Muscle

Skeletal muscle attaches to bones of the skeleton. Skeletal muscles are named according to the following properties: (1) action (e.g., flexor, extensor with regard to movement of the skeleton), (2) shape (e.g., quadrilateral, pennate), (3) origin (i.e., stationary attachment of muscle to skeleton), (4) insertion (i.e., movable attachment of the muscle), (5) number of divisions, (6) location, or (7) direction of fibers (e.g., transverse). The principal muscle groups are shown in Figure A&P6-1.

The contraction of skeletal muscle exerts force on bones or skin and moves them (Figure A&P6-2). Most skeletal muscles are under voluntary control of the nervous system, but some are controlled by the somatic division of the peripheral nervous system, such as those used to maintain balance.

Skeletal muscle is composed of many individual muscle cells called *muscle fibers*. These fibers are held together by thin sheets of fibrous connective tissue *(fascia)*. Fascia also penetrates the muscle, separating it into bundles *(fasciculi)*. Skeletal muscle is attached to the bones of the skeleton by very thin extensions of fascia or by tendons. *Tendons* (fibrous cords) make stronger connections to bone than fascia.

Under microscopic examination, many nuclei of muscle cells are visible and are grouped into thread-like *myofibrils*. A close look at the myofibrils reveals alternating bands of light and dark *(striations)*. Muscle cells can be further divided into smaller segments called *sarcomeres,* delineated by Z bands. The sarcomere is the structure in the muscle where the actual contraction occurs. Two primary myofilaments are present in the sarcomere: thick myosin filaments and thin actin filaments. The *filaments* are proteins that briefly attach and ratchet or slide across one another to cause the muscle to contract.

Cardiac Muscle

Cardiac muscle *(myocardium)* is involuntary and exists only in the heart. It is composed of branched, striated muscle cells connected by gap junctions. Gap junctions are connections between the cells that allow for rapid electrical and chemical communication. Cardiac muscle is controlled by intrinsic factors (e.g., the amount of venous return to the right atrium), hormones, and signals from the autonomic nervous system. Cardiac muscle is discussed in the Unit 13 Anatomy and Physiology Review.

Smooth Muscle

"Smooth" muscle has no visible striations. It contracts involuntarily and is present in the walls of hollow organs (e.g., digestive tract, blood vessels, urinary bladder) and in other areas (e.g., the eye). It is controlled by the autonomic nervous system, hormones, and intrinsic factors in the organ (e.g., stretch caused by food in the intestine). The gap junctions between smooth muscle cells create coordination in movement.

SKELETAL SYSTEM

Humans have an *endoskeleton* that lies *within* the soft tissues of the body. It is composed of living tissue that is capable of growth, adaptation, and repair. The adult body contains 206 bones, which are divided into 2 major categories by position: axial and appendicular. The *axial skeleton* (80 bones) consists of the skull, vertebral column, and thorax. The *appendicular skeleton* (126 bones) includes the bones of the extremities, shoulders, and pelvis (Figure A&P6-3). Bones can also be classified by their shape:

1. *Long bones* are all longer than they are wide and are found in the upper and lower extremities. The humerus, radius, ulna, femur, tibia, fibula, metatarsals, metacarpals, and phalanges are the long bones.

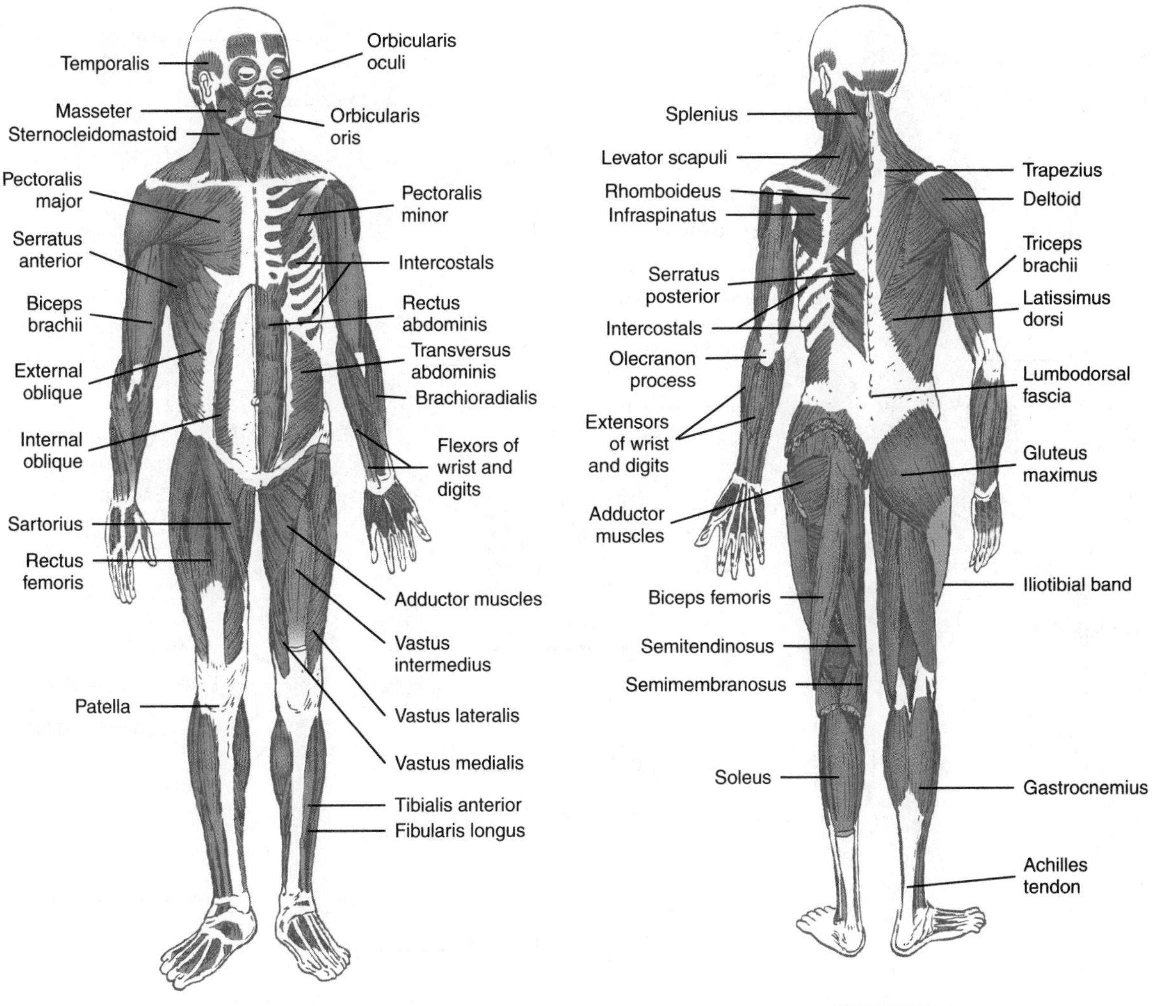

ANTERIOR

Temporalis
Masseter
Sternocleidomastoid
Pectoralis major
Serratus anterior
Biceps brachii
External oblique
Internal oblique
Sartorius
Rectus femoris
Patella

Orbicularis oculi
Orbicularis oris
Pectoralis minor
Intercostals
Rectus abdominis
Transversus abdominis
Brachioradialis
Flexors of wrist and digits
Adductor muscles
Vastus intermedius
Vastus lateralis
Vastus medialis
Tibialis anterior
Fibularis longus

POSTERIOR

Splenius
Levator scapuli
Rhomboideus
Infraspinatus
Serratus posterior
Intercostals
Olecranon process
Extensors of wrist and digits
Adductor muscles
Biceps femoris
Semitendinosus
Semimembranosus
Soleus

Trapezius
Deltoid
Triceps brachii
Latissimus dorsi
Lumbodorsal fascia
Gluteus maximus
Iliotibial band
Gastrocnemius
Achilles tendon

■ **FIGURE A&P6–1**   Principal muscles.

2. *Short bones* (e.g., carpals, tarsals) do not have a long axis; they are cubical.
3. *Flat bones* (e.g., ribs, cranium, scapula, and portions of the pelvic girdle) protect soft body parts and provide large surfaces for muscle attachments.
4. *Irregular bones* have various shapes, such as vertebrae, ear ossicles, facial bones, and pelvis. Irregular bones are similar to other bones in structure and composition.

Gross Anatomy of Bone

A typical long bone (Figure A&P6-4) has a shaft *(diaphysis)* and two ends *(proximal* and *distal epiphyses).* The diaphysis is a hollow cylinder of compact bone that surrounds a medullary cavity *(marrow).* It is lined internally with a thin connective tissue layer called *endosteum.* In children and young adults, the epiphyses are separated from the diaphysis by *epiphyseal cartilage* or plates, where bone grows longer. When bone growth is complete, the epiphyseal cartilage is replaced with

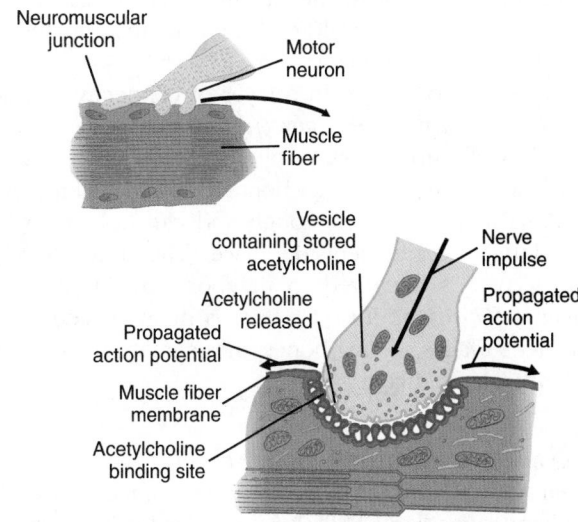

Neuromuscular junction
Motor neuron
Muscle fiber
Vesicle containing stored acetylcholine
Nerve impulse
Acetylcholine released
Propagated action potential
Propagated action potential
Muscle fiber membrane
Acetylcholine binding site

■ **FIGURE A&P6–2**   The neuromuscular junction. When a stimulus, such as a nerve impulse, travels to the neuromuscular junction, acetylcholine is released from storage in vesicles. The acetylcholine diffuses across the cleft and stimulates the muscle to contract.

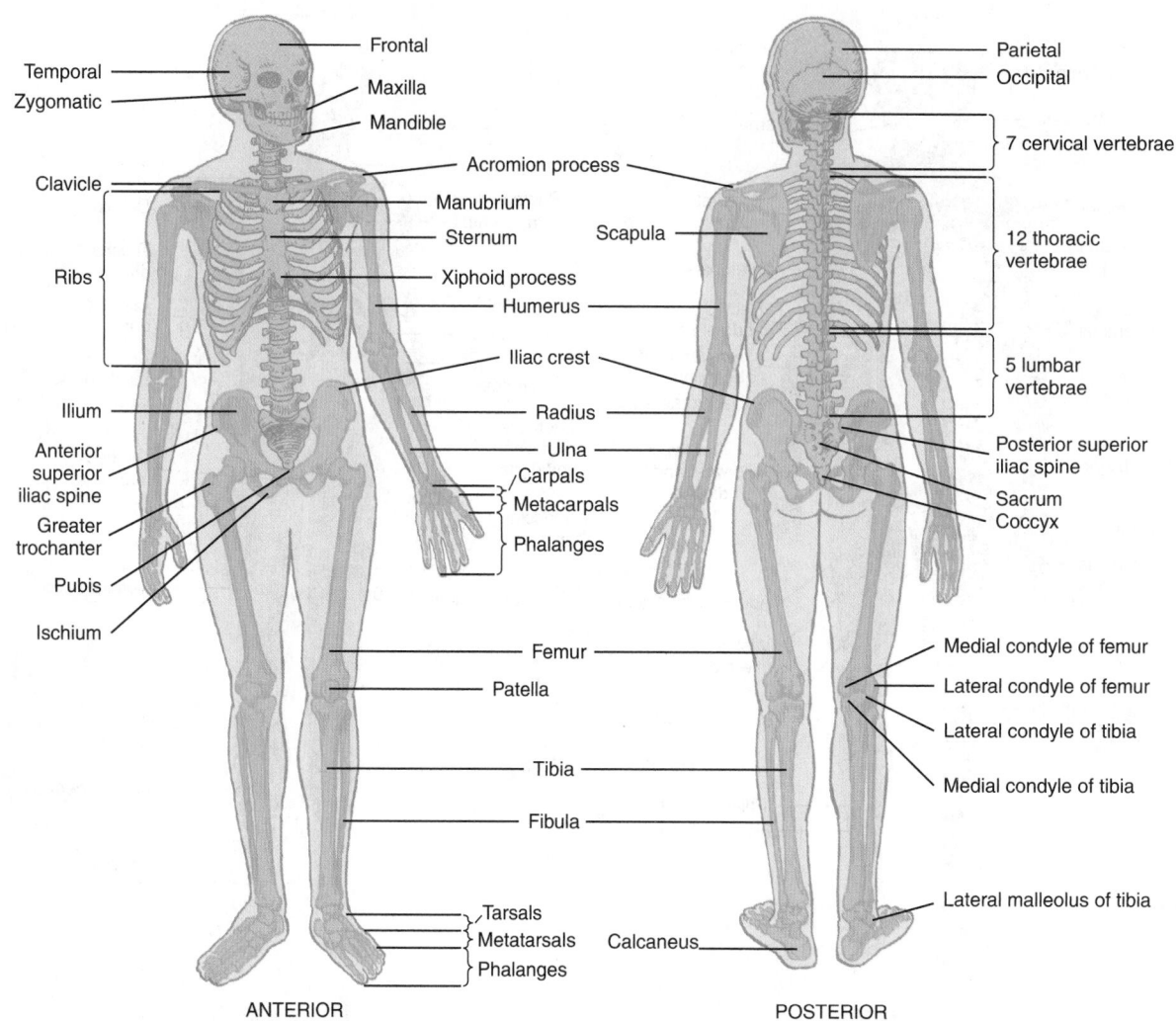

Temporal
Zygomatic
Frontal
Maxilla
Mandible
Clavicle
Acromion process
Manubrium
Sternum
Ribs
Xiphoid process
Humerus
Iliac crest
Ilium
Radius
Anterior superior iliac spine
Ulna
Carpals
Metacarpals
Greater trochanter
Phalanges
Pubis
Ischium
Femur
Patella
Tibia
Fibula
Tarsals
Metatarsals
Phalanges

ANTERIOR

Parietal
Occipital
7 cervical vertebrae
Scapula
12 thoracic vertebrae
5 lumbar vertebrae
Posterior superior iliac spine
Sacrum
Coccyx
Medial condyle of femur
Lateral condyle of femur
Lateral condyle of tibia
Medial condyle of tibia
Lateral malleolus of tibia
Calcaneus

POSTERIOR

■ **FIGURE A&P6–3** The adult human skeleton is composed of 206 bones. The axial skeleton is shown in blue, and the appendicular skeleton is shown in beige.

bone, which joins it to the diaphysis. Fractures of the epiphyseal plates in children can lead to slow bone growth or limb shortening.

Bones are covered with a layer of connective tissue called *periosteum*. The outer *(fibrous)* layer of periosteum is well supplied with blood vessels and nerves, some of which enter the bone through Volkmann's canals. This layer is very tough and can hold nondisplaced fracture fragments in place. The inner *(osteogenic)* layer is anchored to the bone by bundles of collagen *(Sharpey's fibers)*. There is no periosteum on articular surfaces of long bones; these areas are covered with articular cartilage.

Microscopic Anatomy of Bone

When viewed through a microscope, *compact bone* is highly organized and solid. It is organized into structural units called *osteons* or *haversian systems*. An osteon is essentially a cylinder of bone. Each osteon contains (1) vessels in a central canal *(haversian canal);*

(2) concentric layers of bone matrix *(lamellae);* (3) tiny spaces between the lamellae *(lacunae),* which contain osteocytes; and (4) small channels *(canaliculi).* The blood vessels transport nutrients to the bone and carry wastes away from the bone.

Spongy bone does not have such an organized structure. The lamellae are not arranged in concentric circles but rather in directions that correspond to the lines of maximum pressure or tension placed on the bone. Spongy bone has osteocytes embedded in lacunae, and lacunae intercommunicate via canaliculi. Blood reaches the osteocytes by passing through spaces in the bone marrow.

Composition of Bone

Bone's organic framework is formed from protein complexes and fibers, especially collagen (similar to the collagen found in other connective tissues). *Collagen* provides bone with great tensile strength so that it can withstand stretching and twisting. The inorganic salts (calcium and phosphate in crystalline form, termed *hydroxyapatite)*

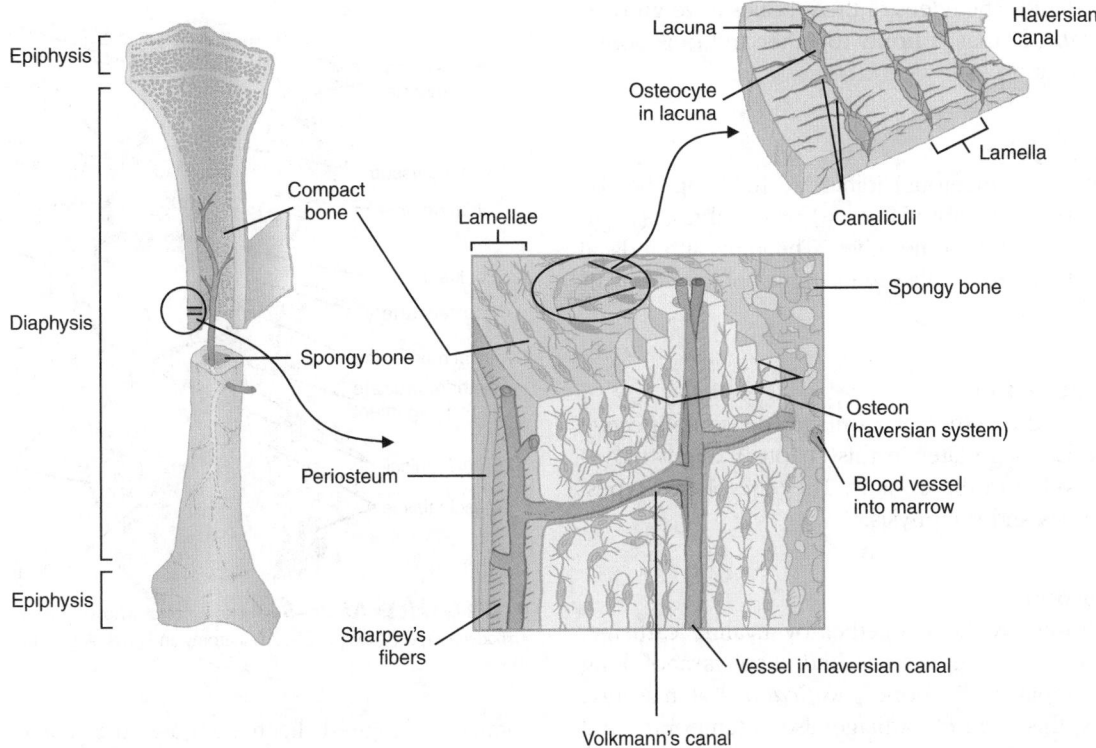

■ FIGURE A&P6–4 A, Longitudinal section of a long bone. **B,** Magnified view of compact bone, with inset showing a section of an osteon (haversian canal).

allow bone to withstand compression. The combination of collagen and salt makes bone exceptionally strong without being brittle. The composition of bone is analogous to that of reinforced concrete, in which steel rods (the collagen) provide tensile strength, and cement, sand, and gravel (the salts) provide compression strength.

Bone contains three types of cells that provide balance and function. *Osteoblasts* are bone-forming cells; they lay down new bone by catalyzing reactions that take calcium and phosphate from the blood and form it into bone matrix in a collagen meshwork. *Osteocytes* are mature osteoblasts that are found in the bone matrix. *Osteoclasts* are cells that resorb (remove) damaged or old bone cells during periods of growth or repair. They are also critical in returning inorganic salts from bone to the bloodstream. These bone cells allow bone to grow, repair itself, and change shape. Even mature bone constantly changes, with new cells being formed and old cells being destroyed.

ARTICULATIONS

Articulations (joints) are places of union between two or more bones. Not all joints permit movement. Joints may be synovial, fibrous, or cartilaginous.

Synovial Joints

Most of the joints in the body are synovial. They are freely movable, permitting position and motion changes.

Synovial joints are capable of various movements, depending on the type of joint. Synovial joints have four characteristics:

1. Each joint is enclosed by an articular *capsule,* resulting in a joint cavity (Figure A&P6-5).
2. The synovial membrane produces *synovial fluid,* which fills the cavity for lubrication and cartilage nourishment.
3. Bone surfaces in the joint are covered by *hyaline cartilage* (articular cartilage).
4. Synovial joints have additional *support* features. *Ligaments* and *tendons* reinforce the capsule and help to limit motion. *Articular disks* are located between the bones in some synovial joints to buffer forceful impact.

Fibrous Joints

Fibrous joints are articulations in which bones are held together by fibrous connective tissue. Very little material separates the ends of the bone, and minimal movement is possible.

Suture Joints

Suture joints include the bones of the skull and sometimes the sutures between the ilium, ischium, and pubic bones. At birth the bones of the skull are separated to facilitate birth. The bones usually fuse by the time a child is 2 years of age. The edges of these bones have grooves *(interdigitations)* that fit firmly together and look somewhat like a suture.

Syndesmosis Joints

Syndesmosis (ligamentous) joints are held together by ligaments (bands of fibrous tissue) or membranes. Syndesmosis joints allow some "give." The joints at the distal end of the tibia and fibula are examples of syndesmosis joints.

Cartilaginous Joints

Bones are held together by cartilage (dense connective tissue; see Cartilage later in this chapter). Slight movement is possible in these joints. They are of two types: synchondrosis and symphysis.

Synchondroses

Synchondroses are held together by hyaline cartilage. Joints between the epiphyses and diaphyses of long bones are replaced by bone *(ossification)* at maturity. In the ribs, this form of cartilage also is temporary and eventually is replaced by bone. In the costal cartilages, synchondroses between ribs and the sternum are not usually replaced by bone.

Symphyses

Symphyses are articular surfaces that have a fibrocartilaginous pad or disk connecting the articulating bones. Slight movement is allowed. Within the joint, the surfaces act as shock absorbers. The vertebrae and pubic bones are separated by symphyses.

CUSHIONING AND SUPPORTIVE STRUCTURES

Bursae and Tendon Sheaths

Bursae are small sacs lined with synovial membrane and filled with synovial fluid (Figure A&P6-5). They act as cushions between structures especially where a muscle or tendon slides across bone. The body has hundreds of bursae. Some are subcutaneous, lying between bone and skin (e.g., the bursa between the olecranon process of the elbow and the skin).

Tendon sheaths are cylindrical synovial structures similar to bursae. They are found where tendons cross joints and may be subject to constant friction, such as the carpal tunnel. The sheath wraps around the tendon, forming a fluid-filled cushion through which the tendon can slide.

Ligaments

Ligaments are bands of fibrous tissue that connect bones at joints and provide stability during movement. Some

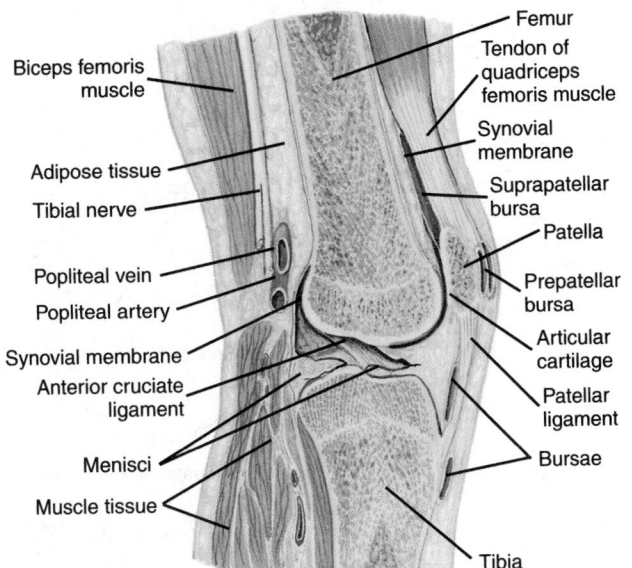

■ **FIGURE A&P6–5** Anatomy of a synovial joint (knee). *(From Thibodeau, G., & Patton, K. [2003]. Anatomy and physiology [5th ed.]. St. Louis: Mosby.)*

commonly injured ligaments are the coracohumeral and the glenohumeral ligaments, which maintain shoulder stability; and the medial, collateral, patellar, and anterior and posterior cruciate ligaments, which support the knee (Figure A&P6-6).

Cartilage

Cartilage is a type of dense connective tissue (type II collagen) that is prevalent throughout the musculoskeletal

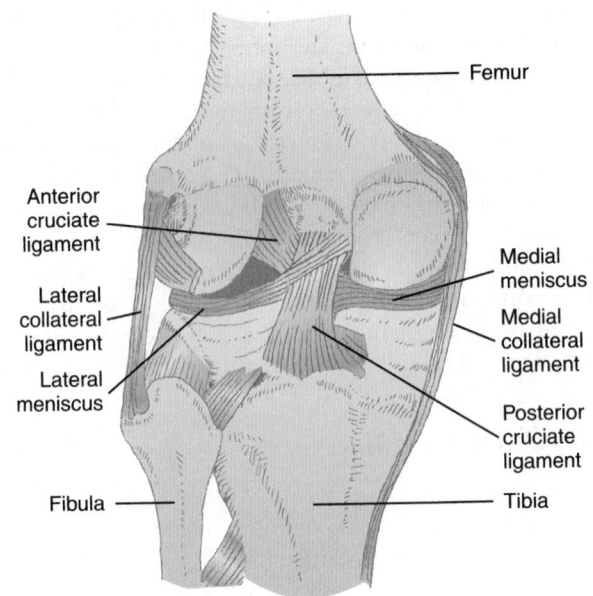

■ **FIGURE A&P6–6** Posterior view of the knee. When the knee is extended, the taut anterior cruciate ligament prevents overextension. When the knee is flexed, the posterior cruciate ligament prevents the tibia from slipping posteriorly.

system. It can resist forces of tension and compression with considerable resilience. It is semi-opaque (bluish white or gray) and has limited nerve and blood supply. Most of the skeleton of an embryo is cartilage that gradually changes into bone *(ossification)*.

Three types of cartilage are found in the body:

- *Hyaline cartilage,* found in the respiratory tract, developing bones, and ends of articulating bones
- *Fibrocartilage,* found in ligaments and intervertebral disks
- *Elastin cartilage,* found in the external ear

FUNCTION OF THE MUSCULOSKELETAL SYSTEM

Muscle

Movement

Skeletal muscle contraction occurs when a stimulus excites an individual muscle fiber (see Figure A&P6-2). The stimulus, a nerve impulse, releases stored acetylcholine (ACh) from the end of the motor neuron in the synapse. ACh crosses the neuromuscular junction and elicits an action potential by binding to a receptor on the muscle cell membrane (e.g., stimulatory electrical impulse). The action potential triggers contraction of the sarcomeres by releasing calcium inside the cell. Nerve fibers can supply more than 100 individual skeletal muscle cells, but an individual muscle cell is controlled by only one nerve. This design provides neural control for precise movement. A continuous flow of stimuli maintains muscle tone (i.e., keeps muscles partially contracted, in a state of readiness for movement).

Calcium binding exposes the active sites on the actin protein. Actin binds to myosin, and the myosin filament heads pivot using previously hydrolyzed adenosine 5′-triphosphate (ATP) as an energy source. The movement releases adenosine 5′-diphosphate (ADP) and allows new ATP to bind to the myosin, detaching the myosin from the actin. Muscle fibers relax between contractions because calcium ions that are released during the action potential are free for only a short time. Calcium quickly returns to storage in the sarcoplasmic reticulum in the muscle. If nerve impulses arrive in rapid succession so that calcium remains free, the muscle will continue to contract (called *spasm* or *tetany*).

To generate power, muscle cells require large amounts of oxygen and glucose. Muscles thus have a rich vascular supply. An oxygen debt develops during exercise if oxygen cannot be delivered to muscles in concentrations great enough to meet the immediate metabolic needs of the cell. Increased oxygen consumption is necessary to relieve oxygen debt during and after exercise.

Skeletal muscle exhibits a length-tension relationship. Before a contraction, stretching the muscle can alter the alignment of the actin and myosin proteins *(preload)*. The maximum tension generated by the contracting muscle comes when the greatest overlap between the actin and myosin proteins occurs, and this is close to the normal resting length of the skeletal muscle.

It is possible to stimulate a muscle but to exert a force so that the muscle does not shorten. This is called *isometric* ("same length") contraction. In contrast, during weight lifting, the muscle generates tension until the tension is sufficient to move the weight, allowing an *isotonic* ("same tension") contraction.

Motor Units and Summation

The *motor unit* is defined as the motor neuron and all skeletal muscle fibers it supplies. The number of muscle fibers involved in each motor unit reflects the degree of control. Small motor units allow fine control, such as in the muscles of the fingers. Large motor units coordinate the response of large muscles, such as those of the trunk.

Strength of contraction is increased by temporal or spatial summation. Temporal summation increases the rate of individual motor unit activity. Spatial summation increases the number of motor units activated. Both spatial and temporal summations can result in *tetany,* a sustained contraction of skeletal muscle.

Propulsion

Smooth muscle is found in the walls of hollow conduits in the body, and its contraction applies pressure that may mix, break up, or move substances forward. For example, smooth muscle of the gastrointestinal (GI) tract propels food through the tract during digestion. Smooth muscle in arterioles regulates arterial blood flow by causing vasodilation and vasoconstriction. Smooth muscle in the uterus contracts during labor, and smooth muscle in the airways can constrict *(bronchospasm)* or dilate to alter air movement.

Heat Production

The activity of skeletal muscle produces heat, some of which can be used to maintain body temperature. During exercise, excess heat is released through sweating and vasodilation. When the body is cold, heat is generated by shivering.

SKELETAL SYSTEM

Bones give form to the body: they support various tissues and organs and permit movement by providing attachments for tendons and muscles. The skeleton is also protective. The rib cage and skull, for example, protect the lungs and the brain and special sense organs, respectively.

Hematopoietic Function

Bone houses the hematopoietic tissues, which manufacture blood cells. In adults, blood cells form in marrow cavities in the skull, vertebrae, ribs, sternum, shoulder, and pelvis. The two types of bone marrow are *yellow* and *red*. Some investigators have noted a third type of bone marrow: brown. *Brown* marrow is generally found in older adults; it is similar to yellow marrow in that it is inactive but lacks adipose tissue. *Yellow* marrow (connective tissue composed of fat cells) is found in the shafts of long bones and extends into the haversian systems. Yellow marrow does not produce blood cells except during times of increased blood cell need. *Red marrow* has a hematopoietic function; it manufactures red and white blood cells and platelets. It is located in the cancellous bone spaces, found in flat bones (see the Unit 17 Anatomy and Physiology Review).

Role of Bone in Homeostasis

Bones also provide a crucial portion of mineral balance; they store calcium, phosphorus, sodium, potassium, and other minerals and release them for cellular metabolism and use by other body systems. When blood levels of calcium fall, the parathyroid gland senses the decrease and releases *parathyroid hormone* (PTH). PTH increases the movement of calcium from bone into the extracellular fluids by stimulating the osteoclasts to break down bone and free calcium. PTH also decreases renal excretion of calcium, increases the excretion of phosphate, and increases the metabolic transformation of vitamin D_3 to its active form to increase calcium absorption from the intestine.

Bone Remodeling

Throughout life, the bone mass continuously undergoes well-regulated processes of bone formation and bone resorption. The process of bone turnover is called *remodeling*, and it is one of the major mechanisms for maintaining calcium balance in the body. As much as 15% of the total bone mass normally turns over each year in a *three-phase process:*

- *Phase 1.* The cycle begins when a stimulus (such as a hormone, drug, or stressor) activates the bone cell precursors to become osteoclasts.
- *Phase 2.* Osteoclasts gradually resorb the bone. They leave behind an elongated cavity *(resorption cavity),* which matches the general structure of the haversian system or trabeculae.
- *Phase 3.* New bone is laid down by the osteoblasts. The osteoblasts follow the path of the osteoclasts to create new haversian systems and trabeculae.

The entire process takes about 4 months. Rebuilding of bone requires normal plasma concentrations of calcium and phosphate and is dependent on vitamin D.

Bone Repair

The remodeling process enables repair of small bony injuries, but breaks *(fractures)* and other wounds of bone heal in a different manner. Initially, the bone heals by forming a hematoma. The fibrin of the hematoma provides a meshwork, which is the initial framework for healing. Granulation tissue *(pro-callus)* is produced, and a fibrocartilaginous callus develops before bony *(osseous)* depositions develop. Osteoblasts deposit disorganized clumps of bone matrix *(callus).* The trabeculae and haversian systems follow. Finally, the bony edges are remodeled to the size and shape of the bone before injury. The callus forms at the site of the fracture and is able to be seen on x-ray, indicating a healed or "old" fracture.

EFFECTS OF AGING

Aging affects bone, muscle, and tendons. Bone tissue is lost because capacity for growth is less than the rate of loss. The haversian systems in compact bone erode. The lacunae enlarge, and cortical bone becomes thin and porous. *Osteoporosis,* a condition of decreased calcium in bone that is highly associated with aging, leads to weak, brittle bones and an increased risk of fracture.

Eventually cartilage becomes more rigid and fragile and muscle bulk decreases. As muscle mass decreases, so does maximal strength, which can decline by 50% between the ages of 20 and 50 years. Several theories have been offered to explain these changes, including changes in activity, reduced circulation, cardiovascular disorders, and nutritional problems.

CONCLUSIONS

The muscles of the body provide movement, propel substances, and produce heat. The three types of muscle—skeletal, cardiac, and smooth—perform distinct functions. Bone provides a framework and a protective structure for the body. The haversian system is the structural unit of bone. The major minerals in bone are calcium and phosphate, which are regulated by parathyroid hormone. Bone is constantly remodeled, and every 4 months it is completely replaced. Joints (articulations) provide connections between bones and allow movement involving more than one bone. Joints may be synovial, fibrous, or cartilaginous.

Musculoskeletal disorders are common. Fractures can occur at any age when forces applied to the bone exceed its tensile or compressive strength. Disorders seen in the articular surfaces (e.g., rheumatoid arthritis, osteoarthritis) develop when the articular cartilage degenerates, leading to pain and decreased movement. Muscle disorders include such conditions as muscular dystrophy (progressive muscle degeneration) and myasthenia gravis (loss of receptors on the muscle for ACh, leading to profound muscle weakness).

BIBLIOGRAPHY

1. Berne, R., et al. (2004). *Physiology* (5th ed.). St. Louis: Mosby.
2. Carroll, R.G. (2007). *Elsevier's integrated physiology.* Philadelphia: Saunders.
3. Kierszenbaum, A.L. (2007). *Histology and cell biology: An introduction to pathology* (2nd ed.). St. Louis: Mosby.
4. Guyton, A., & Hall, J. (2006). *Textbook of medical physiology* (10th ed.). Philadelphia: Saunders.
5. Silverthorn, D. (2006). *Human physiology* (4th ed.). San Francisco, Calif: Pearson Benjamin Cummings.
6. Thibodeau, G., & Patton, K. [2003]. *Anatomy and physiology* [5th ed.]. St. Louis: Mosby.

CHAPTER 25

Assessment of the Musculoskeletal System

ANITA MEEHAN

Assessment of the musculoskeletal system begins with a health history and provides direction for further assessment. Physical examination of the musculoskeletal system can be either general, as in a screening examination, or focused, for a specific problem or injury. Similarly, diagnostic tests can be either general or specific. The resulting data provide information to make judgments about the client's musculoskeletal health. The assessment can include an evaluation of the client's functional status, ability to perform activities of daily living (ADL), and ability to meet self-care needs. This aspect of the assessment evaluates the client's exercise habits and leisure activities that promote musculoskeletal health.

HISTORY

The musculoskeletal history consists of biographical and demographic data, chief complaint, and review of systems information. Collect information to help determine the nature and extent of the client's current disorder. If the chief complaint is related to recent trauma, keep the history brief and focus on the cause of injury. If the injury is extensive, the interview may need to be delayed. Once the client's condition is stable, a more complete history can be obtained. Figures 25-1 and 25-4 provide questions and topic areas to guide a focused musculoskeletal assessment.

Biographical and Demographic Data

Personal information enables individualized care planning. For example, knowing where a client lives and the kind of transportation used helps to understand the energy required for the client to live independently and keep an appointment. Information about the type of employment and hobbies will provide insight into the risk for injury. Knowing the client's social support system is essential in planning care as well.

The client's age and gender may suggest possible causes of musculoskeletal problems. Young or athletic people are more likely to be injured. Osteoarthritis is found in 85% of people over the age of 70 years. Osteoporosis (porous bone) occurs most often in postmenopausal women. Reiter syndrome is most common in men between 20 and 40 years of age. Osteogenic sarcoma is rare after age 40. Paget's disease is rare before the age of 40 and tends to run in families.

Current Health
Chief Complaint

It is important to fully analyze the client's chief complaint. Ask the client to describe the reason for seeking health care. Common musculoskeletal clinical manifestations include pain, joint stiffness, sensory changes, swelling, limited range of motion (ROM)/deformity, and infection (Figure 25-1). These manifestations can affect the ability to perform ADL. Ask the client and significant others to recount their perceptions of the problem and its causes. Answers to these questions can often provide information about areas for further assessment and clues about personal fears and concerns.

---

evolve Web Enhancements

Assessment Terms   English and Spanish

Tables   Assessing Joint Function

Common Laboratory Studies Used in the Diagnosis of Musculoskeletal Conditions

Figures   Assessment of Peripheral Nerves

Be sure to check out the bonus material on the Evolve website and the CD-ROM, including free self-assessment exercises. **http://evolve.elsevier.com/Black/medsurg**

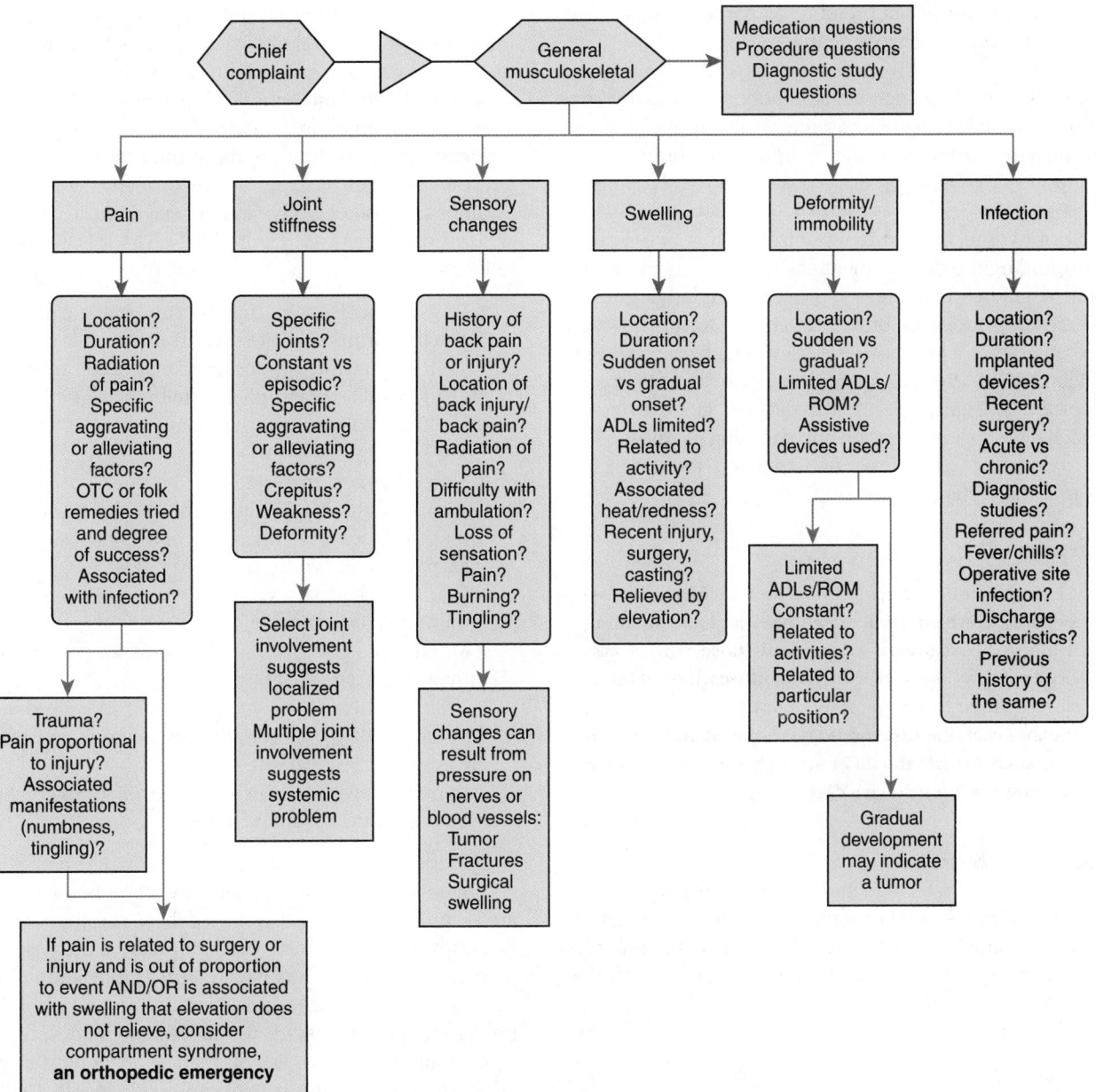

■ FIGURE 25–1 Expanded musculoskeletal assessment.

Clinical Manifestations

Full analysis of the client's chief complaint helps provide the best data for accurate diagnosis and a baseline for comparison of changes in future assessment or after any intervention. Refer to Figure 25-1 as a guide to assess complaints and clinical manifestations of the musculoskeletal system.

Pain. Pain assessment is considered the fifth vital sign. One method of pain assessment is to have the client rate his or her pain on a 0 to 10 (0 = no pain, 10 = worst pain) ascending intensity scale (see Chapter 20 for more detail related to pain assessment and rating scales). The client's description of pain can help to determine the origin of the discomfort. Aches generally indicate a muscle strain, sharp pain may indicate a fracture or infection, and throbbing pain is often bone related.

Joint Stiffness. Joint stiffness can represent local as well as systemic conditions. Associated muscle weakness may indicate a neuromuscular disorder. Crepitus, a grinding sound produced with range of motion, indicates joint irregularity. Locking of the joint is suggestive of underlying cartilage tear or bone malalignment.

Sensory changes. Inquire about tingling, burning, radiating pain, loss of feeling, and weakness. Postoperative swelling, fractures, and tumors are examples of conditions that can put pressure on nerves or blood vessels and produce sensory changes.

Swelling. Swelling and pain commonly accompany bone and muscle injury. Recent cast removal or application may produce temporary swelling of the affected limb.

Surgery may also produce postoperative swelling.

Deformity and Limited Range of Motion. Circumstances surrounding the development of the deformity are important. A gradual onset may indicate an underlying tumor, whereas a sudden deformity suggests a fracture. ROM is measured with a protractor-type device called a *goniometer* (Figure 25-2). Normal range of motion of each joint is depicted in Figure 25-3. For a detailed guide to assessing changes in knee function and choosing diagnostic studies consistent with those findings, see the Integrating Diagnostic Testing feature on p. 464.

Infection

SAFETY
ALERT

Clinical manifestations of infection include redness, swelling, elevated temperature, pain, and foul-smelling drainage. Postsurgical clients and those with a cast need to be evaluated closely for manifestations of infection. If there is any question about the cause of pain under a cast, the cast should be removed and the skin evaluated. Clients should be strongly cautioned against sticking anything down a cast.

Review of Systems

The review of systems includes medical history, surgical history, allergies, medications, dietary habits, social history, and family history. Figure 25-4 on p. 465 identifies topics and questions to guide the collection of information during the review of systems.

In addition to the usual review of systems, ask about musculoskeletal problems such as muscle pain, spasm or tenderness; joint pain, stiffness, swelling, or redness; weakness; limited movement; clumsiness; crepitus; backache; and changes in joints or bones. Investigate each reported problem. Inquire about the effect of the problem on the client's ability to perform ADL. Assessment findings from other body systems may indicate musculoskeletal problems (see Figure 25-4). The following are a few examples:

- Pain or burning on urination can be associated with reactive arthritis (Reiter syndrome).
- Tachycardia and hypertension may accompany gout.
- Conjunctivitis may indicate Reiter syndrome.
- Nongranulomatous uveitis may occur with ankylosing spondylitis.
- Skin changes may indicate musculoskeletal problems, such as wasting of the thenar muscle (palmar surface of hand, base of thumb) suggesting carpal tunnel syndrome.
- Cramping leg pain with activity may indicate intermittent claudication.
- Marked muscle atrophy and weakness accompany hyperparathyroidism.
- Irritable skeletal muscles, cramps, increased deep tendon reflexes, and paresthesias are suggestive of electrolyte imbalances.
- Joint pain with recent chills, fever, or sore throat may indicate rheumatic fever.

Specifically ask the client about any alternative and complementary therapies that may have been tried or are being currently used. Some of these can interact with prescription medications. Two popular nutritional supplements that have received considerable attention in the consumer literature are glucosamine and chondroitin. These substances are found in joint fluid and cartilage. While limited studies show modest benefit in pain relief, these preparations may cause side effects (including mild gastrointestinal upset), and concerns have been raised about their interaction with warfarin.

Some encouraging evidence exists about the potential usefulness of fish oil for relief of inflammation and morning stiffness and for reduction in the use of nonsteroidal anti-inflammatory drugs (NSAIDs) for clients suffering from rheumatoid arthritis. A systematic review of the literature also provides promising evidence for the use of several herbal preparations for the treatment of persistent pain associated with osteoarthritis, such as avocado/soybean unsaponifiables, topical capsaicin, and devil's claw. It is important to remember that herbal preparations are largely unregulated and may present safety issues in their manufacture and potency.

It is also important to inquire about the use of other complementary interventions such as the following: magnet therapy, a therapy believed to provide pain relief by

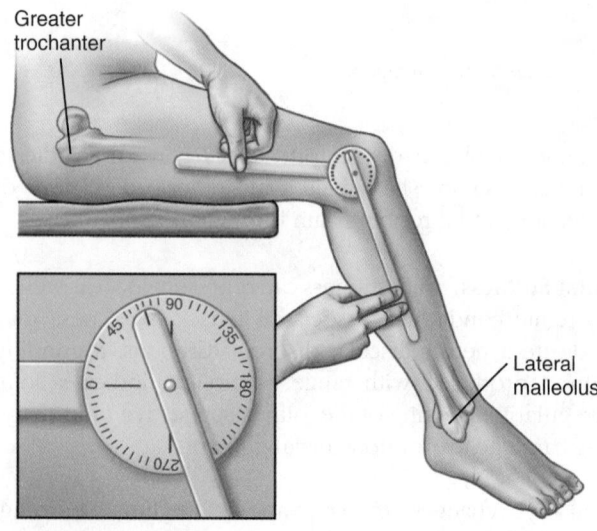

■ **FIGURE 25–2** Use of a goniometer to measure joint range of motion. This knee is flexed at 60 degrees.

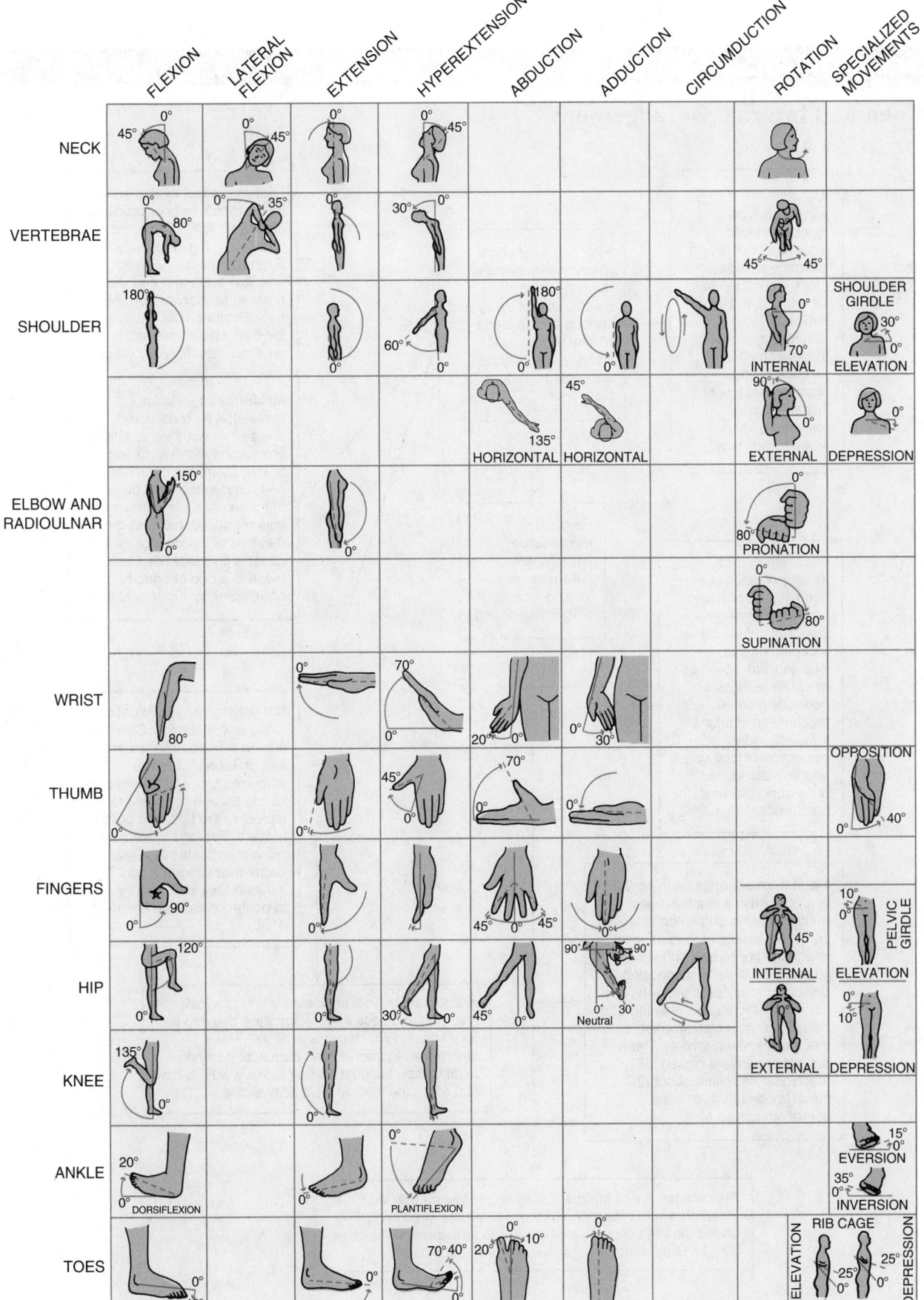

■ FIGURE 25–3 Joint range of motion (ROM). All joints are at 0 degrees when in anatomic position. ROM begins at 0 degrees, as shown by the *solid lines.* Attainment of average normal ROM is shown by the *dotted lines* and the number of degrees in the angle formed by the two lines.

INTEGRATING DIAGNOSTIC TESTING

Knee and Internal Derangement

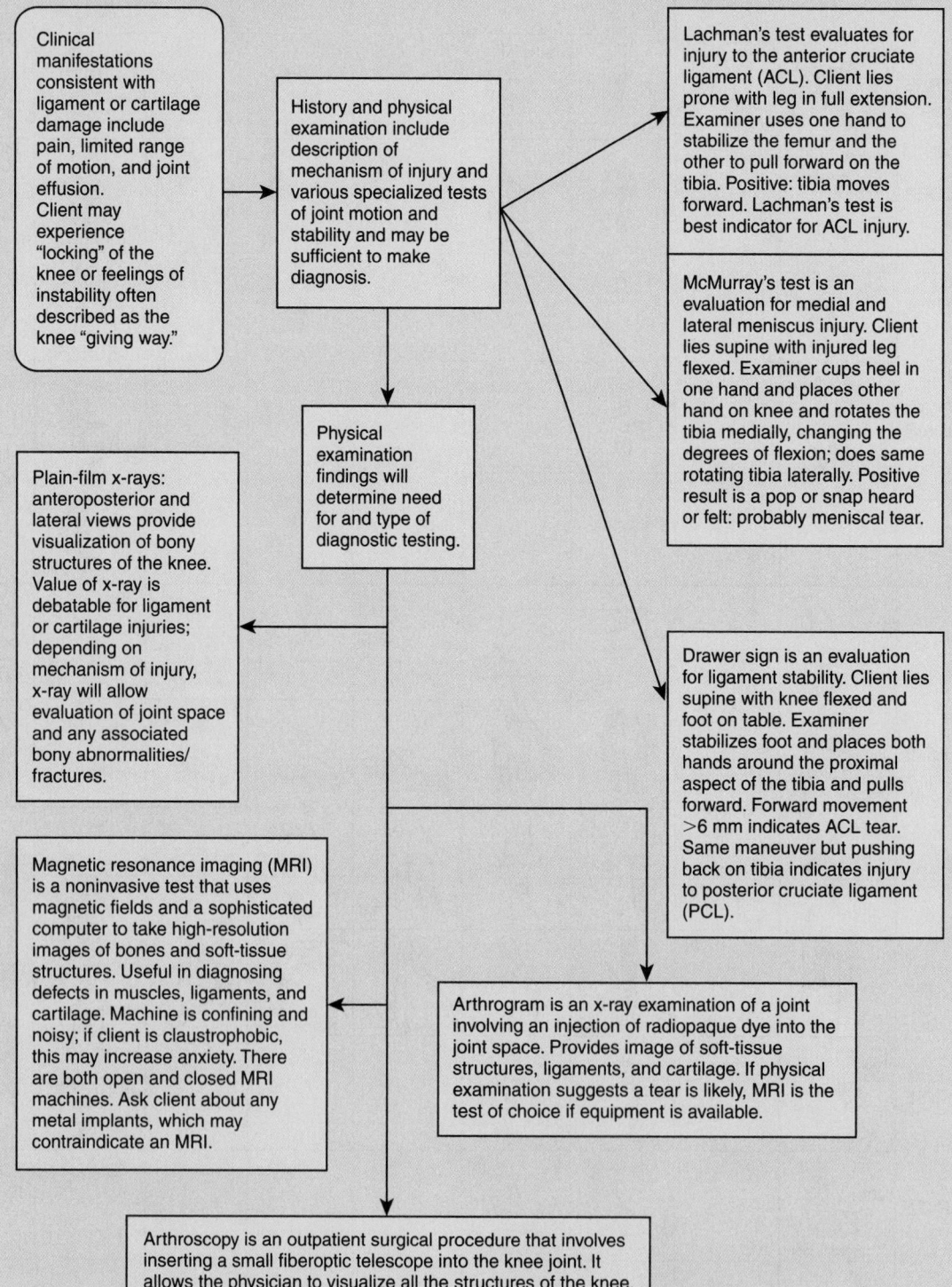

Clinical manifestations consistent with ligament or cartilage damage include pain, limited range of motion, and joint effusion. Client may experience "locking" of the knee or feelings of instability often described as the knee "giving way."

History and physical examination include description of mechanism of injury and various specialized tests of joint motion and stability and may be sufficient to make diagnosis.

Physical examination findings will determine need for and type of diagnostic testing.

Lachman's test evaluates for injury to the anterior cruciate ligament (ACL). Client lies prone with leg in full extension. Examiner uses one hand to stabilize the femur and the other to pull forward on the tibia. Positive: tibia moves forward. Lachman's test is best indicator for ACL injury.

McMurray's test is an evaluation for medial and lateral meniscus injury. Client lies supine with injured leg flexed. Examiner cups heel in one hand and places other hand on knee and rotates the tibia medially, changing the degrees of flexion; does same rotating tibia laterally. Positive result is a pop or snap heard or felt: probably meniscal tear.

Plain-film x-rays: anteroposterior and lateral views provide visualization of bony structures of the knee. Value of x-ray is debatable for ligament or cartilage injuries; depending on mechanism of injury, x-ray will allow evaluation of joint space and any associated bony abnormalities/fractures.

Drawer sign is an evaluation for ligament stability. Client lies supine with knee flexed and foot on table. Examiner stabilizes foot and places both hands around the proximal aspect of the tibia and pulls forward. Forward movement >6 mm indicates ACL tear. Same maneuver but pushing back on tibia indicates injury to posterior cruciate ligament (PCL).

Magnetic resonance imaging (MRI) is a noninvasive test that uses magnetic fields and a sophisticated computer to take high-resolution images of bones and soft-tissue structures. Useful in diagnosing defects in muscles, ligaments, and cartilage. Machine is confining and noisy; if client is claustrophobic, this may increase anxiety. There are both open and closed MRI machines. Ask client about any metal implants, which may contraindicate an MRI.

Arthrogram is an x-ray examination of a joint involving an injection of radiopaque dye into the joint space. Provides image of soft-tissue structures, ligaments, and cartilage. If physical examination suggests a tear is likely, MRI is the test of choice if equipment is available.

Arthroscopy is an outpatient surgical procedure that involves inserting a small fiberoptic telescope into the knee joint. It allows the physician to visualize all the structures of the knee. Can be used to both diagnose and treat a condition.

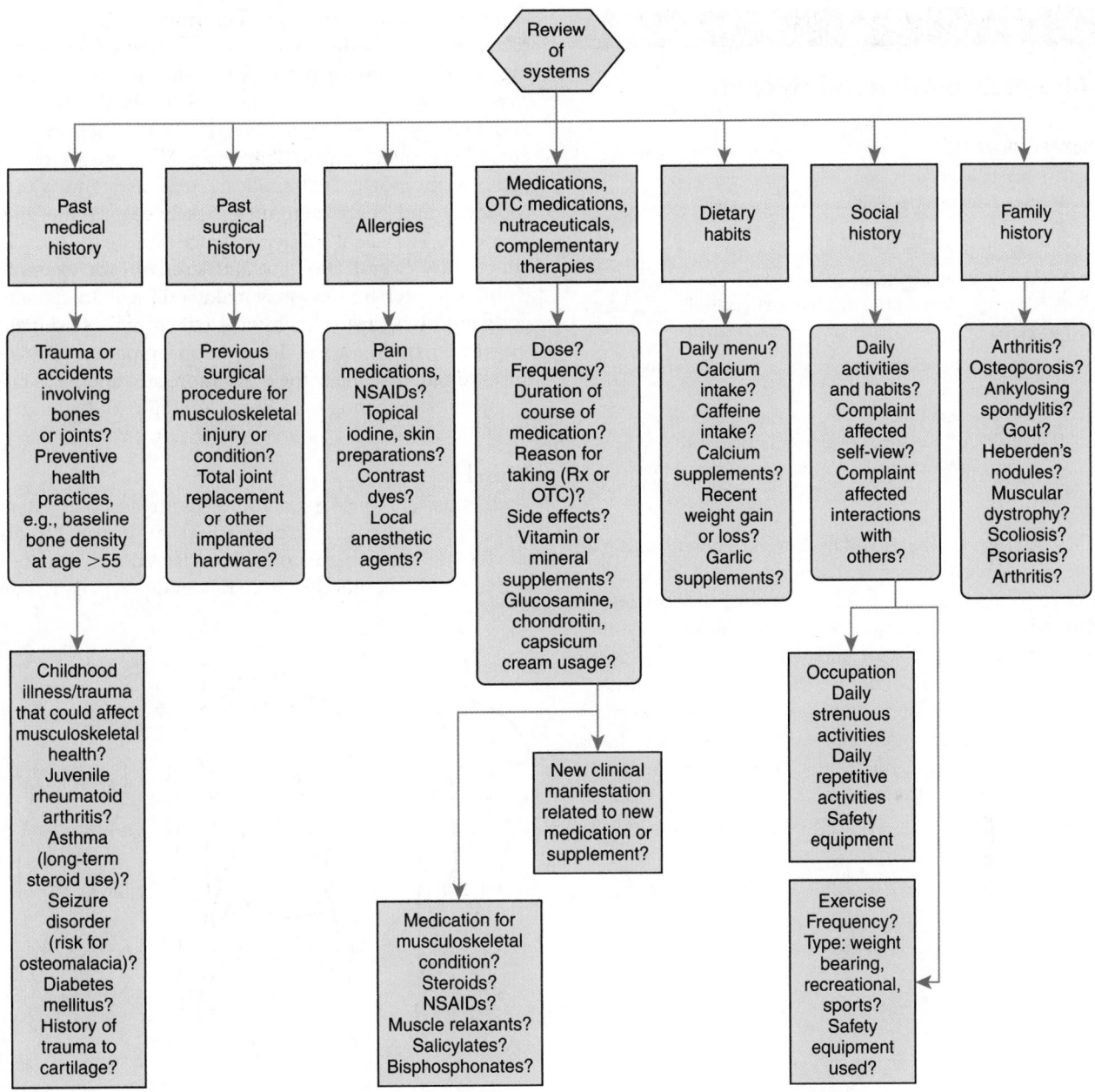

■ **FIGURE 25–4** Expanded musculoskeletal history.

producing energy fields that interfere with the pain pathway; acupuncture, a traditional Chinese medicine technique for pain relief using fine needles inserted along meridians; hydrotherapy, use of water for relief of pain and to increase mobility; homeopathy and mind-body techniques such as *Tai Chi*. Clients should be advised to seek out research evidence to support claims of pain relief or increased mobility and function before investing in these therapies.

PHYSICAL EXAMINATION

Musculoskeletal assessment consists of observing, inspecting, and palpating (1) muscle masses for symmetry, involuntary movements, tenderness, tone, and strength;

(2) joints for symmetry, crepitus, swelling, tenderness or pain, and ROM; and (3) bones for deformity and limb length discrepancy. This assessment should move systematically to avoid missing hidden problems. To evaluate movement it will be necessary to provide sufficient room for the client to sit, stand, and walk, unless a position is contraindicated by their condition. Examination in natural light is preferred. The Physical Assessment Findings in the Healthy Adult box on p. 466 shows how to document normal physical findings when assessing the musculoskeletal system.

General Musculoskeletal Examination

The general musculoskeletal examination includes observation of the client's gait, body mobility, posture, general

---

Physical Assessment Findings in the Healthy Adult

The Musculoskeletal System

INSPECTION

- Joints in alignment; posture straight; gait smooth
- Extremities symmetrical and of equal length
- Muscle groups symmetrical, without atrophy or fasciculations
- Joints without erythema, swelling, or deformities
- Full range of motion (active and passive) in all major joints

PALPATION

- Muscle groups firm, symmetrical, nontender; without masses or spasms
- Joints stable and nontender, without heat, crepitus (palpable or audible), bogginess, or nodules
- Muscle strength in all major muscle groups rated 5/5

---

joint motion, and balance. Observe movement and gait, watching for evidence of discomfort, joint stiffness or muscle weakness, lack of coordination, deformities, or limp, which may indicate a leg length discrepancy. Gait should be evaluated with and without shoes, to assess for coordination and balance. With the client seated, examine the head, neck, shoulders, and upper extremities. With the client standing, examine the chest, back, and pelvis, observing body build, body contours, alignment, and cervical, thoracic, and lumbar spine. With the client supine, examine hips, knees, ankles, and feet for alignment, symmetry, and deformities. Observe the relationship of body parts to one another—feet to legs, legs to hips, hips to pelvis, for instance (Figure 25-5). Note spinal deformities, such as scoliosis, lordosis, and kyphosis (see Figure 25-6, *A,B,C*), which are discussed in greater detail in Chapter 26. Also note abnormalities of the lower extremities, such as genu varum (bowleg) and genu valgum (knock-knee) (Figure 25-6, *D* and *E*). The client's independence and health may be affected by overall mobility and strength; for example, inability to prepare food may make it difficult to maintain good nutrition, or lack of physical activity makes it difficult to prevent osteoporosis. In addition, impaired mobility and strength may make the client more susceptible to falls or injury while caring for a home, toileting, or bathing.

Muscles

Each muscle group is compared with its contralateral side. Palpate muscle groups gently from proximal to distal, feeling the muscle tone. Muscles should feel firm and smooth, nontender, and bilaterally equal in size.

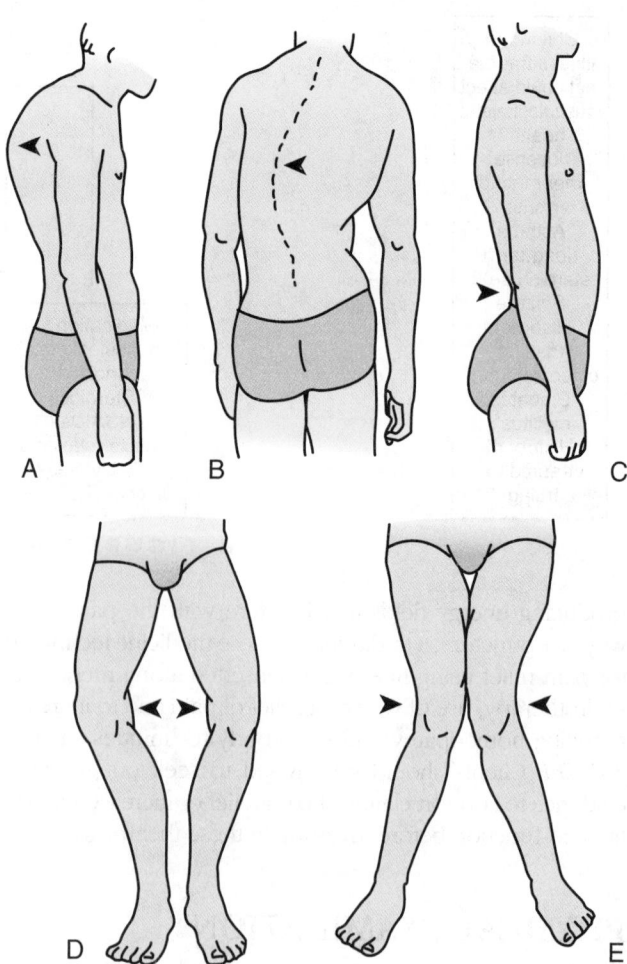

■ **FIGURE 25–6** Musculoskeletal deformities observable during assessment. **A,** Kyphosis. **B,** Scoliosis. **C,** Lordosis. **D,** Genu varum. **E,** Genu valgum.

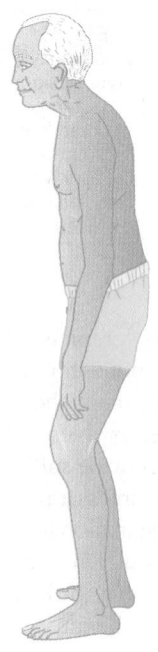

■ **FIGURE 25–5** When performing a musculoskeletal assessment, have the client stand and walk if possible. Observe the client's stance, joint mobility, and posture. If you were to assess this man only while he was reclining, you might not notice his posture, the curvature of his spine, and his limited range of motion.

Hypertrophy, a slight increase in mass, is normal on the dominant side. Atrophy, a decrease in muscle mass, is abnormal. If there is a noticeable inequality in muscle size, a tape measure should be used to assess limb circumferences. Differences of 1 cm or less are considered within normal limits.

Muscle strength is assessed during active ROM. To test muscle strength, ask the client to repeat ROM while applying resistance and note the strength against the resistance (Table 25-1). Note the dominant side before assessing strength; the client's dominant side is usually stronger. Muscle strength is rated on a 0 to 5 scale with 0 for muscle paralysis and 5 for full ROM present against normal resistance and gravity (normal).

Joints and Bones

Inspect the client's joints and bones and compare findings bilaterally. Joints should be symmetrical without evidence of redness, swelling, or deformity. Palpate bones and joints for edema and tenderness, which should be absent. Palpate joints during ROM. They should feel smooth as they move without evidence of crepitus or nodules (see Figure 25-3 on p. 463 and the table Assessing Joint Function on the website). Special assessments to determine whether an injury has occurred in a joint may be performed by an advanced practitioner. The special assessments and other diagnostic tests for the knee are described in the Integrating Diagnostic Testing feature on p. 464.

Related Systems
Neurovascular System

Neurovascular assessment is essential for clients with a past musculoskeletal injury because of the high risk of ischemia, deformity, or loss of function in the affected limb. Assessment involves checking for (1) pain, (2) pallor, (3) pulses, (4) temperature, (5) capillary refill, (6) paresthesia, and (7) mobility of affected joint(s). Rating pain assists in determining if pain is increasing in intensity which may be a possible result of edema or nerve compression. Coolness, pallor, or cyanosis may indicate circulatory compromise. Check pulses and capillary refill bilaterally to determine adequacy of blood supply. Loss of sensation and changes in motor function in a limb can indicate nerve injury. If any of these changes occur suddenly, the doctor must be notified.

Peripheral Nerve Assessment

Testing of nerve function and sensation in major peripheral nerves should be done with the clients eyes closed. See the Assessment of Peripheral Nerves figure on the website for details of peripheral nerve assessment as it *evolve* applies to the musculoskeletal examination.

Light touch should be felt if sensation is normal. The client should be able to demonstrate active range of motion of a specific joint upon request. Perform further assessments such as capillary refill, color, pulses, and skin temperature for assessment of peripheral nerves. If the extremity is immobilized in a cast, splint, or dressings, perform neurovascular assessment, observing for capillary refill and temperature, joint motion, and edema both above and below the level of the immobilizing device or dressing.

DIAGNOSTIC TESTING

The Integrating Diagnostic Studies feature on p. 464 depicts how a client with knee pain and clinical manifestations consistent with ligament or cartilage damage might be evaluated with physical assessment and diagnostic tests.

Noninvasive Tests
Radiography (X-Ray)

Radiography is the most often used noninvasive test for detecting bony abnormalities. Radiographs are used as a screening tool to establish the presence of a skeletal problem; however, they do not show soft tissue/tendon or ligament abnormalities.

TABLE 25-I	**Assessing Muscle Strength**
Muscle Group	**Technique**
Deltoid	Push down client's arm while it is held up and client resists.
Biceps	Hold client's arm in extension while it is fully extended and client flexes arm.
Triceps	Keep client's arm in flexion while it is flexed and client extends arm.
Wrist and finger muscles	Push client's fingers together while client spreads them and resists.
Grip strength	Pull your own crossed index and middle fingers from the client's grasp.
Hip muscles	Hold down client's leg while it is fully extended and while client lifts it off the table (client is supine).
Hip muscles (abduction)	Prevent client from spreading legs apart against resistance applied to the lateral surfaces of the knees (client is supine with legs extended).
Hip muscles (adduction)	Prevent client from bringing legs together against resistance applied to the medial surfaces of the knees (client is supine with legs extended).
Hamstrings	Straighten client's knees while client is supine with knees flexed and resists.
Quadriceps	Flex client's knee while client is supine with knee partially in extension and resists.
Ankle and foot muscles	Dorsiflex client's foot while client resists. Plantar flex client's foot while client resists.

Magnetic Resonance Imaging (MRI)

MRI is a test that uses large magnets to produce a detailed image of soft tissue as well as bone. MRI is used to detect conditions affecting the tendons, ligaments, and muscle.

Computed Axial Tomography (CAT)

A CAT scan allows for a segmental view of the desired area; it is helpful in determining soft tissue tumors and spinal fractures.

Dual-Energy X-ray Absorptiometry (DEXA)

A DEXA scan measures bone loss and is considered the gold standard test for osteoporosis.

Invasive Tests

Arthrocentesis

An arthrocentesis involves needle aspiration of joint fluid using sterile technique. Medication, such as cortisone, may be instilled into the joint after aspiration of fluid. Generally, a compressive dressing is applied after the procedure.

Arthrogram

An arthrogram is an x-ray image of the joint after the injection of dye. This test is useful in evaluating for tears in the joint lining, such as tears in the rotator cuff of the shoulder, or tears of internal structures, such as a meniscal tear in the knee.

Arthroscopy

An arthroscopy is a surgical procedure that involves inserting a small fiberoptic scope into the joint, which provides visualization of the internal structures and allows for surgical intervention at the same time.

Electromyelogram and Nerve Conduction Test (EMG/NCT)

These studies involve inserting small electrodes into the nerve pathway and stimulating the nerve to innervate the muscle while measuring muscle contraction. This test is used to diagnose conditions such as carpal tunnel syndrome.

Other Musculoskeletal Tests

Indium Scan

An indium scan involves the injection of indium 111 that is connected to leukocytes. Because leukocytes naturally accumulate in areas of bone infection, the test is useful to determine bone infection (osteomyelitis) or infections of total joint implants.

Bone Scans

A bone scan requires the injection of a radioisotope, after which the entire body is scanned. A bone scan is used to detect malignancies, stress fractures, and osteomyelitis.

Laboratory Tests

Some of the more commonly used laboratory tests ordered for clients with musculoskeletal complaints include antinuclear antibody (ANA), C-reactive protein (CRP), erythrocyte sedimentation rate (ESR), and rheumatoid factor (RF), which are measures of inflammation, infection, or systemic autoimmune problems. A complete blood cell count (CBC) may be ordered to monitor clients who are taking NSAIDs to detect any manifestations of anemia, a concern for clients on long-term NSAID therapy. Abnormalities in mineral metabolism (levels of calcium, phosphorus, or alkaline phosphatase) are suggestive of musculoskeletal disorders. Elevations in blood levels of muscle enzymes such as creatine kinase, lactate dehydrogenase, and aldolase A are suggestive of muscular dystrophy. The Common Laboratory Studies Used in the Diagnosis of Musculoskeletal Conditions table on the website provides additional descriptions of tests and possible etiologies for abnormal findings. Please refer to a laboratory handbook for the specifics of collecting and handling blood samples.

CONCLUSIONS

Assessment of the musculoskeletal system consists of a complete history, including clinical manifestation analysis and a review of the systems. Physical examination includes evaluation of gait and balance, muscle symmetry and strength, joint symmetry, and range of motion.

Neuromuscular and peripheral vascular systems are also evaluated during the musculoskeletal assessment. In addition, there are a variety of laboratory tests and invasive and noninvasive diagnostic procedures used to diagnose musculoskeletal conditions.

BIBLIOGRAPHY

 Citations appearing in red refer to primary research.

1. Altizer, L. (2004). Compartment syndrome. *Orthopaedic Nursing, 23* (6), 391-396.
2. Hathaway, L. (2004). Pump up your musculoskeletal assessment. *Nursing Made Incredibly Easy, 2*(3), 46-47, 49-50.
3. Kneale, J., & Davis, P. (2005). *Orthopaedic and trauma nursing* (2nd ed). Edinburgh: Churchill Livingstone.
4. Maher, A.B., Salmond, S.W., & Pellino, T.A. (2002). *Orthopaedic nursing* (3rd ed.). Philadelphia: W.B. Saunders.

5. Moore, A., McQuay, H., Derry, S., et al. (2004). Avocado/soybean unsaponifiables for osteoarthritis (electronic version). *Bandolier, April,* 122-123. Retrieved 08/16/06 from www.jr2.ox.ac.uk/bandolier.
6. Schoen, D. (Ed.) (2001). *Core curriculum for orthopaedic nursing* (4th ed). Pitman, NJ: Jannetti.
7. Weiner, D.K., & Ernst, E. (2004). Complementary and alternative approaches to the treatment of persistent musculoskeletal pain. *Clinical Journal of Pain,* 20(4), 244-253.

evolve *Did you remember to check out the bonus material on the Evolve website and the CD-ROM, including NCLEX®-Examination Style Review Questions, Open-Book Quizzes, and Chapter Review Audio Podcasts?*

http://evolve.elsevier.com/Black/medsurg

CHAPTER 26

Management of Clients with Musculoskeletal Disorders

DOTTIE ROBERTS AND JOAN M. LAPPE

The musculoskeletal system allows the human body to maintain its upright posture, to move freely, and to function independently. Bone is a vital, dynamic connective tissue that serves three major functions: (1) it provides a framework for movement and protection of internal organs, (2) it performs a major role in metabolism and mineral homeostasis, and (3) it serves as the primary site of hematopoiesis. Disorders of the musculoskeletal system cause considerable morbidity, lead to decreased quality of life, and often result in reduced life expectancy.

DEGENERATIVE BONE DISORDERS

OSTEOARTHRITIS

Osteoarthritis (OA), or degenerative joint disease, is the most common type of arthritis and has been recognized for centuries. Based on ongoing research on all arthritic disorders, OA is no longer believed to be a wear-and-tear disease that is a normal consequence of aging. Although aging does lead to decreasing quality and quantity of the proteoglycans in articular cartilage, the changes seen in the cartilage of asymptomatic adults are quite different from those found in aging adults with OA. OA is now recognized as a chronic, progressive process in which new tissue is produced in response to joint insults and cartilage deterioration. Systemic involvement and inflammation are not typical of OA, although changes in the joint space may cause a localized inflammatory response that leads to transient joint effusion.

Etiology and Risk Factors

Osteoarthritis has been classified as either *idiopathic* (formerly primary) or *secondary*. *Idiopathic* OA affects people with no history of joint injury, joint disease, or systemic illness that might be associated with the development of arthritis. The most prevalent articular disease in adults 65 years of age and older, idiopathic OA occurs more commonly in women than in men. It accounts for substantial disability as a result of its effects on the large weight-bearing joints and the spine.

Although OA has not historically been considered a genetic disease, a strong familial disposition exists for the development of idiopathic disease. An estimated 10% to 60% of OA cases may be genetically linked, with variance based on the affected joint.[10] Evidence now suggests the existence of an autosomal-recessive trait with gene defects that contribute to early cartilage destruction. In addition, sex hormones and other hormonal factors are believed to play an active part in the development and progression of OA.

Secondary OA occurs more frequently in men than in women. It results from trauma, other inflammatory joint disease, avascular necrosis, or neuropathic disorders such as Legg-Calvé-Perthes disease. Traumatic arthritis can develop after fracture or open joint injury. It can also stem from repetitive injury related to the person's occupation or sport (e.g., wrist arthritis in a keyboard operator, shoulder manifestations in a baseball pitcher).

Because OA is a chronic, incurable disorder, health care providers have focused instead on identifying modifiable risk factors that can decrease the impact of the

---

evolve Web Enhancements

Care Plan The Client with Osteoporosis

Clinical Pathway Total Hip Replacement

Complementary and Alternative Therapy SAM-e Supplements and Osteoarthritis

Be sure to check out the bonus material on the Evolve website and the CD-ROM, including free self-assessment exercises. **http://evolve.elsevier. com/Black/medsurg**

disease. For example, studies have consistently shown that overweight people have higher rates of OA of the knee than peers of normal weight. Although overweight people also appear to be at higher risk for OA of the hip, the association is not as strong or as consistent as for OA of the knee. This risk variation is due to the different amount of force exerted across these joints when a person stands or walks. Up to six times the body's weight is exerted across the knee, whereas only three times the body's weight is exerted at the hip. Weight loss or maintenance is important to minimize the effects of OA.

Clients with OA are also encouraged to follow a regular exercise regimen, which offers benefits in several ways:

- Weight-bearing exercise leads to increased joint mobility and strengthens the joint's supporting muscles, tendons, and ligaments.
- Exercise stimulates cartilage growth by driving synovial fluid through the cartilage matrix. Because articular cartilage lacks blood vessels, the mechanical process of joint movement is essential to cartilage regeneration and continued joint mobility.
- Exercise protects joints indirectly by aiding in weight control.

Pathophysiology

Healthy articular cartilage appears smooth, glistening, and white. It possesses unique viscoelastic and compressive properties that contribute to its shock-absorbing characteristics. *Chondrocytes,* the cells that produce cartilage, constantly remodel and maintain the integrity of articular cartilage that protects the bone ends in a joint. Chondrocytes actually create the cartilage matrix by producing type 2 collagen and proteoglycans. The hydrophilic (water-attracting) properties of the proteoglycans in particular add to the ability of cartilage to resist wear with heavy joint use.

In simplest terms OA can be described as a process of cartilage matrix degradation accompanied by the body's ineffectual attempts at repair. Early pathologic changes include a decrease in proteoglycan content in the matrix, which leads to a softening and loss of elasticity by the cartilage. As the body attempts to compensate, chondrocytes initially proliferate and increase their synthesis of proteoglycans and collagen. Progressive destruction by lysosomal enzymes eventually outweighs production, however, and the cartilage becomes increasingly susceptible to joint friction. Changes in collagen synthesis also occur, minimizing the compressibility of the cartilage. Factors that cause these changes are not clearly understood, but the effect on cartilage is the loss of its ability to resist wear with heavy use.

Fibrillation, erosion, and cracking appear in the superficial layer of cartilage as collagen fibers rupture. Cartilage becomes yellowed and worn over articular

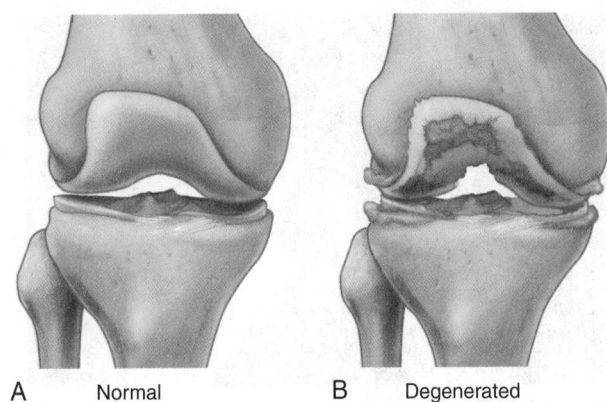

A Normal   **B** Degenerated

■ **FIGURE 26–1** Pathologic changes seen with osteoarthritis. **A,** Normal cartilage-covered bony surfaces for articulation. **B,** Articular cartilage and bony surfaces are altered with loss of joint space and osteophyte formation.

surfaces, bone growth increases at the joint margins, and bony outgrowths (osteophytes) develop (Figure 26-1). Central loss of cartilage, accompanied by buildup of cartilage and bone peripherally, produces inequality in the joint surfaces. The normal distribution of joint stress is changed, resulting in pain and restricted motion. The synovium may also respond with excessive secretion of synovial fluid, creating an inflamed, distended joint capsule.

Clinical Manifestations

The diagnosis of OA is based primarily on history and physical examination. It may be confirmed by radiographic changes that include the presence of osteophytes and of a narrowed joint space caused by erosion of articular cartilage. Because the severity of manifestations does not always correlate with joint changes, however, the American College of Rheumatology (ACR) has established classification criteria for OA that do not rely solely on radiographic findings; criteria vary slightly depending on the affected joint.

Two notable clinical manifestations help in the diagnosis of OA: worsening pain and limitation of movement. Affected joints also may exhibit crepitus, mild tenderness in the area of joint wear, stiffness that increases with activity and decreases with rest, and possibly some joint enlargement. One or more joints may be affected, but joint discomfort is not usually symmetrical. The client may describe weight-bearing joints that "lock" or "give way" as a result of advancing disease. New bone growth in the hands may be evident in the appearance of Heberden's nodes (distal interphalangeal [DIP] joints) or Bouchard's nodes (proximal interphalangeal [PIP] joints) (Figure 26-2).

Although no laboratory test has the capacity to confirm the presence of OA, specific tests may be performed to rule out other conditions that also produce joint pain, such as rheumatoid arthritis (RA), infection, gout, and

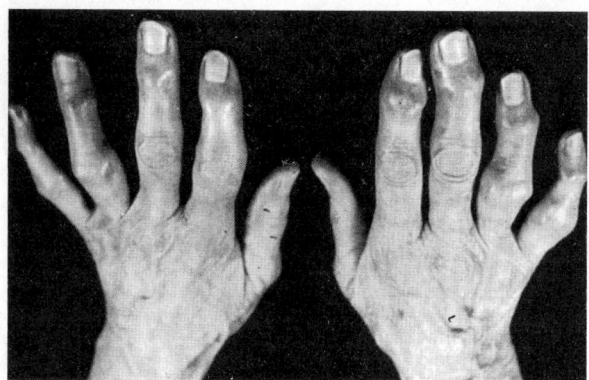

■ **FIGURE 26–2** Osteoarthritis of the distal and proximal interphalangeal joints. *(From Moskowitz, R.W., & Bluestone, R. [2001]. General aspects of differential diagnosis. In R.W. Moskowitz, et al. [Eds.], Osteoarthritis: Diagnosis and medical/surgical treatment [3rd ed.]. Philadelphia: Saunders.)*

tendinitis or bursitis. Differentiation between OA and RA is especially important (Table 26-1). Diagnostic studies may include rheumatoid factor or a serum uric acid determination. Aspiration and analysis of synovial fluid allow the practitioner to rule out infection or crystal deposition. An erythrocyte sedimentation rate (ESR) is useful only if systemic manifestations are present. Depending on the client's clinical presentation, magnetic resonance imaging (MRI) may be ordered to rule out meniscal injury. In practice, the possible diagnoses are usually narrowed greatly after completion of the history and examination.

OUTCOME MANAGEMENT

Medical Management

Goals for medical management of OA include (1) pain management with improvement or maintenance of mobility, (2) functional independence, and (3) maintenance of quality of life. Most people with early OA can be successfully treated with a conservative approach that involves the simultaneous use of several modalities.

All clients benefit from a careful balance between rest and exercise. A sedentary lifestyle can lead to weight gain, which exacerbates arthritic manifestations. Low-impact aerobic exercise, such as brisk walking, does not cause further harm to damaged joints. In fact, walking can relieve pain and improve joint mobility. It also increases muscle tone and enhances joint stability. Exercise can help with weight loss, which should be encouraged in the obese client because obese clients face more rapid destruction of joints in the lower extremities.

TABLE 26–1 Differentiation of Osteoarthritis and Rheumatoid Arthritis

	Osteoarthritis	Rheumatoid Arthritis
Pathology	Progressive process of central cartilage (spurs) destruction Peripheral bone growth in joint	Progressive process marked by exacerbations and remissions Inflammation of synovial membrane with cartilage damage and bone destruction Ligament, tendon, and joint capsule damage
Affected joints	Weight-bearing joints (hips, knees, ankles), spine, DIP and PIP joints* Asymmetric	Small joints (PIP, MCP), wrists, knees Symmetric
Joint effusions	Mild swelling possible from localized inflammatory response	Common
Clinical manifestations	Localized pain and stiffness, mild swelling possible Pain with activity, improves with rest Heberden's and Bouchard's nodules	Pain, swelling, tenderness, redness, and warmth Nodules over extensor surfaces Anemia, fatigue, and muscle aches Pain at rest, especially at night Elevated ESR, often positive rheumatoid factor
Other affected systems	None	Lung, heart, skin
Body size	Possibly overweight	Usually average to below average weight for size
Age at onset	Fourth to fifth decade of life	Young to middle age
Gender	2:1 female-to-male ratio	3:1 female-to-male ratio
Heredity	Genetic factors contribute	Familial tendency
Diagnostic tests	X-rays	Rheumatoid factor (80% positive); x-rays; joint fluid analysis; negative Lyme disease titer
X-ray evidence	Osteophytes, subchondral cysts	Erosions, osteoporosis
Treatment	Exercise and weight control, maintenance of activity level with joint protection Heat or cold applications Relaxation strategies Medication and/or surgery	Inflammation reduction Balanced diet and exercise program with joint protection Relaxation strategies; heat or cold applications Medication and/or surgery

DIP, Distal interphalangeal; *ESR,* erythrocyte sedimentation rate; *PIP,* proximal interphalangeal; *MCP,* metacarpophalangeal.
Modified from Roberts, D. (2002). Degenerative disorders. In A. B. Maher, S. W. Salmond, & T. A. Pellino (Eds.), *Orthopaedic nursing* (3rd ed.). Philadelphia: Saunders.

When even a short exercise session leaves the OA client with sore joints, movement therapies such as *Tai Chi* may be suggested as a low-impact alternative to increase fitness and flexibility within the client's own limits. Instead of pushing the joints to the point of overexertion, the client learns to consider the internal effects of balance and stress reduction to be more important than the physical exercise. Because it gradually increases joint flexibility and muscle strength without loading joints, physicians now recommend *Tai Chi* for clients with varied musculoskeletal conditions.

The client with OA needs to understand the importance of rest if an affected joint becomes painful. The client's use of a cane in the contralateral hand can decrease joint stress during episodes of severe hip or knee pain. A neoprene or elastic brace may also reduce pain and help to stabilize the joint in a functional position. A collar, sling, or corset may be useful for manifestations in the neck, shoulder, or back; however, immobilization should be limited to 1 week to avoid increased joint stiffness.

Some clients also obtain relief by applying heat to affected joints or by alternating applications of heat and cold (contrast baths). Heat applications help with stiffness by increasing collagen elasticity and flexibility. Cold applications are used less frequently than heat but may be beneficial during episodes of acute inflammation, immediately after exercise, or for relief of muscle spasms.

Ionized wrist bracelets are commonly advertised for pain relief; however, as detailed in the Complementary and Alternative Therapy feature at right, research suggests that this form of therapy provides no better relief for musculoskeletal pain than a placebo.

Many clients with OA report good results from topical application of capsaicin cream to affected joints several times a day. The cream is available over-the-counter or can be prescribed in greater concentrations. It can be used alone or as an adjunct to oral medications. Capsaicin is especially effective for OA of the knees and hands. About 50% of capsaicin users describe a cutaneous burning, but this reaction usually declines with continued use.

Nonsteroidal anti-inflammatory drugs (NSAIDs) were previously considered the mainstay of pharmacologic management of OA. Because OA has only a minor inflammatory component, however, NSAIDs may not be the best first-line choice. Furthermore, research suggests that NSAIDs actually disrupt articular cartilage metabolism. Many deaths among older adults are also attributed to NSAID use each year, usually because of gastrointestinal bleeding. Acetaminophen is the drug of first choice for those with hip or knee OA because of its effectiveness, safety, and low cost. It is less likely than NSAIDs to cause gastrointestinal, hepatic, or renal damage. The recommended maximum dose of acetaminophen is 1 g every 6 hours, not to exceed 4 g in a 24-hour period.

COMPLEMENTARY AND ALTERNATIVE THERAPY

Ionized Wrist Bracelets for Musculoskeletal Pain

Researchers found that numerous advertisements support the use of an ionized bracelet to relieve musculoskeletal pain. Therefore they decided to study 610 adults with pain in at least 1 of 12 locations (from the neck to the feet). The mean age of the individuals was 48 years (74.2% female and 87.8% Caucasian). Approximately 80% of the participants believed that the ionized bracelet would work. Participants were randomly assigned to wear either the ionized wrist bracelet or an identical placebo bracelet for 4 weeks. All 610 clients completed the study.

There was no significant difference between the two groups for either end-point of the study (change in pain score or the sum total of pain scores for all locations). The baseline pain score for all body locations for both groups was between 4.2 and 5.8 out of a possible 10; at a 4-week follow-up the scores had decreased 1.3 to 2.6 points. Approximately 77% of the participants in both groups reported an improvement in their maximum pain score, and a similar number had an improved sum of pain scores. Therefore the bracelet did not work better than the placebo.

REFERENCE

Bratton, R., et al. (2002). Effect of "ionized" wrist bracelets on musculoskeletal pain: A randomized, double-blind, placebo-controlled trial. *Mayo Clinic Proceedings, 77,* 1164-1168.

According to ACR guidelines,[5] a person with OA should be switched to an NSAID when severe pain persists despite the maximum acetaminophen dose. Acetaminophen use often continues on an as-needed (prn) basis as an adjunct to the NSAID, which should be started in an over-the-counter (OTC) strength. Progression to prescriptive strengths only occurs when clinical manifestations worsen. To minimize gastrointestinal effects, the NSAID can be prescribed with a synthetic prostaglandin such as misoprostol (Cytotec). The client with a history of gastroesophageal reflux disease (GERD) or peptic ulcer disease may benefit from the use of the cyclooxygenase-2 (COX-2) selective anti-inflammatory drug celecoxib (Celebrex). However, results of the Celecoxib Long-Term Arthritis Safety Study (CLASS) prompted the U.S. Food and Drug Administration (FDA) to require labeling changes for the drug that include presenting information about the risk of serious gastrointestinal and renal effects in older adults who take it. (For more information on osteoarthritis medications, see the Integrating Pharmacology feature on p. 474).[15]

Viscosupplementation is a unique treatment option for knee OA. Hyaluronan, a polysaccharide that is a major component of synovial fluid, can be administered

INTEGRATING PHARMACOLOGY

Medications for Osteoarthritis

Conservative management of osteoarthritis typically focuses on relieving pain and any accompanying inflammation. In early disease in particular, adequate pain management allows the client to continue usual activities.

Unlike aspirin, acetaminophen does not relieve the redness, stiffness, or swelling caused by inflammatory conditions such as rheumatoid arthritis. As a simple analgesic, however, it is now recommended as a first-line treatment for mild osteoarthritis pain. It causes analgesia by inhibiting prostaglandin synthesis. Because of the minimal effects on peripheral prostaglandin synthesis, however, it has no anti-inflammatory effects. Acetaminophen is contraindicated for clients with hepatic disease, and it can cause hepatic toxicity in excess doses (more than 4 g in 24 hours) in clients without previous liver disorders. Because of the hepatic effects of acetaminophen, clients who will be using it regularly for arthritis pain management should be encouraged to avoid alcoholic beverages. The combined effects of acetaminophen and alcohol may be especially damaging to the liver. The client should also be instructed to check the labels of the other over-the-counter medications commonly taken; if acetaminophen is an ingredient in a cold preparation, for example, the client should clarify with a health care provider the amount of additional acetaminophen that may be taken for arthritis pain.

The other major class of medications used for management of arthritis pain is the nonsteroidal anti-inflammatory drugs (NSAIDs). NSAIDs work by interfering with the cyclooxygenase (COX) pathway, ultimately inhibiting prostaglandin synthesis. Prostaglandin causes vasodilation, which allows more blood flow to an affected area and results in the heat and redness of inflammation. Prostaglandin also prolongs pain. By inhibiting prostaglandin synthesis, NSAIDs can decrease inflammation and pain associated with arthritis. The COX-1 enzyme in the stomach wall continuously produces prostaglandins that stimulate mucous formation and protect the stomach lining. Traditional NSAIDs such as ibuprofen and naproxen interfere with the COX-1 enzyme pathway, leading to increased risk of gastrointestinal side effects for clients taking these drugs.

by intra-articular injection into the knee. After injection the joint can produce normal hyaluronan and synovial fluid independently for several months. As it helps to restore the elastoviscosity of the synovial fluid, hyaluronan also provides some relief of arthritic pain. Numerous dietary supplements offer popular alternative therapies for the treatment of OA. Glucosamine reportedly provides the building blocks for the body to make and repair cartilage, and chondroitin is believed to contribute to cartilage elasticity. The client who wishes to take glucosamine and chondroitin must have a realistic approach because it may take weeks for results to become evident. The supplements do not work for everyone, and the

client who has taken them consistently for 2 to 3 months without results may in fact receive no benefit from continued therapy.

SAM-e (S-adenosylmethionine) is a popular European supplement that reached U.S. markets in 1999. SAM-e, which occurs naturally in all living cells, contributes to the production of proteoglycans for cartilage repair. The human body usually makes all the SAM-e it needs, but levels decrease with aging, depression, or deficiencies of B vitamins or methionine. Early research in the United States has shown some positive effects on arthritis pain for people with early OA only, but the supplement does not demonstrate significantly different outcomes than treatment with NSAIDs alone.[1] More research is needed to determine long-term effects of the supplement. (See the Complementary and Alternative Therapy feature on SAM-e Supplements and Osteoarthritis on the website.)

Herbal products are commonly taken by clients with arthritis either to treat their disease or to assist with memory and energy. Many of the most popular herbal products decrease platelet aggregation causing prolonged bleeding time. They may also interact with various prescribed medications. Assessment of the client's use of herbal products is important, particularly if surgery is anticipated. Clients should be cautioned to stop taking herbal products before surgery because of the risk of changes in heart rate, blood pressure, or hemostasis.[6]

Nursing Management of the Medical Client

The goal of nursing management is promotion of a healthy, positive adaptation in the client with OA. Education is the key to successful treatment of the disease, and the nurse plays a major role as a client educator. Clients and their families need accurate information about the disease and about strategies to minimize its impact. Effective education can alter behavior, empowering clients to make a positive change in their health status. Important areas in client education include (1) pain management, (2) rest-activity balance, (3) nutrition and weight loss, and (4) self-care strategies.

Teaching clients about their medications is an important part of the nurse's role in successful long-term pain management. For example, a client who is taking an NSAID must be informed of the manifestations of gastrointestinal bleeding, such as abdominal pain, tarry stools, and hematemesis. Reinforce the client's need to notify the physician immediately if these manifestations occur. Also encourage the client to keep a pain journal to help focus on manifestations and identify cues that signal the need for rest or activity. Suggest nonpharmacologic pain management strategies (e.g., relaxation techniques, guided imagery) to decrease the feelings of anxiety or powerlessness that accompany disease progression.

Other modalities, such as heat or cold, can also be considered to reduce pain.

The client who chooses to use dietary supplements also needs information about known risks and benefits as well as any interactions with established therapies. Although supplements may have a place in arthritis management, the client must understand the implications of delaying medical care or choosing unproven remedies rather than proven treatments.

To assist with self-care deficiencies related to OA, collaborate with an occupational therapist in providing assistive devices to help the client maintain independence with dressing and hygiene. Self-fastening tape (Velcro) closures, zipper pulls, or elastic shoelaces can make dressing easier. Long-handled combs or thick-barreled toothbrushes can also help clients with basic self-care tasks. The client with OA can learn to maintain affected joints in a neutral position at rest to avoid flexion contractures that will affect functional ability.

Also recognize the possible influence of OA on the client's sexual role functioning. Pain and stiffness, along with limited ROM, can create problems with sexual expression. Joint deformities can also negatively affect self-image, leading to reduced libido and depression. Inform the client about alternative sexual positions (e.g., side-by-side) that promote comfort during intercourse, and encourage the client to use analgesics or to take warm baths to alleviate pain and stiffness before sexual activity.

Surgical Management of Hip Osteoarthritis

Osteotomy

Osteotomy is a cut across a bone with resection of a bone fragment either to correct a deformity or to alter stresses on a joint. In early hip OA, when joint congruency still exists and motion is relatively normal, proximal femoral osteotomy may be performed. A wedge of bone is removed from the region of the lesser trochanter to realign the angle of the femoral neck and shaft. Partial weight-bearing is required for at least 3 months after surgery to allow healing of the osteotomy site. Because manifestations of OA generally progress despite this procedure, a large number of clients will require additional surgery. Osteotomy is more frequently performed on clients in their 40s, particularly those with an abnormally shallow acetabulum, with the full expectation that total joint replacement will be needed in the next 10 to 20 years.[4]

Arthrodesis

In an arthrodesis (joint fusion) procedure, the articular joint surfaces, which hold the bone ends together, are removed so that the bone edges unite like a fracture.

Initial fixation may be provided with pins, braces, or casts. Arthrodesis is indicated for irreparable joint damage or instability. The procedure produces a sound, painless limb, but the resulting loss of movement may be a serious disadvantage in large joints such as the hip.

Hip arthrodesis remains the operation of choice for the active client less than 55 years of age with advanced unilateral OA, severe post-traumatic arthritis, or septic arthritis. Hip fusion can result in shortening of the affected extremity by 1 to 1.5 inches, and the client commonly needs a shoe lift postoperatively to help maintain a normal gait. Low back pain and pain in the opposite knee often develop due to an altered gait.

Total Hip Arthroplasty (Replacement)

Total hip arthroplasty (THA) or replacement (THR) is performed to restore joint motion by replacing arthritic bone with metal and plastic components. (See Chapter 77 for a discussion of shoulder, elbow, and hand arthroplasty.)

Indications. Indications for THA include (1) failure of conservative treatments, (2) severe compromise of the client's functional ability, and (3) significant pain. The client's subjective complaints frequently have a greater impact on the decision for surgery than do radiologic changes of the joint. THA may also be performed for complications of femoral neck fractures, congenital disease or deformity, and failure of previous fixations or arthroplasties.

Both *cemented* and *noncemented* hip arthroplasties can be performed. Use of polymethyl methacrylate (PMMA) bone cement allows immediate intraoperative fixation of femoral and acetabular components. Cemented prostheses are used for older clients or for those with compromised bone strength resulting from conditions such as osteoporosis. In younger, active, or heavier clients, loosening of the component at the bone-cement interface may become a problem. For these clients, use of prostheses with porous surfaces allows fixation without cement. Instead, bone grows into the porous surface as the client remains on limited weight-bearing status for a number of weeks after surgery. Although short-term outcomes of the two procedures are equivalent, long-term results must be determined to justify the cost of noncemented surgical technology. Many hospitals and orthopedic surgeons currently use a "demand matching" system to choose appropriately between cemented or noncemented components based on client needs.

Contraindications. Contraindications to THA include (1) recent or active joint sepsis (except in joint revision as a result of infection), (2) neurotrophic joints, or (3) an inability to cooperate with immediate postoperative requirements or long-term joint rehabilitation. In addition, the client's general health must allow tolerance of anesthesia, blood loss, and surgical stress. Heart, lung, liver, and metabolic disorders should be stable before surgery.

Surgical Techniques. A common prosthesis currently in use is a three-component set: (1) the femoral neck and stem, (2) a slide-on femoral head, and (3) a metal acetabulum with or without fixation screw holes. Hip prostheses may be made of several different metal alloys that contribute to the relative lightness and durability of the components (Figure 26-3).

Depending on surgeon's preference and on the type of exposure needed for the procedure, the surgical approach may be (1) anterolateral, (2) direct lateral, (3) transtrochanteric, or (4) posterolateral. The nurse must know the surgical approach to understand the leg position used to dislocate the operative hip. If that position is replicated after surgery, the client's risk for dislocating the hip prosthesis increases.

With an *anterolateral* position, the client lies supine on the table. The operative hip is externally rotated and extended, and the knee is flexed. With the *posterolateral* position, the client lies on his or her side with the operative hip internally rotated, flexed, and adducted. Many orthopedic surgeons use the posterolateral position for the anterior and posterior approaches.

Once the hip has been exposed, the surgeon performs an osteotomy of the femoral neck to expose the acetabulum. Osteophytes and cysts are removed from the acetabulum to prepare it for reaming and for the

prosthesis. Trial prostheses are placed, and their fit is evaluated before the final choice of appropriately sized components. If the prosthesis is to be *press-fit (noncemented),* the bone is prepared for pegs or spikes. The surgeon presses the cup firmly into place and evaluates its apposition to the bone. If a *cemented* prosthesis is used, anchor holes are drilled into the iliac subchondral bone. After cleaning the bone thoroughly with pressure-pulsed lavage, the surgeon cements the cup into position.

To prepare the femur, the surgeon forms a tunnel by reaming the bone's intramedullary canal. After placement of a trial prosthesis, the hip is reduced to assess for motion, stability, and length. If the results are acceptable, the surgeon removes the trial components. For a press-fit prosthesis, the femoral stem is pressed into the reamed intramedullary canal. For a cemented prosthesis, the femur is cleaned and the canal is plugged to prevent the cement from traveling too far distally. The surgeon fills the canal with cement, inserting the femoral stem and then placing the femoral head. After the hip is reduced, the surgeon evaluates the extremity for motion, stability, and length.

Before closing the incision (approximately 10 inches long), the surgeon may place a closed wound drainage system, such as a Hemovac, which may help prevent hematoma. The use of wound drainage systems has decreased in recent years, however, because they have been found to be ineffective in preventing hematomas while possibly increasing the risk of blood loss and contamination of the surgical wound. Instead, wound drainage may be collected for a limited time through a cell-saving device or a suctioned autotransfusion device. The collected blood is returned to the client as a postoperative transfusion, and then the device is discontinued.

A recent trend in THA is to perform the surgery through much smaller incisions. This procedure allows the client to ambulate more quickly with less pain and to be discharged earlier. Candidates for minimally invasive THA are typically thinner, younger, in better health, and more motivated to pursue quick recovery.[4] Risks and benefits of minimally invasive THA have not been documented sufficiently to demonstrate improvement over traditional surgery.

Complications. The in-hospital mortality after THA is very low. Many of the postoperative complications are short-lived and reversible, but some of them can have a great impact on the client's physical and psychological recovery from surgery. The most common and most serious complication is venous thromboembolism, which can occur in as many as 57% of clients if anticoagulant therapy is not administered.[18] Prevention of deep vein thrombosis (DVT) or pulmonary embolism (PE) requires early mobilization, often with a combination of

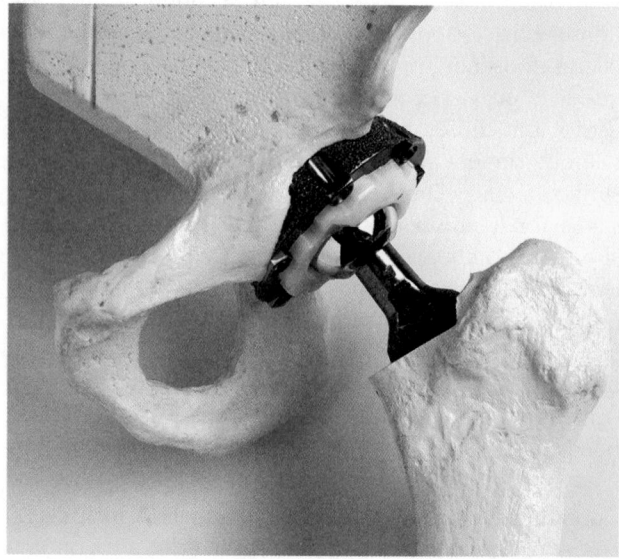

■ **FIGURE 26-3** Hip prosthesis.

pharmacologic and nonpharmacologic methods (see also Chapter 53).

🔖 **Infection following a THA is a serious concern because of the possible development of osteomyelitis. Prophylactic antibiotics are considered essential, and careful wound assessment must begin immediately after surgery. Bladder or urinary tract infection is also possible because of urinary stasis or the presence of an indwelling urinary catheter. Because any localized infection can also spread to the wound, prompt recognition and treatment of clinical manifestations are imperative.**

Postoperative joint instability increases the risk for dislocation or subluxation. The risk is even greater after revision arthroplasty because of the extended surgical exposure and soft tissue deficiencies.

All clients require monitoring and education about the positions that should be avoided while soft tissues heal around the new joint. Positioning precautions are continued for up to 3 months, until the surgical incision has healed and the client's periarticular muscle tone has improved.

🔖 After surgery with the commonly used posterolateral approach, the client must avoid positions of extreme hip flexion (>90 degrees), adduction, or internal rotation. Appropriate postoperative positioning requires an extended hip that is maintained in external rotation and abduction, often by using a foam wedge. An anterolateral approach is used less often. The client must maintain the hip in hyperflexion, adduction, and internal rotation. After this surgical approach, the client can sit up at 90 degrees of hip flexion without increasing the risk of dislocation.

Outcomes. A THA commonly results in immediate reduction of the client's pain. Surgical or incisional pain is often described as substantially less than the "bone-on-bone" pain of OA, and it is frequently more manageable with postoperative analgesia. The client's functional status improves over the course of rehabilitation and usually reaches its optimal level by 1 year after surgery. With the current emphasis on wellness, an increased number of clients now desire to resume sports activities after hip surgery. High activity levels are associated with decreased longevity for replacement components; however, low-impact activities, such as walking or hiking, swimming, bicycling, intermediate snow skiing, doubles tennis, golf, and bowling, are considered fairly safe for client participation and contribute greatly to improved quality of life after surgery.

Revision surgery may be a future consideration because of prosthetic loosening or other complications such as fracture of the femoral shaft, repeated dislocation, osteolysis, or heterotrophic bone formation.

Because of improved techniques for cement insertion and the increased use of press-fit prostheses, loosening now occurs less commonly following THA.

Nursing Management of the Surgical Client: Total Hip Arthroplasty

In the current managed care environment, clients who have undergone THA typically do not remain in the acute care hospital setting for more than 4 or 5 days after a THA. They may be discharged to a rehabilitation unit, extended care facility, or even home. Although there is no universally accepted rehabilitation program after THA, coordination of care in the perioperative period speeds the client's recovery and return to independent living.

Preoperative Care

Assessment. Because most clients are admitted to the hospital on the day of surgery, the preadmission assessment of their physical and psychological readiness is currently accomplished in a variety of ways. Telephone interviews may be used, but many hospitals invite clients into a preoperative clinic for nursing assessment and for laboratory tests or x-rays. Some programs also arrange home visits to allow a physical therapist or nurse to assess the client's ambulation and the safety of the home. Discharge needs can often be identified based on the home environment and the extent of support available to the client.

Diagnosis, Outcomes, Interventions
Diagnosis: Deficient Knowledge. The client's previous inexperience with hospitalization and surgery in general, or with THA and its postoperative restrictions, may be described with the nursing diagnosis of *Deficient Knowledge*. The diagnosis can be written *Deficient Knowledge related to prior inexperience with surgery (total hip replacement)*.

Outcomes. The client will demonstrate understanding of the proposed surgery, postoperative restrictions, and rehabilitation as evidenced by statements and adherence to the postoperative regimen.

Interventions. A common strategy for providing information about the details of hospitalization for THA is the use of a group class or "total joint camp." Clients receive information about various topics, from preoperative strengthening exercises and nothing by mouth (NPO) requirements to postoperative pain management and dietary advances. Topics may include autologous blood donation and other transfusion options. Clients also often have the opportunity to use a walker or crutches for the first time as they are coached by a nurse or physical therapist. Instructors emphasize appropriate positioning precautions to prevent postoperative hip dislocation.

Because poor dentition is also a potential infection source, the client should be encouraged preoperatively to achieve and maintain good oral hygiene.

Evaluation. Clients will provide a simple explanation of the surgery and verbalize their role in recovery. Mild anxiety may heighten the client's receptiveness to information, but severe anxiety can be a powerful barrier to learning. Provide frequent reinforcement of teaching, and encourage the client to ask questions about unclear information.

Postoperative Care

General care of clients after THA does not differ greatly from the usual care provided for any postoperative client. (For a review of general postoperative care, see Chapter 14.) After a THA, however, the client cannot assist with turning or repositioning. Prop up the client with pillows to maintain a side-lying position, and then return the client to a supine position on a 2-hour schedule. Do not turn the client to the operative side unless ordered by the physician. Because of the client's impaired mobility, pay careful attention to maintenance of skin integrity. A pressure-redistribution mattress overlay may be indicated, especially if the client is frail or malnourished. Heels should be floated off the bed to decrease risk of pressure ulcer development.

Indwelling urinary catheters are not routinely used because of the risk of infection, but women are still likely to have a catheter because of the difficulty of positioning on a bedpan or transferring to a bedside commode in the immediate postoperative period. Perform perineal and catheter care carefully, recognizing the client's surgical pain and positioning precautions. Men will often need assistance to sit or stand at the bedside to void.

Assessment. Frequent assessment of neurovascular status is imperative after a THA. Assess both legs for color, warmth, capillary refill, pedal pulses, movement, and sensation. Compare the surgical leg with the unaffected lower extremity. Report any deficits promptly to the surgeon. Ensure that the client's postoperative position is maintained in accordance with specified hip precautions.

The surgical dressing applied at the end of the procedure, used to create pressure and promote hemostasis, is often bulky. It is left in place until removed by the surgeon or with a surgeon's specific order, usually 1 to 3 days after surgery. It should be regularly assessed for excessive drainage, however, and may be reinforced according to the surgeon's preference. After removal of the original dressing, the wound is covered with a light dressing or left open to air as ordered by the surgeon.

Incisions left open to air do need to be covered [?] showering; use a transparent occlusive dressing. Aft[?] ward, carefully examine the wound to be certain t[?] no water has seeped through the dressing becau[?] excessive wetness can interfere with wound healing.

In addition, a closed wound drainage system, such [?] a Hemovac, may be in place. Drainage is usually l[?] than 200 ml/8 hour (or 600 ml/24 hour), but this amou[?] can be increased if the client has been heavily hydrate[?] Measure drain output, and promptly report excessi[?] drainage to the surgeon. If a cell-saver or autotransfusi[?] device has been used, postoperative transfusion will [?] accomplished in accordance with hospital and surge[?] protocols.

Diagnosis, Outcomes, Interventions

Diagnosis: Acute Pain and Chronic Pain. Acute pain [?] expected after any surgery, including THA. The diagn[?] sis can be written as *Acute Pain and Chronic Pa[?] related to local tissue trauma from surgical incision.*

Outcomes. The client will demonstrate comfort as e[?] denced by reporting a tolerable level of pain, usi[?] decreasing amounts of analgesia, being able to mo[?] without grimacing, and stating that the pain is not inte[?] fering with rest or physical therapy.

Interventions. In the immediate postoperative peri[?] the client may experience intense pain and may requi[?] injected opioid analgesics to attain acceptable contr[?] Common interventions include patient-controlled an[?] gesia (PCA) or epidural analgesia. Within 24 to 48 hou[?] the client should be tolerating fluids and able to take o[?] analgesics. Because pain is intensified with moveme[?] the client may attempt to limit activity because of t[?] expected increase in discomfort. Medicate the clie[?] before physical therapy or activities such as showerin[?] and reinforce the importance of ambulation in decrea[?] ing risk for postoperative complications. Although TH[?] can reduce pain in the operative joint, the client wi[?] arthritis in other joints continues to experience chron[?] pain. Once postoperative hemostasis has been achieve[?] the client's usual NSAID may be ordered to addre[?] chronic pain in nonsurgical joints.

Regularly assess for side effects of opioid analgesic[?] Respiratory depression is more likely with PCA or epid[?] ral analgesia than with oral opioids. Use pulse oximet[?] and regular measurement of vital signs to assess the c[?] ent's respiratory status. Constipation, a common prol[?] lem after THA, is related to the client's impaire[?] mobility, opioid use, and progression to a regular die[?] Encourage the client's intake of fluids and dietary fibe[?] In addition, laxatives may be indicated. If the client re[?] ularly uses a bulk-forming laxative or other strategy [?] maintain bowel regularity at home, assist the client [?] continuing that program in the hospital. Stool softene[?] are frequently prescribed; however, they do not actua[?]

aid in elimination of the stool because they are not laxatives. Regular assessment and implementation of a proactive bowel program are important to minimize client concerns about bowel elimination. Interventions should ensure that the client has had a bowel movement before discharge from the acute hospital setting.

Diagnosis: Impaired Physical Mobility. The client's degree of immobility after a THA will be affected by pain and fear of movement as well as by arthritic limitations in other joints. The diagnosis can be written as *Impaired Physical Mobility related to pain or fear of movement.*

Outcomes. The client will demonstrate improved physical mobility as evidenced by the need for less assistance in transfers (bed to chair, bed to standing), by safe use of a walker or crutches, and by the ability to ambulate a functional distance (150 feet).

Interventions. Moving the client after a THA can create much anxiety for both the client and the nursing staff. First, be aware of any weight-bearing limitations ordered for the client before transfer. Following a THA with a cemented prosthesis, the client is often allowed to put as much weight as desired on the operative extremity. This order is written as WBAT (weight-bearing as tolerated) or FWB (full weight-bearing). Although incisional pain may keep the client from putting full body weight on the operative extremity, he or she can safely put weight through the leg without harming the prosthesis. If the surgery was accomplished with a noncemented prosthesis, the physician may order NWB (non–weight-bearing), TTWB (toe-touch weight-bearing), or PWB (partial weight-bearing with a percentage specified, e.g., 25%). If the client is not allowed to bear full weight, pay careful attention to the operative extremity during transfers to ensure that the client avoids placing any weight on the leg.

In addition to postoperative limitations, the client may suffer from arthritis in other joints that increases pain and affects the ability to transfer from the bed to the chair. While in-bed exercises may begin the day of surgery, the client is not usually ready to attempt transfer to a bedside chair until the morning after surgery. When the client stands and transfers for the first time, the assistance of at least two staff members will be required. Use of appropriate technique will ensure a safe transfer for the client and will minimize the risk of injury to the staff member's lower back.

Transferring the Client

All intravenous (IV) lines, urinary catheters, wound drains, and oxygen tubing should be freed for ready movement. Although typically you will determine the side of the bed for transfer, the client usually moves away from the operative side. If the bedside chair has brakes, they should be locked before client transfer is made. The client should also be wearing shoes or slippers with non-skid soles. Staff should assist the client to the edge of the bed, maintaining the operative leg position in accordance with appropriate hip precautions. Encourage the client to push off the bed with his or her arms to reach a sitting position; however, because of weakness in the hip abductors and upper arms, the client may need help to pivot in bed and to sit up.

Once the client is seated at the edge of the bed, apply a gait belt to the client's waist to help with transfer. Use of the gait belt allows you to help with standing and transfer without risking injury to yourself. If the client becomes dizzy or starts to fall, the gait belt also helps you to control the client's movement to the floor or back onto the bed. Place the walker directly in front of the client, ready for use once he or she is standing; however, do not use it to help the client to a standing position because it is not stable.

To help the client to stand, first position your foot in front of the client's foot to keep it from slipping on the floor. Standing close to the client, grasp the gait belt and encourage the client to push off the bed with his or her hands. Once the client is standing, he or she can grasp the walker and pause for a moment to take slow, deep breaths as needed.

Remain aware of the risk for falling, and ask the client about dizziness—a manifestation of orthostatic hypotension—before attempting the final transfer to the chair. To help increase awareness of surroundings, encourage the client to stand erect when using the walker rather than stooping over and looking at the floor. With coaching about weight-bearing status, the client should need no more than a few pivoting movements with the walker to reach the chair. Remind the client not to attempt to sit until he or she can feel the chair seat against the back of his or her legs. Then the client should reach back to grasp the arms of the chair and lower himself or herself slowly to a sitting position. You can assist the client by grasping the gait belt and guiding descent into the chair. Pay close attention to maintaining flexion restrictions. For example, keeping the client's operative leg in a relaxed position, with the knee slightly lower than the hip, allows maintenance of precautions regarding hip flexion related to a posterolateral surgical approach. The gait belt can be loosened after the client is safely settled in the chair.

When the client is ready to return to the bed, coach him or her to slide forward to the edge of the chair, and tighten the gait belt around the client's waist. Again, remind the client to keep the knee slightly lower than the operative hip as a positioning precaution. With the walker in position in front of the chair, the client uses the arms of the chair to push to a standing position before grasping the walker. Using the same ambulation process, return the client to bed and help the client to a supine position. Maintain leg position according to individual hip precautions.

Use appropriately sized equipment for clients who are obese. These devices are designed to move client's safely with less chance of injury for the nursing staff. Monitor the position of the legs when slings are used; adduction of the operative leg must be avoided.

Introduce Additional Client Exercises

If the client is alert postoperatively, in-bed exercises are often begun the afternoon of surgery. Coach the client in the use of ankle pumps and quadriceps and gluteal isometrics ("quad sets" or "glute sets"). Transfers and ambulation with a physical therapist generally begin the morning after surgery. In addition, the therapist may perform gentle active and assisted ROM exercises. The client will continue exercises that improve ROM and strengthen hip muscles, occasionally receiving physical therapy at home or on an outpatient basis after discharge from the acute hospital setting.

Because of its stability, a walker is often used by older clients to assist with ambulation. If the client has arthritis in the shoulders or hands, a special walker with arm platforms may be indicated. Walkers also necessitate less energy expenditure for the client who has respiratory disease. Crutches may be used if the client has no balance problems.

Diagnosis, Outcomes, Interventions

Diagnosis: Risk for Peripheral Neurovascular Dysfunction. Surgery on any joint carries a risk for neurologic or vascular impairment. Be aware of the potential for compartment syndrome and nerve injury related to edema or extremity positioning that places pressure on the peroneal nerve. The diagnosis can be written as *Risk for Peripheral Neurovascular Dysfunction related to lower extremity edema or positioning.*

Outcomes. The client will demonstrate normal neurovascular status as evidenced by adequate peripheral pulses with capillary refill time of 3 seconds or less and by the absence of sensory impairments and motor weakness in the operative extremity.

Interventions. Assess the neurovascular status of the operative extremity at least every 4 hours or as directed by the surgeon. More frequent monitoring may be indicated by the client's condition. Assess the presence and quality of bilateral pedal pulses, skin color and temperature of the extremities, capillary refill in the toes, sensation and movement of the toes, and the client's ability to perform dorsiplantar flexion of the feet. As part of your assessment of motor function, flex and extend the client's toes yourself. If the client feels more pain from passive stretch than active motion, you should be suspicious of compartment syndrome. Compare current assessments to baseline data. Report any new pallor or coolness, numbness or tingling, or inability to move the extremity promptly to the surgeon.

Diagnosis: Risk for Injury. Because the hip is unstable as the surgical incision heals, the risk for dislocation of the prosthesis is a significant concern after a THA. Client education and attention to hip positioning precautions are essential. The diagnosis can be written as *Risk for Injury related to prosthesis dislocation.*

Outcomes. The client will have reduced risk of injury (hip dislocation), as evidenced by verbalization of the risk for hip dislocation, and verbalizing and following positioning precautions while on bed rest and during ambulation or transfers.

Interventions. After a THA, assess the client's position frequently to ensure that precautions related to the specific surgical approach are maintained. Remind the client of appropriate precautions through the use of instructional handouts or fliers that can be posted at the head of the bed. Performance of prescribed exercises, such as gluteal isometrics, also strengthens muscles surrounding the joint capsule and decreases the risk for dislocation.

If the surgeon has used a posterolateral approach, the client should not flex the hip beyond a 90-degree angle, should not bend over to tie or slip on shoes, and should not reach for sheets that are fan-folded at the bottom of the bed. Special attention should be given to precautions when the client is getting in and out of bed or a chair. To avoid extremes of flexion, the client will need an elevated toilet seat (at least 21 inches high). The client should not cross his or her legs and should not inwardly rotate the operative leg.

To help maintain precautions after the posterolateral approach, the client may use a triangular foam abduction pillow placed between the legs and secured with straps (Figure 26-4). Use of the pillow prevents adduction and flexion of the operative hip; however, you must carefully position the straps to avoid placing pressure on the client's peroneal nerve. Instead of an abduction pillow, some surgeons order a knee immobilizer to be worn on the surgical leg. It serves primarily as a reminder to the client of mobility restrictions for that extremity. When using a walker, the client should be coached to point toes outward slightly. This position avoids internal rotation, particularly when the client is turning toward the operative side. Hip precautions must also be followed when the client is turned from back to side. The abductor pillow is left in place, and the client's side-lying position is maintained through the use of pillows at the client's back. Special precautions are needed to prevent the heel from developing a pressure ulcer. Be certain that the heels are free from pressure when the abductor pillow is attached to the legs.

If the surgeon has used an anterolateral approach, precautions are almost the opposite of those for the posterolateral approach. Because the client should avoid active abduction, the legs should be maintained side by side

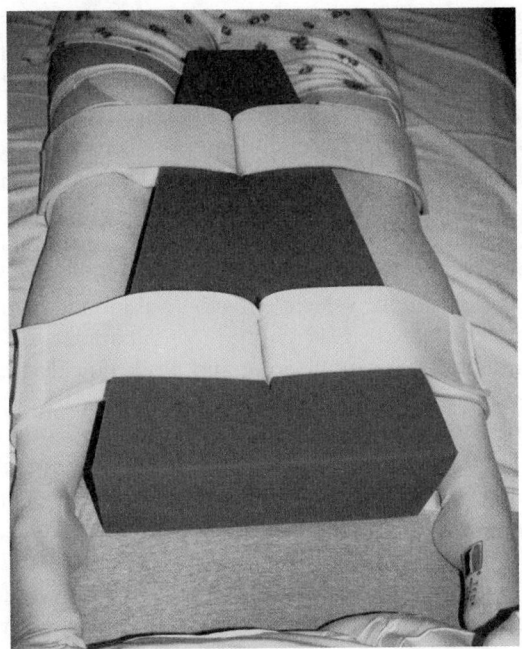

■ **FIGURE 26–4** Abduction wedge is used to prevent hip adduction and flexion after a total hip arthroplasty using a posterior surgical approach.

without a pillow or wedge between them. When walking, the client should avoid turning the toes and knee outward. The operative leg should not be extended backward. To help maintain anterolateral precautions, place the tray table and phone on the client's operative side.

To help the client maintain appropriate hip precautions, an occupational therapist may suggest several assistive devices. Long-handled shoe horns, sock donners, and reachers help the client avoid extreme hip flexion and provide more independence in dressing. The therapist or case manager can also assist the client in acquiring bathroom equipment, such as an elevated toilet seat and shower chair, for use after discharge. Reinforce the importance of using these devices to decrease the risk of hip dislocation.

Diagnosis: Risk for Infection

After a THA, the client is at increased risk for joint infection that may lead to the development of osteomyelitis. Although the incidence of infection is low, it is a great concern as a factor in possible surgical failure, leading to removal of the prosthetic components. Joint replacements that are close to the skin surface or that have limited soft tissue coverage, as in a thin client, are at increased risk for infection. *Revision* THR carries an increased infection rate compared with *primary* THR because of the longer operative time and the larger surgical exposure.

The diagnosis can be written as *Risk for Infection related to alteration in primary defenses, surgical*

incision, and implantation of foreign materials (total hip replacement).

Outcomes. The client will have reduced risk of wound infection as evidenced by normal temperature and white blood cell (WBC) count, the absence of purulent drainage from the wound, and the absence of redness or inflammation at the surgical site.

🪔 Interventions

Prophylactic IV antibiotics are routinely ordered immediately before surgery because of the risk of infection following a THA. The first dose is typically given within 60 minutes before the surgical incision is made, and antibiotics are continued for 24 hours postoperatively.[8] If surgical drains are used to remove wound exudate, they should be emptied at least once each shift using aseptic technique. Because the drainage can harbor pathogens, note its color and odor and promptly report any abnormalities to the surgeon. Also routinely assess the surgical site for redness or purulent drainage. Use of staples is associated with a lower infection rate, but delays in wound healing can suggest superficial infection. Perform dressing changes using strict aseptic technique. Take the client's temperature at regular intervals, and perform careful assessments to determine the cause of any fever.

Increasing joint pain after superficial wound healing is also a possible manifestation of delayed deep infection. Instruct the client to report this manifestation promptly to the physician and to inform other health care providers of the surgery.

SAFETY ALERT

Diagnosis: Risk for Impaired Skin Integrity. After a THA, the client is at high risk for pressure ulcers as a result of decreased physical mobility. Clients are often unable to change positions in bed without a great deal of assistance. Clients are also at risk for tape injury with dressing changes. This risk is due to (1) skin changes that occur in older adults, (2) intraoperative positioning and joint manipulation that lead to soft tissue edema, (3) the type of tape used to secure postoperative dressings, and (4) the method and direction of tape application. The diagnosis can be written as *Risk for Impaired Skin Integrity related to decreased physical mobility or to the application of tape with dressing changes.*

Outcomes. The client will demonstrate intact skin as evidenced by an absence of ulcers over bony prominences and an absence of epidermal stripping beneath the tape used to secure postoperative dressings.

Interventions. To decrease the risk of pressure ulcer development, assist the THA client with position changes on a regular schedule in the immediate postoperative period. As the client regains mobility, he or she will also regain independence in position changes. Carefully assess the skin over bony prominences such as the sacrum and coccyx, scapulae, elbows, and heels. To assess the skin on the heels and feet, any anti-embolism devices will have to be removed. In addition to using a regular turning schedule, assess the need for a pressure-redistribution mattress on the client's bed. Pressure on heels can be relieved, depending on surgeon preference, by using a towel roll for brief periods under the Achilles tendon or by elevating the calf on a thin pillow.

Avoid epidermal stripping by placing postoperative dressings over a skin sealant that is applied wherever the tape touches the skin. Elastic tape should be placed vertically (superior to inferior) without tension to allow for stretching related to postoperative edema. Evaluate any redness, blistering, or epidermal stripping, and consult an enterostomal nurse specialist about the client's care as appropriate.

Collaborative Problem: Risk for Deep Vein Thrombosis. Venous thromboembolism, the most common complication after a THA, can be manifested as DVT. Risk factors include a surgical procedure longer than 30 minutes, advanced client age, previous history of thromboembolism, venous stasis, cardiac conditions such as heart failure or dysrhythmias, lower extremity trauma, obesity, use of oral contraceptives or hormone replacement, sepsis, malignancy, long-term immobilization, stroke, and pregnancy. Clots may form in the calf and travel to the popliteal fossa or the thigh. This collaborative problem can be written as *Risk for Deep Vein Thrombosis related to surgical procedure and immobility* (or other identified risk factors).

Outcomes. The nurse will monitor for the early manifestations of DVT: unilateral calf or thigh pain, redness, or edema.

Interventions. Routinely assess the client for evidence of thrombophlebitis: excessive pain, unilateral edema, or a red vein track. Homans' sign is a more nonspecific indicator. The client may have thrombophlebitis but have a negative Homans' sign. Conversely, a positive Homans' sign can result from other conditions, such as shin splints. Many clients have asymptomatic blood clots.

To decrease the risk of DVT, various pharmacologic and nonpharmacologic interventions are used. Early mobilization is a key factor in decreasing DVT risk. Encourage the client to perform ankle pumps regularly because they contract the calf muscles, simulating the movements of ambulation and encouraging venous blood return to the heart. Physical agents such as pneumatic compression devices and elastic compression stockings are commonly used; these modalities may be used individually or together, and they should be applied to both legs to promote adequate venous return (see Chapter 53). Compression devices or stockings should be worn until the client is fully ambulatory and should be removed only for brief periods for bathing and skin assessment. The pneumatic devices should be applied even when the client is sitting in a chair at the bedside because the dependent position of the lower extremities can contribute to increased venous stasis.

Pharmacologic agents used to decrease the risk of DVT include low-dose unfractionated heparin (UFH), low-molecular-weight heparin (LMWH), warfarin sodium, and the synthetic selective factor Xa inhibitor fondaparinux (Arixtra). LMWH and fondaparinux do not require laboratory monitoring and work quickly to produce anticoagulation. Effects of unfractionated heparin will be monitored with the partial thromboplastin time (PTT). Warfarin is slower to reach therapeutic blood levels but is less expensive and easier for the client to take after discharge. A prothrombin time (PT), with results reported as an International Normalized Ratio (INR), is ordered to monitor the effects of warfarin. Promptly report laboratory results to the surgeon to allow timely ordering of the current day's dose.

In addition, the client who receives UFH or LMWH must be monitored for occurrence of heparin-induced thrombocytopenia (HIT). HIT usually develops after a client has received heparin or LMWH for 5 or more days, but may appear sooner if the client has previous heparin exposure. Heparin-dependent antibodies develop and thrombocytopenia results. HIT is diagnosed by a platelet count <150,000/mm^3 or a drop in platelets of ≥50% from baseline, with no other identified cause of thrombocytopenia. Thromboembolic complications of HIT may include DVT, pulmonary embolism (PE), myocardial infarction or cerebrovascular accident, occlusion of limb arteries (possibly requiring amputation), end-organ damage, or death. If HIT is diagnosed, any form of heparin must be immediately discontinued. The synthetic direct thrombin inhibitor argatroban is then typically prescribed for both prophylaxis and treatment of thrombosis in clients with HIT.[13] Further, LMWH cannot be given to clients with epidural catheters in place for pain control because of the risk of epidural hematoma.

Extensive education about anticoagulants is essential to maximize their effectiveness and to minimize the likelihood of complications. Inform the client of manifestations of internal bleeding, such as tarry stools, rust-colored or tea-colored urine, hematemesis, and abdominal or flank pain. Explain that even a minor cut will bleed for a longer time. Instruct the client to apply direct pressure, for example, following a shaving cut or a cut with a kitchen knife. Urge clients to seek immediate evaluation for any head injury because significant intracranial bleeding can occur in response to even minor trauma if an anticoagulant is being taken. If the client is to take warfarin, reinforce the importance of consistent intake of foods that contain vitamin K (e.g., green, leafy vegetables). Many of these foods are nutritionally important and should not be totally avoided, particularly by clients with a history of heart disease who follow a low-fat diet. If the client will be discharged with a prescription for LMWH, start instruction on injection technique early enough in the hospital to allow ample time for practice and reinforcement.

If you suspect a blood clot, notify the surgeon immediately. Venography or Doppler ultrasound of the leg is commonly used in the diagnosis of DVT. If the test reveals the presence of a clot, the client will be allowed minimal activity for several days (e.g., walking to bathroom) with the leg elevated to promote venous return; heat may be applied locally.[22] A continuous infusion of UFH or subcutaneous administration of LMWH will be initiated immediately. Warfarin is often begun simultaneously, and a warfarin prescription is written for long-term home use to prevent clot recurrence. The surgeon may order calf measurements to aid in the detection of increased swelling related to DVT.

Because of the risk of pulmonary embolism, you must frequently assess the client's respiratory status. A clot in the leg can dislodge and move to the lung, typically causing dyspnea, anxiety, and a pleuritic chest pain. Because pulmonary embolism is often fatal, address suspicious manifestations immediately.

Evaluation. Goals should be mutually established by the client and an interdisciplinary care team that includes a surgeon, a nurse, physical and occupational therapists, and a case manager. A list of goals can be posted in the client's hospital room as a reminder of the focus for each postoperative day. Clinical pathways are commonly used to map the care of clients after a THA because of the consistent postoperative needs of this population. Pathways help providers limit the number of tasks, such as laboratory orders, that may be forgotten or overlooked. Outcomes are often also indicated on the clinical pathway to track client progress consistently. Pathways often extend from admission through acute care to client rehabilitation in another setting. They also allow for later review of discrepancies or "outliers," that is, those clients whose experiences do not conform to the usual postoperative course. See the Clinical Pathway feature on Total Hip Replacement on the website.

Self-Care

The typical acute hospital stay after THA is 4 to 5 days. Because many clients require additional rehabilitation, they are sent from the hospital to rehabilitation centers or skilled nursing facilities until they regain functional independence. Clients can be discharged home if they can transfer independently to and from the bed, walk alone a functional distance of 150 feet on a flat surface, and safely negotiate stairs.

Provide discharge instructions to the client and any family members or friends who will serve as support people during the recovery period. The client must understand the hip precautions indicated by the surgical approach (anterolateral or posterolateral) to avoid dislocation. Precautions may continue for 3 months or longer after surgery, depending on the surgeon's assessment of soft tissue healing around the joint capsule.

Assistive devices, such as a walker or crutches and bathroom equipment, should be available for immediate use at home. The client will progress from walker to crutches or cane as muscle strength increases, perhaps within 4 to 6 weeks after surgery if a cemented prosthesis was used. Clients with a noncemented prosthesis may have limited weight-bearing (e.g., TTWB) for 6 weeks, followed by WBAT with the use of a crutch for another 6 weeks.

Clients frequently have questions about driving or returning to work. Clients with sedentary occupations may be cleared by the surgeon to drive and to return to work within 6 to 8 weeks. They may be counseled, however, to take regular breaks to avoid extended periods of sitting. It may be 3 months before a client can return to an occupation that requires lifting and bending, and activity will remain limited even after going back to work. Low-level physical activity, such as walking or swimming, is usually approved by the surgeon.

Depending on surgeon preference, the client may be allowed to shower after discharge.

Safety measures, such as a nonslip mat and handrails in the shower area, are important. The client should not soak in a tub because water can enter the incision, increasing the risk of infection. Getting in or out of a tub may also violate hip precautions. SAFETY ALERT

 The client can consume a regular diet but should also continue to be aware of any bowel elimination needs. Sexual activity typically can be resumed without discomfort as long as the client observes hip precautions.

The client should understand any medications, such as anticoagulants, that will be taken after discharge and should note follow-up laboratory and surgeon appointments. If the surgeon has ordered home care services or outpatient therapy, provide agency telephone numbers or locations for appointments. After a THA, prophylactic antibiotics are recommended whenever a transient bacteremia is expected, such as with dental work or a minor surgical procedure. The health care provider prescribes oral antibiotic coverage before the procedure.

In addition to bathroom safety features, the client may need other home modifications to aid independent recovery. Ramps, for example, may allow easier access to entrances. If the client lives in a multilevel home, encourage him or her to remain on a ground level until recovery is complete. SAFETY ALERT

Surgical Management of Knee Osteoarthritis

After the hip and the spine, the knee is the third most common site of arthritic involvement. The knee, an extremely complex joint, actually moves in three separate planes. Biomechanical stress during normal walking allows three times a person's body weight to be transmitted through the knee. Going up and down stairs increases the force to four or five times the body weight. The force is unevenly distributed, with the medial side of the knee often receiving the larger amount of stress. OA of the knee is better tolerated than OA of the hip, however, because the knee is not usually painful at rest.

Conservative treatment of OA of the knee is similar to that for the hip. Weight loss, activity modification, use of assistive devices, and use of analgesics or anti-inflammatory medications all help to decrease disease manifestations. Physical modalities such as ice or heat may also offer some pain reduction. Alternative therapies are also similar to those for OA of the hip.

Indications

If conservative interventions no longer control the client's manifestations, surgery may be appropriate. Options for OA management include (1) osteotomy, (2) arthrodesis, (3) unicompartmental knee arthroplasty (UKA), and (4) total knee arthroplasty (TKA). A tibial *osteotomy* may relieve the pain of knee OA by correcting the varus deformity (bow-leg) or valgus (knock-knee) deformity. Knee *arthrodesis* or fusion is indicated for young, active clients who are poor candidates for joint replacement surgery. Knee arthrodesis is often seen as a salvage procedure in response to conditions such as infection, malignant or aggressive tumors, painful Charcot's or neuropathic arthropathy, or severe ligamentous instability. Knee fusion results in shortening of the affected leg by about 0.5 inch, which usually does not create significant postoperative dysfunction; it creates an immobile joint fixed in extension. A recently introduced alternative to tibial osteotomy for the client with medial compartment osteoarthritis of the knee is the UniSpacer. For the client who has intact posterior and anterior cruciate ligaments and meets other clinical criteria, the UniSpacer can be inserted arthroscopically to restore normal knee alignment. An overnight hospital stay may be indicated, but recovery of motion is much quicker than with other invasive procedures.

Unicompartmental knee arthroplasty (UKA) is another alternative to osteotomy for clients who are 60 years or older, not obese, and relatively sedentary. Candidates for UKA must have an intact anterior cruciate ligament, no significant inflammation, and unicompartmental OA with no disease in other compartments of the knee. UKA was actually introduced more than 30 years ago

and until recently has been a controversial surgical alternative. More precise client selection, improved implant design, and better surgical techniques have led to higher initial success rate and fewer complications for UKA compared with osteotomy. The surgery results in less blood loss, and recovery is faster compared with osteotomy or TKA (Box 26-1).

Total knee arthroplasty (TKA), or replacement, allows resurfacing of the arthritic joint with the use of metal and polyethylene prosthetic components. The surgeon attempts to recreate the motions of flexion, extension, rotation, abduction, and adduction that may have been lost with progressive arthritis. TKA also relieves pain and corrects deformity.

Contraindications

Absolute contraindications to TKA include knee sepsis, a remote source of ongoing infection, extensor mechanism dysfunction, and severe vascular disease. Medical conditions that preclude safe anesthesia and the demands of rehabilitation are relative contraindications to surgery.[20] Conditions such as diabetes mellitus in

---

BOX 26-1 Arthroscopic Surgery Versus Placebo for Osteoarthritis of the Knee

A recent randomized, blinded, placebo-controlled trial with a 2-year follow-up was conducted. The setting of the study was a Veterans Affairs medical center in Houston, Texas. A total of 180 clients who were less than or equal to 75 years of age (mean age 52 years, 93% men) were included in this unique study; participating clients had been diagnosed with osteoarthritis of the knee as defined by the American College of Rheumatology, reported at least moderate knee pain despite maximal medical treatment for 6 or more months, and had not received arthroscopy in the previous 2 years. Clients were allocated to 1 of 3 groups: lavage (n = 61), debridement (n = 59), or placebo (n = 60). The placebo group received three 1-cm skin incisions after first taking a short-acting tranquilizer and an opioid and while spontaneously breathing oxygen-enriched air.

Interestingly, lavage and debridement groups did not differ from the placebo group with regard to pain in the study knee at 1 or 2 years or for any secondary outcome measure. Thus in clients with osteoarthritis of the knee, arthroscopic surgery did not relieve pain or improve function more than a placebo procedure. It should be noted that 44% of the eligible participants declined to participate, which raises the possibility of selection bias. The authors noted that, compared with those who declined, participants were younger, more likely to be Caucasian, and had more severe arthritis. It would have been valuable to observe follow-up data on those who declined to be randomized but who subsequently had either debridement or lavage. Regardless, this investigation does question the value of arthroscopic lavage and debridement in active men younger than 65 years of age with osteoarthritis of the knee.

Data from Moseley, J., et al. (2002). A controlled trial of arthroscopic surgery of the knee. *New England Journal of Medicine, 347,* 81–88.

particular increase the client's risk for infection and delayed wound healing. Client obesity may also affect postoperative ambulation and recovery.

Surgical Technique

Knee prostheses most commonly include three components: the femoral component, the tibial plate, and the patellar button (Figure 26-5). These tricompartmental prostheses vary in size to ensure the most accurate fit for each client. Some parts may also be specific for the right or left knee or the femoral and tibial surfaces.

The surgical incision for TKA extends from 4 or 5 inches above the patella to 2 or 3 inches below it. The approach is either medial parapatellar or lateral parapatellar. Soft tissue is balanced across the joint, and the proximal tibia and distal femur are trimmed to fit the chosen prosthesis. Any flexion contractures or deformities (varus or valgus) may also be corrected. After osteotomy the surgeon prepares the bone surfaces to accept the prosthesis based on the use of cemented or press-fit (noncemented) components. The patella is resurfaced with a polyethylene button after the surgeon ensures that the patellar prosthesis will track normally during flexion and extension of the knee.

Wound drains may be placed before closure of the incision, and a bulky pressure dressing is applied. If the client is to start *continuous passive motion* (CPM) immediately, a lighter dressing is used. The Translating Evidence into Practice feature on p. 486 provides further information on the use of CPM after total knee arthroplasty.

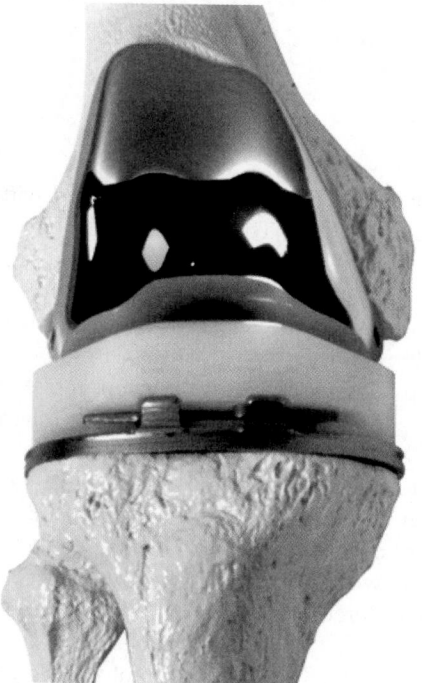

■ FIGURE 26–5 Total knee prosthesis.

Complications

Infection, a potentially severe complication, occurs in 1% to 3% of TKA clients.[26] If it occurs, venous thromboembolism can cause significant morbidity or death. Other complications may include patellar subluxation or dislocation, impaired wound healing, knee stiffness (inability to regain ROM), and loosening of the prosthesis.

Nursing Management of the Surgical Client: Total Knee Arthroplasty

---

Preoperative assessment and care are the same as for the client undergoing THA. Postoperative care concerns are also similar, but emphasis on knee exercise is greater because dislocation is not a significant risk. The goal of knee rehabilitation—to obtain maximal ROM with good muscle control—can be accomplished with consistent physical therapy or use of a continuous passive motion (CPM) machine (Figure 26-6). This apparatus moves the knee slowly through its arc of motion, with settings determined by physician order. The machine, which is placed in a slightly abducted position on the bed, is frequently initiated at 0 degrees of extension and 10 to 40 degrees of flexion. Settings should be gradually and regularly increased, with the client and nurse working collaboratively to achieve the goal of 90 degrees of flexion in the acute care setting.

Depending on surgeon preference, use of the machine can begin immediately after surgery. Some physicians delay initiation of CPM until the evening of surgery or the morning after surgery. The CPM machine should be used a minimum of 6 to 8 hours a day. The client must be supine during use of the CPM machine, with the head of the bed elevated no more than 15 degrees, and should thus be removed from the machine for meals. The client may also find it uncomfortable to use the CPM machine during sleep; this concern should be discussed with the surgeon.

When the client is no longer using the CPM, a knee immobilizer may be ordered to promote knee extension. Make sure that the immobilizer is of the correct length for the client and that it does not rub on the heel or groin. No pillows should be placed under the client's knee while in bed because this promotes flexion contracture.

Both ROM and strengthening exercises are an important part of functional recovery after TKA. Ankle pumps decrease the risk for blood clots in the lower extremities. The physical therapist may lead the client in active ROM exercises or may perform gentle passive ROM and stretching to increase knee flexion or extension. Isometric exercises to strengthen the quadriceps, hamstrings, and gluteal muscles are an important part of the regimen. Straight-leg raises also help with muscle strengthening. A home exercise program after hospital discharge includes ROM exercises and isometrics, with

TRANSLATING EVIDENCE INTO PRACTICE

Use of Continuous Passive Motion After Total Knee Arthroplasty

One of the concerns following total knee arthroplasty (TKA) has been achieving optimal range of motion (ROM) for the client. Continuous passive motion (CPM) machines have been a popular intervention since their development. In recent years, however, research has examined the benefits of CPM versus rehabilitation through physical therapy.

In a study that compared three treatment modalities, the researchers wanted to determine which method of mobilization achieved the maximum ROM in the first 6 months following TKA.[1] Three treatment groups (n = 40/group) were established: standardized exercise and CPM, standardized exercise and slider board therapy, or standardized exercise alone. The three groups were similar with respect to age, gender, and diagnosis at the start of the study. Subjects were examined preoperatively, at the time of hospital discharge, and at 3 and 6 months after surgery. No differences were noted among the groups in knee ROM or in the WOMAC Osteoarthritis Index or the SF-36 scores. Researchers concluded that it is difficult to justify the use of adjunct ROM therapy such as the CPM or sliding board in addition to exercise sessions. As hospital stays continue to decrease for clients who have undergone TKA, their rehabilitation should emphasize active knee movement rather than passive therapy to promote functional independence.

Other researchers examined the effectiveness of CPM in improving postoperative function and ROM after TKA.[2] A group of clients was divided among 3 postoperative treatment regimens: no CPM (n = 19), CPM at 0 to 40 degrees (n = 18), and CPM at 0 to 70 degrees (n = 20). Those clients in the CPM groups used the machines for 48 hours; all clients had identical physical therapy treatment. Clients were assessed preoperatively and at 1 week and 1 year postoperatively. Although clients with CPM at 0 to 70 degrees did experience a significant increase in flexion and ROM at 1 week, no significant differences among the groups were noted at 1 year. In addition, researchers noted that those clients who had CPM had a significant increase in analgesic requirement and in mean postoperative blood drainage. They concluded that CPM had no significant advantage in terms of improving knee function or ROM.

A third group of researchers had similar findings regarding the effects of CPM for clients transferred to a rehabilitation setting following TKA.[3] Knee ROM was measured on admission, on the third and seventh days of hospitalization, and on discharge. One group of clients received CPM for 5 consecutive hours a day plus physical therapy; the other group received only physical therapy. The researchers found neither statistical nor clinical difference between the two groups. They concluded that the use of CPM in a rehabilitation setting has no benefit to clients admitted after a single TKA.

IMPLICATIONS

With decreased lengths of acute hospital stay for clients following TKA, the nurse must be prepared to assist clients to regain functional independence by using strategies that promote knee ROM. The nurse can supplement physical therapy interventions by encouraging early and frequent ambulation to maximize ROM.

REFERENCES

1. Beaupre, L.A., et al. (2001). Exercise combined with continuous passive motion or slider board therapy compared with exercise only: A randomized controlled trial of patients following total knee arthroplasty. *Physical Therapy*, 81(4), 1029-1037.
2. Pope, R.O., et al. (1997). Continuous passive motion after primary total knee arthroplasty. Does it offer any benefits? *Journal of Bone and Joint Surgery. British Volume*, 79(6), 914-917.
3. Chen, B., et al. (2000). Continuous passive motion after total knee arthroplasty: A prospective study. *American Journal of Physical Medicine & Rehabilitation*, 79(5), 421-426.

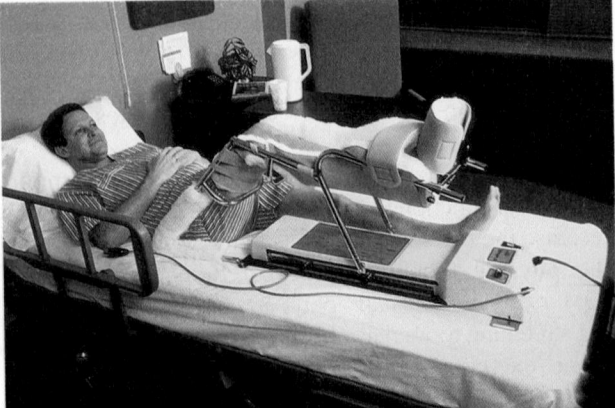

■ **FIGURE 26–6** A continuous passive motion exerciser allows the client to achieve early ROM. *(Courtesy The Chattanooga Group, Inc., Hixson, Tenn.)*

weekly increases in resistance as tolerated without producing joint irritation. To obtain optimal knee function, the client should continue exercises as prescribed after surgery.

The client is usually allowed to transfer from bed to chair within 24 hours after TKA. Carefully supporting the operative extremity, help the client move to a sitting position on the side of the bed. Coach the client to push off from the bed to stand in front of the walker before gripping it. Weight-bearing status is determined by surgeon order based on the use of cemented or noncemented components. The client with a cemented prosthesis is often allowed to bear weight as tolerated; NWB or TTWB is ordered for the client with a noncemented prosthesis. Once the client is in the chair, the operative leg can be elevated slightly for comfort or gently flexed to the floor. When the client has regained enough muscle strength to move the operative leg without assistance, crutch-walking can begin if desired. Use of the assistive device continues until the client has sufficient quadriceps function to ambulate independently.

METABOLIC BONE DISORDERS

Inappropriate functioning of the metabolic processes in bone results in disorders manifested by changes in both physical and chemical structure of the bone. Disorders that alter bony equilibrium and affect bone turnover can be due to estrogen deficiency, parathyroid gland abnormalities, vitamin deficiency, malabsorption, or physical inactivity.

OSTEOPOROSIS

Osteoporosis is defined as a systemic skeletal disorder characterized by compromised bone strength predisposing to an increased risk of fracture. A fracture results when the osteoporotic bone encounters a force greater than it can withstand (e.g., trauma from a fall). The two components of bone strength include bone density and bone quality.

The term *osteopenia* refers to a low *bone mineral density* (BMD) compared with that expected for the person's gender and age. Clients with osteopenia have a greater risk for osteoporotic fracture than those with normal or above-average density. Osteopenia is a risk factor for fracture just as hypertension is a risk factor for stroke.

In an attempt to assess the risk of osteoporotic fracture, the World Health Organization (WHO) has developed several general categories to clarify the definition of osteoporosis. The categories include the following:

1. *Normal*—a value for BMD or *bone mineral content* (BMC) that is not more than 1 standard deviation (SD) below the young adult mean value (Figure 26-7, *A*)
2. *Low bone mass (osteopenia)*—a value for BMD or BMC that lies between 1.0 and 2.5 SD below the young adult mean value
3. *Osteoporosis*—a value for BMD or BMC that is more than 2.5 SD below the young adult mean value (Figure 26-7, *B*)
4. *Severe (established) osteoporosis*—a value for BMD or BMC more than 2.5 SD below the young adult mean value *and* the presence of one or more fragility fractures

Osteoporosis is a major public health problem in many parts of the world, and its scope will increase as the population ages. It affects about 20% of postmenopausal white women in the United States. An additional 52% have osteopenia at the hip. One of every two women will experience a fracture at some point during her life. Nonwhite women and men are also at risk for osteoporotic fractures, although their risk is lower than that for white women.

Osteoporotic fractures also create a heavy economic burden. The annual cost to the health care system associated with osteoporotic fractures has been estimated at $17 billion (2001 dollars). A single hip fracture is estimated to cost $40,000. The number of hip fractures may increase three-fold by the year 2040. Thus any reduction in hip fractures would have a large impact on health care expenditures. The Complementary and Alternative Therapy feature on p. 488 examines bone risks associated with megadoses of vitamin A.

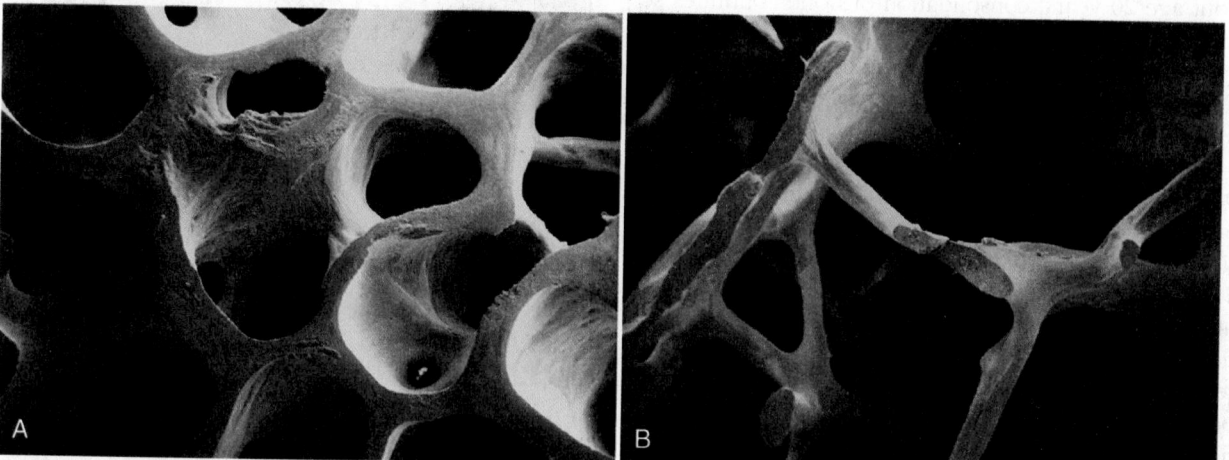

■ **FIGURE 26–7** Electron micrographs of normal **(A)** and osteoporotic **(B)** bone. (From Dempster, D.W., et al. [1986]. A simple method for correlative light and scanning electron microscopy of human iliac crest bone biopsies: Qualitative observations in normal and osteoporotic subjects. *Journal of Bone and Mineral Research, 1*, 15-21.)

Vitamin A and an Increased Risk of Osteoporosis

Several laboratory and epidemiologic studies have suggested an increased risk of fractures in people with a high vitamin A intake. This study enrolled 2322 men, 49 to 51 years of age, in a population-based cohort study. Fractures were found in 266 men during 30 years of follow-up. The risk of fracture was highest among men with the highest serum vitamin A (retinol) levels. Men with the highest levels of retinol had an overall risk of fracture that was greater than that in men with the lowest levels of retinol by a factor of 7 ($p < 0.001$). The level of serum beta-carotene was not associated with the risk of fracture. These initial data in men and previous data in women suggest that megadoses of vitamin A may be associated with a substantially higher risk of fracture. The results of this study and others should encourage immediate normal intakes of vitamin A, especially from supplements, until more clinical studies are completed. In laboratory studies, vitamin A in large doses has been associated with the inhibition of bone-forming cells.

REFERENCE

Michaelsson, K., et al. (2003). Serum retinol levels and the risk of fracture. *New England Journal of Medicine, 348,* 287-294.

Etiology and Risk Factors

Many factors, both genetic and environmental, are involved in the development of osteoporosis. Bone mass, which is measured by bone densitometry and reported as BMC or BMD, is an important risk factor in osteoporosis. To understand the relationship of bone density and risk of fracture, it is helpful to review some facts about bone mass.

Peak bone mass is the highest bone mass attained. Although longitudinal growth usually is complete by about age 20 years, consolidation of bone continues so that peak bone mass is not attained until about age 30 in both men and women. This is noteworthy because it indicates that interventions to increase peak mass can be effective up until about age 30.

What happens to bone mass in women between age 30 and menopause is uncertain. Most likely, bone mass plateaus until menopause or decreases slightly during this period. Bone loss in the hip probably starts as early as age 20. Although it is debated as to when bone loss naturally begins, during perimenopause women experience a marked acceleration in bone loss because of the loss of natural estrogen. Women start to lose bone about 1.5 to 2 years before their last menstrual period and continue rapid loss until about 1.5 years after their last menses. They may lose as much as 15% of their total mass during the perimenopausal period, after which the rate of bone loss slows to a rate of about 1% per year.

Rapid bone loss also occurs in women whose ovaries have stopped functioning, such as women being treated for the prevention and treatment of ovarian and breast cancer.

Although men have larger and stronger skeletons than women, they can experience a marked loss of bone as they age, possibly resulting in fragility fractures. Bone loss in men starts later in life and progresses more slowly. Men do not experience the rapid bone loss associated with the perimenopausal decline in estrogen production seen in women. There are several reasons for loss of bone in men, including declining testosterone levels. In addition, estrogen may play a crucial role in men's bone health and changes in estrogen levels with age may be as important, if not more so, as changes in testosterone levels.

Those who have not gained their maximum peak bone mass have less bone "in the bank" to draw upon once the inevitable bone loss begins. Thus peak bone mass as well as later bone loss is a major determinant of osteoporotic fracture. For this reason, osteoporosis has been described as a pediatric disorder. Strong adult skeletons are built during childhood.

From 60% to 80% of the risk for this disorder is inherited. A history of fracture in a first-degree relative is a risk for fragility fracture. Factors other than heredity known to influence development of osteoporosis are listed in Box 26-2.

Osteoporosis can also result from underlying medical conditions, such as thyrotoxicosis, hyperparathyroidism, anorexia nervosa, and Cushing's syndrome, and from long-term use of medications such as thyroid hormone, anticonvulsants, furosemide, and corticosteroids. A person who has had one osteoporotic fracture is five times more likely to suffer another fracture than a person without a fracture. Thus history of a low-trauma fracture is an important risk factor.

BOX 26-2 Risk Factors for Osteoporosis

MAJOR RISK FACTORS

- Personal history of fracture as an adult
- History of fragility (low-trauma) fracture in a first-degree relative
- Low body weight (less than about 128 pounds)
- Current cigarette smoking
- Use of oral corticosteroid therapy for more than 3 months

ADDITIONAL RISK FACTORS

- Impaired vision
- Estrogen deficiency at any age
- Dementia
- Poor health/frailty
- Recent falls
- Inadequate physical activity
- Low intake of dietary calcium (lifelong)
- Suboptimal levels of serum vitamin D
- Alcohol in amounts of more than two drinks per day

Pathophysiology

Bone is a dynamic tissue that undergoes continuous *remodeling,* the process by which old bone is replaced by new. Bone remodeling serves two principal functions:

1. It replaces old bone with new so that the biomechanical properties of the skeleton are not compromised by continuous use.
2. It plays a role in mineral homeostasis by transferring calcium and other ions into and out of the skeletal reservoir.

The remodeling sequence starts with activation of *osteoclasts,* which resorb a small portion of bone over a relatively short period (as short as 7 to 10 days). Bone formation then takes place as *osteoblasts* form an organic matrix that is subsequently mineralized.

Peak bone mass and the subsequent rate and duration of bone loss are important determinants of whether skeletal integrity will be compromised to the degree that a fragility fracture will result. In addition, as bone tissue is lost, other alterations in the skeleton (e.g., changes in architecture, aging of the bone tissue, accumulation of microdamage) contribute to fracture risk. The supporting structures become so weak that even minimal stress can cause fractures. Spinal fractures occurring with osteoporosis are usually compression fractures that occur when one or more vertebrae collapse from carrying the weight of the upright body.

Clinical Manifestations

In many people, the diagnosis of osteoporosis is made after a fracture, often a vertebral compression fracture. Clinical manifestations of vertebral compression fracture include sudden onset of severe back pain that worsens on movement and is relieved by rest. This acute pain usually subsides within 2 to 6 weeks. Most compression fractures, however, are discovered accidentally on routine x-ray. Progressive vertebral deformities lead to shortened stature and progressive dorsal kyphosis (Figure 26-8). The lower ribs eventually rest on the iliac crests, and downward pressure on viscera causes abdominal distention and bloating. Respiration may also be impaired by restricted lung expansion.

Bone loss can also occur in the mandible, which may lead to loss of teeth or poorly fitting dentures as well as changes in the appearance of the face. Unfortunately, fractures of the wrist in postmenopausal women are often not recognized as osteoporotic fractures.

The many changes in appearance and the difficulty in finding clothing that fits can have a profound negative effect on self-esteem. Quality of life may be affected by chronic pain and functional disability. Fear of subsequent fracture may cause people to reduce their activity.

The "gold standard" for measuring BMD is full-table dual-energy x-ray absorptiometry (DXA). This technique carries low risk and takes only a few minutes. The most commonly measured sites with DXA are the

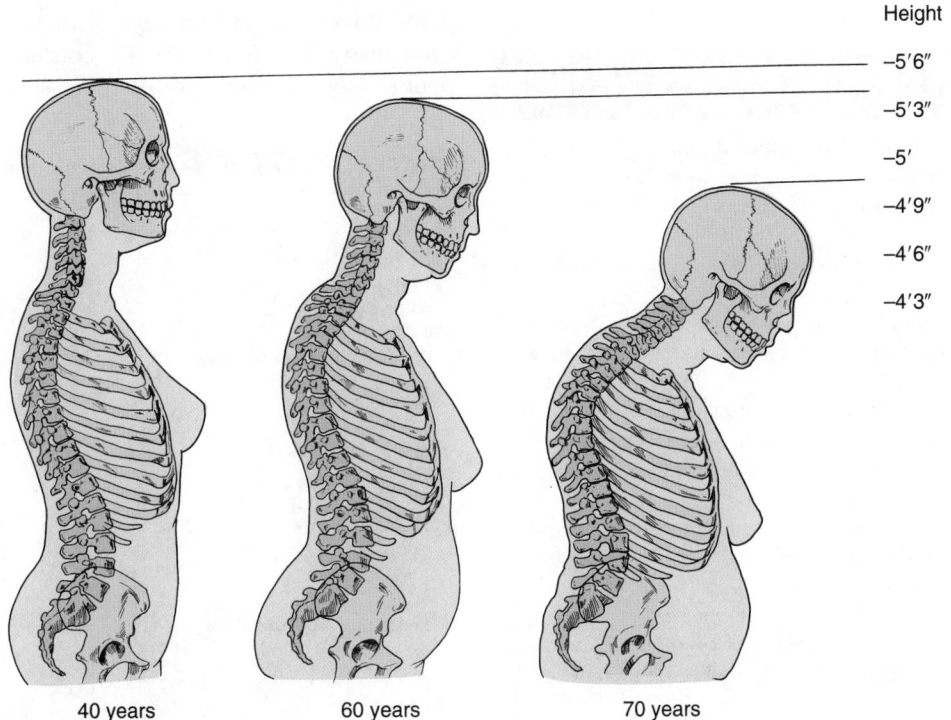

Height

— −5′6″

— −5′3″

— −5′

— −4′9″

— −4′6″

— −4′3″

40 years   60 years   70 years

■ **FIGURE 26–8** Osteoporotic changes: A normal spine at 40 years of age and osteoporotic changes at ages 60 and 70 years. These changes can cause a loss of height and may result in dorsal kyphosis.

spine and the hip. BMD is commonly reported as a "T-score," which is the difference between the client's BMD and the BMD of "young normal adults" of the same gender. The difference between the client's score and the young adult norm is expressed as standard deviation (SD) below or above the average. Thus a person with a T-score of −2.0 would have a BMD that is 2 SD below the average for a young adult of the same gender. Under the WHO criteria, this person would be considered *osteopenic*. Guidelines for BMD testing are shown in Box 26-3.

In recent years, the number of peripheral densitometers has increased dramatically. These devices measure BMD at peripheral sites such as the heel or finger. They include *quantitative ultrasound* (QUS) devices and peripheral DXA. These devices are smaller and less expensive than full-table DXA, and the QUS devices involve no radiation exposure. Criteria for interpreting results with peripheral devices are not well developed, however.

Laboratory tests may be performed to rule out secondary osteoporosis or other metabolic bone diseases. These tests include blood count, urine calcium level, multichannel screen, serum alkaline phosphatase level, serum 25-hydroxyvitamin D level, parathyroid hormone level, ionized calcium level, protein electrophoresis in urine and serum, and thyroid function. Biochemical markers of bone remodeling, such as urinary collagen cross-links, are sometimes used in conjunction with DXA or QUS to monitor the effectiveness of therapy. At this time, however, biochemical markers alone are not appropriate

for diagnosis of osteoporosis or for predicting the risk of fracture in the future.

OUTCOME MANAGEMENT

Medical Management

The goal of medical management is to prevent bone loss and fragility fractures. Lifestyle changes focused on dietary intake of adequate calcium and vitamin D and weight-bearing exercise are prescribed to prevent bone loss. *Hormone replacement therapy* (HRT) is considered for women who are perimenopausal (see later discussion). Cigarette and alcohol cessation is advised.

Preventing Loss of Bone Mass

Osteoporosis is preventable. Strategies for prevention are most effective when they are started in childhood to maximize peak bone mass and to establish lifelong bone-healthy behaviors. Several interventions that maximize and preserve bone mass have general health benefits, including adequate intake of calcium and vitamin D, regular weight-bearing exercise, and avoidance of tobacco and alcohol abuse.

Calcium and Vitamin D Intake

A well-balanced diet containing the recommended level of calcium is an important component of bone health (Table 26-2). The major sources of dietary calcium are dairy products. Calcium can also be obtained from the wide range of calcium-fortified foods that are available (Box 26-4). National surveys of dietary intake indicate that many Americans are not consuming enough calcium. Most women consume less than half of the

---

BOX 26-3 Bone Mineral Density (BMD) Testing Guidelines

BMD testing is recommended for the following:
- All postmenopausal women under age 65 years who have one or more additional risk factors for osteoporosis (besides menopause)
- All women age 65 years and older regardless of risk factors
- Younger postmenopausal women with one or more risk factors (other than being white, postmenopausal, and female)
- Postmenopausal women who present with fractures (to confirm diagnosis and determine disease severity)
- Estrogen-deficient women at clinical risk for osteoporosis*
- Individuals with vertebral abnormalities*
- Individuals receiving, or planning to receive, long-term glucocorticoid (steroid) therapy*
- Individuals with primary hyperthyroidism*
- Individuals being monitored to assess the response or efficacy of an approved osteoporosis drug therapy*

*Medicare covers BMD testing for these individuals age 65 and older.
From the National Osteoporosis Foundation. (1999). *Physician's guide to prevention and treatment of osteoporosis.* Hillsborough, NJ: Excerpta Medica.

TABLE 26–2 Recommended Calcium Intake Levels

Age Levels	Calcium Intake (mg/day)
Infants	
Birth-6 mo	210
7 mo-1 yr	280
Children and Adolescents	
1-3 yr	500
4-8 yr	800
9-18 yr	1300
Adults	
19-50	1000
51-70	1200
>70	1200
Pregnancy and Lactation	
<18	1300
19-50	1000

National Academy of Science. (1999). *Dietary reference intakes for calcium, magnesium, phosphorus, vitamin D, and fluoride.* Washington, DC: Food and Nutrition Board, Institute of Medicine, National Academies Press.

BOX 26-4   Calcium Equivalents of Dietary Sources (300 mg)

- 1 cup of milk
- 1 carton of low-fat yogurt with fruit
- 1¼ cups of frozen yogurt
- 1 cup of vanilla pudding
- 1 cup of baked egg custard
- 1 oz of Swiss cheese
- 1 slice of cheese pizza
- ½ cup of ricotta cheese, part skim
- 1½ oz of cheddar cheese
- 2¼ cups of cottage cheese
- 11 dried figs
- 4 cups of broccoli
- 7 oz of baked wall-eyed pike fillet
- ¾ cup of whole dried almonds

Prepared by Patricia T. Packard, RD, CN, Creighton University Osteoporosis Research Center, Omaha, Neb.

recommended daily levels. As early as age 10, the calcium intake of girls is considerably below that needed for optimal bone health.

People who have difficulty digesting milk because of a lack of the enzyme lactase, which breaks down the milk sugar lactose, may be able to tolerate acidophilus milk, yogurt, and hard cheeses; in addition, milk products may be tolerated if taken in small amounts. Skim milk and low-fat yogurt can be recommended for people who are trying to maintain low-cholesterol diets. Diets high in dairy foods do not cause obesity. In fact, considerable research supports the role of dietary calcium in decreasing the risk of obesity. Dietary calcium is the preferred approach, but calcium supplements should be used when an adequate dietary intake cannot be achieved. All calcium supplements should be taken with food to enhance absorbability. Chewable supplements are preferred over those that are swallowed. Although a high dietary calcium intake is thought to increase the risk of renal calculi (stones), research findings suggest that high-calcium diets actually protect against stone formation.

Vitamin D plays a major role in both calcium absorption and bone metabolism. Vitamin D is made in the skin in the presence of sunlight, or it may be obtained from a few food sources, primarily vitamin D–fortified milk. Although exposure to sunlight is necessary for cutaneous synthesis of vitamin D, prolonged exposure to sunlight does not necessarily increase the amount that is synthesized. An average of 15 minutes a day of sunlight exposure between 10:00 AM and 3:00 PM to hands, and arms probably meets the requirements for most people during the summer or below the 40th latitude. At more Northern latitudes, the angle of the sun is such that sunlight during the winter does not convert vitamin D into the active form. Although the use of sunscreen remains important to reduce photoaging and the risk of skin cancer, when sunscreen is applied the skin receives no sunlight and vitamin D is not synthesized in the skin. Vitamin D supplementation (1000 international units/day) is recommended for institutionalized older people, for people living in high northern or southern latitudes, and for people who have limited sun exposure without sunscreen.

High dietary intake of sodium increases loss of calcium in the urine, and people who consume large amounts of sodium should increase their calcium intake accordingly. Although caffeine modestly increases calcium excretion in the urine, the loss is negligible compared with the effects of protein and sodium. The effect of caffeine can be offset by adding 40 mg of calcium to the diet for each cup of coffee. Phosphorus intake, such as that from drinking carbonated beverages, does not significantly affect calcium balance; however, people who drink a large number of carbonated beverages may not be consuming adequate calcium in the form of milk.

Low protein intake appears to play a distinct detrimental role in the causes and complications of hip fracture. Many older adults have an inadequate protein intake. The clinical outcome after hip fracture is significantly improved with the use of daily oral nutritional supplements or a calcium phosphate pill, which normalize protein intake. Protein supplementation also reduces further bone loss in older clients who have sustained a hip fracture.

Exercise

Weight-bearing exercise, such as walking and running, is necessary for maintaining bone mass because disuse results in bone loss. Swimming and biking have not been found effective in maintaining bone mass, probably because they do not adequately load the bones. The inactivity of older people increases the rate of bone loss and the risk of hip fracture. It has been suggested that regular exercise by older adults would reduce the risk of hip fracture by at least half. In addition to maintaining bone mass by loading the bones, exercise leads to improved physical fitness, which is associated with improved muscle strength, stability, reaction time, balance, and coordination.

All these factors help to decrease the risk of falling and of subsequent fractures. Exercise regimens and weight training increase muscle strength even in people older than 90 years. In light of the positive effects of exercise on bone and on health in general, nurses should recommend regular exercise for all clients. Previously sedentary clients who wish to start a more rigorous exercise program should undergo a physical evaluation before starting.

At least 30 minutes of any physical activity should be incorporated into daily schedules. Even activities such as walking, hiking, gardening, biking, and housework or yard work increase daily energy expenditure and help to promote muscular strength, flexibility, coordination, and endurance, which ultimately may decrease the number and severity of falls.

Alcohol and Tobacco

Alcohol abuse and smoking cigarettes increase the risk of osteoporosis. Current smokers have 2.1 times the risk of hip fractures as nonsmokers. If a woman quits smoking, she reduces her risk of hip fracture by 40%. Excessive alcohol intake reduces bone density and increases the risk of falls. Moderate alcohol intake has no known negative effect on BMD.

Pharmaceutical Prevention and Treatment of Osteoporosis

Medications approved by the FDA to prevent and treat osteoporosis include hormone replacement therapy (HRT), alendronate, raloxifene, risedronate, ibandronate,

zoledronic acid, calcitonin, and teriparatide. Alendronate, risedronate, ibandronate, and zoledronic acid are bisphosphonates. The oral forms are poorly absorbed and must be taken before eating in the morning with a full glass of water and then followed by a 30-60-minute fast. The client should stay in an upright position for 30-60 minutes after taking the medication to avoid reflux and possible irritation to the esophageal mucosa. Ibandronate and zoledronic acid are available in intravenous preparations that are given once every three months and once a year, respectively. These are options for clients who do not tolerate the oral preparations of bisphosphonates. Clients receiving drug therapy for osteoporosis should be taught about the importance of dietary intake and activity as part of any treatment regimen. Treatment should not be limited to people who have had a fragility fracture but should include clients at high risk for osteoporotic fracture. The Translating Evidence into Practice feature below discusses the risks and benefits of HRT for osteoporosis.

TRANSLATING EVIDENCE INTO PRACTICE

Using Hormone Replacement Therapy for Osteoporosis

Although hormone replacement therapy (HRT) has been widely used in prevention and treatment of osteoporosis, new evidence about its benefits and risks requires consideration of its use for bone health. The Women's Health Initiative (WHI), a large randomized primary prevention trial of estrogen and estrogen plus progesterone, found that Prempro (combined estrogen and progesterone) reduced the risk of clinical vertebral fractures and hip fractures by 34%; however, Prempro also increased risks of probable dementia, coronary heart disease, stroke, thromboembolic disorders, breast cancer, and cholecystitis. It is important to note that the WHI used only one type of estrogen preparation at one dose and that a study arm that used estrogen *without* progesterone was not terminated. This raises the question of whether estrogen without progesterone involves fewer risks. Furthermore, the risks of lower doses of estrogen, which have been found to have bone health benefits, were not addressed in the WHI. Based on these findings, when use of HRT is considered solely for prevention of osteoporosis, approved non-estrogen therapies should first be considered. Currently, HRT is recommended for relief of menopausal manifestations and not for long-term prevention of osteoporosis. HRT prevents the estrogen-related bone loss that occurs during the perimenopausal period; however, this bone loss will occur when the HRT is stopped. The skeletal effects of estrogen are obtained with both oral and transdermal preparations.

Marketed as Evista, raloxifene is a member of a class of drugs called *selective estrogen receptor modulators* (SERMs). SERMs provide the benefits of estrogen but avoid the risks.

They prevent bone loss and reduce the incidence of osteoporotic fracture. Their cardioprotective effects are under investigation. SERMs do not increase the risk of breast or uterine cancer. In fact, Evista has been found to decrease the incidence of breast cancer. Evista increases the risk of DVT in a manner similar to that of ERT. Evista also increases hot flashes and is thus not effective in relieving menopausal manifestations.

Drugs that inhibit bone resorption are also prescribed. Alendronate and risedronate are bisphosphonates and are available as Fosamax and Actonel, respectively. These drugs must be taken after a prolonged fast (overnight) with 8 ounces of water, at least 30 minutes before eating or drinking. Clients should remain upright during this 30-minute interval. Calcitonin, a hormone that slows bone resorption, is available as Miacalcin and is delivered as a single daily dose of nasal spray. Calcitonin is less effective than Evista or Fosamax in maintenance of bone mass. Interestingly, calcitonin has analgesic effects, which may help to relieve pain associated with fractures.

Parathyroid hormone (PTH, Forteo) has recently been approved by the FDA for treatment of osteoporosis in postmenopausal women. It is an anabolic (bone-building) agent that is administered daily by subcutaneous injection. Forteo has few side effects, but some clients experience leg cramps and dizziness. The safety and efficacy of Forteo have not been demonstrated beyond 2 years of therapy.

REFERENCE

Writing Group for the Women's Health Initiative Investigators. (2002). Risks and benefits of estrogen plus progestin in healthy postmenopausal women: Principal results from the Women's Health Initiative randomized controlled trial. *Journal of the American Medical Association, 288*, 321-333.

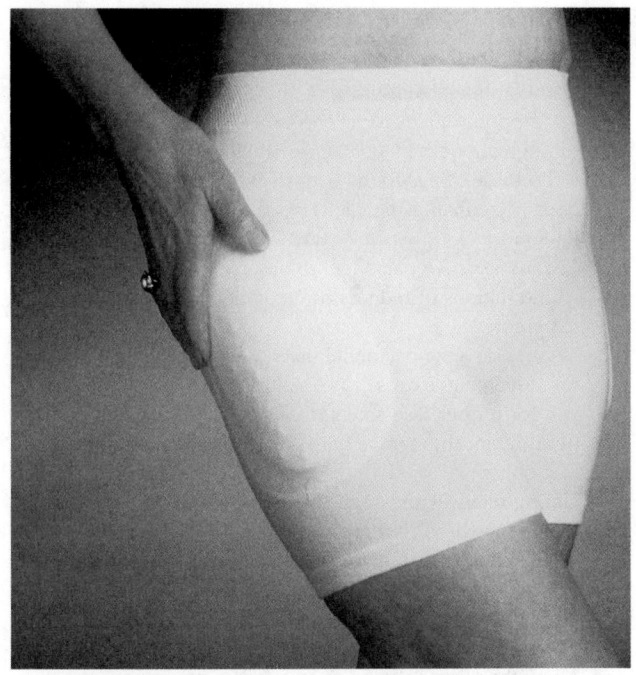

■ **FIGURE 26–9** Safehip. *(Courtesy Tytex Group, Woonsocket, RI.)*

Nonpharmaceutical Prevention of Osteoporosis

People who are at high risk of fracture and falling should be considered for hip protectors (Figure 26-9). These undergarments have protective shields or pads sewn into the area over the greater trochanter on each side. These shields are anatomically designed to shunt the energy of an impact away from the greater trochanter to the soft tissues. Large studies have shown that the rate of hip fracture per fall is 84% lower when hip protectors are worn. The design of the hip protectors is such that the garment is comfortable to wear and is not visibly apparent under slacks or a skirt. The garment has been modified with Velcro fasteners for nursing home clients. The cost of hip protectors is slightly more than the cost of 1 month of anti-resorptive medication.

Promoting Healing After Fracture

The goals of treatment after fracture are to manage pain, regain mobility and strength, promote healing, reduce bone loss, and prevent further fracture. Furthermore, treatment is directed toward limiting the disability associated with existing fractures.

Managing Pain. One of the most important interventions in the care of the client with an osteoporotic fracture is pain management. Often clients present with back pain resulting from vertebral crush fracture syndrome. Strict bed rest for 5 to 7 days is most effective in relieving pain and shortening the course of pain. The client should lie supine or in a side-lying position. After 5 to 7 days of bed rest, the client is instructed to increase activity gradually.

Non-opioid analgesics may be needed for 1 to 2 weeks to aid in pain reduction. If NSAIDs are used, protect the client from gastric ulceration by administering medications with food or antacids.

Flexible corsets with adjustable self-fastening tape (Velcro) may help to relieve back pain and fatigue; however, these corsets cannot correct the underlying problem of bone loss and spinal deformity. Corsets may be worn in bed but are most helpful if worn when the person is in the upright position.

Physical therapy is of utmost importance in the long-term treatment of back pain. Often chronic back pain is associated with decreased ROM, weakness, muscle spasm, postural change, muscle tenderness, and decreased endurance. Physical therapy should be started during the period of bed rest with ROM exercises and mild resistive exercises of the extremities in bed. Heat or ice, ultrasound, and TENS may be used for pain reduction.

Regaining Mobility and Strength. After acute pain subsides, clients should carry out exercises specifically prescribed for them, such as stretching and strengthening. Water aerobics may be initiated early in the treatment before the client can tolerate weight-bearing exercise. A long-term physical activity program should include weight-bearing and aerobic exercise in addition to strengthening and flexibility exercise. Because osteoporotic clients are at risk for subsequent fractures, they should be taught how to move safely while maintaining or increasing their physical activity. The use of splints is addressed in the Management and Delegation feature on p. 494.

Promoting Healing. Good general nutrition should be encouraged after fractures to promote healing. Optimal calcium and vitamin D intake continue to be important, and special attention should be given to adequate protein in the diet, especially in older clients. Calcium phosphate supplements should be considered for people with low protein intake.

Preventing Further Fractures. Medications and treatments used to prevent osteoporosis are continued after a fracture to maintain and improve bone mass in existing bone.

Nursing Management of the Medical Client

Nursing management for the client with osteoporosis is detailed in the Care Plan feature on The Client with **evolve** Osteoporosis on the website.

MANAGEMENT AND DELEGATION

Assisting with Mobility and the Use of Splints

Muscle overuse, traumatic injury, and muscle disuse associated with prolonged bed rest can each contribute to complications of immobility. An important aspect of care is prevention of these unnecessary complications. Interventions to minimize the complications of immobility include passive and active range-of-motion (ROM) exercises as well as the use of splints to maintain normal joint alignment and position. The performance of ROM exercises and the application and removal of splints may be delegated to unlicensed assistive personnel.

Although you may delegate these tasks, as the nurse you remain responsible for the assessment of the client's baseline level of function and development of a plan to prevent the complications associated with immobility. Interdisciplinary collaboration with physical and occupational therapists is often necessary to develop a comprehensive plan of care. Additionally, you will be monitoring the client's progress and response to these interventions and adjusting the plan of care in collaboration with the other involved disciplines.

When delegating these tasks to assistive personnel, emphasize the following:

- Specify any physical limitations that clients may have that would prohibit their ability to move an extremity through its normal ROM.
- Identify the time at which this activity is best performed with a client. Establish a schedule of which the client and assistive personnel are aware. Often ROM activities are incorporated into the morning bath routine, which limits this activity to once per day. Most clients, confined to bed, would be better served if passive or active ROM activities were performed two to three times per day, from the onset of illness. Plan these activity periods to allow for adequate rest intervals.
- Encourage or assist the client to be as independent as possible in performing activities of daily living.

Hair-combing, teeth-brushing, bathing, and eating are all good opportunities for clients to use their extremities through the normal ROM. Care providers are often tempted to do these things for a client to get the job done, but this does not enhance the client's independence, strength, or endurance.

- Remind assistive personnel to observe and report any manifestations of redness or deformity overlying a joint or extremity.
- Instruct assistive personnel that a new complaint of pain on movement is cause to cease the activity and report to you for further assessment. Delegated personnel should put no joint through its full ROM if the client complains of pain.
- During removal and application of splints, observe the skin and involved bony prominence. Any manifestations of redness and irritation are cause for your examination. Revision of the splint, by the appropriate practitioner, may be necessary. Splints are often fitted by occupational therapists, although this may vary.
- Allow the client to stand to transfer from a bed to a chair rather than having the client slide from a bed to a stretcher chair. This action preserves and promotes the function of the quadriceps, pelvis and lower leg muscles; these muscles are essential to the client's ability to resume walking activities. Standing, in contrast to sliding, the client also reduces the incidence of skin shearing that can occur via the slide method. Reserve sliding from bed to chair for clients who lack the mental capacity to follow instructions for standing or for clients who are too weak or unsafe to stand.
- Make sure that ambulation progresses from short to long distances. Assess the client's gait and balance. Instruct assistive personnel to monitor the client's balance and the ability to walk safely.
- Verify the competency of assistive personnel in performing ROM exercises, transfer techniques, and splint application and use during orientation and annually thereafter.

Self-Care

SAFETY
ALERT

Assess clients at high risk for fracture for activity level and dietary adequacy, and perform appropriate teaching to prevent fractures. In addition, assess these clients' risk of falling. Assessment includes visual acuity, medications that may cause dizziness or postural hypotension, and difficulties with balance or coordination as well as the home environment for potential safety hazards.

Evaluation of the home setting is performed via the admission assessment, discussions with the client, consultation with a specialist in social services, and home safety evaluation by a visiting nurse.

Discussion about fall prevention strategies is imperative. Instruct clients who are prone to dizziness to get up slowly from a lying position, first sitting on the side of the bed. The client's eyeglass prescription may need to be updated to improve vision. An aid to ambulation, such as a cane or walker, may also be indicated to prevent falling. Alterations to the home may be recommended. Handrails in the bathroom, removal of scatter rugs, and increased lighting are some of the modifications that may be necessary.

Specific resources in the community that may be helpful to clients with osteoporosis include support groups and exercise programs. The National Osteoporosis Foundation (www.nof.org) is an excellent source of educational resources.

PAGET'S DISEASE

Paget's disease (osteitis deformans) is defined as an idiopathic bone disorder characterized by abnormal and accelerated bone resorption and formation in one or more bones. The normal bone is replaced by abnormal, structurally weaker bone that is prone to fractures. Paget's disease most frequently produces painful deformities of the femur, tibia, lower spine, pelvis, and cranium.

Although the cause of Paget's disease is unknown, research suggests that it may be due to a "slow virus" infection of bone that is present for many years before symptoms appear. A genetic etiology of Paget's disease is also probable because the disease is often present in members of the same family.

Paget's disease is rarely seen in people under the age of 40. Prevalence ranges from 1.5% to 8% of the population, depending on the individual's age and area of the world in which the person lives. Epidemiologic studies suggest that Paget's disease is decreasing both in severity at diagnosis and in prevalence.

In many instances Paget's disease is diagnosed because the client has experienced trauma and x-rays demonstrate the characteristic changes of the disease; 10% to 20% of people with the disease are asymptomatic. Before clinical manifestations occur, x-ray films show increased bone expansion and density. After clinical manifestations have developed, the bone shows a characteristic mosaic appearance (Figure 26-10). Bone scans are the most efficient means of identifying pagetic bone. Laboratory tests include indices of bone turnover such as serum alkaline phosphatase and urinary and serum deoxypyridinoline, N-telopeptide, and C-telopeptide.

In symptomatic Paget's disease, the most common presenting complaints include one or more of the following: deep, aching bone pain; skeletal deformity, such as a barrel-shaped chest, bowing of the tibia or femur, or kyphosis; changes in skin temperature; pathologic fractures through diseased bone; and manifestations related to nerve compression. Diseased bone pressing on the cranial nerves may result in headache, vertigo, hearing loss with tinnitus, and blindness. Osteoarthritis, ankylosing spondylitis, and gout are commonly associated with Paget's disease.

NSAIDs, such as ibuprofen, can often control bone pain. Pain may also be relieved with heat therapy, massage, and bracing. Further orthopedic treatment may be indicated for severe disabling arthritis, severe bowing deformities of the femur or tibia, and pathologic fractures.

Currently, therapies of choice for Paget's disease are three more potent bisphosphonates: pamidronate (Aredia), alendronate (Fosamax), and risedronate (Actonel). Etidronate (Didronel) and tiludronate (Skelid) may be appropriate treatments for some clients but are seldom used. After a course of treatment, bone turnover indices such as alkaline phosphatase return to normal in 60% to 70% of clients, reflecting suppression of abnormal bone turnover. Existing data suggest that effective disease suppression will likely reduce future disabling problems. Unfortunately, deformity and hearing loss are not corrected with these medications. Retreatment is indicated if bone turnover markers exceed the upper limit of normal (once they had decreased to within normal limits).

OSTEOMALACIA

Etiology and Pathophysiology

Osteomalacia is a disease in which the bone becomes abnormally soft because of a disturbed calcium and phosphorus balance secondary to vitamin D deficiency. Osteomalacia is characterized by widespread decalcification and softening of bones, especially in the spine, pelvis, and lower extremities. Bones become bent and flattened as they soften, leading to marked deformities of the weight-bearing bones and to pathologic fractures.

Osteomalacia mainly affects women and it is endemic in Asia, where many people avoid milk and milk products because of allergy or lactose intolerance. The most common cause of osteomalacia is malabsorption or inadequate dietary intake of vitamin D (e.g., strict vegan).[7] It is also seen in Muslim women living in Western countries because their style of dress prevents them from obtaining adequate vitamin D from sunlight exposure. Women who have had multiple pregnancies and who have breast-fed their children also have a higher rate of

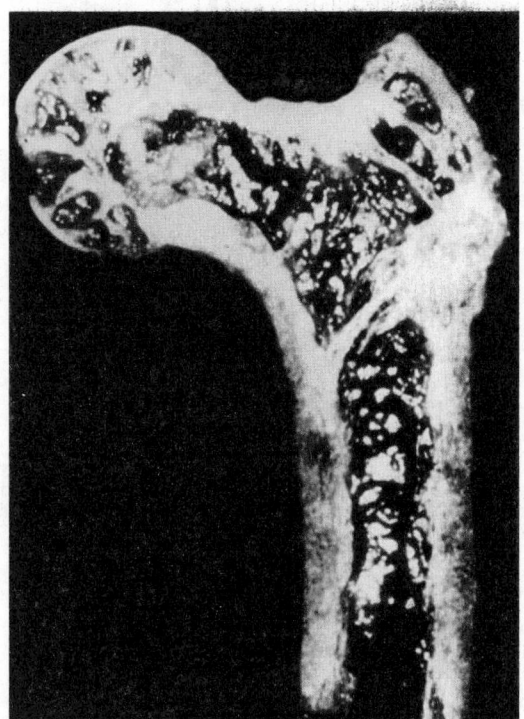

■ **FIGURE 26–10** A pagetoid bone demonstrating the characteristic mosaic pattern seen on x-ray examination. *(From Merkow, R.L., & Lane, J.M. [1990]. Paget's disease of bone. Orthopaedic Clinics of North America, 21[1], 173.)*

the disease. Osteomalacia is similar to rickets, which occurs in children, and the condition is called *adult rickets*.

Additional causes include the following:

- Chronic use of anticonvulsants
- Renal failure or disease
- Hyperthyroid-induced osteopenia
- Phosphate depletion associated with inadequate dietary intake of phosphates

Clients generally report easy fatigability, malaise, and bone pain that is diffuse, poorly localized, and accompanied by a general bony tenderness. Muscular weakness is often seen in severe cases. Serum calcium and phosphorus levels are reduced, and the alkaline phosphatase level is moderately elevated. Radiographs indicate generalized demineralization with trabecular bone loss. Pseudofractures (Milkman syndrome) and cyst formation are common. Bone biopsy may be helpful but is not typically needed for diagnosis.

Intervention for clients with osteomalacia includes daily vitamin D until signs of healing take place, at which time a daily low maintenance dose is continued. Adequate intake of calcium and phosphorus as well as protein should be ensured.

GOUT AND GOUTY ARTHRITIS

Gout is a metabolic bone disorder in which purine (protein) metabolism is altered and the by-product, uric acid, accumulates. Gout is classified as primary or secondary. *Primary* gout is caused by an inherited defect of purine metabolism, leading to increased or decreased renal excretion. It accounts for 85% of all cases, of which 95% affect men. The initial attack of gout occurs in the third or fourth decade of life.

Secondary gout is an acquired condition that occurs following hematopoietic (multiple myeloma, polycythemia vera, and leukemia) or renal disorders. In hematopoietic disorders, cell turnover and uric acid production increase. In addition, gout may develop from the rapid induction of chemotherapy or radiation therapy when there is massive destruction of cells. Renal disorders that decrease the excretion of uric acid also may lead to gout. Hyperuricemia may also result from use of aspirin, thiazide, and mercurial diuretics, and some antituberculosis medications. Alcohol intoxication and starvation increase serum urate levels by inhibiting renal excretion as a result of lactic acidosis and ketosis, respectively. In addition, alcohol ingestion increases urate production by stimulating purine breakdown. Prolonged use of diuretics and other medications (levodopa, nicotinic acid, low-dose salicylates) also reduces the excretion of uric acid and precipitates gout.

In the body, uric acid is made by the enzymatic breakdown of tissue and dietary purines. Hyperuricemia develops because of underexcretion or overproduction of uric acid. In addition to accumulation in the blood, uric acid is concentrated in the synovial fluid, myocardium, kidneys, and ears. When uric acid levels reach a certain level, they crystallize, and the crystals (tophi) are deposited in connective tissue. Because the crystals are deposited in connective tissue, gout is classified as a form of arthritis (Figure 26-11).

Clinical manifestations of gout develop in stages (Table 26-3). The presence of uric acid crystals in an aspirated sample of synovial fluid confirms the diagnosis of gout. Serum uric acid is not reliable in diagnosis of

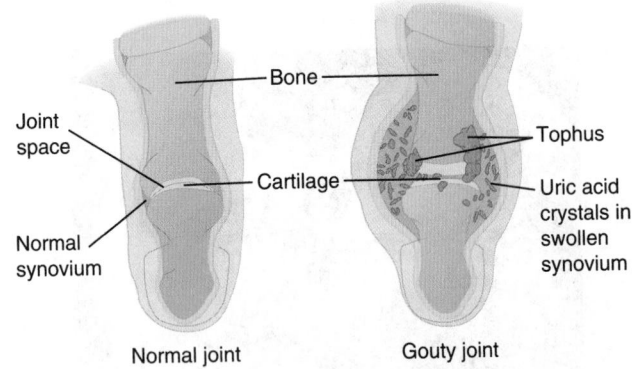

■ **FIGURE 26–11** Comparison of a gouty joint and a normal joint.

TABLE 26–3 Manifestations of Gout by Stage

Stage	Manifestations
Stage I	Asymptomatic hyperuricemia.
Stage II	Acute attack is accompanied by redness, swelling, and exquisite tenderness in one joint (toes, fingers, wrists, ankles, knees, or other joints). Great toe is most common site. First attack develops quickly, often overnight. Fever, tachycardia, malaise, and anorexia may be noted. Acute episode usually subsides within 1 week. As edema subsides, pruritus and local desquamation (tissue loss) may be noted.
Stage III	A period of time between attacks during which affected joint returns to normal and client may be asymptomatic for years. Eventually, other attacks occur.
Stage IV	Permanent changes in multiple joints with restrictions in movement. Tophi may be detected on ears, hands, elbows, feet, and knees. Renal and cardiac disorders may also develop. Client may have uric acid renal stones, renal colic, and hypertension. Atherosclerosis occurs in about 50% of all clients.

gout because 5% to 8% of the population has elevated levels (>7 mg/dl) but only 5% to 20% of clients with hyperuricemia develop gout.[11]

OUTCOME MANAGEMENT

The management of the client with gout has three components: (1) management of the *acute* attack, (2) prophylaxis to prevent acute flare-ups, and (3) *long-term* management of hyperuricemia.

Management of the acute attack includes the use of NSAIDs, corticosteroids, or colchicine (classic treatment now rarely used) to reduce pain and inflammation. Treatment choice is based primarily on the client's other health problems, such as renal insufficiency. NSAIDs are the drugs of choice in most clients without other underlying health problems. Corticosteroids can be given to clients who cannot tolerate NSAIDs or colchicine. They can be given orally, parenterally, intra-articularly, or indirectly via adrenocorticotropic hormone (ACTH). Colchicine is effective during the first 12 to 24 hours of an acute attack, but its effectiveness decreases with the duration of inflammation. It also is related to adverse gastrointestinal effects, particularly diarrhea and vomiting, in 80% of clients.[11] The initial dose of colchicine is 0.6 to 1 mg, followed by 0.5 mg/hour until pain is relieved or manifestations of toxicity develop. Use caution when giving colchicine because the therapeutic dose is close to the toxic dose. Manifestations of toxicity include nausea, vomiting, and diarrhea. Other NSAIDs can be used, such as indomethacin or naproxen. Application of ice over the inflamed joints may also relieve pain.

Medications to lower uric acid level include allopurinol, which blocks formation of uric acid, and probenecid, which promotes resorption of uric acid deposits and excretion of uric acid. Long-term medication is advised in clients who have more than two attacks of gout a year, secondary forms of gout, or persistent hyperuricemia. Salicylates (aspirin) antagonize the action of uricosuric agents and must not be used concurrently.

Opinions differ regarding dietary treatment for gout. In the past, a low-purine intake was used to eliminate many proteins from the diet. Diet modifications may only improve serum uric acid by 1 mg/dl, and are thus rarely able to decrease levels sufficiently to prevent future attacks. Encourage ample fluid intake (2000 to 3000 ml/day) to promote excretion of uric acid. A moderate intake of distilled forms of alcohol does not seem to precipitate gouty attacks; beer, ale, and wine may precipitate them. Excessive alcohol in any form should be avoided; heavy drinkers are much more likely to have recurrent attacks, even with allopurinol therapy.

Gradual weight loss is encouraged after the initial attack. Weight loss alone may reduce the incidence of attacks and uric acid levels; however, a sudden loss of weight may precipitate an attack because of the destruction of cells, which release uric acid.

Clients who can recognize early manifestations of gout may be able to avert the attack by the prompt use of colchicine or indomethacin. Long-term side effects (alopecia, bone marrow suppression, hepatic damage) from these agents, although rare, should be explained to the client.

Nursing management of the client with gout includes pain control. The client is usually placed on bed rest until pain subsides. Once ambulating, the client's need for crutches or a walker should be considered until gait is stable. Explain dietary restrictions, fluid requirements, and long-term self-management.

SPINAL COLUMN DEFORMITIES

The characteristic S curve of the lateral spine develops during fetal life and early childhood. Because other abnormal curves can occur because of defects in the bone, muscles, or nerves, every spinal problem must be considered from both an orthopedic and a neurologic viewpoint.

SCOLIOSIS

In the coronal plane, the spine should appear completely straight. Scoliosis is lateral curvature of the spine in any area—cervical, thoracic, thoracolumbar, or lumbar. It is important to distinguish curvature of *structural* origin from that of *nonstructural* origin. A structural curvature does not correct itself on forced bending against the curvature, and vertebral rotation can be demonstrated. A nonstructural curvature is easily corrected on forced bending or in the supine position, and rotation of the vertebral bodies is not demonstrated.

Idiopathic scoliosis is the most common form, appearing in growing children with no other apparent health problems. Scoliosis occurs most often in preadolescents and adolescents. It was once believed to be primarily a problem in girls, but school screening studies have shown small degrees of abnormal spinal curvature in equal numbers of boys and girls. Both boys and girls should be observed until it is proven that a curve is not progressive. Adult scoliosis may be the progression of a childhood condition that was undiagnosed or untreated when the person was still growing. It can also be caused by degenerative changes in the spine. Continued curve progression is possible even after skeletal maturity if the curvature is greater than 40 or 45 degrees, and excessive curvature can lead to cardiopulmonary problems and pain that prompt the client to seek medical care. The client may also seek help because of cosmetic deformity and loss in height. Skeletally mature clients with a curve less than 20 degrees do not require treatment. Skeletally immature clients with a curve between 20 and 40 degrees require brace management, whereas clients with curves greater than 45 degrees need surgical intervention.

Etiology

The cause of scoliosis can be congenital or neuromuscular. *Congenital scoliosis* results from a malformation of the bony vertebral segment of the spine, either because of failure of (1) formation (the absence of a portion of a vertebra) or because of failure of (2) segmentation (the absence of normal separations between vertebrae). Neuromuscular conditions associated with spinal deformities include cerebral palsy, syringomyelia, polio, myelomeningocele, spinal muscle atrophy, spinal cord tumors, trauma, and myopathic conditions such as muscular dystrophy.

Clinical Manifestations

Clinical manifestations and a family history of spinal deformity are significant, but diagnosis is confirmed by upright posteroanterior and lateral radiographs that reveal a curvature of 10 degrees or more (Figure 26-12, *A*). Curves less than 10 degrees are considered to represent spinal asymmetry rather than scoliosis. X-rays are the only exact tool for monitoring changes in spinal deformity, but excessive radiation exposure is inappropriate in children. Two other noninvasive diagnostic techniques—Moiré topography and the integrated shape-imaging system (ISIS)—produce images on the back surface shape that can be correlated to underlying spinal deformities.

OUTCOME MANAGEMENT

Nonsurgical treatments for clients with spinal deformity consist of observation and bracing. Large trials of other forms of treatment, including electrical stimulation, physical therapy, and chiropractic manipulation, have failed to demonstrate reduced spinal curvature or prevention of curvature progression. Each client needs to be evaluated individually, not only for the medical problem but also for willingness to participate in any suggested therapies. One client may refuse to wear a brace under any circumstances; another may insist on treatment for even a slight curvature.

The decision to proceed with surgical treatment is based not only on the failure of conservative treatments but also on additional factors, such as the client's emotional stability and readiness to undergo a major procedure. Spinal fusion is the ultimate goal in many cases, attaching adjacent vertebrae to each other with a bone graft so the curve will not continue to progress to adulthood. The surgical approach can be posterior or

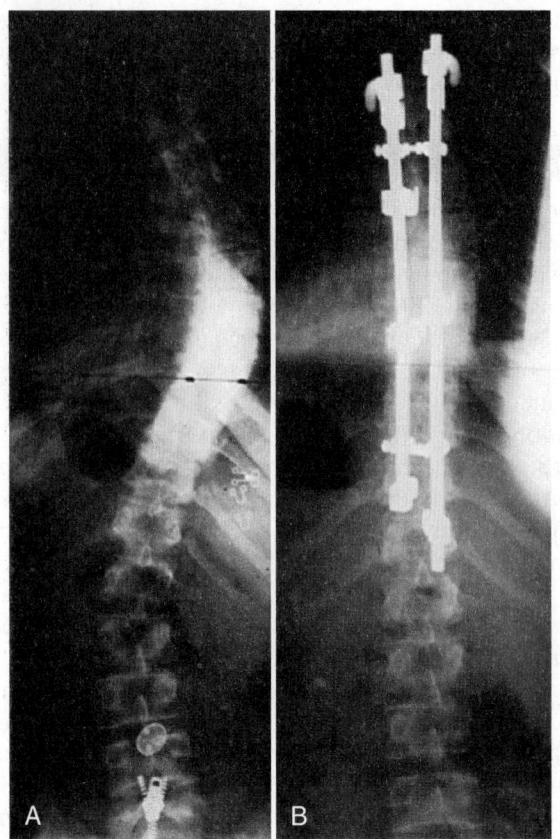

■ **FIGURE 26–12 A,** Scoliosis. **B,** Postoperative x-ray after correction with Cotrel-Dubousset instrumentation. *(From Maher, A.B., Salmond, S.W., & Pellino, T.A. [Eds.]. [2002]. Orthopedic nursing [3rd ed.]. Philadelphia: Saunders.)*

anterior, depending on the location of the deformity. A combined anterior-posterior approach has become increasingly popular for adults with severe thoracolumbar scoliosis.

Various types of instruments can be used to stabilize the spine and correct deformity. The choice of instrumentation is based on the diagnosis, the magnitude of the curvature and the flexibility of the curve, the client's age and inherent bone strength, and the client's ability to wear a postoperative immobilization device. The Cotrel-Dubousset (CD), Texas Scottish Rite Hospital (TSRH), Moss-Miami, and Luque systems are commonly used for a posterior approach (see Figure 26-12, *B*). The Harrington rod system, developed in the 1960s, is still in use because of its availability and because many surgeons are familiar with it. The most common types of instrumentation for an anterior approach are the Zielke and Harris systems.

Complications

Possible complications following scoliosis surgery include neurologic compromise, infection, respiratory problems, spinal fluid leakage, phlebitis, excessive blood loss, implant problems, and pseudarthrosis. The most devastating complications are paralysis and death.

Postoperative Care

Postoperative nursing management focuses on the usual postoperative care (see Chapter 14). Frequent and close assessment of motor and sensory function in the lower extremities is important because the nerves and muscles may have been stretched in surgery. Maintenance of spine immobility is critical. Bending, lifting, and twisting are discouraged in the immediate postoperative period and up to 3 months after hospital discharge, based on physician assessment. Some physicians may prescribe a brace to assist with maintenance of spine precautions. Other postoperative care is discussed in the section on lumbar fusion in Chapter 71.

KYPHOSIS

Also called "humpback" or "dowager's hump," the term *kyphosis* describes a posterior rounding of the thoracic spine. Whereas a certain degree of kyphosis is considered normal, curvatures greater than 45 degrees are believed to be excessive and require additional evaluation as to the cause. Kyphosis is identified as *postural* if the client can voluntarily hyperextend the spine to correct the curvature and if there is no radiographic evidence of structural change. Kyphosis is common in metabolic disorders such as osteoporosis and osteomalacia, but it can also accompany neuromuscular diseases such as cerebral palsy and muscular dystrophy. Severe curvature can affect cardiopulmonary and gastrointestinal function, making intervention essential.

Kyphosis is most often treated with bracing to straighten the spine. Exercises to strengthen muscles and ligaments may also be encouraged. Spinal fusion with or without instrumentation may be required if the curve is severe and progressive, neurologic symptoms exist, and response to other interventions is inadequate.[16]

LORDOSIS

Lordosis is an excessive inward curvature of the lumbar spine that is sometimes seen in pregnant or obese clients or in people with large abdominal tumors. Extreme lordosis may lead to *swayback,* in which the lumbosacral spine curves sharply and the thoracolumbar spine exhibits kyphosis. Lordosis is often associated with sagging shoulders, an exaggerated pelvic angle, and medial rotation of the legs. If necessary, treatment may consist of bracing, spinal fusion, or osteotomy. Hyperlordosis in young children and prepubertal girls is a self-correcting problem thought to be related to rapid skeletal growth without corresponding soft tissue growth.

BONE INFECTIONS

Musculoskeletal system contamination can result either as infection spreads from other sites in the body or from external insults (e.g., puncture, surgery). Infections are often severe and difficult to treat because the bones are relatively inaccessible to protective macrophages and antibodies. Even a small number of microorganisms can be enough to establish a serious infection that can lead to loss of function or even death. For this reason, nurses should be diligent in wound care and alert to any manifestations that suggest infection.

OSTEOMYELITIS

Overview

Osteomyelitis is a severe pyogenic infection of bone and surrounding tissues. Although generally bacterial in origin, osteomyelitis can also be caused by a virus or fungus. *Staphylococcus aureus* is the most common infecting organism, but *Escherichia coli, Pseudomonas, Klebsiella, Salmonella,* and *Proteus* organisms may also be found.

> **Because osteomyelitis can be extraordinarily difficult to cure even with long-term antibiotics, prompt recognition is crucial. Delayed identification or inadequate treatment can result in a chronic infection accompanied by continuing pain, chronically draining sinuses, loss of function, amputation, or death.**
>
> SAFETY ⚠ ALERT

Osteomyelitis occurs most frequently in the femur, tibia, sacrum, and heels. Males are affected more often than females, often as a result of trauma. Susceptibility to infection increases with IV drug use, diabetes, immunocompromising diseases, or a history of bloodstream infections. Osteomyelitis also develops in pressure ulcers and other chronic open wounds. Limiting the spread of osteomyelitis may also be more difficult in clients with a disorder such as malnutrition, alcoholism, or liver failure.

Clinical manifestations may vary slightly according to the site of involvement. Infection in the long bones is generally accompanied by acute localized pain and redness or drainage, often with a history of recent trauma or newly acquired prostheses. However, pain may be absent in debilitated clients (overlying pressure sore that does not heal) or clients with diabetes and osteomyelitis of the foot. Fever and malaise may be present, but adults do not always appear acutely ill with other systemic manifestations. Infection in the vertebrae usually causes pain and mobility difficulties. The client with vertebral osteomyelitis often reports a history of genitourinary infection or drug abuse.

Laboratory studies and x-rays or bone scans are important in the definitive diagnosis of osteomyelitis.

Elevated ESR is common but leukocytosis is variable. Along with clinical manifestations, laboratory results usually allow initial diagnosis and early treatment while the physician waits for further evidence from blood cultures or needle aspirate analysis. Early osteomyelitis can be diagnosed by technetium bone scan or MRI, which can detect lesions within 24 to 72 hours after the onset of infection. Advanced infection can be diagnosed by x-ray, usually 3 to 4 weeks after infection develops.

OUTCOME MANAGEMENT

Elimination of the infecting organism, both locally from the bone and systemically from the body, is the major treatment goal for acute osteomyelitis. Prompt treatment also prevents further bone deformity and injury, increases client comfort, and avoids complications of impaired mobility. Surgery is initially performed on the adult client with osteomyelitis to ensure effective debridement and drainage, elimination of dead space, and adequate soft tissue coverage. Antibiotics alone rarely resolve infection in adults, but they do work more effectively after surgical preparation of the treatment area. High doses of parenteral antibiotics are frequently administered for 4 to 8 weeks to achieve a bactericidal level in the bone tissue. Oral antibiotics are continued for another 4 to 8 weeks, with serial bone scans and ESR measurements performed to evaluate the effectiveness of drug therapy. Open, draining wounds are packed with gauze to promote drainage. Hyperbaric oxygen therapy has been used as an adjunct to antibiotics and surgical debridement. If initial treatment is delayed or inadequate, the necrotic bone separates from the living bone to form *sequestra,* which serve as a medium for additional microorganism growth. Chronic osteomyelitis can result.

SEPTIC ARTHRITIS

Overview

Septic arthritis (also known as pyogenic arthritis, infectious arthritis, septic joint disease, bacterial arthritis, and suppurative arthritis) is a closed-space infection caused by invasion of the synovial membrane by pus-forming bacteria or other pathogens. Joints most commonly affected in adult clients are the knee, hip, shoulder, wrist, and ankle.

A variety of microorganisms may infect the joint, but *Neisseria gonorrhoeae* is the most common causative pathogen in adults under 30 years of age. A significant percentage of staphylococci, the second most common causative organism in adults, is methicillin resistant. *S. aureus* invades the joint through hematogenous spread, as an extension of adjacent soft tissue infection, or from direct inoculation following trauma or an invasive procedure.

Hematogenous spread, in which organisms reach the joint from a remote site, is the most common etiologic mechanism. Because the synovial membrane is very vascular, any microorganism that is circulating in the blood may be easily trapped in the synovial space. Upper respiratory tract infection, otitis media, furuncle, or impetigo may seed a susceptible site such as a previously traumatized or diseased knee joint.

The presence of septic arthritis typically reflects the failure of multiple defense mechanisms. In the early stages of infection, the synovial membrane swells and becomes infiltrated with neutrophils. A purulent effusion distends the joint as the neutrophils release lysosomal proteolytic enzymes that destroy the articular cartilage, subchondral bone, and joint capsule. Enzymatic cartilage destruction can actually occur in 3 to 24 hours, creating a medical emergency that requires prompt treatment to avoid permanent joint damage.

The client often presents with complaints of pain, swelling, warmth, and tenderness in a single joint and also generally experiences an acute systemic reaction. The adult client is more likely than the child to experience only a low-grade fever and malaise; however, high temperatures and shaking chills are generally present in the client who has positive blood cultures.

Assessment focuses on the presence of factors that may predispose the client to joint infection, such as recent surgery or injury, diagnostic procedures, IV drug abuse, or systemic disease. Because effective treatment requires accurate identification of the causative agent, initial laboratory studies attempt to differentiate septic arthritis from autoimmune diseases with joint involvement (such as rheumatoid arthritis). Complete blood cell count (CBC), ESR, the antinuclear antibody (ANA) test, and rheumatoid factor (RF) measurements are often among the studies that are ordered. In addition, joint fluid is aspirated for analysis, and a synovial biopsy is performed. Radioisotope scanning techniques may also be helpful in the early detection of infection.

OUTCOME MANAGEMENT

Antibiotic therapy is a critical part of effective treatment of septic arthritis and must be promptly initiated to prevent permanent joint damage. Choice of antibiotic is empirically based initially on the most common causative organism given the client's age or history. After the specific organism and its sensitivities have been identified from synovial fluid cultures, the antibiotic therapy may be altered. Treatment time varies according to the duration of clinical manifestations, the causative organism, and the status of the client's immune system. For most clients, parenteral antibiotics are administered for 2 to 3 weeks and oral antibiotics continue for another 1 or 2 weeks. Older clients or those with more complex presentations may require parenteral therapy lasting 4 to 6 weeks. Decompression of the infected joint is also necessary, although controversy exists about the best methods. Open synovectomy and debridement or repeated joint aspirations and irrigations may be performed. Arthroscopic drainage and debridement have also been successful.

Effective nursing management requires scrupulous attention to the client's joint position, exercise, and rehabilitation. In the acute phase of septic arthritis, the client is likely to hold the joint in slight to moderate flexion as a position of comfort. Because this can lead to flexion deformities, slings, immobilizers, or splints may be used temporarily to hold the joint in an optimal position. As inflammation begins to resolve, passive ROM exercises are initiated to preserve joint function. CPM has also been used with some success. Active motion and weight-bearing may not be initiated until clinical manifestations and inflammation have almost totally disappeared. Pain management is also important for the client with septic arthritis to provide comfort and to allow greater ease in exercise participation.

BONE TUMORS

A bone tumor *(cancer)* may be benign or malignant (Table 26-4). Benign bone tumors may remain undiagnosed because they often cause no pain. They may be noted as an incidental x-ray finding when the client is being evaluated for another complaint, such as fracture through a bone cyst; however, benign tumors that grow aggressively can cause bone pain, weakness, and destruction.

Malignant Bone Tumors

Primary malignant tumors that originate in bone cells or form within the bone are relatively rare, representing less than 1% of all malignant tumors. Malignant bone tumors include osteosarcoma, fibrosarcoma, chondrosarcoma, and Ewing's sarcoma. Clients typically present with bone pain, particularly at night, and fracture may occur from even slight trauma. Occasionally a mass or lesion may be felt at the tumor site. Clients may also report weight loss, fever, chills, or pulmonary manifestations.

The exact cause of primary bone tumors remains largely unknown, but several factors are believed to play a role in their development. Past trauma has been associated with tumor development, as has exposure to carcinogens such as asbestos, dioxin, and radium. Bone tumors may also develop from benign medical conditions (enchondromatosis, neurofibromatosis) or from metabolic conditions (Paget's disease). Fewer than 5% of clients with malignancies have a hereditary tendency to cancer.

Metastatic bone tumors, which are more prevalent than sarcomas, spread to the bone from primary carcinomas in sites such as the breast, prostate, lung, and kidney. Thyroid, bladder, uterine, colorectal, and vaginal cancers can also metastasize to bone. Cancer cells may spread directly within a body cavity, or they may metastasize by hematogenous or lymphatic spread.

TABLE 26–4 Primary Bone and Cartilage Tumors

Type	Description
Benign Cartilage-Forming Tumor	
Enchondroma	Lesion in mature cartilage but lacking histologic characteristic of chondrosarcoma; found in hands, feet, humerus, ribs, femur; age range, 20-40 yr
Osteochondroma	Most common bone tumor; cartilage-capped bony projection on external bone surface; metaphyses of long bone, especially proximal tibia and distal femur; age range, birth-30 yr
Benign Bone-Forming Tumor	
Osteoid osteoma	Small osteoblastic lesion (less than 1 cm) with demarcated outline and reactive bone formation; femur and tibia; age range, 10-20 yr
Osteoblastoma	Similar to osteoid osteoma but larger (>2 cm); spine, long bones, hand
Giant cell tumor (osteoclastoma)	Aggressive benign bone tumor with richly vascularized tissue consisting of plump spindle-shaped cells and numerous giant cells; distal femur, proximal tibia, distal radius, proximal humerus; age range, 20-40 yr
Malignant Bone-Forming Tumor	
Osteosarcoma	Most common primary malignant bone tumor; formation of bone or osteoid by tumor cell; metaphyses, especially of distal femur, proximal tibia, and proximal humerus; intramedullary region involved; age range, 10-30 yr
Ewing's sarcoma	Composed of densely packed small cells with round nuclei; often confused with osteomyelitis because it presents with fever, anemia, leukocytosis, increased ESR; diaphyseal regions of long and flat bones; age range, 5-15 yr
Fibrosarcoma	Formation of spindle-shaped tumor cells of interlacing bundles of collagen fibers, absence of other types of histologic differentiation; femur, tibia; age range, 5-80 yr
Malignant Cartilage-Forming Tumor	
Chondrosarcoma	Formation of cartilage by tumor cells; higher cellularity and greater pleomorphism than in chondromas; femur, pelvis, ribs, scapula; age range, 30-60 yr

Data from Haynes, K.K. (2001). In D.C. Schoen (Ed.), *NAON core curriculum for orthopaedic nursing* (4th ed.). Pitman, NJ: National Association of Orthopaedic Nurses.

Laboratory studies such as CBC, blood and urine calcium levels, and ESR assist in client evaluation, but they are not diagnostic themselves. Other laboratory tests, however, are used as tumor markers. An elevated serum alkaline phosphatase (AP) level may be noted with osteoblastic tumors, for example, and lactate dehydrogenase (LDH) may mark tumor progression for Ewing's sarcoma. A plain radiograph in anterior and posterior views may provide an initial diagnosis, but other studies—such as a CT scan, MRI, or bone scan—are also commonly performed. A bone biopsy is needed for definitive diagnosis of metastatic bone disease.

OUTCOME MANAGEMENT

The treatment goal for the client with a primary tumor is to eradicate the tumor completely and to promote long-term survival. *Chemotherapy* has dramatically increased the survival of clients diagnosed with primary bone tumors. *Radiation therapy* has become safer because of an increased understanding of cancer and radiobiology; it is also now better tolerated through the use of radiation machines that reduce skin sensitivity. Radiation therapy may be used to decrease tumor size, improve bone strength, and help in pain management. It can be administered alone or in combination with surgery.[2] *Surgery* may be performed to eradicate the disease, either through excision of the tumor and a wide zone of surrounding normal tissue or through amputation. If the tumor is excised, the resulting defect is repaired by using a joint prosthesis or bone graft with internal fixation. The bone graft can be taken from the client at another anatomic site, or an allograft (cadaver) bone may be used.

For the client with metastatic disease, treatment goals include (1) palliation, (2) remission, and (3) extension of life. Pain management requires a collaborative effort of the client, family, and all members of the health care team. Because metastatic tumors can cause severe pain and have the potential to fracture, lesions in the long bones are commonly managed with excision, followed by insertion of intramedullary rods to stabilize the weakened bone. PMMA cement may be used to provide immediate stability, restore function, and supplement poor bone quality.[2] Clients not suitable for surgery are those with limited life expectancy, other severe medical problems, or small lesions treatable with radiation alone. Pain management following surgery is a major focus. Pain should be addressed aggressively and medication effectiveness assessed regularly. Opioids are often delivered by PCA pumps or via epidural catheter. Oral administration facilitates home care management for the client with metastatic tumors, but IV or transdermal medications may be indicated for the client with gastric problems. Other analgesics, such as acetaminophen and anti-inflammatory medications, may also be used because they act on the peripheral pain mechanism. Adjuvant medications, including antidepressants and anticonvulsants, are frequently used to increase the effectiveness of conventional analgesics. The key to pain management is to administer all analgesics on an around-the-clock (ATC) rather than on an as-needed (prn) basis.

Frequent position changes and stimulation of nontumor areas through heat, cold, or massage may be beneficial. Nonpharmacologic strategies, such as music therapy, imagery, and relaxation techniques, may provide powerful adjuncts to opioid administration. Postoperative nursing care also addresses the possible complications related to orthopedic surgery, including infection, DVT, and non-union of grafted bone. Attempts at pain management for the client with a metastatic bone tumor may ultimately lead to a palliative neurosurgical procedure, such as a chordotomy, in which the anterolateral spinal cord tracts are severed to provide relief in the affected areas.

DISORDERS OF THE FOOT

HALLUX VALGUS (BUNIONS)

Bunions, a common foot deformity that involves the first metatarsal and the great toe (hallux), occur nine times more often in women than in men. Bunions may occur as a congenital disorder, or they may be acquired during periods of rapid growth, such as adolescence. They may also occur as a result of local irritation related to restrictive footwear. They result from a pronation abnormality and from hypermobility of the first metatarsal, phalanx, and cuneiform joints. The client typically complains of pain as the bony prominence of the metatarsal head becomes irritated from pushing against the inside of a shoe. *Calluses* under the second and third metatarsal heads occur from a shift in weight-bearing and may also cause pain. Standard anteroposterior and lateral x-rays show exostosis of the first metatarsal head with subluxation or dislocation.

To decrease pressure over the bunion and minimize the likelihood of bursitis, the client may try conservative treatment, consisting entirely of wearing shoes with a larger toe box to allow more space for the forefoot. If a change in footwear does not provide enough relief, orthoses may be ordered or steroid injections administered for acute inflammation. Surgery may be considered if conservative treatment fails, if the client desires cosmetic correction of the deformity, or if functioning of the lateral four toes is also affected. The procedure is designed to realign the great toe through osteotomy of the hallux or through fusion of the metatarsophalangeal joint (Figure 26-13). In addition to routine care, the client who has undergone bunionectomy may use open-toed flat shoes for ambulation.

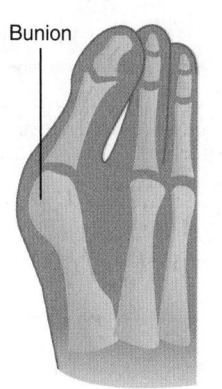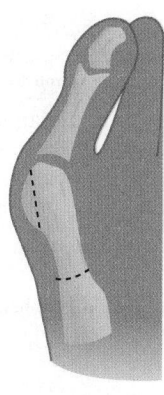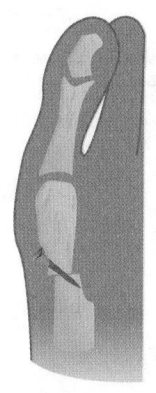

Bunion

Typical cuts in the bone

Typical realignment and screw fixation

■ **FIGURE 26–13** Bunions and their surgical correction.

MORTON'S NEUROMA (PLANTAR NEUROMA)

Athletes commonly experience Morton's neuroma because of excessive pressure placed on the branch of the medial plantar nerve between the third and fourth toes. The pressure causes a *neuroma,* or swelling of the nerve, that leads the client to complain of pain in the ball of the foot. Depending on the extent of the compression, pain may radiate into the toes and be accompanied by numbness. Pain may be increased if the client wears tight-fitting or high-heeled shoes. Hyperextension of the metatarsophalangeal joints or repetitive impact on the forefoot may also increase pain.

The usual treatment involves changing the type of shoe to one with a larger toe box that provides more room for the forefoot. Anti-inflammatory medications are often prescribed. If these are ineffective, steroid injections may be administered. Surgery to remove the neuroma may be considered if other treatments do not produce long-term relief.

HAMMER TOE

Hammer toe is a deformity caused by a flexion contracture of the proximal interphalangeal joint (PIP) with extension or slight hyperextension of the DIP. This deformity often accompanies hallux valgus and may occur in clients with a family history of hammer toe, rheumatoid arthritis (RA), and clawfeet. Hammer toe leads to improper fit of footwear, creating pain with walking and a change in gait patterns. Corns and calluses on pressure areas of the foot may need to be removed.

Treatment centers on choosing footwear with a wide toe box. Pads and inserts can help relieve pressure, but they can also cause previously unaffected areas of the foot to rub against the shoe. Osteotomy of the toe and resection of the proximal phalanx may be required for symptom relief.

MUSCULAR DISORDERS

MUSCULAR DYSTROPHY

Muscular dystrophy (MD) is a term that generally designates a group of genetic disorders involving gradual degeneration of muscle fibers. (For information on myotonic dystrophy, an autosomal-dominant disorder that affects skeletal muscle and smooth muscle as well as other body tissues, see the Genetic Links feature below.) The client experiences progressive weakness

GENETIC LINKS

Myotonic Dystrophy

DESCRIPTION

Myotonic dystrophy is an autosomal-dominant disorder that affects skeletal muscle and smooth muscle as well as other body tissues, including the eyes, heart, endocrine system, and CNS. There are three forms of myotonic dystrophy (DM for Dystrophy: Myotonic): mild, classical, and congenital. Mild DM presents with cataracts and mild myotonia (sustained muscle contraction); life span is normal. Classical DM is characterized by muscle weakness and wasting, myotonia, cataracts, and cardiac dysrhythmias; adults may be physically disabled and have a shortened life span. Congenital DM is associated with hypotonia and severe generalized weakness at birth, often with respiratory insufficiency, mental retardation, and early death. DM is considered the most common muscular dystrophy that affects adults, occurring in approximately 1 in 8000 people.

GENETICS

DM is caused by an unstable inherited mutation in the myotonic dystrophy protein kinase gene (*DMPK* gene) located on chromosome 19. The disease mutation is an expanded CTG trinucleotide repeat that lies in the *DMPK* gene. The number of CTG repeats is strongly correlated with disease severity. Unaffected normal people can have from 5 to 37 CTG repeats. CTG repeat length exceeding 37 repeats is abnormal. The number of repeats often increases through successive generations, accompanied by increasing severity of the disorder and earlier age of onset (a tendency known as *anticipation*). Offspring of an affected individual have a 50% chance of inheriting the disease-causing mutation.

DIAGNOSIS/TESTING

Diagnosis is based on family history and clinical findings and is confirmed by the detection of an expansion of the CTG trinucleotide repeat in the *DMPK* gene. DNA-based testing is essentially 100% sensitive and is clinically available.

MANAGEMENT

No specific treatment for the progressive weakness of DM exists. Treatment can be offered to manage certain manifestations associated with the disease (e.g., medications to counter the effects of myotonia, surgery for cataracts, close monitoring of cardiac status).

TABLE 26–5 Clinical Features in Muscular Dystrophy

Feature	Duchenne MD	Becker MD	Limb Girdle MD
Incidence	Most common type of MD	Less common than Duchenne MD	Less common than Duchenne or Becker MD
Age at onset	Usually <3 yr	Usually 5-15 yr	Usually by second decade
Inheritance	Sex-linked recessive gene, autosomal <10%	Sex-linked recessive gene	Usually autosomal recessive
Pattern of muscle involvement	Onset: Selected symmetrical weakness of proximal pelvic muscles, 3-5 yr Later: shoulder girdle muscle involvement	Similar to Duchenne MD	Proximal shoulder and pelvic girdle
Late muscle involvement	Affects all muscles, including facial, oculopharyngeal, and respiratory	Face spared	Peripheral brachioradialis, hand, and calf
Pseudohypertrophy	Calf muscles	Calf muscles	Occurs in fewer than one third of cases
Contractural deformities	Common	Less common	Occurs in late disease; milder than Duchenne MD
Scoliosis/kyphoscoliosis	Common in late disease	Not severe	Mild in late disease
Heart involvement	Yes	Uncommon in late disease	Rare
Intelligence quotient	Decreased	Normal	Normal
Course	Steady progression	Slow progression	Slow progression, with greater variation among clients

Data from Mason, K.J. (2001). Pediatric and congenital disorders. In D.C. Schoen (Ed.), *NAON core curriculum for orthopedic nursing* (4th ed.). Pitman, NJ: National Association of Orthopaedic Nurses.

and skeletal muscle wasting accompanied by disability and deformity. The various forms of MD are differentiated by the affected muscle groups, the client's age at onset of the disease, the rate of progression, and the inheritance mode (Table 26-5). *Pseudohypertrophic MD* (Duchenne MD) is the most common and severe form of the disease. A sex-linked recessive disorder that affects males almost exclusively, it has been linked to an abnormality of the *Xp21* gene locus. The client experiences wheelchair dependency in early adolescence. Respiratory muscles are eventually involved, and myocardial degeneration leads to cardiomegaly and tachycardia. *Becker MD* is a milder form of the disease that progresses slowly over the course of decades. Some clients with Becker MD need a wheelchair by age 30, although many manage for years with minor aids such as a cane.

Diagnosis of MD is accomplished through use of multiple modalities in an attempt to differentiate the disease from other disorders, such as myasthenia gravis and polymyositis. The most valuable laboratory test is serum creatine kinase analysis; levels are elevated in clients with MD because of an abnormality of striated muscle function. Enzyme levels do decrease, however, as muscle mass decreases. Electromyography may show changes in the pattern of muscle activity consistent with disease.[3] Muscle biopsy is essential to diagnosis of a neuromuscular disease such as Duchenne's MD. Muscle shows degeneration, with fibers replaced by connective tissue and fat in later stages of the disease.

Treatment is largely symptomatic and supportive because there is currently no cure for MD. Care is aimed at increasing the comfort and functional ability through corrective surgery for related deformities or use of braces for the spine or lower extremities. Breathing exercises may also be initiated for respiratory decompensation. Death generally results from respiratory or cardiac failure by late teens or early 20s for the client with Duchenne MD.

RHABDOMYOLYSIS

Rhabdomyolysis is the breakdown of muscle fibers with leakage of potentially toxic cellular contents into the systemic circulation. The most common causes of rhabdomyolysis are trauma and ischemic conditions of the muscle. Traumatic conditions include significant blunt trauma, electrical injury, extensive burns, and prolonged immobilization. Levels of serum creatine kinase (CK) are 5 to 10 times above normal. Hemoglobin and myoglobin may also be found in the urine. Emergency treatment is with large volumes of IV fluids to prevent obstruction of the kidney from the particles of hemoglobin and myoglobin. Hyperkalemia is also present and often requires emergency treatment. Nursing responsibility is to have a high index of suspicion for clients who are at risk, such as those who have had unwitnessed stroke and have been unconscious for an unknown period of time, victims of trauma or assault, or clients who for any reason have remained in one position for many hours, rendering the muscles ischemic.

CONCLUSIONS

The focus of this chapter has been musculoskeletal disorders, including metabolic bone diseases such as osteoporosis. Osteoarthritis is a common degenerative disorder that is often treated with joint replacement surgery. Special nursing care is required after such surgery to maximize the client's outcome. Benign and metastatic bone tumors, common foot disorders, and MD, a hereditary neuromuscular disorder, have also been discussed. An understanding of these disorders is essential for the nurse who provides care for affected clients.

THINKING CRITICALLY

1. You meet an older woman in the total joint class who is considering joint replacement surgery but has not yet scheduled the procedure with her orthopedist. She has osteoarthritis and, because of increasing pain in her hips, she now uses a wheelchair when she goes out in public. She tells you she also has diabetes mellitus. What would you discuss with her to help her prepare appropriately for surgery?

Factors to Consider. What would be the benefit of increased upper arm strength for this client? Is she maintaining tight control of the diabetes? Is weight loss an issue before surgery?

2. A middle-age client is concerned about bone loss resulting from osteoporosis. She tells you that her mother has severe osteoporosis, and she realizes her lifestyle and family history are predisposing factors. She asks you to suggest a lifestyle program for her and her daughters. How should you proceed?

Factors to Consider. What focused assessment should you complete? How should you complete teaching for the client and her daughters?

3. An older woman tells you her physician wants her to eat a diet high in calcium. He wants her to consume 1500 mg of calcium without taking enriched antacids or calcium supplements. This woman is lactose intolerant and has a hiatal hernia. She lives alone on a limited income. What problems might impair her compliance with the prescribed treatment regimen?

Factors to Consider. What dietary sources of calcium are appropriate for the lactose-intolerant client? How does the presence of a hiatal hernia affect dietary intake?

Discussions for these questions can be found on the website.

BIBLIOGRAPHY

Citations appearing in red refer to primary research.

Citations appearing in blue refer to evidence-based practice guidelines and protocols.

1. Agency for Healthcare Research and Quality (AHRQ). (2002). *S-Adenosyl-L-methionine for treatment of depression, osteoarthritis,*
and liver disease. Evidence Report/Technology Assessment No. 64. Retrieved 06/01/07 from www.ahrq.gov/clinic/epcsums/samesum.htm.
2. American Academy of Orthopaedic Surgeons (AAOS). (2005). *Metastatic bone disease.* Retrieved 06/01/07 from www.orthoinfo.aaos.org/indepth/thr_report.cfm?Thread_ID=13&topcategory=Tumors.
3. American Academy of Orthopaedic Surgeons (AAOS). (2004). *Muscular dystrophy.* Retrieved 06/01/07 from www.orthoinfo.aaos.org/fact/thr_report.cfm?Thread_ID=441&topcategory=Children.
4. American Academy of Orthopaedic Surgeons (AAOS). (2004). *Minimally invasive hip replacement.* Retrieved 06/01/07 from www.orthoinfo.aaos.org/fact/thr_report.cfm?Thread_ID=471&topcategory=Children.
5. American College of Rheumatology (ACR) Subcommittee on Osteoarthritis Guidelines. (2001). Recommendations for the medical management of osteoarthritis of the hip and knee: 2000 update. *Arthritis and Rheumatology, 43,* 1905-1915.
6. American Society of Anesthesiologists. (2003). What you should know about herbal and dietary supplement use and anesthesia. Retrieved 06/01/07 from www.asahq.org/patientEducation/herbPatient.pdf.
7. Bratzler, D.W., & Houck, P.M., for the Surgical Infection Prevention Guidelines Writers Workgroup. (2004). Antimicrobial prophylaxis for surgery: An advisory statement from the National Surgical Infection Prevention Project. *Clinical Infectious Diseases, 38,* 1706-1715.
8. Demissie, S., Cupples, L.A., Myers, R., et al. (2002). Genome scan for quantity of hand osteoarthritis: The Framingham Study. *Arthritis & Rheumatism, 46*(4), 946-952.
9. Felson, D.T. (2006). Osteoarthritis of the knee. *New England Journal of Medicine, 354*(8), 841-848.
10. Francis, M.L., & Ranatunga, S.M. (2006). *Gout.* Retrieved 06/01/07 from www.emedicine.com/med/topic924.htm#section~workup.
11. GlaxoSmithKline. (2006). *Heparin-induced thrombocytopenia: One of the most important immunohematologic problems in clinical medicine.* Retrieved 06/01/07 from www.argatroban.com/argatroban_aboutHIT.htm.
12. Gokce-Kutsal, Y., Ozcakar, L., Sekiyurt, N., et al. (2007). Epidemiological multi-center study on osteoporosis. The EDMUSTO study. *Rheumatology International, 13.*
13. Haynes, K. (2002). Neoplasms of the musculoskeletal system. In A.B. Maher, S.W. Salmond, & T.A. Pellino (Eds.), *Orthopaedic nursing* (4th ed.). Philadelphia: Saunders.
14. Iorio, R., Healy, W.L., & Appleby, D. (2004). Preoperative demand matching is a valid indicator of patient activity after total hip arthroplasty. *Journal of Arthroplasty, 19*(7), 825-828.
15. Labeling changes for arthritis drug. (2002). *FDA Consumer, 36*(5).
16. Lowe, T.G. (2006). *Treatment of kyphosis and Sherman's disease.* Retrieved 06/21/07 from www.spineuniverse.com/displayarticle.php/article3095.html.
17. Maher, A.B. (2002). Assessment of the musculoskeletal system. In A.B. Maher, S.W. Salmond, & T.A. Pellino (Eds.), *Orthopaedicnursing* (3rd ed.). Philadelphia: Saunders.
18. O'Reilly, R.F., Burgess, I.A., & Zicat, B. (2005). The prevalence of venous thromboembolism after hip and knee replacement surgery. *The Medical Journal of Australia, 182*(4), 154-159.
19. Pablos, C., Carratala, V., Benavent, J., et al. (2007). Effects of periodized strength training program on bone mineral density in elders with osteoporosis. *Medical and Science Sports and Exercise, 39* (5 Suppl), S422-27.
20. Paget Foundation. (2004). *Paget's disease of bone: Q & A.* Retrieved 06/01/07 from www.paget.org.
21. Palmer, S.H., & Cross, M. (2004). *Total knee arthroplasty.* Retrieved 06/01/07 from www.emedicine.com/orthoped/topic347.htm.
22. Pellino, T.A., et al. (2002). Complication of orthopaedic disorders and orthopaedic surgery. In A.B. Maher, S.W. Salmond, & T.A. Pellino (Eds.), *Orthopaedic nursing* (3rd ed.). Philadelphia: Saunders.
23. Ramzi, D.W., & Leeper, K.V. (2004). DVT and pulmonary embolism: Part II. Treatment and prevention. *American Family Physician, 69* (12). Retrieved 06/01/07 from www.aafp.org/afp/20040615/2841.html.
24. Roberts, D. (2007). Arthritis and connective tissue disorders. In *NAON core curriculum for orthopaedic nursing* (6th ed.). Boston: Pearson Custom Publishing.
25. Roberts, D. (2002). Degenerative disorders. In A.B. Maher, S.W. Salmond, & T.A. Pellino (Eds.), *Orthopaedic nursing* (3rd ed.). Philadelphia: Saunders.

26. Rodts, M.F. (2002). Disorders of the spine. In A.B. Maher, S.W. Salmond, & T.A. Pellino (Eds.), *Orthopaedic nursing* (3rd ed.). Philadelphia: Saunders.
27. Salmond, S.W., & Fine, C. (2002). Infections of the musculoskeletal system. In A.B. Maher, S.W. Salmond, & T.A. Pellino (Eds.), *Orthopaedic nursing* (3rd ed.). Philadelphia: Saunders.
28. Scarfone, R.J. (2006). *Arthritis, septic.* Retrieved 06/01/07 from www.emedicine.com/PED/topic2695.htm#section~workup.
29. Stover, M.D., Beaule, P.F., Matta, J.M., et al. (2004). Hip arthrodesis: A procedure for the new millennium? *Clinical Orthopaedics & Related Research, 418,* 126-133.
30. Ulrich, P.F. (2004). *Understanding idiopathic scoliosis.* Retrieved 06/01/07 from www.spine-health.com/topics/cd/scoliosis/scoliosis01.html.

evolve   *Did you remember to check out the bonus material on the Evolve website and the CD-ROM, including NCLEX®-Examination Style Review Questions, Open-Book Quizzes, and Chapter Review Audio Podcasts?*

http://evolve.elsevier.com/Black/medsurg

CHAPTER 27

Management of Clients with Musculoskeletal Trauma or Overuse

DOTTIE ROBERTS

Anyone who has experienced a broken bone or a ligament strain can appreciate the challenges facing a client who is recovering from musculoskeletal trauma or overuse. Activity restrictions and assistive devices both complicate and facilitate the healing process. Types of fractures and common soft tissue injuries and their medical and nursing management are discussed in this chapter.

FRACTURES

Trauma is the leading cause of death in the United States for those between the ages of 1 and 37, and the fourth leading cause of death for all age groups.[19] Fractures account for a high percentage of traumatic injuries. They can create significant changes in one's quality of life by causing activity restrictions, disability, and economic loss.

A *fracture* is any disruption in the normal continuity of a bone. When fracture occurs, surrounding soft tissue is often damaged as well. A radiograph (x-ray) may confirm the bone injury, but it does not show evidence of the torn muscles or ligaments, severed nerves, or ruptured blood vessels that can complicate the client's recovery. To appropriately care for the client with a fracture, the nurse starts with a concise and accurate description of the injury.

Etiology and Risk Factors

Fracture results from mechanical overload of the bone, when more stress is placed on the bone than it can absorb. The actual amount of force necessary to cause a fracture may vary greatly, depending in part on the characteristics of the bone itself. A client with a metabolic bone disease such as osteoporosis, for example, may fracture with even minor trauma because the bone is weakened by the pre-existing disorder. Fracture may

result from direct force, as when a moving object strikes the body area over the bone. Force may also be applied indirectly, as when a powerful muscle contraction pulls against the bone. In addition, stress or fatigue can lead to fracture because of the bone's decreased ability to withstand mechanical force.

The two types of bone also respond differently to mechanical load. *Cortical* bone, the compact outer layer, is porous and can tolerate more stress along its axis (longitudinally) than across the bone. *Cancellous,* or *spongy,* bone is the dense inner bone material. It contains web-like formations and spaces filled with red marrow that make it better able to absorb force than cortical bone. Bony projections, called *trabeculae,* separate the spaces and are arranged along lines of stress, making cancellous bone even stronger.

Predisposition to fracture results from biologic conditions such as osteopenia (e.g., caused by steroid use or Cushing's syndrome) or osteogenesis imperfecta (a congenital bone disease characterized by defective collagen production by osteoblasts). The bone is brittle and breaks easily. Neoplasms can also weaken bone and contribute to fracture. Postmenopausal estrogen loss and protein malnutrition lead to decreased bone mass and increased risk for fracture. For people with healthy bones, fractures can result from high-risk recreation or employment-related activities (e.g., skateboarding, rock

---

evolve Web Enhancements

Care Plan   The Client in Traction

The Client Following Hip Fracture and ORIF

Case Management   Hip Fracture

Be sure to check out the bonus material on the Evolve website and the CD-ROM, including free self-assessment exercises. **http://evolve.elsevier. com/Black/medsurg**

climbing). Victims of domestic violence are also among people treated for traumatic injuries.

Pathophysiology

The severity of a fracture usually depends on the force that caused the fracture. If the bone's breaking point has been exceeded only slightly, then the bone may crack rather than breaking all the way through. If the force is extreme, such as in an automobile collision or a gunshot wound, the bone may shatter. When fracture occurs, muscles that were attached to the ends of the bone are disrupted. The muscles can undergo spasm and pull the fracture fragments out of position. Large muscle groups can create massive spasms that displace even large bones, such as the femur. Although the proximal portion of the fractured bone remains in place, the distal portion can become displaced in response to both the causative force and the spasm in the associated muscles. Fracture fragments may be displaced sideways, at an angle (angulated), or as overriding bone segments. They may also be rotated or offset.

In addition, the periosteum and blood vessels in the cortex and marrow of the fractured bone are disrupted. Soft tissue damage frequently occurs. Bleeding occurs both from the soft tissue and from the damaged ends of the bone. In the medullary canal, a hematoma forms between the fracture fragments and beneath the periosteum. Bone tissue surrounding the fracture site dies, creating an intense inflammatory response. Vasodilation, edema, pain, loss of function, exudation of plasma and leukocytes, and infiltration of other white blood cells develop. These pathophysiologic responses also are the initial step in bone healing.

Bone Healing

There are only a few tissues in the human body that heal through regeneration rather than formation of scar. Bone is one of these tissues. Fracture repair occurs by the same mechanism as bone formation during normal growth and maintenance, with organized mineralization of newly synthesized bone matrix followed by remodeling into mature bone.

Fracture healing occurs in five stages (Table 27-1). These stages do not occur independently but tend to overlap as bone healing progresses. If fracture healing is altered in any of the five stages, problems with bone union can result.

Factors Affecting Bone Healing

Several factors can change the rate of bone healing. Immediately after the fracture, adequate circulation and proper fragment immobilization are crucial for effective bone healing. Factors such as the presence of systemic or bone diseases, the age and general health of the client, the type of fracture, and the treatment also can affect the speed and success of healing. For example, an impacted fracture may heal within several weeks, but a displaced fracture may take months or even years to heal. A radial or ulnar fracture may heal in 3 months, but fractures in the tibia or femur may require 6 months or longer to heal. A fracture in an infant may heal in only 4 to 6 weeks, but the same fracture in an adolescent may require 6 to 10 weeks to heal. The rate of fracture healing is not significantly decreased in older adults unless the client also has a metabolic disorder such as osteoporosis. Favorable and unfavorable factors that affect bone healing are summarized in Box 27-1.

Clinical Manifestations

Diagnosing a fracture is based on the client's clinical manifestations, history, physical examination, and radiographic findings. Some fractures are immediately obvious; others are detected only on x-ray.

Physical assessment may reveal any of the following clinical manifestations:

- *Deformity.* Swelling from local hemorrhage may cause deformity at the fracture site. Muscle spasms can cause limb shortening, a rotational deformity, or angulation. Compared with the uninjured side, the fracture site may also have obvious deformity.
- *Swelling.* Edema may appear quickly as a result of accumulation of serous fluid at the fracture site and extravasation of blood into surrounding tissues.
- *Bruising* (ecchymosis). Bruising develops from subcutaneous bleeding at the fracture site.
- *Muscle spasm.* Frequently accompanying fractures, involuntary muscle spasm actually serves as a natural splint to decrease further motion of fracture fragments.
- *Pain.* If the client is neurologically intact, pain always accompanies fracture; the intensity and severity of the pain differ from client to client. Pain is usually continuous, increasing in severity until the fracture is immobilized. It results from muscle spasm, overriding of fracture fragments, or damage to adjacent structures.
- *Tenderness.* Tenderness over the fracture site is caused by underlying injuries.
- *Loss of function.* Any loss of function results either from pain caused by the fracture or from loss of the lever-arm function in an affected extremity. Paralysis may be caused by nerve damage.
- *Abnormal mobility and crepitus.* These manifestations are caused by motion in the middle of a bone or by fracture fragments rubbing together to create grating sensations or sounds.
- *Neurovascular changes.* Neurovascular injury results from damage to peripheral nerves or to the associated vascular structures. The client may complain

TABLE 27–1 Stages of Bone Healing

Stage	Description
Stage I: Hematoma stage or inflammatory stage Time: 1-3 days 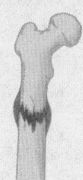	Immediate formation of a hematoma at the site of the fracture. The amount of damage to the bone and to the surrounding soft tissue and blood vessels determines the size of the hematoma. The blood forms a clot among the fracture fragments, providing a small amount of stabilization. Necrosis of adjacent bone occurs in direct relation to the loss of blood supply to the affected region and will extend to the area where collateral circulation begins. Vascular dilation occurs in response to the accumulation of dead cells and debris at the fracture site, and exudation of fibrin-rich plasma initiates the migration of phagocytic cells to the area of injury. If the vascular supply to the fracture site is inadequate, stage I healing will be greatly impaired.
Stage II: Fibrocartilage formation Time: 3 days to 2 weeks 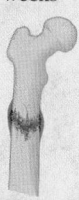	Fibroblasts, osteoblasts, and chondroblasts migrate to the fracture site as a result of the acute inflammation and form fibrocartilage. Organization of the hematoma then offers the foundation for stage II bone and tissue healing. Osteoblastic activity is stimulated by periosteal trauma, and bone formation occurs quickly. The periosteum is elevated away from the bone, and within a few days the combination of periosteal elevation and granulation tissue formation creates a collar around the end of each fracture fragment. As the collars advance, they form a bridge across the fracture site. This early formation of fibrous tissue is sometimes called the *primary callus,* and it results in gradually increasing stability for the fracture.
Stage III: Callus formation Time: 2-6 weeks 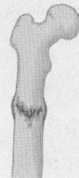	Granulation tissue matures into a provisional callus (procallus) as newly formed cartilage and bone matrix disperse through the primary callus. The procallus is large and loosely woven. It is generally wider than the normal diameter of the injured bone. The procallus secures the bone fragments, extending some distance beyond the fracture site to serve as a temporary splint, but it does not provide strength. If cells are distant from the blood supply and oxygen tensions are relatively low, cartilage is formed. When calcium is deposited in the collagen network of the granulation tissue, fibrous bone forms. Proper bone alignment is essential during stage III. This stage may be the most important in determining successful healing; if it is slowed or interrupted, the final two stages cannot occur. Delayed union or non-union can then result.
Stage IV: Ossification Time: 3 weeks to 6 months 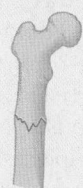	A permanent callus of rigid bone crosses the fracture gap between the periosteum and the cortex to join the fragments. In addition, medullary callus formation occurs internally to establish continuity between the marrow cavities. Trabecular bone gradually replaces the callus along stress lines. Bone union, which can be confirmed by x-ray, is said to have occurred when there is no motion with gentle stress and no tenderness with direct pressure at the fracture site. Weight-bearing in lower extremity fractures is also pain free after bone union.
Stage V: Consolidation and remodeling Time: 6 weeks to 1 year 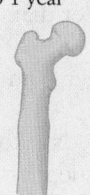	Unnecessary callus is resorbed or chiseled away from the healing bone. The process of bone resorption and deposition along stress lines allows bone to withstand the loads applied to it. The actual amount and timing of remodeling depends on the stresses imposed on the bone by muscles, weight-bearing, and age.

of numbness and tingling or have no palpable pulse distal to the fracture.

■ *Shock.* Bony fragments may lacerate blood vessels. Frank or occult hemorrhage can lead to shock.

Diagnostic Evaluation

Radiography is a common method of assessing for fractures. Use of the correct radiologic view is essential for adequate evaluation of the suspected fracture. Two views (e.g., anteroposterior and lateral) taken at right angles are generally considered the minimal number needed for evaluation, and they should include the joints above and below the suspected fracture to identify additional dislocations or subluxations. Abnormal x-ray findings include soft tissue edema or displacement of air in relation to a shift of the bone after injury. Radiographs of the fractured bone show an alteration in its normal

BOX 27-1 Factors Affecting Bone Healing

FAVORABLE
- Location
  - Good blood supply at bone ends
  - Flat bones
- Minimal damage to soft tissue
- Anatomic reduction possible
- Effective immobilization
- Weight-bearing on long bones

UNFAVORABLE
- Fragments widely separated
- Fragments distracted by traction
- Severely comminuted fracture
- Severe damage to soft tissue
- Bone loss from injury or surgical excision
- Motion/rotation at fracture site as a result of inadequate fixation
- Infection
- Impaired blood supply to one or more bone fragments
- Location
  - Decreased blood supply
  - Midshaft
- Health behaviors such as smoking, alcohol use

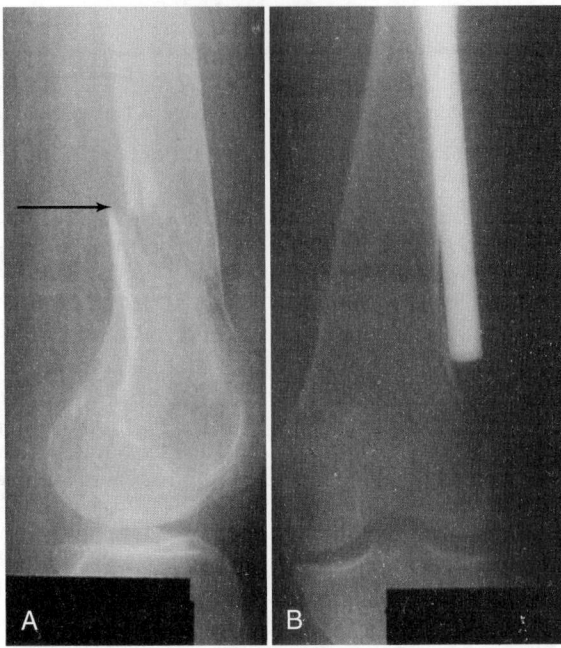

■ **FIGURE 27-1** **A,** Fracture of the supracondylar femur. (Note the radiolucency of the fracture line.) **B,** Reduction of the fracture with traction. The fracture was eventually pinned.

contour and a disruption of the normal joint relationship. The fracture line itself demonstrates increased radiolucency (Figure 27-1). Radiographs are commonly taken before fracture reduction, after reduction, and then periodically during bone healing.

Computerized tomography (CT) can also be used to determine the presence of fractures. An advantage of CT is that other structures (blood vessels) and abnormalities (hematoma) can be seen.

Fracture Classification

The severity of a fracture usually depends on the force that caused the fracture. If the bone's breaking point has been exceeded only slightly, then the bone may crack rather than breaking all the way through. If the force is extreme, such as in an automobile collision or a gunshot wound, the bone may shatter. If the bone breaks in such a way that bone fragments stick out through the skin or a wound penetrates down to the broken bone, the fracture is called an *open* fracture. This type of fracture is particularly serious because once the skin is broken, infection in both the wound and the bone can occur.

Fractures have many descriptors. In fact more than 150 types of fractures have been labeled according to various classification methods. For example, the client may have a compound, transverse fracture of the distal femur. Understanding the forces needed to cause various fractures is helpful. For example, the adult femur does

not fracture easily. Therefore if an adult client is admitted with a fractured femur, thorough assessment for other injuries by reviewing the cause of the fracture is critical. Table 27-2 lists common descriptors of fractures.

The simplest classification method is based on whether the fracture is *closed* or *open* to the environment. A *closed fracture* has intact skin over the site of injury, whereas the *open fracture* is characterized by a break in the skin over the bone injury. Tissue damage can be extensive with open fractures, which are graded according to their severity:

- *Grade I.* The wound is smaller than 1 cm; contamination is minimal.
- *Grade II.* The wound is larger than 1 cm; contamination is moderate.
- *Grade III.* The wound exceeds 6 to 8 cm; there is extensive damage to soft tissue, nerve, and tendon; and there is a high degree of contamination. Because the wound communicates with the external environment, the risk of infection must be promptly recognized and addressed.

OUTCOME MANAGEMENT

Medical Management

The goals of medical management include prompt and thorough assessment of the client to discover all injuries,

TABLE 27-2   **Common Types of Fractures**

Description	Illustration	Description	Illustration
Appearance		Nondisplaced: Fragments aligned at fracture site	
Burst: Characterized by multiple pieces of bone; often occurs at bone ends or in vertebrae			
Comminuted: More than one fracture line; more than two bone fragments; fragments may be splintered or crushed		Oblique: Fracture line occurs at approximately 45-degree angle across longitudinal axis of bone	
Complete: Break across entire section of bone, dividing it into distinct fragments; often displaced		Spiral: Fracture line results from twisting force; forms a spiral encircling bone	
		Stellate: Fracture lines radiate from one central point	
Displaced: Fragments out of normal position at fracture site	Torsion		
		Transverse: Fracture line occurs at a 90-degree angle to longitudinal axis of bone	
Incomplete: Fracture occurs through only one cortex of bone; usually nondisplaced			
		General Description	
		Avulsion: Bone fragments are torn away from body of bone at site of attachment of a ligament or tendon	
Linear: Fracture line is intact; fracture is caused by minor to moderate force applied directly to bone			
Longitudinal: Fracture line extends in direction of bone's longitudinal axis		Compression: Bone buckles and eventually cracks as result of unusual loading force applied to its longitudinal axis	

(Continued)

TABLE 27–2 Common Types of Fractures—Cont'd	
Description	**Illustration**
Greenstick: Incomplete fracture in which one side of cortex is broken and other side is flexed but intact	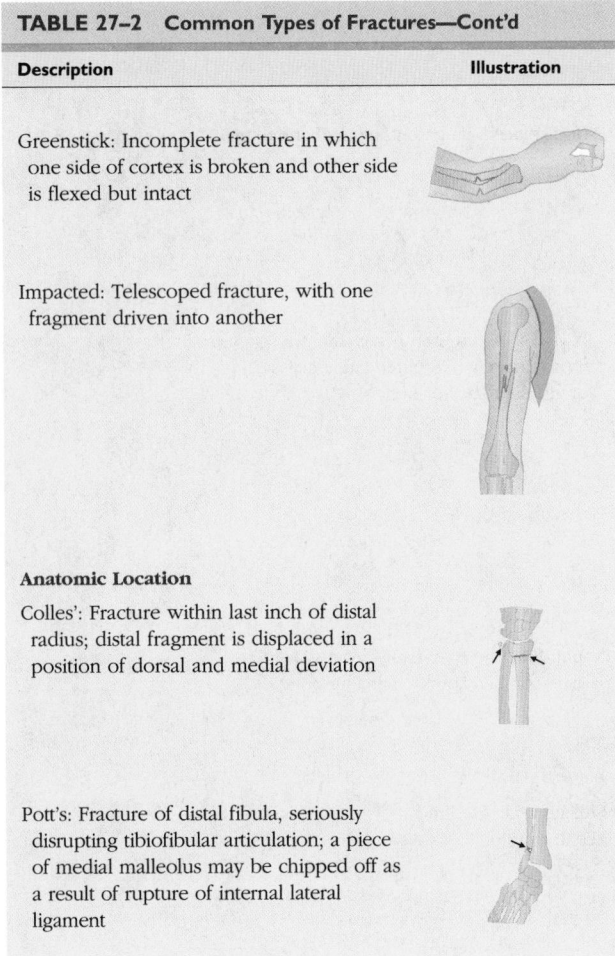
Impacted: Telescoped fracture, with one fragment driven into another	
Anatomic Location	
Colles': Fracture within last inch of distal radius; distal fragment is displaced in a position of dorsal and medial deviation	
Pott's: Fracture of distal fibula, seriously disrupting tibiofibular articulation; a piece of medial malleolus may be chipped off as a result of rupture of internal lateral ligament	

reduction and stabilization of the fracture with immobilization, observation for complications, and eventual remobilization and rehabilitation.

Thorough Initial Assessment

Basic principles of trauma care must be followed during emergency management of fractures. Assessment and treatment are performed simultaneously as the rescuer addresses the general condition of the injured client. During primary assessment, the rescuer focuses on airway management, bleeding, and manifestations of shock. Any potentially life-threatening injuries must be stabilized immediately and emergency assistance summoned to transport the client to a medical facility for additional intervention. An injured client should not be moved unless the current location is not safe.

Because most fractures do not pose a serious threat to life, their management becomes a secondary priority in trauma care. The only exception to this rule is a cervical spine injury; if the client complains of muscle spasm after a cervical spine or head injury, a fracture or dislocation is presumed to be present. The head and neck are immobilized for transportation, and lateral films of the cervical spine are always among the first diagnostic studies.

Suspected injuries to extremities should be carefully splinted and moved as little as possible because multiple fractures frequently occur in the same limb. The rescuer must stabilize the affected area and help the client remain still. An unconscious client should receive emergency management while the rescuer carefully notes any spontaneous movement as well as the client's position, and the condition of the head and extremities. The rescuer performs a neurologic assessment that is based on the type of known or suspected injury. Any soft tissue damage must also be assessed because the injury may indicate a fracture site. Open fractures should be covered with sterile dressings and remain covered to prevent additional contamination until a thorough examination can occur in the nearest hospital.

When the client reaches the emergency department, the neurologic condition and vital signs are closely monitored, and food and fluids are withheld (*nil per os,* nothing by mouth, or NPO) in the event that surgery is needed. Health care providers carefully examine the injured area and obtain the client's history. Details of the injury are helpful in determining the probable type of fracture and associated injuries. If the client was in a motor-vehicle accident, for example, was he or she sitting in the back or front seat? Was the client wearing a seat belt? What was the angle of impact? Was the client pulled from the car after a major collision? Or did the injury occur as a result of a fall on a hip or an outstretched arm?

Arterial damage is a possible early complication after fracture. The arteries may have been contused or lacerated, or they may have been constricted by tightly applied bandages or casts. Indications of arterial damage include a variable pulse rate or absence of a pulse, poor capillary return, swelling, pallor or patchy cyanosis distal to the injury, pain, paresthesias, or coolness of an extremity as a result of poorly filled veins. Blood loss may be considerable, particularly with femur or pelvic fractures, and hypovolemic shock may quickly develop.

Extensive bleeding can occur even with closed fractures, and emergency surgery may become necessary; loss of blood supply to the fracture can result in areas of bone necrosis. With a displaced fracture, a hematoma may develop in the soft tissue as a result of damage to large blood vessels. Soft tissue infection is a high risk with any open fracture; antibiotic therapy should begin as soon as possible after the injury.

Reducing Fractures

The first step in management of a displaced fracture is *reduction:* the manipulation of the bones to restore alignment, position, and length by bringing the bony fragments into close approximation. Reduction, which is also called *bone setting,* alleviates compression or stretching of nerves and blood vessels. Because reduction is generally painful, sedation or local or general anesthesia may be needed.

Not all fractures require reduction. Nondisplaced fractures, for example, are already in proper alignment. Splinting or casting allows the alignment to be maintained as the fracture heals. A few other fractures cannot be adequately splinted and instead are treated simply by resting the affected area until healing occurs (e.g., distal phalangeal fractures).

When a fracture of an extremity divides a bone into two fragments, the fragments are referred to as *proximal* (nearer the trunk) and *distal* (farther from the trunk). Because of its muscle attachment and location, the proximal fragment cannot be manipulated or moved when the fractured bone is being set. Instead, the distal fragment is moved to realign it with the proximal bone segment. Reduction methods can be used alone or in combination.

Closed Reduction. To perform closed reduction, a health care provider applies manual traction to move the fracture fragments and restore bone alignment (Figure 27-2). Closed reduction should be performed as soon as possible after injury to decrease the client's risk for loss of function, to prevent or delay development of traumatic arthritis, and to minimize the possible deforming effects of the injury. Fracture reduction is not an emergency procedure, however, and the client's life should never be jeopardized by attempting early reduction.

Because gravity, weight-bearing, and muscle contraction can again move the fragments, an immobilization device must be applied after x-ray studies have confirmed bone alignment. The immobilizer most commonly used after closed reduction is a *cast*—a temporary device made of synthetic materials such as fiberglass, thermoplastic polymer, or plaster of Paris (anhydrous calcium sulfate). Casts are used for several purposes in addition to immobilization: prevention or correction of deformity; maintenance, support, and protection of realigned bone; and promotion of healing to allow early weight-bearing for ambulation. Casts may be applied in a hospital emergency department, in the operating room, or at the client's bedside in the hospital. They are also commonly applied in a physician's office or clinic.

Synthetic materials are used to construct a strong, light-weight cast that sets in about 5 minutes. They also come in a variety of colors and patterns that can enhance self-esteem in both young and older clients after injury. Synthetic casts maintain their shape and firmness even if they become wet, but they must be dried thoroughly to prevent skin maceration. If there is no incision under the cast, synthetic materials can be dried with a hair blow dryer on a low setting; however, several hours are needed for the cast to dry thoroughly.

Plaster of Paris bandages are individual rolls of precut crinoline impregnated with plaster. They come in various sizes, and the body part to be put in a cast determines the amount of plaster to be used. Plaster casts take at least 24 hours longer than synthetic casts to dry, and they lose their shape if they are allowed to get wet again.

Open Reduction and Internal Fixation. Some fractures have too many pieces of bone, have neurovascular injuries, or would not stay aligned to heal following closed reduction. Open reduction is a surgical procedure where the fracture fragments are realigned. Open reduction is usually performed in combination with internal fixation for femoral and joint fractures. Screws, plates, pins, wires, or nails may be used to maintain alignment of the fracture fragments (Figure 27-3). Rods may also be placed through the fragments or fixed to the side of the bone, or they may be inserted directly into the bone's medullary cavity. Internal fixation provides essential immobilization and helps to prevent deformity, but it is not a substitute for bone healing. If proper healing fails to occur, the internal fixation device may actually loosen or break as a result of stress.

External Fixation. Depending on the client's condition and the physician's judgment, external fixation devices may be used for fracture fragment immobilization (Figure 27-4). If, for example, soft tissue damage precludes the use of a cast, external fixation would be indicated for fracture immobilization. External fixation devices maintain position for unstable fractures and for

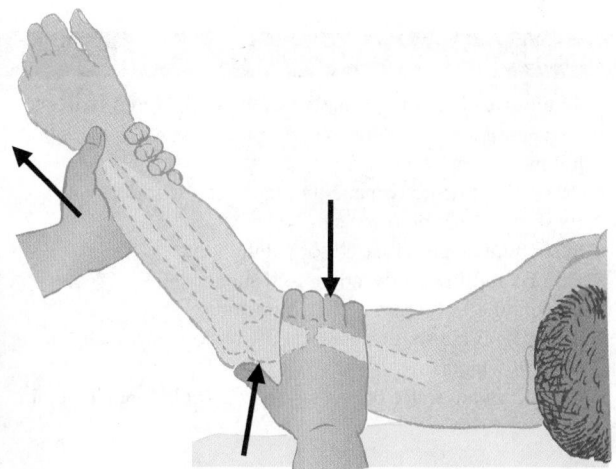

■ **FIGURE 27–2** Closed reduction to realign a supracondylar fracture.

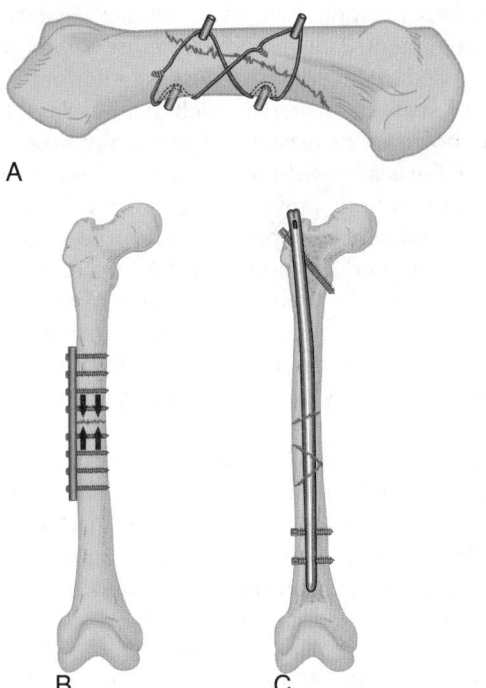

■ **FIGURE 27–3** Examples of different types of internal fixation devices. **A,** Tension band wiring with Kirschner wires for a fracture of the phalanx. **B,** Compression plate and screws in the lateral aspect of the femur. **C,** Sliding hip screw.

weakened muscles, and they support areas with tissue or bone infection. They allow the client to use contiguous joints while the affected area remains immobilized. External fixation may also be indicated for bony non-union if fracture healing has not been successful after a

certain time. Common sites for external fixation include the face and jaw, extremities, pelvis, ribs, fingers, and toes. Pins used in external fixation vary in number, length, and thickness on the basis of the treatment area.

External fixation devices can be cumbersome, and client selection is critical to the successful use of external fixation. Any potential problems with compliance should be discussed thoroughly with the client and family, including the effects of external fixation on the client's lifestyle. Nonadherence with the medical regimen can lead to pin loosening, loss of fracture stabilization, and infection. Specific activity orders are written after the application of an external fixator, with special attention to weight-bearing status when the pelvis or a lower extremity is involved.

Traction. Traction has been used to treat fractures since prehistoric times, and its principles were well known to Hippocrates. Traction is the application of a pulling force to an injured body part or extremity while a countertraction pulls in the opposite direction. The pulling force can be achieved through the use of hands (manual traction) or, more commonly, the application of weights. The purposes of traction are shown in Box 27-2. With improved surgical technique and the development of femoral prostheses and intramedullary rods, traction is not as prevalent as it once was in the treatment of orthopedic injuries. Lower extremity traction, such as Buck or Russell traction, currently has limited application in the preoperative management of a client with a fractured hip, for example. Skeletal traction, however, continues to be an option for multiple trauma clients who are not immediate candidates for open reduction and internal fixation of orthopedic injuries. Various types of traction may also be treatment options before and after surgical reduction of injuries such as cervical fractures.

■ **FIGURE 27–4** External fixation to provide immobilization of a tibial fracture. *(From Stryker Howmedica Osteonics, Mahwah, NJ.)*

BOX 27-2 **Purposes of Traction**
■ Reduce, realign, and promote healing of fractured bones
■ Decrease muscle spasms that may accompany fractures or follow surgical reduction
■ Prevent soft tissue damage through immobilization
■ Prevent or treat deformities
■ Rest an inflamed, diseased, or painful joint
■ Reduce and treat dislocations and subluxations
■ Prevent the development of contractures
■ Reduce muscle spasms associated with low back pain or cervical whiplash
■ Expand a joint space during arthroscopy or before major joint reconstruction

From Theis, L. (2004). Care of patients in traction, casts, or external fixation devices. In *An introduction to orthopaedic nursing* (3rd ed.). Chicago: National Association of Orthopaedic Nurses.

Skin Traction. Skin traction involves the application of a pulling force directly to the skin through the use of skin strips, boots, or foam splints. Buck's traction is the most commonly used form of skin traction. For Buck's traction, a foam boot is applied to the client's affected extremity and attached to a weight that is suspended off the foot of the bed. This type of traction may be used for the client with a hip fracture who is unable to undergo surgical repair until determined to be medically stable. Skin traction bears a low longitudinal force load (5 to 7 pounds), which gives it minimal effectiveness. Because of the risk of skin breakdown, this type of traction should be used only temporarily.

Skeletal Traction. Skeletal traction uses pins to apply force to the bone. With skeletal traction, a direct force can be applied after the physician inserts stainless-steel pins through the bone itself. The most common sites for pin insertion are the distal femur, the proximal tibia, and the proximal ulna. Skeletal traction can be tolerated for longer periods than can skin traction. Weights over 10 pounds are commonly used.

In addition to the mode of application, traction can be categorized as *static* (continuous) or *dynamic* (intermittent). Suspension may also be *running* or *straight* (exerting a direct pull on the affected part) or *balanced* (exerting a pull on the affected part and also supporting the extremity in a splint). Table 27-3 describes major types of traction.

Major disadvantages include the potential need for prolonged bed rest and the resulting effects of extended immobility. Long-term hospitalization is not always indicated if the client in traction can qualify for home care nursing services or, depending on the type of traction, receive additional treatment as an outpatient.

Complications After Fracture

There are several complications with fractures. These include the type of injury, the client's age, the presence of other health problems (co-morbidities), and the client's use of medications that affect bleeding, such as warfarin, corticosteroids, and nonsteroidal anti-inflammatory drugs (NSAIDs). Continuous assessment of the client's neurovascular status for potential complications is critical, as is quick intervention to minimize adverse side effects.

Nerve Injury. Bone fragments and tissue edema associated with the injury can cause nerve damage. Be alert for pallor and coolness of the client's affected extremity, changes in the client's ability to move the digits or the extremity, paresthesia, or complaints of increasing pain.

Compartment Syndrome. Muscle compartments in the upper and lower extremities are enclosed by tough, inelastic fascial tissue that does not expand if the muscle swells (Figure 27-5). Edema that occurs in response to a fracture can lead to an increase in compartment pressure that reduces capillary blood perfusion. When the local blood supply is unable to meet the tissue's metabolic demands, ischemia begins. *Compartment syndrome* is a

---

TABLE 27-3   Major Types of Traction

Traction	Type	Common Conditions Treated	Duration
Cervical			
Chin halter	Skin	Severe strains or sprains; cervical trauma nerve root compression; torticollis	Intermittent
Skeletal tongs: Gardner-Wells, Crutchfield, Vinke	Skeletal	Fractures or dislocations of cervical or high thoracic vertebrae	Continuous
Halo traction	Skeletal	Fractures or dislocations of cervical or high thoracic vertebrae	Continuous
Upper Extremity			
Side-arm	Skin or skeletal	Vertical suspension to forearm	Continuous
Overhead/90-90	Skin or skeletal	Vertical traction to humerus; horizontal suspension to forearm	Continuous
Lower Back			
Pelvic belt or sling	Skin	Low back pain	Intermittent or continuous
Lower Extremity			
Buck	Skin	Hip and knee contracture; preoperative immobilization and muscle spasm relief for hip fractures	Continuous
Balanced suspension: Thomas ring and Pearson and Brady attachment	Skeletal	Used mainly with skeletal pins for supracondylar femur fracture; hip and knee contracture; postoperative positioning and immobilization	Continuous

Modified from Redermann, S. (2002). Modalities for immobilization. In A.B. Maher, S.W. Salmond, & T.A. Pellino (Eds.), *Orthopaedic nursing* (3rd ed.). Philadelphia: Saunders; and from Theis, L. (2004). Care of patients in traction, casts, or external fixation devices. In *An introduction to orthopaedic nursing* (3rd ed.). Chicago: National Association of Orthopaedic Nurses.

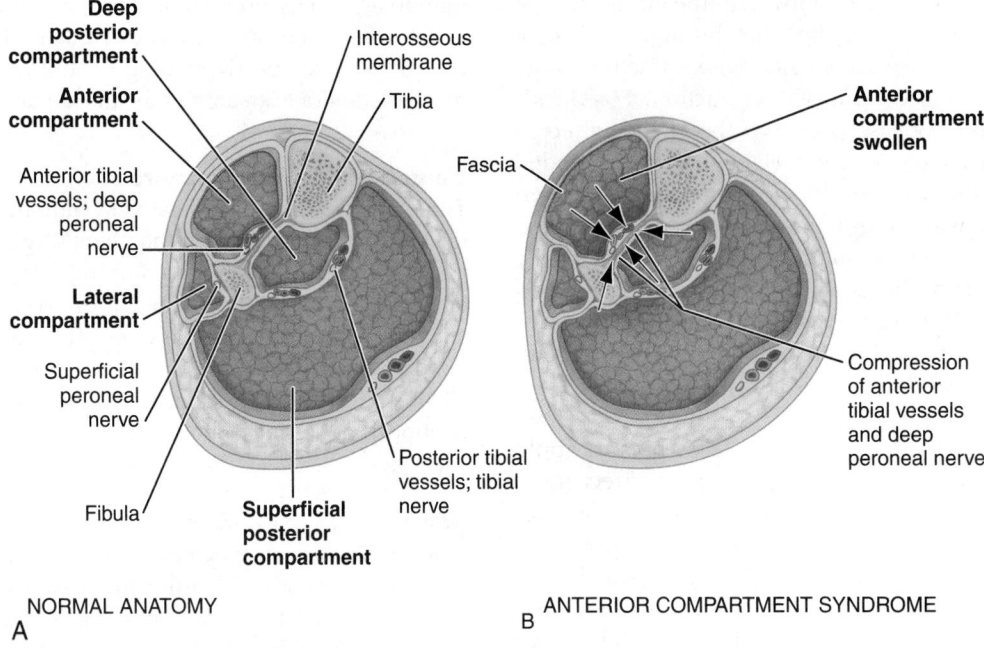

NORMAL ANATOMY
A

ANTERIOR COMPARTMENT SYNDROME
B

■ **FIGURE 27–5　A,** Compartments of the proximal third of the lower leg. The four compartments are (1) anterior, (2) lateral, (3) deep posterior, and (4) superficial posterior. **B,** When swelling occurs in response to injury, the compartment is contained by the inelastic fascia that covers it. Unrelieved pressure compromises nerves and vessels within the compartment.

condition of compromised circulation related to progressively increased pressure in a confined space. It is caused by anything that decreases the compartment size, including external compression forces such as a tight cast or internal factors such as bleeding or edema. Continued ischemia results in histamine release by the affected muscles, leading to even greater edema and a further decrease in perfusion. An increase in lactic acid production causes more anaerobic metabolism and a subsequent increase in blood flow that, in turn, increases the tissue pressure. This leads to a cycle of increasing compartment pressure. Compartment syndrome can occur anywhere in the body but occurs most often in the lower leg and forearm.

SAFETY

⚠

ALERT

If it goes unrecognized or untreated, the client can lose nerve and muscle function. Infection, myoglobinuria, and renal failure may follow, and amputation may become necessary.

A combination of clinical manifestations occurs with compartment syndrome. The classic sign of acute compartment syndrome is pain, especially when the muscle is stretched. The pain may be intensely out of proportion to the injury, especially if no bone is broken.

There may also be a tingling or burning sensation (paresthesias) in the muscle. The muscle may feel tight or full. If the area becomes numb or paralysis develops, cell death has begun and efforts to lower the pressure

in the compartment may not be successful in restoring function.

Compartment syndrome can be diagnosed from the clinical manifestations alone, and intracompartmental pressures can be measured by various monitors. Normal compartment pressure is considered to be 0 to 8 mm Hg. Compartment values that are 10 to 30 mm Hg less than diastolic pressure indicate a possible compartment syndrome because there is not enough perfusion pressure to sustain the muscle. Compartment pressures ranging from 30 to 45 mm Hg historically have been considered high enough to cause tissue necrosis if treatment is not initiated, although exact numbers are still debated.[24]

The primary treatment of compartment syndrome is relief of the source of pressure. To accomplish this, the physician may order a constrictive bandage to be removed or a cast to be bivalved (see Care of the Client in a Cast on p. 519). The affected extremity should be kept at heart level because elevation above the heart actually decreases local arterial perfusion, further compromising blood flow. Cold applications should be avoided with suspected compartment syndrome because they lead to vasoconstriction, which can further compromise circulation. Adequate hydration is important for maintaining the client's mean arterial blood pressure. Pain should be managed to decrease the vasoconstrictive effects of the sympathetic nervous system.

If relief of external pressure is not enough to keep compartment pressures from rising, a fasciotomy may be necessary. An incision through the skin into the fascia of the muscle compartment allows tissue expansion and restores blood flow by relieving pressure on the microcirculation. The incision typically is left open until the swelling decreases; the area is then loosely wrapped and the wrapping is left on for several days. The wound is closed by tertiary intention when edema has subsided.

Volkmann's Contracture. *Volkmann's contracture* is a limb deformity that results from unrelieved compartment syndrome. As prolonged pressure causes ischemia, muscle is gradually replaced by fibrous tissue that traps tendons and nerves. Compartment syndrome following tibial fractures can lead to a painful or numb, dysfunctional, and deformed foot. In the upper extremities, Volkmann's contracture most commonly occurs after fractures of the elbow and forearm or after crushing injuries of the forearm, or it is caused by tight bandages or casts. It can lead to a permanently stiff, claw-like deformity of the hand and arm. Contractures may be avoided through prompt recognition of manifestations of compartment syndrome, followed by limb splinting and compartment decompression as indicated.

Fat Embolism Syndrome. Fat embolism is similar to pulmonary embolism, except that fat is the embolus and the condition is seen in clients with fractures. The highest incidence, up to 90% of all cases, of fat embolism syndrome (FES) occurs following fractures of long bones, such as the femur, tibia, ribs, fibula, and pelvis.[19] Total joint arthroplasty also places the client at risk for FES, and the incidence increases after bilateral procedures. FES increases mortality after fracture by 10% to 20%.[19]

There are two theories of why FES occurs. The mechanical theory states that there is a release of fat globules from the bone marrow into the venous circulation after fracture. The biochemical or metabolic theory suggests that trauma leads to the release of stored fatty acids and neutral fats. Platelet aggregation and fat globule formation then occur. In reality, the pathophysiologic process of FES is unknown; it may include parts of both theories or reflect an entirely different, unknown etiology.

The deposit of embolic fat in the pulmonary circulation can lead to the rapid onset of a disorder similar to adult (acute) respiratory distress syndrome (ARDS). An important aspect of the pathogenesis of FES appears to be endothelial injury caused by fatty acids released from impacted fat droplets, which leads to fluid leakage into interstitial spaces. Perfusion pressure increases, and pulmonary vessels become engorged. As the lung becomes more rigid, the workload of the right side of the heart increases. The fat globules occluding the pulmonary circulation are hydrolyzed into free fatty acids that increase capillary permeability and activate lung surfactant. Hemorrhagic pulmonary edema and patchy alveolar collapse occur, leading to severe hypoxia.

Primary manifestations typically occur within 24 to 72 hours after injury, and include persistent tachycardia, unexplained tachypnea, dyspnea, and hypoxia resulting from ventilation-perfusion abnormalities. Clients can develop fever with high spikes daily. Reddish-brown nonpalpable petechiae develop over the upper body, particularly in the axillae, within 24 to 36 hours of insult or injury. These petechiae occur in only 20% to 50% of clients and resolve quickly, but they are virtually diagnostic when noticed. Agitated delirium is often present and may progress to stupor, seizures, or coma and frequently is unresponsive to correction of hypoxia. A fulminant form of FES can occur within just a few hours of injury and may progress rapidly to death.

Prevention of FES begins with prudent treatment of long bone fractures, including careful handling, appropriate splinting, and avoidance of unnecessary manipulation of the injured area. Prompt surgical fixation after injury (within 24 to 48 hours) is critical. Continuous pulse oximetry for the at-risk client may help in early detection of desaturation, allowing prompt treatment. Early aggressive resuscitation to prevent hypovolemic shock, adequate pain management, blood transfusion through a 20-μm filter, and prevention of sepsis are also considered standard preventive care.

If FES does occur, supportive treatment is directed at preserving the client's respiratory function. Oxygen is administered; intubation and continuous positive airway pressure are sometimes necessary. Steroid use is controversial but may be considered in overt and subclinical forms of FES in an attempt to decrease the inflammatory effects of the fatty acids on the alveolocapillary membrane. Fluid volume replacement is important to prevent circulatory instability.

Deep Vein Thrombosis and Pulmonary Embolism. The client with orthopedic injuries is at high risk for thromboembolic conditions such as *deep vein thrombosis* (DVT) and *pulmonary embolism* (PE). Their elevated risk is due to stasis of blood flow in veins, increased coagulability, and injury to vessels. Stasis of blood increases the contact time between blood and vein wall irregularities. It also prevents naturally occurring anticoagulants from mixing in the blood. Prolonged bed rest or immobility promotes stasis. There is also increased coagulation of blood from the tissue debris, collagen, or fats in the veins. Orthopedic trauma often releases these materials into the blood system. Finally, there may be damage to the vein walls from the fracture fragments, which break intercellular bridges and release substances that promote blood clotting.

Prevention of DVT is a primary goal. Clot prophylaxis is recommended through the use of pharmacologic agents such as an oral anticoagulant or subcutaneous low-molecular-weight (LMW) heparin (fixed dose or weight-adjusted). For appropriately selected clients, physical-mechanical measures such as intermittent pneumatic compression devices or elastic stockings may also have a role in DVT prevention. DVT is discussed fully in Chapter 53.

Infection

SAFETY ALERT

Infection continues to be a cause of morbidity among clients who have open or surgically repaired fractures. Pathogens can contaminate an open fracture at the time of injury or may be introduced at the time of surgery. Surgical wound infection during the postoperative period usually results from *Staphylococcus aureus* or *Staphylococcus epidermidis*. Osteomyelitis, a severe infection of the bone itself, can also result (see Chapter 26).

Cast Syndrome. Cast syndrome (superior mesenteric artery syndrome) occurs only with body spica casts. The duodenum is compressed between the superior mesenteric artery anteriorly and the aorta and vertebral bodies posteriorly, causing a decreased blood supply that can lead to hemorrhage and necrosis of the bowel. Cast syndrome can develop days to weeks after immobilization, especially when the client has lost weight from loss of retroperitoneal fat.

SAFETY ALERT

Untreated cast syndrome can be fatal. Constant assessment is therefore a priority and, because complete gastrointestinal obstruction can develop, immediate nursing intervention is needed.

Long-Term Complications of Fractures

Joint Stiffness or Traumatic Arthritis. After injury or prolonged immobilization, joint stiffness may occur and can lead to joint contracture, ligament tightening or muscle atrophy. Active range-of-motion exercises should be performed to the extent of client tolerance. Also perform passive range-of-motion exercises to decrease the risk for stiffness. The occurrence of traumatic arthritis, which presents with all the symptoms of idiopathic arthritis, is influenced by the severity of the initial injury and the success of bone reduction. Use of acetaminophen or NSAIDs may decrease joint discomfort. Exercise to tolerance may also ameliorate the manifestations of developing arthritis; however, surgical joint replacement may eventually be needed.

Avascular Necrosis. Avascular necrosis (AVN) of the femoral head occurs primarily in fractures proximal to the femoral neck. It results from local circulatory compromise. An x-ray film demonstrates collapse of the femoral head, and the client complains of pain that occurs months to years after fracture repair. Replacement of the femoral head with a prosthesis is required. The best chance for avoiding the development of AVN is prompt surgical repair at the time of fracture.

Nonfunctional Union. Most fractures heal adequately without any problems, but biologic interventions may be employed to stimulate fracture healing.

Malunion. Malunion results when fracture fragments heal in improper alignment as a result of unequal muscle pull and gravity. It can occur if the client bears weight on the affected extremity against medical advice or when an ambulatory device is applied before adequate healing has begun at the fracture site. The primary manifestation is external deformity of the involved extremity. Malunion is diagnosed by radiography. If it is identified early in the course of fracture healing, malunion can be corrected with adjustment of traction or remobilization. Malunion that is diagnosed after healing is complete must be surgically corrected. Prevention is accomplished by adequate fracture reduction and immobilization, and by ensuring that the client understands the importance of any activity or position restrictions.

Delayed Union. Delayed union occurs when healing is slowed but not completely stopped, possibly as a result of distraction of the fracture fragments or a systemic cause such as infection Suspect delayed union if the client complains of continuation or increase in bone pain and tenderness beyond the healing period expected on the basis of the degree of trauma (3 months to 1 year). If the cause can be identified and corrected early, the fracture usually heals.

Non-union. Non-union is identified when fracture healing has not occurred 4 to 6 months after the initial injury and after spontaneous healing is no longer likely to occur. It is generally caused by insufficient blood supply and uncontrolled repetitive stress on the fracture site, possibly as a result of the presence of muscle, tendon, or soft tissue between fracture fragments. Non-union can also result from prolonged or excessive traction; insufficient or inadequate immobilization that allows movement at the fracture site; inadequate internal fixation; or wound infection after internal fixation. On radiograph, non-union is characterized by a relatively narrow gap between fracture fragments. A soft tissue bridge of fibrocartilage and fibrous tissue spans the gap.

Once diagnosed, non-union is treated by bone grafting, internal or external fixation, electric bone stimulation, low-frequency ultrasonography, or a combination of these methods. For example, autogenous or allogeneic bone grafts can be used to stimulate bone growth. Percutaneous injection or implantation of autogenous bone marrow is another intervention that is the subject of current research in fracture healing.[14] A three-dimensional implant or graft can also be used as an aid to bone healing by supporting the attachment, spread, division, and differentiation of bone cells. Osteoinduction involves the use of substances such as platelet-derived growth factor to stimulate bone healing.

Client education is especially important before any of these interventions because weight-bearing on the affected extremity will be contraindicated for a prescribed period of time based on evidence of healing. Weight-bearing on an unstable fracture prolongs healing time.

Fibrous Union. Fibrous tissue is interposed in a wide gap between fracture fragments. Loss of bone through surgery or injury predisposes the client to this type of fracture union. Additional surgical fixation may be required.

Complex Regional Pain Syndrome (CRPS). Formerly known as *reflex sympathetic dystrophy,* this condition is a painful dysfunction and disuse syndrome that is characterized by abnormal pain and swelling of the affected extremity. It is usually precipitated by relatively minor trauma and generally is believed to be related to disorders of the central or peripheral nervous system. The origin may be a small injury commonly in the extremities. Manifestations may include disproportionate pain at the site of injury, edema, muscle spasm or vasospasm, stiffness and decreased joint mobility, increased sweating, atrophy, contractions, and loss of bone mass. Some treatment success has been experienced with sympathetic nerve blocks, especially in early stages of the syndrome. Drug therapies typically involve use of steroids, analgesics, muscle relaxants, and antidepressants, or antiseizure medications. Physical therapy and transcutaneous electric nerve stimulation may also be ordered. Psychological counseling is often suggested for the client living with this chronic condition.

Nursing Management of the Medical Client

Care of the Client in a Cast

Immobilization of a fracture is most often accomplished through the use of a cast or splint (Figure 27-6). Before application of a cast, the nurse's role may entail preparation of the client for casting, including a detailed explanation of the procedure. Skin preparation involves thorough cleansing and assessment of any wounds. The presence of unremovable dirt or foreign particles should be reported to the physician. After the skin preparation, a stockinette is applied over the extremity. It should be cut several inches longer than the expected finished length of the cast so excess portions can be pulled over exposed ends to protect the client's skin. Make sure that the stockinette fits smoothly and without wrinkles to avoid creating pressure points on underlying tissues. Padding or a web roll is then applied to the extremity surrounding the fracture site. Additional padding made be indicated over bony prominences, but too much padding can actually increase pressure. The first layer should be wrapped without stretching the padding, from distal to proximal. Apply the second layer of return wrap a little more tightly, from proximal to distal.

Rolls of plaster casting materials are individually submerged in clean water in a bucket. Excess water is squeezed from the roll, and then the bandage is applied to encircle the injured body part. Synthetic materials do not require submersion. Assist during cast application by supporting the extremity from underneath, using only the palms of your hands to avoid applying pressure to any one area. Fingertips should not be pressed into the cast, and the cast should not be allowed to rest on a hard or sharp surface; these actions might cause flattening or indentations in the cast, which could create pressure. As soon as the casting procedure is complete, the client's skin must be cleansed of excess casting material. Plaster-laden water should never be emptied into an ordinary sink because the plaster sediment solidifies and plugs the plumbing. If a sink with a plaster trap is not available, wait for sediment to settle to the bottom of the bucket, and then drain off the water from the top. The remaining plaster sediment can be scraped from the bottom of the bucket and placed into the garbage container.

Drying a Cast

As the cast dries, a full-strength mature cast develops. Synthetic casts dry to the touch in a few minutes, but they take about 30 minutes to set completely and allow weight-bearing. Plaster casts set quickly but take hours to days to dry completely; a lower extremity plaster cast may not be totally dry for up to 48 hours, and larger casts can take even longer. Because both plaster and synthetic casts generate heat while drying, the client should be instructed to expect the sensation of heat. The cast should not be covered with a blanket or towel while it is drying because the retained heat can burn the client. Several towels may be placed under the cast on the pillow to absorb dampness. While the cast is still damp, the client may feel cold and may experience a decrease in body temperature. Adequate covering is provided for the client while dry, warm air is allowed

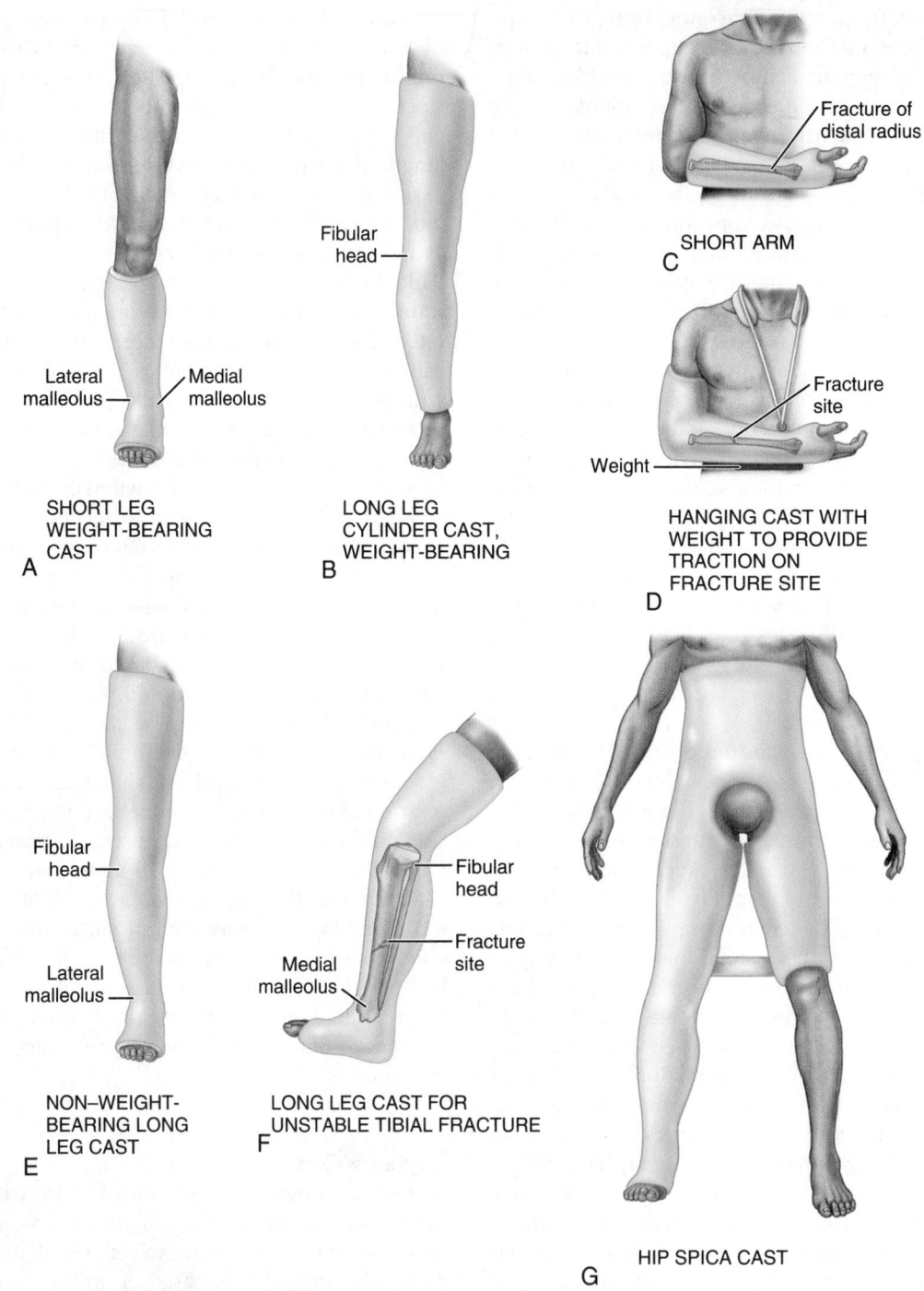

■ **FIGURE 27–6** Common types of casts and possible pressure points.

to circulate around the damp cast. To avoid excessive chilling for the client who is in a large cast, sections of the cast should be exposed for brief periods alternately. Unless it is contraindicated, the client should also be turned regularly to expose more of the new cast to air. Rapid drying through use of a blow dryer is not advised because it can burn the client's skin under the cast and crack the cast.

A wet plaster cast smells musty and is dull on percussion, gray, and cold to the touch. When dry, the plaster cast is odorless, resonant, and white, and it feels close to room temperature when touched. Wet fiberglass casts feel hot and sticky to the touch. A wet fiberglass cast should not be placed over drainage-containing pads, such as incontinence pads, because paper and plaster adhere and the paper will become a permanent part of the cast. Once the cast is completely dry, it can safely be placed on a hard surface (e.g., a casted arm can rest on a table), but the client is usually more comfortable in continuing to rest the casted area on pillows.

Windowing or Bivalving a Cast

Bivalving a cast means cutting the cast along both sides and then splitting it to decrease pressure on underlying tissue. Windows may also be cut into the cast to see wounds under the cast or remove drains. In addition, windows may be cut to allow pulse assessment or to prevent cast syndrome. Bivalving also allows removal of half of the cast for wound care or x-rays. The remaining half of a bivalved cast is often used as an intermittent splint that can be removed and reapplied as the client adjusts to being without a cast. When reapplying a bivalved cast, take care not to pinch the client's skin between the cast halves. When the cast halves are properly fitted, secure them with an elastic wrap.

Neurovascular Assessment. Although casts are protective and therapeutic, they can also cause serious complications. Careful nursing assessment and prompt intervention are necessary to minimize the client's risk for detrimental effects. Be aware of the client's neurovascular status by assessing the following in a casted extremity:

- Color, warmth, pulses distal to the cast, capillary refill (circulatory function)
- Movement of distal fingers or toes, awareness of light touch distal to the cast, changes in sensation (nerve function)

The deep and superficial peroneal nerves and the tibial nerve are most at risk for injury with lower extremity fractures, whereas radial and ulnar nerve function must be assessed with upper extremity injuries. Encourage the client to report any numbness or tingling, although neither may be present even with nerve compression. Pulse, color, and warmth of the injured extremity should also be assessed by comparison with the unaffected extremity. Neurovascular assessment should be performed every 30 minutes for 4 hours after cast or splint application and then every 3 to 4 hours. Table 27-4 describes the technique used for assessment and expected findings.

Assessment of Pain. Careful assessment of pain must be completed regularly, and the client must be encouraged

---

TABLE 27–4 Neurovascular Assessments (CMS)

Parameter Being Assessed	Technique	Expected Finding
Circulation		
Color of affected extremity	Inspect color of affected leg, foot, arm, or hand; compare to opposite side	Color should be the same; it is normal to have some paleness (pallor) in injured tissues; if incisions are present, some redness (erythema) may be noted along incision lines
Capillary refill in nail beds	Compress nail bed and measure time needed for refill (return of color)	Should be 2-3 sec; slowing to 4-6 sec should be reported
Edema	Inspect or palpate for edema in both extremities	No edema should be present; if edema is noted in affected extremity, consider whether it is caused by trauma or surgery or thrombophlebitis; if present in both extremities, consider causes such as heart disease
Pedal pulses	Palpate for pedal pulses on dorsum of foot (dorsalis pedis) or adjacent to medial malleolus (posterior tibialis)	Pulses should be present bilaterally; if dorsal pulse is absent, may be normal variation; absent pulses could also signal compression of vessels from edema
Temperature of affected extremity	Use dorsum (back) of your hand to assess temperature	Temperature should be the same in each extremity; report any coolness or heat in extremity
Movement		
Movement of affected extremity	Ask client to "move your toes/fingers"	Movement should be the same on each side; if decreased movement is noted, determine whether extremity normally moves (e.g., if the client has had a stroke, limited movement may have been present before); if client had surgery on toes or fingers, expect decreased movement as a result of pain and edema; look for even slight movement in area
Sensation		
Sensation of affected extremity	Ask clients which digits they feel you touching; ask specifically if they have a "pins and needles" sensation or if extremity feels as if it is "asleep"	Sensation should be the same on each side; any alterations in sensation should be reported
Pain	Ask clients to rate pain on scale of 0-10 (0 being no pain and 10 being worst pain they have ever felt)	Pain is common in injured extremities; if no pain is reported, client may have recently had pain medication; uncontrollable pain may signal compartment syndrome and should be reported immediately

to verbalize the degree of pain. Inadequate analgesic effects should be reported promptly to the surgeon because an increased dosage or change in medication may be indicated. Unrelieved pain is also a classic manifestation of compartment syndrome; therefore any complaint of pain should be given your full attention. Be especially alert to complaints of progressive pain or pain out of proportion to the injury or treatment.

Assessment of the Cast. The skin around the cast edges should be observed for damage or swelling. Also assess the cast itself.

SAFETY

ALERT

"Hot spots"—areas of the cast that feel warmer than other sections—may indicate tissue necrosis or infection under the cast. "Wet spots" may indicate drainage under the cast or a need for additional drying. Stains can indicate wound drainage or bleeding, and any stained areas should be carefully measured and documented. Also be aware of possible pressure points on underlying structures, such as the lateral malleolus under a short leg cast or the epicondyle under a short arm cast. Closely inspect areas of the cast that are known to cover wounds with the understanding that drainage on the surface of synthetic casts may not wick outward but may go to a dependent area determined by cast position (e.g., beneath the cast if it is flat, posterior and superior if the limb is elevated).

An older cast may develop a sour smell because of perspiration or normal sloughing of outer skin layers. Musty, offensive odors under the cast, however, may indicate tissue necrosis or infection. If the odor of mildew is present, the synthetic cast may have not been thoroughly dried after it became wet; notify the physician because the cast needs to be changed.

Assessment for Complications

Compartment Syndrome. Any client with an extremity fracture should be assessed regularly for compartment syndrome for the first week after injury. Traumatic injury and treatment such as closed reduction usually produce swelling, which progresses for the first 12 to 24 hours after injury. The greatest swelling is likely to be evident in the first 24 to 48 hours.

SAFETY

ALERT

Mild swelling is expected; however, moderate or severe swelling associated with pain or discoloration is abnormal. Excessive swelling constricts the enclosed soft tissues and introduces the risk for compartment syndrome.

The affected extremity should be compared regularly with the uninjured extremity, and current findings should also be compared with baseline assessment data. Manifestations of compartment syndrome can begin as early as 30 minutes after ischemic injury. The primary manifestation is increasing pain or pain that is out of proportion to the injury. Specifically, pain with passive stretching of the muscles in an affected compartment is one of the earliest indicators. Assess for the presence of tingling or paresthesia in the affected extremity; muscle strength and motion; and circulation, including the presence and quality of pulses distal to the injury, capillary refill, skin color, and temperature. Increased tenseness and erythema of the skin also suggest increasing compartment pressures. If the intracompartmental pressure increases to a level above the client's systolic blood pressure, pulses are absent, capillary refill is delayed, and pallor results. Paralysis is a very late sign of compartment syndrome. If compartment syndrome goes unrecognized and tissue pressures are not relieved, muscle damage becomes irreversible after 4 to 6 hours of ischemia; nerve damage becomes irreversible after 12 to 24 hours. The physician must be notified immediately of assessment findings that suggest the development of compartment syndrome. The Critical Monitoring feature below lists additional assessment details.

Fat Emboli. Be alert to manifestations of hypoxemia, such as apprehension, anxiety, agitation, or acute confusion. Petechiae are often noted on the chest, axillae, flanks, abdomen, clavicular fossae, and soft palate. The client with FES also exhibits fever (temperature >103° F [39.4° C]), dyspnea, tachypnea, and tachycardia. Diffuse rales and rhonchi may occur as late signs of FES.

CRITICAL MONITORING

The Client in a Cast

COMPARTMENT SYNDROME
- Diminished or absent pulses; slow nail bed capillary refill (longer than 3 seconds)
- Skin pallor, blanching, cyanosis, or coolness
- Increasing pain, swelling, painful edema peripheral to cast, pain on passive motion
- Paresthesias (tingling, prickling), heightened sensitivity, numbness; hypoesthesia (diminished sensitivity to touch); anesthesia (numbness)
- Motor paralysis of previously functioning muscles
- Infection
- Musty, unpleasant odor over cast or at ends of cast
- Drainage through cast or cast opening
- Sudden unexplained body temperature elevation
- "Hot spot" felt on cast over lesion
- New pain or increased pain

CAST SYNDROME
- Bloated feeling
- Prolonged nausea; repeated vomiting
- Abdominal distention; vague abdominal pain
- Shortness of breath

Deep Vein Thrombosis. The typical manifestations of DVT are unilateral edema, at or below the site of thrombosis, that results from venous inflammation or obstruction. Affected clients often complain of pain and tenderness at the site, which may also be red and warm. Homans' sign (in which dorsiflexion of the foot causes discomfort in the upper calf) is present in fewer than one third of symptomatic clients with DVT. Because Homans' sign is present in more than 50% of symptomatic clients who do not have DVT, it is not considered specific or sensitive to the condition. Venous ultrasonography is a sensitive, accurate, noninvasive examination that has become the standard for diagnosis of DVT.

Infection. The client may describe new pain or an increased level of pain and feelings of increased warmth under a bandage or cast. Assessment may reveal fever or chills, an odor from the area of injury, erythema and warmth around the wound, purulent drainage, and poor wound healing.

Cast Syndrome. If the client is in a body cast, closely attend to any complaints of nausea, abdominal pressure, vague abdominal pain, feelings of bloating or tightness, or inability to take a deep breath. These may be clinical manifestation of cast syndrome, a serious complication that can follow prolonged supine positioning, spinal surgery, or use of a body cast.

Management of suspected cast syndrome includes cutting a window or bivalving the cast to relieve pressure. Nasogastric intubation may be indicated to decompress the intestine, intravenous fluids may be ordered, and the client may be placed on NPO status. Antiemetics should be given sparingly to any client in a body cast because they can mask the manifestations of cast syndrome. The client who is discharged in a body cast should receive careful instruction about the clinical manifestations of cast syndrome and should be encouraged to report any complaints promptly to the surgeon.

Interventions for Clients in Casts. To prevent or relieve swelling, elevate the entire casted extremity higher than the client's heart for the first 24 to 48 hours. Place the affected extremity on pillows. A casted arm may also be elevated in a sling attached to an intravenous (IV) pole. The entire arm, including the elbow, wrist, and hand, must be supported, and the fingers must be kept higher than the elbow to minimize swelling. Also apply ice bags around the cast, and exercise the client's fingers or toes to encourage circulation. Relieve pressure at the cast edges by petaling the cast or loosely padding an uncomfortable area. To prevent footdrop in a cylinder-casted leg, splint or support the client's foot with the ankle in 90 degrees of flexion.

For the client in a hip spica or body cast, the buttocks should be exposed to prevent soiling or dampening of clothing during elimination and to provide adequate skin care. To prevent soiling, incontinence pads can be tucked into the edge of the cast before the client uses a fracture bedpan. Slightly raising the head of the bed facilitates elimination and also prevents excrement from running under the cast; this position is usually allowed unless the client is in shock, is hemorrhaging, or has a spinal injury. Dampness causes skin irritation and may increase the risk of infection if an open wound is present; therefore thorough perineal care must be completed after elimination.

Position changes at least every 2 hours are needed to help prevent complications of immobility, and a turning schedule is useful for ensuring that the client does not remain in one position too long. Give instructions on turning to encourage client activity, but also provide assistance with bed mobility as needed. When mobility assistance is needed, always have adequate staff help to turn a casted client. Three or four people may be needed to turn a client in a body or hip spica cast, for example. Roller boards or mechanical lifts may also be useful.

Depending on the nature of the injury and the physician's orders, clients in casts can often bear weight as soon as the cast is dry. Be aware of the client's weight-bearing status when attempting a transfer.

For client safety, also use a transfer belt when getting the client out of bed. SAFETY ALERT

Weak, older, or debilitated clients may have difficulty with the weight of the cast and may tire rapidly with initial activity. The client should be instructed about the likelihood of increased pain when a casted leg is lowered to a dependent position during initial attempts at ambulation. Help the client lower the leg, reminding the client about the decrease in pain as the leg becomes accustomed to the increased blood flow.

To ensure client cooperation, provide thorough instruction on pain management strategies. Ensure that the client understands the availability of analgesics for treatment of pain and is allowed to voice any concerns about their use, such as fears of addiction. Initiate an honest discussion about any barriers to analgesic use if the client seems hesitant about taking or asking for medication. Administer analgesics as prescribed, and promptly inform the surgeon of inadequate effects. Client instruction should also include alternative methods of pain management, such as distraction, visualization, or massage that might help the client relax.

Itching is a common sensation after the cast dries. Teach the client not to put anything in the cast to scratch the area. These devices (knives, coat hangers, knitting needles, chop sticks) injure the skin. Powders tend to cake inside the cast. Itching can be treated by blowing cool air into the cast, elevating the extremity, applying ice, tapping on the area or taking mild analgesics or antihistamines.

Care of the Client in External Fixation

Assessment. Because external fixation may be used following extensive soft tissue injury, the potential for neurovascular deficit or compartment syndrome is high. Even though the external fixator may be used for treatment of an open fracture, compartment syndrome can nonetheless develop in another compartment of the same extremity. Ongoing neurovascular assessment is critical. Current findings should be compared with baseline data, and the affected extremity should be compared with the unaffected extremity. Instruct the client to report any changes, and address any complaints promptly.

As with the client in a cast, careful assessment of pain must be completed regularly. Analgesia should be assessed, and inadequate effects should be reported promptly to the surgeon because an increased dosage or change in medication may be indicated. Unrelieved pain should raise suspicion of compartment syndrome, and any complaint of pain should be given full attention. Be especially alert to complaints of progressive pain or pain out of proportion to the injury or treatment.

Pin sites and wounds must be regularly assessed for signs of infection, and pins should be checked for loosening. A small amount of bleeding immediately after pin insertion is expected and can be controlled with small pressure dressings; however, bleeding that continues for more than 24 hours should be brought to the surgeon's attention. Wound healing progress must be assessed, and carefully documented. The injury to adipose tissue at the pin sites may produce fatty drainage that looks a great deal like pus. Be alert to more specific signs of infection, such as pin instability, drainage with odor or color, and skin tension or puckering at the insertion site (tenting). If tenting occurs, the surgeon should be notified so that the wound can be extended.

The client's nutritional status greatly affects bone and wound healing; pay attention to the adequacy of food intake as well as the client's ability to eat and swallow. Be aware of complaints of nausea or vomiting. Any abnormal laboratory values should also be assessed as possible evidence of poor nutrition.

If the client smokes, willingness to abstain from smoking should be assessed. It must be emphasized that there is growing evidence that smoking delays or inhibits bone healing after surgery or trauma. 🪔

Interventions. Antibiotics may need to be administered prophylactically for 48 to 72 hours after application of an external fixator. Later, wound care may involve the application of wet-to-dry dressings. Because little consensus has been achieved on pin care methods, follow the surgeon's orders or institutional standards. Loose pins must be reported promptly to the surgeon; they will be removed to prevent osteomyelitis.

The client's sense of balance can be altered by the weight of a fixator frame on the lower extremity. Because the client often also has a prescribed weight-bearing limitation after application of a lower extremity external fixator, be scrupulous in assessing adherence to any weight-bearing restrictions and correct use of ambulatory aids. The amount of support needed from the nurse is determined by the client's ability to control the extremity during movement.

Nausea or vomiting should be addressed aggressively with an antiemetic agent, as ordered, to decrease the risk for nutritional deficits or aspiration. Dietary supplements may be used as needed. Client and family education is critical for achieving a successful outcome with use of external fixation. By the time of discharge, the client should have begun to accept the change in body image that accompanies the use of external fixation. The client should also understand his or her responsibility for pin and wound care. The client should be knowledgeable about manifestations of infection and should be aware of the significance of neurovascular or integumentary changes. The client must also receive instruction on use of analgesics and antibiotics as ordered by the surgeon. Instruction should include alternative methods of pain management, such as distraction, visualization, or massage, that may help the client relax.

Before discharge, teach the client how to meet hygiene needs and discuss any resumption of sexual activity. Clothing may need to be modified with snaps or self-fastening (Velcro) closures before discharge to fit over fixators. Advise the client with a pelvic fixator to reduce intake of gas-producing foods, which can lead to abdominal distention. Once the affected bone is healed, the fixator is removed.

Care of the Client in Traction

Assessment. Before application of traction, assess the client for changes in sensation of the foot and leg seen with diabetes, arterial disease, skin impairments (including allergy to tape), and any history of thrombophlebitis. Obtain a baseline measurement of neurovascular status.

Once traction is in place, both the traction system and the client must be assessed every shift (Box 27-3). A photograph or sketch of the correct traction setup may be useful for nursing staff.

Interventions. If the client's nutritional status becomes a concern, dietary supplements may be ordered. Small, frequent meals may be indicated for the client in a halo

BOX 27-3 Nursing Assessment of a Client in Skeletal Traction

- Check traction equipment every shift and as needed. Full inspection must include:
  - Traction cords aligned in each pulley
  - Cords not stretched and frayed
  - Knots tied tightly and secured with tape
  - Cords hanging free of bed and floor
  - Weights hanging free of bed and floor
  - Correct amount of weights hanging (usually 25-40 pounds)
  - Spreaders, footplates, splints not touching end of bed
  - Overhead frame and bars are intact
  - Bed linen not interfering with line of traction
- Maintain correct body alignment and proper bed position for countertraction, if indicated.
- Do not lift weights without a specific order.
- Check weights after position changes.
- Apply trapeze for ease in moving in bed (if not contraindicated, as in spinal injuries or bilateral upper extremity injuries).
- Assess client for secondary complications of immobility, such as:
  - Thrombophlebitis
  - Constipation
  - Atelectasis
  - Urinary problems
  - Loss of muscle strength
  - Skin breakdown
  - Depression
- Inspect pin entry/exit sites (where applicable) for redness, swelling, odor, bleeding, discharge, tenting.
- Perform pin site care twice a day as ordered.

vest to avoid a feeling of excessive fullness. Bent straws and adapted utensils may be indicated for clients who have limitations on head elevation.

To provide client comfort with elimination, provide a fracture bedpan and ensure privacy when the client needs to use it. The client's diet should include ample fluids and fiber if there are no contraindications. Laxatives may be prescribed and should be administered regularly. Also determine whether the client has regular, effective personal strategies for maintenance of normal bowel elimination and incorporate those methods into the plan of care.

Encourage independence in client activities within the limitations of the traction. The client should be instructed on repositioning techniques, possibly using extended horizontal bars with roller traction to allow movement to a chair at the bedside. Unaffected joints should be exercised regularly through the use of free weights, foam balls, or elastic pull bands. A record book may be used to encourage the client to cross off the exercise session when it is completed.

Immediately after traction removal, the client is often weak and unsteady as a result of muscle atrophy or orthostatic hypotension. The client should be gradually assisted to a sitting position and then to a standing position later as tolerated. Movement of a previously bedridden client to a sitting or standing position may take several days, depending on the effects of previous immobility. Ensure adequate assistance and provide careful physical support when assisting the client with these position changes. An assistive device such as a walker or crutches may be needed for temporary support of weak muscles and stiff joints (see also the Care Plan feature on The Client in Traction on the website).

SPECIFIC FRACTURES

HIP FRACTURES

Approximately 3% to 5% of falls among older adults cause fractures.[9] Hip fractures in particular have become one of the leading causes of morbidity and mortality among the older population. More than 400,000 hospital admissions annually result from hip fractures. More than 60% of people who die from falls are age 75 or older. When compared to younger clients, those age 75 or older who sustain a hip fracture are four to five times more likely to be admitted to a long-term care facility for a year or more. Hip fractures also have a significant impact on health care costs; the annual expense of medical and nursing services is estimated to be $7 billion to $10 billion.

Etiology and Risk Factors

Numerous studies have associated low bone mass and increasing age with an increased risk of hip fracture. Women begin to lose bone about 1.5 years before the last menstrual period; the bone loss continues rapidly until about 1.5 years after the last menses. The rate of bone loss then slows, matching the rate of loss in men by age 65 or 70. The development of low bone mass is known to be influenced by genetic factors. For example, women tend to have lower bone mass if their mothers or fathers have experienced vertebral fractures. Additional factors that can lead to the development of low bone mass include (1) low body weight, (2) physical inactivity, (3) low dietary calcium intake, (4) inadequate levels of serum vitamin D, (5) cigarette smoking, and (6) consumption of alcohol.

More than 90% of hip fractures are caused by falling; however, attempts to decrease the risk of falling through controlled trials have generally been ineffective. Some researchers have concluded that it is the dynamic interaction between the client's physical environment and intrinsic risk factors that actually increases the client's vulnerability to fall and injury.

SAFETY
ALERT

Other factors have been associated with the occurrence of falls that lead to hip fractures. These include the client's orthostatic hypotension, impaired vision, lower limb dysfunction, and neurologic conditions as well as the use of barbiturates or long-acting benzodiazepines. Environmental hazards may also contribute to the older client's tendency to fall. These include loose carpeting or rugs, slippery floors, poor lighting, a slippery tub or shower, irregular pavement, and loose clothing or footwear.

The Translating Evidence into Practice feature below explains how to assess and predict the risk of a fall.

Pathophysiology

Fractures of the hip are either *intracapsular* (located within the joint capsule) or *extracapsular* (located outside the joint capsule). Fractures are also described on the basis of their location in one of the four anatomic areas of the proximal hip (Figure 27-7). *Femoral neck fractures* are more common in frail older adults, especially women, and are often associated with osteoporosis. They generally result from relatively mild trauma. *Intertrochanteric fractures* (between the femoral neck and the greater trochanter) and *subtrochanteric fractures* are more often seen in males and in vigorous older adults; they are likely to be associated with greater traumatic force.

Because blood flow to the hip is an important influence on fracture healing, delayed healing or non-union may occur in areas of the hip where circulation is impaired after injury. Healing of femoral head fractures, for example, is unlikely if AVN develops after local circulatory compromise.

Clinical Manifestations

Hip fracture is often caused by a fall at home that involves only a moderate amount of trauma, such as slipping out of a chair onto the floor. Immediately after the fall, the client is unable to bear weight on the affected

---

☞ TRANSLATING EVIDENCE INTO PRACTICE

Prevention of Falls and Fall-Related Injury

Client falls are a difficult clinical problem that can result in substantial personal, financial, and emotional costs for everyone involved. Accurate fall risk assessment based on research can allow use of appropriate interventions to decrease occurrences in acutely ill populations.

Recognizing the need to validate current tools used for fall risk assessment and to measure the impact of interventions on fall outcomes, McFarlane-Kolb (2004) compared and described differences in fall data within and between two study groups before and after a multitargeted intervention.[1] A 30-bed colorectal/vascular nursing unit was selected for the study, and a fall risk initiative was implemented to include fall risk screening to ensure targeted fall prevention strategies, performance of multitargeted strategies, and training of staff. The researcher utilized the Morse falls scale, with additional risk factors selected from the literature for comparative analysis. The scale was completed retrospectively in a blinded manner (i.e., without knowledge of any falls during the client's hospitalization) for both study groups. The same assessment tool was used to complete the part of the study aimed to accurately profile risk factors for falling within and between groups. Fall data were collected from fall risk assessments, occurrence reports, and medical records.

Comparison of the total sample population of fallers and nonfallers determined that the following variables were significant in predicting falls: male gender, length of stay of 3 days or more, 5 or more medications, 3 or more investigative procedures, and 4 or more medical diagnoses. In addition, sedative/hypnotic use and cognitive impairment showed a trend toward fall risk prediction. History of falling, abnormal gait, cognitive condition, and intravenous therapy were variables found to contribute most to the Morse score in the regression analysis. The author proposed that the Morse scale in combination with the most significant additional risk factors identified (male gender and major tranquilizer use) gives a more accurate risk profile of potential for falling.

With fall risk identified, nurses should implement evidence-based interventions to decrease the likelihood of client injury in the event of a fall. One strategy gaining popularity is the use of hip protectors, which have been described as "crash helmets for the hips."[2] Published research on use of hip protectors has focused on older adults in nursing homes or the community. The strongest evidence to support the use of hip protectors is from studies of nursing home residents; these have demonstrated at least a 50% reduction in falls among residents after implementation of hip protectors. Additional studies have not supported the value of hip protectors in preventing a second fracture. Results of randomized studies thus remain inconclusive on the benefits of hip protectors. For nurses, the important research implication is whether use of hip protectors can be promoted on an individual basis or in selected populations.

REFERENCES

1. McFarlane-Kolb, H. (2004). Fall risk assessment, multitargeted interventions, and the impact on hospital falls. *International Journal of Nursing Practice, 10*, 199-206.
2. Hayes, N. (2004). Hip protectors: Interpreting the evidence and addressing practicalities. *Nursing Older People, 16*(3), 15-20.

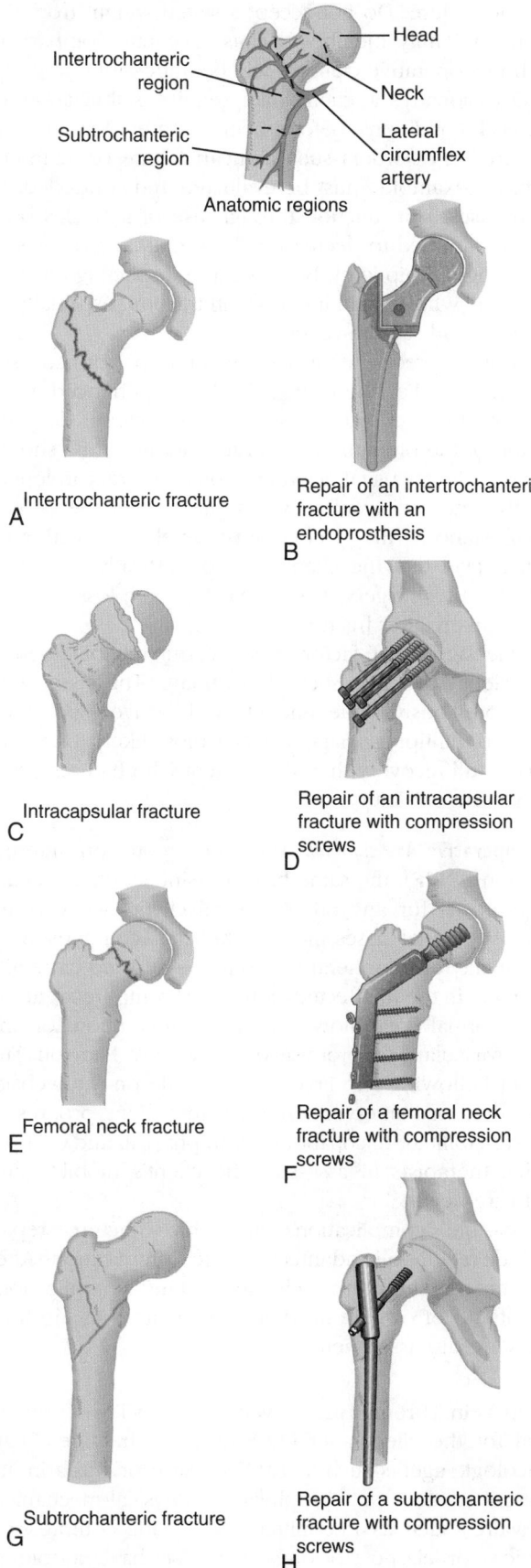

■ **FIGURE 27–7** Anatomic regions of the proximal femur and blood supply. **A-H,** Fracture patterns of the hip and surgical repairs.

leg. Objective findings include a shortened leg and an externally rotated hip. Deformity may also be evident in the lateral hip if the fracture is displaced. Ecchymosis at the hip is most likely to occur with subtrochanteric fractures. Location of pain depends on the specific fracture site (see Figure 27-7, *A, C, E, G*). A femoral neck fracture, for example, is characterized by groin and hip pain that increases with hip movement. Intertrochanteric fractures are accompanied by severe pain over the greater trochanter of the femur, whereas subtrochanteric fractures typically produce pain over the proximal thigh. Additional tissue trauma such as head or hand lacerations may also be evident.

Sometimes hip fracture is not readily noted, so a high index of suspicion often is required for prompt diagnosis and treatment of an occult hip fracture. Even when a client is able to walk and has no documented trauma, localized hip pain, or typical shortening and malrotation deformity, nurses should be alert to the possibility of hip fracture, particularly in a client who is older than 65 years, presents with nonspecific leg discomfort, and complains of difficulty bearing weight on the affected limb. Some clients with hip fracture have normal ambulation and complain only of vague pain in their buttocks, knees, thighs, groin, or back, especially if they also have dementia.

Diagnosis of hip fracture is based on the client's clinical manifestations, history of trauma, and radiologic findings. The presence of a fracture is often confirmed by anteroposterior radiograph, although in some instances additional studies may be ordered. Computed tomographic (CT) scans, bone scans, or magnetic resonance imaging (MRI) may be necessary to identify the fracture site.

OUTCOME MANAGEMENT

Medical Management

For a relatively few clients, nonoperative treatment is the best option following hip fracture. A client who cannot tolerate anesthesia or who was nonambulatory before the fracture may be treated with skeletal traction or spica casting. While the client remains in traction (approximately 8 to 12 weeks), develop a plan of care that will decrease the effects of immobility. For example, excellent skin care must be provided to reduce the risk of pressure ulcer development. Because older clients are at increased risk for skin impairment even before immobilization, a pressure-redistributing mattress and heel elevation are essential. Perform careful frequent assessment of bony prominences such as the heels, sacrum, scapulae, and vertebrae. In addition, instruct the client about leg exercises that will decrease the probability of thromboembolism; pneumatic compression devices or anticoagulant medications will also be used to lessen the likelihood of clot development. Document the presence of intact and/or open skin in high-risk body areas.

Surgical Management

Extensive blood loss can occur after hip fracture, particularly in older clients with other medical conditions. Additional deterioration can occur rapidly if the client is left on bed rest; therefore prompt surgical intervention and early mobilization are keys to successful rehabilitation. The goal of surgical treatment is to achieve a stable reduction and internal fixation of the fracture segments to support early ambulation.

Open Reduction and Internal Fixation

Postoperative treatment goals include the following:

- Complete union of the fracture (4 to 8 months)
- Prevention of deformity and contractures to the hip, knee, or foot
- Restoration of weight-bearing ambulation, with the use of assistive devices if needed
- Relief of pain and fear; prevention of complications
- Maintenance of optimal physiologic function

Fixation may be accomplished through the use of screws, plates, intramedullary pins, or implants (see Figure 27-7, *B, D, F, H*). The term *open reduction* indicates that a surgical incision was made to expose the bone, in contrast to a closed reduction of a fracture (see Reducing Fractures earlier in this chapter). *Internal fixation* indicates that devices such as pins or plates were used to hold the bones in alignment during healing. Perfect anatomic reduction and fixation may be difficult to achieve if the client has decreased bone density as a result of osteoporosis. If the fracture is highly comminuted or the head of the femur has been destroyed, use of an endoprosthesis to replace the entire head of the femur may be necessary. For the client who has an accompanying acetabular fracture, total hip arthroplasty may be indicated (see Chapter 26).

Nursing Management of the Surgical Client

Preoperative Care

Clients who require surgical reduction and fixation of hip fractures most often go directly from the emergency department to the operating room. Delay in repair not only places an older client at risk for additional effects of immobility but also increases the likelihood that AVN will develop as a result of inadequate blood supply to the fracture fragments. Assess routine laboratory tests and the client's baseline weight preoperatively. A bed scale should be used to minimize client discomfort with

this procedure. Do not accept a stated weight from the client or family member because accurate comparison with postoperative changes will be impossible.

Occasionally, a client may require stabilization of medical conditions before being cleared for surgery. Underlying disorders such as heart failure or malnutrition, for example, must be evaluated and controlled. In such cases, skin traction through use of a Buck's boot may be applied to decrease painful muscle spasms surrounding the hip joint. Be diligent in inspecting the skin of clients who remain immobile in traction, especially of the heel and sacrum-coccyx.

Routine preoperative assessment is performed (see Chapter 14). For the client who has experienced a hip fracture, preoperative assessment also includes determination of the preinjury level of functioning. Data should clearly address usual activities, ability to walk independently, and history of previous falls. Under the best of circumstances, the preoperative level of functioning is the level that the client can optimistically expect to achieve after surgery. Unfortunately, some loss of function is likely after fracture repair.

One significant factor in successful rehabilitation is the client's previous social functioning. The client who was previously independent and active and who enjoyed multiple social contacts is more likely to experience a full recovery than is the client who had restricted activity before injury.

Postoperative Assessment. After open reduction, internal fixation (ORIF), the same basic nursing assessments are required as for any other surgical client (see Chapter 14). Additional assessment includes a comparison of the quality of peripheral pulses in the affected extremity with that in the unaffected extremity. Prompt recognition of abnormal data allows for early intervention for any neurovascular compromise (see the Care Plan on The Client Following Hip Fracture and ORIF on the website for additional interventions). As the client progresses into rehabilitation, collaborate with physical and occupational therapists in assessing the client's mobility and self-care needs.

Possible complications after hip fracture repair include fat emboli and infection (see Complications After Fracture earlier in this chapter). Other complications specific to or of high incidence in clients with hip fractures are discussed here.

Deep Vein Thrombosis. Prevention of DVT is a primary goal for the client after ORIF of a hip fracture. Pharmacologic agents such as LMW heparin or warfarin are prescribed for clot prophylaxis. Physical-mechanical measures such as intermittent pneumatic compression devices or elastic stockings may also have a role in DVT prevention. DVT is discussed more fully in Chapter 53.

Pressure Ulcers. A *pressure ulcer* is tissue damage that results from unrelieved pressure, usually over a bony prominence. Its development may have begun as the injured client lay on a hard floor at home, on hard surfaces in an ambulance or in the emergency department, on a table for radiographs or surgery, or in the bed after surgery. Pressure ulcer risk is compounded because the client is unable to turn independently after injury or surgery. Without assistance, the client remains supine or in a semi-Fowler position for most of the hospitalization. Identification of the client's risk for skin impairment can be accomplished through the use of an assessment tool such as the Braden scale, presented in Chapter 49.

A turning schedule is essential for eliminating sustained pressure over bony prominences on the head, scapulae, vertebrae, coccyx, and heels. Other areas such as the elbows, ankles, and medial surfaces of the knees may also be affected by pressure that lasts as little as 15 minutes. Bony areas should be cushioned and supported with each position change. Heels should be elevated with calf pillows or foam boots. Prevention of ischemia can also be accomplished through the use of pressure-reduction bed overlays. An "egg-crate" mattress may contribute to client comfort in the bed, but it does not relieve pressure. Specialty mattresses or air beds are the only appropriate alternatives to assist in pressure redistribution. The client who is using a specialty bed must still be turned on a regular schedule.

Acute Confusion. An acute confusional state (delirium) is characterized by an abrupt onset of numerous global, transient changes in a client's attention, cognition, psychomotor activity, or sleep-wake cycle or in several of these. The client may appear forgetful, inattentive, disoriented, or fearful. Daytime sleepiness and nighttime insomnia may be noticed.

> **In the hospitalized client, confusion creates concerns about safety and dependence on others for self-care needs and can greatly affect the emotional status of the client and family. It can also lead to prolonged hospitalization, possibly contributing to placement in a long-term care facility and definitely increasing costs.**

Some degree of confusion has been identified in up to 60% of hospitalized older clients, although the average incidence of acute confusion is about 20%.[15] Most affected clients have no history of confusion or mental impairment.

Consistent predictors of, or risk factors for, acute confusion have been difficult to identify clearly. The risk for development of confusion may in fact be a cumulative function of the client's biopsychosocial integrity, the level of illness and functional impairment, and the timing and magnitude of added stressors. Known contributors to confusion may be an unfamiliar environment; sensory overstimulation or deprivation; the client's loss of control and uncertain future; a disrupted routine; immobility and pain; and a disrupted elimination pattern. Because use of medications with anticholinergic effects has also been linked to client confusion, carefully monitor all medications.

Careful assessment of the client's attention, memory, orientation, psychomotor behavior, and sleep-wake cycle is needed. The risk for confusion may also be decreased by maintaining appropriate hydration, perfusion, and oxygenation in the client. Attention must be given to managing pain, meeting nutritional requirements, and correcting metabolic imbalances. The client must have easy access to glasses, hearing aids, and other functional devices. Also address environmental factors by reorienting the confused client in a consistent way and minimizing disruption to the usual diurnal rhythms. Companionship of family members or volunteers is helpful, as is the use of calendars, clocks, and newspapers to provide a time reference for the client. Follow institutional guidelines for the use of restraints.

Diagnosis, Outcomes, Interventions

Diagnosis: Acute Pain. Acute pain is expected after ORIF of the hip. The client may also have contusions or abrasions caused by the fall that led to hip fracture. The nursing diagnosis can be written as *Acute Pain related to local tissue trauma from surgical incision or other injuries.*

Outcomes. The client will demonstrate comfort after surgery, as evidenced by moving without grimacing, by requesting analgesics no more frequently than ordered, by using less analgesic each day, and by stating that the pain is tolerable and not interfering with rest or physical therapy.

Interventions. In the immediate postoperative period, the client may experience intense pain and require parenteral or epidural analgesics to attain acceptable control. Common interventions include patient-controlled analgesia (PCA) or epidural analgesia. Ice application over the dressed surgical wound may also increase the client's comfort. The Management and Delegation feature on p. 530 discusses the application of heat and cold.

Within 24 to 48 hours, the client should be tolerating fluids and able to take oral analgesics. Because pain is intensified with movement, the client may attempt to limit activity. Medicate the client before physical therapy or activities such as transferring to the chair, and reinforce the importance of ambulation in decreasing the risk for postoperative complications. Use of non-opioid analgesics can also help with acute pain management, muscle spasms, and other chronic medical problems such as arthritis. Use nonsteroidal anti-inflammatory

MANAGEMENT AND DELEGATION

Application of Heat and Cold

Any equipment used to apply heat or cold may injure the client. Injury may result if the client is unable to perceive discomfort because of decreased peripheral circulation, decreased feeling, decreased sensorium, sedation, or agitation. The client may also be at risk if he or she cannot be left alone safely or if the client alters the controls of the heating pad or cooling device.

The application of heat or cold to an inflamed or painful area that is closed may be delegated to unlicensed assistive personnel. Before delegating the application of heat or cold, consider the following:

- What is the indication for the application of heat or cold? Check the physician's order. The order and indication may be sufficient to tell you whether you can delegate this task or not.
- What is the condition of the affected site? Assess for any areas of redness, swelling, breakdown, or scar tissue. It is important to know the baseline condition of the site before the application of heat or cold. There may be an indication to withhold this treatment or to confer with the physician about the order. You will also need to assess the condition of the site on completion of the treatment.
- What is the client's diagnosis? Is there any history of diabetes mellitus or impairment in sensorium or mentation? This may be an indication for you to perform this treatment yourself. If there is impairment of the client's mental or sensory status, it may be necessary for the unlicensed assistive personnel to remain with the client throughout the treatment.
- What is the competency level of the unlicensed assistive personnel who might perform this task?

Instruct the unlicensed assistive personnel providing the heat or cold application to do the following:

- Perform hand hygiene.
- Assemble the necessary equipment. Advise them as to which method of applying heat or cold is ordered.
- When using ice cubes, they should be placed in an ice bag with a scoop through a funnel; the ice cubes should not be touched with bare hands.
- Check the temperature of the heat or cold device before applying it to the client's skin. A safe range for heat applications is 115° to 125° F [46° to 51° C] for adults.
- Wrap any heat or cold application with a protective cover, such as a towel or a flannel sleeve.
- If using a heating pad, start with the device on the lowest setting to initiate treatment.
- Instruct the client not to adjust the heat setting.
- Check the client's response immediately. If the device is too hot or cold, an adjustment is necessary. Double the protective layer between the device and the skin or allow the temperature of the device to moderate slightly.
- Check the client's skin after 5 minutes. If it is tolerated, leave the heat or cold in place for 20 minutes. If it is not tolerated, the heat or cold should be removed immediately, and the nurse should be notified. Assess the situation and notify the physician as appropriate.
- Remove the heat or cold application at 20 minutes and inform the nurse when the treatment is complete.

You are responsible for examining the affected area and reassessing the client's skin at completion of this treatment. You should document your findings and the client's response to treatment in the medical record. The unlicensed assistive personnel should immediately report any difficulty encountered during the course of treatment.

---

drugs (NSAIDs) cautiously in older adults with impaired kidney function.

Concerns about becoming addicted to opioids should be addressed openly. Many older adults fear that they will become addicted quickly, and they may delay their recovery by tolerating unnecessary pain. Opioid addiction is rare, but the fear is quite intense.

Regularly assess for side effects of opioid analgesics. Confusion and sedation may be seen in the older adult. Respiratory depression is more likely to occur with PCA or epidural analgesia than with oral opioids. Pulse oximetry and regular measurement of vital signs help to assess for hypoxemia that results from shallow or slow breathing. Stimulating the client to deep breathe will raise oximetry values. Naloxone is seldom needed to reverse opioid analgesia, however it should be kept in a convenient place. Constipation can occur after hip fracture and repair as a result of the client's impaired mobility, opioid analgesic use, and slow progression to a regular diet.

Diagnosis: Impaired Physical Mobility. The client's degree of immobility after ORIF of the hip is affected by pain and fear of movement as well as any limitations in other joints. If previous mobility limitations contributed to the fall, the client may have even greater problems with mobilization after surgery. The nursing diagnosis can be written as *Impaired Physical Mobility related to pain, spasms or fear of movement.*

Outcomes. The client will demonstrate improved physical mobility, as evidenced by the need for less assistance in transfers (bed to chair, bed to standing), by safe use of a walker or crutches, and by the ability to ambulate a functional distance (150 feet). For the client with previous mobility limitations, outcomes may focus on bed mobility only.

Interventions. Moving the client after ORIF of the hip can create a great deal of anxiety for both the client and the nursing staff. Physical therapists often assist with moving the client initially. Be aware of any weight-bearing limitations ordered for the client before transfer (Table 27-5

TABLE 27–5 Weight-Bearing Status

Non–weight-bearing	Client does not bear weight on affected extremity; affected extremity should not touch floor.
Touch-down weight-bearing or toe-touch weight-bearing	Client's foot of affected extremity may rest on floor for balance, but no weight is distributed through that extremity.
Partial weight-bearing	Client bears 30-50% of weight on affected extremity.
Weight-bearing as tolerated	Client bears as much weight as tolerable on affected extremity without undue strain or pain.
Full weight-bearing	Client can bear weight fully on affected extremity.

describes weight-bearing limitations). Because the older adult may have balance difficulties that make it difficult to maintain weight-bearing restrictions, the surgeon is likely to prescribe toe-touch or touch-down weight-bearing in which the client rests the foot on the floor for balance but without distributing any weight through the leg. Careful attention must be paid to the operative extremity during transfers to ensure that the client is following weight-bearing requirements. Record the amount of assistance that the client requires for safe transfer. This information provides the benchmark that will determine whether the goal for increased mobility is being met. For example, the client may have needed the assistance of two staff members on the morning after surgery; by the next afternoon, increased mobility was demonstrated when only one nurse was needed to assist with transfer.

In addition to postoperative limitations, the client may suffer from arthritis in other joints or may have residual effects from a previous stroke. These conditions can increase pain and affect the ability to transfer from the bed to the chair. Medicate the client with mild analgesia, such as acetaminophen, early in the morning before activity. When the client stands and transfers for the first time, the assistance of at least two staff members will be needed. Use appropriate technique to ensure a safe transfer for the client and also to minimize the risk of injury to your lower back (see Chapter 26 for additional information on requirements for appropriate mobility assistance).

Diagnosis: Self-Care Deficit. After hip fracture and surgical repair, the client is likely to experience some degree of self-care deficit in hygiene and dressing. Limited mobility may decrease independence in self-care, and assistive devices may be required. The diagnostic statement may read *Self-Care Deficit: Bathing/hygiene, dressing/grooming related to mobility impairment following hip fracture.*

Outcomes. The client will resume pre-injury level of independence in meeting self-care needs.

Interventions. After ORIF of the hip, the client will require assistance to bathe legs, back and buttocks. They will also receive assistance from both physical and occupational therapists. Physical therapists help with ambulation and muscle strengthening. They offer instruction on climbing stairs and on getting in and out of a car. They also provide assistive devices that help in functional independence, such as an elevated toilet seat and a walker. Occupational therapists instruct the client on bathing and dressing techniques. They may suggest use of a tub bench or a long-handled sponge. They may also provide long-handled reachers or sock aids to help the client dress with minimal assistance from others. Nursing staff will reinforce the use of techniques and assistive devices to encourage the client's optimal recovery.

Diagnosis: Risk for Impaired Skin Integrity. If the client has fallen while alone and experienced an extended time on the floor before help arrived, even early assessment may show the development of pressure ulcers over bony prominences. Use a formal pressure ulcer risk assessment tool to determine risk level and specific factors that place the client at risk. After surgery, the client's mobility limitations and pain increase the risk for skin impairment. Malnutrition and dehydration, which may have existed before injury and could be exacerbated postoperatively, may also contribute. Older clients and clients receiving long-term corticosteroid therapy may have especially thin skin that is even more prone to breakdown and tears. The type of tape used to secure postoperative dressings, along with the method and direction of tape application, can also contribute to the development of skin blisters. An appropriate diagnostic statement may be *Risk for Impaired Skin Integrity related to mobility limitations or to the application of tape with dressing changes.*

Outcomes. The client will demonstrate intact skin, as evidenced by the absence of ulcers over bony prominences and heels and absence of epidermal stripping beneath tape used to secure postoperative dressings.

Interventions. After ORIF of the hip, the client should be assisted with position changes at least every 2 hours. The client can be turned to either side but is usually more comfortable on the nonoperative side with a pillow to support the operative leg. Carefully assess the skin over bony prominences such as the sacrum, coccyx, scapulae, elbows, and heels. If areas of skin breakdown are noted, measure and describe them thoroughly. Look carefully for signs of deep tissue injury (purple bruised-like skin) if the client was immobile for a while. Treat the ulcer using institutional protocols or see Chapter 49.

In addition to using a regular turning schedule, place a pressure-reducing mattress on the client's bed. Heels should be "floated" from the bed by placing a pillow under the calves or using soft boots. Assess the fit of the boot each time the client moves in bed. Pressure on the heels also can be relieved by placement of a towel roll for brief periods under the Achilles tendon. Specific skin care products are available to be rubbed gently into affected areas at the first sign of redness. Direct massage of stage I pressure ulcers is contraindicated.

Avoid epidermal stripping by placing postoperative dressings over a skin sealant that is applied wherever the tape would touch the skin. Elastic tape should be placed vertically (superior to inferior) without tension to allow for stretching that is related to postoperative edema. Any redness, blistering, or epidermal stripping should be evaluated, and a wound care nurse specialist should be consulted about the client's care as appropriate. Clients with thin skin should have gauze wraps rather than tape on their skin. Treatment of skin tears is discussed in Chapter 49.

Diagnosis: Risk for Infection. Bone infection is a serious threat and can lead to loss of joint function. Pre-existent poor health also contributes to risk. State this nursing diagnosis as *Risk for Infection related to loss of primary defenses (incision) and malnutrition (if present).*

Outcomes. The client will remain free of manifestations of infection, as evidenced by (1) white blood cell (WBC) count within normal limits, (2) an afebrile state, (3) absence of purulent wound drainage, (4) absence of increasing pain in wound, and (5) no inflammation in wound after 72 hours.

Interventions. Clients often receive prophylactic antibiotics during surgery and in the immediate postoperative period. After ORIF, the physician may prefer to perform the initial dressing change.

SAFETY ALERT **Use strict aseptic technique in performing subsequent dressing changes, carefully assessing the wound each time for signs of healing or infection.**

Diagnosis: Risk for Peripheral Neurovascular Dysfunction. Be aware of the risk for peripheral nerve or vascular impairment after surgery on any joint. Edema or extremity positioning can place pressure on adjacent nerves. The nursing diagnosis can be written as *Risk for Peripheral Neurovascular Dysfunction related to lower extremity edema or positioning.*

Outcomes. The client will demonstrate normal neurovascular function, as evidenced by adequate peripheral pulses with capillary refill time of 3 seconds or less and by the absence of sensory impairments or motor weakness in the operative extremity.

Interventions. Assess the neurovascular function of the operative extremity at least every 4 hours or as directed by the surgeon, and then compare findings to the unaffected extremity. More frequent monitoring may be needed if indicated by the client's condition. Assessment includes the presence and quality of bilateral pedal pulses, skin color and temperature of the extremity, capillary refill in the toes, sensation and movement of the toes, and the client's ability to perform dorsi-plantar flexion of the foot. Any pallor or coolness, numbness or tingling, or inability to move the extremity should be reported promptly to the surgeon.

Diagnosis: Risk for Constipation. Impaired mobility and the use of opioid analgesics can lead to constipation. The risk is increased in older clients who have a pre-existing dependence on laxatives. The nursing diagnosis could be written as *Risk for Constipation related to impaired physical mobility and side effects of opioids.*

Outcomes. The client will maintain a pattern of regular bowel elimination by consuming adequate fluids and high-fiber foods and by having a bowel movement at least every 2 to 3 days.

Interventions. Regular assessment and implementation of a proactive bowel program are important for minimizing clients' concerns about bowel elimination. The client's diet should include ample fluids and fiber if not contraindicated. Stool softeners may have limited usefulness because the client's gastrointestinal motility has been slowed by opioid use. A laxative may be a more appropriate choice to stimulate the return to normal bowel elimination. Also, determine whether the client has regular, effective personal strategies for treating constipation and, if so, use those methods to assist with elimination. The client should be assisted to transfer to a bedside commode or ambulate to the bathroom whenever possible to meet elimination needs. To assist the bedridden client with bowel elimination, offer a fracture bedpan and ensure privacy when the client needs to use it.

Diagnosis: Risk for Imbalanced Nutrition: Less Than Body Requirements. After surgery, the client may experience nausea that delays the progression to a regular diet. Decreased activity may also lead to poor appetite. If the client has experienced blood loss, a nutritional deficit may also occur. Remember that the presence of obesity does not ensure that the client is well nourished. This nursing diagnosis may be stated as *Risk for Imbalanced Nutrition: Less Than Body Requirements related to nausea or poor appetite following hip fracture.*

Outcomes. The client will maintain adequate nutritional intake, as evidenced by energy for participation in physical therapy and by appropriate wound and bone healing.

Interventions. Stress the importance of a high-carbohydrate and high-protein diet for adequate healing, and then assist the client in making food choices as necessary. If the client's appetite remains poor, offer small, frequent meals. Encourage the client to eat at least some of every food at every meal to achieve balanced intake. After blood loss, increased dietary iron or iron supplements may be required. Encourage the client to eat foods high in iron, and administer a supplement as ordered. Inform the client that stool may appear black or tarry as a result of the iron supplement.

Diagnosis: Deficient Knowledge. The identification and treatment of modifiable risk factors, including osteoporosis, is vital to preventing hip fracture. State the diagnosis based on the degree of pre-existent knowledge and adherence to any prior instruction, for example, *Knowledge deficit on the use of calcium replacements related to new diagnosis of osteoporosis and fracture.*

Outcomes. The client will express understanding of how personal risk of fractures with falls can be reduced by maintaining bone health and changing risky behaviors.

Interventions. Various measures are available for treating the underlying causes of bone loss and fragility. See Chapter 26 for plans to reduce risk of osteoporosis. Box 27-4 lists suggestions for reducing hip fractures.

Evaluation. Clinical pathways or care maps are now often used to determine which outcomes have been met for the client with a hip fracture; they often suggest a time frame for meeting each goal. Pain should decrease fairly soon after surgery. Injectable opioid analgesics are not typically required after 24 to 36 hours. The client should advance to oral analgesics as soon as nausea is controlled and liquids are being taken freely. A regular diet should be offered by the first or second day after surgery, again on the assumption that nausea is controlled. Early feeding primes the gastrointestinal

---

BOX 27-4 Reducing Risk of Hip Fractures

- Maintain bone health.
- Maintain proper levels of calcium, vitamin D, bisphosphonates, selective estrogen receptor modulators, and calcitonin.
- Get regular weight-bearing and muscle-strengthening exercise.
- Stop smoking.
- Reduce risk of falls.
- Use assistive devices.
- Fall-proof the house with grab bars in bathroom, stair treads on steps, handrails, and nonslip mats in shower and bathtub.
- Wear sensible shoes that are flat and hard soled.
- Avoid strenuous and dangerous activities; ask for help with moving and lifting objects.
- Keep your vision checked; wear proper glasses.
- Consider side effects of medications, especially dizziness. If dizzy, get up slowly.

---

tract, helping to avoid postoperative ileus. Adequate diet also contributes greatly to the client's physical stamina and to wound healing.

> **If an indwelling urinary catheter has been used, remove it as soon as the client can transfer to a bedside commode to decrease any risk for urinary tract infection (see the Case Management feature on Hip Fracture on the website).**
>
> SAFETY ⚠ ALERT
> *evolve*

A clinical pathway also often describes the involvement of a case manager or social worker in planning the client's discharge. In collaboration with the staff nurse and the physician, the case manager assesses the client's discharge needs on the basis of information about the home environment and social support. An extended-care facility or rehabilitation unit may be one possible destination after acute care hospitalization. The client who can move from bed to chair with minimal or no assistance may go instead directly home with possible visits from a home health aide or nurse to meet other skilled needs, such as hygiene and mobility assistance. When the client is discharged directly to home, the nurse must ensure that the family can safely assist the client with mobility needs and activities of daily living. The case manager assists the client in obtaining any durable medical equipment that may be needed, such as a walker or crutches, and finalizes discharge transportation if necessary. The Bridge to Home Health Care on p. 534 offers advice on Managing the Immobile Client.

PELVIC FRACTURES

The pelvis is a ring-like structure composed mostly of cancellous bone with a thin cortex. This structure provides great strength, allowing the pelvis to offer structural support and also to serve as a shock absorber that protects the abdominal organs. Pelvic fractures have become more common as a result of an increase in high-energy trauma, such as car crashes and gunshot wounds. Most pelvic fractures occur as a result of traffic accidents; pedestrians are injured more often than are the occupants of involved vehicles.

Because fractures of the pelvic ring can vary in stability, their management depends on the severity of the injury. Most cases can be diagnosed correctly with an anteroposterior radiograph. If there is any indication of an unstable fracture, a urethrogram or intravenous pyelogram is used to assess for possible damage to the kidneys and lower urinary tract. Bladder injuries may occur either as an associated injury or as a complication of pelvic ring fracture. Disruption of the pelvic ring leads to hemorrhage in as many as 75% of clients, with the pelvis holding as much as 4 L of blood.[32] Pelvic hemorrhage must be treated immediately by stabilization, either with sheets wrapped around the pelvis or with external

BRIDGE TO HOME HEALTH CARE

Managing the Immobile Client

To prevent skin breakdown and manage other physical and emotional effects of immobility, the multidisciplinary team must collaborate with clients, their family members, and their informal caregivers. The core team members are a nurse, a physical therapist, a social worker, and an occupational therapist.

If the person is expected to spend much time in a chair or wheelchair, good seat cushions can be purchased from most pharmacies and vendors. Heavy foam (4 inches thick) provides pressure reduction for clients with wheelchairs that have sling seats. Cushions of air can be inflated to reduce pressure and prevent posture problems. Pillows or gel should not be used; a pillow allows too much hip adduction and internal rotation and becomes uncomfortable, and gel is expensive and heavy, breaks down, and makes it harder to move a wheelchair.

Evaluate how clients sit and use cushions. Inspect every cushion frequently for signs of wear, which includes seeing an imprint in the foam after the client stands up. Avoid folds, wrinkles, or pockets on surfaces. The proper sitting position includes 90 degrees of flexion at the hips and knees. Clients should sit erect in chairs on their buttocks, not on the sacrum. Place pillows behind a client's back to promote more erect posture.

Teach clients to protect tissue and avoid massaging lotion over bony prominences; massage makes skin soft and susceptible to breakdown or shearing. Minimize friction; avoid having tissue squeezed between two hard surfaces such as bedding and bony prominences. Teach clients, especially those

with paraplegia, to use a mirror to check for friction or pressure. Clients may need assistance with repositioning at least every 2 hours. A footboard, a thoroughly padded plastic crate, or a box can be used to prevent feet from being forced into extreme plantiflexion. The clients' heels, ankles, trochanters, sacrum, scapulae, elbows, and ears need to be checked at least daily. Pillows, blanket or towel rolls, balloons, foam, or rolled-up clothing are useful for padding and positioning. Sheepskin, elbow and heel protectors, and "egg-crate" cushions provide little protection; thick foam is better. Even though good-quality alternating pressure pads are best, there are other options, including air-fluidized beds and low-air-loss beds. When alternating pads are used, watch the skin for several days to ensure that the client is getting enough tissue off-loading (see Chapter 49).

Daily exercise is essential. Passive exercise only increases flexibility, whereas active exercise increases circulation and air exchange, maintains joint lubrication and mobility, and helps prevent contractures. If you feel uncertain about whether to continue the exercise, request assistance from a physical therapist.

After clients progress through the acute stage, they need to consider long-term issues and dramatic lifestyle changes. Provide information about alternative housing options, transportation, yard and housekeeping services, financial assistance, recreation, and stores that deliver prescriptions. Mental health and sexuality issues are important, too. Clients also need to consider and make decisions about nutrition, clothing, informal caregivers, and health care services.

---

fixators. Unstable fractures have been treated aggressively since the mid-1990s with internal fixation in which plates and screws are used to achieve an intact pelvic ring. External fixation is also still used. Less severe pelvic fractures may be treated with bed rest alone. The client needs adequate pain management as well as assessment for neurovascular compromise or the development of complications such as thrombophlebitis or fat embolism.

LOWER EXTREMITY FRACTURES

CONDYLAR FRACTURES

The condyles are bony prominences at the distal end of the femur. Condylar fractures occur most often with high-energy injuries in young clients, or in low-energy injuries in osteoporotic bone of older clients. They may be among several injuries sustained in a motor-vehicle accident, for example, when the client's flexed knee strikes the dashboard. Less severe condylar fractures

are treated with knee immobilizers or casting. For more severe injury, ORIF is indicated. Bone grafting is used for comminuted fractures. Loss of knee mobility is a common outcome, and surgical revision may be needed to improve bony alignment. If the client develops severe pain and disability, *arthrodesis* (fusion) or *arthroplasty* (joint replacement) may be required.

PATELLAR FRACTURES

Fracture of the patella (kneecap) often results from a direct blow to the area. Some separation or splitting of the patella invariably occurs, and the client is unable to extend the knee fully because of pain and related damage to extensor mechanisms. Patellar fractures are usually more evident on a lateral radiograph than on other views. A stellate fracture (cracked patella without fragment displacement) can be managed conservatively by placing the client in a long leg cast for several weeks and then beginning mobilization. Indirect trauma, such as a forced flexion injury sustained in a fall, can result in a transverse fracture. ORIF is often necessary to minimize the potential for later problems with knee motion or chondromalacia. After a comminuted fracture, fragments may be difficult to reduce accurately, and removal of the patella may be best. Surgical repair of extensors such as the quadriceps tendon and the patellar tendon may also be needed.

TIBIAL AND FIBULAR FRACTURES

The fibula can be fractured alone in several ways: from direct trauma to the outer surface of the leg, producing a transverse or comminuted fracture; through twisting injuries, which produce a spiral fracture; or from repeated stress as in long-distance running, which can cause a fatigue fracture usually just above the inferior tibiofibular ligament. Fatigue fractures require immobilization; for other nondisplaced fibular fractures, a cast may be needed to immobilize the ankle.

The tibia can also be broken, leaving the fibula intact. Fracture can result from direct trauma. Repeated stress can lead to a fatigue fracture at the junction of the middle and upper thirds of the tibia. This injury is commonly seen in long-distance runners, hurdlers, and ballet dancers who jump excessively. Twisting injuries rarely result in a lone tibial fracture. Tibial fractures are reduced and treated through cast immobilization, internal fixation, or external fixation. Although it may seem helpful to have the fibula intact, the undamaged bone actually holds the ends of the tibia apart, and it may be necessary to cut the fibula to attain satisfactory alignment of the tibia.

Fractures of both the tibia and the fibula result commonly from motor-vehicle accidents and sports injuries. Treatment concerns include possible problems with fracture union, vascular and soft tissue damage, skin loss, and the development of compartment syndrome. As with lone tibial fractures, fragments may be held in the reduced position through casting from groin to toe. Alternatively, internal fixation would be the treatment of choice for clients with unstable or multiple fractures. External fixation would be necessary if the wound is dirty or if there is skin loss.

The tibial plateau fracture was previously known as a bumper or fender fracture, though only about 25% of these injuries result from impact with an automobile.[30] The most common mechanism of injury is axial loading, as may result from a fall or from a twisting injury. Four fracture patterns can occur: the lateral tibial plateau may be split vertically (common in younger clients); part of the tibial plateau may be thrust downward into the tibia to produce a depressed fracture (common in older or osteoporotic clients); both of these can occur together; or the whole plateau may be depressed. Because the full extent of injury may not be apparent on radiographs, CT scanning or MRI may be needed to determine the fracture anatomy. Any large fragment split

off the tibia must be secured back in place with screws to restore the contour of the bone. Large depressed fragments can be elevated to reconstitute the bone's surface, but the cavity that results below the fracture must be filled with a cancellous bone graft. If only a slight depression occurred in the tibial plateau, more conservative treatment with early mobilization may be appropriate.

FOOT FRACTURES

Because it provides a contact point with the ground and protrudes forward from the body, the foot is especially susceptible to injury. Fracture most often is caused by falls or jumps from great heights, running or twisting, motor-vehicle accidents, or objects dropped on the foot. As with any other injury, the client with open fractures should be taken to the operating room for surgical debridement and repair. Closed fractures of the foot, however, can generally be treated conservatively through cast or brace immobilization or through the use of walking shoes. Weight-bearing is progressively resumed as tolerated.

UPPER EXTREMITY FRACTURES

HUMERAL FRACTURES

Fracture of the proximal humerus is a common traumatic injury in older clients, often caused by a fall on an outstretched arm (Figure 27-8). A fall need not be serious to produce a humeral fracture in an osteoporotic client. Injury to the dominant arm of an older client can lead to dependence and immobility. The risk of falling after the fracture also increases because the sense of balance is impaired as a result of loss of use of the arm. If the fracture is nondisplaced or minimally displaced, the extremity is usually immobilized with a sling. Gentle range-of-motion exercises can be started when shoulder discomfort subsides, usually within 2 or 3 weeks after injury. A displaced fracture is treated by ORIF. Prosthetic replacement is occasionally indicated for an intra-articular fracture or one that is severely comminuted. Prompt, appropriate treatment reduces the risk that AVN of the humeral head will develop.

Fractures of the humeral shaft usually result from a direct blow to the arm, a car crash, a gunshot injury, or a crush injury. Humeral fractures can also result from indirect injuries such as a fall on an outstretched hand or on the elbow. Most humeral shaft fractures can be treated by initial immobilization with a U-shaped splint. Once the swelling has subsided, a commercially available humeral fracture brace may be used in conjunction

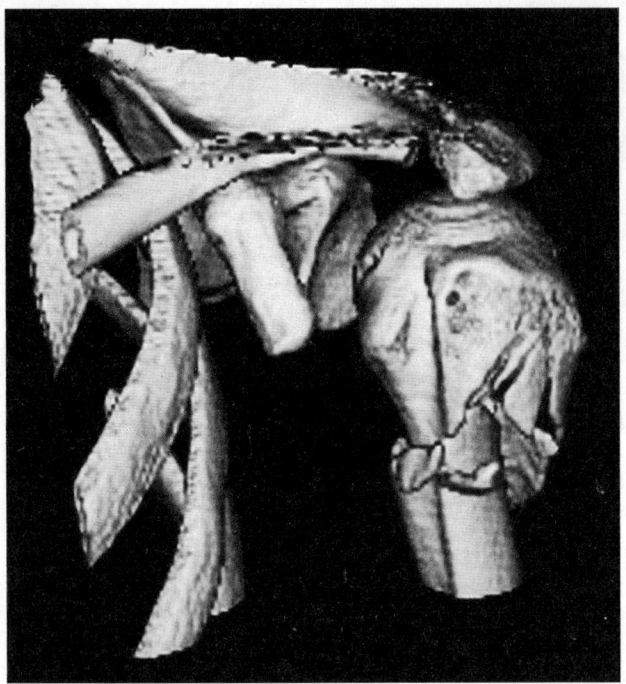

■ **FIGURE 27–8** Fracture of the proximal humerus on CT scan.

with an arm sling. Heavy hanging arm casts should be avoided because they may contribute to fracture non-union. Surgery is indicated for debridement of an open fracture. Surgical stabilization is also required for any fracture associated with a vascular injury.

ELBOW FRACTURES

Intra-articular injuries of the elbow include condylar, olecranon, and radial head or neck fracture. These injuries frequently result from falls on or direct blows to the elbow. Because associated injuries to the three major peripheral nerves (radial, median, and ulnar) are possible, careful neurovascular assessment is critical. A high potential for compartment syndrome also exists after intra-articular fractures of the elbow. Most nondisplaced fractures can be treated with immobilization, followed by early range-of-motion exercises once acute discomfort has diminished (usually after 1 week). A posterior long arm splint may be used with a shoulder sling. Displaced fractures, especially supracondylar fractures, often require ORIF. Repair of the brachial artery may also be necessary after traumatic injury. After surgery, immobilization can be accomplished with a posterior elbow splint, a cast, or traction.

RADIUS AND ULNAR FRACTURES

Fractures of the shafts of the radius and ulna usually result from a direct blow to the forearm, a motor-vehicle accident, or a fall on an outstretched arm. Associated injuries to the nerves (median, ulnar, and radial) and arteries (radial and ulnar) are possible. A sugar-tong splint can be used to provide initial immobilization of forearm fractures. Circumferential cast immobilization is generally not recommended in early treatment because fracture swelling in association with the constriction provided by the cast may lead to compartment syndrome. Immobilization must include the wrist and the elbow to control rotation of the forearm. In adult clients, surgical treatment may be indicated for displaced or open fractures.

As with proximal humeral fractures, fractures of the distal radius are common injuries in older adults. Many older clients have a good outcome even with a residual deformity because their routine activities may not demand full use of the limb; however, deformity and possible resulting arthritic changes in younger clients may lead to inability to perform their current jobs. Colles' fracture is a common injury in which the distal radius fragment is displaced dorsally and proximally. Fracture reduction is greatly enhanced by the use of a nerve block such as the Bier block. This fracture may be treated with 2 weeks of splinting followed by 3 weeks in a short arm cast. Comminuted fractures may require external fixation or ORIF with bone grafting.

HAND FRACTURES

Most fractures of the metacarpals and phalanges are work-related. A delay in seeking evaluation and diagnosis can make fracture reduction difficult because fractures in the hand form early callus within 7 to 10 days and become difficult to manipulate. Treatment involves accurate fracture reduction, movement of the uninvolved fingers to prevent stiffness, and elevation of the extremity to decrease edema. Simple measures such as "buddy taping" or splinting are usually sufficient treatment for stable fractures. Comminuted fractures and those requiring open reduction take longer to consolidate and are not ready for mobilization as quickly. Client motivation plays a critical role in rehabilitation after hand injury and often can be enhanced by a brief course of physical therapy. Motion typically can be started about 21 days after injury for clients with closed, nondisplaced fractures.

Neurovascular assessment is critical for all clients with upper extremity fractures. Carefully compare the color, warmth, movement, sensation, and capillary refill of the affected extremity with those of the unaffected extremity. Elevation of the injured extremity is typically indicated. At night, the client should be observed frequently to be certain that the arm does not move into a dependent position. If a cast or splint has been applied, the client and family should receive careful instruction about cast care and about the clinical manifestations of compartment syndrome.

DISLOCATIONS AND SUBLUXATIONS

Dislocation and subluxation both describe changes in joint relationships. In a dislocation, the opposing joint surfaces are no longer in contact. In subluxation, the joint surfaces are in partial contact, but their relationship is abnormal. Both injuries are caused by acute deforming forces applied to ligaments or tendons from a fall, a blow, or a strong muscle contraction. For example, the client who tries to break a fall down the stairs by holding on to the handrail may dislocate a shoulder. The nurse must identify the mechanism of injury that produced the dislocation so the action is not reproduced during the client's treatment.

Like fractures, dislocations are described in terms of the relationship of the distal bone to the proximal bone. In a posterior dislocation of the knee, for example, the tibia lies posterior to the femur. Although almost any joint can dislocate, some joints are more likely to become dislocated than others. Anterior dislocation of the humerus in the shoulder joint occurs commonly in adults. Anterior dislocation of the knee is the most common lower extremity dislocation. Its occurrence is a medical emergency because of related neurovascular injuries. The adult hip is usually stable, and its dislocation is often associated with severe trauma. Dislocation may also occur following total hip arthroplasty if mobility precautions are not observed.

After dislocation, the client often complains of severe pain that increases with attempted movement. Swelling around or below the joint is likely, along with complete or nearly complete loss of function and a visible deformity that may alter the length of the extremity. Fracture of the joint surface often accompanies dislocation. Neurovascular status of the affected extremity must be assessed carefully because the displaced bone may tear blood vessels and impede circulation, damage nerves, and rupture ligaments or muscle attachments. Immediate reduction is preferred before inflammation and spasm can become significant. If immediate reduction is not possible, analgesics and muscle relaxants must be given before any later attempt to reduce the dislocation. A splint, a harness, or padding should be used for 4 to 8 weeks after acute dislocation or until pain is significantly reduced and muscle function provides adequate support in cases of recurrent dislocation.

After subluxation the client experiences variable pain and the feeling that the joint was out of position briefly. The joint typically feels weak, and pain increases with attempted movement. Because radiographs are often normal with subluxations, the physician must rule out other possible injuries such as sprain, strain, muscle tear, and fracture. Muscle-strengthening exercises can help the client avoid future subluxations. Joint restrictive supports such as a shoulder harness may also be useful.

SPORTS INJURIES

IMPINGEMENT AND ROTATOR CUFF TEARS

The shoulder is a very complex piece of machinery. Its elegant design gives us the ability to do many things. This design gives the shoulder joint great range of motion but not much stability. As long as the parts of this elegant machine are in good working order, the shoulder can move freely and painlessly. Most shoulder injuries involve the soft tissues, and many result directly from repetitive activities such as overhead throwing or overhead motion within the shoulder girdle. The shoulder girdle includes the sternoclavicular joint, the acromioclavicular joint, the glenohumeral joint, the subacromial space, and the scapulothoracic space. Movement at all these articulations allows for the complexity of a pitcher's throwing motion. Four muscles also contribute to the shoulder's varied movements and form the rotator cuff: (1) the subscapularis (anterior), (2) the supraspinatus, (3) the infraspinatus, and (4) the teres minor (posterior). Most tears occur at the supraspinatus.

Normal shoulder movement is a smooth, pain-free activity of the rotator cuff muscles; however, excessive joint activity can lead to repetitive trauma, or muscles can be injured by an external force. Usually, there is enough room between the acromion and the rotator cuff so that the tendons slide easily underneath the acromion as the arm is raised. But each time the arm is raised, there is a bit of rubbing on the tendons and the bursa between the tendons and the acromion. This rubbing is called impingement. Impingement occurs to some degree in everyone's shoulder, caused by day to day activities that use the arm above shoulder level. However, continuously working with the arms raised overhead, repeated throwing activities, or other repetitive actions of the arm can cause impingement to become a problem.

Impingement syndrome presents as generalized aching of the shoulder and pain when raising the arm out from the side or in front of the body. Most clients complain of difficulty sleeping because of pain, especially when they roll over on the affected shoulder. A very reliable sign of impingement is a sharp pain when trying to reach into the back pocket. As the process continues, discomfort increases and the joint may become stiffer. Initial conservative treatment of impingement involves rest with possible sport or job modifications. A sling is not used because adhesive capsulitis can result from shoulder immobilization. NSAIDs and ice applications may relieve pain. Ultrasound, phonophoresis, or iontophoresis may also be used. A subacromial injection of anesthetic and cortisone may be useful as a therapy and also as an aid to differentiating impingement

If the rotator cuff is torn, the client is not able to perform abduction and external rotation. Activity at the glenohumeral joint is also painfully impaired. Confirmation can be gained through use of radiography, arthrography, CT scans, MRI, or arthroscopy.

Treatment of rotator cuff injury often begins conservatively with rest, limited overhead activity, and sling support for the shoulder. NSAIDs may relieve discomfort. Some physicians also advocate intra-articular injection of analgesics or steroids. When acute manifestations subside, the client should begin active exercises that address range of motion and strengthen the rotator cuff muscles. Any elastic graded equipment (e.g., Thera-Band) can be used in a daily program of progressive gentle exercises. Exercise may be preceded by application of heat and followed by ice if discomfort occurs.

Surgery may be necessary if nonoperative treatment does not relieve symptoms, or if the tear is acute and painful, it occurs in the dominant arm of an active individual, or the person needs maximum arm strength for overhead work or sports. Repair will probably be performed on an outpatient basis, although the client may be hospitalized briefly if pain or nausea becomes problematic. Postoperative management includes instruction on the use of a shoulder immobilizer and introduction of a program of gentle exercises such as the pendulum shoulder movement. The neurovascular status of the affected arm should be assessed at regular intervals, and findings should be compared with those of the nonoperative arm. Pain management should also be a focus of postoperative care.

KNEE INJURIES

ANTERIOR CRUCIATE LIGAMENT INJURY

The anterior cruciate ligament (ACL) is a broad ligament joining the anterior tibial plateau to the posterior femoral intercondylar notch. The ACL prevents forward motion of the tibia. Tearing the midportion of the ACL is the most common injury and usually a result of hyperextension, internal rotation, extremes of external rotation, and deceleration. The injured client often describes hearing a loud pop. Severe swelling can occur in the first few hours after injury. The knee feels unstable ("gives way"), particularly in rotation, and full extension is difficult. Knee stability is determined by using the Lachman test. The client rests in a relaxed supine position with the injured knee flexed at 20 to 30 degrees. Placing one hand around the client's distal thigh and the other around the client's proximal tibia, the health care provider attempts anterior-posterior translation. The test result is positive when anterior-posterior sliding occurs. The anterior drawer test is an alternative diagnostic maneuver. The health care provider grasps the tibia just below the joint line and pulls forward with both hands

while assessing the amount of tibial displacement. An intact ACL allows the tibia to move forward only a few millimeters before stopping abruptly. An injured ACL allows greater movement and gives a mushy feel to joint mobility. Routine radiographs may also be used for diagnosis of ACL injury, but the MRI is especially sensitive and specific for difficult cases. Arthroscopy, the most important advance in the diagnosis of knee disorders, can enable the physician to confirm the degree of ACL damage and determine the extent of associated intra-articular injuries. Arthroscopy is also the surgical treatment of choice for ACL reconstruction.

Initial immobilization protects the joint from further injury and decreases pain and swelling. ACL reconstruction can be accomplished within several weeks of injury and still allow a return of joint function and stability. Repair is often accomplished with the use of a portion of the client's patellar tendon. After ACL reconstruction, continuous passive motion (CPM) machines are often used to help the client achieve rapid, satisfactory knee mobility. The CPM machine is generally applied in the recovery area and should be used at least 8 hours a day or until full range of motion is achieved. Sometimes long leg braces with fixed knee flexion are also used, either alone or in combination with the CPM machine. After ACL reconstruction, the client receives instructions on performance of isometric exercises such as quadriceps setting, bent-knee leg exercises, and foot exercises. The exercise program is progressed over the next 4 to 6 months.

MENISCAL INJURY

The meniscus is the fibrous cartilage that lies on top of the tibia, between the tibia and the femur, and acts as the shock absorber of the knee. It is torn less frequently than the ACL, but most longitudinal tears of the meniscus occur in conjunction with ACL or medial collateral ligament injuries (Figure 27-9). Because the meniscus has little blood supply, it heals slowly, if at all, after injury.

Meniscal injuries often result from fixed-foot rotation in weight-bearing with the knee flexed. A combination of compression and rotational forces is thus exerted on the meniscus. Mild swelling may be evident, and the client may complain of joint-line pain. Popping, slipping, catching, or buckling of the knee can also occur, particularly if a piece of the cartilage is torn and floating within the knee capsule.

The McMurray test is the most widely used maneuver for assessing injury of the middle or posterior horn of the meniscus. The client is supine with the injured knee flexed to 90 degrees. The health care provider holds the client's foot with one hand and places the fingers of the other hand at the medial joint line. While applying a varus stress at the knee to compress the medial meniscus, the health care provider externally rotates the lower

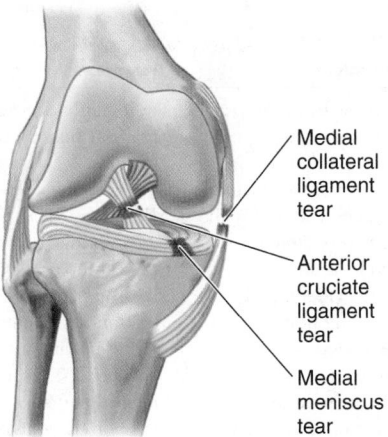

FIGURE 27–9 Common knee injuries: Medial collateral ligament tear, commonly caused by inversion and twisting. Anterior cruciate ligament injury, commonly caused by twisting a hyperextended knee. Medial meniscal injury, commonly caused by twisting an everted knee.

leg, ankle, and foot as a unit. The knee is then extended while the health care provider palpates the medial joint line. The test is considered positive if the client complains of pain localized to the medial or lateral joint line or if a palpable or audible click is produced.

MRI is commonly used to diagnose the injury. Arthroscopy can also be used for diagnosis and at the same time the meniscus can be repaired. After surgery, the leg is elevated and ice is applied. Effective pain management is an initial priority. An exercise program includes quadriceps strengthening and range of motion for the knee.

OVERUSE SYNDROMES

Overuse syndromes are common sports-related problems. They begin insidiously as the result of microtraumas that often do not completely stop the affected person's activity. People who are at greatest risk for overuse include competitive athletes, first-time athletes, "born again" athletes, and those recovering from injury. Other factors may also increase risk (Box 27-5). The client must understand that the manifestations of pain, tenderness, and swelling result from repeated stress on musculoskeletal structures. Nonoperative treatment of stress injuries always includes relative rest. For example, the runner may be restricted from impact-loading activities but still be allowed to cycle or run in the buoyancy of a swimming pool. Ice, compression (when swelling occurs), and NSAIDs are used routinely to reduce inflammation related to the injury.

Prevention should emphasize the importance of stretching to maintain joint flexibility and range of motion. Stretching exercises should be static (i.e., holding muscles in a stretched position for a few moments rather than

repeatedly stretching and relaxing them). Static stretching reduces the danger of overstretching and tissue damage, causes less muscle soreness than a bouncing stretch, and relieves muscle soreness when it occurs. Creatine supplements may also increase strength. This topic is discussed in the Complementary and Alternative Therapy feature below. Common overuse injuries are summarized in Table 27-6.

BOX 27-5   Factors That May Increase Risk for Sports Injury

- Age over 40 years
- Current inactive lifestyle
- Overweight by 20 pounds or more
- Family history of cardiac disease
- Any past experience of pain or pressure in chest, arm, or throat
- Taking medications on a regular basis
- Documented high cholesterol level
- Smokes or has history of pulmonary disease
- History of diabetes or other chronic disorders
- History of joint disease

COMPLEMENTARY AND ALTERNATIVE THERAPY

Oral Creatine Supplementation to Improve Strength

Oral creatine supplements may be the most widely used nutritional supplements among athletes. Therefore a meta-analysis was recently conducted on past studies of these supplements. Researchers found 16 studies for inclusion into their analysis. The summary difference in the maximum weight lifted was 6.85 kg greater after creatine supplements versus placebo for bench press and 9.76 kg greater for squats, but there was no difference for arm curls. In 7 of 10 studies evaluating maximum weight lifted, subjects were younger than 36 years of age and engaged in resistance training. The researchers concluded that oral creatine supplements combined with resistance training increase the maximum weight lifted in young men. There was no evidence of improved performance in older people or women or for other types of strength and power exercises. In addition, the safety of creatine supplements is unknown (one study reported gastrointestinal upset, rash, or headache in subjects taking creatine and no side effects in the three placebo groups.) Therefore these supplements cannot be generally recommended until more trials are concluded.

REFERENCE

Dempsey, R., Mazzone, M., & Meurer, L. (2002). Does oral creatine supplementation improve strength? A meta-analysis. *Journal of Family Practice, 51,* 945-951.

TABLE 27–6   **Sports and Overuse Injuries**

Injury Type	Definition	High Risk Groups	Manifestations	Treatment
Strain	A strain is a twist, pull, and/or tear of a muscle and/or tendon. Caused by direct or indirect trauma (e.g., a fall, a blow to body) that knocks a joint out of position, overstretches, and, in severe cases, ruptures supporting ligaments. Chronic strains are the result of overuse—prolonged, repetitive movement of muscles and tendons.	Athletes, clients with a history of strains and sprains, obese, and people in poor physical condition. Typically, this injury occurs when an individual lands on an outstretched arm, slides into a base, jumps and lands on the side of the foot, or runs on an uneven surface. Chronic strains occur in people who do not have adequate rest breaks during intensive training, people who lift more than they are capable of lifting, those with weak abdominal muscles.	Acute muscle spasm, pain, muscle weakness. Severity of clinical manifestations is related to degree of injury. With more severe strains, ecchymosis and edema may be evident, and range of motion may be quite limited. In severe strains, the muscle or tendon is partially or completely ruptured, often incapacitating the individual. Some muscle function will be lost with a moderate strain, where the muscle/tendon is overstretched and slightly torn.	Radiographs are necessary to rule out possibility of fracture. *R*est, *i*ce, *c*ompression, and *e*levation (RICE) for first 24-48 hours. Surgical repair may be needed if a rupture is present at tendon-bone interface. During healing after strain (4-6 weeks), movement of injured part should be minimized. Activity should never progress to the point that manifestations such as pain or swelling result. After mature scar tissue has formed, the injured part can be gradually and progressively exercised. Overactivity must absolutely be avoided during rehabilitation.
Sprain	A sprain is a stretch and/or tear of a ligament, the fibrous band of connective tissue that joins the end of one bone with another.	Professional and amateur athletes and general public. People at risk for injury have a history of sprains and strains, are overweight, and are in poor physical condition.	Feeling of a tear or a pop in joint. Pain, bruising, and edema. A severe sprain produces excruciating pain at moment of injury, as ligaments tear completely or separate from bone. This loosening makes joint nonfunctional. A moderate sprain partially tears ligament, producing joint instability, and some swelling. A ligament is stretched in a mild sprain, but there is no joint loosening.	Radiographs are necessary to rule out possibility of fracture. *R*est, *i*ce, *c*ompression, and *e*levation (RICE) with protected weight-bearing when client can place some weight on injured extremity. Exercises focus on restoring strength, ankle motion, and proprioception. The third phase of rehabilitation includes activity-specific drills before client is allowed to return to full sports participation. If surgical repair is required for a complete ligament rupture, cast or brace immobilization is needed for 4-6 weeks after injury. Once conventional immobilizer is removed, the injured ankle may be placed in an Aircast to allow dorsiflexion and plantar flexion of the foot while still restricting lateral movement of the ankle.
Stress fracture	Tiny cracks in bones that develop when muscles become fatigued and can no longer absorb shock of repeated impact. When this happens, muscles transfer the stress to the bones, creating a small crack or fracture.	High-impact sports such as track and field, basketball, gymnastics, ballet, or tennis. Adolescents whose bones have not yet fully hardened. Female athletes who have abnormal or absent menstrual cycles that can result in decreasing bone mass. Military recruits.	Pain that develops gradually, increases with weight-bearing activity, and diminishes with rest. Swelling on top of foot or outside ankle. Tenderness to touch at site of fracture. Possible bruising.	Protective footwear for 2-4 weeks. Stiff-soled shoe, a wooden-soled sandal, or a removable short leg fracture brace shoe. Some fractures may require casting, crutches, and surgery.

TABLE 27–6 Sports and Overuse Injuries—Cont'd

Injury Type	Definition	High Risk Groups	Manifestations	Treatment
Plantar fasciitis	Repetitive strain to plantar fascia, which provides support for longitudinal arches of feet. It attaches to plantar surface (sole) of calcaneus (heel bone), and its fibers fan out to attach to forefoot.	Running and jumping athletes. Also develops in clients who are obese, have diabetes, spend most of day on feet, or are flat-footed or have a high arch.	Severe foot pain aggravated by weight-bearing with first steps of morning. Pain then gradually subsides with activity. These clients usually describe a deep ache or bruise at anteromedial portion of calcaneus on plantar surface of foot.	Orthoses, such as heel cups and night exercises for lower leg to improve walking and running form. Ice, anti-inflammatory medications are used. Occasionally steroid injections are needed.
Shin splints or medial tibial stress syndrome	Shin splints result from excessive strain of posterior tibial muscle origin, causing exercise-related pain.	Runners, aerobic dancers, and people in military. Being flat-footed, knock-kneed, or bow-legged. Sudden change in training regimens (longer time, greater distance). Running on concrete. Wearing old shoes.	Pain with activity and residual tenderness at muscle origin for days after running or other repetitive activity. Pain is just behind medial edge of tibia.	Several weeks of rest. Training should resume at a much lower level and progress slowly, with pain providing a guide. Muscle strengthening. Orthotics to correct misalignment and reduce strain. Adequate stretching after training.
Patellar tendinopathy (also known as jumper's knee)	Caused by repetitive stress placed on patellar or quadriceps tendon during jumping.	Specific to athletes who are in jumping sports (basketball, volleyball, high and long jumps).	Pain, tenderness, and sometimes swelling, most commonly at proximal third of patellar tendon near inferior pole of patella. Pain is aggravated by additional jumping.	Rest, ice, stretching and strengthening exercises. Assessment of joint motion and kinematics and sport-specific proprioceptive training. NSAIDs.
Tennis elbow (also known as lateral humeral epicondylitis)	Repetitive use of wrist extensors or flexors leads to small tears of tendons that attach muscles of forearm to humerus at elbow.	People who work with their hands: plumbers, painters, gardeners, carpenters, nurses. Athletes, including racquet sport players, are at risk.	Pain radiating down forearm and over outside of elbow, when lifting objects.	Conservative treatment to reduce pain and gradual stretching and isometric exercises. Counterforce brace can be worn to inhibit full muscle expansion and decrease tension on injured tissue.
Tendinitis and tenosynovitis of hand and wrist	Irritation and inflammation of tendons around wrist joint, where the tendons cross each other or pass over a bony prominence.	Gripping, pinching, pulling, or lifting with repetitive wrist motion.	Pain over area of inflammation. Edema of surrounding soft tissues.	Wrist splint. Ice and anti-inflammatory medications. Steroid injections.

REMOBILIZATION AFTER TRAUMATIC INJURY

Strategies for remobilization are developed to improve joint range of motion, muscle strength, and cardiovascular endurance. Before beginning an exercise program, the client must be aware of limiting factors such as pain and the inability to relax. Exercise should progress at a pace that allows the client to experience no more than a little muscle soreness. Pain in the exercising client may be caused by chronic compartment syndrome and should receive immediate attention.

Passive range-of-motion (PROM) exercises can be performed with the assistance of a therapist or a nurse, or with equipment such as a CPM machine. This type of exercise helps to prevent joint contractures and maintain joint range of motion (ROM). If a CPM machine is ordered, make sure that the device properly fits the client. If, for example, the client is too short for the machine settings, the device may be too tight in the groin. Because the client must be supine when using the machine, assess the skin over pressure points such as the sacrum, scapulae, and heels for signs of impairment. The client should be taught the purpose of the CPM machine and how to stop and start it. The client should also be encouraged to report any manifestations of pressure or irritation.

Active range of motion (AROM) is part of a program that increases muscle strength and endurance. Examples include straight leg raises or knee flexion and extension

COMPLEMENTARY AND ALTERNATIVE THERAPY

Magnet Therapy for Plantar Heel Pain

A randomized, double-blind, placebo-controlled trial of 101 adults with a diagnosis of plantar heel pain for at least 30 days was conducted, and daily pain diaries were kept for a total of 2 months. Cushioned insoles with either active bipolar magnets or sham magnets (placebo) were worn daily by the participants for 2 months. No significant differences were found between the two treatment groups.

REFERENCE

Winemiller, M., et al. (2003). Effect of magnetic vs. sham-magnetic insoles on plantar heel pain: A randomized controlled trial. *Journal of the American Medical Association, 290,* 1474-1478.

when the client is in a sitting position. In active assisted range of motion, the therapist, a mechanical device, or the opposite extremity provides an external force to the affected extremity during joint motion. This type of exercise is often a second step in rehabilitation. It includes isotonic exercise, such as weight lifting, or isokinetic exercise through use of equipment such as Cybex machines.

After an orthopedic injury, the client should ambulate as soon as possible. The client who has been bedridden even for brief periods may exhibit muscle atrophy and weakness, decreased endurance and cardiovascular fitness, and decreased joint flexibility. Orthostatic hypotension is also common after bed rest. A gradual progression of exercise is needed to remobilize the client. Bed exercises may be the first intervention. If the client has been on extended bed rest, a tilt table can be used to assist the client to an upright position.

Be aware of the client's weight-bearing status before attempting to assist with ambulation. The degree of protected weight-bearing is determined by the physician on the basis of the client's injury and any surgical procedure. Ambulatory assistive devices such as canes, a walker, or crutches can be used as needed.

CONCLUSIONS

Traumatic musculoskeletal injuries are common and often have multifactorial causes. Some are self-limiting, with little required besides routine treatment and self-care advice. Other injuries become chronic and present challenges in rehabilitation. Your role is to promote early mobility, prevent possible complications, and teach the client how to prevent further injury.

THINKING CRITICALLY

1. A young college student arrives in the emergency department holding his arm close to his body. His wrist is obviously misshapen, but swelling is minimal. He tells you he was playing basketball with friends and hit the gym wall after running toward the goal to attempt a lay-up shot. He complains of pain with attempted flexion or rotation of the wrist. A radiograph confirms a wrist fracture, and cast application is planned. What intervention should receive priority? What teaching about cast care should be completed?

Factors to Consider. How should you relieve the client's pain? What is involved in the healing process for a fracture? What complications might the client face because of the cast?

2. Friends of a 22-year-old woman assist her into the doctor's office. She twisted her knee on the pitcher's mound during a competitive softball game and says she heard a popping sound. Swelling over her knee is significant. The client states that her knee buckled when she attempted to walk off the field. What is your priority for care? What will be the long-range care goals?

Factors to Consider. What is the initial treatment for this type of injury? What postoperative treatments will be ordered?

3. An 80-year-old woman is brought to the nursing unit to await surgical repair of a femoral neck fracture. She is mildly confused. A neighbor says he found her on her kitchen floor after an apparent fall. What assessment should be performed on an ongoing basis? What will be the treatment goals after an ORIF of the fracture?

Factors to Consider. What possible complications could result after a hip fracture? How can they be prevented?

Discussions for these questions can be found on the website.

BIBLIOGRAPHY

1. Adamo, S.M. (2002). Modalities for mobilization. In A.B. Maher, S.W. Salmond, & T.A. Pellino (Eds.), *Orthopaedic nursing* (3rd ed., pp. 324-350). Philadelphia: Saunders.
2. American Academy of Family Physicians (AAFP). (2005). *Running: Preventing overuse injuries.* Retrieved 07/16/06 from http://familydoctor.org/147.xml.
3. American Academy of Family Physicians (AAFP). (2006). *Plantar fasciitis: A common cause of heel pain.* Retrieved 07/16/06 from http://familydoctor.org/140.xml.
4. American Academy of Orthopaedic Surgeons (AAOS). (2005). *ACL injury: Should it be fixed?* Retrieved 07/16/06 from http://orthoinfo.aaos.org/indepth/thr_report.cfm?Thread_ID=14&topcategory=Knee.
5. American Academy of Orthopaedic Surgeons (AAOS). (2005). *Shin splints.* Retrieved 07/16/06 from http://orthoinfo.aaos.org/fact/thr_report.cfm?thread_id=135&topcategory=Sports%20/%20Exercise.
6. American Academy of Orthopaedic Surgeons (AAOS). (2005). *Rotator cuff tears.* Retrieved 07/16/06 from http://orthoinfo.aaos.org/fact/thr_report.cfm?Thread_ID=127&topcategory=Shou.
7. Barocas, C. (2004). A properly fitted cast starts with a good foundation. *Orthopaedic Technology Review, 4*(6). Retrieved 07/15/06 from www.orthopedictechreview.com/issues/mayjun04/pg36.htm.
8. Bhagia, S.M. (2004). *Meniscal injury.* Retrieved 07/16/06 from www.emedicine.com/pmr/topic75.htm.

9. Centers for Disease Control (CDC). (2006). *Falls and hip fractures among older adults.* Retrieved 07/15/06 from www.cdc.gov/ncipc/factsheets/falls.htm.

10. Childs, S.G. (2002) Athletic performance and injury. In A.B. Maher, S.W. Salmond, & T.A. Pellino (Eds.), *Orthopaedic nursing* (3rd ed., pp. 674-701). Philadelphia: Saunders.

11. Cooper, M.P. (2004). Care of the patient with knee problems. In C.M. Mosher (Ed.), *An introduction to orthopaedic nursing* (3rd ed., pp. 155-167). Chicago: National Association of Orthopaedic Nurses.

12. DeBernardino, T.M. (2006). *Shoulder impingement syndrome.* Retrieved 07/16/06 from www.emedicine.com/sports/topic119.htm.

13. DeNoon, D.J. (2004). *Pre-exercise stretching may not be helpful.* Retrieved 07/16/06 from http://onhealth.webmd.com/script/main/art.asp?articlekey=55782.

14. Einhorn, T.A. (2003). *Basic science of bone graft substitutes.* Retrieved 07/09/06 from www.hwbf.org/ota/am/ota03/bssf/OTA03BG1.htm.

15. Foreman, F.D., Mion, L.C., Trygstad, L., et al. (2003). Delirium: Strategies for assessing and treating. In M. Mezey, T. Fulmer, & I. Abraham (Eds.), *Geriatric nursing protocols for best practice* (2nd ed., pp. 116-140). New York: Springer.

16. Gordon, D.B., & Pellino, T.A. (2002). Assessment and management of pain. In A.B. Maher, S.W. Salmond, & T.A. Pellino (Eds.), *Orthopaedic nursing* (3rd ed., pp. 127-151). Philadelphia: Saunders.

17. Hyman, G. (2005). *Jumper's knee.* Retrieved 07/16/06 from www.emedicine.com/sports/topic56.htm.

18. Kaufmann, R.A. (2003). Managing upper extremity fractures. *Orthopaedic Technology Review, 5*(5). Retrieved 07/16/06 from www.orthopedictechreview.com/issues/sepoct03/pg35.htm.

19. Kirkland, L. (2005). *Fat embolism.* Retrieved 07/15/06 from www.emedicine.com/med/topic652.htm.

20. Kunkler, C.E. (2002). Fractures. In A.B. Maher, S.W. Salmond, & T.A. Pellino (Eds.), *Orthopaedic nursing* (3rd ed., pp. 609-649). Philadelphia: Saunders.

21. Mehallo, C.J. (2004). *Occurrence and prevention of anterior knee pain.* Retrieved 07/16/06 from www.acofp.org/member_publications/0704_1.html#.

22. National Institute of Neurological Disorders and Stroke (NINDS). (2006). *NINDS complex regional pain syndrome information page.* Retrieved 07/15/06 from www.ninds.nih.gov/disorders/reflex_sympathetic_dystrophy/reflex_sympathetic_dystrophy.htm#Is_there_any_treatment.

23. Patel, M. (2004). *Tibial nonunions.* Retrieved 07/15/06 from www.emedicine.com/orthoped/topic569.htm.

24. Paula, R. (2006). *Compartment syndrome, extremity.* Retrieved 07/15/06 from www.emedicine.com/emerg/topic739.htm#section~workup.

25. Rabin, S.I. (2004). *Supracondylar femur fractures.* Retrieved 07/15/06 from www.emedicine.com/orthoped/topic319.htm.

26. Redemann, S. (2002). Modalities for immobilization. In A.B. Maher, S.W. Salmond, & T.A. Pellino (Eds.), *Orthopaedic nursing* (3rd ed., pp. 302-323). Philadelphia: Saunders.

27. Roberts, D. (2004). Care of the patient with hip problems. In C.M. Mosher (Ed.), *An introduction to orthopaedic nursing* (3rd ed., pp. 141-153). Chicago: National Association of Orthopaedic Nurses.

28. Sandor, R., & Brone, S. (2002). Rehabilitating ankle sprains. *The Physician and Sports Medicine, 30*(8), 48-50.

29. Shea, M., & Fields, K.B. (2002). Plantar fasciitis. *The Physician and Sports Medicine, 30*(7), 21-28.

30. Sorenson, S.M. (2004). *Tibial plateau fractures.* Retrieved 07/16/06 from www.emedicine.com/RADIO/topic698.htm.

31. The Cleveland Clinic. (2006). *Fracture, non-union.* Retrieved 07/15/06 from http://cms.clevelandclinic.org/ortho/body.cfm?id=75.

32. Thornton, D.D. (2002). *Pelvic ring fractures.* Retrieved 07/16/06 from www.emedicine.com/RADIO/topic546.htm.

33. Wheeless' Textbook of Orthopaedics. (2005). *Fractures of the patella.* Retrieved 07/16/06 from www.wheelessonline.com/ortho/fractures_of_the_patella.

evolve **Did you remember to check out the bonus material on the Evolve website and the CD-ROM, including NCLEX®-Examination Style Review Questions, Open-Book Quizzes, and Chapter Review Audio Podcasts?**

http://evolve.elsevier.com/Black/medsurg

UNIT 7

NUTRITIONAL DISORDERS

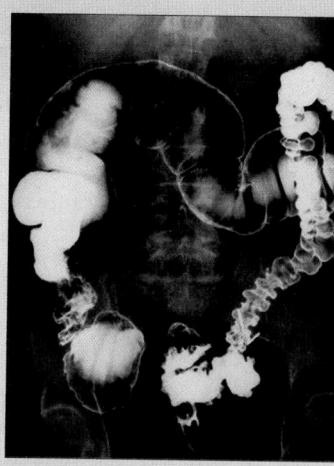

ANATOMY AND PHYSIOLOGY REVIEW:

The Nutritional (Gastrointestinal) System

Robert G. Carroll

The nutritional or gastrointestinal (GI) system is a long, hollow tube that passes through the body, providing an isolated environment for digestion and absorption of nutrients. Ingested contents pass sequentially through the mouth, esophagus, stomach, small intestine (duodenum, jejunum, and ileum), and large intestine (colon) before exiting the body at the anus.

GI tract function is regulated by a complex series of neural, hormonal, and local control systems. The enteric nervous system integrates motor and secretory activities along the GI tract. Ganglia have sensory neurons that respond to temperature, chemical agents, and mechanical deformation (e.g., stretch). Ganglia also have effector neurons to smooth muscle, secretory cells, endocrine cells, and autocrine cells. In general, GI secretion and motility are enhanced by parasympathetic activity and inhibited by sympathetic activity.

GI hormones, which control and integrate both motility and secretion, are distributed in the stomach and small intestine. GI hormones are also important trophic factors, stimulating proliferation of the GI tract to enhance absorptive capacity.

Finally, the GI tract has an extensive immune system. Gut-associated lymphoid tissue (GALT) may account for up to 80% of the immunoglobulin-producing cells in the body. These cells are important because the GI tract is open to the "outside environment."

STRUCTURE OF THE GASTROINTESTINAL TRACT

In cross-section, the GI tract generally has four distinct layers (Figure A&P7-1). The innermost layer is the *mucosa,* where epithelial cells contact ingested food. The mucosa often has microvilli to increase the surface area available for absorption. Beneath the mucosa is the *submucosa (lamina propria),* containing glands, blood vessels, and lymph nodules. Next is a *muscular layer,* with smooth muscle oriented either circularly or longitudinally. The outermost layer is the *connective tissue serosa layer.*

The entrance (mouth, upper esophagus) and exit (external anal sphincter) of the GI tract contain GI-associated skeletal muscle, which is partially under voluntary control. The remainder of the GI tract (Figure A&P7-2) has smooth muscle, which is under involuntary control. GI smooth muscle is electrically connected by gap

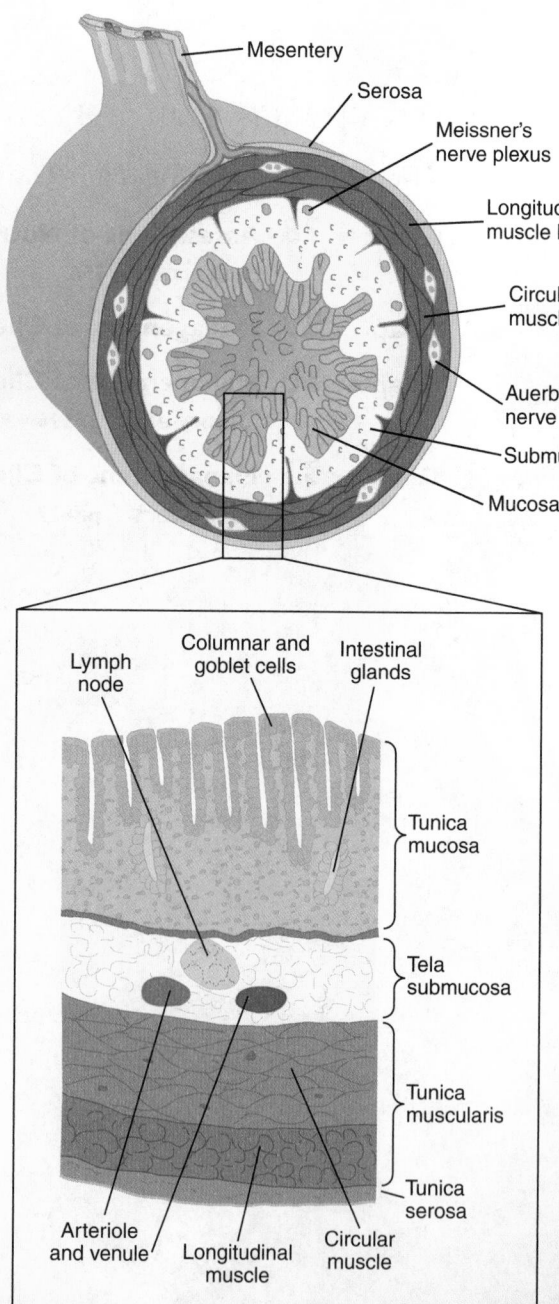

■ **FIGURE A&P7–1** Typical cross-section of the gastrointestinal tract. *Inset* shows enlargement of a cross-section of the small intestine. Microvilli of the mucosa enhance absorption of the diet, and smooth muscle orientation promotes mixing (circular) and peristalsis (longitudinal).

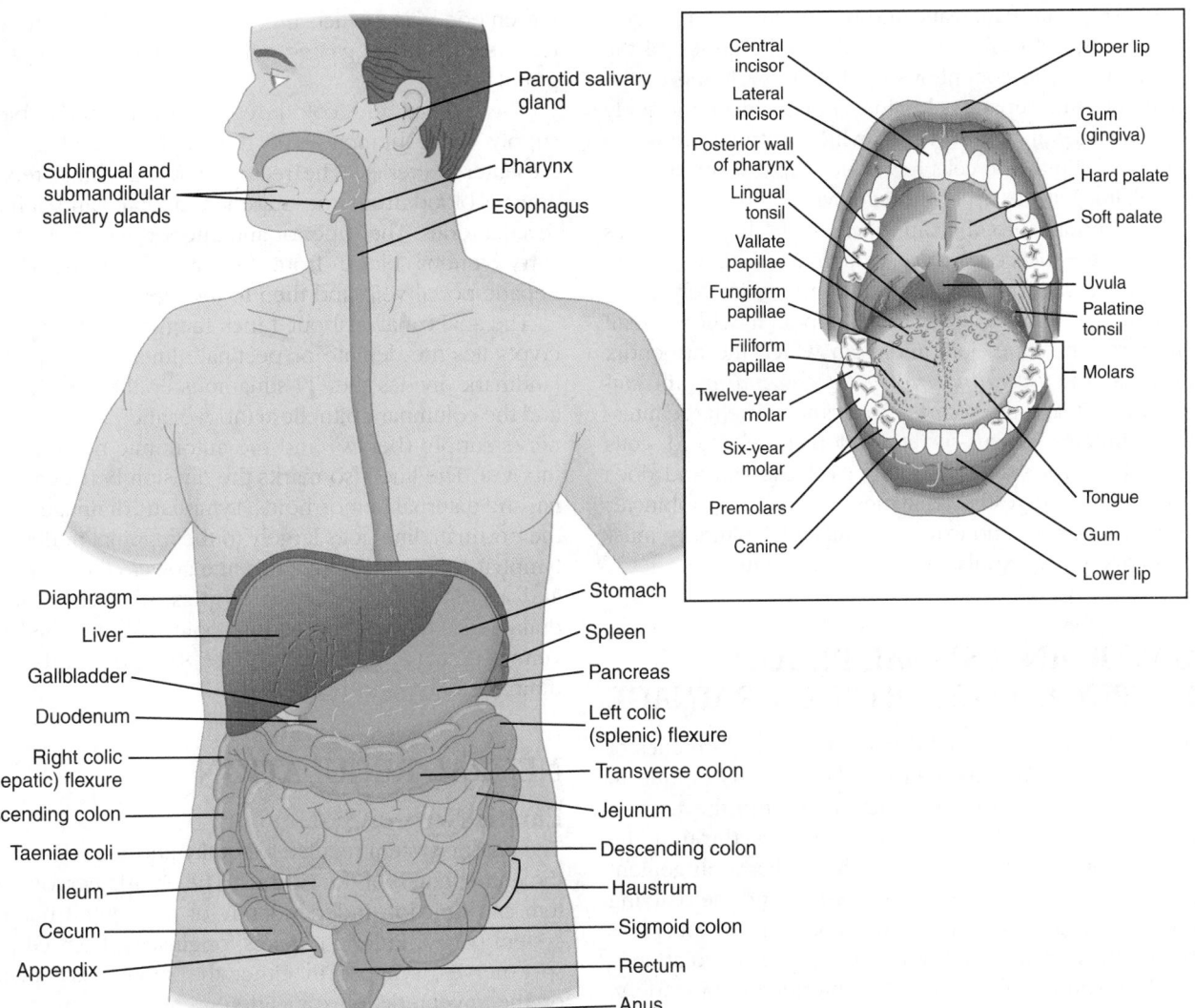

■ FIGURE A&P7–2 The digestive system. Ingested food passes through the mouth, esophagus, stomach, and small and large intestine before exiting at the anus. The liver, gallbladder, and pancreas assist the digestion and absorption of the diet. *Inset* shows the important structures of the oral cavity.

junctions, allowing a wave of depolarization and contraction to spread along the tract (see Motility later in this chapter).

Food is chewed *(masticated)*, mixed with saliva in the mouth, and swallowed. It passes through the pharynx and into the *esophagus.* The upper third of esophagus has striated (voluntary) muscle, the middle third has both types of muscle, and the lower third has only smooth muscle. The vagus nerve innervates both the smooth and the skeletal muscle of the esophagus. Sphincters isolate the esophagus from the remainder of the GI tract. The upper esophageal sphincter prevents entry of tracheal air and the lower esophageal sphincter prevents reflux of gastric contents. Acute failure of the lower esophageal sphincter leads to *esophagitis* (heartburn), and chronic gastric reflux damages the esophagus (Barrett's esophagus) and can lead to cancer. The opposite problem, *achalasia,* occurs if the lower esophageal sphincter does not relax sufficiently to allow food to pass into the stomach.

The stomach is divided into the *fundus, body,* and *antrum.* The fundus and body are highly distensible and act as a reservoir for the ingested meal. Food can be stored unmixed in the fundus and body for up to 1 hour. During this time, there may be a separation because of density, because fats float to the top and liquids accumulate on the bottom. Thus liquids are the first to leave the stomach and be absorbed through the intestine. Gastric contents, called chyme, empty from the antrum through the pylorus into the duodenum. The gastroduodenal junction with the pyloric sphincter sequesters acid in the stomach and bile in the duodenum.

The small intestine is divided into the *duodenum* (25 cm), *jejunum* (2.5 m), and *ileum* (3.6 m). The duodenum and jejunum are the major sites of digestion and absorption. Pancreatic and biliary ducts carry digestive enzymes, bicarbonate, and bile to the lumen of the duodenum. The continuous epithelial cell lining of the small intestine separates luminal contents from the body and provides a barrier across which nutrients must be absorbed. Epithelial cells reproduce rapidly and are lost (exfoliated) at the tip of the microvilli.

The nonabsorbed components of the diet pass through the *ileocecal valve* (a sphincter) to enter the large intestine. The large intestine (approximately 1.5 m in length) includes the *cecum* (a pouch where small and large intestines join and from which the appendix projects); the *ascending, transverse, descending,* and *sigmoid colon;* and the *rectum* (anal canal). The large intestine contains mucus-secreting goblet cells and cells specialized for water absorption; it lacks villi and does not produce digestive enzymes. An internal sphincter (smooth muscle) and external sphincter (voluntary muscle) govern the expulsion of feces (defecation).

GASTROINTESTINAL BLOOD SUPPLY AND LYMPHATIC DRAINAGE

Arterial blood enters the GI tract by various branches of major arteries. Venous drainage, however, is unique in that the veins from the GI tract empty into the hepatic portal vein. Portal venous blood passes through the liver before entering the vena cava. This arrangement allows the liver to begin processing and detoxifying compounds absorbed across the stomach and intestines before those compounds enter the general circulation.

The esophageal arteries, the inferior thyroid artery, and the left gastric artery provide the esophagus with its arterial blood supply. The left gastric and inferior phrenic arteries supply the gastroesophageal area. Venous blood is returned via the azygos, thyroid, and left gastric veins. Lymphatic drainage from the cervical esophagus and from the tracheal and postmediastinal nodes flows to the internal jugular vein, whereas intercostal nodes drain the thoracic esophagus. The lymphatic drainage of the lower esophagus occurs through the diaphragmatic, intracardiac, and left gastric lymph nodes.

The arterial blood supply to the stomach is derived from the celiac artery, which branches off to the lesser and greater curvatures. Two gastric arteries, from the splenic artery, supply the fundus and curvature. The portal vein provides the venous drainage of the stomach. The right and left gastroepiploic veins drain the greater curvature; the right gastric and coronary veins drain the lesser curvature. Lymph nodes of the stomach arise in the submucosa and drain into the thoracic duct.

Except in the duodenum, arterial blood supply to the small intestine is derived from the superior mesenteric artery. Arterial blood from the hepatic artery supplies the duodenum. Venous drainage is via the superior mesenteric vein, which unites with the inferior mesenteric, splenic, and gastric veins and then becomes the portal system.

The cecum and colon receive their arterial blood supply from branches of the superior and inferior mesenteric arteries. The rectum and anal canal receive arterial blood from the superior, middle, and inferior rectal arteries. The superior and inferior mesenteric veins carry venous blood from the large intestine to the hepatic portal vein and then to the liver.

The anal canal is about 1 inch long. At the level of the crypts lies the dentate or pectinate line. This important landmark divides the (1) squamous epithelium (below) and the columnar epithelium (above) and (2) the somatic nerve supply (below) and the autonomic nerve supply (above). The line also marks the division between internal and external hemorrhoids. Lymphatic drainage below the pectinate line goes largely to the inguinal nodes, and lymphatic drainage above this line goes to the pararectal and lateral pelvic (obturator) plexuses. The venous drainage also changes at this point. Above this line, venous drainage is into the portal system. Below this line, drainage is into the vena cava.

NEURAL REGULATION

Enteric Nervous System

The enteric system regulates motility and secretion along the entire length of the GI tract. The enteric nervous system can function independently of the central nervous system (CNS). Enteric reflexes, originating from GI sensory nerves, synapse in either the submucosal plexus or the myenteric plexus. Efferent nerves then supply the smooth muscle or secretory glands. Enteric activity can be modulated by external inputs, particularly by the sympathetic and parasympathetic nerves.

Auerbach's plexus (motor function) and *Meissner's plexus* (sensory function) provide intrinsic innervation for the stomach. Both begin in the esophageal wall and extend the length of the gut. Stimulation of Auerbach's plexus (between the longitudinal and circular muscle layers) generates gastric motility, increasing the intensity and rate of contractions and the release of gastrin from the antrum. Meissner's plexus (in the submucosa) functions with Auerbach's plexus to coordinate the motor and secretory activity of the gastric mucosa.

Sympathetic and Parasympathetic Nervous Systems

Sympathetic nerves supplying the GI tract originate in the celiac, superior mesenteric, inferior mesenteric, and hypogastric ganglia. In general, *sympathetics* inhibit activity in enteric plexuses, constrict GI system blood vessels, and decrease glandular secretions. GI motility is also decreased through contraction of circular muscle and certain sphincters and through indirect inhibition of peristalsis.

The vagus is the primary parasympathetic nerve supplying the GI tract, innervating all structures from the salivary glands to the transverse colon. Nerves from the hypogastric plexus innervate the remainder of the colon. Parasympathetic postganglionic neurons are located in the intramural plexus. In general, *parasympathetics* stimulate motor activity, stimulate secretory activity, and stimulate endocrine secretions.

FUNCTION OF THE GASTROINTESTINAL SYSTEM

The GI system isolates ingested food and provides an environment for digestion and absorption of nutrients. The major functions of the GI tract are (1) motility, (2) secretion, (3) digestion, and (4) absorption.

MOTILITY

Smooth Muscle

Smooth muscle of the GI tract is electrically connected by gap junctions, allowing a wave of depolarization and contraction to spread along the tract. Pacemakers along the length of the GI tract set the slow-wave contraction frequency. Nerves and hormones alter this rate and, therefore, GI motility.

GI smooth muscle produces long, strong contractions. Muscle basal tone provides some tension even at rest, and is influenced by neurotransmitters, hormones, and drugs. Stretching of the GI tract increases action potential frequency (*stress activation*), followed by a decrease back toward the original tension (*stress relaxation*).

Peristalsis is an organized wave of contraction of the longitudinal muscle layer that propels contents aborally (away from the mouth). Distention of a segment of intestine elicits a reflex contraction. The smooth muscle aboral to the contraction relaxes, and the contents move. This sequence repeats, moving contents for a short distance before the wave diminishes and disappears. A descending wave of peristalsis initiates sphincter relaxation, mediated by nitric oxide and vasoactive intestinal peptide (VIP) neurotransmitter in vagal nerves. Decreased vagal cholinergic activity also contributes to relaxation.

Intrinsic motility regulation uses interneurons to coordinate activity. The enteric nervous system has neuromodulators, similar to those in the brain. Intrinsic plexuses inhibit basal activity, and action potentials are thus elicited by less than half of the slow waves.

Contractions of the various layers of smooth muscle propel and mix luminal contents. Contraction of the longitudinal muscle layer accomplishes aboral movement. Contraction of circular muscle mixes luminal contents and increases contact with microvilli.

Mouth Through Esophagus

The process of moving food from the mouth into the esophagus is illustrated in Figure A&P7-3. The esophageal phase of swallowing is involuntary. During swallowing, the larynx is moved to cover the airway and to open the esophagus. Relaxation of the upper esophageal sphincter allows food to enter the esophagus. A primary peristaltic wave, controlled by the swallowing center in the brain, moves food through the esophagus in 10 seconds. Secondary peristalsis is initiated by esophageal distention (enteric nervous system); it propels any food still remaining in the esophagus into the stomach.

Stomach

Gastric contractions after feeding occur at a rate of three per minute. They begin in the middle of the body of the stomach, and increase in force and velocity as they approach the antrum. The antrum has strong contractions that fragment the food into smaller particles and mix the food with gastric secretions to initiate digestion. The rate of contractions is increased by gastrin and decreased by secretin. Sensory afferents from the stomach play a role in satiety. Increased intragastric pressure, gastric distention, gastric acidity, and pain all lessen the desire to eat food.

Gastroduodenal Junction

Gastric contents empty into the duodenal bulb at a controlled rate. The pylorus and terminal end of the antrum contract almost simultaneously (systolic contraction), allowing only a small amount of antral content to enter the duodenum. The remainder of antral contraction moves antral contents backward (retropulsion), causing further mixing. The rate of gastric emptying must match the duodenal buffering ability, or else acid may damage duodenal mucosa and cause duodenal ulcers. The pylorus prevents regurgitation of duodenal contents into the stomach, or else bile may damage stomach mucosa, causing gastric ulcers.

The rate of chyme entry into the duodenum is highly regulated in order to aid digestion. Duodenal acidity (pH <3.5) decreases the rate of gastric emptying. Duodenal acidity causes secretin release, which increases bicarbonate buffer secretion from the pancreas and liver. Chyme becomes more hypertonic as digestion progresses. Duodenal hypertonicity also decreases the rate of gastric emptying by a neural reflex. Fat content in the duodenal chyme also decreases the rate of gastric emptying. Cholecystokinin (CCK) released from the

1.

ORAL PHASE (VOLUNTARY)

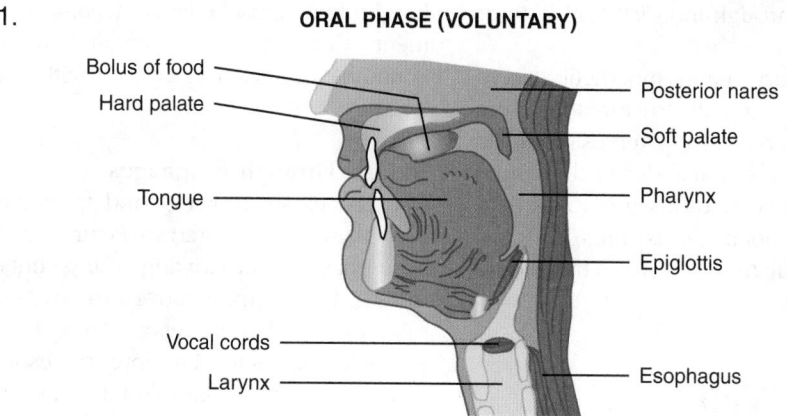

Bolus of food
Hard palate

Tongue

Vocal cords
Larynx

Posterior nares
Soft palate

Pharynx

Epiglottis

Esophagus

2.

PHARYNGEAL PHASE (INVOLUNTARY)

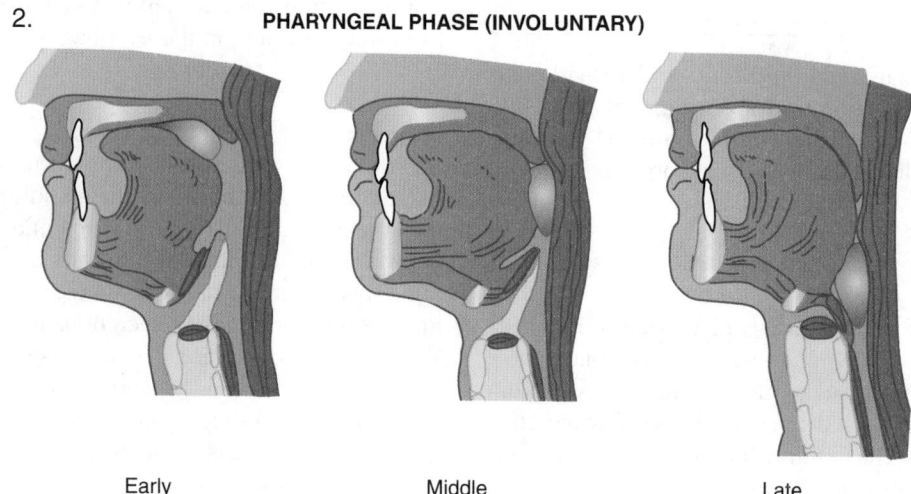

Early　　　　　　　Middle　　　　　　　Late

3.

ESOPHAGEAL PHASE (INVOLUNTARY)

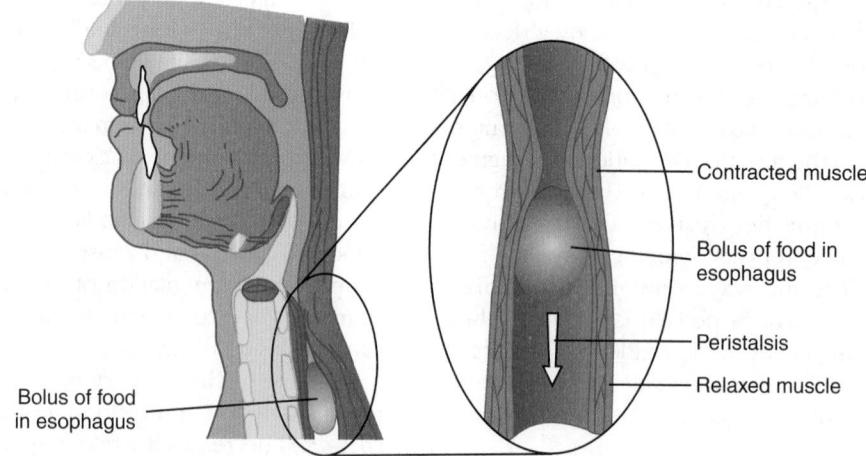

Bolus of food
in esophagus

Contracted muscle

Bolus of food in
esophagus

Peristalsis

Relaxed muscle

■ **FIGURE A&P7–3** Swallowing occurs in three phases: (1) *Voluntary* or *oral* phase. The tongue presses food against the hard palate, forcing it toward the pharynx. (2) *Involuntary* or *pharyngeal* phase. *Early:* Wave of peristalsis forces bolus between tonsillar pillars. *Middle:* Soft palate draws upward to close posterior nares, and respirations cease momentarily. *Late:* Vocal cords approximate and larynx pulls upward, covering the airway and stretching the esophagus open. (3) *Involuntary* or *esophageal* phase. Relaxation of the upper esophageal (hypopharyngeal) sphincter allows a peristaltic wave to move the bolus down the esophagus.

duodenum and jejunum contracts the pyloric sphincter, and glucose-dependent insulinotropic peptide (GIP) may also have a role. Fatty acids (especially long chain and unsaturated) decrease the rate of gastric emptying. Monoglycerides increase contractility of the pyloric sphincter. Amino acids (such as tryptophan) and peptides in the duodenum slow gastric emptying by promoting gastrin release, which constricts the pylorus.

Small Intestine

Peristalsis moves chyme aborally an average of 10 cm per contraction, and chyme takes 2 to 4 hours to move through the 6 meters of small intestine. Segmentation, the most frequent type of intestinal contraction, can be rhythmic, with adjacent sites alternating contraction and relaxation. Eating slows aboral movement of chyme. The enteric nervous system controls the frequency of segmentation and peristalsis. An intrinsic rate of 11 to 13 contractions per minute exists in the duodenum, which decreases to 8 to 9 per minute in the terminal ileum. This rate is modified by extrinsic neural and hormonal inputs.

Migrating Myoelectric Complex

The migrating myoelectric complex generates periods of intense electrical activity, followed by long quiescent periods. The resulting contractions, initiated in the stomach, traverse the entire small intestine. There is evidence for both vagal and hormonal (motilin) roles in initiation, and the enteric nervous system is required for propagation. This process sweeps the intestines clean and inhibits the retrograde movement of bacteria from the colon into the small intestine.

Large Intestine

Segmental contraction divides the colon into numerous haustra. Mass movements occurring three times each day are the most effective propulsion mechanism. Enteric nerves primarily inhibit smooth muscle contraction in the colon. Hirschsprung's disease is the congenital absence of enteric nerves; the colon is obstructed by a tonic contraction.

Although chyme may move through the small intestine in 2 to 4 hours, it takes 1 to 3 days to complete its passage through the large intestine. The colon reabsorbs water and salts as 1500 ml/day enters from the small intestine, and only 50 to 100 ml/day are excreted in feces. Bacteria consume more nutrients and release some vitamins (e.g., vitamin K). Solid wastes (sloughed epithelial cells, bile pigments, unabsorbed food) are prepared for elimination as feces. Colonic water reabsorption is time dependent. Abnormally fast movement of chyme through the large intestine results in diarrhea; abnormally slow movement results in constipation.

The final segments of the large intestine, the rectum and anal canal, extend from the sigmoid colon to the anus. Two sphincter muscles (internal and external) control the opening in the anus. The distal portions of the rectal walls form longitudinal folds, called rectal and anal columns. These folds terminate about 12 inches from the anus and are connected to one another by transverse folds of tissue called valves. Pockets formed by the valves are called sinuses or crypts. Because the external portion of the anal opening is lined with skin that changes at this point to mucosa, this area is sometimes called the *mucocutaneous border.*

Defecation

The rectum is usually nearly empty. Following mass movement, the rectum fills, the internal sphincter relaxes, and the external sphincter reflexively contracts. This process promotes the urge to defecate. The anal canal is normally closed. Voluntary relaxation of the external sphincter allows defecation to proceed, facilitated by increased abdominal pressure.

Vomiting

Vomiting expels gastric (and sometimes duodenal) contents by mouth. Retching, wherein gastric contents are forced into the esophagus but not the pharynx, precedes vomiting. The vomiting reflex follows a set pattern:

1. Reverse peristalsis is initiated in the middle of the small intestine.
2. The pyloric sphincter and stomach relax to receive duodenal contents.
3. Forced inspiration against a closed glottis decreases intrathoracic pressure.
4. Forceful contraction of abdominal muscles increases intra-abdominal pressure.
5. The lower esophageal sphincter relaxes; the pylorus and antrum contract.
6. Gastric contents enter the esophagus.
7. Retching occurs when the upper esophageal sphincter remains closed.
8. Vomiting occurs when the upper esophageal sphincter opens.
9. The trachea closes as in normal swallowing to prevent aspiration.

The medulla has a separate vomiting center and retching center that normally interact. Afferent inputs include stomach and duodenal distention, and pain in the genitourinary system. Dizziness or tickling the back of the throat can also induce the gag reflex and vomiting. Emetics are used to induce vomiting by stimulating receptors in the stomach and duodenum (ipecac) or by activating a chemoreceptive trigger zone (CTZ) in the area postrema of the brain.

SECRETIONS

Most ingested food cannot be absorbed directly. GI secretions digest foods into absorbable components, assist absorption, and help prevent autodigestion (Table A&P7-1). GI secretions are regulated by a series of hormonal and neural feedback mechanisms. In addition to digestive enzymes, secretions include lubricants, ions, absorption facilitators, and bile.

Lubricants

Chewing of foods (mastication) is the initial step in digestion. Chewing mixes the food with salivary mucus, subdivides food, and exposes starches to salivary amylase. Chewing facilitates the mechanical breakdown of food, but chewing is not an essential component of digestion.

Saliva, with both watery and mucous secretions, helps lubricate food as it enters the GI tract. Mucus-secreting cells are located along the entire GI tract, but digestive secretions are limited to the prejejunal GI tract. Salivary glands contribute about 1.5 L/day to the GI tract. The stomach secretes about 2 L/day, and the pancreas secretes 1.5 L/day, helping to liquefy the chyme. The small intestine secretes 1.5 L/day, and the large intestine secretes 400 ml/day. In addition, 0.25 to 1.5 L/day of hepatic secretions enter the duodenum.

TABLE A&P7–1   Gastrointestinal-Associated Secretions

Location	Secretion	Role
Lubricants		
Entire GI tract	Mucus	Lubricant
Salivary gland	Water	Lubricant and solvent
Pancreas	Water	Lubricant
Small intestine	Water	Lubricant
Digestive Enzymes		
Salivary glands	Amylase	Digest starch
	Lingual lipase	Digest triglycerides
Stomach	Pepsin (pepsinogen)	Digest proteins
	Gastric lipase	Digest triglycerides
Pancreas	Amylase	Digest starch
	Lipase	Digest triglycerides
	Colipase	Digest triglycerides
	Phospholipase	Digest phospholipids
	Trypsin	Digest peptides
	Chymotrypsin	Digest peptides
	Nucleases	Digest DNA and RNA
Intestinal epithelium	Disaccharidases	Digest disaccharides
	Peptidases	Digest peptides
Hormones and Neurotransmitters		
Stomach	Gastrin	HCl secretion
Pancreas	Somatostatin	Inhibits insulin, glucagon release
Small intestine	Cholecystokinin	Bile secretion, pancreatic enzyme secretion
	Secretin	Pancreatic bicarbonate secretion
	Glucose-dependent insulinotropic peptide (GIP)	Pancreatic insulin release
	Motilin	GI smooth muscle contraction
	Enteroglucagons	Pancreatic insulin release
Enteric neurons	Vasoactive intestinal peptide (VIP)	GI smooth muscle relaxation
		Pancreatic secretion
	Bombesin	Gastrin release
Ionic Secretions		
Salivary glands	NaHCO$_3$	At high salivary flow rates
	KCl	At low salivary flow rates
Stomach		
Parietal cells	HCl	Activate pepsin
Mucus cells	K$^+$ and HCO$_3^-$	Protect stomach from acid
Pancreas	HCO$_3^-$	Neutralize gastric secretion
Absorption Facilitators		
Stomach	Intrinsic factor	Ileal absorption of vitamin B$_{12}$
Liver	Bile acids	Small intestine lipid absorption

DNA, Deoxyribonucleic acid; *GI*, gastrointestinal; *HCl*, hydrochloric acid; *KCl*, potassium chloride; *NaHCO$_3$*, sodium bicarbonate; *RNA*, ribonucleic acid.

Gastric secretions begin protein digestion and protect the gastric epithelium. After a meal, there are three distinct phases of gastric acid secretion. (1) The *cephalic phase* is due to a neural reflex initiated by the sight, smell, or taste of food. The decrease in antral pH acts directly on the parietal calls to attenuate the cephalic phase. (2) The *gastric phase* is due to gastric distention caused by food in the stomach. (3) The *intestinal phase* is initiated by chyme entry into the duodenum.

Secretion of HCl from the gastric parietal cells involves the interplay of acetylcholine, gastrin, histamine, and a second cell type, the enterochromaffin cell. A powerful synergistic interaction between these stimuli causes difficulty in diminishing acid secretion by blocking only one pathway. HCl secretion can be blocked by atropine or H_2-histamine blocking medications, but a blocker for gastrin is not yet available. Gastric ulcers, although associated with increased HCl secretion, also involve a gram-negative bacterium, *Helicobacter pylori,* that damages the gastric mucosa. Other agents, such as aspirin and nonsteroidal anti-inflammatory drugs (NSAIDs), can damage the gastric mucosa and cause gastric ulcers by reducing the production of protective mucus.

Absorption Facilitators and Ions

Pancreatic enzymes are essential for the normal absorption of lipids, proteins, and carbohydrates. See Table A&P7-1 for a list of important enzymes and ionic pancreatic secretions, and their function.

Bile and the Enterohepatic Circulation

Bile is produced by hepatocytes in the liver, draining through the many bile ducts that penetrate the liver. Bile acids are secreted by liver as bile, stored in the gallbladder, and released into the duodenum in response to food. Bile acts to some extent as a detergent, helping to emulsify fats (increasing surface area to help enzyme action), and thus aid in their absorption in the small intestine. Bile acids are reabsorbed by both diffusion and active transport in the terminal ileum and are returned to the liver by the hepatic portal vein. The liver then actively extracts bile acids from the portal venous blood and secretes the reabsorbed bile acids into bile, thus beginning the process anew. Only about 15% to 35% of the bile acid pool is lost in feces each day and is replaced by new synthesis of bile acids.

Bile acids are normally secreted conjugated to glycine or taurine. In the neutral pH of the small intestine, bile is in the salt form.

With the sphincter of Oddi at the junction of the bile duct and duodenum normally contracted, bile is diverted to and stored in the gallbladder between meals. The gallbladder extracts sodium ions (Na^+) actively, anions via electroneutrality, and water osmotically, thus concentrating bile. CCK is the primary stimulus for the gallbladder

to contract (expel contents) into the duodenum. Vagal nerves also contract the gallbladder and relax the sphincter of Oddi. Sympathetics and VIP do the opposite; they inhibit gallbladder emptying.

Disorders of bile secretions lead to crystal (stone) formation. Gallstones primarily are cholesterol crystals surrounding a bilirubin crystal core. If the cholesterol content exceeds the dissolving capability of the micelles, cholesterol crystals form and act as a nucleus for gallstones. Bile pigment stones, a calcium salt of unconjugated bilirubin, can also form.

DIGESTION AND ABSORPTION

Complex carbohydrates are broken down to absorbable monoglycerides. Poorly absorbed large proteins are broken down into monopeptides, dipeptides, and tripeptides. Pancreatic lipases digest lipids to their fatty acid and triglyceride components, which are then absorbed.

Carbohydrates

Digestion and absorption of carbohydrates occur primarily in the duodenum and the jejunum. The ability to absorb carbohydrates greatly exceeds normal dietary intake. Occasionally, an inability to absorb carbohydrates occurs because of deficiency of digestive enzymes or transport proteins. Microflora metabolize any carbohydrates that pass through to the colon, producing gas, increased motility, and diarrhea. Diagnosis of malabsorption is confirmed by exposure to a specific carbohydrate or a biopsy of jejunal epithelial cells. Treatment involves dietary restriction or supplemental enzyme ingestion.

One common disorder, lactose malabsorption syndrome *(lactose intolerance),* is a genetic lactase deficiency that develops in 50% of adults. This syndrome is almost universal in people with Asian ancestry, and it is common in native Africans and people from Mediterranean areas, but it is relatively infrequent in people of Northern European descent.

Proteins

A protein intake of 0.5 g/kg/day is necessary for normal balance, and a higher intake is required for growth. Dietary intake varies among cultures. Separate from ingestion, the body recycles some protein from the intestines, mostly from digestive secretions (20 g/day) and desquamated epithelial cells (20 g/day). The little protein that is present in the feces is due mostly to colonic bacteria, desquamated cells, and proteins in colonic mucous secretion.

Digestion occurs in the stomach and small intestine, and absorption occurs primarily in the duodenum and jejunum. Large proteins are poorly absorbed. L-Isomers and single amino acids as well as dipeptides and tripeptides are created through enzymatic digestion and absorbed actively by a sodium-coupled process. Genetic malabsorption and intolerance disorders affect both intestinal and renal proximal tubule transport proteins.

Lipids

Triglycerides are the major component of dietary lipids. Other components include sterols, sterol esters, and phospholipids. Lipids are hydrophobic and separate from the remainder of chyme as an oily phase in the stomach. In the duodenum, lipids are emulsified by bile acids and digested to form micelles with bile acids. The micelles are absorbed at the intestinal brush border. Some digestion occurs in the intestine and stomach, but the duodenum, as a result of pancreatic lipases, is the major site of lipid digestion.

Micelles are essential to increase surface contact area for absorption in the duodenum and jejunum. Lipophilic cholesterol, fatty acids, and lysophosphatides diffuse across the cell membrane. The lipids accumulate in the smooth endoplasmic reticulum and are resynthesized to triglycerides, phospholipids, and cholesterol esters. They are then packaged in chylomicrons and extruded by exocytosis. Chylomicrons pass through the lymphatics to enter venous circulation at the thoracic duct.

Fat lost in feces comes primarily from colonic microflora and desquamated cells. Malabsorption of lipids is tied to impaired digestion or absorption. Complete bile deficiency reduces fatty acid absorption by 50% and impairs absorption of other lipids. Complete absence of pancreatic lipases impairs absorption of all classes of lipids. Impaired absorption can also result from epithelial cell damage, such as intestinal mucosal atrophy, tropical sprue, and gluten enteropathy. The addition of nonabsorbable lipids (e.g., Olestra) and lipid absorption inhibitors also impairs the absorption of fat-soluble vitamins (A, D, E, and K).

Water and Electrolytes

The GI tract absorbs 99% of ingested water. Absorption is greatest in the jejunum and least in the colon as a result of the tightness of the "tight junctions" on the epithelial cells. The jejunum is also the primary site of Na absorption, secondary to amino acid and carbohydrate transport. The colon has an active Na absorption. Potassium (K) is reabsorbed in the jejunum and ileum, but net potassium balance is determined in the colon. The colon reabsorbs K if the luminal K concentration is high and secretes K if the luminal K concentration is low. A significant K loss accompanies water loss from diarrhea.

Intestinal chloride load is from ingestion and pancreatic secretions. Chloride is reabsorbed in the jejunum, ileum, and colon. Bicarbonate intestinal load is from pancreatic secretions. It is absorbed in the jejunum and may be secreted in the ileum and colon by HCO_3^-/Cl^-

exchange. There is a net secretion if HCO_3^- levels are high *(alkalosis)* and a net reabsorption if HCO_3^- levels are low *(acidosis)*.

Intestinal Ion and Water Balance

Sympathetic activity enhances water and sodium chloride (NaCl) absorption, and conversely parasympathetic activity decreases water and NaCl absorption. Aldosterone is the primary hormone regulating colonic ion balance, causing Na reabsorption while leading to colonic K loss. Other hormones that influence water and NaCl absorption are enkephalins (opioid peptides), which enhance NaCl and water absorption in the intestine, and somatostatin, which increases colonic NaCl and water absorption.

Excessive GI secretions are a clinically important problem. Na, C, and water secretion in crypts in the small intestine can exceed the absorptive capacity of the remainder of the GI tract. Cholera toxin stimulates crypt cell secretion, as do other cyclic adenosine monophosphate (cAMP) stimulators such as VIP and prostaglandins. Pancreatic cholera results from a pancreatic tumor that secretes VIP. Cholera leads to massive diarrhea.

Diarrhea also results from exposure to excessive osmotic loads, such as the concentrated nutrients used in tube- feeding. The concentrated chyme pulls water to it, leading to diarrhea. Carbohydrate fat malabsorption syndromes have the same effect.

Calcium absorption in the duodenum and jejunum is stimulated by vitamin D. Approximately 50% of ingested magnesium is absorbed along the length of the intestine. Phosphate is absorbed along the length of the intestine, possibly by active transport.

The physical state of iron entering the duodenum greatly influences its absorption. At physiologic pH, ferrous iron (Fe^{2+}) is rapidly oxidized to the insoluble ferric (Fe^{3+}) form. Gastric acid lowers the pH in the proximal duodenum, enhancing the solubility and uptake of ferric iron. When gastric acid production is blocked (for instance, by acid pump inhibitors), iron absorption is reduced substantially. A number of dietary factors influence iron absorption. Ascorbate and citrate increase iron absorption. Conversely, iron absorption is inhibited by plant phytates and tannins. These compounds also chelate iron, and prevent its uptake. Phytates are prominent in wheat and some other cereals, while tannins are prevalent in (nonherbal) teas.

Flora

The small intestine flora are predominantly grampositive lactobacilli, streptococci, and staphylococci. *Aerobacter aerogenes, Bacteroides, Candida albicans, Escherichia coli, Proteus, Pseudomonas,* and *Streptococcus faecalis* are also found. Bile acids and gastric acid may inhibit bacterial proliferation in the intestine. The alkaline environment of the large intestine permits the growth of organisms whose main functions are to break down remaining proteins and indigestible residue. These organisms include *E. coli, S. faecalis, Clostridium perfringens,* and *Lactobacillus.*

Intestinal bacteria convert urea to ammonium salts and ammonia. Bacterial action in the large bowel causes the formation of gases, which provide bulk and help propel feces. This action also synthesizes nutritional factors such as vitamin K, thiamine, riboflavin, vitamin B_{12}, folic acid, biotin, and nicotinic acid.

Vitamins

Vitamins are essential nutrients that must be absorbed from a dietary source. Water-soluble vitamins can be absorbed by membrane transport proteins. Folic acid and nicotinic acid are absorbed by diffusion or facilitated diffusion. Diffusion causes absorption of pyridoxine and riboflavin. Secondary active transport absorbs vitamin C in the ileum, biotin in the duodenum and ileum, and folic acid and thiamine in the jejunum. Vitamin B_{12} absorption across the ileum requires intrinsic factor, a gastric secretion. Lipid-soluble vitamins are absorbed in micelles. These include vitamins A, D, E, and K. Compounds that diminish or impair fat absorption also impair absorption of fat-soluble vitamins.

EFFECTS OF AGING

Physiologic changes in the gastrointestinal tract occur with aging. In the mouth, teeth may loosen from loss of supporting gums and bone. Circulation in the gums is reduced, and aging teeth darken and may become uneven and fracture. Decreased output of the salivary glands leads to dryness of mucous membranes and increased susceptibility to breakdown. This decrease can cause difficulty in swallowing and decreased stimulation of taste buds.

Secretion of digestive enzymes and bile also decreases. In the stomach, atrophy of gastric mucosa leads to a decreased secretion of HCl. A decrease in HCl reduces the absorption of iron and vitamin B_{12}, leading to development of anemia. A resulting proliferation of bacteria in the gut can lead to diarrhea and infection. With a decrease in bile secretion, absorption of fats and fat-soluble vitamins becomes impaired. This decreased absorption of fat can lead to weight loss, and the decrease in fat-soluble vitamins can lead to a variety of problems such as altered calcium metabolism and bleeding from the decrease of vitamin K, which is needed to synthesize clotting factors such as prothrombin.

In the large intestine, peristalsis decreases and nerve impulses are dulled. In addition, the muscular tone of the intestinal wall and abdominal muscle strength are reduced. These changes can result in a decreased sensation to defecate and an increased incidence of constipation.

CONCLUSIONS

A thorough knowledge of the structure and function of the gastrointestinal system helps the nurse provide knowledgeable care to clients. Medical disorders are related to the four major functions of the GI system: digestion, absorption, motility, and secretion. To provide effective interventions, the nurse must understand the normal physiology of this system and the digestive organs.

BIBLIOGRAPHY

1. Berne, R., et al. (2004). *Physiology* (5th ed.). St. Louis: Mosby.
2. Carroll, R.G. (2007). *Elsevier's integrated physiology.* Philadelphia: Saunders.
3. Kierszenbaum, A.L. (2007). *Histology and cell biology: An introduction to pathology* (2nd ed.). St. Louis: Mosby.
4. Guyton, A., & Hall, J. (2006). *Textbook of medical physiology* (10th ed.). Philadelphia: Saunders.
5. Silverthorn, D. (2006). *Human physiology* (4th ed.). San Francisco, Calif: Pearson Benjamin Cummings.

CHAPTER 28

Assessment of Nutrition and the Digestive System

VICKI M. ROSS

Adequate and appropriate nutrition underlies the success of all medical therapies. Nutritional health requires a functional gut that can receive, transport, absorb, and metabolize nutrients. Similarly, adequate and appropriate nutrition is necessary for the gut to function properly. Because of this interdependence, assessment of the gastrointestinal (GI) tract and nutritional status occurs simultaneously or in close succession. A systematic and thorough assessment of the client's nutritional status and upper GI tract can detect a wide range of actual or potential health problems.

This chapter focuses on assessment of nutritional status and the upper GI tract, which includes the mouth, esophagus, stomach, and small intestine. Assessments of the large intestine (colon), rectum, and accessory organs (liver, pancreas, and gallbladder) are presented in Chapters 32 and 42.

SCREENING AND ASSESSMENT OF NUTRITIONAL HEALTH

Nutritional Health

Nutritional health results when the body's nutrient requirements are consistently met.[10] To meet the body's nutrient requirements, adequate and appropriate nutrition must be delivered to, transported by, and absorbed by the GI tract. Furthermore, absorbed nutrients must be metabolized and used at the cellular level. Because of wide variation in factors affecting nutrient requirements, such as age, size, gender, metabolism, and activity level, it is difficult, if not impossible, to determine exact nutrient amounts required for individual clients. However, comparing individual characteristics to published standards or reference groups allows estimation of a client's nutrient requirements.

To determine whether a client is receiving adequate nutrition, begin by collecting information about dietary intake. Ask the client to list the amounts and types of foods and beverages consumed over the past 24 hours and ask whether this is a typical daily intake. If it is not typical, ask the client to describe a typical day of food and beverage intake. Twenty-four hour dietary recalls are quick and relatively easy to obtain; however, the accuracy of the information depends on the client's recall ability. Asking the client to maintain a food diary listing all foods and beverages consumed for 1 to 3 days is a prospective method for collecting diet information. In addition to listing all food and drinks consumed for a specific time period, food diaries should include the amount of each food or drink consumed, how the food or drink was prepared (fried, baked in butter, broiled, steamed), and the time of day the food or drink was consumed.

After obtaining information about dietary intake, assess the adequacy of the client's nutrient intake by comparing it to standard references such as the Food Guide Pyramid or the Dietary Reference Intakes (DRI). The Food Guide Pyramid is a graphic representation of the categories and servings of foods recommended for average, healthy people and is available in nutrition textbooks or on the U.S. Department of Agriculture website.[11] To use the Food Guide Pyramid,

---

evolve **Web Enhancements**

Diversity in Health Care Cultural Influences on Nutrition

Appendix B A Health History Format That Integrates the Assessment of Functional Health Patterns

Tables Food-Borne Poisoning

Common Herbal Supplements

Body Mass Index (BMI)

Be sure to check out the bonus material on the Evolve website and the CD-ROM, including free self-assessment exercises. **http://evolve.elsevier. com/Black/medsurg**

compare the number of servings and types of food (e.g., fruit, bread, dairy) consumed with the recommended number of servings from the respective food group. Clients who consistently omit one or more of the food groups are at nutritional risk, as are clients who consistently eat a disproportionate number of servings from one or more of the food groups.[8]

To determine the adequacy of a client's intake of specific nutrients (e.g., vitamins, minerals, trace elements), consult with a registered dietitian and the DRI.[5] DRI provide research-based information and recommendations for specific nutrients. Table 28-1 lists the average intake (AI) or recommended dietary allowance (RDA) range for nonpregnant adults for selected nutrients.

TABLE 28–1   Recommendations for Daily Intake of Vitamin and Trace Micronutrients

Micronutrient RDA or AI for Nonpregnant Adults	Foods High in Micronutrient	Manifestations of Deficit	Manifestations of Excess
Vitamin A 700-900 mcg RE	Dark green, leafy or yellow-orange vegetables; milk fat; egg yolks; beef liver	Loss of appetite and taste; night blindness; bumpy or scaly skin	Dry lips, eyes, nasal mucosa, and skin; gingivitis; bone pain; hair loss; liver disease
Vitamin B$_1$ (thiamine) 1.1-1.4 mg	Lean meats, egg yolks, legumes, enriched or whole grain cereals, breads	Paresthesias, peripheral neuropathies, mental confusion, heart failure, edema	Dysrhythmias, wheezing, hypotension
Vitamin B$_6$ (pyridoxine) 1.3-1.7 mg	Yeast, wheat germ, pork, liver, whole grain cereals, legumes	Sore, reddened tongue; seborrheic-like dermatitis; paresthesias	Sensory ataxia, impairment of position and vibratory sense
Vitamin B$_{12}$ (cobalamin) 2.4 mcg	Beef, fish, milk, eggs, cheese	Sore, reddened mouth; atrophy of tongue; megaloblastic anemia; paresthesias	None known
Vitamin C (ascorbic acid) 75-90 mg	Oranges, lemons, strawberries, tomatoes, cabbage, green peppers	Gingivitis, dry mouth, alopecia, pruritus, ecchymotic lesions on skin	Gastrointestinal upset, diarrhea
Calcium AI: 1000-1200 mg	Dairy products, sardines; salmon; dark green, leafy vegetables	Osteoporosis, osteomalacia	Calcification of soft tissue; hypercalcemia; constipation; impaired absorption of iron, zinc, or manganese
Copper 900 mcg	Organ meats, legumes, chocolate, nuts	Decreased absorption of iron, anemia, neutropenia, leukopenia	Liver disease, Kayser-Fleischer rings (brown or green ring near corneal limbus and sunflower cataract)
Vitamin D (calciferol) AI: 5-15 mcg	Fish and fish oil, fortified dairy products	Softening of bones, joint pain, fatigue, muscle tetany	Calcification of soft tissue or tympanic membrane, leading to deafness; anorexia; hypotonia
Vitamin E (tocopherol) 15 mg α-tocopherol equivalent	Sunflower, corn, or soybean oil; wheat germ oils	Lipid absorption or transport abnormalities	Pulmonary deterioration, thrombocytopenia, liver and kidney failure
Folate (folic acid) 400 mcg	Legumes, liver, dark green or leafy vegetables, lean beef, potatoes	Sore, reddened tongue and mouth; glossitis; megaloblastic anemia	May decrease availability of zinc
Iron 8-18 mg	Organ meats, shellfish, poultry, legumes, blackstrap molasses, fortified cereals	Hypochromic, microcytic anemia	Vomiting, upper abdominal pain, pallor, cyanosis, shock
Iodine 150 mcg	Seafood, iodized salt	Enlargement of thyroid gland	Goiter, myxedema
Vitamin K AI: 90-120 mcg	Broccoli, cabbage, turnip greens, green tea	Ecchymotic lesions, bruising	Hemolytic anemia, severe jaundice in infants
Manganese 2-5 mcg	Whole grains, legumes, nuts, tea	Magenta tongue, dermatitis	Manifestations of Parkinson's or Wilson's disease
Niacin 14-16 mg niacin equivalents	Organ meats, brewer's yeast, peanuts, fish, poultry, whole grains, beans	Sore, reddened mouth; atrophy of tongue; angular stomatitis; dermatitis	Histamine release, liver toxicity
Riboflavin 1.1-1.3 mg	Liver, milk, cheddar cheese, cottage cheese, yogurt, brewer's yeast	Sore, reddened tongue and mouth; angular stomatitis; seborrhea-like dermatitis	None known
Zinc 12-15 mg	Oysters, wheat germ, beef, cheese	Angular stomatitis, seborrhea-like dermatitis, alopecia	Vomiting, diarrhea, impaired copper absorption

AI, Average intake; *RDA,* recommended dietary allowance; *RE,* retinol equivalents.
From references 5, 8, and 10.

In consultation with a dietitian, calculate the amount of calories and protein consumed by the client in a typical day. In general, the average, healthy person requires about 30 to 35 calories per kilogram and 0.8 to 1.2 g of protein per kilogram of body weight. For example, a woman weighing 55 kg (120 pounds) requires 1650 to 1925 calories and 44 to 66 g of protein. The Food Guide Pyramid and DRI are based on average, healthy populations and may need to be altered for clients who are ill or outside the average height or weight range. In general, protein requirements decrease and nonprotein calorie requirements increase when kidney or liver function is impaired. Dietary fats are restricted for pancreatic exocrine dysfunction and carbohydrates are restricted for pancreatic endocrine dysfunction.

The National Health and Nutrition Examination Surveys (NHANES) are population-based surveys that provide information about dietary intake, nutritional status, and health outcomes related to nutrition. Information from these surveys can be used to assess similar client populations. For example, analyses from population surveys indicate that an increasing percentage of Americans are overweight or obese. Furthermore, obesity is positively associated with increased caloric intake, sedentary lifestyle, and the risk of developing diseases such as diabetes mellitus and heart disease.[2] Therefore it is important to ask questions about the client's physical activity and the presence of diabetes or heart disease when assessing nutritional adequacy.

Malnutrition

Starvation and obesity are forms of malnutrition. Primary and secondary starvation are defined by the inadequate delivery of nutrients over a period of time. Primary starvation occurs when adequate nutrition is not delivered to the upper GI tract (famine, anorexia, mechanical obstructions of the GI tract, fad diets) and secondary starvation occurs when the upper GI tract fails to absorb, metabolize, or use nutrients (ischemic bowel or Crohn's disease). Starvation malnutrition may also be classified based on calorie and/or protein adequacy. Kwashiorkor, marasmus, and mixed-type malnutrition are international terms used to reflect inadequate protein, calorie, and protein-calorie intake, respectively.

Micronutrient malnutrition, another form of starvation malnutrition, occurs when vitamins, minerals, or trace elements are not delivered, absorbed, or used by the body. Because most foods contain more than one micronutrient, inadequate food consumption rarely causes single micronutrient deficits. Instead, clients typically present with multiple nutrient deficits. Because most laboratory tests that measure micronutrients (copper, zinc, manganese) are not sophisticated enough to determine the adequacy of a given micronutrient for a specific client,[10] the best method to identify whether an actual or potential micronutrient deficit exists is a thorough history and meticulous physical examination. See Table 28-1 for foods high in specific micronutrients and clinical manifestations of micronutrient deficits.

Clients with conditions that lead to increased excretion or utilization of micronutrients are at risk for micronutrient deficits. Chronic pancreatitis can lead to fat malabsorption and decreased absorption of fat-soluble vitamins. Because of a reduction in the absorptive surface and shortened transit times, clients with short-bowel syndrome are at increased risk for developing micronutrient deficits. Clients with healing wounds may have increased vitamin C and zinc requirements. Gastric surgery can impair absorption and use of vitamin B_{12}. If dietary intake is inadequate or if the client presents with clinical histories such as these, suspect and assess for micronutrient malnutrition.

Obesity or nutritional excess is also a form of malnutrition that results from nutrient delivery that exceeds the client's nutrient requirements. Chapter 29 contains additional information about malnutrition.

Nutrition Screen or Assessment?

Nutrition screening and nutrition assessment are not the same. Nutrition screening is a method of categorizing clients at high or low risk for malnutrition. In general, nutrition screening takes place within the first few days of the client's encounter with the health care system and includes general questions about nutritional status and upper GI function. Box 28-1 shows an example of a nutrition screening tool. When the nutrition screen indicates a client is at risk for malnutrition, in-depth nutrition and upper GI assessments are performed. Nutrition and upper GI assessments are client-centered and include in-depth histories, physical examinations, and diagnostic testing to determine actual or potential problems involving the upper GI tract, nutritional status, or both.

HISTORY

Assessment of both nutritional status and upper GI tract status begins with collection of health history data. The historical account determines the direction and focus of the physical examination and the required diagnostic testing.

Biographical and Demographic Data

Analyze the client's demographic information (gender, age, religious affiliation, and marital status) as it relates to the client's nutritional status and upper GI function. Because requirements are higher and women are at risk for calcium deficits, specific questions about calcium intake should be incorporated into women's health

---

BOX 28-1   Features of the Admission Nutrition Screening Tool

A. DIAGNOSIS

If the client has one or more of the following conditions, circle it, proceed to section E, and consider the client AT NUTRITIONAL RISK. If the client has none of these conditions, proceed to section B.

- Anorexia nervosa/bulimia nervosa
- Cachexia (temporal wasting, muscle wasting, cancer, cardiac disease)
- Coma
- Diabetes mellitus
- End-stage liver disease
- End-stage renal disease
- Malabsorption (celiac sprue, ulcerative colitis, Crohn's disease, short-bowel syndrome)
- Major gastrointestinal surgery within the past year
- Multiple trauma (closed-head injury, penetrating trauma, multiple fractures)
- Nonhealing wounds
- Pressure ulcers

B. NUTRITION INTAKE HISTORY

If the client has one or more of the following manifestations, circle it, proceed to section E, and consider the client AT NUTRITIONAL RISK. If the client has none of these manifestations, proceed to section C.

- Diarrhea (>500 ml for 2 days)
- Vomiting (>5 days)
- Reduced intake (>½ normal intake for more than 5 days)

C. IDEAL BODY WEIGHT STANDARDS

Compare the client's current weight for height to a chart of ideal body weights. If the client weighs less than 80% of ideal body weight, proceed to section E and consider the client AT

NUTRITIONAL RISK. If the client weighs more than 80% of ideal body weight, proceed to section D.

D. WEIGHT HISTORY

- Any recent unplanned weight loss? No _____ Yes _____
- Amount _____ (lb or kg)
- If yes, within the past _____ weeks or _____ months
- Current weight _____
- Usual weight _____
- Height _____
- Find percentage of weight loss:
- Usual wt − Current wt
- Usual wt × 100 = _____% wt loss

Compare the percentage of weight lost with the values on the following chart; circle the applicable value.

Length of Time	Significant (%)	Severe (%)
1 wk	1-2	>2
2-3 wk	2-3	>3
1 mo	4-5	>5
3 mo	7-8	>8
5 mo	10	>10

If the client has experienced a significant or severe weight loss, proceed to section E and consider the client AT NUTRITIONAL RISK.

E. NURSE ASSESSMENT

Using the above criteria, what is this client's nutritional risk? (check one)

- _____ LOW NUTRITIONAL RISK
- _____ AT NUTRITIONAL RISK

Modified from Kovacevich, D., et al. (1997). Nutrition risk classification: A reproducible and valid tool for nurses. *Nutrition in Clinical Practice, 12,* 22.

---

histories. For older adults living alone, social and financial factors affect their access to and intake of food. When assessing demographic data, be sure to include questions about who prepares and purchases the food.[6]

The risks of GI conditions vary for different ages and gender. For example, in middle age the incidence of esophageal and gastric cancers occurs more often in males than in females but the incidence of these types of cancers rises with age in both genders.[9] Culture and ethnic origin also affect the type, amount, and frequency of dietary consumption (see the Diversity in Health Care feature on Cultural Influences on Nutrition on the website).

Current Health

The client's current health history includes questions about clinical manifestations, medications and dietary supplements, and allergies. Refer to Figure 28-1 for questions to guide an expanded nutrition assessment.

Chief Complaint

Allow the client to describe the chief complaint in his or her own words. Ask questions about the timing and characteristics of the complaint, as well as solicit information related to the aggravating and alleviating factors. Be sure to determine the client's usual nutritional intake, patterns of intake, and whether there has been a change in appetite or weight since the manifestations first appeared. Also determine who is the primary preparer of meals and if anything has changed in meal preparation.

Clinical Manifestations

Clients often present with complaints associated with nutrition or upper GI function such as abdominal pain, nausea and vomiting, indigestion, diarrhea, and changes in weight or appetite. When a client presents with these complaints, conduct an in-depth analysis of clinical manifestations using Figure 28-1 as a guide as well as the questions listed in the following sections.

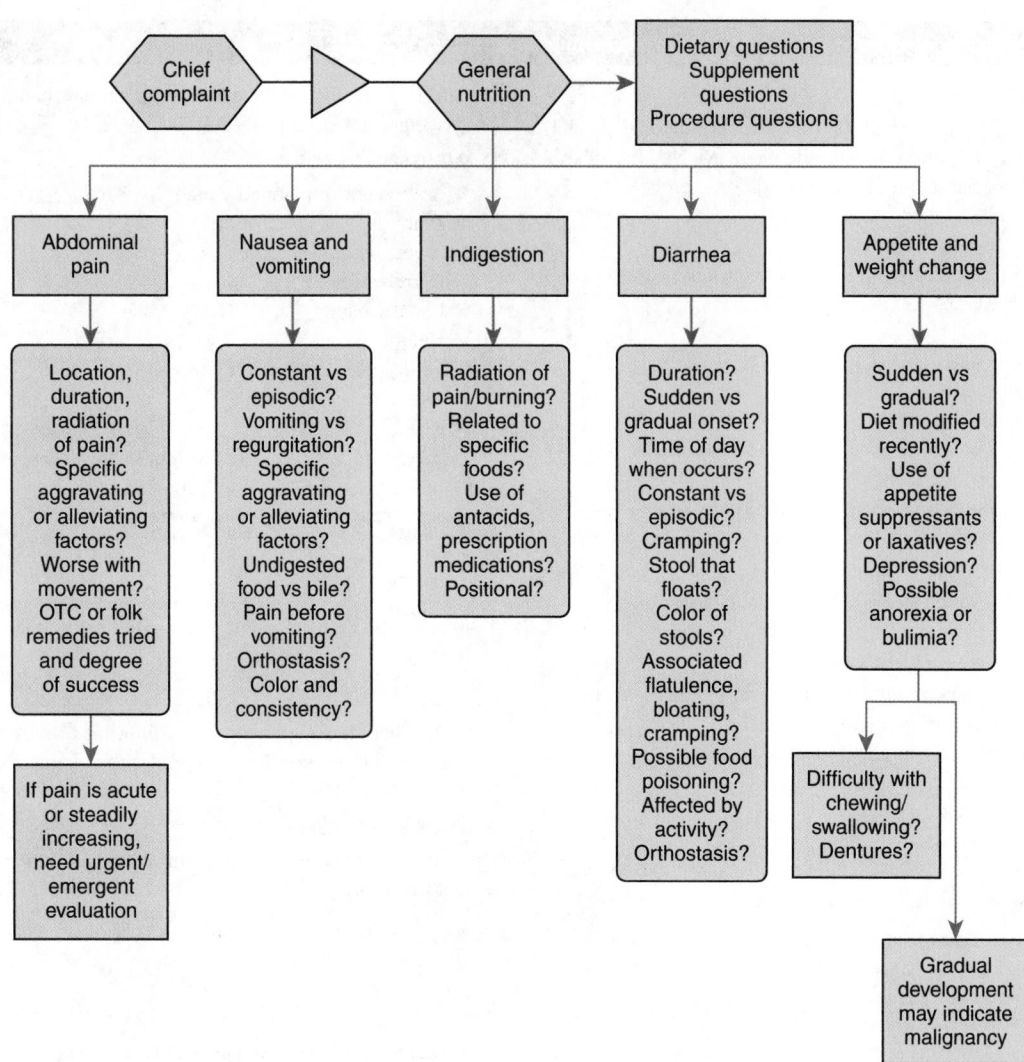

■ **FIGURE 28–1** Expanded nutrition assessment.

Abdominal Pain. Was the pain rapid or gradual in onset? What is the intensity of the pain? Has the pain increased in intensity over the past few hours, days, or weeks? Does the pain radiate? Does the pain worsen or improve with movement? Does food exacerbate or alleviate the pain? What specific foods alter the pain? Abdominal pain is a common presenting manifestation that may be associated with life-threatening conditions. It is important to identify abdominal pain caused by potentially life-threatening conditions. Chapter 32 contains information about differentiating characteristics of abdominal pain.

Nausea and Vomiting. When does nausea or vomiting occur? How long does it last? Is it related to food intake? Does food relieve or worsen the manifestations? Does the vomitus contain undigested food or bile? What does it look like? What is the quantity vomited? Is pain associated with the onset of nausea and vomiting?

Indigestion. Have the client describe the indigestion. Is it a "burping" or burning sensation? Are the manifestations

of indigestion related to food intake? Which foods worsen and which foods relieve the manifestations? Does the client take any medications or antacids for indigestion?

Diarrhea. How many and how much stool is expelled per day? Are stools liquid or solid? What color are the stools? Are the stools black or bloody? Do the stools sink or float? Is there pain with defecation? Does abdominal bloating or cramping accompany the diarrhea? Does diarrhea occur during the day, the night, or both day and night? Is fecal incontinence among the manifestations? How many days or weeks has the diarrhea persisted? Does diarrhea decrease at certain times during the month (indicating a hormonal influence)? Does physical activity change the diarrhea manifestations?

Ask specifically about the relationship of stool output and dietary intake. Bloating and diarrhea that occur after consuming dairy products may indicate lactose intolerance (see Allergies later in this chapter). High-fat diets that result in floating, greasy stools may indicate fat malabsorption. If vomiting or diarrhea persists, assess for fluid and electrolyte deficits (see Chapters 11 and 12).

Nonspecific GI problems, such as nausea, vomiting, and diarrhea, can result from food-borne poisoning. When clients present with these manifestations, ask about the type of food consumed over the past 2 or 3 days, how the food was prepared, and whether anyone else who ate the same food became ill. Chapter 33 contains additional information about food-borne poisoning; refer also to Food-Borne Poisoning: Sources and Manifestations on the website for details.

Appetite and Weight Change. Ask the client to describe his or her appetite. Is it poor, normal, or ravenous? Has there been any change in appetite? Has the usual diet been modified, and, if so, why? If the client has noticed a change in appetite, ask about associated factors such as changes in taste or smell, activity level, or mood states. Ask specific questions about the client's usual weight. Ask whether the client has lost or gained weight and, if so, ask over what period of time this occurred. Was the weight gain or loss intentional? If the weight loss was intentional, ask about the diet plan. Does a specific weight loss organization or health club sanction the client's diet? Does the client take diet pills, such as appetite stimulants or suppressants?

Unintentional changes in weight may stem from psychological or physiologic causes. Ask the following:

- Does the client feel sad or depressed?
- Has there been a change in activity level?
- Has the client experienced early satiety, anorexia, or any changes in the taste of food?
- Does the client have trouble chewing or swallowing or problems with teeth or gums? If the client wears dentures, ask about the fit of the dentures. Ill-fitting dentures can decrease appetite and lead to weight loss.

Review of Systems
Nutrition affects all body systems, and the consequences of malnutrition are not limited to the GI tract. Figure 28-2 provides a guide to the review of systems related to nutrition issues. Refer to Chapter 29 for further discussion of the consequences of malnutrition. Also see Chapters 46 and 47 for questions related to the hepatic and biliary systems. Inquire about the condition of the client's mouth, including the presence of dental caries, number and condition of teeth, condition of the gingivae, and use of dentures:

- Has the client noticed any oral lesions, halitosis, excessive salivation, or mouth dryness?
- How often does the client floss and brush?

- Is the client's water supply fluoridated?
- When was the last visit to the dentist for teeth cleaning?
- Has the client been treated for periodontal disease?
- Does the client have trouble tasting, chewing, or swallowing?
- If pain is reported with eating, is it related to specific foods or associated events?

Past Medical History
The client's history of illnesses or hospitalizations can provide important clues about nutritional status and gut function. For example, a client with a history of bleeding is at increased risk for iron deficiency anemia. A client with liver disease is at increased risk for protein malnutrition. Ask whether the client has been evaluated by a health care provider or if the client has ever been hospitalized for any of the following: peptic ulcer disease, vomiting blood (hematemesis), anemia, jaundice, gallbladder disease, pancreatitis, cancer, a change in bowel habits, tarry stools, or unexplained weight loss or gain. If so, ask if the client had diagnostic tests of the upper GI system, such as a barium swallow, upper GI studies, endoscopic examinations of the upper GI tract, or computed tomography (CT). If so, ask when and where the tests were performed and the results of each test.

Surgical History
Past surgical procedures also provide information about nutritional status and the structure and function of the upper GI tract. Ask specifically about previous surgeries of the mouth, throat, stomach, liver, pancreas, gallbladder, or abdomen (including bariatric procedures). Include dates and results of all tests, procedures, and surgeries performed.

Allergies
To help differentiate food allergies from food intolerances, ask the client about clinical manifestations experienced after eating specific foods. Food allergies typically result in systemic manifestations such as hives or dyspnea, whereas food intolerances are associated with GI manifestations such as abdominal cramping, flatulence, or diarrhea. Although less common than food intolerances, food allergies have been associated with foods such as nuts, shellfish, cow's milk, and food additives such as sulfites.[8]

Food intolerances are common, and lactose is one of the most common causes of food intolerance, especially in adults of Native Americans and non-European descent. When lactase (an enzyme necessary for the breakdown of lactose in the small bowel) is inadequate,

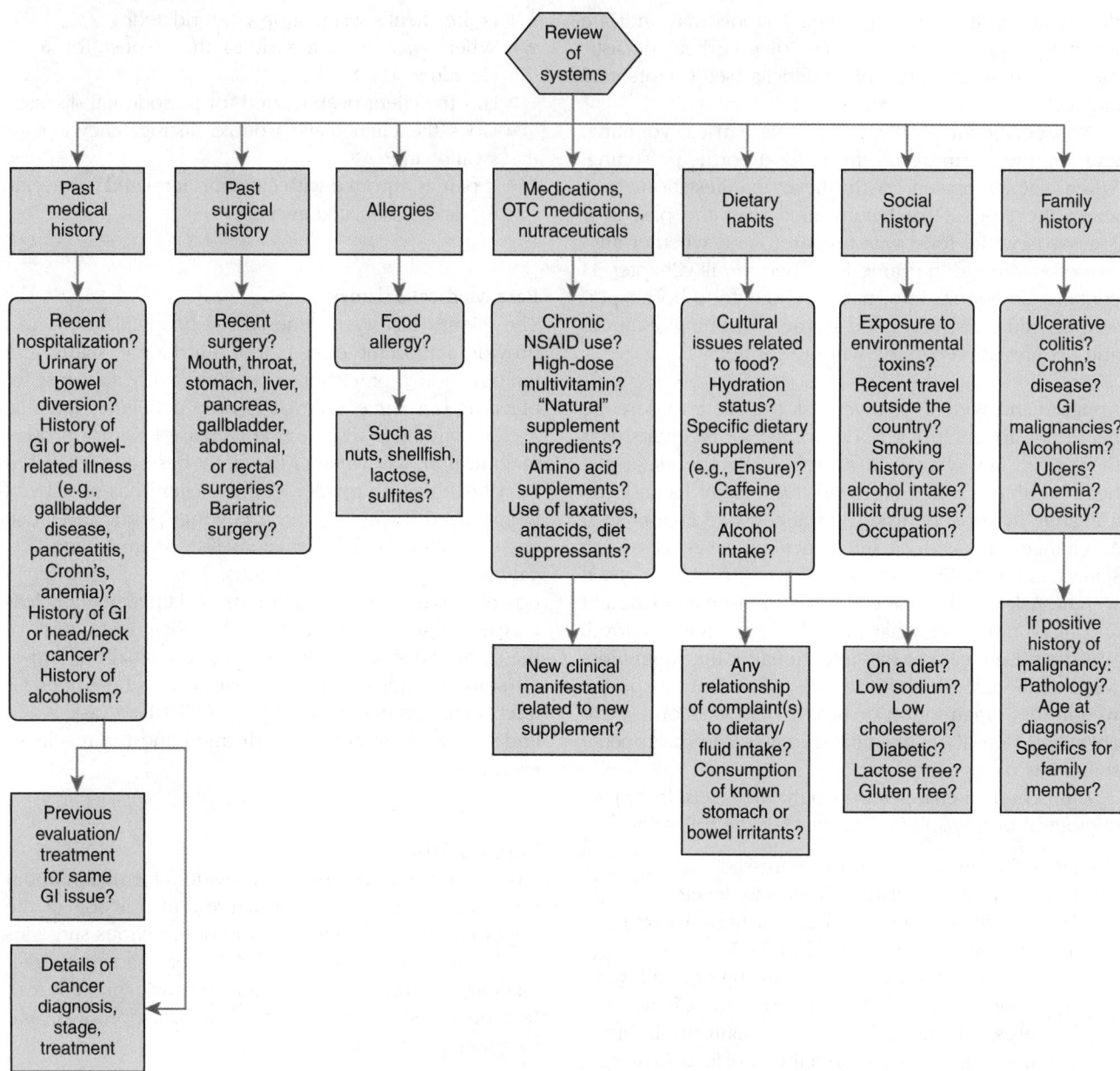

■ **FIGURE 28–2** Expanded nutrition history.

large lactose molecules draw fluid into the small bowel, resulting in abdominal cramping and diarrhea. Reducing or eliminating dairy products from the diet, taking a lactase replacement (Lactaid or SureLac) before eating dairy products, or eating lactase-supplemented products may ease or eliminate the manifestations of lactose intolerance. Because dairy products are high in calcium, it is important to ask the lactose-intolerant client about calcium intake. If the client's dietary intake contains insufficient amounts of calcium, a calcium supplement should be taken.

Medications and Dietary Supplements

Because there are many potential drug-nutrient interactions, it is important to obtain information about the client's drug use. Older clients, especially those who are taking many medications, are at increased risk for drug-nutrient interactions.[6] Obtain detailed information about current or previously prescribed and over-the-counter medications taken by the client. Table 28-2 contains a list of drug classes and potential drug-nutrient interactions.

Dietary supplements sold over the counter are often viewed as harmless. However, taken in excess or with

TABLE 28–2   Drug-Nutrient Interactions

Drug Class	Possible Nutrient Interactions
Antacids	Decreased absorption of calcium, iron, magnesium, zinc
Antibiotics	Cephalosporins: increased vitamin K depletion
Anticoagulants	Vitamin K antagonist
Anticonvulsants	Decreased folate and biotin
Antituberculosis drugs	Interfere with metabolism of vitamins B_6 and B_{12}
Cathartics	Nonrenal losses of calcium, potassium, water
Cholesterol-reducing drugs	Inhibition of fat digestion and absorption
	Simvastatin: grapefruit juice may increase drug level
Diuretics	Increased renal loss of potassium, calcium, magnesium, and zinc
H_2 blockers	Decreased vitamin B_{12} absorption
Monoamine oxidase inhibitors	Interact with tyramine-containing foods (cheese, smoked fish, wine, yeast)

From Skidmore-Roth, L. (2007). *Mosby's nursing drug reference.* St. Louis: Mosby.

other drugs or supplements, dietary supplements can be harmful. Therefore it is important to determine the brand, amount, and frequency of use for all dietary supplements consumed by the client. Dietary supplements include vitamins, minerals, herbs used for medicinal purposes, amino acids, and meal supplements or replacements.

Over half the adult population in the United States consumes some form of vitamin or herbal supplement. Furthermore, evidence supports that most clients have not discussed supplement usage with their health care provider because the provider did not ask.[4] Ask whether the client takes a vitamin supplement and, if so, determine the amount of specific vitamins, minerals, or trace elements contained in each dose. Because vitamin supplements differ in content and dose, it is important to compare the client's dietary requirements with the amount of each micronutrient (vitamins, minerals, trace elements) contained in the supplement. Taken in excess, some vitamins have toxic side effects. For example, beta carotene taken in excess by smokers has been associated with an increased risk of developing lung cancer.[12]

Clients who consume prescribed medications may also take herbal supplements, creating a growing concern about the interaction between prescription drugs and herbal supplements. Ask whether the client consumes any herbs or special products for his or her health. The herbs may be consumed as a tea or in pill, capsule, liquid, or powder form. It is important to note the brand and amount of herbal preparation consumed. Refer to Common Herbal Supplements on the website (also see Chapter 4).

Various forms of amino acids, hormones, and meal supplements are sold as over-the-counter health aids.

Ask clients whether they consume preparations such as glucosamine, melatonin, or dehydroepiandrosterone (DHEA) and, if so, determine the amount consumed. Meal supplements or replacements are usually purchased in a liquid or wafer form and provide a convenient method of increasing nutritional intake. Because of the wide variation in nutritional content and the potential for consuming inadequate or excessive amounts of specific micronutrients, it is important to ask questions about the brand and amount of meal supplement the client consumes each day. See Chapter 29 for additional information about meal supplements.

Dietary Habits

The type, amount, method, and timing of food intake are heavily influenced by psychosocial factors, such as ethnic origin, religion, and family structure. When assessing the client's nutritional status, be sure to ask questions about the relationship of their culture and diet. The Diversity in Health Care feature Cultural Influences on Nutrition on the website contains more information *evolve* about the effect of culture on nutrition.

Psychosocial History

Exposure to environmental toxins and pathogens while at work or traveling increases the client's risk for developing diseases of the GI tract. Ask about the client's occupation and whether toxic substances such as arsenic, lead, mercury, or carbon tetrachloride are present in the workplace. Ask whether the client has recently traveled outside the country. Traveling abroad may increase the client's risk of contracting GI conditions such as nausea, vomiting, or diarrhea caused by pathogenic bacteria, protozoa, helminths, or other parasites.

Family Health History

Genetics and family environment may increase the client's risk of developing certain GI problems. Many diseases, such as ulcerative colitis and Crohn's disease, have a familial component. Similarly, alcoholism and the associated liver disease also have a strong familial link. Inquire about the health status of family members. Is there a family history of cancer, GI ulcers, or colitis? Is there a family history of diabetes, anemia, jaundice, alcoholism, hepatitis, pancreatitis, obesity, peptic ulcers, or irritable bowel syndrome?

PHYSICAL EXAMINATION

Anthropometric Measures

Anthropometric measures provide an assessment of body mass or body compartments. Height, weight, body mass index, frame size, and circumferential measurements are examples of anthropometric measures.

Height and Weight

Use a telescoping ruler and balance scale to measure height and weight. If the client cannot bear weight, consider using a calibrated sling or wheelchair scale. Clothing and shoes affect the obtained height and weight; describe any clothing and accessories (light clothing, shoes with or without heels, orthopedic casts, braces) worn by the client while obtaining the height and weight.

If the client cannot stand, use an arm span measurement to approximate height. To do so, extend the client's arms laterally and measure from the tip of the middle finger on one hand to the tip of the middle finger on the other hand.

Compare the client's current weight to the reported usual weight. A 10% change in weight that is unintentional is significant and the cause of the change in weight should be determined. To calculate the difference as a percentage of usual weight, divide the client's current weight by the usual weight and multiply by 100:

$$\% \text{ of usual weight} = \left(\frac{\text{Current weight}}{\text{Usual weight}}\right) \times 100$$

Body Mass Index

Past methods of determining ideal body weights for individuals have included mathematical formulas or comparison of heights and weights to life insurance tables. Based on numerous independent studies, body mass index (BMI) is gaining favor as the accepted standard for determining desirable body weight. A Body Mass Index table is located on the website for reference. To use the table, find the client's height in the left-hand column, follow the row over to the client's weight, and then up to determine the BMI. The client's BMI can also be calculated by dividing the client's weight in pounds by the height in inches, then dividing by the height in inches again and multiplying by 703.

For example, a 64-inch tall-woman weighing 140 pounds has a BMI of 25.

$$\text{BMI} = ([140 \div 64] \div 64) \times 703 = 24.95$$

The BMI standardizes weight for height. A desirable BMI range associated with good health is between 19 and 24.9. A BMI of less than 18.5 is categorized as underweight or as less than desirable weight for height. A BMI between 25 and less than 30 is considered overweight, and a BMI of 30 or greater is considered obese.

Calculations for BMI are the same for males and females. Muscle mass and bone weigh more than fat and, for a few clients, the BMI may indicate they are overweight or obese when they are not. Therefore clients suspected of having a large frame size or muscle mass (weight lifters, football players) should be assessed for frame size and muscle mass.[10]

Frame Size

Frame size can be estimated by measuring the client's wrist circumference (Box 28-2). Clients who have very small or very large frames may have a BMI at the low or high end of the desirable BMI range, respectively.

Circumference Measurements

Circumference measurements are used to assess the proportion and distribution of muscle mass and body fat. Waist-to-hip ratio and midarm muscle circumference (MAMC) are examples of circumference measurements. Waist-to-hip ratio is determined by dividing the waist measurement at its smallest circumference by the hip measurement at its largest circumference. Waist-to-hip proportions greater than 0.8 for women and 0.9 for men indicate fat distributions associated with negative health outcomes such as cardiovascular disease and diabetes. MAMC measurements require special equipment and standards for comparison. Consult an advanced practice nurse or dietitian for assistance with MAMC assessments.

Mouth

Assessment of the oral cavity includes inspection and palpation. Good illumination is essential. A headlamp provides direct illumination, and a head mirror provides indirect lighting; both items keep your hands free for the physical examination. A penlight and tongue blade may also be used. Always remember to wear gloves and use a gauze pad when palpating the oral cavity and handling the tongue. Although discussed separately, inspection and palpation of the oral cavity usually proceed simultaneously. See Figure 28-3 for the Oral Assessment Guide.

BOX 28-2 Wrist Circumference as a Measure of Body Frame Size

WRIST CIRCUMFERENCE METHOD

1. Measure the client's right wrist (in centimeters) at the point of the smallest circumference, just distal to the styloid process of the radius and ulna.
2. Obtain the client's height (in centimeters) without shoes.
3. Divide the client's wrist circumference into the client's height to obtain the *r* value:

    $$r = \text{Height (in cm)} \div \text{Wrist circumference (in cm)}$$

4. Use the chart below to determine the client's body frame size based on the calculated *r* value and sex:

	Men	Women
Small frame	$r > 10.4$	$r > 10.9$
Medium frame	$r > 9.6\text{-}10.4$	$r > 9.9\text{-}10.9$
Large frame	$r < 9.6$	$r < 9.9$

Category	Scoring		
	1	**2**	**3**
Voice	Normal	Deep or raspy	Difficulty talking or painful
Swallow	Normal swallow	Some pain on swallowing	Unable to swallow
Lips	Smooth, pink, and moist	Dry or cracked	Ulcerated or bleeding
Tongue	Pink, moist, papillae present	Coated or loss of papillae with shiny appearance (with or without redness)	Blistered or cracked
Saliva	Watery	Thick or ropy	Absent
Mucous membranes	Pink and moist	Reddened or coated (increased whiteness) without ulcerations	Ulcerations with or without bleeding
Gingiva	Pink, stippled, and firm	Edematous with or without redness	Spontaneous bleeding or bleeding with pressure
Teeth or dentures or denture-bearing areas	Clean and no debris	Spontaneous bleeding or bleeding with pressure	Plaque or debris generalized along gum line or denture-bearing area

Oral Assessment Guide Total Score: _____ (More than 8 points indicates risk)

■ **FIGURE 28–3** Oral Assessment Guide. *(Copyright © June Eilers 1983/1985. Reprinted with permission of June Eilers, The Nebraska Medical Center, Omaha, Nebraska.)*

Inspection

Begin assessment of the client's mouth by inspecting the lips for symmetry, color, hydration, lesions, or nodules. Put on clean gloves, and instruct the client to open the lips while clenching the teeth. Inspect the position of the upper and lower teeth for malocclusion or missing teeth. If dentures are worn, ask the client to remove them. Note the symmetry of facial movements and the fit of the dentures as the appliance is removed.

Next, ask the client to open and close the mouth and note the symmetry and strength of movement. Ask the client to open the mouth wide, and inspect the structures inside (see Figure A&P7-2 on p. 547). Start at the left side of the mouth and continue in a clockwise fashion. Note any evidence of dental caries, missing or broken teeth, and receding gums. Note the color of the mucosa and gums. Inspect for red lesions (erythroplakia), white lesions (leukoplakia), swelling, bleeding, or ulcers. Survey the pharynx for abnormalities of the tonsils, such as redness, swelling, lesions, ulcers, uvular deviations, drainage, or unusual mouth odor.

Inspect the tongue for symmetry, color, and moisture. Note any areas of atrophy, abnormal coatings, swelling, or lesions. Next, ask the client to stick out the tongue and move it from side to side, upward, and downward. Observe for symmetry of movement and voluntary or involuntary movement. Abnormal tongue movement may result from infiltration of the muscle by tumor or nerve entrapment.[3]

Palpation

Palpate the client's lips, gingivae, and buccal mucosa. Check for loose teeth, masses, swellings, or areas of tenderness. Note the location, size, color, consistency, and presence of tenderness in any lesions.

Gently grasp, extend, and lift the tongue with a gauze pad while inspecting and palpating the underside and the floor of the mouth. Palpate all areas of the tongue and floor of the mouth for masses, swellings, or areas of tenderness. Note any lesions or areas of color change. Scrape all areas of leukoplakia with a tongue blade; if the white patches do not scrape off, refer the client for further work-up, because these areas may be cancerous lesions. Many precancerous oral lesions are pain free and asymptomatic, and all clients with suspicious oral lesions that do not clear within 2 to 3 weeks should be referred for further evaluation.[3]

Release the tongue, and depress it with a tongue blade. Ask the client to say "Aah." Note the symmetry and movement of the uvula and soft palate. If there are no contraindications, give the client a sip of water. As the client swallows, observe for difficulty swallowing (dysphagia) or asymmetrical movement of the oral cavity structures. Oral-pharyngeal dysphagia typically presents as difficulty moving solid foods to the back of the mouth and indicates further assessment and evaluation to rule out cranial nerve involvement (see Chapter 67). Esophageal dysphagia presents as difficulty swallowing solids or liquids and indicates motor disease or obstruction of the esophagus. Both oral-pharyngeal and esophageal dysphagia should be referred for further evaluation.

Abdomen

Because a full bladder can interfere with abdominal assessment, ask the client to void before examining the abdomen. Place the client in a supine position with arms at sides. Place a small pillow under the client's knees to relax the abdominal muscles. Because percussion and palpation can alter intestinal activity, assess the abdomen in the following sequence: inspection, auscultation, percussion, and palpation. Visualize the underlying organs as you assess, and describe the abdomen by anatomic regions or quadrants (Figure 28-4).

Inspection

Stand at the client's right side and begin inspecting the abdomen by noting the condition of the skin and the abdominal contour. The skin should be smooth and intact, with varying amounts of hair. The contour should be flat, concave, or rounded, depending on the client's body type. Note any areas of distention or irregular contour, which may suggest obstruction, hernia, tumor, or previous surgery. Bulging flanks and glistening, taut skin are abnormal findings and suggest ascites (see Chapters 32 and 42).

Inspect the abdomen for rashes, discoloration, scars, petechiae, striae (stretch marks), and dilated veins. Scars on the abdomen should correlate with the client's history of past surgical procedures, and striae, an indication of changes in weight, should correlate with reported changes in weight. Note the shape, position, color, and presence of any discharge at the umbilicus. The umbilicus should be concave, located at the midline, with no evidence of drainage, and the same color as the abdominal skin. Cullen's sign or a bluish periumbilical color suggests intra-abdominal bleeding and may be seen in clients with pancreatitis.[7]

Next, sit at eye level to the client's abdomen and observe for peristaltic movement or abdominal pulsation. Normally, peristaltic movements are not visible but abdominal pulsations may be observed in a very thin client.

Ask the client to raise head and shoulders off the table and observe for a raised ridge or bulge between the rectus abdominal muscles. This raised ridge, known as diastasis recti, is a separation of the rectus muscle caused by conditions of sustained intra-abdominal pressure such as obesity or pregnancy. Diastasis recti is not a true hernia and, for most clients, of no clinical significance.[13]

Inspection and examination of the rectal area occurs after the abdominal examination (see Chapter 32).

Auscultation

Using the diaphragm of your stethoscope, begin auscultating the client's abdomen. Press the diaphragm lightly to the abdominal wall, beginning in the right lower quadrant at the area of the ileocecal valve. Continue in a clockwise fashion, auscultating each quadrant or region. As air and fluid move through the GI tract, soft clicks and gurgles can be heard every 5 to 15 seconds. Note the frequency and character of bowel sounds. Normal bowel sounds occur irregularly at a rate of 5 to 35 per minute.[1] Loud, high-pitched bowel sounds (borborygmi) represent hyperactivity of the GI tract. Borborygmi may be present in clients who are hungry or who have gastroenteritis, or they may be present in early intestinal obstruction.

Hypoactive bowel sounds occur at a rate of one or fewer every minute. To determine the absence of bowel sounds, listen for a total of 5 minutes or at least 1 minute per quadrant. If one does not hear bowel sounds, note the time allotted for auscultation of bowel sounds in the assessment record. Absence of bowel sounds does not mean absence of bowel peristalsis. Hypoactive or absent bowel sounds indicate the need for further assessment of bowel function. Hospitalized clients with nondistended abdomens and no complaints of nausea or vomiting may eat even though bowel sounds are not auscultated. Conversely, clients who have bowel sounds and nausea, vomiting, or abdominal distention should not be fed enterally.

Next, use the bell of your stethoscope to auscultate the abdomen for vascular sounds. A bruit, a venous hum, and a friction rub are examples of abnormal sounds that may be auscultated during the abdominal examination. Bruits auscultated over major blood vessels indicate turbulent blood flow, such as an aneurysm or partial obstruction of a vessel. A continuous venous hum heard in the periumbilical area indicates engorged liver circulation. Friction rubs sound like two pieces of leather rubbing together and suggest a hepatic tumor when heard loudest over the lower right rib cage or splenic inflammation when heard loudest over the lower ribcage in the anterior axillary line.[1]

Percussion

Percuss the abdomen to determine the size and location of abdominal organs and to detect fluid, air, or masses. Percuss all quadrants or regions, and compare the sounds to expected findings. Normally when percussing over the abdomen, high-pitched, loud, or "musical" (tympanic) sounds are heard over gaseous areas and dull (thud-like) sounds are heard over fluid or solid organs. Percussion can be used to determine the size and position of the liver and spleen (see Chapter 42) and to assess the level of a distended bladder (see Chapter 32). Do not percuss the abdomen if you suspect an abdominal aneurysm or if the client has undergone abdominal organ transplantation.

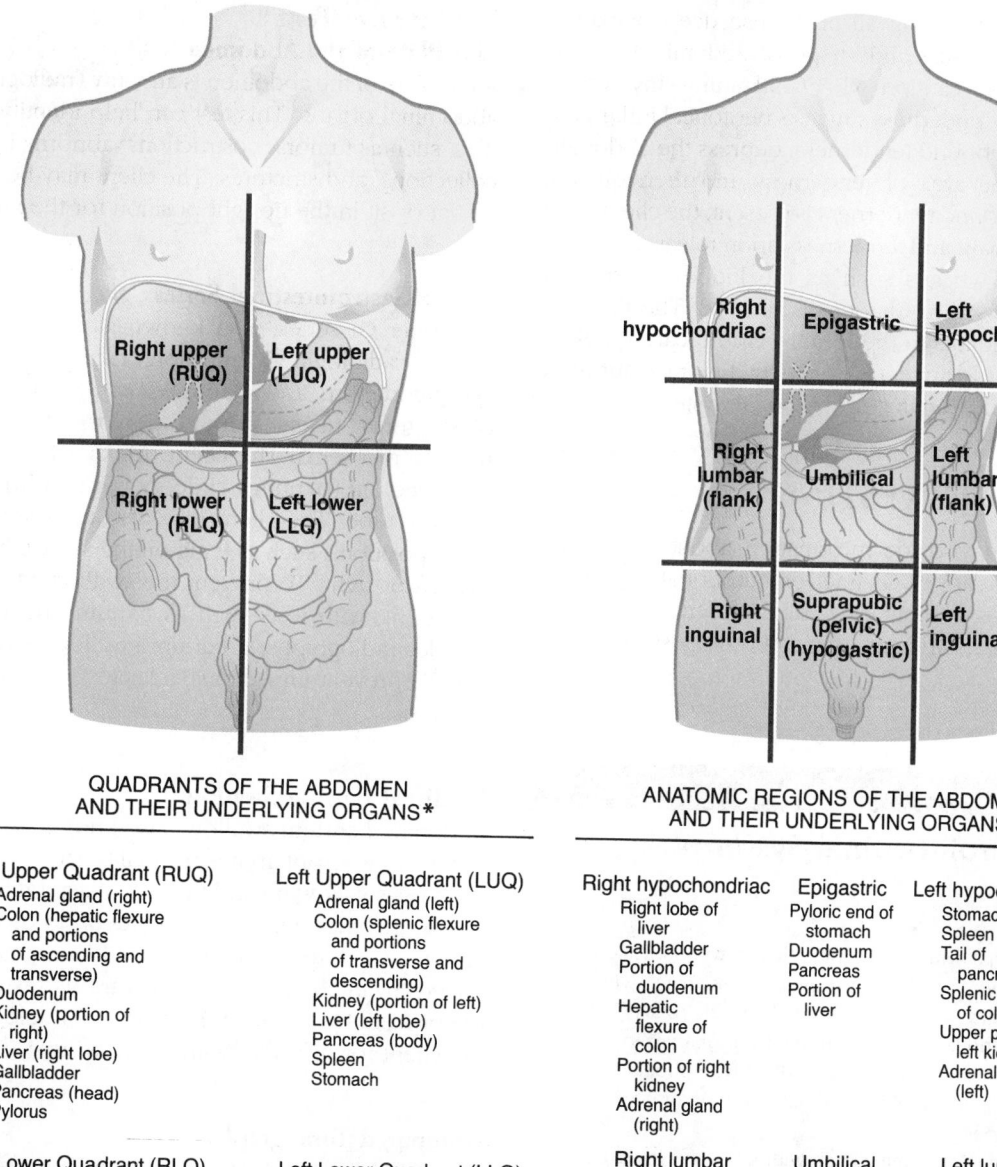

QUADRANTS OF THE ABDOMEN
AND THEIR UNDERLYING ORGANS*

Right Upper Quadrant (RUQ)
Adrenal gland (right)
Colon (hepatic flexure
  and portions
  of ascending and
  transverse)
Duodenum
Kidney (portion of
  right)
Liver (right lobe)
Gallbladder
Pancreas (head)
Pylorus

Left Upper Quadrant (LUQ)
Adrenal gland (left)
Colon (splenic flexure
  and portions
  of transverse and
  descending)
Kidney (portion of left)
Liver (left lobe)
Pancreas (body)
Spleen
Stomach

Right Lower Quadrant (RLQ)
Appendix
Bladder (if distended)
Cecum
Colon (portion of
  ascending)
Kidney (lower pole of
  right)
Ovary (right)
Salpinx (uterine tube;
  right)
Spermatic cord (right)
Ureter (right)
Uterus (if enlarged)

Left Lower Quadrant (LLQ)
Bladder (if distended)
Colon (sigmoid and
  portion of
  descending)
Kidney (lower pole of
  left)
Ovary (left)
Salpinx (uterine tube;
  left)
Spermatic cord (left)
Ureter (left)
Uterus (if enlarged)

*Small intestine loops in all quadrants.

ANATOMIC REGIONS OF THE ABDOMEN
AND THEIR UNDERLYING ORGANS

Right hypochondriac
Right lobe of
  liver
Gallbladder
Portion of
  duodenum
Hepatic
  flexure of
  colon
Portion of right
  kidney
Adrenal gland
  (right)

Epigastric
Pyloric end of
  stomach
Duodenum
Pancreas
Portion of
  liver

Left hypochondriac
Stomach
Spleen
Tail of
  pancreas
Splenic flexure
  of colon
Upper pole of
  left kidney
Adrenal gland
  (left)

Right lumbar
Ascending
  colon
Lower half of
  right kidney
Portion of
  duodenum
  and jejunum

Umbilical
Omentum
Mesentery
Lower
  duodenum
Jejunum and
  ileum

Left lumbar
Descending
  colon
Lower half of
  left kidney
Portions of
  jejunum and
  ileum

Right inguinal
Cecum
Appendix
Ileum (lower
  end)
Right ureter
Right
  spermatic
  cord
Right ovary

Suprapubic
Ileum
Bladder
Uterus (in
  pregnancy)

Left inguinal
Sigmoid colon
Left ureter
Left spermatic
  cord
Left ovary

■ **FIGURE 28–4**   Quadrants and anatomic regions of the abdomen and their underlying organs.

Palpation

Palpate the abdomen in a systematic, quadrant-to-quadrant or region-to-region manner, beginning with nontender areas and progressing to painful ones. Start with light palpation, depressing the abdomen 1 to 2 cm.

Palpate for masses or areas of tenderness. Note any areas of involuntary abdominal rigidity or guarding. McBurney's point is located in the right lower quadrant midway between the umbilicus and the anterior iliac crest. Localization of pain in this area suggests appendicitis.

After lightly palpating all areas, use deep palpation to determine the size and shape of abdominal organs and masses. Use caution when examining any tender areas. Rebound tenderness suggests peritoneal inflammation. To elicit rebound tenderness, depress the abdomen deeply over the area of tenderness and then quickly release it. If rebound tenderness is present, the client feels an increase in pain and tenderness upon release.

Palpation of organs such as the kidney, liver, and spleen is discussed in Chapters 32 and 42. The Physical Assessment Findings in the Healthy Adult feature below shows how to document assessment findings during a normal physical examination of the GI system.

DIAGNOSTIC TESTING

Diagnostic tests provide information about the nature and severity of upper GI tract or nutritional problems. Laboratory tests, radiography, ultrasonography, endoscopy, cytology, gastric analysis, and other tests are commonly used.

Physical Assessment Findings in the Healthy Adult

The Gastrointestinal System

INSPECTION
- **Mouth.** Lips symmetrical, pink, moist, without lesions. Buccal mucosa and gingivae pink, moist, intact, without lesions. Hard and soft palates pink, intact. Tonsils behind pillars, without inflammation. Posterior pharynx pink, without exudate. Uvula rises midline with phonation. Tongue midline, mobile, without deviation or fasciculations.
- **Abdomen.** Flat, symmetrical, with umbilicus inverted, centered, and midline. No scars, lesions, dilated veins, visible peristalsis or pulsations, or separation of rectus muscles at rest or with straining.
- **Anus and rectum.** Perianal area free of lesions, inflammation, fissures, bulges, or external hemorrhoids.

AUSCULTATION
- **Abdomen.** Bowel sounds present in all four quadrants.

PERCUSSION*
- **Abdomen.** General tympany throughout, with liver and splenic dullness. Liver span 10 cm at right midclavicular line.

PALPATION*
- **Abdomen.** Liver and spleen nonpalpable. Abdomen soft, nontender, no masses or rebound tenderness; muscle tone firm, relaxed.
- **Anus and rectum.** Anus and rectum without tenderness, masses, hemorrhoids, or prolapse. Rectal mucosa smooth. Stool negative for blood.

*In assessment of the abdomen, palpation and percussion are performed after auscultation so that the bowel is not stimulated.

Noninvasive Tests
Flat Plate of the Abdomen
A flat plate of the abdomen is an x-ray (radiograph) of the abdominal organs. This test can help identify abnormalities, such as tumors, obstructions, abnormal gas or fluid collections, and strictures. The client may be required to lie flat or sit in the upright position for the x-ray.

Upper Gastrointestinal Series
An upper GI series, also known as a barium swallow, permits radiologic visualization of the esophagus, stomach, duodenum, and jejunum. It can aid in the detection of strictures, ulcers, tumors, polyps, hiatal hernias, or motility problems. The client drinks a radiopaque contrast medium (barium) while standing in front of a fluoroscopy tube. The client may also be asked to assume other positions, such as lying on the x-ray table and turning left or right. To prevent the swallowed barium from interfering with tests such as barium enemas and gallbladder radiographs, a barium swallow is usually done last. To prevent impactions, a laxative is given after barium tests.

Modified Barium Swallow
A modified barium swallow, also known as videofluoroscopy or an oropharyngeal motility study, is performed to assess swallowing and the risk of aspiration. While sitting in a chair equipped with videofluoroscopy, the client is asked to swallow a small amount of barium mixed in liquids and foods of various textures. During the procedure, a speech therapist or radiologist observes the client for difficulty with swallowing.

Computed Tomography
CT scanning is used to identify masses, such as neoplasms, cysts, focal inflammatory lesions, and abscesses of the liver, pancreas, and pelvic areas (Figure 28-5). CT also aids in evaluating local tumor spread, especially if barium studies suggest tumor growth beyond the bowel wall.[14] To distinguish normal bowel from abnormal intraperitoneal masses, contrast media may be administered.

Ultrasonography
Ultrasonography of the GI system helps to identify pathophysiologic processes in the pancreas, liver, gallbladder, spleen, and retroperitoneal tissues. Ultrasound studies can be used to identify fluid, masses (such as tumors), adipose tissue, abscesses, and hematomas. Physical examination is enhanced by ultrasound techniques because palpable masses and areas of tenderness can be correlated with anatomic structures while the client is on the examining table.

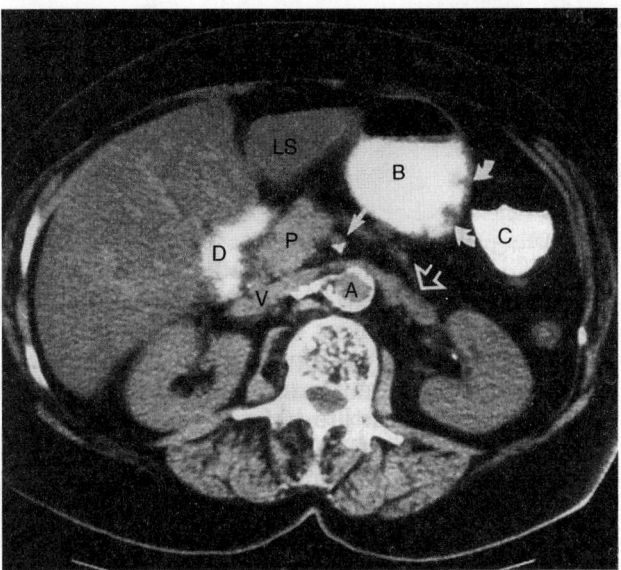

■ **FIGURE 28–5** Normal computed tomography (CT) scan of the stomach. The CT scan is through the body of the stomach (B) at a level just below the spleen. The lateral segment of the left lobe of the liver (LS), head of the pancreas (P), and splenic flexure of the colon (C) are adjacent structures. A, Aorta; D, duodenum; V, inferior vena cava. Solid arrow represents the superior mesenteric artery, and open arrow represents the vein. The rugae (curved arrows) are well visualized. (From Moss, A., Gamsu, G., & Genant, H.K. [1992]. Computed tomography of the body: With magnetic resonance imaging [Vol. 3, 2nd ed.]. Philadelphia: Saunders.)

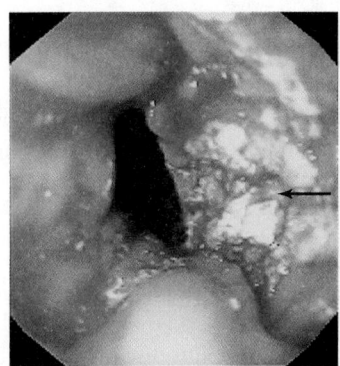

■ **FIGURE 28–6** An endoscopic view of the esophagus showing an esophageal ulcer (arrow).

Invasive Tests

Endoscopy

Endoscopy is the direct visualization of the GI system by means of a lighted, flexible tube. Upper GI tract endoscopy includes esophagoscopy, gastroscopy, and esophagogastroduodenoscopy (Figure 28-6). These procedures are useful for examining clients who have acute or chronic GI bleeding, pernicious anemia, esophageal injury, masses, strictures, dysphagia, substernal pain, epigastric discomfort, or inflammatory bowel disease. Some endoscopes are equipped with a camera that allows the physician to obtain color photographs. If cancer is suspected, cells or tissue can be collected for cytologic examination. Small, single polyps may be removed. Conscious sedation with a sedative, opioid, or tranquilizer may be given before or during the procedure. Anticholinergic medications may be given to decrease oropharyngeal secretions and to prevent reflex bradycardia.

Other Gastrointestinal Tests

Tests of the upper gastrointestinal tract may be conducted to determine the presence of malignant cells, amounts of hydrochloric acid (HCl) or hormones, abnormalities in motor function, or etiology of chest pain. Those tests include exfoliative cytologic analysis, gastric analysis, acid perfusion tests, esophageal manometry, and the Bernstein test.

Exfoliative Cytologic Analysis

Malignant cells exfoliate more readily than normal cells. Exfoliative cytologic analysis is performed to distinguish benign from malignant tissue cells. Areas of the GI tract of interest are lavaged and cells are collected and sent to the laboratory for analysis. Stomach contents may also be examined for the presence of *Helicobacter pylori*, a bacterium that can cause gastritis and peptic ulcer disease.

Gastric Analysis

Gastric analysis is performed to measure secretions of hydrochloric acid (HCl) and pepsin in the stomach. Analysis of gastric contents can aid in the diagnosis of duodenal ulcer, Zollinger-Ellison syndrome, gastric carcinoma, and pernicious anemia. Gastric analysis consists of (1) the basal cell secretion test and (2) the gastric acid stimulation test.

For the basal cell secretion test, a nasogastric tube is inserted and attached to suction. Stomach contents are collected every 15 minutes for 1 hour and then analyzed. If gastric secretion is abnormal, a gastric acid stimulation test is performed. The gastric acid stimulation test measures the amount of gastric acid produced after receiving drugs that stimulate secretion (pentagastrin and betazole). If results are abnormal, radiographic studies or endoscopy may be done to determine the cause. A markedly increased level of gastric acid secretion may indicate Zollinger-Ellison syndrome, whereas a moderately increased level suggests a duodenal ulcer. Decreased levels of gastric acid secretion may indicate gastric ulcer or carcinoma.

Acid Perfusion Test

The acid perfusion test, also known as the Bernstein test, determines whether a client's chest pain is related to acid perfusion across the esophageal mucosa. A nasogastric tube is inserted, and gastric contents are aspirated. Normal saline solution (0.9%) and 0.1% HCl are alternately instilled into the lower esophagus. If the client does not experience pain, the test is considered normal. If pain occurs, normal saline is administered until pain ceases. To ensure that the pain is caused by acid perfusion, 0.1% HCl is readministered. After the test, the nasogastric tube is withdrawn.

Esophageal Manometry

Manometry is used to assess esophageal motor function and can be used to assess and diagnose dysphagia, esophageal reflux, spasm, motility disorders, and hiatal hernia. A special enteric tube with fused small-caliber catheters is inserted into the esophagus. The tube is designed to measure simultaneous pressures of the esophagus and lower esophageal sphincter by infusion of water into the catheters. The client is asked to swallow small amounts of water, and esophageal pressures are recorded during muscular relaxation and contraction.

Ambulatory Esophageal pH Monitoring

Ambulatory esophageal pH monitoring is used to distinguish chest pain caused by gastric acid reflux from chest pain caused by angina or myocardial infarction. Location of the lower esophageal sphincter (LES) is determined by esophageal manometry, and a nasoenteric tube with a pH sensor is inserted 5 cm above the LES. The enteric tube is secured to the client's face and attached to a battery-operated recorder. The client is then instructed to push a button on the recorder at the start and end of specific activities, such as eating, sleeping, and smoking. Tell the client to note when chest pain or indigestion starts and ends.

Because the location of the LES must be determined, inform the client that esophageal manometry may be performed first after which a second enteric tube may be placed for the pH monitoring. You may need to stop giving the client drugs that affect the GI tract (H_2 histamine blockers and motility drugs) before the procedure. Instruct the client about the importance of recording activities and manifestations. The tube must remain securely taped. Tell the client to avoid bumping or pulling the tube when dressing or during face washing.

Laboratory Tests
Nutritional Anemias

Iron deficiency is the most common cause of anemia in world. In addition to iron, normal hematologic func requires adequate intake, absorption, use, and storag nutrients, such as protein, vitamin B_{12}, and cop Assessment of red blood cell function and iron store crucial to nutritional assessment. Chapter 74 descri assessment for hematologic disorders and anemias.

Serum Proteins

Serum proteins are carrier molecules and are also imp tant for maintaining intravascular oncotic pressure. T for serum proteins include albumin, prealbumin, reti binding protein, and transferrin. Table 28-3 lists comn serum proteins, normal values, half-lives, and conditi associated with abnormal values. In general, serum p teins with long half-lives (albumin) tend to be glo indicators of nutritional status, and serum proteins v shorter half-lives (prealbumin and transferrin) sugg acute changes in nutritional status.

Total Lymphocyte Count

Immune function and nutritional status are clo related. Consequently, total lymphocyte count (T an indicator of immune function, provides a gross m sure of nutritional status. To determine TLC, obtai white blood cell (WBC) count with differential f the client's venous blood sample. Next, multiply the centage of lymphocytes by the total WBC count. example, a client with a WBC count of $7000/mm^3$ 30% lymphocytes has a TLC of $2100/mm^3$.

TLCs less than $1800/mm^3$ suggest malnutrition. Beca the TLC is a gross indicator of immune function and n tional status, normally nourished clients may have a TLC after chemotherapy. Alternatively, an elevated may be found in malnourished clients with sepsis.

D-Xylose Absorption Test

D-Xylose, a monosaccharide, is absorbed in the sr intestine and is used to assess malabsorption. After administration of a known quantity of D-xylose, bl

---

TABLE 28–3 Serum Proteins

Protein	Normal Range	Half-Life	Effect of Associated Conditions
Albumin	3.5-5 g/dl	14-20 days	Increased with dehydration
			Decreased with malnutrition, overhydration, trauma, protein loss, liver disea
Prealbumin	20-40 mg/dl	3-5 days	Increased with nutrition intake and renal failure
			Decreased with poor dietary intake
Retinol-binding protein	3-6 mg/L	8-12 hr	Decreased with overhydration, liver disease, zinc and vitamin A deficit
Transferrin	200-400 mg/dl	8-10 hr	Increased with pregnancy, iron deficiency
			Decreased with chronic infection, cirrhosis

and urine levels of D-xylose are measured. Low D-xylose levels in the blood and urine are indicative of malabsorption in the small bowel.

Nitrogen Balance

Nitrogen balance is a measure of the client's anabolic or catabolic state. To determine nitrogen balance, simultaneously record the amount and type of food consumed in a 24-hour period and obtain a 24-hour urine collection for measurement of urine urea nitrogen (UUN). The start and stop times for the food intake record and the 24-hour urine collection must be the same. Consult a registered dietitian to calculate the client's 24-hour protein intake from all sources (oral, tube feeding, parenteral). Protein is approximately 16% nitrogen. To determine the amount of nitrogen consumed over the 24 hours, multiply the amount of protein consumed (in grams) by 0.16. UUN is the major source of nitrogen excretion. Subtract the UUN (in grams) from the amount of nitrogen consumed. Because nitrogen is also lost through the skin, stool, and the GI tract, subtract a correction factor of 3 from the nitrogen consumed, as follows:

$$\text{Nitrogen balance} = (\text{Nitrogen consumed [in grams]} - \text{UUN [in grams]}) - 3$$

A positive nitrogen balance of 4 to 6 g is desirable and an indication of an anabolic state. A negative nitrogen balance suggests a catabolic state.

Fecal Analysis

Fecal lipids are an indication of gut absorption and are discussed in more detail in Chapter 32.

CONCLUSIONS

Nutritional health and a functional upper GI tract are basic to good health. Systematic assessment of the client's nutritional status and upper GI tract can lead to early detection, diagnosis, and treatment of nutrition-related problems and optimal nutrition outcomes.

BIBLIOGRAPHY

Citations appearing in red refer to primary research.

Citations appearing in blue refer to evidence-based practice guidelines and protocols.

1. Barkauskas, V.H., Baumann, L.C., & Darling-Fisher, C.S. (Eds.) (2002). *Health and physical assessment* (3rd ed.). St. Louis: Mosby.
2. Daniels, J. (2006). Obesity: America's epidemic. *American Journal of Nursing, 106*(1), 40-49.
3. Estes, M.E. (Ed.) (2006). *Health assessment and physical examination* (3rd ed.). Delmar Park, NY: Delmar Thomson Learning.
4. Fennel, D. (2004). Determinants of supplement usage. *Preventive Medicine, 39*, 932-939.
5. Food and Nutrition Board—Institute of Medicine. (n.d.). *Food and Nutrition Information Center* [online]. Available at www.nal.usda.gov/fnic/etext/000105.html.
6. Furman, E.F. (2006). Undernutrition in older adults across the continuum of care. *Journal of Gerontological Nursing, 32*(1), 22-27.
7. Jarvis, C. (2004). *Physical examination and health assessment* (4th ed.). Philadelphia: Saunders.
8. Mahan, L., & Escott-Stump, S. (Eds.) (2004). *Krause's food, nutrition, and diet therapy* (11th ed.). Philadelphia: Saunders.
9. Marmo, R., Rotondano, G., Piscopo, R., et al. (2005). Combination of age and sex improves the ability to predict upper gastrointestinal malignancy in patients with uncomplicated dyspepsia: A prospective multicentre database study. *American Journal of Gastroenterology, 100*(4), 784-791.
10. Shils, E., et al. (Eds.) (2006). *Modern nutrition in health and disease* (10th ed.). Baltimore: Williams & Wilkins.
11. United States Department of Agriculture. (n.d.). *Steps to a healthier you* [online]. Available at www.pyramid.gov.
12. Whitworth, A. (2006). Recent research highlights importance of trials halted 10 years ago. *Journal of the National Cancer Institutes, 98*(2), 90-91.
13. Wilson, S.F., & Giddens, J.F. (2005). *Health assessment for nursing practice* (3rd ed.). St. Louis: Mosby.
14. Yamada, T., et al. (Eds.) (2005). *Handbook of gastroenterology* (2nd ed.). Baltimore: Lippincott Williams & Wilkins.

evolve *Did you remember to check out the bonus material on the Evolve website and the CD-ROM, including NCLEX®-Examination Style Review Questions, Open-Book Quizzes, and Chapter Review Audio Podcasts?*

http://evolve.elsevier.com/Black/medsurg

CHAPTER 29

Management of Clients with Malnutrition

VICKI M. ROSS

Malnutrition broadly describes *undernutrition* or *overnutrition*. Undernutrition can develop as a result of acute or chronic diseases and treatments that affect the ability to ingest, digest, or absorb foods. In turn, it can cause such problems as delayed wound healing, impaired immune function, and a decreased functional status. Obesity is an example of overnutrition. Anorexia nervosa and bulimia nervosa are eating disorders that reflect altered nutritional health. Nursing diagnoses pertinent to malnutrition include *Imbalanced Nutrition: More (or Less) Than Body Requirements, Risk for Impaired Skin Integrity, Risk for Infection* and *Feeding Self-Care Deficit.*

PROTEIN-ENERGY MALNUTRITION

Protein-energy malnutrition (PEM), a type of undernutrition, results when the body's need for protein or energy is not supplied in adequate quantity. PEM can be classified as *primary* when the deficits result simply from poor food intake or *secondary,* resulting from decreased nutrient intake or absorption.

Primary PEM is seen most commonly in developing nations or following natural disasters or war, where food supply is disrupted. Although the prevalence of primary PEM has decreased over the past 25 years, there are still an estimated 800 million people worldwide who suffer from PEM. The age groups at greatest risk for PEM are those with increased nutritional needs for growth, reproduction, or milk production—infants, pregnant or lactating women[40]—and older adults.[12]

Over half of all childhood mortality is due directly or indirectly to malnutrition. Thirty-six percent of children in developing nations are underweight and an even higher percent display signs of growth stunting as a result of malnutrition.[41] When a natural disaster, such as drought, flood, earthquake, or famine, occurs, the prevalence of PEM in a developing country may be increased. Similarly, when man-made disasters, such as war, political upheaval, or economic crisis, occur, malnutrition prevalence in the population is exacerbated.[40]

A relatively recent observation in developing countries is the increasing prevalence of obesity or overnutrition concurrently with prevalent PEM. Obesity occurs when caloric supply is excessive but the nutrient content of the diet is poor which promotes chronic diseases (obesity, diabetes mellitus, hypertension, and cancer).[6,35]

Secondary PEM refers to malnutrition associated with acute or chronic disease that causes one or more of the following: (1) decreased food intake, (2) decreased nutrient absorption, (3) increased nutrient losses, or (4) increased nutrient requirements. In developed nations, secondary PEM is more common than primary PEM.

Prolonged deficiencies in energy and protein can result in any of the following clinical syndromes of PEM malnutrition:

- Kwashiorkor, which reflects primarily a chronic deficiency in protein
- Marasmus, which reflects primarily a prolonged deficit in caloric supply
- Marasmic kwashiorkor, which reflects both energy and a protein deficit
- "Kwashiorkor-like malnutrition," which has been coined to describe the abnormally low serum protein concentrations observed in previously well-nourished clients during or after injury or operation

Although severe marasmus, kwashiorkor, and marasmus-kwashiorkor are seen in Western health care facilities, particularly in very ill, older clients, the more common scenario is for clients to be of normal weight or overweight when entering the hospital.

Weight loss during the hospitalization is common, as is rapid development of severely depleted serum protein levels in response to injury, infection, surgical or medical treatments, and prolonged limited intake of protein.[9,17-19] PEM is a significant problem in adult medical and surgical clients in both hospital and home settings. Early studies of malnutrition found PEM in up to 40% of hospitalized medical-surgical clients.[4,5]

Malnutrition remains a problem for hospitalized clients and for clients cared for at home. The epidemiology of malnutrition varies based on individual clients and caregiving situations. Estimates are that over half of hospitalized clients in Europe and North America may be at risk for malnutrition.[6,40]

The older adult population is at particular risk for malnutrition. Decreases in functional capacity, mobility, and independence, which are common in older adults, can result from malnutrition or may contribute to its development.[12,26] The most important changes in body composition associated with aging are a loss of lean body mass and a gain in body fat. The loss of lean body mass is an important factor in the impairment of pulmonary function, immune function, and strength.[40] The Complementary and Alternative Therapy box shown below discusses how protein and energy supplementation may reduce mortality among older adults.

Etiology and Risk Factors

The etiology of PEM is multifactorial and is usually associated with the presence of acute or chronic disease. PEM can be related to socioeconomic factors, physiologic changes in nutrient absorption or nutrient requirements, or medical therapies used to treat disease. Socioeconomic factors that have a negative effect on nutritional status include the following:

- Social isolation
- Limited access to food
- Emotional depression
- Substance abuse
- Poverty

Physiologic factors leading to malnutrition usually result from other diseases that can cause compromised food intake, decreased absorption of nutrients, or increased demand for nutrients. Changes in nutrient intake can result from the disease or from its treatment.

Inadequate food intake is common in hospitals and can lead to malnutrition if diminished intake is prolonged or severe. Many disease processes affect the client's swallowing function and are common reasons for decreased food intake (see Chapter 30).

COMPLEMENTARY AND ALTERNATIVE THERAPY

Oral Protein and Energy Supplements to Reduce Morbidity and Mortality in Older Adults: A Meta-Analysis

Oral supplements (OS) in the form of protein energy drinks are frequently ordered when older clients fail to consume adequate amounts of food. Although frequently prescribed, there has been limited research data to support or dispute the benefits of OS. The limited research data is due in part to the multiple factors associated with OS including the type, amount, and frequency of OS delivered and factors such as client condition, functional ability, and ability to consume OS.[1]

To determine the effectiveness of OS in older clients residing at home, in an institution, or in a hospital, Milne and associates (2006) conducted a meta-analysis of all randomized and quasi-experimental studies that reported comparative results of readily available standard OS (not specialty formulas) to a control group in adults 65 years and older. Of the 55 studies that were included, the evidence suggested a reduction in complications and mortality for people who were undernourished and receiving OS.[2]

The data were statistically significant, showing a reduction in mortality for undernourished clients who received OS in a hospital setting. However, the reduction in mortality risk for undernourished clients in other settings (nursing homes or community) was less obvious, most likely because of the few studies conducted in other settings;

Measures of morbidity varied across all of the studies and included such factors as activities of daily living, grip strength, and different types of infections. Except for weight gain, the data were insufficient to draw any type of conclusions about morbidity factors. For morbidity defined as change in weight, the data consistently supported an increase in weight for those clients receiving OS in the hospital, in a long-term care facility, or at home.

REFERENCES

1. Kayser-Jones, J. (2006). Use of oral supplements in nursing homes: Remaining questions. *Journal of American Geriatrics Society, 54*, 1002-1003.
2. Milne, A., Avenell, A., & Potter, J. (2006). Meta-analysis: Protein and energy supplementation in older people. *Annals of Internal Medicine, 144*, 37-48.

Inadequate absorption of nutrients is the result of various disorders of the gastrointestinal (GI) tract, such as inflammatory bowel disease (see Chapters 31 and 33). In addition, the demand for nutrients increases in response to critical illness and to chronic and infectious diseases.

In your role of preventing and restoring nutritional status, you should take a multidisciplinary approach. Health promotion interventions include activities that support the client's knowledge of normal nutrition and provide nutritional information to maintain optimal health and prevent disease. Such strategies might include diet information related to decreasing cancer risk or identifying sources of support for an older client who cannot prepare meals independently. Health maintenance interventions include targeting specialized diet therapy for a client with an illness (such as diet instruction for a client with Crohn's disease). Health restoration activities can include retraining a client to swallow after a stroke or administering total parenteral nutrition (TPN) to a malnourished client with severe inflammatory bowel disease.

Pathophysiology

PEM can develop gradually over weeks to months, or it can develop more quickly when coupled with severe stress and illness. When the total supply of nutrients is less than the body's requirement over an extended period of time, malnutrition occurs. When the primary deficit is in energy balance, the result is, first, the depletion of adipose tissue or fat stores, with eventual loss of lean body tissue (muscle mass) and fatigue. This deficit is reflected in weight loss. In stressed states protein (mainly from muscle and visceral tissue protein) is used as an energy source.[6] An unintentional weight loss of 5% in 1 month or 10% in 6 months suggests that the client is at significant risk for malnutrition.[2]

When the nutrient deficit is primarily in protein, skeletal muscle is catabolized to meet the body's needs for glucose (in response to hormonal messages), and the liver's synthesis of proteins is altered. The production of serum proteins, such as albumin, transferrin, and prealbumin, is reduced during acute inflammatory conditions, postoperatively, and during significant infections. Rates of protein breakdown are also increased, and serum proteins may shift out of the vascular compartment, resulting overall in low serum protein concentrations. Adequate protein and calorie intake is extremely important during these periods of clinical stress, to enable the production of these serum proteins at adequate levels during the recovery phase. Starvation related to severe stress affects organ function at the cellular level by impairing specific biochemical functions, which increases the risk of mortality and morbidity.[6,40]

Clinical Manifestations

Malnutrition affects all body systems and functions. When performing physical examinations it is important to look for clinical manifestations of malnutrition. Table 29-1 provides information about the pathophysiology and clinical manifestations of malnutrition. See Table 28-1 on p. 557 for information about clinical manifestations of micronutrient deficiencies such as hair loss, dry and bruised skin, brittle nails, bleeding gums, or anemia. As discussed in the Translating Evidence into Practice box on p. 575, malnourished clients are at high risk for developing slow-to-heal wounds.

Abnormal laboratory values that may indicate malnutrition include decreased hemoglobin, albumin, total protein, transferrin, prealbumin, and lymphocyte proliferation. All of these findings are related primarily to a protein deficit. Because of its short half-life of 2 days, prealbumin is the most sensitive indicator of protein deficiency. It can be used to assess improvement in nutritional status with refeeding, and with adequate nutrition support, levels can increase by 1 mg/dl/day. See Chapter 28 for additional information about laboratory assessment of nutrition.

TABLE 29-1 Consequences of Malnutrition

Organ System	Pathophysiology	Clinical Manifestations
Cardiac	Decreased cardiac muscle mass	Postural hypotension Diminished venous return
Pulmonary	Decreased diaphragm strength	Inability to clear secretions
	Decreased respiratory strength	Decreased exercise tolerance
	Decreased endurance	Inability to wean from ventilator
Immune function	Decreased cell-mediated immunity	Increased incidence and severity of infection
	Delayed cutaneous hypersensitivity	
Wound healing	Decreased collagen synthesis	Delayed wound healing
Skeletal muscle strength	Altered muscle contractions	Fatigue
	Relaxation response	Inability to perform activities of daily living
	Decreased muscle endurance	Risk of falling
Gastrointestinal function	Impaired intestinal absorption of lipids	Diarrhea
	Decreased rate of glucose absorption	
	Decreased gastric, pancreatic, and bile production	

TRANSLATING EVIDENCE INTO PRACTICE

Nutrition and Wounds

Nutrition is one of many factors associated with wounds. Because malnourished or highly catabolic trauma clients may develop or have pre-existing wounds, it is tempting to think additional nutrition will prevent or enhance wound healing in these and other clients. However, there is little research to support an association between the delivery of excessive micronutrients and improved wound healing. Small sample sizes and the heterogeneity of studies contribute to the lack of evidence supporting the delivery of specific micronutrients in clients with wounds and have illustrated the need for more research about the associations between nutrition and wounds.[2,3] Even though there are few studies to support the excessive or specific use of micronutrients, experts agree that it is important to provide adequate nutrition.[9]

Unless clients have an underlying condition such as trauma or fever that would require additional calories or protein, there is no evidence to support delivery of calories in excess of 30 to 35 kcal/kg for clients with wounds. In addition, it is important to maintain a euglycemic state for all clients, but especially for clients that have both wounds and diabetes mellitus.[5,7] Similarly, there is no strong evidence to support prevention or healing of wounds with protein delivery in excess of the standard 1.0 to 1.5 g/kg.[1] Although there is some laboratory evidence that specific amino acids such as arginine and glutamine improve wound healing in animal models, the same results have not been consistently obtained in the clinical setting. It is not clear if this inconsistency is due to the true lack of benefit or the heterogeneity of subjects and small sample sizes.[4,8]

Vitamin C, vitamin A, and zinc have a role in healthy skin and under certain conditions may improve wound healing. However, except in the presence of deficient states, there is no consistent evidence to demonstrate that delivery of vitamin C, vitamin A, or zinc in excess of the dietary requirements is of benefit for wound healing. For those clients with specific vitamin or trace element deficits, additional doses in excess of the recommended dietary intake amounts may be appropriate. There is wide variation in the range of recommended amounts for depletion, from 100 to 1000 mg per day, and research is needed to determine the optimal repletion dose. To counteract the effects of glucocorticoids, additional doses of vitamin A in amounts ranging from 10,000 to 25,000 units for up to 7 days have been recommended. Optimal amounts for zinc repletion

have yet to be determined. Some recommend ranges of zinc from 10 to 40 mg/day over 1 to 3 weeks.[1,6,10] It is important to remember all vitamins, minerals, and trace elements may be toxic if delivered to individuals in excessive amounts or over a long period of time.

Typical daily water requirements are 30 to 40 ml/kg per day. Increased water needs resulting from insensible loss through open wounds or fever will need to be calculated based on such factors as underlying condition, size of wound, amount of drainage, and daily weight changes, for example.[9]

IMPLICATIONS

Although there is not strong research evidence to support special nutrition formulations, there is a general consensus that nutrition is an important factor in the development and healing of wounds and that clients who have or at risk of developing wounds should receive a standard nutritional diet (enteral or parenteral) of 30 to 35 kcal/kg and 1.0 to 1.5 g/kg of protein per day. Unless there is evidence of a deficiency, diets and/or dietary supplements should provide 100% of the RDAs for vitamins, minerals, and trace elements. Adequate hydration is an important part of the nutritional program.

BIBLIOGRAPHY

1. Arnold, M., & Barbul, A. (2006). Nutrition and wound healing. *Plastic Reconstructive Surgery, 117*(Suppl), 42S.
2. Benbow, M. (2006). Guidelines for the prevention and treatment of pressure ulcers. *Nursing Standard, 20*(52), 42-44.
3. Langer, G., et al. (2003). Nutritional interventions for preventing and treating pressure ulcers. *The Cochrane Database of Systematic Reviews: Reviews 2003* Issue 4, CD003216.
4. Mandal, A. (2006). Do malnutrition and nutritional supplementation have an effect on wound healing process? *Journal of Wound Care, 16*(6), 254-257.
5. Marston, W.A., & Dermagraft Diabetic Foot Ulcer Study Group. (2006). Risk factors associated with healing chronic diabetic foot ulcers: The importance of hyperglycemia. *Ostomy/Wound Management, 52*(3), 26-32.
6. Patel, G.K. (2005). The role of nutrition in the management of lower extremity wounds. *Lower Extremity Wounds, 4,* 12-22.
7. Rai, N.K., et al. (2005). Effect of glycaemic control on apoptosis in diabetic foot wounds. *Journal of Wound Care, 14*(6), 277-281.
8. Stechmiller, J.K., Childress, B., & Cowan, L. (2005). Arginine supplementation and wound healing. *Nutrition and Clinical Practice, 20,* 52-61.
9. Thompson, C., & Fuhrman, M.P. (2005). Nutrients and wound healing: Still searching for the magic bullet. *Nutrition and Clinical Practice, 20,* 331-347.

OUTCOME MANAGEMENT

Medical Management

Management of PEM starts with identification of clients who are malnourished as well as clients at risk for malnutrition. All clients should be screened for nutritional problems. First-level screening can be done through admission forms or simple questionnaires. Nutritional screening generally focuses on a few key data points (such as a weight change, a change in dietary habits,

and GI manifestations) to identify clients that require a more comprehensive nutritional assessment. A comprehensive nutritional assessment includes a review of the medical history, weight and diet history, anthropometric measurements, biochemical profiles, and physical examination. Quality nutrition support outcomes require identifying early those clients at nutritional risk (see Chapter 28 for an in-depth review of nutritional assessment), determining the appropriate nutrient requirements, and delivering required nutrients via an appropriate route while minimizing or preventing risks of nutrition support.

Determine Nutrient Requirements

Nutrient requirements are calculated to maintain, decrease, or increase weight. Weight maintenance is appropriate for clients within 90% to 120% of a reference weight, whereas depletion of fat stores or weight loss is appropriate for obese clients (>120% of reference weight). Clients with severely depleted fat stores and more than 10% weight loss need calories sufficient to replete these stores and to gain weight.

The energy needs of most clients can be determined with formulas that estimate the basal energy expenditure (BEE). Even though the studies occurred in the early 1900s, the Harris-Benedict equations for basal energy expenditure (BEE) are still the most commonly used formulas:

$$BEE \text{ (men)} = 66 + (13.7 \times \text{Weight in kg})$$
$$+ (5 \times \text{Height in cm}) - (6.8 \times \text{Age})$$

$$BEE \text{ (women)} = 655 + (9.6 \times \text{Weight in kg})$$
$$+ (1.7 \times \text{Height in cm}) - (4.7 \times \text{Age})$$

The BEE represents the basal metabolic rate and is multiplied by a factor that accounts for stress and activity. Table 29-2 outlines targets for daily energy requirements using predictive equations. These equations are most useful in mildly stressed clients and may overestimate or underestimate energy needs during critical illness. Advanced practice nurses or specialized health care providers may use indirect calorimetry to obtain a more precise measurement of energy expenditure for severely stressed clients.

Alternatively, an estimate of 25 kcal/kg body weight is often used when weight maintenance is desired. If weight gain is needed, the caloric goal can be increased to 35 kcal/kg, or an additional 500 kcal/day (to promote a safe rate of weight gain of 1 pound per week) can be added to the caloric estimate for weight maintenance.

The protein needs of a hospitalized client may be nearly twice those of normal needs. The Recommended Daily Allowance (RDA) for protein in healthy people is 0.8 g/kg/day. Protein requirements for the metabolically stressed client range from 1.5 g of protein/kg to as much as 2 g of protein/kg of body weight.

Determine Route of Feeding

In clients with adequate GI tract function, *enteral,* either oral or via a tube, rather than *parenteral* nutrition should

TABLE 29–2 Determining Daily Energy Requirements

Goal for Fat Stores	kcal (in Hospital)	Requirement (kcal/kg/day)
Replete	BEE* × 1.5	30-35
Maintain	BEE × 1.3	25-30
Reduce	<BEE	20-25

* *BEE,* Basal energy expenditure.
From ASPEN Board of Directors and the Clinical Guidelines Task Force. (2002). Guidelines for the use of parenteral and enteral nutrition in adult and pediatric patients. *Journal of Parenteral and Enteral Nutrition, 26*(Suppl 1).

be used. Figure 29-1 presents an algorithm for determining the appropriate route of feeding. Clients may need to alternate between oral, enteral, and parenteral feedings during the course of a hospital admission.

One of the most important benefits of enteral nutrition relates to the value of using the GI tract to maintain and support gut integrity and function and prevent atrophy of the gut mucosa. As compared to parenteral nutrition, the protection offered by using the GI tract can result in a reduction of infectious complications.[2,15] Other factors that make enteral therapy desirable include reduced cost and safer administration.[1]

If the client is able to consume and swallow adequate amounts of nutrition and the gastrointestinal tract is functional, oral nutrition is the route of choice. To prevent or correct existing malnutrition through oral dietary manipulation, a registered dietitian can assist in meal planning or can recommend diet modification to increase oral intake. Supplements to boost the oral intake of calories and protein are available in a variety of forms, such as liquid milk-like drinks, clear juice-like drinks, nutrient bars, and puddings (Table 29-3).

Older adult clients with visual disorders or immobility or clients with neuromuscular impairments such as Parkinson's disease, muscular dystrophy, myasthenia gravis, muscular weakness, or central nervous system tumors may be able to consume adequate amounts of nutrition if environmental factors are altered to accommodate for their disabilities. Interventions should focus on improving nutritional intake, minimizing barriers, and reducing risks of aspiration.

Nursing Management of the Medical Client

Nurses play a vital role in identifying clients with nutritional problems. They are usually the first to assess clients as they enter a health system and provide teaching at dismissal. Nurses also have the most constant contact during a hospitalization.

Improve Nutritional Intake

General strategies to improve nutritional intake relate to choices of menu items and the accessibility of dietitians and food service personnel who can evaluate client food preferences and assist in meal planning. Clients should be able to choose from a menu to avoid food monotony. Dietitians should be accessible during mealtimes to help assess individual preferences. Kitchen facilities and supplies should be available at the unit level to increase client choices. Dedicated refrigeration and microwave equipment for client and family use may encourage the families to bring foods that are appealing to the client and may allow more flexible mealtimes that coincide with the client's appetite.

Increase Appetite

Appetite is often impaired in a hospital setting for a variety of reasons. Several strategies can be used to maximize or

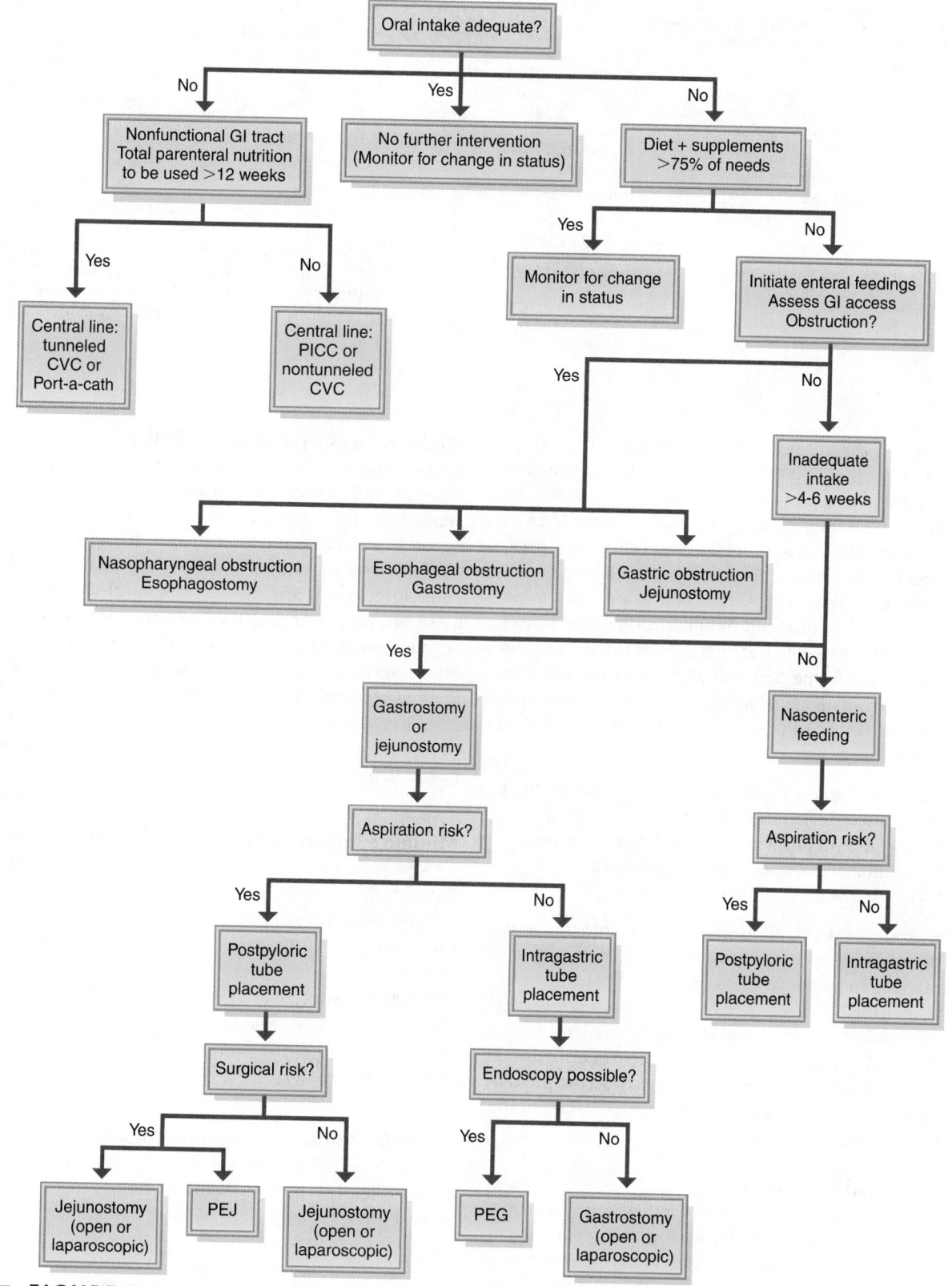

■ **FIGURE 29–1** Algorithm to determine appropriate route of feeding. *CVC,* Central venous catheter; *PEG,* percutaneous endoscopic gastrostomy; *PEJ,* percutaneous endoscopic jejunostomy; *PICC,* peripherally inserted central catheter. *(Data from Mahan, L.K., & Escott-Stump, S.E. [2004]. Krause's food, nutrition, & diet therapy [11th ed., p. 536]. Philadelphia: W.B. Saunders; modified and adapted from Gorman R.C., & Morris, J.B. [1997]. Minimally invasive access to the gastrointestinal tract. In J.L. Rombeau & R.H. Rolandelli [Eds.], Clinical nutrition: Enteral and tube feeding [p. 174]. Philadelphia: Saunders.)*

TABLE 29-3   Oral Nutritional Supplements

Supplement Type	Examples	Calories per Serving	Protein (g per Serving)	Features
Milk based	Nutrashake Carnation Instant Breakfast Ensure Pudding	200-250	8-12	Widely available Economical High calorie/protein
Lactose free	Boost Plus Nutren ProBalance	300-360	13-15	High calorie/protein No lactose
Disease specific	Nepro Resource DiabetiSource	Range dependent on disease focus of supplement (e.g., carbohydrates reduced for client with diabetes mellitus)	Range dependent on disease focus of supplement (e.g., protein restricted for client with renal disease)	Supplement ingredients based on disease (e.g., electrolyte restricted for client with renal disease)
Nutritional bars	Boost Power Bar	180-190	4-10	Candy bar appeal Convenient for travel

enhance a client's desire for food. First, you can create a pleasant environment during mealtime. Clear the area of unsightly bedpans, urinals, suctioning equipment, and dressing supplies. Ensure adequate pain reduction before meals, and avoid invasive procedures or pulmonary treatments just before a meal. Increased activity through regular exercise may also increase the client's appetite.

Appetite can be enhanced by stimulation of the senses of taste, smell, and sight. Taste alterations can occur from injury or surgery to the oral cavity, medications, and oral infections. Oral hygiene is important to support the optimal function of taste buds. Routine mouth care should include the following:

- Cleansing the mouth after each meal and at bedtime
- Using a soft-bristle toothbrush
- Rinsing the mouth with warm saline (salt water)
- Avoiding alcohol-containing mouthwash
- Avoiding glycerin and lemon juice

The aroma of prepared foods may stimulate the appetite. Although clients cannot participate in food preparation, offering them a chance to smell food before a meal may be helpful. On the other hand, noxious odors may negatively affect appetite, and should be avoided.

To help stimulate appetite, let the client see the food, position the food to make it visible, and describe the different foods. Your description is especially important for clients with visual impairment.

Increase Social Interaction

Eating is ordinarily a time for social interaction, yet clients are usually given meals in their own rooms. Creating social contact by feeding clients in a central area or encouraging family and friends to visit during mealtimes may be an option. Client care assignments should be designed so that clients requiring feeding can be assigned to the same caregiver as much as possible. As the client and caregiver develop a therapeutic relationship, the feeding becomes a more pleasurable and successful experience for both.

Minimize Sensory-Perceptual Deficits

Clients with sensory or perceptual deficits require specific nursing actions to ensure adequate food intake. Make sure the client is wearing corrective lenses, if needed, and that they fit properly. If needed, describe the food and its location on the tray. The use of different-colored trays and dishes is helpful to clients with these deficits. Arranging the food in a clock-face pattern is an easy way to orient the client to the position of various foods on the tray. Describing the position of foods is imperative for clients with visual field disturbances. Initially, do not place foods on the client's blind side. However, clients should learn to pan the environment so as to see items placed on their blind side.

Minimize Impact of Neuromuscular Impairments

Various neuromuscular impairments can make the seemingly simple task of eating difficult or impossible. The occupational therapy staff can help in planning the feeding intervention and teaching the correct use of assistive devices. For a client with physical impairment, ensure privacy, allow adequate time for eating, position the client at a 90-degree angle with the meal tray at elbow height, and provide assistive devices, such as plate guards and built-up spoons.

Minimize Impact of Cognitive Impairments

Cognitive impairments can result in the client's misunderstanding the task of eating or being unable to complete the task because of a short attention span. If so, the client requires frequent cues and close supervision. The following nursing actions are useful steps in feeding clients with cognitive impairments:

- Create a quiet, unhurried environment.
- Explain the procedure.
- Orient the client to the purpose of feeding equipment.

- Provide frequent cues to the client (e.g., "Mrs. S, pick up the toast" or "Mr. S, chew the food in your mouth").
- Provide several small meals for clients with short attention spans.

Minimize Fatigue

Another physical factor that can affect a person's ability to feed oneself is endurance. The client may be able to start the task but becomes quickly fatigued and cannot complete it. The client's ability to maintain a level of performance is related to cardiovascular, respiratory, neurologic, and musculoskeletal function. For a client with reduced endurance, plan rest periods before mealtimes, especially when the meal follows an activity, such as physical therapy or ambulation. Help the client conserve energy for eating by helping with meal setup, opening packages, and cutting food.

Minimize Risks of Aspiration

A team approach has been successful in the management of clients with swallowing impairments. Physicians, physical and occupational therapists, and speech pathologists can be helpful in addition to nurses in localizing the impairment and suggesting useful strategies. You must also understand the complexity of normal swallowing mechanisms in order to plan appropriate interventions.

Before feeding a client, test and confirm the following:

- Assess level of consciousness; the client must be alert.
- Assess the client's gag reflex by tickling the back of the throat.
- Have the client produce an audible cough.
- Have the client produce a voluntary swallow.

Feeding should take place in a calm, adequately supervised environment. Place the client in a normal eating position with the feeder clearly visible. Some clients may have trouble moving the food bolus from the front to the back of the mouth. Food should be placed in the unaffected side of the mouth. If the tongue is damaged or impaired, assistive devices, such as adapted feeding syringes, can move food toward the pharynx, where the swallowing reflex (if intact) takes over.

Once the food bolus arrives at the pharynx, the client should tilt his or her chin down to decrease the risk of aspiration. Massaging the throat on the affected side helps stimulate the tactile areas that initiate the swallowing reflex. If the client has difficulty coordinating chewing, breathing, and swallowing, instruct the client to hold his or her head forward and to hold breath before swallowing.

Watch the thyroid cartilage to see whether the client has swallowed, and inspect his or her mouth before placing more food in the oral cavity. Allowing sufficient time between each mouthful helps ensure that the client adequately chews and swallows the food. Stay alert for signs that the client is becoming fatigued, restless, or agitated.

> **Keep suction equipment available in case of an emergency. Also, know how to perform the abdominal thrust (formerly known as Heimlich) maneuver to prevent choking. The Bridge to Home Health Care feature on p. 580 discusses the management of clients with impaired swallowing.**

SAFETY ALERT

Medical Management of the Client Receiving Enteral Nutrition

Enteral Nutrition

Total enteral nutrition (TEN) or tube-feeding refers to a method of infusing nutrient solutions or formulas directly into the GI tract through tubes that enter through the nose, mouth, or abdominal wall. TEN is indicated when the client has impaired ingestion but normal intestinal absorption.

Common indications for TEN are listed in Box 29-1. TEN is contraindicated in clients with complete intestinal

---

BOX 29-1 Indications for Enteral Feeding

NEUROLOGIC AND PSYCHIATRIC
- Anorexia nervosa
- Stroke
- Demyelinating disease
- Failure to thrive
- Inflammation
- Cancer
- Severe depression
- Trauma

OROPHARYNGEAL AND ESOPHAGEAL
- Inflammation
- Cancer
- Trauma

GASTROINTESTINAL
- Fistula (not mid-gut)
- Mild inflammatory bowel disease
- Mild malabsorption
- Mild pancreatitis
- Preoperative bowel preparation
- Short-bowel syndrome (later stages)

MISCELLANEOUS
- Acquired immunodeficiency syndrome (AIDS)
- Burns
- Chemotherapy
- Organ transplantation
- Radiation therapy

Modified from Guenter, P., et al. (1997). Delivery systems and administration of enteral nutrition. In J. Rombeau & R. Rolandelli (Eds.), *Clinical nutrition: Enteral and tube feeding* (3rd ed., p. 240). Philadelphia: W.B. Saunders.

BRIDGE TO HOME HEALTH CARE

Managing Swallowing Difficulties

Swallowing difficulty (dysphagia) can vary in severity and duration. It can be mild to severe, short term (acute), or long term (chronic).

When you feed clients who have dysphagia, use good observational skills and plenty of communication and patience. Observe their responses to what you are doing. They may frown, spit, clamp their jaws together, or cough when food choices are not appealing. Try to adapt meals to their tastes. For example, if a client enjoys bananas, then dice, mash, or blend them into a shake, or even freeze them to offer variety; select the consistency that your client tolerates best.

Promote use of the sense organs during mealtime. Encourage your clients to think or talk about their favorite foods before meals to stimulate saliva flow and to aid in chewing. Ask clients to close their eyes and to visualize tasting and chewing these foods. Provide mouth care before and after the client eats meals and swallows medications to keep the mouth and breath fresh and facilitate saliva production. If your clients find it pleasurable, have them watch the food being prepared, smell the food cooking, and participate in the meal preparation as much as possible. Use an activity such as folding napkins to begin involvement. Play the client's favorite music tapes during mealtime.

The home health nurse should schedule shared visits periodically with the speech or occupational therapist to promote continuity of care. Discuss strategies related to mealtime and food preparation. Work with the therapists to help clients strengthen their mouth muscles by practicing pushing their lips or "puckering," humming, or whistling. Demonstrate the techniques you are trying to teach; hold a mirror so that clients can see their own mouth.

A high Fowler's position with 90-degree flexion of the hips is usually the best position for mealtime. Position your client with shoulders back and torso erect. Slightly flexing the client's head forward may aid in swallowing. Placing a pillow at the lower back and a towel roll behind the neck can facilitate a smooth flow of food from the mouth into the stomach. Observe your clients closely to see which position makes them most comfortable. Cushions, pillows, or bedrolls are used to support any dependent limbs or "weak" sides. Increasing physical comfort decreases distraction and allows more focus on eating.

Maintaining the high Fowler's position, with at least 75- to 80-degree flexion at the hips for at least 30 minutes after a meal, helps reduce reflux and aspiration. Check your client's mouth carefully for lingering food pockets that may become dislodged and cause aspiration long after the meal. For your safety, never place your unprotected fingers in the client's mouth when teeth or dentures are in place.

Close observation, good communication, and a sense of humor will keep mealtime pleasurable for your client and you.

obstruction, severe ileus or pseudo-obstruction, severe diarrhea, intestinal ischemia, or malabsorption syndrome and may be contraindicated in clients with severe acute pancreatitis. In clients with impairments of the proximal GI tract, from fistulae or tumor, TEN feeding may be used if the tip of the tube is positioned distal to the impairment.

The selection of an enteral formula is based on the client's nutrient requirements, the absorptive function of the GI tract, the fluid status, and the level of stress. More than 100 enteral formulas are available on the market today, but most can be placed into one of the following three classifications:

- *Standard formula:* contains intact (nonhydrolyzed) protein; provides 1 to 2 kcal/ml with variable amounts of protein, electrolyte, and fiber.
- *Disease-specific formula:* enhances specific organ function (e.g., kidneys, liver, pulmonary system, or immune system) for clients with organ failure.
- *Predigested semi-elemental formula:* contains hydrolyzed protein in the form of dipeptides, tripeptides, or amino acids. These products are designed for clients with limited digestive function.

Table 29-4 outlines the classification of enteral products and includes brief descriptions of formula characteristics. Standard formulas, which contain 1 kcal/ml, are used most often. Concentrated calorie-dense formulas, which contain 1.5 to 2 kcal/ml, are helpful for clients who are fluid-restricted or unable to tolerate high volumes of formula. High-protein formulas contain more than 50 g/L of protein and are useful for critically ill clients who are hypercatabolic and have a proportionally lower calorie and fluid need with high protein requirements. The addition of fiber to standard formulas can help regulate bowel function and prevent diarrhea and constipation.

Disease-specific formulas contain 1.0 to 2.0 kcal/ml and different amounts of protein, carbohydrates, and fat to address specific disease conditions. For example, formulas for clients who will be undergoing dialysis contain low amounts of protein and electrolytes, while formulas for clients with diabetes mellitus contain a higher proportion of predominantly monounsaturated fat and a lower proportion of simple carbohydrates.

Clients requiring higher proportions of branched-chain amino acids or who have impaired absorption of whole proteins may benefit from predigested semi-elemental formulas.

Because there are so many enteral formulas on the market, it is important to ascertain the amount of vitamins, minerals, trace elements, and water supplied with specific formulas. Typically, enteral formulas provide the RDA of vitamins and trace elements based on an intake of 1500 to 2000 calories/day. Clients receiving lower-calorie regimens with enteral nutrition for extended periods may require supplemental vitamins.

TABLE 29–4   **Classification of Enteral Nutrition (Tube-Feeding) Products**

Classification	Examples	Formula Characteristics
Standard	Osmolite, Isocal, Resource, Entrition	Isotonic, nutritionally complete, average 1 cal/ml, lactose free
	Isocal HCN, Magnacal, TwoCal HN, Nutren	Hyperosmolar, calorically dense (1.5-2.0 cal/ml), nutritionally complete, lactose free
	Fibersource, Jevity, Fiberlan, Ultracal	Isotonic, nutritionally complete, lactose free, contain fiber
Disease-specific	Renal impairment: Suplena, Nepro	Electrolyte, vitamin, and protein content reduced
	Glucose intolerant: Glucerna	Low carbohydrate, high fat
	Trauma stress: TraumaCal, AlitraQ, Impact, Replete, Promote	High protein; some contain fiber, supplemental amino acids, β-carotene
Semi-elemental, predigested	Vivonex T.E.N., Peptamen, Reabilan, Criticare HN	Hyperosmolar, varying in peptide length and amino acids

Fussell, S.T. (2003). Enteral formulations. In L.E. Matarese & M.M. Gottschlich (Eds.), *Contemporary nutrition support practice: A clinical guide* (2nd ed.). Philadelphia: Saunders.

Daily fluid needs of the client receiving enteral nutrition must be calculated to avoid overhydration or underhydration. The most vulnerable client is the one receiving a calorie-dense or concentrated formula, which contains less free water than that in a standard formula. Such a client may require additional water delivered as an intermittent flush or bolus throughout the day to meet fluid needs. A client with excessive GI losses may also require supplemental water to maintain hydration.

Enteral Access

Enteral feeding requires the administration of a liquid solution through a tube into the GI tract. Enteral feedings can be delivered into the stomach (intragastrically) or into the small intestine (duodenally or jejunally). Selection of the type of enteral access device depends on the functional status of the GI tract, the risk for aspiration, and the estimated length of therapy. Figure 29-2 depicts selected enteral access placements.

The functional status of the client's GI tract often defines the site of feeding. Resections, obstructions, motility disorders, or fistulae of the upper GI tract necessitate that the client be fed into the small bowel, distal to the impairment. A client who has aspirated or is at risk for aspiration may benefit from postpyloric feeding. The duration of enteral therapy defines the type of tube placed: temporary tubes for short-term therapy (<4 to 6 weeks) and permanent tubes for long-term therapy (>4 to 6 weeks).

For short-term feeding, nasogastric or nasoenteric tubes are preferred. Performed at the bedside, tubes varying in length and ranging in size from 5 F to 16 F are placed into the stomach or small intestine, and the tip position is then verified with an abdominal radiograph. Smaller diameter tubes (<10 F) are susceptible to blockage with formula and medications and require frequent flushing and/or feeding pump administration of formula. If postpyloric feeding is indicated, the tip of the tube can be advanced under fluoroscopy, or via endoscopy, client positioning, or the administration of prokinetic agents (e.g., cisapride, metoclopramide, or erythromycin). Small-bore enteral feeding tubes are made of polyurethane or silicone plastic and are thus softer and more flexible than a nasogastric tube used for decompression and made of polyvinyl chloride.

For long-term enteral feeding, gastrostomy and jejunostomy tubes are indicated. These tubes can be placed surgically, endoscopically, or radiologically. Surgically placed devices (gastrostomy or jejunostomy tubes) are

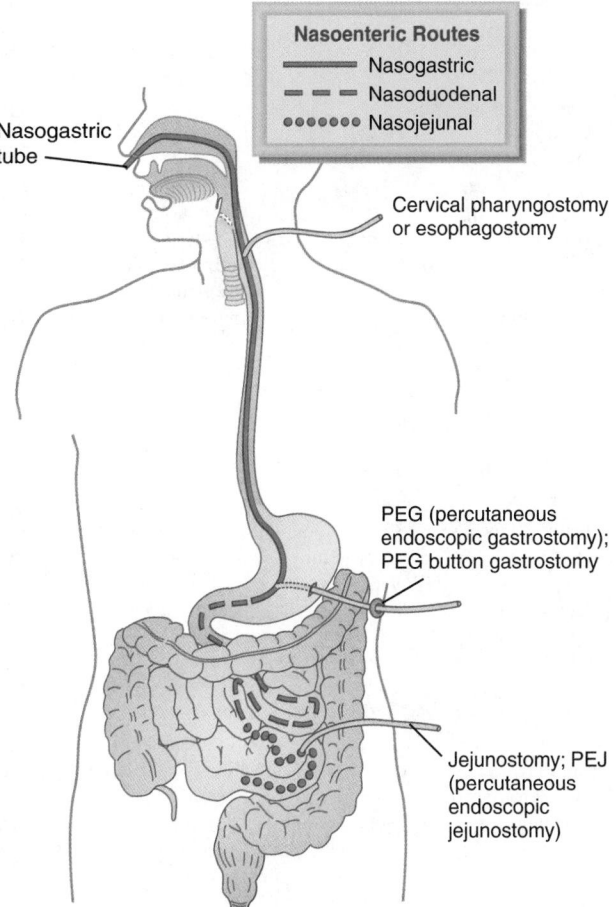

Nasogastric tube

Nasoenteric Routes
— Nasogastric
– – – Nasoduodenal
●●●●●●● Nasojejunal

Cervical pharyngostomy or esophagostomy

PEG (percutaneous endoscopic gastrostomy); PEG button gastrostomy

Jejunostomy; PEJ (percutaneous endoscopic jejunostomy)

■ **FIGURE 29–2** Placements for enteral access. *(From Mahan, L.K., & Escott-Stump, S.E. [2004]. Krause's food, nutrition, & diet therapy [11th ed., p. 538]. Philadelphia: Saunders.)*

used most commonly in clients undergoing a laparotomy, and general anesthesia is required. More recently, the percutaneous endoscopic gastrostomy (PEG) or jejunostomy (PEJ) approach has become the most common method of placing a permanent long-term feeding device. This nonsurgical approach avoids the need for general anesthesia and can be performed on an outpatient basis. Table 29-5 gives more information about specific types of enteral access devices, indications, advantages, or disadvantages.

TABLE 29-5 Enteral Access Devices

Enteral Access	Tube Size and Length	Indications	Advantages	Disadvantages
Nasogastric (small-bore feeding tube)	8-12 F, 17-36 inches	Functional stomach Upper GI tract obstruction Dysphagia to solids Not at risk for aspiration	Placed at bedside Low morbidity Easily inserted Continued use of GI tract	Client discomfort Risk of aspiration
Nasoduodenal	14-18 F, 35-45 inches	Gastric atony Risk of aspiration	Decreased risk of aspiration Continued use of GI tract	Client discomfort Difficult placement Easily malpositioned
Nasojejunal	14-18 F, 36-45 inches	High risk for pulmonary aspiration of gastric contents Functional small bowel	Decreased risk of aspiration Continued use of GI tract	Increased cost of tube and skilled professional to place tube Easily malpositioned
Gastrostomy, surgical	14-30 F	Inability to use percutaneous placement GI surgery Long-term feeding	Continued use of GI tract Can be placed in clients with esophageal or pharyngeal cancers Used in obese clients when unable to transilluminate abdominal wall for PEG placement	General anesthesia Tube migration Easily obstructed Local stoma site complications
Gastrostomy, percutaneous	14-22 F	Long-term feeding tube No history of aspiration	No surgical procedure needed Placement without general anesthesia Continued use of GI tract	Potential for aspiration Cannot be used in obese clients
Low-profile gastrostomy device (G-Button)	18-28 F	Long-term feeding Ambulatory clients Disoriented clients who pull at gastrostomy tube	Increased mobility Decreased cost over time because of device longevity Decreased nursing time compared with time needed for replacement tube change Continued use of GI tract	Skilled professional needed for placement Increased trauma to client compared with replacement tube Increased cost compared with cost of gastrostomy tube change Second procedure required after gastrostomy tube placement
Jejunostomy, temporary	5 F Jejunostomy kit, 14 F	Short-term enteral nutrition Usually ≤2 weeks	Continued use of GI tract	Surgical placement Tube easily obstructed Costly
Jejunostomy, permanent	Whistle tip, 14-18 F	Long-term jejunal feeding	Silicone plastic Continued use of GI tract Easily replaced when fistulous tract is formed Larger-bore Location proximal jejunum, thus elemental products not required	Continuous or slow intermittent tube-feeding required via a pump
Combination tubes for gastric decompression	Gastric port, 16-30 F Jejunal feeding port, 9 F	Long-term feeding Dysfunctional stomach Functional small bowel Short-term postoperative care	Can decompress a dysfunctional stomach and prevent regurgitation of gastric contents during small intestine feeding Continued use of GI tract	Skilled professional needed for placement Expensive process Jejunal feeding needed Can be dislodged from original position Placed during surgery

F, French; *GI*, gastrointestinal; *PEG*, percutaneous endoscopic gastrostomy.
From Lysen, L.K. (2003). Enteral equipment. In L.E. Matarese & M.M. Gottschlich (Eds.), *Contemporary nutrition support practice: A clinical guide* (2nd ed.). Philadelphia: Saunders.

Methods of Administration

Enteral feeding can be administered by either an *intermittent* or a *continuous* drip. The method of delivery is determined by (1) the location of the tube tip and (2) the client's tolerance. Feedings delivered into the stomach may be intermittent or continuous. Feedings delivered directly into the small bowel require a continuous drip.

In *intermittent* or *bolus* feedings, 300 to 500 ml of enteral formula is delivered several times per day. Bolus feedings are usually delivered in 60-ml increments via a syringe over 10 to 15 minutes. Feedings may also be placed into a gravity bag and dripped in over 30 to 60 minutes.

Continuous feedings are administered via an infusion pump to more closely control the rate of infusion. When the tube tip is located in the small intestine, continuous feeding is the desired choice. Continuous feedings are generally infused over 24 hours at rates ranging from 50 to 150 ml. As clients are switched to cycled nocturnal feedings in preparation for discharge, they often require and can tolerate continuous rates slightly greater than 150 ml/hour. However, clients usually cannot tolerate continuous feeding into the small intestine at rates greater than 200 ml/hour.

Continuous feeding into the stomach has been associated with less gastric distention and aspiration compared with bolus or intermittent feeding into the stomach.[11,15,16] In addition, continuous gastric feedings may reduce metabolic complications and protect against stress ulcers more effectively compared with intermittent gastric feedings.

Nursing Management of the Client Receiving Enteral Nutrition

In addition to the nutritional assessment measures described earlier, you should review the type of formula being used; the time, frequency, and amount of feeding; and the specific indications for your client. For clients receiving TEN, nursing interventions should focus on maintaining or improving nutritional health while preventing mechanical, metabolic or infectious complications.

Monitor the client for aspiration of tube-feeding or GI contents. Mechanical complications that have been reported for clients receiving TEN include clogged, dislodged or misplaced tubes, aspiration, skin breakdown, or sinusitis.

The Bridge to Home Health Care feature at right explores the topic of tube feedings in greater detail.

Ensure Delivery of Prescribed Nutrient Requirements

Starter regimens for enteral feedings differ according to tube tip location and the client's clinical status.

Continuous feedings into the small intestine are usually started at 30 to 40 ml/hour and advanced as tolerated every 12 to 24 hours until the daily goal is reached. Intermittent feedings into the stomach are initiated at 100 to 120 ml every 4 hours and advanced every 12 to 24 hours as tolerated. The amount of time continuous tube

BRIDGE TO HOME HEALTH CARE

Managing Tube Feedings

Home health agency nutrition support teams usually consist of a nurse, a registered dietitian, and a pharmacist. When these professionals regularly visit a client who has a new feeding tube, the chances for successfully managing the client and the tube feedings at home are greatly increased. In addition to providing direct care, the team provides instructions to the client and family, communicates with the client's physician, prevents problems if possible, and monitors any problems that develop.

Consistently flushing the tube with water before and after each feeding enhances the longevity of the tube. Although flushing the tube with carbonated beverages has been suggested, studies indicate few or no benefits over flushing with water. Flush all types of feeding tubes with a 50-ml syringe; smaller syringes can create pressure high enough to rupture a tube.

Teach the client and family to secure a nasogastric tube firmly to the nose and to either side of the face or to another position of comfort. To secure the tube, use tape, a transparent occlusive dressing, or a commercial tube holder with a hydrocolloid backing with a self-fastening tape (Velcro) closure.

When the client has a percutaneous endoscopic gastrostomy (PEG) or a percutaneous endoscopic jejunostomy (PEJ), observe daily for tube dislodgment, leaking, skin irritation, and clinical manifestations of infection. Clean the site daily with mild soap and water. Slide the external bridge away for cleaning, then reposition. No dressing is required. Good hand-washing technique is essential for all personnel.

Management of tube feedings varies with the type of infusion: continuous infusion with a pump, bolus infusion, or infusion by gravity. Numerous commercial products are available to meet the client's nutritional needs. The physician and the registered dietitian are responsible for assessing the type of feeding and method of infusion. However, the client may tolerate one formula better than another. Positioning clients at a 45-degree angle or greater helps them tolerate the feeding. Changing the rate and frequency of infusion may decrease or eliminate nausea, diarrhea, or tube displacement. Successful tube-feeding begins in the hospital and continues at home as the client, family, home care nurse, registered dietitian, pharmacist, and physician work together as a team.

feedings are stopped for client activities such as bathing, x-ray, or medication administration should be minimized. Clients often do not receive the prescribed amount of feeding because pumps are turned off for multiple procedures throughout the day.

Assess Tube Location

SAFETY
ALERT

To ensure tips of enteral feeding devices are properly placed, assess tube location before administering an enteral feeding. If a nasoenteric tube is being used to feed a client for the first time, make sure that an abdominal radiograph has verified that the tip is located in the GI tract.

Routinely evaluate the position of the enteral feeding device, and be alert for the possibility of tube migration or dislodgment. Nasoenteric tubes can be marked to indicate the position so that it will be evident if the tube has moved. Nasoenteric tubes can easily migrate when the client coughs or vomits, but more often the tubes are dislodged when a confused or agitated client inadvertently removes the tube.

In addition to determining whether the tube has migrated, you may need to evaluate the location of the tube tip. Is the tube tip in the stomach, small intestine, or respiratory tract? Four methods can be used to evaluate tip location:

- *Aspiration:* observing the fluid that is removed through a large bore feeding tube (this cannot be done with small bore feeding tubes)
- *pH paper testing:* checking the pH of the fluid removed from the feeding tube
- *Measurement:* Measuring and recording the length of the tube outside of the client's nose and then before boluses or every 4-8 hours, checking the measurement.
- *Radiography:* checking the abdominal x-ray film for tube position

Auscultation (injecting air into the feeding tube and listening with a stethoscope) is the least reliable method and should not be used to evaluate the tube tip position. Measuring the length of tube and observing the aspirated fluid and checking its pH are more useful. However, aspiration should not replace a radiographic evaluation after the initial placement or when tube migration is suspected.[23]

An enterostomy (e.g., gastrostomy, jejunostomy) tube can migrate in or out if it is not properly secured at the exit site with sutures or a tube attachment device. Enteral feeding tubes that are not well secured at the exit site can pivot, causing an accumulation of granulation tissue and a widening of the tract. If the tract becomes widened, formula and digestive enzymes can pass through it and excoriate the skin on the abdomen.[10]

Prevent Aspiration

Preventing aspiration during enteral feeding is crucial.[23] The use of postpyloric or small bowel feeding is recommended for a client with a high risk of aspiration. Proper administration and delivery techniques are especially important during gastric feedings. The head of the bed must be elevated 45 degrees for 1 hour before, during, and 1 hour after gastric feeding. Continuous gastric feedings require that the head of the client's bed remain elevated. Gastric residuals can be monitored every 4 hours initially and then as needed to assess gastric emptying and to prevent aspiration. A significant gastric residual is approximately 150 ml, but the volume can be more or less depending on the volumes and rates infused. Feeding into the jejunum theoretically reduces the risk of aspirating enteral formula, particularly for clients with any gastric resection. However, the head of the bed should still be elevated about 30 degrees during continuous jejunal feeding. The addition of blue dye to the enteral feeding should be discouraged. Case reports have documented systemic absorption of the dye in critically ill clients.[21]

Maintain Enteral Access

Nasoenteric tubes most often exit the nose and are secured to the nose or cheek with tape or an adhesive attachment device. To prevent skin breakdown, nasoenteric tubes should exit the nose, hang straight down, and then be gently looped up and secured to the cheek. Tubes that are sharply angled as they exit the nostril can cause necrosis or obstruct the flow of enteral formula through the tube. With any method of securing, the tube should be repositioned and resecured at least every other day to prevent skin irritation.

For tubes that exit the abdominal wall (e.g., PEG, gastrostomy, and jejunostomy tubes), a dressing is required for the first 24 hours after placement. The site care consists of a daily cleaning with mild soap and rinsing with warm water. Dressings are optional for healed enterostomy sites, but a light nonocclusive dressing may help secure the tube as well as contain mucus that commonly drains from the tube tract.

Maintaining the patency of the enteral feeding tube is a critical nursing intervention for the client receiving enteral feeding.

Enteral feeding tubes clog for a variety of reasons, the most common of which is the improper administration of medications through the tube. Medication administration via enteral feeding tubes is probably the most poorly understood part of working with enteral feeding devices and thus is highly susceptible to error. Medications should be given through an enteral access device only when there is an absolute contraindication to taking them by mouth. Problems that can result from incorrect medication

administration via an enteral feeding tube include tube clogging, altered drug availability, and diarrhea. If a client has two tubes in place, such as a gastric tube for decompression and a jejunal or duodenal tube for feeding, consider whether medications could be delivered via the larger gastric tube, as long as the client can tolerate 1/2 hour of postmedication tube clamping. Box 29-2 lists steps to follow for safe administration of medications via an enteral feeding tube.

Tubes of any diameter clog without strict adherence to a flushing protocol. The most effective irrigant for flushing an enteral feeding tube is water. Flush the tube with at least 30 ml of warm water every 4 hours during continuous feedings and before and after each intermittent feeding or medication. Acidic flushing solutions, such as cranberry juice, may precipitate with protein and obstruct the tube; thus they are not recommended.[15]

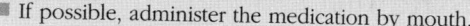

> **BOX 29-2 Guidelines for the Administration of Medications via an Enteral Feeding Tube**
>
> ■ If possible, administer the medication by mouth.
> ■ Use a liquid form of the medication if available.
> ■ If the medication can be crushed, crush it to a fine powder and dissolve it in 30 ml of water.
> ■ Do not crush enteric-coated or time-released tablets or capsules.
> ■ Flush the tube with 30 ml of water before and after giving each medication.
> ■ Do not mix multiple medications or give them together.
> ■ Do not deliver a medication into the small intestine if it must be absorbed in the stomach, such as sucralfate (Carafate) or antacids.
> ■ Hold feedings 1 to 2 hours before and after giving a medication that might have drug-nutrient interactions, such as phenytoin (Dilantin).

Prevent Contamination of Formula and Delivery System

You are primarily responsible for administering and monitoring enteral feeding. The care and handling of the feeding formula and equipment is a key factor in the success of enteral feeding. To prevent contamination of the enteral formula, you must adhere to strict hand-washing before handling the feeding formula and equipment. Open delivery systems, which use cans, syringes, and bags, are the most vulnerable to contamination because of the great degree of manipulation. Formulas administered via an open system should hang for only 4 hours before being changed and the tubing flushed or rinsed. The equipment should be changed every 24 hours. Closed delivery systems, which use a prefilled container with sterile contents, minimize the preparation required by nurses; thus the chance of formula contamination is reduced and the hang time is extended (24 to 48 hours). The Management and Delegation feature on p. 586 outlines the care of selected enteral feeding equipment.

Medical Management of the Client Receiving Parenteral Nutrition

When the gut is not functional or the client cannot be fed enterally, parenteral nutrition (PN) is indicated to maintain nutritional status and prevent malnutrition. Box 29-3 outlines common indications for the use of PN.

Parenteral Nutrition Components

The PN prescription is guided by the nutritional assessment and the definition of nutrient goals for calories and protein. The PN solution contains carbohydrates, fat, protein, fluid, electrolytes, vitamins, and trace elements to meet the client's nutritional requirements.

Carbohydrates. Glucose usually accounts for 50% to 70% of the caloric supply. At least 100 to 150 g of glucose (350 to 500 kcal) should be given daily to prevent catabolism of muscle and to provide glucose for the brain.

Fat Emulsions. Lipid or fat emulsions generally provide about 10% to 30% of the daily caloric need. Fat emulsions (1) provide a calorie-dense (9 kcal/g fat) isotonic energy source and (2) supply fatty acids to prevent essential fatty acid deficiency.

Protein. Crystalline amino acids of differing composition and with concentrations ranging from 3% to 15% are the source of protein in parenteral solutions. The standard commercially available solutions are a mix of essential and nonessential amino acids. Some amino acid solutions have been developed to target specific clinical problems, such as renal failure and liver failure. However, the increase in efficacy over the general amino acid solution is not conclusive, and the cost is considerably greater than for standard formulations.

Fluids, Electrolytes, Vitamins, and Trace Elements. Fluids, electrolytes, vitamins, and trace elements are all equally important in the parenteral nutrient solution. The daily electrolyte regimen should be individualized and should reflect the client's clinical condition (including any ongoing losses) and the function of major organ systems. Like enteral diets, vitamins and trace elements are needed to promote optimal nutritional repletion and support a variety of important metabolic pathways for

MANAGEMENT AND DELEGATION

Nasogastric Tubes

Decompression relieves stomach pressure by removing gas and fluids from the stomach. It can be used to prevent nausea, vomiting, and gastric distention when gastrointestinal (GI) motility is delayed or absent, or when the client has a distal obstruction or recent GI tract surgery. Nasogastric tubes may also be used to initiate enteral feedings upon resumption of bowel motility.

The detailed assessment and potential risks associated with nasogastric tube insertion, maintenance, and removal prevent delegation of these procedures to unlicensed personnel. You may delegate the gathering of equipment and the measurement, recording, and testing of nasogastric drainage to assistive personnel. Delegation of short-term disconnection of nasogastric tubes (for the purposes of toileting or ambulation) may be appropriate under the supervision of a registered nurse (RN). Reconnection of the nasogastric tube to suction requires the RN to verify pressure settings. You may delegate skin care of the client's nose and oral hygiene to unlicensed personnel.

SMALL-BORE FEEDING TUBES AND GASTROSTOMY AND JEJUNOSTOMY TUBES

The most desirable and appropriate method of providing nutrition is via the oral route. For clients who are unable to meet their nutritional needs orally, enteral tube feedings may be an option. Tube feedings may be delivered through large-bore or small-bore gastric tubes that may be inserted by the RN with a physician's order, through gastrostomy tubes, or through jejunostomy tubes. A gastrostomy tube is large and is surgically or endoscopically placed directly into the stomach, exiting through an incision in the left upper quadrant of the abdomen. A jejunostomy tube is also placed surgically (directly into the jejunum for small bowel feedings), or endoscopically (into the gastrostomy tube and passed through to the jejunum).

A physician's order is required for placement of a small-bore nasogastric or nasointestinal feeding tube. Accuracy of feeding tube placement is confirmed by abdominal radiograph. Insertion of nasogastric tubes and verification of placement of nasogastric, gastrostomy, and jejunostomy tubes require problem-solving and knowledge application unique to the professional nurse. For this reason, delegation of these skills is inappropriate. You may delegate skin care of the exit site of the tube to unlicensed personnel.

clients receiving PN. Multivitamin preparations contain both water-soluble and fat-soluble vitamins for daily use. Vitamin K, a fat-soluble vitamin, is not contained in all of these commercial preparations and may be added to the PN formula weekly (10 mg) or daily (1 mg). Other vitamins are sometimes added to the standard vitamin preparation, such as vitamin C to promote wound healing and vitamin B_{12}, thiamine, and folic acid to correct deficiencies commonly associated with alcohol abuse. Guidelines for the administration of trace elements have been outlined by organizations such as the

---

American Society of Parenteral and Enteral Nutrition and are based on age and condition of clients.[24,25]

Combination Systems. In some cases, lipids are infused separately from PN. A total nutrient admixture (TNA) is a single-bag PN delivery system that contains all the required nutrients—glucose, lipids, amino acids, electrolytes, vitamins, and trace elements. The main advantages of the TNA are decreased contamination from fewer manipulations of the IV delivery system, slow continuous infusion of all nutrients supplied, and the need for a single pump for delivery. The main disadvantage is that it is more difficult to detect crystalline precipitates through the TNA. An inline filter is recommended to reduce the risks of TNA precipitates (NOTE: use of inline filter is not a guarantee that precipitates will not be infused).

Vascular Access Devices

Because of the hypertonic glucose concentration, PN is most commonly infused into the central venous circulation where the flow of blood rapidly dilutes the concentration of the solution. Central venous access devices may be inserted percutaneously at the bedside or may be surgically implanted. Catheter tips may be inserted into peripheral veins (e.g., basilic or femoral) or large veins (e.g., subclavian or jugular) and then advanced to the junction of the atrium and superior vena cava. The tip of the catheter must be positioned in a high-flow vein, such as the superior or inferior vena cava, and confirmed by radiograph before PN is infused.

Percutaneous, nontunneled central venous catheters placed via the internal jugular or subclavian veins are often used in acute care settings for a short time. Peripherally inserted central venous catheters (PICC) (see Figure 17-2, C on p. 282) are inserted into a peripheral vein and threaded into the subclavian vein and may be used for months. For extended therapy (>12 weeks), external tunneled central venous catheters or totally implanted ports are the best option (see Figure 17-2, *A* and *B* on p. 282).[14]

For a few clients who can tolerate large volumes of fluid (2 to 3 liters/day), have good peripheral venous access, have low caloric requirements, and require parenteral nutrition for a short time (less than 5 days), *peripheral parenteral nutrition* (PPN) may be used.

> To avoid phlebitis of peripheral veins, it is necessary to keep the osmolarity of the solution less than 900 mOsm/kg, which may require either reduction in glucose and amino acid content or prohibitive fluid administration.

Because of the limitations in glucose and amino acid content, peripheral nutrition may result in caloric and nitrogen underfeeding. Clients who have difficult peripheral venous access, particularly older adults, or those who require parenteral support for more than 5 days should not be treated with PPN. In clients who have excessive caloric or nitrogen needs because of their illness, central access for PN is recommended.

Nursing Management of the Client Receiving Parenteral Therapy

> To ensure optimal nutrition outcomes, nurses must verify PN bags contain the correct nutrients and are infusing at the proper rate. In addition, nurses must intervene to reduce or prevent mechanical, metabolic, and infectious complications associated with PN.

Administer Parenteral Nutrition

> You are responsible for safely administering and monitoring the PN infusion. Just before delivery, check every solution for its expiration date, the correct ingredients (glucose, fat, protein, electrolytes, vitamins, trace elements), leaks or tears in the bag, and the appearance of the solution (separating or cracking of the solution). PN solutions that are past the expiration date or with evidence of leaks or tears in the bag should be destroyed. Check with the pharmacist before destroying PN bags with evidence of cracking or precipitates, as some cases may need follow-up to determine the cause of these types of problems. PN must be delivered using an infusion pump to accurately control the infusion rate and prevent the possibility of a bolus.[39a]

PN solutions are typically infused over 24 hours in the acute care setting. In the home, clients often receive PN at a faster rate so as to infuse all of their nutrients while they are sleeping.

Prevent Mechanical Complications

> **Misplaced and occluded access devices are examples of mechanical complications. Before infusing PN, verify that an x-ray has been done and the tip of the central access device is located at the junction of the vena cava and atrium. Verify the access device is secured by stitches or catheter holders and sterile transparent dressing. You play a pivotal role in ensuring the proper functioning of the vascular access system. Typically, catheter patency is maintained by following a routine heparin or saline flush protocol. However, catheters may differ by manufacturer. Verify the manufacturer's recommendations for the amount and type of solution that should be used to flush the central venous catheter. Report any difficulty with flushing or infusing PN, as this may be indicative of an occlusion, either clot or precipitant. Early detection by you and intervention by physicians or advanced practice nurses may provide an opportunity to salvage a central access device and prevent the client from being exposed to the risks of inserting a new catheter. Assess the area around the catheter insertion site for swelling that might be suggestive of a central vein thrombosis.**

SAFETY ALERT

Prevent Metabolic Complications

Electrolyte disturbances, hyperglycemia, and allergic reactions are examples of metabolic complications. Clients who are severely malnourished and started on PN may develop life-threatening hypokalemia, hypomagnesemia, and hypophosphatemia. To prevent this from occurring, PN rates should be started slowly in severely malnourished clients and electrolytes should be checked frequently before the PN rate is advanced. Acute electrolyte repletion is best accomplished intravenously via a separate infusion bag.

> **The first time PN is administered, blood glucose levels should be monitored every 6 hours to assess the client's response to glucose. If blood glucose level is within the normal range for 24 hours after the client has reached the maximum recommended PN rate, monitoring can be changed to daily.**

SAFETY ALERT

Tight control of hyperglycemia in the PN client has been associated with improved outcomes.[34] Persistent elevations of blood glucose level are managed by delivering regular insulin in the PN solution after the daily requirement for insulin is determined. If the client's clinical status is unstable or the insulin dose cannot be stabilized over a 24-hour period, or both, the insulin should be delivered separate from the PN as an insulin drip or intermittent subcutaneous injections. Most clients can tolerate an acute discontinuation of PN and therefore do not need to be weaned from PN gradually.

SAFETY
⚠
ALERT

Although rare, allergic reactions to lipid preparations or multivitamins have been reported and usually present within 30 minutes. A clinical manifestation of reactions can be any of the following: fever, shaking chills, shortness of breath, chest pain, back pain, or full anaphylaxis. If the client complains of any of these manifestations, stop the PN infusion immediately and inform the health care team of the manifestations to determine appropriate further treatment. Some lipids contain egg lecithin as an emulsifier. Before infusing lipids, verify that the client has no egg allergies.

Prevent Infectious Complications

Prevention of catheter-related infection is the key to the successful use of parenteral nutrition.

SAFETY
⚠
ALERT

🪔 Prevention of infection is also one of The Joint Commission's National Patient Safety Goals. Approximately one quarter of a million infections in hospitalized clients are associated with central venous access devices. For each of those infections, there is an estimated attributable mortality of 12% to 25%.[28] 🪔 Furthermore, the addition of PN through a central venous access device increases the risk of infection two- to nine-fold.[1-3,31] To reduce the risk of infection, you must follow strict guidelines or protocols for the care of the vascular access device before, during, and after its insertion.[8,36,37]

Strict adherence to hand-washing and aseptic technique is clearly the most important way to prevent infection. Masks and sterile gloves should be worn when changing dressings over nontunneled catheters. To minimize manipulations of the catheter, one lumen of a multilumen catheter should be dedicated (and marked) for the infusion of PN. 🪔 The most recent recommendations from the Centers for Disease Control and Prevention (CDC) are to change the tubing for PN solutions every 24 hours.[28]

The dressing change protocol for central venous access devices continues to be controversial. Various protocols exist for skin cleaning and the type and frequency of dressing change. The catheter exit site should be cleaned with an antiseptic agent, such as 70% alcohol and 10% povidone-iodine. A preferred product that has shown positive results in preventing catheter-related infections is chlorhexidine.[28] Antibiotic ointments should not be applied to the catheter exit site.

The type of dressing applied over the catheter exit site should be either a sterile gauze pad or a transparent dressing. Frequency of dressing changes depends on client needs (e.g., more frequent changes are needed for a diaphoretic client) and the type of dressing. Gauze dressings typically are changed every 48 hours, transparent dressings every 3 to 7 days. The most important concept is that the dressing must remain adherent to be effective. Therefore any dressing must be changed immediately if it becomes damp, soiled, or loose. Follow your agency's policy regarding dressing change protocols. Table 29-6 outlines suggested protocols for central catheters that deliver PN.

Evaluation of Nutritional Interventions

When caring for a client receiving enteral or parenteral feedings, you must regularly evaluate the client's response to therapy. Assessing the client's tolerance to the nutrient regimen includes evaluation of the fluid status (intake and output data and weights) and a thorough assessment of the GI system. Evaluation also includes monitoring vital signs, reviewing laboratory tests, and assessing the function of the nutritional access device.

TABLE 29–6 Central Venous Catheter Maintenance

Catheter Type	Site Care	Flushing
Nontunneled central venous catheter	*Dressing:* Transparent or gauze Transparent dressing enhances catheter stability Performed as a sterile dressing Skin antisepsis protocols include one or a combination of the following: 70% alcohol (3 swabs), 10% povidone-iodine (3 swabs), chlorhexidine	*Flush volume:* 3-5 ml *Frequency:* Usually daily
Tunneled, cuffed central venous catheter	*Dressing:* Transparent or gauze until incision healed Dressing commonly discontinued when incision healed and suture removed Performed as an aseptic dressing (skin antisepsis as above)	*Flush volume:* 3-4 ml *Frequency:* Usually daily *Groshong catheters:* 5 ml 0.9% normal saline solution weekly
Peripherally inserted central catheter	*Dressing:* Transparent preferred to enhance catheter stability Performed as a sterile dressing (skin antisepsis as above) Dressings required as long as catheter is in place	*Flush volume:* 2-3 ml *Frequency:* Daily
Ports	*Dressing:* To stabilize Huber needle for port access and infusion of PN Sterile gauze may be placed between needle and skin Huber needle changed at least every 7 days	*Flush volume:* At least 3 ml *Frequency:* Every 4 weeks

From Altman, G.B. (Ed.) (2004). *Delmar's fundamental and advanced nursing skills* (2nd ed.). Delmar Park, N.Y.: Thompson Delmar Learning; and O'Grady, A., et al. (2002). Guidelines for the prevention of intravascular catheter-related infections. *Morbidity and Mortality Weekly Report, CDC 51* (RR-10), 1-31.

Together with a nutritional support team, you will be collecting pertinent data, such as weight, intestinal tolerance, and pertinent laboratory values, to assess the success of the nutrient prescription.

Box 29-4 outlines common parameters used to monitor clients receiving enteral or parenteral nutrition. Comprehensive and routine monitoring can prevent complications related to nutritional support therapies.

Self-Care

Nutritional support therapies, such as enteral and parenteral feedings, are routinely administered in the home setting. Nurses play a pivotal role in determining appropriate candidates for home nutrition support by helping determine the plan of care and providing client and family education.

The nursing assessment includes a comprehensive review of the client and family or caregivers.

To ensure the client or caregiver can carry out complex procedures, the physical and cognitive abilities must be evaluated. Manual dexterity and eyesight are particularly important when care involves programming pumps for infusion and drawing up medication in syringes. The client's home environment must be evaluated to ensure that it is safe for home therapy. The client or caregiver education process should ideally start in the hospital and be reinforced after discharge. Clients receiving either enteral tube feedings or parenteral nutrition need to learn a wide range of related skills (Box 29-5).

EATING DISORDERS

OBESITY

Obesity is characterized by an excess accumulation of fat and reflects, on the most basic level, an overall positive balance between energy intake and expenditure. The causes of obesity are not fully understood, but are recognized as complex and pervasive.

Obesity is defined worldwide by the body mass index (BMI):

$$BMI = Weight\ (kg)/Height\ (m^2)$$

Because BMI greater than $25\ kg/m^2$ is associated with increased prevalence of hypertension and type 2 diabetes mellitus, this level of BMI has been designated as overweight. The prevalence of chronic disease comorbidities is increased further with BMI greater than $30\ kg/m^2$, which is defined as obesity. BMI greater than $40\ kg/m^2$ is accepted as severe obesity.[29] Obesity is a worldwide problem, and by the year 2010 obesity-associated chronic diseases, such as cardiovascular disease, type 2 diabetes mellitus, sleep apnea, and

---

BOX 29-4 Suggested Nutrition Monitoring Protocol

Parameter	Frequency of Assessment
BIOCHEMICAL MEASURES	
Electrolytes	Daily
Magnesium, calcium, phosphorus	Daily
Glucose	Every 6 hours for 48 hours, then daily
Albumin, prealbumin, transferrin	Weekly
Triglyceride	Pre-infusion, post-infusion, then daily
Liver function tests	Pre-infusion, then weekly
Complete blood count, prothrombin time, partial thromboplastin time	Weekly
NURSING ASSESSMENT	
Weight	Daily
Intake/output	Hourly/every 8 hours
Infusion rate	Every 4 hours
Temperature	Every 8 hours
NUTRITIONAL MONITORING	
24-hour urine collection for urinary urea nitrogen	Weekly
Measured resting energy expenditure	Weekly

BOX 29-5 Teaching Topics for Clients Who Need Enteral or Parenteral Feedings at Home

CARE OF THE NUTRITIONAL ACCESS DEVICE
- Flushing the venous access or feeding tube
- Changing the dressing
- Observing for evidence of infection

FORMULA PREPARATION
- Adding medication to the TPN formula
- Placing enteral formula in the feeding bag
- Setting up the enteral or parenteral feeding pump or bag
- Obtaining formula for TPN and related supplies

MONITORING FOR COMPLICATIONS
- Assessing temperature
- Monitoring weight

TPN, Total parenteral nutrition.

---

hypertension, will lead the causes of death in developing countries, far outpacing the current realities of starvation and infectious diseases.

According to the National Health and Nutrition Examination Survey's (NHANES) 2004 data, 66% of Americans are overweight, 32% are obese, and 5% are severely obese. African-American and Hispanic American women are particularly affected, out of proportion to their Caucasian counterparts. Obesity in children in the United States is also growing rampantly, with 18% of all children older than age 2 years being overweight or obese, and greater proportions of minority children than Caucasians being overweight.[29]

Etiology and Risk Factors

The etiology of obesity is multifactorial, making effective prevention and treatment a challenge. Environmental, biologic, and socioeconomic factors are currently seen as key:

1. *Environmental.* Both in the United States and by the evaluation of the World Health Organization, the environment is accepted as a key component of the burgeoning obesity epidemic. The environment impacts both the energy expenditure and the energy intake sides of the energy balance equation.

As cultures become progressively more developed, individuals spend more time sitting (watching television, working with computers) than moving (sports, walking). When the school budgets are tightened, priority is given to electronic resources such as computers and television, and sports programs are eliminated.

Concurrently, the portion sizes of servings of food in restaurants and movie theaters have increased markedly over time, with minimal increment in cost. The end result of the combined effects of reduced energy expenditure and increased energy intake has been termed the "toxic environment," a combination that insidiously promotes weight gain.

2. *Genetic Tendency.* The broad prevalence of obesity in American culture suggests that genetic factors may be less important than previously thought. There are similarities in obesity prevalence within family units, but environment is also a common factor. Many obesity genes have been identified, but none have yet explained the broad prevalence of obesity, even in individuals with severe obesity.

The Pima Indians of Arizona and Mexico have been used historically as an example of a group who may have a thrifty genotype. Severe obesity and type 2 diabetes mellitus are prevalent in the population of Pimas who live in Arizona, who are exposed to an inexpensive, high-calorie food supply. By contrast, those who live in Mexico, with a more traditional diet that is considerably lower in caloric content and that requires considerable expenditure of energy to produce, have much lower prevalence of obesity. These two groups have identical genetic make-up, suggesting that genetic influences may be less important than environmental influences.[29]

3. *Socioeconomic Factors.* Particularly in the United States, obesity is more prevalent in populations with lower socioeconomic status. This trend may reflect a more toxic environment in terms of energy-dense but nutrient-poor food supply and excess television watching. In poorer neighborhoods, outdoor physical activity is limited by concerns for physical safety, and some efforts are underway to provide safe exercise environments in poor neighborhoods.

4. *Ethnic Disparities.* In the United States, Hispanic and African-American women are affected by obesity at greater rates than their Caucasian counterparts or men of the same ethnicity. The reasons for this phenomenon are not clear, necessitating particular sensitivity in dealing with obesity across cultures and possibly requiring different approaches toward prevention.

Pathophysiology and Clinical Manifestations

Obesity is a serious health risk and has been associated with increased risk of mortality and morbidity. Obesity is associated with a series of medical co-morbidities, including type 2 diabetes mellitus, cardiovascular disease, hypertension, hyperlipidemias, stroke, sleep apnea, obesity hypoventilation syndrome, arthritis, and some cancers.[7] Cancers, such as colorectal, breast, and prostate cancer, have been linked to obesity. However, whether this link between cancer and obesity is simply due to the excess weight, to specific dietary factors, or to difficulty in early diagnosis as a result of body build is unclear.

The mechanisms behind the obesity co-morbidities are not completely understood. It is clear, however, that the insulin resistance that is typical of truncal obesity is associated with type 2 diabetes mellitus and hypertriglyceridemia. The sleep and respiratory problems seen with obesity are due to excess fat deposits in the airways and neck. Tendencies toward thrombosis may in part be attributable to reduced physical activity combined with venous stasis.

With loss of 5% to 10% of body weight, significant improvement in co-morbid conditions occurs. Blood pressure and cholesterol levels decrease with resultant reductions in medication use. Type 2 diabetes mellitus improves greatly with weight loss and the sleep disturbances improve markedly.[22]

OUTCOME MANAGEMENT

Medical Management

When a client has severe obesity, the quality of nursing care is key to client and caregiver safety. Oversized equipment may be indicated for safe transfer, transport, and skin management. Clients may require scales calibrated for accuracy at a higher range of body weight, larger blood pressure cuffs and tracheostomies, and oversized gowns for them to be cared for comfortably during a hospital admission or at home. Skin and wound problems are more prevalent in clients with severe obesity and require particular nursing attention for assessment and management.[13]

The medical management of obesity should include a combination of diet, behavior modification, exercise, and occasionally medication. A team, including a psychologist with behavior modification skills and a registered dietitian, can provide the optimal intervention to encourage weight loss. A balanced deficit diet that supplies 500 to 1000 kcal less than total daily energy expenditure should promote the loss of 1 to 2 pounds per week. It is important to note that the focus is on calorie restriction and not the amount of food consumed.[20] To prevent weight regain, it is also necessary to teach clients better diet management skills even if they use meal replacement formulas or very low-calorie diet regimens to begin weight loss. More severe calorie restrictions are difficult to maintain for longer periods and require vitamin and mineral supplementation. Clients consuming low-calorie diets should ingest about 60 g/day of protein (approximately 25% of total calories).

An exercise program should be part of the overall care of the obese client. Exercise is an important way to increase the energy expenditure and to facilitate weight loss. The inclusion of exercise into daily activities (e.g., taking the stairs rather than elevators, parking the car far away from the entrance at work), termed *lifestyle modification,* shows promise. Diet restriction in combination with an exercise program, compared with diet restriction alone, is a more successful way to lose weight and maintain the weight loss.

The role of medications in promoting weight loss is an area of current research. At present, three categories of drugs have FDA approval for the treatment of obesity. Meridia (sibutramine) is an anorectic that targets neurotransmitters to reduce appetite. Phentermine is a thermogenic drug that increases energy expenditure and targets neurotransmitters to reduce appetite. Xenical (orlistat) is a peripheral lipase inhibitor that reduces digestion and absorption of fats.[32] As with all medications, there are side effects associated with each category of drug. Meridia (sibutramine) may be habit-forming and should be used with caution in clients with hypertension or heart disease. Meridia and phentermine may be habit forming and should be used with caution in clients with uncontrolled hypertension or heart disease. They are usually prescribed for 3-6 weeks. Phentermine may induce palpitations or insomnia. Clients taking orlistat may complain of loose stools and flatulence and are risk of fat-soluble vitamin deficiencies because of reduced fat absorption. Although various drugs have been effective in promoting weight loss, any prescribed drug therapy regimen should be under the strict supervision of a qualified health care team to prevent potentially life-threatening complications.

Surgical Management

Surgical treatment of obesity is recommended by the National Heart, Lung, and Blood Institute (NHLBI) for clients who have BMI greater than 40 kg/m^2 or greater than 35 kg/m^2 with co-morbid complications (see www.nhlbi.nih.gov/guidelines/obesity/ob_home.htm). These clients generally have been unsuccessful with multiple diet modifications, behavioral therapy, and drug therapy, and they are so obese that aggressive physical activity is not feasible. Two surgical approaches are currently in use: (1) gastric restrictive and (2) restrictive plus malabsorptive.[22,30] An earlier procedure, the jejunoileal bypass, is no longer performed because of metabolic complications from the extreme malabsorption induced by the procedure.

Gastric Restrictive Procedure

The size of the stomach is reduced by one of two procedures—the vertical banded gastroplasty or the adjustable gastric band. Both involve creation of a small gastric pouch with a restricted outlet to the remaining portion of the stomach. For the adjustable gastric band, a band is placed around the stomach and a subcutaneous port allows for sizing of the band and altering of the outlet size without the need for an additional surgery. Diet instruction must be part of the postoperative care of these clients, focusing on the increased frequency and decreased size of low-calorie meals. In addition, clients are instructed to take a chewable or liquid multivitamin every day.[22,30] Because permanent neurologic changes have occurred from a lack of thiamine, a lifetime of vitamin supplementation must be emphasized.

Malabsorptive Procedure

In addition to the gastric stapling outlined above, the gastric bypass procedure bypasses a segment of duodenum from the food stream, thus inducing the malabsorption of nutrients and dumping manifestations when concentrated sugars are ingested. This gastric bypass procedure is most commonly performed in the United States when substantial weight loss is desired and the client has minimal surgical risk. Approximately 30% of the client's presenting weight is lost in the first year and maintenance of most of the lost weight has been documented for more than 14 years. The diet instruction for gastric bypass is similar to that for gastroplasty alone, but the importance of avoiding sweets to control manifestations of dumping syndrome is emphasized.[22,30]

ANOREXIA NERVOSA AND BULIMIA NERVOSA

Anorexia nervosa is a condition of self-generated weight loss, usually seen in adolescent girls and young women, but also in middle-age women or men.[27,42,43] The criteria for diagnosis of anorexia nervosa include a preoccupation with personal body weight and appearance, behaviors directed at thinness (excess activity and inadequate caloric intake), and the physical results of these behaviors (including extreme weight loss, amenorrhea, osteoporosis, and malnutrition). The psychopathologic presentation dictates the need for psychiatric intervention. A multidisciplinary team approach focused on consistency in addressing the behaviors characteristic of the disease has the greatest success with overall treatment.

Bulimia nervosa is a less serious and entirely separate illness. Clients with bulimia nervosa tend to maintain a relatively normal weight, but go through periods of eating excessively (bingeing) and vomiting (purging) gastric contents to prevent weight gain. It has been suggested that bulimia nervosa is a form of depressive illness.

Etiology and Risk Factors

Anorexia nervosa affects approximately 0.2% to 0.5% of young women. Bulimia nervosa affects 2% to 3% of the same group. Women are 10 times more likely to be affected by an eating disorder than men. These disorders are more prevalent in Western cultures, although their occurrence is increasing in Asian cultures.[42]

Although the cause of eating disorders is not certain, several factors are likely to contribute to development of the disorders. Sociocultural and environmental factors including media and peer influences, family factors including parental discord, and biologic factors including genetics, neurotransmitter regulation, and hormonal functioning have been implicated.[43] Negative affect, low self-esteem, and dieting behavior commonly predate the onset of an eating disorder.

Pathophysiology

The physical changes associated with anorexia nervosa are similar to those seen in starvation. When caloric intake is severely limited, the body adapts by using the body's fat stores and sparing nitrogen stores. With prolonged starvation, significant shifts in fluid and electrolyte balance can occur and can be life-threatening. Alterations in the metabolism of insulin, thyroid hormone, and catecholamines explain common clinical manifestations, including decreases in pulse rate, respiratory rate, blood pressure, cardiac output, and gut motility.[27,42] The hypothalamus responds to the lack of nutrient intake with changes in pituitary function,

resulting in amenorrhea and infertility. Clients with bulimia nervosa may or may not develop these changes. The extent of malnutrition will determine the pathophysiologic changes observed.

Clinical Manifestations

Clients with anorexia nervosa are usually first introduced to the health care system when the disordered eating behavior results in obvious weight loss. Clients may limit themselves to 200 to 500 kcal/day—less than half of the amount needed for ideal body weight. Physical manifestations include dry skin, pallor, bradycardia, hypotension, intolerance to cold, constipation, and amenorrhea (Figure 29-3).

Clinical manifestations of bulimia nervosa include episodes of binge eating followed by self-induced vomiting. The eating and vomiting episodes occur most often in the late afternoon and evening and are done in secret. Some clients may abuse laxatives and diuretics as well.

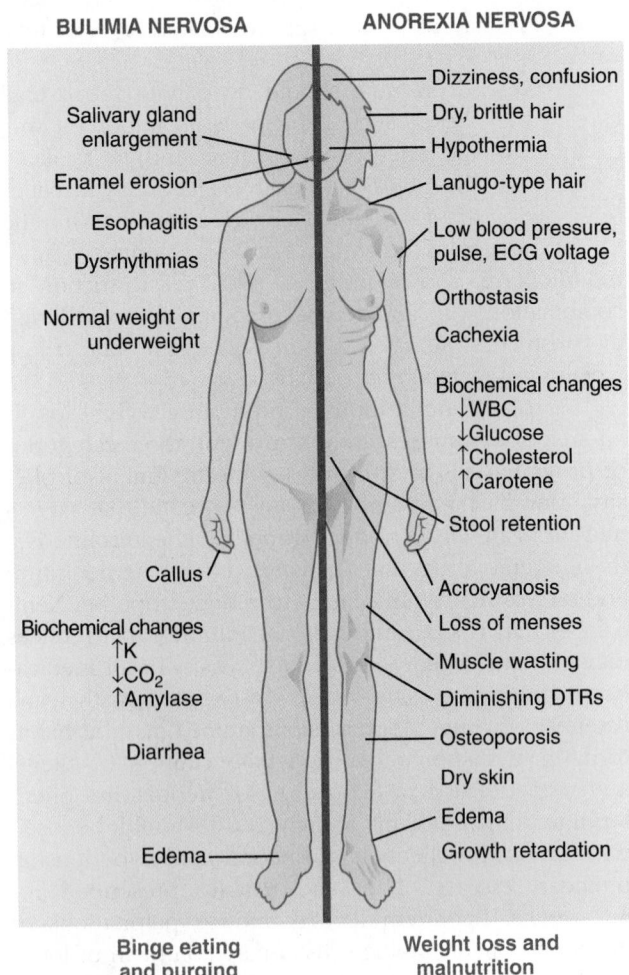

■ **FIGURE 29–3** Physical manifestations of anorexia nervosa and bulimia nervosa. *CO₂*, Carbon dioxide; *DTRs*, deep tendon reflexes; *ECG*, electrocardiograph; *K*, potassium; *WBC*, white blood cell. (*From Mahan, L.K., & Escott-Stump, S.E. [2004]. Krause's food, nutrition, & diet therapy [11th ed., p. 604]. Philadelphia: Saunders.*)

Personality characteristics typical of clients with bulimia are related to depression. Physical manifestations may not be as obvious, because the client with bulimia may be of normal weight without any depletion of fat stores. Less obvious clinical manifestations are erosion of tooth enamel from frequent vomiting and esophageal and throat irritation.

OUTCOME MANAGEMENT

Medical Management

The medical management of eating disorders must include psychological as well as nutritional components. Psychotherapy should focus on the underlying problems causing the disordered eating behavior. The physical rehabilitation of nutritional status targets ways to normalize the client's eating pattern and to help the client begin regaining weight, if needed. Excessive caloric intakes are not necessary in clients with anorexia and can actually be harmful in the severely malnourished client. A registered dietitian should be part of the treatment team and assist in the determination of caloric goals.

Hospitalization is necessary when malnutrition is severe enough to result in serious fluid and electrolyte disturbances. Enteral or parenteral therapy may be needed in extreme cases when the client has not responded to strategies to encourage and improve oral intake, although clients must be taught good eating skills as a part of the therapy. Nutritional support therapies should be introduced slowly in severely malnourished clients to avoid complications of refeeding syndrome. Refeeding syndrome is characterized by precipitous decreases in serum potassium, magnesium, and phosphorus levels when nutrients are administered to depleted clients.

Nursing Management of the Client with Eating Disorders

A comprehensive history helps identify the type of eating disorder. Collect details of weight history and eating patterns to successfully identify the problem and help develop an appropriate plan of care. Have the client describe his or her typical pattern of eating, and ask about the use of appetite-suppressing medication, laxatives, and self-induced vomiting. Other pertinent data include exercise patterns and menstrual history. Interventions are focused on improving the client's self-esteem and body image and on consuming a healthy diet.

Improve Body Image

Recognize that clients suffering from eating disorders typically have low self-esteem. These clients see their self-regulation of food and exercise as ways to prove

they are successful. It is important to involve the client's family and friends to encourage the client as changes are made in the client's eating and physical activity behaviors.

Improve Nutritional Intake

For clients suffering with anorexia nervosa the goal is to induce a safe weight gain of no more than 1 to 2 pounds per week. When caring for a client with anorexia nervosa, help the client select foods from the Food Guide Pyramid for a nutritionally balanced diet. The client is usually allowed to refuse a specific number of foods (such as two or three) so that some sense of control is felt. Observe the client during mealtimes. Be supportive during mealtimes and, if needed, stay with the client following mealtime to prevent the client from purging. Education related to nutrition must include the client's family, caregivers, or co-residents. An accurate calorie count and regular monitoring of weight are other important interventions. Parenteral or enteral nutrition may be needed for refractory clients with extreme malnutrition.

For clients suffering from bulimia, the goal is a safe weight loss of 1 to 2 pounds per week until ideal body weight is achieved and to maintain ideal body weight thereafter. Teach the client how to use the Food Guide Pyramid to select a healthy diet with portions of appropriate size. Encourage the client to eat slowly and develop a regular exercise pattern. Encourage the client to approach food, eating, and self-image in a new way. Provide emotional support and supervision for the client to overcome stressful periods and break the binge-and-purge cycle.

CONCLUSIONS

The nutritional care of the adult medical-surgical client is an important part of a comprehensive treatment plan. Preventing and treating malnutrition is just one way to facilitate recovery from acute and chronic illness. As a nurse, you have a vital role in nutritional assessment as well as in the prevention and treatment of malnutrition. Clients with eating disorders, such as obesity, anorexia nervosa, and bulimia nervosa, may require medical, surgical, or psychological intervention.

THINKING CRITICALLY

1. You are caring for a 62-year-old client in a nursing home. She has had a stroke and is paralyzed, sometimes confused, and incontinent. She refuses to eat and drink after many episodes of coughing and choking at mealtimes. A small-bore feeding tube has been inserted. When you check the tube for aspirate to confirm patency, you are unable to obtain any return aspirate. What

nursing measures should be instituted to determine the problem? What is the priority nursing intervention?

Factors to Consider. What conditions contribute to the lack of aspirate return? What is your decision if the tube remains occluded?

2. You are assigned to care for two clients. One is an older man with a 6-month history of difficulty in swallowing and a weight loss of 25 pounds. The other client, a woman in her mid-30s, has Crohn's disease and has been admitted with an exacerbation of the disease. How should nutritional needs be addressed for each client?

Factors to Consider. How should nutritional needs be met for the client with an upper gastrointestinal tract disorder? With a lower gastrointestinal tract disorder?

3. D.A. is a 20-year-old white woman who is a sophomore in college and living away from home. She is 5 feet 1 inch tall. She has been steadily losing weight, although she participates in the campus meal plan and takes her meals in the dormitory cafeteria. She plays on the college volleyball and basketball teams. Most of the students are excited about Thanksgiving holiday plans, but the dormitory counselor noticed that D.A. has not voiced any plans. She is found unconscious on the floor in the dormitory communal bathroom. She is taken by ambulance to the community hospital. Her college physical health record states that she weighed 98 pounds in June and had no known medical problems. On admission to the hospital, she weighs 79 pounds. What is her percentage of weight loss? What additional data need to be collected?

Factors to Consider. What interventions can be used to increase D.A.'s food intake? Is it feasible for a nurse on a busy medical-surgical unit to stay with D.A. during and after her meals? What alternatives might be used?

evolve *Discussions for these questions can be found on the website.*

BIBLIOGRAPHY

Citations appearing in red refer to primary research.

Citations appearing in blue refer to evidence-based practice guidelines and protocols.

1. Almuneef, M.A., Memish, Z.A., Balkhy, H.H., et al. (2006). Rate, risk factors and outcomes of catheter-related bloodstream infections in paediatric intensive care unit in Saudia Arabia. *Journal of Hospital Infections, 62*(2), 207-213.
2. ASPEN. (2002). Board of directors and the clinical guidelines task force: Guidelines for the use of parenteral nutrition and enteral nutrition in adult and pediatric patients. *Journal of Parenteral and Enteral Nutrition, 26*(Suppl 1).
3. Beghetto, M.G., Victorino, J., Teixeira, L., et al. (2005). Parenteral nutrition as a risk factor for central venous catheter-related infection. *Journal of Parenteral and Enteral Nutrition, 29*(5), 367-373.
4. Bistrian, B., et al. (1974). Protein status of general surgical patients. *Journal of the American Medical Association, 230*, 858-860.
5. Bistrian, B., et al. (1976). Prevalence of malnutrition in general medical patients. *Journal of the American Medical Association, 235*, 1567-1570.
6. Bond, E., & Heitkemper, M. (2003). Protein calorie malnutrition. In V. Carrieri-Kohlman, A. Lindsay, & C. West (Eds.), *Pathophysiological phenomena in nursing: Human responses to illness* (3rd ed.). Philadelphia: Saunders.
7. Casiero, D., & Frishman, W.H. (2006). Cardiovascular complications of eating disorders. *Cardiology in Review, 15*(5), 227-231.
8. CDC. (2005). Reduction in central line-associated bloodstream infections among patients in intensive care units—Pennsylvania, April 2001-March 2005. *MMWR, 54*(40), 1013-1016.
9. Cresci, G.A. (2003). Metabolic stress. In L. Matarese & M. Gottschlich (Eds.), *Contemporary nutrition support: A clinical guide* (2nd ed., pp. 552-559). Philadelphia: Saunders.
10. DeLegge, M.H. (2006). Enteral access in home care. *Journal of Parenteral and Enteral Nutrition, 30*(1), S13-S20.
11. Furhman, M. (2003). Nutrition support: Enteral and parenteral nutrition. In S. Williams & E. Schlenker (Eds.), *Essentials of nutrition and diet therapy* (8th ed., pp. 407-431). Philadelphia: Mosby.
12. Furman, E.F. (2006). Undernutrition in older adults across the continuum of care: Nutritional assessment, barriers, and interventions. *Journal of Gerontological Nursing, 32*(1), 22-27.
13. Gallagher, S. (2002). Obesity and the skin in the critical care setting. *Critical Care Quarterly, 25*(1), 69-76.
14. Grant, J.P. (2006). Anatomy and physiology of venous system vascular access: Implications. *Journal of Parenteral and Enteral Nutrition, 30*(1), S7-S12.
15. Guenter, P., & Silkroski, M. (2001). *Tube feeding: Practical guidelines and nursing protocols.* Silver Spring, Md: Aspen.
16. Haslam, D., & Fang, J. (2006). Enteral access for nutrition in the intensive care unit. *Current Opinions in Clinical Nutrition and Metabolic Care, 9*, 155-159.
17. Kagansky, N., Berner, Y., Koren-Morag, N., et al. (2005). Poor nutritional habits are predictors of poor outcome in very old hospitalized patients. *American Journal of Clinical Nutrition, 82*, 784-791.
18. Kudsk, K., & Sacks, G. (2006). Nutrition in surgery, infection, and trauma. In M.E. Shils, et al. (Eds.), *Modern nutrition in health and disease* (10th ed., pp. 1414-1435). Philadelphia: Lippincott, Williams & Wilkins.
19. Kyle, U.G., Genton, L., & Pichard, C. (2005). Hospital length of stay and nutritional status. *Current Opinions in Clinical Nutrition and Metabolic Care, 8*, 397-402.
20. Ledikwe, J.H., Blanck, H.M., Kettel, K.I., et al. (2006). Dietary energy density is associated with energy intake and weight status in US adults. *American Journal of Clinical Nutrition, 83*(6), 1362-1368.
21. Maloney, J., et al. (2000). Systemic absorption of food dye with sepsis. *New England Journal of Medicine, 343*(14), 1047-1048.
22. Mango, V.L., & Frishman, W.H. (2006). Physiologic, psychologic, and metabolic consequences of bariatric surgery. *Cardiology Review, 14*(5), 232-237.
23. Metheny, N. (2006). Preventing respiratory complications of tube feedings: Evidence-based practice. *American Journal of Critical Care, 15*(4), 360-369.
24. Mirtallo, J. (2001). Introduction to parenteral nutrition. In M. Gottschlich (Ed.), *The science and practice of nutrition support: A case based core curriculum* (pp. 211-224). Dubuque, Iowa: Kendell/Hunt.
25. Mirtallo, J., et al. (2004). Safe practices for parenteral nutrition. *Journal of Parenteral and Enteral Nutrition, 30*(2), S39-70.
26. Mitchell, M. (2003). Aging and older adults. In M. Mitchell (Ed.), *Nutrition across the lifespan* (2nd ed., pp. 429-470). Philadelphia: Saunders.
27. Mitchell, M. (2003). Eating dilemmas: Dietary restraint, binging, purging, excessive consumption, and excessive exercise. In M. Mitchell (Ed.), *Nutrition across the lifespan* (2nd ed., pp. 473-512). Philadelphia: Saunders.
28. O'Grady, A., et al. (2002). Guidelines for the prevention of intravascular catheter-related infections. *Morbidity and Mortality Weekly Report, CDC 51*(RR-10), 1-31.
29. Ogden, C., et al. (2006). Prevalence of overweight and obesity in the United States, 1999-2004. *Journal of the American Medical Association, 295*(13), 1549-1555.

30. Owens, T.M. (2006). Bariatric surgery risks, benefits, and care of the morbidly obese. *Nursing Clinics of North America, 41*(2), 249-263.

31. Oztoprak, N., Cevik, M.A., Akinci, E., et al. (2006). Risk factors for ICU-acquired methicillin-resistant Staphylococcus aureus infections. *American Journal of Infection Control, 34*(1), 1-5.

32. Palamara, K.L., Mogul, H.R., Peterson, S.J., et al. (2006). Obesity: New perspectives and pharmacotherapies. *Cardiology in Review, 14*(5), 238-258.

33. Pichard, C., et al. (2004). Nutritional assessment: Lean body mass depletion at hospital admission is associated with an increased length of stay. *American Journal of Clinical Nutrition, 79*, 613-618.

34. Pittas, A.G., Siegel, R.D., & Lau, J. (2006). Insulin therapy and in-hospital mortality in critically ill patients: Systematic review and meta-analysis of randomized controlled trials. *Journal of Parenteral and Enteral Nutrition, 30*(2), 164-172.

35. Prentice, A., & Webb, F. (2006). Obesity amidst poverty. *International Journal of Epidemiology, 35*(1), 24-30.

36. Rombeau, J.L., & Rolandelli, R.H. (2001). *Clinical nutrition: Parenteral nutrition* (3rd ed.). Philadelphia: Saunders.

37. Ryder, M. (2006). Evidence-based practice in the management of vascular access devices for home parenteral nutrition. *Journal of Parenteral and Enteral Nutrition, 30*(Suppl), S82-93, S98-99.

38. Squires, N. (2006). Dysphagia management for progressive neurological conditions. *Nursing Standard, 20*(29), 53-55.

39. Steiger, E. (2006). Dysfunction and thrombotic complications of vascular access devices. *Journal of Parenteral and Enteral Nutrition, 30*(1), S70-72.

39a. The Joint Commission. (2007). *2008 National Patient Safety Goals Hospital Program*, Retrieved 12/8/07 www.jointcommission.org/PatientSafety/NationalPatientSafetyGoals.

40. Torun, B., & Chew, F. (2006). Protein-energy malnutrition. In M. Shils, et al. (Eds.), *Modern nutrition in health and disease* (10th ed., pp. 881-908). Baltimore: Williams & Wilkins.

41. UNICEF. (2006). *The state of the world's children 2006*. New York: UNICEF.

42. Williams, S., & Schlenker, E. (2003). *Essentials of nutrition and diet therapy* (8th ed.). St. Louis: Mosby.

43. Wolfe, B., & Gimby, L. (2003). Caring for the hospitalized patient with an eating disorder. *Nursing Clinics of North America, 38*(1), 75-99.

evolve **Did you remember to check out the bonus material on the Evolve website and the CD-ROM, including NCLEX®-Examination Style Review Questions, Open-Book Quizzes, and Chapter Review Audio Podcasts?**

http://evolve.elsevier.com/Black/medsurg

CHAPTER 30

Management of Clients with Ingestive Disorders

DAWN P. MURPHY AND JANE HOKANSON HAWKS

The client with an ingestive disorder, regardless of the cause, may have a problem in the oral cavity or esophagus. Common nursing diagnoses for clients with ingestive disorders include *Impaired Oral Mucous Membrane; Pain; Imbalanced Nutrition: Less Than Body Requirements; Impaired Verbal Communication; Impaired Swallowing,* and *Risk for Aspiration.* Usually, the client first experiences pain in the mouth or esophagus, or delay in passage of food, which is evidenced by difficulty with swallowing. Shortly thereafter, oral communication and nutritional intake may be compromised. These complications may also result in the development of personal and family coping problems as well as a lack of knowledge related to the diagnosis and treatment of the disorder. Please refer to Figure 28-3 on p. 565 for detailed oral assessment guidelines.

ORAL DISORDERS

DENTAL DECAY/PERIODONTAL DISEASE

Healthy teeth and gums are important for good general health. Health care providers strive to preserve their clients' healthy gums and natural teeth for as long as possible for the following reasons:

- Natural teeth are almost always more functional in masticating food than are dental prostheses.
- Effective mastication of food helps promote efficient digestion.
- Efficient digestion of food results in healthy gastrointestinal (GI) function and maintenance of general health.

The most common causes of tooth loss are dental decay and periodontal disease. Plaque is the major cause of both caries (decay) and periodontal disease.

Tobacco use may also lead to tooth loss. *The best treatment for dental caries is prevention.* Early in childhood, clients are encouraged to brush and floss frequently and regularly, eat a diet low in simple carbohydrates, use fluoride to increase tooth enamel resistance to bacteria, and schedule regular visits (biannually) to the dentist for examination, cleaning, and treatment of dental caries.

Treatment of dental caries may include drilling out cavities and filling the tooth with material to restore the tooth, extraction (removal) of the entire tooth, and preservation of the tooth by *root canal therapy* (pulpectomy) followed by proper restoration. Any number of teeth can be removed because of tooth or gum disease. Teeth are usually replaced with some type of dental prosthesis (crowns, dentures, dental implants). If only one tooth or a few teeth are removed, local anesthesia is usually used. Removing several teeth or having a full mouth extraction may require sedation or general anesthesia. Potential complications include hemorrhage and abscess formation.

Periodontal disease, caused by plaque formation and bacterial colonization, results in gingival inflammation if the plaque is not removed by proper brushing and flossing. Eventually, inflammation destroys the underlying tissues and separates the gingiva from the tooth. In periodontitis, the inflammation extends from the gums into the alveolar bone and periodontal ligament, destroying the supporting structures of the teeth. As a result, the teeth loosen and fall out or extraction may be required as a result of the severity of the periodontal disease.

MUCOSITIS

Mucositis or stomatitis, an inflammation of the soft tissues of the oral cavity, may be of infectious origin or a manifestation of a systemic condition. It may be caused by *mechanical* trauma, such as injury, or *chemical* trauma, such as drugs used in the treatment of cancer. Jagged teeth, cheek-biting, and mouth-breathing may result in mechanical trauma. Certain foods and drinks as well as sensitivity to mouthwashes or toothpaste may produce chemical trauma. The inflammatory sloughing of tissue allows organisms to multiply, which may lead to infection by viruses, bacteria, yeasts, or fungus.

Mucositis is classified as primary or secondary, depending on the cause. Primary mucositis includes aphthous ulcer (canker sore) (Figure 30-1), herpes simplex (Figure 30-2), and Vincent's angina. Secondary mucositis results when a client's lowered resistance allows an opportunistic infection to develop. Systemic disorders that can affect the oral mucous membranes include (1) allergies, (2) bone marrow disorders, (3) nutritional disorders, (4) immunodeficiency disorders, and (5) chemotherapy, radiation therapy, or immunosuppressive therapy. Table 30-1 compares the most commonly occurring types and manifestations of mucositis.

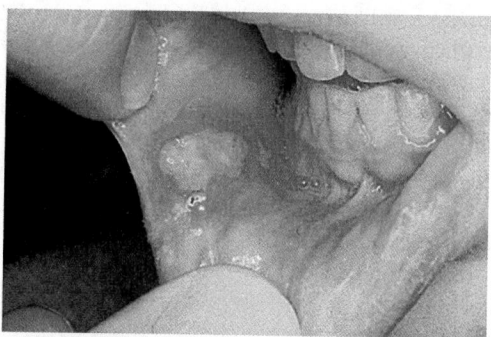

■ **FIGURE 30-1** Major aphthous ulcer (canker sore). *(From Feldman, M., Friedman, L., Brandt, L. [2002]. Sleisenger & Fordtran's gastrointestinal and liver disease: Pathophysiology/diagnosis/management [7th ed.]. Philadelphia: Saunders.)*

CANDIDIASIS

Candidiasis (moniliasis, thrush) is a secondary infection caused by an overgrowth of the organism *Candida*

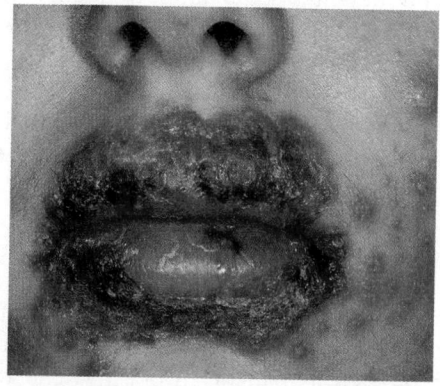

■ **FIGURE 30-2** Herpes simplex of the lip. *(From Habif, T.P. [2004]. Clinical dermatology: Color guide to diagnosis and therapy [4th ed.]. St. Louis: Mosby.)*

TABLE 30-1 Types of Mucositis

Type	Cause	Clinical Manifestations	Prevention and Treatment
Aphthous ulcer (canker sore)	Herpes simplex virus, stress, allergies, endocrine disorders, trauma, vitamin deficiency	Varies widely in size: usually small painful ulcerations on soft tissue of tongue, lips, and buccal mucosa; relatively superficial with raised borders Ulcers may persist for 2-3 weeks, usually non-scarring	Prevention unknown If allergic cause, avoid eggs, citrus foods, chocolate, shellfish, nuts, and milk products Treatment includes topical anesthetic, topical or systemic steroids for shortened healing time
Herpes simplex virus (cold sore)	Herpes simplex virus may lie dormant for extended time, often reactivated by stress or infection	Clear vesicular lesions in oral cavity rupture to form painful ulcerations resembling canker sores Heavy white coating on tongue	Very contagious during vesicular and ulcerative stages Treat pain with oral and topical analgesics Start IV acyclovir for immunocompromised clients If competent immune system administer oral antiviral (acyclovir [Zovirax]) or topical antiviral (penciclovir [Denavir], acyclovir [Zovirax]) Unless secondary infection present, antimicrobials will not affect wound healing
Vincent's angina	Acute bacterial infection of gingiva caused by resident oral flora, fusiform bacteria, and spirochetes Precipitating factors: poor hygiene, increased age, malnutrition, lack of rest and sleep, local tissue damage, and debilitating disease	Sudden onset; erythema and ulceration of gingivae spreading to oropharynx Manifestations include foul taste, pain, choking sensation, fever, thick secretions, anorexia, local lymphadenopathy	Removal of devitalized tissues, rest, improved oral hygiene, bland diet, vitamins Analgesics and saline mouth rinses for comfort measures

albicans, a yeast-like fungus that is part of the normal flora of the oral cavity. Candidiasis of the oral cavity and esophagus is commonly seen in immunosuppressed clients, such as those receiving chemotherapy and/or radiation therapy or those with HIV infection or AIDS. The incidence is also increased in clients with diabetes mellitus and those who are pregnant, under stress, receiving high-dose or long-term antibiotic or steroid-based therapy, or receiving long-term tube-feeding.

Clients at increased risk should be monitored closely. Assessment reveals white patches on the tongue, palate, and buccal mucosa (Figure 30-3). These lesions adhere firmly to the tissues and are difficult to remove. The lesions are often referred to as "milk curds" because of their appearance. Clients describe the lesions as dry and hot and they may complain of frequent sore throat and/or pain on swallowing. Clients who have recurrent candidiasis infections should be examined for a possible systemic cause.

Medical management includes antifungal agents, either nystatin troches or liquid to "swish and spit" or systemic therapy with fluconazole (Diflucan). The antifungal agents alleviate the infection. Prophylactic use of fluconazole is indicated for high-risk and immunosuppressed clients. Topical or oral analgesics, such as acetaminophen or ibuprofen, may also be administered to reduce pain. Mouthwashes of warm saline (or water) are often ordered as part of an oral hygiene regimen. Commercial mouthwashes should be avoided because of the high alcohol level of these products. A liquid or pureed diet may be necessary.

TUMORS OF THE ORAL CAVITY

Benign Tumors of the Oral Cavity

The most common benign tumors of the mouth are fibromas (fibrous tissue), lipomas (fatty tissue), neurofibromas (nerve fiber tissue), and hemangiomas (collection of blood vessels). As with benign tumors in other parts of the body, oral tumors cause problems, primarily by occupying space and causing pressure. Benign tumors are usually excised if the mass causes functional or cosmetic problems.

Premalignant Tumors of the Oral Cavity
Leukoplakia

Leukoplakia, a potentially precancerous, yellow-white or gray-white lesion, may occur in any region of the mouth. The size and shape of lesions vary, but they are usually elevated and have a roughened or leathery surface and clearly defined borders (Figure 30-4).

Leukoplakia is a common disorder of the oral mucous membranes, usually seen in people in their 30s and 40s. Men are affected twice as often as women; however, the incidence in women is increasing because of the increasing number of women who smoke.

Leukoplakia results from chronic irritation of the mucosa by physical, chemical, or thermal factors. Physical factors include poorly fitting dentures, broken teeth, cheek nibbling, and poor alignment of the mandible and maxilla. Chemical and thermal factors arise from the use of tobacco (inhaled, chewed, pipe, cigar) products. Habitual marijuana use is also considered a risk factor. Ingestion of excessively hot food and beverages also places the person at risk. Human papillomavirus (HPV) has recently been identified as a risk factor for leukoplakia and oral cancer.[9] This condition may also develop from systemic factors such as poor nutrition or syphilis. Topical calcipotriol (Dovanex) and topical tretinoin (Retin A) are equally effective therapy when treating oral leukoplakia.

Erythroplakia

Erythroplakia is a red, velvety appearing patch that commonly indicates early squamous cell carcinoma. It occurs most frequently in people ages 50 to 60, with men and women being equally affected. Risk factors are the same as those for squamous cell carcinoma.

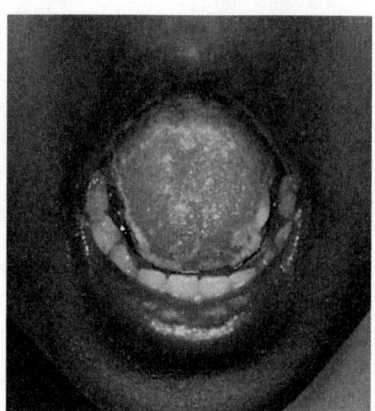

■ **FIGURE 30–3** Oral candidiasis. Note white patches on the upper palate. *(From Jarvis, C. [2004]. Physical examination and health assessment [4th ed]. Philadelphia: Saunders.)*

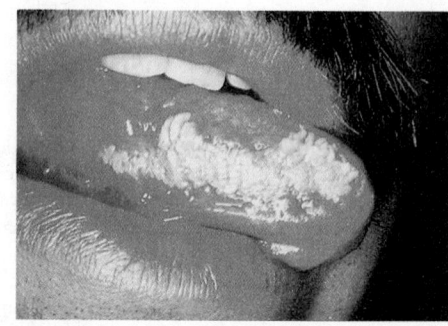

■ **FIGURE 30–4** Leukoplakia of the lateral edge of the tongue. *(Courtesy of The Centers for Disease Control and Prevention, Atlanta.)*

Malignant Tumors of the Oral Cavity

Cancers of the oral cavity account for 2% to 5% of new cancer cases in the United States. Cancers of the oral cavity are most often associated with long-term alcohol consumption and tobacco and marijuana use. HPV infection has recently been identified as a risk factor for development of oral cancers.[1,9]

Health promotion actions include teaching clients to avoid excessive use of tobacco, alcohol, and very hot beverages and foods. Programs at elementary schools and at extracurricular activities encourage individuals to resist peer pressure to start smoking. Encourage clients to maintain meticulous oral hygiene, to eat a well-balanced diet, and to use sunscreen during exposure to sunlight. Health maintenance activities involve oral screening of smokers, tobacco chewers, and drinkers of alcohol and teaching these high-risk individuals to observe for early manifestations of oral cancer. Health restoration interventions include managing chemotherapy and radiation for clients after tumor excision and providing nutritional support as needed. The respiratory and digestive tracts will be affected by treatment with changes in taste, smell, mechanical process of food ingestion, and appearance.

Basal Cell Carcinoma

Basal cell carcinoma of the oral cavity, the second most common oral cancer, occurs primarily on the lips. It starts as a small scab that develops into an ulcer with a characteristic pearly border. Basal cell carcinoma primarily occurs as a result of excessive exposure to sunlight, tending to occur more commonly in fair-skinned individuals who are exposed to sunlight.

Squamous Cell Carcinoma

Squamous cell carcinoma (SCC) is a malignant growth arising from tiny flat squamous cells that line mucous membranes. SCC is the leading type of oral cancer. Most tumors occur in clients older than age 45. Common sites include the lower lip and tongue. About 95% of cancers found on the tongue are squamous cell carcinomas. Malignancies of the tongue represent 1% to 1.5% of all malignancies in the United States.

The primary cause of SCC is chronic irritation of the mucous lining of the mouth and oral cavity. Overuse of alcohol, marijuana, and tobacco (both smoking and chewing) is the primary cause of oral irritation. In combination, tobacco and alcohol are extremely destructive to the oral mucosa.[1]

Manifestations may include a sore or lesion in the oral cavity that does not heal. Red-appearing SCC (erythroplakia), shown in Figure 30-5, may not be well delineated and often bleeds easily. Because SCC usually grows slowly, the lesion may be large before

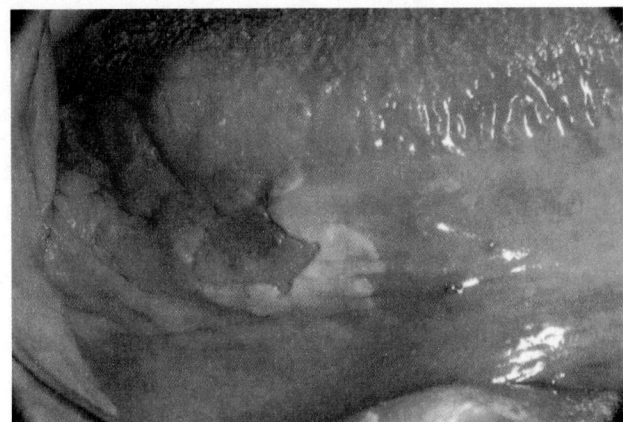

■ **FIGURE 30–5** Oral squamous cell carcinoma. This is an ulcerated lesion with surrounding leukoplakia on the posterior lateral and ventral portions of the tongue. *(From Neville, B.W., et al. [2002]. Oral and maxillofacial pathology [2nd ed]. Philadelphia: Saunders.)*

manifestations are detected. Other manifestations can include a mild irritation of the tongue, sore throat, trouble with wearing dentures, or pain in the tongue or ear.

Only a biopsy with cytology of lesions positively confirms a diagnosis of oral cancer. An excisional, needle, or true-cut biopsy will be obtained using either local or general anesthesia. Fine needle aspiration (FNA) is necessary to evaluate a salivary gland abnormality as well as to provide the tissue diagnosis for lymph node adenopathies. Radiologic studies (CT or MRI) are also important to evaluate tumor size and lymph node spread. To diagnose carcinoma at the base of the tongue, a laryngoscopic examination must be performed. An upper GI endoscopy may be required to visualize laryngeal tumors.

OUTCOME MANAGEMENT

Medical Management

Inhibit Tumor Growth

The survival rate of clients with oral cancer depends on the site and staging of the tumor. The tumor-node-metastasis (TNM) staging system (see Chapter 17) is used to stage oral cancers. Of the oral cancers, cancer of the lip carries one of the highest cure rates. SCC of the tongue carries the poorest prognosis because of the tongue's extensive vascular and lymphatic supply. Management of oral cancers includes surgery, radiation therapy, and chemotherapy, depending on the site and staging of the tumor.

Radiation Therapy. Oral cancers can be treated with *external beam therapy* or *interstitial radiation therapy* *(brachytherapy)*. The external beam passes through the skin or mucous membrane to the tumor. Interstitial radiation involves implanting radioactive seeds into the tissue for a prescribed period of time. Because interstitial radiation affects local tissue, it is used for small lesions that have not infiltrated the surrounding tissue. The client undergoing interstitial radiation is hospitalized and placed on radiation precautions (see Chapter 17) while the materials are active.

Chemotherapy. The effectiveness of chemotherapy for the treatment of oral cancers varies. Several drugs are used to treat head and neck cancers. These drugs include 5-fluorouracil (5-FU), cisplatin (Platinol), methotrexate (Folex), and the taxanes (Taxol, Taxotere). See Chapter 17 for discussion on chemotherapy. 5-FU is also used as a continuous infusion concurrently with radiation for the synergistic effect in a treatment referred to as chemoradiation.

Nursing Management of the Medical Client

Assessment. Carefully question the client about manifestations. A common finding is that of a painful ulcer. Assess the client for difficulty in swallowing, white or red patches on the oral mucosa, bleeding in the mouth, enlarged lymph nodes in the neck, pain referred to the ear, foul odor, and hoarseness. Ask about the use of alcohol and tobacco, oral hygiene habits, and sun exposure. Assess the client's rehabilitative needs. Surgery can cause disfigurement and may alter speech; the client may experience depression from a change in body image and the diagnosis of cancer.

Diagnosis, Outcomes, Interventions

Diagnosis: Impaired Oral Mucous Membrane. A common nursing diagnosis for the client who has oral cancer or who is at risk for oral cancer is *Impaired Oral Mucous Membrane related to irritants such as alcohol or tobacco, chemotherapy, radiation therapy, ill-fitting dentures, poor nutrition, and knowledge deficit of prevention and treatment of oral lesions.*

Outcomes. The client will understand and comply with measures to maintain the oral mucosa, as evidenced by statements of understanding of the substances and activities to avoid. The client will also be able to discuss the treatment regimen.

Interventions

Avoid Oral Irritants. Teach the client about the disease and treatment protocols. Advise the client to avoid chemical, physical, and thermal oral trauma; to perform careful, frequent oral hygiene, preferably three times daily; to see a dentist about ill-fitting dentures; and to see a practitioner about any mouth lesion that does not heal in 2 to 3 weeks.

Promote Comfort. If the client is receiving radiation therapy or chemotherapy, discuss possible side effects of these forms of treatment. Provide the client with comfort measures to minimize side effects, such as frequent oral hygiene and antiemetics to prevent nausea and vomiting. Kepivance (palifermin), a keratinocyte growth factor, before radiation therapy and/or chemotherapy may reduce the severity of mucositis that often occurs.[5]

Diagnosis: Imbalanced Nutrition: Less Than Body Requirements. Clients with oral cancers often have nutritional difficulties, and a usual nursing diagnosis is *Imbalanced Nutrition: Less Than Body Requirements related to oral pain and difficulty eating and swallowing.*

Outcomes. The client will maintain weight or show weight gain before surgery, as evidenced by an increase in intake, maintenance of weight, or a weight gain of 1 pound per week until stable.

Interventions

Promote Nutrition. The location and size of a tumor, and the pain it causes, commonly interfere with a client's ability to eat. Small, frequent feedings can promote intake. Administering an analgesic 30 to 45 minutes before a meal can decrease the pain associated with eating. Provide oral care before and after meals to remove debris and minimize oral odors. A baseline nutrition consult is appropriate and interventions are usually aimed at identifying specific nutritional deficiencies or protein-energy malnutrition. Give the client guidelines for improving the diet including materials for home use as a reference.

Relieve Mouth Dryness. Radiation treatments and some chemotherapy treatments alter salivation and taste perception. *Xerostomia* (dryness of the mouth) usually lessens with the use of pilocarpine and artificial saliva. Teach the client that chewing sugarless gum or sucking on sugar-free sour hard candy will increase saliva production. The client should perform frequent oral rinses with cool water to reduce dryness.

Evaluation. The best outcome is for the client to stop high-risk behaviors for oral cancer, undergo successful treatment, and promote and maintain nutritional status.

Surgical Management

Surgical management of oral cancers ranges from local excision of small tumors to extensive surgery for invasive tumors. Small tumors can be treated in outpatient facilities by local excision, radiation, or laser therapy. Small tumors of the floor of the mouth can be locally excised with or without removing a portion of the mandible. Small tumors in the anterior floor of the mouth can be excised, and the area can be reconstructed with the use of a split-thickness skin graft. In this procedure, a thin layer of skin, usually from the chest or anterior thigh, is aligned onto the surgical site, allowing the client to maintain good mobility and function of the tongue. Xeroform gauze is usually placed over the skin graft and sutured into place. Both the graft and the gauze can restrict tongue movement, causing aspiration of secretions. Because of this packing and as a result of postoperative edema, a tracheostomy tube (see Chapter 60) is usually placed until edema subsides and the oral airway is patent. The client receives nothing by mouth (NPO) for 7 to 10 days after surgery to allow for healing. A nasogastric (NG) feeding tube, gastrostomy, or percutaneous endoscopic gastrostomy (PEG) is used to provide nutrition until the client can resume oral feedings (see Chapter 29).

Clients with invasive tumors require extensive surgical excision, usually involving removal of associated lymph nodes. Depending on the location, glossectomy (removal of the tongue), mandibulectomy (removal of the mandible), hemiglossectomy (removal of part of the tongue), or radical neck dissection may be performed. A radical neck dissection is an extensive procedure that involves removal of all tissue under the skin, from the jaw down to the clavicle, and from the anterior border of the trapezius muscle to the midline. To remove the cervical lymph nodes in this procedure, the surgeon must remove the sternocleidomastoid muscle, the spinal accessory nerve, and the jugular vein. A modified radical neck dissection involves removal of the lymph nodes only and is preferred when the disease is confined to mobile lymph nodes (see Chapter 60 for surgical management of cancer of the larynx).

Nursing Management of the Surgical Client

Assessment. Assessment of the surgical client is similar to assessment of the medical client. Complete routine preoperative and postoperative assessments, and ensure that the client understands the implications of the selected surgical approach and the associated postoperative assessments and treatments. Assessment of rehabilitative needs, such as speech therapy, coping with disfigurement, and depression may also be required.

Diagnosis, Outcomes, Interventions
Diagnosis: Risk for Injury. Surgery for oral cancer involves many potential risks. *Risk for Injury related to surgical procedure (including hemorrhage, ineffective airway clearance, impaired gas exchange, and risk for infection)* is an appropriate nursing diagnosis.

Outcomes. The client will remain free from injury, as evidenced by absence of excessive bleeding, maintenance of a patent airway and gas exchange, and wound healing without manifestations of infection.

Interventions
Maintain Airway

The most critical postoperative intervention is to maintain a patent airway. If the surgical procedure has been extensive, a tracheostomy is usually in place to help prevent respiratory difficulty from edema of the oral and pharyngeal structures. Clients at risk for ineffective airway clearance or impaired gas exchange should be in a semi-Fowler's to a high-Fowler's position after surgery to promote venous lymphatic drainage.   SAFETY ALERT

The client's face may have a dusky appearance from venous congestion. Pulse oximeter readings also should be used to determine whether the client is sufficiently oxygenated.

The client with a tracheostomy may exhibit blood-tinged mucus in tracheal secretions for the first 48 hours after surgery. Bright red bleeding from the tracheostomy tube or site is a manifestation of hemorrhage. Notify the practitioner immediately if this occurs.

Provide Wound Care. The amount of nursing care required by the client after surgery depends on the extent of the procedure. After local excisions, teach the client how to perform hygiene gently. If a dressing and packing are in place, monitor the amount of drainage. After the dressing and packing are removed, the client should rinse the oral cavity with a water or saline solution every 4 hours to remove debris and promote healing. With more extensive surgery, the suture lines must be protected from trauma. Oral hygiene and oral suctioning are usually not implemented until healing has begun and the physician decides that this type of cleaning can be performed without damage to the sutured or incisional area.

Monitor for Bleeding

Hemorrhage may occur at any time after surgery, especially with extensive resection of the tongue. Hemorrhage can be massive because of the large vessels that supply the mouth and oral area. If bleeding occurs, apply pressure on the site until the bleeding stops spontaneously or until medical or surgical intervention occurs.   SAFETY ALERT

Surgical repair may be required to stop the bleeding. If an extensive resection is performed requiring skin grafts, monitor the site every 2 to 4 hours for drainage and manifestations of infection.

Diagnosis: Imbalanced Nutrition: Less Than Body Requirements. After surgical intervention for oral cancers, the client often continues to have difficulties with nutrition. *Imbalanced Nutrition: Less Than Body Requirements related to altered oral mucosa and surgical procedure* is an appropriate nursing diagnosis.

Outcomes. The client will maintain or gain weight after surgery, as evidenced by stabilization of weight and a weight gain of 1 pound per week until weight is stable.

Interventions

Administer Supplemental Nutrition. Immediately after surgery, monitor IV hydration. Assess bowel sounds every shift. The return of bowel sounds is often an indication to begin tube feedings. Assess the client for proper tube placement and measure retention of stomach contents every 4 hours or as ordered. Administer nutritional supplements by pump or bolus feedings as ordered. In addition, the practitioner may order parenteral nutrition (PN) as the first line of nutritional management (see Chapter 29 and discussion of achalasia later in this chapter).

Discuss Eating Modifications. Once the edema has subsided, healing has occurred, and the tracheostomy tube has been removed, the client may resume oral feedings. Caution the client about a decrease in sensation in the oral cavity after surgery. Assess swallowing carefully before eating begins. Instruct the client to avoid putting food directly on the surgical resection site. After meals, the client should always perform oral hygiene to remove any particles that remain and that may cause problems with the incision.

Diagnosis: Impaired Verbal Communication. When the client has a tracheostomy after surgery, a common diagnosis is *Impaired Verbal Communication related to the presence of tracheostomy.*

Outcomes. The client will demonstrate the use of alternative forms of communication to communicate with staff and significant others.

Interventions

Promote Alternate Forms of Communication. Assess the client's literacy, and provide paper and pencil, magic slate, chalkboard, a marker board, or laptop computer for the client to communicate as a substitute for talking. An alternative is to provide the client with a picture board to use for communicating any needs. Ideally, the assessment and instruction are completed preoperatively. The client should be allowed to communicate by gestures or written notes if this approach puts the client at ease. Most important, the nurse's manner should communicate acceptance, compassion, and caring. It is common to treat clients who cannot talk as though they cannot hear or understand. Be alert to any tendency to treat clients as if they are mentally incompetent or deaf. Help the client avoid social isolation by taking the client for walks and meeting others. Friendly social encounters and physical activity can help alleviate depression.

Relieve Anxiety. Help clients who cannot speak to express needs, concerns, and feelings. Check on the client frequently to reduce anxiety and loneliness. Place the call light within easy reach, and respond to the light promptly. If an intercom is used, it should be appropriately labeled regarding the client's limited ability to speak.

Evaluation. The most favorable outcome is that the client heals within 6 weeks to 3 months, according to the extent of the radical surgery, and without complications. Provide the name of the health care provider for the client to call or contact in case complications develop. Evaluate the client's ability to maintain intake of nutrients. If the client can self-feed via a tube until healing occurs and then gradually increase oral intake, then nutritional status should remain adequate. All clients need tremendous emotional support with this type of surgical intervention and need to be evaluated for possible complications related to lack of support from family or significant others.

Self-Care

On discharge, supply the client and family with complete instructions regarding diet, medications, manifestations of complications, and any treatments, such as care of the wound or tracheostomy. Explain how and when to contact health care practitioners. The client needs to be seen by the physician after discharge to ensure complete healing of any extensive surgical wounds. If the client has a tracheostomy, it may be permanent or may be closed at a later date. Clients who have undergone extensive surgery may need a referral to a home health agency for possible assistance with respiratory support (home oxygen), suctioning, nutritional support, and wound and tracheostomy care.

DISORDERS OF THE SALIVARY GLANDS

INFLAMMATION

The parotid gland is the largest salivary gland opening into the oral cavity. *Parotitis* is an inflammation of the parotid glands. It is the most common inflammatory condition affecting the salivary glands and probably results from inactivity of the glands caused by certain medications (such as diuretic and anticholinergic medications), prolonged NG intubation, and lack of oral intake, and dehydration such as that seen in postoperative clients. As secretions of the salivary gland diminish, oral bacteria have an opportunity to invade the gland and multiply. Interventions involve the following:

- Administering antibiotics to treat *Staphylococcus aureus* infection

- Increasing saliva production with the use of sialogogues such as lemon drops
- Keeping the client well hydrated
- Stopping anticholinergic medications

Analgesics and warm compresses may be ordered to alleviate pain. If no improvement is noted in 2 to 3 days, a CT may be completed to rule out abscess, lesion, or impaction of a sialolith (stone). Other differential diagnoses include mumps (if bilateral), Epstein-Barr virus, or HIV.

CALCULI

Stones, or calculi, may form in the salivary glands from inactivity and/or the precipitation of salts. Irritation from the stones causes local inflammation, swelling, and pain when the gland is stimulated to secrete, as during chewing. Intervention requires local excision. Stones occur most commonly in the submaxillary glands, probably because of the longer length of the duct and production of viscous alkaline secretions.

TUMORS

Most tumors in the salivary glands are benign. The most frequently seen malignant tumor is adenocarcinoma. Both benign and malignant tumors are characterized by enlargement of the gland. Pain occurs when expansion within the capsule of the gland creates pressure on sensory nerves. The treatment of choice for both benign and malignant tumors is usually surgical excision. If the tumor has recurred or is highly malignant, radiation therapy may also be used.

DISORDERS OF THE ESOPHAGUS

The most common clinical manifestation of an esophageal disorder is *dysphagia* (difficulty swallowing) that involves the sensation of food sticking in the back of the throat or upper esophagus. If swallowing is painful, it is referred to as *odynophagia*. Dysphagia may be caused by obstructive or motility problems of the esophagus. Obstructive disorders include esophageal tumor while motor disorders are associated with achalasia and neuromuscular disorders such as diabetes mellitus, Parkinson's disease, and stroke. Dysphagia is often accompanied by hesitation in swallowing, the need for repeated attempts to swallow, and throat clearing. Gagging and vomiting may also occur. Other manifestations include regurgitation, pain (which is probably linked with spasm), and heartburn or pyrosis.

DYSPHAGIA

Dysphagia can be caused by any esophageal disorder. Specific causes include neuromotor malfunction, mechanical obstruction, cardiovascular abnormalities, and neurologic diseases.

Dysphagia Caused by Mechanical Obstructions

Mechanical obstructions causing dysphagia include congenital defects, cancer, and acquired conditions such as a hiatal hernia. When an obstruction narrows the esophageal lumen, clients first experience dysphagia only with solid foods. Later, dysphagia becomes associated with semisolid foods and liquids. Finally, clients are unable to swallow their own saliva. Obstructive disorders, particularly esophageal cancer, may be accompanied by weight loss and cachexia.

Dysphagia Caused by Cardiovascular Abnormalities

Dysphagia may result from cardiovascular abnormalities, particularly in older people. Specific conditions causing vascular dysphagia include an enlarged heart, an aortic aneurysm, and calcification of the descending aorta (review the anatomy of the heart and great arteries to the esophagus).

Dysphagia Caused by Neurologic Diseases

Dysphagia also may be caused by certain neurologic diseases, such as stroke, multiple sclerosis, poliomyelitis, and amyotrophic lateral sclerosis (ALS). Stroke is the most frequent cause of dysphagia.

Dysphagia from Other Causes

Dysphagia may be experienced after swallowing, if food gets caught in the esophagus. Clients may obtain relief by drinking liquids to force the impacted bolus through the narrow segment or by retching to dislodge the food. If vomiting does not succeed, endoscopy may be used to remove food lodged in the esophagus.

REGURGITATION

Regurgitation is the ejection of small amounts of chyme or gastric juice from the mouth without antecedent nausea. It is usually caused by an incompetent lower esophageal sphincter (LES). Regurgitation occurring immediately after swallowing results from structural or motor abnormality in the LES. Contributing factors include abnormal motor activity, increased abdominal pressure, and sphincter abnormality. Regurgitation occurs with achalasia, pylorospasm, lesions proximal to the cardia, hiatal hernia, reflux esophagitis, and esophageal ulcer or cancer. Stooping or lying down facilitates the flow of gastric contents into the esophagus, thus exacerbating regurgitation.

ACUTE PAIN

Pain, which may be constant or may occur only with swallowing, suggests diffuse esophageal spasm. Pain may result from alterations of the mucosa from reflux disease, radiation, or viral infection. Pain that affects the esophageal mucosa and occurs with swallowing is called *odynophagia*. The client usually describes the pain as sharp, constricting, sticking, crushing, stabbing, or knife-like. Odynophagia is usually severe, quite distressing, and often associated with a deep and long-lasting pain. The pain, located substernally, may radiate to the neck, back, and shoulder. Pain may occur throughout the day and can be confused with angina. Odynophagia can be triggered by a cold or carbonated beverages or by solid food passing through the esophagus. The most common cause is the reflux of gastric contents into the esophagus.

HEARTBURN OR PYROSIS

Heartburn or pyrosis, also known as indigestion or dyspepsia, is another common manifestation of esophageal disease. Generally, it is a painful sensation of warmth and burning in the lower retrosternal midline. Because clients may use the word "heartburn" to describe very different sensations, it is essential to find out exactly what this term means to the client using it. Heartburn usually means substernal, midline burning that tends to radiate, generally in waves, upward to the neck, resulting from abnormalities of the LES. Clients often describe this discomfort as *cramping* or *knotting*.

Heartburn is commonly experienced with obesity, postural changes (such as bending, stooping, and lifting), gulping of food or liquids, with pregnancy, or ingestion of alcohol. Manifestations often are relieved by standing or eructating. Heartburn also arises in the presence of refluxed gastric or duodenal contents. Disorders most commonly associated with heartburn are reflux esophagitis, hiatal hernia, achalasia, and gastric stasis. Heartburn is common in individuals with pyloric or duodenal ulcers and LES disorders.

ACHALASIA

Achalasia is a motor disorder characterized by progressively incomplete relaxation of the lower esophageal sphincter (LES), and progressive, eventually complete, loss of peristalsis in the esophageal body. Food that has been swallowed has difficulty passing into the stomach and the esophagus above the LES becomes enlarged. Food from one or several meals may lodge in the esophagus and pass slowly into the stomach over time. There is danger of aspiration of esophageal contents into the lungs when the person lies down. The client typically presents with progressive (over months to years) dysphagia, usually expressing the feeling that "something is stuck in the throat." Achalasia commonly occurs in individuals in their 20s and 30s and appears equally often in men and women. Approximately 2 people per 200,000 per year will be diagnosed with achalasia. Clients are frequently treated for gastroesophageal reflux disease (GERD) before the diagnosis of achalasia is made.

Etiology and Risk Factors

The exact cause of achalasia is unknown although several theories of causation exist such as the loss of nerve endings and loss of hormones. Occasionally the client can relate the onset to an episode of acute dysphagia, but more often the onset is obscure. The disease is often not reported until the dysphagia has become severe or the treatment for GERD has been deemed ineffective. Because achalasia is idiopathic, there are no identified risk factors. There may be a familial component.

Scleroderma, an autoimmune disease discussed in Chapter 77, causes fibrosis in many organs and produces severe abnormality of peristalsis of the lower two thirds of the esophagus. The LES becomes incompetent and the combination produces severe esophagitis. The sphincter may become so impaired that the lower esophagus and stomach are visualized as one cavity instead of two entities. Manifestations include heartburn and dysphagia for solids.

Pathophysiology

Achalasia is characterized by impaired motility of the lower two thirds of the esophagus. The LES fails to relax normally with swallowing. Inadequate functioning occurs because nerve impulses cannot pass through the esophagus or sympathetic receptors are absent from the LES. There may be degeneration of the ganglion cells or impairment of impulses from Auerbach's plexus. Impaired propulsion and a constricted LES result in accumulation of food and fluid within the lower esophagus. When hydrostatic pressure exceeds the force of resistance of the LES, the contents pass into the stomach. Reflux esophagitis with resultant ulceration, shown in Figure 30-6, is a possible complication (see Gastroesophageal Reflux Disease later in this chapter). Aspiration of regurgitated esophageal contents may result in atelectasis and other pulmonary problems.

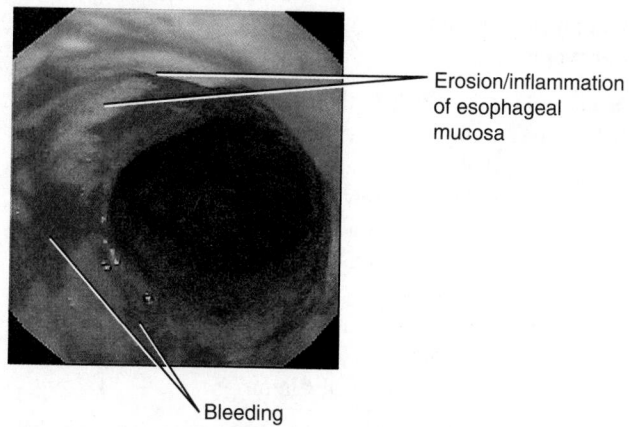

Erosion/inflammation
of esophageal
mucosa

Bleeding

■ **FIGURE 30–6** Endoscopic view of severe esophagitis. Note areas of erosion or inflammation of esophageal mucosa and bleeding.

Clinical Manifestations

The initial manifestation of achalasia is dysphagia. It is difficult for food and fluid to pass through the LES. In the early stages of achalasia, the client may have substernal pain because of spasms of the esophagus or may be unable to eructate (belch). The client may regurgitate undigested food eaten many hours earlier as well as large amounts of mucus that have been stimulated by esophageal irritation. As achalasia progresses, manifestations increase in frequency and severity. Upper respiratory tract infections, emotional disturbances, overeating, obesity, and pregnancy may exacerbate the problem.

Diagnostic tests used to determine the presence of achalasia include barium swallow (Figure 30-7), endoscopy, and manometry. The barium swallow is considered positive for achalasia if it reveals nonpropulsive waves and esophageal dilation. Barium may also be retained in the esophagus. Endoscopy helps determine the status of the LES, the amount of dilation, and the presence of food. Primary diagnosis is based on manometry (measurement of pressure in the esophagus), which confirms the diagnosis with elevated resting pressures in the LES or slow, low-amplitude, or absent peristalsis.

OUTCOME MANAGEMENT

Medical Management

There is no medical or surgical therapy for achalasia that will restore normal esophageal function. Therefore the goal of therapy is to relieve clinical manifestations.

Relieve Manifestations

Management usually begins with medical treatment on an outpatient basis. Often, as the problem progresses,

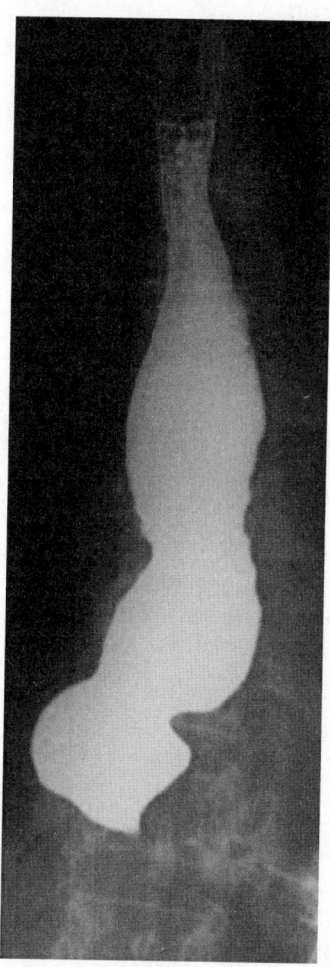

■ **FIGURE 30–7** Esophagram of a client with idiopathic achalasia. Note the dilated esophagus with air-fluid level and distal tapering providing a "bird's beak" deformity in the area of the LES. *(From Feldman, M., Friedman, L., & Brandt, L. [2002]. Sleisenger & Fordtran's gastrointestinal and liver disease: Pathophysiology/diagnosis/management [7th ed.]. Philadelphia: Saunders.)*

hospitalization is required for surgical procedures or for placement of a gastrostomy, percutaneous endoscopic gastrostomy (PEG) tube, or percutaneous endoscopic jejunostomy (PEJ) tube for nutritional support. Medical management also involves dilation of the LES. It may be performed by a gastroenterologist or a surgeon and may be regarded as either a surgical or a medical procedure. Under fluoroscopic guidance, a firm balloon is inflated to a predetermined diameter, thus tearing some of the fibers of the LES. Success is obtained in about 75% of clients in one or two sessions and is determined by more rapid emptying of barium on radiography and cessation of dysphagia. The major complication of balloon dilation is mediastinal tear, which occurs in less than 5% of procedures. Dilation is often used to correct esophageal spasms and stricture.

Administer Medications

Calcium channel blockers are potent smooth muscle relaxants that may help in treatment of achalasia. Botulism toxin is a new therapeutic treatment technique in which the toxin is injected endoscopically into the LES fibers to paralyze the muscle.[19] This treatment is most effective in older adult clients. Unfortunately, the efficacy decreases with repeated treatments because of the development of antibodies by the client.

Modify Diet

Changes in diet may ease the pressure and reflux in the client with achalasia. Small, frequent feedings ease the passage of food, and semisoft, warm foods are better tolerated than cold, hard foods. The client should avoid hot, spicy, and iced foods as well as alcohol and tobacco. Foods should be chewed thoroughly to add saliva to the mixture for lubrication and to allow the bolus to pass more easily from the esophagus to the stomach.

Alternate Positions

The client should experiment with different positions to reduce pressure while eating. Some clients benefit from arching the back while swallowing. After eating, the client should remain upright by standing or sitting. Restrictive or tight clothing, which may increase esophageal pressure and regurgitation, should be avoided.

To prevent nocturnal reflux of food, the client should sleep with the head of the bed elevated. Place the client in semi-Fowler's position, using a wedge pillow to keep the head higher than the LES, or elevate the head of the bed on 4- to 6-inch blocks.

Nursing Management of the Medical Client

Assessment. Obtain a history, noting the manifestations the client is experiencing, the onset and duration of aggravating factors, and any methods the client uses for relief. Assess respiratory manifestations because reflux or regurgitation can affect the respiratory tract. Assess the client's nutritional status, noting any weight changes and the effects of esophageal manifestations on dietary habits.

Diagnosis, Outcomes, Interventions
Diagnosis: Imbalanced Nutrition: Less Than Body Requirements. The client with achalasia experiences a great deal of difficulty swallowing, leading to the nursing diagnosis of *Imbalanced Nutrition: Less Than Body Requirements related to dysphagia.*

Outcomes. The client will maintain an adequate nutritional intake, as evidenced by maintenance of ideal body weight or regaining any weight lost at a rate of 1 pound per week.

Interventions. Consult with the client concerning dietary habits and daily intake of nutrients. Obtain a baseline weight and daily weights. Teach the client about changes in dietary habits that may relieve manifestations, as discussed under Medical Management. A gastrostomy tube, PEG tube, or PEJ tube may be used to provide adequate nutritional support if dysphagia continues to be a problem. Nursing management of tube feedings is discussed in Chapter 29 and later in this chapter under Nursing Management of the Surgical Client.

Diagnosis: Acute Pain. When the client experiences gastric reflux, the acid in the esophagus causes *Acute Pain related to episodes of gastric reflux,* making this an appropriate nursing diagnosis.

Outcomes. The client will experience a decrease in pain or an absence of pain, as evidenced by verbalizing a reduction in or an absence of pain and an ability to maintain oral intake.

Interventions. Pain can be decreased or relieved through the use of medications (such as antacids, histamine H_2-receptor antagonists, and proton pump inhibitors), dietary changes, and repositioning. Assess the client every shift to determine whether medications, changes in diet, and repositioning are effective in controlling or relieving pain.

Evaluation. The most appropriate outcome is that the achalasia is controlled with medical treatment and the client's nutritional status is maintained. If the client's manifestations cannot be controlled with medical treatment, surgical intervention may be necessary.

Surgical Management

The LES may be enlarged surgically by esophagomyotomy (Heller's procedure). The surgeon enlarges the vestibule by incising the circular fibers down to the mucosa over the entire length of the LES (Figure 30-8). At least 80% of clients have improvement in manifestations. A major side effect of the surgery is severe reflux esophagitis.

If a client cannot swallow for long periods, a gastrostomy tube, PEG, or PEJ may be inserted. The tubes may be inserted surgically, laparoscopically, or via percutaneous endoscopy.

For the laparoscopic or surgical method, the physician makes an incision in the wall of the abdomen and the stomach. The feeding tube is inserted through the incisions into the stomach and anchored by balloon or sutures. The client is usually then hydrated and fed by bolus and/or continuous drip feedings.

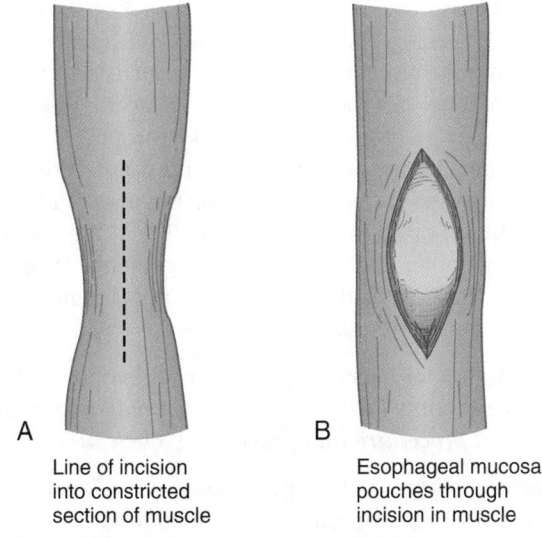

A   Line of incision into constricted section of muscle

B   Esophageal mucosa pouches through incision in muscle

■ **FIGURE 30–8 A** and **B,** Esophagomyotomy (Heller's procedure) is the surgical procedure of choice when a segment of esophagus narrows and causes functional obstruction.

For a percutaneous endoscopic approach, the physician uses local and conscious anesthesia and inserts a cannula into the stomach through a small abdominal incision. The PEG is threaded through and advanced down the esophagus through the abdominal incision and secured by balloon or external or internal crossbars (Figure 30-9). In the jejunostomy procedure, the tube is inserted into the jejunum rather than the stomach. See Chapter 29 for a comparison of enteral feeding routes.

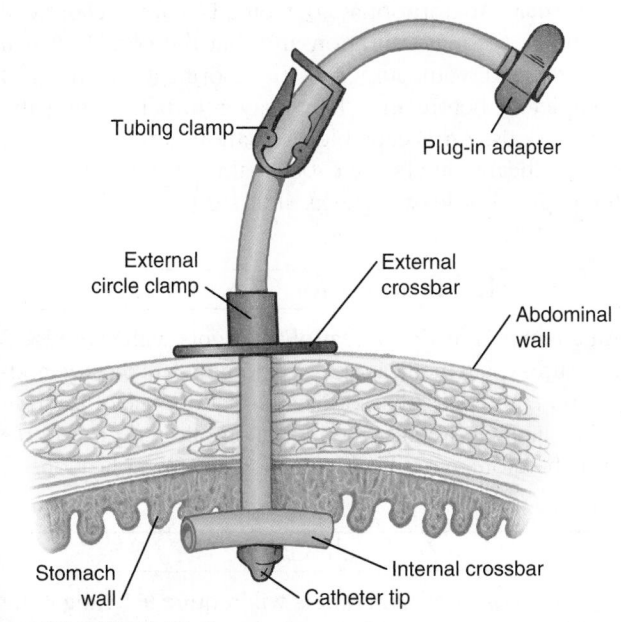

Tubing clamp

Plug-in adapter

External circle clamp

External crossbar

Abdominal wall

Stomach wall

Internal crossbar

Catheter tip

■ **FIGURE 30–9**   Percutaneous endoscopic gastrostomy tube.

Nursing Management of the Surgical Client

Preoperative Care

Assessment. Obtain a history, noting the onset and duration of manifestations the client is experiencing, aggravating factors, and any methods the client uses for relief. Assess the client's respiratory status and nutritional status in addition to the routine preoperative assessments.

Diagnosis, Outcomes, Interventions
Diagnosis: Deficient Knowledge. To prepare the client for surgery, consider the nursing diagnosis *Deficient Knowledge related to preoperative preparation and postoperative care.*

Outcomes. The client will understand and be prepared for surgery, as evidenced by asking questions and expressing statements of understanding.

Interventions
   Teach about Esophageal Dilation. If the client is to undergo esophageal dilation, explain that the client will be awake during the procedure. A local anesthetic solution is sprayed on the throat, and an analgesic or tranquilizer may be given. The client should take long, slow breaths during passage of the bougies. As the bag is inflated, the client may feel brief discomfort. Weighted bougies with increasing weight can also be used for dilation. Esophageal dilation is often performed on an outpatient basis.

   Explain Esophagomyotomy. Esophagomyotomy is a more complex procedure. The client requires a general anesthetic and remains hospitalized for more than 24 hours. Instruct the client undergoing an esophageal procedure about the usual preoperative procedures, such as remaining in an NPO status after midnight and administration of IV fluids and preoperative medications. Discuss pain control, drains, surgical dressings, and the presence of an NG tube, a gastrostomy tube, a PEG tube, or a PEJ tube. The possibility of a thoracotomy approach being used to reach the esophagus requires instruction concerning chest tubes.

   Discuss manifestations of respiratory complications related to esophageal reflux and aspiration. Instruct clients who have undergone an esophagomyotomy to sleep with the head of the bed elevated and to recognize manifestations of respiratory complications. Explain the manifestations of infection and esophageal perforation; urge the client to notify the physician if any of these problems occur.

SAFETY
⚠
ALERT

Postoperative Care
Assessment. Routine postoperative assessments, such as monitoring vital signs, pain, and drainage tubes placed

during surgery, are required. In addition, monitor the client's respiratory and nutritional status and the site of the feeding tube (if placed).

Diagnosis, Outcomes, Interventions

Diagnosis: Imbalanced Nutrition: Less Than Body Requirements. For the client experiencing dysphagia, the nursing diagnosis *Imbalanced Nutrition: Less Than Body Requirements related to dysphagia and placement of a gastrostomy, PEG, or PEJ tube* is appropriate.

Outcomes. The client will maintain an adequate nutritional intake, as evidenced by maintaining ideal body weight or gaining weight at a rate of 1 pound per week to replace previous weight loss.

Interventions. A baseline weight and daily weight measurements should be obtained. Evaluate the need for increased protein in the diet to promote wound healing.

Maintain Feeding Tube. Follow institutional policy regarding care for the client with a gastrostomy, PEG, or PEJ tube. Typically, the client is on NPO status for at least 24 hours before continuous or bolus tube feedings begin. 🛢️ Nursing interventions include checking tube placement via measurement of the tube and checking pH of stomach contents and residual amounts every 4 hours. (Do not assess this via aspiration if the tube is placed in the jejunum, because these tubes are flushed only, not aspirated.) If the gastric return is more than 150 ml or twice the hourly rate, hold the feeding for 1 hour and repeat aspiration before continuing the feeding. After checking placement and administering bolus feedings or medications, flush the tube with 50 to 100 ml of normal saline or water. Keep the head of the bed elevated at least 30 degrees at all times for continuous feedings or for 1 hour after completion of intermittent bolus feedings.

SAFETY
⚠️
ALERT

Change the enteral feeding bag and tubing every 24 hours if an open delivery system is used and rinse with water every 4 hours or after each intermittent feeding to decrease the risk of bacterial contamination. If a closed delivery system is used, the bottle and tubing should be changed every 24 hours.

(See Chapter 29 for additional information about enteral feedings.)

Diagnosis: Risk for Impaired Skin Integrity. When a feeding tube has been placed, the nursing diagnosis *Risk for Impaired Skin Integrity related to placement of a gastrostomy, PEG, or PEJ tube* identifies a potential problem.

Outcomes. The client will maintain or regain normal skin integrity, as evidenced by the absence of exudate, swelling, excoriation, or erythema at the tube insertion site.

Interventions

Provide Feeding Tube Care. Follow your facility's policy regarding routine care. Usually, about 12 to 24 hours after the tube has been surgically placed, the initial dressing may be removed and the skin around the insertion site may be washed with soap and water. A dressing may be applied as needed. Manifestations of infection should be reported to the physician. Teach the client or significant other home care management. (See the Bridge to Home Health Care feature on Managing Tube Feedings in Chapter 29.)

Diagnosis: Risk for Injury. A possible problem in the postoperative client is *Risk for Injury: Pneumothorax related to surgical procedure and presence of chest tubes.*

Outcomes. Injury will be prevented, as evidenced by absence of hemorrhage, absence of manifestations of perforation, normal temperature, and absence of problems associated with chest tubes, such as respiratory distress.

Interventions

Monitor for Complications

After esophageal dilation, monitor the client for manifestations of perforation, such as elevated temperature, chest or shoulder pain, and subcutaneous emphysema. If any of these manifestations are noted, notify the physician immediately. The client will require an x-ray study to determine whether air is in the mediastinum, indicating perforation.

Maintain Chest Tubes. After an esophagomyotomy, a thoracotomy incision and chest tubes are in place. Maintain chest tube drainage and the NG or gastric drainage system, and manage the client's pain. See Chapter 62 for care of the client with chest tubes.

Evaluation. An appropriate outcome is that the client will maintain adequate nutrition and that the condition will be reversed with surgery. The esophagus must heal completely before the client may return to eating the usual foods. An acceptable evaluation is that the client or significant others have been able to continue tube feedings for at least 6 weeks after surgery.

Modifications for Older Clients

An attempt is made to treat older clients with more local measures (pain medications, positioning, and dietary modification) and possibly esophageal dilation. The older adult is less likely to tolerate the more complicated procedures and, therefore, more likely to experience complications.

Self-Care

The client or significant others will require teaching if the feedings are required after discharge. Initially, home visits by a nurse may be necessary to assist the client with any home care needs related to tube feedings, diet, medications, and wound care and to provide an ongoing evaluation of the client's condition. A referral to a social worker may be needed to assist the client with financial assistance, community resources, counseling, and specialized equipment (see Chapter 29).

GASTROESOPHAGEAL REFLUX DISEASE (GERD)

Dyspepsia refers to the heartburn, indigestion, and epigastric pain that affects approximately 50% of the population. GERD can occur in any age group. About 40% of the U.S. population report manifestations of GERD to their primary care provider on a monthly basis. One of the most common causes of dyspepsia is gastroesophageal reflux, a backward flow of gastric contents into the esophagus. Gastroesophageal reflux disease (GERD) is a chronic condition with frequent exacerbations that may result in significant morbidity over time if not appropriately managed. It may range from mild, intermittent manifestations to more severe esophageal erosion and stricture, Barrett's esophagus with precancerous changes, and esophageal carcinoma.

Etiology and Risk Factors

The cause of GERD is unclear. The defense mechanisms of the natural esophageal mucosa become overwhelmed by exposure to hydrochloric acid, pancreatic enzymes, and pepsin in the reflux material. If the LES is affected by drugs, hiatal hernia, or abdominal pressure (pregnancy, obesity), the exposure to reflux material may be enhanced. Researchers have also suggested that motility disorders such as inappropriate relaxation of the LES and delayed gastric emptying are the culprit (Figure 30-10).

When functioning normally, relaxation of the LES is stimulated by swallowing. Relaxation of the LES is a brain stem function that is mediated by the vagus nerve. In the presence of GERD, the LES relaxes independently of peristalsis, thus removing the barrier to reflux. Common triggers for LES relaxation include consumption of foods such as caffeine, alcohol, peppermint, spicy or fried foods, chocolate, and tomatoes. Medications affecting the function of the LES include anticholinergics, beta blockers, estrogen, progesterone, calcium channel blockers, and nitrates.

Other risk factors for GERD include lifestyle and social habits such as alcoholism, smoking, high-fat diet, and obesity, as well as pregnancy and lying in a recumbent position when the stomach is full. Causes of delayed gastric motility are endocrine disorders (diabetes mellitus, hypothyroidism), while autoimmune disorders (scleroderma) and neuromuscular disorders (multiple sclerosis, Parkinson's disease) are associated with esophageal dysmotility. Age and sex are important variables as older adults and men have a 3 to 5 times greater risk of developing Barrett's esophagus and adenocarcinoma of the esophagus.

Risk factors as well as health promotion and maintenance behaviors are important teaching topics. These factors include obesity and weight gain, pregnancy, chewing tobacco, smoking, high-fat foods, theophylline, caffeine, chocolate, and high levels of estrogen and progesterone. Teaching clients to limit or cease smoking and to reduce ingestion of high-fat, acidic, and caffeine- or chocolate-containing food or beverages will help control and prevent GERD. Eating small meals and increasing dietary protein also helps. Losing weight,

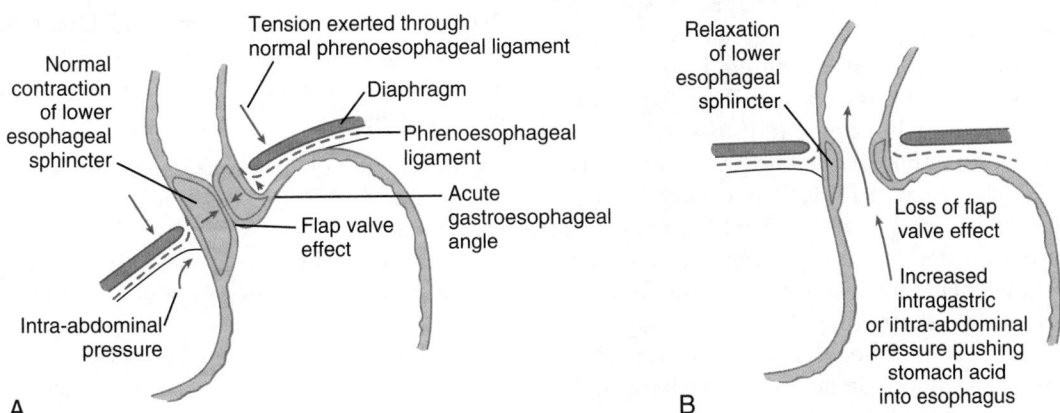

FIGURE 30–10 A, Normal mechanisms preventing esophageal reflux: contraction of lower esophageal sphincter (LES) creating high-pressure zone at the LES, acute gastroesophageal angle causing a flap valve effect, and phrenoesophageal ligament causing a pinchcock valve effect. **B,** Loss of normal mechanisms, creating gastroesophageal reflux disease (GERD): relaxed LES and displaced angle of the gastroesophageal junction allow increased intragastric or intra-abdominal pressure and result in gastric contents leaking into the lower esophagus. (**A** from Price, S., & Wilson, L. [2003]. *Pathophysiology: Clinical concepts of disease processes* [6th ed.]. St. Louis: Mosby.)

elevating the head of the bed for sleeping, and avoiding lifting, straining, bending, and tight or constrictive clothing can further help prevent the problem. Once GERD has developed, a health restoration action is to instruct the client on taking prescribed medications.

Pathophysiology

Normally, a high-pressure zone exists in the region of the gastroesophageal sphincter (LES). High pressure prevents reflux, but permits the passage of food and liquids. When there is relaxation of the LES, pressure decreases and reflux of stomach contents into the lower esophagus occurs. Delayed gastric emptying may also contribute to reflux by increasing gastric volume and pressure. Decreased salivation and buffering from salivary bicarbonate may contribute to impaired clearing of acid reflux from the esophagus. There is also considerable evidence linking GERD and asthma because of aspiration, laryngeal injury, and vagal-mediated bronchospasm.

Reflux esophagitis may occur with gastric or duodenal ulcer, after esophageal or gastric surgery, after prolonged vomiting, or after prolonged gastrointestinal intubation. The reflux most often consists of hydrochloric acid or gastric and duodenal contents containing bile acid and pancreatic juice. Frequent or prolonged reflux results in inflammation of the esophageal mucosa (esophagitis). GERD may present at one of three levels: nonerosive esophagitis (NERD), erosive esophagitis, and Barrett's esophagus. Pathologic GERD is defined as reflux of acid (pH < 4) and evidence of abnormalities such as pathologic biopsies of erosive esophagitis.

Clinical Manifestations

GERD may begin suddenly or gradually. The common subjective manifestations include heartburn, epigastric pain, retrosternal burning, odynophagia, dysphagia, acid regurgitation, water brash (the release of salty secretions in the mouth), eructation, and hoarseness. Less typical manifestations are recurrent laryngitis, sore throat, cough, wheezing, and loss of dental enamel. If the condition is severe, the pain may radiate to the back, neck, or jaw. Pain usually occurs 30 to 60 minutes after meals and is relieved with antacids or fluids other than water. Discomfort sometimes accompanies activities that increase intra-abdominal pressure, such as lifting or straining. The client may state that discomfort occurs when lying supine or when the stomach is distended. Standing and walking may relieve the discomfort. Dysphagia resulting from edema, spasm, or a narrowed lumen is intermittent and worse at the beginning of meals. Responses to pain-relieving measures (such as nitroglycerin) help differentiate between esophagitis and problems of cardiac origin (such as angina pectoris).

Diagnosis is made by history and diagnostic testing. Physical examination is usually normal. There is no standard, but the accepted criterion for diagnosis of GERD is a 24-hour pH probe monitoring. Esophagogastroduodenoscopy (EGD) is the standard for assessing esophageal complications such as esophagitis or Barrett's esophagus. EGD is indicated if the client does not respond to medication or if medication is required for long-term control in a client at high risk for Barrett's esophagus. It is also indicated if manifestations suggest complicated GERD, early satiety, GI bleed, weight loss, severe pain, choking, and chest pain. An additional test is manometry, used to evaluate LES pressure and esophageal motility disorders.

OUTCOME MANAGEMENT

The goals of management are to eliminate or reduce manifestations, heal esophagitis, and prevent recurrences, Barrett's esophagus, esophageal ulcer, and hemorrhage.

Medical Management

Decrease Reflux with Medications

The Integrating Pharmacology box on p. 611 discusses medications used for GERD. For clients receiving long-term therapy with nonsteroidal anti-inflammatory drugs (NSAIDs), misoprostol (Cytotec) is useful for preventing gastric ulcer formation and, in some instances, GERD manifestations. Anticholinergic drugs, calcium-channel blockers, bisphosphonates, and theophylline should be avoided if possible because these drugs appear to decrease LES pressure, delay gastric emptying, or irritate the esophagus.

Decrease Reflux with Lifestyle and Diet Changes

In mild GERD, diet and lifestyle changes may be sufficient to relieve manifestations. Instruct the client to do the following:

- Restrict the diet to small, frequent feedings (four to six per day) to decrease the amount of food in the stomach.
- Drink adequate fluids at meals to assist food passage.
- Eat slowly and chew thoroughly to add saliva to the food.
- Avoid extremely hot or cold foods, spices, fats, alcohol, coffee, chocolate, and citrus juices to decrease acid.
- Avoid eating and drinking for 3 hours before retiring to prevent the common problem of nocturnal reflux.
- Elevate the head of the bed 6 to 8 inches to prevent nocturnal reflux.

Medications for GERD

A variety of medications including antacids, histamine receptor antagonists, cholinergics, gastrointestinal stimulants, and proton pump inhibitors may be used for treatment of GERD.

Drug therapy for GERD often starts with an antacid, which commonly provides prompt relief (about 10 to 30 minutes). Typically, the client takes 30 ml of antacid 1 hour before and 2 to 3 hours after each meal to buffer or neutralize gastric acid secretions and soothe the mucosal lining. Clients typically tolerate combination products such as calcium carbonate/magnesium carbonate (Mylanta) or magnesium hydroxide/aluminum hydroxide (Maalox). Aluminum hydroxide/magnesium carbonate (Gaviscon) is another excellent antacid because of its foaming action. If antacid tablets are taken, they should be thoroughly chewed and taken with a full glass of water.

Two approaches are used in the pharmacologic control of GERD. For mild GERD, first-line therapy consists of histamine receptor antagonists such as ranitidine (Zantac) or famotidine (Pepcid). These medications inhibit histamine at H_2-receptor sites in parietal cells, which decreases gastric acid secretions. If histamine receptor antagonists are used, they should be given an hour before or after antacids. Twice daily dosing is most effective, with the first dose in the morning and the second dose an hour after the evening meal. If relief is obtained (90% of clients), the regimen should be continued for 2 to 3 months and then tapered off until the daily dose is only used on an as-needed basis.

If the client has an inadequate response to histamine receptor antagonists or if manifestations intensify, a proton pump inhibitor (PPI) is prescribed in place of the histamine receptor antagonist. The PPI (lansoprazole [Prevacid], esomeprazole [Nexium]) is initially given twice daily. These drugs are the most effective in treating GERD as they provide more complete control of acid secretion by inhibiting the hydrogen and potassium ATPase enzyme system in the gastric parietal cell. They should be given at least 30 minutes before meals. Treatment will usually continue on a once daily dosage as there is a 75% to 90% recurrence if therapy is discontinued.

If first- and second-line therapies fail, the client is referred to a gastroenterologist for endoscopy. If the endoscopy confirms esophagitis, PPI therapy is initiated immediately because of the superior healing rate of this drug class. If manifestations are eliminated, the client remains on maintenance therapy because a rebound effect is common.

Metoclopramide (Reglan), an antiemetic and cholinergic drug, may also be prescribed because it increases LES pressure by stimulating the smooth muscle of the GI tract and increases the rate of gastric emptying (GI stimulant). This medication is taken 30 to 60 minutes before meals.

- Lose weight, if overweight, to decrease the gastro-esophageal pressure gradient.
- Avoid tobacco, salicylates, and phenylbutazone, which may exacerbate esophagitis.

Endoluminal Gastroplication

Endoluminal gastroplication is a therapy developed for the treatment of symptomatic GERD. The procedure works by creating plications, or pleats, at the LES. Via endoscopy, the physician places two sutures (stitches) near the LES. Two stitches are then tied together to create a pleat near the LES. Only mild sedation is required for this outpatient procedure and clients can resume normal activities the following day.

Nursing Management of the Medical Client

Assess Manifestations

Identify specific manifestations the client has been experiencing. Document onset, frequency and severity, and relationship of manifestations to food and various food products. Assist in maintaining the client's general appearance and nutritional status. Assist the client to identify risk factors for GERD, and instruct the client concerning lifestyle changes to reduce risk factors.

Provide Teaching

Instruct the client in the prescribed diet regimen, and evaluate the client's understanding of both treatment and effectiveness. Administer medications ordered for pain, and document medication effectiveness. Instruct the client in the prescribed medication regimen, and evaluate the client's understanding of the treatment. Teaching to prepare the client for the endoluminal gastroplication is the same as teaching for a client undergoing endoscopic examination of the esophagus.

Surgical Management and Nursing Management of the Surgical Client

---

Clients who do not respond to medical management may undergo one of the surgical procedures discussed under Surgical Management for hiatal hernia.

HIATAL HERNIA

A hiatal hernia (diaphragmatic hernia) is a herniation of a part of the stomach into the thoracic cavity through an enlarged esophageal hiatus in the diaphragm. There are two major types of hernias: *sliding* hernias (type I) and *rolling* or *paraesophageal* hernias (type II). With a sliding hiatal hernia, the upper stomach and the gastroesophageal junction are displaced upward into the thorax (Figure 30-11, *A*). Sliding hiatal hernias account for about 90% of the total cases of esophageal hiatal hernias. With a rolling hiatal hernia, the gastroesophageal junction stays below the diaphragm, but all or part of the stomach pushes through into the thorax (Figure 30-11, *B*).

The incidence of hiatal hernia is estimated as 5 per 1000 in the general population and may be as high as 60% in clients older than age 60 years. Women tend to be affected more often than men, and the incidence increases significantly with age.

Etiology and Risk Factors

Hiatal hernias are related to muscle weakness in the esophageal hiatus, which loosens the esophageal supports and allows the lower portion of the stomach to rise into the thorax. As with other hernias, the muscle weakness is caused by a variety of conditions, such as aging, trauma, congenital muscle weakness, surgery, or anything that increases intra-abdominal pressure such as lifting, coughing, pregnancy, and obesity.

Risk factors are those that weaken the diaphragm and increase intra-abdominal pressure. Pressure may be increased by conditions such as obesity, pregnancy, or ascites.

Health promotion behaviors to prevent or at least delay a hiatal hernia include avoiding any activities that increase intra-abdominal pressure. These activities include heavy lifting and wearing tight constrictive clothing, especially around the waist. Other than these measures, hiatal hernias are not preventable.

Pathophysiology

A hiatal hernia involves protrusion of part of the stomach through a weakness in the diaphragm. The resulting regurgitation and motor dysfunction cause the manifestations associated with hiatal hernia. The major problem with a sliding hiatal hernia is reflux (GERD), which appears to be caused by the exposure of the LES to the low pressure in the thorax.

With a rolling hiatal hernia, the LES remains below the diaphragm and reflux is not a problem. Complications of a rolling hiatal hernia include obstruction, strangulation, and the development of a volvulus.

Clinical Manifestations

Manifestations of hiatal hernia vary in kind and severity. In sliding hiatal hernias, the client may experience heartburn 30 to 60 minutes after meals. Reflux may also result in substernal pain.

The client with a rolling hiatal hernia does not have manifestations of reflux. The client may complain of a feeling of fullness after eating or may have difficulty breathing. Some clients experience chest pain similar to that of angina. Pain is usually worse when the client lies down.

A barium swallow with fluoroscopy can reveal a hiatal hernia by showing the position of the stomach in relation to the diaphragm. A hiatal hernia may also be seen on a chest x-ray.

OUTCOME MANAGEMENT

Medical Management and Nursing Management of the Medical Client

The medical management and nursing management of the medical client with a hiatal hernia is the same as that for the client with GERD. See previous discussion on GERD.

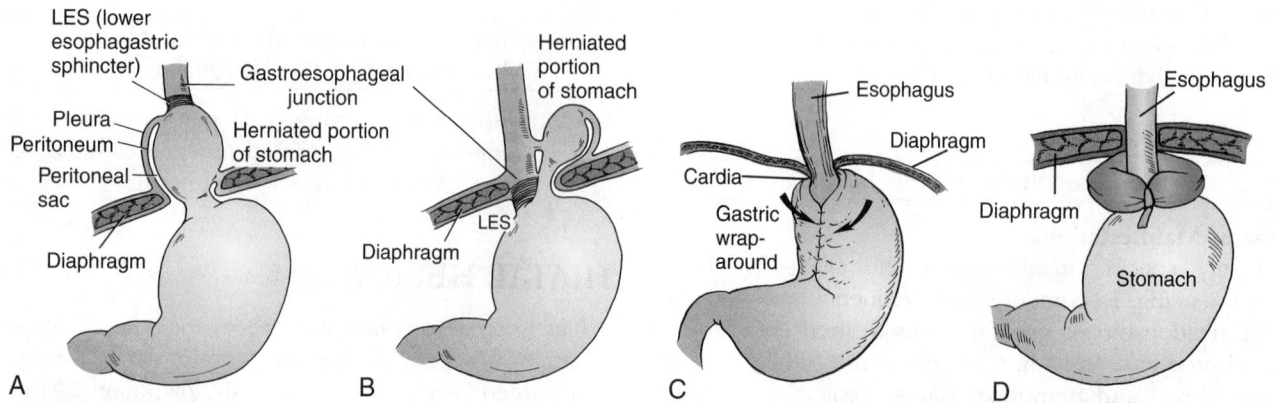

■ **FIGURE 30-11** **A,** A sliding hiatal hernia. **B,** A rolling hiatal hernia. **C,** Nissen fundoplication for hiatal hernia. The gastric fundus is wrapped around the distal esophagus and sutured to itself. **D,** Angelchik antireflux prosthesis in place.

Surgical Management

Clients who do not respond to medical management undergo one of three surgical procedures: the Nissen fundoplication, the Hill operation, or the Belsey operation. The surgeon may use an open surgical approach or a laparoscopic approach that may include robotic-assisted technology to complete these procedures. Recovery is usually faster with the laparoscopic approach.

The *Nissen fundoplication* is most common and involves suturing the fundus around the esophagus (see Figure 30-11, *C*). An abdominal approach is usually used. An increase in pressure or volume in the stomach closes the cardia and blocks reflux into the esophagus. The surgeon creates a valve-like substitute sphincter with inherent contractility.

The *Hill operation* narrows the esophageal opening and anchors the stomach and distal esophagus to the median arcuate ligament (posterior gastropexy). This procedure reinforces the sphincter and recreates the gastroesophageal valve. A partial wraparound (180 degrees) of the stomach around the esophagus is created via an abdominal approach.

The *Belsey (Mark IV) repair* consists of plication of the anterior and lateral aspects of the stomach onto the distal esophagus. The surgeon creates the esophagogastric angle without opening the esophagus or the diaphragm. A 280-degree esophageal wraparound is created via a thoracic approach.

In clients with severe reflux, an Angelchik prosthesis or ring may be inserted. A laparotomy is performed, and a synthetic C-shaped silicone prosthesis is tied around the distal esophagus (see Figure 30-11, *D*). The prosthesis anchors the LES in the abdomen and reinforces sphincter pressure. The success of this procedure is variable, depending on the severity of the problem. In clients with severe reflux, this procedure may be unsuccessful.

Clients undergoing a surgical procedure are encouraged to follow the GERD antireflux medical regimen (medications, diet changes, lifestyle changes) because the recurrence rate is significant.

Nursing Management of the Surgical Client

Postoperative Assessments

The surgical client requires the same assessments as the medical client, as well as routine preoperative and postoperative assessments. If chest tubes are placed postoperatively, monitor the client for respiratory distress.

An abdominal incision results in a greater chance of a wound infection. Assess the wound drainage for manifestations of infection. Clients have an NG tube, and tube patency must be maintained to avoid stomach distention. Always assess postoperative clients for venous thrombus following these types of surgery.

Prevent Respiratory Complications

Teach the client the importance of coughing and deep breathing after surgery to prevent respiratory complications. Because postoperative breathing can be painful, the client must cough and deep breathe to avoid respiratory complications. The use of an incentive spirometer may be ordered by the surgeon. If a thoracic approach is used, explain the purpose of the chest tubes and the care needed (see Chapter 62).

SAFETY
ALERT

Prevent Gas-Bloat Syndrome

Fluids are usually resumed after 24 hours, and the diet is progressively advanced as tolerated when peristalsis returns. Small, frequent meals are provided to avoid overloading the stomach. After fundoplication, the client may experience gas-bloat syndrome if the wrap of the fundus is too tight, causing bloating and an inability to eructate. Clients should avoid carbonated beverages and gas-producing foods. Ambulating can assist peristalsis in removing air from the GI tract. The condition is usually temporary. Instruct clients to report dysphagia, epigastric fullness, bloating, or excessive borborygmi to their physician or practitioner.

DIVERTICULA

An esophageal diverticulum is a sac-like outpouching in one or more layers of the esophagus. As food is ingested, it becomes trapped in a diverticulum and can later be regurgitated. The most common type of esophageal diverticulum is *Zenker's* (esophageal pulsion) diverticulum (Figure 30-12), which occurs above the upper esophageal sphincter. It may be associated with incoordination of the pharynx during swallowing. *Epiphrenic* diverticulum occurs just above the LES and

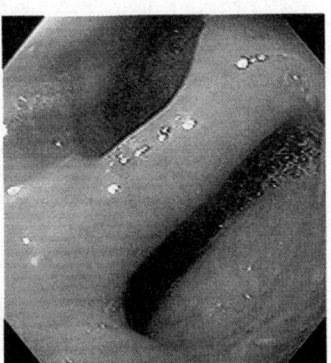

■ **FIGURE 30–12** Endoscopic view of Zenker's diverticulum. Note how difficult it is to distinguish the true lumen of the esophagus from that of the Zenker's diverticulum. *(From Feldman, M., Friedman, L., & Brandt, L. [2002]. Sleisenger & Fordtran's gastrointestinal and liver disease: Pathophysiology/diagnosis/management [7th ed.]. Philadelphia: Saunders; Courtesy D. Langdon, MD.)*

is associated with failure of the LES to relax, and increased amplitude of esophageal contractions. Esophageal diverticula are considered rare. Zenker's diverticula occur three times more often in men than in women.

Etiology and Risk Factors

The cause of esophageal weakness may be a congenital defect, esophageal trauma, scar tissue, or inflammation. There are two categories of diverticula: traction and pulsion. With a *traction* diverticulum, the esophageal mucosa has pulled outward from the esophagus. Traction diverticula are most commonly found in the middle esophagus. With a *pulsion* diverticulum, the esophageal mucosa has pushed outward through a defect in the esophageal musculature. Pulsion diverticula are most commonly found in the upper esophagus. There is no means of prevention.

Pathophysiology

Diverticula in the esophagus often develop in areas of muscle weakness that arise from esophageal trauma, congenital weakness of the esophageal wall, or scar tissue that forms from chronic inflammation of the esophagus. When food becomes trapped in a diverticulum, it may cause a local abscess. Infected diverticula place the client at risk for esophageal perforation because the mucosa is without the protection of the normal esophageal muscle layer.

Clinical Manifestations

Initially, the client usually complains of intermittent or constant difficulty swallowing. As Zenker's pouch enlarges, manifestations progress to aspiration of fluids and regurgitation of food into the mouth. Epiphrenic diverticula may lead to regurgitation of large amounts of accumulated fluid when recumbent. Other manifestations may include halitosis, a sour taste in the mouth, and coughing because of irritation of the trachea from regurgitated food.

A barium swallow is performed to locate the diverticulum. In the case of epiphrenic diverticulum, esophageal manometry may be performed to determine the presence of an associated motility disorder. Endoscopy is usually contraindicated because the diverticulum may be perforated by the endoscope.

OUTCOME MANAGEMENT

Medical Management

Medical management of esophageal diverticula includes dietary management and positioning. Small, frequent meals of semisoft foods often facilitate passage of food.

The client should note which foods ease or worsen the manifestations.

To prevent reflux of food, the caregiver should raise the head of the bed for 2 hours after meals. Sleeping with the head of the bed elevated can often prevent nocturnal reflux. The client also should avoid constrictive clothes and vigorous exercise after eating.

Nursing Management of the Medical Client

Obtain a history from the client, noting the onset and duration of manifestations and whether they occur at mealtimes or at night. Assess the client's respiratory status because regurgitation can cause respiratory complications.

Teach the client how changes in diet and positioning can control manifestations. Encourage the client to try various foods and various positions to evaluate which are most effective.

Surgical Management

When manifestations become severe, surgery may be indicated. A cervical approach is used for Zenker's diverticulum, whereas a thoracic approach is used for diverticula located lower in the esophagus. In both procedures, the diverticulum is excised and the esophageal mucosa is reanastomosed.

Nursing Management of the Surgical Client

Provide Teaching

Discuss the normal preoperative and postoperative routines. Explain that the client will be taking nothing by mouth after surgery and that an NG tube will be present until healing occurs. If a thoracic approach is used, preoperative and postoperative nursing care is similar to that for clients having thoracic surgery and chest tubes (see Chapter 62).

Maintain the Nasogastric Tube

After surgery, the client's NG tube is attached to low intermittent suction to avoid trauma to the stomach lining. Assess the amount and color of drainage during each shift. Check for continued bloody NG drainage as well as for external bleeding. Do not irrigate or reposition the NG tube unless told to do so by the physician. Moving the NG tube can perforate the esophagus or stomach (see Chapter 31 on irrigation of tubes if ordered by the surgeon). Assess the client for manifestations of esophageal perforation, such as chest pain, fever, and subcutaneous emphysema. The client receives IV fluids until tube feedings begin. Once fluids and supplemental feedings begin, record the client's response.

After surgery, the client may be discharged with an NG or a gastrostomy tube in place to allow for esophageal healing. Give the client written and verbal instructions about tube feedings, diet, and positioning. A visiting nurse should see the client at home to ensure that tube feedings are being tolerated well and should continue visits until the feeding tube is removed.

Promote Comfort

Assess the client's pain, and administer and evaluate prescribed analgesics. After surgery, the head of the bed should be elevated 30 degrees to reduce edema around the neck and upper chest. Frequent oral hygiene increases the client's comfort.

ESOPHAGEAL CANCER

Cancer of the esophagus takes the form of either squamous cell carcinoma or adenocarcinoma of the esophageal mucosa (Figure 30-13). An estimated 15,560 new cases of esophageal cancer were projected to be diagnosed in 2007 in the United States.[1] The incidence is three times as high in men as in women, and it is higher in African-American and Asian men than in white men. Squamous cell carcinoma (SCC) is most common in African Americans while adenocarcinoma (AC) of the esophagus is more prevalent in whites. Cancer of the esophagus is much more common in other countries such as Iran, China, South Africa, and India. The most prevalent type of esophageal cancer in these countries is SCC. The rate of AC of the esophagus in Western countries is increasing by 2% yearly while SCC has been decreasing in African-American men and women.

Etiology and Risk Factors

The cause of esophageal cancer is unknown but it is probably multifaceted. The major risk factor for development of SCC is cigarette smoking and alcohol consumption. Human papillomavirus has been found in up to 70% of clients with SCC of the esophagus. The greatest risk factor for AC is Barrett's esophagus. Chronic reflux of gastric contents results in squamous epithelium being replaced by columnar epithelium. Other risk factors for AC may be obesity, ingestion of smoked meats, and poor nutritional intake of vitamins A and C and minerals such as magnesium, selenium, and zinc.

There are no current recommendations in the United States for screening and early detection of esophageal cancer. Once cellular changes of Barrett's esophagus are detected, it is recommended that endoscopic surveillance every 1 to 3 years be initiated. Health promotion and maintenance behaviors involve limiting or stopping smoking and avoiding chronic ingestion of alcohol, hot foods, and hot beverages. Restorative behaviors include advising the client to follow the appropriate medical or surgical regimen for treatment of the specific condition.

Pathophysiology

The esophagus is lined with squamous epithelium, which is continuous until it reaches the gastroesophageal junction. At the junction, columnar tissue lines the esophagus. Most cancers of the esophagus begin as slow-growing tissue changes or dysplasia.

SCC is frequently found in the proximal or mid-esophagus. Cellular changes are usually seen before the development of SCC, and the changes are found more often in smokers than in nonsmokers. SCC of the esophagus can be classified as polypoid, ulcerative, or infiltrative. Infiltrative tumors of the esophagus expand locally and rapidly, causing wall thickening and narrowing of the lumen. A polypoid mass projects into the lumen, obstructing the lumen if undetected. Ulcerative lesions are raised and may expand into the mucosa, elevating until obstructive.

AC frequently arises from the columnar epithelium of the esophagus. The columnar epithelial changes are usually attributed to Barrett's esophagus.

Because the esophagus has no serosal layer, tumors are allowed to spread to adjacent tissues and lymphatic nodes early. The rich lymphatic supply to the mucosa provides an excellent means for the cancer to metastasize widely and quickly, causing the tumor to be unresectable. Common distant metastatic sites are liver, lung, pleura, and kidneys. Other areas include bone, peritoneum, and brain.

Clinical Manifestations

The most common presenting manifestations of esophageal cancer are dysphagia, odynophagia, and pain. Manifestations are usually not apparent until the cancer involves the circumference of the esophagus. By the

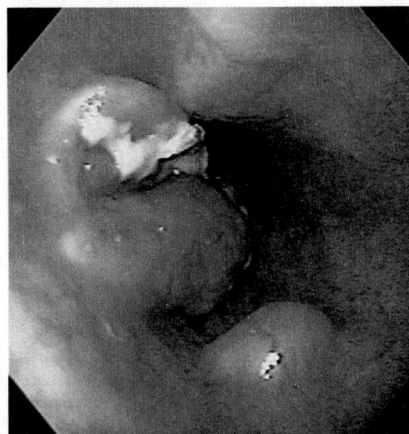

■ **FIGURE 30-13** Squamous cell carcinoma of the esophagus. *(From Wilcox, C.M. [2007]. Atlas of clinical gastrointestinal endoscopy. Philadelphia: Saunders.)*

time the client becomes aware of a swallowing problem and seeks medical care, the cancer frequently has invaded the deeper layers of the esophagus and, sometimes, adjacent structures such as the bronchus and mediastinum.

The dysphagia is usually progressive. Painful swallowing, loss of appetite, and malaise may also be present. As the cancer progresses, dysphagia becomes constant and manifestations of obstruction appear. These manifestations include an increase in salivation and mucus in the throat, nocturnal aspiration, regurgitation, and an inability to swallow even liquids. There may also be pain in the epigastric or sternal area or more distal if bone metastases are present. Liver enzymes will be elevated if liver metastases are present.

Endoscopy with biopsy and cytologic examination is the only definitive method of diagnosing esophageal cancer. Extent of disease may be determined by endoscopic ultrasound and computed tomography (CT). Tumor location, size, depth of invasion, and lymph node involvement are determined as well as the presence of distant metastases. Positron emission tomography (PET) may be used to confirm the presence of metastatic disease seen on CT. Exploratory laparoscopy may be used to visualize and biopsy possible metastatic sites.

OUTCOME MANAGEMENT

Medical Management

Inhibit Tumor Growth
Treatment of esophageal cancer depends on the tumor's location and size, metastases, and the performance status (Karnofsky Performance Scale) of the client. If the cancer is found in an early stage, treatment is directed toward cure; however, it is usually detected in the late stages, when treatment becomes palliative, aimed specifically at allowing the client to continue to live longer with a good quality of life.

Radiation Therapy
Radiation therapy can be used alone as a single therapy, or before surgery (neoadjuvant), after surgery (adjuvant), or concurrently with 5-fluorouracil (5-FU) by continuous infusion (chemoradiation). It reduces tumor size and slows tumor growth. Because radiation therapy may cause stenosis of the esophagus, treatments are usually administered over 6 to 8 weeks to minimize this effect.

Chemotherapy
Chemotherapy may be a single agent or a combination of agents. The goal of therapy is relief of manifestations

and reduction of tumor size. Neoadjuvant chemotherapy can facilitate surgical resection by reducing tumor size and invasiveness of the cancer. Commonly used neoplastic drugs include cisplatin (Platinol) and 5-fluorouracil (5-FU), docetaxel (Taxotere), irinotecan (Camptosar), and oxaliplatin (Eloxatin). Newer agents used in conjunction with chemotherapy are the antiangiogenic (bevacizumab [Avastin], and the anti-EGFR immunoglobulin cetuximab [Erbitux]) in the treatment of esophageal cancer.

Photodynamic Therapy
Photodynamic therapy is a relatively new therapy for treatment of esophageal cancer in clients who are not surgical candidates. The client receives an injection of a light-sensitive drug (Photofrin), which is followed 2 days later with a special fiberoptic probe with a light-bearing tip placed in the esophagus. The light activates the Photofrin and kills only cancer cells. This outpatient procedure uses conscious sedation, takes about 13 minutes to perform, and enables about 1 inch of tumor to be removed. Clients return home the same day and resume their usual activities the next day.

Maintain Nutrition
Maintaining nutrition is a major goal for the client with esophageal cancer. Not only does the cancer itself cause the client to be at risk for malnutrition, but also the treatments (both radiation therapy and chemotherapy) carry a risk of mucositis, nausea, vomiting, and dehydration. Side effects of treatment must be anticipated and management swift. Early in the disease, the client may be able to tolerate small, frequent feedings of soft or semisoft foods. As the disease progresses, a feeding tube may be needed. If necessary, a feeding gastrostomy or jejunostomy may be created. Short-term TPN may be used to improve the client's nutritional status before surgery. Proper positioning after meals is necessary if the client is experiencing frequent regurgitation. The head of the bed should always be elevated 30 degrees.

Nursing Management of the Medical Client

Assessment. Obtain data concerning the client's nutritional status. Most clients complain of dysphagia that is both persistent and progressive. The client initially may have difficulty swallowing solid foods and then may have difficulty swallowing soft foods and liquids.

A careful assessment of dysphagia is important. Other manifestations, such as odynophagia, regurgitation, chronic cough, increased secretions, and hoarseness (from involvement of the larynx), also are important to assess.

Diagnosis, Outcomes, Interventions

Diagnosis: Imbalanced Nutrition: Less Than Body Requirements. Because of the progressively worsening dysphagia, the client with esophageal cancer exhibits the nursing diagnosis *Imbalanced Nutrition: Less Than Body Requirements related to the client's inability to swallow.*

Outcomes. The client will maintain an adequate nutritional status, as evidenced by maintenance of stable body weight or slowed weight loss.

Interventions. Monitor the client's nutritional status throughout treatment, including measurement of daily weight, intake and output, and calories consumed. In the beginning, teach the client about diet changes that can make eating easier. The Translating Evidence into Practice box below examines quality-of-life issues clients face after treatment for esophageal cancer.

As the cancer progresses, tube feedings may need to be provided. Assess the skin around the feeding tube for impairment of skin integrity caused by leakage of gastric juices. Wash the skin around the opening with a gentle soap and dry thoroughly twice daily or as needed. Apply a protective ointment, such as zinc oxide or karaya gum, to the skin for further protection if needed.

Diagnosis: Impaired Swallowing. The client with esophageal cancer experiences increasing dysphagia that may lead to the nursing diagnosis *Impaired Swallowing related to esophageal obstruction from tumor.*

Outcomes. The client will not suffer from impaired swallowing, as evidenced by an absence of choking, the ability to consume oral intake, and the maintenance of a patent airway.

Interventions. Many problems arise when the client is unable to swallow. The client can easily choke on saliva and mucous secretions and must spit frequently or drool. Constant wiping of saliva from the lips can cause irritation, cracking of the skin, and open lesions. Because it is impractical to collect this quantity of secretions in tissues, the client should carry a

---

TRANSLATING EVIDENCE INTO PRACTICE

Quality of Life After Treatment for Esophageal Cancer

The outcomes of treatment for gastroesophageal cancer surgery are important to the client's post-treatment experience and quality of life. Treatment may range from photodynamic therapy for Barrett's esophagus and high-grade dysplasia to complete esophagectomy.[1-4] Dysphagia is the most common manifestation reported after photodynamic treatment[1] and esophagectomy.[4] Other problems reported included hoarseness, reflux, weight loss, diarrhea, fatigue, and loss of physical strength, socialization, and happiness.[2,5,7-9] Treatment with multimodality therapy or surgery only did not affect the postoperative quality of life.[6] These clients reported that these manifestations affected their quality of life by decreasing their ability to perform usual activities of daily living. Clients who had a total gastrectomy reported a better quality of life than clients who had an esophagogastrectomy or esophagectomy.[7] Clients also reported not receiving enough information before treatment regarding the treatment details, side effects, cure, and prognosis.[2] The FACT-E (Functional Assessment of Cancer Therapy-Esophageal) is a tool recently validated that measures quality of life in esophageal cancer clients.[1]

IMPLICATIONS

Nurses need to be aware of the client-reported problems related to treatment. Some clients reported that they would have refused treatment if they knew what the recovery period would entail. The clients asked for more dietary teaching related to eating smaller meals and eating more slowly, and ways to reduce reflux of food.

Nurses must develop teaching plans to fit individualized client's identified needs, especially those related to nutrition, fatigue, and socialization. A nutritional assessment should be performed and a plan developed to facilitate nutrition that includes increased protein for wound and tissue healing and increased energy. Additionally, clients may benefit from a support group to help with meeting socialization needs.

REFERENCES

1. Darling, G., Eton, D., Sulman, J., et al. (2006). Validation of the functional assessment of cancer therapy esophageal cancer subscale. *Cancer, 107*(4), 854-863.
2. Hemminger, L., & Wolfsen, H. (2002). Photodynamic therapy for Barrett's esophagus and high grade dysplasia: Results of a patient satisfaction survey. *Gastroenterology Nursing, 25*(4), 139-141.
3. Magrone, G., Bozzone, A., Romanelli, A., et al. (2006). Rehabilitation and quality of life in patients undergoing surgery for esophageal cancer. *Rays, 31*(1), 13-16.
4. Mills, M., & Sullivan, K. (2000). Patients with operable esophageal cancer: Their experience of information-giving in a regional thoracic unit. *Journal of Clinical Nursing, 9*(2), 236-246.
5. Moraca, R., & Low, D. (2006). Outcomes and health-related quality of life after esophagectomy for high-grade dysplasia and intramucosal cancer. *Archives of Surgery, 141*(6), 545-549.
6. Reynolds, J., McLaughlin, R., Moore, J., et al. (2006). Prospective evaluation of quality of life in patients with localized esophageal cancer treated by multimodality therapy or surgery alone. *British Journal of Surgery, 93*(9), 1084-1090.
7. Spector, N., Hicks, F., & Pickleman, J. (2002). Quality of life and symptoms after surgery for gastroesophageal cancer. *Gastroenterology Nursing, 23*(3), 120-125.
8. Sweed, M., Schiech, L., Barsevick, A., et al. (2002). Quality of life after esophagectomy for cancer. *Oncology Nursing Forum, 29*(7), 1127-1131.
9. Viklund, P., Wengstrom, Y., Rousvelas, I., et al. (2006). Quality of life and persisting symptoms after esophageal cancer surgery. *European Journal of Cancer, 42*(10), 1407-1414.

receptacle to receive the saliva. While hospitalized, clients are often taught to do self-suctioning. Administer or assist with frequent oral care to prevent oral lesions and oral infections.

Diagnosis: Risk for Ineffective Coping. The client with cancer of the esophagus has many problems associated with both the disease and its treatment. This can lead to a nursing diagnosis of *Risk for Ineffective Coping related to changes in body image and potentially terminal prognosis.*

Outcomes. The client will effectively cope with the alterations in body image and potentially terminal prognosis, as evidenced by maintenance of activities and continued social interaction.

Interventions. In addition to meeting the client's physical needs, you must provide emotional support. The gastrostomy tube may cause an alteration in body image and increased dependency. The constant drooling or need to spit may cause the client a great deal of emotional distress. The poor prognosis of esophageal cancer necessitates psychological support and interventions aimed at helping the client and significant others prepare for the client's death (see Chapters 17 and 21).

Evaluation. Successful control of manifestations and prevention of excessive weight loss, and supporting the client to a peaceful death, may be the desired outcomes. Few clients survive for 5 years.

Surgical Management

Esophageal dilation may be necessary throughout the course of the disease to treat strictures and obstruction caused by the tumor. The physician should perform the treatment as often as needed to relieve dysphagia.

In advanced disease, a prosthesis and, more recently, a stent may be inserted to bypass the tumor or to prevent aspiration in clients with fistulae. The prosthesis or stent can maintain esophageal patency, but can perforate the esophagus if it becomes dislodged or the tumor increases in size.

Surgery may be performed for prophylaxis, cure, or palliation, depending on the extent of the disease. For high-risk clients with Barrett's esophagus (a premalignant healing process that occurs in association with GERD), the lower third of the esophagus is removed prophylactically. One of three surgical procedures can be performed:

1. An *esophagectomy* consists of the removal of all or part of the esophagus. The resected esophagus is replaced with a polyester (Dacron) graft. This procedure is usually performed via a thoracotomy, but it may be performed transhiatally, which eliminates the need for a thoracotomy.

2. An *esophagogastrostomy* involves resection of the lower portion of the esophagus and anastomosis of the remainder to the stomach, brought up into the thorax.

3. In an *esophagoenterostomy* (colon interposition), the esophagus is resected and replaced with a segment of the descending colon.

Nursing Management of the Surgical Client

Assessment. Obtain data about the client's nutritional status, ability to swallow, respiratory status, and ability to cope with the diagnosis. In addition, routine preoperative and postoperative assessments are required.

Diagnosis, Outcomes, Interventions
Diagnosis: Risk for Injury. Surgery to treat esophageal cancer is often extensive, necessitating a thoracic approach and leading to the nursing diagnosis *Risk for Injury related to surgical procedure.*

Outcomes. Injury will be prevented, as evidenced by an absence of atelectasis, fever, wound infection, or problems associated with chest tubes.

Interventions

Improve Nutritional Status Before Surgery. Before surgery, clients usually require 2 to 3 weeks of nutritional support. Often, this support includes tube feedings or TPN. The client's weight and fluid and electrolyte status are monitored closely.

Provide Preoperative Teaching. Provide extensive instruction on postoperative respiratory care, including turning, coughing, deep breathing, and chest physiotherapy. Teach the client about all incisions, wound drainage tubes, feeding tubes, and chest tubes that may be present after surgery. Oral care should be performed four times a day to help prevent infection postoperatively. If an esophagoenterostomy is performed, a complete bowel preparation is performed before surgery.

Maintain Airway

After surgery, respiratory care is a high priority. The client may be placed on a ventilator in a critical care unit (see Chapter 63 for care of a client receiving mechanical ventilation). Otherwise, the client must turn, cough, and deep breathe every hour. Carefully assess the client's respiratory status, report any manifestations of atelectasis or pneumonia, and administer supplemental oxygen. Administer pain medication frequently, and assist the client in splinting the incision while coughing. Place the client in a semi-Fowler position to prevent reflux. Continually monitor the chest tube drainage for amount, color, and patency.

Maintain Fluid and Electrolyte Balance. Assess the client's fluid and electrolyte status. Monitor drainage from the NG, gastric, and all drainage tubes at least every shift. The client is NPO for 4 to 5 days until peristalsis returns. During the first 24 hours after surgery, NG or gastric drainage is bloody, but should then change to a greenish yellow color. If bloody drainage continues, it may indicate bleeding at the suture line and should be reported.

Leakage at the site of anastomosis may appear about 5 to 7 days after surgery. Assess the client for early manifestations of shock as well as for fever, fluid accumulation at the wound site, and inflammation. Check all dressings for bleeding, drainage, or separation of the suture lines.

Advance Diet as Tolerated. The client should be started on small sips of water. If this intake is tolerated, the quantity is slowly increased. Supervise the client, making sure the client stays in an upright position, and monitor for manifestations of leakage at the anastomosis site. If this is tolerated, the client gradually progresses to pureed and semisolid foods. Explain the importance of small, frequent feedings, and advise the client to sit upright at meals and for 1 hour after meals to prevent overdistention of the stomach and reflux.

Evaluation. The poor prognosis associated with the diagnosis of cancer of the esophagus means that successful control of manifestations and prevention of extensive weight loss may be the only reasonable outcomes for these clients. Few clients survive for 5 years. Provide support for the client during the process of dying.

Self-Care

Upon discharge, give the client and family written and oral instructions concerning wound healing, nutritional support, respiratory care, and medications. Teach the client about possible wound and respiratory complications, manifestations that should be reported immediately, and how to contact appropriate members of the health care team.

Make appropriate referrals to community agencies. Most clients need a great amount of assistance at home. Provide information about services offered by the American Cancer Society and palliative care (see Chapters 17 and 21) if it becomes apparent that palliative care is necessary.

VASCULAR DISORDERS

The principal vascular disorder of the esophagus is varices. Because esophageal varices result from portal hypertension, this condition is discussed with liver disorders in Chapter 47.

TRAUMA

Major traumatic conditions of the esophagus include chemical burns, the presence of foreign bodies, and injuries from external forces, such as endoscopic equipment. Chemical burns result from the ingestion of acids or alkalis and sometimes from highly spiced foods. Thermal burns can occur after drinking extremely hot liquids, accidentally ingesting foreign bodies that lodge in the natural narrow spots of the esophagus, and self-mutilating related to suicide attempts. Trauma can cause esophageal perforation, with resultant contamination of the mediastinum and stricture formation as complications of the healing process. Treatment of esophageal strictures involves dilation of the esophagus or surgical excision of the diseased portion and reanastomosis or interposition of a piece of gut from the stomach or colon (see Esophageal Cancer earlier in this chapter).

CONCLUSIONS

Disorders of the mouth and esophagus range from fairly simple problems, such as dental caries, to complex and potentially lethal problems, such as cancer of the esophagus. No matter how minor, disorders throughout the oral-esophageal area can interfere with the client's nutritional intake. Always keep this fact in mind when assessing and caring for clients with these disorders.

THINKING CRITICALLY

1. The client is a 72-year-old retired schoolteacher who lives with her 70-year-old sister. She is being evaluated for complaints of chest pain, which have become increasingly more frequent. Yesterday, while she was lifting flats of bedding plants to prepare for planting, she became dyspneic and collapsed. Her sister called the ambulance, and the client was admitted to a medical-surgical unit. This morning, she underwent an abdominal ultrasound before an upper GI series. An electrocardiogram (ECG) followed the tests. When the nurse last checked, the client was sleeping soundly. Now the client's call light is on. When the nurse enters the room, the client is gasping, clutching at her chest, and attempting to get out of bed, saying, "Please help me! I can't catch my breath!" What is your first priority?

Factors to Consider. Is the client experiencing manifestations of a cardiovascular problem or a gastrointestinal one? How can the nurse tell the difference?

2. A 61-year-old woman is being treated as an outpatient for gastroesophageal reflux disease. She tells the nurse that the doctor told her to take Maalox but did not tell her how else to treat her condition. What would the nurse teach this client?

Factors to Consider. What lifestyle changes might help the client manage her condition?

3. An 18-year-old man is seen at a dental clinic following the blow of a soccer ball to the head. Several teeth were loosened by the impact. During the oral examination, the nurse notes that the gums are reddened and tender and bleed easily when probed with a tongue blade. The area under the left premolar is swollen, tender, and abscessed. The client pulls away and tells the nurse to stop because it hurts too much to touch that tooth and states, "It's been hurting for the past several weeks." When questioned, the client states that he brushes his teeth once a day or every other day, has never flossed, and usually eats several candy bars a day. What nursing interventions are appropriate? Why?

Factors to Consider. What might be the problem with the client's tooth? What could be the cause of his gingival problems?

evolve   *Discussions for these questions can be found on the website.*

BIBLIOGRAPHY

Citations appearing in red refer to primary research.

Citations appearing in blue refer to evidence-based practice guidelines and protocols.

1. American Cancer Society. (2007). *Cancer facts and figures.* Atlanta: Author.
2. Annese, V., & Bassotti, G. (2006). Non-surgical treatment of esophageal achalasia. *World Journal of Gastroenterology, 12*(36), 5763-5766.
3. Blair, K., & Beltz, J. (2006). Dyspepsia: Is it gastroesophageal reflux disease or peptic ulcer disease? *Journal of the American College of Nurse Practitioners, 2*(3), 157-163.
4. Bonavina, L. (2006). Minimally invasive surgery for esophageal achalasia. *World Journal of Gastroenterology, 12*(37), 5921-5925.
5. Borges, L., Rex, K., Chen, J., et al. (2006). A protective role for keratinocyte growth factor in a murine model of chemotherapy and radiotherapy-induced mucositis. *International Journal of Radiation, Oncology, Physics, 66*(1), 254-262.
6. Braghetto, I., Csendes, A., Cardemi, G., et al. (2006). Open transthoracic or transhiatal esophagectomy versus minimally invasive esophagectomy in terms of morbidity, mortality, and survival. *Surgical Endoscopy, 20*(11), 1681-1686.
7. Brennan, M., von Bultzingslowen, I., Schubert, M., et al. (2006). Alimentary mucositis: Putting the guidelines into practice. *Supportive Care in Cancer, 14*(6), 573-579.
8. Cerchiettis, L., Navigante, A., Lutteral, M., et al. (2006). Double-blinded, placebo-controlled trial on intravenous L-alanyl-L-glutamine in the incidence of oral mucositis following chemoradiotherapy in patients with head and neck cancer. *International Journal of Radiation Oncology, Biology, Physics, 65*(5), 1330-1337.
9. Cianfriglia, F., DiGregorio, D., Cianfigilia, C., et al. (2006). Incidence of human papilloma virus infection in oral leukoplakia: Indications for a viral aetiology. *Journal of Experimental and Clinical Cancer Research, 25*(1), 21-28.
10. Copstead, L., & Banasik, J. (2005). *Pathophysiology* (3rd ed.). Philadelphia: Saunders.
11. Corley, D., & Kubo, A. (2006). Body mass index and gastroeophageal reflux disease: A systematic review and meta-analysis. *The American Journal of Gastroenterology, 101*(11), 2619-2628.
12. Eisenberg, B. (2006). Combining imatinib with surgery in gastrointestinal stromal tumors: Rational and ongoing trials. *Clinical Colorectal Cancer, 6*(Supp 1), S24-S29.
13. Feldman, M., Friedman, L., & Brandt, L. (2002). *Sleisenger & Fordtran's gastrointestinal and liver disease: Pathophysiology/diagnosis/management* (7th ed.). Philadelphia: Saunders.
14. Goldsmith, H., & Herman, L. (2002). Endoluminal gastroplication. A new therapeutic endoscopic procedure for gastroesophageal reflux disease. *Gastroenterology Nursing, 25*(1), 115-119.
15. Keefe, D., Lees, J., & Horvath, N. (2006). Palifermin for oral mucositis in the high-dose chemotherapy and stem cell transplant setting: The Royal Adelaide Hospital Cancer Centre experience. *Supportive Care in Cancer, 14*(6), 580-582.
16. Keefe, D., Peterson, D., & Shubert, M. (2006). Developing evidence-based guidelines for management of alimentary mucositis: Process and pitfalls. *Supportive Care in Cancer, 14*(6), 492-498.
17. Labenz, J., Nocon, M., Lind, T., et al. (2006). Prospective follow-up data from the ProGERD study suggest that GERD is not a categorical disease. *American Journal of Gastroenterology, 101*(11), 2457-2462.
18. Lehne, R. (2007). *Pharmacology for nursing care* (6th ed.). Philadelphia: Elsevier Saunders.
19. Leyden, J., Moss, A., & MacMathuna, P. (2006). Endoscopic pneumatic dilation versus botulinum toxin injection in the management of primary achalasia. *Cochrane Database of System Reviews, 4,* CD005046.
20. Lopushinsky, S., & Urbach, D. (2006). Pneumatic dilation and surgical myotomy for achalasia. *Journal of the American Medical Association, 296*(18), 2227-2233.
21. McCance, K., & Huether, S. (2006). *Pathophysiology: Biological basis for disease in adults and children* (5th ed.). St. Louis: Mosby.
22. McGuire, D., Correa, M., Johnson, J., et al. (2006). The role of basic oral care and good clinical practice principles in the management of oral mucositis. *Supportive Care in Cancer, 14*(6), 541-547.
23. McGuire, D., Johnson, J., & Migliorati, C. (2006). Promulgation of guidelines for mucositis management: Educating health care professionals and patients. *Supportive Care in Cancer, 14*(6), 548-557.
24. Metheny, N. (2006). Preventing aspiration in older adults with dysphagia. *MEDSURG Nursing, 15*(2), 110-111.
25. Mishra, A., Bharti, A., Varghese, P., et al. (2006). Differential expression and activation of NF-kappa B family proteins during oral carcinogenesis: Role of high risk human papillomavirus infection. *International Journal of Cancer, 119*(12), 2840-2850.
26. Moayyedi, P., Talley, N., Fennerty, M., et al. (2006). Can the clinical history distinguish between organic and functional dyspepsia? *Journal of the American Medical Association, 295*(13), 1566-1576.
27. Nakamura, T., Ota, M., Hayashi, K., et al. (2006). Chemoradiotherapy with and without esophagectomy for advanced esophageal cancer. *Hepato-Gastroenterology, 53*(71), 705-709.
28. Nicolatou-Galitis, O., Velegraki, A., Sotiropoulou-Lontou, A., et al. (2006). Effect of fluconazole antifungal prophylaxis on oral mucositis in head and neck cancer patients receiving radiotherapy. *Supportive Care in Cancer, 14*(1), 44-51.
29. Novistsky, Y., Paton, B., Kercher, K., et al. (2006). Current aspects of surgical management of GERD. *Surgical Technology International, 15,* 53-62.
30. Nguyen, H., Domingues, G., & Lammert, F. (2006). Technological insights: Combined impedance manometry for esophageal motility testing—Current results and further implications. *World Journal of Gastroenterology, 12*(39), 6266-6273.
31. Price, S., & Wilson, L. (2003). *Pathophysiology: Clinical concepts of disease processes* (6th ed.). St. Louis: Mosby.
32. Qadeer, M., Phillips, C., Lopez, A., et al. (2006). Proton pump inhibitor therapy for suspected GERD-related chronic laryngitis: A meta-analysis of randomized controlled trials. *American Journal of Gastroenterology, 101*(11), 2646-2654.
33. Scully, C., Sonis, S., & Diz, P. (2006). Oral mucositis. *Oral Diseases, 12*(3), 229-241.
34. Spector, N., Hicks, F., & Pickelman, J. (2002). Quality of life and symptoms after surgery for gastroesophageal cancer. *Gastroenterology Nursing, 25*(3), 120-125.
35. Stokman, M., Spijkervet, F., Boezen, H., et al. (2006). Preventive intervention possibilities in radiotherapy- and chemotherapy-induced oral mucositis: Results of meta-analyses. *Journal of Dental Research, 85*(8), 690-700.
36. Thor, P., & Blaut, U. (2006). Helicobacter pylori infection in pathogenesis of gastroesophageal reflux disease. *Journal of Physiology and Pharmacology, 57*(Suppl 3), 81-90.
37. Tsujimoto, H., Ono, S., Chochi, K., et al. (2006). Preoperative chemoradiotherapy for esophageal cancer enhances the postoperative systemic inflammatory response. *Japanese Journal of Clinical Oncology, 36*(10), 632-637.

38. Tutuian, R. (2006). Update in the diagnosis of gastroesophageal reflux disease. *Journal of Gastrointestinal and Liver Diseases*, *15*(3), 243-247.

39. Tytgat, G. (2006). Long-term GERD management: The individualized approach. *Drugs of Today*, *42*(Suppl B), 23-26.

40. Wenger, U., Johnsson, E., Arnelo, U., et al. (2006). An antireflux stent versus conventional stents for palliation of distal esophageal or cardia cancer: A randomized clinical study. *Surgical Endoscopy*, *20*(11), 1675-1680.

41. Worthington, H., Clarkson, J., & Eden, O. (2006). Interventions for preventing oral mucositis for patients with cancer receiving treatment. *Cochrane Database of Systematic Reviews*, *2*, CD000978.

42. Youssef, Y., Shekar, N., Lufti, R., et al. (2006). Long-term evaluation of patient satisfaction and reflux symptoms after laparoscopic fundoplication with Collis gastroplasty. *Surgical Endoscopy*, *20*(11), 1702-1705.

43. Zacharoulis, D., O'Boyle, C., Sedman, P., et al. (2006). Laparoscopic fundoplication: A 10-year learning curve. *Surgical Endoscopy*, *20*(11), 1662-1670.

evolve *Did you remember to check out the bonus material on the Evolve website and the CD-ROM, including NCLEX®-Examination Style Review Questions, Open-Book Quizzes, and Chapter Review Audio Podcasts?*

http://evolve.elsevier.com/Black/medsurg

CHAPTER **31**

Management of Clients with Digestive Disorders

DAWN P. MURPHY AND JANE HOKANSON HAWKS

The client with a gastric disorder usually has a problem with nutritional intake. As a result, the most common nursing diagnosis is *Imbalanced Nutrition: Less Than Body Requirements*. Additional nursing diagnoses may include *Acute Pain, Ineffective Therapeutic Regimen Management (Individual) related to dietary changes and pharmacologic management, Fear,* and *Risk for Injury related to complications*.

GENERAL CLINICAL MANIFESTATIONS OF GASTROINTESTINAL DISORDERS

Manifestations of gastrointestinal (GI) tract dysfunction are caused by excessive gastric secretions that can erode stomach mucosa, increase motility, and result in retention of gastric contents. The most prominent clinical manifestations are acute pain, acid reflux, anorexia, belching, flatulence, nausea, vomiting, bleeding, indigestion, and diarrhea.

Pain

Acute pain is the most characteristic clinical manifestation; it usually results from chemical irritation of nerve endings. Nerve irritation occurs when acid comes into contact with the eroded stomach mucosa. It also results from stretching and contracting of the stomach, caused in turn by increased motility and increased smooth muscle tension, as found in an obstruction.

Anorexia

Anorexia, or loss of appetite, is often experienced by clients with malignancy or various other disorders. Hunger is normally caused by several stimuli, including contraction of the empty stomach. When the stomach empties slowly or when gastric stasis occurs because of a gastric disorder, anorexia can result.

Nausea and Vomiting

Nausea is a result of conditions that increase tension on the walls of the stomach, duodenum, or lower end of the esophagus. Unpleasant stimuli, distention, gastritis, and carcinoma of the stomach can produce nausea. Vomiting may follow nausea or occur without it. Vomiting is caused by stimulation of the emetic center, which can occur by the following mechanisms:

1. Stimulation of the chemoreceptor trigger zone (CTZ) in the fourth ventricle. The CTZ is stimulated by various drugs and body chemicals. Conversely, medications of the phenothiazine derivative groups, such as chlorpromazine (Thorazine) and prochlorperazine (Compazine), depress vomiting caused by chemoreceptor stimulation. Selective serotonin receptor antagonists, such as ondansetron (Zofran) and granisetron (Kytril), block serotonin receptors in the vagus nerve and CTZ.
2. Excitation of nerve impulses by any of the following:
   a. Direct mechanical stimuli, as in increased intracranial pressure.
   b. Chemical stimuli from blood-borne metabolites or chemical substances.
   c. Sympathetic and parasympathetic afferent nerve impulses through the vagus, glossopharyngeal, vestibular, and splanchnic nerves (the most sensitive receptors are located in the proximal duodenum).

3. Unpleasant odors, subjects, and sights that stimulate higher center impulses.
4. Distention of stomach or duodenum.
5. Decreased gastric motility.
6. Pain, because the pain centers are close to the vomiting centers in the medulla.
7. Increased intracranial pressure.

Bleeding

Bleeding results from local trauma or irritation that causes erosion or ulceration of the GI tract mucosa. The disorders involved include stomach neoplasms, gastric ulcer, gastritis, anastomotic (marginal) ulcers, and duodenal ulcers. Duodenitis, or inflammation of the duodenum, can also cause bleeding. Although bleeding may have numerous causes, up to 75% of all cases of upper GI tract bleeding result from esophagogastric varices (venous), hemorrhagic gastritis (capillary), or peptic ulcer. Ulcers account for 80% of all upper GI tract hemorrhage.

Diarrhea

Diarrhea can be caused by increased peristalsis resulting from an increased gastrocolic reflex or from the effort of the stomach and intestines to eliminate a local irritant.

Belching and Flatulence

Swallowed air causes most belching and flatulence. It is easy to swallow air during eating and drinking, especially when food is ingested rapidly. Frequently, clients attempt to belch to relieve a vague feeling of distress in the stomach caused by swallowed air. Attempting to belch with the mouth closed sometimes adds more air to the stomach than it removes.

Indigestion

Indigestion or dyspepsia can be caused by such factors as strong emotions, GI tract disease, eating too rapidly, chewing inadequately, gas-forming foods (e.g., beans and cabbage), and food allergy. Eating very large meals and lying down directly after eating can also cause indigestion.

GASTROINTESTINAL INTUBATION

Gastric and duodenal tubes are inserted for several purposes: (1) decompression, (2) lavage, (3) gastric analysis, and (4) tube feedings.

Decompression relieves the pressure caused by contents and gases that remain in the stomach or bowel because of an obstruction. Long intestinal tubes are sometimes used to dilate the lumen or to release an obstruction. Postoperative decompression removes secretions that cannot pass through the GI tract because of edema and decreased gastric motility. The placement of a tube (intubation) helps prevent vomiting, distention, and obstruction.

Lavage is the irrigation or washing out of an organ. Gastric lavage washes out the stomach. It is used most frequently as an emergency treatment in poisoning. Lavage is also used for exfoliative cytology to determine the presence of abnormal cells.

Tube-feeding or *gavage feeding,* referred to as *enteral nutrition,* is a method of giving clients fluids and nutrients via a tube when oral intake is inadequate or impossible.

Types of Tubes

Three types of tubes are used for decompression: (1) *short* nasogastric (NG) tubes are used for the stomach, (2) *medium* tubes extend into the duodenum or jejunum, and (3) *long* tubes are used for the rest of the GI tract (Table 31-1).

Short Tubes

Short tubes include the Levin (single lumen) and Salem sump (double lumen) tubes. Short tubes are long enough to extend into the stomach (about 50 inches) but not into the bowel. These tubes are usually attached to suction, which is set for low intermittent suction for

---

TABLE 31–1 Gastric and Intestinal Tubes

	Length	Size (French)	Lumen	Other Characteristics
Short Tubes				
Levin type (plastic or rubber)	125 cm (50 inches)	12, 16, 18	Single	
Salem sump	120 cm (48 inches)	12, 14, 16, 18	Double	Sump-type suction
Medium Tubes				
Dobhoff (nasoduodenal or nasojejunal)	160-175 cm (60-66 inches)	8, 10, 12	Single	Radiopaque, tungsten weighted
Long Tubes				
Cantor	300 cm (10 feet)	16	Single	Mercury weighted
Harris	180 cm (6 feet)	14, 16	Single	Mercury weighted
Miller-Abbott	300 cm (10 feet)	12, 14, 16, 18	Double	Mercury weighted

the Levin tube. Low continuous suction is used for the Salem sump because the "pigtail" lumen on the Salem sump tube vents the tube and protects gastric mucosa from being sucked against the tube. The pigtail lumen should not be clamped or irrigated and should be kept higher than the client's stomach to prevent drainage. Occasionally, these may be used for short-term enteral feedings over a brief period. However, nasoduodenal tubes are preferred for feedings because of the high rate of aspiration pneumonia associated with NG tube feedings.

Medium Tubes

Medium tubes include a variety of single-lumen naso-duodenal (e.g., Dobhoff) tubes that extend into the duodenum (60 to 66 inches) and are designed for short-term feeding. They are less likely to cause aspiration pneumonia because of their small size and weighted tip. Placement is verified by abdominal x-ray study (radiography).

Long Tubes

The long tubes extend into the small bowel, sometimes for its entire length. These single-lumen tubes are between 6 and 10 feet long and are used to prevent gas and fluid accumulation in the intestine, which is usually caused by intestinal obstruction. Use of long tubes has decreased substantially in the last several years. The more common long tubes are the Miller-Abbott, Cantor, and Harris tubes.

Other Tubes

Long-term enteral feedings—gastrostomy tubes (GTs or G tubes) or jejunostomy tubes (JTs or J tubes)—are often placed surgically. The GT and JT (see Chapter 29) can be inserted surgically or laparoscopically. The percutaneous endoscopic gastrostomy (PEG) approach, which is the most common, and the percutaneous endoscopic jejunostomy (PEJ) approach for tube placement were discussed in Chapter 29.

Inserting Gastrointestinal Tubes

GI tubes are generally inserted through the nose into the stomach or small intestine. These tubes are rarely inserted through the mouth. The following steps are included:
1. Assist the client to a high-Fowler's position.
2. Complete the NEX measurement (distance on the tube from the tip of the nose to the ear lobe plus the distance from the ear lobe to the tip of the xiphoid process) and mark the distance on the tube.
3. Lubricate and gently insert the tube through the nares and posterior nasal pharynx and into the oropharynx.
4. Instruct the client to swallow when the tube is in the oropharynx; sometimes the client is allowed

to drink water at this point to help with tube passage through the sphincter at the proximal end of the esophagus.
5. Advance the tube into the stomach after it passes the sphincter.

To verify placement:
1. Aspirate gastric contents and measure the pH of the aspirant; the pH of the stomach is less than that of the lungs (refer to the Translating Evidence into Practice box on p. 625).
2. Check with an x-ray study for the radiopaque lines on the tube.

Temporarily secure the tube to the nose with hypoallergenic tape. After confirming placement, the tube may be secured with a device designed to secure tube placement or with hypoallergenic tape. (This procedure is used for short tubes only; medium tubes are checked with an x-ray and long tubes need to be able to advance.) Refer to a fundamentals of nursing textbook for additional information related to GI tube insertion and placement verification.

Suctioning Gastrointestinal Tubes

When suction is applied to a GI tube to remove accumulated gas and fluid, ensure that the GI mucosa is not traumatized. Excessive negative pressure causes the mucosa to be sucked into the openings on the tube, impairing suction and injuring the mucosa. Intermittent suction is used to avoid this problem unless a double-lumen tube, such as the Salem sump, is used. Mucus tends to plug the openings of these tubes, making it necessary to irrigate with saline as ordered to maintain or check tube patency (usually every 4 hours) or more frequently if the client complains of nausea.

Nursing Management of Clients
with Gastrointestinal Tubes

Maintain the client's comfort while the tube is in place. Helpful nursing interventions include the following steps:
1. Clean and lubricate external nares. The nares may become sore because of crusted secretions around the tube. Always use a water-soluble lubricant to avoid the possibility of lipid pneumonia when using an oil-based lubricant.
2. Tape or secure the tube in a manner that prevents irritation of the nares.
3. Administer frequent oral hygiene to remove debris, increase comfort, maintain a healthy oral cavity, and stimulate saliva secretion. The client's mouth is usually dry because the absence of chewing prevents the normal stimulus to salivary secretions and the presence of the tube causes mouth breathing.
4. Permit the client, if possible, to chew gum or suck on sour candies or ice chips to help stimulate salivation.

TRANSLATING EVIDENCE INTO PRACTICE

Assessing Gastrointestinal Tube Placement

Norma Metheny is one nursing researcher who has been conducting nursing research related to assessment of gastrointestinal tubes for more than 20 years.[1-14] Placement errors can lead to aspiration pneumonia, vomiting, increased residuals, and other complications.[3,12,14] The greatest error with nasoduodenal feeding tubes is not placing the tubes into the duodenum.[4,13,14] When these tubes are placed in the stomach, the risk of pulmonary aspiration increases.[11] Pulmonary aspiration of tube feedings is a major risk factor for development of pneumonia in critically ill tube-fed clients.[11] Other risk factors included GERD, Glasgow Coma Score <9, use of paralytic agents, and high sedation levels.[11]

Traditionally, checking placement of gastrointestinal tubes was done by nurses who injected air and auscultated to detect proper placement. This method was designed for assessing large nasogastric tubes and has been proven the least effective method for checking placement. Radiologic verification of weighted tubes and aspiration of gastric or duodenal contents for pH testing (using pH paper or tubes with a built-in probe and pH meter) of those contents are the most accurate predictors of gastrointestinal tube placement.[2,7,9,10] In addition, the ability to determine pepsin, trypsin, and bilirubin levels as well as pH at the bedside facilitates assessment of proper position.[2,5,8,10]

Residual volumes of nasogastric, gastric, and nasoduodenal tubes have been researched as well.[1] A common mistake is aspiration of jejunal feeding tubes. These should never be aspirated. In one study, gastric residual volumes (GRVs) were 1.5 times greater from larger diameter feeding tubes versus those from 10F feeding tubes in all clients receiving postpyloric feedings.[6] Findings from another study suggest that nasogastric residuals of more than 200 ml and gastrostomy residuals of more than 100 ml were shown to be of concern,[1] but further research is needed before thresholds can be established.

IMPLICATIONS

Nurses are the health care providers primarily responsible for nasogastric and nasoduodenal tube feedings, and nurses

monitor all other gastrointestinal tubes and feeding tubes. It is imperative that correct assessment for placement (using pH, bilirubin, or enzyme presence) be incorporated into practice. Further research is warranted regarding residual amounts that indicate that a tube feeding should be slowed or discontinued for an hour or more.

REFERENCES

1. Edwards, S., & Metheny, N. (2000). Research for practice: Measurement of gastric residual volume: A state of the science. *MED-SURG Nursing, 9*(3), 125-128.
2. Metheny, N., & Meert, K. (2004). Monitoring feeding tube placement. *Nutrition in Clinical Practice, 19*(5), 487-495.
3. Metheny, N., et al. (1990). Detection of inadvertent respiratory placement of small-bore feeding tubes. *Heart & Lung, 19*(6), 631-638.
4. Metheny, N., et al. (1998). Detection of improperly positioned feeding tubes. *Journal of Healthcare Risk Management, 18*(3), 37-48.
5. Metheny, N., et al. (2000). Development of a reliable and valid bedside test for bilirubin and its utility for improving prediction of feeding tube location. *Nursing Research, 49*(6), 302-309.
6. Metheny, N., et al. (2005). Effect of feeding-tube properties on residual volume measurements in tube-fed patients. *Journal of Parenteral and Enteral Nutrition, 29*(3), 192-197.
7. Metheny, N., et al. (1993). Effectiveness of pH measurements in predicting feeding tube placement: An update. *Nursing Research, 42*(6), 324-331.
8. Metheny, N., et al. (2005). Indicators of tubesite during feedings. *Journal of Neuroscience Nursing, 37*(6), 320-325.
9. Metheny, N., et al. (1999). pH and concentration of bilirubin in feeding tube aspirates as predictors of tube placement. *Nursing Research, 48*(4), 189-197.
10. Metheny, N., et al. (1997). pH and concentrations of pepsin and trypsin in feeding tube aspirates as predictors of tube placement. *Journal of Parenteral Nutrition, 21*(5), 279-285.
11. Metheny, N., et al. (2006). Tracheobronchial aspiration of gastric contents in critically ill tube-fed patients: Frequency, outcomes, and risk factors. *Critical Care Medicine, 34*(4), 1007-1015.
12. Metheny, N., et al. (1994). Visual characteristics of aspirates from feeding tubes as a method for predicting tube location. *Nursing Research, 43*(5), 282-287.
13. Metheny, N., & Stewart, B. (2002). Testing feeding tube placement during continuous tube feedings. *Nursing Research, 15*(4), 254-258.
14. Metheny, N., & Titler, M. (2001). Assessing placement of feeding tubes. *American Journal of Nursing, 101*(5), 36-46.

Excessive use stimulates gastric secretions and causes electrolyte loss through the suction.

5. Brush the client's teeth or assist the client in brushing teeth.

6. Request an order for anesthetic mouth rinses or lozenges because the presence of the tube frequently causes sore throat.

Placement of the tube in the throat may result in cricoid chondritis (irritation of the cricoid cartilage of the larynx) and laryngeal injuries. Presenting clinical manifestations include localized odynophagia, pain radiating to the ears, sore throat, stridor, bloody sputum, and mild hoarseness.

Assess for these potential complications and report the findings immediately. An order for anesthetic lozenges or gargles to relieve manifestations may be needed. Frequent assessment of secretions for color, odor, and quantity is essential. Report any changes to the physician or health care provider. It may be necessary to send samples of these secretions to the laboratory for analysis. Measure the contents of the suction containers to maintain an accurate record of GI losses. Metabolic alkalosis may result from a major loss of water and electrolytes through gastric suction. Monitor potassium levels, because potassium is one of the major electrolytes lost through suctioning.

The irrigating solution instilled into a GI tube is counted as intake if it is not removed when contents are aspirated. Keep accurate records of the amount instilled and the amount aspirated from the tube during irrigations. Normal saline is the preferred irrigating solution because water, a hypotonic solution, increases electrolyte loss through osmotic action if the tube is irrigated frequently.

GASTRITIS

Gastritis is a term that encompasses a series of conditions that present with inflammation of the gastric mucosa. It is classified based on time course (as either acute or chronic), histologic features (biopsy), and proposed pathogenic mechanism. The incidence of gastritis is highest in the fifth and sixth decades of life as a result of natural thinning of the gastric mucosa with aging; men are more frequently affected than women. Clients who are heavy drinkers and smokers are also more likely to develop gastritis.

ACUTE GASTRITIS

Etiology and Risk Factors

The acute form of gastritis may be seen with nausea and vomiting, epigastric discomfort, bleeding, malaise, and anorexia. It usually stems from ingestion of a corrosive, erosive, or infectious substance. Aspirin and other non-steroidal anti-inflammatory drugs (NSAIDs), digitalis, chemotherapeutic drugs, radiation therapy, steroids, acute alcoholism and cocaine use, food poisoning (typically caused by *Staphylococcus* organisms), and HIV/AIDS are common causes. In addition, food substances, including excessive amounts of tea, coffee, mustard, paprika, cloves, and pepper, can precipitate acute gastritis. Foods with a rough texture or those eaten at an extremely high temperature can also damage the stomach mucosa. Ingestion of corrosive agents, such as lye or drain cleaner, also causes acute gastritis with the damage/loss of the mucosal layer.

Disorders linked with acute gastritis include uremia, shock, central nervous system lesions, hepatic cirrhosis, portal hypertension, and prolonged emotional tension. Acute gastritis is usually of short duration unless the gastric mucosa has suffered extensive damage, or is untreated, in which case it may evolve into chronic gastritis.

Health promotion behaviors include limited use of NSAIDs, alcohol, and caffeine and avoidance of nicotine products, both smoking and chewing. Health maintenance behaviors include use of enteric-coated aspirin, cytoprotective agents (sucralfate [Carafate], misoprostol [Cytotec], and bismuth subsalicylate [Pepto-Bismol]) to protect the stomach lining, histamine-receptor antagonists to decrease gastric acidity, or proton pump inhibitors to block gastric acid production. Clients with medical disorders that may lead to gastritis should follow orders for prescribed medications to minimize stomach irritation.

Pathophysiology

The most common causes of acute gastritis are infectious. The pathogens include *Helicobacter pylori, Escherichia coli, Proteus, Haemophilus,* streptococci, and staphylococci. Bacterial infection of the stomach is rare but may be life-threatening. The mucosal lining of the stomach normally protects it from the action of gastric acid, and gastric acid may protect the stomach from bacterial infection. If this barrier is penetrated by inflammation and necrosis, infection occurs, with resultant injury to the mucosa. When hydrochloric acid comes into contact with the mucosa, injury to small vessels occurs with edema, hemorrhage, and possible ulcer formation. The damage associated with acute gastritis is usually limited if treated promptly.

Clinical Manifestations

Assessment typically reveals epigastric discomfort usually described as burning or aching, abdominal tenderness, cramping, belching, reflux, severe nausea and vomiting, and sometimes hematemesis. Sometimes GI bleeding is the only manifestation. When contaminated food is the cause of gastritis, diarrhea usually develops within 5 hours of ingestion of the offending substance.

Diagnosis is based on a detailed history of food intake, medications taken, and any disorders related to gastritis. The physician may also perform a gastroscopic examination with a biopsy to determine histologic (cell) changes as well as epithelial degeneration (response to injury).

OUTCOME MANAGEMENT

Medical Management

Intervention involves removing the cause and treating the manifestations. Vomiting frequently responds to medications of the phenothiazine group; pain responds to antacids or histamine (H_2) receptor antagonists. These topics are discussed in the Integrating Pharmacology box on p. 627. If ingestion of NSAIDs is a problem, a prostaglandin E_1 (PGE_1) analog may be prescribed to protect the stomach mucosa and inhibit gastric acid secretion.

Initially, foods and fluids are withheld until nausea and vomiting subside. Once the client tolerates food, the diet includes decaffeinated tea, gelatin, toast, and simple, bland foods. The client should avoid spicy foods,

Medications for Peptic Ulcer Disease

Because most peptic ulcers are caused by *H. pylori* bacteria, a triple therapy aimed at eliminating the bacteria and reducing gastric secretions is prescribed. Triple therapy consists of two anti-infective agents (clarithromycin [Biaxin] or amoxicillin and metronidazole [Flagyl]) and a proton pump inhibitor (lansoprazole [Prevacid], pantoprazole [Protonix], omeprazole [Prilosec]). These are usually given for 1 week but may be repeated if necessary. Levofloxacin may be substituted for clarithromycin or amoxicillin when there has been a treatment failure with either of those antibiotics. In addition, research findings suggest that a 10-day course of medications may be warranted if there has been a treatment failure as well as the change in antibiotics used. Sometimes a quadruple therapy consisting of a proton pump inhibitor, tetracycline, metronidazole, and a bismuth salt may be administered.

Other medications prescribed include hyposecretory agents that reduce or inhibit acid secretions. These agents include H_2-receptor antagonists (ranitidine [Zantac]; cimetidine [Tagamet]; famotidine [Pepcid]), prostaglandin analogs (misoprostol [Cytotec]), proton pump inhibitors (omeprazole [Prilosec], esomeprazole [Nexium]), and antacids. H_2-receptor antagonists inhibit the action of histamine on the H_2 receptors that trigger parietal cell response to chemical stimulation, which results in reduced gastric acid output and concentration. Prostaglandin analogs, in addition to decreasing acid secretion, stimulate production of cytoprotective mucus. Proton pump inhibitors act by inhibiting the gastric enzyme (H^+, K^+)-ATPase, which catalyzes the final step of HCl production at the secretory surface of the gastric parietal cells. Antacids neutralize gastric acid for approximately 30 minutes.

Another medication for short-term treatment of peptic ulcers is known as a mucosal barrier fortifier (sucralfate [Carafate]. These drugs prevent hydrogen ion back-diffusion into the mucosa and stimulate mucus production, which results in accelerated peptic ulcer healing.

caffeine, and large, heavy meals. In the continued absence of nausea, vomiting, and bloating, the client can slowly return to a normal diet.

Nursing Management of the Medical Client

Nursing management of the medical client with acute gastritis is described in the section on chronic gastritis.

CHRONIC GASTRITIS

This condition appears in three stages:

- *Superficial gastritis*—Inflammatory changes are limited to the surface mucosa, which causes an erythemic, edematous mucosa with small erosions and hemorrhages. Gastric glands are intact at this stage.

- *Atrophic gastritis*—Inflammation extends deeper into the mucosa with progressive glandular destruction. It is invariably present in pernicious anemia; it is characterized by a decreased number of parietal and chief cells (chief cells secrete the digestive enzymes [pepsins] of the stomach).

- *Hypertrophic gastritis or gastric atrophy*—Inflammatory infiltrates produce a dull and nodular mucosa with irregular, thickened, or nodular rugae; mucosa may be thin with blood vessels clearly visualized. Hemorrhages occur frequently. Gastric glands undergo transformation at this stage, and the metaplastic changes are an important predisposing factor for gastric cancer.

Etiology and Risk Factors

Chronic gastritis is classified into two types according to the area involved. **Type A** *(autoimmune gastritis)* refers to gastritis of the fundus and body of the stomach, and is frequently associated with loss of parietal cells and pernicious anemia. **Type B** is the most common form of gastritis and is caused by *H. pylori* infection. Peptic ulcer disease (PUD) or gastric surgery may lead to chronic gastritis. Other risk factors are similar to those for acute gastritis. After gastric resection with a gastrojejunostomy, bile and bile acids may reflux into the remaining stomach, causing gastritis. *H. pylori* infection has become acknowledged as an independent risk factor for gastric cancer, as it can lead to chronic atrophic gastritis. Worldwide epidemiologic studies have identified a higher incidence of *H. pylori* infection in clients with adenocarcinoma of the stomach as well as a three-fold to six-fold increased risk for gastric cancer. Age is also a risk factor; chronic gastritis is more common in older adults.

Pathophysiology

The initial pathophysiologic changes associated with chronic gastritis are the same as with acute gastritis. The stomach lining first becomes thickened and erythematous and then becomes thin and atrophic. Continued deterioration and atrophy lead to loss of function of the gastric glands containing parietal cells. When the acid secretion decreases, the source of intrinsic factor is lost. This loss results in inability to absorb vitamin B_{12} and the development of pernicious anemia. Gastric atrophy with metaplasia has been observed in chronic gastritis with *H. pylori* infection. These changes may lead to an increased risk for adenocarcinoma of the stomach.

Clinical Manifestations

Manifestations vary greatly; they include a gnawing or burning ache or pain, nausea, vomiting, loss of appetite, belching, and weight loss. They may be vague or absent (because the problem does not cause an increase in hydrochloric acid). Assessment may reveal anorexia, a feeling of fullness, dyspepsia, belching, vague epigastric pain, nausea, vomiting, and intolerance of spicy or fatty foods.

Complications of Gastritis

The clinical course of clients with chronic gastritis may include such complications as bleeding, pernicious anemia, and gastric cancer. Bleeding can be a complication of gastritis, especially when the stomach mucosa becomes denuded or erosive. Bleeding is common with use of alcohol, aspirin, or NSAIDs. The client should undergo an endoscopic examination to determine the source of the bleeding. Another possible complication of atrophic gastritis is diminished ability of the stomach to secrete intrinsic factor, resulting in malabsorption of vitamin B_{12}, which is confirmed by the Schilling test. Gastric cancer may be suspected in a client whose gastritis does not heal with therapy. (See Gastric Cancer later in this chapter.)

OUTCOME MANAGEMENT

Medical Management

Intervention begins when the health care provider rules out cancer as a causative factor. Discomfort may lessen with a bland diet, small frequent meals, antacids, H_2-receptor antagonists, proton pump inhibitors, and avoidance of foods that cause manifestations. If *H. pylori* bacteria are present, antibiotics and other medications are administered to eliminate the bacteria although eradication of *H. pylori* as a preventive measure for gastric cancer is not recommended. (see the Integrating Pharmacology feature on Medications for Peptic Ulcer Disease, p. 627). If 1 week of this regimen does not succeed in eliminating the bacteria, the regimen may be repeated for an additional week. If pernicious anemia develops, intramuscular injections of vitamin B_{12} may be administered monthly for the remainder of the client's life.

Nursing Management of the Medical Client

When assessing the client with acute or chronic gastritis, carefully focus on risk factors. Consider the client's diet, eating patterns, use of prescription and over-the-counter drugs, and lifestyle, including alcohol consumption and cigarette smoking.

Reduce Pain

Focus on teaching the client about the causes of gastritis and foods that may worsen the disease. Help the client assess factors that increase manifestations, such as stress or fatigue, taking certain medications on an empty stomach, ingestion of foods and beverages, alcohol consumption, and smoking. Encourage the client to avoid these factors.

Aluminum hydroxide with magnesium carbonate (Gaviscon), which produces a soothing foam, is the best antacid for gastritis. H_2-receptor antagonists, proton pump inhibitors, antisecretory agents, and drugs that enhance mucosal defenses also provide pain reduction (see the Integrating Pharmacology feature on Medications for GERD in Chapter 30).

If the nausea and vomiting are severe, the client may be restricted to nothing by mouth (NPO) until these problems decrease in severity. When the pain and nausea associated with gastritis have subsided, the client is instructed to have a well-balanced diet and avoid irritating foods and beverages.

Promote Self-Care

Cases of acute and chronic gastritis are managed at home unless complications develop. Instruct the client with chronic gastritis to see the health care provider at regular intervals. This is particularly important if the diagnosis is *H. pylori* infection and atrophic gastritis, because these problems are closely related to gastric cancer. Teach the client to use medications correctly, to maintain adequate nutrition, and to control risk factors that contribute to gastritis.

Surgical Management

If conservative measures have not controlled bleeding, surgery may be necessary. Subtotal gastrectomy, pyloroplasty, vagotomy, or total gastrectomy may be indicated with severe erosive gastritis. These procedures are discussed in the following section on peptic ulcer disease (PUD).

PEPTIC ULCER DISEASE

PUD involves a disruption in the continuity of the lower esophageal, gastric, or duodenal mucosa, leading to a local defect resulting from inflammation. An ulcer may occur in any part of the GI tract that comes into contact with gastric juices (hydrochloric acid and pepsin). The ulcer may be found in the esophagus, stomach, duodenum, or the jejunum after gastroenterostomy.

Peptic ulcers are fairly common in the United States, occurring in 4 million individuals yearly with an estimated cost of treatment exceeding 10 billion dollars yearly. Lifetime prevalence of PUD in the United States is approximately 12% in men and 10% in women. An estimated 15,000 deaths occur per year as a result of complications of PUD. Gastric ulcers are more likely to occur during the fifth and sixth decades of life; duodenal ulcers more commonly occur during the fourth and fifth decades for men. For women, the occurrence is about 10 years later in life. Men are more likely to have both gastric and duodenal ulcers.

DUODENAL ULCERS

Duodenal ulcers have a higher incidence than gastric ulcers but the incidence of malignancy is much less. These ulcers usually occur within 3.0 cm of the pylorus and are usually characterized by high gastric acid secretion. They are usually less than or equal to 1.0 cm in diameter, but may reach 3.0 to 6.0 cm. The ulcers are sharply demarcated, and depth may reach the muscularis propria (layer of muscle below mucosa). Some are associated with normal gastric secretion but rapid emptying of the stomach. Hypersecretion of acid is attributed to a greater mass of parietal cells. Stimuli for acid secretion include protein-rich meals, alcohol consumption, calcium, and vagal stimulation.

Clients with a duodenal ulcer experience low pH levels in the duodenum for longer periods. This may be due to a significant decrease in bicarbonate secretion in the duodenum, in which *H. pylori* infection is thought to play a role.

Finally, clients with duodenal ulcers have more rapid gastric emptying. The combined effect of hypersecretion of acid and rapid emptying of food from the stomach reduces the buffering effect of food and results in a large acid load in the duodenum. Within the duodenum, inhibitory mechanisms and pancreatic secretion (an alkaline solution) may be insufficient to control the acid load.

GASTRIC ULCERS

Gastric ulcers are found most often distal to the junction between the antrum and the acid secretory mucosa; they are usually within 1 inch (2.5 cm) of the pylorus of the stomach, in an area where gastritis is common. Gastric ulcers are defined as a break in the mucosal surface >5 mm in size with depth to the submucosa. The mucosal barrier, which differs from the layer of glycoprotein mucus that overlies the gastric epithelium, normally allows hydrochloric acid to be secreted into the stomach without injury to the epithelial cells. An incompetent pylorus may decrease production of mucus, the usual gastric defense. The reflux of bile acids through an incompetent pylorus into the stomach may break the mucosal barrier. Decreased blood flow to the gastric mucosa may also alter the defensive barrier and may make the duodenum more susceptible to gastric acid and pepsin trauma. The recurrence rate of gastric ulcer is lower than that of duodenal ulcer. However, gastric ulcers, in contrast to duodenal ulcer, may be malignant.

STRESS-INDUCED AND DRUG-INDUCED ULCERS

Besides peptic ulcers, acute gastric erosion, frequently called *stress ulcers* or *stress erosive gastritis,* can occur after an acute medical crisis. Major assaults that give rise to gastroduodenal ulcerations include severe trauma or major illness, severe burns (may cause what is known as Curling's ulcers), head injury or intracranial disease (frequently called Cushing's ulcers), ingestion of a drug (e.g., aspirin, NSAIDs, steroids, or alcohol) that acts on the gastric mucosa (Figure 31-1), shock, and sepsis.

Etiology and Risk Factors

The causal factor in more than 90% of all peptic ulcers has been attributed to *H. pylori*. *H. pylori* is the only bacteria classified by the World Health Organization as a Class I carcinogen. Eradication of the organism usually results in resolution of gastritis and decreased risk of developing gastric cancer. The vaccine HELIVAX, approved by the FDA in 2003 for the prevention and treatment of *H. pylori* infection, induces the generation of *Helicobacter*-specific antibody secreting cells in the gastric antrum and duodenum where the infection usually occurs.

The occurrence of PUD depends on the defensive resistance of the mucosa in relation to the aggressive force of secretory activity. The defensive resistance of the mucosa depends on mucosal integrity and regeneration, the presence of a protective mucus barrier, adequate blood flow to the mucosa, ability of the duodenal inhibitory mechanism to regulate secretion, and the presence of adequate gastromucosal prostaglandins. The aggressive factors of PUD are related to the presence of *H. pylori* and the volume of hydrochloric and biliary acids. Ulceration occurs when aggressive factors exceed the defensive barrier. The aggressive nature of the gastric juice may be the result of hypersecretion of gastric juices, increased stimulation of the vagus nerve, decreased inhibition of gastric secretions, increased

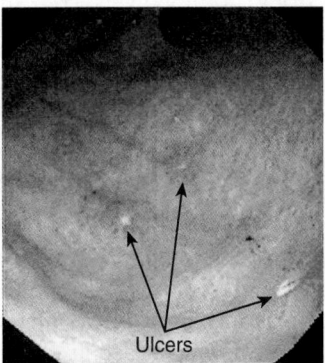

Ulcers

■ **FIGURE 31–1**   Gastric ulcerations caused by nonsteroidal anti-inflammatory drugs.

capacity or number of parietal cells secreting hydrochloric acid, or increased response of the parietal cells to stimulation.

Risk factors that contribute to PUD include smoking (nicotine), chewing tobacco, steroids, aspirin, NSAIDs, caffeine, alcohol, and stress. Certain medical conditions, including Crohn's disease, Zollinger-Ellison syndrome, and hepatic and biliary disease, may also play a role.

Health promotion and health maintenance actions for clients with PUD are the same as those discussed for acute gastritis. Because smoking is often found to be the cause of failure of *H. pylori* eradication therapy, clients are encouraged to stop smoking before beginning another course of treatment. Health restoration for clients involves treating medical disorders that cause secondary PUD. Ensure that the client complies with the prescribed medication regimen to minimize stomach irritation. Treat aggressively any disorders that result in the development of PUD, for example, long-term use of steroids, severe burns, and chronic renal failure.

Pathophysiology

In addition to *H. pylori* inflammation as the primary pathophysiologic change, two different mechanisms for the development of PUD have been proposed. In the stomach, it is thought that a breakdown of the normally protective epithelial lining causes gastric ulcers. Under normal circumstances, flow of hydrochloric acid from the lumen of the stomach is prevented by the presence of tight, nonpermeable junctions between the epithelial cells and by the slightly alkaline layer of mucus that coats the surface of the gastric epithelium.

NSAIDs are one of the most commonly used medications in the United States, and are the second most frequent cause of PUD. As many as 3% to 4% of NSAID users develop PUD each year, but up to 80% of clients with serious NSAID-related complications do not present with previous dyspepsia-related manifestations.

In the formation of a gastric peptic ulcer, the diffusion barrier may be interrupted by the chronic presence of such injurious substances as aspirin, NSAIDs, cortisone, adrenocorticotropic hormone (ACTH), caffeine, alcohol, chemotherapeutic agents, and hypersecretory conditions. These substances may stimulate acid production, cause local mucosal damage, and suppress mucus secretion. The substances strip away surface mucus and cause degeneration of epithelial cell membranes with massive diffusion of acid back into the gastric epithelial wall.

The pathogenesis of duodenal peptic ulcers has a different proposed mechanism, because excess acid secretion is responsible for ulcer development. Activity of the vagus nerve is increased in people with duodenal ulcers, particularly during a fasting state and at night. The vagus nerve stimulates the pyloric antrum cells to release gastrin, which travels via the bloodstream and acts on the gastric parietal cells to stimulate the release of hydrochloric acid.

Another factor in PUD is emotional stress, which can cause an increase in gastric secretion, blood supply, and gastric motility by thalamic stimulation of the vagal nerves. Hormonal influence takes place via the hypothalamus through the pituitary-adrenal route. In clients with stress reactions, the sympathetic nervous system causes the blood vessels in the duodenum to constrict, which makes the mucosa more vulnerable to trauma from gastric acid and pepsin secretion. On activation of the adrenal cortex, mucus production decreases and gastric secretion increases. Together, these factors result in increased vulnerability to ulceration. Stress reactions thus upset the aggressive-defensive balance. Prolonged stress associated with burns, severe trauma, and other conditions can produce stress ulcers, or stress erosive gastritis, in the GI tract.

Zollinger-Ellison syndrome is characterized by abnormal secretion of gastrin by a rare islet cell tumor in the pancreas. Pathophysiologic changes associated with this syndrome include hypergastrinemia and diarrhea secondary to fat malabsorption resulting from decreased duodenum-inactivating pancreatic lipase or acid-induced injury of the villi. In addition to increased gastric secretion, hyperplasia of the gastric mucosa is induced by the trophic effects of gastrin. Treatment of Zollinger-Ellison syndrome is aimed at suppression of acid secretion.

Treated ulcers usually heal without difficulty. Untreated ulcers or those that do not respond to treatment can result in perforation, hemorrhage, or obstruction, which may require surgical treatment. Some ulcers recur after healing, particularly if the risk factors associated with their development are not modified.

Critically ill clients are susceptible to *stress ulcers*. For example, gastric mucosal changes caused by stress develop within 72 hours in 78% of clients with greater than 35% burns on their body. Stress ulcers manifest with superficial gastric erosions, often accompanied by painless massive gastric hemorrhage. The client characteristically has multiple lesions, usually small and superficial, that do not extend through the muscularis mucosae. These lesions may appear to ooze blood. The mechanism causing stress ulcerations is unknown, but it probably involves ischemia. In the presence of acid, ischemia can produce erosive gastritis and ulcerations. Increased hydrogen ion back-diffusion and decreased mucosal perfusion may also contribute to stress ulcer formation. Low gastric pH (high acidity) is necessary for development of stress ulcers.

Researchers continue to seek the precise mechanism by which stress ulcers occur. Few manifestations accompany stress ulcers. These ulcerations are typically painless unless perforation occurs, which is rare. Upper GI tract hemorrhage is the major manifestation of stress ulcers. About 10% of clients experience dyspepsia before hemorrhage, but typically there are no warning manifestations. When stress ulcers cause profound hemorrhage, the mortality rate increases to about 50%.

Clinical Manifestations
Acute Pain
The principal manifestation of ulcers is an aching, burning, cramp-like, gnawing pain. The pain has a definite relationship to eating. With gastric ulcers, food may cause the pain and vomiting may relieve it. Clients with duodenal ulcers have pain with an empty stomach, and discomfort may be relieved by ingestion of food or antacids. Clients usually describe the pain as circumscribed in an area 2 to 10 cm (0.8 to 4 inches) in diameter, between the xiphoid cartilage and the umbilicus. Gastric ulcer pain often occurs in the upper epigastrium, with localization to the left of the midline, whereas duodenal pain is in the right epigastrium. Ulcer pain also varies with the site, size, or penetration of the ulcer or the amount of surrounding fibrotic tissue.

In duodenal ulcers, steady pain near the midline of the back between the sixth and tenth thoracic vertebrae with radiation to the right upper quadrant may indicate perforation of the posterior duodenal wall. Fullness or hunger may also be present. Distention of the duodenal bulb produces epigastric pain, which may radiate to the back and thorax. Hydrochloric acid secretion may produce edema and inflammation, with resultant pain, or may activate motor changes with increased spasm, intragastric pressure, and increased motility, also with resultant pain. In addition, ulcer pain tends to occur in distinct periods (periodicity).

Nausea and Vomiting
Clients with a duodenal ulcer usually have a normal appetite unless pyloric obstruction is present. Carcinoma, gastric ulcers, or gastritis may be associated with anorexia, weight loss, and dysphagia. Vomiting occurs more often with gastric ulcer than with uncomplicated duodenal ulcer. It also occurs more frequently when the ulcer is in the pylorus or antrum of the stomach. Vomiting results from gastric stasis or pyloric obstruction, and the client typically vomits undigested food. Severe retching and vomiting may suggest an esophageal tear.

Bleeding
Clients with ulcers often bleed when the ulcer erodes through a blood vessel. Bleeding may occur as massive hemorrhage or may be occult, with slow oozing. Approximately 25% of clients with gastric ulcers may experience bleeding.

The diagnosis of ulcers is confirmed on the basis of manifestations, radiographic evidence, and endoscopy. The history and physical examination do not yield much

significant information in a client with uncomplicated peptic ulcer. A complete blood cell count with decreased hematocrit and hemoglobin values may indicate bleeding. Stool testing for occult blood will usually be positive if bleeding is present. Testing for the presence of *H. pylori* can be done via urea breath tests or identification of *H. pylori* serum antibodies in addition to esophagogastroduodenoscopy (EGD) with biopsy. Monoclonal stool antigen testing may also be used to diagnose the presence of *H. pylori* as well as to evaluate the client for cure after the use of pharmacologic eradication measures have been instituted.

The major diagnostic tests include EGD and an upper GI tract x-ray series. The EGD has several advantages. It allows the physician to take tissue specimens and to treat the ulcer with either multipolar electrocoagulation (MPEC) or heater-probe therapy (see complications under Medical Management).

OUTCOME MANAGEMENT

Medical Management
The primary objective of interventions for peptic ulcer is to provide stomach rest and depends largely on the cause. Approaches include neutralizing or buffering hydrochloric acid, inhibiting acid secretion, decreasing the activity of pepsin and hydrochloric acid, and eradicating *H. pylori* from the GI tract. Specific measures include medications (see the Integrating Pharmacology feature on Medications for Peptic Ulcer Disease, p. 627), physical and emotional rest, dietary management, and stress reduction. The HELIVAX vaccine may be used to treat the client and could be added to the list of routine immunizations in children in the future. It is also being tested as an alternative to antibiotics in those already infected with *H. pylori*.

Response to the therapeutic program varies with clients' perception of their health status and the degree to which lifestyle influences the ulcer disease. The following list outlines the hallmarks of successful interventions:

- The client experiences a decrease in pain with eventual elimination of all ulcer pain and related manifestations.
- The client eats a nutritionally sound diet and reports increased tolerance of food.
- The client complies with the medication schedule.
- The client identifies stressors and develops ways to modify stress and make necessary lifestyle changes.

Modify Diet
For uncomplicated ulcer disease, few physicians or advanced practitioners favor strict dietary changes. There is scant evidence that diet treatment promotes or

accelerates healing. Foods known to increase gastric acidity or cause discomfort should be avoided, such as coffee, alcohol, protein foods, and milk.

Prevent and Treat Complications

Hemorrhage, perforation, and obstruction are the main complications that develop after PUD.

Hemorrhage

Assess Bleeding. Hemorrhage varies in degree from minimal, manifested by the presence of occult blood in the stool (melena), to massive, manifested by vomitus containing bright red blood (hematemesis). The usual manifestation of GI tract bleeding is either vomiting of coffee ground–like material or passing of tarry stools. Acid digestion of blood in the stomach results in a granular dark emesis, whereas digestion in the duodenum or below may result in a black stool. Hemorrhage tends to occur more often with gastric ulcers, especially in the older adult population (Figure 31-2). Although the onset of hemorrhage may be associated with fatigue, nervous tension, upper respiratory tract infection, dietary indiscretion, alcoholism, or irritating drugs, there may be no known precipitating factor.

Manifestations depend on the severity of the hemorrhage. With mild bleeding (<500 ml), the client may experience only slight weakness and diaphoresis. Severe loss of more than 1 L of blood in 24 hours may cause manifestations of shock (see Chapter 81).

Prevent Shock. Intervention for massive bleeding aims to treat hypovolemic shock, prevent dehydration and electrolyte imbalance, and stop the bleeding. The client, who should be fasting, receives intravenous fluids until the bleeding subsides. The nurse or the physician may insert an NG tube in the presence or absence of blood in the stomach to assess the rate of bleeding and prevent gastric dilation; subsequent administration of room temperature saline can then remove blood from the stomach. The room temperature saline is cooler than the body temperature, which creates mild vasoconstriction.

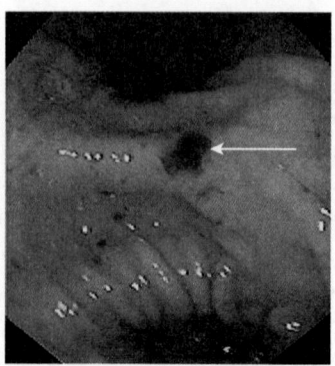

■ **FIGURE 31–2** Bleeding ulcer on gastric mucosa.

Gastric cooling may also be promoted by cool saline lavage, which, although controversial, further curtails hemorrhage through its vasoconstrictive effect. Iced saline is rarely used because it may lead to more mucosal damage by decreasing perfusion to the gastric mucosa and may cause a vagal response, decreasing systemic perfusion.

Replace Fluids. Blood volume depletion is a major problem for the client with severe hemorrhage. For those who have suffered a massive upper GI tract hemorrhage, a primary objective of intervention is to replace blood volume.

Restlessness and tachycardia are the earliest manifestations of hypovolemia. The client has a greatly decreased urine output, which should be monitored with a Foley catheter and hourly urine measurement. This is important because fluids must be replaced to prevent damage to the kidneys. A urine output of less than 0.5 ml/kg/hour should be reported to the physician.

Administer Vasopressin. Arterial administration of vasopressin (via an infusion pump) can also control acute hemorrhage. Vasopressin produces few complications if given intravenously for less than 36 hours to control bleeding.

Inject Artery with Emboli. Another approach to control bleeding is selective arterial embolization with angiography. The emboli may consist of autologous blood clots with or without an absorbable gelatin sponge. A modified clot may be made with a mixture of the client's own blood, aminocaproic acid, and platelets. Fibrin glue has also been used.

Maintain Rest. The client must have minimal activity for several days after bleeding has subsided. Rest decreases blood pressure and GI tract activity. When bleeding stops, the client is allowed bathroom privileges. If the client requires opioids, administer with caution. Morphine sulfate can cause nausea and vomiting; however, the drug may calm the client who is extremely restless and apprehensive. A better alternative is to manage anxiety with non-opioid alternatives.

Maintain High Gastric pH. During the first few days of hemorrhaging, gastric pH should be maintained between 5.5 and 7.0. To maintain the pH at this level, administer H_2-receptor antagonists intravenously for 4 days or as prescribed and advance to oral administration. Monitor gastric pH at least each shift. Anticholinergics are not recommended. Administer antacids for 1 week to complement the H_2-receptor antagonists. Give antacids 1 hour before or 2 hours after the H_2-receptor antagonists so that the antacids do not interfere with absorption of drugs. The client may require antacids every 30 minutes after starting intake of food or fluids.

Stop Bleeding Surgically. If bleeding continues beyond 48 hours, recurs, or is associated with perforation or obstruction, surgery may be indicated. Increased surgical risk is associated with prolonged bleeding, multiple transfusions, debilitation, electrolyte imbalances, and increased age. Surgical procedures include partial gastric resection, excision of the ulcer, and vagotomy and pyloroplasty.

Perform Multipolar Electrocoagulation or Heater-Probe Therapy. Two endoscopic procedures have been effective in treating bleeding ulcers: MPEC and heater-probe therapy. When using MPEC, a bipolar electric current cauterizes the bleeding lesion; with heater-probe therapy, direct heat cauterizes the lesion.

Perforation

Perforation is usually a surgical emergency. When the ulcer perforates, gastroduodenal contents escape through the anterior wall of the stomach into the peritoneal cavity, resulting in chemical peritonitis, bacterial septicemia, and hypovolemic shock. Peristalsis diminishes, and paralytic ileus develops. Posterior perforation is not as clear and often results in pancreatitis, because the pancreas plugs the perforation.

Assess Pain. Perforation occurs most frequently with duodenal ulcers (Figure 31-3). It occurs when the ulcer erodes through the tunica muscularis. The client experiences sudden, sharp, severe pain beginning in the midepigastrium. As peritonitis develops, the pain spreads over the entire abdomen, which becomes tender, hard, and rigid. (See discussion of peritonitis in Chapter 33.)

The degree of pain depends on the amount and type of contents that are spilled into the peritoneal cavity. The pain often causes the client to bend over or draw the knees up to the abdomen in an effort to decrease the tension on the abdominal muscles. If the perforation occurs on the posterior gastric wall, it may erode through to adjacent organs and become sealed, causing few manifestations. When a perforation erodes into the pancreas, manifestations of pancreatitis develop (see Chapter 46).

Replace Fluids. If perforation occurs, the client needs immediate replacement of fluids, electrolytes, and blood as well as administration of antibiotics. Nasogastric suction should be instituted to drain gastric secretions and thus prevent further peritoneal spillage. A small perforation that closes immediately by adhering to adjacent tissues causes only a small loss of gastric contents.

Correct Perforation Surgically. When surgery is necessary, the surgeon evacuates the escaped gastric contents, cleans the peritoneal cavity by flushing it out with normal saline or an antibiotic (or both), and closes the perforation by patching it with omentum. Vagotomy and hemigastrectomy or vagotomy and pyloroplasty provide definitive control of both the ulcer and the complications (see the Case Study feature on Perforated Ulcer Managed Surgically on the website). After surgery, antibiotics are given to combat peritonitis. The NG tube remains in the stomach until peristalsis returns. Postoperative complications include subphrenic abscess, hemorrhage, duodenal or gastric fistula, atelectasis, and pneumonia.

Obstruction. Long-standing ulcer disease causes scarring because of repeated ulcerations and healing. Scarring at the pylorus frequently causes pyloric obstruction, manifested most often by pain at night, when the stomach cannot be emptied by peristalsis. Pyloric obstruction can also lead to vomiting. Surgery (pyloroplasty) is usually required to correct the problem.

Nursing Management of the Medical Client

Assessment. Nursing assessment involves gathering both psychosocial and pathophysiologic data concerning the client. To assess psychosocial aspects of ulcer disease, ask the client about a familial incidence of ulcer, ingestion of medications that cause gastric irritation, cigarette smoking, alcohol intake, stressors, and coping patterns. Questions about lifestyle, occupation, work, and leisure activities can yield valuable information.

Physical assessment includes accurately observing and immediately reporting manifestations that help pinpoint the diagnosis or that might indicate the presence of a complication. Manifestations include pain, vomiting, and, occasionally, bleeding and changes in appetite. Always obtain a complete history of previous ulcer

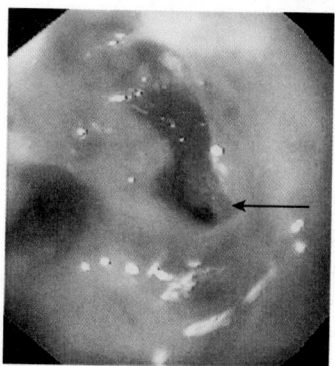

■ **FIGURE 31-3** Perforation of a duodenal ulcer.

attacks, including frequency, duration, manifestations, and response to intervention.

SAFETY

⚠️

ALERT

Monitor for the development of complications of ulcers, such as hemorrhage, perforation, or obstruction. Assessment also involves ascertaining a description of the bleeding, including hematemesis and melena. Note such factors as color, amount, consistency, and frequency. Bright red blood usually signifies new bleeding; dark red blood indicates old bleeding. If bleeding is severe, always maintain a current and accurate record of the client's hemoglobin, hematocrit, red blood cell count, and fluid intake and output. Monitor the client closely for the development of manifestations of shock that might occur if bleeding is present.

Because of shock, the client may experience decreased renal blood flow, which causes a decrease in the glomerular filtration rate and in renal excretion. As the body absorbs the by-products of erythrocyte destruction and renal blood flow decreases, watch for an increase in blood urea nitrogen (BUN), creatinine, and ammonia levels. An elevated BUN may follow dehydration from vomiting.

Monitor the client for the development of perforation. Assess the abdomen for pain, tenderness, or rigidity. Report suspected perforation to the physician immediately, and prepare the client for possible surgery.

Monitor the client for the development of gastric obstruction. If the client vomits, record the frequency and the consistency (digested or undigested food or hematemesis) of the vomitus. If pyloric obstruction is present, nasogastric tube and intravenous fluids and electrolytes are needed until the problem is corrected surgically.

Diagnosis, Outcomes, Interventions

Diagnosis: Acute Pain or Chronic Pain. One of the most common nursing diagnoses for the client with a peptic ulcer is acute or chronic pain: *Acute Pain or Chronic Pain related to gastric mucosal injury.*

Outcomes. The client's pain will be relieved, as evidenced by healing of gastric or duodenal mucosal injury and the client's statement of decreased pain on a pain scale of 1 to 10 with the pain being less than 2 or 3.

Interventions

Administer Prescribed Medications. Administer medications as ordered to relieve the client's pain. The medications are discussed in the Integrating Pharmacology feature on Medications for Peptic Ulcer Disease. Assess the effectiveness of the medications that the client is taking, and notify the physician if the pain is not relieved by the medications used in the treatment regimen.

Promote Rest and Relaxation. Avoidance of strenuous physical activity decreases gastric secretions and peristalsis. Help the client achieve rest, both physically and mentally. Be alert for factors that interfere with the client's rest. Arrange the environment to encourage relaxation. If certain visitors or telephone calls agitate the client, discourage these visits or calls until the client improves.

Encourage clients who attempt to carry on their normal work routine (despite prescribed rest) to schedule physical and mental relaxation. Explore with the client and significant others or co-workers ways to reduce work responsibilities temporarily.

Modify Diet. The diet must meet basic nutritional needs. Because an empty stomach stimulates gastric acid secretion, advise the client to eat small amounts at frequent, regular intervals. Discourage ingestion of alcohol, cola, tobacco, caffeine, milk, and foods that cause discomfort. The client may drink decaffeinated beverages.

During the acute phase, the client often requires a bland, nonirritating, low-fiber diet. Clients and their significant others need to learn the modifications in the diet. Have the dietitian review the home diet with the client or whoever will be cooking for the client.

Diagnosis: Ineffective Therapeutic Regimen Management (Individual). For the client with an uncomplicated ulcer, most of the care must be done by the client at home. Write the nursing diagnosis as *Risk for Ineffective Therapeutic Regimen Management (Individual) related to lack of knowledge of cause of ulcer and measures to treat and prevent recurrence.*

Outcomes. The client will understand and be able to discuss the cause of the ulcer and the treatment and ways to prevent recurrence.

Interventions

Provide Teaching. Treatment of PUD places the responsibility for self-care on the client. To maintain self-care, the client must understand the process underlying ulcer development and the rationale underlying interventions.

Help the client to do the following:

- Understand the pathogenesis of the ulcer and the significance of the pain.
- Realize that healing takes place rapidly when the irritating effect is removed.
- Understand what caused the condition to develop and what must be done to lessen the stimulation.
- Discover which substances cause pain by stimulating secretion of gastric juices and eliminate the substances from the diet to promote ulcer healing.

■ Stop smoking as smoking is considered a risk factor for treatment failure when *H. pylori* bacteria cannot be eradicated with usual pharmacologic treatment.

■ Understand the importance of continuing the medical regimen, although the pain is gone, until healing is completed.

■ Recognize that once maintenance therapy stops, the ulcer may recur.

Instruct the client to use acetaminophen instead of aspirin preparations when these medications are needed. Teach the client to examine the labels of all nonprescription medications, particularly cold remedies, for aspirin (acetylsalicylic acid), other salicylates, NSAIDs (ibuprofen), adrenocorticosteroids, and ACTH. These medications are ulcerogenic (ulcer causing), particularly used in combination. If any of these medications must be taken, advise the client to check with the physician first, to eat between meals, and to use H_2-receptor antagonists or antacids to protect the stomach lining.

Provide Support. Helping clients with PUD cope with psychosocial problems is a vital part of intervention. Encourage the client to learn about the stressors that may be causing the development of ulcers. Discussing coping and relaxation techniques may enable clients to better deal with problems.

Evaluation. Medical management usually controls PUD, often within a few weeks. Many clients must continue treatment to remain ulcer-free. The client must follow the therapeutic regimen and practice appropriate health maintenance and restoration behaviors to avoid complications and prevent future recurrence of PUD.

Surgical Management

Gastric Surgical Procedures

Indications. Various types of gastric surgery are performed to reduce the stomach's acid-secreting ability or to remove a malignant or potentially malignant lesion. Surgical intervention is usually viewed as being either elective, to treat clients who do not respond to medical intervention, or urgent/emergent, to treat an ulcer-related complication such as hemorrhage or perforation. Most chronic, recurring ulcers are eventually managed surgically. Many of the procedures described herein can be performed laparoscopically or with open surgical methods.

Surgery for prevention of ulcer recurrence is performed to do the following:

■ Facilitate enterogastric regurgitation of mucus secretions, bile, and pancreatic juice

■ Decrease the secretory capacity of the stomach by removing parietal cells

■ Remove stimuli for hydrochloric acid secretion by cutting the vagus nerve (vagotomy)

■ Eliminate the gastrin hormone mechanisms by antrectomy

Contraindications. Most contraindications to gastric surgery involve the client's age and physical condition. Any life-threatening disease process, such as chronic obstructive pulmonary disease (COPD) or heart failure, may be a contraindication to surgery.

Complications. Complications are discussed in the section following the types of surgeries.

Outcomes. The outcomes desired from the various surgeries are that the client will survive and recover from the surgery without further injury related to surgery. After most procedures, the client will return home in 7 days or less and resume the previous lifestyle within 6 to 12 weeks. It may take 3 months to a year before the client can eat normally.

Types of Operations

Vagotomy. Vagotomy is performed to eliminate the acid-secreting stimulus to gastric cells. There are three types of vagotomy (Figure 31-4, *A*):

1. *Truncal vagotomy.* Each vagus nerve is completely cut.
2. *Selective vagotomy.* The surgeon partially severs the nerves to preserve the hepatic and celiac branches.
3. *Proximal vagotomy.* Partial cutting is performed, but only the parietal cell mass is denervated; innervation of both the antrum and the pyloric sphincter is preserved.

Cutting the vagal nerve fibers selectively avoids the problems of impaired emptying and diarrhea that follow the truncal vagotomy. It also eliminates the necessity for a drainage anastomosis to offset gastric stasis. Proximal vagotomy also reduces acid secretion and preserves the function of the antrum.

Vagotomy with Pyloroplasty. Vagotomy with pyloroplasty involves cutting the right and left vagus nerves and widening the existing exit of the stomach at the pylorus. This procedure prevents stasis and enhances gastric emptying, thereby preventing belching, weight loss, and feelings of fullness (Figure 31-4, *B*).

Gastroenterostomy. A simple gastroenterostomy (Figure 31-4, *C*) permits regurgitation of alkaline duodenal contents, thereby neutralizing gastric acid. A drain is made in the bottom of the stomach and sewn to an opening made in the jejunum. Because this neutralization interferes with the inhibition of gastrin release, a net increase in acid secretion may result. If the

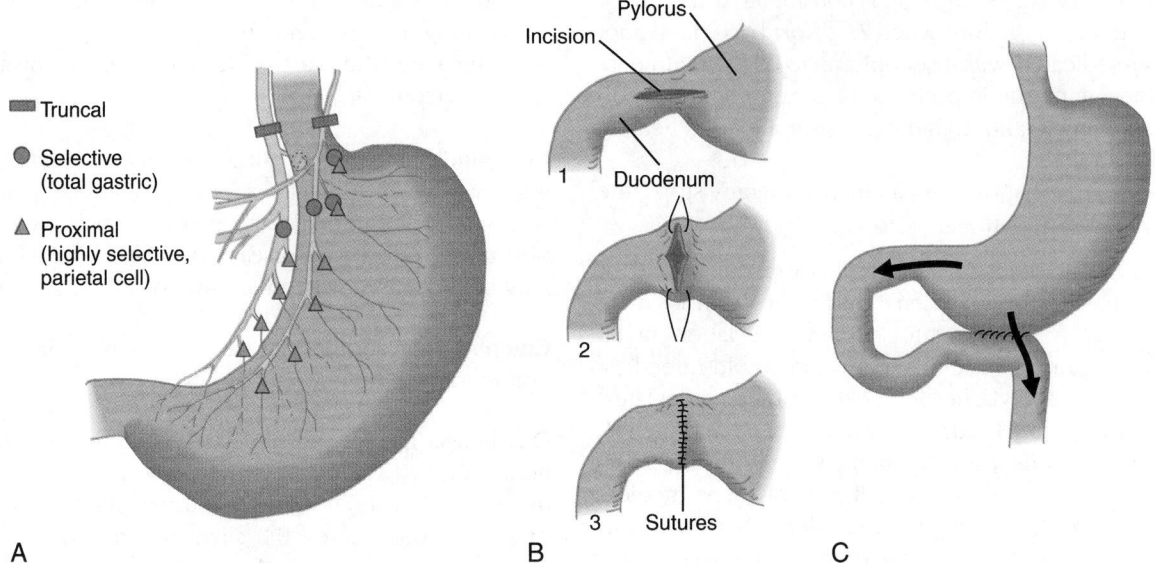

■ **FIGURE 31-4** Vagotomy and drainage. **A,** Sites at which the three types of vagotomy are performed. **B,** Pyloroplasty provides a larger opening from stomach to duodenum to enhance emptying after vagotomy. **C,** Gastroenterostomy, another associated surgical procedure, creates a passage between the body of the stomach and the jejunum.

gastroenterostomy drains the stomach, it reduces motor activity in the pyloroduodenal area. Drainage also diverts acid away from the ulcerative area, which facilitates healing. A gastroenterostomy does not reduce the secretory capacity of the parietal cell mass, and the gastrin mechanism continues to function. Gastroenterostomy should be combined with vagotomy to reduce vagal influences.

Antrectomy. Antrectomy is performed to reduce the acid-secreting portions of the stomach. The procedure removes the entire antrum of the stomach; thus the cells that secrete gastrin are excised. This delays or eliminates the gastric phase of digestion by withdrawing the source of stimulation for acid release and slows the direct response to protein. The surgeon then anastomoses the remaining portion of the stomach to the duodenum.

Antrectomy is often accompanied by vagotomy; thus the cephalic and gastric phases of gastric secretion are eliminated and GI tract motor activity is decreased. This surgical procedure usually prevents recurrence and is probably superior to more extensive operations.

Subtotal Gastrectomy. Subtotal gastrectomy, a generic term referring to any surgery that involves partial removal of the stomach, may be accomplished by either a Billroth I or a Billroth II procedure (Figure 31-5). In a *Billroth I* procedure, the surgeon removes part of the distal portion of the stomach, including the antrum. The remainder of the stomach is anastomosed to the duodenum. This combined procedure is more properly called *gastroduodenostomy*. It decreases the incidence of

dumping syndrome that often occurs after a Billroth II procedure.

A *Billroth II* resection involves reanastomosis of the proximal remnant of the stomach to the proximal jejunum. Pancreatic secretions and bile continue to be secreted into the duodenum, even after gastrectomy. Because these secretions are necessary for digestion, a

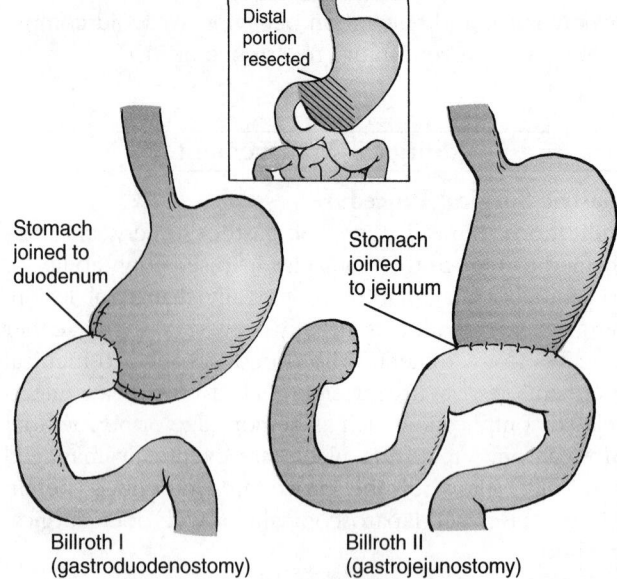

■ **FIGURE 31-5** Subtotal gastrectomy removes acid-secreting portions of the stomach. After removing the distal stomach *(inset)*, a surgeon sutures the remaining portion of the stomach to the duodenum (Billroth I procedure) or to the proximal jejunum (Billroth II procedure). The proximal duodenum is left with the Billroth II to allow bile and pancreatic secretions to flow into the duodenum to aid digestion and neutralize acid from the stomach.

route to the intestine must be preserved. Surgeons prefer the Billroth II technique for treatment of duodenal ulcer because recurrent ulceration develops less frequently after this surgery.

Total Gastrectomy. Total resection of the stomach is the principal intervention for extensive gastric cancer. This surgery involves removal of the stomach, with anastomosis of the esophagus to the jejunum, an esophagojejunostomy (Figure 31-6). To perform total gastrectomy, the surgeon may enter the chest; thus the client returns from surgery with chest tubes. Newer procedures that eliminate opening the chest are beginning to be used.

Complications of Gastric Surgeries

Marginal Ulcers. A marginal ulcer can develop where gastric acids come in contact with the operative site, either at the site of the anastomosis or in the jejunum. Ulceration may cause scarring and obstruction. Hemorrhage and perforation can also occur at the surgical site.

Hemorrhage. The reported incidence of hemorrhage after gastric surgery is 1% to 3%. Bleeding is usually caused by a splenic injury or slippage of a ligature. Assess the client postoperatively for manifestations of bleeding and intraperitoneal hemorrhage.

Alkaline Reflux Gastritis. Alkaline reflux gastritis caused by duodenal contents occurs after gastric surgery in which the pylorus has been bypassed or removed. It also occurs after pyloroplasty and gastrojejunostomy. Usually, an associated vagotomy has been performed, which

decreases gastric motility, allowing reflux of duodenal contents into the stomach.

Acute Gastric Dilation. In the immediate postoperative period, distention of the stomach produces epigastric pain, tachycardia, and hypotension. The client complains of a feeling of fullness, hiccups, or gagging. Gastric dilation rapidly improves after insertion of a nasogastric tube or clearing of a plugged nasogastric tube.

Nutritional Problems. Nutritional problems common after stomach removal include vitamin B_{12} and folic acid deficiency, calcium metabolism disorders, and reduced absorption of calcium and vitamin D. Such problems result from a shortage of intrinsic factor and inadequate absorption because of rapid entry of food into the bowel. With the Billroth II gastric resection, pancreatic juice and bile secretion are reduced because the usual stimulus of food passing through the duodenum is missing.

Dumping Syndrome. This postprandial problem occurs after gastrojejunostomy because ingested food rapidly enters the jejunum without proper mixing and without the normal duodenal digestive processing. It usually subsides in 6 to 12 months. Early manifestations, which occur 5 to 30 minutes after eating, involve the vasomotor disturbances of vertigo, tachycardia, syncope, sweating, pallor, palpitation, diarrhea, and nausea with a desire to lie down. The client's blood pressure and pulse rate may either rise or fall.

Dumping syndrome is most common after the Billroth procedures. Intestinal manifestations include epigastric fullness, distention, abdominal discomfort, abdominal cramping, nausea (with only occasional vomiting), and borborygmi (rumbling sounds in the bowel). The client may experience tenesmus (ineffectual and painful straining to defecate). Pain is not present.

Early manifestations are probably caused by rapid movement of extracellular fluids into the bowel to convert the rapidly entering hypertonic bolus into an isotonic mixture. This rapid fluid shift decreases the circulating blood volume. A jejunum distended with food and fluid increases intestinal peristalsis and motility. Late manifestations, which occur 2 to 3 hours after eating, are a result of rapid entry of high-carbohydrate food into the jejunum, an increase in blood glucose level, and excessive insulin levels.

Management involves decreasing the amount of food ingested at one time and maintaining a high-protein, high-fat, low-carbohydrate, dry diet. Gastric emptying can be delayed by eating in a recumbent or semi-recumbent position, lying down after meals, increasing the fat content in the diet, and avoiding fluids 1 hour before, with, or 2 hours after meals. (See the Client

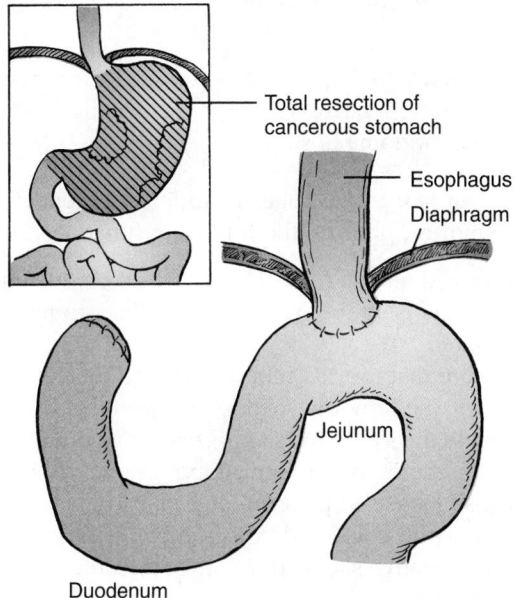

Total resection of cancerous stomach

Esophagus

Diaphragm

Jejunum

Duodenum

■ **FIGURE 31–6** Total gastrectomy *(inset)* with anastomosis of esophagus to jejunum (esophagojejunostomy), which is the principal intervention for extensive gastric cancer.

Education Guide feature on Diet for Dumping Syndrome on the website.)

The client may also be given sedatives and antispasmodic agents to delay gastric emptying. When manifestations persist, surgical intervention may include reducing the size of the gastroenterostomy or converting a Billroth II resection to a Billroth I by inserting a short segment of jejunum between the duodenal stump and the stomach.

Gastrojejunocolic Fistula. This postoperative complication follows recurrent PUD. The fistulae arise from perforation of a recurrent ulceration at the gastrojejunal anastomosis site. The perforation forms a fistula between the ulcer and adjacent bowel. Manifestations are variable but include fecal vomiting, diarrhea, weight loss, and anorexia. Belching of gas that has a fecal odor may also occur. The manifestations are caused by bacterial overgrowth in the small intestine.

Pyloric Obstruction. Pyloric obstruction, manifested by vomiting, occurs at the pylorus and is caused by scarring, edema, inflammation, or a combination of these conditions. When vomiting persists, alkalosis tends to develop because large quantities of acid gastric juice are vomited. A client who vomits persistently is usually hospitalized to receive intravenous fluids with electrolytes added.

Pyloroduodenal obstruction can cause gastric dilation, gastritis, and gastric stasis. These mechanisms create manifestations that gradually make it more difficult for the stomach to empty. Assess the client for feelings of fullness, distention, or nausea after eating, with loss of appetite and weight loss.

Management of obstruction focuses on restoring fluid and electrolytes and decompressing the dilated stomach; if necessary, surgical intervention is instituted.

Nursing Management of the Surgical Client

Preoperative Care

Provide Support. Surgical intervention for gastric and duodenal conditions may be either a planned procedure or an emergency. When emergency surgery is required (e.g., for acute obstruction, perforation, or hemorrhage), the client is very ill and is usually frightened. Provide calm, efficient, knowledgeable care, and explain what is being done. Note and respond to the client's nonverbal behavior. Help significant others provide the client with empathy and emotional support.

When cancer is suspected, the client may want to talk about fears and concerns. Listen to the client carefully, respond to cues, and offer support and understanding. The client may wish to attend to personal matters before surgery (e.g., review a will, see a member of the clergy).

When elective surgery is done, the client has an extensive series of preoperative tests, such as a GI tract x-ray series, endoscopy, and perhaps acid secretion studies (see Chapter 28).

Provide Teaching. Preoperative teaching should include an explanation of the surgery. Explain that the client will have either an NG tube or a gastrostomy tube with suction. An intravenous infusion line is placed in the client's hand or arm for fluids until the surgical site heals. Thoroughly demonstrate and discuss the importance of deep-breathing exercises or use of an incentive spirometer or both. Warn clients that the high abdominal incision makes deep breathing uncomfortable and that the high incision increases the risk of respiratory complications.

Postoperative Care

Assessment. Assess the client with surgical management of PUD in the same way as for the client being managed medically. In addition, perform routine preoperative and postoperative assessments (see Chapter 14).

Diagnosis, Outcomes, Interventions

Diagnosis: Risk for Injury. After surgery, the client is susceptible to postoperative complications. The nursing diagnosis is *Risk for Injury: Postoperative complications (immediate and delayed) related to bleeding, distention, and atelectasis.*

Outcomes. The client will not suffer injury related to postoperative complications (immediate and delayed) as evidenced by decreasing bloody drainage from the NG tube, absence of abdominal distention, and normal breath sounds.

Interventions. Nursing care after gastric surgery is the same as postoperative care for any client recovering from major abdominal surgery.

Maintain Nasogastric Tube. In addition to general postoperative care, perform the following functions:

- Assess drainage from the NG tube and document.
- Maintain NG tube patency with saline irrigations, as ordered.
- Ensure that the NG tube is attached to suction, and maintained on low suction as ordered.
- Assess the operative site for excessive drainage; too much fluid in the remaining gastric stump may cause increased pressure and injury.
- Assess the color and consistency of drainage from the operative site, and report or document bleeding or hemorrhaging.

After surgery, the client has an NG or gastrostomy tube to prevent retention of gastric secretions. Carefully assess for abdominal distention. Do not reposition the NG or gastrostomy tube after gastric surgery because it may be placed directly over the suture line. Gently irrigate with saline *only* if specifically ordered to do so by the physician.

The color of the drainage in the NG tube may be bright red during the early hours after surgery, but it should become dark red by the end of 24 hours. The drainage has the appearance of coffee grounds for several days after surgery.

Monitor for Complications

Immediate complications after gastric surgery include hemorrhage, gastric distention, obstruction, and disruption of the suture line. Assess for general surgical complications, such as shock, hemorrhage, pulmonary problems, thrombosis, infection (peritonitis), evisceration, and paralytic ileus. Nausea and vomiting should not occur if the nasogastric tube is patent. Carefully measure and document intake (oral and intravenous) and output (urine, suction, and wound drainage).

Promote Comfort. Keep the client comfortable with liberal administration of pain medications; this helps the client to cooperate more fully during deep-breathing and coughing exercises. Give fluids by intravenous infusion, as ordered, until edema and swelling have diminished enough to allow fluids to pass the operative area (seen as a decrease in the gastric tube output and return of bowel sounds).

Diagnosis: Imbalanced Nutrition: Less Than Body Requirements. After surgery the client is at risk for *Imbalanced Nutrition: Less Than Body Requirements related to decreased nutrient absorption secondary to dumping syndrome.*

Outcomes. The client will maintain adequate nutrition, as exhibited by maintaining weight and with no evidence of dumping syndrome.

Interventions. When healing has occurred, clamp the NG or gastrostomy tube and begin oral intake by giving the client clear water, usually 30 ml at a time. Aspirate the tube after 1 hour to determine whether the fluid has been retained. When GI function has returned (e.g., active bowel sounds, passage of flatus) and the client tolerates clear water, the NG tube is usually removed and the diet progresses to soft foods; eventually, a regular diet of five or six small meals a day is given. The diet should not begin too early or progress too rapidly. At first, the client may experience discomfort if too much food is taken at one time.

Evaluation. Postoperatively, some clients need help to reduce the number of stressors in their lives. Strategies for altering lifestyle may be an important part of the rehabilitation and recovery plan. Clients need to know that convalescence after gastric surgery tends to be slow. It may be 3 months before clients regain strength and even partially begin to eat in a more normal manner. It may take a year or more before clients can eat three normal meals per day, and they may need to eat five times per day to accommodate changes in the anatomic structures. When complications such as dumping syndrome occur, clients may feel disappointed. Many clients expect a rapid recovery and may be unprepared when complications develop. Most clients can learn to control manifestations and lead a fairly normal life.

GASTRIC CANCER

Gastric cancer refers to the malignant neoplasms found in the stomach, usually adenocarcinoma, although there may be malignant lymphomas. The American Cancer Society estimated that 21,260 new cases of gastric cancer would be diagnosed in 2007, with 11,210 deaths attributed to gastric cancer.[1] Stomach cancer is twice as common in men as in women, more common in whites in the United States, and more frequent in clients who have pernicious anemia.

Etiology and Risk Factors

Although no specific cause of gastric cancer has been identified, several factors are associated with the development of the disease. The latest research indicates that the presence of *H. pylori* in the stomach increases the incidence of gastric cancer. Gastric cancer often develops in conjunction with chronic atrophic gastritis and affects individuals who live in urban areas, have a low socioeconomic status, eat smoked fish or meats, and have a history of exposure to background radiation or trace metals in soil. The changes in the mucosa may lead to an increase in absorption of carcinogens from the diet, such as pickled foods, salted fish, and nitrates. Other etiologic factors include achlorhydria, pernicious anemia, and smoking. There may also be a genetic factor because the disease seems to run in families. Coal miners, bakers, workers employed in metal crafts, and those working in dusty, smoky, and sulfur dioxide–containing environments are at increased risk. Wood or tobacco smoke, nitrite food preservatives, and overheated fat products may predispose clients to gastric cancer.

Avoidance of the carcinogenic agents is important, especially in clients with other risk factors, such as chronic gastritis, *H. pylori* infection, and pernicious anemia. Cessation of smoking is an excellent health promotion behavior. The American Cancer Society recommends screening for Cag A strain of *H. pylori* bacteria in people with a family history of gastric cancer.

Pathophysiology

Gastric cancer most often arises from the mucous lining of the stomach. Most of these cancers occur in the lesser curvature of the stomach in the pyloric and antral regions. Prognosis is best for stomach cancer involving polypoid lesions; it is poor for ulcerating cancers and poorest for infiltrating forms. Stomach cancer spreads by direct extension into the pancreas, via the lymphatics, and by hematogenous infiltration of the liver, lungs, and bones. The particular route depends on the location and the type of tumor. Some tumors penetrate, some ulcerate, and some spread along the tissue planes.

Gastric cancer is staged using the tumor, node, and metastasis (TNM) classification with stages I to IV (see Chapter 17). The cancer is resectable in early stages before it has invaded the wall of the stomach. The 5-year survival rate is about 90% for local disease while it falls to below 10% for stage III disease. In advanced gastric cancer, the survival rate is almost zero.

Clinical Manifestations

Because clinical manifestations occur late in the course of the disease, stomach cancer is seldom detected in an early stage. Unless hemorrhage or perforation occurs, manifestations are vague and indefinite. The presence of a palpable mass, ascites, or bone pain caused by metastasis may be the first manifestation. Manifestations vary, depending on the location of the tumor in the stomach. If the cancer grows near the cardia, the client may experience dysphagia because of early involvement of the esophagus. If the cancer is near the pylorus, manifestations may result from obstruction.

Assessment reveals weight loss, vague indigestion, anorexia, or a feeling of fullness or mild discomfort so insidious that the client does not recognize it as abnormal or seek medical assistance. Discomfort may be caused or relieved by eating. Anemia from blood loss commonly occurs, and occult blood may be present in the stool. The presence of lactic acid and a high lactate dehydrogenase (LDH) level in the gastric juice suggests carcinoma.

The diagnosis of gastric cancer is confirmed by upper GI tract x-ray examination and gastroscopy. Gastroscopy allows direct visualization and permits cytologic brushing or biopsies to facilitate retrieval of cells for cytologic examination.

OUTCOME MANAGEMENT

Medical Management

Little effective medical treatment is available for gastric cancer. Clients may receive chemotherapy and radiation therapy, but the primary treatment is surgical resection. At present, best results are achieved with multiple drug combinations. Chemotherapy includes the oral agent imatinib mesylate (Gleevec) for gastrointestinal stromal tumors (GIST). Imatinib mesylate (Gleevec) selectively inhibits c-kit tyrosine kinase. Conventional drugs used in gastric cancer include 5-fluorouracil, mitomycin C, cisplatin, etoposide, leucovorin, and doxorubicin (Adriamycin). Studies are showing a benefit in long-term survival with the use of radiation and chemotherapy after surgery. Total parenteral nutrition (TPN) (see Chapter 29) is a method for providing nutrition to the client intravenously, bypassing the GI tract.

Surgical Management

Surgery is the intervention that most effectively treats stomach cancer. Unfortunately, because the diagnosis is usually late, surgery is more often palliative than curative. Gastrectomy, either partial (with Billroth I or II reconstruction) or complete depending on tumor location, is the usual procedure. Ideally, the surgeon removes all local growth and associated lymph nodes. When an extensive tumor makes resection impractical or impossible and the pylorus is obstructed, the surgeon may perform a palliative gastroenterostomy (surgical creation of a passage between the stomach and small intestine).

Nursing Management of the Surgical Client

Assessment. Clients may present with manifestations similar to those of PUD, but frequently manifestations are not present until the tumor is advanced. While assessing the client, note any history of risk factors predisposing to the development of gastric cancer. These include a history of chronic gastritis, pernicious anemia, previous gastric surgery, presence of *H. pylori* infection, or smoking. Ask the client if there is a history of ingestion of large amounts of nitrates, smoked fish, salty foods, or pickled foods.

Diagnosis, Outcomes, Interventions

Diagnosis: Acute Pain. Both before and after surgery, a primary nursing diagnosis for the client is *Acute Pain related to gastric erosion and postoperative pain related to high surgical incision.*

Outcomes. The client will have pain controlled or experience a reduction in pain, as evidenced by the client's use of a pain scale of 1 to 10 and stating a pain score of less than 2 or 3.

Interventions. It is important that the client experience pain reduction. Pain that is not controlled can interfere with sleep and eating and contributes to overall physical and mental deterioration. (Chapter 20 describes pain control in detail.) The client should have verbal and written instructions regarding medications, treatments, and follow-up care.

Diagnosis: Imbalanced Nutrition: Less Than Body Requirements. An important nursing diagnosis for the client with gastric cancer is *Imbalanced Nutrition: Less Than Body Requirements related to decreased appetite, pain, possible gastric obstruction, and nausea and vomiting.*

Outcomes. The client will maintain nutritional intake to meet metabolic requirements, as evidenced by maintenance of normal body weight.

Interventions. Nutritional therapy is an important aspect of management of the client with gastric cancer. TPN or jejunostomy tube feedings may be used postoperatively (or for clients with inoperable disease) to maintain the nutritional status (see Chapter 29).

Diagnosis: Fear. Because of the uncertainty of the disease, an appropriate nursing diagnosis for the client with gastric cancer is *Fear related to knowledge deficit, body image changes, treatment, and life-threatening illness.*

Outcomes. The client will have reduced or controlled fear, as evidenced by the client's ability to understand and discuss disease and treatment options.

Interventions. The client needs an explanation of the disease and all treatment options. Reinforce information to the client as needed. The client also needs information concerning operative procedures and postoperative interventions (NPO status, NG tubes, other drains, intravenous infusions). This information helps decrease the client's fear.

Postoperative complications include hemorrhage, obstruction, anemia, nutritional deficiency, dumping syndrome, duodenal stump leakage, gastric dilation, and delayed gastric emptying. A home health care referral can assist the client with emotional support and treatments and provide an ongoing assessment of the client's condition. Referring the client to a dietitian, member of the clergy, and hospice team may also be necessary. Various community support groups are also available (e.g., I Can Cope). For terminal cancer care, see Chapters 17 and 21.

Evaluation. The prognosis for clients with gastric surgery for cancer is poor. Generally, surgery is performed to provide a palliative means of assisting the client to be more comfortable, rather than a cure of the stomach cancer. Therefore the only appropriate outcome may be as good a quality of life as possible and adequate control of manifestations.

CONCLUSIONS

Gastric disorders are common; unless treated promptly and completely, gastric disorders can continue to cause problems throughout the client's life. Assist clients to learn a new way to achieve and maintain health and to make necessary lifestyle changes. This may be a difficult task; however, unless the client is willing to modify behaviors, many of the gastric disorders recur. The foci of nursing interventions are education and modifications of the client's behavior to promote a healthier lifestyle pattern.

THINKING CRITICALLY

1. A young female executive comes to the health clinic with complaints of epigastric pain and malaise. She works under stress and smokes heavily. She is in a hurry and wants quick action. The physician or advanced health practitioner recommends ranitidine (Zantac) for pain reduction and an upper gastrointestinal x-ray film to rule out a duodenal ulcer. What further nursing assessment is required? What nursing interventions should be planned?

Factors to Consider. What places the client at risk for a duodenal ulcer? What teaching is required for medication and dietary management? How should changes in lifestyle be addressed?

2. A 43-year-old male client is being evaluated for intractable peptic ulcer disease (PUD). He has a history of recurrent duodenal ulcers. Last night he awakened at 2:00 AM and requested an antacid. This morning after breakfast, he passed a large, dark, liquid stool that tests positive for occult blood. Just before receiving his 11:00 AM H_2-receptor antagonist, he turns on his call light. When the nurse enters the room, he is lying on his side with his knees drawn up, moaning and holding his pillow against his abdomen. He is diaphoretic, pale, and breathing rapidly and shallowly. The client states, "It's never hurt like this before. I feel as though I've been stabbed." What should the nurse's first actions be? What has probably happened to this client? Will he need surgery?

Factors to Consider. If surgery is needed, what type of surgery may need to be performed? What are the expected nursing assessments postoperatively? Is he at risk for complications? What discharge teaching will be needed to enhance his health maintenance and prevent future recurrence of PUD?

3. A 52-year-old man who had a subtotal gastrectomy for stage III gastric cancer 10 weeks ago is having difficulty maintaining his body weight. His usual body weight is 190 pounds; he currently weighs 165 pounds. His wife reports that her husband is depressed, will not eat, and sleeps all day in his chair. She states, "I don't know what to do anymore! I think he just wants to die." She then starts crying. What should the nurse say to the client's wife? Whom should the nurse contact to assist the family?

Factors to Consider. Why is the client at nutritional risk? What is his percentage of weight loss? What measures might be initiated to facilitate nutrition?

Discussions for these questions can be found on the website. **evolve**

BIBLIOGRAPHY

Citations appearing in red refer to primary research.

Citations appearing in blue refer to evidence-based practice guidelines and protocols.

1. American Cancer Society. (2007). *Cancer facts and figures*. Atlanta: Author.
2. Ang, T., & Fock, K. (2006). Nocturnal acid breakthrough: Clinical significance and management. *Journal of Gastroenterology and Hepatology, 21*(Suppl 5), S125-128.
3. Braga, M., et al. (2002). Feeding the gut early after digestive surgery: Results of a nine-year experience. *Clinical Nutrition, 21*(1), 59-65.
4. Copstead, L., & Banasik, J. (2005). *Pathophysiology: Biological and behavioral perspectives* (3rd ed). Philadelphia: Saunders.
5. Davies, A., Froomes, P., French, C., et al. (2006). Randomized comparison of nasojejunal and nasogastric feeding in critically ill patients. *Critical Care Medicine, 30*(3), 586-590.
6. Edwards, S., & Metheny, N. (2000). Research for practice: Measurement of gastric residual volume: A state of the science. *MEDSURG Nursing, 9*(3), 125-128.
7. Ford, A., Delany, B., Forman, D., et al. (2006). Eradication therapy for peptic ulcer disease in *Helicobacter pylori* positive patients. *Cochrane Database of Systematic Reviews, 2*, CD003840.
8. Gisbert, J., de la Morena, F., & Abraira, V. (2006). Accuracy of monoclonal stool antigen test for the diagnosis of *H. pylori* infection: A systematic review and meta-analysis. *The American Journal of Gastroenterology, 101*(8), 1921-1930.
9. Gisbert, J., & Morena, F. (2006). Systematic review and meta-analysis: Levofloxacin-based rescue regimens after *Helicobacter pylori* treatment failure. *Alimentary Pharmacology and Therapeutics, 23*(1), 35-44.
10. Graham, D., & Genta, R., (2004). Gastritis and *Helicobacter pylori*. In L. Goldman & D. Ausiello (Eds.), *Cecil textbook of medicine* (22nd ed., pp. 823-827). Philadelphia: Saunders.
11. Griffin-Sobel, J., & Suozzo, S. (2002). Nursing research priorities for the care of the client with a gastrointestinal disorder. *Gastroenterology Nursing, 25*(5), 188-191.
12. Hatakeyama, M. (2006). The role of *Helicobacter pylori CagA* in gastric carcinogenesis. *International Journal of Hematology, 84*(4), 301-308.
13. Lehne, R. (2004). *Pharmacology for nursing care* (5th ed.). Philadelphia: Saunders.
14. Leontidadis, G., Sharma, V., & Howden, C. (2006). Proton pump inhibitor treatment for acute peptic ulcer bleeding. *Cochrane Database of Systematic Reviews, 1*, CD002094.
15. Louw, J. (2006). Peptic ulcer disease. *Current Opinion in Gastroenterology, 22*(6), 607-611.
16. Marzio, L., Cellini, L., & Angelucci, D. (2003). Triple therapy for 7 days vs. triple therapy for 7 days plus omeprazole for 21 days in treatment of active duodenal ulcer with *H. pylori* infection: A double blind placebo controlled study. *Digestive and Liver Disease, 35*(1), 20-23.
17. Metheny, N., & Meert, K. (2004). Monitoring feeding tube placement. *Nutrition in Clinical Practice, 19*(5), 487-495.
18. Metheny, N., et al. (2005). Effect of feeding-tube properties on residual volume measurements in tube-fed patients. *Journal of Parenteral and Enteral Nutrition, 29*(3), 192-197.
19. Metheny, N., et al. (2005). Indicators of tubesite during feedings. *Journal of Neuroscience Nursing, 37*(6), 320-325.
20. Metheny, N., et al. (2006). Tracheobronchial aspiration of gastric contents in critically ill tube-fed patients: Frequency, outcomes, and risk factors. *Critical Care Medicine, 34*(4), 1007-1015.
21. Metheny, N., & Stewart, B. (2002). Testing feeding tube placement during continuous tube feedings. *Nursing Research, 15*(4), 254-258.
22. Orloff, S., & Debas, H. (2004). Peptic ulcer disease: Surgical therapy. In L. Goldman & D. Ausiello (Eds.), *Cecil textbook of medicine* (22nd ed., pp. 834-838). Philadelphia: Saunders.
23. Pritchard, D., & Crabtree, J. (2006). *Helicobacter pylori* and gastric cancer. *Current Opinion in Gastroenterology, 22*(6), 620-625.
24. Raudonis, B. (2003). Palliative care update for gastroenterology nurses. *Gastroenterology Nursing, 26*(1), 26.
25. Rustgi, A. (2004). Neoplasms of the stomach. In L. Goldman & D. Ausiello (Eds.), *Cecil textbook of medicine* (22nd ed., pp. 1208-1211). Philadelphia: Saunders.
26. Saad, R., Shoenfeld, P., Kim, H., et al. (2006). Levofloxacin-based triple therapy versus bismuth-based quadruple therapy for persistent *Helicobacter pylori* infection: A meta-analysis. *The American Journal of Gastroenterology, 101*(3), 488-496.
27. Spratto, G., & Woods, A., (2005). *PDR nurse's handbook*. New York: Thompson Delmar Learning.
28. Suzuki, T., Matsuo, K., et al. (2006). Smoking increases the treatment failure for *Helicobacter pylori* eradication. *The American Journal of Medicine, 119*(3), 217-224.

evolve **Did you remember to check out the bonus material on the Evolve website and the CD-ROM, including NCLEX®-Examination Style Review Questions, Open-Book Quizzes, and Chapter Review Audio Podcasts?**

http://evolve.elsevier.com/Black/medsurg

UNIT 8

ELIMINATION DISORDERS

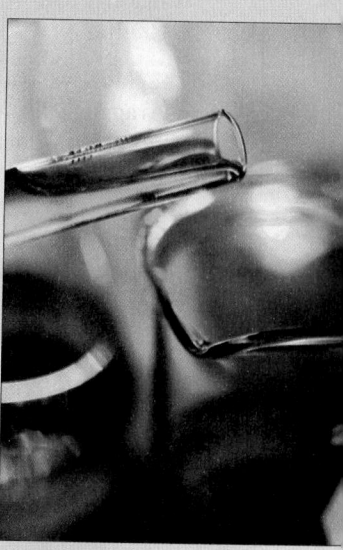

ANATOMY AND PHYSIOLOGY REVIEW:

The Elimination Systems

Robert G. Carroll

The urinary tract is composed of the following four structures:

- Kidneys
- Ureters
- Bladder
- Urethra

The kidneys balance the urinary excretion of substances against the accumulation within the body through ingestion or production. Consequently, they are a major controller of fluid and electrolyte homeostasis. The kidneys also have several non-excretory metabolic and endocrine functions, including blood pressure regulation, erythropoietin production, insulin degradation, prostaglandin synthesis, calcium and phosphorus regulation, and vitamin D metabolism.

Filtration at the renal glomerulus is the first step in urine formation. Normally, a volume equal to plasma volume is filtered every 45 minutes, and a volume equal to total body water is filtered every 6 hours. *Glomerular filtrate* is similar to plasma but lacks cells and large-molecular-weight proteins. The glomerular filtrate is modified by active transport, diffusion, and osmosis as it passes through the renal tubules. *Reabsorption* of filtrate components enhances conservation of glucose, peptides, electrolytes, and water. *Secretion* of plasma components enhances elimination of organic acids and bases (and some drugs). The remnants of the glomerular filtrate exit the kidney through the ureters.

The *ureters* conduct urine from the kidneys to the bladder by peristaltic contraction. The *bladder* is a distensible chamber that stores urine until it is eliminated. The *urethra* is the exit passageway from the bladder, and it carries urine for elimination from the body.

STRUCTURE OF THE ELIMINATION SYSTEM

KIDNEYS

The kidneys are located retroperitoneally, in the posterior aspect of the abdomen, on either side of the vertebral column (Figure A&P8-1). They lie between the twelfth thoracic and the third lumbar vertebrae. The left kidney is usually positioned slightly higher than the right because of the position of the liver. Adult kidneys average 11 cm in length, 5 to 7.5 cm in width, and 2.5 cm in thickness. Affixing the kidneys in position behind the parietal peritoneum is a mass of perirenal fat (adipose capsule) and connective tissue called *Gerota's* (subserosa) *fascia*. A fibrous capsule (renal capsule) forms the external covering of the kidney itself, except the hilum. The kidney is further protected by layers of muscle of the back, flank, and abdomen as well as by layers of fat, subcutaneous tissue, and skin.

The kidney has a characteristic curved shape, with the convex distal edge and a concave medial boundary. In the innermost part of the concave section is the hilus, through which pass the renal artery, renal vein, lymphatics, nerves, and the renal pelvis (the natural upper extension of the ureter). A fibrous capsule surrounds and adheres to the renal parenchyma. Each kidney is divided into three major areas: (1) cortex, (2) medulla, and (3) pelvis (Figure A&P8-2).

The cortex of the kidney lies just under the fibrous capsule, and portions of it extend down into the medullary layer to form the renal columns (columns of Bertin) or cortical tissue that separates the pyramids. The medulla is divided into 8 to 18 cone-shaped masses of collecting ducts called *renal pyramids*. The bases of the pyramids are positioned on the corticomedullary boundary. Their apices extend toward the renal pelvis, forming *papillae*. Each papilla has 10 to 25 openings on the surface, through which the urine empties into the renal pelvis (see Figure A&P8-2, *inset*). Eight or more groups of papillae are present in each pyramid; each empties into a minor calix, and several minor calices join to form a major calix. The two to three major calices are outpouchings of the renal pelvis. They channel the urine from the pyramids to the renal pelvis. The renal pelvis cavity is lined with transitional epithelium. The combined volume of the pelvis and calices is about 8 ml. Volumes in excess of this amount damage the renal parenchymal tissue. The renal pelvis narrows as it reaches the hilus and becomes the proximal end of the ureter.

Within the cortex lies the nephron, the functional unit of the kidney, which consists of both vascular and tubular elements (Figure A&P8-3). Filtration begins at the renal glomerulus. The glomerular tuft (glomerulus) contains capillaries and the beginning of the tubule system, called *Bowman's capsule*. Filtrate from the glomerulus enters Bowman's capsule and then passes through a series of tubule segments that modify the filtrate as it passes

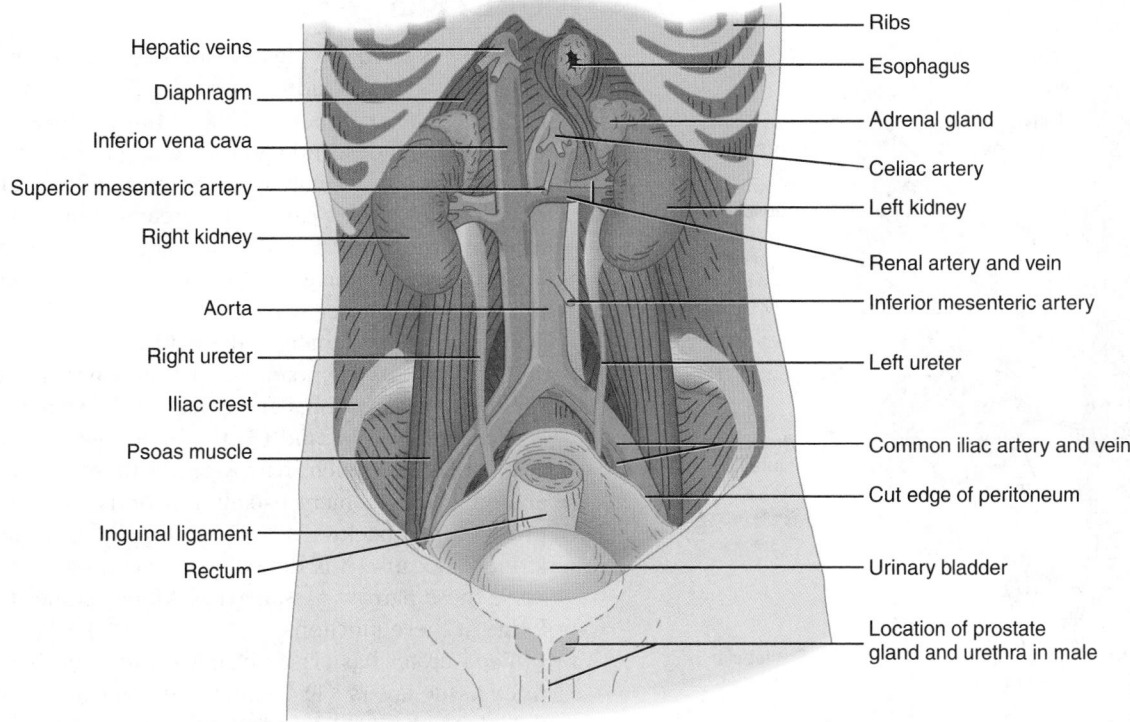

Hepatic veins
Diaphragm
Inferior vena cava
Superior mesenteric artery
Right kidney
Aorta
Right ureter
Iliac crest
Psoas muscle
Inguinal ligament
Rectum

Ribs
Esophagus
Adrenal gland
Celiac artery
Left kidney
Renal artery and vein
Inferior mesenteric artery
Left ureter
Common iliac artery and vein
Cut edge of peritoneum
Urinary bladder
Location of prostate
gland and urethra in male

■ **FIGURE A&P8–1** Anatomic relationship of the kidneys and related structures.

through the renal cortex and medulla and finally flows into the renal calyces. A second capillary bed, the peritubular capillaries, carries the reabsorbed water and solute back toward the vena cava.

Renal Blood Flow and Glomerular Filtration

The kidneys receive 20% to 25% of the cardiac output under resting conditions, averaging more than 1 L of arterial blood per minute. The renal arteries (see Figure A&P8-2) branch from the abdominal aorta at the level of the second lumbar vertebra, enter the kidney, and progressively branch into *lobar arteries,* interlobar arteries, *arcuate arteries,* and interlobular arteries. Blood flows from the interlobular arteries through the afferent arteriole, the glomerular capillaries, the efferent arteriole, and the peritubular capillaries. Some of the peritubular capillaries carry a small amount of blood (approximately 5% of renal blood flow) to the renal medulla in the vasa recta (long, straight blood vessels)

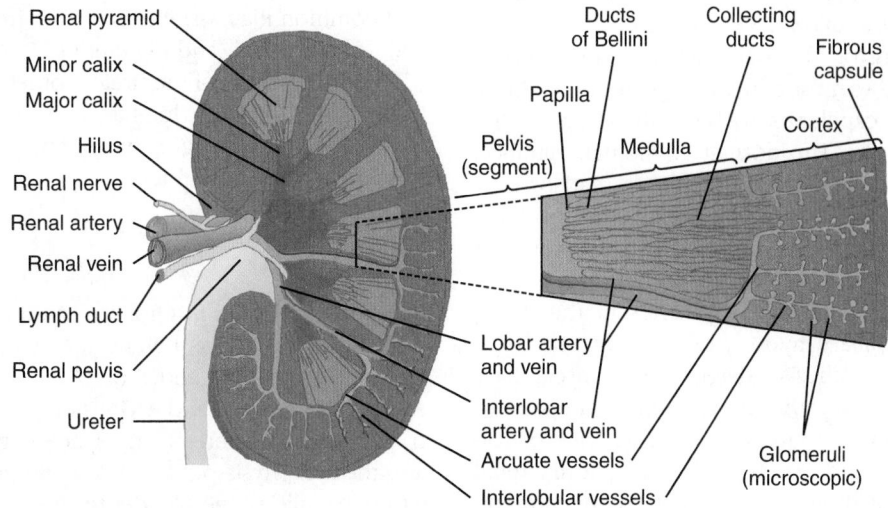

Renal pyramid
Minor calix
Major calix
Hilus
Renal nerve
Renal artery
Renal vein
Lymph duct
Renal pelvis
Ureter

Ducts of Bellini
Collecting ducts
Fibrous capsule
Papilla
Cortex
Pelvis (segment)
Medulla
Lobar artery and vein
Interlobar artery and vein
Arcuate vessels
Interlobular vessels
Glomeruli (microscopic)

■ **FIGURE A&P8–2** Anatomy of the kidney. *Inset,* Enlargement of a segment of the kidney.

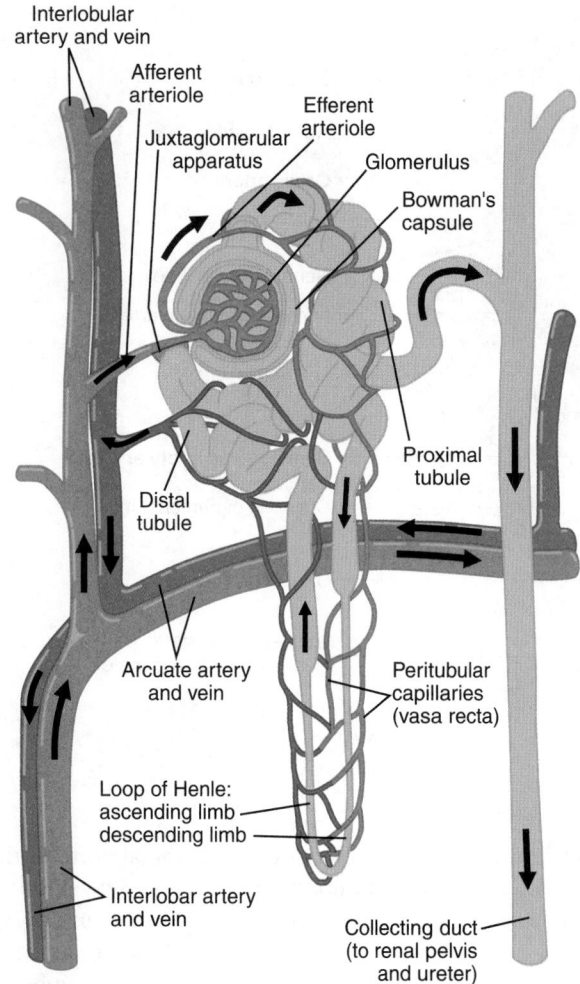

Interlobular
artery and vein

Afferent
arteriole

Efferent
arteriole

Juxtaglomerular
apparatus

Glomerulus

Bowman's
capsule

Proximal
tubule

Distal
tubule

Arcuate artery
and vein

Peritubular
capillaries
(vasa recta)

Loop of Henle:
ascending limb
descending limb

Interlobar artery
and vein

Collecting duct
(to renal pelvis
and ureter)

■ **FIGURE A&P8–3** Diagram of a nephron and associated vascular structures. From Carroll, R.G, (2007). *Elsevier's integrated physiology*, Philadelphia: Mosby.

before entering the venous drainage. The blood leaves the kidney in a venous system that closely corresponds to the arterial system: interlobular veins, arcuate veins, interlobar veins, and the renal vein. The renal circulation then empties into the inferior vena cava.

The arrangement of the two capillary beds in series in the nephron allows most of the large volume of filtrate at the glomerular capillaries to be reabsorbed by the peritubular capillaries. The normal glomerular filtration rate is 125 ml/min, but because of filtrate reabsorption at the peritubular capillaries, only about 1 ml of urine flows from the kidneys each minute. If this volume of reabsorption did not occur, blood pressure could not be maintained. As with other capillaries in the body, the balance of capillary hydrostatic and oncotic pressures (Starling's hypothesis) determines transcapillary fluid movements. Also, the long, straight vessels of the vasa recta permit a countercurrent exchange of solute and allow blood to perfuse the hypertonic renal medulla without disrupting the osmotic concentration gradient.

URETERS

The ureters form the medial tapering of the renal pelvis at the hilus of the kidney. Usually 25 to 35 cm long in the adult, the ureters lie in the extraperitoneal connective tissue and descend vertically along the psoas muscle toward the pelvic cavity (see Figure A&P8-1). After dipping into the pelvic cavity, the ureters course anteriorly to join the bladder in its posterolateral aspect. At each ureterovesical junction, the ureter runs obliquely through the bladder wall for about 1.5 to 2 cm before opening into the lumen of the bladder.

Three points of potential obstruction exist: (1) the ureteropelvic junction, (2) the pelvic brim (where ureters cross iliac arteries), and (3) the ureterovesical junction. The ureter is much narrower at these points. This anatomic arrangement usually functions as a valve that prevents the backward flow (reflux) of urine into the kidney. Because it is difficult for calculi (stones) to traverse these narrow passageways, kidney stones typically lodge at these junctions.

Each ureter has elastic characteristics and is made of three tissue layers: (1) an inner mucosa (transitional epithelial membrane) lining the lumen, (2) a muscular layer, and (3) a fibrous outer layer. The musculature is generally designated as *inner longitudinal* and *outer circular*. Along most of the ureter, however, the muscle fibers actually run obliquely and blend with one another to form a mesh-like tissue. The muscle arrangement allows urine to be propelled down the ureter by peristaltic action. This peristalsis is regulated by a myogenic pacemaker located near the renal calices.

Blood is supplied to the ureters by one or more vessels that run longitudinally along the tube. The number and assortment of arteries anastomosing with the ureteric vessels vary with each individual. Because the ureters travel through several anatomic areas, the ureteral vessels are fed by several of the following arteries: (1) renal (frequently), (2) testicular or ovarian, (3) aorta and common iliac, (4) internal iliac (frequently), (5) vesical, (6) umbilical, and (7) uterine.

The innervation of the ureter comes from the eleventh thoracic to the first lumbar nerves. The network of nerves becomes progressively more dense toward the terminal end of the ureters.

BLADDER

The urinary bladder is a hollow organ located in the anterior half of the pelvis behind the symphysis pubis. (See the Unit 9 Anatomy and Physiology Review and Figures A&P9-1, *B* on p. 841 and A&P9-4 on p. 849 for a discussion of anatomic structures.) The space between the bladder and the symphysis pubis is filled with a loose connective tissue that allows the bladder to stretch cranially as it fills. The peritoneum covers the top border of the bladder, and the base is held loosely in place by the true ligaments. The bladder is also enveloped by a loose fascia.

The bladder wall has several tissue layers. The internal lining of the vesical wall is transitional epithelium with some mucus-secreting glands. Then there are three ill-defined muscle layers: the inner and outer layers (longitudinal) and the middle layer (circular). The fibers from these layers interweave to form a mesh-like muscle layer called the *detrusor muscle.* This arrangement allows the bladder wall to be elastic while maintaining strength. Bundles of these smooth muscle layers come together at the base of the bladder to form the *internal sphincter,* or opening into the urethra. The *trigone* describes the triangular area formed by the ureterovesical junctions and the internal sphincter.

The superior and lateral aspects of the bladder are served by the superior vesical artery, which branches from the umbilical artery and internal iliac artery. The inferior vesical artery, which supplies the underside of the bladder, may arise independently or in common with the middle rectal artery. The veins draining the bladder pass to the internal iliac trunk.

Innervation for the bladder comes from the hypogastric sympathetic, pelvic parasympathetic, and pudendal somatic nerves. Ganglia are most commonly found in the bladder base and around the urethral orifice. These areas tend to act in continuity with each other, and their functions seem to be coordinated by both the sympathetic and the parasympathetic nervous systems (Figure A&P8-4).

URETHRA AND MEATUS

The urethra is a tube that extends from the base of the bladder to the surface of the body. The female and male urethras differ greatly.

Female Urethra

The female urethra is about 4 cm long and curves slightly forward as it reaches the external opening, or *meatus,* located between the clitoris and the vaginal orifice. The urethra is lined with epithelium, which contains some mucus-secreting glands. The longitudinal muscle layer is a continuation of the longitudinal layer of bladder muscle. The circular muscle fibers encompass the urethra and meet with the circular bladder muscle. This muscle thins out near the meatus. As the urethra passes through the urogenital diaphragm, the circular muscle fibers form the external sphincter. The short urethra is one of the reasons that urinary tract infection is more common in women.

Male Urethra

In males, the urethra is a common outlet for the reproductive system and urinary elimination. The prostate gland, although not a direct part of the urinary system, is a major cause of urinary dysfunction in men. Located below the bladder neck, the prostate completely surrounds the urethra. Normally, this relationship causes no problem, but if the prostate enlarges it constricts the urethra and obstructs the outflow of urine.

The male urethra is about 20 cm long and is divided into three main sections. The prostatic urethra extends about 3 cm below the bladder neck, through the prostate gland, to the pelvic floor. The ejaculatory ducts of the reproductive system empty into its posterior wall. The membranous urethra is about 1 to 2 cm long and ends where the muscle layer forms the external sphincter. The distal portion is the cavernous, or penile, urethra. About 15 cm long, it travels through the penis to the urethral orifice at the tip of the penis. It is also lined with epithelial cells.

■ **FIGURE A&P8–4** ■ Innervation of the urinary bladder and associated structures involved in the micturition reflex. Bladder-wall stretch receptors send afferent projections along sensory nerves to the spinal cord. In the spinal cord, the sensory nerves stimulate parasympathetic activity and inhibit sympathetic activity. The resultant bladder contraction further increases pressure in the bladder. Decreased activity of the pudendal nerve relaxes the external sphincter, allowing expulsion of urine. *(From Guyton, A.C., & Hall, J. [2006]. Textbook of medical physiology [11th ed.]. Philadelphia: Saunders.)*

Ureter
Body
Trigone
Bladder neck (posterior urethra)
External sphincter
Sympathetics
Parasympathetics
Pudendal
L1 L2 L3 L4 L5 S1 S2 S3 S4

FUNCTION OF THE ELIMINATION SYSTEM

TRANSCAPILLARY FLUID EXCHANGE

Fluid movement at each capillary bed depends on the balance of fluid pressures and osmotic pressures. Glomerular capillary blood pressure reflects resistance to flow at afferent and efferent arterioles. Preglomerular contraction (primarily afferent arteriole), such as caused by renal sympathetic nerves, decreases the flow of blood into the glomerular capillaries and decreases glomerular capillary blood pressure and glomerular filtration rate (GFR). Postglomerular contraction (primarily efferent arteriole), such as caused by angiotensin II, traps blood in the glomerulus and increases glomerular capillary pressure and GFR. Peritubular capillary blood pressure decreases after either afferent or efferent arteriolar contraction. A decrease in peritubular capillary pressure facilitates reabsorption of glomerular filtrate.

Plasma oncotic pressure, which results primarily from albumin, attenuates filtration at the glomerular capillaries. If the glomerular barrier is damaged, the permeability of the glomerular capillary to protein decreases the normal oncotic reabsorptive forces, and so GFR is increased. The primary barrier to protein filtration is the negatively charged endothelium and basement membrane of the glomerular capillaries, which repel negatively charged proteins. A loss of this negative charge, such as occurs in diabetes, allows some proteins to pass into the urine (proteinuria).

TUBULAR MECHANISMS FOR SECRETION AND REABSORPTION

The renal tubules are lined with epithelial cells that selectively secrete or reabsorb compounds (Table A&P8-1). The process of secretion and reabsorption is very energy intensive. This blind-ended tubular segment originates at the glomerulus. Transport proteins and tightness of tight junctions help to define functionally the segments of the tubules. Because the renal tubules and urinary tract are lined with epithelial cells, tubular fluid is functionally outside of the body (similar to the gastrointestinal [GI] tract).

Modification of ultrafiltrate occurs by diffusion and selective transport in tubules (Figure A&P8-5). Diffusion is quantitatively the most important process. Some compounds are absorbed by carrier-mediated transport, such as sodium-coupled glucose transport.

Glomerular filtrate travels progressively through Bowman's capsule, the proximal tubules, the loop of

TABLE A&P8–1 Kidney Reabsorption and Secretions

Compound	Mechanism	Blocker
Proximal Tubule Reabsorbed		
Na^+	Facilitated diffusion	Amiloride
HCO_3^-	Na^+/H^+ antiport	Carbonic anhydrase inhibitors
Cl^-	Electrical charge	
K^+	Diffusion	
Water	Osmosis	
Glucose	Na-coupled transport	
Amino acids	Na-coupled transport	
Urea		
Urate		
Proximal Tubule Secreted		
Penicillin	Active transport	Probenecid
PAH (p-aminohippuric acid)		
Quinine, choline, thiamine, others		
Creatinine		
H^+		
Thick Ascending Limb of the Loop of Henle Reabsorbed		
Na^+	Na/K/2Cl transporter	Furosemide and bumetanide
K^+	Na/K/2Cl transporter	Furosemide and bumetanide
Cl^-	Na/K/2Cl transporter	Furosemide and bumetanide
Mg^{2+}		
NH_4^+	Na/K/2Cl transporter	Furosemide and bumetanide
Thick Ascending Limb of the Loop of Henle Secreted		
H^+	H^+ ATPase	
Distal Tubule Reabsorption		
Na^+/Cl^-	NaCl symport	Thiazides
Na^+	Electrogenic (aldosterone)	Amiloride, spironolactone
H^+ or HCO_3^-	Intercalated cells	Carbonic anhydrase inhibitors
Distal Tubule Secretion		
K^+	Aldosterone Na reabsorption	Amiloride, spironolactone
H^+	H^+ ATPase	
Collecting Duct Reabsorption		
Urea	Transporters (ADH control)	
Water	Osmosis (ADH control)	
NaCl	NaCl symport	Thiazides

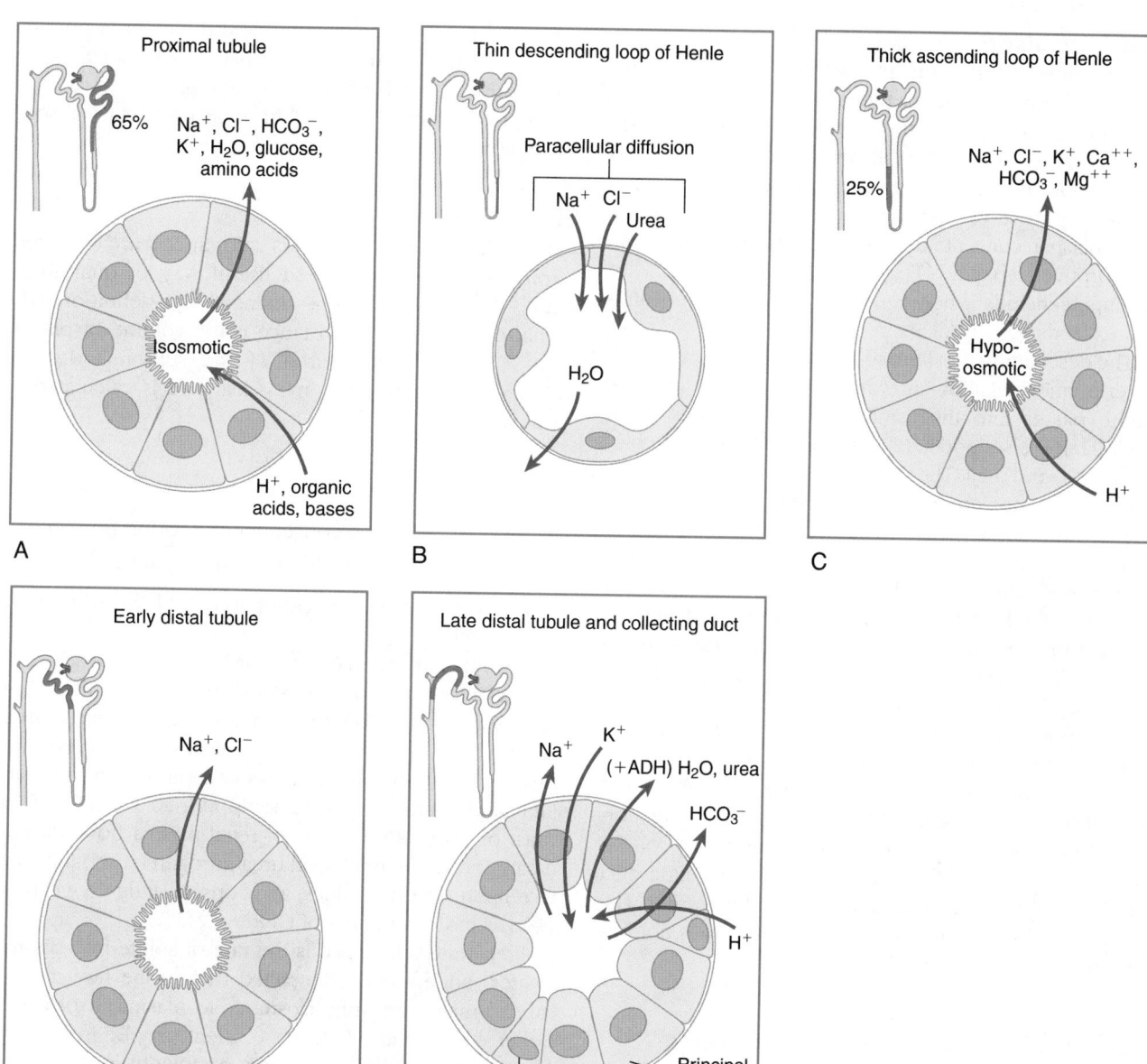

■ **FIGURE A&P8–5** Reabsorption and secretion of compounds in the different renal tubule segments. Reabsorption is movement from the lumen into the body, and secretion is movement from the body into the lumen.

Henle, distal tubules, the connecting segment, and the collecting duct; it then enters renal medullary space, passes into the ureter, and is stored in the bladder before exiting the body as urine. The tubule segments are anatomically adjacent to the vascular supply for that nephron, so that most of the filtrate is reabsorbed back into the blood at each nephron. The juxtaglomerular apparatus consists of the glomerulus and the distal tubule that originated from that glomerulus. This arrangement allows negative feedback control of glomerular filtrate formation at the individual nephron level.

Water reabsorption is driven by osmotic gradients just like everywhere else in the body. The osmolarity of the renal cortex is 300 mOsm, also similar to that in most areas of the body. The osmolarity of the renal medulla, however, can reach 1500 mOsm because of the high concentrations of urea, sodium, and chloride in the interstitial spaces. Two tubular segments, the loop of Henle and collecting ducts, pass through the renal medulla and consequently play a major role in determining urine volume and osmolarity by regulation of water reabsorption.

Renal Tubular Segments

The proximal tubules are "the workhorse of the nephron"; they reabsorb 65% of filtered water, Na^+, Cl^-, and K^+. They also reabsorb 100% of filtered hexoses (glucose), amino acids, and small peptides by Na^+ coupled co-transport. Because this mechanism exhibits saturation kinetics, glucose can pass into the urine if the filtered load (plasma concentration × GFR) exceeds the renal reabsorptive capacity (T_{max}). This occurs in diabetes mellitus, generally when the plasma glucose concentration exceeds 300 mg/dl.

The descending thin limb of the loop of Henle is highly water permeable, allowing water to exit the tubule as the filtrate passes into the osmotically concentrated renal medulla. It is also moderately permeable to sodium chloride (NaCl) and urea. The thick ascending limb of the loop of Henle is water impermeable, as are the remaining segments of the urinary system, unless antidiuretic hormone is present. In the ascending loop, the Na/K/2Cl transporter reabsorbs electrolytes, and this solute transport without water movement results in hypotonic filtrate (100 mOsm); so this tubule segment is sometimes called the *diluting segment*. The thick ascending limb of the loop of Henle is the site of action for "loop" diuretics.

Transport in the distal tubule and collecting duct represent the final chance to modify the tubular fluid before it is lost as urine. Aldosterone promotes K secretion and Na reabsorption in the distal tubule, and antidiuretic hormone (ADH) increases water reabsorption in the collecting duct. The filtrate that flows from the collecting duct into the ureter is the final excretory product: urine. The bladder stores urine for elimination, but it does not further modify urine composition.

Renal Mechanisms in Acid-Base Balance

Renal acid/base excretion of acids complements pulmonary carbon dioxide (CO_2) elimination to regulate body acid-base status. Renal acids are hydrogen (H^+), ammonium (NH_4^+), phosphate, and sulfate buffers. The renal base is predominantly bicarbonate (HCO_3^-). Because of the high HCO_3^- filtered load, reabsorption of bicarbonate is the primary task of the tubule segments. This is accomplished in the proximal and distal tubules by H^+ secretion and carbonic anhydrase–mediated CO_2 formation. Ultimately, urinary acid secretion is determined by plasma CO_2 levels.

Ammonium (NH_4^+) formation in the proximal tubule augments acid secretion, particularly in chronic acidosis. The proximal tubule cells metabolize glutamine to form ammonia (NH_3). NH_3 is uncharged and diffuses into the tubular lumen, where it combines with secreted H^+ to form NH_4^+. Ionic NH_4^+ does not freely diffuse, and it remains in the lumen in a process called *ammonia trapping*.

Distal nephron pH is regulated by intercalated cells. There are two populations of intercalated cells. One is oriented for HCO_3^- secretion, and the other is oriented for H^+ secretion. An increased plasma CO_2 level causes net $NaHCO_3$ reabsorption, correcting the acidosis. A decreased plasma CO_2 level promotes net HCl reabsorption, correcting the alkalosis.

Clearance

The rates at which various substances are "cleared" from the plasma provide a useful way of quantifying the effectiveness of the kidney. By definition, the renal clearance of a substance is the volume of plasma that is completely cleared of the substance by the kidneys in a period of time. Clearance is calculated as follows:

$$C_x = \frac{U_x[V]}{P_x}$$

$$\text{Clearance} = \frac{(\text{Urine concentration})\ (\text{Urine flow rate})}{\text{Plasma concentration}}$$

where U_x is urine concentration and [V] is urine minute volume.

Clearance of inulin (not insulin) is an ideal substance to use because inulin is a substance that is only filtered by kidneys. It is not excreted or absorbed, so it is a perfect substance to test clearance. In clinical settings, creatinine provides a noninvasive measurement of an estimate GFR, and clearance of *p*-aminohippuric acid (PAH) or Diodrast provides an estimate of renal plasma flow. Plasma creatinine levels and blood urea nitrogen (BUN) increase as renal function declines, and consequently they can be used as indirect indices of GFR.

Free water clearance is the rate of solute-free plasma (water) added to or subtracted from urine flow necessary to make the urine isosmotic to plasma. It provides a measure of water balance. A client may be in positive free water clearance if urine osmolarity is less than plasma osmolarity or in negative free water clearance if urine osmolarity is greater than plasma osmolarity.

Urinary Concentration and Dilution

Urine osmolarity reflects the balance of water and solute reabsorption rates. It is determined by the medullary osmolarity and the amount of antidiuretic hormone (ADH) acting on the collecting ducts because these dictate water reabsorption. Glomerular filtrate is isosmotic with plasma (300 mOsm), and the filtrate osmolarity remains unchanged in the proximal tubule. Osmolarity increases in the descending loop of Henle. The ascending loop of Henle, where the Na/K/2Cl transporter removes ions, but not water, causes the filtrate osmolarity to drop to 100 mOsm. This value is close to the lower limit of urine osmolarity. ADH acts on the distal tubule and collecting duct to increase water and urea permeability, allowing the filtrate to become isosmotic with the cortex (300 mOsm); if a large amount of ADH is present, it becomes isosmotic with the inner medulla (1500 mOsm). The inner medulla osmolarity represents the upper limit on urine osmolarity.

REGULATION OF URINE FORMATION

Renal perfusion pressure is the dominant long-term regulator of glomerular filtrate formation and urine production (pressure diuresis and pressure natriuresis). Other mechanisms also alter the rate of filtrate formation and the efficiency of filtrate reabsorption.

Tubuloglomerular feedback at the juxtaglomerular apparatus provides negative feedback control of GFR. The juxtaglomerular apparatus is formed by the junction of the glomerular afferent arteriole and the macula densa of the distal convoluted tubule. A decrease in distal tubule NaCl delivery causes a reflex increase in GFR, both by afferent arteriolar dilation and by angiotensin II–mediated efferent arteriolar constriction. Blockade of angiotensin II formation reduces the effectiveness of this system and may cause a drop in GFR. Many medications for the treatment of hypertension block angiotensin-converting enzyme (ACE), and may cause a decline in GFR.

Neural regulation by the sympathetic nervous system also controls urine formation. Sympathetic contraction of afferent arterioles reduces filtrate formation, enhances salt and water conservation, and diverts blood flow from the kidneys. Renal sympathetics are activated in response to hypotension sensed by arterial baroreceptors and in response to hypovolemia sensed by cardiopulmonary volume receptors.

RENAL ENDOCRINE AND METABOLIC ACTIONS

Most endocrine actions of the kidney are tied to the cardiovascular system. The kidneys synthesize and secrete erythropoietin, the hormone that increases red blood cell synthesis in the bone marrow. Renin release from the juxtaglomerular apparatus ultimately leads to the formation of vasoconstrictor angiotensin II and the release of aldosterone. Intrarenal prostaglandin production assists the regional distribution of renal blood flow. One exception to the renal-cardiovascular connection is vitamin D. The kidneys convert vitamin D into its active form, 1,25-dihydroxycholecalciferol. Activated vitamin D enhances intestinal Ca^{2+} absorption.

Second only to the liver, the kidney has a powerful gluconeogenesis capacity. Urine represents a possible loss pathway for nutrients, especially in disease. Proteinuria may cause a greater loss of protein than may be offset by ingestion. The glucosuria of diabetes may also represent a significant loss of potential calories and increase the risk of urinary tract infection.

MICTURITION

Urine production by the kidneys is relatively constant ($\approx$1 ml/min), but it can vary from 0.5 to 20 ml/min. The flow through the ureters is intermittent and is controlled by the rate of peristaltic wave generation. The peristalsis that forces the urine into the bladder for storage occurs every 10 to 150 seconds. Parasympathetic activation increases the frequency of peristalsis, and sympathetic stimulation decreases the frequency. Afferent (pain) nerves initiate the ureterorenal reflex. This reflex, activated by obstruction, causes ureter constriction and also causes afferent arteriolar constriction to decrease urine production. Lodging of kidney stones in the ureter is a major cause of this reflex.

Both sensory and motor components of the pelvic nerves supply the bladder. Activation of the parasympathetic nerves causes a contraction of the detrusor muscle (bladder). The internal sphincter at the neck of the bladder is normally contracted, but it is relaxed when the bladder muscle contracts. The external sphincter is skeletal muscle under voluntary control, innervated by pudendal nerves. These nerves are tonically active, but activity can be decreased when controlled from higher central nervous system (CNS) centers.

The micturition reflex is initiated when bladder filling increases wall tension above a threshold point, which is felt as the urge to void. Sensory nerves transmit tension information to the spinal cord, where an increase in parasympathetic activity causes contraction of the detrusor muscle. This contraction further increases wall tension, increasing reflex parasympathetic activity and enhancing the contraction. The process repeats until (1) tension plateaus (for about 1 minute), (2) the reflex fatigues, or (3) the external sphincter is relaxed and the bladder empties. If emptying does not occur, the process will begin again after a few minutes.

Urination is facilitated by abdominal contraction, which compresses the bladder and increases wall tension, initiating the reflex. The micturition reflex is modulated by descending inputs from higher CNS structures. The pons has both strong facilitatory and inhibitory centers. The cerebral cortex also can modulate the reflex, allowing voluntary control of the timing of urination.

EFFECTS OF NUTRITION AND AGING

Aging causes shrinking of the kidneys and a progressive loss of renal function. This change is usually not critical because the kidneys have an excess function capacity.

Damage or loss of one kidney, however, may allow the age-related changes to significantly alter overall renal function in the remaining kidney. The increased capillary hydrostatic pressure caused by hypertension, hypotension, or protein ingestion causes progressive damage to glomeruli and accelerates the age-related decrease in renal function. Low-protein diets attenuate the age-related decrease in renal function and are recommended for clients with damaged kidneys.

The aging process also affects the act of micturition. The bladder becomes funnel shaped as a result of alterations in the connective tissue and weakening of the pelvic floor muscles. Irritability of the bladder wall often increases, adding more urgency to the normal desire to void. Finally, impairment of the detrusor muscle's ability to elongate results in decreased bladder capacity. Because of these changes, older adults may have problems with incontinence, frequency, urine retention, or dysuria.

Dietary components can alter renal function at the glomerulus and tubule levels. Ingestion of a protein-rich meal dilates the afferent arteriole, and increases renal blood flow. The increase in glomerular capillary pressure increases GFR. These responses are termed *postprandial renal hyperemia*.

BIBLIOGRAPHY

1. Berne, R., et al. (2004). *Physiology* (5th ed.). St. Louis: Mosby.
2. Carroll, R.G. (2007). *Elsevier's integrated physiology.* Philadelphia: Saunders.
3. Guyton, A., & Hall, J. (2006). *Textbook of medical physiology* (10th ed.). Philadelphia: Saunders.
4. Kierszenbaum, A.L. (2007). *Histology and cell biology: An introduction to pathology* (2nd ed.). St. Louis: Mosby.
5. Nielsen, S., et al. (2002). Aquaporins in the kidney: From molecules to medicine. *Physiology Review, 82,* 205-244.
6. Silverthorn, D. (2006). *Human physiology* (4th ed.). San Francisco, Calif: Pearson Benjamin Cummings.

CHAPTER 32

Assessment of Elimination

KAREN A. HANSON AND SUSANNE A. QUALLICH

Despite advanced technology for diagnosing problems of elimination, every diagnostic evaluation is guided by an accurate, thorough, and documented assessment. Assessment of elimination is fundamental to the evaluation of the client.

Taking a health history requires exceptional skills in speaking, listening, observing, and interpreting the client's communication because anxiety and embarrassment often accompany the discussion of bowel, urinary, or genital problems. Language and semantic barriers can interfere with communication, especially with the variety of terms used to describe bowel and urinary elimination. Differences in educational background can result in fear and poor communication when the client has difficulty understanding medical terminology. A calm, caring, and accepting atmosphere during the interview promotes communication. The client may wish to have a family member present to assist with describing the details of the problem or health history.

BOWEL ELIMINATION

HISTORY

Assessment of the lower gastrointestinal (GI) system begins with the health history, followed by physical examination of the abdomen, anus, and rectum and diagnostic studies. Review previous hospitalizations, surgery, potential exposure to infection, recent travel, current medications, habits, and family history. Explore family risk factors for lower GI disorders, such as a history of colon cancer. Determine whether the client has had recommended screening for colon cancer.

Biographical and Demographic Data

A thorough review of biographical and demographic characteristics helps elicit data related to disorders that are most likely to occur. Colorectal cancer is due to hereditary and lifestyle factors, and it has been estimated that 75% of colon cancers result from modifiable dietary and lifestyle factors.[26] Gastric carcinomas are much more common in the Far East but have been steadily declining overall since World War II, especially in developed countries.[9] In recent years, the incidence of esophageal adenocarcinoma has increased fivefold in the United States and Europe, exceeding that of any other cancer.[9] Ulcerative colitis occurs typically between the second and fourth decades of life and more frequently in whites and in those of Jewish descent. Diverticular disease incidence rises in societies with low dietary fiber intake. In the United States and other developed countries, the prevalence is nearly 10%.[19]

Current Health

An open-ended question such as "How are you feeling?" can elicit concerns about health problems. Explore potentially relevant areas such as the client's social situations, life events, and difficulties surrounding the health problem. Many lower GI manifestations are vague and have various causes.

---

evolve Web Enhancements

Appendix B A Health History Format That Integrates the Assessment of Functional Health Patterns

Tables Causes of Urine Discoloration

Be sure to check out the bonus material on the Evolve website and the CD-ROM, including free self-assessment exercises. **http://evolve.elsevier. com/Black/medsurg**

Chief Complaint

Allow clients to describe the chief complaint in their own words. Elicit information about and learn to recognize a wide variety of manifestations that are potentially associated with a specific GI disorder. Gather information about timing and characteristics of the complaints, as well as the aggravating and alleviating factors. Explore all manifestations, because a health problem related to the GI system rarely occurs in the absence of other manifestations or etiologic events. Clients may be aware of other relevant manifestations. Review the client's health status and discuss general health, diet, lifestyle, and health risk factors. It is an opportune time to assess the client's health awareness and implement health promotion teaching. Refer to Chapter 28 for discussions of diet history and nutritional assessment and refer to this chapter for assessment of elimination patterns. Obtain more specific information about the problem by means of a review of clinical manifestations. Figure 32-1 provides information to guide assessment of common manifestations associated with gastrointestinal complaints.

Clinical Manifestations

Review possible GI manifestations. Does the client have dyspepsia, abdominal pain, nausea, or vomiting? Has there been a change in characteristics of bowel movements? Are clinical manifestations of excessive bloating, flatulence, or belching present? Does the client experience rectal pain or tenesmus? Have there been associated manifestations of weight loss or appetite changes?

Abdominal Pain. Abrupt onset of abdominal pain could indicate emergent conditions such as appendicitis, volvulus, or bowel obstruction. Pain of gradual onset may be related to acute inflammation of the colon or

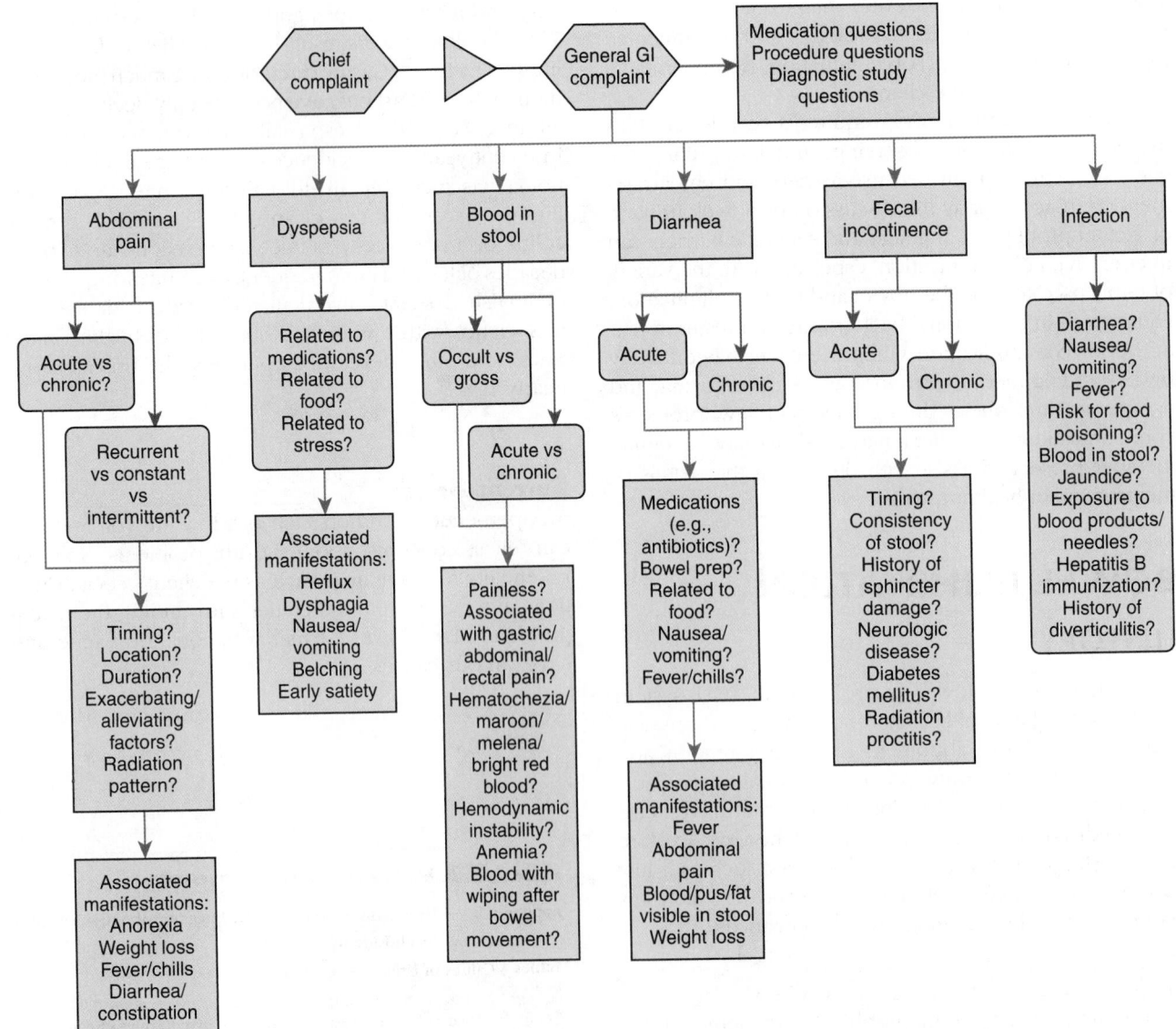

■ **FIGURE 32–1** Expanded gastrointestinal assessment.

diverticula, severe gastroenteritis, or constipation and gas. Is the problem related to food intake? If the complaint is lower abdominal pain, determine whether it is sharp, dull, aching, burning, intermittent, or spasmodic. If the pain is deep, dull, and diffuse, it is probably visceral in origin, that is, the result of localized inflammation or ischemia.

Right upper quadrant pain may be hepatic in origin, resulting from disorders such as hepatitis, liver abscess, or perihepatitis. Right lower quadrant pain may indicate appendicitis. Left upper quadrant pain may result from a splenic rupture, infarct, or abscess. Pain in the left lower quadrant suggests a left colon origin and may indicate diverticulitis or ischemic colitis. Generalized abdominal pain suggests a number of possible causes such as appendicitis, intestinal obstruction, inflammatory bowel disease, or generalized peritonitis.

Dyspepsia. This type of discomfort or pain is located in the upper part of the abdomen, and is common in the general population. Dyspepsia is described using many terms, such as a "gnawing," "aching," or "hunger-like" pain. It can be an indicator for duodenal ulcer or gastric ulcer, although both are marked by episodic complaints of discomfort. Clients may describe the pain as intermittent, occurring in intervals of weeks to months, lasting for several weeks, and there may also be complaints of nausea and vomiting. Refer to Chapter 28 for more assessment information related to upper GI disorders.

Blood in the Stool (Hematochezia). Is there evidence of hematochezia or melena? If the client has noticed bloody stools, ask whether bleeding occurs with every bowel movement or only on occasion. Ask whether the blood is mixed in with the stool or present only on the surface. Some clients will have an upper gastrointestinal source for their bleeding. Diverticular hemorrhage, colitis, neoplasms, hemorrhoids and angioectasias can cause blood in the stool. The Integrating Diagnostic Testing feature on p. 656 details further evaluation of this complaint.

Diarrhea. If diarrhea is present, ask about nighttime complaints, which may indicate inflammatory bowel disease (IBD) rather than irritable bowel syndrome (IBS). The Integrating Diagnostic Testing box on p. 657 describes further evaluation of the client who complains of diarrhea. Abdominal pain that accompanies diarrhea is frequently associated with infectious gastroenteritis, inflammatory bowel disease, diverticulitis, and early intestinal obstruction. Excessive ingestion of synthetic, nonabsorbable sugars such as sorbitol may cause diarrhea.

Fecal Incontinence. This is the involuntary passage of stools through the anus, and can take the form of well-formed stools to liquid bowel movements. It is commonly underreported, as clients suffer emotionally. It is socially devastating, resulting in silent suffering, anxiety, fear of embarrassment, and isolation. Many factors contribute to this condition, including impaired neurologic function and decreased rectal sensation. Clients should be asked if this condition worsens with activity or changes with intra-abdominal pressure, such as with sneezing.

Infection. Clients suffering from an infection of the GI tract can suffer a variety of manifestations that range from nausea, vomiting, and diarrhea to bloating or cramping. It is important to ask about the onset and duration of any of these issues. The client should be assessed for other manifestations, such as risk of hepatitis and possible jaundice.

Review of Systems

Review other organ systems. Has there been weight loss despite a good appetite? Does the client complain of facial flushing or bronchospasm? This can be seen with carcinoid syndrome. Inflammatory arthritis can be seen with inflammatory bowel disease and Whipple's disease. Are there manifestations related to the accessory organs of digestion, such as the development of jaundice, ascites, peripheral edema, generalized intractable pruritus, clay-colored stools, or dark urine? Skin manifestations are often present with gastrointestinal disorders. Ecchymosis resulting from vitamin K deficiency can be seen with malabsorption of fat-soluble vitamins and celiac sprue. Dermatomyositis is a cutaneous manifestation seen commonly with gastric cancer, particularly in clients older than 50. Epidermoid cysts (inclusion cysts) of the face, scalp, and extremities occur in more than 50% of clients affected with familial adenomatous polyposis or Gardner's syndrome. Figure 32-2 on p. 658 offers a guide to taking the history of a client with a gastrointestinal complaint.

Past Medical History

The past health history includes information about the general state of health, past illnesses, immunizations, injuries, hospitalizations, radiation treatments, surgeries, current medications, and allergies. Abdominal or pelvic radiation treatments for malignancy can result in radiation enteritis or proctitis. In addition to common childhood and adult infectious diseases, question the client about hepatitis and intestinal infections, and chronic intestinal disorders such as inflammatory bowel disease, celiac disease, or gastrointestinal cancers. Clients who are immunodeficient because of human immunodeficiency virus (HIV) or immunosuppressive medications are at risk for gastrointestinal infections from cytomegalovirus, herpes simplex virus, *Clostridium difficile, Cryptosporidium,* adenovirus, and rotavirus.[2] Ask whether the client has received routine childhood and adult immunizations and

INTEGRATING D I A G N O S T I C   T E S T I N G

Hematochezia

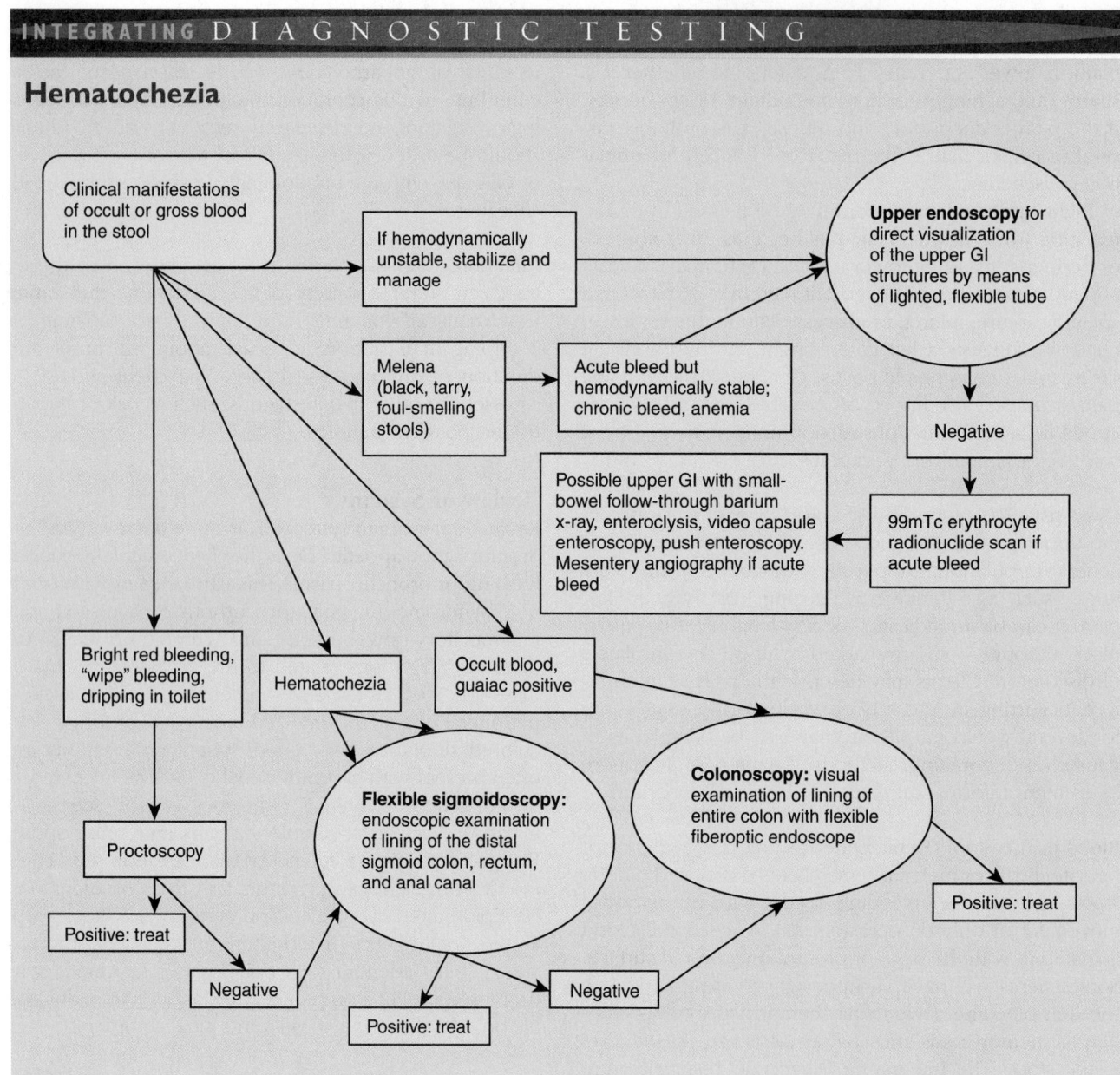

boosters including combined tetanus, diphtheria, and pertussis (Tdap) vaccine. For clients at risk, ask about vaccinations for hepatitis A and B, *Haemophilus influenzae,* and pneumococcal disease. If the client has been recently hospitalized, ask for a hospital summary, including laboratory and diagnostic study results.

Past Surgical History
Ask about previous surgeries, particularly those involving the GI tract or accessory organs. Cholecystectomy

can result in postoperative diarrhea. Abdominal and pelvic gastrointestinal, genitourinary, and gynecologic surgeries can result in abdominal pain syndromes, possibly attributable to adhesions and scarring. Small intestine resections can lead to chronic malabsorption of fat-soluble vitamins, as well as electrolyte disturbances and dehydration. Bariatric surgery for obesity increases the risk of gallstones; internal hernias; vitamin B_{12}, folate, and iron deficiencies; hypocalcemia; dysrhythmias; dumping syndrome; dairy intolerance; constipation or diarrhea; hair loss; and depression.[4]

INTEGRATING DIAGNOSTIC TESTING

Diarrhea

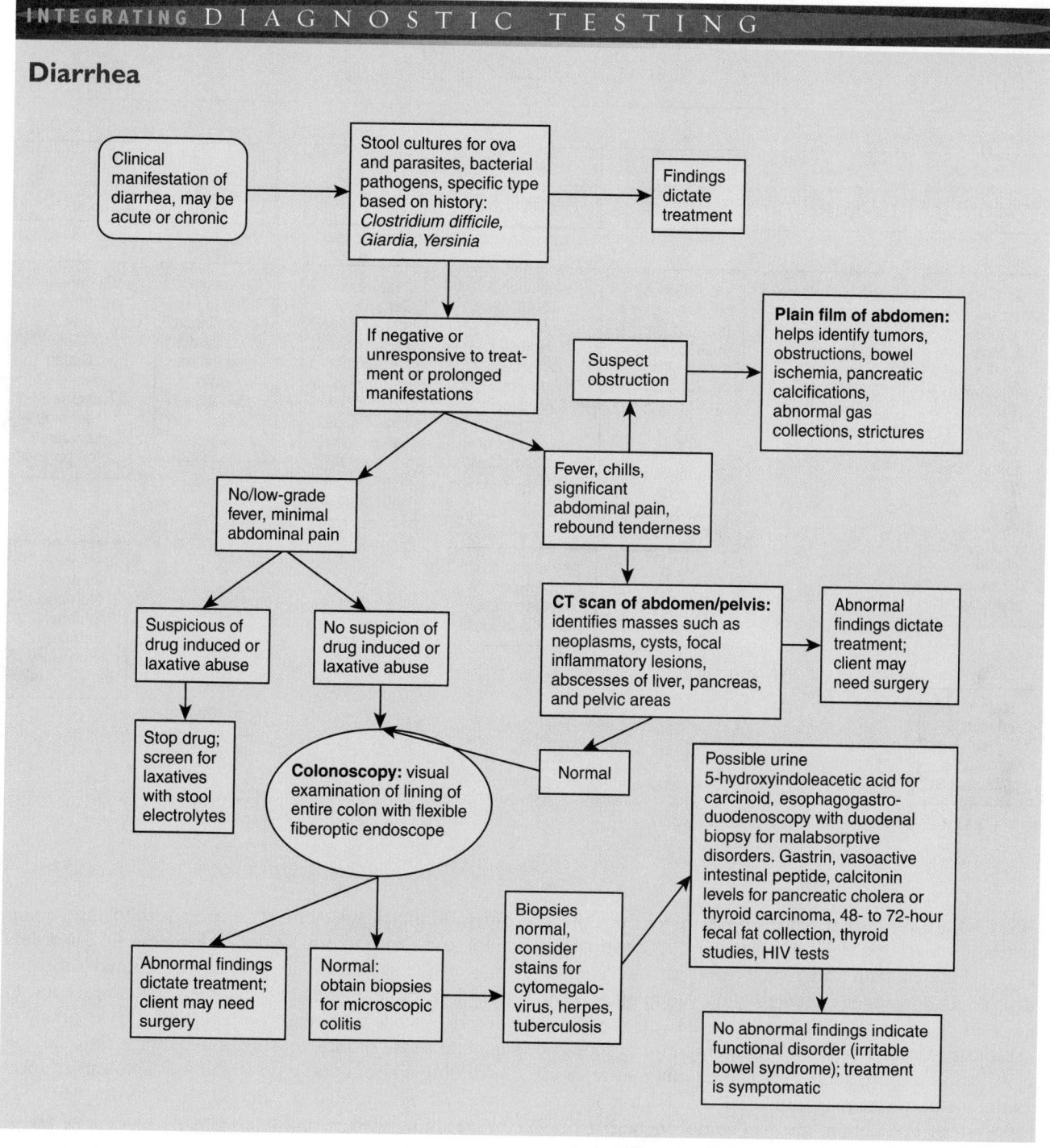

Allergies

Seek specific details to determine the client's allergic response, such as hives, abdominal pain, nausea, vomiting, diarrhea, or lip and tongue swelling. For food allergies, distinguish between foods that are merely difficult to tolerate and those that induce an actual allergic reaction. Ask about the specific food, amount, clinical manifestations, and timing of manifestations after ingestion of a particular food.

Medications

Most oral medications have potential for gastrointestinal side effects. Ask about prescription and over-the-counter (OTC) medications, such as vitamins, antacids, laxatives, enemas, pain relievers, herbal remedies, and nutraceuticals (health food supplements). Ask when medications were started and obtain details of recent dose changes. Clients may not mention OTC medications and herbal remedies. High-dose nonsteroidal anti-inflammatory drugs

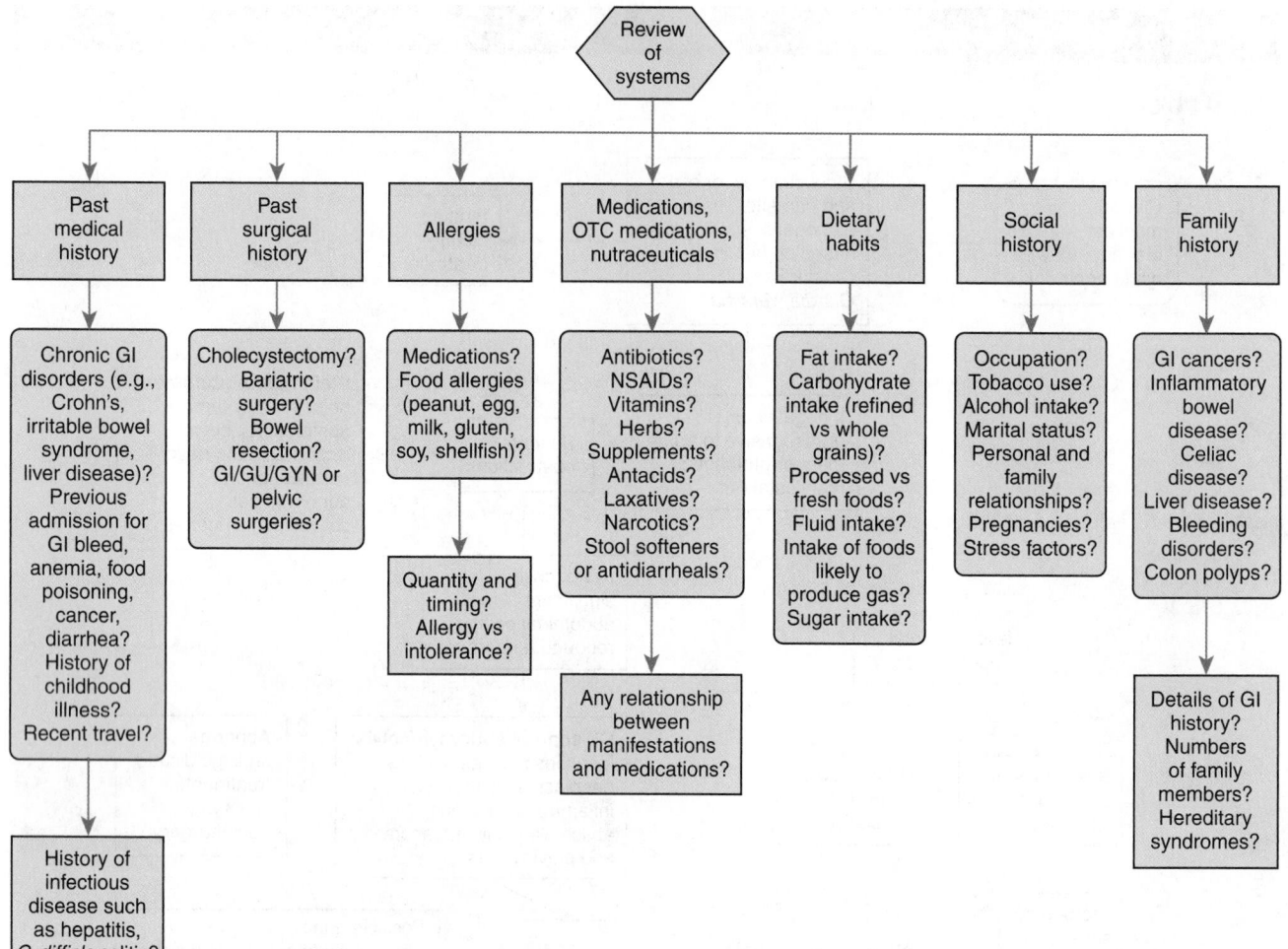

■ **FIGURE 32–2** Expanded gastrointestinal history.

(NSAIDs) are associated with serious upper and lower gastrointestinal toxicity and bleeding.[17] Constipation and abdominal pain can result from narcotic agents. Magnesium-containing antacids and antibiotics may result in diarrhea. Weight loss agents such as orlistat can cause steatorrhea while phentermine and sibutramine cause constipation. Traditional alternative and complementary therapies are used by at least 30% of the Western population, and spending on herbal products is said to exceed $5 billion annually in the United States.[24] About 10% of complementary therapies are used for GI disorders.[24]

Dietary Habits

Thorough assessment of dietary habits is essential when evaluating GI elimination disorders. The diet may be a causative factor, or it may have been altered to help ameliorate the manifestations. Clients often report self-imposed elimination diets because of perceived intolerance to certain foods such as lactose, gluten, and fiber. Artificial sweeteners such as sorbitol and mannitol can lead to an osmotic diarrhea. GI disorders may cause significant impairment of normal digestive function. When assessing the diet, ask the client to describe what was eaten on a typical day to obtain a general sense of intake. Ask about average fluid intake, including amount and type. Ask about amounts of food eaten if suspicious of an eating disorder such as anorexia nervosa or bulimia nervosa. Questions about how the client feels about his/her current weight and what the perceived ideal body weight should be can lend clues to anorexia. Body image distortions are also common in bulimia but are associated with binge eating behavior.

Social History

Determine the nature of the client's social environment and family interactions. Studies have shown that gastrointestinal functions such as the motility of the gallbladder, stomach, and intestine as well as the secretion of digestive juices can be affected by family interactions.[8] Does the client enjoy work, school, and free time socializing with friends and family? What is the client's understanding of the illness? Where does the client obtain information about the illness? Social and cultural beliefs play a major role in how clients interact with the health care system. As many as 70% to 90% of illnesses in ethnic groups, including African Americans, Asians, Hispanics, and Native Americans, in Western societies are managed outside traditional medical facilities.[8] Additionally, one in three Caucasians seeks alternative therapies.[8] It is important to identify the client's beliefs about the illness and expectations of treatment. Have there been any stressful life or work events? Determine any occupational and environmental exposure to diseases or toxins. Has there been potential exposure to food or water contamination through travel? Travel to countries with poor sanitation can lead to diarrhea from *Escherichia coli* and from parasites such as *Giardia, Entamoeba histolytica,* rotavirus, and the Norwalk virus. Ask whether the client has a regular exercise program and whether physical activity is part of the daily routine.

Family History

A number of GI disorders have a familial association. Ask about family history of inflammatory bowel disease, colon polyps, celiac disease, and gastrointestinal cancers, particularly colon cancer. Familial adenomatous polyposis (FAP) is an autosomal dominant disease that leads to hundreds to thousands of adenomatous polyps in the large intestine and development of colon cancer is inevitable. Gastric polyps can also occur with FAP although they are usually benign. A number of liver disorders are familial including hemachromatosis, alpha$_1$-antitrypsin deficiency, and porphyria. Pernicious anemia has no known genetic basis, although clustering in families is found.

PHYSICAL EXAMINATION

Physical examination of the lower GI tract includes the abdomen, anus, and rectum. Discussions of upper GI tract, liver, pancreas, and spleen assessment appear in Chapters 28 and 42. An example of an abdominal assessment recording can be found on p. 568 in Chapter 28.

Abdomen

Lower GI tract assessment begins with the abdomen. The abdomen is divided into either four quadrants or nine regions for descriptive purposes. Be familiar with the abdominal structures located in each of these areas (see Figure 28-4 on p. 567).

The equipment for the examination of the abdomen includes a stethoscope. The client should be supine, with the abdomen fully exposed. The arms should be at the sides and the knees flexed. Stand at the client's right side. If the current problem is one of abdominal pain, examine the area of pain last to avoid stimulating tightening of the abdominal muscles (guarding). Proceed as follows: inspection, auscultation, percussion, and palpation.

Inspection

Inspect the abdominal contour and note whether it is flat, rounded, or scaphoid. Look for evidence of distention, masses, asymmetry, or visible peristaltic waves, which are abnormal and should be reported. Note scars, petechiae, and the presence of dilated veins. Note the shape, position, and color of the umbilicus. A protruding umbilicus may indicate an umbilical hernia. Dilated veins around the umbilicus *(caput medusae)* are indicative of cirrhosis.

Auscultation

Auscultation of bowel sounds provides information about the motion of liquid and air through the intestinal tract. While the client is supine, place the diaphragm of the stethoscope gently over the mid-abdomen. Normal bowel sounds are heard every 5 to 10 seconds and generally range from 5 to 35 per minute. If no sounds are heard after listening for at least 2 minutes in one quadrant, bowel sounds are considered absent. Listening in one area of the abdomen, such as the lower right quadrant, is usually sufficient because bowel sounds are widely transmitted. The absence of bowel sounds suggests a paralytic ileus that may be related to diffuse peritoneal irritation or due to the effects of anesthesia. Rushes of rapid, high-pitched musical or metallic bowel sounds may mean early intestinal obstruction.

Auscultate for abdominal bruit. Abdominal bruit may be a normal finding in a thin young client but may indicate vascular disease. Place the diaphragm of the stethoscope in the midline of the abdomen 2 inches above the umbilicus, and listen carefully for an aortic bruit. Bruit is discussed further in Chapter 51.

Percussion

Percussion is used to detect the presence of fluid, gaseous distention, or solid masses and to determine the location and size of abdominal organs, primarily the liver and spleen. At times, it may be preferable to palpate before percussion, especially if the client is complaining of abdominal pain.

The client should be supine. Percuss the abdomen lightly in all four quadrants. The most common percussion note heard in the abdomen is *tympany* (high pitched, loud, or musical), which is due to the presence of gas in the stomach, small bowel, and colon. The presence of feces and fluid can cause areas of dullness.

Observe any areas of dullness that might indicate mass or an enlarged organ such as a distended bladder, ovarian tumor, or enlarged liver or spleen. This observation will guide the palpation. If the bladder is full, the suprapubic area may sound *dull* (thud-like sounds over fluid or solid organs) when percussed (see the discussion of bladder percussion later in this chapter). Percussion of the liver and spleen is discussed in Chapter 42.

Palpation

Abdominal palpation usually proceeds from light to deep and then to the liver, spleen, and kidneys. The client is supine, and the examination begins with the area of the abdomen that is farthest from the area of pain, if pain is present.

Light palpation is used to detect masses, areas of muscular spasm or rigidity, and areas of direct tenderness. Deep palpation is used to determine the size and shape of abdominal organs and masses. Palpable findings are correlated with those found on percussion.

Perform a test for *rebound tenderness* if the client has abdominal pain. Palpate slowly and deeply away from the area of suspected inflammation, and then quickly withdraw the palpating hand. The feeling of pain on the side of the inflammation that occurs when the palpating hand is withdrawn is called *rebound tenderness*. Because this maneuver may induce generalized pain, perform the test at the end of the abdominal examination. Palpation of the liver and spleen is discussed in Chapter 42, and palpation of the kidneys is discussed later in this chapter.

DIAGNOSTIC TESTING

Diagnostic tests provide information about the nature and severity of lower GI tract problems. Laboratory tests, radiography, ultrasonography, endoscopy, cytology, and other tests are commonly used. Refer to a diagnostic testing manual for more specific information related to the nursing care and implications for the tests identified in the following discussion.

Noninvasive Tests
Flat Plate of the Abdomen

A flat plate of the abdomen is an x-ray film of the abdominal organs. It is used to help identify tumors, obstructions, bowel ischemia, pancreatic calcifications, abnormal gas collections (which may indicate bowel obstruction), and strictures.

Lower Gastrointestinal Barium Studies

A barium enema is administered for the radiographic examination (with or without fluoroscopy) of the large intestine. Barium sulfate (single-contrast technique) or barium sulfate and air (double-contrast technique) are instilled rectally. The test is indicated for clients with a history of altered bowel habits; lower abdominal pain; or passage of blood, mucus, or pus in the stools. The test helps to detect tumors, diverticula, stenosis, obstructions, inflammation, ulcerative colitis, and polyps. Defecating proctography is used to further assess the cause of constipation by providing information about the ability to empty the rectum, the rate of emptying, the width of the anal canal, and the movement of the pelvic floor. Structural abnormalities such as a rectocele can be identified.

Computed Tomography

Computed tomography (CT) is used to assess for acute diverticulitis and abscess formation, diagnose colorectal cancer, and stage rectal tumors. CT is a useful alternative to barium enema for clients who are unable to retain barium. CT colonography or "virtual" colonoscopy uses helical CT scanning of the colon after bowel preparation and colon distention for polyp and cancer detection. The technology is evolving and not currently recommended as a primary screening method for colorectal cancers. It may be useful in clients who refuse colonoscopy or have had an incomplete examination, and may be able to detect extracolonic abnormalities. CT enterography uses a combination of a neutral oral contrast agent with a small amount of barium added and CT imagining to identify luminal bowel and bowel wall disease in addition to extraintestinal disease. It is used primarily to diagnose and manage Crohn's disease.

Scintigraphy

Scintigraphy is used for diagnosing delayed gastric emptying as well as small bowel and colon transit. The client ingests a radiolabeled meal (technetium [Tc] 99 m sulfur colloid in low-fat eggs) and a gamma camera takes images of the gastrointestinal tract at 2-, 4-, 6-, and 24-hour intervals. Scintigraphy can identify dysmotility syndromes when mechanical obstruction has been ruled out.

Ultrasonography

Ultrasonography is used to identify pathophysiologic processes in the pancreas, liver, gallbladder, spleen, and retroperitoneal tissues. Nonalcoholic fatty liver disease (NAFLD or NASH) is suspected when fatty infiltration of the liver is seen on ultrasonography of the abdomen in obese clients with minimal alcohol use. Endoscopic ultrasonography combines the use of linear endoscopy and radial echoendoscopy to identify perianal or periesophageal lesions and is used as a guide for fine needle aspirations for identified submucosal lesions. Doppler ultrasonography using color flow duplex sonography is used to detect changes in blood flow in the mesentery vessels when mesentery ischemia or ischemic colitis is suspected.

Manometry

Rectal manometry is used to measure the resting and squeeze pressures of the internal and external sphincters as well as rectal sensation and function in clients with suspected pelvic floor dysfunction or fecal incontinence. Positive manometry findings suggest neurogenic deficit or sphincter injury. A microballoon or water-perfused or solid-state transducer measures resting and squeeze pressures throughout the length of the anal canal. Rectal sensation tests are done by volumetric measurements of first detectable sensation, sensation of fullness, and maximum tolerated volume by balloon distention.

Invasive Tests
Endoscopy

Endoscopy is the direct visualization of the GI system by means of a lighted, flexible tube. The physician can directly observe sources of bleeding and surface lesions and determine the status of healing tissues. Endoscopy of portions of the small intestine that cannot be directly visualized with a scope can be achieved by use of video capsule.

Proctosigmoidoscopy

Proctosigmoidoscopy is the endoscopic examination of the lining of the distal sigmoid colon, the rectum, and the anal canal using two instruments: a proctoscope and a sigmoidoscope. Indications include a recent change in bowel habits, lower abdominal and perineal pain, rectal prolapse on defecation, anal pruritus, and passage of mucus, blood, or pus in the stool. Sigmoidoscopy is not as thorough as colonoscopy because only half of the colon is visualized; however, it is considered safer.

Colonoscopy

Colonoscopy is the visual examination of the lining of the entire colon with a flexible fiberoptic endoscope. The procedure is indicated for clients with a history of constipation and diarrhea, persistent rectal bleeding, or lower abdominal pain when results of proctosigmoidoscopy and a barium enema are negative or inconclusive. Colonoscopy is also used to screen clients at high risk for colon cancer. Colonoscopy every 10 years is recommended for average risk clients for colorectal cancer surveillance.[6]

Video Capsule Endoscopy

Video capsules became available in 2001. The first system consisted of an ingestible capsule endoscope, a data recorder, and a workstation.[13] The capsule device captures two images per second and has a battery life of 8 hours. After the client swallows the capsule, the images are transmitted by a digital radiofrequency communication channel to an external data recorder unit worn around the waist. This allows for direct visualization of the small intestine when occult gastrointestinal bleeding or lesions are suspected and traditional endoscopy is unrevealing. After an overnight fast, the client swallows the video capsule and wears the data recording unit for the subsequent 8 hours. This test is often indicated for obscure small intestine bleeding not explained through standard studies.

Double Balloon Enteroscopy

This is a system of an endoscope and an overtube outfitted with inflatable balloons that allow advancement of the endoscope through the entire small bowel. If the ileocecal valve is not reached with the antegrade endoscopy, then a retrograde approach can be employed. With a retrograde approach, a colon preparation is necessary. This technology allows visualization and therapeutic intervention of small intestine pathology.

Laboratory Tests

Diagnostic tests are performed to determine the nature of the lower GI disorder. The general methods of diagnosis include laboratory tests, radiographic studies, ultrasonography, and endoscopy. Hematologic and chemistry panels are valuable in determining anemia that may be due to blood loss or malabsorption and hypoalbuminemia caused by protein malabsorption or liver disease. Leukocytosis is seen with inflammatory and infectious conditions. Detailed information regarding laboratory tests used when evaluating GI disorders can be found in specific procedure texts.

Cancer Antigens

Carcinoembryonic antigen (CEA) is a glycoprotein secreted on the glycocalyx surface of cells lining the GI tract and is normally produced during the first or second trimester of fetal life. High CEA levels are characteristic of various malignant conditions such as cancer of the colon, lung, or breast and of certain nonmalignant conditions such as liver disease, cirrhosis, pancreatic cysts, heavy smoking, and IBD. CEA is not useful for colorectal cancer screening. CEA is used as a preoperative test for comparison with postoperative levels as a prognostic indicator. Failure to normalize indicates incomplete resection, and a sustained and progressive rise after postoperative normalization indicates cancer recurrence.

CA 19-9 is a serologic tumor marker defined by monoclonal antibodies and may be elevated in clients with colorectal cancer, gastric cancer, and pancreatic cancer.[18] If elevated above 100 units/ml in the presence of weight loss (>20 pounds) and hyperbilirubinemia (>3 mg/dl), it may be predictive of pancreatic cancer even if other imaging modalities are inconclusive.[21]

Celiac Sprue Serologic Tests

Gliadin antibody tests, both immunoglobulin G (IgG) and IgA, are often performed for complaints of diarrhea, although sensitivity varies between laboratories and with severity of the disease. Gliadin antibody tests lack specificity for celiac disease and are no longer used for screening purposes but can be used to follow response to a gluten-free diet. Endomysium is a connective tissue protein in human tissue. Clients with celiac sprue disease have IgA antibodies against the endomysium. The endomysial antibody test is less sensitive than gliadin but more specific. Tissue transglutaminase is an enzyme released by fibroblasts when the small intestine is inflamed. Positive results with endomysial antibody or tissue transglutaminase tests should be followed by a small intestine biopsy and ultimately human leukocyte antigen (HLA) typing to confirm diagnosis of celiac sprue.

Fecal Occult Blood Tests

🫖 A fecal occult blood test (FOBT) should be performed with a home-based guaiac-based test, immunochemical test, or fluorometric quantitative assay. Two samples from each of three consecutive stools should be tested annually, and if positive, complete colonoscopy is recommended by the American Society of Gastrointestinal Endoscopy (ASGE) and the American Cancer Society (ACS). Samples that are taken by digital rectal examination in the office setting are less sensitive and therefore a poor screening method for colorectal cancer.[5]

Stool Examination for Ova and Parasites and Bacterial Pathogens

Examination of a stool specimen can detect intestinal infection caused by several types of parasites and their ova (eggs). Bacteriologic examination of the stool identifies pathogens that may cause overt GI disease. Identifying these organisms is necessary to treat the client and thereby prevent potentially serious complications. A sensitivity test may follow isolation of the pathogen.

Clostridium difficile toxin is suspected in diarrhea following the use of antibiotics or chemotherapy or after invasive procedures such as surgery or colonoscopy. Clinical manifestations range from mild diarrhea to toxic megacolon and even death. Hospital data from the CDC provide evidence of an increased frequency of *C. difficile* infections from 31 per 100,000 in 1996 to 61 per 100,000 in 2003.[12] Most of these cases were in clients older than age 65. Further studies have identified the emergence of an epidemic strain that is fluoroquinolone resistant.[22]

Some viruses may also cause GI manifestations but can be detected only by immunoassay or electron microscopy.

Other Stool Studies

Quantitative fecal fat studies can detect malabsorptive disorders. Dietary lipids, emulsified by bile, are almost completely absorbed in the small intestine, provided biliary and pancreatic secretions are adequate; however, both digestive and malabsorptive disorders may cause *steatorrhea* (excessive secretions of fecal lipids). A 72-hour stool collection for fecal fat after ingestion of a diet containing 80 to 100 g of fat is useful in confirming steatorrhea and can guide further evaluation for pancreatic insufficiency or celiac sprue.

Fecal leukocytes are present in infectious colitis and inflammatory bowel disease. *Fecal lactoferrin* is an iron-binding glycoprotein secreted by most mucosal membranes and is fairly sensitive (86%) and highly specific (100%) for inflammatory bowel disease versus irritable bowel syndrome.[12]

Stool electrolyte tests can differentiate between secretory and osmotic diarrhea. Secretory diarrhea has a vast differential but is quite rare. Osmotic diarrhea is more common, is often watery, and is caused by carbohydrate malabsorption, particularly poorly absorbed carbohydrates, or ingestion of exogenous magnesium.[16] The stool osmotic gap, which is the difference between stool osmolality and twice the stool sodium (Na^+) and potassium (K^+) concentrations, is normally between 50 and 125 mOsm/kg. In secretory diarrhea (increased water in the stool), the osmotic gap is <50 mOsm/kg; in osmotic diarrhea (lack of absorption of electrolytes or increased ingestion of nonabsorbable solutes), the osmotic gap is >125 mOsm/kg.

URINARY ELIMINATION

HISTORY

Assessment of the genitourinary (GU) system of a male or female client includes evaluation of urinary elimination, as well as sexual and reproductive function. This chapter describes assessment relative to urologic function; Chapter 37 describes assessment of the reproductive systems.

Biographical and Demographic Data

Collection of biographical and demographic data forms the basis of the assessment for any body system. This includes such information as age, gender, marital status, race, and the geographic location where the client spends the majority of his/her time.

There are diseases and health conditions that are more prevalent in particular groups of people. Urinary incontinence affects approximately 13 million Americans, with the highest prevalence in the older adult population.[1] It is more common in women than in men (10% to 30% versus 1.5% to 5%)[1] and often presents in older multiparous women as stress incontinence. Testicular cancer is most frequently diagnosed in young men between ages 25 and 35. Benign prostate hyperplasia (BPH) can be seen in men older than 40 years, and becomes increasingly common with advancing age. BPH is a common cause of both irritative and obstructive voiding complaints in adult men (see Chapters 37 and 38 for further discussion of BPH and testicular cancer). Bladder cancer occurs more often in men than women, and more often in white males than African-American or Hispanic males. There can be a familiar pattern to some genitourinary (GU) diseases as well, such as nephrolithiasis and autosomal dominant polycystic kidney disease (ADPKD).

Current Health

Discussion of GU complaints can make many clients uncomfortable, as most clients do not routinely discuss their patterns of elimination. Every effort should be made to make the client as comfortable as possible by encouraging a relaxed atmosphere that is also private (this is also a necessary part of maintaining compliance with Health Insurance Portability and Accountability Act [HIPAA] regulations) when obtaining the GU history. It is also important to assess both verbal and nonverbal feedback as the discussion progresses, and to converse in a manner that indicates you understand and respect the client.

Chief Complaint

When discussing GU complaints, ask about common urologic complaints (Figure 32-3). Clients who have a urologic complaint can describe one or more problems that can be categorized as generalized questions regarding medications or diagnostic studies, pain, hematuria, urine volume issues, lower urinary tract symptoms (LUTS), incontinence, or infection.

Clinical Manifestations

Often clients have many questions regarding general GU issues. Their primary complaint may simply be that they are requesting additional information regarding a diagnosis, medication change, proposed treatment, or inquiry into whether a concern they have is urology-related. They should be questioned as completely as possible to detail the nature of their concern and provide appropriate direction. Figure 32-3 may be used to guide the GU assessment of clinical manifestations.

Pain. When discussing pain and the GU system, the client must be asked if voiding, elimination, sexual activity, or specific movements contribute to the pain. Refer to Table 32-1 for clues to the specific presentation of pain in the GU system at specific spinal cord levels, as this can help decode patterns of referred pain. See also the male and female reproductive chapter for additional discussion for some of these pain syndromes.

Clients with interstitial cystitis and chronic prostatitis are unique groups, and may have pain as the main GU manifestation. They can suffer from chronic pain syndromes that include suprapubic pain, chronic pelvic pain, dyspareunia, and dysuria, as well as multiple irritative voiding manifestations.

Hematuria. When a client presents with a complaint of hematuria, it should first be determined if it was gross hematuria (sufficient red blood cells [RBCs] to change the color of the urine) or a previous diagnosis of microscopic hematuria (RBCs seen only under the microscope). Urine that is pinkish or red can be quite startling, and clients should be asked if there is pain with urination and about any recent GU procedure. See the Integrating Diagnostic Testing feature on p. 666. Clients with gross hematuria should be asked if the hematuria is present during the start of the urinary stream, or if it is noticeable during the entire urinary stream.

Microscopic hematuria can be the result of multiple urologic and medical/renal disorders.[10,11] Clients may have a history of persistent or chronic microscopic hematuria, which can be the presenting manifestation of their disease. See the following chapters for additional details: urologic (Chapter 34) and renal (Chapters 35 and 36).

Alteration in Urine Volume Output. The adult bladder typically has a volume of approximately 400 ml, and most adults (depending on their fluid intake) will void about six times a day. This pattern of urine output can be affected by multiple factors, including illness, level of activity and perspiration, and kidney function. Each client should be asked about the onset and duration of the complaint, and assessed for daily fluid intake and color of urine as a way to support low- or high-volume urinary output (lighter color urine is less concentrated, darker color urine is more concentrated).

Anuria is a total urine output of less than 100 ml in 24 hours and is most commonly seen with chronic renal failure clients. Oliguria is present when the total urine output is less than 400 ml/day. Older adult clients are considered oliguric if the urine output is less than 600 ml/day. If the ability to concentrate urine is severely

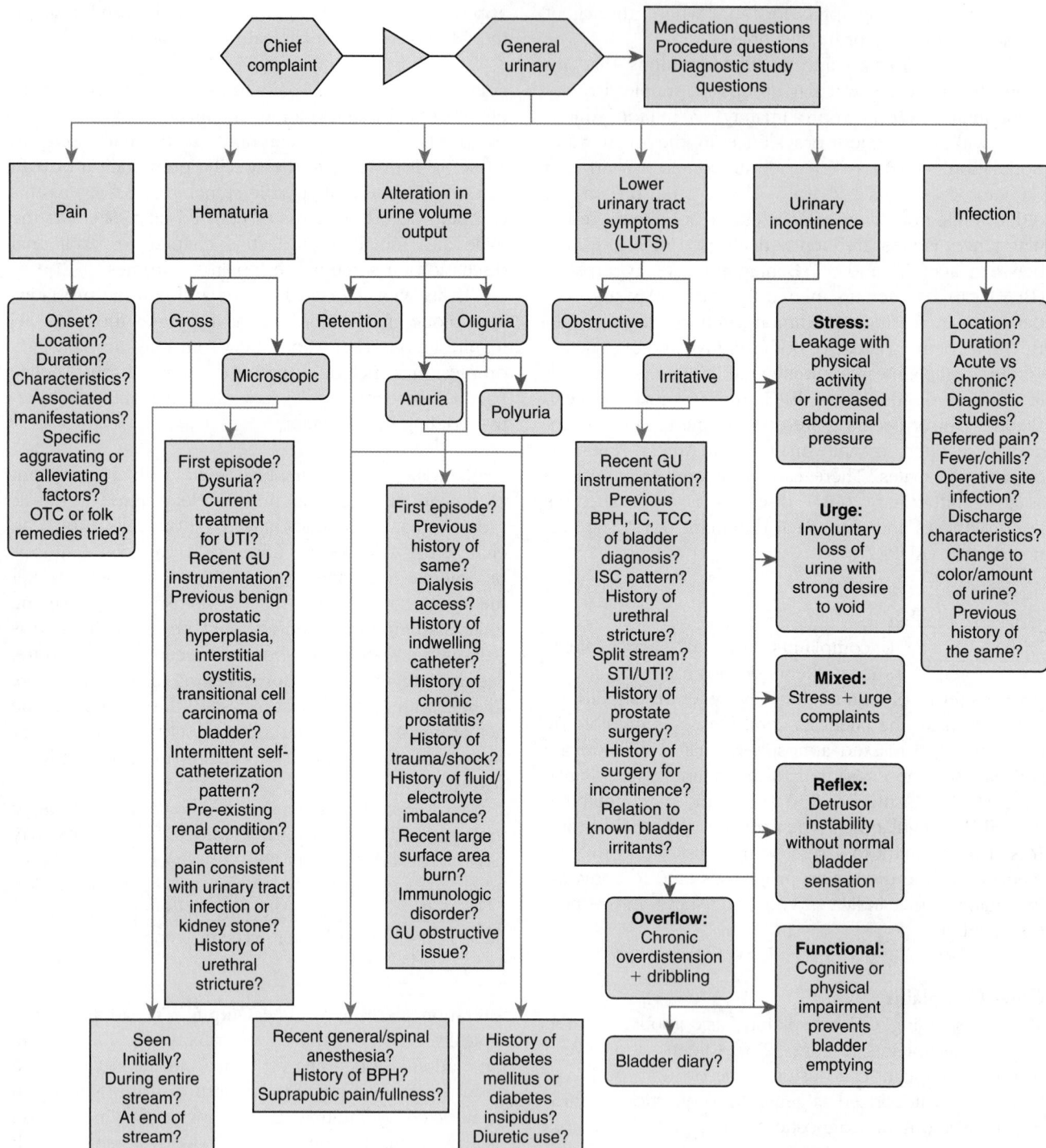

■ **FIGURE 32–3** Expanded genitourinary assessment. *BPH,* Benign prostatic hypertrophy; *IC,* interstitial cystitis; *ISC,* intermittent straight catheterization; *STI,* sexually transmitted infection; *TCC,* transitional cell carcinoma; *UTI,* urinary tract infection.

impaired, oliguria can be described as less than 1000 to 1500 ml/day. Oliguria can be a temporary condition seen after acute events or secondary to systemic events that alter the body's overall fluid status. Decreased urine output occurs with shock, dehydration, and reduced cardiac output, resulting in decreased blood flow to the kidney. Renal injury caused by infection, trauma (including vascular insults), or some manner of postrenal obstruction (such as stones) can also present as a decrease in urinary output.

Polyuria describes frequent voiding, and commonly large amounts. This is due to some derangement in the fluid status of the body that causes the kidneys to excrete more urine, usually with a low specific gravity. Diabetes mellitus, use of diuretics, and diabetes insipidus are only some of the causative factors.

TABLE 32–1 Patterns of Genitourinary Pain

Source of Pain	Autonomic Innervation	Sensory Innervation	Organs with Similar Innervation	Presentation
Kidney/renal pain *Caused by distention of renal capsule*	T10-12, L1	Thoracic and lumbar cord Also some S2-4	Autonomic: suprarenal medulla, colon, spleen Sensory: visceral organs	Dull, constant ache to CVA,* lateral to sacrospinalis muscle and just below 12th rib Can spread to subcostal area toward umbilicus or LLQ Can see nausea, vomiting, abdominal distention
Pseudorenal pain *Mimics renal pain or ureteral colic*	T10-12	Thoracic and lumbar cord	Autonomic: suprarenal medulla, colon, spleen Sensory: visceral organs	Caused by mechanical derangement of costovertebral or costotransverse joints, which results in pressure on costal nerves Can cause costovertebral pain that radiates to ipsilateral LQ Pain positional, acute, absent on arising, and increases during day Exacerbated with heavy work
Ureteral pain *Caused by hyperperistalsis and smooth muscle spasm as ureter tries to overcome obstruction*	*Upper ureter:* T11-12 *Mid-left ureter:* T12, L1	Thoracic and lumbar cord	Autonomic: T11-12 colon, spleen, ascending colon, T12-L1 descending colon Sensory: visceral organs	Caused by acute obstruction Back pain from renal capsular distention and colicky pain Radiates to CVA, toward LQ, along course of ureter In men: also pain to bladder, scrotum, testicle In women: also pain to vulva *Upper ureter stone:* pain radiates to testicle *Mid-right ureter stone:* pain referred from McBurney's point; can look like appendicitis *Mid-left ureter stone:* mimics pain to descending or sigmoid colon *Stone close to bladder:* edema and inflammation to ureteral outlet, with resulting bladder irritability
Vesical (bladder) pain *Pain most likely secondary to spasms*	S2-4	S2-4	Autonomic: colon	Overdistention: suprapubic pain; other suprapubic pain likely not bladder in origin Pain with UTI: usually referred to distal urethra
Prostatic pain *Pain directly from prostate uncommon*	S2-4	S2-4	Autonomic: colon	Acute inflammation: may have discomfort or fullness to perineal or rectal area Possible lumbosacral backache Can cause dysuria, frequency, urgency
Epididymal pain *Results from acute infection*	S2-4	S2-4	Autonomic: colon	Pain in scrotum Begins as pain in groin or LQ abdomen Can reach costal angle and mimic stone pain Inflammation of testicle possible
Testicular pain/labial pain *Can be difficult to distinguish from epididymal pain in men*	S2-4	S2-4; also some T10-11	Autonomic: colon Sensory: kidney	Testicular pain very severe, felt locally Can radiate along spermatic cord to lower abdomen or CVA (men) Can radiate lower abdomen or CVA (women) Can be due to inguinal hernia or varicocele (men)

* *CVA, Costovertebral angle; LLQ, left lower quadrant; LQ, lower quadrant.*

Clients who have significant amounts of postvoid residual urine or experience urinary retention (>100 ml) may describe a sense of incomplete bladder emptying. This is noted either as bladder fullness after urinating or more commonly as "double voiding," a second urination within 5 to 15 minutes after the initial void. This voiding pattern can occur in the client who has undergone general or spinal anesthesia, particularly the older client. A bladder scan device can be very helpful in assessing the amount of fluid in a client's bladder.

Long-standing high residual urine volumes, sometimes in excess of 1000 ml, are considered chronic urinary retention. Clients experience little or no pain but may demonstrate other obstructive manifestations and lack organized control over bladder function. Overflow incontinence is common in these clients because the bladder remains full to capacity at all times.

In the case of a comatose, confused, or other client that cannot communicate these volume changes, nursing assessment plays a vital role. Tracking a client's daily fluid intake and urinary and other fluid output may be the only way that these alterations are noticed.

Acute urinary retention is a sudden inability to void, and can be accompanied by severe suprapubic pain

INTEGRATING DIAGNOSTIC TESTING

Hematuria

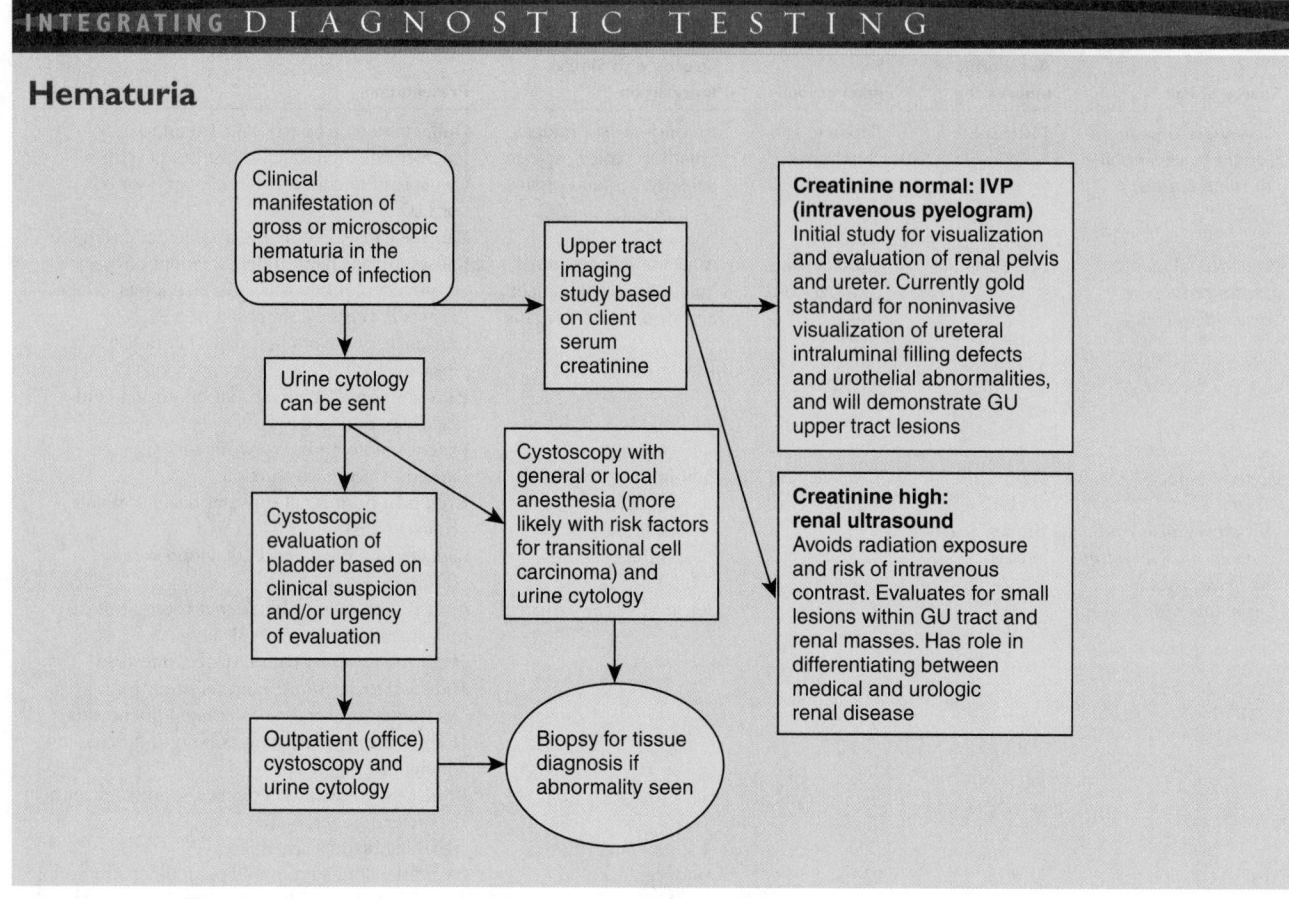

and urgency. It may occur postoperatively or postpartum, with use of certain medications, or with worsening of bladder outlet obstruction, such as seen with acute prostatitis. It is a medical emergency requiring immediate intervention (urethral or suprapubic catheterization).

Lower Urinary Tract Symptoms (LUTS). Irritative complaints are the result of the bladder being subjected to prolonged bladder outlet obstruction. These include urgency, frequency (repetitive voiding every 2 hours or less), nocturia, and dysuria. They can be seen with a variety of conditions that include infection, BPH, inflammation of the bladder (such as that seen with interstitial cystitis), malignancy, bladder stones, or any neurogenic dysfunction of the lower urinary tract. Irritative complaints can also be seen with some psychological conditions. Nocturia can also be a symptom of clients that suffer from dependent edema. When they are recumbent while sleeping, the fluid returns to the circulation and can be filtered by the kidney, resulting in increased urine output.

Obstructive complaints are the result of obstruction of the bladder outlet from the growing prostate, bladder stones, urethral stricture, or neurologic disease that prevents the proper function of the bladder. They include hesitancy (a delay of 10 seconds or more when beginning to urinate), intermittency (interrupted stream when urinating), weak stream, dribbling at the end of urination, and a sensation of having incompletely emptied the bladder. Assessment of a client's ability to empty the bladder can be quickly and easily accomplished with the use of a bladder scanner.

In men, the International Prostate Symptom Score (IPSS), shown in Figure 32-4, or American Urologic Association (AUA) symptom index can be used to quantify complaints of LUTS. Both scales specifically ask about incomplete bladder emptying, frequency, intermittency, urgency, weak stream, straining when beginning to urinate, and nocturia as well as overall inconvenience because of these issues. The resulting score can then be used to chart the progression of prostate conditions or the success of interventions. There is no equivalent scale for women, although scales to evaluate interstitial cystitis manifestations are similar. Further details of issues related to the prostate can be found in Chapter 38.

	Not at all	Less than 1 time in 5	Less than half the time	About half of the time	More than half the time	Almost always	Your score
Incomplete emptying Over the past month, how often have you had a sensation of not emptying your bladder completely after you finish urinating?	0	1	2	3	4	5	
Frequency Over the past month, how often have you had to urinate again less than 2 hours after you finished urinating?	0	1	2	3	4	5	
Intermittency Over the past month, how often have you found you stopped and started again several times when you urinated?	0	1	2	3	4	5	
Urgency Over the last month, how difficult have you found it to postpone urination?	0	1	2	3	4	5	
Weak stream Over the past month, how often have you had a weak urinary stream?	0	1	2	3	4	5	
Straining Over the past month, how often have you had to push or strain to begin urination?	0	1	2	3	4	5	

	None	1 time	2 times	3 times	4 times	5 times or more	Your score
Nocturia Over the past month, how many times did you most typically get up to urinate from the time you went to bed until the time you got up in the morning?	0	1	2	3	4	5	
Total IPSS score							

	Delighted	Pleased	Mostly satisfied	Mixed—about equally satisfied and dissatisfied	Mostly dissatisfied	Unhappy	Terrible
Quality of life due to urinary symptoms							
If you were to spend the rest of your life with your urinary condition the way it is now, how would you feel about that?	0	1	2	3	4	5	6

Total score: 0-7, Mildly symptomatic; 8-19, moderately symptomatic; 20-35, severely symptomatic.

■ **FIGURE 32–4** International Prostate Symptom Score (IPSS) for assessment of the effects of benign prostate hyperplasia. *(From Cockett, A.T. K., et al. [Eds.] [1994]. The Second International Consultation on Benign Prostatic Hyperplasia [BPH]. Paris: Scientific Communication International.)*

Urinary Incontinence. Urinary incontinence is the involuntary loss of urine, and it can have a variety of causes: urge, reflex, stress, mixed, overflow, and functional. Incontinence of any type can lead to clients who avoid social interactions and physical activity, for fear of increasing the degree of incontinence as well as fear of odor. It can have a profound impact on a client's self-esteem, and the client can shy away from sexual intimacy because of embarrassment. Each complaint of incontinence should be questioned thoroughly as to the specifics of the situations in which the incontinence occurs. Detailing the specifics of an incontinence complaint will enable an accurate evaluation; refer to the detailed discussion of incontinence in Chapter 34 for further information.

Infection. When assessing the client with a suspected GU infection, establish the duration of the infection and any pattern of pain that accompanies it (see the previous Pain section). It is also vital to determine if the client has recently been treated for the same issue, and for how long. Clients should be asked about the presence of any discharge, particularly if there is concern regarding a wound, suprapubic tube, or incision site. Any suspicion of sexually transmitted infections (STIs) should be thoroughly investigated (refer to Chapter 41).

A urinary tract infection (UTI) is a common cause of dysuria, but is rarely accompanied by pain and constitutional complaints unless the client has a compromised immune system or bladder dysfunction that prevents complete emptying. Infection of the epididymis or testicle can have a sudden onset with few constitutional complaints, and possible radiation of the pain. Prostatic pain is possible but uncommon, and is seen with acute or chronic prostatitis, along with possible systemic manifestations. Untreated bladder stones and kidney stones can also increase the incidence of infection.

Certain groups are at risk for complicated UTIs (a UTI with a high risk of treatment failure). This includes clients with abnormalities of GU anatomy or functional abnormalities, the very young or very old, and immunocompromised clients. A complicated UTI creates a risk for progression of the infection into pyelonephritis. Refer to the Integrating Diagnostic Testing feature on p. 668 for further details on the evaluation of a client with a suspected UTI.

Systemic Manifestations. Systemic manifestations of common urologic diseases can include weight loss, general malaise, and unexplained fever. As with any infection, clients may complain of manifestations such as nausea, vomiting, fever, or chills. There are also well-documented patterns of referred pain for many GU conditions (refer to Table 32-1 on p. 665).

Not all clients will present with textbook-common presentations. In some cases, the clients may have manifestations that more closely mimic neurologic, GI, or musculoskeletal complaints. For instance, renal pathology causes GI complaints because the kidneys

INTEGRATING DIAGNOSTIC TESTING

Urinary Tract Infection

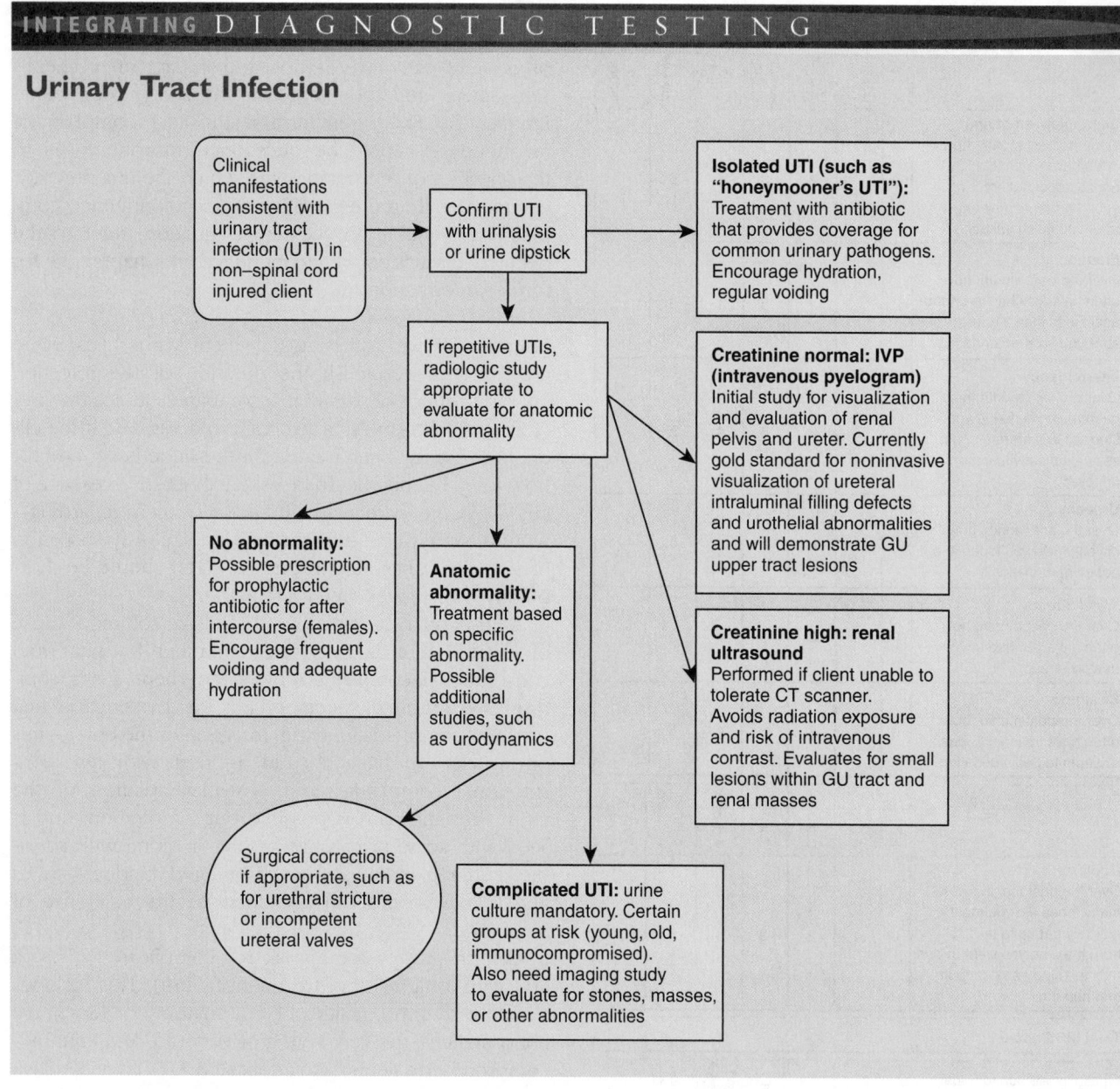

Clinical manifestations consistent with urinary tract infection (UTI) in non–spinal cord injured client

Confirm UTI with urinalysis or urine dipstick

Isolated UTI (such as "honeymooner's UTI"): Treatment with antibiotic that provides coverage for common urinary pathogens. Encourage hydration, regular voiding

If repetitive UTIs, radiologic study appropriate to evaluate for anatomic abnormality

Creatinine normal: IVP (intravenous pyelogram) Initial study for visualization and evaluation of renal pelvis and ureter. Currently gold standard for noninvasive visualization of ureteral intraluminal filling defects and urothelial abnormalities and will demonstrate GU upper tract lesions

No abnormality: Possible prescription for prophylactic antibiotic for after intercourse (females). Encourage frequent voiding and adequate hydration

Anatomic abnormality: Treatment based on specific abnormality. Possible additional studies, such as urodynamics

Creatinine high: renal ultrasound Performed if client unable to tolerate CT scanner. Avoids radiation exposure and risk of intravenous contrast. Evaluates for small lesions within GU tract and renal masses

Surgical corrections if appropriate, such as for urethral stricture or incompetent ureteral valves

Complicated UTI: urine culture mandatory. Certain groups at risk (young, old, immunocompromised). Also need imaging study to evaluate for stones, masses, or other abnormalities

---

are anatomically related to many of the intra-abdominal organs, and inflammation of the kidneys can lead to patterns of referred pain in sites such as the colon. Kidney conditions in particular can lead to nausea, vomiting, and abdominal distention because of the "renointestinal reflex," which refers to the common sensory and autonomic innervation of these two systems (see Table 32-1 on p. 665).

In clients with chronic GU diagnoses such as chronic kidney disease (CKD), systemic manifestations are due to the long-term consequences inherent in the disease process. Along with the expected electrolyte derangements,

CKD clients will demonstrate complaints that are consistent with fatigue, anorexia, neurologic changes, and hypogonadism in men. Renal failure can also mimic peptic ulcer disease, gallbladder complaints, or the clinical presentation of appendicitis. As the process becomes more severe, manifestations of end-stage disease will present, such as increasing edema and mental status changes, as well as manifestations that are specific to electrolyte disturbances. However, many GU conditions can present in a similar manner; it is possible for a man with advanced prostate cancer to present with fatigue, dysuria, electrolyte imbalances, dehydration, and anorexia.

Review of Systems

It is vital to approach the assessment of the GU system in an orderly fashion that includes consideration of both anatomic and physiologic conditions that could contribute to the current complaint. Figure 32-5 demonstrates a systematic approach for obtaining an expanded GU history. When beginning the history of the complaint, it is important to distinguish among acute, persistent, chronic, and recurrent complaints.

Begin with questions that will detail any complaints that the client may have, trying to encourage that the client narrow the complaints as much as possible to those

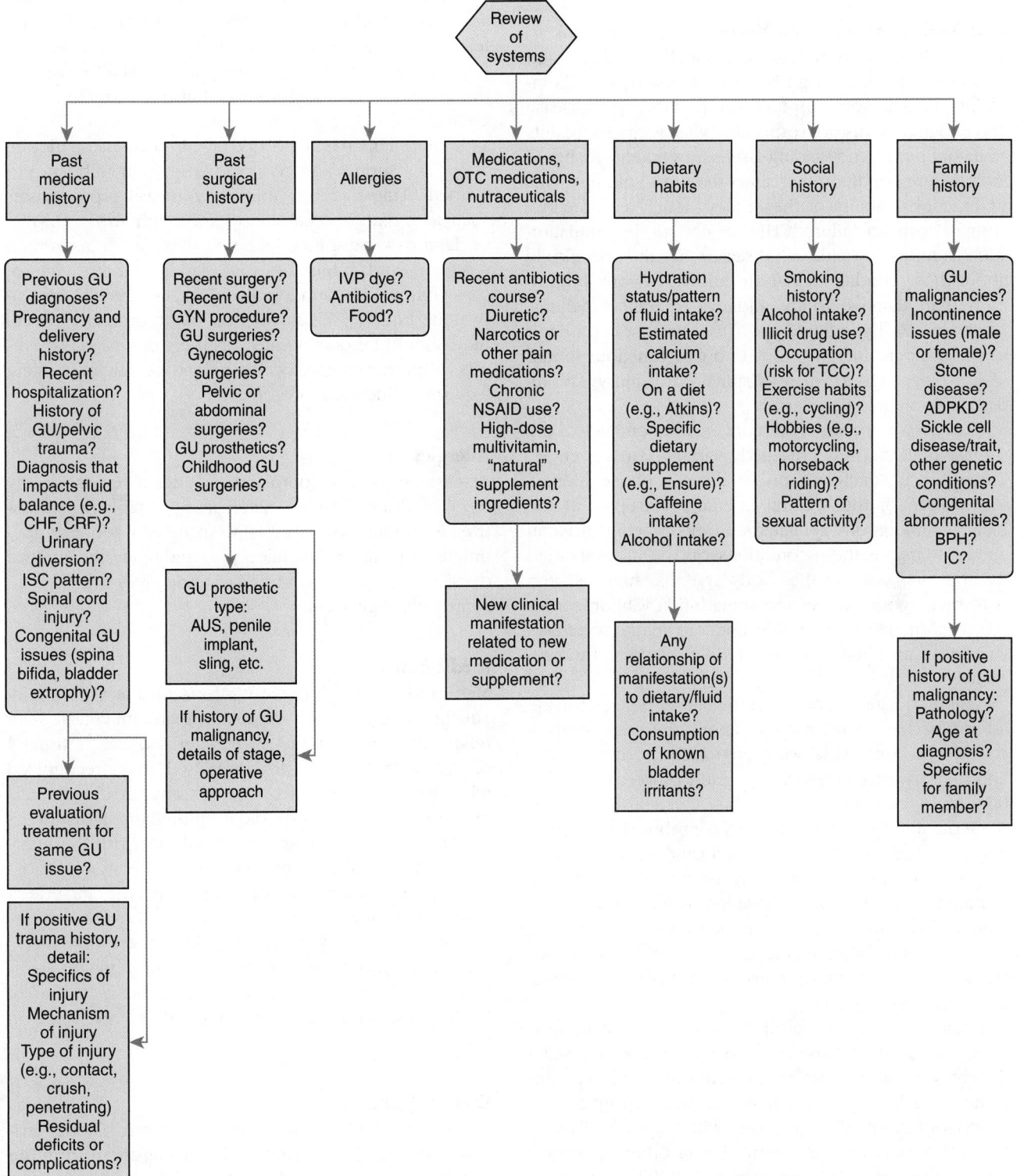

■ **FIGURE 32–5** Expanded genitourinary history. *ADPKD*, Autosomal dominant polycystic kidney disease; *AUS*, artificial urinary sphincter; *BPH*, benign prostatic hypertrophy; *CHF*, congestive heart failure; *CRF*, chronic renal failure; *IC*, interstitial cystitis; *ISC*, intermittent straight catheterization; *IVP*, intravenous pyelogram; *TCC*, transitional cell carcinoma.

that are relevant to the GU system. This includes questions about possible GI complaints, weight loss or gain, clinical manifestations of infection, pain, edema, fatigue or lethargy, headaches, and changes in mental acuity. Include questions that detail the client's occupation and hobbies (such as sports or patterns of exercise).

Past Medical History and Recent Hospitalizations

The baseline history should always include a discussion of previous medical diagnoses. In the case of a GU complaint, this can focus around any previous GU disease and pregnancy history (especially vital with complaints of incontinence and voiding issues in women). It should include any condition that alters the fluid volume status or functional ability of the kidneys (such as infection, congestive heart failure [CHF], or chronic inflammation such as lupus or sickle cell disease). Inquire specifically about those conditions that are known to contribute to end-organ damage to the kidneys (diabetes mellitus, hypertension, hyperlipidemia). Diseases that can impair the neurologic integrity of GU organ function should also be investigated, such as spinal cord injury, stroke, diabetes, or multiple sclerosis.

There is a wide variety of congenital anomalies of the urinary tract that have distinctly varying consequences. There can be malformation or absence of the kidney, malposition of the urethral opening, extrophy of the bladder, ambiguous genitalia, and incompetent ureteral valves. Many of these conditions can be accompanied by abnormalities of other body systems, such as seen with meningomyelocele and spina bifida. Children with GU abnormalities commonly undergo many corrective surgeries, and many have chronic bladder function issues.

Childhood infections can have consequences for the adult GU client. Most notable among these are streptococcal infections, which can lead to kidney dysfunction, and mumps orchitis, which can lead to subfertility/infertility in the adult male.

Geographical location can also contribute to GU complaints. Clients who spend a significant amount of time in a hot climate many be more prone to dehydration. Certain living conditions or locations can raise the suspicion for infection from larva-infested water; for example, infection with flukes of the genus *Schistosoma* causes schistosomiasis, which predisposes to urinary obstruction and bladder cancer.

If there is a history of abdominal or pelvic trauma, establish the mechanism of injury whenever possible. Specific GU injuries can be expected in certain circumstances, such as with a pelvic fracture, during contact sports, or the straddle injury seen with bicycling. Trauma to the GU tract can also result during other occasions, such as the urethral trauma seen with childbirth or inadvertent urethral trauma during GU instrumentation.

These types of injury can result in voiding complaints or a higher incidence of UTI and dysuria complaints.

Surgical History

A thorough surgical history is vital to the assessment of GU complaints. Both abdominal and retroperitoneal surgery can result in damage or scarring to both the sensory and the overall neurologic components of the GU system, resulting in such varied manifestations as erectile dysfunction, incontinence, and chronic pain. Surgery to the vertebrae or spinal cord can also contribute to GU complaints.

If the client has a history of GU diagnoses, inquire about any surgical procedures that may have been performed. This includes minimally invasive procedures such as extracorporeal sound wave lithotripsy (ESWL) or laparoscopic procedures, as well as transurethral resection and fulguration of bladder tumors, radical cystectomy with urinary diversion, or cryoablation of prostate tumors. Whenever possible, the precise procedure should be documented, as there are various methods for performing a specific procedure, such as a sling for urinary incontinence.

Allergies

Assessment of any complaint includes a review of any food or drug allergies. Since many radiologic studies used to evaluate GU complaints include IV contrast, document any history of allergy to radiographic contrast dyes as well as to iodine, as iodine dyes are used in some radiologic tests.

Medications

Medications can have many effects on the GU system; anticholinergics and alpha-sympathomimetics can relieve urinary incontinence but can also lead to urinary retention. There are specific GU risks recognized with certain categories of medications. In older adults or chronic users, nonsteroidal anti-inflammatory drugs (NSAIDs) can result in interstitial nephritis.[17] Heavy consumption of acetaminophen has been associated with an increased risk of renal cancer.[14] Include a generalized question to confirm that the medications are being taken as intended. With prescription medications, socioeconomic status alone may make it difficult for a client to take the medication as intended. Medications with recognized GU effects are listed in Box 32-1.

Dietary Habits

Some foods and supplements are known bladder irritants (Box 32-2), and simply eliminating these from the diet can correct or reduce GU manifestations, such as those seen with interstitial cystitis.[3] Nutritional status

BOX 32-1	Medications That Affect Urinary Elimination
Medication Type	**Effect on Urination**
Anticholinergics	Decreased detrusor contractility (oxybutynin, methantheline), urinary retention, hesitancy
Antispasmodics	Decreased detrusor contractility (dicyclomine, belladonna), urinary retention, urinary hesitancy
Tricyclic antidepressants	Decreased detrusor contractility (imipramine), urinary retention, less incontinence
Cholinergics	Increased detrusor contractility (bethanechol chloride), incontinence, urgency
Alpha-sympathomimetics	Increased sphincter resistance (pseudoephedrine), urinary retention, dysuria
Alpha-blockers	Reduced sphincter resistance (prazosin, terazosin), frequency, incontinence
Estrogens (women)	Increased urethral muscle tone (progestin, estriol), reduced incontinence
Anti-androgens (men)	Improved urinary flow (flutamide, bicalutamide)
Sedatives-hypnotics	Urinary incontinence
Nonsteroidal anti-inflammatories	Renal papillary necrosis (long term)
Diuretics	Polyuria, urinary incontinence (hydrochlorothiazide)
Aminoglycoside antibiotics	Nephrotoxicity (gentamicin, amikacin)
Calcium channel blockers	Urinary retention (diltiazem, verapamil)
Alcohol	Polyuria, frequency, urgency

BOX 32-2 Foods That Are Known or Likely Bladder Irritants

- Alcoholic beverages
- Aspartame (NutraSweet)
- Caffeine-containing beverages
- Carbonated beverages
- Chocolate
- Citrus fruits/juices
- Cranberries
- Mayonnaise
- Milk/milk products
- Nicotine
- Nuts (e.g., peanuts, pecans, pistachios, walnuts)
- Onions
- Other fruits (e.g., mango, strawberries, plums, peaches, guava)
- Processed meats (e.g., ham, pepperoni, smoked meats)
- Salt/sodium
- Soy milk/soybeans/tofu
- Soy sauce
- Spicy foods/spices
- Tomato juice/products
- Vinegar

can impact fluid and electrolyte balance; high-protein diets create ketosis and predispose a client to kidney stone formation. Other dietary habits can increase the risk for urinary stones, such as a diet high in dairy products. High-fat diets have recently been linked to an increased risk for prostate cancer. Herbal supplements used for prostate health include saw palmetto (*Serenoa repens*), pygeum (*Pygeum africanum*), pumpkin (*Cucurbita pepo*), and nettle root (*Urtica dioica*).[19] Megadose vitamins (40,000 units of vitamin A, 100 mg of vitamin B_6, 2000 mg of vitamin C, 400 units of vitamin E, and 90 mg of zinc) were shown in one small study to have secondary prevention benefits over RDA vitamins in clients with bladder cancer.[25] Nutraceuticals that men diagnosed with prostate cancer or trying to prevent prostate cancer may take include vitamin E, lycopene, dehydroepiandrosterone (DHEA) (to boost testosterone if treated for prostate cancer), and selenium.[23] Evaluate the medication or supplement along with its

dose, route of administration, recent dosage changes, and frequency of use to establish a potential relationship to the onset of the chief complaint.

Psychosocial History

Psychosocial assessment should be continual during the interview process. The client should be assessed for level of knowledge regarding the GU system as a whole, functional mobility, manual dexterity, and impairments in vision, hearing, or speech. Assess the client's knowledge of the impact of such factors as fluid intake, toileting facilities, and social support systems on the present complaint.

When assessing young adults with urinary complaints, investigate childhood experiences with toilet training and accessibility of lavatory facilities during the school day that may have had a long-term effect on urination patterns. Determine the anxiety level regarding voiding in a public place, and overall stress level in daily life.

If there is a current or previous cancer diagnosis that factors into the current complaint, observe body language for a clue to any depression that may contribute to the client's complaint or complicate treatment.

Occupation can provide a clue to a particular client's risk for a GU diagnosis. Both aromatic amines and diesel exhaust have been implicated as risk factors for bladder cancer. Occupations such as teaching and nursing have been shown to have an increased risk for bladder dysfunction because of the potential for limited breaks for toileting.

Physical exercise should rarely be discouraged. But some types of activities can predispose a client to GU complaints. Long-distance runners sometimes have microscopic or gross hematuria, which, although typically temporary and self-limiting, can indicate underlying glomerular disease. Long-distance bicyclists may develop urethral and vulvar trauma, prostatic complaints, or pudendal neuropathy that can cause perineal pain, erectile dysfunction in men, and sexual dysfunction in women.

Complete assessment for the GU system includes detailing any history of tobacco, alcohol, and recreational drug use. Cigarette smoking is a well-established risk factor for bladder, renal, and urothelial cancers. Smoking has also been implicated as an independent risk factor for erectile dysfunction. Alcohol is a well-established bladder irritant and will contribute to increased urinary output. Chronic alcoholism may lead to autonomic and peripheral neuropathy that impairs urinary function, impairs sexual function, and creates secondary hypogonadism in men.

Specifically question the pattern of sexual activity, as this can contribute to the risk for urinary tract infection in both genders, as well as possible prostatitis in men (this can also provide insight into risk for HIV; this is detailed more in Chapter 41).

Family Health History

Questions regarding the family health history should evaluate for any genetic disease that has GU manifestations (such as autosomal dominant polycystic kidney disease [ADPKD], tuberous sclerosis, von Hippel-Lindau disease, and cystinuria), GU malignancies, siblings with congenital abnormalities, or first-degree relatives with a GU malignancy.[7,15] Some conditions are genetically linked, such as stone disease, hypertension, diabetes, and BPH.

PHYSICAL EXAMINATION

The urologic physical examination will be tailored to the client's specific complaint or condition. Instruct the client to attempt to empty the bladder before the examination. When the physical examination has been completed, document findings using the feature above, right, as a guide.

Abdomen

Inspection

Have the client lie in a supine position with arms at the sides and knees slightly flexed to relax the abdominal muscles. If the client has complained of abdominal, back, or flank pain, note whether there is guarding or restlessness in this position. Inspect the abdomen for symmetry and contour. Asymmetry or a mass in the

---

Physical Assessment Findings in the Healthy Adult

The Urinary System

Inspection	Lower abdomen flat, nondistended; external urethral orifice pink without discharge
Auscultation	No renal bruit noted anteriorly or posteriorly over right or left costovertebral angle
Percussion	Flat note over symphysis pubis and tympany over lower abdomen; no tenderness posteriorly over right or left costovertebral angle
Palpation	Lower pole of right kidney palpable, smooth, nontender; left kidney nonpalpable

---

upper quadrants may indicate a renal tumor or hydronephrosis, although only a very large renal or adrenal mass in a very thin client is usually visible. Fullness in the suprapubic area may indicate a distended bladder.

Note any surgical or traumatic scarring that may have affected the urinary or GI tract or caused adhesions, especially if the client presents with abdominal complaints. Inspect carefully for surgical scars as this is a common point of omission for any clients. Note any herniation, either at the site of surgical scarring, around a stoma, or in the ventral area (epigastric or umbilical region), particularly with straining (see discussion under lower GI elimination physical examination).

Auscultation

Auscultation is performed before palpation to avoid disruption of vascular murmurs and bowel sounds. Renal artery bruits are heard just above and slightly left of the umbilicus and can indicate renal artery stenosis, aneurysm, or arteriovenous malformation. If a bruit is heard, avoid deep palpation. Evaluate bowel sounds in all four quadrants for frequency, intensity, and pitch, especially in the presence of GI manifestations.

Percussion

Percussion is valuable in identifying a bladder containing at least 150 ml of urine. The percussion sound changes from tympanic to dull over a full bladder. Blunt percussion can also be valuable if performed anteriorly and posteriorly to identify renal masses or tenderness when renal trauma and hemorrhage prevent deep palpation. See an assessment text for details regarding this technique.

Palpation

Begin palpation with a light touch, depressing the skin no deeper than 1 to 2 cm, to assess tenderness and muscle resistance or guarding, which might be a sign of peritoneal irritation. Light palpation allows examination of tender abdominal areas with minimal production of pain, as pain may cause voluntary muscle rigidity.

Examine each of the four quadrants, noting areas of muscle resistance, which may indicate a superficial or large pelvic mass, either infectious or neoplastic, or bladder distention if it is in the suprapubic area. It can also indicate a collection of serum or urine, a hematoma, or a pocket of infection, particularly if the client had a recent surgical procedure. Involuntary muscle rigidity is usually unilateral, whereas voluntary rigidity is symmetrical. Describe identified masses in terms of location, size, consistency, surface characteristics, tenderness, mobility, and pulsation. Assess rebound tenderness to determine the presence of peritoneal inflammation. Last, palpate any region under suspicion on the basis of the health history and previous inspection.

Deep palpation follows light palpation and should be performed only by an advanced practitioner. It is used primarily to detect renal enlargement or masses. The technique is similar to that of light palpation, but the depth is 4 to 5 cm. The kidneys are normally well protected by the diaphragm and lower ribs and cannot be palpated easily, except in the case of ADPKD.

An empty bladder cannot be palpated or percussed. In acute or chronic urinary retention, the bladder rises up out of the pelvis at the midline toward the umbilicus. It may be seen and usually felt. When there is chronic urinary retention, the bladder is atonic and difficult to palpate, making evaluation with a bladder scanner necessary.

Genitalia

Use inspection and palpation to examine the genitalia; specifics of both the male and female examination are detailed in Chapter 37. Clients tend to be anxious about examination of the genitalia, so it is vital to remain straightforward and professional when performing this portion of the examination.

Male Clients

This examination is best performed in a warm room. While the male client lies supine, inspect the perineum and groin area for manifestations of skin irritation or excoriation, especially if he has reported urinary incontinence. Examine the glans meatus. Circumcised males have a dry glans, whereas uncircumcised males have a relatively moist and pink glans. Examine the urethral meatus after carefully retracting the foreskin if the male is uncircumcised. The foreskin should retract easily; if it is somewhat stenotic, this is known as *phimosis*. The meatus is located centrally on the glans and its mucosa is pink and moist, readily separating when the glans is pressed between the thumb and forefinger.

Female Clients

Urologic examination of the female genitalia includes examination of the external genitalia and in some cases a complete pelvic examination. Inspect for the presence of urethral or vaginal discharge indicative of infection. Ask the client to cough or strain, and observe for any bulging of the vaginal walls. Bulging of the anterior vaginal wall can indicate a *cystocele* and bulging of the posterior vaginal wall can indicate a *rectocele*. Cystocele is a result of the relaxation of the pelvic floor musculature (commonly as a result of childbirth) and may be the source of irritative voiding manifestations and stress incontinence.

Lymph Nodes

Inspect and palpate the supraclavicular and inguinal groups of lymph nodes if metastatic cancer of the prostate or testis is suspected. Chapter 74 describes examination of the inguinal lymph nodes.

Related Body Systems

Assess pertinent information about other body systems, such as blood pressure, temperature, fluid balance, evidence of peripheral edema, and neurologic or vascular changes that affect the lower extremities. Document your findings, as they may be related to disorders of the urinary tract.

DIAGNOSTIC TESTING

Diagnostic tests provide information about the nature and severity of lower GI tract problems. Laboratory tests, radiography, ultrasonography, endoscopy, cytology, and other tests are commonly used. Refer to a diagnostic testing manual for more specific information related to the nursing care and implications for the tests identified in the following discussion.

Noninvasive Tests
KUB (kidney, ureters, bladder)

This is the simplest of the available uroradiologic studies. It is used as a screening or preliminary test, often to assess for renal or ureteral lithiasis. KUB often shows calcified abnormalities and can demonstrate large soft tissue masses in the abdomen. KUB is routinely used to track the progress of ureteral stones as they progress the length of the ureter.

Intravenous Pyelogram (IVP)

This is the initial study for the visualization and evaluation of a client's renal pelvis, collecting system, and ureter. Is it currently considered the gold standard for noninvasive visualization of ureteral intraluminal filling defects and urothelial abnormalities, and will demonstrate GU upper tract lesions. Its major drawback is that it is less sensitive in the visualization of small lesions within the GU tract.

Renal Ultrasound

The ultrasound test is recommended if the client is unable to tolerate the CT scanner or if the serum creatinine level is too high to permit an IVP. It avoids radiation exposure and risk of intravenous contrast. A renal ultrasound is used primarily to evaluate for small lesions within the GU tract and renal masses.

Computerized Tomography (CT)

The CT scan is the preferred study for staging malignancies of the GU tract. CT has a rapid scanning time, is well-tolerated by most clients, and detects subtle differences in tissue density. CT scan is an excellent imaging method for the evaluation of renal and retroperitoneal pathology, and is indicated when an IVP or ultrasound indicates a mass. Unenhanced helical CT scan is also superior for the evaluation of suspected or actual stone disease.

CT urography is available at some facilities, and offers a combination of the routine CT scan and an IVP study. It may be superior at detecting renal cell carcinomas, and in the future may replace the IVP as the preferred study.

Magnetic Resonance Imaging (MRI)

MRI has multiple uses in the evaluation of GU conditions, as it provides excellent images of the retroperitoneum, bladder, prostate, testes, and even the penis. The use of gadolinium as the contrast medium allows this test to be used with clients who have suffered a decline in renal function. MRI studies include images in all three planes and provide excellent soft tissue characterization. There is no exposure to radiation, but many clients find the MRI machine and slow scanning time can result in claustrophobia.

Invasive Tests

Refer to Chapter 34 and the discussion of the incontinence evaluation for a discussion of the unique diagnostic testing and fluorourodynamic studies that evaluate bladder function, capacity, and sensation.

There are several invasive biopsy options that can have a part in the diagnosis of bladder and renal pathology, such as the renal biopsy. Refer to Chapter 35 for a thorough discussion of the suspected pathologies that would require such a biopsy for evaluation.

Transurethral Biopsy

Biopsy of a suspicious lesion in the bladder that is discovered during cystourethroscopy is done with the client under regional or general anesthesia. Biopsy specimens of surrounding bladder tissue are also taken randomly to evaluate the rest of the bladder. Care of the client is the same as for the client undergoing endoscopy but also involves preparation for anesthesia.

Intervention includes assisting the client in anesthesia recovery as well as using comfort measures for urethral pain, bladder spasms, flank pain, and dysuria, which are commonly experienced after biopsy. Instruct the client to watch for clinical manifestations of urinary tract infection or infection of the puncture site and to report these promptly after the procedure.

Transrectal Biopsy

Biopsy of the prostate gland is performed via a rectal approach after a urine specimen confirms that there is no infection. The biopsy specimen is usually obtained with a multiple-core biopsy needle guided by ultrasonography. For a detailed discussion of the procedure and its indications, refer to Chapter 38.

Endoscopy

Endoscopy (see Chapter 34) is utilized in urology most commonly in *cystourethroscopy*. Cystoscopy allows diagnostic inspection of the urinary tract for evidence of urinary calculi, infection, vesicoureteral reflux, prostatic obstruction, bladder tumor, and urethral stricture (Figure 32-6). For a complete discussion of these procedures and their indications, refer to a procedure textbook. Endoscopic procedures for the upper urinary tract (see Chapter 34) include the following: ureteroscopy, flexible ureteropyeloscopy, and nephroscopy. For details on these and other procedures, such as

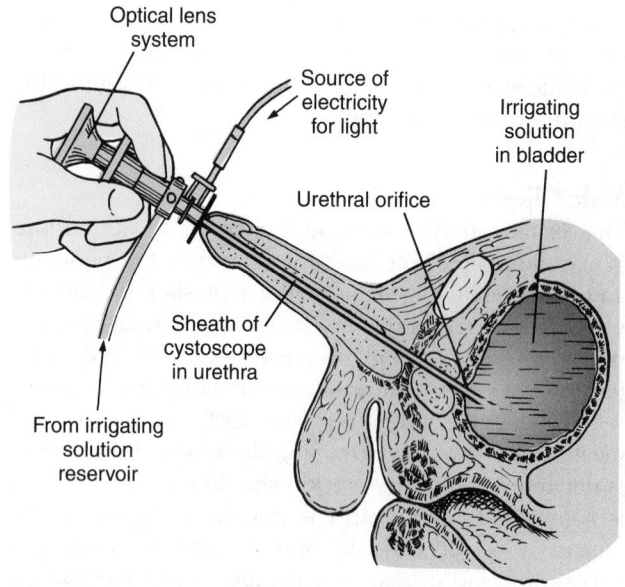

■ **FIGURE 32-6** Cystoscope in the male bladder.

urodynamic studies, common to the care of urologic clients, refer to a diagnostic test textbook.

Laboratory Tests

Laboratory tests for the urinary system consist primarily of urine and blood studies. See a diagnostic testing book for additional information.

Urine Studies

Clients who describe changes in their urine should be asked to detail the color, clarity/opacity, and any noted odor (other than ammonia). Urine should be pale yellow and clear and have the faintest odor of ammonia. These characteristics can change, depending on disease states and hydration status. For instance, UTI can cause hematuria in both genders.

The most significant color change that a client can report is that of gross hematuria; often this is the only indication of a GU malignancy. Other instances of color change can also be significant, but can be false positives influenced by such factors as dietary intake of certain foods or multivitamins. The timing of hematuria can aid in narrowing the potential causes. Clients should be asked to describe when during the stream blood occurs: initial (urethral causes), terminal (prostatic), or total hematuria (any site in the GU tract, anatomic or physiologic cause). There should also be a question regarding the presence of clots, and whether or not the client has to strain to initiate the stream. If straining is a new manifestation, it can indicate retained clots.

The clarity of urine is most commonly affected by infection or inflammation that results in the presence of WBCs or bacteria in the urine. It can be the result of amorphous phosphates in alkaline urine, or semen caused by retrograde ejaculation. Less common causes include crystals, mucus (such as with a urinary diversion or neobladder), or fecal material. Urine with a strong odor is a common indicator of concentrated urine, but can also signal infection. Urine can degrade if left standing at room temperature and become increasingly ammonia-rich in odor.

Urinalysis. Clients who present with urinary tract manifestations typically undergo a urinalysis. Urinalysis performed by dipstick provides a wide variety of information (Table 32-2 on p. 676). Microscopic urinalysis quantifies white and red blood cells and indicates the presence of casts, crystals, bacteria, or epithelial cells. Microscopic urinalysis differentiates between actual RBC presence in the sample and a false positive on the dipstick test.

Depending on the test ordered, urinalysis may be performed on a clean catch specimen, midstream specimen, fresh urine specimen, first morning specimen, 12- or 24-hour collection, multiple bottle voidings (serial urine collections), or a specimen obtained with a catheter. Refer to a nursing fundamentals book for details on the collection of these specimens.

When urinary tract infection is suspected from the client's history or the presence of bacteria or significant white blood cells on urinalysis, a urine culture is necessary. This test identifies the offending organism and quantifies the amount of colonization. Generally, the presence of organisms at a concentration greater than 100,000 colony-forming units (cfu)/ml indicates infection, although treatment is recommended for 10,000 to 100,000 cfu/ml if clinical manifestations consistent with infection are present.[20] Urine cultures are particularly important for recurrent UTIs, for a complicated UTI, or in the client with a UTI that seems refractory to treatment.

Urinalysis collection technique is the same as that for midstream clean catch or catheter specimens. Determining the sensitivity of the organism to specific antibiotics is not usually necessary because *E. coli,* known to cause 85% of routine infections, is sensitive to most oral antibiotics. Identifying the drugs to which the bacteria are sensitive is done in cases with recurrent or persistent manifestations of urinary tract infection.

When urothelial carcinoma or inflammatory disease of the bladder, renal pelvis, ureters, or urethra is known or suspected, urine cytologic evaluation is performed. The specimen may be clean voided or a bladder washing obtained either by catheterization or cystoscopically. If a voided specimen is obtained, the ideal is to send the first voided specimen of the day. This test is also helpful in diagnosing cytomegalovirus or other viral disease.

Quantitative Urine Studies. Urine creatinine clearance is most often part of quantitative urine studies. Creatinine determines the glomerular filtration rate and tubular excretion ability of the kidney. Creatinine is a byproduct of muscle energy metabolism and is excreted in the urine at a fairly constant rate. Creatinine level in the urine is equivalent to the glomerular filtration rate, and may be diminished in renal disorders. Excretion rates of other urinary components and the completeness of the collection can be interpreted when measured with creatinine clearance. For determination of creatinine clearance or other quantitative urine studies, the urine specimen is collected for 12 or 24 hours as ordered (see the Quantitative Urine Studies table on the website **evolve** for more information).

Blood Studies

Blood Urea Nitrogen. Blood urea nitrogen (BUN) is a measure of renal function because urea is the primary end product of protein metabolism and is excreted by the kidneys. An elevated BUN level may indicate renal insufficiency, although it is not specific for the kidneys.

TABLE 32–2 Discussion of Urinalysis Components

Urinalysis Component	Interpretation
Normal Findings	
Color	Bright red if urologic or anatomic cause
Pale yellow or amber	Tea-colored or brown urine may be due to old clots, glomerulonephritis, or other medical (physiologic) cause
Crystalluria	May indicate stone disease
Negative	As urine cools additional crystals can precipitate out
Presence does not always indicate disease, but can form in urine left at room temperature	Cystinuria caused by inborn error of metabolism that results in abnormal metabolism of amino acids
	Sulfa crystals have pathologic significance; tend to form renal calculi that may damage renal tubules
	X-ray dye crystals possible after contrast study
Direct bilirubin	Early sign of extrahepatic biliary tract obstruction, intrinsic hepatic disease
Negative	
Glucose	Indicates that serum glucose level exceeds resorptive capacity of kidneys (>180 mg/dl)
Negative	
Ketones	If positive, indicates body fat is metabolized for energy
Negative	Seen with diabetic ketoacidosis, fasting, pregnancy, vomiting, diarrhea
Leukocyte esterase	If positive, suggests infection within urinary tract (does not localize source of infection); 80–90% sensitive;
Negative	approximately 95% specific
Nitrite	If positive, suggests infection within urinary tract (does not localize source of infection); 50% sensitive;
Negative	approximately 95% specific
Osmolality	Indicates concentrating ability of kidney
Average range 500-800 mOsm, but can be 50-1400 mOsm	Increased: hypernatremia, acidosis, shock
	Decreased: diabetes insipidus, hypercalcemia, excessive hydration, renal tubular acidosis
pH	Measures free hydrogen ion in urine
4.5-8.0	Indicates ability of renal tubules to maintain normal hydrogen ion concentration
	Aids in diagnosis of metabolic or respiratory acid-base disorders and maintenance of alkaline or acidic urine for stone disease
Protein	3–4+ may indicate glomerulonephritis or other decline in kidney function
Negative	Transient elevation possible with prolonged fever and excessive physical exertion
	False positive possible if urine is concentrated, contains WBCs or vaginal secretions
Casts	*RBC casts:* indicate renal disease, glomerular source (medical hematuria); indicate bleeding from renal parenchyma
Absent	*Leukocyte casts:* indicate renal disease
	Hyaline casts: can be seen in a urinalysis after exercise
	Granular casts: indicate renal tubular disease
	WBC casts: seen with acute pyelonephritis; characteristic of tubulointerstitial disease
Specific gravity	Concentration of urine as compared with water
1.003-1.030	Indicates hydration status
	Decreased renal function: decreased ability to concentrate urine
	May see low specific gravity with hydronephrosis, intrinsic renal disease
Urobilinogen	Small amount excreted in urine daily
0-4 mg/24 hours	Increased levels indicate liver disease, hemolytic disorders
	Low/absence represents obstruction of biliary tract

BUN may be elevated because of systemic factors such as sepsis, excess protein consumption, starvation, dehydration, and cardiac failure. Two thirds of the renal function must be compromised before an elevation in BUN level is seen.

The normal ratio of BUN to creatinine values is 10:1. This can be elevated (20:1) if the client is dehydrated or has bilateral urinary obstruction. This ratio can be decreased if the client is overhydrated or in advanced hepatic insufficiency.

Serum Creatinine

Serum creatinine level is more specific for renal function because it is not affected by dietary intake or hydration status. It can be elevated in cases of glomerulonephritis, pyelonephritis, acute tubular necrosis, nephrotoxicity, renal insufficiency, and renal failure. Elevations are also seen in clients who have renal failure secondary to outlet obstruction. Elevated serum creatinine levels can occur with systemic disease such as hypertension or diabetes, but this value will remain normal until 50% of the renal function has been compromised.

Creatinine Clearance

This test is the most accurate measurement of renal function that does not require the injection of dye or radiologic testing. The normal value is 90 to 110 ml/min and declines with age.

CONCLUSIONS

A thorough knowledge of the potential causes of elimination disorders is essential to obtain a pertinent health history and to perform an accurate physical assessment. Careful assessment facilitates formulation of accurate nursing and medical diagnoses and planning for the optimal treatment of the client. Knowledge of diagnostic testing is necessary to prepare the client for the tests and to facilitate the diagnostic process.

BIBLIOGRAPHY

Citations appearing in red refer to primary research.

Citations appearing in blue refer to evidence-based practice guidelines and protocols.

1. Agency for Health Care Policy and Research. (1992). *Clinical practice guideline: Urinary incontinence in adults.* Washington, DC: U.S. Department of Health and Human Services.
2. Baden, L., & Maguire, J. (2001). Gastrointestinal infections in the immunocompromised host. *Infectious Disease Clinics of North America, 15*(2), 639-670.
3. Bryant, C., Dowell, C., & Fiarborther, G. (2002). Caffeine reduction education to improve urinary symptoms. *British Journal of Nursing, 11*(8), 560-565.
4. Buchwald, H. (2005). Bariatric surgery for morbid obesity: Health implications for patients, health professionals, and third-party payers. *Journal of the American College of Surgeons, 200*(4), 593-604.
5. Collins, J., Lieberman, D., Durbin, T., et al. (2005). Accuracy of screening for fecal occult blood on a single stool sample obtained by digital rectal examination: A comparison with recommended sampling practice. *Annals of Internal Medicine, 142*(2), 81-85.
6. Davila, R., Rajan, E., & Baron, T. (2006). ASGE guideline: Colorectal cancer screening and surveillance. *Gastrointestinal Endoscopy, 63*(4), 546-557.
7. Droller, M.J. (2004). Primary care update on kidney and bladder cancer: A urologic perspective. *Urologic Clinics of North America, 88*(2), 309-328.
8. Drossman, D. (2006). A biopsychosocial understanding of gastrointestinal illness and disease. In Feldman (Ed.), *Sleisenger & Fordtran's gastrointestinal and liver disease* (7th ed.). St. Louis: Saunders.
9. Ginsberg, G., & Fleischer, D. (2006). Esophageal tumors. In Feldman (Ed.), *Sleisenger & Fordtran's gastrointestinal and liver disease* (7th ed.). St. Louis: Saunders.
10. Grossfeld, G.D., Litwin, M.S., Wolf, J.S., et al. (2001). Evaluation of asymptomatic microscopic hematuria in adults: The American Urological Association best practice policy—Part I: Definition, detection, prevalence, and etiology. *Urology, 57*(4), 599-603.
11. Grossfeld, G.D., Litwin, M.S., Wolf, J.S., et al. (2001). Evaluation of asymptomatic microscopic hematuria in adults: The American Urological Association best practice policy—Part II: Patient evaluation, cytology, voided markers, imaging, cystoscopy, nephrology evaluation, and follow-up. *Urology, 57*(4), 604-610.
12. Headstrom, P., & Surawicz, C. (2005). Chronic diarrhea. *Clinical Gastroenterology and Hepatology, 3*, 734-737.
13. Iddan, G., & Swain, C. (2004). History and development of capsule endoscopy. *Gastrointestinal Endoscopy Clinics of North America, 14*, 1-9.
14. Kaye, J.A., Wald Myers, M., & Jick, H. (2001). Acetaminophen and the risk of renal and bladder cancer in the general practice research database. *Epidemiology, 12*(6), 690-694.
15. Kolettis, P.N. (2003). Genetic diseases in adults. *Urologic Clinics of North America, 30*(1), 153-160.
16. Langmead, L., & Rampton, D. (2006). Review article: Complementary and alternative therapies for inflammatory bowel disease. *Alimentary Pharmacology & Therapeutics, 23*(3), 341-349.
17. Lewis, J., Kimmel, S., Localio, A., et al. (2005). Risk of serious upper gastrointestinal toxicity with over the counter nonaspirin nonsteroidal anti-inflammatory drugs. *Gastroenterology, 129*, 1865-1874.
18. Minghini, A., Weireter, L.J., & Perry, R. (1998). Specificity of elevated CA 19-9 levels in chronic pancreatitis. *Surgery, 124*, 103-105.
19. Simmang, C., & Shires, G.I. (2006). Diverticular diseases of the colon. In Feldman (Ed.), *Sleisenger & Fordtran's gastrointestinal and liver disease* (7th ed., pp. 2100-2111). St. Louis: Saunders.
20. Tanagho, E.A., & McAninch, J.W. (2003). *Smith's general urology* (16th ed.). New York: McGraw-Hill Medical.
21. Tessler, D., Catanzaro, A., Velanovich, V., et al. (2006). Predictors of cancer in patients with suspected pancreatic malignancy without a tissue diagnosis. *American Journal of Surgery, 191*(2), 191-197.
22. Todd, B. (2006). Clostridium difficile: Familiar pathogen, changing epidemiology: A virulent strain has been appearing more often, even in patients not taking antibiotics. *American Journal of Nursing, 106*(5), 33-36.
23. Uzzo, R.G., Brown, J.G., Horwitz, E.M., et al. (2004). Prevalence and patterns of self-initiated nutritional supplementation in men at high risk of prostate cancer. *BJU International, 93*(7), 955-960.
24. Vickers, A., & Zollman, C. (1999). ABC of complementary medicine: Herbal medicine. *British Medical Journal, 319*, 1050-1053.
25. Walsh, P.C., et al. (2002). *Campbell's urology* (8th ed). Philadelphia: Saunders.
26. Young, M. (2003). Prevention of colon cancer. In K. Rakel (Ed.), *Integrative medicine* (pp. 549-554). Philadelphia: Saunders.

evolve *Did you remember to check out the bonus material on the Evolve website and the CD-ROM, including NCLEX®-Examination Style Review Questions, Open-Book Quizzes, and Chapter Review Audio Podcasts?*

http://evolve.elsevier.com/Black/medsurg

CHAPTER 33

Management of Clients with Intestinal Disorders

DAWN P. MURPHY AND JANE HOKANSON HAWKS

The client with an intestinal disorder usually has a problem with bowel elimination. Hence the most common nursing diagnoses are *Constipation, Bowel Incontinence,* and *Diarrhea.* Additional nursing diagnoses are *Acute Pain, Chronic Pain, Imbalanced Nutrition: Less Than Body Requirements, Deficient Fluid Volume,* and *Disturbed Body Image.*

GENERAL CLINICAL MANIFESTATIONS

The epithelial cells of the gastrointestinal (GI) tract are specialized for absorption and secretion. These cells facilitate digestion and nutritional intake, while repelling harmful pathogens and mutagens. The latter is accomplished by maintenance of the integrity of the mucosal surface and the presence of immune cells that take residence within the bowel. Disorders of the intestine cause manifestations through the physical disruption of the mucosal layer (blood loss, fluid loss, infection) or nutritional abnormalities caused by impaired digestion and nutrient absorption. The function of the gastrointestinal tract is also dependent on the coordinated propulsion of food through the lumen by smooth muscle contraction.

Disruption of normal motility may be direct (obstructing mass) or indirect (inflammatory mediators that affect muscle movement). The movement of intestinal contents *(chyme)* through the intestine may be slowed, obstructed, or accelerated, or the secretion, motility, and absorption of intestinal contents may be disrupted. Manifestations of intestinal disorders are related to the organ involved, and vary according to which function (motility, digestion, or absorption) is disturbed. The major manifestations of dysfunction are hemorrhage, pain, nausea and vomiting, distention, constipation, diarrhea, and abnormal fecal contents.

Hemorrhage

Bleeding can be caused by trauma, ulceration, inflammation, or a growth that erodes through a blood vessel. The usual manifestation is blood in the stool *(hematochezia)* rather than in vomitus *(hematemesis).* The amount of bleeding varies from a minute quantity that is undetectable except by testing *(occult blood)* to large quantities that cause stools to be bright red to tarry black *(melena).* The stool color is affected by (1) the digestive processes acting on the blood and (2) the rapidity with which chyme passes through the bowel. For instance, slow bleeding from the duodenum may not increase peristalsis and may produce a tarry stool. If the rate of bleeding or peristalsis increases, subsequent stools may become brighter red. Bleeding may be caused by trauma, ulceration, inflammation, or a mass that erodes through the wall of a blood vessel. Gastrointestinal bleeding is divided into upper and lower GI with the ligament of Treitz in the upper duodenum being the anatomic dividing line. Bleeding may be *acute,* with hematemesis, melena, or hematochezia, or *chronic,* presenting as guaiac-positive stool or iron deficiency anemia. The stool color and presentation is determined by the rapidity with which the stool passes through the intestine and the location of the source of bleeding

---

evolve Web Enhancements

Client Education Guide   Ostomy Supplies (English Version and Spanish Translation)

Colostomy Irrigation (English Version and Spanish Translation)

Ethical Issues in Nursing   Short-Staffing

Management and Delegation   Application and Care of Rectal Pouches and Rectal Tubes

Be sure to check out the bonus material on the Evolve website and the CD-ROM, including free self-assessment exercises. **http://evolve.elsevier. com/Black/medsurg**

within the bowel. For instance, a source of bleeding located in the small intestine or ascending colon will present with darker color of "old blood" than a source in the descending or rectal area, which will present as brighter red, frank blood.

Pain

Pain may be acute or chronic, and is mediated by the autonomic nervous system. Mechanical, inflammatory, or ischemic changes cause pain by stimulating the nerve endings in the muscular or submucosal layers of bowel wall. Mechanical factors cause pain by stretching and distending the bowel; these actions then activate nerve endings. For example, edema, vascular congestion, and bloating cause painful stretching. Biochemical mediators that are released during the inflammatory process cause pain by stimulating nerve endings.

Obstruction of blood supply to the intestine *(ischemia)* may also cause pain. Acute or partial occlusion of the mesenteric artery causes intermittent pain during digestion because of the greater need for blood at that time. Occlusion can occur in the major artery or in one of the smaller branches.

Abdominal pain occurs in varying degrees and may be localized or difficult for the client to pinpoint. It is characterized by onset, duration, radiation, and character. There are four characterizations:

Visceral pain arises from a stimulus acting on the involved portion of the bowel. It results in a diffuse, poorly localized pain that clients describe as gnawing, burning, or cramping. The cause may be chemical irritation, mechanical stimulation, contraction against resistance, or sudden distention.

Somatic pain arises from irritation of the parietal peritoneum. It is more localized sharp pain, resulting in abdominal tenderness and rigidity on palpation.

Referred pain is visceral pain that is felt at a distance from the affected organ.

Rebound pain is visceral pain that is felt on *release* of pressure when palpating the client's abdomen.

Nausea and Vomiting

In intestinal disorders, nausea results from distention of the duodenum. Vomiting occurs from changes in the integrity of the intestinal wall (as in gastroenteritis) or from changes in the motility of the bowel (such as caused by an obstruction). Vomitus that contains fecal matter usually indicates a distal obstruction in the small intestine.

Distention

Distention is caused by excessive gas or trapped gas in the intestines. It may be due to the inability to digest adequately a specific nutrient (such as lactose), it may result from a defect in intestinal motility, or it may be caused by complete obstruction of the intestine. *Flatus* (passing of bowel gas) in excess may be another clinical manifestation.

Diarrhea

Diarrhea is defined as an increase in the frequency, volume, and fluid content of stool. Rapid propulsion of intestinal contents through the small bowel results in diarrhea and may lead to a serious fluid volume deficit. Common causes are infections, malabsorption syndromes, medications, allergies, and systemic diseases.

Constipation

Constipation is the infrequent or difficult passage of stools or the passage of hard or pellet stools. It is a common manifestation that can be caused by inadequate fluid or bulk, mechanical blockage of the passage of intestinal contents (by a tumor), or slow peristalsis.

Abnormalities in Fecal Content

The presence of fats or other abnormal constituents, normally absorbed from the stool, indicates malabsorption. Other fecal abnormalities that can aid in diagnosis are bacteria, parasites, pus, blood, and abnormal quantities of mucus from the colon.

INFLAMMATORY DISORDERS

Inflammation can occur in any portion of the bowel and can be caused by organisms, toxins produced by organisms, infiltration of the bowel wall by granulomatous processes, trauma, medications, and injury from radiation.

VIRAL AND BACTERIAL INFECTIONS: GASTROENTERITIS

Gastroenteritis is an inflammation of the stomach and intestinal tract that primarily affects the small bowel. The major clinical manifestations are diarrhea of varying degrees and abdominal pain and cramping. Associated clinical manifestations are nausea, vomiting, fever, anorexia, distention, *tenesmus* (straining on defecation), and *borborygmi* (hyperactive bowel sounds).

Gastroenteritis occurs throughout the world, often in epidemic outbreaks. Contaminated food and water are major sources of these diseases and cause thousands of deaths yearly. The incidence of infections caused by food-borne diseases is rising. These diseases cost society billions of dollars each year. According to the Centers for Disease Control and Prevention (CDC), 33,000,000 cases of food-borne diseases occur annually in the

United States, about 1 of every 10 Americans; about 9000 die. *Salmonella* and related strains cause an estimated 4 million cases of food-borne illnesses each year, and *Campylobacter* causes an estimated 2 million illnesses each year. Another bacterium, *Escherichia coli* 0157:H7, causes an estimated 30,000 infections and 250 deaths annually.

Infection with *Clostridium difficile (C. difficile),* also known as pseudomembranous colitis, is a bacterial dysentery commonly seen in clients who have been receiving large doses of antibiotics or who have taken antibiotics for longer than 7 days. Other medications that may predispose individuals to *C. difficile* are H2 blockers, preoperative bowel preparations, and chemotherapy. *C. difficile* occurs most often in clients 65 years of age and older, in immunocompromised clients, in clients with chronic lung disease or chronic renal failure, in clients undergoing GI procedures, and in clients who use enemas, stool softeners, and GI stimulants. It is also more common in clients who undergo prolonged hospital stays, especially in intensive care units (ICUs), in clients transferred from small hospitals to tertiary care centers, and in clients placed in semiprivate rooms or wards. The condition is the most common cause of nosocomial infections in hospitalized clients, especially those undergoing surgical procedures.

Traveler's diarrhea primarily occurs in clients who are visiting developing countries whose sewer systems are inadequate. High-risk areas include India, Mexico, Africa, Southeast Asia, and portions of Latin America and the Middle East. Traveler's diarrhea is acquired through consumption of contaminated food or drink (tap water, ice, uncooked vegetables and salad, and unpeeled fruit). The pathogens most commonly isolated are *Campylobacter, E. coli,* and *Shigella.* Less common are *Salmonella, Aeromonas,* and *Vibrio.*

Etiology and Risk Factors

Pathogens that cause GI disease are transmitted by the fecal-oral route, from person to person, and through ingestion of fecally contaminated food and water. GI infections are often referred to as "food poisoning" because food is frequently the vehicle for transmission of actively growing microbes or their toxins. Common bacterial sources of contaminated foods are eggs *(Salmonella),* fresh greens and raw or undercooked meat *(E. coli),* and chicken *(Campylobacter jejuni).* Outbreaks of food-borne viral infections are almost entirely caused by fecally contaminated shellfish. Unpasteurized milk, apple juice, ice cream, and mayonnaise are also sources of food-borne infection. Other causative organisms are *Vibrio cholerae* (cholera), *Shigella* bacilli (dysentery), *Staphylococcus aureus* (staphylococcal food poisoning), and *Listeria.* The incubation period for all viral and bacterial infections ranges from 6 hours to 4 or 5 days.

Also see the Food Borne Poisoning Table on the website for Chapter 28.

Health promotion actions for avoiding such GI infections involve (1) instructing clients about good handwashing technique after defecation and before handling food and (2) obtaining available vaccinations against bacterial and viral gastroenteritis. Encourage cleanliness and sanitation as well as proper food handling, preparation, and storage techniques, such as cooking meats to 150° F, cooking chicken to 170° F, and not allowing food to sit at room temperature for long periods. Warn clients not to eat food containing raw eggs and to refrain from buying cans, boxes, or jars that are damaged. Advise clients to avoid the use of antibiotics over a long time. Teach travelers going to developing countries about safe food practices, such as avoiding tap water, ice cubes, milk products, raw meat or seafood, salads, and foods that cannot be cooked or peeled.

Health maintenance activities include the assessment of clients who are receiving high or continued doses of antibiotics for manifestations of *C. difficile* infection and other manifestations of GI infection secondary to antibiotic use. Health restoration interventions involve client self-management of manifestations. Instruct clients to follow their medication regimen and to call their health care provider if (1) manifestations continue for several days, (2) they might be dehydrated, or (3) body temperature is higher than 100° F. Promote bowel rest and replacement of fluids and electrolytes as needed.

Pathophysiology

Normally, human intestinal flora protects the bowel from colonization of pathogens; however, the intestinal flora can be (1) disrupted by harmful bacteria and viruses that cause tissue damage and inflammation or (2) depressed by antibiotic therapy, administered either orally or parenterally. Antibiotics most often implicated in the depression of normal flora are clindamycin, penicillins, cephalosporins, and aminoglycosides.

Pathogens cause tissue damage and inflammation by releasing endotoxins that stimulate the mucosal lining of the intestine, resulting in greater secretion of water and electrolytes into the intestinal lumen. The active secretion of chloride and bicarbonate ions in the small bowel leads to inhibition of sodium reabsorption. To balance the excess sodium, large amounts of protein-rich fluids are secreted into the bowel, overwhelming the large bowel's ability to reabsorb the fluid and leading to diarrhea. Pathogens also cause damage and inflammation by invading and destroying the mucosal lining of the bowel, resulting in bleeding and ulceration. When the integrity of the GI tract is impaired, its ability to carry out digestive and absorptive functions can be affected. Figure 33-1 illustrates the pathophysiology of *C. difficile*–associated diarrhea (CDAD).

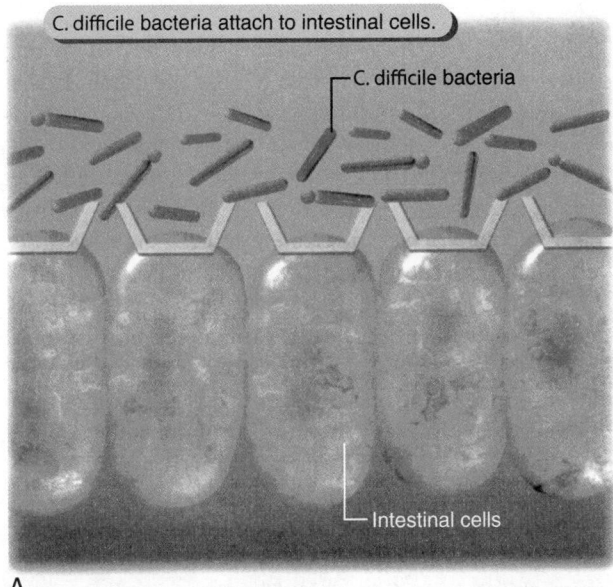

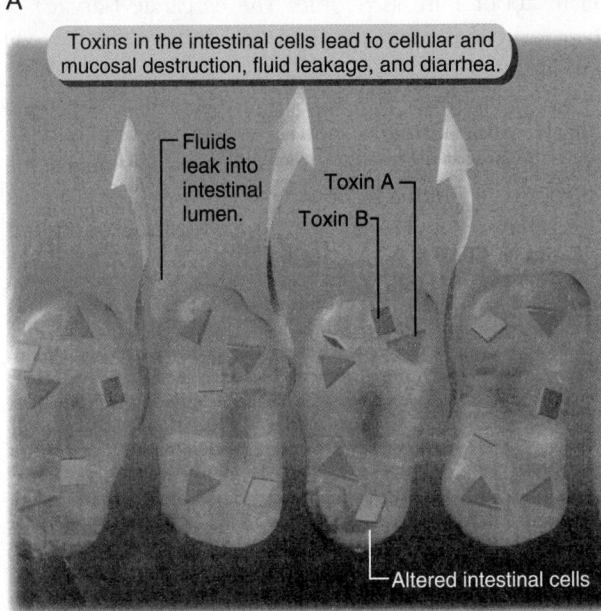

■ **FIGURE 33–1** How *Clostridium difficile*–associated diarrhea (CDAD) develops. **A,** *C. difficile* bacteria attach to intestinal lining and begin to secrete toxins A and B. **B,** Toxin A, an enterotoxin, causes hemorrhaging and fluid leakage into the gut. Toxin B, a potent cytotoxin, decreases cellular protein synthesis. A third substance secreted by toxins A and B inhibits gut motility. *(From Sheff, B. [1999]. Minimizing the threat of* C. difficile. *Nursing, 99, 33-39.)*

Clinical Manifestations

The universal manifestation of gastroenteritis is diarrhea, which occurs in varying intensity, depending on the organism involved and the health status of the individual client. The diarrhea may be mild (two to three stools per day) or intense (more than 10 watery stools per day). Nausea, vomiting, and anorexia may occur from abdominal distention caused by increased fluid content and undigested food. Abdominal pain, cramping, and

borborygmi may occur from gas released from undigested food, irritation of bowel mucosa, and distention of the intestines. The client may have a fever, depending on the causative organism. The stool may test positive for leukocytes and may contain the causative organism as well as mucus and varying amounts of blood.

The gold standard for *C. difficile* is the cytoxan neutralization test that confirms the presence of toxins in the stool. Other stool tests for confirming the diagnosis of *C. difficile* are the latex agglutination test, which is less sensitive than the previous test, and the newest test, enzyme-linked immunosorbent assay (ELISA), which is rapid and reliable. An endoscopic examination will reveal a bowel mucosa that is inflamed, edematous, and containing numerous plaques. Diagnosis can be confirmed by biopsy of the intestine (Figure 33-2).

Prognosis

Most cases of gastroenteritis are temporarily disabling and self-limiting, with resolution in 1 to 5 days; however, gastroenteritis can be fatal in debilitated, older, or very young people. Early detection and treatment with fluids and electrolytes are critical to prevent death or disability in such cases. Up to 16% of clients infected with *E. coli* 0157:H7 develop hemolytic uremic syndrome (HUS), which causes death in 3% to 5% of the people it affects. Of the clients who survive HUS, 10% to 50% develop chronic sequelae that include chronic renal failure, cardiomyopathy, pulmonary problems, chronic hypertension, and encephalopathy. HUS is the major cause of renal failure in children.

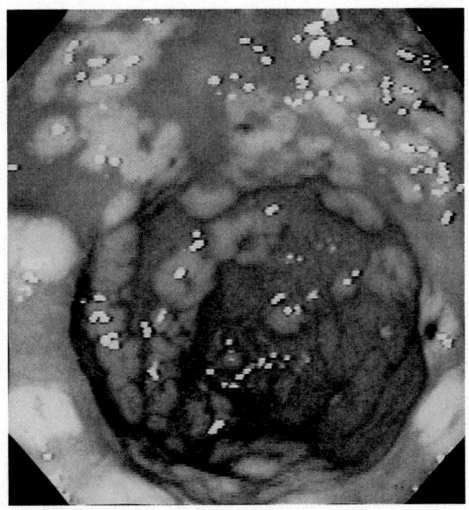

■ **FIGURE 33–2** Colonoscopy findings in *Clostridium difficile* colitis. Note the multiple yellow coalescent plaques throughout the rectum. In some areas around the yellow plaques, edema is present, manifested by loss of the normal vascular pattern. In other areas, the vascular pattern is preserved. *(From Feldman, M., Friedman, L., & Sleisenger, M. [2002]. Sleisenger & Fordtran's gastrointestinal and liver disease: Pathophysiology/diagnosis/management [7th ed., p. 1916]. Philadelphia: Saunders.)*

PARASITIC INFECTIONS

More than two million cases of parasitic illnesses are recorded annually in the United States. An increasing number of people in the United States are being exposed to parasitic diseases because of increased international travel, international food trade, and consumption of raw and undercooked foods. Currently more than 100 parasites are known to cause food-borne disease, and many have only recently been identified.

Protozoa

Protozoa organisms are parasites that replicate in the intestines of infected hosts and are excreted in the feces. They are transmitted in the same way as bacterial and viral pathogens; however, fewer numbers or organisms are needed to produce clinical manifestations. Enteric protozoa are the leading cause of water-borne disease and are becoming more frequently implicated as causes of food-borne infections. Several new protozoa have been identified, for example, *Cyclospora,* which has been linked to contaminated raspberries. Some protozoa are becoming resistant to methods used to eliminate them, such as chlorination.

Giardiasis, the most common protozoal diarrheal illness in the United States, is caused by the protozoan *Giardia lamblia.* It generally spreads through spoiled food or surfaces contaminated with feces from infected animals or humans. It can also be spread by swallowing contaminated recreational water found in swimming pools, hot tubs, Jacuzzis, and lakes. Most infected people are asymptomatic; however, those with manifestations may present several weeks after exposure with nausea, vomiting, excessive foul flatulence, and malabsorption, which results in weight loss and copious, foul-smelling, greasy stools. Organisms infect the small intestine mucosa and submucosa and are found in the stool. The medications used for treatment include metronidazole (Flagyl), quinacrine (Atabrine), and furazolidone (Furoxone). A new vaccine may be available in the near future; however, at present no agent is effective in preventing giardiasis.

Cryptosporidium is associated with water-borne and food-borne outbreaks in nursing homes and day care centers. It is spread by drinking contaminated water or swimming in infected lakes or swimming pools. The organism attaches itself to the intestinal epithelium, causing surface damage, inflammation, and watery diarrhea.

Amebiasis produces diarrhea when a protozoan *(Entamoeba histolytica)* invades the lining of the colon. Manifestations include rectal inflammation as well as blood, pus, and amebae in the stool. Metronidazole (Flagyl) is the drug of choice for treatment.

Helminths

The intestinal tract may be infested with any of several species of helminths or parasitic worms, including *Ascaris* (roundworms), *Enterobius* (pinworms), *Trichinella spiralis* (which causes trichinosis), and various species of *Cestoda* (tapeworms). These parasites are found worldwide. Worm infestations, contracted through the skin or from ingesting contaminated food or water, can cause serious, even fatal disease if the parasites are not eradicated from the intestinal tract. Worms also may cause urinary tract infections or pruritus ani. Fortunately, most of these parasites are susceptible to medications such as mebendazole and pyrantel pamoate. Piperazine and quinacrine hydrochloride also may be used, but they have more side effects. Treatment of all household members may reduce reinfection.

Schistosomiasis is caused by a blood fluke (a parasitic flatworm). The infection is prevalent worldwide, occurring in about 1 in 30 people. The cercariae (larvae) of the parasite penetrate the skin, migrate to the liver via the lungs, and remain in intrahepatic portal venules until the worm matures. The mature worm, which does not multiply within humans, then moves into its final habitat. Depending on the species involved, the worm may settle in the veins of the large bowel, small bowel, or bladder, where it lays eggs. These eggs, which form pseudotubercles (small, knobby prominences), have been found in every system of the body. Schistosomiasis may have mild or severe manifestations, depending on the species of worms involved and the number present. Laboratory studies to identify the species are completed before pharmacologic treatment with oxamniquine, metrifonate, praziquantel, or niridazole is started.

OUTCOME MANAGEMENT

Medical Management

Treatment for food-borne illnesses is usually supportive as most infections are self-limiting. Most infected clients do not benefit from antibiotics. An exception to this is traveler's diarrhea that is usually caused by *E. coli,* rotavirus, or *Salmonella.* Treatment with a fluoroquinolone has proven to be effective.

Rest the Bowel

Rest, with nothing by mouth (NPO [from the Latin *nil per os*]) until the vomiting has stopped, is the best intervention.

Decrease Diarrhea

When diarrhea is severe and does not resolve within 2 to 3 days, the infecting organism needs to be identified from stool specimens and blood samples. Medications to decrease intestinal motility are usually not administered because the infecting agents need to be eliminated, particularly *C. difficile* infection, because the bacteria multiply if GI motility is slowed and the bacteria are retained. For severe cases of *C. difficile* infection, the client receives metronidazole and vancomycin orally or intravenously.

Restore Fluids and Electrolytes

The client is started on small amounts of clear liquids as tolerated. An electrolyte replacement beverage may be given. The diet is advanced after 24 hours as tolerated. If the client becomes dehydrated because of severe fluid depletion, an intravenous fluid such as normal saline may be administered. A potassium supplement may be ordered if the client's serum potassium level is low.

Nursing Management of the Medical Client

Most clients present with an acute onset of diarrhea. Carefully note a description of the diarrhea, including (1) onset; (2) number, color, and consistency of stools; and (3) accompanying manifestations, such as nausea and vomiting. Ask the client about recent foreign travel and antibiotic use. Obtain a diet history that includes all foods the client has eaten in the past 5 days. Ask especially about foods known to be at high risk for causing infection.

Assess the client's abdomen. Examination may reveal hyperactive bowel sounds, distention, and tenderness. Dehydration and electrolyte imbalance may be present, depending on the amount of fluids and electrolytes lost. Assess muscle weakness and fatigue that are caused by hypokalemia. Metabolic alkalosis from bicarbonate loss (manifested in part by hypochloremia and hypokalemia) is also a potential problem. Carefully examine all stools for blood and mucus, and record intake and output. Examine the client's anal area for irritation. After cleaning the area, apply a protective moisture barrier product for clients with irritation. Be especially cautious in caring for a client with a colostomy or ileostomy.

Administer anti-infective medications, such as antibiotic and antiparasitic agents, to treat the specific cause of the diarrhea if appropriate. Antidiarrheals may be ordered if the diarrhea is uncontrollable. If manifestations of fluid and electrolyte imbalance are noted, start IV fluids until oral fluids are tolerated. Begin clear liquids with electrolytes in small amounts until the client can tolerate toast and crackers. Advance the diet as tolerated.

Prevent spread of the disease to others. Remind the client to wash hands and maintain absolute cleanliness. If the client is hospitalized, transfer the client to a private room and initiate contact isolation precautions. Follow the facility's protocol. Spores from *C. difficile* live for months on environmental surfaces, for example, toilets, bedpans, and floors. **Therefore ensure meticulous cleaning of the environment and use dedicated equipment when possible. Follow the facility's guidelines for the disposal of contaminated equipment. Never use an electronic rectal thermometer because of the potential for spreading bacteria. Provide written and oral instructions regarding medications, diet, and rest as well as about when and how to report any continued problems. Teach family and visitors about precautions and how to follow procedures. Ensure them that their chance of becoming infected is remote.**

Relapses and reinfection are common. Therefore the client should be closely monitored for any clinical manifestations of recurring disease.

APPENDICITIS

Appendicitis is an inflammation of the vermiform appendix that develops most commonly in adolescents and young adults (Figure 33-3). It can occur at any age but is rare in clients younger than 2 years and reaches a peak incidence in clients between 20 and 30 years. It is not common in older adults; however, when it does occur in such clients, rupture of the appendix is more common. Appendicitis affects 7% to 12% of the population.

Etiology and Risk Factors

Appendicitis can be caused by the following:

- A fecalith (a fecal calculus, or stone) that occludes the lumen of the appendix
- Kinking of the appendix
- Swelling of the bowel wall
- Fibrous conditions in the bowel wall
- External occlusion of the bowel by adhesions
- Infection with *Yersinia* organisms has been found in up to 30% of cases

No particular risk factors for appendicitis have been identified. Because it is not preventable, early detection of the condition is important.

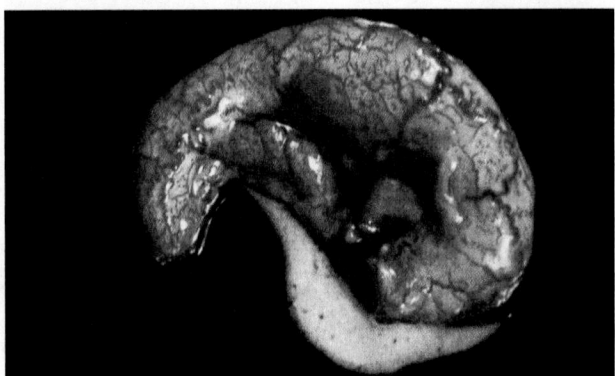

■ **FIGURE 33–3** Appendicitis. This appendix is inflamed and distended with yellowish pus. *(From Price, S.A., & Wilson, L.M. [2003]. Pathophysiology: Clinical concepts of disease process [6th ed.]. St. Louis: Mosby. Courtesy of Gerald D. Abrams, MD, Department of Pathology, University of Michigan—Ann Arbor.)*

Pathophysiology

When the appendix becomes obstructed, the intraluminal pressure increases, leading to decreased venous drainage, thrombosis, edema, and bacterial invasion of the lumina. Arterial compromise occurs, with necrosis and invasion of the bowel wall. If the process develops slowly, the infection may be walled off by the adjacent structures, forming an abscess. Rapid progression of vascular impairment may lead to rupture and fistula formation between the appendix and adjacent structures (bladder, small intestine, sigmoid, or cecum).

Clinical Manifestations

The classic manifestations of appendicitis begin with acute abdominal pain that comes in waves *(visceral)*. At first, the pain may be perceived merely as discomfort that makes the client feel that passing flatus or having a bowel movement will bring relief. Unfortunately, many clients take a laxative during this period, which may lead to rupture of the appendix and peritonitis.

The pain typically starts in the epigastrium or periumbilical region. It then shifts to the right lower quadrant as the inflammatory process spreads to involve the parietal peritoneal surface, thereby bringing the inflammatory process into contact with the peritoneum. The pain becomes more severe and steady rather than intermittent; the client often *guards* or protects the area by lying still and drawing the legs up to relieve tension on the abdominal muscles.

Assessment also may reveal vomiting that begins after the pain starts, anorexia, low-grade fever, coated tongue, and halitosis (fetid breath). Mild leukocytosis is usually present, with the white blood cell (WBC) count between 10,000 and 18,000/mm^3. Diagnosis is confirmed with tenderness at McBurney's point, which lies midway between the right anterior superior iliac crest and the umbilicus, or any location that corresponds to the location of the appendix. Abdominal radiography is usually not of value in diagnosis of appendicitis.

OUTCOME MANAGEMENT

Surgical Management

Appendectomy

There is no medical treatment for appendicitis. Preoperatively, IV fluids and antibiotics are administered. Pain medication is withheld until the diagnosis is confirmed.

Indications. Surgical intervention involves removal of the appendix *(appendectomy)* within 24 to 48 hours of onset of the manifestations. The surgery can be performed through a small open incision or a laparoscope (a lighted scope used to visualize and remove the appendix). When the operation is performed in time the mortality rate is less than 0.5%. Delay usually cause rupture of the organ and resultant peritonitis (se Peritonitis).

Complications. Perforation of the bowel is the mos common complication. Antibiotics and surgical drainage are required if perforation occurs. Peritonitis ma develop after perforation.

Outcomes. Following a laparoscopic procedure, the cli ent is usually discharged in 24 to 48 hours. Another da of hospitalization may be indicated after an open surgi cal procedure. Lifting is restricted for 2 to 4 weeks. The client can resume all activities 4 to 6 weeks after surgery

---

Nursing Management of the Surgical Client

Assessment. The client is usually admitted with sever abdominal pain. Carefully assess the pain, especially to determine its location. Also assess the client for reboun tenderness (sharp pain when pressure is released o abdomen after deep palpation) and the presence of peri tonitis (see Peritonitis). Carefully assess the client's vita signs, fluid and electrolyte status, and laboratory data The client with appendicitis should fast preoperatively.

Diagnosis, Outcomes, Interventions
Diagnosis: Acute Pain. One of the most appropriate nursing diagnoses for the client with acute appendiciti is *Acute Pain related to inflammation.*

Outcomes. The client describes decreased postoperative pain.

Interventions

> An abrupt change in the character of the pain preoperatively may indicate perforation. Postoperatively, pain control, as described in Chapters 14 and 20, should be practiced. Sometimes pain medication is not given until the client is actually ready for surgery. Never give an enema or a laxative or apply heat to the abdomen of the client with appendicitis because any one of these actions may lead to bowel perforation.

Diagnosis: Risk for Deficient Fluid Volume. Another appro priate nursing diagnosis for the client with acute appen dicitis is *Risk for Deficient Fluid Volume related to vomiting.*

Outcomes. The client maintains fluid and electrolyte bal ance, as evidenced by balanced intake and output and electrolyte levels within normal limits.

Interventions. As soon as the client is admitted, IV fluids are started to maintain fluid balance, with electrolytes added as needed. If the client is vomiting, a nasogastric

(NG) tube may be inserted. Carefully measure intake and output.

Diagnosis: Risk for Infection. The diagnosis *Risk for Infection related to rupture of appendix* is common.

Outcomes. An infection will not develop, or rupture will be diagnosed early, as evidenced by (1) removal of the appendix before rupture or (2) prompt treatment of the rupture.

Interventions. Check the client's vital signs regularly, monitoring closely for an increase in temperature and a change in pulse rate and blood pressure measurements, which may signify a ruptured appendix. Preoperative antibiotics are usually administered to reduce risk of infection. Monitor pain closely. If the pain becomes generalized throughout the abdomen and the abdomen becomes rigid and board-like, the appendix may have ruptured.

After surgery, monitor vital signs, urine output, level of consciousness, and IV therapy; also assess the client's respiratory status and the surgical wound. The client may have a drain, and if the appendix ruptured, packing may be present. Assess the dressings, provide wound care, reposition the client approximately every 2 hours, and adequately manage the client's pain.

The client who has had a ruptured appendix with an infected wound needs to be taught appropriate care of the wound. Wound care usually involves irrigation of the wound with sterile saline and application of a sterile dressing at least three to four times a day. Assess the client's ability to function at home and to care for the wound. A home health care referral should be initiated to assist the client with physical needs and to ensure that the wound is healing properly.

Evaluation. The usual outcome after an uncomplicated appendectomy is healing within a few weeks. If the appendix has ruptured, however, healing takes longer. With a ruptured appendix, healing cannot occur until the infection has cleared and the wound is clean. A secondary closure may be required after the wound is clean. Some incisions are left open to heal through granulation *(regeneration)* of tissue.

PERITONITIS

Peritonitis is inflammation of the peritoneal membrane. The *peritoneum* is a semipermeable two-layered sac filled with about 1500 ml of fluid. This sac covers all the organs in the abdominal cavity. Because it is well supplied with somatic nerves, stimulation of the parietal peritoneum that lines the abdominal and pelvic cavities causes sharp, well-localized pain. The visceral peritoneum is relatively insensitive.

Etiology and Risk Factors

Peritonitis is a localized or generalized inflammatory process that may be acute or chronic. Acute peritonitis is caused by a decrease in the motor activity of the bowel, causing the intestinal lumen to become distended with gas and fluid. Inability of the intestine to reabsorb fluid causes an accumulation in the peritoneal cavity. Bacteria may enter through a perforation in the GI tract, from the external environment, and through the bloodstream. Normal flora of the intestine become a source of infection when they enter the sterile peritoneal cavity. The most common organism is *E. coli,* although streptococci, staphylococci, and pneumococci also may be involved. The peritoneum may produce a more local reaction by walling off of the inflammatory process. If the stimulus is overwhelming, however (bowel obstruction or perforation), allowing the source of infection to proliferate, an abscess will result.

There are no primary risk factors for peritonitis because the condition is a result of another problem. Causes include ruptured or gangrenous gallbladder, perforated peptic ulcer, perforated stomach or intestine secondary to cancer or inflammatory bowel disorders, bowel obstruction, penetrating wounds, and other conditions (such as acute pancreatitis and mesenteric thrombosis). The major preventive measures are early diagnosis of clients at risk for peritonitis and initiation of early treatment to help prevent spread of the infection.

Pathophysiology

Peritonitis produces severe systemic effects. Circulatory alterations, fluid shifts, and respiratory problems can cause critical fluid and electrolyte imbalances. The inflammatory response shunts (diverts) extra blood to the inflamed area of the bowel to combat the infection. Peristaltic activity of the bowel ceases. Fluids and air are retained within its lumen, raising pressure and increasing fluid secretion into the bowel. Thus circulating blood volume diminishes. The inflammatory process increases oxygen requirements at a time when the client has difficulty ventilating (breathing) because of abdominal pain and increased abdominal pressure, which elevates the diaphragm.

Clinical Manifestations

Manifestations of peritonitis vary according to the cause. Pain may be localized or generalized. Well-localized pain that causes rigidity of abdominal muscles and pain that increases with any pressure or motion of the abdomen are characteristic of peritonitis. Also, the client usually experiences nausea, vomiting, and, possibly, a low-grade fever. Assessment reveals absence of bowel sounds and shallow respirations because the client is trying to avoid the pain caused by body movement.

The client with peritonitis commonly has an elevated WBC count (20,000/mm^3) with a high neutrophil count. Abdominal x-ray studies are performed, which may show dilation and edema of the intestines or free air or fluid in the abdominal cavity. If the client is vomiting, manifestations of imbalanced fluid and electrolyte balance also may be present.

OUTCOME MANAGEMENT

Medical Management

Maintain Fluid and Electrolyte Balance

If peritonitis is advanced and if surgery is contraindicated by shock and circulatory failure, oral fluids are prohibited. IV fluids are necessary for the replacement of electrolyte and protein losses. A nasogastric (NG) tube or a long intestinal tube may be inserted to reduce pressure within the bowel. See Chapter 31 for nursing care of a client with an NG or intestinal tube.

Control Infection

Once the infection has been isolated and the client's condition improves, surgical drainage and repair can be attempted. The other major treatment of peritonitis is IV antibiotic therapy with potent broad-spectrum agents.

Surgical Management

Surgery may be performed to prevent peritonitis, such as an appendectomy for an inflamed appendix or a colon resection (surgical removal) for inflamed diverticulum. If the perforation is not prevented, the major surgical intervention is incision and drainage of the abscess once it is walled off.

Nursing Management of the Surgical Client

Preoperatively, obtain a thorough history, including specific information about the client's pain. Assess the abdomen, noting the presence or absence of bowel sounds. Palpate the abdomen, noting whether the abdomen is firm, distended, or rigid. Note areas of rebound tenderness.

Clients with peritonitis are acutely ill and are given broad-spectrum antibiotics immediately. The perforated organs are usually repaired as soon as the client is stable enough to withstand the stress of surgery. During surgery, any leakage can be sampled for culture so that specific antibiotic therapy can be implemented. The peritoneal cavity is irrigated with an antibiotic solution to reduce the bacterial count. Often the wound is packed open or drains are placed so that infection can be treated.

Postoperatively, carefully monitor clients for the development of postoperative complications, such as acute respiratory distress syndrome (ARDS), sepsis, and shock. Closely monitor the client's fluid balance by assessing vital signs, bowel sounds, urine output, skin turgor, mucous membranes, and weight. Immediately report any manifestations of sepsis, such as a drop or rise in temperature or a drop in blood pressure. IV fluids are administered along with antibiotic therapy.

On discharge, provide the client with oral or written instructions regarding wound care, medications, activity restrictions, and follow-up visits.

INFLAMMATORY BOWEL DISEASE

Inflammatory bowel disease (IBD) consists of two chronic inflammatory disorders: Crohn's disease (regional enteritis) and ulcerative colitis. The incidence rate of ulcerative colitis (UC) is about 11 per 100,000 and that of Crohn's disease is 7 per 100,000. The United States, United Kingdom, Sweden, and Norway have the highest rates in the world. Each year, 30,000 people learn that they have a moderate to severe form of IBD. It is estimated that IBD costs between $2 and $3 billion annually in lost wages and disability and health care payments.

These chronic, recurrent diseases can occur in people at any age but peak onset is in young adults between 15 and 30 years of age. A definitive diagnosis is hard to make because the manifestations mimic other conditions and because there may be long periods of remission. There is no known cure. Treatment is symptomatic. Responses are often unpredictable and clients with IBD frequently require surgery to remove diseased sections of the bowel and to repair holes in the intestine. Because of the similarities between Crohn's disease and ulcerative colitis, the two conditions are compared throughout the following discussion.

Etiology and Risk Factors

The cause of IBD remains unclear, but it probably involves a combination of genetic predisposition, environmental conditions, and defects in immune regulation. Chromosome 16 recently was strongly linked to Crohn's disease, but not ulcerative colitis. No specific dietary factor has been linked in studies to IBD. Some believe that the disease is of bacterial origin because many clients have a history of bacterial infection before the onset of the condition. It is believed that any one of these factors weakens the intestinal wall, allowing it to become more susceptible to inflammation and tissue breakdown when in contact with disease-producing organisms. Other theories suggest that destructive enzymes and a lack of protective substances in the bowel wall cause the inflammatory process. An emotional disturbance can precipitate an exacerbation or prolong an attack, but it is not the primary cause.

The only risk factors identified for IBD are genetic. Genetic studies have uncovered a link between Crohn's disease and variants of the *CARD15* (also known as *NOD2*) gene on chromosome 16q. Recently, the interleukin-23 receptor gene (*IL-23R*) on chromosome 1p31 has been found to have a large effect on IBD as well as other inflammatory disorders such as rheumatoid arthritis, multiple sclerosis, and psoriasis. These findings will be used to drive future treatment modalities.

IBD is reported to be 4-fold higher among the Ashkenazi Jewish population of Europe. IBD runs in families. The lifetime risk for the first-degree relative of a client with IBD is approximately 10%. If both parents have IBD, each child will have a 36% chance of being affected. Relatives of clients with IBD are more likely to experience IBD than the general population. A 20-fold to 50-fold increase in occurrence among siblings and a 50-fold to 100-fold increase in children have been noted in families of clients with IBD. There are no preventive measures.

Crohn's Disease

Crohn's disease (CD) is a chronic relapsing disease that can develop segmentally (without sequence and skipping sections) in the alimentary tract. The most common locations are the terminal ileum and colon although any part of the gastrointestinal tract may be affected. Unlike ulcerative colitis, the rectum is frequently not involved. Crohn's disease more characteristically involves the entire thickness of the bowel wall *(transmural)*, particularly the submucosa. Perirectal fistulae, fissures, abscesses, and anal stenosis are present in 33% of clients with CD. The liver and pancreas may also be affected. The mortality rate is not high, but recurrences and complications can result in disability. The client feels well between attacks; however, each bout leaves the intestine more scarred and less able to absorb nutrients.

Ulcerative Colitis

Ulcerative colitis is a disease that spans the entire length of the colon and involves only the mucosa and submucosa of the large intestine. The disease usually starts in the rectum and distal colon, spreading upward beyond the rectosigmoid valve to involve most of the sigmoid and descending colon. The disease extends in a contiguous manner with distinct demarcations between normal and unhealthy areas. Ulcerative colitis causes inflammation, thickening, congestion, edema, and blood

loss through minute lacerations that eventually develop into abscesses. The edema can lead to extreme friability of the mucosa, and bleeding and perforation can thus occur from any minor trauma. It occurs at all ages, but the incidence is higher among young adults, women, and Jews.

Pathophysiology
Crohn's Disease

Lesions typically develop in several separated segments of bowel. They are visible on gross examination (without aid of a microscope), and their color differs dramatically from that of normal tissue (Figure 33-4). Examination of the bowel tissue by endoscopy reveals edematous, heavy, reddish purple areas. Granular spots also may be present. Enlarged lymph nodes appear in the submucosa, and Peyer's patches are seen in the intestinal mucous membrane. These areas undergo small superficial ulcerations with granulomas and fissures. Fissures may completely penetrate the bowel wall, leading to fistulae and abscesses. Fistulae, in turn, release toxic substances from the intestine into the bloodstream, the abdominal cavity, and other organs. Collections of lymphocytes throughout the mucosa, submucosa, and serosa are the only microscopic features of Crohn's disease. The small bowel wall becomes congested and thickened, narrowing the lumen.

Extraintestinal complications include malabsorption, kidney stones, hydronephrosis, stomatitis, peripheral arthritis, and pyoderma gangrenosum, an inflammatory, ulcerative condition of the skin. Gallstones occur in 13% to 34% of clients. Anorectal problems include internal fistulae and abscesses. Anal fissure (see later discussion) is common and is directly related to the severity of the diarrhea, which produces ulceration of the

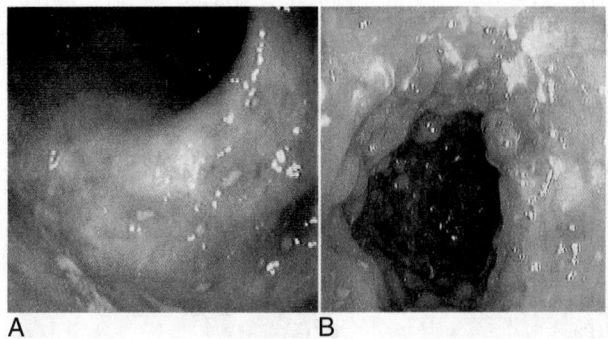

A   B

■ **FIGURE 33–4** Endoscopic appearance of Crohn's disease. **A,** Typical aphthous ulcers consisting of a central white depression surrounded by a slightly elevated, erythematous rim only a few millimeters in diameter. **B,** Findings more typical of advanced disease, with erythema, edema, and a cobblestone appearance. *(From Feldman, M., Friedman, L.S., & Sleisenger, M.H. [2002]. Sleisenger & Fordtran's gastrointestinal and liver disease: Pathophysiology/diagnosis/management [7th ed., Vol. 2]. Philadelphia: Saunders.)*

perianal skin. Pain is aggravated by walking, sitting, and defecation.

Ulcerative Colitis

Ulcerative colitis is a disease that spans the entire length of the colon and involves only the mucosa and submucosa of the large intestine. The disease usually starts in the rectum and distal colon, spreading upward beyond the rectosigmoid valve to involve most of the sigmoid and descending colon. The disease extends in a contiguous manner with distinct demarcations between normal and unhealthy areas. Ulcerative colitis causes inflammation, thickening, congestion, edema, and blood loss through minute lacerations that eventually develop into abscesses. The edema can lead to extreme friability of the mucosa, and bleeding and perforation can thus occur from any minor trauma. It occurs at all ages, but the incidence is higher among young adults, women, and Jews.

The appearance of the colon depends on the stage, activity, and severity of the disease (Figure 33-5). The most characteristic lesion of ulcerative colitis is an inflammatory infiltrate called a *crypt abscess*. This abscess consists of polymorphonuclear leukocytes, lymphocytes, red blood cells, and cellular debris appearing at the base of the crypts of Lieberkühn. Secretions from crypt abscesses result in purulent discharge from the bowel mucosa. Abscesses may become necrotic and may ulcerate.

Infections secondary to ulcerative colitis produce further inflammatory reactions in the mucosa and submucosa. When the inflammatory lesions heal, scarring and fibrosis, with narrowing, thickening, and shortening of the colon, and loss of haustral folds, may follow.

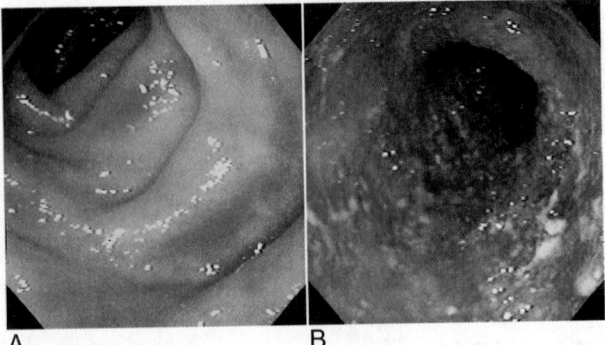

■ **FIGURE 33–5** Spectrum of severity of ulcerative colitis. **A,** Colonoscopy in mild ulcerative colitis demonstrated by edema, loss of vascularity, and patchy subepithelial hemorrhage. **B,** Colonoscopy in severe ulcerative colitis with loss of vascularity, hemorrhage, and mucopus. *(From Feldman, M., Friedman, L.S., & Sleisenger, M.H. [2002]. Sleisenger & Fordtran's gastrointestinal and liver disease: Pathophysiology/diagnosis/management [7th ed., Vol. 2]. Philadelphia: Saunders.)*

Cancer of the colon is more common among clients with ulcerative colitis than in the general population. The incidence is greatly increased when ulcerative colitis develops before the client is 16 years of age and in clients who have had the condition for more than 20 years.

Toxic megacolon is an extreme dilation of a segment of the diseased colon (often the transverse segment) that results in complete obstruction. Toxic megacolon usually occurs during an acute exacerbation of ulcerative colitis, and it may follow hypokalemia, a barium enema, or the use of anticholinergics, opioids, corticosteroids, or antibiotics. Bacterial overgrowth contributes to this complication. Perforation and peritonitis may complicate the condition.

Clinical Manifestations

Crohn's disease and ulcerative colitis produce similar manifestations. Clients suffer from abdominal pain, diarrhea, fluid imbalances, and weight loss. Severe diarrhea or vomiting may cause metabolic acidosis. Remissions are followed by exacerbations of acute disease. When the disease is acute, the client has a fever. The general appearance of clients with IBD varies from reasonably healthy to wasted, drawn, and malnourished, with varying degrees of pallor. Clients usually report a steady and progressive weight loss. Inspection reveals a flat or concave shape to the abdomen, with visible peristaltic activity. Palpation of the abdomen reveals tenderness over the area of inflamed bowel. Increased bowel sounds are heard on auscultation. Hemorrhoids and, in Crohn's disease, perianal abscesses, fistulae, and ulcers may be apparent.

Hematocrit and hemoglobin values are usually decreased. A barium enema study with air contrast is often performed to differentiate ulcerative colitis from Crohn's disease. The client with suspected IBD routinely undergoes colonoscopy. Biopsy and cytologic studies also help to distinguish among carcinoma, ulcerative colitis, and Crohn's disease.

Crohn's Disease

Diarrhea in Crohn's disease is usually less severe than that in ulcerative colitis. Stool consistency is typically soft or semiliquid. Urgency to expel stools may awaken the person at night. The client rarely passes gross blood unless ulceration is present. Malabsorption, associated with steatorrhea, may develop. If so, stools may be foul-smelling and fatty.

The client with severe steatorrhea, diarrhea, or longstanding enteritis may have associated nutritional deficits, weight loss, anorexia, pain, anemia, debility, fatigue, and metabolic disturbances. Nutritional deficits arise from (1) a reduction in the intestinal absorptive surface; (2) malabsorption of protein and carbohydrates;

and (3) impaired absorption of fat, folic acid, iron, calcium, and vitamins A, B$_{12}$, C, D, E, and K. Alterations in bile salt and vitamin metabolism may result from surgery or mucosal defects. Metabolic requirements increase because of the inflammatory process and infection, the decrease in food intake, and the loss of nutrients in the feces because of rapid GI transit time. Electrolytes lost from diarrhea include sodium, potassium, chloride, the trace elements (magnesium, zinc, copper), and minerals. Nitrogen excretion remains normal if there is no loss of protein from the inflammatory exudate. The consequences of malnutrition include the following:

- Loss of immunocompetence
- Decreased resistance to infection
- Diminished wound healing
- Reduced pancreatic enzyme output
- Impaired healing (fistulae and surgical wounds)
- Decreased iron-binding capacity resulting from chronic infection or blood loss

Ulcerative Colitis

The predominant manifestation of ulcerative colitis is diarrhea (20 or more stools per day) and passage of blood in the stool. The severity and frequency of diarrhea depend on the extent of involved colon. Severe diarrhea can cause a loss of 500 to 17,000 ml of water in 24 hours. Liquid stools occur with tenesmus and may contain blood, mucus, and pus. A sense of urgency and cramping abdominal pain may occur with the diarrhea. The client typically experiences cramping, pain, and tenderness in the lower left quadrant.

Nausea, vomiting, anorexia, fever, weight loss, and decreased serum potassium concentration may occur with severe disease. In addition, the client loses plasma proteins, prothrombin, and fluids. Anemia may develop with severe blood loss and decreased dietary iron intake.

Physical findings include tenderness in the lower left quadrant, guarding, and (in severe ulcerative colitis) abdominal distention. Following remissions, ulcerative colitis may recur after bouts of emotional stress, dietary indiscretion, or the ingestion of irritants such as laxatives and antibiotics. Physical exertion, respiratory tract infections, and fatigue also may instigate an attack.

Prognosis

Both types of IBD usually follow a chronic, intermittent course with remissions and exacerbations. Disease severity will affect presentation of manifestations as well as management and prognosis. The only known cure for ulcerative colitis is surgical removal of the colon. Surgical procedures and medication therapy can control the manifestations in Crohn's disease, but currently there is no known cure.

OUTCOME MANAGEMENT

Medical Management

Decrease Diarrhea

Medical treatments, which aim primarily to control the manifestations, are similar for ulcerative colitis and Crohn's disease. Because the inflammatory process in Crohn's disease involves deeper layers of the bowel wall and is more chronic, healing may occur more slowly than in ulcerative colitis. Thus anti-inflammatory therapy, including steroids, is required for longer periods in Crohn's disease than in ulcerative colitis.

Fluids, electrolytes, and blood are replaced as needed to maintain the client's homeostasis. Physical activity should be kept to a minimum during an acute attack to decrease intestinal motility. The client with a mild attack can work but will need extra rest. The client with fever, toxemia, frequent bowel movements, bleeding, or pain requires bed rest. Failure of the inflamed colonic mucosa to reabsorb water and electrolytes, bile salts, and lactose interferes with the control of diarrhea. The extent of large bowel involved by the disease influences the severity of diarrhea. The client should keep a record of the number of stools and their consistency and color as well as the presence or absence of blood.

Bowel rest and parenteral hyperalimentation may result in restored immunocompetence, greater resistance to infection, correction of nutritional deficiencies, and relief of edema and bowel inflammation.

Pharmacologic Agents

Once inflammatory bowel disease has been diagnosed, the client receives pharmacologic agents with the hope of bringing the disease into remission. A variety of pharmacologic agents are used to control diarrhea, reduce inflammation, and treat pain. These agents are summarized in the Integrating Pharmacology feature on p. 690.

Increase Nutritional Intake

Nutritional deficiencies are the most common complications of IBD. These deficits derive from decreased intake, increased losses, greater nutritional requirements, and side effects of certain medications. Diarrhea leads to fluid and electrolyte losses with resultant muscle wasting and edema. Malabsorption resulting from bacterial overgrowth or mucosal involvement of the bowel may cause further problems. Deficiencies of fat-soluble vitamins (A, D, E, and K) and folate may develop. Vitamin K deficiency causes bleeding tendencies.

INTEGRATING PHARMACOLOGY

Medications for Inflammatory Bowel Disease

Inflammatory bowel disease (IBD) cannot be cured with medications. However, medications that target the inflammatory process are usually effective in controlling active IBD in most clients (up to 80%) and sustaining remission for prolonged periods. The primary goal of therapy is to reduce inflammation in the gut. Most health care providers use a stepped approach to therapy in which more potent agents are added to the regimen if less active drugs fail to achieve an adequate response. Combination therapy of the drugs discussed below is frequently used. Periods of exacerbation will require additional or increased dosages of medications while periods of remission will require less. The client is considered to be in remission when the mucosal lining is healed and manifestations such as diarrhea, abdominal cramps, and tenesmus are controlled.

The 5-aminosalicylate-based compounds have remained the mainstays of treatment for clients with mild to moderate active ulcerative colitis and Crohn's disease. These drugs block the production of prostaglandins and leukotrienes to decrease the inflammatory process. Examples include sulfasalazine (Azulfidine), 5-aminosalicylic acid (5-ASA), mesalamine (Asacol, Pentasa, Rowasa), olsalazine (Dipentum), and balsalazide (Colazal). Sulfasalazine is metabolized by intestinal bacteria into 5-ASA and sulfapyridine, a sulfa component that accounts for up to 30% of adverse side effects associated with sulfasalazine (allergic reactions, cramping, diarrhea, dizziness, fever, rash). Mesalamine has fewer side effects than sulfasalazine because of the absence of sulfapyridine when it is metabolized. Mesalamine is also available in delayed-release formulations such as Pentasa and Asacol. Because folate absorption may be impaired, clients should be supplemented with folic acid. Clients who are allergic to aspirin should not take the 5-ASA drugs. Oral formulations should be used for more proximal disease in the small bowel or ileum while suppositories and enemas should be used for distal colonic disease.

Clients whose IBD fails to respond to the salicylates may require glucocorticoid medications. These may be administered orally or rectally as well as intravenously. They should only be taken during exacerbations and have not been shown to be effective as maintenance therapy. Antacids or histamine receptor antagonists should be given during steroid therapy to prevent gastric ulceration. Steroids reduce adrenal function and may impair resistance, causing defective healing of abscesses and fistulae. Steroids do not cure IBD, but they modify its course. Clients should be tapered off steroids as soon as remission is achieved to prevent long-term complications.

A new, nonsystemic steroid, budesonide (Entocort), has been shown to be effective in treating active Crohn's disease, but it is not effective in preventing remissions of the disease. Budesonide has fewer systemic side effects than other steroids and can be administered topically as an enema and orally in a controlled release form.

When salicylates and corticosteroids are not successful, management of the disease with more toxic, secondary-line agents becomes crucial. These immunomodulators include 6-mercaptopurine (6-MP) (Purinethol), methotrexate (Folex), and azathioprine (Imuran). These drugs have many toxic side effects, however, including blood dyscrasias, infection, pancreatitis, and digestive intolerance. Methotrexate is used in Crohn's disease but is not effective for ulcerative colitis. Cyclosporine (Sandimmune) is used in Crohn's disease accompanied by severe fistulae. It alters T-cell response more rapidly than 6-MP or azathioprine but is not beneficial for long-term maintenance therapy as toxicity includes hypertension, tremors, and renal dysfunction. Tacrolimus is being studied for short-term treatment of severe disease. Mycophenolate mofetil (CellCept) is under study for Crohn's clients who cannot tolerate azathioprine or mercaptopurine.

Infliximab (Remicade) is a monoclonal antibody that has been extremely effective in treating moderate to severe Crohn's disease by inhibiting tumor necrosis factor (TNF) response. TNF is a natural protein that causes intestinal inflammation. It is the only drug used specifically for Crohn's disease and is given by a single IV infusion that may be repeated every 2 to 3 months. Of active Crohn's disease clients refractory to glucocorticoids, 6-MP, or 5-ASA, 65% will respond to intravenous infliximab. Studies suggest that up to 80% of clients respond initially and about one third of all clients remain in remission after a single infusion.

The newest immune medication used for IBD is natalizumab (Antegren), which attaches to immune cells and stops them from leaving the bloodstream and going to the site of inflammation.

Other medications that may be given during acute exacerbations include anticholinergic and antidiarrheal medications to relieve abdominal cramps and help control diarrhea. Anticholinergic, antidiarrheal, and antispasmodic agents allow the colon to rest. Antibiotics may be used to prevent or control infections and to treat anal fistulae and perianal disease. The sulfonamides and antibiotics such as metronidazole (Flagyl) and ciprofloxacin (Cipro) are the medications of choice.

Diet and Supplements. A diet high in protein and calories is given in an attempt to restore normal nutritional levels but is not always well tolerated. Liquid supplements are residue free, low in fat, and digested mainly in the upper jejunum.

Anemia and vitamin deficiencies should be corrected nutritionally or with supplements. Folate deficiency, which may be due to the therapeutic use of sulfasalazine, may be prevented by (1) increasing dietary intake of folate, (2) having the client take sulfasalazine between meals, or (3) supplementing the intervention regimen with folic acid.

Total Parenteral Nutrition. Total parenteral nutrition (TPN) is indicated when a client has not responded to medical intervention, is being prepared for surgery, or has undergone intestinal resection. TPN provides bowel rest by removing all stimulation of secretion and by decreasing fecal bulk. Weight gain, positive nitrogen balance, and a temporary remission of manifestations can occur. TPN appears to be more useful in Crohn's disease than in ulcerative colitis.

When oral food and fluids are resumed, they should be chemically and mechanically nonirritating and high in calories, protein, and minerals. The client should avoid cocoa, chocolate, citrus juices, cold or carbonated drinks, nuts, seeds, popcorn, and alcohol.

Nursing Management of the Medical Client

Assessment. Assess the client's bowel elimination pattern, noting the number of stools and their color and consistency, and also the presence or absence of blood or steatorrhea. Also assess the client's abdomen. Note bowel sounds and the location of pain. Complete a nutritional assessment, as directed in Chapter 28.

Diagnosis, Outcomes, Interventions
Diagnosis: Diarrhea. Diarrhea is the most common manifestation of IBD, and so the primary nursing diagnosis is *Diarrhea related to inflamed intestinal mucosa.*

Outcomes. The client will experience a decrease in diarrhea, as evidenced by a decrease in number and a more solid consistency of stools.

Interventions. Antidiarrheal medications may be administered to control the client's diarrhea. Perianal excoriation often occurs with diarrhea. After every bowel movement, gently clean the skin with warm water and apply a protective moisture barrier product. (See the Management and Delegation feature on the Application and Care of Rectal Pouches and Rectal Tubes on the website.)

Diagnosis: Imbalanced Nutrition: Less Than Body Requirements. The client with inflammatory bowel disease has many difficulties with nutrition, making *Imbalanced Nutrition: Less Than Body Requirements related to diarrhea and malabsorption* a common nursing diagnosis.

Outcomes. The client will increase nutritional intake to meet metabolic requirements as evidenced by weight stabilization and possibly weight gain.

Interventions. Monitor the client's nutritional intake. The type of diet ordered depends on the client's condition. If the client can tolerate a diet, encourage intake of fluids and food. Because eating stimulates the gastrocolic reflex and the urge to defecate, many people are afraid to eat; small servings may enable the client to avoid this problem. Foods should be easily digested to promote absorption during the short time the food remains in the bowel.

Clients with Crohn's disease are often receiving home TPN because as a result of disease exacerbation they cannot tolerate foods for long periods (see Chapter 29). These clients also may have undergone multiple bowel resections, resulting in short-bowel syndrome and problems of malabsorption.

Diagnosis: Acute Pain. Another common nursing diagnosis for the client with inflammatory bowel disease is *Acute Pain related to inflamed mucosa.*

Outcomes. The client will experience a relief in abdominal pain as evidenced by the client's statement that pain has been relieved.

Interventions. Assess the client's pain, and give pain medications as ordered. Note any changes in the client's complaints of pain because they may indicate the development of complications. Opioids are generally used sparingly so that they do not mask manifestations.

Diagnosis: Risk for Ineffective Coping. Stress is associated with IBD and clients frequently report a poor quality of life. Write the nursing diagnosis as *Risk for Ineffective Coping related to stress of disease and exacerbations related to stress.*

Outcomes. The client will cope effectively with the disease as evidenced by fewer exacerbations and an improved coping style. The client will report an improved quality of life. The Translating Evidence into Practice box on p. 692 discusses quality of life for clients with IBD.

Interventions. Although emotional factors may not contribute to the cause of the disease, they do influence its course. Prolonged stress often precedes the onset of IBD and exacerbations. Recommend that the client schedule a follow-up physical examination and colonoscopy every 1 to 2 years. Refer clients with IBD to the Crohn's and Colitis Foundation of America (www.ccfa.org) to learn about the condition and about meetings of local support groups. Instruct the client to call the physician at the first manifestation of IBD recurrence.

Evaluation. It is hoped that the client's disease will respond to medical management and that the client will achieve remission, improved coping, and adequate nutritional intake. If the client's IBD does not respond to medical management, surgical intervention may be required.

Surgical Management

Surgery, the only cure for ulcerative colitis, is usually indicated when medical management fails and the condition is intractable. Of clients with ulcerative colitis, 25% to 40% must undergo proctocolectomy with a

Quality of Life with Inflammatory Bowel Disease

Inflammatory bowel disease (IBD) is a chronic disorder with no known cure. It is characterized by remissions and exacerbations. Clients with IBD suffer from physical and psychological symptoms and must live with the uncertainty of the disease course. As a result, many clients report a poor quality of life.

Nursing and medical research studies, both quantitative and qualitative, have assessed the quality of life in clients with IBD. Research participants included clients in an outpatient clinic,[7] parents with IBD,[5] young adults with the disease,[2] and women undergoing loop ileostomy surgery.[6] In addition, one experimental research study examined the effects of nursing-led counseling sessions to help clients cope with the disease.[7] Data were collected by means of questionnaires and interviews.

Findings from these studies were that clients have maladaptive coping skills and suffer from life-disrupting challenges that profoundly affect their peers, families, and individuals in their social support systems. Surgery to create a loop ileostomy for women with ulcerative colitis proved to be a disappointment as the dream of full recovery was unrealized and women learned to cope with changes to their body, pain, and problems with the loop ileostomy.[6] One study found that parents with IBD have difficulty with parenting and suffer from guilt, worry, and depression in regard to effective parenting. Participants in this study reported that their children became angry, anxious, and frustrated when their social activities were interrupted because of the disease. On a positive note, parents with IBD reported closer relationships with their children as a result of the disease and children who were caring and understanding.[5]

Recommendations from the studies were that any co-morbid psychiatric illnesses be treated and that risk factors for psychological distress be identified early.[4] Those at particularly high risk for psychological distress are those who lack family support, those with severe manifestations, and those with young children. Nurses should strive to understand the disease from each client's perception.[2,3] Clients need help with determining problem-solving coping strategies, reducing stress, dealing with uncertainty, and gaining personal control and self-responsibility.[3,4,7] Both clients and people in their support system need social support and education about the disease. They also need assistance with recovering and maintaining physical strength during periods of remission.[7]

IMPLICATIONS

Clients with IBD often suffer from poor quality of life because of the chronic nature of the disease and its clinical manifestations. Learning how to manage the disease and gain personal control is essential to a good quality of life. Nurses are in an ideal situation to help these clients achieve good quality of life through education, counseling, and support.

REFERENCES

1. Casellas, F., et al. (2001). Influence of inflammatory bowel disease on different dimensions of quality of life. *European Journal of Gastroenterology and Hepatology, 13*(5), 567-572.
2. Daniel, J. (2002). Young adults' perceptions of living with chronic inflammatory bowel disease. *Gastroenterology Nursing, 25*(3), 83-94.
3. Delmar, C., Boje, T., Dylmer, D., et al (2006). Independence/dependence—A contradictory relationship? Life with a chronic illness. *Scandinavian Journal of Caring Sciences, 20*(3), 261-268.
4. Dudley-Brown, S. (2002). Prevention of psychological distress in persons with inflammatory bowel disease. *Issues in Mental Health Nursing, 23*(4), 403-422.
5. Mukherjee, S., et al. (2002). An insight into the experiences of parents with inflammatory bowel disease. *Journal of Advanced Nursing, 37*(4), 355-363.
6. Notter, J., & Burnard, P. (2006). Preparing for loop ileostomy surgery: Women's accounts from a qualitative study. *International Journal of Nursing Studies, 43*(2), 147-159.
7. Smith, G., et al. (2002). Impact of a nurse-led counseling service on quality of life in patients with inflammatory bowel disease. *Journal of Advanced Nursing, 38*(2), 152-160.
8. Tanaka, M., & Kazuma, K. (2005). Ulcerative colitis: Factors affecting difficulties of life and psychological well being of patients in remission. *Journal of Clinical Nursing, 14*(1), 65-73.

permanent ileostomy (Brooke's end ileostomy) or a continent ileostomy such as an ileal pouch–anal anastomosis. A Kock pouch may be performed but generally requires multiple surgeries. Partial or subtotal colectomy is not usually recommended in ulcerative colitis, as colitis will usually reoccur in the remaining colon. Surgery is not indicated in Crohn's disease except to treat complications. Surgery may be indicated in either or both conditions, however, for complications such as perforation, hemorrhage, obstruction, toxic megacolon, abscess, fistula, and disease intractability.

Total Proctocolectomy

In a total proctocolectomy, the colon and rectum are removed and the anus is closed. The terminal ileum is brought out through the abdominal wall, and a permanent ileostomy (Brooke's end ileostomy) is formed.

Kock Pouch

Indications. A Kock pouch is a procedure in which a reservoir or pouch is constructed from the distal 45 cm of the ileum. This allows stool to be stored intra-abdominally until it is drained through a nipple valve made from an intussuscepted portion of ileum (prolapse of one part of intestine into an adjacent section) (Figure 33-6). The client has a flat stoma on the right side of the abdomen. Advantages of the continent ileostomy are (1) no need to wear an external pouch, (2) minimal skin problems, and (3) usually no flatus or leakage of stool. The client drains the pouch several times a day by intubation with a catheter through the nipple valve, usually in response to a feeling of fullness.

Contraindications. A Kock pouch should not be performed for Crohn's disease because of the likelihood of recurrent disease in the ileal pouch. If the client has malnutrition, TPN may be required to improve the outcome of surgery and promote wound healing.

Complications. After the formation of the Kock pouch, suture line leakage with local or generalized peritonitis may occur in the early postoperative period. The client may be unable to intubate the pouch because of slippage of the nipple valve. Other complications that may occur later in the recovery period include pouchitis, fistula formation, and obstruction by food residue.

Outcomes. The client resumes usual activities within 4 to 6 weeks. Nutritional status also improves. The client experiences improved quality of life without the necessity of frequent trips to the bathroom.

Ileal Pouch–Anal Anastomosis

Indications. Ileal pouch–anal anastomosis involves several surgical procedures that result in the creation of a pelvic pouch, an internal reservoir created from the distal ileum, and sutured into the anorectal canal. The most common procedure is the J pouch. Clients who choose this procedure avoid an ostomy.

Surgery is usually performed in two steps. During the first step, the rectal mucosa is excised and the colon removed. An ileoanal reservoir (pouch) is then created in the anal canal, and a temporary loop ileostomy is formed to divert fecal contents until the pouch heals. After healing has taken place, usually in 2 to 3 months, the ileostomy is reversed so that stool drains into the reservoir, which is created by suturing two loops of bowel together (Figure 33-7). Some surgeons are completing this procedure in one surgery so that a temporary ileostomy is not required.

Contraindications. This anastomosis should not be performed for Crohn's disease. If malnutrition is a problem, TPN may be needed to improve the outcome of surgery and promote wound healing.

Complications. Complications include anastomotic leakage, pouchitis (inflammation of the pouch), and bowel obstruction.

Outcomes. The client resumes regular activities in 4 to 6 weeks after the second procedure or after the first procedure if a temporary ileostomy has not been performed.

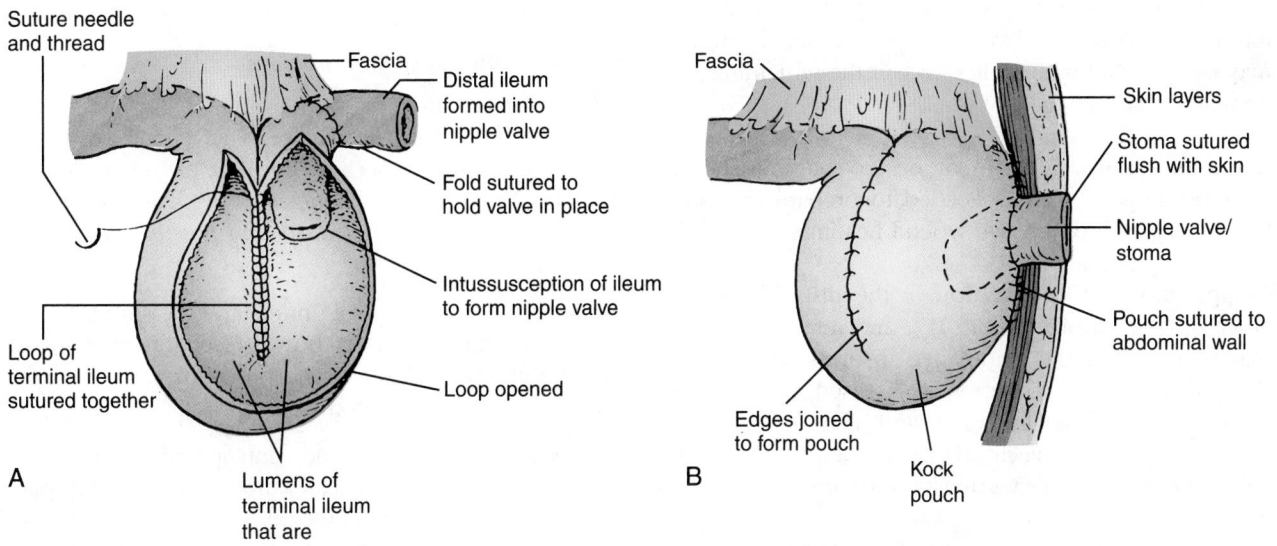

■ **FIGURE 33–6** Continent ileostomy (Kock pouch). **A,** Loop of terminal ileum is sutured together and cut open. Using forceps, the surgeon intussuscepts the distal ileum to form a nipple valve. **B,** Free edges are sutured together to form the reservoir, the stoma is sutured flush with the skin, and the pouch is sutured to the abdominal wall.

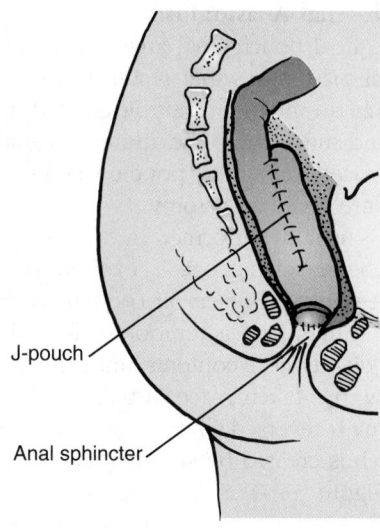

J-pouch

Anal sphincter

■ **FIGURE 33–7** Ileal J pouch–anal anastomosis. The two-loop ileal pouch is simple to construct, provides adequate storage capacity, and is evacuated spontaneously and fully.

Nutritional status improves, and the client experiences improved quality of life with nearly normal bowel movements and fewer trips to the bathroom.

Surgical Resection of the Small Bowel

Indications. In Crohn's disease, surgery is used only to treat the complications because even when the diseased portion is removed, the incidence of recurrence is 50%. The physician may prescribe antibiotics to control infection. During surgical resection for Crohn's disease, attempts are made to preserve as much of the small intestine as possible. Two thirds of the small intestine may be removed with no ill effects if the remaining portion is normal.

Contraindications. Clients may be too malnourished to undergo surgery. TPN is needed to prepare the client for surgery and to improve wound healing.

Complications. With resection of the distal ileum, the client cannot absorb vitamin B_{12}, and removal of more than 6 to 8 feet results in impaired absorption of glucose, fat, and protein. If the colon is diseased, an ileotransverse colectomy (right colon and ileum), segmental colectomy, or total colectomy may be performed. A total colectomy with ileorectal anastomosis may be the surgery of choice.

For 1 to 3 weeks after extensive small bowel resection, the client may be unable to tolerate oral intake and may experience further losses in body protein or lean body mass. TPN is given until oral intake is resumed. Diarrhea usually occurs during the first 6 weeks after

surgery. Anemia (from iron deficiency, steatorrhea, or decreased protein absorption) also may ensue. Paralytic ileus (see discussion later) is another possible complication.

Clients with either irreversible intestinal failure or short-bowel syndrome resulting from multiple bowel resection may be candidates for small bowel transplantation (SBT). This procedure is an alternative therapy for clients who might otherwise face the prospect of lifelong TPN. In the past, cadaver donors were used, but more recently a living-related intestinal transplantation has been accomplished. Clients undergoing SBT have a difficult postoperative course and long-term complications of immunosuppression, and they are at risk for graft rejection (see Chapter 80).

Outcomes. It is hoped that the client can return to regular activities with complete wound healing and adequate nutrition 4 to 6 weeks after surgery.

Nursing Management of the Surgical Client

Assessment. Assessment of the surgical client is similar to assessment of the medical client; however, routine preoperative and postoperative assessments as discussed in Chapter 14 are also necessary. Recently, assessment of bowel sounds has been questioned as an indicator of bowel motility. Rather, the return of flatus; the absence of abdominal pain, distention, bloating, nausea, and vomiting; and the return of appetite were found to be better indicators of returning GI motility in postoperative abdominal surgery clients.[31] If the client is malnourished, TPN may be required preoperatively to improve nutritional status.

Diagnosis, Outcomes, Interventions

Preoperative Care

Diagnosis: Deficient Knowledge. The client who is to undergo surgical resection for IBD has many learning needs. The nursing diagnosis is *Deficient Knowledge related to surgical procedure and possible ileostomy or other bowel resection.*

Outcomes. The client will understand the surgical procedure and implications of bowel resection as evidenced by the ability to describe the procedure and perform a demonstration of ileostomy care.

Interventions. Describe the anticipated postoperative course, including the types of tubes that will be in place. Ostomy care must be fully explained to the client scheduled for ileostomy surgery. A preoperative visit from a member of any ostomy association may be helpful. An enterostomal therapy nurse should assist with the preoperative preparation. Before surgery, the site of the ileostomy is selected, with consideration being given to the location of the disease, body contours, convenience, and type of clothing the client wears. The client may wear the pouch for 1 to 2 days before surgery to ensure comfort with the site selected. To provide assistance and support, assess the client's body image as well as feelings about loss of a major body part and wearing a pouch for a lifetime.

If the client is having a continence-sparing surgery, extensive teaching is still required. The client needs to understand the type of bowel resection to be performed and the implications of the surgery. With some procedures, a temporary ileostomy (ileal pouch–anal anastomosis) may be necessary; with other procedures (e.g., the Kock pouch), the client's method of waste elimination is imbalanced permanently.

Postoperative Care

Diagnosis: Risk for Injury. The client undergoing stoma formation is prone to complications. The nursing diagnosis is *Risk for Injury related to postoperative complications of stomal necrosis, retraction, prolapse, stenosis, or obstruction.*

Outcomes. The client will not suffer injury, as evidenced by minimal distention, rapid return of normal peristalsis, and absence of fluid and electrolyte imbalance.

Interventions

Monitor Stoma. Monitor the stoma after surgery. Ensure that there is no pressure on the stoma that could interfere with circulation. Assess the color of the stoma frequently (see Figure 33-13 for appearance of a normal stoma).

> **If the stoma becomes pale, dusky, or cyanotic, notify the physician immediately. When blood supply to the stoma is compromised, surgical revision is required.**

Advance Diet. An NG tube is in place for several days after surgery to remove gases and fluids that would increase intestinal distention and put pressure on the suture line. The drainage must be accurately noted. The passage of flatus indicates return of peristalsis. As bowel sounds return, clamp the tube as prescribed, and give the client ice chips and water. When the client has tolerated ice chips and water for a minimum of 24 hours, the tube is usually removed, and clear liquids are given.

Monitor for Complications. Although the postoperative course for most clients with ileostomy is uneventful, several complications can occur. The most common is an intestinal obstruction, which may be caused by obstruction of the lumen, adhesions, food, or stomal edema. Early manifestations of obstruction are (1) anorexia;

(2) abdominal cramps; (3) absence of ileostomy drainage or a foul, brown, watery discharge in the pouch; and (4) visible peristalsis. Other early postoperative complications are hemorrhage, hypoxia, and fluid and electrolyte imbalance. If severe or prolonged problems with absorption occur, parenteral nutrition may be necessary.

Diagnosis: Risk for Disturbed Body Image. The client with an ostomy has to face alterations in self-concept and body image. Write the nursing diagnosis as *Risk for Disturbed Body Image related to alteration of lifestyle secondary to ostomy.*

Outcomes. The client experiences a positive body image and self-concept as evidenced by the client's statements and the ability to care for the ostomy without embarrassment.

Interventions. A few days after surgery, the client needs to begin to (1) confront the stoma and (2) integrate its function and appearance into his or her body image. Help the client to look at and touch the stoma as soon as possible. Always use proper terms for the stoma and equipment.

Because clothing can be a concern for the client with an ostomy, clothing options should be discussed. Discourage the client from wearing a tight waistband, which might rub on the stoma. Encourage the client to try on various outfits to ensure that the stoma and pouch are not visible. A visit from another person with an ostomy, usually available through the local chapter of the American Cancer Society, often helps the client realize that the ostomy can be easily hidden beneath clothing.

Encourage the client to verbalize feelings about the stoma and its appearance. The client may be accepting of the stoma because the illness (ulcerative colitis) is now gone and the client's life can be more normal and productive than it had been with the disease. Young men and unmarried women may express the greatest concern about body image. Find out how family or significant others now view the client. Their response might be positive because the client may have been chronically ill before surgery and now appears much healthier.

Diagnosis: Effective Therapeutic Regimen Management. The client with a new stoma has much to learn about self-care. The nursing diagnosis is *Effective Therapeutic Regimen Management related to ileostomy care, care following ileorectal anastomosis, care of an ileal pouch–anal anastomosis, or care of a continent ileostomy.*

Outcomes. The client will understand proper care of the chosen surgical procedure as evidenced by (1) the ability to apply the appliance correctly, without leakage, and to empty the pouch appropriately; and (2) the absence of perianal breakdown.

Interventions

Ileostomy

Teach Ostomy Care. The client must master the skills needed to provide self-care. Stoma care is the area of greatest concern to the client with an ileostomy. The Management and Delegation feature below discusses stoma care and the use of ostomy appliances. Refer to a fundamentals of nursing text for more information related to ostomy care. Consultation with an enterostomal therapy nurse, if available, may enhance teaching and care.

The frequency with which the ileal pouch needs to be emptied varies with each client. It should be emptied whenever it is approximately one third to one half full. Instruct the client to empty the pouch during times of low output, usually before meals, at bedtime, and on arising in the morning. It is best to change the pouch when the ileostomy is the least active, usually first thing in the morning. Coating the pouch with drops of vegetable oil before using it prevents the contents from sticking to the sides and helps it to slide out easily.

Teach Stoma Assessment. When changing the pouch, the client should learn to check the size and color of the stoma, assess the odor of the drainage, and observe for manifestations of irritation. When the ileostomy begins to function, the output is minimal. As the client takes in more food, the drainage becomes thicker and has a weak odor. Because an ileostomy may drain continuously (drainage is related to eating patterns), a pouch must be worn continuously, and the stoma must be covered with gauze when the pouch is being changed.

MANAGEMENT AND DELEGATION

Stoma Care and Application of Ostomy Appliances

The care of a mature stoma and the application of an ostomy appliance may be delegated to unlicensed assistive personnel. The assessment and care of a newly created ostomy, however, should be performed only by a registered nurse. Before delegating stoma care and applying an ostomy appliance, consider the following:

- The age of the ostomy. Is this a postsurgical client with a new ostomy or a client with an ostomy that is several weeks, months, or years old? For the client with a new ostomy, you or a trained ostomy nurse should provide care. For the client with a long-standing ostomy, assess the ostomy to ensure that the client is caring for it properly and that the stoma and surrounding skin are intact before you delegate ostomy care to assistive personnel.
- The client's need to learn self-care of the stoma and ostomy. You or a trained ostomy nurse should provide this instruction for a client needing to learn self-care.
- The client's acceptance of the ostomy, altered appearance, and bowel function. Clients having difficulty accepting their altered body image would benefit from having you or an ostomy nurse help them increase the acceptance and their ability to cope with the new ostomy.
- The competency level of the unlicensed assistive personnel who will potentially perform this task.

The assistive personnel providing stoma care and applying ostomy appliances should be instructed to do the following:

- Provide privacy for the client.
- Place a waterproof pad around the ostomy or under the client to protect the skin and bed linens.
- Empty the contents of the ostomy bag before removing the bag, noting the consistency, color, volume, and odor of the feces.
- Gently remove the skin barrier and bag while supporting the client's skin. An adhesive remover may be applied if necessary to remove adhesive residue from peristomal skin. This should be avoided if there is evidence of skin irritation or excoriation.
- Place a gauze pad or tissues over the exposed stoma to avoid soiling from leakage.
- Wash the skin around the stoma with warm water and a mild soap, and wash the stoma with clear water.
- Thoroughly rinse the area with water and pat it dry.
- Note the color, moisture, and protrusion of the stoma and the condition of the surrounding skin.
- Create a circle ⅛ to ¼ inch larger than the size of the stoma on the back of the appliance. A stoma-measuring guide may be helpful for this procedure. The appliance wafer may have to be cut in an irregular shape to accommodate a noncircular stoma.
- Prepare the wafer and appliance as a unit.
- Smooth the wafer to remove all air bubbles.
- Fill in irregular stoma borders with skin paste applied around the opening in the wafer before applying it to the skin.
- Apply the unit, appliance, wafer, and bag around the stoma. Position the bag to hang in a dependent position. If the client is ambulatory, remember to position the bag for optimal drainage while the client is upright.
- Dispose of the soiled bag and appliance properly. Do this outside the client's room to prevent embarrassment about any odors.

Assistive personnel should report immediately to you if they find black, tarry stools or overt signs of blood in the bag or bleeding from the stoma. Reddened, inflamed skin surrounding the stoma should also be brought to your attention. Information pertaining to the care and condition of the stoma should be recorded.

Prevent Skin Irritation. The pouch should be cut to fit the stoma, allowing only $\frac{1}{16}$ inch of room around the stoma. If the pouch does not fit well, severe skin irritation can occur because of the alkalinity of the effluent. Skin irritation can vary from redness to weeping dermatitis or ulceration. Irritation also can result from adhesives or frequent removal of the appliance. Any hair around the stoma should be cut with small scissors or cut with an electric clipper following the grain of hair. This helps prevent folliculitis and soreness. The skin should be washed and rinsed thoroughly between removing one pouch and applying another. Some appliance companies suggest using an adhesive remover wipe each time the pouch is changed, followed by washing with a mild soap and thoroughly rinsing with water. Then towel- or air-dry. With a two-piece setup, a pouch is snapped onto the faceplate, which is applied to the skin. This arrangement allows easy emptying of the pouch. The faceplate usually remains adherent to the skin for 5 to 7 days but may need to be changed sooner if it becomes loose or if leakage occurs.

Treat Skin Problems. If skin irritation occurs, first check the fit of the pouch. The best initial treatment for this problem would be to reapply the ostomy appliance, ensuring a proper fit and seal. The skin barrier of the appliance is usually sufficient to protect and heal the skin. If this method does not work, other barriers must be used. A wide variety of skin care products are available. If the problems continue, consult an enterostomal therapy nurse for further assistance.

Skin infection also can occur. *Candida* is the most common cause. The peristomal skin takes on a rash-like appearance. An antifungal powder should be rubbed onto the affected skin area. The barrier can then be applied over the powder.

Reduce Odor. Foods such as eggs, fish, onions, cabbage, and some greens cause stool odor; therefore deodorizing solutions and tablets may be placed in the pouch. Spinach, parsley, yogurt, and buttermilk reduce drainage odor.

Discuss Medications. The client also needs special instructions regarding prescription and over-the-counter medications. Enteric-coated tablets, such as iron preparations, vitamins, hormones, multilayer tablets, timed-release capsules, and gelatin capsules may not be absorbed in the small intestine. The client should note whether any medications are obvious in pouch drainage; if so, the physician must prescribe different medications or different forms of medication.

Emphasize Fluid Intake. The client who has had an ileostomy needs to pay close attention to fluid intake. It is easy for such a client to become dehydrated. The approximate output from an ileostomy is 1200 to 1500 ml/day. The client must monitor this output for any increase that could lead to severe fluid and electrolyte imbalance.

Explain Dietary Recommendations. A low-residue diet that is high in protein, carbohydrates, and calories is recommended after ileostomy surgery. Supplemental vitamins A, D, E, K, and B_{12} may be needed. Berries, whole-grain cereals, and raw fruits and vegetables can cause problems for the client with an ileostomy. Any foods that cause discomfort or diarrhea should be omitted. Ingested foods pass through the ileostomy within 4 to 6 hours. It is not advisable to eat a large meal close to bedtime.

The client with an ileostomy must learn to chew food well (20 to 25 chews for each bite) because the shortened bowel transit time would cause poorly chewed food to be passed undigested. High-fiber and high-cellulose foods may absorb excessive moisture, leading to swelling and possibly constipation or even obstruction. Foods that should be avoided or limited, at least initially, include popcorn, peanuts, tough fibrous meats, vegetables with skins, rice, bran, and coconuts.

Clients may find that the postoperative diet is less restrictive than the diet they followed before the surgery. The diet required by the presence of the disease was often restricted because so many foods increased the diarrhea and other manifestations. Clients with ileostomies often gain weight after surgery, sometimes to the point of having to restrict caloric intake.

Prevent Urolithiasis. Some clients with ileostomies tend to have calcium oxalate, uric acid, or urinary calculi because greater amounts of fluid are lost through the ileostomy, leading to decreased urine output. Uric acid stones tend to form when urine volume is low and the urine is persistently acidic. Ingestion of sodium bicarbonate or potassium citrate alkalinizes the urine. Allopurinol may be used if uric acid levels remain elevated. Fluid intake should be at least 2000 ml daily.

Ileal Pouch–Anal Anastomosis. The client with an ileal pouch–anal anastomosis has no need to learn about stoma or pouch care unless a temporary ileostomy was created. The client will learn to prevent leakage by responding to the sensation to defecate. After the bowel adapts to the surgical alteration, the stool becomes more formed, although it will always be loose. Most clients have between two and eight stools per day. Kegel exercises, to strengthen the tone of the anal sphincter muscles, will facilitate continence. Teach the client to tighten the anal sphincter muscles as if stopping a bowel movement. Hold for a count of 10 while squeezing tightly and then relax for a count of 10. These exercises should only be carried out when approved by the surgeon. Perianal skin irritation is likely to occur as a result of seepage and the enzyme content of liquid stool. The client should be taught to gently wipe the perianal area after each bowel movement. A moisture-barrier ointment such as Desitin can provide comfort. Pouchitis occurs in about 30% of clients. Clinical manifestations are an increase in number of stools, malaise, bleeding, and fever. Pouchitis is treated with metronidazole (Flagyl); ciprofloxacin, mesalamine, or steroids are used for severe cases. The client should maintain an adequate fluid intake.

Kock Pouch (Continent Ileostomy)

Maintain Ileal Drainage. During surgical formation of the Kock pouch, an evacuation catheter is inserted. A skin barrier and special gauze dressing are then applied. These hold the catheter in an upright position to avoid stress on a healing nipple valve. It is imperative to avoid distention of the ileostomy reservoir in the early postoperative period because of the pressure it would put on the suture line. Thus the reservoir is attached to straight drainage for several days after surgery. Then it is emptied every 2 hours for about 2 weeks.

Carefully observe for the start of ileal drainage, which usually begins 3 or 4 days postoperatively. About 2 weeks after surgery, the catheter is removed from the pouch. The catheter may then be used to drain the pouch. The intervals between draining are gradually increased each week until the ileostomy is emptied four to six times per day and once or not at all at night.

Teach Reservoir Catheterization. Explain the following procedure for emptying the reservoir, which should be performed with the client sitting on the toilet:

1. Lubricate the catheter with a water-soluble lubricant, and insert it into the stoma through the valve.
2. Allow the contents to drain by gravity through the catheter into the bathroom toilet; drainage should be complete in 3 to 5 minutes.
3. Apply a small gauze dressing over the stoma.
4. Clean the equipment with mild soap, and rinse it; the equipment can be carried in a plastic case.

The reservoir volume continues to increase to a maximum of around 600 ml in 6 months.

Explain Dietary Recommendations. The client needs an oral intake of at least eight 8-ounce glasses of fluid per day. Foods that could cause a blockage of the valve and the stoma, including mushrooms and nuts, may need to be avoided. All foods need to be chewed thoroughly because partly digested food may occlude the stoma.

Diagnosis: Risk for Sexual Dysfunction. In the client with an ileostomy, there are no physiologic reasons for sexual dysfunction; however, after J pouch surgery, both men and women may experience alterations in sexual function because of injury to nerves in the pelvic region. Men might experience impotence or retrograde ejaculation. Women may experience vaginal dryness and painful intercourse. Psychological reasons may also lead to dysfunction. Therefore the nursing diagnosis is *Risk for Sexual Dysfunction related to concern about ileostomy and disturbed body image and self-concept.*

Outcomes. The client will not have sexual dysfunction as evidenced by the ability to resume presurgery sexual functioning and role.

Interventions. The client with an ileostomy or pouch may be concerned about sexual activity and pregnancy. Encourage the client to express any such concerns and to discuss them with the sexual partner. Clients can be taught activities to lessen the intrusiveness of the pouch during intercourse, such as emptying the pouch before intercourse, wearing a soft flannel pouch cover, and being open to using different positions for intercourse. If problems arise, a sexual therapist should be consulted for further information and assistance. Impotence is uncommon; psychological reasons should be explored if it does occur.

Pregnancy and normal vaginal delivery are possible for a client with an ileostomy. The United Ostomy Association has a wide variety of booklets available for clients with an ostomy. Titles include *Sex, Pregnancy and the Female Ostomate; Sex, Courtship and the Single Ostomate; Sex and the Male Ostomate;* and *Insight into the Emotional Aspects of Ileostomies and Colostomies.* Similar resources are available from the American Cancer Society.

Evaluation. If teaching is adequate, the client should be able to care for the ostomy and to handle the altered elimination. Preoperative activities can usually be resumed within 6 weeks.

Self-Care

Postoperative care and care of the stoma or diversion should be reinforced before the client is discharged. The client with an ileostomy should be encouraged to join the United Ostomy Association. This organization often helps clients regain self-esteem and improve self-concept and body image. The successful rehabilitation of others helps clients believe that they, too, can return to a normal lifestyle.

See the Client Education Guide on Ostomy Supplies on the website for the equipment needed to care for an ileostomy. The client should be aware of the nearest ostomy supply center so that equipment will be easy to obtain. If the client experiences difficulty with self-care, a visiting nursing or enterostomal therapy nurse should visit the client at home to follow up on learning needs. Clients with J pouches can find information on the Internet at www.ccfa.org.

No long-term restrictions are placed on physical activities. Tell the client to wear a medical alert identification bracelet and to carry a brief description of the pouch and drainage procedure in case of an emergency.

NEOPLASTIC DISORDERS

BENIGN TUMORS OF THE BOWEL

Various types of benign tumors are found in the bowel. Polyps, lesions that project into the lumen of the bowel, are the most commonly found benign tumor (Figure 33-8). Some polyps have stems (*pedunculated*) whereas others do not (*sessile*). Polyps are usually benign lesions, but some types are precursors of cancer (i.e., premalignant tumors). Polyps are dangerous because (1) they can mask the presence of a malignant tumor, and (2) they may serve as the focus for bowel obstruction or intussusception. Benign bowel tumors have clinical manifestations similar to those of malignant tumors. Some benign tumors bleed profusely and cause abdominal discomfort. Bleeding benign tumors are usually removed surgically.

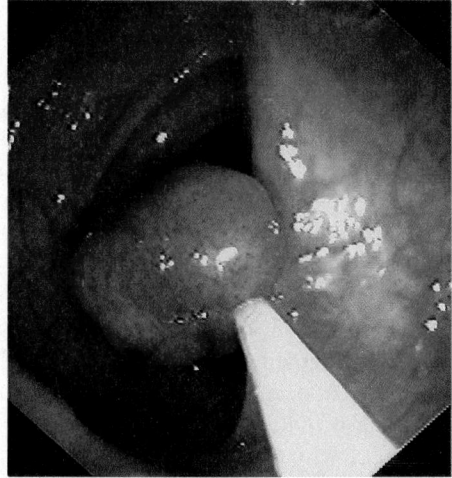

■ **FIGURE 33–8** Colonic polyps. *(From Copstead, L.C., & Banasik, J.L. [2005]. Pathophysiology: Biological and behavioral perspectives [3rd ed.]. Philadelphia: Saunders. Courtesy of L.E. Copstead.)*

CANCER OF THE SMALL BOWEL

Fewer than 5% of all GI cancers involve tumors of the small bowel. It was estimated that in 2007, about 5637 people had cancer of the small bowel and of these, estimated deaths were 1070.[1] The average age at onset is 53 to 58 years. Most tumors are in the ileum, with the remainder almost equally divided between the duodenum and jejunum. Manifestations are vague and nonspecific; they include weight loss, pain, anemia, nausea, vomiting, obstruction, a palpable mass, and hemorrhage.

Surgery is the only intervention that offers hope of cure. Unfortunately, even with early diagnosis and bowel resection, only about 20% of clients with small bowel cancer survive 5 years. With late diagnosis, the 5-year survival rate decreases to about 5%.

COLORECTAL CANCER

Colon and rectal (colorectal) cancer is the most common GI cancer in the United States. Colon cancer is three times more common than rectal cancer. Colorectal cancer occurs equally in men and women, is the third most common cancer, and is the second leading cause of death from cancer in the United States. It is estimated that about 154,000 new cases of colorectal cancer were diagnosed in 2007 with a mortality rate of 10% to 15% (approximately 52,000).[1] The probability of developing colorectal cancer at some point in one's lifetime is roughly 6%, or 1 of 17 people. With early detection, the 5-year survival rate for clients with stage I and II colon cancer is 91%. Once the cancer has spread to lymph nodes (stage III), the survival rate at 5 years is 60%. The 5-year survival rate drops to 6% once the cancer has metastasized to other organs (stage IV). Colorectal screening and detection decreases the incidence and mortality of colorectal cancer by leading to early removal of precancerous lesions. Although low-cost screening methods have been available for decades, the screening rate remains low. Most tumors are found in the distal portion of the large bowel. Survival following diagnosis correlates with the stage of tumor invasion (Figure 33-9).

Etiology and Risk Factors

The cause of colorectal cancer is not definitely known. It occurs equally in men and women and occurs in all ethnic groups; however, the highest prevalence and mortality rates occur in those of African-American descent. It may be related to low-residue, high-fat diets and highly refined foods with an inadequate intake of fruits and vegetables. There is a higher incidence in cities, in industrialized countries, and among obese clients and those

■ **FIGURE 33-9** Stages of colon cancer: tumor (T), node (N), metastasis (M) system. **A,** Dukes A or TNM I. Cancer is confined to bowel mucosa. **B,** Dukes B or TNM II. Cancer extends into muscle, serosa, and connective tissue or adheres to or invades adjacent organs. **C,** Dukes C or TNM III. Cancer penetrates the bowel wall and adheres to or invades adjacent organs; lymph nodes are positive. **D,** Cancer metastasizes to distant organs.

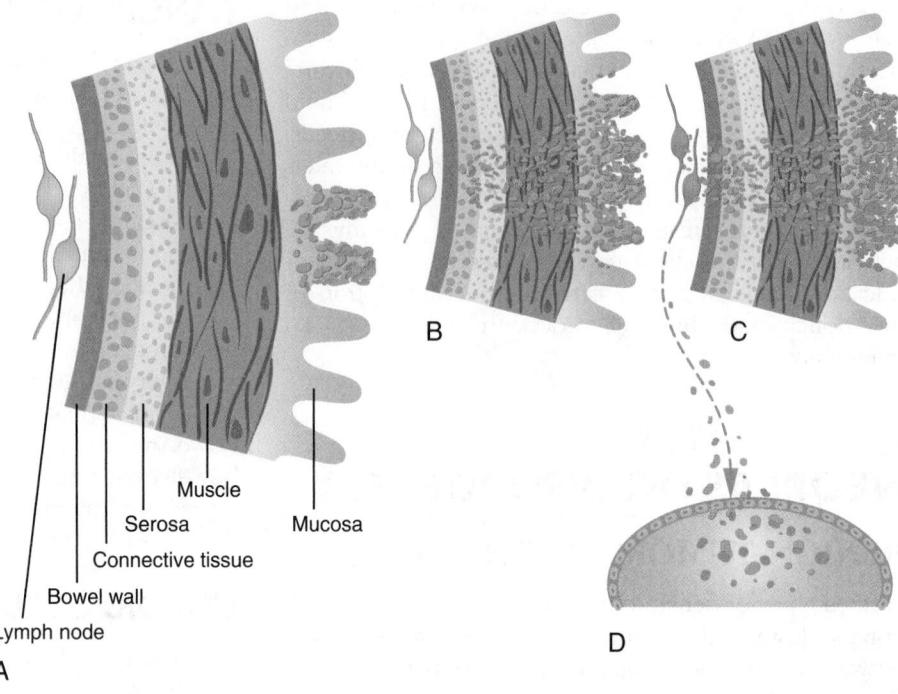

with sedentary lifestyles. ⚱ Two types of hereditary forms of colorectal cancer are caused by genetic mutations (see the Genetic Links feature on Hereditary Colorectal Cancer on p. 701). Gene mutations found in people with hereditary nonpolyposis colorectal cancer (HNPCC) suggest a predisposition for the development of colon cancer to be 90%, with the typical age of onset occurring in the 40s. Those with a genetic disposition to familial adenomatous polyposis (FAP) also have a higher risk of developing colorectal cancer. Only about 5% to 10% of clients with colorectal cancer have a hereditary basis for the disease, however. The risk of cancer increases sharply with age, with 90% of colorectal cancers developing after 50 years of age. Other risk factors are a history of breast, ovarian, or endometrial cancer; or IBD, especially ulcerative colitis. The Complementary and Alternative Therapy feature on p. 702 discusses the relationship between iron deficiency and gastrointestinal cancer.

⚱ Epidemiologic studies indicate that diet may be a major factor in the development of cancer of the large bowel. Studies on bulk in stool and the rate of transit of fecal matter have so far given mixed results. Some researchers propose that metabolic and bacterial end products are carcinogenic and that constipation allows a longer contact with the bowel wall, thus raising the probability that cancer will develop. Increasing fiber in the diet may reduce exposure to carcinogens by speeding stool transit through the intestines. The Complementary and Alternative Therapy feature on p. 702 explores the use of a low-fat, high-fiber diet to reduce

rectal mucosal proliferation. Studies of dietary fat intake and risk of colorectal cancer have also resulted in mixed results. Long-term consumption of red meat has also been implicated in increased risk of colorectal cancer in the distal large intestine. Folate, calcium, magnesium, and selenium have been found to possibly prevent colon cancer.

⚱ Some studies have indicated that regular use of aspirin, nonsteroidal anti-inflammatory drugs (NSAIDs), and COX-2 inhibitors (celecoxib) may reduce the risk of colon cancer. The chemoprevention of colorectal cancer is discussed in the Complementary and Alternative Therapy feature on p. 702. ⚱ However, recent studies have also shown a link between use of these medications and cardiovascular disease, so the benefits of using these drugs must be weighted against the risks. Use of aspirin, NSAIDs, or COX-2 inhibitors is health promotion action, as well as the dietary inclusion of fiber, fruits, and vegetables, especially cruciferous vegetables such as cauliflower, broccoli, Brussels sprouts, and cabbage. ⚱ Recent studies suggest that regular physical exercise may be protective against colon but not rectal cancer.

⚱ Health maintenance activities include yearly screening with fecal occult blood test (FOBT) and digital rectal examination (DRE) for people at average risk for colorectal cancer who are 50 years of age and older. A flexible sigmoidoscopy, colonoscopy, or double-contrast barium enema study should be performed every 5 to 10 years in clients with normal screening results and more frequently in clients from whom polyps have been

GENETIC LINKS

Hereditary Colorectal Cancer

Currently there are two well-described hereditary colorectal cancer syndromes.

HEREDITARY NONPOLYPOSIS COLON CANCER (HNPCC)

Description. Colorectal cancer associated with HNPCC typically develops in a single colonic lesion, with most occurring in the proximal (right side) colon. Affected people are also at risk for extracolonic malignancies including carcinoma of the endometrium, ovary, stomach, small bowel, pancreas, upper renal tract, and the hepatobiliary tract. Mean age of onset is 45 years. Affected individuals have an 80% lifetime risk of colon cancer and affected women have a 20% to 60% lifetime risk of endometrial cancer.

    Incidence. About 1% to 6% of all colorectal cancer is thought to be due to HNPCC.

    Genetics. Autosomal dominant pattern of inheritance; each offspring of an affected parent has a 50% chance of inheriting the HNPCC genetic mutation. HNPCC results from a germ-line mutation in one of several DNA mismatch repair genes *(MLH1, MSH2, MSH6,* and *PMS2).*

    Diagnosis/Genetic Testing. A hallmark of HNPCC colorectal tumors is microsatellite instability (MSI). The presence of MSI in the tumor suggests the presence of a germ-line mutation. Testing generally begins with MSI testing of tumor tissue, followed by mutation analysis of the four genes if the tumor is positive for microsatellite instability. Mutations in *MSH1* and *MLH1* account for *90%* of mutations found in HNPCC families.

    Management. Close surveillance with annual colonoscopy is recommended for clients with strong clinical evidence of HNPCC or those with a known germ-line mutation. Annual screening for extracolonic malignancies is recommended, including transvaginal ultrasonography and endometrial aspiration for pathologic assessment beginning at age 30 years.

FAMILIAL ADENOMATOUS POLYPOSIS (FAP)

Description. FAP is a heritable colon cancer syndrome in which hundreds, if not thousands, of precancerous colonic polyps begin to develop from 7 to 36 years of age. Without a total colectomy, the risk of cancer is almost 100%. Extracolonic manifestations include polyps of the gastric mucosa and duodenum, osteomas, dental anomalies, congenital hypertrophy of the retinal pigment epithelium (CHRPE), soft tissue tumors, desmoid tumors, and associated cancers. A milder variant known as *attenuated FAP* has been described in which fewer polyps develop at a later age (around 50 to 55 years).

    Incidence. Estimated to be responsible for 1% of all colorectal cancer.

    Genetics. FAP is inherited in an autosomal dominant manner. About 75% to 80% of clients with FAP have an affected parent. Offspring of an affected parent have a 50% risk of inheriting the altered *APC* gene.

    Diagnosis/Testing. FAP is caused by mutation in the *APC* gene, but the diagnosis primarily relies on clinical findings by colonoscopy. Molecular genetic testing is clinically available and detects about 95% of the disease-causing mutations.

    Management. Management involves close surveillance of clients who carry an *APC* mutation or clients who are at risk but whose genetic status has not yet been determined. Recommended treatment for individuals with classic FAP is often colectomy.

---

removed or when a close relative (sibling, parent, or child) was affected by colorectal cancer or an adenomatous polyp before age 60.

    Large clinical trials are currently underway to compare stool-based molecular screening with FOBT and colonoscopy. Colorectal epithelial DNA can be extracted from stool samples to assist in detection of cancer cells. A positive test indicates the presence of early cancer cells or precancerous polyps.

    The virtual colonoscopy is a new technique that remains under investigation. It involves use of computerized imaging to produce a three-dimensional image of the colon. The colon is scanned after the bowel is filled with fluid. It is less costly and less invasive than a colonoscopy; however, polyps cannot be removed or biopsies performed. Magnetic resonance colonography is an alternative to colonoscopy. It detects endoluminal masses and lesions and is used to screen clients who are at high risk for colon cancer. However, with both of these techniques, if an abnormality is detected, a flexible sigmoidoscopy or colonoscopy must still be performed for further visualization and biopsy. Finally, the pill camera is a large pill containing a tiny camera that the client swallows. It takes pictures of the bowel lining every few seconds and is most effective in filming the small bowel.

    Clients who have a family or personal history of colorectal cancer, polyps, IBD, or genetic indicators for colorectal cancer should begin colorectal cancer screening at a younger age and should undergo screening more frequently.[1] It is vital to explain to all clients the necessity for early detection and the importance of reporting manifestations such as rectal bleeding and a change in bowel habits to a health care provider.

Pathophysiology

More than 95% of colorectal cancers develop from adenomatous polyps (adenomas). The three types of adenomas are tubular, tubulovillous, and villous. The last type has the highest risk of becoming cancerous. The polyps grow slowly, and most take 5 to 10 years or longer to

Iron Deficiency and Gastrointestinal Cancer

A cohort study with 2 years of follow-up was conducted in the United States. A total of 9024 civilian, non-institutionalized people 25 to 74 years of age (60% women, 83% Caucasian) were included. Men and postmenopausal women (n = 6227) with iron deficiency alone (n = 223) and iron deficiency anemia (n = 51) had an increased risk for gastrointestinal malignancy (any malignancy of the esophagus, stomach, small intestine, colon, or rectum). Similar results were found in individuals 50 or older (n = 4447) and in individuals 65 or older (n = 2733). The researchers concluded that men and postmenopausal women with iron deficiency (with or without anemia) had an increased risk for gastrointestinal cancer within 2 years. One potential recommendation from this study is that any individual over 50 years of age who is found to have an iron deficiency should at least be encouraged to have a colonoscopy.

REFERENCE

Ioannow, G., et al. (2002). Iron deficiency and gastrointestinal malignancy: a population-based cohort study. *American Journal of Medicine, 113,* 267-280.

Low-Fat and High-Fiber Diet to Reduce Rectal Mucosal Proliferation

Diets high in fiber, fruits, and vegetables and low in fat have long been recommended for reduction of colorectal cancer and cardiovascular disease, However, recent research findings have not shown high-fiber, low-fat diets as a prevention intervention for colorectal polyps and cancer. Researchers evaluated the effects of a 4-year low-fat, high-fiber, fruit- and vegetable- enriched dietary intervention on colorectal epithelial cell proliferation among 399 clients from the Polyp Prevention Trial.[3] This trial is a randomized, multicenter trial with adenoma recurrence as the primary end-point. Rectal biopsies were performed on clients at baseline, after 1 year, and after 4 years. No significant differences occurred between the dietary intervention group and control group.[3] These observations are similar to the findings in later studies in which dietary intervention did not appear to reduce risk of colorectal cancers.[1,2] In the study by Park and colleagues (2005), dietary fiber intake was not found to be statistically inversely related to the risk of colorectal cancer in a pooled analysis of 13 studies. Low-fat intake did not reduce the risk for colorectal cancer in postmenopausal women in the Beresford et al. (2006) findings.

REFERENCES

1. Beresford, S., Johnson, K., Ritenbaugh, N., et al. (2006). Low-fat dietary pattern and risk of colorectal cancer: The women's health initiative randomized controlled dietary modification trial. *Journal of the American Medical Association, 295*(6), 643-654.
2. Park, Y., Hunter, D., Spiegelman, D., et al. (2005). Dietary fiber intake and risk of colorectal cancer: A pooled analysis of prospective cohort studies. *Journal of the American Medical Association, 294*(22), 2849-2857.
3. Pfeiffer, R., et al. (2003). The effect of a low-fat, high-fiber, fruit and vegetable intervention on rectal mucosal proliferation. *Cancer, 98,* 1161-1168.

become malignant. As a polyp becomes malignant, it increases in size within the lumen and begins to invade the bowel wall (Figure 33-10). Tumors in the right intestine tend to be bulky and to cause necrosis and ulceration. Tumors in the left intestine start as small, button-like masses that cause ulceration of the blood supply. Clients with FAP develop hundreds to thousands of polyps in their colons at an early age and have an almost 100% chance of developing cancer by the age of 40. As a result, some elect to have a prophylactic colectomy as a preventive measure.

Colon cancer is staged using the TNM (tumor-node-metastasis) classification system. The Dukes classification system is an older, less commonly used system. The TNM system is described in Chapter 17. Figure 33-9 compares the TNM system with the Dukes system. Dukes classifications (A, B, C, D) correlate with the TNM stage groupings (I, II, III, IV).

Malignant bowel tumors spread by (1) direct extension to a nearby organ, such as to the stomach from the transverse colon; (2) lymphatic and hematogenous channels, usually to the liver; and (3) seeding of, or implanting of cells into, the peritoneal cavity. The urinary bladder, ureters, and reproductive organs are frequently involved by direct extension. Blood-borne metastasis extends most commonly to the liver but also may involve the lungs, kidneys, and bones.

Clinical Manifestations

Manifestations of colon cancer include rectal bleeding, changed bowel habits, abdominal pain, weight loss, anemia, and anorexia. In general, tumors in the small bowel and right colon are more likely to cause abdominal pain and cramping, nausea, and vomiting. Because the large intestine distends, cancer located there has fewer early manifestations. At this location, lesions often ulcerate, resulting in anemia and dark, reddish brown stools. Anorexia, weight loss, weakness, debility, and a palpable mass in the right lower quadrant may be present at the time of diagnosis. Lesions of the ascending colon and transverse colon often manifest as progressive obstruction.

Tumors in the descending colon and rectum frequently cause obstructive manifestations, ribbon-like stools containing bright red blood and mucus, altered bowel habits, and tenesmus, but not weight loss,

Chemoprevention of Colorectal Cancer

Findings indicate that some medications may have a role in the prevention of polyps and/or colorectal cancer. These agents include aspirin, NSAIDs, and celecoxib (a COX-2 inhibitor).

In a study of 82,911 women enrolled in the Nurses' Health Study from 1980 to 2000, the risk of colorectal cancer was reduced in women who had taken aspirin regularly for more than a decade. Maximal risk reduction was seen with aspirin doses greater than 14 tablets per week, which is substantially higher than doses recommended for prevention of cardiovascular disease. Compared with nonregular users,[3] there was a significantly lower risk reduction for colon cancer but not rectal cancer among women taking 2 or more aspirin or NSAID tablets per week

COX-2 inhibitors have also been studied for prevention of colorectal polyps. In one study, more than 1500 clients received once-daily celecoxib or placebo in a randomized, placebo-controlled, double-blind study.[1] At 3 years, the celecoxib recipients were significantly less likely than the placebo recipients to have developed any colorectal adenoma (34% vs 49%) or an advanced adenoma (5% vs 10%). Serious cardiovascular events occurred in 2.5% and 1.9% of the celecoxib and placebo groups, respectively (a nonsignificant difference).[1] In another randomized, placebo-controlled, stratified-dose study, more than 2000 clients received celecoxib at one of two doses (400 or 200 mg twice daily) or twice-daily placebo.[2] At 3 years, the proportions of clients who had developed any colorectal adenoma were 38%, 43%, and 61% with higher-dose celecoxib, lower-dose celecoxib, and placebo, respectively. Advanced adenomas also developed less often in the celecoxib groups than in the placebo group (6% and 8% versus 17%). Serious cardiovascular events occurred significantly more often with celecoxib than with placebo (3.4% and 2.6% versus 1%).[2]

Prevention of colorectal polyps or adenomas might be warranted particularly in clients who have an increased risk of colorectal cancer. However, before recommending regular aspirin, NSAID, or celecoxib usage for prevention of colorectal cancer, the risk of gastrointestinal bleeding and cardiovascular events must be considered. Health professionals should continue to follow the data on these drugs.

REFERENCES

1. Arber, N., Eagle, C., Spicak, J., et al. (2006). Celecoxib for the prevention of colorectal adenomatous polyps. *New England Journal of Medicine, 355*(9), 885-895.
2. Bertagnolli, M., Eagle, C., Zauber, A., et al. (2006). Celecoxib for the prevention of sporadic colorectal adenomas. *New England Journal of Medicine, 355*(9), 873-884.
3. Chan, A., Giovannucci, E., Meyerhardt, J., et al. (2005). Long-term use of aspirin and nonsteroidal anti-inflammatory drugs and risk of colon cancer. *Journal of the American Medical Association, 294*(8), 914-923.

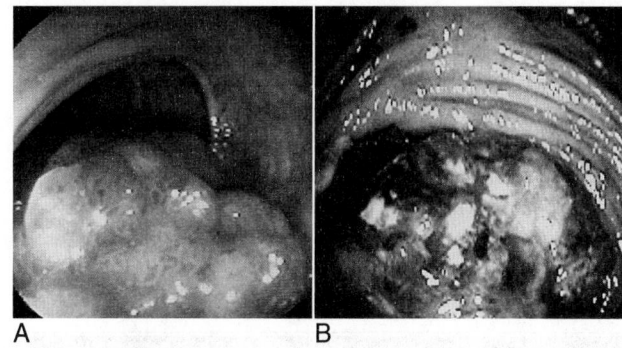

■ **FIGURE 33-10** Carcinomas of the cecum seen at colonoscopy. Carcinomas of the proximal colon are often large and bulky polypoid lesions **(A)** and may outgrow their blood supply and become necrotic **(B)**. *(From Feldman, M., Friedman, L.S., & Sleisenger, M.H. [2002]. Sleisenger & Fordtran's gastrointestinal and liver disease: Pathophysiology/diagnosis/management [7th ed., Vol. 2]. Philadelphia: Saunders.)*

anemia, or dyspepsia. Bleeding is the manifestation that often prompts the client to seek health care.

One third of malignant tumors of the distal colon and rectum can be felt with an examining finger, which makes DRE one of the most important screening methods. A stool guaiac test is performed to check for gastrointestinal bleeding. Serum carcinoembryonic antigen (CEA) is the tumor marker that may be elevated in colorectal cancer and may aid in determining the progress of the disease. CA 19-9 is the tumor marker for pancreatic cancer and not reliable for colorectal cancer. Radiographic studies of the colon may show either a filling defect or a stricture. Colonoscopy and computed tomography (CT), which help establish tumor size and metastasis, identify more than half of colorectal tumors. Flexible fiberoptic colonoscopies permit better visualization into the right colon, extend the diagnostic capabilities of the procedure, and enable collection of biopsy specimens (see Chapter 32). A new screening test that detects DNA shed from precancerous colon polyps and early-stage colon cancer in the stool is in the developmental stages.

Prognosis

The prognosis for the client with colorectal cancer depends on (1) the grade of the cancer, (2) the depth of penetration, (3) the number of lymph nodes evaluated and the number of nodes positive for tumor, and (4) the margin status. Favorable histologic features include grade 1 or 2 with no lymphatic invasion and negative surgical margins (no tumor within 2 mm of margin). The College of American Pathologists recommends that no fewer than 12 lymph nodes be excised and tested for accurate staging.

The 5-year survival rates, listed according to TNM staging, vary depending on the adjuvant therapy received. For example, the MOSAIC trial reported disease-free survival (DFS) for stage III clients at 4 years to be 61% in clients who received 5-fluorouracil (5-FU)/ leucovorin and 69% in clients who received FOLFOX4 (5-FU, leucovorin, and oxaliplatin) chemotherapy. For stage II clients, DFS varied between 81% and 86%, depending on the chemotherapy regimen. Early diagnosis and treatment are essential for a good outcome; however, only 37% of colorectal cancers are identified in the early stages.

OUTCOME MANAGEMENT

Medical Management

Decrease Tumor Growth

The primary treatment for colon cancer is surgery; however, chemotherapy is used as an adjunct to improve survival in tumors that cannot be completely removed. Chemoembolization may be used to destroy solitary tumors that have metastasized to the liver. Radiation therapy and chemotherapy are given alone or together. The combination can increase the survival of clients with rectal cancer; there is less evidence that the combination increases survival of clients with colon cancer. Vaccine therapy continues to be studied in the treatment and prevention of colorectal cancer.

Radiation Therapy. Radiation therapy is often used before surgery to reduce the size of the tumor and make it more resectable. Local interventions at the tumor site after surgery include implantation of radioactive isotopes into the tumor area. Isotopes used include radium, cesium, and cobalt. Iridium has been used in the rectum. Postoperatively, radiation therapy is used for clients classified with Dukes B or C tumors. It may also be used for clients with Dukes D cancer. Radiation therapy is not begun until surgical healing has taken place.

Chemotherapy. Chemotherapy may be used to reduce metastasis and control its manifestations; however, drug resistance limits the effectiveness of chemotherapy in colorectal cancer. Entire classes of cytotoxic drugs are rendered ineffective.

There are effective drugs that are not influenced by these multi-drug resistance mechanisms. For example, the combination of leucovorin (folinic acid) and 5-fluorouracil (5-FU) has improved survival in stage III tumors. Recent studies demonstrated that adding irinotecan (Camptosar) to the first-line therapy has been effective in treating metastatic cancer. The combination of irinotecan, 5-FU, and leucovorin is known as IFL, or the Saltz regimen. Toxic effects (nausea, vomiting, diarrhea) are more frequent with IFL, and the regimen has been modified from its original formula.

Newer regimens contain oxaliplatin (Eloxatin) along with 5-FU and leucovorin. These combinations, which have different doses for each drug, are known as either FOLFOX4 or FOLFOX6. The FOLFOX combinations have been approved by the FDA for metastatic colon cancer and may be given with or without the new anti-angiogenic drug such as bevacizumab (Avastin) or the epidermal growth factor (EGFR) inhibitor cetuximab (Erbitux). All of these combinations have been shown to increase time to progression and overall survival.

Nursing Management of the Medical Client

Care of the client undergoing medical treatment for colon cancer revolves around care of a client undergoing chemotherapy and, occasionally, radiation therapy. See Chapter 17 for further information about the care of these clients.

Surgical Management

About three of four clients undergo surgery and about 60% are cured. Intervention depends on the type of

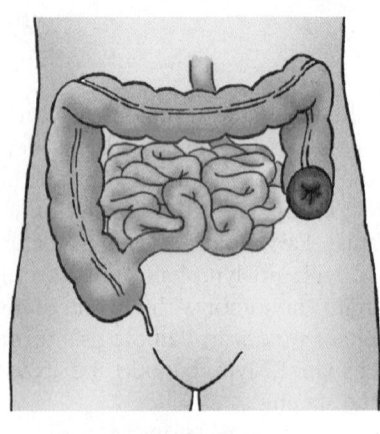
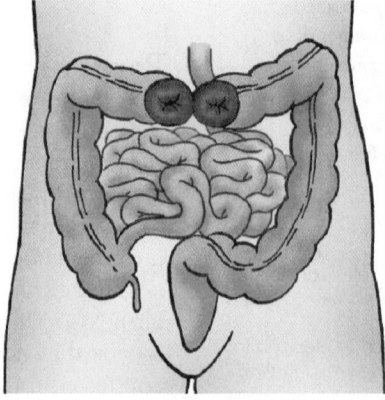
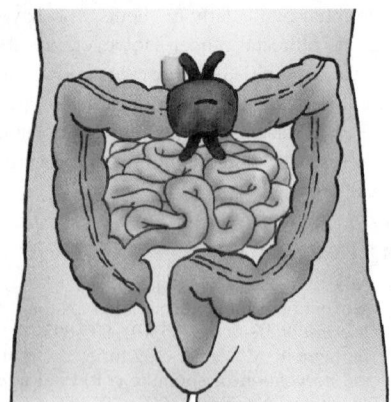

Single-barrel   Double-barrel   Loop

■ **FIGURE 33–11** Types of colostomies. Single-barrel colostomies are usually permanent. Double-barrel colostomies are usually temporary, and stomas may be adjacent or several inches apart. Loop colostomies are temporary and are formed by bringing a loop of colon through the abdominal wall and supporting it with a plastic brace.

tumor, its location and stage, and the client's general condition. The basic goal of surgery is to remove the tumor with proximal and distal margins of the normal bowel tissue that contain blood vessels. Adjacent lymph nodes are also removed, usually 10-20 to determine invasion of tumor and possibility of spread of tumor to other organs. Poor surgical margins with rectal biopsy or resection indicate that there are remaining tumor cells at the surgical site. As a result, radiation therapy may be indicated.

A variety of surgical procedures are performed to treat colorectal cancer (Figures 33-11 and 33-12). Early colorectal cancers can be excised and removed through a colonoscope; however, most procedures entail colon resection, which can be completed laparoscopically or through an open surgical procedure. The tumor is removed with several inches of colon on either side of the tumor. An end-to-end anastomosis is performed, if possible. A sleeve resection may be performed for clients with advanced disease; it is a less involved procedure in which segments of the intestine are resected to relieve obstruction and bleeding.

Several different procedures are used for rectal cancer, depending on tumor location. It may be possible to preserve sphincter function by resecting tumors located in the proximal area. It may not be possible, however, to preserve sphincter function if tumors are less than 8 cm from the anal opening.

Colostomy

Indications. A colostomy may need to be performed for colorectal cancers. This procedure involves creating an opening between the colon and abdominal wall, from which fecal contents will pass. Because the main function of the large bowel is to absorb water, the colostomy is easier to manage nearer the sigmoid colon because the stool is more formed here than in the transverse or right colon. A colostomy can be located in the ascending, transverse, descending, or sigmoid colon and can be permanent or temporary.

A temporary colostomy allows the bowel to rest and later may be reanastomosed. The temporary colostomy also can be used to treat inoperable bowel cancer, with the ostomy placed proximal to the cancer. A temporary colostomy is made most commonly at the midpoint of the left colon or transverse colon, whereas a permanent colostomy is usually placed in the sigmoid colon. When creating a temporary loop colostomy, the surgeon brings a loop of bowel out through a wound that is separate from the surgical incision. To keep the loop from slipping back into the abdominal cavity, the surgeon places a rod or bridge beneath it. Although the bowel is usually opened by cauterization during surgery, the surgeon may wait 2 or 3 days postoperatively to open the bowel. Because there are no sensory nerve endings in the bowel wall, this procedure is essentially painless, except for some cramping. The surgeon usually indicates which is the proximal loop and which is the distal loop.

A colostomy may also be single-barreled or double-barreled. When only one loop end of bowel is opened onto the abdominal surface, the result is called an *end* or *single-barreled colostomy;* the client has only one stoma. An end colostomy is permanent if the bowel distal to it has been resected. A *double-barreled colostomy* is one in which both loops, distal and proximal, are open onto the abdominal wall. It may be closed later, depending on the disease present. A double-barreled colostomy can be two separate stomas, a loop with one stoma and two openings, or one stoma and a mucus fistula. The fistula expels mucus and is covered with a gauze dressing or pouch.

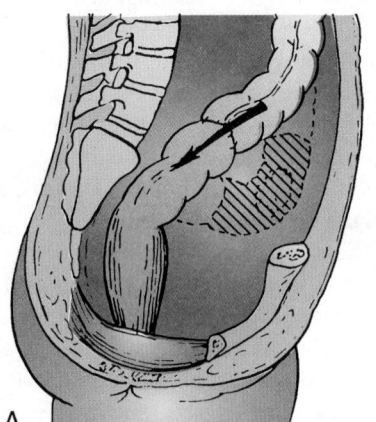 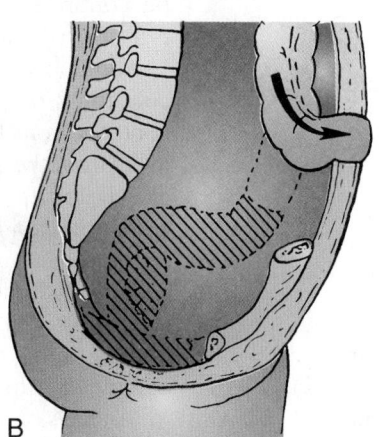 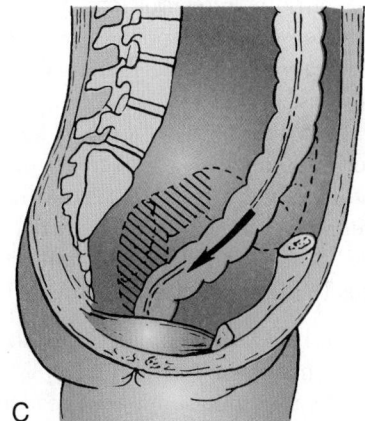

A   B   C

■ **FIGURE 33–12** Resecting malignant tumors in the rectosigmoid segment of the bowel. **A,** Anterior resection with primary anastomosis is used for cancer at any point in the bowel except the terminal rectum. Associated lymph nodes are resected. **B,** Abdominoperineal (anteroposterior) resection with formation of permanent colostomy (Miles' operation) for cancer involving the anus and terminal portion of the rectum. **C,** Proctosigmoidectomy with pull-through and preservation of external sphincter muscles is appropriate when the tumor is in the proximal rectum and unlikely to metastasize further.

Contraindications. Any health condition that makes the client a poor surgical risk is a contraindication to a colostomy procedure.

Complications. Suture line leakage with local or generalized peritonitis may occur in the early postoperative period. Other complications are hemorrhage and stomal necrosis, retraction, prolapse, and stenosis. Stomal complications may require additional surgery to revise the stoma.

Outcomes. The client resumes usual activities within 4 to 6 weeks and is able to perform self-care of the stoma. If needed, radiation therapy and chemotherapy are initiated.

Abdominal-Perineal Resection

Rectal tumors may require an abdominal-perineal resection, with the formation of a permanent or end colostomy. The affected colon and entire rectum are excised, and the anus is closed. The colon is removed through an abdominal incision, and the rectum through a perineal incision. Newer surgical techniques allow removal of low sigmoid tumors while leaving the rectal sphincter intact; normal bowel elimination is maintained.

Nursing Management of the Surgical Client

Preoperative Care

The client often presents with weight loss and a change in bowel habits. Obtain accurate descriptions of manifestations as well as an assessment of major risk factors, such as a family history of colon cancer, ulcerative colitis, or familial polyposis. Assess the abdomen, noting any abnormalities, such as pain, distention, and masses.

Preoperatively, a diet high in calories, protein, and carbohydrates but low in residue may be given to provide nutrition and reduce peristalsis. TPN may be necessary to provide nutrients and vitamins the client requires.

The bacteria level in the bowel must be lowered preoperatively to decrease the risk of infection. Clients needing a bowel resection must undergo a bowel preparation to minimize bacterial growth in the bowel and postoperative wound infection. This preparation usually involves the following:

- A low-residue or liquid diet to reduce the fecal contents of the bowel
- Oral administration of cathartics, such as polyethylene glycol–electrolyte solution (GoLYTELY) or a preprocedure bowel evacuator (Fleet Prep Kit), which is started at least 12 to 24 hours preoperatively

- Administration of antibiotics, such as sulfonamides and possibly neomycin and cephalexin, usually by mouth, for 12 to 48 hours preoperatively
- Administration of enemas to clean the bowel (the inside of the bowel lumen should be as clean and as bacteria free as possible)
- Blood transfusions to correct severe anemia and enhance wound healing

Identify the client's level of anxiety and provide supportive efforts. Explain all treatments and procedures fully. Clarify and reinforce the information provided by the physician. Encourage clients to ventilate their feelings and meet with health team members to discuss treatments and prognosis. The client also needs to know how treatment decisions will be made when the results of pathologic study are available and what to expect after the operation, such as placement of tubes and measures to prevent postoperative complications.

If a colostomy is necessary, an enterostomal therapy nurse should be asked to educate the client about the ostomy, answer questions, and advise about the optimal placement of the stoma. If an enterostomal therapy nurse is not available, assume the responsibility for teaching the client about the stoma. The risk of sexual dysfunction should be explained to the client in a supportive atmosphere.

Postoperative Care

Assessment. Immediate postoperative assessments are as discussed in Chapter 14. Assess for the return of peristalsis and GI motility indicated by passage of flatus; absence of abdominal pain, distention, bloating, nausea, and vomiting; and return of appetite. Recently, assessment of bowel sounds has been questioned as an indicator of bowel motility in postoperative abdominal surgery clients.[131] Gastric suction may be continued until peristalsis returns. Make sure the NG tube is patent.

Additionally, if a colostomy was created, monitor the colostomy output, and use special care to keep fecal contents from the colostomy (which contains bacteria) away from the surgical incision. Assess the client's stoma closely for the presence of stomal ischemia. The stoma should be red and moist. If it becomes dark or dusky, report this change to the surgeon immediately.

If an abdominoperineal resection with creation of an end colostomy is performed, assess both the abdominal and perineal wounds. The incision may be sutured completely closed; however, sometimes drains are left in the incision and may be attached to a suction device such as a Hemovac. When suction is not used, a Penrose drain can be placed in the wound. Change the dressing frequently or as ordered. A large amount of serous drainage can be expected from the perineal wound. It often takes several weeks to months for the wound to heal completely because of its size.

Diagnosis, Outcomes, Interventions
Diagnosis: Risk for Injury. The postoperative client is at risk for the development of postoperative complications. The nursing diagnosis is *Risk for Injury related to postoperative complications, including infection, hemorrhage, wound disruption, thrombophlebitis, and abnormal stomal function.*

Outcomes. The client does not experience an injury as evidenced by absence of manifestations of infection, bleeding, and evidence of wound disruption, thrombophlebitis, stomal ischemia, and bowel spillage.

Interventions
Monitor Vital Signs. Immediate postoperative interventions are the same as those used for any major abdominal procedure; they involve monitoring vital signs for manifestations of infection and shock.

Advance Diet as Tolerated. An NG tube is usually in place until peristalsis returns. It is usually several days before the NG tube is discontinued and the client begins to consume fluids and food. However, recent research findings suggest that clients may be started on foods earlier than previously considered feasible. Chewing gum has also been found to increase saliva production, which triggers gastrointestinal reactions that restore bowel function faster. As the client tolerates food, he or she is slowly advanced to a regular diet.

Decrease Cramping. Abdominal cramps commonly occur after surgery, as does distention of the bowel. Distention is uncomfortable and may put pressure on suture lines. The insertion of a rectal tube for 20 to 30 minutes per physician order will help if the rectum contains gas. Early ambulation helps to relieve distention and promotes peristalsis.

Apply Rectal Dressing. Prepare the client to wear a rectal dressing throughout the healing period. The character, volume, and odor of the drainage should be assessed. If the drainage in any way suggests a developing infection, arrange for a culture of the wound to identify the organism.

Occasionally, in the immediate postoperative period, sump drainage is placed in the perineal wound. This is also indicated if the wound becomes infected. The sump tube is attached to suction, allowing the wound to heal from its deepest portion without forming an abscess.

Reduce Pain. The perineal wound can be very painful, and the client should receive sufficient medication to control the pain. Once the packing is removed, the wound is irrigated, and the client should take a sitz bath three or four times a day. The client will find a side-lying position in bed most comfortable.

Monitor Stoma Drainage. There may be a colostomy pouch over the stoma. Make sure that this pouch is not applying pressure to the stoma, which would interfere with its blood supply. When changing or emptying the pouch, prevent contamination of the surgical wound by fecal discharges. Monitor the return of bowel function by observing the type and quantity of discharges from the stoma.

Prevent Thrombophlebitis

The high lithotomy position associated with the abdominoperineal resection is associated with an increased risk of development of postoperative phlebitis. To prevent this problem, subcutaneous injections of heparin, usually 5000 units every 12 hours after surgery, are often prescribed. Sequential pressure stockings or thigh-high anti-embolic hose also must be worn. The client must perform leg exercises before and after surgery. Monitor the client for manifestations of thrombophlebitis.

SAFETY

ALERT

Diagnosis: Risk for Disturbed Body Image. The client with an ostomy must face alterations in self-concept and body image. Write the nursing diagnosis as *Risk for Disturbed Body Image related to colostomy and lifestyle changes.*

Outcomes. The client adjusts to changes in body image as evidenced by the ability to identify and use effective coping methods in dealing with the disease and losses experienced.

Interventions. Give emotional support while the client begins the process of adjusting to the colostomy. It is also important to provide extensive teaching about how to care for the colostomy. The client's significant others also must adjust to the colostomy; help them by listening to their reactions and explaining the client's problems to them.

A client's reactions to a new colostomy may range from apparently easy acceptance to total withdrawal from social contacts. How well clients adjust depends partly on their attitudes toward excretory functions, previous knowledge about colostomies, and general ability to adjust to stressful situations.

Some clients refuse to look at the stoma and find it difficult to accept its presence, whereas others begin to participate in stoma care almost immediately. Your reactions to and manner toward the client and the care required can affect the client's adjustment. For some clients, the colostomy represents a "cure"; for others, it is palliation when the cancer has spread.

Continuing sexual relationships is a major concern for the client with a colostomy and the significant other. There is no physical reason that a client cannot enjoy normal sexual relations, although a small number of men become impotent after a radical perineal dissection. If this complication occurs, the physician may recommend a urology consultation to discuss treatment options for impotence (see Chapter 38). Psychological barriers may cause problems. With love, patience, understanding, and good hygienic practices, there should be no problem; however, it may be several months after surgery before a couple manages to reestablish a satisfactory sexual relationship. Referral to a social worker, counselor, psychiatric liaison, sex therapist, or registered nurse with a counseling background may be beneficial.

Diagnosis: Effective Therapeutic Regimen Management. The client with a colostomy needs to learn about self-care. The nursing diagnosis is *Effective Therapeutic Regimen Management related to colostomy care, irrigation, and possible complications associated with colostomies.*

Outcomes. The client understands care of the colostomy, as evidenced by the ability to (1) apply the pouch; (2) care for peristomal skin; (3) irrigate the colostomy, if applicable; and (4) prevent or treat any associated problems.

Interventions. Carefully assess the client's physical condition and emotional and mental attitudes toward the colostomy before attempting to teach ostomy self-care. Pace the teaching to the client's level of acceptance of the colostomy and ability to manage it.

Teach Ostomy Care. Teach the client how to apply the pouch to the stoma correctly. The client first should be taught how to examine the stoma. A healthy stoma is red and slightly raised. Figure 33-13 shows a colostomy during the application of an appliance. The skin around the stoma *(peristomal skin)* should be clear, without evidence of irritation. The peristomal area should be cleaned well with a mild soap and water and dried well before the new pouch is applied. The skin should be treated with a skin barrier and the new pouch applied, cut about $\frac{1}{16}$ to $\frac{1}{8}$ inch larger than the stoma. The pouch should be changed every 4 to 5 days or when leakage occurs. If a two-piece system is used, the faceplate may stay in place for 7 days.

Teach the client to empty the pouch when it is about half full and how to clean out the pouch when emptying it. The client should demonstrate the ability to empty and change the pouch independently before being discharged. See the earlier discussion of ileostomy care for further information.

Teach Stoma Irrigation. Clients with end sigmoid colostomies can be taught to regulate the colostomy

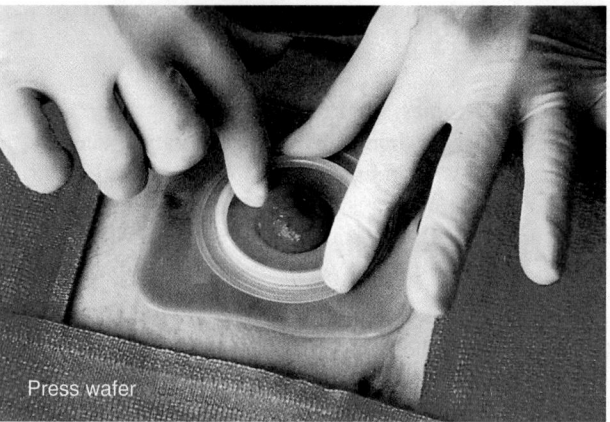

Press wafer

■ **FIGURE 33–13** Healthy stoma during application of wafer. Note that the stoma is red, moist, and healthy looking. The nurse is pressing the wafer onto the skin. The temperature of the client's skin warms the wafer to help it adhere to the client. *(Courtesy ConvaTec, Bristol-Myers Squibb, Skillman, NJ.)*

through regular irrigation. Clients who are physically, mentally, and emotionally capable should be encouraged to attempt irrigation and regulation. Some clients, despite irrigation, may never achieve regularity of elimination. If they have not achieved regularity within 6 months, they probably never will.

See the Client Education Guide on Colostomy Irrigation on the website for the steps involved in irrigation. The best time for irrigation is when the client formerly had a daily bowel movement because the bowel is already "trained" to evacuate at this time. If inserting the catheter proves difficult, let a little solution flow in and rotate the catheter. If the catheter will not go in, teach the client to apply gloves or a finger cot, lubricate the finger, and gently pass it into the stoma. This method often dislodges any feces that might be near the stoma. If the client cannot pass a catheter and no obstruction is felt digitally, the client should notify the health care provider.

If cramping occurs, the client should stop the solution temporarily, take a few deep breaths, and restart the solution slowly. The client should *never* (1) use more than 1000 ml, (2) irrigate the colostomy more than once a day, or (3) irrigate the colostomy if diarrhea is present.

If there is no return after irrigation, the client should ambulate, gently massage the abdomen, and try drinking some warm water. If there is still no return, the client should apply a pouch and try the irrigation again the next day. If there is no return the second day, the client should notify the health care provider.

Minimize Flatus. Flatus is an embarrassing problem because the client may have no control over its passage and no sensations to indicate when it is about to pass. Flatus can make clients avoid social situations. Clients can be taught how to muffle the passage of gas from their colostomies. Women may hold their purses or arms, and men their folded jackets or hats, over the stoma to muffle the noise. Odor-proof pouches and pouches with charcoal filter disks are available, but the most satisfactory way to control flatus is through diet. Because everyone is different, clients must learn by trial and error which foods cause gas. In general, nuts, corn, cabbage, sauerkraut, broccoli, cauliflower, and legumes are gas-forming foods. Swallowing air by eating too rapidly, chewing gum, and drinking carbonated beverages also cause intestinal gas.

Evaluation. The client should recover from surgery without complications and should resume usual activities within 6 weeks. When a colostomy has been performed, the client should be able to manage it within 2 months. If the client is unable to accomplish self-care, the need for further teaching should be explored.

Self-Care

In preparation for discharge, clients need support and knowledgeable advice as they learn to live with their colostomies. The client needs to know the nearest location for purchase of ostomy supplies (see the Client Education Guide on Ostomy Supplies on the website). *evolve* Immediately after dismissal, home delivery of supplies may be necessary. The enterostomal therapy nurse can help the client learn to manage and accept the ostomy and to achieve a smooth transition from the health care facility to the home. Some cities have established ostomy rehabilitation clinics to help clients, and most large communities have an ostomy association that maintains contact with the American Cancer Society. These support groups are helpful because clients can share their ostomy concerns with others who have similar problems. A home health care referral can add to the client's peace of mind, identify problems that might not otherwise be known, and ensure necessary follow-up care. The Bridge to Home Health Care feature below explores how to help clients adjust to having a colostomy.

BRIDGE TO HOME HEALTH CARE

Adjusting to Life with a Colostomy

When you visit a client who has a new colostomy, assess the stoma and peristomal skin thoroughly before selecting a pouch. The stoma should be beefy red; a pale red or pale pink stoma indicates a limited blood supply. A healthy stoma is moist; dryness suggests dehydration. Note whether the outer edges are intact and attached to the peristomal skin. The stoma should be round and raised; it will shrink during the next 4 to 6 weeks. Assess the stoma when the pouch is off and the client is lying down; repeat when the client sits. Watch for (1) changes in stoma shape, (2) skin folds, (3) creases, and (4) dimpling of the peristomal skin.

Clients and caregivers are more likely to manage a colostomy independently if they understand and follow your instructions and participate in care. Demonstrate how to clean the stoma; request return demonstrations. Some bleeding is normal; applying pressure should stop the bleeding. Excessive bleeding is abnormal; if this happens, a physician should be called immediately. Tell the client and caregiver to expect output (effluent) daily. The effluent will be runny initially but will thicken within 2 to 4 weeks. Expect excessive flatulence (bowel gas) for 4 to 8 weeks. Teach clients and caregivers to watch for manifestations of intestinal obstruction that require immediate medical care, such as nausea or vomiting, body temperature exceeding 101° F, severe abdominal pain, distention, limited or no output, and decreased bowel sounds.

Leakage is a common problem. To minimize leakage, provide detailed instructions about pouch fit and care; the pouch should be changed twice a week. *Do not* assume that the appliance the client took home from the hospital will fit when the stoma

shrinks. If the peristomal skin retracts, the client needs a pouch with a convex wafer, not a flat wafer. If the stoma is round, you may use a precut pouch; if it is not round, use a cut-to-fit pouch. Make and date a pattern of the stoma by tracing the outline of the stoma on a clear piece of rigid plastic with an indelible marker. Cut out the pattern and check it for proper fit against the stoma; it may not fit when the stoma shrinks. Use an ostomy belt that is snug but not tight to improve the bond between the pouch and peristomal skin. If the client is using a two-piece pouch system, make sure that there is a good seal between the pouch and the wafer.

To reinforce instructions between your visits, leave simple, step-by-step directions for pouch changing for clients and caregivers. Also leave written details about purchasing ostomy supplies locally or by mail order. Provide verbal and written diet and hydration information. Suggest that the client avoid foods high in fiber initially, such as corn, popcorn, mushrooms, peanuts, and Chinese foods; these foods can cause the bowel to swell and become obstructed. When the swelling decreases in 4 to 8 weeks, clients should be able to gradually resume eating a regular diet. At this time, clients should also increase fluid consumption to prevent constipation.

Refer clients with a colostomy and their family members to organizations that can help them cope with the colostomy diagnosis and changed body image, such as the United Ostomy Association of America (1-800-826-0826); the American Cancer Society (1-800-227-2345); and the Wound, Ostomy, and Continence Nurses Society (1-888-224-9626). Nurse members of the last group can provide valuable information about resuming a normal lifestyle and can help manage complicated ostomies.

Before discharge, advise clients that it may take several weeks for them to regain their strength after major bowel surgery; further, when segments have been removed from the bowel, bowel habits may alter until the body adjusts to the situation. You may need to teach the client and his or her significant others how to change dressings at home because wounds may not be healed totally by the time the client is discharged. In general, teaching should cover (1) dressing changes, (2) dietary or activity restrictions, (3) colostomy care if applicable, and (4) manifestations of intestinal obstruction and perforation.

The client who is having a problem with the colostomy should see an enterostomal therapy nurse. The client with an abdominoperineal resection needs follow-up from the surgeon to ensure that the perineal wound is healing properly.

OTHER DISORDERS OF THE LARGE AND SMALL BOWEL

HERNIATIONS

A *hernia* is the abnormal protrusion of an organ, tissue, or part of an organ through the structure that normally contains it. Hernias most commonly occur in the abdominal cavity when a section of the bowel protrudes through as a result of a congenital or acquired weakness of abdominal musculature. Hernias can occur at any age and in either gender. About 700,000 inguinal herniorrhaphies are performed in the United States each year. Indirect inguinal hernias, the most common type, typically occur in men. Direct inguinal hernias are found more commonly in older people. Incisional or ventral hernias occur most often in clients who had poor wound healing after surgery. Obese or pregnant clients are more likely to develop umbilical hernias.

Etiology and Risk Factors

Hernias develop when there is a defect in the integrity of the muscular wall accompanied by increased intra-abdominal pressure. Congenital muscle weakness is one risk factor, as are any factors that increase intra-abdominal pressure. The muscle weakness cannot be prevented, but exercises can be performed to strengthen weak muscles. Because obesity is one cause of increased intra-abdominal pressure, such an increase can be prevented by weight control. Avoiding heavy lifting and straining also reduces intra-abdominal pressure. Early diagnosis is important to prevent incarceration and strangulation of the herniated tissue.

Pathophysiology

Defects in the muscular wall may be congenital and caused by weakened tissue or a wide space at the inguinal ligament, or may be caused by trauma. Intra-abdominal pressure increases with pregnancy, obesity, heavy lifting, coughing, and traumatic injuries from blunt pressure. When two of these factors coexist with some tissue weakness, a hernia may occur. Increased pressure without a weakness is not likely to cause a hernia. Weakness, in addition to being present from birth, is acquired as part of the aging process. As clients age, muscular tissues become infiltrated and are replaced by adipose and connective tissues.

When the contents of the hernial sac can be replaced into the abdominal cavity by manipulation, the hernia is said to be *reducible*. *Irreducible* and *incarcerated* are terms that refer to a hernia in which the contents of the sac cannot be reduced or replaced by manipulation.

When pressure from the hernial ring (the ring of muscular tissue through which the bowel protrudes) cuts off the blood supply to the herniated segment of bowel, the bowel becomes *strangulated*. Incarcerated hernias usually become strangulated. This situation is a surgical emergency because unless the bowel is released, it soon becomes gangrenous because of the lack of blood supply.

Hernias can penetrate through any defect in the abdominal wall, through the diaphragm, or through some internal structure within the abdominal cavity (Figure 33-14). This discussion covers only the more common types of hernias: inguinal (both indirect and direct), femoral, umbilical, and incisional. (Hiatal hernia is discussed in Chapter 30.)

Indirect Inguinal Hernia

An indirect inguinal herniation occurs through the inguinal ring and follows the spermatic cord through the inguinal canal. It is more common in males than females because of the space allowed for the testicles to descend. There is a high incidence of indirect inguinal hernia in young people. The incidence is also high among clients 50 to 60 years of age and then gradually decreases in older age groups. These hernias can become extremely large and often descend into the scrotum.

Direct Inguinal Hernia

In a direct inguinal hernia, bowel passes through the abdominal wall in an area of muscular weakness, not through a canal, as do indirect inguinal and femoral hernias. This type of hernia is more common in older clients. Direct inguinal hernia gradually develops in an area that is weak because of a congenital deficiency in the number of fibers it contains.

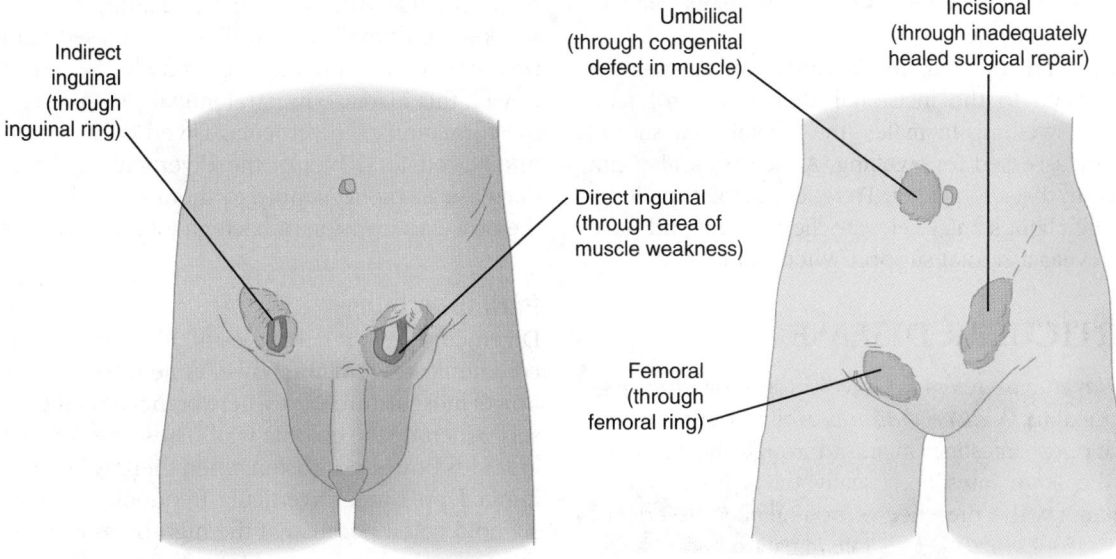

■ **FIGURE 33–14** Common types of herniation.

Femoral Hernia

A femoral hernia occurs through the femoral ring and is more common in females than in males. It begins as a plug of fat in the femoral canal that enlarges and gradually pulls the peritoneum, and almost inevitably the urinary bladder, into the sac. There is a high incidence of incarceration and strangulation with this type of hernia.

Umbilical Hernia

Umbilical herniation in the adult is more common in women and is due to increased abdominal pressure. It usually occurs in obese clients and in multiparous women.

Incisional or Ventral Hernia

The incisional or ventral hernia occurs at the site of a previous surgical incision that has healed inadequately because of a postoperative problem, such as infection, inadequate nutrition, extreme distention, or obesity.

OUTCOME MANAGEMENT

Medical Management

Hernias that are not strangulated or incarcerated can be mechanically reduced. A truss, a firm pad held in place by a belt, also can be used to keep the hernia reduced. The pad is placed over the hernia after it has been reduced and is left in place to prevent the hernia from recurring. The client is taught to apply the truss daily before arising. The client should carefully inspect the skin under the truss for any manifestation of breakdown. "Watchful waiting" is an acceptable option for men with inguinal hernias that are minimally symptomatic.

Surgical Management

Inguinal hernia repairs (herniorrhaphies) are common, occurring in an estimated 28 of every 10,000 population in the United States. A hernia repair is performed using a small incision directly over the weakened area. The intestine is then returned to the perineal cavity, the hernia sac is excised, and the muscle is closed tightly over the area. Mesh may facilitate healing and prevent recurrence. Hernias in the inguinal region are usually repaired with the use of spinal or local anesthesia. Most hernia repairs are now performed as outpatient procedures. Laparoscopic extraperitoneal (LEP) herniorrhaphy is a newer technique that results in higher success rates with less recurrence, less pain, and shorter postoperative recovery periods.

Some repairs are difficult because there is insufficient muscle mass to keep the intestines in place. In this case, mesh grafts are used to reinforce the area of herniation. Clients with difficult repairs are usually hospitalized for 1 to 2 days to receive prophylactic antibiotics.

Nursing Management of the Surgical Client

Make certain the client voids after hernia surgery because urinary retention is a common problem, especially in males. Return the client to a general diet as soon as the client can tolerate food. When general anesthesia is used, postoperative progress is slower. Assure the client that during the immediate postoperative period, the hernia will not recur. Some clients hesitate to become active because of this fear. The client should be told not to engage in any lifting for 4 to 6 weeks after surgery. Obese clients progress more slowly, heal more slowly, and may need more encouragement to participate in postoperative activities.

Following an inguinal hernia repair, an ice pack is usually applied to the incisional area to control pain and reduce swelling. In males, the scrotal area should be carefully assessed for swelling. An ice pack also can be applied to the scrotal area. To reduce scrotal swelling, position the client so as to elevate the scrotum and have the client wear a scrotal support when out of bed.

DIVERTICULAR DISEASE

Diverticular disease refers to two disorders: diverticulosis and diverticulitis. A *diverticulum* is a blind out-pouching or herniation of intestinal mucosa through the muscular coat of the large intestine, usually the sigmoid colon. *Diverticulosis* is the presence of noninflamed diverticula (Figure 33-15). *Diverticulitis* is inflammation and obstruction of a colonic diverticulum. Perforation may occur because of the increased intraluminal pressure. Diverticulitis is common in obese clients and affects 50% of men and women over 50 years of age and almost 75% of those over 80 years of age. It is estimated, however, that only 20% of those with diverticulitis will develop manifestations of disease. Although diverticula may be found all through the bowel, 85% of diverticulitis arises in the sigmoid and descending colon.

Etiology and Risk Factors

Low-fiber diets have been implicated in the development of diverticula because such diets decrease bulk in the stool and predispose to constipation. The etiology of diverticular disease is related mainly to two factors: weakening of the bowel wall and increased intraluminal pressure. In the presence of muscle weakness in the bowel, this increase in intraluminal pressure can lead to the formation of diverticula. Diverticulitis occurs when undigested food blocks the diverticulum, leading to a decrease in blood supply to the area and predisposing the bowel to invasion of bacteria into the diverticulum.

Pathophysiology

Diverticula have a narrow neck, like that of a flask, that communicates with the bowel lumen. Weak points in the bowel musculature exist where branches of the blood vessels penetrate the colonic wall. These weak points create areas for bowel protrusion when there is increased intraluminal pressure. Diverticula frequently develop in the sigmoid colon because of the high pressures required in this area to move the stool into the rectum.

Diverticulitis may be acute or chronic. If the diverticulum is not infected, it causes few problems. When fecaliths do not liquefy and drain from the diverticulum, however, they may become trapped, causing irritation and inflammation (diverticulitis). The inflamed area becomes congested with blood and may bleed or perforate. Chronic diverticulitis results in increased scarring and eventual narrowing of the bowel lumen, potentially causing obstruction.

Diagnosis of acute diverticulitis can be confirmed by plain film of the abdomen if free perforation is present, and computed tomography (CT) with contrast may identify an abscess or fistula. Sigmoidoscopy is of little diagnostic value since the disease is usually extraluminal.

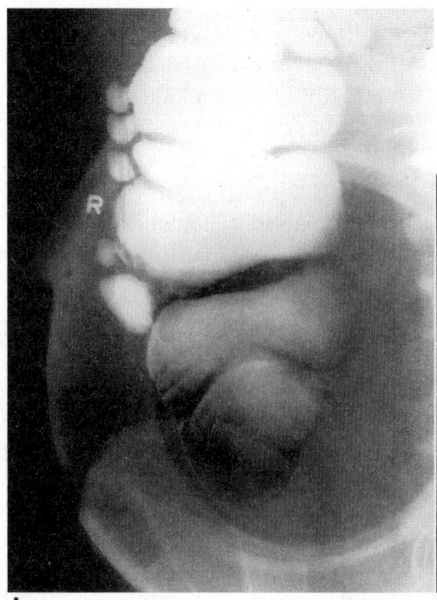
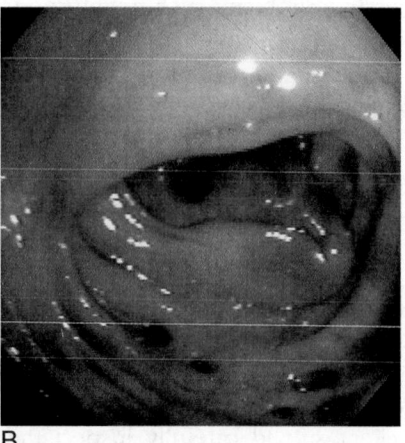

A   B

■ **FIGURE 33–15 A,** A barium enema showing right-sided diverticulosis. **B,** Endoscopic appearance of a diverticulum in the right colon. *(A courtesy of Mark Feldman, MD; B from Feldman, M., Friedman, L.S., & Sleisenger, M.H. [2002]. Sleisenger & Fordtran's gastrointestinal and liver disease: Pathophysiology/diagnosis/management [7th ed., Vol. 2]. Philadelphia: Saunders.)*

Clinical Manifestations

The manifestations of diverticulitis depend on the extent of the inflammation and the site of occurrence. Discomfort consists of dull, episodic, or steady left lower quadrant or midabdominal pain. Assessment also reveals alteration in bowel habits (constipation, diarrhea, or both), increased flatus, anorexia, abdominal distention, and low-grade fever. Localized tenderness may occur in the left lower quadrant. A mass may be palpable on abdominal examination. The inflammatory process usually subsides within several weeks.

Although free perforation is rare, if the infection penetrates the pelvic floor or retroperitoneal tissues, abscesses may result. The client may present with manifestations of sepsis including hemodynamic compromise and deterioration of mental status. Extension of the inflammation to adjacent organs can lead to fistulae of the bladder or vagina and peritonitis. Repeated inflammation can result in narrowing and obstruction of the bowel.

Trace blood may be found in the stools, but profuse bleeding is uncommon. Stools also may contain mucus. Urinary frequency can occur if the inflammation is in the proximity of the bladder. Straining, coughing, or lifting causes an increase in intra-abdominal pressure and manifestations such as diarrhea, constipation, pain, mucus, and flatus. The clinician may palpate a tender mass on digital rectal examinations.

OUTCOME MANAGEMENT

Medical Management

Asymptomatic diverticular disease requires no specific therapy other than diet modification. Mild disease can be treated by adherence to a high-fiber diet and prevention of constipation with bran and bulk laxatives (hydrophilic colloids). Advise clients to notify the physician of any change in bowel movement pattern (constipation or diarrhea) or character (the presence of mucus or blood) or if fever, abdominal pain, or urinary manifestations develop.

Diverticulitis may be treated conservatively with medical intervention by allowing the colon to rest. Clients with acute diverticulitis are assigned to NPO status, may have an NG tube, and receive parenteral fluids and antibiotics until pain, inflammation, and temperature decrease. If opioids are required for pain management, meperidine is the drug of choice. Morphine sulfate should be avoided because it has been shown to cause spasm of the colon. When the acute episode subsides, oral liquids and, later, a progressively more inclusive diet can be added. Nursing care involves the preceding interventions and teaching the client about diet changes.

Surgical Management

About 20% of clients with diverticulitis will require surgery. Surgery is indicated for diverticular disease with complications such as hemorrhage, obstruction, abscesses, and perforation. Surgical procedures usually involve ligation and removal of the sac or resection of involved bowel if complications develop. With abscess or obstruction, the surgeon performs a colon resection with a temporary colostomy, which is left in place until the client's condition improves. For some clients, the temporary colostomy alone allows the bowel to rest and heal. For nursing care, see the earlier discussion of bowel resection.

MECKEL'S DIVERTICULUM

Meckel's diverticulum is a congenital sacculation on the antimesenteric border of the ileum. It is the most common and significant congenital anomaly of the small intestine. It occurs within 60 to 100 cm from the ileocecal valve in adults, is approximately 5 cm in length, and has a diameter smaller than that of the ileum but significantly larger than that of the appendix. The diverticulum has all the layers of the normal intestine and the mucosa is similar to that of the adjoining ileum. Of the Meckel's diverticula that become symptomatic, half contain ectopic gastric, duodenal, pancreatic, biliary, or colonic tissue.

The gastric mucosal lining sometimes ulcerates and bleeds or perforates. In addition, the diverticulum may become inflamed and may mimic appendicitis. Meckel's diverticulum is sometimes attached to the umbilicus by a fibrous band and may be the focus around which the bowel twists, causing obstruction. Treatment involves surgical excision of the diverticulum.

INTESTINAL OBSTRUCTION

Partial or complete impairment of the forward flow of intestinal contents is known as an *intestinal obstruction*. About 90% of bowel obstructions occur in the small bowel, especially in the ileum, which is the narrowest segment.

> **Obstructions of the small intestine are a common surgical emergency. Large bowel obstructions usually occur in the sigmoid colon. The mortality rate for acute obstruction in the small bowel is 10% and in the large bowel, 30%. Obstruction produces nausea, vomiting, dehydration, and severe pain. Intestinal obstruction has a high mortality rate if it is not diagnosed and treated within 24 hours.**

SAFETY ⚠ ALERT

Etiology and Risk Factors

Obstruction of the small intestine may be caused by narrowing of the intestinal lumen as a result of inflammation, cancer, adhesions, hernia, volvulus, intussusception, food blockage, or compression from outside the intestine. Paralytic ileus (see later discussion), vascular problems such as mesenteric embolus and thrombus, and hypokalemia from diuretics or antihypertensive agents also may result in small bowel obstructions. Lobar pneumonia, peritonitis, and pancreatitis frequently produce an ileus (see later discussion) of infectious origin.

Cancer accounts for about 80% of obstructions of the large intestine, with most occurring in the sigmoid colon. Other causes are diverticulitis, ulcerative colitis, and previous abdominal surgery. Factors that cause intestinal obstructions may be mechanical, neurogenic, or vascular.

Mechanical Factors

Adhesions

Adhesions are probably the most common cause of obstruction in both the small and large intestines. Adhesions form after abdominal surgery, and for unknown reasons, some clients have massive adhesions. Irritants that remain in the abdomen following surgical procedures enhance the formation of adhesions. These fibrous bands of scar tissue can become looped over a portion of the bowel. The loops then can become either the focus around which the bowel can twist *(volvulus)* (Figure 33-16) or the band that mechanically obstructs the bowel by external pressure. The presence of multiple adhesions increases the risk of obstruction.

Hernia

An incarcerated hernia may or may not cause obstruction, depending on the size of the hernial ring; however, the potential for obstruction is always present in any hernia. A strangulated hernia is always obstructed because the bowel cannot function when its blood supply is cut off.

Volvulus

Volvulus is a twisting of the bowel that commonly occurs about a stationary focus (e.g., tumor or Meckel's

diverticulum) in the abdominal cavity (see Figure 33-16). It can cause infarction of the bowel and can occur in either the large or the small bowel. Volvulus sometimes can be corrected without surgical intervention. Successful decompression of the bowel with a long tube (Cantor or Miller-Abbott tube) releases pressure against the proximal end of the loop, thus allowing a small bowel volvulus to relax.

Intussusception

Intussusception, which sometimes complicates IBD, is a telescoping of the bowel (slipping of a section of bowel into an adjacent section) (Figure 33-17). The condition is often associated with tumor of the large bowel. Peristaltic action telescopes the proximal bowel into the bowel distal to it. Intramural lesions often cause intussusception.

Cancers

Cancer accounts for about 80% of mechanical obstructions in the large bowel and mostly affects the sigmoid colon. Carcinogenesis is slow and, because of the large lumen of the bowel, may become advanced before a fecal mass lodges at the constricted site and precipitates an acute obstructive process. In the small bowel, obstructive manifestations are frequently the first indication of a tumor. Even though the lumen of the small bowel is smaller, manifestations do not appear early in the process because the intestinal contents are liquid.

Neurogenic Factors

Neurogenic factors are responsible for an adynamic (or functional) obstruction, the most common type of intestinal obstruction. An adynamic obstruction, also called *paralytic ileus,* is caused by lack of peristaltic activity and commonly occurs after abdominal surgery. The bowel ceases to function for longer than 72 hours as a result of the sympathetic nervous system's response to an insult to the peritoneum. Extensive surgical procedures in the bowel and in the retroperitoneal area may cause a postoperative neurogenic problem. Additional

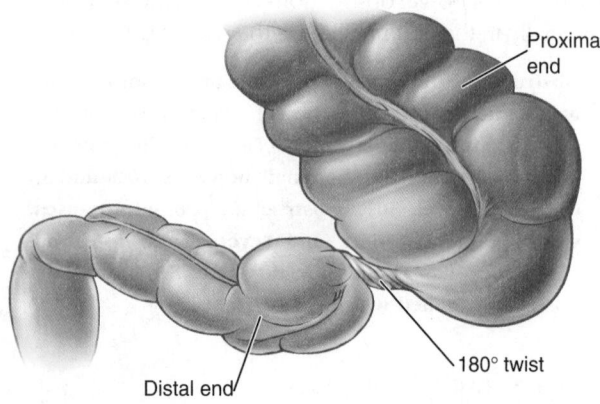

■ **FIGURE 33–16** Volvulus. Intestine twists at least 180 degrees, causing obstruction and ischemia.

Proximal end

Distal end

180° twist

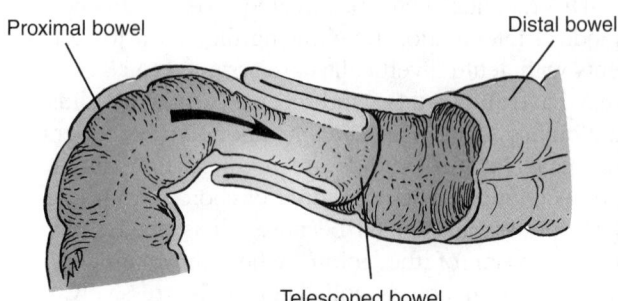

■ **FIGURE 33–17** Intussusception. A portion of bowel telescopes into adjacent (usually distal) bowel.

Proximal bowel

Distal bowel

Telescoped bowel

causes of adynamic ileus are trauma, hypokalemia, myocardial infarction, and vascular insufficiency. Treatment involves aspiration of secretions by NG suction until the bowel begins to function.

Vascular Factors

When the blood supply to any part of the body is interrupted, the part ceases to function and pain occurs. Blood is supplied to the bowel by way of the celiac and superior and inferior mesenteric arteries. These vessels have anastomotic intercommunications at the head of the pancreas and along the transverse bowel. Obstruction of blood flow can arise as a result of complete occlusion *(mesenteric infarction)* or partial occlusion *(abdominal angina)*.

Complete Occlusion (Mesenteric Infarction)

Any occlusion of arterial blood supply to the bowel, as in mesenteric thrombosis, effectively stops bowel function. The usual cause is an embolus. An acute occlusion, at its onset, causes intense abdominal pain. Usually, there are no manifestations of advanced intestinal obstruction because the pain results from ischemic tissue rather than from obstruction. Ischemia is the most serious result of intestinal obstruction because as the process advances, fever, leukocytosis, shock, peritonitis, and other manifestations of bowel gangrene appear. Ischemia renders the bowel more permeable, allowing *E. coli* and *Klebsiella,* part of the normal bowel flora, to penetrate the intestinal wall and enter the peritoneal cavity.

> **Acute mesenteric obstruction constitutes a surgical emergency and carries a high mortality rate (about 75%). Surgical intervention must be initiated early. Sometimes an embolectomy can restore circulation. The surgeon also must resect necrotic (dead) segments of the bowel.**

Partial Occlusion (Abdominal Angina)

Abdominal angina usually results from atherosclerosis of the mesenteric arteries, a common although often asymptomatic problem found in 33% of routine autopsies. Because there is a greater need for oxygenation during the digestive process, pain may develop 15 to 30 minutes after eating in a client with abdominal angina. Initially, pain may occur only after ingestion of a large meal. As the atherosclerosis becomes more widespread, however, it may occur even after a small meal, and eventually the pain becomes almost continuous.

Manifestations arise only when interruption of blood supply is sufficient to compromise bowel function. At this time, in addition to pain after eating, assessment reveals a change in bowel habits, nausea and vomiting, and weight loss as a result of the client's restriction of intake to avoid the discomfort of eating. Vascular or bypass grafts can sometimes improve the blood supply to the affected portion of the bowel.

Pathophysiology

Normally, the bowel secretes 7 to 8 L of electrolyte-rich fluid, and most of the fluid is reabsorbed. When the bowel is obstructed, this fluid is partially retained within the bowel and partially eliminated by vomiting, causing severe reduction in circulating blood volume, which results in hypotension, hypovolemic shock, and diminished renal and cerebral blood flow. Because fluid is lost but blood cells are not, hematocrit and hemoglobin values rise, thus increasing the potential for vascular occlusive disorders such as coronary, cerebral, and mesenteric thromboses.

For instance, with the onset of an obstruction, fluids and air collect proximal to the site of the problem, causing distention. Compared with the large bowel, manifestations occur sooner and are more intense in a small bowel blockage because the small bowel is narrower and normally more active. The large volume of secretions from the small bowel adds to the distention. The only significant secretion from the large bowel is mucus.

Distention causes a temporary increase in peristalsis as the bowel attempts to force the material through the obstructed area. Within a few hours, the increased peristalsis ends and the bowel becomes flaccid, thus reducing pressure within the lumen and slowing the process caused by the obstruction. Greater pressure within the bowel reduces its absorptive ability, which increases the fluid retention still further. Soon the intraluminal pressure reduces venous return, increasing venous pressure, congestion, and vessel fragility. This process in turn raises capillary permeability and allows plasma to extravasate (escape) into the bowel lumen and the peritoneal cavity. The bowel wall becomes permeable to bacteria, and bowel organisms enter the peritoneal cavity. Rising pressure in the bowel wall soon slows arterial blood flow, causing necrosis and, in some cases, toxemia and peritonitis.

Strangulation of the bowel results in decreased arterial blood supply. Necrosis and perforation may force the intestinal contents into the peritoneal cavity, causing peritonitis. Bacteria proliferate in the strangulated bowel and may form endotoxins. When the endotoxins are released into the peritoneal cavity or systemic circulation, there is rapid circulatory collapse with endotoxic shock, accounting for the high mortality rate associated with this condition. These complications are especially likely to occur in older adults, who tend to have atherosclerotic narrowing of these vessels, making thrombosis more likely.

Clinical Manifestations

Manifestations of intestinal obstruction depend on the level and length of bowel involved, the extent to which the obstruction interferes with blood supply, the completeness of the obstruction, and the type of lesion producing the obstruction. Local changes in the bowel wall include congestion, fragility, reduced circulation, and increased pressure. Increased pressure leads to reverse peristalsis, producing vomiting that helps prevent overdistention of the bowel. These local effects result from (1) loss of fluids, electrolytes, and plasma; (2) bacterial proliferation; and (3) perforation. Systemic effects include a reduction in extracellular fluid and circulating blood volume, toxemia, and peritonitis.

The client with small bowel obstruction typically experiences abdominal pain in rhythmically recurring waves. The pain results from distention and the small intestine's peristaltic efforts to push its contents past the obstruction. Small intestinal pain is felt in the upper and midabdomen, whereas colonic pain is experienced in the lower abdomen. Soon after the small intestine becomes distended, the peristaltic waves are visible, accompanied by high-pitched tinkling sounds. Vomiting is almost always present, with the frequency corresponding to the anatomic location of the obstruction. Vomiting often brings some relief from the pain if the obstruction is high or proximal to the ileum.

If the obstruction is distal to the ileum, vomiting fails to empty the bowel completely, allowing the accumulation of fluids, residue, and gases. As the muscles become atonic, loops of small bowel dilate, compounding the problem of distention. Eventually, severe distention may raise the diaphragm, thereby inhibiting respirations. Hypoxia (resulting from inadequate respirations, decreased circulating blood volume, and hypotension) often develops. Vomiting is more severe if the obstruction is located high in the small bowel. At first, vomitus is composed of semidigested food and chyme; later, it becomes watery and contains bile. Finally, the client vomits dark fecal material, the result of bacterial growth in the fluid that has stagnated in the obstructed bowel.

When the colon is obstructed, the competent ileocecal valve prevents regurgitation (and vomiting), and pressure within the lumen increases, resulting in distention. The cecum may perforate. Obstruction of the colon results in imbalanced bowel habits, lower abdominal pain, a desire to defecate, distention, and borborygmi. In the presence of an incompetent ileocecal valve, distention progresses to the small intestine. Vomiting that accompanies large intestine obstruction is a very late manifestation that occurs only from a distended small intestine.

Clients with vomiting may experience severe fluid and electrolyte imbalances. They lose not only water but also sodium, chloride, potassium, and bicarbonate. The result is an acute extracellular volume deficit (dehydration), which in turn lowers the circulating blood volume. Hydrogen ion imbalances frequently occur in intestinal obstructions, with metabolic acidosis being the most common problem. Initially vital signs may be normal, but tachycardia suggests not only dehydration but possible bowel ischemia as well.

Specific diagnostic tests for possible bowel obstruction consist of a plain x-ray film (which shows gas shadows), barium or radiopaque x-ray studies, and complete blood studies. Increased hemoglobin and hematocrit values may indicate dehydration. Leukocytosis may point to a strangulated bowel. A decrease in sodium, potassium, and chloride levels and a rise in nonprotein nitrogen and blood urea nitrogen (BUN) levels may indicate small bowel obstruction.

OUTCOME MANAGEMENT

Medical Management

Decompress the Bowel

The major treatment for an intestinal obstruction is the insertion of an intestinal tube (see Chapter 31). Often an intestinal tube both decompresses the bowel and breaks up the obstruction.

In adynamic ileus, the best intervention is bowel rest and prevention of distention by gastric suction. Medications are not effective in stimulating bowel activity. The bowel will respond when it recovers completely from the effects of obstruction.

Nursing Management of the Medical Client

Assessment. Obtain a complete history of the onset of manifestations, eating patterns, food tolerance, vomiting episodes, stools (number per day and appearance), distention, and factors that increase or decrease pain.

During physical assessment, note abdominal distention, the quality of bowel sounds, the presence and extent of dehydration, and manifestations of abdominal pain, such as muscle guarding. A lack of bowel sounds indicates peritoneal irritation or adynamic ileus. Usually, in the case of bowel obstruction, auscultation reveals high-pitched peristaltic rushes with high, metallic tinkling sounds.

Diagnosis, Outcomes, Interventions

Diagnosis: Deficient Fluid Volume. A priority nursing diagnosis for the client with an intestinal obstruction is *Deficient Fluid Volume related to vomiting, decreased intestinal reabsorption of fluid, and decreased intestinal secretions.*

Outcomes. The client maintains fluid balance, as evidenced by balanced intake and output, no manifestations of dehydration, and blood pressure measurements within the client's normal range.

Interventions

Maintain Fluid Balance. Maintain good fluid balance in the client with an obstruction by carefully replacing fluids and electrolytes. Administer parenteral fluids with sodium chloride, bicarbonate, and potassium added as ordered.

Decompress the Bowel. An intestinal tube is inserted and attached to suction to relieve the vomiting and distention. If the obstruction is not mechanical, an intestinal tube can achieve decompression. If the obstruction is due to adhesions, hernia, or tumors, the tube stops at the point of obstruction and keeps the bowel decompressed above the obstruction.

Note the progress of an intestinal tube, the amount and type of drainage, and whether or not relief of distention and nausea occurs. Assess and measure drainage from the intestinal tube; document color, odor, consistency, and volume. Inform the physician of blood levels of sodium, potassium, and bicarbonate, and the pH of the blood, all of which reflect fluid and electrolyte balance.

Provide Discharge Teaching. For dismissal following medical resolution of the obstruction, the client needs to learn ways to prevent recurrence and to maintain bowel elimination. The client must be seen by a primary health care provider at intervals after the obstruction is relieved to confirm that it has not recurred. The client's nutritional status also should be monitored to ensure that adequate nutrition is maintained.

Evaluation. Once the obstruction is relieved medically, bowel function should return to normal within a matter of days. If the obstruction cannot be relieved medically, surgery is required.

Surgical Management

If intestinal intubation does not relieve the obstruction, surgery is the only remaining option. The major objective in treating bowel obstruction is to relieve the cause and thus eliminate the problem; however, the cause is not always immediately obvious. Diagnosis of the cause of the acute abdominal condition may be difficult and commonly can be made only during surgery. Document specific observations to aid in the diagnosis.

In most vascular and mechanical obstructions, surgical excision of the cause is the only intervention. Surgery relieves the obstruction and removes any ischemic bowel. Relieving the obstruction should reestablish bowel patency. The type of surgery depends on the location and type of obstruction. The surgeon may perform bowel resection, colostomy, or a bypass procedure.

Nursing Management of the Surgical Client

Assessment of the surgical client is the same as assessment of the medical client. In addition, routine preoperative and postoperative assessments are required. Additional nursing interventions are the same as those discussed for other GI procedures.

IRRITABLE BOWEL SYNDROME

Irritable bowel syndrome (IBS) is a functional disorder of motility in the intestine. There is no organic disease or anatomic abnormality, nor are there any genetic markers. It is not life-threatening, nor is it associated with development of cancer. Other descriptive names for this condition are spastic colon, irritable colon, nervous indigestion, spastic colitis, intestinal neurosis, and laxative or cathartic "colitis." IBS is the most common GI disorder in Western society with a prevalence of 10% to 15%, accounting for 50% of subspecialty referrals and the writing of more than five million prescriptions annually. In the United States, three of every four of those affected are women. It is most often diagnosed between the ages of 30 and 50, although 50% of those affected report that they had clinical manifestations in childhood. Although approximately 70% of the clients who meet diagnostic criteria do not seek medical care, it still accounts for 12% of primary care visits and is the second leading cause of missed workdays.

Etiology and Risk Factors

The exact mechanism of IBS is not clear, but it is believed to be a result of an abnormality in the communication between the enteric nervous system and the central nervous system. Other factors that are believed to contribute to development of the syndrome include altered gut motility (exaggerated response to stimuli) and visceral hypersensitivity, psychosocial factors, and neurotransmitter imbalance. Clients at risk for IBS are those who consume diets high in fat, gas-producing foods, lactose, carbonated beverages, caffeine, and alcohol. Also at risk are clients who smoke, are lactose intolerant, have high stress in their lives, or complain of alterations in sleep and rest. Recent studies have suggested a relationship between childhood sexual abuse and IBS in women and overgrowth of bacteria in the small intestine in clients with IBS.

Health promotion strategies are to instruct clients to consume a high-fiber, low-fat, well-balanced diet that avoids problematic foods and carbonated beverages. Also encourage clients to reduce stress, limit smoking and alcohol consumption, engage in regular exercise, and get 8 hours of sleep each night. To promote health maintenance, advise clients to stop smoking and to follow the diet and fluid recommendations previously described. Encourage clients to practice stress relaxation techniques. Health restoration actions are to administer sedative and antispasmodic medications. Encourage clients to follow diet, exercise, and relaxation regimens and to increase fiber in their diets.

Pathophysiology

Three components appear to be involved in the development of IBS: GI motility, visceral hypersensitivity, and neurotransmitter imbalance. Motility can be altered by any number of factors including diet and emotional state as well as neurotransmitter imbalance and visceral hypersensitivity. The visceral hypersensitivity is the result of an exaggerated response to varied stimuli in the ileum, colon, and rectum. Balloon-distention studies of the ileum have indicated that IBS clients experience distention and pain at lower volumes and pressures than control subjects. In these studies, correlation with differences on functional MRI and positron emission tomography

(PET) suggests a primary central defect of visceral pain processing. Neurotransmitter imbalance may be implicated. Studies have shown that serotonin, 95% of which is located in the gastrointestinal tract, can be found in increased quantities in clients with IBS. Serotonin elevations cause peristaltic reflex and intestinal secretion, which results in nausea, vomiting, abdominal pain, and bloating (Figure 33-18). Other neurotransmitters under investigation may provide a link between bowel contractility and visceral sensitivity as well as between the enteric and central nervous systems.

Psychosocial factors, specifically stress, have been shown to alter motility in the gut in both IBS and normal clients. Psychological disturbances are not directly associated with IBS but are overrepresented in these clients. Additional factors that may contribute to the development of IBS include diet, genetics, drugs, smoking, hormones, and other lifestyle choices. Food intolerance is common in clients with IBS but true allergies are rare. Estrogen level, lack of sleep and exercise,

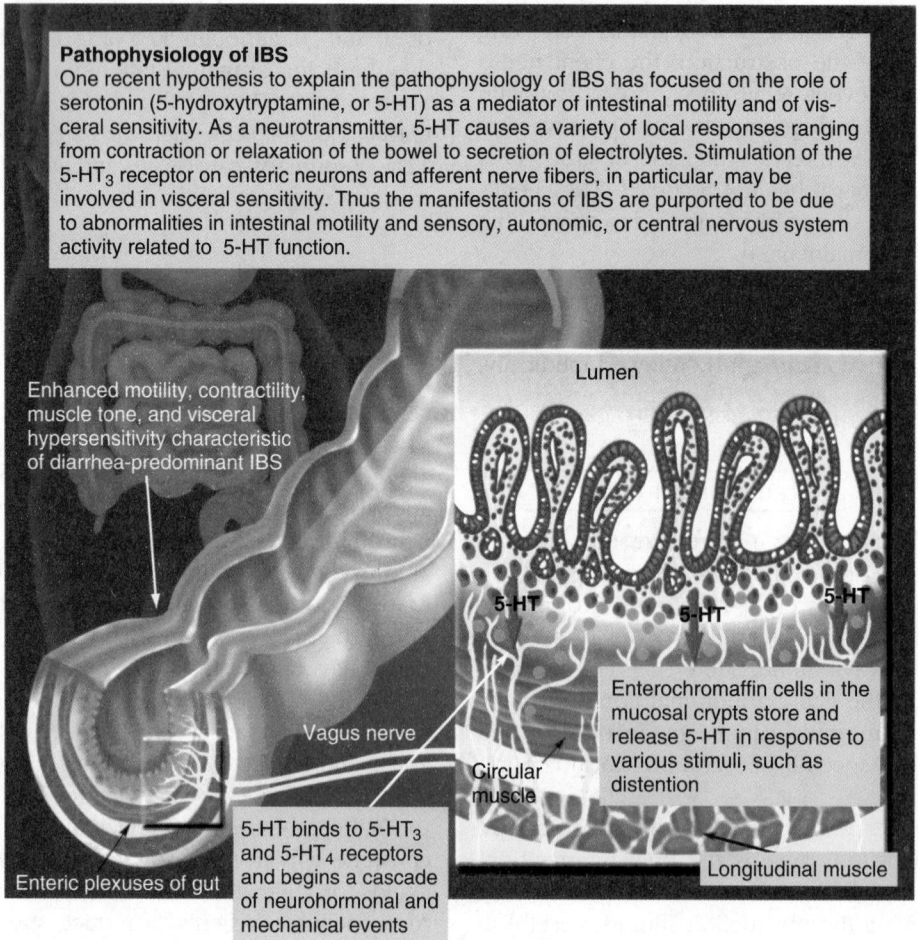

Pathophysiology of IBS
One recent hypothesis to explain the pathophysiology of IBS has focused on the role of serotonin (5-hydroxytryptamine, or 5-HT) as a mediator of intestinal motility and of visceral sensitivity. As a neurotransmitter, 5-HT causes a variety of local responses ranging from contraction or relaxation of the bowel to secretion of electrolytes. Stimulation of the 5-HT$_3$ receptor on enteric neurons and afferent nerve fibers, in particular, may be involved in visceral sensitivity. Thus the manifestations of IBS are purported to be due to abnormalities in intestinal motility and sensory, autonomic, or central nervous system activity related to 5-HT function.

Enhanced motility, contractility, muscle tone, and visceral hypersensitivity characteristic of diarrhea-predominant IBS

Lumen

5-HT

5-HT

5-HT

Enterochromaffin cells in the mucosal crypts store and release 5-HT in response to various stimuli, such as distention

Vagus nerve

Circular muscle

Longitudinal muscle

5-HT binds to 5-HT$_3$ and 5-HT$_4$ receptors and begins a cascade of neurohormonal and mechanical events

Enteric plexuses of gut

■ **FIGURE 33-18** Pathophysiology of irritable bowel syndrome (IBS). The manifestations of IBS are thought to be related to abnormalities in serotonin (5-hydroxytryptamine or 5-HT), which is a mediator of intestinal motility and visceral sensitivity. *(From Heitkemper, M., & Jarrett, M. [2001]. It's not all in your head: Irritable bowel syndrome.* American Journal of Nursing, *101[1], 26-33.)*

and a history of eating disorders may also affect GI motility. Dietary agents vary among clients; however, most clients can clearly identify them.

Clinical Manifestations

The manifestations of IBS are thought to be related to abnormalities in bowel motility and visceral sensitivity caused by the action of 5-hydroxytryptamine (5-HT). The client with IBS usually has some combination of the following manifestations: crampy abdominal pain usually located in the lower abdomen, change in bowel function, constipation or diarrhea, hypersecretion of colonic mucus, dyspeptic manifestations (flatulence, nausea, anorexia), and some level of anxiety or depression. There is usually relief after defecation. Women report that manifestations are often worse around the time of menses. Manifestations vary in intensity. Fiber, fruits, alcohol, caffeine, and fatigue may aggravate or precipitate manifestations. Clients complain about interference with activities of daily living and a poor quality of life.

Emotional disturbances affect the autonomic nervous system (ANS) and its innervation of the bowel. Disturbances of ANS function probably alter motor activity and bowel transit time. Manifestations may mimic various organic and systemic diseases. Pain may be steady or intermittent, and there may be a dull, deep discomfort with sharp cramps in the morning or after eating. The typical pattern consists of lower left quadrant abdominal pain and constipation or diarrhea. Tenderness over the sigmoid area also may be present.

Diarrhea tends to be the major problem but does not usually occur at night; nocturnal diarrhea tends to be associated with organic disease of the bowel. Examination of the stool reveals mucus but not blood. Eating may aggravate pain and defecation, and passing flatus or stool may provide temporary relief. Spastic contractions sometimes occur with stools that are small, dry, hard, and pellet-like. Other manifestations are abdominal disturbances such as nausea, distention, dyspepsia, eructation (belching), and borborygmi as a result of aerophagia (swallowing of air) and decreased gas motility. Anorexia, foul breath, sour stomach, flatulence, and cramps also may be present. Associated behavioral disturbances are anxiety, tension, nervousness, depression, sleep disturbances, weakness, and difficulty concentrating.

Because there are no confirmatory diagnostic tests for or histologic features of IBS, diagnosis generally is made by excluding other diseases. A thorough history (including diet and medications) and physical examination are crucial. Diagnostic techniques must eliminate the possibility that the client has organic GI disease. The Rome II symptom-based criteria for IBS, published in 2002, state that the abdominal discomfort or pain must last for at least 12 consecutive weeks within 12 months along with two of the following: discomfort or pain relieved with defecation, onset associated with a change

in frequency of stool, or onset associated with a change in form or appearance of stool. Clients older than 50 years in whom IBS is suspected must be carefully evaluated to rule out malignancy and diverticular disease. When functional bowel disease develops, the client usually gives a history of nervousness and emotional disturbance. The client also may be bowel conscious and a frequent user of cathartics and enemas. Palpation may demonstrate abdominal tenderness, particularly along the course of the colon.

Flexible sigmoidoscopy and colonoscopy are not recommended for diagnosis in the absence of alarming complaints such as weight loss, refractory diarrhea, onset after age 50, GI blood loss, or fever. Sigmoidoscopy or colonoscopy may be utilized to exclude cancer, IBD, infection, diverticular disease, celiac disease, or autoimmune diseases. A complete blood count and stool examination are needed to rule out occult blood, ova, parasites, and pathogenic bacteria.

OUTCOME MANAGEMENT

Medical Managemeont

Encourage Lifestyle Changes

Treatment is supportive. Advise the client to limit responsibilities, seek rest, and adopt measures to reduce stress, such as progressive relaxation, biofeedback, and a regular exercise routine. The client can control manifestations through diet, medication, and regular physical activity. The client must continue with routine followup assessment and care.

Administer Medications

No specific class of medications is universally effective, although new drugs that block or modulate 5-HT receptors are being developed. Tegaserod (Zelnorm), a 5HT4 receptor blocker, has been FDA approved for the treatment of constipation in clients with IBS. Alosetron (Lotronex) was originally approved by the FDA for treatment of IBS with severe diarrhea. It was later pulled and has since been reintroduced with approval by the FDA. Antidiarrheals such as loperamide (Imodium) slow bowel transit, enhance water absorption, and strengthen anal sphincter tone, resulting in fewer stools. Antispasmodics (Bentyl), especially anticholinergics, are commonly prescribed to relax smooth muscle. Calcium channel blockers have been proposed for the treatment of IBS because of their ability to relax GI smooth muscle by reducing calcium influx. Antidepressant drugs have been used successfully in management of IBS. Tricyclic agents delay bowel transit, and serotonin reuptake inhibitors improve pain manifestations. Vegetable mucilages, such as psyllium hydrophilic mucilloid (Metamucil), can increase stool bulk.

Modify Diet

A high-fiber diet helps control IBS through the production of bulkier stools and reduction of tension in the walls of the sigmoid colon. Fiber helps to manage both constipation and diarrhea. In constipation, the softer, bulkier, and heavier stools produced by dietary fiber tend to decrease transit time. In diarrhea, the fiber diet helps absorb water, giving form to the stool and increasing transit time.

Sources of fiber include bran cereals, whole wheat, other whole grains such as brown rice, and fresh vegetables. Clients should drink six to eight 8-ounce glasses of water daily because water helps to regulate stool consistency and frequency. If diarrhea is a problem, the client needs to avoid foods that may cause it, such as carbonated and caffeinated beverages, and to drink liquids between meals rather than at mealtime.

Nursing Management of the Medical Client

Reinforce the physician's explanation of the nature of the disorder, the intervention plan, and the prognosis. Make it clear to the client that the bowel responds to stress, foods, and medications. Emphasize the importance of regular hours, nourishing meals, and adequate sleep, exercise, and relaxation. Help the client to establish a regular bowel routine. Advise the client with diarrhea to limit foods that produce gas or irritate the bowel and to avoid (1) caffeinated and carbonated beverages, (2) alcohol, (3) foods containing indigestible carbohydrates, such as beans, and (4) milk and milk products. Provide empathy and support.

CELIAC DISEASE

Celiac disease, also known as *nontropical sprue,* is a disorder that causes severe malabsorption. The disorder is characterized by marked atrophy of the villi in the proximal small intestine induced by ingestion of gluten-containing foods. *Gluten* is a high-molecular-weight protein found in rye, oats, barley, and wheat. It is found in bread, bread products, beer, and many other processed foods. Clients present with diarrhea, steatorrhea, and weakness, which is relieved when the client begins a gluten-free diet. Corticosteroids may be required if the gluten-free diet is not successful in relieving manifestations.

DISORDERS OF THE ANORECTAL AREA

The major function of the rectum is to store feces until evacuation. When feces enter the rectum, peristalsis occurs. Many disorders in the rectal area result from

constipation or failure to empty the rectum when peristalsis occurs.

At the mucocutaneous border of the anal canal, the mucous membrane changes to skin with cutaneous somatic nerve endings. Because of this anatomic structure, lesions of the external anal canal are very painful. The two most common manifestations are bleeding and pain. Drainage of mucus and fecal matter and irritation of the skin by organisms can cause intense itching.

Hemorrhoids and skin tags may protrude from the anal opening, and there may be drainage of pus from abscesses. Bright-red blood per rectum usually indicates a lesion of the left colon or anorectal region. Blood on the toilet paper alone usually indicates perianal disease, whereas blood on the surface of a formed stool may suggest a polyp or carcinoma of the left colon or rectum. Blood mixed with the stool suggests inflammatory bowel disease or carcinoma of the proximal colon. Blood in the toilet bowl after the passage of formed stool suggests hemorrhoidal bleeding, the most common source of bright-red blood in the stool. All rectal bleeding must be evaluated by a health care provider.

HEMORRHOIDS

Hemorrhoids are perianal varicose veins. They may be internal or external (Figure 33-19). Internal hemorrhoids are varicosities of the superior hemorrhoidal plexus occurring above the mucocutaneous border (pectinate line); they are covered by mucous membrane and are innervated by the autonomic nervous system. Hemorrhoids are a common disorder, affecting both men and women of any age, but the incidence is higher in people between 20 and 50 years of age.

Etiology and Risk Factors

By the age of 50, almost half of the population has hemorrhoids. Enlargement of hemorrhoids is caused by increased intra-abdominal pressure. Pregnancy, constipation with prolonged straining, obesity, heart failure, prolonged sitting or standing, and cirrhosis with portal hypertension also raise the incidence of hemorrhoids.

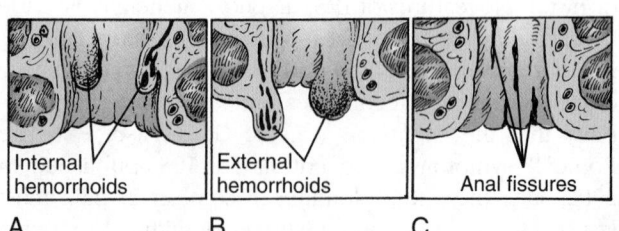

■ **FIGURE 33–19 A,** Internal hemorrhoids. **B,** External hemorrhoids. **C,** Anal fissures.

Any condition that increases constipation, intra-abdominal pressure, or hemorrhoidal venous pressure raises the risk of development of hemorrhoids. Prevention of constipation through more fiber in the diet is an excellent measure to reduce the risk of hemorrhoids.

Pathophysiology

Tenesmus increases intra-abdominal and hemorrhoidal venous pressures, leading to distention of the hemorrhoidal veins. When the rectal ampulla (pouch) is filled with formed stool, venous obstruction is believed to occur. As a result of the repeated and prolonged increase in this pressure and the obstruction, hemorrhoidal veins become permanently dilated. As a result of the distention, thrombosis and bleeding also may occur.

Clinical Manifestations

The major manifestation of external hemorrhoids is an enlarged mass at the anus. Internal hemorrhoids are characterized by bleeding and prolapse (protrusion outside the anus). Other manifestations are rectal itching and constipation. Pain may be present if there is associated thrombosis. The blood is bright red and may be seen in the stool or on toilet tissue. A prolapse may occur in severe cases after exercise or after prolonged standing. Hemorrhoids may prolapse during defecation and spontaneously return, or the client may need to replace them manually. In some clients, hemorrhoids are prolapsed at all times.

External hemorrhoids are diagnosed by visual examination; internal hemorrhoids are diagnosed through history; digital palpation; anoscopy, which is using a hollow, lighted tube to view the rectum; and proctoscopy, which is useful for a more complete examination of the rectum. Asking the client to strain during assessment causes the veins to enlarge, thus aiding diagnosis.

Complications of hemorrhoids are bleeding, thrombosis, and hemorrhoidal strangulation. Severe bleeding from prolonged trauma to the vein during defecation can cause iron deficiency anemia. Blood oozes or may even spurt out following a bowel movement. Thrombosis within the hemorrhoids can occur at any time and manifests as intense pain. Strangulated hemorrhoids, which are prolapsed hemorrhoids in which the blood supply is cut off by the anal sphincter, can result in thrombosis when blood within the hemorrhoid clots. Assessment reveals severe pain, extreme edema, and inflammation.

OUTCOME MANAGEMENT

Medical Management

Medical therapy is used for small, uncomplicated hemorrhoids with mild manifestations.

Prevent Constipation

Dietary changes used to treat constipation include increasing fluids and fiber in the diet. Constipation unrelieved by diet may require use of a stool softener (docusate sodium) or a hydrophilic psyllium preparation (e.g., Metamucil).

Relieve Pain

For pain, an initial application of cold packs, followed by warm sitz baths three or four times a day, should help. A topical anesthetic or steroid preparation, such as lidocaine (Xylocaine) or steroid cream, also reduces pain and itching.

Nursing Management of the Medical Client

Prevent Constipation

The client with hemorrhoids should take measures to avoid constipation. The anal area is very painful, and the client may avoid defecating, resulting in hard stool or fecal impaction. Encourage the client to take bulk laxatives, stool softeners, or mineral oil as prescribed to promote stool passage. Monitor the stool for consistency and blood.

Counsel the client to (1) eat fiber-containing foods and drink ample fluids to prevent straining and (2) avoid laxatives as much as possible. Remind the client not to sit on the toilet longer than necessary; this position impairs blood flow and puts added pressure on anal vessels.

Relieve Pain

Encourage 15-minute warm sitz baths three or four times per day for 15 minutes. Witch hazel compresses are soothing to the mucosa. Other over-the-counter preparations may temporarily relieve pain.

Surgical Management

Several surgical procedures are used to treat hemorrhoids. Most are performed as outpatient or clinic procedures. Botox injections into the internal sphincter of clients who have just undergone hemorrhoidectomy have been used to reduce pain postoperatively.

Sclerotherapy

Sclerotherapy is performed by the injection of a sclerosing agent (a substance that causes formation of scar tissue) between and around the veins. This produces an inflammatory reaction that leads to thrombosis and fibrosis. This procedure can be performed on an outpatient basis but requires one to four injections 5 to 7 days apart. The sclerosing agent can scar the anal canal.

Ligation

Ligation, a common procedure for internal hemorrhoids, is performed in the office setting. The client can usually resume normal activities immediately after the treatment. Unfortunately, the procedure cannot be used for external hemorrhoids and may be only temporarily effective. The surgeon inserts a ligator, a small, double-lumen cylinder with a small rubber band on the inner layer, through an anoscope. The hemorrhoid is then grasped with forceps and pulled through the ligator. The rubber band is placed around the neck of the hemorrhoid. Although bleeding can occur, the most common problem is some pain during ligation. The client takes a bulk laxative after the procedure to avoid local trauma from a hard fecal mass. In 8 to 10 days, the rubber band cuts through the neck of tissue, and the tissue sloughs.

Cryosurgery

Cryosurgery (freezing) of hemorrhoids is an outpatient procedure that is performed less commonly today. The freezing of the tissue leads to necrosis and sloughing of the hemorrhoids. The problems associated with this procedure are the prolonged periods of drainage, the amount of foul drainage, the presence of large residual skin tags, and possibly incomplete destruction of the hemorrhoids.

Laser

Laser removal of hemorrhoids also is performed on an outpatient basis. The hemorrhoid is burned off with the laser. There is minimal bleeding, although the procedure causes some pain.

Hemorrhoidectomy

With a hemorrhoidectomy, the vein is excised, and the area either is left open to heal by granulation or is closed with sutures. The open method is very painful but has a high rate of success. The suture method, although far less painful, is more likely to cause infection and result in poor healing. Complications include infection, stricture formation as the lesion heals, and hemorrhage. Hemorrhage may occur immediately after surgery or about 10 days later as a result of sloughing of tissue. Also, bleeding may not be evident because it can occur into the rectum without being passed immediately.

Nursing Management of the Surgical Client

Promote Healing

After the client has undergone a procedure to remove hemorrhoids, stress the importance of keeping the area clean and the stool soft but formed to help prevent strictures. Encourage the client to wash the area after defecation and to pat it dry. Local moist heat, applied with a washcloth or piece of cotton to the anal opening for a few minutes, cleans, soothes, and promotes healing. Never apply heat in the immediate postoperative period because of the increased risk of hemorrhage. Beginning 12 hours after surgery, sitz baths three or four times a day, as the client desires, and after each bowel movement are encouraged. A sanitary napkin is the most convenient perianal dressing if one is required.

Prevent Complications

Postoperative complications requiring nursing assessment include hemorrhage and urinary retention. The proximity of the bladder and tenderness in the area sometimes make urination difficult. Reestablishment of bowel habits is another potential postoperative problem. The client may need instruction on the relationship of proper diet and adequate fluid intake to bowel regularity, the physiology of defecation, and the importance of establishing a regular bowel routine.

Relieve Pain

Postoperative pain can be controlled with parenteral and then oral analgesics. Warn the client to avoid vigorous perianal wiping during the immediate postoperative period. The client is usually given a stool softener and mineral oil to soften and lubricate the first stool. Warn clients that fainting can occur, from pain and vagal stimulation, during the first postprocedure bowel movement.

ANAL FISSURE

An *anal fissure* is an ulceration or tear of the lining of the anal canal, usually the posterior wall, that occurs as a result of excessive tissue stretching and possibly from passage of a hard or large stool. The skin tear is tender and tends to reopen at subsequent defecation.

Chronic fissures are usually secondary to infectious material retained in the anal crypts. Sharp pain accompanies defecation, followed by burning. Severe muscle spasm of the sphincter usually accompanies chronic conditions. The client may try to avoid defecation, aggravating the condition.

If the acute lesion does not heal with local dilations, cleaning, and control of constipation, the tract can be excised surgically. A chronic fissure usually does not heal spontaneously and requires surgery.

Advise the client to (1) keep the stool soft with psyllium hydrophilic mucilloid (Metamucil), mineral oil, or docusate sodium, as prescribed; (2) have a daily bowel movement, assisted by laxative use as needed; and (3) clean the area after defecation, preferably with warm water. Sitz baths aid healing and may relieve pain. Suppositories with a local anesthetic may relieve constipation. Some colorectal surgeons are using Botox injections for treatment of chronic anal fissures.

ANAL FISTULA

A *fistula* is a sinus tract that develops between two body cavities or between a body cavity and the surface of the body. A rectal fistula is a tract that leads from the anal canal to the skin outside the anus or from an abscess to either the anal canal or the perianal area. It usually is preceded by an abscess. A fistula may heal temporarily and then open and drain periodically.

Anal fistula is a chronic condition for which surgery is the only cure. The surgeon excises the tract and cleans the area, leaving it open to heal by granulation. It may heal very slowly and be very painful. Advise the client to keep the area clean, especially after a bowel movement.

ANORECTAL ABSCESS

Anorectal abscesses form in several locations. Most abscesses begin as cryptitis, with the formation of cysts that extend through the tubular ducts into the submucosal spaces. They also can originate from abrasions of the local tissues, with entry of a virulent organism. Anal intercourse may also cause a rectal abscess. Treatment involves drainage of the abscess and surgical excision of any associated fistulae. Two stages of surgery may be required to accomplish the needed resection.

CANCER

Carcinoma and melanoma can occur at the anus but are rare, constituting fewer than 5% of anorectal cancers. They spread by local extension into the perirectal spaces and then to the inguinal nodes. Cancer of the anal canal or lower rectum can coexist with other rectal conditions, and the client may falsely attribute bleeding to a hemorrhoid instead of carcinoma. Anal cancers are more common in African Americans, in clients infected with human papillomavirus (HPV) or HIV, and in clients with pre-existing anal and perianal problems, such as fistulae. Bleeding, local pain and itching, and tenesmus are characteristic manifestations. The client is usually aware of a lump near the anus that has bled and that gradually becomes more and more painful, particularly during or just after a bowel movement. Many cancers are not diagnosed until they are large, and by then the prognosis is poor. Tumors are treated with chemoradiation (continuous infusion of 5-fluorouracil while receiving radiation) and chemotherapy, and usually require surgical excision. Surgical intervention varies according to the tumor stage (degree of invasiveness) and involves excision of the anus with a possible abdominoperineal resection.

BOWEL INCONTINENCE

Bowel incontinence may develop in clients as a result of aging, trauma, diabetes mellitus, rectal prolapse, or childbirth injuries or from a neurogenic cause, such as spina bifida. Clients with cancer in the lower pelvic and rectal areas or with a history of radiation therapy to the rectal region are also at risk for bowel incontinence. A rectal pouch may be applied to collect feces, to protect the skin from prolonged contact with fecal material, and to prevent subsequent skin breakdown. FlexiSeal FMS is latex-free device that uses a soft, flexible silicone catheter that conforms to sphincter anatomy. The catheter is inserted into the rectum and a low-pressure balloon is filled with water or saline and connected to a closed-end collection bag that helps eliminate fecal contact with skin surfaces. See the Management and Delegation feature Application and Care of Rectal Pouches and Rectal Tubes on the website. *evolve*

As an aid to promote continence, a device called an artificial rectal sphincter (ARS) has been used successfully to promote bowel continence in almost all clients except those who have a history of cancer or radiation and who would be unable to activate the pump. The device mimics the natural process of bowel control and elimination.

The ARS consists of three parts: (1) a cuff, placed under the skin to fit around the anal canal for an artificial rectal sphincter; (2) a pressure-regulating balloon placed in the abdominal wall and filled with liquid such as a contrast agent that can be seen on x-ray; and (3) a control pump placed in the scrotum or labia to inflate the cuff. The cuff inflates like a balloon to prevent the passage of stool and to promote continence. To evacuate the rectum, the client deflates the plastic ring and stool is able to pass. After a bowel movement, the cuff automatically inflates in 10 minutes.

General or spinal anesthesia is used for surgical implantation of the ARS, and the procedure takes about 1 hour. The bowel is cleaned with antibiotics, laxatives, and enemas.

Postoperatively the client is given IV antibiotics for several days to prevent infection. The nurse teaches the client how to deflate the cuff for bowel evacuation, monitors the client's bowel patterns, and observes for complications such as mechanical failure, infection, and ulceration. If mechanical failure is suspected, manometry is used to measure the closing pressure of the ARS. Client satisfaction has been reported. (See also the Management and Delegation feature on Application and Care of Rectal Pouches and Rectal Tubes on the website for clients with diarrhea.) *evolve*

PILONIDAL CYST

A *pilonidal cyst* occurs at the base of the sacrum, usually contains hair, and becomes infected, forming an abscess and then a sinus tract. It is most common in young adults, especially men. It may result from hairs that penetrate the skin and cause sinus tracts to form. Constant irritation (e.g., from clothing and perspiration from activity) can cause hair to become embedded and then infected. Acute pain, erythema, and swelling result, followed by drainage from the abscess. Treatment involves surgical excision of the abscess. Healing is slow, and the client is usually given antibiotics to clear the infection, preventing recurrence.

Blunt or Penetrating Trauma

Blunt or penetrating trauma to the abdomen refers to accidental or intentional trauma causing internal injuries. Most blunt abdominal trauma is caused by automobile steering wheel or pedestrian accidents, whereas most penetrating trauma is caused by gunshot wounds or stabbings.

Etiology and Risk Factors

Almost any kind of injury can cause blunt trauma to the abdomen. In automobile accidents, rapid, uncontrolled deceleration is the force that produces the trauma, when the client's body hits the steering wheel or some other object. Penetrating trauma commonly results from gunshot wounds, which cause a great deal of internal damage. Stabbings are the next most common cause of penetrating abdominal wounds, although the wounds are less traumatic.

Trauma is the leading cause of death in adults younger than 40 years and the fifth leading cause of death in all adults. Although not all cases of trauma involve abdominal trauma, abdominal injuries are common with motor-vehicle accidents. One method of prevention is wearing seat belts, which could decrease abdominal trauma during accidents.

Pathophysiology

Blunt trauma to the abdomen can cause shearing, crushing, or compressing forces that rupture the bowel and other abdominal structures. Gunshot wounds can damage every structure in the abdomen. The bullets may perforate the stomach or bowel, causing peritonitis and sepsis.

Stab wounds produce fewer traumas to internal abdominal structures because the abdominal organs have more time to shift out of the way of the penetrating instrument.

Clinical Manifestations

Assessment of the client first involves obtaining a thorough history of the accident so that the extent of blunt trauma can be estimated. For penetrating trauma, careful assessment of the position of entry and possibly exit wounds is vital.

The client may show manifestations of an acute abdomen with either type of trauma. With both injuries, either internal or external hemorrhage may occur. If the bowel is ruptured, manifestations of peritonitis are present. All abdominal drainage is closely assessed for the presence of bowel contents.

Abdominal lavage is commonly used to assess the presence of bleeding in all abdominal wounds. This procedure involves instillation of a crystalloid solution into the peritoneal cavity followed by paracentesis (drainage of contents). Note and record the color and amount of the drainage.

A CT scan of the abdomen is now considered the base assessment of intra-abdominal injury. Angiography, intravenous pyelography (IVP), and other studies may be performed to assess different organs and the degree of trauma suffered.

OUTCOME MANAGEMENT

Medical Management

If minimal blunt trauma was sustained without severe injury to any abdominal organs, the client may simply be observed for problems once the diagnostic tests have been performed. Penetrating trauma always requires surgical intervention. The major complications of trauma are hemorrhage, shock, peritonitis, and sepsis.

The client's pain is treated conservatively until the severity of trauma has been determined. If the bowel has been ruptured, large doses of IV antibiotics are given to control infection. If hemorrhage and shock are present, IV fluids, colloids, and vasopressors may be used. The client is assigned to NPO status until the abdomen has been assessed and found to be intact.

Surgical Management

The treatment of choice for abdominal trauma with injury is an exploratory laparotomy. Depending on the injury, the surgery may be as simple as a closure of tears or as complex as a bowel resection and temporary colostomy.

Nursing Management of the Medical-Surgical Client

Careful assessment of the client's injury is vital. The client often must be prepared for immediate emergency surgery. Prepare the client as quickly as possible, knowing that postoperatively much more teaching and support will be required.

Usually, once the injuries and repair have had sufficient time to heal and the infection has been adequately treated, the client returns to the hospital so that the temporary ostomy may be closed and the bowel returned to normal.

Discharge Teaching

Before discharge, the client may need education regarding home health care, which may include ostomy care and extensive wound care. The client or his or her significant others may have to learn to change dressings and to care for an open, draining wound. Follow-up care from a visiting nurse may also be required for the administration of antibiotics at home, further ostomy teaching, or wound care for an open, draining wound.

CONCLUSIONS

Intestinal disorders are common; however, if they are not treated promptly and completely, they may cause problems throughout the client's life. Even with early treatment, many clients require ostomies for treatment of large and small bowel disorders. The resultant body image changes are the focus of nursing interventions to educate the client and to facilitate behavior modifications that will promote health and adaptation to the changes.

THINKING CRITICALLY

1. A young man is admitted with an exacerbation of inflammatory bowel disease. He reports frequent watery stools, general weakness, lack of appetite with a loss of 5 pounds in a week, and cramping abdominal pain. What nursing history and physical assessment are required? How will his exacerbation be treated?

Factors to Consider. What are the clinical manifestations of inflammatory bowel disease? What are priority nursing interventions?

2. An older client has undergone a bowel resection with placement of a temporary transverse colostomy for treatment of colon cancer. He lives with his wife of 25 years. She is very interested in learning how to help her spouse manage care for the stoma and how to change the colostomy bags. What is your priority assessment? What teaching methods should you use to teach the client and his wife?

Factors to Consider. What is the appearance of a healthy stoma and healthy skin around the stoma? What dietary management is important?

3. A woman in her 50s schedules an appointment with her health care provider because she has found blood in her stool and has noticed a change in bowel habits. She states that her father died of colon cancer and she has been afraid to see her health care provider because she fears she might also have colon cancer. What are priority nursing interventions? What teaching methods should be used for this woman?

Factors to Consider. What are the causes of colorectal cancer? What are its clinical manifestations? How is it treated?

Discussions for these questions can be found on the website. **evolve**

BIBLIOGRAPHY

Citations appearing in red refer to primary research.

Citations appearing in blue refer to evidence-based practice guidelines and protocols.

1. American Cancer Society. (2007). *Cancer facts and figures*. Atlanta: Author.
2. Amerine, E. (2006). Celiac disease goes against the grain. *Nursing 2006, 36*(2), 46-48.
3. Banks, N., & Razor, B. (2003). Preoperative stoma site assessment and marking. *American Journal of Nursing, 103*(3), 64A-64D.
4. Beaven, A. (2006). Adjuvant therapy for colorectal cancer: Yesterday, today, and tomorrow. *Oncology, 20*(5), 461-473.
5. Beitz, J. (2004). Continent diversions: The new gold standards of ileoanal reservoir and neobladder. *Ostomy/Wound Management, 50*(9), 26-35.
6. Beresfor, S., Johnson, K., Ritenbaugh, N., et al. (2006). Low-fat dietary pattern and risk of colorectal cancer: The women's health initiative randomized controlled dietary modification trial. *Journal of the American Medical Association, 295*(6), 643-654.
7. Cahill, B. (2005). Colorectal cancer—Which test is best? *Advances for Nurse Practitioners, 13*(1), 71-75.
8. Chao, A., Thun, M., Connell, C., et al. (2005). Meat consumption and risk of colorectal cancer. *Journal of the American Medical Association, 293*(2), 172-182.
9. CCO Formulary. (2006). *Folfox4.* Accessed 12/03/06 at www.cancercare.on.ca/pdfchemo/Folfox4-adv-col.pdf.
10. CCO Formulary. (2006). *Folfox6.* Accessed 12/03/06 at www.cancercare.on.ca/pdfchemo/Folfox6-adv-col.pdf.
11. Chung, D., & Rustgi, L. (2003). HNPCC syndrome: Genetics and clinical implications. *Annals of Internal Medicine, 138*(7), 560-570.
12. Cobrin, G., & Korsten, M. (2005). It's getting easier to pin down and treat IBS. *The Clinical Advisor, April,* 19-25.
13. Colorectal Cancer Collaborative Group. (2001). Adjuvant radiotherapy for rectal cancer: A systematic overview of 8507 patients from 22 randomized trials. *Lancet, 358*(9290), 1291-1304.
14. Cotton, P., Durkalski, V., & Pineau, B. (2004). Computed tomographic colonography (virtual colonoscopy): A multicenter comparison with standard colonoscopy for detection of colorectal neoplasia. *Journal of the American Medical Association, 291*(14), 1713-1719.
15. Crohn's & Colitis Foundation of America. (2006). *About Crohn's disease.* Accessed 12/03/06 at www.ccfa.org/info/crohns.
16. Crohn's & Colitis Foundation of America. (2006). *About ulcerative colitis and proctitis.* Accessed 12/03/06 at www.ccfa.org/info/ucp.
17. Crohn's & Colitis Foundation of America. (2006). *Treatment options.* Accessed 12/03/06 at www.ccfa.org/info/treatment.
18. Crohn's & Colitis Foundation of America. (2006). *Major genetic link to Crohn's and colitis found.* Accessed 12/03/06 at www.ccfa.org/about/press/il23.
19. Dial, S., Delany, J., Barkun, A., et al. (2005). Use of gastric acid-suppressive agents and the risk of community-acquired *clostridium difficile*-associated disease. *Journal of the American Medical Association, 294*(23), 2989-2995.
20. Duerr, R., Taylor, K., Brant, S., et al. (2006). A genome-wide association study identifies IL23R as an inflammatory bowel disease gene. *Science, 314*(5804), 1461-1463.
21. Fakih, M. (2004). 5-Fluorouracil leucovorin and oxaliplatin (FOLFOX) in the treatment of metastatic colon cancer with severe liver dysfunction. *Oncology: International Journal for Cancer Research and Treatment, 67,* 222-224.
22. Feldman, M., Friedman, L., & Sleisenger, M. (2002). *Gastrointestinal and liver disease: Pathophysiology/diagnosis/management* (7th ed.). Philadelphia: Saunders.

23. Fitzgibbons, R., Giobbie-Hurder, A., Gibbs, J., et al. (2006). Watchful waiting vs repair of inguinal hernia in minimally symptomatic men: A randomized clinical trial. *Journal of the American Medical Association, 295*(3), 285-292.

24. Fuss, U., Becker, C., Yang, Z., et al. (2006). Both Il-12 and IL-23 are synthesized during active Crohn's disease and are down-regulated by treatment with anti-IL-12 p40 monoclonal antibody. *Inflammatory Bowel Diseases, 12*(1), 9-15.

25. Giovannucci, E. (2003). Diet, body weight and colorectal cancer: A summary of epidemiologic incidence. *Journal of Women's Health, 12*(2), 173-182.

26. Goldman, L., & Ausiello, D. (2004). *Cecil textbook of medicine* (22nd ed.). Philadelphia: Saunders.

27. Heitkemper, M., & Jarrett, M. (2005). Overlapping conditions in women with irritable bowel syndrome. *Urologic Nursing, 25*(1), 25-31.

28. Larsson, S., Bergkvist, L., & Wolk, A. (2005). Magnesium intake in relation to risk of colorectal cancer in women. *Journal of the American Medical Association, 293*(1), 86-89.

29. Lin, H. (2004). Small intestinal bacterial overgrowth: A framework for understanding irritable bowel syndrome. *Journal of the American Medical Association, 292*(7), 852-858.

30. Lotronex. (2006). Accessed 12/04/06 from www.fda.gov/cder/drug/infopage/lotronex/lotronex.htm.

31. Madsen, D., Sebolt, T., Cullen, L., et al. (2005). Listening to bowel sounds: An evidence-based practice project. *American Journal of Nursing, 105*(12), 40-50.

32. McCance, K., & Huether, S. (2006). *Pathophysiology: The biologic basis for disease in adults and children* (5th ed.). St. Louis: Mosby.

33. Milburn Jessup, J., Stewart, A., Greene, F., et al. (2005). Adjuvant chemotherapy for stage III colon cancer: Implications of race/ethnicity, age, and differentiation. *Journal of the American Medical Association, 294*(21), 2703-2711.

34. Mitka, M. (2003). Colon cancer screening guidelines stress initial test's importance. *Journal of the American Medical Association, 289*(9), 1089-1090.

35. Molbach, K., Mead, P., & Griffin, P. (2002). Antimicrobial therapy in patients with *E. coli* 0157:H7 infection. *Journal of the American Medical Association, 288*(8), 1014-1016.

36. Park, S., Sung, J., Han, S., et al (2005). Oxaliplatin, folinic acid and 5-fluorouracil (Folfox-4) combination chemotherapy as second-line treatment in advanced colorectal cancer patients with irinotecan failure: A Korean single center experience. *Japanese Journal of Clinical Oncology, 35*(9), 531-535.

37. Park, Y., Hunter, D., Spiegelman, D., et al. (2005). Dietary fiber intake and risk of colorectal cancer: A pooled analysis of prospective cohort studies. *Journal of the American Medical Association, 294*(22), 2849-2857.

38. Pearson, C. (2004). Inflammatory bowel disease. *Nursing Times, 100*(9), 86-90.

39. Peluso, I., Pallone, F., & Monteleone, G. (2006). Interleukin-12 and Th1 immune response in Crohn's disease: Pathogenetic relevance and therapeutic implication. *World Journal of Gastroenterology, 12*(35), 5606-5610.

40. Price, S., & Wilson, L. (2003). *Pathophysiology: Clinical concepts of disease processes* (6th ed.). St. Louis: Mosby.

41. Schottenfeld, D., & Beebe-Dimmer, J. (2006). Chronic inflammation: A common and important factor in the pathogenesis of neoplasia. *CA—A Cancer Journal for Clinicians, 56*(2), 69-83.

42. Stein, P. (2004). Ulcerative colitis—Diagnosis and surgical treatment. *Association of Operating Room Nurses Journal, 80*(2), 243-258, 261-262.

43. Todd, B. (2006). *Clostridium difficile:* Familiar pathogen, changing epidemiology. *American Journal of Nursing, 106*(5), 33-36.

44. Walsh, J., & Terdiman, J. (2003). Colorectal cancer screening: Scientific review. *Journal of the American Medical Association, 289*(10), 1288-1296.

45. Weber, C. (2005). Update on foodborne disease. *Urologic Nursing, 25*(2), 126-128.

46. Weeks, J., et al. (2002). Short-term quality-of-life outcomes following laparoscopic-assisted colectomy vs open colectomy for colon cancer. *Journal of the American Medical Association, 287*(3), 321-328.

47. Whiteford, M., et al. (2002). The evolving treatment of anal cancer: How are we doing? *Archives of Surgery, 136*, 886-891.

48. Wichmann, M., Hutti, T., Winter, H., et al. (2005). Immunological effects of laparoscopic versus open colorectal surgery: A prospective study. *Archives of Surgery, 140*, 692-697.

evolve *Did you remember to check out the bonus material on the Evolve website and the CD-ROM, including NCLEX®-Examination Style Review Questions, Open-Book Quizzes, and Chapter Review Audio Podcasts?*

http://evolve.elsevier.com/Black/medsurg

CHAPTER 34

Management of Clients with Urinary Disorders

Francie Bernier and Terran Warren Sims

Nurses commonly provide the initial assessment, diagnosis, and outcome management of altered urinary elimination and related nursing diagnoses. *Impaired urinary elimination* is a nursing diagnosis used for dysfunction involving the urethra, bladder, or ureters. More specific nursing diagnoses include *Stress Urinary Incontinence, Reflex Urinary Incontinence, Functional Urinary Incontinence,* and *Urinary Retention.* Several additional nursing diagnoses are discussed throughout the chapter.

Because of the personal nature of the urinary system, its proximity to the reproductive system in females, and the shared urinary and reproductive system of males, urinary disorders commonly lead to feelings of shame, isolation, and embarrassment. It is vital that nurses be sensitive to the psychosocial needs of any client with a urinary disorder.

It is also important to recognize that urinary diagnoses may signal that other medical conditions coexist. Long-term sequelae or conditions occurring as a consequence of altered urinary elimination may include such problems as impaired kidney function, changes in fluid volume and electrolytes, skin breakdown, changes in quality of life, and other associated conditions.

INFECTIOUS AND INFLAMMATORY DISORDERS

CYSTITIS

The diagnosis of a *urinary tract infection* (UTI) is typically confirmed on the basis of a certain number of microorganisms in the urinary system (usually 10^5 organisms), although manifestations may begin with many fewer organisms. The infectious process usually affects the bladder, but the urethra, ureters, and kidneys may be involved. *Cystitis,* the most common type of UTI, is an inflammation of the bladder wall, usually caused by ascending bacteria or obstructive voiding patterns that lead to decreased flow or stasis of urine. UTI is one of the most common infections treated by primary care providers. Untreated, it has the potential for serious consequences, such as pyelonephritis (inflammation of the kidney) (see Chapter 35) and bacteremia (bacteria in the blood). On rare occasions, complications of a UTI can lead to death.

The prevalence of UTIs is about eight times higher in women than in men, probably because the female urethra is shorter and lies closer to the anal and vaginal openings. This position increases the risk of bacterial contamination of the lower urinary tract. About 6 to 7 million young women see physicians for UTIs each year, second in frequency only to upper respiratory tract infections. In 5% to 10% of cases, the UTI recurs after initial treatment.

The incidence of UTIs increases during hospitalization, usually from catheterization procedures and possibly from inadequate catheter care. 🪔 Nosocomial (hospital-acquired) UTIs occur in about 2% of inpatients. About 1% of nosocomial UTIs (5000 each year) become life-threatening. Catheter-associated urinary *tract* infections account for about 40% of all nosocomial infections and increase the duration of hospital stay, the cost, and mortality risk.

Etiology and Risk Factors

The most common UTI-causing bacteria are gram-negative organisms found in the intestine. *Escherichia coli* probably causes about 80% of UTIs, and *Klebsiella* causes about 5% of reported UTIs. *Enterobacter* and *Proteus* are found in about 2% of reported cases.

Women with vaginal *candidiasis* commonly complain of UTI manifestations. Other causative organisms, such as *Chlamydia trachomatis, Trichomonas vaginalis, Neisseria gonorrhoeae,* and herpes simplex, may be responsible for UTI manifestations as well. Therefore ask female clients about any gynecologic manifestations when clients present with potential UTIs.

🪔 Besides the shorter urethra and its proximity to the vagina and anus, other risk factors for women may be related to sexual intercourse, poorly fitting diaphragms, spermicides, pregnancy, poor hygiene, dysfunctional voiding patterns, or a history of female genital mutilation (see Chapter 39). Additionally, synthetic underwear and pantyhose, tight jeans, wet bathing suits, and allergens or irritants in perfumed toilet paper or feminine hygiene products can also foster the development of cystitis. Colonization of the vaginal opening and urethral meatus with *E. coli* is characteristic of women who have recurrent UTIs. 🪔 Hormonal changes in pregnant and postmenopausal women alter the vaginal pH, change the vaginal flora, and may allow abnormal levels of normal bacteria to grow. In addition, shrinkage of the mucosal layer of the lower urogenital system of postmenopausal women increases the risk of urethral irritation during intercourse. In fact, sexual intercourse may increase the risk of UTI in all women. The thrusting motion during coitus can push organisms up the urethra and into the bladder, which can lead to cystitis if the woman does not void after intercourse. The term "honeymoon cystitis" is frequently used to describe this phenomenon.

Diabetes mellitus, tumors, calculus, or the presence of indwelling urethral catheters or kinked catheters that prevent proper drainage dramatically increase the occurrence of UTIs.

SAFETY ALERT **UTIs are the most common nosocomial infection, making it one of the infections targeted in the TJC National Patient Safety Goals. Among catheterized clients, the rates for UTIs in most hospitals are greater than 50%, with some rates reported as high as 100%. Indwelling catheters can introduce bacteria into the urinary tract, possibly from poor insertion technique, irritation and consequent inflammation of the urethra, and ascension of bacteria along the length of the catheter. The rate of infection increases significantly if the drainage system does not remain closed.**

Health promotion and health maintenance strategies are discussed under Nursing Management of the Medical Client.

Pathophysiology

The most common mechanism by which a UTI develops is via ascending and invading bacteria. The organism triggers an inflammatory response in the lining of the urinary tract. This irritation leads to pain, frequent voiding, and other clinical manifestations.

Clinical Manifestations

Any change in a client's voiding habits should be assessed as a possible UTI. The most common clinical manifestations of cystitis are burning pain on urination (dysuria), frequency, urgency, voiding in small amounts, an inability to void, incomplete emptying of the bladder, cloudy urine, and hematuria (blood in the urine). Asymptomatic bacteriuria (bacteria in urine) is seen in about 10% of cases, most often in older adults. 🪔 The only reported manifestation of asymptomatic bacteriuria in an older client may be a change in the mental status with or without fever.

🪔 A urine culture is the most accurate diagnostic tool. Initially, a dipstick test for leukocyte esterase and nitrite activity may detect bacteriuria, allowing for immediate broad-spectrum antibiotic therapy to begin. However, the dipstick test should not be used as the exclusive diagnostic tool for a UTI. Some bacteria, such as enterococci, do not convert from nitrites to positive nitrites. Therefore a urine culture is essential for all clients with evidence of cystitis or a positive dipstick test. Sensitivity testing can determine which antibiotic will respond to specific bacteria. 🪔 A urine specimen drawn by catheter yields a more accurate test than does a voided specimen. See the Integrating Diagnostic Testing feature on p. 668 for more information related to diagnosis of UTI.

OUTCOME MANAGEMENT

Medical Management

Inhibit Bacterial Growth

To promote comfort and decrease complications, broad-spectrum antibiotics typically begin before the culture and sensitivity results are known. Later, on the basis of the sensitivity report, a more specific antibiotic may be prescribed. The Integrating Pharmacology feature below describes medications used to treat urinary tract infections.

A client who reports continued manifestations after completing an antibiotic course or who complains of recurrent UTIs should return for a follow-up culture after antibiotic therapy. If the urine is not yet sterile, antibiotic therapy may be continued with the same or another antibiotic, based on the sensitivity report of the repeated culture.

Chronic or recurrent infections are a frustrating problem. Each infection must be treated with antibiotics. Persistent infections may call for suppression to keep the urine sterile. This measure consists of a small dose of antibiotic taken once daily or several times a week. Clients should be educated to avoid self-diagnosis and self-treatment with over-the-counter products, such as phenazopyridine. Each infection necessitates culture and sensitivity testing with specific treatment. The primary caregiver either may prescribe continuous suppression therapy or may continue episodic administration of antibiotics when a UTI recurs.

INTEGRATING PHARMACOLOGY

Medications for Urinary Tract Infection

The primary medication for the treatment of acute urinary tract infection is an antibiotic aimed at targeting the specific bacteria causing the infection. The specific bacteria should be cultured from a clean or sterile urine specimen. Each of the most commonly prescribed antibiotics and urinary antiseptics acts in a specific way to inhibit bacterial growth. Most commonly used pharmacologic agents include urinary antibiotics such as sulfonamides (trimethoprim-sulfamethoxazole [Bactrim]) and fluoroquinolones (ciprofloxacin [Cipro] and nitrofurantoin [Macrobid]). In addition, medications containing azo dyes, such as phenazopyridine (Pyridium), may also be prescribed to minimize the burning sensation often felt with cystitis. Pyridium turns urine bright orange and makes the client feel better after one dose. However, the client needs to understand that the complete course of the prescribed antibiotic must be taken to eradicate the bacteria.

The preferred course of treatment is a 7- to 10-day antibiotic regimen. If the client remains symptomatic following antibiotics, the urine should be cultured again. In some cases, the same bacteria are present despite the initial course of antibiotics. Therefore a second urine culture will report the presence of bacteria that may be more sensitive to a more specific or different antibiotic. In some clients, treatment must be extended for 14 days. This is especially true if the client is medically compromised, such as a hospitalized client with an indwelling catheter or a client with a history of diabetes mellitus or immunosuppression.

There is a growing trend to provide self-care for medication administration in clients with chronic infections. For example, women who experience UTIs in relation to sexual activity may receive a prescription for an antibiotic and instructions to take the medication after coitus. Other clients with frequent recurrences are:

- Offered a prescription for medication
- Taught to recognize early manifestations of a UTI
- Instructed to begin antibiotic therapy at the first hint of infection
- Reminded to complete the full course of antibiotics even if the manifestations disappear

Treating the client with asymptomatic bacteriuria is yet another problem. Some clinicians suggest that an asymptomatic infection be treated only if intervention is certain to prevent further morbidity or if the client is medically compromised. Others suggest immediate antibiotic treatment to reduce the risk of damage to the upper urinary tract.

Modify Diet

Certain foods are known to irritate the bladder, such as caffeine, alcohol, tomatoes, spicy food, chocolate, and some berries. Clients should be encouraged to avoid bladder irritants during the acute phase of the UTI.

Cranberry juice and ascorbic acid (vitamin C) have been used to acidify the urine. The use of these various dietary measures is under investigation, as explained in the Translating Evidence into Practice feature on p. 730. The tannin proanthocyanidins is thought to block bacteria from attaching to the bladder wall, thus flushing it from the urinary system.

Increase Fluid Intake

To treat and prevent UTI, encourage increased fluid intake, especially water, if the client is not required to restrict fluids. The desired amount is 3 to 4 L/day. Research suggests that calculating 0.5 ounce of fluid per pound of body weight (or dividing body weight in half to find the ounces of fluid needed) is an easy way to individualize fluid intake. Increased fluids flush the urinary system and are important in preventing *urolithiasis* (urinary calculi, or stones) in clients treated with sulfa drugs. Fluids containing alcohol and caffeine should be avoided because they increase mucosal irritation.

Prevent Complications

Broad-spectrum antibiotic therapy may destroy normal flora in the body and allow an overgrowth of opportunistic organisms. On occasion, diarrhea, associated bowel problems, and vaginal candidiasis may develop. Some antibiotics may reduce the effectiveness of oral

Cranberry-Based Products in the Prevention/Treatment of Urinary Tract Infections

Urinary tract infections (UTIs) account for more than 11 million visits to physicians' offices annually. Additionally, UTIs have been noted to become increasingly resistant to first-line antibiotic therapy.[4] Recently, evidence has suggested that the ingestion of cranberry juice or cranberry products has been effective in the prevention of UTIs or to decrease the manifestations of UTIs.[1,2,5-10] Cranberry juice, a red tart juice, is available in juice concentrations of 10% to 25%. The pure cranberry juice is acidic and is often unpalatable to clients even when mixed with a sweetener. Although the berry when harvested before it is ripe produces a milder and clear juice, no studies have discussed the evaluation of red cranberry juice versus white cranberry juice in the treatment of UTIs.[3]

According to earlier studies, the active ingredient—proanthocyanidins (condensed tannins)—found in cranberries and blueberries acidifies the urine, inhibiting certain urinary pathogens to adhere to the epithelial cells of the bladder. When the urinary pH increases from 4.5 to 5.0 and urine osmolarity is elevated, the proanthocyanidins affect the adherence of *Escherichia coli (E. coli)* to the bladder epithelial wall.[1,7] The evidence suggests that this phenomenon is most effective in the presence of *E. coli* and *Enterococci fecalis*. However, it has not been tested for other bacteria such as *Pseudomonas aeruginosa, Staphylococcus epidermidis,* or *Candida albicans*.

Kontiokari and colleagues compared cranberry and lingonberry juice with *Lactobacillus* GG drink and no intervention to determine which was most effective in preventing recurrent UTIs in women.[5] Their findings indicated that cranberry and lingonberry juice prevented recurrence of UTIs in women, whereas *Lactobacillus* GG drink or no intervention did not prevent recurrence of UTIs.[5] Another study by Dignam and colleagues found a decrease in institutional UTI rates from 27.2 per month to 20 per month after all residents were given 4 ounces of cranberry juice per day.[2] Similarly, McMurdo and colleagues found that the UTI rate in hospitals was twice as high in older clients receiving placebo versus older clients receiving 300 ml of cranberry juice per day.[6] Regal and colleagues reviewed double-blind, placebo-controlled studies from 1980 to 2005 on prevention of UTIs and concluded that cranberry juice and topical estrogen were effective in preventing UTIs in extended-care facilities but vitamin C was not effective.[8]

Additionally, cranberry tablets are available in strengths of 400 to 500 mg for dietary supplementation. The recommended dosing of cranberry tablets is from 1 to 2 tablets per day to 1 to 2 tablets with each meal.[3] McGuinness and colleagues conducted a study that used placebo and cranberry tablets containing 8000 mg of cranberry concentrate.[7] They found that UTIs developed in 32% of the placebo control group and in

34% of the cranberry tablet group.[7] The failure of the cranberry tablets was thought to be related to the inability to ensure that proanthocyanidins (the active ingredient in cranberries) were actually present in the cranberry tablets. They recommended that clients drink cranberry juice or eat cranberries. When studying the effects of cranberry tablets, Stothers[10] found that both cranberry juice and cranberry tablets statistically reduced the number of UTIs compared to placebo, with tablets being cheaper ($624 for tablets versus $1400 for juice per year).[10] Use of the tablets and use of the juice both decreased the use of antibiotics during the year as well.

IMPLICATIONS

Recent evidence supports the use of cranberry products to prevent UTIs. Evidence supports the use of cranberries or cranberry juice but is mixed with regard to cranberry tablets. Hence additional research is warranted before conclusions regarding cranberry tablets can be made. Nurses should offer supplemental cranberry juice as a preventive measure for those who are at risk for UTIs, especially those in long-term care facilities. In addition, teaching clients with UTIs about the preventive properties of cranberry juice or cranberries is appropriate.

REFERENCES

1. Chambers, S.T., et al. (1999). Inhibitors of bacterial growth in urine: What is the role of betaines? *International Journal of Antimicrobial Agents, 11,* 2933-2936.
2. Dignam, R., et al. (1998). The effect of cranberry juice on urinary tract infection rates in a long-term care facility. *Annals of Long Term Care, 6*(5), 163-167.
3. Gray, M. (2002). Are cranberry juice or cranberry products effective in the prevention or management of urinary tract infection? *Journal of Wounds, Ostomy and Continence, 29,* 122-126.
4. Howell, A.B., & Foxman, B. (2002). Cranberry juice and adhesion of antibiotic-resistant uropathogens. *Journal of the American Medical Association, 287*(230), 3083-3084.
5. Kontiokari, T., et al. (2001). Randomized trial of cranberry-lingonberry juice and *Lactobacillus* GG drink for the prevention of urinary tract infection in women. *British Medical Journal, 322,* 1571-1573.
6. McMurdo, M., et al. (2005). Does ingestion of cranberry juice reduce the symptoms of urinary tract infection in older people in a hospital? A double-blind placebo controlled study. *Age & Aging, 34*(3), 256-261.
7. McGuinness, S., Krone, R., & Metz, L. (2002). A double-blind, randomized, placebo-controlled trial of cranberry supplements in multiple sclerosis. *Journal of Neuroscience Nursing, 34*(1), 4-7.
8. Regal, R., Pham, C., & Bostwick, T. (2006). Urinary tract infections in extended care facilities: Preventive management strategies. *The Consultant Pharmacist: The Journal of the American Society of Consultant Pharmacists, 21*(5), 400-409.
9. Robbins, B., & Bondi, S. (2003). Does cranberry juice prevent or treat urinary tract infection? *Journal of Family Practice, 52*(2), 154-156.
10. Stothers, L. (2002). A randomized trial to evaluate effectiveness and cost effectiveness of naturopathic cranberry products as prophylaxis against urinary tract infections in women. *Canadian Journal of Urology, 9*(3), 1558-1562.

contraceptives and estrogen, whereas sulfa drugs increase sensitivity to the effects of the sun.

Complications can also occur if the infection is not completely eradicated. An ascending infection can

migrate from the bladder to the kidneys, resulting in pyelonephritis. Recurrent pyelonephritis can predispose the client to renal scarring and chronic renal failure if damage to the kidneys is severe enough. In clients with a history of recurrent or chronic infections, diagnostic testing is necessary to prevent complications associated with recurrent UTIs.

Nursing Management of the Medical Client

Assessment. Direct the initial nursing assessment at the history and clinical manifestations, as described earlier, to determine whether the problem is acute or chronic. Also, take a gynecologic, sexually transmitted infection (STI), and contraceptive history from female clients. Question male clients about presenting manifestations and take an STI history.

A key nursing responsibility is to instruct the client about clean-catch urine collection to minimize contamination from surface organisms. Appropriate collection of a clean-catch urine specimen for a dipstick test and culture and sensitivity should be included in the assessment. The urine specimen should initially be checked for leukocytes, blood, and nitrites. Color, odor, and clarity should also be evaluated. The urine specimen should then be sent for culture and sensitivity testing. If a client presents with chronic manifestations, additional radiologic diagnostic testing may be ordered to locate the origin of the disease process.

Diagnosis, Outcomes, Interventions

Diagnosis: Impaired Urinary Elimination. The primary nursing diagnosis when a client is experiencing problems related to cystitis is *Impaired Urinary Elimination related to irritation and inflammation of the bladder mucosa.*

Outcomes. The client will have return of normal voiding habits within 3 days of starting antibiotic treatment as evidenced by an absence of fever, pain, burning, frequency, and urgency.

Interventions

Inhibit Bacterial Growth. Give adequate instructions to the client regarding antibiotic therapy and dietary and activity restrictions needed during antibiotic therapy. Make sure the client understands the drug, its side effects, whether to take it with or without food, and the importance of taking the full course of the drug even after manifestations disappear. Have the client restate the antibiotic instructions by asking questions to ensure that the instructions have been understood.

Modify Diet. Provide information about dietary changes needed to keep the urine acidic and to reduce bladder irritation, such as avoiding alcohol and caffeinated beverages. Caffeine is found in coffee, tea, chocolate, some carbonated beverages, and some over-the-counter medications. Spicy foods and tomatoes are also associated with increased bladder irritation. Encourage clients with chronic UTIs to drink 10 ounces of cranberry juice daily to acidify the urine and decrease the likelihood of bacterial attachment to the bladder wall.

Increase Fluid Intake. To control the urgency and frequency caused by a UTI, clients may limit rather than increase fluid intake. Instruct your client to eliminate fluids that increase urgency and frequency, such as caffeinated beverages, and to increase the intake of other fluids to 3 to 4 L/day to flush the urinary system. To treat infection and prevent recurrence, teach the client how to calculate an appropriate fluid intake: 0.5 ounce of fluid per pound of body weight per day unless this amount is contraindicated.

Prevent Complications. Tell the client about the increased manifestations that might result from infection of the upper urinary tract and what to do if those manifestations occur.

 You should maintain a closed urinary drainage system and provide meticulous perineal care with mild soap and water for clients with an indwelling catheter. Keep the catheter bag below the level of the bladder at all times. These interventions help to achieve the TJC National Patient Safety Goal related to health care associated infections.

SAFETY

ALERT

Teach Health Promotion Strategies. Encourage the client to engage in health promotion activities to prevent UTIs. For example, encourage a fluid intake of at least 3 L/day, especially of water and acid-ash items to acidify the urine (such as cranberry juice). Advise clients to avoid caffeinated and alcoholic beverages or any of the foods that may irritate the bladder lining.

An important health promotion activity centers on client teaching to prevent recurrence of UTI. Female clients should learn the risks associated with chemical irritants such as spermicides, intercourse, and poorly fitted vaginal devices, and the additional risk of lowered estrogen levels associated with menopause. A review of correct hygienic practices should also be included. Alert both male and female clients that STIs can cause manifestations similar to those of a UTI. Inform male clients about obstructive voiding problems caused by benign prostatic hypertrophy (BPH) that lead to urinary stasis.

Emphasize the importance of increased fluids and avoidance of foods and fluids that increase irritation. Also, remind the client to void every 2 to 4 hours during the day (unless the bladder program is planned otherwise) to keep the urinary system flushed. Pregnant women should be encouraged to void every 2 to 3 hours.

Encourage women to void before and after coitus. Suggest that sexually active women use positions that minimize pressure on the anterior vaginal wall during intercourse. Also emphasize the need to maintain good perineal hygiene. For example, instruct women to wipe the urinary meatus from front to back. Encourage women who experience frequent UTIs to shower rather than take tub baths, and urge them to avoid bubble baths, salts, and scented feminine hygiene products. Wearing cotton underpants, which are more absorbent and breathable or porous than synthetic undergarments, and avoiding pantyhose with slacks, a practice that can trap moisture in the perineal region, are additional ways to lower the risk of UTI in women.

The application of vaginal estrogen increases circulation to the lower urogenital system and increases the mucosal layer of atrophic tissues commonly seen in postmenopausal women. Because the lower urogenital system is heavily enriched with estrogen receptors and blood supply before menopause, women should be informed about the need for topical estrogen and systemic estrogen in the postmenopausal period. Using a vaginal lubricant during intercourse is helpful as well.

Health maintenance activities include (1) monitoring pregnant women and older male clients (especially those with BPH) for the presence of UTI, (2) teaching high-risk clients the clinical manifestations of infection, and (3) monitoring clients with an indwelling catheter for the presence of infection. Many postoperative clients receive prophylactic antibiotics while an indwelling catheter is in place.

Finally, clients with a UTI are managed with antibiotics and increased fluid intake. To restore health, clients should be taught ways to prevent recurrence and the importance of taking all antibiotics, followed with repeated cultures and sensitivity testing as ordered.

Diagnosis: Acute Pain. Another common nursing diagnosis for clients with cystitis is *Acute Pain related to irritation and inflammation of bladder and urethral mucosa.*

Outcomes. The client will be able to urinate with minimal or no discomfort within 24 hours after treatment begins and will return to normal voiding habits within 3 days, as evidenced by an absence of pain and burning on urination.

Interventions. Medications prescribed specifically to treat pain, such as phenazopyridine (Pyridium), should be administered. Other comfort measures include forcing fluids to dilute urine and taking a warm sitz bath to decrease urethral smooth muscle spasms. Some clients find a heating pad applied to the suprapubic area helpful in reducing bladder spasms and suprapubic pain.

Evaluation. After the first 24 hours of treatment, the client should be able to report a reduction in pain, burning, urgency, and frequency. Antibiotic therapy usually brings about complete resolution of irritation and pain within 3 days. If indicated, urine culture specimens should be negative after 1 week of treatment or after the course of antibiotics is completed.

Surgical Management

The need for surgery is rare; operations are performed only to address structural anomalies that cause repeated infections. Strictures of the bladder neck or urethra are the most common problems requiring surgical intervention. BPH may also be treated surgically (see Chapter 38). Nursing care after surgery is discussed under the specific disorder. Chapter 38 describes nursing care of men after surgery for BPH.

Self-Care

Promotion of self-care for a client with a UTI includes recognition of lifestyle changes needed to decrease risk factors, the ability to restate the medication protocol, and return for follow-up urine cultures, if indicated. Explain risk factors for UTIs and health promotion strategies to prevent recurrence. These strategies include increased fluid intake, fluid and diet modifications, voiding every 2 hours, and lifestyle modifications, as previously discussed. Advise the client to seek care if manifestations recur.

Modifications for Older Clients

In older people, cystitis may occur more often than in younger people but for different reasons. Causes might include immobility, constipation, fecal and urinary incontinence, urinary retention (incomplete voiding), altered mental status, or systemic disease.

In older women, atrophic changes resulting from decreased estrogen affect the vagina and urethra. In older men, increased size of the prostrate gland can increase their risk for UTI. These alterations cause bladder dysfunction, which may predispose older clients to infection.

When administering medications to older or compromised clients, you must consider their renal and hepatic status. Many drugs used to treat UTIs necessitate that the client have adequate renal and hepatic function, particularly with long-term administration. Also, consider any changes in cardiovascular status that might prevent an increase in fluid intake.

URETHRITIS

Urethritis, or inflammation of the urethra, is commonly associated with STIs or sexually transmitted infections (see Chapter 41) and is an associated manifestation of cystitis. The most common causes of urethritis are gonorrhea, chlamydial infection, and other bacterial infections. Among women, common causes also include feminine hygiene sprays, scented toilet paper, sanitary napkins, spermicidal jellies, UTIs, and changes in the vaginal mucosal lining. In short, any irritant that comes into contact with the urethra can cause urethritis.

Exposure to irritants causes the mucosal lining of the urethra to become inflamed. The mucosal lining becomes swollen, painful, red, and irritated. Pus may be produced. *Pyuria,* the presence of pus in the urine, is a common indication of urethritis. Manifestations are similar to those described for cystitis. Frequently, women reveal a history of chemical irritant exposure. Male clients frequently exhibit a urethral discharge.

The diagnosis is often confirmed on the basis of the client's history and clinical manifestations. Culture and sensitivity testing of the urine should be performed, and culture specimens should be obtained to exclude STIs if indicated.

Management of urethritis includes removing the etiologic mechanism. If a microorganism is the cause, administration of systemic and topical antibiotics is essential. Sitz baths and an increased fluid intake are also encouraged. Advise the client to avoid coitus until the manifestations subside or treatment of the STI is completed. The use of lubricants with intercourse decreases irritation in women who have had frequent episodes. Common medications are the same as those used to treat cystitis. The physician may also prescribe topical estrogens for a menopausal woman.

Prevention of urethritis by decreasing exposure to STIs is essential. Inform women about the increased risk of urethritis from spermicides and about the need to avoid feminine hygiene sprays, perfumed toilet paper, and scented sanitary napkins.

URETERITIS

Ureteritis, or inflammation of the ureter, is commonly associated with pyelonephritis (see Chapter 35). Once the kidney infection is treated, ureteral inflammation usually subsides. Chronic pyelonephritis can cause the ureter to become fibrotic and narrowed by strictures, which in turn can continue to foster this condition.

UROSEPSIS

Urosepsis is a gram-negative bacteremia originating in the genitourinary tract. It has become more prevalent among institutionalized clients, especially if the client has an underlying condition. The most common predisposing factors are an indwelling catheter or an untreated UTI in a medically compromised client. Two other primary risk factors for urosepsis are immunosuppression therapy and chemotherapy.

The most common organism responsible for gram-negative bacteremia is *E. coli,* which has the ability to develop resistant strains. Traditionally, gram-negative bacteria have always been recognized as the causative organism of urosepsis. However, there is increasing evidence to suggest that gram-positive bacteria, fungi, viruses, and parasites may also be responsible. Therefore more research, better diagnostic testing, and better and more aggressive implementation of a therapeutic program directed at eliminating bloodstream invasion of the bacteria with correction and prevention of the pathophysiologic events that cause urosepsis are essential.

The pathophysiologic mechanisms of urosepsis are complex and not fully understood. The disorder can lead to septic shock and death if it is not treated immediately and aggressively (see Chapter 81). The cell wall of the gram-negative bacillus is composed of a lipid-carbohydrate complex. Bacteria release endotoxins, which damage cells. The cells release lysosomes, which further damage tissues and instigate kinins and the complement cascade. Cellular metabolism becomes anaerobic, and lactic acidosis develops. Fever and altered mental status are the most common early manifestations. Additionally, research indicates that hyperventilation is often observed before fever begins in clients suffering from urosepsis.

Clients at increased risk for urosepsis should be monitored closely to prevent development of irreversible shock. To prevent sepsis and shock, treatment of urosepsis must be instituted immediately after specimen collection for culture and sensitivity testing.

SAFETY

⚠

ALERT

Initial treatment consists of intravenous (IV) aminoglycosides, beta-lactam antibiotics (such as aztreonam), or third-generation cephalosporins until culture results are available. As soon as culture and sensitivity results are available, the antibiotic may be changed if necessary. IV treatment is directed by the status of the client and continued for 3 to 5 days once the client becomes afebrile. Oral antibiotics are continued for the duration of therapy.

INTERSTITIAL CYSTITIS

Cystitis may be noninfectious or abacterial. One type, interstitial cystitis (IC), is also called painful bladder disease (PBD), Hunner's ulcer, urethral syndrome, pseudomembranous trigonitis, and other names. This greatly underdiagnosed condition involves urgency, frequency, and a painful bladder despite a lack of bacteria in the urine culture. The most severe forms of this disease involve ulcerations and hemorrhages in the bladder wall. The cause of these ulcers is unknown, but the ulcers may stem from a defect in the epithelial molecular layer of the bladder wall.

Etiology and Risk Factors

IC occurs mainly in young women (90% to 95% of all cases), usually white but occasionally African American women. 🔦 Clients with inflammatory and irritable bowel disorders also have a higher incidence of IC.

Pathophysiology

IC is a poorly understood disorder with an unclear pathophysiology. It may be a local autoimmune phenomenon. Despite clinical manifestations, the urine is usually sterile. The most current theory seems to be associated with a breakdown in the permeability of the glycosaminoglycan layer of the bladder mucosa, which is usually impermeable to urea and bacteria. This theory has been questioned in some studies that suggest that the permeability of the bladder in clients with IC is no greater than that in normal people.

Characteristic pathologic changes are found in more severe forms of IC, including nonspecific chronic inflammatory infiltrate, edema, vasodilation, and eventually fibrosis of the submucosa and detrusor layers of the bladder wall. The fibrosis of the submucosa seems to decrease the elasticity of the detrusor muscle, which decreases bladder capacity.

Mast cell infiltrates have been identified in the bladders of clients with IC, particularly in the detrusor layer. Because mast cells are associated with allergic reactions, it is worth noting that about half of clients with IC are reported to have allergies and 30% have inflammatory bowel disease. Finally, another hypothesis is that bacteria are found only in the mucosal wall of the bladder and not in the urine.

Clinical Manifestations

The clinical manifestations of IC are tenderness in the area of the bladder trigone during anterior palpation in a vaginal examination, complaints of lower abdominal or pelvic pain, urinary urgency and frequency (up to 60 times a day), *nocturia* (excessive urination at night), and, in some women, dyspareunia (painful intercourse). Presenting manifestations and their severity vary from client to client. Some women find the disorder debilitating. Manifestations may be present for years and treated as bacterial cystitis before an appropriate diagnosis is made.

🔦 The National Institute of Diabetes, Digestive, and Kidney Diseases recommends specific diagnostic criteria for identifying clients with clinical manifestations. These criteria include the following:

- A detailed client history with physical examination
- A completed bladder diary
- Urine cytology
- Urodynamic evaluation to determine bladder capacity and evaluate bladder function
- Cystoscopy with the client under anesthesia and with hydrodistention of the bladder
- Bladder biopsy

During cystoscopy and hydrodilation of the bladder, the presence of outpouches in the bladder wall, Hunner's ulcers, and a severely decreased bladder capacity are considered by many physicians to be the clinical diagnostic features of IC. Others believe that IC may be present even without these findings.

OUTCOME MANAGEMENT

Medical Management

Reduce Pain

The treatment of IC is controversial, with no single accepted treatment. Anti-inflammatory, antispasmodic, antidepressant, and antihistamine medications and, occasionally, tranquilizers or opioids may be used.

🔦 Pentosan polysulfate sodium (Elmiron) is the newest oral medication of choice. This drug increases the bladder defense mechanism or detoxifies irritants in urine that might break down the bladder lining. The mechanism of action is like heparin, with anticoagulant and antifibrin effects. Relief of manifestations may take up to 3 months.

Other treatments include instillation of a variety of agents into the bladder to promote healing and pain reduction, such as sodium oxychlorosene (Clorpactin), silver nitrate, and dimethyl sulfoxide (DMSO). Heparin has been instilled in the bladder, initially daily for 3 to 4 months. Therapy is continued three times a week for 3 to 6 months. Some clients may not notice any improvement in manifestations until after the first 2 to 4 months of treatment. All of these treatments are designed to decrease the permeability of the bladder mucosa so that the causative agent has more difficulty penetrating the lining.

Although the mechanism of action is unclear, bacille Calmette-Guerin (BCG) has been effective as an intravesical agent administered weekly. BCG instillations for 6 weeks have led to a decreased need for pain medications, a doubling of cystometric capacity, and sometimes a decrease in client discomfort.

Referrals to centers providing conservative management programs with behavioral intervention, electrical stimulation, and biofeedback to the pelvic floor musculature may also alleviate manifestations of IC. Because of the chronic nature of the disorder, physicians are reluctant to offer opioids for pain reduction. During severe exacerbations, however, opioids may be appropriate.

Improve Coping

Many clients with IC complain of exhaustion and depression. The exhaustion usually stems from poor sleep patterns caused by nocturnal urgency, frequency, and pain. Depression can result from frustration, exhaustion, chronic pain, and difficulty in obtaining effective medical care.

During the acute phase, these clients may require medications to improve sleep as well as antidepressant therapy to increase coping ability. Referrals to social workers or other health care professionals to improve coping strategies and mental status may be needed. You also may need to refer the client to a center that specializes in treating IC.

Nursing Management of the Medical Client

Reduce Pain

Nurses provide a great deal of education about drug therapy. Many of the medications have a cumulative effect, making long-term therapy necessary for maximal results. You may need to continuously reinforce this point if the client grows frustrated with pharmacologic intervention. You also should counsel the client before opioid intervention. Because IC is a chronic problem, inform the client about risk factors associated with opioids.

Improve Coping

Your major responsibility is to support the client through diagnosis and treatment. Because the cause of IC is unclear, few nursing interventions are aimed at prevention. IC is a chronic disorder requiring long-term client support. Clients may need additional psychological counseling to help with stress-related coping strategies. Become familiar with national and local resources for clients with IC or painful bladder disease (Interstitial Cystitis Association), and refer clients as appropriate.

Bladder retraining with conservative management programs can help reduce clinical manifestations. Teaching clients to void by the clock rather than by urge gently and slowly increases bladder capacity. Biofeedback-directed pelvic floor exercises teach the client the urge suppression technique. This process decreases episodes of urgency and frequency and promotes control of manifestations. The additional use of transvaginal or transanal electrical stimulation may help override bladder spasms and can increase the quality of pelvic floor contractions.

Surgical Management

Surgery is rarely used to manage the client with IC. The traditional therapy is hydraulic distention of the bladder, with or without instillation of DMSO to increase the bladder's functional capacity. Clients with severely reduced bladder capacity and incapacitating manifestations may be candidates for a transurethral resection (TUR), laser surgical resection of the lesions, a partial or complete *cystectomy* (resection of the bladder), and *urinary diversion* (surgical rerouting of the normal urinary flow) (see Bladder Cancer).

OBSTRUCTIVE DISORDERS

BLADDER CANCER

Most bladder cancers are transitional or papillary tumors in the bladder urothelium. These tumors may infiltrate the bladder wall. Bladder cancer is the most frequent neoplasm of the urinary tract, accounting for about 6% of all cancer cases in men and 2% in women.[2] The American Cancer Society estimated 67,160 new cases of bladder cancer in 2007 and 13,750 associated deaths.[2] Bladder cancer is rarely seen in adults younger than 40 years of age and occurs most frequently in 50- to 60-year-old adults. Now the fourth most common cancer in men and the tenth most common cancer in women, it affects whites twice as often as blacks.[2]

Etiology and Risk Factors

The disease process has several possible causes. There is a strong correlation between cigarette smoking and bladder cancer. Hence a health promotion and health maintenance strategy is to encourage smokers to stop smoking and to be screened regularly after age 50 years for hematuria and other manifestations of bladder cancer. The use of supplements to reduce the risk of bladder cancer is considered in the Complementary and Alternative Therapy feature on p. 736.

Industrial exposure to certain substances, such as aniline dyes, asbestos, and aromatic amines (e.g., benzidine and 2-naphthylamine), may also result in bladder cancer. The latency period of industrial exposure can be as long as 18 to 45 years. Workers in this high-risk group should also be screened regularly after age 50 for hematuria and other manifestations of bladder cancer.

Artificial sweeteners have been weakly linked to the development of bladder cancer. Attempts to connect coffee consumption and bladder cancer have produced contradictory findings because of the increased use of artificial sweeteners and cigarettes associated with coffee consumption. Other risk factors may be chronic cystitis, pelvic radiation, the chemotherapeutic drug cyclophosphamide (Cytoxan), and low fluid intake. Increasing fluid intake to reduce the risk of cancer is discussed in the Complementary and Alternative Therapy feature on p. 736.

Clients who have undergone transurethral resection or removal of superficial bladder cancer should return for regular cystoscopic follow-up as a health maintenance and restoration activity. Teaching clients to care for a urinary diversion is a health restoration activity provided by nurses.

Pathophysiology

Bladder cancer appears to result from exposure of the bladder wall to a *carcinogen* (a cancer-causing agent).

Supplements to Reduce the Risk of Bladder Cancer

A large epidemiologic study found somewhat similar results to the Health Professionals Follow-up Study. Researchers investigated the association between individual vitamin C and vitamin E supplements and bladder cancer mortality among more than 991,000 U.S. adults in the Cancer Prevention Study II cohort. This data set covered 16 years of follow-up, and 1289 deaths (962 men and 327 women) from bladder cancer were recorded.

Regular vitamin C supplement use was not related to bladder cancer mortality during any follow-up period. However, regular vitamin E supplement use for 10 or more years (but not of shorter duration) was associated with a reduced risk of bladder cancer mortality (RR = 0.60). A reduction in bladder cancer mortality was found in adults who never smoked (RR = 0.84) and in ex-smokers (RR = 0.69), but the reduction was most evident in current smokers (RR = 0.31).

The authors of this study did not endorse the use of vitamin E supplements for smokers because of the large impact on overall disease risk in current smokers from other studies. The primary recommendation, which seems most appropriate, was to stop smoking completely to prevent both bladder cancer and early morbidity and mortality from other diseases. Thus the preliminary data so far indicate that current smokers may not benefit from individual vitamin C and vitamin E supplements in terms of overall disease morbidity and mortality reduction, but ex-smokers and those who have never smoked may derive some benefit (mostly from vitamin supplements), especially in regard to bladder cancer reduction.

REFERENCE

Jacobs, E., et al. (2002). Vitamin C and vitamin E supplement use and bladder cancer mortality in a large cohort of U.S. men and women. *American Journal of Epidemiology, 156*, 1002-1110.

RR, Relative risk.

Cigarette smoking or second-hand smoke may result in carcinogenic metabolites produced by abnormal tryptophan metabolism, with the metabolite excreted in the urine. Cigarette smoke also contains nitrosamines as well as 2-naphthylamine (both carcinogens), which are also excreted in the urine. 🗫 Deletion in chromosome 9 is the most consistent chromosomal finding. Deletions in chromosomes 3, 8, 11, and 18 are often associated with high-grade disease.

Premalignant proliferative changes are often found in the transitional cell layer. These changes are called *dysplasia* and refer to abnormal cell configuration found in several degrees of severity. The extent of dysplasia may be described as mild, moderate, or severe, leading to carcinoma in situ (localized). Most bladder cancers start as papillary or transitional cell tumors and account for 70% of bladder tumors. These tumors are most

Fluid Consumption to Reduce the Risk of Bladder Cancer

Increased fluid consumption from numerous sources may reduce the risk of bladder cancer. The largest cohort study attempting to determine the relationship between fluid intake and bladder cancer risk was taken from the Health Professionals Follow-up Study. Approximately 48,000 male health professionals were followed for 10 years, with a total of 252 cases of bladder cancer found during this time period. Men in this study updated their diet and medical history every 2 years. Data on total fluid intake were taken from the reported intake frequency of 22 beverage types on a diet questionnaire.

Age and smoking were found to have a major relationship with bladder cancer risk. Total fluid consumption was inversely related with the risk of bladder cancer (RR = 0.51) for the highest quintile of intake (>2531 ml/day) versus the lowest (<1290 ml/day). Water intake was responsible for a significantly lower risk (*p* for trend = 0.001) when comparing 6 or more cups/day versus 1 cup (RR = 0.49). This risk decreased by 7% for each 240-ml daily increment of fluid consumption.

The baseline questionnaire used in this study could not provide insight regarding the source of water (tap and/or bottled) consumed on a regular basis. Thus the investigators in this study could not clearly comment on the effect of the water source and any potential risk. However, data from approximately one third of the cohort found that the majority of these men (78%) consumed municipal water. In addition, the inverse relationship for water and risk was consistently observed in all regions of the United States and was also observed for the individuals who reported drinking water from municipal sources.

This investigation suggests that a greater consumption of water could decrease the risk of bladder cancer by an average of 50%. No beverage except water demonstrated a significant inverse relationship with bladder cancer, but the consumption of all other types of fluids, with the exception of fruit juice, was also related to a lower risk (RR = 0.63). Other fluids that reduced the risk included milk, sodas, lemonade, coffee, tea, and alcoholic beverages. Whether or not greater fluid intake affects risk remains to be determined, but if it does it may be a partial explanation of why certain regions of the world experience lower rates of bladder cancer despite a higher rate of smoking.

REFERENCE

Michaud, D., et al. (1999). Fluid intake and the risk of bladder cancer in men. *New England Journal of Medicine, 340*, 1390-1397.

RR, Relative risk.

commonly found in the trigone of the bladder and lateral wall of the bladder.

Staging of a tumor indicates the depth of penetration into the bladder wall and degree of *metastasis*. Staging must be done to determine the treatment modality. Clinical staging includes the results and review of an excretory urogram, cystoscopy, biopsy, and bimanual examination with the client under anesthesia. For evaluation of specific areas of metastasis as well as for staging, chest radiography, lymphangiography, isotope bone scans, computed tomography (CT), and liver function analysis are needed. The most frequently used staging systems are the Jewett-Marshall-Strong System and the tumor-node-metastasis (TNM) classification. The stages refer to the depth of invading tumor found during biopsy (Figure 34-1).

Superficial tumors have a good chance of being eradicated or stabilized; however, recurrence is frequent. Therefore it is crucial to do follow-up cystoscopic examinations every 3 months for 2 years, with additional cystoscopic examinations every 6 months for 2 years, then yearly. Most recurrences of superficial tumors represent lesions that can be controlled by transurethral resection.

Metastasis to other organs begins once the invading cancer penetrates the submucosal and muscular layers of the bladder. The invasion progresses through pelvic lymph nodes and spreads to liver, bones, and lungs. As metastasis progresses, it can extend into the rectum, vagina, other pelvic soft tissues, and retroperitoneal structures. The prognostic "dividing line" lies between stages B1 and B2; stage C and D tumors portend a much poorer prognosis. Clients with superficial bladder tumors have a survival rate of 70% after 5 years. Other clients with muscle invasive disease experience tumor recurrence within 18 to 24 months of the diagnosis.

Clinical Manifestations

Gross painless hematuria is most frequently the first manifestation of bladder cancer, occurring in 85% of all cases. Initially, the bleeding is usually intermittent, which may lead a client to delay seeking health care. As the disease becomes more invasive, the client may experience frequent bladder irritability with dysuria, frequency, and urgency. Frequently, gross hematuria or obstruction in voiding forces the client to seek help. The amount of hematuria does not correlate with stage of disease. See the Integrating Diagnostic Testing feature on p. 666 for diagnostic evaluation of hematuria.

Numerous attempts have been made to identify other screening tests including the BTA (bladder tumor antigen) test, NMP22 (nuclear matrix protein) test, and TRAP (telomeric repeat amplification protocol) assay, but all lack sufficient sensitivity. Newer techniques under investigation include assays designed to detect hyaluronic acid, hyaluronidase or survivin, a substance that inhibits cellular apoptosis.

Another examination, intravenous pyelogram (IVP), is a dye-enhanced x-ray examination that allows one to evaluate not only the bladder but also the ureters and kidneys. CT, magnetic resonance imaging (MRI), and ultrasonography also may be done to assess the bladder and surrounding structures, such as the rectum or uterus, possible sites of spread. A tumor marker, serum carcinoembryonic antigen (CEA), which is present with adenocarcinomas of the bladder, can also be evaluated.

OUTCOME MANAGEMENT

Medical Management

The outcome desired with medical management is to eradicate the bladder of transitional or papillary cell carcinoma in situ in the early stages. This is best achieved with alkylating intravesical chemotherapy or BCG instillations, which are the first-line and most common therapies. Advanced cancer that has invaded muscle is usually treated surgically with a radical cystectomy. Radiation therapy is rarely used in cases of advanced disease or as palliative treatment. Radiation therapy may be used in combination with chemotherapy for a bladder-sparing approach to invasive bladder cancer if surgery is not elected.

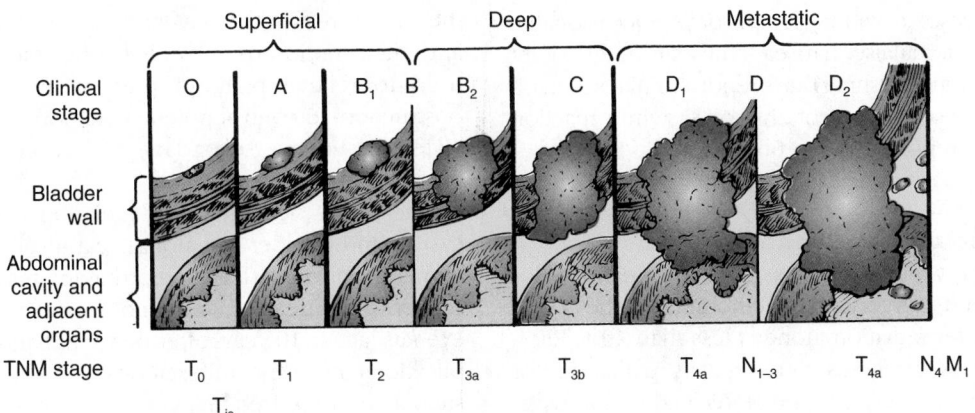

■ **FIGURE 34–1** The Jewett-Marshall-Strong clinical staging of bladder cancer. The diagram shows the degree of tumor infiltration at each stage and compares it with the tumor, node, metastasis (TNM) system. *(Modified from Karlowicz, K. [Ed.] [1995]. Urologic nursing: Principles and practice. Philadelphia: Saunders.)*

Chemotherapy Administration

Intravesical therapies can be administered for superficial tumors, such as transitional cell, papillary cell, or stage 0-A tumors. Intravesical BCG therapy appears to be successful in treating carcinoma in situ. The best results have been obtained with BCG as an intravesical agent for transitional cell tumors, although it has also been used for papillary tumors, adenocarcinoma, and squamous cell carcinoma.

Usually, BCG is instilled into the bladder through a urethral catheter. The catheter is clamped or removed. The client is directed to retain the fluid for 2 hours, with side-to-side position changes or supine-to-prone changes required every 15 to 30 minutes. Once the 2 hours have passed, the client voids in a sitting position or the catheter is unclamped to allow drainage. Finally, the client is instructed to drink two glasses of water to help flush the bladder. Steroids and ciprofloxacin (Cipro) have sometimes been given after intravesical BCG treatment to prevent recurrence. If two treatment cycles of intravesical BCG have been ineffective, most urologists recommend a cystectomy (see the Complementary and Alternative Therapy feature on Combination Mega-Dose Supplement and the Recurrence of Bladder Cancer at right).

Intravesical instillation of an alkylating chemotherapeutic agent, another common practice, provides concentrated topical treatment with relatively little systemic absorption. Gemcitabine (Gemzar), mitomycin (Mutamycin), doxorubicin (Adriamycin), valrubicin (Valstar), and cyclophosphamide (Cytoxan) are all used for low-grade, superficial papillary tumors. Systemic chemotherapy drugs are used for more advanced disease, to treat the metastasis of the bladder tumor, and to prolong life. However, surgical removal of the bladder is the most common approach in advanced disease when tumor has invaded muscle.

The major side effects or complications of intravesical chemotherapy or BCG instillation include bladder irritation, frequency, urgency, and dysuria. These manifestations usually resolve within 1 or 2 days. Occasionally, hematuria, fever, malaise, nausea, chills, arthralgia (joint pain), and pruritus (itching) are reported. These manifestations are more representative of systemic reaction and should be reported to the physician.

Radiation Therapy

Radiation therapy alone is not as effective a treatment for bladder cancer as surgery and chemotherapy; the 5-year survival rate after radiation alone is less than 40%. Radiation therapy is rarely used except as palliation for advanced disease that cannot be eradicated by intravesical chemotherapy or radical surgery. Most bladder cancers are poorly radiosensitive, and high doses of radiation are necessary.

COMPLEMENTARY AND ALTERNATIVE THERAPY

Combination Mega-Dose Supplement and the Recurrence of Bladder Cancer

An older trial that has yet to be duplicated included 65 clients with transitional cell carcinoma (TCC) of the bladder and BCG (bacille Calmette-Guérin) immunotherapy. Clients were randomly assigned to a group that received by mouth either the recommended daily allowance (RDA) of several vitamins and a mineral or the RDA of several vitamins and a mineral plus 40,000 international units of vitamin A, 100 mg of vitamin B_6, 2000 mg of vitamin C, 400 international units of vitamin E, and 90 mg of zinc.

No difference in the time to recurrence was noted in the first 10 months of the study, but significant differences occurred after that time period. The overall follow-up was a mean of 45 months (40 months for the RDA group and 49 months for the RDA-plus-other-vitamins group). The 5-year estimates (Kaplan-Meier interval) of recurrence were 91% in the RDA group ($n = 30$) and 41% in the RDA-plus-other-vitamins group. This difference was statistically significant, and mild nausea was the most common side effect.

This study obviously requires a larger randomized trial to confirm its findings, but the initial result is interesting and should probably at least be discussed with clients undergoing a similar conventional treatment protocol. Some questions concerning the individual clients in this study were not addressed, such as nutritional or vitamin and mineral deficiency status and other lifestyle and genetic differences between the groups. These issues need to be addressed in future studies.

REFERENCE

Lamm, D., et al. (1994). Megadose vitamins in bladder cancer: A double-blind clinical trial. *Journal of Urology, 151,* 21-26.

External supervoltage radiation, somewhat unsuccessful by itself, is effective when used in combination with surgery or chemotherapy. Hyperbaric radiation therapy increases the oxygen tension of the tumor cells and their radiosensitivity. Palliative radiation may be used to relieve pain, to prevent and relieve bowel obstruction, to control potential hemorrhage, and to alleviate leg edema secondary to venous or lymphatic obstruction.

The major side effects of radiation are hemorrhagic cystitis and bladder irritation. Local instillation of formalin may control bladder hemorrhaging resulting from the cancer or the treatments. Hemorrhagic cystitis may occur even as late as 10 years after pelvic radiation. Other complications include manifestations of cystitis and proctitis, such as dysuria, frequency, urgency, nocturia, and diarrhea. Delayed adverse effects, such as ileitis, colitis, persistent cystitis, bladder ulceration, and fistula formation, may occur as late as 6 to 12 months after radiation.

Nursing Management of the Medical Client

Assessment. Begin your assessment of a client being evaluated for bladder cancer with a careful health, medical, and surgical history. Because this client will be undergoing extensive diagnostic evaluation, be sure to collect additional information about drug, chemical, and food allergies. Explain risk factors from exposure to known carcinogens. Ask the client about changes in urine or urination patterns, noting changes in color, frequency, and amount.

Diagnosis, Outcomes, Interventions

Diagnosis: Powerlessness and/or Decisional Conflict. The client with bladder cancer may experience *Powerlessness and/or Decisional Conflict related to lack of knowledge of disease process, options, treatment, and side effects of therapy; difficulty in deciding on treatment options; fear of the disease process and treatment; and loss of control following the diagnosis and decisions regarding treatment offered.*

Outcomes. The client will learn about the medical management of the disease process, with a full understanding of client responsibilities during the treatment. The client and family will be involved with decisions about therapies and care. The client will also be encouraged to help direct care with involved health care professionals.

Interventions

Provide Education. To increase knowledge, educate the client and family about the use, rationale, risks, side effects, and expected outcomes of intravesical chemotherapy, BCG instillation, radiation, and surgery. You play an important role in client education of treatment modalities and complications that may accompany them.

Encourage Decision Making. Encourage the client to discuss and make decisions about care. Provide opportunities for the client to express desires for care as well as time to discuss what the diagnosis and treatment mean personally.

Diagnosis: Impaired Urinary Elimination. *Impaired Urinary Elimination related to urgency, frequency, dysuria, and hematuria resulting from chemotherapy, radiation, or BCG instillation for treatment of bladder cancer.*

Outcomes. Normal voiding will resume by day 3 after removal of the catheter, and the client will not experience sequelae to BCG instillation, chemotherapy, or radiation therapy.

Interventions. Nursing management of intravesical chemotherapy includes client education, administration of the chemotherapy agent, care of the client throughout the procedure, and monitoring for complications after administration.

Provide Education. Preparation before BCG or chemotherapy bladder instillation requires fluid restriction for 4 hours before the procedure to decrease the need to void for 2 hours afterward. Tell the client that a catheter will be inserted before the instillation and that it will be necessary to rotate and change positions every 15 to 30 minutes during treatment. After the 2-hour instillation, fluids are encouraged to flush the urinary system. Explain that treatments are typically repeated weekly for 4 to 8 weeks and then monthly for varying periods. Follow-up cystoscopy is required to monitor tumor growth.

Promote Safety

Because of the toxicity of the intravesical chemotherapy or BCG instillation, it is important to provide a safe environment for health care workers who may come in contact with the chemotherapeutic agent. For 6 hours after treatment, all urine and the toilet bowl must be disinfected with bleach.

SAFETY

ALERT

Promote Comfort. Dysuria or irritation while voiding may result from the side effects of chemotherapy, placement of an indwelling catheter, and the presence of the tumor, and it must be managed. Tumor pain is managed with analgesics. Irritative problems of dysuria, frequency, and urgency from the catheter will diminish when the catheter is removed. Irritation from the chemotherapy will decrease after about 2 days.

Reassure the client that dysuria, frequency, and urgency from catheter placement and intravesical treatment will diminish over 2 days. Discuss prescribed analgesics, antispasmodics, or anticholinergics, and explain how they should be taken.

Diagnosis: Risk for Injury. The client who undergoes chemotherapy, BCG instillation, or radiation therapy is at *Risk for Injury from side effects of these treatments.*

Outcomes. Complications resulting from these treatments will be minimized. The client will verbalize an understanding of risk and side effects following the selected treatment option.

Interventions. Explain expected and unexpected outcomes of BCG instillation, chemotherapy, or radiation therapy. Inform the client and family how and when to alert medical staff to potential complications. Interventions for side effects include administering antispasmodics, increasing fluid intake, and administering urinary tract antiseptics or analgesics.

If a high temperature develops after BCG instillation, treatment with isoniazid or other medications used to treat tuberculosis may be indicated.

For radiation proctitis, the client requires a low-residue diet and drugs to decrease intestinal motility. For complete information on nursing care for clients receiving radiation therapy, see Chapter 17.

Evaluation. Complications that arise from medical treatment may be difficult to manage, but they typically resolve after the treatment has ended. Evaluation of the nursing management of radiation therapy and intravesical BCG and chemotherapy is based on the client's ability to restate personal responsibilities, to verbalize an understanding of the disease process, and to participate in care.

Because clients with bladder cancer require long-term follow-up care and continuous evaluation, they must understand the disease process and long-term follow-up responsibilities needed to maintain optimal health. If medical therapies are unsuccessful, surgical removal of the bladder may be required.

Surgical Management

Several surgical options may be used to treat bladder cancer that has not responded to medical therapies or that has invaded the bladder muscle. Surgical intervention ranges from local resection and fulguration of the tumor (destruction of tissue by electrical current through electrodes placed in direct contact with the growth) to total cystectomy, which requires diversion of normal urinary flow. Most of the surgical procedures can be performed via traditional open, laparoscopic, or robotic-assisted methods.

Transurethral Resection

The simplest procedure is transurethral resection of the bladder tumor and fulguration done for low-grade, superficial, isolated papillary tumors or, sometimes, for inoperable tumors for palliation. The bladder is accessed through a cystoscope, which has been inserted through the urethra. This procedure is commonly followed by intravesical BCG or chemotherapy to prevent recurrence from reattachment of loose bladder cancer cells. Assess for hematuria, stenosis, and other complications after surgery. Hematuria, a common problem after transurethral resection, is controlled with a three-way indwelling catheter and, if necessary, bladder irrigation.

After transurethral resection of the bladder, the client usually has hematuria. A three-lumen, indwelling urethral catheter is attached to a continuous or intermittent closed bladder irrigation system to facilitate urine flow, minimize blood clots, and monitor for postoperative bleeding. Nursing care is similar to that after transurethral resection of the prostate (see Chapter 38). Bright red or pink urine fades to clear in about 3 days.

Partial Cystectomy

A segmental or partial cystectomy may be done if the client cannot tolerate a radical cystectomy and for an isolated tumor that cannot be treated by transurethral resection. Up to half the bladder can be removed. This procedure is appropriate for 10% to 15% of clients. The recurrence rate can be high.

During the initial postoperative period, bladder capacity is markedly reduced. The postoperative bladder may be able to hold no more than 60 ml. Over several months, bladder tissue expands, increasing its capacity from 200 to 400 ml.

Cystectomy and Urinary Diversion

A radical cystectomy with urinary diversion is the procedure of choice when potentially curable stage B disease is too advanced for transurethral resection or intravesical chemotherapy. The procedure may also be performed for treatment of the following:

- Neurogenic bladder (see later discussion)
- IC or radiation-induced cystitis with severely reduced bladder capacity
- Congenital anomalies of the lower urinary tract, such as bladder exstrophy

Radical cystectomy entails removal of the bladder, urethra, uterus, fallopian tubes, ovaries, and anterior segment of the vagina in women. In men, the bladder, urethra, and usually the prostate and seminal vesicles are removed. Cystectomy also involves removal of perivesical fat and dissection of the pelvic lymph nodes. This procedure is necessary when the tumor has invaded the bladder wall, involves the trigone, or cannot be treated adequately by less radical methods. When the bladder and urethra are removed, permanent urinary diversion is required. The entire surgical procedure is done in one step, with urinary diversion and cystectomy performed at the same time.

Ileal Conduit

An ileal conduit (also called ureteroileostomy, ileal bladder, or Bricker's procedure) is one type of urinary diversion. Using a segment of the intestine as a conduit, the surgeon constructs a system in which urine empties through an artificial opening in the skin called a *stoma* (Figure 34-2). Usually a portion of the terminal ileum, which has the least reabsorptive power, is used for the conduit. After the continuity of the remaining intestine is reestablished with end-to-end anastomosis, the proximal end of the segment is closed. The distal end is brought out through a hole created in the abdominal wall, folded back, and sutured to the skin to form a stoma. The ureters are then implanted into the ileal segment. Urine flows into the conduit and is continually propelled out through the stoma by peristalsis. Mucous shreds are present in the urine because of the mucus produced by the lining of the bowel.

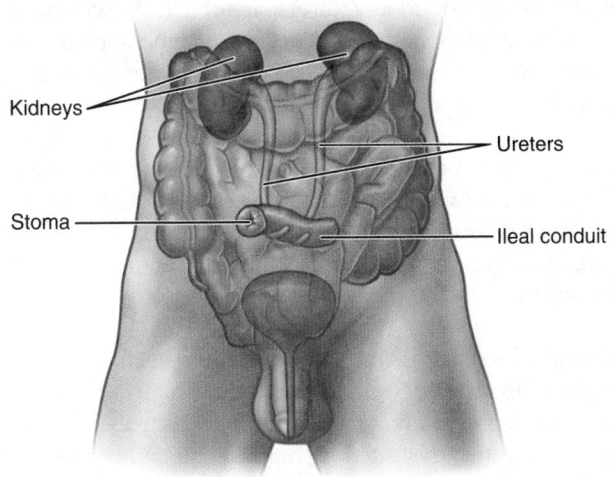

■ FIGURE 34–2 Ileal conduit. A segment of the terminal ileum is used to create an artificial bladder to which the ureters are attached. Urine continually drains from the ileal conduit through a stoma and into an ostomy pouch.

Indications. The client who has undergone an ileal conduit must wear an appliance over the stoma to collect the urine. This procedure involves less time and the conduit is easier to construct compared with other diversion procedures, which makes it an excellent choice for older clients who are unable to tolerate a lengthy surgery because of other medical conditions. Because the ileal segment is not a reservoir, absorption of electrolytes and the frequency of other complications are minimal.

Contraindications. Clients with chronic bowel disease or colon cancer may not be candidates. Any medical condition that prevents a major surgical procedure is also a contraindication.

Complications. Several complications related to stoma management (e.g., skin irritation, stomal defects, and stomal pouching problems) may arise. Leakage at the anastomosis site, stenosis, peristomal hernia, ulceration, and obstruction at the ureteroileal anastomosis may develop. Finally, clients who have undergone an ileal conduit procedure are at increased risk for pyelonephritis, hydronephrosis (distention of renal pelvis and calices with urine), and formation of calculi.

Outcomes. About 6 to 8 weeks after surgery, it is expected that the client will adjust to the stoma and appliance, maintain stoma and appliance care, and return to most previously enjoyed activities.

Indiana Pouch

Other diversionary procedures are the Indiana pouch, Florida pouch, Kock pouch, and continent internal ileal reservoir. A reservoir is created from the ascending colon and terminal ileum. The Indiana pouch is an improved and larger version of the original Kock pouch (Figure 34-3). Other continent reservoir operations vary slightly regarding surgical technique and the portion of the colon and ileum used.

Once the reservoir has been created, the ureters are implanted into the side of the diversion. A special nipple valve is then constructed and used to attach the reservoir to the skin. Several weeks after surgery, the client is taught to use a catheter to drain the reservoir at 3- to 4-hour intervals. Long-term goals suggest internal storage of up to 800 ml of urine is possible, with a daytime continence rate of up to 96% and a nighttime continence rate of up to 86%.

Indications. Because this procedure involves no appliance for collecting urine, it is used for clients with a life expectancy of more than 2 years. Creation of the reservoir and nipple valve requires 1 to 3 more hours of surgical time compared with the time needed to construct an ileal conduit. The client's serum creatinine level should be 2.5 mg/dl or less. The client will need gross and fine

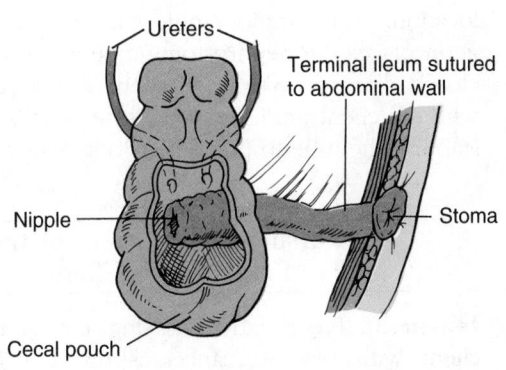

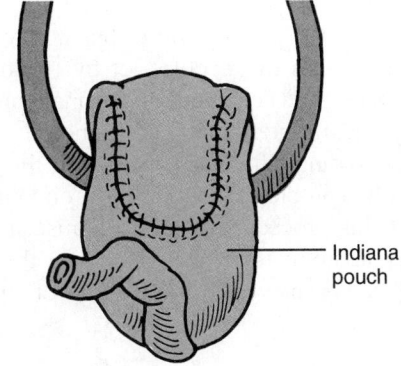

■ FIGURE 34–3 Indiana pouch procedure.

motor coordination to catheterize the nipple valve and must be willing and able to participate in self-care. Electrolyte reabsorption is minimal with this diversion technique as long as the urine is drained regularly.

Contraindications. Clients with a history of significant bowel resection and malabsorption related to diarrhea, irritable bowel syndrome, ulcerative colitis, diverticular disease, bowel cancer, Crohn's disease, progressive neurologic disorders, morbid obesity, kidney disease (creatinine level >2.5 mg/dl), and pelvic radiation are not candidates for an Indiana pouch. Clients who have poor manual dexterity or are not capable of self-care may not be candidates for this procedure.

Complications. Possible complications include incontinence, difficult catheterization, urinary reflux, anastomotic leaks, pyelonephritis, obstruction, bacteriuria, calculi, erectile dysfunction, electrolyte imbalances, malabsorption of bile salts or vitamin B_{12}, and rupture of the reservoir.

Outcomes. It can be normal for clients to experience urinary incontinence intermittently for months postoperatively. About 8 to 10 weeks after surgery, the client will have improving urinary continence, will remain free of UTI, and will return to activities pursued before surgery. Self-catheterization should begin 2 to 3 weeks postoperatively.

Neobladder

Sometimes the urethra can be spared, allowing the creation of a *neobladder,* also known as an ileal W-bladder. This operation can be the treatment of choice for a client with bladder cancer requiring cystectomy. Although this procedure differs from one in which the reservoir empties through an abdominal stoma, a neobladder empties via a pelvic outlet to the urethra. If the urethra is resected, a reconstructed neourethra together with an artificial sphincter is created. This procedure is more successful in males because of the longer urethra.

Several weeks after surgery, the catheter is removed and the client empties the neobladder by relaxing the external sphincter and creating abdominal pressure. The client must learn intermittent self-catheterization to cope with any voiding difficulties. Even with the potential postoperative problems that may be encountered, acceptance of this procedure is high because it allows a more normal anatomy to be maintained for the client. Total continence is achieved in 84% to 96% of clients at 5 years.

Indications. Because an appliance is not required and normal anatomy is maintained, the neobladder technique is the preferred urinary diversion for clients with a life expectancy of more than 2 years and with no contraindications. Other indications are as described for an Indiana pouch.

Contraindications. In addition to the contraindications listed for an Indiana pouch, clients with bladder tumors in the trigone region of the bladder, diffuse carcinoma in situ, multifocal tumors, or bladder cancer involving the prostate are not candidates for this procedure.

Complications. Possible complications include pouch rupture from hypercontinence, inability to empty the bladder completely, incontinence, electrolyte imbalances, erectile dysfunction, and calculi. With resection of the ileum, possible metabolic changes include the following: (1) malabsorption of bile salts, vitamin B_{12}, fat, and fat-soluble vitamins A, D, E, and K; (2) increased risk of biliary and kidney stones and steatorrhea.

Outcomes. The client will go home 4 to 8 days after surgery with a catheter in place. The catheter will be removed about 4 weeks after surgery, and the client will be taught to "strain to void" (see later discussion on strain voiding or "Valsalva voiding" and self-catheterization). After 2 to 3 months, the client is expected to have urinary continence, to be able to empty the bladder completely, and to return to previously pursued activities.

PALLIATIVE PROCEDURES

Percutaneous Nephrostomy or Pyelostomy

For the client with inoperable bladder cancer, a percutaneous nephrostomy or pyelostomy may be performed to prevent obstruction. A catheter is inserted into the renal pelvis by surgical incision or, more likely, by a percutaneous puncture procedure. In the surgical approach, a balloon-tipped or mushroom-tipped catheter is connected to an external drainage system.

In the percutaneous nephrostomy procedure, a trocar is inserted under fluoroscopy by direct puncture into the renal pelvis or calyx. A flexible small-gauge needle is then used to instill contrast material to verify proper location. Using angiographic wire as a guide, the surgeon places the nephrostomy tube and connects it to a closed drainage system. The entire procedure is done with the client under local anesthesia. It is important to stabilize the tube to prevent dislodgment.

Nursing Management of the Preoperative Client

Assessment. Preoperative nursing management of the client with bladder cancer is directed at educating the client and family. Assess the client and family's understanding of pending diagnostic testing, bladder cancer, and the proposed surgical procedure. Evaluate the client's anxiety level by providing opportunities to talk about feelings and to ask questions about the upcoming surgery, the potential for distorted body image, and support systems outside the hospital.

In addition to educating and counseling the client, obtain physical assessment findings. Check for (1) costovertebral tenderness and masses in the upper abdomen and flank, (2) distention before and after urination, (3) vaginal or rectal masses, and (4) manifestations of discharge in urethral meatus and perianal areas. Assessment of other body systems includes (1) monitoring vital signs, (2) measuring intake and output, (3) examining skin for color, bruises, petechiae, and hydration, and (4) auscultating heart and lung sounds.

Complete a self-care or functional assessment to determine whether the client can manage drains and indwelling catheters and is able to catheterize a continent stoma or urethra. Finally, determine whether a family member can provide care or whether home health care is available to the client.

Diagnosis, Outcomes, Interventions

Diagnosis: Deficient Knowledge. The most common nursing diagnosis preoperatively is *Deficient Knowledge related to bladder cancer and diagnostic testing, possible bowel preparation prior to surgical intervention, and surgical intervention with associated expected course of treatment.*

Outcomes. Preoperative education will result in an increased awareness of the procedure and lowered anxiety preoperatively and postoperatively. The client will understand diagnostic tests, bowel preparation, surgical intervention, and the anticipated postoperative course, as evidenced by statements and demonstrations of self-care.

Interventions

Provide Preoperative Teaching. Assess the client's educational deficits surrounding bladder cancer, the proposed treatment, and expected outcomes by encouraging discussion. Include the family in the discussion to review diagnostic evaluation, preoperative treatment, and postoperative expectations. Explain the purpose of various tubes, such as IV lines, the nasogastric (NG) tube, stents, drains, and catheters that will be present after surgery and when they will be discontinued. As needed, discuss support services available after discharge.

Discuss Bowel Preparation. If a diversion or pouch procedure has been chosen as the appropriate surgical intervention, discuss the preoperative bowel preparation ("bowel prep"). Because a segment of bowel will be used to create the conduit or reservoir, this measure relates to the segment of intestine to be used in the procedure.

Bowel preparation calls for a clear liquid diet for 1 to 3 days, laxatives and enemas to clear the bowel, and antibiotics to lower the bacterial count in the bowel. Because this step takes several days and includes enemas, dietary restrictions, and medications, it is extremely important to teach the client and family to strictly adhere to the directions.

Arrange for Wound, Ostomy, and Continence Nurse Visitation. If the client will have a pouch or diversion procedure, a visit from a wound, ostomy, and continence (WOC) nurse may be reassuring for the client and family. This visit allows the client and family to interact and learn the expected postoperative course with a nurse with expertise in this field.

Before surgery, the WOC nurse selects and marks the best site for ostomy placement if the surgeon plans to construct a stoma. The main criterion for stomal placement is finding a site that allows the faceplate of the drainage appliance to bind securely to the surface of the abdomen. The stoma must be clearly visible to the client. This means that the surgeon should avoid the umbilicus, rib margins, pubis, iliac crests, and pre-existing scars, wrinkles, or crevices. Placing the stoma directly on the client's waistline can cause excessive pressure from clothing.

The client is observed in the supine, standing, and sitting positions during the selection process. Stoma placement is usually on the right lower quadrant of the abdomen, in the abdominal rectus muscle, about 2 inches below the waist and 2 inches from the midline. Explain the proper way to care for the urinary diversion.

Diagnosis: Risk for Disturbed Body Image. The client is at *Risk for Disturbed Body Image related to surgery, possible stoma formation, possible sexual dysfunction, and potential change in urinary elimination.*

Outcomes. The client will not experience body image disturbance postoperatively, as evidenced by the ability to discuss concerns regarding altered body image, stoma placement, change in urination pattern, risk of sexual dysfunction, and verbalization of fears.

Interventions. Identify factors that reveal the client's difficulty in coping with anticipated changes in body image. If a diversion procedure is necessary, in addition to a preoperative visit from an enterostomal nurse, you may want to suggest a visit from a client with a similar diagnosis and procedure. These visits provide the client with a comfortable opportunity to ask questions, to experience a sense of comfort and support, and to receive information.

Preoperative teaching should include explanations of the expected anatomic and physiologic alterations and possible effects for the client. Because of the lifestyle changes that are required by diversion or pouch surgery, be sure to offer support and refer the client for additional counseling if indicated. Community associations, such as the United Ostomy Association and the American Cancer Society, provide tremendous help for clients undergoing urinary diversion.

Radical bladder surgery may cause a disturbance in sexual function. Because of the private and personal nature of this surgery, you should use this opportunity to discuss the risk for sexual dysfunction following radical surgery for bladder cancer. Although nerve-sparing procedures and vaginal reconstruction procedures can reduce sexual dysfunction, clients should be prepared to take advantage of available resources in case impotence or difficulty with intercourse develops after surgery.

Evaluation. It is expected that the client will be prepared for and will undergo the selected surgery successfully. The client should restate information about bladder cancer, diagnostic testing, bowel preparation, and surgical intervention. In addition, the client should voice concerns about body image disturbance and sexual dysfunction after surgery. The client should be aware of outside resources available following discharge.

Nursing Management of the Postoperative Client

Assessment. Routine postoperative evaluation and care involve the usual assessments for a client after major abdominal surgery. The Critical Monitoring feature at right describes specific assessments to be completed.

Peristalsis in the intestinal tract is absent for several days because of the manipulation and resection of the bowel. The client continues to receive nothing by mouth (i.e., remains on NPO status) with IV lines and a nasogastric tube in place until peristalsis returns. Assessment of bowel sounds and nasogastric contents is required as well as passing of flatus.

Urine flow never stops after surgery. Ureteral stents originating in the renal pelvis extend through the ureters and through the reservoir, conduit, or neobladder. The stents that exit through a stoma are contained in the pouch. With continent reservoirs, a catheter is placed through the nipple valve to drain the internal reservoir for 2 to 3 weeks until healing occurs. For an Indiana pouch and neobladder, a suprapubic catheter may be placed through the abdominal wall into the reservoir to keep it drained while another catheter is placed through the urethra and is used as a stent. This protects the anastomosis of the urethra and neobladder.

CRITICAL MONITORING

Postoperative Monitoring After Urinary Diversion Procedures

- **Measure urine output every hour for the first 24 hours, and at least every 8 hours thereafter; report any amount less than 0.5 ml/kg/hour (≈30 ml/hour) or no output for more than 15 minutes.**

- Check the ostomy pouch for leaks and the skin under it for irritation every 4 hours initially, then every 8 hours.
- Inspect the stoma every hour for the first 24 hours after surgery. (This gives a baseline from which you can quickly detect deviations. The stoma should be red and moist.) If you find no problems, extend intervals to every 4 hours, then to every 8 hours.
- Note the size, shape, and color of the stoma. Peristomal sutures may be seen adhering to the skin and mucosal bowel edge. Expect it to be edematous in the immediate postoperative period. The edema diminishes within a few weeks. However, other changes may indicate complications, warranting immediate action from the surgeon.

- **A dusky or cyanotic stoma color may denote an insufficient blood supply and the onset of necrosis. This is an emergency.**

- The reduced blood supply may result from surgical technique, from an appliance faceplate that is too small or improperly centered, or from peristomal protective materials that have been poorly applied. Other complications with the stoma include prolapse (protrusion from the skin) or retraction into the abdomen beneath the skin.
- Watch for manifestations of peritonitis, such as fever and abdominal pain and rigidity. Leakage at the site of the anastomosis or ureteral separation from the conduit may allow urine to seep into the peritoneal cavity, leading to peritonitis.
- Observe for bleeding. Although bleeding from the stoma may indicate a surgical defect, it is also common for the intestinal mucosa, which is fragile, to bleed during a change of appliance or because of a poorly fitted collection pouch.

In some instances, ureteral stents or catheters may drain urine after neobladder or continent reservoir surgery. The stents and suprapubic catheter are removed once adequate healing has occurred, usually in 3 to 4 weeks. The suprapubic catheter is usually the last tube to be discontinued. Constantly monitor the tubes for patency and continuous drainage, usually in separate closed gravity systems, with irrigation as prescribed to maintain patency. For the first 24 to 48 hours, hourly intake and output records may be required. Clients should be kept from manipulating tubes immediately after surgery.

Complications. The greatest potential problems after any diversion or pouch procedure are infection, wound dehiscence, skin irritation, ulceration, and stomal defects. Monitor the client for other complications as well following a radical cystectomy. Cystectomy is a very invasive surgery that puts the client at risk for most of the usual postoperative complications, including shock and hemorrhage. The extensive pelvic dissection associated with this surgery can increase the risk of thrombophlebitis. Additionally, pelvic lymph node dissection can predispose the client to lymphedema in the lower limbs. You may need to assess calf circumference during each shift for clinical manifestations of deep venous thrombosis (DVT).

Later complications are renal deterioration caused by reflux, stenosis of the stoma, strictures at the site of the anastomosis, hydronephrosis, calculi, incontinence, urinary retention, and peristomal hernia. Stenosis of the stoma may occur from scarring during stomal maturation. If the opening on the faceplate is too large, epithelial hyperplasia or thickening of the peristomal skin may contract the stoma. Clients with urinary diversion are also susceptible to uric acid and calcium stone disease. The onset of urinary stone development usually occurs at least 2 years postoperatively and sometimes as long as 5 to 10 years later. Obstruction anywhere in the urinary tract may interfere with normal urine flow.

Other potential complications of continent reservoirs or pouch procedures include incontinence, difficult catheterization, urinary reflux, and possible pyelonephritis, obstruction, bacteriuria, electrolyte imbalances, urolithiasis, or absorptive problems. The reservoir may leak if the client does not comply with the self-catheterization protocol.

Diagnosis, Outcomes, Interventions

Diagnosis: Risk for Injury: Occlusion of Urinary Drainage. A potential problem for the postoperative client is *Risk for Injury: Occlusion of urinary drainage device related to hematuria, clot formation, and swelling following the surgical procedure.*

Outcomes. Catheters and other drainage tubes will not become obstructed, and urine will flow freely.

Interventions. Nursing care after segmental bladder resection centers on maintaining constant urinary drainage to ensure that the remaining bladder does not become distended, putting strain on the suture line. The client usually has both urethral and suprapubic catheters. The client is discharged with the catheters in place, and they remain in place for about 2 weeks or until complete healing has occurred.

As with any major abdominal surgery, clients who undergo a radical cystectomy and urinary diversion are at an increased risk for hemorrhage. Monitor the client's vital signs, the incision, and the drainage tubes closely for early signs of excessive bleeding. If an ileal conduit is formed, the client has a pouch in place to collect urine from the ileal conduit or ureteral catheters or stents.

After a continent diversion, make sure that the catheter is draining urine freely. If any obstruction occurs, the newly created reservoir can become damaged and internal leakage along the suture line can occur. Monitor the catheter output closely, and perform irrigations at regular intervals as directed. Perform catheter irrigation gently in the immediate postoperative period, using about 30 to 60 ml of normal saline solution. Irrigation is necessary to prevent obstruction from clots or mucus.

After neobladder surgery, one catheter and one suprapubic drain will be in place to prevent overdistention of the newly created bladder. These are treated as closed drainage systems. Carefully monitor the neobladder for possible obstruction. Regular irrigation is needed to rid the neobladder of mucus.

When ureteral stents or catheters are placed, patency is important to prevent hydronephrosis and pyelonephritis. Because there is no mucus in urine from the kidney, irrigation is usually not required and is kept to a minimum to prevent pyelonephritis and hydronephrosis.

Do not irrigate ureteral catheters unless you have a specific order to do so, and then only use 5 to 10 ml of sterile saline solution. Urine output from each ureteral catheter should be 0.25 ml/kg/hour or roughly half of the 0.5 ml/kg/hour normally expected from a urethral catheter. SAFETY ALERT

Ureteral catheters may drain into a pouch when a stoma is present (see the Critical Monitoring feature on Postoperative Monitoring After Urinary Diversion Procedures).

If the client has a stoma, a temporary, clear urostomy pouch over the stoma is connected to a gravity drainage system. Sometimes ureteral stents are used to splint the ureters while they heal. These stents, usually removed before the client is discharged from the hospital, may extend through the stoma.

Label all catheters, stents, and drainage tubes to prevent errors in irrigation and output calculations. Secure all tubes. Use a separate closed gravity drainage system for each tube unless, as with an ileal conduit, ureteral catheters exit into the pouching system until they are discontinued. A separate system for each tube minimizes the risk and extent of bacterial infection. SAFETY ALERT

Diagnosis: Readiness for Enhanced Self-Care and Effective Therapeutic Regimen Management. Clients undergoing any type of urinary diversion need to learn new self-care strategies. The nursing diagnoses of *Readiness for Enhanced Self-Care* and *Effective Therapeutic Regimen Management related to complexity of therapeutic regimen* are applicable for this client.

Outcomes. The client will effectively manage the urinary diversion or neobladder, as evidenced by the ability to describe the regimen and to perform the required care successfully.

Interventions

Ileal Conduit. For a client with an ileal conduit, teach stoma care and skin care, promote self-care of the collection device, prevent odor, promote independence, and encourage follow-up.

Teach Stoma and Skin Care. The client needs to learn to care for the stoma and skin with proper application of a urinary pouch. See the Bridge to Home Health Care feature at right, a fundamentals of nursing textbook, and *evolve* the figure on the website: Applying a disposable ostomy pouch. An opening, no more than 3 mm larger than the stoma, must be cut in the skin barrier to fit over the stoma. This opening should be remeasured after the edema in the stoma recedes. The barrier is then applied to the skin before attaching the pouch or faceplate. Skin irritation or breakdown is a constant threat to a client with a urinary diversion. The pouch may be left on as long as it is not leaking for a maximum of 7 days. Nystatin creams or powders are effective against topical yeast infections around the stoma.

Promote Self-Care of the Collection Device. Urine pouches have a valve in the bottom for intermittent urine drainage. Alternatively, the pouch may be drained by gravity into a leg or bedside bag, especially at night. The self-contained pouch drainage system allows the client to resume most, or all, former activities with little or no change in style of dress. Instruct clients to empty the pouch when it is one-third to one-half full. The weight of accumulating urine may pull the faceplate away from the skin and cause leakage. Advise clients to check the seal often if they are perspiring heavily.

Prevent Odor. Urine odor is a common problem with urinary stomas. Noxious odors result mostly from poor hygiene, alkaline urine, normal breakdown of urine (ammonia), concentrated urine from insufficient fluid intake, and the ingestion of certain foods, such as asparagus. Because diluted urine has less odor, adequate fluid intake is helpful. Reusable appliances can be washed with mild soap and lukewarm water. Rinse the pouch and allow it to dry.

Promote Independence. Long-term nursing intervention aims to maintain a functional urinary system and prevent complications. It takes time for clients and significant others to adjust to a urinary diversion. Even though counseling may have been excellent during the preoperative period, the reality of the diversion commonly produces anxiety, depression, and anger. The

🏠 BRIDGE TO HOME HEALTH CARE

Managing an Ileal Conduit

When clients first come home from the hospital, they need your help to get organized and feel in control. Use a small plastic basket, such as one purchased at a discount store, to store small supplies, such as adhesive tape, stoma adhesive, a pen, and a small scissors. A wash basin, a small box, or a small organizer on wheels works well for the larger items, such as faceplate or wafers, skin barriers, pouches, and paper towels.

Typically, clients are taught about stoma care before discharge, but they may have been so overwhelmed that they did not hear or remember instructions. Once home, they may have many questions. While you change the appliance, have your clients lie down with a mirror positioned so they can become accustomed to seeing the stoma and can learn to care for the stoma without experiencing side effects such as faintness or dizziness. Eventually, the client should face the toilet while sitting comfortably on a stool or chair.

Before removing the original wafer, cut the new faceplate or wafer to size, and make certain that everything is ready. Some clients may need a circular insert in the wafer to form a convex angle that makes a tighter seal around the small stoma. Once you take off the old appliance, cover the stoma; peristalsis causes urine to squirt out spontaneously.

Do not make your client laugh; pressure will cause urine to leak out. It is frustrating to repeatedly clean the area. Use thick, absorbent paper towels to cover the stoma; they are also inexpensive and readily available.

Before cleaning the skin surface, make sure that the stoma is open and not becoming filled with mucus from the bowel. Quickly cover the stoma with a paper towel to absorb urine. To keep the skin healthy, wash around the stoma with soap and water. Once you are ready to secure the appliance, remove the paper towel quickly and apply the wafer. Place your warm hands on the faceplate or wafer for a few minutes to help it adhere to the skin. Assess skinfolds before applying the wafer; consider shifting the wafer to a diamond position to decrease the bend at the fold and the potential for leaking.

Leakage is one of the most distressing aspects of the ileal conduit. Instruct clients to attach an overnight Foley bag to the pouch at bedtime and to be sure that there are no kinks in the tubing. Back-pressure and overflow into the pouch cause the faceplate or wafer to pop off or leak. Until they feel confident, clients may decide to awaken about 2:00 am to check the pouch. During the day, they need to empty the pouch often because the tension of a full pouch causes leakage. Clients should change the pouch every 5 to 7 days.

Clients may call on WOC nurses at local hospitals, the United Ostomy Association, and the American Cancer Society for help in adjusting to an ileal conduit.

client may need help at first to look at or even talk about the stoma. As soon as possible after surgery, the client must begin to help care for the stoma, peristomal skin, and drainage system, gradually assuming more responsibility until achieving independence (see the Client Education Guide feature on Learning to Care for a Urinary Diversion on the website).

Encourage Follow-Up. A client with bladder cancer and complications such as calculi and stenosis must receive follow-up at regular intervals to assess for a recurrence of the cancer. The client should also continue to be seen by a WOC nurse to check for problems with the ostomy.

Continent Diversion. Postoperative care for the client with an Indiana pouch is similar to that for any client with a urinary diversion, except there is no external pouch. The client has a catheter and suprapubic drain in place to drain urine continuously until the pouch heals. The reservoir is irrigated through the catheter with about 50 to 60 ml of normal saline every 4 hours to wash out clots or mucus, which may cause obstruction.

Teach Reservoir Catheterization. After a radiographic study, remove the catheter at 2 to 4 weeks after surgery to make sure that the continent reservoir is functioning properly. The client must learn to empty and irrigate the reservoir at regular intervals. The principles of catheterization of a urinary reservoir are the same as for clean, intermittent urinary self-catheterization.

Using a 16F to 20F catheter with a generous amount of water-soluble lubricant, show the client how to insert the catheter into the nipple valve. Warn against forcing the catheter into the reservoir. If resistance occurs, tell the client to pause and apply only gentle pressure while slightly rotating the catheter. If this does not work, the client should call the physician. Advise the client to insert the catheter every 2 to 3 hours to drain the reservoir. Each week thereafter, the interval is increased by 1 hour, until finally catheterization is completed every 4 to 6 hours during the day and every 6 hours at night.

Teach Reservoir Irrigation. Once the urine has stopped flowing, the client should take several deep breaths and move the catheter in and out 2 to 3 inches to be sure that the pouch is fully emptied. The catheter should be withdrawn slowly so additional urine can drain.

After urine has been drained from the reservoir, tell the client to leave the catheter in place and to use 50 to 60 ml of normal saline solution to irrigate the reservoir and to prevent excess mucus buildup, which may cause obstruction. The fluid can be either gently aspirated or allowed to drain from the catheter. Once the irrigant is drained, the catheter is removed and the end of the catheter is pinched before removal to prevent dripping. The irrigations may be repeated until the drainage returns free of mucus. If the mucus is viscous (thick), increasing fluid intake and drinking cranberry juice can decrease the viscosity. Usually, mucus production lessens over time.

Because the catheterization procedure can be unpredictable, advise clients to carry catheterization supplies with them. Most clients develop a sensation of abdominal pressure when catheterization is needed. Regular fluid intake and adherence to the catheterization schedule are important. A full reservoir puts pressure on the nipple valve, making catheterization much more difficult. Clients should be taught to practice these skills before discharge. They may need follow-up with a visiting nurse for additional help.

Teach Strain Voiding and Intermittent Self- Catheterization. With a neobladder, the client must learn how to *strain void,* relaxing the external sphincter and increasing abdominal pressure to start the urine stream. Show the client how to perform clean self-catheterization in case the bladder cannot be emptied by regular voiding.

Encourage Follow-Up. Following urinary diversion, the client should be monitored at 3, 6, 9, and 12 months. The assessment includes electrolyte values, serum creatinine and blood urea nitrogen (BUN) values, and renal function studies. Renal damage may occur in noncompliant clients who neglect to empty the pouch and who then develop infection. These clients often experience severe kidney infections and damage, and an ileal conduit may be created to replace the neobladder or Indiana pouch so that urine will drain freely.

Diagnosis: Risk for Sexual Dysfunction. Extensive surgical dissection may alter the reproductive anatomy, creating a *Risk for Sexual Dysfunction related to potential postoperative impotence in men or painful intercourse in women following a radical cystectomy and changes in body image affecting sexuality.*

Outcomes. The client will accept and adopt alternative methods of sexual expression and will obtain additional information about sexuality through questions and statements.

Interventions. Male clients have a risk of impotence after a radical cystectomy related to the prostate removal. Offer counseling both before and after the surgery to help the client adjust to any alterations (see Chapter 38 for information about alterations in male sexuality). PDE-5 inhibitors, given three times weekly, are offered to most male clients immediately after the catheter is removed to maintain blood flow to the corpora cavernosa, so that when sexual intercourse can be resumed the client will have fewer problems with impotence. Other medications and devices are available to increase blood flow in the penis.

For women who have had a total abdominal hysterectomy, bilateral salpingo-oophorectomy, and anterior vaginal resection, the result can be shortening and tightening of the vagina, leading to painful intercourse. Alternative positions, lubricants, topical estrogen, and vaginal dilators may decrease the discomfort. Booklets discussing both female and male sexual dysfunction are available from the American Cancer Society.

For partners of any client, encourage holding, touching, kissing, and other activities to promote intimacy. Partners are often afraid to touch the client for fear of inflicting pain; embarrassment may also be an issue. Encourage open discussions.

Evaluation. Carcinoma in situ is considered curable with a simple transurethral resection. Intravesical chemotherapy or BCG may be combined to decrease the risk of recurrence. If the postoperative care of the client has been successful, the client will be able to make the transition to self-care with minimal difficulty. Even with a radical cystectomy, however, the 5-year survival rate for clients with muscle-invasive tumor (stage C or greater) is only 40% to 50%.

Self-Care

Motivation to promote preoperative self-care may influence the postoperative course. Direct the client toward self-care by improving knowledge, encouraging independence, and fostering participation in care and treatment. When the client increases self-care, the need for nursing care decreases and health promotion activities increase.

For reservoir irrigation or intermittent self-catheterization, the client may need referrals to durable medical equipment companies for ostomy supplies or catheters. These items can be delivered to the client's home. If the client lives alone, it may be necessary to arrange home delivery of groceries and medications.

Housekeeping and lifting are limited for the first 6 to 8 weeks after surgery. Evaluate the client's ability to engage in self-care, and identify the need for additional care from home health nurses. If the client cannot provide care and if a family member is involved with care, respite services may be required. Also consider directing the client and family to local support groups.

Modifications for Older Clients

The major modification for older clients with urinary diversion stems from difficulties with self-care. Changing an appliance is one area of difficulty because some dexterity is required. Older clients commonly have arthritis and other disabilities, including decreased visual acuity, that may limit their ability to manipulate catheters and pouches. These concerns must be closely assessed and appropriate assistance offered.

URETERAL TUMORS

Primary tumors of the ureter are rare. Ureteral cancer occurs mainly in men in their 50s and 60s. This form of cancer rarely affects women. Ureteral neoplasms usually extend from renal or bladder neoplasms or from tumors originating in the bowel, uterus, or ovary. Those primary neoplasms usually occur first as a papillary, transitional cell, or squamous cell carcinoma. These tumors are most frequently found in the lower third of the ureter. In later stages of ureteral cancer, the tumor extends outside the ureter to adjacent structures and regional lymph nodes or to distant sites. Common sites for metastasis include the lungs and liver.

Usually, the first manifestation of ureteral malignancy is gross hematuria. The tumor normally develops painlessly until obstruction occurs. At this point, the client may experience flank pain with or without hydronephrosis. Diagnosis is made through urine cytology, IVP, cystoscopy, ultrasonography, and CT scanning.

Treatment of ureteral cancer almost exclusively involves surgical excision and resection. Radiation may also be used in advanced cases with local extension. When the lesion is located in the middle or proximal third of the ureter, the surgical procedure usually involves nephroureterectomy—removal of the kidney, ureter, and attached segment of the bladder on the affected side. If the tumor is in the distal third of the ureter and noninvasive, a more conservative procedure may be used; in this case, just the distal portion of the ureter is resected with ureteral reimplantation.

Silicone rubber (Silastic), polytetrafluoroethylene (Teflon), and bovine carotid heterograft are used to replace the resected ureter, facilitating reimplantation in the bladder. A ureter-ureter anastomosis also may be performed. Preoperative and postoperative intervention is similar to that for clients undergoing nephrectomy, ureteral reimplantation, or segmental resection of the bladder.

If the decision is made not to perform any of these procedures, some palliative measure may be needed to prevent or alleviate ureteral obstruction. Percutaneous nephrostomy tube placement may be a temporary or permanent palliative option. Urinary diversion may be performed, as described previously, or a ureteral stent catheter may be placed into the ureter during cystoscopy to maintain its patency. The older catheter—a flanged, winged stent (Gibbon's stent)—or the newer double **J** stent prevents migration up the ureter or dislodgment by ureteral peristaltic waves or gravity.

URINARY CALCULI

Urinary calculi (*urolithiasis*) are calcifications in the urinary system. Commonly called stones, calculi form primarily in the kidney (*nephrolithiasis*), but they can form in or migrate to the lower urinary system. They are typically asymptomatic until they pass into the lower urinary tract. Stones are usually managed by a urologist. Primary bladder calculi are rare and usually develop from a history of urinary stasis from obstruction or chronic infection.

Up to 4% of the population in the United States have urolithiasis. About 12% of the male population have a renal stone by age 70 years. More than 200,000 Americans require hospitalization for treatment of stones each year. Many more people pass stones spontaneously with only minor manifestations that require no treatment, whereas others are treated in an ambulatory setting. The recurrence rate for calcium oxalate stones is about 50% within 5 years.

Etiology and Risk Factors

The two primary causative factors are (1) urinary stasis and (2) supersaturation of urine with poorly soluble crystalloids. Increased solute concentration occurs because of fluid depletion or an increased solute load. This increased concentration leads to the precipitation of crystals, such as calcium, uric acid, and phosphate. Urinary pH influences the solubility of certain crystals, with some crystal types precipitating readily in acid urine and some in alkaline urine. Abnormal pH levels occur in renal tubular acidosis with the administration of carbonic anhydrase inhibitors, in the presence of urea-splitting bacteria, and in severe, chronic diarrhea. Stasis of urine from bladder neck obstruction, continent urinary diversion, and immobilization increases the risk for development of stones because the crystals in unmoving urine precipitate more readily.

Infection, foreign bodies, failure to empty the bladder completely, metabolic disorders, obesity and weight gain, and obstruction in the urinary tract contribute to the formation of calculi as well. The presence of precipitators has been noted in the urine (such as protein matrix and bacteria or inflammatory elements).

Inhibitor substances, such as citrate and magnesium, appear to keep particles from aggregating and forming crystals; a lack of inhibitors increases risk of stone development. Not only does the deficiency of inhibitors predispose the client to calculi, but there may be "anti-inhibitors" in the urine, such as aluminum, iron, and silicon. Certain medications may induce calculus formation, such as acetazolamide, absorbable alkalis (e.g., calcium carbonate and sodium bicarbonate), and aluminum hydroxide. Massive doses of vitamin C increase urinary oxalate levels.

There is an increased risk of calculus formation in the southeast part of the United States—an area known as "the stone belt." Men between ages 30 and 50 years have three times the risk of calculi. Stones are also more common among people of European or Asian descent. Once

a client has had calculi, there is an increased risk of additional ones.

Urolithiasis results not from any single factor but from multiple phenomena. One unanswered question is "Why do some clients form calculi when others do not?" This problem is particularly important with recurrent "stone formers."

Risk factors for stone formation include anything that causes either stasis or supersaturation of the urine, such as the following:

- Immobility and a sedentary lifestyle, which increase stasis
- Dehydration, which leads to supersaturation
- Metabolic disturbances that result in an increase in calcium or other ions in the urine
- Previous history of urinary calculi
- Living in stone-belt areas
- High mineral content in drinking water
- A diet high in purines, oxalates, calcium supplements, animal proteins
- UTIs
- Prolonged indwelling catheterization
- Neurogenic bladder
- History of female genital mutilation

Health promotion and health maintenance activities are discussed under Nursing Management of the Medical Client.

Pathophysiology

The exact mechanism of stone formation has not been clearly defined. Some researchers believe that a low dietary calcium intake contributes, whereas others contend that a high calcium intake contributes. Both groups agree on the role of supersaturation, however. Crystallization appears to be the primary factor in calculus development from the following:

- Supersaturation of urine with increased solutes
- Matrix formation caused when mucoproteins bind to the mass of the stone
- Lack of inhibitors caused by increased or absent protectors against stone formation
- A combination of these conditions

In general, crystal growth involves *nucleation,* in which crystals are formed from supersaturated urine. Growth continues by aggregation to form larger particles. One of these particles may travel down the urinary tract until it is trapped at some narrow point where stone formation occurs.

Inhibitor substances (e.g., citrate, pyrophosphate, and magnesium) have been identified as *chelating agents.* When present in adequate amounts, they act to keep crystals from aggregating and forming stones. When inhibitors are absent, stone formation following crystal aggregation is more likely. Also, a fibrous matrix of urinary organic material (mostly mucoproteins) may form in the kidney or bladder, producing a substance into which crystallites are deposited and trapped. This, then, becomes the nidus of the stone. The excessive production of this mucoprotein may, in part, account for a family history of urolithiasis in clients with calculi.

Types of Calculi

Stones may be of one crystal type or a combination of types.

Calcium

Calcium is the most common substance and is found in up to 90% of stones. Calcium stones are usually composed of calcium phosphate or calcium oxalate. They may range from very small particles, often called "sand" or "gravel," to giant staghorn calculi, which may fill the entire renal pelvis and extend up into the calyces (Figure 34-4). The peak onset is during a person's 20s, and these stones affect primarily males.

Hypercalciuria (an increased solute load of calcium in the urine) is caused by four main components:

■ A high rate of bone reabsorption, which liberates calcium, as in Paget's disease, hyperparathyroidism, Cushing's disease, immobility, and osteolysis caused by malignant tumors of the breast, lung, and prostate
■ Gut absorption of abnormally large amounts of calcium, as in milk-alkali syndrome, sarcoidosis, and excessive intake of vitamin D
■ Impaired renal tubular absorption of filtered calcium, as in renal tubular acidosis
■ Structural abnormalities, such as "sponge kidney"

About 35% of all clients with calcium stones do not have high serum levels of calcium and demonstrate no apparent cause of hypercalciuria.

There are two variants of hypercalciuria:

■ The primary abnormality is increased intestinal absorption of calcium or increased bone reabsorption. The resulting higher serum calcium level triggers increased renal filtration of calcium and parathyroid hormone (PTH) suppression. This in turn decreases tubular reabsorption, thereby increasing the concentration of calcium in the urine.
■ "Renal leak" of calcium, the other abnormality, is caused by a tubular defect. The resulting hypocalcemia stimulates PTH production, which increases intestinal absorption of calcium. This cycle fits into the previous one, causing an increased solute load of calcium. Clients with this problem are often called "calcium wasters."

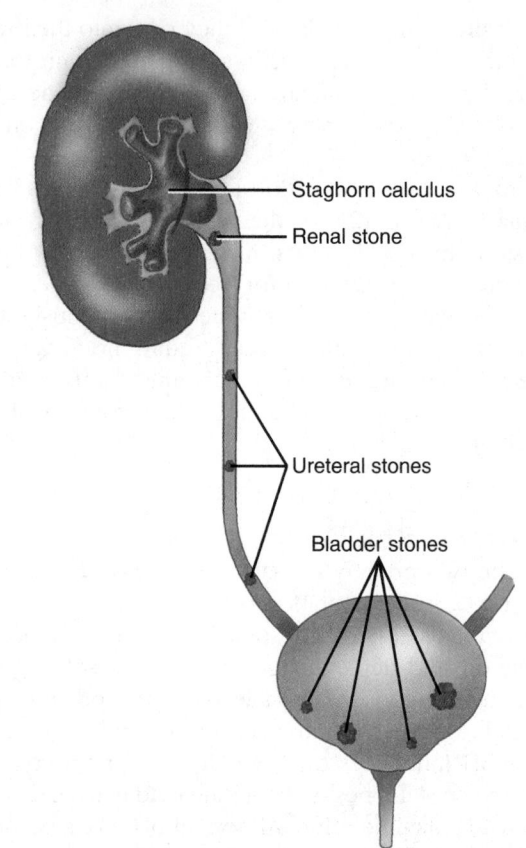

■ **FIGURE 34–4** Staghorn calculus (stone) and other locations of calculi in the urinary tract.

Oxalate

The second most frequent stone is oxalate, which is relatively insoluble in urine. Its solubility is affected only slightly by changes in urinary pH. The mechanism of oxalate availability is unclear but may be closely related to diet. The disease is most common in areas where cereals are a major dietary component and least common in dairy farming regions.

An increased incidence of oxalate stones may be related to the following:

■ Hyperabsorption of oxalate, seen with inflammatory bowel disease and a high intake of soy-based products
■ Postileal resection or small bowel bypass surgery
■ Overdose of ascorbic acid (vitamin C), which metabolizes to oxalate
■ Familial oxaluria (oxalate in the urine)
■ Concurrent fat malabsorption, which may cause calcium binding, thus freeing oxalate for absorption

Struvite

Struvite stones, also called triple phosphate, are composed of carbonate apatite and magnesium ammonium phosphate. Their cause is certain bacteria, usually

Proteus, which contain the enzyme urease. This enzyme splits urea into two ammonia molecules, which increases the urine pH. Phosphate precipitates in alkaline urine. This action is responsible for the label "urea-splitter" characterizing these organisms.

Stones formed in this manner are staghorn calculi (see Figure 34-4). Abscess formation is common. Struvite stones are difficult to eliminate because the hard stone forms around a nucleus of bacteria, protecting them from antibiotic therapy. Any small fragment left after surgical removal of the stone begins the cycle again.

Uric Acid

Uric acid stones are caused by increased urate excretion, fluid depletion, and a low urinary pH. *Hyperuricuria* is the result of either increased uric acid production or the administration of uricosuric agents. Approximately 25% of people with primary gout and about 50% of people with secondary gout develop uric acid stones. A high dietary intake of foods rich in *purine* (a crystalline base) may predispose clients to uric acid stone formation. Also, treating neoplastic disease with agents that cause rapid cell destruction may increase the urinary uric acid concentration. Moreover, a link between hyperuricuria and calcium stone formation may exist. It is hypothesized that uric acid crystals absorb some of the crystal inhibitors normally found in urine.

Cystine

Cystinuria is the result of a congenital metabolic error inherited as an autosomal recessive disorder. Cystine stones typically appear during childhood and adolescence; development in adults is very rare.

Xanthine

Xanthine stones occur as a result of a rare hereditary condition in which there is a xanthine oxidase deficiency. This crystal precipitates readily in acid urine.

Summary

Despite the type of stone that forms, the potential damage is essentially the same: (1) pain, spasm, or colic from peristalsis movements of the ureter contracting on the stone; (2) obstruction with possible hydronephrosis or hydroureter; (3) tissue trauma with secondary hemorrhage; and (4) infection.

Clinical Manifestations

The most characteristic manifestation of renal or ureteral calculi is a sharp, severe pain of sudden onset caused by movement of the calculus and consequent irritation. Depending on the site of the stone, this pain may be either *renal colic* or *ureteral colic.* Renal colic originates deep in the lumbar region and radiates around the side and down toward the testicle in the male and the bladder in the female. Ureteral colic radiates toward the genitalia and thigh.

When the pain is severe, the client usually has nausea, vomiting, pallor, grunting respirations, elevated blood pressure and pulse, diaphoresis, and anxiety. Visceral pain such as renal colic is mediated by the autonomic nervous system via celiac ganglia, which causes nausea, vomiting, decreased intestinal motility, and possibly paralytic ileus. Some people, especially those with bladder stones, experience manifestations of urgency, frequency, hematuria, and chronic cystitis. Pressure against the bladder neck during micturition (voiding) may cause a heavy feeling in the suprapubic region, obstruction in voiding, a decreased bladder capacity, and an intermittent urinary stream. If the stone enters the urethra, urine flow is obstructed. The pain lasts for minutes to days and can be somewhat resistant to opioid intervention.

Pain may be intermittent, which usually means that the stone has moved. Physicians hypothesize that the ureter dilates just proximal to the calculus, which allows urine to pass, relieving the ureteral distention. Then, as the stone moves into a new obstruction site, the pain returns. The pain subsides when the stone reaches the bladder.

Pain caused by renal stones is not always severe and colicky. It may be dull or aching or may be experienced as a heavy feeling. This is particularly true during the early stages of hydronephrosis. Other manifestations of calculi include infection with an elevated temperature and white blood cell (WBC) count and urine obstruction that causes hydroureter, hydronephrosis, or both. The Integrating Diagnostic Testing feature on p. 752 provides more information related to the diagnosis of urinary stones. Once the stone is retrieved, its components must be analyzed. Additional studies of blood and urine may be required to determine whether metabolic problems predispose the client to stone formation. Other possible disease processes, such as metastatic bone cancer, must be ruled out as possible causes of calculi.

OUTCOME MANAGEMENT

Determining the size of the calculus is essential in selecting the treatment. Stones smaller than 4 or 5 mm can pass without intervention.

Medical Management

Conservative or medical management is appropriate if there is no obstruction, if the pain can be managed, if the client can be hydrated with oral fluids, and if the stone

INTEGRATING D I A G N O S T I C   T E S T I N G

Nephrolithiasis/Urolithiasis

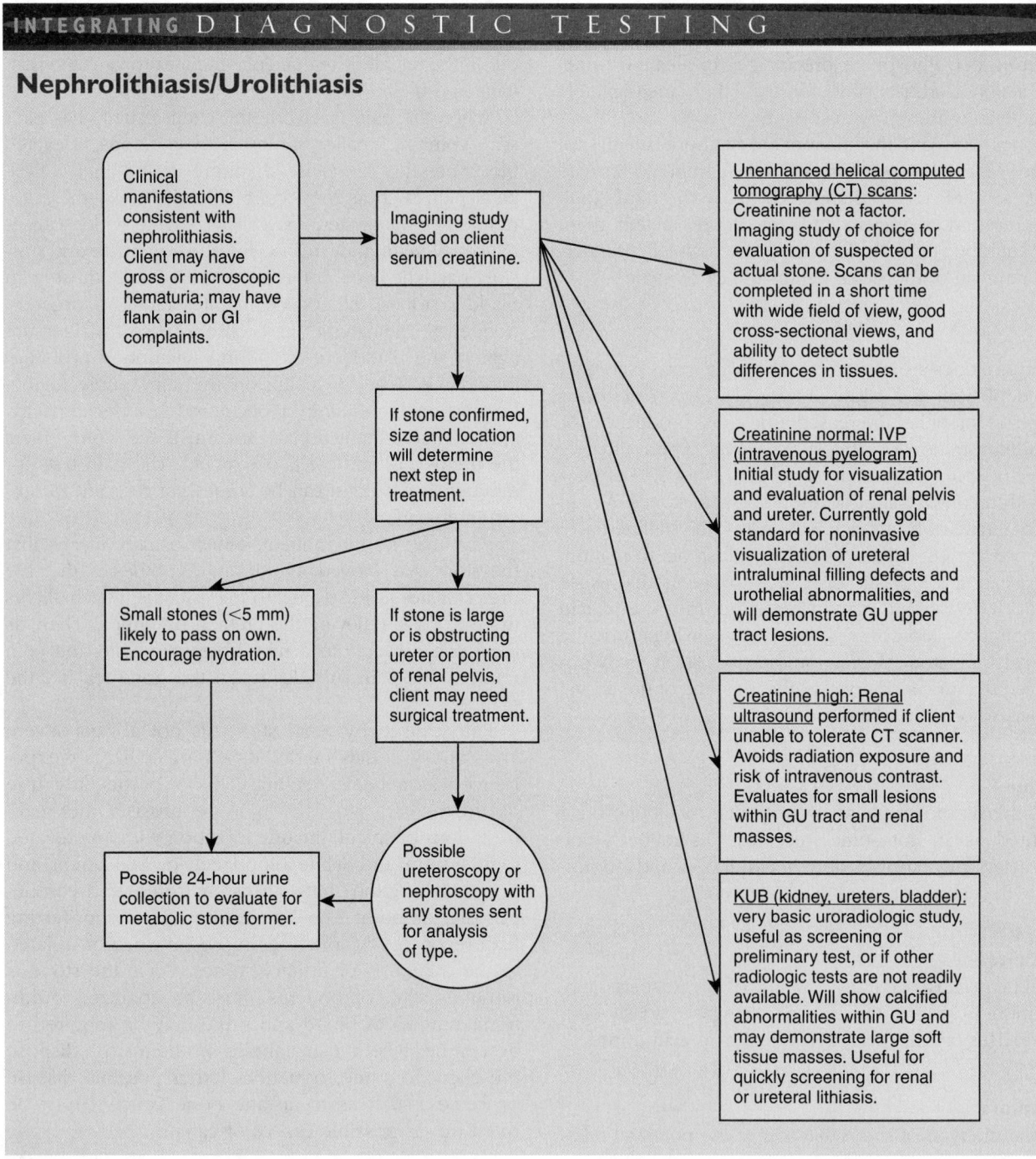

Clinical manifestations consistent with nephrolithiasis. Client may have gross or microscopic hematuria; may have flank pain or GI complaints.

Imagining study based on client serum creatinine.

If stone confirmed, size and location will determine next step in treatment.

Small stones (<5 mm) likely to pass on own. Encourage hydration.

If stone is large or is obstructing ureter or portion of renal pelvis, client may need surgical treatment.

Possible 24-hour urine collection to evaluate for metabolic stone former.

Possible ureteroscopy or nephroscopy with any stones sent for analysis of type.

Unenhanced helical computed tomography (CT) scans: Creatinine not a factor. Imaging study of choice for evaluation of suspected or actual stone. Scans can be completed in a short time with wide field of view, good cross-sectional views, and ability to detect subtle differences in tissues.

Creatinine normal: IVP (intravenous pyelogram) Initial study for visualization and evaluation of renal pelvis and ureter. Currently gold standard for noninvasive visualization of ureteral intraluminal filling defects and urothelial abnormalities, and will demonstrate GU upper tract lesions.

Creatinine high: Renal ultrasound performed if client unable to tolerate CT scanner. Avoids radiation exposure and risk of intravenous contrast. Evaluates for small lesions within GU tract and renal masses.

KUB (kidney, ureters, bladder): very basic uroradiologic study, useful as screening or preliminary test, or if other radiologic tests are not readily available. Will show calcified abnormalities within GU and may demonstrate large soft tissue masses. Useful for quickly screening for renal or ureteral lithiasis.

is less than 5 mm. Medical management is directed at relieving the acute manifestations while facilitating the passage of small stones. The desired outcomes of medical management are to increase fluids, reduce pain, and minimize calculus formation by implementing diet changes and administering medications. Most clients pass the stone naturally from the ureter and bladder. If the stone does not move, if it causes obstruction, or if x-ray studies suggest that the calculus is too large to pass safely to the

urethra, more invasive treatment is necessary. After the acute phase, medical management is directed toward preventing recurrence of stone formation.

Increase Fluids

The most effective management strategy is to increase fluid intake to facilitate passage of small stones and to prevent the development of new ones. Encourage clients to increase fluids to 3 to 4 L daily, unless contraindicated, to ensure a urine output of 2.5 to 3 L daily. The increased urine volume resulting from this high fluid intake decreases the concentration of solutes and alleviates urinary stasis. Increased fluids may also decrease pain, prevent an increase in stone size, and prevent infection. The kind of fluid the client drinks depends on dietary restrictions, but at least one half of the fluid should be water.

Reduce Pain

Pain is most severe in the first 24 hours. In addition to pain control with increased fluids, the client usually requires treatment with opioids and antispasmodic agents. Opioids such as morphine sulfate are given intravenously or intramuscularly (IV or IM) to control moderate to severe pain. Nonsteroidal anti-inflammatory drugs (NSAIDs) may also be effective.

Antispasmodic agents, such as oxybutynin chloride (Ditropan), are very effective for relieving and controlling colic pain associated with spasms of the ureter. Clients with repeated stone formation may have a family member drive them to a clinic, ambulatory care center, or emergency department for administration of opioid analgesics and antispasmodic agents so that they can relax, go home, and pass the stone naturally. Other clients may require admission to an acute care setting for administration of these medications. For nausea and vomiting associated with colic, antiemetics may also be necessary.

Prevent Stone Recurrence

Diet modifications and medications may be required to prevent further calculus formation in clients who return with repeated stones. Increased fluid intake is still the primary prevention measure. Results of a stone analysis are essential before these recommendations are implemented.

Implement Dietary Changes

Some controversy exists over dietary restrictions because of their uncertain effectiveness and the problems clients experience in following the regimen. In the past, calcium stones and hypercalciuria were controlled by limiting excessive calcium intake to 800 mg daily. However, more recent research has supported increasing dietary intake of calcium-rich foods. This research is explored in the Translating Evidence into Practice feature on p. 754.

Clients with oxalate stones should avoid high-oxalate foods, such as tea, tomatoes, instant coffee, cola drinks, beer, rhubarb, green beans, asparagus, spinach, cabbage, celery, chocolate, citrus fruits, apples, grapes, cranberries, peanuts, and peanut butter. Megadoses of vitamin C increase oxalate excretion in the urine and should be avoided. If the stone is composed of uric acid, the client should follow a low-purine diet, which involves limiting such foods as aged cheeses, wine, bony fish, and organ meats.

Administer Medications

Following recurrent stone formation, analysis of the stone, or abnormal metabolic findings, medications may be required. For hypercalciuric clients, a thiazide diuretic such as hydrochlorothiazide promotes calcium resorption from the renal tubules, thereby preventing excess calcium loads in the urine. Potassium citrate is commonly added to the thiazide diuretic to replace potassium as needed.

For low urine citrate levels, potassium or sodium citrate may be ordered. Because these medications can be expensive, many urologists encourage the client to drink a quart of lemonade for both the increased fluid and citrate benefits.

Calcium oxalate stones may be treated with vitamin B_6 (pyridoxine), magnesium oxide, or cholestyramine. For clients with hyperuricosuria and calcium oxalate stones, allopurinol (Zyloprim) is prescribed only if a reduced purine diet fails and stones persist.

Uric acid stones are treated with drugs to lower uric acid concentration, such as allopurinol. In addition, sodium bicarbonate or citrate may be indicated to increase urinary pH because uric acid stones form in acidic urine. This treatment is also effective for xanthine stones, which are inhibited in alkaline urine. Cystine stones are treated with tiopronin (Thiola) and d-penicillamine, which make cystine more soluble for excretion. Long-term antibiotics are used to control the infection that leads to struvite stone formation.

Nursing Management of the Medical Client

Assessment. Ask the client about any family history of calculi, previous UTIs, immobility, and recent dietary habits. For instance, a large intake of purines may be significant, as would be drinking a large amount of fruit juice or tea, which could cause oxalate precipitation. Also assess the amount, pattern, and types of fluids consumed.

Assess the client for the clinical manifestations described earlier. Use rating scales to measure the severity of pain. Many clients describe renal or ureteral colic as "the worst pain I've ever had." Vital signs should be monitored. A decreasing blood pressure may indicate severe pain and impending shock; increased pulse rate and temperature may result from infection. A sudden onset of little or no urine output suggests obstruction, which is an emergency that must be treated immediately to preserve kidney function. Frequency and dysuria commonly occur when a stone reaches the bladder.

All urine voided should be strained through several layers of gauze or through a commercial urine strainer.

TRANSLATING EVIDENCE INTO PRACTICE

Calcium Intake and Its Relationship to Kidney Stone Formation

In the past, clients with a history of calcium oxalate kidney stones have been advised to decrease their intake of calcium-rich foods to 800 mg/day to reduce the recurrence of kidney stones. However, more recent literature contradicts these previous dietary instructions. New theories propose that calcium stone formation in the kidney may be linked to a diet high in protein. A high-protein diet increases urinary calcium, oxalate, and uric acid secretion and increases the probability of stone formation in normal subjects.

Study findings by Curhan and colleagues questioned previous research findings and treatment of kidney stones.[3] Their results suggest that a higher intake of dietary calcium was strongly associated with a decreased risk of calcium-based renal stones.[3] Curhan et al. reported the incidence of kidney stones was lower by 50% in men with a calcium intake of up to 1326 mg/day compared with the incidence in those who took 516 mg of calcium/day.[3] The men who ingested up to two glasses of milk per day had half the risk of stone formation as those who drank less than one glass per month. Another study reported a similar diet of high calcium, low protein, and low sodium reduces the risk of reoccurrence of kidney stones.[2]

In women, it has been reported that increased dietary intake of calcium was not associated with risk of kidney stone formation. However, the intake of supplemental calcium was related to an increased risk of kidney stones. Additionally, an increased intake of sucrose and sodium increased the risk of stone formation, whereas increased fluids or potassium decreased the incidence.[4] Sodium citrate preparations and cranberry juice were found to decrease the risk of calcium oxalate stone formation in two separate studies.[1,5]

IMPLICATIONS

Nurses should encourage clients who have had at least one calcium oxalate kidney stone to increase fluids and dietary calcium intake and to reduce protein and sodium intake. Intake of dietary calcium should be encouraged in all clients to prevent osteoporosis and to prevent calcium oxalate kidney stones. Other dietary adjustments to lower oxalate intake, take sodium citrate, or ingest cranberry juice may also be recommended.

REFERENCES

1. Allie-Hamdulay, S., & Rogers, A. (2005). Prophylactic and therapeutic properties of a sodium citrate preparation in the management of calcium oxalate urolithiasis: A randomized, placebo-controlled trial. *Urological Research, 33*(2), 116-124.
2. Borghi, L., et al. (2002). Comparison of two diets for the prevention of recurrent stones in idiopathic hypercalciuria. *New England Journal of Medicine, 346,* 77-84.
3. Curhan, G.C., et al. (1993). Prospective study of dietary calcium and other nutrients and the risk of symptomatic kidney stones. *New England Journal of Medicine, 328,* 833-838.
4. Curhan, G.C., et al. (1997). Comparison of dietary calcium with supplemental calcium and other nutrients as factors affecting the risk of kidney stones in women. *Annals of Internal Medicine, 126,* 497-504.
5. McHarg, T., Rogers, A., & Charlton, K. (2003). Influence of cranberry juice on urinary risk factors for calcium oxalate kidney stones formation. *British Journal of Urology, 92*(7), 765-768.

Carefully examine all debris caught by straining. Save any stone material so that the stone's composition can be analyzed as a basis for treatment and to show how much has passed through the urinary tract. A routine urinalysis, urine for culture and sensitivity testing, and a 24-hour urine specimen may be needed.

Diagnosis, Outcomes, Interventions

Diagnosis: Acute Pain. The priority nursing diagnosis is *Acute Pain related to irritation and spasm from stone movement in the urinary tract.*

Outcomes. The client will report pain reduction or control.

Interventions. During the acute phase of treatment, offer pain medications, antispasmodics, and antiemetics, if necessary. For severe pain, give the medications on a regular schedule. Use a rating scale to help evaluate the client's pain.

Once pain is controlled, the client should force fluids and ambulate, which facilitates passage of the stone. Relaxation techniques, such as guided imagery or therapeutic or healing touch, can help relieve pain. Help the client find a comfortable position to alternate with ambulation.

Diagnosis: Effective Therapeutic Regimen Management. More than half of clients with a urinary calculus experience another episode within 5 years. As a result, an important nursing diagnosis is *Effective Therapeutic Regimen Management related to prevention of recurrent calculi.*

Outcomes. The number of recurrences will be reduced, and the interval between stones will increase.

Interventions

Increase Fluids. Teach the client to drink 3 to 4 L of fluid daily to flush the urinary system. At least half the fluid consumed should be water. Intake should be as consistent as possible throughout the 24-hour period.

As a rule, encourage the client to drink a full glass of water every hour during the day and two large glasses just before going to bed. This schedule may create the need to void during the night, at which time the client should drink another glass of water.

Teach Stone Prevention Measures. Besides increased fluid intake, teach the client about other measures to prevent stone recurrence, such as diet modifications, medications if required, and avoidance of urinary stasis (see the Client Education Guide feature on Preventing Recurrence of Urinary Stones on the website). Prompt treatment of UTIs and early recognition of manifestations of stone recurrence are also important.

Health promotion activities include frequent turning and range of motion for immobilized clients, increased fluid intake, and decreased intake of stone-forming solutes in the diet, such as oxalates, purines, and animal proteins. Health maintenance interventions include monitoring high-risk clients with indwelling catheters or obstructions for calculi.

Evaluation. If medical management is successful, the client's pain is controlled, the stone passes unaided, and the client has no complications of obstruction or infection. The client is able to describe factors that increase the risk of developing stones and is able to identify self-care strategies to prevent stone recurrence.

Surgical Management

About 20% of stones require additional treatment with shock wave lithotripsy or endourologic or surgical procedures. Open surgery is used only for the small percentage of clients who cannot be successfully treated with lithotripsy or endourologic procedures.

Endourologic Procedures

Depending on the position of the calculus, cystoscopy may be done. Small stones may be removed transurethrally with a cystoscope, ureteroscope, or ureterorenoscope. Additionally, one or two ureteral catheters or stents may be inserted past the stone. From this point, several different interventions are appropriate. The catheters may be left in place for 24 hours or longer to drain urine trapped proximal to the stone and to dilate the ureter, which may prompt spontaneous movement of the calculus. Otherwise, the catheter may mechanically guide the stone downward as it is removed.

At times, a continuous chemical irrigation may be used to dissolve uric acid, struvite, and cystine stones. Finally, an attempt may be made to manipulate or dislodge the stone with a variety of special catheters with loops and expanding baskets used to snare the stone. Care is the same as that following cystoscopy.

Larger stones may be crushed with an instrument called a *lithotrite* (stone crusher) to facilitate removal. *Cystolitholapaxy* is performed when a bladder stone is soft enough to be crushed. In cystoscopic lithotripsy, an ultrasonic lithotrite is placed to pulverize the stone, followed by extensive flushing of the bladder. Possible complications associated with this procedure include

hemorrhage, urinary retention, infection, bladder perforation, and possibly retained stone fragments.

A flexible ureteroscope, passed through a cystoscope, is used to collect stones in the ureter. This procedure, called *ureteroscopy,* is used to retrieve 4- to 5-mm stones or, combined with ultrasonic lithotripsy, to remove fragments after treatment. Minimal sedation or anesthesia is necessary, and postoperative complications are usually few.

A flexible ureterorenoscope can be passed for access to the entire upper urinary tract, including the distal ureter and intrarenal collecting system so that stones or lesions in the lower pole or lateral calices can be reached.

A nephroscope may be inserted to retrieve free-lying renal stones. Figure 34-5, *A* shows a nephroscope in place. The stone may be removed with alligator forceps or a stone basket followed by irrigation. Electrohydraulic, laser, or ultrasound lithotripsy may be completed through the nephroscope. After this procedure, a nephrostomy tube remains in place for 1 to 5 days. The client can go home with it in place. Increased fluids are essential to achieve a urine output greater than 3000 ml (3 L). The tube is removed after diagnostic studies determine that all stone fragments have been removed.

Lithotripsy

Laser Lithotripsy

A newer treatment for calculi is laser lithotripsy. Lasers are used together with a ureteroscope to remove or loosen impacted stones. Constant water irrigation of the ureter is required to dissipate the heat. Complications resulting from this procedure are the same as those of any endourologic procedure.

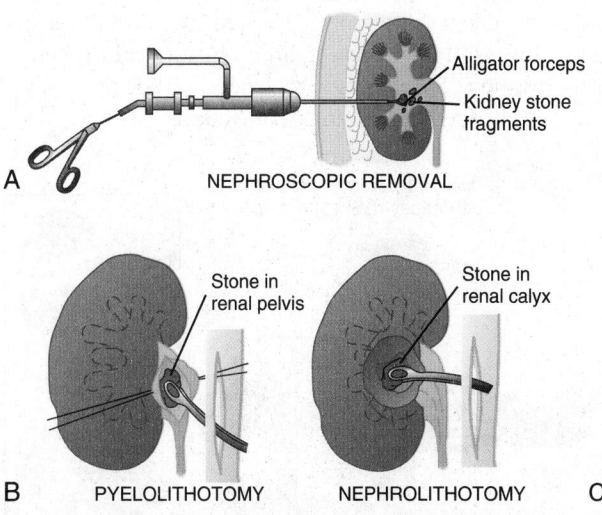

■ **FIGURE 34–5** Surgical techniques for removal of kidney stones. **A,** Percutaneous nephroscopic removal of kidney stones. **B,** Pyelolithotomy—open surgical procedure to retrieve stones from renal pelvis. **C,** Nephrolithotomy—open surgical procedure to remove stones from renal calyx.

Extracorporeal Shock Wave Lithotripsy

Extracorporeal shock wave lithotripsy (ESWL) is the use of sound waves applied externally to break up stones in the kidney or ureter (Figure 34-6). High-energy shock waves, aimed by fluoroscopy, are transmitted to the stone. The shock waves break the stones into small fragments, which are passed or retrieved endoscopically. The client may be strapped to a frame in a water bath or secured on a table, depending on the type of lithotripsy equipment used. The client is usually offered conscious sedation or general anesthesia.

The procedure lasts 30 to 50 minutes with administration of 500 to 1500 shock waves. Cardiac monitoring is required to synchronize shock waves with the R wave to prevent cardiac dysrhythmias. Complications of ESWL include ecchymosis on the affected flank, retained fragments, urosepsis, perinephric hematoma, and hemorrhage.

Stone fragments may collect in the distal ureter, obstructing the kidney. To prevent this accumulation and obstruction, a double J stent is commonly placed via cystoscopy before ESWL for stones larger than 6 mm. The stent is removed during a follow-up visit.

After ESWL, the client may experience renal or ureteral colic that needs to be treated with antispasmodics. Early ambulation and increased fluid intake are important for flushing out stone fragments. The fragments may be passed for up to 3 months after the procedure.

Percutaneous Lithotripsy

Percutaneous lithotripsy involves the insertion of a guide percutaneously (through the skin) under fluoroscopy near the area of the stone. An ultrasonic wave is aimed at the stone to break it into fragments.

Open Surgical Procedures

If the stone is too large or if endourologic and lithotripsy procedures fail to remove it, an open surgical procedure is performed. Surgery is rarely needed because of the success of modern, less invasive options.

A *ureterolithotomy* is the surgical removal of a stone from the ureter through a flank incision for higher stones or an abdominal incision for lower ones. A Penrose drain and ureteral catheter are usually placed postoperatively for healing and drainage of urine.

Cystolithotomy, removal of bladder calculi through a suprapubic incision, is used only when stones cannot be crushed and removed transurethrally. A stone is removed from the renal pelvis by *pyelolithotomy* and from the renal calyx by a *nephrolithotomy.* Figure 34-5, *B* and *C* on p. 755 illustrates these procedures.

Rarely, a partial or total *nephrectomy* (see Chapter 35) is necessary because of extensive kidney damage, overwhelming renal infection, or abnormal renal parenchyma, which can be responsible for stone formation.

Nursing Management of the Surgical Client

Assessment. Preoperative assessment includes the general condition of the client, including the presence of conditions that may present problems postoperatively. It is a priority to assess the client's understanding of the condition and the procedure to be performed. Other assessments are similar to those described under Nursing Management of the Medical Client.

Diagnosis, Outcomes, Interventions
Diagnosis: Risk for Injury. With any endourologic procedure, lithotripsy, or surgery, the client has a *Risk for Injury related to postoperative complications.*

Outcomes. The client will remain free from injury, as evidenced by absence of hemorrhage, by vital signs within preoperative limits, by normal WBC count and temperature, and by a total urine output of at least 0.5 ml/kg/hour from all sources.

Interventions

Increase Fluids. Increase the client's IV or oral fluids to 3 to 4 L daily as described earlier, unless contraindicated.

Monitor Urine Output

🪔 **Maintain the client's urine output at 0.5 ml/kg/hour or more. Assess any indications of hemorrhage, stone retention, urinary retention, or infection. As needed, irrigate the client's bladder to wash out possible stone fragments. See Chapter 38 for discussion of continuous bladder irrigation (CBI). Continue to strain all urine.**

Nursing care after a ureterolithotomy may involve care of a ureteral catheter.

🪔 **Output of at least 0.25 ml/kg/hour from the ureteral catheter should be expected and closely monitored. Because the renal pelvis holds only 5 ml, ureteral catheters must be kept patent (open) and are never clamped. Institute prompt intervention with**

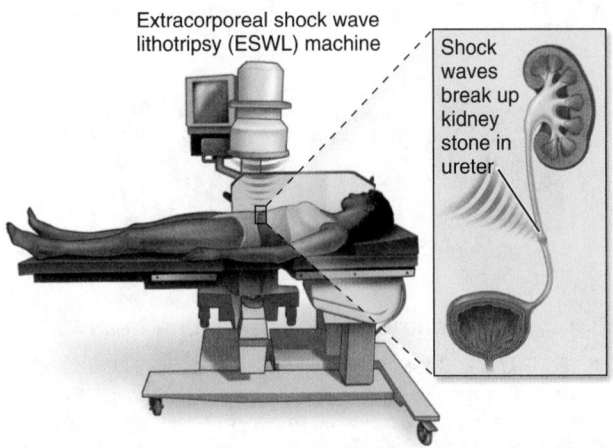

Extracorporeal shock wave lithotripsy (ESWL) machine

Shock waves break up kidney stone in ureter

■ **FIGURE 34–6** Extracorporeal shock wave lithotripsy (ESWL).

any unexpected reduction in urine flow. Several conditions—such as mucus shreds, blood clots, and chemical sediment—can interfere with the flow of urine through these catheters. Plus, ureteral peristalsis occasionally pushes the catheters out of the ureter into the bladder.

Closely monitor the catheter output. Each ureteral, suprapubic, and urethral catheter should drain into its own collection bag so that the source of the reduced urine flow is noticed immediately. Each tube or bag should be labeled. Measure and record the output of each catheter every hour for the first 24 hours. Output from each catheter should be monitored every 4 to 8 hours until removal. Most of the urine will drain from the ureteral catheters for the first 48 to 72 hours postoperatively. As the inflammation decreases, urine flows around ureteral catheters and is drained by the urethral or suprapubic catheters. Report a total urine output of less than 0.5 ml/kg/hour or a lack of output from ureteral catheters for more than 15 minutes to the physician immediately.

If the physician orders ureteral catheter irrigation, use strict sterile technique. A maximum of 3 to 5 ml of irrigating solution, usually sterile saline solution, should be allowed to flow in by gravity. Very gentle force should be used. If you cannot confirm patency, notify the physician immediately. Use extreme care to ensure that the catheter is not dislodged. If it is not sutured in place, secure it carefully to the client's skin with tape.

Drainage from a nephrostomy tube should also be carefully monitored and cared for with interventions similar to those used for ureteral catheters. Irrigation amounts, if ordered, are no more than 3 to 5 ml. Because the tube goes directly into the kidney, maintain sterile technique to prevent infection.

Clients with any type of catheter must be taught how to care for the catheter before returning home. Clients should learn how to clean around catheters, empty them, prevent kinking, and irrigate them if necessary. A home health nurse may be required to assist with these activities.

Prevent Complications. If the client has a flank incision, care is similar to that needed after nephrectomy (see Chapter 35). To prevent pneumonia, the client should cough and deep breathe 10 to 20 times each hour. To facilitate this, administer opioids regularly to control incisional pain. Other postoperative interventions are similar to those for a client with any major abdominal incision, such as monitoring bowel sounds, vital signs, and output from drains and nasogastric tubes. Antibiotics may be given prophylactically or at the first sign of infection.

Evaluation. It is expected that surgical intervention for stone removal would be completed with the least invasive procedure possible and before renal damage occurs. In most instances, the client can go home the day of the procedure and does not need to be hospitalized. Clients may go home with catheters in place for about a week; they need to learn catheter care or have home health follow-up. For major surgical intervention, the client is dismissed 3 to 4 days after the procedure.

Self-Care

A client with urolithiasis is at risk for recurrence. You have a major role in helping the client develop and maintain an effective, individual regimen to prevent stone recurrence. The main components of prevention are (1) increased fluids, (2) dietary modifications, (3) medications as ordered, and (4) prompt treatment of UTIs. The client must understand that these are lifelong changes in lifestyle. If catheters are in place after surgical intervention, client management of the tubes is necessary before discharge from the hospital.

URINARY REFLUX

Urinary reflux is the backward flow of urine in the urinary tract. It usually begins at the vesicoureteral junction. Urine flows back into the ureter and upward into the renal pelvis. The severity of vesicoureteral reflux is stated as grade I, which is least severe, through grade V, which is most severe. There is an increase in the development of reflux in men older than 50 years of age because of chronic bladder neck obstruction from BPH. Reflux typically occurs in younger children or in young adults from congenital abnormalities of the vesicoureteral junction.

Etiology and Risk Factors

Reflux can be caused by a congenital abnormality, such as ectopic ureter, chronic bladder infections secondary to dysfunctional bladder, or outlet obstruction in the bladder neck. Urinary reflux is more frequently seen as a result of another condition. Reflux contributes to the increase of intravesical pressure (within the bladder) until it finally overwhelms the resistance of the intramural ureteral sphincters, allowing reflux to occur. Clients with obstructions must be evaluated to have the cause identified and treated to prevent and relieve intravesical pressure.

Pathophysiology

In bladder outlet obstruction, the main result is the continuous presence of residual urine, which leads to chronic UTIs. Continual overdistention of the bladder can also decrease detrusor tone, increasing the bladder's capacity and raising the threshold needed to start the micturition reflex.

Renal damage and pyelonephritis are the two primary problems resulting from vesicoureteral reflux. Because the capacity of the renal pelvis is only 5 ml, larger amounts of urine can cause renal parenchymal changes, hydronephrosis, or hydronephroureterosis if they result from ureteral obstruction or reflux. The increased hydrostatic pressure leads to renal cortical atrophy from ischemia and hypoxia and then to calicectasis (dilation of the renal calices). The destruction of kidney tissue, often asymptomatic and undetected, can progress to end-stage renal disease. The kidneys are usually protected from ascending infections by the intramural portion of the distal ureter. With reflux, however, any pathogens in the bladder are carried through the ureters to the kidney. This problem leads to recurrent pyelonephritis. Chronic pyelonephritis leads to renal failure.

Clinical Manifestations

The major manifestation of reflux in the bladder neck is pyelonephritis. When the obstruction is in the vesicoureteral junction or higher, renal failure may be clinically evident. The major diagnostic studies are (1) the voiding cystourethrogram (VCUG) to visualize the lower urinary system during voiding, (2) cystoscopy to evaluate manifestations of obstruction, (3) ureteroscopy to assess the vesicoureteral junction, (4) ultrasound to assess for hydronephrosis, and (5) IVP to evaluate the entire collecting system. Blood studies of BUN and creatinine levels are also done to assess renal function.

OUTCOME MANAGEMENT

Surgical Management

Because there are no medical regimens to prevent or treat reflux caused by ectopic ureter, the primary therapy is surgical. Renal damage from the reflux usually calls for surgical intervention. Surgery is also indicated for obstruction at the ureteropelvic junction, for intractable infection, and for a problem not resolved by maturation. Because the most common causes of reflux are ureteral defects, surgical procedures focus on reimplantation or other treatments for the ureter.

Postoperatively, a urethral or suprapubic catheter keeps the bladder empty to reduce tension on the suture line. A ureteral catheter is also inserted into the ureter involved in the surgical procedure. The tip of this tiny, semi-rigid catheter usually rests in the renal pelvis. The distal end extends through the bladder and out through the urethra or through an abdominal incision.

A ureteral catheter provides three benefits: it splints the ureter to facilitate healing, it prevents obstruction from edema after surgery or other trauma in the area, and it drains urine.

Nursing Management of the Surgical Client

Carefully assess any client with a high risk of obstruction for any manifestation of urinary reflux. The client being evaluated for urinary reflux requires support during this diagnostic process. Preoperative preparation for ureteral surgery is similar to that required by any client who needs surgery (see Chapter 14).

Postoperative care is similar to that discussed earlier for urinary calculi. Assess the color of the client's urine frequently. Expect it to progress from bright red to clear yellow over a matter of days. Discharge teaching depends on a variety of factors, including the cause of the reflux, the treatment or procedure done, and the amount of renal damage present. For the client with kidney damage, renal function must be monitored at regular intervals to evaluate any changes in status.

VOIDING DISORDERS

URINARY RETENTION

Urinary retention is the inability of the bladder to empty partially or completely during voiding. Treatment is directed at relieving the cause of the problem.

Etiology and Risk Factors

Detrusor failure is the most common cause of urinary retention in women. Failure of the bladder to contract is often associated with neurologic conditions. In men, obstructive voiding resulting from an enlarged prostate is the frequent cause of retention. Other disorders, urethral strictures, medications, detrusor-sphincter dyssynergia, calculi, blood clots, tumors, bladder neck contractures, and history of female genital mutilation may also cause retention. Neuropathies affecting bladder function include diabetes mellitus, strokes, and spinal cord injuries. These long-term problems affect the neurologic status of the bladder and interfere with the micturition reflex. Remember, urinary retention is a manifestation of another pathologic condition.

Retention may be caused by decreased sensory input to and from the bladder, muscle tension, anxiety, or other neurologic conditions affecting the bladder. Surgery has traditionally been a factor; spinal anesthesia causes retention more often than does general anesthesia. After surgery, 10% to 15% of clients who received general anesthesia require catheterization because of an inability to void, and 20% to 25% of those who received spinal anesthesia require a catheter.

In women, prolapse of the back wall of the vagina (rectocele or enterocele) increases the risk of retention by exerting pressure against the urethra. Also, a large cystocele may cause kinking of the bladder neck, decreasing the bladder's ability to empty.

More than half of men older than age 50 experience BPH, a common cause of retention. This is not a preventable problem, although the client with an enlarged prostate should be monitored closely for obstruction secondary to the enlargement. Neurologic injury or disease, such as diabetes mellitus, spinal cord injuries, or multiple sclerosis, may lead to urinary retention as well. Other risk factors are a history of structural abnormalities and use of certain medications, such as tricyclic antidepressants. In some clients, a psychogenic origin may be found.

Pathophysiology

Retention of urine is hazardous because the resulting urinary stasis contributes to UTIs, stone formation, and eventual complications of long-term structural damage to the bladder, ureters, or kidneys. Additionally, continued bladder distention leads to loss of bladder tone.

The pathologic process of retention produces a snowball effect. Retained urine increases hydrostatic pressure against the bladder wall, which results in hypertrophy of the detrusor muscle, formation of trabeculae (connective tissue in the bladder wall), or development of diverticula. At the same time, peristalsis in the ureteral musculature increases against the pressure of the accumulating urine. The ureter may gradually become elongated, tortuous, and fibrotic. Increasing pressure is also transmitted through the renal pelvis and calices into the renal parenchyma. The resulting hydronephrosis exerts pressure on the blood vessels, causing ischemia and increasing the renal damage. If the process is not interrupted, it can proceed to renal failure and death. Figure 34-7 demonstrates the sequence. Even after the retention is relieved, when the alterations caused by increased pressure reach the renal parenchyma, the damage may be permanent and irreversible.

Medications, such as opioids, tricyclic antidepressants, sedatives, antispasmodics, anti-Parkinson drugs, beta-adrenergic blockers, and psychotropic agents, can interfere with normal neurologic function and the micturition reflex. Diseases with neurologic effects, such as stroke, multiple sclerosis, diabetes mellitus, tabes dorsalis, and spinal cord lesions, also disrupt the micturition reflex.

Urinary retention may result in chronic UTIs or a series of UTIs and dysfunctional voiding. Conversely, chronic UTIs and dysfunctional voiding may result in urinary retention. The detrusor muscle may become irritated and fail to function correctly, leading to incomplete bladder emptying. Irritation and scarring of the bladder neck or urethra may develop, thus placing these clients at greater risk for urinary retention.

A disorder of psychogenic origin, such as anxiety or fear of voiding in a public restroom, may lead to distention of the bladder and urinary retention. Inability to relax the urethra because of anxiety or neurologic deficit may lead to urinary retention as well.

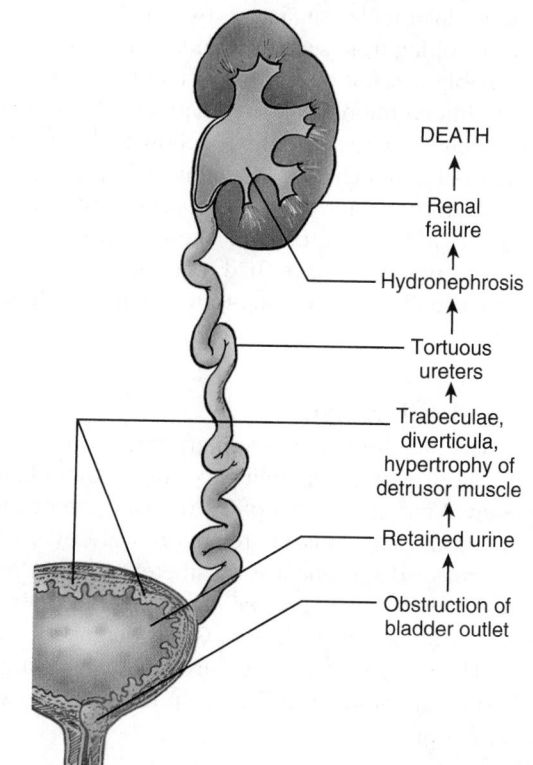

■ FIGURE 34–7 Potential effects of urinary tract obstruction.

DEATH

↑

Renal failure

↑

Hydronephrosis

↑

Tortuous ureters

↑

Trabeculae, diverticula, hypertrophy of detrusor muscle

↑

Retained urine

↑

Obstruction of bladder outlet

Anorectal problems, such as hemorrhoids, abscess, fecal impaction, and vaginal prolapse, can be contributing factors, either from obstruction or from secondary spasms of the perineal musculature that interfere with the urethra during voiding.

Decreased oral or IV fluid intake reduces the glomerular filtration rate (GFR), which causes very slow urine production and overfilling of the bladder. The slow increase allows the detrusor muscle to accommodate the increased volume until the muscle's fibers are stretched beyond their ability to contract, hampering micturition.

Urinary retention with overflow incontinence results from the following events. As the bladder continues filling, the intravesical pressure increases. Eventually, this pressure overcomes the resistance of the sphincter. Urine flows out of the bladder until it reduces the intravesical pressure, but only to the level at which the external sphincter can again control the flow of urine. Most clients report that the bladder does not feel empty. It overfills again, and the cycle is repeated.

Prolonged obstruction leads to increased pressures in the urinary tract and may predispose the client to bladder diverticula. A *diverticulum* is a pouch or sac resulting from the herniation of the mucous membrane lining caused by weakness in the muscular wall of an organ. Bladder diverticula are most common in men. Many diverticula are asymptomatic and are usually discovered by chance during assessment of other conditions.

Bladder diverticula can cause two major problems: (1) UTIs, resulting from stasis of urine, and (2) malignancies, probably a result of chronic irritation by persistent infection. Intervention involves removing the obstruction and relieving the retention, followed by surgical excision of the pouch and reestablishment of normal patency of the urinary tract. Postoperatively, catheter drainage of urine is required to allow complete tissue healing. Clients who have had chronic or recurring infections usually require long-term antibiotic therapy after surgery.

Clinical Manifestations

The primary manifestation of urinary retention is a distended bladder or an inability to empty the bladder completely. Voided amounts of 25 to 50 ml one or more times an hour may indicate retention with overflow. The major diagnostic test is catheterization. A postvoid residual amount greater than 100 ml after an attempt to void signals retention. Other diagnostic measures, such as cystoscopy and urodynamic testing to include pressure voiding studies, help identify the cause of the retention.

OUTCOME MANAGEMENT

Medical Management

Identifying the cause of urinary retention is the first step in determining treatment. Finding the underlying neurologic problem or obstructive disorder is crucial in selecting a treatment plan.

Administer Medications

In some cases, cholinergic medications have been known to help stimulate bladder contractions. If a mechanical obstruction is present, however, cholinergic drug therapy should not be used. In this instance, intravesical pressure increases against an obstructed outlet, causing ureterovesical reflux or a ruptured bladder.

Although their effects are somewhat controversial, bethanechol (Urecholine) and neostigmine (Prostigmin) are commonly administered. Bethanechol not only improves detrusor tone but also increases bladder outlet and urethral resistance. To counteract this, bethanechol is sometimes combined with phenoxybenzamine (Dibenzyline), prazosin (Minipress), and terazosin (Hytrin), which are potent alpha-adrenergic blockers.

Urethral Dilations

In some instances, urinary retention is relieved by dilation of the urethra by means of the placement of progressively larger urethral sounds (see the table on the **evolve** website titled Urologic Instruments Most Commonly

Encountered in a Clinical Setting for examples of sounds). Local or sometimes general anesthesia is used for sedation during sound placement.

Nursing Management of the Medical Client

Interventions described next are appropriate for the nursing diagnosis *Urinary Retention*.

Assess Urine Output Patterns

It is important to distinguish retention from *oliguria* (diminished urinary secretion) and *anuria* (complete suppression of urinary secretion). In urinary retention, the kidneys are producing a normal amount of urine but the bladder does not function properly. It fills with urine and rises above the level of the pubic symphysis, sometimes being displaced to either side of midline. Percussion over the bladder produces a dull sound. The client may experience increasing discomfort and the need to urinate. The client also may complain of restlessness, sweating, anxiety, bladder pain, and feelings of bladder fullness. A bladder scan estimates urine amounts in the bladder accurately.

Implement Measures to Stimulate Independent Voiding

Nursing interventions may be used initially to treat retention. Provide privacy, and place the client in a normal sitting or standing position, using gravity and increased intra-abdominal pressure to help relieve an acute problem. Running the water or flushing the toilet within earshot of the client may encourage voiding. Tape-recorded aquatic sounds may be effective. A warm bath or pouring warm water over the perineum often promotes muscle relaxation. Immersing the client's hands in water sometimes works. Applying ice or gently stroking the inner thigh sometimes works as well. These measures may stimulate trigger points of the micturition reflex. If the client is tense and anxious, any measure that induces relaxation may aid in relieving the situation, even a back rub or soothing music.

The client should not be catheterized unless urine amounts by bladder scan are greater than 300 ml or the client complains of discomfort. For clients with persistent urinary retention, a straight or retention catheter may be inserted through the external meatus, into the urethra beyond the internal sphincter, and into the bladder. A straight catheter is removed after the bladder drains. An indwelling (Foley) catheter is usually inserted after two straight catheterizations. The catheter is kept in place for continuous or intermittent drainage by inflating a balloon near the catheter's tip. Strict sterile techniques are used for insertion except for clients on an intermittent self-catheterization program; these clients may use clean technique.

The indwelling catheter is attached to either a bedside drainage bag or a leg bag. A leg bag may be used for long-term catheterization, especially for a client going home with the catheter in place. A newer belly bag is also available for clients with long-term catheter placement. These devices allow the client more mobility and eliminates the embarrassment of carrying a drainage bag in public view.

Because of the bag's small capacity, the leg bag must be emptied frequently. A conventional drainage system is used at night to avoid the need to empty the leg bag at night. (The change in bags is not necessary with the belly bag.) Instruct the client to avoid attaching the rubber straps too tightly, because doing so may cause skin irritation, thrombophlebitis, and ulcer formation. Loose straps tend to tighten as the bag fills. Recent improvements have led to the use of nylon self-fastening tape (Velcro) leg straps for clients with circulatory problems, those with latex allergy, and those at high risk for skin breakdown. Meticulous skin care and periodic removal of the bag help prevent these problems. Cleanliness and odor control are managed by washing the apparatus with mild soap and water and allowing the bag to air dry.

Prevent Infection

Minimizing hospital-acquired infections is one of the TJC National Patient Safety Goals. Prolonged **use of an indwelling catheter increases the risk of UTI and tissue trauma. More than 80% of people who develop nosocomial (hospital-acquired) UTIs have undergone urologic instrumentation. The risks of bacteriuria leading to urosepsis increases in direct relationship to duration of catheter placement; estimates of infection rates range from 4% (within 24 hours) to 95% (within 4 weeks). Organisms enter the catheter through any contamination or break in the system or intrude via the thin layer of fluid and exudate that forms around the outside of the catheter.**

Catheter insertion should be avoided unless necessary to monitor urine output. Wash your hands **thoroughly before and after handling a catheter or drainage system. In addition, do the following:**

1. **Maintain a closed drainage system.**
2. **Avoid backflow of urine.**
3. **Avoid unnecessary manipulation of the catheter during perineal cleaning.**
4. **Prevent microbial invasion and colonization in the urine collection bag.**
5. **Maintain patency of the catheter.**
6. **Encourage a high fluid intake.**

On occasion, prophylactic antibiotics are given to clients with catheters in place. The practice is not routine, however, because of the threat of resistant organisms and possible adverse reactions.

Prevent Tissue Injury

Tissue trauma may occur during catheterization. Tissue irritation or necrosis may result from the following:

- Use of an oversized catheter
- Continuous pressure and pulling of the catheter between the meatus and the site of taping on the leg or abdomen
- Friction caused by the continuous movement of the catheter, causing tissue breakdown and enhancing encrustation on the outside of the catheter
- Local or systemic allergic reactions to rubber in clients with a history of latex allergy; silicone catheters may be used in these clients

The subject of bladder decompression drainage is still misunderstood. In the past, it was incorrectly assumed that rapid emptying of a distended bladder through a catheter could result in bladder hemorrhage and hypotension. Consequently, the catheter was clamped after 1000 ml of urine had been drained, reopened after an hour to drain another 1000 ml, and clamped and reopened again until the bladder was decompressed. Cystometric studies have shown that this problem does not occur with retention. It is currently thought that any amount of urine can be drained. Drainage does not occur rapidly, because the usual size of a catheter does not allow rapid drainage.

Surgical Management

Surgical intervention is usually done when a structural defect is found. Intervention may include (1) removal of an enlarged prostate gland or urethral stricture or (2) correction of a structural abnormality.

Bladder Neck Repair

Surgical intervention is sometimes needed for obstructions below the bladder. If the bladder neck becomes rigid as a result of inflammation, cystoplasty may be done by insertion of an elastic wedge into the area. A transurethral incision of the bladder neck might also be performed. Excision of urethral strictures, sometimes with a *urethroplasty* (plastic repair of the urethra), helps return proper functioning. Alternatively, a meatotomy may be performed to open the urethral meatus.

Suprapubic Cystotomy

Indications. Suprapubic catheterization is sometimes used to relieve urinary retention. Placement of the catheter allows postoperative clients to begin a bladder training program. The catheter is placed when urethral catheterization is difficult, as in clients with a severely enlarged prostate, urethral strictures, or quadriplegia. Local anesthesia is used, although general anesthesia may be used if another surgical procedure is also performed. To facilitate proper placement of the catheter, the bladder must be distended with urine or water before insertion. If the bladder is insufficiently distended with urine, additional fluid is instilled through a catheter or cystoscope.

The suprapubic skin is prepared. Under sterile technique, the suprapubic catheter is inserted through a small surgical incision or by passing a trocar through the skin into the bladder. Once the trocar is in place, the pointed core of the cannula is removed. The catheter is threaded through the cannula and attached to a closed drainage system. The catheter is commonly sutured in place or secured with a commercially made retention seal. When the catheter is removed, the muscle layers of the bladder immediately contract over the puncture site and shrink the surface wound.

Contraindications. Short-term catheter placement may be a possible contraindication.

Complications. Potential complications of a suprapubic catheter include dislodgment of the catheter, hematuria (especially after the use of a large-bore catheter), bowel perforation during trocar insertion, and failure of the wound to close, which results in a urinary fistula.

Outcomes. When a suprapubic catheter is used instead of a urethral catheter, a lower rate of UTIs, increased comfort, and easier implementation of a bladder training protocol are expected.

Nursing Management of the Surgical Client

The client with a suprapubic catheter requires care similar to that needed for clients with a urethral catheter. The most frequent problem is catheter obstruction caused by (1) twisting or kinking or (2) sediment or clots. Disconnecting the catheter from the drainage tubing can disrupt the siphon drainage. When the catheter is removed, dressing changes may be needed to protect the skin from urinary leakage from the site. The suprapubic catheter site usually closes completely immediately or within 24 hours of removal.

Self-Care

The client who is discharged with an indwelling suprapubic or urethral catheter needs to know how to care for the catheter at home. The family and significant others should learn how to empty the drainage bag and how to prevent infection. They should also be taught the clinical manifestations of UTI and instructed to call the physician if they occur. When the client is discharged with a catheter in place, follow-up care is required. Removal of the catheter depends on the cause of the retention.

Modifications for Older Clients

Older clients are more susceptible to urinary retention because of a chronic decrease in bladder tone. Retention leading to infection may also be worse in older clients. Treatment, however, remains the same.

URINARY INCONTINENCE

Urinary incontinence has been defined by the International Continence Society (ICS) as "a condition in which involuntary loss of urine is a social or hygienic problem and is objectively demonstrable."[1] Approximately 13% to 56% of noninstitutionalized adults older than age 60 years and at least half of nursing home residents have problems related to incontinence.[1] The annual cost of incontinence exceeds $15 million.[1] Yet most people avoid seeking treatment because they feel shame and embarrassment, which means that the problem is severely underreported and underdiagnosed. Many health care providers do not understand the effects of urinary incontinence on quality of life. Affected people may forfeit their active lifestyles and turn to a reclusive existence because they fear embarrassment.

There are three major types of incontinence: (1) *stress urinary incontinence,* (2) *detrusor overactivity,* and (3) *overflow urinary incontinence.*[1] Under each of these types are many subtypes that may present in clients as an individual diagnosis or a combination of diagnoses.

Etiology and Risk Factors

Urinary incontinence commonly results from many factors, including anatomic defects and physical, physiologic, psychosocial, and pharmacologic factors. Anatomic and physiologic incontinence results from sphincter weakness or damage, urethral deformity, altered muscle tone at the urethrovesical junction, and detrusor instability.

Stress urinary incontinence is the complaint of involuntary leakage on effort or exertion.[1] It commonly results from obstetric or surgical trauma, the loss of estrogen associated with menopause, repeated straining, urogenital prolapse, and congenital weakness. After a suprapubic prostatectomy and transurethral prostatectomy, men may experience some exertional urine loss after the postoperative catheter is removed. Surgical interventions may cause bladder neck damage, with possibly permanent incontinence. A radical perineal or retropubic prostatectomy may cause permanent incontinence if the bladder neck is partially damaged during surgery.

Dysfunction of the urethrovesical junction (the area where the bladder meets the urethra) occurs mainly in women. Common causes include pregnancy, vaginal delivery, menopause, and surgical procedures that damage nerves leading to muscles of the pelvic floor. These injuries may lead to stress incontinence of varying degrees. A change in the angle of greater than 30 degrees from a horizontal plane during straining indicates hypermobility resulting from relaxation of the urethrovesical junction.

A simple diagnostic test for a hypermobile urethrovesical junction is a *Q-tip test*. A sterile, well-lubricated cotton applicator is placed in the urethra. The client is asked to strain as if to have a bowel movement. More than a 30-degree difference in a horizontal plane indicates a positive result or urethral hypermobility of the urethrovesical junction (Figure 34-8).

Detrusor overactivity (referred to as *Urge Incontinence* by NANDA-I) has many possible causes, although in many cases the cause remains unknown. On occasion, the cause can be identified as a bladder lesion, lower or upper spinal cord lesion, complication of pelvic surgery, or neurologic deficit. The ICS offers two descriptions to characterize bladder overactivity. In the first, the bladder contracts either spontaneously or with provocation while the client attempts to inhibit micturition. These contractions are seen during the filling phase of a cystometrogram in a neurologically intact client. In the second, detrusor overactivity results from disturbances of the nervous control mechanism. These clients have objective evidence of bladder dysfunction from a neurologic disorder. This type of bladder overactivity, known as *detrusor hyperreflexia* (called *Reflex Incontinence* by NANDA-I), is commonly seen in the client with a history of a stroke or neurologic impairment.[1]

Incontinent episodes of *detrusor overactivity* (called *Urge Incontinence* by NANDA-I) occur randomly. Those who have this diagnosis often report they experience involuntary urination that is preceded by a warning of a few seconds to a few minutes. It is caused by uncontrolled contraction or overactivity of the detrusor muscle. It is sometimes observed in clients who have central nervous system disorders (Alzheimer's disease, brain tumor, Parkinson's disease, multiple sclerosis), bladder disorders (interstitial cystitis, radiation effects, carcinoma in situ), and spinal cord interference with spinal inhibitory pathways (spondylosis, cancer growth in spinal cord). However, it is diagnosed in clients who do not have these central neurologic disorders.

Overflow urinary incontinence, as defined by ICS and NANDA-I, is an involuntary urine loss associated with overdistention of the bladder. The bladder is able to store urine but does not empty completely, causing urine loss as a result of diminishing resistant pressures.

Functional incontinence may be the result of physical, psychosocial, or pharmacologic causes unrelated to the status of the urinary system. Physical causes of incontinence independent of disorders of the urinary tract are often related to physical immobility, especially with older adults. These clients are often physically unable to get to the toilet independently because of stroke, fractures, or weakness. Failing vision and distances from the bathroom can also contribute to incontinence if the client cannot see the commode or bedpan.

Psychosocial causes of incontinence range from true psychological problems, such as dementia, to simple confusion. Clients may be unaware of the need to void or may be unable to respond appropriately when they feel the urge to empty the bladder. Other possible causes include regression, dependence, insecurity, sensory deprivation, and the disturbance of conditioned reflexes.

Drugs can also contribute to incontinence, especially overflow incontinence. Examples include the following:

- Opioids, tranquilizers, sedatives, and hypnotic agents, all of which may affect sensory perception
- Alcohol
- Rapid-acting diuretics
- Antihistamines
- Atropine and atropine-like substances
- Hypotensive agents
- Alpha-adrenergic blockers
- Beta-adrenergic agents
- Ganglionic blockers

Other causative factors include fecal impaction, bladder scarring, urethral adhesions, diabetes mellitus, and obesity. Frequent voiding by clients who fear "accidents" leads to decreased bladder capacity, increased detrusor tone, and thickening of the bladder wall, which only fosters the dysfunction.

Incontinence health promotion activities involve preventing impaired mobility and UTIs, exercising to minimize muscle weakness, and assisting clients to the

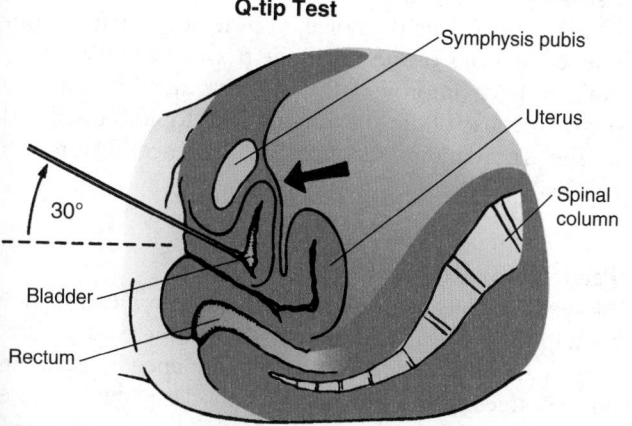

Q-tip Test

Symphysis pubis

Uterus

Spinal column

30°

Bladder

Rectum

■ **FIGURE 34–8** Diagnostic "Q-tip test" determines the descent of the normal urethrovesical junction contributing to stress incontinence in women. More than a 30-degree increase during exertional activities indicates a hypermobile urethrovesical junction.

bathroom by the clock to prevent accidents. Health maintenance measures are to thoroughly assess clients who report incontinence and monitor high-risk clients for development of incontinence. Teaching clients to perform pelvic muscle exercises (Kegel exercises) to improve muscle tone, to follow bladder training protocols, and to decrease incontinence by regulating fluid intake (e.g., not drinking large amounts of fluid at bedtime) are examples of health restoration interventions.

Pathophysiology

Pathophysiologic changes associated with incontinence vary with the specific cause of the disorder. In *stress incontinence,* increased vesical pressure commonly stems from such activities as sneezing, coughing, laughing, and exertion. There may be some dysfunction of the urethral sphincter or, in women, changes in the urethrovesical junction caused by weakness of periurethral muscles. Muscle weakness from childbirth, menopause, or other problems loosens the pelvic floor. In addition to the loss of muscle tone supporting the urethrovesical junction, there is increased descent, with a funneling effect of the bladder neck during exertion. In men, the pathophysiologic change usually results from BPH, which causes retention, overflow, and stress incontinence.

Detrusor overactivity (*Urge Incontinence* according to NANDA-I) is associated with several pathophysiologic changes, and in some cases, the pathophysiologic cause is unknown. One problem is uninhibited detrusor contraction associated with motor disorders. Another cause is decreased mobility from an upper motor neuron spinal lesion combined with an inability to stop voiding once the impulse is felt.

Overflow urinary incontinence stems from overdistention of the bladder and eventual overflow of the excessive amount of urine. Usually, this problem results from obstruction at the bladder outlet, as with BPH.

If incontinence is not controlled, it can lead to both psychological and physical problems. The psychological consequences of incontinence are serious. Clients may isolate themselves, and the fear of embarrassment may lead to depression. Incontinence is also a leading cause of nursing home admissions. The physical complications of incontinence include infection, skin breakdown, and permanent voiding dysfunctions.

Clinical Manifestations

The major manifestation of urinary incontinence is involuntary urine loss. Manifestations vary from client to client. An excellent diagnostic tool, the *bladder diary,* reveals voiding frequency, fluid intake, patterns of urinary urgency, and number and severity of incontinent episodes. The Integrating Diagnostic Testing feature on p. 765 illustrates additional information related to diagnostic testing of urinary incontinence.

OUTCOME MANAGEMENT

Successful management of urinary incontinence requires appropriate diagnostic testing. Treatments include pelvic floor exercises and behavioral interventions, drug therapy, and surgery. The least invasive treatment should be tried first. Many therapies aimed at improving incontinence can be implemented without risk to the client. Success is based on motivation, competency, and willingness to add these changes to one's lifestyle. Surgery should be performed only when a structural or anatomic defect is found.

The goals of treatment for a client with urinary incontinence include the following:

- Careful evaluation
- Treatment decisions based on the specific abnormalities identified for each client
- Treatment modalities that coordinate with the client's personality, expectations, environment, and clinical status
- A treatment plan that includes ways to circumvent environmental constraints
- Ability of the client to make an informed choice among treatment options

Medical Management

Many noninvasive, behavior-based therapies may be effective in controlling some types of incontinence. The International Continence Society provide numerous algorithms that detail the diagnosis and treatment of various forms of incontinence.[1] Injectable agents such as Botox are being explored for medical treatment of incontinence.

Pelvic Muscle Exercises

Originally designed for postpartum women, these exercises—commonly known as Kegel exercises—have long been the technique of choice for reducing urinary incontinence. Reports of success range from 30% to 90%. New devices have improved the success rate by fostering the correct use of these exercises. This topic is discussed in the Translating Evidence into Practice feature on p. 766.

Pelvic Floor Reeducation

Biofeedback has been used for clients with incontinence to help them learn to reuse the pelvic floor musculature. Clients are educated to control incontinence by isolating and contracting the pelvic floor muscles. The use of biofeedback has been successful in eliminating incontinence in about 54% to 77% of clients who try it.

Biofeedback provides a "relay-like" system by which the client can visualize the isolation and contraction

Urinary Incontinence

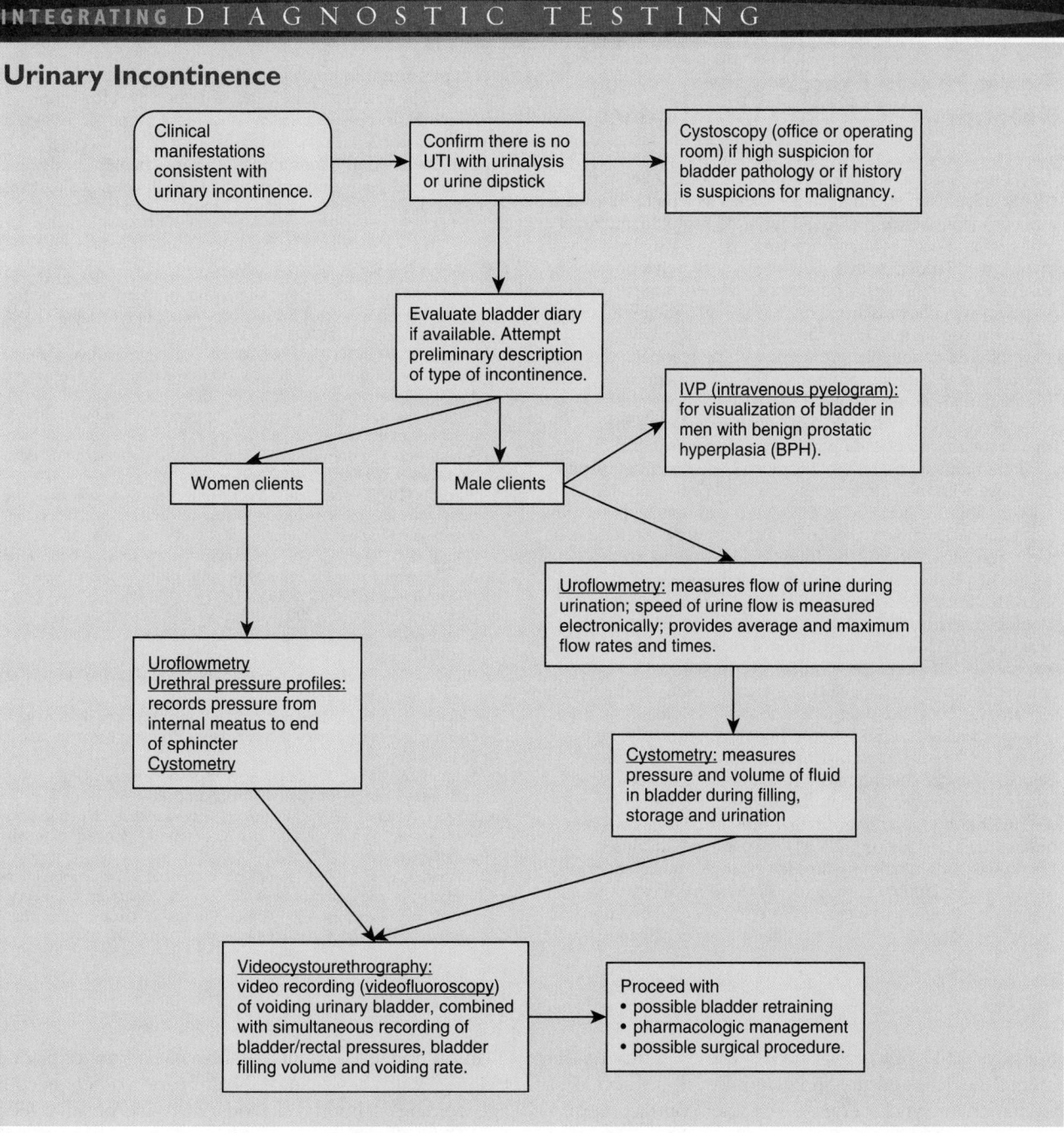

the pelvic floor musculature. Either pressure manometry or electromyographic (EMG) monitoring records the muscle strength or muscle activity.

Clients are taught to use the pelvic floor muscles to override the sense of urgency in an effort to retrain the bladder. They can also be taught to contract the correct muscle group to inhibit urine loss caused by exertion. Biofeedback can also be used to teach clients to relax the pelvic floor if they have problems with urinary retention.

Electrical Stimulation

Electrical stimulation of the pelvic floor can be used to inhibit the micturition reflex and to contract the pelvic floor muscles. Delivery of a weak electrical current helps to close the urethra more tightly by direct and reflexogenic contraction of the striated periurethral muscles. Electrical stimulation also helps increase bladder volume through bladder inhibition and stabilized detrusor activity.

The most common method of delivery is by insertion of a vaginal or anal sensor. The procedure can be done

TRANSLATING EVIDENCE INTO PRACTICE

Pelvic Muscle Exercises for Treatment of Urinary Incontinence

Kegel exercises, first introduce by Dr. Arnold Kegel in the 1940s, have been encouraged for clients as a method to treat urinary incontinence. Dr. Kegel reported symptomatic relief of stress and urge incontinence (urge is now usually called overactive bladder) with a daily regimen of pelvic muscle exercise. Over the years, physicians have encouraged clients to perform pelvic muscle exercise as the first-line treatment of urinary incontinence. Over the past 20 years, many nurses have offered continence programs with biofeedback-directed pelvic muscle exercise programs. These instructional rehabilitation programs have repeatedly demonstrated cost-effective care while decreasing or eliminating the manifestations associated with urinary incontinence.

Although surgery and medications have been developed for those with incontinence, the cost and risk associated with surgery and the side effects associated with medications are not treatments chosen by clients. Pelvic muscle exercise has been recommended by the International Continence Society as the first-line treatment for urinary incontinence.[7] It provides improved continence with little risk. Studies have demonstrated that verbal instructions are not adequate in teaching clients correct performance of pelvic muscle exercise.[1-6,8-11] Continence nurses use biofeedback to help clients recognize the specific events that initiate incontinence episodes. Clients are then taught to contract the pelvic floor muscle quickly to eliminate the urgency, frequency, and urine loss associated with overactive bladder. The quick squeezes excite the inhibitory reflex to relax the bladder while the squeezes associated with stress incontinence close the urethra by increasing urethral pressure. During a stress incontinent episode, urine loss is experienced during increased abdominal pressure, for example, while sneezing, coughing, or laughing. To decrease these manifestations, clients are taught to squeeze before the specific exertional activities that precede the incontinent episode. Eventually, clients perform these pelvic muscle contractions automatically to control their incontinence manifestations. Additionally, these specifically educated continence nurses offer a well-rounded program consisting of emotional support, behavioral interventions, dietary changes, and individualized plans that are specific to each client's diagnosis and clinical manifestations.

REFERENCES

1. Bump, R.C., et al. (1991). Assessment of Kegel pelvic performance after brief verbal instruction. *American Journal of Obstetrics & Gynecology, 170*(2), 208-212.
2. Burgio, K., et al. (1998). Behavioral vs drug treatment for urge urinary incontinence in older women. *Journal of the American Medical Association, 280*(23), 1995-2000.
3. Burgio, K., et al. (2003). Behavioral training with and without biofeedback in the treatment of overactive bladder in older women: A randomized, controlled trial. *Journal of the American Medical Association, 288*(18), 2293-2299.
4. Burns, P. (1993). A comparison of effectiveness of biofeedback and pelvic muscle exercise treatment of stress incontinence in older community-dwelling women. *Journal of Gerontology, 48*(4), 167-174.
5. Dougherty, M., et al. (2002). A randomized trial of behavioral management for continence with rural older women. *Research in Nursing and Health, 25*(1), 3-13.
6. Filocamo, M., et al. (2005). Effectiveness of early pelvic floor treatment for post prostatectomy incontinence. *European Urology, 48*(5), 734-738.
7. Hunskaar, S., et al. (2003). Epidemiology and natural history of urinary incontinence. *Urology, 62*(4), 16-23.
8. Kincade, J., et al. (2005). Self-monitoring and pelvic floor muscle exercise to treat urinary incontinence. *Urologic Nursing, 25*(5), 353-363.
9. Milne, J., & Moore, K. (2006). Factors impacting self-care for urinary incontinence. *Urologic Nursing, 26*(1), 41-51.
10. Russell, A., et al. (2005). Evaluating performance of pelvic floor exercises in women with urinary incontinence. *Journal of Reproductive Medicine, 50*(7), 529-532.
11. Wyman, J., et al. (1998). Comparative efficacy of behavioral interventions in the management of female urinary incontinence. Continence Program for Women Research Group. *American Journal of Obstetrics and Gynecology, 179*(4), 999-1007.

in a physician's office or at home. The client inserts the internal device, and the stimulation level is directed at maintaining a synchronous pelvic floor contraction during an on-and-off cycle. See the website for a figure that shows the computerized systems used for biofeedback and electrical stimulation.

Bladder Training and Behavioral Training

The client who uses bladder and behavioral training to address incontinence first voids at short intervals throughout the day—once an hour or less, if necessary. The client then tries to gradually lengthen the time between voiding up to 3 hours. Behavioral training with biofeedback or verbal feedback to teach pelvic floor muscle control showed a 63% to 69% improvement in continence in community-dwelling older women.

Institutionalized clients can also use a form of bladder training. With these clients, health care workers encourage voiding at hourly intervals and give positive feedback. The time between voiding can then be gradually increased to 2 hours.

Medications

Drug therapy for incontinence is guided primarily by the following events. During the bladder filling phase, the detrusor relaxes because of beta-adrenergic activity. At the same time, the bladder outlet contracts in response to alpha-adrenergic stimulation. If these actions are insufficient to keep urine in the bladder, drugs can be prescribed to supplement or replace them. The pharmacologic treatment of urinary incontinence is described in the Integrating Pharmacology feature on p. 767.

Medications for the Treatment of Urinary Incontinence

Medication is often the first treatment offered to clients with incontinence. These medications are diagnosis specific. Overactive bladder is treated with anticholinergic agents such as oxybutynin (Ditropan) and tolterodine (Detrol). Anticholinergics work by increasing the volume in the bladder that can be tolerated before an involuntary bladder contraction occurs, decreasing the strength of the involuntary bladder contraction, and increasing the total bladder capacity. Extended-release formulas of these drugs are available. Additionally, Ditropan has an antispasmodic action as well. It has an inhibitory effect on the smooth muscle of the bladder and has a local anesthetic effect. Tolterodine has an antimuscarinic property that has fewer side effects than other anticholinergics.

Tricyclic antidepressants such as imipramine (Tofranil) and amitriptyline (Elavil) are also often prescribed for overactive bladder as well as for interstitial cystitis. The tricyclics act by increasing the synaptic concentration of serotonin or norepinephrine in the central nervous system. This leads to bladder wall relaxation and increased bladder capacity.

A commonly prescribed medication for incontinence in women is vaginal estrogen. Recent studies have not found oral estrogen to be effective for treatment of incontinence and it is not recommended. Before the menopausal years, the urogenital system is enriched with estrogen receptors that bring an excellent blood supply to the vaginal mucosa. During the perimenopausal years and through the postmenopausal years, the decreasing circulating estrogens lead to atrophic changes of the vagina, urethra, and bladder trigone. As the mucosal layers atrophy, the tissues become less elastic as the urethra loses its ability to close properly. The application of vaginal estrogen increases the circulation, leading to improved function of the lower urogenital system.

Fluid Intake and Dietary Changes

The major nutritional aspect of management involves controlling fluid intake. Decreasing fluid intake, especially after dinner, may help decrease nocturia. For obese clients, weight reduction may help decrease stress incontinence by decreasing pressure against the bladder neck during exertion. The client should also avoid bladder irritants, such as alcohol, chocolate, and caffeinated drinks.

Nursing Management of the Medical Client

Multiple nursing diagnoses can be used, depending on the specific type of incontinence: *Stress Urinary Incontinence, Reflex Urinary Incontinence, Urge Urinary Incontinence* (Detrusor Overactivity according to ICS), and *Functional Urinary Incontinence*. All of the following interventions may be implemented as appropriate. Nurses often offer the first intervention for the client with urinary incontinence. The primary intervention is asking about bladder health with sensitivity. Many clients feel shame and embarrassment about incontinence, and they may be reluctant to acknowledge the existence of a bladder control problem that affects their quality of life.

Implement a Bladder Training Program

A successful bladder training program requires patience. The client must accept the program and be a willing and active participant. The first step is to discuss all procedures, expectations, and anticipated outcomes with the client. Do your best to inspire a sense of hope and a positive attitude when discussing the client's prognosis.

A bladder training program involves (1) adequate fluid intake, (2) accessibility to a toilet, (3) muscle-strengthening exercises, and (4) carefully scheduled voiding times. Implementing the program also requires well-organized teaching guidelines. The client also may need behavioral modification or intermittent catheterization.

Monitor Fluid Intake

Many clients with incontinence reduce their fluid intake to decrease urine production and increase control. Actually, adequate fluid intake and adequate urine production are necessary to stimulate the micturition reflex. Unless the client's physical status is a contraindication, encourage a daily fluid intake of 0.5 ounce of fluid for every pound of body weight. Carefully space these fluids throughout the day, limiting fluids in the evening to allow longer sleep periods at night. Fluids should be free of caffeine and alcohol, both of which may irritate the bladder.

Teach Kegel Exercises

Performed diligently, Kegel exercises strengthen the pubococcygeal muscle, help resolve stress incontinence, and decrease urgency and frequency. Instruct the client to contract the pelvic floor muscles as if to hold back intestinal gas. Do not ask the client to start and stop the urine stream as a way to isolate the correct muscle group. Stopping and starting the urine stream may cause dysfunction of the micturition reflex and may encourage urinary retention.

Once the client can isolate the correct muscle group, he or she should contract these muscles 10 times in sitting, standing, and lying positions, three times a day, working up to 10-second contractions. Then encourage the client to contract the pelvic floor muscles to learn the urge suppression technique or before any exertion that might cause incontinence. As with any exercise program, the program takes a conscious effort and may take months for the muscles to become adequately toned.

Develop a Voiding Schedule
At the same time that the client is strengthening pelvic floor muscles, the nurse should develop a voiding schedule with the client. Determine how often the client urinates during the day by asking the client to maintain a voiding record. Depending on the voiding pattern, help the client to the toilet or commode every 30 minutes, increasing the time to 2 hours. As the program progresses, encourage the client to hold the urine longer. This increases voiding intervals, which increases bladder capacity.

Implement Biofeedback Techniques
Biofeedback and behavior modification may improve the outcome of the bladder training program. Use biofeedback techniques to help the client regain control over the external urethral sphincter and pelvic floor musculature. An internal probe is placed to measure the pelvic floor muscle activity. As the client contracts the pelvic floor, a visual analog scale or video graphs indicate the activity, strength, and duration of the muscle contraction. The system gives immediate feedback of progress. The therapy can be offered in the practitioner's office or with the use of a home unit.

Use Behavior Modification
Behavior modification is a variation of the voiding schedule. This program conditions the bladder to empty when the client attempts to void. The client is encouraged to void by the clock rather than by urge. The initial time between voiding is based on a completed bladder diary before therapy is begun. The time between voiding may be as little as every 30 minutes, with weekly increases of 15 to 30 minutes between. The gradual increase in time between voiding helps to decrease detrusor overactivity and to increase bladder capacity.

Explore Obstructive Devices
Obstructive devices are sometimes used for women with stress incontinence and vaginal prolapse (Chapter 39). For example, certain types of vaginal pessaries can reduce incontinence by supporting the descending urogenital angle at the bladder neck. When a pessary is fit properly, the client should be able to void completely without urethral obstruction. Women using such devices should have the dexterity to remove the device for cleaning several times a week or when not in use. If the client is unable to remove the pessary, she should return to the clinic every 3 weeks to have the pessary removed, cleaned, and reinserted, and she should undergo a vaginal inspection for infection and irritation.

Recommend Counseling
A mental health consultation may help clients with depression that stems from incontinence. Talking to a counselor can help clients manage the fear of embarrassment, sense of increased dependence, and self-image problems accompanying incontinence. Avoid medications such as antidepressants because of the potential for more bladder dysfunction.

Use Other Incontinence Products
Disposable Pads. Sometimes none of the measures described are effective. Nursing interventions must then be aimed at protecting the client's skin, clothing, and bed linen. Adult-sized disposable pads or briefs help protect and increase the social mobility of clients with chronic incontinence. These commercially available undergarments have elastic legs and cellulose padding that draws fluid away from the skin by capillary action. Some brands include an odor-reducing agent.

Skin Care. If the skin becomes wet, it must be meticulously cleaned with a pH-balanced cleaner and dried to prevent serious rashes and skin breakdown from maceration and ammonia. The skin should then be carefully moisturized. Indwelling catheters to drain urine should be used only to avoid skin breakdown.

Condom Systems. External condom catheter drainage involves placing a thin rubber or plastic sheath over the penis and connecting it to either a leg bag or a bedside drainage bag. When the bladder releases urine, it runs down the tube into the collecting device. Problems include leakage (with or without detachment of the condom), twisting of the condom, and stasis of urine, which can macerate the penis.

Select the correct size of sheath, attaching it to stay in place without compromising circulation to the distal penis. Make sure that the sheath is not too tight, particularly at the ring. You may need to remove some of the client's pubic hair before preparing the skin. Wash the penis with soap and water and allow it to dry thoroughly to remove skin oils. If appropriate, apply an adhesive paste or commercial skin barrier.

Many commercially prepared condom systems contain a double-sided adhesive liner that is applied to the penis before the condom. Many newer devices are self-adhesive.

When rolling the condom sheath over the penis, allow at least 1.5 cm between the distal end of the penis and the internal end of the sheath. This reduces skin irritation. Make sure that the foreskin is over the glans.

Use only elastic tape to allow for expansion or erection. Apply this tape in a spiral only. To avoid impaired circulation, never encircle the penis completely with tape. Frequently monitor the patency of the system, and remove the condom daily to clean and dry the skin.

Encourage Follow-Up

The client should be seen at regular intervals to make sure that interventions are adequate and continence is improved. Referral to a continence clinic may sometimes be appropriate to ensure close follow-up of continuing problems. The National Association for Continence and the Simon Foundation for Continence both publish newsletters containing important information for the incontinent client and family. The Management and Delegation feature below discusses delegation of responsibility while caring for clients with urinary incontinence.

Surgical Management

Surgical procedures are performed only to correct or compensate for anatomic defects leading to incontinence. After an injury to the bladder neck, the surgeon can resuspend the bladder neck and attempt to recreate normal anatomy. Implantation of an artificial sphincter can bring about opening and closing of the urethra to

---

MANAGEMENT AND DELEGATION

Helping Clients with Urinary Incontinence

Various underlying conditions can result in urinary incontinence. Although women are at greater risk than men, incontinence also affects men. You and the physician assess and evaluate the client to determine the appropriate interventions to manage incontinence, possibly using a bladder record or voiding diary to document patterns and trends. Pelvic muscle rehabilitation, behavior therapy, pharmacologic interventions, and surgical procedures are the recommended treatments. For many, incontinence is an acute problem; for others, it is a chronic one.

Bladder training, assistance with toileting, and providing good skin care are duties that may be delegated to unlicensed assistive personnel. These measures are necessary for improving continence and for keeping clients dry and clean to prevent complications associated with skin irritation and ulceration.

Helping the incontinent client who cannot get out of bed is crucial in preventing skin breakdown and pressure ulcers. Utilizing a bedpan, a bedside commode, or a raised toilet seat may be helpful at times. If the client uses a walking aid to ambulate, ensure that the wheelchair, walker, or cane is near the bed and that the pathway to the bathroom is well lit and clear. Indicate which modality is appropriate for each client.

Instruct unlicensed assistive personnel to:

- Respond promptly to all call lights in their assigned area.
- Closely measure and record urine output. Cloudy, foul-smelling, or dark urine should be reported immediately to you.
- Give each client plenty of time to void. Create privacy by closing the door or pulling the bedside curtain.
- Never scold a client who is wet. The client may be upset or feel ashamed about incontinence.

With bladder training instruction, direct unlicensed assistive personnel to:

- Assist or prompt the client to the bathroom on a scheduled interval, usually every 1 to 2 hours at the beginning of the training period.
- Increase the interval of time to assist or prompt the client to the bathroom as the client begins to achieve dryness.

Ask unlicensed assistive personnel to:

- Explain when the next bathroom time will be before they leave the room.
- Offer positive reinforcement to the client who can successfully void or asks for assistance to the bathroom to urinate, or has a dry absorbent pad.
- Assist clients with exercises to strengthen pelvic muscles to help minimize incontinence, reinforcing your previous instruction.

Direct unlicensed assistive personnel about which toileting methods to use:

- *Scheduled toileting:* Assist the client to the bathroom every 2 to 4 hours whether or not the client is wet or dry.
- *Prompted voiding:* Check whether the client is wet or dry; ask the client whether he or she needs to void, and help the client to the bathroom if the client answers "yes."
- *Habit training:* Once the client's voiding times each day are determined, help the client to the bathroom at the same times each day.

Maintaining clean, dry, and intact skin is necessary to prevent skin breakdown and unnecessary complications associated with wet skin. Instruct unlicensed assistive personnel to provide proper skin care and to identify any changes such as red, excoriated, or tender skin to you. The regimen may include the following:

- Cutting back on evening or night fluid intake to decrease voiding accidents during the night
- Changing disposable wet pads or diapers every time the client is wet
- Using ointments or creams to protect the skin and to serve as a barrier after cleaning the client
- Applying absorbent pads or diapers that are not chafing to the skin

Have unlicensed assistive personnel communicate and report (1) any changes in skin or urine, (2) the client's inability to follow the toileting plan, and (3) any other questions that arise. You are responsible for assessing, implementing, evaluating, and making all changes to the client's plan of care.

allow voiding. Other procedures, such as collagen or fat injections, are used to fill or occlude a urethra that cannot close completely.

Bladder Neck Suspensions

Bladder neck suspensions restore the normal urethrovesical junction or lengthen and support the urethra. Resuspending the bladder neck allows the urethrovesical junction to function correctly.

The *Burch colposuspension* is a popular surgical procedure for women with stress incontinence. This surgical intervention is a modification of an older procedure known as the MMK (Marshall, Marchetti, Krantz). In the Burch procedure, a surgeon fixes the periurethral tissue to Cooper's ligament, whereas in the MMK procedure, the surgeon sutures the periurethral tissue to the symphysis pubis. After surgery, a suprapubic catheter must usually be in place for up to 14 days. The drainage system must remain patent because the pressure of a filling bladder can inhibit the healing process.

A *sling procedure* is used for intrinsic sphincter deficiency, a severe type of stress incontinence. Material is placed beneath the urethra to elevate it and to increase urethral compression. The sling material may be synthetic or autologous (from one's self), such as fascia from another part of the client's abdomen. There are many variations of the procedure; some present a significant risk of voiding dysfunction and others present risk of rejection of the synthetic material used for urethral support.

One type of *sling procedure* is called a *TVT*, or transvaginal tape. When a TVT procedure is placed in a woman, a synthetic material made of Prolene is loosely positioned under the urethra at the bladder neck. It supports the urethra and bladder neck during the activities that trigger a stress incontinent episode. The procedure is done as an outpatient surgery and the client is often discharged within several hours of completion of the TVT.

Other surgical procedures provide an intact, patent route for the transport of urine. Scar tissue that interferes with normal bladder neck function must be removed.

Implantation of an Artificial Urinary Sphincter

Implantation of an artificial urinary sphincter may help some clients achieve continence. This procedure usually is avoided until all other treatments have failed. Figure 34-9 shows a sphincter device, which consists of an inflatable cuff, a reservoir, and a control pump. The surgeon implants the cuff around the bladder neck or urethra, the deflation (or control) pump in the scrotum or labia, and the fluid reservoir in the abdomen.

The cuff keeps the urethra closed until the client manually squeezes the pump. This moves the fluid from the cuff to the reservoir. The bladder then drains. The cuff

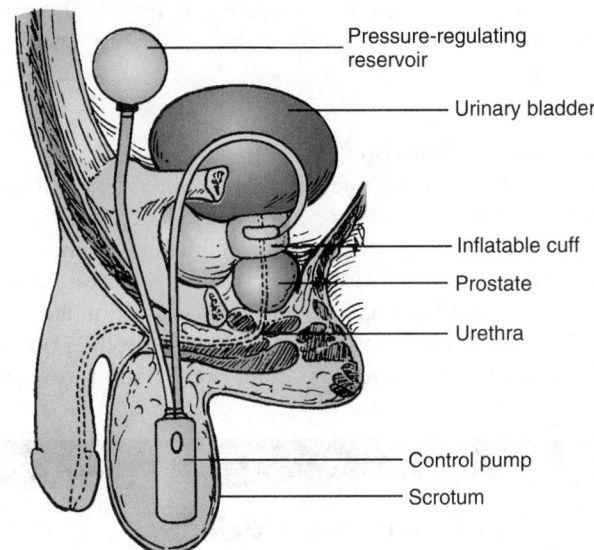

■ **FIGURE 34-9** Artificial urinary sphincter. This surgically implanted urethral sphincter restores continence. To urinate, the client deflates the cuff around the bladder neck by squeezing the control pump within the scrotum. The cuff reinflates automatically.

automatically refills after 3 to 5 minutes, again occluding the urethra.

Candidates for this treatment must not have an obstructed lower urinary tract, detrusor hyperreflexia, or progressive neurologic disease affecting bladder function. Clients must have adequate manual dexterity and motivation to manage the system. Failure of the device poses a long-term risk that the client will need more surgery. Clients must be absolutely compliant, or else the upper tracts of the urinary system can be damaged by obstruction.

Nursing Management of the Surgical Client

Nursing care of clients undergoing surgery focuses on maintaining adequate urinary drainage. With bladder suspension, preventing distention is a priority to help avoid excessive pressure on the healing surgical site. During the immediate postoperative period, a bladder training program is initiated to help the client regain detrusor muscle tone. Clamp the catheter for lengthening intervals while urine collects in the bladder, unclamping it periodically to empty the bladder. If the client reports severe pressure, the catheter should be unclamped immediately.

If a suprapubic catheter is used, the client should try to void every 2 to 3 hours. After voiding is attempted, the catheter is drained to measure the residual urine and determine the effectiveness of bladder emptying.

Self-Care

The expected outcome is that the client will resume control over bladder function. Many strategies to achieve continence may be tried, and the client selects what is most comfortable and best able to support preferred activities. Management options can be expensive, such as multiple biofeedback sessions. If continence is achieved with any of the described therapies, however, treatment to achieve continence is cheaper than the purchase of adult briefs for daily use; in addition, the client would be free to engage in desired activities. Teach the client about continence options, and help the client make decisions about treatment options.

Modifications for Older Clients

Incontinence is not a normal part of the aging process, but it is a common problem among older adults. Older clients can be treated with any of the previously mentioned treatments. Because older people are more sensitive to many medications, care should be used when drugs are administered.

NEUROGENIC BLADDER

The term *neurogenic bladder* refers to several bladder dysfunctions caused by lesions of the central or peripheral nervous systems (Figure 34-10). Their manifestations depend on the site of the lesion. A neurogenic bladder may involve a combination of one or more nervous system dysfunctions. There are five major types of neurogenic bladder dysfunction:

- Uninhibited
- Sensory paralytic (detrusor muscle hyperreflexia)
- Motor paralytic (detrusor muscle areflexia)
- Autonomous
- Reflex

Neurogenic bladder dysfunctions may also be classified according to the level of the lesion in the central nervous system.

Upper motor neuron lesions occur above the sacral segments of the spinal cord. They produce bladders that are spastic or characterized by exaggerated reflexes (hyperreflexia).

Lower motor neuron lesions occur at or below the sacral vertebrae. They produce bladders that are lacking reflexes (areflexic) or tone (atonic).

The incidence of neurogenic bladder dysfunction reflects the incidence and etiology of neurologic injuries or disorders. With certain disorders, a neurogenic bladder may develop in 100% of clients, as with transection of the spinal cord. Clients with conditions such as multiple sclerosis are affected with varying degrees of manifestations.

Etiology and Risk Factors

Risk factors for neurogenic bladder disorders include tumors, neurologic disorders, and trauma to the nervous system. Accidents are the only preventable cause of this problem. The uninhibited neurogenic bladder produces "infantile" or uninhibited voiding. The urge to void causes urine to flow. The primary cause is a lesion in the corticoregulatory tracts, as from a stroke or multiple sclerosis. A sensory paralytic bladder results from an interruption in the lateral spinal tracts, as occurs in tabes dorsalis, diabetic neuropathy, and pernicious anemia. Because of the sensory loss, the client cannot sense the bladder filling. This lack of perception leads to atonic bladder, retention with possible overflow incontinence, and upper tract involvement. A motor paralytic bladder is the most uncommon type and is caused by lesions in the motor outflow from vertebrae S2 to S4. Disease processes causing this dysfunction include poliomyelitis, tumor, trauma, spina bifida, and infection. This dysfunction may be temporary if a bacterial or viral infection is the cause. Although there is full sensation of bladder filling, even to the point of pain, the client cannot initiate micturition. Clients with an autonomous neurogenic bladder cannot perceive bladder fullness, or they cannot start and maintain urination without some type of exertional pressure. Retention and incontinence are common

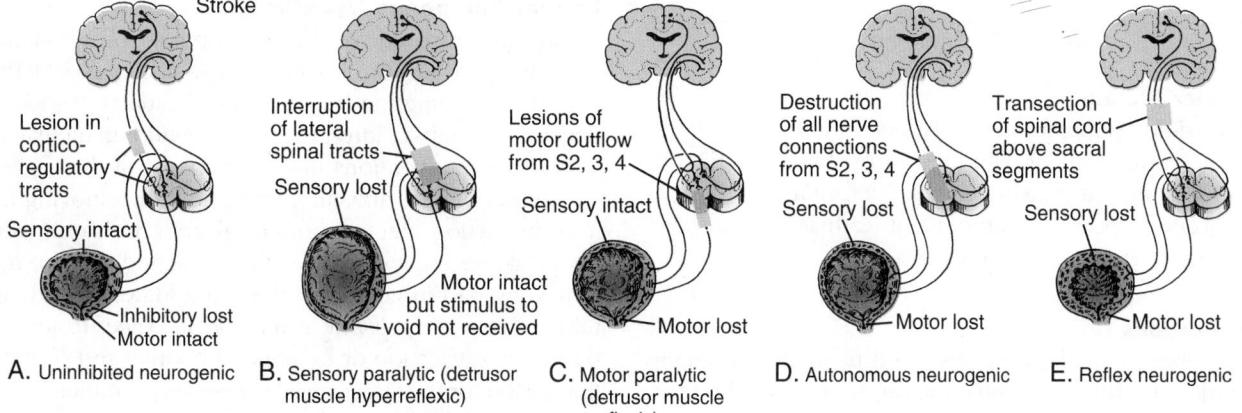

■ **FIGURE 34-10** Types of neurogenic bladder dysfunction.

problems. The autonomous type of dysfunction occurs after destruction of all nerve connections between the bladder and the central nervous system at vertebra S2, S3, or S4 following trauma, inflammatory processes, spinal anesthesia, or malignancy. Transection of the spinal cord above the sacral segments causes a reflex neurogenic bladder. There is no sensation, and the bladder contracts reflexively but does not empty completely.

Pathophysiology

Lesions at the lower motor neuron level of the spinal cord often directly interfere with the reflex arc, leading to inappropriate interpretation of efferent and afferent impulses. When the bladder fills, the message is transmitted through afferent fibers to the brain cortex. The injury keeps these impulses from being correctly interpreted, leading to loss of the micturition reflex. A flaccid bladder with urinary retention is the result.

With upper motor neuron lesions, impulses are not transmitted to or from the lower spinal areas to the cortex. When the bladder distends, no sensation is transmitted. Because the lower cord is intact, activity of the reflex arc can occur. The client would have reflex incontinence as a result.

When the damage is to the cortical area itself, as with a stroke or trauma, the client cannot correctly interpret the impulses that are being transmitted. Unless the client is evaluated and treated appropriately, serious UTIs, skin breakdown associated with incontinence, and even renal failure resulting from chronic overdistention of the bladder are more likely to develop.

Clinical Manifestations

The major clinical manifestation of neurogenic bladder dysfunction is retention with or without incontinence. The client may or may not feel a need to void or feel a sense of bladder distention. The diagnosis is made from the location of neurologic dysfunction.

OUTCOME MANAGEMENT

Medical Management

Bladder Training

If possible, some form of bladder training should be attempted for a client with neurogenic bladder dysfunction. This measure includes a bladder training program, medication, possible intermittent catheterization, and sometimes surgical intervention.

Medications

A number of medications are used to treat neurogenic bladder dysfunction. Antispasmodics and anticholinergics (such as tolterodine [Detrol], oxybutynin [Ditropan], solifenacin [Vesicare], and propantheline [Pro-Banthine])

are given to relieve uninhibited or reflex bladder contractions. Phenoxybenzamine and other alpha-adrenergic blockers may be used. Bethanechol may help stimulate an atonic bladder. Other medications described in the discussion of incontinence may be useful as well.

Preventing Complications

Autonomic dysreflexia **is a serious, potentially life-threatening complication affecting clients who have spinal cord injuries. It may occur during bladder training programs if the urinary system or bowel becomes obstructed. The most frequent cause is bladder distention or feces in the rectum, although autonomic dysreflexia can be triggered by visceral distention or stimulation of pain receptors in the skin. This condition results from an excessive autonomic response to normal stimuli and affects primarily clients with upper motor neuron lesions.**

The most common manifestations are severe hypertension, bradycardia, a throbbing headache, flushing, diaphoresis above the level of the lesion, blurred vision, nasal congestion, nausea, and pilomotor spasm ("goose bumps") above the lesion. If left untreated, this problem can lead to retinal hemorrhage, seizures, or stroke. It is important for the client to recognize the earliest manifestations and summon help immediately. Preventing bladder distention is one way to prevent this emergency. If stool is accumulating in the rectum, careful evacuation should be done to avoid either overdistention or overstimulation.

Medications such as diazoxide (Hyperstat), phenoxybenzamine (Dibenzyline), guanethidine monosulfate (Ismelin), propantheline bromide (Pro-Banthine), phentolamine mesylate (Regitine), and mecamylamine (Inversine) relieve both acute manifestations and the chronic recurrence of episodes.

Nursing Management of the Medical Client

Prevent Autonomic Dysreflexia

Always be prepared for the development of autonomic dysreflexia. If severe hypertension (sometimes 300/180 mm Hg), flushing, and a pounding headache suddenly develop, you must address the manifestations immediately.

Nursing interventions involve removal of the triggering stimuli by reestablishing urine flow or removing the fecal impaction. Remove any fecal impaction only after a topical anesthetic agent has been inserted into the rectum to avoid further stimulation. In addition, a catheter may be necessary; if one is already in place, restore its patency by irrigation or by removing kinks and obstructions. Monitor the client's vital signs every 5 minutes, and raise the head of the bed to the semi-Fowler's position. Administer medications as ordered.

Teach Methods to Stimulate Micturition

Neurogenic bladders are difficult to control, but you can teach many clients how to stimulate the micturition reflex and maintain urination. Assist the client by providing external pressure on the abdomen. The client can lean forward or press on the abdomen. Have the client breathe deeply to push the diaphragm downward. Wearing a corset or girdle can provide an extra source of external pressure. The Valsalva maneuver is another method of increasing intra-abdominal pressure on the urinary bladder.

Another method that helps the client learn to empty the bladder is the Credé maneuver. The client places the fingers over the bladder and presses downward slowly toward the symphysis pubis, as though "milking" the urine out of the urinary system. This should be done with great caution. If the client has sphincter dyssynergia (failure of muscle coordination) or if the sphincter does not readily relax, the Credé maneuver can lead to sphincter damage and may cause ureteral reflux if there is any obstruction of outflow. The Credé maneuver is often combined with intermittent self-catheterization.

The client can use several other methods to initiate and maintain micturition. Locate trigger points on the body (lower abdomen, inner thighs, and pubic area), and explain how to stimulate them by stroking, pinching, or applying ice. Stretching the anal sphincter also relaxes the reflexes of the external urethral sphincter because they are both innervated by the pudendal nerve. The client leans forward while sitting on the toilet and inserts two gloved fingers into the anus. The fingers are then either widened apart or pulled posteriorly. Men must be careful to avoid touching the glans penis, which stimulates the bulbocavernosus reflex, contracting the external sphincter.

Perform Intermittent Catheterization

For the treatment of long-term or short-term bladder atony (lack of tone), an intermittent catheterization program is an alternative to indwelling catheterization. A straight urethral catheter is inserted into the bladder at specified intervals, the urine is drained, and the catheter is removed. This may be done in a health care facility or in the client's home (see a fundamentals' textbook to review catheterization and see the Bridge to Home Health Care feature on Inserting Urinary Catheters on the website).

Teach Intermittent Self-Catheterization

Clients with bladder atony should be encouraged to learn self-catheterization because it increases independence and mobility. The client or any other person who has been properly educated about the technique may insert the catheter.

Sterile technique is necessary in health care facilities because of the high risk of nosocomial infections. At home, *clean technique* can be used for catheterization without increasing the rate of UTIs. Clean technique is also easier and less expensive for the client. To reduce the risk of bacteriuria, urinary antiseptics and acidification or bladder irrigation with antibiotics and antiseptics are used with each catheterization.

There are several procedural differences between clean and sterile techniques. For clean technique:

1. Gloves are not worn. The client must perform thorough hand-washing before starting the procedure.
2. A clean (rather than a sterile) catheter is used.
3. The catheter can be washed and reused indefinitely.
4. Lubricant should be used because the urethra is susceptible to traumatic urethritis.

The catheter should be washed thoroughly with mild soap (like Ivory) and water, rinsed, and allowed to air dry. It should be stored in a brown paper bag or other clean container such as a clean dry towel to allow air to dry inside the catheter.[73a]

During self-catheterization, the client may sit or stand. When a female client stands, she should separate her legs or place one leg on a toilet seat. After separating the labia, she can use a mirror to find the meatus.

Timing is important for successful catheterization programs. Catheterization should be carried out at specified intervals throughout the day until bedtime. The interval between catheterization is set according to the degree of continence. The average interval for adults is every 3 to 4 hours, but the client usually has to start at intervals of 2 to 3 hours. Clients should use the catheter to remove 350 to 400 ml of urine each time. A client who cannot follow a schedule is not an appropriate candidate for the program.

The amount of fluid intake allowed is under debate. Some programs allow fluid as desired; others restrict fluid intake to varying degrees. This aspect of the program requires systematic investigation. Clinicians generally recommend that the client drink about 250 ml of fluid at about 2-hour intervals. Ingestion of large amounts of fluid within a short period can cause bladder distention and reflux. Most clients are urged to drink up to 2 L of fluid daily at regular intervals.

A catheter-free bladder and absence of bacteriuria indicate a successful intermittent catheterization program. Controversy exists about the treatment of asymptomatic bacteriuria. A successful catheterization program may be due to several factors, including intermittent bladder distention, which causes stimulation of the normal micturition reflex and reactivation of the bladder's normal antibacterial properties. Other advantages include continence, independence, good hygiene, prevention of complications arising from urinary stasis or a retention catheter, decreased cost, and comfortable sexual relations.

Intermittent catheterization is not a panacea. The program requires the client to assume a great deal of personal responsibility. Some clients are not sufficiently motivated to fulfill the responsibilities involved in self-catheterization. Also, some problems can occur when the client is away from home.

Clients with high resting pressures in the bladder who are incontinent between catheterizations are likely to have difficulty with intermittent self-catheterization. All clients should be evaluated before starting the program. If urodynamic evaluation reveals high resting pressures, anticholinergic medications are administered.

Surgical Management

Surgery is not the primary treatment option for the client with neurogenic bladder. However, if conservative measures are ineffective in treating the neurogenic bladder, surgical intervention may be necessary. External sphincterotomy or incision of the bladder neck may restore normal bladder emptying. Interrupting innervation to the bladder reflex can aid an uninhibited bladder. Injection of alcohol into the subarachnoid space or rhizotomy (cutting) of the sacral nerves increases bladder capacity by inhibiting reflex bladder contractions, without interfering with normal sphincter function. Sometimes a temporary sacral nerve block is performed before surgery to evaluate the potential candidate. Electrodes may be implanted at thoracic or cervical levels of the spinal epidural space and attached to a percutaneous stimulator. As soon as the client learns to regulate the electrical stimulation properly, the device can be used to inhibit or interrupt reflex bladder contractions.

Continuous intrathecal baclofen administered through an implanted infusion pump is another method of treating a neurogenic bladder. Baclofen helps decrease spasms and detrusor sphincter dyssynergia. Clients report improvement in bladder compliance and capacity. Finally, if all else fails, urinary diversion may be performed to provide the client with a more manageable urinary system.

Nursing Management of the Surgical Client

Nursing care of the client undergoing surgery for a neurogenic bladder with either an external sphincterotomy or a revision of the bladder outlet is the same as for any client undergoing bladder surgery. Urine output maintenance is the priority of these clients. A suprapubic or urinary catheter may be needed until healing occurs.

As with the other surgical procedures, focus care on teaching the client self-care. The client needs to learn to regulate electrical stimulation appropriately to inhibit or interrupt the reflex bladder contractions.

Proper care of the implantable infusion pump is another important area of client education. Care of clients undergoing urinary diversion has been discussed under Bladder Cancer.

Self-Care

The focus of discharge teaching for the neurogenic bladder client is intermittent self-catheterization. Teach the client and significant others a bladder training program and, possibly, a catheterization program. Assess the client's ability to understand and perform self-care procedures, and ensure that the client understands the self-catheterization program. Written materials, teaching videos, and diagrams can be used to reinforce the teaching.

Clients need to be assessed in the home setting to make sure they can function as well as in the hospital. A visiting nurse may be included to help in the discharge planning of the self-catheterization or bladder training program. The client's urinary function should be monitored at regular intervals, including renal function tests and yearly renal ultrasound studies. Teach the client to call the health care provider if manifestations of a UTI develop.

Modifications for Older Clients

Older clients are more likely to have other medical problems, such as arthritis and visual changes, that can interfere with their ability to use the self-catheterization program. However, they may still be able to use this method if they have adequate help.

TRAUMATIC DISORDERS

BLADDER TRAUMA

Bladder trauma is defined as a blunt or penetrating injury to the bladder that may cause bladder rupture. Bladder trauma often results from automobile accidents, when the seat belt compresses the bladder. A bladder distended by urine can rupture with a direct blow to the lower abdomen. The bladder may also be punctured by a bullet, knife, bony splinter from a fractured pelvis, or internal medical instrumentation. When the bladder ruptures, urine spills into the peritoneal cavity. Complications of peritoneal urine accumulation from a ruptured bladder are peritonitis and pelvic cellulitis.

Clinical Manifestations

Bladder injuries usually produce hematuria and pain low in the abdomen or pain referred to a shoulder. The client also may have trouble voiding. Manifestations of peritonitis may develop as well. Fever is usually present as the peritonitis and pelvic cellulitis continue to develop. If the client has had an injury or blow to the abdomen, suspect bladder injury as the cause of the manifestations.

Medical Management

The first treatment for suspected bladder injury is insertion of an indwelling or suprapubic catheter to monitor for hematuria or urine production and to keep the bladder decompressed during healing. Any injury other than a simple contusion or very small perforation requires surgical repair.

Nursing Management of the Medical Client

Immediately assess for a suspected bladder injury if the client has had blunt trauma to the lower pelvis or abdomen. Closely monitor the client's urine output for both amount and the presence of hematuria. Report any decrease in urine output in relation to fluid intake to the physician immediately. Careful catheter insertion is necessary for the client with suspected bladder trauma.

Surgical Management

Clients with bladder injuries usually require surgical intervention. After a urethral or suprapubic catheter has been inserted, surgical repair of the damaged bladder wall is performed. The extravasated urine in the perivesical area is drained. It is important to maintain urinary drainage through a patent catheter to promote healing and to avoid the potential development of fistulae or leakage.

Nursing Management of the Surgical Client

Postoperatively, maintain urinary drainage to prevent tension on the sutures in the bladder. A Penrose drain is left in place to allow drainage of any urine remaining in the pelvis. This may necessitate dressing changes.

Because the client may be discharged with an indwelling or suprapubic catheter, teach catheter care to the client and significant others. Assess the client's self-care abilities to determine a possible need for assistance at home. If the client or significant others cannot care for the catheter, arrange for a home health visit.

Follow-up care is essential after discharge to assess healing. A cystogram may be done before the catheter is removed. If a suprapubic catheter has been placed, the client can begin bladder training before the catheter is removed. If the client has a urethral catheter, the catheter is removed before the client can attempt to void. If clients do not void within 4 to 6 hours after removal, the catheter should be reinserted.

URETHRAL TRAUMA

The urethra as well as the bladder may be injured in a pelvic fracture. Falling astride an object, such as the bar on a boy's bike, with sudden force to the groin may cause urethral contusion and laceration. Injury may also occur during medical or surgical interventions, may be self-inflicted, or may occur after female genital mutilation (see Chapter 39). Penetrating wounds also cause urethral damage.

Evaluation of urethral damage is indicated if the client cannot void, has an altered urine stream, or has visible blood at the meatus. Even if the client can pass some urine through the urethra, voiding causes urinary extravasation, resulting in swelling of the scrotum or inguinal areas, which can lead to sepsis and necrosis. Blood may appear at the external meatus and may also extravasate into the surrounding tissues, giving the area an ecchymotic appearance.

The two most common complications of urethral trauma are (1) development of urethral strictures and (2) risk of impotence in men. Impotence occurs because the corpora cavernosa of the penis, blood vessels, or nerves supplying this area are damaged.

Proper management of urethral injuries is controversial. Clinicians generally agree that urinary drainage must first be established with either a urethral or a suprapubic catheter. Some physicians suggest an immediate primary surgical repair of the urethra. Others prefer to wait 2 to 3 weeks to see whether the urethra will heal around the urethral catheter without surgery. During any waiting period, the client must be monitored for developing infection and continuing extravasation of urine.

URETERAL TRAUMA

The ureters are located deep within the abdomen and are protected by the spine and surrounding musculature. Thus most ureteral trauma takes place accidentally during surgery. Perforation or tearing may occur during manipulation of intraureteral catheters or other instruments. The ureters may be occluded by ligating sutures or a misplaced clamp, or they may be transected during pelvic surgery. Many surgeons insert ureteral stents before pelvic procedures to easily identify the ureters and prevent trauma. Gunshot and stab wounds may also traumatize the ureters. On occasion, blunt trauma from a car accident can tear these structures.

Trauma is often not discovered until a clinical manifestation develops, such as hematuria, flank pain, or the presence of extravasated urine. As the urine seeps out into the tissues, pain may occur in the lower abdomen and flank. As extravasation continues, there may be sepsis, paralytic ileus, a palpable intraperitoneal mass, and the appearance of urine in an external wound. IVP and ultrasonography are the most definitive means of diagnosis.

Surgical intervention is used to repair the defect, preferably with end-to-end anastomosis. More radical procedures may be needed, such as cutaneous ureterostomy, transureteroureterostomy, and reimplantation.

The surgeon may use prosthetic ureteral implants. A nephrectomy is performed if obstruction or sepsis causes severe renal damage. It is essential to treat sepsis aggressively. Significant extravasation of urine may necessitate that the surgeon open the abdomen and drain the urine.

CONGENITAL ANOMALIES

A congenital anomaly of the bladder is exstrophy of the bladder that develops when the symphysis pubis fails to close in utero. The lower anterior abdominal wall and anterior bladder wall are absent, allowing the bladder to protrude through the defective abdominal wall. These conditions are often treated with urinary diversion in childhood, but additional revisions may be needed as the child grows. Children who have had a diversion may be candidates for continent reservoir revisions.

Although congenital anomalies of the ureter are uncommon, several types are described:

1. *Ectopic ureter* occurs when a ureter follows an abnormal course or has an abnormal distal opening. It is the most common congenital ureteral anomaly. An ectopic ureter occurs as a result of the abnormal embryologic development of the ureter. During micturition, this anomaly often results in a back-flow of urine. Misplacement of the meatus (hypospadias and epispadias) is discussed in Chapter 38.
2. *Duplicate ureters,* arising from the same renal pelvis, may develop when the ureters on one side unite at some point; both may open in the normal portion of the trigone or both may open into the urethra or vagina. This anomaly is not usually recognized unless a radiographic study is done for another reason. Pyelonephritis develops, and an evaluation reveals the anomaly. Surgical intervention is usually not necessary unless complications occur.
3. *Abnormal dilation of the ureter (megaureter)* is characterized by dilation and pouching of the ureteral wall just adjacent to the vesicoureteral junction. Resulting manifestations are seen as reflux or obstructive effects, which predispose the client to recurrent UTIs.
4. *Congenital ureteropelvic obstruction* occurs at the junction of the renal pelvis and the ureter. This anomaly is usually bilateral. A mild obstruction may never cause manifestations of a urinary tract disorder. As long as the kidney produces urine at a rate less than 6 ml/min, the ureter can generally handle the flow; however, urine production greater than this rate causes urinary stasis in the kidney,

which results in hydronephrosis. If the condition is symptomatic, treatment consists of surgical repair of the narrowed section at the ureteropelvic junction.

CONCLUSIONS

Urinary system disorders can be extremely problematic for clients. Nurses play a major role in the diagnosis, prevention, and treatment of these disorders. Many of the disorders of the urinary system are chronic or become chronic problems, leading to renal disease or incontinence. Some of the manifestations of these disorders can drastically alter the client's self-concept and lifestyle. Problems of the lower urinary tract may become life-threatening, and the nurse must ensure that the client receives prompt and adequate treatment of disorders within the lower urinary system.

THINKING CRITICALLY

1. A 28-year-old newlywed woman has been experiencing pain and burning with urination for the past 24 hours. This is the third episode of urinary manifestations she has had in the past 3 months. What is the probable cause of the urinary manifestations? What further information do you need to assess her problem? What can you do to help her treat this problem and prevent further difficulties?

Factors to Consider. For what urinary tract problems does the client's status as a newlywed place her at risk? Which tests would help differentiate an infectious problem from a noninfectious one?

2. The client had a radical cystectomy with formation of an Indiana pouch 12 hours ago. He has a catheter in place, which has drained 10 ml in the last hour. The stoma is a very pale pink. His vital signs are elevated from their preoperative levels. His pulse rate is 100 beats/min, and his temperature is slightly increased. What actions would be appropriate at this point in the client's care?

Factors to Consider. Is the client's urine output within expected limits? What color should a fresh stoma normally be?

3. A 69-year-old man with diabetes mellitus is admitted with severe left flank pain, nausea, vomiting, and diarrhea. His abdomen is soft and only slightly tender. His urinalysis reveals increased red blood cells, and his KUB shows a large staghorn calculus in the left kidney with hydronephrosis of the left kidney. What would be a priority assessment for this client?

Factors to Consider. What other diagnostic tests should be done? What are the treatment options for large renal stones?

Discussions for these questions can be found on the website.

BIBLIOGRAPHY

Citations appearing in red refer to primary research.

Citations appearing in blue refer to evidence-based practice guidelines and protocols.

1. Abrams, P., Cardozo, L., Fall, M., et al. (2002). The standardization of terminology of lower urinary tract function: Report from the standardization sub-committee of the International Continence Society. *Neurology & Urodynamics, 21,*167-178.
2. American Cancer Society. (2007). *Cancer facts and figures.* Atlanta: Author.
3. Appell, R. (2002). Injection therapy for urinary incontinence. In P. Walsh, et al. (Eds.), *Campbell's urology* (8th ed., pp. 1172-1186). Philadelphia: Saunders.
4. Atala, A., & Keating, M. (2002). Vesicoureteral reflux and megaureter. In P. Walsh, et al. (Eds.), *Campbell's urology* (8th ed., pp. 2053-2116). Philadelphia: Saunders.
5. Bassi, P. (2002). BCG therapy of high-risk superficial bladder cancer. *Surgical Oncology, 11*(12), 77-83.
6. Bates, F. (2002). Assessment of the female patient with urinary incontinence. *Urologic Nursing, 22*(5), 305-314.
7. Baumgartner, R., et al. (2002). Causes of increased length of stay following radical cystectomy. *Urologic Nursing, 22*(5), 319-323.
8. Benson, M., & Olsson, C. (2002). Cutaneous urinary diversion. In P. Walsh, et al. (Eds.), *Campbell's urology* (8th ed., pp. 3789-3834). Philadelphia: Saunders.
9. Bernier, F., & Jenkins, P. (1997). The role of vaginal estrogen in the treatment of urogenital dysfunction in postmenopausal women. *Urologic Nursing, 17*(3), 92-95.
10. Blaivas, J., & Groutz, A. (2002). Urinary incontinence: Pathophysiology, evaluation, treatment overview, and nonsurgical management. In P. Walsh, et al. (Eds.), *Campbell's urology* (8th ed., pp. 1027-1043). Philadelphia: Saunders.
11. Blumenfeld, J., & Vaughn, E. (2002). Renal physiology and pathophysiology. In P. Walsh, et al. (Eds.), *Campbell's urology* (8th ed., pp. 169-227). Philadelphia: Saunders.
12. Boyd, L. (2003). Intravesical bacillus Calmette-Guérin for treating bladder cancer. *Urologic Nursing, 23*(3), 189-192, 199.
13. Burgess, A.W. (2005). Death by catheterization?. *American Journal of Nursing, 105*(4), 56-59.
14. Burgio, K., et al. (2002). Behavioral training with and without biofeedback in the treatment of overactive bladder in older women: A randomized controlled trial. *Journal of the American Medical Association, 288*(18), 2293-2299.
15. Chancellor, M.B., & Yoshimura, N. (2002). Physiology and pharmacology of the bladder and ureter. In P. Walsh, et al. (Eds.), *Campbell's urology* (8th ed., pp. 831-886). Philadelphia: Saunders.
16. Colella, J., Kochis, E., Galli, B., & Munver, R. (2005). Urolithiasis/nephrolithiasis: What's it all about? *Urologic Nursing, 25*(6), 427-449.
17. Cunningham, E., & Marcason, W. (2002). Are there special dietary guidelines for interstitial cystitis? *Journal of the American Dietetic Association, 102*(3), 379.
18. Dalbagni, G., Russo, P., Bochner, B., et al. (2006). Phase II trial of intravesical gemcitabine in bacille Calmette-Guérin-refractory transitional cell carcinoma of the bladder. *Journal of Clinical Oncology, 24,* 2729-2734.
19. Epstein, L., & Goldberg, R. (2005). The overactive bladder and quality of life. *Journal of Fertility, 50*(1), 30-36.
20. Fitzgerald, M. P., Brensinger, C., Brubaker, L., et al. (2005). What is the pain of interstitial cystitis like? *International Urogynecology Journal, 17*(1), 69-72.
21. Francis, P., & Winfield, H. (2006). Care of the patient undergoing robotic-assisted laparoscopic pyeloplasty. *Urologic Nursing, 26*(2), 110-116.
22. Francis, P., & Winfield, H. (2006). Medical robotics: The impact on perioperative nursing practice. *Urologic Nursing, 26*(2), 99-109.
23. Gontero, P., & Kirby, R. (2004). Proerectile pharmacological prophylaxis following nerve-sparing radical prostatectomy (NSRP). *Prostate Cancer and Prostatic Diseases, 7,* 223-226.

24. Gray, M. (2002). Are cranberry juice or cranberry products effective in the prevention or management of urinary tract infection? *Journal of Wound, Ostomy & Continence Nursing, 29,* 122-126.
25. Gray, M. (2002). Continence nursing at the dawn of the 21st century: A futurist perspective. *Urologic Nursing, 22*(4), 233-236.
26. Gray, M., & Krissovich, M. (2003). Does fluid intake influence the risk for urinary incontinence, urinary tract infection, and bladder cancer? *Journal of Wound, Ostomy and Continence, 30*(3), 126-131.
27. Gray, M., & Moore, K. (2008). *Urologic disorders.* St. Louis: Mosby.
28. Grossman, H., Soloway, M., Messing, E., et al. (2006). Surveillance for recurrent bladder cancer using a point-of-care proteomic assay. *Journal of the American Medical Association, 295*(3), 299-305.
29. Hampton, T. (2004). Chemicals linked to bladder cancer in smokers may play a wider role. *Journal of the American Medical Association, 292*(17), 2072.
30. Hanno, P. (2002). Interstitial cystitis and related disorders. In P. Walsh, et al. (Eds.), *Campbell's urology* (8th ed., pp. 631-670). Philadelphia: Saunders.
31. Hanson, K. (2002). BCG installations for bladder cancer and latent tuberculosis infections. *Urologic Nursing, 22*(2), 132-134.
32. Hanson, K. (2005). Minimally invasive and surgical management of urinary stones. *Urologic Nursing, 25*(6), 458-465.
33. Hanson, K. (2005). Urinary stones and Crohn's disease. *Urologic Nursing, 25*(6), 466-468.
34. Harrahill, M. (2004). Bladder trauma: A review. *Journal of Emergency Nursing, 30*(3), 287-288.
35. Hendriksen, K., & Witjes, J.A. (2006). Intravesical gemcitabine: An update of clinical results. *Current Opinions in Urology, 16,* 361-366.
36. Hendrix, S., Cochrane, B., Nygaard, I., et al. (2005). Effects of estrogen with and without progestin on urinary incontinence. *Journal of the American Medical Association, 293*(8), 935-948.
37. Herschorn, S., & Carr, L.K. (2002). Vaginal reconstructive surgery for incontinence and prolapse. In P. Walsh, et al. (Eds.), *Campbell's urology* (8th ed., pp. 1092-1139). Philadelphia: Saunders.
38. Hooton, T., Scholes, D., Gupta, K., et al. (2005). Amoxicillin-clavulanate vs ciprofloxacin for the treatment of uncomplicated cystitis in women: A randomized trial. *Journal of the American Medical Association, 293*(8), 949-955.
39. Howell, A., & Foxman, B. (2002). Cranberry juice and adhesion of antibiotic-resistant uropathogens. *Journal of the American Medical Association, 287*(23), 3083-3084.
40. Hunskaar, S., et al. (2003). Epidemiology and natural history of urinary incontinence in women. *Urology, 62*(4), 16-23.
41. Jiminez, V., & Marshall, F. (2002). Surgery of the bladder cancer. In P. Walsh, et al. (Eds.), *Campbell's urology* (8th ed., pp. 2809-2844). Philadelphia: Saunders.
42. Krieg, K. (2005). The role of diet in the prevention of common kidney stones. *Urologic Nursing, 25*(6), 451-457.
43. Kielb, S. (2005). Stress incontinence: Alternatives to surgery. *International Journal of Fertility, 50*(1), 24-29.
44. Lehmann, S., & Dietz, C. (2002). Double-J stents: They're not trouble free. *RN, 65*(1), 54-60.
45. Li-Ming, S., & Sosa, R.E. (2002). Ureteroscopy and retrograde ureteral access. In P. Walsh, et al. (Eds.), *Campbell's urology* (8th ed., pp. 3306-3318). Philadelphia: Saunders.
46. Lingeman, J.E., Lifschitz, D.A., & Evan, A.P. (2002). Surgical management of urinary lithiasis. In P. Walsh, et al. (Eds.), *Campbell's urology* (8th ed., pp. 3361-3451). Philadelphia: Saunders.
47. MacDiarmid, S. (2006). *Therapeutic management of overactive bladder: A CME/CE initiative.* Hasbrouck Heights, NJ: Veritas Institute for Medical Education.
48. Malkowicz, S.B. (2002). Management of superficial bladder cancer. In P. Walsh, et al. (Eds.), *Campbell's urology* (8th ed., pp. 2785-2802). Philadelphia: Saunders.
49. McDougall, E.M., et al. (2002). Percutaneous approaches to the upper urinary tract. In P. Walsh, et al. (Eds.), *Campbell's urology* (8th ed., pp. 3320-3360). Philadelphia: Saunders.
50. McGuire, E.J., & Clemens, J.Q. (2002). Pubovaginal slings. In P. Walsh, et al. (Eds.), *Campbell's urology* (8th ed., pp. 1151-1172). Philadelphia: Saunders.

51. McDougall, W. (2002). Use of intestinal segments and urinary diversion. In P. Walsh, et al. (Eds.), *Campbell's urology* (8th ed., pp. 3745-3788). Philadelphia: Saunders.

52. Menon, M., & Resnick, M.I. (2002). Urinary lithiasis: Etiology, diagnosis, and medical management. In P. Walsh, et al. (Eds.), *Campbell's urology* (8th ed., pp. 3229-3305). Philadelphia: Saunders.

63. Messing, E. (2002). Urothelial tumors of the urinary tract. In P. Walsh, et al. (Eds.), *Campbell's urology* (8th ed., pp. 2732-2784). Philadelphia: Saunders.

54. Middelton, L., & Lessick, M. (2003). Inherited urologic malignant disorders: Nursing implications. *Urologic Nursing, 23*(1), 15-29.

55. Morris, R. (1999). Female genital mutilation: Perspectives, risks, and complications. *Urologic Nursing, 19*(1), 13-19.

56. Mulhall, J., Land, S., Parker, M., et al. (2005). The use of an erectogenic pharmacotherapy regimen following radical prostatectomy improves recovery of spontaneous erectile function. *Journal of Sexual Medicine, 2*(4), 532-540.

57. Newman, D. (2004). Incontinence products and devices for the elderly. *Urologic Nursing, 24*(4), 316-334.

58. Newman, D., & Palmer, M. (Eds.) (2003). The state of the science on urinary incontinence. *American Journal of Nursing, 3*(Suppl), 1-58.

59. Overstreet, D., & Sims, T. (2006). Care of the patient undergoing radical cystectomy with a robotic approach. *Urologic Nursing, 26*(2), 117-125.

60. Overstreet, D., & Sims, T. (2006). Robotic-assisted laparoscopic cystectomy with ileal conduit for urinary diversion. *Urologic Nursing, 26*(2), 126-128.

61. Palmer, M. (2004). Physiologic and psychologic age-related changes that affect urologic clients. *Urologic Nursing, 24*(4), 247-257.

62. Park, S., & Davila, G.W. (2005). Overactive bladder: Treatment options for the aging woman. *Journal of Fertility, 50*(1), 37-44.

63. Parsons, C.L. (2005). Argument for the use of the potassium sensitivity test in the diagnosis of interstitial cystitis. *International Urogynecology Journal, 60*(6), 30-31.

64. Parsons, C.L., & Newman, D. (2005). Chronic pelvic pain of bladder origin: A focus on interstitial cystitis. *Clinical Courier, 23*(38), 1-15.

65. Payne, C.K. (2002). Urinary incontinence: Nonsurgical management. In P. Walsh, et al. (Eds.), *Campbell's urology* (8th ed., pp. 1069-1091). Philadelphia: Saunders.

66. Polt, C. (2006). Taking the pressure off for women with stress incontinence. *Nursing 2006, 36*(2), 49-51.

67. Ratner, V., & Perilli, L. (2003). Interstitial cystitis: An updated overview. *Urologic Nursing, 23*(2), 107-111.

68. Rosser, M. (2002). Alarming rise in bladder cancer seen in UK: Incidence increased 34% in women vs. 8% men in 25 years, possibly because of smoking. *Urology Times, 5*, 1.

69. Sanchinin, M., Gunelli, R., Nanni, O., et al. (2005). Relevance of urine telomerase in the diagnosis of bladder cancer. *Journal of the American Medical Association, 294*(16), 2052-2056.

70. Sasso, K. (2003). Case study: Challenges of pessary management. *Journal of Wound, Ostomy and Continence Nursing, 30*(3), 152-158.

71. Schaeffer, A. (2002). Infections and inflammations of the genitourinary tract. In P. Walsh, et al. (Eds.), *Campbell's urology* (8th ed., pp. 515-602). Philadelphia: Saunders.

72. Schoenberg, M. (2002). Management of invasive and metastatic bladder cancer. In P. Walsh, et al. (Eds.), *Campbell's urology* (8th ed., pp. 2803-2817). Philadelphia: Saunders.

73. Smith, J.J., & Barrett, D.M. (2002). Implantation of the artificial genitourinary sphincter in men and women. In P. Walsh, et al. (Eds.), *Campbell's urology* (8th ed., pp. 1187-1194). Philadelphia: Saunders.

73a. Society of Urologic Nurses and Associates (2006). Clinical practice guidelines: Adult clean intermittent catheterization. Accessed 12/13/07 from www.suna.org/members/adultcic.pdf.

74. Specht, J. (2005). 9 myths of incontinence in older adults. *American Journal of Nursing, 105*(6), 58-69.

75. Taylor, E., Stampfer, M., & Curhan, G. (2005). Obesity, weight gain, and the risk of kidney stones. *Journal of the American Medical Association, 293*(4), 455-462.

75a. The Joint Commission (2007). 2008 National patient safety goals hospital program. Accessed 12/13/07 from www.jointcommission.org/PatientSafety/NationalPatientSafetyGoals/08_hap_npsgs.htm.

76. Toughill, E. (2005). Indwelling urinary catheters: Common mechanical and pathogenic problems. *American Journal of Nursing, 105*(5), 35-37.

77. Vogelzang, N. (2004). Tumors of the kidney, bladder, ureters, and renal pelvis. In L. Goldman & D. Ausiello (Eds.), *Cecil textbook of medicine* (22nd ed., pp. 1226-1230). Philadelphia: Saunders.

78. Webster, G., & Gurlnick, M.L. (2002). Retropubic suspension surgery for female sphincteric incontinence. In P. Walsh, et al. (Eds.), *Campbell's urology* (8th ed., pp. 1140-1150). Philadelphia: Saunders.

79. Wein, A. (2002). Neuromuscular dysfunction of the lower urinary tract and its treatment. In P. Walsh, et al. (Eds.), *Campbell's urology* (8th ed., pp. 931-1026). Philadelphia: Saunders.

80. Wein, A. (2005). New theories in interstitial cystitis. *Journal of Urology. 174*(5), 1902-1903.

81. Wein, A. (2002). Pathophysiology and categorization of voiding dysfunction. In P. Walsh, et al. (Eds.), *Campbell's urology* (8th ed., pp. 887-899). Philadelphia: Saunders.

evolve *Did you remember to check out the bonus material on the Evolve website and the CD-ROM, including NCLEX®-Examination Style Review Questions, Open-Book Quizzes, and Chapter Review Audio Podcasts?*

http://evolve.elsevier.com/Black/medsurg

CHAPTER 35

Management of Clients with Renal Disorders

ANITA E. MOLZAHN

The kidneys regulate the body's fluid, electrolyte, and acid-base balances while removing toxic substances from the blood and excreting them in urine. The kidneys also play a significant role in erythropoietin and prostaglandin synthesis, in insulin degradation, and in the renin-angiotensin-aldosterone system.

Many common disease processes and injuries can interfere with normal renal function. Some of these disorders can result in renal failure (see Chapter 36). Because of the potential seriousness of any renal problem, the client and his or her significant others have physical as well as psychological needs. You need to know about the whole person and the person's family and maintain awareness of appropriate interventions.

EXTRARENAL CONDITIONS

Many conditions located primarily in other parts of the body affect the kidneys, such as diabetes mellitus, hypertension, and sepsis. This chapter provides a brief description of the renal implications of these extrarenal conditions. For further discussion, see Chapters 45, 52 and 81.

DIABETES MELLITUS

One of the most common extrarenal diseases affecting the kidney is diabetes mellitus. *Diabetic nephropathy,* a progressive process, commonly leads to renal failure. About 30% of clients with end-stage renal disease (ESRD) (also known as stage 5 chronic kidney disease [CKD]) have diabetes mellitus. Researchers estimate that 25% to 50% of clients with insulin-dependent diabetes mellitus (IDDM, or type 1 diabetes mellitus) develop ESRD within 10 to 20 years of beginning insulin therapy. Renal disease also occurs in the non–insulin-dependent or type 2 diabetic client. The incidence of proteinuria is about 25% after 20 years of diabetes mellitus.

Several pathologic changes lead to renal failure in clients who have diabetes mellitus. The most common is a characteristic intercapillary *glomerulosclerosis,* or scarring of the capillary loops. Progressive microangiopathy, called *nephrosclerosis,* affects the afferent and efferent arterioles and eventually scars the glomerulus, tubules, and interstitium. *Pyelonephritis* (kidney infection) can scar the renal parenchyma and lead to ischemia. It may also lead to renal papillary necrosis and sloughing of the papillae. *Neurogenic bladder* dysfunction may contribute to renal failure. The high incidence of urinary tract infection or the increased pressure in the kidney caused by the backup of urine may also contribute to renal dysfunction.

Initially, the sclerotic, or hardening, process of glomerulosclerosis increases renal vascular resistance, contributing to systemic hypertension. This does not cause renal insufficiency. Indeed, the glomerular filtration rate (GFR) may increase as much as 20% to 50% above the normal GFR during this early "silent" phase. It is now recognized that microalbuminemia (measurable by assay) occurs quite some time before clinical proteinuria. If it is diagnosed, it may be a much earlier indicator of eventual renal failure. As more nephrons are destroyed, available functioning renal tissue decreases and the client begins to show clinical proteinuria (a key manifestation), hypertension, edema, and evidence of renal failure.

The kidney metabolizes 30% to 40% of insulin, and as renal function declines the degradation of insulin also decreases, resulting in a lower insulin requirement.

---

evolve **Web Enhancements**

Table Less Common Renal Infectious Processes

Be sure to check out the bonus material on the Evolve website and the CD-ROM, including free self-assessment exercises. **http://evolve.elsevier. com/Black/medsurg**

Renal failure may be initially identified when the client is evaluated for recurrent insulin reactions. Researchers hope the sclerotic process can be slowed by the following:

- Carefully controlling hypertension (see the Translating Evidence into Practice feature on Managing Hypertension in Diabetic Clients to Slow Progression of Renal Disease below)
- Adjusting insulin therapy and carefully monitoring blood glucose level to maintain euglycemia
- Restricting dietary protein (see the Complementary and Alternative Therapy feature on Slowing the Progression of Diabetic Nephropathy with a Unique Diet, p. 781)

Regardless of diabetic control, however, renal failure inevitably develops within 5 to 10 years after the appearance of significant proteinuria.

HYPERTENSION

Because the kidneys receive a large share of cardiac output, renal function can affect or be affected by cardiovascular changes. Renal blood flow determines the GFR, which directly affects renal function. Hypertension is one condition that can either cause or be affected by renal disease. For example, renovascular hypertension results from renal artery stenosis or renal infarction. The reduction in renal blood flow activates the renin-angiotensin-aldosterone system and increases systemic blood pressure.

Renal hypertension associated with parenchymal renal disease (e.g., glomerulonephritis, polycystic disease, pyelonephritis) usually results from the kidney's decreasing ability to excrete salt and water. Other causes include increased renin release from increased glomerular perfusion and inadequacy of renal vasodilating substances, as occurs with analgesic nephropathy. Among clients with renal failure, 80% to 85% of hypertension results from excess salt and water retention; renovascular hypertension accounts for up to 15% of all systemic hypertension.

On the other hand, sustained systemic high blood pressure adversely affects the kidneys. Researchers report that nephrosclerosis can be seen microscopically in clients who have had uncontrolled hypertension for more than 5 years, although all other renal diagnostic tests may be normal. Kidney damage is the direct result of

TRANSLATING EVIDENCE INTO PRACTICE

Managing Hypertension in Diabetic Clients to Slow Progression of Renal Disease

Both diabetes mellitus and hypertension can result in renal failure. One third of hypertensive males lose renal function over 7 years. It has been estimated that 5% of hypertensive clients with elevated serum creatinine levels will require dialysis therapy.[1-4,6] Diabetic nephropathy may reduce glomerular filtration rate by 10 to 12 ml/min/year if hypertension is untreated. It has been found that lowering blood pressure to less than 130/80 mm Hg in clients with chronic kidney disease slows renal disease progression.[1,2,4] Clients with proteinuria of greater than 1 g/24 hour benefit from even tighter control of blood pressure to levels of less than 125/75 mm Hg. Lowering blood pressure reduces mortality in those at risk for cardiovascular events, including diabetic clients.[1,3]

Despite this evidence, management of blood pressure in diabetic clients is less than optimal. Chronic disease management focusing on care processes and intermediate outcomes such as glycemic control found positive outcomes in type 2 diabetic clients. A recent randomized trial of a specialized clinic focusing on intensified multiple risk factor intervention showed improved microvascular disease and a trend toward improved macrovascular disease in diabetic clients within 4 years.[7] Similar benefits were seen in a before-and-after study of diabetic clients with more advanced chronic kidney disease.[8] Multidisciplinary clinics offering care by nurses and physicians, and sometimes other professionals, have demonstrated improved outcomes.[8]

IMPLICATIONS

Control of blood pressure in diabetic clients and good disease management can improve outcomes and can slow progression of renal disease in diabetic clients.[5] Nurses, in their roles as primary health care providers and as members of specialized disease management teams, can reduce the morbidity and complications associated with diabetes mellitus and hypertension. Further research should address the specific interventions and strategies that are most effective.

REFERENCES

1. American Diabetes Association. (2005). Diabetes, hypertension, and cardiovascular disease: An update. *Diabetes Care, 28*(Suppl 1), S4-S36.
2. Berl, T., Hunsicker, L.G., Lewis, J.B., et al. (2005). Impact of achieved blood pressure on cardiovascular outcomes in the Irbesartan Diabetic Nephropathy Trial. *Journal of the American Society of Nephrology, 16*, 2170-2179.
3. Chobanian, A., et al. (2003). The Seventh Report of the Joint National Committee on Prevention, Detection, Evaluation, and Treatment of High Blood Pressure: The JNC 7 Report. *Journal of the American Medical Association, 289*(19), 2560-2572.
4. Hajjar, I., & Kotchen, T. (2003). Trends in prevalence, awareness, treatment, and control of hypertension in the United States, 1988-2000. *Journal of the American Medical Association, 290*(2), 199-206.
5. Norris, S.L., et al. (2002). The effectiveness of disease and case management for people with diabetes: A systematic review. *American Journal of Preventative Medicine, 22*, 15-38.
6. Russell, T.A. (2006). Diabetic nephropathy in patients with type 1 diabetes mellitus. *Nephrology Nursing Journal, 33*, 15-28.
7. Sidorov, J., et al. (2002). Does diabetes disease management save money and improve outcomes? *Diabetes Care, 25*, 684-689.
8. Wagner, E.H., et al. (2001). Chronic care clinics for diabetes in primary care: A system wide randomized trial. *Diabetes Care, 24*, 695-700.

Slowing the Progression of Diabetic Nephropathy with a Unique Diet

In general, clients with end-stage renal disease are encouraged to follow a low-protein diet to slow the progression of their disease. However, a recent study challenged this notion by using a carbohydrate-restricted, low-iron, polyphenol-enriched diet. Foods rich in polyphenols include olive oil, cranberries, green tea, red wine, and grapes.

A total of 191 clients with type 2 diabetes mellitus and impending renal failure were included (men and women 49 to 62 years of age). Clients had a history of diabetes mellitus for 5 to 15 years and a glycosylated hemoglobin level of 6.0% to 9.3%. Current medications for both hypertension and glucose control were continued. Clients were assigned to either the low carbohydrate diet or a conventional protein-restricted diet (0.8 g/kg). The main features of the low-carbohydrate diet were a 50% reduction of carbohydrates; replacement of iron-enriched meats with iron-poor meats and foods known to inhibit iron absorption; elimination of all liquids except tea, water, and red wine; and the use of olive oil for frying and dressings. Unfortunately, compliance was not assessed.

Clients were followed for an average of 3.9 years. No significant differences were seen in the baseline characteristics of the two groups. Serum creatinine levels doubled in 21% of the clients following the lower carbohydrate diet versus 39% of the control group ($p < 0.01$). Thus a polyphenol-enriched diet with 50% carbohydrate reduction and low iron availability was better than a conventional protein-restricted diet in slowing the progression of diabetic nephropathy. More studies are needed, but the results are interesting.

REFERENCE

Facchini, F., & Saylor, K. (2003). A low-iron-available, polyphenol-enriched, carbohydrate-restricted diet to slow progression of diabetic nephropathy. *Diabetes, 52*, 1204-1209.

degenerative changes in the arterioles and interlobular arteries caused by increased blood pressure.

There is a direct correlation between the duration and degree of elevated blood pressure and the severity of renal vascular disease. Progression of the disease usually can be halted or slowed by controlling blood pressure (see the Translating Evidence into Practice feature on Managing Hypertension in Diabetic Clients to Slow Progression of Renal Disease, p. 780). Client teaching is vital to managing the hypertension and preventing renal failure.

HYPOTENSION

Cardiovascular shock, or hypotension, also affects renal function. Renal vasoconstriction reduces renal blood flow. Because of the autoregulation capabilities of the kidneys (see Chapter 11, 12, 13, 32 and 81), however, GFR remains at a functional level until the advanced stages of systemic shock, at which time acute renal failure develops. Restoring systemic blood pressure usually reverses the renal vasoconstriction, and kidney function returns, typically within 2 to 8 weeks provided prolonged ischemia has not occurred. A period of polyuria (excessive urination) may follow the correction of hypovolemia, although the mechanisms for this are unclear.

Before renal function returns to normal, another oliguric period may occur, followed by a "mobilization phase" in which sequestered fluid is shifted into the intravascular space. This shift may cause some hypertension until the kidneys can remove the extra fluid. Careful assessment of the client's fluid status and meticulous fluid management are crucial during these recovery phases.

RHABDOMYOLYSIS

Rhabdomyolysis is a disorder usually associated with traumatic injury of skeletal muscle tissue, which releases myoglobin and intracellular substances into the blood. It can also occur after serious crush injuries, strenuous exercise, seizures, heat stroke, prolonged coma, drug overdose, and as a side effect of the use of statins for treatment of hyperlipidemia.[20] The resulting acute renal failure is usually reversible with treatment.

Clinical evidence of rhabdomyolysis includes fever, malaise, nausea, vomiting, muscular weakness, muscle pain, and swelling. The release of substances from damaged muscles results in myoglobinemia, myoglobinuria (which can be seen as brown urine and confirmed through urinalysis), hyperkalemia, hyperphosphatemia, hyperuricemia, and elevated creatine kinase levels. Hypocalcemia occurs initially because of the precipitation of calcium with phosphate. Later, in the diuretic phase of acute renal failure, hypercalcemia can occur as calcium is mobilized.

Treatment is typically symptomatic, including bed rest to reduce muscle metabolism and steps to correct acidosis and electrolyte imbalances and maintain normal fluid volume. In severe cases, dialytic therapy may be necessary.

CARDIOVASCULAR DISEASE

Cardiac disease influences kidney function primarily through its effect on cardiac output and circulating blood volume. The hemodynamic and hormonal changes of cardiac disease may decrease the kidneys' ability to excrete sodium and water. This, in turn, increases intravascular congestion and edema and establishes a pathologic cycle.

Hemodynamic changes also occur with normal aging. Blood flow to the kidneys decreases by up to half by age 70 years, and GFR can decrease by 40% to 50% as well. Renal function deteriorates as glomeruli become sclerotic and atrophy.

PERIPHERAL VASCULAR DISEASE

Thromboembolic disease can affect the renal circulation and cause infarction of the tissue supplied by the affected blood vessel. In clients with sickle cell disease, the interstitial hypertonicity and low oxygen pressure found in the renal medulla seem to favor sickling of red blood cells in the kidney's juxtamedullary region. These cell masses cause gross hematuria (from rupture of venules), papillary necrosis, renal infarction, concentration disturbances (from interference with the countercurrent mechanism), nephrotic syndrome, pyelonephritis, and, finally, renal failure.

In disseminated intravascular coagulation (DIC), in which diffuse clotting consumes clotting factors and causes hemorrhage in affected areas throughout the body, the kidney is the organ most affected.

SEPSIS

Extrarenal sepsis may affect kidney function either through its effect on systemic circulation or by stimulating the immune system. Renal reactions to septic shock are similar to those in hypotension. Immunologic injury can lead to glomerulonephritis (see Glomerulonephritis later in this chapter). Occasionally, pathogens may break away from extrarenal foci of infection and travel to the kidney to establish additional sites.

PREGNANCY

Pregnancy has a definite influence on kidney function. During the first trimester, the collecting system dilates and the kidneys enlarge; this may persist 9 to 12 weeks after delivery. Renal blood flow and GFR increase by 30% to 50% during pregnancy, contributing to increased creatinine clearance and decreased uric acid excretion. These normal changes (such as lower serum creatinine level) must be taken into account in interpreting laboratory findings for pregnant women. Pregnancy also increases the likelihood of proteinuria (usually transient), polyuria, and nocturia (excessive urination at night). These disorders may be caused by external bladder compression and alterations in antidiuretic hormone metabolism.

OTHER CAUSES

Kidney function is influenced by many other extrarenal disease processes, such as cancer, connective tissue disorders, and metabolic disturbances. Many systemic diseases produce clinical manifestations like those of glomerulonephritis, although they typically have other systemic features characteristic of the disease (see Glomerulonephritis). These diseases include systemic lupus erythematosus (SLE), systemic scleroderma, polyarteritis nodosa, thrombocytopenic purpura, Wegener's granulomatosis, hemolytic-uremic syndrome, gout, amyloidosis,

and Henoch-Schönlein syndrome. Diagnosis can be confirmed by renal biopsy.

Renal disease has become an increasingly common complication for people infected with the human immunodeficiency virus (HIV). Among the several renal disorders associated with HIV and acquired immunodeficiency syndrome (AIDS) are renal tuberculosis and cytomegalovirus, such malignancies as lymphoma and Kaposi's sarcoma, and HIV-associated nephropathy, a focal glomerulosclerosis that is manifested by nephrotic syndrome (see Nephrotic Syndrome later in this chapter).

NEPHROTOXINS

Nephrotoxins have specific, destructive effects on renal cells. They can cause the following types of renal injury: acute tubular necrosis, defects in the tubular transport system, interstitial nephritis, vasculitis, and nephrotic syndrome. Box 35-1 presents some common nephrotoxic substances. Acute tubular necrosis is the most frequent injury resulting from exposure to nephrotoxins. Some nephrotoxins also cause tubular transport defects and nephrotic syndrome.

BOX 35-1 Nephrotoxins

ANTIBIOTICS
- Aminoglycosides
- Tetracyclines
- Amphotericin B
- Cephalosporins
- Sulfonamides (co-trimoxazole)
- Bacitracin
- Polymyxin

HEAVY METALS
- Lead
- Mercury
- Bismuth
- Arsenic
- Copper
- Cadmium
- Gold
- Lithium

POISONS
- Mushrooms
- Insecticides
- Herbicides
- Snake venom (bites)

ANESTHETICS

CONTRAST DYES

ORGANIC SOLVENTS
- Ethylene glycol
- Gasoline
- Kerosene
- Turpentine
- Tetrachloroethylene
- Carbon tetrachloride
- Trichloroethylene
- Chlorinated hydrocarbons

ANALGESICS
- Salicylates
- Acetaminophen
- Phenacetin
- NSAIDs (nonsteroidal anti-inflammatory drugs)

OTHER DRUGS
- Probenecid
- Phenytoin
- Heroin
- Dextran
- Mannitol
- Interleukin-2
- Cisplatin
- Amphetamines
- Aristolochic acid (Chinese herb)

All five types of kidney damage may result from nephrotoxic reactions to medications. You must know about the possible adverse effects of any medication a client takes so that you can assess and intervene appropriately. Two types of medications well-known to cause renal damage are antibiotics and certain analgesics (see Box 35-1). Because the kidneys are the major route of excretion for many antibiotics and analgesics, renal tissue is directly exposed to these compounds. Researchers estimate that 5% to 10% of clients with ESRD have analgesic nephropathy. Diuretics may have nephrotoxic effects as well and, when used aggressively, can cause hypovolemia. The longer the exposure, the higher the risk of renal toxic effects. Pre-existing renal disease, decreased renal blood flow, electrolyte imbalances, and concurrent use of other nephrotoxic medications enhance a medication's nephrotoxic effect.

Carefully monitor renal function tests to identify early nephrotoxic reactions so that causative medications can be discontinued or the dose decreased. Closely monitor drug levels to ensure that dosages stay in the therapeutic range. Besides using these medications as briefly as possible and at as low a dose as possible, maintaining a high fluid intake may help prevent nephrotoxic effects. A high urine output keeps the medication diluted in the kidney and helps prevent crystallization.

Anesthesia reduces the kidney's vasoconstrictive ability, which helps protect it against systemic blood pressure drops; thus the kidney is made more vulnerable to the effects of shock. In addition, certain anesthetics, particularly methoxyflurane, have a direct nephrotoxic effect. Administration of this general anesthetic agent can cause acute tubular necrosis and has been associated with fatal acute renal failure. Halothane may also adversely affect renal function.

Radioiodinated contrast agents used in radiographic and computed tomographic (CT) studies have been associated with acute tubular necrosis. Risk factors include age older than 60 years, pre-existing renal insufficiency (especially diabetic nephropathy), dehydration, low cardiac output with pre-existing renal disease, proteinuria, hypoalbuminemia, multiple myeloma, and multiple contrast studies within a 24-hour period. See the Complementary and Alternative Therapy feature below.

COMPLEMENTARY AND ALTERNATIVE THERAPY

Oral Acetylcysteine Supplements for Preventing Acute Deterioration in Renal Function After Coronary Angiography in Moderate Renal Insufficiency

Acetylcysteine tablets already play several roles in medicine. For example, they seem to reduce hepatic damage from acetaminophen overdose and have a role in clearing lung function in cystic fibrosis. Other roles for this supplement are being explored. Many procedures in medicine are life-saving, but require contrast or some type of dye to help identify abnormalities in the human body. However, if the dye is given in large amounts during a procedure, it can damage the kidneys. For example, large amounts of dye are needed for visualization of the arteries during angiography and angioplasty. Those same clients do not pump blood as well from the left ventricle, which means the dye does not get diluted easily because circulation is not good.

A randomized, blinded, placebo-controlled trial with a 7-day follow-up was conducted in a university hospital in Hong Kong.[1] A total of 200 clients (mean age 68 years, 61.5% men, 100% Chinese) with moderate chronic renal insufficiency and upcoming elective coronary angiography were studied. Clients received either oral acetylcysteine (600 mg twice daily, n = 102) or a placebo (n = 98) both the day before and the day of angiography (total treatment duration of 2 days). All clients received a nonionic, low-osmolality contrast agent (iopamidol).

Kay et al. found that in clients with moderate chronic renal insufficiency, oral acetylcysteine was safe and effective in preventing acute deterioration in renal function after elective coronary angiography.[1] In fact, acute contrast media–induced reduction in renal function was reduced by 68% in the supplement group compared to the placebo group (NNT = 12).[1]

Similarly, acetylcysteine was also found to be helpful for reducing renal deterioration in at-risk clients 62 years of age with histories of renal insufficiency, diabetes mellitus, elevated cholesterol, and/or smoking in Milan, Italy, who were scheduled to undergo angioplasty and possible stent placement.[2] In a randomized study, 354 clients having angioplasty were assigned to 3 groups. One group received the standard acetylcysteine dose of 600 mg IV before the procedure and 600 mg orally twice a day for 48 hours after the procedure for a total of 3000 mg. Another group received twice that amount in the same manner. The third or control group received a placebo. Serum creatinine levels increased by 25% or more in 33% of the control group, in 15% of the standard dose group, and in 8% of the double dose group.

Therefore acetylcysteine should be considered for high-risk clients who have diabetes mellitus or chronic renal disease and are about to undergo coronary angiography.

REFERENCES

1. Kay, J., et al. (2003). Acetylcysteine for prevention of acute deterioration of renal function following elective coronary angiography and intervention: A randomized controlled trial. *Journal of the American Medical Association, 289*, 553-558.
2. Marenzi, G., et al. (2006). N-Acetylcysteine and contrast-induced nephropathy in primary angioplasty. *New England Journal of Medicine, 254*(26), 2773-2782.

NNT, Number needed to treat.

Using non-dye studies whenever possible and keeping the client well hydrated throughout the test will reduce the risk of acute renal failure. Baseline renal function tests before the contrast study should be available to compare with post-test findings. Monitor the client's urine output carefully for several hours after the study is completed.

ACQUIRED DISORDERS

NEPHROLITHIASIS

Although calculi (stones) can form anywhere in the urinary tract, the most frequent site is the kidney. These stones may travel down the urinary tract, lodge anywhere along the tract, and cause obstruction and tissue damage, or they may stay in the kidney. Urolithiasis is described in detail in Chapter 34.

Treatment and nursing care of clients with renal calculi is similar to that for clients with calculi lower in the urinary tract. Damage to the kidney caused by calculi can be permanent, however, and may require nephrectomy (described later).

PYELONEPHRITIS

Pyelonephritis is an inflammation of the renal pelvis and parenchyma caused by a bacterial infection. The cause may be an active infection in the kidney or the remnants of a previous infection. The two main types of pyelonephritis are acute and chronic. They differ primarily in their clinical picture and long-term effects.

Etiology and Risk Factors
Sometimes an infection may be a primary disease, as happens with reduced host resistance (e.g., calculi, malignancy, hydronephrosis, or trauma). Most kidney infections, however, are extensions of infectious processes located elsewhere, especially the bladder. In Chapter 34, the etiologic mechanism and pathogenesis of infections in the lower urinary tract are discussed.

The bacteria spread to the kidney primarily by ascending the ureter to the kidney. Blood and lymphatic circulation also provide channels for the organisms. Ureteral reflux, which allows infected urine back into the ureter, and obstruction, which causes urine to back into the ureter and allows organisms to multiply, are the most common causes of ascending urinary tract infections. *Escherichia coli* is the most common bacterial organism that causes pyelonephritis.

Health promotion is key to preventing the recurrence of infection and further renal damage. The nurse provides information to clients about health and lifestyle measures to prevent urinary tract infections, including (1) perineal hygiene measures (such as wiping from front to back), (2) acidification of the urine (by drinking cranberry juice or taking ascorbic acid), and (3) ensuring adequate fluid intake. Early detection and adequate treatment of lower urinary tract infections greatly reduce the incidence of pyelonephritis.

After infection, health maintenance includes education about the importance of completing the course of antibiotics. Follow-up cultures are important with recurrent pyelonephritis to ensure that the infection has been eradicated. Health restoration measures depend on the extent of renal damage and the cause of the disease. If obstruction precipitated the infection, the cause of the obstruction must be treated.

Acute Pyelonephritis
Acute pyelonephritis often occurs after bacterial contamination of the urethra or after introduction of an instrument, such as a catheter or a cystoscope.

Chronic Pyelonephritis
Chronic pyelonephritis is more likely to occur after chronic obstruction with reflux or chronic disorders. It is slowly progressive and usually is associated with recurrent acute attacks, although the client may not have a history of acute pyelonephritis.

Pathophysiology
Pyelonephritis occurs when bacteria enter the renal pelvis, causing an inflammatory response and an increase in white blood cells (WBCs). The inflammation leads to edema and swelling of the involved tissue, beginning at the papillae and sometimes spreading to the cortex. The infection can be either ascending, as occurs after cystitis or prostatitis, or descending, as from a streptococcal infection in the bloodstream.

As the infection is treated and the inflammation recedes, fibrosis and scar tissue may develop. The calices become blunted with scarring in the interstitial tissues. If the infection recurs, more scar tissue develops; fibrosis and altered tubular reabsorption and secretion lead to decreased renal function.

Acute Pyelonephritis
Acute pyelonephritis is associated with the development of renal abscesses, perinephric abscesses, emphysematous pyelonephritis, and chronic pyelonephritis, which can lead to renal failure. Acute pyelonephritis is usually brief. It often recurs, however, either as a relapse of a previous infection not eradicated or as a new infection; 20% of these recurrences take place within 2 weeks after completion of therapy. A client must be treated adequately to prevent the development of chronic pyelonephritis.

The infection may also progress to bacteremia and urosepsis.

Chronic Pyelonephritis

This disease is characterized by a combination of caliceal abnormalities and overlying cortical scarring. The kidney becomes contracted, and the number of functioning nephrons decreases as they are replaced by scar tissue. Renal failure may ensue, although uremia is less common than once thought.

Clinical Manifestations

Acute Pyelonephritis

Acute pyelonephritis is characterized by enlarged kidneys, focal parenchymal abscesses, and accumulation of polymorphonuclear lymphocytes around and in the renal tubules. Typically, the client seems to be in acute distress, although in some cases this disorder causes minimal or no manifestations.

Assessment usually reveals high fever, chills, nausea, flank pain on the affected side (costovertebral angle [CVA] tenderness), headache, muscle pain, and general prostration. The pain commonly radiates down the ureter or toward the epigastrium and may be colicky if the infection is complicated by calculi or sloughed renal papillae. Commonly, the client has experienced dysuria, frequency, urgency, and other evidence of cystitis for several days. The urine may be cloudy or bloody, is foul smelling, and shows a marked increase in WBCs and casts. See Chapter 32 and Figure 32-8 for more information related to assessment of urinary tract infections.

Chronic Pyelonephritis

This disease has no specific manifestations of its own. Thus it is usually discovered incidentally when the client is being evaluated for hypertension or its complications. Hypertension is the most frequent manifestation of the disease. Abnormal laboratory studies may show azotemia, pyuria, anemia, acidosis, and proteinuria. They may also demonstrate poor urine-concentrating ability.

OUTCOME MANAGEMENT

Medical Management

Acute Pyelonephritis

Ideal outcomes of medical management include (1) elimination of the pathogenic organisms with appropriate antibiotics, as identified by urine culture and sensitivity studies, and (2) removal of any factor or disease contributing to decreased host resistance. If calculi or other obstructions are found to be the cause of recurrent infection, appropriate treatment must be instituted.

Inhibit Bacterial Growth. Antibiotic therapy is based on the results of urine culture and sensitivity tests. Typically, a broad-spectrum antibiotic is prescribed; it may be changed after the results of the culture are available. Sulfonamides or the combination of sulfamethoxazole and trimethoprim is commonly used as first-line therapy unless the client is allergic to one of these drugs. Typically, antibiotic therapy continues for 10 days to 2 weeks. In severe cases of acute pyelonephritis, intravenous antibiotics may be administered. With oral therapy, the client must understand that completing the full course of antibiotic therapy is important to prevent recurrence of the infection. Recurrent infections are commonly treated with long-term prophylactic antibiotic therapy. Additional pharmacologic therapy may be needed to correct any predisposing factors.

Relieve Pain. Analgesic or urinary antiseptic medications can be prescribed to reduce discomfort. Antibiotics quickly reduce discomfort as well.

Chronic Pyelonephritis

The desired outcome of medical management is prevention of further renal damage. If bacteria are found, appropriate antibiotics are given, as in acute pyelonephritis. Chronic pyelonephritis tends to be less painful. Above all, hypertension must be controlled. Additional intervention depends on the degree of renal failure that has already occurred. Although high fluid intake may be advisable in acute pyelonephritis, it may be contraindicated in chronic pyelonephritis if the degree of renal dysfunction is significant.

Inhibit Bacterial Growth. Antibiotics specific to the bacteria present are given to treat chronic pyelonephritis (see Acute Pyelonephritis and Chapter 34).

Control Hypertension. Renal damage can cause hypertension, which can cause further renal damage. Thus it is important to control the client's blood pressure. Reduction of dietary sodium and pharmacologic therapy may be indicated. Management of hypertension is discussed in Chapter 52.

Nursing Management of the Medical Client

Assessment. Assessment of the client with pyelonephritis begins with a thorough history and physical examination, giving close attention to the presence of risk factors, previous urinary tract infections, hypertension, and CVA tenderness. Look for evidence of pyelonephritis.

Diagnosis, Outcomes, Interventions

Diagnosis: Risk for Deficient Fluid Volume. A common diagnosis is *Risk for Deficient Fluid Volume related to fever, nausea, vomiting, and possible diarrhea.*

Outcomes. The client will maintain fluid balance as evidenced by balanced intake and output, maintenance of adequate hydration, and an absence of manifestations of dehydration.

Interventions. Prepare the client for the diagnostic tests and probable antibiotic therapy. Clients with severe nausea and vomiting may require intravenous fluids. Keep in mind that overhydration may dilute antimicrobials, diminishing their effectiveness. See Chapter 34 on the nursing care of the client with cystitis.

Diagnosis: Acute Pain. Another common nursing diagnosis is *Acute pain related to an inflammatory process in the kidney and possible colic.*

Outcomes. The client will report either that there is no pain or that pain is controlled.

Interventions. Medications can be given to control pain caused by calculi. CVA tenderness should decrease as the antibiotics control the infection. Medication for nausea can be given as needed with antipyretics for high fevers. Adequate treatment of the infection quickly reverses the dysuria, pyuria, and frequency. Urinary analgesics (see Chapter 34) can also help the client with these problems. Fluid intake of 3 to 4 L daily is recommended. This fluid helps to dilute the urine and to reduce irritation and burning. The continual flow of urine serves to prevent stasis and discourage multiplication of bacteria in the urinary tract.

Diagnosis: Readiness for Enhanced Self-Care. Client teaching is important to promote self-care and to prevent recurrent infections. Write the diagnosis *Readiness for Enhanced Self-Care to prevent recurrent infections.*

Outcomes. The client will have knowledge of the treatment regimen and understand how to prevent recurrent infections as evidenced by the client's statements and no recurrence of infection.

Interventions. The preventive measures for acute and chronic pyelonephritis are similar to those for cystitis (see Chapter 34). It is important to prevent permanent renal damage. Ensure that the client can recognize the manifestations of a urinary tract infection and knows to seek prompt medical attention when these manifestations do occur.

When the acute infection subsides, instruct the client to continue follow-up care. This care includes completing the full course of antibiotic therapy and having repeated urine cultures. Also, teach ways to prevent further infections in the urinary tract, including ensuring a high fluid intake (see Chapter 34).

It is vital that the client return for follow-up urine cultures and possibly other diagnostic tests if the cause of the pyelonephritis is not clear. Emphasize that follow-up cultures are important because bacteriuria may be present without producing any manifestations. Advise the client to report any manifestations of recurrence immediately so that retreatment can begin.

Evaluation. The infection should subside with adequate antibiotic treatment. Successful management results in reduced pain and negative findings on follow-up urine cultures. The client must also be made aware of the cause of this infection and ways to prevent further infections (see Chapter 34).

Modifications for Older Clients

In older clients, the kidneys may be less able to recover from a severe infection. Antibiotic therapy should be monitored closely because older adults often vary in their sensitivity and response to the medication. Older adults may also have altered blood levels of antibiotics because renal perfusion decreases with age, reducing the kidney's ability to excrete drugs.

OTHER INFECTIOUS PROCESSES

Bacteria cause most cases of pyelonephritis, but renal candidiasis, a fungal infection, is becoming more prevalent. Renal tuberculosis, renal abscesses, and perinephric abscesses are other less common infectious processes. They are briefly described in the Less Common Renal Infectious Processes table on the website.

HYDRONEPHROSIS

Hydronephrosis is distention of the renal pelvis and calices caused by an obstruction of normal urine flow. Urine production continues, and the urine is trapped proximal to the obstruction. Causes of occlusion include calculus, tumor, scar tissue, congenital structural defects, and a kink in the ureter.

Whatever the cause, the accumulating urine exerts pressure on the renal pelvis wall. At low to moderate pressures, the kidney may dilate with no obvious loss of function. Over time, sustained or intermittent high pressure causes irreversible nephron destruction. In addition to pressure-related problems, pyelonephritis is always a risk because of urinary stasis.

OUTCOME MANAGEMENT

Medical Management

Treatment aims to relieve the obstruction and prevent infection. Depending on the location of the obstruction, it may involve placement of a ureteral catheter or stent above the point of obstruction. Typically, surgery is required (see Chapter 34) to relieve the obstruction and restore adequate drainage of the urinary system.

Removal of the obstruction results in sudden release of the pressure on the renal parenchyma caused by the trapped urine, which leads to diuresis. Thus postobstructive diuresis occurs and can lead to fluid and electrolyte imbalances, including dehydration. The kidney gradually begins to concentrate urine appropriately.

Nursing Management of the Medical Client

Assessment of a client with hydronephrosis includes monitoring for the presence, location, intensity, and character of pain. Monitor urine output, and report manifestations of renal failure (oliguria, anorexia, lethargy), hematuria, and dysuria. Reduced urine output could indicate obstruction. Scan the client's bladder to assess for any manifestations of distention or urinary retention. The kidneys, if palpated, may be tender.

Make frequent assessments, including hourly outputs; daily weights; vital signs every 30 minutes for the first 4 hours and then every 2 hours; urine for specific gravity, albumin, and glucose; and edema. Also make periodic serum electrolyte and glucose determinations, and consider the expected presence of severe fatigue caused by urinary losses and the need for frequent observation. Fluid management during this period is crucial; hourly fluid replacement is based on the previous hour's output.

Clients who have had hydronephrosis should watch for manifestations of infection and obstruction, such as pain and reduced urine output. Avoiding urinary tract infections is important in preventing pyelonephritis and preserving renal function (see Chapter 34).

Surgical Management

Surgery is commonly required to relieve the obstruction causing hydronephrosis. Management of the surgical client is discussed under urolithiasis in Chapter 34.

RENAL CANCER

Benign kidney tumors are rare. Classifications include lymphangioma, lipoma, medullary fibroma, adenoma, leiomyoma, and oncocytoma. When large benign tumors occur, it is relatively impossible to distinguish them from a malignant tumor by x-ray examination. At least 85% of all renal tumors are malignant, and about 12,890 people die of kidney cancer each year. The tumors are most common in people 50 and 70 years of age. They affect men more often than women. About 51,190 new cases of renal cancer were expected to be diagnosed in the United States in 2007.[1]

Etiology and Risk Factors

The exact cause of renal tumors is unknown. Some links have been established between renal cancer and smoking, hypertension, and obesity. Exposure to lead, cadmium, and phosphates also increase the risk of developing renal cancer. An inactivation of a critical gene on the short arm of chromosome 3 is thought to be related to the development of renal cancer.

Because of the possible association between smoking and renal cancer, one means of avoiding renal cancer may be to quit or not to start smoking. Avoiding exposure to chemicals such as lead, phosphate, and cadmium may also prevent some renal cancers. A lifestyle that minimizes the development of obesity and hypertension may also be helpful (see the Complementary and Alternative Therapy feature below). The cause of many renal cancers is not established, however, and prevention may not be possible.

After surgery, most clients have difficulty in dealing with cancer and the risk of recurrence. If nephrectomy is required, clients are often concerned about living with only one kidney. Assure clients that one kidney can meet the body's needs but that care should be taken to protect that kidney. The care includes preventing injuries and infections, controlling blood pressure if necessary, and maintaining overall health and well-being through adequate nutrition and rest, for example.

Pathophysiology

Renal cell carcinoma (RCC), or adenocarcinoma, is the most common tumor type; it accounts for 90% of all kidney cancer. Tumor growth begins in the renal cortex and

---

COMPLEMENTARY AND ALTERNATIVE THERAPY

Fatty Fish Consumption and Renal Cell Carcinoma

The epidemiologic evidence that fatty fish consumption may be associated with lower risk of several cancers is not consistent, and no studies of renal cell carcinoma (RCC) exist. This study examined the association between fatty fish and lean fish consumption and risk of RCC in 61,433 women in the Swedish Mammography Cohort study. During a mean follow-up between 1987 and 2004 (15.3 years for a total of 940,357 person-years), 150 incident RCC cases were diagnosed. After adjustment for potential confounders, an inverse association of fatty fish consumption with the risk of RCC was found, but no association was found with lean fish consumption. Compared with no consumption, the multivariate rate ratio (RR) was 0.56 (95% confidence interval [CI], 0.35-0.91) for women eating fatty fish once a week or more. The findings suggest that consumption of fatty fish may reduce the risk of RCC in women.

REFERENCE

Wolk, A., Larsson, S., Johansson, J.E., et al. (2006). Long-term fatty fish consumption and renal cell carcinoma incidence in women. *Journal of the American Medical Association, 296*(11), 1371-1376.

usually continues for some time before it produces manifestations. The tumor can grow very large and tends to compress the adjacent renal parenchyma rather than infiltrate it. The tumor, usually avascular, tends to surround blood vessels and constrict them. The lungs and mediastinum are the most frequent metastatic sites of occurrence. Liver, bone, skin, spleen, renal vein, and brain are other common sites of metastases.

Other types of renal cancer include (1) nephroblastoma, (2) sarcoma, and (3) epithelial tumors in the renal pelvis. Nephroblastoma, or Wilms' tumor, is primarily a childhood disease, although it occasionally occurs in adults. The prognosis for adults is worse than that for children, with some sources reporting only a 25% survival rate. Sarcoma is infrequent and typically arises in the renal capsule. Most tumors of the renal pelvis are primarily urothelial in origin and include three tissue types: transitional cell, squamous cell, and adenocarcinoma.

Spontaneous regression of renal adenocarcinoma reportedly occurs in less than 1% of all cases. Most of these regressions occur after nephrectomy and involve metastatic areas. Authorities consider these episodes as evidence that the disease is associated with immunologic or hormonal factors.

Clinical Manifestations

Manifestations of renal malignancies vary, and tumor growth may advance significantly before the disease is discovered. It is not uncommon for the client to have clinical manifestations apparently unrelated to renal disease. Frequently, a palpable abdominal mass found during a routine physical examination arouses the first suspicion. The average time between the onset of hematuria and the onset of pain is 9 months and that between initial pain and diagnosis is 14 months. Extrarenal manifestations are commonly found before a diagnosis of renal cancer is confirmed. Up to 35% of clients have metastasis when the final diagnosis of a renal cancer is made.

The common triad of manifestations consists of hematuria, flank pain, and a palpable abdominal or flank mass. The hematuria is usually gross and intermittent, which helps to explain the client's delay in seeking medical advice. The clinical picture also contains a combination of the following usual findings: fever, weight loss and cachexia, fatigue, hypertension, amyloidosis, thrombophlebitis, anemia, erythrocytosis, hypercalcemia, abnormal serum liver profile, and an elevated erythrocyte sedimentation rate (ESR). Less frequent findings include peripheral neuropathy, inferior vena cava obstruction, priapism, and varicocele. Hydronephrosis may occur if the tumor obstructs the ureteropelvic junction. The incidence of pulmonary embolus as a presenting manifestation may be higher than previously thought because of the high rate of vena cava and renal vein

involvement. Plasma erythropoietin, renin, and chorionic gonadotropin levels are elevated, and prostaglandin production increases in renal cell carcinoma.

Several diagnostic tests help confirm a diagnosis of renal cancer. Intravenous pyelogram (IVP) is probably the most helpful in identifying a space-occupying lesion. Ultrasonography helps differentiate a cyst from a solid mass. Other noninvasive procedures include CT scan, nephrotomography, and radioisotope studies. Arteriography is used to evaluate the renal vascular system. Renal biopsy, usually done percutaneously, provides definitive data about the lesion.

OUTCOME MANAGEMENT

Staging of the tumor helps delineate the appropriate treatment and can suggest the client's prognosis (Figure 35-1). Five-year survival rates for stage 1 are about 65%; for stage 2, about 40%; 10-year rates drop to 40% and 35%, respectively. Five-year survivals are rare in stages 3 and 4.[1]

Medical Management

Radiation Therapy

Radiation may be used as an adjunct with chemotherapy and surgery. Irradiation is most useful in preoperative preparation of the tumor. It is sometimes also used postoperatively to destroy residual or recurrent tumor cells, treat lymphatic involvement, and treat metastatic sites, such as bones, palliatively.

Chemotherapy

Clinical investigators continue to search for an effective chemotherapeutic regimen. Medroxyprogesterone and testosterone have been used as hormonal therapy, but

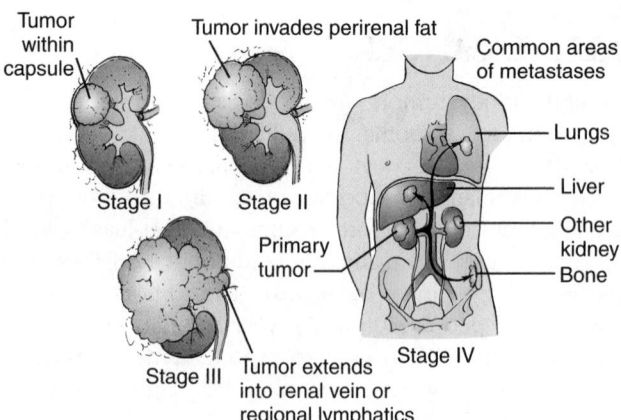

■ **FIGURE 35–1** Staging system for renal carcinoma. Stage 1 tumor is confined within the renal capsule. Stage 2 tumor extends beyond the renal capsule to invade local perinephric fat but has no metastasis. Stage 3 tumor extends into the renal vein or involves local lymphatics. Stage 4 tumor has metastasized to other parts of the body.

their effectiveness has been limited. 🪔 Vinblastine seems to be the most effective single agent, with response rates of 25%. Combination regimens seem to increase toxic effects without improving response rates. Many agents are being studied, but renal cancer cells seem insensitive to chemotherapeutic or hormonal agents, possibly because of their slow growth rate.

Immunotherapy

🪔 Immunotherapy holds some promise in the treatment of renal cancer. Stimulants of the immune system have led to some positive results as long as the tumor is not too large and the immunosuppression is not too severe. There has also been some response to natural and recombinant interferon-alfa. Interleukin-2 has been approved by the Food and Drug Administration for treating renal carcinoma. Studies using vaccines are underway.[15] Clients are immunized with irradiated tumor cells and evaluated for immune responses and clinical tumor regression. Nonmyeloablative allogeneic stem-cell transplantation is another new approach. This may induce sustained regression of metastatic renal cell carcinoma in clients who have had no response to conventional immunotherapy, but further studies are required.[9]

Nursing Management of the Medical Client

Nursing management of the client with renal cancer must include general aspects of care for any cancer (see Chapter 17).

Surgical Management

Nephrectomy

For renal cell carcinoma, the surgical procedure of choice is generally radical nephrectomy, which includes removal of the kidney, the adrenal gland, and perinephric fat with the retroperitoneal lymphatics. Several surgical approaches can be used to remove the diseased kidney. Transabdominal and thoracoabdominal approaches are preferred to secure the renal artery and vein and to prevent the spread of malignant cells.

A retroperitoneal approach is also possible. An incision of 6 to 10 inches is made, usually in the flank area; muscle layers are divided; and tissues are excised. The renal artery and vein are clamped and cut, and the ureter is dissected. When the tumor is in the renal pelvis, a nephroureterectomy is usually performed because of a tendency for transitional cell cancer to "seed" down the ureter into the bladder. With nephroureterectomy, a cuff of the adjacent bladder is removed.

Lymphadenectomy remains controversial. Even in advanced cases, when the prognosis is poor, nephrectomy is sometimes done to relieve pain and hematuria.

If the neoplastic disease is bilateral or if there is a solitary functioning kidney, a partial nephrectomy can be done on at least one kidney, leaving enough renal tissue to support life without long-term dialysis. If partial nephrectomy is not possible in either instance, the entire kidney is removed and the client undergoes dialysis. These clients may be candidates for renal transplantation, but they are usually maintained with dialysis for about a year to watch for recurrence of the disease.

Although open nephrectomy remains the procedure of choice for many urologists, laparoscopic and robotic-assisted laparoscopic nephrectomy are being performed in a number of centers with considerable success. Four small incisions are made through fewer muscle layers. A special laparoscope is inserted through one of the incisions, and laparoscopy instruments are placed in the others. Carbon dioxide is passed through a tube in one incision to inflate the abdominal cavity, which enables the surgeon to see the organs and provides room for manipulation of instruments. At the end of the procedure, the kidney is removed through a small 2- to 3-inch incision below the navel.

🪔 The laparoscopic surgical procedure with or without robotic assistance tends to be longer (6.9 versus 2.2 hours), but clients who undergo the laparoscopic procedure require fewer analgesics, resume oral intake earlier, are discharged home earlier, and return to work sooner than those undergoing open surgery. Increasingly, removal of a kidney for organ donation is being performed laparoscopically.

Indications. Nephrectomy or heminephrectomy is indicated with tumors of the kidney.

Contraindications. As with any surgery, nephrectomy is contraindicated in clients with systemic or respiratory tract infections. General health must be satisfactory to withstand anesthesia, blood loss, and surgical stress. Any metabolic and systemic disorders should be stabilized before surgery.

Complications. Because the kidney is a very vascular organ, the risk of hemorrhage is high. Renal artery embolization of the affected kidney may be done to obstruct the tumor's blood supply and reduce its vascularity, thereby reducing the risk of hemorrhage. Embolization is usually accomplished by occluding the renal artery using an absorbable gelatin sponge (Gelfoam), metal coil, barium, subcutaneous fat, isobutyl-2-cyanoacrylate, absolute ethanol, or a balloon. This procedure may also be performed to control hemorrhage in an inoperable kidney. In addition, some researchers believe that embolization may stimulate an immune response against the dying cancer cells. Other possible complications include those associated with any major surgery, such as atelectasis, pneumonia, thromboembolism, and infection of the surgical wound.

Outcomes. Nephrectomy reduces pain and hematuria caused by the tumor. The hospital stay is typically 4 to 6 days, with a return to work in 4 to 8 weeks. With laparoscopic nephrectomy (with or without robotic assistance), hospitalization is reduced and return to work after 2 to 4 weeks is common. Living with one kidney has few, if any, negative effects. Long-term outcomes, however, depend on the stage of the cancer.

Nursing Management of the Surgical Client

Preoperative Care
Preoperative preparation of the client having renal surgery includes the general guidelines described in Chapter 14. Increase fluid intake, if indicated, to ensure adequate excretion of waste products before surgery. Give emotional support because the client may be anxious, not only about the surgery but also about postoperative renal function and possible recurrence of the disease. If the remaining kidney functions adequately, assure the client that this kidney can fully meet the body's needs.

Postoperative Care
Assessment. Postoperatively, monitor the client's vital signs frequently and watch for any manifestations of bleeding or hemorrhage. Bleeding may be through the incision or internal.

Surgically induced or spontaneous pneumothorax occurs occasionally after nephrectomy; monitor for this complication by assessing for sudden shortness of breath and loss of breath sounds on the affected side.

Diagnosis, Outcomes, Interventions
Diagnosis: Risk for Injury: Postoperative Complications. The nursing diagnoses are likely to include *Risk for Injury: Postoperative complications related to surgical procedure*. Although postoperative care is similar to that for a laparotomy, one of the greatest challenges is reestablishing effective breathing patterns. Deep breathing and coughing are difficult because the incision is very close to the diaphragm. Also, if the jackknife position is used during the operative procedure, pain and soreness in the thoracic region are increased, limiting respiratory excursion. Paralytic ileus is a common problem. Urine output must be maintained.

Outcomes. The client will maintain normal respiratory excursion and have no additional breath sounds and no signs of atelectasis or infection. There will be normal bowel sounds within 2 to 3 days. Urine output will be at least 0.25 ml/kg/hour if one kidney is removed and 0.5 ml/kg/hour if a partial nephrectomy is performed.

Interventions. Liberal use of opioids (including patient-controlled analgesia) to reduce pain and external mechanical support of the chest and abdomen with pillows or hands help the client to perform deep-breathing and coughing exercises more effectively. An incentive spirometer provides immediate feedback about the effectiveness of deep breathing.

> 🦴 **Other interventions include carefully assessing the client's urine output and gastrointestinal status postoperatively and beginning oral intake only after adequate bowel function has resumed. Total urine output from all urine collection tubes should total 0.25 ml/kg/ hour if one kidney is removed or 0.5 ml/kg/hour if a partial nephrectomy is performed. Notify the physician of lesser amounts.**

Other wound drainage tubes also need to be monitored. Early ambulation is indicated.

Diagnosis: Acute Pain. A nursing diagnosis of *Acute Pain related to surgery* is common because the nephrectomy incision is extensive and causes significant discomfort. Muscle pain may develop from the prolonged position maintained during surgery.

Outcomes. Comfort will be attained and pain will be reduced, as indicated by the client's reports of reduced discomfort or tolerable pain, as well as by nonverbal indications of reduced discomfort, particularly during movement.

Interventions. The pain may be reduced by opioid analgesics (including the use of patient-controlled analgesia) and proper positioning. Epidural fentanyl or morphine sulfate can provide effective analgesia.

Evaluation. The client should be able to resume regular activities within 6 to 8 weeks after surgery. Long-term survival is dependent on the stage of cancer diagnosed.

Self-Care

With shorter hospitalizations, clients who have undergone nephrectomy may require home care and support. Clients are weakened by surgery and possibly by other treatments. Activity should increase gradually; typically, 6 weeks must elapse before clients are ready to return to work or lift more than 10 pounds.

Concern about recurrence of the cancer is common. The American Cancer Society and other support groups may be helpful in the client's adjustment to cancer. People with one kidney can lead normal lives. There is, however, a need to protect the remaining kidney by prevention of infection and trauma.

TUBULOINTERSTITIAL DISEASE

Traditionally, the term *interstitial nephritis* has been applied to renal disease characterized by the presence of inflammatory cells in the spaces between the renal tubules. Not all disease processes included in this classification are inflammatory, however. Therefore the term *tubulointerstitial disease* is being advocated for this category of renal disorders.

Tubulointerstitial diseases are commonly classified as either acute or chronic. The acute form usually represents an allergic reaction and has a rapid onset. Assessment findings are typically related to tubular injury. Manifestations often include fever, skin rash, eosinophilia, oliguric renal failure, and occasionally gross hematuria. The disease may progress along any of three courses:

- Complete recovery
- Rapid progression to renal failure and death
- Movement to the chronic form

Although corticosteroids are commonly prescribed, their value is unclear. Treatment is similar to that for acute renal failure (see Chapter 36).

Chronic tubulointerstitial disease is characterized by progressive interstitial fibrosis and usually chronic inflammatory cell infiltration with tubular atrophy. In the terminal stages, the altered renal vasculature and renal structure make the disease virtually indistinguishable from chronic pyelonephritis.

Morphologic findings in tubulointerstitial disease include interstitial edema, cellular infiltration of the interstitium, tubular cellular atrophy and flattening, and interstitial fibrosis. As the disease progresses, renal involvement extends beyond the tubules to progressive fibrosis of Bowman's capsule with secondary involvement of the glomeruli.

Potential causes of this pathologic process include acute pyelonephritis, septicemia, analgesic abuse (especially with phenacetin, aspirin, and acetaminophen), immunologic mechanisms (for example, renal allograft, SLE, and Sjögren's syndrome), heavy metal toxicity, drug toxicity, hypercalcemia, and hypocalcemia. In addition, several medication hypersensitivities can contribute. The medications involved include rifampin, penicillin and its analogs, sulfonamides, cephalosporins, allopurinol, captopril, cimetidine, azathioprine, phenytoin, thiazide, lithium, NSAIDs, and possibly furosemide.

An early manifestation of tubulointerstitial disease is a sudden, unexplained decrease in renal function that may be mild to severe. Specifically, there may be inability to concentrate urine, salt wasting, and poor acidification of the urine leading to metabolic acidosis. Finding a variety of urine sediment abnormalities is also common. Because glucose, uric acid, phosphates, amino acids, and bicarbonate are not effectively reabsorbed in the tubules, they appear in the urine. Severe bicarbonaturia is an indicator of renal tubular acidosis. Proteinuria is less severe than with other renal disease. Systemic hypertension is a common finding.

GLOMERULONEPHRITIS

Glomerulonephritis encompasses a variety of diseases, most of which are caused by an immunologic reaction that results in proliferative and inflammatory changes in glomerular structure. Glomerulonephritis can be acute or chronic. It is usually manifested by either a nephrotic syndrome or a nephritic syndrome. Percutaneous renal biopsy is typically used to identify the type of glomerulonephritis, and the findings assist in planning interventions and determining the prognosis.

NEPHROTIC SYNDROME

Nephrotic syndrome is a set of clinical manifestations caused by protein wasting secondary to diffuse glomerular damage. Manifestations include proteinuria (>3.5 g/day), hypoalbuminemia, and edema. Abnormal permeability of the glomerular basement membrane (especially to albumin) results in loss of protein in the urine. The resulting hypoalbuminemia alters oncotic pressure in the vascular tree, and fluid moves into the interstitial spaces, causing edema. This movement stimulates plasma renin activity and augments aldosterone production; as a result, the kidney retains sodium and water, thus adding to the accumulation of extracellular fluid.

Hyperlipidemia usually occurs also, probably because of increased hepatic lipoprotein synthesis in response to decreased levels of serum albumin. Depending on the degree of renal failure, some level of normocytic anemia is common.

The causes of nephrotic syndrome are numerous. Besides glomerulonephritis, certain systemic disorders can cause it, such as diabetes mellitus, SLE, amyloidosis, hepatitis B, syphilis, carcinoma, leukemia, infectious disease, and preeclampsia. Other predisposing factors include allergic reactions, reactions to drugs (such as penicillamine, anticonvulsants, probenecid, captopril, gold salts, heroin, and NSAIDs), renal vein thrombosis, sickle cell disease, and heart failure.

Potential complications of nephrotic syndrome include the effects of extracellular fluid accumulation and the progressive development of renal failure. The client may also experience severe hypovolemia, thromboembolism, secondary aldosteronism, abnormal thyroid function, osteomalacia, and increased susceptibility to infections.

Usually, edema is the client's chief problem. Although its onset may be insidious, it becomes massive. The client's skin typically assumes a characteristic waxy pallor resulting from the edema rather than anemia. Other manifestations include anorexia, malaise, irritability, and abnormal or absent menses. Large amounts of protein appear in the client's urine along with granular and epithelial cell casts and fat bodies; proteinuria may account for losses of 4 to 30 g/day. Some hematuria may be present. Serum albumin concentrations may drop as low as 1 to 2.5 g/dl.

The primary aim of treatment for nephrotic syndrome is to heal the leaking glomerular basement membrane, stop the loss of protein in the client's urine, and break the cycle of edema. Interventions typically include maintaining the client's fluid and electrolyte balance, reducing inflammation, preventing thrombosis, and minimizing protein loss.

Maintain Fluid and Electrolyte Balance

Unless the client is hyponatremic, fluids are not usually restricted. The client's fluid balance, however, should be carefully monitored via daily weights, girth measurements, and intake and output determinations. These data are important because weight loss may represent true tissue loss involving protein rather than fluid.

Loop diuretics (i.e., those that work on the loop of Henle), such as furosemide (Lasix), are typically prescribed. Plasma volume expanders, such as albumin, plasma, and dextran, may be administered to raise the oncotic pressure in the vascular tree. The increased pressure pulls fluid from the extracellular spaces, making it available for kidney filtration. Diuresis in older clients must be handled with particular caution because of their reduced ability to tolerate sudden shifts in intravascular volume.

Because the kidneys have a reduced capacity to excrete sodium, mild sodium restriction usually is instituted. The diet should be as palatable as possible, however, because the client must consume adequate protein and calories. Potassium may also be restricted as serum potassium levels rise.

Because edema disrupts cellular nutrition, the client is at increased risk for skin breakdown. Thus skin care is vital. Interventions include good hygiene, massage, position changes, and possibly special mattresses. Use research-based tools to assess the client's risk of breakdown (see Chapter 18).

Reduce Inflammation

Steroid therapy helps some clients, depending on the cause of disease. Cytotoxic agents such as cyclophosphamide and chlorambucil, indomethacin, anticoagulants, and antiplatelet agents may be used as well.

Prevent Thrombosis

Because clients with nephrotic syndrome are vulnerable to renal vein thrombosis, some are given long-term anticoagulation therapy. Teach such clients how to monitor for hemorrhage, and encourage them to carry identification that lists the drugs they take.

Minimize Protein Loss

For clients with nephrotic syndrome, most physicians recommend a protein intake of 1 to 1.5 g/kg/day with more than 35 kcal/kg/day to prevent further protein breakdown.

Twenty-four-hour urine collections are used to measure urinary protein losses and monitor the success of treatment. Treatment to reduce inflammation ultimately reduces protein loss.

An important nursing role is to help the client with nephrotic syndrome maintain health and cope with the illness. Teach the client to take prescribed medications regularly, follow the prescribed diet, and report changes in health status, such as increasing edema, reduced urine output, weight gain, respiratory distress, and signs of infection. Explain that the amount of exercise allowed is based, at least in part, on the severity of the edema. Bed rest is imposed only during severe edema. As the fluid level moves toward normal, the client is allowed more activity. Other important areas of teaching include nutrition, prevention of infection, and methods of careful self-assessment.

NEPHRITIC SYNDROME

Nephritic syndrome refers to a set of clinical manifestations that includes hematuria and at least one of the following: oliguria (urine output <400 ml/24 hour), hypertension, elevated blood urea nitrogen (BUN) level, or decreased GFR. Nephritic syndrome is common with many types of glomerulonephritis, including immunoglobulin A (IgA) nephropathy and Henoch-Schönlein purpura. Treatment includes management of the underlying disease (usually through immunosuppressive drugs, as noted later) and symptomatic treatment of blood pressure and uremia.

TYPES OF GLOMERULONEPHRITIS

There are many types of glomerulonephritis, most of which involve either nephrotic syndrome or nephritic syndrome. The diagnosis of the specific type can be made by assessment of clinical manifestations and through renal biopsy. Box 35-2 presents a classification system based on etiology. Table 35-1 describes the onset, diagnostic findings, and prognosis for various types of glomerulonephritis.

Pathophysiology

Glomerulonephritis is an immunologic disorder that causes inflammation and increased cells in the glomerulus. Because the primary function of the glomerulus is to filter blood, most cases result when antigen-antibody complexes produced by an infection elsewhere in the body become trapped in the glomerulus. This entrapment causes inflammatory damage and impedes glomerular function, reducing the glomerular membrane's capacity for selective permeability. The source of the antigens

BOX 35-2 Classification of Glomerulonephritis Based on Etiology

PRIMARY GLOMERULONEPHRITIS—IMMUNE RESPONSE TO PATHOGENS

- Acute glomerulonephritis
- Postinfectious glomerulonephritis
- Group A beta-hemolytic streptococcus
- Other infectious conditions such as cytomegalovirus infection, measles, mumps, staphylococcus, or pneumococcal bacteremia
- Infectious glomerulonephritis
- Membranoproliferative glomerulonephritis
- Rapidly progressive glomerulonephritis
- Idiopathic membranous glomerulonephritis
- Immunoglobulin A (IgA) nephropathy
- Chronic glomerulonephritis
- Lipoid nephrosis
- Focal glomerular sclerosis

SECONDARY GLOMERULONEPHRITIS—RELATED TO SYSTEMIC DISEASE

- Goodpasture's syndrome
- Hemolytic-uremic syndrome
- Henoch-Schönlein purpura
- Polyarteritis
- Progressive systemic sclerosis
- Systemic lupus erythematosus
- Wegener's granulomatosis
- Thrombocytopenic purpura
- Postpartum renal failure

TABLE 35–1 Types of Glomerulonephritis Onset, Findings, and Prognosis

Type	Onset	Diagnostic Findings	Prognosis
Poststreptococcal glomerulonephritis	1-3 weeks after beta-hemolytic streptococcal infection of throat or skin Nephritic syndrome	Underlying infection Elevated antistreptolysin O titer Microscopic urinalysis, urine with many casts	Variable Complete recovery to end-stage renal disease
Membranoproliferative glomerulonephritis	Nephrotic syndrome sometimes preceded by a streptococcal infection	Proteinuria Hematuria (microscopic or gross)	Gradual progressive chronic renal failure
Rapidly progressive glomerulonephritis	Nephritic syndrome Sudden May follow antigen or infection Peak ages 40-60 yr	Hematuria Edema Hypertension Proteinuria Oliguria Acidosis	Progresses to renal failure within weeks or months
Idiopathic membranous glomerulonephritis	Insidious Peak ages 40-70 yr Unknown antigen	Asymptomatic proteinuria or nephrotic syndrome	Mixed: 25% have spontaneous remission, 25% have renal failure, 25% have persistent proteinuria, 25% have deteriorating renal function
Immunoglobulin A (IgA) nephropathy (also called Berger's disease)	Most common in young adults Nephritic syndrome	Hematuria Red blood cell casts on microscopic urinalysis	Usually progresses slowly over 10-20 yr; a small proportion progress to renal failure
Lipoid nephrosis (also called minimal change glomerulonephritis)	Nephrotic syndrome	Found on biopsy	Generally good May be relapses and spontaneous remission
Focal glomerular sclerosis	Peaks between ages 30 and 50 yr Nephrotic syndrome	Found on biopsy May be few symptoms	Poor, although rate of deterioration varies widely Recurs after transplantation
Membranous glomerulonephritis	Commonly secondary to drug therapy toxins or systemic autoimmune disease Nephrotic syndrome Insidious onset	Heavy proteinuria	Variable 30% have spontaneous remission
Hemolytic-uremic syndrome	Follows infection with *Escherichia coli* (01571 H7 serotype) History of eating undercooked hamburger Children and older adults particularly vulnerable	Hemorrhagic manifestations, such as bleeding and bruising Purpura manifestations, such as acute renal failure, hemolytic anemia, and thrombocytopenia	Recovery rate 95% but may leave residual renal damage

may be either *exogenous* (e.g., after streptococcal infection) or *endogenous* (as in SLE). Evidence also indicates that some antigen-antibody complexes may form in the kidney itself.

Glomerulonephritis may also result from antibodies affixed to the glomerular basement membrane. For example, Goodpasture's syndrome involves pulmonary hemorrhage and glomerulonephritis.

The primary pathologic processes in glomerulonephritis, lipoid nephrosis, and focal glomerular sclerosis are proliferation and inflammation; however, lipoid nephrosis and focal glomerular sclerosis are characterized by degeneration. Figure 35-2 depicts the pathophysiologic mechanisms of glomerulonephritis.

Clinical Manifestations

Acute glomerulonephritis may develop insidiously or suddenly, varying considerably with the pathophysiology involved. Classic manifestations of sudden onset include hematuria with red blood cell casts and proteinuria. Fever, chills, weakness, pallor, anorexia, nausea, and vomiting may be present. Generalized edema, particularly facial and periorbital swelling, is a typical finding. The client may have ascites, pleural effusion, and heart failure.

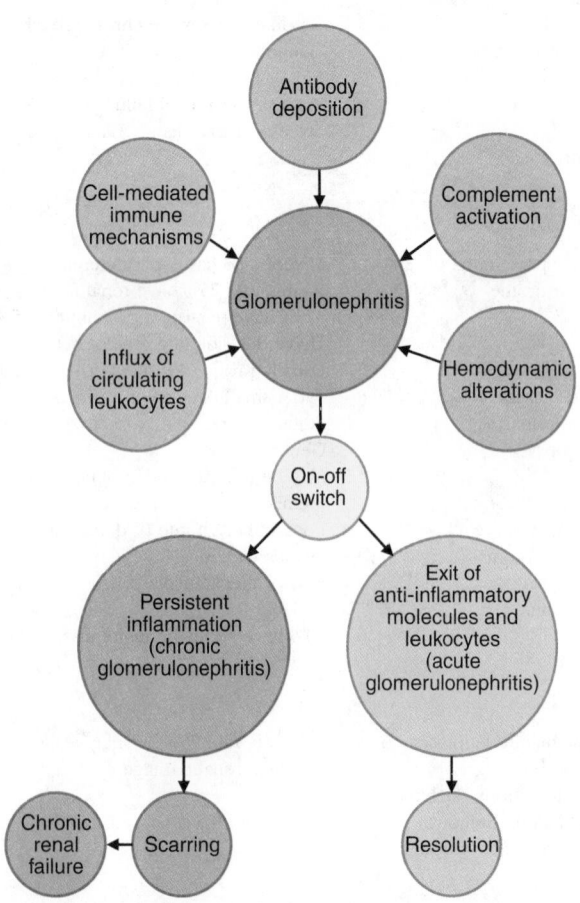

■ **FIGURE 35–2** Pathophysiologic mechanisms of glomerulonephritis.

The client is likely to have a headache and moderate to severe hypertension. Visual acuity may be reduced because of retinal edema. Abdominal or flank pain may develop, probably because of kidney edema and distention of the renal capsule. Oliguria, even anuria, may be present for several days; the longer it persists, the more irreversible the kidney damage. In contrast, the disease may be so mild that the client reports only vague weakness, anorexia, and lethargy.

Acute glomerulonephritis can become a fulminant process, proceeding quickly to uremia or chronic glomerulonephritis. Most clients, however, start to recover within 14 days. Most clinical manifestations disappear within several weeks, although hematuria and proteinuria may be present for longer periods. If complete recovery does not occur within 2 years, it probably will not occur at all.

Some clinicians use the term *subacute glomerulonephritis* to describe disease persisting longer than 6 to 8 weeks. Although most of the manifestations of the acute disease have disappeared, the client is still at high risk for exacerbation of glomerulonephritis. The term *latent glomerulonephritis* refers to an asymptomatic condition characterized by significant albumin levels and casts in the urine for more than 1 year after acute onset. These findings indicate continued but slow parenchymal changes.

Most types of glomerulonephritis can progress to a chronic state. Sometimes, glomerulonephritis is first seen as a chronic process. Chronic glomerulonephritis progresses over an extended period, often as long as 30 years. When it progresses to end-stage renal failure, dialysis must begin or the client will die.

As the glomeruli and tubules are destroyed by the pathologic process, the kidneys shrink and become severely contracted. Fibrous and scar tissue replaces functioning renal tissue. Sclerosis of renal blood vessels also occurs. The destruction rates vary.

Common manifestations include malaise, weight loss, edema, increasing irritability and mental cloudiness, a metallic taste in the mouth, polyuria and nocturia resulting from the kidney's inability to concentrate urine, headache, dizziness, and digestive disturbances. As the disease progresses, these manifestations intensify, and the client may experience respiratory difficulty and angina.

The cardinal manifestation of this disease is hypertension. It is not uncommon for the client to experience such complications as nosebleed, manifestations of arteriosclerosis, cardiomegaly, and hemorrhage into the kidneys, lungs, retina, or cerebrum. Edema increases as heart failure becomes more severe and the serum albumin level decreases. Examination of the eyegrounds shows vascular changes and edema of the discs. Urinalysis shows a fixed specific gravity, small amounts of proteinuria except during exacerbation, casts, WBCs, renal tubular cells, and consistent hematuria. Anemia tends to be severe.

Examining the urine usually provides the information necessary for a diagnosis of glomerulonephritis (see Chapter 32). Gross hematuria and proteinuria are the cardinal findings. The client's urine, which may be scant, usually has a dark, smoky, cola-colored, or red-brown hue. The proteinuria produces a persistent and excessive foam. The urine may have a low pH and a specific gravity in the midnormal to high-normal range if there is enough renal damage to affect the kidneys' ability to concentrate.

Other studies may assist in the diagnosis as well. Serum urea nitrogen and creatinine levels may be elevated, and creatinine clearance rates may be decreased. C-reactive proteins and antistreptolysin O titer are usually elevated in poststreptococcal glomerulonephritis, and the serum complement level is low in many forms of glomerulonephritis. Hematocrit and hemoglobin studies may indicate anemia, particularly if renal failure is imminent.

OUTCOME MANAGEMENT

Medical Management

Medical intervention aims to eliminate antigens, to alter the client's immune balance, and to inhibit or alleviate inflammation to prevent further renal damage and improve kidney function. Although some clients may require initial hospitalization, treatment is typically on an outpatient basis.

Reduce Inflammation

Plasmapheresis has been used in some research protocols to reduce the number of antigens in certain types of glomerulonephritis, including rapidly progressive glomerulonephritis. This intervention is usually administered in conjunction with corticosteroids and immunosuppressive agents (azathioprine, cyclophosphamide). The technique is designed to remove the specific circulating antibody or mediators of the inflammatory response. Large volumes of the client's plasma are cyclically removed and replaced with fresh frozen plasma through a continuous-flow blood cell separator.

Antibiotic therapy (such as penicillin for streptococcal organisms) is used to treat poststreptococcal glomerulonephritis. It is also used prophylactically after streptococcal infections to prevent further damage.

Maintain Fluid and Electrolyte Balance

Volume overload and hypertension are treated with diuretics, antihypertensives, and restriction of dietary sodium and water. Common complications of fluid overload include heart failure with pulmonary edema and increased intracranial pressure. Renal failure may develop (see Chapter 36). Appropriate monitoring is

essential and should include vital signs, intake and output, and weight. Recognizing complications early facilitates prompt medical intervention.

Nursing Management of the Medical Client

Assessment. For any client with suspected glomerulonephritis, take a comprehensive history that includes upper respiratory tract infection (such as strep throat), skin infections, scarlet fever, or a history of glomerulonephritis. Also question the client about systemic disorders that might be present, such as SLE, scleroderma, amyloidosis, and hypertension. Any recent invasive procedures should also be noted.

Physical examination may reveal ascites, pleural effusion, and manifestations of heart failure with pulmonary edema. Examine the urine closely for color, amount, and abnormal substances. In particular, microscopic analysis of the urine can be a valuable diagnostic tool with glomerulonephritis; urinary casts are commonly seen under high magnification (see Chapter 32). Check the client's vital signs closely, especially the blood pressure.

Diagnosis, Outcomes, Interventions
Diagnosis: Imbalanced Nutrition:
Less Than Body Requirements. If the client has a reduced appetite or an aversion to food, the nursing diagnosis *Imbalanced Nutrition: Less Than Body Requirements related to anorexia and increased metabolic demands* is appropriate.

Outcomes. The client will maintain adequate nutritional intake, as evidenced by no weight loss, an absence of a negative nitrogen balance, and normal electrolytes.

Interventions. It is important to protect the kidneys while they are recovering their function. The prescribed diet is likely to be high in calories and low in protein. This diet is designed to avoid protein catabolism and enables the kidney to rest because it handles fewer protein molecules and metabolites.

The degree to which protein is restricted depends on the amount excreted in the urine and the client's individual requirements. Sodium is also restricted, depending on the amount of edema present. Anorexia, nausea, and vomiting may interfere with adequate intake, requiring creative intervention on your part. A dietitian can help plan the client's diet around these restrictions.

Diagnosis: Excess Fluid Volume. A common nursing diagnosis in glomerulonephritis is *Excess Fluid Volume related to reduced urine output*.

Outcomes. The client will maintain balanced intake and output, as evidenced by no manifestations of edema or fluid overload.

Interventions. Appropriate fluid balance is important. Careful monitoring of daily weight and intake and output helps determine the progress of the edema and thus provides an estimate of renal function. Daily measurement of edematous parts (especially legs and abdomen) also provides useful, objective data. The client's allowable fluid intake is based on the intake and output measurements. Fluid intake is usually restricted. Thirst may be relieved by offering hard candies, lemon slices, or ice chips rather than a glass of water. Assist the client to "plan" fluid distribution during the day to make the best use of allowed fluids.

Diagnosis: Fatigue. Another common nursing diagnosis is *Fatigue related to increased metabolic demands and anemia.*

Outcomes. The client will conserve energy through an adequate balance of rest and activity, as evidenced by absence of complaints of fatigue.

Interventions. Rest is essential—both physical and emotional. As mentioned, activity level correlates directly with the amount of hematuria and proteinuria. Exercise also increases catabolic activity. The allowable amount of activity depends on the results of serial urinalyses. Bed rest interspersed with periods of limited activity may continue for several weeks to months. Therefore the client may need help in arranging personal matters, such as family, home, job, finances, and community responsibilities.

Encourage the client to talk about any fears or concerns, and, if necessary, help the client deal with the emotional reactions expected during a long-term illness with a questionable prognosis. Only after handling these problems can the client rest emotionally. Appropriate diversionary activities may help the client cope with prolonged physical immobility.

Diagnosis: Risk for Impaired Skin Integrity. A typical nursing diagnosis is *Risk for Impaired Skin Integrity related to edema.*

Outcomes. The client will maintain tissue integrity; skin will remain intact.

Interventions. Edema interferes with cellular nutrition, which makes the client more susceptible to skin breakdown. Take precautions to prevent this complication. Interventions include good hygiene, massage, and position changes as well as other prophylactic measures, such as mattress devices. Use research-based tools to assess the client's risk of breakdown (see Chapter 18).

Diagnosis: Risk for Infection. Another diagnosis after immunosuppressive therapy is *Risk for Infection related to altered immune response secondary to treatment.*

Outcomes. The client will maintain a healthy immune status, free of infection, as evidenced by normal temperature and an absence of local or systemic manifestations of infection.

Interventions. Glomerulonephritis markedly diminishes a client's natural defenses to infection, especially to streptococcal organisms. Immunosuppressive medications and corticosteroids further reduce host resistance. Although isolation is not necessary, take care to protect the client from people with obvious infectious processes. General supportive measures help boost the client's defense mechanisms. Client teaching should involve appropriate ways to avoid infections, especially respiratory and urinary tract infections.

Evaluation. The client must be able to understand the condition and the reasons for limitations, including dietary and fluid restrictions. Stress the importance of follow-up treatments to minimize the risk of recurrence.

Self-Care

Clients with glomerulonephritis are followed as outpatients, often for many years. Self-care activities should include attending regular follow-up appointments, adhering to recommended medications and dietary restrictions, and monitoring for changes in condition. These are discussed further later in this chapter under Chronic Kidney Disease. It is vital that blood pressure be controlled to prevent further renal damage; many clients learn to monitor their own blood pressure at home. Because the disease may progress to renal failure, there are numerous quality-of-life issues, as discussed in Chapter 36.

Modifications for Older Clients

The older client is at greater risk for renal damage because of the pre-existing effects of age on the kidneys. The older client is also more likely to have concurrent chronic diseases—such as hypertension and diabetes mellitus—that may have affected the kidneys, although treatment is the same.

CHRONIC KIDNEY DISEASE

Chronic kidney disease (CKD) is a rapidly growing health problem. Estimates are that 11% of the U.S. population or 19.2 million people have CKD.[10] The Centers for Disease Control and Prevention in Atlanta has recently established a chronic kidney disease program to enhance surveillance and prevention programs for CKD at the federal and state levels.

The many diseases described in this chapter can lead to CKD, and the etiology will differ by disease. Recognition of the type of kidney disease and etiology may be useful to prevent or slow progression of the disease.

Etiology and Risk Factors

The increasing incidence of CKD partially reflects increased obesity-related hypertension and diabetes mellitus in sedentary, well-nourished populations. Since cardiovascular disease and diabetes mellitus are frequently co-morbid conditions associated with CKD, aggressive treatment of the disease and risk factors can slow progression of the illness and limit morbidity and mortality (See the Translating Evidence into Practice feature Managing Hypertension in Diabetic Clients to Slow Progression of Renal Disease on p. 780).

The National Kidney Foundation (NKF) Kidney Disease Outcome Quality Initiative (K/DOQI) defined CKD as kidney damage with a glomerular filtration rate (GFR) <60 ml/minute/1.73 m² for more than 3 months. The NKF developed a classification system for the stages of CKD (Table 35-2). Traditionally, the classification of the type of kidney disease has been focused on pathology and etiology. The K/DOQI classification system focuses on the GFR, but it remains important to diagnose the cause of CKD.

Pathophysiology

There are many diseases that cause CKD; each has its own pathophysiology. However, there are common mechanisms for disease progression. Pathologic features include fibrosis, loss of renal cells, and infiltration of renal tissue by monocytes and macrophages. Proteinuria, hypoxia, and excessive angiotensin II production all contribute to the pathophysiology. In an attempt to maintain GFR, the glomerulus hyperfiltrates; this results in endothelial injury. Proteinuria results from increased glomerular permeability and increased capillary pressure. Hypoxia also contributes to disease progression. Angiotensin II increases glomerular hypertension, which further damages the kidney.

Clinical Manifestations

The clinical manifestations of CKD are highly variable. Many people with CKD have few if any complaints. In stage 1, clients usually have normal blood pressure, no laboratory test abnormalities, and no clinical manifestations. Clients in stage 2 are generally asymptomatic, but may develop hypertension, and laboratory test abnormalities exist. In stage 3, clients are still usually asymptomatic but laboratory values suggest abnormalities in several organ systems, and hypertension is frequently present. By stage 4, clients begin to experience clinical manifestations associated with CKD such as fatigue and poor appetite. At stage 5, full-blown clinical manifestations of end-stage renal disease (ESRD) are evident (see Chapter 36).

Proteinuria is one of the strongest predictors of progression of CKD. As the GFR declines, clients may show not only proteinuria but also hypertension, a wide range of lab abnormalities, and manifestations resulting from disorders in other organs. These disorders include anemia, metabolic acidosis, dyslipidemia, bone disease, protein-energy malnutrition, and neuropathy; alterations in health status are described in more detail in Chapter 36 in relation to ESRD.

OUTCOME MANAGEMENT

The focus of management of CKD is on slowing the progression of the disease and in preventing risk factors that lead to complications.

Medical Management

Ideal outcomes of medical management include the following:

- Controlling blood pressure (BP) to below 130/80 mm Hg
- Managing blood glucose level to maintain HbA$_{1c}$ below 7%
- Managing hyperlipidemia with diet and cholesterol-lowering drugs (usually statins)
- Managing and treating emerging manifestations of renal failure including anemia, hyperphosphatemia and hyperparathyroidism, hyperkalemia, and metabolic acidosis
- Preparing clients for renal replacement therapy when necessary (see Chapter 36)

Reduce Blood Pressure

Hypertension in CKD increases the risk of loss of kidney function. The lower the BP, the lower the risk of cardiovascular disease. At blood pressures above 115/75 mm Hg, the risk of cardiovascular mortality doubles for each increase of 20 mm Hg systolic and 10 mm Hg diastolic BP. Clinical practice guidelines suggest

TABLE 35–2 National Kidney Foundation Classification of Chronic Kidney Disease

Stage	Description	Other Terms Used	GFR (ml/min/1.73 m²)
1	Kidney damage with nomal glomerular filtration rate (GFR)	At risk	>90
2	Kidney damage with mild decrease in GFR	Chronic renal insufficiency (CRI)	60-89
3	Moderate decrease in GFR	CRI, chronic renal failure (CRF)	30-59
4	Severe decrease in GFR	CRF	15-29
5	Kidney failure	End-stage renal disease (ESRD)	<15

Modified from National Kidney Foundation: *K/DOQI (Kidney/Dialysis Outcomes Quality Initiative) clinical practice guidelines for chronic kidney disease: Evaluation, classification and stratification.* Accessed 01/30/04 at www.kidney.org/professionals/doqi/kdoqi/toc.htm.

that systolic BP should be maintained below 130 mm Hg and diastolic BP below 80 mm Hg in people with less than 1 g of proteinuria/day and <125/75 mm Hg in people with >1 g of proteinuria/day.[38]

There are currently more than 125 antihypertensive agents available for the treatment of hypertension. Although many of them are very effective, control of BP is challenging. Further discussion of treatment for hypertension is included in Chapter 52. Numerous large, randomized control trials have shown that angiotensin-converting enzyme inhibitors (ACEIs) are superior to non-ACEI agents in reducing progression of renal disease, reducing ischemic heart disease and congestive heart failure event rates, and reducing mortality. ACEI and angiotensin receptor blockers (ARBs) either alone or in combination are the preferred agents for both diabetic and nondiabetic kidney disease.[38] Current thinking is that combination therapy is more effective than stepped therapy.[40] Because these agents carry the risk of hyperkalemia, potassium levels require close monitoring.

Reduce Serum Lipids

Cardiovascular mortality is elevated among people with CKD. For this reason, low-fat diets and administration of cholesterol-lowering medications, particularly statins, are indicated. The NKF recommends maintaining LDL <100 mg/dl, non-HDL <130 mg/dl, and triglycerides <500 mg/dl.[37] Hyperlipidemia should be managed aggressively to reduce the risk of atherosclerotic cardiovascular disease.

Control Blood Glucose Level

Diabetic nephropathy can be ameliorated with aggressive control of blood glucose levels and management of hypertension. The goal is to maintain preprandial blood glucose values of 80 to 120 mg/dl in the morning and 100 to 140 mg/dl at bedtime and HbA_{1c} levels less than 7%.

Control Phosphorus Intake

Elevations in the levels of serum phosphorus, calcium-phosphorus product, and parathyroid hormone substantially increase the risk of death. The NKF recommends that serum phosphorus level be maintained between 2.7 and 4.6 mg/dl for those with stage 3 or 4 CKD, dietary phosphorus intake should be limited, and phosphorus binders started if necessary.[36]

Nursing Management of the Medical Client

Assessment. For any client with CKD, take a comprehensive history that includes medications and diet currently prescribed. Check blood pressure regularly. Monitor

urine studies including microalbumin and albumin levels as well as blood creatinine level, GFR, red blood cell count, and levels of electrolytes, glucose, and lipids for changes suggesting increasing renal failure. Physical assessment findings that suggest progressing renal failure may include fatigue, peripheral edema, shortness of breath, adventitious lung sounds, heart murmurs or gallops, bruising, memory loss, GI disturbances, impaired wound healing, and increased infections.

Diagnosis, Outcomes, Interventions

Diagnosis: Effective Therapeutic Regimen Management and Readiness for Enhanced Self-Care. The nursing goals for the client with CKD are to minimize the risk of progression of the disease and prevent or manage risk factors associated with morbidity and mortality. For this reason, two nursing diagnoses are *Effective Therapeutic Regimen Management* and *Readiness for Enhanced Self-Care*.

Outcomes. The client will control risk factors through self-management of medications, diet, and exercise, as evidenced by normal blood pressure and normal or stabilized laboratory values including blood glucose and creatinine levels and reduced or stabilized proteinuria.

Interventions. Nursing interventions include health education and mutual goal setting to address risk factors such as high blood pressure, poor glycemic control, proteinuria, and smoking. Blood pressure management can include dietary therapy (reduced sodium), exercise, and antihypertensive medications. Many clients are taught to monitor their blood pressure at home.

Control Blood Glucose Level. Glycemic control is addressed further in Chapter 45. Dietary management, exercise, antidiabetic agents, and insulin therapy are essential aspects of managing blood glucose levels.

Encourage Smoking Cessation. Smoking cessation assistance is another important area for prevention of risk factors. The mechanisms of the effect of smoking on kidney disease progression are unclear, but studies have shown an association between smoking and decreasing renal function. Smoking increases the risk of developing type 2 diabetes mellitus and microalbuminuria, and furthering progression of diabetic nephropathy. Smoking was related to the development of kidney disease in a longitudinal study of 2585 people with no previous history of kidney disease with a mean follow-up of 18.5 years.[16] There are many nursing strategies to facilitate smoking cessation, but this is a difficult addiction to overcome and repeated and varied interventions may be necessary.

Diagnosis: Imbalanced Nutrition: More Than Body Requirements. Excess weight can contribute to the development of CKD. As a result, the nursing diagnosis is often

Imbalanced Nutrition: More Than Body Requirements related to sedentary lifestyle and calorie intake greater than energy used.

Outcomes. The client will demonstrate weight control as exhibited by a near-normal body weight and a body mass index (BMI) of <35 kg/m^2.

Interventions. Health education about both exercise and diet is a vital part of weight reduction programs. Exercise programs can vary considerably based on the client's interests, current level of activity, and present health status. Asking clients to keep a food diary can be very useful in assessing specific dietary problems. Teaching about healthy food choices is an important nursing role. Referral to a dietitian can be very helpful, particularly in complex cases. Dietitians can provide individualized instruction and sample diet plans and instruct the client further about many possible diet modifications necessary at various stages of CKD. These modifications might include reduced sodium, reduced phosphorus, low fat, low potassium, and reduced protein intake as well as reduced calories, depending on the stage of kidney disease and the laboratory value abnormalities.

Evaluation. Evaluation of interventions will involve assessing GFR to determine whether the disease has been stabilized and the progression of the disease slowed. Blood pressure, proteinuria, and body weight will be within normal limits.

Self-Care

Self-management of CKD is key to control of CKD and its complications. Clients typically feel well, so it is important to help them understand the treatment goals and risks for complications. Self-management often involves home monitoring of blood pressure, dietary modifications, medications, exercise, weight reduction, and smoking cessation.

RENAL TRAUMA

Serious kidney injury is relatively rare because of the protection afforded by the rib cage, the heavy muscles of the back, and the tough capsule surrounding the kidney. Traffic accidents and falls in which the client lands on the abdomen, flank, or back are the most common cause of injury, usually from blunt trauma. Kidney lacerations can result from fractures of the spine and ribs as well as penetrating injuries from bullets and knives.

Pathophysiology

Five categories of traumatic injury can affect the kidney:

- Contusion with intrarenal hemorrhage
- Minor laceration (rupture with subcapsular hemorrhage)
- Major laceration (rupture into the renal pelvis)
- "Fractured" kidney (shattered rupture)
- Vascular (pedicle) injury, which damages renal blood supply (Figure 35-3)

In a contusion, a hematoma develops and remains confined within the renal parenchyma. Rupture of the kidney may cause hemorrhage between the capsular walls; bleeding may or may not reach into the renal pelvis. A shattered or fractured kidney causes hemorrhage throughout the renal tissue. The pedicle holds the renal artery and other vital circulatory and nervous system connections to the kidney. Injury to the pedicle may jeopardize the life of the kidney and may occur with or without intrarenal hemorrhage.

Clinical Manifestations

The type of injury the client has suffered gives the first real key to identifying renal trauma. Commonly, the client has multiple serious injuries, and renal trauma may not be immediately apparent. Hematuria (gross or microscopic) is a cardinal manifestation and is found in about 80% of cases. However, serious renal injury can

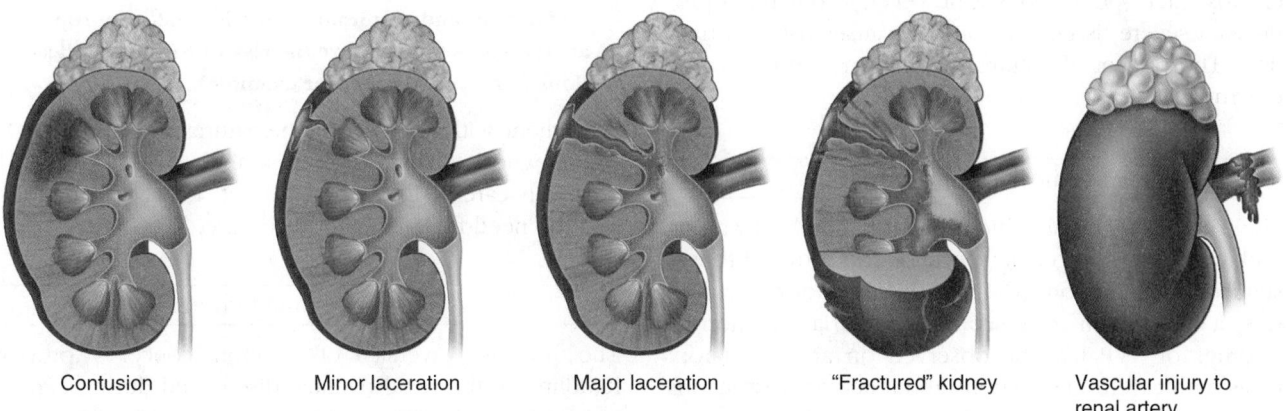

| Contusion | Minor laceration | Major laceration | "Fractured" kidney | Vascular injury to renal artery |

■ **FIGURE 35-3** Categories of renal trauma.

occur without hemorrhage, and clear urine does not automatically rule out renal trauma. Other findings include shock, flank pain, and a palpable mass in the affected flank area or over the 11th or 12th rib. Paralytic ileus may also occur. You may see bruises over the client's flank and lower back secondary to retroperitoneal hemorrhage, a development known as Grey Turner's sign. A KUB film, IVP, retrograde pyelography, renal scan, ultrasonography, CT scan, and renal arteriography all help confirm the type and degree of kidney injury.

Complications

In addition to the immediate problems of hemorrhage and loss of functioning renal tissue, kidney trauma makes the client highly susceptible to a number of other problems. Even in closed injuries, there is a high risk of sepsis leading to kidney and perinephric abscesses. Secondary hemorrhage is not uncommon. Other complications include hypertension resulting from fibrosis and ischemic kidney, renal artery thrombosis, arteriovenous aneurysms, fistula formation from extravasation of urine, urinomas, and pseudocysts.

OUTCOME MANAGEMENT

Whether conservative or surgical treatment should be used for renal trauma is controversial. Most physicians agree that kidney contusion calls for conservative treatment. Other minor injuries, such as small subcapsular hematomas and minor lacerations without extravasation, may also be better followed conservatively.

Clients with major injuries (e.g., renal fracture, parenchymal injury with major arterial occlusion, avulsion injuries, tears in the renal artery or vein, and parenchymal lacerations with extending perirenal hematomas or urinary extravasation) may require surgical exploration. Possible indications include continued moderate to severe hemorrhage and continued urinary extravasation. Urinary extravasation itself is not a definite reason for surgery because sterile urine usually resolves or is encapsulated spontaneously; however, it sometimes produces a severe tissue reaction and causes fistula formation. The pocket of extrarenal urine may also become obstructive.

Medical Management

Medical management, which primarily involves waiting and watching, is possible because the retroperitoneal space allows tamponade. In the absence of other injuries, a client with microscopic hematuria and normal findings on IVP may be observed on an ambulatory basis with careful instructions about activity restrictions and the need for adequate hydration. If there is gross hematuria, bed rest is required until the urine clears.

Serial observations of the urine, hematocrit level, and vital signs are made to watch the progress of the hemorrhage. Sequential urine specimens may be collected to compare current and previous urine color and turbidity.

Even if replacement fluids are not needed, a prophylactic intravenous line may be established, and a type and crossmatch for blood may be done. If a hematoma is present or IVP shows urine extravasation, the client may receive antibiotics to prevent sepsis. The physician prescribes blood transfusions if the hematocrit is low. After the urine clears, the client can be more active. After discharge, the client needs follow-up blood pressure checks and IVP studies to rule out secondary hypertension and anatomic changes in the renal system.

Nursing Management of the Medical Client

Nursing management of the client with renal trauma varies considerably, depending on extent of injury. The goals of nursing care are to prevent further bleeding and injury and to alleviate the client's anxiety.

Assessment includes checking for tenderness at the CVA. Watch for bleeding, which may occur as hematuria or may be internal, depending on the nature of the injury. Assess the client's vital signs for evidence of shock. Make serial observations of urine, hematocrit level, and vital signs to watch the progress of hemorrhage. Sequential urine specimens may be collected to compare current and previous urine color and turbidity.

Nursing interventions during conservative treatment center on monitoring urinary elimination patterns and helping the client to cope and comply with the medical regimen. If there is gross hematuria, bed rest is required until the urine clears. Monitoring includes assessment of vital signs as well as intake and output.

Notify the physician if urine output drops below 0.5 ml/kg/hour. Because bed rest can cause problems with bowel elimination and adequate fluid intake, circulation, and respiratory function, take appropriate measures to minimize the risk of these complications (passive exercise, for example).

A client with microscopic hematuria and normal IVP results who is observed on an ambulatory basis should be given careful instructions about activity restrictions and the need for adequate hydration.

Surgical Management

The greatest diversity of opinion concerns proper handling of the renal damage discovered during exploration. When the other kidney is functioning effectively, some physicians recommend free use of nephrectomy to avoid later sequelae, whereas others believe that the goal should be salvaging maximal renal function. The latter group advocates giving the conservative approach a fair trial and, if surgery is necessary, attempting to repair the kidney before deciding to remove it. With renal vascular injury, fewer than half of kidneys can be salvaged if the injury is 18 hours old; there is virtually no chance of renal recovery after 24 hours.

Renal hemorrhage may be controlled by injection of an autologous clot into the secondary arteries supplying the bleeding site. Blood is drawn from the client and allowed to clot. The clot is then injected angiographically. Because normal endothelium has a strong clot-lysing effect, the clot disappears from the normal adjacent vasculature after several hours and affects only the damaged portion.

If kidney repair is attempted rather than nephrectomy, the surgical procedure is designed to debride devitalized tissue, achieve hemostasis, establish a watertight seal of the collecting system, approximate the renal parenchymal edges, and drain the renal fossa.

Two surgical techniques improve the outcome of repair:

- *Extracorporeal,* or *bench, surgery* allows the kidney to be removed from the body for better visualization and manipulation of the organ during the repair process; the kidney is returned by autotransplantation. During its time outside the body, the kidney is maintained by hypothermia or by a perfusate mechanically pulsed through it.
- The *slush technique,* in which the kidney is immersed in iced saline slush, slows the metabolism and oxygen requirement of renal tissue, allowing longer intraoperative ischemic times. This technique causes some systemic hypothermia, but it is not significant. Pedicle vascular injury may also be repaired.

If either technique fails, nephrectomy is necessary.

Nursing Management of the Surgical Client

Nursing management of the client undergoing surgery for renal trauma is similar to that for other surgical procedures on the kidney (see Nephrectomy earlier in this chapter).

Self-Care

The client being observed on an ambulatory basis requires an appropriate teaching plan covering health maintenance activities and the need for a follow-up program. The client should promptly report any change in condition or recurrence of bleeding or pain to the physician. Strenuous activity should be avoided for several weeks or more, depending on the extent of the injury. The client must also maintain adequate hydration.

RENAL VASCULAR ABNORMALITIES

The kidneys depend on adequate blood circulation to nourish tissues and provide blood for filtration so that they can perform their intended functions. Anything that interferes with the normal circulatory flow significantly reduces renal function.

RENAL ARTERY DISEASE

Etiology and Risk Factors

Of all cases of renal artery disease, 90% are caused by atherosclerosis or fibromuscular dysplasia. Atherosclerosis affects males more often than females and usually involves the proximal third of the artery. Health promotion activities are the same as those for atherosclerosis as discussed with circulatory and cardiac disorders. Fibromuscular dysplasia is an alternating stenosis and dilation; arteriographic studies demonstrate a "string-of-beads" appearance of the artery. This condition affects females four to five times as often as males. Because the cause is unknown, there are no health promotion actions.

There are several other, less common, causes of renal artery disease. Cancer may obstruct the vessels. Embolism or thrombosis can cause acute obstruction. Trauma, as described earlier, can interrupt blood flow. The renal artery may be purposely occluded to produce a "medical nephrectomy" or total renal infarction; the occlusion may be done preoperatively in the case of renal adenocarcinoma or to control proteinuria or hypertension. Shredded Gelfoam can be used, or a liquid substance that polymerizes instantly when it comes in contact with blood may be injected into the renal artery. A dissecting aneurysm in the renal artery may also interrupt renal circulation.

Pathophysiology

The end result of any of these conditions, if severe enough, is reduced renal blood flow. The reduced flow causes renal parenchymal ischemia and, finally, renal atrophy. The role of renal artery disease in renovascular hypertension is also well documented, and hypertension alone may indicate treatment of the condition.

Clinical Manifestations

Because of the kidney's compensatory mechanisms, the gradual development of renal artery stenosis from atherosclerosis and cancer may lead to few manifestations, at least until the resulting hypertension and decreasing renal function become evident. Acute obstruction makes itself known relatively quickly, however. Manifestations of this sudden episode include flank pain over the affected kidney or abdominal pain and fever. Atrial dysrhythmias are a frequent finding; however, because they commonly alternate with periods of normal sinus rhythm, this manifestation can be missed. Urinalysis may be normal, and blood chemistry profiles may show elevated levels of aspartate aminotransferase and lactate dehydrogenase. IVP shows a nonfunctioning kidney, and a renal scan shows no arterial blood flow.

In response to reduced renal circulation, collateral circulation helps preserve the kidney if sufficient development takes place before total obstruction. Collateral circulation, in addition to a marked reduction in filtration, renal work, and oxygen requirements, allows the kidney to tolerate ischemic periods for up to several weeks. In acute total occlusion, a normal kidney can remain viable for about 2 hours before infarction and tissue necrosis begin.

OUTCOME MANAGEMENT

Surgical Management

Treatment of the ischemic kidney usually involves surgical revascularization. Arterial endarterectomy may be done with follow-up anticoagulant or antiplatelet therapy. In the technique known as *percutaneous transluminal renal angioplasty* (PTRA), the vessel is cleared with a balloon catheter. If it cannot be recanalized, a renal artery resection with end-to-end anastomosis or an aortorenal bypass graft procedure may be performed.

Percutaneous Transluminal Renal Angioplasty
In clients undergoing PTRA, a balloon-tipped catheter is inserted, usually through the femoral artery, and threaded under radiologic guidance to the obstructed renal artery. The physician inflates the balloon and pulls it through the obstructed area, stretching it and increasing the size of the arterial lumen. A stent may be placed at the site of occlusion to maintain the size of the lumen, prevent restenosis, and minimize the risk of abrupt vessel reclosure. If a stent is placed, antiplatelet agents or anticoagulants may be prescribed to minimize the risk of acute thrombosis.

Indications. Renal artery angioplasty is usually the first intervention for renovascular hypertension. If angioplasty is unsuccessful or if the condition recurs, more invasive surgical approaches are considered.

Contraindications. Angioplasty may be contraindicated if there is previous damage to the femoral artery or severely impaired circulation to the limb.

Complications. Renal artery angioplasty is considered a relatively safe procedure. The overall complication rate is about 10%. The most common complications include renal artery dissection, renal artery thrombosis or occlusion, segmental renal infarction, and hematoma formation or puncture trauma.

Outcomes. About one third of clients with renovascular hypertension do not respond to this therapy. A significant number are cured, and about half improve significantly. The treatment can be repeated if necessary. Clients usually return home in 24 to 48 hours.

Nursing Management of the Surgical Client

Preoperative Care
Because the length of stay is limited for most clients undergoing PTRA, it is a challenge to coordinate their care during the diagnostic and intervention phases of treatment. Typically, diagnostic tests such as angiograms and blood work are completed during the week before the procedure. Teaching about angioplasty and discharge instructions must be provided in a short period.

Postoperative Care
Care after PTRA is similar to other care after any angioplasty. Just after the procedure, vital signs are monitored every 15 minutes for 1 hour, every 30 minutes for 2 hours, hourly for 3 hours, and then regularly according to the established protocol. Check the dressing at these times for manifestations of bleeding or hematoma formation, and check peripheral pulses to assess circulation in the affected limb. Bed rest for up to 24 hours may be ordered.

In the longer term, the client's blood pressure should be monitored because hypertension can indicate recurrence of the lesion. Control of hypertension is crucial to preserving renal function.

After renal artery bypass graft surgery, nursing care is similar to other care after any kidney surgery, such as nephrectomy (discussed earlier in this chapter); however, in the postoperative period after an aortorenal bypass graft procedure, the client may experience an initial exacerbation of hypertension. Its cause is unclear, but it is thought to be related to systemic vasoconstriction secondary to general anesthesia and intraoperative hypothermia, severe pain, or transient renin secretion caused by clamping the aorta and manipulating the kidney. This episode usually lasts no more than 48 hours, but it can be significant and may require medical intervention. You must monitor blood pressure frequently.

RENAL VEIN DISEASE

The primary pathologic process involving the renal vein is thrombosis. Obstruction of venous drainage increases interstitial pressure, which reduces renal function. Findings include severe lumbar pain, renal enlargement, proteinuria, and hematuria. If the obstruction is bilateral, oliguria and azotemia occur. Contributing factors include diabetic nephropathy, chronic glomerulonephritis, and renal amyloidosis.

Kidney survival depends largely on the development of collateral circulation before the vessel is fully occluded. Embolectomy or ligation of the renal veins may be done, and anticoagulants may be prescribed. Intravenous streptokinase is used to lyse the occluding clot. If enough renal damage has occurred, nephrectomy is an option.

CONGENITAL DISORDERS

Renal congenital anomalies usually involve abnormalities in the number, position, form, size, or structure of the kidneys. Blood supply may be abnormal, although malformations that significantly affect renal function are rare. Anomalies of the ureteropelvic junction usually obstruct at that point and result in hydronephrosis. Typically, this situation is discovered and treated during childhood.

ANOMALIES INVOLVING KIDNEY NUMBER AND POSITION

Renal agenesis is the absence of one or both kidneys. Having only one kidney presents no difficulty if this kidney functions adequately. A client can live normally with one properly functioning kidney, as kidney donors aptly demonstrate. Bilateral agenesis, however, is fatal. Even in unilateral agenesis, the functioning kidney is at high risk for development of additional anomalies.

Supernumerary kidneys (more than two kidneys) are usually asymptomatic and are discovered during IVP. The extra ureter enters either the ipsilateral ureter or the bladder.

Ectopic, or malpositioned, kidneys are usually found in the pelvis, although thoracic kidneys have been documented. Problems associated with this anomaly include respiratory difficulties, pain caused by pressure on nerves or surrounding structures, and difficulty in childbirth.

Occasionally, one kidney may be across the midline so that both kidneys are on the same side. This condition usually remains undiscovered until infection or obstruction indicates a need for x-ray examination.

ANOMALIES INVOLVING KIDNEY FORM AND SIZE

Anomalies of kidney form and size include aplasia, hypoplasia, dysplasia, and *horseshoe kidney*. Aplastic kidneys are small and contracted and contain no

functioning renal tissue. Renal hypoplasia produces miniature kidneys with some functioning tissue. Although clinically this condition may be asymptomatic, it may cause hypertension and recurrent urinary tract infection.

Horseshoe kidney results when two kidneys are joined into a single organ whose shape somewhat resembles that of a horseshoe (Figure 35-4). The kidneys are connected, usually at the lower poles, by an isthmus of tissue. Because the developmental error interferes with normal ascent and medial rotation, the kidney is usually located in the lower lumbar region with its pelvis facing anteriorly. Although clients with horseshoe kidney may be asymptomatic, they are susceptible to hydronephrosis, infection secondary to ureteropelvic junction obstruction, and calculus formation.

ANOMALIES INVOLVING CYSTIC DISEASE

Cystic disease in renal tissue can range from a simple, solitary fluid-filled mass to almost complete replacement of renal structures by cystic tissue. A simple renal cyst commonly originates superficially in the renal parenchyma. It grows slowly and usually produces no manifestations until adulthood, when it may cause heaviness and pain in the abdomen and become a palpable mass. Arriving at a diagnosis may be complicated because renal cysts closely resemble malignant tumors; naturally, differentiation between the two is vital. As long as a simple renal cyst remains asymptomatic, intervention is usually unnecessary. If intervention is necessary, the cyst may be aspirated with a needle, or a partial nephrectomy may be performed to remove it.

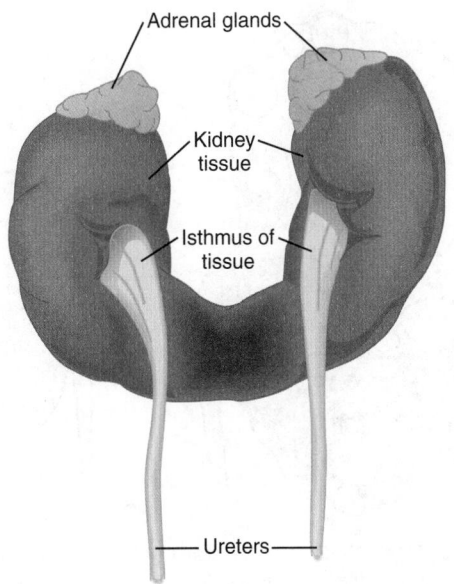

■ **FIGURE 35–4** A horseshoe kidney is usually created by tissue joining the lower poles.

Polycystic Kidneys

Polycystic disease of the kidney is a hereditary disorder in which grape-like cysts containing serous fluid, blood, or urine replace normal kidney tissue (Figure 35-5). The condition may develop at any age.

Infantile polycystic kidney disease is inherited as an autosomal recessive trait, and both parents must have carried the gene. It is a rare disorder that affects both kidneys and often the liver. In an infant, the disease usually causes death within days. Milder forms of the disease do not appear until childhood.

Adult polycystic disease accounts for about 10% of the clients receiving dialysis or transplantation. It is inherited as an autosomal dominant trait (see the Genetic Links feature at right). It usually appears after age 40, although it may begin as early as age 20 or as late as age 80. There are diverse manifestations; the most common are dull, aching lumbar or flank pain, which may be colicky, and hematuria. Other common findings are proteinuria, palpable kidney masses, pyuria, calculi, and uremia. Early in the disease, the ability to concentrate urine decreases. Hypertension develops along with cardiac enlargement and heart failure.

Polycystic liver disease occurs in about one third of cases, and cystic lesions are sometimes found in the thyroid, lung, pancreas, spleen, ovary, testis, epididymis, uterus, and bladder. Cerebral aneurysms occur in about 2% of clients with polycystic kidney disease.

The cystic kidney can become so enlarged that it causes severe pressure on other organs, with production of additional extrarenal manifestations. The ultimate result of this disease is ESRD (see Chapter 36). As the disease slowly progresses, renal nephrons are destroyed,

renal function deteriorates, and uremia ultimately results. The mean duration of polycystic kidney disease from onset of manifestations to development of uremia varies a great deal and may be 15 to 30 years or longer.

Because there is no known way to arrest the progress of the destructive cysts, conservative medical treatment is designed to preserve kidney function. Urinary tract infection is the most common complication because of the distorted renal architecture; chronic infection can occur if resistant bacteria develop. Aggressive control of hypertension is essential.

Unlike clients with decreasing creatinine clearance rates caused by other kidney diseases, those with polycystic kidney disease seem to waste rather than retain sodium. Thus they may need increased sodium and water intake. However, if they are hypertensive, which is often the case, dietary sodium is restricted. Dietary restrictions should be individualized for all clients with chronic kidney disease. When ESRD develops, dialysis or renal transplantation is required. Nursing

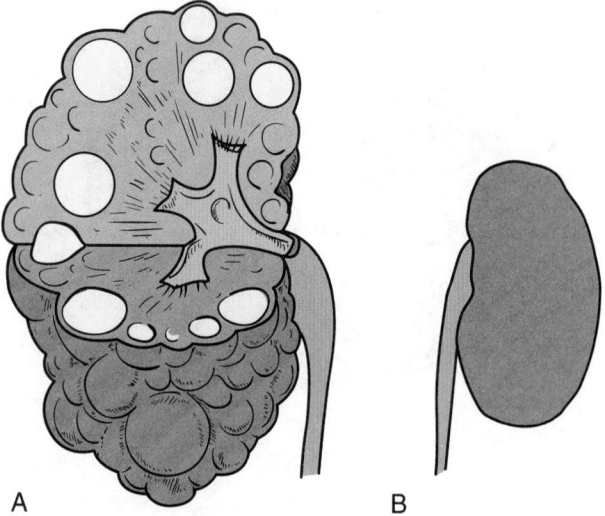

■ **FIGURE 35–5** Polycystic kidney **(A)** filled with fluid or blood-filled cysts that alter the architecture of the kidney. Notice how much larger it is in size compared to a normal kidney **(B)**.

A B

GENETIC LINKS

Autosomal Dominant Polycystic Kidney Disease Description

Autosomal dominant polycystic kidney disease (ADPKD) is an adult-onset disorder characterized by progressive cyst development and bilaterally enlarged polycystic kidneys. Clinical features include renal function abnormalities, hypertension, pain, and renal insufficiency. About 50% of clients develop end-stage renal disease by about age 60. Cysts can also occur in other organs (e.g., liver, pancreas). The prevalence of ADPKD in live births ranges from 1:400 to 1:1000 with approximately 400,000 affected people in the United States.

GENETICS

ADPKD is caused by mutations in the *PKD1* gene (~85% of cases) located on chromosome 16 or the *PKD2* gene (~15% of cases) located on chromosome 4. Molecular genetic testing of the *PKD1* and *PKD2* genes is available clinically. As an autosomal dominant condition, offspring of an affected individual with ADPKD have a 50% chance of inheriting the disease-causing mutation. Most clients have a parent with ADPKD, but de novo mutations (new or spontaneous mutations) occur in about 10% of families.

DIAGNOSIS/TESTING

Diagnosis is established by imaging studies of the kidneys or by molecular genetic testing of the *PKD1* and *PKD2* genes.

MANAGEMENT

As yet there is no treatment specifically directed towards the disease. Current therapy is aimed at reducing morbidity and mortality from renal and other complications of the disease.

interventions for clients with renal failure are discussed in Chapter 36.

Genetic counseling (see Chapter 15) is advisable because of the hereditary nature of the disease, especially if the disease is diagnosed during childbearing years. Because the disease typically appears after the childbearing period, however, the likelihood of transmitting the disease to another generation is high. Therefore counseling the extended family is essential when the disease has been identified.

Adult-Onset Medullary Cystic Disease

Adult-onset medullary cystic disease, sometimes called *uremic sponge kidney* or *medullary polycystic disease,* is also an autosomal dominant disorder. It is similar to polycystic disease in all aspects except that it progresses to uremia rapidly after its onset in the teenage years or between ages 20 and 29. Hemodialysis and renal transplantation are likely to be required.

Medullary Sponge Kidney

Medullary sponge kidney is a cystic disorder in which spaces are produced at the apex of the renal pyramids. Onset peaks during adolescence or between ages 30 and 40 years. Infection, calculi, pain, and hematuria are potential complications. Renal function usually remains adequate unless the client has uncontrolled infection or calculi.

OTHER HEREDITARY RENAL DISORDERS

Other hereditary renal disorders include some types of chronic nephritis (such as Alport's syndrome), congenital nephrotic syndrome, distal renal tubular acidosis, idiopathic hypercalciuria, and nephrotic diabetes insipidus. Many of these conditions are fatal during childhood, but some persist into adulthood and are discussed in the appropriate parts of this text.

CONCLUSIONS

Renal disorders are highly complex. You must have a clear understanding of the structure and function of the renal system to care for clients with these conditions. The outcomes of successful treatment include preservation of renal function.

THINKING CRITICALLY

1. A 35-year-old newlywed woman enters the emergency department with acute abdominal pain and a temperature of 101.8° F. Her abdomen is distended, and she has not had a bowel movement today, even though she is usually regular. The abdominal pain is diffuse and on the right side. She has no rebound tenderness and no pain at McBurney's point. Her WBC is 15,000/mm³. What problems other than appendicitis might she be experiencing? What other assessments should be made?

Factors to Consider. What type of renal problem might she be experiencing? What teaching would she need once the diagnosis is made? What medication might be prescribed and why? What follow-up is needed?

2. L.S. is a 22-year-old male college student with a diagnosis of acute glomerulonephritis. Three weeks ago, he received oral antibiotic therapy for strep throat. He is scheduled for a renal biopsy to confirm a diagnosis of acute poststreptococcal glomerulonephritis. What other diagnostic assessments should be made? What is the expected course of treatment?

Factors to Consider. What teaching does this client need when the diagnosis is confirmed? What medication might be prescribed, and how will it be delivered? What follow-up is needed?

3. C.H. is a 68-year-old retired mail carrier who lives with his wife. They spend 6 months living in their home state in the Midwest and spend the winter months in Arizona. The client is admitted with a diagnosis of suspected renal cell carcinoma. Diagnostic tests confirm the diagnosis. What surgical procedure will be scheduled? What nursing interventions are associated with this procedure?

Factors to Consider. What diagnostic tests were used to confirm the diagnosis of renal carcinoma? What tests will be used to determine whether radiation, chemotherapy, and immunotherapy are needed? Describe the postoperative assessments you should make for pain management, vital signs, surgical dressings, drainage tubes, and urine output. If Mr. and Mrs. H. plan to drive to Arizona a month after surgery, what should you discuss with them about their travel plans?

Discussions for these questions can be found on the website.

BIBLIOGRAPHY

 Citations appearing in red refer to primary research.

 Citations appearing in blue refer to evidence-based practice guidelines and protocols.

1. American Cancer Society. (2007). *Cancer facts and figures.* Atlanta: Author.
2. American Diabetes Association. (2004). Nephropathy in diabetes. *Diabetes Care, 27,* S79-S83.
3. Avery-Lynch, M. (2004). The genetic role in autosomal dominant polycystic kidney disease and nephrology clinical practice. *CANNT Journal, 14*(4), 26-30.
4. Brenner, B.M., & Levine, S.A. (Eds.) (2004). *Brenner and Rector's the kidney* (7th ed.). Philadelphia: Saunders.
5. Burrows-Hudson, S. (2005). Chronic kidney disease: An overview. Early and aggressive treatment is vital. *American Journal of Nursing, 105*(2), 40-49.

6. Campese, V.M., Mitra, N., & Sandee, D. (2006). Hypertension in renal parenchymal disease: Why is it so resistant to treatment? *Kidney International, 69*, 967-973.

7. Campoy, S., & Elwell, R. (2005). Pharmacology and CKD. *American Journal of Nursing, 105*(9), 60-72.

8. Chadban, S.J., & Atkins, R.C. (2005). Glomerulonephritis. *Lancet, 365*(9473), 1797-1806.

9. Coppin, C., Prozolt, F., Awa, A., et al. (2004). Immunotherapy for advanced renal cell cancer. *Cochrane Database of Systematic Reviews, 3*, CD001425.

10. Coresh, J., Astor, B.C., Greene, T., et al. (2003). Prevalence of chronic kidney disease and decreased kidney function in the adult US population: Third National Health Nutrition Examination Survey. *American Journal of Kidney Diseases, 41*(1), 1-12.

11. Dinwiddie, L., Burrows-Hudson, S., & Peacock, E. (2006). Stage 4 chronic kidney disease. *American Journal of Nursing, 106*(9), 40-52.

12. Eknoyan, G. (2004). On the central role of studies on the kidney in the recognition, conceptual evolution and understanding of hypertension. *Advances in Chronic Kidney Disease, 11*, 192-196.

13. Eknoyan, G. (2004). Alternative and complementary medicine and chronic kidney disease. *Advances in Chronic Kidney Disease, 12*, 245-338.

14. Fisher, M., Lehnerz, S., Hebert, J., & Parikh, C. (2004). Kidney disease is an independent risk factor for adverse fetal and maternal outcomes in pregnancy. *American Journal of Kidney Disease, 43*, 415-423.

15. Fishman, M., & Antonia, S. (2004). Specific antitumor vaccine for renal cancer. *Lancet, 363*(9409), 583-584.

16. Fox, C.S., Larson, M.G., Larson, M.G., et al. (2004). Predictors of new-onset kidney disease in a community based population. *Journal of the American Medical Association, 291*, 844-850.

17. Fried, L.F., Orchard, T.J., & Kasiske, B.L. (2001). The effect of lipid reduction on renal disease progression: A meta analysis. *Kidney International, 59*, 260-269.

18. Goldman, L., & Ausiello, D. (Eds.) (2004). *Cecil textbook of medicine* (22nd ed.). Philadelphia: Saunders.

19. Goodman, W.G. (2004). The consequences of uncontrolled secondary hyperparathyroidism and its treatment in chronic kidney disease. *Seminars in Dialysis, 17*(3), 209-216.

20. Graham, D.J., Staffa, J.A., Shatin, D., et al. (2004). Incidence of hospitalized rhabdomyolysis in patients treated with lipid-lowering drugs. *Journal of the American Medical Association, 292*, 2585-2590.

21. Guyton, A.C., & Hall, J.E. (2005). *Textbook of medical physiology* (11th ed.). Philadelphia: Saunders.

22. Hansberry, M.R., Whittier, W.L., & Krause, M.W. (2005). The elderly patient with chronic kidney disease. *Advances in Chronic Kidney Disease, 12*(1), 71-77.

23. Harriston, S. (2004). A review of rhabdomyolysis. *Dimensions of Critical Care Nursing, 23*, 155-161.

24. Holcomb, S.S. (2005). Evaluating chronic kidney disease risk. *Nurse Practitioner, 30*(4), 12-14, 17-18.

25. Johansen, K.L. (2005). Exercise and chronic kidney disease: Current recommendations. *Sports Medicine, 35*(6), 485-499.

26. Karnik, J., & Chertow, G.M. (2000). Analgesic-related renal disease: Causes, patients at risk, management. *Journal of Critical Illness, 15*(1), 49-51, 55-58.

27. Kausz, A.T. (2004). Chronic kidney disease in the older patient with diabetes. *Clinical Geriatrics, 12*(7), 39-47.

28. Koeppen, B.M., & Stanton, B.A. (2007). *Renal physiology* (4th ed.). St. Louis: Mosby.

29. Kramer, H., & Molitch, M.E. (2005). Screening for kidney disease in adults with diabetes. *Diabetes Care, 28*, 1813-1816.

30. Legg, V. (2005). Complications of chronic kidney disease: A close look at renal osteodystrophy, nutritional disturbances, and inflammation. *American Journal of Nursing, 105*(6), 40-49.

31. McCarley, P.B., & Salai, P.B. (2005). Cardiovascular disease in chronic kidney disease: Recognizing and reducing the risk of a common CKD morbidity. *American Journal of Nursing, 105*(4), 40-53.

32. McClellan, W.M. (2006). The epidemic of renal disease—What drives it and what can be done? *Nephrology Dialysis and Transplantation, 21*, 1461-1464.

33. Meister, J., & Reddy, K. (2002). Rhabdomyolysis: An overview: This rare disease may be on the rise. *American Journal of Nursing, 102*(2), 75, 77, 79.

34. Molzahn, A.E., & Butera, E. (2006). *Contemporary nephrology nursing: Principles and practice.* Pitman, NJ: American Nephrology Nurses Association.

35. Morey, A.F., & McAninch, J.W.R. (1996). Renal trauma: Principles of evaluation and management. *Trauma Quarterly, 13*(1), 79-94.

36. National Kidney Foundation. (2003a). K/DOQI clinical practice guidelines for bone metabolism and disease in chronic kidney disease. *American Journal of Kidney Diseases, 42*(Suppl 3), S1-S201.

37. National Kidney Foundation. (2003b). K/DOQI clinical practice guidelines for managing dyslipidemias in chronic kidney disease. *American Journal of Kidney Diseases, 41*(Suppl 3), S1-S91.

38. National Kidney Foundation. (2004). K/DOQI clinical practice guidelines on blood pressure management and use of antihypertensive agents in chronic kidney disease. *American Journal of Kidney Diseases, 42*(Suppl 3), S1-S201.

39. Nelson, D.B. (2003). Minimal change glomerulopathy in pregnancy. *Nephrology Nursing Journal, 30*, 45-57.

40. Neutel, J.M. (2006). The role of combination therapy in the management of hypertension. *Nephrology Dialysis and Transplantation, 21*, 1469-1474.

41. Palmieri, P.A. (2002). Obstructive nephropathy: Pathophysiology, diagnosis and collaborative management. *Nephrology Nursing Journal, 29*, 15-23.

42. Ramakrishnan, K., & Scheid, D.C. (2005). Diagnosis and management of acute pyelonephritis in adults. *American Family Physician, 71*, 933-942.

43. Rosenstein, D., & McAninch, J.W. (2003). Update on the management of renal trauma. *Contemporary Urology, 15*(7), 42-44.

44. Rule, A.D., Larson, T.S., Bergstralh, E.J., et al. (2004). Using serum creatinine to estimate glomerular filtration rate: Accuracy in good health and in chronic kidney disease. *Annals of Internal Medicine, 141*(12), 929-937.

45. Russell, T.A. (2005). Acute renal failure related to rhabdomyolysis: Pathophysiology, diagnosis, and collaborative management. *Nephrology Nursing Journal, 32*, 409-419.

46. Russell, T.A. (2006). Diabetic nephropathy in patients with type 1 diabetes mellitus. *Nephrology Nursing Journal, 33*, 15-28.

47. Sarnak, M.J., Greene, T., Wang, X., et al. (2005). The effect of a lower target blood pressure on the progression of kidney disease: Long term follow-up of the Modification of Diet in Renal Disease Study. *Annals of Internal Medicine, 142*(5), 342-351.

48. Scholes, D., Hooton, T.M., Roberts, P.L., et al. (2005). Risk factors associated with acute pyelonephritis in healthy women. *Annals of Internal Medicine, 142*(1), 20-27.

49. Schrier, R.W. (2005). *Manual of nephrology* (6th ed.). Philadelphia: Lippincott, Williams & Wilkins.

50. Schrier, R.W. (2002). *Renal and electrolyte disorders* (6th ed.). Philadelphia: Lippincott, Williams & Wilkins.

51. Shoham, D.A., Vupputuri, S., & Kshirsagar, A.V. (2005). Chronic kidney disease and life course socioeconomic status: A review. *Advances in Chronic Kidney Disease, 12*(1), 56-63.

52. Sica, D. (2004). Optimizing hypertension and vascular health: Focus on ethnicity. *Clinical Cornerstone, 6*(4), 28-38.

53. Strauss, W., & Zimmerman, R.W. (2004). Advisor forum. The latest on renal cancer. *Clinical Advisor for Nurse Practitioners, 7*(1), 57.

54. Tanagho, E.A., & McAninch, J.W. (2004). *Smith's general urology* (16th ed.). Norwalk, Conn: Lange Medical Books/McGraw-Hill.

55. Then, K.L., & Rankin, J.A. (2004). Hypertension: A review for clinicians. *Nursing Clinics of North America, 39*, 793-814.

56. Thomas-Hawkins, C., & Zazworsky, D. (2005). Self-management of chronic kidney disease. *American Journal of Nursing, 105*(10), 40-49.

57. Thorp, M.L., Eastman, L., & Smith, D.H. (2006). Managing the burden of chronic kidney disease. *Disease Management, 9*, 115-121.

58. Toto, R.D., Rinner, S., & Ram, C.V.S. (2004). Symposium on hypertension. ACE inhibitors and target organ protection: An expanded role for these antihypertensive agents. *Postgraduate Medicine, 116*(2), 11-16.

59. Vupputuri, S., Batumen, V., Muntner, P., et al. (2004). The risk for mild kidney function decline associated with illicit drug use among hypertensive men. *American Journal of Kidney Diseases, 43*, 629-635.

60. Walsh, P., & Retik, A.B. (2002). *Campbell's urology* (8th ed.). Philadelphia: Saunders.

evolve   *Did you remember to check out the bonus material on the Evolve website and the CD-ROM, including NCLEX®-Examination Style Review Questions, Open-Book Quizzes, and Chapter Review Audio Podcasts?*

http://evolve.elsevier.com/Black/medsurg

CHAPTER 36

Management of Clients with Renal Failure

Anita E. Molzahn

A disruption in renal function impairs the body's ability to maintain fluid, electrolyte, and acid-base balance. Reduced renal function interferes with erythropoietin and prostaglandin synthesis. Insulin degradation and the renin-angiotensin-aldosterone system are also affected by decreased renal function.

The most common diseases and problems that cause renal failure are described in Chapter 35. In this chapter, manifestations of acute and chronic renal failure and treatments used to replace or restore renal function, such as dialysis and transplantation, are outlined. Psychosocial needs may arise from the physiologic problems caused by stage 5 chronic kidney disease (CKD) (also known as end-stage renal disease [ESRD]). You have a key role in helping promote quality of life and rehabilitation for these clients.

UREMIC SYNDROME

The terms uremia, uremic syndrome, and renal failure are used synonymously. *Uremia* literally means "urine in the blood." This term and the term *uremic syndrome* describe a set of manifestations that result from loss of renal function. This loss may be of sudden onset or may develop over a long period. It may be self-limiting or irreversible. Sudden loss of kidney function, as occurs with damage from trauma, shock, toxins, or acute glomerulonephritis, brings on uremia rapidly and usually causes severe deterioration of the client's condition. Gradual loss of kidney function over an extended period may occur with glomerulonephritis, hypertension, chronic pyelonephritis, and other diseases.

Because the kidneys perform a wide variety of functions, the effects of uremia occur not only in the kidneys but also in other organ systems. Because of the time involved, CKD causes more degenerative changes throughout the body than acute uremia does. However, both types

of renal failure have many of the same consequences. Unless the process can be halted or replacement therapy initiated, coma, seizures, and death result.

ACUTE RENAL FAILURE

Acute renal failure (ARF) refers to the abrupt loss of kidney function. Over a period of hours to a few days, the glomerular filtration rate (GFR) decreases. Serum creatinine and urea nitrogen or blood urea nitrogen (BUN) levels increase. A healthy adult who eats a normal diet needs a minimum urine output of about 400 ml over 24 hours to excrete the body's waste products through the kidneys. Any lower amount indicates a decreased GFR. *Oliguria* refers to daily outputs of urine between 100 and 400 ml; *anuria* refers to urine output of less than 100 ml.

Etiology and Risk Factors

There are many possible causes of ARF, the most common of which are hypotension and prerenal hypovolemia. The etiologic mechanisms of these disorders are discussed in Chapter 35.

Classification

The numerous causes of ARF can be categorized into three major areas: prerenal, intrarenal, and postrenal (Figure 36-1).

Prerenal Causes

Prerenal causes of ARF are those that interfere with renal perfusion. The kidneys depend on adequate delivery of blood to be filtered by the glomeruli. 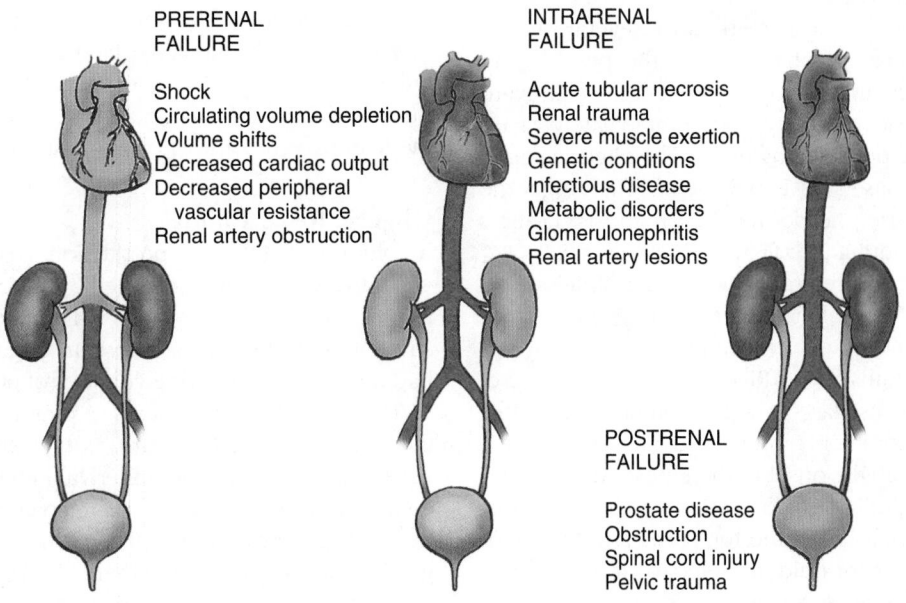 Therefore reduced renal blood flow lowers the GFR and can lead to ARF. Conditions that contribute to decreased renal blood flow include the following:

- Circulatory volume depletion, as may occur with diarrhea, vomiting, hemorrhage, excessive use of diuretics, burns, renal salt-wasting conditions, or glycosuria
- Volume shifts, as from third-space sequestration of fluid, vasodilation, or gram-negative sepsis
- Decreased cardiac output, as during cardiac pump failure, pericardial tamponade, or acute pulmonary embolism
- Decreased peripheral vascular resistance, as from spinal anesthesia, septic shock, or anaphylaxis
- Vascular obstruction, such as bilateral renal artery occlusion or dissecting aneurysm

Intrarenal Causes

Intrarenal (or renal) causes of ARF involve parenchymal changes caused by disease or nephrotoxic substances. Acute tubular necrosis is the most common intrarenal cause of ARF and accounts for about 75% of cases. This destruction of the tubular epithelial cells results from impaired renal perfusion or direct damage by nephrotoxins. In addition to the nephrotoxins described in Chapter 35, acute tubular necrosis may be caused by heme pigments, such as myoglobin and hemoglobin, which are liberated from damaged muscle tissue. This release may result from trauma (rhabdomyolysis), such as surgery, crush injury, and electric shock, or from nontraumatic conditions, such as severe muscle exertion, genetic conditions (such as diabetes mellitus or malignant hyperthermia), infectious disease, metabolic conditions (such as hypokalemia, phosphatemia, or heat stroke), and rejection of a transplanted kidney.

Other intrarenal causes of ARF include glomerulonephritis; microvascular and large vascular lesions, as in hemolytic-uremic syndrome; thrombosis; vasculitis; scleroderma; trauma; atherosclerosis; tumor invasion; and cortical necrosis, which is caused by prolonged vasospasm of the cortical blood vessels.

Postrenal Causes

Postrenal causes of ARF arise from an obstruction in the urinary tract, anywhere from the tubules to the urethral meatus. Common sources of obstruction include prostatic hypertrophy, calculi, invading tumors, surgical accidents, ureteral or urethral strictures or stenosis, and retroperitoneal fibrosis. Spinal cord injury may lead to decreased bladder emptying and a functional obstruction.

General Considerations

In management of the client with ARF, it is important to determine whether the disorder originates from prerenal, intrarenal, or postrenal causes before intervention begins. Appropriate interventions require determining the cause of the disorder.

One health promotion strategy is to teach clients about the risks of nephrotoxic agents identified in Chapter 35. Other health promotion and health maintenance actions include monitoring of vital signs and urine output and early identification and reversal of hypotension and hypovolemia, the two causes of ARF

PRERENAL FAILURE

Shock
Circulating volume depletion
Volume shifts
Decreased cardiac output
Decreased peripheral
    vascular resistance
Renal artery obstruction

INTRARENAL FAILURE

Acute tubular necrosis
Renal trauma
Severe muscle exertion
Genetic conditions
Infectious disease
Metabolic disorders
Glomerulonephritis
Renal artery lesions

POSTRENAL FAILURE

Prostate disease
Obstruction
Spinal cord injury
Pelvic trauma

■ **FIGURE 36–1** Causes of acute renal failure: prerenal, intrarenal, and postrenal.

associated with the highest mortality rates. Prevention of urinary obstruction is another health promotion and maintenance action.

Pathophysiology

The pathogenesis of ARF is not clear. One hypothesis is that the damaged tubules cannot conserve sodium normally, which activates the renin-angiotensin-aldosterone system. The effect is to redistribute the renal vascular supply by increasing the tone of both the afferent and efferent arterioles. The resulting ischemia may cause an increase in vasopressin, cellular swelling, inhibition of prostaglandin synthesis, and further stimulation of the renin-angiotensin system. The reduced blood flow decreases glomerular pressure, GFR, and tubular flow; thus oliguria occurs.

Another theory is that cellular and protein debris in the tubule obstructs the lumen, which raises the intratubular pressure. The increasing oncotic pressure opposes filtration pressure until glomerular filtration stops. A biochemical theory claims that decreased renal blood flow leads to decreased oxygen delivery to the proximal tubules; this causes a reduction in cellular adenosine triphosphate, which increases cytosolic and mitochondrial calcium concentrations. The result of this process is cell death and tubular necrosis. Vasomotor nephropathy, which causes spasms of peritubular capillaries, may result in tubular damage. Other possible pathogenic mechanisms include leakage of filtered urine through damaged tubules back into the peritubular capillaries and chemical or morphologic changes in the basement membrane of the glomerular capillary, which decrease nephron filtration. The reversibility of this mechanism depends on the level of destruction of the basement membrane.

Clinical Manifestations

The clinical course of ARF is marked by several phases. The onset (or initiating) phase covers the period from the precipitating event to the development of renal manifestations. Manifestations may begin immediately or up to a week after the precipitating event. The oliguric-anuric (or nonoliguric) phase lasts 1 to 8 weeks. The longer the oliguric-anuric phase, the poorer the prognosis. Dialysis may be required during the oliguric-anuric phase.

A gradual or abrupt return to glomerular filtration and leveling of the BUN signal the diuretic phase. Urine output may be 1000 to 2000 ml/day, which may lead to dehydration; 25% of the deaths from ARF occur during this phase.

The recovery phase lasts 3 to 12 months. During this time, the client commonly returns to an activity level similar to that before the onset of the illness. Mild tubular abnormalities, including glycosuria and decreased concentrating ability, may continue for years, and the client is continually at risk for fluid and electrolyte imbalance, especially during times of stress.

The effects of ARF are widespread. The major consequences include the following:

- Fluid and electrolyte imbalances (fluid overload or depletion, hyperkalemia, hyponatremia, hypocalcemia, and hypermagnesemia)
- Acidosis
- Increased susceptibility to secondary infections
- Anemia
- Platelet dysfunction
- Gastrointestinal complications (anorexia, nausea, vomiting, diarrhea or constipation, and stomatitis)
- Increased incidence of pericarditis
- Uremic encephalopathy characterized by apathy, defective recent memory, episodic obtundation, dysarthria, tremors, convulsions, and coma
- Impaired wound healing

Other manifestations are usually a result of these sequelae. The most common overall manifestation of ARF is alteration of the expected urine output. Usually, oliguria or anuria is found, but polyuric ARF accounts for 30% of the cases. There are two varieties of ARF: nonoliguric and oliguric.

Nonoliguric Renal Failure

Although nonoliguric, or polyuric, ARF is being recognized more often, its status remains controversial. It may be an independent entity or may be a phase of oliguric ARF.

Clients with nonoliguric renal failure may excrete as much as 2 L/day, and this must be recognized as a possible manifestation of ARF. The urine produced is dilute and nearly iso-osmolar, reflected in a low urine specific gravity indicating that not all nephrons have stopped filtering. Hypertension and tachypnea, with manifestations of fluid overload, are commonly found. The client may also demonstrate manifestations of extracellular fluid depletion, such as dry mucous membranes, poor skin turgor, and orthostatic hypotension. Nonoliguric renal failure is usually associated with less morbidity and mortality than the oliguric form, probably because of the lesser degree and shorter duration of azotemia.

Oliguric Renal Failure

In oliguric ARF, urine production is usually less than 400 ml/day. However, the aging kidney normally loses its concentrating ability, and renal function becomes more susceptible to insult. Therefore an older client may have had oliguria even at urine volumes of 600 to 700 ml/day.

The clinical manifestations of oliguric ARF depend on the cause. In prerenal failure, assessment findings are diverse, depending on the underlying condition. The client commonly has a history of a precipitating event, such as hemorrhage or cardiac insult. The urine has a high specific gravity and osmolarity, and there is little or no proteinuria. Urine sediment is usually normal, although it may contain a few hyaline and granular casts. There is little urinary sodium excretion. The BUN/creatinine ratio is significantly elevated, reaching levels between 10:1 and 40:1.

Systemic manifestations of intrinsic renal failure may include edema, weight gain, hemoptysis resulting from elevated left ventricular end-diastolic pressure, weakness from anemia, and hypertension. The urine has a fixed specific gravity, a high sodium concentration, and definite proteinuria. The client with glomerulonephritis has hematuria and red blood cell and hemoglobin casts. Acute tubular necrosis causes muddy brown granular casts. If there has been significant tissue damage, expect elevated levels of serum creatinine, phosphokinase, and potassium.

Urine produced in postrenal failure may have fixed specific gravity and elevated sodium concentration with little or no proteinuria. Urine sediment is generally normal. The most definitive manifestations are those indicating obstruction, as described with calculi and neoplasms. Wide fluctuations between anuria and polyuria may indicate intermittent urinary tract obstruction. The Integrating Diagnostic Testing feature on p. 812 summarizes diagnostic tests used to evaluate acute renal failure.

Prognosis

The mortality rate in ARF may be as high as 50%; the highest mortality rates occur when failure is caused by trauma or surgery. The lowest mortality rate is in ARF caused by nephrotoxic substances (see Chapter 35). When obstruction or glomerulonephritis is the cause, the mortality rate is low.

OUTCOME MANAGEMENT

Medical Management

Prevent Acute Renal Failure

The medical management of ARF is largely based on preventing and treating its effects. As with any disease process, prevention is the primary intervention. Attaining and maintaining adequate hydration and diuresis in high-risk clients are crucial, as is the prevention of contributing factors.

Once ARF has developed, prompt recognition and action facilitate restoration of optimal renal function. Correction of the underlying condition, such as hydration for a client with hypovolemic shock, may be all that is necessary in ARF caused by prerenal disorders. Postrenal causes must be rectified. In the meantime, the sequelae of ARF require specific intervention.

Maintain Fluid and Electrolyte Balance

In ARF, maintenance of fluid and electrolyte balance is key to survival. Imbalances are common and pose significant challenges to the clinician.

Fluid replacement must be done carefully to avoid fluid overload. Fluid replacement volumes are usually calculated on the basis of some fraction of the previous day's urine output plus an amount (commonly 400 ml) to account for the usual insensible losses that occur during a 24-hour period. Amounts lost in other ways, such as vomiting and diarrhea, are added to the daily allotment. Unless the client is receiving total parenteral nutrition (TPN), some physicians use a daily weight loss of 0.2 to 0.5 kg/day as a measure of the success of the fluid replacement program. This amount represents the usual daily weight loss through catabolism and loss of lean body mass.

Diuretic therapy may be used cautiously. Furosemide and mannitol are the drugs used most often, but furosemide can be nephrotoxic, increasing the risk of further renal damage. It is also important to avoid dehydration, and fluids should be replaced as needed to maintain adequate blood flow to the kidneys.

Electrolyte replacement is based primarily on urine and serum electrolyte concentrations. Hyperkalemia is probably the most dangerous imbalance because of its contribution to cardiac dysrhythmias and arrest. In addition to the kidney's inability to excrete potassium, this electrolyte is released in greater quantities from the body cells when acidosis is present and is further increased by rapid tissue catabolism.

Electrocardiographic monitors are commonly used to check for effects of hypokalemia or hyperkalemia. Treatment of hyperkalemia is described in the Integrating Pharmacology box on p. 813. Hyponatremia usually results from dilution rather than true lack of sodium. Therefore intervention is a matter of proper fluid replacement (i.e., fluid restriction and self-correction).

Because magnesium is normally excreted by the kidneys, it can accumulate in renal failure. Dark green vegetables, unrefined grains, seeds, nuts, legumes, and antacids and osmotic laxatives containing magnesium should be avoided because they increase serum magnesium levels.

Metabolic acidosis usually results from the accumulation of acid waste products. Sodium bicarbonate, sodium lactate, or sodium acetate may be used in the short term to correct this condition. Dialysis is usually used for severe acidosis.

The Integrating Pharmacology feature highlights some of the common medications used in ARF.

Replace Renal Function

Dialysis (detailed later in the chapter) is frequently required for treatment of ARF. Indications for dialysis include significant volume overload, uncontrolled hyperkalemia or acidosis, progressive uremia as evidenced by rising BUN and creatinine concentrations, altered central nervous system function, and pericarditis.

Acute Renal Failure

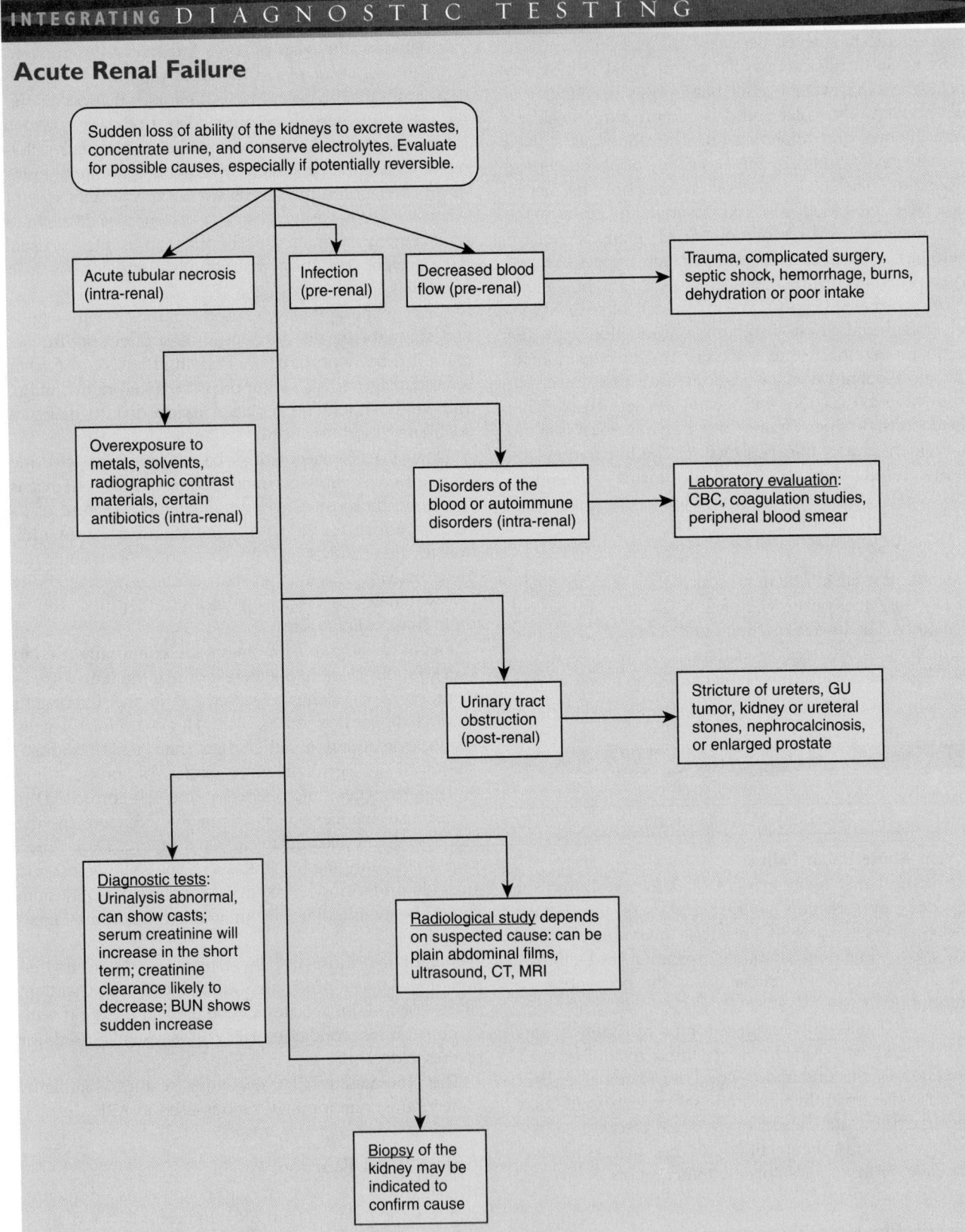

Medications for Acute Renal Failure

Treatment of acute renal failure (ARF) depends on the cause of the renal failure. For instance, in some autoimmune diseases, immunosuppressive agents may be prescribed. Generally, treatment is based on manifestations. Low doses (1 to 5 mcg/kg/min) of dopamine hydrochloride (Intropin) may be given to activate dopamine receptors in the kidney. Dopamine, a sympathomimetic, can dilate renal blood vessels, which improves renal function, increases urine flow, and increases sodium excretion to improve renal function.

Metabolic acidosis is common and is typically treated with sodium bicarbonate. Hypertension is also a common manifestation of ARF. Where hypertension is a result of fluid volume excess, fluid removal through renal replacement therapy is generally preferable to the administration of antihypertensive medications. In other cases, hypertension is caused by an excess of renin production by the kidneys (starting the renin-angiotensin system); aggressive antihypertensive therapy is then needed to control blood pressure effectively. Diuretic therapy may be used cautiously. Furosemide and mannitol are the drugs used most often, but furosemide can be nephrotoxic, increasing the risk of further renal damage. Diuretics are typically not very effective in clients with advanced renal failure.

Hyperkalemia is potentially life-threatening because of the risk of cardiac arrest; it should be treated immediately and aggressively. Treatment may include administration of calcium, which antagonizes membrane actions. Cation exchange resins may be administered orally or rectally to facilitate excretion of potassium through the gastrointestinal tract. Cation exchange resins (e.g., Kayexalate) that exchange potassium for other electrolytes can be administered orally or rectally. They start to act within 2 to 3 hours. Sorbitol, an osmotic cathartic, is given with cation exchange resins to induce a diarrhea to eliminate the potassium ions that were exchanged for sodium ions in the resins. Sorbitol can be given orally, as an enema, or by nasogastric tube. Potassium-containing foods and medications should be avoided. In an emergency, administration of 50% glucose and regular insulin, with sodium bicarbonate if necessary, can temporarily prevent cardiac arrest by moving potassium into the cells and reducing serum potassium levels. Insulin and glucose (beta$_2$-adrenergic agonists) and sodium bicarbonate force potassium into the cells; these three types of medications work within 30 to 60 minutes and last several hours.

Infection is one of the most frequent complications of ARF and occurs in as many as 70% of cases. Prophylactic use of antibiotics is sometimes indicated and treatment of infections is based on culture and sensitivity reports.

In ARF, particular care should be taken to avoid nephrotoxic agents to prevent further injury to the already damaged kidneys. The absorption, distribution, metabolism, and elimination of medications must be considered before medications are prescribed or administered. If the kidneys are not functioning, drugs that are normally excreted by the kidney can accumulate to toxic levels. Some drugs are removed by dialysis; others are not. All these factors should be considered when determining dosage, route, and time of administration. Also, drugs that are nephrotoxic (e.g., aminoglycosides, intravenous pyelogram [IVP] dye) may cause further damage to a dysfunctional organ and should be avoided.

There are some special considerations for dialysis of clients with ARF. First, heparin is generally decreased to reduce the risk of bleeding. Because hypotension is common, clients must be carefully monitored and replacement fluids provided as appropriate.

For clients with ARF, continuous renal replacement therapy (CRRT) has benefits. Box 36-1 summarizes the various types of CRRT: (1) continuous arteriovenous hemofiltration, (2) continuous venovenous hemofiltration, (3) continuous venovenous hemodialysis, (4) continuous arteriovenous ultrafiltration, and (5) slow continuous ultrafiltration. In essence, these methods involve removal of plasma water and dissolved contents from the client's blood across a membrane. In contrast, in dialysis, particles are removed by diffusion. Slow continuous removal of waste products and water through CRRT is less stressful to the client than shorter, more efficient dialysis treatments.

Prevent Infections

Secondary infections are a significant cause of death in clients with ARF. The client must be monitored carefully for infectious processes; if these occur, they should be treated aggressively. Except for monitoring urine output during ARF, indwelling urethral catheters are usually avoided because of their great potential for introducing infection. If a catheter is placed, meticulous catheter care is essential.

Monitor the Client

Treatment of ARF may take place in an intensive care unit or other critical care unit, depending on the cause. Much of the care consists of physiologic monitoring and assessment. In addition to monitoring fluid and electrolyte balance, you should monitor the progression of manifestations associated with renal failure. Pericarditis occurs in as many as 18% of clients with renal failure. Assessment findings include pleuritic pain (which may subside when the client assumes an upright position), pericardial friction rub, tachycardia, and fever. Treatment usually starts with steroids or nonsteroidal anti-inflammatory drugs (NSAIDs). Pericardiocentesis and pericardiectomy may be necessary if cardiac function is compromised.

SAFETY
⚠
ALERT

Other problems call for relief of manifestations. The increasing BUN level decreases the seizure threshold, resulting in an increase in the number of seizures. These seizures may be relieved by intravenous phenytoin or phenobarbital. Anemia is treated by transfusions or the use of recombinant erythropoietin. Erythropoietin is a hormone produced by the kidney that stimulates red blood cell production. Erythropoietin is used in CKD, but its use in ARF has not been studied extensively. Bleeding tendencies may be minimized by correcting vitamin K deficiencies as well as by reducing the serum BUN level, because BUN interferes with platelet aggregation.

Maintain Nutritional Status

Proper nutrition is crucial. A high-calorie, low-protein diet is usually prescribed. The diet may also be low in sodium, magnesium, phosphate, and potassium. The protein must be of high biologic value (complete), containing the essential amino acids to reduce nitrogenous waste products. Adequate carbohydrate intake reverses the process of gluconeogenesis. During the acute phases, intake should be 135 to 150 nonprotein kilocalories (kcal) for each 6.25 g of protein ingested; this ratio is considered adequate for preventing protein catabolism. Liquid supplements, low in potassium, may also be used. If oral intake is not sufficient to meet requirements, tube feedings or TPN, including lipids, may be instituted.

Nursing Management of the Medical Client

Assessment. Carefully monitor any client with risk factors for ARF. It is important to assess fluid balance in any hospitalized or seriously injured client. Because hypovolemia is a common cause, assess the client closely for this problem. When the diagnosis is ARF, carefully assess for such complications as pleural effusion, pericarditis, acidosis, and uremia. The Case Study feature on p. 815 addresses acute renal failure and abdominal aortic aneurysm resection.

Diagnosis, Outcomes, Interventions
Diagnosis: Deficient Fluid Volume or Excess Fluid Volume. A common nursing diagnosis in ARF is *Deficient Fluid Volume related to fluid loss from a variety of causes*. Another common nursing diagnosis is *Excess Fluid Volume related to inability of the kidneys to produce urine secondary to ARF*.

Outcomes. The client will maintain fluid balance, as evidenced by a balanced intake and output. If fluid volume excess occurs, it will be managed with dialysis or CRRT.

Interventions. Careful monitoring of fluid balance indicators is crucial to the management of ARF. Accurate intake and output measurements guide the fluid replacement regimen. Compare these values and look for 24- to 48-hour trends. Check the client's vital signs (including measurements of postural blood pressure and apical pulse rate), skin turgor, and mucous membranes about every 4 hours, depending on the severity of the illness.

BOX 36-1   Types of Renal Replacement Therapies

Modalities of continuous renal replacement therapies (CRRT) are similar in that they slowly remove water from the body. However, they differ in the way they remove solutes.

Diffusion is the process where particles move from an area of high concentration through a semipermeable membrane to a solution of low concentration. *Convection* is the process whereby replacement fluid pulls waste through the semipermeable membrane. High flow rates of fluid (e.g., 1000 to 2000 ml/hour) drag more particles across the membrane than slower flow rates.

Ultrafiltration is a process of removal of fluid from the extracorporeal circuit by creating pressure across the membrane.

Continuous arteriovenous hemofiltration (CAVH) was the first slow renal replacement procedure. CAVH involved circulation of blood from an artery through a hemofilter and returned through a vein. It requires a blood pressure high enough to circulate the blood. More recently, other forms of CRRT use pumps to circulate blood and replacement fluids and dialysate and a double-lumen catheter is inserted into a large vein rather than using both an artery and a vein.

Slow continuous ultrafiltration (SCUF) is used to remove fluid; it involves convection through a process called ultrafiltration. It is used when fluid removal is the prime therapeutic goal. While some urea is removed with plasma water, the rate of urea removal is low.

Continuous venovenous hemofiltration (CVVH) works by convection. Blood is removed and returned through venous access. Fluid is infused into the extracorporeal circuit and removed rapidly by the hemofilter. As a result, wastes and toxins are removed by convection.

Continuous venovenous hemodialysis (CVVHD) is a slow form of dialysis in which blood is removed and returned through a venous access. Diffusion is the process used to remove wastes and electrolytes. However, the flow rate of blood and dialysate is slower than in conventional hemodialysis.

Continuous venovenous hemodiafiltration (CVVHDF) uses both convection and diffusion to remove fluids, waste particles, inflammatory mediators, and other toxins. Like dialysis, a dialysate solution runs counter to the blood and particles are removed by diffusion. In addition, an electrolyte solution is pumped into the blood to promote convection. It has the best clearances but is more expensive and technically challenging.

Continuous arteriovenous ultrafiltration (CAVU) is a process of fluid removal from the blood whereby blood is removed from an artery through an extracorporeal circuit where fluid is removed and then returned through a vein. Ultrafiltration is the process used to remove fluid.

Acute Renal Failure and Abdominal Aortic Aneurysm Resection

Mr. Carlson is a 70-year-old retired farmer who is brought in by squad to a small rural hospital. He complains of boring-type abdominal pain that radiates through to the back. A computed tomography scan of the abdomen reveals a dissecting abdominal aneurysm. Mr. Carlson is flown to an urban hospital for emergency resection of the aneurysm. Complications encountered in surgery require that the aorta be cross-clamped for a number of hours. Multiple blood products are administered to replace those lost through hemorrhage. Mr. Carlson is admitted to the surgical intensive care unit for postoperative care and monitoring. . . . *Case Study continued on the website and the CD-ROM with discussions, multiple-choice questions, and a nursing care plan.*

Carefully obtain daily weight measurements using the same scale at the same time of day. Obtain blood pressure measurements via an arterial line, if one is in place.

Urine specific gravity, usually an indication of fluid balance, may not be useful with intrinsic renal disease. Abnormalities in heart sounds, breath sounds, and mental status may indicate the presence of fluid and electrolyte imbalances.

When the physician has determined the client's fluid allotment, make sure that intake amounts for each shift are followed. This means carefully monitoring fluid intake to ensure that the prescribed amount is taken. Often, this amount represents a significant fluid restriction for the client, which causes a problem with thirst. Help the client stay within the prescribed restriction with careful oral hygiene and judicious use of ice chips, lip ointments, and appropriate diversionary activities. Placing the allotted water in a spray bottle may help spread out the amount taken. Fluid from foods must be taken into account as well. To conserve fluids for the client, administer medications with meals, if possible.

Diagnosis: Imbalanced Nutrition: Less Than Body Requirements. Another common nursing diagnosis for clients with this disorder is *Imbalanced Nutrition: Less Than Body Requirements related to anorexia and altered metabolic state secondary to renal failure.*

Outcomes. The client will maintain adequate nutritional status, with sufficient nutrients to meet metabolic needs.

Interventions. A client with renal failure commonly experiences anorexia, nausea, stomatitis, and taste changes. These manifestations, combined with a generally less palatable diet, make adequate nutrition a challenge for nurse and client. Critically ill clients with ARF will be unable to eat. Work with the client and dietitian to plan a diet that is acceptable.

Provide a pleasant environment at mealtime. Preparing foods in an attractive manner and presenting them in small amounts may help. Medications to alleviate the discomfort of nausea and stomatitis may be useful. Enteral or parenteral nutrition may be instituted if the client's nutritional status cannot be maintained with oral intake.

Diagnosis: Risk for Impaired Skin Integrity. You may need to use the diagnosis *Risk for Impaired Skin Integrity related to poor cellular nutrition and edema.*

Outcomes. The client will maintain skin integrity, as evidenced by intact skin and mucous membranes.

Interventions. The poor systemic nutrition and edema that accompany renal failure may cause skin breakdown. Meticulous skin care, frequent turning, and special mattresses are important. Range-of-motion exercises facilitate movement and increase circulation.

Diagnosis: Risk for Infection. Renal failure makes clients more susceptible to infection, resulting in a nursing diagnosis of *Risk for Infection related to lowered resistance.*

Outcomes. The client will maintain immune status, resisting infection. This will be evidenced by normal vital signs, a normal white blood cell count, and no outward manifestations of infection.

Interventions. The client with ARF is immunocompromised and susceptible to secondary infection. Nursing interventions must be designed to prevent infection in the usual high-risk sites (e.g., respiratory tract, wounds, central catheters, and mouth). Urethral catheters are avoided if possible. If they must be used, provide meticulous catheter care. Also, be alert to early manifestations of infection so that aggressive medical treatment may be instituted.

Diagnosis: Anxiety. Inevitably, the client experiences *Anxiety related to unknown outcome of disease process.*

Outcomes. The client will manage the anxiety, as evidenced by calmness and an ability to focus.

Interventions. Because the client's physical needs are obvious, it is easy to forget that the client as well as significant others will be anxious and frightened. Give frequent, careful explanations, and provide emotional and psychological support.

Evaluation. Fluid balance must be maintained. If fluid volume excess develops, it is managed with dialysis or CRRT to reduce body weight and to balance intake and output. Intact skin should be maintained. The client and family will be less anxious, and able to cope with the information provided.

Although ARF manifestations may continue, most clients with ARF recover within 4 to 10 weeks of correction of the underlying problem. Renal function may continue to improve for up to 12 months after the onset of ARF. The client is particularly vulnerable to additional renal injury during this time.

Self-Care

It is important for the client to understand the implications of ARF and the importance of following the therapeutic regimen. The client and significant others have to understand how to prevent further renal damage. The client must be closely observed by a nephrologist for at least a year after ARF is reversed so that deterioration of renal function can be monitored. The client and significant others require knowledge of renal failure and an understanding of the possible need for ongoing treatment.

Modifications for Older Clients

Older clients are at increased risk for ARF because of reduced cardiac contractile function, vascular compliance, renal plasma flow, and renal mass. The older adult has more difficulty maintaining a homeostatic fluid balance. The ability to retain sodium declines with age, as does the ability to concentrate urine. Older clients are also more likely to have pre-existing renal damage from such diseases as hypertension, diabetes mellitus, and benign prostatic hypertrophy in men. Dosages of medications that are nephrotoxic or excreted by the kidney may need to be adjusted.

CHRONIC KIDNEY DISEASE (STAGE 5)

Chronic kidney disease (CKD) (see Chapter 35) is irreversible and progressive reduction of functioning renal tissue. When the remaining kidney mass can no longer maintain the body's internal environment, renal failure is the result. This is labeled stage 5 CKD and is also called end-stage renal disease (ESRD). CKD can develop insidiously over many years, or it may result from an episode of ARF from which the client has not recovered.

The incidence of ESRD or stage 5 CKD varies widely by state and country. In the United States, the incidence is 338 new cases per million people. According to the U.S. Renal Data System, at the end of 2003 a total of 441,051 people were being treated for end-stage renal disease (ESRD); approximately 28% have a functioning transplant, 66% receive hemodialysis, and 5.7% are undergoing a form of peritoneal dialysis (for some people, data were not available).[54] This pattern of treatment varies widely globally.

Etiology and Risk Factors

The causes of stage 5 CKD (ESRD) are numerous. In Chapter 35, various injuries and disease processes that may result in kidney failure were discussed. Chronic glomerulonephritis, ARF, polycystic kidney disease, obstruction, repeated episodes of pyelonephritis, and nephrotoxins are examples of causes. Systemic diseases, such as diabetes mellitus, hypertension, lupus erythematosus, polyarteritis, sickle cell disease, and amyloidosis, may produce CKD. Diabetes mellitus is the leading cause and

accounts for more than 30% of clients who receive dialysis. Hypertension is the second leading cause of ESRD.

To reduce the risk of CKD, the client should be closely observed and should receive adequate treatment to control or slow the progress of these problems before they progress to ESRD. Some conditions, such as lupus and diabetes mellitus, can progress to kidney failure despite close treatment.

Pathophysiology

The pathogenesis of ESRD involves deterioration and destruction of nephrons with progressive loss of renal function. As the total GFR decreases and clearance is reduced, serum urea nitrogen and creatinine levels increase. Remaining functioning nephrons hypertrophy as they filter a larger load of solutes. A consequence is that the kidneys lose their ability to concentrate urine adequately. To continue excreting the solutes, a large volume of dilute urine may be passed, which makes the client susceptible to fluid depletion. The tubules gradually lose their ability to reabsorb electrolytes. Occasionally, the result is salt wasting, in which urine contains large amounts of sodium, which leads to more polyuria.

As renal damage advances and the number of functioning nephrons declines, the total GFR decreases further. Thus the body becomes unable to rid itself of excess water, salt, and other waste products through the kidneys. When the GFR is less than 10 to 20 ml/min, the effect of uremic toxins on the body becomes evident. If the disease is not treated by dialysis or transplantation, the outcome of ESRD is uremia and death.

Clinical Manifestations

The clinical manifestations of the early stages of renal failure depend on the disease process and contributing factors. As nephron destruction progresses to ESRD, the manifestations are described as uremic syndrome. Recently, the National Kidney Foundation proposed a set of clinical practice guidelines outlining a uniform classification system for CKD (see Table 35-2 on p. 797 and discussion in Chapter 35). This classification and stratification system has replaced less precise terms such as "chronic renal insufficiency" and "chronic renal failure."

The clinical manifestations of CKD stage 5 are present throughout the body. No organ system is spared. The Concept Map on pp. 818-819 illustrates the treatment of stage 5 chronic kidney disease. Renal alterations (described previously) include the inability of the kidney to concentrate urine and regulate electrolyte excretion. Polyuria progresses to anuria, and the client loses normal diurnal patterns of voiding. In addition, all normal functions of the kidney, such as regulation of acid-base balance, regulation of blood pressure, synthesis of 1,25-dihydroxycholecalciferol, biogenesis of erythropoietin, degradation of insulin, and synthesis of prostaglandins, are impaired.

Electrolyte Imbalances

Electrolyte balance may be upset by impaired excretion and utilization in the kidney. Although many clients maintain a normal serum sodium level, the salt-wasting properties of some failing kidneys, in addition to vomiting and diarrhea, may cause hyponatremia. Apparent hyponatremia may be a dilutional effect of water retention. Late in the disease, salt and water retention often contributes to hypertension and heart failure.

Because the kidneys are efficient at excreting potassium, potassium levels usually remain within normal limits until late in the disease. However, hyperkalemia then becomes a challenging problem. Catabolism, potassium-containing medications, trauma, blood transfusions, and acidosis contribute to potassium excess. The Complementary and Alternative Therapy feature below explores the efficacy of noni juice in the prevention and treatment of renal disease.

Several mechanisms contribute to hypocalcemia. Conversion of 25-hydroxycholciferol to 1,25-dihydroxycholecalciferol (necessary to absorb calcium) is decreased, which results in reduced intestinal absorption of calcium. At the same time, phosphate is not excreted, which causes hyperphosphatemia. Because calcium and phosphate are inversely related, a high phosphate level results in a reduced calcium level. This combination stimulates the parathyroid glands to secrete parathyroid hormone to facilitate phosphate excretion and increase the serum calcium level by resorbing calcium from bone. Osteomalacia, osteitis fibrosa, and osteosclerosis are commonly seen in clients with stage 5 CKD as a result of these metabolic alterations in calcium, phosphorus, parathyroid hormone, and vitamin D. In some clients, hypercalcemia may develop because of persistent secretion of parathyroid hormone.

Mildly elevated serum magnesium levels are found early in the disease. Magnesium does not usually reach a dangerous level unless the client is receiving magnesium-containing laxatives or antacids.

Metabolic Changes

In advancing renal failure, levels of BUN and serum creatinine increase as waste products of protein metabolism accumulate in the blood. The serum creatinine level is the most accurate measure of renal function. The normal ratio of BUN to creatinine is 10:1, and it remains the same as both the creatinine level and BUN level increase.

The proteinuria accompanying renal disease and sometimes inadequate dietary intake of proteins causes hypoproteinemia, which lowers the intravascular oncotic pressure. Serum uric acid level is often high but is not commonly associated with manifestations of gout.

Carbohydrate intolerance results from impaired insulin production and metabolism. Four mechanisms are responsible: (1) peripheral insulin antagonism, (2) impaired insulin secretion, (3) a prolonged insulin half-life, which is directly related to kidney malfunction, and (4) abnormalities in levels of circulating insulin. Therefore special care is needed in adjustment of insulin doses for clients with diabetes mellitus complicated by renal failure. Even short-acting regular insulin functions as a longer-acting insulin, resulting in a need for lower dosages or fewer injections per day. Blood glucose levels must be monitored closely.

Elevated triglyceride levels are found almost universally. This type IV hyperlipidemia is thought to be caused by increased production of lipids by the liver in response to elevated blood glucose and insulin levels. At the same time, assimilation of lipids in the peripheral tissues appears to be reduced, possibly because of the blockage of lipoprotein lipase activity. This contributes to a secondary complication of cardiovascular disease.

Metabolic acidosis occurs because of the kidney's inability to excrete hydrogen ions. Decreased reabsorption of sodium bicarbonate and decreased formation of dihydrogen phosphate and ammonia contribute to this problem. Acidosis accentuates hyperkalemia and the reabsorption of calcium from the bones.

Pericarditis is usually related to the accumulation of uremic toxins, rarely to infection. Manifestations include pericardial pain (often reduced by an upright position), tachycardia, pleural friction rub, and fever. The condition may progress to pericardial effusion and cardiac tamponade, a life-threatening complication.

COMPLEMENTARY AND ALTERNATIVE THERAPY

Noni Juice and Renal Disease

Noni juice (*Morinda citrifolia*) is a popular drink in some alternative medicine circles. It has been advertised by some as promoting health and as helping to cure many types of conditions. However, no good research studies have been completed to see if this is true. The general recommended dose for noni juice (as found on the Internet) is approximately 1 ounce/day, but some websites promote higher intakes. Individuals with kidney disease whose blood levels of potassium get too high may experience irregular heart rhythms or even a heart attack. Noni juice contains moderate levels of potassium in small doses. Therefore clients should be careful and find out the potassium level of their brand, or they should just play it safe and stay away from this alternative medicine until more studies are concluded.

REFERENCES

1. Burrowes, B.A., & Van Houten, G. (2005). Use of alternative medicine by patients with stage 5 chronic kidney disease. *Advances in Chronic Kidney Disease, 12*, 312-325.
2. Mueller, B., Scott, M.K., Sowinski, K.M., & Prag, K.A. (2000). Noni juice (*Morinda citrifolia*): Hidden potential for hyperkalemia? *American Journal of Kidney Disease, 35*, 310-312.

CONCEPT MAP

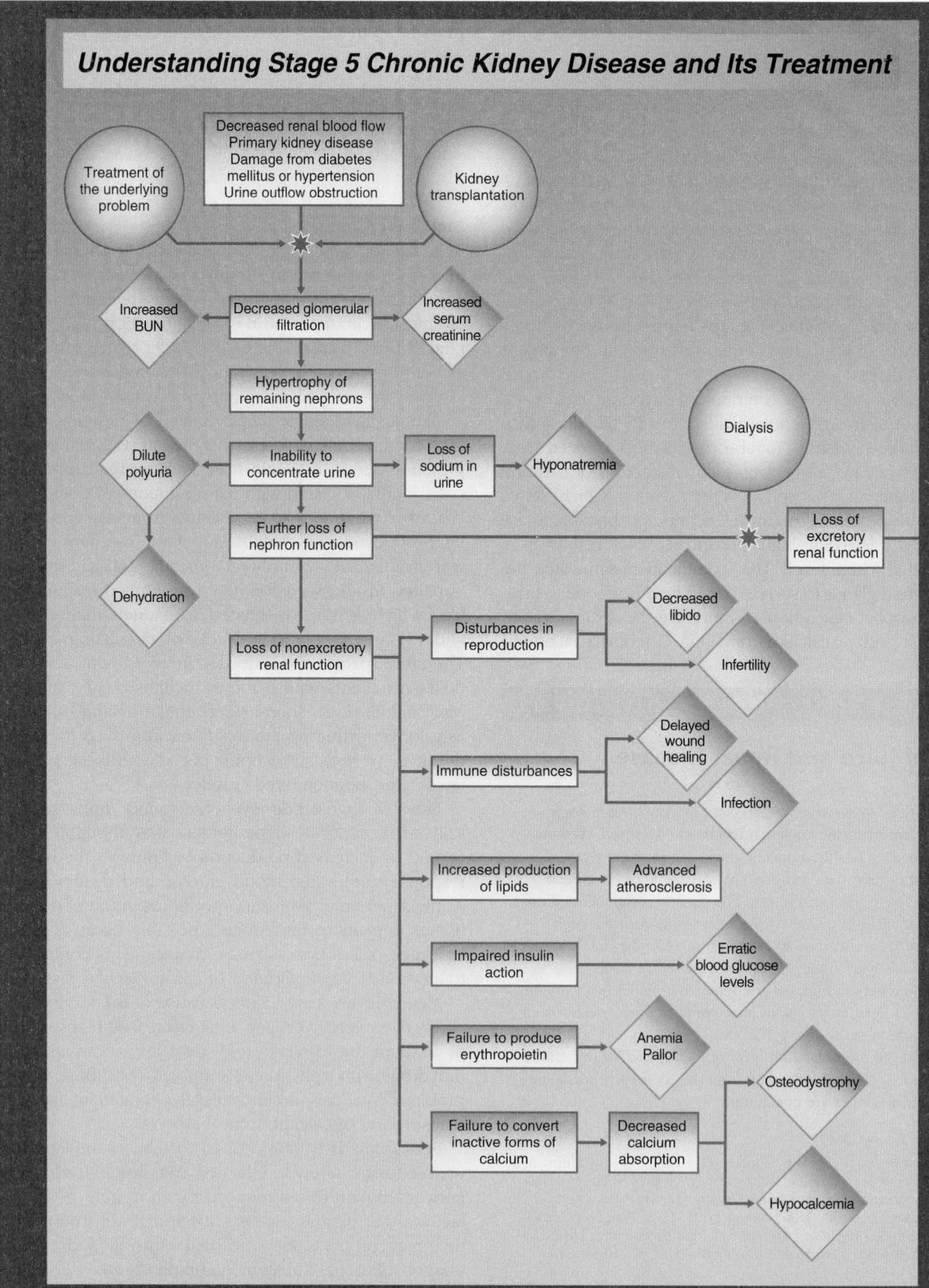

Understanding Stage 5 Chronic Kidney Disease and Its Treatment

CONCEPT MAP

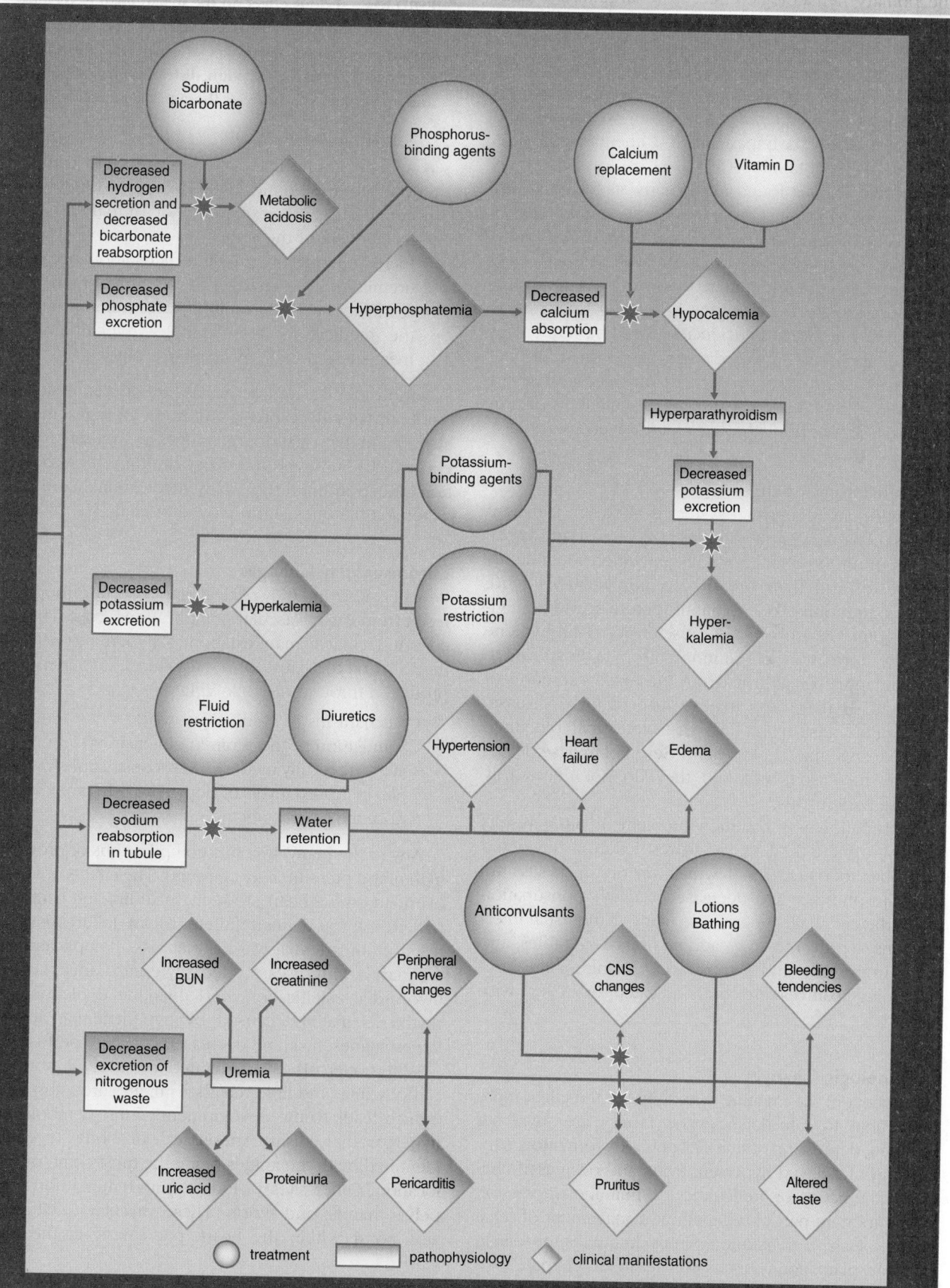

Hematologic Changes

The primary hematologic effect of renal failure is anemia, usually normochromic and normocytic. It occurs because the kidneys are unable to produce erythropoietin, a hormone necessary for red blood cell production. If it is left untreated, hematocrit levels can decrease to less than 20%. Frequently the fatigue, weakness, and cold intolerance accompanying the anemia lead to a diagnosis of renal failure.

The mild anemia found in the early stages is usually due to reduced production of the hormone erythropoietin, which results in decreased production of red blood cells. Later, hemolysis, gastrointestinal losses, and clotting abnormalities contribute to the severity of the condition. Occasionally, the client has iron or folate depletion because of nutritional deficiencies. Bleeding tendencies become apparent as the disease progresses. Platelet abnormalities are the primary defect responsible for bleeding in the uremic client. The accumulation of uremic toxins interferes with platelet adhesiveness.

Gastrointestinal Changes

The entire gastrointestinal system is affected. Transient anorexia, nausea, and vomiting are almost universal. Clients often experience a constant bitter, metallic, or salty taste, and their breath commonly smells fetid, fishy, or ammonia-like. Stomatitis, parotitis, and gingivitis are common problems because of poor oral hygiene and the formation of ammonia from salivary urea. Accumulations of gastrin (from increased secretion of gastric acid) may be a major cause of ulcer disease. Esophagitis, gastritis, colitis, gastrointestinal bleeding, and diarrhea may be present. Serum amylase levels may be increased, although they do not necessarily indicate pancreatitis.

Constipation is a common problem. It often results from phosphate-binding agents, restriction of fluids and high-fiber foods (many of which are rich in potassium and phosphorus), and decreased activity. Constipation is a particular challenge because many of the usual interventions to prevent it (e.g., adding fruits, vegetables, and grains to the diet) and to treat it (e.g., using magnesium-containing laxatives) are contraindicated for a client with ESRD.

Immunologic Changes

Impairment of the immune system makes the client more susceptible to infection. Several factors are involved, including depression of humoral antibody formation, suppression of delayed hypersensitivity, and decreased chemotactic function of the leukocytes. Immunosuppression is an important part of the medical management of renal diseases such as glomerulonephritis. Immunosuppression after transplantation is discussed later in this chapter.

Changes in Medication Metabolism

ESRD has a serious effect on the metabolism of medications. The uremic client is at high risk for medication toxicity because of the effect of renal changes on the pharmacokinetics (absorption, distribution, metabolism, and excretion) of otherwise therapeutic medications.

There are three main causes of this toxicity:

- A high plasma level of the medication caused by low serum albumin level, decreased binding sites, impaired renal excretion, or impaired hepatic metabolism of the drug
- Increased sensitivity to the medication because of uremia-induced changes in the target organ
- A metabolic load resulting from administration of the medication; for example, hypoalbuminemia means less protein available for binding

Various tables and formulas are available to help guide dosage decisions. Medication dosages must be altered and the usual dosage ranges are not safe for a client with CKD. Assess the client carefully for toxic reactions. Keep in mind that many medications, particularly water-soluble ones, are removed by dialysis.

Cardiovascular Changes

Between 50% and 65% of deaths that occur during ESRD result from cardiovascular complications. The most common clinical manifestation is hypertension (which may also be the cause of renal failure). Hypertension is produced through the following:

- Mechanisms of volume overload
- Stimulation of the renin-angiotensin system
- Sympathetically mediated vasoconstriction; for example, increased levels of dopamine β-hydroxylase
- Absence of prostaglandins

Any of the many systemic complications of prolonged high blood pressure may be found. The effects of volume overload on the heart are seen, including left ventricular hypertrophy and heart failure. Heart failure may also result from anemia, vascular access, complications of coronary artery disease, electrolyte imbalance, acidosis, myocardial calcification, and thiamine depletion. Dysrhythmias may be caused by hyperkalemia, acidosis, hypermagnesemia, and decreased coronary perfusion.

Atherosclerosis is accelerated because of abnormal carbohydrate and lipid metabolism, impaired fibrinolysis (which leads to the development of microemboli), and hyperparathyroidism. Arterial calcifications have been identified, with the ankles being the most common early location. Other sites include the abdominal aorta, feet, pelvis, hands, and wrists. These vascular calcifications also occur within the heart, particularly at the mitral valve.

Respiratory Changes

Some of the respiratory effects, such as pulmonary edema, can be attributed to fluid overload. Pleuritis is a frequent finding, especially when pericarditis develops. A characteristic condition called *uremic lung* is a type of pneumonitis that responds well to fluid removal. Metabolic acidosis causes a compensatory increase in respiratory rate as the lungs work to eliminate excess hydrogen ions.

Musculoskeletal Changes

The musculoskeletal system is affected early in the disease process, and up to 90% of clients with ESRD experience renal osteodystrophy. This condition develops insidiously and takes several forms: osteomalacia, osteitis fibrosa, osteoporosis, and osteosclerosis. The etiologic mechanism involves the kidney-bone-parathyroid and calcium-phosphate-vitamin D connections. As the GFR decreases, phosphate excretion decreases and calcium elimination increases. Abnormal levels of calcium and phosphate stimulate the release of parathyroid hormone, which mobilizes calcium from the bones and facilitates phosphate excretion.

As renal failure progresses, the kidney no longer converts vitamin D to its active form, 1,25-dihydroxycholecalciferol. The lack of this substance interferes with calcium absorption from the intestine and paradoxically facilitates phosphate retention. Thus mineralization of the bone with calcium and phosphate is impaired. Demineralization of the bone frees more calcium and phosphorus into the blood. As the disease progresses, the parathyroid gland may become unresponsive to the normal feedback system and continue to produce parathyroid hormone, accelerating renal osteodystrophy. Partial parathyroidectomy is the treatment of choice when hypercalcemia and high plasma levels of parathyroid hormone cannot be controlled with medication.

In addition to bone demineralization, this process leads to deposition of calcium in subcutaneous, vascular, and visceral tissues throughout the body. In advanced stages, joint pain is severe. The client may also report diffuse and generalized bone and muscle pain. Bone deformities and frequent fractures are common. In children, bones fail to calcify, causing growth retardation. Tissue calcifications may be lethal if they develop in vital tissues, such as cerebral, coronary, or pulmonary vessels.

Some clients complain of muscle cramps. These may result from osmolar changes in the body fluids or sometimes from hypocalcemia.

Integumentary Changes

Integumentary problems are particularly uncomfortable for some clients with ESRD. The skin is also often very dry because of atrophy of the sweat glands. Severe and intractable pruritus may result from secondary hyperparathyroidism and calcium deposits in the skin. Pruritus can lead to excoriated skin caused by continued scratching.

Several color changes affecting the skin are found in clients with renal failure. A bleeding tendency often results in increased bruising, petechiae, and purpura. These do not usually cause problems themselves, but their presence may be alarming to the client. The pallor of anemia is evident. Retained urochrome pigments make the skin orange-green or gray in color.

Hair is brittle and tends to fall out; nails are thin and brittle as well. Characteristic red bands that develop on the nails are called Muehrcke's lines. Another nail pattern that has been observed is a "half-and-half" nail, with the proximal half normally white and the distal portion brown.

Neurologic Changes

Although dialysis has reduced the incidence of neurologic changes, some clients experience these problems early in the disease process. Peripheral neuropathy causes many manifestations, such as burning feet, inability to find a comfortable position for the legs and feet (restless legs syndrome), gait changes, footdrop, and paraplegia. These manifestations move up the legs and may extend to include the arms. Initially, it is primarily a problem of the sensory system; however, if left untreated, it may progress to the motor system. Nerve conduction becomes slower, and deep tendon reflexes and vibratory sense are diminished.

Central nervous system involvement is demonstrated through forgetfulness, inability to concentrate, short attention span, impaired reasoning ability and judgment, impaired cognitive functioning, increased nervous irritability, nystagmus, twitching, dysarthria, seizures, central nervous system depression, and coma. Involvement of the cranial nerves may alter any of the senses. Hearing threshold levels show a high-frequency deficit early in the disease, and hearing progressively deteriorates. Uremic amaurosis is the sudden onset of bilateral blindness, which seems to be reversed in hours to days. The eyes often contain calcium salts, which give them an irritated appearance.

Reproductive Changes

Women commonly experience menstrual irregularities, particularly amenorrhea (absence of menstrual periods), and infertility. However, some women with ESRD have conceived and had successful full-term pregnancies. Men commonly report impotence of both physiologic and psychological causes. They may also experience testicular atrophy, oligospermia (decreased sperm count), and reduced sperm motility. Both genders report decreased libido, possibly from both physiologic and psychological factors.

Endocrine Changes

ESRD also affects the endocrine system, including insulin utilization and parathyroid function discussed previously. Pituitary hormones, such as growth hormone and prolactin, may be increased in some clients. The levels of luteinizing hormone and follicle-stimulating hormone vary greatly from client to client. Thyroid-stimulating hormone level is usually normal, but it may show a blunted response to thyrotropin-releasing hormone; this commonly results in hypothyroidism.

Psychosocial Changes

Psychosocial changes probably result from both the physiologic alterations and the extreme stress experienced by a client who has a chronic, life-threatening disease. Common stressors include feelings of powerlessness and lack of control over the illness and treatment, intrusive therapy, restrictions imposed by the medical regimen, changes in body image, and changes in sexuality.

Clients commonly experience role reversal, loss or reduction of work, financial strain, and many lifestyle changes. Scheduling dialysis can create many difficulties. The client's self-concept and body image may be altered, leading to further problems.

Clients cope with these stressors in various ways, and not all coping strategies are positive. They can range from obtaining support from family and friends and seeking more information about the condition to depression and thoughts of suicide. Indeed, helping a client cope with psychosocial changes can be very challenging.

Prognosis

The survival rate of clients with ESRD has improved with the advent and improvement of dialysis and transplantation. At 1 year after dialysis begins, the survival rate is about 78%. After 5 years, the rate decreases to 39%.[54]

OUTCOME MANAGEMENT

Medical Management

Conservative treatment does not cure CKD, but it may slow the progress of the disease. Eventually, many clients need renal replacement therapy. However, even successful dialysis and transplantation does not preclude the potential for death from complications of renal failure or its treatment.

After correcting causative factors, control of blood pressure, managing lipids, fluid and dietary adjustments, and blood sugar control for diabetic clients are the mainstays of conservative intervention for a client with CKD. The following are the five goals of medical management:

1. To preserve renal function
2. To delay the need for dialysis or transplantation as long as feasible
3. To alleviate extrarenal manifestations as much as possible
4. To improve body chemistry values
5. To provide an optimal quality of life for the client and significant others

Preserve Renal Function and Delay Dialysis

Preservation of renal function can delay the need for dialysis therapy. It can be accomplished by controlling the disease process (see Chapter 35), by controlling blood pressure, and by reducing dietary protein intake and catabolism.

CKD commonly causes hypertension, which accelerates kidney damage. Good blood pressure control helps to preserve renal function. Blood pressure can be controlled through diet, weight control, and medications (see Chapters 35 and 52).

Specific adjustments of dietary elements often depend on the results of the client's blood chemistry studies. Although there is some debate over whether and how to restrict proteins, keeping the daily intake of protein of high biologic value below 50 g may slow the progression of renal failure. Generally, recommendations range from no restriction other than avoiding high-protein fad diets to a restriction to 1 g/kg/day. This protein must be of high biologic value so that the essential amino acids can be used more efficiently with less nitrogenous waste. This restriction of proteins also limits accumulation of acid, potassium, and phosphate.

It is also important to provide adequate nonprotein calories to prevent or reduce catabolism. One recommendation is a carbohydrate and fat intake of 40 to 50 kcal/kg/day. As the renal disease progresses, the client's ability and willingness to consume adequate nutrition diminish and the challenge becomes not only to maintain appropriate intake of nonprotein calories but also to satisfy protein needs. In these instances, elemental diets, enteral feedings, or TPN may be used instead of or in addition to regular food intake.

Alleviate Extrarenal Manifestations

Pruritus can be annoying. Many interventions have been tried, including topical emollients and lotions, antihistamines, intravenous lidocaine, and ultraviolet B light, but relief has been inconsistent and usually temporary. Subtotal parathyroidectomy has sometimes helped, but there have been reports of recurrence. Effective dialysis seems to relieve the manifestations for many clients.

Neurologic manifestations require measures to protect the client from injury. Anticonvulsants and sedatives may be used. Phenothiazines are potentiated by uremia and should be avoided. The increase of uremic toxins causes a reduction in cognitive functioning, and patience is required in explanations of the disease or treatment plan to the client.

The hematologic changes can also be treated medically. 🪔 Therapy with epoetin alfa three times a week (or weekly as darbepoetin alfa) helps stimulate the production of red blood cells. Supplemental iron, vitamin B_{12}, and folic acid are usually administered as well.

🪔 Cardiovascular disease is the major cause of mortality in clients with CKD. Increasingly, hyperlipidemia is being treated with statins to minimize the risk of myocardial infarction and stroke.

Sleep disturbances are common, sometimes as a result of restless legs syndrome and other times for a variety of other reasons. Assessment and treatment by a sleep clinic may result in better sleep patterns and less daytime fatigue.

Improve Body Chemistry

The client's body chemistry can be improved through dialysis, medications, and diet. Dialysis removes excess water and nitrogenous wastes, reducing the manifestations of renal failure. Dialysis can be used temporarily if the client has ARF or as a permanent, life-sustaining treatment if the client has ESRD. In the latter case, dialysis must continue for the rest of the client's life unless a successful kidney transplant is performed.

Dialysis is also used to control uremia and to physically prepare the client to receive a transplanted kidney. Dialysis is usually necessary to keep the client alive until a suitable donor kidney is found. If the transplanted kidney does not immediately function adequately, dialysis may help prevent uremia until the kidney begins functioning sufficiently.

🪔 The following are the four basic goals of dialysis therapy:
1. To remove the end products of protein metabolism, such as urea and creatinine, from the blood
2. To maintain a safe concentration of serum electrolytes
3. To correct acidosis and replenish the bicarbonate levels of the blood
4. To remove excess fluid from the blood

Principles of ultrafiltration and diffusion are used to accomplish the goals of dialysis. *Ultrafiltration* refers to removal of fluid from the blood using either osmotic or hydrostatic pressure to produce the necessary gradient. *Diffusion* is the passage of particles (ions) from an area of high concentration to an area of low concentration. Both processes occur across a semipermeable membrane with pores large enough to allow certain particles (such as urea, creatinine, and electrolytes) to pass through but too small to allow the passage of larger particles (such as protein and red blood cells). When the two solutions are separated by a semipermeable membrane, solute particles move toward the solution of lower concentration. Simultaneously, water moves toward the solution of higher solute concentration.

Solute particles and water can move freely across the membrane in either direction between the blood and the dialysate. Thus if the blood has a higher concentration of urea, creatinine, and certain electrolytes than does the prepared dialysate solution, these particles move into the dialysate solution, lowering the level in the blood. If the blood is deficient in a substance, such as bicarbonate, the higher concentration of this substance in the dialysate causes it to move into the blood, raising the blood level.

There are two types of dialysis: *peritoneal dialysis* and *hemodialysis*. The semipermeable membrane used in the dialyzer or "artificial kidney" is either the peritoneal membrane (for peritoneal dialysis) or an artificial membrane (for hemodialysis). The blood and a specially prepared electrolyte solution, called the *dialysate,* are placed in compartments on opposite sides of the membrane. Equalization of the concentrations of the two solutions results.

Peritoneal Dialysis. Peritoneal dialysis involves repeated cycles of instilling dialysate into the peritoneal cavity, allowing time for substance exchange, and then removing the dialysate. The procedure is useful for both ARF and ESRD and for fluid and electrolyte imbalances. It has been used to treat overdoses of drugs and toxins, but because its clearance is much slower than that with hemodialysis, it may not be adequate for that purpose.

One of the primary advantages of peritoneal dialysis is its relative ease, which allows it to be used in community health care facilities without the sophisticated equipment needed for hemodialysis. It can be easily managed at home and commonly allows the client more independence and mobility than hemodialysis does.

🪔 Peritoneal dialysis is typically used for clients with severe cardiovascular disease, especially those whose problems would be worsened by the rapid changes in urea, glucose, electrolytes, and fluid volume that occur during hemodialysis. Some physicians prescribe peritoneal dialysis for diabetic clients to reduce the risk of retinal hemorrhage associated with the heparin used during hemodialysis and because good blood glucose control can be achieved by adding insulin to the dialysate. Peritoneal dialysis is the dialysis treatment of choice for children because it seems to have less effect on growth.

Contraindications to peritoneal dialysis include hypercatabolism, in which peritoneal dialysis cannot adequately clear uremic toxins, and poor condition of the peritoneal membrane because of adhesions or scarring. Relative contraindications to peritoneal dialysis include obesity, a history of ruptured diverticula, abdominal disease, respiratory disease, recurrent episodes of peritonitis, abdominal malignancies, severe vascular disease, back problems (because the increased weight of fluid may increase back strain), and extensive abdominal surgery with drains or tubes that may increase the risk of infection.

Types of Peritoneal Dialysis. Several types of peritoneal dialysis are in use. The most common are continuous ambulatory and automated peritoneal dialysis.

Continuous Ambulatory Peritoneal Dialysis (CAPD). In the continuous type of peritoneal dialysis, 1.5 to 3 L of dialysate is instilled into the abdomen and left in place for a prescribed period of time. The solution is then drained by gravity flow. When drained, the bag is changed and new dialysate is instilled into the abdomen as the process continues.

CAPD usually uses four dialysis cycles every 24 hours, including an 8-hour dwell overnight. There are two major advantages. First, because there is no need for machinery, electricity, or a water source, the client can go about almost any desired activity during dialysis. Second, because the continuous exchange process closely resembles normal renal function, the body more easily maintains homeostasis, allowing fewer dietary and fluid restrictions. For management of diabetic clients, insulin can be added to the dialysate.

See the Bridge to Home Health Care feature on Living with Peritoneal Dialysis on the website.

Automated Peritoneal Dialysis. Automated peritoneal dialysis necessitates use of a peritoneal cycling machine. This method can be performed as continuous cyclic, intermittent, or nightly intermittent peritoneal dialysis.

Continuous Cyclic Peritoneal Dialysis. In this variation, there are usually three cycles at night and one cycle with an 8-hour dwell in the morning. The advantage of this procedure is that the peritoneal catheter is opened only for the on-and-off procedures, which reduces the risk of infection. Another advantage is that the client does not require exchanges at work or school.

Intermittent Peritoneal Dialysis. This is not a continuous dialysis procedure. Instead, dialysis is performed for 10 to 14 hours, three to four times a week, by the same peritoneal cycling machine as in continuous cyclic peritoneal dialysis. Hospitalized clients may be dialyzed for 24 to 48 hours at a time if they are catabolic and require additional dialysis time.

Nightly Intermittent Peritoneal Dialysis. Dialysis is performed for 8 to 12 hours each night with no daytime dwells.

Peritoneal Dialysis Procedures. Several steps are involved.

Peritoneal Catheter Insertion. For a client who needs peritoneal dialysis, one of several types of soft catheters is inserted through the abdominal wall and into the peritoneal cavity. Usually, the catheter is inserted in the operating room, with the client under local anesthesia, although it may be inserted at the client's bedside. The client is medicated before the procedure to provide relaxation and to reduce discomfort.

The preferred insertion site is 3 to 5 cm below the umbilicus, an area that is relatively avascular and has relatively low fascial resistance. Figure 36-2 illustrates three types of peritoneal catheters. The Tenckhoff catheter has two polyester (Dacron) felt cuffs bonded to the catheter. Over a period of 1 to 2 weeks, there is an ingrowth of fibroblasts and blood vessels into the cuffs, which fix the catheter in place and provide an effective barrier against dialysate leakage and bacterial invasion. Note in Figure 36-3 that a subcutaneous tunnel is created for the catheter to reduce direct bacterial invasion into the peritoneum. The other catheters illustrated have cuffs to provide stability.

Dialysate. The dialysate is usually allowed to run into the peritoneal cavity by gravity flow. It is warmed slightly to avoid chilling the client and to dilate the peritoneal blood vessels, thus facilitating substance exchange. In an adult, 2 L is usually instilled, although smaller amounts are generally used at first until the wound heals. Throughout the procedure, care must be taken to prevent air from entering the peritoneal cavity.

The *dwell time* is the period during which the dialysate is left in the peritoneal cavity. In intermittent peritoneal dialysis, equilibrium between the dialysate and the

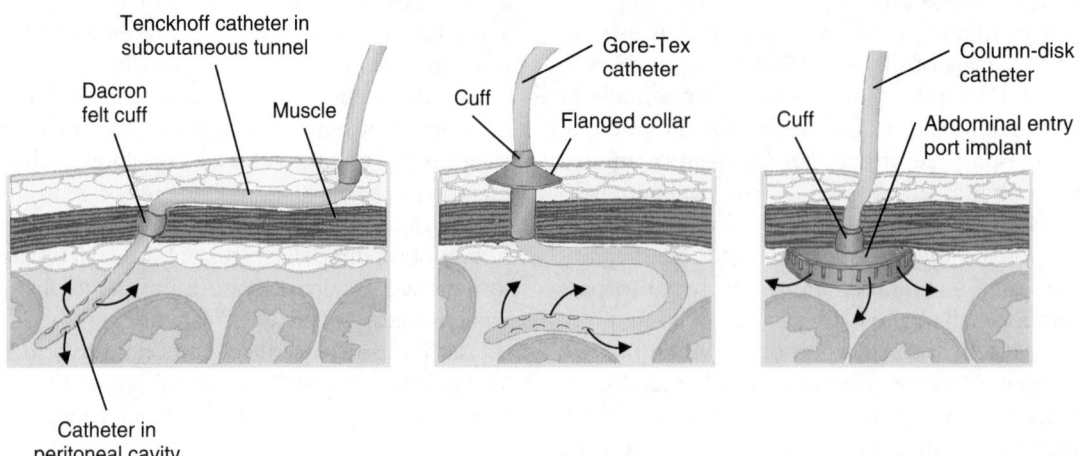

■ **FIGURE 36–2** Three types of peritoneal dialysis catheters. The Tenckhoff catheter has two polyester (Dacron) felt cuffs that hold the catheter in place and prevent dialysate leakage and bacterial invasion; a subcutaneous tunnel also helps prevent infection. The Gore-Tex catheter has a Dacron cuff above a flanged collar. The column-disk catheter has a cuff and a large abdominal entry port implant.

body fluids usually occurs within 15 to 30 minutes, with the maximum exchange occurring during the first 5 minutes. Therefore the solution is typically left in place 30 to 45 minutes for manual dialysis or 10 to 20 minutes when an automatic cycler is used. The fluid is then allowed to run out through the catheter by gravity. In continuous ambulatory and automated peritoneal dialysis procedures, the dwell time is prolonged to 4 to 8 hours with a solution that allows continuous exchange and better clearance of certain elements.

Cycles. The number of dialysis cycles depends on the normalization of body fluids and blood chemistries, as indicated by laboratory studies. Peritoneal clearance is influenced by several factors, including the size of the membrane area, blood flow to the peritoneum, and alterations in the permeability of the peritoneal membrane.

Complications of Peritoneal Dialysis. Although peritoneal dialysis is considered a safe procedure, a number of complications can be attributed to it.

Peritonitis. Peritonitis is the major concern; therefore meticulous aseptic technique must be maintained during handling of the catheter, tubing, and dialysate solution. Bacteria may enter the peritoneal cavity through contaminated dialysis fluid, a contaminated catheter lumen, or the catheter insertion site.

Clinical evidence of peritonitis includes fever, rebound abdominal tenderness, nausea, malaise, and a cloudy dialysate output. Laboratory tests routinely used to diagnose peritonitis include white blood cell counts with differential, culture and sensitivity, and Gram's stain of the peritoneal fluid. Peritonitis is the diagnosis when the dialysate white blood cell count exceeds $100/mm^3$ and neutrophils are greater than 50%. The causative organism does not always grow in routine cultures, but Gram's stain is positive in up to 40% of the samples.

If peritonitis develops, appropriate antibiotics are added to the dialysate; in addition, systemic antibiotics may be used.

Catheter-Related Complications. Catheter problems include displacement and obstruction. Obstruction may be due to malposition, adherence of the catheter tip to the omentum, or infection. Constipation can reduce catheter flow, possibly because peristalsis facilitates outflow. A bisacodyl suppository may be used prophylactically even if the client is not constipated. Fluid leakage may indicate improper catheter function, incomplete healing of the insertion site, or excessive instillation.

Especially in the early stages, it is sometimes necessary to use small-volume instillations. Bloody effluent is usually insignificant and disappears spontaneously. Heparin may be added to the dialysate to prevent fibrin clot formation in a new catheter or after treatment for peritonitis. Also be aware of the possibility of bowel perforation, which is most likely to occur in cachectic (profoundly ill and malnourished) clients or those who

have abdominal adhesions. Fecal material returned in the dialysate or massive diarrhea after instillation may also signal perforation. Bladder perforation can also occur if the bladder has not been emptied before catheter insertion.

Dialysis-Related Complications. Pain during dialysis may result from rapid instillation, incorrect dialysate pH or temperature, dialysate accumulation under the diaphragm, or excessive suction during outflow. Some pain is expected in the early stages but should disappear after 1 to 2 weeks. Low back pain may develop with continuous dialysis procedures because the abdominal weight affects posture; appropriate exercises help relieve this problem. Hernias may develop. Systemic cardiovascular and neurologic effects are usually the result of fluid and electrolyte imbalances. Especially during small-volume exchanges, a significant amount of dialysate fluid may be absorbed by the body.

Hypotension may result from too rapid removal of fluid. Overhydration, from insufficient fluid removal, may manifest as heart failure and pulmonary edema. Hypoalbuminemia leading to hypovolemia often occurs because the peritoneal membrane allows the passage of albumin, as much as 100 g/day if the client is infected. It is especially a problem if dietary intake of protein is poor, the client is infected, or dialysis treatment is used for several consecutive days. Hyperglycemia may occur in diabetic clients as a result of absorption of glucose from the dialysate and electrolyte changes. These clients require extra insulin. Respiratory difficulties may occur during dwell time because of pressure on the diaphragm. Weight gain may occur because of the high concentration of glucose in the dialysate.

Outcomes. Long-term outcomes associated with peritoneal dialysis are considered good. The treatment is usually effective for years. However, scarring of the peritoneum and repeated infections may require a change to hemodialysis.

Hemodialysis. Hemodialysis is used for clients with acute or irreversible renal failure and fluid and electrolyte imbalances. It is usually the treatment of choice when toxic agents, such as barbiturates after an overdose, need to be removed from the body quickly.

Historical Overview. The first artificial kidney was developed in 1943 in The Netherlands. In 1960 the first successful treatment of clients with ESRD was reported. In the early years, although the technology was available, the exorbitant cost and lack of equipment required a stringent selection process in choosing clients for hemodialysis. Clients were screened on the basis of their motivation, intelligence, emotional stability, and rehabilitative potential. In essence, it had to be decided who among the many potential candidates would best be able to cope with the program and who would make the biggest contribution to society.

In 1972 an amendment to the Social Security Act required that anyone with ESRD be able to have any life-saving treatment needed. In 1973 Medicare assumed the financial responsibility for many clients receiving hemodialysis. Thus this treatment for clients with ESRD has become widely available and the population receiving hemodialysis represents a wide cross-section of age, rehabilitative potential, and socioeconomic status. There continue to be debates about selection of appropriate candidates, when to start, and when and how to stop.

Hemodialysis Procedure. In hemodialysis, the client's toxin-laden blood is diverted into a dialyzer, cleaned, and then returned to the client (Figure 36-3). While the blood is in the dialyzer, a mechanical proportioning pump causes dialysis fluid to flow on the other side of the membrane (Figure 36-4). Toxins diffuse across the membrane from the blood to the dialysate. Strict asepsis must be maintained throughout the procedure.

One of the vital aspects of hemodialysis is the establishment and maintenance of adequate blood access. Without it, hemodialysis cannot be done. The major routes of access are central venous catheters for short-term access and internal arteriovenous fistulae and grafts for chronic dialysis.

Central venous catheters for hemodialysis are large-bore double-lumen catheters that are inserted percutaneously into the jugular, femoral, or subclavian vein. They are used when immediate access to the bloodstream is needed. These access sites can be easily placed at the

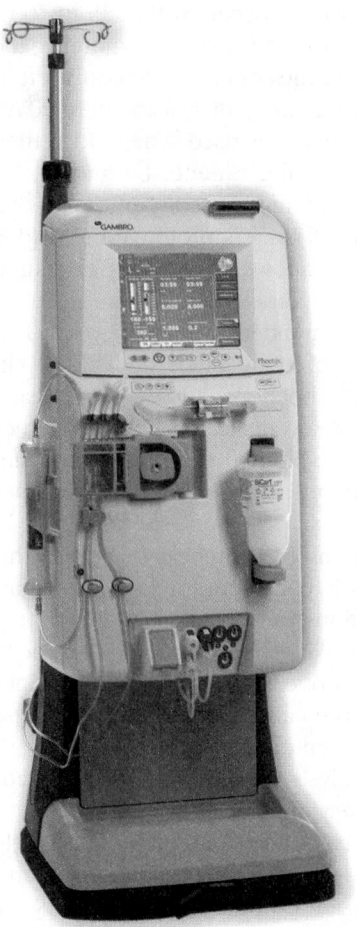

■ **FIGURE 36–4** Gambro Phoenix dialysis system. *(Courtesy Gambro Renal Products, Lakewood, Colo.)*

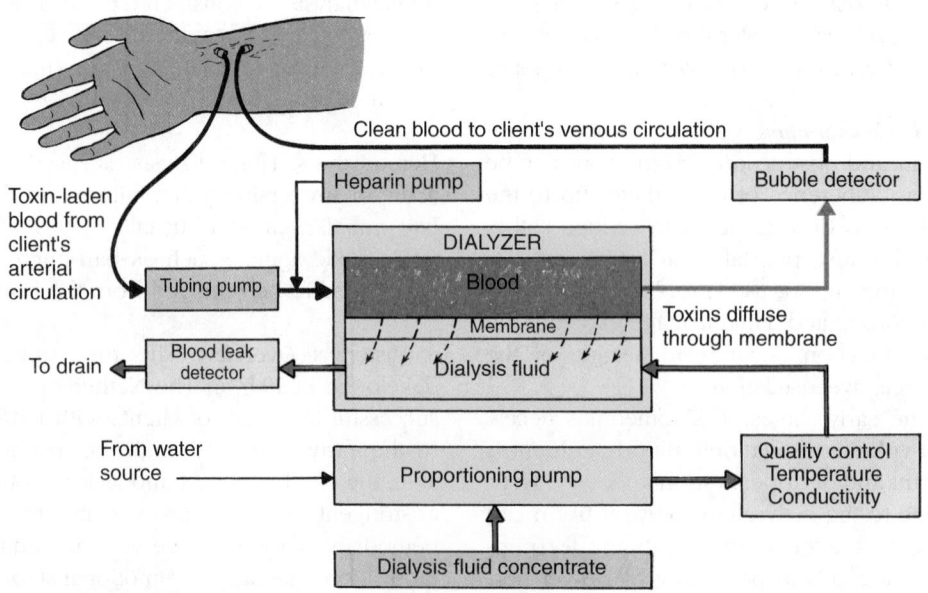

■ **FIGURE 36–3** Typical hemodialysis system. Toxin-laden blood from the client diffuses across the membrane within the dialyzer into the dialysis fluid. Clean blood is returned to the client.

bedside and used immediately after placement is confirmed by x-ray. Longer term catheters, that are tunneled and cuffed, are used if temporary access is required for longer than 3 weeks. Unfortunately, they are easily infected and are associated with a high incidence of venous stenosis. Strict aseptic technique must be used during insertion, and dressing changes are usually performed by a limited number of trained nurses. Thrombosis and infection are the most common complications. Subclavian vein placement is the least preferred because of the risk of pneumothorax.

External arteriovenous shunts are seldom used today but were the most commonly used access sites in the early days of dialysis. Surgery is done to place two rubber-like silicone (Silastic) cannulae into the forearm or leg. The two cannulae are connected to form a U shape. Blood flows from the client's artery through the shunt into the vein. This access can be created quickly and thus is particularly suitable when dialysis must be started immediately. However, infection at the insertion site and clotting are complications that often necessitate removal. Other problems that occur with shunts are accidental dislodgment, hemorrhage, and skin erosion.

The internal arteriovenous fistula (AVF) is the access of choice for clients receiving chronic dialysis.

According to current practice guidelines, 50% of all clients new to dialysis should have an AVF placed. The AVF is created through a surgical procedure in which an artery in the arm is anastomosed to a vein in an end-to-side, side-to-side, side-to-end, or end-to-end fashion (Figure 36-5, A). The result is an opening or fistula between a large artery and a large vein. The flow of arterial blood into the venous system causes the veins to become engorged (Figure 36-5, B). These fistulae require up to 6 weeks to mature before they can be used, which makes this approach inappropriate for immediate hemodialysis. Peritoneal dialysis or large venous access catheters may be used while the fistula is maturing. External arteriovenous shunts are rarely used.

The internal arteriovenous graft is used for chronic dialysis when the AVF is not possible. In this approach, an artificial graft (made of various synthetic and biologic materials) is used to create an artificial vein for blood flow. One end of the artificial graft is anastomosed to an artery, tunneled under the skin, and anastomosed to a vein. The graft can be used 2 weeks after insertion. Complications include clotting, aneurysms, and infection.

Once the fistula or graft is placed and ready for use, two 15- or 16-gauge needles are placed in the access at each dialysis treatment (Figure 36-5, C). A pump pulls

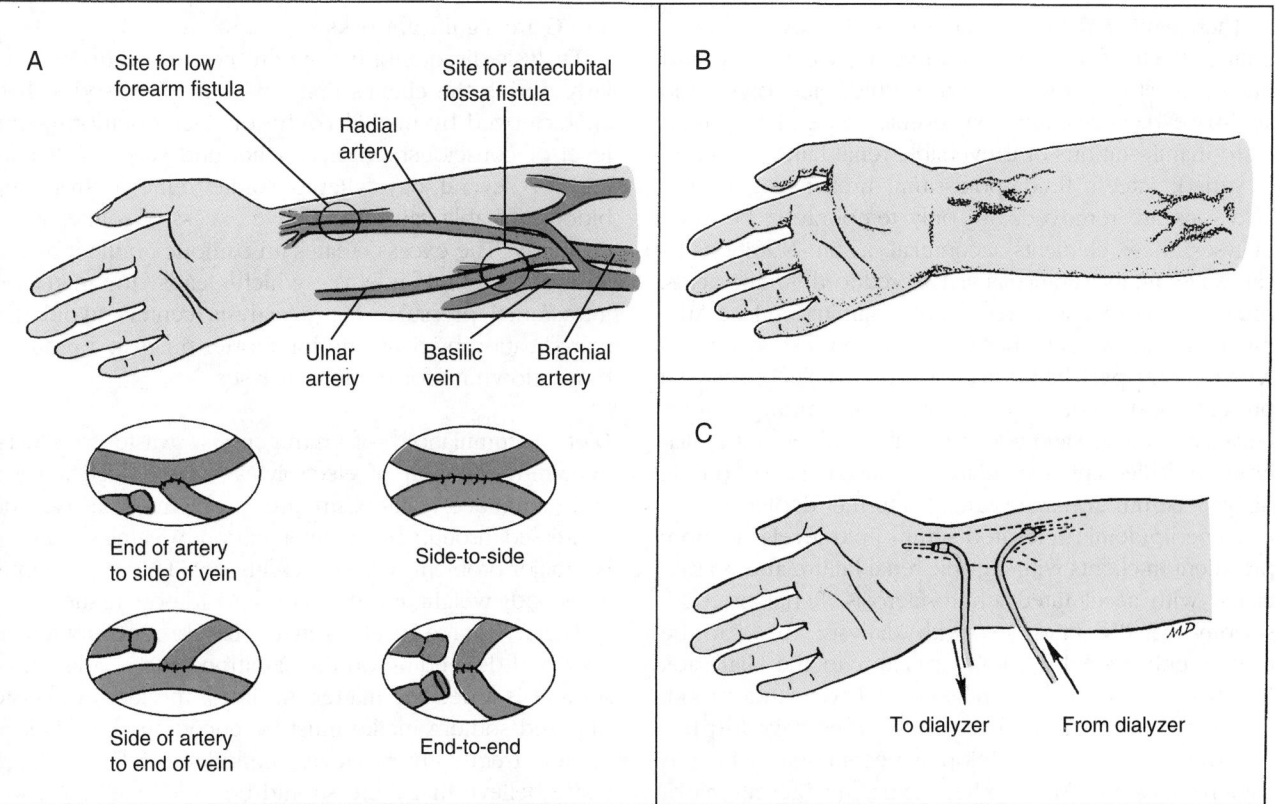

A, Site for low forearm fistula   Site for antecubital fossa fistula   Radial artery

Ulnar artery   Basilic vein   Brachial artery

End of artery to side of vein   Side-to-side

Side of artery to end of vein   End-to-end

B

C   To dialyzer   From dialyzer

■ **FIGURE 36–5** Internal arteriovenous fistula. Surgical creation of an arteriovenous anastomosis provides easy access to blood for hemodialysis. This method reduces the risk of infection and makes external shunts unnecessary except during hemodialysis. The internal fistula must be created 2 to 6 weeks before it can be used. **A,** Types of fistulae. **B,** Appearance of arm with fistulae. **C,** Dialysis needles in place. Red = artery, blue = vein.

arterial blood out by way of the fistula and into the hemodialyzer. Blood returns to the client by a tube connected to the other needle. Alternatively, single-needle dialysis may be used. With this device, only one puncture is required each time, but there may be significant recirculation of dialyzed blood, meaning that clearance rates are decreased. Internal arteriovenous grafts may cause hand swelling or ischemia (steal syndrome), carpal tunnel syndrome, hemorrhage, thrombosis, and aneurysms. Besides the arm, the subclavian, thigh, and ankle areas may be used as sites for hemodialysis access.

Dialyzers. Several types of dialyzers are available, including flat plate and hollow fiber mold devices. Choice of a particular system is mostly a matter of preference. There are differences in solute clearance rates (e.g., urea, creatinine, larger molecules) as well as ultrafiltration rates. Many centers that perform long-term dialysis disinfect and reuse the dialyzer for the same client to reduce costs. The dialysate solution is altered to fit the client's need.

Hemodialysis Schedules. Hemodialysis for ESRD must be continued intermittently for the client's lifetime unless successful kidney transplantation is performed. A typical schedule is 3 to 4 hours of treatment 3 days per week. This schedule varies with the size of the client, the type of dialyzer used, the rate of blood flow, and other factors.

Therapeutic Effects of Hemodialysis. The overall therapeutic effects of hemodialysis are to (1) clear waste products from the body; (2) restore fluid, electrolyte, and acid-base balances; and (3) reverse some of the untoward manifestations of irreversible renal failure. Success is varied. Excess fluid, potassium, urea nitrogen, and acid ions are removed, but only temporarily; between dialyses, these elements accumulate again. Nutritionally, carbohydrate intolerance is usually reduced. Amino acids, protein, glucose, and water-soluble vitamins are lost. Anemia generally worsens because of blood loss associated with the therapy. The predialysis causative factors are still present, and additional losses occur during dialysis because of blood sampling, residual blood left in the dialyzer, and bleeding secondary to anticoagulation during dialysis. Serum iron stores are also further depleted.

Hyperlipidemia (elevated serum lipid levels) is more prevalent in clients with chronic renal failure and is associated with accelerated atherosclerosis. Renal osteodystrophy usually improves with dialysis; this can be further enhanced by adding calcium to the dialysate. Pruritus may occur for reasons not yet understood. Men who have maintenance dialysis often have low testosterone levels and develop gynecomastia, which is usually transient. Many other sexual manifestations of uremia are reversed after a period of adaptation.

The usual effect of hemodialysis on serum concentration of medications is increased clearance, which is therapeutic in the case of overdose. Dosage schedules are altered to prevent, as much as possible, loss of medications through dialysis. Supplemental doses may be necessary to maintain therapeutic levels of certain medications.

Complications of Long-Term Hemodialysis. In addition to its therapeutic effects, chronic hemodialysis can cause a number of complications:

- Technical problems, such as blood leaks, overheating of the dialysate solution, insufficient loss of fluid, improper concentration of salts in the dialysate, and clotting
- Hypotension or hypertension
- Cardiac dysrhythmias from potassium imbalance
- Air embolus
- Hemorrhage resulting from heparinization with particular concern for subdural, retroperitoneal, pericardial, and intraocular bleeding
- Restless legs syndrome
- Pyrogenic reactions

Gastrointestinal ulcer disease is often complicated by hemorrhage. Muscle cramps may occur as a result of hyponatremia or hypo-osmolality and too rapid removal of fluid. Infection is a significant complication. Common infectious processes include local access infection, bacteremia, and infectious endocarditis, and hepatitis B and C are significant risks.

Dialysis disequilibrium syndrome can occur, particularly during the client's first few dialysis episodes. It is characterized by mental confusion, deterioration of the level of consciousness, headache, and seizures. It may last for several days. Rapid solute removal from the blood probably causes a relative excess of solutes intracellularly. The excess creates an osmotic gradient resulting in cerebral edema, which leads to increased intracranial pressure. Many dialysis centers avoid this complication by dialyzing for shorter times at a reduced blood flow rate for the first dialyses.

Diet. Accumulation of nitrogenous waste products, impaired excretion of electrolytes, vitamin deficiencies, and continued catabolism are problems that can be addressed through dietary intervention. Wasting syndrome is a major problem. The client with renal failure constantly loses body weight, muscle mass, and adipose tissue.

Dietary intake of electrolytes may be encouraged or restricted depending on the situation. The regulation of sodium is a delicate matter. At times, the kidneys waste salt, and sodium intake must be encouraged to replace it. More frequently, however, the kidneys retain sodium. Some believe that there should be moderate restriction with careful monitoring of urinary sodium excretion as a guideline. Serial monitoring of fluid status also gives important information about sodium needs.

Potassium is frequently restricted. Clients must be reminded not to use salt substitutes because they contain potassium chloride. When hyperkalemia becomes evident, restriction of potassium in food and fluids is instituted. In an emergency situation, when the serum potassium level is greater than 7 mEq/L, the client may require emergency treatment (see the Integrating Pharmacology feature on Medications for Acute Renal Failure, p. 813). Dialysis is also effective in removing potassium from the blood.

If serum calcium levels are low, adequate calcium intake is important. Dietary sources may be supplemented with calcium carbonate, calcium lactate, or calcium gluconate. If serum calcium levels are high, however, dietary restriction may be recommended. Phosphorus is restricted. In addition, calcium carbonate may be used to reduce phosphorus levels further. Finally, mild magnesium restriction may be imposed.

Medications. Medications commonly prescribed for clients with CKD are described in the Integrating Pharmacology feature below.

Promote Quality of Life

Renal failure and its therapies significantly affect the quality of life of the client and family members. As noted earlier, there are numerous stressors and life changes. Much of the care required by dialysis clients and their families concerns the psychosocial aspects of dialysis.

Clients receiving maintenance dialysis often have ambivalent feelings. They realize that dialysis therapy is their tie to life, but the many restrictions and lifestyle changes it imposes make adherence to the regimen extremely difficult. Clients often report that they feel in limbo between the worlds of life and death.

The process of adaptation to loss is part of adjustment. It is not uncommon for clients to feel grateful and optimistic at the start of dialysis treatments. Usually, they have felt ill for some time, and they view the intervention as a route to survival and feeling well again. It takes a few days or weeks for them to realize fully the permanent place of dialysis in their lives. Depression during this period is expected. The suicide rate among clients receiving dialysis has been estimated as 100 times that of the general population.

INTEGRATING PHARMACOLOGY

Medications for Stage 5 Chronic Kidney Disease

Clients with chronic renal failure typically take numerous medications to manage manifestations of their illness. Many factors must be considered before administering these drugs, including absorption, distribution, metabolism, and elimination of the medication. Because the kidneys are not functioning, drugs that are normally excreted by the kidney can accumulate to toxic levels. Some drugs are removed by dialysis; others are not. All these factors should be considered when determining dosage, route, and time of administration. Also, drugs that are nephrotoxic (e.g., aminoglycosides, intravenous pyelogram [IVP] dye) may cause further damage to a dysfunctional organ and should be avoided.

All clients with renal failure need vitamin supplements and folic acid, because water-soluble vitamins are dialyzed out, and because dietary restrictions may preclude adequate dietary intake. Also, in renal failure, there are significant disturbances in calcium and phosphorus balance. This is because vitamin D is normally activated in the kidney, and when kidneys are not functioning properly, calcium is not absorbed in sufficient quantities. Vitamin D analogs, such as calcitriol, help with the absorption of calcium. These drugs require close monitoring of serum calcium and phosphorus levels. Furthermore, many clients with renal failure take calcium supplements. Calcium carbonate and calcium acetate are relatively inexpensive and are useful both as calcium supplements and as phosphate binders. Because phosphorus is not excreted normally, serum phosphorus level is high and serum calcium level tends to be low. This can result in severe bone disease, known as osteitis fibrosa. Phosphate binders lower serum phosphorus level by binding with phosphates in the gut. However, they also tend to cause constipation. As a result, many people also take stool softeners or cathartics. Laxatives with magnesium should be avoided because of the risk of toxicity.

Hypertension is common in clients with renal failure. In some cases this is a result of fluid volume excess, and in other cases it can be caused by an excess of renin production by the kidneys (starting the renin-angiotensin system). Fluid volume removal through dialysis is one strategy to manage hypertension, but many clients need antihypertensives to control blood pressure effectively. There are many classifications of antihypertensives including angiotensin-converting enzyme inhibitors (e.g., captopril, enalapril, benazepril), beta-adrenergic blockers (e.g., propranolol, atenolol, metoprolol, labetalol), calcium channel blockers (e.g., nifedipine, verapamil), alpha$_1$-receptor blockers (e.g., prazosin), alpha$_2$-agonists (e.g., methyldopa, clonidine), and vasodilators. Each has a different mechanism of action, and, typically, considerable monitoring and adjustment of dosage and types of medication takes place before normotension is attained. Diuretics are typically not effective in clients with stage 5 CKD.

Erythropoietin is a hormone that is produced by the kidney and stimulates the production of red blood cells. A common manifestation of renal failure is anemia. Since 1989 this deficiency has been treated with epoetin alfa (EPO), a recombinant erythropoietin that increases hematocrit to near-normal levels. It can be administered intravenously, after hemodialysis, or subcutaneously. This results in significant improvements in the energy level and quality of life of clients with the illness. If iron levels are low, oral or intravenous iron treatment should also be initiated to optimize treatment with EPO. Long-acting forms of EPO (e.g., Aranesp) have recently been made available.

TRANSLATING EVIDENCE INTO PRACTICE

Quality of Life in End-Stage Renal Disease

Many aspects of renal replacement therapy have a negative impact on the quality of life of clients with ESRD.[1-6] Numerous manifestations, a restricted diet, and a demanding dialysis schedule prevent clients from living normal lives. However, in recent years, there has been considerable research addressing factors to enhance quality of life in this population. It has been recognized that a positive outlook, social support, and higher subjective health status[5,6] as well as sleep disturbances, pain, erectile dysfunction, client satisfaction with care, depressive affect, symptom burden, and intrusiveness of illness are related to quality of life.[3] It has also been noted that renal transplantation offers a higher quality of life than dialysis therapy.[3,5]

In recent years, there has been increasing emphasis on rehabilitation of clients with end-stage renal disease. In a study of 226 clients at approximately 60 days after the initiation of treatment, exercise activity was the most important predictor of quality of life.[4]

Qualitative research approaches have been used to explore why some clients live long and live well on dialysis. In one study, 18 clients who had been receiving dialysis therapy for more than 15 years were interviewed.[2] Life on dialysis was described as a transformation into comprehensive, active self-management of the disease, its treatment, and its manifestations. Participants in the study described affirmations such as self-preservation (i.e., I want to live), self-identity (i.e., I am still me), self-worth (i.e., I am still valuable), and self-efficacy (i.e., I am in control).[3]

Management of their illness included selective manifestation report and management, vigilant oversight of care,

proposal of treatment, confrontation of the system through active self-advocacy, and independent adoption of treatment and use of alternative therapies.[2] Similarly, others have found that love from others, accepting it as part of life, and trust in God were important strategies.[1]

IMPLICATIONS

Chronic renal failure and its treatment can severely compromise quality of life of people affected by the disease. Self-management is integral to ensuring a good quality of life. This requires considerable time and energy on the part of the client affected by the disease. Nurses can support self-management through education of clients, planning for exercise programs, and through supportive communication.

REFERENCES

1. Al-Arabi, S. (2006). Quality of life: Subjective descriptions of challenges to patients with end stage renal disease. *Nephrology Nursing Journal, 33,* 285-292.
2. Curtin, R.B., & Mapes, D.L. (2001). Health care management strategies of long-term dialysis survivors. *Nephrology Nursing Journal, 28,* 385-394.
3. Curtin, R.B., et al. (2002). Long-term dialysis survivors: A transformational experience. *Qualitative Health Research, 12,* 609-624.
4. Kimmel, P., & Patel, S.S. (2006). Quality of life in patients with chronic kidney disease: Focus on end-stage renal disease treated with hemodialysis. *Seminars in Nephrology, 26*(1), 68-79.
5. Kutner, N.G., Zhang, R., & McClellan, W.M. (2000). Patient reported quality of life early in dialysis treatment: Effects associated with usual exercise activity. *Nephrology Nursing Journal, 27,* 357-367.
6. Molzahn, A.E., Northcott, H.C., & Hayduk, L. (1996). Quality of life of patients with ESRD: A structural equation model. *Quality of Life Research, 5,* 426-432.
7. Molzahn, A.E., Northcott, H.C., & Dossetor, J.B. (1997). Perceptions of physicians, nurses, and patients regarding quality of life of patients with end stage renal disease. *American Nephrology Nurses Association Journal, 24,* 325-335.

Common psychosocial problems include changes in body image, dependence on technology, and uncertainty regarding the future. The client's own feelings of weakness and the presence of the AVF and dialysis equipment are constant reminders of the illness. Relationships with relatives and friends, job, and community roles and responsibilities are often altered. The client's need for independence is continually threatened by dependence on the dialysis equipment and care providers. This is especially true of adolescents and young adults. The stress on marital relationships and with significant others is extreme.

Research suggests that the quality of life of clients with ESRD is influenced positively by transplantation, erythropoietin therapy, social support, a positive outlook on life, and the ability to function (including work and activities of daily living). The Translating Evidence into Practice box above addresses quality-of-life issues faced by clients with end-stage renal disease. Providing an optimal quality of life involves a concerted effort by all members of the health care team with the client and family members as active partners. Many dialysis facilities have established active rehabilitation

programs. Elements of these programs include education, exercise, encouragement, employment, and evaluation.

Nursing Management of the Medical Client

Assessment. When a client is thought to have ESRD, take a complete history and look closely for risk factors. Question the client about past and present medications, diet and weight changes, energy levels and unexplained fatigue, and the pattern of urinary elimination.

Assess the client for the multiple effects of CKD on all body systems, such as the presence of cardiovascular or respiratory abnormalities, neurologic changes, gastrointestinal problems, or skin changes.

Assess the client's understanding of CKD, the diagnostic tests that will be done, and the possible treatment regimens. Evaluate the client's level of anxiety and ability to cope. Involve the family in the assessment to determine their ability to cope with the disease and treatments.

When a client has stage 5 CKD, the client and significant others, the nephrologist, the nephrology nurse, and often other members of the health care team discuss the use of dialysis and decide which type best meets the client's needs. If the client is to receive dialysis, assess the client's and significant others' understanding of the treatment regimen and the client's ability to cope with the treatment regimen. The family's ability to cope and their ability to support the client are also important considerations.

When the client begins peritoneal dialysis, assess for infection. Inspect the insertion site carefully for redness or other problems. Carefully assess the drained dialysate or effluent for cloudiness, fibrin streaks, or blood. Monitor the client's vital signs and weight closely.

If the client is undergoing hemodialysis, assess the patency of the vascular access site. In a patent AVF or graft, a "thrill" or vibrating sensation should be palpable and a bruit should be audible with a stethoscope. It is vital that this site be assessed for possible occlusion or, if it is an external site, for infection. Also ascertain the client's understanding of the access site and its care.

Diagnosis, Outcomes, Interventions

Diagnosis: Deficient Fluid Volume or Excess Fluid Volume. As with all renal disorders, a common nursing diagnosis is *Deficient Fluid Volume* or *Excess Fluid Volume related to impaired renal function, fluid shifts between dialysate and blood, and blood loss during hemodialysis.*

Outcomes. Fluid balance will exist, as evidenced by the absence of edema or dehydration.

Interventions

Monitor Fluid Volume Status. A fluid volume deficit or overload is a serious problem. The current fluid status must be known and fluid intake carefully regulated accordingly. Monitor the client's fluid status by observing daily weights, orthostatic blood pressure, skin turgor, and mucous membrane moistness and by meticulous intake and output comparisons.

Give written instructions to outpatients that explain how to weigh themselves properly and how to interpret the relationship of daily weight loss or gain to their need for sodium and water. Help the client understand that vomiting, diarrhea, and working or playing in a hot environment may cause excessive fluid loss and must be prevented or controlled. Teach the client how to take his or her blood pressure and record it daily.

Follow Fluid Restrictions. When the fluid allowance for the day has been determined, help the client follow the recommendation. Fluid restrictions are difficult for most clients. Offer suggestions about reducing thirst and moistening lips by using lip balms, performing frequent oral hygiene, and eating ice chips or using spray bottles rather than drinking. Spread out fluid intake over a longer time. If intravenous fluids are used, carefully attend to them to ensure proper administration rates.

Water may be restricted so that the client can drink more nutritious liquids.

Monitor Fluid Status During Dialysis. During dialysis, carefully monitor the client's vital signs, including postural blood pressure, pulse rate, weight, and intake and output. Watch for hypovolemia and retention of dialysate. The amount of desired fluid loss may be ordered by the dialysis physician. Alternatively, a "dry" or "ideal" weight is established and you select appropriate solutions to remove additional fluid.

If fluid does not drain properly during peritoneal dialysis, check the system for kinks or other obstructions. Inform the physician about fluid accumulations that exceed the limit set in the dialysis orders. If the client is undergoing hemodialysis, hypotension and excess fluid removal are risks; monitor carefully.

Diagnosis: Imbalanced Nutrition: Less Than Body Requirements. Another common nursing diagnosis in stage 5 CKD is *Imbalanced Nutrition: Less Than Body Requirements related to anorexia and nausea.*

Outcomes. The client will maintain adequate nutrition, as evidenced by maintenance of weight without loss of muscle mass.

Interventions. Dietary management is vital to the conservative management of stage 5 CKD. Anorexia results from many of the manifestations of irreversible renal failure, emotional depression, and a frequently unpalatable diet. Thus a major nursing challenge is to help the client consume adequate nutrition while minimizing uremic toxicity. This problem escalates as the disease progresses, and the client may develop an aversion to meat and other sources of protein.

To help stimulate the client's appetite, take measures to relieve nausea and vomiting, stomatitis, and other gastrointestinal manifestations. Diet counseling is essential. Teaching aids (such as those found on the National Kidney Foundation website at www.kidney.org or the Kidney School website at www.kidneyschool.org) may be helpful. Arrange for dietary consultation if possible. The client needs to know how to translate the dietary regimen into palatable, understandable menus. Help the client select and prepare foods and learn where to obtain special foods if necessary. Exercise may also improve appetite.

Diagnosis: Constipation. The treatment of stage 5 CKD leads to the predictable nursing diagnosis of *Constipation related to medications, fluid and dietary restrictions, and decreased activity level.*

Outcomes. The client will have less difficulty with bowel elimination.

Interventions. Constipation is a major problem for clients with stage 5 CKD. Because of fluid restrictions, inability to eat most high-fiber foods, constipating medications, and limited activity, it is difficult to use customary measures for preventing constipation.

Bran, which is limited in potassium or phosphorus, can be used. Stool softeners are often administered regularly, although care should be taken to avoid those that contain calcium and sodium. If necessary, bulk laxatives (such as psyllium hydrophilic mucilloid) may be given. The recommended amount of fluid should be taken with the powder and subtracted from the day's fluid allotment.

Stimulant and lubricant laxatives should be used only if necessary, especially compounds containing magnesium or phosphorus, such as sodium biphosphate–sodium phosphate (Fleet) enemas. If none of these measures is effective, small-volume, gentle stimulant enemas may be used sparingly, but large-volume enemas should be avoided because of possible fluid and saline absorption. Clients with ESRD are at risk for diverticular disease because of the constipation and straining.

Diagnosis: Fatigue. Physiologic alterations can ensure a nursing diagnosis of *Fatigue related to anemia and altered metabolic state.*

Outcomes. The client will have greater energy, activity tolerance, and endurance.

Interventions. Anemia should be treated with iron and erythropoietin therapy to increase energy levels. Exercise is an important strategy to reduce fatigue and improve quality of life. Many dialysis units are implementing exercise programs with stationary bicycles. It is important to have the physician assess the client first and reinforce the need for exercise. Physiotherapists or exercise physiologists can be very helpful to develop programs for debilitated clients. Resource materials for exercise programs can be found at www.kidneyschool.org/pdfs/KS-Module_12.pdf or www.lifeoptions.org/catalog/pdfs/booklets/exercise.pdf.

Rest is also important to any client whose body is under a great deal of stress. Insomnia is frequently a problem, and you may need to make suggestions about how to solve this problem (as by observing a presleep quiet time and establishing a presleep routine). Assessment in a sleep center may be helpful. Hypnotics and sedatives must be used cautiously because they may alter mentation and may be metabolized differently by a client with renal failure.

Diagnosis: Risk for Impaired Skin Integrity. Edema and skin changes create a *Risk for Impaired Skin Integrity related to edema, dry skin, and pruritus.*

Outcomes. The client will maintain tissue integrity, as evidenced by intact skin.

Interventions. Dry skin is a common problem. Use of soap may need to be eliminated. Because of the increased risk of secondary infection, the client's skin needs to be kept clean. Moisturizing oils in the bath water or applied directly to the skin help to correct dryness. Avoid any products that contain alcohol or perfumes; they increase dryness and pruritus. If edema is present, avoid sustained pressure on the area. The potential for skin breakdown is particularly acute in clients with diabetes mellitus. Observe for poor circulation and areas of breakdown or infection. Assess feet of diabetic clients daily and teach them foot care (see Chapter 45).

Diagnosis: Readiness for Enhanced Self-Care. An important diagnosis is *Readiness for Enhanced Self-Care related to learning to live with a chronic illness, uncertain future, many stressors, role reversal, and effects of long-term dialysis.*

Outcomes. The client and family will adapt to the chronic illness, as evidenced by acceptance of the client's condition and ability to support the client. The client and family will effectively adapt to the effects of long-term dialysis, as evidenced by the client's level of activity, feelings of self-worth, and participation in dialysis treatment.

Interventions

Involvement in Decision Making. Assistance for the client and significant others must begin before dialysis is started. A client with CKD faces a future of continued deterioration but with an unknown course and timetable. In addition, the disease itself produces manifestations that contribute to the client's susceptibility to stress.

Many clients must make important decisions about the choice of treatment modes at a time when they do not feel well. It is often difficult for the client to voice concerns about discontinuing dialysis, and it may be difficult for care providers and families to accept the client's decision to stop treatment and choose death instead. For these reasons, you need to assess how the client handled change and stress before the illness began. The client and significant others need to be actively involved in the care planning process because they will be living with the disease for many years.

Provide Support. The client and significant others will have many questions about issues such as family functioning, job or school demands, dependence, and sex. The client may experience reduced self-esteem. Significant others commonly report a decline in their quality of life that correlates directly with changes in the client's quality of life. Encourage the client and significant others to discuss their feelings and concerns, together and individually, using therapeutic communication techniques. Support groups and peer counseling programs are often helpful.

Offer Home Dialysis. About 15% of all clients who receive dialysis do so at home. The cost of this type of program is less than that of in-center dialysis, and it usually improves the client's quality of life. Home dialysis offers the client more access to significant others and greater feelings of independence and control. However, this type of treatment also produces stress on personal relationships, especially on the person who becomes the "dialysis helper" during home hemodialysis. Some spouses have voiced concern about lack of free time and increased responsibility; others see it as an opportunity to give something back to their spouse or loved one. Some states have funding available to pay for a non–family member to serve as dialysis helper. In some instances, this may reduce tension and improve the quality of life for the family.

Clients for home dialysis programs must be selected carefully. Criteria might include stability of relationships, psychological stability, financial support, and lack of severe physical complications. A successful program requires care providers who are advocates of home dialysis, a good training program, and good support services, including nursing, medical, and social services; provision of supplies; equipment maintenance; dietary counseling; home visits; and retraining as necessary.

Provide Information. Teaching is a crucial part of the nursing management plan. Usually, the client is observed on an outpatient basis and is responsible for following the recommended treatment regimen. The client and significant others must know about normal renal function and how the disease has altered it, the details of the management protocol and how to follow it, a number of self-assessment skills as described earlier, and when to seek professional consultation for possible complications. Teaching aids are available from many sources, such as the National Kidney Foundation, the National Association of Patients on Hemodialysis and Transplantation, various corporations, and the Internet. The Life Options Rehabilitation Program offers an award-winning website known as Kidney School (see www.KidneySchool.org).

Explain Dialysis. The client and significant others need to understand dialysis and its ramifications. With peritoneal dialysis, most clients continue the treatment mode in their homes; hence their knowledge needs to be complete and detailed. They participate in a complete training program so that they can handle the entire dialysis process independently.

Continuous monitoring during hemodialysis provides vital information about the progress of the treatment and allows early diagnosis of potential complications. There should be a well-organized plan for observing and recording vital signs, dialysate composition and temperature, and functioning of the entire dialysis system and blood flow. The client should also be alert to early manifestations of potential complications, as listed earlier. The nurse often serves as case manager and coordinates the services provided by the nephrology team, which includes the physician, social worker, dietitian, and nurses. In addition, the disease interferes with normal cognitive functioning; memory deficits and a short attention span may necessitate simple presentations and frequent repetition of information. Although the client is readily available during dialysis treatment, this may not be the best time to teach about the therapy, because of cognitive changes that accompany shifts in levels of electrolytes and nitrogenous wastes. Significant others need reassurance that this is common and that the client will be more capable of learning after institution of regular dialysis and outside of dialysis treatments. Retained learning must be continually evaluated.

Reduce Anxiety. Although clients with renal disease must learn about their disorder, they may not always be ready to learn. Anxiety itself interferes with learning.

Diagnosis: Risk for Infection. Indwelling catheters carry a high *Risk for Infection related to the presence of an indwelling peritoneal catheter and instillation of dialysate or related to venipuncture and connection of tubing during hemodialysis.*

Outcomes. The client will remain free of infection, as evidenced by a normal white blood cell count, absence of fever, and clear dialysate.

Interventions

Because peritonitis is the main complication of peritoneal dialysis, strict aseptic technique must be used throughout the procedure. Masks are normally worn by the nurse and client when the peritoneal dialysis circuit is opened. Gloves are worn by anyone touching the catheter during all connection and disconnection procedures. The catheter is soaked before and after these procedures in a povidone-iodine or other disinfecting solution. Dressing changes around the catheter site are performed according to the specific unit protocol. Be sure dressings are kept dry at all times.

With hemodialysis, strict aseptic technique is used during venipuncture and when attaching the tubing and solution.

SAFETY

⚠

ALERT

Diagnosis: Risk for Ineffective Breathing Pattern. Peritoneal dialysis also creates a *Risk for Ineffective Breathing Pattern related to pressure from dialysate.*

Outcomes. The client will have normal respiratory status, as evidenced by an absence of shortness of breath.

Interventions. Because dialysate presses on the diaphragm, full excursion may be reduced and an immobilized client may be at risk for respiratory problems. Encourage the client to cough and deep breathe regularly. Keep the client in the semi-Fowler position to ease breathing. Also, remind the client to stay alert for early manifestations of compromised respiratory function.

Diagnosis: Risk for Injury. Trauma and complications associated with the vascular access for hemodialysis may occur, leading to the nursing diagnosis of *Risk for Injury related to trauma to hemodialysis vascular access site*.

Outcomes. Risk will be controlled; the client will not experience injury to the vascular access site, as evidenced by continued patency of the site.

Interventions

SAFETY
ALERT

Careful attention to prevention of infections and clotting is important to the life expectancy of the access site. A dressing is used to protect central venous catheters from infection. The access site must also be protected from trauma that could cause clotting, bleeding, or physical disruption of the site. For example, warn the client against wearing tight sleeves or carrying a purse over the access site. The limb that contains the access site should not be used to take blood pressure measurements or to draw blood.

Between dialysis treatments, the skin over the fistula or graft requires only routine care with soap and water. The site of a fistula should be carefully assessed. To assess patency, palpate over the fistula for a thrill and auscultate for a bruit at regular intervals. The client must also learn to assess the access site for patency.

Evaluation. The client is expected to improve physically and mentally when dialysis begins. The client's weight and blood pressure should begin to stabilize if dietary and fluid restrictions are followed and as fluid balance stabilizes.

Normal electrolyte and albumin levels reflect adequate nutrition and adherence to diet. The client should report regular, normal bowel movements. The client should report less fatigue and increased energy and activity as hematocrit values approach normal levels. Skin should remain intact.

The client should understand and adapt to the treatment regimen and be successfully maintained with peritoneal dialysis or hemodialysis. Clients receiving peritoneal dialysis (and some receiving hemodialysis) should be able to demonstrate successful performance of the dialysis procedure and care of the vascular access site or peritoneal catheter. They should remain free from complications associated with dialysis. As long as venous or peritoneal access can be maintained, the client can be managed with dialysis until transplantation (if the client is a candidate) is completed, the client elects to stop dialysis, or other complications result in death.

Significant others will exhibit coping mechanisms to deal with the client's chronic illness and dialysis, show acceptance of problems, support the client, and report improved satisfaction with their own quality of life. The family and significant others are important sources of support for the client.

Self-Care

Clients must learn to adhere to dietary and fluid intake modifications and take prescribed medications as ordered. In many cases, they must monitor and record weight and blood pressure measurements daily. Care of the vascular access or peritoneal catheter is necessary. Lack of adherence to the regimen may lead to serious complications.

Modifications for Older Clients

The type of dialysis selected for older clients is based on an assessment that includes the presence of other disorders. Older clients may have had multiple abdominal surgical procedures with the development of adhesions that limit the usefulness of peritoneal dialysis. They are more likely to have pre-existing cardiovascular problems that may limit selection of vascular access sites.

RENAL TRANSPLANTATION

Surgical Management

Indications

Renal transplantation is the surgical implantation of a human kidney from a compatible donor in a recipient. This procedure is performed as an intervention in stage 5 CKD. The kidney is surgically placed extraperitoneally in the iliac fossa. The renal artery is anastomosed to the recipient's hypogastric internal or external iliac artery (occasionally the aorta) and the renal vein is anastomosed to the recipient's iliac vein (Figure 36-6). Usually, the kidney begins to function immediately.

Selection of a transplant recipient is based on careful evaluation of the client's medical, immunologic, and

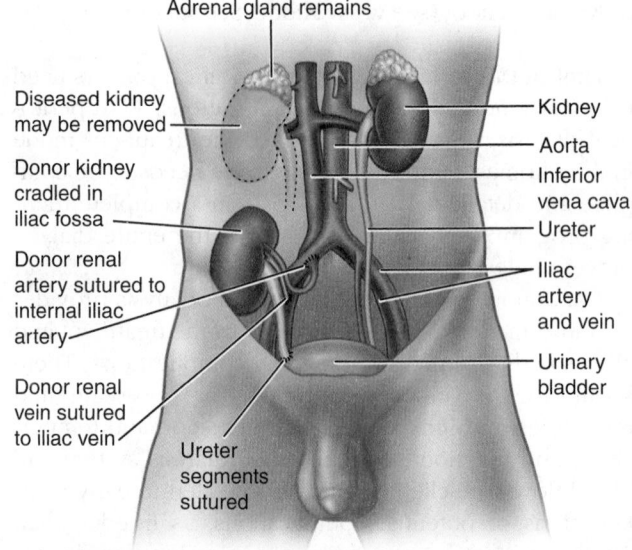

■ **FIGURE 36–6** Transplanted kidney placement in the right iliac fossa.

psychosocial status (see Chapter 80). Usually, a recipient is younger than age 70, has an estimated life expectancy of 2 years or more, and is expected to have an improved quality of life after transplantation. Conservative management and dialysis should have the client in the best possible health. Bilateral nephrectomy may be performed before the transplantation procedure for persistent or active bacterial pyelonephritis, uncontrolled renin-mediated hypertension, polycystic kidneys, or rapidly progressive glomerulonephritis.

Successful transplantation prolongs life and markedly improves its quality. The client is freed from the restrictions of dialysis and from the reversible manifestations of uremia.

Because graft survival rates are higher, the most desirable source of kidneys for transplantation is a living related donor who matches the client closely. Willing family members are evaluated for physical and mental health and screened for ABO blood group, tissue-specific antigen, and human leukocyte antigen histocompatibility (see Chapter 80). Some centers transplant kidneys from emotionally related donors, such as friends or spouses; a few transplant centers have 'paired exchange' programs where two kidney donors who are unable to donate to a relative (for reasons related to blood type or immunological incompatibility) donate to another person on the wait list in exchange for a similar donation to their loved one. In recent years, a few centers have accepted 'altruistic living donations' from donors who do not know who the recipient will be, but wish to help others. In recent years, the number of living donations is close to or has exceeded the number of cadaveric donations, because of the limited supply of the latter.

Contraindications

Infection and active malignancy are the only absolute contraindications to transplantation. However, some physical conditions markedly increase the risk for the client, primarily because long-term immunosuppressive medications are necessary to avoid graft rejection. Clients with liver disease, psychological disorders, advanced atherosclerosis, hypertension, respiratory disease, and gastrointestinal bleeding need particular consideration. Despite this, the primary factor limiting transplantation is the availability of kidneys.

Complications

Major complications of transplantation, such as graft rejection (and antirejection therapy), infection, skin and gastrointestinal problems, and other complications, are discussed in Chapter 80.

Graft Rejection. The manifestations of renal transplant rejection include fever, graft tenderness at the site of the transplanted kidney, anemia, and malaise.

Urinary Tract Complications. Several complications may occur in the urinary tract. Although it is rare, spontaneous rupture of the kidney may occur because of rejection or ischemic damage. Leaking of urine from the ureter-bladder anastomosis causes the development of a urinoma, which eventually puts pressure on the kidney and ureter, reducing renal function. Long-term uremia and steroid therapy may predispose the client to ureteral, bladder, or caliceal-cutaneous fistulae. Other urinary tract complications include ureteral, bladder, or pelvic leaks, as well as obstruction, reflux, and lymphoceles.

Cardiopulmonary Complications. Hypertension occurs in 50% to 60% of adult recipients and may be caused by renal artery stenosis, acute tubular necrosis, acute and chronic graft rejection, hydronephrosis, hyperaldosteronism, large-dose steroids, and cyclosporine. Cardiac dysrhythmias and heart failure may result from fluid and electrolyte imbalances.

Pneumonia caused by bacteria and fungi is the most frequent respiratory complication. Other respiratory problems include pulmonary edema, pulmonary emboli, and reactivated tuberculosis.

Other Complications. The reproductive problems associated with stage 5 CKD commonly disappear after transplantation. The incidence of gynecologic malignancies is higher than in the general population, with cervical cancer dominating. Successful pregnancies have occurred after transplantation, but there is a risk for both the fetus and the mother with a transplanted kidney.

Outcomes

Over the years, both recipient and graft survival rates have greatly improved. One-year graft survival rates are 85% to 90% with transplants from living related donors and 75% to 80% with cadaver kidneys. The overall mortality rate 2 years after transplantation is about 10%. This represents a dramatic decrease; 2 decades ago, the 2-year survival rate was 40% to 50%.

In particular, the decrease in the death rate related to infection in the first 2 years after transplantation has been dramatic. Advances in immunosuppressive therapy and the treatment of infectious diseases have contributed to the overall improvement. Cardiovascular problems remain the leading cause of death in the late transplantation period. Myocardial infarction, stroke, and heart failure are the primary causes of death.

Nursing Management of the Surgical Client

Preoperative Care

Before kidney transplantation, assess the client's understanding of the procedure and follow-up regimen. Also, assess the client's ability to cope with a complex medication regimen after transplantation. The client needs to understand the transplantation and therapeutic regimen. Preoperative preparation of both the living donor and the recipient includes all aspects of general preoperative care as outlined in Chapter 14.

Postoperative Care

Assessment for renal transplant recipients is similar to that for most other postoperative clients (see Chapter 14), with the exception of the focus on renal function. Give particular attention to fluid balance, and carefully monitor intake and output (every 30 to 60 minutes) and weight (daily). To monitor renal function and maintain electrolyte balance, obtain serial laboratory determinations of hemoglobin, hematocrit, BUN (urea nitrogen), creatinine, electrolytes, white blood cell count, and platelets. Auscultate the kidney regularly to check for bruits, which might indicate stenosis at the site of anastomosis. Monitoring of vital signs is key, because even a slight temperature increase may indicate an infection.

The function of the transplanted kidney is a primary concern after surgery. A kidney from a cadaver may not function immediately, and the client may be maintained with hemodialysis until it functions adequately. Postoperatively, manage intravenous fluids carefully; the amount of fluid infused is typically based on the previous hour's output. A high urine output is usually desired. The additional care required by the recipient is related to potential complications. Care of the client with a transplant is discussed in more detail in Chapter 80.

Psychologically, the client must be helped to incorporate the new kidney as a part of the whole being. Provide education and counseling to enhance changes in lifestyle that promote health-seeking behaviors and compliance with transplantation medications. If the graft fails, expect the client to feel anger, hostility, guilt, and helplessness/hopelessness. Relatives and friends may mirror these feelings. Role changes may occur; for example, a family member may no longer feel needed. Similarly, the client may have difficulty giving up the sick role.

Self-Care

Failure to follow the prescribed regimen is a major problem after transplantation, and your knowledge and creativity are needed to help the client follow the recommended regimen. Many clients—particularly adolescents—miss doses of their immunosuppressive medications (see Chapter 80). This practice contributes to early loss of renal function and possible graft loss.

Clients may be reluctant to take medications for many reasons. For some, the side effects disrupt their lives. Others may believe that they no longer need the medications because their condition is stable. Economic concerns also need to be addressed. Work with the client to provide needed information and to develop strategies that fit the client's lifestyle.

Overall, transplantation offers clients with stage 5 CKD a much better quality of life than dialysis therapy. Renal function returns and many of the clinical manifestations of ESRD disappear. Complications do occur, and care must be taken to prevent graft loss. Renal transplant recipients are monitored regularly at transplantation clinics. The visits become less frequent as renal function stabilizes and time passes. Blood tests are done regularly to monitor serum creatinine levels and cyclosporine levels. Every transplantation center has protocols for routine follow-up tests.

Modifications for Older Clients

Clients older than 60 years are evaluated on an individual basis; clients 75 years of age have had successful transplantations. In older clients, a less effective immune system in conjunction with immunosuppressants can lead to further complications.

 CONCLUSIONS

Caring for the client with kidney failure, whether acute or chronic, involves many challenges. Numerous physical and psychosocial manifestations are associated with renal disease and its treatment. The nurse can significantly impact the client's quality of life through the provision of education, encouragement, promotion of exercise, and ongoing assessment of the client and family as well as evaluation of programs offering treatment for ESRD. The nurse, in collaboration with the multidisciplinary team, can facilitate positive outcomes.

 THINKING CRITICALLY

1. You are caring for a 74-year-old man 1 day after coronary artery bypass surgery. His urine output is about 15 ml/hour. He has a long history of hypertension (controlled), and his blood pressure usually ranges from 180 to 190 over 90 to 100 mm Hg. His blood pressure since surgery has ranged from 120 to 130 over 70 to 76 mm Hg. His serum sodium concentration is 145 mEq/L and potassium concentration is 4.9 mEq/L. His skin turgor is poor, and his mucous membranes are dry. What is your first assessment and action?

Factors to Consider. What has his intake been since surgery? What are the possible causes of his low blood pressure, increased electrolytes, and decreased urine output? If he has renal failure, what is the probable cause? What other assessments should you make?

2. You are caring for a 60-year-old woman with diabetes mellitus, hypertension, and chronic renal failure. She has had hemodialysis for over a year and has decided that she no longer wants to continue living this way. She has informed her physician and family that she no longer wishes to continue dialysis. Her family is trying to

persuade her that she should go for her next treatment. She asks your opinion, "Would you want to live this way?" How would you respond? How would you ensure that she is making the right decision?

Factors to Consider. What is the client's cognitive and emotional status? How have the client and her family members coped with the illness and its treatment? Given the information you have, what is her prognosis? Do people have the right to refuse life-sustaining therapy? Knowing that health care resources are finite, what is the best use of resources for all members of society?

Discussions for these questions can be found on the website.

BIBLIOGRAPHY

Citations appearing in red refer to primary research.

Citations appearing in blue refer to evidence-based practice guidelines and protocols.

1. Abbott, E.C., Cruess, D.F., Agodoa, L.Y.C., et al. (2004). Early renal insufficiency and late venous thromboembolism after renal transplantation in the United States. *American Journal of Kidney Diseases, 43,* 120-130.
2. Arduino, M.J., & Tokars, J.I. (2005). Why is an infection control program needed in the hemodialysis setting? *Nephrology News and Issues, 19*(7), 44, 46–49.
3. Audrain, J., & Vesely, T.M. (2004). Vascular access for hemodialysis. *Journal of the Association for Vascular Access, 9,* 214-217.
4. Ayanian, J.Z., Clearly, P.D., Keogh, J.H., et al. (2004). Physicians' beliefs about racial differences in referral for renal transplantation. *American Journal of Kidney Diseases, 43,* 350-357.
5. Baldwin, D., & Jensik, S. (2005). Posttransplant diabetes mellitus in renal transplantation. *Graft, 7*(2), 74-84.
6. Bernardini, J. (2004). Peritoneal dialysis: Myths, barriers and achieving optimum outcomes. *Nephrology Nursing Journal, 31,* 494-498.
7. Bloe, C. (2004). Acute medical emergency: Acute renal failure. *Nurse 2 Nurse, 4*(9), 26-27.
8. Borkan, S.C. (2002). Extracorporeal therapies for acute intoxications. *Critical Care Clinics, 18*(2), 393-420.
9. Brenner, B.M., & Levine, S.A. (Eds.) (2004). *Brenner and Rector's the kidney* (7th ed.). Philadelphia: W.B. Saunders.
10. Bresnahan, B.A. (2005). Renal transplantation: Long term renal function and the stable patient. *Graft, 7,* 156-167.
11. Burrows-Hudson, S., & Prowant, B.F. (Eds.) (2005). *Nephrology nursing: Standards of practice and guidelines for care.* Pitman, NJ: American Nephrology Nurses Association.
12. Burrowes, J.D. (2004). Incorporating ethnic and cultural food preferences in the renal diet. *Advances in Renal Replacement Therapy, 11,* 97-104.
13. Caimi, G., Carollo, C., & Presti, R.L. (2005). Pathophysiological and clinical aspects of malnutrition in chronic renal failure. *Nutrition Research Reviews, 18*(1), 89-97.
14. Campoy, S., & Elwell, R. (2005). Pharmacology and CKD. *American Journal of Nursing, 105*(9), 60-72.
15. Carson, C.C. (2005). 50 years of renal transplantation: A major milestone, but miles still to go. *Contemporary Urology, 17*(4), 9.
16. Chang, G., Wu, C., Pan, S., et al. (2004). The diagnosis of pneumonia in renal transplant recipients using invasive and noninvasive procedures. *Chest, 125,* 541-547.
17. Chuang, S., Sung, J., Kuo, S., et al. (2005). Oral and dental manifestations in diabetic and nondiabetic uremic patients receiving hemodialysis. *Oral Surgery, Oral Medicine, Oral Pathology, Oral Radiology & Endodontics, 99,* 689-695.
18. Curtin, R.B., Mapes, D., Schatell, D., et al. (2005). Self-management in patients with end stage renal disease: Exploring domains and dimensions. *Nephrology Nursing Journal, 32,* 389-398.
19. Curtin, R.B., Johnson, H.K., & Schatell, D. (2004). The peritoneal dialysis experience: Insights from long-term patients. *Nephrology Nursing Journal, 31*(6), 615-625.
20. Danovitch, G.M. (Ed.) (2004). *Handbook of kidney transplantation* (4th ed.). Philadelphia: Lippincott Williams & Wilkins.
21. Daugirdas, J.T., Blake, P.G., & Ing, T.S. (2001). *Handbook of dialysis* (3rd ed.). Philadelphia: Lippincott Williams & Wilkins.
22. Davison, S.N., & Jhangri, G.S. (2005). The impact of chronic pain on depression, sleep and the desire to withdraw from dialysis in hemodialysis patients. *Journal of Pain and Symptom Management, 30,* 465-473.
23. Diaz-Buxo, J.A., & Crawford-Bonadio, T.L. (2005). Impact of peritoneal dialysis technology on patient care. *Advances in Peritoneal Dialysis, 21,* 112-114.
24. Druml, W. (2005). Nutritional management of acute renal failure. *Journal of Renal Nutrition, 15*(1), 63-70.
25. Fowler, C., & Baas, L. (2006). Illness representations in patients with chronic kidney disease on maintenance hemodialysis. *Nephrology Nursing Journal, 33,* 173-186.
26. Gillies, M., & Sims, K. (2005). Renal and diabetes nursing education: Peritoneal leak risk assessment tool. *Australian Nursing Journal, 13*(5), 24.
27. Giri, M. (2004). Choice of renal replacement therapy in patients with diabetic end stage renal disease. *EDTNA/ERCA Journal of Renal Care, 30*(3), 138-142.
28. Hagren, B., Pettersen, I., Severinsson, E., et al. (2005). Maintenance hemodialysis: Patients' experiences of their life situation. *Journal of Clinical Nursing, 14,* 294-300.
29. Hamdan, A., Medawar, W., Younes, A., et al. (2005). The effect of hemodialysis on voice: An acoustic analysis. *Journal of Voice, 19,* 290-295.
30. Harwood, L., Locking-Cusolito, H., Spittal, J., et al. (2005). Preparing for hemodialysis: Patient stressors and responses. *Nephrology Nursing Journal, 32,* 295-303.
31. Hiewe, S., & Dahlgren, M.A. (2004). Living with chronic renal failure: Coping with physical activities of daily living. *Advances in Physiotherapy, 6*(4), 147-157.
32. Hossli, S.M. (2005). Clinical management of intradialytic hypotension: Survey results. *Nephrology Nursing Journal, 32,* 287-292.
33. Kasinskas, C., & Piazza, D. (2004). Chronic renal failure—A clinical pathway. *Acute Care Perspectives, 13*(3), 3-4.
34. Kinnel, K. (2005). Should patients eat during hemodialysis treatments? *Nephrology Nursing Journal, 32,* 513-515, 568.
35. Lameire, N., VanBiesen, W., & Vanholder, R. (2005). Acute renal failure. *Lancet, 365*(9457), 417-430.
36. Locking-Cusolito, H., Harwood, L., Wilson, B., et al. (2005). Prevalence of risk factors predisposing to foot problems in patients on hemodialysis. *Nephrology Nursing Journal, 32,* 373-384.
37. Ly, J., Marticorena, R., & Donnelly, S. (2004). Red blood cell survival in chronic renal failure. *American Journal of Kidney Diseases, 44,* 715-719.
38. Mapes, D. (2005). Nurses' impact on the choice and longevity of vascular access. *Nephrology Nursing Journal, 32,* 670-674.
39. Molzahn, A.E., & Butera, E. (2006). *Contemporary nephrology nursing: Principles and practice.* Pitman, NJ: American Nephrology Nurses Association.
40. Monroe, J., & Raiz, L. (2005). Barriers to employment following renal transplantation: Implications for the social work professional. *Social Work in Health Care, 40*(4), 61-81.
41. Nakamura, A.T., Btaiche, I.F., Pasko, D.A., et al. (2004). In vitro clearance of trace elements via continuous renal replacement therapy. *Journal of Renal Nutrition, 14*(4), 214-219.
42. Nelson, S.L., Shouten, J.M., & Valentine, L.O. (2005). Reducing vascular access complications: An evidence-based approach. *Journal of Vascular Access, 6,* 167-170.
43. Radhakrishnan, J., & Kiryluk, K. (2005). Acute renal failure outcomes in children and adults. *Kidney International, 69,* 17-19.
44. Redmond, A., & Doherty, E. (2005). Peritoneal dialysis. *Nursing Standard, 19*(40), 55-66, 68.

45. Redmond, A., McDevitt, M., & Barnes, S. (2004). Continuing professional development. Acute renal failure: Recognition and treatment in ward patients. *Nursing Standard, 18*(22), 46-55.

46. Ronsberg, F., Isles, C., Simpson, K., et al. (2005). Renal replacement therapy in the over 80s. *Age and Aging, 34*(2), 148-152.

47. Russell, T.A. (2005). Acute renal failure related to rhabdomyolysis: Pathophysiology, diagnosis, and collaborative management. *Nephrology Nursing Journal, 32,* 409-419.

48. Savey, A., Simon, F., Izopet, J., et al. (2005). A large nosocomial outbreak of hepatitis C virus infections at a hemodialysis center. *Infection Control and Hospital Epidemiology, 26,* 752-760.

49. Schrier, R.W. (2005). *Manual of nephrology* (6th ed.). Philadelphia: Lippincott Williams & Wilkins.

50. Schrier, R.W., & Wang, W. (2004). Mechanisms of disease: Acute renal failure and sepsis. *New England Journal of Medicine, 351* (2), 159-169, 201–204.

51. Strippoli, G.F.M., Tong, A., Johnson, D., et al. (2004). Antimicrobial agents to prevent peritonitis in peritoneal dialysis: A systematic review of randomized controlled trials. *American Journal of Kidney Disease, 44*(4), 591-603.

52. Thomas-Hawkins, C., & Zazworsky, D. (2005). Self-management of chronic kidney disease. *American Journal of Nursing, 105*(10), 40-49.

53. Thorp, M.L., Eastman, L., & Smith, D.H. (2006). Managing the burden of chronic kidney disease. *Disease Management, 9,* 115-121.

54. U.S. Renal Data System. (2006). *Annual data report: Atlas of end-stage renal disease in the United States.* Bethesda, Md: National Institutes of Health, National Institute of Diabetes and Digestive and Kidney Diseases. Retrieved 07/15/06 from www.usrds.org.

55. Vale, L., Cody, J., Wallace, S., et al. (2005). Continuous ambulatory peritoneal dialysis versus hospital or home haemodialysis for end-stage renal disease in adults. *Cochrane Library, 4.*

56. Ward, K. (2005). Kidneys, don't fail me now! *Nursing Made Incredibly Easy, 3*(2), 18-23, 25-27, 42.

57. Zorzanello, M.M. (2004). Clinical consult. Peritoneal dialysis and hemodialysis: Similarities and differences. *Nephrology Nursing Journal, 31,* 588-589.

evolve *Did you remember to check out the bonus material on the Evolve website and the CD-ROM, including NCLEX®-Examination Style Review Questions, Open-Book Quizzes, and Chapter Review Audio Podcasts?*

http://evolve.elsevier.com/Black/medsurg

UNIT 9

SEXUALITY AND REPRODUCTIVE DISORDERS

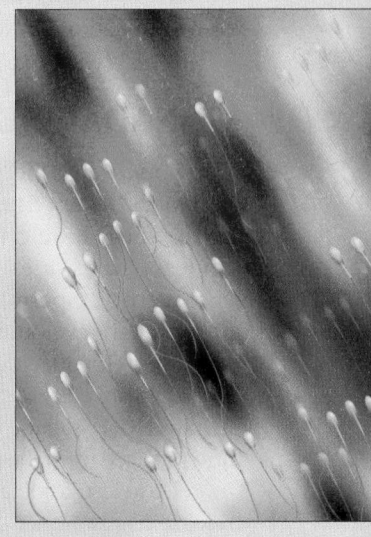

ANATOMY AND PHYSIOLOGY REVIEW:

The Reproductive Systems

Robert G. Carroll

The human reproductive system is specialized for the production and joining of *germ* cells—the ovum, or egg (female), and the sperm (male). The female reproductive system is also specialized to nurture and protect the fertilized ovum during the 9-month gestation period. Gonadal development begins in utero, but maturation of the reproductive system *(puberty)* is delayed until adolescence. At 45 to 60 years of age, fertility gradually decreases, ending at *menopause* (permanent cessation of menstruation) in women.

GONADAL DEVELOPMENT

The *gonads* are the sex glands of the female *(ovaries)* and male *(testes)*. Their primary function is to form germ cells, which have half the normal number of chromosomes. The ovaries produce ova; the testes produce spermatozoa (sperm).

Gonadal development begins during the fifth week of fetal life. Gonadal differentiation occurs in the seventh and eighth weeks of gestation. Human chorionic gonadotropin (HCG) is made by the embryo soon after conception and released from the placenta, stimulating the fetal ovaries to release estradiol and progesterone and the testes to release testosterone. In males, the wolffian ducts develop into the epididymis, vas deferens, and seminal vesicles, and the müllerian ducts regress. In females, the wolffian ducts regress and the müllerian ducts develop into the fallopian tubes, uterus, and upper vagina. The external genitalia, the glans penis and scrotum, are complete in the male by 14 weeks of gestation from the stimulation of testosterone. The clitoris, labia majora, and labia minora are complete in the female by 11 weeks of gestation. In the absence of testosterone, female genitalia develop.

FEMALE REPRODUCTIVE SYSTEM

GENITAL STRUCTURES

External Structures

The female reproductive organs consist of both external and internal structures. The external structures, collectively termed the *vulva* or *pudendum,* play a role in sexual stimulation and provide a barrier to protect the body from foreign materials (Figure A&P9-1, *A*). External female genital structures consist of the mons pubis, labia majora, labia minora, clitoris, vestibule, and vestibular bulbs. The *perineum* is the area posterior to the vestibule, between the vestibule and the anus.

Internal Structures

The internal female genital structures produce and release the reproductive cell or ovum, transport ova to the potential site of fertilization, and provide an appropriate environment for the implantation, growth, and delivery of the fetus (Table A&P9-1).

Ovaries are the female gonads, producing the female germ cell (ovum) and hormones (estrogen and progesterone). Normally two ovaries are located in the pelvis, one on either side of the uterus, and connected by the fallopian (uterine) tubes (Figure A&P9-1, *B*). The ovaries are contained in the posterior surfaces of the broad ligaments. They are also supported by the suspensory ligament (to the side of the pelvis) and by the utero-ovarian ligament (to the uterus). Each ovary is about the size, shape, and weight of an almond. In young females, ovaries are smooth; with age, they become pitted as a result of multiple ovulations.

Ova, in various stages of development, together with their surrounding tissue, make up the *ovarian follicles.* Each follicle contains a developing ovum; it grows and matures in the stroma, close to an abundant blood and lymphatic supply. A mature follicle (a mature ovum and its surrounding tissues) is an endocrine gland secreting estrogen hormones (see Estrogens later in this chapter). At birth, several hundred thousand follicles, each containing an oocyte (end-stage ovum), are present. They decrease in number as puberty approaches (the onset of functional reproductive capability), and they gradually disappear up to and around menopause.

As ovarian follicles grow larger they become discernible to the naked eye; these large ovarian follicles are sometimes called graafian follicles. An ovarian follicle that is larger than about 2 cm is called an ovarian cyst. The *corpus luteum* is a glandular body that produces the hormones progesterone and estrogen. It develops from a graafian follicle after ovulation (see Secretory [Luteal] Phase later in this chapter).

Two *fallopian tubes* connect the uterus to the ovaries and are the usual site of fertilization (Figure A&P9-1, *C*). Each fallopian tube is about 10 cm long.

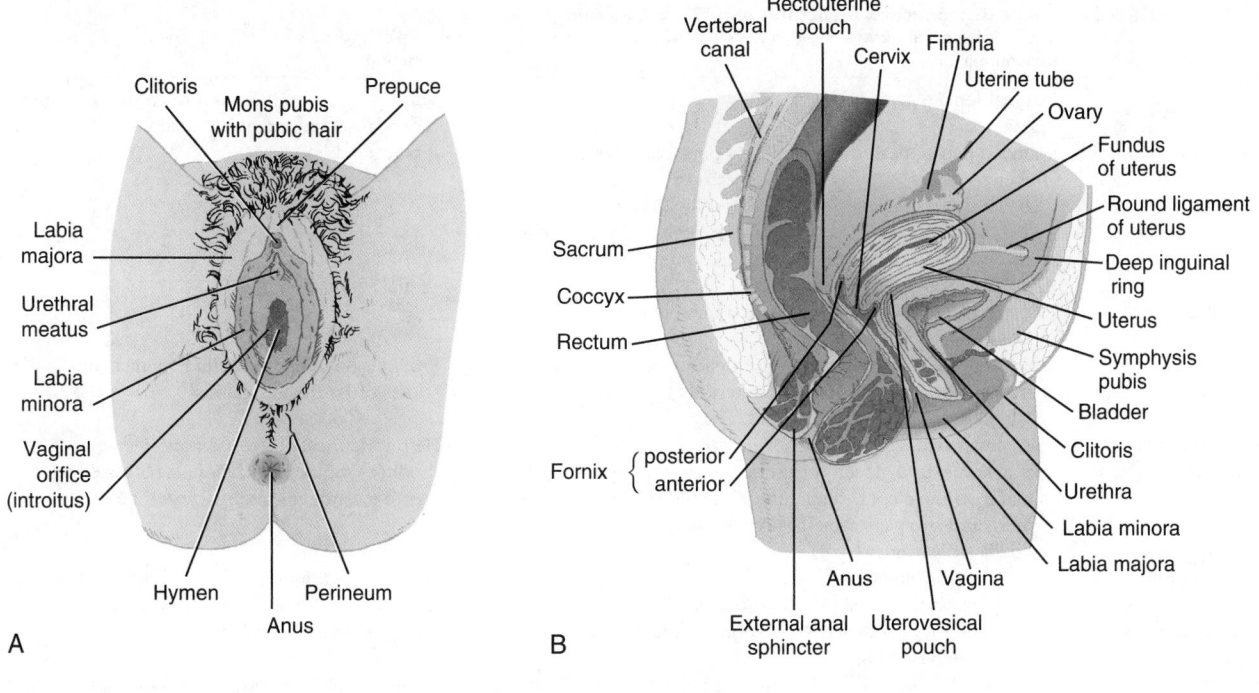

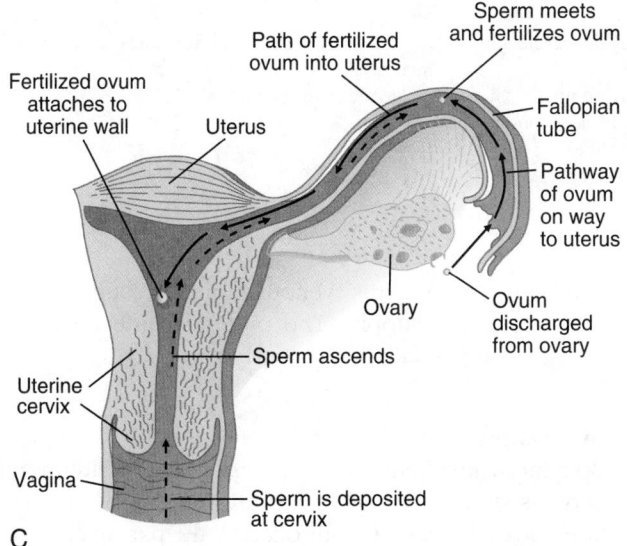

■ **FIGURE A&P9–1** **A,** Anatomic landmarks of external female genitalia. **B,** Midsagittal section of the female pelvis. **C,** Pathways of sperm and ovum in the female reproductive organs.

The *uterus* is located in the pelvic cavity slightly below and between the fallopian tubes, almost at a right angle to the vagina. The normal uterus is movable in all directions. However, it maintains a normal position in the body cavity through the action of various ligaments and the pelvic floor. The cardinal (lateral cervical) ligaments run between the pelvic wall and the cervix and vagina and provide the most support and a route for blood supply. Round ligaments extend from the external genitalia to the uterus, just below the fallopian tubes. If these ligaments are weak, the uterus is likely to prolapse (drop) into the vagina.

The uterus has three functional layers: (1) the *parametrium,* the thin peritoneal and fascial covering of the uterus; (2) the *myometrium* (bulk of the uterus), a muscular layer composed of three layers, mainly of involuntary muscles; and (3) the *endometrium,* the mucous membrane lining the inner surface of the uterus. The superior two thirds of the endometrium responds cyclically to hormones. A fertilized ovum normally implants in the endometrium. When the ovum is not fertilized, the endometrial lining is shed (see Menstrual Cycle later in this chapter).

The *vagina* is a musculomembranous canal connecting the uterus with the external genitalia. The mucosa

TABLE A&P9–1   **Female Reproduction Structures and Their Function**

Structure	Description	Function
Vulva	External female genitalia	Vulva protects body from foreign materials and plays a role in sexual stimulation
Mons pubis	Rounded pad of flesh over symphysis pubis; hair-covered after puberty	Protects pubic bone
Labia majora	Two elongated folds of tissue separated by a cleft	
Labia minora	Two thin folds of tissue between labia majora and vaginal opening; they divide and unite to form hood-like prepuce of clitoris	
Clitoris	Homologous to penis	Sexual stimulation
Vestibular bulbs	Two sacculated collections of veins; homologous to corpus spongiosum	
Vestibule of vagina	Almond-shaped space, consisting of delicate mucous membranes, between labia minora; bounded anteriorly by clitoris and posteriorly by fourchette	Provides opening for urethra, vagina, and two ducts of Bartholin's glands
Bartholin's glands	Two mucus-secreting glands	Help to lubricate tissues during intercourse
Ovaries	Two almond-sized glands consisting (outer to inner layers) of surface germinal epithelium, tunica albuginea (dense connective tissue), and stroma; stroma has cortex (dense outer layer) and medulla (loose inner layer)	Produce ova for fertilization; synthesize and secrete estrogens and progesterone
Ovarian follicle	Ovum plus surrounding tissue	Develops ovum from primary to mature (graafian)
Ovum	Female reproductive cell (23 chromosomes)	Combines with sperm to form zygote
Fallopian tubes	Thin-walled tubes with serosal covering, muscular layer, and ciliated mucous lining	Transport ova to uterus for implantation
Uterus	Pear-shaped, hollow muscular organ in pelvic cavity (2-5 cm thick, 5 cm long, 5 cm at widest point to 2 cm at narrowest point with opening to vagina [cervix])	Environment for implantation, development, and delivery of fetus; cervix allows entry of sperm for fertilization
Vagina	Canal between uterus and vestibule having three layers: epithelium, fibrous connective tissue, and muscular layer	Route of entry for sexual intercourse; exit for menstrual blood and birth canal
Breasts	Modified sebaceous glands and skin appendages lying within superficial fascia of anterior chest wall (vertically from second to sixth rib, horizontally from sternum to midaxillary line); parenchyma consists of ductular, lobular, and acinar epithelial structures; stroma is made of fibrous and fatty tissue	Produce milk to feed infants

of the inner surface of the vaginal wall folds over in small ridges (rugae) extending laterally upward. This rugal pattern adds to the elasticity of the vagina, making it very distensible. The rectum is posterior to the lower two thirds of the vagina. The smooth rugal pattern and elasticity of the vagina diminish with age during the menopausal and postmenopausal years. Because of its proximity to external openings, the vagina can easily become infected from urethral or rectal secretions.

Pelvic Blood Supply, Innervation, and Lymphatic Drainage
Blood Supply
The most important *blood supply* to the external genitalia comes from the internal iliac artery. This artery branches to supply the pelvic floor, pelvic walls, and pelvic viscera. The principal vessels supplying the internal female pelvic genitalia are the *uterine arteries* from the internal iliac artery and the *ovarian arteries,* which stem directly from the aorta. The uterine artery provides a rich vascular bed to the uterus and anastomoses the arterial supply to the vagina (vaginal arteries). The ovarian artery supplies blood to the ovaries, fallopian tubes,

and body of the uterus. Venous drainage roughly parallels the arterial supply. The pudendal artery supplies the external genitalia with blood.

Innervation
Both the sympathetic and the parasympathetic autonomic nervous systems provide innervation to the pelvic structures. Sexual arousal is controlled by the parasympathetic dilation of blood vessels in the vestibular bulbs and clitoris. The uterine myometrium is innervated only by sympathetic nerve fibers. The perineum is supplied principally by the pudendal nerve, which is somatic innervation.

Lymphatic Drainage
The pelvic *lymphatics* are a rich network of superficial and deep systems that roughly parallel the blood supply. The intermingling of the pelvic lymphatics and blood vessels is significant for the potential spread of cancer.

THE BREASTS

Breasts have an important role in modern culture. Because breasts are visible, their size and shape are often viewed as a measure of sexuality, femininity, and attractiveness. However, breasts are a secondary sex characteristic; that is, reproduction can occur without them. The physiologic function of female breasts is milk secretion to feed infants. An average nonlactating breast weighs between 150 and 250 g, and a lactating breast weighs 400 to 500 g.

The *parenchyma* of a breast consists of ductular, lobular, and acinar epithelial structures. The stroma of a breast is made of fibrous and fatty tissue, the proportion of which changes during pregnancy and lactation. The upper lateral quadrant of the breast, which is mostly glandular, is the most common site of breast cancer occurrence. A breast consists of 12 to 20 *lobes,* subdivided into *lobules,* made up of acini. Breast lobes are arranged like the spokes of a wheel around the nipple. Each lobe is drained by a duct, 12 to 20 of which open independently on the surface of the nipple.

The *nipple,* normally located at the fourth intercostal space, is surrounded by a circular pigmented area, called the areola. Estrogen increases pigmentation of the areola at any age and particularly during pregnancy. The areolar epithelium contains some small hairs and sebaceous glands, sweat glands, and accessory mammary glands. The sebaceous glands (Montgomery's glands) enlarge to lubricate the nipple during pregnancy and lactation.

Blood and Nerve Supply
The three main sources of the breast's blood supply are the internal thoracic artery, lateral thoracic artery, and posterior intercostal arteries. These arteries form an extensive network of anastomoses. The main veins follow the arterial pattern. The nerve supply is derived from the anterior and lateral branches of the fourth to sixth intercostal nerves.

Lymphatic Drainage
Lymphatic pathways, in general, follow the pathways of the veins. There are three types of lymphatic drainage of the breast (Figure A&P9-2):

- Cutaneous or superficial lymphatic drainage from the skin
- Areolar lymphatic drainage from the areola and nipple
- Glandular lymphatic drainage from deep glandular tissue

Lymphatic drainage pathways and lymph nodes are important in the prognosis and treatment of breast cancer (see Chapter 40).

Functions of the Breast
The following physiologic changes affect the breast:

- Growth and development
- The menstrual cycle
- Pregnancy and lactation

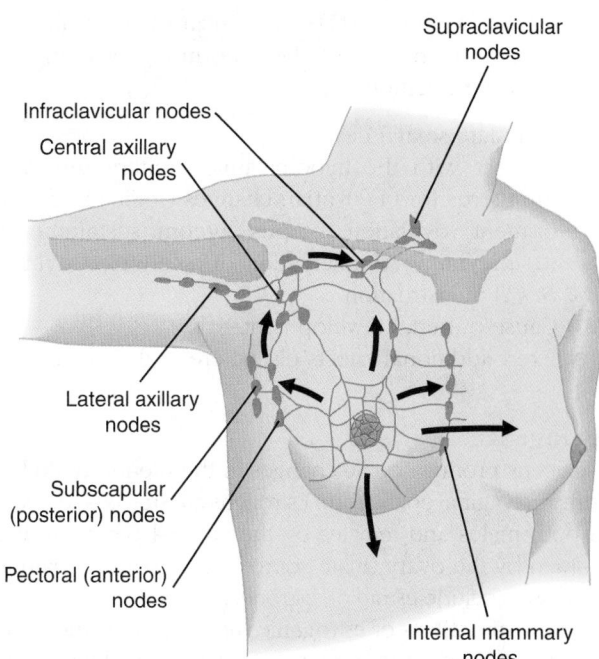

■ **FIGURE A&P9-2** Routes of lymphatic drainage from the breast. These routes are important routes of spread of breast cancer.

Estrogen and progesterone act synergistically with the pituitary growth hormones prolactin and corticotropin to produce breast development and function. Breast development usually occurs between 9 and 16 years of age and takes 4 to 5 years. Estrogen is responsible for the growth of the breast and periductal stroma. Progesterone promotes the development of lobular and acinar structures.

During pregnancy, estrogen, progesterone, and pituitary hormones increase, increasing breast vascularity and the permeability and dilation of breast lymphatics and ducts. When pregnancy ends, prolactin initiates lactation. Prolactin and corticotropin help maintain lactation. The "letting down" (flow) of milk is a complex response involving a mother's subjective response and the mechanical stimulation of suckling. Suckling releases the pituitary hormone oxytocin into the bloodstream, which causes the mammary acini to contract and release milk into the duct system.

After menopause, the ovaries stop producing estrogen and progesterone. Estrogen is then produced only by the adrenals through stimulation from the anterior pituitary. During this life stage, there is a continuous involution of the breast with loss of glandular elements and tissue atrophy. They are replaced largely with fibrous tissue and increase in laxity, resulting in ptosis. There is also a reduction in areolar pigmentation.

FEMALE REPRODUCTION

Role of Hormones
Under control of the hypothalamic releasing factors and anterior pituitary follicle-stimulating hormone (FSH) and

luteinizing hormone (LH), the ovaries manufacture estrogens and progestins. These hormones accomplish the following functions:

- Stimulate sexual desire
- Interact with the hypothalamic-pituitary unit and the uterus for (1) ovarian changes (follicular development, ovulation, corpus luteum sustainment), (2) pregnancy (implantation of a fertilized ovum), or (3) menstruation
- Cause pubertal development
- Exert additional effects elsewhere in the body

Estrogens

Estrogens produce cyclic changes in the uterine endothelium and vaginal epithelium. Estrogens are steroids secreted in both males and females by the adrenal cortex and in women by the ovary (main source) and placenta. Natural estrogens include estradiol, estrone, and estriol.

The main effects of estrogenic stimulation on the body occur at puberty and include breast growth (fatty tissue deposition, pigmentation), fat deposition in the vulva, pubic and axillary hair growth, bony pelvis growth and broadening, closure of the epiphyseal plates of long bones, vaginal epithelial changes, and general growth. The effects of hormones on menstruation are discussed later in this chapter.

It is not known precisely how the trophic actions of estrogen interact with other endocrine systems. Thus whether estrogen replacement should be given during menopause is under investigation. Osteoporosis (increased bone porosity) is associated with estrogen deficiency in perimenopausal women.

Progesterone

Progesterone is a steroid hormone that helps prepare the endometrium to receive and implant the fertilized ovum; it also promotes development of the placenta (a spongy structure in the uterus that provides nourishment for a developing fetus) and the mammary glands.

Progesterone is used therapeutically to treat threatened abortion and such menstrual problems as dysmenorrhea or amenorrhea. It is secreted from the placenta and the corpus luteum under control of the anterior pituitary hormone LH in order to sustain an implanted embryo. Progesterone plays a minor role in sodium and water balance. It also influences nitrogen balance, breast function, and body temperature during the menstrual cycle, raising body temperature by 1° F in the postovulatory phase of the cycle.

Menarche

The onset of menstruation (menarche) is a biologic, psychological, and social milestone. Psychosocial support, education about the physical changes that are happening, and knowledge about self-care are essential at this stage of life.

The average age for menarche in the United States is 12.8 years. Menarche is preceded by characteristic body changes (such as breast development) occurring between ages 9 and 16 years. The age at which menarche occurs is affected by many factors. Menarche may be delayed by poor nutrition, high levels of exercise (athletes or dancers), and several medical conditions, such as diabetes mellitus, congenital heart disease, and ulcerative colitis. Early menarche can occur with other conditions, such as hypothyroidism, central nervous system (CNS) tumors, and head trauma. Girls usually show an increase in height of only 2 to 3 inches after the onset of regular menstruation.

Early menstrual cycles are often irregular and anovulatory (menstrual flow is not preceded by ovulation, production, and discharge of an ovum). Although regular menstrual cycles may not occur for several years, the woman is still potentially fertile.

Menstrual Cycle

The menstrual cycle is a complex set of recurrent changes in the uterus, ovaries, cervix, and vagina (Figure A&P9-3). For the uterus, the menstrual cycle consists of the following stages:

- Proliferation
- Secretion
- Premenstrual phase
- Menstruation

Each phase is characterized by specific histologic changes in the endometrium. The length of the menstrual cycle is calculated from the first day of menstrual flow. The cycle generally runs 25 to 32 days but can vary from month to month and especially from one female to another.

The menstrual cycle depends on interactions between the CNS, anterior pituitary, ovaries, and uterus. Variations in the length of the proliferative phase (which ends with ovulation) typically cause a change in the length of the entire cycle (but do not change the luteal phase). Environmental influences, climatic changes, emotionally traumatic experiences, stress, or acute or chronic illness also may affect the menstrual cycle.

Proliferative Phase

The proliferative phase of the menstrual cycle depends on the ratio of FSH to LH. In the ovary, after menstrual flow has begun, primary follicles (containing oocytes, or primitive ova) and follicular cells begin to develop under the influence of FSH from the anterior pituitary gland (see Figure A&P9-3). The thecal (stromal) cells surrounding ova produce estrogens. The increased level of estrogen signals the pituitary to inhibit FSH production and to stimulate secretion of LH. Acting together, the two pituitary hormones stimulate further estrogen production. Estrogens further inhibit FSH release from the anterior pituitary. LH becomes dominant, stimulating further maturation of the follicle.

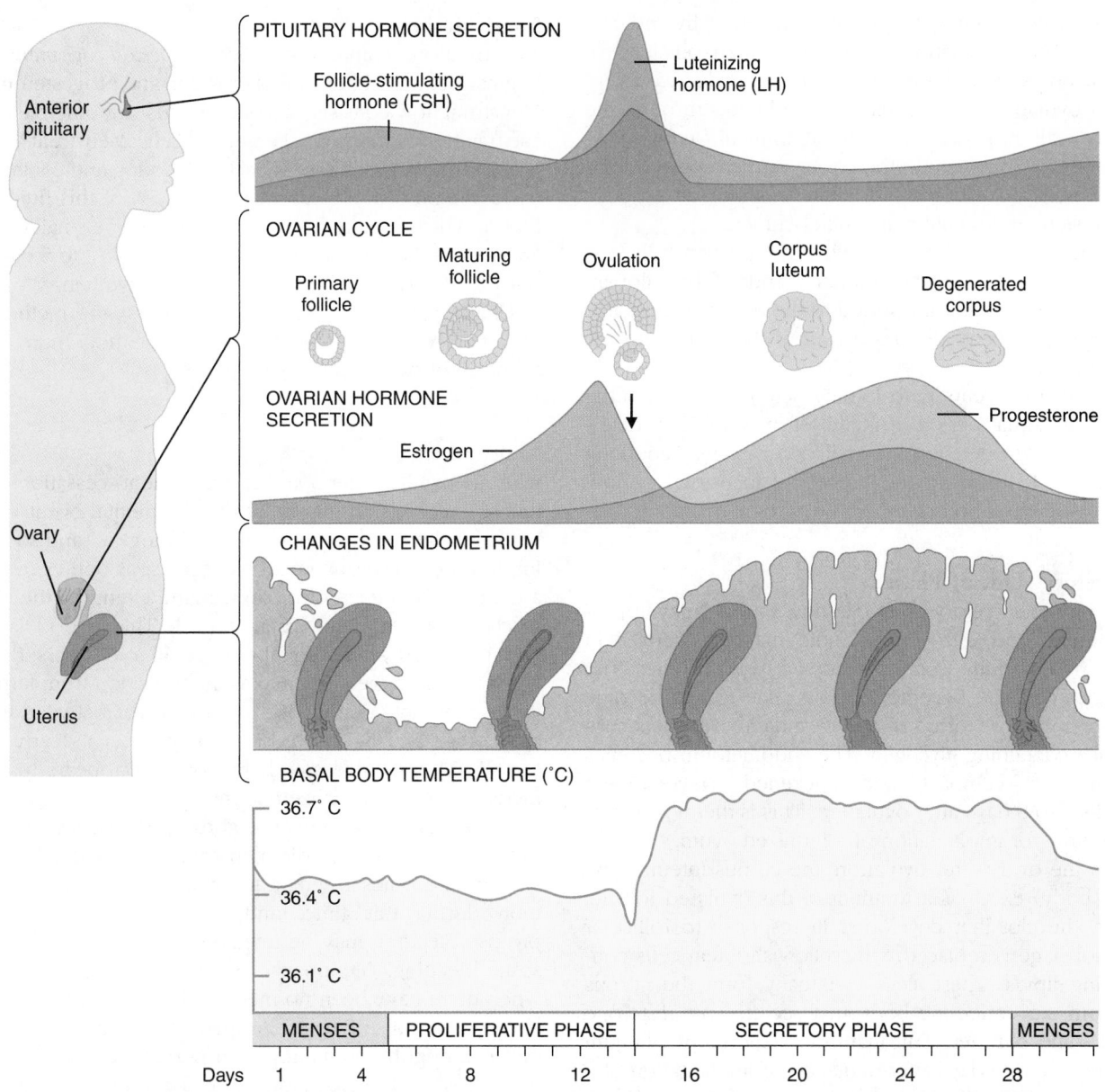

■ **FIGURE A&P9–3** Menstrual (uterine) cycle. Note hormonal control of the menstrual cycle and the effects on the ovaries *(center)* and endometrium *(bottom)*.

About 2 days before ovulation, a graafian follicle reaches full maturity and the remaining primary follicles degenerate. Ovulation is caused by a large surge of LH instigated by estrogen via a positive feedback loop and occurs when the graafian follicle migrates to the cortex of the ovary, where it ruptures through the ovary wall.

In the uterus, meanwhile, related changes occur, largely in response to increased estrogen from the developing follicle. At the end of a menstrual flow, the uterine endometrium (containing surface epithelium, glands, connective tissue, spaces, and blood vessels) is thin because much of it has sloughed off during menstrual flow. Estrogen stimulates growth of a new endometrial surface layer and restores the uterine epithelium (hence

the word "proliferative"). Glands and stroma grow, and the epithelium becomes thicker and more vascular. Endometrial proliferation peaks about 2 days before ovulation.

The cervix also undergoes cyclic changes. Most importantly, the secretion of mucus, a clear fluid that is receptive to sperm, greatly increases just before ovulation. Vaginal changes during this phase include proliferation and thickening of the vaginal epithelium caused by estrogen. This change is greatest at the time of ovulation.

Ovulation

Increasing levels of estrogen cause a decrease in FSH secretion, allowing a sharp increase in LH to occur. Over a 24-hour period, this process causes the thecal and granulosa cells lining the follicle to hypertrophy and proliferate. When ovulation occurs, the ovarian follicle involutes and estrogen production temporarily decreases.

At ovulation, the graafian follicle breaks through the ovary wall and passes into the abdominal cavity. Some hemorrhage occurs into the center of the ruptured follicle, where a clot quickly forms. Ovulation may produce a transient abdominal pain (mittelschmerz).

Once in the abdominal cavity, the graafian follicle is usually picked up by the fimbriated ends of the fallopian tube and is slowly transported to the uterus. Unless it is fertilized, it eventually passes out of the body with the menstrual flow.

Ovulation occurs 12 to 15 days before the onset of the next menstrual period. It is almost impossible to determine exactly when ovulation will occur, even by counting from the first day of the preceding menstrual period. However, basal body temperature rises at ovulation.

Secretory (Luteal) Phase
During the secretory phase (lasting 10 to 14 days), progesterone and estrogen promote marked changes in the endometrium. Connective tissue hypertrophies. The arteries coil and become tortuous. The glands become larger and more tortuous, and abundantly secrete a substance containing glycogen. The endometrium becomes edematous, compact, and thickened. Development peaks 7 to 8 days after ovulation. This is the most favorable time for implantation of a fertilized ovum.

In the ovary after ovulation, the corpus luteum (yellow body) exists as a remnant of this ovulated follicle. First, the clot that developed in response to follicular hemorrhage is replaced with yellowish luteal cells containing lipids. These cells eventually form the corpus luteum, an endocrine body that secretes progesterone and some estrogen. Full maturity of the corpus luteum occurs about 9 days after ovulation. If implantation of a fertilized ovum (pregnancy) does not occur, then the corpus luteum begins to degenerate.

Premenstrual (Ischemic) Phase
Degeneration (involution) of the corpus luteum occurs about 2 to 4 days before menstruation. A concurrent decrease in progesterone and estrogen production occurs, causing endometrial retraction and degeneration. The endometrium becomes heavily infiltrated with leukocytes. The coiled arteries constrict and ischemia results. The endometrium shrinks. At the same time, production of cervical mucus decreases, with mucus becoming more opaque and somewhat resistant to sperm.

The premenstrual phase ends as the constricted arteries open. Small patches of necrotic endometrium break off, and menstrual flow begins. The LH and FSH ratio changes; the pituitary is stimulated to increase its production of FSH; and the cycle begins again.

Menstruation
Menstruation, commonly called a *period* or *menses,* begins with the withdrawal of estrogen and progesterone. Menstrual flow consists of blood, mucus, endometrial tissue fragments, and vaginal epithelial cells. Menstrual flow is usually dark red, has a characteristic odor, and contains 60 to 150 ml of fluid. About 50% to 75% of this fluid is blood, which usually does not clot, but some small clots are normal. Menstruation usually lasts about 4 to 5 days, but 1 to 10 days may be normal for some women.

Chapter 39 covers menstrual disorders, and methods of contraception (prevention of pregnancy) may be found in obstetrics nursing texts.

Menopause
Like menarche, menopause (permanent cessation of menstruation) is an important developmental event in a woman's life that has physical, psychological, and social implications for the woman. Menopause is one event of a complex sequence of biologic aging events of the climacteric or perimenopausal period. This period lasts about 15 to 20 years from about age 40 to 60 years, during which time the body makes the transition from fertility to infertility. Menopause usually occurs between the ages of 48 and 54 years, but it may occur as early as age 35. The average age at menopause appears to be increasing in industrialized countries.

Menstrual cessation may be abrupt, but usually occurs over 1 to 2 years. Periodic menstrual flow gradually lessens and becomes irregular. Anovulatory cycles are common during this time, and occasional episodes of profuse bleeding may be interspersed with episodes of scant bleeding. Menopause is said to have occurred when there have been no menstrual periods for 12 consecutive months. Because unplanned pregnancy may occur during the premenopausal period, sexually active women should use contraception for at least 6 months after menses have ceased. Any spontaneous uterine bleeding after menopause is abnormal and should be investigated aggressively.

Although the cause of menopause is not known, certain predictable physiologic changes and experiences occur. During the climacteric period, a gradual decrease in the number of maturing ovarian follicles and a parallel decline in the production of ovarian estrogen occur. Over time, as the ovaries become unresponsive to pituitary hormones, and toward the end of the climacteric period, the ovaries atrophy. Other changes associated with menopause, such as hot flashes and vaginal atrophy, are related to decreased estrogen production.

Menopause is not a disease. Most women pass through menopause with minimal or no problems. The modern menopausal woman is younger-looking, more active, and has more positive attitude about menopause than in the past. The stereotype of the menopausal woman who is miserable and who seeks medical assistance for a wide range of symptoms has been disproved. Research shows that menopause itself does not cause poorer health or greater use of health care facilities. Menstrual variation (irregular menses, skipped periods, and occasional scanty or moderately heavy menses) usually do not warrant any intervention.

Although further study of the psychosexual changes associated with the perimenopausal period is needed, any changes that occur are the result of the complex interaction of anatomic, physiologic, psychological, and social factors. Vaginal lubrication may be reduced in the perimenopausal years, and this dryness may cause discomfort or bleeding with intercourse. Estrogen or hormone replacement therapy (HRT) can usually relieve this discomfort. Some studies have reported lessened interest in sexual activity among menopausal women, but other authors claim freedom from pregnancy allows women to relax and enjoy intercourse more. With increased life expectancy, the typical woman can spend more than one third of her life in the postmenopausal years.

During the menopausal years, many women are faced with life situations that affect mood, such as growing older, adjusting to children leaving home, and accepting increased responsibility for aging parents. Diseases such as cardiovascular disease and osteoporosis increase after menopause and do require medical management. Many women's health initiatives have been developed. Nurses can help counter some misconceptions and negative connotations associated with menopause by stressing the normal and positive aspects of the experience, clarifying misconceptions about menopause, and differentiating the physiologic manifestations of menopause from midlife developmental changes.

MALE REPRODUCTIVE SYSTEM

STRUCTURES

The male reproductive organs consist of paired *testicles* lying within the scrotum, epididymides, seminal ducts (vas deferens), spermatic cords, seminal vesicles, ejaculatory ducts, bulbourethral (Cowper's) glands, the prostate gland, and the penis (Table A&P9-2 and Figure A&P9-4). The penis and scrotum are external, visible genitalia, whereas the other structures are internal. The male perineum is the external area between the scrotum and the anus.

Penis and Related Structures

The *penis* is both a sexual organ (organ of copulation) and an organ for urination. This cylindrical, pendulous structure suspends from its attachment to the pubic arch. The skin of the penis is dark, hairless, thin, and loose (permitting considerable distention).

The portion of the penis between its end or head and its attachment to the pubic bone is the *shaft*. In males, the external opening of the urethra (*meatus* or orifice) is in the glans (*glans penis*), the cone-shaped end or

TABLE A&P9–2 Male Reproductive Structures and Their Functions

Structure	Description	Function
Penis	Erectile tissue arranged in three columns, each enclosed in a fascial sheath (tunica albuginea): two lateral columns (corpora cavernosa) and a median column (corpus spongiosum) that contains urethra; all are surrounded by a thick, fibrous envelope (Buck's fascia)	Ejects semen for fertilization; excretes urine
Bulbourethral (Cowper's) glands	Two small glands above corpus spongiosum; homologous to Bartholin's glands	Enhances lubrication during intercourse
Scrotum	Double pouch of muscular contractile tissue between root of the penis and perineum; bisected by a ridge; each half contains a testicle and epididymis and part of a spermatic cord made up of nerves, testicular vessels (spermatic artery, vein, lymph vessels), and vas deferens	Provides protective environment for production of sperm
Testicles	Two smooth, solid, ovoid structures (4 cm × 2-2.5 cm) with outer coat of inelastic fibrous tunica albuginea; lobules in testicles contain tubules composed of germ cells (develop into sperm) and Sertoli cells (support spermatogenesis); between tubules are Leydig cells (source of testosterone)	Produce testosterone and sperm
Sperm	Germ cell with flattened, broad, oval head with a nucleus, protoplasmic middle piece or neck, and a hair-like tail (flagellum); has 23 chromosomes	Fertilizes ovum
Epididymis	Small oblong structure consisting of a convoluted tube 4-6 m long; attaches to upper end of testicle	Transports sperm
Vas deferens	Smooth muscle tube about 46 cm long	Stores and transmits sperm from testicles
Prostate gland	Partly muscular, partly glandular structure posterior to symphysis pubis; urethra and ejaculatory ducts pass through it	Contributes to liquefaction of semen
Seminal vesicles	Two sac-like structures 5 cm long; they connect to vas deferens	Secretions contribute to sperm nutrition and activation

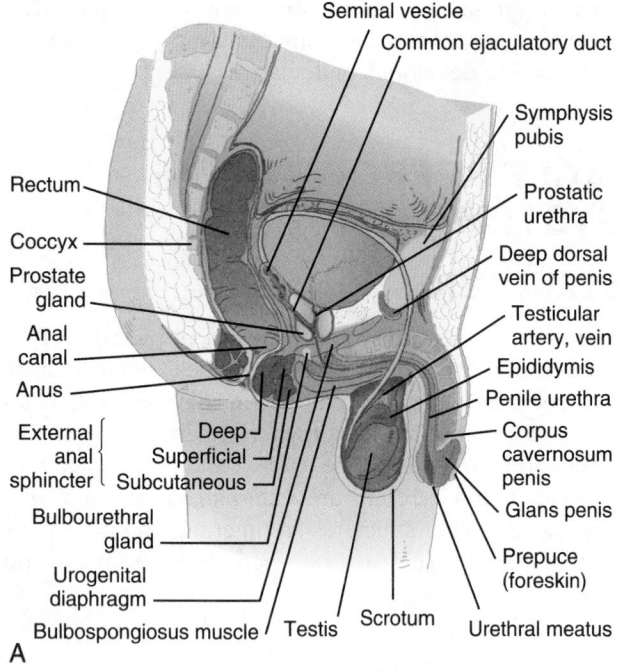

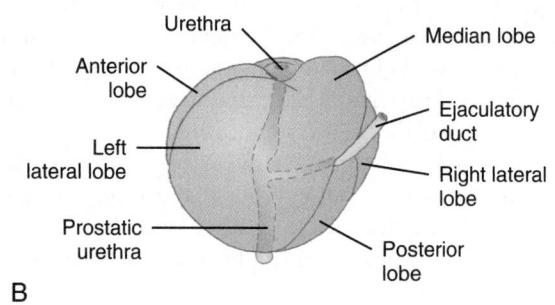

■ **FIGURE A&P9–4** **A,** Midsagittal section of the male pelvis and external genitalia. **B,** Anatomy of the prostate gland.

head of the penis. The glans is the conical expansion of the corpus spongiosum. The expanded posterior border of the glans is the *corona*. At its junction with the shaft is the *coronal sulcus*. A flap of movable skin (*foreskin* or *prepuce*) covers the glans before circumcision. *Smegma* is a cheesy, thick, odoriferous secretion of sloughed-off epithelial cells that collects under the prepuce. (In females, smegma is the secretion of the apocrine glands of the clitoris, together with epithelial cells.)

The penis is embryologically homologous to the female clitoris. The penis is usually flaccid. However, when stimulated (physically or during sexual excitement), it becomes rigid. An *erection* occurs when the corpora cavernosa fill with blood. The tissue becomes congested (hyperemic) with blood. Following *orgasm* (climax of sexual excitement) and *ejaculation* (emission of semen), the blood leaves. An erect penis is larger than a flaccid penis. Penis size, however, does not physically influence sexual pleasure. The secretion of the bulbourethral (Cowper's) glands forms part of the semen.

Scrotum and Testes

The *scrotum* is a double pouch hanging from the base of the penis. It is separated into halves internally by muscular contractile tissue *(tunica dartos)* and externally by a *raphe* (ridge) that runs over the scrotum from the base of the penis to the anus. Each half of the scrotum contains (1) a testicle with its epididymis and (2) part of a spermatic cord held together by spermatic fascia.

The *vas deferens* (ductus deferens, seminal duct) is the excretory duct of the testicle. It is the target and namesake of vasectomy. It is the continuation of the epididymis and conveys sperm from the testicle. The *ejaculatory duct* then conveys semen to the urethra.

The spermatic cord goes through the inguinal canal, and the vas deferens continues into the abdominal cavity. It passes behind the bladder, anterior to the rectum, to join the duct of the seminal vesicle, becoming the ejaculatory duct. The spermatic cord is movable for protection from trauma and facilitates optimal production of mature, functional sperm.

Testicles produce the male hormone *(testosterone)* and the male reproductive cells *(sperm)*. Many lobules, separated by septa, divide a testicle. Each lobule contains one to three seminiferous tubules where sperm are produced. Each testicle contains 600 to 1200 seminiferous tubules (90% of the mature testis). Between the seminiferous tubules are interstitial cells called *Leydig cells,* the source of testosterone. The lobules of the testicles lead to straight ducts that join a plexus, from which efferent ducts lead to the epididymis.

The *epididymis* rests on and beside the posterior surface of the testicle. Its head caps the upper end of the testicle and its tail becomes continuous with the vas deferens, which joins other vessels to form the spermatic cord. The head of the epididymis contains 12 to 20 testicular efferent ducts.

Sperm

Sperm are mature male sex or germ cells that develop after puberty. Resembling tadpoles, sperm self-propel themselves by flagella. A normal sperm has a flattened, broad, oval head with a nucleus. A middle piece or protoplasmic neck connects to the tail. During fertilization, the sperm's head pierces an ovum. The sperm's tail is lost when fusion of two cells occurs. Sperm are produced in the seminiferous tubules of the testicles. Sperm develop in great quantities from spermatids (spermoblasts) and are stored in the epididymis.

Prostate and Related Structures

The prostate gland surrounds the neck of the male urinary bladder and urethra. In children, the prostate is small, but during puberty, it grows to the size of a chestnut. The adult prostate gland (see Figure A&P9-4) lies like a flattened cone in the pelvis, about 2 cm posterior to the symphysis pubis. A normal adult male's prostate weighs 15 to 20 g and is 4 to 6 cm long. The prostate is inverted, so its apex is inferior, and is suspended by the urogenital diaphragm. The base of the prostate is superior and, at the bladder neck, anterior to the rectum. A firm, fibrous capsule containing smooth muscle fibers in its inner layer encloses the prostate. The bladder overlies the basal surface of the prostate. The posterior surface of the prostate is in close contact with the rectal wall. This is the surface of the prostate available for digital examination.

The portion of the urethra that passes through the prostate is called the *prostatic urethra*. Prostatic muscle fibers encircle the urethra and separate the prostate's glandular tissue.

The seminal vesicles are sac-like structures whose secretion, a component of semen (seminal fluid or ejaculate), may contribute to sperm nutrition and activation. They lie behind the bladder. The seminal vesicles connect to the vas deferens on each side.

Male Breasts
The male breast is similar to that of a preadolescent girl. It contains a few ducts surrounded by connective tissue. Estrogen can cause a man's breast to enlarge (gynecomastia) (see Chapter 40). Accumulation of fat in obese men can also make the breasts appear large.

MALE SEXUAL DEVELOPMENT AND FUNCTION

Development of the male genitalia requires two hormones: (1) müllerian duct inhibitory factor, secreted by Sertoli cells, and (2) testosterone, secreted by Leydig cells (see Gonadal Development earlier in this chapter). Germ cells develop into spermatozoa, and Sertoli cells support spermatogenesis.

The hypothalamus and pituitary gland regulate testicular function. The hypothalamus secretes gonadotropin-releasing hormone (GnRH) in a pulsatile fashion. GnRH stimulates the anterior pituitary gland to produce LH and FSH. LH stimulates Leydig cells to produce testosterone, which modulates the secretion of GnRH and, therefore, LH through negative feedback to the hypothalamus and pituitary gland. FSH and testosterone stimulate Sertoli cells and germ cells to start and complete spermatogenesis. Inhibin, released from Sertoli cells, provides negative feedback on FSH by the anterior pituitary.

Testosterone is the primary androgen secreted by the testis. The testis also secretes androstenedione and estradiol. Estradiol may be important for skeletal maturation in the male.

Spermatogenesis
Spermatogenesis is the process of sperm production and development that occurs within the seminiferous tubules during and following puberty. This process begins at puberty as a result of stimulation by the gonadotropic hormones from the anterior pituitary.

Spermatogonia are the germinal epithelial cells found in the outer border of the tubular epithelium. These cells are continually formed to replenish themselves, while a portion continue to develop into sperm. During the first stage of spermatogenesis, the spermatogonia divide and migrate toward the Sertoli cells. The spermatogonia penetrate the membranes of Sertoli cells and become enveloped within the cytoplasm of these cells. The spermatogonia continue this close relationship with Sertoli cells throughout their development.

During the 24 days when it is in contact with Sertoli cells, the spermatogonium changes and enlarges to form a primary spermatocyte. After this development, the spermatocyte splits into 2 secondary spermatocytes, each with only 23 chromosomes—half the original number. After 2 to 3 days, the spermatocytes undergo a second division to form 4 spermatids, each with 23 chromosomes. The sperm that eventually fertilizes the female ovum contains half the genetic material, while the ovum contains the other half.

The period of spermatogenesis from germinal cell to sperm takes about 74 days. During this time, the spermatocytes lose some cytoplasm, the chromatin material of the head reorganizes to form a compact head, and the remaining cytoplasm and cell membranes collect at one end of the cell to form the tail of the sperm.

Role of Hormones
Testosterone is essential to the growth and division of the germinal cells that form the sperm. LH stimulates Leydig cells to secrete testosterone. FSH stimulates Sertoli cells, promoting spermatogenesis. Estrogens, formed from testosterone when Sertoli cells are stimulated by FSH, appear to be essential in spermatogenesis. Growth hormone promotes early division of spermatogonia.

Maturation in the Epididymis
After the sperm are formed in the seminiferous tubules, they spend several days passing through the epididymis. After the sperm have spent about 24 hours in the epididymis, they become motile and capable of fertilization (i.e., they are mature). Sperm are stored in small amounts in the epididymis but are mainly stored in the vas deferens and the ampulla of the vas deferens. With low levels of sexual activity, the sperm can be stored there up to a month, maintaining their motility and fertility. When sexual activity is frequent, sperm may be stored only a few days.

Prostatic Fluid
The prostate gland secretes a milky fluid that forms part of the semen. This fluid aids the passage of sperm and

helps keep them alive, supplying them with food, if needed. Prostatic secretion is manufactured in a network of branching glands embedded in muscle within the prostate. This muscle contracts during ejaculation, and prostatic secretions are ejected through the ejaculatory ducts into the urethra.

Semen

Semen is a thick, opalescent secretion discharged by males at the climax of sexual excitement or orgasm. It contains sperm and other secretions. About 10% of the semen is composed of sperm and fluid from the vas deferens, with about 60% made up of fluid from the seminal vesicles. The remaining 30% is composed of prostatic fluid and small amounts of mucoid secretion from the bulbourethral glands.

Semen is slightly alkaline, with a pH of about 7.5. The prostatic fluid contains a clotting enzyme, which causes the fibrinogen of the seminal vesicle fluid to form a weak coagulum. This coagulum holds the semen near the uterine cervix. The coagulum dissolves in about 15 to 30 minutes, at which time the sperm become highly motile. The sperm can live within the vagina for 24 to 48 hours after ejaculation.

Intercourse and Orgasm

Intercourse deposits sperm in the vagina to allow fertilization of the ovum. Preparation for intercourse involves an often complex set of physical and psychic stimulation, and is influenced by social values. Sensory inputs are primarily from the glans penis, but also the adjacent genital areas and the perineal region.

Sympathetic, parasympathetic, and somatic nerves contribute to the male sexual response. Erection is mediated by the pelvic parasympathetic nerves. The parasympathetic nervous system (PNS) mediates relaxation of the corpora cavernosa and corpus spongiosum vascular smooth muscle, allowing an increase in blood flow and engorgement of the tissue. Acetylcholine activates nitric oxide synthase, causing cGMP-mediated smooth muscle relaxation.

Parasympathetic activation results from a spinal reflex caused by sensory stimulation and can be modified (enhanced or blunted) from descending autonomic control. At the same time, penile sympathetic activity (which normally vasoconstricts) is diminished. Penetration and friction increase sensory input.

Continuing stimulation leads to emission: the movement of sperm from the vas deferens and into the urethra. Prostate and seminal gland secretions are also moved into the urethra. Emission is under sympathetic control, and sympathetic activity also contracts the internal bladder sphincter, isolating the bladder from the urethra.

Continued stimulation leads to a climax, with male ejaculation Sympathetics mediate ejaculation, with successive contraction of the vas deferens and ampulla, the prostate, and finally the seminal vesicles. Ejaculation is supplemented by contraction of abdominal muscles in a thrusting motion. Climax is followed by a period of resolution, with reversal of the events that preceded intercourse.

CONCLUSIONS

The human reproductive system is tremendously complex, and reproductive and sexual characteristics can have a great physical and emotional impact on a person's life from conception. Changes initiated at the fetal stage cause differentiation between male and female. Sexual maturation, starting between the ages of 9 and 13 years, alters both external and internal structures. A thorough knowledge of the structure and function of the female and male reproductive systems is important so the nurse can provide safe, effective care for clients with associated problems. The nurse must be sensitive to the delicate nature of reproductive problems because many disorders affect sexuality.

BIBLIOGRAPHY

1. Berne, R., et al. (2004). *Physiology* (5th ed.). St. Louis: Mosby.
2. Carroll, R.G. (2007). *Elsevier's integrated physiology*. Philadelphia: Elsevier.
3. Kierszenbaum, A.L. (2007). *Histology and cell biology: An introduction to pathology* (2nd ed.). St. Louis: Mosby.
4. Guyton, A., & Hall, J. (2006). *Textbook of medical physiology* (11th ed.). Philadelphia: Elsevier Saunders.
5. Silverthorn, D. (2006). *Human physiology* (4th ed.). San Francisco, Calif: Pearson Benjamin Cummings.

CHAPTER 37

Assessment of the Reproductive Systems

LIANNE F. HERBRUCK AND SUSANNE A. QUALLICH

The ability to assess the reproductive system competently and compassionately is important to clients on physical as well as psychosocial levels. Sound assessment skills in combination with a nonjudgmental attitude that is both professional and empathic are required in order to provide an environment that promotes the client's comfort, cooperation, and participation in health care.

Besides providing a history and physical examination, an adequate reproductive assessment should include an in-depth review of the client's lifestyle, health habits, self-perception, body image, and developmental stage, along with cultural, religious, socioeconomic, and educational factors. These factors can help the nurse understand the client's health-seeking behaviors and perceptions of health care. They may also define clinical interactions with the client; respect for the client's values facilitates effective care.

Because of the close association between the reproductive, urinary, and bowel elimination systems, be prepared for some overlap in their assessment (see Chapter 32). Be prepared for some difficulty when discussing reproduction and elimination, as clients may be uncomfortable, or embarrassed, with the subject matter. Educational or cultural barriers may also inhibit a client from discussing a problem. Remain sensitive and nonjudgmental, and try to put the client at ease. Assess the client's understanding of health care information, and explore what the client perceives as needs and problems. If a client is anxious or feeling stressed, for example, during a pelvic or prostate examination, there may be the need to repeat teaching and/or counseling information to promote health maintenance. By providing a sensitive, humane orientation to reproductive health care, clients will be reassured and motivated to continue health-seeking behaviors.

THE FEMALE REPRODUCTIVE SYSTEM

Many women receive most, if not all, of their primary health care from obstetric and gynecologic health care providers, not only for gynecologic conditions but also for general health. An annual gynecologic examination gives the provider the opportunity to discuss health maintenance activities and answer health-related questions. Take this opportunity to teach breast self-examination (BSE) and discuss risk factors associated with gynecologic cancer and heart disease. Discuss lifestyle factors that affect health maintenance, such as diet, exercise, adequate sleep and rest, stress management, cessation of smoking, and general risk factor identification. If appropriate, provide information about protection against sexually transmitted infections (STIs) (refer to Chapter 41).

---

evolve **Web Enhancements**

Assessment Terms English and Spanish

Appendix A Religious Beliefs and Practices Affecting Health Care

Appendix B A Health History Format That Integrates the Assessment of Functional Health Patterns

Web Tables Sexual Health Assessment

Findings on the Internal Speculum Examination

Web Figures Positions for Breast Examination

Collection of Cervical Cytology Specimens

Pelvic Examination and Insertion of the Vaginal Speculum

Rectal-Prostatic Assessment

Web Boxes Disease as a Factor in Oral Contraceptive Pill Use and Pregnancy

Be sure to check out the bonus material on the Evolve website and the CD-ROM, including free self-assessment exercises. **http://evolve.elsevier.com/Black/medsurg**

After establishing rapport, perform a comprehensive gynecologic nursing assessment appropriate to the situation. Follow the health history with a systematic physical examination. Diagnostic tests may be ordered, some of which may be performed by the nurse. The resulting data are the basis for subsequent intervention.

HISTORY

The health history for the female reproductive system includes data related to the genitals, the reproductive system, the breasts, and the woman's overall health status. Conduct the interview portion of the examination in private, while the woman is clothed, to maintain her level of comfort.

The health history interview gives the care provider the opportunity to focus on client needs. Because the genital organs and their reproductive capacity have symbolic significance for many women, problems in this area may result in psychological consequences. Do not insist on obtaining information the client is hesitant to reveal. Empathic listening is supportive and may lessen any stress the woman may feel. Keep in mind that the woman herself may not fully understand her responses.

Deep, powerful feelings can prevent women from seeking gynecologic care. The opportunity to express and discuss feelings with a nurse who is skilled in therapeutic communication may help these women cope more effectively and follow through with appropriate care. A supportive conversation can provide opportunities for clarifying a woman's misconceptions about her diagnosis, proposed treatment, and preventive care. Always be alert to opportunities to educate your client and make her feel safe and at ease.

Biographical and Demographic Data

Biographical and demographic data can help to establish the client's health risk status. For example, the risk of breast cancer rises with age. Ethnicity may also be a risk factor for certain gynecologic cancers, such as cancer of the cervix. Information regarding the client's living and working environments is important as questions exist regarding the influence of environmental factors on the development of reproductive disorders.

Current Health

Obtain a comprehensive overview of the current health status of the client's reproductive system. Assess the regularity of the client's menstrual cycle, including length of each cycle, as well as number of days and amount of flow. Ask about premenstrual symptoms (PMS) and how they impact the client's lifestyle. Ask about current sexual practices, birth control method(s), and potential exposure to sexually transmitted infections (STIs).

Chief Complaint

Ask the client to describe her reason for seeking gynecologic care. Be alert to the possible nature of the problem and the woman's level of understanding of the problem. This information will direct the health history interview and your health teaching. If the client's visit is for a specific problem rather than for a routine examination, ask her to relate the history of the problem and conduct an analysis of her clinical manifestations.

Clinical Manifestations

Elicit a detailed report from the client regarding the clinical manifestations that relate to her chief complaint (Figure 37-1 on p. 853). This will help to focus the examination on the issues that are most important to the client. Some common gynecologic complaints that cause women to seek medical care include pelvic pain, breast pain, abnormal uterine bleeding, infertility, and infection.

General Pelvic Pain. Complaints of pelvic pain can be difficult to assess because of the number of body systems that are present in the pelvic area. Questions such as onset, duration, timing, aggravating/alleviating factors, and the presence of fever or chills provide baseline data. Clients should be asked to try and localize the pain as much as possible, in an attempt to narrow the potential etiologies. Pelvic pain includes such varied causes as ectopic pregnancy, interstitial cystitis, ovarian torsion, appendicitis, pelvic inflammatory disease, and painful intercourse.

Breast Pain. Many women experience breast tenderness before menstruation in relation to hormonal changes. Ask the client about breast pain or tenderness and its occurrence in relation to the menstrual cycle. If a lump is present, ask the woman to describe its location, onset, size, degree of tenderness, and whether she notices change during the menstrual cycle. Ask about any nipple discharge and determine the color, consistency, amount, and odor if present.

Abnormal Uterine Bleeding. Abnormal bleeding can refer to the absence of menstrual flow (amenorrhea), painful menstruation (dysmenorrhea), irregular bleeding (metrorrhagia), or excessive uterine bleeding (menorrhagia). The client should be asked to detail the condition as completely as possible, including any contributing factors. Abnormal bleeding can be an indication of such diverse conditions as perimenopause, uterine or cervical cancers, bleeding disorders, and endocrine dysfunctions. Refer to Chapter 39 for additional details on the evaluation of a client with this complaint.

Infertility. Female clients may present with a history of the inability to conceive after 12 months or more of

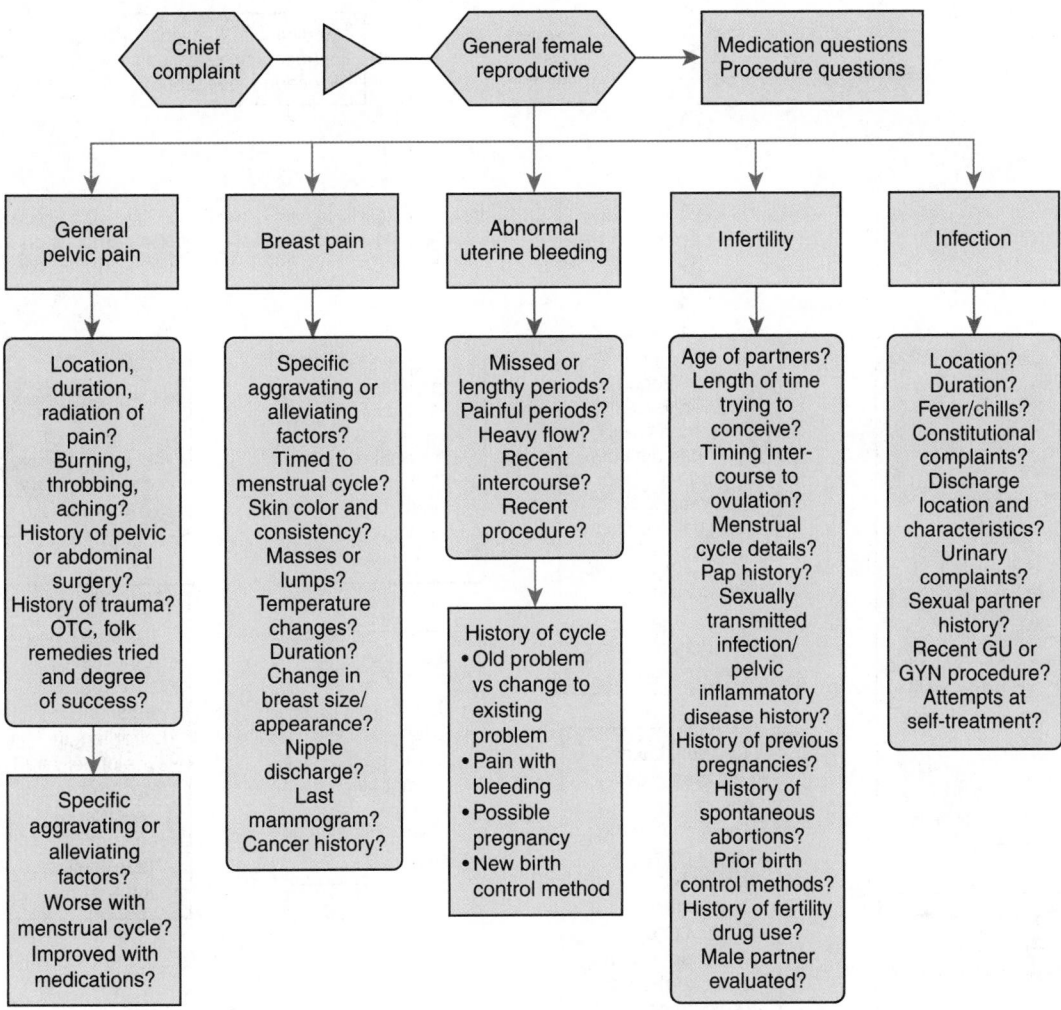

■ **FIGURE 37-1**   Expanded female reproductive assessment.

unprotected intercourse, the inability to conceive a second or third time, amenorrhea, or multiple miscarriages. There are many possible factors that can contribute to fertility complaints, including endocrine factors such as polycystic ovarian syndrome, endometriosis, and diabetes mellitus.

Infection. Ask about previous problems with genitourinary infections and vaginitis. Discuss the specifics of the client's current presentation, including such manifestations as pain, itching, or discharge. Determine whether the woman has a history of previous pelvic infection or STI, treatment, or related complications. See Chapter 41 for clinical manifestations of various STIs and Chapter 39 for other gynecologic infections.

Gynecologic and Obstetric History

A gynecologic history includes questions about breasts, menstruation, contraceptives, sexual practices, obstetric problems, genitourinary problems, and reproductive health practices (see Figure 37-2 on p. 854).

Breast History

Ask the client about breast pain or tenderness, and determine whether the woman has breast lumps or masses, either presently or in the past. Ask if the woman performs monthly breast self-examination (BSE). Determine history of breast cancer in the client's blood-related female relatives (mother, sisters, maternal grandmother, or maternal aunts), as breast cancer in these relatives indicates an increased risk of breast cancer for the client. Also inquire about genetic testing for BRCA1 or BRCA2 if there is a known family history.

Menstrual History

Important factors to include in a menstrual history include age menses began, first day of last menstrual period, regularity of cycles, and clotting or unusually heavy flow. Pain during the menstrual cycle should be assessed, including a description of the pain, duration, and relief measures. Ask the client about any mid-cycle bleeding or spotting. Determine the occurrence of clinical manifestations of Premenstrual Syndrome (PMS) and

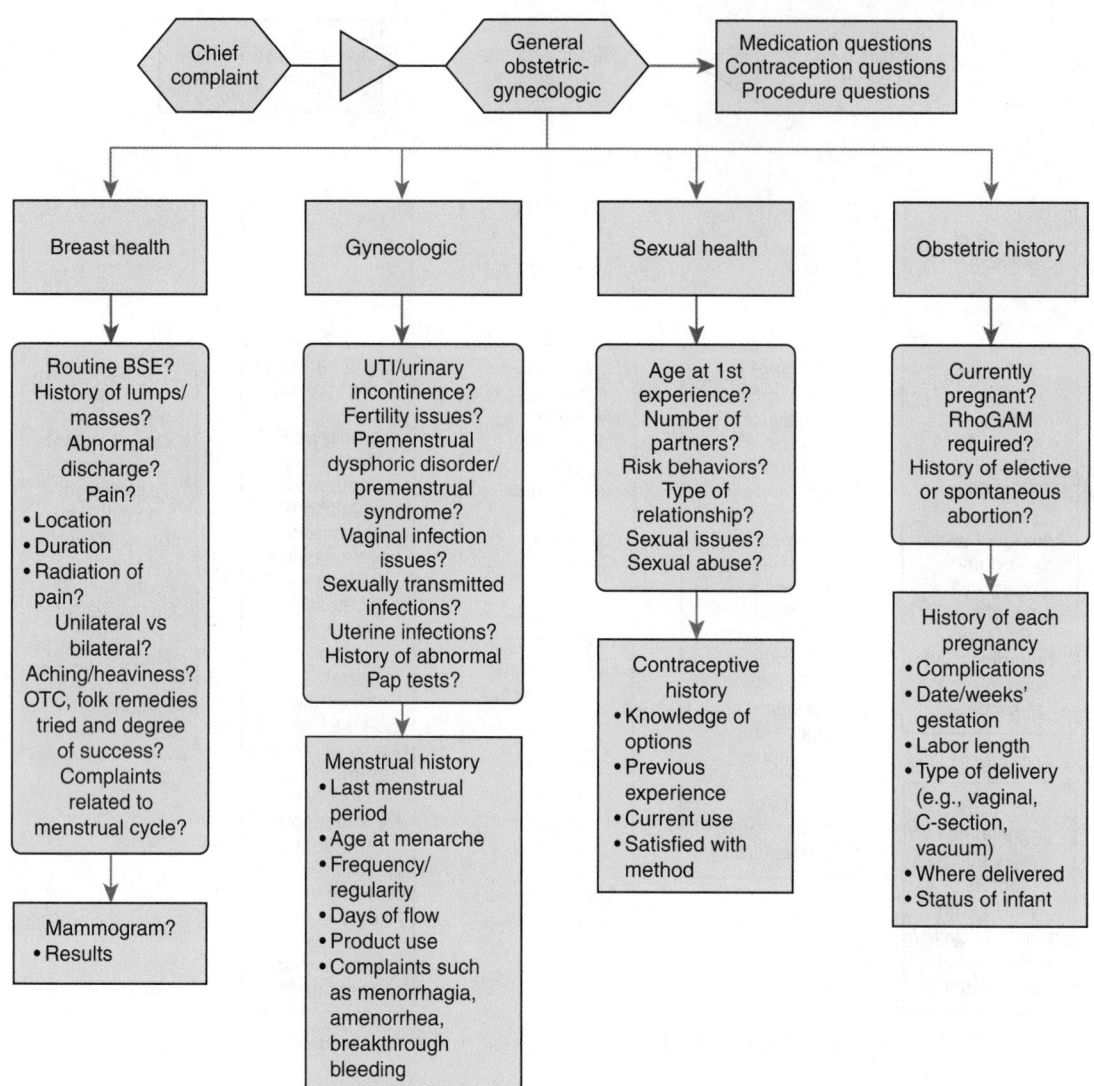

■ FIGURE 37–2 Expanded gynecologic and obstetric history.

their impact on the client's lifestyle. Also ask if the client takes any medications to control bothersome manifestations of PMS. In the middle-age woman, ask about any menopausal changes she may be experiencing.

Sexual History

The purpose of a sexual history is to identify sexual problems as well as to give the woman an opportunity to ask questions or express concerns. Encourage client participation by ensuring the client understands why the questions are asked and re-emphasizing client confidentiality. A nonjudgmental approach is essential. Determine the date of the most recent Papanicolaou (Pap) smear and its results.

Begin with general questions about whether the woman is satisfied and comfortable with her current sexual activity (refer to the Sexual Health Assessment on the *evolve* website). Respond to any concerns or issues raised in terms the client can understand. Be alert for any risk-

taking behaviors, especially those that increase the risk of STIs. Determine whether the woman had a previous pelvic infection or STI exposure, and subsequent treatment or complications. Some of these diseases, left unrecognized or untreated, can damage the reproductive system, particularly the fallopian tubes. The result may be problems with fertility and achieving pregnancy. See Chapter 41 for further information on STIs. Ask if the client has received the HPV vaccine series. Some strains of human papillomavirus (HPV) increase a woman's risk of developing cervical dysplasia and cancer.

Contraception

Document the current contraceptive method, satisfaction with the method, duration of use, any problems, and any desire to change methods. Also document previous contraceptive methods, including any problems and reasons for discontinuing the method. If the client is sexually active, but not using birth control, examine her feelings towards pregnancy, as well as her desire to achieve, or avoid, getting pregnant at this time.

Obstetric History

If the woman is in her childbearing years, ask whether she thinks she could be pregnant. Pregnancy may contraindicate radiologic studies, as well as certain medications. If the woman has been pregnant, obtain a history of each pregnancy, including the delivery and postpartum period. Document details of difficulties or complications (physical or psychosocial). It is important to include spontaneous or planned abortions in this history. See the website for detailed questions to assess the obstetric history.

Review of Systems

The review of systems is a process to gather information regarding the different organ systems of the body. The review is generally done from head to toe. Note especially

cardiovascular disorders (hypertension, angina [pain], myocardial infarction [MI], thrombophlebitis), endocrine disorders (hypothyroidism, hyperthyroidism), disorders of the pituitary gland, liver disorders, and cholecystitis. Ask about problems involving the urinary tract and reproductive system, such as urinary tract infection, urinary incontinence, vaginitis, and any bleeding disorders associated with menstruation (amenorrhea, dysmenorrhea, breakthrough bleeding, menorrhagia, or postcoital bleeding). Figure 37-3 includes questions to ask to obtain the general female reproductive history.

Past Medical History

To investigate the client's past health history, review her childhood and infectious disease history, major illnesses, surgeries, and hospitalizations, as well as current medications, vaccination history, and known allergies. Take this opportunity to review the client's diet and exercise habits, as well as social and family history.

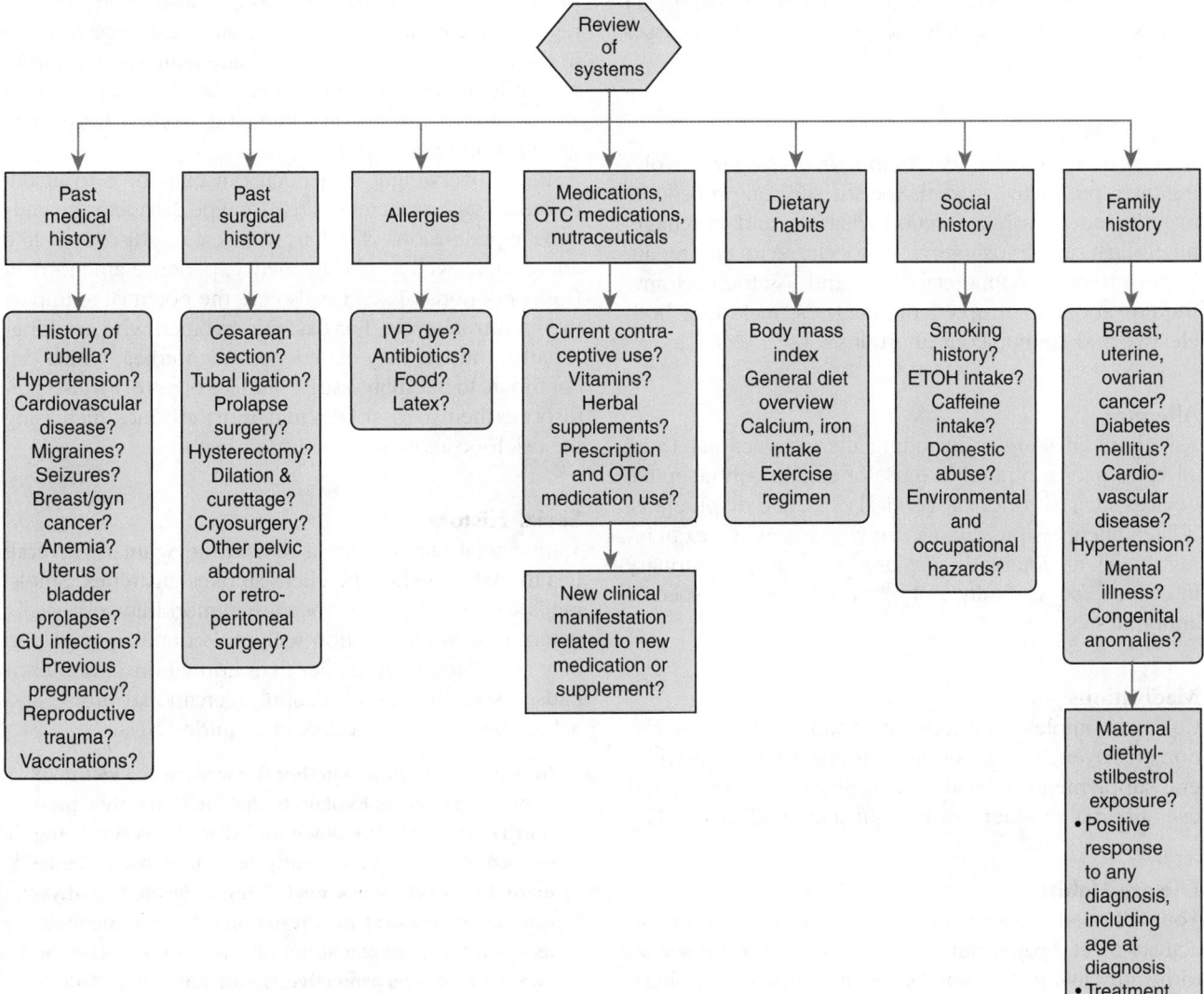

■ **FIGURE 37–3** Expanded female reproductive history.

Childhood diseases, such as rubella, can prove dangerous to unexposed women if they are contracted during pregnancy. Maternal rubella during the first trimester increases fetal risk for congenital disorders. Ask the client whether she had rubella or has known immunity to it. If she is contemplating pregnancy, suggest that a rubella titer be drawn to determine her immunity status. If immunity is lacking (negative titer), encourage the woman to be vaccinated. Advise newly immunized women to avoid pregnancy for at least 3 months. A pregnant woman should not be vaccinated.

Ask about major illnesses and hospitalizations. In women of childbearing age, certain disease processes are negatively linked to the use of oral contraceptives and pregnancy outcomes (see the box titled Disease as a Factor in Oral Contraceptive Pill Use and Pregnancy on the website).

Discuss previous problems with genitourinary infections and vaginitis. Determine whether the woman experiences urinary or fecal incontinence and the circumstances surrounding the incontinence (Chapter 34 discusses urinary incontinence; Chapter 33 discusses fecal incontinence).

Surgical History

Review past surgeries, with emphasis on surgery involving the reproductive system. Specific surgical procedures may include cesarean section, dilation and curettage, tubal ligation, cryosurgery, cystocele/rectocele repair, hysterectomy, oophorectomy, and salpingectomy. Inquire about interrupted pregnancies, including both elective and spontaneous abortions.

Allergies

Ask about all allergies, including allergic reactions. Latex allergies may contraindicate use of certain contraceptive devices such as condoms, cervical caps, and diaphragms. If latex allergy is present, use vinyl gloves while examining the client. Antibiotics are used to treat genitourinary infections, so carefully note any allergies to specific antibiotics.

Medications

Collect a complete medication history, including prescription and over-the-counter medications, vitamin and mineral supplements, recreational or illegal substances, and use of herbal or other "natural" substances (Table 37-1).

Dietary Habits

You will need to assess the client's general nutrition and activity level. Proper nutrition and exercise are essential to healthy living. An appropriate diet, along with physical activity, can improve severity of compounding disease and decrease risk factors for long-term health

TABLE 37–1 Common Herbs Used for Female Reproductive Issues

Herb	Use
Black cohosh (*Cimicifuga racemosa*)	Menstrual irregularity, PMDD, and menopausal problems
Chamomile (*Matricaria recutita, Chamaemelum nobile*)	Menstrual cramps
Chaste tree (*Vitex agnus-castus*)	PMDD and menopausal problems, possibly for mastalgia
Evening primrose (*Oenothera biennis*)	PMDD
Feverfew (*Tanacetum parthenium*)	Menstrual problems
Sage (*Salvia officinalis*)	Menstrual irregularity
Soybeans and legumes	Phytoestrogens, which may help to prevent breast cancer

PMDD, Premenstrual dysphoric disorder.

problems. Appropriate body weight also contributes to regular functioning of the menstrual cycle. Women in their childbearing years need adequate calcium, iron, and folic acid as part of proper nutrition (see Chapter 28 for further discussion). Pregnant women have even greater nutritional needs.

Being overweight in general can contribute to health disorders such as increased risk for type 2 diabetes mellitus and hypertension. Women with eating disorders like anorexia, as well as obesity, may experience amenorrhea (loss of periods). Exercise also has the potential to impact the menstrual cycle. For example, women who are long-distance runners may experience amenorrhea, which can contribute to infertility issues. The loss of estrogen also predisposes them to loss of calcium from the bones, increasing the risk for osteoporosis and stress factures.

Social History

Many social factors play a role in the woman's overall health. Ask whether the client smokes cigarettes. Smoking is associated with an increase in morbidity, especially when used in conjunction with oral contraceptives, and may be related to an earlier than normal onset of menopause. Note the use of alcohol, recreational drugs, and habits that increase the risk of acquiring STIs.

In private, ascertain whether the woman is a victim of domestic violence. Explain to the client that this question is asked of all women and that she is not being singled out. Clients frequently deny domestic violence many times before acknowledging it. Be alert to physical and behavioral manifestations that are inconsistent with the explanation of their cause. Also be aware of an overprotective significant other. This is an appropriate place to educate women about available options if violence is, or becomes, a problem.

Ask the woman about any exposures to hazards encountered at work, including toxins or radiation, as many substances can affect overall health status generally, and reproductive function specifically.

Family Health History

A comprehensive family history is always an important part of the client's medical history. Any family history of diabetes, cardiovascular disease, or cancer of a reproductive organ may indicate a higher risk for development of those diseases. If the woman's mother received diethylstilbestrol (DES) while pregnant with the client, the woman might be at risk for reproductive tract cancer or structural and functional abnormalities.

PHYSICAL EXAMINATION

After speaking with the woman and obtaining the appropriate medical history, the woman will need to prepare for the physical portion of the examination. She should be given privacy, and ample time, to disrobe necessary garments. If a full physical with breast examination is planned, request that the woman disrobe completely and have her put on a gown.

The examination should flow from head to toe, with the more invasive pelvic procedures performed at the end of the examination. Elements of a standard gynecologic examination can vary slightly but usually include the following physical assessment and general laboratory data:

- Vital signs (temperature, pulse, respiration, and blood pressure)
- Height
- Weight
- Urinalysis
- Physical assessment of skin, heart, lungs, breasts and axillae, thyroid, and abdomen
- Pelvic examination and Pap smear

If unusual or abnormal findings are obtained during the gynecologic history or physical examination, the client should be referred for additional data, such as ultrasound, mammography, or blood work. Normal findings are described in the Physical Assessment feature above, right.

Breasts and Axillae

Examination of the breasts and axillae is an important part of the gynecologic examination. Good lighting is essential. There is generally a nice flow to examining the breasts, axillae, heart, and lungs together while the client is sitting up. She may then be helped to a supine position for the remainder of the examination. Always remember to maintain client privacy. A good time to instruct the client on breast self-examination (BSE) is during the physical examination of the breasts (Box 37-1 on p. 858). The American Cancer Society recommends that women begin BSE at age 20.

Physical Assessment Findings in the Healthy Adult

The Female Reproductive System

INSPECTION
Breasts and Axillae. Breasts symmetrical, full, rounded, smooth in all positions, without dimpling, retractions, or masses. Faint, even vascular pattern and striae are noted. Nipples everted, areolae even. Axillae even color, without masses or rash.

Genitalia. Pubic hair distribution varies with stage of sexual development; clean, coarse. Labia majora covered with pubic hair in adult women; may gape open slightly. Labia minora pink, smooth. Clitoris midline, smooth. Urethral meatus pink, discharge absent. Vaginal orifice clean, without bulges.

PALPATION
Breasts and Axillae. Breasts firm without masses, lumps, local areas of warmth, or tenderness. Nipples without discharge. Axillae smooth, nodes nonpalpable.

Genitalia. Pelvic floor musculature firm. Skene's glands without discharge or tenderness. Bartholin's glands without masses or tenderness. No bulges in vaginal wall with straining.

Inspection

A thorough breast examination requires exposure of both breasts for comparison. Breasts are best inspected in three positions. Begin breast inspection while the client is seated with her arms at her sides. Next, ask her to raise her hands over her head while you examine the lateral and undersurfaces of each breast. Finally, have her press her hands firmly on her hips to tighten the pectoral muscles. Pectoral contraction exaggerates manifestations of retraction or skin flattening. Examine women who have large or pendulous breasts while they bend at the waist and face forward with the breasts hanging down (see the Positions for Breast Examination **evolve** figure on the website).

Breasts should be symmetrical, although it is not unusual for one breast to be slightly larger than the other. Their contour is even, without dimpling (retraction) or masses. Stretch marks (striae) may be present. Areas of edema or hyperpigmentation should be absent. Inspect the areolae and nipples for size, shape, contour, symmetry, surface characteristics, and masses or lesions. Axillae should be free of rashes or masses.

Palpation

Palpate the axillae while the client is seated. Examine the five sets of axillary lymph nodes (Figure 37-4, p. 858). The client's arm should be relaxed to ease palpation. Nodes should be nonpalpable, though detection of one or two small, nontender, mobile nodes is often a normal finding. Abnormal findings include firm, fixed nodes that may or may not be tender. If nodes are palpated, note

BOX 37-1   Breast Self-Examination

Breast self-examination (BSE) is a simple technique that women can use to assess for changes in their breasts that may signal breast cancer. The risk is highest in women older than 50 but women in their 20s should begin BSE. The woman should become familiar with the normal appearance and feel of her breasts to be confident of her ability to perform BSE. Advise the woman to schedule a regular time each month to assess her breasts. The best time is approximately 1 week after the onset of the menstrual cycle each month.

Teach the woman to perform BSE as follows:

1. Lie down and place your right arm behind your head. The examination is done while lying down, not standing up, because breast tissue spreads evening over the chest wall and is as thin as possible, making it easier to feel all the breast tissue.
2. Use the finger pads of the three middle fingers on your left hand to feel for lumps in the right breast. Use overlapping dime-sized circular motions of the finger pads to feel breast tissue.
3. Use three different levels of pressure to feel all the breast tissue. Light pressure is needed to feel the tissue closest to the skin; medium pressure to feel a little deeper; and firm pressure to feel the tissue closest to the chest wall and ribs. A firm ridge in the lower curve of each breast is normal.
4. Move around the breast in an up and down pattern starting at an imaginary line drawn straight down your side from the underarm and moving across the breast to the middle of the sternum (chest or breast bone). Be sure to check the entire breast area, going up and down until you feel only ribs and up to the neck or clavicle (collar bone).
5. Repeat the examination on your left breast using the finger pads of the right hand.
6. While standing in front of a mirror with your hands pressing firmly down on your hips, look at your breasts for any changes of size, shape, contour, dimpling, pulling, or redness or scaliness of the nipple or breast skin. Continue to look for changes with your arms down at your sides and then with your arms raised up over your head with you palms pressed together.
7. Examine each underarm while sitting up or standing and with your arm only slightly raised so you can easily feel in this area.

Modified from the American Cancer Society: *How to perform a breast self-examination.* Accessed 10/12/06 from www.cancer.org/docroot/cri_2_6x_how_to_perform_a_breast_self-exam.

the number of nodes felt, their location, size, shape, mobility, tenderness, and consistency.

Breast palpation is best facilitated with the client supine, with the arm of the breast being palpated behind the head. Clients with large, pendulous breasts, as well as those with a history or risks for breast cancer, should be palpated in both seated and supine positions. Conduct breast palpation systematically to examine all breast tissue, including the tail of Spence in the upper outer quadrant. Palpate the areola and nipple gently.

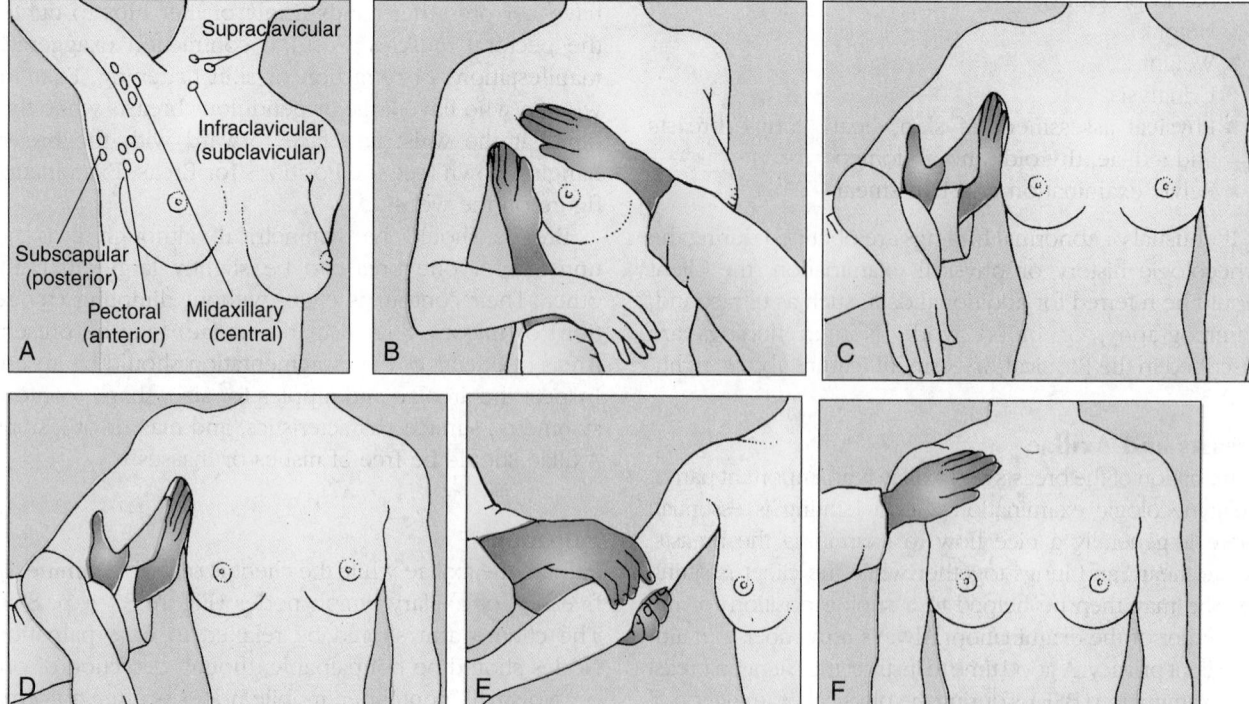

■ FIGURE 37–4   Assessment of axillary lymph nodes. **A,** Location of the groups of nodes examined. **B,** Pectoral (anterior) nodes. **C,** Midaxillary (central) nodes. **D,** Subscapular (posterior nodes). **E,** Brachial (lateral) nodes. **F,** Infraclavicular (subclavicular) nodes. Axillary nodes are also palpated for male clients.

Compress the nipple between thumb and index finger. The nipple may become erect with manipulation. In the nonpregnant or non-nursing client there should be no discharge present.

If the client reports a mass or tenderness, begin palpation with the unaffected breast so that you have a basis for comparison. If you feel a lump or mass, note its characteristics (exact location, size, shape, contour, consistency, mobility, and tenderness), and the position the client was in for palpation. Use the areola as a reference point.

Pelvis

Women often find pelvic examinations embarrassing, humiliating, and anxiety provoking, especially if it is performed roughly or in a perfunctory and hurried manner. Protect the woman's dignity, and communicate with her before, during, and after the examination. Remain professional and promote comfort at all times by being nonjudgmental, relaxed, and open to questions, concerns, and feelings. Avoid actions or remarks that might be misconstrued by the client as demeaning or sexually provocative. Explain all actions to the client before proceeding, and use a gentle, but firm touch during the examination. A pelvic examination will be less dreaded when the woman can participate and learn while retaining a sense of power and control.

Ask about previous experiences with pelvic examinations, and acknowledge any feelings the woman may have. If this is the client's first examination, explain the procedure fully. Tell the woman when and where she will be touched to help her avoid tensing up, which produces discomfort. Provide the opportunity for her to empty her bladder if needed.

Help the client to assume a dorsal recumbent or lithotomy position, and keep her draped until it is time for the examination. Do not keep a woman exposed any longer than necessary.

External Genitalia

Start with a general inspection of the external genitalia (see Figure A&P9-1, *A* for a review of the anatomy of the female peritoneum and genitalia). Place one hand on the client's thigh before touching the perineum. Inspect the mons pubis (mound of tissue superior to the labia), labia majora, and labia minora. The labia majora are symmetrical, rounded, and full, and may gape slightly if the client has had a previous vaginal delivery. The labia minora are thinner than the labia majora, and one side may be larger than the other side. Use the thumb and index finger to separate the labia minora for inspection of the vulva and remaining external structures. All areas should be free of edema, malodor, inflammation, and lesions.

The urethral meatus, a small slit just above the vaginal opening, can be difficult to locate, particularly in women

who have had a vaginal delivery. The meatus should be free of discharge, inflammation, or swelling. If a discharge is present, collect a specimen for culture. Inspect the clitoris, hymen (mostly absent in a sexually active client), and vaginal orifice (introitus). Discharge, inflammation, edema, or lesions should be absent. If inflammation and edema are present near the posterior introitus, palpation of Bartholin's glands is indicated (Figure 37-5, *A*). Discharge from the urethral meatus indicates palpation of Skene's glands (Figure 37-5, *B*).

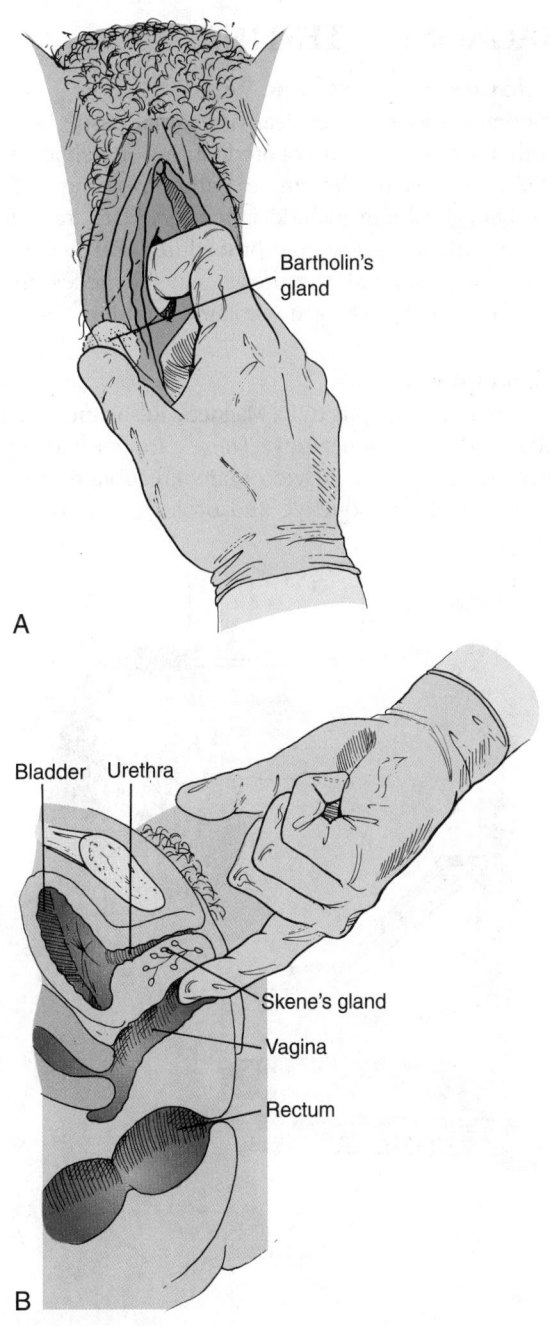

■ **FIGURE 37–5 A,** Palpation of Bartholin's glands. **B,** Palpation of Skene's glands.

Vaginal Speculum, Bimanual, and Rectovaginal Examination

The internal vaginal examination, which includes use of the vaginal speculum and the bimanual and rectovaginal examination, is usually performed by an advanced practice nurse or physician and will not be discussed in depth. Please consult a physical assessment textbook for more information related to the pelvic examination. See the Collection of Cervical Cytology Specimens and Pelvic Examination and Insertion of the Vaginal Speculum figures, as well as the Internal Speculum Examination table located on the website.

DIAGNOSTIC TESTING

Noninvasive Gynecologic Tests

Sometimes abnormal cervical or vaginal tissue, a mass, or other problem is discovered during a pelvic examination. Studies to determine pathophysiology of the underlying problem include laboratory data, radiology, ultrasound, and endoscopic procedures. Further examination using general anesthesia may be necessary for exploration of a mass or unexplained tenderness.

Radiography

Computed Tomography (CT), Magnetic Resonance Imaging (MRI), and Ultrasonography. These are modalities in which images of the pelvic organs are obtained in the assessment of reproductive and urologic disorders (see Chapter 32). There is no special preparation for CT scan or MRI unless a contrast agent (dye) is given. Pregnancy and morbid obesity are contraindications for both tests.

> Ask the woman whether she has a copper-containing intrauterine device in place, the presence of which may contraindicate MRI.

When performed with a vaginal probe, an *ultrasound* examination enhances the view of the adnexae and is used to evaluate ovarian cancer, cysts, and ovaries that have been stimulated with fertility-enhancing drugs. *Sonohysterography* utilizes a saline infusion in conjunction with transvaginal ultrasound to enhance the endometrial imaging and aid in the diagnosis of uterine and endometrial abnormalities.

Noninvasive Breast Tests
Radiography

Two radiographic tests for breast screening are ultrasound and mammography. Presently, only mammography has been shown to be useful for widespread breast cancer screening. Ultrasonography is not specific enough to identify lesions suggestive of cancer, but it can differentiate cystic from solid lesions. Other methods of testing are being investigated.

Mammography. A mammogram is a soft-tissue radiographic breast examination used to detect small invasive and noninvasive tumors and benign lesions (Figure 37-6).

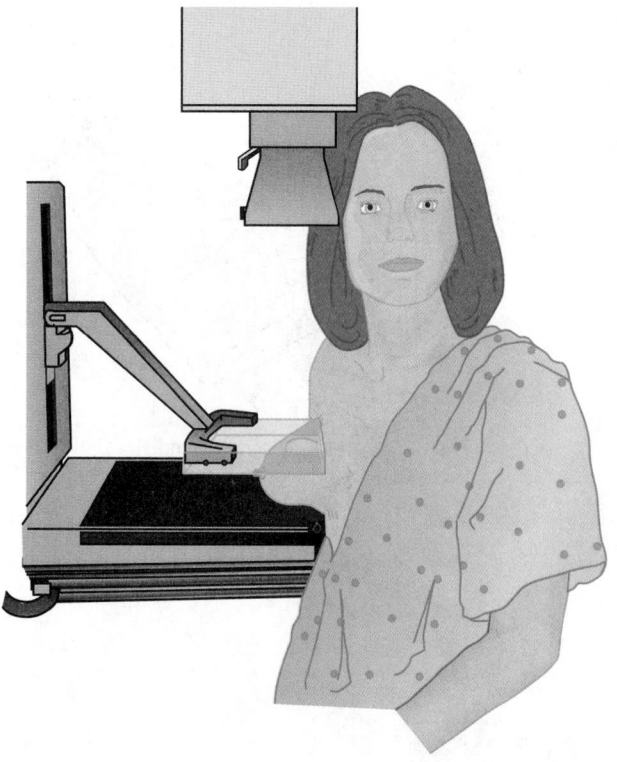
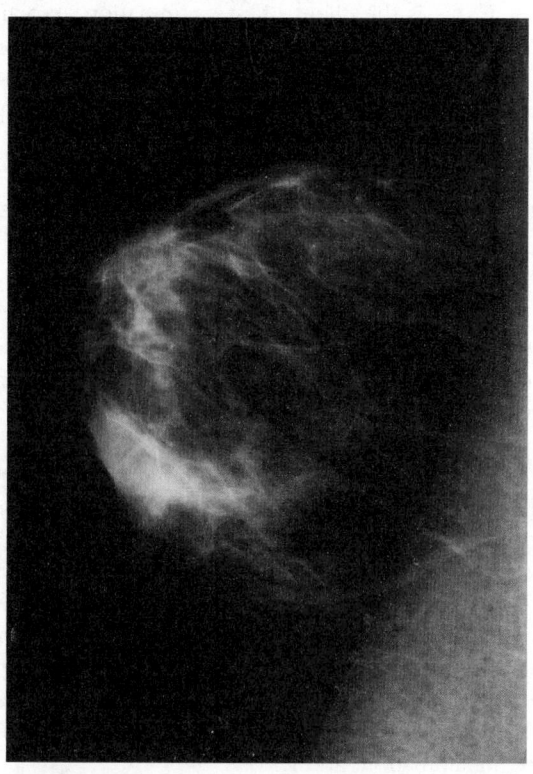

A   B

■ **FIGURE 37–6 A,** Mammography, a technique for obtaining an x-ray image of the breast, is a reliable mechanical method of detecting breast cancer before it can be felt. This technique is also used to help diagnose breast cancer. **B,** A normal mammogram of the left breast.

It can identify some breast cancers before they are palpable (Box 37-2 below). During a mammogram, the breast is placed between an x-ray plate and a compression paddle that is adjusted so the breast is compressed between the two plates to obtain the best image possible. For screening mammograms, two views of each breast are taken from different angles (cranial-caudal and oblique).

Though some controversy exists about the age at which to begin routine screening, the ACS recommends a baseline mammogram for all women by 40 years of age, and routine screening of asymptomatic women 40 and older every year.[1] Women are encouraged to begin breast self-examinations (BSE) at age 20. Women of all ages with an increased risk for breast cancer will need to discuss further recommendations with their care provider. Box 37-3 lists questions commonly asked about mammograms.

Ultrasonography. Ultrasonography is useful in determining the consistency of breast masses and differentiating cystic (fluid-filled) from solid lesions. It can help to confirm fluid consistency of cystic-appearing lesions seen on a mammogram. It cannot, however, differentiate solid benign from solid cancerous lesions. It is also useful in guiding fine-needle aspiration of cysts and other breast masses.

Invasive Gynecologic Tests
Endoscopy

Endoscopic procedures for assessing the female reproductive system include colposcopy, hysteroscopy, and laparoscopy. As this review of the procedures is brief, please reference a diagnostic testing textbook for more in-depth discussion of endoscopic procedures and related nursing care.

Colposcopy. Coloscopy involves the use of a stereoscopic binocular microscope (colposcope) to examine the cervical epithelium, vagina, and vulva. It is indicated for all women whose Pap smears show dysplasia. It also

---

> **BOX 37-2 Indications for Mammography**
>
> Indications for mammography include the following:
> - Diagnosis of potentially curable cancer and follow-up treatment
> - Evaluation of questionable breast masses or other abnormal physical findings
> - Determination of whether/where a biopsy should be performed
> - Detection of breast cancer in a woman with metastatic cancer if the primary site is unknown
> - Routine screening

> **BOX 37-3 Common Questions About Mammography**
>
> Common questions and possible answers about mammography include the following:
> 1. *How often should I have a screening mammogram?* Use the ACS or National Cancer Institute (NCI) guidelines for the age and risk group. Typically, baseline by age 40, and every year after 40. However, it can be based on provider and client preference.
> 2. *What is the cost?* Prices vary. Inquire at the facility where the mammogram will be performed. Tell the client that it is worthwhile to compare prices. However, the client should ensure that the facility meets the necessary quality standards.
> 3. *How much time is involved?* About 15 to 30 minutes. Results are usually available within 1 to 21 days, depending on the facility.
> 4. *What preparation is required?* The woman should not wear any body powder, creams, or deodorant on the torso the day of the procedure.
> 5. *Is there pain?* Discomfort may be experienced because of the compression needed to obtain the best image. Some women find it helpful to schedule a mammogram for the week after the end of their menses, when the breasts are less tender. Women who have tender breasts may take a nonsteroidal anti-inflammatory drug, if not contraindicated, about 1 hour before the procedure.
> 6. *Is there a risk in the exposure to the radiation?* Mammography uses the smallest dose possible. The long-term effects of an annual mammogram are considered to be harmless.

---

may be used to examine suspected lesions in the lower genital tract. Colposcopy increases diagnostic accuracy and reduces the need for biopsy, though biopsy can be performed at this time if a lesion is present. The procedure is safe and painless, and it can be performed in pregnant women.

Hysteroscopy. Hysteroscopy, the procedure by which the intrauterine cavity is viewed directly through a hysteroscope (Figure 37-7, p. 862), has multiple uses. They include ruling out organic causes in abnormal uterine or postmenopausal bleeding, examining suspected leiomyomas or polyps, removing an intrauterine device with a missing string, evaluating infertility, and performing surgical techniques for uterine abnormalities. It is contraindicated if the client has acute pelvic inflammatory disease, recurrent chronic upper genital tract infection, or recent uterine perforation. It also is contraindicated in pregnancy.

Laparoscopy

Laparoscopy is a safe, convenient procedure that can be performed in hospitals, offices, or clinics equipped for outpatient surgery. The laparoscope is a telescope with an illuminated optical system. It is inserted into the abdomen through a small incision in, or near, the umbilicus to visualize abdominal and pelvic organs. Laparoscopy may be performed diagnostically for conditions such as pelvic pain, pelvic masses, infertility, suspected ectopic pregnancy, and endometriosis. It also may be performed therapeutically for such procedures as tubal ligation, lysis of adhesions, and treatment of endometriosis. The main contraindications to laparoscopy are serious cardiac or pulmonary disease. Severe obesity may also preclude its use.

Gynecologic Biopsy

The two most common biopsies performed in gynecologic testing are cervical and endometrial. This overview is brief; refer to a diagnostic testing textbook for more detailed information regarding pre- and post-procedure care.

Cervical Biopsy. When suspicious lesions are identified on the cervix, either with the naked eye or by colposcopic magnification, cervical biopsy can be performed to rule out malignancies. A biopsy may be done when a cervical lesion is first noted, or it may be delayed until about 1 week after the menstrual period, when the cervix is least vascular. Areas of the cervix that are dysplastic, metaplastic, or malignant will undergo color change when a solution of 3% acetic acid solution is applied to the cervix. Those areas are biopsied and specimens are sent for further testing. Cervical biopsy is contraindicated in the pregnant woman.

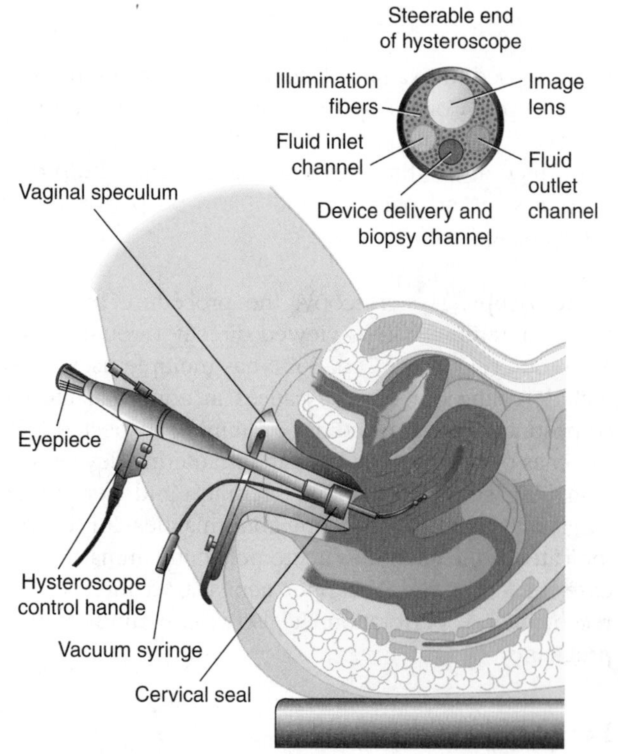

Endometrial Biopsy. Endometrial tissue samples necessary for histologic study are obtained through endometrial biopsy. Samples of the endometrium may be used to analyze endometrial cancer, dysfunctional uterine bleeding, and, occasionally, infertility. After a bimanual examination of the uterus, the cervix is dilated under sterile conditions, and a uterine sound is inserted to measure the depth of the uterine cavity. An aspirating instrument is passed into the uterus, and a small amount of tissue is removed from the endometrium for further examination.

Breast Biopsy

Biopsy is essential to the diagnosis of breast cancer. No treatment should be undertaken without an unequivocal histologic diagnosis of cancer. Core needle biopsy and fine needle aspiration (FNA) are two methods of tissue gathering. Both tests involve taking only a small amount of cells and tissue from a lesion. Open biopsy may be required if neither test produces an adequate diagnostic result.

Core Needle Biopsy. Core needle biopsy is a relatively simple procedure that takes just a few minutes. A core of tissue is obtained, fixed in preservative, and sent for histologic diagnosis.

Fine Needle Aspiration. With FNA, a needle and syringe are used to aspirate cells from a breast mass or fluid from a cyst. The cells are fixed on a slide (as in a Pap smear), and a cytologic diagnosis is made. The cytologic examination is useful for confirming the diagnosis of clinical and mammographic findings of fibroadenoma (a fibrocystic condition), intramammary lymph nodes, fat necrosis, subareolar papillomatosis, chronic subareolar abscess, and cancer.

Open Biopsy. About 35% of clients who require an open biopsy for a breast lesion have a malignancy. Excisional biopsy involves removal of the entire palpable mass; incisional biopsy only removes a portion of the mass. In both cases, the tissue removed is sent to the pathologist for histologic assessment. Frozen-section examination may be done for rapid diagnosis.

Percutaneous needle localization determines the area for an open biopsy if a mass is very small. The lesion is localized in the radiology department, and a thin needle is passed into the area identified by mammography. A second mammogram confirms the position of the lesion. The needle is secured in place with tape, and the woman is taken to the operating room, where an open biopsy is immediately performed.

■ **FIGURE 37-7** Hysteroscopy. An endometrial biopsy may be obtained during hysteroscopy.

Laboratory Tests

At this time, no reliable laboratory tests have been found for breast cancer screening. Identifying a reliable biologic tumor marker for breast cancer could possibly aid in the detection or treatment of the disease. Genetic screening of women at increased risk for breast cancer, including BRCA1 and BRCA2 testing, is discussed in Chapter 40.

Cytology

Cytology is the examination of structure, function, pathology, and chemistry of the cell. The most common gynecologic laboratory studies are the Pap smear, wet smear, and cervical culture. These specimens are obtained during the speculum examination. The woman should not be menstruating at the time specimens are collected. Instruct her to avoid sexual intercourse, douching, or using vaginal hygiene sprays or deodorants for 2 to 3 days before a test.

Papanicolaou Smear

In gynecology the most common cytologic test is the Papanicolaou (Pap) smear, named after George Papanicolaou, its developing physician. The Pap smear is a painless test that can identify pre-invasive and invasive cervical cancer. The principle of the Pap test is based on the fact that both normal and abnormal cells are shed from the uterine and cervical linings and pass into their secretions. When a cytologic smear of these secretions is examined under a microscope, early cellular changes can be detected before disease becomes clinically apparent.

The American Cancer Society recommends an annual Pap test for women who are or have been sexually active, or who have reached 21 years of age. After a woman has had three or more consecutive normal annual examinations, the Pap smear may be performed less often at the discretion of the health care provider. The Pap test should be continued after menopause, and vaginal smears are obtained for Pap smear in women who have had a hysterectomy with removal of the cervix.

If the Pap smear result reveals a vaginal infection, the woman may be treated for vaginitis and the Pap test repeated later. If the Pap test result shows dysplasia or abnormal tissue, treatment will vary according to extent of the lesion, grade of the dysplasia, and preference of the woman and her health care provider. The Pap test can be difficult to interpret. Make sure the client knows how to access a caregiver in the event she does not fully understand her results. For more information on cervical cancer, see Chapter 39.

Wet Smear and Cervical Culture

The wet smear is used to detect vaginal infection with *Candida albicans, Trichomonas vaginalis,* or organisms that cause bacterial infections. The test is performed with secretions collected from the vaginal vault. A cervical culture or antigen detection test can be done to detect infection with *Neisseria gonorrhoeae* or *Chlamydia trachomatis.* Secretions are taken from the endocervical canal and placed on various culture mediums, depending on the organism. Because of the asymptomatic nature of these infections, sexually active women are often tested routinely during regular examinations.

THE MALE REPRODUCTIVE SYSTEM

Disorders of the male reproductive system and urinary tract (which is closely associated with the reproductive tract) occur in men of all ages. Assessing these disorders requires expertise in conducting the health history interview and physical examination. Young men may have limited contact with the health care environment unless they perceive a problem with their sexual or reproductive function. Many men, regardless of age, are uncomfortable discussing issues associated with these body systems.

HISTORY

A complete health history, including the sexual and reproductive system, and physical examination are necessary for men experiencing reproductive disorders. History-taking provides an opportunity to allow men to express sensitive concerns, identify and dispel myths and misinformation, teach correct health information, offer referrals, and facilitate further communication.

Biographical and Demographic Data

Review the client's biographical and demographic data to determine his health risk status. Age, race, and occupation all have health risk implications. Men older than 50 years of age may have benign prostatic hypertrophy (BPH), an enlargement of the prostate gland. Men younger than age 40 who have manifestations that resemble those of BPH are more likely to have prostatitis. African-American men and those older than 40 years of age are at increased risk for adenocarcinoma of the prostate. Younger men, particularly those between ages 25 and 35, have a higher incidence of testicular cancer. Occupations and activities that involve prolonged, strenuous lifting or straining can provoke hernias. Exposure to some chemicals and pesticides may be linked to fertility and reproductive disorders.

Current Health

Discuss with the client his primary reason for seeking care. It may be for a yearly prostate check, he may need refills on medications that help manage his urinary or sexual function, or he may have noticed a new manifestation that has caused him concern.

Chief Complaint

The male client may present with problems related to the genitourinary or reproductive system or to sexuality. Common complaints may be related to pain, testicular or scrotal problems, sexual function issues, lower urinary tract symptoms/complaints (LUTS), infertility, or infection.

Clinical Manifestations

Refer to Figure 37-8 for a guide to assessing a man's chief complaint or clinical manifestations related to the male

reproductive system. Men may complain of urologic complaints, which were discussed in Chapter 32.

Pain. The client can describe pain in the testicles or scrotum in a variety of ways including acute, nauseating pain; a dull ache with a progressive onset; or sharp, focused pain. If there is a history of trauma, it is vital to establish the mechanism of injury. There may be a history of a sudden onset of acute pain and elevation of the affected testicle. The onset of the discomfort may also have occurred over time, and could be associated with lesions or drainage from the scrotum, as well as a history of recurrent scrotal infections and current constitutional complaints. Is the pain the result of a prolonged erection? Is there pain while urinating?

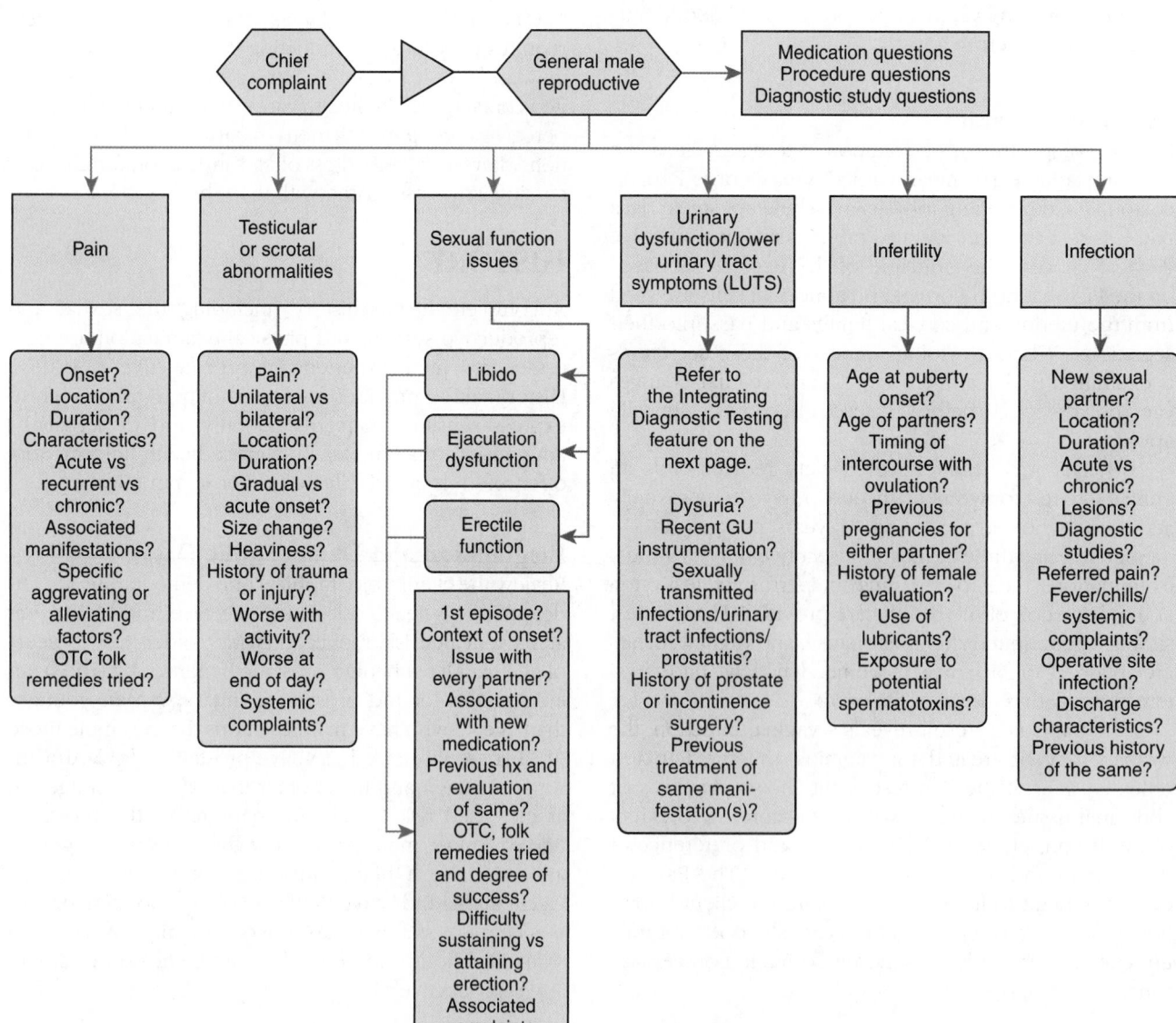

■ **FIGURE 37-8** Expanded male reproductive assessment.

Testicular or Scrotal Abnormalities. A client may have noticed a painless swelling of the testicle, a distinct nodule, or other asymmetry of the testes on testicular self-examination (TSE). Testicular abnormalities may be firm, smooth, nodular, or fixed. There may have been some minor trauma to the affected side that predates the onset of swelling. The testicle may have gradually enlarged over time, with some associated heaviness. The client may describe a distinct mass or diffuse enlargement of the affected testicle or scrotum or he may be unable to report the length of time any abnormality has been present. Refer to the Integrating Diagnostic Testing feature below for details of the evaluation of a testicular or scrotal complaint.

INTEGRATING D I A G N O S T I C T E S T I N G

Testicular or Scrotal Complaints

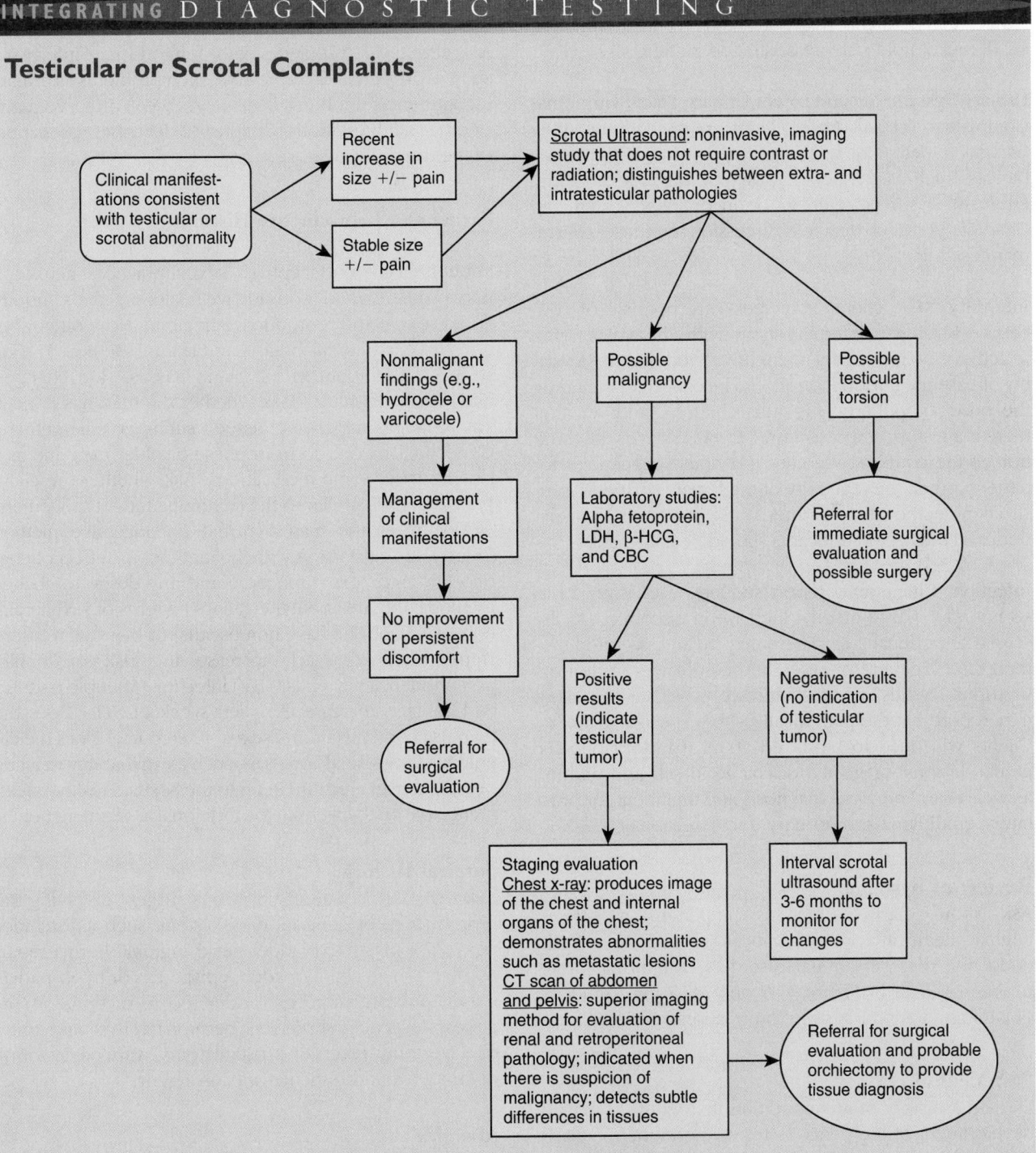

CBC, Complete blood cell count; *β-HCG,* beta-human chorionic gonadotropin; *LDH,* lactic dehydrogenase.

Sexual Function Issues. The client may present with concerns regarding declining erectile function that may have occurred over several years. There could be a history of relatively rapid or recent onset of decline in overall sexual function, which could result from a new medication or a surgical procedure. The nature of the complaint should be discussed as completely as possible, detailing the nature of the dysfunction (attaining versus sustaining an erection, libido or ejaculation issues) and the conditions of the complaint (whether the problem is constant or only with certain partners). Has there been erectile dysfunction (ED), loss of libido, depressed mood, or fatigue?

Urinary Dysfunction and Lower Urinary Tract Symptoms/ Complaints (LUTS). Male clients, particularly as they become older, may report a variety of voiding disturbances, such as frequency, polyuria, oliguria, nocturia, enuresis, dysuria, urgency, or incontinence. Refer to Chapter 32 for a detailed discussion of these clinical manifestations.

Infertility. Male clients may seek care because of concerns regarding their fertility status, with a history of trying to achieve pregnancy for a lengthy period of time. A variety of baseline information should be collected, including the onset of puberty, previous children, and whether there is a history of a vasectomy. Details such as the duration of the couple's infertility, previous pregnancies for either partner, the regularity of the female partner's menstrual cycle, the timing of intercourse in relation to ovulation, and the use of lubricants should be collected.

Infection. Clients may report sudden onset (over 24 to 48 hours) versus a gradual increase in discomfort to the scrotal or perineal area. There may be an associated urethral discharge and/or fever, and complaints of dysuria, urethritis, cystitis, or prostatitis are possible. The client may report that the pain localizes to a specific structure. Clients will need to be asked about a history of STIs, genital lesions, or genital discharge in self and partner, as well as any previous diagnosis and treatment for prostatitis, epididymitis, or urinary tract infections (UTIs).

Review of Systems

Ask about diabetes mellitus, hypertension, stroke, angina, heart attack (or myocardial infarction [MI]), endocrine disorders, renal disorders, and urinary tract problems. Refer to Figure 37-9 on p. 867 for a guide to obtaining additional history information from a man.

Past Medical History

Discuss a history of any condition that would affect the development of the penis, testes, or hormones status of the client (including cryptorchidism, hypothyroidism, pituitary malfunction). The most significant childhood infectious disease to affect male fertility is mumps. Its occurrence in young men is associated with sterility. Ask whether the client has ever had mumps or been immunized against it. ⬥ Ask about major illnesses, such as diabetes mellitus, hypertension, stroke, and heart attack or MI; men who have been diagnosed with these conditions can have difficulties with erectile function as a result of neurologic and vascular changes. Ask about spinal cord injuries or back problems; these can contribute to both erectile and ejaculatory problems. Detail previous treatment for testicular or genitourinary (GU) malignancies. Ask about past problems with genitourinary infections, such as prostatitis. Does he have such problems as urinary incontinence, dribbling, hesitancy, a weak urinary stream, or other manifestations? Chapter 32 describes assessment of the urinary system.

Sexual and Reproductive History

A sexual and reproductive history includes questions about breasts, contraceptives, sexual practices, genitourinary problems, and reproductive health practices. Inquire about sexual and reproductive hygiene. How often does the man examine his breasts and testes (see Box 37-4 on p. 868)? Ask about breast pain, masses, skin changes, and nipple discharge. Ask whether the man has noticed any changes in breast tissue, such as enlargement. Gynecomastia can occur in obese or older men and as a side effect of some medications. Ask whether the client performs BSE, similar to the technique taught to women.

Document the man's current contraceptive method (if any), his satisfaction with the method, the effect of contraception on sexual function, and any desire to change methods. Inquire about the client's patterns of sexual relationships. Does he have homosexual or bisexual relationships, both of which increase the risk of human immunodeficiency virus (HIV) infection? Multiple partners and contacts increase the client's risk of STIs. Does the man use condoms during sexual intercourse? Does the client have any sexual concerns, such as an inability to attain or maintain an erection? Refer to the Sexual Health Assessment table on the website for additional assessment points.

Surgical History

Ask the client about any previous surgery involving the reproductive or genitourinary system, such as orchidopexy; Y-V plasty to bladder neck; inguinal hernia repair as infant, small child, or adult; epispadias or hypospadias repair; prostate surgery; bladder reconstructions or surgeries; testicular surgeries; herniorrhaphy; vasectomy or vasectomy reversal; prostatectomy; varicocelectomy; orchiopexy; and testicular torsion repair.

Allergies

Ask the client about allergies to antibiotics, rubber, or latex. Establish if there is an allergy to radiologic contrast media.

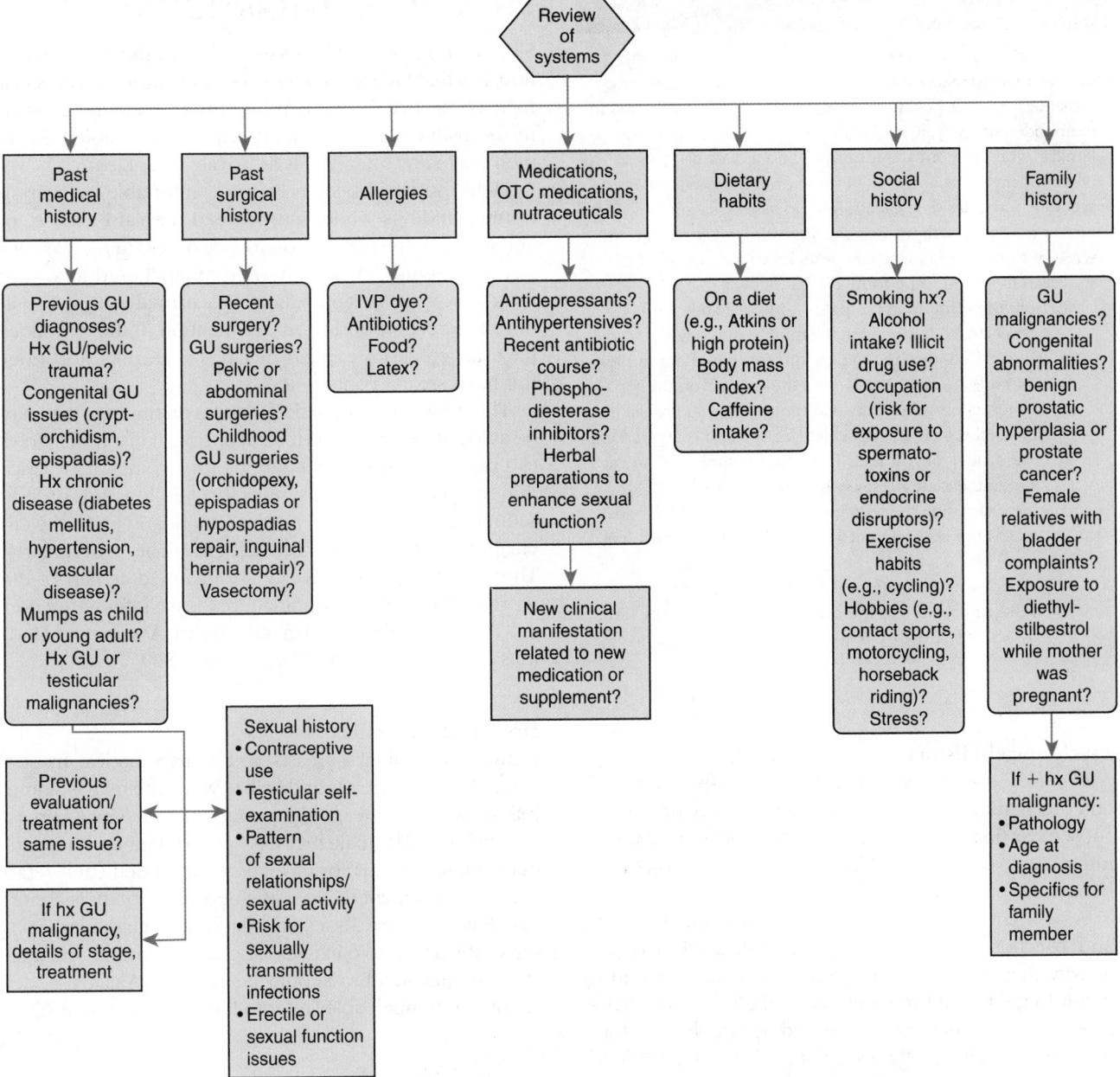

■ **FIGURE 37–9** Expanded male reproductive history.

Medications

Obtain a complete medication history for prescription, over-the-counter, and recreational drugs; nutritional supplements; and herbal remedies. Some medications prescribed for hypertension (methyldopa, clonidine, hydralazine, and beta blockers), for depression, and for the treatment of prostate cancer can cause sexual function difficulties. Other medications can decrease sperm count and motility. Inquire as to whether the client has used phosphodiesterase inhibitors either with or without a prescription. Recreational drugs (marijuana and hallucinogens) that alter behavior can also affect physiologic reproductive function and may raise the risk of STIs. Herbs frequently used to treat reproductive disorders include saw palmetto *(Serenoa repens)* for BPH and yohimbe *(Pausinystalia yohimbe)* for erectile dysfunction. Yohimbe is being monitored by the FDA and nurses should encourage men to avoid it (see Table 4-2 on p. 53).

Dietary Habits

Review the client's overall diet, and include assessment of any specific diets (such as a diet for clients with diabetes, or one designed to encourage muscle growth with the use of high-protein supplements). Discuss the client's body mass index (BMI) (see Chapter 28) in the context of his overall health and risk for diseases such as obesity and cardiovascular disease.

BOX 37-4 Testicular Self-Examination

Testicular self-examination (TSE) is a simple technique that men can use to assess for changes in their testicles that may signal testicular cancer. The risk is highest in adolescents and in men under age 35 years. As with BSE, the man should become familiar with the normal appearance and feel of his genitals to be confident of his ability to perform TSE. Advise the man to schedule a regular time each month to assess his genitals. The best time is after bathing, because the warm water causes the scrotum to relax and makes the testicles easier to examine.

Teach the client to perform TSE as follows:

1. Hold the scrotum in the palms of your hands, and examine each testicle with the thumbs and fingers of both hands. The index and middle fingers should be on the underside of each testicle with the thumbs on the top.
2. The testicle is rolled between the thumb and fingers. A normal testicle is shaped like an egg and is about 4 cm (1⅗ inches) long. It feels firm but not hard (like an ear lobe) and should be smooth without lumps.
3. After examining the testicles, examine the epididymides (behind the testicles); they should be soft and may feel sponge-like.
4. Examine the spermatic cords, which ascend from the epididymides up into the body. They are normally firm, smooth tubular structures.

Psychosocial History

Assess the client's use of caffeine, alcohol, tobacco, and recreational drugs, including marijuana. These substances may affect the sperm count, contribute to impotence, decrease libido, or encourage risk-taking behaviors.

Assess the man's occupation, environment, habits, and psychosocial factors. Include a discussion of any activity that would put the groin area at risk for trauma or prolonged pressure (such as football, hockey, marathon cycling, motorcross, or riding three- or four-wheeled vehicles). Determine the client's risk for exposure to pesticides, heat, heavy metals, hormones, and radiation. These materials can potentially directly affect male fertility. Assess the degree of stress the client reports at home, at work, and in his relationships.

Family Health History

Ask whether the client has a family history of testicular or other genitourinary malignancies, infertility, diabetes mellitus, hypertension, stroke, heart disease, endocrine disorders, and prostate or bladder problems (including female relatives with bladder conditions). As with women whose mothers took DES during pregnancy, men who have been exposed to DES in utero are at increased risk for congenital anomalies, including structural defects of the genitourinary system and reduced semen quality.

PHYSICAL EXAMINATION

Skillful history-taking helps to establish a therapeutic relationship that facilitates physical examination and aids in a focused history. Many men find physical examination of the reproductive system stressful and embarrassing. Some men may view the genitals as private or unclean.

Help the client become more comfortable by sharing normal findings while you proceed. Explain each step, and increase the client's comfort by maintaining eye contact, proceeding in an unhurried manner, and involving the client in self-examination. Occasionally, a man will have an erection during an examination. If the man does have an erection, explain that this is normal and does not have sexual connotation.

The physical examination focuses on findings that may be associated with reproductive or sexual disorders. Refer to a physical assessment textbook for a complete description of the physical examination. Follow an orderly sequence for the physical examination, and teach the client how to perform similar self-examinations regularly. The male breasts and axillae are included as part of the reproductive system examination. Please refer to the normal findings as described in the Physical Assessment Findings in the Healthy Adult feature on p. 869.

Breasts and Axillae

Examine the client's breasts and axillary nodes. Inspect and palpate the breasts and axillae while the man is sitting, following the same guidelines as for the female breast examination. The male breast is flat and symmetrical, without nodules, edema, or ulceration. One-sided (unilateral) breast enlargement that persists beyond puberty is abnormal. Palpation reveals a small, flat disk of glandular tissue under the areola. No masses, discharge, or breast enlargement (gynecomastia) should be present. Axillary nodes should be nonpalpable (refer to Figure 37-4 on p. 858).

External Genitalia

The client may be supine or lying on his side with his legs spread slightly for the first portion of the genital examination; ask him to stand during the assessment for inguinal herniation. Alternatively, the client might stand for the entire examination of the genitals. Because the male urethra is the common conduit for both urine and semen, examination of the male reproductive tract also includes assessment of the urinary system. Inspect the external genitalia and perineum (see Figure A&P9-4, A on p. 848), observing the pubic hair and skin. Knowledge of the normal growth and age-appropriate development of the male genitalia aids in assessment of the male reproductive system. Observe general appearance and body build, noting the hair distribution. Pubic hair distribution in men is triangular, with hair covering the symphysis pubis, base of the penis, and inner aspects of the thighs.

The Male Reproductive System

INSPECTION

Breasts and Axillae. Breasts symmetrical, smooth in all positions, without retractions or masses. Vascular pattern and striae absent. Nipples everted and areolae even. Axillae even color, without masses or rash.

Penis. Penis size and shape vary among individuals. Foreskin may or may not be present. Head of penis slightly rounded without discharge (if client is circumcised). Smegma under the foreskin (normal if client is uncircumcised). Urinary meatus at the tip of the head of the penis, free of discharge or drainage. Shaft smooth.

Scrotum. Scrotal size and shape vary normally. Hangs below the penis with the left side lower than the right. Scrotal skin thin and rugose. Sparse hair on the scrotum. Transillumination shows no masses or areas of thickness.

Inguinal-Femoral Area. Coarse hair covers symphysis pubis, inner thighs, extending toward umbilicus. No bulges over the inguinal or femoral area either at rest or with coughing or straining.

PALPATION

Breasts and Axillae. Breasts firm without masses, lumps, local areas of warmth, or tenderness. Nipples even, without discharge. Axillae smooth, nodes nonpalpable.

Penis. Masses along the penile shaft and head of the penis absent. Firm, nontender.

Testis. Two testicles present, smooth, oval, and similar in consistency. Mobile and equal in size. Slight tenderness with palpation.

Epididymis. Present at the posterior of the scrotum (found in the anterolateral or anterior area of the testis in a small percentage of men). No tenderness.

Vas Deferens. Cord-like, mobile, smooth, and nontender. No masses.

Inguinal Canal. No bulge or mass in inguinal canal either at rest or with straining.

Hair distribution may also spread toward the umbilicus in a diamond pattern. Inspect hair for nits and the skin for parasites, rashes, excoriation, and lesions.

Penis

The penis includes the penile shaft, prepuce (foreskin), glans, and urethral meatus. Inspect and palpate these structures for lesions, nodules, swelling, inflammation, atrophy, and discharge. The foreskin, if present, covers the glans. The foreskin is absent in a circumcised client. The foreskin must be retracted to expose the glans, and a small amount of cheesy, thick, white, odoriferous smegma between the glans and the foreskin is normal. The area is normally free of lesions; if any are present, palpate them for tenderness, size, shape, and consistency. If other discharge is noted, a specimen may be obtained

for culture. The area between the glans and foreskin is a common site of yeast infection and venereal lesions. Palpate the penile shaft gently between your thumb and first two fingers. It is smooth and semifirm, and the skin should move easily over underlying structures. The penis should be free of nodules, thickened or hard areas, or tenderness.

The urethral meatus should be noted at the tip of the glans, and should appear as a slit. Malposition of the meatus on either the underside of the penile shaft (*hypospadias*) or the upper side (*epispadias*) is a congenital condition, but may be noted in adult males. The meatus is pink and without ulcers, scars, inflammation, or discharge. The glans is compressed gently between thumb and index finger to open the meatus, and inspect for discharge or lesions. If a discharge is noted, a culture may be sent; refer to Chapter 41 or a laboratory textbook for details.

Scrotum

Inspect the scrotum and palpate for symmetry, size, shape, and swelling. Size and shape vary from one individual to another. Scrotal skin is darker than other skin surfaces and is loose and wrinkled. The scrotum has a right and a left half, each containing a testis, epididymis, spermatic cord, and vas deferens. The left testis often hangs lower than the right. Scrotal size varies with ambient temperature; cold results in contraction, warmth in relaxation. Scrotal skin should be loose, without tension. The testes are ovoid, and vary in size in adult males, averaging 2 × 4 cm. On palpation the testes are smooth, firm, and rubbery and without nodules, masses, or tenderness. Older clients may have smaller, less firm testes. Compare the testes bilaterally for similarity.

If a testis is not apparent, palpate the femoral and inguinal area; it is possible to find that an adult male client has an undescended testes. Nodules to the testes are never normal and are concerning for malignancy. These nodules may be firm, tender, nodular, mobile, or fixed.

The epididymis is located on the superior aspect of the testis and extends down the posterior surface. Each epididymis is palpated between thumb and index finger, and feels soft, resilient, and tender. Compare for similarity. Swelling, nodularity, and hardness are abnormal, but may be noted in the client who underwent a vasectomy many years ago.

The vas deferens (spermatic cord) begins at the superior, lateral aspect of the testis. It is differentiated from the epididymis by its firmer, tubular feel. Compare findings bilaterally. Palpate the vas deferens along its length toward the inguinal canal. Note any thickening and asymmetry, which are abnormal. The client should be instructed to bear down (Valsalva) during the examination as this can provoke a varicocele if one is present.

If swelling, nodules, or other abnormalities are noted during the scrotal examination, transillumination may be performed (Figure 37-10 on p. 870). In a darkened room

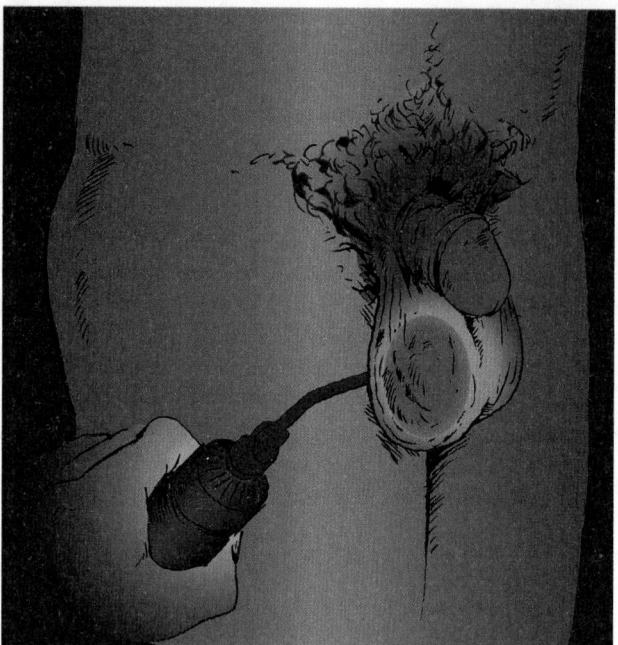

■ **FIGURE 37-10** Transillumination of the scrotum. In a darkened room, place a strong, lighted flashlight or transilluminator next to the scrotum, as shown. Light normally passes through the scrotum (transillumination), but this does not occur with testicular tumor. A hydrocele shines red.

a flashlight is shined through the scrotum from behind the mass. 🪔 A scrotum filled with serous fluid will transilluminate as a red glow. More solid lesions, such as a hematoma or a mass, do not transilluminate and may be seen as a dark shadow.

Inguinal Region

While the client is standing, examine for an inguinal hernia (a prolapse or protrusion of a loop of intestine through the inguinal wall or canal). Inspect the inguinal areas for bulges while the client stands quietly and again after he bears down and strains (Valsalva) as though attempting a bowel movement. Bulges should be absent. Refer to Table 37-2 for a description of the various types of hernias and associated physical examination maneuvers.

Prostate

Assess the anus, rectum, and prostate gland. A rectal-prostatic examination should be performed annually in men older than 50 (over 40 in high-risk clients) to look for manifestations of an STI, changes in the size and consistency of the prostate gland, and evidence of a tumor or acute or chronic infection. The normal prostate is located 2 to 5 cm beyond the anal sphincter along the anterior wall of the rectum. It is normally about 4 cm long and 5 cm wide (Figure A&P9-4, *B*, p. 848). An empty bladder makes the examination more comfortable and more accurate. Explain that it is normal to experience sensations of having to urinate or defecate during the examination.

The rectal-prostatic examination is usually performed by an advanced-practice nurse or physician. Please see a physical assessment textbook for more information related to this examination or go to the figure depicting rectal-prostatic assessment on the website.

DIAGNOSTIC TESTING

Various diagnostic tests are available to assess for disorders of the male reproductive system. There is often anxiety regarding the results of these tests; careful explanations before and during the tests can aid in alleviating some of this anxiety. Physiologic preparations may be required, such as fasting or an enema. During the test, tell the client what is happening. Help him maintain the required positions. Observe him during and after the test for adverse reactions, such as pain, excessive anxiety, pallor, or nausea.

TABLE 37-2   Hernia Descriptions

Hernia Type	Description	Assessment Technique
Direct inguinal hernia	Enters inguinal canal behind external ring because of weakened abdominal wall Does not pass through inguinal canal	Gently insert index finger into loose scrotal skin over external inguinal ring. Finger does not enter to external ring. Client must bear down in order to provoke any bulging, which should be absent.
Indirect inguinal hernia	Enters inguinal canal through internal ring and can remain in canal or pass down through external ring and into scrotum	Gently invaginate scrotal skin with index finger, following vas deferens to where it passes into external ring. Advance palpating finger as far as possible. Client must bear down in order to provoke any bulging, which should be absent. Any palpated mass should retreat up the canal when client relaxes.
Femoral hernia	Occurs inferiorly and more laterally compared with inguinal hernia Has appearance of an enlarged inguinal lymph node More common in women	Palpate inguinal area directly for femoral hernia while client is relaxed after instructing to bear down. Palpable mass should be absent.

Noninvasive Tests
Radiography
Both CT scanning and MRI are used to assess male reproductive and urologic disorders. The use of these studies includes clinical staging of testicular and prostate cancers and imaging to aid in identification of undescended testes or hernias.

Ultrasonography
Scrotal Ultrasound. Ultrasound is a noninvasive, inexpensive, and widely available imaging study. There is no need for contrast or exposure to radiations. Ultrasound is excellent for examination of the scrotum and its contents, and distinguishes between extra- and intratesticular pathologies.

Transrectal Ultrasound. Ultrasound is also used to image the prostate and seminal vesicles. A well-lubricated transducer is inserted into the rectum. The probe is covered with a water-filled condom to enhance sound-wave transmission; a full bladder may also improve sound transmission. The examiner moves the probe along the prostate to complete the scan.

Radionuclide Imaging
Radioisotope scans may be used to assess testicular abnormalities, such as torsion, epididymitis, abscess, tumors, hydroceles, varicoceles, and spermatoceles. A radioactive substance is administered intravenously, and several scans are taken.

> **Before a scan is taken, ask the client whether he has a history of allergies.**

Invasive Tests
Urodynamic Assessment
Urodynamic studies measure pressure from the bladder or urethra, urinary flow, and striated muscle activity. Common tests include uroflowmetry, cystometry, electromyography, and a urethral pressure profile. They are useful in determining the cause of frequency and decreased urinary stream in men (as from prostatic obstruction).

Cystoscopy
Cystoscopy is indispensable for assessing and treating prostate and urologic problems. It is used to determine the cause of urinary manifestations, such as those related to prostatic hypertrophy, and to obtain specimens, such as in a transurethral prostatic biopsy. Cystoscopy can be done in a urologist's office or in an operating room before surgery. Inspection of the bladder interior includes looking for trabeculation, diverticula, and bladder neck contracture, and checking the size and contours of the prostatic lobes.

Prostatic Biopsy
Biopsy of the prostate allows cytologic examination for the presence of cancer. The tissue may be obtained by a transurethral, transrectal, or perineal approach. Preparation includes an enema, and the client must void before the procedure. The transrectal approach is the most common; the client is placed in the Sims position. A rectal examination is performed to identify any hard nodules. The biopsy is performed with ultrasound guidance for the needle position. From 6 to 12 cores may be removed for microscopic examination.

Testicular Biopsy
There are very precise indications for a testicular biopsy, and they are primarily in the context of a male-factor infertility evaluation. This biopsy can provide information regarding spermatogenesis and the suitability of sperm for in vitro fertilization. Suspected testicular cancer is not an indication for a testicular biopsy.

Laboratory Tests
PSA Testing
Prostate cancer screening has been revolutionized by the prostate-specific antigen (PSA) assay. PSA, a glycoprotein produced by the prostate gland and found in prostatic fluid, aids the liquefaction of semen. Normal PSA levels are less than 2.6 ng/ml[4] independent of race. The PSA level increases with age, but can be elevated with BPH or prostatitis. When a PSA is 2.6 to 10 ng/ml, the likelihood of prostate cancer is judged as moderate, but values greater than 10 ng/ml indicate a high level of suspicion.

Prostatic massage, urethral instrumentation (such as catheterization or cystoscopy), ejaculation, or rectal examination within 48 hours before the assay can cause elevated PSA levels.[4,7]

Several additional tests are available: (1) PSA *density* (PSAD), (2) PSA *velocity* (PSAV), and (3) fractionated PSA. PSA density relates PSA level to prostate size.[3] The PSA density test is combined with transrectal ultrasonography (TRUS) to determine prostate volume. Scores are calculated by dividing the PSA by the prostate volume. Men who have PSA density levels less than 0.15 ng/ml are considered unlikely to have significant prostate cancer. As PSA levels rise, however, the presence of cancer cells is more likely. PSA velocity involves the rate of change in PSA level over time. Men who have a PSA velocity that rises more than 0.7 ng/ml per year or that increases 20% or more a year are considered at high risk of having prostate cancer. Fractionated PSA measures free versus protein-bound PSA in blood. Men with prostate cancer have a higher proportion of PSA bound to protein; the proportion of free PSA is higher in men with BPH.

Semen Examination

Semen testing is used to evaluate fertility, and the success of a vasectomy. To provide an adequate sample, the client should abstain from ejaculation for 2 to 5 days before the test. Prolonged abstinence may decrease sperm quality and motility, whereas more frequent ejaculations reduce sperm concentration and volume. The sample is collected via masturbation, and should be processed within 60 minutes.

Culture Analysis

Secretions from the throat, penis, and anus or lesions from the oral, pharyngeal, and perineal areas may be examined for microorganisms. A sterile, cotton-tipped applicator is placed on or in the affected area, and the specimen is transferred to a sterile tube or slide for culture and identification. Refer to a laboratory handbook for the specifics of culture collection.

 CONCLUSIONS

Assessment of the female and male reproductive systems requires knowledge of the physiologic and psychological implications associated with reproductive and selected endocrine disorders. Exhibit a concerned, caring attitude when assessing any client with a potential reproductive disorder, as these disorders are laden with psychosocial overtones. Assess the client in a thorough but matter-of-fact manner to put the client at ease and to expedite a complete assessment.

 BIBLIOGRAPHY

Citations appearing in red refer to primary research.

Citations appearing in blue refer to evidence-based practice guidelines and protocols.

1. American Cancer Society. (2007). *Cancer facts and figures.* Atlanta: ACS.
2. American Urological Association. (2000). *Prostate-specific antigen (PSA) best practice policy.* Linthicum, Md: Author.
3. Clark, N. (2002). *Women and nutrition: Tips for athletes with amenorrhea.* Accessed 10/12/06 from www.naturalstrength.com/nutrition/.
4. Gretzer, M., & Partin, A. (2003). *Campbell's Urology Updates: PSA and PSA Molecular Derivatives, 1*(1), 1-12.
5. Krane, J.F., et al (2001). Papanicolaou smear sensitivity for the detection of adenocarcinoma of the cervix. *Cancer Cytopathology, 93*(1), 8-15.
6. Quallich, S.A., & Rupp, P. (2005). Genitourinary system. In M. Goolsby & L. Grubbs (Eds.), *Advanced assessment: Interpreting findings and formulating differential diagnoses.* Philadelphia: F.A. Davis.
7. Tanagho, E.A., & McAninch, J.W. (2003). *Smith's general urology* (16th ed.). New York: McGraw-Hill Medical.
8. Varney, H., Kriebs, J.M., & Gegor, C.L. (2004). *Varney's midwifery* (4th ed.). Sudbury, Mass: Jones & Bartlett.

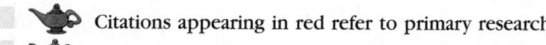 **evolve** *Did you remember to check out the bonus material on the Evolve website and the CD-ROM, including NCLEX®-Examination Style Review Questions, Open-Book Quizzes, and Chapter Review Audio Podcasts?*

http://evolve.elsevier.com/Black/medsurg

CHAPTER 38

Management of Men with Reproductive Disorders

MIKEL GRAY

Today men are more actively involved in health maintenance as evidenced by their increased interest in fitness and exercise, increased attainment of lifestyle factors related to fitness (such as smoking cessation), and increased participation in childbirth and parenting. With the recent emphasis on prostate health and prostate cancer, these interests have expanded to incorporate issues of reproductive and urinary health maintenance. Armed with knowledge about risk factors, preventive measures, and improvements in disease management, men are more likely to engage in preventive health-promoting behaviors and participate in health screening and early detection programs designed to avoid the morbidity and mortality associated with delayed diagnosis and management of common chronic diseases.

This increased attention to health promotion behaviors in adult males has provoked health care professionals, including nurses, to champion the concept of "men's health" services or clinics using similar strategies to those that have evolved in women's health services. Disorders of the genitourinary system are an important component of men's health. Nevertheless, men are often reluctant to ask for help because they regard such problems as a potential threat to their sexuality or identity as a man. Some men may also fear negative reactions from their health care providers because of their age or sexual preference.

Because of this reluctance to seek help, skillful therapeutic interaction is essential to help men express their concerns. Sensitivity to fear and embarrassment, respect for privacy and confidentiality, careful history taking, and addressing information needs help to put male clients at ease. When the client allows, partners should be brought into management plan discussions because most reproductive and genital disorders affect relationships.

Statements such as "Many men are concerned about how this problem will affect their sex lives," "It is common to worry about how your partner might feel about this problem," and "What are some of your concerns?" may help the client begin to talk about his concerns.

Giving men permission to express their feelings and their health-related concerns draws them and their significant others into the process of health care. Having topic-related brochures visible may provide the impetus for a man to ask questions.

PROSTATE DISORDERS

BENIGN PROSTATIC HYPERPLASIA

The prostate is the genital organ most commonly affected by benign and malignant neoplasms. Benign enlargement of the prostate gland is an extremely common process that occurs in nearly all men with functioning testes. The term benign prostatic enlargement is defined as prostate growth sufficient to obstruct (block)

---

evolve **Web Enhancements**

Case Study Cancer of the Prostate at the End of Life

Complementary and Alternative Therapy Flaxseed and a Low-Fat Diet for Men with Prostate Cancer

Korean Red Ginseng for Erectile Dysfunction

Non-Bacterial Chronic Prostatitis and Quercetin

Prostate Cancer Prevention with Finasteride

Selenium Supplements and Prostate Cancer Risk

Zinc Supplements and Prostate Cancer Risk

Bridge to Home Health Care Intermittent Self-Catheterization for Men

Table Urologic Instruments Most Commonly Encountered in a Clinical Setting

Be sure to check out the bonus material on the Evolve website and the CD-ROM, including free self-assessment exercises. **http://evolve.elsevier.com/Black/medsurg**

the urethral outlet, resulting in bothersome lower urinary tract symptoms (LUTS), urinary tract infection (UTI), hematuria, or compromised upper urinary tract function. Nevertheless, the term benign prostatic hyperplasia (BPH), defined as a nonmalignant histologic growth of the glandular elements of the prostate, is more commonly used and will be used throughout this chapter. Histologic evidence of prostate enlargement begins about the third decade of life and increases proportionally with aging. Specifically, about 43% of men in their 40s will have evidence of BPH, as will 50% of men in their 50s, 75% to 88% in their 80s, and nearly 100% of men reaching the ninth decade of life. The prevalence of BPH of sufficient magnitude to produce moderate to severely bothersome LUTS is lower, however, varying from about 17% of men in their 50s, 27% of men in their 60s, and 35% of men in their 70s. Europeans and African Americans have similar prevalence rates of BPH, but Asian Americans tend to have lower rates of BPH. The incidence of BPH is lowest among immigrants, however, and it increases with subsequent generations, suggesting environmental as well as possible racial differences.

Etiology and Risk Factors

The etiology of BPH is only partly understood. Whereas prostate enlargement is nearly universal in men with functioning testes, it is arrested following bilateral orchiectomy. Although androgens, and particularly testosterone, are not direct causes of BPH, their presence is critical to the normal growth and development of the prostate as well as BPH. Within the prostate, testosterone is converted to dihydrotestosterone (DHT) under the influence of an enzyme called 5α-reductase. DHT is the locally active form of testosterone that supports prostate growth and development throughout life, and the prostate remains sensitive to androgen production throughout life to maintain both prostate size and function. As a man ages and prostate enlargement occurs, 5α-reductase and DHT levels remain similar to those seen in younger men, but recent evidence has shown that the balance between two forms of this enzyme may be compromised, contributing to prostatic enlargement. Additional factors associated with BPH include a defect in local substances that regulate the programmed cellular death (apoptosis) common to many tissues within the body, including the skin and gastrointestinal tract. Imbalances of local growth factors, local inflammation, and genetic factors are also thought to influence the risk of BPH and the timing of its onset.

Multiple possible risk factors for BPH have been studied. For example, dietary factors have been examined, and lycopene in cooked tomatoes, green and yellow vegetables, and other elements of a traditional Japanese diet appear to provide some protection against BPH. Obesity (particularly increased abdominal girth) may increase the risk for BPH. The effect of diabetes mellitus on BPH appears to be minimal. Prospective analysis of a group of 2115 men from Olmstead County, Minnesota, demonstrated that while men with diabetes mellitus were more likely to develop bothersome LUTS than non-diabetic men, they demonstrated equivocal increase in prostate size. Physical activity has been shown to exert a protective effect against prostatic enlargement, possibly because of its indirect effects on obesity. Smoking has been hypothesized to exert a protective effect on BPH because it reduces serum testosterone levels, but epidemiologic studies have shown that it has only a slight effect on BPH risk compared with the well-documented and severe adverse health risks associated with cigarette use. Heavy alcohol use and cirrhosis of the liver impede prostate enlargement. Frequent use of α-adrenergic agonists commonly found in over-the-counter cold medications or diet pills increases the severity of bothersome LUTS associated with BPH and the risk for acute urinary retention.

Pathophysiology

Histologic evidence of prostate enlargement alone does not constitute a clinically relevant problem. Instead, the clinical disorders associated with BPH occur when this enlargement obstructs the bladder outlet, leading to bothersome LUTS, an increased risk of urinary tract infection, and compromised upper urinary tract function. Two processes produce this obstruction: hyperplasia and hypertrophy. Hyperplasia originates in the glandular (stromal) cells near the urethra—the transitional zone. On the microscopic level, prostatic hyperplasia is nodular, but the effect on palpation is a symmetrically enlarged gland free from the palpable nodes characteristic of prostate cancer. Obstruction occurs when hyperplasia narrows the lumen of the segment of the urethra coursing through the prostate. Obstruction also occurs when the prostate encroaches upon the bladder neck, reducing its ability to funnel in response to micturition, and when growth of the so-called median lobe of the prostate extends into the prostatic urethra. BPH is also influenced by the prostatic capsule (connective tissue covering the gland); in some men the capsule allows hyperplasia to expand outward, increasing the size of the prostate rather than the severity of urethral compression and urinary obstruction. Hypertrophy of the smooth muscle of the prostate also contributes to urethral obstruction via both active and passive forces. Hyperplasia of the prostate is accompanied by hypertrophy of the smooth muscle of the gland. Smooth muscle hypertrophy exacerbates urinary obstruction by increasing muscle tone at the bladder neck and proximal (prostatic) urethra and by mechanically adding to the tissue constricting the urethral lumen.

Our understanding of the effects of urethral obstruction on the lower urinary tract remains incomplete, but it has grown significantly over the past several decades (Figure 38-1). The bladder's initial response to increasing urethral resistance to outflow is to amplify the strength of the detrusor contraction. This strategy is often initially successful, leading many men to report relief from bothersome LUTS that may persist for a period of months to years. Further growth of the prostate and exacerbation of urethral obstruction, however, ultimately overwhelm the detrusor muscle's ability to ensure effective bladder evacuation by micturition. The result may be a decline in the force of the urinary stream, and feelings of incomplete bladder emptying despite urination. In addition to these LUTS, men tend to note bothersome LUTS that affect bladder storage, daytime voiding frequency, nocturia, and urgency. These LUTS are often associated with overactive detrusor contractions that may lead to urgency, and urge urinary incontinence in some cases. It is these clinical manifestations that typically provoke men to seek help from a health care professional. (See Figure 32-2, Expanded Genitourinary Assessment, on p. 658, for more information related to the diagnosis of LUTS.) If the man does not seek help for his bothersome LUTS and the process of prostatic enlargement continues, the detrusor may eventually decompensate, leading to urinary residual volumes and, ultimately, to a weakened muscle contraction, even after relief from urethral obstruction.

> **Alternatively, decompensation of the detrusor muscle may lead to an episode of acute urinary retention, defined as the complete inability to urinate. This condition is a medical emergency because uremia or bladder rupture and peritonitis will occur if the bladder is not relieved. In addition, acute urinary retention is associated with an increased risk of postoperative complications following surgical management of BPH.**

SAFETY
ALERT

A minority of men do not experience the bothersome LUTS described above, or they do not interpret these manifestations as indicating the need to seek care. When the obstruction associated with BPH is prolonged and severe, the client will experience compromised renal function or renal failure. Fortunately, this condition, sometimes referred to as silent prostatism, affects only a very small portion of men who experience BPH (i.e., fewer than 1%).

Urinary tract infection and hematuria also may be associated with BPH. Obstruction of the bladder outlet and urinary retention increase the risk of UTI (see Integrating Diagnostic Testing: Urinary Tract Infection on p. 668). This risk is greatest when catheterization, cystoscopy, or transurethral surgery is performed, which enables bacteria contained within the prostatic acini to reach the bladder. Urinary retention and obstruction also complicate the treatment of a UTI because incomplete bladder emptying compromises the complete evacuation of urine, bacteria, and toxins from the bladder.

The pathophysiology of hematuria caused by BPH is not entirely understood. It is known that angiogenesis (growth of blood vessels) is a part of hyperplasia and that these vessels may be prone to disruption and bleeding. Prolonged bleeding also may occur after catheterization, cystoscopy, or transurethral prostate surgery. The incidence of hematuria among men with BPH is unknown, but it has been noted that hematuria is the primary indication for transurethral surgery for BPH in 12% of all men diagnosed with BPH (see Integrating Diagnostic Testing: Hematuria on p. 666).

Clinical Manifestations

Bothersome LUTS (see Figure 32-3 Expanded Genitourinary Assessment and discussion of LUTS in Chapter 32, p. 666). provoke men with BPH and urethral obstruction to seek care. These manifestations usually develop slowly and may persist for months or years before the man defines them as sufficiently bothersome to seek help. Bothersome LUTS associated with bladder storage include nocturia (awakening from sleep because of the desire to urinate). Men younger than 65 years normally

Dilated pelvis

Normal kidney and ureter

Hydronephrosis

Hydroureter

Urine retention and reflux

"Fishhooking" of ureter

Thickening, diverticulation

Normal urinary bladder and prostate

Impeded outflow of urine

Enlarged prostate

■ **FIGURE 38–1** Complications of benign prostatic enlargement. *Left,* Normal kidney, ureter, bladder, and prostate. *Right,* Potential complications.

experience no nocturia or one episode of nocturia, and up to two episodes of nocturia are normal in men over age 65. In contrast, men with BPH often experience three or more episodes of nocturia per night that may lead to chronic sleep deprivation. Men with BPH also tend to report daytime voiding frequency, defined as urination more often than every 2 hours while awake, and urgency (a sudden and strong desire to urinate that is difficult to defer). LUTS associated with voiding include hesitancy, a decline in the force of the urinary stream, intermittent urinary stream, and feelings of incomplete bladder emptying. The severity of obstruction and LUTS caused by BPH is not related to the size of the enlargement. This lack of correlation occurs because physical assessment of prostate size is based on palpation of the exterior of the gland while the severity of obstruction and related BPH reflect a combination of active and passive factors.

Acute urinary retention is the complete inability to urinate. The client may report no urine output at all or dribbling leakage, called overflow urinary incontinence (see Chapter 34). Suprapubic discomfort and restlessness crescendo as the bladder fills beyond physiologic capacity (the volume at which a strong desire to urinate is perceived) and approaches anatomic capacity (the maximum volume the bladder can safely hold without imminent risk of rupture or other damage).

History-taking includes specific questions about daytime voiding frequency, nocturia, urgency, urinary incontinence, the force of the urine stream, hesitancy, need to strain, perception of bladder emptying, and prior episodes of acute urinary retention. The American Urological Association's International Prostate Symptom Score (IPSS) is a short questionnaire commonly used by urologists to assess the client's opinion about the severity of these manifestations (the IPSS appears in Figure 32-4 on p. 667). This instrument provides a reliable and valid description of bothersome LUTS associated with BPH, but it fails to differentiate LUTS caused by BPH from those caused by other, nonobstructive etiologies. It demonstrates good predictive validity (it accurately reflects the success of various treatments for the relief of bothersome LUTS).

A digital rectal examination (DRE) is performed to assess prostate size and to differentiate BPH from prostate enlargement caused by adenocarcinoma or infection. BPH reveals a symmetrically enlarged prostate with an obliterated central sulcus. Prostatic infection (prostatitis) is associated with symmetric enlargement, a boggy consistency, and discomfort on palpation. Adenocarcinoma of the prostate is associated with asymmetric enlargement, hardened nodules, or induration. Urinalysis and blood tests for kidney function (urea nitrogen or blood urea nitrogen [BUN] and creatinine levels) are routinely performed, and a urine culture or serum prostate-specific antigen (PSA) measurement to assess for cancer is

performed in selected cases. Chemistry panels, such as electrolyte levels, liver function, and blood coagulation studies, may be added if surgery is being considered.

Uroflowmetry may be completed to assess the voiding pattern and measure maximum and average flow rates. A man starts this test with a full bladder and then voids into a specific toilet or container, emptying his bladder to the best of his ability. Residual urine is determined after the urine flow either by catheterization or by ultrasonography (bladder scan). A maximum urinary flow of 12 ml/sec or greater in a man age 55 years or older greatly reduces the likelihood of urethral obstruction associated with BPH, but a voiding pressure flow study must be completed to measure definitively the severity of obstruction and to determine its cause. Depending on the severity of the client's manifestations and general medical condition, cystourethroscopy, intravenous pyelography (IVP), or urodynamic studies may be done (see Chapter 32 and the Integrating Diagnostic Testing: Urinary Incontinence in Chapter 34 on p. 765).

OUTCOME MANAGEMENT

Medical Management

Medical management has become a common initial approach for BPH because it is noninvasive and effective in cases of mild to moderate obstruction. "Watchful waiting" is a relatively new approach to BPH, particularly for the client with mild LUTS assessed by IPSS. Ongoing assessment, including repeated measurement of a symptom score such as the IPSS, is necessary to determine whether the magnitude of bothersome LUTS increases or other complications (such as acute urinary retention) occur. An increase in IPSS score (reflecting exacerbation of voiding problems or high symptom score at baseline) indicates the need for more definitive treatment, as does the occurrence of a complication such as UTI, hematuria, or an episode of acute urinary retention.

Relax Prostate Muscle/Slow Prostate Growth
More aggressive medical treatment is aimed at reducing urethral obstruction by relaxing smooth muscle within the prostate, proximal urethra, and bladder neck or blocking the action of 5α-reductase, the enzyme that converts testosterone to DHT, allowing local growth of the prostatic stroma. The Integrating Pharmacology box on p. 877 summarizes medications used to treat benign prostatic hyperplasia.

In addition to the U.S. Food and Drug Administration (FDA)-approved drugs listed in the preceding Integrating Pharmacology box, a growing number of men use phytotherapeutic agents (use of herbs for healing purposes) to manage BPH. The most widely used agent is *Serenoa repens* (saw palmetto). See the Complementary and

Medications for Benign Prostatic Hyperplasia

Medical management of benign prostatic hyperplasia (BPH) involves the use of medications that slow prostate growth or relax prostate muscle. Alpha$_1$-adrenergic blockers relax the smooth muscle of the prostate, bladder neck, and proximal urethra. These drugs are often also used in the treatment of hypertension. Examples of medications in this category include terazosin (Hytrin), doxazosin (Cardura), tamsulosin (Flomax), and alfuzosin (Uroxatral). A 4-week treatment trial is needed to evaluate the maximum efficacy of these drugs. Terazosin and doxazosin require titration and are typically taken at bedtime because peak serum levels occur approximately 2 hours after administration, increasing the risk for orthostatic hypotension or dizziness. Tamsulosin and alfuzosin are less likely to cause these side effects, and they do not routinely require titration. Other side effects associated with this class of drugs include tachycardia, nasal congestion, and retrograde ejaculation. Alfuzosin carries less risk for retrograde ejaculation than do other drugs in this class.

5α-Reductase inhibitors slow prostate growth by inhibiting the conversion of testosterone into dihydrotestosterone (DHT) in the prostate gland. They also lower serum PSA levels and may mask the occurrence of prostate cancer. Examples of medications in this category include finasteride (Proscar) and dutasteride (Avodart). These drugs must be taken for 6 to 12 months to assess maximum ability to relieve bothersome LUTS. Because 5α-reductase also acts on hepatic tissue and finasteride is primarily metabolized by the liver, hepatic function tests are important before therapy is started. Side effects are mild and include a decrease in ejaculatory volume, decreased libido, and erectile dysfunction in about 1% to 5% of men taking either of these medications. Both agents can cause abnormal development of a male fetus. Hence pregnant women should not handle the medication without gloves or come in contact with the semen of a man taking this drug.

A major randomized clinical trial, the Medical Therapy of Prostate Symptoms (MTOPS) study, demonstrates that combination therapy (alpha$_1$-adrenergic antagonist plus 5α-reductase inhibitor) relieves LUTS and prevents progression of BPH more effectively than treatment with a single agent.[1]

Anti-androgens and LHRH antagonists, agents used to treat prostate cancer, have been tried in the treatment of BPH but the side effects outweigh the benefits for most men.

REFERENCE

Logan, Y.T., & Belgeri, M.T. (2005). Monotherapy versus combination drug therapy for the treatment of benign prostatic hyperplasia. *American Journal of Geriatric Pharmacotherapy, 3*(2), 103-114.

Alternative Therapy feature on *Serenoa repens* and *Pygeum africanum* Supplements for Benign Prostate Hyperplasia on p. 878. β-Sitosterol is extracted from *Hypoxis rooperi* (South African star grass) to form the primary active ingredient in Harzol and Azuprostat. Its actions on BPH are unknown, but it is hypothesized to inhibit one or more growth factors involved in prostatic hyperplasia. Nevertheless, at least two randomized, controlled trials show symptom relief among men taking these preparations compared with those taking placebo. Other agents purported to relieve bothersome LUTS associated with BPH include couch grass, pumpkin, pipsissewa, and pygeum. Of these, pipsissewa is not recommended because dosages and its side effect profile have not been determined. Pumpkin has not been shown to be beneficial for managing BPH manifestations. The efficacy of pygeum compared with finasteride or saw palmetto has not been documented, and it should not be used in combination with other medications for BPH until studies assessing its safety in combination with these agents have been completed.

Relieve Retention

Acute urinary retention is initially managed by an indwelling catheter. It is usually left in place for 2 to 4 weeks to allow the bladder to recover from injury caused by the acute overdistention of the bladder wall associated with acute retention. Following this period, the client may be given a voiding trial. The bladder is filled with sterile water or saline, preferably heated to body temperature, and the catheter is removed. The client is then asked to urinate and the voided volume is compared with the infused volume to determine the efficiency of micturition. Alternatively, the client may be taught to perform clean intermittent catheterization, particularly if long-term retention occurs (see the Bridge to Home Health Care feature on Intermittent Self-Catheterization for Men on the website.) Men *evolve* who are not candidates for surgery or intermittent catheterization may require long-term indwelling catheterization.

Nursing Management of the Medical Client

Assessment. Ask the client to describe all urinary manifestations, focusing on lower urinary tract symptoms (LUTS) including storage LUTS, such as daytime and nighttime voiding frequency, urgency, and urinary incontinence; voiding LUTS, such as a reduced force of intermittency or hesitancy; and post-void LUTS, such as a post-void dribble. Ask about the presence of hematuria (blood in the urine).

Clients often consume herbal agents in the belief that they are safer than physician-prescribed medications. You should ask your clients whether they are taking saw palmetto, couch grass, pipsissewa, pumpkin, or pygeum or other preparations for BPH. Client teaching for the man using phytotherapy includes information about the actions of these agents, their efficacy, and the safety of their use in combination with prescribed drugs.

SAFETY

⚠

ALERT

COMPLEMENTARY AND ALTERNATIVE THERAPY

Serenoa repens (Saw Palmetto) and Pygeum africanum Supplements for Benign Prostatic Hyperplasia

Saw palmetto (*Serenoa repens*) has the most evidence to date of any supplement for improving the manifestations of benign prostatic hyperplasia (BPH) or noncancerous enlargement of the prostate.[2] This posting included 3 new trials involving 230 additional men. In this update, 3193 men from 21 random trials lasting 4 to 48 weeks reported improved urinary symptom scores when compared with placebo and similar improvements when compared with finasteride. Saw palmetto is derived from a dwarf palm tree that grows in the southwest United States; it contains a mixture of fatty acids, sterols (alcohol-based steroid), and flavonoids. Its principal action in relationship to BPH appears to be inhibition of 5α-reductase enzyme activity, similar to the action of finasteride.

An analysis of all studies that included extracts of the African plum tree, or *Pygeum africanum,* was recently conducted.[1] Researchers found that 18 studies met the selection criteria that included 1562 clients.[1] However, only 5 trials (n = 430) provided information on a global assessment of improvement of clinical manifestations after treatment with this supplement, which was rated by physicians and not clients. In addition, most trials were short and did not compare this herbal product to standard prescription drugs. Therefore it is possible that this herb is providing nothing more than a placebo effect. Regardless, more men in the supplement versus placebo group had an overall improvement in manifestations rated by their physician. The increase in peak urine flow was 23% greater, and the reduction in residual urine volume was 24% greater in the *Pygeum africanum* versus placebo group. The groups did not differ in dropout rates and side effects. Thus very limited evidence suggests that *Pygeum africanum* extract is more effective than a placebo for improving clinical manifestations and urodynamic study results in men with BPH.

REFERENCES

1. Wilt, T., et al. (2006). Pygeum africanum for benign prostatic hyperplasia. *Cochrane Database System Retrieval, 1,* CD001044.
2. Wilt, T., et al. (2006). Serenoa repens for benign prostatic hyperplasia. Cochrane Prostatic and Urologic Cancers Group. *Cochrane Database of Systematic Reviews, 2,* CD001423. Posted 10/01/06.

Diagnosis, Outcomes, Interventions
Diagnosis: Readiness for Enhanced Self-Care. The nurse has a major teaching role to help the client manage BPH. Hence the nursing diagnosis is *Readiness for Enhanced Self-Care related to desire to learn more about BPH, manifestations, and medical treatments.*

Outcomes. The client will understand BPH, manifestations, and medical treatment, as evidenced by client statements, increased fluid intake, and ability to follow medication regimen.

Interventions
Provide Teaching About BPH. Men often have only a vague understanding of what an enlarged prostate is, much less where the gland lies. Many men fear they have prostate cancer or that BPH is a precursor of prostate cancer. Beliefs about treatment affecting their sexual functioning are also a concern. Show the client and significant other a picture of the reproductive organs and prostate, and explain the effects of enlargement on urine excretion.

Encourage Fluids. Many clients limit their fluid intake to combat the manifestations of BPH. Explain that concentrated urine acts as an irritant to the bladder. Caffeine and alcohol also can exacerbate bothersome LUTS, and their intake should be reduced or avoided.

> **Clients increase their risk of UTI with limited fluid intake. Unless otherwise contraindicated, the client should maintain an intake of 30 ml/kg/day or ½ ounce per pound of body weight.**

Explain Medications. If medications are being used to treat BPH, men need a thorough explanation of how the medications work, their side effects, and precautions. Warn the client to increase dosage only under the physician's orders because more medication may not help manifestations and may cause serious cardiovascular problems. Encourage clients to be patient because the effects of medication on the prostate may take time.

> **Discourage clients from taking medications that contain alpha-adrenergic agonists (e.g., cold medicines and diet pills) because they can cause a man with BPH to experience acute urinary retention, which can be a medical-emergency. Clients are also discouraged from taking over-the-counter cold remedies containing diphenhydramine (Benadryl), which has strong anticholinergic properties that may relax the decompensated detrusor muscle and precipitate acute urinary retention. Clients are counseled to inform all health care providers of their BPH because multiple medications (including antimuscarinics, certain antidepressants, antipsychotics, and calcium channel blockers) may adversely affect bladder function and increase the risk for acute urinary retention.**

Diagnosis: Impaired Urinary Elimination. The client with BPH usually experiences manifestations such as frequency, urgency, hesitancy, change in urinary stream, incontinence, retention, and nocturia. Write the nursing diagnosis as *Impaired Urinary Elimination related to increasing urethral occlusion.*

Outcomes. The client will remain free of manifestations of BPH or those manifestations will decrease with treatment, as evidenced by absence of frequency, urgency, hesitancy, change in stream, incontinence, retention, or nocturia.

Interventions

Catheterize. When the client has urinary difficulties, such as obstruction, urinary retention, or diminished renal function, some form of catheterization may be necessary. See the table on the website, Urologic Instruments Most Commonly Encountered in a Clinical Setting, which shows various types of urethral catheters. (The Bridge to Home Health Care feature on the website explains intermittent self-catheterization for men.)

> **Never force a urinary catheter. If it cannot be inserted with gentle pressure, notify the urologist, who may need special instruments to get the catheter past the obstruction.**

Bladder spasms are common with indwelling catheters. If bladder discomfort and leakage are significant, medications can be ordered to reduce them (see Chapter 34). Clean the meatus several times a day with water and mild soap.

Monitor Urine Output.

> **If an indwelling catheter is placed for acute retention, observe the client for hourly urine output (should be at least 0.5 ml/kg/hour), hematuria, and shock caused by postobstructive diuresis.**

Hematuria can occur because of the sudden release of pressure on the blood vessels supplying the bladder or mild trauma resulting from catheterization. Postobstructive diuresis means increased urine output caused by inability of the renal tubules to absorb water and electrolytes after prolonged urinary obstruction. It is usually self-limiting but can cause sodium depletion in some clients, which leads to vascular collapse and death if not detected and treated.

Evaluation. The client should be able to manage the manifestations of the disease and to take the medication appropriately. Clients should also continue follow-up so that the usefulness of the medical treatment can be assessed. Surgical intervention may be needed if medical management fails.

Surgical Management

Surgery is indicated in cases of high-magnitude obstruction (particularly when complicated by an episode of acute urinary retention), severe LUTS, recurrent UTI, hematuria, bladder stones, or upper urinary tract distress. The part of the gland causing the obstruction is removed in a procedure called a prostatectomy. The term prostatectomy is a misnomer because the procedure is actually removal of new tissue growth. Figure 38-2 on p. 880 illustrates various surgical approaches. The method used depends on the size of the prostate, the health of the client, and surgeon preference. Robotic assistive devices may be used for laparoscopic prostatectomy procedures in major medical centers.

Regrowth of prostate tissue after prostatectomy for BPH occurs over a period of 1 to 15 years, and it occasionally requires a repeat procedure. In addition, prostate cancer may still develop because the total prostate is not removed. These clients need the same follow-up as other men who have not had prostate surgery.

Operative Technique

Transurethral Resection of the Prostate. Transurethral resection of the prostate (TURP) remains a widely used technique for managing BPH, and it continues to be the "gold standard" against which all other procedures are measured. A resectoscope is inserted through the urethra (see Figure 38-2, *A*). The surgeon visualizes the inside of the bladder by inserting a cystoscope (telescopic lens) through the resectoscope. A movable loop is inserted through the resectoscope that cuts tissue and coagulates bleeding vessels with high-frequency electric current. (A cold-punch resectoscope that punches out tissue, piece by piece, with a circular knife blade is rarely used today.)

Irrigating fluid is infused into the bladder via the cystoscope, allowing visualization of the resection. Repeated irrigation and drainage of this fluid ensure that resected tissue and debris are removed from the bladder. Sterile irrigation fluid is used for transurethral surgery that allows the electrical conductance needed for resection and coagulation. An isotonic fluid is selected; however, normal saline is avoided because of its suboptimal conductivity properties. In addition, a hypotonic solution such as water must never be used because it will readily absorb into the bloodstream and creates a high risk for transurethral resection (TUR) syndrome. TUR syndrome is characterized by hyponatremia, hypervolemia, hemolysis, and acute renal failure. Clinical manifestations of TUR syndrome include agitation, acute delirium, bradycardia, tachypnea, and vomiting. Although unusual, it can occur even when isotonic solutions are used, particularly if resection involves surgical times longer than 60 to 90 minutes, allowing extensive absorption of irrigation into the vascular system. If manifestations of TUR syndrome occur, the physician is notified immediately and fluid and other supportive measures are initiated promptly. Bleeding is common after this procedure, and constant or intermittent irrigation is necessary.

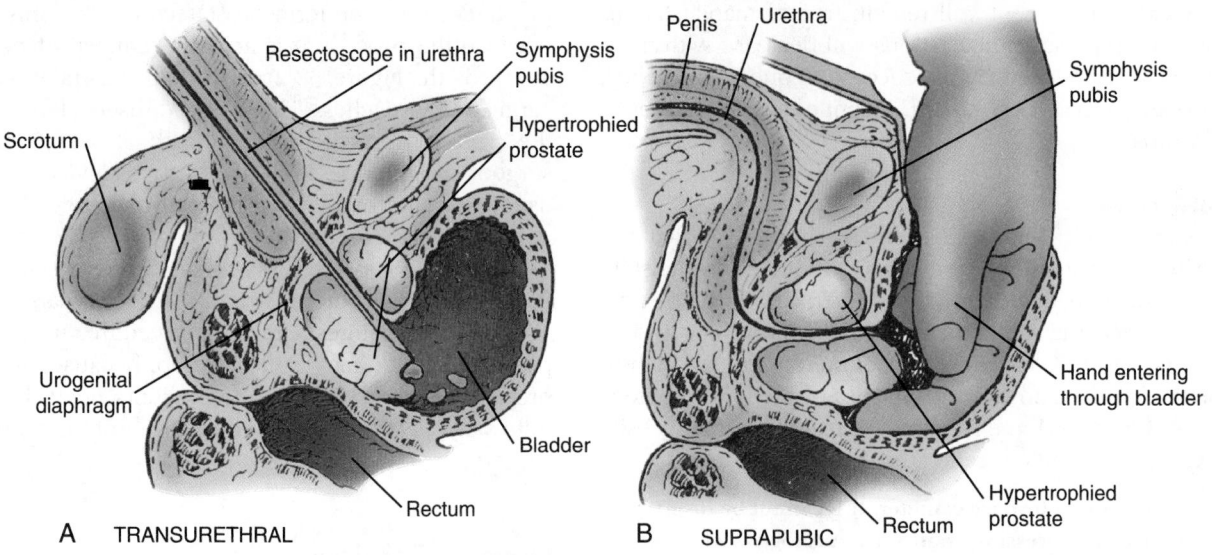

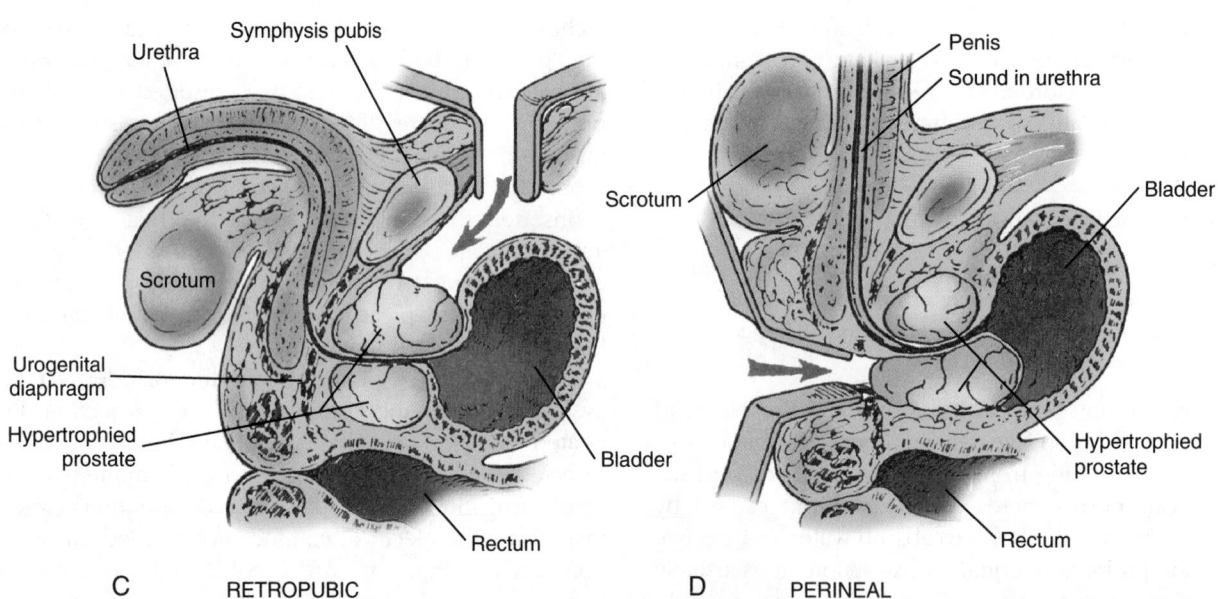

■ **FIGURE 38–2**   Surgical approaches to the prostate. **A,** Transurethral resection of the prostate (TURP) is a closed method of treatment; no incision is made, and the hyperplastic prostate tissue is removed through a resectoscope (like a cystoscope), which is inserted through the urethra. **B,** Suprapubic (transvesical) prostatectomy is an open method of treatment in which the hyperplastic prostatic tissue is enucleated through the anterior walls of the abdomen and bladder. **C,** Retropubic (extravesical) prostatectomy is an open method of treatment; a low abdominal incision is made between the pubic arch and the bladder. **D,** Perineal prostatectomy is an open method of treatment involving an incision between the anus and the scrotum.

Suprapubic Prostatectomy. Suprapubic prostatectomy is a surgical approach that involves a lower abdominal incision (Figure 38-2, *B*). It may be the operation of choice when (1) the prostate is too large to be resected transurethrally; (2) a large, pedunculated middle prostatic lobe or lateral lobes are present; (3) a bladder abnormality needs correction; or (4) an abdominal surgical exploration is necessary. An incision is made into the bladder, and the enlarged tissue is enucleated by blunt dissection. Both suprapubic and urethral catheters are inserted. Bladder abnormalities can be treated concurrently with this procedure, and complete

tissue removal is facilitated; however, hemostasis can be difficult to achieve.

The client may experience more bladder spasms, urinary leakage into the abdominal wound around the suprapubic catheter, and a relatively prolonged and uncomfortable convalescence. Incontinence and erectile dysfunction (ED) (impotence) can occur after this procedure.

Retropubic Prostatectomy. In the retropubic prostatectomy (see Figure 38-2, *C*), the surgeon approaches the prostate through a low abdominal incision without entry into the bladder. This is the operation of choice when the prostate is very large and a severe urethral stricture is present. Advantages include direct visualization of the prostate and direct hemostasis in the prostatic fossa. Disadvantages are that associated bladder problems cannot be treated and osteitis pubis (pubic bone inflammation) may occur.

Perineal Prostatectomy. An incision is made into the perineum between the anus and the scrotum (see Figure 38-2, *D*). This operation is rarely used for treating BPH because of the great potential for ED. The client must be in a lithotomy position, which is contraindicated for clients with severe arthritis or cardiopulmonary disease. Other complications include rectourethral fistula, UTI, epididymitis, and urinary retention.

Minimally Invasive Therapies. A number of procedures have been developed that offer potential advantages compared with open surgery or TURP. Collectively, these techniques have been termed minimally invasive therapies. Although the morbidity and need for hospitalization vary among these procedures, they are generally associated with less bleeding and minimal or no need for hospitalization compared with the gold standard for surgical management for BPH, the TURP.

Transurethral Incision of the Prostate. Transurethral incision of the prostate (TUIP) is an option for men with a small prostate that is causing outlet obstruction. Incisions are made into the prostatic tissue to enlarge the lumen of the prostatic urethra. This procedure is associated with relatively few postoperative complications and can be performed with local anesthesia for high-risk clients. High client satisfaction has also been reported with this procedure; many clients report no change in ejaculation, which makes this an excellent procedure for younger men with a small prostate gland.

Transurethral Electrovaporization. Transurethral electrovaporization of the prostate (the VaporTrode procedure) uses similar equipment as that required for TURP, with the exception of a specially designed ball or bar that is inserted through a working port of the resectoscope and attached to an electrocautery power source. Tissue vaporization requires electric power of 200 to 300 W, compared with the 80 to 150 W used to cauterize blood vessels during TURP. It vaporizes prostatic tissue and offers the potential advantage of reducing bleeding. It also destroys tissue samples that are sent for pathologic analysis following traditional TURP. A prospective randomized clinical trial comparing the VaporTrode to TURP demonstrated comparable results up to 5 years following the procedure. Electrovaporization may be combined with traditional TURP, particularly when prostate size is considerable or tissue protrudes into the proximal urethra.

Laser-Assisted Procedures. Transurethral ultrasound-guided laser incision of the prostate (TULIP) is a minimally invasive procedure in which a laser is used to make the incision into the prostate. It is associated with minimal blood loss, no irrigation is necessary, and the client does not always need a catheter after surgery. Laser ablation of prostatic tissue gained some popularity in the 1980s but its use subsequently declined because of the need for prolonged catheterization following the procedure and the length of time required to resect enough prostatic tissue to effectively relieve bladder outlet obstruction. More recently, laser-assisted procedures have re-emerged because of the evolution of two newer procedures: holmium laser enucleation of the prostate (HoLEP) and photoselective vaporization of the prostate (Green Light Laser). HoLEP uses holmium: yttrium-aluminum-garnet laser energy to resect relatively large sections of prostate tissue. Although the time required to complete the procedure is longer than that required for TURP, postoperative bleeding is minimized, and it is expected to provide long-term results that are comparable, or possibly even superior, to TURP. HoLEP is also favored because of its efficacy in the management of larger prostate sizes, a limitation of older laser-assisted techniques. Photoselective vaporization uses potassium-titanyl-phosphate laser energy to ablate prostatic tissue. Unlike other laser procedures, sterile water for irrigation is used for photoselective vaporization, because of its optimal qualities. Clinical experience with the procedure indicates that most clients can be discharged on the day of surgery without an indwelling catheter. The ability to remove the catheter on the procedure day represents a significant advantage for clients.

Laser-assisted procedures continue to evolve, and alternative forms of laser energy have led to the development of two new procedures that have overcome multiple limitations associated with older forms of therapy used during the 1980s. Nevertheless, a complete evaluation of the long-term efficacy of both of these laser-assisted procedures must be completed before their clinical role in the management of BPH can be determined.

Hyperthermia and Thermal Therapy. Hyperthermia and thermal therapies are newer procedures. Hyperthermia refers to the administration of temperatures below 45° C; thermal therapy refers to administration of higher temperatures. Three techniques—microwaves, radiofrequency, or high-intensity ultrasound waves—may be used to heat the prostate and destroy prostate tissue. Transurethral microwave thermotherapy requires passage of a catheter into the urethra that is used to deliver microwave energy. A temperature probe is placed in the rectum, and water is circulated through the system to prevent urethral or rectal heat injury. The transurethral needle ablation (TUNA) system uses radiofrequency energy to destroy prostatic tissue. Special needles are placed into the prostate, and radiofrequency energy is used to provoke tissue coagulation and necrosis. A shield is used to protect the urethra, and multiple treatments are usually required. Water-induced thermotherapy (WIT) uses heated water to destroy obstructive prostate tissue; it is delivered via a 20F catheter in a single 30- to 45-minute session.

🪔 Each of these therapies can be completed in an outpatient setting using local anesthesia only. The initial magnitude of relief from obstruction and the durability of results, however, are less than those achieved by TURP.

Prostatic Stent. Traditionally, prostatic stent insertion is indicated for clients who are extremely poor operative risks. The mesh-like tube (a coil-shaped device has also been used) can be inserted through an endoscope into the prostatic urethra, where it holds the urethra open mechanically. Over time, usually about 3 to 6 months, epithelial cells grow over the stent, which is permanent in most cases. Irritative LUTS are common, but they usually subside within several months. The stents have to be removed when they migrate, become encrusted or infected, or cause persistent perineal discomfort. Removal may be difficult. To prevent complications, clients are cautioned to avoid catheterization through the stent for 3 months after placement.

Complications

Complications after treatment vary between treatments. They may include bleeding (particularly associated with TURP), infection, persistent obstruction (particularly seen with minimally invasive therapies), accidental displacement of the catheter, stenosis of the urethra or bladder neck, epididymitis, urinary incontinence, ED, or retrograde (backward) ejaculation. Urethral stricture or bladder neck contracture is usually treated with dilation, although urethroplasty may be required in severe or refractory cases. Persistent incontinence after TURP affects 1% to 2%. Clients with overactive detrusor contractions (overactive bladder), voiding frequency, and sensory urgency initially may note an increase in the frequency of urinary leakage or de novo incontinence. 🪔 Pharmacotherapy combined with pelvic muscle rehabilitation and fluid and dietary control may be required to control overactive bladder that has been "unmasked" by removal of obstructive prostatic tissue.

Erectile dysfunction occurs in 5% to 10% of clients and only when nerves are damaged during surgery for prostate resection. Of major concern to clients is the occurrence of retrograde ejaculation. Because the verumontanum is destroyed during most prostate surgery, antegrade (forward) ejaculation cannot occur. Instead, semen goes into the bladder during ejaculation and is

voided with the next urination, creating cloudy urine. This effect is harmless, but sexual function may be impaired unless the client is advised of this anticipated effect and reassured that it is expected to alter fertility potential but not libido or erectile function.

Outcomes

It is expected that the client will achieve significant relief from bothersome LUTS without complications. In addition, objective measures of lower urinary tract function should reveal alleviation of obstruction and urinary retention.

Nursing Management of the Surgical Client

Preoperative Care

Assess the client's ability to empty his bladder. The bladder should be percussed for distention. If the client cannot void, a urethral catheter may have to be placed. Clients taking any drug or supplement with anticoagulant effects must discontinue these substances before surgery. The nurse should carefully review all prescription drugs, over-the-counter medicines, and herbal agents for anticoagulant properties. 🪔 This review also incorporates high-dose vitamin E or multivitamins because daily supplementation with vitamin E of 400 international units or higher exerts a dose-dependent anticoagulant effect. Preoperative assessment should also include attention to expectations about the procedure, such as anticipated changes in voiding and sexual function. You are often able to lessen the client's fear and anxiety during the nursing history by reinforcing preoperative teaching provided by the urologist and by ensuring that the client (and partner if possible) understands the anticipated outcomes of the procedure. Respond to the concerns of the client and significant others with empathic listening, accurate information, and ongoing support. Restating the explanations given by the surgeon and anesthetist when securing informed consent is particularly helpful because stressed clients frequently forget what they have been told.

Informed consent requires that the man understand the risks (e.g., possible sexual dysfunction, including ED; retrograde ejaculation; and infertility) and short-term and long-term benefits (e.g., relief of urinary manifestations and promotion of optimal renal function). It is important for the client to receive honest answers to questions concerning sexuality and reproduction.

Postoperative Care

Assessment. Immediately after surgery, your major task is to observe the vital signs and maintenance of urinary drainage. Indwelling catheters are used to facilitate urinary drainage after many types of prostate procedures. Document the urine color, including the presence of blood clots, each time urine output is recorded.

Various types of catheter irrigation systems may be used with these catheters. Closed irrigation, or closed bladder irrigation (CBI), permits either constant or intermittent irrigation without the hazard of violating aseptic technique. Refer to a fundamentals textbook for more information related to CBI and see Figure 38-3. Isotonic fluid is used to maintain the outflow of clear or slightly pink urine. Pay close attention to the irrigation rate, and never reduce the rate until directed to do so because premature reduction of the irrigation rate will predispose the client to stasis of debris or blood, leading to catheter blockage. Ensure that the catheter drainage bag is emptied regularly and when it is approximately 75% full to avoid stasis or interruption of urinary drainage.

Frequently assess the client's urine output. Documentation of output must include records of intake and output, and it should include the amount instilled with the irrigation. Differentiation of urine output versus output from the irrigation process is important because it is possible for the client to have a urine output of less than 0.5 ml/kg/hour that is easily missed if irrigation drainage is not subtracted to calculate true urine output.

Ensure catheter patency frequently to make sure the catheter is draining; blockage of an irrigated bladder rapidly leads to overdistention, secondary hemorrhage, and formation of blood clots or infection. Proper positioning of the catheter and drainage system is important to maintain good drainage and prevent obstruction of the system. Blood clots, prostatic debris, mucus plugs, kinked tubing, or catheter displacement may obstruct urinary flow.

Diagnosis, Outcomes, Interventions

Diagnosis: Risk for Injury. A common problem after all procedures is *Risk for Injury related to presence of urinary catheters, hematuria, irrigation, or suprapubic drains.*

Outcomes. The client will not experience hemorrhage, as evidenced by absence of gross bleeding, infection, catheter obstruction, and water intoxication and maintenance of urine output of at least 0.5 ml/kg/hour.

Interventions

Maintain Irrigation. Closed bladder irrigation decreases the development of obstruction. If obstruction is suspected, manual (hand) irrigation may be necessary. After prostatectomy for BPH, at least 60 ml of irrigant must be used, with some force, to dislodge and evacuate

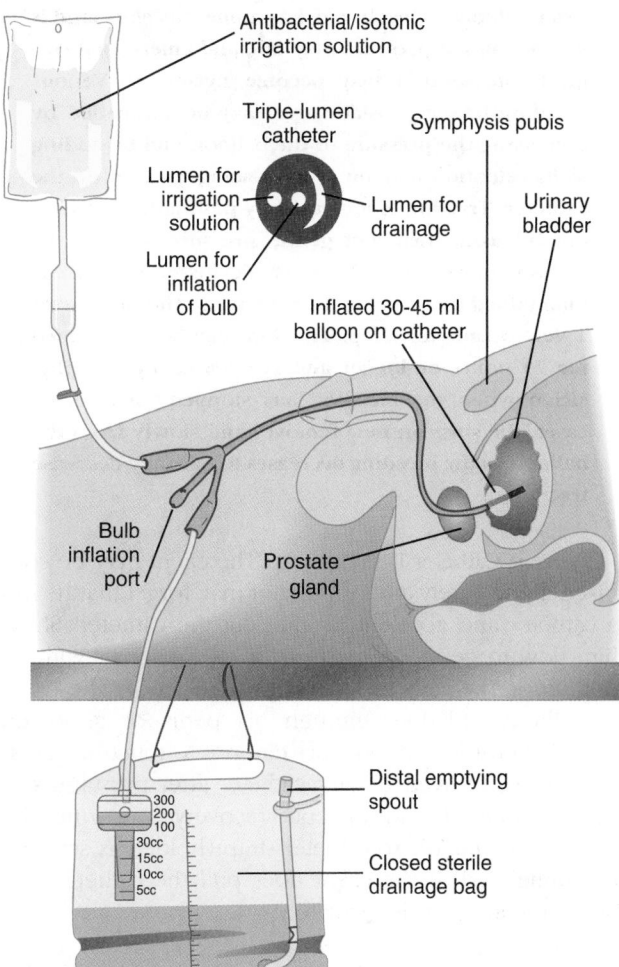

■ **FIGURE 38–3** A closed bladder irrigation system.

blood clots and other debris. If there is resistance to the introduction of irrigating fluid into the catheter or if there is no return of irrigating fluid, do not force the fluid. Instead, notify the surgeon immediately. Never remove a catheter that is occluded; instead, determine a plan for re-catheterization in close consultation with the physician.

Catheters and the procedures themselves cause increased urethral mucus production. Practice good meatal care. Keep the penis and meatal area clean by washing them with soap and water at least twice a day. Antibacterial ointments were formerly used, but they are no more effective than cleansing with a perineal cleanser or soap and water. Antibacterial soaps or antiseptics may dry out skin.

Monitor for Bleeding. Some hematuria is usual for several days after surgery; however, frank bleeding, arterial or venous, may occur during the first day after surgery.

Arterial blood is bright red, has numerous clots, and is viscous. Blood pressure may fall, and emergency surgical intervention may become necessary. Venous bleeding in the prostatic area may be controlled by increasing the pressure in the balloon end by adding to its retention balloon or by placing traction on the catheter. Traction is increased by pulling the catheter out by using firm but gentle pressure so that the balloon moves into the prostatic fossa. Traction is maintained by securing the catheter to the thigh with a Velcro catheter strap. Traction may be maintained for 24 hours or longer and is released by the physician when the bleeding has stopped. In selected cases, the surgeon may remove fluid slowly from the balloon as the bleeding decreases to partially decrease traction.

Prevent Catheter Dislodgment. The client may be confused immediately after surgery or may forget that he has a catheter and accidentally pull out the catheter. Show him how to get in and out of the bed or chair without pulling on the catheter. Remind the client that he has a tube in his bladder through his penis or abdomen (whichever it is), and instruct him not to touch it. A displaced or removed urinary catheter after prostatic surgery is painful and disrupts recovery. Securing the catheter with a Velcro catheter strap (holder) is strongly recommended. If the client does pull the catheter out, notify the surgeon immediately.

Prevent Infection. Observe the client carefully for local or systemic indications of infection. Handle catheters, drainage apparatus, and urine collection carefully to avoid introducing microorganisms into the urinary tract. Maintain a closed urinary drainage system unless manual irrigation is absolutely required. Encourage increased fluid intake, ambulation, and deep-breathing exercises.

Wound drains are usually removed earlier than suprapubic catheters. Keep skin around the drain and catheter sites clean, dry, and protected. Observe for redness, edema, or infection.

In some cases, a suprapubic catheter may remain in place until voiding function has returned. When the client is voiding well, the suprapubic catheter can be removed. Expect urinary leakage from the suprapubic catheter site, mostly on the day the catheter is removed, until the wound is completely healed. Frequent dressing changes are necessary at first. If a suprapubic catheter is removed before the client has returned to normal voiding, the wound may not heal properly, leading to fistula formation.

Monitor for Retention. The length of time urethral catheters are left in place varies according to the surgeon's judgment, the type of surgery, and the client's preoperative lower urinary tract function. Removal of the catheter is associated with a risk for urinary retention because of changes in detrusor contractility, transient obstruction resulting from urethral edema or local discomfort, or urethral blockage caused by clots or other debris. A voiding trial may be completed to evaluate voiding function after a TURP or similar procedure. While this procedure assesses the client's immediate ability to urinate, it does not exclude the possibility of urinary retention occurring hours to 1 day following catheter removal. Therefore the client is informed of the possibility for delayed retention and instructed about management of this unanticipated outcome.

Manage Temporary Incontinence. Advise the client that storage LUTS such as daytime voiding frequency, urgency, leakage, and dysuria are anticipated and will persist until complete healing occurs. Keep reminding him that these problems are temporary but may take some time to resolve. Be understanding of the man's feelings, and assist him to cleanse the perineal area after urine loss without embarrassing him. Counsel him about the use of containment devices, urethral clamps, or absorbency products that may be needed temporarily. They vary in size, shape, and absorbency capacities. Pelvic muscle exercises may help to reduce this problem. Additional surgery is occasionally required for persistent incontinence.

Diagnosis: Acute Pain. A common nursing diagnosis is *Acute Pain related to surgery and bladder spasms.*

Outcomes. The client's pain will be under control, as evidenced by the client's report.

Interventions. Pain control after surgery is discussed in Chapters 14 and 20. Bladder spasms frequently occur after prostate procedures, and incisional pain will occur if an open surgery (prostatectomy) is completed. Incisional pain is usually described as continuous, dull, boring pain of moderate to severe intensity; bladder spasms are typically described as periods of intense cramping discomfort or pressure. When bladder spasms are suspected, ensure that the drainage system is not blocked because obstruction as well as bladder irritation causes bladder spasms. Antispasmodic medications, such as belladonna and opium (B&O) suppositories, propantheline bromide (Pro-Banthine), or immediate-release oxybutynin (Ditropan IR), may be prescribed to achieve prompt relief of bladder spasm. Side effects associated with these medications include dry mouth, drowsiness (especially with B&O suppositories), or acute confusion in older clients. Because antispasmodic drugs can cause constipation, and straining at stool can precipitate bleeding from the operative site, stool softeners such as docusate sodium (Colace) are often given. Men with severe cardiac disease or narrow-angle glaucoma should not receive these agents.

Evaluation. It is expected that the client will be discharged without complications and resume regular activities within 4 to 6 weeks. Depending on the procedure performed, some clients return home the same day. The client who has undergone TURP is usually discharged about 2 to 3 days after the operation. Clients who had open procedures are discharged after 4 to 6 days. Voiding of urine improves, and complications such as urgency, frequency, and dribbling end within 3 months.

Self-Care

Provide Teaching

In addition to teaching the client verbally, give him written materials to take home after discharge. If applicable, review catheter and wound management. Clients who go home with a catheter may have a leg bag for day use and a Foley bag for use at night.

Some activities are limited after prostatectomy. The surgeon's orders should be followed regarding heavy lifting, strenuous activity, prolonged sitting, sexual activity, and driving or riding in an automobile. Because prolonged sitting increases intra-abdominal pressure and may precipitate bleeding, the man should avoid sitting except during meals. Clients should avoid driving an automobile or taking prolonged automobile rides until at least 2 weeks after surgery, when the risk of bleeding lessens. Strenuous exercise is also contraindicated for 4 to 6 weeks.

Prevent Injury

Advise the client not to strain during defecation for at least 6 weeks after surgery because this can lead to bleeding from the operative site. Docusate sodium, prune juice, and milk of magnesia are usually satisfactory bowel stimulants during this time. Increasing the amount of fluids also helps to prevent constipation. The client should avoid or limit intake of alcohol and other bladder irritants such as caffeine. Smoking should be discouraged because coughing puts strain on the surgical area.

Teach Pelvic Muscle Rehabilitation

Activity-induced incontinence (stress urinary incontinence) is typically a transient problem, although 1% to 2% of men may have long-term urinary incontinence (UI) following prostate surgery. Transient urine loss may be managed by containment products such as a pad that inserts into the underclothing. Simultaneously, men should be taught the principles of pelvic floor muscle rehabilitation or referred to a nurse specialist or physical therapist who specializes in this type of treatment. Pelvic muscle rehabilitation comprises three components: (1) biofeedback to promote muscle identification and isolation; (2) muscle training to improve maximal strength,

endurance, and function; and (3) neuromuscular reeducation to enable the client to contract the muscles strategically in a way that maximizes continence. Biofeedback methods are usually needed to help the client identify the pelvic muscles. Options include contracting the muscles during DRE, contraction while seated in a chair with a firm seat, or interruption of the urinary stream. If the latter strategy is used, it is critical to differentiate this biofeedback strategy from an exercise and instruct the man to practice this no more than once daily or every other day over a period of 1 to 3 days until effective muscle identification is learned. Muscle training consists of a graded exercise program of repeated pelvic muscle contractions. Teach the client to tighten the pelvic muscles for 6 to 10 seconds followed by a rest period of equal duration. Begin with 5 to 10 exercises daily and gradually increase to 25 to 35 daily exercises over a period of 6 to 12 weeks. Neuromuscular reeducation focuses on teaching the knack. Teach the client to contract his pelvic floor muscles consciously whenever he coughs, sneezes, or lifts a heavy object. Although this is a conscious effort initially, eventually it will be incorporated by most clients as a subconscious response to activities likely to provoke urinary leakage over time. Clients who are unable to identify the pelvic floor muscles or who do not respond to treatment after 4 to 6 weeks should be referred to a specialist for clinician-directed rehabilitation. The Translating Evidence into Practice feature on p. 886 describes pelvic muscle rehabilitation after prostatectomy.

Treat Erectile Dysfunction. Erectile dysfunction is an uncommon complication of prostatectomy, and the greatest risk is associated with open surgical procedures. Sildenafil (Viagra) may be given to post-prostatectomy clients postoperatively in an attempt to maintain blood flow to the corpora cavernosa during the recovery period and prevent or reverse apoptosis (programmed cellular death) caused by prolonged disuse of the erectile mechanism. Research has shown that this strategy is beneficial for men undergoing radical prostatectomy, but its efficacy in men undergoing TURP or prostatectomy for BPH is not known.

Information and supportive care for the client and his partner are extremely important. The client needs to know that he can still please a partner and that lovemaking techniques other than intercourse may be necessary. The partner should be reassured that sexual intimacy will not harm the client. The couple may need information about alternatives to intercourse, such as cuddling, stroking, or manual or oral stimulation to orgasm. Vacuum erection devices, intracorporeal injections, and intraurethral or oral medications are also topics that sexual counselors can discuss. A penile implant may be considered in selected cases (see Erectile Dysfunction later in this chapter), and referral for sexual counseling is often helpful.

TRANSLATING EVIDENCE INTO PRACTICE

Pelvic Muscle Rehabilitation Following Prostatectomy

Urinary incontinence can be a complication of radical prostatectomy procedures. Despite improvements in surgical approaches, many men experience moderate to severe urinary incontinence postoperatively. The treatment of this condition varies widely from medications or additional surgery to progressive therapy programs to increase the activity of the muscles of the pelvic floor and improve urinary leakage experienced by prostatectomy clients.

Men with postprostatectomy incontinence who practiced repeated pelvic muscle contractions with or without behavioral biofeedback (to assist with correct muscle identification) or electrical stimulation several times per day reported decreased incontinence following treatment in more than 75% of the cases. By instituting biofeedback sessions with pelvic floor muscle exercises before radical prostatectomy, even better outcomes were achieved. Clients who received the sessions and performed the exercises before surgery had significantly better outcomes than clients who received the sessions and performed the exercises after the radical prostatectomy.

IMPLICATIONS

Nurses have an important role in providing teaching and interventions related to pelvic floor muscle strengthening exercises before radical prostatectomy procedures to improve client outcomes related to urinary continence following surgery. Completing the biofeedback sessions with pelvic floor muscle exercises before surgery increases the nurse's role in educating the prostatectomy client to achieve continence. It gives the client knowledge about exactly what is involved in doing the pelvic muscle exercises and what to expect after surgery. Additionally, a rapport can be established between the nurse and client that can be carried through the postoperative period.

REFERENCES

1. Burgio, K., et al. (2006). Preoperative biofeedback assisted behavioral training to decrease post-prostatectomy incontinence: a randomized, controlled trial. *Journal of Urology, 175*(1), 196-201.
2. Burgio, K., Stutzman, R., & Engle, B. (1989). Behavioral training for post-prostatectomy urinary incontinence. *Journal of Urology, 141,* 303-306.
3. Jackson, J., et al. (1996). Biofeedback: A noninvasive treatment for incontinence after radical prostatectomy. *Urologic Nursing, 16*(2), 50-54.
4. Moore, K., Griffiths, D., & Hughton, A. (1999). Urinary incontinence after radical prostatectomy: A randomized controlled trial comparing pelvic muscle exercises with or without electrical stimulation. *British Journal of Urology International, 83,* 57-65.
5. Moorhouse, D., et al. (2001). Behavioral treatments for post-prostatectomy incontinence. *Ostomy/Wound Management, 47*(12), 30-31, 33–38, 40.
6. Moul, J. (1999). Pelvic muscle rehabilitation in males following prostatectomy. *National Association for Continence, 17*(2), 1-3.
7. Nahon, I., et al. (2006). Systematic review of the treatment of post-prostatectomy incontinence. *Urologic Nursing, 26*(6), 461-475, 482.
8. Shell, J. (2002). Evidence-based practice for symptom management in adults with cancer: Sexual dysfunction. *Oncology Nursing Forum, 29*(1), 53-69.
9. Sueppel, C., Kreder, K., & See, W. (2001). Improved continence outcomes with preoperative pelvic floor muscle strengthening exercises. *Urologic Nursing, 21*(3), 201-210.
10. Van Kampen, M., et al. (2000). Effect of pelvic floor re-education on duration and degree of incontinence after radical prostatectomy: A randomized controlled trial. *The Lancet, 355,* 98-102.
11. Wisinski, C., Rolf-Carbaugh, L., & Bangs, K. (2001). Physical therapy treatment for urinary incontinence utilizing rectal weights following radical prostatectomy. *Journal of the Section on Women's Health, 25*(4), 9-11.

Arrange Follow-Up

Be sure the client knows when and where to reach the surgeon and how to get in touch with health care professionals if he has concerns. He should especially report any elevated temperature, unusual bleeding, manifestations of wound infection or urinary tract infection (UTI), and obstructed urinary flow. He should know the date and time of his follow-up appointment with the surgeon.

PROSTATE CANCER

Prostate cancer is the second most commonly diagnosed cancer in men (following skin cancer) and has recently emerged as the leading cause of cancer-related deaths in American men. In 2007 approximately 219,000 men in the United States will be diagnosed with prostate cancer, and about 27,000 will die because of this malignancy.[4]

Etiology and Risk Factors

The cause of prostate cancer is unknown, but it is known that two types of tumors are diagnosed in the clinical setting. A latent form can be identified in as many as 30% of men during the fifth decade of life and about 60% to 70% of men in their 80s. Clinically aggressive prostate cancer affects about one in six American men, and it demonstrates the local invasion and metastatic properties of other forms of cancer. Therefore researchers must determine the mechanisms that cause prostate cancer to develop as well as those factors that cause it to progress to the clinically aggressive form that causes men to die of the disease. While these factors are not yet known, a discussion of the risk factors associated with both forms of prostate cancer provides clues that are likely to solve this persistent mystery.

 Men with a family history of prostate cancer are at high risk for developing adenocarcinomas, and 10% of all cases are believed to be inherited. For example, a focus for prostate cancer susceptibility at a young age has been located on the long arm of chromosome 1, and the *PCAP* and *CAPB* genes (both components of chromosome 1) have been identified as leading to an increased risk for prostate cancer. Additional research has identified a gene on the X chromosome (*HPCX*) that appears more often in men with prostate cancer, suggesting that the familial predisposition may exhibit heterogeneity (susceptibility based on the expressions of more than one gene). Of note, genetic predisposition to breast cancer has progressed along similar lines, and shared susceptibility loci on chromosome 1 suggest a possible biologic linkage to breast cancer in the women of certain families as well as prostate cancer in the men of these families. This topic is explored further in the Genetics Links box below.

Although 10% are thought to be inherited, the remaining 90% must be classified as sporadic. Nevertheless, it is postulated that sporadic and inherited cancers have similar etiologies from a biochemical perspective. Research into noninherited prostate cancer has led to hypotheses that these tumors may arise from damage or loss of genes that control essential cellular processes such as replication (cell replacement) or apoptosis (programmed cellular death).

In addition to increases in our understanding of possible causes of the initiation of prostate malignancies, research during the past decade has greatly increased our understanding of the processes that cause a prostate tumor to progress from a slow growing to a clinically relevant (and potentially deadly) cancer. Genetic factors associated with this progression include damage to chromosome 10q, affecting the *PTEN/MMAC* suppressor gene; abnormalities of chromosome 12, resulting in loss of the tumor suppression of gene *p27,* and overexpression of gene *MYC,* because of alterations in the long arm of chromosome 8q. In addition, an abnormality of the AR locus of the X chromosome has been identified that is hypothesized to contribute to the progression of advanced stage prostate cancers from hormone-sensitive to hormone-independent tumors, an ominous event that greatly limits effective treatment options.

Prostate cancer risk increases with age, particularly as men reach the sixth decade of life. Approximately three

GENETIC LINKS

Prostate Cancer

Prostate cancer is the most common cancer diagnosed in American men, and the leading cause of cancer deaths. Approximately 220,000 new cases will be diagnosed each year, and about 27,000 men will die annually from the disease. One of every six men will be diagnosed with prostate cancer in his lifetime. Three definitive risk factors have been established for prostate cancer, including age, ethnic background, and family history. Prostate cancer affects primarily older men, with men over 65 at highest risk. The incidence of prostate cancer is highest among African Americans, and lowest in Asian populations. Studies show that a family history of prostate cancer is strongly and consistently associated with increased risk. Men with one first-degree relative with prostate cancer have a two- to three-fold increased risk of developing prostate cancer compared to men with no family history. The risk is significantly higher for men with multiple affected relatives, or an affected relative who was diagnosed under 65 years of age.

GENETICS
While the majority (approximately 75% to 85%) of cases of prostate cancer in the general population are sporadic (those with no family history), studies suggest that about 5% to 10% of all prostate cancer cases are hereditary. Men with hereditary prostate cancer (HPC) represent families which meet at least one of the following criteria: three or more first-degree relatives with prostate cancer, prostate cancer occurring in three generations through the paternal or maternal side of the family, or at least two first-degree relatives diagnosed with prostate cancer at age 55 or younger. Studies suggest that the hereditary form of prostate cancer is associated with dominantly inherited susceptibility genes with high penetrance.

The first prostate cancer susceptibility gene, called *HPC1* (Hereditary Prostate Cancer 1), was mapped (localized) in 1996 to the long arm of chromosome 1. Subsequently, several other prostate cancer susceptibility genes have been linked to various chromosome regions (e.g., regions on chromosomes 1, 8, 17, and 20 and the X chromosome). Three of these susceptibility genes have been cloned and mutations identified. However, research to date has shown that the genetic mechanisms of inherited susceptibility to prostate cancer are very complex and not well understood.

DIAGNOSIS/TESTING
Genetic testing for detecting inherited susceptibility to prostate cancer is not yet clinically available. Currently, genetic testing is only performed within the context of research studies.

Screening for early detection of prostate cancer includes annual measure of prostate-specific antigen (PSA) and digital rectal examination (DRE). Diagnosis is based on clinical manifestations; family history; digital rectal examination to palpate enlargement, firmness, or unusual lumps in the prostate; and the level of PSA in the blood. PSA is an enzyme secreted by the prostate epithelium that can be detected in the blood. If the PSA or DRE is abnormal, a transrectal ultrasound (TRUS) is commonly performed with needle biopsy of any suspicious area.

MANAGEMENT
Treatment depends on the point of diagnosis and the severity of the disease. Small clusters of early stage prostate cancer can be found in millions of men in an apparently harmless, latent form. It is not unusual for physicians to take a "watch and wait" approach to these early cancers, and monitor the progression of disease by PSA levels and physical examinations. Other treatment options include surgery, radiation, hormonal therapy, and chemotherapy.

of four men diagnosed with prostate cancer will be age 65 years or older. In contrast to this trend, the risk for clinically aggressive tumors appears to be greater among younger men, especially among those diagnosed during their 50s or earlier.

Race also acts as a risk factor for developing prostate cancer as well as the likelihood of experiencing a clinically aggressive tumor 🪔 For example, African-American men are at greatest risk for developing prostate cancer compared with any other group, and this risk incorporates a greater likelihood of having an advanced stage tumor at initial diagnosis or dying of prostate cancer (refer to the Community-Based Practice feature on Prostate Cancer, below). 🪔 In contrast, Asian Americans have a lower risk for prostate cancer when compared with Caucasians or African Americans. This

COMMUNITY-BASED PRACTICE

Prostate Cancer

Prostate cancer is especially concerning in ethnic minorities. Data show that African-American men have higher death rates from prostate cancer yet are ill-informed about the disease, testing, and treatment; and do not typically seek out prostate cancer testing. Men from other minority groups also suffer from a lack of knowledge and are not as likely as Caucasian men to get tested for prostate cancer. Large-scale screening events would seem to be an easy solution to this problem, but research shows that screenings are often unsuccessful. To address this disparity, nurses could devise and implement a community-based program to reach minority men where they are in the community.

To be successful, a program designed to improve knowledge of and screening for prostate cancer must be culturally relevant and convenient. It must also address the root causes of the failures of other, similar programs. Men from many ethnic minorities believe that the health care provider should initiate conversations on health care issues; hence they may believe that if it is not brought up, prostate cancer is not an important topic for them. Having an event where nurses provide information about prostate cancer without the men having to ask for it is one way to increase their knowledge. Going a little further, nurses could partner with several local doctors or clinics and schedule appointments at the educational event for prostate screening. If held during office hours, the nurses could even call the client's own physician (if he has one) and schedule an appointment there.

If assessment of the population reveals that most men do not have health care providers or transportation (or time off from work), nurses could design a program that would include on-site screening too. Nurses would have to help the client create a plan for getting test results (if not delivered on-site) and following up with treatment recommendations. This would be especially true for new immigrants who may not be aware of services available for transportation in their communities.

Many men from ethnic minorities believe that a diagnosis of cancer equals a death sentence. This fatalistic attitude may influence their intent to follow up an educational event with actual screening. Including a cancer survivor from the ethnic group being served would help dispel this notion and would be a source of support for the men.

Nurses can ensure that the program is culturally relevant in other ways, too. Educational materials should be written in the predominant language of the group with which they are working. The program must appeal to cultural values; for instance, the Hispanic attribute of machismo includes a component of taking care of one's family. Ensuring good health is one way to support loved ones. Including health care providers from the same minority community and referrals to physicians (or other health care providers) also in the same minority community help create trust from the participants. It would also be important to include male health care providers.

Getting the word out about a screening activity should include media that men of color prefer. Research has shown that radio and television are favored over newspapers and the Internet. Where to have an educational or screening event is also an important decision. Nurses need to look to the respected institutions in the community. Many African-American and Hispanic people indicate that the church is an important part of their lives. Holding an event in a church, with the clergy's enthusiastic support, would improve outcomes. Similarly, holding an event at a work site, with employer encouragement, would also improve outcomes. This has been identified as especially important for agricultural workers. Other possible sites include barber shops, sports events, and technical programs where the majority of participants are male.

Nurses have a major role to play in primary and secondary prevention of many diseases. There is a great opportunity for nurses to be instrumental in decreasing the negative outcomes from prostate cancer in minority men. By thinking creatively, nurses can design and implement a culturally relevant screening or educational event for prostate cancer in our communities of color.

REFERENCES

1. Centers for Disease Control and Prevention. *Prostate cancer statistics.* Available at www.cdc.gov/nchs/data/hus/hus05.pdf#053.
2. Chan, E., et al. (2003). Cultural sensitivity and informed decision making about prostate cancer screening. *Journal of Community Health, 28,* 393-405.
3. Clarke-Tasker, V.A., & Dutta, A. (2005). African American men and their reflections and thoughts on prostate cancer. *The American Black Nurses Foundation Journal, 3,* 56-60.
4. Gordin, S.S., & Heck, J.E. (2005). Cancer screening among Latino subgroups in the United States. *Preventative Medicine, 40,* 515-526.
5. Kleier, J. (2006). Language adaptation and testing of the prostate health questionnaire for Jamaican and Haitian men. *Urologic Nursing, 26*(4), 304-310.
6. Maliski, S., Heilemann, M., & McCorkle, R. (2002). From "death sentence" to "good cancer": Couples' transformation of prostate cancer diagnosis. *Nursing Research, 51,* 391-397.
7. McCorkle, R., et al. (2007). Comparison of depressive symptoms, sexual function, and marital interaction in men and their spouses after radical prostatectomy. *Urologic Nursing, 27*(1), 65-77
8. Meade, C.D., et al. (2003). Focus groups in the design of prostate cancer screening information for Hispanic farm workers and African American men. *Oncology Nursing Forum, 30,* 967-975.
9. Ward-Smith, P. (2006). Cultural disparities in the diagnosis and treatment of prostate cancer. *Urologic Nursing, 26*(5), 397-399, 405.

difference is greatest in Asians residing in Asia, and it diminishes when Asian men migrate to the United States, reflecting the contribution of environmental and dietary risk factors.

The greatest dietary risk factor for prostate cancer is the consumption of a diet that is high in saturated animal fats. In contrast, consumption of green and yellow vegetables or lycopene contained in tomatoes is associated with a reduced risk of prostate cancer, indicating a probable protective effect (see the Complementary and Alternative Therapy feature on Lycopene and Prostate Cancer Risk, below). Green tea may prevent and diminish the progression of prostate cancer (see the Complementary and Alternative Therapy feature on Green Tea and Prostate Cancer, below, right). It should be noted that green tea supplements may contain high doses of vitamin K that could interfere with the blood thinner warfarin (Coumadin). Vitamin D deficiency also may increase the risk for prostate cancer, but this risk may be reduced with adequate exposure to sunlight, a critical component of vitamin D metabolism in the human. Other supplements such as selenium and zinc may lower the risk of development of prostate cancer. (See the Complementary and Alternative Therapy features on Selenium Supplements and Prostate Cancer Risk and on Zinc Supplements

and Prostate Cancer Risk on the website.) There is also *evolve* preliminary evidence that pomegranate juice may reduce the rise in prostate-specific antigen (PSA) levels in men who have failed localized therapy for prostate cancer, as explained in the Complementary and Alternative Therapy feature on p. 890. Statin drugs to lower serum lipid levels have been found to improve survival following brachytherapy for localized prostate cancer, which suggests that dietary fat and lipid levels may play a role in prostate cancer development and progression.[44]

Testosterone and DHT, essential to the growth and development of the prostate, play an important but poorly understood role in prostate cancer initiation and progression. High levels of testosterone have been linked to development of prostate cancer. Absence of functioning testes is associated with absence of BPH or prostate cancer, and consumption of a low-fat, high-fiber diet (known to reduce circulating testosterone levels) diminishes prostate cancer risk. Male pattern baldness (associated with increased levels of testosterone) is also associated with an increased risk of prostate

---

Lycopene and Prostate Cancer Risk

Mixed evidence exists suggesting that the antioxidant lycopene (found in abundance in tomatoes) may reduce prostate cancer risk. A recent review of the literature demonstrates multiple cell culture, animal, and case-control studies have shown that lycopene is inversely associated with prostate cancer risk.[1] A study of 1338 men with prostate cancer among a group of 29,361 men participating in a study of early detection methods for cancer and associated risk factors found no association between lycopene intake and cancer risk.[2] The data also failed to detect any association between total tomato servings or most tomato-based foods and prostate cancer risk. However, a protective effect was found in men with a family history of prostate cancer. The results of this study and the review of the literature reinforce the urgent need for additional research to determine the relationship between lycopene intake and prostate cancer risk.

REFERENCES

1. Ansari, M.S., & Ansari, S. (2005). Lycopene and prostate cancer. *Future Oncology, 1*(3), 425-430.
2. Kirsh, V.A., et al. (2006). A prospective study of lycopene and tomato product intake and risk of prostate cancer. *Cancer Epidemiology, Biomarkers & Prevention, 15*(1), 92-98.

Green Tea and Prostate Cancer

Green tea may prevent and diminish the progression of prostate cancer, because of catechins that are thought to possess antioxidant, antiangiogenesis, and antiproliferative properties. Two studies provide weak evidence that regular consumption of green tea may reduce cancer risk. A group of 130 community-dwelling men in southeast China who had biopsy-confirmed adenocarcinoma of the prostate were compared to 274 case controls without any malignancy.[2] Men who consumed green tea were less likely to develop prostate cancer than were those who did not consume tea, and those who consumed a higher daily volume of green tea were less likely to develop prostate cancer than those who consumed smaller amounts. A second, pilot study reported on the results of a green tea catechin pill, consumed as three 200-mg tablets daily by 60 men prospectively randomized to catechin or a placebo. Statistically significant differences in prostate cancer were measured after 1 year of measurement.[1] Nevertheless, definitive results await findings from a properly powered clinical trial.

REFERENCES

1. Bettuzzi, S., et al. (2006). Chemoprevention of human prostate cancer by oral administration of green tea catechins in volunteers with high-grade prostate intraepithelial neoplasia: A preliminary report from a one-year proof-of-principle study. *Cancer Research, 66*(2), 1234-1240.
2. Jian, L., et al. (2004). Protective effect of green tea against prostate cancer: A case-control study in southeast China. *International Journal of Cancer, 108*(1), 130-135.

Pomegranate Juice and Prostate Cancer

A phase II, two-stage clinical trial for men with rising PSA levels after surgery or radiotherapy was conducted with men who had PSA >0.2 ng/dl and Gleason score ≤7. The men were treated with 8 ounces (570 total polyphenol gallic acid equivalents) of pomegranate juice daily. The mean PSA doubling time significantly increased with treatment from a mean of 15 months at baseline to 54 months post-treatment ($p < 0.001$). In vitro assays comparing pretreatment and post-treatment serum showed a 12% decrease in cell proliferation and a 17% increase in apoptosis ($p = 0.0048$ and 0.0004, respectively). Although these results are promising, further research using a placebo-controlled trial is warranted before further conclusions can be generated. Also, the cost, increased calories of pomegranate juice, and possible drug interactions must also be considered for clients with prostate cancer.

REFERENCE

Pantuck, A., et al. (2006). Phase II study of pomegranate juice for men with risking prostate-specific antigen following surgery or radiation for prostate cancer. *Clinical Cancer Research, 12*(13), 4018-4026.

cancer. Also, see the Complementary and Alternative Therapy feature on Prostate Cancer Prevention with Finasteride on the website. More ejaculations were found to lower the risk of prostate cancer development in the ongoing Health Professionals Follow-Up Study (HPFS) of 29,342 U.S. men ages 46 to 81 who provided information on the history of the frequency of ejaculation from sexual intercourse, nocturnal emission, and masturbation on a self-administered questionnaire every 2 years from 1992 to 2000. Men reporting 21 or more ejaculations per month versus men reporting 4 to 7 ejaculations per month had a lifetime 33% reduction in prostate cancer risk.[33] Additional studies of ejaculations and prostate cancer risk are needed before this association can be confirmed.

Environmental and occupational risk factors include living in an urban area and specific occupations such as fertilizer, textile, and rubber industries and work with batteries containing cadmium.

Several potential risk factors have been identified but largely disproved when further research was completed. For example, neither BPH nor vasectomy has been associated with prostate cancer. Sexually transmitted virus-like organisms have been found in prostate cancer tissue, suggesting that viruses may act as a risk factor; however, the magnitude of this risk remains unclear.

Pathophysiology

More than 90% of all cancers arising from the prostate are adenocarcinomas. They typically arise from the peripheral zone of the prostate gland, in contrast to BPH that originates in the transitional zone. A tumor becomes clinically relevant when local invasion or distant metastasis interrupts the function of the urinary tract and other organ systems, producing morbidity or death. Whereas no premalignant lesion has been definitely associated with prostate cancer, high-grade prostatic intraepithelial neoplasia (PIN) has been found to occur in the same location as adenocarcinomas.

The magnitude of local invasion or metastasis is evaluated according to a staging system. The tumor, node, metastases (TNM) (see Chapter 17) or Jewett systems (see Chapter 34) are used to stage prostate cancers. Applied to prostate cancer, stage T1 and T2 (Jewett stages A and B) tumors have remained contained within the prostatic capsule and are diagnosed as localized prostate cancer. In contrast, stage T3 and T4 (Jewett stages C and D) tumors have spread beyond the prostatic capsule and are classified as advanced stage prostate cancers. They are associated with metastatic spread to lymph nodes (N1) or spread to distant organs (M1).

The likelihood that an individual tumor will behave in a clinically aggressive manner is evaluated as grade. The Gleason system is typically used to grade prostate cancers. It is based on how well-differentiated tumor cells appear on microscopic analysis. Poorly differentiated (anaplastic) cells are associated with a greater risk of aggressive behavior, whereas more highly differentiated cells are less aggressive. Gleason scores are calculated by adding the most common grade of a tumor present in the man's biopsy or surgical specimen with the grade of the second most common tumor grade. Gleason scores of 6-7 are associated with a 40% chance of metastasis; Gleason scores of 8 to 10 are associated with a 75% chance of metastasis.

Clinical Manifestations

Men with localized prostate cancer typically have no clinical manifestations, and early detection relies on measurement of the serum PSA combined with DRE because these tests have about 50% accuracy when performed in isolation. The American Cancer Society and American Urological Association recommend regular testing on all men between 50 and 70 years of age and routine testing beginning at age 40 years for African Americans or any man with one or more first-order relatives with prostate cancer. Screening may be completed annually, but more recent research has led to recommendations that men whose PSA is less than 1 should be retested every 5 years and men whose PSA is between 1 and 2 should undergo annual testing. DRE and PSA measurement in men older than 70 must be judged on an individual basis; it is not recommended in men whose life expectancy is less than 10 years.

Prostate-specific antigen (PSA) is a glycoprotein produced by the prostate gland, and it is elevated in men with certain prostate conditions such as prostate cancer, BPH, or prostatitis. Normal PSA levels are less than 2.6 ng/ml. When the PSA is 2.6 to 10 ng/ml, the likelihood of prostate cancer is judged as moderate, but values greater than 10 ng/ml indicate a high level of suspicion. A variety of factors other than prostate cancer may elevate the PSA. DRE elevates the PSA only slightly, and it may be measured before or after the DRE has been completed. Prostatitis sharply elevates the PSA, and a period of 6 weeks or longer should pass before PSA is measured in a man with a recent history of a prostate infection. Recent urethral instrumentation such as catheterization or cystoscopy acutely elevates the PSA, and they should not be performed immediately before PSA measurement.

Several techniques have been developed to increase the PSA test's ability to predict the presence of prostate cancer. A fractionated PSA measures free versus protein-bound PSA in the blood. Men with prostate cancer have a higher proportion of their PSA bound to protein, whereas the proportion of free PSA is higher in men with BPH. Measurements of PSA density (PSAD) are useful in men whose original values fall in the moderate suspicion range (2.6 to 10 ng/ml). PSAD combines the serum PSA value and prostate volume assessed via transrectal prostatic ultrasound. Scores are calculated by dividing the PSA by the prostatic volume; men with a score above 0.15 are more likely to have cancer than men with lower values. PSA velocity (PSAV) involves the rate of change in PSA level over time. Men who have a PSAV that rises more than 0.7 ng/ml/year or that increases 20% or more a year are considered at high risk of having prostate cancer.[24]

Digital rectal examination requires careful palpation of the prostate and seminal vesicles; it is typically performed by a physician or nurse practitioner. The man may be examined while supine, in a lithotomy position, or in stirrups, based on the examiner's preference. The client is warned that the examination will cause mild discomfort and pressure in the rectum. A DRE that reveals one or more hardened nodules, asymmetry between the palpable lobes, induration, or a stony gland fixed to the rectal wall is suspicious for prostate cancer.

Abnormality of the PSA or DRE indicates the need for more definitive evaluation with a transrectal ultrasound (TRUS) and biopsy. An isolated elevation in PSA should be confirmed several weeks later before proceeding with further testing, including prostate biopsy.[12] Preparation for the procedure includes careful explanation of the procedure. The client is counseled that the probe will produce a sensation of rectal pressure and may cause a desire to defecate. Tissue biopsy generates a sudden noise, but no sensation of a needle stick.

All anticoagulant medications, including prescribed agents, over-the-counter drugs such as aspirin, or dietary supplements such as high-dose vitamin E, should be discontinued 7 days before and 1 day following transrectal ultrasound (TRUS) with biopsy. Bowel cleansing using an enema or stimulant may be required in selected clients. Antimicrobial therapy may be given on the day of the procedure. Following ultrasound and biopsy, the client is instructed to monitor the stool for excessive bleeding.

SAFETY

ALERT

Pathologic analyses of biopsies are used to determine the presence of a malignancy and its stage. If prostate cancer is found, additional tests are ordered to clarify the stage of the cancer. A bone scan, chest x-ray, and computed tomography (CT) or magnetic resonance imaging (MRI) of the abdomen and pelvis are completed to identify the presence of nodal or distant organ metastasis. A specific imaging scan can be used to locate metastases of prostate cancer in soft tissue. Capromab pendetide (ProstaScint) targets prostate-specific membrane antigen (PSMA), which is found in prostate cancer cells. Two sessions 4 days apart are required. The ProstaScint scan is especially useful in finding "skipped" metastases (i.e., abdominal lymph node involvement without pelvic lymph node involvement), but it is expensive.

OUTCOME MANAGEMENT

Nursing Management of Clients Undergoing Diagnosis

Provide Support

Men with prostate cancer and their significant others need ongoing sensitive support and accurate information to make the difficult decisions required of them. Their concerns are considerable and may include the choices of available treatments, fear of death, anxiety about residual disability and illness, feelings of loss of control, and the possible effects of the illness on people in their social network and in their marriage. After diagnosis, prostate cancer can affect their masculinity and self-esteem. Depression and fatigue are common after many treatments for prostate cancer.

Suggest Resources

Increased awareness of prostate cancer has led to the development of many resources, including books, articles, and Internet websites in the public sector. Local and national prostate cancer support groups have organized. Information is also available from the American Cancer Society (Man to Man program), the American Urological Foundation in Baltimore (866-746-4282), and

US TOO International in Hinsdale, Illinois (800-808-7866).

Be sure to include the client's partner or spouse in planning care at the time of diagnosis and when the client is choosing treatment as well as when he is adapting to the treatment. The partner usually takes on essential support responsibilities when the client is gathering information and coping with the disease and treatments.

Surgical Management of Localized Prostate Cancer

Radical Prostatectomy

Radical prostatectomy is the treatment of choice for localized prostate cancer, provided the client's health is adequate to undergo the physical stress of anesthesia and surgery, he has a life expectancy of 10 to 15 years, and he elects surgery when presented with a fair and balanced explanation of all the available treatment options. Radical surgery involves removing the entire prostate gland (rather than just enucleation), its outer capsule, the seminal vesicles, sections of the vas deferens, adjacent lymph nodes, and (in many cases) the bladder neck. Bilateral prostatic lymph node dissection (BPLND) is usually limited to clients with higher PSA values and Gleason scores. Open surgical approaches include the retropubic (see Figure 38-2, *C*, p. 880) and perineal (see Figure 38-2, *D*) approaches. Radical retropubic surgery is the most commonly performed procedure; it offers several potential advantages to alternative approaches. Specifically, preservation of one or both neurovascular bundles of the prostate reduces the risk for ED and may moderate incontinence risk. In contrast, the perineal approach is associated with a reduced risk for urinary incontinence, but preservation of the neurovascular bundles cannot be achieved with this approach, and it may increase the risk for anal sphincter damage and fecal incontinence.

Laparoscopic radical prostatectomy with robotic assistance is gaining popularity. Four to five small incisions are made and 5- to 10-mm trocars are placed to gain access to the prostate. Anatomic manipulations are similar to those used for traditional radical prostatectomy, and the prostate, capsule, and seminal vesicles are removed. Advantages include absence of the larger incision required for open surgery with reduced operative time and a potentially faster recovery period. Disadvantages include prolonged anesthesia time and a greater risk for positive margins compared with open surgery, indicating incomplete tumor removal.

Complications following radical prostatectomy include bleeding, infection, urinary incontinence, ED, rectal injury, and anal sphincter damage with fecal incontinence. The risk of urinary incontinence (UI) is greatest immediately following catheter removal; it will gradually subside over the first 2 postoperative years to 35% to 50%. The vast majority will have only occasional, mild UI, but about 8% will have significant, chronic UI requiring continuous use of containment pads or devices. The risk of ED exists for all techniques, but preservation of at least some spontaneous erectile activity may be as high as 70% when radical retropubic prostatectomy is combined with preservation of both neurovascular bundles in otherwise healthy men with good sexual function before surgery. The risk of anal sphincter damage and fecal incontinence may be higher in men undergoing radical perineal prostatectomy and the risk for rectal damage requiring temporary diversion is higher for laparoscopic procedures.

Cryosurgical Ablation

In cryosurgical ablation of the prostate, the surgeon uses guided TRUS to insert cryoprobes into desired areas of the prostate to freeze and thereby destroy the tissue. A warming tube in the urethra keeps the urethral tissue from freezing. Cryosurgery may be an option for clients with localized cancer and other serious medical conditions that preclude them as candidates for radical surgery. Complications associated with cryoablation include urinary incontinence and ED.

Nursing Management of the Surgical Client

Prevent Injury

The physical nursing care for the client with prostatic cancer is based on the same principle applied to all clients undergoing other major abdominopelvic surgery (see Chapter 14). The client will return from surgery with an indwelling catheter and a midline incision (retropubic approach) or U-shaped perineal incision (perineal approach).

> **Monitor urine output closely for the first several days; reddish-colored urine is anticipated during the immediate postoperative period, but a yellow hue should return by postoperative day 2. Notify the physician immediately if brisk bleeding or passage of clots occurs. If catheter blockage occurs, promptly contact the urologist but avoid irrigation that may compromise delicate anastomoses.**

Compression devices for the lower extremities are maintained over the first 1 to 2 postoperative days, particularly if the client has undergone perineal prostatectomy requiring placement stirrups.

Incisional pain is usually managed by nonpharmacologic interventions, oral opioid drugs, and nonsteroidal anti-inflammatory drugs (NSAIDs). Bladder spasms are managed using the same interventions described for the surgical management of BPH. Constipation is avoided because it places potentially harmful stress against the delicate urethral anastomosis. Maintain the client on a low roughage diet, combined with regular ambulation to encourage peristalsis and stool softeners as directed.

Enemas should be avoided, particularly if the client has undergone radical perineal prostatectomy.

Men are typically discharged 2 to 3 days after surgery. The indwelling catheter can be removed as early as postoperative day 3, but it is more often left in place for 2 to 3 weeks. While the catheter remains indwelling, special care must be taken to avoid traction against the urethra while the anastomotic site heals.

Provide Support

The psychosocial and emotional care of these clients differs from care of clients with BPH because issues such as cancer and sexual image must be addressed. Thoughts of postoperative self-care at home can be overwhelming. Both the client and significant other need detailed instructions, much reassurance, and resources for supplies and advice if concerns surface at home. Sildenafil (Viagra), vardenafil (Levitra), tadalafil (Cialis) or intraurethral alprostadil (MUSE) is given to many clients after prostatectomy to maintain blood flow to the corpora cavernosa and prevent apoptosis during recovery, thus reducing the risk or severity of ED.

Medical Management of Localized Prostate Cancer

Options for localized prostate cancer include watchful waiting, external beam or interstitial radiation therapy, and hormone deprivation. Controversy exists regarding the most effective management of prostate cancer.

Watchful waiting requires DRE, serum PSA measurement, and completion of a lower urinary tract symptom (LUTS) score such as the IPSS every 6 to 12 months. The physician also monitors the man's constitutional manifestations of disease progression, including unintended weight loss, hematuria, bone pain, or pathologic fracture. Watchful waiting is reserved for highly selected cases; strong indications are men age 70 years or older with well-differentiated, small-volume tumors and a life expectancy of less than 10 years. Men older than 70 with low-volume, moderately differentiated tumors are strong candidates if their life expectancy is 5 years or less. Watchful waiting can be combined with dietary measures designed to slow tumor progression. Men are advised to reduce their intake of saturated fats and to increase their intake of lycopene, selenium, and soya-containing foods. (See the Complementary and Alternative Therapy feature on Flaxseed and a Low-Fat Diet for Men with Prostate Cancer on the website.)

Decrease Tumor Growth

Radiation Therapy. Two techniques are used to deliver radiation to prostate tumors. External-beam radiation irradiates the prostate and pelvic region using a machine that resembles diagnostic x-ray machines. It is delivered over multiple treatments during a period of 6 weeks or longer. Traditional radiotherapy is being replaced with newer, conformal techniques that generate three-dimensional CT images to focus the radiation and limit the exposure of adjacent structures. Conformal techniques allow the delivery of a higher radiation dose without increasing the risk of complications. Proton-beam radiotherapy combines conformal imaging and charged protons to target more specifically prostate cancer cells while limiting damage to the overlying skin or adjacent structures including the bladder and rectum.

Brachytherapy requires the implantation of radioactive iodine-125 or pallidium-103 seeds directly into the prostate. They emit highly localized radiation energy to kill localized cancer cells without excessive harm to nearby healthy cells. Proper placement of these seeds is critical, and a preprocedural map of the prostate gland, using ultrasound or CT, is obtained. A grid is then placed over the perineum and ultrasonic or CT imaging is used to deliver seeds to the prostate alone. These seeds remain in the body, but their radioactivity declines over a period of months.

Hormonal Deprivation Therapy. Hormone therapy is used in highly selected cases of localized prostate cancer. Treatment is associated with significant adverse side effects, however, and its use is limited primarily to men with advanced stage disease as discussed below.

Medical Management of Advanced Prostate Cancer

Hormonal Deprivation/Chemotherapy

Medical management involves hormonal deprivation therapy and chemotherapy, as described in the Integrating Pharmacology feature on p. 894. Hormonal deprivation therapy is designed to block androgen (testosterone) production and includes a selection or combination of bilateral orchiectomy, estrogens, gonadotropin-releasing hormone analogs, and anti-androgens. The greatest amount of androgen (about 90%) is produced in the testicles, and small amounts are produced in the adrenal glands (10%). As explained in the Complementary and Alternative Therapy box on p. 895, strength training may be useful for men who are receiving androgen-deprivation therapy for prostate cancer.

Androgen deprivation can be achieved by several techniques. Orchiectomy is a technically simple procedure that removes both testes. It is also irreversible, however, and associated with profound adverse psychological effects. Thus when presented with options for managing advanced prostate cancer, the vast majority of men prefer medical castration using hormonal agents or similar drugs.

INTEGRATING P H A R M A C O L O G Y

Medications for Prostate Cancer

Hormonal deprivation therapy is the most common medical treatment for men with advanced prostate cancer. Hormonal deprivation is designed to block androgen (testosterone) production and includes estrogens, gonadotropin-releasing hormone analogs, and anti-androgens. Chemotherapy is used primarily for palliation.

HORMONAL DEPRIVATION THERAPY

Luteinizing hormone–releasing hormone (LHRH) agonists (also called gonadotropin-releasing hormone analogs) are used as first-line therapy for advanced stage prostate cancer. These drugs act by causing an initial surge in luteinizing hormone (LH) and testosterone levels, rapidly followed by a decline in testosterone levels similar to that achieved by castration. The primary forms of LHRH agonists are leuprolide (Lupron) and goserelin (Zoladex). Leuprolide acetate is administered as a deep intramuscular injection every 1 to 4 months, leuprolide acetate for injectable suspension (Eligard) is administered subcutaneously every 3 to 4 months, and goserelin is administered subcutaneously every 1 to 3 months. Viadur is a newer technique for delivering leuprolide. A cylindrical device implanted in the upper arm delivers a small dose of leuprolide over a period of 12 months. Hot flashes, erectile dysfunction, loss of libido, and minor weight gain caused by water retention are common side effects.

Alternatives to LHRH agonists include oral nonsteroidal anti-androgens (drugs that block androgenic effects at the level of the tumor cell such as cyproterone acetate and medroxyprogesterone acetate). Examples of anti-androgens include bicalutamide (Casodex), flutamide (Eulexin), and nilutamide (Nilandron). These medications block androgens produced by the adrenal glands and are often combined with LHRH therapy called maximal androgen blockade (MAB). The nonsteroidal anti-androgens are administered orally. Gynecomastia, diarrhea, and erectile dysfunction are common side effects.

The beneficial effects associated with estrogen (diethylstilbestrol, or DES) are not yet understood. Oral therapy is avoided because of the high risk for adverse cardiovascular side effects. Several trials throughout the world have investigated parenteral DES and found it to be beneficial while avoiding the unacceptable side effects associated with oral administration.

Intermittent hormone deprivation therapy using the MAB technique is an alternative to ongoing therapy. Potential advantages include periods of "rest" between treatments, allowing relief from adverse side effects; however, definitive studies comparing this technique to ongoing therapy are not available and initial results do not favor the efficacy of this technique as compared to ongoing hormone deprivation.

CHEMOTHERAPY

Chemotherapy is used for palliation (alleviation of manifestations) when prostate cancer is hormone-resistant or independent. Chemotherapeutic agents may be given singly or in combination, depending on protocols. Examples of agents sometimes used are cyclophosphamide (Cytoxan), fluorouracil, estramustine phosphate (Emcyt), doxorubicin (Adriamycin), mitomycin (Mutamycin), paclitaxel (Taxol), and etoposide (VP-16, Etopophos). Mitoxantrone (Novantrone) is a chemotherapeutic drug used in combination with corticosteroids to relieve pain in hormone-resistant prostate cancer. This treatment is often successful after just one dose. Zoledronic acid (Zometa) is a bisphosphonate that may be administered for prostate cancer bone metastases. It delays or reduces bone metastases by improving bone strength.

Nursing Management of the Medical Client

Provide Education

Nursing care depends on the type of medical therapy. Explain how treatments help prostate cancer, their side effects, and expected outcomes. Repetitive explanations are often necessary because clients must absorb much information and make decisions during a period when they may be in a state of shock. Provide information in a variety of formats, and include telephone numbers to be called when the client or partner has questions.

Explain Side Effects

Educate the man undergoing external-beam radiation about the rationale for radiation treatments, the necessity for multiple treatments, and the need to strictly attend all sessions to maximize the likelihood of success. Advise clients about possible adverse side effects, including radiation-induced cystitis or proctitis. Radiation cystitis is defined as inflammation of the bladder wall in response to unavoidable irradiation needed to treat a prostate malignancy. Tell the client that he may note dysuria (discomfort with voiding), daytime voiding frequency, an increase in the number of times he awakens to void, and suprapubic discomfort. The physician may prescribe an antimuscarinic agent such as tolterodine or oxybutynin or a urinary analgesic such as phenazopyridine. Reassure the client that radiation cystitis usually subsides within 4 to 6 weeks of radiation therapy.

Inform the client that radiation proctitis, characterized by frequent defecation, bowel cramping or urgency, and the defecation of blood and mucus, may occur. Reassure the client that, like radiation cystitis, it peaks during the latter stages of treatment but usually subsides within 4 to 6 weeks of the end of therapy. Mild manifestations can be managed by frequent defecation and antimuscarinic

Weight Lifting for Men Receiving Androgen Deprivation Therapy for Prostate Cancer

A total of 155 men with prostate cancer who were scheduled to receive androgen deprivation therapy for at least 3 months were randomly assigned to a weight-lifting program 3 times a week for 12 weeks (n = 82) or to a control group (n = 73). Men assigned to the weight-lifting program experienced less fatigue with activities of daily living ($p = 0.002$) and had higher quality of life scores ($p = 0.001$) compared to men in the control group. Men who lifted weights had higher levels of upper body ($p = 0.009$) and lower body ($p < 0.001$) muscular fitness versus men in the control group. The 12-week weight-lifting intervention did not improve body weight, body mass index, waist circumference, or subcutaneous skinfolds. However, lifting weights should be advocated for men receiving androgen deprivation therapy because of the profound impact on fatigue and quality of life.

REFERENCE

Segal, R., et al. (2003). Resistance exercise in men receiving androgen deprivation therapy for prostate cancer. *Journal of Clinical Oncology, 21,* 1653-1659.

medications similar to those used for acute cystitis. In addition, counsel men to avoid or reduce their intake of foods or beverages likely to irritate the bowel or bladder, including caffeine and heavily spiced or fatty foods. The man is advised to avoid any rectal biopsies because of the risk of subsequent bleeding or fistula formation.

Advise the client that external-beam radiation therapy may irritate the perineal skin. Teach him to cleanse the perineal skin with a mild cleanser and lukewarm water, paying special attention to skin folds, followed by dusting with a very small amount of cornstarch-based or talcum-based powder. Wearing loose cotton clothing also may relieve skin irritation. Radiation treatments also produce fatigue and loss of appetite. Counsel the client and partner that consumption of as many as six small meals per day, concentrating on foods that are high in protein and carbohydrates, will reduce these manifestations. A multivitamin should be taken daily throughout radiation therapy.

Preparation for brachytherapy typically includes bowel cleansing and administration of prophylactic antibiotics. An oral bowel stimulant such as magnesium citrate may be combined with a cleansing enema to prepare the bowel. Advise the client to maintain a clear liquid diet 12 to 24 hours preceding the study as directed. Instruct the client that the procedure is likely to produce rectal pressure or mild discomfort when the ultrasound probe is placed, but pain is not associated with implantation of radioactive seeds. A catheter is left in place that may be removed on the day of the procedure. Complete a voiding trial when removing the catheter (refer to the discussion of BPH earlier in this chapter). Teach the client that seed implantation will cause inflammation of the prostate that is likely to provoke bothersome LUTS, including daytime voiding frequency, an increase in nocturia, and difficulty initiating a urinary stream. These manifestations are typically transient and subside as prostatic inflammation diminishes.

Although rectal bleeding is uncommon after brachytherapy, you should instruct the client to monitor his stool for passage of large volumes of bright red blood, and advise him about how to manage radiation cystitis and proctitis. In addition, advise the client to avoid rectal biopsies that may cause excessive bleeding or fistula formation.

Teach the client and partner the principles of radiation safety following brachytherapy in consultation with the radiation oncologist and based on institutional policies. Advise the client that his semen is likely to have a brownish color over the first 1 to 2 months following implantation, and intercourse should be avoided during this period. In addition, intercourse with the intention of bearing children is strictly contraindicated unless cleared by the urologist or radiation oncologist. Clients are also taught to refrain from having children (or adults) sit in their lap for a prolonged period of time during the first 2 months following therapy.

Provide Support

Encourage men with prostate cancer and their significant others to attend relevant support groups or to subscribe to publications by organizations mentioned earlier. The best ways for clients to control fear and to keep a positive attitude are to learn as much as they can about treatments and to meet other men with prostate cancer. A health care provider who specializes in ED can best counsel a couple about ways to achieve sexual satisfaction.

Relieve Pain

When a client has metastases, assess pain levels (see Chapter 20) as well as activities of daily living. Keeping a pain diary is useful for the client's and the provider's awareness. Men tend to be stoic about pain and may have misconceptions about taking opioids. Carefully explain that addiction and decreasing drug effectiveness are not problems when cancer pain is being treated. Better pain control helps a man stay active and in control of his life. These issues are explored in the Case Study on p. 896.

CASE STUDY   *evolve*

Cancer of the Prostate at the End of Life

Everett Larson is a 72-year-old man who has been widowed for 15 years. Mr. Larson is being visited at this time to be admitted into hospice for end-stage prostate cancer. Mr. Larson lives alone in his own home and would like to stay there indefinitely . . . *Case Study continued on the website and CD-ROM with discussions, multiple-choice questions, and a nursing care plan.*

Prostatitis

Prostatitis (inflammation of the prostate gland) is a common and often perplexing problem. Traditionally, prostatitis was classified into four categories: acute bacterial, chronic bacterial, abacterial, and prostatodynia. This system has now been replaced by the National Institutes of Health (NIH) taxonomy with the following categories: category 1, acute bacterial prostatitis; category 2, chronic bacterial prostatitis; category 3, chronic pelvic pain syndrome (includes abacterial prostatitis and prostatodynia); and category 4, asymptomatic inflammatory prostatitis.[57] Category 1 is defined as an acute bacterial infection of the prostate causing intense local inflammation and pain as well as systemic illness or sepsis. Category 2 is a localized bacterial infection of the prostate that produces moderate localized discomfort but no systemic illness. Category 3 is diagnosed when men experience chronic pelvic pain in the absence of objective evidence of bacterial infection of the prostate. The NIH defines two subtypes of category 3: category 3A is diagnosed when manifestations are associated with objective evidence of prostatic inflammation, and category 3B is diagnosed when manifestations occur in the absence of such findings. Category 4 is diagnosed when pathologic analysis of a prostate biopsy or TURP specimen reveals evidence of infection and inflammation despite absence of reported manifestations.

Prostatitis is the most common urologic disorder in men younger than 50 years. About two million American men seek care for manifestations of prostatitis each year.

Etiology and Risk Factors

Category 1 (acute bacterial) prostatitis is typically caused by gastrointestinal or sexually transmitted bacteria. It causes severe localized prostatic inflammation that may interfere with the client's ability to urinate. Most men also experience systemic illness that may require hospitalization in severe cases. Although most cases have no apparent causes, risk factors include a recent bout of epididymitis, unprotected penetrative anal intercourse,

urethral stricture or meatal stenosis, and recent catheterization or cystoscopy.

The etiology of category 2 (chronic bacterial) prostatitis is not known. It is uncommon and accounts for less than 10% of all men with nonacute manifestations of prostatitis. Gastrointestinal (gram-negative) organisms are the most common cause of chronic prostatitis. Possible causes of bacterial invasion in men with chronic prostatitis include poor relaxation of the pelvic floor muscles during urination, causing turbulence and movement of bacteria from the urethra to prostatic ducts.

Category 3 prostatitis accounts for the remaining 90% of men with nonacute manifestations. Its etiology remains unknown.

Category 4 prostatitis is a pathologic diagnosis. Whether its presence predisposes clients to prostatitis or prostate cancer is not known.

Pathophysiology

Category 1 (acute bacterial) prostatitis leads to sepsis (bacterial invasion of the bloodstream) and a systemic immunologic response. Local immunologic responses include a rapid rise in the levels of immunoglobulin A (IgA), IgG, and PSA protein. The PSA level will return to normal within 6 weeks of treatment, but IgA and IgG levels remain elevated for 6 to 12 months. The reasons why some patients with a bacterial infection develop systemic responses while others experience only local inflammation with mild to moderately bothersome manifestations remain unknown.

Little is known about the pathophysiology of category 3 prostatitis. Some researchers speculate that the pain produced by this syndrome arises from pelvic muscle myalgia rather than prostatic inflammation, whereas other research reveals indirect evidence that turbulence of urine causes reflux of urate into the prostatic ducts with subsequent inflammation. Recent research has attempted to link category 3 prostatitis with interstitial cystitis, a chronic abacterial inflammation of the bladder predominant in women.

Clinical Manifestations

The client's manifestations depend on the category of prostatitis. The client with acute bacterial prostatitis presents with abrupt onset of urinary urgency, frequency, nocturia, and dysuria, and he may have urinary retention. Fever, chills, and malaise are present, and the client complains of low back and perineal pain. He appears quite ill and may be experiencing nausea and vomiting. The prostate is extremely tender and boggy when examined. Prostate massage (expression of prostate secretions via digital rectal examination) is avoided because it is painful to the client and may exacerbate bacteremia. Bacteriuria and pyuria will reveal infection, and a urine culture is used to guide antibiotic therapy in category 1 prostatitis.

Many clinical manifestations of categories 2 and 3 prostatitis are similar. Bothersome LUTS include frequent daytime urination, nocturia, and a seemingly paradoxic combination of urinary urgency and hesitancy when micturition is attempted. Localized pain manifestations include the perineum (area between the rectum and scrotum), testes, and tip of the penis, as well as dysuria and pain during or after ejaculation.

Assessment of category 1 prostatitis relies on urinalysis and urine culture; a blood culture may also be obtained. The client is evaluated for urinary retention, and vital signs are taken to determine the severity of systemic illness.

Assessment of categories 2 and 3 prostatitis relies on examination of the urine and expressed prostatic secretions. A four-glass test was traditionally used to diagnose prostatitis, but this procedure has largely been replaced with a two-specimen technique. The client is instructed to arrive at the clinic with a comfortably full bladder. He washes the glans penis and retracts the foreskin (if uncircumcised). A midstream urine specimen is collected and analyzed via dipstick, microscopy, and culture when indicated (specimen 1). Immediately following urination, the physician will perform a DRE and any urethral discharge will be collected for microscopic analysis and culture (if feasible). This second specimen is the expressed prostatic secretion (EPS).

OUTCOME MANAGEMENT

Medical Management

Reduce Inflammation

Clients with category 1 (acute bacterial) prostatitis may be so ill that they need hospitalization and intravenous (IV) antibiotics. Practically all antibiotics diffuse into the prostate when it is acutely inflamed, and a broad-spectrum fluoroquinolone is the drug of choice. An oral antibiotic is given when feasible, but clients with severe systemic illness may require parenteral drugs initially. Transurethral instrumentation is avoided unless absolutely necessary for urinary retention. The client should have at least 4 weeks of antibiotic therapy to eradicate the infection completely and to prevent chronic prostatitis.

The choice of antibiotic for chronic bacterial prostatitis is limited to those able to penetrate the fat and cholesterol internal environment of the chronically inflamed prostate. Regular prostatic massage has been advocated in an attempt to mechanically remove bacteria and toxins from the gland and to optimize penetration by antimicrobials, but a comparatively small randomized clinical trial involving 62 men randomized to treatment with massage alone, massage plus antimicrobials, and antimicrobials alone failed to demonstrate any advantage for massage. Fluoroquinolones, such as ciprofloxacin, remain the drug of choice, and trimethoprim-sulfamethoxazole (Bactrim or Septra) is a good alternative. Long-term therapy (usually 30 days) is necessary, particularly when trimethoprim-sulfamethoxazole is administered.

Several treatment options can be used in men with category 3 prostatitis. Alpha-adrenergic blockers may be prescribed to reduce turbulence within the prostatic urethra and relieve urinary hesitancy. NSAIDs, hot sitz baths, and regular sexual activity (ejaculation) may provide transient relief from pelvic pain. In addition, an empirical trial of a fluoroquinolone has provided relief in some clients. Pelvic floor muscle rehabilitation, particularly focusing on muscle relaxation, may be taught to relieve myalgia. Surgery may be considered for the client with chronic bacterial prostatitis when medical therapy does not improve manifestations that affect the man's quality of life. (See the Complementary and Alternative Therapy feature on Non-Bacterial Chronic Prostatitis and Quercetin on the website.)

Nursing Management of the Medical Client

Teach all clients with prostatitis techniques of pelvic muscle relaxation to relieve discomfort associated with pelvic muscle hypertonicity and urinary hesitancy. Constipation can be a painful problem for clients with prostatitis. It should be managed by adequate fluid intake combined with adequate intake of dietary fiber and exercise.

The client may be uncomfortable, frustrated, and fearful that the manifestations will never go away or may lead to something more serious than infection. He may have sexual or fertility concerns or may believe that the infection can be sexually transmitted. Clients need much reassurance and teaching. They should understand the importance of complying with the total treatment course and know the side effects of prescribed medications. Clients should also be taught that recent research suggests that increasing sexual activity or masturbation may help to decrease prostatic gland congestion.

TESTICULAR AND SCROTAL DISORDERS

See the Integrating Diagnostic Testing feature on Testicular or Scrotal Complaints on p. 865 for more information related to the diagnosis of scrotal and testicular disorders.

TESTICULAR CANCER

Testicular cancer is the most common and serious solid tumor cancer in men between 15 and 35 years of age. It rarely occurs in men younger than age 15 or older than age 40. It is uncommon, with about 7900 cases diagnosed and 400 deaths in the United States in 2007.[4] In many cases it is curable, sometimes even in an advanced stage. Testicular cancer is less common in African-American and Asian men. The incidence is about the same in Hispanic men as in Caucasian men. In Israel, the rate is three times higher in Jewish men than in non-Jewish men. Testicular cancer is about twice as frequent in high socioeconomic groups.

Etiology and Risk Factors

The cause of testicular cancer is unknown. Family history, exogenous estrogen, and cryptorchidism (undescended testicles) are known risk factors. Cryptorchidism is the major risk factor. Surgery (orchiopexy) is recommended soon after birth, but it does not completely eliminate the risk of cancer.

The male offspring of women who used estrogen in the form of diethylstilbestrol (DES) during the first trimester of pregnancy (called DES sons) or who were exposed to estrogen-progestin combinations (frequently used in diagnostic tests to confirm pregnancy) are at greater risk for testicular cancer. Between 1940 and 1970, DES was given to pregnant women who had a high risk of spontaneous abortion. DES sons also have an increased risk of genitourinary abnormalities such as micropenis, meatal stenosis, varicocele, hypoplastic testicles, infertility, and abnormal semen.

Children with an undescended testicle should be closely observed. Men ages 15 to 45 should practice monthly testicular self-examination (see Chapter 37 and the Integrating Diagnostic Testing feature entitled Testicular and Scrotal Disorders). Men at high risk for testicular cancer should see a physician for yearly examinations. Early detection can lead to early diagnosis and cure.

Pathophysiology

Most testicular cancers (90% to 95%) are germinal cell tumors, such as seminoma (about 30% to 40% of all tumors), embryonal carcinoma (about 20%), teratocarcinoma, or choriocarcinoma. Seminomas generally carry a favorable prognosis (about a 90% 5-year survival rate) because they are usually localized, metastasize late, and are radiosensitive.

Nongerminal tumors make up the remainder of testicular tumors and are classified as either interstitial cell tumors or testicular adenomas. They arise from interstitial cells or cells that compose the fibrous and vascular networks. They are usually benign.

Metastasis occurs primarily through lymphatic spread. Drainage from the right testis is to the inter-aortocaval nodes, whereas the left drains to the preaortic nodes. Rectoperineal nodes are commonly affected. Distant metastasis occurs most commonly to the lung and rarely to the liver, viscera, bone, or brain.

Choriocarcinoma spreads via the bloodstream. Even after surgical removal, testicular cancer can occur in the other testicle. Carcinoma in situ (localized), although rare, frequently involves both testes. Rarely, testicular tumors are secondary to cancers in another primary site.

Clinical Manifestations

Most commonly, men with testicular tumors experience a painless enlargement, noted as heaviness, in the testicle (in about 75% of cases). Some men describe it as a dragging sensation (see Chapter 37 and the Integrating Diagnostic Testing feature entitled Testicular and Scrotal Disorders). Pain is rarely felt; however, the tumor is often found after an injury because the testicle is examined as a result of the injury. A thorough description of family and birth histories and manifestations is the first step in assessment.

Assessment findings suggesting metastasis to the retroperitoneal lymph nodes include back pain, vague abdominal pain, nausea and vomiting, bowel and bladder changes, anorexia, and weight loss. If the lungs are involved, manifestations may include cough, dyspnea, and hemoptysis.

The next step is physical examination of the scrotum and testicles, in which the health care provider determines the location and size of any nodule. If there is a nodule, a light may be held against the scrotum to see whether it is transilluminated (to see whether light passes through) (see Figure 37-10, p. 870). Whereas cysts and hydroceles are transilluminated, tumors and hernias are not.

Ultrasonography of the testes follows. If tumor is suspected, chest x-ray studies and CT scans are ordered to detect metastases. An IVP may be ordered to detect urinary tract involvement.

Blood tests are ordered. Alpha-fetoprotein (AFP), beta human chorionic gonadotropin (beta-HCG), and lactic acid dehydrogenase (LDH) are the tumor markers used to detect testicular cancer. Elevated AFP level is not seen in clients with testicular seminomas. Beta-HCG can be elevated in either seminomas or nonseminomas and, when elevated, may cause gynecomastia in men with testicular cancer. LDH is often elevated in germinal testicular cancers because of the cancer's cell activity, and this elevation also suggests metastasis because LDH is produced in the liver, kidney, and brain.

Testicular cancer is verified by inguinal exploration. If a definite mass is not found, a frozen biopsy may be done. If there is still suspicion, a radical orchiectomy is performed. The testis, epididymis, and vas deferens are removed. The spermatic cord is ligated just inside the internal inguinal ring to prevent seeding of the cancer. Any testicular mass is considered malignant until proved otherwise.

Staging testicular tumors helps to guess at prognosis and to determine treatment options. Testicular tumors are staged as follows:

- Stage I$_a$: Tumor confined to testicle (T1 N0 M0)
- Stage I: Metastasis to para-aortic or iliac nodes (T1 N1 M0)
- Stage II: Tumor spread to retroperitoneal nodes but disease limited to below the diaphragm (T2-3, N2, M0)
- Stage III: Tumor above the diaphragm or spread to body organs (usually the lungs) (T4, N3-4, M+)

OUTCOME MANAGEMENT

Surgical Management

Radical orchiectomy, performed to diagnose testicular cancer, is also the primary treatment. Retroperitoneal lymph node dissection (RPLND) may be done when there is lymph node involvement. The primary use of this procedure is controversial in advanced stage cancer because treatment with chemotherapy for nonseminomas is very successful. Impotence rates are high after RPLND because many of the autonomic nerves necessary for ejaculation are located in this area. RPLND is performed when testicular cancer is embryonal because this type of cancer metastasizes rapidly.

In other types of testicular cancer, surgeons who perform RPLND believe that it limits the amount of chemotherapy needed. This approach may be used as an adjunct to chemotherapy when only a partial response is achieved. A thoracoabdominal or transabdominal incision is made, and modified dissection techniques are used. The newest approach is a laparoscopic node dissection. A smaller incision and fewer complications (especially retrograde ejaculation) result after laparoscopic surgery.

Nursing Management of the Surgical Client

Clients undergoing radical orchiectomy usually require a short hospital stay and experience few complications. The scrotal area is tender and slightly swollen after surgery. Ice bags are applied to the scrotum, and a scrotal support is worn when the client is ambulating. Teach the client self-care strategies and how to monitor for the development of complications. Provide written instructions, a resource he can call if questions or concerns arise, and a follow-up appointment with the surgeon. The client needs to be aware that testicular cancer can recur in the other testicle, and he should know how to perform testicular self-examination.

If the client undergoes RPLND, hospitalization is longer, depending on the approach used. Counseling about potential infertility problems and sperm banking takes place before the procedure.

Postoperatively, the client must be monitored closely for possible problems associated with major abdominal surgery. The client requires adequate pain control to comply with ambulation and vigorous coughing and deep breathing to prevent respiratory complications. Anxiety and fear about cancer, sexuality, quality of life, and life expectancy are issues that must frequently be addressed. Be sure that follow-up appointments are made with the surgeon and oncologist for further treatment if appropriate.

Medical Management

Medical management follows radical orchiectomy during the treatment of testicular cancer. A period of close follow-up and observation is necessary to detect recurrence and plan future care.

Destroy Cancer Cells

Radiation Therapy. Low-grade seminomas are particularly radiosensitive. The perineum and pelvis are irradiated, as are the mediastinal and supraclavicular nodes if peritoneal nodes are positive for cancer. Side effects include common complications associated with pelvic radiation: irritable bowel and bladder problems, skin reactions, fatigue, nausea, and anorexia. Radiation may also cause temporary or permanent infertility. Side effects are usually minimal because the dose and number of treatments required are low. Almost 95% of clients with low-stage seminomas survive more than 5 years.

Chemotherapy. Nonseminomatous tumors are not radiosensitive, and they and high-grade seminomas are therefore treated with chemotherapy. The major agent used is cisplatin in combination with vinblastine and bleomycin. Cisplatin in combination with other agents dramatically increases the long-term survival rate for men with testicular cancer. These agents, in combination with a variety of others, have been used to treat metastatic disease or refractory tumors with some success. (Complications of these chemotherapeutic agents are covered in Chapter 17.) Cisplatin has nephrotoxic effects, bleomycin causes pneumonitis, and vinblastine causes peripheral neuropathy.

Nursing Management of the Medical Client

During assessment of a man born between 1940 and 1971, ask whether his mother took any medication during pregnancy to prevent pregnancy or miscarriage. If he appears at particular risk but does not know these details, it may be necessary to obtain the mother's medical history. Information and referral are available through DES Action, Long Island Jewish-Hillside Medical Center, New Hyde Park, NY 11040.

Supportive nursing care for these young men is important during both diagnosis and treatment. Be aware of the threat to sexuality that this condition and its treatment pose to young men. Chapter 17 reviews the care of clients undergoing chemotherapy and radiation therapy.

TESTICULAR TORSION

Testicular torsion (Figure 38-4, *A*) occurs when a testicle is mobile and the spermatic cord twists, cutting off the blood supply. It is the most common testicular disorder in children. It can occur at any age but is most usual at puberty, and about 30% of cases occur in men in their 20s. Manifestations usually arise suddenly with acute scrotal swelling and severe pain as blood supply to the testicles is interrupted.

If testicular torsion is suspected, a testicular scan and Doppler ultrasonography are performed to assess the blood supply. While blood flow is decreased in testicular torsion, it is increased with epididymitis.

Testicular torsion is an emergency requiring immediate surgical intervention. The spermatic cord is untwisted and the testicle is immobilized by suturing it to the scrotum (orchiopexy). Without prompt surgery, the testicle may atrophy or develop an abscess. If the testicle is necrotic, it is removed. Because there is a risk that the other testicle will be susceptible to torsion, it is also affixed to the scrotum at the time of surgery.

ORCHITIS

Orchitis is a rare, acute testicular inflammation, usually caused by a viral infection. Mumps orchitis, which occurs in about 30% of men who develop mumps after puberty, is usually bilateral.

Assessment reveals edematous and extremely tender testicles, reddened scrotal skin, fever, and prostration. Treatment includes bed rest, scrotal support, local heat to the scrotum, and medications for pain reduction, fever, and infection. An acute phase may last about a week. Permanent sterility may occur if both testicles are affected, whereas decreased fertility may result if only one is affected.

EPIDIDYMITIS

Epididymitis is more common than orchitis. Infections in the urethra, prostate, or bladder can spread along the vas deferens; infections also spread through the lymphatic and vascular systems. Bladder outlet obstruction can cause reflux of infected urine. Epididymitis can occur as a complication related to urethral instrumentation, such as catheterization or instrumentation in transurethral surgeries, but its frequency has decreased since prophylactic antibiotics have been prescribed after such procedures. Sexually transmitted organisms frequently cause the condition in younger men, and urinary pathogens cause epididymitis in older men. Trauma is a noninfectious cause.

Epididymitis is almost always unilateral. Early in the disease, a client has local pain and swelling. As epididymitis progresses, the testis becomes involved (epididymo-orchitis), the entire scrotum becomes reddened and painful, and an inflammatory hydrocele can occur. After the acute phase, fibrosis and occlusion may result, with subsequent sterility. Recurrences are common when other conditions are unresolved. Treatment is the same as for orchitis.

HYDROCELE, HEMATOCELE, AND SPERMATOCELE

Hydrocele (see Figure 38-4, *B*) is a painless collection of clear, yellow fluid in the scrotum caused by an opening between the peritoneum and the tunica vaginalis or by an imbalance in production and reabsorption of fluid within the tunica vaginalis. The soft intrascrotal mass is translucent to light. Often, if the hydrocele is due to a communication with the peritoneum, it decreases in size when the man lies down. If constant discomfort,

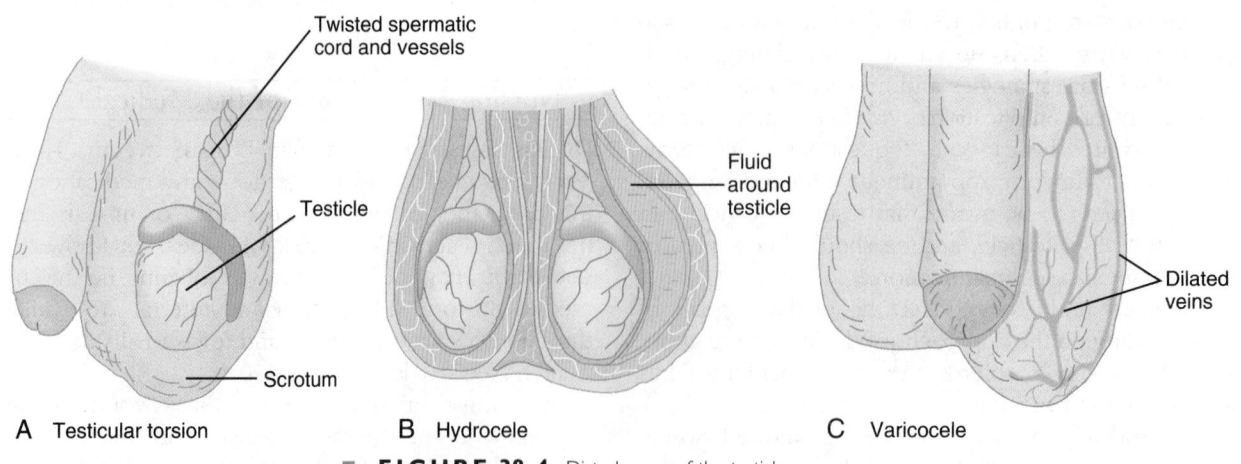

Twisted spermatic cord and vessels

Testicle

Scrotum

Fluid around testicle

Dilated veins

A Testicular torsion **B** Hydrocele **C** Varicocele

■ **FIGURE 38–4** Disturbances of the testicles.

embarrassment, or impaired circulation occurs, aspiration or surgical drainage may be performed. Hydroceles can conceal a testicular tumor or inguinal hernia.

A hematocele is a collection of blood in the tunica vaginalis caused by trauma. Hematoceles are less likely than hydroceles to be transilluminated on light examination. They require only drainage.

A spermatocele is a cystic dilation of part of the epididymis that contains a milky fluid and dead spermatozoa. It is typically painless, and surgery is usually not required.

VARICOCELE

Varicocele (see Figure 38-4, *C* on p. 900) is a dilation and varicosity of the pampiniform plexus (the network of veins supplying the testicles) within the scrotum. They usually arise slowly. Ninety percent of varicoceles are left-sided because the left spermatic vein enters the renal vein at a 90-degree angle, causing back pressure. Pain may be relieved by masturbation or sexual intercourse. Varicoceles are found in 19% to 41% of men who are evaluated for infertility. A right-sided varicocele suggests tumor or retroperitoneal fibrosis.

On palpation, with the man standing, a varicocele feels like a mass of tortuous veins above and posterior to the testicle. When the man lies down, the mass abates. Treatment includes the use of a scrotal support. Surgery is performed if there is severe pain or if the varicocele is thought to contribute to infertility.

VASECTOMY (ELECTIVE STERILIZATION)

A vasectomy is an elective surgical procedure to ensure a permanent method of contraception. It is sometimes performed after a prostatectomy to prevent retrograde epididymitis. The surgery is usually performed in the urologist's office or in an outpatient setting with the use of local anesthesia. The procedure, performed through a small incision in the scrotum, involves cutting out a segment of the vas deferens, ligating the ends, and tucking them into different tissue planes to prevent reanastomosis (Figure 38-5).

Slight pain, swelling, and bruising occur postoperatively, but discomfort is controlled with ice, a mild analgesic such as acetaminophen (aspirin is avoided to prevent bleeding), and rest for a few days. A scrotal support also increases client comfort. The client can resume heavy lifting and sexual intercourse about a week after surgery. The client must continue to practice other means of birth control until the follow-up semen analysis shows azoospermia (absence of sperm) because live sperm are left in the ampulla of the vas deferens. Bleeding, infection, and mild chronic pain (rare) are complications that can occur after vasectomy.

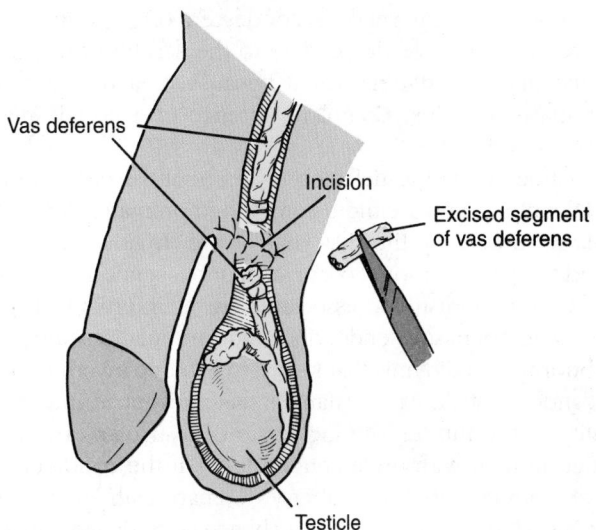

■ **FIGURE 38–5** Vasectomy.

The client must consider vasectomy a permanent means of contraception. Vasovasostomy, which is a surgical reversal of a vasectomy, can be done; however, it is expensive and fertility is not guaranteed.

UNDESCENDED OR MALPOSITIONED TESTICLES

The most common congenital testicular condition is malpositioned undescended testes (cryptorchidism) (Figure 38-6). Testes normally descend from the abdomen into the scrotum before birth, but sometimes they do not. One or both testicles may be arrested in the abdomen, inguinal canal (canalicular), low pelvis, or high scrotum. An ectopic testicle descends to the wrong

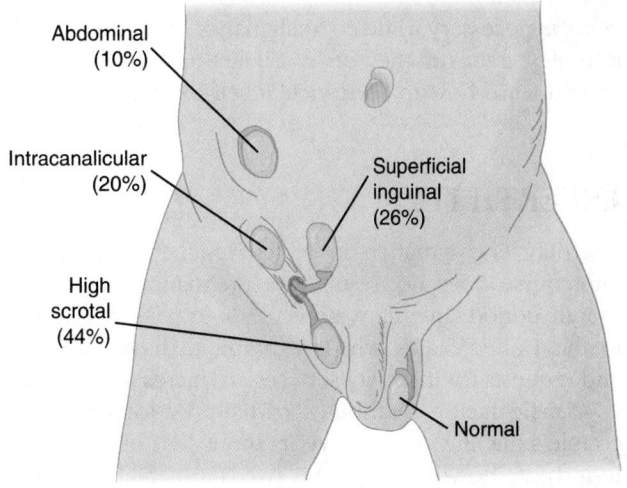

■ **FIGURE 38–6** Undescended or malpositioned testis (cryptorchidism).

area outside the normal path of descent (e.g., perineum). A retractile testicle descends into the scrotum but pulls back into the inguinal canal because of a hyperactive cremasteric reflex. Complete absence of a testicle may also occur.

Undescended testicles occur in about 4% of full-term male infants and are more common in premature infants. Many resolve by the first year of life. Inguinal hernias and torsion commonly occur with undescended testicles.

Cryptorchidism is associated with infertility. High body temperature, endocrine understimulation, and an abnormal epididymis that seems to accompany an undescended testicle cause changes that prevent normal fertility in the future. The incidence of testicular cancer is high in men with undescended testes if the condition is not corrected before puberty. A man with an undescended testicle has a 1 in 80 chance of testicular cancer development. Correction, reduces, but does not remove, the increased risk of cancer, and lifelong monitoring is recommended.

Treatment, which is surgical, is performed when the child is between 9 and 12 months old and certainly by 18 months, not only to allow time for spontaneous descent but also to decrease the risk of total infertility and testicular cancer. An inguinal incision is used so that additional repair (i.e., hernia repair or excision of connective tissue bands) or orchiectomy (should the testicle look abnormal) can be done.

Retractile testes usually descend and stay in the scrotum by puberty, but surgery is not required. HCG has sometimes been used to promote passage of the testicle into the scrotum. Luteinizing hormone–releasing hormone (LHRH) is administered as a nasal spray in Europe, but it has not been approved for use in the United States.

If the cryptorchidism is bilateral, the child should be assessed for intersexuality (an intermingling of female and male characteristics with external characteristics often contradictory to internal characteristics), especially if the condition is associated with other genital abnormalities. Continuous follow-up through the childbearing years is necessary to detect malignancy and to deal with infertility issues if they arise. Clients and their parents should learn how to do testicular self-examination.

INFERTILITY

Infertility is a situation in which regular, unprotected intercourse does not result in a pregnancy over a 12-month period. Infertility affects 20% to 35% of couples in the United States who are trying to have children, and requests for infertility services are increasing rapidly.

A male factor contributes partially or totally to the couple's inability to conceive in about 50% of the cases. It is best, however, that the two partners be treated together. Minimal fertility (subfertility) in one partner can be offset by strong fertility in the other. If both partners are minimally fertile, infertility is more likely. Awareness of these statistics alerts health care professionals to clients who may have concerns about infertility but who have difficulty expressing them. Male factors for infertility are discussed in this chapter.

Etiology and Risk Factors

Pretesticular (hormonal) causes involve endocrine dysfunction and account for about 3% to 25% of cases. Examples are pituitary and adrenal tumors, thyroid disorders, diabetes mellitus, and cirrhosis.

Testicular causes are most common. Varicoceles are found in 19% to 41% of infertility cases. Other testicular causes include congenital abnormalities, torsion, genitourinary infection, trauma, and exposure to substances known to interfere with spermatogenesis (sperm formation). Cryptorchidism is directly related to infertility.

Post-testicular causes include congenital blockage of the vas deferens and other malformations of structures distal to the testes. Additional causes include epididymitis, emotional factors, surgical procedures that cause retrograde ejaculation, and some medical conditions such as renal disease or paraplegia.

Infection of the prostate, epididymis, or testicle can affect fertility. The mumps virus attacks the testicle in 5% to 37% of adults who acquire the infection. Of these men, 16% to 65% have bilateral involvement. Although rare in the Western world, tuberculosis is a genital infection seen in other countries and in immigrants to the United States.

Whether testicular trauma and infertility are related is a matter of controversy. The formation of anti-sperm antibodies is one theory. Some surgical procedures cause retrograde ejaculation.

Chemicals, drugs, and other substances that affect spermatogenesis are called gonadotoxins (e.g., heavy use of alcohol, marijuana, and anabolic steroids). Many medications, including allopurinol, cimetidine, nitrofurantoin, sulfasalazine, and chemotherapeutic drugs, have been related to infertility. Alpha-adrenergic blockers and ganglion blockers can cause retrograde ejaculation and may thus be a secondary cause of inability to conceive. Exposure to agricultural, industrial, and warfare agents is an increasing concern. Lead, agent orange (a herbicide used as a defoliant in Vietnam), and some pesticides affect fertility. Tobacco smoke has been investigated as a cause of infertility, but a clear link has not been established; data suggest that smoking may be involved in subfertility. Radiation and hyperthermia also affect fertility.

Problems with intercourse are responsible for infertility in about 5% of couples. These include ED, premature ejaculation, unfavorable timing or frequency of intercourse, excessive masturbation, and aberrant sexual behaviors. Many water-soluble lubricants used during intercourse can be toxic to sperm.

Pathophysiology

The pathophysiologic mechanisms involved in infertility vary, and the problem is often complex. Hormonal imbalance between the hypothalamus, pituitary gland, and testicles can interfere with the production and maturation of sperm. Hypoxia of the testicle and elevated scrotal temperature cause germ cell damage. Seminal WBCs present in genitourinary infections are believed to release bioactive cytokines that affect spermatogenesis.

Some viruses and bacteria directly destroy cells or cause enough inflammation to cause tissue necrosis. Sexually transmitted infections (STIs), particularly gonorrhea and infection with *Chlamydia trachomatis,* may account for cases of infertility because they can cause testicular atrophy, but a clear relationship has not been proved. Immune responses may prevent the formation of normal sperm. Gonadotoxins can decrease the number of sperm, decrease motility (the forward movement of sperm), or cause abnormal morphology. Congenital factors and trauma can impair patency of the ductal system that extends from the testicles through the prostate.

Clinical Manifestations

Assessment of infertility includes obtaining a detailed occupational, sexual, medical, and reproductive history and conducting a thorough physical examination. During an examination, the presence of testicles and their size, varicocele or other scrotal and penile abnormalities, and secondary sex characteristics are noted. A prostate massage and specimens of secretions may be obtained for culture to check for infection. A post-ejaculatory urine specimen may also be checked for the presence of sperm, which suggests retrograde ejaculation.

Semen analysis is performed on more than one specimen. Semen volume and viscosity, number and concentration of sperm, motility, and morphology are analyzed. The presence of white blood cells or agglutination of sperm is noted. A normal semen analysis would show the following values:

- Semen volume, 1.5 to 5 ml
- Concentration, >20 million sperm/ml
- Total sperm count, >50 to 60 million
- Motility, 60% grade 2 or higher (on a scale of 1 to 4)
- Morphology, 60% normal

Motility refers to the forward movement of sperm; morphology refers to sperm form and size. Normally, sperm have one head and one tail. Abnormal sperm may be immature, may have misshapen heads, or may have two tails. Some infertility specialists consider slightly lower percentages for sperm count, motility,

and morphology to be adequate when evaluating semen quality. Other more specific tests may be done to evaluate semen, such as checking for viscosity, coagulation, and the presence of fructose.

Serum endocrine studies are conducted to assess testosterone, prolactin, luteinizing hormone (LH), and follicle-stimulating hormone (FSH). For example, if testosterone levels are normal, nonhormonal causes are pursued. If testosterone levels and prolactin levels are low but LH levels are high, primary testicular disease may be suspected. If FSH levels are high, spermatogenesis is probably arrested. If FSH levels are normal, azoospermia (absence of sperm) or oligospermia (scarcity of sperm) is probably caused by obstruction in the post-testicular ducts, which may be corrected by microsurgery.

If anatomic abnormalities are suspected, imaging techniques such as Doppler ultrasonography, MRI, cavernosography, and color flow Doppler imaging are ordered. A testicular biopsy may be performed if sperm are absent or scarce along with normal hormone levels. Clients are carefully selected for such studies because the tests are costly and, when invasive, may cause testicular damage.

OUTCOME MANAGEMENT

Medical Management

Pretesticular Causes

Treatment of male infertility with pretesticular causes varies. No treatment is available for primary testicular failure or hypogonadism. Testosterone may be prescribed to correct low testosterone levels. A testosterone patch is applied directly to the scrotum (Testoderm) or to the torso or extremities (Androderm). Scrotal skin is five times more permeable, and there is concern about too much absorption and side effects. With both transdermal methods, skin irritation or contact dermatitis is experienced in about 9% of clients. Testosterone is contraindicated for men with prostate cancer or severe bladder outlet obstruction. Hyperprolactinemia may be treated by surgical removal of a pituitary tumor or by administration of bromocriptine (Parlodel).

Treatment of male sexual dysfunction is discussed under Erectile Dysfunction later in this chapter. For oligospermia caused by excessive frequency of ejaculation, recommend that the couple have intercourse only once every 36 hours during the woman's periovulatory period because it takes 24 hours for a normal sperm count to be generated after ejaculation.

Testicular Causes

Treatment of male infertility with testicular causes also varies. Instruct the client to avoid factors that depress spermatogenesis such as heat, drugs, alcohol, and marijuana. He should keep the testicles cool by avoiding hot baths and tight clothing or by using a commercially prepared, water-dampened scrotal-cooling device; keeping the testes cool appears to improve the sperm count. Advise the client to maintain good nutrition. Medications such as HCG or testosterone (Depo-Testosterone) are sometimes prescribed as hormonal treatments. Nonhormonal therapy may consist of kallikrein, steroids, indomethacin, arginine, zinc, or vitamins. Varicocele is treated surgically.

Post-Testicular Causes

Treatment of male infertility with post-testicular causes involves correcting ejaculatory abnormalities and obstruction. Ejaculatory abnormalities may be corrected by the split-ejaculate technique. The first half of the ejaculate contains more sperm than the second half. The first half may be used for artificial insemination or may be deposited in the vagina during intercourse, followed by withdrawal of the penis. Absence of ejaculation or retrograde (backward) ejaculation may be treated with drugs such as ephedrine, imipramine, or antihistamines. When the client experiences retrograde ejaculation, artificial insemination may be performed using sperm from urine obtained by centrifugation. Obstructive infertility is treated by surgery.

Appropriate antimicrobial drugs are used to treat genitourinary infections. Male infertility with immunologic causes may be treated with steroids and artificial insemination of sperm that have been washed to remove antibodies contained in the sperm.

Nursing Management of the Medical Client

Provide Support

The client and his partner are often highly emotional in the diagnostic phase, and your sensitivity can ease their concerns somewhat. Both may need help and support to express their feelings and concerns about infertility. Failure to conceive may make several demands on the couple, threatening their individual self-concepts, gender roles, relationship, and sexual interaction. Guilt and blame about previous sexual activity, STIs, or abortion may come between them. Some men find masturbation (necessary to obtain a semen sample) difficult for personal, cultural, or religious reasons. Many men do not know what chemicals they have been exposed to at the workplace or elsewhere. Fear and anxiety may be lessened during your assessment and teaching sessions. This provides you with the opportunity to support, respond to questions, and explain diagnostic and treatment procedures. Emphasize the need for consistent follow-up to evaluate progress.

Referral for counseling or support groups, or both, for infertile couples may be appropriate. A nationally known support group in the United States is RESOLVE (Department P, Box 474, Belmont, MA 02178).

Provide Education

Because thorough and complete fertility assessment is expensive and can be ineffective, the client needs to understand the testing and the reasons for the various examinations. Explain fully how to collect a specimen for sperm analysis so that results are accurate. Written as well as verbal instructions are important because anxiety levels may be high. The man should refrain from sexual activity for 3 days before collecting a semen sample and should take the specimen immediately (within 1 hour) to the laboratory for analysis. Masturbation is the preferred method because some semen is lost during intercourse. Condoms and lubricants may make the sperm immotile. The specimen should be kept close to the body to maintain normal temperature. Two to three interval specimens are required for evaluation because results can vary. Ensure that the client understands the medical regimen suggested and the importance of following it closely.

Prevent Infertility

If possible, it is more effective to prevent infertility than to treat it. Clients who want to conceive at present or in the future can try to prevent infertility by doing the following:

1. Avoiding gonadotoxins, as discussed earlier
2. Decreasing exposure to occupational and environmental hazards
3. Keeping the scrotum cool by avoiding excessive heat, hot baths, and tight clothing
4. Avoiding transmission of STDs by limiting the number of sexual partners and by using condoms
5. Developing effective means of stress reduction
6. Eating a well-balanced, nutritious diet

PENILE DISORDERS

PHIMOSIS

Phimosis occurs when the penile foreskin (prepuce) is constricted at the opening, making retraction difficult or impossible. The condition can be congenital or a result of inflammation, infection, or local trauma. It is not usually painful, but it can lead to obstructive uropathy if it is severe enough. Prolonged phimosis, caused by chronic inflammation and irritation, predisposes to penile cancer. Assessment reveals edema, erythema, tenderness, and purulent discharge. Intervention includes controlling infection with local treatment and broad-spectrum antimicrobial drugs.

Effective genital hygiene is essential to prevent acquired penile disorders. In uncircumcised males, the man cleans the penis by pulling the foreskin back gently and washing the area with a washcloth. This technique should be done daily to eliminate the normally accumulated smegma, and the foreskin should be returned to its normal position.

Routine circumcision (surgical removal of the foreskin) of male infants has not been considered medically necessary by the American Academy of Pediatrics and other health professionals and health organizations. Some parents have religious or cultural reasons for continuing the practice of circumcision. The operation may be indicated for clients with penile infection, phimosis, or paraphimosis. The rate of penile cancer is almost nil in circumcised men. The procedure should be done with the client under general anesthesia. Potential risks include excessive bleeding, infection, and penile trauma.

PARAPHIMOSIS

Paraphimosis (Figure 38-7) occurs when a tight foreskin, once retracted, cannot be returned to its normal position. This sometimes happens after rigorous cleaning, masturbation, sexual intercourse, catheter insertion, or cystoscopy if the foreskin is not returned to its normal position. Circulation is thus impeded, and the glans swells rapidly. It is painful and edema is common. The foreskin can be gently compressed either manually or with an elastic wrap. The client can then attempt manual reduction by gently pulling the foreskin. Surgical incision of the foreskin with local anesthesia may be necessary if the condition does not resolve.

POSTHITIS AND BALANITIS

Posthitis (foreskin inflammation) and balanitis (inflammation of the glans penis and the mucous membrane beneath it) are caused by irritation and invasion of microorganisms. Good hygiene and thorough drying of the penis are recommended. It is important to assess for diabetes mellitus, which predisposes the client to secondary infection. Antibiotics may help control local infection. Circumcision may be necessary.

URETHRITIS

Urethritis, an acute urethral inflammation, is discussed under STIs and urinary disorders (see Chapters 34 and

41). It is mentioned throughout this chapter because it predisposes to other genitourinary disorders.

URETHRAL STRICTURE

Urethral stricture is caused by urethral scarring or narrowing. It may be congenital or caused by untreated or severe urethritis or urethral injury (including urologic instrumentation, e.g., cystoscopy). Manifestations are caused by obstruction and include: small-caliber urinary stream, hyperdistended bladder, infection, fever, and dysuria. Urethral strictures are released surgically by urethral dilation or urethroplasty. See Chapter 34 for further information.

PEYRONIE'S DISEASE

Fibrous plaques develop in the connective tissue in Peyronie's disease, usually near the dorsal midline of the penile shaft in middle-age and older men. Although the etiologic mechanism is unknown, one theory is that the disease is caused by an abnormal fibrotic reaction to trauma. The disease has two phases: acute and chronic. Pain is more likely during the initial phase, and plaques begin to develop. This phase can last about 12 to 18 months. Pain usually subsides during the chronic phase, but fibrosis is increased.

Diagnosis may be made during history-taking, although men usually seek a physician because of concern about penile lumps (fear of cancer), painful erection, or ED. The man may have penile curvature on erection, painful erection, and unsatisfactory vaginal penetration. Peyronie's disease is often associated with Dupuytren's contracture of the hand tendons.

Some cases improve spontaneously. Reassure the client that this is not a malignant condition and does not lead to development of cancer. If a client is not having discomfort and has soft plaques and minimal curvature, the physician may advise waiting several months before instituting therapy. Medical treatment includes vitamin E, para-aminobenzoic acid, tamoxifen, and colchicine. Intralesional injections, local radiation, and ultrasonography have also been used. Surgical correction is necessary when previous treatments have failed and the client is unable to perform sexually.

PRIAPISM

Priapism is a prolonged, persistent penile erection without sexual desire. It can last hours or even days and may be very painful. The condition is sometimes associated with leukemia or sickle cell anemia. Self-injection of medications (mainly papaverine) to treat impotence is the other common cause. It may also result from some

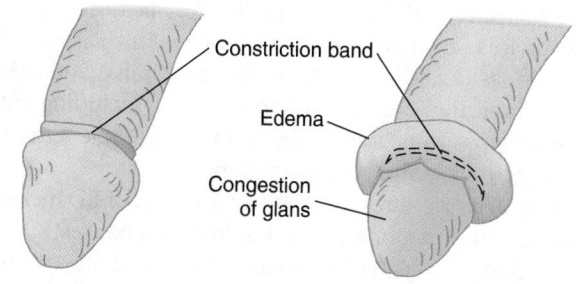

FIGURE 38–7   Paraphimosis.

medications, such as anticoagulants, alcohol, phenothiazine, alpha-adrenergic blockers, and marijuana.

Two major types of priapism have been defined according to a physiology-based system. High-flow arterial priapism, the less common type, usually occurs after trauma and is less painful. Low-flow veno-occlusive priapism, the more common form, is an emergency situation and is extremely painful.

In the client with low-flow priapism, circulation to the penis is compromised, predisposing to ischemia and permanent ED. The client may also be unable to void. Treatment in most cases consists of aspiration of blood from the penis followed by serial intracavernosal injections of phenylephrine.

Low-flow priapism must be resolved within 24 hours to prevent penile ischemia, gangrene, fibrosis, and ED. If the more conservative treatments are unsuccessful, more invasive therapy is required to prevent permanent damage. Surgical treatment is designed to drain the congested blood from the corpora cavernosa.

High-flow priapism can often be treated with ice and compression. If these measures are not successful, the client may require selective embolization or ligation of the traumatized artery.

Be sensitive to the embarrassing nature of this problem. Men are often reluctant to admit that this problem has occurred and yet may be in severe pain. Be understanding, and try to make the client comfortable while decreasing the client's embarrassment about the problem.

PENILE CANCER

Penile cancer is rare. In 2007 less than 1300 cases were diagnosed and less than 300 men died of penile cancer.[4] It usually affects the foreskin in older, uncircumcised men who have suffered chronic irritation and have poor hygiene practices. Human Papillomavirus (HPV) increases the risk of penile cancer. Associated genital cancer sometimes develops in sexual partners (e.g., cervical cancer in females). Any dry, wart-like, painless growth on the penis or foreskin that fails to respond to antibiotics should be assessed for cancer. If an early diagnosis is made, excision and circumcision may be all that is necessary.

Many men find penile problems embarrassing and consequently do not seek medical attention for months. By this time, a lesion may be ulcerated, involve the foreskin and penile shaft, and have metastasized to the inguinal nodes. Penile shaft resection or sometimes penectomy and dissection of enlarged inguinal nodes may be necessary. Dissection of the pelvic lymph nodes carries a risk of long-term lymphedema affecting one or both lower extremities.

ERECTILE DYSFUNCTION

Our understanding of ED (impotence) has expanded significantly over the last 2 decades, as have the options for managing this common disorder. ED is defined as an inability to achieve or maintain an erection sufficient for sexual activity. Occasional erectile failure may occur because of a variety of self-limiting factors, but consistent failure that affects 50% of attempts at sexual activity is considered clinically relevant.

Etiology and Risk Factors

Both psychological and physiologic factors typically combine to cause ED. Important psychological factors include performance anxiety, stress and fatigue, low self-esteem, depression, and changes in a relationship. After experiencing failure once, a man may be so anxious that he "fails" again and again, worsening the problem.

A variety of physiologic factors may contribute to ED. Although aging does not cause ED, multiple age-related factors increase the risk of ED. For example, an increase in local nerves (both adrenergic and cholinergic receptors) may promote penile flaccidity while reducing the penile response to nitric oxide (the primary neurotransmitter responsible for a penile erection). Diminished testosterone levels, combined with increases in the levels of estradiol and serum prolactin, may reduce libido, leading to a decline in the number of erections in older men, an increase in the time needed to achieve sexual arousal, and an increase in the interval between successful erections. Nevertheless, it must be emphasized that none of these changes inevitably leads to ED, and many older men enjoy successful erections and intercourse throughout their lifetimes. Other endocrine disorders associated with sexual dysfunction include hyperprolactinemia and thyroid dysfunction. An increased level of prolactin blocks testosterone effectiveness and decreases the desire for sexual activity; both hyperthyroidism and hypothyroidism predispose to ED.

Major medical risk factors for ED include cardiovascular disease, hypertension, diabetes mellitus, long-term cigarette smoking, renal failure, neurologic disorders affecting the spinal cord, stroke, and chronic obstructive pulmonary disease. Congenital defects affecting gonadal development and testosterone production predispose men to erectile dysfunctions, although surgical castration does not necessarily lead to impotence. Illicit drugs, such as cannabis, cocaine, and hallucinogens, impair erectile function, as does alcohol. Multiple prescriptive and over-the-counter medications may produce ED, including antihypertensives, anticholinergics, alpha-adrenergic agonists (decongestants), and certain antidepressants.

Surgical procedures associated with a risk of ED include extensive abdominopelvic and spinal procedures. Open prostatectomy and TURP occasionally produce erectile dysfunction, but radical prostatectomy carries a high risk for impotence. Urethral stricture or injury, genital trauma, pelvic bone fracture, or Peyronie's diseases (painful curvature of the penis) are also associated with ED.

Pathophysiology

A normal erection comprises two phases. When the penis is flaccid, local arterioles provide enough blood flow to meet nutritional needs of penile tissues but not enough for rigidity. A variety of sensory and psychological stimuli may trigger the release of neurotransmitters and paracrines from local nerve receptors and blood vessels, producing an erection. The erection begins with relaxation of smooth muscle of local arterioles and sinusoids (blood-filled sinuses) within the corpora cavernosa. As arterial blood fills the sinusoids, tumescence (an increase in penile length and circumference) occurs initially. When the cavernous bodies reach the limits imposed by their fibrous outer covering (the tunica albuginea), however, veins and venules within are compressed and the erection achieves sufficient rigidity for vaginal penetration. Following a period of rigidity, the penis returns to a flaccid state. This requires increased tone in the smooth muscle of the arterioles and sinusoids of the cavernous bodies and reversal of venous compression. Although the endocrine system influences erectile function via effects on the development of secondary sex characteristics and libido, individual erections are controlled by neurovascular mechanisms. Interruption of any one of these physiologic events as a result of a physiologic disorder or psychological dysfunction leads to erectile failure and may cause ED unless it is corrected.

Clinical Manifestations

A detailed medical and sexual history is the first step in determining the cause of ED. A focused physical examination is performed to identify contributing factors such as congenital defects of the male reproductive system, neurologic deficits, or cardiovascular disease such as hypertension. Laboratory tests often include serum testosterone and LH levels as well as prolactin levels and thyroid function. A nocturnal penile tumescence study may be completed to identify the presence of nocturnal erections and their quality. Specialized tests such as color duplex Doppler ultrasonography or dynamic infusion cavernosometry are completed in highly selected cases when potentially reversible vascular problems are suspected as the principal cause of erectile dysfunction.

OUTCOME MANAGEMENT

Medical Management

Correct Psychological Problems

Sometimes just giving accurate information about normal sexual function, alternative sexual activity, and dispelling myths is all that is necessary for a client to deal with ED. Myths about sexual activity greatly influence outcome success. Behavioral modification techniques (the best known were developed by Masters and Johnson in the 1960s) may be used when psychogenic causes are identified as the principal cause of ED, and counseling is often invaluable as part of a multimodal management plan.

Correct Physiologic Problems

When physiologic causes are involved, several approaches may be used. Medications may be altered and recreational drugs such as cigarette smoking or alcohol consumption stopped. Medical conditions causing ED need to be treated if possible. Low serum testosterone levels can be augmented using a parenteral or transcutaneous delivery system, provided hypogonadism or deficiency of endogenous testosterone has been identified during evaluation.

Stimulate Erection

Medications. The Integrating Pharmacology feature on p. 908 outlines medications used for erectile dysfunction. The website provides a Complementary and Alternative Therapy box on the use of Korean red ginseng for erectile dysfunction.

Vacuum Erection Devices. Vacuum erection devices are legitimate medically prescribed pumps that mechanically achieve an erection. A cylinder is placed over the penis and a pump is used to create vacuum suction, thus drawing blood into the corpora cavernosa. When an erection is achieved, a compression ring is applied to the base of the penis and the cylinder is removed for intercourse. The ring must be removed within about 30 minutes to prevent tissue damage caused by interrupted circulation. Bruising and cold penile skin and a lack of spontaneity are minor problems that may result. Priapism occurs rarely.

Nursing Management of the Medical Client

Provide Support

A sensitive, caring approach is vital for nurses who work with these clients because embarrassment may cause many men to avoid treatment. Just knowing that ED is common and treatment alternatives are available can be reassuring to the client. Involve the sexual partner when the client permits.

Provide Education

Teach the client about normal erectile physiology, factors that interfere, and how different approaches correct the problem. Inform the client about public or

INTEGRATING PHARMACOLOGY

Medications for Erectile Dysfunction

Several oral agents, one intraurethral suppository, and several injectable drugs are available for the management of erectile dysfunction.

The oral drugs are phosphodiesterase-5 (PDE5) inhibitors. Specific agents include sildenafil (Viagra), vardenafil (Levitra), and tadalafil (Cialis). These drugs block the action of PDE5, a substance that promotes the metabolism of cyclic GMP and nitric oxide. Blockade of this drug prolongs and enhances the actions of these substances within the corpora cavernosa. The drugs do not generate an erection as do the injectable agents; instead, they enhance the client's ability to achieve and sustain an erection that must be stimulated by psychological, visual, tactile, and other factors. Side effects may include headache, a flushed feeling, dyspepsia, nasal congestion, and a color tinge or other mild visual disturbances. Clients taking PDE5 inhibitors should not take nitrates in any form as they may lead to a dramatic and dangerous reduction in blood pressure. Caution must be observed when men are taking alpha-adrenergic blockers or have a peptic ulcer.

Intracavernosal vasodilating drugs such as papaverine, phentolamine, and prostaglandin E_1 (PGE_1) (Casodex) can be injected. Combinations of these drugs may be given in a single injection. Because pain, bruising, and fibrosis at the injection site and priapism are possible side effects, it is recommended that injections be given not more than two or three times per week.

Intraurethral instillation of an alprostadil (PGE_1) pellet (MUSE) has been successful. This approach eliminates injection of the penis, but the technique must be accurately performed to achieve erection. This approach can be a good one for a client who is obese or has problems with dexterity or vision. The drug should not be given more than twice in a 24-hour period. Side effects are the same as described previously; intraurethral pain and minor bleeding may occur. PGE_1 administration is contraindicated if penile anatomy is abnormal or the client has urethritis. A gel version and a creme version of alprostadil are in final phase III trials in the United States. These versions are topically applied to the head of the penis before intercourse.

Yohimbe, an alpha-adrenergic blocking agent, causes vasodilation of the corpora cavernosa and may alleviate erectile dysfunction in some cases. Side effects include fluid retention, nausea, orthostatic hypotension, and diaphoresis; studies have shown that yohimbine is often ineffective for men with moderate to severe erectile dysfunction.

dispose of equipment. He should know that bruising might occur. Injections should be given at the 2 o'clock or 10 o'clock position, and sites should be rotated to minimize fibrotic changes. Intraurethral pellets require using the applicator correctly, careful insertion, and waiting about 10 minutes for an erection to occur. Standing or walking during this time and stimulation are important.

Surgical Management

Surgical management of ED includes implantation of a penile prosthesis, revascularization procedures, and incision of Peyronie's plaques. Penile prostheses are most common if medical therapy is not effective and if the client is a good surgical candidate.

Penile Prosthesis

The following are the two basic categories of penile prostheses (Figure 38-8):

1. Inflatable prostheses come in one-piece, two-piece, and three-piece units that are hydraulic devices. In the one-piece prosthesis, the reservoir, pump, and cylinders fit within the penis. Two-piece units have a reservoir-pump system within the scrotum. The reservoir on the three-piece devices is implanted in the abdominal cavity and the pump is implanted in the scrotum.
2. Semirigid prostheses can be malleable, with spring-like mechanisms that help make the penis more erect for intercourse, or mechanical, with cable strands in the device that can be bent to make the penis more erect.

Ice and penile or scrotal elevations are used postoperatively to minimize swelling. Pain should be well controlled with medication. Sexual activity can usually be resumed 6 to 8 weeks after surgery when healing is complete and pain is controlled. Infection, extrusion of the prosthesis, and mechanical failure are some of the complications after surgery.

Revascularization

Revascularization surgical procedures attempt to restore circulation to the corpora cavernosa. Although initially successful, these techniques are uncommon because they lack durability.

Nursing Management of the Surgical Client

Care of the client having surgery for ED is the same as that of any surgical client. Penile circulation and dressing should be observed consistently as ordered. Encourage the client to use pain medication before the pain becomes severe. All clients are given antibiotics before and after surgery. The client is taught preoperatively how to use the prosthesis and cautioned not

community resources. If medication is used, explain how to administer the medication and caution the client to follow directions as prescribed and not to use the medication more often than directed.

The client who must use intracorporeal injections needs to know how to draw up medication into a syringe, cleanse the site, inject the medication, and safely

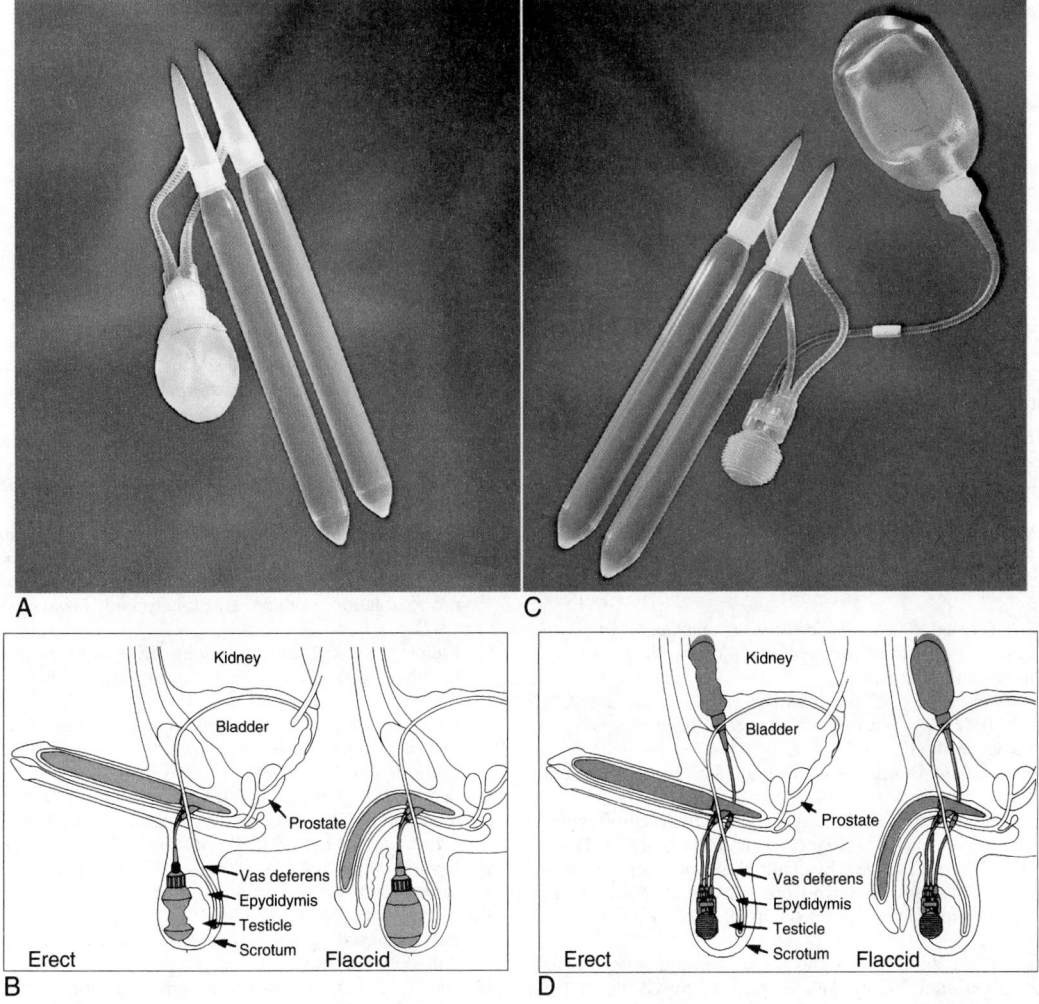

■ **FIGURE 38–8** Penile prostheses. **A,** Mark II (two-piece inflatable penile prosthesis). **B,** Mark II prosthesis erect and flaccid. **C,** Alpha I (three-piece inflatable penile prosthesis). **D,** Alpha I prosthesis erect and flaccid. (Courtesy Mentor, Santa Barbara, Calif.)

to use it before healing has occurred. These men need a great deal of emotional support because of secrecy with friends, emotional issues with partners, and sometimes doubt about the decision to have surgery related to pain.

CONCLUSIONS

Male genital and reproductive disorders can be complex problems for both the client and the nurse. The client often finds that these disorders threaten sexuality and sexual function or normal urinary elimination. These effects may be physiologic, but complex psychosocial problems also arise.

Prostate disorders are among the most common problems experienced by men throughout their lifetime. Cancers of the male reproductive tract can be life-threatening, but if they are detected early, they can be cured or at least controlled for long periods. Problems such as ED and infertility directly affect both partners, who experience the diagnostic and treatment phases together. The nurse acts as a caregiver, educator, support, and resource person.

THINKING CRITICALLY

1. Your client underwent a laser-assisted TURP yesterday. Closed bladder irrigation is being used, and his urine is dark to bright red with multiple clots. He is complaining of intense cramping pain in the lower abdomen. What further assessments should you make? What could be causing the cramping pain? What nursing action should you take?

Factors to Consider. Is the dark to bright red urine output normal at this stage? What does the nature of the client's pain tell you about its likely cause?

2. A young man in his early 20s is given a diagnosis of testicular cancer, and he is very concerned about the treatment's effects on his

ability to perform sexually and to father children. What issues should you discuss with him?

Factors to Consider. What impact might a bilateral orchiectomy or a radical lymph node dissection have on erectile function and fertility? What might be the effect of a unilateral orchiectomy? What options for fathering children are important to consider before the client undergoes treatment?

evolve *Discussions for these questions can be found on the website.*

BIBLIOGRAPHY

Citations appearing in red refer to primary research.

Citations appearing in blue refer to evidence-based practice guidelines and protocols.

1. Albaugh, J. (2006). Intracavernosal injection algorithm. *Urologic Nursing, 26*(6), 449-453.
2. Albaugh, J., et al. (2002). Health care clinicians in sexual health medicine: Focus on erectile dysfunction. *Urologic Nursing, 22*(4), 217-232.
3. Albaugh, J., & Lewis, J. (2005). *Understanding erectile dysfunction: Patient evaluation and treatment options.* Pitman, NJ: Society of Urologic Nurses and Associates.
4. American Cancer Society. (2007). *Cancer Facts & Figures 2007.* Downloaded 01/21/07 from www.cancer.org/downloads/STT/CAFF2006PWSecured.pdf.
5. Ateya, A., et al. (2006). Evaluation of prostatic massage in treatment of chronic prostatitis. *Urology, 67*(4), 674-678.
6. Bodell, A., & Shore, D. (2002). Prostate cancer screening in asymptomatic men in a community setting. *Urologic Nursing, 22*(1), 31-37.
7. Broderick, G., & Lue, T. (2002). Evaluation and nonsurgical management of erectile dysfunction and priapism. In P. Walsh, et al. (Eds.), *Campbell's urology* (8th ed., pp. 1619-1672). Philadelphia: Saunders.
8. Burke, J.P., et al. (2006). Diabetes and benign prostatic hyperplasia progression in Olmsted County, Minnesota. *Urology, 67*(1), 22-25.
9. Cox, B., et al. (2002). Vasectomy and risk of prostate cancer. *Journal of the American Medical Association, 287*(23), 3110-3115.
10. Dal Maso, L., et al. (2006). Lifetime occupational and recreational physical activity and risk of benign prostatic hyperplasia. *International Journal of Cancer, 118*(10), 2632-2635.
11. DiMeo, P. (2006). Psychosocial and relationship issues in men with erectile dysfunction. *Urologic Nursing, 26*(6), 442-446, 453.
12. Eastham, J., et al. (2003). Variation of serum prostate-specific antigen levels: An evaluation of year-to-year fluctuations. *Journal of the American Medical Association, 289*(20), 2696-2700.
13. Eastham, J., & Scardino, P. (2002). Radical prostatectomy. In P. Walsh, et al. (Eds.), *Campbell's urology* (8th ed., pp. 3080-3106). Philadelphia: Saunders.
14. Eisenburger, M., & Carducci, M. (2002). Chemotherapy for hormone-resistant prostate cancer. In P. Walsh, et al. (Eds.) Campbell's urology (8th ed., pp. 3209-3226). Philadelphia: Saunders.
15. el-Sakka, A.I. (2006). Lower urinary tract symptoms in patients with erectile dysfunction: Analysis of risk factors. *Journal of Sexual Medicine, 3*(1), 144-149.
16. Elzayat, E.A., & Mostafa, M. (2006). Holmium laser enucleation of the prostate (HoLEP): The endourologic alternative to open prostatectomy. *European Urology 2006, 49*(1), 87-91.
17. Gaines, K. (2002). Zoledronic acid (Zometa): Bisphosphonate for prostate cancer/bone metastases. *Urologic Nursing, 22*(6), 398-400.
18. Goldstein, M. (2002). Surgical management of male infertility and other scrotal disorders. In P. Walsh, et al. (Eds.) *Campbell's urology* (8th ed., pp. 1475-1530). Philadelphia: Saunders.
19. Gray, M. (1998). Psychometric analysis of the international prostate symptom score. *Urologic Nursing, 18,* 175-183.
20. Gray, M. (2001). Etiology of erectile dysfunction. *Clinician Reviews, 11*(Suppl), 9-14.
21. Gray, M. (2002). Prostate cancer primer. *Urologic Nursing, 22,* 151-169.
22. Gray, M., & Brown, K.C. (2002). Genitourinary system. In J. Thompson, G. McFarland, J. Hirsh, et al. (Eds.), *Clinical nursing* (5th ed., pp. 917-999). St. Louis: Mosby.
23. Grayhack, J.T., McVary, K.T., & Kozlowski, J.A. (2002). Benign prostatic hyperplasia. In J. Gillenwater, et al. (Eds.), *Adult and pediatric urology* (4th ed., pp. 1402-1470). Philadelphia: Lippincott, Williams & Wilkins.
24. Gretzer, M., & Partin, A. (2003). *Campbell's Urology Updates: PSA and PSA Molecular Derivatives, 1*(1), 1-12.
25. Han, M., Alfert, H., & Partin, A. (2002). Retropubic and suprapubic open prostatectomy. In P. Walsh, et al. (Eds.), *Campbell's urology* (8th ed., pp. 1423-1434). Philadelphia: Saunders.
26. Hewitt, A. (2001). Early catheter removal following radical perineal prostatectomy: A randomized clinical trial. *Urologic Nursing, 21*(1), 37-44.
27. Incrocci, L., & Slob, A. (2002). Incidence, etiology, and therapy for erectile dysfunction after external beam radiotherapy for prostate cancer. *Urology, 60*(1), 1-7.
28. Jarow, J., et al. (2002). Male infertility evaluation guidelines. *The Journal of Urology, 167*(5), 2138-2144.
29. Joseph, A. (2001). Male pelvic anatomy/post-prostatectomy incontinence. *Urologic Nursing, 21*(1), 25-29.
30. Joseph, A. (2006). Noninvasive therapies for treating post-prostatectomy urinary incontinence. *Urologic Nursing, 26*(4), 271-276.
31. Kattan, M. (2006). Measuring hot flashes in men treated with hormone ablation therapy: An unmet need. *Urologic Nursing, 26*(1), 13-21.
32. Kleier, J. (2006). Language adaptation and testing of the prostate health questionnaire for Jamaican and Haitian men. *Urologic Nursing, 26*(4), 304-310.
33. Leitzmann, M., et al. (2004). Ejaculation frequency and subsequent risk of prostate cancer. *Journal of the American Medical Association, 291*(3), 1578-1586.
34. Lepor, H., & Lowe, F. (2002). Evaluation and nonsurgical management of benign prostatic hyperplasia. In P. Walsh, et al. (Eds.), *Campbell's urology* (8th ed., pp. 1337-1378). Philadelphia: Saunders.
35. Lessick, M., & Katz, A. (2006). A genetics perspective on prostate cancer. *Urologic Nursing, 26*(6), 454-460.
36. Lewis, R., & Jordon, G. (2002). Surgery for erectile dysfunction. In P. Walsh, et al. (Eds.), *Campbell's urology* (8th ed., pp. 1673-1708). Philadelphia: Saunders.
37. Lue, T. (2002). Physiology of penile erection and pathophysiology of erectile dysfunction and priapism. In P. Walsh, et al. (Eds.), *Campbell's urology* (8th ed., pp. 1591-1617). Philadelphia: Saunders.
38. Lynch, D.F., & Pettaway, C.A. (2002). Tumors of the penis. In P. Walsh, et al. (Eds.), *Campbell's urology* (8th ed., pp. 2945-2981). Philadelphia: Saunders.
39. Marks, L., et al. (2002). Herbal formulation for prostate cancer. *Urology, 60*(3), 369-377.
40. McCallum, T., Moore, K., & Griffiths, D. (2001). Urinary incontinence after radical prostatectomy: Implications and urodynamics. *Urologic Nursing, 21*(2), 113-119, 124.
41. Middelton, L., & Lessick, M. (2003). Inherited urologic malignant disorders: Nursing implications. *Urologic Nursing, 23*(1), 15-30.
42. Moul, J., & Civitelli, K. (2001). Managing advanced prostate cancer with Viadur (leuprolide acetate implant). *Urologic Nursing, 21*(6), 385-396.
43. Moyad, M. (2003). Osteoporosis part III—Not just for bone loss: Potential benefits of calcium and vitamin D for overall general health. *Urologic Nursing, 23*(1), 69-74.
44. Moyad, M., et al. (2006). Statins, especially atorvastatin, may improve survival following brachytherapy for clinically localized prostate cancer. *Urologic Nursing, 26*(4), 298-303.
45. Nahon, I., et al. (2006). Systematic review of the treatment of post-prostatectomy incontinence. *Urologic Nursing, 26*(6), 461-475, 482.
46. Naspro, R., et al. (2005). Update of the minimally invasive therapies for benign prostatic hyperplasia. *Current Opinion in Urology, 15*(1), 49-53.
47. Ng, C., et al. (2006). Hormone ablation for the treatment of prostate cancer: The lived experience. *Urologic Nursing, 26*(3), 204-212.
48. Nuhoglu, B., et al. (2005). Transurethral electrovaporization of the prostate: Is it any better than standard transurethral prostatectomy? 5-year follow-up. *Journal of Endourology, 19*(1), 79-82.

49. Ohl, D., & Quallich, S. (2006). Clinical hypogonadism and androgen replacement therapy: An overview. *Urologic Nursing, 26*(4), 253-260, 269.

50. Parrott, B. (2003). TUNA of the prostate in an office setting: Nursing implications. *Urologic Nursing, 23*(1), 33-40.

51. Plowden, K. (2006). To screen or not to screen: Factors influencing the decision to participate in prostate cancer screening among urban African-American men. *Urologic Nursing, 26*(6), 477-482.

52. Quallich, S. (2006). Examining male infertility. *Urologic Nursing, 26*(4), 277-289.

53. Quallich, S., & Ohl, D. (2002). Penile prosthesis case study. *Urologic Nursing, 22*(2), 91-95.

54. Quallich, S., & Ohl, D. (2002). Penile prosthesis: Patient teaching and perioperative care. *Urologic Nursing, 22*(2), 81-90.

55. Roehrborn, C.G., & McConnell, J.D. (2002). Etiology, pathophysiology, epidemiology and natural history of BPH. In P. Walsh, et al. (Eds.), *Campbell's urology* (8th ed., pp. 1297-1336). Philadelphia: Saunders.

56. Sattelle, K. (2002). Men's health in focus. *Professional Nurse, 17* (11), 633.

57. Schuster, T. (2006). Premature ejaculation. *Urologic Nursing, 26*(4), 245-250.

58. Shinohara, K., & Carroll, P. (2002). Cryotherapy for prostate cancer. In P. Walsh, et al. (Eds.), *Campbell's urology* (8th ed., pp. 3171-3181). Philadelphia: Saunders.

59. Shiri, R., et al. (2005). Association between the bothersomeness of lower urinary tract symptoms and the prevalence of erectile dysfunction. *Journal of Sexual Medicine, 2*(3), 4384-4400.

60. Sigman, M., & Jarow, J. (2002). Male infertility. In P. Walsh, et al. (Eds.), Campbell's urology (8th ed., pp. 1475-1531). Philadelphia: Saunders.

61. Shoskes, D., Katske, F., & Kim, S. (2001). Diagnosis and management of acute and chronic prostatitis. *Urologic Nursing, 21*(4), 255-264.

62. Starnes, D., & Sims, T. (2006). Care of the patient undergoing robotic-assisted prostatectomy. *Urologic Nursing, 26*(2), 129-137.

63. Starnes, D., & Sims, T. (2006). Robotic prostatectomy surgery. *Urologic Nursing, 26*(2), 138-140.

64. Stipetich, R., et al. (2005). Nursing considerations in brachytherapy-related erectile dysfunction. *Urologic Nursing, 25*(4), 249-259.

65. Tan, A., & Gilling, P. (2005). Lasers in the treatment of benign prostatic hyperplasia: An update. *Current Opinion in Urology, 15*(1), 55-58.

66. Thompson, I. (2006). Adjuvant radiotherapy for pathologically advanced prostate cancer: A randomized clinical trial. *Journal of the American Medical Association, 296*(19), 2329-2335.

67. Wallace, M., & Powel, L. (2002). *Prostate cancer: Nursing assessment, management and care.* New York: Springer-Verlag.

68. Ward-Smith, P., & Kapitan, D. (2005). Quality of life among men treated with radiation therapy for prostate cancer. *Urologic Nursing, 25*(4), 263-268.

69. Weingard, K. (2006). Nursing implications of androgen deprivation therapy-associated bone loss. *Urologic Nursing, 26*(4), 261-270.

70. Willener, R., & Hantikainen, V. (2005). Individual quality of life following radical prostatectomy in men with prostate cancer. *Urologic Nursing, 25*(2), 88-100.

71. Wojcik, M., & Dennison, D. (2006). Photoselective vaporization of the prostate in ambulatory surgery. *AORN Journal, 83*(2), 330-334, 337-340, 343-345, 347-350.

72. Wong, Y., et al. (2006). Survival associated with treatment vs observation of localized prostate cancer in elderly men. *Journal of the American Medical Association, 296*(22), 2683-2693.

evolve *Did you remember to check out the bonus material on the Evolve website and the CD-ROM, including NCLEX®-Examination Style Review Questions, Open-Book Quizzes, and Chapter Review Audio Podcasts?*

http://evolve.elsevier.com/Black/medsurg

CHAPTER 39

Management of Women with Reproductive Disorders

Lianne F. Herbruck

Gynecologic disorders and their treatments often lead to temporary, and sometimes permanent, change in sexual functioning or sexual identity. They also have the potential to change a woman's perceived, or actual, body structure. Alterations in sexuality and body image have a major effect on some women's feminine identity, including feelings of shame, embarrassment, and other negative emotions. In the 19th century, the common medical view was that the reproductive organs dominated a woman's body. Some aspects of this view, which reduces women's identity to the functioning of their body parts, persist in modern culture. Nurses caring for women with reproductive disorders need to understand these implications in order to give adequate and supportive care to the client.

Pelvic pain is one of the most common problems experienced in women with disorders of the female reproductive system. See the Integrating Diagnostic Testing feature on p. 914 for an overview of possible causes of pelvic pain and related diagnostic tests and treatment.

MENSTRUAL DISORDERS

CULTURAL INFLUENCES

Attitudes toward menstruation are often culturally based, and adolescent girls may be taught a variety of folk beliefs and practices at the time of puberty. Some Hispanic cultures, for example, discourage menstruating females from walking barefooted, washing their hair, or taking showers or baths. In various cultures, menstruating women may be subject to restrictions on work and physical activities as well as rules related to the disposal of menstrual fluid and the proper disposal of sanitary napkins. Many cultures do not permit intercourse during menstruation as women are seen to be "unclean" at this time. Religions, including Islam and some forms of Judaism, require or encourage women to engage in certain practices during and after menstruation. There are also some religions that are strictly against use of contraceptives, sterilization, and abortion. As a result of various cultural and religious influences, one can understand that reproductive disorders can have far-reaching effects on women. The nurse must be aware of, and sensitive to, different beliefs and respect cultural practices.

REACTIONS TO MANIFESTATIONS

Many women experience some menstrual problems during the 30 or more menstrual years of their reproductive life. Obvious abnormalities, such as excessive and irregular vaginal bleeding, cause women to seek medical care. Less obvious menstrual problems are often not brought to the attention of health care providers. And, for various reasons, some women do not seek care at all. For example, one woman may be unable to discuss menstruation as she views the subject as a personal and intimate problem that should be kept private. Another woman may have low self-esteem and may dismiss her own complaints as unimportant. Some women may not seek help, expecting the problems will disappear in time.

INTEGRATING DIAGNOSTIC TESTING

Pelvic Pain

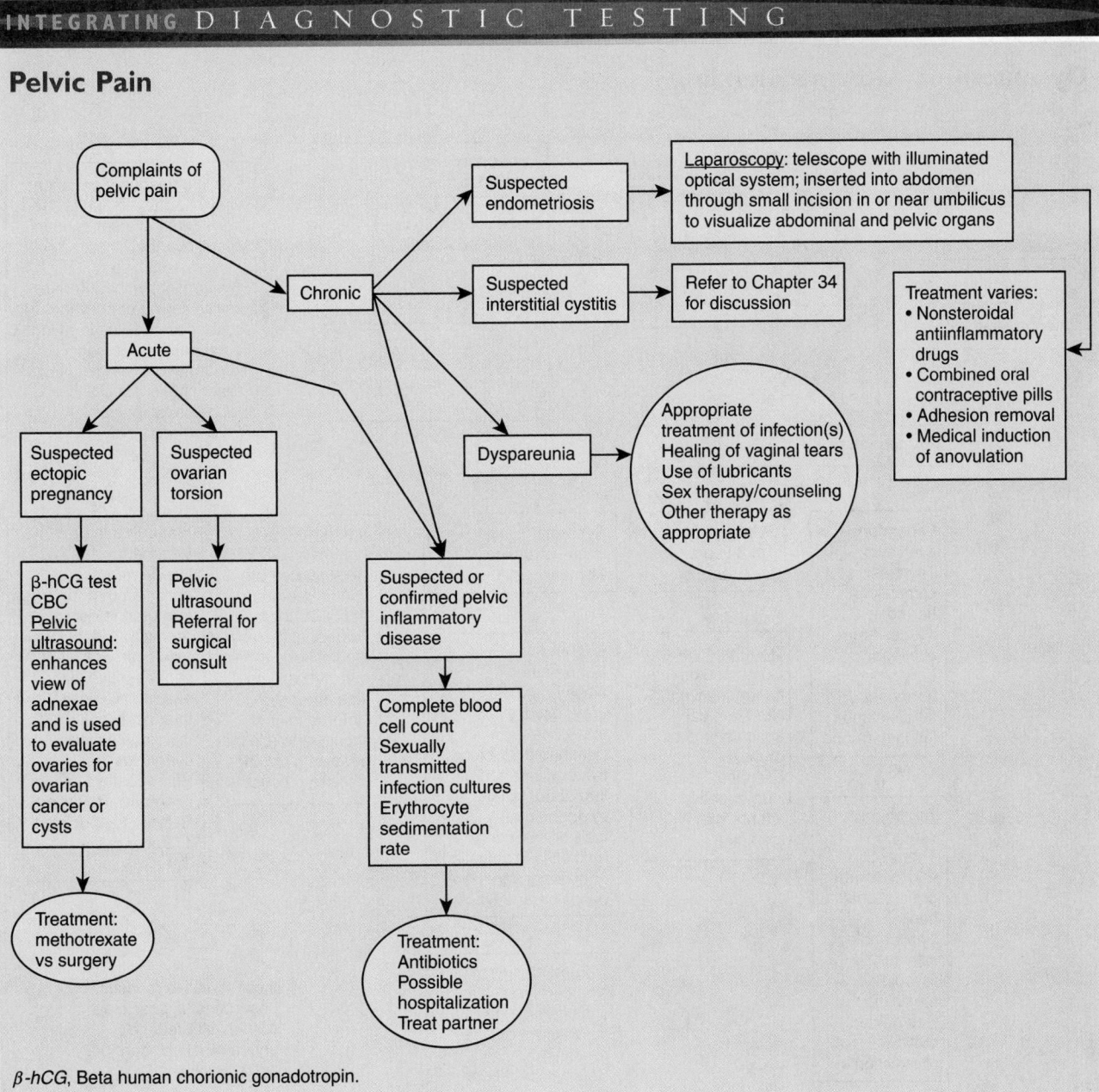

β-hCG, Beta human chorionic gonadotropin.

Others may desire a relief of manifestations, but may fear the potential treatment and/or diagnosis.

Opportunities for discovery of menstrual disorders may occur during a discussion of contraception or other client needs. It is not uncommon for menstrual problems to remain undetected unless the nurse is skillful and sensitive in assessment.

COMMON MENSTRUAL DISORDERS

Changes in menstrual patterns and associated manifestations can disrupt activities of daily living and create anxiety in many women. The presence of abnormal uterine bleeding necessitates careful assessment by a qualified health care provider as it may indicate underlying pathologic disease (see the Integrating Diagnostic Testing feature on p. 914).

Common menstrual disorders include dysmenorrhea, abnormal uterine bleeding, and premenstrual syndrome (PMS), which is discussed in the Complementary and Alternative Therapy feature on p. 915. Abnormal uterine bleeding encompasses a wide variety of menstrual disorders, including amenorrhea (Figure 39-1), menorrhagia, and metrorrhagia. Typical manifestations and treatments of these disorders are listed in Table 39-1. For a complete and in-depth review of menstrual disorders, please consult a women's health (obstetrics and gynecology) textbook.

INTEGRATING DIAGNOSTIC TESTING

Dysfunctional Uterine Bleeding

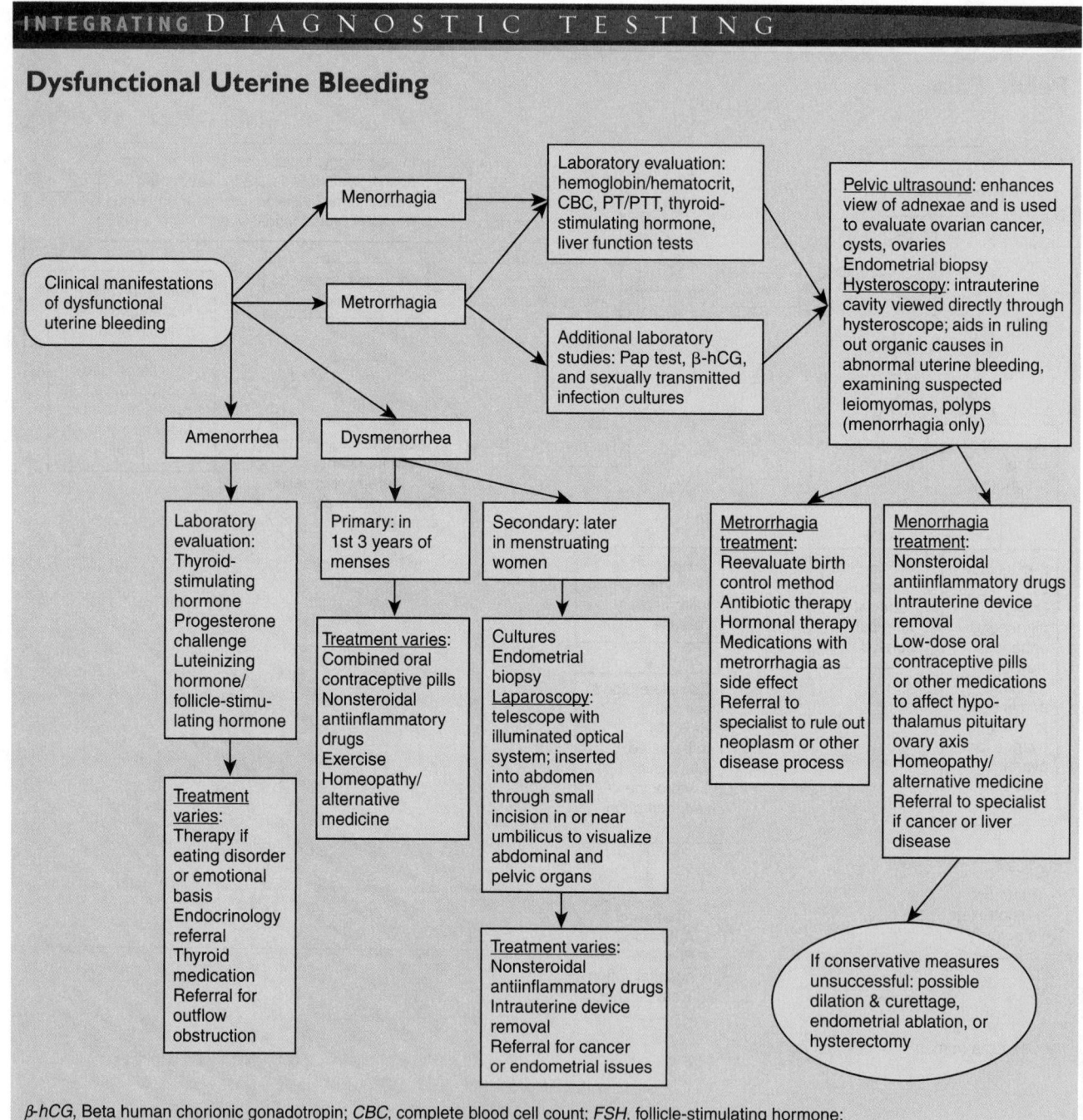

β-hCG, Beta human chorionic gonadotropin; *CBC*, complete blood cell count; *FSH*, follicle-stimulating hormone; *LFT*, liver function testing; *LH*, luteinizing hormone; *PT*, prothrombin time; *PTT*, partial thromboplastin time; *TSH*, thyroid-stimulating hormone.

MENOPAUSE

Physiologic menopause (cessation of menstruation) is discussed in the Unit 9 Anatomy and Physiology Review.

SURGICAL MENOPAUSE

Menopause may be induced at any age by surgical removal of the ovaries, ablation with chemicals, or pelvic irradiation. Removal of the uterus alone (hysterectomy) does not usually cause surgical menopause, although side effects from hysterectomies may produce menopausal manifestations.

PERIMENOPAUSAL CHANGES

A follicle-stimulating hormone (FSH) level greater than 40 milliunits/ml combined with a low serum

COMPLEMENTARY AND ALTERNATIVE THERAPY

Calcium Supplements and PMS

Calcium and vitamin D are known to reduce manifestations of premenstrual syndrome (PMS). Ovarian hormones, particularly estrogen, exhibit regulatory effects on calcium and vitamin D levels. As ovarian hormones increase during the menstrual cycle, calcium levels drop and this calcium dysregulation has been linked to PMS. Studies have shown that adding calcium supplements to the daily diet improves PMS manifestations in many women.[2,3] A new study assessed the role of daily calcium and vitamin D in decreasing the initial risk of PMS development. The study followed 3000 women over a period of 10 years. The study showed that women who had a daily intake of vitamin D and calcium equivalent to four servings had a lower risk of PMS development. A daily, balanced diet including skim milk, cheese,

yogurt, fortified orange juice, and spinach may reduce initial development of PMS.[1] Further study is warranted, but the results are promising. Other benefits of adequate calcium and vitamin D consumption are a decreased risk of osteoporosis and some cancers.

REFERENCES

1. Bertone-Jacobs, E., et al. (2005). Calcium and Vitamin D intake and risk of incident premenstrual syndrome. *Archives of Internal Medicine, 165*(11), 1246-1252.
2. Thys-Jacobs, S. (2000). Micronutrients and the premenstrual syndrome: The case for calcium. *Journal of the American College of Nutrition, 19*(2), 220-227. Retrieved 11/11/06 from www.jacn.org/cgi/content/full/19/2/220#R37.
3. Thys-Jacobs, S., et al. (1998). Calcium carbonate and the premenstrual syndrome: Effects on premenstrual and menstrual symptoms. *American Journal of Obstetrics and Gynecology, 179*, 444-452.

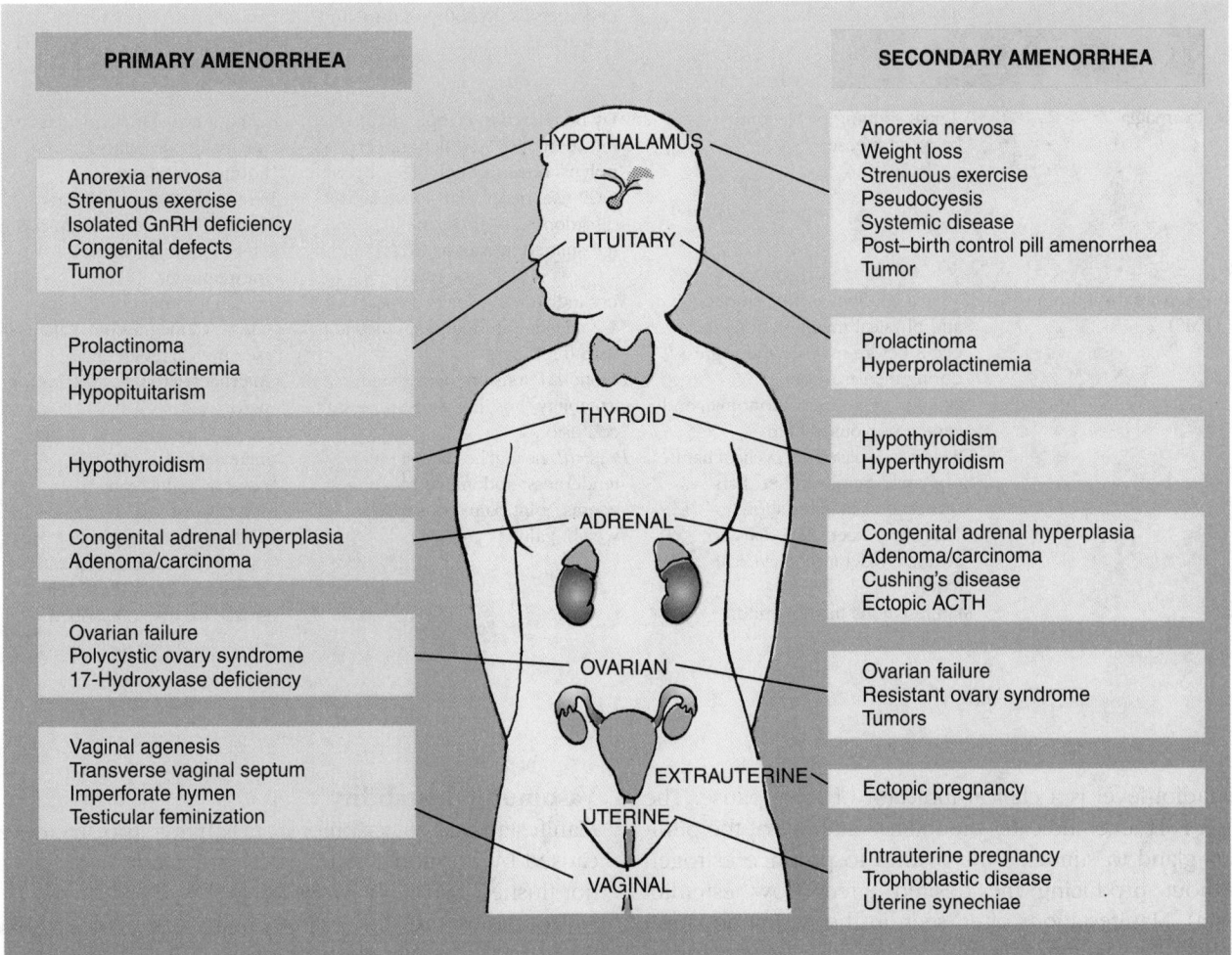

■ **FIGURE 39–1**   Primary and secondary causes of amenorrhea. *ACTH*, Adrenocorticotropic hormone; *GnRH*, gonadotropin-releasing hormone.

TABLE 39-1 Common Menstrual Disorders

Disorder	Definition	Manifestations	Management
Amenorrhea	Absence of menses *Primary amenorrhea* is diagnosed if woman has not begun to menstruate by age 16	Commonly results from pregnancy	Rule out pregnancy
Both primary and secondary have a number of potential causes, many of which can overlap (see Figure 39-3)	*Secondary amenorrhea* is absence of menses for 6 months in woman who previously had regular cyclic bleeding or 12 months in woman with history of irregular bleeding	Also associated with defects along hypothalamic-pituitary-ovarian-uterine axis, strenuous exercise, eating disorders, oral contraceptive pill (OCP) use, illness, and outflow obstructions	Refer to endocrinologist if underlying hormonal problem suspected Counsel and educate regarding weight control, body image, excessive exercise and stress; psych consult if necessary
Dysmenorrhea	Painful periods *Primary* begins 1-2 days before menses and subsides within 24 hr of flow; related to excess prostaglandin *Secondary* usually associated with underlying pathology or disease such as endometriosis	Sharp, crampy pain in suprapubic area that may radiate to thighs or back Nausea, vomiting, diarrhea; related to ovulatory cycles Dull pain in lower abdomen, back, and thighs Bloating and pelvic fullness occasionally with heavy flow	Primary and secondary manifestations are treated same NSAID therapy, OCP use, prostaglandin synthesis inhibitors, ibuprofen, naproxen Treat or remove underlying pathology to improve outcome with secondary
Menorrhagia	Excessive vaginal bleeding at normal cyclical intervals Difficult to accurately define "excessive blood," 3-4 saturated pads or tampons in 4 hr usually excessive	Hemoglobin/hematocrit may show anemia Related to anovulatory cycles, uterine fibroids, lesions, spontaneous abortions, IUD use, endometritis, hypothyroidism, and cancer	Accurate diagnosis; rule out pregnancy, IUD removal; use of estrogen and progestins, OCPs, NSAID therapy, antifibrinolytic agents. Endometrial biopsy to determine cause, endometrial ablation to destroy tissue (may cause sterility)
Metrorrhagia	Vaginal spotting or bleeding between menses	May be related to ectopic pregnancy, infections, IUD, ovulation, cervical polyps, breakthrough bleeding with OCP use, neoplasias, coagulation disorders, cancer, sexually transmitted infections (STIs)	Rule out pregnancy, malignant/nonmalignant tumors, hormonal abnormalities Treat underlying conditions Change OCP course or dosing Refer to appropriate specialist for treatment
Premenstrual syndrome (PMS)	Cyclical combination of emotional and physical manifestations that occur before menses and regress during menstruation Involves endocrine, autonomic, and central nervous systems Diagnosis is based on cyclical nature of manifestations rather than presence of manifestations Clients may keep PMS diary to accurately determine cyclical nature Manifestations may be mild, moderate, or severe	Very individual, usually appear 1-2 days before menses, relieved with full flow *Emotional:* tension, depression, irritability, hostility, forgetfulness, confusion *Physical:* headache, breast tenderness, abdominal bloating, edema, joint pain, constipation, weight gain	Vitamin and mineral therapy (B_6, A, C, magnesium, calcium) (see the Complementary and Alternative Therapy feature on p. 915) Decrease caffeine and alcohol, increase water Analgesics, aldactone to decrease edema OCPs may reduce physiologic and psychological elements Sometimes Zoloft, Paxil, or Prozac may be prescribed

estradiol level is a clinical indicator of menopause. The high FSH level indicates the intense attempt of the pituitary gland to stimulate the ovaries to produce estrogen without producing the desired effect (low estradiol level). Manifestations often seen in the perimenopausal period are vasomotor instability, menstrual irregularities, and vaginal changes (Box 39-1).

Vasomotor Instability

Manifestations of vasomotor instability appear to be caused by hormonal changes. They include hot flashes, hot flushes, and night sweats.

Hot flashes are sudden involuntary waves of heat that begin in the upper chest or neck and proceed up the face and head. They can be mild, moderate, or severe

BOX 39-1   Clinical Manifestations of Menopause

- Hot flashes
- Night sweats
- Changes in menstrual bleeding, culminating in complete cessation of menses
- Mood swings
- Fatigue
- Insomnia
- Irritability
- Anxiety
- Depression
- Incontinence
- Vaginal dryness
- Dyspareunia
- Decreased libido
- Memory loss
- Pelvic organ prolapse
- Headaches
- Increased risk of cardiovascular disease
- Osteoporosis and increased hip fracture risk
- Brittle nails, thinning hair, and dry skin
- Water retention and weight gain
- Joint pain
- Backache

and are experienced by 68% to 92% of perimenopausal women. The sensations last from a few seconds to an hour and are exacerbated by anything that increases heat production in the body. Severe hot flashes can be extremely disruptive to daily activities. A hot flash may be accompanied by a hot flush, which is defined by measurable change in skin temperature, visibly flushed skin, and perspiration. A night sweat is a hot flash that occurs in the night, is accompanied by perspiration, and is often followed by chills.

Atrophic Vaginitis and Other Changes

Atrophic vaginitis is defined as an inflammation of the vagina. The decrease in estrogen during, and following, menopause thins vaginal mucosal tissue and decreases lubrication, which can result in increased vaginal sensitivity and susceptibility to infection. Common clinical manifestations are vaginal irritation, burning, pruritus, increased leukorrhea (vaginal discharge), bleeding, and dyspareunia (difficult or painful intercourse).

Urogenital changes related to the loss of the estrogen-rich mucosal layer of the urethra might play a role in the higher incidence of cystitis and urethritis. The pubococcygeus muscles tend to lose their tone, and stress incontinence (see Chapter 34) may occur.

Estrogen has been shown to inhibit bone breakdown and loss. The decrease or absence of estrogen during menopause, in conjunction with other risk factors, such as loss of bone calcium, predisposes women to osteoporosis. Complaints of depression or other emotional changes at menopause are common in some women more than at any other time in their lives, though no relationship between depression and menopause has been clinically demonstrated.

OUTCOME MANAGEMENT

Medical Management

Evaluate Use of Hormone Replacement Therapy (HRT)

HRT may be part of the medical management of perimenopausal, menopausal, and postmenopausal manifestations. HRT can alleviate vasomotor instability, vaginal and urinary tract atrophy, and dyspareunia. However, women must be educated about the advantages and risks of HRT so that they can make informed decisions about treatment.[62] Several studies, described in the Translating Evidence into Practice feature on p. 918, report the benefits and risks of long-term use of HRT.

Fears related to HRT use and potential increases in the incidence of breast and uterine cancer cause confusion for many women trying to adequately alleviate their menopausal manifestations. In the middle to late 1970s, an association between unopposed (estrogen without progestin) estrogen replacement therapy (ERT) and endometrial cancer was discovered. This association has been studied extensively and ERT is no longer recommended for a woman with an intact uterus. Instead, estrogen is given with progestin as progestin provides a protective effect against endometrial cancer.

For the client whose uterus has been surgically removed, ERT is recommended because progestin may unfavorably alter the ratio of high-density-lipoprotein (HDL) and low-density-lipoprotein (LDL) cholesterol. Transdermal estrogen patches are an alternative when oral estrogens cannot be tolerated. Vaginal estrogen is indicated for any woman experiencing urogenital manifestations of menopause. Box 39-2 lists contraindications and possible uses for ERT.

Recent research findings suggest that hormone replacement therapy be taken for only 5 years.[15] ERT or HRT use must be individualized according to the client's needs, wishes, risks, and individual manifestations. In clients opting for ERT or HRT, risks should be assessed for osteoporosis, cardiovascular disease, and breast or endometrial cancer. Clients should be monitored for the development of breast cancer with annual breast examinations and mammography. Women must receive adequate education regarding anticipated effects of HRT, as well as manifestations of potential complications.

Hormone Replacement Therapy

The clinical manifestations that occur during perimenopause and menopause and their long-term sequelae often make women anxious about entering this phase of their reproductive life. Because estrogen deprivation has been associated with these changes, hormone replacement has been used and advocated to decrease or eliminate the annoying manifestations, improve cardiovascular health, and lessen the incidence of osteoporosis.

For the woman with an intact uterus, the common therapy is HRT, which is a hormone therapy consisting of both estrogen and progestin. The presence of progestin in this combined regimen protects the woman from endometrial hyperplasia, which is a potentially precancerous condition that is the forerunner to uterine cancer. Women who do not have a uterus are able to take estrogen only as replacement therapy (ERT). With the elimination of vasomotor manifestations, reduced pelvic floor dysfunction, and improvement in cardiovascular and osteoporosis risk, hormone replacement appeared to significantly improve clinical manifestations of menopause, while offering some protection from the risks of life-threatening conditions associated with menopause.

However, HRT and ERT have not come without their own set of associated risk factors and negative side effects. This has raised many questions surrounding the risks versus benefits of prescribing hormonal therapy to menopausal women. The Heart and Estrogen/Progestin Replacement Study (HERS) reported observational data that suggest no overall benefit to HRT with an unexpected excess of cardiovascular events.[3,5] In the Women's Health Initiative (WHI) Estrogen with Progestin trial, researchers found an increased risk of breast cancer, heart attack, stroke, and blood clots in the women taking HRT as opposed to women taking placebo. The trial was stopped in 2002 as these risks outweighed the benefits of reduced hip fracture and decreased risk of colorectal cancer.[11-13]

The WHI also ran a trial to evaluate estrogen replacement alone. In contrast to the HRT study, estrogen alone does not appear to increase the risk of breast cancer, particularly early stage and ductal, in postmenopausal women. However, this study was stopped in 2004 as researchers found ERT to be associated with a higher risk of stroke, and had no significant impact on overall cardiovascular health.[4,12] Data also showed that women who had lower overall risks for breast cancer had fewer incidences of breast cancer when taking estrogen, while women who were at higher risk were more likely to have breast cancer while taking estrogen when compared to their counterparts receiving placebo. Women receiving estrogen were also more likely to have abnormal mammograms and a higher incidence of biopsy than women administered placebo.[11,12]

Other data suggest that estrogen and progestin increase the incidence of dementia and do not prevent mild cognitive impairment in postmenopausal women.[7,8] Both ERT and HRT decrease the risk of osteoporosis and are considered preventive measures against osteoporosis but neither is as effective as alendronate (Fosamax) alone.[2] Combination therapy with HRT and alendronate was the most effective in prevention of bone loss in older women.[2] The optimal duration of therapy for osteoporosis prevention is not known but is considered lifelong. Raloxifene (Evista), an estrogen receptor modulator, prevents osteoporosis and may provide cardioprotective effects without increasing cancer risk. Raloxifene cannot be given to women who are taking HRT and ERT.

Alternative supplements for the treatment of menopause have been under consideration. Phytoestrogens are a group of chemicals found in plants that mimic estrogen. They may offer protection against a wide range of human conditions, including breast cancer, cardiovascular disease, cognitive dysfunction, osteoporosis, and menopausal manifestations. High concentrations of phytoestrogens can be found in legumes, such as soybeans, soy products, chickpeas, red clover, sweet potatoes, carrots, garlic, and green beans. Clinical application must be fully established. Adding phytoestrogens to the diet may offer a safe, and less expensive, alternative to HRT and ERT therapy.[1,6,10]

IMPLICATIONS

Much controversy exists in the literature regarding whether women should begin, or continue, to take hormone replacement therapy with the onset of menopause. This important decision, made cooperatively by the client and health care professional, must be individualized, and based on the client's health and familial risks, as well as her specific clinical manifestations of menopause. The best use of HRT or ERT would be a regimen that relieves manifestations of menopause using the smallest dose possible for the shortest duration. HRT should not be used to combat chronic disease. Nurses have the opportunity to discuss and provide the necessary education regarding choices in treatment of menopausal manifestations and menopausal disease prevention.

REFERENCES

1. Ewies, Anyman. (2002). Phytoestrogens in the management of the menopause. *Obstetrics & Gynecology Survey, 57*(5), 306-311.
2. Greenspan, S., Resnick, N., & Parker, R. (2003). Combination therapy with hormone replacement and alendronate for prevention of bone loss in elderly women: A randomized controlled trial. *Journal of the American Medical Association, 289*(19), 2525-2533.
3. Grady, D., et al. (2002). Cardiovascular disease outcomes during 6.8 years of hormone therapy: Heart and estrogen/progestin replacement study follow-up (HERS II). *Journal of the American Medical Association, 288*(1), 49-57.
4. Hsia, J., et al. (2006). Conjugated equine estrogens and coronary heart disease. *Archives of Internal Medicine, 166*(3), 357-365.
5. Hlatky, M.A., et al. (2002). Quality-of-life symptoms in postmenopausal women after receiving hormone therapy: Results from the Heart and Estrogen/Progestin Replacement Study (HERS) trial. *Journal of the American Medical Association, 287*(5), 591-597.
6. Marsden, J., & A'Hern, R. (2003). Progestogens and breast cancer risk: The role of hormonal contraceptives and hormone replacement therapy. *Journal of Family Planning and Reproductive Health Care, 29*(4), 185-187.
7. Rapp, S., et al. (2003). Effect of estrogen plus progestin on global cognitive function in postmenopausal women. The Women's Health Initiative Memory Study: A randomized controlled trial. *Journal of the American Medical Association, 289*(20), 2663-2672.
8. Shumacher, S., et al. (2003). Estrogen plus progestin and the incidence of dementia and mild cognitive impairment in postmenopausal women. The Women's Health Initiative Memory Study: A randomized controlled trial. *Journal of the American Medical Association, 289*(20), 2651-2662.
9. Tagliaferri, M., Cohen, I., & Tripathy, D. (2006). *The new menopause book*. New York: Avery.
10. Tsourounis, C. (2001). Clinical effects of phytoestrogens. *Clinical Obstetrics & Gynecology, 44*(4), 836-842.
11. Women's Health Initiative. (2006). *Effects of conjugated equine estrogens on breast cancer and mammography in postmenopausal women with hysterectomy.* Retrieved 11/16/06 from www.whi.org/findings/ht/ealone_bc.php.
12. Women's Health Initiative. (2006). *Women's Health Initiative updated analysis: No increased risk of breast cancer with estrogen alone.* Retrieved 11/16/06 from www.nhlbi.nih.gov/new/press/06-04-11a.htm.
13. Writing Group for the Women's Health Initiative Investigators. (2002). Risks and benefits of estrogen plus progestin in healthy postmenopausal women: Principal results from the Women's Health Initiative randomized controlled trial. *Journal of the American Medical Association, 288*, 321-333.

BOX 39-2   Estrogen Use and Contraindications

ABSOLUTE CONTRAINDICATIONS

- Known or suspected breast or uterine cancer, or any estrogen-dependent cancer or strong family history of the same
- Undiagnosed abnormal uterine bleeding
- Previous or present thrombophlebitis
- Impaired liver function
- Acute liver disease
- Pregnancy

USE WITH CAREFUL EVALUATION AND MONITORING

- Vascular disease, including phlebitis
- Diabetes mellitus
- Hypertension
- Uterine fibroids
- Migraine headaches
- Endometriosis
- Gallbladder disease
- Obesity and heavy smoking, especially in combination with vascular disease or hypertension

---

Nursing Management of the Medical Client

Provide Education

Nurses have a unique role in providing support, education, and assistance for women going through menopause and their partners or significant others. Accurate information about menopause and what to expect can be helpful and reassuring. Provide educational information about the risks and benefits of hormone therapy. Offer advice and adjuvant therapies to help clients cope with minor discomforts of menopause. This topic is addressed in the Complementary and Alternative Therapy box below.

POSTMENOPAUSAL BLEEDING

Postmenopausal bleeding (vaginal bleeding occurring after menopause) is a manifestation, not a diagnosis, and is never a normal finding. Careful assessment is necessary because it may indicate one of many conditions of the lower reproductive tract (Figure 39-2).

COMPLEMENTARY AND ALTERNATIVE THERAPY

Alternative Medicines for Hot Flashes and Minor Discomforts of Menopause

Phytoestrogens are plant estrogens and can be found in soy products, flaxseed, nuts, and brown rice. Their estrogen is similar to a woman's natural estrogen and they have a mild estrogenic effect on the body. One analysis of randomized controlled trials for hot flashes or reduction of menopausal manifestations showed that soy provided some benefit in 6 of the 11 randomized trials.[3] However, a recent review of the literature concluded no clear benefit of soy food or extracts or red clover in reducing hot flashes or other manifestations of menopause.[1,2] Further clinical study is needed to evaluate usefulness and safety of these products. Other natural hormones (estriol, progesterone, and androgens) have the potential to relieve manifestations of menopause without the negative side effects of synthetic hormones, but also need further clinical study.[4]

Relaxation techniques such as yoga, meditation, and imagery may help menopausal manifestations. Yoga has the potential to increase flexibility and strengthen bones, as well as balancing the endocrine system, which can help restore balance to the hormonal changes taking place. Yoga may also help women deal with the emotional stress of the transition.[4]

Performance of Kegel exercises can increase pelvic floor muscle tone. Intercourse and masturbation aid circulation and keep vaginal tissues flexible. Using water-soluble vaginal lubricants, topical estrogen creams, or other vaginal estrogen preparations reduces or improves vaginal manifestations.

Remind women experiencing menopause of the value of good health habits. Balanced nutrition, adequate sleep, and rest are important. Regular exercise improves bone and cardiovascular health. Participation in weight-bearing exercises, increase of calcium intake, cessation of smoking, and reduction of alcohol and caffeine intake all may help decrease risks of osteoporosis as well as manifestations of menopause. Maintaining a good sense of humor can also help women through the transition.

REFERENCES

1. Dennehy, C.E. (2006). The use of herbs and dietary supplements in gynecology: An evidence-based review. *Journal of Midwifery and Women's Health, 51*(6), 420-409.
2. Krebs, E.E., et al. (2004). Phytoestrogens for treatment of menopausal symptoms: A systematic review. *Obstetrics and Gynecology, 104*, 824-836.
3. Kronenberg, F., & Fugh-Berman, A. (2002). Complementary and alternative medicine for menopausal symptoms: A review of randomized, controlled trials. *Annals of Internal Medicine, 137*, 805-813.
4. Tagliaferri, M., Cohen, I., & Tripathy, D. (2006). *The new menopause book*. New York: Avery.

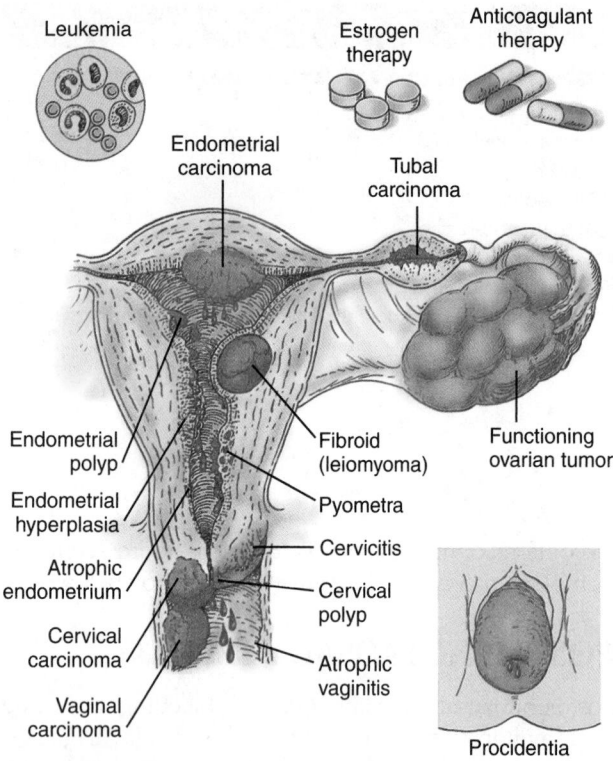

FIGURE 39–2 Causes of postmenopausal bleeding.

PELVIC INFLAMMATORY DISEASE

The term pelvic inflammatory disease (PID) refers to ascending pelvic infection that involves the upper genital tract. The most common complication seen with PID is a pelvic abscess.

Etiology and Risk Factors

Common causes of PID include *Chlamydia trachomatis,* gonococci, staphylococci, streptococci, and other pus-producing (pyogenic) organisms as well as untreated bacterial infections. Most infections are sexually transmitted infections (STIs), and lack of condom use increases the risk of passing bacteria between partners.

Health promotion advice for clients includes avoiding (1) unprotected intercourse, (2) an intrauterine device (IUD) for birth control, (3) sex with multiple partners, especially with use of an IUD, and (4) douches. Immunization with the vaccine to prevent human papillomavirus is another health promotion activity. To maintain health, clients should seek treatment immediately when manifestations of PID appear, or if a sexual partner has a known STI.

Health restoration activities include advising clients to complete the full course of medications used to treat PID and to follow health promotion recommendations to prevent reinfection.

Pathophysiology

Bacterial infections in the upper genital tract may travel along several routes. *C. trachomatis,* gonococcal and staphylococcal organisms tend to spread across the endometrium to the fallopian tubes, causing acute salpingitis (inflammation of the fallopian tubes). If the tubes become occluded, they may drain pus, leukocytes, and other debris into the pelvic cavity, causing pelvic peritonitis. This material may also form a pocket around the ovary, causing a tubo-ovarian abscess.

Streptococci spread similarly, but tend to travel via the uterine or cervical lymphatics across the parametrium to the tubes or ovaries. Pelvic cellulitis and occasional thrombophlebitis of the major pelvic veins may occur. Another route of infection is from the pelvic cavity itself. Organisms such as *Escherichia coli* may come from a ruptured bowel, causing peritonitis.

Scarring of the fallopian tubes by the inflammatory process causes more than 50% of women with a history of PID to have difficulty becoming pregnant or to experience an ectopic pregnancy.

Clinical Manifestations

PID may be "silent" (asymptomatic), especially in its early stages. Clinical manifestations of PID include malaise, fever, chills, anorexia, nausea and vomiting, aching, and tachycardia. The woman usually experiences acute, sharp, severe aching pain on both sides of the abdomen or pelvis that is worsened by urination or defecation and may be accompanied by a heavy, purulent, and, possibly, odorous discharge. Occasionally, vaginal bleeding occurs. Onset of PID depends on (1) the virulence (degree of severity) of the infecting organism, (2) the status of the client's pelvic organs, and (3) the client's general health.

Significant historical information related to PID includes any acute lower genital tract infection and choice of contraception (IUD use correlates with a higher incidence of PID). A thorough sexual history is important.

The long-term sequelae of untreated, silent PID may be detected when attempts to achieve a pregnancy are unsuccessful. During a clinical evaluation of the client, routine screening tests, such as cultures, may yield positive results. Cultures of any drainage may be tested for infection, and histologic examination of endometrial biopsy specimens, colposcopy (examination with use of a large color-filtering, magnifying instrument), or ultrasonography to identify an abscess may also be used in the diagnosis of PID.

OUTCOME MANAGEMENT

Medical Management

Eliminate Causative Organism

Most clients with PID are treated as outpatients, receiving antibiotics appropriate to the specific organism causing the infection. Hospitalization may be necessary for a client with PID who is acutely ill. During hospitalization, antibiotics are administered in maximal doses if the cause of PID is bacterial.

Surgical Management

Some abscesses must be removed by surgical intervention. The type of surgical intervention and its timing, either acute or after initial medical management, vary with the health care provider's philosophy. Risk of surgery must be balanced against that of continuing unsuccessful medical therapy, which often leads to chronic PID.

Nursing Management of the Medical-Surgical Client

Promote Drainage and Comfort

Pain management is important. Sitz baths or heat applied to the lower back or abdomen, along with analgesic use, may reduce pain. The nurse must assist with frequent perineal care, as well as documenting any vaginal discharge. The woman should maintain a semi-Fowler's position in bed to promote drainage.

Provide Support

Psychosocial support of the client is imperative. Feelings of guilt and emotional stress are common as PID is often caused by STIs. Some women are infertile after PID. This loss of fertility may be difficult for the client and her significant other to accept. Plan time for and encourage the expression of client feelings.

Provide Education

Education is important for the client with PID. Discuss the infection and recognizing clinical manifestations of recurrence. The client should be instructed in general hygienic practices, such as regular washing of the perineal area with soap and water, wiping from front to back after elimination, changing tampons and pads several times a day during menses, and washing hands before and after changing tampons or pads. Inform clients when sexual activity can be resumed, and discuss safe sexual practices.

CHRONIC PELVIC INFLAMMATORY DISEASE

Chronic PID can occur if the acute phase of the illness does not respond to treatment or if treatment is inadequate. Clinical manifestations of chronic PID include chronic pelvic discomfort, menstrual disturbances or dysfunctional uterine bleeding, constipation, malaise,

and periodic return of acute manifestations. Sterility, which results from destruction of part of the fallopian tubes and loss of their patency, is one of the more serious complications.

Treatment of chronic PID is aimed at removing the offending organism and improving the client's general health. If treatment is unsuccessful, surgical removal of the pelvic organs may be necessary.

UTERINE DISORDERS

ENDOMETRIOSIS

Endometriosis is an abnormal condition in which endometrial tissue is found in internal sites other than the uterus. The most common site of tissue relocation is the pelvic cavity, especially the ovaries and dependent portions of the pelvic peritoneum. Rarely, tissue may lie outside the pelvis, such as in surgical scars and the lungs (Figure 39-3). Overall incidence in women of reproductive age is 5% to 10%. However, it may be more prevalent as up to 25% of cases are asymptomatic and can be a secondary finding during pelvic surgery or exploration for other reasons. Women in their mid-30s are most commonly affected, though it can appear anytime from first menses to menopause. There is a familial predisposition.

Etiology and Risk Factors

The cause of endometriosis is unknown, although several theories have been proposed. Retrograde menstruation, the most accepted theory, asserts that menstrual secretions flow backward through the fallopian tubes and deposit particles of viable endometrial tissue outside the uterine cavity. The endometrial tissue then reproduces itself on pelvic structures. The vascular and lymphatic dissemination theory contends that the metastasis of endometrial tissue occurs through the lymphatic and vascular systems to locations outside the uterus. This may explain some of the distant sites of metastasis, such as the lungs and kidneys.

Pathophysiology

However endometriosis reaches its destination, the translocated endometrial tissue responds to hormonal stimulation, regardless of location, and bleeds, producing a variety of manifestations. Scarring, inflammation, and adhesions occur at extrauterine sites, causing organs and peritoneal surfaces to become fixed to each other.

Infertility is a major complication of endometriosis. Usually, the infertility is due to scarring, which leads to obstruction of the fallopian tubes.

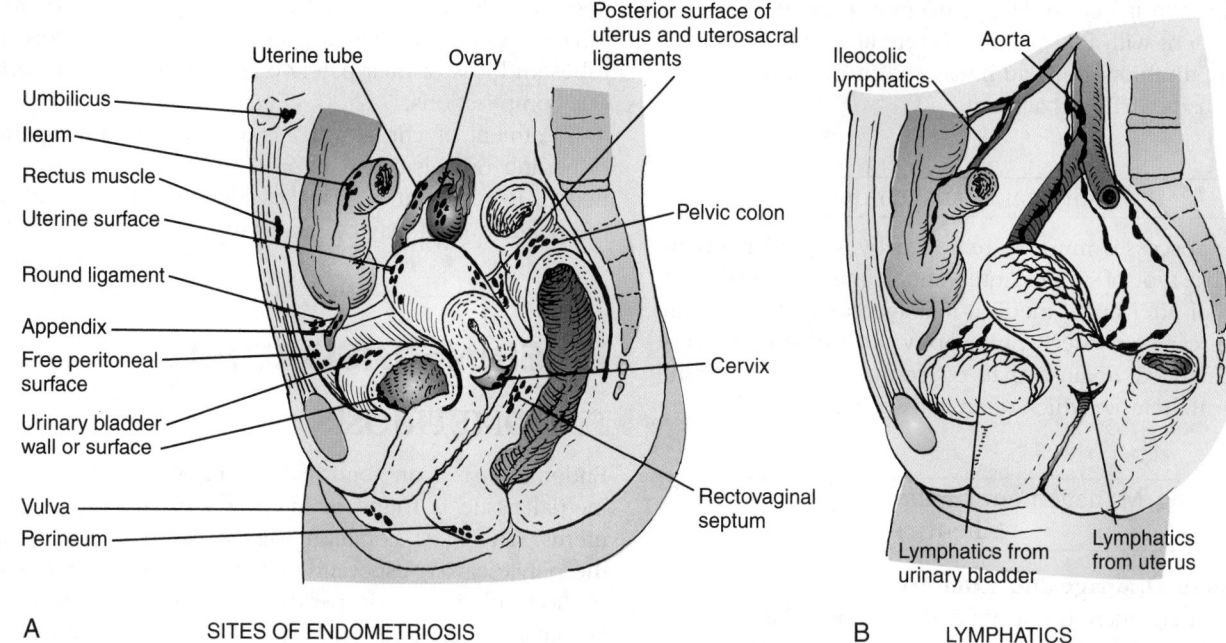

A   SITES OF ENDOMETRIOSIS   B   LYMPHATICS

■ **FIGURE 39–3** Endometriosis. **A,** Sites of endometriosis. The locations most frequently affected are the ovaries and the dependent pelvic peritoneum. However, many other sites may be involved. **B,** Pelvic and lymph nodes are important.

Clinical Manifestations

Manifestations of endometriosis relate more to the site than to the extent of disease present. Pain is the most characteristic manifestation. Pain typically begins before the menstrual period, reaching its peak just before onset, or during the first 1 to 2 days of the flow. Pain can last for the duration of menstruation and sometimes for several days afterward. Pain may be located in several areas, making the diagnosis more difficult to confirm.

Other manifestations of endometriosis are dyspareunia, menstrual irregularities, and infertility. Endometriosis inside the ovary can produce a "chocolate" cyst, or endometrioma. Severe pain is associated with the presence, or rupture, of this cyst. Implants of endometrium on the ureters may cause urinary obstruction. Bowel involvement may cause painful defecation, bleeding, diarrhea, or obstruction.

History and pelvic examination are important. Direct observation of lesions through laparoscopy or surgery is necessary for a definitive diagnosis.

 OUTCOME MANAGEMENT

Medical Management

Appropriate treatment of endometriosis depends on the client's manifestations, age, number of children (parity), and extent of disease. With mild manifestations, the client is given support, information, and coping strategies. Additional treatment is generally necessary if manifestations become severe or the disease progresses. If the client desires pregnancy, nonsteroidal anti-inflammatory drug (NSAID) therapy during menstruation is often her best option.

Reduce Manifestations

Hormonal medications that suppress estrogen production in order to reduce lesion growth can be used to relieve manifestations in women with severe disease, or who do not desire pregnancy. Continuous use of a low ratio estrogen-to-progestin oral contraceptive (OCP) may shrink endometrial tissue and reduce its function in abnormal sites. This type of treatment is not successful in all women.

Other hormonal treatments are geared to medically induce menopause. The gonadotropin-releasing hormone (GnRH) agonists leuprolide (Lupron) and nafarelin (Synarel) suppress secretions of the pituitary gonadotropins luteinizing hormone (LH) and FSH. This suppression ultimately decreases ovarian function. Although these medications effectively help shrink endometrial tissue, relieve pain, and prevent further tissue growth, they produce menopausal side effects.

Danazol (Danocrine) is an androgenic synthetic steroid and its use ultimately causes anovulation and hypogonadotropism, resulting in amenorrhea and regression of endometriosis. Androgenic side effects may include acne, hirsutism (excess hair), weight gain, decreased breast size, hot flashes, and vaginal dryness. Danazol may not fully suppress ovulation, so contraception is indicated.

Surgical Management

Surgical management is also dictated by severity of disease, age of client and desire for childbearing. The only definitive cure is total abdominal hysterectomy with bilateral salpingo-oophorectomy (TAH-BSO), which is the removal of uterus, cervix, fallopian tubes, and ovaries. This causes surgically induced menopause and permanent sterility. TAH-BSO is used when other measures have failed and the client does not wish to preserve fertility.

Conservative surgical intervention is available for women who desire childbearing capabilities. The goal of conservative surgery is to restore normal anatomy and remove adhesions and endometrial implants.

Nursing Management of the Medical-Surgical Client

Nursing care of the client with endometriosis consists of support during the diagnostic process as the client considers the various treatment options. Psychosocial support is a priority as issues related to pain and infertility can affect self-esteem and take an emotional toll on the client. Nursing interventions should include discussion of information about the nature of endometriosis, its treatment, and ways to cope with the manifestations.

Surgical management is similar to that discussed for abdominal hysterectomy, tubal ligation, or laparoscopy (see later discussion).

BENIGN UTERINE TUMORS (LEIOMYOMAS)

Leiomyomas (fibroids, fibromas, fibromyomas, fibroleiomyomas, and myomas) are benign uterine tumors that arise from the uterine muscle tissue. They are the most common tumors of the female genital tract and occur in 20% to 30% of women. They are seen more often in African-American women, and are more common in women approaching menopause.

Etiology and Risk Factors

The cause of leiomyomas is unknown. However, their growth seems to be related to estrogen stimulation as the fibroids often enlarge with pregnancy and OCP use, and shrink with menopause. There may also be a genetic component.

Pathophysiology

Leiomyomas develop from the uterine myometrium. A leiomyoma begins as a simple proliferation of smooth muscle cells. It is suggested that this proliferation occurs at points of maximal stress within the myometrium. Because there are many points of stress within the uterus resulting from contractions, fibroids are often multiple (Figure 39-4).

Classification

Leiomyomas are classified according to their location, with those occurring in the uterine body the most common (Box 39-3).

Clinical Manifestations

Frequently, leiomyomas are asymptomatic. Manifestations relate to tumor size, location, and number. The most common clinical manifestation is abnormal uterine bleeding, which may be excessive in amount or duration. Anemia may result from the hypermenorrhea with manifestations of tiredness, weakness, and lethargy. Other common manifestations may include dysmenorrhea, pelvic pressure, urinary frequency or retention, and back pain. Less common manifestations include constipation, abdominal pain, and dyspareunia (painful intercourse). The tumor may or may not be palpable.

Clients with leiomyomas may experience sterility, or have a history of one or more spontaneous abortions. Because manifestations regress with the lowered estrogenic state of menopause, any new manifestations developing during these years, must be carefully assessed to rule out other disease processes, such as cancer.

Diagnosis is generally established via a characteristic history, and confirmed by findings of abdominal and pelvic examinations. Ultrasonography may demonstrate an abnormal uterine shape.

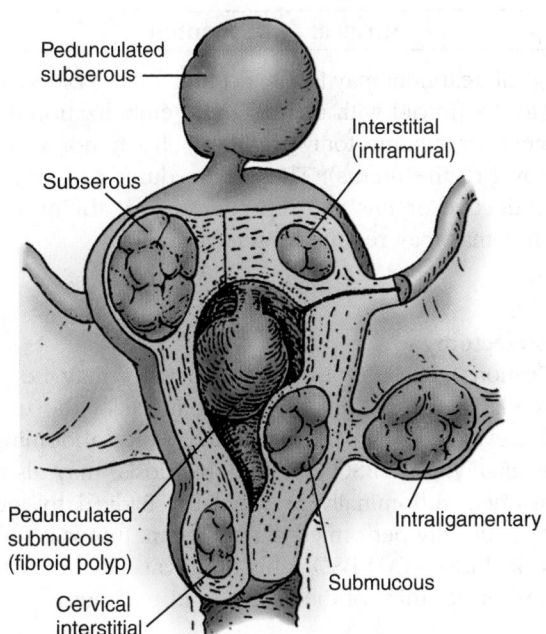

■ **FIGURE 39–4** Sites of leiomyomas (fibroids). Uterine leiomyomas, depending on their location and size, may interfere with passage of sperm and implantation of a fertilized ovum.

BOX 39-3	Types of Uterine Leiomyomas
Type	**Description**
Intramural	In uterine wall, surrounded by myometrium
Submucosal	Under endometrium, involving endometrial cavity; may become pedunculated (grow on a stalk)
Subserosal	On outer surface (under serosa) of uterus; tend to become pedunculated, wandering, multiple, and large
Wandering or parasitic	Pedunculated leiomyoma that breaks off pedicle and attaches to other tissue, particularly omentum
Intraligamentous	Implants on pelvic ligaments
Cervical	Infrequent, may obstruct cervical canal

OUTCOME MANAGEMENT

Medical Management

Asymptomatic leiomyomas can be observed every 6 months by a practitioner if (1) the client is not pregnant, (2) there is no excessive bleeding or pressure on the bladder, bowel, or ureters, and (3) the tumor is not rapidly growing.

GnRH analogs (see Endometriosis earlier in this chapter) may be administered to reduce size and inhibit growth of tumors. Malignant degeneration is rare.

Surgical Management

Surgical treatment may involve cutting off the blood supply to the fibroid with uterine artery embolization, laser surgery, or myomectomy (removal of a tumor without removal of the uterus). These procedures preserve the reproductive organs and reproductive capability. Large leiomyomas may require hysterectomy.

Hysterectomy

Indications. Three types of hysterectomy may be performed. Total hysterectomy is a removal of the uterus and cervix, and can be performed either abdominally or vaginally. TAH-BSO (see Endometriosis) may also be performed abdominally or vaginally. Radical hysterectomy is usually performed if a malignant tumor is found and includes TAH-BSO plus removal of the lymph nodes, upper third of the vagina, and parametrium.

Contraindications. Contraindications to hysterectomy include health conditions that prevent surgery.

Complications. Hemorrhage and infection are the primary complications.

Outcomes. Pain, abnormal bleeding, and anemia, if present, will cease. For all procedures except myomectomy, menstruation ends.

Nursing Management of the Surgical Client

Preoperative Care

Obtain a thorough history from the client, especially if there are complaints of irregular bleeding, and assess the client's knowledge of her condition and her surgical options. Make sure she understands her options and the differences among proposed procedures. Listen carefully for any questions she has about sexuality after treatment.

Reduce Pain. Before surgery is performed, pain medications, sitz baths, or application of heat to the lower abdomen may be helpful in reducing discomfort.

Provide Education. If a hysterectomy is planned, be sure to discuss the loss of fertility. If TAH-BSO or radical hysterectomy is planned, discuss surgical menopause and its implications. Discuss how sexual intercourse may be affected after a (radical) hysterectomy because of the shortening of the vagina and possible scar tissue. This may cause dyspareunia, the pain of which may be felt deep in the pelvis. Tell the client that once healing has occurred, intercourse should be pain free. Let her know that there are methods to help women achieve this goal. Answer any questions, and encourage the client and her significant other to express their feelings and concerns about sexuality.

Postoperative Care

Assessment. The proximity of the bladder to the female reproductive organs increases the risk of urinary problems, which must be monitored postoperatively. A Foley catheter is usually inserted at the time of surgery and left in place for 24 hours. Catheterization comes with potential postoperative problems including urinary tract infection (UTI) and temporary urinary retention as a result of voiding dysfunction.

Assess gastrointestinal (GI) function by palpating the abdomen, listening for bowel sounds, noting distention, and observing for the passing of flatus. After an abdominal hysterectomy, assess the abdominal incision for bleeding and intactness.

Assess vaginal bleeding. One saturated pad in 4 hours after abdominal or vaginal hysterectomy is acceptable. Excessive bleeding should be considered if one sanitary napkin is saturated in 1 hour or less.

Diagnosis, Outcomes, Intervention

Diagnosis: Risk for Complicated Grieving. Some women experience grief about their loss of the female reproductive organs, making *Risk for Complicated Grieving related to loss of reproductive capacity and perceived loss of femininity* an appropriate nursing diagnosis for a client undergoing hysterectomy.

Outcomes. The client can be expected to go through a grieving process over her loss of reproductive capabilities and may express her feelings about the loss.

Interventions. When reproductive ability is lost, the client may undergo a grief response. It is important for the nurse to understand the grieving process and to be able to help the woman understand that this response is normal. Some women experience relief rather than grief. Support normal grieving, including temporary denial, which is a part of the grieving process. If the client continues to experience grief beyond the normal degree or time expected, she may require counseling.

Diagnosis: Risk for Infection. During surgery for a hysterectomy, a Foley catheter is inserted, leading to the nursing diagnosis *Risk for Infection related to surgical intervention and presence of a urinary catheter.*

Outcomes. The client will remain free of infection, or will report any infection immediately for proper diagnosis and treatment.

Interventions

Prevent Urinary Tract Infection. When a Foley catheter is in place, instruct the client to keep the urinary drainage catheter below the level of the bladder, drink at least 2 to 4 L of liquid daily, and report any urinary pain or discomfort. Check the urinary drainage system closely for leaks and kinks in the system, provide complete perineal care every shift, and report any change in color or odor of the urine. When a Foley catheter is discontinued, monitor the client for the first void. Voiding frequently in small amounts, inability to void, and bladder distention or hematuria should be reported to the physician.

Prevent Urinary Retention. Often, a suprapubic catheter is placed instead of a Foley catheter. This allows the client to clamp the catheter and attempt to void as soon as she is ambulatory. If the suprapubic area becomes distended when the catheter is clamped and the client is unable to void, the suprapubic catheter can be opened and drained. Using a suprapubic catheter avoids the need for recatheterization of a client who cannot void.

Monitor Temperature. The woman's temperature should be assessed every 4 hours postoperatively. In addition, assess any incisional sites for warmth, redness, or moisture, and document any changes or increases in vaginal discharge.

Diagnosis: Constipation. Because of bowel manipulation during surgery, the nursing diagnosis *Constipation related to bowel manipulation during surgery* is appropriate.

Outcomes. The client will not become constipated, and bowel distention will be treated, as evidenced by return to a normal bowel pattern and absence of abdominal distention.

Interventions

Promote Peristalsis. Pain and discomfort after abdominal hysterectomy usually center on the incision and postoperative gas pains. After abdominal hysterectomy, GI functioning returns slowly. Uncomfortable gas pains are often experienced during the early postoperative period. Early, frequent ambulation helps improve GI function. If gas pains persist, a small enema may be prescribed to facilitate peristalsis and prevent constipation. Continue to encourage frequent ambulation to facilitate the return of normal GI functioning. Drinking warm fluids may encourage the return of peristalsis.

Evaluation. It is expected that the client will recover from a hysterectomy without complications. She should be able to return to normal activities within 4 to 6 weeks without permanent problems.

Self-Care

The client should understand the type of surgery she had, and the necessary surgical follow-up. Discharge teaching should include a reminder that menses will have ceased, but menopause will not have been induced unless the ovaries have been removed. The client must be instructed to eat a well-balanced diet, drink six to eight glasses of water daily, and get plenty of rest. To reduce stress on abdominal muscles and surgical sites, heavy lifting should be avoided for 6 weeks. The client must also avoid activities that increase pelvic congestion (aerobic activity or prolonged standing), as optimal circulation is necessary to promote healing of tissues. To ensure healing of the vaginal cuff and reduce risk of infection, clients should avoid intercourse for 6 weeks until healing is complete. Any fresh bleeding or abnormal vaginal discharge must be reported to the surgeon.

ENDOMETRIAL (UTERINE) CANCER

Endometrial cancer is the most common malignancy of the female genital reproductive system. In 2007 the American Cancer Society estimated that 39,080 new cases of uterine cancer would be diagnosed in the United States with an estimated 7400 women dying of uterine cancer. The 5-year survival rate is 96% if the cancer is discovered at an early stage.[1]

Etiology and Risk Factors

Endometrial cancer is most strongly related to an imbalance between estrogen and progesterone levels, resulting in excessive circulating estrogen. Common sources of excessive estrogen include unopposed ERT (see earlier discussion), early onset of menarche, and late menopause. Other risk factors for endometrial cancer include obesity, nulliparity, other reproductive cancer, tamoxifen use for breast cancer, family history, diabetes mellitus, and hypertension. Pregnancy and OCP use offer some protection. Women with an intact uterus who choose hormone therapy after menopause should use combined HRT to minimize the risk for developing uterine cancer.

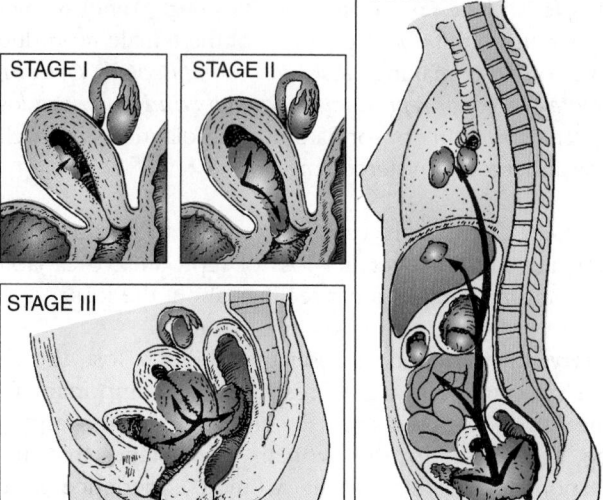

■ **FIGURE 39–5** Staging uterine cancer. *Stage I:* The tumor is confined to the uterine corpus. *Stage II:* The cancer has also invaded the cervix. *Stage III:* The cancer has spread beyond the uterus but remains confined to the pelvis, such as in the bladder or rectum. *Stage IV:* Highest level of invasiveness because the cancer has spread beyond the pelvis, causing metastatic disease and large masses, such as in the liver or lungs.

Pathophysiology

Nearly all (95%) uterine cancers are adenocarcinomas, a tumor involving the glands.[1] Adenocarcinomas are slow-growing tumors that invade the uterus, causing uterine enlargement. The cancer may then spread to the myometrium, cervix, and other reproductive and peritoneal structures. Metastasis through the lymphatics may bring the cancer to distant sites such as the brain and lungs.

Clinical Manifestations

The most significant manifestation of uterine cancer is abnormal uterine bleeding. Any bleeding in a post-menopausal woman should be considered a sign of potential cancer. Other manifestations, such as pain, are usually related to late stage disease and metastasis to other organs (Figure 39-5). A diagnosis of endometrial cancer is usually established by pelvic examination and pathologic analysis of an endometrial biopsy specimen.

OUTCOME MANAGEMENT

Surgical Management

Endometrial cancer is generally treated with surgery, radiation, or a combination. Early endometrial cancer is surgically treated with a TAH-BSO. Surgical management is the same as that described for benign uterine tumors (leiomyomas).

Medical Management

Surgery may be preceded, or followed, by external or internal irradiation. External irradiation is discussed in Chapter 17. Internal (intracavity) radiation therapy (IRT) begins by placing an applicator into the woman's uterus via the vagina. After correct placement is verified by x-ray study, the client is taken to a hospital room where a radioactive isotope is placed in the applicator. This may be done on an inpatient (1 to 3 days) or outpatient basis.

Precancerous endometrial changes may be treated with the hormone progesterone. Chemotherapy and hormonal therapy with tamoxifen (Nolvadex) are used to treat late stages of endometrial cancer.

Nursing Management of the Medical-Surgical Client

Nursing care of the surgical client is the same as that described for the client with benign uterine tumors (leiomyomas).

For the radiation treatment, the client is isolated in a private room while the radioactive implants are in place.

She must remain on bed rest, with the head of the bed flat or elevated no more than 20 degrees. Movement is restricted and a Foley catheter is inserted to prevent implant dislodgment. Increased fluid intake, to prevent urinary stasis, is encouraged. You may also administer antiemetics, broad-spectrum antibiotics, sedatives, analgesics, antidiarrheal medications, and heparin (to prevent thrombophlebitis).

> **Radiation precautions are enforced while a radioactive implant is in place. Organize care so you spend minimal time at the bedside. Visitors should keep visits brief. Radiation therapy is detailed in Chapter 17.**

The high dose of radiation may cause vaginal shrinkage, vaginal adhesions, and stenosis. Such changes can make vaginal sexual activities uncomfortable or painful. Discuss use of vaginal dilators and water-soluble lubricants to encourage recovery of the tissue and sexual functioning. Support for the woman experiencing body image changes is extremely important at this time.

CERVICAL CANCER

About 11,150 new cases of invasive cervical cancer are expected to be diagnosed in 2007, with approximately 3670 cases resulting in death.[1] Because of the prevalence of screening with the Papanicolaou test (Pap smear), the incidence of invasive cervical cancer has steadily decreased over the years. More women are being diagnosed with pre-invasive cancerous lesions, resulting in fewer mortalities as there is virtually a 100% cure rate when detected at a pre-invasive stage.[1] Recent advances in human papillomavirus (HPV) vaccines are offering hope for use in HPV therapy and prophylaxis (see the Translating Evidence into Practice feature Human Papillomavirus Screening for Women with Abnormal Pap Smear Results on p. 988 in Chapter 41).

Etiology and Risk Factors

HPV is the leading cause of cervical cancer, with a notable relationship between the presence of HPV strains 16 and 18 and cervical intraepithelial neoplasia (CIN).[25] CIN has the potential to progress to carcinoma in situ and invasive cervical cancer. Other risk factors include multiple sexual partners (client or her partner), early age (<20 years) of first intercourse, history of STIs, smoking tobacco, immunosuppression, low socioeconomic status, and poor access or use of health care.[7]

Annual Pap smears should be encouraged in all sexually active women, especially those at high risk. Clients should also be instructed to seek early treatment of vaginal or cervical infections, to limit the number of sexual partners, and to use condoms to limit the

transmission of HPV and other STIs. Since 5 to 15 years may elapse between the pre-invasive and invasive stages of cervical cancer, early detection is crucial to diagnosis at the pre-invasive stage when the cancer is practically 100% curable.

Pathophysiology

Cervical dysplasia (an abnormal alteration in cell structure), the earliest premalignant change noted in cervical epithelium, is further divided into several levels: mild dysplasia (CIN 1), moderate dysplasia (CIN 2), severe dysplasia (CIN 3), and carcinoma in situ. The Pap smear is the primary diagnostic tool for cervical cancer. Any abnormal Pap smear result indicates the need for further assessment (see Chapter 37 for more information on Pap screening).

Approximately 90% of cervical cancers are squamous cell carcinomas, beginning at the squamocolumnar junction near the external end of the cervix. The spread of squamous cell cervical cancer occurs by direct extension to the vaginal mucosa and pelvic cavity structures. Metastasis to the liver, lungs, or bones occurs through the lymphatic and circulatory systems. Cervical adenocarcinomas originate in endocervical glands. They are less common, but are increasingly being detected in routine screening and are now known to be directly related to HPV strains 16 and 18.[8]

Clinical Manifestations

There are no early indications of carcinoma in situ or early cervical cancer. The classic manifestation of invasive cancer is the presence of abnormal vaginal bleeding, especially after intercourse. Metrorrhagia, postmenopausal bleeding, and polymenorrhea (increased frequency of menstrual bleeding) may be present. As the disease advances, or the neoplastic area becomes infected, vaginal discharge becomes dark, profuse, and foul smelling.

Other assessment findings that develop as the disease progresses relate to the areas involved in the malignant process. They include pressure on the bowel and/or bladder, bladder irritation, rectal discharge, anemia, and heavy, aching abdominal pain. Fistulae may form as the malignancy erodes through the walls of adjacent organs. Pain is often a late manifestation

OUTCOME MANAGEMENT

Medical Management

Irradiation is used as primary therapy for early cervical cancer. It is usually curative, but it induces menopause. Intracavity radiation was described previously (see Endometrial [Uterine] Cancer earlier in this chapter), and external irradiation is discussed in Chapter 17. Chemotherapy may be used in conjunction with irradiation.

Treatment of clients with cervical cancer during pregnancy varies depending on the stage of the cancer, the gestational age of a pregnancy, and the client's wish to preserve fertility. A client can usually complete the pregnancy if CIN or carcinoma in situ is diagnosed.

Nursing Management of the Medical Client

Prevent Complications

For the care of a client with radiation implants, see Endometrial (Uterine) Cancer earlier; external radiation is discussed in Chapter 17.

Prevent Recurrence

Encourage clients who have been treated conservatively for cervical cancer to have frequent health examinations to identify manifestations of recurrence. Pelvic examinations and Pap smears should be scheduled every 3 months for the first 2 years, or as advised by the physician.

Surgical Management

Treatment may range from conization, loop electrocautery excision procedure (LEEP), and cryosurgery or laser surgery for localized tumors, to a radical hysterectomy for invasive cancer.

Cold Conization

Cold conization is a procedure during which a cone-shaped biopsy of the cervix is obtained. The procedure may be performed when colposcopic examination is not considered adequate. Cold conization is particularly helpful if the endocervical glands are involved and are not readily visualized. Occasionally, the excised area contains the entire malignancy surrounded by a wide margin of normal tissue. In these cases, conization serves not only as the diagnostic procedure but also as the treatment. Conization allows women to maintain reproductive capacity.

Loop Electrocautery Excision Procedure

LEEP is the newest, and most common, procedure. LEEP is performed to excise the cervical areas causing concern. Under local anesthesia, the lesions are totally removed by a low-voltage diathermy loop (an electrical current causing burning). Rapid healing and less tissue damage are benefits of LEEP.

Cryosurgery and Laser

Cryosurgery is the freezing of diseased cervical tissue. The treatment has minimal side effects, though post-

treatment discharge lasts 2 to 4 weeks. Laser surgery uses a direct beam (heat) to remove diseased tissue. Although women experience less discharge after laser surgery, there is often more discomfort after the procedure.[54]

Hysterectomy

A total abdominal hysterectomy is used to treat carcinoma in situ in women who have finished childbearing or to treat invasive cancer. Pelvic exenteration (Figure 39-6) is a radical procedure involving removal of pelvic organs including the uterus, fallopian tubes, ovaries, and vagina. The bladder, rectum, or colon may be removed if the cancer has spread. An ileal conduit or ileostomy may be performed if removal of the bladder or colon is indicated.

Nursing Management of the Surgical Client

For care of the client with a hysterectomy, see Benign Uterine Tumors (Leiomyomas). For care of the client with an ileal conduit, see Chapter 34. For care of the client with a colostomy or ileostomy, see Chapter 33.

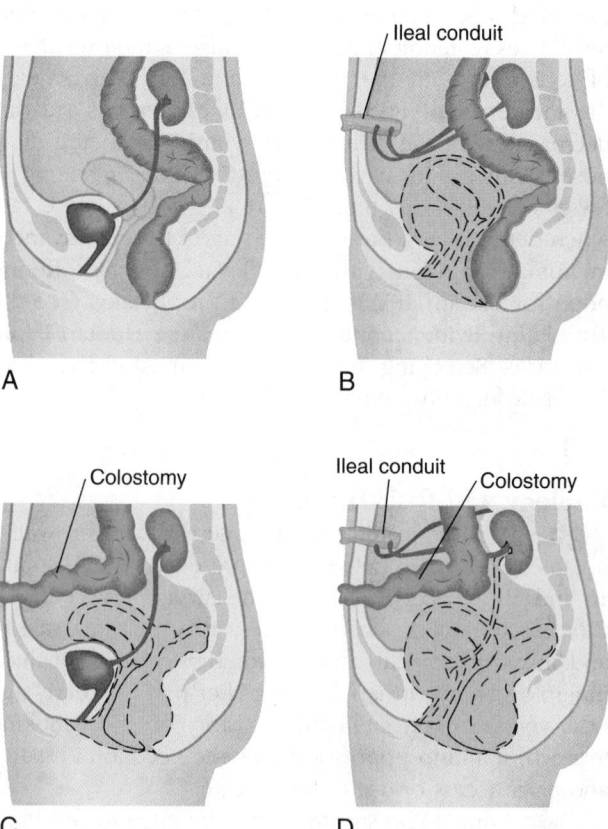

FIGURE 39–6 Pelvic exenteration. **A,** Natural pelvic structures. **B,** Anterior exenteration: formation of the ileal conduit. **C,** Posterior exenteration: formation of colostomy. **D,** Total exenteration: formation of both ileal conduit and colostomy.

Cryosurgery, LEEP, Laser Surgery, and Conization

Explain Procedure. To prepare a client for cryosurgery, laser therapy, or a LEEP, explain that the procedure will be performed with a vaginal speculum in place, and that no surgical incision will be made. With conization, there will be a surgical incision. During treatment, clients may experience headaches, dizziness, flushing, and some cramping.

Provide Support. During the procedure, support the client by staying with her and informing her of what is to be done. Acknowledge her presence during the procedure by talking, listening, and facilitating expression of her concerns, and allow her to retain as much self-control as possible.

Promote Comfort. Assess the client's discomfort during the procedure. Mild analgesics may be prescribed for pain following the procedure. Educate her about post-procedure discomfort and what to expect afterward. Mild cramping may continue for several days.

Encourage Perineal Hygiene. Healing takes 4 to 6 weeks. The client may expect a clear, watery discharge up to several weeks, followed by a malodorous discharge from the sloughing of dead cells. If discharge continues longer than 8 weeks, suspect infection. Meticulous perineal hygiene minimizes the risk of infection and makes the client more comfortable. The client should take showers during this time, avoiding tub and sitz baths.

Despite vigorous treatment, some women with cervical cancer become terminally ill (see Chapter 21 for palliative care). In this situation, the goals of care change and are directed toward physiologic and psychosocial comfort. Pain reduction (see Chapter 20) may be accomplished through use of opioid analgesics. Palliative irradiation may also be used as a pain reduction measure in some cases.

UROGENITAL DISPLACEMENT AND PROLAPSE

Urogenital displacement and prolapse occur when the pelvic organs relax and descend into the vagina. The organs generally involved are the urethra, bladder, uterus, bowel, and rectum. Surgery is one successful measure to reduce prolapse. Other, nonsurgical techniques include use of a pessary, a vaginal support device that holds the organs in correct position, and increasing pelvic floor support with Kegel exercises (Chapter 34, p. 766). The Colpexin sphere, a new tool that facilitates proper pelvic floor muscle exercise (PFME)

technique, may provide the extra support women need to attain maximum benefits of PFMEs and reduce the need for surgical intervention.[48]

Etiology and Risk Factors

The biggest risk factor for pelvic organ prolapse, particularly uterine, is childbearing. Even the most nontraumatic birth can result in some loss of pelvic muscle tone. The decrease in levels of circulating estrogens during menopause can cause the supporting structures of the pelvic floor to lose their elasticity and strength, resulting in relaxation and organ prolapse.[48] Other factors that put a woman at risk for urogenital prolapse are multiparity, childbirth trauma, chronic straining, previous pelvic surgeries or radiation, abdominal masses, and effects of gravity and age.

Improvements in obstetric care, including better labor preparation for women and less traumatic assisted delivery techniques, have decreased prolapse occurrence. Encouraging pregnant clients to seek qualified obstetric care and instructing them in proper Kegel exercise technique (see Chapter 34, p. 766) are activities that may help prevent prolapse.

Clinical Manifestations
Cystocele and Rectocele

A cystocele is descent of the bladder into the vagina (Figure 39-7, *A* and *B*), and may cause urinary disturbances such as incontinence, urinary tract infections, and urinary retention. A rectocele is the protrusion of the rectum into the vagina (Figure 39-7, *C* and *D*), and may result in constipation, incomplete emptying of the rectum, fecal incontinence, and rectal or vaginal pressure. To completely empty the rectum, some women find it necessary to support the posterior wall of the vagina with a finger while having a bowel movement.

Cystoceles and rectoceles may be asymptomatic. Common complaints include a feeling of "something in my vagina," or a pulling sensation, and women may experience low backache. The cystocele is seen as a bulging of the anterior vaginal wall, while the rectocele is seen as a bulging of the lower end of the posterior vaginal wall.

Vaginal or Uterine Prolapse

Vaginal or uterine prolapse is the descent of the uterus into the vagina (Figure 39-8). With complete prolapse, the cervix protrudes through the vagina, and the vagina becomes inverted. Bleeding from irritation or ulcerations on the prolapsing cervix may occur. Other manifestations are increasing vaginal pressure, dyspareunia, and backache.

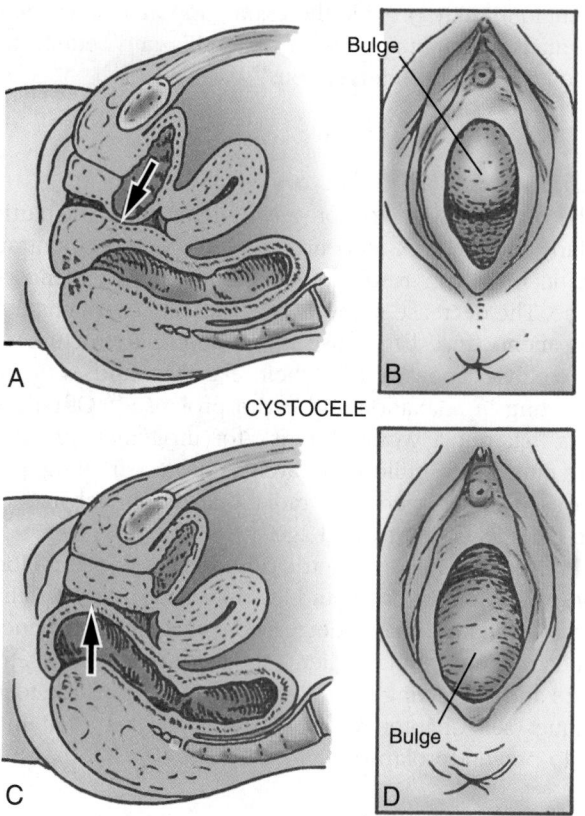

■ **FIGURE 39–7 A,** Cystocele. Note the bulging of the anterior vaginal wall. The urinary bladder is displaced downward. **B,** The cystocele pushes the anterior vaginal wall downward into the vagina. **C,** Rectocele. **D,** Note the bulging of the posterior vaginal wall.

OUTCOME MANAGEMENT

Surgical Management

Treatment of prolapse depends on the extent of prolapse and the client's health status. Reconstructive surgery is one option, but tends to be used only when medical management does not relieve clinical manifestations.

Surgical repair of cystocele and rectocele involves cutting the vaginal wall(s). The exposed tissue between the vagina and bladder or rectum is then tightened so the pelvic or rectal organs will no longer push through.

Hysterectomy may be performed at the same time as the reconstructive surgery if the uterus has descended into the vagina and the client does not want to preserve fertility. The uterus is removed from its supporting broad, round, and uterosacral ligaments. Those ligaments are then attached to the vaginal cuff to maintain vaginal length.

Nursing Management of the Surgical Client

Prevent Bladder Distention

During the operation, and for at least the first 24 hours afterward, the bladder is kept decompressed. A Foley catheter is usually removed as soon as the client is ambulatory. To avoid placing pressure along the suture line, the client must keep her bladder empty by voiding every 2 hours. If a suprapubic catheter is placed, bladder retraining is begun once the client is ambulatory.

Monitor Bleeding

Postoperatively, it is normal to see a small to moderate amount of frank vaginal bleeding.

> **Heavy vaginal bleeding accompanied by a rapidly distending, rigid abdomen, referred shoulder pain, and indications of shock may indicate immediate surgery.**

Medical Management

The vaginal pessary, a device to support prolapsing organs, has been used successfully as an alternative to surgery.[14] Pessaries come in different sizes and styles, and are fitted to the individual woman. Clients should be able to void normally with the pessary in place, and it should be comfortable. Postmenopausal women may also be offered HRT to improve tissue tone.

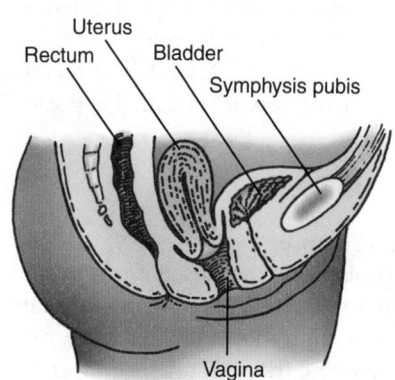

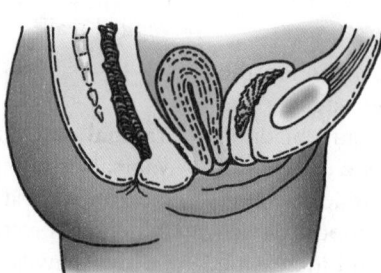

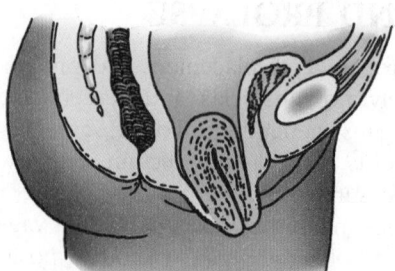

FIRST-DEGREE PROLAPSE   SECOND-DEGREE PROLAPSE   THIRD-DEGREE PROLAPSE

■ **FIGURE 39–8** Uterine prolapse. Note the progressive prolapse of the uterus into the vagina until it is visible externally.

Nursing Management of the Medical Client

Teach Pelvic Floor (Kegel) Exercises

See Chapter 34, p. 766, for Kegel instruction. Kegel exercises can be performed frequently during the day, whenever the client thinks of doing them, or for a specified number of times two or three times a day. 🕯️ The Colpexin sphere may facilitate proper Kegel technique and improve pelvic floor tone in some women.[48]

Teach Pessary Care

Pessaries have the potential to irritate vaginal mucosa, especially if left in place too long. The client should learn to remove and reinsert the device daily after cleaning with a mild, unscented soap and water. Some clients with poor manual dexterity need help with its removal and cleaning.

Follow-up care is important. Within 2 weeks after fitting the pessary, the client needs professional reassessment. The clinician will perform a pelvic examination to assess the vaginal mucosa for irritation, comfort of the device, and normal urinary function. Estrogen cream may be inserted into the vagina at bedtime to maintain tissue integrity. Any vaginal bleeding should be reported immediately.

POLYPS

Polyps are pedunculated tumors that are most commonly seen in the endometrium and on the cervix (Figure 39-9). Uterine polyps may cause hypermenorrhea, or intermenstrual, postmenopausal, and postcoital bleeding. They are the most common, benign lesions of the uterus that occur during the reproductive years. Asymptomatic polyps should be monitored as they may undergo malignant changes, particularly in postmenopausal women.

Cervical polyps are easily removed by ligation, a procedure usually performed in the physician's office without anesthesia. Because of their location within the uterus, endometrial polyps are not as easily removed.

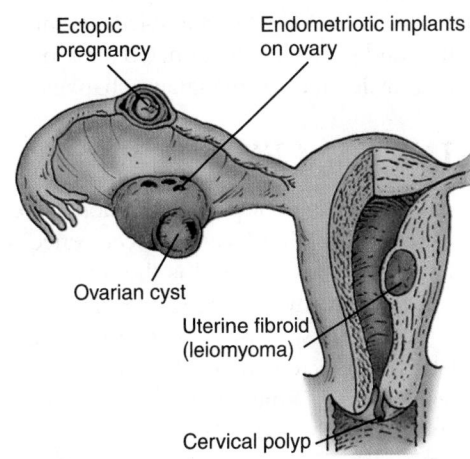

■ **FIGURE 39-9** Common sites of common benign gynecologic lesions.

If they become symptomatic and require removal, hysteroscopy is usually performed. All polyps are sent for pathologic examination.

OVARIAN DISORDERS

BENIGN OVARIAN TUMORS

Early detection of ovarian tumors is difficult as they are often asymptomatic until they are large enough to cause discomfort. Common benign ovarian tumors include follicular cysts, corpus luteum cysts, polycystic ovarian syndrome, dermoid cysts, and ovarian fibromas (Box 39-4).

Typical manifestations include constipation, urinary frequency, full feeling in the abdomen, vague pelvic aching, painful defecation, and dyspareunia. Late manifestations of benign tumors may include marked abdominal distention with dyspnea, peripheral edema, and anorexia. Pelvic pain may present with rapid tumor growth, and acute pain may be experienced during menses or with rupture. Sometimes the tumor can impact regular menstruation and impair fertility.

BOX 39-4	Ovarian Cysts/Benign Ovarian Conditions	
Type of Cyst	**Characteristics**	**Management**
Follicular	Unruptured follicle at time of ovulation May grow with hormonal stimulation	Manage presenting symptoms Weight loss may help obese clients
Corpus luteum	Corpus luteum fails to regress after ovulation	OCPs used if cyst is small
Polycystic ovary syndrome	One or both ovaries enlarged with multiple follicles; oligomenorrhea or amenorrhea; women usually hyperandrogenic with LH hypersecretion	Surgical excision may be necessary if cyst continues to grow or is unresponsive to treatment
Dermoid	Asymptomatic, unilateral ovarian tumors	
Teratomas	Germ cell tumor; mature form benign, immature form malignant; may contain skin, bone, hair, or teeth	
Fibromas	Benign, solid tumors; can be extremely large and may fill pelvic cavity	

Complications include (1) hemorrhage into a cyst, with rupture and possible infection, (2) torsion (twisting) of a cystic pedicle, and (3) malignant changes.

OVARIAN CANCER

Ovarian cancer, the second most common gynecologic cancer, accounts for 3% of cancer occurrence and 6% of cancer deaths in women and is the leading cause of death from reproductive malignancies in women. An estimated 22,430 new cases of ovarian cancer are expected to be detected in the United States in 2007, with 15,280 deaths.[1] White women show higher rates of ovarian cancer than do African-American women. Early diagnosis of ovarian cancer is uncommon.

Etiology and Risk Factors

Although the cause of ovarian cancer is unknown, identified risk factors include nulliparity, history of infertility, family history of ovarian or breast cancer (mutations in *BRCA1* or *BRCA2* genes have been observed in families),[1,42] family history of hereditary nonpolyposis colorectal cancer (HNPCC), ERT, and age older than 50 years. Use of ovulation-stimulating medications in fertility treatments may be linked to an increase in risk. Interruption of ovulatory cycles, such as more than one full-term pregnancy, oral contraceptive use, and breastfeeding offer some protective benefits.

Health maintenance activities include routine pelvic examinations, though ovarian masses are usually undetectable at early stages. In women at high risk, determinations of CA-125 antigen levels and performance of transvaginal ultrasound and bimanual pelvic examination should be routinely completed. Prophylactic oophorectomy may be performed in women with *BRCA1* or *BRCA2* mutations as a way of increasing life expectancy.[1] Early detection offers a 94% 5-year survival rate.[1] However, only 19% of ovarian malignancies are diagnosed early, when they are asymptomatic.

Pathophysiology

Most ovarian cancers are epithelial tumors, although some are adenocarcinomas. The cancer tends to grow and spread silently until pelvic pressure on adjacent organs or abdominal distention cause the woman to seek medical care. By this time, the malignancy has often spread to the other ovary, fallopian tubes, uterus, and ligaments (Figure 39-10), and may also invade bowel surfaces, the omentum, liver, and other organs. The usual routes of metastasis are lymphatic spread, hematogenous spread (through blood), local extension, and peritoneal seeding.

Clinical Manifestations

Late stage ovarian cancer generally presents with persistent GI disturbances, including abdominal distention

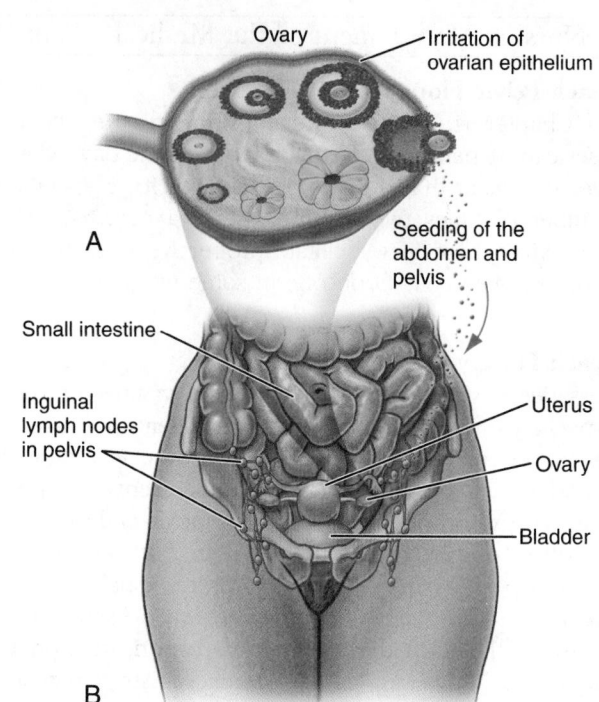

■ **FIGURE 39–10 A,** Etiology of ovarian cancer shown by irritation of the ovarian epithelium. **B,** Metastasis occurs through the lymphatic system or by direct seeding of the abdomen and pelvis.

with ascites, increasing abdominal girth, urinary frequency and urgency, pain and pressure caused by the growing tumor or effects of urinary and bowel obstruction, malnutrition with weight loss, and, ultimately, general severe pain.

Identification of any palpable ovarian mass should always be considered an abnormal finding and followed up with pelvic sonogram to rule out abnormalities. Serum CA-125, a tumor marker thought to be useful in early detection of ovarian cancer, may be more beneficial in tracking identified tumor growth and regression.[47] New diagnostic blood tests, including lysophosphatidic acid (LPA) and soluble epidermal growth factor receptor (SEG-FR), have potential for improved diagnostic evaluation of ovarian cancer, but studies are continuing.[4,5,42]

OUTCOME MANAGEMENT

Surgical Management

Ovarian cancer is treated aggressively, as it is often found at an advanced stage. The only definitive way to diagnose ovarian cancer is with exploratory surgery. During the surgical procedure, physicians can obtain biopsy specimens of adjacent structures, and perform resection if the mass is malignant. TAH-BSO is considered the typical treatment, with a more radical internal structure resection (debulking) used in advanced disease. The less residual tumor left, the better the prognosis.

Medical Management

Adjuvant therapy varies with the stage of the disease. Surgery alone may be effective for women presenting with low-risk, stage I disease.[1] Systemic chemotherapy (see Chapter 17) may be administered to women with high risk, stage I ovarian cancer. Stage II or higher ovarian cancers typically receive the same treatment as those with stage I disease, with the inclusion of pelvic and, possibly, abdominal radiation.

Nursing Management of the Medical-Surgical Client

For the nursing care of the client who has undergone TAH-BSO, see the discussion earlier in this chapter; for care of the client with cancer, see Chapter 17; for palliative care, see Chapter 21.

VAGINAL DISORDERS

The vagina is an acidic cavity with a normal protective population of flora, including various bacteria. Normal vaginal function depends on a delicate balance between hormones and bacteria. Disturbance of this balance can precipitate infection. Disorders include vaginal discharge and pruritus, vaginitis, and vaginal cancer. Other, more uncommon disorders and manifestations that can affect the female genitalia may include toxic shock syndrome, fistulae (Figure 39-11), bartholinitis, and female genital mutilation (see Table 39-2).

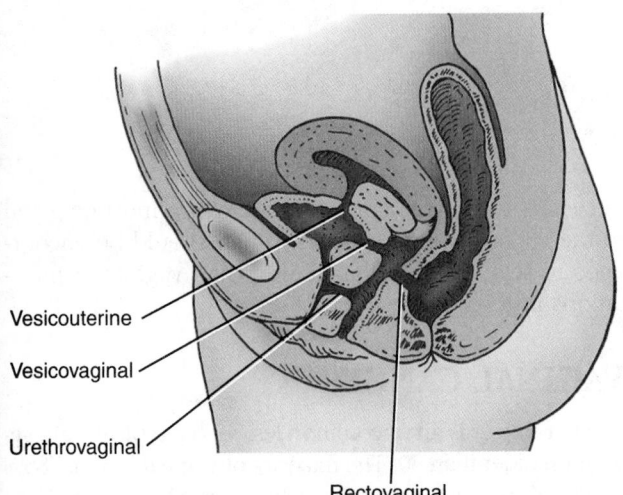

Vesicouterine

Vesicovaginal

Urethrovaginal

Rectovaginal

■ **FIGURE 39–11** Locations of main types of vaginal fistulae.

VAGINAL DISCHARGE AND PRURITUS

Vaginal discharge and itching are some of the most common reasons women seek health care. The female reproductive tract maintains its integrity through various natural defense mechanisms. Inflammation and infection occur when organisms disrupt or overcome these natural defenses. Leukorrhea is the normal, white, vaginal discharge, secreted by the endocervical glands for the purpose of keeping vaginal mucous membranes moist. Changes in the amount, color, character, or odor of discharge may indicate a problem.

The most common causes of vaginal discharge and irritation are vaginal infections, parasites (such as pinworms), STIs (see Chapter 41), and mechanical or allergic irritants. Most inflammatory and infectious vaginal problems are accompanied by pathologic vaginal discharge. The discharge can cause itching, irritation, and redness of the vulva and surrounding areas, and may be accompanied by burning and frequency of urination, anal discomfort, and pain in the lower abdominal region.

Douching has been used as a way to control normal vaginal discharge and odor. There is evidence in medical literature that douching not only is unnecessary but also can be detrimental. Douching washes away protective vaginal mucus and normal bacterial flora. This may lead to overgrowth of undesirable bacteria and yeast, thereby increasing the risk of vaginal irritation and infection.

VAGINITIS

Vaginitis is an inflammation of the vagina characterized by a change in vaginal discharge, which may be profuse, odorous, and purulent and may be accompanied by dysuria and vaginal bleeding. There is often vulvar itching, and clients commonly complain of discomfort when voiding as well as dyspareunia.

Candidiasis *(Candida albicans)*, *Trichomonas vaginalis,* and bacterial vaginosis are the most common causes of vaginitis. Other causes include changes in normal vaginal flora and pH and invasion of the vagina by virulent organisms, conditions that can be caused by mechanical irritation, overmedication with antibiotics, long-term steroid therapy, uncontrolled diabetes mellitus, and acquired immunodeficiency syndrome (AIDS). Health promotion actions related to vaginitis are described in the Client Education Guide on Preventing Vaginitis on the website.

Diagnosis is confirmed by a speculum examination and microscopic examination of the discharge. Specimens may be obtained for culture if manifestations indicate an STI or bacterial infection. Women tend to self-diagnose manifestations of vaginitis, often believing they have a yeast infection. Attempts to treat with

TABLE 39–2   Less Common Vaginal Disorders

	Definition and Causes	Manifestations	Treatments
Toxic shock syndrome	Acute local infection caused by *Staphylococcus aureus* May become systemic Related to prolonged placement of tampons or barrier contraceptives	Sudden high temperature, vomiting, severe, watery diarrhea Characteristic rash and hypotensive shock develop within 48 hr	Antibiotics to treat causative organism, fluid replacement Hygiene counseling including changing tampons more frequently, good hand-washing, and appropriate removal of diaphragm (within 24 hr) and sponge (within 30 hr) after intercourse
Vaginal fistulae (see Figure 39-11)	Abnormal tube-like passages between vagina and bladder (vesicovaginal), rectum (rectovaginal), or urethra (urethrovaginal) May result from injury or surgery	Urine or flatus and feces leak into vagina Vaginal and vulvar tissues excoriate Client feels "unclean" and may experience offensive odors Clients may exhibit psychosocial problems because of embarrassing nature of problem Rarely heal spontaneously	Diagnosis is often difficult, and surgical correction is often unsuccessful, even under optimal conditions Provide support and acceptance to client Teach manifestation management and care Postsurgery, prevention of constipation and infection is paramount Adequate fluid intake is critical Any stress on surgical site could cause fistulae to reopen
Bartholinitis	Inflammation of Bartholin's glands caused by organisms (i.e., Staphylococci, Streptococci, and *E. coli*) May become palpable painless cyst (Bartholin's cyst)	Often relate to size of cyst and include dyspareunia and pain when walking	Systemic antibiotics for causative organism Local heat and sitz baths to help drainage Surgery indicated if cancer suspected or for repeated infections or abscess formation
Female genital mutilation (FGM) (female circumcision)	Unnecessary surgical modification of female genitalia Practiced in African countries mainly; seen in immigrant populations in U.S. and Europe; 2 million new cases each year, though many countries are seeing drop in rate Type I is excision of clitoral prepuce and all or part of clitoris Type II includes removal of labia minora; accounts for 85% of FGM procedures Type III (infibulation) is type II with removal of interior labia majora and suturing together of two sides of vulva, leaving a small opening for urine and menstrual flow Type IV includes other procedures like pricking or burning of clitoris[35,64,65]	Done for religious and social reasons Also to ensure marital fidelity, distinguishing local women, or procuring bride price Some think it makes women cleaner and less sexually promiscuous Complications include sexual complications, labor complications (including fetal and maternal death), chronic vaginal and pelvic infections, hemorrhage, shock and death during procedure, psychological trauma, and altered psychosexual beliefs	Relief of clinical manifestations Cesarean or de-infibulation (anterior episiotomy) may be required to enable birth Nonjudgmental attitude and trusting relationship necessary Intervention of counseling may be necessary to deal with unresolved grief FGM involving girl under 18 must be reported as it is considered child abuse

over-the-counter medications, such as those for *Candida,* can complicate the diagnostic process.

Atrophic vaginitis occurs in postmenopausal women and is attributed to estrogen deficiency. Long-term use of estrogen cream is the typical medical treatment. Engaging in normal sexual activities may also help to prevent clinical manifestations. An appropriate antibiotic is used to treat any secondary infection.

Vaginitis can be a stubborn, discouraging problem. Treatments are aimed at correcting the cause and ameliorating the manifestations. Early treatment may be necessary to prevent chronicity. Attention must be given to the client's overall health. Women should be encouraged to seek professional care for their vaginal manifestations instead of trying to self-treat.

VAGINAL CANCER

Vaginal cancer is an uncommon lesion that typically affects women older than 50. The majority of vaginal lesions (85% to 90%) are squamous cell. Clear-cell adenocarcinomas account for about 10%. It was estimated that 2140 new cases of vaginal cancer would be diagnosed in the United States in 2007, with an estimated 790 deaths. Although rare, vaginal cancers account for about 3% of all cancers of the female reproductive system.[1]

Etiology and Risk Factors

Etiology of vaginal cancer is unknown. Vaginal squamous cell carcinomas develop over many years from precancerous changes called vaginal intraepithelial neoplasias (VAIN).[1] Clear-cell adenocarcinomas have a direct relationship to maternal ingestion of DES, or in utero exposure to DES in girls and women between menarche and age 30 years. Other risks for vaginal cancer include a history of STI or infection with herpes virus or HPV, smoking, vaginal irritation, and cervical cancer.

Pathophysiology

Primary invasive vaginal cancer tends to involve the anterior or posterior vaginal wall, or both. Complications may involve the urinary bladder or bowel, including fistula formation (see Figure 39-11). Because of a rich vaginal lymphatic supply, metastasis can occur early in the disease process. The prognosis for vaginal cancer is generally poor. Low survival rates can be attributed to the rarity of the cancer, typically advanced stage at diagnosis, and difficulty treating the cancer with radiation or surgery because of proximity of important structures.

Clinical Manifestations

Lesions of vaginal cancer are often well advanced before manifestations appear. Indications of vaginal cancer include foul vaginal discharge, painless vaginal bleeding, and the presence of a vaginal mass or lesion. Urinary bladder manifestations, such as pain and frequency, may occur if a vaginal mass compresses the bladder.

Women exposed to DES in utero should receive careful examination of the vagina and cervix, including cytologic examination of any questionable areas. Colposcopy may be used to identify areas to be sampled for biopsy.

OUTCOME MANAGEMENT

Medical Management

The usual treatment for vaginal cancer is either external or intravaginal radiation therapy. The type and amount depend on the tumor staging at time of treatment. Chemotherapy may be used in conjunction with radiation. Side effects may include shrinking of the vagina and irritation of internal structures.

Surgical Management

For earlier stages, radical hysterectomy, lymphadenectomy, and vaginectomy are performed. Pelvic exenteration is used in more advanced cancer if the bladder or rectum is involved, and it is also indicated in a client with recurrent metastases. The client with radiation treatment failure may also have surgical removal of the tumor.

Nursing Management of the Medical-Surgical Client

Provide Support

Vaginal surgery may be anxiety-promoting and frightening. Ostomies (see Chapters 33 and 34) may need to be performed, which can add to the client's fears. A supportive and therapeutic nurse is a valuable tool for these clients.

Discuss Sexuality

A therapeutic environment, which allows your client to feel comfortable discussing sexual concerns and problems, is essential. Postoperatively, vaginal sexual activity is not possible unless there has been vaginal reconstruction. After surgery or radiation therapy, sex may be difficult because of changes in the size and shape of the vagina. Try to assure the client that she may still enjoy normal vaginal sexual activity. The use of vaginal dilators and lubricants can prevent vaginal fibrosis and tightening, while encouraging stretching of the tissue. A warm bath, back rub, alternative positioning, relaxation techniques, and pain medication may also help.

VULVAR DISORDERS

VULVITIS

Vulvitis is an inflammation of the vulva and is caused by direct irritation of vulvar tissues. Vulvitis is a clinical manifestation rather than a condition, and its risk is increased in women who have skin disorders, inflammatory problems, infections, allergies, low estrogen level, incontinence, and poor perineal hygiene. It is also related to sensitivities to soaps, detergents, spermicides, and vaginal sprays or perfumes.

Vulvitis is characterized by redness and swelling of the labia, and severe pruritus. Blisters may be seen as well. Medical treatment is based on the specific cause of the condition. Itching may be relieved with local or systemic antipruritic or antihistamine agents, including hydrocortisone cream or diphenhydramine hydrochloride (Benadryl).

The client may use cold compresses and should avoid feminine hygiene sprays. She should wear light, nonrestrictive clothing, including well-washed and well-rinsed cotton underpants. Keeping the vulva clean and dry, and applying the prescribed ointment, will also help healing and prevent recurrence.

VULVAR CANCER

Vulvar cancer is found mainly in women older than 50. It was estimated that, in 2007, approximately 3490 cases would be reported in the United States with 880 cases resulting in death.[1]

Etiology and Risk Factors

Vulvar disorders (including lichen sclerosus), smoking, and other genital cancers increase the risk of vulvar cancer. Contracting certain STIs, especially HPV, also increases the risk. Recent increases in the numbers of younger women presenting with vulvar cancer is thought to be attributed to HPV exposure.[1]

Pathophysiology

Approximately 90% to 95% of vulvar cancers are squamous cell carcinoma. The remaining 5% to 10% are adenocarcinoma, Paget's disease, malignant melanoma, or sarcoma.

Vulvar cancer typically starts as vulvar intraepithelial neoplasia (VIN), which progresses to invasive cancer. Vulvar cancer grows slowly and remains localized for a long time. Lesions are located in the labia. Metastasis is local (by direct extension) and lymphatic. Vulvar cancer prognosis is generally good, unless there is lymph node involvement.

Lichen sclerosus (LS) is a chronic, inflammatory skin disorder that affects the vulva. LS is characterized by gray patches of epithelium that may crack and become infected, causing tissue to ulcerate and macerate. These areas may eventually become malignant.

Clinical Manifestations

The labia majora are the most common site for vulvar cancer. Initially, the client may be asymptomatic. When the lesion grows to 1 to 2 cm, the client may experience itching and soreness or pain. Some women may experience bleeding and dysuria, and there may be raised bumps or a wart-like growth. Because the manifestations are similar to those of nonmalignant vulvar lesions, the potential seriousness may not be recognized by the client or caregiver. As the cancer progresses, clinical manifestations of vulvar edema and pelvic lymphadenopathy develop. Secondary infection may cause a foul-smelling discharge. Biopsy of the affected area confirms the diagnosis.

OUTCOME MANAGEMENT

Medical Management

When lichen sclerosus is present, a biopsy to rule out cancer is indicated. Infection is treated with an appropriate systemic or topical antibiotic, steroid creams, and hormone cream. Other manifestations are treated symptomatically. Itching can be treated symptomatically with antipruritic creams such as hydrocortisone.

Irradiation and chemotherapy are not generally used, as involved tissues do not tolerate them well.

Nursing Management of the Medical Client

Nursing management of the client with lichen sclerosus is mainly supportive care throughout the diagnostic period. Educating the client about the infectious process, treatment regimens, and proper self-care is important.

Surgical Management

A vulvectomy may be performed to remove abnormal tissue. Procedures include a skinning technique, local wide excision, and simple or radical vulvectomy (Figure 39-12).

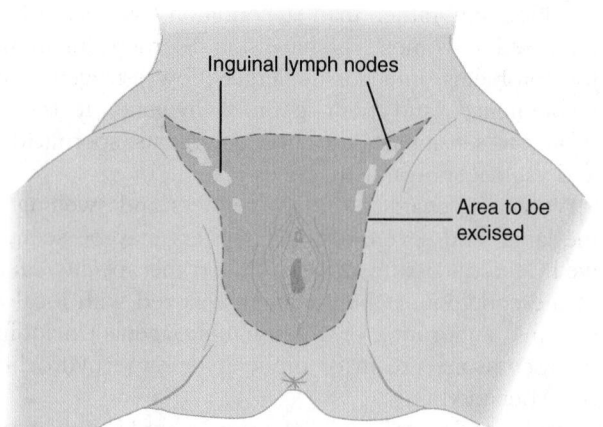
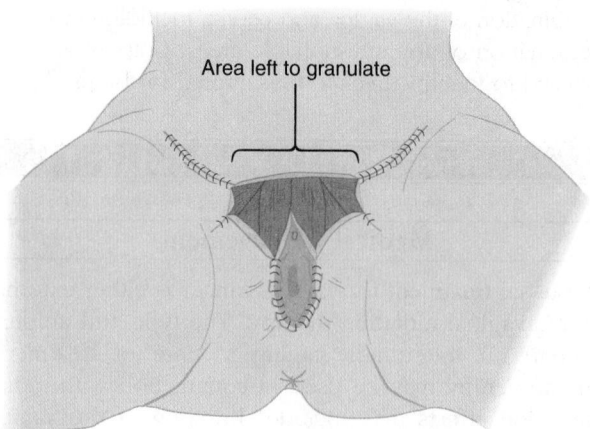

A

B

■ **FIGURE 39–12** Radical vulvectomy. **A,** Area to be excised and line of incision (dashed line). The vulvar skin, underlying subcutaneous tissue and muscles, and regional lymph nodes are excised. If the anus is involved, the incision also continues around it. Inguinal and femoral lymph nodes are resected en bloc. **B,** Completed surgery. Perineal skin is approximated to the vagina, and a large area is left open to heal gradually by filling in with granulation tissue. A simple vulvectomy (not shown) does not remove the lymph nodes. Hence the incision does not extend into the groin.

A laser may be used in conjunction with these procedures to destroy specific abnormal tissue. Extensive surgery is avoided if the client's condition allows a simpler procedure.

Nursing Management of the Surgical Client

Preoperative Care

For a woman having vulvar surgery, psychosocial support is especially important and must begin preoperatively. Problems you might anticipate are fear of disfigurement, grief over the loss of a body part, fear of death, and sexual concerns.

Preoperative preparation includes client teaching aimed at understanding the surgery, preoperative procedures, and what to expect in the postoperative period. See the Client Education Guide on Recovering from Radical Vulvectomy on the website.

Postoperative Care

Clients undergoing a radical vulvectomy are susceptible to many postoperative complications because of the extensive nature of the operation. Wound infections and delayed wound healing may lead to numerous problems. Careful monitoring of the amount of bleeding is critical in the postoperative period.

Prevent Thrombophlebitis. Antiembolism or sequential compression stockings are worn postoperatively to prevent leg edema and thrombophlebitis. Resuming ambulation and performing leg exercises as early as possible postoperatively will improve circulation. Clients should avoid sitting with the legs dependent, standing, and crossing the legs. A low-dose anticoagulant, such as heparin, warfarin (Coumadin), or aspirin, may be used prophylactically.

Prevent Infection. A Foley catheter is usually in place for 7 to 14 days, and a suction device (e.g., Hemovac) will be in the incision to facilitate drainage and reduce the risk of infection.

> **Prevent infection in the incisional area through frequent dressing changes, perineal care or sitz baths after voiding and bowel movements, and meticulous wound care.**

Promote Voiding. Some women experience unpredictable voiding difficulties following a radical vulvectomy. A client may present with complaints of incontinence, retention, or a dysfunctional voiding pattern (see Chapter 34).

Provide Support. Psychosocially, a vulvectomy can be a devastating experience for a woman because of its direct effect on the external genitalia. The surgery, and disfigurement secondary to the surgery, especially a radical vulvectomy, can lead to body image distortion. Physically, the client may experience stenosis of the introitus, loss of sensation within the vagina, and inability to orgasm, all of which make intercourse painful or difficult.

Sexual counseling should be considered for all women undergoing vulvectomy, and their partners. Assist the client and her partner by communicating openly with them, answering their questions, explaining structural vulvar changes, and suggesting alternative forms of sexual arousal for the client. Nursing care involves helping the woman redefine her self-image to include the physical changes of vulvectomy. Create an environment in which she can express her feelings. Provide opportunities for her to mourn the loss and its effect on her sexuality. Encourage her to resume her normal activities as soon as possible to reinforce her feelings of self-worth.

CONCLUSIONS

Female reproductive disorders can occur at any time throughout a woman's life. These problems range from menstrual disorders to life-threatening malignancies. Nurses can provide much of the needed education to help clients become more aware of preventive measures. Physical and psychosocial care of the client undergoing diagnosis and treatment is important and the skillful, empathic nurse can positively assist the woman through what can be an extremely distressing diagnosis and treatment.

Nurses who need more information on reproductive issues should consult a women's health (obstetrics and gynecology) textbook. More complete and in-depth information on women's reproductive health can be found there.

THINKING CRITICALLY

1. The client, a 52-year-old woman, comes into the clinic stating, "I can't put up with it any longer!" Her last menstrual period was 4 months ago, and she has had severe hot flashes and night sweats for almost 6 months with no abatement. Vaginal intercourse has become so painful that she and her husband have refrained from sexual activity for 3 months. She states that the night sweats are so bad that she has had very few nights of uninterrupted sleep.

Factors to Consider. What are your priorities for her care? What interventions might be used?

2. A 38-year-old woman enters the clinic with a complaint of acute, sharp, severe bilateral pelvic pain. She has a temperature of 102.2 °F, a pulse rate of 100 beats/min, a respiratory rate of 20 breaths/min, and chills. Her cervical culture shows gonococcal infection. She uses oral contraceptives for birth control.

Factors to Consider. Besides teaching her about antibiotic medication, what is your priority in caring for her, and what interventions are necessary?

3. The client, a 61-year-old woman, had a TAH-BSO 2 days ago for early endometrial cancer. Her Foley catheter was removed yesterday. Her temperature is 101.1 ° F, her pulse rate is 96 beats/min, and her respiratory rate is 16 breaths/min. Her blood pressure is 128/74 mm Hg. She complains of flank pain and urinary hesitancy. Her urine output for the past 4 hours is 120 ml, which is the total from three separate voidings. Her urine is cloudy and has a slightly foul odor.

Factors to Consider. What is your priority, and what interventions are needed?

 Discussions for these questions can be found on the website.

BIBLIOGRAPHY

🏮 Citations appearing in red refer to primary research.

🏮 Citations appearing in blue refer to evidence-based practice guidelines and protocols.

1. American Cancer Society. (2007). *Cancer facts and figures.* Atlanta: Author.
2. Anonymous. (2002). Menstrual pain severely affects almost half of U.S. women. *American Journal of Operating Room Nurses, 75*(4), 788.
3. Anonymous. (2002, July). Newer not necessarily better for treating dysmenorrhea. *PR Newswire, 16,* 1.
4. Baron, A., et al. (2003). Soluble epidermal growth factor receptor (SEGFR/sErbBl) as a potential risk, screening and diagnostic serum biomarker of epithelial ovarian cancer. *Cancer Epidemiology Biomarkers and Prevention, 12*(2), 103-113.
5. Baron, A., et al. (2005). Soluble epidermal growth factor receptor (SEG-FR) and cancer antigen 125 (CA125) as screening and diagnostic tests for epithelial ovarian cancer. *Cancer Epidemiology Biomarkers and Prevention, 14*(2), 306-318.
6. Bensaid, C., et al. (2006). Performance of laparoscopy in identifying malignant ovarian cysts. *Surgical Endoscopy, 20*(9), 1410-1414.
7. Boyer, et al. (2001). Hispanic women's perceptions regarding cervical cancer screening. *Journal of Obstetric, Gynecologic and Neonatal Nursing, 30*(2), 240-245.
8. Castellsague, X., et al. (2006). Worldwide human papillomavirus etiology of cervical adenocarcinoma and its cofactors: Implications for screening and prevention. *Journal of the National Cancer Institute, 98*(5), 303-315.
9. Centers for Disease Control and Prevention. (2007). *DES update.* Retrieved 01/26/07 from www.cdc.gov/des/consumers/about/index.html.
10. Clark, T., et al. (2002). Accuracy of hysteroscopy in the diagnosis of endometrial cancer and hyperplasia: A systematic quantitative review. *Journal of the American Medical Association, 288*(13), 1610-1621.
11. Davida, G. (2006). Treating vaginal prolapse. *American Journal for Nurse Practitioners, 10*(5), 49-55.
12. DeLancey, J. (2005). The hidden epidemic of pelvic floor dysfunction: Achievable goals for improved prevention and treatment. *American Journal of Obstetrics and Gynecology, 192,* 1488-1495.
13. Dennehy, C.E. (2006). The use of herbs and dietary supplements in gynecology: An evidence-based review. *Journal of Midwifery & Women's Health, 51*(6), 402-409.
14. Fernando, R., Thaker, R., Sultan, A., et al. (2006). Effect of vaginal pessaries on symptoms associated with organ prolapse. *Obstetrics and Gynecology, 108*(1), 93-99.
15. Grady, D., et al. (2002). Cardiovascular disease outcomes during 6.8 years of hormone therapy: Heart and estrogen/progestin replacement study follow-up (HERS II). *Journal of the American Medical Association, 288*(1), 49-57.
16. Greenspan, S., Resnick, N., & Parker, R. (2003). Combination therapy with hormone replacement and alendronate for prevention of bone loss in elderly women: A randomized controlled trial. *Journal of the American Medical Association, 289*(19), 2525-2533.
17. Harris, L. (2002). Ovarian cancer: Screening for early detection. *American Journal of Nursing, 102*(10), 46-53.
18. Hlatky, M.A., et al. (2002). Quality-of-life symptoms in postmenopausal women after receiving hormone therapy: Results from the heart and estrogen/progestin replacement study (HERS) trial. *Journal of the American Medical Association, 287*(5), 591-597.
19. Jae-Hoon, K., et al. (2002). Osteopontin as a potential diagnostic biomarker for ovarian cancer. *Journal of the American Medical Association, 287*(13), 1671-1680.
20. Janssens, K., Bosmans, M., & Temmerman, M. (2005). *Sexual and reproductive health and rights of refugee women in Europe; Rights, policies, status and needs: Literature review.* Retrieved 01/12/07 from www.icrh.org/Documents/literature.pdf.
21. Johnson, M., et al. (2006). *NANDA, NOC, and NIC linkages: Nursing diagnoses, outcomes, & interventions* (2nd ed.). St. Louis: Mosby.
22. Kellogg-Spadt, S., & Albaugh, J. (2003). Herbs, amino acids, and female libido. *Urologic Nursing, 23*(2), 160-161.
23. Kennedy, A., Sculpher, M., Coulter, A., et al. (2002). Effects of decision aids for menorrhagia on treatment choices, health outcomes, and costs: A randomized controlled trial. *Journal of the American Medical Association, 288*(21), 2701-2708.
24. King, J. (2006). Polycystic ovary syndrome. *Journal of Midwifery and Women's Health, 51*(6), 415-422.
25. Kulasingam, S., et al. (2002). Evaluation of human papillomavirus testing in primary screening for cervical abnormalities: Comparison of sensitivity, specificity, and frequency of referral. *Journal of the American Medical Association, 288*(14), 1749-1757.
26. Lacey, J., et al. (2002). Menopausal hormone replacement therapy and risk of ovarian cancer. *Journal of the American Medical Association, 288*(3), 334-341.
27. Larson, U., & Okonofua, F. (2002). Female circumcision and obstetric complications. *International Journal of Gynecology and Obstetrics, 77,* 255-265.
28. Lightner, D. (2002). Female sexual dysfunction. *Mayo Clinic Proceedings, 77*(7), 698-702.
29. Lowdermilk, D., & Perry, S. (2004). *Maternity and women's health care* (8th ed.). St. Louis: Mosby.
30. Mailhot, T., & Richard, A. (2007). *Uterine prolapse.* Retrieved 01/12/07 from www.emedicine.com/emerg/topic629.htm.
31. Maloney, C. (2002). Estrogen and recurrent UTIs in the postmenopausal woman. *American Journal of Nursing, 102*(8), 44-52.
32. Mandelblatt, J., et al. (2002). Benefits and costs of using HPV testing to screen cervical cancer. *Journal of the American Medical Association, 287*(18), 2372-2381.
33. Martin, V. (2005). Straight talk about ovarian cancer. *Nursing 2005, 35*(4), 36-41.
34. Marinkovic, S., & Stanton, S. (2004). Incontinence and voiding difficulties associated with prolapse. *Journal of Urology, 171,* 1021-1028.
35. Mashburn, J. (2006). Etiology, diagnosis and management of vaginitis. *Journal of Midwifery and Women's Health, 51*(6), 423-430.
36. Morrison, L., Scherf, C., Ekpo, G., et al. (2001). The long-term reproductive health consequences of female genital cutting in rural Gambia: A community-based survey. *Tropical Medicine and International Health, 6*(8), 643-653.
37. Narvane, A., et al. (2001). Serotypes of *Chlamydia trachomatis* and resistance for development of cervical squamous cell carcinoma. *Journal of the American Medical Association, 285*(1), 47-52.
38. Nelson, H., et al. (2002). Postmenopausal hormone replacement therapy. *Journal of the American Medical Association, 288*(7), 872-881.
39. Pasacreta, J., Jacobs, L., & Cataldo, J. (2002). Genetic testing for breast and ovarian cancer risk: The psychosocial issues. *American Journal of Nursing, 102*(12), 40-48.
40. Pearlstein, T. (2002). Selective serotonin reuptake inhibitors for premenstrual dysphoric disorder: The emerging gold standard? *Drugs, 62*(13), 1869-1885.
41. Price, S., & Wilson, L. (2003). *Pathophysiology: Clinical concepts of disease processes* (6th ed.). St. Louis: Mosby.

42. Otto, S. (2001). Gynecologic cancers. In S. Otto (Ed.), *Oncology nursing* (4th ed., pp. 248-284). St. Louis: Mosby.

43. Rapp, S., et al. (2003). Effect of estrogen plus progestin on global cognitive function in postmenopausal women. The Women's Health Initiative Memory Study: A randomized controlled trial. *Journal of the American Medical Association, 289*(20), 2663-2672.

44. Rexrode, K.M., & Mason, J.E. (2002). Postmenopausal hormone therapy and quality of life: No cause for celebration. *Journal of the American Medical Association, 287*(5), 641-642.

45. Robinson, J. (2006). Anatomical and hormonal influences in women's dermatologic health. *Journal of the American Medical Association, 295*, 1443-1445.

46. Rosen, T. (2003). Update on genital lesions. *Journal of the American Medical Association, 290*, 1001-1005.

47. Rustin, G., et al. (2001). Use of CA-125 to define progression of ovarian cancer in patients with persistently elevated levels. *Journal of Clinical Oncology, 19*(20), 4054-4057.

48. Sasso, K. (2005). The Colpexin sphere: A new conservative management option for pelvic organ prolapse. *Journal of Urologic Nursing, 26*(6), 433-441.

49. Shumacher, S., et al. (2004). Conjugated equine estrogens and incidence of probable dementia and mild cognitive impairment in postmenopausal women: Women's Health Initiative Memory Study. *Journal of the American Medical Association, 291*(24), 2947-2958.

50. Shumacher, S., et al. (2003). Estrogen plus progestin and the incidence of dementia and mild cognitive impairment in postmenopausal women. The Women's Health Initiative Memory Study: A randomized control trial. *Journal of the American Medical Association, 289*(20), 2651-2662.

51. Solomon, D., et al. (2002). The 2001 Bethesda system: Terminology for reporting results of cervical cytology. *Journal of the American Medical Association, 287*(16), 2114-2119.

52. Sorg, D. (2001). Vulvodynia: More than just pain. *American Journal of Nursing, 101*(2), 24AAA-24DDD.

53. Spies, J. (2002). Leiomyomata treated with uterine artery embolization: Factors associated with successful symptom and imaging outcome. *Journal of the American Medical Association, 287*(10), 1241.

54. Stearns, V., et al. (2003). Paroxetine controlled release in the treatment of menopausal hot flashes: A randomized controlled trial. *Journal of the American Medical Association, 289*(21), 2827-2834.

55. Stenchever, M., et al. (2001). *Comprehensive gynecology* (4th ed.). St. Louis: Mosby.

56. Stewart, F., et al. (2001). Clinical breast and pelvic examination requirements for hormonal contraception. *Journal of the American Medical Association, 285*(17), 2232-2240.

57. Stoler, M. (2002). New Bethesda terminology and evidence-based management guidelines for cervical cytology findings. *Journal of the American Medical Association, 287*(16), 2141-2142.

58. Stone-Godena, T. (2006). Vulvar pain syndromes: Vestibulodynia. *Journal of Midwifery and Women's Health, 51*(6), 502-509.

59. Todd, A. (2002). An alternative to hysterectomy. *RN, 65*(3), 30-33.

60. UNICEF. (2005). *Changing a harmful social convention: Female genital mutilation/cutting.* Retrieved 01/26/07 from www.unicef.org/childrenandislam/events/changing_fgm_press.html.

61. UNICEF. (2005). *Female genital mutilation/cutting: A statistical exploration.* Retrieved 01/12/07 from www.unicef.org/publications/files/FGM-C final 10 October.pdf .

62. Varney, H., Kriebs, J., & Gegor, C. (2004). *Varney's midwifery* (4th ed.). Boston: Jones & Bartlett.

63. Vleck, J., & Safranek, S. (2002). What medications are effective for treating symptoms of premenstrual syndrome (PMS)? *Journal of Family Practice, 51*(10), 894.

64. World Health Organization. (2005). *The World Health Report: Make every mother and child count.* Geneva: World Health Organization.

65. World Health Organization. (2006). Female genital mutilation and obstetrical outcome: WHO collaborative prospective study in six African countries. *The Lancet, 367*, 1835-1841.

66. Wright, T., et al. (2002). Consensus guidelines for the management of women with cervical cytological abnormalities. *Journal of the American Medical Association, 287*(16), 2120-2129.

67. Wright, T., Holinka, C., Ferenczy, , et al. (2002). Estradiol-induced hyperplasia in endometrial biopsies from women on hormone replacement therapy. *American Journal of Surgical Pathology, 10*, 1269-1275.

68. Writing Group for the Women's Health Initiative Investigators. (2002). Risks and benefits of estrogen plus progestin in healthy postmenopausal women. Principal results from the Women's Health Initiative: Randomized controlled trial. *Journal of the American Medical Association, 288*(3), 321-333.

69. U.S. Preventive Services Task Force. (2003). Postmenopausal hormone replacement therapy for the primary prevention of chronic conditions: Recommendations and rationale. *American Journal of Nursing, 103*(6), 83-91.

evolve   *Did you remember to check out the bonus material on the Evolve website and the CD-ROM, including NCLEX®-Examination Style Review Questions, Open-Book Quizzes, and Chapter Review Audio Podcasts?*

http://evolve.elsevier.com/Black/medsurg

CHAPTER 40

Management of Clients with Breast Disorders

MELISSA CRAFT

A woman who finds a breast lump or other breast problem will probably first suspect cancer, even though 8 of 10 lumps are benign. Despite many misconceptions regarding the etiology of breast cancer, public awareness about this health threat has grown dramatically. In the past, the subject was avoided, or if information was shared, it was often inaccurate. Now breast cancer is openly discussed, and information about this topic is frequently presented in mass media. With the recent media focus on breast cancer awareness and early detection, the public is becoming more aware of the roles that breast self-examination, clinical examination, and especially routine mammograms have in the early detection of a breast mass.

Nurses have a responsibility to teach the public about breast lesions and cancer, to correct misconceptions, and to provide accurate information concerning normal breasts and breast disease, detection, and treatment. Facts about the disease, treatment, and prognosis need to be shared openly with all members of society, particularly the underserved. If women understand the importance of early detection and treatment, they are more likely to have regular mammograms and less likely to delay seeking medical care when an abnormality is found. Delay in seeking medical care is often due to (1) fear that the problem is cancer and (2) lack of knowledge that breast cancer can be curable if caught early.

BREAST CANCER IN WOMEN

Breast cancer is the most common malignancy in women in the United States and is second only to lung cancer as a cause of cancer death.[2,22] The incidence of breast cancer in the United States had been increasing gradually for the past 30 years. However, from 2006 to 2007, the number of new cases of invasive breast cancer diagnosed in women in the United States was estimated to decrease from 212,920 (2006) to 178,480 (2007), with 41,430 (2006) and 40,910 (2007) deaths caused by the disease.[2] The sharp decrease from 2006 is thought to be related to fewer women taking hormone replacements for menopause following the sudden termination of the Women's Health Initiative (WHI) study in 2002.[48] At age 85 years, a woman's risk for breast cancer is one in eight, depending on where she lives. The highest incidence of breast cancer occurs in the United States and Europe.

Before 1990 there was little evidence of any decrease in the United States age-standardized death rate from breast cancer. Currently, breast cancer mortality appears to be declining among all women. Between 1990 and 2002, death rates decreased by 2.3% annually for all races combined.[2,22] (Breast cancer in men is rare and is discussed later in this chapter.) The decrease in mortality may be ascribed to the combined benefits of early detection and better treatment.[18] There is some evidence that the death rate is reduced when practitioners follow evidence-based practice guidelines.[11,43] The increase in early diagnosis attributable to mammography and the generally increased awareness of breast cancer among women and their physicians have resulted in

---

evolve **Web Enhancements**

Case Study Breast Cancer with Mastectomy

Client Education Guide Arm Care After Axillary Lymph Node Dissection (English Version and Spanish Translation)

Postmastectomy Exercises (Spanish Translation)

Ethical Issues in Nursing Communication Problem or Ethical Dilemma?

Tables TNM Staging System for Breast Cancer

Complementary and Alternative Therapy Multivitamins, Alcohol, and Breast Cancer

Be sure to check out the bonus material on the Evolve website and the CD-ROM, including free self-assessment exercises. **http://evolve.elsevier. com/Black/medsurg**

detection of smaller tumors, which are more likely to be localized and to be treated successfully.[22]

Probably the most important encouragement to breast cancer detection has been the discovery that screening mammography reduces breast cancer deaths by 30%.[1,60] The Breast and Cervical Cancer Mortality Act of 1990 was enacted to ensure that underinsured or uninsured women receive mammograms and appropriate treatment services.[15] In 2000 the Breast and Cervical Cancer Treatment and Prevention Act (BCCTP) was passed to help provide treatment to women diagnosed with breast and cervical cancer. Women need to understand the importance of mammography in detecting breast cancers while tumors are small. Likewise, they should understand that the treatment is less toxic and more effective for all modalities used when the disease is detected early, even before the tumor is palpable. With regard to surgery, less tissue is removed when the tumor is small; therefore better cosmesis is possible. With irradiation of a smaller volume of diseased tissue, cure is more likely and a lower dose is needed for radiation therapy. With adjuvant treatment, a small tumor burden means that systemic therapy may not be needed; if it is needed, then drug treatment is more successful. Smaller tumors also mean less regional node involvement and fewer complications associated with axillary node dissection.[59]

Nurses need to provide current and accurate information concerning the latest approaches to breast cancer treatment and related complications. Encouraging the client to participate in research, if appropriate, is especially important, so that critical questions regarding breast cancer therapy can be addressed. Clients and their families are required to make many difficult decisions. The nurse can be especially helpful by ensuring that the client understands treatment options and by providing clarification when appropriate.

Etiology and Risk Factors

The cause of breast cancer is not known. Many women are anxious about their risk for breast cancer, and many tend to overestimate their risk. Even though genetic, hormonal, or biochemical factors are likely to be involved, 70% of women with breast cancer have no known risk factors.

Age and Ethnicity

All women are at risk for breast cancer, and the most important single risk factor is age. Risk increases with age, although the rate of increase slows after menopause. Since 1987 incidence rates have continued to increase for women age 50 and over; however, rates have decreased for women age 40 to 49, and stayed essentially unchanged for women under 40.[3] Compared to Caucasian women, African-American women younger

than 50 have a higher age-specific incidence of breast cancer.[47]

Edwards and colleagues, in their examination of the impact of race on survival in breast cancer, found not only that African-American women are less likely to be cured than their non–African-American counterparts, but also that they survive for a shorter time until death from breast cancer.[22] Even when matched for tumor stage, they are more at risk for micrometastatic disease and early death. It is not clear whether these findings are related to tumor biology, host response, or variability in treatment. Psychosocial and socioeconomic factors have a major role in governing access to medical care. Uninsured clients and those insured by Medicaid present with more advanced disease, have a higher risk of death, and have lessened survival compared with privately insured clients.[10,47]

Breast cancer incidence among Hispanic women living in North America is only 40% as great as that among non-Hispanic Caucasian women. Asian women born in Asia have a very low lifetime risk of breast cancer, but their daughters born in North America have the same lifetime risk of breast cancer as for American Caucasian women.[10] Overall incidence rates in Caucasians, African Americans, and Hispanic/Latinos did not change much during 1992 to 2002; however, there continues to be disparity between stage-specific incidence, with African-American women more likely to be diagnosed with larger tumors.[3] The Community-Based Practice box on p. 942 addresses disparities in the incidence of breast cancer.

Ovarian and Hormonal Function

Early menarche (first menses) and late menopause (cessation of menses) lead to an increased total lifetime number of ovulatory menstrual cycles and a corresponding 30% to 50% increase in breast cancer risk. The woman who experiences natural menopause before age 45 years has a risk for breast cancer that is half that of the woman whose menopause occurs after age 55 years.[1] Likewise, oophorectomy before a woman reaches menopause lowers her risk of breast cancer by approximately two thirds. Both nulliparity (no births) and age older than 30 years at first live birth are associated with a nearly doubled risk of subsequent breast cancer.[3]

The use of hormone replacement therapy (HRT) has also demonstrated a small but significant increase in risk for breast cancer in women who have used it for more than 10 years. The Women's Health Initiative (WHI) study, which included women randomized to receive hormones or placebo, was conducted by the National Heart, Lung, and Blood Institute (NHLBI).[48] Increased risk of breast cancer was observed for women in the estrogen plus progesterone arm but only after approximately 4 years. No increased risk was observed in the estrogen

COMMUNITY-BASED PRACTICE

Breast Cancer

The presence of nursing when planning for the health needs of the community is relevant. Nursing's underpinnings with serving people in need and using a holistic focus in a nonjudgmental manner are why it is imperative to include our profession.

The Interfaith Health Project, a multi-denomination group that is composed of nine ministries within the city of Omaha, Nebraska, initiated informal data collection of its congregation. They found that Hispanic women were interested in exercise classes. The Douglas County Health Department (in Omaha, Nebraska) became involved shortly thereafter and developed the "Latinas en Accion" (Latin Women in Action) group. In addition, The Douglas County Health Department desired to enlarge the focus of the initial project and is currently performing a formalized data collection to better understand the complete health care needs of this rapidly growing Hispanic population.

To enhance cultural competence during data collection, the Douglas County Health Department sought the assistance of one of its natives, Dr. Madelyn Leininger, a nursing leader with a doctorate in anthropology who is renowned for her work in developing transcultural nursing theory.[3] In this nursing model, patterns and practices of health care (including holistic health, illness, and death) are influenced by technology, religion and philosophy of life, kinship/families/social links, cultural views, and beliefs. These factors were actively incorporated in the development of a three-part open-ended questionnaire.

This questionnaire, to elicit transcultural assessment with Hispanic women, is administered during scheduled exercise classes. Senior nursing students are responsible for collecting data about family backgrounds, including the following: which members provide "caring" behaviors within the family, which members provide health care within the home, definitions and meaning of health and illness, strategies used to adapt to stress and life in the United States, and use of religion as a means of coping. Sophomore nursing students are responsible for collecting physical signs of health (e.g., body mass index [BMI], balance, waist measurements, blood pressure, and pulse rate).

A 3-year federal grant was approved based on this model and the "Latinas en Accion" group was started in August of 2006. Dr. Leininger held a workshop before data collection to facilitate understanding of the theoretical tenets and mission of this project for the staff (at all levels) of the Douglas County Health Department and its various community members that form this project's team.

Actual health care topics identified by Hispanic women have been skin health and healthy diet. Potential topics to be covered in the future will be breast health and diabetes mellitus. Although African American women have the highest rate of breast cancer, Hispanic women have had the fewest clinical breast examinations compared to other ethnic groups.[1] They are the third most likely ethnic group to develop breast cancer.[1] This connotes a negative outcome when diagnosing breast cancer in its early stages and increases the risk of later diagnosis and metastasis of the disease. A contributing factor to the preference Latina women have for women health care providers results in the avoidance of breast examination if the provider of health care is a male.

A reduction in breast cancer has been noted in women who exercise on a regular basis.[2] Information about breast self-examination and the relationship of exercise to decreasing breast cancer rates should be disseminated in conjunction with "Latinas en Accion" exercise classes. This relationship could help reinforce attendance at these exercise classes and encourage women to start performing self breast-examinations. A listing of female health care providers (including certified nurse-midwives [CNMs] and advanced practice registered nurses [APRNs]) and medical doctors [MDs]) could be distributed to class participants to encourage annual breast examinations.

REFERENCES

1. Coughlin, S.S., et al. (2004). Breast cancer screening practices among women in the United States, 2000. *CDC Cancer Causes and Control, 15*(2), 159-170.
2. Gilliland, F.D., et al. (2001). Physical activity and breast cancer risk in Hispanic and non-Hispanic white women. *American Journal of Epidemiology, 154*(5), 442-450.
3. Leininger, M. (1995). *Transcultural nursing: Concepts, theories, research and practices.* New York: McGraw-Hill and Greyden Press.

only arm after 7 years of follow up.[37] Previous studies have indicated that using HRT for less than 5 years (or short-term use) is considerably less likely to increase the risk of breast cancer.[48] Therefore it is possible that, for short-term use, there may be more benefit than risk.[45,48]

It has been recommended that combination HRT not be prescribed for long-term use.[46] The American Heart Association has recommended making HRT decisions based on noncoronary benefits and risks. The choice for each woman must be individual and frequently involves a formal risk-benefit analysis including the possibility of increased risk of breast cancer.

At present there is no convincing evidence that oral contraceptive use affects the risk of breast cancer.[23] However, women who have a strong family history of breast cancer may have an increased risk, especially if they use oral contraceptives before the age of 30.[32,42]

Benign Breast Disease

Benign breast disease is not more common in women with other risk factors for breast cancer. Nonproliferative lesions (e.g., cysts, duct ectasia, mild hyperplasia, and fibroadenoma) do not increase the risk of breast cancer; however, cellular atypia or atypical hyperplasia (a proliferative disease) is an example of a histologic change associated with a higher risk. Complex fibroadenomas, sclerosing adenosis, epithelial calcification, and papillary apocrine changes increase the relative risk of breast cancer two-fold to three-fold, but the exact incidence and factors that influence malignant transformation are not well determined.[1] Studies indicate that women with a family history of breast cancer and atypical hyperplasia have at least a three-fold increased risk of breast cancer.[65]

Family History

Family history is one of the known risk factors for breast cancer. Breast cancer attributable to the inheritance of a specific germ line mutation from either maternal or paternal relatives is rare. In fact, the breast cancer susceptibility genes *BRCA1* and *BRCA2* and the *p53* tumor suppressor gene have been identified in fewer than 10% of all women with breast cancer. The Genetic Links box at right explores familial breast cancer susceptibility. Certain populations have a higher incidence of *BRCA* mutations than the general population (e.g., native Icelanders and Ashkenazi Jews).[1] Depending on the familial context, the lifetime risk of breast cancer, ovarian cancer, or both associated with carrying a mutation ranges from 50% to 85%.[1] Families with several affected first-degree relatives and clients with early-onset disease have been found to harbor mutations at a higher frequency. Commercial testing for mutations in *BRCA1* and *BRCA2* as well as for less common mutations that predispose to breast cancer, such as HNPCC (hereditary nonpolyposis colon cancer) and Li-Fraumeni, are available.[1] The decision to undergo genetic testing is individual and carries both benefits and limitations. Comprehensive breast cancer screening and high-risk counseling centers are ideal mechanisms for providing women with individualized evaluation, education, screening, and, when appropriate, genetic testing.[4]

In addition to hereditary breast cancer, it is estimated that approximately 15% to 20% of breast cancer cases are familial. Like hereditary cancer, a clustering of two or more relatives is affected; however, the ages of onset are older and a clear inheritance pattern may not be demonstrated. Familial breast cancer is probably related to a combination of genetic and environmental factors, and studies on these families may yield discovery of additional breast cancer genes. Newer multigene assays such as ONCOVUE BRE may be helpful in uncovering minor genetic changes that predispose women to breast cancer in the absence of strong family history.[6]

Environmental and Dietary Factors

An increased incidence of breast cancer has been reported in women who received mantle radiation for

---

GENETIC LINKS

Breast Cancer Susceptibility Genes: *BRCA1* and *BRCA2*

DESCRIPTION

Major cancer susceptibility genes may account for 5% to 10% of breast cancer cases. Two genes (*BRCA1* and *BRCA2*) have been identified and are thought to account for approximately 75% of all hereditary breast cancer. Other breast cancer susceptibility genes exist and contribute to a much smaller amount of breast cancer cases. Disease-causing mutations result in a predisposition to breast and ovarian cancer and other cancers, including prostate, colon, and others. Features suggestive of a *BRCA1/BRCA2* family include multiple affected family members, early age of onset, and bilateral disease.

GENETICS

BRCA1 and *BRCA2* mutations are estimated to occur in 1 of every 300 individuals. Persons who are Ashkenazi Jewish have a much higher incidence of these mutations: 1 of every 40 individuals. These mutations are inherited in an autosomal dominant manner, with each offspring of an affected parent having a 50% risk of inheriting the mutation.

DIAGNOSIS/TESTING

Clinical molecular testing for *BRCA1/BRCA2* is available for an affected individual who is at high risk for having a *BRCA1/BRCA2* mutation or for at-risk family members of an individual who has an identified mutation. Multiple molecular laboratory methods are used to identify mutations, but identification of all disease-causing mutations cannot be guaranteed.

MANAGEMENT

Education and counseling of affected individuals and family members are essential. Recommendations are made for cancer screening of individuals who have a *BRCA1* or *BRCA2* mutation. Some women choose to have prophylactic mastectomy and oophorectomy to reduce the risk of cancer.

---

the treatment of Hodgkin's disease, particularly if they were younger than 20.[31,34] The latency period is between 10 and 25 years. The disease in this group typically presents more aggressively, with a high rate of nodal involvement and bilaterality. It is for this reason that all clients who receive mantle radiation for Hodgkin's disease, especially those treated before age 20 years, receive a regular mammography follow-up examination to detect these lesions early.[34] Based on a review of high risk imaging protocols, the American Cancer Society published guidelines in Spring 2007 recommending annual MRI for these women as well as an annual mammogram.[57] Sophisticated, modern radiation therapy techniques have lowered the incidence of breast cancer and other long-term complications in these clients.[34]

Alcohol intake is the best-established dietary risk factor for breast cancer in epidemiologic studies. The positive correlation of alcohol intake with breast cancer risk has been established, and it appears that moderate alcohol intake (one to two drinks per day) increases the risk of breast cancer by altering estrogen metabolism.[21] Drinking in moderation, defined as about one drink per day, is an example of a modifiable risk factor for breast cancer. Folic acid has been shown in previous research to reduce the risk of breast cancer in women who consume alcohol; however, in a recent study, it was found to actually increase risk.[63] (See the Complementary and Alternative Therapy feature on Multivitamins, Alcohol, and Breast Cancer on the website.)

Many women and clinicians question the role of diet in breast cancer development. As is commonly observed, Japanese women living in Japan have a very low incidence of breast cancer. When they move to the United States, their risk for breast cancer approximates that of native Caucasian women within one generation. It is unclear if this is due to environmental or dietary factors although most researchers favor dietary factors. A recent prospective study found no significant difference between an intervention group of women on a low-fat diet versus a control group.[53] There is, however, a possibility that the influence of dietary fat, obesity, and high caloric intake may impact postmenopausal breast cancer differently than premenopausal breast cancer. The Complementary and Alternative Therapy box at right addresses the link between diet and breast cancer. Identification of separate risk factors for premenopausal and postmenopausal women may determine a role for fat intake in the future.[64]

Epidemiologic evidence does not support any substantial increase in breast cancer risk associated with caffeine consumption, and in fact a recent study indicates that drinking coffee might have a beneficial effect for premenopausal women and breast cancer reduction.[7] Studies have shown that consumption of fruits and vegetables is not significantly related to a reduction in breast cancer risk.[29] Passive cigarette smoking has been thought to be unrelated to breast cancer risk, but a new study suggests that passive and active smoking may impart a small risk for premenopausal breast cancer, especially when smoking is initiated at young ages.[33] More importantly, for nurses in particular, several recent studies have suggested that working at night may increase the relative risk of breast cancer by 60%.[19] The risk appeared to be related to the amount of time spent working at night. Working night shifts increased risk by about the same amount as alcohol use and delayed childbirth.[58] This could have obvious implications for nursing both individually and collectively.

Nurses have a unique role in fostering health promotion and in teaching women about breast cancer as well

COMPLEMENTARY AND ALTERNATIVE THERAPY

Diet and Breast Cancer: Everything in Moderation?

Researchers in this study were motivated by the observation that in many studies there seems to be a U-shaped association of body mass index and survival in breast cancer. In other words, moderate and healthy weight may be associated with a better survival rate as opposed to extremes in weight (too thin or too heavy). The researchers wanted to see if this relationship is true for diet. A total of 477 women with surgically resected T1 to T3, N0/1, M0 breast cancer completed a food frequency questionnaire approximately 9.3 ± 4.6 weeks after diagnosis (reporting their intakes of food over the previous 12 months). Median follow-up of the survivors was 6.1 years.

Researchers found a nonlinear survival association for protein, oleic acid, cholesterol, polyunsaturated-saturated fat ratio, and percentage of calories from fat and percentage of calories from carbohydrates. Their data suggest that the midrange (moderation) intake of most major energy or food sources was associated with the most favorable outcomes, whereas extremes in diet were associated with less favorable outcomes. In summary, moderate diets or lifestyles that produce a normal body mass index may be associated with the best breast cancer outcomes.

REFERENCE

Goodwin, P., et al. (2003). Diet and breast cancer: Evidence that extremes in diet are associated with poor survival. *Journal of Clinical Oncology, 21*, 2500-2507.

as in identifying a woman's individual risk for breast cancer. Because most women—especially those with any family history of breast cancer—greatly overestimate their risk for breast cancer, it is helpful to instruct women about the known risk factors and, as indicated, provide support to lessen some of their fears (Table 40-1). Counseling, with appropriate referrals when required, should always accompany specific recommendations for clients with significant risks. The American Cancer Society published new screening guidelines in May 2003 and updated them in 2007. These guidelines help women determine the appropriate screening for their individual risk. The new guidelines also state that women who are at increased risk for breast cancer may benefit from more frequent screenings and additional imaging modalities (e.g., ultrasound and magnetic resonance imaging [MRI]).[4,11,57,62]

Health Promotion Activities

Although no known agent or practice guarantees that a woman will remain free of breast cancer, methods are under investigation that may alter the risk and therefore can be considered health promotion activities.

TABLE 40–1   **American Cancer Society Guidelines for Early Breast Cancer Detection**

Women at average risk	Begin mammography at age 40.
	For women in their 20s and 30s, it is recommended that clinical breast examination be part of a periodic health examination, preferably at least every 3 years. Asymptomatic women ages 40 and older should continue to receive a clinical breast examination as part of a periodic health examination, preferably annually.
	Beginning in their 20s, women should be told about the benefits and limitations of breast self-examination (BSE). The importance of prompt reporting of any new breast symptoms to a health professional should be emphasized. Women who choose to do BSE should receive instruction and have their technique reviewed on the occasion of a periodic health examination. It is acceptable for women to choose not to do BSE or to do BSE irregularly.
	Women should have an opportunity to become informed about the benefits, limitations, and potential harms associated with regular screening.
Older women	Screening decisions in older women should be individualized by considering the potential benefits and risks of mammography in the context of current health status and estimated life expectancy. As long as a woman is in reasonably good health and would be a candidate for treatment, she should continue to be screened with mammography.
Women at increased risk	Women who have a lifetime risk of breast cancer exceeding 20%-25% including women who have a strong family history of breast and/or ovarian cancer and women who were treated for Hodgkin's disease should be screened with annual mammogram and annual MRI.

From American Cancer Society. (2007). *American Cancer Society guidelines for the early detection of cancer.* Retrieved 01/27/07 from www.cancer.org/docroot/PED/center/ PED_2_3x_ACS_Cancer_Detection_Guidelines_36.asp?sitearea=PED; and Saslow, D., Boates, C., Burke, W., Harms, S., et al. (2007) American Cancer Society guidelines for breast screening with MRI as an adjunct to mammography. *CA Cancer Journal for Clinicians, 57,* 75-89.

Chemoprevention. Chemoprevention is the use of a drug to prevent the development of a certain malignancy. Two agents have been found to decrease the risk of breast cancer: tamoxifen (Nolvadex) and raloxifene (Evista). These agents are discussed in the Integrating Pharmacology feature on p. 946. Tamoxifen is an agent commonly used in clients who have breast tumors with receptors for estrogen. Fisher and colleagues[25] looked at tamoxifen and its role in decreasing the incidence of breast cancer in high-risk clients. In this study, 13,388 high-risk women were randomized to receive either placebo or tamoxifen 20 mg/day. Tamoxifen reduced the risk of invasive breast cancer by 49% overall; however, endometrial cancer developed in twice as many women in the tamoxifen group as in the placebo group. In another study, 7705 women with osteoporosis were randomized to receive either a placebo or raloxifene.[17] Over 33 months, nearly twice as many invasive breast cancers were seen in the placebo group as in the raloxifene group.

In contrast to the tamoxifen trial, there was no increase in the incidence of endometrial cancer in women who received raloxifene. Because raloxifene had never been compared with tamoxifen as a chemopreventive agent and had not been studied in women at high risk for breast cancer, the National Surgical Adjuvant Breast Project (NSABP) conducted a double-blind study that compared these 2 drugs in 19,747 high-risk women. Results from this trial, first reported in April 2006, indicated that although breast cancer chemoprevention was equal between the two drugs, raloxifene did appear to have fewer side effects. These findings, however, were not statistically significant for any side effect except for the development of cataracts requiring

surgery.[44] The FDA approved raloxifene (Evista) in September 2007 for the prevention of breast cancer in postmenopausal women.

Prophylactic Mastectomy. The only other measure that may predictably prevent the occurrence of breast cancer and be considered a method of health promotion is prophylactic mastectomy. All of the breast tissue is removed in a woman who does not have evidence of breast cancer. Women who may benefit from this procedure are those who have a strong family history of breast cancer, a history of breast cancer in the other breast, a history of atypical hyperplasia on repeated surgical biopsies, or the presence of a mutated *BRCA1* or *BRCA2* gene. Breast cancer incidence may be reduced as much as 90% in women who have a prophylactic mastectomy.[55] However, it is not known whether prophylactic mastectomy is superior to careful clinical and radiologic screening of high-risk women, especially with the emergence of the role of MRI in the screening of high-risk breast cancer clients.

Lifestyle Changes. Women can also be encouraged to make changes in lifestyle to lower their potential risk for breast cancer. For instance, they can decrease their consumption of alcohol. Although a moderate decrease in dietary fat intake does not appear to reduce the risk of breast cancer, decreasing fat intake to 20% of dietary calories is a worthwhile goal for many chronic diseases.[1]

Exercise may have an indirect role in the prevention of breast cancer. Exercise leads to a decrease in body fat, thereby reducing the amount of free estrogen stored in body fat. Hence it is another health promotion activity.

Medications for Breast Cancer

Many women with breast cancer receive a hormonal agent as one part of their treatment. Generally it is the last modality used in their multimodality regimen. Drugs used include tamoxifen or an aromatase inhibitor. Some women will receive one agent for 2 to 3 years followed by the other. Dosing for tamoxifen (Nolvadex) is 20 mg/day for 5 years, for anastrozole (Arimidex) 1 mg/day, for letrozole (Femara) 2.5 mg/day, and for exemestane (Aromasin) 25 mg/day.

Tamoxifen is a drug classified as a selective estrogen receptor modulator. It works by competing for the binding site normally occupied by estrogen. By blocking the ability of estrogen to bind with estrogen receptor–positive breast cancer cells, it controls and even prevents the growth of breast cancer cells. Tamoxifen is usually well tolerated and has limited potential for drug interactions. There are side effects, however, and some may affect the breast cancer survivor's quality of life. Side effects include hot flashes, mood swings, depression, and anecdotal reports of memory changes. Other side effects include an increased risk for stroke, pulmonary emboli, cataracts, endometrial cancer, and vaginal dryness. Women should be followed up by their oncologist and family practitioner and gynecologist to monitor for any negative sequelae of taking tamoxifen.

Aromatase inhibitors block the synthesis of estrogen from adrenal androgens. They are useful in postmenopausal women who are not producing estrogen from their ovaries. For this reason tamoxifen is the hormonal agent given to premenopausal women. Aromatase inhibitors may cause musculoskeletal disorders such as myalgia, joint stiffness, and osteoporosis. Other side effects include hypercholesterolemia, stroke, and pulmonary emboli. Women should be monitored for osteoporosis and treated appropriately.

IMPLICATIONS

With increasing numbers of premenopausal women taking tamoxifen, it is important to recognize that amenorrhea, although likely, is not guaranteed, and that the woman could become pregnant. Tamoxifen is thought to be teratogenic, so premenopausal women should practice some form of birth control while taking it. Risks and benefits of both of these hormonal agents need to be addressed with clients so they can make informed decisions.

REFERENCES

1. American Cancer Society. (2007). *Cancer facts and figures 2007*. Atlanta: Author.
2. Breast Cancer Guidelines. (2007). *Clinical Practice Guidelines in Oncology, version 2*. National Comprehensive Cancer Network. Retrieved 09/20/07 from www.nccn.org/professionals/physician_gls/PDF/breast.pdf.
3. Buzdar, A.U., & Cuzick, J. (2006). Anastrozole as an adjuvant endocrine treatment for postmenopausal patients with breast cancer: Emerging data. *Clinical Practice Research, 1*(12), 1037s-1048s.
4. Cataliotti, L., et al. (2006). Comparison of anastrozole versus tamoxifen as preoperative therapy in postmenopausal women with hormone receptor-positive breast cancer: The preoperative "Arimidex" compared to tamoxifen (PROACT) trial. *Cancer*, Apr 5, Epub

Health Maintenance Activities

Health maintenance involves optimal screening and early detection of breast cancer. Regardless of the method used, regular and careful physical examination is the key to identifying asymptomatic cancerous lesions. When combined with mammography, physical examination decreases mortality, especially in women older than age 50. According to the National Cancer Advisory Board (NCAB), a committee that advises and consults with the director of the National Cancer Institute (NCI), data presented at the Consensus Development Conference showed that regular screening mammography of average-risk women in their 40s reduces deaths from breast cancer by about 17% to 24%.[9] On the basis of this finding, the NCAB recommended to the NCI that women between the ages of 40 and 49 years have screening mammograms every 1 to 2 years if they are at average risk for breast cancer. In November 2000, the American College of Radiology (ACR), the American Cancer Society, the American Medical Women's Association, and numerous women's groups issued a statement that supports annual screening mammography starting at age 40 years. The ACR believes that clinical trials have shown that having screening mammograms every year, compared to every 1 to 2 years, allows the detection of cancers at an earlier stage.[11] In January 2002, the U.S. Preventive Services Task Force (USPSTF) reaffirmed the value of mammography for women older than 40 years. Once a mammogram reveals an area suggestive of cancer, an ultrasound study is a useful complement to diagnostic mammography as a means for distinguishing cystic from solid masses. For women with particularly dense breasts or with implants, MRI scanning and digital mammography provide improved sensitivity. It is hoped that better mammography technology, including digitized radiography, routine use of magnified views, and greater skill in interpretation, combined with MRI and positron emission tomography (PET) scanning, will make it possible to identify breast cancers at an earlier stage. The results of a large prospective trial comparing digital mammography and film-screen mammography reported that digital mammography is superior to film mammography in women with dense breast tissue, in women under age 50, and in premenopausal/perimenopausal women.[52]

Health care professionals and health care advocates have for many years promoted breast self-examination (BSE) as a key component of early cancer detection because most breast cancers are detected by the woman herself, usually after the mass has grown to the size of 2.5 cm or larger. The only reason the cancer is detected then is that the mass is large enough to be felt. A better goal would be to detect the cancer while it is still small, before it can be felt (Figure 40-1). The only way to do this is by regular mammography and physical examination by a trained clinician (see Chapter 37). BSE

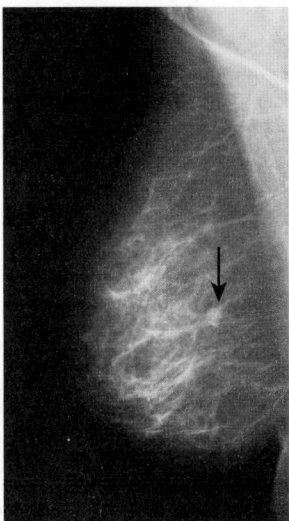

FIGURE 40–1 Screening mammogram of a 56-year-old woman with a strong family history of breast cancer, right mediolateral oblique view. The mammogram shows a small, irregular, nonpalpable mass *(arrow)*, which was highly suggestive of malignancy. Refer to Figure 37-6 on p. 860 for a view of a normal mammogram.

has not been proven to save lives or to increase survival. There is insufficient evidence to recommend for or against the teaching of BSE; however, teaching a woman to examine her breasts is an important strategy for increasing her awareness of the risk of breast cancer.[3]

Health Restoration Activities

Using arm exercises and proper positioning after surgery to prevent lymphedema, obtaining a prosthesis, and undergoing breast reconstruction are health restoration activities. If lymphedema develops despite exercises and positioning, referral to a physical therapist or specialized nurse for lymphedema management is recommended. The Complementary and Alternative Therapy box at right explores the benefits of exercise for breast cancer survivors.

Pathophysiology

Breast cancers are malignant tumors that typically begin in the ductal-lobular epithelial cells of the breast and spread via the lymphatic system to the axillary lymph nodes. The tumor may then metastasize to distant regions of the body, including lungs, liver, bone, and brain. The finding of breast cancer in the axillary lymph nodes is an indicator of the tumor's ability for potential distant spread and is not merely contiguous growth into the adjacent region of the breast. Most primary breast cancers are adenocarcinomas located in the upper outer quadrant of the breast (Figure 40-2).

Carcinoma In Situ

Malignant-appearing cells confined to the ductal or lobular units without permeation of the basement membrane

Exercise for Breast Cancer Survivors

A total of 53 postmenopausal breast cancer survivors were randomly allocated to an exercise group (n = 25) or control group (n = 28). The exercise group trained on cycle ergometers 3 times a week for 15 weeks, and the control group did not train. Peak oxygen consumption increased significantly in the exercise group, as did overall quality of life scores compared to the control group.[2]

Until recently, many doctors told women who had lymph node dissection and/or radiation treatment as treatment for breast cancer that weight lifting might increase the risk of lymphedema. However, in a recent study 45 breast cancer survivors participated in the Weight Training for Breast Cancer Survivors study.[1] In the study by Ahmed and colleagues, these women, including 13 who already had lymphedema, lifted weights 2 times a week for 6 months. None of the women that lifted weights had a change in arm circumference of 2 cm or more after the 6 months of weight lifting. It was concluded that exercise may actually increase lymph flow and decrease lymphedema manifestations.

Thus exercise training should be advocated in postmenopausal breast cancer survivors (and possibly all survivors) because of a significant effect on cardiopulmonary function and quality of life and a way to minimize lymphedema.

REFERENCES

1. Ahmed, R., et al. (2006). Randomized controlled trial of weight training and lymphedema in breast cancer survivors. *Journal of Clinical Oncology, 24*(18), 2765-2772.
2. Courneya, K., et al. (2003). Randomized controlled trial of exercise training in postmenopausal breast cancer survivors: Cardiopulmonary and quality of life outcomes. *Journal of Clinical Oncology, 21*, 1660-1668.

represent carcinoma in situ. *Ductal carcinoma in situ* (DCIS) is a precursor of infiltrating carcinoma. Pathologists classify DCIS as high-grade, intermediate-grade, or low-grade according to the growth pattern of cells occupying the ducts, their nuclear features, mitotic activity, presence of necrosis, and type of microcalcifications. Low-grade DCIS tends to be the most common and is typically multifocal; high-grade DCIS is second in prevalence and tends to be architecturally contiguous and associated with prominent microcalcifications. High-grade DCIS tends to be estrogen receptor–negative, shows increased expression for human epidermal growth factor receptor (HER-2)/neu protein (c-erbB2), and has a mutated *p53* tumor suppressor gene.

Ipsilateral (affecting the same side) invasive carcinoma develops within 10 years in approximately 30% of cases of DCIS. Left untreated, intraductal carcinoma transforms into invasive ductal carcinoma.

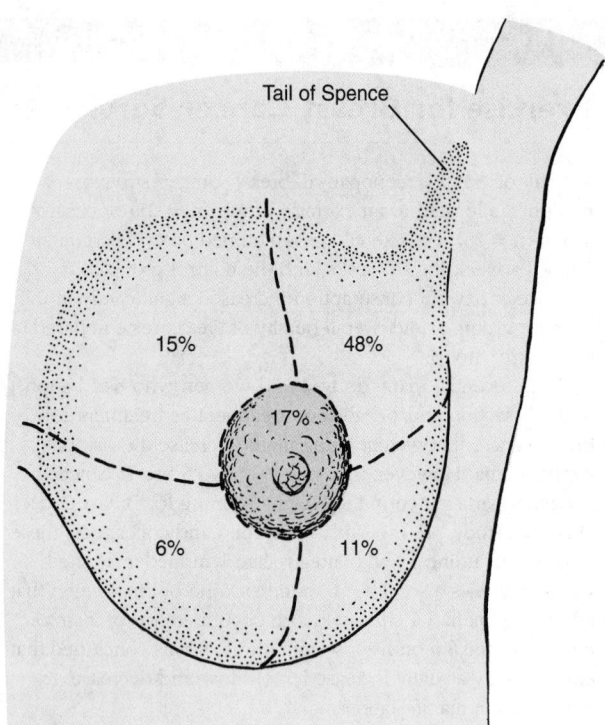

Tail of Spence

15% 48%

17%

6% 11%

■ **FIGURE 40–2** Frequency of occurrence of breast cancer according to location. The highest occurrence is in the upper outer quadrant and in the tail of Spence.

Lobular carcinoma in situ (LCIS) is characterized by a solid proliferation of atypical cells expanding as lobular units. In contrast to DCIS, LCIS is usually found incidentally and is not typically associated with microcalcifications. Long thought of as merely a risk factor for breast cancer in either breast, research is beginning to suggest that LCIS is actually a precursor of breast cancer similar to DCIS and may require focused treatment such as wide excision.[39]

Invasive Breast Cancer

Most breast cancers (75%) are infiltrating ductal carcinomas. They typically metastasize to regional lymph nodes and beyond. Lobular carcinomas account for about 5% to 10% of cases and usually present as a generalized thickening. Tumor types that are associated with a favorable prognosis include tubular (accounting for 2% of cases), medullary (5% to 7%), and mucinous (colloid) carcinoma (3%). These histologic types tend to have low-grade histology, positive estrogen and progesterone receptor status, diploid deoxyribonucleic acid (DNA) content, low S phase fraction (discussed later under Prognosis and Defining Extent of Disease), and no oncogenic markers. Tumors with poor clinical prognosis are those associated with high-grade histology and dermal lymphatic invasion, designated as "inflammatory carcinoma." Inflammatory breast cancer is characterized

by skin redness and induration. Edema and warmth are other common associated findings. Frequently, palpable axillary and supraclavicular nodes and distant metastases are involved.

Clinical Manifestations

Most breast cancers present as painless, nontender, hard, irregularly shaped, nonmobile masses. About 60% of cancers are somewhat movable, 40% have regular borders by palpation, and 40% can feel soft or cystic. Even when no mass is present, other physical findings, such as nipple discharge, induration, and dimpling, can suggest malignancy. Heat and erythema of the breast skin may be related to inflammation but may also indicate inflammatory carcinoma. Skin edema is characteristic of malignant disease. The edema is due to the invasion and obstruction of dermal lymphatics by the tumor. If a tumor is suspected on the basis of the physical findings, a diagnostic mammogram is indicated.

Radiographic Findings

Additional diagnostic films of the affected breast, as well as localized compression and magnification views, increase the specificity of identifying the abnormality. Digital mammography and computer-assisted diagnosis (CAD) may be useful to evaluate the lesion, because these tests allow more variations in exposure and show the differences in tissue contrast more clearly. CAD uses a software program to target lesions suspected to be malignant. The specificity of the image is enhanced by on-screen evaluation, which improves detection.

Fine-Needle Aspiration

Fine-needle aspiration (FNA) is performed on an outpatient basis. The purpose is to determine whether a solid lump is a cyst or to confirm a clinically apparent diagnosis. If the mass turns out to be a cyst, the lump should disappear after the aspiration. If a lump is solid, a cytologic specimen may be obtained by making several passes into the lesion to retrieve small cell samples; this technique can reduce the incidence of false-negative results. If the FNA results are negative and the physician suspects cancer from the clinical findings, excisional biopsy (open) is indicated.

Stereotactic Needle-Guided Biopsy

Stereotactic needle-guided biopsy (SNB) is used mainly to target and identify nonpalpable lesions in the breast that have been detected with mammography. The basic goal is to immobilize the breast from fixed horizontal and vertical coordinates to calculate the exact position of the lesion within a three-dimensional field. SNB permits biopsy diagnosis of benign disease without the trauma or scarring of an open biopsy.

Ultrasound Core Biopsy

Ultrasound-guided breast biopsy is used when the lesion can be seen on ultrasound. It is easier for the client than a stereotactic biopsy because she can lie on her back and does not have to have her breast immobilized during the procedure. A local anesthetic is used to anesthetize the area and a biopsy is performed using a large-bore biopsy needle.

Open Biopsy

Excisional or open biopsy may be chosen when the lesion is determined to be solid and indeterminate in nature, when results of cytologic or histologic analysis are insufficient, or when the clinical or mammographic findings suggest malignancy. A wire-localized biopsy procedure similar to the stereotactic method can be used; the aim of this procedure is to assist the surgeon in locating the nonpalpable lesion for the purpose of excisional biopsy and to minimize the volume of tissue removed to avoid unnecessary deformity.

Prognosis and Defining Extent of Disease

Once a diagnosis of cancer is made, the cancer needs to be evaluated further to determine the most appropriate therapy. For example, if breast-conserving surgery (lumpectomy) is being considered, the presence of microcalcifications must be evaluated further to determine whether the disease in the breast is multifocal.

The tumor is staged according to the extent of local, regional, and distant spread. *Staging* permits an accurate definition of the extent of the disease and therefore a more accurate prognosis. The American Joint Committee on Cancer (AJCC) staging system for breast cancer is based on the tumor-node-metastasis (TNM) system, presented on the website. Prognosis for breast cancer is associated primarily with the extent of disease at detection. The tumor staging is based on (1) the size of the primary tumor; (2) whether it extends to the chest wall or skin; (3) the presence of axillary lymph nodes; (4) whether they are matted, fixed, or mobile; and (5) the presence of distant metastases (Figure 40-3). The

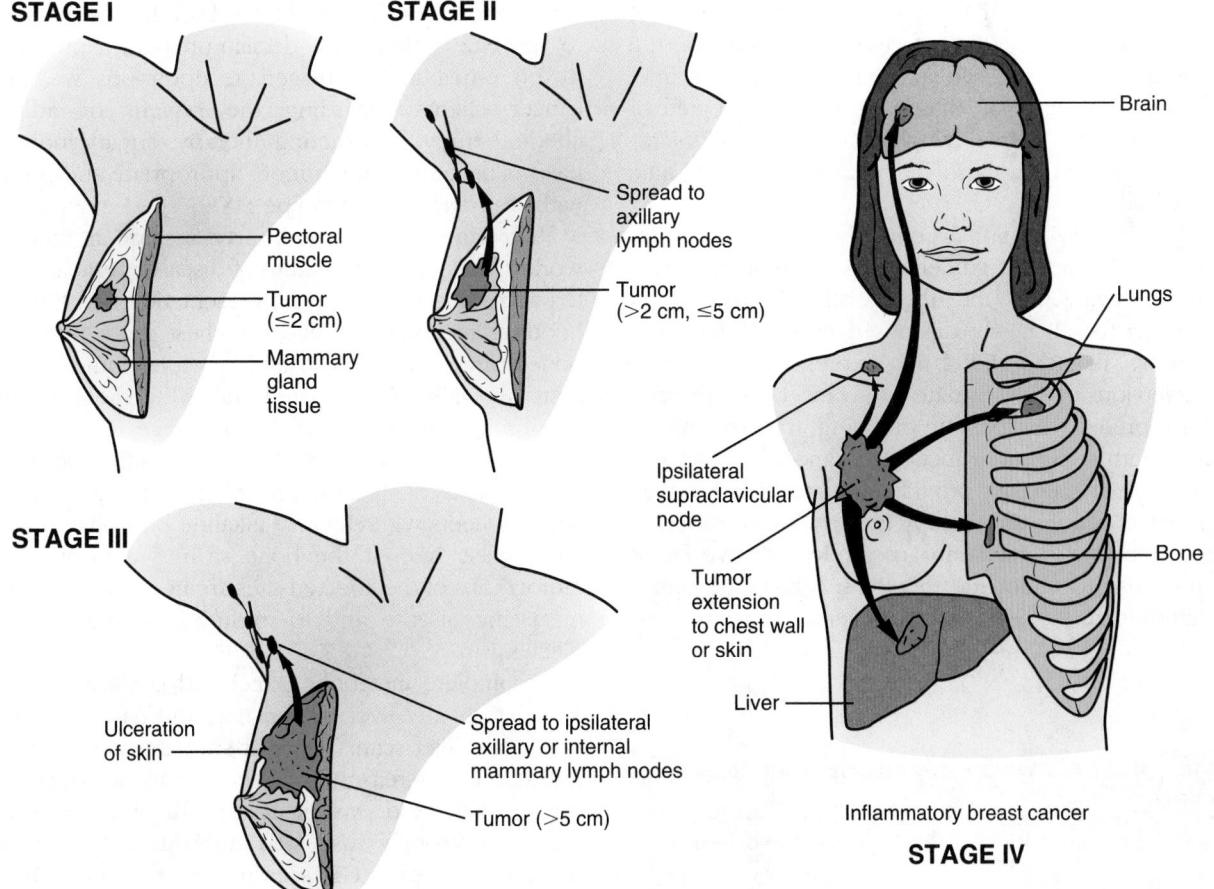

FIGURE 40–3 Clinical staging of breast cancer. *Stage I:* Tumor 2 cm or less in diameter and confined to the breast. *Stage II:* Tumor up to 5 cm, or early metastasis to axillary lymph nodes. *Stage III:* Tumor larger than 5 cm with involvement of the ipsilateral axillary or internal mammary lymph nodes. *Stage IV:* Distant metastasis, such as to brain, bone, or liver; ipsilateral supraclavicular lymph node; skin or extension to chest wall; or inflammatory breast cancer.

5-year survival rate for breast cancer based on stage of disease is presented in Table 40-2.

Prognostic factors are used to determine prognosis or the natural history of breast cancer. At present, only pathologic lymph node status, tumor size, estrogen and progesterone receptor status, level of HER-2/neu expression, histologic grade, and histopathology are considered to be independent prognostic indicators and therefore appropriate to consider in determining therapy and prognosis. Another factor that is often taken into consideration is the DNA content of the tumor. *DNA ploidy* refers to the degree of multiplication of chromosome sets. *Diploid* and *euploid* signify an exact multiple of the haploid number of chromosomes. *Aneuploid* indicates a deviation from an exact multiple of the haploid number and a poorer prognosis. The S phase index identifies the percentage of tumor cells in S phase (start of DNA synthesis) of the cell growth cycle. The higher the percentage of cells in S phase, the more aggressive the cancer.

The tumor is generally graded to determine the degree of differentiation and therefore prognosis. Tumors are classified as *well differentiated* (grade I), *moderately well differentiated* (grade II), or *poorly differentiated* (grade III) according to the degree of anaplasia observed. Other factors identified on the pathology report include nucleus size and shape, presence or absence of mitotic figures, and degree of tubule formation. Dermal lymphatic invasion and microvascular invasion may also be predictive of metastatic disease.

The 2007 National Comprehensive Cancer Network (NCCN) practice guidelines for breast cancer recommend evaluation of the level of HER-2/neu expression for all newly diagnosed clients.[11] Research has shown that the HER-2/neu expression is used in the selection of appropriate adjuvant chemotherapy and to predict the benefit of using trastuzumab in women with recurrent or metastatic cancer.[30] It has also been demonstrated to provide a survival advantage when used as adjuvant therapy in early breast cancer.[51] Steroid receptor status is an accepted predictive factor for response to endocrine therapies. If the tumor is determined to be estrogen receptor positive and progesterone receptor positive, anti-estrogen therapy is an appropriate therapeutic option with or without chemotherapy. Selective aromatase inhibitors (AIs) such as anastrozole (Arimidex), letrozole (Femara), and exemestane (Aromasin) have been shown to provide both an alternative to tamoxifen for estrogen receptor-positive postmenopausal women and an adjunct to therapy when both are used sequentially.[66] Ongoing research studies will help establish the appropriate synergy of these agents and provide data for decision making regarding long-term risk/benefit because of side effects such as the increased risk of osteoporosis presented by AIs.[35]

Tumor markers are not considered useful preoperatively when adjuvant therapy for cure is planned. Tumor markers are assessed as part of the work-up of advanced disease and generally have significance only in a woman with metastatic disease. Carcinoembryonic antigen (CEA), CA-125, and CA 15-3 are substances produced by the tumor and are present in the serum of the woman with breast cancer. A tumor marker is expected to be present only in metastatic disease, in which case it is assessed on a monthly basis to monitor response to therapy. A 21-gene Recurrence Score Assay (Oncotype DX) has been shown to provide additional decision-making information in node-negative, estrogen receptor-positive breast cancer clients regarding the benefit of adjuvant chemotherapy.[16] Targeting therapy on an individual basis is becoming much more appropriate and possible with tests such as Oncotype DX.

Pretreatment assessment may include a metastatic work-up to determine extent of disease. Tests are selected according to the clinical presentation and the likelihood of metastatic disease. A chest x-ray film and a bone scan are possible useful baseline studies. A bone scan is usually not indicated unless the client has invasive breast cancer that is at least stage II or III. Only 30% to 60% of clients with a true-positive bone scan have increased alkaline phosphatase levels, and only 20% of clients with elevated alkaline phosphatase levels are disease free. If the bone scan is abnormal, then radiographs of the affected sites are necessary to confirm metastatic disease and to exclude a benign etiologic mechanism.

A complete metabolic panel and physical examination detects any liver dysfunction and may identify the need for a liver scan. The liver scan is usually not done unless there is reason to suspect that the disease has spread or if the disease is at stage III. When metastatic disease is strongly suspected, an MRI study or a computed tomography (CT) scan may be ordered to further define and measure the extent of disease. A PET scan is not usually indicated unless results of the MRI or CT scan are indeterminate and metastatic disease is strongly suspected.

TABLE 40–2   **Five-Year Survival Rate for Breast Cancer by Stage**

Stage	5-Year Survival (% of Clients)
Localized	96
Regional	80
Distant	58

Data from *Surveillance Epidemiology End Results (SEER)*, National Cancer Institute. Retrieved 01/27/07 from www.seer.ims.nci.nih.gov.

OUTCOME MANAGEMENT

In the past, management of the client with breast cancer typically included a modified radical or a radical mastectomy. Postoperatively, the surgeon would assure the woman that all the cancer was removed and that treatment was ended. The current management approach to localized breast cancer is much more complicated, because much more is known about the systemic nature of breast cancer and the need for local control as well as appropriate adjuvant therapy. Historically, it was believed that cancer spread locally to the lymph nodes in an orderly, defined manner. If this was true, radical mastectomy should eliminate the disease. However, breast cancer does not spread in an orderly manner and cancer cells metastasize through the bloodstream and lymphatic system to other tissues and organs such as skin, regional lymph nodes, or more distant sites, including bone, lung, liver, and brain. Because breast cancer is a systemic disease, less radical, more breast-conserving surgical procedures are done in combination with radiation therapy, hormonal therapy, or chemotherapy.

Soon after a biopsy-proven diagnosis of breast cancer, the client should consult with a team of interdisciplinary consultants before deciding on the definitive approach to management of her breast cancer. Most insurance companies encourage this consultation because there are numerous approaches to the management of breast cancer and an interdisciplinary approach is not only most advantageous for the client but also most efficient and cost-effective. The interdisciplinary team generally includes a medical oncologist, a radiation oncologist, and a surgical oncologist. An oncology nurse, a nutritionist, and a psycho-oncologist are also vital members of the team, because many clients have questions concerning quality of life, how to maintain nutrition, and ways to promote communication among family members.

Primary Breast Cancer

Carcinoma in situ (meaning that the cancer has not invaded the tissue of origin) is becoming more of an issue in local control of breast cancer, because of the success of mammography in detecting these small cancers. DCIS is generally managed by local excision with or without radiation. The risk of local recurrence following breast-sparing surgery is approximately 10% at 10 years. Whether radiation therapy is necessary for all clients is uncertain. Some clients with DCIS may be appropriately treated with excision alone. Selection criteria relate to the client's age and the tumor size, grade, and margin as well as the client's other health problems and willingness to accept potential increased risk of local recurrence.[11] The addition of tamoxifen as therapeutic as well as prophylactic treatment following local treatment is gaining acceptance. (See the Integrating Pharmacology feature on Medications for Breast Cancer, p. 946.) Women require scheduled diagnostic follow-up mammograms along with physician examination every 6 to 12 months.

LCIS has historically been considered a risk factor for breast cancer rather than a precursor lesion. However, recent studies suggest that LCIS may actually carry more risk for a subsequent invasive cancer in the affected breast than was previously thought and that wide local excision may be more appropriate than watchful waiting.[50] Following local excision, options for management range from careful observation and mammography at 6- to 12-month intervals to bilateral prophylactic mastectomy—options that for many women appear either too conservative or too extreme. The physician-nurse team needs to explain the options carefully and permit time for the client to understand her risks and choices for management.

Management of localized invasive breast cancer has changed dramatically since the mid-1980s. Approximately 40% of women with breast cancer are currently managed with breast-conserving surgery. Many more women are candidates for this procedure, but treatment decisions are complex and involve how both the woman and her physician view pros and cons of each choice. Several studies have indicated that breast-conserving treatments, consisting of the removal of the primary tumor by some form of lumpectomy with or without irradiation to the breast, result in survival that is equal to that of more extensive procedures, including mastectomy and modified radical mastectomy.[11] Similarly, the addition of radiation therapy to mastectomy does not improve 10-year survival rates and is not indicated if the surgical margins are clear and if no other factors place the client at high risk for local recurrence. However, recent studies have suggested a survival advantage for women with positive axillary nodes even after mastectomy and axillary node dissection. The current NCCN guidelines call for consideration of postmastectomy irradiation in these women.[11]

At the time of the initial consultation, a plan of care is devised and the goal of therapy is determined. It is crucial to identify clients at substantial risk for recurrence because they benefit from systemic therapy. Likewise, in a woman with a tumor smaller than 1 cm with no evidence of axillary node involvement, there is little justification for adjuvant chemotherapy. When the tumor is larger than 1 cm and there is evidence of axillary lymph node involvement, other parameters are assessed, such as estrogen receptor status and measures of tumor growth rate. These help determine not only the need for adjuvant chemotherapy but also whether a doxorubicin-containing regimen is appropriate. For example, tumors with a high proportion of cells in the S phase of cell division are associated with a greater risk of relapse, and chemotherapy offers a greater survival benefit. Cancers that lack either estrogen or progesterone receptors are more likely to recur within 5 years than those that are estrogen receptor positive and progesterone receptor positive. Tumors with a poor nuclear grade have a higher degree of recurrence than tumors with a good nuclear grade.

🔸 Tumors that overexpress HER-2/neu protein (c-erbB2) or that have a mutated *p53* gene have a poorer prognosis and may benefit more from chemotherapy containing doxorubicin or taxane. These women also benefit from treatment with trastuzumab following chemotherapy.

Surgical Management

The extent of the surgical intervention is determined by the clinical presentation and by the possibility of resecting the tumor with clean margins. The goal is to preserve the breast, because there is no evidence that a mastectomy is more beneficial than a lumpectomy plus radiation therapy. However, because of size or the multifocal or multicentric extent of disease, a mastectomy may be necessary to provide adequate tumor removal.

Breast-Preserving Procedures

Indications. Breast-preserving procedures are selected for stage I and stage II breast cancers. Such conservative surgical approaches may be appropriate, depending on the size of the primary tumor. Clients with small invasive cancers generally require a wide local excision under local or general anesthesia for partial mastectomy involving removal of the tumor plus a 1- to 2-cm margin of normal tissue (lumpectomy). A variation of the procedure is the quadrantectomy (removal of the quadrant of the breast in which the cancer is located).

🔸 Radiation therapy is begun once healing is confirmed, as long as the client is not receiving a doxorubicin- or taxane-containing regimen. If the individual is to receive either of these two chemotherapeutic agents plus radiation, then the radiation therapy commences 3 weeks after the last course of chemotherapy. If the client is to receive methotrexate (Mexate) and 5-fluorouracil (5-FU) with or without cyclophosphamide (Cytoxan), the radiotherapy may begin with the chemotherapy, may be sandwiched in after the third course and continued for 5 to 6 weeks, or may begin a few weeks after the last course of chemotherapy.

Contraindications. Breast-conserving surgery is not performed when women cannot tolerate irradiation because of prior radiation therapy to the breast or chest wall, pregnancy, or pre-existing rheumatic disorders, such as arthritis, lupus, and scleroderma. Other contraindications are extensive intraductal involvement requiring a wide incision, the presence of two cancers simultaneously i the same breast, diffuse malignant microcalcification throughout the breast, and large, aggressive tumors. Clie preference for a complete breast removal, client fear c radiation side effects, and inability to travel to and from radiation therapy facility are additional contraindication

Complications. Although rare, infection, cellulitis, hem; toma, and, less commonly, lymphedema may occur afte the surgery.

Outcomes. After breast-conserving surgery with radi; tion therapy or chemotherapy or both, the client wi remain free of cancer and its recurrence.

Mastectomy

Indications. Mastectomy is the treatment of choice whe the following apply:

- The tumor involves the nipple-areola complex.
- The tumor is larger than 7 cm.
- The tumor exhibits extensive intraductal diseas involving multiple quadrants of the breast.
- The woman cannot comply with radiation therapy

A *modified radical mastectomy* is an en bloc remov; of the breast, axillary lymph nodes, and overlying skir with the muscles left intact. Because of more sophist cated diagnostic techniques that detect breast cancer of a smaller size and at an earlier stage, this procedur is done much less frequently than it was 10 to 15 year ago. In a *total* or *simple* prophylactic *mastectomy,* use most commonly to prevent cancer in high-risk women breast tissue and some skin are removed, including th nipple and areola complex. Lymph nodes are no removed in a prophylactic mastectomy.

Contraindications. Although not contraindicated fc treatment of small tumors, mastectomy is usually nc used for stage I and stage II tumors unless the client pre fers this approach.

Complications. Possible complications of breast surger include lymphedema, infection, seroma, hematom; and cellulitis. Because clients are often discharged from the hospital within a few days of surgery, they shoul be taught to report any unusual manifestations early Any evidence of infection, such as fever, chills, or a area of redness or inflammation along the incision lin should be reported to the physician. Any increase i drainage, foul odor, or separation at the incision sit should be reported immediately.

Outcomes. After surgery and adjuvant chemotherapy c radiation therapy, the client will remain free of cance and its recurrence. If a cancer-free state cannot b achieved, the focus is on promoting quality of life for the client.

Axillary Dissection

The role of axillary dissection is in transition. In women with clinically negative node disease and a primary tumor that is 1 to 2 cm in size, a node dissection is probably not necessary.[1] The NCCN Practice Guidelines state that in clients who have particularly favorable tumors, those in whom the selection of adjuvant systemic therapy will not be altered, and older clients or those with serious co-morbid conditions, axillary node dissection could be considered optional.[11] Sentinel node biopsy—biopsy only of the node(s) responsible for draining the affected area of the breast—is considered the preferred method of axillary node sampling by the NCCN if the client is an appropriate candidate and there is a sentinel node team available.[11] Information regarding nodal status is valuable in determining prognosis and eligibility for research protocols and targeting treatment regimens.

Recognizing that most women with breast cancer benefit from adjuvant chemotherapy, hormonal therapy, or both, some authorities claim that it is no longer necessary to determine the status of the axillary lymph nodes in clients with breast cancer. However, the lymph node status in clients with early breast cancer remains the most powerful predictor of recurrence and survival. Furthermore, nearly one third of clients with clinically negative nodes are found to have pathologically involved nodes. Information obtained from pathologic examination of axillary lymph nodes frequently changes the adjuvant therapy plan for women with nonpalpable axillary lymph nodes.[67]

In some cases, axillary node dissection is not necessary because its findings would not affect the choice of therapy. For example, a client presenting with a large primary cancer or evidence of metastatic disease that requires extensive surgery does not need an axillary dissection, nor does a client undergoing mastectomy for a tumor larger than 5 cm or a client in whom the surgical margins are positive for residual tumor. In both of these cases, the risk of local recurrence is sufficiently high to warrant the use of postmastectomy radiotherapy to the chest wall and supraclavicular areas. Women who have four or more positive axillary lymph nodes also are at increased risk for local recurrence; chest wall and regional lymph node irradiation is recommended in this setting and has been shown to substantially reduce the risk of local recurrence.[11]

Sentinel Node Biopsy

Nodal assessment may be conducted using the sentinel node biopsy, a diagnostic test to determine the status of regional lymph nodes. The sentinel node is the first lymph node to receive lymphatic drainage from a tumor. The node can be detected by injection of a blue dye or radioactive colloid around the primary tumor, which travels to and identifies the first draining (sentinel) node.

The procedure is technically challenging but has been rapidly adopted into clinical practice because of the advantages it offers over traditional axillary node dissection. Clients who have sentinel node procedures versus axillary node dissections may have less lymphedema, numbness, pain, and arm stiffness; increased arm mobility and arm strength; and better quality of life scores.[59] The AJCC staging guidelines were revised in 2002 to reflect sentinel node information, and the specific use of these results to plan care is continuing to be evaluated.[41]

Nursing Management of the Surgical Client

Preoperative Care

Assessment. The preoperative time, before the biopsy for breast cancer and before a woman knows whether she has cancer in her breast or not, is extremely stressful, constituting a psychological emergency. To put off the biopsy for more than just a few days is often impossible for the woman once a cancer is suspected. Once the diagnosis is established, the woman can return to the routines of her life, or if the biopsy result is positive, she can begin to mobilize her resources to determine the next step. Initially, the woman may be in shock and perhaps even denial, because her decision to undergo the biopsy procedure may have been based largely on her recognition that 8 of 10 breast masses are benign. A few days are often needed for the woman to recover from the diagnosis of cancer before beginning the consultation process.

Most women do not sign consent for an immediate surgical resection or mastectomy upon evidence of a positive biopsy result. Generally, women are given ample time to evaluate the options for management once the diagnosis is confirmed. Most authorities recommend that definitive surgery be performed within 2 weeks of the biopsy, but some women need more time to sort through the copious literature before deciding on a course of treatment. Physicians are required to present the risks and benefits of each of the numerous treatment options for breast cancer and to allow the woman to choose her course of treatment. The options include (1) mastectomy alone, (2) mastectomy with immediate reconstruction, and (3) breast-conserving treatment. Because there is no absolute right answer for many women, each option must be fully considered. Every woman with breast cancer deserves time to deliberate and to participate actively in the decision-making process. Because the possibilities for treatment may be overwhelming, it is appropriate to refer the woman to a comprehensive breast center in which all disciplines are available to address her concerns regarding therapy. Many women say this time is the most stressful period for them following their diagnosis. The nurse can be very helpful in ensuring that information is presented in an understandable format and support autonomous decision making while reducing the overwhelming nature of the experience.

The plan for treatment, which may include surgery, radiation therapy, chemotherapy, hormone therapy, or biologic immunomodulation therapy, is laid out before treatment is begun. In addition, clients should be offered a research protocol if they are eligible. It is an enormous challenge to help clients understand and feel confident in their decisions regarding therapy. To be knowledgeable about the client's options for therapy, make every effort to be present for the initial discussion between the physicians and the client and family. Then clarify any misconceptions the client and family members may have, and reinforce what they have been told regarding the therapy.

Diagnosis, Outcomes, Interventions

Diagnosis: Deficient Knowledge. The nursing diagnosis may be expressed as *Deficient Knowledge related to inexperience and new information regarding available options for treatment.*

Outcomes. The client will understand the available treatment options, as evidenced by her questions and statements concerning options and her ability to explain her choice.

Interventions

Explain Options. The woman should receive information about recommendations and treatment options before surgery or treatment is initiated. The nurse can help women understand treatment options.

Initiate Teaching Plan. Because the typical hospital stay for a modified radical mastectomy or lumpectomy and axillary node dissection surgery is 1 to 3 days, preoperative teaching is done on an outpatient basis, usually in the physician's office. Give clients written instructions regarding postoperative care, including wound care and hand and arm care. Some clients may even go home the day of their surgery. With appropriate support at home and visits from home care nurses, this may be an excellent option for some clients. Nursing assessment provides data about knowledge deficits for use in formulating a teaching plan. This plan includes preoperative activities, explanations of surgery, postoperative care, discharge planning, and a discussion of any limitations the woman may have as a result of surgery. Encourage the woman to question her physicians about lymph node dissection versus sentinel lymph node sampling. Because the woman's anxiety level may be so high that she cannot remember new

information, it is important to provide written as well as oral instructions. Give instructions in the presence of a family member. Because clients are discharged early postoperatively, they also need emergency phone numbers and written instructions regarding whom to call if they have a question or a problem after discharge. Evaluate the client's and family members' learning, and repeat information as often as is necessary.

Diagnosis: Risk for Ineffective Individual Coping and Risk for Compromised Family Coping. The nursing diagnosis may be expressed as *Ineffective Individual Coping and Compromised Family Coping related to diagnosis of cancer and surgical changes in breast.*

Outcomes. The client will cope with the diagnosis of cancer and surgical changes in the breast, as evidenced by her statement of acceptance and decisions about treatment. Family members will also cope effectively, as evidenced by support given to the client.

Interventions. Preoperatively or before any treatment, assess the client's and significant others' coping ability and concerns. Do not rush the assessment. Identify the coping mechanisms usually used by the client and her significant others. Are there any potentially disabling coping patterns? Use this information as the basis of support. The woman may fear pain, mutilation, death, loss of control, and the hospital environment. Use these findings to establish a plan of care to help the client use positive, growth-producing coping and to avoid disabling coping.

Evaluation. For a positive outcome, the client will be adequately prepared for surgery and its outcomes. Recovery from the surgical procedure is usually uncomplicated. Delayed grieving, even months following mastectomy, is not uncommon, because intellectually the woman knows the surgery is necessary and because her grief is overshadowed at first by fear of dying.

Postoperative Care

Assessment. Assess the client's psychological reaction to the surgery. Also, inspect the wound and drains, assess for the presence of clinical manifestations of infection and pain, and perform routine postoperative assessments as discussed in Chapter 14.

Diagnosis, Outcomes, Interventions

Diagnosis: Disturbed Body Image. A nursing diagnosis of *Disturbed Body Image related to impending changes in breast and sexuality* may be appropriate.

Outcomes. The client will begin to exhibit her presurgical or baseline positive body image, as evidenced by wearing usual make-up and using her own nightgown or other feminine attire after surgery.

Interventions

Initiate Referral. Because the hospital stay is short (1 to 3 days) or that of an outpatient, there may be little opportunity for the woman to express her usual feelings regarding her femininity and the manner in which she might display a positive adaptation to her surgery. In this case, it is appropriate merely to ask the woman if she feels that she or family members might benefit from a consultation with the psycho-oncologist, social worker, or sex therapist. Ask whether she would like to talk to someone who has had a similar surgical procedure, possibly someone from the American Cancer Society's Reach for Recovery program. The Case Study on the website deals with issues related to mastectomy.

Assess Coping Strategies. Women who undergo surgery for breast cancer experience a sense of loss—changes in life routines, social interactions, self-concept, and body image—and fear of death. Recovery during the postoperative period after mastectomy requires a great deal of energy. Fatigue is a persistent complaint for 6 months or more after surgery. A client's usual coping strategies may not be effective. Not everyone perceives or handles stress in the same way. Displacement, projection, denial, hope, prayer, meditation, stoicism, fatalism, and any combination of these reactions may be used as coping mechanisms. Clients who have surgically lost a breast may adapt in the same way as they would to any loss.

Encourage Self-Care Activities. Effective postoperative care is essential for successful psychosocial and physical rehabilitation. During the 1- to 3-day hospital stay, the focus of nursing care is on recovery from surgery and anesthesia as well as on discharge planning for self-care postoperative management. The client's self-image improves with self-care activities.

Explain Possible Body Image Concerns After Discharge. The full impact of losing a breast or having breast cancer may not be felt until a while after the client goes home. Many women are surprised by events such as the amount of pain and discomfort, fatigue, slow incision healing, and arm swelling. Ordinary motions, such as shifting to a comfortable position in bed, may be difficult and painful. As time passes, however, the woman and her significant others reorganize and restructure their lives. During this time, the woman resumes her role in society. Important changes in this role may be necessary. Individual women cope differently; feelings of sexual inadequacy, poor body image, and loss of a sense of femininity are common. Because body image is further altered by weight gain and alopecia if the woman is undergoing chemotherapy, she should be encouraged to purchase a wig and other hair coverings before hair loss. Fatigue, decreased libido, and periods of depression are common in women receiving chemotherapy and radiation therapy. Treatment for cancer may hasten menopause in perimenopausal women or bring the return of manifestations in women who are menopausal but have had to discontinue hormone replacement therapy. Hence women want to discuss quality-of-life concerns such as osteoporosis, hot flashes, and mood swings. Black cohosh, as well as other phytoestrogens, has been studied as a means of reducing hot flashes in women undergoing breast cancer treatment, as explained in the Complementary and Alternative Therapy feature below.

Discuss Strategies to Improve Body Image. Gradually the woman will decide whether to conceal her incision from significant others or let it be seen. The incision may be camouflaged for a woman by an appropriately fitted brassiere or a special bathing suit or evening dress, but doubts and fears about her attractiveness may affect even the most secure woman. You can offer understanding and facilitate communication between the client and significant others. The woman may wish to talk with other breast cancer survivors who have faced similar problems as a result of breast cancer. Breast cancer support groups may also be beneficial, but they should be composed of women in similar stages of illness. A woman who is undergoing adjuvant therapy for curative breast cancer, for example, may be overwhelmed and frightened by the discussions and concerns of women with advanced metastatic breast cancer.

COMPLEMENTARY AND ALTERNATIVE THERAPY

Black Cohosh and Hot Flashes

Black cohosh, also known as *Cimicifuga racemosa*, has been studied as a means of reducing hot flashes in women undergoing breast cancer treatment. Sales of black cohosh in the United States have exceeded over $80 million per year. Remefemin is one of the most popular black cohosh products sold in the United States. However, black cohosh 40 mg/day did not work any better than placebo in reducing hot flashes in women with and without a history of breast cancer treatment.[1,2] It is possible that higher doses of black cohosh may help, but in the meantime, low-dose antidepressants may be better options for the reduction of hot flashes.

REFERENCES

1. Jacobsen, J., et al. (2001). Randomized trial of black cohosh for the treatment of hot flashes among women with a history of breast cancer. *Journal of Clinical Oncology, 19,* 2739-2745.
2. Pockaj, B., et al. (2006). Phase III double-blind, randomized, placebo-controlled crossover trial of black cohosh in the management of hot flashes: NCCTG Trial N01CC. *Journal of Clinical Oncology, 24*(18), 2836-2841.

Diagnosis: Risk for Impaired Skin Integrity. The nursing diagnosis may be expressed as *Risk for Impaired Skin Integrity related to surgery or radiation therapy.*

Outcomes. The client will remain free of impairment in skin integrity after surgery or radiation therapy, as evidenced by healing skin without redness, infection, hematoma formation, or breakdown.

Interventions

Provide and Explain Dressing and Drain Care. Postoperatively, a pressure dressing is usually used initially. Explain that a drain, connected to gentle suction, prevents blood or serum collection in the operative space after a modified radical mastectomy or axillary node dissection. Instruct the woman about emptying the drain and recording the amount of drainage.

SAFETY ⚠ ALERT

Advise her to notify the physician if the drain becomes plugged or dislodged, or shows any sign of infection, or if frank bleeding develops.

When changing the dressing, gently encourage the woman to look at the incision. Seeing the incision for the first time is often difficult, but the nurse's matter-of-fact approach can help. In future dressing changes, teach methods of cleaning the incision at home and of watching for manifestations of infection.

Prevent Skin Complications Following Radiation Therapy. During radiation therapy, scaling, flaking, dryness, itching, erythema, rash, or dry desquamation of the involved skin may occur.

SAFETY ⚠ ALERT

Careful treatment of the skin is important in minimizing the skin effects of radiation therapy. Instruct women not to wash the area with soap but to rinse it with water only. No lotion or powder is to be put on the skin that overlies the radiation port. If the area under the arm becomes reddened because of friction, moisture, or radiation damage, place soft, clean gauze pads between skinfolds to prevent skin breakdown.

Diagnosis: Risk for Injury. The nursing diagnosis may be expressed as *Risk for Injury related to increased risk of infection and lymphedema secondary to axillary node dissection.*

Outcomes. The client will not experience injury, as evidenced by absence of infection or lymphedema.

Interventions. Arm edema (e.g., lymphedema) occurs less commonly than in the past because of the performance of less extensive mastectomy procedures and less extensive axillary dissection. Lymphedema results from insufficient transport of water and protein from the skin and subcutaneous tissue because of an inadequate development or eradication of lymphatic vessels. Lymphedema following axillary dissection has been reported in as many as 70% of cases, although probably a more accurate estimate of the average occurrence of lymphedema as a significant consequence of local therapy for breast cancer is 20% in the United States and Europe.[1] Clearly, the major risk for lymphedema exists when complete axillary dissection with stripping of the axillary vein and nodal irradiation is combined with mastectomy.

Older age, obesity, and lifting of heavy objects such as grocery bags and suitcases are also thought to increase the risk of lymphedema. Arm edema, stiffness, pain, and numbness have been reported in 40% to 50% of clients approximately 1 month after beginning radiation therapy to the axilla. Lymphedema occurring years after surgery or radiation therapy is generally the result of infection, inflammation, or recurrent tumor.

Administer Antibiotics for Infection.

If a woman complains of redness, swelling, and a generalized area of warmth on the affected arm with or without fever, she should be examined for possible infection in the hand or arm. If an infection is present, the woman may need to be admitted to the hospital for intravenous antibiotics to treat the infection. Such infections can occur from a slight cut on the hand, and even though they may seem innocuous, they pose a serious threat to these clients.

Prevent Lymphedema. 🪔 In the early postoperative period, encourage arm exercises, and elevate the arm on a pillow so that the elbow is level with the heart and the hand rests just higher than the elbow. The goal is to promote lymphatic drainage and prevent infection. The Client Education Guide on p. 947 presents postmastectomy exercises (see also the Complementary and Alternative Therapy feature on p. 955).

Do not perform venipunctures or take blood pressure measurements on the affected arm to reduce the risk of lymphedema and infection.

Minimize Lymphedema. Wearing an elastic bandage or a custom-fitted pressure-gradient elastic sleeve may be helpful in the months following surgery if lymphedema is present. Some women think that wearing a sleeve while they are on an airplane minimizes swelling caused by pressure changes in the airplane, although no studies have confirmed the efficacy of this practice.

Emphasize that it is important to prevent lymphedema. Once lymphedema occurs, it is more likely to occur again and be progressive. This is because the tissue, like a balloon, is a potential space that, once expanded, will expand again to that size and beyond with little provocation.

Available treatments include application of compression garments, use of intermittent pneumatic compression, and

Postmastectomy Exercises

When to Begin	Purpose	Exercises: Perform Exercises 5-10 Times Each, Three Times a Day
Postoperative days 1-5	Prevent and/or reduce swelling	Position arm against your side in a relaxed position. Elbow should be level with your heart, with the wrist just above the elbow when resting. Rotate wrist in a circular fashion. Touch fingers to shoulder and extend arm fully.
After drains are removed	Promote muscle movement without stretching	While standing, brace yourself with your other arm and bend over slightly, allowing your affected arm to hang freely. Swing the arm in small circles and gradually increase in size. Make 10 circles—rest—repeat in the opposite direction. Swing arm forward and back as far as you can without pulling on the incision. While standing, bend over slightly and swing arms across the chest in each direction. While sitting in a chair, rest both arms at your side. Shrug both shoulders, then relax. While sitting or standing, pull shoulders back, bring the shoulder blades together.
After sutures are removed	Stretch and regain full range of motion. To gain mobility of your shoulder, you must move it in *all* directions, several times a day	While lying in bed with arm extended, raise arm over your head and extend backwards. While lying in bed, grasp a cane or short pole with both hands across your lap. Extend arms straight up and over your head and return. Repeat, rotating the cane clockwise and then counterclockwise while over your head. While standing, extend arm straight over your head and down. Extend your elbow out from your side at a 90° angle—hold it for 10 seconds—relax. Extend your arm straight out from your side even with your shoulder—extend arm straight up toward the ceiling. Stand at arm's length facing a wall. Extend arms so your fingertips touch the wall. Creep fingers up the side of the wall, stepping forward as necessary. Repeat the procedure going down the wall—keep arms extended. Stand sideways to the wall. Extend arm out so fingers touch the wall. Creep up the wall a little more each day. Use hand and arm normally.
After 6 weeks	Strengthen arm and shoulder and regain total use of arm and shoulder	Begin water aerobics. Begin overall fitness program. Begin aerobics, Jazzercise, or other resistive exercises. Avoid using weights, as these may increase arm edema and subsequent swelling.

massage by a trained physiotherapist. Clients can obtain more information from the National Breast Cancer Coalition, the International Society of Lymphology, and the Oncology Nursing Society.

Evaluation. The client who has undergone breast surgery for cancer will be discharged from the hospital 24 to 72 hours postoperatively. The surgical wounds may be healed within 4 weeks. Regaining complete use of the affected arm and shoulder may take as long as weeks to several months, depending on the extent of the surgical procedure, rate of healing, compliance with exercises, and the degree of postoperative complications.

Self-Care

To promote self-care, the client needs to learn about postoperative arm exercises, postoperative care, and care of the breast prosthesis. A referral to Reach for Recovery may also be helpful.

Teach Arm Exercises

In the early postoperative period (days 1 and 2), encourage the client to focus on the elbow, wrist, and hand of the affected side. The client performs active elbow flexion and extension, gently squeezes a soft rubber ball, and does deep breathing to facilitate lymph flow. Shoulder shrugs and active range of motion, including flexion and abduction, can be added on the second postoperative day. Encourage self-care activities (e.g., feeding, combing hair, washing face) and other activities that use the arm, with care taken not to abduct the arm or to raise the arm or elbow above shoulder height until the drains are removed.

Approximately 10 days after surgery, the client can begin active assisted range-of-motion exercises (see Client Education Guide on Postmastectomy Exercises). Tell the client to do these exercises at least twice a day as tolerated. Provide pain medication 30 minutes before exercises to permit the client to perform exercises with reduced pain. ✎ Women who do not carry out these exercises as instructed are at greater risk for lymphedema and loss of shoulder joint mobility. (Arrangements for a physical therapist to assist with range-of-motion and strengthening exercises may need to be made at the same time surgery is planned because of the shortened hospital stay.) Always provide written and oral instructions about arm precautions. (See the Client Education Guide feature on Arm Care After Axillary *evolve* Lymph Node Dissection on the website.)

Refer to Reach for Recovery

The Reach for Recovery program of the American Cancer Society is a rehabilitation program for breast cancer survivors, specifically those who have had breast surgery. This program helps women meet common psychosocial, physical, and cosmetic needs. With authorization of the physician and the client's permission, volunteers from this program visit the hospital or the home and give the woman information and help, including the following:

1. A kit, ball, book, rope, and temporary soft cotton prosthesis for women who have had a mastectomy
2. Instruction sheet for and demonstration of postoperative axillary node dissection exercises
3. Discussion of brassiere comfort, various breast prostheses, clothing adjustments, and personal problems as appropriate

Provide Breast Prosthesis

Women who have had a mastectomy may wear a temporary lightweight prosthesis immediately after the sutures and drains are removed. This may facilitate adjustment to the loss of the breast. A soft cotton breast form may be supplied by the Reach for Recovery visitor; cotton padding inserted into a pocket sewn into a lightweight brassiere is also a good temporary substitute. A permanent prosthesis should not be purchased until the wound has healed completely because the contours of the incision site may change. Cocoa butter may be rubbed into the incision once healing has occurred to help soften the scar and prevent scar contracture.

Some women choose breast reconstruction. If a woman chooses to have a prosthesis, even temporarily while considering breast reconstruction, she should choose one that is appropriate for her. A breast prosthesis may be purchased in foundation departments in most large stores or at medical-surgical supply stores that sell durable medical equipment. Most of these stores have experienced sales associates to help women obtain the proper fit. Most private and government insurance plans pay for at least the first breast prosthesis and brassiere, as long as a written prescription from the physician accompanies the receipt. Many plans also pay for yearly replacements.

Surgical Management for Breast Reconstruction

Many women have feelings of loss, depression, and alterations in body image after mastectomy. Breast reconstruction is an accepted component of the treatment plan. In the 1990s improvements were made to surgical prostheses and surgical techniques, helping women become more confident in their choice to have reconstructive surgery and retain their self-confidence and body image, thereby enhancing their quality of life. The goal for clients having reconstructive surgery is to "feel whole again." This includes appearing "normal" in a bathing suit as well as in the nude.

The only contraindications to breast reconstruction are the client's need for chest wall irradiation and the physical inability to withstand additional surgery because of a co-morbid condition. Breast reconstruction is not contraindicated by a woman's age, her need for adjuvant chemotherapy, a poor prognosis, or even the presence of metastatic disease. The timing of the breast reconstruction may be immediate (at the time of the mastectomy) or delayed, even until years after mastectomy. When adjuvant chemotherapy is planned, the surgeon may prefer to wait until the chemotherapy is completed to begin reconstructing the breast.

Several surgical techniques can be used to reconstruct the breast mound and nipple-areola complex. The choice of technique is based upon the client's wishes, the amount of tissue available, and whether the woman has had radiation therapy in the past. The simplest method of reconstruction involves the insertion of an implant into a pocket of skin purposely left by the surgeon. This approach is best for women with small or moderate-size breasts, in whom the implant is of a size similar to the remaining breast. Other methods of reconstruction include the following.

Tissue Expanders

A tissue expander is a deflated silicone envelope that is inserted under the chest muscles and expanded slowly over 6 to 8 weeks by adding 60 to 200 ml of saline per week via a remote percutaneous injection port. When the skin overlying the breast mound is sufficiently over inflated to accommodate the implant comfortably, the expander is removed and the implant is inserted.

Transverse Rectus Abdominis Muscle Flap

The transverse rectus abdominis muscle (TRAM) flap procedure is commonly referred to as the "tummy tuck." A low transverse elliptical incision is made, and abdominal muscle and fat are tunneled under the abdominal skin to the mastectomy site. Tissue viability and perfusion are retained by the superior epigastric vessel. The tissue can also be transferred as a free flap. The donor site in the abdomen is closed as for a modified abdominoplasty (Figure 40-4). Contraindications to the TRAM flap are the presence of abdominal scars and inadequate abdominal tissue.

Latissimus Dorsi Muscle Flap

The latissimus dorsi muscle, a large fan-shaped muscle beneath the scapula, is used when inadequate skin is available at the mastectomy site. It is considered an expendable muscle because alternative muscle groups are able to adduct the humerus and rotate the shoulder posteriorly. An ellipse of skin along with the latissimus dorsi muscle is tunneled through the axilla and rotated onto the

mastectomy site. The viability of the tissue is maintained through the thoracodorsal vessels (Figure 40-5).

Gluteal Muscle Free Flaps

A less common form of breast reconstruction involves the use of the gluteus muscle (superior gluteal artery perforator free flap or GAP flap). The muscle and overlying skin are lifted from their bed and connected to the chest wall using an operating microscope. Although TRAM flaps are still most commonly used for autogenous reconstruction, the GAP flap provides an excellent alternative that may gain in popularity with the ability to reconstruct both breasts at the same time.[20]

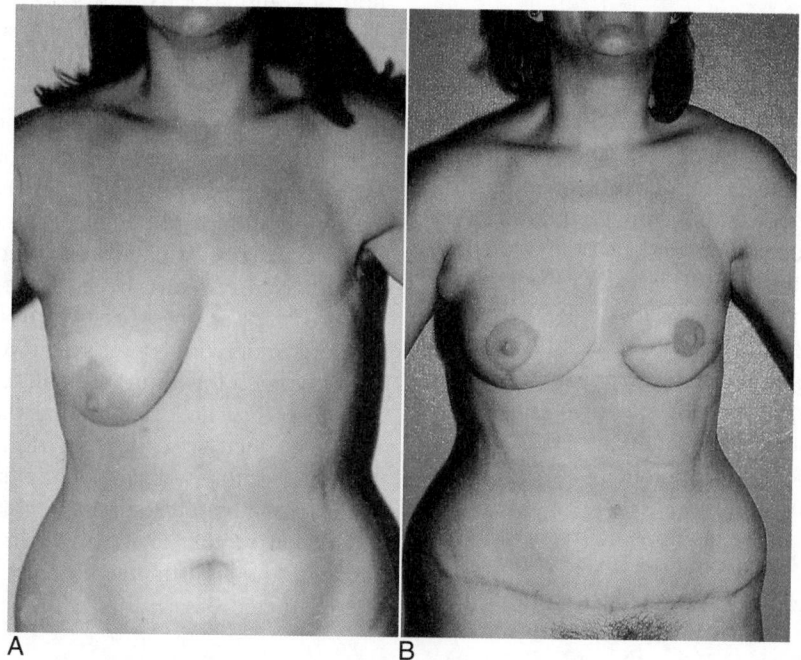

■ **FIGURE 40–4** Breast reconstruction using transverse rectus abdominis myocutaneous flaps. **A,** Preoperative appearance. **B,** Postoperative appearance.

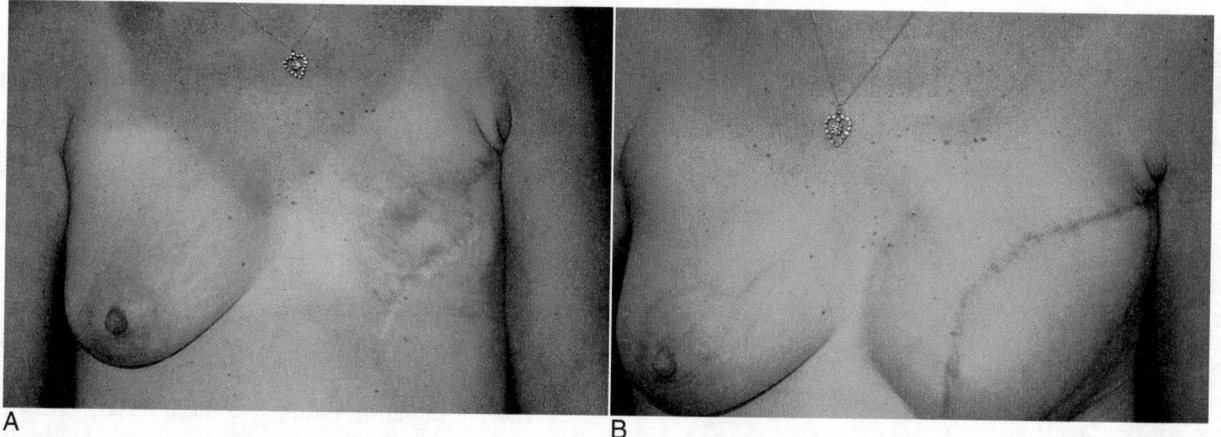

FIGURE 40–5 An ideal result of reconstructive surgery using a latissimus dorsi myocutaneous flap and an implant. **A,** Preoperative appearance. **B,** Postoperative appearance. A subpectoral implant is used in the right breast for symmetry.

Nipple-Areola Reconstruction

Some women elect also to have the nipple-areola reconstructed. To achieve symmetry, nipple reconstruction should be delayed for several months following breast reconstruction. During the healing process, the contour of the reconstructed breast may change as the incisions heal and edema subsides. Areola can be reconstructed with a tattoo or by nipple sharing. The dark tissue of the areola is most commonly reconstructed by tattooing. Nipple projection is constructed with a skate flap (Figure 40-6). Many years ago, the nipple was removed from the breast before amputation and stored ("banked") on the inner thigh. This procedure is no longer performed because of the risk of cancer spread.

Nursing Management of the Client with Breast Reconstruction

Preoperative Care

Preoperatively, the nurse reinforces the physician's instructions regarding the goals of reconstruction and any postoperative care needs. It is important that the client have realistic expectations of the outcome of the surgery. The client may be shown pictures of reconstructed breasts to familiarize her with what can be achieved. The client may express anger, disbelief, and fear related to the surgery, especially if the reconstruction is being combined with a mastectomy for a known carcinoma. Many women will at the same time express relief that the cancer surgery is being done and the cancer is being removed. Some will find comfort in discussing their feelings of disbelief at this time. Periods of depression are normal.

Encourage clients to express their feelings and fears with family members and to seek assistance from the psycho-oncology service or chaplain if appropriate. Assess risks for anesthesia-related problems and operative blood loss before surgery. Advise any client who smokes cigarettes to stop, because smoking compromises flap and skin circulation.

Postoperative Care

In addition to providing the postoperative nursing care required by any person having surgery, after reconstructive breast surgery you will assess the flap or breast area for color, temperature, and capillary refill. If any area appears dusky and congested with blood, the flap may be suffering from venous obstruction. A flap that is pale is not receiving blood and may be experiencing arterial constriction. Whenever circulation or perfusion is in question, notify the physician immediately. The success of this surgical procedure is directly dependent on astute nursing assessment and proper physician notification of complications. Laser Doppler flow may be used to monitor skin perfusion after free flap transfer.

Inform a woman with a recent subpectoral implant that initially the implant feels very firm and is higher on the chest than a normal breast. Over time, the muscle stretches, allowing the implant to drop and soften. Women with subpectoral implants do not wear bras because the implant needs to move into the pocket created in the chest wall. Women who undergo other types of surgery may return from the operating room wearing a bra to support the breasts. A front-closing support bra without underwire is preferred. Wearing a bra also helps some women feel more normal, encouraging a return to wellness. Psychosocial readjustment to breast reconstruction, including incorporation of the reconstructed breast into the woman's body image, usually occurs 3 to 4 months after surgery. A recent study indicated that writing letters to their new/lost breasts may facilitate the adjustment of breast cancer clients to their reconstructed breasts.[54]

Medical Management

Eliminate or Prevent Spread of Cancer

After surgery or instead of surgery, it may be possible to prevent further extension of cancer or to completely eliminate the cancer cells by using radiation therapy, chemotherapy, or hormonal therapy.

Radiation Therapy. Radiation therapy is used in breast cancer treatment as follows:

- The breast and underlying chest wall are irradiated after lumpectomy or quadrantectomy as adjuvant therapy for stage I or II breast cancer.
- Women who are poor surgical candidates because of health problems such as heart disease typically receive radiation therapy to the affected breast.
- The chest wall is irradiated if it is involved or for local control after mastectomy with positive margins.

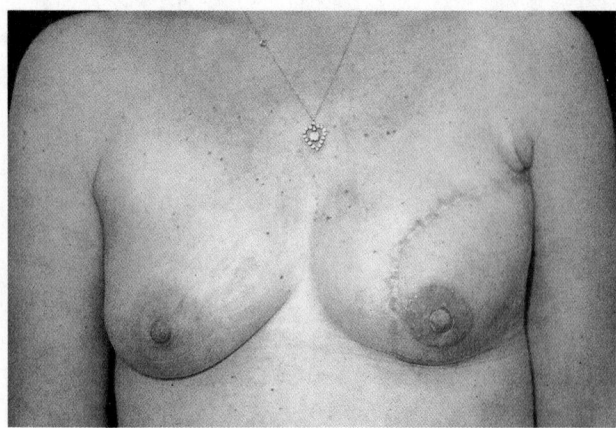

■ **FIGURE 40–6** Nipple-areola reconstruction.

- The axilla is irradiated in women at high risk for axillary metastases who are poor surgical candidates for axillary dissection or who have gross disease that was not surgically excised.
- The supraclavicular region is irradiated if positive axillary nodes are found.
- Additional areas are irradiated for management of metastatic disease to the brain, bone, or skin.

Radiation in combination with lumpectomy or quadrantectomy is an accepted treatment for early-stage breast cancer. An axillary dissection or a sentinel node biopsy is usually done for staging purposes. Radiation therapy, when used to treat micrometastatic disease following mastectomy, successfully reduces the risk of local recurrence and therefore of distant metastases. The utility of radiation therapy following mastectomy or modified radical mastectomy comes into question when the client is also receiving adjuvant chemotherapy, tamoxifen, or both. (See the Integrating Pharmacology feature on Medications for Breast Cancer.) Recent studies indicate a survival advantage for radiation therapy in postmastectomy node-positive women.[11] However, the use of postoperative radiation therapy is not indicated in clients with negative axillary nodes except when there is evidence of disease at the deep margins of the tumor.

When chemotherapy is given with radiation therapy, the radiotherapy may be given concomitantly or sandwiched with the chemotherapy, or given sequentially after completion of the chemotherapy. Concomitant therapy results in a greater incidence of skin reactions than has been reported with sequential treatment. The only situation in which external beam radiation therapy might be given before chemotherapy is in a case in which there are negative axillary nodes (and therefore low risk for distant disease) and positive surgical margins, when the risk for local recurrence is great. The real risk to women with breast cancer is systemic disease. Therefore chemotherapy is critically important to eradicate any micrometastatic disease wherever it may be, including the chest.

Radiation therapy can be administered through an external beam or via brachytherapy, or iridium implants. For external beam irradiation, the radiation is administered on an outpatient basis 5 days a week for 5 to 6 weeks to the entire breast (and possibly the lymphatics), usually with a boost to the tumor bed. The total dose of radiation is approximately 5000 rad. Regional lymph nodes may be treated if they have not been removed.

Brachytherapy is given for a much shorter period of time, twice a day for 5 days. Therefore this type of radiation may be performed before chemotherapy with little delay to the systemic treatment. An alternate method of administering brachytherapy involves using a tiny bag that is inflated inside the surgical cavity (MammoSite brachytherapy device). The radiation source is placed and the client is finished with her radiation in a week. Studies show that in a select group of screen-detected, node-negative women with early stage breast cancer, the MammoSite brachytherapy device may reduce the time, inconvenience, and toxicity associated with traditional radiotherapy.[56]

Interstitial implant therapy using iridium-192 is an outpatient procedure using high dose rate brachytherapy. The insertion of the iridium (Ir) implant may be done using local anesthesia. Stainless-steel guide needles are threaded through the tumor area at l-cm intervals. Flexible plastic tubes are inserted in the guide needles. The guide needles are then removed, leaving the tube in place. Strands of radioactive iridium seeds are threaded through each tube (Figure 40-7). The seeds, at 1-cm intervals, form a grid with those above and below to cover the tissues evenly with radiation. At the end of the insertion procedure, a button is attached to the end of the tubes and the ends are crimped and cut to prevent the seeds from falling out. An x-ray film confirms the location of the implant. The implant usually must remain in place for 2 or 3 days. The procedure is mildly uncomfortable.

Side effects of radiation therapy to the breast include the following:

- Temporary skin changes such as itching, dryness, tenderness, redness, swelling, and dry desquamation
- Moist desquamation, especially in skinfolds
- Fatigue

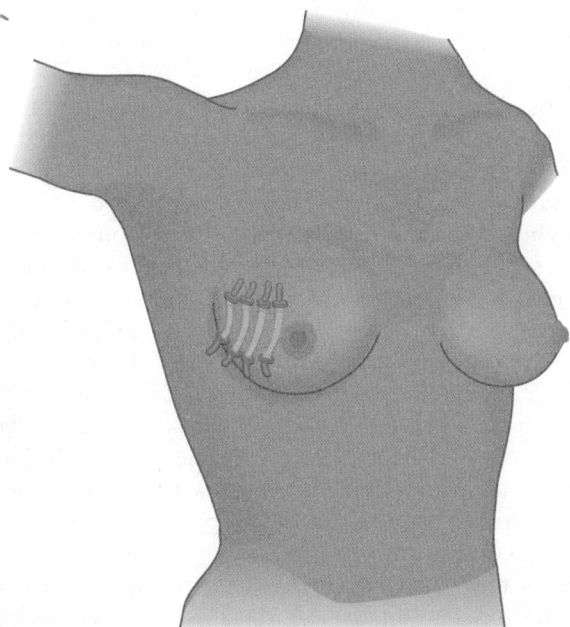

■ FIGURE 40–7 Radiation therapy given via iridium implants.

■ Dry throat may occur as a result of radiation scatter, especially if the supraclavicular area is irradiated
■ Pneumonitis (rare), which may present as a dry cough and dyspnea, a result of inflammatory changes in the irradiated underlying lung
■ Arm edema (rare), occurring more commonly with axillary irradiation
■ Increased susceptibility to rib fracture in the irradiated field
■ Difficulty in obtaining optimal doses of chemotherapy in women receiving chemotherapy concurrently with radiation therapy because of the effect of radiation on bone marrow

Radiation therapy can be emotionally taxing and physically fatiguing. Nursing support is needed during the 5- to 7-week treatment period. Women receiving radiation therapy have many of the same fears as those having a mastectomy: fear of death, fear of mutilation, and feelings of sexual inadequacy. These are compounded by the stress of daily treatment and the fatigue that occurs with coping with a chronic illness, often while recovering from the side effects of chemotherapy.

Systemic Chemotherapy

Localized Breast Cancer. Adjuvant systemic chemotherapy for early stage I and stage II breast cancer generally follows local surgical intervention and includes combinations of cyclophosphamide (Cytoxan), doxorubicin (Adriamycin), methotrexate (Mexate), 5-fluorouracil (5-FU), paclitaxel (Taxol), and docetaxel (Taxotere). Both six cycles of cyclophosphamide, methotrexate, and 5-fluorouracil (CMF) and four cycles of doxorubicin and cyclophosphamide with methotrexate, 5-fluorouracil, or leucovorin (Wellcovorin) are standard adjuvant (curative) therapy for breast cancer.

For the most part, clients are divided into three groups: those who have no involved axillary lymph nodes, those with one to three involved nodes, and those with four or more involved nodes. Adjuvant systemic therapy is usually not given to women whose largest tumors are 0.5 cm or less in diameter and without lymph node involvement. Clients whose tumors are larger than 0.5 cm but less than 1 cm and without lymph node involvement may be divided into those with a low risk of recurrence and those who have unfavorable prognostic features that warrant consideration of adjuvant therapy. Unfavorable prognostic features include lymphatic invasion, high S phase fraction, high nuclear and histologic grades, and HER-2–positive status.

Clients with lymph node involvement or with tumors larger than 1 cm in diameter are appropriate candidates for adjuvant systemic therapy. Cytotoxic chemotherapy using CMF; or a regimen of cyclophosphamide, doxorubicin, and 5-FU (CAF); or just cyclophosphamide and doxorubicin (AC) is appropriate for node-negative clients. For those clients who have positive lymph nodes, chemotherapy regimens that contain an anthracycline (doxorubicin) are preferred. The addition of paclitaxel may be superior to AC alone for node-positive women who are estrogen receptor negative, particularly in clients who overexpress HER-2/neu.[11] For women who have receptor-positive tumors, hormonal therapy for 5 years is also recommended. The hormonal therapy used may be tamoxifen alone, aromatase inhibitor alone, or a combination of tamoxifen and aromatase inhibitor. Recent studies suggest an additive benefit when an aromatase inhibitor is used either immediately, or after 2 to 3 years of tamoxifen, or after completing a 5-year course of tamoxifen.[12] (See the Integrating Pharmacology feature on Medications for Breast Cancer.) The addition of hormonal therapy significantly improves the 10-year survival outlook for this population.[18] The benefit of the addition of hormonal therapy to chemotherapy is less clear for women younger than 50 years with hormone receptor–positive tumors.[28] It is clear that aromatase inhibitors are not appropriate for the premenopausal client. Aromatase inhibitors work by blocking the conversion of androgens into estrogen. Since premenopausal women are still producing estrogen via the ovary, an aromatase inhibitor not only would be ineffective for reducing endogenous estrogen level but also might actually increase circulating levels of estrogen because of a negative feedback loop. The additive benefit of chemotherapy to tamoxifen therapy for women 50 or older with hormone receptor–positive tumors may not provide a large absolute benefit. Therefore the decision to give both adjuvant treatments should be individualized, especially in those women with an already favorable prognosis or in older women with co-morbidities.[11]

The decision to use hormonal therapy with or without chemotherapy in women with estrogen receptor–positive disease should be based on the absolute magnitude of risk reduction expected with the systemic therapy and the individual client's willingness to experience toxicity in order to achieve that incremental risk reduction. For women with estrogen receptor–negative disease, the choice is for adjuvant chemotherapy. Adjuvant combination chemotherapy on the average produces an absolute improvement of 7% to 11% in 10-year survival rates for women younger than 50 and 2% to 3% for those ages 50 to 69.[13]

In some instances, the physician may recommend primary, induction, or "neoadjuvant" chemotherapy (i.e., given before surgery). Primary chemotherapy is beneficial because the physician can evaluate response to chemotherapy directly, which is impossible once the cancer is removed. Therefore the physician can know whether the choice of chemotherapy is optimal. In addition, the tumor may actually shrink so much that the disease may be "downstaged," permitting a breast-preserving procedure.

However, although preoperative chemotherapy is as effective as postoperative chemotherapy, the results have not demonstrated higher cure rates or influenced survival for stage I and II breast cancers. It does, however, offer the opportunity to observe the biologic response of the tumor to the effects of chemotherapy. Hormonal therapy has also been used in neoadjuvant settings and early studies demonstrate promising results.[14]

Advanced Localized Breast Cancer. When a client has more extensive (stage III) yet curable disease, her options and decisions for therapy are even more difficult and controversial. Women with unfavorable stage IIIA or IIIB breast cancers generally require a more aggressive management approach. Affected women typically have larger tumors (>5 cm), direct invasion of the skin of the breast or the chest wall, or fixed or matted axillary lymphadenopathy. Usually, these women undergo preoperative chemotherapy, with or without hormone therapy, followed by surgery and radiotherapy. An alternative approach involves the use of high-dose combination chemotherapy, followed by an additional combination of agents that are also active in breast cancer. The concept is to minimize the risk of drug resistance and to attempt to kill cells before they have an opportunity to mutate to resistance. The addition of paclitaxel every 3 weeks for four cycles following the standard doxorubicin (Adriamycin) and cyclophosphamide regimen every 3 weeks for four cycles for women with node-positive breast cancer is associated with increased relapse-free survival.

Other adjuvant treatments include the combination of paclitaxel and the monoclonal antibody trastuzumab (Herceptin). When these two agents are combined, there appears to be significant synergy with little increased toxicity.[51] The most common side effects are acute fever or chills and the potential for cardiac dysfunction. The combination of trastuzumab and anthracyclines is associated with more incidents of cardiac dysfunction; therefore combination chemotherapy with anthracyclines and trastuzumab is not recommended.[40] HER-2 is overexpressed in 25% to 30% of human breast cancers and indicates a worse prognosis in clients who have positive axillary lymph nodes. Despite the association of HER-2 overexpression with poor prognosis, a clinical response to taxanes was three times more likely to occur in HER-2–positive clients than in HER-2–negative clients.[8] Several large, randomized controlled trials have demonstrated the effectiveness of trastuzumab and paclitaxel as single and combined agents for adjuvant breast cancer, leading to the recommendation to add trastuzumab to the adjuvant therapy of HER-2–positive clients.[51]

Dose intensification requiring the use of autologous hematopoietic support is not considered standard therapy in adjuvant breast cancer. Research conducted by the National Surgical Adjuvant Breast Project included two randomized trials (NSABP B22 and NSABP B25) of dose intensification, and neither one to date has demonstrated that higher doses of drug given in a compressed time period are superior to standard dosing of the same drugs (doxorubicin and cyclophosphamide).[5,24] Newer studies support the investigational and unproven nature of dose-intense treatment for breast cancer and the toxicity associated with dose intensification is significant.[38] Trials on dose-dense chemotherapy, however, which is based on mathematical models of tumor growth, have demonstrated efficacy and provide an option for treating node-positive women.[49,36] Dose-dense chemotherapy involves giving standard doses of standard regimens more frequently with supportive growth factors to reduce side effects and increase tumor cell kill. Theoretically, this allows recovery of normal tissue while overcoming tumor resistance.

Nursing Management of the Medical Client

Assessment. Nursing management of the woman receiving chemotherapy for breast cancer centers on her need for information and instructions regarding self-care procedures. Because in most cases the woman undergoes breast surgery in the hospital and goes home 1 to 3 days later, there is often little time to discuss her concerns regarding chemotherapy and radiation therapy. Even though the client does not start these treatments until complete healing has taken place (usually 3 to 4 weeks after surgery), the nurse has an important role in providing the client and family members with information regarding the side effects of chemotherapy and radiation therapy. In planning care, be sure to consider the emotional, social, cognitive, spiritual, and physical impact of the diagnosis and treatment on the woman and her family.

Diagnosis, Outcomes, Interventions

Diagnosis: Effective Therapeutic Regimen Management. The nursing diagnosis may be expressed as *Effective Therapeutic Regimen Management* and *Readiness for Enhanced Self Care related to chemotherapy and radiation therapy.*

Outcomes. The client will understand the purpose and goals of chemotherapy and radiation therapy as evidenced by her statements concerning the necessity for treatment and possible side effects associated with that treatment.

Interventions

Teach About Radiation Therapy. Teaching is a major role of the nurse who is caring for clients receiving radiation therapy. Include in the teaching plan instructions regarding skin care, sun protection, and management of fatigue. If the client is receiving chemotherapy concurrently, there is heightened risk for infection because of neutropenia. Therefore instruct clients to report any evidence of infection. Monitor blood counts on a weekly basis. Tell the client that written materials, including the booklet *Radiation Therapy and You,* are available from the NCI free of charge by calling 1-800-4-CANCER. See Chapter 17 for further information on radiation therapy.

Teach About Chemotherapy. Nurses are responsible for teaching clients about the side effects of chemotherapy. The booklet *Chemotherapy and You* (also available free of charge from the NCI) explains the purpose of chemotherapy and possible side effects. Once the regimen is selected, discuss side effects. Teach the client the names of the drugs, how the drugs are given, expected side effects and their management, preventive measures, and complications that need to be reported to the physician or nurse (e.g., infection, fever, bruising, bleeding, mouth sores).

Vary the teaching plan, depending on the drug regimen selected, because the side effects are different for each of the drugs. For example, not all chemotherapy agents cause hair loss. Women receiving methotrexate and 5-FU do not experience hair loss, whereas women receiving doxorubicin and cyclophosphamide have complete hair loss at 2 to 3 weeks after their first injection. Cyclophosphamide taken orally for 14 days and methotrexate and 5-FU given by injection twice a month cause a gradual thinning of the hair, but generally the woman can get by without a wig, especially if her hair is kept short. Methotrexate and 5-FU can cause diarrhea and stomatitis, which may interrupt therapy. Advise women taking cyclophosphamide by mouth for the 14-day regimen to drink eight glasses of water a day to prevent hemorrhagic cystitis. Paclitaxel may cause neurologic toxicity; therefore clients need to be assessed for difficulty with gait, constipation, and fine motor movements.

Diagnosis: Imbalanced Nutrition: Less Than Body Requirements. The nursing diagnosis may be expressed as *Imbalanced Nutrition: Less Than Body Requirements related to nausea, vomiting, and stomatitis secondary to chemotherapy.*

Outcomes. The client will maintain adequate nutrition, as evidenced by absence of nausea and vomiting, control of stomatitis, intake of adequate calories, and no or minimal weight loss.

Interventions. Nausea, vomiting, anorexia, stomatitis, and taste change are common side effects of chemotherapy agents. Some drugs, specifically doxorubicin and methotrexate, cause stomatitis 4 to 5 days after the injection.

Provide Oral Hygiene. To minimize the severity of the stomatitis, the client is instructed to perform oral hygiene three to four times a day and to rinse with baking soda and water to maintain a basic environment in the oral cavity. Bacteria thrive in an acidic environment. If a client experiences any mouth soreness, she should suck on ice during injection of the chemotherapy agent. This simple form of cryotherapy helps to minimize exposure of the oral cavity to the irritating effects of chemotherapy agents.

Prevent Nausea and Vomiting. Nausea and vomiting are usually preventable when antiemetic medications are taken on a schedule rather than just as needed. A combination of a dopamine antagonist, a serotonin antagonist, and a steroid is usually adequate to prevent nausea and vomiting from chemotherapy. Because chemotherapy slows colonic transit time, clients often experience epigastric distress and bloating after administration of these agents. In addition, the serotonin antagonists can be constipating. For these reasons, encourage clients to eat lightly, taking primarily liquids for the 3 days following chemotherapy. Drugs such as metoclopramide (Reglan) are useful to enhance gastric emptying and to reduce bloating. Most women who receive chemotherapy for breast cancer do not lose weight; in fact, they gain weight. Women receiving CMF therapy may gain between 15 and 25 pounds during their therapy. Counsel clients to control their weight and to watch what they are eating.

Evaluation. Many factors affect the duration of the chemotherapy regimen. The following are some considerations:

- Whether the chemotherapy is adjuvant
- Stage at which the breast cancer was diagnosed
- Co-morbidities
- Whether the disease remains stable during chemotherapy

Self-Care

Teach About Follow-Up Surveillance

The highest risk factor for breast cancer is a history of breast cancer. Therefore instruct clients that they require follow-up cancer surveillance for the rest of their lives. Most women are emotional and apprehensive after completing their adjuvant therapy. For the most part, they are happy to be finished but nervous that they are no longer receiving any therapy to oppose the cancer. If they are receiving tamoxifen or an aromatase inhibitor, remind them that it is treatment for their cancer as well as a medicine to help prevent breast cancer. Women express fear that the cancer will come back. It is important to acknowledge and discuss the fact that they will worry and feel afraid, so that they can realize that such feelings are normal.

Explain that the physical examination by the physician every 3 to 4 months is designed to detect any problem early and that they should make every effort to keep their appointments. The surveillance schedule involves a physical examination every 3 to 4 months for 3 years, every 6 months for 2 years, and then once a year. A mammogram and a chest film (optional) are obtained every 12 months. Breast MRI may be used on an annual or semi-annual schedule for follow-up. Routine chemistry screening is done every year. For women taking tamoxifen who still have their uterus, a pelvic examination is done every year.

Routine liver, bone, and brain scans are not indicated as surveillance tests for recurrent disease. Until research determines that early institution of therapy is critical to the outcome, the goal of surveillance is to detect the disease just as the disease becomes symptomatic.

Promote Acceptance of Body Image

For the woman who has had a mastectomy, acceptance of the change in body image takes time. Evaluate adaptation to this loss by asking the woman how she feels about the loss and whether she thinks it would be helpful to see a social worker or psycho-oncologist to discuss strategies for coping. Adaptation and acceptance of the loss may be evident by her ability to discuss plans for a permanent prosthesis or by her questions regarding breast reconstruction. Do not insist that a woman look at her incision; she needs to wait until she is ready. A woman's reluctance to look at the incision is in no way evidence of inability to accept her loss.

Inform women of outside resources that can help them adapt to the changes imposed by the disease. For example, breast cancer support groups and other resources help the woman and her significant other learn to cope. Information about where to buy a prosthesis and a wig is helpful. Even having the telephone number and name of a person who can help with a wig or prosthesis can make a difficult time more bearable. (See the Complementary and Alternative Therapy feature on Exercise for Breast Cancer Survivors.)

OUTCOME MANAGEMENT

Local Recurrence

Nearly 80% of local recurrences appear within 5 years of mastectomy.[1] Local recurrence after mastectomy generally presents as an isolated nodule in or under the skin of the chest wall, usually near the mastectomy scar. Breast reconstruction does not interfere with early detection of a local recurrence. A complete staging work-up is conducted to define the extent of recurrence. Wide local excision and radiation therapy have been the standard form of local treatment for clients with local recurrence after mastectomy. Hormone therapy is appropriate if the tumor is estrogen receptor positive, or chemotherapy is recommended in view of the very high risk for distant metastases. The goal of therapy is control of local and distant disease.

Local recurrence after breast-preserving surgery and radiation therapy carries a better prognosis than that associated with local recurrence after mastectomy. Mastectomy is the standard form of therapy for local recurrence, as long as there is no evidence of supraclavicular node involvement or distant metastases.

Metastatic Breast Cancer

Medical Management

Determine Extent of Disease

Despite adjuvant therapy, after varying periods of disease-free survival, nearly half of clients who have received treatment for apparently localized breast cancer develop metastatic disease. The majority of cases occur within 2 years of definitive surgery, but several initial breast cancer recurrences occur more than 5 years after initial therapy.[1] In general, the clinical course and presentation of metastatic disease are variable in terms of growth rate and responsiveness to systemic therapy. As a result of the heterogeneous nature of breast cancer, the disease may present as aggressive visceral disease in multiple organs, as a small skin recurrence such as in a supraclavicular lymph node, or as metastatic bone disease.

Selection of therapy depends on the extent of disease and whether any visceral organs are involved. The goal of therapy is control of disease and optimal palliation with prolongation of life and minimal disruption of the woman's lifestyle and quality of life. Life expectancy after breast cancer recurrence is variable. If disease recurs in the liver, most women die within 3 years of the recurrence. Others with disease in bone or skin may survive for many years. Women with more aggressive disease tend to be *premenopausal,* with estrogen receptor–negative, HER-2–positive disease that recurs in liver or lung. Women with less aggressive disease tend to be *postmenopausal,* with estrogen receptor–positive disease that is HER-2–negative and recurs in bone and skin.

All clients with suspected metastatic disease undergo a metastatic work-up to determine the extent of disease. Typically, a physical examination, serum chemistry profiles, a complete blood count, chest radiograph, and a bone scan are obtained initially. If the client has clinical manifestations associated with organ dysfunction, a CT scan of the area is appropriate. A CT scan or MRI study of the chest, abdomen, or pelvis may also be done if the client is being considered for a research protocol. Serum markers may be ordered and include CEA, CA-125, and CA 15-3. Serum markers that are elevated are monitored monthly to evaluate response to therapy.

Prevent Further Extension of Cancer

Once the extent of disease is determined, an overall therapeutic approach is established based on the client's age, disease-free interval, hormone receptor status, and location and extent of disease. For older women with limited and non–life-threatening disease, no significant manifestations of disease, and estrogen receptor–positive tumors, hormone therapy is the initial treatment of choice. If the disease involves liver or lung or if the tumor is estrogen receptor negative, the choice of treatment is chemotherapy, with or without trastuzumab if the tumor is HER-2 positive. Radiation therapy is instituted only if the disease is symptomatic.

The basic philosophy of management for metastatic breast cancer is to use all therapies to their fullest worth, but not to the point of toxicity, when the treatment becomes worse than the disease. A treatment that creates a stable condition is still a worthwhile treatment. Treatments are not abandoned until their utility is fully spent. The emphasis is on the need for therapeutic options.

Endocrine Therapy. As stated earlier, when a woman is known to have breast cancer, her tissue sample is tested for the presence of estrogen and progesterone receptors. Estrogen and progesterone receptor assays are performed using radio immunoassay and immunohistochemical techniques. The more strongly estrogen receptor positive the tumor, the more likely it is that the disease will respond to hormone therapies. Yet although more than 60% of human breast cancers are estrogen receptor positive, no more than two thirds of them will respond to endocrine therapy.

Hormone therapies are generally classified as *ablative* (removal of the hormone) or *additive* (addition of a hormone); both types change the hormonal environment sufficiently to affect tumor growth. The response rates for all hormonal manipulations are basically similar. Women who have a response to one hormonal intervention often have a response to a second after the first becomes ineffective.

In general, the least toxic intervention is chosen first. Once the disease is no longer controlled with a specific approach, the next least toxic agent is selected, and so forth. There is no therapeutic benefit to combining hormone therapies. It is generally accepted practice to continue each therapy for as long as it provides benefit before instituting other therapy. Even withdrawing a hormone manipulation may result in a therapeutic response.

Anti-estrogens. If the woman has not previously received an aromatase inhibitor or tamoxifen, it is typically the first hormonal agent given because of its limited toxicity. Aromatase inhibitors work well in postmenopausal clients and are not cross-resistant. Therefore if an agent worked in the adjuvant period, a different aromatase inhibitor or tamoxifen could be given for recurrent or metastatic disease. Tamoxifen works in premenopausal women, but it is more active in the absence of ovarian function and is therefore especially effective in postmenopausal women. Other anti-estrogens include toremifene (Fareston), raloxifene (Evista), and long-acting ICI 182,780 (Faslodex).

Ablative Endocrine Procedures. Ablative endocrine procedures have been replaced by specific, well-tolerated hormone treatments. In premenopausal women, it is possible to administer goserelin (Zoladex), a luteinizing hormone–releasing hormone (LHRH) agonist that causes a medical oophorectomy. Injections are given every 1 to 3 months depending on the preparation. The only difference between surgical oophorectomy and medical oophorectomy is that results with surgical intervention are immediate and permanent.

If initial hormone ablation therapy fails, administration of either megestrol acetate (Megace) or an aromatase inhibitor is an option. Aromatase inhibitors prevent the peripheral conversion or aromatization of other steroids (namely, androgens to estrogen), primarily in body fat. The efficacy of aromatase inhibitors is limited to postmenopausal women. In clinical trials it appears that anastrozole (Arimidex), exemestane (Aromasin), and letrozole (Femara) as aromatase inhibitors are associated not only with less toxicity but also with greater efficacy and even survival than have been reported for megestrol acetate.[1]

Chemotherapy. Eventually, all hormone-responsive tumors become refractory to hormone manipulation, and chemotherapy becomes the treatment of choice. The selection of combination chemotherapy again is guided by the toxicity of the regimen and the extent of disease. A doxorubicin-containing regimen is usually selected if the client has lung or liver disease, because the response is usually prompt and durable. CMF is also a good option and is somewhat less toxic. The taxanes with or without trastuzumab are excellent options, as is vinorelbine (Navelbine). All of these drugs and drug combinations are options for the woman with metastatic disease, and each offers some degree of response and tumor control.

For the most part, metastatic breast cancer is considered an incurable disease; however, women may live for years with only a single site of metastasis, such as bone metastases. A promising treatment option for women with bone metastases is a bisphosphonate added to the chemotherapeutic or hormonal therapy regimen. Pamidronate (Aredia), clodronate (Ostac), and zoledronic acid (Zometa) not only reduce pain and the incidence of complications but also help the bone to heal and prolong survival of the client without complications associated with bone metastases. The drugs improve bone strength and make the bone more resistant to bone metastasis.[23] Pamidronate and zoledronic acid are given intravenously over 2 hours every month. Adjuvant clodronate therapy has been shown to decrease the risk of bone metastases.[1,26]

BREAST CANCER IN MEN

Breast cancer in men is rare, with approximately 2030 new cases diagnosed and nearly 450 deaths attributable to breast cancer projected for 2007.[2] The number of new cases has been rising in men for the last several years. The average age at onset is about 60 years (10 years older than the average for women). Factors associated with an increased risk of breast cancer in men include the following:

- A first-degree male or female relative with breast cancer
- Presence of the *BRCA2* gene
- Klinefelter's syndrome
- Hepatic schistosomiasis
- Exposure to ionizing radiation
- Prolonged heat exposure

Breast cancer in men tends to be identified at a more advanced stage, possibly because of the unexpected nature of the disease and the fact that the mass is usually painless and located beneath the nipple-areola complex. Generally, the mass is detected when it becomes large, ulcerates, or becomes fixed to underlying muscle. Assessment findings indicating male breast cancer include a painless lump beneath the areola or, more often, nipple discharge, retraction, crusting, or ulceration.

Biopsy is necessary for diagnosis of male breast cancer. The most common histologic type is infiltrating ductal carcinoma. Most male breast cancers are estrogen receptor positive and respond to endocrine therapy. Staging of disease is the same as for women. Axillary dissection is done to determine nodal status and prognosis.

A modified radical mastectomy is usually required to obtain clear margins. Radiation therapy may be indicated, depending on the size of the primary tumor. Chemotherapy, usually a doxorubicin-containing regimen, may be administered as adjuvant therapy and followed by radiation. Tamoxifen therapy is appropriate for adjuvant therapy. In the presence of metastatic disease, an LHRH agonist (goserelin) is appropriate hormonal manipulation and takes the place of orchiectomy. The pattern of metastasis is similar to that of female breast cancer.

BENIGN BREAST DISEASE

Most women have a profound underlying fear of breast cancer. For some women the fear is so great that they are immobilized and ignore the problem altogether. This is why some women who see a physician because of a lump, pain, or nipple discharge present with breast cancer at an advanced stage. Mastalgia, or breast pain, is frequently linked emotionally to the fear of breast cancer. Become sensitive to the emotional aspects associated with breast problems, take clients' fears seriously, provide reassurance through discussion, and perform appropriate evaluation.

The basic techniques of breast evaluation consist of the following:

- A breast-oriented medical history, including the woman's age, menstrual history, family and personal history of breast cancer, last mammogram, and current or past history of hormone therapy
- Clinical breast examination
- Mammography
- Biopsy of a persistent palpable mass

Table 40-3 summarizes common benign breast problems.

MAMMAPLASTY

Mammaplasty is the surgical revision in the size or shape of the breast. It is often performed electively for cosmetic reasons to enlarge or reduce breast size.

Breast Augmentation

Clients seeking breast augmentation are often young women who have had chronic feelings of inadequacy and self-consciousness because of small or undeveloped breasts. Some clients are mature women who have postpartum breast atrophy. Current prostheses are durable, seamless, silicone rubber envelopes filled with saline or silicone. The prosthesis is inserted beneath existing breast tissue or the pectoralis muscle (called subpectoral placement) through an inframammary (under the breast), transaxillary (through the axilla), or periareolar (around the nipple) incision (Figure 40-8).

Thorough preoperative breast assessment is essential to rule out breast cancer. Mammography is generally not recommended in women younger than 35 years unless they have a positive family history of cancer or a suspicious lump. Surgery is performed on an outpatient basis. Nurses provide teaching and support, mostly over the telephone.

Early complications of breast augmentation include changes in breast or nipple sensation, hematoma (collection of clotted blood), infection, or leakage from the prosthesis. The most frequent complication is capsule formation (development of fibrous sacs of scar tissue enclosing the implant), followed by contracture of the scar. These complications cause excessive breast firmness and distortion of the breast into a hard, round ball. Possible causes of capsular contracture include infection and formation of a seroma (a collection of serosanguineous

TABLE 40–3 Benign Breast Disorders

Benign Breast Problem	Definition	Presentation	Treatment
Mastalgia	Breast pain	Cyclical or persistent Focal or generalized	Based on presentation Dietary changes such as reducing caffeine intake
Fibrocystic breasts	Most common pathologic problem in female breast	Fluid-filled cysts, tender nodular breast tissue with cyclical variation	Cyst aspiration if painful Dietary modifications such as reducing caffeine intake
Hyperplasia and atypical hyperplasia	Cellular proliferation ranging from normal cells to abnormal cells	Hyperplasia present in 20% of biopsy specimens Atypical hyperplasia in 1% of biopsy specimens: represents risk factor for breast cancer	No additional treatment for hyperplasia Atypical hyperplasia usually requires excisional biopsy with possible chemopreventive treatment with tamoxifen or raloxifene
Fibroadenoma	Benign tumor	Common breast tumor occurring in young women 15-30 Nontender, round, firm or rubbery mass 1-3 cm in diameter	May require no treatment If large or if woman desires, can be surgically removed
Papilloma	Lesion growing in terminal portion of duct	Typically occurs in women in 40s; may present with serous or serosanguineous nipple discharge Multiple papillomas may be indicative of increased breast cancer risk	Ductogram for nipple discharge Surgery for removal of ducts as indicated
Duct ectasia	Disease of ducts in subareolar zone	Palpable dilated duct; thick, sticky nipple discharge; burning pain; itching and inflammation	No increased risk for cancer; no surgical intervention required
Gynecomastia	Hypertrophy of one or both male breasts	Increased breast size in male	Caused by some drugs including estrogen, tumors, thyroid conditions, and hepatic problems Thorough evaluation to determine cause and then appropriate interventions

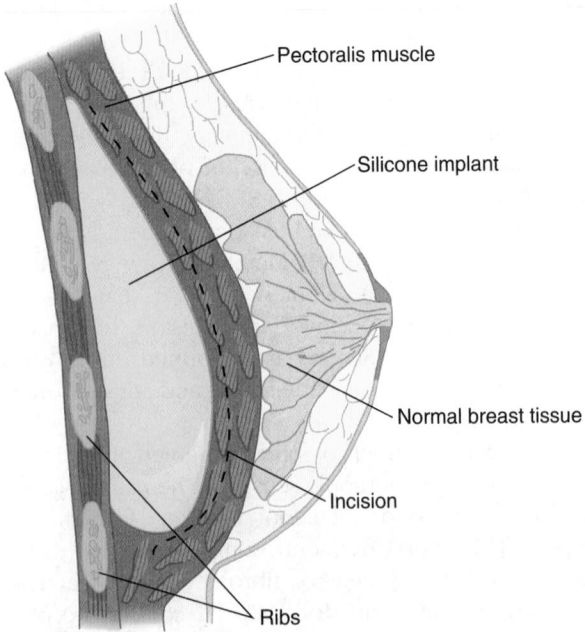

■ **FIGURE 40–8** Augmentation mammaplasty is achieved by insertion of a saline-filled implant beneath the pectoral muscle. The incision is represented by a *dashed line*.

fluid) or hematoma. The basic problem in these processes is that the body's defense mechanisms respond to the prosthesis as a foreign body, and scar tissue forms around the prosthesis to wall it off. Capsule formation is usually treated with open (surgical) capsulotomy. Open capsulotomy, performed under general anesthesia, involves incising the capsule.

Breast massage may be prescribed postoperatively with smooth-walled implants or after capsulotomy to reduce capsule formation. Breast massage typically begins postoperatively according to the surgeon's instructions. Teach the woman to push each breast up, to the side, and toward the middle of the chest, supporting the breast in each position for a count of 10. Discharge instructions usually include the following:

- To reduce edema, maintain a head-elevated position for a week when in bed.
- To reduce hematoma formation, get plenty of rest for a week (no excessive activity; take it easy).
- To avoid moving the pectoralis muscle and irritating the surgical site, do not raise the arms above the head for 3 weeks (e.g., while washing or brushing hair), do not play golf or tennis or swim for 6

weeks, sleep on the back and not on the stomach or sides, and be careful when closing car doors.

- Because of their anticoagulant effect, do not use aspirin or aspirin-containing compounds.
- Notify the physician if bleeding occurs or if a fever with temperature greater than 37.6° C (99.6° F) develops.

Reduction Mammaplasty

Reduction mammaplasty surgically reduces the size of large, pendulous breasts. Women usually seek such surgery to reduce the physical and psychosocial discomforts of large breasts, such as back pain, the presence of bra strap indentations in the shoulders, inability to wear normal clothing styles, intertriginous dermatitis (skin breakdown under large breasts), and distress from others' comments about breast size.

Excess breast tissue is removed through incisions under the breast (Figure 40-9). The nipple is transposed on a pedicle of tissue or grafted onto the newly formed breast. A possible complication is loss of blood supply to the nipple-areola complex. Any duskiness or pallor around the nipple-areola complex should be reported to the physician. Altered sensation and the inability to perform breast-feeding are common findings after this procedure.

Mastopexy

Mastopexy is the correction of mammary ptosis (drooping) to achieve an improved breast contour and position. Mastopexy may be performed with subcutaneous mastectomy or on normal breasts to improve contour. Postoperative care is similar to that with other types of breast surgery.

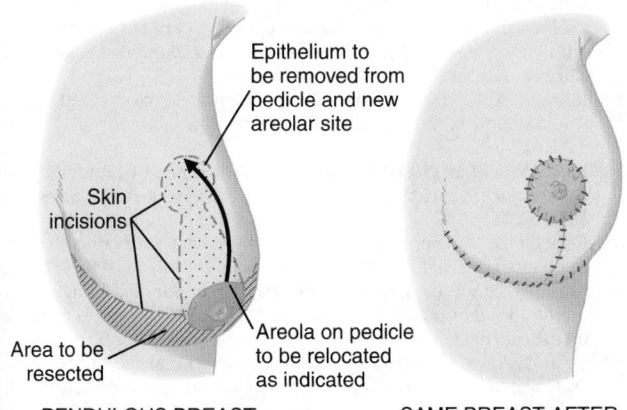

Epithelium to be removed from pedicle and new areolar site

Skin incisions

Area to be resected

Areola on pedicle to be relocated as indicated

PENDULOUS BREAST BEFORE SURGERY

SAME BREAST AFTER RECONTOURING

■ **FIGURE 40–9** Reduction mammaplasty, in which breasts are surgically reduced. Excess breast tissue is removed, and the breast is recontoured. The nipple is relocated (e.g., moved higher) on a pedicle of tissue. The pedicle supplies the nipple with blood until new blood vessels form.

 CONCLUSIONS

Diseases of the breast are usually benign conditions that occur throughout the life cycle. Breast cancer, however, has greatly increased in incidence over the past 30 years. The nurse has a vital role in teaching clients early detection methods so that breast cancer can be detected at a curable stage.

All diseases of the breast potentially pose problems in body image and sexuality. Even benign fibrocystic changes can cause breast tenderness and possibly interfere with sexual functioning. Breast cancer and the possibility of mastectomy as treatment can be extremely threatening to a woman's body image. The nurse can help the client cope with these potential threats and successfully adapt to any changes that occur.

THINKING CRITICALLY

1. The pathology report of your client's breast biopsy reads: "8 mm invasive ductal carcinoma, invasive carcinoma to the margins, estrogen receptor–positive and progesterone receptor–positive." The client is considering further treatment and asks you what her options are. How would you respond?

Factors to Consider. What treatment options might the client have? What interventions might be required?

2. Your client has come to the surgery clinic 10 days after a modified radical mastectomy. The breast incision line is clean and intact. A Jackson-Pratt drain is sutured in place in the axilla. The skin around the drain is clean and intact. Drainage is serosanguineous, and the client has recorded 25 ml and 20 ml, respectively, of drainage per 24 hours for the last 2 days. The client looks at the incision and the drain and asks questions while you examine her incision and drainage site. She asks when the drain will come out, when she can drive her car, when she can shower and resume her normal activities, and when she can be fitted for a prosthesis. What would you tell her? What else should you assess? What medical and nursing care does this client need during her appointment? What other teaching needs does she have?

Factors to Consider. Think about what structures are removed as part of the modified radical mastectomy. What are the functions of these structures? What functional limitations can be expected to affect the client's self-care needs? Consider the client's needs in this immediate postoperative period, in a few months, and over the long term.

3. Two years ago, your client's stage II cancer of the right breast was treated with a quadrantectomy (margins negative), axillary lymph node dissection (8 of 19 nodes positive), radiation therapy of the chest and axilla, and six courses of CAF (Cytoxan [cyclophosphamide], Adriamycin [doxorubicin], 5-fluorouracil) chemotherapy. Today, she presents with pain, tingling, and swelling of her right hand and arm. She states that although she noticed intermittent problems with slight swelling over the past 6 months, it has

become severe over the past 2 weeks and is affecting her ability to work as a court stenographer. What further information should you assess? What are your priority interventions?

Factors to Consider. What do pain, tingling, and swelling of the hand and arm suggest in a client who has undergone lymph node dissection? Should a referral to a physical therapist for lymphedema management be made?

 Discussions for these questions can be found on the website.

BIBLIOGRAPHY

Citations appearing in red refer to primary research.

Citations appearing in blue refer to evidence-based practice guidelines and protocols.

1. Abeloff, M., et al. (2006). Breast. In M. Abeloff, et al. (Eds.), *Clinical oncology* (3rd ed.). New York: Churchill Livingstone.
2. American Cancer Society. (2007). *Cancer facts and figures 2007*. Atlanta: Author.
3. American Cancer Society. (2002). *Breast cancer facts and figures 2001-2002*. Atlanta: Author.
4. American Cancer Society. (2007). *American Cancer Society guidelines for the early detection of cancer*. Retrieved 01/27/07 from www.cancer.org/docroot/PED/center/PED_2_3x_ACS_Cancer_Detection_Guidelines_36.asp?sitearea=PED.
5. Anonymous. (2002). Benefit of a high-dose epirubicin regimen in adjuvant chemotherapy for node-positive breast cancer clients with poor prognostic factors: 5-year follow-up results of French Adjuvant Study Group 05 randomized trial. *Journal of Clinical Oncology, 19*(3), 602-611.
6. Aston, C., et al. (2005). Oligogenic combinations associated with breast cancer risk in women under 53 years of age. *Human Genetics, 116*(3), 208-221.
7. Baker, J.A., et al. (2006). Consumption of coffee, but not black tea, is associated with decreased risk of premenopausal breast cancer. *Journal of Nutrition, 6*(1), 166-171.
8. Baselga, J.B., et al. (1997). HER-2 overexpression and paclitaxel sensitivity in breast cancer. Therapeutic implications. *Oncology, 11*(3), 43-48.
9. Berns, E.A., Hendrick, R.E., & Cutter, G.R. (2002). Performance comparison of full-field digital mammography to screen-film mammography in clinical practice. *Medical Physics, 29*(5), 830-834.
10. Bradley, C.J., Given, C.W., & Roberts, C. (2002). Race, socioeconomic status, and breast cancer treatment and survival. *Journal of the National Cancer Institute, 94*(7), 490-496.
11. Breast Cancer Guidelines. (2007). *Clinical practice guidelines in oncology, version 2, 2006*. National Comprehensive Cancer Network. Retrieved 9/20/07 from www.nccn.org/professionals/physician_gls/PDF/breast.pdf.
12. Buzdar, A.U., & Cuzick, J. (2006). Anastrozole as an adjuvant endocrine treatment for postmenopausal patients with breast cancer: Emerging data. *Clinical Practice Research, 1*(12), 1037s-1048s.
13. Carlson, R.W., et al. (2006). NCCN Task Force report: Adjuvant therapy for breast cancer. *Journal of the Comprehensive Cancer Networks*, Suppl 1, s1-s26.
14. Cataliotti, L., et al. (2006). Comparison of anastrozole versus tamoxifen as preoperative therapy in postmenopausal women with hormone receptor-positive breast cancer: The pre-operative "Arimidex" Compared to Tamoxifen (PROACT) trial. *Cancer*, Apr 5, Epub.
15. Centers for Disease Control and Prevention. (2002). *Breast and cervical cancer fact sheet*. Retrieved 10/20/03 from www.cdc.gov/cancer/nbccedp.
16. Cobleigh, M.A. (2005). Tumor gene expression and prognosis in breast cancer patients with 10 or more positive lymph nodes. *Clinical Cancer Research, 11*, 8623-8631.
17. Cummings, S.R., et al. (1999). The effect of raloxifene on risk of breast cancer in post menopausal women: Results from the Multiple Outcomes of Raloxifene (MORE) trial. *Journal of the American Medical Association, 281*(3), 2189-2197.
18. Cuzick, J., Sasieni, P., & Howell, A. (2006). Should aromatase inhibitors be used as initial adjuvant treatment or sequenced after tamoxifen? *British Journal of Cancer, 94*(4), 460-464.
19. Davis, S., & Mirick, D.K. (2006). Circadian disruption, shift work and the risk of cancer: A summary of the evidence and studies in Seattle. *Cancer, Causes, Control, 17*, 539-545.
20. Dellacroce, F.J., & Sullivan, S.F. (2005). Application and refinement of the superior gluteal artery perforator free flap for bilateral simultaneous breast reconstruction. *Plastic Reconstruction Surgery, 116*(1), 97-103.
21. Dumitrescu, R.G., & Shields, P.G. (2005). The etiology of alcohol-induced breast cancer. *Alcohol, 35*(3), 213-225.
22. Edwards, B.K., et al. (2005). Annual report to the nation on the status of cancer, 1975-2002, featuring population based trends in cancer treatment. *Journal of the National Cancer Institute, 97*, 1407-1427.
23. *Facts about menopausal hormone therapy* (NIH Pub. No. 05-5200). (2005). Bethesda, Md: U.S. Department of Health and Human Services.
24. Fisher, B., et al. (1999). Further evaluation of intensified and increased total dose of cyclophosphamide for the treatment of primary breast cancer: Findings from National Surgical Adjuvant Breast and Bowel Project B-25. *Journal of Clinical Oncology, 17*(11), 3374-3388.
25. Fisher, B., et al. (1998). Tamoxifen for prevention of breast cancer. Report of the National Surgical Adjuvant Breast and Bowel Project: Project P-1 Study. *Journal of the National Cancer Institute, 90*, 1371-1388.
26. Gaines, K. (2002). Zoledronic acid (Zometa): Bisphosphonate for prostate cancer/bone metastases. *Urologic Nursing, 22*(6), 398-400.
27. Genetic-familial high risk assessment: Breast and ovarian cancer. (2006). *National Comprehensive Cancer Network's clinical practice guidelines in oncology, version 1, 2006*. Retrieved 01/27/07 from www.nccn.org/progessionals/physician_gls/PDF/genetics_screening.pdf.
28. Goldstein, L.J. (2006). Controversies in adjuvant endocrine treatment of premenopausal women. *Clinical Breast Cancer, 6*(Suppl 2), s36-40.
29. Gonzalez, C.A. (2006). The European prospective investigation into cancer and nutrition (EPIC). *Public Health Nutrition, 9*(1A), 124-126.
30. Hurley, J., et al. (2006). Docetaxel, cisplatin, and trastuzumab as primary systemic therapy for human epidermal growth factor receptor 2 positive locally advanced breast cancer. *Journal of Clinical Oncology, 24*, 1831-1838.
31. Itami, J. (2002). Hodgkin lymphoma. *Nippon Acta Radiologica, 62*(5), 215-220.
32. Jernstrom, H., et al. (2005). Impact of teenage oral contraceptive use in a population-based series of early onset breast cancer cases who have undergone BRCA mutation testing. *European Journal of Cancer, 41*, 2312-2320.
33. Johnson, K.C. (2005). Accumulating evidence on passive and active smoking and breast cancer risk. *International Journal of Cancer, 117*, 619-628.
34. Kaste, S.C., et al. (1998). Breast masses in women treated for childhood cancer: Incidence and screening guidelines. *Cancer, 82*, 784-792.
35. Koberle, D., & Thurlimann, B. (2005). Adjuvant endocrine therapy in postmenopausal breast cancer patients. *Breast, 14*, 446-451.
36. Kummel, S., et al. (2006). Randomised trial: Survival benefit and safety of adjuvant dose-sense chemotherapy for node-positive breast cancer. *British Journal of Cancer*, April 11, Epub.
37. LaCroix, A.Z. (2005). Estrogen with and without progestin: Benefits and risks of short-term use. *American Journal of Medicine, 118*(12, Suppl 2), 79-87.
38. Leonard, R.C., et al. (2004). Conventional adjuvant chemotherapy versus single-cycle, autograft-supported, high-dose, late intensification chemotherapy in high-risk breast cancer patients: A randomized trial. *Journal of the National Cancer Institute, 96*, 1076-1083.
39. Li, C.I., Malone, K.E., Saltzman, B.S., et al. (2006). Risk of invasive breast carcinoma among women diagnosed with ductal carcinoma

in situ and lobular carcinoma in situ, 1998-2001. *Cancer,* Apr 10, Epub.

40. McKeage, K., & Perry, C.M. (2002). Trastuzumab: A review of its use in the treatment of metastatic breast cancer overexpressing HER-2. *Drugs, 62*(1), 209-213.

41. McReady, D.R., et al. (2004). Influence of the new AJCC breast staging system on sentinel lymph node positivity and false-negative rates. *Journal of the National Cancer Institute, 96,* 8731-8735.

42. Narod, S.A., et al. (2002). Oral contraceptives and the risk of breast cancer in BRCA1 and BRCA2 mutation carriers. *Journal of the National Cancer Institute, 94,* 1773-1779.

43. National Cancer Institute. (2005). *Annual report to the nation on the status of cancer 1975-2002, with a special feature on treatment trends. Questions and answers.* Retrieved from www.cancer.gov/ newscenter/pressreleases/ReportNation2005QandA.

44. National Cancer Institute. (2006). *Initial results of the Study of Tamoxifen and Raloxifene (STAR) releases: Osteoporosis drug raloxifene shown to be as effective as tamoxifen in preventing invasive breast cancer.* Retrieved 01/27/07 from www.cancer.gov/newscenter/pressreleases/STARresultsApr172006.

45. Nelson, H.D. (2002). Assessing benefits and harms of hormone replacement therapy: Clinical applications. *Journal of the American Medical Association, 288*(7), 882-884.

46. Nelson, H.D., et al. (2002). Postmenopausal hormone replacement therapy: Scientific review. *Journal of the American Medical Association, 288*(7), 872-881.

47. Newman, L.A., et al. (2002). Ethnicity related differences in the survival of young breast carcinoma patients. *Cancer, 95*(1), 21-26.

48. NIH. (2002). *NHLBI stops trial of estrogen plus progestin due to increased breast cancer risk, lack of overall benefit.* Retrieved from www.nih.gov.

49. Orzano, J.A., & Swain, S.M. (2005). Concepts and clinical trials of dose dense chemotherapy for breast cancer. *Clinical Breast Cancer, 6,* 402-411.

50. Page, D.L., et al. (2003). Atypical lobular hyperplasia as a unilateral predictor of breast cancer risk: A retrospective cohort study. *Lancet, 361,* 125-129.

51. Piccart-Gebhart, M.J., et al. (2005). Trastuzumab after adjuvant chemotherapy in HER2-positive breast cancer. *New England Journal of Medicine, 353,* 1659-1672.

52. Pisano, E.D., et al. (2005). Diagnostic performance of digital versus film mammography for breast cancer screening. *New England Journal of Medicine, 353,* 1773-1783.

53. Prentice, R.G., et al. (2006). Low-fat dietary pattern and risk of invasive breast cancer: The Women's Health Initiative Randomized Controlled Dietary Modification Trial. *Journal of the American Medical Association, 295,* 629-642.

54. Rancour, P., & Brauer, K. (2003). Use of letter writing as a means of integrating an altered body image: A case study. *Oncology Nursing Forum, 30,* 841-846.

55. Rebbeck T.R., et al. (2004). Bilateral prophylactic mastectomy reduces breast cancer risk in BRCA1 and BRCA2 mutation carriers: The PROSE Study Group. *Journal of Clinical Oncology, 22,* 1055-1062.

56. Sarin, R. (2005). Partial-breast treatment for early breast cancer: Emergence of a new paradigm. *National Clinical Practice in Oncology, 2*(1), 40-47.

57. Saslow, D., Boates, C., Burke, W., Harms, S., et al. (2007) American Cancer Society guidelines for breast screening with MRI as an adjunct to mammography. *CA Cancer Journal for Clinicians, 57,* 75-89.

58. Schernhammer, E.S., Kroenke, C.H., Laden, F., et al. (2006). Night work and risk of breast cancer. *Epidemiology, 17*(1), 108-111.

59. Schulze, T., et al. (2006). Long term morbidity of patients with early breast cancer after sentinel lymph node biopsy compared to axillary lymph node dissection. *Journal of Surgical Oncology, 93*(2), 109-119.

60. Screening for Breast Cancer. (2002). *Guide to clinical preventive services: Periodic updates* (3rd ed.).Rockville, Md: U.S. Preventive Services Task Force.

61. Singletary, K.W., & Gapstur, S.M. (2001). Alcohol and breast cancer. Review of epidemiologic and experimental evidence and potential mechanisms. *Journal of the American Medical Association, 286,* 2143-2152.

62. Smith, R.A., et al. (2003). American Cancer Society guidelines for breast cancer screening: Update 2003. *CA: Cancer Journal for Clinicians, 53,* 141-169.

63. Stolzenberg-Solomon, R.Z., et al. (2006). Folate intake, alcohol use, and postmenopausal breast cancer risk in the prostate, lung, colorectal, ovarian cancer screening trial. *American Journal of Clinical Nutrition, 83,* 895-904.

64. Vogel, V.G. (2000). *Management of people at high risk for breast cancer.* Boston: Blackwell Scientific Publications.

65. Webb, P.M., et al. (2002). History of breast cancer, age and benign breast disease. *International Journal of Cancer, 100*(3), 375-378.

66. Winer, E.P., et al. (2005). American Society of Clinical Oncology technology assessment on the use of aromatase inhibitors as adjuvant therapy for postmenopausal women with hormone receptor-positive breast cancer: Status report 2004. *Journal of Clinical Oncology, 23,* 619-629.

67. Wong, S.L., et al. (2002). Optimal use of sentinel lymph node biopsy versus axillary node dissection in patients with breast carcinoma. *Cancer, 95*(3), 478-486.

evolve *Did you remember to check out the* *bonus material on the Evolve website and the CD-ROM, including NCLEX®-Examination Style Review Questions, Open-Book Quizzes, and Chapter Review Audio Podcasts?*

http://evolve.elsevier.com/Black/medsurg

CHAPTER 41

Management of Clients with Sexually Transmitted Infections

MEG BLAIR

SEXUALLY TRANSMITTED INFECTIONS: AN OVERVIEW

The term *sexually transmitted infection* (STI) refers to any infection contracted primarily through sexual activities or contact. *STI* has replaced the older term *venereal disease* (VD), which referred to diseases transmitted only by sexual intercourse. STI is also known as sexually transmitted disease (STD). More than 50 organisms are known to be spread through sexual activity. The five most widely known STIs in the United States are chlamydia, gonorrhea, syphilis, genital herpes, and genital warts. Other infections are chancroid, lymphogranuloma venereum, granuloma inguinale, trichomoniasis, human immunodeficiency virus (HIV), hepatitis, and some enteric and ectoparasitic infections. The number of STIs is increasing as new agents are implicated in the sexual transmission of disease.

STIs share the following characteristics:

- STIs can be transmitted by any sexual activity between opposite-sex or same-sex partners (not only vaginal-penile sex but also oral and anal sex).
- Having one STI confers no immunity against future reinfection with that STI or with any other STI (except, possibly, for hepatitis B).
- Sexual partners of infected clients need to be assessed for treatment (see individual infections for specific recommendations).
- STIs affect people from all socioeconomic classes, cultures, ethnicities, and age groups.
- Women bear a disproportionate number of the effects of STIs.
- Frustration, anger, anxiety, fear, shame, and guilt are common emotions associated with an STI diagnosis.
- STIs frequently coexist in the same client.

The last fact may be responsible for some treatment failures. Current treatment guidelines for STIs are available from the Centers for Disease Control and Prevention (CDC) in Atlanta and on the CDC website (www.cdc.gov).

STIs are a serious public health problem. Recognized since the beginning of recorded history, these diseases have been associated with substantial morbidity and, in some cases, mortality. The incidence of STIs continues to increase worldwide, and infections are becoming more severe. STIs also facilitate infection with HIV/AIDS. Thus the scope of health and other problems they create is increasing rather than decreasing. It is a matter of public concern that treatments for STIs be easy to obtain, safe, inexpensive, and effective.

Except for the common cold and influenza, STIs are the most prevalent communicable diseases in the United States, which has the highest STI rate in the industrialized world. Most sources describe STI rates as epidemic. Although HIV/AIDS is probably the best publicized and most dangerous, the most common STIs are chlamydia, gonorrhea, genital herpes, and genital warts. Symptomatic STIs are diagnosed in more than 15 million people in the United States annually (not including HIV/AIDS) and 86% of affected people are between 15 and 29 years of age. Another 40 million people are infected with human papillomavirus (HPV), which causes genital warts.

---

evolve Web Enhancements

Bridge to Home Health Care   Teaching About Sexually Transmitted Infections

Client Education Guide   Sexually Transmitted Infections (English Version and Spanish Translation)

Ethical Issues in Nursing   Does the Right to Privacy of Clients with Sexually Transmitted Infections Supersede the Right to Know of Potentially Infected Partners?

Be sure to check out the bonus material on the Evolve website and the CD-ROM, including free self-assessment exercises. **http://evolve.elsevier.com/Black/medsurg**

It is estimated that 50% of all Americans will have been exposed to or will contract an STI by age 30 years.

Official national incidence statistics for STIs are published by the CDC and by local health authorities, but the actual incidence is unknown. Accurate statistics are difficult to compile for a number of reasons. Statistics reflect the accuracy of case reporting, and reporting is not mandatory for all STIs. Rates for some STIs, such as genital herpes and genital warts, are based on estimates derived from local studies and physicians' reports. These estimates are thought to be low. Even rates developed from mandatory case reporting are believed to be low. There are several causes for physician and clinic underreporting, including poor compliance with screening recommendations.

The costs of STIs are staggering, both in medical expense and in emotional suffering. Up to $17 billion a year is spent to treat STIs and their sequelae (consequences), including at least $2 billion a year to treat subsequent infertility. These figures, like statistics, can be misleading. For instance, women, who are two times more likely to be infected with an STI than men, are less likely to receive treatment, often because the STI is asymptomatic. Also, STIs can lead to infertility. The cost of treating infertility caused by STIs is an indirect cost of the STI. Many couples in lower socioeconomic classes cannot afford infertility treatments. Hence infertility services are used most often by middle-class and upper-class couples.

Etiology and Risk Factors

STIs can be caused by bacteria, viruses, protozoa, fungi, and ectoparasites. Although younger people have the highest rates for STIs, all age groups are at risk. Anyone who engages in intimate physical contact can contract and transmit an STI. Many health care providers do not always acknowledge that fact, especially in regard to middle- or upper-class clients. Health care providers often fail to consider that adolescents or older adults are sexually active. Research shows that health care professionals are unskilled and uncomfortable taking a client's sexual history, which can lead to underscreening (Box 41-1).

The fetus or neonate can be infected across the placenta or during vaginal birth. Infants and children can be infected through child abuse. Children and adolescents are particularly vulnerable because of biologic variables and because they are more likely to have more frequent unprotected sex and shorter term relationships, leading to multiple partners, and they face obstacles in obtaining health care services. In adolescents, peer group pressure and the belief that they are invincible also are factors when considering the presence of STIs. Older adults can be infected or can experience residual effects from infections contracted earlier in life. Some manifestations of STIs can be mistaken for other age-related diseases. When a client complains of manifestations that could be an STI, then STIs should be part of the differential diagnosis.

The worldwide increase in the incidence of STIs is a result of many factors. Antibiotic-resistant strains of bacteria have become more common. For example, the incidence of gonorrhea has risen since the evolution of penicillinase-producing *Neisseria gonorrhoeae*. Some strains of gonorrhea are also resistant to quinolone antibiotics. The use of intrauterine devices (IUDs) and oral contraceptives may lower women's resistance to infection and facilitate transmission of STIs. Women may not think to use an infection barrier *in addition to* effective contraception. Sterilized women often do not use condoms. Many people have a cavalier attitude about STI infections because of advances made in antimicrobial therapy, and thus do not consider STIs to be serious diseases with possible complications.

Lack of knowledge also plays a role in the incidence of STIs. Clients may find it difficult to obtain accurate information, even from health professionals. Politics and religion continue to affect the controversy over sex education in schools. Accurate information about sex and STIs is not always presented in a manner designed for young people. Information presented to children and adolescents must take into account their age, developmental level, and culture, as explained in the Translating Evidence into Practice feature on p. 976. Research continues on the best ways to educate individuals and encourage them to change risky behaviors.

The following are specific risk factors for acquiring STIs:

- Intravenous (IV) drug use
- Other substance abuse
- High-risk sexual activity (use of prostitutes or sex worker, multiple or casual sexual partners, sex with IV drug users and infected people, unprotected sex, exchanging sex for money or drugs)
- Younger age
- Younger age at *sexarche* (the beginning of sexual activity)
- Inner city residence
- Poverty or lower socioeconomic status
- Poor nutrition
- Poor hygiene

According to the CDC, STI prevention and control of STIs should focus on five major concepts:

- Education (particularly on risky behaviors) and counseling
- Identification of people with asymptomatic infections and infections in people not likely to seek medical care
- Accurate diagnosis and effective treatment when infection is present
- Evaluation and treatment of sexual partners (see CDC guidelines; generally all partners in the last 60 days, or most recent)
- Pre-exposure vaccination if available

Sex education in schools, risk-reduction counseling, promotion of safer sex, and an open, accepting attitude from health professionals can increase knowledge levels. Health professionals must be comfortable asking clients about sexual activity and must provide information in a way that does not "turn off" the client or cause embarrassment. See Box 41-1 How to Take a Sexual History for more information and tips on providing this essential, but sensitive, service.

Other control measures for STIs include maintaining a high index of suspicion for sexually transmitted infections, providing screening according to established

---

BOX 41-1 How to Take a Sexual History

Nurses provide holistic care to clients in all settings. Sexuality is one of the basic human needs, as explained by Maslow (1954). To care for clients in a holistic fashion, nurses must include assessment of sexuality and sexual functioning as a routine part of health care. This becomes even more important when considered in light of the current epidemic of sexually transmitted infections and HIV/AIDS.

Unfortunately, most health care professionals do not incorporate assessment of sexual functioning and sexuality into their daily practice. There are several reasons for this. Discomfort with the process and language used is one reason frequently cited as a barrier. Another barrier is lack of knowledge regarding appropriate timing and pertinent topics to be included. Yet another barrier is health care providers' attitudes towards certain groups in the population. Older adults, for example, are often not seen as sexual beings (see step 8). "Good" teenagers are not sexually active, and sexual discussions may "give them ideas." Health care professionals may have biases against homosexual activity that may influence their ability to discuss these sex acts.

Following are steps nurses can take to increase their proficiency with sexual history-taking:

Step 1. *Realize that questioning clients about sexuality is an important part of nursing care, not an intrusion.* Sexual dysfunction is often an early manifestation of systemic illness. Sensitivity to this topic may lead to an early diagnosis and better control of a disease process. Many medications have sexual side effects, which may lead to clients not taking them. Some physical conditions (such as spinal cord injury) have a direct impact on sexual functioning and quality of life. It is helpful to remember that nurses learn to be comfortable asking about other private matters, such as bowel and bladder function, menstrual cycles, drug and alcohol use, and domestic violence. Sexuality is just one more arena to include.

Step 2. *Examine and clarify your own values and beliefs.* Having a clear knowledge of your own positions allows you to set these feelings aside and to care for clients whose values, beliefs, and practices may vary greatly from your own.

Step 3. *Ask general or specific questions based on the client's needs.* In a visit for routine health care, general questioning may be all that is needed. When a client seeks health care for specific problems related to sexuality or has clinical manifestations suggestive of sexual disease or dysfunction, more detailed questions are warranted.

One model frequently used by health care providers is the PLISSIT model, which consists of four parts: **P**ermission giving, **L**imited **I**nformation, **S**pecific **S**uggestions, and **I**ntensive **T**herapy.

PLISSIT MODEL

Permission giving: Professionals should ask for and give their clients permission to speak with them about sexually oriented issues. An open atmosphere and general statements can set the stage for permission. A good opening statement is "I always ask my clients about sexuality and sexual functioning. If it is OK with you, I will ask you some questions about this now." This allows the nurse to question the client without seeming too abrupt, and also gives the client permission either to talk about sexual issues or to decline. It also sets the stage that this is an expected part of health care. All health care professionals should function at this level.

Limited Information: This level includes discussing anatomy and physiologic functioning of the body systems involved in sexuality. Nurses functioning at this level also provide basic information about diseases affecting sexual organs and functioning and help clear up myths and misconceptions related to sex and sexual functioning. All nurses have a working knowledge of anatomy and physiology and should be functioning at this level. An example might be teaching an adolescent female about menstrual cycles.

Specific Suggestions: All nurses should be able to provide sexually oriented specific suggestions to the group of clients they see most frequently. An orthopedic nurse should be able to counsel post–joint replacement surgery clients about positions to avoid during sexual activity. A nurse caring for clients with cardiac problems should be able to teach when sexual activity can be safely resumed after a heart attack or bypass surgery. An example of an appropriate statement for this level is "Some men who take this medication have trouble having erections. If this is a concern for you, let's discuss it, because there are other medications that might work for you without causing this problem."

Intensive Therapy: This may be too time-consuming for the typical nurse, who may need to refer clients to licensed sex therapists. Topics covered under intensive therapy can include relationship problems, depression, sexual dysfunction, or body image problems. All nurses should have access to resources for clients if they themselves are not able to provide this level of service.

BOX 41-1   How to Take a Sexual History—Cont'd

When the nurse needs to take a more detailed sexual history, the model provided by the California Chlamydia Action Coalition is a helpful way to organize questions. Use the "5 Ps" to ask about the following:

1. Partners
2. Prevention of pregnancy
3. Protection from STIs
4. Practices
5. Past STIs

Their website has an excellent tool available for use. Visit www.stdhivtraining.org, click "Resources," and enter "A Guide to Sexual History Taking" in the search box. More information, including a PowerPoint presentation on sexual history-taking, can be found at the website of the Association of Reproductive Health Professionals, at www.arhp.org.

Step 4. *Make an effort to gather reproductive health information about each of your clients.* You should know when a female client's last menstrual period was, her pregnancy history, and when she last had screenings such as mammograms, Pap smears, and breast self-examinations. For the male client, inquire about prostate health, digital rectal examinations, prostate-specific antigen tests, and testicular self-examinations. Reproductive health can be considered the "first tier" of knowledge for all clients.

Step 5. *Learn how client's medications and health care problems can affect sexuality.* Look for "natural openings" in your conversations with clients. An opportune time to discuss medication side effects is while taking the medication history. If a client has a medical condition that causes fatigue, general questions such as "How does this affect your ability to work? Does it affect your relationship with your (significant other)?" can lead to a discussion of sexuality. This can be considered the "second tier" of knowledge needed to care for clients.

Step 6. *When discussing the "third tier" or specific sexual activities and issues, use nonjudgmental language.* Instead of asking "Are you a homosexual or a heterosexual?" a better question is "Do you have sex with men, women, or both?" Not only does this avoid making the client feel judged, but also it will result in more accurate information. For a myriad of cultural, religious, or personal reasons, many people who have had same-sex partners do not identify themselves as "gay" or "homosexual." They may be bisexual, they may have an occasional same-sex encounter, or they may be living "on the down low," meaning living a lifestyle that appears to be heterosexual but having frequent sex with same-sex partners. The important factor is the activity that carries the risk for acquiring sexually transmitted infections, not the label given to the person.

Step 7. *Use language the client understands.* Many clients will use slang for body parts and sexual activities. If you have to use the same terms to ensure the client understands, then do so, but also take the time to teach the client the correct wording. This will help the client understand other health care professionals, written material, or other resources he or she may access regarding sexual health.

In addition, be specific about what you say and be clear about what the client means. Many people think the word "sex" only refers to vaginal intercourse. If you ask clients "Do you have sex?" they may say no when, in fact, they are participating in very risky sexual behaviors.

Step 8. *Be sensitive to the client's age, but avoid stereotyping.* For adolescents, know current trends and common slang. Keep your message tailored to specific risks you and the teen identify. Maintain a present-oriented approach involving the teen instead of lecturing on vague consequences that may occur years from now. Let the teen practice specific skills and communication techniques. Then help the adolescent see responsible sexual behavior as part of achieving some near-term goals as well, such as attending college. Assure the teen you will keep their confidentiality. And do not assume the teenager has knowledge. Many teens portray themselves as very sophisticated about sexual matters, when their information may be very inaccurate. Reputable sources of information about sex are limited for teens.

When working with older adults, do not assume they are not sexually active. Studies show older adults often remain sexually active well into their later years. Older adults often do not believe they are at risk of catching sexually transmitted infections from their partners and may not have experience buying and using condoms. In one recent study, an entire focus group denied ever having seen a condom. Older adults from minority cultural groups may be more comfortable getting sexually oriented information from a cultural peer who speaks their native language. Older adults may believe that sexuality issues are private and may not be comfortable discussing them at all.

In summary, nurses are responsible for caring for the entire client, and this includes sexuality. To help stem the exploding epidemic of sexually transmitted infections, nurses need to incorporate taking sexual histories into their repertoire.

Role-play with peers you are comfortable with. Practice asking specific sexually oriented questions or teaching on a sexual topic. The more often you use the language required for this discussion, the more comfortable you will become.

REFERENCES

1. Albaugh, J.A., & Kellogg-Spadt, S. (2003). Sexuality and sexual health: The nurse's role and initial approach to patients. *Urologic Nursing, 23,* 227-228.
2. Annon, J. (1974). *The behavioral treatment of sexual problems.* Honolulu: Enabling Systems.
3. Association of Reproductive Health Professionals. *Mature sexuality.* Available at www.arhp.org/files/MatureSexuality_sexual%20history%20taking.ppt.
4. Brooks, R.A., Etzel, M.A., Hinojos, E., et al. (2005). Preventing HIV among Latino and African American gay and bisexual men in a context of HIV-related stigma, discrimination, and homophobia: Perspectives of providers. *AIDS Patient Care and STIs, 19,* 737-744.
5. California Chlamydia Action Coalition. (2001). *A guide to sexual history taking.* Available at www.stdhivtraining.org/educ/training_module/docs/08v2-Guide-SexHist_Taking.pdf.
6. Halpern-Felsher, B.L., Cornell, J.L., Kropp, R.Y., et al. (2005). Oral versus vaginal sex among adolescents: Perceptions, attitudes, and behavior. *Pediatrics, 115,* 845-851.
7. Maslow, A.H. (1954). *Motivation and personality.* New York: Harper and Row.
8. Perlman, S.E., Postlethwaite, D., Stump, S., et al. (2001). Taking a sexual history from and counseling women on teratogenic drugs. *Journal of Reproductive Medicine, 46*(2), 163-168.
9. Rose, M.A. (2004, March). Planning HIV education programs for older adults: Cultural implications. *Journal of Gerontological Nursing,* 34-39.
10. Skelton, J.R., & Matthews, P.M. (2001). Teaching sexual history taking to health care professionals in primary care. *Medical Education, 35,* 603-608.
11. Tsai, Y. (2004). Nurses' facilitators and barriers for taking a sexual history in Taiwan. *Applied Nursing Research, 17,* 257-264.

TRANSLATING EVIDENCE INTO PRACTICE

Adolescents and Sexually Transmitted Infections—What Works for Education and Screening?

Adolescents and young adults have the highest rates of STIs in America today. One in four teens acquires an STI each year and half of all new STI cases are seen in people 15 to 24 years of age. Forty percent of all *Chlamydia* cases are seen in children age 15 to 19. The new vaccination for HPV is recommended for girls starting at age 9. Clearly adolescents are at great risk for STIs, yet they are the group of people most likely to encounter barriers to receiving accurate health information and to have access to medical services. Even when access to service exists, teens often receive substandard care. Even though screening young women for STIs is extremely cost-efficient and reduces disease incidence, a recent study found that only one third of physicians would screen adolescents known to be sexually active for STIs.

The goal of educating people about STIs is to convince them to change their behavior when it comes to risky sexual practices. This is difficult in all populations, but presents special challenges when working with adolescents. Besides being biologically more susceptible to STIs, many social and developmental influences create barriers to safe behavior in this age group. Teens use concrete reasoning and have a present-oriented and short-term view of events. An adolescent girl might not be able to conceptualize acquiring a disease that has no manifestations and that may affect her fertility in 10 to 15 years. A teen may say she is in a "long-term" relationship, when, in reality, the relationship may endure a matter of weeks. Some teens cannot complete a task requiring multiple steps (physically using a condom correctly). Egocentrism often leads teens to believe they can "tell" who has an STI and who is "safe."

Recent research shows that while teens have positive views toward using condoms, they perceive their risk of acquiring an STI to be low, especially with their "main partner," making condom use inconsistent. Adolescent women may not be able to engage in sophisticated negotiations over condom use. Teens also have different attitudes towards sex that may be somewhat based on inaccurate knowledge: in surveys large numbers of teens engage in oral sex, believing it is less risky than other sexual activities.

IMPLICATIONS

There are ways to improve STI services delivered to teens. Foremost would be increasing knowledge. Politics, religion, cultural norms, and parental views all influence traditional methods of delivering information. While school-based programs do decrease STI incidence, it would also seem prudent to increase available knowledge delivered outside of the usual formal structures. The Internet and "street medicine" initiatives are potential avenues to reach teens. Alternative health care delivery sites, such as job training programs, have been used to educate, screen, and treat teens. Newer urine tests being used in these arenas are much more acceptable testing methods for teens than cultures and should be provided whenever possible.

Teens in recent surveys focused on the negative impact having an STI would have on their social lives rather than on the serious complications that may occur. Outreach can emphasize this point while delivering accurate information about the medical consequences of specific STIs. Teaching methods must appeal to the audience and should focus on individualizing the message to specific risky behaviors and present-oriented consequences, rather than providing broad information. Teens need help dealing with peer pressure and improving their communication skills. Help the teen formulate ways of avoiding the risk and allow the teen to practice needed skills. Use terms the teen can understand. Ask concrete but open-ended questions about behaviors that do not require the teen to formulate a judgment about behavior.

However, even accurate knowledge does not guarantee a desired behavior change. Teens are struggling with establishing their own identities and competing priorities and may not see a way to translate an abstract decision into concrete action. Examining the pros and cons of a proposed change along with a sexual partner may help the adolescent make specific changes in sexual behavior.

REFERENCES

1. Banikarim, C., Chacko, M, Wiemann, C.M., & Smith, P.B. (2003). Gonorrhea and chlamydia screening among young women: Stage of change, decisional balance, and self-efficacy. *Journal of Adolescent Health, 32,* 288-295.
2. Chacko, M.R., Von Sternberg, K., & Velasquez, M.M. (2004). Gonorrhea and chlamydia screening in sexually active young women: The processes of change. *Journal of Adolescent Health, 34,* 424-427.
3. DiClement, R.J., Wingood, G.M., Crosby, R.A., et al. (2004). A descriptive analysis of STI prevalence among urban pregnant African-American teens: Data from a pilot study. *Journal of Adolescent Health, 34,* 376-383.
4. Ford, C.A., Jaccard, J., Millstein, S.G., et al. (2004). Young adults' attitudes, beliefs, and feelings about testing for curable STIs outside of clinic settings. *Journal of Adolescent Health, 34,* 266-269.
5. Halpern-Felsher, B.L., Cornell, J.L., Kropp, R.Y., & Tschann, J.M. (2005). Oral versus vaginal sex among adolescents: Perceptions, attitudes, and behavior. *Pediatrics, 115,* 845-851.
6. Hu, D., Hook, E.W., & Goldie, S.J. (2004). Screening for *Chlamydia trachomatis* in women 15-29 years of age: A cost-effectiveness analysis. *Annals of Internal Medicine, 141,* 501-513.
7. Koniak-Griffin, D., Lesser, J., Nyamathi, A., et al. (2003). Project CHARM: An HIV prevention program for adolescent mothers. *Family & Community Health, 26*(2), 94-107.
8. Moss, N.J., Gallaread, A., Siller, J., & Klausner, J.D. (2004). "Street Medicine": Collaborating with a faith-based organization to screen at-risk youths for sexually transmitted diseases. *American Journal of Public Health, 94,* 1081-1084.
9. VanDevanter, N.L., Messeri, P., Middlestadt, S.E., et al. (2005). A community-based intervention designed to increase preventive health care seeking among adolescents: The Gonorrhea Community Action Project. *American Journal of Public Health, 95,* 331-337.

guidelines, performing follow-up after treatment when indicated, and reporting confirmed cases of STIs. The CDC recommends that women recently treated for some STIs (particularly chlamydia and gonorrhea) be retested 3 months after treatment or the next time they seek care within the following 3 to 12 months. This is not for test-of-cure, but rather because women recently treated for some STIs show very high rates of subsequent infection. Clients tested for any STI should be tested for all other common STIs, including HIV/AIDS.

Examination and treatment of sex partners has been a difficult issue. Partner notification and treatment has been proven to reduce disease incidence, but the effectiveness of current methods remains unclear. Alternatives to traditional partner notification and treatment include client-delivered therapy. Medication and education are given to the index client to supply to his/her partners, who can then be treated without the inconvenience of having to see a health care provider. Evidence from three research studies shows that this method increases the likelihood of sexual partners getting effective treatment.[4,9,14] Medications or prescriptions need to be accompanied by written information. Client-delivered therapy should not be used in cases of trichomoniasis, syphilis, or with men who have sex with men. In certain areas, there are legal barriers to this practice.

Health restoration includes measures to reverse the effects of disease, such as infertility (see Chapters 38 and 39). Although some STIs can be passed nonsexually, most are transmitted sexually because the causative organisms thrive in a warm, dark, moist environment within the body and survive only very briefly outside that environment. Therefore their transmission requires intimate contact. Prevention and control must focus on breaking the chain of sexual transmission of infection.

Pathophysiology

An STI occurs when an individual is infected by an organism through sexual contact. Some STIs remain localized; others spread and become systemic. Some STIs present as an acute episode; others are chronic illnesses. See sections on specific STIs for more detailed information.

Clinical Manifestations

Clinical manifestations vary among the STIs and depend on the organism involved and the location of the infection (local or systemic). Infections may be grouped according to their primary manifestation (e.g.,

those that cause vaginal discharge). Diagnostic testing is individualized for each condition. See specific STIs for more detailed information and also refer to the Integrating Diagnostic Testing feature below.

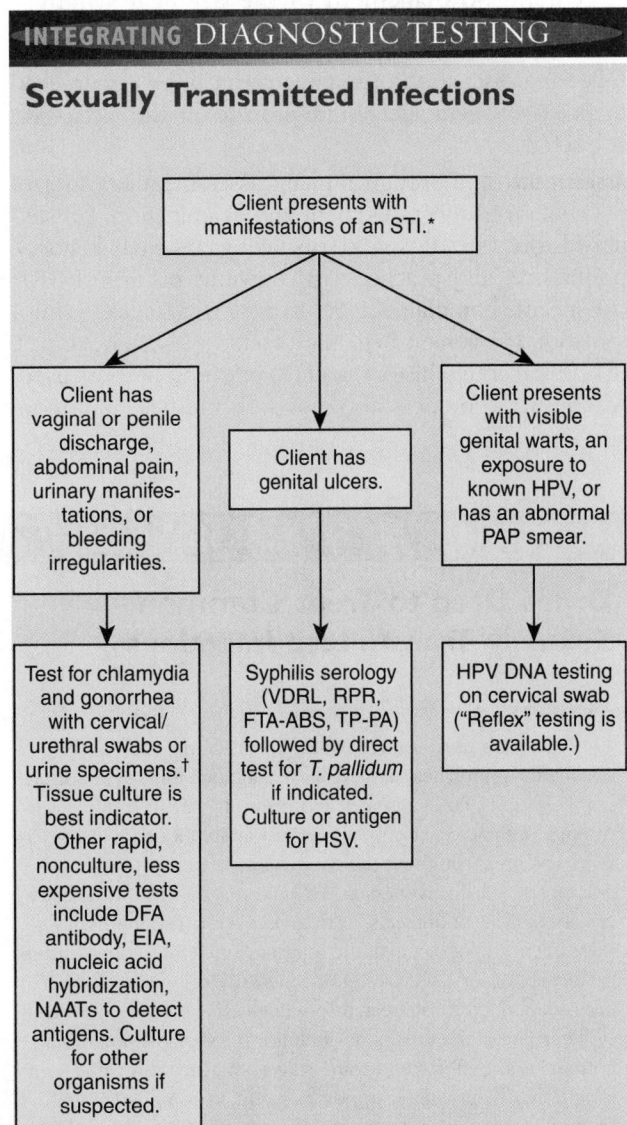

INTEGRATING DIAGNOSTIC TESTING

Sexually Transmitted Infections

Client presents with manifestations of an STI.*

Client has vaginal or penile discharge, abdominal pain, urinary manifestations, or bleeding irregularities.

Client has genital ulcers.

Client presents with visible genital warts, an exposure to known HPV, or has an abnormal PAP smear.

Test for chlamydia and gonorrhea with cervical/urethral swabs or urine specimens.† Tissue culture is best indicator. Other rapid, nonculture, less expensive tests include DFA antibody, EIA, nucleic acid hybridization, NAATs to detect antigens. Culture for other organisms if suspected.

Syphilis serology (VDRL, RPR, FTA-ABS, TP-PA) followed by direct test for *T. pallidum* if indicated. Culture or antigen for HSV.

HPV DNA testing on cervical swab ("Reflex" testing is available.)

DFA, Direct immunofluorescent antibody microscopy; *EIA*, enzyme immunoassay; *FTA-ABS*, fluorescent treponemal antibody absorption; *HPV*, human papillomavirus; *HSV*, herpes simplex virus; *NAATs*, nucleic acid amplification tests to detect *C. trachomatis* or *N. gonorrhoeae*; *RPR*, rapid plasma reagin, which uses an antigen to detect the antibody relatively specific for *T. pallidum*; *TP-PA*, *T. pallidum* particle agglutination; *VDRL*, Venereal Disease Research Laboratory.

*Clients presenting with one STI should be offered testing for other STIs and HIV. Follow CDC guidelines for screening asymptomatic women.
†Testing for chlamydia and gonorrhea should be done together.

OUTCOME MANAGEMENT

Medical Management

Medical management focuses on eradicating the offending organism, if possible, or managing a chronic condition. The Integrating Pharmacology feature below provides a concise pharmacologic overview.

Nursing Management of the Medical Client

Nursing outcomes are similar to medical outcomes. The following discussion of nursing care can be generalized to all STIs. Specific details are provided in the discussion of each STI.

Assessment. A thorough nursing assessment consists of (1) general health assessment and examination, (2) sexual history (see Box 41-1 on taking a sexual history), preference, and practices, (3) previous history of STIs, (4) specific complaints (60% to 80% of STIs are asymptomatic), (5) genital hygienic practices (i.e., douching), (6) contraceptive history, and (7) infection barriers used. A holistic approach also assesses lifestyle, nutrition, stress, and sexuality. High-risk clients should be screened for STIs regardless of whether manifestations are present at the time of a visit to a health care provider. Never assume that a client is not sexually active and make sure that the client understands questions exactly.

Nurses need to know about the variety of sexual activities, their effect on transmission of STIs, and the common manifestations for which to assess. Separate personal views of morality from appropriate nursing activities. Judgmental attitudes may deter clients from seeking care and may interfere with therapeutic relationships. Bias and prejudice can be communicated in obvious and subtle ways that make the client feel uncomfortable, judged, and discounted. A prejudiced health professional cannot provide comprehensive care. An accepting attitude may ensure treatment and prevent infection transmission.

STIs are associated with a social stigma. Ashamed, many clients try to keep the diagnosis secret or may refuse to seek care. Many relate STIs with low social status and immorality, and many have misconceptions and fears about the dangers of STIs. Other problems may surface with discovery of an STI. For example, a newly

INTEGRATING PHARMACOLOGY

Drugs Used to Treat Common Sexually Transmitted Infections

ANTIBIOTICS

Antibiotics are used for STIs caused by bacteria, such as chlamydia, gonorrhea, and syphilis. Antibiotic therapy eradicates manifestations, cures disease, and prevents spread of infection through antimicrobial properties. Oral antibiotics should be taken evenly throughout the day. Doxycycline may lessen contraceptive effectiveness and should not be taken with dairy products, iron, or antacids. Ceftriaxone is reconstituted with lidocaine to reduce pain at the injection site. Quinolone-resistant gonorrhea occurs; see CDC guidelines. Clients treated for gonorrhea need to be treated for chlamydia also and vice versa.

Penicillin is the treatment of choice for syphilis. Some oral antibiotics are effective in some stages, but they must be taken long term. Clients need support to maintain compliance with therapy. Treatment in latent syphilis is primarily directed toward preventing or slowing complications. Transmission is not affected. Antibiotic treatment of bacterial vaginosis alleviates irritating vaginal manifestations and cures infection. Clients should avoid alcohol during oral therapy and for 24 hours afterward.

Chancroid is treated with either oral azithromycin or an injection of ceftriaxone. Granuloma inguinale is treated with oral doxycycline, and another bacterial infection, bacterial vaginosis, is treated with metronidazole.

ANTIVIRAL AGENTS

Antiviral therapy is used for human papillomavirus (HPV) infection and for herpes. The main goal of therapy in HPV infection is to remove symptomatic warts. Each topical drug has specific directions regarding frequency of application, duration of treatment, and adjunct skin care. Topical ointments should be applied wearing a glove.

Podofilox/podophyllin prevents cell division. Imiquimod is an immune-enhancer that stimulates local immune response. Cryotherapy causes cell lysis. Acid application causes protein coagulation and wart destruction. Interferons inhibit viral replication and may have an immunostimulating effect. Systemic interferons have no effect, but can be injected directly into the wart.

Antiviral therapy used in herpes offers partial control and more rapid resolution of manifestations in acute episodes and provides suppressive therapy for clients who suffer frequent recurrences. All drugs interfere with viral replication. Treatment for recurrent episodes should begin with the prodromal phase. No drug is curative. Commonly used drugs for herpes include acyclovir, famciclovir, and valacyclovir. The new once-daily regimen should improve compliance and quality of life.

ANTIPROTOZOAN THERAPY

Treatment for trichomoniasis with oral metronidazole relieves manifestations, cures infection, and halts transmission. Topical metronidazole does not reach therapeutic levels for treatment for this condition, so it is given orally.

 Modified from the *2006 Sexually Transmitted Diseases Treatment Guidelines* with further information from *Mosby's Nursing Drug Reference.*

infected client may be angry with the presumed responsible sexual partner or may hesitate to identify or inform the sexual partner or partners about the STI. When a marital or committed relationship is involved, questions about infidelity or infertility may arise.

Clients can seek treatment from various sources: health department STI clinics, physician offices, emergency departments, Planned Parenthood clinics, and other community-based clinics. All points of service must be prepared to deal with STIs and have staff sensitive to the needs of these clients. Strict confidentiality is essential. It is especially, but not exclusively, important to homosexual men and lesbians, who may be at risk for discrimination if their sexual orientation is disclosed.

Diagnosis, Outcomes, Interventions

Diagnosis: Ineffective Health Maintenance. The client with an STI needs to improve health behaviors, which makes *Ineffective Health Maintenance related to lack of understanding of the causes, treatments, and prevention of STIs* the priority nursing diagnosis.

Outcomes. The client will understand the cause, treatment, and prevention of specific STIs, as evidenced by client's statements, the client's avoidance of STIs, successful treatment of an STI, and, if possible, the absence of recurrence of the STI.

Interventions

Teach About STIs. Provide accurate, specific, factual information about the transmission, prevention, and treatment of STIs in terms the client can understand (see the Client Education Guide on Sexually Transmitted Infections on the website). Clarify any misinformation the client has about STIs; for example, many people erroneously believe that oral contraceptives protect them against STIs and do not use condoms in conjunction with their contraceptives. Often women who have been surgically sterilized, who have IUDs, or who are postmenopausal (and who do not need birth control) fail to consider condom use for disease protection. Teaching methods should consider religious and cultural concerns. (See the Bridge to Home Health Care website feature Teaching About Sexually Transmitted Infections for information on teaching clients about STIs in a sensitive manner.) The Community-Based Practice box on p. 980 suggests ways nurses can educate clients about STI prevention and treatment in the community. Include the following topics in teaching sessions about specific STIs:

1. Name, nature, and seriousness of the condition
2. Mode of transmission
   a. Any sexual activity can spread STIs, not just penile-vaginal contact.
   b. High-risk activities include certain sexual acts and/or sexual relations with new or multiple partners.
3. Actions the client should take to prevent the spread of infection to others
   a. Clients should always use a new condom for each sexual act (male and female condoms are available).
   b. Clients should finish all prescribed medications.
   c. Sexual partners should be evaluated and treated if needed.
   d. Clients should refrain from sexual actions until both partners have been treated.
   e. Clients should refrain from sexual relations if either partner has any manifestations of an STI.
4. Incubation periods
5. Manifestations of infection
6. Asymptomatic problems
7. When and how to seek treatment. Be sure the client understands the difference between Papanicolaou (Pap) smears and STI examinations; both are not always done at the same time. (Most people seeking treatment or screening for STIs assume the Pap smear and testing for all infections is being done. A client seeking a Pap smear may believe that STI screening is being done at the same time. Explain to clients if this is not the case.)
8. Treatment methods. Teach clients about medication or other treatments.
9. Follow-up care (when and how to obtain it)
10. Consequences of not completing treatment
    a. Infertility
    b. Chronic abdominal pain
    c. Higher risk of ectopic pregnancy or spontaneous abortion
11. Risks and consequences of recurrent infections, for example, STIs increase the risk of acquiring HIV infection

Teach Condom Use. Promote the use of a new condom for every act of penetrating sexual activity. The latex condom (called a *rubber* in lay terms) is the most effective mechanical barrier to STIs, and its use by sexually active people who are at risk should be promoted. Sexually active men and women should learn to use condoms properly, effectively, and consistently. Condom failure is primarily a result of improper or inconsistent use rather than product defect. Visit the website of the American Social Health Association for information on proper use of both male and female condoms at www.ashastd.org.

There are several barriers to using condoms. Women may not believe they are empowered to make healthy choices. Condoms require male cooperation, and many women are in relationships defined by an imbalance of power in which they cannot insist on condom use. Some studies have shown that the fear of losing a sexual partner is greater for some women than the fear of contracting an STI, even AIDS. Older people may

COMMUNITY-BASED PRACTICE

Sexually Transmitted Infections and HIV/AIDS

Bringing nursing care to nontraditional community settings is a particularly relevant activity for impacting the health and well-being of people who have, or who are at risk for, sexually transmitted infections (STIs) and HIV/AIDS. Some of the people most at risk for STIs and HIV/AIDS are the least likely to have access to appropriate health care or to use it if available. Providing education, screening, counseling, and even treatment for positive results at alternative delivery sites can decrease the incidence of these infections and improve health outcomes.

Several health initiatives, including *Project CHARM* for pregnant and childbearing adolescents and *Check Out That Body* for adolescents and young adults, have partnered with community organizations such as schools, after-school programs, and job training sites to provide comprehensive health care for targeted populations. However, even well-designed and implemented programs often fail to lead participants to increased screening and health care seeking activities, so the impetus now is to find less structured sites for spontaneous interventions that do not rely on pre-planning. Using sites where the population of interest is likely to be found can increase the numbers of people who take advantage of the services being offered.

Many alternative health care sites may not be appropriate for activities related to STIs and HIV/AIDS. While supermarkets and malls may be attractive sites for blood pressure screening or for flu shots, the sensitive nature of these infections may make finding locations more difficult. Literally taking health care to the streets can provide an avenue for reaching at-risk individuals. An excellent example of this can be seen in the recent initiative by the San Francisco Department of Public Health (SFDPH).

Partnering with a local faith-based organization (the Providence Foundation, associated with the Providence Baptist Church), the SFDPH sent staff into the community to recruit adolescents to educational and screening activities held in various locations such as a barber college, some local restaurants, the YMCA, and after-school and employment programs. The staff was careful to divide the geographic areas so that members of rival gangs could be included. At the sessions, staff provided education and participants could participate in urine screening. For positive results, the staff contacted the individuals, treated them, and gave them treatment packs for their partners. There were also rallies at the church parking lot complete with education, screening, and food and entertainment. The adolescents were encouraged to bring their partners to any of these events. Four percent (4%) of adolescents screened had positive test results for STIs and were treated.

This program is an excellent example of creative, community-based thinking. Using workers from the local community and providing services free of the bias health care workers sometimes have toward people with STIs were important components of the program. Partnering with a respected local organization (a church), respecting cultural influences (gang affiliations), and providing convenient testing and treatment ensured the success of this outreach activity.

REFERENCES

1. Koniak-Griffin, D., Lesser, J., Nyamathi, A., et al. (2003). Project CHARM: An HIV prevention program for adolescent mothers. *Family and Community Health, 26*(2), 94-107.
2. Moss, N.J., Gallaread, A., Siller, J., et al. (2004). "Street Medicine": Collaborating with a faith-based organization to screen at-risk youths for sexually transmitted diseases. *American Journal of Public Health, 94*, 1081-1084.
3. Sieverding, J., Boyer, C.B., Siller, J., et al. (2005). Youth united through health education: Building capacity through a community collaborative intervention to prevent HIV/STI in adolescents residing in a high STI prevalent neighborhood. *AIDS Education and Prevention, 17*, 375-385.
4. VanDevanter, N.L., Messeri, P., Middlestadt, S.E., et al. (2005). A community-based intervention designed to increase preventive health care seeking among adolescents: The gonorrhea community action project. *American Journal of Public Health, 95*, 331-338.

not have experience with condoms. Condoms may not be acceptable to some clients for religious, cultural, or ethnic reasons. Tips on negotiating condom use with sexual partners can also be found at www.ashastd.org.

Use Therapeutic Communication. When caring for clients with STIs, nurses obtain privileged or private information and provide instruction about these diseases. Both activities require sensitivity and skillful interaction. The successful nurse needs to be adept in interpersonal communication. Such clients need encouragement, support, and accurate information.

Identify Resources. Nurses play a pivotal role in identifying community and national resources available to clients. Most public health agencies have STI education, prevention, and treatment programs that are open to the public. Clients can also obtain information anonymously from the National STI Hotline (1-800-227-8922) or the National HIV/AIDS Hotline (1-800-342-AIDS), or at www.ashastd.org.

Diagnosis: Anxiety. The client with an STI often experiences a great deal of uncertainty, which makes *Anxiety related to threat to biologic integrity and threat to self-concept* an important nursing diagnosis.

Outcomes. The client will experience a decrease in anxiety, as evidenced by verbal statements, showing acceptance of the condition, and demonstrating appropriate coping methods.

Interventions

Provide Support. STIs can threaten a client's self-concept and pose potential physical problems, such as infertility and fetal damage. The client may express guilt, apprehension, and fear of rejection. Help the client reduce anxiety by being warm and supportive, facilitating the expression of feelings, and encouraging effective coping strategies.

Help with Problem-Solving. Assist the client with learning and problem-solving once anxiety is reduced. Role-playing and practicing negotiation skills may help the client become more assertive in being able to ensure sexual health.

Other Diagnoses. *Risk for Situational Low Self-Esteem, Acute Pain, Impaired Tissue Integrity,* and *Risk for Ineffective Therapeutic Regimen Management* are other diagnoses to consider.

Evaluation. It is expected that the STI will be successfully treated and, if possible, eradicated. The client will be able to state the cause, manifestations, treatment, and prevention of STIs and will remain free of STIs.

INFECTIONS CHARACTERIZED BY URETHRITIS OR CERVICITIS

CHLAMYDIAL INFECTIONS

Chlamydia is the nation's most common bacterial STI. In 2004 the number of *reported* new cases was nearly 930,000.

Etiology and Risk Factors

The causative organism, *Chlamydia trachomatis,* is a nonmotile, gram-negative bacterium. This organism is the most common cause of what was previously diagnosed as nonspecific vaginitis in women and as nongonococcal urethritis (NGU) in men.

C. trachomatis is transmitted by intimate sexual contact. Women usually acquire the infection during vaginal intercourse with an infected man, but it can also be transmitted through oral-anal contact, anal penetration, or oral sex. The infection does not cross the placenta, but passage through the birth canal of an infected mother can cause conjunctivitis and pneumonia in a newborn. The incubation period is 7 to 21 days.

Pathophysiology

Chlamydial infection is known as "the great sterilizer" and is considered the most important cause of pelvic inflammatory disease (PID) and tubal infertility. Undetected and untreated cases can have serious, irreversible consequences. *C. trachomatis* causes inflammation that leads to scarring and ulceration of involved tissue. In women, the infection can extend to the endometrium and salpinx (fallopian tube); the major consequence is salpingitis (inflammation of the fallopian tubes) with subsequent infertility or high risk of ectopic (tubal) pregnancy. Secondary extension to the peritoneum can cause PID (see Chapter 39). In men, the infection can cause a urethral stricture that may extend to the *epididymis.* Sterility can result from the ensuing epididymitis (see Chapter 38). A serious systemic complication more common in men is Reiter syndrome, which consists of urethritis, polyarthritis, and conjunctivitis.

Clinical Manifestations

Chlamydial infections primarily affect the cervix, urethra, and rectum. In most cases, the infection is asymptomatic for an extended period. In women, the primary site of infection is the endocervix. The cervix becomes edematous and produces a yellow, mucopurulent vaginal discharge. This discharge may be accompanied by spotting at menstrual midcycle or with sexual intercourse. *C. trachomatis* also causes urethritis with dysuria (painful or difficult urination) and urinary frequency in women. Often these clinical manifestations lead to an inaccurate diagnosis and treatment for urinary tract infection. Involvement of Bartholin's duct produces a purulent discharge.

In males, the chief manifestation is urethritis with dysuria (painful and difficult urination) and clear to mucopurulent discharge. In both sexes, proctitis (rectal inflammation) and pharyngitis (inflammation of the pharynx) may develop with rectal and orogenital contact.

Because chlamydia may produce few or no manifestations (especially in women), clients often do not seek medical treatment and the diagnosis is difficult and often missed. Because chlamydial and gonorrheal infections frequently coexist, diagnostic tests and treatment are recommended for both when either condition is suspected. Presumptive treatment for chlamydia in clients being treated for gonorrhea is appropriate and cost-effective, particularly when testing for *C. trachomatis* is not performed.

The definitive test for the fast and accurate diagnosis of chlamydial infection has yet to be developed. The best and most sensitive diagnostic test is tissue culture of cellular material from the urethra, endocervix, or rectum. This test, however, is expensive and technically difficult. Rapid nonculture detection tests performed on urogenital secretions are readily available. See the Integrating Diagnostic Testing: STIs feature. These tests are more convenient, less expensive, and quicker than the standard culture. Nucleic acid amplification tests (NAATs) to detect *C. trachomatis* antigens are the most sensitive tests for *C. trachomatis* in endocervical and urethral specimens and have been FDA-cleared for use in urine samples. Many clients find urine testing more acceptable than endocervical or urethral swabbing. Screening is recommended for all asymptomatic, high-risk clients in whom chlamydia might be present. Priority groups for testing are (1) high-risk pregnant women,

(2) adolescents, and (3) women age 20 to 24 years who have new or multiple sexual partners or who do not use condoms routinely. Many sources also recommend testing any woman with a history of infertility, ectopic pregnancies, or spontaneous abortions.

OUTCOME MANAGEMENT

Medical Management

Eradicate Infection and Manifestations

The treatment of choice for chlamydial infection is doxycycline (Vibramycin) given orally for 7 days or one dose of azithromycin (Zithromax). To prevent complications, it is imperative that treatment be aggressive and started when the infection is suspected (before test results are back), and that the entire course of antibiotics be completed. Antibiotics are almost always effective; therefore test of cure is not necessary unless manifestations persist or recur. If testing is not done, treatment is prescribed on the basis of clinical diagnosis only or as co-treatment for gonorrhea. All sexual partners within the last 60 days should be examined and treated. When the client's last sexual contact occurred more than 60 days before diagnosis, the last partner should be treated. The CDC recommends that medications be dispensed on-site and that the first dose be directly observed to improve compliance. This is especially important for the single-dose regimen as clients may not be willing to take the time to fill a prescription for only one pill.

Nursing Management of the Medical Client

Eradicate Infection and Manifestations

Instruct clients about the greater risk of infection with multiple sexual partners and inform them of the serious danger of sterility, particularly for women. Also emphasize that this infection may have a long latency period. Infected clients should scrupulously avoid all sexual activity until both partners are cured, and they should use condoms thereafter.

GONORRHEA

Gonorrhea (also known as *clap, white, drips, strain,* and *dose* in lay terms) can be divided into two categories: local and disseminated. *Local infection* can involve the mucosal surfaces of the cervix, urethra, and rectum; vestibular glands; pharynx; or conjunctiva. *Systemic infection (disseminated gonococcal infection)* involves bacteremia with polyarthritis, dermatitis, endocarditis, and meningitis. Systemic infection is more common in women.

Etiology and Risk Factors

Gonorrhea is one of the most prevalent STIs in the United States with over 330,000 cases reported yearly. Some studies show that gonorrhea may be grossly underreported. Teenagers and young adults are at highest risk. Most cases of gonorrhea occur in people age 15 to 29 years, with the highest rate in those age 20 to 24 years.

Pathophysiology

Gonorrhea is caused by the gram-negative diplococcus *Neisseria gonorrhoeae.* The causative organism is highly contagious, but does not survive long outside the body. Gonorrhea, therefore, is almost always transmitted by direct sexual contact. The few rare exceptions are infection in infants, who can contract gonorrhea during vaginal birth, and infection of medical personnel through broken skin. The incubation period is 3 to 8 days.

Clinical Manifestations

The endocervical canal is the primary site of gonorrheal infection in women. In most women, the urethra is also infected. Infection can also involve the vestibular glands and anus. The vagina is highly vulnerable to the infection before puberty. The infection may be asymptomatic in women. There is a large *carrier population* (people who carry the organism and have no manifestations but can transmit the infection) for gonorrhea. Manifestations of gonorrhea include (1) heavy, yellow-green, purulent vaginal discharge, (2) cervical erythema, (3) a red, swollen, sore vulva, (4) abnormal menstrual bleeding, and (5) dysuria and urinary frequency.

The most common complication of gonorrhea in women is salpingitis, which can progress to PID. Both PID and salpingitis can produce infertility secondary to scarring and occlusion of the fallopian tubes. The first recognizable manifestations of gonorrhea in women may arise from PID.

Manifestations of gonorrhea are usually evident earlier in men than in women. The infection is principally one of the anterior urethra that produces a purulent discharge, dysuria, and urinary frequency. Complications include epididymitis and prostatitis, but these are not common with early and complete antibiotic therapy. In addition to the gender-specific manifestations, both men and women may have conjunctivitis or pharyngitis because of orogenital contact or proctitis from anal contact.

Disseminated infection results from gonococcal bacteremia and is often manifested by septic arthritis, skin lesions, asymmetrical arthralgias, and tenosynovitis (inflammation of the tendon and synovial membrane). Rarely, hepatic adhesions (Fitz-Hugh–Curtis syndrome), endocarditis, or meningitis occurs.

Diagnosis of gonorrhea can be made through history, physical examination, identification of the gonococcus on a smear, or culture of the exudate from infected areas. Culture remains the test of choice for non-genital specimens. See the Integrating Diagnostic Testing: STIs feature. NAAT is FDA approved for all secretions, including urine, which may increase client willingness to be tested and/or screened.

OUTCOME MANAGEMENT

Medical Management

Eradicate Infection and Manifestations
All sexually active men and women in high-risk groups should be screened for gonorrhea on a regular basis. All clients in whom gonorrhea is detected should also be tested for chlamydial infection.

Gonorrhea is treated aggressively with antibiotics, without waiting for test results, on the basis of clinical manifestations. Before the advent of resistant organisms, penicillin was the treatment of choice. The current recommended regimen for uncomplicated gonorrhea is a single intramuscular (IM) dose of ceftriaxone (Rocephin), or a single oral dose of cefixime (Suprax), ciprofloxacin (Cipro), ofloxacin (Floxin), or levofloxacin (Levaquin). Quinolone antibiotics should not be used to treat gonorrhea in men who have sex with men, or in geographic areas where quinolone-resistant infections are found. They should also not be used in infections acquired abroad. The CDC and state health departments maintain current information about quinolone-resistant gonorrhea. Before using these antibiotics, check with local authorities or the CDC website www.cdc.gov/std/gisp.

A single IM injection of spectinomycin (Trobicin) can be used for clients who cannot tolerate ceftriaxone. All clients treated for gonorrhea need to be treated concurrently for chlamydial infection (see the Integrating Pharmacology feature on Drugs Used to Treat Common Sexually Transmitted Infections on p. 978).

For clients with disseminated gonococcal infection, the recommended regimen is administration of ceftriaxone, given IM or IV every 24 hours and continued 24 to 48 hours after improvement begins, followed by cefixime or ciprofloxacin, given orally for a full week. There are alternative regimens available with quinolones.

After therapy for uncomplicated gonorrhea is completed, a follow-up examination and culture are not necessary because treatment failure is rare. Recurring or unresolved cases should be evaluated with a follow-up culture. Any gonococcal organisms on the second culture should be tested for antibiotic sensitivity and possible resistant organisms. As with chlamydia, health care providers are encouraged to re-test clients recently treated for gonorrhea, as reinfection is common. Screening should be done after 3 months, or the next time the client seeks care within 12 months after treatment.

Nursing Management of the Medical Client

Eradicate Infection and Manifestations
Discuss the importance of identifying and treating all sexual partners, because there seems to be a reservoir population of asymptomatic men. Recurrence due to reinfection may indicate the need for improved client education and sexual partner referral. Investigation of the client's sexual contacts is essential for the prevention and control of gonorrhea. All sexual partners within the 60 days before diagnosis (or the last contact if greater than 60 days) should undergo examination, testing, and treatment. Reporting sexual contacts can be difficult and frightening for an infected client. Ask for contact information in a positive, nonthreatening way.

Warn pregnant clients of the danger of infecting their newborns during delivery. Clients receiving treatment for gonorrhea must understand the importance of taking the *complete* course of prescribed medication.

INFECTIONS CHARACTERIZED BY ULCERATIONS

SYPHILIS

Syphilis (lay terms are *bad blood, lues, pox,* and *syph*) is a systemic, highly infectious STI. Unlike the other STIs, it is always a systemic disease. It became less prevalent after the advent of penicillin, but the infection has not been eradicated. The incidence of syphilis peaked in the early 1990s and declined for a few years. In 1997, 75% of all U.S. counties reported no new cases, which has led the CDC to call for its complete eradication. However, the incidence is now increasing in many areas; this is worrisome because syphilis is often a "herald" disease for HIV infection. In 2002 there were more than 32,000 new cases reported, half of which are in 16 counties and 1 city in the United States. Much of this increase has been seen in men who have sex with men (MSM).

Etiology and Risk Factors
Syphilis is caused by the delicate motile (self-moving) spirochete *Treponema pallidum*. Although *T. pallidum* cannot survive long outside the body, it is highly infectious. Sexual transmission of *T. pallidum* occurs only when the mucocutaneous lesions of primary and secondary syphilis are present. Adolescents, young adults, and MSM are at greatest risk. Syphilis is a known cofactor for development of HIV infection.

Pathophysiology

T. pallidum enters the body through intact mucous membranes or abraded skin, almost exclusively by direct sexual contact. After entry, the organisms multiply locally and disseminate systemically through the bloodstream and lymphatics. The infection can also be passed transplacentally from an untreated pregnant woman to her fetus during any stage of the disease *(congenital syphilis)*.

In rare instances, syphilis has been contracted through nonsexual personal contact, accidental inoculation, or blood transfusion from a syphilitic donor. Syphilis can progress to irreversible blindness, mental illness, paralysis, heart disease, and death without treatment.

Clinical Manifestations

Syphilis is characterized by well-defined sequential stages that occur over years: primary, secondary, latent (early latent and late latent), and tertiary.

Primary Stage

The principal manifestation of primary syphilis is the appearance of a genital chancre. A *chancre* is an oval ulcer with a raised firm border that does not bleed readily and is painless unless infected (Figure 41-1). The chancre develops at the site of inoculation, usually the genitalia, anus, or mouth. Most commonly, a single chancre occurs about 4 weeks after initial infection. Chancres in women often remain unnoticed.

Lymphadenopathy may occur as lymph glands near the chancre become enlarged. Nodes are painless, firm, and discrete. If untreated, a chancre heals spontaneously in 4 to 6 weeks, leaving a thin, atrophic scar.

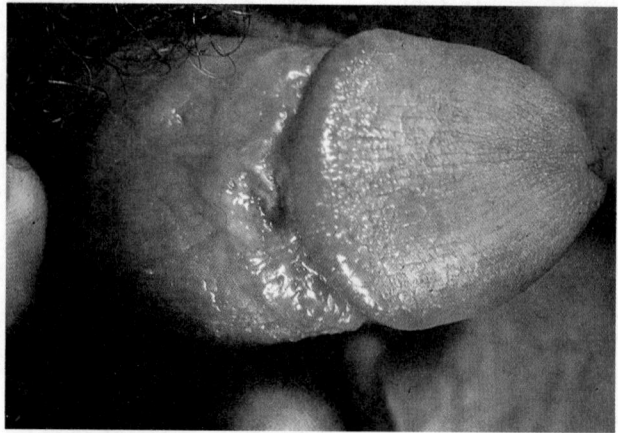

■ **FIGURE 41–1** Ulcer of primary syphilis. *(Courtesy Dr. Rodney M.S. Basler.)*

Secondary Stage

If the primary infection is untreated, secondary syphilis develops 6 to 8 weeks after infection. The following are indications of the second stage:

1. *Generalized rash.* Typically, a maculopapular and nonpruritic rash appears; the rash can be anywhere but often appears on the palms of the hands and soles of the feet (few other diseases cause a rash in these locations); the rash is highly infectious.
2. *Generalized, nontender, discrete lymphadenopathy.*
3. *Mucous patches.* Gray, superficial patches occur on the mucous membranes in the mouth and may be accompanied by a sore throat.
4. *Condylomata lata.* Broad-based, flat papules usually can be easily distinguished from the typical narrow-based, pedunculated growth of condylomata acuminata (genital warts). Condylomata lata may develop in warm, moist body areas—most commonly on the labia or anus or at the corners of the mouth. They are highly contagious.
5. *General flu-like manifestations,* including nausea, anorexia, constipation, headache, a chronically elevated temperature, and muscle, joint, and bone pain.
6. *Patchy hair loss* from eyebrows and scalp (alopecia).

Secondary stage manifestations usually disappear after 2 to 6 weeks. A latency period then begins.

Latent Stage

Latent syphilis is defined as that period after infection with *T. pallidum* when a client is seroreactive (with a positive blood test) but shows no other evidence of disease. During this stage, syphilis is noninfectious except via transplacental spread or blood transfusion. Syphilis is not transmitted by sexual contact during the latent phase unless a secondary syphilitic mucocutaneous skin lesion reoccurs during early latent syphilis. Latent syphilis acquired during the previous 12 months is called "early latent syphilis." All other cases are considered "late latent" or "latent of unknown duration." About 66% of those infected remain in this stage without further problems.

Tertiary Stage

In 1 to 35 years after the primary infection, about 33% of clients with untreated syphilis experience devastating, irreversible complications, such as chronic bone and joint inflammation, cardiovascular problems (for example, valvular involvement, aneurysms), granulomatous lesions *(gummas)* on any part of the body, and ophthalmic, auditory, and central nervous system problems. This stage, although not infectious, may be terminal if untreated (see Chapter 71 for manifestations of neurosyphilis [syphilis affecting the central nervous system]).

Diagnosis

The diagnosis of syphilis is based on health assessment and various direct and indirect laboratory studies. A *direct test* identifies the causative organism; an *indirect test* identifies antibodies of the causative agent. *T. pallidum* cannot be grown in culture. Primary or secondary stage lesions can be scraped and the causative organism identified directly with dark-field microscopy (DFA) testing. Dark-field examination must be done by an expert, because other spirochetes closely resembling *T. pallidum* are present in oral and genital mucosa. This test confirms a diagnosis of syphilis in the primary stage (when other tests are generally negative) and the secondary stage.

Serologic tests for syphilis are indirect tests that detect antibodies. These antibodies are not present in the serum until 4 weeks *after* the appearance of the chancre. See the Integrating Diagnostic Testing: STIs feature.

The Venereal Disease Research Laboratory (VDRL) test for nonspecific antibodies is the most commonly used screening test. The fluorescent treponemal antibody absorption (FTA-ABS) serologic test is more specific because it measures antibodies specific to *T. pallidum*. It is used when the VDRL result is positive but the diagnosis of syphilis is still uncertain. The FTA-ABS test result usually becomes positive 3 to 4 weeks after infection. Once positive, FTA-ABS test results usually remain positive for the client's life, regardless of treatment or cure. Cerebrospinal fluid may be examined for characteristic findings in late neurosyphilis.

Syphilis often coexists with other infections. The CDC recommends that all clients with syphilis be counseled on the risks of HIV infection and encouraged to undergo HIV testing, plus screening for other common STIs.

OUTCOME MANAGEMENT

Medical Management

Eradicate Infection and Manifestations

Parenteral penicillin remains the treatment of choice for all stages of syphilis; however, the structural changes present in late syphilis are irreversible despite successful treatment. The dosage schedule and length of therapy are determined by the stage of the infection and current guidelines for treatment. For primary, secondary, and early latent syphilis, the treatment of choice is benzathine penicillin G, given IM in one dose. Late latent syphilis (or latent of unknown duration) and tertiary syphilis are treated with three weekly penicillin injections. Neurosyphilis is treated with IV aqueous crystalline penicillin G. Health care providers should be vigilant about using the correct preparation of penicillin as Bicillin C-R (benzathine-procaine penicillin) is a common product and has been used inappropriately to treat syphilis.

Use of penicillin to treat syphilis in clients with penicillin allergy is a complicated issue. Clients who are pregnant or noncompliant with therapy or who have neurosyphilis should undergo desensitization and treatment with penicillin. Desensitization guidelines are available from the CDC. For nonpregnant clients who are allergic to penicillin, doxycycline or tetracycline may be given, but they are not as effective as penicillin and require a much longer treatment time, potentially affecting compliance.

Treatment failure can occur with any given regimen. Compliance is often a problem. Clients should be reexamined clinically and evaluated with serologic testing at 6, 12, and 24 months after treatment. No definitive criteria for cure exist. With successful treatment, ideally, no evidence of infection should be present and serial serologic test values should decline.

Treating sexual partners is also a complex issue; treatment is best guided by information available from the CDC. All people who have had sexual contact with the client who has primary syphilis must be identified and evaluated. Most practitioners treat sexual contacts as if they have primary syphilis whether or not they show evidence of infection.

Nursing Management of the Medical Client

Eradicate Infection and Manifestations

A client with syphilis needs information and psychosocial support to deal with this complex illness. Individualize health teaching to meet the client's particular needs and psychosocial situation. A diagnosis of syphilis can be frightening and difficult to accept.

Clients with primary or secondary syphilis should abstain from sexual contact for at least 1 month after treatment. Adequate treatment should be curative, but reinfection is possible and can be detected with clinical examinations and monitoring of serologic test values. Proper follow-up, although essential, is time-consuming and difficult. Many clients do not understand the severe consequences of not obtaining adequate treatment.

GENITAL HERPES

Genital herpes is a chronic, systemic viral infection. Although recognized for centuries, genital herpes has received renewed attention because of its epidemic incidence. Now one of the most common STIs (at least 50 million cases in the United States), it is the most frequent cause of genital ulceration. Its peak incidence is among adolescents and young adults.

Etiology and Risk Factors

Caused by herpes simplex virus (HSV) type 2, the infection is closely related to other herpes infections, such as the classic cold sore caused by HSV type 1. HSV type 1 infection is mainly nongenital, occurring above the waist (often on the lips or nose). HSV type 2 infection occurs primarily below the waist as a sexually transmitted genital infection. It is possible for HSV type 1 to cause genital infections and for HSV type 2 to cause oral lesions (Figure 41-2).

Pathophysiology

The HSV organism is present in the exudate of the lesion. Herpes can be transmitted while a lesion is present and for 10 days after a lesion has healed. Genital herpes is usually transmitted by direct contact with the exudate during sexual activity, but transmission is possible by *fomites* (objects that can harbor pathogenic microorganisms), such as towels used by an infected person. Many cases of genital herpes are acquired from people who do not know they have an infection or who are asymptomatic at the time of sexual contact. Newborns can be infected during vaginal delivery when active genital lesions are present. Cesarean section prevents this transmission.

Clinical Manifestations

Many people with HSV type 2 infection have mild or unrecognized disease. Manifestations of genital herpes usually occur 3 to 7 days after contact. Initially, a burning sensation (paresthesia) is noted at the site of inoculation. Next, numerous small vesicles with an erythematous border form painful, shallow ulcers that then crust and heal with a scar in about 2 to 4 weeks.

The major problem with HSV is recurrence. Up to 75% of clients have a recurrent infection within 1 year of the first episode. The virus is believed to lie dormant in the body, probably in nerve ganglions, until it is activated, at which point another episode of genital herpes, with

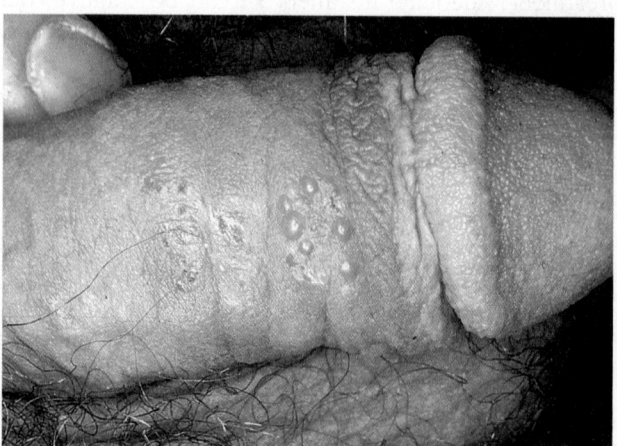

■ **FIGURE 41–2** Typical herpes vesicles. *(Courtesy Dr. Rodney M.S. Basler.)*

characteristic lesions, occurs. Stress, infection, trauma, menses, or sexual activity may trigger recurrent episodes.

Characteristically, recurrent genital herpes causes only local manifestations. Prodromal (pre-onset) manifestations of a burning sensation may occur before the vesicles erupt. The vesicles tend to reappear at the sites of previous infection, but they can involve new sites. Manifestations are similar to, but usually less severe than, those in the primary infection. Vesicles rupture in 24 to 48 hours, and the syndrome generally lasts 7 to 10 days.

Potential complications of HSV infections include disseminated infections, meningitis, and transverse myelitis. Women are at risk for spontaneous abortion, and it has been suggested that HSV type 2 predisposes to carcinoma of the cervix.

A diagnosis of genital herpes is often made visually. The diagnosis is confirmed by a viral culture, direct immunofluorescence staining, or antigen detection testing of the vesicular exudate. A Pap smear can also be performed; the presence of multinucleated giant cells in the Pap smear, with or without inclusion bodies, is characteristic of a herpes infection.

OUTCOME MANAGEMENT

Medical Management

Reduce Manifestations

Genital herpes is a chronic disease without a cure. Treatment does not cure HSV infection or prevent its spread. Management focuses on preventing or lessening occurrences and giving palliative care. The recommended treatment for an acute primary infection is acyclovir (Zovirax), famciclovir (Famvir), or valacyclovir (Valtrex) taken orally for 7 to 10 days. Famciclovir has recently been approved by the FDA for a single-day treatment regimen. The same antiviral medications can be used for 5 days to treat recurrent outbreaks.

Clients with frequent recurrences (six or more episodes in 1 year) take daily suppressive therapy. Daily acyclovir taken for 4 months to 3 years may prevent or reduce the frequency and severity of recurrence in most people. Clients should begin oral suppressive therapy when they first recognize the prodromal sensations or first become symptomatic. The need for daily suppressive therapy should be reevaluated after 1 year. Severe disease is treated with IV acyclovir.

Nursing Management of the Medical Client

Prevent Reinfection

When the vesicles of herpes rupture, they release a highly contagious exudate. Clients and health care providers should wash their hands thoroughly after any contact with the herpetic lesions to avoid further spread. HSV infections of the eye are particularly serious.

Infected clients should have separate towels and other personal items and avoid touching their eyes. Clients should avoid sexual contact when vesicles are present and use condoms during latent periods because the possible risk of transmission exists even when lesions are not present. Women should have annual pelvic examinations and Pap smears.

Provide Support

Coping with genital herpes may cause tremendous psychosocial stress. Although recurrence cannot always be predicted, nurses can help clients identify possible triggers. Reappearance of the infection can significantly affect sexual activity. Support groups may help clients deal with the anger, guilt, and shame that many commonly feel. Stress reduction techniques may be helpful. Sexual partners should be offered counseling, evaluation, and treatment if needed.

Reduce Pain

The pain of herpes lesions is problematic. Palliative measures include (1) keeping the involved area clean and dry, (2) wearing loose-fitting, nonsynthetic undergarments, and (3) using sitz baths, cooling applications, and analgesic medications, such as aspirin, for pain reduction.

CHANCROID

Several other STIs are common outside of the United States, but may be seen here with more frequency because of immigration or travel abroad. They are chancroid, lymphogranuloma venereum, and granuloma inguinale. Chancroid is a highly contagious infection caused by the gram-negative bacillus *Haemophilus ducreyi*. Chancroid presents with multiple painful, irregular, and deep genital ulcers often accompanied by tender inguinal lymphadenopathy (Figure 41-3). There is a high rate of HIV and syphilis infection in clients with

chancroid. Clients with chancroid should also be tested for HIV infection, HSV infection, and syphilis.

Definitive diagnosis requires a culture, which is not widely available. A clinical diagnosis may be made based on client presentation if the client does not have evidence of syphilis or genital herpes. Recommended treatment is oral azithromycin or ceftriaxone given IM in a single dose. Sexual partners need to be treated.

LYMPHOGRANULOMA VENEREUM

Lymphogranuloma venereum is a systemic infection caused by certain strains of *C. trachomatis*. The primary lesion is a small, painless papule on the glans penis or the vaginal mucosa that heals spontaneously and may go unnoticed.

The most common clinical manifestations are markedly tender, enlarged, and inflamed inguinal lymph nodes (*buboes*) that can drain, ulcerate, and scar; lymphatic obstruction; and marked external genital deformity. Definitive diagnosis is made with a positive culture for *C. trachomatis*. Recommended therapy is doxycycline, given orally for 21 days. Oral erythromycin is an alternative.

GRANULOMA INGUINALE

Granuloma inguinale (donovanosis) is a chronic infection caused by the small gram-negative bacillus now known as *Klebsiella granulomatis*.

Granuloma inguinale is characterized by genital and perianal papular lesions without lymphadenopathy. These become painless, gradually enlarging, ulcerating granulomatous lesions that cause tissue destruction. The lesions are highly vascular, bleed easily, and have a beefy-red appearance. Diagnosis is made with microscopic smears taken from edge scrapings of the lesion.

Treatment consists of a long course of an antibiotic such as trimethoprim-sulfamethoxazole or doxycycline but relapses can occur despite adequate treatment. All partners who have had sexual contact with an infected client within 60 days before diagnosis need evaluation and treatment.

INFECTION WITH HUMAN PAPILLOMAVIRUS

GENITAL WARTS (CONDYLOMATA ACUMINATA)

Etiology and Risk Factors

There are at least 20 million people who have genital warts in the United States. Caused by human papillomavirus (HPV), they are usually transmitted by sexual contact. Genital warts have become epidemic (6.2 million new

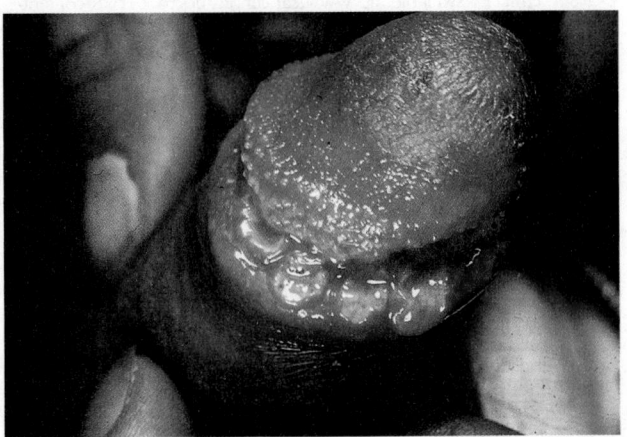

■ FIGURE 41-3 Chancroid lesions. (*Courtesy Dr. Rodney M.S. Basler.*)

infections yearly), in part because they are often asymptomatic and undiagnosed. At least 50% of individuals who are sexually active have it and by the age of 50, 80% of all women have it. Factors that may favor their development include HIV, pregnancy, smoking, drug or alcohol use, poor nutrition, and fatigue.

Pathophysiology

More than 30 types of HPV affect the genital tract. The natural history of HPV is complex and poorly understood. Infection with certain strains of HPV is strongly associated with carcinomas of the genitals, including the cervix.

Human papillomavirus screening for women with abnormal Pap smear results is considered in the Translating Evidence into Practice feature below.

Clinical Manifestations

Genital warts are benign growths that typically occur in multiple, painless clusters on the vulva, vagina, cervix, perineum, anorectal area, urethral meatus, or glans penis 1 to 2 months after exposure (Figure 41-4). Oral, pharyngeal, and laryngeal lesions can also occur. HPV can cause laryngeal papillomatosis in infants born to mothers with vaginal warts.

TRANSLATING EVIDENCE INTO PRACTICE

Human Papillomavirus Screening for Women with Abnormal Pap Smear Results

Cervical cancer is the second most common cancer affecting women worldwide and is a significant cause of morbidity and mortality, particularly in the developing world where more than 288,000 women will die of this disease each year. Rates of cervical cancer deaths have plunged in the United States because of the use of the Papanicolaou (Pap) smear, but there are still large areas where the death rate from this preventable cancer is unacceptably high. The American Cancer Society estimates that 11,150 women will be diagnosed with cervical cancer in 2007 and that 3670 women will die.

Although the Pap smear is recognized as an invaluable tool, there are several well-known problems with it. Many women are not routinely screened and may go years without a Pap smear. This is a particular problem for older women. Whatever the cause, more than half the women with cervical cancer have not had a Pap smear in at least 3 years, despite repeated contacts with health care providers.

The link between cervical cancer and the human papillomavirus (HPV) is well established; at least 90% of all cervical cancers are known to be caused by HPV and the other 10% of cases may reflect false-negative test results for the virus. Several types of HPV are strongly oncogenic; subtypes 16 and 18 are responsible for as much as 68% of all cancers. DNA testing can be done on cervical samples. "Reflex HPV testing" is done on previously collected Pap smear samples; if a Pap smear returns with abnormalities, the remaining fluid can be tested for HPV without the client needing to return for another examination.

Women whose test results are negative for high-risk HPV can be managed with a conservative approach. Women whose test results are positive for high-risk HPV can have treatment decisions tailored to their increased risk of developing advanced lesions and cancer. HPV DNA testing has a sensitivity for detecting high-grade lesions and invasive cancers that is equal to or superior to that of Pap smears.

According to the 2001 Consensus Guidelines for the Management of Women with Cervical Cytological Abnormalities, three treatment options exist for atypical squamous cells of undetermined significance (ASCUS): serial

repeat testing, colposcopy, or HPV DNA testing. The preferred option is to collect the HPV DNA sample with the Pap smear and analyze it only if the Pap result is abnormal ("reflex testing"). Women whose tests are positive for high-risk HPV should be referred for colposcopy. HPV DNA testing is also recommended for women with low-grade squamous intraepithelial lesions (LSIL) after colposcopy shows no cancer, and HPV DNA testing is in the algorithm for postmenopausal women. Two negative tests for high-risk HPV lend an almost 100% negative predictive value for invasive disease.

One of the most important advances in the prevention of cervical cancer has been the development of the vaccine for HPV, Gardasil. Gardasil is effective against four HPV subtypes, including types 16 and 18. The FDA has approved the vaccination, which is given as a series of three injections, for girls age 9 to 26. The vaccine will be most effective when given before a young woman has any sexual contact. Although effective, it will not protect against all types of HPV and will not prevent all cases of cervical cancer, so routine Pap testing is still required. Research continues on other HPV vaccines and on vaccinating men, who serve as the vector for HPV in most infected women.

REFERENCES

1. American Cancer Society. (2007). *Cancer facts and figures 2007.* Atlanta: Author.
2. American Cancer Society. (2006). *HPV vaccine approved; prevents cervical cancer.* Available at www.cancer.org/docroot/NWS/content/NWS_1_1x_HPV_Vaccine_Approved_Prevents_Cervical_Cancer.
3. American Society for Colposcopy and Cervical Pathology. (2001). *Consensus guidelines for the management of women with cervical cytological abnormalities.* Available at www.asccp.org.
4. Brotzman, G.L. (2005, July). Evaluating the impact of HPV-related diseases. Special Edition of *The Journal of Family Practice*, s3-s9.
5. Bosch, F.X., & de Sanjose, S. (2003). Human papillomavirus and cervical cancer—Burden and assessment of causality. *Journal of the National Cancer Institute Monographs,* No. 31. Oxford University Press: Journal of the National Cancer Institute.
6. Centers for Disease Control and Prevention. (2006). *HPV vaccination questions and answers.* Available at www.cdc.gov/std/health comm/fact_sheets.htm.
7. Geipert, N. (2005). Vaccinating men for HPV: New strategy for preventing cervical cancer in women? *Journal of the National Cancer Institute, 97,* 630-631.
8. National Cancer Institute. (2006). *Human papilloma virus and cancer: Questions and answers.* Available at www.cancer.gov/cancertopics/factsheet/Risk/HPV.

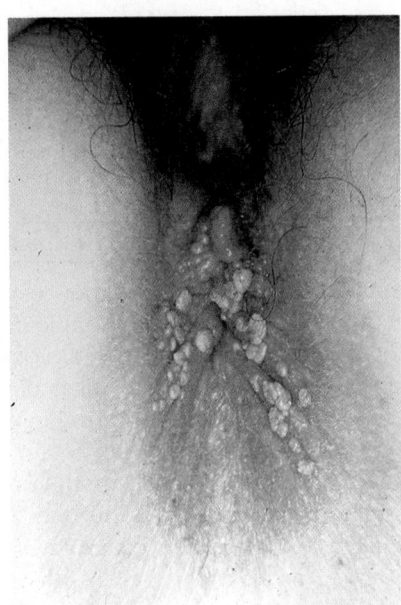

■ **FIGURE 41–4** Genital warts (condylomata acuminata). *(Courtesy Dr. Rodney M.S. Basler.)*

Diagnosis is typically made visually. Subclinical (asymptomatic or not visible) warts can be identified through Pap smear and colposcopy (examination of vagina and cervical tissues with a scope containing a magnifying lens) of the cervix. Acetic acid applied to tissue infected with HPV turns a characteristic whitish color. Biopsies may be performed to differentiate warts from carcinoma or condylomata lata of the secondary stage of syphilis.

OUTCOME MANAGEMENT

Medical Management

Remove Visible Warts

There is no cure for genital warts. A variety of chemical, mechanical, and ablative techniques are used for visible lesions, but no specific antiviral therapy for the HPV is available, and no treatment is considered optimal. Treatment varies according to the site and severity of the warts and is guided by client and provider preference. Treatment is more successful if the warts are small and have been present for less than a year. Treatment of subclinical cases is not recommended if the client does not also have cervical squamous cell lesions. Treated warts may resolve, show no change, or worsen despite therapy. Treatment does not eliminate the infection and clients usually need a series of treatments. Experts consider the "watch and wait" approach an acceptable treatment option in uncomplicated cases.

Topical Therapy

The most common client-applied treatments are podofilox solution mixture or imiquimod cream, both of which are applied directly to the visible warts. Podophyllin resin, trichloroacetic acid (TCA), or bichloroacetic acid (BCA) are available for provider administration. The CDC also lists trichloroacetic acid as an alternative to BCA. For safe application of client-applied treatments, the client must be able to see and reach the warts easily. Podofilox is contraindicated during pregnancy. If warts persist, other modes of therapy should be considered (see the Integrating Pharmacology feature on Drugs Used to Treat Common Sexually Transmitted Infections on p. 978).

Other Treatment

Warts can be treated with cryotherapy, carbon dioxide lasers, and electrocautery, and simple surgical excision can be used on extensive warts. The antiviral drug interferon has been used both systemically and intralesionally, but is not considered effective given systemically and should be avoided. Warts found in the vagina, urethral meatus, or anus can be treated following more extensive guidelines from the CDC.

It is not necessary to evaluate and treat sexual partners of clients with genital warts, because treatment is not effective in eradicating the infection or its spread. Female partners should be referred for a Pap smear, and all sexual partners should be offered the opportunity to be examined and tested for other STIs.

Nursing Management of the Medical Client

Inform clients with genital warts that no cure exists and that female clients are at increased risk for genital malignancy. HPV infections are strongly associated with cancer of the cervix and vulva in women and squamous cell carcinoma of the penis in men. All women with genital warts should receive a Pap smear and, when indicated, cervical colposcopy and biopsy. Encourage condom use. See the Translating Evidence into Practice feature on Human Papillomavirus Screening for Women with Abnormal Pap Smear Results on p. 988.

INFECTIONS CHARACTERIZED BY VAGINAL DISCHARGE

Infections manifested by vaginal discharge include trichomoniasis and vaginitis (bacterial and yeast). Although occasionally transmitted sexually, candidiasis (vaginal yeast infection) is generally not considered an STI. Recurrent vaginal yeast infections are a common manifestation of HIV infection in women and can also be seen frequently in clients with uncontrolled diabetes mellitus (vaginitis is discussed in Chapter 39).

TRICHOMONIASIS

Etiology and Risk Factors

Trichomoniasis is a protozoal infection causing vulvovaginitis. Although not life-threatening, the incidence is high worldwide and the infection remains a major health problem. Often asymptomatic, trichomoniasis affects 3 million people annually, and its role in PID and infertility may be greatly underestimated.

Pathophysiology

Trichomoniasis is caused by the anaerobic, flagellated, parasitic protozoan *Trichomonas vaginalis*. The organism is almost always transmitted sexually. *T. vaginalis* prefers an alkaline environment (pH 6 to 7), and alterations in the vaginal *flora* (the usual bacteria and fungi)—from douching, for instance—make a woman more susceptible to infection. Trichomoniasis can be resistant to treatment, and recurrence is common.

Clinical Manifestations

Manifestations may be minor, especially in men. In women, manifestations include a copious, malodorous, yellow-green vaginal discharge. This is irritating to the vulva and causes severe itching, burning, and excoriation and maceration of the vulvar tissues. Occasionally, the cervix is covered with punctate (point-like) hemorrhages ("strawberry cervix"). The vaginal mucosa appears reddened and slightly edematous. Some women experience dyspareunia (pain during sexual intercourse).

If trichomoniasis extends to the urethra, urinary frequency and burning with urination may occur. This is the most common manifestation in a man. Anal involvement may also occur, either asymptomatically or with a slight discharge. Bladder and anal involvement are more common when the infection becomes chronic.

The diagnosis can be made by examining a fresh, warm specimen of vaginal exudate in a saline wet mount under a microscope in which the highly motile organisms are seen. Cultures are rarely necessary. The vaginal speculum used during the examination must be inserted without lubrication to avoid destroying the organism. If possible, instruct the client not to douche before the vaginal examination.

OUTCOME MANAGEMENT

Medical Management

Eradicate Infection and Manifestations

The preferred treatment of trichomoniasis is a single oral dose of metronidazole (Flagyl) or tinidazole (Tindamax) with simultaneous treatment of all sexual partners for a cure. Metronidazole should not be taken during the first trimester of pregnancy because it may adversely affect fetal development. *T. vaginalis* itself does not affect the fetus. Single-dose metronidazole therapy is usually curative, but recurrence is common. Instruct clients to seek prompt treatment if manifestations return. Metronidazole may be given in a 7-day regimen for recurrent infection.

Nursing Management of the Medical Client

Advise clients taking metronidazole not to drink alcoholic beverages for 24 hours after completing therapy, because doing so might cause nausea, vomiting, and headaches. This prohibition includes all alcohol-containing products, such as cough syrup. Emphasize the importance of good perineal hygiene. Treatment should continue through the client's menstrual period because the vagina is more alkaline during this time and a flare-up is more likely to occur. Metronidazole can be taken without regard to meals. Advise clients that urine may turn dark, reddish brown.

BACTERIAL VAGINOSIS

Bacterial vaginosis, formerly known as nonspecific or *Gardnerella* vaginitis, is a common condition in adults. It is the most common cause of vaginal discharge in women, although many clients are asymptomatic.

Etiology and Risk Factors

Bacterial vaginosis is linked to sexual activity, particularly having multiple sex partners, although not all cases are caused by sexual activity. It is often seen in women who douche, and it can occur after other genital infections and invasive gynecologic procedures.

Pathophysiology

Like the organisms responsible for vulvovaginal *Candida* (yeast) infections, the causative bacteria are found in the normal vagina. The infection is caused by the overgrowth of a number of different organisms, including *Gardnerella vaginalis* and vaginal anaerobes. Overgrowth may occur when the normal flora and pH of the vagina are altered and replaced with high numbers of anaerobic bacteria.

Clinical Manifestations

The vulvovaginitis produced by bacterial vaginosis is mild or asymptomatic. The main manifestation is a mild to moderate, malodorous vaginal discharge. The discharge is usually thin, watery, and grayish white and tends to adhere to the vaginal wall. The odor is described as "fishy" and is often more noticeable after sexual intercourse. Manifestations are almost always confined to the vulvovaginal area. Mild vaginal burning and irritation may occur, but redness and pruritus are not common.

Evaluation is mainly by physical examination of the vagina, microscopic examination of the discharge, and determination of the pH of the discharge. The diagnosis is determined by the presence of at least three of the following manifestations:

- A homogeneous gray or white discharge that adheres to the vaginal wall
- Vaginal fluid pH above 4.5 (normal pH is 4.0 to 4.5)
- Positive result of the "whiff" test—a fishy odor elicited when potassium hydroxide (KOH) is added to the vaginal fluid
- Presence of *clue cells* (desquamated vaginal epithelial cells characteristically stippled by the adherence of coccobacilli to their surfaces) on either a saline wet mount or a Gram stain of vaginal fluid

OUTCOME MANAGEMENT

Medical Management

The recommended treatment of bacterial vaginosis in nonpregnant women is metronidazole (Flagyl), given orally or intravaginally for 7 days. Single-dose regimens can be used to improve compliance, but they are less effective than the 7-day regimen. Pregnant women are treated with lower doses of metronidazole to minimize exposure to the fetus. Alternative treatment includes metronidazole in a high, single dose, or clindamycin orally or intravaginally.

Nursing Management of the Medical Client

Bacterial vaginosis is not necessarily transmitted sexually, although its occurrence is associated with sexual activity. Treatment of male partners is recommended only with recurrent or resistant infection. Recurrence is common.

ACQUIRED IMMUNODEFICIENCY SYNDROME

AIDS is a viral STI that develops from HIV infection. HIV/AIDS has reached epidemic proportions worldwide. HIV infection has had an effect on the transmission of STIs, and vice versa. People with AIDS are more susceptible to other STIs. These coexistent STIs require more aggressive therapy and tend to recur. Conversely, people infected with an STI, especially those with genital ulcerations, are more susceptible to HIV infection. On the positive side, national campaigns to prevent and control the transmission of HIV have had a beneficial effect on the

incidence of some STIs (e.g., reduced incidence of hepatitis B in the homosexual population). AIDS is discussed in Chapter 78.

VACCINE-PREVENTABLE INFECTIONS

Vaccines for STIs are receiving increasing attention as possible strategies for control of STIs. Currently, vaccines are available for hepatitis A and B, and for HPV. Trials are under way for vaccines against other STIs. Every person seeking screening or treatment of STIs should be offered the hepatitis B vaccine, and certain high-risk groups (men who have sex with men, people who have sex with IV drug users) should be offered the hepatitis A vaccine. Gardasil, the vaccination for HPV, is approved for girls and women ages 9 to 26.

HEPATITIS

Hepatitis A is caused by a virus and is most commonly transmitted through oral-fecal contamination. The virus is also found in serum and saliva. Risk factors for hepatitis A include (1) household or sexual contact with people who have the virus, (2) homosexual activity, and (3) IV drug abuse or sexual contact with an IV drug user. Measures that are typically used to decrease the spread of other STIs do not stop the transfer of this virus.

Sexual contact is the most frequently reported mode of transmission for the hepatitis B virus (HBV) (50% of all cases), although blood-borne and perinatal transmission also occur. Clients at high risk for sexually transmitted hepatitis B are (1) heterosexuals with multiple sexual partners, (2) sexual partners of IV drug users, and (3) men who have sex with men. The incidence of sexually transmitted hepatitis B has decreased dramatically in the homosexual population, probably as a result of the modification of high-risk sexual behaviors to prevent AIDS.

Hepatitis C is associated with sexual activity (20% of cases). Sexually oriented risk factors include having multiple partners, having sex with an IV drug user, and engaging in sexual activities that cause trauma. See Chapter 47 for further discussion of hepatitis A and B.

DISEASES CAUSED BY INFESTATIONS

PEDICULOSIS PUBIS AND SCABIES

Cutaneous infestation with pubic lice (pediculosis pubis) or mites (scabies) results either from close physical contact with an infected person or from contact with contaminated objects of an infected person, such as linens and clothing. Because sexual transmission is possible, these conditions are included in any list of STIs. For further discussion, see Chapter 49.

SEXUALLY TRANSMITTED ENTERIC INFECTIONS

Gastroenteritis caused by enteric pathogens is typically acquired from food or water contaminated with fecal matter. Since the mid-1970s, it has been recognized that these pathogens can also be transmitted by oral and anal sexual contact. Sexually transmitted enteric infections include shigellosis, salmonellosis, amebiasis, and giardiasis. Men who have sex with men are at highest risk for these infections. See Chapter 33 for a discussion of gastroenteritis.

MANAGEMENT OF CLIENTS REPORTING SEXUAL ASSAULT

Victims of sexual assault need immense support from health care professionals, a discussion of which is beyond the scope of this chapter. Regarding STIs, a sexual assault victim needs an immediate physical examination, including tests for pregnancy, gonorrhea, chlamydial infection, trichomoniasis, HIV, hepatitis A and B, and syphilis. Follow-up testing should be repeated in 2 weeks; syphilis and HIV testing should also be repeated at 6, 12, and 24 months. Prophylaxis for HIV infection is described in Chapter 78.

CONCLUSIONS

STIs are more prevalent than ever before. This phenomenon is attributable to many factors. Sexual activity, especially among adolescents and young adults, has increased. Many STIs are asymptomatic and go undetected. Nurses are in a unique position to help clients protect, salvage, or restore their sexual health and have an ever-increasing responsibility and role in the prevention, early detection, and treatment of STIs.

THINKING CRITICALLY

1. A 20-year-old unmarried man comes to a walk-in STI clinic with a purulent urethral discharge. The diagnosis is uncomplicated gonorrhea. The client has no known allergies. He is sexually active with multiple partners. He gives a temporary address. What are the priorities of care? What are the priority interventions?

Factors to Consider. What effect would the client's status as a walk-in client have on your planning? Consider the fact that gonorrhea often leads to PID in women. What effect would the temporary address have on your planning and need for identification of partners? What infections are likely to coexist with gonorrhea?

2. Your client is a 65-year-old widowed woman who comes for treatment of acute, symptomatic genital herpes. Her male sexual contact told her when their sexual relationship began that he had a history of genital herpes but that, because he had no active lesions, there was no risk of her becoming infected. She is humiliated by having contracted herpes and tells you that she feels dirty and contaminated. She also states that she knows nothing about condoms and, furthermore, that she "wouldn't be caught dead buying them." What are the goals of her care? What interventions might be used?

Factors to Consider. How accurate is the client's knowledge about the transmission of genital herpes? What are her psychosocial needs? What obstacles to buying condoms can you identify, and how will you help this client control her sexual health?

3. A 25-year-old monogamous woman seeks outpatient treatment for the irritating, malodorous vaginal discharge of trichomoniasis. She has had trichomoniasis before, and metronidazole (Flagyl) was prescribed. What interventions should the care of this client include?

Factors to Consider. Knowing that metronidazole is usually curative, consider what might have caused this recurrence.

Discussions for these questions can be found on the website.

BIBLIOGRAPHY

🛢 Citations appearing in red refer to primary research.

🛢 Citations appearing in blue refer to evidence-based practice guidelines and protocols.

1. Adderley-Kelly, B., & Stephens, E.M. (2005, May-June). Chlamydia: A major threat to adolescents and young adults. *ABNF Journal*, 52-55.
2. American Cancer Society. (2006). *HPV vaccine approved: Prevents cervical cancer.* Available at www.cancer.org/docroot/NWS/content/NWS_1_1x_HPV_Vaccine_Approved_Prevents_Cervical_Cancer.asp.
3. Burstein, G.R., Snyder, M.H., Conley, D., et al. (2005). Chlamydia screening in a health plan before and after a national performance measure introduction. *Obstetrics & Gynecology, 106*, 327-334.
4. Centers for Disease Control and Prevention. (2006). *Expedited partner therapy in the management of sexually transmitted diseases.* Atlanta, Ga: U.S. Department of Health and Human Services.
5. Centers for Disease Control and Prevention. (2006). Sexually transmitted diseases treatment guidelines, 2006. *Morbidity and Mortality Weekly Report, 55*(RR-11), 1-95.
6. Centers for Disease Control and Prevention. (2005). *Trends in reportable sexually transmitted diseases in the United States, 2004.* Atlanta, Ga: Author.
7. Centers for Disease Control and Prevention. (2004). Brief report: Azithromycin treatment failures in syphilis infections, San Francisco, California, 2002-2003. *Annals of Emergency Medicine, 44*, 232-234.
8. Chesson, J.M., Blandford, T.L., Gift, T.L., et al. (2004). The estimated direct medical cost of sexually transmitted diseases among American youth, 2000. *Perspectives on Sexual and Reproductive Health, 36*, 11-19.

9. Golden, M.R., Whittington, W.L.H., & Handsfield, H.H. (2005). Effect of expedited treatment of sex partners on recurrent or persistent gonorrhea or chlamydial infection. *New England Journal of Medicine, 352,* 676-685.

10. Gupta, R., Wald, A., Krantz, E., et al. (2004). Valacyclovir and acyclovir for suppression of shedding of herpes simplex virus in the genital tract. *Journal of Infectious Diseases, 190,* 1374-1381.

11. Hammarlund, K., & Nystrom, M. (2004). The lived experience of genital warts: The Swedish example. *Health Care for Women International, 25,* 489-502.

12. Hu, D., Hook, E.W., & Goldie, S.J. (2004). Screening for *Chlamydia trachomatis* in women 15 to 29 years of age: A cost-effectiveness analysis. *Annals of Internal Medicine, 141,* 501-513.

13. Kane, B.G., Degutis, L.C., Sayward, H.K., et al. (2004). Compliance with the Centers for Disease Control and Prevention recommendations for the diagnosis and treatment of sexually transmitted diseases. *Academic Emergency Medicine, 11,* 371-377.

14. Kissinger, P., Mohammed, H., & Richardson-Alston, G. (2005). Patient-delivered partner treatment for male urethritis: A randomized, controlled trial. *Clinical Infectious Diseases, 41,* 623-629.

15. Miller, W.C., Ford, C.A., Morris, M., et al. (2006). Prevalence of chlamydial and gonococcal infections among young adults in the United States. *Journal of the American Medical Association, 291,* 2229-2236.

16. Sparks, R., Helmers, J.R.L., Handsfield, H., et al. (2004). Rescreening for gonorrhea and chlamydial infection through the mail: A randomized trial. *Sexually Transmitted Diseases, 31*(2), 113-116.

17. Tyler, I. (2005, May/June). Herpes simplex type 2 virus: A new horizon. *ABNF Journal,* 63-64.

evolve *Did you remember to check out the bonus material on the Evolve website and the CD-ROM, including NCLEX®-Examination Style Review Questions, Open-Book Quizzes, and Chapter Review Audio Podcasts?*

http://evolve.elsevier.com/Black/medsurg

UNIT 10

METABOLIC DISORDERS

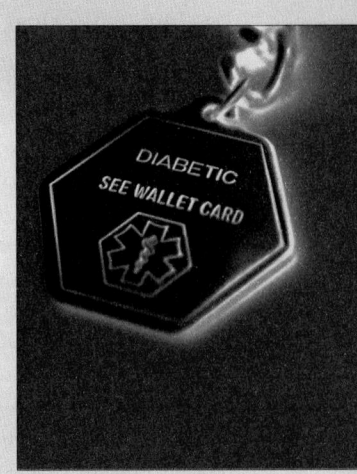

ANATOMY AND PHYSIOLOGY REVIEW:

The Metabolic Systems

Robert G. Carroll

Metabolism is the entire collection of chemical reactions that occur in all living cells. These processes are the basis of life, allowing cells to grow and reproduce, maintain their structures, and respond to their environments. Metabolism depends on the availability of fuel (glucose and fatty acids) and oxygen, and on the balance of *anabolic* (building) against *catabolic* (breakdown) processes. Regulation of this balance is dynamic and is one function of the endocrine and neuroendocrine systems. Metabolic processes affect all cells of the body, and whole-body metabolic regulation involves numerous endocrine structures, the liver, muscle, fat, and brain cells.

Endocrine secretions, together with the nervous system, coordinate the balance of metabolism, reproduction, water and electrolyte balance, and nutrient absorption. Metabolism is closely regulated by thyroid hormone, with some influence exerted by cortisol and epinephrine. Growth and development are regulated by growth hormone (also called *somatotropin*), with thyroid hormone, insulin-like growth factors, and the sex hormones providing significant effects. Plasma glucose is closely regulated by insulin, with glucagon and the metabolic hormones cortisol, growth hormone, and epinephrine having a role. Endocrine agents involved in water and electrolyte balance, nutrient absorption, and reproduction are described in Units 7, 8 and 9.

The liver and pancreas have both endocrine and exocrine roles. The exocrine secretions assist the digestion and absorption of the diet (see the Unit 7 Anatomy and Physiology Review). The endocrine role is tied closely to metabolism, particularly the regulation and storage of plasma glucose. Plasma glucose represents the balance of glucose absorption from the diet, movement into and out of storage pools, new glucose synthesis from amino acids *(gluconeogenesis)*, and, finally, glucose consumption by the tissues. The liver plays a central role in these processes and is a good point to begin the discussion of metabolism.

STRUCTURE OF THE METABOLIC SYSTEMS

LIVER

The liver is the largest gland in the body, representing about 2.5% of body weight. It lies in the right upper quadrant of the abdomen, just below the diaphragm. The rib cage encloses the liver except for the lower margin. The lungs extend over the liver's upper portion. The lower portion of the liver provides a "roof" for the stomach and intestines. A peritoneal covering blankets most of the liver and also the adjacent gallbladder. The liver divides at the falciform ligament into two major lobes, right and left (Figure A&P10-1). These two lobes, in turn, divide into superior and inferior portions of the posterior, anterior, medial, and lateral segments.

Liver blood flow represents about 20% of the cardiac output, about 1 L/min. The hepatic artery supplies the liver with about one third of its blood, and the portal vein supplies the other two thirds (see Figure A&P10-1, *B*). The hepatic artery carries oxygenated blood; the portal vein carries nutrient-rich deoxygenated blood. The superior and inferior mesenteric veins and the splenic vein, which receive blood from the pancreas, spleen, stomach, intestines, and gallbladder, join to form the portal vein. The portal vein carries nutrients, metabolites, and toxins from the digestive organs to the liver for processing, detoxification, or assimilation. Blood pressure in the portal system sinuses is low; hence any process elevating central venous pressure causes liver engorgement. Similarly, any process impeding blood flow through the liver causes engorgement of vessels draining the digestive organs. The liver is an important reservoir for blood, with contraction of the hepatic venules and veins moving about 500 ml into the circulation.

The functional unit of the liver is the *lobule,* and the *hepatocyte* is the major cell. Hepatocytes are arranged in a hub-like fashion around a central vein. One side of the polyhedral hepatocyte faces the *hepatic sinusoids* (the capillary system of the liver); another side faces the bile canaliculi. As incoming blood from the portal vein and the hepatic artery enters the sinusoids and passes through the liver lobules, many substances are exchanged between the blood and the hepatocytes. Lymphatic ducts drain excess interstitial fluid. Bile is formed in the hepatocytes, is secreted into the *bile canaliculi,* and travels through bile ductules to the gallbladder for storage. Endothelial and *Kupffer cells* form the walls of the sinusoids.

Kupffer cells are an important part of the mononuclear phagocyte system (formerly the reticuloendothelial system). This system is so effective that less than 1% of the bacteria entering the portal system from the intestine pass through the liver. This process prevents bacteria from directly entering the bloodstream. After leaving the sinusoids, blood flows into the central vein, the hepatic veins, and the inferior vena cava.

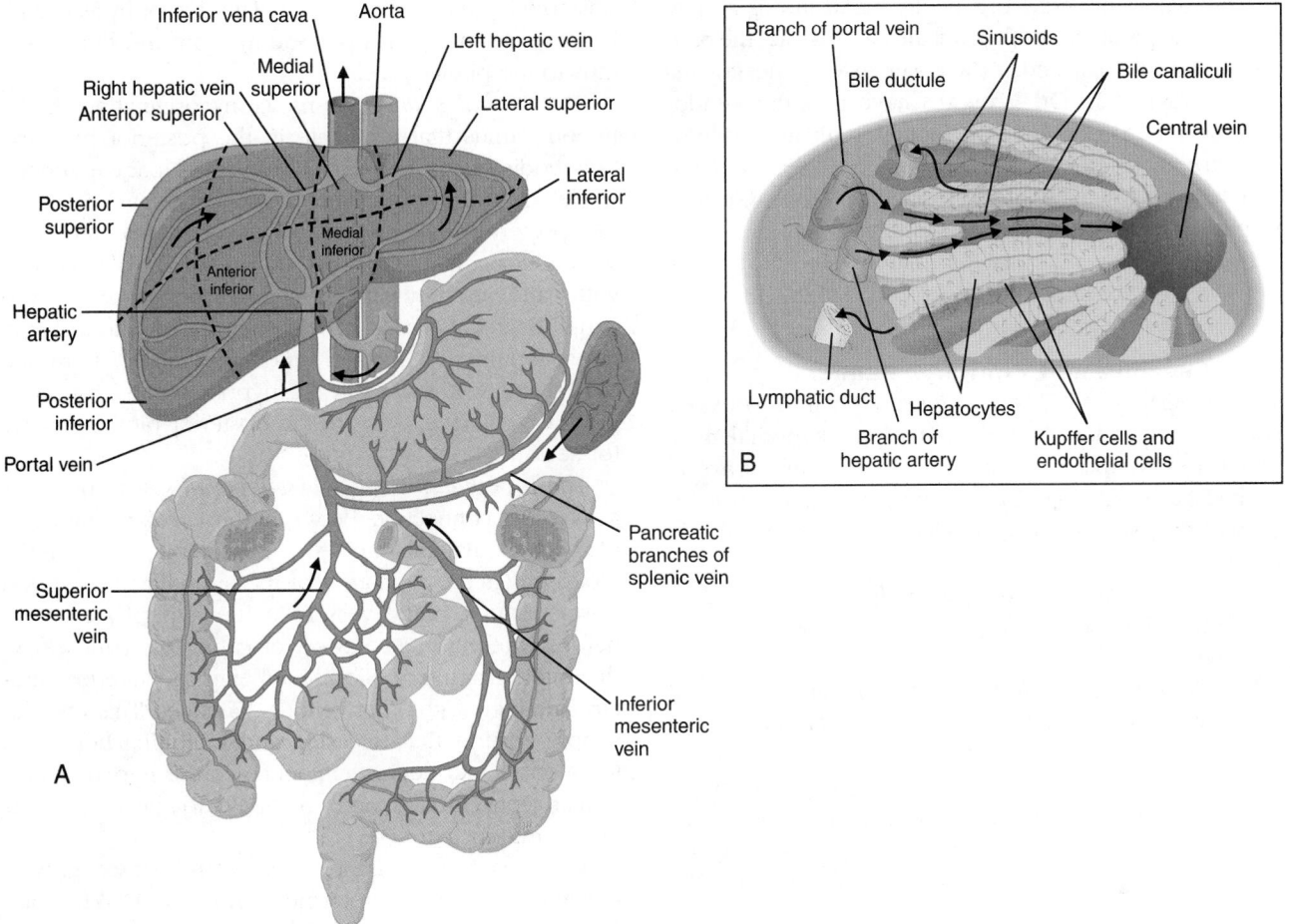

■ **FIGURE A&PI0–I** The liver and vascular drainage systems. Blood enters the liver from the hepatic artery, and the hepatic portal vein supplies the liver with blood from the digestive organs. *Inset,* Liver lobule. Blood from the hepatic artery and portal vein is processed by the hepatocytes as it flows through the sinusoids into the central vein. Lymphatics and bile ducts leave the liver through separate pathways.

ENDOCRINE SYSTEM

The endocrine glands are distributed throughout the body. *Endocrine* tissues (*endo,* "within") secrete a compound (hormone) that is carried by the blood to act on a target tissue. This is in contrast to *exocrine* (*exo,* "outside") tissues, which secrete across an epithelium, such as sweat and pancreatic peptidases (the lumen of the gastrointestinal [GI] tract is "outside" the body); and *paracrine* (*para,* around) cells, whose secretions do not need to be transported in the blood to reach their target tissue because they communicate with nearby cells.

Hormones are generally classified on the basis of molecular structure as follows:

■ *Steroids.* Steroids are derived from cholesterol and are consequently poorly soluble in water. After secretion, steroids are transported in the blood by carrier proteins. Steroids diffuse across the cell membrane of the target tissue and bind to a cytoplasmic-binding protein. The steroid-binding protein complex enters the nucleus, where it alters deoxyribonucleic acid (DNA) transcription. There is usually a lag of minutes to hours before steroids exert their effects.

■ *Peptides.* Proteins and *polypeptides* are synthesized in the endoplasmic reticulum of the endocrine tissue and are secreted in vesicles. After transport in the blood, they bind to cell membrane receptors on the target tissues and activate either second messenger systems within the cell or ion channels. Peptide hormones, such as insulin, generally have rapid response times.

■ *Amino acid derivatives.* The derivatives of tyrosine include thyroid hormone and the catecholamines epinephrine, norepinephrine, and dopamine. Thyroid hormone alters DNA synthesis through a pathway similar to that for steroids, but the catecholamines bind cell membrane receptors, similar to the mechanism of peptides.

The major endocrine organs described in this review include the pituitary, the thyroid, the parathyroid, the pancreas, the adrenal, and, to a lesser extent, the gonads (Figure A&P10-2). Other organs have important endocrine secretions, including the kidney (renin and erythropoietin), the heart (atrial natriuretic peptide), and the placenta of a pregnant female (human chorionic gonadotropin, estrogen, progesterone, and the growth hormone somatomammotropin). See the Anatomy and Physiology Reviews for Units 8, 9, and 12.

Hypothalamus and Pituitary Gland

The pituitary gland *(hypophysis)* is a small (1 g) extension on the dorsal surface of the hypothalamus, connected to the hypothalamus by the hypophyseal stalk (Figure A&P10-3). The pituitary has three histologically distinct sections, two of which secrete hormones in humans:

1. The *anterior pituitary (adenohypophysis)* is glandular tissue that contains a variety of secretory cell types.
2. The *posterior pituitary (neurohypophysis)* is neural tissue that contains glia cells and terminal axons from cells of the hypothalamus.
3. The *pars intermedia* is a vestigial remnant in humans, with little physiologic significance.

The hypothalamus lies dorsal to the pituitary gland and regulates secretion of both the anterior and the posterior pituitary hormones. The hypophyseal stalk has two distinct pathways leading from the hypothalamus to the pituitary.

The *neural stalk* contains axons originating in the hypothalamus that terminate in the posterior pituitary. Cell bodies are in the supraoptic and paraventricular nuclei of the hypothalamus, and axons terminate in the posterior pituitary, where the synaptic terminals secrete hormones rather than make synaptic connections with another neuron. The *posterior pituitary* also contains glia-like cells, which support and nourish the nerve endings. Oxytocin and antidiuretic hormone (ADH) are synthesized in the hypothalamus and transported within the axons to the posterior pituitary gland for secretion.

The *hypothalamo-hypophyseal portal system* provides a vascular connection between the median eminence of the hypothalamus and the anterior pituitary. Arterial blood enters the capillaries of the hypothalamus. Blood flows through portal vessels in the hypophyseal stalk before entering a second set of capillaries (sinuses) in the anterior pituitary. Blood then exits the anterior pituitary and joins with other venous drainages. This vascular supply ensures that releasing and inhibiting hormones secreted in the median eminence of the hypothalamus remain concentrated until delivered to the target cells of the anterior pituitary.

The *anterior pituitary* secretes and stores growth hormone, adrenocorticotropic hormone (ACTH), follicle-stimulating hormone, thyroid-stimulating hormone, luteinizing hormone, and prolactin.

Thyroid and Parathyroid

The thyroid gland is located in the neck, just below the cricoid cartilage, and is somewhat H-shaped (Figure A&P10-4). The right and left lateral lobes lie on either side of the trachea. The lobes are connected by a thin mass of tissue (the *isthmus*), which stretches over the surface of the trachea. Each lobe is composed of irregularly shaped lobules, which consist of a multitude of tiny sacs (follicles) filled with a jelly-like, iodine-containing substance called *colloid* (see Figure A&P10-4, *inset*). The main component of colloid is thyroglobulin—the storage form of the hormone thyroxine. The *parathyroid glands* are four small glands near, attached to, or embedded in the thyroid gland.

Endocrine Pancreas

The pancreas (see Figure A&P10-2) contains islets of Langerhans, which secrete three hormones that regulate blood glucose level: (1) *alpha* cells secrete *glucagons,* (2) *beta* cells secrete *insulin,* and (3) *delta* cells secrete *somatostatin,* identical to the growth hormone inhibitory hormone secreted by the hypothalamus. The close proximity of these cells within the islets allows a coordinated

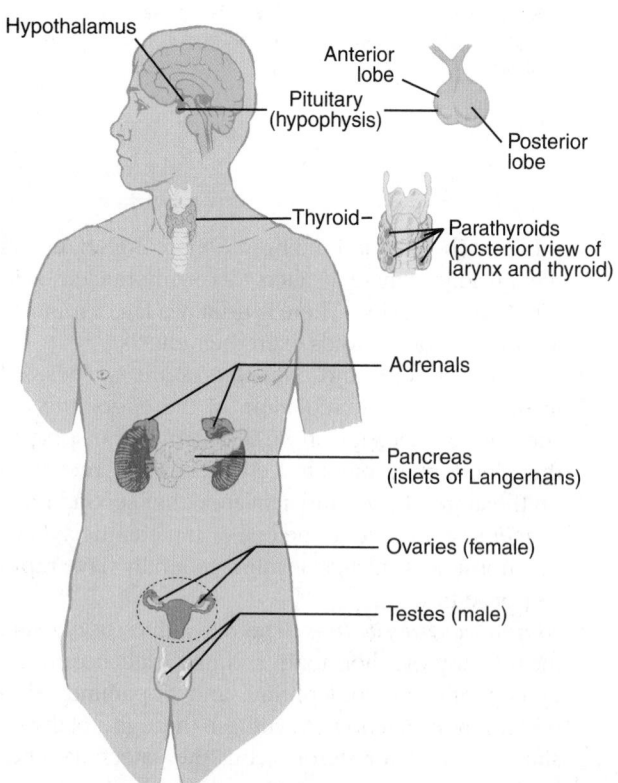

■ **FIGURE A&P10–2** Major organs of the endocrine system.

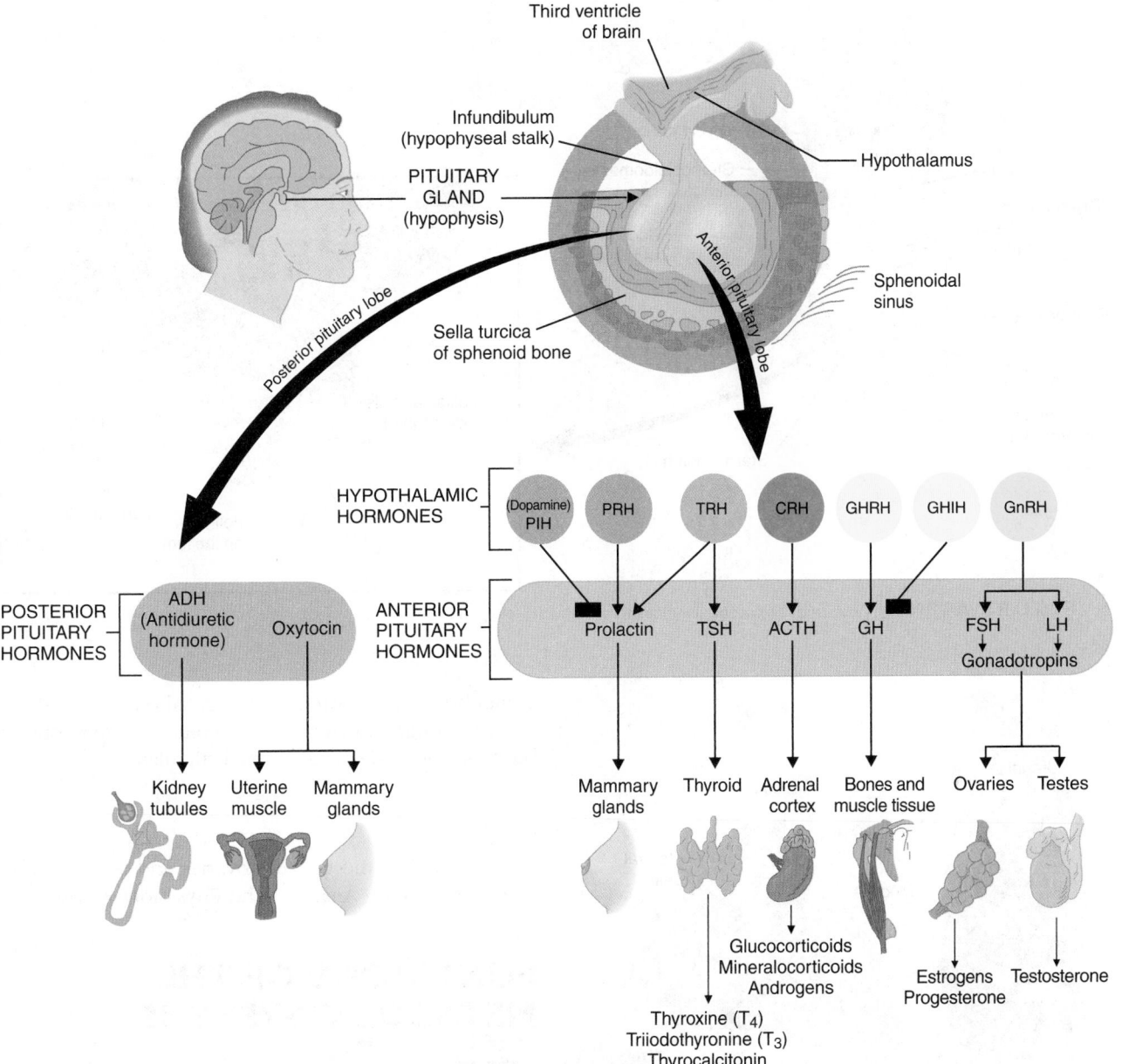

■ **FIGURE A&P10–3** Hypothalamus, pituitary gland, and target tissues. The pituitary gland is suspended from the hypothalamus by the infundibulum or hypophyseal stalk. Hormones released from the hypothalamus travel in a portal vascular system to the anterior pituitary gland, where they stimulate (or inhibit) the release of anterior pituitary hormones. Posterior pituitary hormones are synthesized in the hypothalamus and are released from axons in the posterior pituitary gland.

paracrine regulation of pancreatic secretion because insulin inhibits glucagon release and somatostatin inhibits both insulin and glucagon release.

Adrenal Glands

The adrenal glands are paired endocrine organs situated on top of the kidneys. The adrenal gland is divided into an outer cortex and an inner medulla (Figure A&P10-5). The *cortex* has three zones. The outer *zona glomerulosa* secretes the mineralocorticoids aldosterone and corticosterone. The inner *zona fasciculata* and *zona reticularis*

secrete the glucocorticoids cortisol and corticosterone as well as androgen sex hormones. Corticosterone and deoxycorticosterone are secreted in small amounts and exert both glucocorticoid and mineralocorticoid effects. Adrenal cortical hormones are steroids formed from a cholesterol nucleus. Deficits in synthetic enzymes often lead to overproduction of other adrenal hormones. Stimuli that enhance adrenal cortical secretions also cause hypertrophy of the appropriate cortical zones.

The *adrenal medulla* functions as a postganglionic sympathetic nerve, secreting the catecholamines

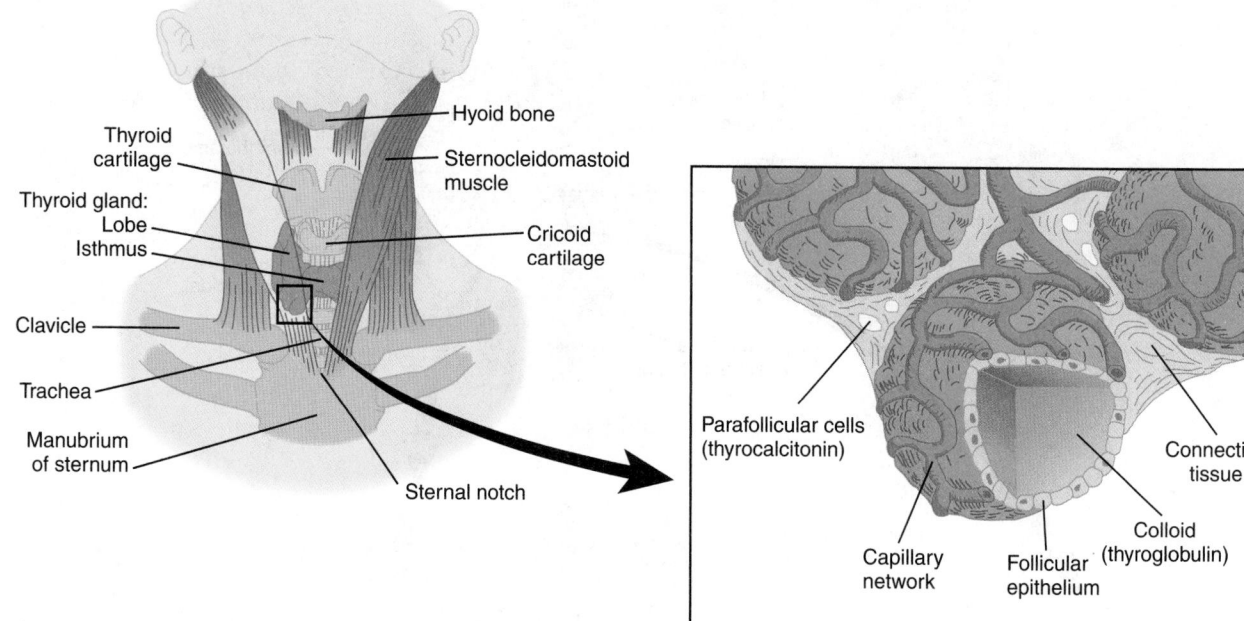

■ **FIGURE A&PI0–4** Gross and microscopic (inset) anatomy of the thyroid gland.

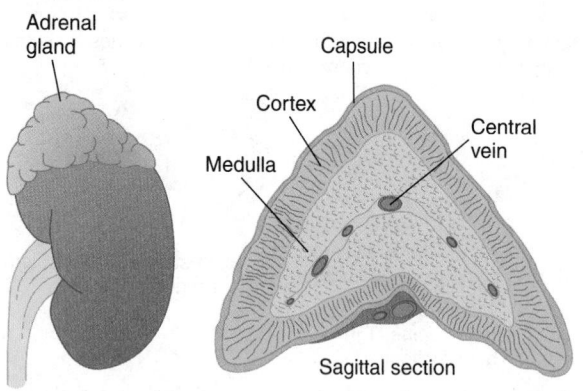

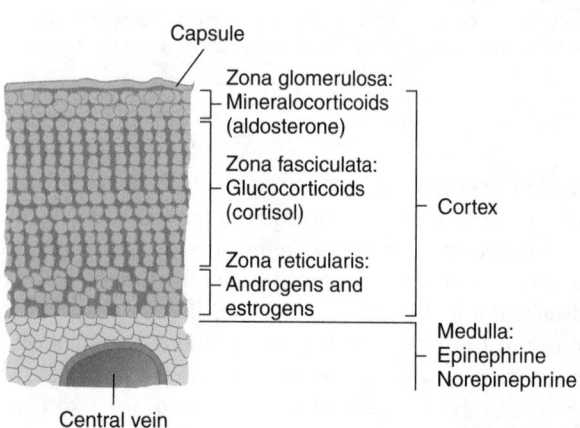

■ **FIGURE A&PI0–5** Gross and microscopic anatomy of the adrenal gland.

epinephrine and norepinephrine. About 80% of the basal (resting) catecholamine secretion is epinephrine, but this ratio varies with adrenal stimulation.

Gonads

The structure of the gonads (ovaries and testes) is covered in the Unit 9 Anatomy and Physiology Review.

FUNCTIONS OF THE METABOLIC SYSTEMS

LIVER

The liver plays a central role in the regulation of metabolic substrates, glucose, and fatty acids. Additionally, hepatic synthesis provides most of the proteins circulating in the plasma.

The liver is also the major storage organ for *glycogen,* a polymer of glucose. In addition to storage, the liver converts glucose to glycogen *(glycogenesis),* breaks down glycogen into glucose *(glycogenolysis),* and forms glucose from other sugars *(galactose* and *fructose)* or amino acids *(gluconeogenesis).* The regulation of these processes is discussed later.

The major functions of the liver in relation to fat metabolism are as follows:

■ Oxidation of fatty acids for energy
■ Formation of most lipoproteins

- Synthesis of cholesterol and phospholipids
- Synthesis of fats from proteins and carbohydrates

The liver provides energy from fats by splitting them into glycerol and fatty acids; when the fatty acids are oxidized, tremendous amounts of energy are released.

Most of the cholesterol synthesized in the liver is converted into bile salts; the remainder is transported in the lipoproteins, which deliver fat for energy to cells, throughout the body. Phospholipids are also synthesized in the liver and transported in lipoproteins. The cholesterol and phospholipids help form cell membranes and intracellular structures and are involved in cellular function.

The primary functions of the liver in relation to protein metabolism are as follows:

- Deamination of amino acids
- Formation of urea for removal of ammonia from the body
- Formation of plasma proteins
- Biotransformation of hormones, drugs, and other substances

Degradation is the process of excess amino acid catabolism. This process begins in the liver with deamination, the removal of amino groups ($-NH_2$). Ammonia (NH_3), which results from deamination, is converted into urea by the liver and is excreted by the kidneys and intestines. Ammonia can also be formed in the intestines by bacterial action. In severe liver disease or damage, ammonia that is normally converted to urea by the liver accumulates to dangerously high levels in the blood. As a result, a severe toxic state *(hepatic encephalopathy)* develops.

The liver also synthesizes plasma proteins, such as albumin, prothrombin, fibrinogen, and clotting proteins (factors V, VI, VII, IX, and X). Albumin is essential for maintaining plasma oncotic pressure; the other proteins contribute to blood clotting. Plasma oncotic pressure prevents intravascular fluid from moving out into the extravascular spaces, where it manifests as *ascites* and varying degrees of peripheral edema. Vitamin K, a fat-soluble vitamin, must be present for synthesis of several clotting proteins. Assimilation of vitamin K depends on the presence of bile in the intestine. Gamma-globulins are the only major plasma proteins not synthesized by the liver.

The liver primarily detoxifies and biotransforms hormones, drugs, and other chemicals. Some substances are deactivated by deamination, hydroxylation, oxidation, or reduction. Through conjugation, other substances become soluble in water, resulting in their excretion through the bile and, therefore, in feces or urine.

Clients with compromised liver function are at high risk for untoward reactions to many medications, all opiates, and many chemicals. The two major problems that result are prolonged action and toxicity from failure to excrete the medication or its by-products.

ENDOCRINE SYSTEM

Regulation of endocrine secretions is generally by a negative feedback loop, linking the hormone to a response, to another hormone, or to glucose or some other plasma compound. Endocrine agents also have significant trophic effects on the target tissues, with high hormone levels often causing hypertrophy and inadequate hormone levels causing atrophy. Regulation of the endocrine system is often integrated with the nervous system. When the distinction between endocrine and nervous systems is blurred, the system is described as the *neuroendocrine system*.

Hypothalamus and Pituitary Gland

The hypothalamus regulates secretion of anterior and posterior pituitary hormones. Five hypothalamic-releasing hormones and two hypothalamic-inhibitory hormones regulate secretion of the six anterior pituitary hormones (see Figure A&P10-3).

Growth Hormone (Somatotropin)

Growth hormone is secreted by the anterior pituitary; it exerts several effects:

- Stimulates growth in almost all body tissues, causing both an increase in cell size *(hypertrophy)* and an increase in cell number *(hyperplasia)*
- Diverts amino acids into protein synthesis *(anabolism)* and decreases protein breakdown *(catabolism)*
- Enhances the use of free fatty acids as metabolic substrates, which depletes body fat stores
- Increases plasma glucose levels but protects amino acid pools (discussed later)

Insulin has an important permissive, or facilitatory, role in growth hormone–mediated growth. It enhances the entry of both glucose and amino acids into cells. Growth hormone exerts some of its effects through an intermediary, the somatomedins, or insulin-like growth factors.

Growth hormone secretion is enhanced by various stressful and normal stimuli, including starvation, chronic protein deficiency, hypoglycemia, low plasma levels of free fatty acids, exercise, and the first hours of sleep. Hypothalamic secretion of growth hormone releasing and inhibitory hormones is the primary regulator of growth hormone release.

Prolactin

The hypothalamus also produces prolactin. Hypothalamic control of prolactin is unique in that the normal control of prolactin release is by hypothalamic prolactin inhibitory hormone. Consequently, interruption of the hypothalamo-hypophyseal portal system increases pituitary prolactin release. Prolactin-releasing hormone is important in the suckling reflex (see the Unit 9 Anatomy and Physiology Review).

Antidiuretic Hormone and Oxytocin

Nerve endings in the *posterior pituitary* secrete oxytocin and antidiuretic hormone (ADH), also known as *vasopressin*. Oxytocin, formed primarily in the paraventricular nucleus of the hypothalamus, promotes uterine contraction during parturition and causes expression of milk ("letdown") following suckling (see the Unit 9 Anatomy and Physiology Review). ADH is formed primarily in the supraoptic nucleus and is released by increases in plasma osmolarity or by low blood pressure. Stress, trauma, and anesthetics can also promote ADH release. A common cause of premature labor is dehydration caused by the proximity of these two hormones in the pituitary. The mechanism of ADH control of water and electrolyte balance is discussed in the Unit 8 Anatomy and Physiology Review.

Thyroid Gland

Thyroid hormone is a composite of three (T_3) or four (T_4) iodinated tyrosine residues. Triiodothyronine (T_3) and thyroxine (T_4) are both called *thyroid hormone*. Thyroid hormone is lipid soluble, and 99% of thyroid hormone in the plasma is bound to thyroid-binding globulin. Of the two thyroid hormones, T_3 has the most rapid effect on target tissues, requiring 3 days for peak effect; T_4 (the more common) requires 11 days for peak effect (and is therefore referred to as the inactive form).

Thyroid hormone has several functions:

- It increases metabolism, enhancing carbohydrate consumption and increasing the size and density of mitochondria.
- It assists in acclimatization to cold environments by increasing metabolic rate (heat production is a byproduct of metabolism).
- It increases DNA translation and transcription.
- It increases protein synthesis but also has protein catabolic effects.
- It promotes growth and is required for normal growth in children.

Finally, thyroid hormone has a permissive effect to increase other endocrine secretions.

Thyroid hormone is formed in epithelium-lined follicles that contain the glycoprotein thyroglobulin. Thyroglobulin can contain five to six thyroid hormone molecules. Dietary iodine is required for thyroid hormone synthesis. Iodine is oxidized within the follicles and binds a tyrosine residue (T_1) of thyroglobulin. Iodinated tyrosines are coupled while still part of the thyroglobulin molecule, forming T_2, T_3, and T_4. The mature hormone is released by digestion of thyroglobulin, with recycling of unused iodine, T_1, and T_2.

Release of thyroid hormone is regulated by negative feedback by T_4 on thyroid-stimulating hormone (TSH) release at the anterior pituitary. TSH stimulates proteolysis of thyroglobulin, releasing T_3 and T_4. TSH also stimulates iodine uptake by the thyroid for new thyroid hormone synthesis, increasing the activity of thyroid gland cells and increasing thyroid hormone synthesis. TSH release is controlled by the hypothalamic tripeptide thyrotropin-releasing hormone (TRH). Cold exposure is a potent stimulus for TRH release, but the feedback loop for the effect of temperature on TRH is not yet established.

Parathyroid Glands

The endocrine secretion of the parathyroid glands is the polypeptide parathyroid hormone (PTH). A fall in serum calcium levels causes release of PTH: PTH acts on bone to release calcium, the GI tract via vitamin D to increase intestinal calcium absorption, and the kidneys to decrease urinary calcium excretion. These effects all act to restore circulating plasma calcium levels.

Endocrine Pancreas

The islets of Langerhans of the pancreas secrete three hormones that regulate blood glucose level: (1) insulin, (2) glucagon, and (3) somatostatin.

Insulin

Insulin is a small protein derived successively from a pre-prohormone and a prohormone. Insulin circulates as a free hormone, has a short plasma half-life of about 6 minutes, and is cleared from the plasma primarily by the liver and kidneys. Insulin binds to receptors on the surface of target tissues and enhances glucose transport across the membrane. Insulin decreases blood glucose level by enhancing uptake, use, and storage of glucose in hepatic, muscle, and adipose tissues (discussed later). Insulin enhances amino acid transport into cells; it acts synergistically with growth hormone to promote cell hypertrophy and hyperplasia.

C-peptide is a fragment of the prohormone that remains after insulin is cleaved. The concentration of C-peptide can be used to distinguish between the amount of insulin being produced naturally (generating C-peptide) from the amount being administered from an injection (which does not have C-peptide).

Note that the brain is refractory to insulin and must use glucose for a metabolic substrate. The brain is prioritized to receive glucose and its glucose transporter has a much higher glucose affinity than the insulin-sensitive transporter, so only a severe decline in the blood glucose level can lead to hypoglycemic shock.

Insulin is released after ingestion and absorption of carbohydrates. The initial phase, due to the release of stored insulin, peaks in 5 minutes. A delayed phase, from synthesis of new insulin, persists until blood glucose concentration returns to fasting levels. The ability of insulin to control plasma glucose levels is the basis of the glucose tolerance test (GTT) used to diagnose diabetes mellitus.

In the absence of insulin, fats are used as metabolic substrates. The incomplete oxidation of fatty acids results in the ketoacidosis that is characteristic of untreated diabetes mellitus. The lack of insulin elevates blood glucose level, causing an osmotic diuresis (see the Unit 8 Anatomy and Physiology Review). Finally, the lack of insulin promotes protein catabolism and inhibits growth.

Glucagon

Glucagon is an extremely potent hormone that is released when blood glucose levels drop below 90 mg/dl. Glucagon acts on the liver to elevate plasma glucose levels, an action opposite that of insulin. The second messenger for glucagon is cyclic adenosine monophosphate (cAMP); it allows excessively high glucagon levels to affect other tissues (enhancing cardiac contractility, enhancing bile secretion, and inhibiting gastric acid secretion). Protein ingestion enhances glucagon release as well as insulin release. This simultaneous secretion of insulin and glucagon allows cells to use and store glucose without severely decreasing plasma glucose levels. Glucagon is also released during exercise and helps prevent hypoglycemia despite enhanced glucose use by muscle. Glucagon can also be given by injection for the treatment of hypoglycemia.

Somatostatin

Somatostatin is a small polypeptide with a short (2-minute) half-life; it has many inhibitory actions. Somatostatin is released after ingestion of a meal and inhibits the release of both insulin and glucagon. The net action of somatostatin is to delay nutrient absorption by the GI tract, thus prolonging the duration of intestinal food absorption after a meal.

ADRENAL GLANDS

Adrenal Cortex
Aldosterone

The primary mineralocorticoid secreted by the adrenal cortex is aldosterone. About 50% of aldosterone is free in the plasma; the remainder is bound. Aldosterone is degraded in the liver and is excreted in the urine and feces as a glucuronide or sulfate. Infusion of aldosterone causes a drop in plasma potassium levels by increasing renal excretion of potassium in exchange for sodium. Plasma potassium concentration is the primary regulator of aldosterone release through a negative feedback control mechanism. Angiotensin II can also promote aldosterone synthesis and release, and adrenocorticotropic hormone (ACTH) has a permissive role in aldosterone production and secretion.

Cortisol

The primary glucocorticoid secreted by the adrenal cortex is cortisol. Following secretion, 94% of cortisol is bound in the plasma to transcortin, a cortisol-binding globulin, and 6% is free. Cortisol is degraded in the liver and is excreted in the urine and feces as a glucuronide or sulfate. Cortisol is a potent metabolic regulatory hormone, increasing plasma glucose level and promoting use of alternate metabolic substrates for energy (discussed later). Cortisol stimulates appetite and leads to deposition of fat in some central adipose tissues despite the use of fat from peripheral tissues (see the clinical description of Cushing's syndrome). Metabolic changes in cortisol assist the transition to nonglucose support of metabolism in starvation.

Cortisol release is regulated by a hypothalamus-pituitary-adrenal cascade. The hypothalamus secretes corticotropin-releasing hormone (CRH), which is carried by the hypothalamo-hypophyseal portal system to the anterior pituitary gland, where it stimulates ACTH release. ACTH travels in the blood to the adrenal gland, where it promotes conversion of cholesterol to pregnenolone, the rate-limiting step in adrenal glucocorticoid and androgen secretion. Because of a common synthetic pathway, pituitary ACTH also stimulates adrenal androgen production.

The release of ACTH coincides with the release of other compounds formed from the same pre-prohormone. These include (1) melanocyte-stimulating hormone (which stimulates pigment production in epidermal cells), (2) beta-lipotropin (which may stimulate aldosterone release), and (3) the opiate beta-endorphin.

Cortisol is generally described as a stress hormone. Painful stimuli promote release of CRH from the hypothalamus. Emotional stress generated in the limbic system also promotes hypothalamic release of CRH. Cortisol has significant anti-inflammatory effects, retarding the development and enhancing the resolution of the inflammatory response. Therefore glucocorticoids are used as anti-inflammatory agents. Glucocorticoid secretion exhibits a strong diurnal rhythm, which is highest in the early morning and lowest in the late evening.

Adrenal Medulla

The adrenal medulla secretes the catecholamines epinephrine and norepinephrine, whose actions mimic those of the sympathetic nervous system but have a longer duration. Epinephrine and norepinephrine have strong beta$_1$-adrenergic effects and are potent stimulators of heart rate and contractility. Epinephrine has strong metabolic effects and increases the metabolic rate by up to 100%. These effects include increasing metabolic substrates in the plasma by lipolysis and glycogenolysis (discussed later).

Gonads

The sex hormones have important trophic and metabolic effects. The synthetic pathways for estrogens and androgens share many common precursors with each other and with the adrenal cortical steroids. Consequently, sex hormones originate predominantly from the gonads but are secreted in lower amounts from the adrenal glands.

Androgens, primarily testosterone, have a potent anabolic action and are the primary "steroid" abused by athletes. Testosterone is controlled by the hypothalamic-pituitary axis. Gonadotropin-releasing hormone (GnRH) causes luteinizing hormone (LH) to be released from the hypothalamus, and LH acts on the Leydig cells of the testes to promote testosterone synthesis and release. The reproductive significance of testosterone is discussed in the Unit 9 Anatomy and Physiology Review. A secondary effect of testosterone is to promote protein synthesis as well as the musculoskeletal growth that accompanies puberty.

In the female, LH also stimulates androgen production in the ovarian thecal cells, but the aromatase enzyme of the ovarian granulosa cells converts the androgens into the estrogen estradiol. The puberty-related increase in musculoskeletal growth and the onset of menstruation are results of increases in the cyclic release of estrogen and progesterone (see the Unit 9 Anatomy and Physiology Review).

METABOLIC SUBSTRATES

Plasma Glucose

Glucose is the primary metabolic substrate for the body. The plasma glucose level is normally about 100 mg/dl in both the fed and fasted states. Glucose entry into most cells is insulin dependent. One notable exception is the brain; cerebral glucose utilization is independent of insulin and requires a plasma glucose level of only 60 mg/dl; levels below this will disrupt brain function and stimulate the sympathetic nervous system to restore blood flow to the brain.

Plasma glucose represents the balance between glucose absorption from the diet, movement into and out of storage pools, and utilization by the tissues. Glucose storage pools include glycogen, the glycerol component of fat, and amino acids. Although only insulin acts to decrease plasma glucose levels, the hormones glucagon, cortisol, growth hormone, and epinephrine all can elevate plasma glucose levels. This multiple endocrine control allows protection of one or more glucose storage pools (Figure A&P10-6). For example, glucagon mobilizes all storage pools, resulting in increased plasma glucose level. Growth hormone prevents gluconeogenesis but increases glucose level by the other mechanisms. Cortisol preserves glycogen and fat stores in the center of the body but mobilizes all other glucose pools, including gluconeogenesis. Epinephrine mobilizes fat and glycogen pools.

After a meal, excess plasma glucose is moved into storage, facilitated by insulin. During periods of fasting, glucose is moved from the storage pools, first from glycogen, then from fats, and—if the fast is sufficiently long—then from the amino acid pools.

Plasma Amino Acids

Plasma amino acid levels are not controlled by a tight negative feedback mechanism. Ingestion of a protein-rich meal, however, increases both insulin and growth

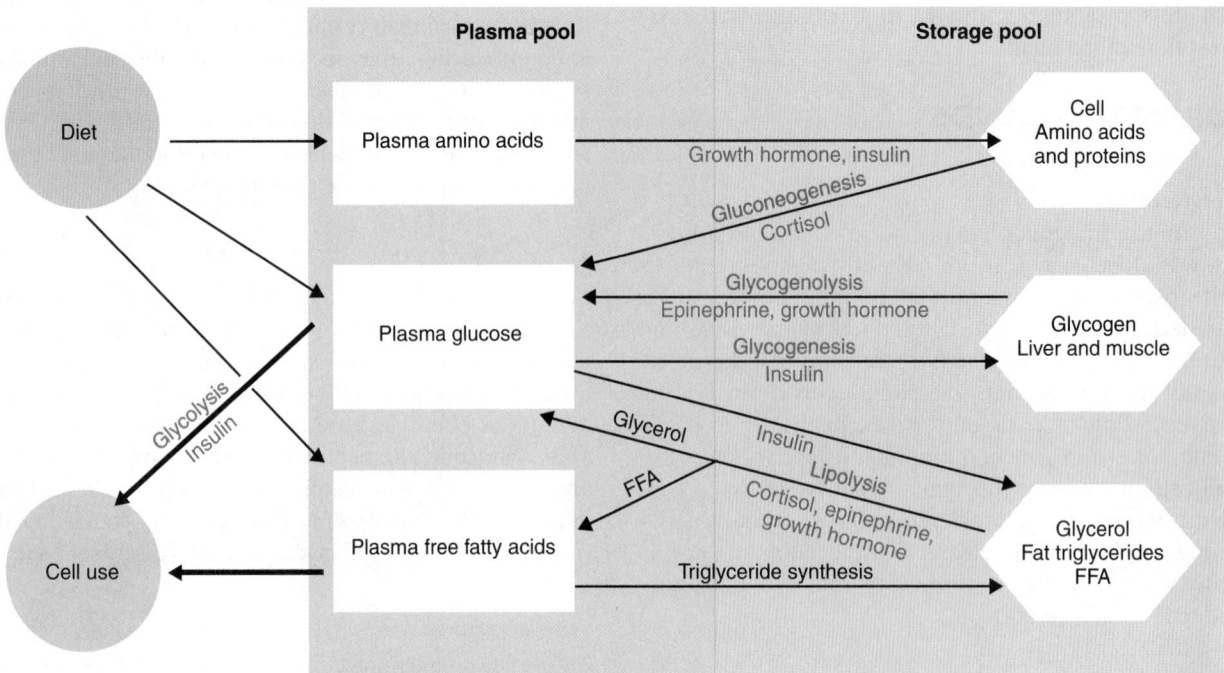

■ **FIGURE A&P10–6** Regulation of metabolic substrates. Cells consume glucose or fatty acids to support metabolism. Plasma glucose is regulated by multiple endocrine mechanisms, which act primarily on the movement into and out of storage pools. Glucose is stored if the plasma glucose level is greater than 110 mg/dl; glucose is mobilized from storage pools if the plasma glucose level is less than 90 mg/dl. *FFA*, free fatty acid.

hormone levels. Growth hormone alone enhances cellular uptake of amino acids and preserves amino acid stores (by blocking gluconeogenesis) when insulin level is not elevated. When insulin level is also elevated, the combined action of growth hormone and insulin greatly enhances uptake of amino acids.

Plasma Free Fatty Acids

Free fatty acids are the baseline metabolic substrate and are used unless insulin shifts metabolism to glucose as a metabolic fuel. The heart in particular can oxidize free fatty acids and thus is not as dependent as the remainder of the body to use glucose as a metabolic substrate. In the American diet, food is ingested with sufficient frequency that insulin levels are high, and glucose is normally used as the metabolic fuel. When metabolized, fatty acids are incompletely oxidized, however, with ketone bodies produced as a metabolic by-product.

Plasma levels of free fatty acids are not controlled by a tight negative feedback mechanism. A drop in plasma glucose levels, however, causes the release of epinephrine, cortisol, and growth hormone, all of which promote lipolysis. This results in the movement of fatty acids from the storage pool in fat cells into the plasma pool, providing an alternative substrate for metabolism when glucose availability is limited.

Plasma Calcium

The plasma calcium level (Ca^{2+}) is tightly regulated around 9.4 mg/dl, with a normal range of 9 to 10 mg/dl. About 40% of plasma Ca^{2+} is tightly bound to plasma proteins, and an additional 10% is combined in non-ionized salts with citrate and phosphate. About 5 mg/dl (50%) of plasma Ca^{2+} is free.

More than 99% of calcium within the body is stored in bone, most of it combined with phosphate in hydroxyapatite crystals. Regulation of plasma calcium levels involves balancing dietary absorption, renal excretion, and exchange between the plasma and storage areas. PTH and vitamin D_3 are the major regulators of plasma calcium levels, with a minor role for the hormone calcitonin.

Infusion of PTH results in elevated plasma calcium levels and decreased plasma phosphate levels. The increase in plasma calcium level occurs by enhancing dietary calcium absorption (via vitamin D_3), by decreasing renal calcium excretion, and by mobilizing calcium from the bone storage pools. Plasma calcium concentration is the primary regulator of PTH release. PTH synthesis and release are stimulated by a drop in plasma calcium level and help to regulate calcium levels during pregnancy and lactation. PTH also decreases phosphorus levels by increasing its renal excretion.

Dietary absorption of calcium requires activated vitamin D. Vitamin D can be absorbed from the diet or synthesized through ultraviolet (sun) light action on 7-dehydrocholesterol. Vitamin D is then converted successively in the liver and then in the kidney to 1,25-hydroxycholecalciferol, the active form.

Calcitonin is a polypeptide secreted by the parafollicular C cells of the thyroid gland. Although infusion of calcitonin decreases the plasma calcium concentration, its role in regulating plasma calcium levels is minor.

Alterations in plasma calcium levels produce physiologic changes. Hypocalcemia increases neuronal excitability. Motor neurons exhibit spontaneous depolarizations, leading to tetanic muscular contractions. The hand is particularly susceptible, resulting in carpopedal spasm. Severely low calcium levels can lead to tetany of the heart and dysrhythmias. Hypercalcemia depresses neuronal and muscle activity.

EFFECTS OF AGING

With aging, the functions of the liver, biliary system, and exocrine pancreas all begin to deteriorate. In the liver, the number and size of hepatic cells are reduced, leading to a decreased weight and mass. Fibrotic tissue also increases, leading to a decrease in protein synthesis, liver enzymes, and cholesterol synthesis. The decrease in enzyme activity diminishes the liver's ability to detoxify drugs and increases the risk of toxic levels of a variety of medications in older adults.

The pancreas is also affected by the process of aging, with calcification of the pancreatic vessels, and by changes in the size of the ducts through distention and dilation. These changes lead to decreased production of lipase, resulting in reduced fat absorption and digestion. Older people also may experience a decreased absorption of fat-soluble vitamins and an increase of fat excreted through the feces (steatorrhea).

CONCLUSIONS

Metabolic regulation is a complex body function. The multiple endocrine systems that regulate the availability of metabolic fuels reflect the essential role of glucose and fatty acids in survival. The process is complicated by the fact that the body must cope both with periods of excess nutrients (after a meal) and with prolonged fasting.

BIBLIOGRAPHY

1. Berne, R., et al. (2004). *Physiology* (5th ed.). St. Louis: Mosby.
2. Carroll, R.G. (2007). *Elsevier's integrated physiology*. Philadelphia: Saunders.
3. Kierszenbaum, A.L. (2007). *Histology and cell biology: An introduction to pathology* (2nd ed.). St. Louis: Mosby.
4. Guyton, A., & Hall, J. (2006). *Textbook of medical physiology* (11th ed.). Philadelphia: Saunders.
5. Silverthorn, D. (2006). *Human physiology* (4th ed.). San Francisco, Calif: Pearson Benjamin Cummings.

CHAPTER 42

Assessment of the Endocrine and Metabolic Systems

DIANNE M. SMOLEN

Clients with endocrine or metabolic system disorders may have specific complaints such as nausea, diarrhea, or fatigue. These clients may also have vague, intermittent, generalized manifestations. Because of the different functions of the endocrine glands and the organs of metabolism, and because most glands and organs are relatively inaccessible, there is no single, uniform assessment for clients with endocrine or metabolic disorders. Assessment of clients with such disorders usually focuses on the manifestations of hormone excess or deficiency or metabolic dysfunction. For these reasons it is important to assess the client's presenting clinical manifestations, health history, physical examination, diagnostic tests, and family and social history. After completing a thorough assessment, analyze the data related to the client's current situation.

HISTORY

During the health history interview, help the client sequence the recalled experiences and manifestations. Linking events and clinical manifestations may aid in the diagnostic process.

Biographical and Demographic Data

Note biographical and demographic data, such as the client's age, gender, ethnic background, and geographical residence. Some disorders, such as gallbladder disease, diabetes mellitus, and hepatitis, are associated with age or gender as well as where a person lives. For example, as a person ages, fewer hormones and metabolic secretions may be produced or their effect on target organs may diminish.

Current Health
Chief Complaint

Thorough investigation of the client's chief complaint is necessary for accurate assessment. Ask the client to indicate when the problem began; the onset, duration, intensity, and characteristics of the problem; and any alterations in usual health status. Like gastrointestinal disorders, common manifestations related to endocrine and metabolic disorders may be ambiguous with a puzzling origin.

Clinical Manifestations

During the assessment ask the client about pain, infection/inflammation, gastrointestinal manifestations, skin changes, perfusion problems (bleeding, bruising, or vital sign changes), sensory/mental status changes, visual changes, and urinary/reproductive changes. Figure 42-1 depicts a systematic approach to completion of an expanded assessment of a client with an endocrine or metabolic disorder.

Pain. The client's perception of pain and its description are often helpful in diagnosing the origin of the problem. When discussing pain with a client with a suspected liver, biliary, or endocrine disorder, the pain is often associated with the abdomen. Abdominal pain may be formally described as visceral, parietal, or referred. It is important to have the client describe the character of the pain, location, duration, and any aggravating or alleviating factors.

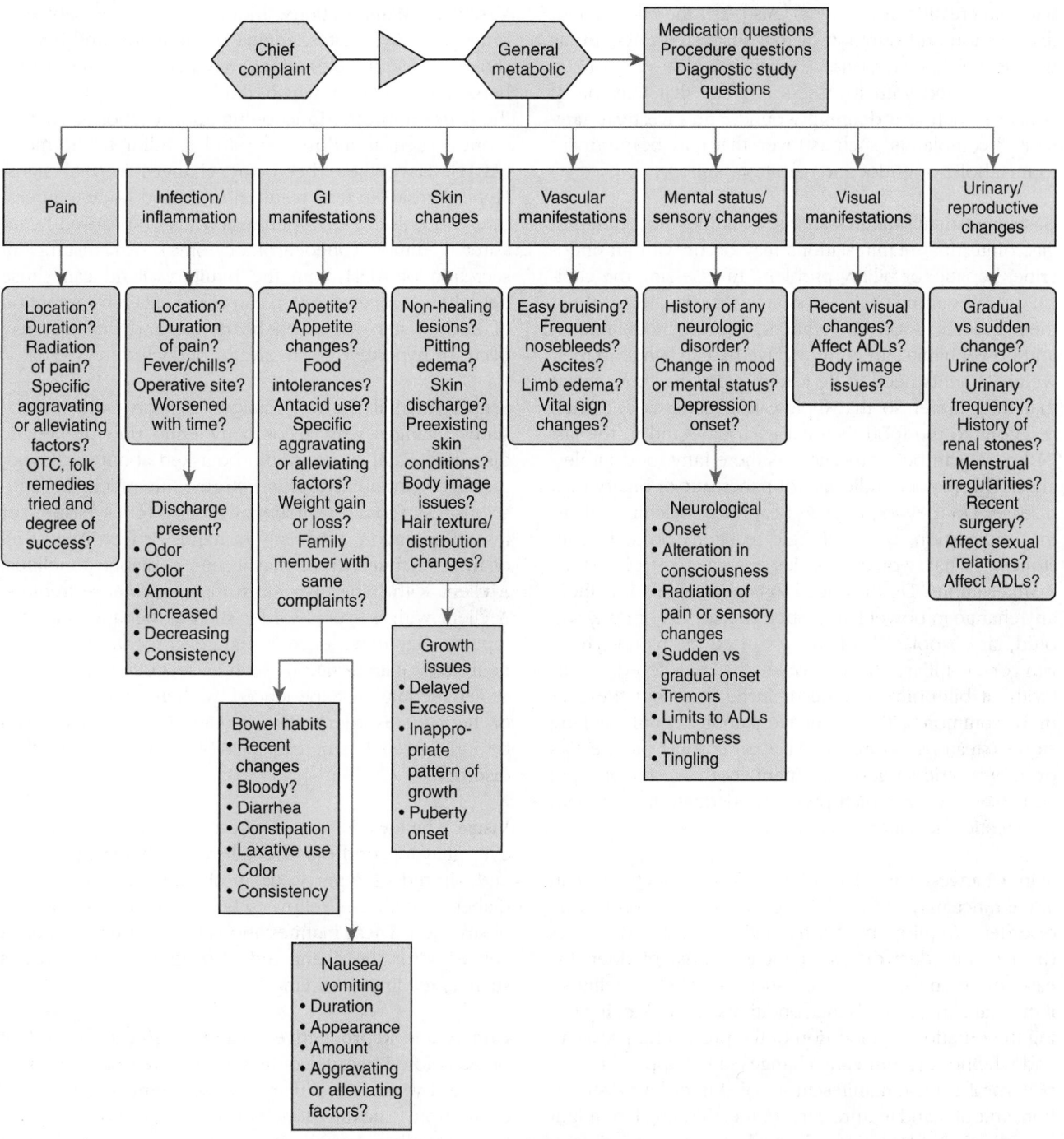

■ **FIGURE 42–1** Expanded metabolic assessment.

If pain is radiating to the back, it can be a manifestation of a pancreatic, gallbladder, or biliary tract disorder.

Visceral pain is characterized as dull, aching, burning, cramping, or colicky. Visceral pain is poorly defined or localized and occurs when the intestines become distended or contract forcefully. It may also occur when the capsules of solid organs such as the liver and spleen are stretched. Parietal pain occurs when the parietal peritoneum becomes inflamed such as in peritonitis or appendicitis. Parietal pain is characterized by more severe and

steady pain. Referred pain is the type of pain that travels or is referred from the primary site to a distant site. Referred pain occurs at a distant site that is innervated at approximately the same levels as the disrupted abdominal organ.

Infection/Inflammation. An infection (involves a pathogenic agent) or inflammation (tissue reaction to injury) may involve the gallbladder, pancreas, or liver. Ask the client if an infection or inflammation is suspected and if there has been a previous similar problem (such as with pancreatitis or hepatitis). Also, ask the client about the location and duration of that suspected infection as well as the character, onset, duration, and severity of factors associated with it. Assess any site that may be of concern, such as a draining wound, and investigate any related complaints, such as fever, that may be pertinent to metabolic or endocrine manifestations.

Gastrointestinal Manifestations. Multiple and different gastrointestinal manifestations may occur with an endocrine, hepatic, or biliary problem. In assessing the clinical manifestations it is important to ask clients about their appetite, food intolerances, nausea and vomiting, and bowel habits, and if they have had a change in their weight. Clients need to be asked questions about foods that they prefer so that their eating patterns and their reactions to the food they eat each day (and in the last 24 hours) can be established. Is there fatty food intolerance? This may be indicative of pancreatic or biliary tract disease. Do they experience heartburn, belching, bloating, indigestion, or an allergic reaction (possible gallstones)? What worsens or lessens the gastrointestinal manifestations? Do they need to take an antacid? Is there any change in bowel habits such as diarrhea or dark-colored, tarry stools? This may be caused by hyperthyroidism or a biliary tract problem. Clay-colored stools (without bilirubin) may occur in hepatitis but they are more common with obstructive jaundice. Foul-smelling stools (steatorrhea) may occur with chronic pancreatitis or after gastric surgery; it is partially the result of rapid gastric emptying, which prevents adequate mixing with pancreatic and biliary secretions.

Skin Changes. Disorders of the skin with changes in appearance may occur with hepatic, biliary, or endocrine disorders. Inquire about a history of systemic disorders (liver or bile duct disease, pancreatitis, gallbladder disease, or an endocrine disease such as diabetes mellitus); if there are any pre-existing conditions of the skin, including the duration and location of the presenting problem; and whether there are any changes in the appearance or pattern of clinical manifestations of skin or hair distribution, amount, and texture. Dry, brittle, thinning hair might be indicative of hypothyroidism while soft, silky hair may indicate hyperthyroidism. The Integrating Diagnostic Testing feature on p. 1009 provides a flow chart for further diagnostic evaluation of the client with metabolic condition–related skin changes. Ask the client if the skin has been jaundiced (viral hepatitis, cirrhosis, and obstructive or cholestatic liver disease), if blisters have appeared, or if a lesion has not healed (diabetes mellitus). Note any changes in pigmentation of the skin (hyperpigmentation suggests Addison's disease; hypopigmentation is vitiligo, an endocrine condition) or if the hands, head, feet, and face have enlarged (may suggest acromegaly, an endocrine problem).

Vascular Manifestations. Inquire about nosebleeds, bruising easily, ascites, edema of the limbs, and hemorrhoids. These manifestations may occur as a result of a hepatic disorder in which fluid overload results from the liver's improper functioning and metabolism of hormones, such as aldosterone and antidiuretic hormone (ADH). Have there been any changes in vital signs? Hyperthyroidism may result in increased body temperature and pulse rate. Hypertension may be caused by an adrenal tumor (pheochromocytoma). An insufficient secretion of ADH from the pituitary gland can cause dehydration; oversecretion can cause excessive retention of body water. Increased heart rate and flushing may occur in hyperthyroidism and in pheochromocytoma.

Sensory/Mental Status Changes. Sensory and mental status changes may accompany endocrine or hepatic disorders. Each client should be asked about weakness, increased irritability, any extreme alteration in consciousness (coma), emotional lability (cries easily), or loss of sensation, especially in hands or feet. Any or all of these manifestations may occur in diabetes mellitus. A client with hyperthyroidism may experience tremors. A client with a liver disorder such as hepatic encephalopathy may experience a change in mental status and neurologic manifestations such as seizures or coma.

Fatigue may be experienced by clients with endocrine or hepatic disorders. Pain radiating to the back can be indicative of pancreatic, gallbladder, or biliary tract disorder.

Visual Changes. Visual manifestations such as bulging eyes may occur from the effects of hyperthyroidism, and blurred or other visual problems may occur from diabetes mellitus. Yellow sclera may indicate biliary obstruction. These manifestations may cause body image concerns for the client and also affect daily activities such as reading or driving.

Urinary and Reproductive Changes. Urine may be dark or tea colored because of impaired excretion of bilirubin caused by hepatocellular disease. Renal calculi may occur from calcium stone formation caused by hyperparathyroidism. Irregularities in the menstrual cycle, loss of libido, impotence or infertility, and loss or premature development of secondary sexual characteristics may occur with an endocrine disorder. Increased frequency of urination may be caused by diabetes mellitus or diabetes insipidus.

Review of Systems

If an endocrine or metabolic disorder is suspected, a thorough assessment is important because endocrine and metabolic disorders can affect multiple areas of the body. During the review ask about questions relevant to past

INTEGRATING DIAGNOSTIC TESTING

Skin Disorders

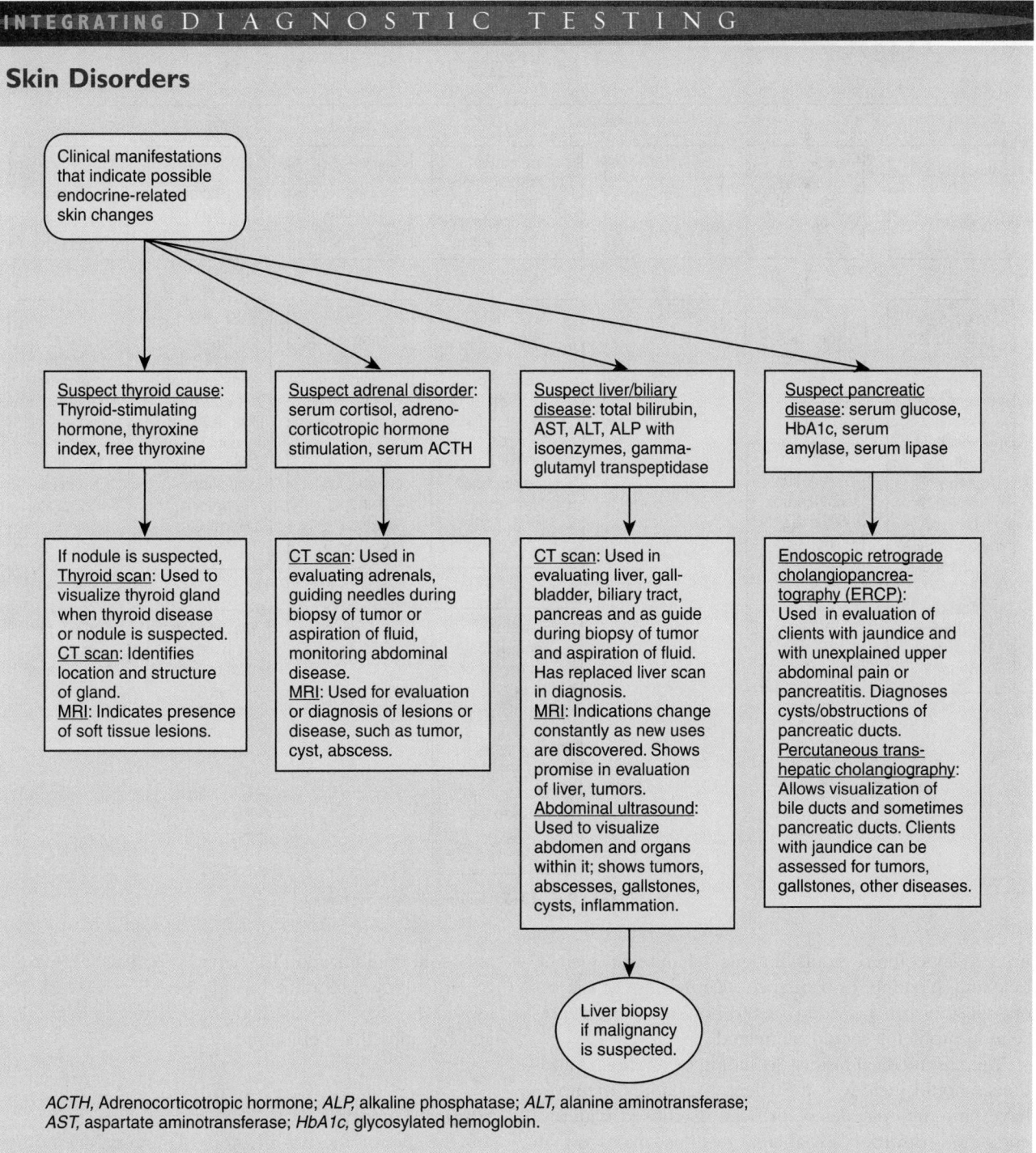

Clinical manifestations that indicate possible endocrine-related skin changes

Suspect thyroid cause: Thyroid-stimulating hormone, thyroxine index, free thyroxine

Suspect adrenal disorder: serum cortisol, adrenocorticotropic hormone stimulation, serum ACTH

Suspect liver/biliary disease: total bilirubin, AST, ALT, ALP with isoenzymes, gamma-glutamyl transpeptidase

Suspect pancreatic disease: serum glucose, HbA1c, serum amylase, serum lipase

If nodule is suspected, <u>Thyroid scan</u>: Used to visualize thyroid gland when thyroid disease or nodule is suspected. <u>CT scan</u>: Identifies location and structure of gland. <u>MRI</u>: Indicates presence of soft tissue lesions.

<u>CT scan</u>: Used in evaluating adrenals, guiding needles during biopsy of tumor or aspiration of fluid, monitoring abdominal disease. <u>MRI</u>: Used for evaluation or diagnosis of lesions or disease, such as tumor, cyst, abscess.

<u>CT scan</u>: Used in evaluating liver, gallbladder, biliary tract, pancreas and as guide during biopsy of tumor and aspiration of fluid. Has replaced liver scan in diagnosis. <u>MRI</u>: Indications change constantly as new uses are discovered. Shows promise in evaluation of liver, tumors. <u>Abdominal ultrasound</u>: Used to visualize abdomen and organs within it; shows tumors, abscesses, gallstones, cysts, inflammation.

<u>Endoscopic retrograde cholangiopancreatography (ERCP)</u>: Used in evaluation of clients with jaundice and with unexplained upper abdominal pain or pancreatitis. Diagnoses cysts/obstructions of pancreatic ducts. <u>Percutaneous transhepatic cholangiography</u>: Allows visualization of bile ducts and sometimes pancreatic ducts. Clients with jaundice can be assessed for tumors, gallstones, other diseases.

Liver biopsy if malignancy is suspected.

ACTH, Adrenocorticotropic hormone; *ALP,* alkaline phosphatase; *ALT,* alanine aminotransferase; *AST,* aspartate aminotransferase; *HbA1c,* glycosylated hemoglobin.

medical history, past surgical/procedure history, allergies, prescription medications, over-the-counter (OTC) medications, nutraceuticals, dietary habits, social history, and family history.

Specifically, inquire about clinical manifestations that are related to the metabolic and endocrine disorders that could contribute to the current chief complaint. Investigate any reported complaint and inquire about the effect of the problem on the client's daily life. Figure 42-2 offers a guide to collecting an expanded metabolic or endocrine history.

Past Medical History and Recent Hospitalizations

It is important to know if a client has a history of hospitalizations or treatment for metabolic disorders involving the liver, gallbladder, or exocrine pancreas (such as jaundice, abdominal swelling [ascites] or pain, dark-colored

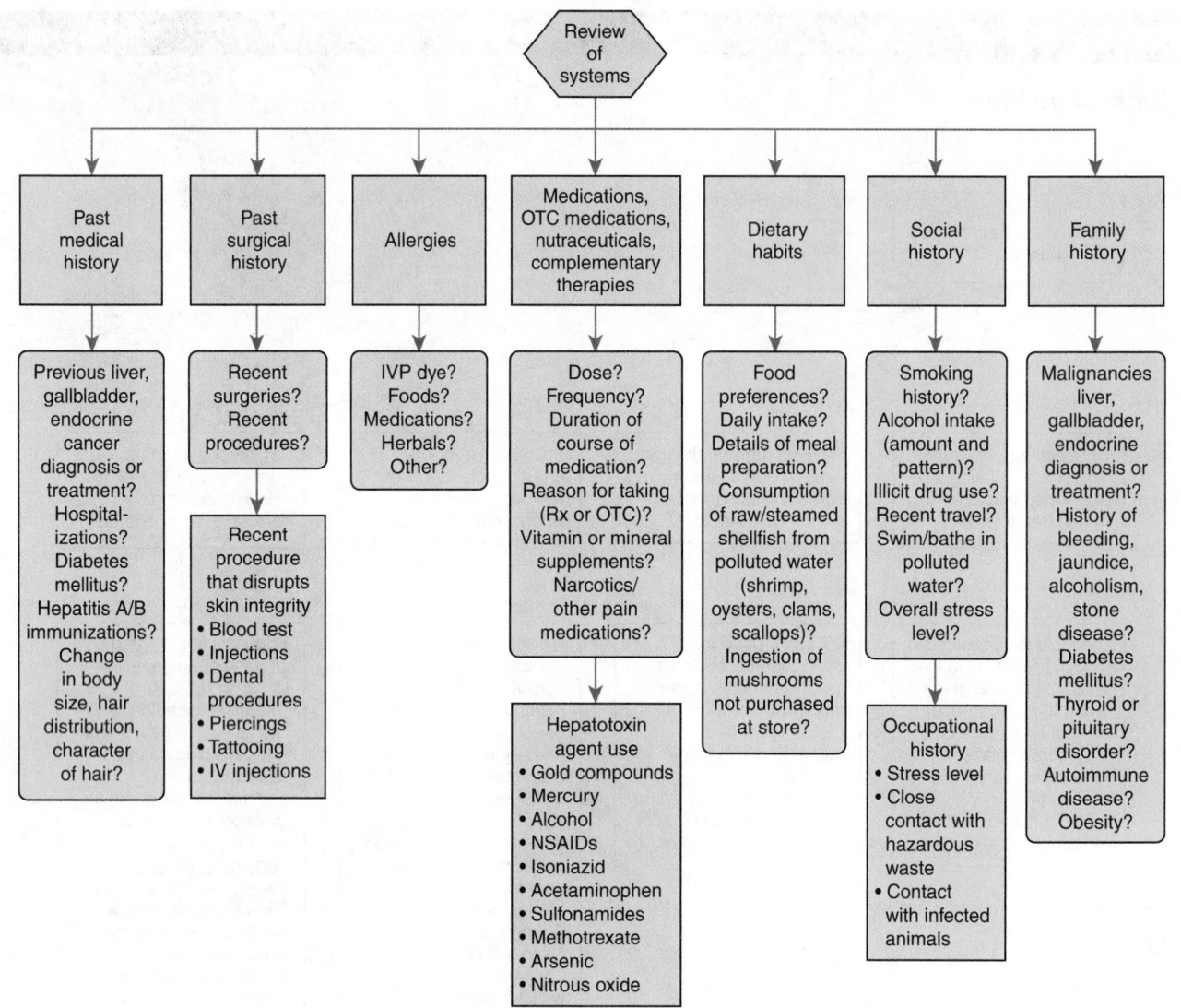

■ **FIGURE 42–2** Expanded metabolic history.

urine, clay-colored stools, fatigue, change in weight, belching, bloating, or flatulence). Knowledge of the client's history can provide clues to how the current presenting problems should be treated.

The past medical history, including recent hospitalizations, should include if the client and family members have had any episodes of or been diagnosed with any endocrine disorders. Diabetes mellitus may run in families. A history of trauma as a child or adolescent is important in that trauma to the head can lead to hypopituitarism. A history of excessive urination and thirst (diabetes mellitus), growth patterns that were different from those of other members of the family, changes in the amount and distribution of hair, or excessive growth in extremities (hands, feet, or head) may all indicate endocrine disorders.

The client's immunization status is important. It is important to know if the client has been immunized against hepatitis A or B or has ever received post-

exposure immunization for hepatitis A. This information is particularly important for any health care worker or those who live in areas of the world where hepatitis A and hepatitis B are epidemic.

Surgical History

Ask the client if there is a history of surgery, chemotherapy, or radiation therapy for a metabolic or endocrine disorder, especially to the head or neck. Radiation, in particular, may cause functional problems with the thyroid gland. If any disorder involved surgery or a biopsy, this information is important in order to assess for recurrences. Information about any diagnostic procedures that were performed can be helpful. Procedures such as scans (hepatoiminodiacetic acid [HIDA]), blood work, and endoscopic retrograde cholangiopancreatography (ERCP) may be helpful in deciding if more invasive treatment, such as surgery, is indicated. It is also helpful to know if any of the procedures (for example, biopsies, ultrasounds, or other procedures) caused problems. For example, a procedure such as ERCP may cause pancreatitis.

Has the client had recent blood tests, transfusions of blood products, dental procedures, ear or other body piercing, tattooing, or any intravenous injection with a potentially contaminated needle? Note such procedures in an assessment, because breaks in the skin may be the route of entry for hepatitis virus (type B or C) or other pathogens.

Allergies

The client needs to identify any known allergies to food or medications. Specifically ask about reactions to iodine. Iodine is contained in contrast media used in some diagnostic studies of the metabolic system.

Medications

Ask specifically about the use of hormones and steroids, including name, dose, and duration of use. Does the client have a history of taking anabolic steroids? Ask about medications that the client is currently taking or has taken previously, including over-the-counter drugs. Many drugs and chemicals are potentially hepatotoxic, such as alcohol, gold compounds, mercury, phosphorus, anabolic steroids, acetaminophen, isoniazid, halothane, sulfonamides, arsenic, thiazide diuretics, zidovudine (azidothymidine), and anticancer drugs, such as methotrexate. Other medications to ask about are oral contraceptives, anesthetic agents, and antipsychotic agents. If the client abruptly stopped taking corticosteroids, the client may be at risk for acute adrenal insufficiency.

Ask about the use of alternative therapies, such as herbal medicines. Herbal medicines used in the treatment of type 1 diabetes mellitus include aloe vera juice, beans (*Phaseolus* species), bitter gourd, karela (*Momordica charantia*), black tea (*Camellia sinensis*), fenugreek (*Trigonella foenum-graecum*), gurmar (*Gymnema sylvestre*), macadamia nut, and Madagascar periwinkle (*Catharanthus roseus*). Effects of some herbs include lowering of blood pressure (fenugreek), a boosting of insulin production (gurmar), and increased use of available insulin (black tea).

Kelp (*Fucus vesiculosus*) may help with weight loss in hypothyroid disorders. Milk thistle (*Silybum marianum*) is used for treatment and prophylaxis of chronic hepatotoxicity, inflammatory liver disorders, and certain types of cirrhosis.

Dietary Habits

A review of dietary habits can point out potential precipitating and aggravating factors as well as alleviating factors. Certain foods are known to cause bloating (gaseous abdominal distention), flatulence (passage of intestinal gas through the anus), belching (eructation or gas through the mouth), heartburn (a sensation of burning or warmth in the retrosternal region between the xiphoid and the manubrium), and indigestion (involves reflux esophagitis). For example, acidic food, large meals, and fatty foods are known to be a precipitating cause of bloating, flatulence, belching, indigestion, and heartburn as well as pain in the gallbladder area.

Social History

The client's use and pattern of alcohol intake, cigarette smoking, and recreational drug use is important information to assess. Pay attention to alcohol use because alcoholism often accompanies liver and pancreatic disease. Use of any items with the blood or body fluids of a person with hepatitis B and hepatitis C viruses is a known risk factor. The sexual history of a client may also reveal the possible sources of infection with the hepatitis virus.

Ask about the client's occupation and work environment. Does the client report being exposed to factors that are known to cause liver damage (hepatotoxins) such as mercury and lead, anesthetic agents such as nitrous oxide, and chemicals such as carbon tetrachloride and certain pesticides? Does the client engage in activities that increase the risk of exposure to substances that cause hepatitis or pancreatitis?

Ask the client about the home and work environment. Assessment of the psychosocial history and lifestyle patterns provides data about the client's physical and psychological status. Working or living in a stressful environment may increase the severity of disorders such as diabetes mellitus. Does the client report engaging in a healthy lifestyle that includes exercise and adequate sleep? Diet and physical activity are important in the management of both type 1 and type 2 diabetes mellitus (see Chapter 45). Specifically ask about food, alcohol, illicit drugs, or tobacco products used in order to relax.

Family Health History

When assessing a client with an endocrine or metabolic disorder, inquire about the family history. A number of endocrine disorders are inherited or tend to run in families. Also, ask the client about any malignancies that have occurred. Has any family member had problems similar to those of the client? Do autoimmune problems run in the family, such as Addison's disease?

PHYSICAL EXAMINATION

Physical assessment of endocrine or metabolic (liver, biliary, or pancreatic) dysfunction involves careful examination of the entire body and is integrated throughout the interaction with the client. Refer to an assessment textbook for more specific information on assessing the client with a metabolic and/or endocrine disorder.

The assessment covers general health and nutritional status along with the skin, head, neck, thorax, abdomen, upper and lower extremities, and genitalia. Examine all body systems in a systematic manner from head to toe using inspection, auscultation, percussion, and palpation. Table 42-1 provides details related to the physical assessment of the endocrine and metabolic systems. Before the examination, ask the client to point to any painful area; examine that area last. As stated earlier, hepatic or biliary pain is often located in the right upper quadrant (Figure 42-3).

TABLE 42–1   Key Points of a Physical Examination: *Endocrine and Metabolic Disorders*

Steps	Normal or Common Findings	Significant or Abnormal Findings
Inspection		
Note:		
Color of skin	Same as or lighter than other areas	Redness, cyanosis, jaundice, lesions, ecchymosis, needle marks, or hematomas
Eyes	White sclerae	Sclerae: yellow tint
Symmetry, contour, shape of abdomen	Flat, rounded abdomen	Distended, asymmetrical, masses
Surface of abdomen	Smooth	Tight, shiny; engorged, prominent veins, spider angiomas
Rectal area	No dilated veins (hemorrhoids)	Presence of distended veins (hemorrhoids)
General nutritional state Weigh Observe for ascites	Adequate for height and build	Obesity or malnutrition
Auscultation		
Place stethoscope (warmed) over right upper quadrant; listen for vascular sounds or friction rubs	No venous hums No friction rubs	Venous hum with both diastolic and systolic components
Percussion		
Abdomen: Note percussion sounds in four quadrants	Tympany over abdomen, bladder, intestines, and aorta; dull over liver, spleen, pancreas, kidneys, and uterus	Dullness over enlarged organs; indicates need for further assessment for ascites
Liver: Span; percuss upward from below client's umbilicus on right midclavicular line (MCL) until dullness is heard; mark this point; percuss downward from lung resonance in right MCL to dullness and measure distance between two marks	Liver span is 6-12 cm; no tenderness	Liver span is greater than 12 cm
Note if tender, soft, or firm; smooth or nodular	Slightly tender, soft, smooth surface	Nodular, more than slightly tender, hard
Spleen: Note size; percuss downward in left posterior axillary line, beginning with lung resonance until dullness is heard	Dullness between ribs 6 and 10	Dullness extends above sixth rib or covers large area—indicates enlargement
Palpation		
Use palmar surface of extended fingers		
Liver: Palpate lightly on right side, and then palpate deeply	No tenderness, pain, masses	Tenderness, rigidity, nodules, enlarged
Spleen: Note: If spleen can be percussed, it is best not to palpate it; palpate lightly on left side, distal to MCL	No tenderness, pain, masses	Tenderness, rigidity, nodules, enlarged
Adaptations for Older Adults		
Inspection		
Contour	Sagging and rounded because of loss of muscle tone and accumulation of fat	Right upper quadrant or epigastric pain from liver and biliary tract
Palpation		
Note liver span and borders	Span may be shortened, but border is more easily palpated	Epigastric pain from pancreas, stomach, or duodenum

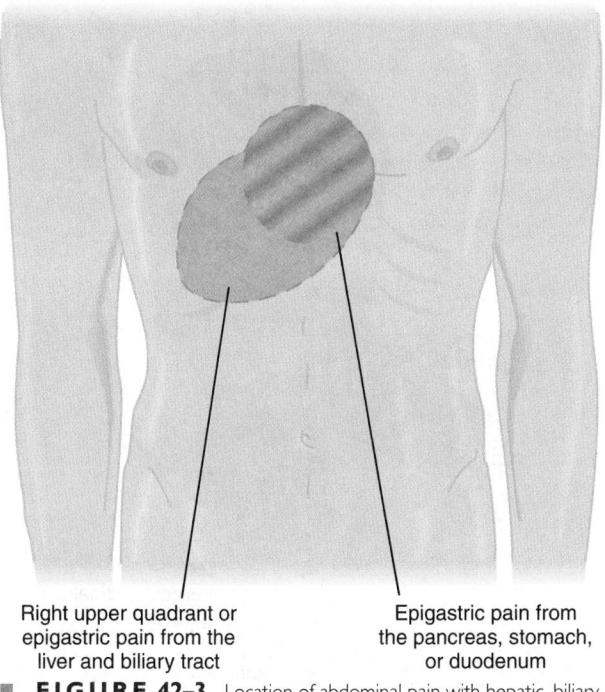

Right upper quadrant or epigastric pain from the liver and biliary tract

Epigastric pain from the pancreas, stomach, or duodenum

■ **FIGURE 42–3**   Location of abdominal pain with hepatic, biliary, or pancreatic disorders.

General Appearance and Nutritional Status

Begin by assessing general appearance and health status. Is the client alert and responding appropriately to questions? Observe the client's mood, level of consciousness (orientation, alertness), verbal and nonverbal behavior, memory, affect, and speech patterns. Note any anxiety or nervousness, depression, apathy, or anger.

Assess nutritional status. Weigh the client and note if the client is very thin or overweight. Obesity may accompany gallbladder disease. Ask whether the client has a pattern of right upper quadrant pain after eating certain high-fat foods (e.g., nuts, chocolate). Chapter 28 describes the assessment of nutrition.

Vital Signs

Measure and assess vital signs. Temperature is elevated in hyperthyroidism or may be low-normal or below normal in hypothyroidism. Observe respirations for altered rate and rhythm. Blood pressure may be elevated or decreased in certain metabolic and endocrine disorders.

Skin (Integument)

Observe hair texture and distribution over body surfaces. Note brittleness or loss of hair (alopecia). Inspect the skin for color, pigmentation, striae, ecchymoses, or mottling. Palpate the skin for texture, thickness, moisture, and diaphoresis. Inspect and palpate the nails for color, texture, brittleness, presence of ridges, and peeling.

Head/Eyes/Nose/Mouth/Neck

Inspect the head for contour, shape, symmetry, and proportion, along with the facial features. Observe skin color for erythema or rash over the cheeks. Observe facial expression for anxiety.

Inspect and palpate the eyebrows, noting hair distribution. Observe eye position, symmetry, shape, and eyelid lag. Note color of sclerae: Are they yellowish or white? If an ophthalmic exam is required, see Chapter 64 for a discussion of how to use an ophthalmoscope and Chapter 45 for a description of retinal changes associated with diabetes mellitus.

Inspect mucosa of the nose for swelling and color. Listen for noisy or labored breathing.

For the mouth, inspect the color of the oral mucosa and the condition of the client's teeth. Note malocclusion. Observe if the client has difficulty chewing.

Listen to the client's voice for hoarseness or huskiness. Note clarity, pitch, and volume of speech. Ask the client to swallow and observe for difficulty or pain in swallowing. Inspect the neck for symmetry, alignment, or bulging over the thyroid gland. For more complete information about examination of the neck, consult a health assessment textbook. See Figure 42-4 for a description of how to palpate the thyroid gland. Refer to the Physical Assessment Findings in the Healthy Adult feature on p. 1014 for an example of documentation for a normal thyroid examination.

Upper and Lower Extremities

Examine the arms and legs for size, shape, and symmetry. Note peripheral edema. Palpate and note peripheral pulse amplitude (see Chapter 2). Assess deep tendon reflexes and observe their relaxation time (see Chapter 67).

For the upper extremities ask the client to extend the hands with palms down; observe for fine tremors and for reddened palms (palmar erythema). Note the size of the hands in proportion to the rest of the body. For the lower extremities note the color and distribution of hair. Assess the size of the client's feet in proportion to the rest of the body. Separate the toes, and observe for deformities and skin changes, such as thickening, fissures, and nail thickening.

Thorax

In males, inspect for gynecomastia (breast enlargement), which can develop because of decreased metabolism of estrogen when the liver is dysfunctional. Auscultate for extra heart sounds, such as a systolic murmur (see Chapter 54).

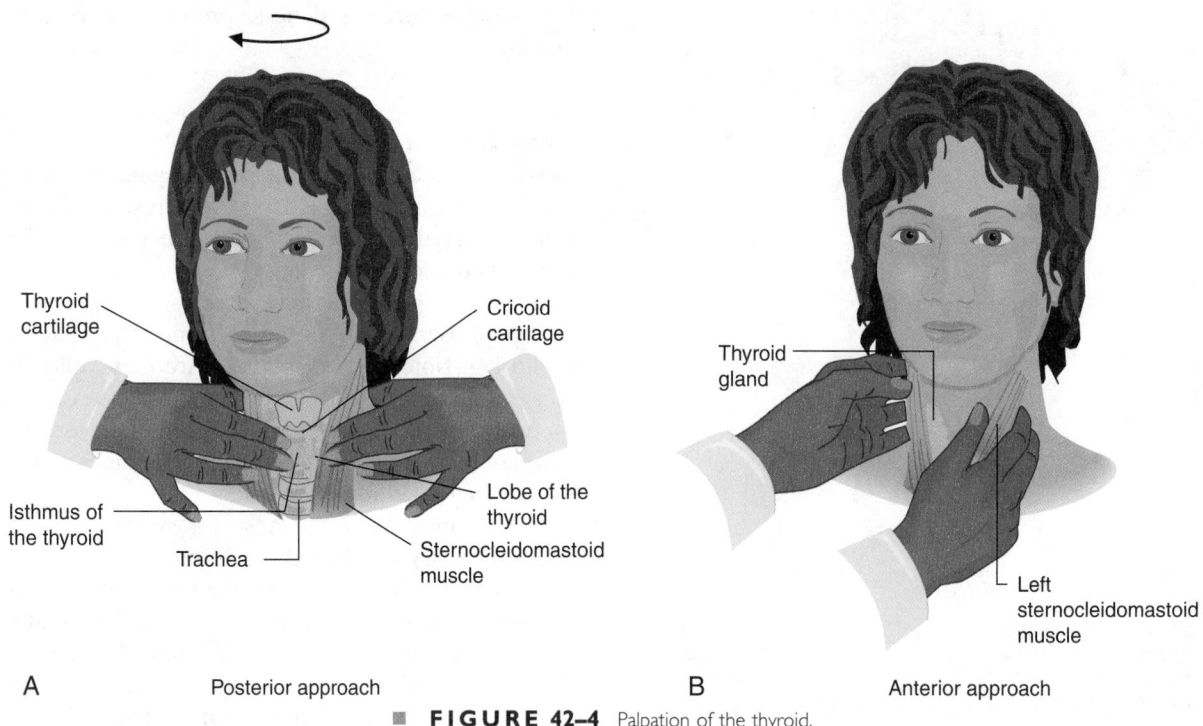

Thyroid cartilage

Cricoid cartilage

Isthmus of the thyroid

Trachea

Lobe of the thyroid

Sternocleidomastoid muscle

Thyroid gland

Left sternocleidomastoid muscle

A   Posterior approach   B   Anterior approach

■ **FIGURE 42–4** Palpation of the thyroid.

Abdomen

Assessment of the abdomen includes inspection, auscultation, percussion, and palpation. As noted previously, examine painful areas last. The key points of a physical examination for endocrine and metabolic disorders, including the abdominal assessment, are detailed in Table 42-1. For more advanced assessment techniques (such as testing for shifting dullness or the fluid wave test), consult a health assessment textbook. Chapter 28 includes a recording of a normal abdominal assessment.

Genitalia and Rectum

Observe the pattern of pubic hair distribution, particularly in women. A diamond-shaped (male) pattern is indicative of a masculinizing tumor. Note the size of the testes in male clients and the clitoris in female clients for comparison with expected norms. The remainder of the endocrine assessment consists of diagnostic studies, because the only endocrine glands accessible to physical examination are the thyroid gland and gonads (see Chapter 37 for further information about assessment of the reproductive system).

Inspect the rectal area for dilated veins (hemorrhoids). These may be present in clients with cirrhosis and portal hypertension.

Modifications for Older Adults

When assessing the older adult client for possible endocrine or metabolic disorders, remember to divide the physical assessment into several parts to avoid fatigue. Allow adequate time for the physical examination so that the information needed is clearly communicated to the client. Speak clearly and distinctly when asking for specific information or giving instructions so that the request is understood and heard.

When inspecting the abdomen, note the contour and color. A rounded, sagging abdomen is a normal finding because of the tendency for fat to accumulate in the lower abdomen and hips and for the abdominal muscles to weaken. Note any areas of tenderness or discomfort because old age may blunt the manifestations of pain caused by peritoneal inflammation, for example (see Table 42-1).

Physical Assessment Findings in the Healthy Adult

The Thyroid Gland*

INSPECTION

The thyroid gland is not normally seen on inspection.

PALPATION

The gland rises and falls with swallowing. Isthmus at midline, soft. Right lobe slightly larger than the left lobe. Texture rubbery without nodules. Nontender.

AUSCULTATION

No bruits heard over either lobe.

*Findings for the metabolic system are found in Chapter 28 as part of the abdominal assessment.

DIAGNOSTIC TESTING

For more detailed information about endocrine function studies and metabolic function studies, please refer to the table on the website titled Diagnostic Imaging and Other Tests for Endocrine and Metabolic Function or to a diagnostic testing textbook.

Noninvasive Endocrine Function Tests
Tests of Thyroid Structure and Function

The thyroid gland can be assessed for size, shape, position, and function by scanning, ultrasound, magnetic resonance imaging (MRI), computed tomography (CT), radionuclide imaging, fine needle aspiration, and testing the Achilles tendon reflexes.

Radioiodine Uptake

The body cannot distinguish between radiolabeled ("tagged") iodine and nonradiolabeled iodine. Consequently, the thyroid absorbs radioactive iodine and processes it just as it does regular iodine. Radioiodine is excreted in the urine just as is ordinary iodine. The laboratory may measure the client's urine output of radioactive iodine after the test. Many factors can distort findings. Consult a diagnostic testing textbook to determine what questions need to be asked of the client.

Tests of Adrenal Structure and Function

The adrenal cortex can be assessed for lesions or disease by CT, MRI, adrenal venogram, and angiography.

Tests of Pituitary Structure and Function

The structure of the pituitary gland can be assessed by skull x-ray study, CT, or MRI. Tumors of the pituitary may be visualized with these studies.

Metabolic Function Studies

Abdominal Ultrasonography. Ultrasonographic examination provides valuable diagnostic information about liver, pancreatic, and biliary tract conditions. The technique is rapid, and little or no preparation is required. Depending on the area to be examined, the client may or may not fast before the procedure. Reassure the client that the test is painless and safe. There are no specific precautions or observations after ultrasonography.

Radiography. Many procedures used to diagnose disorders of the liver, pancreas, and biliary tract involve the use of x-rays. Plain x-ray films of the abdomen may show diaphragm elevation caused by hepatic enlargement or calcification in the abdominal organs. Upper or lower gastrointestinal series using barium contrast medium also provide important information about the accessory organs of digestion (liver, gallbladder, and pancreas). Spot x-ray films are obtained to detect pancreatic and duodenal diseases (tumor at the head of the pancreas or a stricture caused by chronic pancreatitis).

Radiologic studies with iodinated contrast media permit visualization of tubes and vessels. Before any of these procedures are performed, question the client about known hypersensitivity to iodine.

Computed Tomography. CT is used to identify and evaluate liver, biliary tract, gallbladder, and pancreatic disorders. It is useful for distinguishing cysts or tumors and differentiating obstructive from nonobstructive jaundice (Figure 42-5). The client is instructed to fast, except for having water, before the test.

Invasive Endocrine Function Tests
Angiography

Angiography allows visualization of the hepatic, biliary, and pancreatic arterial vessels after administration of contrast medium. It is used to identify abnormalities of vascular structure and function, observe masses, and note bleeding sites in the pancreas, spleen, and portal system.

Portal Pressure Measurement

Measurements of portal pressure and flow help to (1) diagnose portal hypertension, (2) indicate the severity of portal hypertension, and (3) guide decisions about appropriate intervention, which may include surgery. Also, the indirect calculation of sinusoid pressure helps determine the location of an obstruction in the liver and thus identify the underlying disorder. Normal portal pressure is 5 to 10 mm Hg.

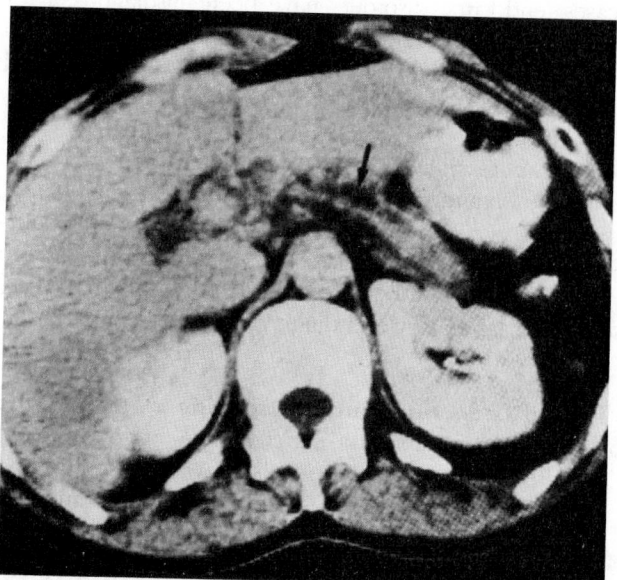

■ **FIGURE 42–5** Computed tomography scan showing chronic pancreatitis.

Biopsy

Biopsy is the single most valuable diagnostic study because it is often the determining factor for the final diagnosis. It involves removal of a sample of living tissue for analysis. Biopsies may be open or closed procedures. An open biopsy necessitates a general anesthetic and a major abdominal incision. A closed biopsy, or percutaneous liver biopsy, is performed to aspirate a core of tissue via needle for histologic study. The biopsy is usually a "blind" procedure (Menghini's technique) performed using local anesthesia and a transpleural or subcostal approach. The primary disadvantage of Menghini's technique is that the surgeon cannot see where the needle is going.

Paracentesis

Paracentesis is used to (1) extract fluid accumulation in the peritoneum (ascites), (2) relieve intra-abdominal tension, which can impair the client's respiratory status, or (3) obtain fluid for culture. See a diagnostic testing textbook for specific information on this test.

Laboratory Tests

A client with an endocrine dysfunction may need several general types of diagnostic tests. Blood levels of various hormones specific to the endocrine glands are measured. Some hormones are measured for specific levels; others, such as thyroid hormone, are measured according to how well they combine with plasma proteins or radioactive iodine. The Laboratory Tests for Endocrine and Metabolic Function table on the website describes common laboratory tests of endocrine function (pancreas, thyroid, parathyroid, adrenal, and pituitary), and metabolic function (liver, biliary, and exocrine pancreas). The client may be anxious about the tests and the possible results. In many cases, endocrine disorders have been misdiagnosed for years because of the nonspecific manifestations of the disorders. After the correct diagnosis is made, the client and family may need help coping with ongoing care.

Similarly, a client with a metabolic dysfunction (exocrine pancreas, liver, or biliary tract) frequently requires multiple diagnostic measures. No single laboratory test, radiographic study, or surgical procedure yields sufficient data to confirm a diagnosis or establish the degree of malfunction. For the specifics of sample handling, consult a laboratory and diagnostic testing textbook.

Tests of Endocrine Pancreas Function

Diagnostic assessment of pancreatic endocrine function is related to blood glucose levels. Elevated fasting blood glucose concentration is usually the first indication of hyperglycemia. Glycosylated hemoglobin (HbA_{1C}), or glycohemoglobin, is a measure of the average blood glucose level over 3 months and can be obtained in the nonfasting state. A more detailed presentation of diagnostic tests related to diabetes mellitus can be found in Chapter 45.

Tests of Thyroid Function

Several tests are available to assess thyroid function. A brief overview of the most common laboratory tests follows. For more details, refer to the Laboratory Tests for Endocrine and Metabolic Function on the website.

Serum Thyroid-Stimulating Hormone. Measurement of the basal serum thyroid-stimulating hormone (TSH) concentration is useful in differentiating primary and secondary hypothyroidism. In primary hypothyroidism, the thyroid gland compensates for a functional abnormality that impairs the ability to synthesize hormones. This results in hypersecretion of TSH. In contrast, the serum TSH concentration is almost always low or undetectable in secondary and tertiary hypothyroidism.

Antithyroid Antibody Tests. Many thyroid disorders are presumed to have an autoimmune basis, such as Hashimoto's thyroiditis, some types of myxedema, and Graves' disease (a form of hyperthyroidism). Serologic tests may be performed to determine whether the client's blood contains antithyroid antibodies.

Serum Thyroxine and Triiodothyronine. Radioimmunoassay can be used to measure triiodothyronine (T_3). Hyperthyroidism, viral hepatitis, pregnancy, and oral contraceptives increase the levels of serum thyroxine (T_4); hypothyroidism, strenuous exercise, heparin, and lithium decrease serum T_4 levels.

Analysis of T_3 and T_4 concentrations has largely replaced the older technique of estimating basal metabolic rate (BMR). BMR is calculated by measuring the amount of oxygen the body consumes when in a state of complete mental and physical relaxation.

T_3 Resin Uptake. If thyroid function is below normal or if serum protein levels are high, resin uptake of T_3 is depressed. If thyroid function is above normal or serum protein levels are low, resin uptake of T_3 is elevated.

Serum Cholesterol. The serum cholesterol level may be elevated in primary hypothyroidism, which may explain why this condition is accompanied by a marked tendency toward atherosclerosis. People with hyperthyroidism usually have a lower serum cholesterol level. Serum cholesterol level is not a specific test of thyroid function, however, because its levels are influenced by many factors other than thyroid hormone levels.

Tests of Parathyroid Function

Measurements of serum calcium, phosphorus, serum alkaline phosphatase, parathyroid hormone, and osteocalcin concentrations are important to evaluate because of the relationship between the parathyroid and thyroid glands.

Tests of Adrenal Function

Adrenal function tests may be used to evaluate medullary and cortical hormones and their metabolites by assessing both serum and urine specimens. Adrenocortical hormones include cortisol (glucocorticoid), aldosterone (mineralocorticoid), and small amounts of sex hormones (androgens). Adrenal medullary hormones include epinephrine and norepinephrine (catecholamines).

Aldosterone Levels. Plasma levels of aldosterone, angiotensin II, and renin can be measured at any time. Plasma levels of aldosterone can be increased by administering potassium, restricting sodium, or having the client assume an upright position. Plasma levels of aldosterone can be decreased by infusion of saline.

Serum Cortisol Test/Dexamethasone Suppression. Serum cortisol is measured in clients suspected to have hyperfunctioning or hypofunctioning adrenal glands. Cortisol levels usually increase and decrease during the day in a pattern called the diurnal variation. Cortisol levels are highest around 6 to 8 AM and gradually decrease during the day, reaching their lowest point around midnight.

Consult a laboratory and diagnostic testing textbook for specific information about this test.

Serum Adrenocorticotropic Hormone (ACTH). Serum levels of ACTH can be assessed after infusion of synthetic ACTH. Urine levels of ketosteroid would be expected to increase to 25 mg in 24 hours; plasma levels of cortisol should increase to 10 to 40 mcg/dl. Urine levels of ketosteroid can be measured with 24-hour urine specimens. Ketosteroids are metabolites of the hormones produced by the adrenal cortex. A preservative is required for the collection bottle. If the client has an indwelling catheter, the urinary drainage bag is emptied frequently and the urine is refrigerated.

Plasma Renin Assays. Plasma levels of renin can be used in the differential diagnosis of primary versus secondary hyperaldosteronism.

Urinary Catecholamines. Adrenal medullary function can be assessed through urine levels of catecholamines and their metabolites (vanillylmandelic acid).

Tests of Pituitary Function

Hormone Assays. Hormonal disorders caused by malfunction of the pituitary gland can lead to a wide variety of clinical manifestations, depending on which hormone is involved. Growth hormone (GH) and ADH are presented as examples of hormones secreted by the anterior (GH) and posterior (ADH) lobes of the pituitary gland. See Chapter 44 for further discussion.

Growth Hormone Levels. GH is secreted in a diurnal pattern, and its level can be assayed. Consult a diagnostic and laboratory testing textbook and Chapter 44 for more information.

Metabolic Function Tests

The most common laboratory tests for metabolic function (liver, biliary, and exocrine pancreas) include those used to measure levels of serum enzymes, including bilirubin, proteins, antigens, antibodies, fats, bleeding and clotting factors, and related urine and stool studies. Details on hepatitis virus infection are presented in Chapter 47.

CONCLUSIONS

Once you have gained a thorough knowledge of the structure and function of the endocrine and metabolic organs, you must examine the diagnostic assessment of these organs. Systematic assessment of the client with possible disorders of the endocrine and metabolic organs can lead to prompt diagnosis and treatment. The diagnostic process can be facilitated by adequately preparing the client for diagnostic procedures and by assisting with, or collecting, assessment data.

BIBLIOGRAPHY

1. Barkauskas, V.H. (2002). Abdomen. In V.H. Barkauskas, L.C. Baumen, & C.S. Fisher (Eds.), *Health and physical assessment* (3rd ed., pp. 384-414). St. Louis: Mosby.
2. Bickley, L.S., & Szilagyi, P.G. (2007). *Bate's guide to physical assessment and history taking* (9th ed.). Philadelphia: Lippincott Williams & Wilkins.
3. Bringhurst, F.R., Demay, M.B., Krane, S.M., et al. (2005). Bone and mineral metabolism in health and disease. In D. Kasper, et al. (Eds.), *Harrison's principles of internal medicine* (16th ed., pp. 2238-2249). New York: McGraw-Hill.
4. Friedman, L.S. (2004). Liver, biliary tract & pancreas. In L.M. Tierney, S.J. McPhee, & M.A. Papadakin (Eds.), *Current medical diagnosis and treatment 2002* (43rd ed., pp. 629-678). New York: Lange Medical Books/McGraw-Hill.
5. Ganong, W.F. (2003). *Review of medical physiology* (19th ed.). Norwalk, Conn: Appleton & Lange.
6. Ghany, M., & Hoglnagle, J.H. (2005). Liver and biliary tract disease. In E. Braunwald, et al. (Eds.), *Harrison's principles of internal medicine* (16th ed., pp. 1808-1813). New York: McGraw-Hill.
7. Greensberger, N.J., & Paumgartner, G. (2005). Diseases of the gallbladder and bile ducts. In D. Kasper, et al. (Eds.), *Harrison's principles of internal medicine* (16th ed., pp. 1880-1891). New York: McGraw-Hill.
8. *Healthy people 2010: Understanding and improving health* (2000). Sudsbury, Mass: Jones & Bartlett.
9. Jameson, J.L. (2005). Principles of endocrinology. In D. Kasper, et al. (Eds.), *Harrison's principles of internal medicine* (16th ed., pp. 2067-2075). New York: McGraw-Hill.
10. Jameson, J.L., & Weetman, A.P. (2005). Diseases of the thyroid. In D. Kasper, et al. (Eds.), *Harrison's principles of internal medicine* (16th ed., pp. 2104-2127). New York: McGraw-Hill.

11. Jarvis, C. (2004). *Physical examination and health assessment* (4th ed.). Philadelphia: Saunders.

12. Kee, J.L. (2002). *Laboratory and diagnostic tests with nursing implications* (6th ed.). Stamford, Conn: Appleton & Lange.

13. Lichtenstein, D. (2004). Diseases of the pancreas. In T.E. Andreoli, et al. (Eds.), *Cecil essentials of medicine* (6th ed., pp. 379-387). Philadelphia: Saunders.

14. Melmed, S. (2005). Disorders of the anterior pituitary and hypothalamus. In D. Kasper, et al. (Eds.), *Harrison's principles of internal medicine* (16th ed., pp. 2076-2097). New York: McGraw-Hill.

15. Monkemuller, K.E., Garcia-Gallont, R., & Fallon, M.B. (2004). Disorders of the gallbladder and biliary tract. In T.E. Andreoli, et al. (Eds.), *Cecil essentials of medicine* (6th ed., pp. 423-428). Philadelphia: Saunders.

16. Pagana, K.D., & Pagana, T.J. (2006). *Mosby's manual of diagnostic and laboratory tests* (3rd ed.). St. Louis: Mosby.

17. Pratt, D.S., & Kaplan, M.M. (2005). Evaluation of liver function. In D. Kasper, et al. (Eds.), *Harrison's principles of internal medicine* (16th ed., pp. 1813-1821). New York: McGraw-Hill.

18. Price, S., & Wilson, L. (Eds.) (2003). *Pathophysiology* (6th ed.). St. Louis: Mosby.

19. Robertson, G.L. (2001). Disorders of the neurohypophysis. In D. Kasper, et al. (Eds.), *Harrison's principles of internal medicine* (16th ed., pp. 2097-2104). New York: McGraw-Hill.

20. Seidel, H.M., et al. (2006). *Mosby's guide to physical examination* (6th ed.). St. Louis: Mosby.

21. Sommers, M.S., & Johnson, S.A. (2002). *Diseases and disorders: A nursing therapeutics manual* (2nd ed.). Philadelphia: F.A. Davis.

22. Swearingen, P.L. (2006). *Manual of medical-surgical nursing care* (6th ed.). St. Louis: Mosby.

23. Williams, G.H., & Dluhy, R.G. (2005). Disorders of the adrenal cortex. In D. Kasper, et al. (Eds.), *Harrison's principles of internal medicine* (16th ed., pp. 2127-2148). New York: McGraw-Hill.

evolve **Did you remember to check out the bonus material on the Evolve website and the CD-ROM, including NCLEX®-Examination Style Review Questions, Open-Book Quizzes, and Chapter Review Audio Podcasts?**

http://evolve.elsevier.com/Black/medsurg

CHAPTER 43

Management of Clients with Thyroid and Parathyroid Disorders

ALLEN HANBERG

THYROID DISORDERS

Many terms describe normal and abnormal states of thyroid function. *Euthyroidism* means that the thyroid gland is functioning normally. Like other endocrine disorders, the two primary thyroid disorders are related to increased secretion *(hyperthyroidism)* and decreased secretion *(hypothyroidism)* of the gland's hormones.

GOITER

Enlargement of the thyroid gland may be seen with both hyperthyroidism and hypothyroidism. It generally results from a lack of iodine, inflammation, or benign or malignant tumors. Enlargement may also appear in hyperthyroidism, especially Graves' disease, in which the client typically has exophthalmos as well.

Etiology and Risk Factors

The two major forms of simple goiter are endemic and sporadic.

Endemic goiter is caused principally by nutritional iodine deficiency. It typically occurs in fall and winter months and is twice as prevalent in women as it is in men. Also, because the need for thyroid hormone (TH) is particularly great during growth spurts, pregnancy, and lactation, goiter commonly develops in adolescents, pregnant women, and nursing mothers who live in iodine-deficient regions such as the Midwest, Northwest, and Great Lakes regions. This issue is explored in the Translating Evidence into Practice feature on p. 1020.

Sporadic goiter is not restricted to any geographical area. Major causes include the following:

- Genetic defects resulting in faulty iodine metabolism
- Ingestion of large amounts of nutritional *goitrogens* (goiter-producing agents that inhibit thyroxine [T_4] production), such as cabbage, soybeans, or spinach

- Ingestion of medicinal goitrogens, such as glucocorticoids, dopamine, or lithium

Health promotion practices include the ingestion of iodized salt and avoidance of goitrogens.

Pathophysiology

If there is a lack of sufficient dietary iodine or if production of TH is suppressed, the thyroid enlarges in an attempt to compensate for hormonal insufficiency. Goiter is essentially an adaptation to a deficiency of TH, but may also occur in response to increased pituitary secretion of thyroid-stimulating hormone (TSH).

Clinical Manifestations

Diagnosis of simple goiter is confirmed by history, clinical findings (Figure 43-1), and laboratory tests. The client may be euthyroid as a result of the gland's attempt to compensate.

OUTCOME MANAGEMENT

Medical Management

 When enlargement is a compensatory reaction to iodine deficiency and consequent suppression of T_4 secretion, the client can be treated with preparations of iodine and thyroid hormones. Either a strong iodine

---

ᴇᴠᴏʟᴠᴇ Web Enhancements

Case Study   Hyperthyroidism and Postmenopausal Osteoporosis

Client Education Guide   Thyroid Supplements (English Version and Spanish Translation)

Be sure to check out the bonus material on the Evolve website and the CD-ROM, including free self-assessment exercises. **http://evolve.elsevier. com/Black/medsurg**

Increasing the Recommended Dietary Allowance of Iodine

Iodine is a trace element. Unlike larger amounts of minerals such as sodium and potassium, the actual requirements for trace elements are less than 100 mg/day. Many of the trace elements are metals and many are a part of some enzyme system. The recommended dietary allowance of iodine in the United States is about 150 mcg/day for adults and adolescents and about 200 mcg/day in pregnant and breast-feeding women. This figure is also recommended by the World Health Organization (WHO). The WHO believes that about 2 billion individuals have iodine deficiency, which is defined as iodine in the urine of less than 100 mcg/L.

Iodine is used to make thyroid hormones. The main natural dietary source of iodine comes from seafood, meats, and some vegetables. Countries that are located far from the sea or ocean used to have some of the largest deficiencies but that has changed because iodine has been added back to some commercial products, usually salt. Some countries, such as Canada, have made it mandatory to put iodine in salt. In the United States, iodination of salt is not mandatory, but iodized salt (40-80 mcg of iodine per gram of salt) is used by about 70% to 75% of homes in the United States. However, iodine intake by various individuals in the United States and other countries has actually decreased because of a variety of reasons, including a reduced intake of table salt, the reduced use of iodate and iodine in various commercial food industries, and the use of non-iodized salt in processed food.

Iodine deficiency can lead to numerous problems from pregnancy complications to short stature, mental abnormalities, neurologic problems, learning issues, and increase in size of the thyroid gland (goiter). Excessive iodine intake can lead to similar problems. A recent, large study from three regions in China outlines the current problems with iodine where intakes were poor, adequate, or too high for at least 5 years.[1] The researchers found that excessive intake of iodine was correlated with higher rates of thyroid problems including hypothyroidism and autoimmune reactions against the thyroid gland itself. This is a troubling finding, but equally or even more troubling was the finding in the same study that a deficient iodine intake was associated with mental abnormalities and pregnancy complications.

IMPLICATIONS

Some researchers[2] are recommending an intake of 300 to 400 mcg of iodine per day, especially for children and pregnant or breast-feeding women. The best way to do this is to increase the iodination of salt or make it mandatory in countries around the world. Nurses should encourage clients and their families to use iodized salt and to be certain they are getting the right amount of this important trace element.

REFERENCES

1. Teng, W., et al. (2006). Effect of iodine intake on thyroid diseases in China. *New England Journal of Medicine, 354*(26), 2783-2793.
2. Utiger, R. (2006). Iodine nutrition—more is better. *New England Journal of Medicine, 354*(26), 2319-2821.

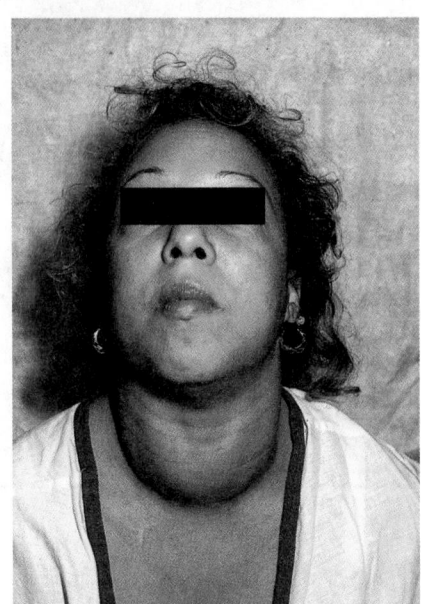

■ **FIGURE 43-1** Massive thyroid enlargement caused by diffuse toxic goiter. (*From Swartz, M.H. [2002]. Textbook of physical diagnosis [4th ed.]. Philadelphia: Saunders.*)

solution (Lugol's solution) or saturated solution of potassium iodide (SSKI) drops can be administered. Iodine reduces the size and vascularity of the enlarged gland.

The client's diet should also be higher in iodine. The client may switch to iodized salt. Dietary goitrogens should be avoided.

⚱ Endemic goiter can be prevented with the use of iodized salt. Adults require at least 50 mg of iodine per day; however, 200 to 300 mg/day is considered the minimum adequate intake needed to prevent goiter.

Surgical Management

Surgical management of goiter is discussed in detail under Hyperthyroidism.

HYPOTHYROIDISM

Hypothyroidism is a deficiency of TH resulting in slowed body metabolism, decreased heat production, and decreased oxygen consumption by the tissues. Underactivity of the thyroid gland may result from primary thyroid dysfunction, or it may be secondary to anterior pituitary dysfunction.

Etiology and Risk Factors

In *primary hypothyroidism,* TH levels are low and TSH levels are elevated, indicating that the pituitary is attempting to stimulate the secretion of thyroid hormones but the thyroid is not responding. This is the most common form of primary-autoimmune hypothyroidism known as *Hashimoto's disease.*

Secondary hypothyroidism develops when there is insufficient stimulation of a normal thyroid gland, resulting in decreased TSH levels. It may also start as a malfunction of the pituitary or hypothalamus or by peripheral resistance to TH. When this occurs, both TSH and TH levels are low in the serum.

Tertiary or *central hypothyroidism* develops if the hypothalamus cannot produce thyroid-releasing hormone (TRH) and subsequently does not stimulate the pituitary to secrete TSH. It may be due to a tumor or other destructive lesion in the hypothalamic region. When this occurs, both TSH and TH levels are again low in the serum.

Subclinical hypothyroidism is defined as hypothyroidism that is diagnosed with an elevated TSH level but a normal to low-normal T_4 level. Manifestations resemble those of mild hypothyroidism with subtle cardiac defects.

Pathophysiology

The thyroid gland needs iodine to synthesize and secrete thyroid hormones: T_4, triiodothyronine (T_3), and thyrocalcitonin (calcitonin). Production of thyroid hormones depends on the secretion of TSH from the anterior pituitary and the ingestion of adequate protein and iodine. The hypothalamus regulates the pituitary secretion of TSH.

Decreased levels of thyroid hormones lead to overall slowing of the basal metabolic rate. This slowing of all body processes leads to *achlorhydria* (decreased secretion of hydrochloric acid in the stomach), decreased gastrointestinal tract motility, bradycardia, slowed neurologic functioning, and a decrease in heat production resulting in a decreased basal body temperature.

The most important changes caused by reduced levels of thyroid hormones are those that affect lipid metabolism. The reduction in thyroid hormones causes an increase in serum cholesterol and triglyceride levels and an increase in atherosclerosis, arteriosclerosis, and coronary heart disease in clients with hypothyroidism.

Because thyroid hormones play a role in the production of red blood cells, people with hypothyroidism also show evidence of anemia, with possible vitamin B_{12} and folate deficiency.

Clinical Manifestations

Manifestations of hypothyroidism depend on whether it is mild, severe (myxedema), or complicated (myxedema coma).

Mild Hypothyroidism

Clients with mild hypothyroidism (the most common form) may be asymptomatic or may experience vague manifestations that escape detection such as cold,

lethargy, dry skin, forgetfulness, depression, and some weight gain. Constipation related to slowed peristaltic action and lack of normal physical activity may also be reported (Table 43-1).

As hypothyroidism worsens, the thyroid enlarges in an attempt to produce enough T_4. Typically, clients seek medical advice when the goiter grows large enough to distort the appearance of the neck. Diagnostic tests for hypothyroidism confirm the clinical picture of hypometabolism and depressed thyroid activity. The serum TSH level is elevated and radioactive iodide uptake is decreased.

Myxedema

Myxedema may develop in clients with undiagnosed or undertreated hypothyroidism that experience stress such as infection, drug use, respiratory failure, heart failure, and trauma. It is characterized by a dry, waxy type of swelling with abnormal deposits of mucin in the skin and other tissues. The edema is non-pitting and is common in the pretibial and facial areas.

Clients with myxedema may also have hypercholesterolemia, hyperlipidemia, and proteinemia as a result of T_4 changes in the synthesis, mobilization, and degradation of serum lipids. Elevated lipid levels may contribute to the later development of cardiac problems. Dilutional hyponatremia may develop as a result of the marked impairment of water excretion because of decreased delivery of sodium and volume to the distal renal tubules associated with decreased renal blood flow.

Myxedema Coma

The most severe complication of hypothyroidism is myxedema coma, an extremely rare condition with a mortality rate of nearly 100%. This emergency state is characterized by a drastic decrease in metabolic rate, hypoventilation leading to respiratory acidosis, hypothermia, and hypotension. Complicating conditions include hyponatremia, hypercalcemia secondary to adrenal insufficiency, hypoglycemia, and water intoxication. It may be triggered by stress—as from surgery or infection—or by noncompliance with thyroid treatment.

SAFETY

ALERT

  OUTCOME MANAGEMENT

Hypothyroidism is rarely a primary diagnosis. Usually, the diagnosis is made after the development of another medical problem. Clients with hypothyroidism are typically managed on an outpatient basis with TH replacement. Treatment is an ongoing, lifelong process. Clients with myxedema or myxedema coma are managed as a medical emergency.

TABLE 43–1   Manifestations of Hypothyroidism and Hyperthyroidism

System	Hypothyroidism	Hyperthyroidism
Cardiovascular	↓ HR + ↓ SV: ↓ CO	↑ HR + ↑ SV: ↑ CO
	↓ Myocardial O_2 demand	↑ O_2 consumption
	↑ Peripheral vascular resistance	Systolic BP ↑ 10-15 mm Hg
	Possible hypertension	Diastolic BP ↑ 10-15 mm Hg
	Hyperlipidemia	Palpitations
	Hypercholesterolemia	Rapid, bounding pulse
	Distant heart sounds	Possible heart failure, edema
Gastrointestinal	↓ Peristalsis	↑ Peristalsis
	Anorexia	↑ Appetite
	Possible weight gain	Weight loss
	Constipation	Diarrhea
	↓ Protein metabolism	↑ Use of adipose and protein stores
	↑ Serum lipids	↓ Serum lipids
	Delayed glucose uptake	↑ Gastrointestinal secretions
	↓ Glucose absorption	
Musculoskeletal	Slow movements	Fatigue
		Muscle weakness
		Tremors
Integumentary	Dry, coarse, scaly skin	Profuse sweating
	Hair that falls out	Moist skin
	Thick, brittle nails	Flushed, warm skin
	Expressionless face	Hair: fine, soft, straight, possible hair loss
	Periorbital edema	Heat intolerance
	Thick, puffy skin: face and pretibial areas	
	Cold intolerance	
Neurologic	↓ Deep tendon reflexes	↑ Deep tendon reflexes
	Fatigue, somnolence	Nervousness, restlessness
	Slow, deliberate speech	Emotional instability: anxiety, worry, paranoia
	Apathy, depression, paranoia	
	Impaired short-term memory	
	Lethargy	
Reproductive	Females: menorrhagia, anovulation, irregular menses, decreased libido	Females: amenorrhea, irregular menses, ↓ fertility, ↑ tendency for spontaneous abortion
	Males: decreased libido, impotence	Males: impotence, decreased libido
		↓ Sexual development prepuberty
Other	Myxedema	Exophthalmos

BP, Blood pressure; *CO*, cardiac output; *CO_2*, carbon dioxide; *HR*, heart rate; *O_2*, oxygen; *SV*, stroke volume.

Medical Management

The desired outcomes of the medical management of hypothyroidism are to correct TH deficiency, reverse manifestations, and prevent further cardiac and arterial damage.

For hypothyroidism to be reversed permanently, the client must take TH for life.

Levothyroxine sodium is the principal form of replacement therapy. Dosages vary with the client's age, the severity of the hypothyroidism, general medical condition (particularly regarding cardiovascular disorders), and response to medical treatment at the initiation of TH therapy. Children and older adults receive smaller doses.

Clients who respond to TH therapy receive a maintenance dose of T_4 daily for life. Pharmacologic goitrogens are replaced by drugs that do not interfere with TH function. The drug of choice for thyroid replacement is levothyroxine sodium, which is converted in the body to both T_4 and T_3 (see the Integrating Pharmacology feature on p. 1023).

Clients with hypothyroidism of long duration notice an improvement in manifestations within 2 to 3 weeks of starting medication; however, hoarseness, anemia, and changes in hair and skin may take many months to resolve.

Myxedema Coma

The desired outcome of the medical management of myxedema coma is to reverse the condition to save the client's life. Supportive measures begin immediately and include maintaining a patent airway, giving oxygen, and replacing fluids intravenously. The client is kept warm, and vital signs are closely monitored until the client begins to recover. Vasopressors are used to maintain tissue perfusion and levothyroxine sodium is given intravenously with glucose and corticosteroids.

Medications for Thyroid Disorders

Medications used in the treatment of hyperthyroid conditions are used to reduce thyroid hormone levels. Medications used in the treatment of hypothyroid conditions are used to increase thyroid hormone levels.

Two medical treatment options exist for hyperthyroidism. First, the client may be temporarily treated with anti-thyroid drugs such as propylthiouracil (PTU), which inhibits thyroid hormone synthesis. Second, radioactive iodine (^{131}I) offers a more permanent option because it destroys thyroid tissue. Radioactive iodine is not given to pregnant women because it may enter the fetal circulation and destroy fetal thyroid tissue.

Clients with hypothyroidism must receive lifelong thyroid hormone replacement therapy such as Synthroid (levothyroxine). Thyroid hormone levels are routinely monitored to ensure adequate dosage prescription. Thyroid hormone replacement therapy is also prescribed for clients with goiters because it promotes shrinkage of the gland.

Clients with thyrotoxicosis may receive additional drug therapy for palliative treatment. For example, beta-adrenergic blockers may be prescribed to control heart rate and tremors. Acetaminophen may be prescribed for fever.

Nursing Management of the Medical Client with Myxedema

Assessment. Monitor for the physical manifestations of myxedema, such as periorbital and facial edema, a blank facial expression, a thick tongue, and generalized slowing of all muscle movement. Vital signs are also affected and must be monitored closely. The client is hypothermic. Depressed respirations precipitate respiratory acidosis. Alterations in heart rate and blood pressure follow.

Diagnosis, Outcomes, Interventions

Diagnosis: Risk for Injury: Myxedema Coma. A client with acute hypothyroidism is susceptible to the development of myxedema coma, leading to the nursing diagnosis *Risk for Injury: Myxedema coma related to hypersensitivity to anesthetics, sedatives, and opioids secondary to decreased metabolic rate.*

Outcomes. The client will not receive the usual doses of anesthetics, sedatives, and opioids so that development of myxedema coma will be prevented and the client will not be injured.

Interventions. The client should not receive sedatives unless absolutely necessary. If a sedative or opioid must be given, administer no more than one third to one half of the usual dose. Then assess the client carefully for respiratory depression or a decreased level of consciousness.

Evaluation. It is expected that after successful treatment the client will demonstrate no evidence of heart failure, edema, or skin impairment; temperature and urine output will be normal; and no further evidence of myxedema will be seen. After the client is out of danger and alert, long-term management begins (see the following section).

Self-Care

Hypothyroidism is a lifelong disease that must be managed with the client's full participation. The client should understand the pharmacologic regimen, nutrition, and follow-up required to control the condition.

To promote self-care, focus your teaching on the client's need to understand the manifestations of hyperthyroidism and hypothyroidism, to follow the medication regimen and diet, and to seek medical attention appropriately. Evaluate the client's level of knowledge about the disorder and the importance of taking TH daily for life. Develop and implement a teaching plan based on the client's particular needs. Also provide a written list (such as the one in the Client Education Guide feature on Thyroid Supplements on the website) of the manifestations of thyroid deficiency or excess. Instruct the client and his or her significant others to contact the physician if those manifestations develop.

Monitor the client's weight weekly. Physical manifestations of hypothyroidism should decrease over 3 to 12 weeks as TH levels increase. Emphasize the need for iodized salt. Advise the client to drink sufficient fluids, increase physical activity, and eat a high-fiber diet to prevent constipation. Remind the client to have TH levels checked routinely until they stabilize and then at regular intervals to ensure that they remain normal.

Modifications for Older Clients

Subclinical hypothyroidism refers to a combination of elevated TSH levels, normal T_3 and free thyroxine (FT_4) levels, and no clinical manifestations. Subclinical hypothyroidism occurs in up to 15% of postmenopausal women. The most common causes are autoimmune thyroiditis, Hashimoto's disease, previous thyroid surgery or treatment with radioactive agents, and noncompliance with prescribed T_4 replacements.

Clients with generalized complaints may benefit from small doses of T_4, which indicates that their condition is symptomatic rather than subclinical.

Remember that a principal hazard in giving T_4 to an older client is the development of ischemic heart disease as evidenced by angina. The response to therapy and serum levels must be observed closely. The client's pulse rate should be monitored daily.

SAFETY

ALERT

The difficulty in diagnosing hypothyroidism in older adults is that the manifestations are usually vague and generic to other disease processes.

HYPERTHYROIDISM

Hyperthyroidism (excessive secretion of TH) is a highly preventable endocrine disorder. Like most thyroid conditions, it is a disorder that predominantly affects women (in a female-to-male ratio of 4:1), especially women between ages 20 and 40 years.

Etiology and Risk Factors

Hyperthyroidism may be due to overfunctioning of the entire gland or, less commonly, to single or multiple functioning adenomas of thyroid cancer. The most common form of hyperthyroidism is Graves' disease (toxic, diffuse goiter), which has three principal hallmarks: hyperthyroidism, thyroid gland enlargement (goiter), and *exophthalmos* (abnormal protrusion of the eyes). Graves' disease is an autoimmune disorder mediated by immunoglobulin G (IgG) antibody that binds to and activates TSH receptors on the surface of the thyroid cells.

Health maintenance and restoration activities include monitoring TH levels if TH replacement is given, removal of thyroid tumors, and administration of antithyroid medications.

Pathophysiology

Hyperthyroidism is characterized by loss of the normal regulatory controls of TH secretion. Because the action of TH on the body is stimulatory, hypermetabolism results, with increased sympathetic nervous system activity. Excessive amounts of TH stimulate the cardiac system and increase the number of beta-adrenergic receptors, leading to tachycardia and increased cardiac output, stroke volume, adrenergic responsiveness, and peripheral blood flow. Metabolism increases greatly, leading to a negative nitrogen balance, lipid depletion, and a state of nutritional deficiency and weight loss.

Hyperthyroidism also results in altered secretion and metabolism of hypothalamic, pituitary, and gonadal hormones. If hyperthyroidism occurs before puberty, sexual development is delayed in both genders. After puberty, hyperthyroidism results in diminished libido in both men and women. Women also have menstrual irregularities and decreased fertility.

Clinical Manifestations

Because hyperthyroidism is caused by excessive secretion of TH, the clinical picture of Graves' disease is opposite to that of hypothyroidism. Assessment reveals a client who appears extremely agitated and irritable, with hand tremors at rest. Despite a ravenous appetite, weight loss occurs as a result of the hypermetabolic state. Manifestations include loose bowel movements, heat intolerance, profuse diaphoresis, tachycardia, and incoordination related to tremors. The skin becomes warm, smooth, and moist, and hair appears thin and soft.

Moreover, the client's emotions are adversely affected by the turbulent activity within the body. Moods may be cyclic, ranging from mild euphoria to extreme hyperactivity to delirium. The excessive hyperactivity in turn leads to extreme fatigue and depression, again followed by episodes of overactivity.

Goiter, the second characteristic of Graves' disease, is due to hyperplasia and hypertrophy of the thyroid cells. The gland may grow to three or four times its normal size. Cellular overgrowth results in the release of excessive amounts of TH into the blood.

The diagnosis of Graves' disease is confirmed on the basis of the client's often striking physical appearance (enlarged neck, protruding eyes [exophthalmos], agitated expression); the manifestations of agitation, restlessness, and weight loss; and laboratory findings. Serum TH levels are usually all elevated, although they are occasionally euthyroid. Serum cholesterol levels are usually depressed. See the tables on the website for Chapter 42—Diagnostic Imaging and Other Tests for Endocrine and Metabolic Function and Laboratory Tests for Endocrine and Metabolic Function—for the usual laboratory findings.

Complications

The three major complications of Graves' disease are exophthalmos, heart disease, and thyroid storm (thyroid crisis, thyrotoxicosis).

Exophthalmos

Exophthalmos is the third major manifestation of Graves' disease. The cause of ophthalmologic changes in Graves' disease seems to be autoimmunity against retro-orbital tissues. The client who develops exophthalmos has protruding eyes and a fixed stare (Figure 43-2). It develops as a result of proptosis, lid retraction, muscle swelling, and tissue edema from a prolonged hyperthyroid condition. Manifestations may include a gritty sensation in the eye, photophobia, lacrimation, inflammatory changes, and dyslogia.

Unlike the manifestations of goiter and hyperthyroidism, exophthalmos does not necessarily regress with therapy. Diuretics may alleviate some periorbital edema. Glucocorticoids such as prednisone are given in large doses to reduce inflammation of the periorbital tissues, but may produce many undesirable side effects. Methylcellulose eye drops help reduce eye irritation. Radiation therapy to the retro-orbital tissues may help in severe cases. Surgical decompression of the orbits may be

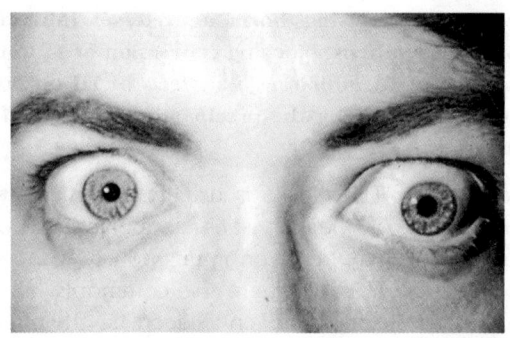

■ **FIGURE 43–2** Extreme exophthalmos in hyperthyroidism. Because the eyes are surrounded by unyielding bone, fluid accumulation in the fat pads and muscles behind the eyeballs causes protruding eyes and a fixed stare in the client with exophthalmos. Without intervention, the client with severe exophthalmos may be unable to close the eyelids and may develop corneal ulceration or infection. Eventually, this can result in total loss of vision. *(From Scheie, H.G. [1977]. Textbook of ophthalmology [9th ed.]. Philadelphia: Saunders.)*

performed when all other measures fail to correct exophthalmos. This procedure may save the client's vision when eye changes are severe.

A number of general nursing interventions also help to reduce eye discomfort and prevent corneal ulceration and infection. Instruct a client with exophthalmos to wear dark eyeglasses. Warn the client to avoid getting dust or dirt in the eyes. If the eyelids cannot be closed easily or at all, have the client wear a sleeping mask or lightly tape the eyes shut with non-allergic tape. Elevate the head of the bed at night, and have the client restrict salt intake to relieve edema.

Heart Disease

Heart disease poses a serious threat. Tachycardia and atrial fibrillation almost always accompany thyrotoxicosis. Heart failure is found among older clients with long-standing thyrotoxicosis.

Treatment of these cardiac complications is covered in Unit 13.

Thyroid Storm (Thyrotoxicosis)

Thyroid storm (thyrotoxicosis) is a potentially fatal acute episode of thyroid overactivity characterized by high fever, severe tachycardia, delirium, dehydration, and extreme irritability. Thyroid storm is a clinical diagnosis; no laboratory tests differentiate hyperthyroidism from thyroid storm in general.

OUTCOME MANAGEMENT

Medical Management

The desired outcomes of medical management for clients with Graves' disease are to curtail the excessive secretion of TH and to prevent and treat complications. Choice of intervention is based on age, goiter size, and whether the client has other health problems. The three major forms of therapy are antithyroid medication, radioiodine therapy, and surgery.

Curtail Excessive Secretion of Thyroid Hormone

Antithyroid medication is recommended for clients younger than 18 years of age and for pregnant women. The major medications used to control hyperthyroidism include iodide, propylthiouracil, and methimazole (Tapazole). Adrenergic blocking agents may be administered as adjunctive therapy.

Propylthiouracil is the most commonly used antithyroid medication. It corrects hyperthyroidism by impairing TH synthesis. With the usual dosage regimen, propylthiouracil ameliorates Graves' disease within 4 to 8 weeks. Several months may pass before manifestations completely abate, however. When euthyroid, the client is advanced to a maintenance dose three times a day (see the Integrating Pharmacology feature on Medications for Thyroid Disorders on p. 1023). The most serious toxic effect of propylthiouracil is agranulocytosis (see Chapter 75). Less severe adverse reactions include mild allergies (rash and pruritus).

Iodine therapy is prescribed for two reasons: (1) to reduce the vascularity of the thyroid gland before subtotal or total thyroidectomy and (2) to treat thyroid storm. Iodine preparations act temporarily to prevent the release of TH into the circulation by increasing the amount of TH stored in the gland. The stored TH is eventually released back into the circulation, however, once again producing hyperthyroidism. For this reason, iodine preparations are usually given only for 10 to 14 days before surgery. If iodine is given for a longer period or if it is given alone (not in combination with propylthiouracil), the thyroid gland may no longer be capable of maintaining TH storage. As a result, TH floods the circulation, and hyperthyroidism becomes more severe than before.

The iodine medication of choice is potassium iodide. Lugol's solution is also used but is more expensive than potassium iodide and tends to inactivate antithyroid preparations in the bowel.

Therapy with radioactive iodine (^{131}I) is prescribed mainly for middle-age and older clients. This intervention offers many advantages: it is economical, is simple to administer, and can be prescribed on an outpatient basis, as described in the Case Study on p. 1026. Radiotherapy is contraindicated for pregnant women and is rarely used for children.

The rationale behind ^{131}I therapy for Graves' disease is simple. The thyroid gland is unable to distinguish between regular iodine atoms and radioiodine atoms. Consequently, when the client receives a dose of ^{131}I,

CASE STUDY   *evolve*

Hyperthyroidism and Postmenopausal Osteoporosis

Mrs. Gonzales is a 55-year-old Hispanic woman who presents at a free clinic for migrant farm workers. She is dressed in a lightweight sundress and sandals despite outdoor temperatures around 50 ° F. Mrs. Gonzales complains of pounding in her chest and shortness of breath without exertion. She relates that she has lost 20 pounds in the last 6 weeks even though she has been eating more than usual. A thyroxine (T_4) level determined at the clinic is twice the normal value. The nurse practitioner has arranged for additional outpatient diagnostic studies.... *Case Study continued on the website and the CD-ROM with discussions, multiple-choice questions, and a nursing care plan.*

the thyroid gland picks up the radioiodine and concentrates it just as it would regular iodine. As a result, the cells that concentrate ^{131}I to make T_4 are destroyed by the local irradiation, TH secretion diminishes, and the manifestations of hyperthyroidism and goiter disappear. Because radioiodine destroys thyroid cells, however, one of the major possible complications of ^{131}I therapy is hypothyroidism. Therefore assess for manifestations of hypothyroidism after instituting ^{131}I therapy.

The manifestations of hyperthyroidism usually subside within 6 to 12 weeks after ^{131}I administration. Sometimes resistant clients require a second or, in rare instances, a third dose of radioiodine. The client who becomes euthyroid still needs regular medical examinations because hypothyroidism may develop several years after radiotherapy.

Prevent and Treat Complications

Adrenergic blocking agents are sometimes given as adjunctive therapy to control the activity of the sympathetic nervous system. Evidence now exists that these agents are of great benefit to the "hyperthyroid heart," which has increased sensitivity to catecholamines and an increased number of beta-adrenergic receptor sites. Therefore these agents help lessen manifestations such as palpitations and tachycardia, tremors, and nervousness. The most commonly used medication is propranolol.

The client with hyperthyroidism requires a high-calorie (4000 to 5000 calories), high-protein diet to compensate for the hypermetabolic state and prevent a negative nitrogen balance and weight loss.

SAFETY ⚠ ALERT **Thyroid storm is considered a medical emergency. The high fever is treated with hypothermia blankets; dehydration is reversed with the administration of intravenous fluids. Management of thyroid storm**

involves suppressing hormone release, inhibiting hormone synthesis, blocking conversion of T_4 to the more active T_3, inhibiting the effects of TH on body tissues, and treating the precipitating cause, if it is known.

Blockade of TH release is usually achieved by oral administration of iodides, such as potassium iodide. Sodium iodide may be given intravenously. Glucocorticoids and propylthiouracil, are also commonly used oral drugs. Beta-blockers are given to decrease the effects of sympathetic nervous system stimulation and to treat tachycardia.

Nursing Management of the Medical Client

Assessment. By obtaining a complete history and asking questions concerning weight, appetite, activity, heat intolerance, and bowel activity, you can assess for the presence of typical manifestations of hyperthyroidism. Also ask about mood alterations (see the Critical Monitoring feature below).

Diagnosis, Outcomes, Interventions
Diagnosis: Imbalanced Nutrition: Less Than Body Requirements. A client with hyperthyroidism is hypermetabolic, leading to the nursing diagnosis *Imbalanced Nutrition: Less Than Body Requirements related to accelerated metabolic rate resulting in weight loss and decreased energy levels.*

Outcomes. The client's weight loss will end as evidenced by an ability to consume sufficient calories to return to ideal body weight.

Interventions. Provide the client with a well-balanced diet high in calories, protein, carbohydrates, and minerals. Discourage the ingestion of foods that increase peristalsis and thus result in diarrhea, such as highly seasoned, bulky, or fibrous foods.

CRITICAL MONITORING

Thyrotoxicosis/Thyroid Storm

These manifestations should be monitored in a client who is believed to be at risk for thyroid storm:
- Anxiety, short attention span, irritability
- Hyperreflexia
- Increased temperature (as high as 106° F)
- Increased pulse rate (as high as 200 beats/min)
- Systolic hypertension
- Dyspnea
- Augmentation of other disorders, such as atrial fibrillation, heart failure, angina pectoris (chest pain), paranoia, and anxiety

The client should be weighed daily; weight losses of more than 4.4 pounds (2 kg) should be reported. If the client continues to appear malnourished despite an ample diet, supplemental vitamins, particularly vitamin B complex, may be needed.

Evaluation. The client with Graves' disease should recover from the hyperthyroidism without difficulty when the medication regimen has begun.

Surgical Management

Thyroidectomy

Thyroidectomy (removal of the thyroid gland) may be total or partial. *Total* thyroidectomy is performed to remove thyroid cancer. Clients who undergo this operation must take thyroid hormones permanently. *Subtotal* thyroidectomy is performed to correct hyperthyroidism and extreme cases of simple goiter. About five sixths of the gland is removed. Because one sixth of the functioning gland is left intact, hormone replacements may not be necessary.

Indications and Contraindications. Ideally, clients selected are young and free of any condition that makes them poor operative risks (e.g., diabetes, heart disease, renal disease).

Preoperative preparation for a subtotal thyroidectomy is extremely important. If possible, the client must be euthyroid before the operation. Preoperative care for a client with Graves' disease includes administration of antithyroid drugs to suppress secretion of thyroid hormones and iodine preparations to reduce the size and vascularity of the organ, thereby diminishing the chance of hemorrhage (see Medical Management earlier in this chapter). Adequate preoperative preparation may take as long as 2 to 3 months.

Complications. Besides the usual complications of any surgery, which include hemorrhage and infection, the client after thyroidectomy is at risk for thyroid storm, tetany, respiratory obstruction, laryngeal edema, and vocal cord injury. If the client is not euthyroid, the risk of intraoperative or postoperative thyroid storm is greatly increased.

> **Although uncommon, respiratory obstruction may result from swelling related to the surgical site. Rarely, vocal cord paralysis may result from nerve damage. Hypoparathyroidism may result from inadvertent removal of parathyroid gland tissue. The parathyroid glands lie just behind the lobes of the thyroid and are commonly disturbed and sometimes inadvertently removed during surgery. Careful postoperative monitoring of neurologic irritability and serum calcium levels is performed for this reason.**

Outcomes. Surgical treatment is effective in most people with Graves' disease. A small percentage will remain hyperthyroid, and hypothyroidism develops in some.

Nursing Management of the Surgical Client

Preoperative Care

Assess the client for typical manifestations of Graves' disease. A hypermetabolic state may be obvious from apparent weight loss, and exophthalmos may be obvious as well. Also, question the client about visual difficulties, fatigue, weakness, tremors, and insomnia.

Promote Preoperative Euthyroid State. The client must be carefully prepared for a thyroidectomy to avoid complications (e.g., thyroid storm and hemorrhage). Outcomes of successful preparation for thyroid surgery are as follows:

- The client is euthyroid before entering the operating room. Tests of thyroid function are within normal limits.
- Manifestations of thyrotoxicosis are greatly diminished or absent. The client appears rested and relaxed.
- Weight and nutritional status are normal; any weight lost earlier has been regained.
- Cardiac problems are under control, pulse rate is normal, and preoperative electrocardiograms show no dangerous dysrhythmias.

Postoperative Care

Assessment

Monitor for Postoperative Complications. Assemble the needed equipment at the bedside before the client returns from surgery.

> **The equipment includes a blood pressure cuff and stethoscope, additional pillows, oxygen, suction equipment, intubation supplies, and a tracheostomy set. Ampules of calcium gluconate should be on hand in the medicine room or on the emergency cart (see the Critical Monitoring feature on p. 1028).**

SAFETY ALERT

Monitor and Treat Hypocalcemia

> **Muscle twitching and hyperirritability of the nervous system may indicate hypocalcemic tetany. Hypocalcemia can develop after thyroidectomy if the parathyroid glands are accidentally removed during surgery. Manifestations may develop 1 to 7 days after surgery. Monitor the client for Chvostek's and Trousseau's signs (see Figure 12-3 on p. 159); report positive responses to the physician immediately. Also call a physician if the client develops numbness and tingling around the mouth, fingertips, or toes; muscle**

SAFETY ALERT

CRITICAL MONITORING

Intravenous Calcium Infusion

Measures for safe administration of intravenous calcium include the following:

- Dilute to reduce vein irritation and venospasm.
- Administer into a large central or deep vein.
- Confirm patency of the IV before administration.
- Monitor vital signs and serum calcium levels.
- Observe for hyperchloremic acidosis if calcium carbonate is administered.
- Observe for extravasation. Necrosis and sloughing may occur.
- If extravasation occurs, inject 1% procaine hydrochloride and hyaluronidase using a 25- to 27-gauge needle to reduce vasospasm.

spasms; or twitching. Make sure calcium gluconate ampules are available at the bedside and that the client has a patent intravenous line.

Diagnosis, Outcomes, Interventions. Postoperative management of the client with a thyroidectomy is outlined in the care plan on pp. 1030-1031.

Evaluation. The client should be discharged within several days of surgery without difficulty. The wound should heal within 6 weeks without infection.

Self-Care

Hyperthyroidism is a chronic disease that must be managed with the client's full participation. When the immediate postoperative period and its dangers have passed, turn your attention to teaching. Several important areas should be included.

Neck Exercises

Teach the client how to support the weight of the head and neck when sitting up. Show the client how to place the hands at the back of the head when flexing the neck or moving.

Medications

SAFETY
⚠
ALERT
evolve

If a total thyroidectomy has been performed, explain self-administration of thyroid medications (see the Client Education Guide feature on Thyroid Supplements on the website and the Integrating Pharmacology feature on Medications for Thyroid Disorders). Teach the client the medication regimen and the need for lifelong replacement therapy.

Follow-up Monitoring

Make an appointment for the client with the physician after discharge. Serum thyroid levels must be determined to monitor treatment. Emphasize the importance of seeing the physician at least twice a year to avoid complications related to hormone replacement.

SAF
⚠
AL

Promote Wound Healing

Teach the client how to care for the incision when it has healed by using lanolin or vitamin E cream to soften the wound and minimize scarring.

Modifications for Older Clients

Hyperthyroidism in older clients is also notorious, however, for atypical or minimal manifestations. It is often overlooked because the manifestations are atypical.

Indeed, manifestations are commonly attributed to aging. Weight loss, lack of ocular findings, and normal-sized thyroid glands are commonly found on assessment. Many clients actually appear apathetic instead of hyperactive. Cardiovascular abnormalities, such as heart failure, atrial dysrhythmias (usually digoxin resistant), and various degrees of heart block, may be caused by hyperthyroidism. If the cardiac condition is pre-existing, it may be exacerbated by hyperthyroidism.

The diagnosis of hyperthyroidism is established by appropriate laboratory tests. It is usual to find elevated T_4 and suppressed TSH levels. Hyperthyroidism in older clients is treated with radioactive iodine.

THYROIDITIS

Thyroiditis (inflammation of the thyroid gland) appears in three basic forms: acute suppurative, subacute thyroiditis (either granulomatous [painful thyroiditis] or lymphocytic [silent or painless thyroiditis]), or chronic thyroiditis (also known as Hashimoto's disease).

Etiology and Risk Factors

Acute suppurative thyroiditis is an uncommon inflammatory disease usually caused by bacterial invasion in the form of an abscess of the thyroid gland. *Streptococcus pyogenes, Staphylococcus aureus,* and *Pneumococcus pneumoniae* are the most common etiologic agents. Usually, it affects women between 20 and 40 years of age, but it also occurs in children and older people. Most affected clients have a pre-existing thyroid disorder.

Subacute granulomatous thyroiditis is a self-limiting inflammatory condition. No etiologic agent has been identified, although the condition may be viral in origin and commonly follows a respiratory tract infection. Autoimmune abnormalities have been described. There also appears to be a genetic predisposition to the development of both subacute granulomatous and lymphocytic thyroiditis. Of people with subacute granulomatous thyroiditis, 80% are women between 40 and 50 years of age.

Chronic thyroiditis (Hashimoto's disease) is the most common form of thyroiditis. It is more prevalent in women than in men and usually occurs between 20 and 50 years of age. Hashimoto's disease is a long-term inflammatory disorder. It is most commonly caused by autoimmune destruction of the thyroid gland. Genetic predisposition also plays a role in its causation.

Pathophysiology

Acute thyroiditis is a state of acute infection and inflammation. Usually, one lobe of the thyroid is more affected than the other. Follicular destruction, cell infiltration, and colloid depletion occur. Microabscesses form.

Subacute thyroiditis has three phases:

- *Phase 1:* The condition begins with a 3- to 4-week prodromal viral illness. Fever and malaise precede the sudden onset of a tender goiter. The thyroid gland may become two to three times its normal size. Mild hyperthyroidism may be present because of sudden release of thyroid hormones into the circulation as a result of the inflammation and destruction of the thyroid gland.
- *Phase 2:* Mild hypothyroidism develops because of incomplete recovery of the injured gland and exhaustion of stored thyroid hormones. Relapse may occur. Hypothyroidism is rarely permanent.
- *Phase 3:* The recovery phase may begin 2 to 4 months after onset.

Hashimoto's disease is manifested by an enlarged thyroid gland that may produce hypothyroid manifestations if the gland is destroyed by the autoimmune system. A euthyroid state may prevail if the gland is not destroyed.

Clinical Manifestations

Manifestations of acute thyroiditis include abrupt onset of unilateral anterior neck pain with possible radiation to the ear or mandible on the affected side. Fever, diaphoresis, and other manifestations of bacterial toxicity may also be present.

Subacute granulomatous thyroiditis is usually painful, whereas subacute lymphocytic thyroiditis is usually painless. Assessment data may include characteristic anterior, unilateral neck pain that may have an abrupt onset, usually after a respiratory tract infection or viral episode. Radiation to the ear on the ipsilateral side may occur. Manifestations of viral infection, such as myalgia, low-grade fever, lassitude, and sore throat, may occur. About 50% of clients present with thyrotoxicosis.

Subacute lymphocytic thyroiditis is characterized by occasional hyperthyroidism and a painless goiter. The goiter is firm, diffuse, and mildly enlarged.

Manifestations of chronic thyroiditis include painless, asymmetrical enlargement of the gland, which causes pressure on the surrounding structures and can lead to dysphagia and respiratory distress. Most clients are euthyroid, about 20% are hypothyroid, and fewer than 5% are hyperthyroid.

The diagnosis of thyroiditis may be confirmed by evaluation of levels of serum T_3, FT_4, ^{131}I uptake, TSH, erythrocyte sedimentation rate, and thyroid antibodies. Clients with acute thyroiditis are typically euthyroid according to laboratory tests.

For subacute granulomatous thyroiditis, laboratory findings reveal hyperthyroidism in about 50% of clients. With subacute lymphocytic thyroiditis, laboratory diagnosis includes decreased radioactive iodine uptake, elevated T_3 and T_4 levels, and frequently positive thyroid antibodies.

In chronic thyroiditis, immune antibodies are usually positive. Other thyroid function levels may be normal, increased, or decreased.

OUTCOME MANAGEMENT

Medical Management

Acute thyroiditis usually responds to parenteral antibiotic therapy. Treatment of subacute granulomatous thyroiditis is supportive. Therapy may include salicylates, nonsteroidal anti-inflammatory drugs (NSAIDs), and oral glucocorticoids such as prednisone. The desired outcome of treatment in subacute lymphocytic thyroiditis is to provide relief of manifestations of hyperthyroidism with beta-adrenergic blocking agents. Antithyroid medications are not indicated.

The course of Hashimoto's disease varies. Some clients experience spontaneous remission, whereas others remain stable for years. In about one third of cases, hypothyroidism develops from gradual atrophy of the gland. Intervention is intended to reduce the size of the gland and correct any thyroid function abnormalities. Immunologic tests are not useful in monitoring these clients.

Surgical Management

Clients with acute thyroiditis that does not respond to medical treatment may require incision and drainage of the affected gland. Depending on the size of the thyroid area to be incised and concurrent medical problems, the procedure can be done in the physician's office or during a short stay in the hospital. A fine needle biopsy may be performed to rule out malignancy in chronic thyroiditis.

CARE PLAN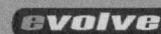

Postoperative Management of the Client with a Thyroidectomy

Nursing Diagnosis: Imbalanced Nutrition: Less Than Body Requirements (NANDA) related to hypermetabolic state and impaired utilization and storage of nutrients.

Outcomes: Appetite, Nutritional Status, Weight: Body Mass (NOC). Client will maintain or increase body weight to ideal weight and will consume adequate nutrients.

Interventions	(NIC)	Rationales
1. Weigh daily.	Nutrition Management Nutritional Monitoring	Monitors weight gain or loss.
2. Monitor nutritional intake.	Nutrition Management Nutrition Therapy Nutritional Monitoring	Monitors intake of nutrients.
3. Provide oral hygiene before meals.	Nausea Management	Improves taste of food.
4. Assess for difficulty swallowing.	Airway Management Nutritional Management	Monitor for difficulty swallowing.
5. Administer antiemetics as ordered.	Nausea Management	Relieves nausea and vomiting.
6. Give fluids by mouth as tolerated as ordered.	Nutrition Therapy Nausea Management	Promotes adequate hydration.
7. Provide small, frequent meals.	Nausea Management Nutrition Therapy	Prevents feeling of fullness and ensures adequate nutritional intake.
8. Monitor electrolytes, hemoglobin, and hematocrit.	Electrolyte Management Laboratory Data Interpretation	Inadvertent removal or devascularization of the parathyroid glands can cause postoperative hypoparathyroidism.

Evaluation: With interventions, the client will maintain weight and body mass or begin to gain weight by consuming adequate nutrients.

Nursing Diagnosis: Suffocation, Risk for (NANDA) related to potential respiratory obstruction due to hemorrhage, edema of glottis, laryngeal nerve damage, or tetany.

Outcomes: Respiratory Status: Airway Patency (NOC). Client will maintain a patent airway and adequate gas exchange.

Outcomes: Respiratory Status: Ventilation, Vital Signs (NOC). Client will breathe with minimal difficulty; no manifestations of hypoxia will be seen.

Interventions	(NIC)	Rationales
1. Continuously assess for manifestations of airway obstruction such as increasing restlessness, tachycardia, apprehension, cyanosis, stridulous respiration, and retraction of neck tissues.	Airway Management	Prevent or minimize risk factors in the client at risk for aspiration.
2. Cough and deep breathe every hour.	Airway Management Respiratory Monitoring	Ensure airway patency and adequate gas exchange.
3. Suction mouth and trachea if necessary.	Airway Management Aspiration Precautions	Facilitate patency of airway passages.
4. Use semi-Fowler position when client is conscious, unless client is hypotensive.	Airway Management Positioning	Promote physiologic and/or psychological well-being. Immobilization of head and neck is essential to prevent flexion and hyperextension of neck with resultant strain on suture line. Semi-Fowler position used for comfort.
5. Have tracheostomy set, endotracheal tube, laryngoscope, and oxygen on hand. Equipment for establishing an airway and administration of oxygen must be available for immediate use.	Airway Management	Acute respiratory obstruction caused by hemorrhage, edema of glottis, laryngeal nerve damage, or tetany is an emergency.
6. Give continuous mist inhalation as ordered.	Airway Management	Humidification of air promotes easier breathing and helps to liquefy mucous secretions.
7. Administer oxygen as ordered.	Oxygen Therapy Intravenous Therapy	Improves gas exchange.
8. Place the client in the semi-Fowler or Fowler position with arms supported with pillows.	Positioning	Relieves pressure on the diaphragm.
9. Assess for crackles and increased respirations.	Respiratory Monitoring Vital Signs Monitoring	Identifies fluid in lungs.
10. Administer oxygen and blood products as ordered.	Oxygen Therapy Intravenous Therapy	Improves gas exchange.

Evaluation: With interventions, the client will maintain a patent airway and adequate gas exchange.

Nursing Diagnosis: Pain, Acute (NANDA) related to actual postoperative tissue damage.
Outcomes: Comfort Level (NOC). Client will maintain adequate comfort for optimal recovery.

Interventions	(NIC)	Rationales
1. Assess pain and respiratory status every 1-2 hours or as needed.	Pain Management Vital Signs Monitoring	After thyroidectomy, hemorrhage and respiratory obstruction may develop. Elevated pulse rate and hypotension may be indicative of hypovolemic shock. Postoperative clients commonly experience pain related to tissue damage around the surgical site.
2. Administer pain medications as ordered. Do not oversedate. Give opioids judiciously.	Pain Management	Meperidine and morphine sulfate are both used during early postoperative period to relieve pain and promote rest. Do not give opioids if respirations fall below 12 breaths/min or with profuse respiratory secretions.
3. Support head and neck with pillows and sandbags.	Pain Management	Immobilization of the head and neck is essential to prevent flexion and hyperextension of neck with resultant strain on suture line.
4. Use semi-Fowler position.	Pain Management	Semi-Fowler position used for comfort.

Evaluation: With interventions, the client will maintain adequate comfort for optimal recovery.

Nursing Diagnosis: Impaired Skin Integrity (NANDA) related to surgical incision.
Outcomes: Tissue Integrity: Skin and Mucous Membranes (NOC). Client will maintain skin integrity to promote optimal wound healing.

Interventions	(NIC)	Rationales
1. Keep dressings to neck clean and dry.	Wound Care	Prevent infection.
2. Assess wound dressing for tautness. Keep dressings loose.	Wound Care	Tight wound dressing may be indicative of bleeding into the tissues.
3. Apply emollients (mineral oil, baby oil, lanolin).	Pruritus Management Wound Care	Emollients reduce evaporation and keep skin moist.
4. Use cool, light cotton clothing, which promotes evaporation.	Pruritus Management	Minimizes irritation and itching.
5. Keep clothing and bedding dry.	Pruritus Management	Minimizes itching.
6. Keep the environment cool (65°-70° F).	Pruritus Management	Minimizes itching and vasodilation.
7. Avoid activities that promote sweating.	Pruritus Management	Minimizes itching and vasodilation.
8. Keep nails short and smooth.	Pruritus Management	Prevents breaking skin integrity when scratching.
9. Administer diphenhydramine HCl (Benadryl).	Pruritus Management Medication Administration	Antihistamine that has antipruritic and sedative effect; itching is worse at night.
10. Encourage diversional activities.	Pruritus Management	Decreases perception of itching and improves coping.

Evaluation: With interventions, the client will maintain skin integrity for optimal wound healing.

Nursing Diagnosis: Risk for Injury (NANDA).
Outcomes: Thyroid Storm, Hypocalcemia, or Hemorrhage. Thyroid storm will be recognized and treated early. Client will maintain normal calcium levels. Hypocalcemia will be recognized early and treated appropriately. Bleeding from surgical wound will be recognized and treated early.

Interventions	(NIC)	Rationales
1. Check dressing and vital signs every 15 minutes, or per postoperative orders/protocols.	Bleeding Precautions: Wound Electrolyte Management: Hypocalcemia	After thyroidectomy, hemorrhage and respiratory obstruction may develop.
2. Observe for bleeding at front, sides, and back of neck.	Bleeding Precautions: Wound	After thyroidectomy, hemorrhage may develop. Elevated pulse rate and hypotension are indicative of hemorrhagic shock.
3. Examine back of neck and shoulders for bleeding because blood tends to drain posteriorly.	Bleeding Precautions: Wound	Alkaline soap dries skin.
4. Check dressing for tightness; uncomfortable tautness may indicate bleeding into the tissue; loosen dressing and call physician immediately.	Bleeding Precautions: Wound	Dyspnea, stridulous respirations, and retraction of neck tissues indicate respiratory obstruction. After thyroidectomy, respiratory obstruction may develop.
5. Assess client for hypocalcemia and monitor calcium, magnesium, and phosphate levels.	Electrolyte Management: Hypocalcemia	Inadvertent removal or devascularization of the parathyroid glands can cause postoperative hypoparathyroidism.
6. Carefully assess for manifestations of thyroid storm: elevated temperature, extreme restlessness, agitation, and tachycardia. Report abnormal vital signs and laboratory values to physician immediately.	Electrolyte Management: Hypocalcemia	These are early manifestations of thyroid storm.

Evaluation: With interventions, the client will maintain normal calcium levels. Hypocalcemia will be recognized early and treated appropriately.

Nursing Management of the Medical-Surgical Client

Nursing care of a client with thyroiditis is usually supportive until the diagnosis is made. Then, as with other thyroid disorders, care revolves around helping the client learn correct medication administration. If surgery is necessary, care is the same as discussed earlier.

Discharge teaching focuses on ensuring that the client understands the medication and how to take it. Thyroid function is monitored at regular intervals after client discharge for development of hyperthyroidism or hypothyroidism and for testing the effectiveness of medication.

THYROID CANCER

The incidence of thyroid cancer is rising. One reason may be the maturation of people who were exposed to low-dose radiation early in life. Thyroid cancer estimates in the United States for 2007 were more than 33,550 new cases and nearly 1530 deaths.[1] Women are three times more likely to develop thyroid cancer than men. Its incidence peaks during the 60s, but it may arise from infancy to old age. Mortality is lowest in the young if the cancer is well differentiated.

Etiology and Risk Factors

Benign adenomas are usually not dangerous, although they occasionally grow large enough to cause respiratory problems by pressing against the trachea. Malignant transformation sometimes occurs, and the benign nodules become cancerous. Other risk factors include genetic predisposition, a family history of thyroid cancer, and a history of radiation therapy 10 to 20 years following cancer treatment elsewhere in the body.

Pathophysiology

Papillary and follicular carcinomas are the two most frequent types of thyroid cancers, with papillary forms accounting for about 75% of those. Both are slow-growing firm tumors that are palpable, and they may spread to regional lymph nodes in 15% (follicular) to 50% (papillary) of cases.[4-6,17,21]

Clinical Manifestations

The major manifestation of thyroid cancer is the appearance of a hard, irregular, painless nodule in an enlarged thyroid gland. The nodule itself is typically solitary, rapidly enlarging, and "cold" (i.e., it does not absorb radioactive iodine, in contrast to benign adenomas, which may absorb radioactive iodine). This is determined by giving a tracer dose of ^{131}I and performing a thyroid scan 24 hours later to assess ^{131}I uptake by any nodules. "Hot" nodules absorb more isotope than normal tissue and are usually benign.

If the tumor has metastasized, the lymph nodes are sometimes palpable. The diagnosis of thyroid cancer is confirmed by fine needle aspiration biopsy.

OUTCOME MANAGEMENT

Medical Management

Without prompt, aggressive therapy, a client with thyroid cancer risks death. Chemotherapy, ^{131}I external radiation, or TSH suppressive therapy may be used for metastasis, as discussed earlier. A client with a benign nodule is likely to undergo long-term suppression therapy with levothyroxine. The desired outcome is to suppress serum TSH level without causing hypothyroidism.

Surgical Management

Treatment usually includes removal of all or part of the thyroid. Neck resection may be done for metastases to the neck (see section on Thyroidectomy). As with a thyroidectomy for noncancerous lesions, the major postoperative complications are respiratory distress, recurrent laryngeal damage, hemorrhage, and hypoparathyroidism.

Nursing Management of the Medical-Surgical Client

Nursing care of the client with thyroid cancer is similar to the care of any client undergoing a thyroidectomy. The client also needs the support and teaching that a client with cancer requires. If the client is to have chemotherapy, additional teaching is needed.

PARATHYROID DISORDERS

HYPERPARATHYROIDISM

Hyperparathyroidism, a disorder caused by overactivity of one or more of the parathyroid glands, is classified as primary, secondary, or tertiary. It usually occurs in clients older than 60 and affects women twice as often as men, and clients with renal failure. The overall incidence of hyperparathyroidism is 27 per 100,000.[18,21]

Etiology and Risk Factors

Primary hyperparathyroidism develops when the normal regulatory relationship between serum calcium levels and parathyroid hormone (PTH) secretion is interrupted. The interruption occurs when an adenoma or hyperplasia of the gland exists without an identifying injury.

Secondary hyperparathyroidism occurs when the glands are hyperplastic because of malfunction of another organ system. It is usually the result of renal failure but may also occur as a result of cancers such as multiple myeloma, or carcinoma with bone metastasis.

Tertiary hyperparathyroidism occurs when PTH production is irrepressible (autonomous) in clients with normal or low serum calcium levels.

Pathophysiology

The normal function of PTH is to increase bone resorption, thereby maintaining the proper balance of calcium and phosphorus ions in the blood. Excessive circulating PTH leads to bone damage, hypercalcemia, and kidney damage.

Primary Hyperparathyroidism

The severity of hypercalcemia reflects the quantity of hyperfunctioning parathyroid tissue. Excessive PTH stimulates transport of calcium into the blood from the intestine, kidneys, and bone. Nephrolithiasis is secondary to calcium phosphate kidney stones and deposition of calcium in the soft tissues of the kidney. Pyelonephritis may complicate the nephrolithiasis. Bone resorption related to hypercalcemia may develop.

Secondary Hyperparathyroidism

Chronic renal failure and hyperphosphatemia cause secondary hyperparathyroidism. As the glomerular filtration rate (GFR) decreases in chronic renal failure, serum phosphorus levels rise, which causes the serum calcium level to fall. PTH secretion is stimulated. This increase decreases renal tubular absorption of phosphorus, causing serum phosphorus levels to return to normal. As the GFR continues to decrease, PTH is secreted in increased amounts to decrease tubular reabsorption of phosphorus and maintain serum phosphorus level at or close to normal limits.

Clinical Manifestations

While some clients with hyperparathyroidism may be asymptomatic, there exists a myriad of manifestations arising from skeletal disease, renal involvement, gastro-intestinal tract disorders, and neurologic abnormalities, as outlined in the Critical Monitoring feature above, right, and in Figure 43-3.

Manifestations of bone disease range from backache, joint pain, and bone pain to pathologic fractures of the spine, ribs, and long bones. In long-standing cases, assessment reveals deformity and bending of the bones. Osteitis fibrosa with supraperiosteal resorption or bone cysts, arthritis, or radiologic osteoporosis may also exist.

Manifestations of renal involvement include polyuria and polydipsia; the appearance of sand, gravel, or stones (calculi) in the urine; azotemia; and hypertension resulting from renal damage. Without intervention, renal

---

CRITICAL MONITORING

Hyperparathyroidism and Hypoparathyroidism

These manifestations should be monitored in a client who is thought to have a diagnosis of hyperparathyroidism or hypoparathyroidism.

Hyperparathyroidism	Hypoparathyroidism
Increased bone resorption	Decreased bone resorption
Elevated serum calcium levels	Depressed serum calcium levels
Depressed serum phosphate levels	Elevated serum phosphate levels
Hypercalciuria and hyperphosphaturia	Hypocalciuria and hypophosphaturia
Decreased neuromuscular irritability	Increased neuromuscular activity, which may progress to tetany

---

insufficiency may progress to fatal renal hypertension and uremia.

Hypercalcemia produces mainly gastrointestinal manifestations such as thirst, nausea, anorexia, constipation, ileus, and abdominal pain. Decreased neuromuscular

Clinical Manifestations of Hyperparathyroidism:
"Bones, Stones, Moans, and Groans"

Bones	Stones
Osteitis fibrosa with: • Subperiosteal resorptions • Osteoclastomas • Bone cysts Radiological "osteoporosis" Osteomalacia or rickets Arthritis	Renal stones Nephrocalcinosis Polyuria Polydipsia Uremia
Abdominal groans	**Psychic moans**
Constipation Indigestion, nausea, vomiting Peptic ulcer Pancreatitis	Lethargy, fatigue Depression Memory loss Psychoses-paranoia Personality change, neuroses Confusion, stupor, coma
Other	
Proximal muscle weakness Keratitis, conjunctivitis Hypertension Itching	

■ **FIGURE 43–3** Clinical manifestations of primary hyperparathyroidism.

irritability is also common. Often, clients have a history of peptic ulcer or gastrointestinal bleeding. Assessment may also reveal psychiatric manifestations; listlessness, depression, and paranoia are sometimes associated with high levels of serum calcium.

Major complications include the manifestations associated with hypercalcemia and those associated with treatment, such as dehydration, hypocalcemia, and gastrointestinal problems.

The diagnosis of hyperparathyroidism mainly rests on laboratory and x-ray findings. Serum calcium levels are elevated, serum phosphate levels are depressed, and both urine calcium and urine phosphorus levels are high. In addition, alkaline phosphatase level is elevated in the 25% of clients who have associated bone disease (see the Laboratory Tests for Endocrine and Metabolic Function for Chapter 42 on the website). Clients with skeletal damage generally present with diffuse demineralization of bones, bone cysts, subperiosteal bone resorption, and loss of the lamina dura around the teeth.

OUTCOME MANAGEMENT

Medical Management

The desired outcomes of the medical treatment of hyperparathyroidism include lowering severely elevated calcium levels and long-term management of hypercalcemia with drugs to increase bone resorption of calcium.

Serum calcium levels are lowered by hydration and calciuria. Hydration can be achieved with an infusion of normal saline solution. Normal saline is the fluid of choice because it both expands the volume and acts in the kidney to inhibit the resorption of calcium. Furosemide (Lasix), a loop diuretic, may also be used to promote calciuria after rehydration has occurred. Thiazide diuretics are not used because they promote calcium retention in the kidneys. A client with hypercalcemia should have a diet low in calcium and vitamin D.

Drugs that inhibit bone resorption include plicamycin (Mithracin), gallium nitrate (Ganite), phosphates, and calcitonin. Plicamycin is a chemotherapeutic drug that is effective in lowering serum calcium levels. The hypocalcemic effect occurs after 24 hours and lasts about 1 to 2 weeks. The dose is about one tenth that used for cancer treatment, and the adverse effects are proportionally lower.

Gallium nitrate, a newer drug, is now being used more often because it has even fewer side effects. Glucocorticoids may be used to reduce hypercalcemia by decreasing the gastrointestinal absorption of calcium. Etidronate (Didronel) or calcitonin can be used to decrease the release of calcium by bones (see the Integrating Pharmacology feature above, right).

INTEGRATING PHARMACOLOGY

Medications for Parathyroid Disorders

The desired outcomes of the medical treatment of hyperparathyroidism include lowering severely elevated calcium levels and long-term management of hypercalcemia with drugs to increase bone resorption of calcium.

Serum calcium levels are lowered by hydration and calciuria. Furosemide (Lasix), a loop diuretic, may be used to promote calciuria. Drugs that inhibit bone resorption include plicamycin (Mithracin), gallium nitrate (Ganite), phosphates, and calcitonin. Plicamycin is a chemotherapeutic drug that is effective in lowering serum calcium levels. The hypocalcemic effect occurs after 24 hours and lasts for about 1 to 2 weeks. Gallium nitrate may be used because it has fewer side effects.

Glucocorticoids may be used to reduce hypercalcemia by decreasing gastrointestinal absorption of calcium. In addition, Didronel (etidronate) or calcitonin may be used to decrease the release of calcium by bones.

For clients with chronic hypoparathyroidism, the desired outcome of intervention is to restore the serum calcium level to normal concentrations. In clients with acute hypoparathyroidism, 10% calcium gluconate solution in an intravenous infusion is ordered. In chronic hypoparathyroidism, the client is given oral calcium salts (calcium gluconate, calcium lactate, or calcium carbonate) to maintain normal serum calcium levels. The client may also be given vitamin D to maintain serum calcium levels. Some clients may receive replacement of the absent hormone.

Nursing Management of the Medical Client

Assessment. Obtain a thorough history from the client to determine whether any risk factors are present. The client may exhibit psychological changes, such as lethargy, drowsiness, memory loss, and emotional lability, all manifestations seen in hypercalcemia.

Diagnosis, Outcomes, Interventions
Diagnosis: Impaired Urinary Elimination. The development of urinary lithiasis in clients with hyperparathyroidism may lead to the nursing diagnosis *Impaired Urinary Elimination related to renal involvement secondary to hypercalcemia and hyperphosphaturia resulting in urolithiasis, painful urination, hematuria, and spasms.*

Outcomes. The client will resume a normal urine output as evidenced by urine production of 0.5 ml/kg/hour without development of stones.

> **Amounts less than 0.5 ml/kg/hour should be reported to the physician.**

Interventions

Encourage Fluids. The client should consume at least 3000 ml of fluid each day. Dehydration is dangerous in clients with hyperparathyroidism because it increases the serum calcium level and promotes the formation of renal stones.

Prevent Urolithiasis. Cranberry juice or prune juice may help make the urine more acidic. Acidification helps to prevent renal stone formation because calcium is more soluble in acidic urine than in alkaline urine.

Strain Urine of Stones. If a kidney stone is present, strain all urine to detect gravel and stones. Save any specimens of abnormal urine for the physician to examine and for laboratory analysis. Also, observe the urine for blood and assess the client for renal colic (see Chapter 34).

Evaluation. Depending on the cause of the hypercalcemia, medical management may be able to control primary hypercalcemia. If it does not, surgery may be required. If the condition is secondary to renal failure, management is more chronic.

Surgical Management

Parathyroidectomy

Indications. Definitive treatment of primary hyperparathyroidism is surgical removal of the gland or glands causing hypersecretion of PTH. Intraoperative, rapid parathyroid hormone assay measurement affords the ability to ensure removal of all hyperfunctioning parathyroid tissue.

Autotransplantation of the parathyroid glands is a useful modality for the management of certain forms of hyperparathyroidism and radical neck surgery. After partial parathyroidectomy, it is possible to transplant the remaining healthy parathyroid tissue to a safer location, such as the brachioradial muscle of the forearm. Re-exploration of the neck in the future may cause laryngeal nerve damage and influence complications of the original surgery. Transplantation procedures take some time to come to full effect. In the meantime, the client must supplement the diet with calcium and vitamin D to prevent hypoparathyroidism and hypocalcemia.

If hyperparathyroidism is surgically treated early in its course, the chance of total recovery is good. Bone pain may disappear within 3 days after removal of parathyroid tissue, and bone lesions may heal completely. Unfortunately, serious renal disease might not be reversible by parathyroid surgery.

Complications. Complications after parathyroidectomy are similar to those following thyroidectomy and rarely occur.

Hypocalcemia is a potentially life-threatening complication even if some parathyroid glands are left untouched because edema reduces their function. The client may also experience respiratory distress related either to hemorrhage or to recurrent laryngeal nerve damage. SAFETY ALERT

Outcomes. The cure rate for primary hyperparathyroidism after surgical removal is greater than 95%.

Nursing Management of the Surgical Client

Assessment. The client undergoing surgery may have long-standing hyperparathyroidism and thus should be assessed for complications of the disease. Renal function should be carefully assessed preoperatively.

Diagnosis, Outcomes, Interventions

Diagnosis: Risk for Injury. The client undergoing surgery for hyperparathyroidism is at risk for a number of complications. An important nursing diagnosis is *Risk for Injury related to preoperative drug sensitivities and postoperative complications.*

Outcomes. The client will not suffer injury as evidenced by the absence of medication reactions preoperatively and by the absence of respiratory distress, hemorrhage, and hypocalcemia postoperatively.

Interventions

Administer Digitalis

If the client is receiving digitalis, administer this medication with extreme caution. Clients with hypercalcemia are hypersensitive to digitalis, and toxic manifestations may develop quickly. SAFETY ALERT

Monitor for Postoperative Complications

During the postoperative period, new problems arise, some of which are the reverse of those found preoperatively. During the immediate postoperative period, nursing care is similar to that after thyroidectomy; that is, assess the client carefully for hemorrhage, airway obstruction, injury to the recurrent laryngeal nerve, and tetany. Also watch for manifestations of hormonal imbalance.

Mild tetany resulting from a drop in the serum calcium level is expected after removal of parathyroid tissue. Typically, the uncomfortable tingling of the hands and around the mouth that follows parathyroid resection is temporary. If it persists or is severe, however, calcium gluconate is administered intravenously.

Evaluation. If hypercalcemia remains unrelieved by medical management, surgery is usually therapeutic. If a partial parathyroidectomy is unsuccessful, the remaining gland may need to be transplanted to the forearm to reduce absorption of the hormone. This measure usually eliminates the problem. As long as the client is closely observed in the immediate postoperative period, complications of hypocalcemia are usually controllable.

Modifications for Older Clients

Hyperparathyroidism in older adults is an overlooked disease. It is estimated that 1 of 1000 men and 2 of 1000 women older than 60 years experience hyperparathyroidism.[18] This disease often goes undiagnosed in older people because manifestations in the early stages are subtle and attributed to old age, depression, or anxiety. The manifestations intensify as the serum calcium level continues to rise and other physiologic and functional changes occur. Laboratory diagnosis is the same as for a younger client, but treatment may be complicated by medical problems and medication.

HYPOPARATHYROIDISM

Hyposecretion of the parathyroid glands produces hypoparathyroidism. That is, serum calcium levels are abnormally low, serum phosphate levels are abnormally high, and pronounced neuromuscular irritability (tetany) may develop.

Hypoparathyroidism is diagnosed in women more often than men. The incidence is related to thyroid surgery. The incidence of temporary hypoparathyroidism after total thyroidectomy ranges from 6.9% to 25%. The incidence after subtotal thyroidectomy is 1.6% to 9%.[18]

Etiology and Risk Factors
The causes of hypoparathyroidism are either *iatrogenic* (treatment-induced) or *idiopathic* (without a specific cause). Iatrogenic causes include accidental removal of the parathyroid glands during thyroidectomy, infarction of the parathyroid glands because of an inadequate blood supply to the glands during surgery, and strangulation of one or more of the glands by postoperative scar tissue. Health maintenance actions include monitoring of PTH, calcium, and phosphorus levels. Calcium supplements are required for life to prevent tetany.

In rare occurrences idiopathic hypoparathyroidism may exist. Like Graves' disease and Hashimoto's disease, it may be an autoimmune disorder with a genetic basis. *Pseudohypoparathyroidism* (Albright's hereditary osteodystrophy) is an inherited form of hypoparathyroidism that involves a lack of end-organ responsiveness to PTH.

Pathophysiology
Normally PTH acts to increase bone resorption, which maintains proper serum calcium levels. PTH also regulates phosphate clearance by the renal tubules, thereby maintaining the correct inverse balance between serum calcium and serum phosphate levels. Consequently, when parathyroid secretion is reduced, bone resorption slows, serum calcium levels fall, and severe neuromuscular irritability develops. Somewhat paradoxically, calcifications form in various organs, such as the eyes and basal ganglia. Also, without sufficient PTH, fewer phosphorus ions are secreted by the distal tubules of the kidney, renal excretion of phosphate falls, and serum phosphate levels rise.

The client may fully recover from the effects of hypoparathyroidism if the condition is diagnosed early, before serious complications begin. Unfortunately, cataracts and brain calcification, once formed, are irreversible.

Clinical Manifestations
The manifestations of hypoparathyroidism result mainly from low serum calcium levels. Manifestations are always more severe in clients with an elevated serum pH (alkalosis) of any cause (e.g., hyperventilation, ingestion of antacids). They worsen because, when the pH of the blood rises, the amount of ionized calcium drops, although total serum calcium remains the same. With less ionized calcium available to the body, the manifestations resulting from hypocalcemia become more severe until the alkalosis is corrected.

Acute Hypoparathyroidism
Acute hypoparathyroidism is caused by accidental damage to parathyroid tissues during thyroidectomy. It is characterized by greatly increased neuromuscular irritability, which results in tetany. Clients with tetany experience painful muscle spasms, irritability, grimacing, tingling of the fingers, laryngospasm, and dysrhythmias. Assessment also reveals Chvostek's and Trousseau's signs. In some cases, tetany is so severe that a tracheostomy is required to correct acute respiratory obstruction secondary to laryngospasm.

Chronic Hypoparathyroidism
Chronic hypoparathyroidism is usually idiopathic, resulting in lethargy; thin, patchy hair; brittle nails; dry, scaly skin; and personality changes. Ectopic or unexpected calcification may appear in the eyes and basal ganglia. Thus cataracts and permanent brain damage, accompanied by psychosis or convulsions, may develop. In addition, severe persistent hypocalcemia adversely affects the heart, causing dysrhythmias and eventual cardiac failure.

The diagnosis of hypoparathyroidism is based on the following physical examination findings related to hypocalcemia:

- Presence of Chvostek's sign (see Figure 12-3)
- Presence of Trousseau's sign (see Figure 12-3)
- Hyperactive deep tendon reflexes (DTRs)

- Circumoral paresthesia
- Numbness and tingling of fingers

The diagnosis of hypoparathyroidism also stems from the following findings:

- Laboratory findings showing low calcium level, low PTH level, high phosphorus level, decreased urine calcium level
- Radiographic studies of the skull or computed tomography (CT) of the head showing areas of calcification
- Ophthalmic examination revealing calcification of the ocular lens, which may lead to cataract formation

Complications

If treatment is not started rapidly in acute hypoparathyroidism, death can result from the respiratory obstruction secondary to tetany and laryngospasms. In chronic hypoparathyroidism, the complications are calcifications in the eye and basal ganglia.

OUTCOME MANAGEMENT

Medical Management

Acute hypoparathyroidism (with its major manifestation of acute tetany) is a life-threatening disorder. The desired outcomes of emergency care are to elevate serum calcium levels as rapidly as possible, to prevent or treat seizures, and to control laryngeal spasm and consequent respiratory obstruction.

For clients with chronic hypoparathyroidism, the desired outcome of intervention is to restore the serum calcium level to normal concentrations. Calcium levels are increased more gradually than in acute hypoparathyroidism.

Elevate Serum Calcium Levels

In clients with acute hypoparathyroidism, to elevate serum calcium levels quickly, the physician prescribes 10% calcium gluconate solution in an intravenous infusion. While administering the calcium gluconate, instruct the client to inhale carbon dioxide by breathing into a paper bag. Carbon dioxide inhalation causes a mild metabolic acidosis, which elevates the amount of ionized calcium in the blood.

When the condition has stabilized and the dangers of tetany have passed, the client is given oral calcium salts to maintain normal serum calcium levels. The desired outcome of therapy for chronic hypoparathyroidism is to keep the client asymptomatic with a serum calcium level of about 8.5 to 9.2 mg/dl. The client is given oral calcium salts (calcium gluconate, calcium lactate, or calcium carbonate).

The client is given vitamin D in addition to calcium supplements to maintain serum calcium levels. Commercially available forms of vitamin D include ergocalciferol (vitamin D_2) and dihydrotachysterol (Hytakerol). All three forms of vitamin D are effective in correcting hypocalcemia. They are available as either tablets or oily liquids. Aluminum hydroxide gel (Amphojel) is also prescribed.

The ideal treatment of this PTH-deficient condition is replacement of the absent hormone. A pure form of PTH has now been synthesized and is available (see the Integrating Pharmacology feature on Medications for Parathyroid Disorders).

A client with hypoparathyroidism should receive a diet high in calcium but low in phosphorus. Again, vitamin D is needed to maintain serum calcium levels, and clients should be encouraged to select foods or supplements enriched with vitamin D.

Tetany and laryngeal spasms may occur suddenly and without warning in clients at risk for acute hypoparathyroidism. Calcium gluconate should be readily available at the bedside, and in many cases an order is left to have a tracheotomy tray available at the bedside. SAFETY ALERT

Nursing Management of the Medical Client

Assessment. Carefully assess the client at risk for acute hypoparathyroidism (e.g., the post-thyroidectomy client) for development of hypocalcemia. Question the client about any numbness or tingling around the mouth or in the fingertips or toes. Check for Chvostek's and Trousseau's signs (see Figure 12-3). In addition, assess for any manifestation of respiratory distress secondary to laryngospasm.

In a client with chronic hypoparathyroidism, assess for obvious physical changes, such as dry skin and hair. Also assess for a parkinsonian syndrome or cataracts. Assess the teeth because pits may encircle them, indicating enamel hypoplasia.

Diagnosis, Outcomes, Interventions
Diagnosis: Risk for Injury: Muscle Tetany. A client with hypoparathyroidism is susceptible to hypocalcemia, which can lead to the nursing diagnosis *Risk for Injury: Muscle Tetany related to decreased serum calcium levels.*

Outcomes. The client will remain free from injury as evidenced by a return of calcium levels to normal range, a normal respiratory rate, and blood gases within normal limits.

Interventions
Prevent Respiratory Arrest. When caring for a client with severe hypoparathyroidism, always be prepared for laryngeal spasm and respiratory obstruction. Have an endotracheal tube, laryngoscope, and tracheostomy set available when caring for a client with acute tetany.

Monitor and Prevent Tetany. When a client is at risk for sudden hypocalcemia, as after thyroidectomy, an ampule of intravenous calcium carbonate is usually kept at the bedside for immediate use if necessary. When the intravenous tubing is removed, it is sometimes capped so that rapid venous access is available. Sometimes clients are encouraged to ingest a ready source of calcium carbonate, such as Tums.

Evaluation. If hypocalcemia is transient after a thyroidectomy, it usually resolves as edema decreases. If it is chronic, the client is usually able to manage the therapeutic regimen with minimal difficulty.

Self-Care

Because hypoparathyroidism can be a chronic condition, the client must be able to provide self-care. Teaching is important for the client with chronic hypoparathyroidism because this client requires lifelong medication and dietary modification.

Medications

When teaching the client about take-home medications, make sure the client knows that all forms of vitamin D, except dihydroxycholecalciferol, are slowly assimilated by the body. Therefore it may take a week or longer for the manifestations to improve.

Modifications

Teach the client about a diet high in calcium but low in phosphorus. Remind the client to omit cheese and milk products, which have a high phosphorus content. Explain that calcium supplements may be obtained in either tablet or solution form, depending on preference. Oral calcium administration is usually discontinued when the client responds to vitamin D preparations.

Emphasize the importance of lifelong medical care for the client with chronic hypoparathyroidism. Instruct the client to have serum calcium levels checked by a physician at least three times a year. Normal blood serum calcium levels must be maintained to prevent complications. If hypercalcemia or hypocalcemia develops, the physician will adjust the treatment regimen to correct the imbalance.

CONCLUSIONS

You must make careful assessments of clients with thyroid or parathyroid disorders. These disorders can be controlled and the manifestations reversed if they are discovered in a timely manner and prompt and proper treatment is begun. You are an important resource for these clients, who require considerable education. You are also responsible for closely monitoring any client who needs surgery for either the thyroid or the parathyroid gland.

The client is particularly vulnerable during this postoperative period, and high-level nursing surveillance and intervention facilitate successful recovery.

THINKING CRITICALLY

1. A 64-year-old man comes to the clinic with a 6-month history of progressive fatigue, weakness, and dyspnea. On further questioning, you find that he has had an unintentional weight loss of 30 pounds despite an increased appetite. Your physical examination reveals an alert and oriented man who looks his stated age. He is somewhat anxious. His attention span is short, and you must repeat many questions. His heart rate is 118 beats/min, blood pressure 154/98 mm Hg, temperature 101° F; the skin is warm and moist; deep tendon reflexes are hyperactive. What are priorities for care?

Factors to Consider. What additional subjective and objective data should you collect to confirm a diagnosis? What medication might be started after the diagnosis is made?

2. The client is a woman with a long history of chronic renal failure. She receives dialysis three times a week. She is currently hospitalized for a complicated pneumonia. On reviewing her laboratory values, you note that her serum calcium level is 6.8 mg/dl. What are the implications for care?

Factors to Consider. What is the relationship of calcium metabolism to renal function? What are the dangers associated with this serum calcium level? What treatments should be initiated to treat this, and what should be done to prevent recurrence?

3. A middle-age woman comes to the clinic with manifestations of weight gain, lethargy, fatigue, and severe constipation. After diagnostic evaluation, the client is given Synthroid, 0.1 mg, for hypothyroidism. What general information should you give the client about hypothyroidism? About the medication?

Factors to Consider. What should you teach the client about the expected therapeutic response to this medication? About side effects? How often are blood studies required for the client being treated with thyroid medications?

Discussions for these questions can be found on the website.

BIBLIOGRAPHY

Citations appearing in red refer to primary research.

Citations appearing in blue refer to evidence-based practice guidelines and protocols.

1. American Cancer Society. (2007). *Cancer facts & figures 2007.* Atlanta: Author.
2. Cappola, A., et al. (2006). Thyroid status, cardiovascular risk, and mortality in older adults. *Journal of the American Medical Association, 295*(9), 1033-1041.
3. Clyde, P., Harari, A., Getka, E., et al. (2003). Combined levothyroxine plus liothyronine compared with levothyroxine alone in primary hypothyroidism: A randomized controlled trial. *Journal of the American Medical Association, 290*(22), 2952-2958.

4. Davies, L., & Welch, H.G. (2006). Increasing incidence of thyroid cancer in the United States, 1973–2002. *Journal of the American Medical Association, 295*(18), 2164-2167.

5. Deftos, L., & Gagel, R. (2004). Medullary thyroid carcinoma and calcitonin. In L. Goldman, et al. (Eds.), *Cecil textbook of medicine* (22nd ed., pp. 1571-1574). Philadelphia: Saunders.

6. Dillman, W. (2004). The thyroid. In L. Goldman, et al. (Eds.), *Cecil textbook of medicine* (22nd ed., pp. 1391-1411). Philadelphia: Saunders.

7. Franklyn, J., Sheppard, M., & Maisonneuve, P. (2005). Thyroid function and mortality in patients treated for hyperthyroidism. *Journal of the American Medical Association, 294*(1), 71-80.

8. Gahart, B., & Nazareno, A. (2007). *Intravenous medications* (23rd ed.). St. Louis: Mosby.

9. Gussekloo, J., et al. (2004). Thyroid status, disability and cognitive function, and survival in old age. *Journal of the American Medical Association, 292*(21), 2591-2613.

10. Holcomb, S. (2002). Thyroid disease. *Dimensions of Critical Care Nursing, 21*(4), 127-133.

11. Imaizumi, M., et al. (2006). Radiation dose-response relationships for thyroid nodules and autoimmune thyroid diseases in Hiroshima and Nagasaki atomic bomb survivors 55-58 years after radiation exposure. *Journal of the American Medical Association, 295*(9), 1011-1022.

12. Johnson, M., et al. (2006). *NANDA, NOC, and NIC linkages: Nursing diagnosis, outcomes, & interventions* (2nd ed.). St. Louis. Mosby.

13. Larsen, R., et al. (2003). *Williams textbook of endocrinology* (10th ed.). Philadelphia: Saunders.

14. Kumrow, D., & Dahlen, R. (2002). Thyroidectomy: Understanding the potential for complications. *MEDSURG Nursing, 11*(5), 228-236.

15. Malchiodi, L. (2002). Thyroid storm. Recognizing the signs and symptoms of this life-threatening complication. *American Journal of Nursing, 102*(5), 33-35.

16. Miller, F., et al. (2006). Risk factors for the development of hypothyroidism after hemithyroidectomy. *Archives of Otolaryngology—Head and Neck Surgery, 132*, 36-38.

17. Schultz, P. (2002). Providing information to patients with a rare cancer: Using internet discussion forums to address the needs of patients with medullary thyroid carcinoma. *Clinical Journal of Oncology Nurses, 6*(4), 219-222.

18. Spiegel, A. (2004). The parathyroid glands, hypercalcemia, and hypocalcemia. In L. Goldman, et al. (Eds.), *Cecil textbook of medicine* (22nd ed., pp. 1562-1570). Philadelphia: Saunders.

19. Steingrimsdottir, L., et al. (2005). Relationship between serum parathyroid hormone levels, Vitamin D sufficiency, and calcium intake. *Journal of the American Medical Association, 294*(18), 2336-2340.

20. Surks, M., et al. (2004). Subclinical thyroid disease: Scientific review and guidelines for diagnosis and management. *Journal of the American Medical Association, 291*(2), 228-244.

21. Weigel, R., et al. (2004). Cancer of the endocrine system. In M. Abeloff, et al. (Eds.), *Clinical oncology* (3rd ed., pp. 1611-1648). Philadelphia: Churchill Livingstone.

evolve **Did you remember to check out the bonus material on the Evolve website and the CD-ROM, including NCLEX®-Examination Style Review Questions, Open-Book Quizzes, and Chapter Review Audio Podcasts?**

http://evolve.elsevier.com/Black/medsurg

Management of Clients with Adrenal and Pituitary Disorders

ALLEN HANBERG

ADRENOCORTICAL DISORDERS

Glandular hypofunction and hyperfunction characterize the major disorders of the adrenal cortex. Underactivity of the adrenal cortex results in a deficiency of glucocorticoids, mineralocorticoids, and adrenal androgens. The person with adrenal hypofunction is a prime candidate for injury, deficient knowledge, and feelings of powerlessness. Overactivity of the adrenal cortex results in excessive production of glucocorticoids, mineralocorticoids, and androgens or estrogens. The person with adrenal hyperfunction needs to focus on preventing injury and infection, acquiring effective coping mechanisms, and learning about the disease process.

ADRENAL INSUFFICIENCY

Hypofunction of the adrenal cortex can originate from a disorder in the adrenal gland itself (primary adrenal insufficiency), or it may result from hypofunction of the pituitary-hypothalamic unit (secondary adrenal insufficiency).

PRIMARY ADRENAL INSUFFICIENCY

Commonly known as *Addison's disease*, primary adrenal insufficiency results from idiopathic atrophy or destruction of the adrenal glands by an autoimmune process or other disease. Thomas Addison first described this disorder in 1849.

Etiology and Risk Factors
Primary adrenal insufficiency is caused by hypofunction of the adrenal glands. It is a rare disorder, and its incidence and prevalence in the United States are unknown. An autoimmune process accounts for 75% of primary adrenal insufficiency. It is commonly seen in people with

acquired immunodeficiency syndrome (AIDS). Tuberculosis is the cause in about 20% of cases of Addison's disease. Adrenal metastasis from the lung, breast, or gastrointestinal tract; melanoma; or lymphoma may also cause primary adrenal insufficiency. Additional causes include bilateral adrenalectomy and hemorrhagic infarction with necrosis of the adrenal gland.

Risk factors for primary adrenal insufficiency include (1) a history of other endocrine disorders, (2) taking glucocorticoids for more than 3 weeks with sudden cessation, (3) taking glucocorticoids more than once every other day, (4) adrenalectomy, and (5) tuberculosis. Ingestion of glucocorticoids may also result in secondary adrenal insufficiency as discussed later in the chapter.

Health promotion and health maintenance activities for clients receiving glucocorticoids include instruction on the risks and benefits of this therapy and on the proper means of withdrawing glucocorticoids. Health maintenance activities for those receiving long-term steroid therapy include education about the need for supplemental steroids to prevent acute adrenal insufficiency and having parenteral steroids available for use when the client is unable to take oral steroids. Health restoration activities include ensuring that the client is mindful of the need for follow-up with the physician to monitor steroid levels.

Pathophysiology
Autoimmunity is the most common cause of adrenal insufficiency. Lymphocytic infiltration of the adrenal

---

evolve **Web Enhancements**

Concept Map Understanding Hypercortisolism (Cushing's Disease) and its Treatment

Be sure to check out the bonus material on the Evolve website and the CD-ROM, including free self-assessment exercises. **http://evolve.elsevier. com/Black/medsurg**

cortex is the characteristic feature. Addison's disease is frequently accompanied by other immune disorders. Gradual destruction leads to chronic adrenal insufficiency. Continued loss of cortical tissue accompanies a deficiency of mineralocorticoids as well as glucocorticoids. Adrenocortical hypofunction results in decreased levels of mineralocorticoids (aldosterone), glucocorticoids (cortisol), and androgens.

Clinical Manifestations

The onset of Addison's disease is usually insidious. The client experiences mild fatigue, languor, irritability, weight loss, nausea, vomiting, and postural hypotension, usually weeks or months before the diagnosis is confirmed. As the disorder progresses, manifestations intensify. By then, the client has lost more than 90% of both adrenal cortices.

Diagnosis of Addison's disease depends primarily on blood and urine hormonal assays. Primary adrenal insufficiency is characterized by a low cortisol production rate and a high plasma adrenocorticotropic hormone (ACTH) concentration.

Other diagnostic tests that may be ordered to evaluate the effects of hypofunction of the adrenals on the body are the following: (1) serum electrolyte levels (especially hyponatremia and hyperkalemia in primary adrenal insufficiency and hyponatremia alone in secondary disease); (2) blood glucose level; (3) complete blood count (to assess for anemia); (4) x-ray studies; (5) computed tomography (CT); and (6) magnetic resonance imaging (MRI) of the adrenals and pituitary.

OUTCOME MANAGEMENT

Addisonian crisis is an emergent condition that requires careful monitoring in the critical care unit. Thereafter the rate of recovery is client specific. Normally, Addison's disease can be managed on an outpatient basis if the client receives and follows proper self-care instructions.

Medical Management

Addisonian Crisis

Addisonian crisis, or *acute adrenal insufficiency,* may occur when the client has been under stress without appropriate hormone replacement. Stressors include pregnancy, surgery, infection, states of dehydration or anorexia, fever, and emotional upheaval. Manifestations are related to the degree of hormone deficiency and electrolyte imbalance and include sudden, penetrating pain in the back, abdomen, or legs; depressed or changed mentation; volume depletion; hypotension; loss of consciousness; and shock.

Correct Fluid and Electrolyte Imbalances

The overall desired outcome of treatment is prevention of the morbidity and mortality associated with the addisonian crisis.

> **Untreated, addisonian crisis is fatal. The cause of the crisis must be determined and treated immediately. Hypotension and electrolyte imbalance need to be corrected quickly. Rapid rehydration is essential. An isotonic solution usually corrects the volume depletion, salt depletion, and hypotension. The client may also need oxygen, vasopressors, or volume expanders. Sodium polystyrene sulfonate (Kayexalate) may be administered orally or as an enema in combination with sorbitol for treatment of hyperkalemia. Kayexalate is a resin that releases sodium ions in exchange for potassium ions.**

SAFETY ALERT

Correct Hypoglycemia

Hypoglycemia must be evaluated and corrected with intravenous (IV) glucose (5% dextrose [D$_5$] solution IV or IV glucose push bolus).

Replace Steroids

Hydrocortisone 100 mg is administered as an intravenous (IV) bolus followed by 100 mg IV every 8 hours for 24 hours. The IV hydrocortisone is tapered as the client's status dictates. Oral hydrocortisone is initiated. The Integrating Pharmacology feature on p. 1042 provides additional details on steroid hormone replacement.

Addison's Disease

At one time Addison's disease was fatal within months. Today, with the availability of synthetic corticosteroids, clients with Addison's disease can live normal, active lives, provided they receive adequate glucocorticoid replacement. Use corticosteroids with caution. Carefully assess clients for manifestations of hypercortisolism, which can result from excessive long-term cortisol therapy. Most clients receive glucocorticoid and mineralocorticoid replacement.

Osteoporosis is a complication that may develop with excessive use of glucocorticosteroids because the protein matrix in the bones is broken down and therefore calcium cannot be retained. Closely observe clients with other medical problems that may be worsened with steroid use.

Nursing Management of the Medical Client

Addisonian Crisis

Assessment. Monitor the client's vital signs closely while the disease is being diagnosed. Check the pulse carefully, at least every 4 hours. Take orthostatic blood

INTEGRATING PHARMACOLOGY

Corticosteroids

Glucocorticoids may be prescribed for a variety of reasons and disorders because of the anti-inflammatory and immune-response suppression properties of these drugs. Glucocorticoids are categorized in three categories based on duration of action: long, intermediate, or short. Attention must also be given to the sodium-retaining capabilities of this class. For example, dexamethasone (Decadron) is a long-acting glucocorticoid that is often prescribed for head injuries because it suppresses inflammation and also has a low sodium-retaining ability, which is important in averting cerebral edema.

For clients with adrenal insufficiency, steroid hormone replacement therapy is essential. Most often, short-acting glucocorticoids such as hydrocortisone (Hydrocortone) are prescribed in a divided dose regimen with two thirds of the daily dose taken in the morning and one third taken in the afternoon. This practice simulates the body's normal ebb and flow of cortisol activity. Clients must be instructed on the essential nature of this therapy and the need to comply with the drug regimen. Wearing a drug alert identification device is essential and clients must also be advised to inform all health care providers regarding their steroid dependence. Adjustments in dosages may be expected during times of stress and clients should be taught to contact their primary health care provider as needed during these situations.

Mineralocorticoids such as fludrocortisone (Florinef) are also prescribed for a variety of reasons. Primarily mineralocorticoids act to conserve sodium and therefore water, resulting in increased circulating blood volume. This makes this class of drug an ideal choice for clients with chronic syncope related to orthostatic hypotension. Clients with adrenal insufficiency typically are prescribed a single daily dose of a mineralocorticoid.

If the steroid dose is too high, excessive amounts of sodium and water are retained and potassium excretion is high.

Diagnosis, Outcomes, Interventions

Diagnosis: Risk for Injury: Addisonian Crisis. The client must be diligent in self-care, or the nursing diagnosis may be *Risk for Injury: Addisonian Crisis related to adrenal insufficiency.*

Outcomes. The client will not exhibit injury as evidenced by the absence of hypotension, shock, or other manifestations of acute adrenal insufficiency.

Interventions

Monitor for Manifestations of Crisis. Addisonian crisis usually develops over 24 to 48 hours. Closely monitor for sudden profound weakness; severe abdominal, back, and leg pain; hyperpyrexia (although this may be suppressed by steroids) followed by hypothermia; hypotension associated with high cardiac output, normal wedge pressure, and low systemic resistance; coma; renal shutdown; and death.

> **An adrenal crisis is a medical emergency that must be treated rapidly and vigorously. The three major desired outcomes of intervention are (1) reversal of shock, (2) restoration of blood circulation (the client usually has a deficit of at least 20% of extracellular fluid volume), and (3) replenishment with essential steroids.**

Correct Fluid, Electrolyte, Steroid Imbalances. Immediately on admission, 1000 ml of normal saline with water-soluble glucocorticoid (hydrocortisone phosphate or hydrocortisone sodium succinate) added is rapidly infused. The dosage of the prescribed glucocorticoid is gradually reduced. It is administered intramuscularly (IM) or IV every 8 hours on days 1 and 2 of the crisis and gradually reduced thereafter. Hypoglycemia is controlled by a glucose infusion, either an IV bolus or an IV drip as part of rehydration. Hyperkalemia is controlled or corrected with Kayexalate. The precipitating event must be corrected. Plasma, oxygen, and vasopressor medications may be indicated.

> **Throughout the emergency period, monitor BP, administer IV infusion and medications, monitor hourly urine output, report oliguria (a manifestation of shock), and minimize exposure to emotional and physical stress. Observe for manifestations of glucocorticoid overdose and overhydration, such as generalized edema from fluid retention, hypertension, flaccid paralysis from hypokalemia, psychosis, and loss of consciousness. Also evaluate electrolyte levels for hyperkalemia, hyponatremia, and hypoglycemia, and correlate these findings with the client's manifestations.**

---

pressure (BP) readings and pulse rate measurements. Report drops in BP or orthostatic changes.

As rehydration occurs and electrolyte imbalances are corrected, assess increased physical vitality and emotional well-being. Assess bony prominences for pressure ulcers in immobilized clients. With therapy, listlessness and exhaustion should gradually disappear.

Monitor for exposure to cold and infections. Immediately inform the physician if evidence of infection develops. Remember, a client with Addison's disease cannot tolerate stress. Infection imposes additional stress on the body, and cortisol levels need to be higher during infectious illnesses.

Carefully assess for manifestations of sodium and potassium imbalance (see Chapter 12). Obtain daily weights for objective measurement of fluid gain or loss. If steroid replacement therapy is inadequate, sodium loss and potassium retention will continue to be uncorrected.

With rapid, efficient intervention, addisonian crisis usually resolves within 12 hours. The client's condition stabilizes, and the convalescent period begins. When the client can tolerate food and fluids by mouth, steroid replacement can be administered orally.

Prevent Future Crises. After the immediate crisis is over, help the client avoid further development of adrenal insufficiency. Obtain a medical identification (Medic-Alert) bracelet and an emergency kit before discharge from the hospital. Instruct the client to carry these items at all times. The client's name and diagnosis should appear on the identification bracelet, and a wallet card should state that the client receives daily hydrocortisone and that the medication must be administered by injection in an emergency.

Dexamethasone can be kept in a prepared syringe in an emergency kit with sterile alcohol wipes for cleaning the injection site. The kit should also contain written information about the client's diagnosis, prescribed drugs, dosage schedules, and emergency phone numbers, including the physician's name and phone number.

Adrenal insufficiency is a potentially life-threatening condition, but when properly recognized and treated, it has little or no effect on life span. There are no dietary or activity restrictions.

Evaluation. The outcome of treatment for addisonian crisis is easily evaluated, usually within 12 hours of treatment. By this time, the client should no longer exhibit any manifestations of addisonian crisis or death would have occurred.

Self-Care

Management of Addison's disease takes place in the community with regular medical follow-up of the client's status. Hence, the focus of management is on self-care. Carefully assess the client's ability to understand and perform self-care. The client needs extensive instruction in self-care activities to achieve independence. Appropriate outcomes for the client with Addison's disease are that the client's weight remains stable, the vital signs and cortisol levels remain within normal limits, and the client states that fatigue has decreased.

Steroid Replacement

The client must learn how to take steroids correctly. Provide the client and the client's significant others with written instructions on self-administration of steroids. (The client and significant others should have demonstrated their ability to prepare and administer injections.) The client needs to know the following information:

- Actions of prescribed hormones (hydrocortisone, fludrocortisone)

- Importance of taking medications daily, without fail, exactly as prescribed
- Principles of self-administration of oral medications (e.g., the client must check the label on the bottle before taking the medication and document medications taken and their side effects)
- Manifestations of overdosage and underdosage
- Importance of hydrocortisone self-injection when unable to tolerate oral medication (because of nausea and vomiting) and during times of acute stress (motor vehicle accident, trauma) because the body is unable to provide the needed additional glucocorticoid coverage
- Need for an IM self-injection kit to be available at all times
- Need for a Medic-Alert bracelet showing the diagnosis and the need for cortisol replacement
- Need for the client to call a health care provider if questions arise after discharge from the medical center

Emphasize that the client who takes glucocorticoids must call the physician to obtain a dosage increase when experiencing stressful situations (e.g., emotional upheavals, dental extractions, minor surgery, upper respiratory tract infections). The general rule is to double the glucocorticoid dosage for up to 1 week, depending on manifestations, and then resume normal dosage. In addition, temporary mineralocorticoid dosage is reduced by 50% to avoid excessive salt retention and hypertension. Encourage the client to consult the physician for dosage adjustment. The medication must be administered IM when nausea and vomiting prevent oral administration. SAFETY ALERT

Follow-Up Monitoring

Remind clients to keep semi-annual appointments with the physician, even when their health is good and self-medication is proceeding smoothly. As with diabetes mellitus, the control of Addison's disease is a lifelong responsibility.

Modifications for Older Clients

Adrenal diseases are uncommon in older people. The effects of normal aging on the adrenals are unclear. It appears, however, that ACTH and cortisol production remains constant throughout life. Older people may be more sensitive to the side effects of steroid therapy because these problems (e.g., osteoporosis, hypertension, diabetes mellitus) already exist.

SECONDARY ADRENAL INSUFFICIENCY

Secondary adrenal insufficiency results from dysfunction of the hypothalamic-pituitary-adrenal (HPA) axis (see the

Unit 10 Anatomy and Physiology Review). The most common cause is chronic treatment with glucocorticoids for non-endocrine uses. Other causes include the following:

- Hypopituitarism resulting in decreased ACTH secretion by the pituitary gland, which causes decreased secretion of cortisol and androgens by the adrenal gland
- Pituitary tumor or infarction
- Radiation
- Suppression of hypothalamic-pituitary secretion of ACTH related to hypercortisolism caused by either exogenous administration of corticosteroids or oversecretion of corticosteroids by an adrenal tumor (in both cases, the adrenal glands atrophy and become filled with lipids)

Secondary adrenal insufficiency is characterized by low cortisol production and low plasma ACTH levels. Because circulating levels of corticosteroids remain high, these clients do not experience manifestations of adrenocortical insufficiency unless steroid therapy is discontinued suddenly or the tumor is resected. If corticosteroid therapy is tapered gradually, with the dose reduced each day, adrenal gland function usually returns to normal.

Assessment reveals that clients with secondary adrenal insufficiency experience cortisol deficiency. Aldosterone continues to be secreted in sufficient amounts. Treatment involves administering glucocorticoids, as in Addison's disease. Mineralocorticoid replacement is unnecessary. Instruct the client to wear an emergency identification bracelet and to carry an emergency kit for hydrocortisone injection in case of an adrenal crisis.

ADRENOCORTICAL HYPERFUNCTION

Hyperfunction of the adrenal cortex can result in excessive production of glucocorticoids, mineralocorticoids, and androgens. Major conditions of adrenocortical hyperfunction are hypercortisolism (glucocorticoid excess) and primary aldosteronism (aldosterone excess).

HYPERCORTISOLISM

Hypercortisolism (Cushing's syndrome) was first described by Harvey Cushing in 1932. It results from overactivity of the adrenal gland, with consequent hypersecretion of glucocorticoids. Cushing's syndrome is relatively rare, and its incidence is unknown. It occurs mainly in women 20 to 40 years of age; however, it can occur up to age 60.

Etiology and Risk Factors

Iatrogenic hypercortisolism (resulting from medical interventions) accounts for most cases because of the frequent therapeutic use of high-dose glucocorticoids. Hypersecretion of cortisol can be caused by a cortisol-secreting adrenal tumor or adrenal hyperplasia, resulting from overproduction of ACTH. Adrenal tumors are responsible for about 30% of cases of Cushing's syndrome. Most (85%) are benign, but 15% are malignant. There are two sources of excessive ACTH secretion:

- Pituitary hypersecretion and pituitary tumors, which cause about 70% of cases of Cushing's syndrome. These usually benign tumors are either small basophil adenomas or large chromophobe adenomas. Pituitary hypersecretion of ACTH that results in glucocorticoid excess is called *Cushing's disease*.
- Ectopic secretion of ACTH (or *ectopic ACTH syndrome*). ACTH-secreting tumors located outside the pituitary gland are a rare cause of Cushing's syndrome. The tumors that most frequently cause ectopic ACTH syndrome are oat cell carcinoma of the lung; pancreatic islet cell carcinoma; and carcinoid tumors of the lung, gut, thymus, and ovary.

Iatrogenic Cushing's syndrome, another form of the disorder, results from exogenous (originating outside the body, e.g., taking supplemental medication) administration of synthetic glucocorticoids in supraphysiologic amounts. Thus educating clients to avoid unnecessary use of exogenous steroids is an important health promotion activity. Health maintenance activities include (1) educating clients who are at risk for manifestations of Cushing's syndrome; (2) treating clinical manifestations of hypernatremia, hypokalemia, hyperglycemia, and hypertension; and (3) teaching clients about adrenalectomy and steroid replacement. Health restoration activities include making sure that clients understand the importance of surgery, lifelong steroid replacement, and recognizing disease complications that may have already developed (such as osteoporosis or "buffalo hump," a fat pad on the neck).

Pathophysiology

When Cushing's syndrome develops, the normal function of the glucocorticoids becomes exaggerated and the classic picture of the syndrome emerges (Figure 44-1). This exaggerated physiologic action of glucocorticoids appears as follows:

- Persistent hyperglycemia (or "steroid diabetes").
- Protein tissue wasting, which results in muscle wasting and weakness; capillary fragility, which results in ecchymosis; and osteoporosis from bone matrix wasting. Osteoporosis can become so severe that even mild trauma can cause fractures. Com-

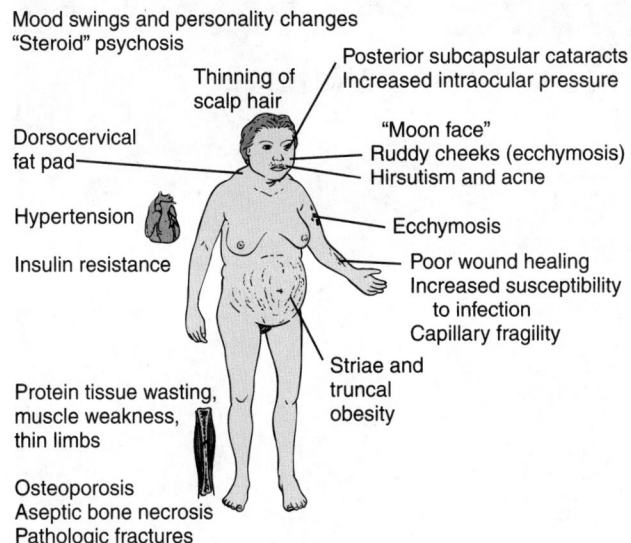

Mood swings and personality changes
"Steroid" psychosis

Thinning of scalp hair

Posterior subcapsular cataracts
Increased intraocular pressure

Dorsocervical fat pad

"Moon face"
Ruddy cheeks (ecchymosis)
Hirsutism and acne

Hypertension

Ecchymosis

Insulin resistance

Poor wound healing
Increased susceptibility to infection
Capillary fragility

Protein tissue wasting, muscle weakness, thin limbs

Striae and truncal obesity

Osteoporosis
Aseptic bone necrosis
Pathologic fractures

■ **FIGURE 44–1**   Clinical manifestations of Cushing's syndrome.

pression fractures can develop in the osteoporotic spine, leading to kyphosis and loss of height.

■ Potassium depletion, leading to hypokalemia, dysrhythmias, muscle weakness, and renal disorders.

■ Sodium and water retention, which causes edema and hypertension.

■ Hypertension, which eventually predisposes the client to left ventricular hypertrophy, heart failure, and stroke.

■ Abnormal fat distribution (in conjunction with edema), which results in a moon-shaped face, a dorsocervical fat pad on the neck (buffalo hump), and truncal obesity with slender limbs. Also, pink and purple striae appear on the breasts, axillary areas, abdomen, and legs because of thinning of the skin. Striking changes in appearance occur after the development and cure of Cushing's syndrome. Old photographs can be useful in showing changes over time.

■ Increased susceptibility to infection and lowered resistance to stress increase vulnerability to microorganisms of all types. Because of suppression of the inflammatory response, people with Cushing's syndrome show few manifestations of infection. They also demonstrate poor wound healing.

■ Possible increased production of androgens can cause virilism (masculine characteristics) in women. Manifestations of virilism include acne, thinning of scalp hair, and hirsutism (excessive bodily and facial hair in a male pattern).

■ Mental changes include memory loss, poor concentration and cognition, euphoria, and depression. Sometimes a condition called "steroid psychosis" develops. Depression can predispose the client to suicidal thoughts. About 80% of the clients meet the criteria for a major affective disorder: 50% with

unipolar depression, 30% with bipolar illness. The Concept Map on pp. 1046-1047 illustrates the pathophysiology, treatment, and clinical manifestations of this disorder.

Clinical Manifestations

Even for clients who have a classic cushingoid appearance, it is important to perform diagnostic studies for confirmation. Laboratory tests for Cushing's syndrome reflect hyperglycemia, fluid and electrolyte disturbances, and immunosuppressive responses that characterize excessive glucocorticoid secretion. Thus in Cushing's syndrome glucose tolerance decreases and glucosuria appears.

In the plasma ACTH test, low ACTH levels point to an adrenal tumor as the cause of hypercortisolism. Overproduction of cortisol by the adrenal tumor provides negative feedback to the pituitary gland, which responds by reducing ACTH release. The high cortisol level also provides feedback to the hypothalamus, which reduces release of corticotropin-releasing hormone.

An ectopic ACTH-producing tumor usually yields a normal or elevated ACTH level. ACTH production by the tumor is independent of pituitary production of ACTH. Thus despite negative feedback to the hypothalamic-pituitary unit, ACTH levels remain high.

If ACTH levels from the petrosal sinuses are greater than ACTH levels from a peripheral site (the arm), a pituitary tumor is identified as the source of hypercortisolism. If central ACTH levels (petrosal) and peripheral ACTH levels (arm) are equivalent, an ectopic ACTH-secreting tumor is likely.

OUTCOME MANAGEMENT

Surgical Management

Surgical removal of even one adrenal gland requires careful inpatient monitoring because the remaining adrenal gland may have atrophied and stopped producing adrenocortical hormones. For Cushing's syndrome caused by an adrenal tumor, an adrenalectomy can be performed to remove the gland containing the tumor. In case of ectopic ACTH-secreting tumors, the tumor can be difficult to localize. If no source is found, a bilateral adrenalectomy can be performed to interrupt the production of cortisol in response to the ACTH produced by the tumor, or the client can be treated with anti-glucocorticoids while the search for the tumor continues. ☜ Laparoscopic adrenalectomy is being evaluated as an alternative to traditional adrenalectomy. Early studies indicate that it may reduce postoperative morbidity.

After successful surgical removal of the adrenals, the client receives lifelong glucocorticoid and mineralocorticoid replacement. Most physical manifestations of Cushing's syndrome resolve after bilateral adrenalectomy.

Understanding Hypercortisolism (Cushing's Disease) and Its Treatment

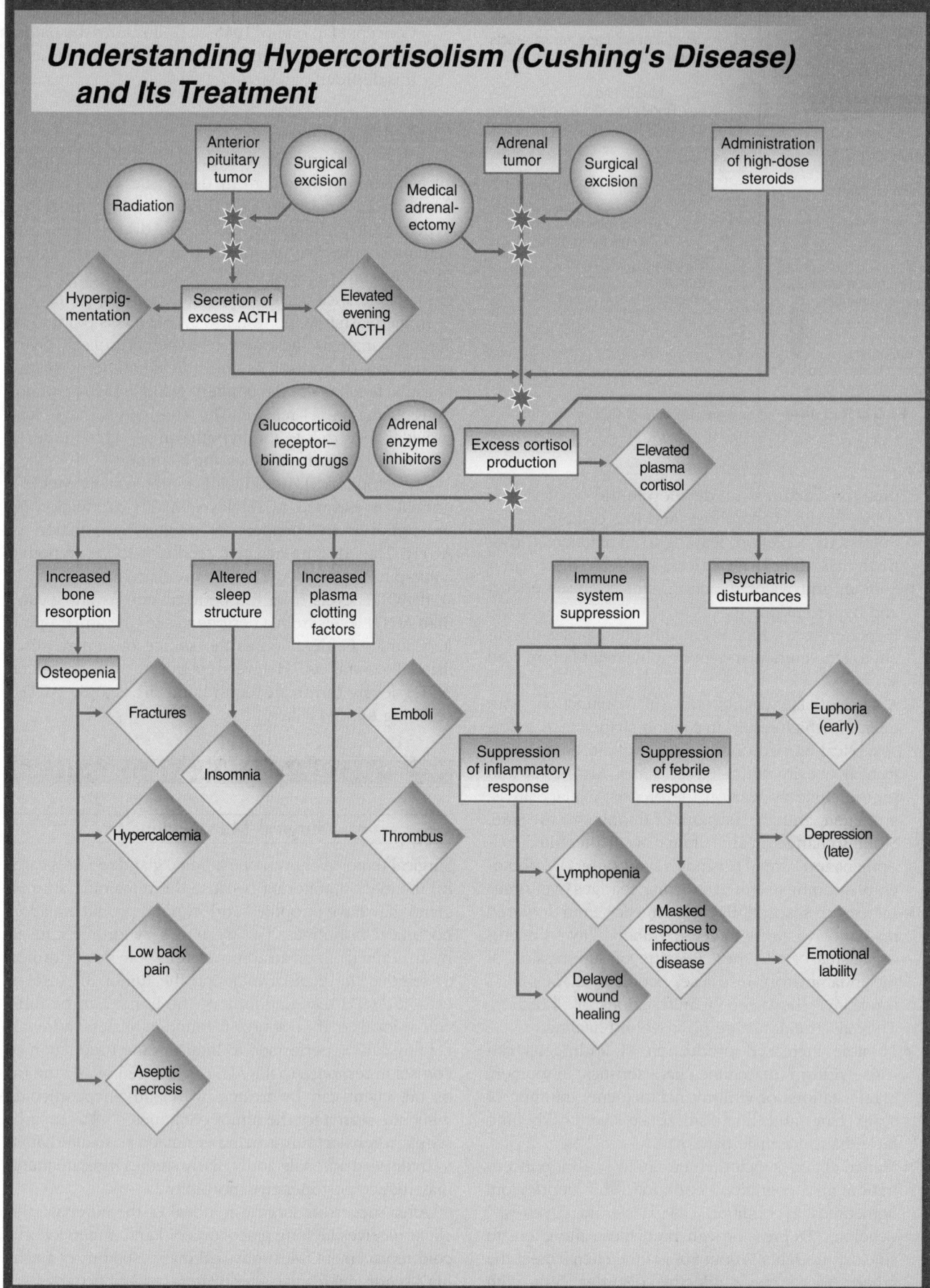

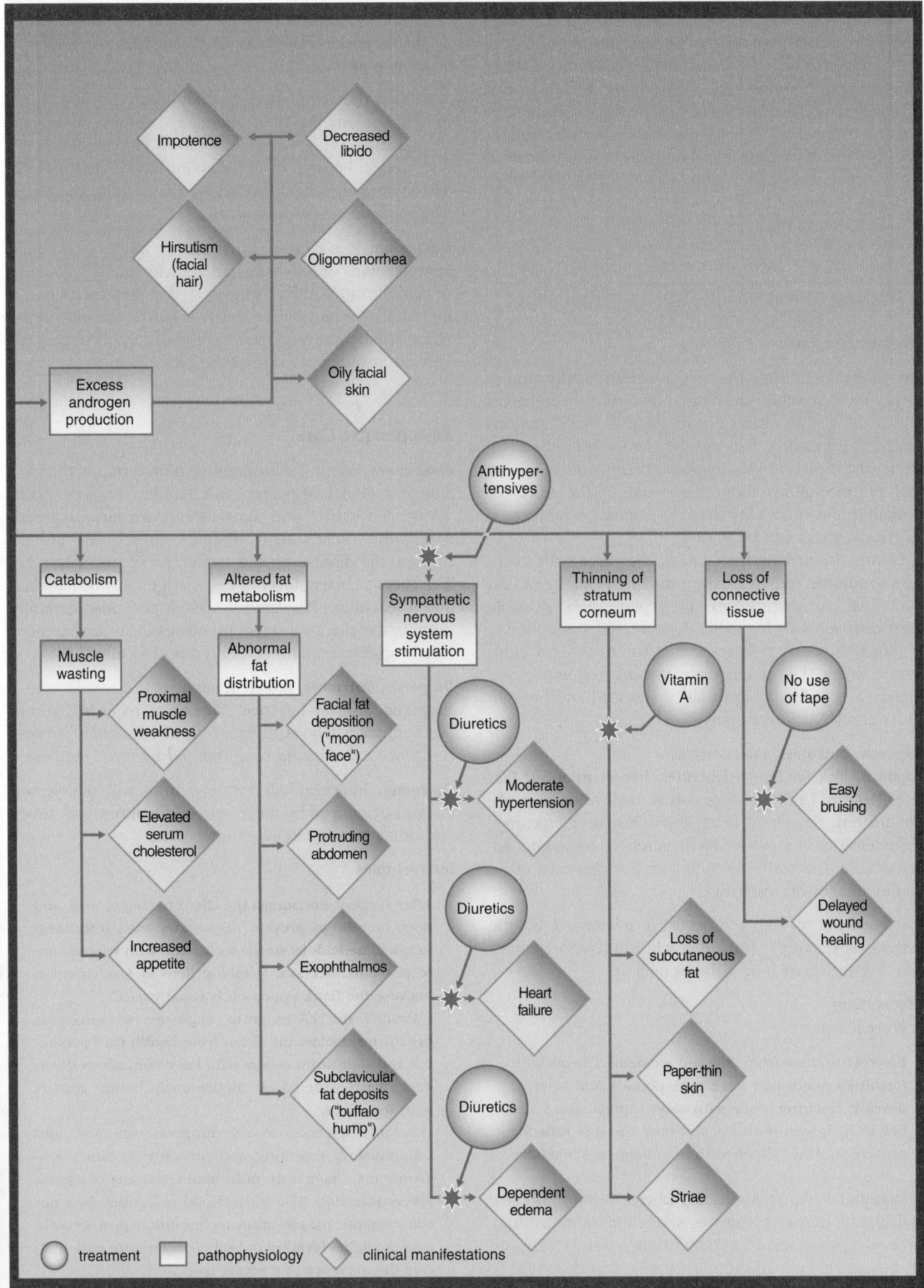

Resection of most pituitary tumors causing Cushing's disease is performed via transsphenoidal hypophysectomy (see Chapter 69). Occasionally, large or anatomically complex tumors are excised via a transfrontal approach (see later discussion of hypophysectomy). A surgical cure rate of 85% to 90% has been documented. Because the HPA axis has been suppressed, adrenal insufficiency develops postoperatively. The axis takes 12 to 24 months to recover. Replacement steroids are indicated during this time.

Nursing Management of the Surgical Client

Preoperative Care

Assessment. Begin by obtaining a careful history from a client with possible Cushing's syndrome. The client may exhibit the characteristic clinical manifestations identified previously. Support the client during the diagnostic phase of care. At this point, there is often a great deal of uncertainty about the cause of the disorder. Explain to the client why these tests must be performed before treatment can be started.

During the preoperative phase, the client with Cushing's syndrome requires expert nursing assessment and care. The crucial problems of hypertension, possible heart disease, diabetes mellitus, increased susceptibility to infection, decreased resistance to stress, and emotional lability (i.e., a tendency toward frequent mood changes) or instability must all be assessed and brought under control before surgery.

Diagnosis, Outcomes, Interventions
Diagnosis: Risk for Injury: Fractures, Hypertension, or Diabetes Mellitus. Until the diagnosis is made and the problem treated, the client is at Risk for Injury: Fractures, Hypertension, or Diabetes Mellitus related to osteoporosis, sodium and water retention, or the presence of an insulin antagonist, respectively.

Outcomes. Injury will not occur as evidenced by the absence of fractures. The client will not have hypertension, hyperglycemia, or diabetes mellitus.

Interventions
Prevent Injury

SAFETY
ALERT

Protect the client from falls and accidents. Clients with Cushing's syndrome have osteoporosis and tend to develop fractures even with mild trauma. Keep the bed in its lowest position, and raise the side rails for protection. Assist clients with ambulation to avoid falls.

Monitor for Hypertension and Diabetes Mellitus. Monitor vital signs at frequent intervals. Assess the client carefully for evidence of severe hypertension, such as elevated BP, headache, failing vision, irritability, and dyspnea.

Check for postural hypotension (but have the client change position slowly to avoid injury from a sudden drop in BP).

Obtain the client's weight daily in a consistent manner. If sodium intake is reduced, edema and weight should diminish. Obtain daily blood glucose levels via finger stick. Positive results may indicate diabetes mellitus (steroid diabetes) caused by the insulin antagonist action of the excessive cortisol.

Evaluation. It is expected that clients will have minimal complications or will have had appropriate management of complications before surgery so that they can undergo the adrenalectomy successfully. A glucocorticoid preparation will be given on the morning of surgery to prevent adrenal insufficiency during the procedure.

Postoperative Care

Assessment Routine postoperative monitoring of the incision and special assessments for manifestations of shock, addisonian crisis, and renal shutdown are required. Assess the client's ability to perform self-care and to manage the disease for the remainder of his or her life. The client's current level of knowledge must be assessed and a teaching plan carefully developed. Also carefully monitor the client's thought processes including memory loss, cognitive impairment, and mood swings.

Diagnosis, Outcomes, Interventions
Diagnosis: Risk for Infection. The client receiving steroid replacement will be at *Risk for Infection related to lowered resistance to stress and compromised immune response.*

Outcomes. Infection will not develop or will be detected early as evidenced by the absence of leukocytosis, fever, and other manifestations of infections.

Interventions

After surgery, encourage the client to cough, turn, and deep breathe to prevent respiratory tract infections. Employ meticulous sterile technique with wound care to prevent infection. Paralytic ileus is less common because the flank approach is usually used.

Protect the client from exposure to infectious organisms. Isolate the client from health care personnel and significant others who have contagious disorders. Wash your hands meticulously before contact with the client.

Because glucocorticoids suppress immune and inflammatory reactions, a client with Cushing's syndrome may have only mild manifestations of even a severe infection. The white blood cell count does not show significant elevation in immunosuppressed clients. A slight elevation in body temperature may indicate the presence of a severe infection.

Evaluation. If the surgical management of Cushing's disease is successful, neither injury related to the surgery nor addisonian crisis will develop. If complications do occur, desired outcomes may be related to successful management of the complications, such as control of hemorrhage, prevention of shock, and control of addisonian crisis.

Appropriate outcomes also include the control of side effects of the steroid therapy. Because these cannot be completely avoided, the client's ability to control them is an appropriate area to evaluate. The client should be able to differentiate complications from the side effects of medications.

Medical Management

Usually, a client with primary adrenal hyperplasia is treated surgically as an inpatient. Medical management is reserved for clients with inoperable tumors or metastatic tumors that warrant palliative care (Table 44-1). The outcome, therefore, is related to achieving comfort versus cure. Medical management options include radiation therapy and administration of adrenal blocking agents or ACTH-reducing agents to decrease the effects of the adrenal hyperplasia.

Radiation Therapy

Radiation therapy can be used to treat primary pituitary tumors and other ACTH-secreting adenomas. Radiation can be applied to the pituitary gland either internally or externally. Internally, the radiation is applied through a transsphenoidal implant. Radiation is not always effective in even palliative treatment of tumors and may destroy normal tissue. For ACTH-secreting adenomas, such as lung tumors, palliation is possible. Radiation therapy is commonly used concurrently with surgical or pharmacologic management to enhance its effectiveness and reduce long-term side effects.

Adrenal Blocking Agents

Medications that interfere with ACTH production or adrenal hormone synthesis are available. Mitotane (Lysodren) is a cytotoxic antihormonal agent that inhibits corticosteroid synthesis without destroying cortical cells. Aminoglutethimide (Cytadren) and trilostane (Modrastane) are other cytotoxic agents that block the synthesis of glucocorticoids and adrenal steroids.

ACTH-Reducing Agents

Cyproheptadine (Periactin), bromocriptine, or somatostatin is used to treat hypersecretion caused by pituitary abnormalities and resulting in increased ACTH levels. These agents appear to interfere with ACTH production, thereby reducing the effect on the adrenals.

Self-Care

The client with a bilateral adrenalectomy needs to learn self-care because lifelong glucocorticoid replacement is essential. If only one adrenal gland has been removed, daily cortisol replacement continues until the remaining

---

TABLE 44-1   Therapies for Cushing's Syndrome, Cushing's Disease, and Ectopic ACTH Syndrome

Condition	Responsible Lesion	Therapies	Remarks
Cushing's syndrome	Adrenal tumor (benign or malignant)	Adrenalectomy	Adrenalectomy for benign unilateral tumor; usually curative Bilateral adrenalectomy must be followed by lifelong administration of corticosteroids
	Adrenal carcinoma with widespread metastases	Surgery and chemotherapy (mitotane)	Chemotherapy largely unsuccessful
Cushing's disease	Pituitary tumor (or unidentified lesion) that secretes excessive amounts of ACTH	Microsurgical resection of pituitary adenoma	Pituitary surgery successful in 95% of cases
		Irradiation of pituitary gland	Irradiation successful in 75% of cases; therapeutic effects not apparent for months after initiation of therapy
		Total bilateral adrenalectomy (corrects adrenal hyperplasia caused by excessive ACTH stimulation)	Total bilateral adrenalectomy must be followed by lifelong replacement therapy with glucocorticoid and mineralocorticoid
Ectopic ACTH syndrome	Extra-adrenal malignant tumor	Surgical removal of ectopic malignant tumor; chemotherapy used to control hypercortisolism and promote remission in clients with inoperable cancer	Surgery rarely successful because metastasis usually occurs before diagnosis; chemotherapy purely palliative

ACTH, Adrenocorticotropic hormone.

gland functions normally (usually after 6 to 12 months). Before discharge, the client and the client's significant others need instruction on self-administration of replacement hormones (hydrocortisone). They should successfully demonstrate the injection technique before discharge. The client should also be able to repeat and comply with instructions and to remain free of addisonian crisis or adrenal insufficiency.

Modifications for Older Clients

Older clients may exhibit excessive manifestations of Cushing's syndrome because these clients may already have osteoporosis, hypertension, and diabetes mellitus. Older clients are also more susceptible to the side effects of steroid replacement therapy.

HYPERALDOSTERONISM

Aldosterone is the most powerful of the mineralocorticoids. Its primary role is to conserve sodium, and it also promotes potassium excretion. The incidence of primary hyperaldosteronism in the hypertensive population is unknown, affecting about 1% of the population. It affects women twice as often as men and appears most frequently in middle-age people.

Etiology and Risk Factors

Primary hyperaldosteronism refers to hypersecretion of aldosterone resulting from an adrenal lesion, which is usually benign. The disease, which produces secondary hypertension, hypokalemia (in most), and hypernatremia, is also known as *Conn's syndrome*.

Secondary hyperaldosteronism results from a variety of conditions that cause overproduction of aldosterone. These conditions include sodium-wasting renal disease, laxative or diuretic abuse, dehydration, cirrhosis with ascites, heart failure, and a decrease in intravascular volume. Hypertension is uncommon.

There are no particular risk factors for primary hyperaldosteronism. Risk factors for secondary hyperaldosteronism include chronic heart failure, cirrhosis with ascites, nephrotic syndrome, and hypertension caused by destructive renal artery disease. Health promotion measures, therefore, are successful treatment and control of the causative disease process. The more successfully these factors are controlled, the less secondary hyperaldosteronism is present.

Pathophysiology

Aldosterone affects tubular reabsorption of sodium and water and excretion of potassium and hydrogen ions in the renal tubular epithelial cells. These effects lead to the development of hypernatremia, hypervolemia, hypokalemia, and metabolic alkalosis. With hypervolemia and hypernatremia, BP increases, often to very high levels, and renin production is suppressed. The hypertension can lead to cerebral infarcts and renal damage.

Secondary hyperaldosteronism is a result of continuous secretion of aldosterone secondary to high levels of angiotensin II, resulting from high plasma renin activity. Decreased renal perfusion of a variety of causes is the underlying mechanism.

Clinical Manifestations

Clients with primary hyperaldosteronism may be asymptomatic, but incidental findings include hypertension, hypernatremia, and hypokalemia. Without intervention, all of the complications of chronic hypertension, such as visual disturbances, heart failure, renal damage, and stroke, may occur. Unfortunately, the renal complications resulting from long-term hypertension tend to be progressive. Therefore clients with primary hyperaldosteronism need to be identified and treated early in the course of the disease.

Hypokalemia results from excessive urinary excretion of potassium ions. This problem in turn causes muscle weakness, paralysis, or cardiac dysrhythmias because potassium loss reduces normal neuromuscular irritability. In addition, excessive potassium excretion results in polyuria. The large urine output leads to polydipsia (excessive thirst).

> **Finally, hypokalemia leads to metabolic alkalosis because of shifting of hydrogen ions into the cells in exchange for potassium and exchange of hydrogen ions in the tubular cells for sodium ions from the tubular urine. Metabolic alkalosis causes a decrease in ionized calcium levels, which can result in tetany and respiratory suppression.**

Despite sodium retention, clients with hyperaldosteronism rarely develop overt edema. Although extracellular fluid increases moderately, excessive water is normally excreted in the urine with potassium ions. Over time, the kidneys tend to adjust physiologically to excessive secretion of aldosterone, and water excretion reaches an equilibrium with sodium intake. The kidneys' eventual "escape" from the sodium-retaining and water-retaining action of aldosterone is sometimes called the *escape phenomenon.*

The diagnosis of primary hyperaldosteronism is based on low serum potassium levels, alkalosis, and elevated urinary or plasma aldosterone levels with low plasma renin levels (elevated in secondary hyperaldosteronism). In addition, radiographic studies may reveal cardiac hypertrophy resulting from chronic hypertension.

Radionuclide scanning techniques using radiolabeled iodocholesterol allow visualization of the tumors.

OUTCOME MANAGEMENT

Surgical Management

Surgery is the treatment of choice for the client with primary hyperaldosteronism. A unilateral or bilateral adrenalectomy must be performed. A client undergoing a unilateral adrenalectomy may need temporary replacement of glucocorticoids. A client who requires a bilateral adrenalectomy needs permanent replacement (see Addison's disease discussion). Clients usually receive glucocorticoids preoperatively to prevent adrenal hypofunction. In two thirds of cases, removal of the aldosterone-secreting tumor completely resolves the hypertension, hypokalemia, and hypernatremia. Most clients have normal BP readings by the third postoperative month.

Nursing Management of the Surgical Client

Help prepare the client for the diagnostic assessment so that the diagnosis of hyperaldosteronism can be achieved rapidly and the treatment performed before permanent damage occurs. Administer prescribed medications, and closely monitor the client for hypertension or renal damage. Preoperative and postoperative management is the same as that described for hypercortisolism.

Discharge planning must include client education about a low-sodium diet, medications, and manifestations of hypokalemia if the client is to be medically treated. The client should also understand the disease process and manifestations.

Medical Management

A client who cannot be treated surgically may receive spironolactone (Aldactone) to increase sodium excretion and to treat the hypertension and hypokalemia. Hypertension may take 4 to 8 weeks to correct. Potassium levels should be carefully monitored for the development of hyperkalemia, especially if the client has been receiving potassium supplements or a high-potassium diet. The Integrating Pharmacology feature above, right, lists complications of spironolactone therapy. Amiloride is the drug of choice for clients who cannot tolerate spironolactone.

Nursing Management of the Medical Client

Assess the client's ability to manage the complex therapeutic regimen. Plan and implement a teaching program for self-care.

Complications of Spironolactone Administration

Spironolactone is the drug of choice for primary hyperaldosteronism. It effectively lowers blood pressure and improves hypokalemia. The administration of spironolactone is complicated by the following:
1. Side effects such as gastrointestinal discomfort, impotence, decreased libido, gynecomastia, and menstrual irregularities.
2. Increase in the half-life of digoxin. The client's digoxin dosage may be reduced based on serum levels.
3. Concomitant therapy with salicylates. Salicylates increase renal tubular excretion of canrenone, the major active metabolite of spironolactone, thus decreasing its effectiveness.

ADRENOMEDULLARY DISORDERS

Two important tumors occur in the adrenal medulla: *pheochromocytoma,* a tumor that causes hyperactivity of the gland, and *neuroblastoma,* a malignant tumor made up of cells resembling a neuroblast. For a complete description of neuroblastoma, an important tumor in children, consult a pediatric textbook.

PHEOCHROMOCYTOMA

A pheochromocytoma is a catecholamine-secreting tumor of the chromaffin cells of the sympathetic nervous system; it is usually found in the adrenal medulla. Pheochromocytomas are rare. In autopsy series, the incidence of pheochromocytoma is 0.1% in clients with diastolic hypertension. The condition is equally common in women and men. Although the disease can occur at any age, it is most common in middle age and rarely occurs after age 60 years.

Etiology and Risk Factors
The cause of pheochromocytomas is unknown. In some cases, they appear to have a familial basis. They often occur together with neuroectodermal diseases and with multiple endocrine neoplasia type IIA. There are no known risk factors for pheochromocytoma.

Pathophysiology
Usually weighing less than 200 g, a pheochromocytoma is composed of chromaffin cells, so named (Latin *affinis, affinitas,* affinity) because these cells stain brownish yellow with chromic salts. In 85% to 95% of cases,

pheochromocytomas arise within the adrenal medulla. Occasionally, however, they develop from the chromaffin tissues found in the sympathetic paraganglia. Pheochromocytomas are typically benign; fewer than 10% are malignant. Because of the excessive amounts of epinephrine and norepinephrine they secrete, they can produce severe manifestations and even death (Table 44-2).

Once a pheochromocytoma is diagnosed, certain risk factors are known to influence catecholamine release. Catecholamine release occurs with various frequencies and intensities and is called a *paroxysm*. Risk factors that may stimulate a paroxysm include the following:

- Smoking
- Micturition (voiding reflex)
- Activities that displace abdominal organs, such as bending, exercising, straining, vigorous palpation of the abdomen, and pregnancy
- Certain drugs, such as histamines, anesthetics, atropine, opiates, fentanyl, steroids, and glucagon

Without early intervention, the client is at risk for cerebral hemorrhage and cardiac failure. If a pheochromocytoma is discovered early in its development, it can usually be removed surgically.

Clinical Manifestations

A client with pheochromocytoma may present with manifestations of diabetes mellitus (elevated blood glucose level and glucosuria), hypertension (elevated BP, headaches), hyperthyroidism (increased metabolic rate, diaphoresis, agitation, rapid pulse rate, palpitations, emotional outbursts), and psychoneurosis (emotional instability).

Hypertension is the principal manifestation of pheochromocytoma, and it can be persistent, fluctuating, intermittent, or paroxysmal (rapid onset and abrupt cessation). Typically, the client has episodes of high BP accompanied by pounding headaches. Other manifestations of sympathetic overactivity include sweating, apprehension, palpitations, nausea, and vomiting. Excessive release of catecholamines also results in excessive conversion of glycogen into glucose in the liver. Consequently, hyperglycemia and glucosuria occur during attacks. Such manifestations can develop spontaneously or may be precipitated by emotional stress, physical exertion, or change in body position.

Acute attacks may be associated with profuse diaphoresis (perspiration), dilated pupils, and cold extremities. Severe hypertension can precipitate a stroke or sudden blindness.

Because pheochromocytoma is curable, early and accurate diagnosis is essential. Current methods of diagnosis include the history and physical examination, chemical tests for catecholamines and metabolites, direct assay of catecholamines in the blood, and radiologic imaging.

TABLE 44–2 Effects of Epinephrine and Norepinephrine

Epinephrine	Norepinephrine
Cardiovascular System	
Constricts superficial blood vessels; in small doses, dilates muscle, brain, and coronary vessels, thus shunting blood supply to organs; essential for "fight or flight"	Constricts blood vessels (especially peripheral), causing increased peripheral resistance
Raises blood pressure	Raises blood pressure greatly
Increases cardiac output	Decreases cardiac output because of increased peripheral resistance
Increases pulse rate dramatically	Increases pulse rate moderately
Constricts spleen, shunting stored red blood cells into general circulation	
Increases coagulability of blood	
Respiratory System	
Increases rate and depth of respirations	
Dilates bronchi	
Nervous System	
Stimulates central nervous system, increasing alertness and producing a feeling of fright, excitation, and impending doom	
Dilates pupils	Dilates pupils
Inhibits gastrointestinal tract	
Metabolism	
Increases nonesterified fatty acid level of blood	Inhibits gastrointestinal tract
Promotes conversion of glycogen to glucose	Increases nonesterified fatty acid level of blood
Increases body metabolism	Increases body metabolism slightly

Data from DeGroot, L., & Jameson, J. (2001). *Endocrinology* (4th ed.). Philadelphia: Saunders.

OUTCOME MANAGEMENT

Surgical Management

Adrenalectomy

Indications. The primary treatment of a pheochromocytoma is surgical removal of one or both adrenal glands, depending on whether the tumor is unilateral or bilateral. The procedure is the same as that described for Cushing's syndrome.

Contraindications. The presence of complications of pheochromocytoma may make the client a poor surgical risk. Ideally, surgery is performed before complications develop; however, high BP and vascular complications may necessitate treatment before surgery can take place. Alpha-adrenergic blocking agents, such as phentolamine (Regitine), can be used in an IV bolus or IV drip for hypertensive crisis. Oral phenoxybenzamine (Dibenzyline) is used at least 7 days preoperatively to control BP, reduce manifestations, and eliminate paroxysms before surgical removal of the affected gland.

Complications associated with pheochromocytoma that may delay surgery include hypertensive retinopathy, hypertensive nephropathy, myocarditis, increased platelet aggregation, stroke, and heart failure. Death may result from myocardial infarction, stroke, dysrhythmias, irreversible shock, renal failure, or dissecting aortic aneurysm.

Complications. The surgical procedure for pheochromocytoma is not without danger. There are two serious hazards.

> **First, excessive discharge of pressor hormones during induction of anesthesia or manipulation of the tumor can cause extreme increases in BP and cardiac dysrhythmias. Second, after resection of the tumor, BP can fall precipitously.**

Outcomes. Surgical removal of the pheochromocytoma can be curative in most cases if the growth is discovered before cardiovascular damage becomes permanent. Some clients may receive less medication at discharge after surgery. Lifelong steroid replacement must be initiated after a bilateral adrenalectomy.

Nursing Management of the Surgical Client

Preoperative Care

Assessment. Assess and control the client's BP preoperatively. Closely monitor the client for the development of stressful episodes before treatment has begun. Evaluate the client's neurologic status in case the client has a stroke because of the extremely elevated BP.

Diagnosis, Outcomes, Interventions

Diagnosis: Risk for Injury. The client with a pheochromocytoma is at great risk for injury preoperatively. Write the nursing diagnosis *Risk for Injury related to excessive release of epinephrine and norepinephrine preoperatively.*

Outcomes. Injury will not occur or will be detected early as evidenced by absence of hypertensive episodes and cardiovascular or cerebral damage.

Interventions. During the preoperative phase, the desired outcome of treatment is preventing attacks of acute paroxysmal hypertension, thereby lowering the risk of further damage to the cardiovascular system.

Important nursing interventions include (1) promoting rest and relief from stress; (2) administering prescribed sedatives; (3) providing a diet high in vitamins, minerals, and calories; (4) prohibiting beverages containing caffeine, such as coffee, tea, and colas; and (5) monitoring vital signs. In most cases, the physician prescribes an alpha-adrenergic blocking agent, such as phenoxybenzamine.

Postoperative Care

Assessment

> **The first 24 to 48 hours after surgery is a critical period demanding vigilant nursing assessment. After surgery, the client should be closely monitored for adrenal insufficiency, hypotension, hemorrhage, and shock. Urine output and BP are assessed hourly.**

SAFETY

ALERT

Diagnosis, Outcomes, Interventions

Diagnosis: Risk for Injury. The client is at increased risk for such problems as hypotension postoperatively. Write the nursing diagnosis as *Risk for Injury related to postoperative hypotension, hemorrhage, and shock.*

Outcomes. Injury will not occur or will be detected early, as evidenced by a normotensive state and an absence of hemorrhage, shock, or addisonian crisis.

Interventions

Monitor and Prevent Shock

> **During the immediate postoperative period, observe for manifestations of shock and hemorrhage. After removal of the tumor, profound shock can develop as catecholamine levels drop. Hypotension can persist for 24 to 48 hours. Hemorrhage can occur because of the high vascularity of the adrenal glands.**

SAFETY
ALERT

To prevent postoperative shock, do the following:
1. Give IV fluids as prescribed, such as blood, plasma, dextran, or glucose in water to maintain blood volume.
2. Administer IV pressors as prescribed at a rate sufficient to maintain BP within a safe range. Check BP as often as necessary to titrate the medication.
3. Carefully measure hourly urine output. If the client voids less than 0.5 ml/kg/hour, notify the physician. Oliguria can signify impending shock and consequent renal shutdown.
4. Assess the client for manifestations of hemorrhage. Check the dressing every half hour for bloody drainage. If the client is bleeding internally, an abdominal hematoma can develop, resulting in paralytic ileus or nonmechanical bowel obstruction (see Chapter 33). Manifestations of paralytic ileus include abdominal pain, distention, severe

nausea, vomiting, and diminished or absent bowel sounds.

5. If cortical tissue has been resected during surgery, assess the client closely for manifestations of adrenal insufficiency (see addisonian crisis discussion). If both adrenal glands have been removed, the client must receive cortisol replacement for life.

Evaluation. It is expected that the client will have no complications postoperatively or that complications that occur will be managed successfully so that the client is discharged within 4 to 5 days postoperatively. Self-care outcomes are evaluated by the client's ability to manage steroid replacement after surgery. Although side effects of steroids cannot be avoided, there are ways to minimize them, and the client's ability to control these and avoid complications can be evaluated.

Self-Care

After a bilateral adrenalectomy, the client must learn self-care measures. When the critical postoperative period is over, most clients experience an uneventful convalescence. A client who will be self-administering corticosteroids needs instruction concerning the administration and side effects (see Addison's disease discussion).

Modifications for Older Clients

Damage related to hypertensive episodes associated with the pheochromocytoma tends to affect older clients, whose cardiovascular and cerebrovascular systems may be weak and thus susceptible to damage by elevated BP.

ANTERIOR PITUITARY DISORDERS

Disorders of the pituitary gland occur most frequently in the anterior lobe. Major causes of pituitary disease include functioning tumors, nonfunctioning tumors, pituitary infarction, genetic disorders, and trauma. The three principal pathologic consequences of pituitary disorders are (1) hyperpituitarism, (2) hypopituitarism, and (3) local compression of brain tissue by expanding tumor masses.

HYPERPITUITARISM AND HYPERPROLACTINEMIA

Etiology and Risk Factors

Hyperpituitarism is defined as oversecretion of one or more of the hormones secreted by the pituitary gland.

It is caused primarily by a hormone-secreting pituitary tumor, typically a benign adenoma. Syndromes associated with hyperpituitarism are Cushing's syndrome, acromegaly, amenorrhea, galactorrhea, hyperthyroidism, and, rarely, hypergonadism in the male.

Pathophysiology

Prolactin and growth hormone are the hormones most commonly overproduced by adenomas. They lead to hyperprolactinemia and acromegaly (Figure 44-2), respectively. Increased amounts of growth hormone lead to rapid growth of all body tissues. This increased growth leads to gigantism (Figure 44-3) if it occurs before closure of the epiphysis and acromegaly if it occurs after epiphyseal closure.

Clinical Manifestations

Pituitary tumors produce both systemic and local effects. Systemic effects include excessive or abnormal growth patterns related to overproduction of growth hormone, abnormal milk secretion (galactorrhea), and overstimulation of one or more of the target glands, resulting in release of excessive thyroid, sex, or adrenocortical hormones.

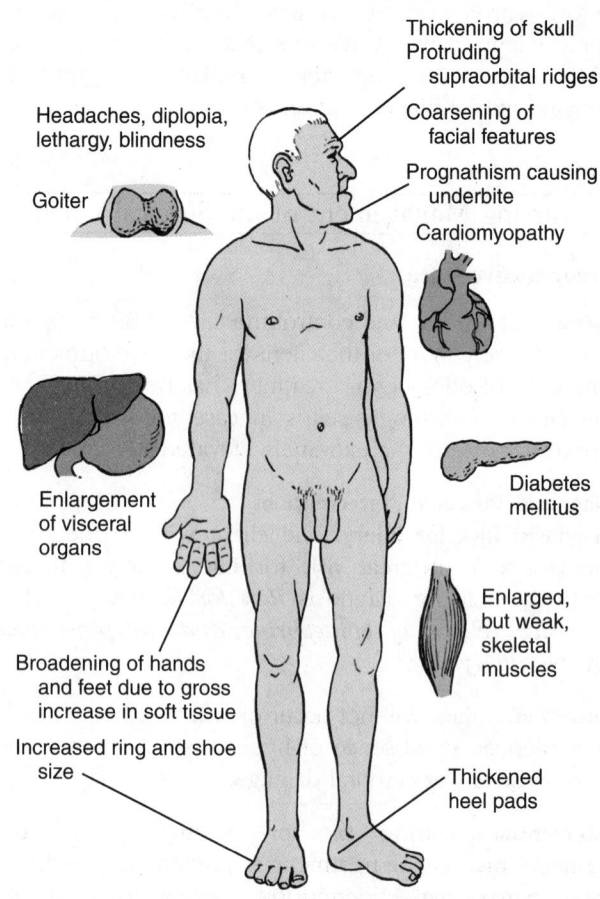

Headaches, diplopia, lethargy, blindness

Goiter

Thickening of skull
Protruding supraorbital ridges

Coarsening of facial features

Prognathism causing underbite

Cardiomyopathy

Enlargement of visceral organs

Broadening of hands and feet due to gross increase in soft tissue

Increased ring and shoe size

Diabetes mellitus

Enlarged, but weak, skeletal muscles

Thickened heel pads

■ **FIGURE 44–2** Clinical manifestations of acromegaly.

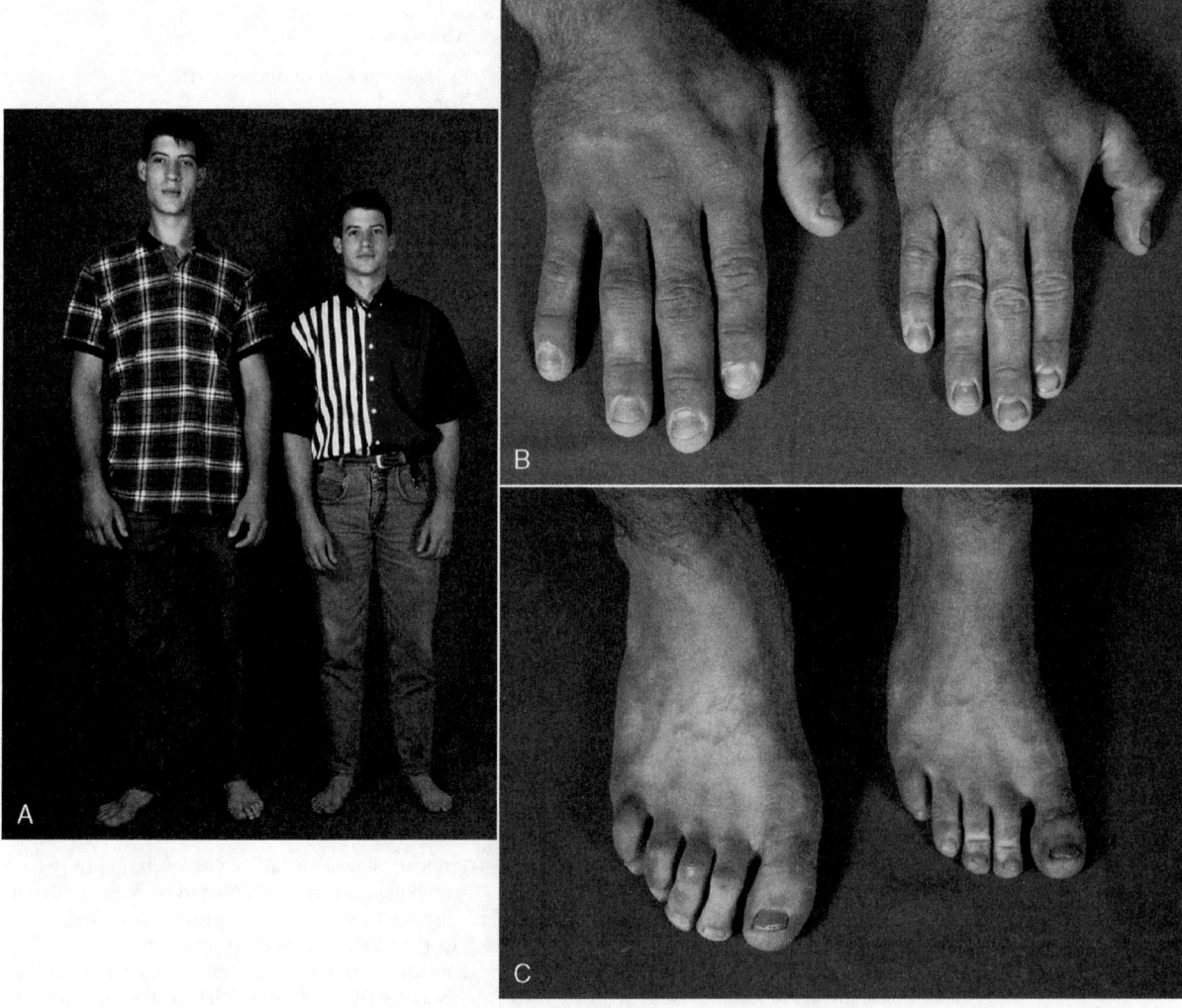

■ **FIGURE 44–3** Primary gigantism. **A,** A 22-year-old man with gigantism resulting from excess growth hormone is shown to the left of his identical twin. The increased height **(A),** enlarged hand **(B),** and enlarged foot **(C)** of the affected twin are apparent. Their height and features began to diverge at the age of approximately 13 years. *(Courtesy Robert F. Gagel, MD, and Ian McCutcheon, MD, University of Texas M.D. Anderson Cancer Center, Houston, Tex.)*

Locally, pituitary tumors produce manifestations because the bony cranium that houses the tumor cannot expand to accommodate a growing mass. Local manifestations include visual field abnormalities resulting from pressure on the optic chiasm, headaches, and somnolence. Table 44-3 provides additional information related to hyperprolactinemia and acromegaly.

OUTCOME MANAGEMENT

Surgical Management

A client with a pituitary tumor must have the tumor resected. A variety of approaches can be used to remove a pituitary tumor. Usually, a transsphenoidal hypophysectomy is performed (see Chapter 69).

Nursing Management of the Surgical Client

Assessment. Most clients are frightened by the prospect of having the pituitary gland removed. Provide the client and the client's significant others with emotional support and comfort throughout the preoperative period.

The initial manifestations are vague; therefore the client may have seen many physicians and may have had multiple examinations and tests while seeking a diagnosis. The client and family may be fearful, skeptical, or relieved with the final diagnosis of pituitary tumor. Assess the client's reaction to the diagnosis, expectations for the surgery, educational needs related to the diagnosis and treatment plan, and available support network after discharge.

Physical assessment includes baseline vital signs and weight as well as neurologic assessment. The client should also have a preoperative eye examination by an ophthalmologist. These findings are essential to establish

TABLE 44-3 Hyperprolactinemia and Acromegaly in Hyperpituitarism

	Hyperprolactinemia	Acromegaly
Hormone secreted	Excessive prolactin (PRL) causes prolactinoma	Excessive growth hormone (GH)
Risk factors	Hyperprolactinemia; estrogen therapy; oral contraceptive use; pregnancy may increase tumor size and dysfunction	None
Etiology	Pregnancy; hypothalamic-pituitary disorders; hypothyroidism; drug ingestion (estrogen or oral contraception)	Anterior pituitary adenoma; abnormal hypothalamic function (rare)
Pathophysiology	PRL-producing tumors deliver excess PRL systemically	GH-producing adenomas deliver excess GH systemically, leading to rapid growth in other body tissues (with exception of the CNS), causing organomegaly; increase in tumor size within confined space can result in destruction of entire pituitary and cause hypopituitarism
Clinical manifestations related to hormone oversecretion	Abnormal lactation (galactorrhea) in nonlactating breast; amenorrhea; decreased vaginal lubrication; decreased libido in men; impotence; depression; anxiety; headache; visual loss	Local overgrowth of bone: skull and mandible; soft tissue overgrowth; lethargy; weight gain; paresthesias; glucose intolerance; coarse facial features; irregular or absent menses; enlargement of hands and feet over 1-10 yr; depression; headache; visual field impairment; osteoarthritis; paresthesias; impotence
Complications related to tumor growth	Headaches; visual disturbances affecting cranial nerves III, IV, VI; hypopituitarism; infertility; decreased bone growth	Hypopituitarism; cancers of gastrointestinal tract; increased mortality secondary to cardiovascular atherosclerosis, cerebral atherosclerosis, congestive heart failure, respiratory disease, hypertension, diabetes mellitus
Pharmacologic intervention	Bromocriptine is treatment of choice; bromocriptine can reduce PRL levels in 90% of clients; adverse reactions may contribute to noncompliance: nausea, headaches, dizziness, nasal stuffiness, hypotension, depression	Somatostatin analog octreotide is very effective in reducing GH levels; pharmacologic treatment may cause cholelithiasis; bromocriptine is effective in 60-80% of clients
Surgical intervention	Transsphenoidal microsurgery; complications: residual tissue may produce elevated hormone levels, visual loss, diabetes insipidus, postoperative infection	Transsphenoidal microsurgery is treatment of choice; complications: same as in hyperprolactinemia
Radiation treatment	May decrease adenoma, but local complications are common because of tissue scarring and impairment of anterior pituitary function (hypopituitarism)	Produces slower decline of GH levels, implying higher morbidity related to atherosclerotic disease, respiratory disease, hypertension, diabetes mellitus, and gastrointestinal cancer; hypopituitarism
Diagnosis	Measurement of GH, ACTH, FSH, LH, PRL, testosterone, gonadotropins; thyroid function tests (T$_3$, T$_4$, FT$_4$, TSH); liver function tests (LDH, CPK, AST, alkaline phosphatase); coagulation studies; kidney function tests (serum creatinine, BUN, 24-hr urine collection for protein, creatinine clearance, GFR); urinalysis; pregnancy testing; CT or MRI for pituitary adenoma localization	Radioimmunoassay or enzyme-linked immunosorbent assay for GH level; serum GH level; insulin-like growth factor; CT scan or MRI for pituitary edema localization; oral GTT may demonstrate hyperglycemia; usually, GTT suppresses normal GH release 1-2 hr after ingestion, but in acromegaly GH level remains elevated

ACTH, Adrenocorticotropic hormone; *AST*, aspartate aminotransferase; *BUN*, blood urea nitrogen; *CNS*, central nervous system; *CPK*, creatine phosphokinase; *CT*, computed tomography; *FSH*, follicle-stimulating hormone; *FT$_4$*, free thyroxine; *GFR*, glomerular filtration rate; *GH*, growth hormone; *GTT*, glucose tolerance test; *LDH*, lactate dehydrogenase; *LH*, luteinizing hormone; *MRI*, magnetic resonance imaging; *PRL*, prolactin; *TSH*, thyroid-stimulating hormone; *T$_3$*, triiodothyronine; *T$_4$*, thyroxine.

a baseline for postoperative comparison. To perform the neurologic assessment, check the following:

- Pupil equality and reactivity to light
- Hand grip for strength, equality, and ability to release on command
- Level of consciousness
- Orientation to time, place, person, and location
- Appropriate response to stimuli
- Visual acuity and visual fields

Diagnosis, Outcomes, Interventions

Diagnosis: Risk for Injury. A typical postoperative nursing diagnosis would be *Risk for Injury related to postoperative complications.*

Outcomes. Injury will not result from surgery as evidenced by absence of addisonian crisis, balanced intake and output, no manifestations of increased intracranial pressure, normal temperature, and absence of manifestations of cerebrospinal fluid (CSF) leakage or meningitis.

Interventions

Prevent Adrenal Insufficiency. Before surgery, the client usually receives an IV injection of cortisol. Glucocorticoids help the client tolerate the stress of an operation that can result in loss of adrenocortical function.

Monitor Intracranial Pressure

Treatment after transfrontal hypophysectomy resembles that for any craniotomy (see Chapter 69). Immediately after surgery, assess for cerebral edema and rising intracranial pressure (elevated BP, widened pulse pressure, low pulse rate, pupil changes, altered respiratory pattern, decreasing level of consciousness).

Monitor for Hormonal Insufficiencies

Because the pituitary gland no longer produces tropic hormones, watch for target gland deficiencies, such as adrenal insufficiency and hypothyroidism. In addition, diabetes insipidus can occur temporarily because of antidiuretic hormone (ADH, vasopressin) deficiency, as outlined in the Critical Monitoring feature at right. This deficiency is related to surgical manipulation. Maintain strict documentation of intake and output. Notify the physician if urine output is more than 200 ml/hour with a specific gravity below 1.005.

Provide Oral Hygiene. The client who has undergone transsphenoidal hypophysectomy requires frequent oral hygiene with a gauze sponge; the lips should be lubricated with petroleum jelly. The client should not brush the teeth for 2 weeks after surgery.

Evaluation. Appropriate outcomes after a hypophysectomy include the absence of postoperative complications and the client's ability to manage lifetime hormone replacement. If complications occur, the appropriate outcome would be that these complications are controlled without permanent problems.

Self-Care

After a hypophysectomy, the client must take replacement hormones for life. Instruct the client to avoid gastric irritation by taking cortisone with milk, food, or an antacid. Advise the client to notify the physician about gastritis, tarry stools, or frank blood in the stools. Some clients may also require thyroid or sex hormone replacement. In addition, some need vasopressin replacement to treat *diabetes insipidus*. As a result of deficient ADH, clients may experience polyuria (large urine output) and low urine specific gravity readings. Diabetes insipidus is usually transient after surgery but can persist, indicating the need for chronic hormone replacement.

SEXUAL DISTURBANCES

Excess secretion of gonadotropic hormones, such as luteinizing hormone (LH) and follicle-stimulating hormone (FSH), from pituitary tumors can produce sexual precocity in children. Excess prolactin secretion can cause amenorrhea or galactorrhea (excessive flow of milk) in women.

CRITICAL MONITORING

Does Your Client Have an Antidiuretic Hormone (ADH) Imbalance?

	Diabetes Insipidus	Syndrome of Inappropriate Secretion of Antidiuretic Hormone
ADH	↓	↑
Urine output	↑	↓
Urine osmolality	↓	↑
Urine specific gravity	↓	Value insignificant
Serum Na⁺	↑	↓
Urine Na⁺	↓	↑
Plasma osmolality	↑	↓
Daily weights	↓	Sudden ↑ (without edema)
Mentation changes	Related to electrolyte imbalance and hypotension	Related to degree of hyponatremia

---

Physicians consider surgical removal the treatment of choice for radiologically demonstrable tumors.

Clients with increased prolactin secretion and no radiologic or neurologic evidence of a pituitary tumor often respond to bromocriptine, an ergot-like compound. Clients with prolactinomas can be successfully treated with bromocriptine. A dopamine agonist, bromocriptine inhibits prolactin secretion. Surgery is no longer the treatment of choice in most cases.

HYPOPITUITARISM

In contrast to hyperpituitarism, hypopituitarism is a deficiency of one or more of the hormones produced by the anterior lobe of the pituitary. When both the anterior and posterior lobes fail to secrete hormones, the condition is called *panhypopituitarism*. Hypopituitarism and panhypopituitarism are rare disorders.

Etiology and Risk Factors

The nine most important causes of hypopituitarism are known as the "nine *I*'s":

- Invasion (most common)—pituitary tumors, central nervous system tumors, carotid aneurysm
- Infarction—postpartum necrosis (Sheehan's syndrome), pituitary apoplexy

- Infiltration—sarcoidosis, hemochromatosis
- Injury—head trauma, child abuse
- Immunologic—lymphocytic hypophysitis
- Iatrogenic—surgery, radiation therapy
- Infectious—mycoses, tuberculosis, syphilis
- Idiopathic—familial
- Isolated—deficiency of an anterior pituitary hormone, such as growth hormone, LH, FSH, thyroid-stimulating hormone (TSH), ACTH-lipotropic pituitary hormone (ACTH-LPH), or prolactin

Clinical Manifestations

The pituitary gland has enormous functional reserve; therefore manifestations of hypopituitarism usually do not appear until 75% of the pituitary has been obliterated by tumor or thrombosis. Manifestations depend on age of onset as well as the hormones that are deficient. The onset of hypopituitarism is usually gradual. The classic course of progressive hypopituitarism is an initial loss of growth hormone and gonadotropin, followed by deficiencies of TSH, then ACTH, and finally prolactin.

Specific disorders resulting from pituitary hyposecretion include the following:

- *Short stature*. Severely stunted growth results from either a congenital lack of growth hormone or the development of a space-occupying intracranial tumor, meningitis, or brain injury during early childhood.
- *Sexual and reproductive disorders*. Deficiencies of the gonadotropins (LH and FSH) can produce sterility, diminished sex drive, and decreased secondary sex characteristics. Decreased FSH and LH lead to infertility and amenorrhea, diminished spermatogenesis, and testicular atrophy.
- *Hypothyroidism*. Because the synthesis of thyroid hormone depends on TSH, therapeutic ablation or pathologic destruction of the pituitary gland causes hypothyroidism unless the client receives thyroid hormone (see Chapter 43).
- *Secondary adrenocortical insufficiency*. Adrenal insufficiency can follow diminished synthesis of ACTH by the pituitary gland, which in turn causes diminished secretion of adrenocortical hormones by the adrenal cortex.
- *Prolactin deficiency*. This deficiency is indicated by absence of lactation in the postpartum woman.

Diagnosis of growth hormone deficiency rests on the inability of stimulating agents—such as levodopa, arginine, and insulin—to increase plasma growth hormone levels. ACTH levels can be measured to diagnose secondary adrenal insufficiency. Cortisol levels are low in both primary and secondary hypothyroidism; however, when it is a primary deficiency, ACTH levels are high.

In a client with secondary hypopituitarism, ACTH levels are low. Low serum thyroid hormone levels, together with low serum TSH levels, establish the diagnosis of hypothyroidism. Sexual and reproductive disorders are diagnosed by low levels of sex steroids and low levels of plasma FSH and LH. Skull x-ray studies may reveal enlargement of the sella turcica, erosion of the sphenoid bone, or calcification of a suprasellar mass. CT or MRI may provide an enhanced view of an x-ray finding.

OUTCOME MANAGEMENT

Treatment of hypopituitarism involves removal, if possible, of the causative factor (such as a tumor) and permanent replacement of the hormones secreted by the target organs.

Medical Management

Injections of human growth hormone successfully treat growth hormone deficiency. Previously, human growth hormone was scarce and available for only a few clients. Now it is produced by recombinant deoxyribonucleic acid (DNA) technology and is readily available. Medications prescribed to replace hormones include corticosteroids to correct secondary adrenocortical insufficiency, thyroid hormone to treat myxedema, and sex hormones to correct hypogonadism.

Assessment of the client with hypopituitarism focuses on target organs that depend on pituitary secretions (see specific disorders such as Addison's disease and hypothyroidism). Nursing interventions are also directed at problems resulting from deficiency at the target organ. See the appropriate secretions for specific interventions.

POSTERIOR PITUITARY (NEUROHYPOPHYSEAL) DISORDERS

Unlike the adenohypophysis, the neurohypophysis is rarely destroyed by disease. Even if the posterior lobe becomes damaged or is surgically destroyed with the anterior lobe, hormonal deficiencies usually do not develop because the hypothalamus continues to synthesize oxytocin and ADH. If the hypothalamus suffers damage, however, deficiencies of oxytocin and ADH develop even if the neurohypophysis is healthy and intact.

The major disorder of the posterior lobe is ADH deficiency, also known as *diabetes insipidus*. Excessive ADH causes a condition called the *syndrome of inappropriate antidiuretic hormone* (SIADH), which can occur with lung cancer, head injuries, cranial surgery, pituitary tumors, encephalitis, poliomyelitis, and myxedema. Table 44-4 compares diabetes insipidus and SIADH.

TABLE 44–4   Comparison of Diabetes Insipidus and Syndrome of Inappropriate Secretion of Antidiuretic Hormone

	Diabetes Insipidus (DI)	Syndrome of Inappropriate Secretion of Antidiuretic Hormone (SIADH)
Definition	Deficiency of antidiuretic hormone (ADH, vasopressin) results in inability to conserve water	Excessive amounts of ADH secreted from posterior pituitary and other ectopic sources
Incidence	Unknown; DI idiopathic in about 30% of all clients with DI; tumors can be related to 25% of DI cases; head injury accounts for 16%; cranial surgery for 20% of DI cases	Approximately 80% of clients with small cell carcinoma have evidence of impaired ability to excrete water secondary to ectopic production of vasopressin
Etiology	Central or neurogenic DI: CNS interruption of anatomic integrity of posterior pituitary; localized or generalized edema from head trauma, vascular lesions, centrally acting drugs, or CNS infections may also cause central DI; ADH synthesis or release is affected; may be transient or permanent Complete DI occurs when there is disruption of hypophyseal tract and complete absence of ADH Nephrogenic DI: rare hereditary disorder; acquired structural or functional change in kidney occurs; ADH produced normally, but distal and collecting tubules cannot respond Idiopathic DI	Ectopic production of vasopressin by malignancy is most common cause (degree of vasopressin impairment is relative to extent of malignant disease); see Risk factors below
Risk factors	Head injury, neurosurgery, hypothalamic tumors, pituitary tumors, brain infections or inflammation; drugs that inhibit vasopressin release: ethanol, glucocorticoids, adrenergic agents, phenytoin, narcotic antagonists, lithium	Vasopressin overuse (from DI); malignant conditions that may contain ectopic sources of vasopressin-like hormone: bronchogenic carcinoma; lymphoma of duodenum, brain, bladder; pancreatic cancer; prostatic cancer; increased intracranial pressure secondary to infectious processes or brain trauma; infectious processes—viral or bacterial pneumonia; drugs that may stimulate vasopressin release: vincristine, cyclophosphamide, thiazides, phenothiazines, carbamazepine, vinblastine, cisplatin, oxytocin; endocrine disorders: adrenal insufficiency, myxedema, anterior pituitary insufficiency; analgesics; vomiting
Pathophysiology: normally ADH increases kidneys' permeability to water to promote water reabsorption and decrease urinary output; ADH is normally released in response to ↑ serum osmolality and ↓ extracellular volume	With ADH deficiency: permeability of water is diminished, resulting in excretion of large volumes of hypotonic fluid Three patterns may develop: (1) transient DI—abrupt onset within first few days after neurosurgery, resolves within several days; (2) permanent DI (prolonged DI)—abrupt and early onset, persists for several weeks or forever, usually occurs after damage to hypothalamus or neurohypophyseal stalk; (3) triphasic DI—immediate postinjury increase in urine volume with decrease in urine osmolality lasting 4-5 days; interphase occurs over next 5-7 days when urine volume decreases to normal and is followed by permanent phase of polyuria	Key features of ADH excess: (1) water retention, (2) hyponatremia, (3) hypo-osmolality; a continual release of ADH causes water retention from renal tubules and collecting ducts; extracellular fluid volume increases with dilutional hyponatremia; hyponatremia suppresses renin and aldosterone secretions, causing decrease in proximal tubule reabsorption of Na^+
Physical examination	Integumentary: dry, cool skin, dry mucous membranes Cardiovascular: tachycardia Physical manifestations related to specific electrolyte imbalance	Physical manifestations related to hyponatremia: decreased deep tendon reflexes, fatigue, headache, anorexia, nausea, decreased mental status, seizures, coma Physical manifestations related to fluid volume excess: weight gain without edema, jugular venous distention, tachycardia, tachypnea, rales
Clinical manifestations	Genitourinary: polyuria—a few liters to 18 L/day; clear urine; urinary frequency; nocturia Gastrointestinal: weight loss; polydipsia (if thirst mechanism intact) Integumentary: dry skin and mucous membranes Neurologic: mentation changes as electrolyte imbalance and hypotension worsen	Related to degree of hyponatremia: confusion, lethargy, irritability, seizures, coma Gastrointestinal: decreased motility with anorexia, nausea, vomiting; abrupt weight gain *without edema* of 5-10%
Complications	Electrolyte imbalance; hypovolemia; hypotension; shock	Seizures; coma; permanent brain damage; disease processes already in progress may be complicated

(Continued)

TABLE 44-4 Comparison of Diabetes Insipidus and Syndrome of Inappropriate Secretion of Antidiuretic Hormone—Cont'd

	Diabetes Insipidus (DI)	Syndrome of Inappropriate Secretion of Antidiuretic Hormone (SIADH)
Diagnosis	Urine: output—a few liters to 18 L/day; specific gravity 1.005; osmolality <200 mOsm/kg H_2O Plasma osmolality ↑ secondary to hypovolemia and dehydration Serum Na^+ ↑ secondary to hypovolemia and dehydration Serum osmolality >290 mOsm/kg H_2O Serum Na^+ ↓ secondary to volume depletion Water deprivation study: positive results Hypertonic saline test: positive for DI if there is little or no ↑ in plasma ADH levels	Serum Na^+ ↓; urine Na^+ ↑; blood urea nitrogen ↑; serum osmolality ↓; urine osmolality ↑; absence of hypotension, hypovolemia, or edematous states; water load test: positive for SIADH, abnormal water excretion; serum Na^+ remains ↓; serum osmolality remains ↓; urine osmolality remains ↑
Surgical management	Hypophysectomy to remove posterior pituitary tumor	None
Medical management	IV fluids; ADH replacement with DDAVP (desmopressin) IV, subcutaneous, or intranasal; nasal solution bid is drug of choice; onset of action is 1 hr, 6-24 hr duration; Pitressin tannate in oil is given IM; aqueous Pitressin is used for acute, transient form of DI	Hypertonic IV fluids to correct hyponatremia; sodium restriction; diuretics to correct low plasma osmolality; monitor urine electrolyte loss; replace electrolyte loss; demeclocycline to facilitate free water clearance; treat underlying cause
Nursing management	1. Know which clients are at risk 2. Monitor intake and output 3. Monitor for excessive thirst or urination 4. Assess serum and urine values: ↓ specific gravity, ↓ urine osmolality, ↑ serum osmolality are early indicators of DI 5. Observe effects of DI on concurrent medical and surgical disorders 6. Client and family teaching	1. Know which clients are at risk 2. Monitor appropriate urine and serum laboratory tests 3. Assess for manifestations of hyponatremia by evaluating neurologic status 4. Monitor daily weights and intake and output 5. Observe for changes in concurrent disorders 6. Administer demeclocycline as ordered to interfere with ADH action; monitor for possible nephrotoxicity 7. Monitor for hypernatremia with fluid over-correction 8. Client and family teaching
Prognosis	Excellent if there is compliance with vasopressin therapy	Depends on cause and sodium level and serum osmolality; poor for client with bronchogenic carcinoma; seizures and coma contribute to chronic brain dysfunction

IM, Intramuscular; *IV,* intravenous.

GONADAL DISORDERS

Testicular dysfunction can be primary, a disorder of testicular function, or secondary to a disorder of hypothalamic-pituitary function. Primary testis dysfunction can involve the seminiferous tubules (germ cells or Sertoli cells), Leydig cells, or both. Germ cell abnormalities cause infertility by disrupting spermatogenesis. Secondary sexual development and virilization are normal because testosterone production is not interrupted. When Leydig cell function is impaired, testosterone production falls, and virilization is impaired.

Causes of primary hypogonadism include genetic defects, malnutrition, trauma, infection, renal failure, radiation, chemotherapy, and environmental toxins (such as lead or alcohol). The cause, however, is usually unknown. Klinefelter's syndrome, caused by a chromosomal anomaly with a 47,XXY chromosome constitution, is an example of a genetic disorder causing primary testicular failure.

Secondary testicular dysfunction, frequently referred to as *hypogonadotropic hypogonadism,* results from inadequate secretion of gonadotropins. This complication leads to infertility and hypoandrogenism. The extent of LH and FSH deficiency and the age of onset determine the clinical manifestations. Prepubertal hypogonadism leads to eunuchoid body proportions (resulting from deficiency in male hormones), small testes, and lack of virilization.

Causes of secondary hypogonadism include hypothalamic or pituitary tumors, trauma, degenerative lesions, and radiation. Kallmann syndrome, which involves a deficiency of gonadotropin-releasing hormone (GRH) production by the hypothalamus, is an example of congenital secondary testicular dysfunction. People with Kallmann syndrome do not mature normally because of gonadotropin deficiency. Midline defects, such as cleft lip or palate, color blindness, anosmia, and ataxia, are common findings.

CONCLUSIONS

Adrenal, pituitary, and gonadal disorders are not common but are extremely complex and diverse. Obtaining a thorough understanding of the adrenal, pituitary, and gonadal anatomy and physiology can help you care for clients with these disorders. Most of these conditions (such as hypopituitarism) are acute and affect many body systems, whereas others become chronic and lead to a wide variety of other problems, such as Addison's disease. Teaching is vital to the care of these clients; understand these conditions so that appropriate teaching plans can be initiated.

THINKING CRITICALLY

1. The client is a woman with a 9-year history of Addison's disease. Normally she takes her prescribed doses of a glucocorticoid (dexamethasone [Decadron]) and a mineralocorticoid (fludrocortisone [Florinef]) without fail. She is 29 years old and is otherwise in good health. The client stayed home from work today because she began to experience nausea, vomiting, diarrhea, and fever with diaphoresis. Because of the nausea and vomiting, she did not take her medications. When her husband returned home at 5:30 PM, he found her unconscious. What events led to the client's unconsciousness? How might missing her medications have affected the client?

Factors to Consider. What acute disorder do the nausea, vomiting, diarrhea, and fever suggest? How might they affect a person with Addison's disease?

2. A 50-year-old woman has been taking glucocorticoids for 10 years for asthma. She is admitted to the hospital for sudden onset of severe low back pain. What factors may have contributed to her back pain?

Factors to Consider. What are the potential long-term effects of oral glucocorticoid therapy? What are their manifestations?

3. A 23-year-old man is admitted for a head injury related to an automobile accident. While doing your hourly checks, you note that his urine output has been 800 ml since the last check. Over the next 3 hours, the client excretes an additional 3000 ml of very clear urine. His blood pressure has dropped, and urine specific gravity is less than 1.005. What are your priorities for care?

Factors to Consider. Is the urine output within normal limits? How might his urine output be related to his head injury?

Discussions for these questions can be found on the website.

BIBLIOGRAPHY

  Citations appearing in red refer to primary research.

1. Burt, M.G., & Ho, K.K.Y. (2006). Newer options in the management of acromegaly. *Internal Medicine Journal, 36*(7), 437-444.
2. Coursin, D., & Wood, K. (2002). Corticosteroid supplementation for adrenal insufficiency. *Journal of the American Medical Association, 287*(2), 236-240.
3. Gaines, K. (2004). Desmopressin (DDAVP) for enuresis, diabetes insipidus, and…. *Urologic Nursing, 24*(6), 520-523.
4. Jones, R., & Huether, S. (2006). Alterations of hormonal regulations. In K. McCance & S. Huether (Eds.), *Pathophysiology: The biologic basis for disease in adults and children* (5th ed., pp. 683-734). St. Louis: Mosby.
5. Heffernan, M., et al. (2006). Prevention of osteoporosis associated with chronic glucocorticoid therapy. *Journal of the American Medical Association, 295*(11), 1300-1303.
6. Holcomb, S.S. (2006). Do the clues add up to Addison's disease? *Nursing 2006, 36*(3), 64hn1-3.
7. Kreutzer, J., & Fahlbusch, R. (2004). Diagnosis and treatment of pituitary tumors. *Current Opinion in Neurology, 17*(6), 693-703.
8. Labeur, M., Arzt, E., Stalla, G.K., et al. (2004). New perspectives in the treatment of Cushing's syndrome. *Current Drug Targets— Immune, Endocrine & Metabolic Disorders, 4*(4), 335-342.
9. Lenders, J., et al. (2002). Biochemical diagnosis of pheochromocytoma. Which test is best? *Journal of the American Medical Association, 287*(11), 1427-1434.
10. Li Voon Chong, J., et al. (2002). Elderly people with hypothalamic-pituitary disease and untreated GH deficiency: Clinical outcome, body composition, lipid profiles and quality of life after 2 years compared to controls. *Clinical Endocrinology, 56*(2), 175-181.
11. Loriaux, D.L. (2004). The adrenal cortex. In L. Goldman, et al. (Eds.), *Cecil textbook of medicine* (22nd ed., pp. 1412-1418). Philadelphia: Saunders.
12. Maite, A., et al. (2004). Pituitary adenoma. In M. Abeloff, et al. (Eds.), *Clinical oncology* (3rd ed., pp. 1395-1399). Philadelphia: Churchill Livingstone.
13. Mattke, A., Vender, J., & Anstadt, M. (2002). Pituitary apoplexy presenting as Addisonian crisis. *Texas Heart Institute Journal, 29*(3), 293-300.
14. Moltich, M. (2004). Anterior pituitary. In L. Goldman, et al. (Eds.), *Cecil textbook of medicine* (22nd ed., pp. 1367-1385). Philadelphia: Saunders.
15. O'Connor, D.T. (2004). The adrenal medulla, catecholamines, and pheochromocytoma. In L. Goldman, et al. (Eds.), *Cecil textbook of medicine* (22nd ed., pp. 1419-1424). Philadelphia: Saunders.
16. Raisbeck, E. (2002). Recognizing adrenal insufficiency. *Emergency Nurse, 10*(4), 24-26.
17. Robinson, A. (2004). Posterior pituitary. In L. Goldman, et al. (Eds.), *Cecil textbook of medicine* (22nd ed., pp. 1385-1391). Philadelphia: Saunders.
18. Salvatori, R. (2005). Adrenal insufficiency. *Journal of the American Medical Association, 294*(19), 2481-2488.
19. Serri, O., Chik, C.L., Ur, E., et al. (2003). Diagnosis and management of hyperprolactinemia. *Canadian Medical Association Journal, 169*(6), 575-581.
20. Simm, P.J., McDonnell, C.M., & Zacharin, M.R. (2004). Primary adrenal insufficiency in childhood and adolescence: Advances in diagnosis and management. *Journal of Pediatrics and Child Health, 40*(11), 596-599.
21. Weigel, R., et al. (2004). Cancer of the endocrine system. In M. Abeloff, et al. (Eds.), *Clinical oncology* (3rd ed., pp. 1611-1648). Philadelphia: Churchill Livingstone.
22. Weiss, G., et al. (2004). Menopause and hypothalamic-pituitary sensitivity to estrogen. *Journal of the American Medical Association, 292*(24), 2991-2996.
23. Zhu, X., et al. (2005). Genetic control of pituitary development and hypopituitarism. *Current Opinion in Genetics & Development, 15* (3), 332-340.
24. Zelena, D., Mergl, Z., & Makara, G. (2006). The role of vasopressin in diabetes mellitus-induced hypothalamo-pituitary-adrenal axis activation: Studies in Brattleboro rats. *Brain Research Bulletin, 29*(1), 9.

evolve *Did you remember to check out the bonus material on the Evolve website and the CD-ROM, including NCLEX®-Examination Style Review Questions, Open-Book Quizzes, and Chapter Review Audio Podcasts?*

http://evolve.elsevier.com/Black/medsurg

CHAPTER 45

Management of Clients with Diabetes Mellitus

JAMES A. FAIN

Diabetes mellitus is a chronic, progressive disease characterized by the body's inability to metabolize carbohydrates, fats, and proteins, leading to hyperglycemia (high blood glucose level). Diabetes mellitus is sometimes referred to as "high sugars" by both clients and health care providers. The notion of associating sugar with diabetes mellitus is appropriate because the passage of large amounts of sugar-laden urine is characteristic of poorly controlled diabetes mellitus. While hyperglycemia plays an important role in the development of diabetes-related complications, high levels of blood glucose are only one component of the pathologic process and clinical manifestations associated with diabetes mellitus. Other pathologic processes and risk factors are just as important, and sometimes independent factors. Diabetes mellitus can be associated with serious complications, but people with diabetes mellitus can take preventive measures to reduce the likelihood of such occurrences.

Diabetes mellitus has become an epidemic in the United States with 21 million people (e.g., 7% of the U.S. population) having this disease. Approximately 15 million people are diagnosed with diabetes mellitus, with nearly an additional 6 million estimated to have the disease but who are undiagnosed. As a significant public health problem, diabetes mellitus is the sixth leading cause of death in the United States.[16] In addition, total estimated diabetes mellitus costs in the United States in 2002 were $132 billion (direct and indirect costs) with direct medical costs accounting for $92 billion and $40 million in indirect costs (e.g., disability, work loss, and premature mortality).[16] While the increasing burden of diabetes mellitus is alarming, much of the burden of this major public health problem can be prevented by early detection, improved delivery of care, and better education for diabetes self-management.

CLASSIFICATION OF DIABETES MELLITUS

Diabetes mellitus is classified as one of four different clinical states including type 1, type 2, gestational, or other specific types of diabetes mellitus. Box 45-1 gives an overview of the various types of diabetes mellitus.[19] Type 1 diabetes mellitus is the result of autoimmune beta-cell destruction, leading to absolute insulin deficiency. Type 2 diabetes mellitus is the result of a progressive insulin secretory defect along with insulin resistance, usually associated with obesity. Gestational diabetes mellitus is a type of diabetes mellitus diagnosed during pregnancy. Other types of diabetes mellitus may occur as a result of genetic defects in beta-cell function, diseases of the pancreas (e.g., cystic fibrosis), or disease induced by drugs.

In 1979 the National Diabetes Data Group[29] (NDDG) developed criteria for the classification and diagnosis of diabetes mellitus. By 1997, and again in 2003, the Expert Committee on the Diagnosis and Classification

---

evolve **Web Enhancements**

Case Study Diabetes Mellitus and Pneumonia

Case Management Diabetes Mellitus

Client Education Guide Self-Injection of Insulin (Spanish Translation)

Sick Day Management for Diabetes Mellitus (Spanish Translation)

Visual Complications of Diabetes (English and Spanish Translations)

Complementary and Alternative Therapy Lifestyle Interventions to Reduce the Risk of Type 2 Diabetes Mellitus

Concept Map Understanding Diabetes Mellitus and Its Treatment

Ethical Issues in Nursing How Do Nurses Teach Compliance to Clients with Diabetes Mellitus?

Be sure to check out the bonus material on the Evolve website and the CD-ROM, including free self-assessment exercises. **http://evolve.elsevier. com/Black/medsurg**

> **BOX 45-1   Types of Diabetes Mellitus and Abnormal Glucose Metabolism**
>
> **DIABETES MELLITUS**
> 1. Type 1 diabetes mellitus
> 2. Type 2 diabetes mellitus
> 3. Causes of secondary diabetes mellitus
>   a. Genetic defects
>   b. Diseases of the pancreas (such as pancreatitis, neoplasia, trauma/pancreatectomy)
>   c. Endocrinopathies (such as acromegaly, Cushing's syndrome, pheochromocytoma, hyperthyroidism)
>   d. Drug/chemical-induced (as from glucocorticoids, thyroid hormone, diazoxide, thiazides, phenytoin sodium [Dilantin], nicotinic acid)
>   e. Infections (such as congenital rubella, cytomegalovirus infection)
>   f. Genetic syndromes associated with diabetes mellitus (such as Down syndrome, Klinefelter's syndrome, Huntington's chorea)
> 4. Gestational diabetes mellitus
>
> **PRE-DIABETES MELLITUS**
> 1. Impaired glucose tolerance (IGT) (2-hour post-glucose load 140 to 199 mg/dl)
> 2. Impaired fasting glucose (IFG) (fasting blood glucose 100 to 125 mg/dl)
>
> Modified from American Diabetes Association. (2003). Report of the Expert Committee on the Diagnosis and Classification of Diabetes Mellitus. *Diabetes Care, 26*(Suppl 1), S5-S20.

of Diabetes Mellitus[19] proposed changes to the original NDDG classification. Such changes were supported by the American Diabetes Association (ADA) and the National Institute of Diabetes and Digestive and Kidney Diseases (NIDDK). Previously, diabetes mellitus was classified as either insulin-dependent diabetes mellitus (IDDM) or non–insulin-dependent diabetes mellitus (NIDDM). With the use of insulin therapy commonplace with both types of diabetes mellitus, IDDM is now referred to as type 1 diabetes mellitus and NIDDM is referred to as type 2 diabetes mellitus. The ADA also recommended using Arabic numerals, type 1 and type 2, rather than Roman numerals in referring to the two types of diabetes mellitus.[19]

Clients who do not have type 1 or type 2 diabetes mellitus may be classified as having an *impaired fasting glucose (IFG)* or *impaired glucose tolerance (IGT)*. An IFG is a glucose concentration between 100 and 125 mg/dl while an IGT is defined as a 2-hour oral glucose tolerance test (75-g glucose load) with a glucose concentration between 140 and 199 mg/dl. Both IFG and IGT refer to a metabolic state between normal and diabetes mellitus, referred to as *prediabetes*.[13,16]

Diabetes mellitus may also result from other disorders or treatments. Genetic defects in the beta cells can lead to the development of diabetes mellitus. Several hormones, such as growth hormone, cortisol, glucagon, and epinephrine, can antagonize or counteract insulin. Excess amounts of these hormones (as in acromegaly, Cushing's syndrome, glucagonoma, and pheochromocytoma) cause diabetes mellitus. In addition, certain drugs (e.g., glucocorticoids and thiazides) may cause diabetes mellitus. Such types of secondary diabetes mellitus account for 1% to 2% of all diagnosed cases of diabetes mellitus.

Gestational diabetes mellitus is a diagnosis of diabetes mellitus that applies to women in whom glucose intolerance develops or is first discovered during pregnancy. Gestational diabetes mellitus develops in 2% to 5% of all pregnant women but usually disappears when the pregnancy is over. It occurs more frequently in African Americans, Hispanic Americans, Native Americans, and women with a family history of diabetes mellitus or babies over 9 pounds at birth; obesity is also a risk factor.

Etiology and Risk Factors
Type 1 Diabetes Mellitus

Type 1 diabetes mellitus, previously called IDDM or *juvenile-onset diabetes mellitus,* is characterized by destruction of pancreatic beta cells, leading to absolute insulin deficiency. Type 1 diabetes mellitus affects 10% of all people in the United States who have diabetes mellitus and is usually diagnosed before the age of 30. The incidence of type 1 diabetes mellitus is 12 to 14 cases per 100,000 people younger than 20 years, with an incidence of 1 case per 500 people younger than 16 years.[16] Type 1 diabetes mellitus is one of the most common childhood diseases, being three to four times more common than such chronic childhood diseases as cystic fibrosis, juvenile rheumatoid arthritis, and leukemia. The incidence of type 1 diabetes mellitus in males is similar to that in females with the condition more commonly seen among African Americans, Hispanic Americans, Asian Americans, and Native Americans than in whites.[13,16] Risk factors are less well-defined for type 1 diabetes mellitus than for type 2 diabetes mellitus.

Type 1 diabetes mellitus is inherited as a heterogeneous, multigenic trait. Identical twins have a risk of 25% to 50% of inheriting the disease, whereas siblings have a 6% risk and offspring a 5% risk. Despite this strong familial influence, 90% of people in whom type 1 diabetes mellitus develops do not have a first-degree relative with diabetes mellitus. An association also exists between type 1 diabetes mellitus and several human leukocyte antigens (HLAs). Environmental factors such as viruses appear to trigger an autoimmune process that destroys beta cells. Islet cell antibodies (ICAs) then appear, increasing in amount over months to years as beta cells are destroyed.[13] Fasting hyperglycemia (elevated blood glucose level) occurs when 80% to 90% of beta-cell mass has been destroyed.

Identification of ICAs has made it possible to detect type 1 diabetes mellitus in its preclinical stage.

Autoantibodies directed against insulin are found in 20% to 60% of clients with type 1 diabetes mellitus before initiation of exogenous insulin therapy. The combination of large amounts of ICAs, presence of insulin autoantibodies, and decreased first-phase insulin secretion (representing insulin stored in beta cells) can predict the onset of type 1 diabetes mellitus within 5 years.[13]

There are no known health promotion activities to prevent type 1 diabetes mellitus; however, physical activity and adherence to a prescribed meal plan may limit the development of diabetes-related complications.

In some instances, high-risk individuals (i.e., first-degree relatives of people with type 1 diabetes mellitus) are screened and appropriate counseling and follow-up instituted.[6]

Health maintenance activities involve the following:

- Maintaining blood glucose at levels as normal as possible
- Preventing hypoglycemia and hyperglycemia with stress, illness, or exercise by closely monitoring blood glucose levels and taking early action
- Performing daily foot care
- Preventing complications of diabetes mellitus by removing or treating coexisting risk factors such as smoking, hypertension, hyperlipidemia, and use of nephrotoxic drugs

Health restoration actions include the following:

- Prompt treatment of foot abrasions or infections
- Follow-up visits to assess for complications of diabetes mellitus and to reinforce learning needs
- Yearly funduscopic examinations by an ophthalmologist with treatment as needed
- Treatment of coexisting risk factors as described previously

Type 2 Diabetes Mellitus

Type 2 diabetes mellitus, previously called NIDDM or *adult-onset diabetes mellitus,* is a disorder involving both genetic and environmental factors. Type 2 diabetes mellitus is the most common type of diabetes mellitus, affecting 90% of all people who have the disease. Type 2 diabetes mellitus is usually diagnosed after the age of 40 and is more common among older adults, obese adults, and certain ethnic and racial populations. However, the diagnosis of type 2 diabetes mellitus in children and adolescents is on the increase, particularly in African Americans and Hispanic/Latino Americans.[16] On average, people diagnosed with type 2 diabetes mellitus have had the diagnosis for about 6.5 years before clinical identification and treatment.[16]

The prevalence of type 2 diabetes mellitus is markedly higher in Native Americans, African Americans, and Hispanic Americans, as well as in older and obese people.[13,16] Diabetes mellitus is the leading cause of new

blindness in adults 20 to 74 years of age and is the leading cause of chronic renal failure, accounting for about 40% of new cases. Likewise, diabetes mellitus is responsible for more than half the number of nontraumatic amputations in the United States.[13,16]

Type 2 diabetes mellitus is not associated with HLA tissue types, and circulating ICAs are rarely present. Heredity plays a major role in the expression of type 2 diabetes mellitus. It is more common in identical twins (58% to 75% incidence) than in the general population.

Obesity is a major risk factor, with 85% of all people with type 2 diabetes mellitus being obese. It is unclear whether impaired tissue (liver and muscle) sensitivity to insulin or impaired insulin secretion is the primary defect in this type of diabetes mellitus.[13] In addition, the prevalence of coronary artery disease in people with type 2 diabetes mellitus is twice that in the non-diabetic population, and cardiovascular and total mortality rates are two-fold to three-fold greater than in non-diabetic people.[13] These issues are explored in the Translating Evidence into Practice feature on p. 1065. Also see the Community-Based Practice feature on p. 1066 for a discussion of diabetes mellitus health promotion and maintenance activities.

Health promotion actions for type 2 diabetes mellitus include the following:

- Following eating habits based on "MyPyramid" (as noted later)[36]
- Avoiding foods high in refined sugars and saturated fats
- Maintaining ideal body weight, starting in childhood
- Exercising regularly
- Returning to pre-pregnancy weight or ideal body weight postpartum

Health maintenance activities involve the following:

- Screening high-risk individuals (i.e., people with family history of diabetes mellitus in first or second generation; members of certain racial or ethnic backgrounds [African American, Native American, Mexican American, Asians/Pacific Islanders]; people older than age 45 with any other risk factor; people with hypertension or hyperlipidemia; clients with previous impaired glucose tolerance; women with previous gestational diabetes mellitus or those who have had a baby weighing more than 9 pounds; and people with a history of recurrent infection, habitual physical inactivity, or polycystic ovary syndrome) by measuring a fasting blood glucose level[7]
- Performing periodic assessments to determine the client's learning needs and to assess glycemic control
- Using strategies shown to reduce complications of diabetes mellitus by removing or treating coexisting risk factors such as smoking, hypertension, hyperlipidemia, and use of nephrotoxic drugs

■ Performing daily foot care

■ Preventing hypoglycemia or hyperglycemia by closely monitoring blood glucose levels and taking early action

🏮 Health restoration actions include the following:

■ Teach meal planning and physical activity programs to reduce obesity
■ Prompt treatment of foot abrasions or infections
■ Follow-up visits to assess for complications of diabetes mellitus and reinforce learning needs
■ Yearly funduscopic examinations by an ophthalmologist with treatment as needed
■ Treatment of previously described risk factors
■ Control of angina and peripheral vascular disease

Pathophysiology
Type 1 Diabetes Mellitus

Type 1 diabetes mellitus does not develop in all people who have a genetic predisposition. Of those in whom gene markers (DR3 or DR4 HLA) indicate risk, diabetes mellitus ultimately develops in less than 1%. 🏮 Environmental triggers have long been suspected in type 1 diabetes mellitus. Incidence is increased in both spring and fall, and onset is often coincidental with epidemics of various viral diseases. Active autoimmunity is directed against the beta cells of the pancreas and their products. ICAs and insulin antibodies progressively decrease the effective circulating insulin level.[13]

This slow, progressive insult to the beta cells and endogenous insulin molecules can result in an abrupt onset of diabetes mellitus. Hyperglycemia can result from acute illness or stress (see the Case Study on p. 1067), which increases insulin demand beyond the reserves of the damaged beta-cell mass. When the acute illness or stress resolves, the client may revert to a compensated state of variable duration in which the pancreas once again manages to produce adequate amounts of insulin. This compensated state, referred to as the *honeymoon period,* typically lasts for 3 to 12 months. The process ends when the diminishing beta-cell mass cannot produce

---

🏮 TRANSLATING EVIDENCE INTO PRACTICE

Can We Prevent Type 2 Diabetes Mellitus?

In the United States in 2005, the prevalence of diabetes mellitus among adults (20 and older) was 20.6 million people or 9.6%, which is up sharply from 1995 when the prevalence was 7.4%.[2] In adults over the age of 60 the prevalence is 10.3 million people or 20.9%.[2] Results of several research studies over the past few years have indicated that lifestyle approaches can effectively prevent or delay the onset of type 2 diabetes mellitus.[3-9] Characteristics associated with an increased risk of type 2 diabetes mellitus include elevated fasting glucose levels (IFG) and postload oral glucose tolerance test (OGTT) concentrations, increased body mass index, central obesity, certain ethnic and racial backgrounds, family history of diabetes mellitus, and gestational diabetes mellitus.[1,5] Clinical trials of diabetes mellitus prevention among high-risk individuals have demonstrated the association between lifestyle interventions and decreased progression to type 2 diabetes mellitus.[3-9]

IMPLICATIONS

Knowledge of characteristics associated with an increased risk of type 2 diabetes mellitus is very useful in identifying appropriate population subgroups to target screening efforts aimed at identifying high-risk individuals and those individuals with undiagnosed type 2 diabetes mellitus. Several studies[4-9] have provided evidence that there is an association between successfully implemented lifestyle intervention (diet, physical activity, or both) and a decrease in progression to type 2 diabetes mellitus. The Diabetes Prevention Program[3] showed reduction in incident rates of diabetes mellitus among racially and ethnically diverse group of males with IGT and a body mass index greater than 24 kg/m[2]. The effectiveness of the lifestyle intervention group in reducing the incidence of type 2 diabetes mellitus was significantly greater than that of the medication group (metformin).[3] In addition, lifestyle education programs about diet and exercise lowered plasma glucose levels and reduced the incidence of type 2 diabetes mellitus.[5-7,9] Weight loss also reduced the incidence of type 2 diabetes mellitus.[4] Therefore the focus of future research needs to identify the most effective lifestyle intervention in terms of clinical outcomes, time required, and cost.

REFERENCES

1. American Diabetes Association. (2004). Screening for type 2 diabetes (position statement). *Diabetes Care, 27*(Suppl 1), S11-S14.
2. Centers for Disease Control and Prevention. (2005). *National diabetes fact sheet for the United States in 2005.* Retrieved 02/13/07 from www.cdc.gov/diabetes/pubs/pdf/ndfs_2005.pdf.
3. Diabetes Prevention Program Research Group. (2002). Reduction in the incidence of type 2 diabetes with lifestyle intervention or metformin. *New England Journal of Medicine, 346,* 393-403.
4. Hamman, R., et al. (2006). Effect of weight loss with lifestyle intervention on risk of diabetes. *Diabetes Care, 29,* 2102-2107.
5. Johnson, R., Williams, S., & Spruill, I. (2006). Genomics, nutrition, obesity, and diabetes. *Journal of Nursing Scholarship, 38*(1), 11-18.
6. Lindstrom, J. (2006). Sustained reduction in the incidence of type 2 diabetes by lifestyle intervention: Follow-up of the Finnish diabetes prevention study. *Lancet, 368,* 1673-1679.
7. Tuomilehto, J., Lindstrom, J., & Eriksson, J.G. (2001). Prevention of type 2 diabetes mellitus by changes in lifestyle among subjects with impaired glucose tolerance. *New England Journal of Medicine, 344,* 1343-1350.
8. Weinstein, A., et al. (2004). Relationship of physical activity vs body mass index with type 2 diabetes in women. *Journal of the American Medical Association, 292,* 1188-1194.
9. Yamaoka, K., & Tango, T. (2005). Lifestyle education programmes lower glucose concentrations and reduce the incidence of type 2 diabetes: A meta-analysis of randomized controlled trials. *Diabetes Care, 28,* 2780-2786.

COMMUNITY-BASED PRACTICE

Diabetes Mellitus

Diabetes mellitus has become a global health concern, and has now reached pandemic status. Most cases of diabetes mellitus are type 2, which is amenable to intensive lifestyle changes. The Diabetes Prevention Program has demonstrated that exercise and weight loss contribute to the delay and prevention of type 2 diabetes mellitus. Opportunities for students to engage in diabetes mellitus focused community-based activities exist in all communities.

Most nursing curricula have traditionally focused on diabetes mellitus management but now the time is right to change the focus. The priority for community-based intervention programs should now be health promotion through teaching about the risk factors and preventive measures for type 2 diabetes mellitus. Nursing educators can embrace the challenges of this public health threat by designing clinical experiences for nursing students to take primary prevention into the community. There is research that shows the benefits of such efforts in reducing the incidence of type 2 diabetes mellitus. Students can provide education at public locations or in their places of worship, teach children the benefits of exercise and food portion control in schools, or participate in exercise classes for people in groups at high risk to develop the disease.

Secondary prevention can include providing blood glucose screening in public locations. Churches, shopping malls, movie theaters, and grocery stores are all examples of places where a clinical experience could bring secondary prevention to the community.

Baccalaureate nursing students in Houston, Texas, participate in community-based service-learning through collaboration with other community partners: faculty from the University of Texas Health Science Center (UTHSC)—Houston School of Medicine and School of Nursing and school nurses and physical education teachers from the community. Students participate in screenings for diabetes mellitus and other diseases.

Nursing students in Omaha, Nebraska, take primary and secondary prevention activities into the community by participating in health fairs, by providing blood glucose checks at shopping malls, and by presenting educational seminars at middle schools aimed at getting students to improve their eating habits and increase their participation in exercise. Students also participate with a local agency to provide exercise classes for Hispanic women.

There are multiple opportunities for nurses to take diabetes mellitus education and prevention into the community at a variety of locations and events. Partnering with agencies that serve populations who are at highest risk for diabetes mellitus and consulting respected members of the community will help increase community participation. Nurses need to take advantage of any opportunity they find. An example of this "out of the box" thinking occurred in Fond du Lac, Wisconsin, where the public health nurse working with inhabitants of the local reservation worked with tribal leaders who were also Master Gardeners to plant communal vegetable gardens, coordinated cooking classes that respected and promoted the use of traditional foods, and helped organize the first Diabetes Powwow.

REFERENCES

1. Beem, S.E., et al. (2004). Aiming at "De Feet" and diabetes: A rural model to increase foot examinations. *American Journal of Public Health, 94*(10), 1664-1666.
2. Brosnan, C.A., et al. (2005). Student nurses participate in public health research and practice through a school-based screening program. *Public Health Nursing, 22*(3), 260-266.
3. Hjelm, K., et al. (2003). Preparing nurses to face the pandemic of diabetes mellitus: A literature review. *Journal of Advanced Nursing, 41*(5), 424-434.
4. Keltner, B., Kelley, F.J., & Smith, D. (2004). Leadership to reduce health disparities: A model for nursing leadership in American Indian communities. *Nursing Administration Quarterly, 28*(3), 181-190.
5. Tierney, A.J. (2003). This issue of JAN. *Journal of Advanced Nursing, 41*(50), 419-420.
6. Walker, E.A., et al., for the Diabetes Prevention Program Research Group. (2006). Adherence to preventive medications: Predictors and outcomes in the Diabetes Prevention Program. *Diabetes Care, 29*(9), 1997-2002.

enough insulin to sustain life. The client then becomes dependent on exogenous insulin (produced outside the body) administration to survive.[13]

Type 2 Diabetes Mellitus

The pathogenesis of type 2 diabetes mellitus differs significantly from that of type 1. A limited beta-cell response to hyperglycemia appears to be a major factor in its development. Beta cells chronically exposed to high blood levels of glucose become progressively less efficient when responding to further glucose elevations. This phenomenon, termed *desensitization,* is reversible by normalizing glucose levels. The ratio of *proinsulin* (a precursor to insulin) to insulin secreted also increases.[13]

A second pathophysiologic process in type 2 diabetes mellitus is resistance to the biologic activity of insulin in both the liver and peripheral tissues. This state is known as *insulin resistance.* People with type 2 diabetes mellitus have a decreased sensitivity to glucose levels, which results in continued hepatic glucose production, even with high blood glucose levels. This is coupled with an inability of muscle and fat tissues to increase glucose uptake. The mechanism causing peripheral insulin resistance is not clear; however, it appears to occur after insulin binds to a receptor on the cell surface (Figure 45-1).

Insulin is a building (anabolic) hormone. Without insulin, three major metabolic problems occur: (1) decreased glucose utilization, (2) increased fat mobilization, and (3) increased protein utilization (see Concept Map feature on Understanding Diabetes Mellitus and Its Treatment).

Decreased Glucose Utilization

Cells that require insulin as a carrier for glucose can take in only about 25% of the glucose they require for fuel. Nerve tissues, erythrocytes, and the cells of the intestines, liver, and kidney tubules do not require insulin for glucose

Diabetes and Pneumonia

Ms. Washington is a 44-year-old African-American woman who has been sick for the past week. She has been treated with erythromycin (E-Mycin) 500 mg q 6 hr and phenylpropanolamine-guaifenesin (Entex LA) q 12 hr as an outpatient after being seen in the clinic for a persistent cough, loss of voice, chest pain from coughing, fever, chills, and mild nausea without vomiting. She now reports that she has been coughing sputum that is brown to green, with small amounts of red blood present. Ms. Washington is also complaining of left shoulder pain for the past 3 days, fatigue, sinus pressure, congestion, fullness in the ears, and postnasal drainage. She also reports frequent urination without dysuria or urgency and feeling thirsty all the time. ... *Case Study continued on the website and the CD-ROM with discussions, multiple-choice questions, and a nursing care plan.*

transport. However, adipose tissue, along with skeletal and cardiac muscle, requires insulin for glucose transport. Without adequate amounts of insulin, much of the ingested glucose cannot be used.[22]

With inadequate amounts of insulin, blood glucose levels rise. This elevation continues because the liver cannot store glucose as glycogen without sufficient insulin levels. In an attempt to restore balance and return blood glucose levels to normal, the kidney excretes the excess glucose. Glucose appears in the urine *(glucosuria)*. Glucose excreted in the urine acts as an osmotic diuretic and causes excretion of increased amounts of water, resulting in fluid volume deficit.[13,22]

Increased Fat Mobilization

In type 1 diabetes mellitus and occasionally with severe stress in type 2 diabetes mellitus, the body turns to fat stores for energy production when glucose is unavailable. Fat metabolism causes breakdown products called *ketones* to form. Ketones accumulate in the blood and are excreted through the kidneys and lungs. Ketone levels

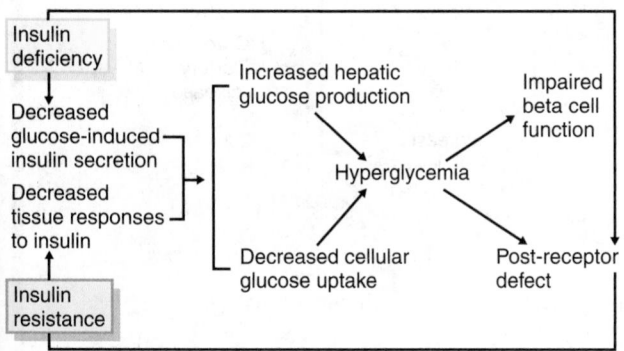

■ FIGURE 45-1   Relationship between insulin resistance and insulin secretion in type 2 diabetes mellitus. *(Modified from American Diabetes Association. [1998]. Medical management of non-insulin dependent [type 2] diabetes [4th ed., p. 18]. Alexandria, Va: Author.)*

can be measured in the blood and urine; high levels can indicate uncontrolled diabetes mellitus.[13,22]

Ketones interfere with the body's acid-base balance by producing hydrogen ions. The pH can decrease, and metabolic acidosis can develop. In addition, when ketones are excreted, sodium is also eliminated, resulting in sodium depletion and further acidosis. The excretion of ketones also increases osmotic pressure, leading to increased fluid loss. Also, when fats are the primary source of energy, body lipid levels can increase to five times normal, leading to increased atherosclerosis.[13,22]

Increased Protein Utilization

Lack of insulin leads to protein wasting. In healthy people, proteins are constantly being broken down and rebuilt. In people with type 1 diabetes mellitus, without insulin to stimulate protein synthesis, the balance is altered, which leads to increased catabolism (destruction). Amino acids are converted to glucose in the liver, further elevating glucose levels. If this condition goes untreated, clients with type 1 diabetes mellitus appear emaciated. The pathophysiologic processes of diabetes mellitus continue, leading to many acute and chronic complications, discussed later in the chapter.[13,22,26]

Clinical Manifestations

An elevated blood glucose level, called *hyperglycemia,* leads to common clinical manifestations associated with diabetes mellitus. In type 1 diabetes mellitus, the onset of clinical manifestations may be subtle with the possibility of life-threatening situations likely to happen (i.e., diabetic ketoacidosis). In type 2 diabetes mellitus, the onset of clinical manifestations may develop so gradually that clients may notice few or no clinical manifestations for a number of years.

The clinical manifestations of diabetes mellitus are increased frequency of urination *(polyuria)*, increased thirst or fluid intake *(polydipsia)*, and, as the disease progresses, weight loss despite hunger and increased food intake *(polyphagia)*. Tables 45-1 and 45-2 list common clinical manifestations and distinguishing features of diabetes mellitus.

Diagnosis of Diabetes Mellitus

Physical examination, medical history, and laboratory tests are employed to evaluate clients with diabetes mellitus. Clinical manifestations suggest the presence of diabetes mellitus, but laboratory tests are needed to make a definitive diagnosis.

Fasting Blood Glucose Level

A fasting blood glucose sample is drawn when the client has not ingested any nutrients other than water for at least 8 hours. This blood sample generally reflects glucose level from hepatic production. If the client is receiving a dextrose intravenous (IV) solution, results of the test must be

Understanding Diabetes Mellitus and Its Treatment

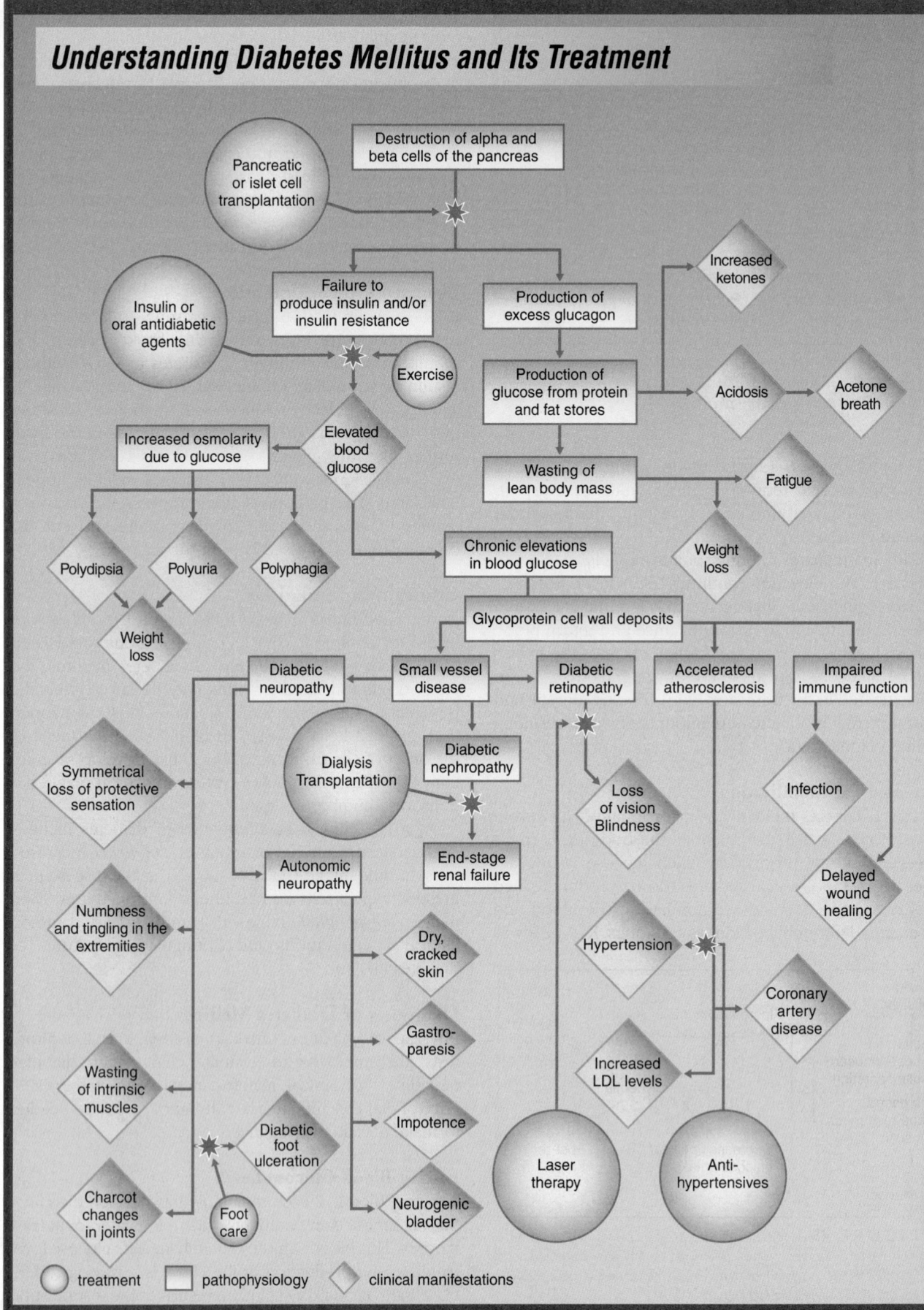

TABLE 45–1   Selected Clinical Manifestations of Diabetes Mellitus at Diagnosis

Clinical Manifestation	Pathophysiologic Basis	Type 1 Diabetes Mellitus	Type 2 Diabetes Mellitus
Cardinal manifestations			
Polyuria* (frequent urination)	Water not reabsorbed from renal tubules secondary to osmotic activity of glucose; leads to loss of water, glucose, and electrolytes	++[†]	+
Polydipsia* (excessive thirst)	Dehydration secondary to polyuria causes thirst	++	+
Polyphagia* (excessive hunger)	Starvation secondary to tissue breakdown (catabolism) causes hunger	++	+
Weight loss*	Initial loss secondary to depletion of water, glycogen, and triglyceride stores; chronic loss secondary to decreased muscle mass as amino acids are diverted to form glucose and ketone bodies	++	–
Recurrent blurred vision	Secondary to chronic exposure of ocular lens and retina to hyperosmolar fluids	+	++
Pruritus, skin infections, vaginitis	Bacterial and fungal infections of skin seem to be more common; research conflicting	+	++
Ketonuria	When glucose cannot be used for energy in insulin-dependent cells, fatty acids are used for energy; fatty acids are broken down into ketones in blood and excreted by kidneys; in type 2 diabetes mellitus, sufficient insulin is present to depress excessive use of fatty acids but not enough to permit use of glucose	++	–
Weakness and fatigue, dizziness	Decreased plasma volume leads to postural hypotension; potassium loss and protein catabolism contribute to weakness	++	+
Often asymptomatic	Body can "adapt" to a slow rise in blood glucose level to a greater extent than it can to a rapid rise	–	++

* Often referred to as *classic manifestations* of diabetes mellitus.
[†] +, Sometimes seen; ++, usually seen; –, not usually seen.

TABLE 45–2   Distinguishing Features of Diabetes Mellitus

Feature	Type 1	Type 2
Synonyms	Insulin-dependent diabetes mellitus (IDDM), juvenile diabetes, labile or brittle diabetes	Non–insulin-dependent diabetes mellitus (NIDDM), adult- or maturity-onset diabetes, mild diabetes
Age at onset	Usually occurs before age 30 yr, but may occur at any age	Usually occurs after age 30 yr, but can occur in children
Incidence	~10%	~90%
Type of onset	Usually abrupt, with rapid onset of hyperglycemia	Insidious, may be asymptomatic or mildly asymptomatic; body adapts to slow onset of hyperglycemia
Endogenous insulin production	Little or none	Below normal, normal, or above normal
Body weight at onset	Ideal body weight or thin	85% of clients are obese; may be of ideal body weight
Ketosis	Prone to ketosis, usually present at onset, often present during poor control	Resistant to ketosis, can occur with infection or stress
Manifestations	Polyuria, polydipsia, polyphagia, fatigue	Often none, may be mild manifestations of hyperglycemia
Dietary management	Essential	Essential
Exercise management	Essential	Essential
Exogenous insulin administration	Dependent on insulin for survival	20%-30% of clients may require insulin
Oral hypoglycemic agents	Not effective	Effective
Teaching needs	At diagnosis and ongoing	At diagnosis and ongoing

analyzed with that variable in mind. In clients who are known to have diabetes mellitus, food and insulin are withheld until after the specimen is obtained. 🪔 The diagnosis of diabetes mellitus is made when a client's fasting blood glucose level is greater than 126 mg/dl. Values between 110 and 125 mg/dl indicate an IFG.[13,19] The fasting blood glucose measurement provides the best indication of overall glucose homeostasis and is the preferred method of diagnosing diabetes mellitus.

Casual Blood Glucose Level

🪔 Clients may also be diagnosed with diabetes mellitus based on clinical manifestations and a casual (random) blood glucose level greater than 200 mg/dl.[13,19] A casual blood glucose sample can be drawn any time of day without regard to fasting. Elevated blood glucose levels may occur after meals, after stressful events, in samples drawn from an IV site, or in cases of diabetes mellitus.

Postload Blood Glucose Level

A postload or postprandial (after a meal) glucose level can also be drawn and used to diagnose diabetes mellitus. Postload blood glucose samples are drawn 2 hours after a standard meal and reflect the efficiency of insulin-mediated glucose uptake by peripheral tissues. Normally, blood glucose level should return to fasting levels within 2 hours. A 2-hour postload glucose level greater than 200 mg/dl during an oral glucose tolerance test (OGTT)[13,19] is confirmation for a diagnosis of diabetes mellitus (Box 45-2).

BOX 45-2 Screening and Diagnosis Guidelines for Diabetes Mellitus

GUIDELINES FOR TESTING FOR DIABETES MELLITUS

Testing for diabetes mellitus should be considered in all adults at age 45. If results are normal, testing should be repeated at 3-year intervals.

Testing should be considered at a younger age or performed more often for clients with the following risk factors:

- Obesity (>120% of desirable body weight or a body mass index above 25 kg/m^2)
- Habitual physical inactivity
- Polycystic ovary syndrome
- Diabetes mellitus in a first-degree relative
- Racial predisposition (as in African-American, Hispanic, Native American populations)
- In women who have given birth to a baby weighing more than 9 pounds or who have a history of gestational diabetes mellitus
- Hypertension (blood pressure >130/80 mm Hg)
- A high-density lipoprotein level <35 mg/dl or triglyceride level >250 mg/dl
- On previous testing, impaired glucose tolerance or impaired fasting glucose levels

GUIDELINES FOR DIAGNOSIS OF DIABETES MELLITUS

Fasting plasma glucose level above 126 mg/dl (7.0 mmol/L). Fasting is defined as no caloric intake for at least 8 hours.

Or

Manifestations of diabetes mellitus plus casual plasma glucose concentration above 200 mg/dl (11.1 mmol/L). *Casual* is defined as any time of day without regard to time since last meal. Classic manifestations include polyuria, polydipsia, and unexplained weight loss.

Or

A 2-hour postload glucose level above 200 mg/dl during an oral glucose tolerance test. This test should be performed using a glucose load containing the equivalent of 75 g of anhydrous glucose dissolved in water.

Plasma Glucose Values

Fasting plasma glucose	<110 mg/dl	Normal fasting glucose
	110-125 mg/dl	Impaired fasting glucose
	>126 mg/dl	Diagnosis of diabetes mellitus
Oral glucose tolerance test, 2 hours after eating	<140 mg/dl	Normal glucose tolerance
	140-199 mg/dl	Impaired glucose intolerance
	>200 mg/dl	Diagnosis of diabetes mellitus

Modified from American Diabetes Association. (2003). Report of the Expert Committee on the Diagnosis and Classification of Diabetes Mellitus. *Diabetes Care, 26*(Suppl 1), S5-S20.

In older adults, postload levels are higher, typically increasing by 5 to 10 mg/dl per decade after age 50 years because of the normal decline in glucose tolerance associated with aging. Smoking and drinking coffee can lead to falsely elevated values at 2 hours, whereas strenuous exercise can lead to falsely decreased values.

Laboratory Tests Related to Diabetes Mellitus
Glycosylated Hemoglobin Level

Glucose normally attaches itself to the hemoglobin molecule on a red blood cell. Once attached, it cannot dissociate. Therefore the higher the blood glucose levels, the higher the levels of glycosylated hemoglobin (HbA$_{1C}$).[22] The term HbA$_{1C}$ is referred to as an A1C. The A1C is an average blood glucose level measured over the previous 3 months. It is stated as a percentage and is useful in evaluating long-term glycemic control. To avoid diabetes-related complications, the ADA recommends keeping the A1C level below 7%.[8]

The ADA recommends that A1C testing be done routinely on all people with diabetes mellitus. The A1C test should be done semiannually in clients who have met the primary target goal for glycemic control (<7%) and quarterly in clients who have not met the primary goal for glycemic control.[8] Conditions that increase erythrocyte turnover, such as bleeding, pregnancy, or asplenia (absence of the spleen as after splenectomy), lead to falsely low A1C concentrations. High aspirin doses, alcohol ingestion, uremia, elevated hemoglobin levels, and heparin therapy can cause falsely elevated A1C levels.[22]

Glycosylated Albumin Level

Glucose also attaches to proteins, primarily albumin. The concentration of glycosylated albumin (fructosamine) represents the average blood glucose level over the previous 7 to 10 days.[22] This measurement is useful when short-term determinations of average blood glucose level are desired. The reliability and clinical applicability continue to be evaluated.

Connecting Peptide (C-Peptide) Level

When the proinsulin produced by pancreatic beta cells is broken apart by an enzyme, two products are formed, insulin and connecting peptide, commonly called *C-peptide*. Because C-peptide and insulin are formed in equal amounts, this test indicates the amount of endogenous insulin production.[22] Clients with type 1 diabetes mellitus usually have no or low concentrations of C-peptide. Clients with type 2 diabetes mellitus tend to have normal or elevated levels of C-peptide.

Ketonuria

Urine levels of ketones can be tested by clients' use of dipstrips or tablets. The presence of ketones in the urine (a condition called *ketonuria*) indicates that the body is using fat as a major source of energy, which may result in ketoacidosis. Test results are indicated by the presence of color changes, indicating the presence of ketones. All clients with diabetes mellitus should test their urine for ketones during acute illness or stress, when blood glucose levels are elevated (>240 mg/dl), and when they are pregnant or have evidence of ketoacidosis (e.g., nausea, vomiting, or abdominal pain).

Some testing strips detect ketones as well as glucose. Although urine testing is important for checking ketones, urine testing for glucose is not a reliable method for monitoring.

Proteinuria

Microalbuminuria measures microscopic amounts of protein in the urine *(proteinuria)*. The presence of protein *(microalbuminuria)* in the urine is an early manifestation of kidney disease. Testing the urine for microalbuminuria shows early nephropathy, long before it would be evident on routine urinalysis. The ADA recommends that all clients with diabetes mellitus be tested for microalbuminuria annually.[8] Some clients, however, require more frequent testing to detect progression of kidney disease related to the adverse effects of certain medications on the kidneys.

Self-Monitoring of Blood Glucose (SMBG)

The key to managing diabetes mellitus is to keep the blood glucose level as close to normal as possible or within a target range that is agreed upon between the client and health care provider. Self-monitoring of blood glucose (SMBG) provides immediate feedback and data on blood glucose levels. SMBG is recommended for all clients with diabetes mellitus, regardless of whether they have type 1, type 2, or gestational diabetes mellitus. SMBG is a way to know how the body responds to food, insulin, activity, and stress.[15]

The frequency and timing of SMBG depend on the needs and goals of each individual client. For most clients with type 1 diabetes mellitus and pregnant women taking insulin, SMBG is recommended three or more times daily. Testing should be done before each meal, before bedtime, and possibly in the middle of the night (e.g., 3:00 AM). For clients with type 2 diabetes mellitus, the frequency and timing of SMBG are mutually agreed upon by the client and health care provider. If clients with type 2 diabetes mellitus are taking oral medications, they usually do not have to monitor as often as someone with type 2 diabetes mellitus taking insulin. Extra times to SMBG level should include the following:

- When starting a new drug (oral agent) or insulin
- When starting an over-the-counter medication that affects blood glucose levels (e.g., steroid)
- When you are sick/under a lot of stress

- When you think your glucose level is too high or too low
- When you lose or gain weight
- When there is a change in your medication dose, eating plan, or physical activity plan

OUTCOME MANAGEMENT

Medical Management

Medical management for clients with diabetes mellitus includes restoring and maintaining blood glucose levels to as near normal as possible by balancing diet, exercise, and the use of oral hypoglycemic agents or insulin.[1,13,15,38] In general, when diabetes mellitus is successfully managed, clients avoid the complications of hypoglycemia and hyperglycemia. However, complications may develop in some clients with diabetes mellitus despite their vigorous efforts to carefully control the disease.

Initial as well as ongoing client education is vital in helping the client manage this chronic condition. Interventions must be individualized to the client's goals, age, lifestyle, nutritional needs, maturation, activity level, occupation, type of diabetes mellitus, and ability to independently perform the skills required by the management plan. Incorporation of psychosocial aspects into the overall plan is vital.[13,15]

Promote Proper Nutrition

Dietary management is an essential component of diabetic care and management. The general goal of dietary management is to help clients with diabetes mellitus improve metabolic control by making changes in nutrition habits. Specific goals include (1) improving blood glucose and lipid levels, (2) providing consistency in day-to-day food intake (in type 1 diabetes mellitus), (3) facilitating weight management (in type 2 diabetes mellitus), and (4) providing adequate nutrition for all stages of life. Lifestyle interventions are further explored in the Complementary and Alternative Therapy feature on p. 1072 and on the website.

Achieving nutrition-related goals requires a team approach that includes the client. Effective self-management requires an individualized approach, taking into account the client's personal lifestyle and diabetes management goals. A nutritional assessment is used to determine the nutrition prescription on the basis of what the client with diabetes mellitus is able and willing to do.[1,3] SMBG, lipid levels, blood pressure, and renal status are all essential aspects of nutrition-related management.

Alcohol. Other dietary concerns involve alcohol consumption and use of artificial sweeteners. Clients with diabetes mellitus do not need to give up alcoholic beverages entirely, but health care providers must be aware of the potential adverse effects of alcohol specific to diabetes mellitus and teach clients accordingly. Alcohol calories

Lifestyle Intervention or Metformin to Prevent or Delay Type 2 Diabetes Mellitus

A unique randomized, placebo-controlled trial with a mean follow-up of 2.8 years was conducted with a total of 3234 participants from 27 centers in the United States. The mean age of the participants was 51 years and 68% were women. Individuals had a body mass index (BMI) greater than or equal to 24 and a blood glucose level 5.3 to 6.9 mmol/L in the fasting state and 7.8 to 11 mmol/L 2 hours after a 75-g oral glucose load. Follow-up was 93%. Participants were allocated to an intensive program of lifestyle changes ($n = 1079$), standard lifestyle recommendations plus metformin (850 mg twice daily) for glucose control ($n = 1073$), or placebo ($n = 1082$). The intensive lifestyle change consisted of a combined intervention that would maintain a 7% or greater reduction in body weight through a low-calorie, low-fat diet and moderate physical activity. The incidence rates of diabetes mellitus were 4.8, 7.8, and 11 clients per 100 person-years for the intensive lifestyle changes, metformin, and placebo groups, respectively. Thus the lifestyle intervention reduced the risk of being diagnosed with type 2 diabetes mellitus by 50% and metformin reduced the risk by 25% compared to placebo. In overweight individuals with elevated fasting and postload blood glucose concentrations, an intensive lifestyle change or metformin treatment plus standard lifestyle recommendations was more effective than standard lifestyle recommendations alone for preventing or delaying the onset of type 2 diabetes mellitus.

REFERENCE

From Diabetes Prevention Program Research Group. (2002). Reduction in the incidence of type 2 diabetes with lifestyle intervention or metformin. *New England Journal of Medicine, 346,* 393-403.

must be figured into total caloric intake to prevent weight gain. Alcohol does not require insulin for absorption and it is generally absorbed before other nutrients. Alcohol can impair the process of gluconeogenesis, especially if the alcohol is consumed on an empty stomach. Hypoglycemia may occur, especially in clients who use insulin to manage their disease. Alcohol can also impair the client's ability to recognize and treat the hypoglycemia. Hence moderate consumption (1 drink per day in women and no more than 2 drinks per day in men) and ingestion of food with the alcohol are recommended.[1]

Artificial Sweeteners. Artificial sweeteners may help clients achieve desired caloric intake restrictions. Nutritive sweeteners such as fructose, sorbitol, and xylitol contain calories similar to sucrose but they cause less elevation in blood glucose levels. These products may have a laxative effect as well. Non-nutritive sweeteners have minimal or no calories and no elevation in blood glucose levels. Saccharine, aspartame (NutraSweet), and sucralose (Splenda) are examples of non-nutritive sweeteners

that have been approved by the U.S. Food and Drug Administration (FDA) for clients with diabetes mellitus.

Promote Regular Physical Activity

A program of planned physical activity is a crucial part of the treatment plan for a client with diabetes. Physical activity lowers blood glucose level by increasing carbohydrate metabolism, fosters weight reduction and maintenance, increases insulin sensitivity, increases high-density lipoprotein (HDL) levels, decreases triglyceride levels, lowers blood pressure, and reduces stress and tension.[4]

The primary side effect of acute physical activity is hypoglycemia (low glucose level). Occasionally, hyperglycemia (elevated glucose level) and ketosis can occur in clients with type 1 diabetes mellitus. Hypoglycemia is a significant risk for clients who exercise while taking insulin or oral hypoglycemics. Adjustments are sometimes needed to prevent hypoglycemia in the client taking insulin, because hepatic glucose production is blocked or partially inhibited by exogenous insulin. For example, a reduction in short-acting insulin of 30% to 50% can decrease the risk of hypoglycemia. Clients who use meal planning and physical activity alone to control type 2 diabetes mellitus are not at risk for hypoglycemia when exercising.

Administer Medications

Pharmacologic interventions should be considered when the client cannot achieve normal or near-normal blood glucose levels with nutrition and exercise therapies.[38]

Oral Antidiabetes Drugs. Oral antidiabetes agents are available in the United States for the management of diabetes mellitus (see the Integrating Pharmacology feature on Medications for Clients with Diabetes Mellitus on p. 1073). The major classes of oral antidiabetes drugs include sulfonylureas, biguanides, meglitinides, thiazolidinediones, alpha-glucosidase inhibitors, incretin mimetics, and amylinomimetics.

Many of the oral medications are aimed at only one aspect of the underlying pathogenesis of type 2 diabetes mellitus. Thus multiple medications are often needed to achieve optimal glycemic control. Given that type 2 diabetes mellitus is a progressive disease complicated by side effects associated with various pharmacologic interventions (e.g., hypoglycemia and weight gain), newer medications, such as incretin mimetics and amylinomimetics, have been developed that target multiple aspects of the underlying pathogenesis of type 2 diabetes mellitus.

Insulin Therapy. Clients with type 1 diabetes mellitus do not produce enough insulin to sustain life. They depend on exogenous insulin administration on a daily basis. In contrast, clients with type 2 diabetes mellitus are not dependent on exogenous insulin for survival. However, clients with type 2 diabetes mellitus may need to take

Medications for Clients with Diabetes Mellitus

Clients with type 1 diabetes mellitus must take insulin. Type 2 diabetes mellitus clients are managed with drugs in several chemical classes: alpha-glucosidase inhibitors, biguanides, meglitinides, sulfonylureas, thiazolidinediones, incretin mimetics, and amylinomimetics. The main actions of many of these drugs are either to stimulate beta cells of the pancreas to produce more insulin or to increase tissue response to insulin. Sulfonylureas and meglitinides are oral hypoglycemic agents that stimulate beta cells of the pancreas to secrete insulin. Second-generation sulfonylureas also increase tissue response to insulin (insulin sensitizer) and decrease glucose production by the liver. Biguanides increase tissue response to insulin (insulin sensitizer), decrease hepatic production of glucose, decrease absorption of glucose from the small intestine, and decrease triglyceride and low-density lipoprotein levels. Thiazolidinediones increase insulin action at receptors and postreceptors in hepatic and peripheral tissue to decrease insulin resistance and often decrease triglyceride levels. Alpha-glucosidase inhibitors delay the digestion of complex carbohydrates and certain sugars to blunt the peak of blood glucose and insulin levels after meals.

A new therapeutic class of medications based on incretin hormones has been developed. Incretin hormones are gastrointestinal hormones that are released following food ingestion. Two major incretin hormones that have been identified include a glucagon-like peptide (GLP-1) and glucose-dependent insulinotropic polypeptide (GIP).[18] Both hormones play a major role in stimulating insulin secretion and facilitating homeostasis following food ingestion. Byetta (exenatide), an incretin mimetic, is a GLP-1 receptor agonist. This medication is indicated for use in people with type 2 diabetes mellitus who are not adequately controlled with a sulfonylurea, metformin, or a combination of both. Exenatide is an analog of GLP-1 and is derived from a compound found in the saliva of the Gila monster, a lizard located in the southwestern part of the United States. This analog enhances insulin secretion in response to elevated blood glucose levels.[18] There is a risk of hypoglycemia when exenatide is used with a sulfonylurea, or with a combination of a sulfonylurea and metformin. Exenatide also is associated with mild to moderate GI manifestations, such as nausea, vomiting, and diarrhea. Several other new incretin-based medications are currently in development and undergoing clinical testing.[32]

Symlin (pramlintide) is another new class of diabetes medication referred to as an amylinomimetic or antihyperglycemic. Pramlintide is an injectable diabetes mellitus medication for use in people with type 1 and type 2 diabetes mellitus. It acts primarily by regulating glucose concentrations in the postprandial state; enhances satiety, leading to weight loss; decreases mealtime insulin requirements; and improves glycosylated hemoglobin levels.[24] In addition to regulating post-meal increases in glucose concentrations, pramlintide slows gastric emptying and suppresses glucagon secretion.[24] Symlin (pramlintide) is a synthetic analog of the hormone amylin. Amylin is a naturally occurring hormone located in the beta cells of the pancreas and secreted with insulin in response to food intake. Like insulin, amylin is absent or deficient in people with diabetes mellitus. Amylin and insulin work together with glucagon to maintain normal glucose concentrations. Insulin and amylin concentrations normally increase while glucagon levels decrease after meals. Amylin slows gastric emptying and suppresses glucagon secretion.[25] The most common side effect associated with taking pramlintide is nausea, and this side effect can be reduced by ingesting amylin with 30 grams of carbohydrate or 250 calories.[25,32] When used with insulin there is an increased risk of hypoglycemia, particularly in people with type 1 diabetes mellitus. If hypoglycemia does occur, the insulin dose, not pramlintide, is the cause. Lowering the bolus insulin (mealtime insulin) amount by 30% to 50% is recommended to help resolve hypoglycemia. Pramlintide is not recommended for clients who do not follow their current insulin regimen or check their blood glucose levels three or more times a day; have a history of hypoglycemia requiring assistance; or have been diagnosed with gastroparesis and use medications that stimulate gastrointestinal motility; this medication is also contraindicated in pediatric clients or pregnant women.[25]

In addition to insulin or antidiabetic medications, many diabetic clients take an angiotensin-converting enzyme (ACE) inhibitor to decrease blood pressure and minimize nephropathic changes and take aspirin or ticlopidine to decrease the risk of thrombus formation. Calcium channel blockers and diuretics may also be used to manage hypertension. Antilipemic drugs may be added to prevent or treat microvascular and macrovascular complications of diabetes mellitus. Lyrica (pregabalin) may be ordered to treat diabetic peripheral neuropathy pain. Reglan (metoclopramide) may be administered to clients with gastroparesis, and PDE-5 drugs may be ordered for men with erectile dysfunction.

insulin for adequate glucose control, especially in times of stress or illness.

Insulin Sources. Insulin is made chemically by recombinant DNA technology (human insulin) with different durations of action (rapid-, short-, intermediate-, and long-acting).

Each type of insulin has different peak and duration times. Nurses must be certain that they are administering the proper dose of the correct type of insulin ordered.

Most clients who require insulin therapy receive human insulin produced by recombinant deoxyribonucleic acid (DNA) technology (Table 45-3).[38] Compared with animal insulins, human insulin peaks more precisely and predictably, has a shorter duration of action, and has reduced antigenicity (ability to produce antigen response), and it does not cause lipoatrophy (loss of subcutaneous fat) or lipodystrophy (fat metabolism disturbance leading to loss of subcutaneous fat) at the injection site.

Insulin works to lower blood glucose level by promoting the transport of glucose into cells, and by

TABLE 45–3 Types of Human Insulin and Comparative Actions

Action	Preparation	Appearance	Onset	Peak	Duration
Rapid-acting	Humalog (insulin lispro)	Clear	5-10 min	1 hr	2-4 hr
	NovoLog (insulin aspart)	Clear	5-10 min	1 hr	2-4 hr
Short-acting	Humulin R (regular)	Clear	0.5-2 hr	2-4 hr	4-6 hr
	Novolin R (regular)	Clear	0.5-2 hr	2-4 hr	4-6 hr
Intermediate-acting	Humulin N (NPH)	Cloudy	2-4 hr	4-10 hr	10-16 hr
	Humulin L (Lente)	Cloudy	2-4 hr	4-10 hr	10-16 hr
	Humulin 70/30 (premixed) (70% NPH, 30% regular)	Cloudy	0.5-1 hr	Dual	10-16 hr
Long-acting	Humulin U (Ultralente)	Clear	6-10 hr	None	18-20 hr
	Lantus (insulin glargine)	Clear	1 hr	None	24 hr

inhibiting the conversion of glycogen and amino acids to glucose. The type and species of the insulin used, injection technique, site of injection, level of insulin antibodies, and individual client response all can affect the onset, peak, and duration of action of insulin. The normal secretory pattern of endogenous insulins follows a basal-level secretion, with increased production in response to an incoming carbohydrate load. In clients with type 1 diabetes mellitus, the goal is to mimic this increase with injections of exogenous insulin.

Rapid-Acting Insulin. The development of rapid-acting insulin analogs was approved in 1996 to minimize the absorption limitations of regular human insulin. The rapid-acting insulin analogs insulin lispro (Humalog) and insulin aspart (NovoLog) have become the foundation in the management of clients with type 1 and type 2 diabetes mellitus.

SAFETY ALERT
The action and potency of Humalog and NovoLog are similar to those in regular human insulin. However, the onset of action begins to work about 5 minutes after they are injected, peaking in 1 hour and with a duration of action lasting about 2 to 4 hours. Both insulin analogs are approved for subcutaneous injection or with the continuous insulin infusion pump and should be taken immediately before eating.

Both analogs provide many benefits in achieving glucose control and may ultimately prevent or delay diabetes-related complications.

SAFETY ALERT
Remind clients that because insulin analogs work so quickly, hypoglycemia can develop rapidly if they do not consume adequate calories immediately after injection.[31]

Humalog and NovoLog are available as premixed insulins containing both a rapid-acting and an intermediate-acting component. Humalog Mix 75/25 contains 75% insulin lispro in a crystalline protamine form (intermediate-acting) and 25% soluble (rapid-acting) insulin lispro. NovoLog Mix 70/30 contains a mixture of 70% insulin aspart as the crystalline protamine form (intermediate-acting) and 30% soluble (rapid-acting) insulin aspart.[31]

 Administration of a mixture of insulin produces a more normal glycemia in clients than use of a single insulin. When a rapid-acting insulin is mixed with an intermediate- or long-acting insulin, the insulin should be injected within 15 minutes before a meal.

Insulin Dosage. Insulin therapy should be individualized. For a client with newly diagnosed diabetes mellitus, a simple regimen with fixed doses may be used at first. The starting dose of insulin is 0.5 unit/kg/day. Two thirds of the dose is commonly given in the morning, and one third is given in the evening. The health care team works to adjust the numbers and timing of injections to smooth out normal patterns. Then the dose can be increased. Algorithms are detailed guidelines to help clients self-adjust the daily insulin dose, based on SMBG levels, food intake, exercise, and departures from normal routine (e.g., added stress or illness). These guidelines use a prospective (predictive) approach to blood glucose control.[2,38]

Insulin dosage varies greatly because of the effects of the various types of insulin. Figure 45-2 depicts examples of various insulin regimens. In determining the dosage, the health care team must consider both the client's requirements and the client's response to the insulin. After initial stabilization, the team helps the client learn how to make adjustments in insulin doses, timing, food intake, and exercise. Unexplained fluctuations in blood glucose level often occur. The team needs to help the client feel confident in his or her ability to control the diabetes mellitus.

Insulin Pump Therapy. Small portable pumps for the continuous administration of regular insulin are sometimes used (Figure 45-3). The small pump, worn externally, injects insulin subcutaneously into the abdomen through an indwelling needle site that is changed every 1 to 3 days. Insulin is normally infused at a low basal rate (a rate that matches the client's basal metabolic needs), with additional infusion of larger amounts (boluses) of insulin before meals.

Insulin pumps commonly improve blood glucose control by means of continuous subcutaneous insulin infusion. However, they do not have a built-in feedback mechanism for monitoring blood glucose levels. To benefit from use of an insulin pump, the client must

Rapid acting

Insulin effect

B L D HS

Meals

Regular

Insulin effect

B L D HS

Meals

NPH

Insulin effect

B L D HS

Meals

Regular NPH

Insulin effect

B L D HS

Meals

Regular NPH NPH

Insulin effect

B L D HS

Meals

Regular Regular Regular

Insulin effect

Ultralente

B L D HS

Meals

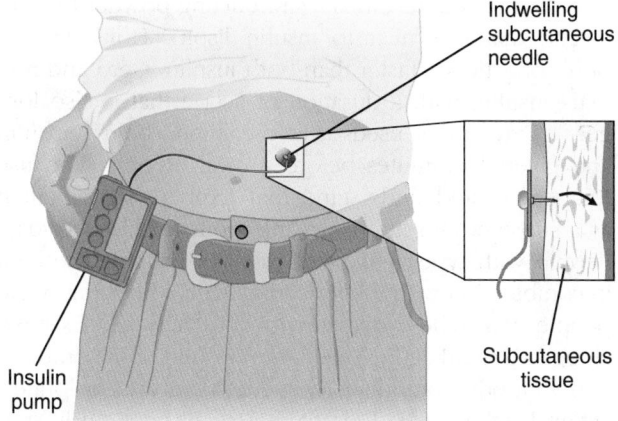

Indwelling subcutaneous needle

Insulin pump

Subcutaneous tissue

■ **FIGURE 45–3** Insulin pumps are worn externally and connected to an indwelling subcutaneous needle, usually inserted in the abdomen.

comply with dietary requirements and usually must deliver the correct premeal bolus of insulin. The client must also monitor blood glucose levels four times a day and make decisions about dosages by using problem-solving skills. Complications from use of insulin pumps include infection at the injection site, hypoglycemia from pump malfunction or mistakes in calculating the insulin dosage, and diabetic ketoacidosis from injecting too little insulin to meet regular or increased metabolic needs.

At the start of insulin pump therapy, the client must be supervised carefully in either an inpatient or an outpatient setting. During this time, the clinician adjusts the pump for basal and bolus doses before meals, according to the client's usual diet and exercise regimen and previous insulin requirements. Researchers are trying to produce an implantable pump that not only administers insulin but also monitors blood glucose levels, much as a normal pancreas does.

Inhaled Insulin. Inhaled insulin, an alternative to insulin injections, has been tested for safety and efficacy and approved by the FDA in January 2006 for use with people who have type 1 or type 2 diabetes mellitus over the age of 18. Exubera is the first inhaled insulin product to be approved for use in the United States.

Recent technological advances have made it possible to deliver insulin to the alveolar space through use of an inhaler-type device. Insulin is then rapidly absorbed into the alveolar capillaries and dispersed throughout the systemic circulation. The Exubera inhaler is about the size of an eyeglass case, weighing about 4 ounces.

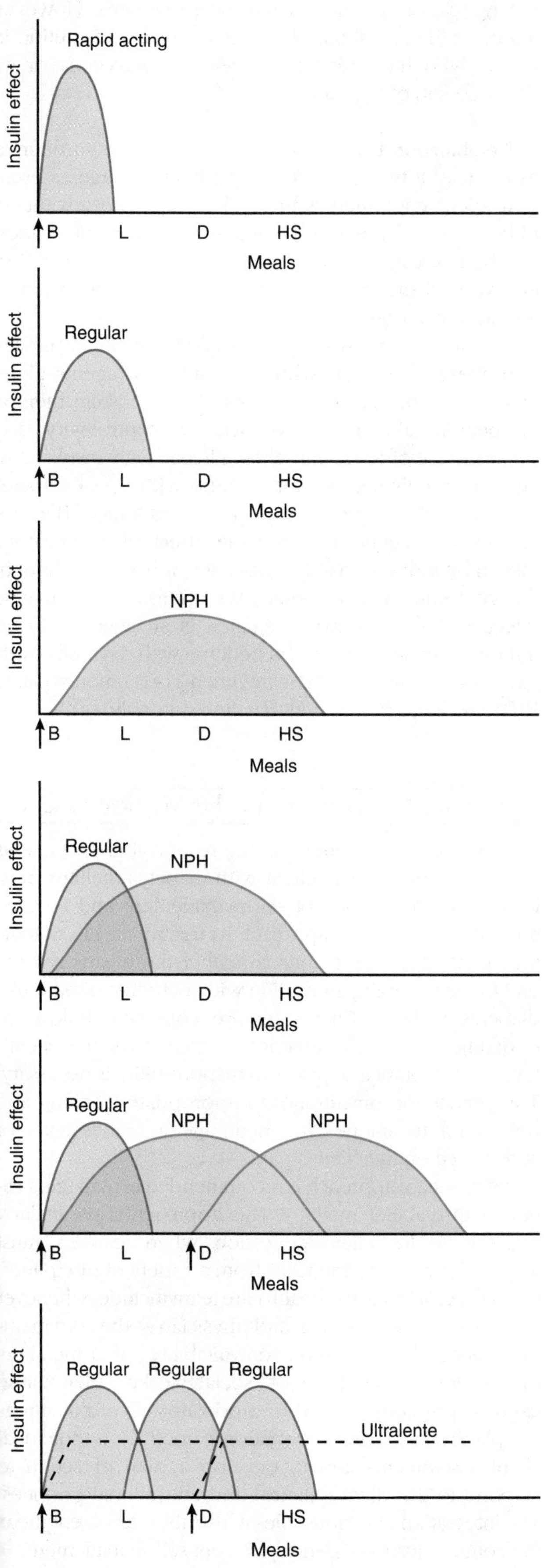

■ **FIGURE 45–2** Insulin regimens. Only a few of a variety of possible regimens are shown here. Some clients require only one injection per day, whereas others may require split mixed doses (such as mixtures of NPH or Ultralente and regular or rapid-acting insulin) or several doses of the same type of insulin (such as NPH insulin). Insulin regimens must be individualized for each client. *B,* Breakfast; *D,* dinner; *HS,* bedtime; *L,* lunch.

Inhaled insulin is a short-acting powder form of insulin that is similar to insulin lispro. However, the onset of action is faster than both insulin lispro and regular insulin, with a duration of action that is also longer.[30] Exubera is used as a mealtime (bolus) insulin and given 10 minutes before a meal. People who use Exubera should understand that Exubera is not taken as a substitute for all insulin injections taken every day. People with type 1 diabetes mellitus will use Exubera in combination with longer-acting injected insulin, while people with type 2 diabetes mellitus may use Exubera alone as a rapid-acting (mealtime) insulin or in combination with other oral diabetes medications and/or longer-acting insulins. Data from a small pilot study suggested that when oral diabetes medications failed in people with type 2 diabetes mellitus, adding premeal inhaled insulin improved glycemic control.[37]

As with all forms of insulin, a possible side effect of Exubera is hypoglycemia. Use of Exubera may likewise cause a cough, dry mouth, sore throat, chest discomfort, or shortness of breath.

SAFETY
⚠
ALERT

Exubera is not recommended in people who smoke or have stopped smoking in the past 6 months; have unstable or uncontrolled lung disease; or are allergic to insulin.

Intensive Diabetes Mellitus Therapy. In 1983 the NIDDK launched a 10-year, randomized clinical trial to assess the safety and determine the benefits of intensive diabetes mellitus therapy. The most comprehensive diabetes mellitus study ever conducted, it compared the effects of two different treatment methods on the long-term development of diabetes-related complications.[17] Clients were randomly assigned to either an intensive treatment group or a conventional treatment group.

Clients in the intensive treatment group learned to adjust their insulin doses to keep their blood glucose levels as close to normal as possible. Treatment included three or more insulin injections a day or the use of an insulin pump; SMBG levels four or more times a day; a special meal plan; an initial hospital stay; and weekly to monthly clinic visits. Clients in the conventional treatment group followed a regimen that included insulin injections once or twice a day; daily SMBG; and clinic visits every 3 months. Researchers monitored clients in both groups for manifestations of diabetic eye disease (retinopathy) as well as kidney (nephropathy) and nerve (neuropathy) disease. Results of the trial indicated that intensive therapy delayed the onset or slowed the progression of chronic complications of diabetes mellitus by 35% to more than 70%. The risk of hypoglycemia was three times higher in the intensive treatment group than in the conventional treatment group. However, the risk of hypoglycemia was believed to be greatly outweighed by the reduction in microvascular and neurologic complications. Based on these results, it is recommended that clients with type 1 diabetes mellitus

receive closely monitored intensive regimens. However, intensive therapy should be implemented with caution in clients who have repeated severe hypoglycemia or an unawareness of hypoglycemia.[17]

Combination Therapy. Combination therapy is defined as the use of two or more oral antidiabetes agents or an oral agent combined with insulin. The advantage of combination therapy is that in some instances an additive benefit can be demonstrated from taking two different types of medications that can complement and even augment each other.

In some clients with type 2 diabetes mellitus (mostly non-obese clients) in whom sulfonylurea agents alone failed to normalize blood glucose levels, insulin therapy has been required to achieve metabolic control very early in the course of disease. In these clients, daily insulin dosage is markedly higher than in clients with type 1 diabetes mellitus. This is attributed to insulin resistance. Because sulfonylurea agents enhance the effect of endogenous insulin by reducing insulin resistance, it has been thought that combining insulin therapy with sulfonylureas may be effective. One prescribed regimen is an injection of an intermediate-acting insulin at bedtime with daytime coverage by a sulfonylurea. This regimen is commonly called BIDS (*b*edtime *i*nsulin with *d*aytime *s*ulfonylurea).[33]

Nursing Management of the Medical Client

Diabetes self-management is the responsibility of clients and their families. The client with diabetes mellitus must be empowered to accept self-management and become the focus of the team approach to treatment. Physiologic treatment of manifestations is neither the means nor the end of responsibility in dealing with a chronic disease like diabetes mellitus. Clients require consistent follow-up, updating, and reinforcement. Assessment of the client's level of acceptance of personal responsibility is necessary. This guides the practitioner to appropriate teaching and behavioral techniques to encourage a higher level of acceptance on the client's part.

A team approach is recommended in managing clients with diabetes mellitus. This approach is particularly appropriate for client education when learners must acquire knowledge and skills from a variety of disciplines. Crucial members of the health care team include, whenever possible, a nurse, dietitian, and physician as the core members. Depending on need and availability, other members may include a psychologist, social worker, pharmacist, exercise physiologist, and/or a podiatrist. Team meetings are planned to share information gained from individual client assessments and to develop a plan of action to respond to the client's clinical and educational priorities. The integration of various roles within the team strengthens the communication essential to client self-management.

There are two approaches to diabetes mellitus education:[9-11,21]

- The *compliance-based approach* is intended to improve client adherence to the treatment recommendations of health care professionals. It is based on the assumption that health care professionals are diabetes mellitus care experts and that, in general, clients should comply with their recommendations regarding diabetes mellitus self-management.
- In the *empowerment-based approach,* the primary purpose of diabetes mellitus education is to prepare clients to make informed decisions about their own diabetes care. This approach assumes that most clients with diabetes mellitus are responsible for making important and complex decisions.[9-11,21]

Health care professionals use some combination of the two approaches based on their own values and understanding of the purposes of education. For example, clients with newly diagnosed diabetes mellitus may wish to have the health care team make most of the decisions until they become familiar with the costs and benefits of various options in diabetes self-management.

Survival education includes the crucial information necessary to meet the client's immediate survival needs. These vary widely from client to client. For example, insulin injection is a survival skill for a client with newly diagnosed type 1 diabetes mellitus but is unlikely to be a necessary skill in a client with newly diagnosed type 2 diabetes mellitus. Survival information varies in content, depending on the type of diabetes mellitus and age of the client, but tends to focus on skills such as insulin injection, treatment of hypoglycemia, glucose self-monitoring, sick day management, diabetic ketoacidosis, and basic dietary information. When clients are comfortable with survival skills, they can progress to more in-depth information.[13,15] Box 45-3 presents essential diabetes mellitus education content.

Assessment. Clients with diabetes mellitus must be closely assessed for level of knowledge and ability to perform self-care. The type of diabetes mellitus, clinical status of the client, and plans for treatment are also important assessments. Ask clients whether they take any vitamin, mineral, or herbal supplements to decrease blood glucose levels or for other purposes. The Complementary and Alternative Therapy features at right and on p. 1078 provide additional information on the relationship of these substances to diabetes mellitus. Chromium and garlic may lower blood glucose and cholesterol levels and magnesium may increase insulin sensitivity. Blueberries, especially European bilberries, may also decrease blood glucose levels. Niacin may impair glucose tolerance.

BOX 45-3 Education Content for Clients with Diabetes Mellitus

A. Function and structure (anatomy and physiology) of the pancreas
B. Definition of diabetes mellitus and relationship to abnormal function of pancreas
C. Manifestations of hyperglycemia
D. Methods to control hyperglycemia
   1. Diet
   2. Exercise
   3. Oral antidiabetic agents
   4. Insulin
      a. How/when/where/why to give insulin
      b. Storage/disposal of insulin and needles
E. Daily self-monitoring of blood glucose levels
F. Sick day rules
   1. Testing for ketones in urine
G. Complications of diabetes mellitus (definition, cause, manifestations, treatment)
   1. Acute: hypoglycemia, diabetic ketoacidosis, HHNS
   2. Chronic: microvascular and macrovascular

COMPLEMENTARY AND ALTERNATIVE THERAPY

Multivitamin and Mineral Supplement and the Risk of Infection in Clients with Type 2 Diabetes Mellitus

A randomized, double-blind, placebo-controlled trial was conducted in which 130 community-dwelling adults were allocated to a multivitamin and mineral supplement or placebo daily for 1 year. More individuals taking placebo than those taking the multivitamin supplement reported an infectious illness over the year of study (73% versus 43%; $p < .001$). Infection-related absenteeism (e.g., missing work) was also higher in the placebo group (57% versus 21%; $p < .001$). The individuals with type 2 diabetes mellitus ($n = 51$) were responsible for this finding. Among diabetes mellitus clients receiving placebo, 93% reported an infection, whereas 17% of those receiving supplements ($p < .001$) reported an infection. A larger clinical trial is needed, but this study does initially support the use of a daily inexpensive multivitamin for clients with type 2 diabetes mellitus to reduce the risk of infections (upper respiratory tract infection, lower respiratory tract infection, influenza-like syndrome, gastrointestinal infection, and urinary tract infection). Participants without diabetes mellitus ($n = 79$) did not experience any change in reported infections compared to those taking placebo in this study.

From Barringer, T., et al. (2003). Effect of a multivitamin and mineral supplement on infection and quality of life: A randomized, double-blind, placebo-controlled trial. *Annals of Internal Medicine, 138,* 365-371.

Diagnosis, Outcomes, Interventions
Diagnosis: Readiness for Enhanced Self-Care. The client with diabetes mellitus must be able to perform self-care to keep the condition well controlled, leading to the nursing

COMPLEMENTARY AND ALTERNATIVE THERAPY

Cinnamon and Blood Glucose Levels

Research related to cinnamon consumption and weight loss, cholesterol level reduction, and serum glucose level reduction is mixed. A 2003 study[1] in Pakistan consisted of 60 type 2 diabetic clients (30 men and 30 women) with an average age of 52 years who were randomized into 1 of 6 groups. Groups 1 through 3 respectively consumed 1, 3, and 6 g of cinnamon daily for 40 days and groups 4 to 6 were given placebos for 40 days. After 40 days, all levels of cinnamon consumption decreased fasting blood glucose levels by 18% to 29%, total cholesterol by 12% to 26%, LDL (bad cholesterol) levels by 7% to 17%, and triglycerides by 23% to 30%; however, there was no change in HDL (good cholesterol) levels. No significant changes were found in the placebo group for any of the values.

However, two other studies in 2006 had somewhat opposing results. A study in Germany[2] looked at 79 clients with type 2 diabetes mellitus taking prescription oral antidiabetic medications but no insulin. They were randomly assigned to take a placebo or a 3-g cinnamon capsule 3 times per day for 120 days. There was a significantly greater reduction in blood glucose levels in the cinnamon group compared to the placebo group (−3.4%). Clients with higher blood glucose levels had greater responses than clients with lower levels. However, there were no significant differences in HbA$_{1C}$ or cholesterol levels between the cinnamon and placebo groups.

In the third study from The Netherlands,[3] a total of 25 type 2 diabetic, postmenopausal women with an average age of 63 years and a BMI of 30 were given either 1.5 g of real cinnamon or a placebo for 6 weeks. Insulin sensitivity, glucose levels, and cholesterol levels did not change in either group.

All three studies have small sample sizes and limited timeframes for cinnamon consumption. Hence additional randomized, controlled trials with larger sample sizes are needed before conclusions related to cinnamon consumption via capsule or powder can be determined.

REFERENCES

1. Khan, A., et al. (2003). Cinnamon improves glucose and lipids of people with type 2 diabetes. *Diabetes Care, 26*(12), 3215-3218.
2. Mang, B., et al. (2006). Effects of cinnamon extract on plasma glucose, HbA, and serum lipids in diabetes mellitus type 2. *European Journal of Clinical Investigations, 36*(5), 340-344.
3. Vanschoonbeck, K., et al. (2006). Cinnamon supplementation does not improve glycemic control in postmenopausal type 2 diabetes patients. *The Journal of Nutrition, 135*(4), 977-980.

COMPLEMENTARY AND ALTERNATIVE THERAPY

Coffee Consumption and Risk of Type 2 Diabetes Mellitus

Emerging epidemiologic evidence suggests that higher coffee consumption may reduce the risk of type 2 diabetes mellitus. A MEDLINE review examined 9 cohort studies of coffee consumption and risk of type 2 diabetes mellitus including 193,473 participants and 8394 incident cases of type 2 diabetes mellitus.[1] The relative risk (RR) of type 2 diabetes mellitus was 0.65 (95% confidence interval [CI], 0.54–0.78) for the highest coffee consumers (≥6 or 7 cups per day) and 0.72 (95% CI, 0.62–0.83) for the second highest (4 to 6 cups per day) coffee consumers compared with the lowest consumption category (0 or ≤2 cups per day). The associations did not differ substantially by sex, obesity, or region (United States and Europe). In the cross-sectional studies conducted in northern Europe, southern Europe, and Japan, higher coffee consumption was consistently associated with a lower prevalence of newly detected hyperglycemia, particularly postprandial hyperglycemia.

REFERENCE

van Dam, R.M., & Hu, F. (2005) Coffee consumption and risk of type 2 diabetes: A systematic review. *Journal of the American Medical Association, 294* (1), 97-104

diagnosis *Readiness for Enhanced Self-Care related to desire to learn about diabetes mellitus and management options, physical activity for diabetes mellitus management, and dietary management of diabetes mellitus.*

Outcomes. The client will relate the basic pathophysiologic mechanism of diabetes mellitus, explain the need for physical activity and meal planning in the treatment, and list the clinical manifestations of acute and chronic complications. The client will plan a physical activity program to maintain blood glucose levels at preset levels and will identify strategies to monitor for and prevent complications associated with exercise.

The client will state the relationship of dietary management to blood glucose control, and will choose foods that meet caloric needs and offer a well-balanced diet. The client will recognize the times at which it is necessary to substitute a food or reduce portion size to maintain blood glucose control. The client will discuss with the health care team difficulties seen in compliance with plans for diet, maintain blood glucose levels within preset parameters, and maintain weight within preset parameters.

Interventions

Explain the Pathophysiology of Diabetes Mellitus. You or a diabetes educator should explain to the client and family the basic pathophysiologic mechanism of diabetes mellitus and how the disorder is managed. Sometimes the information is given through classes or by videotape. The client should also receive some form of written information to reinforce the material. Also, the client should be monitored for denial or anger about the diagnosis as part of a coping response.

Plan a Physical Activity Program. Clients with diabetes mellitus must consult the clinician before starting an exercise program. Pre–physical activity screening may include a history, physical examination, A1C, exercise stress test, foot evaluation, and laboratory determination of blood glucose level. The client with diabetes mellitus may not be able to exercise intensely to achieve a calculated heart rate because of a pre-existing cardiac condition, advanced age, or joint problems. The client should be helped to choose an exercise regimen and to set reasonable goals, because any increase in activity level is beneficial. Walking is usually well tolerated. Using a stationary bicycle or swimming is possible for clients with foot problems.

Clients with diabetes mellitus must start any new activity at a well-tolerated intensity level and duration, with gradual (over a period of weeks or months) increases in intensity and duration until preset exercise goals are reached. Exercise should include warm-up and cool-down periods before and after the activity. It is best to exercise at the same time of day, if possible. Because regular exercise is very important, have the client plan an alternative activity in case environmental or other factors make the usual exercise difficult. Unplanned exercise can be dangerous for clients taking insulin or oral hypoglycemic agents. During periods of exercise, the muscles are stimulated to use glucose. Therefore blood glucose levels can fall abruptly.[4]

Prevent Complications from Physical Activity. Clients should make sure they are adequately hydrated before starting exercise. They should eat 15 to 30 g of carbohydrate before exercise if the blood glucose level is less than 100 mg/dl and should carry a carbohydrate snack as well as their diabetes mellitus identification. If the blood glucose level is 100 to 150 mg/dl, the client may exercise and have a snack later. If the blood glucose level is greater than 250 mg/dl and the client has not just eaten, ketone levels should be checked. Clients with this glucose level should wait to exercise, because vigorous activity can raise blood glucose levels by releasing stored glycogen. Alcohol and beta-blockers should be avoided because they may increase the risk of hypoglycemia or hyperglycemia.[4]

Plan Nutrition Therapy to Achieve Target Blood Glucose Level. A balanced nutritional plan is important for all clients, whether or not they have diabetes mellitus. Emphasize to the client and family members that they are not eating a "diabetic diet" but, rather, are following a balanced meal plan. Adherence to nutrition principles is one of the most challenging aspects of diabetes mellitus management. It requires a team effort. For an effective plan, assessment of the person's present eating patterns, knowledge of a healthy eating plan, and willingness and ability to modify patterns and nutritional needs is vital. Specific nutritional information should include the following:[1,4]

- Appetite
- Alcohol use
- Use of artificial sweeteners
- Food allergies
- Ethnic and cultural influence on food habits

- Ability to obtain and prepare food (including financial ability)
- Community resources currently used
- Amount and type of physical activity
- Chronic disease requiring dietary modification
- Gastrointestinal disease
- Vitamin, mineral, or food supplements used
- Weight patterns
- Current eating patterns
- Dietary concerns of client
- Dental and oral health
- Medications with nutritional implications

The results of this assessment form a personal profile used to arrive at individualized goals. As a member of the health care team, you must have a knowledge base of both nutritional assessment and appropriate interventions. Basic nutritional assessment includes anthropometric measures, biochemical tests, physical assessment, and dietary evaluation. No single parameter can measure the client's nutritional status or determine problems or needs. Figure 45-4 shows how assessment fits into the total nutritional plan for the collaborative management of diabetes mellitus. After the assessment, individualized goals are determined. Nutritional assessment and the client's understanding that optimal nutrition can lead to reduction of risk factors for chronic health problems and improve overall health constitute the starting point for goal selection.

For example, if the client has type 2 diabetes mellitus and is obese, emphasize that nutritional changes can help to lower blood glucose levels, decrease lipid levels, and lower blood pressure as well as help in losing weight. Weight loss also appears to increase insulin sensitivity and to normalize liver glucose production. The client should understand that dietary treatment is the best and initial treatment. If nutritional status does not improve, glucose-lowering medications, insulin, lipid-lowering agents, or antihypertensives may be required.

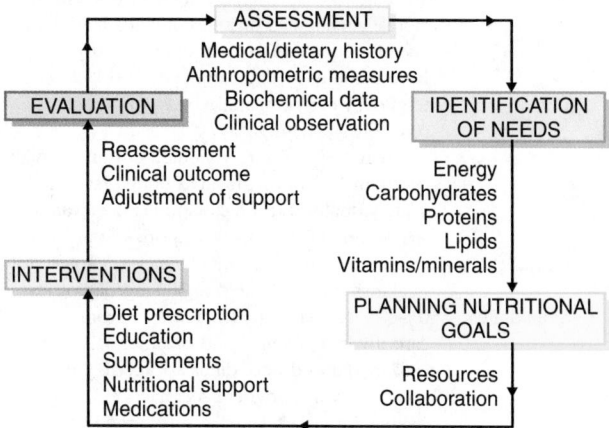

FIGURE 45-4 Assessment as part of the total nutritional plan for the collaborative management of diabetes. *(Data from Copstead, L.C., & Banasik, J.L. [2000]. Pathophysiology: Biological and behavioral perspectives [2nd ed.]. Philadelphia: Saunders.)*

A standard "diabetic diet" is no longer prescribed for all clients with diabetes mellitus; instead, many dietary options exist (Table 45-4). Basically, the client with diabetes mellitus should strive to follow the Dietary Guidelines for Americans ("MyPyramid") issued by the U.S. Department of Agriculture (USDA) and U.S. Department of Health and Human Services (USDHS) in 2005 for current recommended nutritional guidelines.[36]

Calories. Caloric restrictions, especially for people with lifelong obesity, may be perceived negatively. Obesity is a complex interaction between genetic and environmental factors. The most successful approach to weight reduction is unclear, but the client should understand caloric restriction, regular exercise, behavior modification; and accept peer and professional support. Moderate caloric reduction is described as a reduction of 250 to 500 calories per day less than usual. Reduction of fat calories may be a good initial modification. Regular exercise (three to five times weekly) enhances weight loss and is a predictor of successful weight maintenance.[1,4]

Protein. In general, Americans with and without diabetes mellitus consume more protein than needed to meet nutritional needs. Protein should be incorporated into the diet through a variety of foods. Very-low-calorie diets are often deficient in protein and may result in accelerated protein breakdown. High protein intake increases renal workload and glomerular filtration rate. Some studies in people with diabetes mellitus indicate that reducing protein intake may delay progression of nephropathy. At present, the lower end of the recommended scale for protein intake (about 10% of daily calories) is sufficiently restricted and is recommended for clients with nephropathy. In certain cases, protein requirements vary from the adult recommended daily allowance; this is true for infants, children, adolescents, and pregnant women.[1]

Fat. The USDA national food consumption surveys reveal that most Americans eat too much fat. About 36% of calories in the average adult diet comes from fat, with about 13% being from saturated fat. The general recommendation for Americans is to decrease total dietary fat to 30% or less of total calories, with saturated fat being decreased to less than 10%. This reduction is consistent with a diet to reduce cardiovascular disease.

Carbohydrates. For most of the 20th century, the most widely held belief about dietary treatment of diabetes mellitus was that sugar was to be avoided. Little or no scientific evidence supports this assumption. When fed as a single nutrient, sucrose produces a glycemic response similar to that for bread or pasta. In the United States, the average diet obtains almost half of total carbohydrate intake in the form of simple sugars. Clinical guidelines suggest that 50% to 60% of the diet should consist of carbohydrates, in either simple or complex form. An occasional high-sucrose dessert poses no problem for the client with diabetes mellitus when it is accounted for in the day's total caloric and carbohydrate plan. Because some desserts are also high in fat, however, they should be limited.[1]

Diet Management for Clients with Type 1 Diabetes Mellitus. Meals should be adjusted to match insulin action. Breakfast should be eaten within 1 hour after the morning insulin dose (immediately after injection when rapid-acting insulin is used) and a carbohydrate should be eaten about 3 hours later; lunch should be eaten about 4 to 5 hours after the morning insulin dose. When multiple insulin injections are used, greater flexibility with meal timing is possible.

Examples of dietary approaches when working with type 1 diabetes mellitus are the following:

- Handouts available from government sources, such as the USDA's "MyPyramid"[36] and the USDHS publication, which uses the four-basic-food-groups approach[35]
- Individualized menus developed by collaboration between the client and dietitian
- The exchange system, last revised in 1986, that helps with uniform meal planning; available from the ADA in a simple pamphlet called *Healthy Food Choices* or in an expanded version called *Exchange Lists for Meal Planning*
- Counting components of the diet, such as counting calories and grams of fat
- A point system that uses lists of foods with point values and a prescribed number of total points
- The total available glucose system, which looks at foods in terms of their metabolic effects (highly motivated clients who desire flexibility may like this system)

TABLE 45–4 Recommended Nutritional Guidelines for Clients with Diabetes Mellitus	
Calories	Sufficient to achieve and maintain reasonable weight
Protein	Adequate to ensure maintenance of body protein stores; clients with diabetes mellitus have same protein requirements as people who do not have diabetes mellitus; in general, 10%-20% of total daily calories should be from protein (equal to ~0.8 g/kg/day)
Fats	Less than 30% of calories should be from fat, with less than 10% of that from saturated fat sources; if individualized risk factors indicate elevated VLDL and LDL levels, total calories from saturated fat may be reduced to 7%; cholesterol intake should be limited to 300 mg/day or less
Carbohydrates	50%-60% of total calories should be from carbohydrates; simple and complex carbohydrates do not differ appreciably in their ability to worsen hyperglycemia
Fiber	Clients with diabetes mellitus are urged to consume 20-35 g of fiber per day, same as recommendation for all Americans

LDL, Low-density lipoprotein; *VLDL,* Very-low-density lipoprotein.

Diagnosis: Risk for Unstable Blood Glucose. A client with diabetes mellitus must understand and be able to self-monitor glucose levels and learn self-injection of insulin, leading to the nursing diagnosis of *Risk for Unstable Blood Glucose related to lack of knowledge and lack of previous experience with testing blood and urine and lack of knowledge and lack of experience with self-injection of insulin.*

Outcomes. The client will state personal goals for urine ketone and blood glucose testing parameters, demonstrate correct techniques for blood glucose testing (including timing), and demonstrate correct technique for urine ketone testing (including timing). The client will test blood glucose levels at regular times (including during illnesses and when traveling), and will prick the side of the finger, where nerve endings are fewer and more blood is available. The client will test urine for ketones when the glucose level is high (>240 mg/dl) or during illnesses; keep a record of all tests performed and bring this record to regular, scheduled follow-up visits; and store testing materials away from heat, light, and moisture.

The client will state that insulin lowers blood glucose level, and will name the type or types of insulin prescribed and the onset, peak, and duration of each. The client will administer injections at regular times, 10 to 60 minutes before meals, every day, even when ill. The client will wash hands before preparing insulin injections, demonstrate proper mixing of insulin, and withdraw prescribed dosage using sterile technique.

When taking two types of insulin, the client will withdraw the prescribed dosage of each insulin into one syringe without contaminating either bottle (regular insulin is drawn up first). A client who uses insulin glargine (Lantus) must draw up the insulin glargine in a separate syringe and not mix it with any other insulin. The client will demonstrate the correct technique of insulin injection. The client will store at least one extra bottle of insulin in the refrigerator, not use insulin past the expiration date, and will purchase insulin syringes before all of the current supply has been used.

The client will wear medical identification (Medic-Alert) bracelet or necklace, or carry a diabetic identification card. The client will state manifestations and describe treatment of hypoglycemia, and will always carry something to treat hypoglycemia.

Interventions

Provide Instruction on Blood Glucose Monitoring. All clients with newly diagnosed diabetes mellitus require teaching about urine and blood glucose monitoring. All clients with diabetes mellitus may require review or update of information for self-care. Newer, more accurate blood glucose meters that are easier to use are constantly being made available. Only the basics are covered in this discussion; you must keep up-to-date on each meter's advantages and disadvantages.

Many kinds of meters are available. Each client needs to be evaluated so that the proper meter is obtained. The client's ability to calibrate the meter and to visually interpret the digital reading must be considered. Some meters can be connected to a computer, which can convert blood glucose results into bar graphs or other printouts. Glucose meters are available for the visually impaired that give audio commands for use of the device and announce the blood glucose reading.

In addition to demonstrating the techniques of blood glucose self-monitoring, discuss the normal blood glucose range, goals for good control (individualized for each client), when to test, how to record test results, and what to do when abnormal results are obtained. Consult a diabetes educator for assistance in helping the client choose an optimal meter.

Clients can use blood glucose strips if they are unable or unwilling to purchase a meter. Make sure the client is not color blind and can read the results accurately. Compare the client's results with blood glucose meter readings to check for accuracy. With some meters and strips, a 15% difference is seen between capillary blood and venous blood glucose levels. The capillary blood reading is lower. When insulin is being adjusted, make sure to account for this difference. As long as the source of blood is consistent, no adjustment is required.

> **Both health care agencies and clients need to verify the accuracy of their blood glucose determinations. The Joint Commission (TJC) and other regulating bodies dictate the procedure and frequency for quality control of meters used in health care agencies.**
>
> SAFETY
> ALERT

The usefulness of many glucose meters is technique-dependent. Because treatment is based on results, correct methods of use must be ensured. Clients can perform a self-test and simultaneously send a blood specimen to the laboratory to compare results. Manufacturers of meters also provide quality-control testing solutions, which clients should be instructed to use routinely (weekly, for example).

> **Quality control of glucose monitors is a constantly changing area; nurses and clients must keep up-to-date (see the Management and Delegation feature on Measuring and Recording Blood Glucose Levels on p. 1082).**
>
> SAFETY
> ALERT

Provide Instruction on Urine Testing. Urine testing for glucose is rarely done; however, urine can be tested for ketones (beta-hydroxybutyric acid, acetoacetic acid, and acetone). These substances appear in the urine of clients who are fasting, clients with poorly controlled type 1 diabetes mellitus, and clients with type 1 or type 2 diabetes mellitus who have a secondary illness. Ketones result from fat metabolism and are therefore present during fasting.[13,34] In a client with diabetes

MANAGEMENT AND DELEGATION

Measuring and Recording Blood Glucose Levels

The measurement and recording of blood glucose levels may be delegated to unlicensed assistive personnel. Delegate the data collection only to those who have demonstrated competency in performing this task. Consider the following issues:

- Initial orientation and demonstration of competence in the performance of blood glucose monitoring, including quality control and equipment management requirements
- Instruction on the time schedule and frequency to obtain blood glucose levels
- Proper method of recording and reporting of the blood glucose level
- Rotation of sites from which to obtain samples in order to minimize client discomfort

You are responsible for defining those blood glucose levels that are immediately reportable to you (e.g., levels outside the range of 70 to 180 mg/dl). Instruct assistive personnel to report any difficulty in obtaining the sample or concerns the client may raise during the process of obtaining a sample.

Verify the competency of assistive personnel in performing blood glucose level testing during orientation and annually thereafter.

mellitus, however, the presence of ketones may indicate the serious complication of diabetic ketoacidosis (see later discussion).

Provide Instruction on Insulin Administration. When administered correctly, insulin acts as a life-saving medication for the insulin-dependent client. When administered incorrectly, it may cause complications ranging from tissue damage to lethal hypoglycemia (*insulin shock*). To administer insulin properly, the client must be familiar with insulin concentrations, syringes, storage, preparation for injection, and techniques for self-injection. The Client Education Guide feature below lists guidelines for self-injection of insulin.[2]

Insulin Concentrations. Insulin is prescribed in units.

Only administer insulin with an insulin syringe, pen, jet, or inhaler.

The most commonly prescribed strength in the United States is U-100. U-100 insulin contains 100 units of insulin per milliliter. It is the insulin of choice for nearly all clients. Those who require large amounts of insulin may benefit from using U-500 insulin, which contains 500 units of insulin per milliliter.[4,38]

Insulin Syringes. The most commonly used syringe can deliver a maximum of 100 units of insulin in 1 ml. However, insulin syringes are manufactured with capacities

CLIENT EDUCATION GUIDE

Self-Injection of Insulin

PROCEDURE

1. Wash hands.
2. Clean site with soap and water or 70% isopropyl alcohol (optional).
3. Store insulin vial in original carton to keep clean (or wipe top of insulin vial with 70% isopropyl alcohol).
4. Check insulin for any residue. Mix insulin by rolling the vial between your palms or by shaking the vial to resuspend all but short-acting insulins.
5. Pull air into syringe to the number of units needed.
6. Inject air into the insulin vial.
7. Invert insulin vial and draw insulin into syringe.
8. Aspirate prescribed amount of short-acting insulin into syringe first, intermediate- or long-acting insulin second.
9. Inspect syringe for air bubbles.
10. Never mix insulin glargine (Lantus) with another insulin because it has a pH of 4 and will cause precipitation when mixed with other insulins.
11. Pinch up and hold skinfold and inject at 90-degree angle.
12. If you are thin or have loose skin, inject insulin at 45-degree angle to avoid an intramuscular injection, which is absorbed faster.
13. Routine aspiration is not necessary.
14. Inject insulin.

DISPOSAL

State laws require that needles and syringes be disposed of as a single unit in a puncture-resistant container. It is unsafe to recap, bend, or break the needle.

SYRINGE REUSE

The manufacturer intends that the insulin syringe and needle be disposed after one use. Research demonstrates that most people with diabetes mellitus reuse the needle and syringe until the needle becomes dull or bent or comes in contact with any surface other than skin. Most insulins have a bacteriostatic agent in them. If you reuse syringes and needles, recap the needle after each use; reusing may carry increased risk for infection, especially if you have poor personal hygiene, acute concurrent illness, or open wounds on hands. Discuss the practice of reuse with your practitioner before initiating:

- Can you safely recap the needle?
- Can you see clearly enough?
- How is your manual dexterity?
- Do you have a visible tremor?

Store syringes at room temperature. The potential benefit of using alcohol on the needle is unknown. It may remove the silicone coat on the needle and contribute to pain at the puncture site.

of 0.25, 0.30, 0.50, and 1 ml. For smaller prescriptions (50 units, 30 units, or less), smaller syringes are used.[3] A smaller syringe enables a more precise insulin dosage. Two lengths of needles are available: short (8 mm) and long (12.7 mm). Short needles are not recommended for obese clients because of variability of insulin absorption when injected into adipose tissue. See the figure on the website for examples of sizes of insulin syringes such as a 50-unit syringe, 100-unit syringe, and a syringe that has ½-unit markings.

Insulin Pens. Insulin pens for multiple injections are another insulin delivery method. The pen-like holders are loaded with prefilled cartridges holding 150 to 300 units of insulin. A disposable needle is attached to the pen for each insulin injection, so clients must carry needles for each injection but they do not have to carry extra syringes or bottles of insulin. The insulin dose is dialed or entered into the pen. Each new needle may require priming before the desired insulin dose is dialed or entered into the pen for administration.

Needle-Free Technology. Jet injectors, which are pen-like devices, can be used in place of insulin syringes for delivery of insulin. The needle-less devices supply sufficient force to propel a fine liquid jet of insulin through the skin and to disperse the insulin into subcutaneous tissue. Devices introduced from the 1970s through the mid-1990s were large, heavy, and expensive. Newer devices as shown in Figure 45-5 are much lighter, cheaper, and easier to clean than earlier models. The problem of safe disposal of needles is avoided with needle-less injectors.

Insulin Storage. Although manufacturers recommend storing vials of insulin in the refrigerator, injecting cold insulin can sometimes make the injection more painful. When beginning use of a vial of insulin, remove it from the refrigerator.

> **Avoid temperature extremes of less than 36° F or greater than 86° F. Vials in use may be kept at room temperature for about 1 month. A slight loss of potency may occur after 30 days at room temperature. Humalog, regular insulin cartridges, or prefilled regular insulin pens may be kept unrefrigerated for 28 days. Because of potential variations in temperature, insulin should not be left in a car or checked in airline baggage. Mark the date on the vial when it was initially opened. Do not use any insulin beyond its expiration date. Inspect each vial of insulin before each use for changes (i.e., clumping, frosting, or change in clarity or color) that may affect its potency. Visual inspection should show rapid- and short-acting insulin as well as insulin glargine to be clear and all other insulin types to be uniformly cloudy.[2] The client should always have a spare vial on hand.[2,38]**

Insulin Preparation and Injection. Experts once thought that insulin vials should be rolled between the hands to resuspend the insulin without creating air bubbles. Now they believe that vials containing NPH

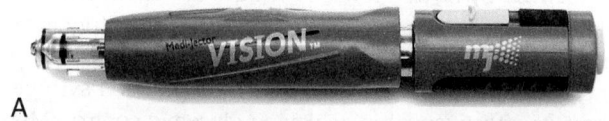

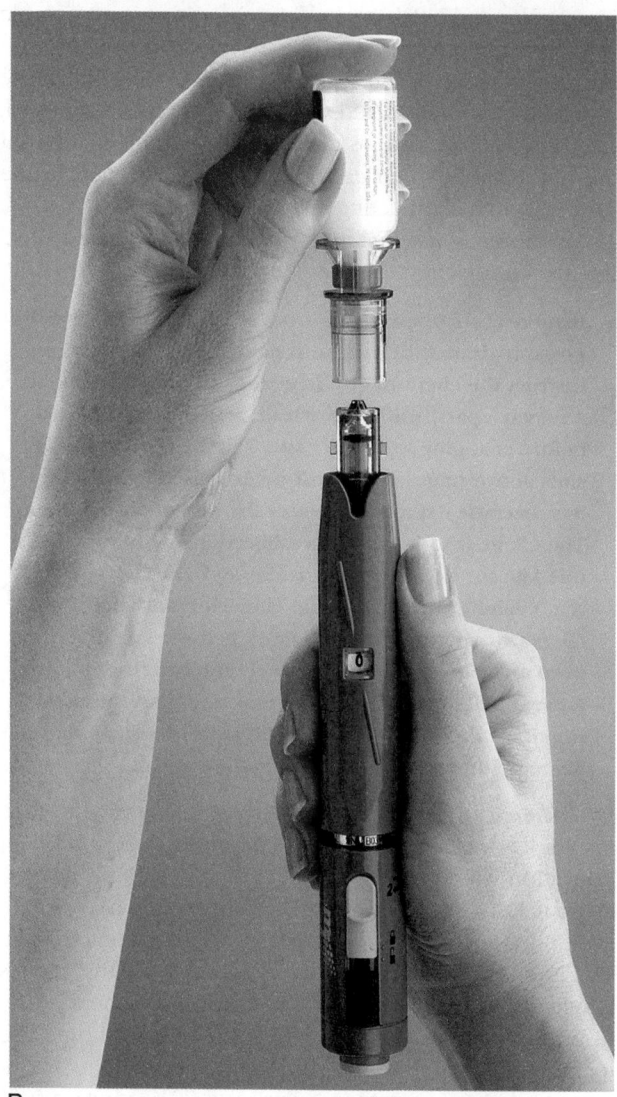

■ **FIGURE 45–5 A,** Medi-Jector VISION needle-less device for insulin injection. **B** shows how the jet apparatus is refilled with insulin. *(Courtesy Antares Pharma, Inc., Exton, Penn.)*

and Lente suspensions should be agitated vigorously to mix the insulin to deliver consistent insulin concentrations.

To minimize the discomfort of subcutaneous insulin injection, administer the insulin at room temperature. The number of bacteria carried through a small-gauge needle is insufficient for infection to occur, and alcohol preparation is no longer considered necessary. If alcohol is used to clean the site, wait until it has evaporated completely. Have the client try to relax. Penetrate the skin quickly. Do not change the direction of the needle once it has entered the subcutaneous tissue or while it is being withdrawn.[2]

Prefilled Syringes. Prefilled syringes are chemically stable for up to 3 weeks when stored in the refrigerator. SMBG may need to be performed more frequently to check whether storage of the insulin in prefilled syringes alters its effectiveness in achieving glycemic control. Mixing regular and NPH insulins in one syringe is acceptable and convenient (insulin glargine cannot be mixed with any other insulin because it has a pH of 4.0 and will cause precipitation when mixed with other insulins). Premixed, fixed-proportion insulins are available commercially, but are not suitable when daily variations are needed in the dose or when short-acting insulin is required.[38]

Site Selection and Rotation. Certain sites are best used for insulin injection (Figure 45-6).

SAFETY ⚠ **ALERT**

Insulin absorption varies from site to site. To avoid possibly dramatic changes in daily insulin absorption, instruct the client to give injections in one area, about an inch apart, until the whole area has been used, before changing to another site. Tell the client to avoid sites above muscles that will be exercised heavily that day, because exercise increases the rate of absorption. The client who is taking two injections daily may use one site for the morning insulin and another site for the evening insulin. Some clinicians instruct their clients to use only the abdomen because of its more even and rapid absorption rate. Emphasize the importance of adhering to a definite injection plan for avoiding tissue damage. Rotate injection sites in one area to decrease the variability of absorption.

Techniques for Self-Injection. Most clients who take insulin learn to give themselves injections (see the Client Education Guide on Self-Injection of Insulin). It is primarily your responsibility to instruct clients with diabetes mellitus in the techniques for preparing and injecting insulin. The amount of teaching needed depends on the client's familiarity with insulin and the injection equipment.

Equipment that the client will purchase for home use includes insulin of the type prescribed, absorbent cotton, approved syringes with needles, and 70% ethyl or 91% isopropyl alcohol (optional). As noted, alcohol preparation of the injection site is no longer considered necessary, and cleansing of the top of the insulin vial may increase the risk of infection by transferring resident bacteria from fingers to the vial unless gloves are worn. Storing insulin in its original carton or in a container that will keep it clean may be a more practical option.

Although the prospect of daily injections for life is far from pleasant, the client's attitude toward this intervention may be largely influenced by your own attitude. A matter-of-fact approach helps the client understand and accept responsibility for self-care. Schedule a teaching session for self-injection techniques. Some clients find it difficult to inject the needle into their own skin. For these clients, you might select the site and insert the needle. Then, as the first step in self-injection, have the client push in

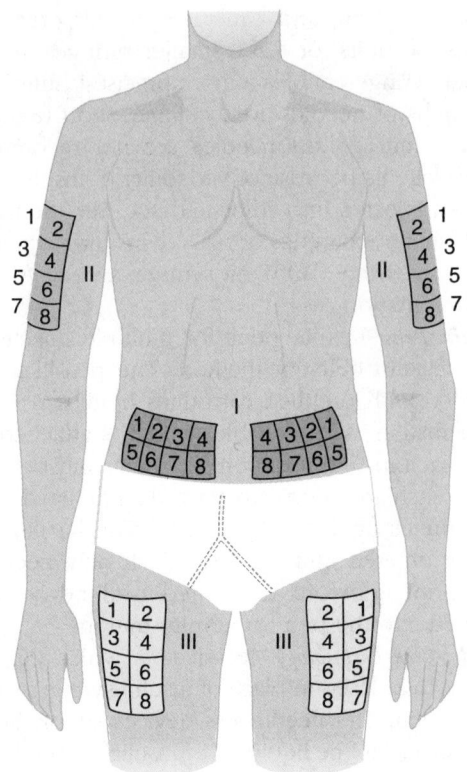

■ **FIGURE 45–6** Sites used for insulin injection. The injection site can affect the onset, peak, and duration of action of the insulin. Insulin injected into the abdomen (area I) is absorbed fastest, followed by insulin injected into the arm (area II) and the leg (area III).

the plunger and remove the needle. As the client gains confidence, self-injecting will be less traumatic.

See the Case Management feature on Diabetes Mellitus on the website.

Evaluation. It is expected that clients with type 1 or type 2 diabetes mellitus will learn about the disease process and methods of control. If management is successful, complications of diabetes mellitus will be avoided as much as possible. For a client with newly diagnosed type 1 diabetes mellitus, return demonstration should be expected for all activities with increasing proficiency over time. The client should not be expected to accomplish complete self-care after a single teaching session. The amount of time required varies from client to client. Follow-up visits must be initiated to make sure that the client is following recommendations and has not experienced problems with the therapeutic regimen. Over time, periodic follow-up visits will help you monitor the client's ability to perform self-care and anticipate any potential difficulties.

Self-Care

Before hospital discharge, the client and family must have a basic understanding of diabetes mellitus and its management with blood glucose monitoring, insulin injections, foot care, nutrition, and exercise. Because diabetes mellitus is a chronic disorder, the client needs time to adapt to as well as to learn about the many changes that are occurring. The client should be encouraged to anticipate a usual day at work, school, or home and should be taught how and when to give insulin, how to monitor blood glucose level, and what types of foods to eat.

Clients with diabetes mellitus need ongoing monitoring of their self-care ability. A1C levels are usually checked, as is the client's log of daily glucose levels and insulin. Chronic changes that result from diabetes mellitus should also be assessed on an ongoing basis by checking the client's vision, kidney function, degree of neuropathy, blood pressure, and skin condition. If the client is older or debilitated, home nurse visits may be an excellent asset. A referral to a visiting nurse organization or home health care agency should be initiated before discharge.

Modifications for Older Clients with Diabetes Mellitus

Diabetes mellitus is common among older adults and represents an important health problem for this population. Currently, 6.3 million (19%) of all people over the age of 65 years have diabetes mellitus. Many changes that occur with normal aging affect glucose levels. Blood glucose levels increase with age; fasting levels increase by about 1 mg/dl per decade and postprandial values by 6 to 13 mg/dl per decade. It is believed that peripheral receptor sites become less sensitive to insulin with time. A decline also takes place in levels of glucose-regulating hormones (glucagon and epinephrine) and in lean body mass. These changes may be accompanied by decreased physical activity and a poor diet. Older adults with diabetes mellitus are more susceptible to stroke, myocardial infarction (MI), angina, or seizures. Diminished sensations may mask the manifestations of hyperglycemia. Accompanying changes in liver and kidney function and multidrug regimens may exacerbate hypoglycemia.

In general, nutritional guidelines for older clients with diabetes mellitus are no different than those for older clients without diabetes mellitus. However, older people with diabetes mellitus are at increased risk for problems that can cause functional limitations, such as pain, urinary incontinence, decreased vision (i.e., retinopathy, glaucoma, cataracts), decreased proprioception, and postural hypotension.

Impairments in mental status, functional abilities, and sensory function may interfere with the client's ability to understand and follow the treatment plan. In the older client, the risk of acute complications from hypoglycemia may outweigh the benefits of strict glucose control. The older client may enjoy good health and do very well on an individualized treatment plan. A team approach, aimed at maximizing health through optimal diet and exercise, may improve the client's quality of life as well as achieve adequate glucose control.

Surgical Management of Diabetes Mellitus

Pancreas Transplant

Indications. Some clients with type 1 diabetes mellitus receive pancreas transplants. The first pancreas transplant was completed in 1966. Eighty percent of pancreas transplantation procedures are now done concurrently with kidney transplantation. This is usually because the antirejection medication cyclosporine has such severe side effects, including hyperglycemia and nephrotoxicity, that adequate renal function unaffected by nephropathy must be present. The client's own pancreas is left intact (98% of its function is exocrine in nature), and the new pancreas is usually anastomosed (attached) to the iliac artery and vein, through which insulin can enter the systemic pathway. The new pancreas is placed in the lower pelvic cavity, and the duct is connected to the urinary bladder. The exocrine secretions of the new pancreas drain into the bladder and are not absorbed. The surgical procedure generally lasts from 4 to 6 hours. Pancreas-after-kidney transplants and pancreas-only transplants account for the remaining 20% of pancreas transplantation procedures.

Contraindications. Clients with type 1 diabetes mellitus must have well-functioning kidneys to receive only a pancreas transplant. If not, the pancreas and kidney must be transplanted simultaneously, or the pancreas must be transplanted following a successful kidney transplant. Other contraindications include problems that make the client unable to withstand the stress of surgery. Clients with type 2 diabetes mellitus do not benefit from pancreas transplantation. Type 2 diabetes mellitus results from a failure of insulin action, which cannot be improved by adding a pancreas.

Complications. Major complications of pancreas transplantation include vessel thrombosis, rejection, and infection. To help prevent thrombosis, the volume of blood flowing through the pancreas is kept at a high rate for 72 hours. Careful monitoring of laboratory values, fluid and electrolyte status, physical manifestations, and vital sign changes can alert you to possible complications.

A sharp and sudden decrease in urine amylase levels, rapid increases in blood glucose levels, gross hematuria (blood in urine), severe pain in the iliac fossa, and tenderness in the graft area are manifestations of vessel thrombosis.

Manifestations of acute and chronic graft rejection include fever, increased serum creatinine and blood urea nitrogen (BUN) levels, weight gain, and graft tenderness. Proteinuria is a primary manifestation of chronic rejection. In addition, fever, decreased urine amylase levels, increased serum amylase levels, hyperglycemia, and graft tenderness are manifestations of graft rejection.

SAFETY

ALERT

To prevent graft rejection, immunosuppressive therapy with monoclonal antibodies (OKT3) or polyclonal antibody preparations (cyclosporine [Sandimmune], and azathioprine [Imuran] and prednisone) is administered. See Chapter 80 for further discussion of immunosuppressive agents.

Outcomes. It is expected that the client will recover from the pancreas or pancreas-kidney transplant surgery and will be discharged from the hospital within 7 to 10 days without the need for insulin. Within 3 to 4 months, the client resumes a normal life as long as medication and health care regimens are followed closely. Complications such as rejection and infection slow postoperative progress. The client's quality of life is improved as a result of freedom from the need for insulin and the return to a normal diet and a less restricted lifestyle. Successful transplantation is indicated by improvement in blood glucose control (levels between 60 and 110 mg/dl) and C-peptide levels.

Islet Cell Transplant

Islet cell transplant is also being investigated as a treatment for type 1 diabetes mellitus. Less toxic antirejection drugs are required for this procedure but the desired outcomes have been limited.

Nursing Management of the Surgical Client

Once the client has chosen transplantation as an alternative to medical care and is placed on the recipient waiting list, he or she needs to undergo an extensive physical and psychological evaluation (see Chapter 80). Nursing care focuses on assessing the client's needs for knowledge and information.

The major focus of care is to monitor for rejection, adverse effects of immunosuppressive agents, infection, and occlusion of vessels. Careful monitoring for changes in vital signs, laboratory values, fluid and electrolyte status, and physical manifestations is important to determine the onset of complications: thrombosis, infection, and rejection. Blood glucose levels range between 60 and 110 mg/dl, without administration of exogenous insulin. Urine amylase levels remain constant, with urine pH between 7.0 and 8.5.

Immunosuppressive therapy started before surgery must be continued on a regular schedule postoperatively to prevent rejection of the new pancreas. Nursing implications for immunosuppressive agents to prevent rejection and treat rejection are described in Chapter 80.

Self-Care

The self-care regimen following pancreas or pancreas-kidney transplantation is complex for the client and significant others. Teach the client and significant others about long-term, ongoing care, which includes frequent follow-up to monitor the status of the new organs. Discuss self-care involved in managing medications, diet, physical activity, and manifestations of rejection and infection. Explain why continuing the present medication regimen is important and why the client should never miss a dose. Explain the manifestations of rejection and infection if the client cannot remember, needs a review, or did not receive complete information. See Chapter 80 for additional information related to transplantation.

MANAGEMENT OF THE CLIENT WITH DIABETES MELLITUS UNDERGOING OTHER TYPES OF SURGERY

Surgery is a stressful experience for anyone; for a client with diabetes mellitus, however, surgery imposes several additional stressors. Surgery interrupts the client's usual therapeutic regimen. The diet must be temporarily changed and the dosage of insulin or oral hypoglycemic agent readjusted.

> **The stress of surgery raises blood glucose levels. The client is susceptible to infection. The surgical incision itself becomes a new potential portal of entry for pathogens. Furthermore, postoperative healing in these clients may be slower than normal.**

To offset these problems, clients with diabetes mellitus require special interventions, both preoperatively and postoperatively. They may vary, depending on whether the client has type 1 or type 2 diabetes mellitus and whether the surgery is elective or performed on an emergency basis.

Preoperative Care

The goal of preoperative care for clients with diabetes mellitus is thorough regulation of blood glucose levels before surgery. Clients with type 1 diabetes mellitus need to be closely monitored for several days or even weeks before elective surgery to stabilize their condition and, thereby, to decrease surgical risk. If a client with type 1 diabetes mellitus and poor glucose control requires emergency surgery, the surgeon must choose between operating on a hypoglycemic or hyperglycemic client and postponing an emergency operation until the diabetes mellitus is controlled. In either case, the client needs constant monitoring of vital signs, frequent laboratory and bedside glucose studies, and vigilant nursing intervention. Clients with well-controlled type 2 diabetes mellitus usually undergo surgery with only slightly more risk than that for the general population.

Typically, preoperative preparation for clients with type 1 and type 2 diabetes mellitus includes the following:

- Preoperative laboratory tests, including fasting and preprandial blood glucose levels; glycosylated hemoglobin level; serum electrolytes, BUN, and serum creatinine levels; complete blood count; ECG and cardiac enzymes; and chest radiograph
- Early-morning scheduling of surgery so that the client's diet and insulin regimen undergo as little disruption as possible
- Omission of food, water, and oral hypoglycemic agents on the morning of surgery (one long-acting hypoglycemic agent, chlorpropamide, is discontinued 1 to 2 days before surgery because of its long half-life)
- IV infusion of insulin for insulin-dependent or insulin-requiring clients, usually with glucose (5%) to prevent hypoglycemia (if the surgery is relatively minor, such as for cataract removal, the surgeon may order a 5% dextrose solution infusion and half the usual dose of intermediate-acting insulin; the anesthesiologist can monitor blood glucose levels in the operating room)
- A blood glucose determination performed and reported to the physician within 1 hour before the operation to ensure that the client (who has taken nothing by mouth since midnight) will not develop hypoglycemia during surgery

Intraoperative Care

Once the client arrives in surgery, management again depends on the severity of the diabetes mellitus and the extent of the surgery. Regular insulin, in a dose based on the client's blood glucose levels and a sliding scale or an insulin protocol, can be given by the IV route. Continuous insulin infusion therapy is preferred. Subcutaneous insulin should not be given intraoperatively because its absorption is affected by body temperature, circulatory blood volumes, and certain anesthetics.

Postoperative Care

After surgery, the goals of postoperative management are to stabilize the client's vital signs, correct fluid and electrolyte imbalances, reestablish control of the diabetes mellitus, prevent wound infection, and promote wound healing.

The following are important postoperative interventions:

- Administer prescribed IV infusions and regular insulin or continuous insulin infusion therapy until the client can take oral nourishment.
- Once the client can tolerate fluids, offer those that contain calories to prevent hypoglycemia. Once the client can eat, make food available. Discuss the client's calorie level with a dietitian to ensure that enough calories are provided for postoperative wound healing.
- Obtain a blood glucose level four to six times daily.
- Resume the client's prescribed preoperative insulin type and dosage once blood glucose control is reestablished, foods are being consumed at adequate levels, and it has been reordered by the physician.
- Observe for evidence of hypoglycemia after surgery, such as a decrease in blood pressure or an increase in heart rate in a client who is still unresponsive from anesthesia.
- Avoid catheterization, if possible, to prevent bladder infection.
- Change wound dressings with meticulous sterile technique to prevent wound infection.
- Assess the client's wound and incision frequently for signs of infection. Be alert for abnormal amounts of drainage or foul-smelling drainage.
- Observe for and treat manifestations of skin breakdown, especially if the client has peripheral vascular disease or neuropathy.

MANAGEMENT OF A SICK CLIENT WITH DIABETES MELLITUS

The Client Education Guide on p. 1088 presents guidelines for the client to follow during illnesses.

ACUTE COMPLICATIONS OF DIABETES MELLITUS

HYPERGLYCEMIA AND DIABETIC KETOACIDOSIS

Hyperglycemia results when glucose cannot be transported to the cells because of a lack of insulin. Without available carbohydrates for cellular fuel, the liver converts its glycogen stores back to glucose (glycogenolysis) and increases the biosynthesis of glucose (gluconeogenesis). Unfortunately, however, these responses worsen the situation by raising the blood glucose level even higher.[13,34]

In type 1 diabetes mellitus, as the need for cellular fuel grows more critical, the body begins to draw on its fat and protein stores for energy. Excessive amounts of fatty acids are mobilized from adipose tissue cells and transported to the liver. The liver, in turn, accelerates the rate at which it produces ketone bodies (ketogenesis) for catabolism by other body tissues, particularly muscle. As fat metabolism increases, the liver may produce too many ketone bodies. Ketone bodies accumulate in the blood (ketosis) and are excreted in the urine (ketonuria).

CLIENT EDUCATION GUIDE ⓔ

🫖 Sick Day Management Guidelines for Diabetes Mellitus*

You should have an individualized plan of care prescribed by the health care team to use during illness.

Monitoring is an essential part of diabetes management, but this is even more vital during the stress of illness. Insulin requirements may be increased secondary to reduced activity and increased secretion of counterregulatory hormones. To prevent diabetic ketoacidosis, you should know the following:

Self-Monitoring of Blood Glucose Level. It is important to self-monitor blood glucose levels more frequently during illness, often every 2 to 4 hours. If pre-meal blood glucose values stay greater than 250 mg/dl, then test for urine ketones and contact your health care provider.

Ketones. Urine ketones should be monitored when you feel sick or when blood glucose level is greater than 250 mg/dl. Test for ketones every 2 to 4 hours.

Insulin. Do not stop taking insulin, even if you are vomiting and unable to eat. Additional regular insulin may be required, based on self-monitored blood glucose levels.

Nutrition/Fluids. Adequate fluid intake and carbohydrates are essential during illness. Eating 10 to 15 g of carbohydrate every 1 to 2 hours and small quantities of fluid every 15 to 30 minutes is usually sufficient to prevent dehydration and ketoacidosis. Clear broth, tea, and ice chips are usually well tolerated.

Examples of foods and beverages containing about 15 g of carbohydrate are as follows:

- 1 regular whole Popsicle
- ½ cup applesauce
- ¾ cup regular soft drink
- ½ cup ginger ale
- ½ cup orange juice or apple juice
- 1 cup Gatorade
- ½ cup regular gelatin

Notify your health care provider when you have any of the following problems:

- Illness that persists more than 24 hours
- Severe abdominal pain
- Temperature greater than 100° F, oral
- Persistent diarrhea
- Vomiting with inability to consume fluids for more than 4 hours
- Blood glucose levels difficult to control or moderate to high levels of ketones in urine
- Shortness of breath or chest pain
- Acute visual loss
- Other unexplained health problems

*Most applicable to clients with type 1 diabetes mellitus and those with type 2 diabetes mellitus receiving insulin therapy.

Metabolic acidosis develops from the acidic (pH-lowering) effect of the ketones acetoacetate and beta-hydroxybutyrate. This condition is called *diabetic ketoacidosis*. Severe acidosis may cause the diabetic client to lose consciousness, a condition called *diabetic coma*. Diabetic ketoacidosis always constitutes a medical emergency and requires immediate medical attention.[13,22,34]

Diabetic ketoacidosis is the most serious metabolic disturbance in type 1 diabetes mellitus and is a common cause of hospital admission.

Diabetic ketoacidosis is identified in about 40% of clients with previously undiagnosed diabetes mellitus and is responsible for more than 160,000 hospital admissions each year. It occurs most frequently in teenagers and older adults.

Etiology and Risk Factors

Common causes of diabetic ketoacidosis include the following:

- Taking too little insulin
- Skipping doses of insulin
- Inability to meet an increased need for insulin created by surgery, trauma, pregnancy, stress, puberty, or infection
- Developing insulin resistance through the presence of insulin antibodies

Pathophysiology

Diabetic ketoacidosis is marked by a relative or absolute lack of insulin. Insulin may be present, but not in sufficient amounts for the increased need for glucose attributable to the stressors present (such as infection). When the body lacks insulin and cannot use carbohydrates for energy, it resorts to using fats and proteins. Excess production of counterregulatory hormones (glucagon, catecholamines, cortisol, and growth hormones) secondary to stress appears to play an important role in the development of diabetic ketoacidosis. These hormones antagonize the effects of insulin and foster diabetic ketoacidosis by promoting hyperglycemia, osmotic diuresis, lipolysis with secondary hyperlipidemia, and acidosis. Figure 45-7 summarizes the pathophysiologic mechanisms involved. The process of catabolizing fats for fuel leads to three pathologic events: ketosis and acidosis; dehydration; and electrolyte and acid-base imbalance.

Ketosis and Acidosis

The metabolic effect of insufficient insulin on fat metabolism was examined previously. In diabetic ketoacidosis, buffering of acid by bicarbonate, which is excreted as carbon dioxide and water, fails to compensate for ketosis.

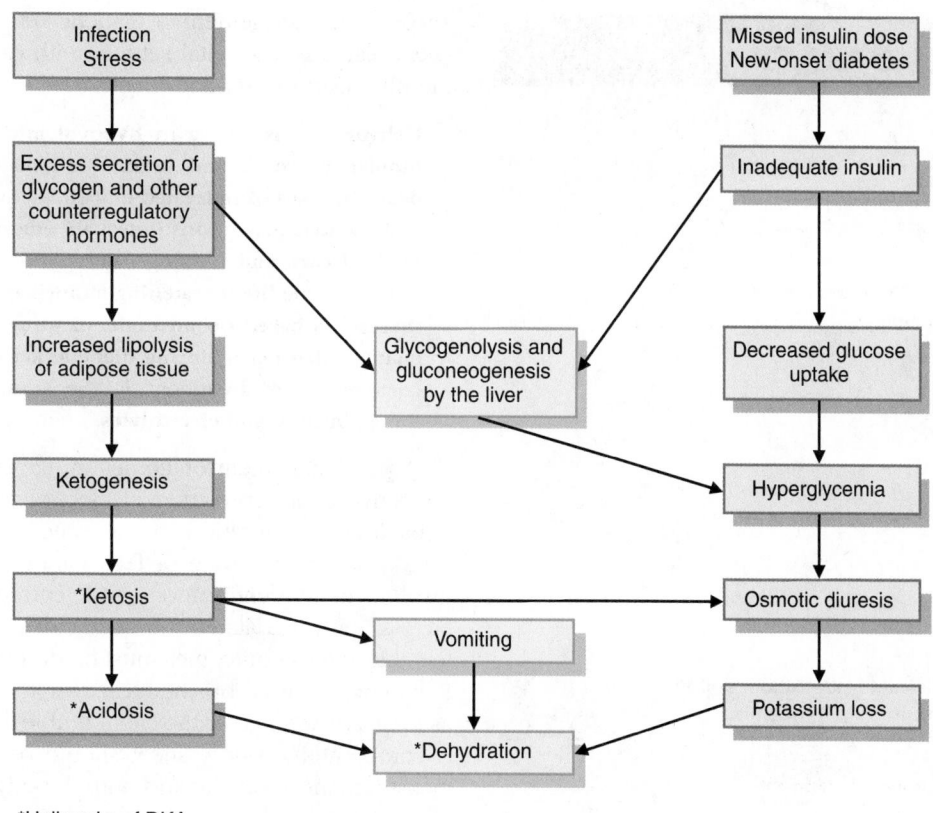

*Hallmarks of DKA

■ **FIGURE 45–7**   The pathophysiology of diabetic ketoacidosis. *(Modified from White, N.H., & Henry, D.N. [1996]. Special issues in diabetes management. In D. Haire-Joshu [Ed.], Management of diabetes mellitus: Perspectives of care across the lifespan [2nd ed., p. 344]. St. Louis: Mosby.)*

Respirations increase in rate and depth (Kussmaul's respirations), and the breath has a "fruity" or acetone-like odor.

Dehydration

Clients with ketoacidosis lose fluids from several sources. They excrete large amounts of urine in the body's attempt to eliminate excessive glucose and ketones. Second, acidosis can cause severe nausea and vomiting, with further losses of fluid and electrolytes (notably sodium and chloride). Finally, water is lost in the breath as the body attempts to rid itself of excess acetone and carbon dioxide.

Typically, clients in diabetic coma lose an amount of water equivalent to 10% of body weight, plus about 40 g of sodium. Severe dehydration resulting from these fluid losses may be followed by hypovolemic shock and lactic acidosis.

Electrolyte Imbalance

As the pH of the blood decreases (acidosis), the accumulating hydrogen ions move from the extracellular fluid to the intracellular fluid. The movement of hydrogen ions into the cells promotes the movement of potassium out of the cells into the extracellular fluid, which results in severe intracellular potassium depletion and elevated extracellular potassium levels. Initially, the intracellular potassium loss may go unrecognized because serum potassium levels are often normal or elevated. As the resulting osmotic diuresis continues, however, much potassium is excreted in the urine. If the client becomes severely dehydrated, hemoconcentration and oliguria may cause the serum potassium levels to increase even higher, which may be life-threatening and result in cardiac dysrhythmias.

In addition to potassium losses, the client in metabolic acidosis loses excessive amounts of sodium, phosphate, chloride, and bicarbonate in the urine and vomitus.

Clinical Manifestations

Common presenting manifestations of the client in diabetic ketoacidosis are listed in Box 45-4. Clinical manifestations and assessment priorities common with acute hyperglycemia are listed in Table 45-5.

OUTCOME MANAGEMENT

Medical Management

Assessment priorities and clinical manifestations for the client with acute hyperglycemia are presented in

BOX 45-4 Common Manifestations of Diabetic Ketoacidosis

- Abdominal pain
- Anorexia
- Dehydration
- Fruity odor of ketones on breath
- Hyperpnea or Kussmaul's respirations
- Hypotension
- Impaired level of consciousness or coma
- Nausea and vomiting
- Polyuria
- Somnolence
- Tachycardia
- Thirst
- Visual disturbances
- Warm, dry skin
- Weakness
- Weight loss

TABLE 45–5 Clinical Manifestations and Priority Assessments for Acute Hyperglycemia

Clinical Manifestations	Priority Assessments
Dehydration	Assess skin for dryness, flushed color, and "tenting." Assess mucous membranes for dryness. Monitor urine output for polyuria followed by oliguria. Monitor vital signs for hypotension and tachycardia. Monitor for fluid overload during treatment for hyperglycemia.
Electrolyte imbalances	Monitor for hyperkalemia: peaked T waves on ECG, ectopic beats, changes in heart rate, hypotension, diarrhea and hyperactive bowel sounds, muscle cramps, nausea and vomiting, hypotension. Monitor for hypokalemia: flattened T waves and U wave on ECG, ectopic beats, hypotension, ileus, nausea and vomiting, fatigue, lethargy, muscle weakness and cramps. Monitor for hyponatremia: nausea, vomiting, diarrhea, tachycardia, hypotension, lethargy, confusion, seizures, muscle weakness.
Hyperglycemia	Monitor blood glucose levels and check urine for ketones. Monitor for polyuria, polyphagia, and polydipsia. Monitor for hypoglycemia during treatment for hyperglycemia.
Hyperosmolality	Monitor serum osmolality, blood urea nitrogen, serum creatinine. Assess for lethargy, disorientation, and behavioral changes.
Metabolic acidosis	Monitor for hypotension, dysrhythmias, hyperventilation, lethargy, confusion, coma, headache, acetone breath.

Table 45-5. Management of diabetic ketoacidosis usually takes place in a hospital setting, with care managed by the physician, nurse, and pharmacist.

Dehydration resulting in hypovolemic shock, acute tubular necrosis, and uremia are major causes of death in cases of untreated diabetic ketoacidosis. Diabetic ketoacidosis constitutes an emergency. Rapid medical care and nursing intervention are essential to correct the life-threatening abnormalities. Effective therapy is based on an understanding of metabolic changes that occur during diabetic ketoacidosis. The cornerstone of treatment is the administration of fluids, insulin, and electrolytes.

Management outcomes in diabetic ketoacidosis are rehydration, correction of electrolyte and acid-base imbalances, restoration to a state of carbohydrate catabolism from a state of fat catabolism by providing insulin, and identification and correction of those factors that precipitated the ketoacidosis. The measures to achieve these outcomes must be done with great care. Fully correcting all biochemical abnormalities may take as long as 1 week after the client is able to eat solid food. A comprehensive flow sheet should be kept to record measurements of intake and output, body weight, fluids, electrolytes, insulin, and ketones.

Rehydrate

Intravenous rehydration is required for all clients who are vomiting, are unable to drink, and have acidosis. IV infusions of isotonic or normal saline (0.9% sodium chloride) are started immediately. Usually, the client receives 1000 ml of isotonic solution by the IV route during the first hour (10 to 20 ml/kg), followed by an additional 2000 to 8000 ml of solution over the next 24 hours. Clients with compromised cardiovascular function may require slower IV fluid replacement, as shown in the Critical Monitoring feature on p. 1091 and in Box 45-5.

A nasogastric tube may be necessary if the client is comatose or is vomiting and likely to aspirate the vomitus. The client's mouth may be dry because of the nasogastric tube and the dehydration. Frequent oral care is important. Assess bowel sounds frequently for changes. Encourage the client to drink once he or she can tolerate fluids. Drinking salted broth is beneficial to replenish needed sodium.

Record intake and output accurately. Most clients require a urinary catheter to monitor urine output. Report a urine output less than 0.5 ml/kg/hour. Because clients with diabetes mellitus are susceptible to infection, aseptic catheter care is essential.

The Rehydration Process

- The best indication of the degree of dehydration is weight loss, which may be determined when the client's baseline weight is known; loss may be 10% of total body weight.
- Other clinical indices to monitor are tissue turgor, pulse rate, condition of mucous membranes, level of consciousness, thirst, hematocrit, and positional blood pressure changes (to check for orthostatic hypotension).
- For older adults and clients with heart disease, fluid replacement should be determined according to central venous pressure measurement.
- Too aggressive fluid replacement (particularly with normal saline) may induce heart failure; frequent auscultation of the lungs is vital.

Reverse Shock

If the client is in circulatory collapse, the physician may order blood, albumin, or other plasma volume expanders, such as dextran, to be administered alternately with normal saline solution. Also, the client may receive combinations of colloids and saline solution that raise serum levels of both sodium chloride and plasma protein.

Restore Potassium Balance

Because of the lowered pH in untreated ketoacidosis, potassium leaves the intracellular space, and transient hyperkalemia develops. The total body potassium level is depleted, despite a normal or elevated serum potassium level.

Correct potassium replacement requires caution and timely action. Once intervention begins with fluids and insulin, dangerous hypokalemia may develop, manifested by weakness, extreme dyspnea, and even cardiac arrest. Hypokalemia occurs because potassium reenters the cells (along with glucose) after insulin administration and then is excreted in the urine with rehydration and restoration of renal function.

 SAFETY ALERT

General agreement exists on the following points of assessment and intervention:

- **Frequently assess and measure urine output. Do not administer potassium to a client with low urine output; dangerous hyperkalemia may develop. Notify the physician promptly if urine output declines dramatically or is less than 0.5 ml/kg/hour.**
- **Assess the client continuously for evidence of hyperkalemia (bradycardia, cardiac arrest, weakness, flaccid paralysis, oliguria) or hypokalemia (weakness, flaccid paralysis, paralytic ileus, cardiac arrest). Hyperkalemia may be present during the first 4 hours of intervention. Hypokalemia usually develops 4 to 24 hours after the initial intervention.**
- **Replace potassium carefully following protocols (Box 45-6).**

BOX 45-5   Intravenous Fluid Replacement in Diabetic Ketoacidosis*

HOUR 1
- Provide 15-20 ml/kg of isotonic sodium chloride (0.9%) (normal saline) or full-strength Ringer's lactate (lactated Ringer's solution).

HOUR 2
- Continue fluid as above at 15 ml/kg. If the client is hypernatremic, has heart failure, or is a child, consider half-strength sodium chloride (0.45% normal saline).

HOUR 3
- Reduce fluid intake to 7.5 ml/kg in adults. Fluid should be 0.45% normal saline.

HOUR 4
- Adjust fluid intake to meet clinical need. Consider urine output rate in calculation.

*When blood glucose level approaches 250 mg/dl, change fluid to 5% dextrose in half-strength sodium chloride (D₅/0.45% normal saline). Continue intravenous fluids until client can ingest food and drink without vomiting.
Modified from Bode, B. (2003). *Medical management of type 1 diabetes* (4th ed.). Alexandria, Va: American Diabetes Association.

BOX 45-6   Potassium Replacement in Diabetic Ketoacidosis

In clients with adequate urine output, lead II of the 12-lead electrocardiogram may be used as a guide for plasma potassium (K^+) concentration. Flattening or inversion of the T wave with U wave and prolongation of the QT interval indicate hypokalemia. Peaking of T waves, loss of P wave, and a disrupted QRS complex indicate hyperkalemia.

Intravenous replacement of potassium is based on plasma K^+ concentration. If K^+ concentration is:

- <3 mEq/L, infuse ≥0.6 mEq/kg/hour
- 3-4 mEq/L, infuse 0.6 mEq/kg/hour
- 4-5 mEq/L, infuse 0.2-0.4 mEq/kg/hour
- 6 mEq/L, withhold until K^+ concentration is <6.0 mEq/L

Add K^+ to replacement fluid therapy. If concentration is 20-40 mEq/L and infusion into peripheral vein causes irritation, infuse into central vein.

Recheck plasma K^+ concentration every 2 hours if previous value was <4 or >6 mEq/L.

Modified from Bode, B. (2003). *Medical management of type 1 diabetes* (4th ed.). Alexandria, Va: American Diabetes Association.

- Plan to begin potassium administration within 1 to 2 hours after starting insulin therapy and after adequate urine output is ensured.
- When the client has recovered sufficiently to resume eating and drinking, give foods and liquids that are high in potassium, such as bananas or orange juice.
- Monitor sodium chloride and phosphate levels. Sodium is replaced by normal saline. Phosphate levels can also vary to the same degree noted for potassium levels. Sometimes the physician alternates potassium chloride with potassium phosphate in the IV fluid.

Correct pH and Administer Insulin

Clients presenting in diabetic ketoacidosis usually have phosphate depletion from a combination of decreased food intake, excessive catabolism, and increased urinary excretion.

SAFETY ALERT

As with administration of potassium, administration of insulin enhances movement of phosphate into the cells, which further reduces plasma phosphate concentration. However, administering too much phosphate can induce hypocalcemia. Calcium levels should be checked before phosphate (as potassium phosphate) is given.

Clinicians usually administer sodium bicarbonate only to clients with a blood pH of 7.1 or less. Such replacement therapy partially corrects the metabolic acidosis. As the client's condition improves, normal body mechanisms restore the blood pH to normal.

Low-dosage insulin therapy (5 to 10 units/hour) is ordered for the client in diabetic ketoacidosis. Although the blood glucose concentration is usually sharply elevated in diabetic ketoacidosis, a blood glucose level less than 300 mg/dl does not exclude the diagnosis. The client in ketoacidosis may receive an initial IV bolus of regular insulin (0.15 unit/kg) in the emergency department. Before starting an infusion of insulin, ask whether the client has already received insulin that day. Insulin should never be given subcutaneously to someone in diabetic ketoacidosis, because the subcutaneous tissues are dehydrated and poorly perfused as a result of dehydration and hypovolemic shock.[34]

Traditionally, the hyperglycemia associated with diabetic ketoacidosis is treated with an IV bolus of regular insulin. Then an insulin drip should be started. Either 0.9% (normal) saline solution or 0.45% saline may be used, depending on the degree of dehydration and concurrent medical problems. Prepare the last amount of insulin in the smallest IV bag available (e.g., 100 units of regular insulin in 100 ml of IV fluid). This gives a 1:1 ratio of regular insulin to IV fluid. Prime the IV tubing with the IV solution first, and then add the regular insulin, because insulin adheres to the IV tubing. Label the IV bag clearly with the dose and type of insulin added. The IV regular insulin must be administered meticulously by a control pump and checked frequently.

After the bolus, infuse insulin at a rate of 0.1 unit/kg/hour. If no improvement in the acidosis occurs within 2 to 4 hours, the infusion rate should be doubled. Severe insulin resistance may be precipitated by severe stress. The glucose level is normalized more quickly than pH.

Blood glucose levels need to be monitored every 30 minutes initially, preferably with a blood glucose meter. Rapid blood glucose test results allow you to adjust the insulin infusion rapidly and correctly. When the blood glucose levels approach 250 mg/dl, the insulin infusion should be reduced and 5% dextrose added to the infusion so that the blood glucose level can be maintained at about 250 mg/dl for the first 12 to 24 hours. Faster correction of hyperglycemia can lead to cerebral edema. Monitor the client's level of consciousness closely to assess for this uncommon complication. Monitor blood glucose levels every 1 to 2 hours after reaching 250 mg/dl until they are stable.[34]

As the client improves, decisions must be made about when to discontinue IV insulin and fluids and begin subcutaneous insulin administration. Normalization of the client's vital signs, correction of acidosis, and ability to take oral fluids are important considerations. Short-acting insulin is usually administered subcutaneously every 4 to 6 hours, with the first dose given 15 to 30 minutes before stopping IV insulin. The initial dose is about 0.2 unit/kg. Subsequent doses are determined by blood glucose levels.

While any metabolic abnormalities are being corrected, the cause of the client's diabetic ketoacidosis must be pursued aggressively. Cultures of urine, throat, sputum, and blood; chest x-ray films; and an electrocardiogram (ECG) may reveal the source of stress. Before discharge of the client from the hospital, the health care team reviews the situation that led to diabetic ketoacidosis and institutes teaching for risk factor reduction.

Prevent Recurrence

Primary prevention of diabetic ketoacidosis is through client education. Preventing diabetic ketoacidosis is the long-term goal of good diabetes management. Clients and their families should understand enough about ketoacidosis to avoid potential causes, to recognize its approach, to slow down or minimize its development, and to seek help fast if it begins to occur. To prevent diabetic ketoacidosis, clients with diabetes mellitus should learn to do the following:

- Take insulin in appropriate doses at appropriate times.
- Monitor blood glucose level frequently, at least before each meal and at bedtime.

■ Monitor urine ketone levels when blood glucose levels increase to greater than 250 mg/dl.

■ Schedule regular appointments with a health care provider to review blood glucose levels, weight gains or losses, and general state of health and well-being. Recognize manifestations of infection—a major cause of diabetic ketoacidosis. The first clinical manifestations of infection (upper respiratory tract, urinary tract, or vaginal infection) should be reported immediately to the health care provider; other stressors, such as family or emotional problems, can also precipitate diabetic ketoacidosis.

The client should telephone for assistance if any of the following develop:

■ Anorexia, nausea, vomiting, or diarrhea
■ Ketonuria persisting for more than 8 hours
■ Fever or infection
■ Any manifestation of acidosis

Emphasize that the greatest weapons against diabetic ketoacidosis are regular, daily SMBG; adherence to the diabetes management program; and early recognition of and intervention in mild ketosis.

HYPERGLYCEMIC HYPEROSMOLAR NONKETOTIC SYNDROME

Hyperglycemic hyperosmolar nonketotic syndrome (HHNS) is a variant of diabetic ketoacidosis characterized by extreme hyperglycemia (600 to 2000 mg/dl), profound dehydration, mild or undetectable ketonuria, and the absence of acidosis. HHNS most commonly occurs in older clients with type 2 diabetes mellitus (Box 45-7).

Mortality with HHNS is greater than with diabetic ketoacidosis (10% to 40%), primarily because clients typically are older and commonly have significant medical problems. HHNS sometimes occurs in people with undiagnosed diabetes mellitus and in known diabetic clients after a long period of uncontrolled hyperglycemia. The precipitating factors for HHNS may be the same as those for diabetic ketoacidosis. There is almost always an identifiable precipitating factor.

The major difference between HHNS and diabetic ketoacidosis is the lack of ketonuria with HHNS. Because some residual ability to secrete insulin remains in type 2 diabetes mellitus, the mobilization of fats for energy usually does not occur. In the absence of adequate insulin, the blood becomes loaded with glucose. Glucose molecules are too large to pass into cells; therefore osmosis of water occurs from the interstitial spaces and cells to dilute the glucose in the blood. Osmotic diuresis occurs. Eventually, the cells become dehydrated.[13]

The client's fluid intake can initially balance the loss of fluid and glucose through the urine. The imbalance gradually becomes more severe as the client cannot

---

BOX 45-7 Factors Associated with Hyperglycemic Hyperosmolar Nonketotic Syndrome (HHNS)

THERAPEUTIC AGENTS
■ Glucocorticoids
■ Diuretics
■ Diphenylhydantoin
■ Beta-adrenergic blocking agents
■ L-Asparaginase
■ Immunosuppressive agents
■ Chlorpromazine
■ Diazoxide

THERAPEUTIC PROCEDURES
■ Peritoneal dialysis
■ Hemodialysis
■ Hyperalimentation
■ Surgical stress

CHRONIC ILLNESS
■ Renal disease
■ Heart disease
■ Hypertension
■ Previous stroke
■ Alcoholism
■ Psychiatric diagnosis
■ Loss of thirst

ACUTE ILLNESS
■ Infection
■ Gangrene
■ Urinary tract infection
■ Septicemia
■ Burns
■ Gastrointestinal bleeding
■ Myocardial infarction
■ Pancreatitis
■ Stroke

From American Diabetes Association. (2004). Screening for type 2 diabetes (position statement). *Diabetes Care, 27*(Suppl 1), S11-S14.

---

match intake to output. In time, the client becomes obtunded and is unable to respond to thirst. At this point, the process is self-perpetuating.

The following are the four major clinical features of HHNS:[13]

■ Severe hyperglycemia (600 to 2000 mg/dl)
■ No or only slight ketosis
■ Profound dehydration (10% to 15% loss of body water)
■ Hyperosmolality (increased concentration) of plasma and elevated blood urea nitrogen level

Typically, the client experiences excessive thirst, altered level of consciousness (coma or confusion), and manifestations of dehydration. The precipitating event should be determined and corrected as soon as possible, even during resuscitation. HHNS is treated with vigorous fluid replacement and administration of insulin and electrolytes.

SAFETY ALERT

A common initial intervention is infusion of normal saline solution over a 2-hour period, followed by administration of hypotonic (0.45%) saline solution. As in diabetic ketoacidosis, potassium, sodium, chloride, and phosphates are administered intravenously.

Insulin is given via an infusion pump, but usually at lower dosages, because the client is producing some insulin. Because of severe dehydration, blood glucose levels decrease rapidly with fluid administration. Dextrose is added to the IV fluid when the blood glucose level reaches about 250 mg/dl, to prevent hypoglycemia. Because many clients who have HHNS are older and have other cardiovascular or renal disorders, fluid volume and electrolyte changes must be carefully assessed, especially if acute or chronic renal failure complicates the course.

As the population ages, an increasing number of clients will experience HHNS and you need to be alert for its manifestations. Before discharge, review the causes of HHNS with the client and family, including insulin injection (if necessary) and blood glucose testing techniques. Help the client understand how serious these acute complications are and how to prevent them in the future.

HYPOGLYCEMIA

Hypoglycemia (also known as an *insulin reaction* or hypoglycemic reaction) is a common feature of type 1 diabetes mellitus and can also be seen in clients with type 2 diabetes mellitus treated with insulin or oral agents. The precise blood glucose level at which clients have manifestations of hypoglycemia varies, but they usually do not occur until the blood glucose level is less than 50 to 60 mg/dl.

Etiology and Risk Factors
Hypoglycemic reactions may result from the following:

- An overdose of insulin or, less commonly, a sulfonylurea
- Omitting a meal or eating less food than usual
- Overexertion without additional carbohydrate compensation
- Nutritional and fluid imbalances caused by nausea and vomiting
- Alcohol intake

Inadvertent or deliberate errors in insulin dose are a frequent cause of hypoglycemia. Other changes in the schedule of meals or insulin administration, vigorous unexpected exercise, or sleeping later than usual in the morning can also cause hypoglycemia. The effects of alcohol, marijuana, or other drugs can mask a client's awareness of hypoglycemia in its earliest stages.

Hypoglycemia can also occur secondary to administration of an oral hypoglycemic agent. Most recorded cases have been in clients receiving chlorpropamide (Diabinese), which has a duration of action of 24 to 72 hours. Clients at risk for hypoglycemia while taking an oral hypoglycemic are older than age 60 years, have poor nutritional intake, use alcohol, have hepatic or renal dysfunction, and are on multi-drug regimens. Hypoglycemic reactions can be severe and prolonged.

Pathophysiology
Normally, hypoglycemia triggers counterregulatory hormones, primarily glucagon and epinephrine, to promptly increase blood glucose levels by stimulating glucose release from the liver and inhibiting insulin secretion. Under usual conditions, this leads to normoglycemia.[22]

In contrast, clients with type 1 diabetes mellitus have abnormalities in this feedback system. Typically, within the first 2 to 5 years of diabetes mellitus, the secretion of glucagon becomes deficient. Later, the secretion of epinephrine may become impaired secondary to subclinical neuropathy. The regulation of insulin absorption from subcutaneous fat also becomes impaired.

The combination of these abnormalities makes the client with type 1 diabetes mellitus susceptible to frequent development of hypoglycemia. In this respect, hypoglycemic shock is more dangerous than diabetic ketoacidosis. About 1 in 10 clients with type 1 diabetes mellitus suffers one severe reaction per year that requires emergency treatment. Untreated or prolonged hypoglycemia can cause permanent brain damage, memory loss, decreased learning ability, paralysis, and death.

Clinical Manifestations
Hypoglycemic manifestations are generally divided into two major categories (Box 45-8).

Adrenergic
Adrenergic (autonomic) manifestations are associated with increasing epinephrine levels and are considered "mild" reactions. Cognitive deficits usually do not occur, and affected people are capable of self-treatment. Diaphoresis, although not mediated via adrenergic nerve endings, is usually grouped with the adrenergic manifestations of hypoglycemia. Adrenergic reactions usually occur during rapid decreases in blood glucose levels. They have been reported by clients with poorly controlled diabetes mellitus when the decrease in blood glucose level is rapid, even in the absence of hypoglycemia. These manifestations can also occur during other stressful or anxiety-provoking events. These mild reactions may produce only minimal disruptions of daily activities.[15,22]

Neuroglycopenic
Neuroglycopenic manifestations are associated with lack of glucose availability to the brain and resultant decrease in cognitive functioning.

BOX 45-8   Manifestations of Hypoglycemia

ADRENERGIC (INCREASED EPINEPHRINE)

- Shakiness
- Irritability
- Nervousness
- Tachycardia, palpitations
- Tremor
- Hunger
- Diaphoresis
- Pallor
- Paresthesias

NEUROGLYCOPENIC (DECREASED GLUCOSE TO BRAIN)

- Headache
- Mental illness
- Inability to concentrate
- Slurred speech
- Blurred vision
- Confusion
- Irrational behavior
- Lethargy, severe
- Loss of consciousness
- Coma
- Seizure
- Death

These reactions typically produce longer lasting and more severe manifestations than those characteristic of mild reactions. Common manifestations are headache, irritability, drowsiness, weakness, and tremor. The client may need assistance in treatment. Severe hypoglycemic reactions render the client unable to self-treat. The client may be awake and alert, semicomatose, or comatose.[15,22]

Hypoglycemia can occur at any time of day or night. It seems to occur most commonly during exercise, 8 to 24 hours after strenuous exercise, and in the middle of the night. Severe hypoglycemia seems to occur more often in clients who have hypoglycemic unawareness, defective glucose counterregulation, and autonomic neuropathy as well as in clients receiving intensive diabetes therapy.

The period during which the client is most likely to experience an insulin reaction depends on the type of insulin given, the client's response to that type of insulin, and the timing of the insulin injection in relation to food intake.

When insulin is given in the morning, short-acting preparations tend to produce reactions before lunch; intermediate-acting insulins, 2 or 3 hours before dinner; and long-acting insulins, between 2:00 AM and breakfast. NPH or Lente insulin injected before dinner (5:00 PM) can cause hypoglycemia around 2:00 AM, when the normal blood glucose level is lowest because of the decrease in metabolism, and again at around 8:00 AM, when the insulin peaks if breakfast is not eaten on time.

OUTCOME MANAGEMENT

Medical Management

Return Blood Glucose to Normal Levels

Management of hypoglycemia depends on the severity of the reaction (Table 45-6). To reverse mild hypoglycemia, 15 g of simple carbohydrate is given and works quickly to increase blood glucose levels. Reactions that occur during the night should be treated with a carbohydrate followed by a longer-acting mixture of carbohydrate and protein (8 ounces of milk, for example).

> **A blood glucose test (with a glucose meter) should be performed as soon as manifestations begin. If a meter is not available, it is safer to assume and treat hypoglycemia. Blood glucose level is retested in 15 to 30 minutes, and treatment is repeated if the level is not more than 100 mg/dl. Moderate reactions may need two or more treatments with 15 g of carbohydrates.**
>
> **Never force an unconscious or semiconscious client to drink liquids, because fluid may be aspirated into the lungs. The unconscious client with severe hypoglycemia needs glucagon or IV glucose immediately. Family members of clients with diabetes mellitus can administer glucagon at home in the event of a serious hypoglycemic reaction. Glucagon, administered**

SAFETY
ALERT

TABLE 45–6   Interventions for Hypoglycemia

Clinical Manifestations	Interventions
Mild Hypoglycemia	
Tremors	10-15 g of carbohydrate, contained in the following:
Tachycardia	4 oz orange juice
Diaphoresis	6 oz regular soda
Paresthesias	6-8 oz 2% milk
Excessive hunger	6-8 Lifesavers candies
Pallor	1 small (2-oz) tube of cake icing
Shakiness	4 tsp granulated sugar
Moderate Hypoglycemia	
Manifestations listed above plus	20-30 g of carbohydrate
Headache	Glucagon, 1 mg subcutaneous or IM
Mood swings	
Irritability	
Inability to concentrate	
Drowsiness	
Impaired judgment	
Slurred speech	
Double or blurred vision	
Severe Hypoglycemia	
Disorientation	50% dextrose, 25 g IV
Seizures	Glucagon, 1 mg IM or IV
Unconsciousness	

IM, Intramuscularly; IV, intravenously.

intramuscularly or subcutaneously in the amount of 1 mg for adults, may eliminate the need for emergency department intervention.

The pharmacy dispenses glucagon in the form of a powder, with the diluent in a separate vial. Instruct family members how and when to mix and inject glucagon, and let them know that the client may experience nausea or vomiting on awakening. Even though glucagon is effective in most clients, its effect is transient and slower than that of dextrose. Hypoglycemia often recurs. Medical assistance is advisable if hypoglycemia recurs, vomiting prevents oral intake, or the client's status does not improve.

A client who experiences severe hypoglycemia in the hospital usually receives 10 to 25 g of IV glucose (as 50% or 25% dextrose) over 1 to 3 minutes. This is followed by an infusion of 5% dextrose at 5 to 10 g/hour until the client is fully recovered and able to eat.

Prevent Hypoglycemia

 Because insulin reactions are common, clients with newly diagnosed diabetes mellitus must understand the following:

- Why hypoglycemia occurs
- When it is most likely to occur
- The early clinical manifestations of hypoglycemia
- The danger of severe or repeated reactions
- The importance of early intervention
- How to prevent insulin reactions

Whenever administration of insulin or an oral hypoglycemic agent begins, the client must be taught to identify clinical manifestations and to manage hypoglycemia. Once a client experiences and then fully recovers from an episode of hypoglycemia, thoroughly reassess the intervention program. In some cases, insulin reactions develop because the client carelessly prepares insulin dosages, fails to eat, or exercises excessively.

SAFETY ALERT **Explain the dangers of repeated insulin reactions to a client who is careless in maintaining a normoglycemic balance. These dangers include loss of consciousness, trauma caused by falling after losing consciousness, injury from poor decision making, seizures, loss of brain cells, and eventual death. Emphasize conscientious adherence to the therapeutic program.**

In other cases, hypoglycemia develops because the prescribed insulin dosage is too large or the client's dietary intake is too small. Instruct the client to record the time and probable cause of any hypoglycemic episodes on the blood test record. The health care team and the client can then evaluate the record together, making appropriate changes. Teach the client with type 1 diabetes mellitus to adjust diet and insulin by monitoring results.

Finally, be certain that the client with diabetes mellitus obtains a diabetic identification tag or medical identification bracelet or necklace and a diabetic identification card. Sometimes, a client who is experiencing an insulin reaction behaves as if intoxicated or mentally disturbed. By carrying proper identification, the client can avoid being arrested at a time when emergency care is desperately needed.

Table 45-7 compares the data and interventions for diabetic ketoacidosis, HHNS, and hypoglycemia.

As in many chronic disorders, the client needs to develop a positive self-concept and a feeling of control. Help the client and significant others understand the complications associated with diabetes mellitus. Equally important, help the client develop and maintain self-care skills that meet emotional and social needs as well as physical ones.

OTHER HYPOGLYCEMIC DISORDERS

Other manifestations of altered counterregulatory mechanisms in type 1 diabetes mellitus are (1) hypoglycemic unawareness, (2) hypoglycemia with rebound hyperglycemia (Somogyi effect), and (3) the dawn phenomenon.

Hypoglycemic Unawareness

Hypoglycemic unawareness refers to a syndrome in which people with diabetes mellitus are unaware they are hypoglycemic and therefore do not initiate treatment. In the Diabetes Control and Complications Trial, about one third of all episodes of severe hypoglycemia seen in awake, intensively treated clients were not accompanied by manifestations of sufficient severity that clients could effectively prevent neuroglycopenia.[17] In the past, this condition was incorrectly viewed as being rare and associated only with advanced neuropathy.

Repeated episodes of hypoglycemia seem to blunt the hormonal defense mechanisms that prevent it (blunted epinephrine response) and the client's ability to perceive early manifestations.

Beta-adrenergic–blocking agents (such as propranolol) can cause hypoglycemic unawareness and blunt adrenergic (epinephrine) effects in clients with diabetes mellitus, because these effects are primarily mediated by beta-adrenergic receptors. Therefore beta-blockers are contraindicated in clients with diabetes mellitus.

Clients with hypoglycemic unawareness (absence of manifestations of hypoglycemia when glucose level is less than 55 mg/dl) require consultation with an experienced physician. Increasing the frequency of SMBG levels particularly before driving and after exercise, should be encouraged. Clients may wish to choose a slightly higher blood glucose target before meals and during the night.

TABLE 45–7 Acute Complications of Diabetes Mellitus

	Diabetic Ketoacidosis (DKA)	Hyperglycemic, Hyperosmolar, Nonketotic Syndrome (HHNS)	Hypoglycemia
Type of diabetes	Usually type 1; may occur in type 2	Type 2	Type 1 or type 2
Clinical manifestations	Warm/dry skin, nausea, vomiting, flushed appearance, dry mucous membranes, soft eyeballs, Kussmaul's respirations or tachypnea, abdominal pain, impaired consciousness, hypotension, tachycardia, acetone breath, acute weight loss Polyuria (early) Oliguria/anuria (late)	Same as for DKA, except Kussmaul's respirations and acetone breath usually not present Alterations in level of consciousness, severe dehydration Nausea and vomiting not present Tachypnea, shallow respirations	Mild reaction: tremors, palpitations, pallor, sweating, hunger Moderate reaction: headache, irritability, drowsiness, weakness, visual disturbances, decreased mental acuity Severe reaction: loss of consciousness, seizures
Precipitating factors	Undiagnosed diabetes Omission of insulin dose Puberty Infection Cardiovascular disorder Other physical or emotional stress, such as pregnancy or surgery Trauma	Undiagnosed diabetes Infection or other stress Medications: phenytoin sodium (Dilantin), thiazide diuretics, steroids, chlorpromazine Dialysis GI bleed Hyperalimentation, myocardial infarction Acute pancreatitis Central nervous system disorders Major burns rehydrated with high volumes of glucose	Delay or omission of meal Insulin overdose Excessive exercise Improper timing of insulin and food
Onset of manifestations	Slow (hours to days) or quickly	Slow (hours to days)	Rapid (minutes to hours)
Laboratory findings			
Plasma glucose	300-1500 mg/dl	600-2000 mg/dl	60 mg/dl or less
Serum sodium	Normal or decreased	Normal or increased	Normal
Serum potassium	Normal or elevated at first, then decreased	Same as for DKA	Normal
Blood urea nitrogen	Elevated	Elevated	Normal
Serum ketones	Elevated	Absent	Absent
White blood cells	Elevated	Elevated	Normal or elevated
Hematocrit	Elevated	Elevated	Normal
Urine glucose	Elevated	Elevated	Absent
Urine ketones	Elevated	Absent	Absent
Arterial blood gas	Metabolic acidosis with compensatory respiratory alkalosis	Normal (metabolic acidosis of shock is profound and prolonged)	Normal or slight respiratory acidosis
pH	Less than 7.3	Usually normal or slightly decreased	Normal
Osmolality	300-350 mOsm/L	Usually over 350 mOsm/L	Normal
Acute intervention	IV regular insulin IV fluids such as normal saline or half normal saline Potassium when urine output is adequate Sodium bicarbonate, rarely Phosphate, usually Electrocardiogram Correct underlying problem	Correct underlying problem IV regular insulin IV fluids such as normal saline or half normal saline Potassium when urine output is adequate	Mild reaction: 10-15 g of simple carbohydrate Moderate reaction: one or more simple carbohydrates, glucagon may be needed, 0.5-1 mg Severe reaction: glucagon IM or subcutaneously, repeat × 1 in 10 min prn, may need IV glucose
Preventive measures	Prompt medical attention when necessary Plan ahead for illness care Frequent SMBG checks during illness or stressful events	Frequent SMBG checks during illness or stressful events Prompt medical attention when necessary	Sleeping late should be planned in advance; if oversleeping >45 min is planned, changes in insulin or food intake may be necessary Have short-acting carbohydrate available when exercising or reduction of insulin dose before exercise Restrict alcohol intake Double-check insulin type and dosage before administration

GI, Gastrointestinal; IM, intramuscularly; IV, intravenously; SMBG, self-monitored blood glucose.

Self-management education and follow-up must be intensified for these clients. For clients with type 1 diabetes mellitus, maintaining good control is as much of a problem during the night as at any other time of day.

Hypoglycemia with Rebound Hyperglycemia (Somogyi Effect)

Hypoglycemia followed by rebound hyperglycemia, known as the *Somogyi effect* or *Somogyi phenomenon,* may complicate diabetes mellitus management. This phenomenon was implicated in the past as a common cause of fasting morning hyperglycemia. Studies have found it to be a rare occurrence. It usually results from excessive evening insulin dosing. The pathophysiology involves hypoglycemia, leading to counterregulatory hormone secretion and resultant liver production of glucose. This increase in glucose level, along with insulin resistance secondary to increased hormone levels, is thought to contribute to rebound hyperglycemia.

Nocturnal rebound hyperglycemia should be investigated by SMBG levels between 2:00 and 4:00 AM and again at 7:00 AM. If early-morning levels are less than 50 to 60 mg/dl and those at 7:00 AM are greater than 180 to 200 mg/dl, rebound hyperglycemia may have occurred. Decreasing the intermediate-acting insulin dose at supper time, moving the intermediate-acting insulin dose to bedtime, or increasing the size of the bedtime snack should prevent this phenomenon.

Dawn Phenomenon

The dawn phenomenon refers to an early-morning (4 to 8 AM) increase in blood glucose level without preceding nocturnal hypoglycemia. Dissipation of insulin does not appear to be the sole cause of this phenomenon. It has been found in people with both type 1 and type 2 diabetes mellitus and probably occurs in people without diabetes mellitus. Growth hormone, increased insulin clearance, and diurnal variation in counterregulatory hormone levels seem to play a role.

The key clinical implication of the dawn phenomenon is that attempts to normalize pre-breakfast glucose levels often result in early-morning hypoglycemia. SMBG and education about bedtime snacks, manifestations of nocturnal hypoglycemia, and the importance of avoiding hypoglycemia are vital. Investigation has shown positive effects with the use of Ultralente instead of NPH insulin in the elimination of this phenomenon.

CHRONIC COMPLICATIONS OF DIABETES MELLITUS

Clients with diabetes mellitus are living longer, with an increased risk for development of chronic complications (Box 45-9). Chronic complications are the major causes of morbidity and mortality in clients with diabetes mellitus. These changes affect many body systems and can be devastating to clients and their families; they affect clients with both type 1 and type 2 diabetes mellitus. Diabetes-related complications are classified as one of two types:[26]

- *Macrovascular,* including coronary artery disease, cerebrovascular disease, hypertension, peripheral vascular disease, and infection
- *Microvascular,* including retinopathy, nephropathy, and neuropathy

Sustained increases in glucose levels create an imbalance of substances used for making the matrix between cells. Enzyme systems normally convert glucose to other sugars, such as sorbitol and fructose, to lower blood glucose level. Sorbitol, fructose, and glucose accumulate in the basement membrane of the cell and between the cells. Intracellular accumulations of sorbitol cause intracellular edema and affect function.

The microcirculation is affected by extracellular accumulation of glucose, sorbitol, and fructose. The thickened basement membrane increases the distance over which nutrients and waste products must travel to and from the cell. As a result, the cells receive inadequate oxygen and nutrition and cannot rid themselves of waste. Unfortunately, the process starts as early as 2 years after the onset of diabetes mellitus.

Clinicians often see clients with diabetes mellitus in the hospital with an MI, with loss of cognitive or physical function as a result of a stroke, or with a lower limb amputation necessitated by peripheral vascular disease. Prevention of these all-too-common macrovascular health problems should be a major focus of nurses working with clients with diabetes mellitus (Table 45-8).

BOX 45-9 Chronic Complications of Diabetes Mellitus

MACROVASCULAR COMPLICATIONS
- Coronary artery disease
- Cerebrovascular disease
- Hypertension
- Peripheral vascular disease
- Infection

MICROVASCULAR COMPLICATIONS
- Retinopathy
- Nephropathy
- Leg and foot ulcers
- Sensorimotor neuropathy
- Autonomic neuropathy
  - Pupillary
  - Cardiovascular
  - Gastrointestinal
  - Genitourinary

TABLE 45–8 Macrovascular Disease in Diabetes Clinical Manifestations, Diagnosis, and Interventions

Clinical Manifestations	Diagnosis	Interventions
Cerebrovascular Disease		
Atherothromboembolic infarctions *(transient ischemic attacks and cerebral vascular accidents)* are more severe, have higher mortality rate, have higher recurrence rate	History Manifestations Physical examinations Computed tomography scan Magnetic resonance imaging	Same as for non-diabetic clients, plus improved glucose control, aspirin, dipyridamole, ticlopidine; ongoing education and support
Heart Disease (Coronary Heart Disease)		
Diabetic clients have higher incidence of coronary artery changes that influence decreased oxygen and nutrients to myocardium	History Manifestations Physical examinations Electrocardiogram Cardiac enzymes Cardiac catheterization Stress test Autopsy	Same as for non-diabetic clients with cerebrovascular disease, plus improved glucose control, exercise, diet Hypertension control: use of diuretics may worsen hyperglycemia if hypokalemia exists and may adversely affect lipid levels Beta-adrenergic blockers (may cause hypoglycemia), calcium-channel blockers, thrombolytic agents, aspirin, angioplasty, bypass surgery
Clients have more *angina* and higher mortality with *myocardial infarction;* manifestations are often "silent"		
Clients with a history of diabetes mellitus and myocardial infarction have higher incidence of *heart failure, shock,* and *dysrhythmias*		
Cardiomyopathy may occur secondary to small vessel infarctions, causing myocardial fibrosis and hypertrophy		
Additional coronary artery disease manifestations: *Exertional weakness, peripheral edema, orthopnea, fatigue*		
Features such as female gender, which normally protects from premature heart disease, do not pertain to individuals with diabetes		
Peripheral Vascular Disease (PVD)		
The incidence of *carotid bruits, intermittent claudication, absent pedal pulses,* and *ischemic gangrene* is increased in diabetes mellitus	History Manifestations Physical examinations Doppler studies Angiogram Neuropathy identification	Daily foot inspection aimed at prevention and early intervention; meticulous foot care, padded sport socks, well-fitting shoes; weight reduction; smoking cessation; safe exercise programs; ongoing education
PVD and neuropathy augment morbidity associated with trauma and infection in lower extremity		
Hypertension		
Usually asymptomatic	History Physical examinations Orthostatic blood pressures with pulse recordings Elevated blood pressure readings at 2-3 recordings Urinalysis: 24-hr urine collection for protein, creatinine clearance, and GFR Renal angiogram to evaluate for renal artery stenosis from atherosclerotic disease	Eliminate risk factors; educate client on this silent but deadly disease; diet education: low protein, low salt Pharmacologic intervention dependent on blood pressure readings: diuretics, angiotensin-converting enzyme inhibitors, calcium-channel blockers, alpha-blockers
Infection		
Diabetic clients have higher incidence of *Pseudomonas external otitis* and *monilial skin infections;* common sites of infection in diabetic client include *urinary tract and skin*	History Manifestations Physical examinations Laboratory data: serum, increased WBCs and blood glucose; urine, increased WBCs	Improved glucose control; antibiotics, antifungals as required; follow-up with laboratory data; ongoing client education

GFR, Glomerular filtration rate; *WBC,* white blood cell.

MACROVASCULAR COMPLICATIONS

Coronary artery disease, cerebrovascular disease, and peripheral vascular disease are more common, tend to occur at an earlier age, and are more extensive and severe in people with diabetes mellitus. Macrovascular disease (disease of large arteries) reflects atherosclerosis with deposits of lipids within the inner layer of vessel walls. The risk for development of macrovascular complications is higher in those with type 1 diabetes mellitus than in clients with type 2 diabetes mellitus.

Macrovascular disease, especially coronary artery disease, is the most common cause of death in diabetic clients, accounting for 40% to 60% of all cases of diabetes-related macrovascular disease. The most common reason for hospitalization in diabetic clients is for treatment of macrovascular complications. Diabetes mellitus not only is an independent risk factor for these complications but also is a major risk factor for hypertension and hyperlipidemia. Typically, levels of very-low-density and low-density lipoproteins are increased and levels of high-density lipoproteins are decreased. The most characteristic lipid abnormality in diabetes mellitus is an elevated triglyceride level. Therefore the influence of diabetes mellitus in these diseases is multiplicative, not additive.

Macrovascular disease tends to occur years before the onset of clinical diabetes mellitus and to occur in people with impaired glucose tolerance at a rate similar to that in people with type 2 diabetes mellitus. This phenomenon, called *syndrome X,* further establishes the need for disease prevention and health promotion.

Health promotion activities include (1) managing obesity and maintaining ideal body weight, (2) exercising, (3) not smoking, and (4) achieving normal blood lipid levels. Health maintenance actions include (1) prompt recognition and treatment of hyperglycemia with exercise, food, and medication; (2) aggressive management of hypertension, including regular blood pressure checks; and (3) screening high-risk clients (e.g., those with a family history of diabetes mellitus). Health restoration activities involve (1) controlling angina, (2) treating peripheral vascular disease, (3) using SMBG to keep track of manifestations, (4) controlling risk factors for macrovascular disease, (5) stressing medication compliance and follow-up, and (6) working closely with the client.

Some speculate that type 2 diabetes mellitus may be one piece of a syndrome caused by insulin resistance. A well-established association has been demonstrated among hyperglycemia, hyperinsulinemia, dyslipidemia, and hypertension, which leads to coronary artery disease and stroke. The acronym CHAOS (*c*oronary artery disease, *h*ypertension, *a*dult-onset diabetes mellitus, *o*besity, and *s*tress) has been used to remind health care providers to look at the client's entire risk profile for cardiovascular disease when determining treatment for diabetes mellitus.

Successful weight reduction with a balanced diet improves lipid profiles, lessens glucose intolerance, lowers blood pressure, and eliminates obesity; otherwise, successful treatment of macrovascular disease in clients with diabetes mellitus parallels that in the non-diabetic population.[1,3,8]

Coronary Artery Disease

Clients with diabetes mellitus are two to four times more likely than non-diabetic clients to die of coronary artery disease, and the relative risk factor for cardiovascular disease in women with type 2 diabetes mellitus is three to four times greater. Female gender does not protect the diabetic woman from premature macrovascular disease. In many clients with diabetes mellitus, macrovascular events or processes such as coronary artery disease are atypical or silent, and they often present as indigestion or unexplained heart failure, dyspnea on exertion, or epigastric pain. Coronary artery disease is common in clients younger than age 40 years if diabetes mellitus is of long duration. Clients with diabetes mellitus who have had an MI have an increased chance of complications or of having a second infarction, compared with that in non-diabetic clients who have had an MI. After an MI, diabetic clients also experience a higher incidence of heart failure, shock, and dysrhythmias. It has been suggested that insulin therapy in type 2 diabetes mellitus may actually increase the incidence of atherosclerotic disease, because such therapy often leads to weight gain and increased blood pressure.

Cerebrovascular Disease

Prevention of cerebrovascular disease includes the same strategies as for prevention of coronary artery disease, including (1) control of hypertension, lipid levels, and obesity; (2) smoking cessation; (3) exercise; and (4) good nutritional practices.

Cerebrovascular disease, particularly atherothromboembolic infarctions manifested by transient ischemic attacks and cerebrovascular accidents (strokes), is more common and severe in clients with diabetes mellitus. The incidence is two to three times greater in diabetic clients. The relative risk is higher in females, highest in the fifth and sixth decades of life, and much higher in clients with hypertension. In the United States, the southeastern states are often referred to as the "Stroke Belt" because of the sizable African-American population in that region with its increased prevalence of hypertension. Many clients presenting with stroke have undiagnosed diabetes mellitus. In clients with diabetes mellitus, strokes are more serious and carry higher recurrence and mortality rates, especially with type 2 diabetes mellitus.

It is speculated that the increased prevalence of stroke in clients with diabetes mellitus may be related to the development of diabetic nephropathy and resultant proteinuria, hypertension, and platelet adhesiveness. Clients who present with stroke and high blood glucose levels have a much poorer prognosis than that in clients with normoglycemia. Ticlopidine, a platelet aggregation inhibitor, may be more effective than aspirin in lowering the risk of stroke, especially in clients with diabetes mellitus. This drug may also cause increased cholesterol levels and neutropenia (decreased neutrophils).

Hypertension

A 40% increased rate of hypertension has been noted in the diabetic population. Hypertension is a major risk factor for stroke and nephropathy. Inadequately treated hypertension augments the rate at which nephropathy develops. Individualized pharmacologic treatment for hypertension greater than 130/80 mm Hg is suggested for clients with diabetes mellitus. Angiotensin-converting enzyme (ACE) inhibitors and calcium-channel blockers are the agents of choice for treatment. Beta-blockers and diuretics may increase glucose tolerance and lipid levels.

Peripheral Vascular Disease

In diabetes mellitus, the incidence and prevalence of carotid bruits (abnormal sound or murmur), intermittent claudication, absent pedal (foot) pulses, and ischemic gangrene are increased. More than half of nontraumatic lower limb amputations are associated with diabetic changes such as sensory and autonomic neuropathy, peripheral vascular disease, an increased risk and rate of infection, and poor healing. This chain of events, which may lead to amputation, is illustrated in Figure 45-8.

Infections

Clients with diabetes mellitus are susceptible to infections of many types. Once infections occur, they are difficult to treat. Three factors that may contribute to the development of an infection are impaired polymorphonuclear leukocyte function, diabetic neuropathies, and vascular insufficiency. Poor glycemic control augments the importance of these factors. Infected areas heal slowly because the damaged vascular system cannot carry sufficient oxygen, white blood cells, nutrients, and antibodies to the injured site. Infections increase the need for insulin and enhance the possibility of ketoacidosis.[3,15]

Urinary tract infections are the most common type of infections affecting clients with diabetes mellitus, particularly women. One factor may be the inhibition of polymorphonuclear leukocyte activity while glucosuria is present. Glucosuria is associated with hyperglycemia. The development of a neurogenic bladder, which results in incomplete emptying and urinary retention, may also contribute to the risk of a urinary tract infection.

Diabetic foot infections are common. Their occurrence is directly related to the three factors just listed, plus hyperglycemia. Up to 40% of diabetic clients with foot infections may require amputation, and 5% to 10% will die despite amputation of the affected area. With proper education and early intervention, foot infections are usually eliminated in a timely manner.[5] Effective foot care can be the initial break in the chain of events that leads to amputation, as shown in Figure 45-8 and described in the Bridge to Home Health Care feature on p. 1103.

MICROVASCULAR COMPLICATIONS

Microangiopathy refers to changes that occur in retinal, renal, and peripheral capillaries in diabetes mellitus. The Diabetes Control and Complications Trial has made it clear that consistent and tight glycemic control may prevent or stop microvascular changes.[17]

Diabetic Retinopathy

Diabetic retinopathy is the major cause of blindness among clients with diabetes mellitus; about 80% have some form of retinopathy 15 years after diagnosis. The exact cause of retinopathy is not well understood but is probably multifactorial and associated with protein glycosylation, ischemia, and hemodynamic mechanisms. Stress from increased blood viscosity is a hemodynamic mechanism that increases permeability and decreases elasticity of capillaries.[22]

There are three types of diabetic retinopathy:

- *Nonproliferative* diabetic retinopathy is the early phase of retinopathy. It is characterized by microaneurysms (outpouching) and intraretinal "dot and blot" hemorrhages. It occurs in most clients with long-term diabetes mellitus and in many cases it does not progress or affect visual acuity.
- *Preproliferative* diabetic retinopathy involves further progression of the hemorrhages and decreasing visual acuity. It usually progresses to proliferative diabetic retinopathy.
- *Proliferative* diabetic retinopathy is the final and most vision-threatening type. The weakened and damaged vessels that have proliferated, or formed, in response to ischemia may rupture, causing retinal hemorrhage and exudates.

The retina, which is the most essential structure of the eye, has the highest rate of oxygen consumption of any tissue in the body. Consequently, if the retina is deprived of oxygen-carrying blood secondary to destruction of its capillaries, tissue anoxia (lack of oxygen) develops swiftly.[22]

Diabetic retinopathy is the leading cause of blindness in the United States among adults 20 to 74 years of age and causes from 15,000 to 24,000 new cases of blindness each year. Risk factors under investigation that may affect the development of retinopathy include chronic hyperglycemia, poor glycemic control, disease duration, hypertension, pregnancy, puberty, polyuria, and smoking (see the Client Education Guide feature on Visual Complications of Diabetes on the website).

Clinical manifestations of retinopathy typically do not develop until the later stages, when clients have acute vision problems. Blurred vision is a common manifestation that results from an abnormally high blood glucose level. In addition, seeing "floaters" or flashing lights may

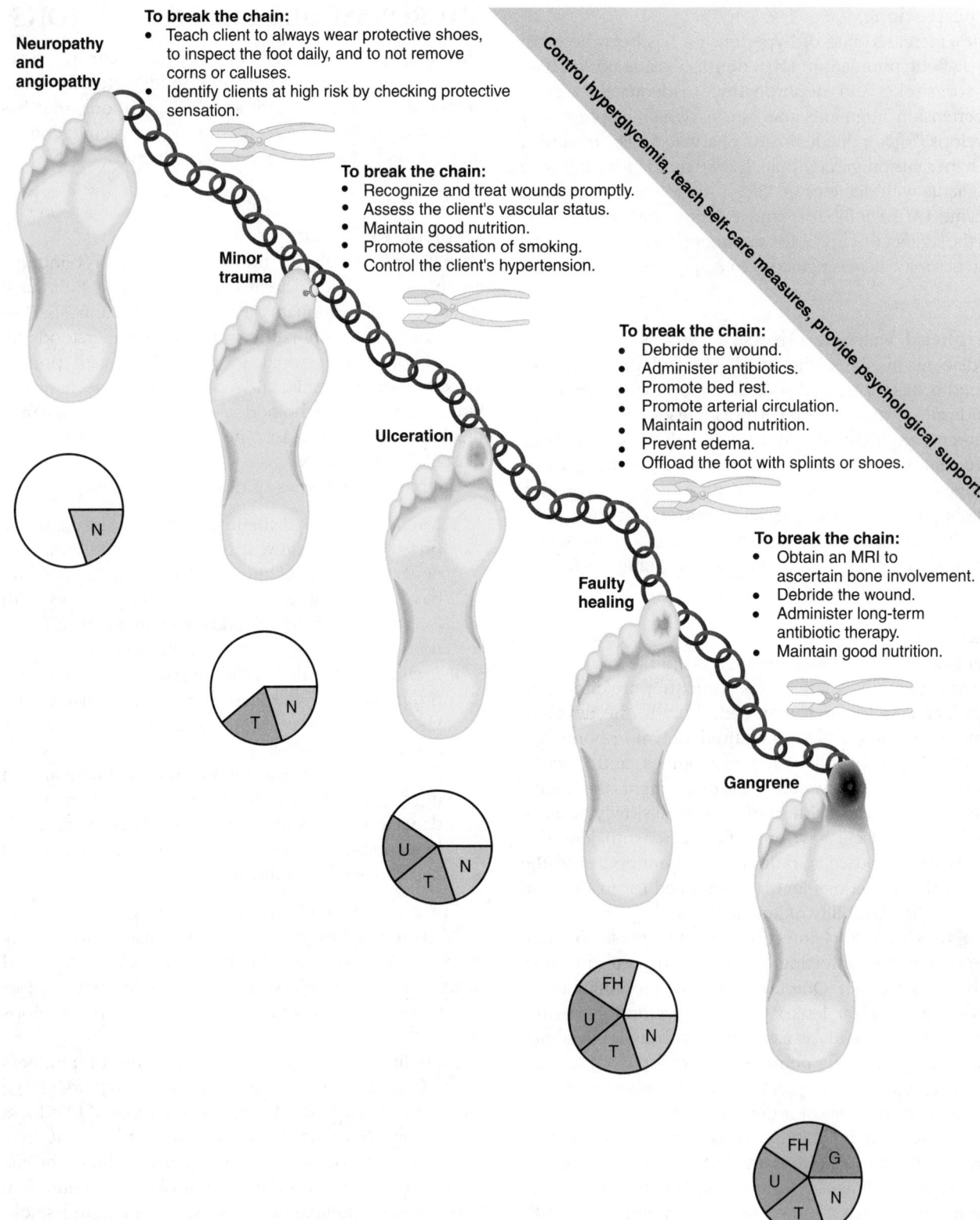

Neuropathy and angiopathy

To break the chain:
- Teach client to always wear protective shoes, to inspect the foot daily, and to not remove corns or calluses.
- Identify clients at high risk by checking protective sensation.

Minor trauma

To break the chain:
- Recognize and treat wounds promptly.
- Assess the client's vascular status.
- Maintain good nutrition.
- Promote cessation of smoking.
- Control the client's hypertension.

Ulceration

To break the chain:
- Debride the wound.
- Administer antibiotics.
- Promote bed rest.
- Promote arterial circulation.
- Maintain good nutrition.
- Prevent edema.
- Offload the foot with splints or shoes.

Faulty healing

To break the chain:
- Obtain an MRI to ascertain bone involvement.
- Debride the wound.
- Administer long-term antibiotic therapy.
- Maintain good nutrition.

Gangrene

Control hyperglycemia, teach self-care measures, provide psychological support.

■ **FIGURE 45–8** Breaking the chain of events that leads to amputation in high-risk clients with diabetes mellitus. High-risk clients (those with neuropathy, vascular disease, structural deformities, abnormal gait, skin or nail deformities, or a history of previous diabetic ulcers or amputations) need frequent monitoring by the health care team. *CT,* Computed tomography. *(Modified from Pecoraro, R.E., & Burgess, E.M. [1992]. Pathways to diabetic limb amputation: Basis for prevention. Diabetes Spectrum, 5, 329-334.)*

Foot Care for Clients with Diabetes Mellitus

People who have diabetes mellitus often develop minor foot problems that progress to major problems, and even amputation. Many foot problems can be prevented or resolved at an early stage. The most important responsibilities of the nurse in foot care for diabetic clients are assessment, education, and direct care measures.

The nurse who initially works with the client in the community needs to do a thorough diabetic assessment that includes evaluation of the client's knowledge, self-care ability, physical status, and needs. Refer the client to a physician if anything abnormal is noted. Physical assessment of the feet includes the following:

- Observation of the dermatologic condition, to detect absence of hair, diminished turgor, dry or rough skin, hyperpigmentation, fissures, calluses, ulcers, and lesions or nail problems, such as thickness or discoloration
- Evaluation of the vascular status by checking peripheral pulses, blood return after blanching, skin temperature, consistency (to rule out edema), and color
- Examination for evidence of orthopedic problems such as hammer toes or bunions
- Evaluation of the neurologic status by testing the deep tendon reflexes and response to pain, vibration, and touch

Clients who have diabetes mellitus must receive specific education about circulation, self-inspection, protection, and daily foot care. If clients cannot safely perform the necessary tasks independently, it is imperative that other caregivers accept responsibility. Some clients need a combination of helpers, including the home health care nurse, the community health nurse at a foot care clinic, family members, and informal caregivers. Medicare reimbursement for foot care and other home health services is limited. Nurses must advocate for clients and help them obtain the most appropriate and cost-effective services.

Clients who have diabetes mellitus need to maximize the circulation of their feet. Teach them to maintain good nutrition and adequate fluid intake. Instruct them not to smoke, cross their legs, or wear restrictive clothing. Demonstrate how to do foot and ankle range-of-motion exercises by writing the alphabet with their feet. Teach them to inspect all areas of their feet daily, looking for open areas, warmth, redness, discharge, formation of calluses or corns, or anything unusual.

Encourage clients to use protective measures, such as (1) always wearing good-fitting, high-quality shoes, (2) avoiding temperature extremes, and (3) seeking immediate medical attention for any injury or problem. Teach daily care of the feet that includes washing with a mild soap; drying thoroughly, especially between the toes; moisturizing feet, except between the toes; and keeping toenails trimmed. If it is necessary to soak feet before trimming toenails, do not soak for longer than 5 to 10 minutes.

Routine foot care performed by nurses in the community may include care of the skin (washing, drying, lubricating, massaging), removal of corns and calluses (shaving to healthy skin with a file or blade), and cutting the toenails. Toenails should be cut straight across or with a slight curve following the shape of the toe and filed smooth to prevent pressure or cutting of adjacent toes.

As with any nursing procedure, appropriate infection control measures should be followed. Cleanse supplies properly, wear gloves and protective eye wear, and dispose of used blades following adequate disposal protocols for sharps.

---

indicate hemorrhage or retinal detachment. Because of a lack of early clinical manifestations, it is important to assess the potential for visual problems in all clients with diabetes mellitus, including the date of their last dilated pupil examination.

OUTCOME MANAGEMENT

Major interventions, particularly in the early phases, include achievement of euglycemia and normalization of blood pressure. When retinopathy threatens vision, outpatient laser therapy (photocoagulation) is usually recommended. It halts or slows the decline in vision in most diabetic clients if it is used before too much damage has occurred. Although extensive photocoagulation usually diminishes peripheral vision and may decrease night vision, its success in preserving good visual acuity makes it worthwhile despite these side effects.

If the extent or location of the damage makes photocoagulation ineffective, or if the vitreous is too scarred or clouded with blood, vision may be improved with a vitrectomy, a surgical procedure that removes the vitreous and replaces it with saline solution. About 70% of clients who have vitrectomies notice an improvement in or stabilization of their sight, and some recover enough to resume reading and driving.

Nephropathy

Diabetic nephropathy is the single most common cause of stage 5 chronic kidney disease, formerly known as end-stage renal disease (ESRD). About 35% to 45% of clients with type 1 diabetes mellitus are found to have nephropathy 15 to 20 years after diagnosis. About 20% of clients with type 2 diabetes mellitus are found to have nephropathy 5 to 10 years after diagnosis. A consequence of microangiopathy, nephropathy involves damage to and eventual obliteration of the capillaries that supply the glomeruli of the kidney. This damage leads in turn to a complex of pathologic changes and manifestations (intercapillary glomerulosclerosis, nephrosis, gross albuminuria, and hypertension).[23] Risk factors include poor glycemic control, duration of disease, and hypertension.

 Some clients self-check microalbumin levels at home. This test can detect very small quantities of urinary albumin, which can indicate very early renal disease. With worsening of the nephrosis, stage 5 chronic kidney disease or ESRD ensues. Unless the client can be maintained with hemodialysis or receives a renal transplant, uremia eventually causes death.[23]

Clients with nephropathy monitor their blood glucose levels and blood pressure at home. ACE inhibitors can be used to decrease the microalbuminuria. Hypertension should be treated aggressively, as it can be the catalyst for the progression of nephropathy. Clients with nephropathy are taught to eat a low-protein diet and to avoid nephrotoxic drugs (e.g., gentamicin).

SAFETY ALERT

If contrast dye is required for radiographic study, mannitol may be ordered, but the client must drink fluids after the test to clear the dye from the kidneys. Serum creatinine levels should be assessed before the administration of the contrast dye or other nephrotoxic agents.

Like diabetic retinopathy, diabetic nephropathy cannot be cured. However, prompt and adequate interventions for renal and bladder infections can prevent these causes of renal failure. Control of hypertension and tight glycemic control can contribute to a delay in the development of nephropathy or a decrease in its progression. Unsuccessfully treated nephropathy progresses to stage 5 chronic kidney disease also known as ESRD. Treatment at this point includes hemodialysis, peritoneal dialysis, or kidney transplantation.

Neuropathy

Neuropathy is the most common chronic complication of diabetes mellitus. Nearly 60% of diabetic clients experience it. Because nerve fibers do not have their own blood supply, they depend on the diffusion of nutrients and oxygen across the membrane. When axons and dendrites are not nourished, their transmission of impulses slows. In addition, sorbitol accumulates in nerve tissue, further diminishing both sensory and motor function. Both temporary and permanent neurologic problems may develop in clients with diabetes mellitus during the course of the illness. The neuropathy may be mild (causing minor inconveniences) or so severe that the quality of life is affected. Identified causes of diabetic neuropathy include (1) vascular insufficiency, (2) chronic elevations in blood glucose level, (3) hypertension, and (4) cigarette smoking. Clients may present with mononeuropathy or polyneuropathy and may have sensory or motor impairment, depending on which nerves are involved.[15]

Clients with high blood glucose levels often experience nerve pain. Nerve pain is different from other types of pain you may feel, such as pain from a sprained ankle or muscle ache. Nerve pain often feels like a numbness, stabbing, tingling, or burning sensation that may keep clients up at night or stop them from doing daily tasks. This is often referred to as *diabetic peripheral neuropathy* (DPN). Pregabalin (Lyrica) is the first medication approved by the FDA to treat pain that occurs with DPN and postherpetic neuralgia (phn), two of the most common forms of nerve pain. Lyrica is also approved as an adjunctive treatment for partial onset of seizures in adults. The most common side effects include dizziness, sleepiness, dry mouth, swelling of hands and feet, and blurred vision.

Mononeuropathy

Mononeuropathy, or focal neuropathy, usually involves a single nerve or group of nerves. Mononeuropathies produce sharp, stabbing pains and are usually caused by an infarction of the blood supply. The muscles innervated by nerves affected by focal neuropathies are painful and are at risk for atrophy from disuse. Treatment may include surgical decompression for compression lesions.

Polyneuropathy

Polyneuropathy, or diffuse neuropathy, involves the sensory and autonomic nerves. Sensory neuropathy is the most common type. It is commonly assessed as bilateral, symmetrical, and affecting the lower extremities. The client describes tingling, numbness, burning, and mild to total sensory loss. This complication is a major factor in injuries to the legs. Treatment includes foot care education to prevent trauma and ulcers. Painful neuropathy may be treated with tricyclic antidepressants, phenytoin, or carbamazepine. Polyneuropathy also may simply resolve spontaneously.

Autonomic Neuropathy

Autonomic neuropathy manifests itself in its effect on pupillary, cardiovascular, gastrointestinal, and genitourinary functions.

Pupillary. Autonomic neuropathy of the pupil interferes with the pupil's ability to adapt to the dark. Pupil dilation is inadequate. Clients are at risk for accidents when driving at night. The environment should be well lighted at night.

Cardiovascular. Autonomic neuropathy of the cardiovascular system is evidenced by an abnormal response to exercise. A fixed heart rate may be noted. Orthostatic hypotension may occur, which is dangerous. Resting tachycardia is another possible cardiovascular effect.

Gastrointestinal. Autonomic neuropathy commonly affects the gastrointestinal tract. The client may have dysphagia, abdominal pain, nausea, vomiting, malabsorption, postprandial hypoglycemia, diarrhea, constipation, or fecal incontinence. Gastroparesis (delayed stomach emptying) may give the client the feeling of stomach fullness. This may contribute to anorexia, decreased intake, weight loss, and labile blood glucose levels related to food malabsorption. About 20% to 30% of diabetic clients have gastroparesis, manifestations of which may be alleviated with metoclopramide (Reglan).

Genitourinary. Bladder hypotonicity, or neurogenic bladder, is a common manifestation of autonomic neuropathy. Manifestations may include straining with urination, infrequent urge to urinate with long periods of time between voiding, and a decreased urine stream. Urinary stasis may occur, leading to urinary tract infection. In the male client, autonomic neuropathy can contribute to erectile dysfunction and retrograde ejaculation. Penile injections, implantable devices, or sildenafil (Viagra) may improve function (see Chapter 38 on male reproductive problems). Women with autonomic neuropathy may experience painful intercourse, which estrogen-containing lubricants can resolve (see Chapter 39 on female reproductive problems).

CONCLUSIONS

Diabetes mellitus is a chronic disease characterized by abnormalities in carbohydrate, fat, and protein metabolism. The two major categories of diabetes mellitus are type 1 and type 2. Meal planning, exercise, and medication are the main forms of treatment. Acute complications include hyperglycemia with diabetic ketoacidosis and hypoglycemia. Chronic complications are relentlessly progressive and result from multiple changes in small and large vessels. Because diabetes mellitus is chronic, nursing management focuses on teaching the client and family how to manage the disorder on a day-to-day basis and how to assess for complications.

THINKING CRITICALLY

1. A client with type 1 diabetes mellitus takes 14 units of regular insulin and 32 units of NPH insulin subcutaneously at 7 AM and 5 PM every day. He is now hospitalized for pneumonia and nausea. It is 9:30 AM. On entering his room, you observe the client talking to his plants. What is your priority intervention? How will his confusion be resolved?

Factors to Consider. When does regular insulin level peak? What might be the underlying cause of the client's confusion? How might you confirm the presence of hypoglycemia?

2. An older woman with type 1 diabetes mellitus calls the clinic and tells the nurse that she has the flu. She tells the nurse that she

usually takes Humulin N, 12 units, and Humulin R, 8 units, every morning. She has not taken her insulin this morning because of vomiting, nausea, and an inability to eat. She tells the nurse she lives alone. What telephone advice is appropriate? How often should she monitor her blood glucose levels while she is ill?

Factors to Consider. What learning needs does the client exhibit? When should the insulin be given? Is a clinic visit warranted?

3. The client is a 72-year-old woman who has a 25-year history of type 2 diabetes mellitus. She has managed her care adequately over the years; with the advent of home glucose monitoring, her blood glucose levels have been very well controlled. Her main problem is a history of significant hypertension, controlled with a daily antihypertensive. Lately, she finds that small cuts and bruises take longer than usual to heal. What are the chronic complications of diabetes mellitus? What teaching should you consider for this client?

Factors to Consider. What risks does this client face as a result of her long-term diabetic history? How would you approach teaching about complications?

Discussions for these questions can be found on the website. evolve

BIBLIOGRAPHY

Citations appearing in red refer to primary research.

Citations appearing in blue refer to evidence-based practice guidelines and protocols.

1. American Diabetes Association. (2004). Nutrition principles and recommendations in diabetes (position statement). *Diabetes Care, 27*(Suppl 1), S36-S46.
2. American Diabetes Association. (2004). Insulin administration (position statement). *Diabetes Care, 27*(Suppl 1), S106-S109.
3. American Diabetes Association. (2004). Management of dyslipidemia in adults with diabetes (position statement). *Diabetes Care, 27*(Suppl 1), S68-S71.
4. American Diabetes Association. (2004). Physical activity/exercise and diabetes mellitus (position statement). *Diabetes Care, 27* (Suppl 1), S58-S62.
5. American Diabetes Association. (2004). Preventive foot care in people with diabetes (position statement). *Diabetes Care, 27*(Suppl 1), S63-S64.
6. American Diabetes Association. (2004). Prevention of type 1 diabetes mellitus (position statement). *Diabetes Care, 27*(Suppl 1), S133.
7. American Diabetes Association. (2004). Screening for type 2 diabetes (position statement). *Diabetes Care, 27*(Suppl 1), S11-S14.
8. American Diabetes Association. (2006). Standards of medical care for patients with diabetes mellitus (position statement). *Diabetes Care, 29*(Suppl 1), S4-S42.
9. Anderson, R., et al. (2003). Diabetes Empowerment Scale-Short Form (DES-SF). *Diabetes Care, 26*(5), 1641-1642.
10. Anderson, R., & Funnell, M. (2000). *The art of empowerment: Stories and strategies for diabetes educators*. Alexandria, Va: American Diabetes Association.
11. Anderson, R., et al. (1995). Patients' empowerment: Results of a randomized clinical trial. *Diabetes Care, 18*(7), 943-949.
12. Asp, A. (2005). Diabetes mellitus. In L. Copstead & J. Banasik (Eds.), *Pathophysiology* (3rd ed., pp. 1000-1025). Philadelphia: Saunders.
13. Bardsley, J., & Ratner, R.E. (2006). Pathophysiology of the metabolic disorder. In C. Mensing (Ed.), *The art and science of diabetes self-management: A desk reference for healthcare professionals* (pp. 143-161). Chicago: American Association of Diabetes Educators.

14. Barnett, A., et al. (2006). An open, randomized parallel-group study to compare the efficacy and safety profile of inhaled human insulin (Exubera) with metformin as adjunctive therapy in patients with type 2 diabetes poorly controlled on a sulfonylurea. *Diabetes Care, 29*, 1282-1287.

15. Bode, B. (2003). *Medical management of type 1 diabetes* (4th ed.). Alexandria, Va: American Diabetes Association.

16. Centers for Disease Control, U.S. Department of Health and Human Services. *National Diabetes Fact Sheet* 2005. Accessed 02/13/07 from www.cdc.gov/diabetes/pubs/factsheet05.htm.

17. Diabetes Control and Complications Trial Research Group. (1993). The effect of intensive treatment of diabetes on the development and progression of long-term complications in insulin-dependent diabetes mellitus. *New England Journal of Medicine, 329*(14), 977-998.

18. Drucker, D.J. (2006). Incretin-based therapies: A clinical need filled by unique metabolic effects. *Diabetes Educator, 32*(Suppl 2), S65-S71.

19. Expert Committee on the Diagnosis and Classification of Diabetes Mellitus. (2003). Report of the Expert Committee on the Diagnosis and Classification of Diabetes Mellitus. *Diabetes Care, 26*(Suppl 1), S5-S20.

20. Foley, S. (2006). Investing in diabetes management. *American Journal of Nursing, 106*(4), 19-20.

21. Funnell, M.M., & Anderson, R. (2003). Patient empowerment: A look back, a look ahead. *Diabetes Educator, 29*(3), 454-458, 460.

22. Guyton, A., & Hall, J. (2004). *Textbook of medical physiology* (11th ed.). Philadelphia: Saunders.

23. Jones, R., & Huether, S. (2006). Alterations of hormonal regulation. In K. McCance & S. Huether (Eds.), *Pathophysiology: The biologic basis for disease in adults and children* (5th ed., pp. 683-734). St. Louis: Mosby.

24. Karl, D.M. (2006). Learning to use pramlintide. *Practical Diabetology, 25*(1), 42-46.

25. Kruger, D. (2006). Symlin and Byetta: Two new antihyperglycemic medications. *Practical Diabetology, 25*(1), 49-52.

26. Lorber, D. (2006). Macrovascular disease in diabetes. In C. Mensing (Ed.), *The art and science of diabetes self-management: A desk reference for healthcare professionals* (pp. 475- 510). Chicago: American Association of Diabetes Educators.

27. Mitka, M. (2004). Metabolic syndrome recasts old cardiac, diabetes risk factors as a "new" entity. *Journal of the American Medical Association, 291*(17), 2062-2063.

28. Monnier, L., et al. (2006). Activation of oxidative stress by acute glucose fluctuations compared with sustained chronic hyperglycemia in patients with type 2 diabetes. *Journal of the American Medical Association, 295*(14), 1681-1687.

29. National Diabetes Data Group. (1979). Classification and diagnosis of diabetes mellitus and other categories of glucose intolerance. *Diabetes, 28*, 1039-1057.

30. Rave, K., Bott, S., Heinemann, L., et al. (2005). Time-action profile of inhaled insulin in comparisons with subcutaneously injected insulin lispro and regular human insulin. *Diabetes Care, 28*, 1077-1082.

31. Rolla, A.R. (2002). Insulin analog mixes in the management of type 2 diabetes mellitus. *Practical Diabetology, 21*(4), 36-43.

32. Siminerio, L. (2006). Challenges and strategies for moving patients to injectable medications. *Diabetes Educator, 32*(Suppl 2), S82-S90.

33. Steil, C.F. (2006). Pharmacologic therapies for glucose management. In C. Mensing (Ed.), *The art and science of diabetes self-management: A desk reference for healthcare professionals* (pp. 321-355). Chicago: American Association of Diabetes Educators.

33a. The Joint Commission. (2007). 2008 National Patient Safety Goals Hospital Program. Accessed 12/26/07 from www.jointcommission.org/PatientSafety/NationalPatientSafetyGoals/.

34. Umpierrez, G.E., Murphy, M.B., & Kitabchi, A.E. (2002). Diabetic ketoacidosis and hyperglycemic hyperosmolar syndrome. *Diabetes Spectrum, 15*(1), 28-36.

35. U.S. Department of Agriculture, U.S. Department of Health and Human Services. (2005). *Dietary guidelines for Americans.* Hyattsville, Md: USDA Human Nutrition Information Service.

36. U.S. Department of Agriculture. (2005). *MyPyramid.* Accessed 02/12/07 from www.mypyramid.gov

37. Weiss, S.R., Cheng, S.L., Kourides, I.A., et al. (2003). Inhaled insulin provides improved glycemic control in patients with type 2 diabetes mellitus inadequately controlled with oral agents: A randomized controlled trial. *Archives of Internal Medicine, 163*, 2277-2282.

38. White, J.R., & Campbell, R.K. (2003). Pharmacologic therapies for glucose management. In M.J. Franz (Ed.), *A core curriculum for diabetes education: Diabetes management therapies* (5th ed., Book 2, pp. 95-154). Chicago: American Association of Diabetes Educators.

evolve *Did you remember to check out the bonus material on the Evolve website and the CD-ROM, including NCLEX®-Examination Style Review Questions, Open-Book Quizzes, and Chapter Review Audio Podcasts?*

http://evolve.elsevier.com/Black/medsurg

CHAPTER 46

Management of Clients with Exocrine Pancreatic and Biliary Disorders

DIANNE M. SMOLEN

Some disorders of the exocrine pancreas and the biliary tract are acute, and others are chronic. Manifestations are often similar to those of other conditions. The nurse plays an important role in assessing the client's manifestations and in managing the outcomes of medical and surgical treatment.

DISORDERS OF THE EXOCRINE PANCREAS

A client with a pancreatic disorder may have problems with both digestion and utilization of glucose. The relative inaccessibility of the pancreas to direct examination and the nonspecificity of manifestations associated with pancreatic disorders make the diagnosis of some conditions difficult. In addition, more than 90% of the pancreas must be damaged before fat and protein digestion problems become apparent.[7]

ACUTE PANCREATITIS

Pancreatitis (inflammation of the pancreas) may be acute or chronic. Acute pancreatitis, an inflammation of the pancreas resulting in autodigestion of the pancreas by its own enzymes, is fairly common. However, it is a potentially lethal inflammatory process associated with edema, various amounts of autodigestion, fat necrosis, and sometimes hemorrhage.

Although the frequency is about 5000 new cases per year in the United States, with a mortality rate of about 10%, the number of clients who have recurrent acute pancreatitis or chronic pancreatitis is not known.[21]

The incidence of pancreatitis varies in different countries and depends on the cause (e.g., alcohol, gallstones, metabolic factors, drugs). In the United States, acute pancreatitis is related to alcohol consumption more commonly than to gallstones (second most common); in England, the opposite is true.

Etiology and Risk Factors

Acute pancreatitis has many causes, such as alcohol (ethanol) abuse, cholelithiasis (gallstones), abdominal trauma, virus infection, drugs, and metabolic factors. The mechanisms by which these conditions trigger pancreatic inflammation have not been identified.

Acute pancreatitis is thought to result from inappropriate intrapancreatic activation of proteases, which causes autodigestion of the pancreas. Exactly how this occurs is not known. It is thought that alcohol-induced pancreatitis may include a physiochemical alteration of protein that results in plugs that block the small pancreatic ductules. Biliary pancreatitis occurs when edema or an obstruction blocks the ampulla of Vater, resulting in reflux of bile into pancreatic ducts or direct injury to the acinar cells. Other causes include the following:

■ Hyperlipidemia, which may occur secondary to nephritis, castration, or exogenous estrogen administration, or as hereditary hyperlipidemia
■ Hypercalcemia arising as a result of hyperparathyroidism
■ Cholecystitis and cholelithiasis
■ Familial cases with no definite mechanism defined
■ Pancreatic tumor
■ Pancreatic trauma or pancreatic duct obstruction, such as penetrating or blunt external trauma, intraoperative manipulation, or ampullar manipulation and pancreatic ductal overdistention during endoscopic retrograde cholangiopancreatography (ERCP)

- Pancreatic ischemia during episodes of hypotensive shock, cardiopulmonary bypass, visceral atheroembolism, or vasculitis
- Drugs; although azathioprine and estrogens have been directly linked with the disease, many other drugs are believed to have an association (e.g., antibiotics, anticonvulsants, thiazide diuretics, sulfonamides, valproic acid)
- Other general causes, such as pancreatic duct obstruction, obesity, duodenal obstruction, viral infection (e.g., mumps), carcinoma, scorpion venom, ERCP, peritoneal dialysis, and factors still to be determined

Avoidance of alcohol is the best way to promote health and to reduce the risk of pancreatitis. Limiting or completely stopping ingestion of alcohol may be a health promotion, health maintenance, or health restoration activity, depending on a diagnosis or potential diagnosis of pancreatitis. Recent studies found that obesity is a major risk factor for severe pancreatitis. It is thought that increased deposits of fat around the pancreas may predispose people with pancreatitis to more extensive pancreatic necrosis. Correction of these risk factors, such as cholecystectomy for gallstones, is a health maintenance or restoration action. Risk of pancreatitis may be reduced by administration of somatostatin or gabexate mesylate, a protease inhibitor.[5]

Pathophysiology

The etiologic mechanism of pancreatic damage remains unclear. The pathologic changes occurring in the pancreas may be due to premature activation of proteolytic and lipolytic pancreatic enzymes. These enzymes are normally activated in the duodenum. The pancreas normally releases protease in an inactive form. Once protease is in the intestine, the action of intestinal enterokinase converts pancreatic trypsinogen (one of the proteases) into trypsin. In pancreatitis, however, activation of the proteases and lipases occurs before secretion into the intestine. When these enzymes are activated before they are secreted into the intestine, pancreatic tissue damage occurs.

Exactly how the enzymes become active in the pancreas is unknown, but they may be triggered by reflux of bile from the duodenum into the pancreatic duct or by pancreatic duct obstruction, as noted previously. The net effect of this enzymatic activation is autodigestion of the pancreas. Once pancreatic inflammation begins, a vicious circle continues the process of further tissue damage and enzyme activation. As the process becomes chronic, the pancreatic parenchyma is destroyed.

In most clients, acute pancreatitis is a mild disease; in 10% to 15% of clients, however, a severe form of illness develops that leads to a lengthy hospitalization, complications, and significant rates of morbidity and mortality. Such clients present a major medical challenge because

they require an intensive care setting, hemodynamic monitoring, and frequent laboratory and radiographic evaluation. It is important to predict the severity of acute pancreatitis and increased risk of dying on presentation. Several predictive scoring systems exist. However, physicians do not always use them because they are not useful predictors. The key indicators of a severe attack are identified in Box 46-1.

Clinical Manifestations

Manifestations in clients with acute pancreatitis are largely the result of activation of proteases and lipases and the resulting autodigestion of the pancreas. Manifestations vary from mild, nonspecific abdominal pain to profound shock with coma and death. The predominant clinical feature is abdominal pain caused by edematous distention of the pancreatic capsule, local peritonitis resulting from enzyme release into the peritoneum, ductal spasm, or pancreatic autodigestion stimulated by increased enzyme secretion when eating.

Pain normally begins in the mid-epigastrium as steady and boring and achieves maximal intensity several hours later. In most clients extreme epigastric or umbilical pain radiates to the back as well as to the chest, flanks, and lower abdomen. In clients with alcohol-associated pancreatitis, pain often begins 12 to 48 hours after an episode of inebriation. Clients with gallstone-associated pancreatitis typically experience pain after a large meal. Nausea and vomiting are frequently present because

---

BOX 46-1 Risk Factors That Indicate a Severe Attack of Pancreatitis

1. Organ failure*
   a. Cardiovascular hypertension (systolic blood pressure <90 mm Hg) or tachycardia (heart rate >130 beats/min)
   b. Pulmonary: Po_2 <60 mm Hg[†]
   c. Renal: oliguria (<50 ml/hr) or increasing BUN or creatinine level
   d. Gastrointestinal bleeding
2. Pancreatic necrosis
3. Obesity (BMI >29)
4. Hemoconcentration (hematocrit >44%)
5. C-reactive protein >150 mg/L
6. Trypsinogen activation peptide
   a. >3 Ranson criteria (not fully utilizable until 48 hr)[‡]
   b. APACHE II score >8 (cumbersome)[‡]
7. Age: >70 years

* Most useful.
[†] BUN, Blood urea nitrogen; Po_2, partial pressure of arterial oxygen.
[‡] Often cited, but less useful.
Data from Greenberger, N.J., & Toskes, P.P. (2005). Acute and chronic pancreatitis. In D. Kasper, et al. (Eds.), *Harrison's principles of internal medicine* (16th ed., pp. 1895-1906). New York: McGraw-Hill.

pain stimulates the vomiting center and gastric and intestinal hypomotility. Pain may be relieved by sitting with the trunk flexed and knees drawn up.

Physical examination reveals a distressed, anxious client with abdominal distention and tenderness and fever caused by paralytic ileus of the small bowel resulting from localized peritonitis. Severe hemorrhagic pancreatitis may produce two distinctive manifestations: (1) Turner's sign (bluish discoloration of the left flank) and (2) Cullen's sign (bluish discoloration of the periumbilical area). These manifestations, which occur in fewer than 3% of cases, are the result of tissue catabolism and blood-stained retroperitoneal fluid, respectively. Jaundice, caused by common bile duct obstruction by pancreatic edema, may be present in clients with gallstone-associated pancreatitis but otherwise is uncommon in the initial phase of the disease.

Clients with severe pancreatitis may exhibit severe circulatory complications, such as hypotension; pallor; cool, clammy skin; hypovolemia; hypoperfusion; obtun-

dation; and shock. Shock is not unusual; it may result from the following:

- Hypovolemia secondary to loss of blood and plasma proteins into the retroperitoneal space
- Increased formation and release of kinins, which cause vasodilation and increased vascular permeability
- Systemic effects of proteolytic enzymes released into the circulation

As many as 10% to 20% of clients have evidence of left pleural effusion or left hemidiaphragmatic elevation. Other clinical findings include subcutaneous fat necrosis and cerebral abnormalities, such as belligerence, confusion, psychosis, and coma; these are caused by hyperosmolality, hypoperfusion, and hypoxia, cerebral fat embolism, or disseminated intravascular coagulopathy. Diabetes mellitus may develop secondary to the disease.

Diagnostic evaluation discloses abnormal findings. The Integrating Diagnostic Testing feature below provides a description of these findings.

INTEGRATING DIAGNOSTIC TESTING

Pancreatitis

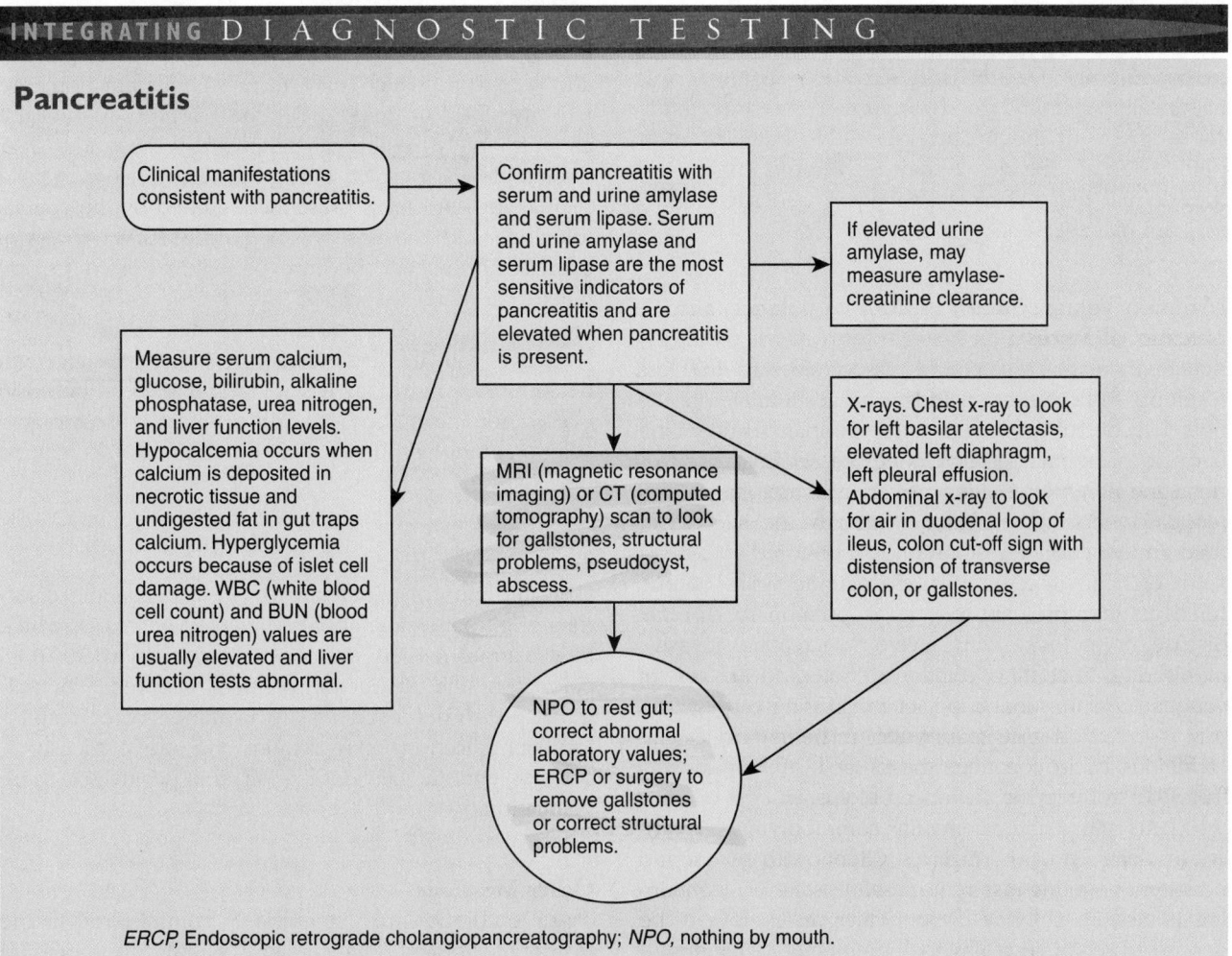

ERCP, Endoscopic retrograde cholangiopancreatography; *NPO,* nothing by mouth.

Pancreatitis in Clients with Acquired Immunodeficiency Syndrome

Pancreatitis has a higher incidence among people with acquired immunodeficiency syndrome (AIDS) because of the high prevalence of infections involving the pancreas, such as cytomegalovirus, and the frequent use of certain medications administered for treatment of AIDS, such as didanosine, pentamidine, and trimethoprim-sulfamethoxazole.

Prognosis

The mortality rate for severe acute pancreatitis is high, especially when cardiovascular, renal, or hepatic impairment is present or when pancreatic necrosis develops. Recurrences of acute pancreatitis are common in clients with alcoholic pancreatitis. See Box 46-1 for risk factors that adversely affect survival in acute pancreatitis.[7]

OUTCOME MANAGEMENT

Medical Management

Reduce Pain

Pain is usually treated with opioid analgesics, and meperidine has been the drug of choice. Morphine was historically contraindicated because it was thought to cause spasm of the sphincter of Oddi, but now morphine is an acceptable alternative.[5] Buprenorphine and transdermal fentanyl have also been used successfully for pain management.[9,11]

Maintain Volume Status, Electrolyte Balance, and Nutritional Status

Acute pancreatitis is commonly associated with fluid loss resulting from emesis. Fluids can accumulate in the bowel secondary to ileus or in the peripancreatic region because of edema. Management of the client involves replacing lost body fluids, correcting hypovolemia, and restoring electrolyte balance. Normally the success of fluid and electrolyte restoration is monitored by assessment of heart rate, blood pressure, and urine output. In clients with pre-existing cardiac, pulmonary, or renal disease or in those with severe pancreatitis, invasive monitoring, including urinary catheterization, central venous pressure monitoring, or monitoring cardiac output, is indicated. Clients with severe hemorrhagic pancreatitis may require transfusions of blood or clotting factors to correct coagulation problems.

Clients with acute pancreatitis commonly have a variety of electrolyte abnormalities. Clients with severe and persistent vomiting may require saline solutions containing potassium chloride. Serum calcium levels may be depressed secondary to hypoalbuminemia. Calcium gluconate must be given intravenously if there is evidence of hypocalcemia with tetany. Mild hyperglycemia is usually corrected with fluid volume replacement, but marked hyperglycemia or glycosuria calls for careful insulin administration.

Treatment may involve attempts to suppress pancreatic exocrine function even though they may not change the course of the disease. Therapy to decrease these enzymes may include nasogastric (NG) suction to prevent gastrin from entering the duodenum. Controlled trials, however, have indicated that NG suction may not help in treatment of mild to moderately severe acute pancreatitis. In addition, anticholinergics as well as histamine (H_2) blockers, protease inhibitors such as aprotinin, glucocorticoids, calcitonin, nonsteroidal anti-inflammatory drugs (NSAIDs), and glucagon have not been effective in treating pancreatitis. Pancreatitis may also be associated with nutritional problems when the client has been allowed nothing by mouth (NPO; *nil per os*), has nausea and vomiting, or has undergone NG suction. Nutritional problems are detailed later in this chapter.

Maintain Pancreatic Rest

Pancreatic rest involves withholding food and liquids by mouth initially because food ingestion increases pancreatic secretion, which may increase inflammation and pain. No food or fluids should be given orally until the client is largely free of pain and has bowel sounds. Clear liquids are then given, and gradual advancement to a regular low-fat diet is prescribed, guided by the client's tolerance and the absence of pain. Caution must be exercised, however, because premature return to oral intake has been associated with development of pancreatic abscess and reactivation of inflammation.

Clients with moderate to severe pancreatitis need to be supported nutritionally with total parenteral nutrition (TPN). Administration of a carbohydrate and amino acid solution along with lipids as a source of calories may be necessary.

Treat Complications

Complications of pancreatitis include pancreatic disorders (e.g., pancreatic abscess, infected necrosis), which may warrant surgery, or nonpancreatic disorders (e.g., colonic or bile obstruction or metabolic, renal, or pulmonary disorders). Clients with pulmonary or respiratory complications may require supportive measures, such as endotracheal intubation and positive-pressure ventilation.

Other Measures

Antibiotics are not routinely administered in the treatment of acute pancreatitis of mild to moderate severity because they are without proven benefit; they are generally reserved for documented infections including necrotizing acute pancreatitis.[7]

It may be necessary to perform peritoneal dialysis to rid the peritoneum of potentially toxic compounds commonly found in exudate from acute pancreatitis. Histamine, vasoactive kinins, elastase, prostaglandins, phospholipase A, trypsin, and chymotrypsin may mediate adverse systemic effects, such as hypotension, pulmonary failure, hepatic failure, and altered vascular permeability. This form of therapy is usually reserved for clients who show early clinical deterioration despite maximal intensive care support.

Nursing Management of the Medical Client

Assessment. Until a confirmed diagnosis is made, concentrate on preparing clients for diagnostic procedures and on assessing and treating manifestations of disease (see earlier discussion). Assess the location, severity, and character of the pain as well as the onset, duration, and precipitating or relieving factors. Evaluate the client's response to pain and the therapies used to relieve discomfort. Much of your role focuses on educating the client and the client's significant others about procedures and their rationales and monitoring of the client's pain level and respiratory status.

Diagnosis, Outcomes, Interventions
Diagnosis: Acute Pain. A common nursing diagnosis for the client with pancreatitis is *Acute Pain related to inflammation of the pancreas and surrounding tissue, biliary tract disease, obstruction of pancreatic ducts, and interruption of the blood supply.*

Outcomes. The client will demonstrate an absence or a decrease in pain level as evidenced by verbalizing this fact and resting quietly and showing fewer expressions of pain (e.g., grimacing, guarding of the area of discomfort, and crying).

Interventions
Administer Pain Medications. Administer pain medications in a timely manner. Other drugs are often ordered (e.g., anticholinergics, histamine receptor antagonists) to quiet the pancreas and to decrease enzyme secretion.

Promote Pancreatic Rest. The pancreatic rest program includes withholding foods and liquids by mouth and encouraging bed rest; in clients with moderately severe pain or ileus and abdominal distention or vomiting, nasogastric suction is also recommended. NG suctioning can be used to decrease gastrin release from the stomach, prevent gastric contents from entering the duodenum, remove hydrochloric acid (a powerful stimulant to the release of pancreatic enzymes), decrease distention, and promote comfort. NG suction should be considered elective rather than mandatory. Check the

system frequently to ensure that NG suction is functioning properly.

Provide Comfort Measures. Nonpharmacologic measures are often helpful in relieving pain, relaxing the client, and enhancing the effects of opioids. Correct positioning (particularly a side-lying position with the knees curled up to the chest and a pillow pressed against the abdomen or upright in a sitting position with the trunk flexed), back rubs, relaxation techniques, and a quiet environment all help to promote comfort and rest.

Diagnosis: Risk for Imbalanced Fluid Volume. A possible complication of acute pancreatitis is *Risk for Imbalanced Fluid Volume related to vomiting, nasogastric suctioning, NPO status, shifting of body fluids, fever, and diaphoresis.*

Outcomes. The client will remain in fluid balance, will be hydrated, and will maintain electrolyte levels within normal limits.

Interventions

> **Monitor vital signs for changes in pulse rate and blood pressure measurements (fluid volume changes) as well as respiratory rate (acid-base imbalance). If necessary, use hemodynamic monitoring to check for changes in fluid and electrolyte status. Electrocardiographic (ECG) findings of cardiac rhythm changes may be the first indication of electrolyte imbalance.**
>
> **Check laboratory values for significant changes, and observe for physical manifestations of hyperglycemia, hypocalcemia, and hypokalemia. Monitor the client's response to fluid administration and blood products by monitoring intake and output and assessing for edema, adventitious lung sounds, skin turgor, and mucous membrane alterations. Measure abdominal girth and monitor urine output (at least 0.5 ml/kg/hour). Report significant changes promptly because these clients are at increased risk.**

SAFETY

ALERT

Diagnosis: Imbalanced Nutrition: Less Than Body Requirements. Pancreatitis leads to many gastrointestinal manifestations, making *Imbalanced Nutrition: Less Than Body Requirements related to inability to ingest or digest food or absorb nutrients, nausea and vomiting, NPO status, and nasogastric suctioning* a common nursing diagnosis for this client.

Outcomes. The client will maintain adequate nutritional status as evidenced by maintaining normal body weight, keeping blood glucose within normal limits, and showing no evidence of muscle wasting.

Interventions. Depending on the severity of illness, these clients may be kept on NPO status until the client is largely free of pain and has bowel sounds. Nutrition may be provided through hyperalimentation and lipids (see Chapter 29).

Assess the overall nutritional status of the client by checking daily weights, tissue integrity, and the presence of adequate body fat and muscle mass. If oral intake is resumed too soon, re-exacerbation of manifestations may occur. Therefore monitor the client's response to oral intake carefully, and begin intake slowly with liquids before the client progresses to a normal diet. As noted previously, administration of antispasmodics, anticholinergics, histamine receptor antagonists, and antacids to reduce gastric and pancreatic secretions may provide some relief, but none of these therapies have been proven effective in shortening the duration of the disease, in reducing complications, or in reducing mortality.

If the pancreas has been severely damaged, it may be necessary to administer replacement pancreatic enzymes to replace the enzyme deficit and aid digestion. These drugs are discussed in the Integrating Pharmacology feature below.

Diagnosis: Ineffective Breathing Pattern. The client with acute pancreatitis has the potential for development of many problems. One appropriate nursing diagnosis is *Ineffective Breathing Pattern related to abdominal distention or ascites, pain, or respiratory complications.*

Outcomes. The client will maintain an effective breathing pattern as evidenced by a respiratory rate within normal limits, relaxed respiratory effort, absence of cyanosis, clear lungs, and a breathing pattern that supports blood gas or pulse oximetry results within normal limits.

Interventions. Assess the client's respirations for rate and effort. Your assessment should include lung auscultation for decreased lung sounds (potential for atelectasis), rales, or rhonchi (potential for pneumonia and pleural effusion), and for cyanosis. Many times, these clients have been given a prescription of bed rest, which precludes the need for prophylactic nursing interventions of pulmonary hygiene (e.g., turning, coughing, deep breathing, incentive spirometry). Keeping the client comfortable with analgesics enhances full inspiration and normal breathing patterns. Positioning, such as placing the client in the semi-Fowler or a side-lying position, may facilitate normal respiration.

Reducing anxiety, especially if alcohol abuse is known, will also improve breathing patterns. The client must be encouraged to face the problem that alcohol is causing if it is the source of the pancreatitis. Encourage the client to talk about the problem and to explore ways to cope with the illness. Recommend groups such as Alcoholics Anonymous, and encourage the client to join such a program. Discuss supportive services available with the client and the client's significant others.

Evaluation. Within a few days of treatment, the client is expected to experience less pain and gradually resume eating and drinking. For more severe cases, the client must remain on NPO status and rest the pancreas for a much longer time. If this occurs, the client will require TPN to maintain adequate nutrition.

INTEGRATING PHARMACOLOGY

Pancreatic Enzyme Replacement Therapy in Chronic Pancreatitis

Chronic pancreatitis leads to decreased pancreatic protease secretion. Proteases break down protein into basic building blocks to be used by the body for maintenance of health. Lack of proteases leads to pancreatic stimulation, causing abdominal pain. In addition, a decrease in lipase secretion results in steatorrhea (fatty stools). Proteases and lipases are necessary to help prevent maldigestion, steatorrhea, and malnutrition. In clients with chronic pancreatitis, supplementation with pancreatic enzymes provides the serine proteases and lipases necessary to correct the defects.

Pancreatic enzyme therapy is not complex and has few side effects. The effectiveness with which it works depends on factors such as enzyme formulation, dosage, frequency, and other therapies in the client's overall treatment plan. Several enzyme products are available that are enteric coated and nonenteric coated and that contain differing amounts of protease, lipase, and amylase.

Digestive enzymes such as gastric acid may alter the usual physical and chemical nature of lipase. In addition, duodenal pH can be lower than normal in chronic pancreatitis because of reduced bicarbonate secretion. Therefore acid-suppressing medications and enteric-coated enzyme preparations are often used in a client's treatment. A minimum of 30,000 international units of lipase and 10,000 international units of trypsin are needed within 4 hours postprandial to achieve adequate digestion of protein, fat, and carbohydrates.

Surgical Management

Indications
Operative intervention is indicated in four specific circumstances:

- Uncertainty of diagnosis; relief of pain
- Treatment of secondary pancreatic infection: pancreatic necrosis and pancreatic abscess
- Correction of associated biliary tract disease
- Progressive clinical deterioration despite optimal supportive care

If clients with severe pancreatitis do not respond to medical management, operative intervention may be indicated to debride necrosis or, again, to exclude other possible diagnoses as causative factors. A laparotomy with sump drainage will facilitate drainage of a pancreatic abscess.

It is usually necessary to resect necrotic tissue because undrained pancreatic abscesses are associated with a high mortality rate. Treatment of pancreatic abscess combines medical therapy with antibiotic therapy, operative debridement to remove infected necrotic material, and surgical drainage.

If the client has extensive disease of the entire gland, a subtotal pancreatectomy may be performed. The surgical procedure involves attaching a small remnant of the remaining head of the pancreas to the duodenum. A more extensive procedure, Whipple's surgical procedure (pancreaticoduodenectomy), may be necessary if the pancreatitis is confined to the head of the pancreas. In this instance, the distal third of the stomach, the duodenum, common bile duct, gallbladder, and head of the pancreas are removed.

Because it is sometimes difficult to identify acute pancreatitis, exploratory laparotomy may be indicated to eliminate processes such as perforated viscus or acute mesenteric ischemia. If uncomplicated acute pancreatitis is present, no manipulation is needed and the surgery is terminated. In presumed gallstone-associated pancreatitis, cholecystectomy and intraoperative cholangiography are favored. In clients with severe hemorrhagic pancreatitis with necrosis, debridement of necrotic tissue is performed and retroperitoneal drainage is established.

Contraindications

In the past, biliary tract surgery for gallstone-associated pancreatitis was deferred for up to 8 weeks; however, up to 35% (range, 11% to 48%) of clients awaiting elective surgery experienced a recurrence of pancreatitis. Today most surgeons proceed with surgery as soon as the initial manifestations of pancreatitis resolve.

Complications

Ileus, abdominal distention, and vomiting are possible postoperative complications that require NG suction if they occur. A serious complication of acute pancreatitis is adult (acute) respiratory distress syndrome (ARDS), which can occur within 3 to 7 days of the onset of pancreatitis and after the administration of large volumes of fluid and colloids given to sustain blood pressure and adequate urine output. See the Critical Monitoring feature above for findings mandating early intervention in these clients.

Outcomes

Clients are expected to recover from the surgical procedure and not experience postoperative complications.

CRITICAL MONITORING

Manifestations of Adult (Acute) Respiratory Distress Syndrome Secondary to Acute Pancreatitis

- Acute respiratory distress: tachypnea, dyspnea, accessory muscle breathing, and cyanosis
- Fever and dry cough that develop over a short period
- Fine crackles heard throughout lung fields on auscultation
- Possible confusion and agitation
- Hypoxemia with partial pressure of oxygen (Po_2) 50 mm Hg
- Early—hypocapnia and respiratory alkalosis
- Late—hypercapnia and respiratory acidosis

Once bowel sounds have returned, about 3 days after surgery, the NG tube is discontinued. If tube removal is tolerated and pain is relieved, the client will begin liquids within the next 24 to 72 hours. The client is discharged once a low-fat diet is tolerated.

Nursing Management of the Surgical Client

Preoperative Care

Preparing a client for pancreatic surgery requires the usual preoperative care. In addition, close monitoring of white blood cell (WBC) count, hematocrit, serum electrolytes, serum calcium, serum creatinine, urea nitrogen or blood urea nitrogen (BUN), aspartate aminotransferase (AST), lactate dehydrogenase (LDH), and arterial blood gases (ABGs) is essential. Other measures may be necessary, depending on the severity of the client's illness, such as insertion of an NG tube, continued replacement of fluids, and monitoring central venous pressure and blood culture results.

Preoperative nursing management of the client with acute pancreatitis is similar to that described under Nursing Management of the Medical Client. Pay special attention to the nutritional status of the client as well as to the breathing pattern, fluid volume and electrolyte levels, control of pain, and possible complications as the client is prepared for surgery. The client will require preoperative teaching about the procedure and what to expect postoperatively (see Chapter 14). Encourage clients to ask questions about their condition, treatment, and progress.

Postoperative Care

Assessment. After pancreatic surgery, you should have achieved the following:

1. Have a clear idea of the surgical procedure performed and its purpose, steps, and dangers.

2. Be aware of the location and purpose of each drain inserted during surgery. If there are multiple drains, especially external drains, assess each for proper function.

SAFETY

⚠

ALERT

3. Continually assess tubes or drains that are in place for decompression. If a T tube or internal stent becomes nonfunctional, alert the surgeon immediately to prevent leakage at the internal insertion site. Leakage may lead to peritonitis or fistula formation. Assess for placement, location (internal or external), and proper function and patency of the drains. If the drains do not appear to be functioning, notify the physician immediately.

After pancreatic excision, it is important to know how much pancreatic tissue was removed. When there is a decrease in endocrine tissue, control of blood glucose level with insulin and diet becomes necessary. Exocrine loss does not pose immediate postoperative problems but does necessitate lifelong enzyme replacement when oral ingestion is resumed. Assess the functional ability of remaining pancreatic tissue after excision of the pancreas, determining both endocrine and exocrine functioning and its long-term implications. If the client has lost all endocrine function, insulin administration will be necessary (see Chapter 45). Continue to monitor the client for manifestations of hypoglycemia and hyperglycemia.

With the loss of exocrine function, replacement of pancreatic enzyme function with medications such as pancrelipase (Pancrease) becomes necessary (see the Integrating Pharmacology feature on Pancreatic Enzyme Replacement Therapy in Chronic Pancreatitis on p. 1112). When the client begins to eat, watch for the development of diarrhea and steatorrhea (fatty stools), which indicate that insufficient pancreatic enzymes are present.

Diagnosis, Outcomes, Interventions. See the nursing diagnoses discussed under Nursing Management of the Medical Client (in the section on acute pancreatitis) relating to pain, fluid and electrolyte balance, ineffective breathing pattern, and nutrition. All are applicable in the postoperative situation. In addition, the following nursing diagnoses are specifically related to the postoperative period.

Diagnosis: Ineffective Therapeutic Regimen Management/ Effective Therapeutic Regimen Management. After pancreatectomy, the client will have many and complex learning needs, leading to the nursing diagnosis *Ineffective Therapeutic Regimen Management/Effective Therapeutic Regimen Management related to care, postoperative pain, nutritional needs, diabetic care, pancreatic enzyme replacement, or alcohol abuse and need for follow-up care.*

Outcomes. The client will understand discharge instructions, as evidenced by the ability to describe and demonstrate appropriate wound care, diet, proper diabetes care, activity and exercise level, and correct administration and side effects of the medication regimen. In addition, the client will collaborate with health providers to decide on a therapeutic regimen that is congruent with health goals and lifestyle and treatment of alcoholism, if present. If alcoholism is present, encourage the client to seek help with stopping drinking before irreversible damage is done.

Interventions. Assess the knowledge of the client and the client's significant others before providing appropriate learning guidelines preceding the client's discharge. Provide instructions for wound care. The client will require changes in diet as necessitated by diabetes mellitus. Provide guidelines for nutritional needs and an appropriate low-fat diet.

Provide the client with important information concerning diabetes mellitus, including information about hyperglycemia (polyuria, polydipsia, and polyphagia) and hypoglycemia (see Chapter 45). Explain medications (pancreatic enzymes), including action, side effects, and when to notify the physician. If the client has had surgery, routine postoperative teaching (see Chapter 14) and education about the care of drains (if still in place) will be needed.

Evaluation. If no complications arise, the client can be discharged about a week after surgery. Hence a visiting nurse may visit the client after discharge to assess the client's ability to follow the postoperative regimen. The client will need to be seen at regular intervals to ensure adherence to the regimen.

The client's ability to abstain from alcohol should be assessed carefully and further counseling provided as needed. In the short term, the client should recover from acute pancreatitis without complications. Long-term recovery, however, often depends on the client's willingness and ability to alter lifestyle.

Self-Care

Because of the complex nature of pancreatitis and the importance of the client's understanding of how to lower the risk of recurrence, clients must become knowledgeable about the causes of the disease, treatment, possible complications, and home health care. Before discharge home, ask the client and significant others to verbalize home health care needs related to diet; medications, including indications, dosage, frequency, and side effects; and the manifestations of recurrence.

Medications. Assess the client's level of understanding and learning needs. Discuss the medication regimen with the client, including its purpose, dosage, frequency, and possible side effects. Explain that an insulin supplement may be required because of pancreatic damage.

Begin your teaching as soon as possible to ensure that the client and the client's significant others are fully prepared to cope with glucose monitoring, diet, and insulin administration (see Chapter 45).

Diet Modifications. Instruct the client about dietary restrictions, such as avoiding alcohol, tea, coffee, spicy foods, and heavy meals, which stimulate pancreatic secretions and produce attacks of pancreatitis. Clients should understand the benefit of eating small, frequent meals high in protein, low in fat, and moderate to high in carbohydrate.

Teach Manifestations of Recurrence. Ensure that the client is aware of the manifestations of recurrence of pancreatitis and the importance of reporting these manifestations immediately. These manifestations include steatorrhea; severe back or epigastric pain; persistent gastritis, nausea, and vomiting; weight loss; elevated temperature; and evidence of hyperglycemia.

CHRONIC PANCREATITIS

Chronic pancreatitis is a progressive, inflammatory, destructive disease of the pancreas most often caused by alcoholism (70% to 80% of all cases).[5]

Pathophysiology

Chronic pancreatitis involves progressive fibrosis and degeneration of the pancreas. Characteristically, the pancreas is progressively destroyed by repeated flares of usually mild attacks of pancreatitis. After repeated attacks of acute pancreatitis, this inflammatory process results in scarring and calcification of pancreatic tissue. The damage is irreversible, affecting both endocrine and exocrine pancreatic functions.

In the United States and in other industrial countries, chronic alcoholism is the most frequent cause of chronic calcifying pancreatitis. In up to 25% of American adults, chronic pancreatitis is of unknown or idiopathic cause; it may also be hereditary. A gene for hereditary pancreatitis (cystic fibrosis transmembrane conductance regulator [CFTR]), transmitted as an autosomal dominant trait with variable penetrance, has been identified on chromosome 7. Protein malnutrition is a cause in other parts of the world. Other causes include untreated hyperparathyroidism, congenital anomalies, and pancreatic trauma.

Clinical Manifestations

In chronic pancreatitis, as in acute pancreatitis, pain may be continuous, intermittent, or absent; clients with severe pain may also experience vomiting, constipation, fever, and jaundice. The client may reduce pain or experience some pain relief by sitting in bed with the knees flexed and pressing a pillow to the abdomen. The client

generally experiences more pain when supine. Attacks may last only a few days or as long as 2 weeks.

Because food may worsen the pain, the client usually reduces food intake, resulting in weight loss. Reduction in digestive enzyme secretion eventually causes malnutrition and contributes to the weight loss. Ultimately, because of involvement of islet tissue, hyperglycemia develops with manifestations of diabetes mellitus. Type 1 diabetes mellitus occurs in up to one third of clients.

The client also suffers from (1) abdominal distention with flatus and cramps, (2) the presence of scattered calcification throughout the pancreas as noted radiographically, and (3) frequent passage of foul fatty stools (steatorrhea). Thus the clinical group of manifestations that serves as a classic presentation of chronic pancreatitis is abdominal pain, weight loss, pancreatic calcification, diabetes mellitus, and steatorrhea. In addition, many clients present with a history of opioid analgesic abuse in an effort to control pain. Pain or digestive disturbance may motivate a person with chronic pancreatitis to seek help.

See the Integrating Diagnostic Testing feature for specific information on diagnostic testing. Also, see the Translating Evidence into Practice feature on p. 1116.

OUTCOME MANAGEMENT

Medical Management

Relieve Pain

The control of pain can be a major problem and is generally the sole indication for surgical intervention. Attempts to control pain pharmacologically should begin with non-opioid analgesics and should progress to opioid analgesics, if needed. Surgical procedures may also be an option.[7] For alcohol-related pancreatitis, total abstinence from alcohol is imperative and sometimes successful in itself for pain reduction. The diet should be low in fat according to one source,[5] although another source advocates a diet moderate in fat (30%), high in protein (24%), and low in carbohydrate (40%).[7]

Steatorrhea may be treated with pancreatic supplements selected for their high lipase activity. See the Integrating Pharmacology feature on Pancreatic Enzyme Replacement Therapy in Chronic Pancreatitis on p. 1112. Concurrent administration of sodium bicarbonate H$_2$-receptor antagonists (e.g., ranitidine) or a proton pump inhibitor (e.g., omeprazole) may decrease the inactivation of lipase by acid and thereby may further decrease steatorrhea.

Treat Endocrine Insufficiency

Exogenous insulin therapy may be necessary because of destruction of islet tissue.

TRANSLATING EVIDENCE INTO PRACTICE

Chronic Pancreatitis, Pain, Malabsorption, and Poor Nutritional Status

The causes of chronic pancreatitis include prolonged alcohol use, pancreatic duct obstruction, pancreas divisum, hereditary pancreatitis, hypertriglyceridemia, hypercalcemia, trauma, and occasionally cystic fibrosis. In about 25% of affected people, no cause is identified.[1]

Chronic pancreatitis is characterized by a gradual and irreversible loss of pancreatic tissue structure and function. There is a loss of pancreatic acinar cells and progressive scarring of pancreatic tissue that result in a decrease in enzyme output. Enzymes that are diminished include lipase, amylase, and proteases. A lack of these enzymes leads to maldigestion, malabsorption of nutrients, and eventually malnutrition if untreated. Steatorrhea, which is the passage of fat in the stool, is the primary manifestation of malabsorption. It occurs when greater than 90% to 95% of pancreatic function is lost.[2] In addition, eating induces abdominal pain, and this causes poor oral intake, weight loss, and poor nutritional status. How can these clients be managed properly to avoid weight loss, reduce their risk for nutritional deficiencies, and still be treated effectively for the pain?

According to current research, treatment for clients with chronic pancreatitis is directed toward two major problems: abdominal pain and malabsorption.[2] The pain is often severe enough to require the use of opioids, further reducing the appetite. Clients with severe and persistent pain need to avoid alcohol completely as well as large meals rich in fat. When the pain is severe enough to require opioids (and hence addiction), a number of surgical procedures may be performed to relieve that pain. One procedure, an ERCP, may provide some pain reduction with a sphincterotomy of the pancreatic sphincters, dilation of strictures, removal of calculi, or stenting of the pancreatic ducts. In some clients, pain reduction may come only as a result of a pancreatic resection, although these clients tend to develop pancreatic endocrine and exocrine insufficiency and must be treated with enzyme replacement therapy. Recent studies have indicated that administration of pancreatic enzymes may decrease abdominal pain in selected clients with chronic pancreatitis.[2] The clients most likely to benefit are those with mild to moderate exocrine pancreatic dysfunction.

For managing maldigestion, treatment with pancreatic enzyme replacement therapy may be helpful.[1,2] Diarrhea and steatorrhea may be improved with this treatment, although steatorrhea may not be completely corrected.[1] The use of pancreatic enzymes to reduce the pain of chronic pancreatitis has been variable and has presented somewhat controversial results.[3] Overall, pancreatic enzyme supplementation is safe, well tolerated, and beneficial for clients with chronic pancreatitis.[4]

IMPLICATIONS

Nurses caring for clients with chronic pancreatitis on a gastroenterology unit or in the outpatient setting should carefully monitor the client's weight, height, and serum pre-albumin and albumin levels as a part of the routine nursing assessment. These measures are effective screening methods to detect clients at risk for poor nutritional status. Documentation of the results of the assessment is also important to establish a baseline of information and to monitor the client's progress. Nurses should be aware that therapy could be individualized by the physician to meet each client's nutritional needs.

REFERENCES

1. Greenberger, N.J., & Toskes, P. (2005). Acute and chronic pancreatitis. In D. Kasper, et al. (Eds.), *Harrison's principles of internal medicine* (16th ed., pp. 1895-1906). New York: McGraw-Hill.
2. Lichtenstein, D.R. (2004). Diseases of the pancreas. In T.E. Andreoli, et al. (Eds.), *Cecil essentials of medicine* (6th ed., pp. 379-387). Philadelphia: Saunders.
3. Steer, M.L. (2004). Exocrine pancreas. In C.M. Townsend, et al. (Eds.), *Sabiston textbook of surgery* (17th ed., pp. 1643-1678). Philadelphia: Saunders.
4. Trolli, P.A., Conwell, D.L., & Zuccaro, G. (2001). Pancreatic enzyme therapy and nutritional status of outpatients with chronic pancreatitis. *Gastroenterology Nursing*, 24(2), 84-87.

Treat Exocrine Insufficiency

Exocrine insufficiency is treated with exogenous pancreatic enzyme therapy. See the Integrating Pharmacology feature on Pancreatic Enzyme Replacement Therapy in Chronic Pancreatitis on p. 1112. This therapy may include lipase, trypsin, or H_2-receptor antagonists.

Surgical Management

Several surgical approaches are available. The major surgical procedures are depicted in Figure 46-1. The four major goals of surgical intervention for chronic pancreatitis are to achieve the following:

1. Correct the primary tract disease (ampullar procedure)
2. Relieve ductal obstruction (ductal drainage procedure)
3. Alleviate pain (ablative procedure)
4. Alleviate pain (denervation procedure)

Endoscopic or surgical drainage is indicated for pseudocysts that cause manifestations. Pancreatic ascites or pancreaticopleural fistulae resulting from a disrupted pancreatic duct can be managed by endoscopic placement of a stent across the disrupted duct. Breaking up stones (calculi) in the pancreatic duct by lithotripsy is rarely done today, but endoscopic removal of stones from the duct at ERCP or placement of a stent across pancreatic duct strictures may reduce pain. For clients with chronic pain and nondilated ducts, a percutaneous celiac plexus nerve block may be ordered, although results are often disappointing.

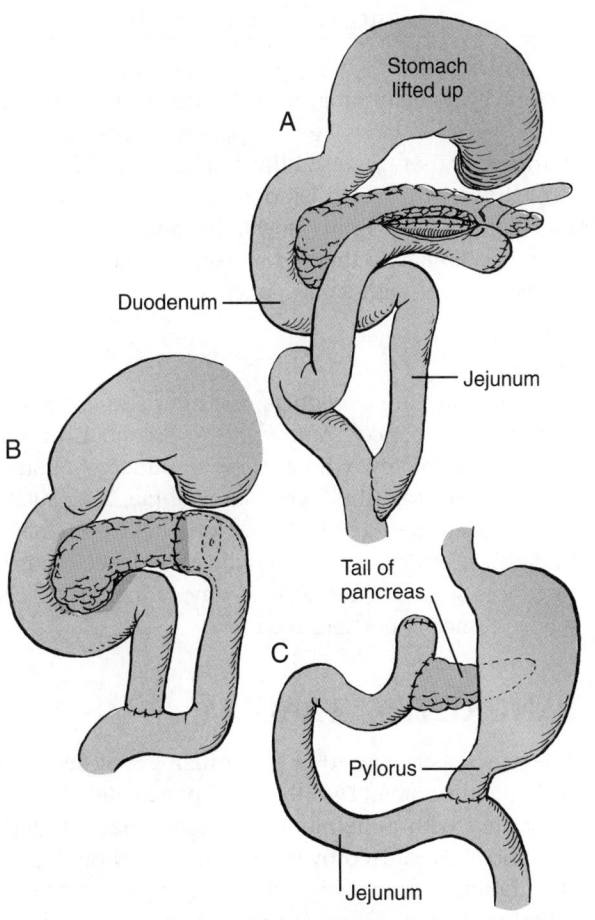

Stomach
lifted up

A

Duodenum

Jejunum

B

Tail of
pancreas

C

Pylorus

Jejunum

A. **Side-to-side pancreaticojejunostomy (ductal drainage)**
Indicated when gross dilation of pancreatic ducts is
associated with septa and calculi. The most successful
procedure, with rates of 60% to 90%.

B. **Caudal pancreaticojejunostomy (ductal drainage)**
Indicated for the uncommon cases of isolated proximal
pancreatic ductal stenosis not involving the ampulla.

C. **Pancreaticoduodenal (right-sided) resection (ablative)
(with preservation of pylorus) (Whipple procedure)**
Indicated when major changes are confined to head of
pancreas. Preservation of pylorus avoids usual sequelae
of gastric resection.

■ **FIGURE 46–1** Surgical procedures for chronic pancreatitis and pancreatic cancer.

The prognosis for the client with chronic pancreatitis is good if acute attacks decrease in frequency. Replacement therapy for chronic fat indigestion permits a fairly normal life. If the client continues to drink alcohol, the prognosis is poor. Repeated attacks eventually cause death from shock or renal failure. The most common complication is addiction to narcotics.[7]

PANCREATIC PSEUDOCYSTS

Pancreatic pseudocysts are localized collections of pancreatic secretions (high concentrations of amylase, lipase, and trypsin) in a cystic structure usually adjacent to the pancreas rather than within the parenchyma. Pseudocysts account for up to 75% of all cystic lesions of the pancreas. They develop in up to 15% of clients after an attack of acute alcoholic pancreatitis, but they may be associated with acute pancreatitis of other causes, chronic pancreatitis, trauma, and pancreatic cancer.

The most common clinical picture of a client with pancreatic pseudocyst involves abdominal pain, early satiety, nausea, and vomiting. Less common manifestations include pruritus, jaundice, sepsis, and hemorrhage. Diagnosis of pseudocyst is made through the same assessment as that used for pancreatitis.

Treatment is based on the presence or absence of manifestations, the client's age, and the size of the cyst. Cysts smaller than 6 cm in diameter often resolve spontaneously. Clients with such cysts are followed up with frequent ultrasound studies to determine whether the cyst is decreasing in size. Clients with persistent manifestations or pseudocyst-related complications, such as infection, require operative intervention. Erosion of an inflammatory process into a blood vessel can result in a major hemorrhage into the cyst.

Surgical procedures include internal drainage of the pseudocyst (cystojejunostomy, cystogastrostomy, and cystoduodenostomy), pancreatic resection, distal pancreatectomy, and, least often, percutaneous or endoscopic drainage.

PANCREATIC CANCER

Cancer is the most common neoplasm affecting the pancreas. About 75% of cancers occur in the head of the pancreas, and 25% are in the body and tail of the pancreas.[5] Pancreatic cancer is the fourth most common cause of death from cancer, exceeded only by lung, colorectal, and breast (in women) or prostate (in men) cancer.[5] Of clients with pancreatic cancer, 90% die within the first year of diagnosis. Mutations in *K-ras* genes have been found in specimens of human pancreatic cancer and associated with mutation of the *p16INK4* gene located on chromosome 9.[11] Cancer of the pancreas is more common in blacks than in whites, in smokers, and in men. It appears to be linked to diabetes mellitus, the use of alcohol, a history of previous pancreatitis, smoking, ingestion of a high-fat diet, obesity, and organic chemicals, such as coke, coal, gas, and benzidine.

Risk factors include age, obesity, prior abdominal radiation, and family history. Research indicates that obesity significantly increases the risk of pancreatic cancer, but physical activity appears to decrease this risk, especially among overweight people. Health promotion actions include avoidance of risk factors and pancreatitis. Health maintenance and health restoration activities are limited because of the poor prognosis associated with pancreatic cancer.

Duct cell adenocarcinoma accounts for more than 90% of cell types of malignant pancreatic exocrine tumors. Less common types of pancreatic exocrine cancer include cystadenocarcinoma and acinar cell carcinoma. Periampullary adenocarcinomas originate in the region of the ampulla of Vater. Clients typically present with jaundice, significant unexplained weight loss, and abdominal pain. Many clients are managed operatively by either resection (approximately 30%) or palliative therapy to relieve manifestations such as jaundice.[11]

Carcinomas of the tail and body of the pancreas usually present with significant weight loss and abdominal pain. Because of their location, these tumors generally grow to a large size before manifestations occur and the diagnosis is made. Therefore the resectability rate is low (<7%), and the prognosis is poor (a 5- to 6-month mean survival). The response to chemotherapy (fluorouracil) that has been most promising has been achieved through use of radiation therapy combined with either 5-fluorouracil or gemcitabine.[18]

OUTCOME MANAGEMENT

Medical Management

Medical treatment for pancreatic cancer includes radiation therapy (e.g., high-dose external beam, interstitial seed of iodine-125 or iridium-192, brachytherapy, and intraoperative radiation therapy) and drugs (e.g., 5-fluorouracil alone or with radiation therapy and nitrosourea, mitomycin-C, and doxorubicin).

Surgical Management

Surgical treatment is Whipple's surgical procedure, when lesions are strictly limited to the head of the pancreas. The operation involves a pancreaticoduodenectomy with removal of the distal third of the stomach, pancreaticojejunostomy, gastrojejunostomy, and choledochojejunostomy (see Figure 46-1). Nursing care for these clients is similar to that for Nursing Management of the Surgical Client with acute pancreatitis.

Prognosis

Mortality rates are as high as 15% after surgical resection of pancreatic cancer. Although the potential for cure is restricted to the few who are able to undergo a complete surgical resection, the 5-year survival rate after such surgical procedures is only 10%. Nonetheless, clients who undergo resection and eventually experience recurrence of cancer survive three to four times longer than clients whose tumor is not removed.[11]

PANCREATIC TRAUMA

The pancreas is injured in fewer than 2% of people with abdominal trauma. Two thirds of pancreatic injuries are associated with penetrating abdominal trauma, and the remainder are caused by blunt trauma. Although pancreatic trauma occurs somewhat infrequently, it is associated with high morbidity and mortality rates because of the difficulty in detecting these injuries and the likelihood of massive injury to nearby organs. Because the pancreas is retroperitoneal, clinical indicators of injury are often not obvious for several hours. Clients with penetrating abdominal trauma show manifestations of hemorrhage, progressive peritonitis, and hypovolemia.

The presentation of blunt pancreatic trauma is varied. Most people with blunt trauma have injuries to surrounding organs and vascular structures, and pancreatic trauma is discovered on treatment of these other injuries. In clients without injury to other areas, the only findings may be mild epigastric pain and tenderness; progressive deterioration yields the diagnosis of pancreatic injury. Treatment involves surgery to control hemorrhage, to debride nonviable tissue, to preserve viable tissue, and to provide drainage of pancreatic secretions.

CYSTIC FIBROSIS

Cystic fibrosis (CF) is a hereditary, chronic disease characterized by abnormal secretions of the exocrine glands. It is genetically transmitted as an autosomal recessive trait. See the Genetics Links box on Cystic Fibrosis in Chapter 62 for more information. More than 25,000 Americans have CF, and 850 new cases are diagnosed annually in the United States. CF is the most common fatal genetic disease of children of European-American heritage. It is diagnosed and managed in childhood, but improvements in care have allowed many clients to survive into adulthood.

Improvements in the management of infants and children with CF have led to a greater number of adults with CF. Typically, these adults have a small stature and appear somewhat emaciated with a barrel chest and clubbing of fingers. Pulmonary complications are the most physically visible. See Chapter 62 for a discussion of management of the respiratory problems. Because the digestive problems encountered with CF are generally managed with diet and oral administration of pancreatic enzymes and fat-soluble vitamins, clients are hospitalized for treatment of respiratory complications rather than for pancreatic or intestinal problems. In addition to pulmonary problems, clients experience impaired pancreatic exocrine function because of decreased lipase released into the bowel. The result is malabsorption of lipids with blockage of the pancreatic ducts by thick mucus. Pancreatic fibrosis, degeneration, and atrophy of tissues follow, with eventual development of fatty infiltration and loss of function. The intestines have thick, viscous mucus, which may cause a thick mass within the bowel. The lack of pancreatic enzymes causes steatorrhea.

Nursing management of the client with CF focuses on two major nursing diagnoses: (1) *Ineffective Airway Clearance* and (2) *Imbalanced Nutrition: Less Than Body Requirements*. Interventions for clients with CF include promoting the following:

- Clearance of secretions and control of infection in lungs (expectorants, postural drainage, antibiotics)
- Administration of pancreatic enzymes
- Adequate nutrition
- Absence of intestinal obstruction

BILIARY TRACT DISORDERS

Disorders of the gallbladder and ducts are extremely common. In the United States alone, it is estimated that 20 million people have gallstones with approximately 1 million new cases developing each year.[6]

The two most common conditions are gallstones and associated cholecystitis (inflammation of the gallbladder). About 98% of clients who present with symptomatic gallbladder disease have gallstones. Malignancies and congenital anomalies of the biliary tract are relatively uncommon.

Before beginning this discussion, note the list of terms used in association with these conditions (Table 46-1).

CHOLELITHIASIS (GALLSTONES)

The incidence of gallstones increases with age, as do the risks associated with cholelithiasis. In the United States,

TABLE 46-1 Biliary Tract Terminology	
Term	**Definition**
Chole-	Pertaining to bile
Cholang-	Pertaining to bile ducts
Cholangiography	X-ray study of bile ducts
Cholangitis	Inflammation of bile duct
Cholecyst-	Pertaining to gallbladder
Cholecystectomy	Removal of gallbladder
Cholecystitis	Inflammation of gallbladder
Cholecystography	X-ray study of gallbladder
Cholecystostomy	Incision and drainage of gallbladder
Choledocho-	Pertaining to common bile duct
Choledocholithiasis	Stones in common bile duct
Choledochostomy	Exploration of common bile duct
Cholelith-	Pertaining to gallstones
Cholelithiasis	Presence of gallstones
Cholescintigraphy	Radionuclide imaging of biliary system

more than 10% of men and 20% of women have gallstones by 65 years of age. Women account for nearly 70% of those treated for gallstones, although the mortality rate may be higher in men. Twice as many white Americans as black Americans are affected, and although gallstones are less common in blacks, cholelithiasis attributable to hemolysis occurs in more than one third of people with sickle cell anemia.

The prevalence of gallstones is much the same in Europe and Australia. Clients with diabetes mellitus, obesity, Crohn's disease, and cirrhosis show an increased incidence.

Most of our present knowledge of cholesterol gallstones comes from the study of Pima Native American women in south-central Arizona, in whom the occurrence is 75% in those over 25 years of age. Pigment stones are dominant in Asians and in African Americans.

Etiology and Risk Factors

Gallstones are crystalline structures formed by concretion (hardening) or accretion (adherence of particles, accumulation) of normal or abnormal bile constituents. According to various theories, there are four possible explanations for stone formation.

First, bile may undergo a change in composition. Studies of subjects with cholesterol gallstones indicate that their bile is supersaturated with cholesterol but deficient in bile salts. The cholesterol saturation of bile seems to increase with age. Changes in bile composition, however, do not completely explain why gallstones form.

Second, gallbladder stasis may lead to bile stasis. Bile stasis may (1) change the composition of bile, (2) supersaturate bile with cholesterol, and (3) precipitate some bile constituents. Gallbladder stasis may result from decreased contractility and emptying of the gallbladder and from spasm of the sphincter of Oddi. Circumstances in which gallbladder stasis occurs (e.g., TPN; low-fat, weight-reduction diets; spinal cord injury; pregnancy) are associated with a high rate of gallstone formation. More specifically, TPN without oral intake for longer than 1 month is associated with gallbladder sludge formation and cholelithiasis. Delayed emptying of the gallbladder may correlate with hormonal factors. In pregnant women, the female sex hormone estrogen increases, which increases dietary uptake of cholesterol and biliary cholesterol secretion. This may explain why gallstones seem to be associated with pregnancy. In addition, one of the precautions for administering estrogen substances to postmenopausal women is gallbladder disease.

Third, infection may predispose a person to stone formation. Inflammatory debris can form a nidus (point of origin) for stone growth. The related tissue injury may alter the composition of bile by increasing the reabsorption of bile salts and lecithin. Certain organisms may also play a part in stone formation by altering the composition of bile. For example, *Escherichia coli* increases the amount of bilirubin available for pigment stones and *Streptococcus faecalis* reduces bile salts.

Fourth, genetics and demography can affect stone formation, as shown by the higher prevalence in American Indians, Chilean Indians, Chilean Hispanics, Northern Europeans, and South Americans than in Asians.

Health promotion activities to minimize gallstone formation include maintaining a low-fat diet, maintaining ideal body weight, and limiting the number of pregnancies. Clients receiving TPN for longer than 1 month should be monitored closely as health maintenance and restoration actions. In addition, a low-carbohydrate diet and physical activity may help prevent gallstones, and it has been shown that women who consume caffeinated coffee appear to be protected against gallstones.[5]

Pathophysiology

Gallstone formation involves several factors:
1. Bile must become supersaturated with cholesterol or calcium.
2. The solute must precipitate from solution as solid crystals.
3. Crystals must come together and fuse to form stones.

Gallstones are generally of three types: (1) cholesterol, (2) pigment, and (3) mixed. Because the incidence of pure stone formation is rare, stones are generally classified by the predominant substance.

Cholesterol stones are the most common type; the incidence increases with age, and the prevalence is higher in women. Stones are usually smooth and whitish yellow to tan.

Pigment stones are present in about 30% of people with cholelithiasis in the United States. In these people,

bile contains an excess of unconjugated bilirubin. Pigment stones may be black (associated with hemolysis and cirrhosis) or earthy calcium bilirubinate (associated with infection in the biliary system).

Mixed stones may be a combination of cholesterol and pigment stones or either of these with some other substance. Calcium carbonate, phosphates, bile salts, and palmitate make up the more common minor constituents.

Most gallstones are formed in the gallbladder, but they may also form in the common duct or hepatic ducts of the liver. The actual incidence is not known, however, because some stones do not cause manifestations and they pass through the ducts into the bowel unnoticed. Occasionally, a stone is discharged into the small intestine. If the stone is large enough, it can obstruct the narrow terminal ileum, causing gallstone ileus.

The pathologic findings are best interpreted from the clinical manifestations of the disease, which may be acute or chronic. Once a client becomes symptomatic, treatment and follow-up are essential to prevent progression to a more severe, sometimes fatal, complication of gallbladder disease. About one third of these complications are due to free perforation, which occurs when a gangrenous area becomes necrotic and bile breaks into the peritoneal cavity. The mortality rate is about 20% for peritonitis with systemic distribution of pepsin.

Clinical Manifestations

Manifestations of biliary tract disorders are similar to those of several other conditions. Box 46-2 lists some

---

BOX 46-2 Disorders with Manifestations Similar to Those of Chronic and Acute Cholecystitis

CHRONIC CHOLECYSTITIS
- Angina pectoris
- Chronic pancreatitis
- Esophagitis
- Hiatal hernia
- Peptic ulcer
- Pyelonephritis
- Spastic colitis

ACUTE CHOLECYSTITIS
- Acute appendicitis
- Acute hepatitis
- Acute myocardial infarction
- Acute pancreatitis
- Acute pyelonephritis
- Intercostal neuritis
- Intestinal obstruction
- Perforated ulcer
- Pleurisy
- Renal calculus
- Right lower lobe pneumonia

common diseases that must be differentiated from acute and chronic cholecystitis.

Fewer than half of the people with gallstones report any distress because gallstones cause no manifestations unless complications develop. The most specific and characteristic manifestation of gallstone disease is pain or biliary colic, which is caused by spasm of the biliary ducts as they try to dislodge the stones. This pain usually follows the temporary obstruction of the gallbladder outlet. Characteristically, the pain starts in the upper midline area, radiates around to the back and right shoulder blade, and, for some clients, passes straight through to the back and substernal areas. The client is often restless, changing positions frequently to relieve the intensity of the pain. Pain may persist for only a few hours or several days, and the interval between attacks is variable.

If the stone is blocking the cystic duct, manifestations of acute cholecystitis (see Acute Cholecystitis) may occur. If the stone lodges in the common duct, gallstones can be complicated by cholangitis (inflammation of the bile duct) and pancreatitis. Jaundice appears only when common duct obstruction is present.

Nausea and vomiting may occur; occasionally, self-induced vomiting alleviates the manifestations. Assessment may further reveal a history of flatulence, bloating, epigastric pain, belching, intolerance for fatty foods, and vague upper abdominal sensations. Occasionally, clients who have these problems still have them after cholecystectomy.

Assessment of these clients becomes important in that manifestations of biliary colic and coronary artery disease are remarkably similar. Considering the prevalence of both these problems, accurate diagnosis is essential. Many times the diagnosis is based on the manifestations alone. Physical findings are present only during an attack with pain, with pain being the cardinal manifestation. The right upper quadrant or epigastric area is tender to palpation with voluntary muscle guarding, but manifestations of peritonitis are absent. The gallbladder is not palpable, and the temperature is normal.

Blood test results are unremarkable. For confirmation of the presence of gallstones and acute cholecystitis, several diagnostic tests are performed. The Integrating Diagnostic Testing feature below provides a description of these tests.

OUTCOME MANAGEMENT

Medical Management

Reduce Pain

Pain may arise from contraction of the gallbladder during transient obstruction of the cystic duct by gallstones. Analgesics may be administered intramuscularly (IM) or intravenously (IV) on a schedule, with a patient-controlled analgesia (PCA) pump, or as needed for pain. Antacids, H_2 blockers, or proton pump inhibitors are

INTEGRATING DIAGNOSTIC TESTING

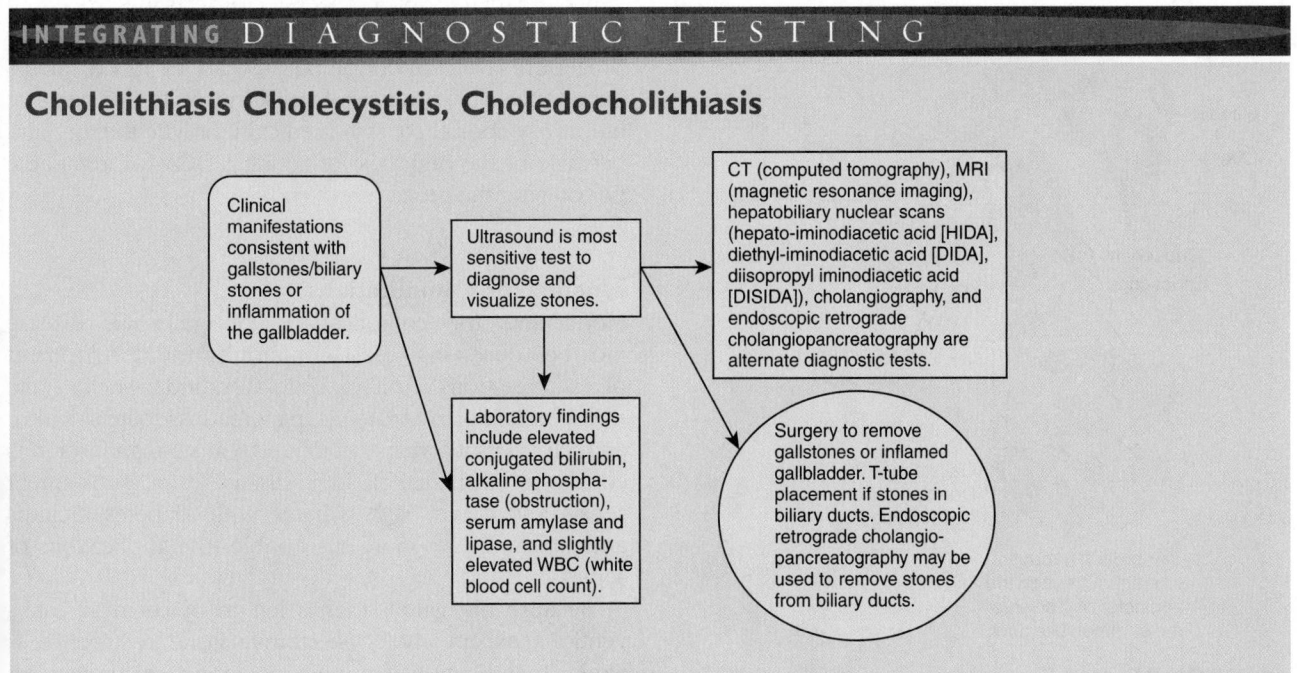

Cholelithiasis Cholecystitis, Choledocholithiasis

Clinical manifestations consistent with gallstones/biliary stones or inflammation of the gallbladder.

Ultrasound is most sensitive test to diagnose and visualize stones.

CT (computed tomography), MRI (magnetic resonance imaging), hepatobiliary nuclear scans (hepato-iminodiacetic acid [HIDA], diethyl-iminodiacetic acid [DIDA], diisopropyl iminodiacetic acid [DISIDA]), cholangiography, and endoscopic retrograde cholangiopancreatography are alternate diagnostic tests.

Laboratory findings include elevated conjugated bilirubin, alkaline phosphatase (obstruction), serum amylase and lipase, and slightly elevated WBC (white blood cell count).

Surgery to remove gallstones or inflamed gallbladder. T-tube placement if stones in biliary ducts. Endoscopic retrograde cholangiopancreatography may be used to remove stones from biliary ducts.

given to neutralize gastric hyperacidity and to reduce associated pain, and antiemetics are given to minimize nausea and vomiting. Antibiotics are administered to reduce the likelihood of infection. Nitroglycerin may reduce biliary colic as well.

Monitor Fluid and Electrolyte Balance

During an acute attack of biliary colic, the client remains on NPO status, with IV fluids administered to maintain hydration. The client may lose fluids if an NG tube has been inserted for symptomatic relief of vomiting or if pancreatitis is a probable diagnosis.

The diet progresses according to the client's tolerance. The client is advised to avoid foods that precipitate biliary colic. Instructions may include avoiding a fatty meal or a large meal after fasting.

Nonsurgical Approaches to Eradicate Stones

Endoscopy. Retrograde endoscopy for stone removal is an important nonsurgical alternative. To remove a gallstone from the common bile duct, the physician passes an endoscope orally into the duodenum and then passes a wire snare into the common bile duct through the ampulla of Vater, securing and removing the obstructing stone (Figure 46-2). The physician may choose to enlarge the ampulla of Vater by endoscopic papillotomy to allow passage of stones. If stones remain in the common bile duct after cholecystectomy and a T tube is still in place, the physician may pass a stone-retrieving basket or other device through the T-tube tract to remove the stone.

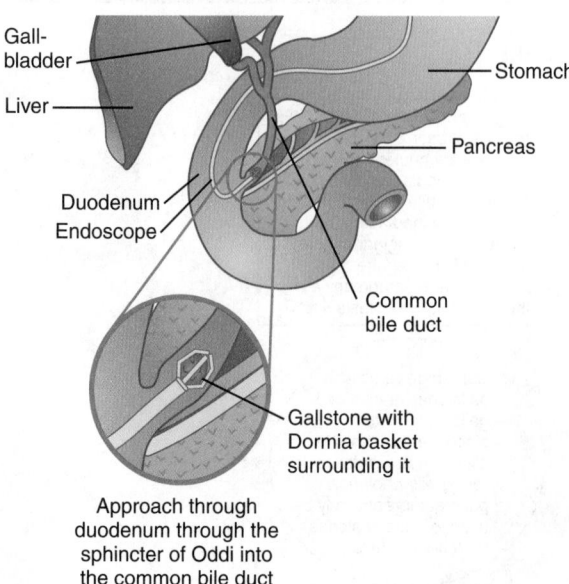

Gallbladder
Liver
Stomach
Pancreas
Duodenum
Endoscope
Common bile duct
Gallstone with Dormia basket surrounding it

Approach through duodenum through the sphincter of Oddi into the common bile duct

■ **FIGURE 46–2** Retrograde cholendoscopic removal of gallstones.

Gallstone Dissolution (Cholesterol-Dissolving Agents). The oral administration of agents for dissolving cholesterol gallstones—chenodeoxycholic acid (CDCA), or chenodiol; and ursodeoxycholic acid, or ursodiol (UDCA)—may be used in selected clients who refuse cholecystectomy or who are not good candidates for surgery, which accounts for fewer than 10% of clients with these manifestations. The dose is 7 mg/kg daily of each agent or 8 to 10 mg/kg of ursodeoxycholic acid in divided doses daily. Both drugs act to reduce the amount of cholesterol in bile; however, each drug uses a different mechanism. The highest success rate occurs in clients with small floating, radiolucent gallstones. Stones tend to reoccur (30% to 50% of clients over 3 to 5 years of follow-up), and taking medication for an indefinite time can be costly. Because of these disadvantages and the success of laparoscopic cholecystectomy, the use of oral cholesterol-dissolving agents is limited.[6]

Extracorporeal Shock Wave Lithotripsy. Extracorporeal shock wave lithotripsy (ESWL), where up to 1500 shock waves are directed at stones until they are crushed, may be used as an ambulatory treatment in some cases. The client should have symptomatic cholelithiasis with fewer than four stones, each smaller than 3 cm in diameter, and no history of liver or pancreatic disease.

Contraindications to the procedure are the presence of common duct stones, recent acute cholecystitis, cholangitis, and pancreatitis.

Lithotripsy is used infrequently as an option for treatment in the United States today because of the emergence of laparoscopic cholecystectomy as the procedure of choice for symptomatic cholelithiasis. In addition, the procedure is less an option because about 30% of clients experience a recurrence of gallstones within 5 years of lithotripsy combined with medical litholytic therapy and because of the high cost of taking UDCA for a variable period after the procedure.[5,6]

Monitor for Complications

Monitoring for complications of gallstone disease includes observing, most commonly, for development of manifestations of biliary colic. Conditions such as bile duct obstruction, cholangitis, pancreatitis, acute calculus, and cholecystitis may occur and cause manifestations consistent with gallbladder disease and subsequent sepsis and death. Clients with diabetes mellitus and gallstones are more susceptible to complications of sepsis.

Because the gallbladder is left in place in all interventions except cholecystectomy, stone recurrence is likely. Investigation continues on long-term prevention of gallstone recurrence.

Nursing Management of the Medical Client

Assessment. If the client is being admitted for evaluation and treatment of manifestations, your assessment should focus on collecting subjective and objective data and noting the client's response to medications. Assess the client's manifestations carefully to help determine the diagnosis. Check vital signs at regular intervals to document inflammation associated with stones. Also assess the client's knowledge of the diagnostic process. Closely monitor the client for manifestations of obstruction from the gallstones.

Diagnosis, Outcomes, Interventions
Diagnosis: Acute Pain or Chronic Pain. Because one of the major manifestations of the disease is pain, *Acute Pain or Chronic Pain related to biliary spasms* is the major nursing diagnosis.

Outcomes. The client will demonstrate absence of or a decrease in pain as evidenced by the client's verbalizing that pain is absent or decreased and by the client resting quietly.

Interventions
Administer Pain Medications. Administer pain medication as ordered; document and note the client's response to the medication. Encourage the client to verbalize the effectiveness of the medication by describing whether the pain is absent or decreased.

Provide Comfort Measures. Other comforting measures may be helpful. Providing a quiet environment and using relaxation techniques, such as a back rub, may promote rest and enhance the effects of the analgesics.

Diagnosis: Risk for Imbalanced Fluid Volume. Because of the associated gastrointestinal manifestations, write the nursing diagnosis as *Risk for Imbalanced Fluid Volume related to vomiting and nasogastric suctioning.*

Outcomes. The client will maintain adequate hydration and electrolyte balance as evidenced by normal skin turgor, moist oral mucous membranes, urine output greater than 0.5 ml/kg/hour, and no manifestations of electrolyte imbalance.

Interventions
Insert a Nasogastric Tube. If the client continues vomiting, obtain an order for an NG tube with a suction attachment to relieve distention and vomiting. Suction also removes the gastric juices that stimulate cholecystokinin, which in turn causes painful contractions of the gallbladder. NG suction is usually maintained on a low intermittent setting when a single-lumen tube (e.g., Levin) is used or on a low continuous setting when a double-lumen tube (e.g., Salem sump) is used.

Administer IV Fluids and Electrolytes. Assess and document intake, output, and electrolyte laboratory values, communicating discrepancies to the physician. Assess the client for manifestations of dehydration, such as dry mucous membranes, poor skin turgor, and urine output less than 0.5 ml/kg/hour.

Diagnosis: Risk for Injury. The client undergoing endoscopic retrograde stone removal is assigned the nursing diagnosis *Risk for Injury related to medication during the procedure and possible introduction of bacteria into common bile duct.*

Outcomes. The client will remain free from injury and infection following endoscopic retrograde stone removal as evidenced by the airway remaining patent without aspiration and the absence of manifestations of infection, such as elevated temperature.

Interventions. For the client undergoing endoscopic retrograde papillotomy or stone removal, a local anesthetic solution is sprayed on the back of the throat. This intervention facilitates the passing of the endoscope.

> **SAFETY ALERT**
>
> **After the endoscopic procedure, carefully check for the return of the gag reflex before allowing oral intake. If the client receives sedation, raise the side rails on the bed for protection and keep the call light within reach. Antibiotics are often administered during the procedure to minimize the risk of infection from introduction of bacteria from the intestine into the common bile duct.**

Evaluation. Most clients recover from acute cholecystitis in a few days without complications. Once the biliary system is allowed to rest, inflammation decreases and recovery progresses. Clients should be monitored for the development of chronic cholecystitis.

Self-Care

The client and the client's significant others will need to learn about the suggested therapeutic regimen; diet changes; indications for drugs and their side effects, dosage, and administration instructions; and ways to prevent recurrence. Clients who undergo gallstone dissolution most frequently receive UDCA. CDCA administration may result in mild to moderate elevation in liver function test values and serum cholesterol levels. In addition, clients receiving CDCA may experience disabling diarrhea.

Medications
After assessing the level of understanding and learning needs, educate the client about the purpose of oral dissolution therapy, expected responses, and possible untoward reactions. Because oral dissolution medication must be taken over a long period, help the client to

devise ways to remember to take the medication daily. For example, a pillbox that is divided into the days of the week clearly indicates whether the client has missed a dose.

The client who is being treated medically may be sent home with oral analgesics or other medications for comfort as well as with an oral dissolution agent. Be sure that the client and the client's significant others can relate all necessary information to the nurse before discharge.

Diet Modifications

Diet instructions may be necessary if ingestion of food precipitated the attack; that is, if a fatty food caused the biliary colic, inform the client about the need for a low-fat diet.

Prevent Recurrence

Advise the client about what to do if another attack occurs. The client has probably been encouraged by the physician to consider elective cholecystectomy or other surgical intervention before gallbladder disease progresses. Provide written material on gallbladder disease at this time to aid the client in understanding and in making decisions.

Surgical Management

Whether to operate on a client with asymptomatic chole-lithiasis ("silent gallstones") is an area for debate. The potential for serious complications (e.g., acute cholecystitis, sepsis, and choledocholithiasis) can pose a significant risk. Older adults and clients with type 1 diabetes mellitus have a high incidence of gallstones. Because these population groups are at high risk during acute biliary attacks and emergency procedures, surgeons may recommend that they undergo elective cholecystectomy to avoid later emergency surgery. Other procedures that may be performed include percutaneous cholecystolithotomy and laparoscopic cholecystectomy.

Laparoscopic Cholecystectomy

Indications. Laparoscopic cholecystectomy has become the treatment of choice for symptomatic gallbladder disease. The procedure is suitable for most clients, even those with acute cholecystitis, because there is minimal trauma to the abdominal wall. This makes it possible for clients to go home within 24 hours after the procedure and return to work within a few days instead of a few weeks, as is the case with a cholecystectomy performed with an abdominal incision.

With the client under general anesthesia, carbon dioxide is used to create pneumoperitoneum through a needle inserted near the umbilicus. Near the umbilicus, an endoscope is inserted through a small incision to view the gallbladder and to determine the feasibility of success associated with this procedure. Three other small incisions are created: one for grasping the gallbladder, one for suction and irrigation, and one for dissection instruments and applying clips (Figure 46-3).

Contraindications. Laparoscopic cholecystectomy is contraindicated if stones are known to exist in the common bile duct. Laparoscopic cholecystectomy does not allow exploration or removal of stones from the common duct.

Complications. Possible complications of surgery or anesthesia include pneumonia or atelectasis, deep vein

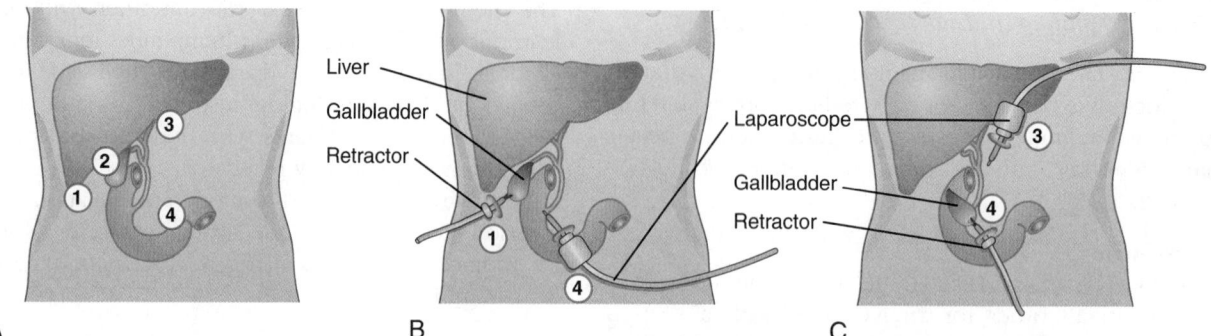

■ **FIGURE 46–3** Laparoscopic cholecystectomy. **A,** Standard sites of four ports used in laparoscopic cholecystectomy. *1,* The lateral port is used to retract the gallbladder. *2,* The subcostal port is used for suction/irrigation. *3,* The superior midline port is used to insert the laparoscope later in the procedure while the gallbladder is being withdrawn from the umbilical port. *4,* The umbilical port is most often used to insert the laparoscope for most of the procedure and then is used to withdraw the gallbladder after the laparoscope is moved to the superior midline port. **B,** Preparing the gallbladder for removal by ligating it from attachments (e.g., cystic duct, artery, vein). *1,* The gallbladder is retracted through the lateral port. *4,* A laparoscope is inserted through the umbilical port to visualize the gallbladder. **C,** Removal of the gallbladder. *3,* Laparoscope through the superior midline port. *4,* Removal of the gallbladder through the umbilical port.

thrombosis or pulmonary embolism, and damage to the biliary tract and hemorrhage. Operative cholangiography is a protective procedure for complications of cholecystectomy. The advantages of small scars and a short hospital stay, however, have influenced surgeons to opt for this procedure more often. Clients who undergo this procedure are at less risk because they are ambulatory sooner and usually require only oral analgesia. Because of the carbon dioxide pressing on the diaphragm, nausea, vomiting, and shoulder pain are more frequent if the client's head and torso are elevated too soon after surgery.

Outcomes. Most clients are discharged on the day of surgery or the day after. In most cases, they can resume normal activities and return to work after 3 to 4 days.

Cholecystectomy

Indications. A cholecystectomy consists of excising the gallbladder from the posterior liver wall and ligating the cystic duct, vein, and artery. The surgeon usually approaches the gallbladder through a right upper paramedian or upper midline incision. If necessary, the common duct may be explored through this incision. When stones are suspected in the common duct, operative cholangiography may be performed (if it has not been ordered preoperatively). The surgeon may dilate the common duct if it is not already dilated as a result of a pathologic process. Dilation facilitates stone removal. The surgeon passes a thin instrument into the duct to collect the stones, either whole or after crushing them.

After exploring the common duct, the surgeon usually inserts a T tube to ensure adequate bile drainage during duct healing (choledochostomy). The T tube also provides a route for postoperative cholangiography or stone dissolution, when appropriate (Figure 46-4).

A conventional open cholecystectomy is indicated when a laparoscopic cholecystectomy does not allow for retrieval of a stone in the common bile duct and when the client's physique does not allow access to the gallbladder. Occasionally, when a client is very obese, the gallbladder is not retrievable via laparoscopic instruments. Further, a surgeon may have difficulty accessing the gallbladder in an adult with a small frame and may need to perform the conventional open cholecystectomy.

Contraindications. A client's physical condition may not be able to withstand the stress of surgery, including loss of fluids and electrolytes and the stress of anesthesia. Cholecystotomy, incision, and drainage of the gallbladder may be performed as an alternative procedure.

Complications. After cholecystectomy, monitor the client for the usual postoperative complications, such as

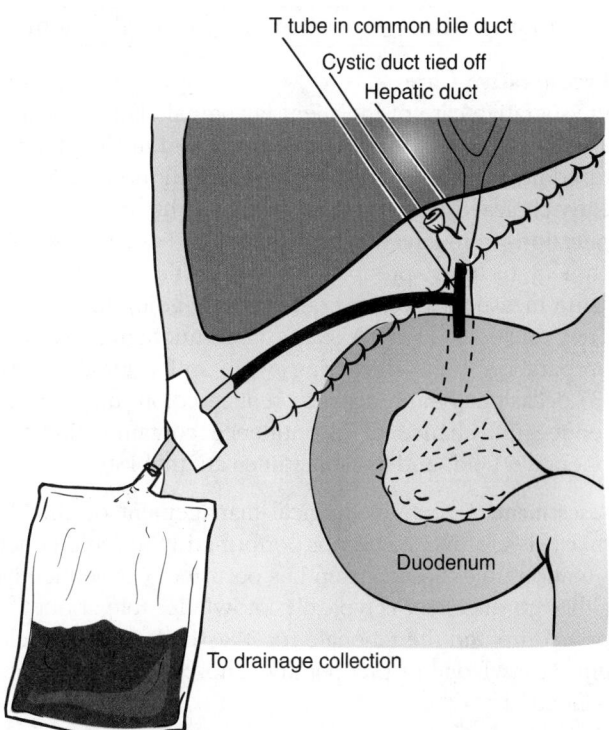

T tube in common bile duct
Cystic duct tied off
Hepatic duct

Duodenum

To drainage collection

■ **FIGURE 46–4** Placement of a T tube. The surgeon ties off the cystic duct and sutures the T tube to the common bile duct with the short arms of the T tube toward the hepatic duct and duodenum. The long arm of the T tube exits the body near the incision site. Skin suture and tape secure placement.

hemorrhage, pneumonia, thrombophlebitis, urinary retention, and ileus. The risk of bile leakage into the abdominal cavity is more applicable to surgeries involving the gallbladder. With hemorrhage and bile leakage, the client feels severe pain and tenderness in the right upper quadrant, abdominal girth increases, bile or blood may leak from the wound, blood pressure drops, and tachycardia develops.

Outcomes. Cholecystectomy results in immediate cessation of pain in most clients and prevents development of complications such as acute cholecystitis, choledocholithiasis, and cholangitis. Persistence of manifestations after removal of the gallbladder indicates (1) a possible misdiagnosis or functional bowel disorder, such as esophagitis, peptic ulceration, pancreatitis, or irritable bowel syndrome; (2) a technical error; (3) a retained or recurrent common bile duct stone; or (4) spasm of the sphincter of Oddi. Clients must be hospitalized for about 3 days before dismissal. They may be sent home with a T tube in place for 1 to 2 weeks. 🪔 When stones are present in the common bile duct, research indicates that both complications and cost can be saved if preoperative ERCP performed for suspicion of uncomplicated common bile duct stones is replaced by intraoperative cholangiography (IOC).[2]

Nursing Management of the Surgical Client

Preoperative Care

Preoperative care of the client facing gallbladder or biliary surgery is the same as that described in Chapter 14. In addition, preparation involves careful monitoring for early clinical findings that may indicate the onset of complications from infection or obstruction. For laparoscopic cholecystectomy, preoperative preparation involves the same measures taken for other clients going to surgery. They include (1) NPO status after midnight, (2) skin preparation (i.e., showering with antibacterial soap), (3) occasionally an enema to reduce colon mass and to reduce the chance of incontinence contaminating the operative field, and (4) sometimes an antibiotic.

Assessment. Generally, surgical management of cholelithiasis is elective and is not performed in an emergency situation unless obstruction has occurred. Consequently, although the client is typically knowledgeable about the procedure and the rationale for it, assessment of the client's knowledge of preoperative and postoperative care is needed.

Diagnosis, Outcomes, Interventions

Diagnosis: Deficient Knowledge. The preoperative client may not be completely knowledgeable about surgical procedures, particularly gallbladder surgery. The nursing diagnosis, therefore, can be *Deficient Knowledge related to gallbladder surgery and recovery.*

Outcomes. The client will verbalize an understanding of the procedure; will demonstrate an ability to carry out coughing, deep-breathing, and leg exercises; and will verbalize knowledge regarding the immediate postoperative course.

Interventions. Reinforce information given to the client about the surgical procedure. Determine the level of understanding and the learning needs of the client and the client's significant others. Provide material that can be read or viewed at the client's own pace. Give verbal instructions and a demonstration to ensure that the client can perform postoperative exercises (turning, coughing, deep breathing, and wound splinting) properly and can understand their importance.

Clients also need some knowledge of what to expect postoperatively, such as IV fluids, T-tube placement and drainage, pain control, and activity. Studies have shown that preoperative client education significantly reduces the risk for development of postoperative complications.

Postoperative Care

Respiratory status is carefully monitored after surgery of the gallbladder or biliary tract because of the potential for development of atelectasis and pneumonia. Closely monitor drainage from all biliary tubes and drainage from the incision site, for amount, character, and color. Carefully assess cardiovascular status and manifestations of hemorrhage or shock. Hemorrhage, although rare, can occur if an inflamed gallbladder has adhered to the liver.

Analgesia for pain management is important and should be given on a regular basis to promote comfort and rest as well as to enhance the client's ability to cough and deep breathe.

Maintain hydration and fluid balance IV until the client is no longer on NPO status and can receive fluids orally. When the client is allowed oral intake, the amount of fluid and food should be sufficient and well balanced enough to maintain renal function and body weight (minimal loss of weight). Clients are generally allowed to progress to a regular diet, with fat content included as tolerated.

Assessment. Postoperative assessment of the client is important; it includes careful monitoring of vital signs, breath and bowel sounds, and general level of responsiveness to check for complications such as hemorrhage, respiratory problems, or infection. In addition, intake is monitored to reflect renal function, and output is carefully measured, including wound drainage, vomiting, or nasogastric suctioning.

Assess the client's incision for redness or swelling. Monitor the level of pain as well as the location, severity, and the effectiveness of any interventions.

After a laparoscopic cholecystectomy, referred pain to the shoulder is a common postoperative pain pattern. Shoulder pain occurs because of the carbon dioxide that has not been released or absorbed by the body. Carbon dioxide causes irritation of the phrenic nerve and diaphragm and may decrease respiratory excursion.

Diagnosis, Outcomes, Interventions

Diagnosis: Risk for Injury. The postoperative client is at risk for the development of many complications leading to the nursing diagnosis *Risk for Injury related to postoperative complications of hemorrhage, infection, fluid and electrolyte imbalance, pulmonary changes (atelectasis, pneumonia), urinary retention, ileus, and decreased gastrointestinal motility.*

Outcomes. The client will receive appropriate assessments and interventions for early detection and prevention of injury from postoperative complications as evidenced by stable vital signs; normal pulmonary function; normal gastrointestinal function; laboratory values within normal limits; urine output of at least 0.5 ml/kg/hour; an intact incision that does not exhibit redness, odor, or purulent drainage; and no manifestations of thrombus or embolus.

Interventions

Assess Postoperatively. Take routine postoperative vital signs and assess for manifestations of shock, such as cyanosis; diaphoresis; cold, clammy skin; decreased blood pressure; and increased pulse rate. As vital signs are checked, check dressings and drainage tubes at the same time for unusual amounts of bleeding or drainage. If any of the aforementioned manifestations or changes occurs, check vital signs frequently and notify the physician.

Prevent Pneumonia. The client should change position at least every 2 hours. While the client is awake for turning, help the client to cough and deep breathe. Some hospitals use devices such as incentive spirometry to encourage lung expansion and spontaneous coughing. When these devices are used, it is helpful to demonstrate their use before surgery.

Auscultate the lungs for rales, rhonchi, and diminished breath sounds every 4 hours for the first 24 hours and every 8 hours thereafter. If the client had a cholecystectomy, it will be even more difficult for the client to take deep breaths and cough because of the location of the incision. Take extra care to ensure that the client is comfortable enough to breathe normally. Many physicians and nurses believe that smaller doses of opioid given more frequently are beneficial. Splinting the incision helps as well.

Monitor Fluids and Electrolytes. Measure intake and output every 4 hours or more frequently if ordered. Assess amounts for discrepancies. Because it is not unusual for new postoperative clients to be behind on fluids for the first few hours, do not expect output to equal intake initially. Assess the client for edema along with the lung sounds every 4 hours as another assurance that the client is tolerating the fluids that are being infused.

Unless the client is otherwise compromised, such as being acutely ill at the time of surgery or having a history of other health problems (e.g., heart disease or diabetes mellitus), laboratory work probably will not be ordered until the following day. Monitor these values for indications of fluid and electrolyte imbalance (see Chapters 11 and 12).

Monitor Urine Output. Generally, the client can void within 6 hours after surgery; if not, assess the bladder for distention. The client may not to be able to void because of pain, discomfort, and position or because of an absence of feeling the need to void as a result of the effects of anesthesia and opioids. The client may need to be catheterized to empty the bladder initially.

Maintain Nasogastric Tube. Occasionally, after gallbladder surgery, the client may return with an NG tube attached to suction. Check the tube frequently to ensure that it is patent and that placement is correct for adequate drainage. A plugged or displaced tube not only causes distention, nausea, and vomiting, but also may place undue stress on the surgical site. Auscultate bowel sounds every 4 hours to note return of normal bowel activity. Depending on the surgery, the client may or may not be allowed oral intake before bowel sounds return.

Offer oral care at least every 2 hours while the client is on NPO status. This may consist of rinsing the mouth with water, using nonalcoholic mouthwash, swabbing with a moist swab, or assisting the client with brushing the teeth. Assess the oral mucous membranes at least every 8 hours for integrity, color, and moistness. While the client is taking nothing orally, it may be helpful to place a wet washcloth over the lips to humidify the air. Offering ice chips or sips of liquid as soon as allowed also provides much relief.

Advance Diet as Tolerated. For the more involved surgical procedure, such as a cholecystectomy, clients are usually not allowed a normal diet until they have begun to pass flatus and until bowel sounds are heard. After the client is allowed to have fluids or food, continue to assess the client for abdominal distention and normal bowel sounds to ensure that the intake is being tolerated. Because early activity also helps the return of intestinal motility, the client should be encouraged to begin progression of regular activities as soon as possible.

Prevent Infection. If the nurse is to change the dressings, the incision should be checked simultaneously for redness, swelling, drainage characteristics and amounts, and odor. If drains such as a T tube are present, observe the drainage for its characteristics and amount. Check the client's temperature at least every 4 hours or more frequently if necessary. Keep the dressing and incision clean and dry because moisture enhances bacterial growth. Subjective complaints of increased pain may be the first manifestation of an infectious process taking place.

> **For this reason, it is important to document the location, type, and amount of pain routinely so that comparison can be made and a significant change in condition can be noted immediately. Many times it is your assessment that alerts the physician and facilitates the diagnosis of infection.**

SAFETY ALERT

Diagnosis: Acute Pain. The client may have problems with postoperative pain. Therefore the nursing diagnosis *Acute Pain related to surgical procedure and incision* is applicable.

Outcomes. The client will feel reduction of pain, as evidenced by resting comfortably and quietly, a blood pressure and heart rate within normal limits, and the ability to tolerate postoperative exercises and activities.

Interventions. Assess and document the level, location, and type of pain as well as the client's response to pain medication. You may need to intervene and obtain new medication orders if the ordered medication is ineffective. It may be necessary to administer medication to coincide with activity to keep the client active. Nonpharmacologic measures are also helpful. Providing a quiet environment (even limiting visitors if necessary), changing the client's position, and rubbing the client's back are all important in relaxing the client and in enhancing the effects of the pain medication. Assist the client in splinting the incision, and instruct the client on the best way to get out of bed and to lie down.

Evaluation. The client should heal without difficulty and may be discharged within about 3 to 4 days after cholecystectomy. The client will be able to resume normal activities in 4 to 6 weeks. After laparoscopic cholecystectomy, the client is usually discharged the day of or the day after surgery and can return to normal activities within 3 to 4 days.

Self-Care

Because the client will be faced with early discharge from the health care setting, the client should be able to verbalize and accurately demonstrate home health care needs and skills, for example, (1) identifying manifestations of infection; (2) demonstrating wound care; (3) naming medications, their purpose, side effects, and administration instructions; and (4) stating activity and dietary restrictions.

Teach the client about home health care as soon after surgery as possible to assess the client's learning potential and learning needs. Instruction should include wound care, dressing changes with a return demonstration, and assessing for manifestations of infection.

Teach Manifestations to Report
Be sure the client is knowledgeable about which manifestations should be reported to the physician and how to contact the physician.

SAFETY
ALERT

Advise the client to report fever, chills, nausea and vomiting, jaundice, dark-colored urine, pale-colored stools, and pruritus. If the client is discharged with a drain or T tube in place, the client should know the purpose of the tube, how to secure it, how to empty it, what amounts of drainage can be expected, and abnormal characteristics of drainage.

Diet and Activity Modifications
Explain and reinforce activity and dietary restrictions thoroughly. Advise that heavy lifting (>10 pounds) or strenuous work or sports should be avoided for as long as prescribed by the physician. Instruct and question

clients regarding their discharge medications, the possible adverse medication side effects, and the dosage of the medications. Explain that a low-fat (to be increased gradually), high-carbohydrate, high-protein diet is needed and that alcohol should be avoided to minimize the risk of pancreatic involvement.

Modifications for Older Clients

In older clients, gallstones do not necessarily cause pain, fever, or jaundice. Mental confusion, shakiness, and an elevated alkaline phosphatase level may be the only manifestations of gallstones in the older population. Nonsurgical decompression techniques may be preferred in high-risk older clients.

> **An older client that undergoes a cholecystectomy is at greater risk for injury related to anesthesia, pain medications, and sometimes the response to the trauma of surgery. Postoperative care should be modified to prevent injury. Especially in the immediate postoperative period, the side rails should be up, the bed in low position, and the call light within easy reach.**
>
> **Depending on the client's response to anesthesia and pain medication, frequent reorientation to the environment and circumstances may be necessary. In particular, be alert to the fact that older clients tend to become confused after surgery, especially at night. Remind the older client how to summon help and why it is important to not get up alone. Be sure that all IV lines and drainage tubes are secure to prevent the client from inadvertently disconnecting them.**

ACUTE CHOLECYSTITIS

Acute cholecystitis refers to acute inflammation of the gallbladder wall. The incidence of cholecystitis is increased in clients who are overweight, especially those with a sedentary lifestyle. Certain ethnic groups, including Chinese, Jewish, and Italians, have a higher rate of the disease.

Etiology and Risk Factors
Cholecystitis is associated with gallstones and obstruction of the cystic duct by a stone in 90% of cases.[5] Obstruction of a cystic duct by a stone is the usual cause of acute cholecystitis. In 5% to 10% of clients, however, calculi obstructing the cystic duct are not found during surgery (acalculous cholecystitis, or cholecystitis without stones). In more than 50% of such cases, an underlying cause of the inflammation is not found.[7]

The major preventable risk factors are sedentary lifestyle and obesity. If the client increases activity level and maintains a low-fat diet, the risk of cholecystitis can be reduced. Encourage clients to engage in exercise and to follow healthy dietary habits.

Pathophysiology

Acute calculous cholecystitis, which appears to be caused by obstruction of the cystic duct, in turn causes distention of the gallbladder. Subsequently, (1) venous and lymphatic drainage is impaired, (2) proliferation of bacteria occurs, (3) localized cellular irritation or infiltration (or both) takes place, and (4) areas of ischemia may develop. The inflamed gallbladder wall is edematous and thickened, it may have areas of gangrene, or necrosis may be present. The term empyema describes a gallbladder that contains pus, which is the equivalent of an intra-abdominal abscess and may be associated with severe sepsis. Recurrent episodes of acute cholecystitis cause fibrosis of the wall of the gallbladder.

Complications of untreated acute cholecystitis are usually associated with septic complications. Others are consequences of ischemia, inflammation, adhesions, and gangrene: perforation, pericholecystic abscess, and fistula.

Acalculous cholecystitis (cholecystitis without stones) is far less common than cholecystitis attributable to gallstones. It can be triggered by (1) multiple blood transfusions, (2) gram-negative bacterial sepsis, or (3) tissue damage after burns, trauma, or extensive surgery. Other possible contributing factors include hyperalimentation, prolonged fasting, hypotension, anesthesia, opioid analgesics, and mechanical ventilation with positive endexpiratory pressure. Clients with diabetes mellitus and systemic arteritis are also susceptible.

Clinical Manifestations

Inflammation of the gallbladder may be acute or chronic. The most common and reliable finding on physical examination is tenderness in the right upper quadrant, epigastrium, or both. Although clients with chronic and acute cholecystitis may complain of the same type of pain, the distinguishing factor is the severity and persistence of the pain. Chronic cholecystitis rarely lasts more than a few hours, whereas acute cholecystitis may last several days.

Pain in acute cholecystitis may be located in the epigastric, subscapular, or right upper quadrant regions. Sometimes the pain is referred to the right scapula. The pain usually starts suddenly, increases steadily, and reaches a peak in about 30 minutes. Abdominal examination may disclose a tender abdomen with right upper quadrant guarding. Murphy's sign may be elicited when the client is asked to take a deep breath. About 60% to 70% of clients with acute cholecystitis have experienced biliary colic episodes in the past from ductal spasm when a stone moves from the gallbladder into ducts, causing waves of pain (biliary colic).

In addition to pain, the following problems may be divulged in clients with acute cholecystitis:

- Nausea and vomiting occur in about 75% of clients as a result of impulses transmitted to the vomiting center from distention of bile ducts.
- A low-grade fever is often present from the response to inflammation, but this may be absent in older clients, immunocompromised clients, and clients receiving steroidal therapy.
- Mild jaundice occurs in only 10% of cases.
- Right upper quadrant tenderness, fever, and leukocytosis suggest acute cholecystitis, particularly if other assessment data support this diagnosis.

For the diagnostic evaluation of acute cholecystitis, see the Integrating Diagnostic Testing feature Cholelithiasis, cholecystitis, and choledocholithiasis on p. 1121.

OUTCOME MANAGEMENT

Medical Management

Clients thought to have acute cholecystitis may need to be hospitalized, and initial management should include administration of antibiotics effective against organisms found in the bile in about 80% of the cases. These organisms include both gram-positive and gram-negative aerobes and anaerobes: *Escherichia coli*, *Klebsiella* species, *Clostridium* species, and *Streptococcus* species.[6]

Antibiotics that are effective given singly include ampicillin, ureidopenicillins such as piperacillin or mezlocillin, third-generation cephalosporins, or aminoglycosides. A combination of these drugs may be more effective in clients with diabetes mellitus or with debilitated conditions. Further medical management is the same as for symptomatic cholelithiasis (see Cholelithiasis [Gallstones]).

Nursing Management of the Medical Client

Assessment becomes extremely important because several other disease entities may produce the same manifestations (see Box 46-2). Collect subjective and objective data, and note the client's response to all medications.

Nursing care is the same as that for the medical management of cholelithiasis except for the certainty that these clients will receive a course of antibiotics. Observe the client for the development of complications, which may include increased pain in the right upper quadrant or jaundice (from an obstruction) and decreased or absent bowel sounds (from peritonitis). For additional information on nursing management, see Nursing Management of the Medical Client under Cholelithiasis.

Surgical Management

Once the diagnosis of acute cholecystitis is made, the decision for early or delayed cholecystectomy depends on the risk factors. Delayed surgery is usually the correct decision for clients who have unstable angina, significant carotid artery disease, heart failure, cirrhosis, and other conditions that would increase their risk.

Cholecystectomy for the client with acute cholecystitis is more difficult than elective surgery because of the distended, inflamed gallbladder. Usually, the gallbladder must be decompressed first to allow complete visualization of all surrounding structures and to avoid injury to the extrahepatic bile ducts.

Cholecystotomy (surgical drainage of the gallbladder) is usually performed only when cholecystectomy is too dangerous, given all the risk factors. Although the procedure relieves the obstruction, the cure depends on the ability of the client's immune system to resolve the inflammatory process. Treatment of complications of cholecystotomy is usually cholecystectomy. See Nursing Management of the Surgical Client under Cholelithiasis.

ACUTE ACALCULOUS CHOLECYSTITIS

Acute acalculous cholecystitis (without stones) accounts for about 4% to 8% of all cases of acute cholecystitis. Although data are inconclusive, this condition is said to be occurring increasingly. It tends to occur after or in association with other conditions, especially major trauma, burns, or surgery. Other pre-existing conditions include the postpartum period after a prolonged childbirth, bacterial sepsis, and debilitating systemic diseases, such as cardiovascular disease, tuberculosis, and sarcoidosis. No apparent precipitating factor is present, however, in as many as 50% of the clients.

The pathologic process does not differ from that of the calculous type, although the incidence of gangrene and perforation is higher. It is debatable whether this is an inherent feature of the disease or the result of delayed diagnosis.

Recognition of the disease may be delayed when the client cannot communicate well because of concomitant disease or post-traumatic or postoperative states. The manifestations are the same as those of acute calculous cholecystitis: pain in the right upper quadrant, epigastrium, or both and vomiting. Although pain is the cardinal manifestation in the calculous type, it may be obscured or absent in acalculous cholecystitis because of opioid administration, a decreased level of consciousness, or abdominal pain from an incision or from another disease process. Significant physical findings are the same as those in acute calculous cholecystitis, and the same diagnostic procedures are used.

The standard treatment is emergency cholecystectomy because of the increased risk of gangrene and perforation.

CHRONIC CHOLECYSTITIS

Chronic cholecystitis sometimes arises as a sequela to acute cholecystitis. Typically, however, it develops independently of acute cholecystitis. In addition, it is almost always associated with gallstones. Chronic cholecystitis principally affects middle-age and older obese women. The female-to-male ratio is 3:1.

Assessment data for chronic cholecystitis are similar to those of acute cholecystitis with certain exceptions. In chronic states, (1) the pain is less severe, (2) the temperature is not as high, and (3) the leukocyte count is lower. Vague manifestations of indigestion, epigastric pain, fat intolerance, heartburn, and flatulence accompany chronic cholecystitis. The client has usually experienced these manifestations as well as repeated attacks (mild or severe) of acute cholecystitis for a long time. Eventually fibrous tissues begin to replace the normal muscle and mucosal tissues of the gallbladder. As a consequence, the gallbladder loses its ability to concentrate bile.

Diagnosis depends largely on ultrasonography, and other diagnostic procedures provide supplementary information. Diagnostic findings include (1) cholelithiasis, (2) gallbladder wall thickening (>3 mm), and (3) delayed visualization or nonvisualization of the gallbladder on radionuclide scanning. Scarring from chronic inflammation may partially or completely obstruct the cystic duct and thus account for this delay in visualization or nonvisualization. It may be difficult to differentiate chronic cholecystitis from other disorders. Conditions that produce manifestations similar to the manifestations of cholecystitis (acute and chronic) are listed in Box 46-2. The diagnostic process serves to rule out these conditions.

Conservative interventions include (1) eating a low-fat diet; (2) losing weight; and (3) administering anticholinergics, sedatives, and antacids. When medical intervention is ineffective, cholecystectomy may be the treatment of choice. About 90% of clients obtain relief of manifestations after cholecystectomy. Of the gallbladders removed, 95% contain stones.

CHOLEDOCHOLITHIASIS AND CHOLANGITIS

Choledocholithiasis is defined as stones in the common duct. Common bile duct calculi can arise from the gallbladder or hepatic ducts. Thus common duct stones can occur in the absence of a gallbladder and are classified as primary. Cholangitis is inflammation of the bile duct.

Common duct stones are found in about 10% to 15% of clients with cholelithiasis. The incidence increases with age, and the frequency of gallstones in the common duct in the older population may be as high as 25%.[6] Frequently, inflammation or bacteria are present, and cholangitis may develop.

Etiology and Risk Factors

The cause is essentially the same as that for cholelithiasis. This condition is sometimes combined with a narrowing of the papilla, which traps stones. The risk factor for choledocholithiasis is that a small stone may pass from the gallbladder and lodge in the common bile duct.

Pathophysiology

The pathophysiology is essentially the same as that for cholelithiasis. Most bile duct stones are cholesterol or mixed stones. They form in the gallbladder and move into the biliary tree through the cystic duct.

Clinical Manifestations

Common duct calculi may be asymptomatic or cause biliary colic, bile duct obstruction, cholangitis, or pancreatitis. Early manifestations of choledocholithiasis are not easily distinguished from gallbladder colic or acute cholecystitis. Pain may be mild or severe and cannot be differentiated from gallbladder pain. Jaundice is intermittent if obstruction is intermittent but may be progressive if the stone becomes impacted in the cystic duct or bile duct. Chills and fever, frequently recurring attacks of severe right upper quadrant pain, and a history of jaundice are manifestations of cholelithiasis.

Infrequently, manifestations of cholangitis are accompanied by shock and confusion, coma, or other central nervous system manifestations. These manifestations signal the presence of acute toxic cholangitis, a condition in which the infected bile or pus is under pressure within the duct system. Emergency decompression of the duct system is necessary to prevent death.

OUTCOME MANAGEMENT

Medical Management

Medical management of pain is based on its severity and frequency and is similar to medical management described for cholelithiasis. Management of inflammation involves antibiotic therapy when cholangitis is present.

Surgical Management

Indications

Indications for surgical management of common duct calculi may include emergency intervention, which is rare unless severe ascending cholangitis is present. Usually, however, surgical management in some form is necessary for symptomatic choledocholithiasis.

Treatment includes hospitalization, treatment of infection, and removal of stones. The removal of stones may be accomplished surgically in clients with an intact gallbladder by cholecystectomy and choledochotomy. As many as 20% of clients undergoing cholecystectomy will prove to have common bile duct stones in addition to stones in the gallbladder. With the development and refinement of laparoscopic cholecystectomy, the management of common bile duct stones in the presence of gallstones is becoming more easily defined. To remove common bile duct stones, preoperative ERCP with endoscopic papillotomy and stone extraction followed by laparoscopic cholecystectomy is the preferred approach. Postoperative ERCP may also be done if necessary, but research indicates that when dealing with potential stones of the common bile duct, intraoperative cholangiography reduces complications and is more cost-effective than performing ERCP preoperatively.

Common duct stones in a client who has previously had a cholecystectomy are best treated by endoscopic papillotomy with stone extraction, as opposed to transabdominal surgery. The surgeon opens the sphincter of Oddi and allows passage of gallstones up to 1 cm in diameter. The success rate is about 90%. Extracorporeal shock wave lithotripsy is used when stones are too large to extract via the endoscopic approach. Success can be achieved in 70% to 85% of these complicated cases. Most common duct stones are found and removed at the time of cholecystectomy.

Liver function should be thoroughly evaluated preoperatively by measuring the prothrombin time. If results are abnormal, function should be restored to normal with administration of vitamin K. Antimicrobial agents (e.g., mezlocillin IV along with either metronidazole or gentamicin IV) should be given.

Another procedure, choledochostomy, consists of opening the common duct surgically, removing stones, and inserting a T tube for drainage. Choledochostomy may be performed in conjunction with cholecystectomy. Otherwise, cholecystectomy may be necessary at a later date.

Postoperative antibiotics are not usually given after biliary tract surgery unless specimens of the bile obtained for culture during the surgery are positive for organisms.

Contraindications

Contraindications to surgical management of choledocholithiasis include older clients and those who are poor surgical risks.

Complications

Surgical traumas or the presence of stones may result in ductal edema after choledochostomy. Inserting a T tube prevents bile from spilling into the peritoneal cavity and maintains patency of the duct (see Figure 46-4). T tubes may be attached to continuous gravity drainage or to collapsible bags in the dressing site.

Avoid tension on long tubing and obstruction by kinking. Carefully measure drainage from the T tube. The tube usually drains 300 to 500 ml in the first 24 hours. This amount decreases to less than 200 ml after 3 to 4 days. Record the volume and color of the drainage. To prevent excessive loss of bile, place the drainage bag for the T tube at the level of the abdomen rather than hanging the bag below the bed. At this height, bile flows into the bag only when pressure is high in the biliary tree.

Excessive T-tube drainage may indicate obstruction. Occasionally, it signals development of a biliary fistula. Excessive bile losses may necessitate recycling the client's bile drainage. The bile may be returned to the client through an NG tube or orally in fruit juice.

Thick bile or bile containing blood clots may prevent drainage or cause inadequate amounts of drainage from the T tube. Without intervention, bile may begin to leak from the choledochotomy site instead of through the T tube. To prevent this problem, the physician may decide to irrigate the tube with sterile saline.

On rare occasions, tube dislodgment causes failure of the T tube to drain. The tube may dislodge from the common duct when the client moves from a supine to a sitting position. This complication may result from excessive tension during T-tube insertion in surgery.

After a few days, the T tube will probably be clamped during meals to aid fat digestion. The tube remains in place for about 10 days. A T-tube cholangiogram should be done on or about the seventh or eighth postoperative day to assess for bile duct obstruction. When the T-tube cholangiogram indicates absence of obstruction, the surgeon may decide to remove the T tube. If a retained stone is discovered during cholangiography, the client may go home with the T tube in place. The surgeon may remove the stone through the T-tube tract with a catheter later.

Outcomes

When stones are extracted, the client is likely to experience a reduction in pain and a general increase in well-being and quality of life. Encourage the client to increase the level of activity and maintain a low-fat diet to reduce the risk of forming additional future stones.

Nursing Management of the Surgical Client

Nursing management is the same as that for the client with a cholecystectomy.

SCLEROSING CHOLANGITIS

Sclerosing cholangitis is an uncommon inflammatory disease of the bile ducts that causes fibrosis and thickening of their walls and multiple short, concentric strictures. The disease is progressive and gradually causes cirrhosis, portal hypertension, and death from hepatic failure. It may also predispose the client to the development of cholangiocarcinoma. Some cases are associated with inflammatory bowel disease, especially ulcerative colitis. Sclerosing cholangitis and papillary stenosis are important complications of acquired immunodeficiency syndrome (AIDS). In addition, cytomegalovirus and *Cryptosporidium* are observed frequently in such clients, indicating that these organisms may be involved in causing primary sclerosing cholangitis.

The cause has been linked to altered immunity, toxins, and infectious agents. Clients often have the hepatocompatible antigen human leukocyte antigen-B (HLA-B), suggesting that genetic factors may play a role. The disease is most common in men 20 to 40 years of age. The male-to-female ratio is 3:2.

Usually clients present with fatigue, anorexia, weight loss, jaundice, and pruritus. They sometimes complain of vague upper abdominal pain. The diagnosis is usually made by endoscopic retrograde cholangiography, clinical findings, and liver biopsy.

Medical management consists of corticosteroids and broad-spectrum antimicrobial therapy with inconsistent, unpredictable results when cholangitis is a recurrent problem. Immunosuppressants, bile acid binding agents, colchicine, and penicillamine have also been used with inconsistent and unpredictable results. These agents do not alter the slow, progressive course of the disease. Recent experience shows that ursodiol, in a high dose of 20 mg/kg/day, may reduce cholangiographic progression and liver fibrosis. Cholestyramine may help control the pruritus.

The success of surgical intervention is limited by the progressive nature of the disease and the recurrent cholangitis. Surgery is generally limited to stent procedures to open the ducts. Cholecystectomy should not be performed unless there is definite evidence of cholecystitis or cholelithiasis. Although surgical therapy may be life saving in some circumstances, it has to be considered palliative in the overall context of the disease. The definitive management of these clients is liver transplantation, which is the procedure of choice. Survival rates with transplantation are 85% at 3 years.[5]

CARCINOMA OF THE GALLBLADDER

Although cancer of the gallbladder is the most common malignant lesion of the biliary tract, it accounts for only 5% of all cancers at autopsy. Most cancers of the gallbladder develop in conjunction with stones rather than polyps. Of all clients with this malignancy, the mean age is approximately 70 years and the female to male ratio is 4:1[4]; however, the incidence of bile duct cancer is predominant in men. Native Americans, Hispanics, northeastern Europeans, Israelis, and Japanese immigrants to the United States are at greatest risk for cancer of the gallbladder. At least 70% of these clients have gallstones. Adenocarcinoma accounts for the vast majority of all cases.

The clinical presentation differs according to stage of the disease. There is no distinct pattern because the manifestations depend on the site of the lesion, its extent, and the presence or absence of pre-existing biliary manifestations. Usually, however, the clinical manifestations are unrelenting right upper quadrant pain, weight loss, jaundice, and a palpable right upper quadrant mass.

Treatment modalities and their effectiveness are widely debated. Treatment varies from radical resection, to palliative relief of duct obstruction, to chemotherapy or radiation. None of the treatments have been found to increase survival.

The prognosis for cancer of the gallbladder is poor. About 95% of clients with unresectable disease die within the first year, and fewer than 5% are alive at 5 years.[4] Trials of radiation and chemotherapy in clients with primary gallbladder cancer have been disappointing. The long-term survivors are generally those in whom the diagnosis of cancer had not been made before cholecystectomy was performed and was determined by pathologic study.

CONCLUSIONS

Biliary and exocrine pancreatic disorders are common but are extremely complex and diverse. Some of these conditions are treated without further difficulty, such as cholecystitis, whereas others can become chronic and lead to a wide variety of other problems, such as pancreatitis. Teaching is vital to the care of these clients, and the nurse must understand these conditions to initiate appropriate teaching plans.

THINKING CRITICALLY

1. You are assigned to care for a 45-year-old executive who has been admitted with recurrent vomiting and severe upper abdominal pain radiating to his back. This is his first admission for pancreatitis. He admits to drinking 1 pint of whiskey over a weekend and having several beers nightly on weekdays. His alcohol intake has been greater in the past. Laboratory data include the following: amylase, 750 units/L (normal, 25 to 125 units/L); lipase, 5.6 units/ml (normal, 10 to 140 units/L); aspartate aminotransferase (AST), 150 units/L (normal, 5 to 40 units/L); and alanine aminotransferase (ALT), 60 units/L (normal, 1 to 45 units/L). How do you feel about caring for this client?

Factors to Consider. Are you comfortable with the client's lifestyle? Do the biochemical studies support a diagnosis of pancreatitis? What do you need to consider if he complains of pain? What should you do if you discover he is allergic to meperidine? Should a nasogastric tube be inserted?

2. A 45-year-old woman is admitted to the hospital complaining of colicky pain in the right upper abdominal quadrant. She states that the pain is worse when she eats fried foods. She also states that she has vomited on several occasions, and it seems to relieve her manifestations. What are your priorities in assessing and caring for the client?

Factors to Consider. What types of diagnostic procedures should be scheduled? Why is an accurate assessment of the clinical manifestations important? What indications warrant insertion of a nasogastric tube?

3. A 70-year-old woman comes to the emergency department with complaints of recurrent episodes of epigastric pain during the past 9 months. Chills, fever, and jaundice have occurred for the first time and have persisted for 4 days. Her white blood cell count is normal. Serum bilirubin and alkaline phosphatase values are elevated. There is no history of alcoholism, blood transfusions, or hepatitis. The client takes no medications except an occasional "Bufferin for my arthritis." Her past medical history is unremarkable except for a cholecystectomy 10 years ago after an episode of cholecystitis. What are the priorities for care?

Factors to Consider. What are the client's clinical manifestations? Would surgical treatment alleviate the problem? What might cause stricture of the bile ducts?

Discussions for these questions can be found on the website.

BIBLIOGRAPHY

Citations appearing in red refer to primary research.

1. Ackley, B.J., & Ladwig, G.B. (2006). *Nursing diagnosis handbook* (7th ed.). St. Louis: Mosby.
2. Barwood, N.T., et al. (2002). Changing methods of imaging the common bile duct in the laparoscopic cholecystectomy era in western Australia: Implications for surgical practice [Abstract]. *Journal of the American Medical Association*, 287(14), 1779.
3. Boucher, R. (2005). Cystic fibrosis. In D. Kasper, et al. (Eds.), *Harrison's principles of internal medicine* (16th ed., pp. 1543-1546). New York: McGraw-Hill.
4. Dienstag, J.L., & Isselbacher, K.J. (2001). Tumors of the liver and biliary tract. In E. Braunwald, et al. (Eds.), *Harrison's principles of internal medicine* (15th ed., pp. 588-591). New York: McGraw-Hill.
5. Friedman, L.S. (2005). Liver, biliary tract, and pancreas. In L.M. Tierney, S.J. McPhee, & M.A. Papadakis (Eds.), *Current medical diagnosis and treatment* (44th ed., pp. 627-678). New York: Lange Medical.
6. Greenberger, N.J., & Baumgartner, G. (2005). Diseases of the gallbladder and bile ducts. In D. Kasper, et al. (Eds.), *Harrison's principles of internal medicine* (16th ed., pp. 1881-1891). New York: McGraw-Hill.
7. Greenberger, N.J., & Toskes, P.P. (2005). Acute and chronic pancreatitis. In D. Kasper, et al. (Eds.), *Harrison's principles of internal medicine* (16th ed., pp. 1895-1906). New York: McGraw-Hill.
8. Guyton, A.C., & Hall, J.E. (2006). *Textbook of medical physiology* (11th ed.). Philadelphia: Elsevier Saunders.

9. Hubbard, G., & Wolfe, K. (2003). Meperidine misuse in a patient with sphincter of Oddi dysfunction. *The Annals of Pharmacotherapy*, 37(4), 534-537.

10. Lichtenstein, D.R. (2004). Diseases of the pancreas. In T.E. Andreoli, et al. (Eds.), *Cecil essentials of medicine* (6th ed., pp. 379-387). Philadelphia: Elsevier Saunders.

11. Mayer, R.J. (2005). Pancreatic cancer. In D. Kasper, et al. (Eds.), *Harrison's principles of internal medicine* (16th ed., pp. 537-539). New York: McGraw-Hill.

12. McCance, K.L., & Huether, S.E. (2006). *Pathophysiology: The biologic basis for disease in adults and children* (5th ed.). St. Louis: Mosby.

13. Monkemuller, K.E., Garcia-Gallont, R., & Fallon, M.B. (2004). Disorders of the gallbladder and biliary tract. In T. Andreoli, et al. (Eds.), *Cecil essentials of medicine* (6th ed., pp. 423-428). Philadelphia: Saunders.

14. Pagana, K.I., & Pagana, T.J. (2006). *Manual of diagnostic and laboratory tests* (3rd ed.). St. Louis: Mosby.

15. Schlapman, N. (2001). Spotting acute pancreatitis. *RN*, 64(11), 55-59.

16. Schull, P.D. (2006). *Nursing spectrum drug handbook*. Dallas: Nursing Spectrum.

17. Sommers, M.S., & Johnson, S.A. (2002). *Diseases and disorders: A nursing therapeutic manual* (2nd ed.). Philadelphia: F.A. Davis.

18. Steer, M.L. (2004). Exocrine pancreas. In C.M. Townsend, et al. (Eds.), *Sabiston textbook of surgery* (17th ed., pp. 1643-1678). Philadelphia: Saunders.

19. Stevens, M., Esler, R., & Asher, G. (2002). Transdermal fentanyl for EB management of acute pancreatitis pain. *Applied Nursing Research*, 15(2), 102-110.

20. Topazian, M. (2005). Gastrointestinal endoscopy. In D. Kasper, et al. (Eds.), *Harrison's principles of internal medicine* (16th ed., pp. 1730-1739). New York: McGraw-Hill.

21. Toskes, P.P., & Greenberger, N.J. (2005). Approach to the patient with pancreatic disease. In D. Kasper, et al. (Eds.), *Harrison's principles of internal medicine* (16th ed., pp. 1891-1895). New York: McGraw-Hill.

evolve *Did you remember to check out the bonus material on the Evolve website and the CD-ROM, including NCLEX®-Examination Style Review Questions, Open-Book Quizzes, and Chapter Review Audio Podcasts?*

http://evolve.elsevier.com/Black/medsurg

CHAPTER 47

Management of Clients with Hepatic Disorders

DIANNE M. SMOLEN

The liver plays a central role in many essential physiologic processes. It is the primary organ of lipid synthesis, and it detoxifies endogenous and exogenous substances such as hormones, drugs, and poisons. When the normal physiologic processes are altered, numerous hepatic and extrahepatic manifestations of liver disease appear. These manifestations offer the initial clue to liver disease, regardless of the cause.

This chapter describes the clinical features of liver diseases, their medical and surgical management, and measures the nurse can take to assist clients with such nursing diagnoses as *Impaired Skin Integrity, Excess Fluid Volume, Fatigue, and Imbalanced Nutrition: Less Than Body Requirements*.

JAUNDICE

Jaundice, or icterus, is the yellow pigmentation of the sclerae, skin, and deeper tissues caused by excessive accumulation of bile pigments in the blood. It is a common manifestation of a variety of liver and biliary diseases and serves as a starting point for evaluating many of these disorders. Bilirubin (bile pigment), a product of red blood cell (RBC) breakdown, is deposited in the skin and excreted in the urine when present in the blood in excessive amounts (hyperbilirubinemia). This characteristic makes jaundice a valuable indicator of a variety of disorders involving either hemolysis or biliary obstruction. When there is an obstruction blocking the flow of bile into the intestine, jaundiced clients also may have clay-colored stools because of the lack of bilirubin and its metabolites in the intestine (Table 47-1).

Bilirubin is formed from the breakdown of hemoglobin from RBCs by macrophages. This unconjugated bilirubin, measured as "indirect bilirubin," is not water soluble, cannot be filtered in the kidney, and thus is not excreted in the urine. Normally the unconjugated bilirubin returns to the liver via the bloodstream and is conjugated with glucuronic acid to form conjugated bilirubin (measured as "direct bilirubin"), which is water soluble. The conjugated bilirubin travels to the gallbladder and eventually to the intestines. In the bowel, bacterial action converts bilirubin to urobilinogen. A small amount of urobilinogen is absorbed into the bloodstream to be returned to the liver or excreted in the urine.

Etiology and Risk Factors

The cause of jaundice may be described according to the location of the pathologic change. It may occur because of a problem (1) outside the liver (resulting in unconjugated hyperbilirubinemia, in which the accumulated bilirubin is predominantly of the unconjugated type) or (2) in the liver or biliary tract (resulting in conjugated hyperbilirubinemia, with predominantly conjugated bilirubin). When the problem is in the liver or biliary tract, the cause may be hereditary cholestatic syndromes, hepatocellular dysfunction, or biliary obstruction.

Pathophysiology

The underlying pathophysiologic mechanism in jaundice relates to whether the jaundice results from the accumulation of predominantly unconjugated or conjugated bilirubin in the serum.

TABLE 47–1   Types of Jaundice

Types of Jaundice	Location and Cause
Unconjugated hyperbilirubinemia (predominant indirect-acting bilirubin)	**Increased Bilirubin Production**
	Hemolysis (e.g., spherocytosis, autoimmune disorders)
	Ineffective erythropoiesis (e.g., megaloblastic anemias, hematoma)
	Decreased Hepatic Uptake
	Gilbert syndrome
	Drugs (e.g., rifampin, radiographic contrast agents)
	Neonatal
	Decreased Conjugation
	Gilbert syndrome
	Crigler-Najjar syndrome types I and II
	Neonatal jaundice
	Hepatocellular disease
	Drug inhibition (e.g., chloramphenicol)
Conjugated hyperbilirubinemia (predominant direct-acting bilirubin)	**Impaired Hepatic Excretion**
	Familial disorders (e.g., Dubin-Johnson syndrome, Rotor's syndrome, benign recurrent cholestasis, cholestasis of pregnancy)
	Hepatocellular disease
	Drug-induced cholestasis
	Primary biliary cirrhosis
	Sepsis
	Postoperative
	Extrahepatic ("Mechanical") Biliary Obstruction
	Gallstones
	Tumors of head of pancreas
	Tumors of bile ducts
	Tumors of ampulla of Vater
	Biliary strictures (postcholecystectomy, primary sclerosing cholangitis)
	Congenital Disorders
	Biliary atresia

Data from Sheikh, A.M., Fallon, M.B., et al. (2004). Jaundice. In T.E. Andreoli, et al. (Eds.), *Cecil essentials of medicine* (6th ed., pp. 399-407). Philadelphia: Saunders; and Friedman, L.S. (2002). Liver, biliary tract, and pancreas. In L.M. Tierney, S.J. McPhee, & M.A. Papadakis (Eds.), *Current medical diagnosis and treatment* (43rd ed., pp. 626-668). New York: Lange Medical.

Unconjugated Hyperbilirubinemia

Unconjugated hyperbilirubinemia may result from the overproduction of bilirubin as a result of hemolysis, from impaired hepatic uptake of bilirubin caused by certain drugs, or from impaired conjugation of bilirubin by glucuronide, as in Gilbert syndrome, Crigler-Najjar syndrome, or drug reactions.

Conjugated Hyperbilirubinemia

Conjugated hyperbilirubinemia may result from the impaired excretion of bilirubin from the liver resulting from hepatocellular disease, drugs, sepsis, hereditary disorders such as Dubin-Johnson syndrome, or extrahepatic biliary obstruction. The pathologic mechanism in conjugated hyperbilirubinemia varies according to the type of jaundice (mechanisms are summarized in Table 47-1).

See the Chapter 42 website table Laboratory Tests for Endocrine and Metabolic Function for laboratory test results pertinent to liver disorders.

Hereditary Cholestatic Syndromes

Jaundice related to hereditary cholestatic syndromes or intrahepatic cholestasis (stagnation of bile in liver or bile ducts) results from faulty excretion of bilirubin conjugates, as in conditions such as Dubin-Johnson syndrome or Rotor's syndrome.

Hepatocellular Disease

Hepatocellular jaundice is due to defective uptake, conjugation, or transport of bilirubin by the liver. Liver cell dysfunction or necrosis caused by hepatitis, for example, or defective bile transport in the bile canal and small bile duct can cause hyperbilirubinemia. Unknown channels absorb the pooled bile components into the bloodstream. Although obstructive jaundice usually refers to jaundice caused by an obstruction, such as a stone, hepatic cellular damage can also result in obstruction sufficient to cause jaundice.

Biliary Obstruction

Biliary obstruction, the cause of obstructive jaundice, results from impaired bilirubin transport and excretion in the biliary system. In this case, the problem arises from obstruction of an extrahepatic bile duct by gallstones.

Clinical Manifestations

Manifestations of jaundice include yellow sclerae, yellowish orange skin, clay-colored feces, tea-colored urine, pruritus (itching), fatigue, and anorexia. Features of laboratory diagnostic tests used to identify the underlying cause and type of jaundice are found on the Chapter 42 website table Laboratory Tests for Endocrine and Metabolic Function.

OUTCOME MANAGEMENT

Medical Management

Determine the Cause of Jaundice

An early goal in managing jaundice is to determine which category of disease explains the client's jaundice. The clinical evaluation is an important element in this determination and includes a carefully documented health history, physical examination, basic tests of liver function, and a complete blood count (CBC). Additional tests, such as imaging studies, serologic tests, and laboratory pathologic evaluation, may be required.

The health history should focus on specific manifestations, including the presence and character of pain, fever, or other manifestations of active inflammation and change in appetite, weight, and bowel habits. The clinical evaluation should focus on features of the client's illness that point to hereditary cholestatic syndromes, hepatocellular disease, or biliary obstruction.

Reduce Pruritus and Maintain Skin Integrity

Pruritus, caused by an accumulation of bile salts in the skin, results from obstructed biliary excretion. Some clients experience only mild itching; others suffer such extreme itching that they tear at their skin or scratch during sleep. If skin lesions develop and become infected, antibiotics may be ordered.

Oral cholestyramine resin provides some relief by binding bile salts in the intestine so that they can be excreted. Antihistamines and phenobarbital (which enhances bile flow) may also relieve itching.

Nursing Management of the Medical Client

Assessment. The client should be observed closely for development of jaundice. Often the first manifestation the client notices is a change in taste, manifested as a distaste for a food or drink the client previously liked, such as coffee. Pruritus is another early manifestation of incipient jaundice. Check the sclerae daily for the development of yellow coloration.

Diagnosis, Outcomes, Interventions
Diagnosis: Impaired Skin Integrity. The most common nursing diagnosis for the client with jaundice is *Impaired Skin Integrity related to pruritus.*

Outcomes. The client's itching will be controlled as evidenced by the client's statements of relief, decreased dryness of skin, maintenance of skin and mucous membrane integrity, and a decrease in scratching.

Interventions. Administer antihistamines and phenobarbital as prescribed to relieve the itching. For clients with extreme itching, administer oral cholestyramine resin to bind with bile salts in the intestine so that they can be excreted. Suggest other interventions, including tepid water or emollient baths, avoidance of alkaline soap, and frequent application of lotions.

Encourage the client to wear loose, soft clothing. Provide soft bed linens (cotton is best), and change soiled linens as soon as possible. Keep the room cool.

Diagnosis: Disturbed Body Image. Clients with jaundice often experience problems associated with the nursing diagnosis *Disturbed Body Image related to yellowing of skin and sclerae.*

Outcomes. Clients will cope with body image disturbance as evidenced by clients not isolating themselves, verbalizing and demonstrating acceptance of appearance (grooming, dress, posture, eating patterns, and self-presentation), and initiating or reestablishing support systems.

Interventions. Reassure the client that the discoloration is usually temporary. Assist the client in personal hygiene as needed, and promote activity as tolerated. Encourage clients to express their feelings about their self-image.

Evaluation. Jaundice should resolve with treatment of the underlying condition. It usually begins to disappear within 4 to 6 weeks. The return of normal stool and urine color is an indication of resolution. As the jaundice lessens, the client's appetite and body image improve and the pruritus subsides.

Surgical Management

Surgical exploration of the common bile duct (choledochostomy) enables the diagnostician to differentiate choledocholithiasis (stone in the common bile duct) from tumor. If carcinoma (usually of the head of the pancreas) is discovered during exploration, the surgeon may perform a palliative anastomosis of the gallbladder to the jejunum to bypass the common bile duct. Chapter 46 describes surgical management of the client undergoing a choledochostomy.

HEPATITIS

Simply stated, hepatitis is inflammation of the liver. This inflammation may be caused by viruses, toxins, or chemicals (including drugs). Jaundice usually develops, and the liver is tender. Other manifestations depend on the causative agent and the degree of organ disruption. There are several types of hepatitis, such as viral, toxic, chronic, and alcoholic.

VIRAL HEPATITIS

Viral hepatitis occurs worldwide. It is the most common blood-borne infection in the United States and many parts of the world. The most common types of hepatitis are hepatitis A virus (HAV), hepatitis B virus (HBV), hepatitis C virus (HCV), hepatitis D virus (delta agent), and hepatitis E virus—which cause hepatitis A through E, respectively. A sixth agent, hepatitis F virus, and a seventh agent, hepatitis G virus plus TT virus, have been identified, but do not cause hepatitis. Agents other than hepatitis A through G that may cause viral hepatitis include rubella virus, varicella virus, retroviruses, yellow fever virus, adenoviruses, and Marburg virus. Epstein-Barr virus (which causes infectious mononucleosis), cytomegalovirus, and herpes simplex virus are other possible causes of viral hepatitis, especially in immunocompromised people.

Although the manifestations of infection are similar in hepatitis A through E, the conditions differ related to incubation period, mode of transmission, severity, and prevention. Table 47-2 describes basic information about the various hepatitis viruses, and additional information is presented in the following paragraphs.

TABLE 47–2 Comparison of Types of Viral Hepatitis

Feature	Hepatitis A Virus (HAV)	Hepatitis B Virus (HBV)	Hepatitis C Virus (HCV)	Hepatitis D Virus (HDV)	Hepatitis E Virus (HEV)
Incubation (days)	15-45, mean 30	30-180, mean 60-90	15-160, mean 50	30-180, mean 60-90	14-60, mean 40
Onset	Acute	Insidious or acute	Insidious	Insidious or acute	Acute
Age preference	Children, young adults	Young adults (sexual and percutaneous), babies, toddlers	Any age, but more common in adults	Any age (similar to HBV)	Young adults (20-40 years)
Risk factors/high-risk groups	Infected feces, fecal-oral route; may be airborne if copious secretions; shellfish from contaminated water; no carrier state	Most U.S. cases now result from heterosexual transmission; contact with blood and body fluids; carrier state	Contact with blood and body fluids; source of infection uncertain in many clients; carrier state	Co-infects with hepatitis B; close personal contact; carrier state	Fecal-oral route, food- or water-borne; no carrier state
Transmission Fecal-oral	+++	-	-	-	+++
Percutaneous	Unusual	+++	+++	+++	-
Perinatal	-	+++	+[a]	+	-
Sexual	+	++	-[a]	++	-
Clinical severity	Mild	Occasionally severe	Moderate	Occasionally severe	Mild
Fulminant	0.1%	0.1%-1%	0.1%	5%-20%[b]	1%-2%[e]
Progression to chronicity	None	Occasional (1%-10%) (90% of neonates)	Common (50%-70% chronic hepatitis; 80%-90% chronic infection)	Common[d]	None
Carrier	None	0.1%-30%[c]	1.5%-3.2%	Variable[f]	None
Cancer	None	+ (neonatal infection)	+	+	None
Prognosis	Excellent	Worse with age, debility	Moderate	Acute, good Chronic, poor	Good
Prophylaxis	IG Inactivated vaccine	HBIG Recombinant vaccine	None	HBV vaccine (none for HBV carriers)	Experimental vaccine being tested
Therapy	None	Interferon Lamivudine Adefovir	Pegylated interferon plus ribavirin	Interferon +	None

[a] Primarily with HIV co-infection and high-level viremia in index case; risk ≈5%.
[b] Up to 5% in HBV/HDV co-infection; up to 20% in HDV superinfection of chronic HBV infection.
[c] Varies considerably throughout the world and in subpopulations within countries.
[d] In acute HBV/HDV co-infection, the frequency of chronicity is the same as that for HBV; in HDV superinfection, chronicity is invariable.
[e] I0%-20% in pregnant women.
[f] Common in Mediterranean countries, rare in North America and western Europe.
Modified from Dienstag, J.L., & Isselbacher, K.J. (2005). Acute viral hepatitis. In D. Kasper, et al. (Eds.), *Harrison's principles of internal medicine* (16th ed., pp. 1822-1838). New York: McGraw-Hill.

Etiology, Risk Factors, and Transmission

The etiologies of hepatitis A through E that cause acute viral hepatitis are all characterized at the molecular level. All except hepatitis B are RNA viruses. Hepatitis B is a DNA virus. Information about the risk factors and transmission of hepatitis can be seen in Table 47-2.

Pathophysiology

The pathophysiologic features in viral hepatitis are similar regardless of the cause. Hepatocytes undergo pathologic changes and are damaged in two distinct ways: through direct action of the virus (as occurs in HCV) or through cell-mediated response to the virus (as occurs in HBV). Inflammation of the liver with areas of necrosis occurs, and the resultant damage leads to impairment of function. The degree of functional impairment depends on the amount of hepatocellular damage. The endoplasmic reticulum—responsible for protein and steroid synthesis, glucuronide conjugation, and detoxification—is the first cellular organelle (a specialized part of a cell that performs a definite function) to undergo change, and liver functions that depend on these processes are altered. Kupffer cells (fixed phagocytic cells found in sinusoids of liver) increase in both size and number. Vascular and ductular tissues undergo inflammatory changes. Healing of the damaged hepatic tissue generally occurs in 3 to 4 months. Complications of hepatitis occur, although rarely (see Complications of Hepatitis).

Prevention

Prevention of viral hepatitis depends primarily on the form of the virus and its mode of transmission.

> Maintaining good personal hygiene and proper sanitation are the best ways to prevent HAV infection. At-risk clients should be advised to wash their hands after bowel movements or changing diapers as well as before cooking or eating. For HBV and HCV infection, prophylactic measures are similar. Latex condoms should be worn during sex. Drug users should be warned against sharing needles, drugs, and syringes. At-risk clients should avoid sharing personal items such as razors and toothbrushes. (See Table 47-2.)

Hepatitis A

> Household and personal contacts of clients with HAV should be given immune globulin. Administration of immune globulin (gamma globulin [Gammar]) is helpful prophylaxis both before and after exposure. Immune globulin is administered intramuscularly after exposure but not after the development of clinical manifestations. Clients who live in or visit high-risk areas can be protected for up to 3 months by immune globulin.

The earlier in the incubation period that the prophylactic immune globulin is given, the greater the protection.

SAFETY
ALERT

> Two effective inactivated hepatitis A vaccines are available and recommended for people living in or traveling to endemic areas, people with chronic liver disease, people with clotting-factor disorders who are treated with concentrates, animal handlers, military personnel, bisexual and homosexual men, health care workers, sewage workers, illicit drug users, food handlers, and day care center caregivers. In states with a high incidence of hepatitis A, routine vaccination of all children has been recommended. For adults, recommended HAV vaccines are either 1 ml of Havrix or 1 ml of Vaqta intramuscularly, followed by a second 1-ml dose at 6 to 12 months.[5]

Hepatitis B

Until 1982 prevention of hepatitis B (HB) was based on passive immunization either with standard immunoglobulin (Ig) containing a moderate level of anti-HBs or with hepatitis B immune globulin (HBIG) containing a higher level of anti-HBs. Whereas immune globulin (IG) and HBIG may have reduced the frequency of clinical illness, it was never proved that either globulin prevented infection. In 1987 a genetically engineered vaccine was developed to provide active immunity. Current recommendations for immunization against HBV can be divided into those for pre-exposure and those for post-exposure prophylaxis.

SAFETY
ALERT

> For pre-exposure prophylaxis (active immunity) against HBV in settings of frequent exposure and for those at high risk, three intramuscular injections (given in the deltoid, not gluteal, muscle) of HBV vaccine are recommended at 0, 1, and 6 months. Adverse reactions include headache, fever, nausea, vomiting, abdominal cramps, local soreness, redness, and swelling. Authorities strongly recommend this killed virus vaccine for all people.
>
> Despite the availability of safe and effective vaccines, a strategy for vaccinating people in the high-risk groups has not been successful. After introduction of the vaccines, the incidence of new hepatitis B cases continued to increase in the United States; fewer than 10% of all individuals in the high-risk group have been vaccinated. Therefore to have an impact on the incidence of HBV infection in the United States, hepatitis B vaccine is now included in the routine vaccination schedule for children (see Chapter 19). It is also recommended for adolescents and adults not previously immunized with the HBV vaccine.[5]
>
> For post-exposure prophylaxis in people who are not vaccinated and who sustained an exposure to HBV, a combination of hepatitis B immune globulin (HBIG) and HBV vaccine is recommended.

Hepatitis C

The transmission and prevention of HVC is similar to that of HVB. Immune globulin (IG) is ineffective in preventing hepatitis and is no longer recommended for post-exposure prophylaxis. In addition, hepatitis C vaccination is not a possible option. As shown in the Integrating Pharmacology feature shown here, drug therapy includes interferon (IFN) or pegylated interferon (PEG-IFN), a longer-acting form of interferon than IFN. More commonly, a combination therapy with IFN or PEG-IFN and ribavirin (Rebetol) is administered. Interferon is given three times a week subcutaneously; oral ribavirin is given daily. ⚗ For clients with HCV, genotype 1, PEG-IFN alfa combined with ribavirin is now replacing conventional IFN alfa combined with ribavirin as the treatment of choice for chronic HCV.

Hepatitis D

Because hepatitis D coexists with HBV, the vaccine for HBV can help to prevent hepatitis D also. The precautions that help prevent hepatitis B also are useful in preventing delta hepatitis.

Hepatitis E

General hygiene precautions are necessary for prevention of hepatitis E. Experimental recombinant vaccines have been developed and are undergoing clinical testing for prevention of hepatitis E. It is not known whether IG prevents hepatitis E or not.

Clinical Manifestations

Clients with viral hepatitis all experience liver inflammation and other pathologic changes that are similar. HBV, HCV, and hepatitis D are usually the most severe, although they may be asymptomatic in some clients. The onset of manifestations ranges from abrupt to insidious according to the incubation period and the degree of infectivity. Manifestations of viral hepatitis are systemic and vary from client to client.

Manifestations that occur during the earlier (prodromal) phase may include jaundice, lethargy, irritability, myalgia, arthralgia, anorexia, nausea, vomiting, abdominal pain (caused by stretching of Glisson's capsule surrounding the liver as a result of inflammation), diarrhea or constipation, fever, and other flu-like manifestations. Fever is caused by the release of pyrogens in the inflammatory process. Fatigue and malaise are the result of reduced energy metabolism by the liver. Pruritus, the result of bile salt accumulation in the skin, is typically mild and transient and may be more intense at its onset and termination. Jaundice, caused by impaired excretion of conjugated bilirubin, may or may not be present; when it is, it is first seen in the sclerae of the eyes and mucous membranes.

INTEGRATING PHARMACOLOGY

Interferons

Interferons (IFNs) are highly purified proteins and a natural product of human leukocytes within 4 to 6 hours after viral stimulation. IFNs exhibit a broad spectrum of antiviral and cytotoxic activity as well as immunomodulating properties (i.e., it favorably adjusts the immune system to combat foreign invasion of antigens and viruses better). As an immunomodulating agent, IFN enhances the phagocytic activity of macrophages and augments specific cytotoxicity of lymphocytes for target cells. IFN is species specific but not viral specific, meaning that it partially inhibits the reproduction of a virus immediately when a virus enters a cell. Thus the immune system and the IFN system of defense complement each other.

The several types of IFN include four types of alpha IFN: IFN alfa-2a, IFN alfa-2b, IFN alfa-n1, and IFN alfacon-1. The two types of beta IFN are IFN beta-1a and IFN beta-1b, but they are not used in the treatment of hepatitis. All types are produced by DNA recombinant techniques. The IFNs have been evaluated in a variety of viral infections, particularly in the treatment of chronic hepatitis B and C infections. IFN alfa-2a has been used effectively in hepatitis C and in chronic hepatitis B. IFN alfa-2b is used in chronic hepatitis B or C, IFN alfa-n1 is used in chronic hepatitis C, and IFN alfacon-1 is used in chronic hepatitis C.

The IFNs are not available for oral administration but must be given intramuscularly, subcutaneously, or intravenously. Adverse effects may differ slightly between types of IFN but primarily include flu-like manifestations: headache, fatigue, fever, chills, injection site reaction (pain, edema, hemorrhage, inflammation), pain, myalgia, arthralgia, and some central nervous systems effects such as depression and anxiety, dizziness, confusion, insomnia; respiratory effects such as cough; gastrointestinal effects such as nausea, diarrhea, and abdominal pain; and skin conditions such as rash, alopecia, pruritus, and urticaria.

Nursing implications include monitoring for and reporting any untoward clinical manifestations noted previously, withholding the IFN if manifestations of hepatitis worsen (i.e., jaundice or ascites), and monitoring laboratory tests that indicate liver, kidney, and thyroid function (e.g., serum albumin, bilirubin, alanine aminotransferase, hemoglobin and hematocrit).

Anicteric (without jaundice) hepatitis may or may not precede jaundice. Children with hepatitis are usually anicteric. Adults often note the appearance of darker urine (the color of tea or mahogany) and clay-colored stools a few days before clinical jaundice develops. The darker urine is from the presence of urobilinogen, which is excreted through the kidneys instead of through the bowel as normally occurs. Other manifestations often abate when jaundice appears, but they also may worsen.

If irritability and drowsiness become severe, assess for the possibility of hepatic encephalopathy. ⚗

Deterioration of handwriting is an early manifestation of hepatic encephalopathy; thus at each shift ask clients to write their name and observe their writing closely for changes. Asterixis, an abnormal muscle tremor sometimes called "liver flap," may accompany encephalopathy. This manifestation is easily elicited by applying a blood pressure cuff on the upper arm and noting whether the tremor is present when the cuff is released. Mild depression is not uncommon because of (1) the nature of the illness (weakness, jaundice, itching, and nausea), (2) its long duration and the expense of treatment, (3) the need for confinement, and (4) forgetfulness and the inability to concentrate on completion of activities of daily living (ADLs).

Bleeding tendencies may develop either from reduced prothrombin synthesis by injured hepatic cells or from reduced absorption of the fat-soluble vitamin K as a result of reduced levels of bile in the intestines. Anemia may occur because of the decreased life span of erythrocytes (RBCs). Erythrocyte destruction results from liver enzyme alterations. A transient hyperglycemia sometimes develops, and a client with diabetes mellitus may need to increase insulin dosage at this time.

The liver is larger than normal in hepatitis and is tender to palpation. Some people with viral hepatitis have spider angiomas, palmar erythema, and gynecomastia, which disappear during the recovery period. A small percentage (5% to 15%) of clients experience splenomegaly or enlargement of the posterior cervical lymph nodes. Occasionally hepatitis B is accompanied by arthralgias, rash, vasculitis, or glomerulonephritis.

Occasionally cholestatic viral hepatitis syndrome may develop. This uncommon disease process resembles mechanical obstruction; it is difficult to differentiate cholestatic viral hepatitis from biliary tract obstruction resulting from gallstones, strictures, and tumors.

The cause and pathophysiology of this hepatitis variant are unclear. Cholestatic viral hepatitis syndrome causes jaundice, itching, and the typical flu-like and gastrointestinal problems of hepatitis, but the manifestations often last longer and are more severe. Serum bilirubin reaches levels of 10 to 15 mg/dl. Diagnostic studies reveal elevations in the levels of serum lipoproteins, globulins, cholesterol, and alkaline phosphatase. Rarely the liver progressively enlarges.

Fulminant viral hepatitis may develop. This life-threatening form resembles acute liver failure with manifestations of encephalopathy (increased excitability, insomnia, somnolence, and impaired mentation). The liver rapidly decreases in size. Other problems include gastrointestinal bleeding, disseminated intravascular coagulation (DIC), fever with leukocytosis and neutrophilia, hepatorenal problems of oliguria and azotemia, edema and ascites, hypotension, respiratory failure, hypoglycemia, bacterial infection of the respiratory or urinary tract

or both, and thrombocytopenia and coagulopathy. The prognosis is poor, and death may occur before jaundice appears. Liver transplantation may be performed to save the client's life.

The presence of hepatitis B surface antigen (HBsAg) in the blood usually indicates that the person is infectious. Another antigen, hepatitis B early antigen (HBeAg), is often associated with progression of acute hepatitis to chronic hepatitis and indicates a highly infectious state.

Levels of serum aminotransferases first rise and then begin to fall as bilirubin starts to increase. Levels that rise, peak, drop, and then rise again indicate severe liver damage and a poor prognosis. Jaundice may not be clinically recognizable until levels are about 3 mg/dl. Levels of bilirubin that increase above 20 mg/dl and remain elevated for a long period may indicate severe liver necrosis, which has a poor prognosis. Mild prolongation of the prothrombin time (PT) sometimes occurs. The gamma globulin fraction and alkaline phosphatase levels are elevated in some clients. If HBV is responsible, detection of HBsAg is possible before the level of aspartate aminotransferase (AST) (formerly serum glutamic-oxaloacetic transaminase [SGOT]) rises.

Prognosis

By 3 to 6 weeks, nearly all clients with acute viral hepatitis demonstrate normal results on liver function tests; however, the clinical course, morbidity, and mortality of viral hepatitis may vary considerably. In most cases, clients recover in 3 to 16 weeks, although results on liver function testing are abnormal for a longer time. Most clients recover completely. The mortality rate is less than 1%; this rate is reportedly higher in older adults.[9]

OUTCOME MANAGEMENT

Medical Management

The acute manifestations of hepatitis generally subside over 2 to 3 weeks. Complete clinical and laboratory recovery occurs in hepatitis A by 9 weeks and in hepatitis B and hepatitis C by 16 weeks. Severe complications develop in fewer than 1% of clients with hepatitis. Clients who have severe nausea and vomiting and difficulty maintaining normal fluid balance need to be hospitalized if progressive deterioration occurs.

Reduce Fatigue

Rest is advisable in proportion to the severity of manifestations. Bed rest is usually not necessary but is recommended on an as-needed basis during the initial prodromal, anicteric phase of the disease, when the infection is most active and there is decreased metabolism by the liver. Return to normal activity during the convalescent period should be gradual. If pruritus disturbs rest, cholestyramine, antihistamines, emollients, and lipid creams may be prescribed.

Maintain Nutritional and Fluid Balance

No specific dietary measures are indicated, but most clients find a high-calorie, low-fat, high-carbohydrate diet more easily digested and more palatable. Small, frequent meals and high-calorie snacks are recommended. During the most severe phase of the illness, when changes occur in the stomach or bowel, anorexia and nausea may be so extreme that oral intake of any kind is greatly reduced. In such cases, IV administration of 10% glucose is indicated. As the client's manifestations abate and appetite improves, food and fluid intake may be resumed as tolerated. All alcoholic beverages should be avoided.

Reduce Effects of Hepatitis

Few medications are available for treating viral hepatitis. Antibiotics are not prescribed. Antiemetics control nausea and vomiting, but phenothiazines should not be used because they are biotransformed in the liver and are therefore potentially toxic. Parenteral vitamin K may be given to clients with prolonged prothrombin time (PT). Antihistamines may provide relief of pruritus but may cause sedation. Glucocorticoid therapy has no effect on viral hepatitis and is of no value in its treatment. Although glucocorticoids may reduce serum aminotransferase and bilirubin levels, they have no effect on liver necrosis or regeneration. Use of interferon-alfa for 6 to 24 weeks appreciably decreases the risk of chronic hepatitis but may be reserved for clients whose serum HCV RNA levels fail to clear after 1 to 2 months.

Bile Acid Sequestrants

The administration of the bile acid sequestrants cholestyramine (Questran) or colestipol (Colestid) can relieve pruritus associated with elevated levels of bile acids that may result from severe cholestatic liver disease. Both drugs bind bile acids in the gastrointestinal tract, forming an insoluble complex that is excreted in the feces. The result of this action is increased clearance of cholesterol.

Immune Globulin

Immune globulin, although not used to treat viral hepatitis, does provide prophylaxis for family and friends. If given early, standard immune globulin (a preparation of proteins capable of acting as antibodies, formerly termed immune serum globulin) may prevent hepatitis A or mitigate the severity of manifestations. HAV does not remain in the blood long; therefore there is no healthy carrier state for HAV as there is for HBV.

Vaccines

Vaccines are available to promote immunity to HAV and HBV. Vaccines for HEV are being tested. In addition to immune globulin, they may be administered prophylactically in people exposed to infected clients.

Medications to Avoid

Clinicians administer few medications to clients with hepatitis. Medications such as chlorpromazine, aspirin, acetaminophen, and a variety of sedatives are given as infrequently as possible because of their hepatotoxic properties.

Nursing Management of the Medical Client

Assessment. To determine the type of hepatitis present, always begin by questioning the client about possible exposure to risk factors. Ask about common manifestations, especially jaundice, and about manifestations of disease progression, such as hepatic encephalopathy (see Hepatic Encephalopathy under Complications of Cirrhosis). Assess the results of liver function studies, and monitor them to ascertain progression of the disease. Also assess the ability of the client and the family to provide home and self-care. Their understanding of the disease and its implications is vital to its successful management in the home setting.

Diagnosis, Outcomes, Interventions

Diagnosis: Fatigue. The client with hepatitis has tremendous metabolic demands, leading to the nursing diagnosis *Fatigue related to decreased metabolic energy production secondary to liver dysfunction.*

Outcomes. The client will convey reduced fatigue and heightened energy as evidenced by compliance with activity restrictions and a gradual increase in activity to the pre-illness level.

Interventions. Fatigue associated with hepatitis may interfere with ADL. Most clients experience the greatest fatigue during the anicteric phase (before jaundice occurs) and begin to feel stronger during the icteric phase. Fatigue may persist, however, even after the jaundice clears. Clients with severe jaundice may suffer pruritus (see Jaundice for nursing interventions for *Impaired Skin Integrity related to pruritus*). During the period of severe fatigue, advise the client to rest in bed. Most clients who feel capable of being up and around can do so without harm if they rest after meals and do not engage in any activity to the point of becoming overly tired. Because prolonged bed rest itself can lead to weakness, a reasonable activity level is more conducive to recovery than enforced bed rest.

Encourage ADLs such as exercise of bathroom privileges, performance of personal hygiene measures, and self-feeding unless these activities cause excessive fatigue. Advise the client to plan rest periods while jaundice is present, especially after meals. Clients who engage in excessive activity too early in the recovery phase sometimes experience a relapse, potentially leading to liver failure.

Diagnosis: Imbalanced Nutrition: Less Than Body Requirements.

For the liver to heal properly and to regenerate, nutrition is important. Clients with hepatitis often have a decreased appetite, leading to a common nursing diagnosis of *Imbalanced Nutrition: Less Than Body Requirements related to anorexia, nausea, bile stasis, and altered absorption and metabolism.*

Outcomes. The client will maintain an intake of the required calories to maintain weight as evidenced by having no weight loss and possibly having weight gain.

Interventions

Modify Diet. To help the client meet the nutritional requirements associated with hepatitis, perform the following:

- Provide a nutritious breakfast. Because anorexia usually worsens during the day, breakfast may be the best-tolerated meal.
- Encourage the client to avoid fatty foods, which can induce nausea.
- Include the optimal amount of protein and carbohydrates to allow recovery of injured liver cells without overfeeding. If the client has no problem with protein metabolism, a normal intake is helpful for tissue repair. Clients with severe hepatitis who are at risk for developing hepatic encephalopathy, however, require a low-protein diet (to prevent the buildup of ammonia in the blood from incomplete clearing of protein metabolic wastes). Alterations in fat metabolism differ according to the degree of interruption of bile production and excretion.
- Suggest multiple small meals. This approach allows the client with anorexia to ingest a diet of 2500 to 3000 calories more comfortably. Also, candy, juice, sweetened tea, and carbonated drinks can supply calories when nausea is a problem.

Avoid Alcohol. Remind the client to avoid alcohol, which is an extremely hepatotoxic agent.

Provide Vitamin Supplements. Explain that vitamin supplements are not generally necessary in uncomplicated hepatitis if the diet is adequate in nutrients.

Vitamin K supplements, as ordered, may be administered if the PT is longer than normal.

Relieve Nausea and Vomiting. Clients who experience severe nausea and vomiting may obtain relief with antiemetics. Before administering these medications, review their effect on liver function. Phenothiazines such as prochlorperazine (Compazine) are usually contraindicated. If the client cannot tolerate any oral intake, provide IV nutrition.

Diagnosis: Anxiety. Because predicting the outcome of hepatitis is difficult, the nursing diagnosis *Anxiety related to uncertainty of the effects of hepatitis* is common.

Outcomes. The client will experience a decrease in anxiety as evidenced by the ability to discuss his or her feelings about the disease.

Interventions. Encourage clients with hepatitis to express their feelings concerning the following:

- The illness
- The duration and cost of the illness
- Alterations in home life and financial status (especially for the parent of young children or for the sole family earner)
- The effect of the illness on future health problems
- The possibility of death in clients who are very ill

Suggest psychosocial and financial counseling for the client who is disturbed. Increase the client's knowledge and understanding of the illness by teaching the facts about the illness and its management. Increased knowledge can reduce anxiety.

Evaluation. Because the clinical course of acute viral hepatitis varies considerably from one client to another, the nurse must assess outcomes carefully to determine whether they have been met. Recovery without permanent liver damage is expected to occur within 1 to 4 months. Permanent damage may result if the therapeutic regimen is not followed.

Self-Care

Most clients recover from acute viral hepatitis, do not require hospitalization, and are appropriately managed at home. Clinical and biochemical relapses may occur before full recovery, however. In addition, complications of acute viral hepatitis may develop, necessitating careful monitoring, especially in older clients.

Avoid Hepatotoxins

There is no specific ongoing pharmacologic management of clients recovering from acute viral hepatitis. Advise the client to avoid alcohol and medications such as aspirin, acetaminophen, and sedatives because of their hepatotoxicity.

Promote Nutrition

Encourage clients to continue eating a well-balanced, nutritional diet. A low-fat, high-carbohydrate diet is generally tolerated best. A well-balanced diet promotes liver healing, leading to improved tolerance for activity.

Promote Rest

Help the client understand the need for adequate rest so that the liver can heal on its own. The client needs to be active enough to prevent complications of immobility but not so active to risk relapse. Discuss with the client the need for help at home after discharge (such as with housework or shopping) because limits on activity will still have to be maintained. The client is also expected to resume pre-hepatitis activities and to remain free from complications.

Prevent Infection and Reinfection

Teach the client to avoid reinfection or possible spread of the infection to other family members. You may recommend vaccination for HAV and HBV to promote health maintenance. Caution the client and the client's significant others to avoid sexual activity until there is no longer a chance of disease transmission (generally after liver function tests have returned to normal) and to check with the physician before resuming sexual relations. The client will need to see a physician at regular intervals after discharge to ensure that the liver is healing and no further damage has occurred.

COMPLICATIONS OF HEPATITIS

Clients with viral hepatitis typically recover completely from the illness in 3 to 16 weeks. Clients who are otherwise healthy usually recover from hepatitis A without major sequelae. Although hepatitis A is associated with a low mortality, relapses weeks to months after apparent recovery may occur. Hepatitis A does not progress to chronic liver disease. Fulminant hepatitis resembling acute liver failure may occur and is primarily seen in hepatitis B and D as well as in hepatitis E and rarely in hepatitis A. Clients with hepatitis B tend to experience more complications; 1 in 10 people develops chronic active hepatitis as a result of hepatitis B, often leading to destruction of the liver. Cirrhosis may follow a severe case of hepatitis B or chronic active hepatitis.

Primary hepatocellular carcinoma is a potential complication of chronic hepatitis. Other possible complications of hepatitis include chronic persistent hepatitis, chronic carrier state, and aplastic anemia.

Fulminant Hepatitis

Fulminant hepatitis (massive hepatic necrosis) is rare and, as noted previously, is seen primarily in hepatitis B and D as well as in hepatitis E and A. Fulminant hepatitis causes severe illness and is fatal in 1% to 2% of all cases and in up to 20% of cases occurring in pregnant women. Fulminant hepatitis involves a progression of manifestations that include jaundice, hepatic encephalopathy, and ascites. The death rate varies with age but approaches 90% to 100%, especially in people older than age 60.

Chronic Hepatitis

Chronic hepatitis exists when liver inflammation continues beyond a period of 3 to 6 months. Acute viral hepatitis in the end may lead to chronic hepatitis, with the exception of hepatitis A and E. Causes of chronic hepatitis are listed in Box 47-1.

Several categories of chronic hepatitis have been noted in the past. These categories were based on histologic criteria and included chronic persistent hepatitis (CPH), chronic lobular hepatitis (CLH), and chronic active hepatitis (CAH). CPH and CLH were thought to be milder and have a good prognosis; progression to more serious lesions was considered rare. CAH was thought to have a more serious prognosis with significant risk for progression to cirrhosis and liver failure.

More information is now available about the causes, natural history, pathogenesis, serologic features, and therapy of chronic hepatitis. The former categories have been replaced by categories based on (1) its cause or etiology; (2) its histologic activity or grade of injury as determined by the numbers and location of inflammatory cells; and (3) its degree of progression or stage as determined

---

BOX 47-1   Causes of Chronic Hepatitis

VIRAL
- Hepatitis B
- Hepatitis B with superimposed hepatitis D
- Hepatitis C

DRUGS AND TOXINS
- Methyldopa
- Nitrofurantoin
- Amiodarone
- Isoniazid

AUTOIMMUNE
- Presence of *HLA-B8* and *HLA-DR3* following hepatitis A, Epstein-Barr infection, or measles

GENETIC AND METABOLIC DISORDERS
- Wilson's disease
- Alpha$_1$-antitrypsin deficiency
- Nonalcoholic steatohepatitis

Data from Sheikh, A.M., Fallon, M.B., et al. (2004). Acute and chronic hepatitis. I T.E. Andreoli, et al. (Eds.), *Cecil essentials of medicine* (6th ed., p. 400 Philadelphia: Saunders.

TABLE 47–3 Comparison of Old and New Nomenclature of Chronic Hepatitis

| Old Classification | New Classification | |
	Grade (Activity)	Stage (Fibrosis)
Chronic persistent hepatitis	Minimal or mild	None or mild
Chronic lobular hepatitis	Mild or moderate	Mild
Chronic active hepatitis	Mild, moderate, or severe	Mild, moderate, or severe

Data from Dienstag, J.L., & Isselbacher, K.L. (2005). Chronic hepatitis. In D. Kasper, et al. (Eds.), *Harrison's principles of internal medicine* (16th ed., pp. 1844-1855). New York: McGraw-Hill.

by degree, location, and distortion of normal architecture by fibrosis (Table 47-3).

In clients with what was formerly known as CPH, cirrhosis is absent or rare. As a general rule, clients are asymptomatic or have mild manifestations such as fatigue, anorexia, or nausea and some liver enlargement. Clients with CPH generally have an excellent prognosis. In the new nomenclature, CPH is classified by grade as minimal or mild chronic hepatitis and by stage as absent or mild fibrosis.

In clients with what was formerly known as CLH, portal inflammation with foci of necrosis and inflammation in the liver lobule occur. Progression to CAH and cirrhosis is rare. CLH corresponds in the new nomenclature to a mild or moderate grade and a stage of absent or minimal fibrosis.

CAH is characterized by elevation of serum transaminase levels for more than 6 months. CAH is a progressive disorder that can lead to cirrhosis, liver failure, and death. Although some clients are asymptomatic, most clients tend to have mild to severe constitutional clinical manifestations, especially fatigue. Jaundice and hyperbilirubinemia are more common in CAH. In the new nomenclature for chronic hepatitis, what used to be CAH spans the entire spectrum of activity grade from minimal, to mild, to severe chronic hepatitis; the grade of portal, periportal, and lobular inflammation; and the stage of fibrosis that can be mild, moderate, or severe fibrosis as well as cirrhosis.

With the new classification and criteria for identification of chronic hepatitis, both serologic studies and liver biopsies are used in the diagnosis and in planning treatment (Figure 47-1). This next section addresses briefly three types of chronic hepatitis: chronic hepatitis B, chronic hepatitis C, and autoimmune hepatitis.

Chronic Hepatitis B

Chronic hepatitis B primarily affects males; nearly 400 million people worldwide and 1.25 million in the United States are affected.[6] Chronic hepatitis B follows acute HBV in about 5% of adults in the United States. Clients who are HBsAg and HBeAg positive are considered to be in a high replicative phase compared with those who are HBsAg and HBeAb positive (low replicative phase). Onset of the disease tends to be insidious. Clinical manifestations include fatigue and intermittent or persistent jaundice. Treatment of chronic HBV depends on the level of virus replication but generally includes lamivudine 100 mg orally daily. This medication can be given instead of IFN for the treatment of chronic hepatitis B and is tolerated much better. Other antiviral

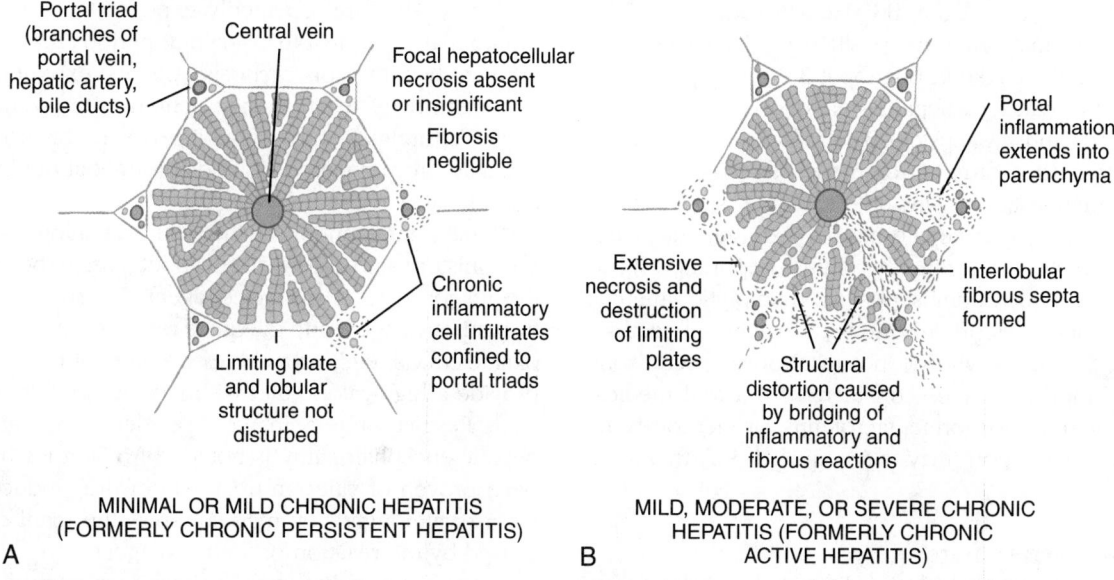

MINIMAL OR MILD CHRONIC HEPATITIS
(FORMERLY CHRONIC PERSISTENT HEPATITIS)

A

MILD, MODERATE, OR SEVERE CHRONIC
HEPATITIS (FORMERLY CHRONIC
ACTIVE HEPATITIS)

B

■ **FIGURE 47–1** Comparison of structural changes with chronic hepatitis. **A,** Inflammation is confined to portal triads in minimal or mild chronic hepatitis (formerly known as chronic persistent hepatitis). **B,** Inflammation extends into the parenchyma in mild, moderate, or severe hepatitis (formerly known as chronic active hepatitis).

agents such as adefovir dipivoxil may be given. Strategies using multiple drugs are likely to be tried in the future. IFN may be administered also, but the medication may not be tolerated well and has not been effective in immunosuppressed people. Short-term treatment with glucocorticoids may be helpful, but glucocorticoids are not effective for long-term therapy.

Chronic Hepatitis C

Chronic hepatitis C follows acute hepatitis C in 50% to 70% of cases. Many cases of hepatitis C are identified in asymptomatic clients who have no known history of acute hepatitis C. They discover they have chronic hepatitis C when they decide to donate blood or as a result of routine laboratory screening tests. Chronic hepatitis C tends to be slowly and insidiously progressive with approximately one fourth of the cases progressing eventually to end-stage cirrhosis. Progression to cirrhosis is variable and depends on multiple factors, such as degree of liver histology, age when infected, and duration of infection. Clinical manifestations are similar to those for chronic hepatitis B and include fatigue, depression, weight loss, and arthralgia. Jaundice is rare. Treatment of chronic hepatitis C is generally considered in clients under age 70 with elevated serum aminotransferase levels and more than minimal inflammation or fibrosis on liver biopsy. Standard therapy is a combination of recombinant interferon-alfa (IFNa) and ribavirin (see the Integrating Pharmacology feature on Interferons on p. 1152).[6,12,15,19]

Autoimmune Hepatitis

Autoimmune liver disease is generally a disease of young women and is characterized by hepatic inflammation with plasma cells and fibrosis but can occur in either gender at any age. Affected people often are positive for human leukocyte antigen B8 (HLA-B8) and HLA-DR3 and older clients often are positive for HLA-DR4. The onset is usually insidious, but about 25% of cases present as an acute attack of hepatitis or follow a viral illness such as hepatitis A, Epstein-Barr infection, or measles or exposure to a drug or toxin such as nitrofurantoin. Clinical manifestations include multiple spider nevi, acne, hirsutism, and hepatomegaly. Extrahepatic manifestations include arthritis, thyroiditis, nephritis, ulcerative colitis, and Coombs'-positive hemolytic anemia. Treatment includes prednisone with or without azathioprine. Clients who do not respond to prednisone and azathioprine may be considered for a trial medication regimen: cyclosporine, tacrolimus, or methotrexate. Liver transplantation may be required for treatment failures.[9]

Chronic Carrier State

A carrier state is possible in clients who demonstrate persistent HBsAg without clinically evident disease but who are able to transmit the disease. Carriers of HBsAg

are at increased risk for development of hepatocellular carcinoma, especially if they were infected during infancy or early childhood. A carrier state may also develop for hepatitis C; blood donated by apparently healthy clients may transmit hepatitis C when transfused.

Aplastic Anemia

Aplastic anemia, although rare, carries a high death rate when it occurs after acute viral hepatitis. No treatment has been demonstrated to be effective in reversing this condition although bone marrow transplant has been successful for some clients. Management is supportive and palliative. Therapy includes (1) IV fluids to provide hydration, (2) correction of electrolyte abnormalities, (3) medications for reduction of pain and nausea, and (4) adequate caloric intake.

TOXIC HEPATITIS

Toxins and drugs can produce a wide variety of pathologic lesions in the liver. Some agents cause toxic hepatitis, whereas others produce necrosis, cholestasis, or cancers. The extent and type of hepatitis produced by the toxin depend on the degree of exposure, the chemical properties of the hepatotoxin, and the genetic makeup of the individual. Most commonly, the causative agent is a toxic metabolite formed by the drug-metabolizing enzymes within the liver. Table 47-4 lists some hepatotoxic agents. Liver necrosis occurs within 2 or 3 days after acute exposure to a dose-related hepatotoxin; however, several weeks may pass before manifestations of idiosyncratic reactions appear. People experiencing either type of hepatotoxicity demonstrate abnormal results on liver function testing.

People who are repeatedly exposed to hepatotoxins in minimal amounts but over long periods may develop chronic hepatitis or cirrhosis. Clients experiencing a hypersensitivity reaction may demonstrate eosinophilia, fever, arthralgia, and sometimes xanthomatosis (an excessive accumulation of lipids brought about by faulty lipid metabolism).

Nursing intervention begins with obtaining a detailed drug history and information about past exposure and the response to a suspected agent. Ensure removal of the causative agent and adequate rest, promote alleviation of side effects (e.g., with cholestyramine for pruritus), and provide a high-calorie diet with fats and protein as tolerated. Restrict protein intake if evidence of impending hepatic encephalopathy is noted. Steroids have not been proven of value in treatment of drug-induced liver disease, although they may suppress the manifestations caused by the reaction of the toxic agent.

Renal failure sometimes appears as a complication of toxic hepatitis. Assessment and interventions for renal failure are discussed in Chapter 36.

TABLE 47-4 Known Hepatotoxic Substances (Cause Alteration in Liver Morphology)

Principal Morphologic Change	Class of Agent	Example of Substance
Cholestasis	Anabolic steroid	Methyl testosterone
	Antithyroid	Methimazole
	Antibiotic	Erythromycin
		Nitrofurantoin
		Rifampin
		Amoxicillin-clavulanic acid
	Oral contraceptive	Norethynodrel with
	Oral hypoglycemic	mestranol
	Tranquilizer	Chlorpropamide
	Immunosuppressive	Chlorpromazine
	Calcium channel blocker	Cyclosporine
		Verapamil, nifedipine
Hepatitis	Oncotherapeutic	Methotrexate
	Anesthetic	Halothane
	Antihypertensive	Methyldopa, captopril
	Antibiotic	Isoniazid, rifampin
	Diuretic	Chlorothiazide
	Antidepressant	Isoniazid, amitriptyline, imipramine
	Anti-inflammatory	Ibuprofen, indomethacin
	Antifungal	Ketoconazole, fluconazole
Toxic (necrosis)	Hydrocarbon	Carbon tetrachloride
	Metal	Yellow phosphorus
	Mushroom	*Amanita phalloides*
	Analgesic	Acetaminophen

Data from Dienstag, J.L., & Isselbacher, K.L. (2005). Toxic and drug-induced hepatitis. In D. Kasper, et al. (Eds.), *Harrison's principles of internal medicine* (16th ed., pp. 1838-1844). New York: McGraw-Hill.

ALCOHOLIC HEPATITIS

Alcoholic hepatitis may be acute or chronic. It is caused by parenchymal necrosis resulting from heavy alcohol ingestion. Although sometimes reversible, this condition is the most frequent cause of cirrhosis. This fact is important because cirrhosis of the liver is a common cause of death among adults in the United States.

Clinical manifestations of alcoholic hepatitis usually develop after a bout of heavy drinking. Assessment reveals anorexia, nausea, abdominal pain, splenomegaly, hepatomegaly, jaundice, ascites, fever, and encephalopathy. Laboratory studies typically show anemia, leukocytosis, and an elevated serum bilirubin level. Liver biopsy reveals fatty hepatic tissue. Hepatitis resulting from excessive alcohol intake carries a poor prognosis, particularly if the client continues to ingest alcohol.

Nursing interventions include providing a high-vitamin, high-carbohydrate diet, administering folic acid and thiamine supplements, and giving parenteral fluids as ordered. Administration of liquid formulas may be useful in increasing caloric intake. Steroids sometimes have a beneficial effect, although their use remains controversial.

CIRRHOSIS

Cirrhosis of the liver is a chronic, progressive disease characterized by widespread fibrosis (scarring) and nodule formation. Cirrhosis occurs when the normal flow of blood, bile, and hepatic metabolites is altered by fibrosis and changes in the hepatocytes, bile ductules, vascular channels, and reticular cells.

The following are the four major types of cirrhosis:

- Alcoholic (historically called Laënnec's cirrhosis or micronodular or portal cirrrhosis)
- Postnecrotic (macronodular or toxin-induced cirrhosis)
- Biliary
- Cardiac

The types are compared in Table 47-5. The two major clinical problems in cirrhosis are (1) decreased liver function and (2) portal hypertension. The latter problem develops in severe cirrhosis.

Cirrhosis is the eighth leading cause of death in the United States.[9] Men are more likely than women to have alcoholic (Laënnec's) cirrhosis. Worldwide, postnecrotic cirrhosis is the most common form; it is also more common in women. Mortality is higher from all types of cirrhosis in men and nonwhites.

Etiology and Risk Factors

The causes of cirrhosis have not been clearly identified, although the relationship between cirrhosis and excessive alcohol ingestion is well established. Countries with the highest incidence of cirrhosis have the greatest per capita consumption of alcohol. Genetic predisposition with a familial tendency, as well as a hypersensitivity to alcohol, is seen in alcoholic cirrhosis.

The primary risk factor for cirrhosis is alcohol ingestion, especially in the absence of proper nutrition. Any client with a family history of alcoholism should avoid alcohol because of the increased risk. Hence cessation of alcohol consumption may be a health promotion, health maintenance, or health restoration activity. The amount of alcohol consumed daily appears to be a more important factor than the pattern of drinking (binge versus daily) or the type of alcoholic beverage consumed. If the client is in a poor nutritional state, the likelihood of damage is greater and the damage is more severe. Viral hepatitis is the primary risk factor for postnecrotic cirrhosis, which makes prevention of hepatitis through vaccination and good hygiene the most important health promotion activity.

Other risk factors for cirrhosis of the liver are biliary cirrhosis with intrahepatic cholestasis or obstruction of bile

TABLE 47–5 Comparison of Postnecrotic, Biliary, Cardiac, and Alcoholic Cirrhosis

Definition	Etiology	Pathology	Assessment Data	Diagnosis and Prognosis	Intervention(s)
Postnecrotic (Macronodular) Cirrhosis					
Most common worldwide form Massive loss of liver cells, with irregular patterns of regenerating cells	Postacute viral (types B and C) hepatitis Postintoxication with industrial chemicals Some infections and metabolic disorders	Liver small and nodular	As in alcoholic cirrhosis except less muscle wasting and more jaundice	Needle biopsy of liver establishes pathologic processes Within 5 years, 75% die of complications ↑ serum aminotransferases ↑ gamma globulins	Treat complications as needed
Biliary Cirrhosis					
Bile flow decreased with concurrent cell damage to hepatocytes around bile ductules	*Primary:* Chronic stasis of bile in intrahepatic ducts Cause unknown Autoimmune process implicated	Early-stage biopsy reveals inflammatory process with necrosis of cells and ducts Hepatocytes are lost and scar tissue remains	Fatigue Generalized pruritus Dark urine Pale stools Jaundice Impaired bile flow	Elevated serum bilirubin levels *Early:* 3-10 mg/100 ml *Late:* >50 mg/100 ml High elevations of alkaline phosphatase ↑ gamma globulins ↑ blood lipids	*Primary:* Ursodiol Treatment is symptomatic (e.g., high-calorie diet, lower intake of fats by 30-40 g/day if problems develop) Cholestyramine for pruritus Supplement of fat-soluble vitamins
	Secondary: Obstruction of bile ducts outside of liver	End stage similar to postnecrotic type	Steatorrhea ↓ absorption of fat-soluble vitamins Elevated serum lipids ↑cholesterol deposits in subcutaneous tissues Signs of portal hypertension	Presence of lipoprotein X ↑ serum bile salts Hypoprothrombinemia ↑ antimitochondrial antibody in primary cases ↑ serum copper in primary cases	*Secondary:* Treatment to relieve mechanical obstruction
Cardiac Cirrhosis					
Chronic liver disease associated with severe right-sided long-term heart failure (fairly rare)	Atrioventricular valve disease Prolonged constrictive pericarditis	*Early:* Dark-colored liver enlarged by blood and edema fluid	Slight jaundice, enlarged liver, and ascites in person with severe cardiac impairment over 10-year span RUQ pain during acute congestion	↑ conjugated bilirubin in serum ↑ sulfobromophthalein ↓ albumin in serum ↑ serum aminotransferases ↑ alkaline phosphatase Liver biopsy *Prognosis:* Depends on course of cardiac disease	Cause of chronic heart failure is treated if possible
	Decompensated cor pulmonale	*Late:* Liver capsule thickens and nodular scarring occurs	Cachexia Fluid retention Circulatory problems		
Alcoholic Cirrhosis					
Alcoholic cirrhosis (Laënnec's, micronodular) Small nodules form as result of persistence of some offending agent	Associated with alcohol abuse	Scarring and collagen tissue deposits Regenerating nodules are very small Normal lobular structure is destroyed	May produce no symptoms for long periods Onset of symptoms may be insidious or abrupt *Early:* Weakness, fatigue, weight loss *Later:* Anorexia, nausea, and vomiting Abdominal pain Ascites Menstrual irregularities Impotence Enlarged breasts in men Hematemesis Spider angiomas	Liver biopsy; history of alcohol abuse; high AST; high bilirubin (slight); anemia Prognosis depends on presence of complications and continued abuse of alcohol	Primarily supportive Correction of vitamin and mineral deficiencies if any (e.g., folate, thiamine, pyridoxine, vitamin K, and minerals [magnesium and phosphate]); treat complications as needed (e.g., ferrous sulfate for anemia, IV vasopressin for esophageal varices, reduce or withhold dietary protein for hepatic encephalopathy or vitamin K for hemorrhagic tendency)

AST, Aspartate aminotransferase; *IV,* intravenous; *RUQ,* right upper quadrant.

Data from Chung, R.T., & Podolsky, D.T. (2005). Cirrhosis and its complications. In E. Braunwald, et al. (Eds.), *Harrison's principles of internal medicine* (16th ed., pp. 1858-1869). New York: McGraw-Hill.

ducts; use of drugs (such as acetaminophen, methotrexate, or isoniazid); hepatic congestion from severe right-sided heart failure; constrictive pericarditis; valvular disease; alpha$_1$-antitrypsin deficiency; infiltrative disease (such as amyloidosis, glycogen storage diseases, or hemochromatosis); Wilson's disease; and nutritional deficits related to jejunal bypass. Acetaminophen overdose was determined as the most frequent cause of acute liver failure.[17]

Pathophysiology

Cirrhosis is the final stage in many types of liver insults. The cirrhotic liver usually has a nodular consistency, with bands of fibrosis (scar tissue) and small areas of regenerating tissue. There is extensive destruction of hepatocytes. This alteration in the architecture of the liver alters flow in the vascular and lymphatic systems and bile duct channels. Periodic exacerbations are marked by bile stasis, precipitating jaundice.

Portal vein hypertension develops in severe cirrhosis. The portal vein receives blood from the intestines and spleen. Thus an increase of pressure in the portal vein causes (1) a retrograde increase in pressure resistance and enlargement of the esophageal, umbilical, and superior rectus veins, which may result in bleeding varices; (2) ascites (the result of osmotic or hydrostatic shifts leading to fluid accumulation in the peritoneum); and (3) incomplete clearing of protein metabolic wastes with a resultant increase in ammonia, thus leading to hepatic encephalopathy.

Continuation of the process as a result of unknown causes or of alcohol abuse usually results in death from hepatic encephalopathy, bacterial (gram-negative) infection, peritonitis (bacterial), hepatoma (liver tumor), or complications of portal hypertension. The Concept Map feature, pp. 1150-1151, on Understanding Cirrhosis and Its Treatment summarizes pathophysiologic changes, clinical manifestations, and treatment of cirrhosis.

Clinical Manifestations

Manifestations of cirrhosis diminish if the process is arrested at an early stage. Cirrhosis is a disease that initially progresses slowly. Thus people with cirrhosis often discover the condition incidentally when seeking health care for other problems. In the early stages of cirrhosis, findings include hepatomegaly (enlarged liver), vascular changes, and abnormal results of laboratory tests. Palpation reveals a firm (scarred), lumpy (nodular), usually enlarged liver (although the liver becomes hard and shrunken in late cirrhosis).

In advanced cirrhosis, assessment reveals the following severe complications with their physiologic bases: ascites caused by malnutrition, portal hypertension, hypoalbuminemia, and hyperaldosteronism; gastrointestinal bleeding arises from esophageal varices (swollen veins), hypoprothrombinemia, thrombocytopenia, and portal hypertension and often results in encephalopathy.

Splenomegaly (enlargement of the spleen) indicates severe portal hypertension. Anemia, leukopenia, or thrombocytopenia may result from splenomegaly. Portal hypertension may cause prominent abdominal wall veins and internal hemorrhoids.

Infections may be present as a result of an enlarged, overactive spleen, causing leukopenia. In addition, the bacteria that remain in the portal venous blood bypass the liver and are not removed by Kupffer cells and hence may cause infection. Ammonia no longer removed by the liver accumulates to levels toxic to the brain, resulting in encephalopathy. Renal failure occurs with rapidly failing hepatic function. Laboratory determinations reveal impaired hepatocellular function: elevated serum levels of liver enzymes (AST, alanine aminotransferase [ALT], and lactate dehydrogenase [LDH]), hypoalbuminemia, anemia, and prolonged PT. Liver biopsy allows a definitive diagnosis and demonstrates the associated pathologic changes.

OUTCOME MANAGEMENT

Medical Management

Monitor for Complications
Ascites, bleeding esophageal varices, and hepatic encephalopathy are discussed in depth later in this chapter. They are the most feared complications of cirrhosis. Renal failure (hepatorenal syndrome) and infection also are deadly. Family members and the client are taught manifestations of progressive liver failure. The family members should know what manifestations they need to report to the physician and when to seek immediate assistance, such as when variceal bleeding or a decrease in the level of consciousness occurs. Clients with encephalopathy may need extensive home care.

Maximize Liver Function
Although cirrhosis is a progressive, degenerative disorder, steps are taken to minimize the risk of trauma and maximize regeneration, thereby slowing the course of the disease and prolonging life. A nutritious diet is recommended for clients with cirrhosis. The diet should be palatable, with adequate calories and protein (75 to 100 g/day) unless hepatic encephalopathy is present, in which case protein is limited. A list of foods to be included in the diet is given to the client and family. Fat intake need not be restricted. If edema or fluid retention is present, restrict sodium and fluids. If the client is receiving a thiazide diuretic, the diet should be high in potassium. The B vitamins and fat-soluble vitamins (vitamins A, D, E, and K) are commonly given to clients with alcoholic cirrhosis. Adequate rest also is important to maximize regeneration of the liver. In

CONCEPT MAP

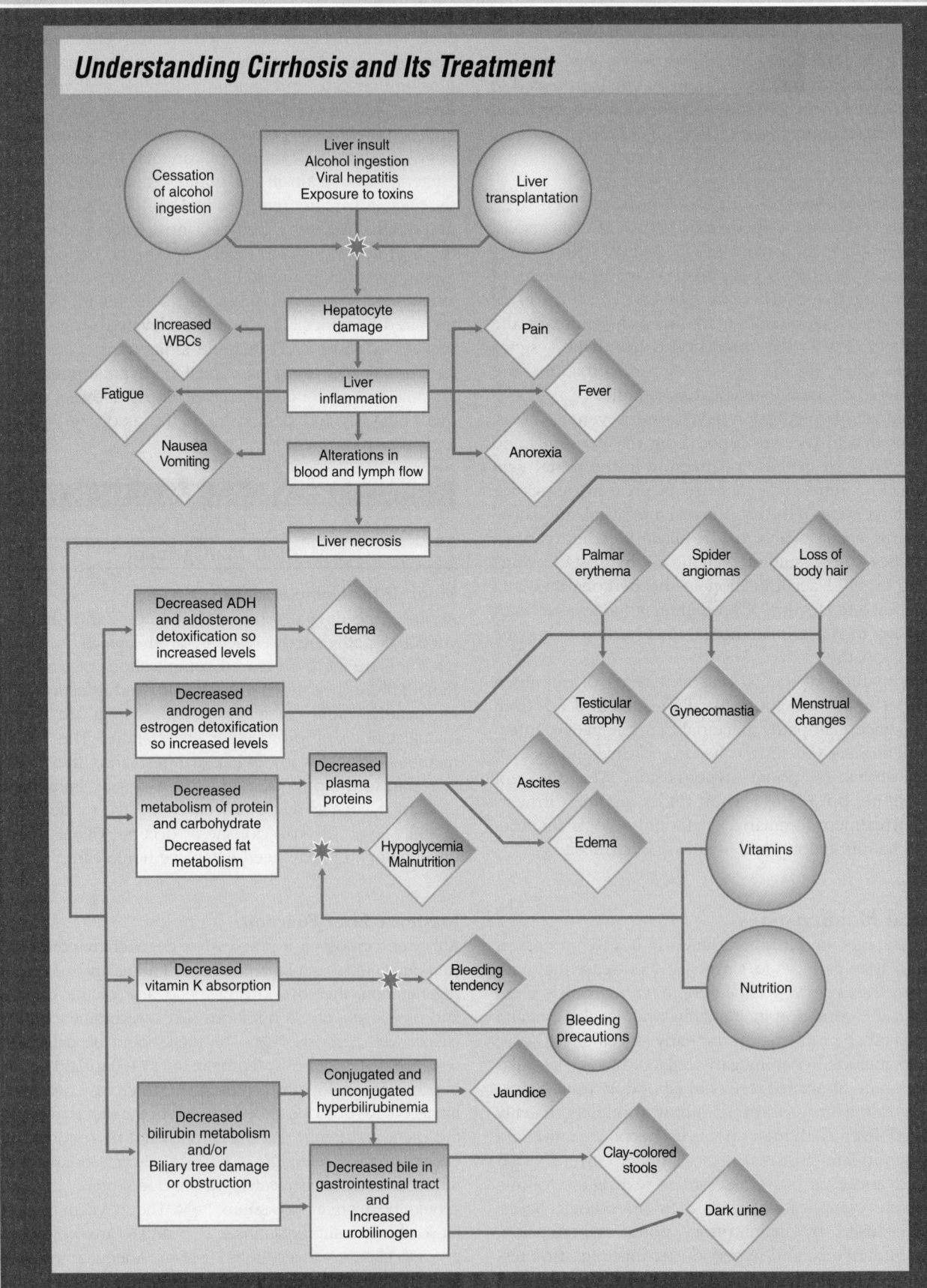

Understanding Cirrhosis and Its Treatment

C O N C E P T   M A P

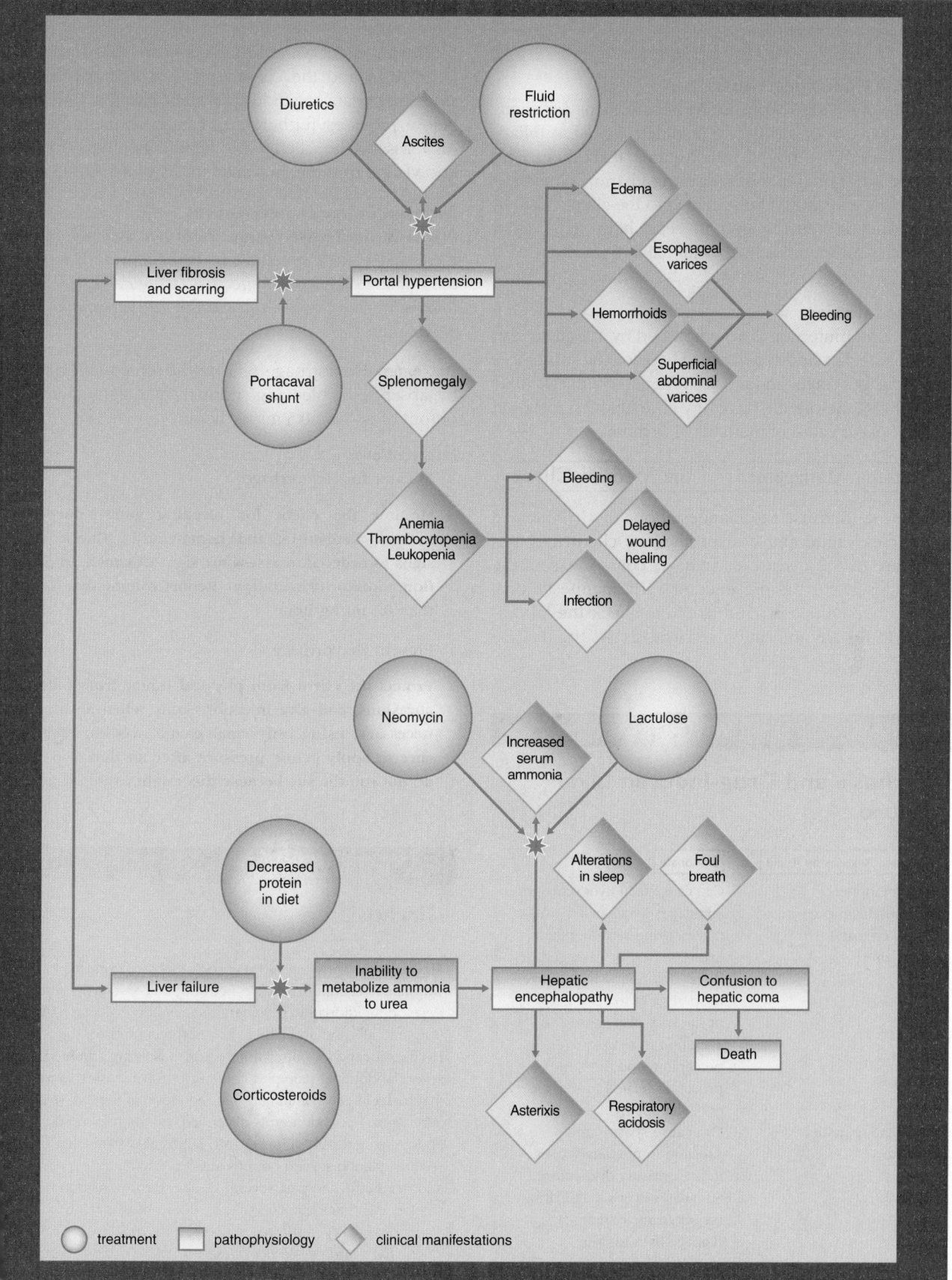

postnecrotic or posthepatic cirrhosis, the clinician may prescribe corticosteroids to reduce manifestations of cirrhosis and improve liver function. Other medications may be used to treat the complications.

Treat the Underlying Causes

It is important that exposure to hepatotoxins be eliminated, that use of alcohol be avoided, and that biliary obstruction be removed. Medications that should be avoided are shown in the Integrating Pharmacology feature below and should be specified to the client. The client should be encouraged to seek help (e.g., from Alcoholics Anonymous [AA]) with alcohol abstinence.

Prevent Infection

Prevention of infection is accomplished by adequate rest, appropriate diet, and avoidance of hepatotoxic substances (alcoholic beverages and medications and chemicals toxic to the liver). Before the discovery of antibiotics, infection was the major cause of mortality in cirrhosis.

Nursing Management of the Medical Client

Assessment. Because the manifestations of cirrhosis are sometimes vague and nonspecific, the client may not be aware of the disease early in its course. Assess the client closely for the presence of early manifestations, such as hepatomegaly, and carefully check the laboratory data for any indication of cirrhosis. As the disease progresses, assess for manifestations of complications of cirrhosis, such as ascites, portal hypertension, or hepatic encephalopathy. These are discussed later in the chapter.

When a client with cirrhosis is hospitalized, use laboratory data and the client's physical and psychosocial assessment data to guide care planning. The Case Study below provides further information about these tests. Also assess the client and family members for their knowledge of the important aspects of self-care.

Diagnosis, Outcomes, Interventions

Diagnosis: Ineffective Tissue Perfusion. Because of the increased risk of bleeding in the client with cirrhosis, the nursing diagnosis *Ineffective Tissue Perfusion related to bleeding tendencies and varices that may hemorrhage* is common.

Outcomes. Hemorrhage will be prevented as evidenced by absence of bleeding, normal vital signs, and urine output of at least 0.5 ml/kg/hour.

Interventions

Monitor for Hemorrhage

Monitor the client for bleeding gums, purpura, melena, hematuria, and hematemesis. Check vital signs as ordered to assess for signs of shock. In addition, monitor urine output. Report volume that is less than 0.5 ml/kg/hour.

Prevent Hemorrhage

Protect the client from physical injury from falls or abrasions, and give injections only when absolutely necessary, using only small-gauge needles. Be sure to apply gentle pressure after an injection, but do not rub the site because this might cause bruising.

INTEGRATING PHARMACOLOGY

Cirrhosis and Drug-Induced Liver Failure

Drugs to Restrict or Avoid	Rationale
Acetaminophen	Can cause fatal liver damage
Phenobarbital, phenytoin, chlorpromazine (Thorazine)	Stimulates liver's major drug-metabolizing system; when liver diseased or damaged, drugs may not be metabolized properly and toxicity may occur; may also cause alteration in sensory perception and thought processes related to hepatic encephalopathy
Morphine, paraldehyde, codeine	Can cause spasms and pressure in the biliary tract, thus increasing discomfort
Alcohol	Stimulates liver's major drug-metabolizing system; can damage liver further

---

CASE STUDY *evolve*

Cirrhosis

Mr. James is a 53-year-old man on disability from his job as a warehouse forklift driver. He became unable to work after developing idiopathic peripheral neuropathy, which resulted in frequent falls and an inability to run the controls of the forklift. He uses a cane to ambulate. Mr. James is being admitted with severe abdominal pain and coffee-grounds emesis. He reports that he had been vomiting bright red blood in the 2 days before admission. His abdomen is distended, with a measured abdominal girth of 52 inches. Mr. James also states that he has recently gained several pounds and has had shortness of breath and fatigue for the past several weeks. He reports that he smokes cigarettes but says that he does not use alcohol . . . .

. . . Case Study continued on the website and the CD-ROM with discussions, multiple-choice questions, and a nursing care plan.

Provide Client Teaching. Instruct the client to avoid vigorous nose-blowing and straining with bowel movements. Sometimes stool softeners are ordered to prevent straining with rupture of varices. Antidiarrheal agents may be administered to control diarrhea. If bleeding gums are noted, advise the client to use a soft toothbrush and to refrain from flossing until the bleeding has ceased.

Diagnosis: Imbalanced Nutrition: Less Than Body Requirements. For the liver to regenerate, the client must have adequate levels of vital nutrients; otherwise, the unmet requirements lead to the nursing diagnosis *Imbalanced Nutrition: Less Than Body Requirements related to anorexia, impaired liver function, decreased absorption of fat-soluble vitamins, and diarrhea.*

Outcomes. The client will receive adequate nutrition as evidenced by no weight loss and no manifestations of malnutrition.

Interventions

Modify Diet. The diet should provide ample protein to rebuild tissue but not enough protein to precipitate hepatic encephalopathy (75 g of high-quality protein per day). The diet should supply sufficient carbohydrates to maintain weight and to spare protein stores. A low-fat and low-sodium (200 to 1000 mg/day) diet is also suggested. Total daily calories should range between 2500 and 3000. Place the client on daily weight, intake and output, and calorie counts to assess fluid and nutritional balance.[3]

Closely monitor the laboratory and nutritional panels for manifestations of improvement or further deterioration. If ammonia levels rise (normal levels are 70 to 200 mg/dl in whole blood and 56 to 150 mg/dl in plasma), foods high in protein may be restricted.

If the client has ascites or edema, fluids as well as sodium should be restricted in the diet. Small, frequent meals make it easier for clients with anorexia to eat enough food. Adequate rest and a stable environmental temperature should be ensured to allow optimal use of calories. Administer prescribed medications, such as antacids, antiemetics, antidiarrheals, or cathartics, to decrease gastric distress, but avoid antiemetics such as phenothiazines.

Provide Vitamin Supplements. The physician usually prescribes a maintenance multivitamin preparation or, in severe malnutrition, therapeutic levels of vitamins. Also, vitamins A, D, E, and K are supplied if fat absorption is adequate. Frequently vitamin K injections are ordered to improve blood clotting factors. The client with severe malabsorption may require IV vitamins with calcium gluconate supplementation. Encourage family or friends to provide desirable foods as permitted.

Diagnosis: Activity Intolerance. The client with cirrhosis often experiences severe fatigue, leading to the nursing diagnosis *Activity Intolerance related to bed rest, fatigue, lack of energy, and altered respiratory function secondary to ascites.*

Outcomes. The client will maintain a balance between rest and activity as evidenced by the absence of fatigue and problems associated with immobility.

Interventions. Clinicians often prescribe rest for clients with cirrhosis, but how much rest is necessary is debated. During periods of acute malfunction, rest reduces metabolic demands on the liver and increases circulation. Long-term planning should include counseling the client to rest frequently and to avoid unnecessary fatigue.

Diagnosis: Risk for Injury. Because the liver is in a very precarious state, intake of alcohol or other hepatotoxins should cease immediately. Otherwise the nursing diagnosis *Risk for Injury related to continued intake of hepatotoxins* becomes appropriate.

Outcomes. The client will not suffer injury from continued intake of hepatotoxins as evidenced by cessation of drinking and avoidance of medications that may cause further damage.

Interventions. Ensure that all known hepatotoxic medications (including alcohol) are removed from therapeutic regimens and that dosages of all drugs thought to be metabolized by the liver have been lowered. Avoid the administration of sedatives and opiates.

Diagnosis: Ineffective Protection. Because of portal hypertension and decreased filtering capability of the liver, the nursing diagnosis *Ineffective Protection related to alcohol abuse and inadequate nutrition* may be appropriate.

Outcomes. The client will not experience systemic infection or spontaneous bacterial peritonitis with ascites.

Interventions. Clients with cirrhosis may experience spontaneous bacterial peritonitis with ascites; mortality is high when this occurs. Your role as nurse is to monitor for manifestations of infection and to administer antibiotics as prescribed. Antibiotics may be required to control intestinal flora that aggravate encephalopathy.

Evaluation. The outcome in cirrhosis depends on the client's ability to stop the intake of alcohol or any other substances toxic to the liver early enough to prevent irreparable liver damage. If biliary obstruction is the cause of the cirrhosis, the client must seek further medical or surgical treatment. Once extensive damage has occurred, the client will not recover and the disease will progress with manifestations of liver failure.

Self-Care

Clients with cirrhosis are managed at home unless they encounter complications or are in the end stage of the disease process. Hence it is important to teach them how to maintain adequate nutrition, to alternate rest and activity, and to avoid hepatotoxic substances. Refer the client to the appropriate agency or support group for assistance with alcohol cessation, such as AA, Al-Anon, or Alateen. See Chapter 24 for further information on alcoholism. Provide referrals to community nursing support agencies as needed. If the client is exposed to hepatotoxic agents in the workplace, suggest that the client try to change jobs. Emphasize that regular checkups and blood tests to follow the progress of the disease are needed.

COMPLICATIONS OF CIRRHOSIS

PORTAL HYPERTENSION

Portal hypertension exists when there is a persistent increase in blood pressure in the portal venous system occurring as a result of increased resistance to or obstruction of blood flow through the portal venous system into the liver.

Etiology and Risk Factors

Most cases of portal hypertension in the United States are associated with cirrhosis. The portal vein is likely to be obstructed by a thrombus; a tumor is the next most common cause. Box 47-2 lists factors that may cause portal hypertension.

BOX 47-2 Factors in the Pathogenesis of Cirrhotic Portal Hypertension

- Increased resistance to flow
- Presinusoidal obstruction
- Portal or splenic vein occlusion (thrombosis, tumors)
- Schistosomiasis
- Congenital hepatitis fibrosis
- Sarcoidosis
- Sinusoidal
- Cirrhosis (all causes)
- Alcoholic hepatitis
- Postsinusoidal
- Veno-occlusive disease
- Budd-Chiari disease
- Constrictive pericarditis
- Increased portal blood flow
- Splenomegaly not caused by liver disease
- Arterioportal fistula

Data from Arguedas, M.R., & Fallon, M.B. (2004). *Cecil essentials of medicine* (6th ed.). Philadelphia: Saunders.

Pathophysiology

The normal blood flow to and from the liver depends on proper functioning of the portal vein (70% of inflow), the hepatic artery (30% of inflow), and the hepatic veins (outflow). Disease processes that damage the liver or its major vessels or alter the flow of blood through these structures are responsible for the development of portal hypertension. Portal hypertension results either from increased blood flow in the portal vein or from an increased resistance to flow within the portal venous system.

The most common cause of portal hypertension is cirrhosis. The pathophysiologic mechanism in cirrhosis is increased resistance, which is intrahepatic and primarily sinusoidal. Portal hypertension may also arise from presinusoidal obstruction, either outside the liver (as in portal vein thrombosis) or within it (as in schistosomiasis). In addition, lesions leading to portal hypertension may be postsinusoidal, either within the liver (as in veno-occlusive disease) or distal to it (as in Budd-Chiari syndrome or right-sided heart failure). Rarely, portal hypertension occurs in the normal liver from markedly increased inflow beyond the capacity of the compliant portal vessels to absorb. Arterial-portal venous fistulas and massive splenomegaly resulting from infection or cancer are examples of causes of this type of portal hypertension. The degree of liver dysfunction varies with the causative process, the duration of the process, and individual client characteristics.

Normal portal venous blood pressure is 5 to 10 mm Hg. Portal hypertension exists when the pressure rises 5 mm Hg higher than the inferior vena cava pressure. Collateral vessels develop in an effort to equalize pressures between the two venous systems. The spleen and other organs that empty into the portal venous system also begin to undergo the effects of congestion. See the Concept Map feature on Understanding Cirrhosis and its Treatment.

Clinical Manifestations

In clients with portal hypertension, assessment reveals a network of slightly tortuous epigastric vessels that branch off the area of the umbilicus and lead toward the sternum and ribs (caput medusae); an enlarged, palpable spleen; internal hemorrhoids; bruits, which may be heard over the upper abdomen; and ascites, which typically appears when there is concurrent liver disease.

Direct measurement of portal venous blood pressure is possible only during laparotomy. The diagnosis of portal hypertension often relies on indirect measurements of portal pressure—obtained at liver scanning, splenoportography, abdominal angiography, or liver biopsy—and on other laboratory data (see Chapter 42). Radiography and endoscopy procedures may be used to differentiate variceal hemorrhage from other types of gastrointestinal bleeding.

OUTCOME MANAGEMENT

Medical Management

One of the most serious disabling complications of portal hypertension is dilation of the superior rectal veins, abdominal wall veins, and esophagogastric veins. With conditions such as cirrhosis, portal venous blood pressure increases, causing esophageal veins to swell and distend. These swollen, dilated veins are called varices. Several factors can contribute to the rupturing of varices (Figure 47-2): increased portal venous blood pressure, increased intrathoracic pressure (coughing and straining at stools), irritation by food or alcohol, and erosion by gastric juices. The veins of the stomach and esophagus are most subject to rupture; when rupture occurs, it constitutes a medical emergency.

Another mechanism that leads to hemorrhage involves the spleen. The splenic vein merges with the superior mesenteric vein to form the portal vein. When pressure increases in the portal venous system, damage to the spleen occurs. Damage to the spleen is not proportional to the increase in portal venous blood pressure. As the spleen enlarges, it destroys blood cells, especially platelets, which increases the risk of hemorrhage and anemia.

Hepatic encephalopathy is an extremely dangerous complication of portal hypertension. This problem usually arises following a period of bleeding into the gastrointestinal tract. Digestion of this blood takes place in the intestines. Because blood is a protein, this process increases ammonia in the gut and bloodstream. In turn, the excessive ammonia disturbs brain function. The Critical Monitoring feature above lists assessment findings that mandate early intervention in esophageal bleeding secondary to portal hypertension. Hepatic encephalopathy is discussed later in this chapter.

Death often follows rupture of esophageal varices if the hemorrhage is not immediately controlled. To stop hemorrhage, health practitioners perform

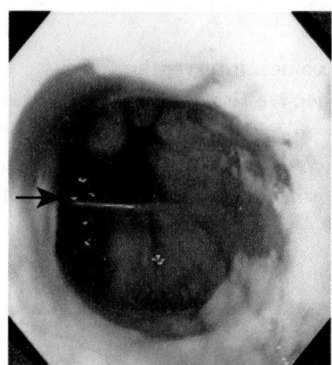

■ **FIGURE 47–2** A bleeding esophageal varix. *(Courtesy Martin Sears, MD, Internal Medicine and Diagnostic Problems, Fremont, Neb.)*

emergency measures: injection sclerotherapy, transjugular intrahepatic portosystemic shunt, administration of vasopressin, balloon tamponade, beta-adrenergic blocking agents, endoscopic electrocautery, direct ligation of the bleeding varices, transhepatic embolization of the left gastric vein, or even urgent portacaval shunt surgery.

Cold saline lavage is probably ineffective but is occasionally done while the client is awaiting transport to surgery or the gastrointestinal laboratory. Fluids, especially volume expanders and blood products, are administered to maintain volume.

Control Hemorrhage

Sclerotherapy. To perform sclerotherapy, the operator passes an endoscope into the esophagus and injects a sclerosing agent (e.g., morrhuate sodium) that flows into the varices. The sclerosing agent initially causes inflammation of the vein wall and then fibrosis. The operator may give repeated injections over a period of weeks until the varices are no longer prominent.

Transjugular Intrahepatic Portosystemic Shunt. For years, surgical decompression procedures were used to lower portal pressure in clients with bleeding esophageal varices. Survival rates in clients with hepatitis were not, however, improved with portal vein-systemic (portosystemic) shunt surgery. Decompression can now be accomplished without surgery through the percutaneous placement of a portosystemic shunt, called a transjugular intrahepatic portosystemic shunt (TIPS). In this procedure, an expandable metal stent is advanced with the aid of fluoroscopy to the hepatic veins during an angiogram and then through the liver to create a direct portacaval channel. Physiologically TIPS is similar to a side-to-side surgical shunt. Placement is successful in more than 90% of the clients, and bleeding is controlled in 90% to 95% of clients. This method offers an alternative to surgery for refractory bleeding caused by portal hypertension.

This procedure does have some difficulties, however. Stents frequently undergo stenosis or occlude over a period of months, prompting the need for another TIPS or another approach. Also, encephalopathy may develop. TIPS should be reserved for individuals who are considered poor surgical risks or who fail endoscopic or medical management.

Vasopressin. When varices rupture, IV vasopressin is routinely administered to stop variceal bleeding. Administration of vasopressin achieves temporary lowering of portal pressure. These agents reduce portal venous blood flow by constricting afferent arterioles. Direct infusion of vasopressin into the superior mesenteric artery is most effective. Serious side effects include hypothermia, myocardial and gastrointestinal tract ischemia, and acute renal failure. It is therefore contraindicated in clients with a recent myocardial infarction. Vasopressin may be given in conjunction with nitroglycerin, which is administered intravenously, sublingually, or by patch to minimize vasoconstrictive side effects. Alternatively, somatostatin is at least as effective as vasopressin. Drug therapy may stop bleeding, but it has no effect on survival.

Beta-Adrenergic Blocking Agents. The effectiveness of beta-adrenergic blocking agents (e.g., propranolol [Inderal], metoprolol [Lopressor], or nadolol [Corgard]) in the management of acute variceal bleeding is limited because they reduce the heart rate (and hence the blood pressure) and mask the early manifestations of hypoglycemia; however, studies suggest that such therapy has been effective in preventing a first episode of variceal bleeding or subsequent episodes after an initial bleed.

Balloon Tamponade. Applying pressure to ruptured varices via balloon tamponade may stop hemorrhage. For this intervention the clinician inserts a Sengstaken-Blakemore or Minnesota tube into the stomach and inflates the esophageal and gastric balloons (Figure 47-3). The pressure of the esophageal balloon against the varices may stop the bleeding. It is important to release this pressure periodically to prevent tissue necrosis. The esophageal balloon is not left inflated for more than 24 hours. Also, it is important to remove secretions and saliva that accumulate above the balloon to prevent aspiration.

   The Minnesota tube has an additional port for aspiration of secretions above the esophageal balloon. Ensure that the gastric balloon is inflated to prevent migration of the tube. You should also have scissors at the bedside to be able to remove the tube in an emergency. Complications of balloon tamponade may occur in 15% or more of clients and include aspiration pneumonitis as well as

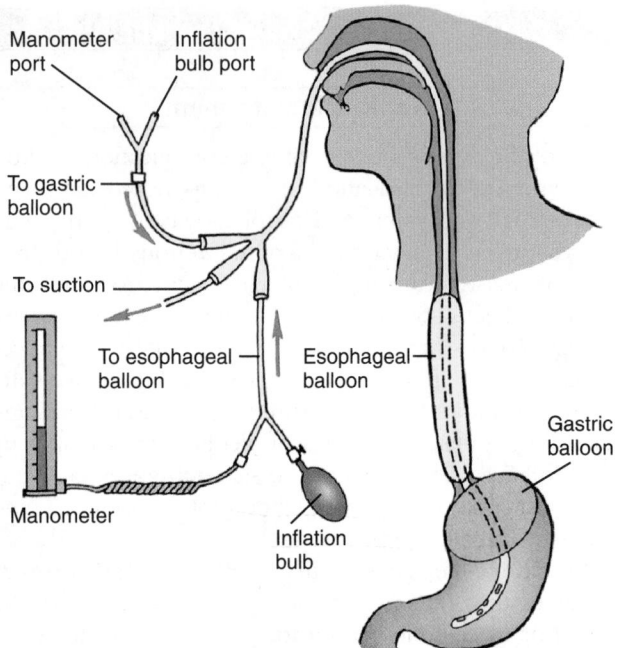

■ **FIGURE 47–3** A Sengstaken-Blakemore tube may be used to control ruptured esophageal varices, a potential complication of portal hypertension.

esophageal rupture. This intervention is performed less frequently today now that other treatment is available. However, use of tamponade may achieve stabilization of a client so that sclerotherapy or surgery becomes a treatment option.

Nursing Management of the Medical Client

Assessment. The major assessment for you to make is for the presence of hemorrhage. The other important aspect of assessment is to check for indicators of the client's clinical status after any intervention to treat the hemorrhage, such as assessing tube function after placement of a Sengstaken-Blakemore or Minnesota tube. Monitor the client's vital signs continuously for any significant changes.

Diagnosis, Outcomes, Interventions
Diagnosis: Ineffective Tissue Perfusion. With rupture of varices, the nursing diagnosis that must be addressed immediately is *Ineffective Tissue Perfusion related to portal hypertension and rupture and hemorrhage of esophageal varices.*

Outcomes. Hemorrhage will be controlled as evidenced by the return of vital signs to normal and no further bleeding.

Interventions. The client can learn activities to help reduce the risk of rupture of esophageal varices.

Prevent Hemorrhage. The nurse should instruct the client as follows:

- Avoid straining maneuvers that increase intra-abdominal or intrathoracic pressure.
- Avoid rough foods, which may traumatize the esophagus, and spicy foods, which may irritate the esophageal mucosa.
- Develop an emergency plan in case severe esophageal varices should rupture.

Include in this plan a list of all emergency telephone numbers. Discuss the plan with both the client and the client's family members.

Monitor for Hemorrhage

If hemorrhage from ruptured varices occurs, monitor blood pressure, pulse rate, respiration, and urine output continuously, and assist with interventions to restore circulating blood volume. Monitor vital signs closely throughout this period. This is a critical time for nursing intervention and can be a stressful time for the client, family members, and nurse.

Further information on the assessment and treatment of shock and hemorrhage can be found in Chapter 81.

Diagnosis: Impaired Gas Exchange. The client with ruptured varices is susceptible to many problems. A major potential problem is addressed in the nursing diagnosis *Impaired Gas Exchange related to decreased oxygen supply secondary to aspiration pneumonitis or obstruction occurring after balloon tamponade with the Sengstaken-Blakemore tube.*

Outcomes. The client will not suffer injury related to the Sengstaken-Blakemore tube as evidenced by the absence of respiratory distress, the absence of aspiration, and the absence of esophageal ischemia.

Interventions

Prevent Esophageal Necrosis. The pressure of the esophageal balloon on the esophagus not only stops hemorrhage but also may cause esophageal necrosis. As noted earlier, you must release the pressure on the esophagus periodically to prevent tissue damage. Consult the physician about how often to release balloon pressure because practices vary widely.

Prevent Aspiration Pneumonia. Aspiration pneumonia is another complication of balloon tamponade. The inflated balloon in the esophagus prevents saliva and secretions from reaching the stomach. Ascertain whether the tube used for tamponade has a suction port above the esophageal balloon. If not, insert a nasogastric tube to the upper balloon level or perform suctioning frequently to remove accumulating fluid.

Prevent Nares Erosion. Tubes inserted through the nose may cause erosion of the nares, especially if traction is applied to the tamponading tube (practices differ). To prevent this complication, clean and lubricate the external nares. Provide padding if necessary.

Prevent Airway Obstruction. Airway obstruction, another complication of balloon tamponade, occurs when the gastric balloon deflates or breaks and traction on the tube pulls the esophageal balloon up into the oropharynx. Keep scissors at the bedside. If this emergency arises, cut the tube and pull it out to restore airway patency. To prevent airway obstruction, label each port of the tube to prevent accidental deflation of the gastric balloon.

Diagnosis: Acute Confusion. Because of the potential buildup of ammonia, the client with bleeding varices is likely to have the nursing diagnosis *Acute Confusion related to portosystemic encephalopathy and hepatic coma occurring in conjunction with gastrointestinal bleeding and accumulation of ammonia.*

Outcomes. The client will be oriented to person, place, and time. Serum ammonia levels will not increase, and the level of consciousness will not decrease.

Interventions

Monitor Level of Consciousness

Assess the client's level of consciousness and orientation on a regular basis (after performing a baseline assessment). Ask clients to write their name each day, and assess for writing deterioration and possible rising ammonia levels. Also assess the client regularly for the development of asterixis (liver flap or flapping tremor). Monitor for evidence of gastrointestinal bleeding, including melena or hematemesis, because bleeding can precipitate hepatic coma. Report the bleeding promptly to the physician.

SAFETY ⚠ ALERT

Protect from Injury

Protect the client from injury by keeping the side rails up and the bed in the lowest position. Assist the client with ambulation as needed. Use caution when administering sedatives, antihistamines, and other agents that affect the central nervous system (CNS).

SAFETY ⚠ ALERT

Evaluation. Although the acute episode of bleeding from esophageal varices can usually be controlled, the development of varices is a clinical manifestation of deterioration of the liver and increasing portal hypertension. The client will need careful and continued follow-up to prevent recurrence or further complications.

Surgical Management

Endoscopic Band Ligation

In this procedure esophageal varices are ligated and strangulated with small elastic O-rings placed in the appropriate place during endoscopy. Band ligation has proved at least as effective as sclerotherapy in controlling acute variceal bleeding and preventing rebleeding. Because treatment-related complications occur less frequently with band ligation, this procedure is recommended for long-term obliteration of varices that have bled.

Transjugular Intrahepatic Portosystemic Shunt

Transjugular intrahepatic portosystemic shunt has emerged as a technique to create a portal-systemic shunt via a percutaneous approach. (See the previous section on TIPS.)

Portosystemic Shunt

Several surgical procedures can be used to reduce the danger of hemorrhage from varices caused by portal hypertension. These procedures involve anastomosing the high-pressure portal venous system to the low-pressure systemic venous system. This creates a portosystemic shunt.

Surgical creation of a portosystemic shunt reduces portal hypertension by sending portal venous blood directly into the inferior vena cava, bypassing the liver. Other vessels may be altered, depending on the type of shunt selected.

Such a procedure lowers portal venous blood pressure, thus decreasing the risk of rupture of esophageal varices. Figure 47-4 illustrates some portosystemic (portal vein-vena cava) shunt procedures.

Overall, clients who require portosystemic shunts are poor surgical candidates because of their suboptimal nutritional status, their increased risk of infection, and their deteriorating liver function. Usually such surgery is used only as a last resort because the risk of death is high in the early operative period. The role of portosystemic shunt surgery in the management of bleeding esophageal varices after initial medical control of bleeding is uncertain.

Indications. Although surgical shunting reduces the risk of recurrent hemorrhage, the overall mortality of clients undergoing such surgery is comparable to that of clients managed medically. The similarity of outcomes is related to the increased incidence of encephalopathy in surgically managed clients when the shunted blood is not cleared of toxic substances and to the higher incidence of death from progressive liver failure with their increased longevity. For these reasons, the surgical creation of a portosystemic shunt is reserved for clients who have not responded to other treatment and who, despite periodic endoscopic sclerotherapy, continue to bleed.

Contraindications. The main contraindication to portosystemic shunt procedures is poor general health so that the client is not able to withstand the trauma, blood and fluid loss, and anesthesia of surgery.

Complications. Major complications after a shunt procedure are bacteremia and DIC, heart failure, shunt clotting, and hepatic encephalopathy. Clients must be monitored closely to detect the onset of these complications, and corrective measures need to be implemented quickly if they arise.

Outcomes. Clients who undergo portosystemic shunt procedures require surgery because other methods of controlling bleeding have been unsuccessful. The goal of these procedures is (1) to reduce portal venous blood flow enough to prevent variceal hemorrhage, (2) to preserve enough blood inflow to the liver to prevent hepatic encephalopathy and hepatic failure, and (3) to increase client comfort (the shunting is a palliative procedure).

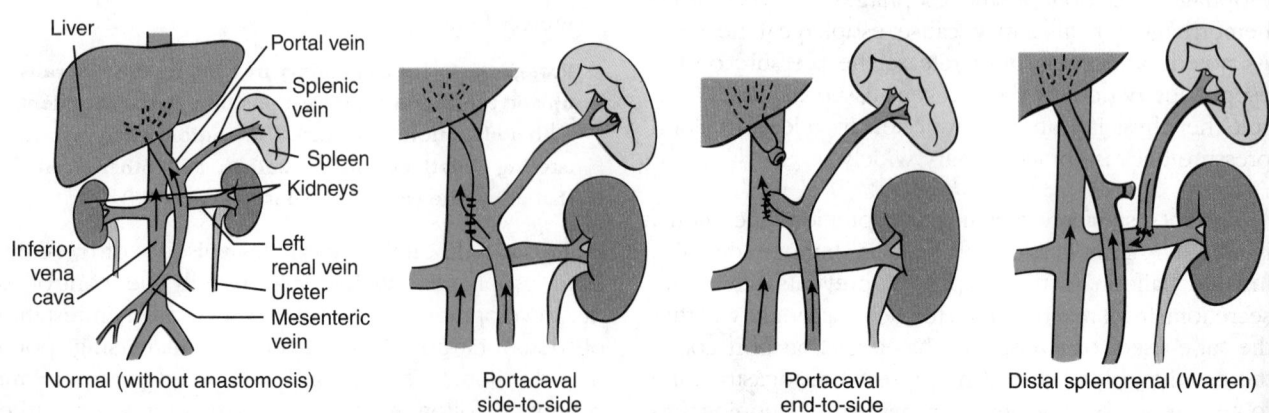

Normal (without anastomosis)   Portacaval side-to-side   Portacaval end-to-side   Distal splenorenal (Warren)

■ **FIGURE 47–4** Some types of portacaval or portosystemic shunt procedures used to reduce portal hypertension.

Nursing Management of the Surgical Client

Preoperative Care

Preoperative management of the client undergoing a portosystemic shunt procedure includes an appraisal of the client's general physical condition and readiness for surgery along with assessment of the client's neurologic, respiratory, and renal systems to establish a baseline. Blood and urine may be examined for the presence of infectious organisms, and an arterial blood gas analysis may be performed to assess general respiratory function.

Blood-clotting mechanisms are analyzed as are the client's fluid and electrolyte status and levels of ammonia, protein, bilirubin, and liver enzymes. If the client has an inappropriate level of any one of these substances, measures are taken to correct the problem. If the hemoglobin and hematocrit levels are low, the client may receive a blood transfusion. The client's general nutritional status is important, and protein hydrolysates are administered by total parenteral nutrition (TPN) if indicated.

Postoperative Care

Assessment. After portosystemic shunt surgery, assess the client's respiratory, renal, and hemodynamic status. In addition, observe the client and inspect the operative site carefully for any manifestations of shunt clotting, such as pain, distention, or nausea. Assess the client after portosystemic shunt surgery by monitoring for the following:

- Presence of hemorrhage, hypovolemia, and oliguria
- Fluid and electrolyte imbalance (dilutional hyponatremia, ascites)
- Respiratory rate and rhythm (rales, atelectasis, labored breathing, pneumonia)
- Hypoalbuminemia
- Hypoglycemia
- Manifestations of infection (fever, increased white blood cells [WBCs])
- Pain levels
- Mental status (alertness)

Diagnosis, Outcomes, Interventions. Nursing diagnoses associated with care of the client after portosystemic shunt surgery include *Ineffective Tissue Perfusion, Impaired Gas Exchange, and Acute Confusion* (see Nursing Management of the Medical Client). In addition, *Excess Fluid Volume* is a pertinent nursing diagnosis for the client undergoing portosystemic shunt surgery.

Diagnosis: Excess Fluid Volume. The client who has undergone portosystemic shunt surgery often retains excess fluid, leading to the nursing diagnosis *Excess Fluid Volume related to retention of fluids secondary to portal hypertension, liver failure, and hemodilution of blood related to the new portosystemic shunt.*

Outcomes. A normovolemic state will be maintained as evidenced by a stable or decreasing abdominal girth and a regular respiratory rate and rhythm.

Interventions

Assess for Excess Fluid Volume. Assess the client for retention of fluid, which is likely to occur because of hemodynamic fluid shifts. Measure abdominal girth to obtain a baseline, and then recheck daily or every shift, as appropriate, to detect development of ascites. Also, monitor weight and intake and output. Output should not be less than intake. Assess for the presence of edema and document its degree, from 1+ (barely noticeable) to 4+ (deep and pitting). Be sure to check for clinical indicators of pulmonary edema, including dyspnea and orthopnea. See that appropriate pulmonary and respiratory therapy is initiated if the client has any respiratory involvement.

Monitor and Treat Postprocedure Complications. Assess the client for hepatic encephalopathy. If portal hypertension is due to liver disease, carefully monitor for postoperative hemorrhage because bleeding tendencies often arise from liver cell malfunction. Assess cardiovascular function carefully because the shunt increases venous return to the heart, thus increasing the workload of the heart and placing the client at risk for heart failure.

After surgery carefully monitor laboratory data, including hemoglobin, hematocrit, PT, ammonia level, blood urea nitrogen (BUN) level, bilirubin level, blood gas concentrations, and fluid and electrolyte levels. If the hemoglobin and hematocrit levels are below normal, you may need to administer a blood transfusion; however, many times the low hematocrit and hemoglobin levels occur because of hemodilution that results after the shunt is completed. If clotting time (PT) is not within normal limits, administer vitamin K. If the client is having difficulty breathing because of ascites, it is doubly important after surgery to implement measures that improve respirations (turning, coughing, and deep breathing; respiratory treatments; and maintaining any chest drainage system). Other areas in which you may need to intervene for clients who have undergone portosystemic shunt surgery include the following:

- Administering IV fluids plus blood or volume expanders such as dextran and maintaining line patency and prescribed flow rates
- Monitoring blood and urine values and noting any manifestations of infection (such as increased WBCs and elevated erythrocyte sedimentation rate)
- Eliminating medications that sedate, depress the CNS, or are known hepatotoxins (e.g., acetaminophen)
- Maintaining nutrition: While the client is receiving nothing by mouth, that is, is on *nil per os* (NPO) status, usually for several days postoperatively,

administer TPN; when food intake begins, protein intake may be limited and increased slowly if BUN and ammonia levels and mental status remain within normal limits

■ Maintaining sterile technique when changing dressing(s)

■ Maintaining patency if a gastrointestinal tube is in place

■ Assisting the client and the client's family to cope with postoperative discomfort and with issues pertinent to chronic liver disease and its sequelae

When emergency shunt surgery is performed, little time may be available to complete preoperative teaching of appropriate information to the client and the client's significant others. Present careful explanations postoperatively to compensate for the lack of preoperative teaching.

Evaluation. Although shunt procedures may decrease the bleeding, the long-term prognosis for the client is poor. Severe encephalopathy often develops, followed by coma and death.

ASCITES

Etiology and Risk Factors

Ascites is the accumulation of fluid in the peritoneal cavity that results from the interaction of several pathophysiologic changes. Portal hypertension, lowered plasma colloidal osmotic pressure, and sodium retention all contribute to this condition. Disease processes that lead to these events include cirrhosis of the liver, right-sided heart failure, tuberculous peritonitis, cancer, and complications of pancreatitis.

Pathophysiology

Any process that blocks the flow of blood through the liver sinusoids to the hepatic veins and vena cava causes an increase in hydrostatic pressure in the portal venous system. Most commonly, this problem develops in cirrhosis of the liver or right-sided heart failure. As portal pressure increases, plasma leaks directly from the liver capsule and the congested portal vein into the peritoneal cavity. Congestion of lymph channels occurs, leading to the leakage of more plasma into the peritoneal cavity. Loss of plasma proteins into ascitic fluid from the portal venous system reduces oncotic pressure in the vascular compartment. Reduction in oncotic pressure limits the vascular system's ability to hold onto or collect water.

In addition, hepatocellular damage reduces the liver's ability to synthesize normal amounts of albumin. Decreased albumin synthesis leads to hypoalbuminemia, which is exacerbated by leakage of protein into the

peritoneal cavity. The circulating blood volume decreases from loss of colloid osmotic pressure. The secretion of aldosterone increases to stimulate the kidneys to retain sodium and water. As a result of hepatocellular damage, the liver is unable to inactivate aldosterone. Thus sodium and water retention continue. More fluid is held, and the volume of ascitic fluid grows.

Clinical Manifestations

Ascitic fluid typically produces abdominal distention, bulging flanks, and a downward-protruding umbilicus. Although large accumulations of ascitic fluid are obvious, small or moderate amounts may be more difficult to detect. See Chapter 42 for a discussion of the assessment of a client with ascites.

Diagnostic tests to confirm the presence of ascites include paracentesis, abdominal x-ray studies, ultrasonography, and computed tomography (CT) scan. These tests may locate fluid in the peritoneal cavity. Paracentesis provides samples of fluid for analysis. Findings help determine the underlying cause of the ascites; for example, the finding of malignant cells may indicate a tumor.

OUTCOME MANAGEMENT

Medical Management

Correct Fluid and Electrolyte Imbalance

Fluid and electrolyte balance is corrected by improving renal sodium excretion and restricting sodium and water intake. This involves discontinuing medications that inhibit prostaglandin synthesis and thus impair renal sodium excretion (e.g., aspirin, ibuprofen, indomethacin).

Paracentesis. Repeated large-volume paracentesis, in combination with IV administration of albumin to maintain plasma volume, is used to manage clients with ascites resulting from cirrhosis; however, repeated removal of fluid, protein, and electrolytes from the body causes severe disturbances in homeostasis. It is becoming more common to remove the least amount of fluid, such as 100 ml, sufficient to relieve manifestations such as shortness of breath. Clients must be monitored for rupture of the umbilicus.

Albumin. The physician may prescribe IV administration of albumin to replace each liter of ascitic fluid that is removed.

Diet Modifications. The diet is low in sodium with restriction of fluids. Protein intake is moderate unless the client has manifestations of hepatic encephalopathy

Promote Effective Breathing Pattern

Edema in the form of ascites, besides compressing the liver and thus affecting its function, may also cause shallow breathing and impaired gas exchange, resulting in respiratory compromise. When ascites is present, potassium-sparing diuretics (e.g., spironolactone) are prescribed. Oxygen may be prescribed, and arterial blood gas analysis and pulse oximetry may be ordered. Semi-Fowler or high-Fowler position, as well as daily or every-shift measurement of abdominal girth, is often prescribed.

Maintain Skin Integrity

When edema is present in liver disease, the client is at increased risk for development of skin impairment and possibly infected skin lesions. If jaundice is present, tepid water or emollient baths may be ordered, along with the use of non-alkaline soaps and application of emollient lotions. If antihistamines are prescribed, observe for excessive sedation.

Transjugular Intrahepatic Portosystemic Shunt

The TIPS procedure is described earlier as a treatment choice for esophageal varices; however, TIPS also is useful in selected clients for the management of ascites. Even though mobilizing ascitic fluid may precipitate severe hepatic encephalopathy in some clients, TIPS remains a promising treatment for ascites.

Nursing Management of the Medical Client

Assessment. Some simple assessments to perform at the bedside are the following:

- Percussion of the abdomen; if the client has ascites, the sound will be dull
- Measurement of circumference (abdominal girth)
- Assessment of the client for ascites (see Chapter 42)

Assess the amount of distress caused by the ascites. Ask whether the fluid is interfering with sleeping, eating, and breathing. Assess for the presence of a hydrothorax or misplaced point of maximal impact (PMI). The Care Plan feature on pp. 1162-1164 provides more detailed interventions and rationales for this type of client.

Diagnosis, Outcomes, Interventions
Diagnosis: Excess Fluid Volume and Deficient Fluid Volume. The client with ascites has a combination of volume problems leading to the nursing diagnoses *Excess Fluid Volume* and *Deficient Fluid Volume related to fluid shifts secondary to portal hypertension, hypoalbuminemia, and hyperaldosteronism.*

Outcomes. A normal balance of fluid between the intracellular and extracellular spaces will be maintained as evidenced by absence of hypovolemia, normal serum albumin levels, decreased abdominal girth, and normal blood pressure measurements.

Interventions

Restrict Fluids. Restriction of the client's fluid intake must be strictly followed. Give medications with meals, if possible, so that mealtime fluids can be used for taking medications.

Monitor Intake and Output. Measure abdominal girth daily (sometimes twice a day), and weigh the client daily. Monitor intake and output daily. Output should be equal to or exceed intake.

Administer Albumin and Diuretics. Administer albumin and diuretics as ordered.

> **Give the albumin first to pull fluid back into the blood vessels. Give the diuretics second to promote excretion of the extra fluid. Assess the client for electrolyte imbalance and heart failure.**

SAFETY

ALERT

Avoid Hepatotoxins. Avoid administering aspirin and nonsteroidal anti-inflammatory drugs (NSAIDs) because they inhibit prostaglandin synthesis and, as noted previously, impair sodium excretion by the kidney.

Monitor After Paracentesis. Monitor the client closely after a paracentesis procedure. Check vital signs frequently to ensure that the client has tolerated the procedure well, and check the dressing carefully to ensure that excessive amounts of fluid are not lost. Sometimes a pouch is placed to collect leaking fluid. If too much fluid is lost, the physician may suture the site closed to prevent excess loss.

Diagnosis: Ineffective Breathing Pattern. Ascites leads to many other problems. *Ineffective Breathing Pattern related to increased intra-abdominal pressure on the diaphragm* is a common nursing diagnosis in clients with ascites.

Outcomes. The client will not experience an ineffective breathing pattern as evidenced by the absence of shortness of breath and the presence of normal respiratory excursion.

Interventions. Position the client in the high-Fowler position to facilitate breathing, and monitor the client's respiratory status for the development of atelectasis or pneumonia. To maintain respiratory function, ask the client to cough and deep breathe hourly, use an incentive spirometer, or receive ultrasound treatments if the cough does not loosen to expectorate respiratory secretions.

Diagnosis: Impaired Skin Integrity. In clients with ascites, severe edema as well as other problems may develop, leading to the nursing diagnosis *Impaired Skin Integrity related to immobility, edema, and pressure from the abdomen.*

C A R E   P·L A N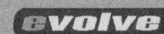

Management of the Client with Hepatic Failure

Nursing Diagnosis: Activity Intolerance (NANDA) related to anemia from poor nutrition and bleeding, ascites, dyspnea from pressure of ascites on diaphragm, muscle wasting.

Outcomes: Activity Tolerance, Energy Conservation, Self-Care: Activities of Daily Living; Blood Loss Severity; Fluid Balance, Fluid Overload Severity (NOC). Client will feel rested with fewer complaints of fatigue and increased tolerance for activities.

Interventions	(NIC)	Rationales
1. Alternate rest and activity.	Energy Management	Conserves energy and reduces demands on liver.
	Activity Therapy	Increases activity tolerance and endurance.
2. Assist with activities of daily living (ADL).	Self-Care Assistance	Conserves energy and reduces demands on liver.
3. Monitor hemoglobin and hematocrit. Assist with treatment of GI bleeding.	Bleeding Reduction: GI	Allows detection and treatment of gastrointestinal bleeding.
4. Administer blood transfusions or iron supplements as ordered to treat anemia.	Blood Products Administration Medication Administration	Decreased production of clotting factors can lead to hemorrhage and anemia.
5. Assist with measures to decrease edema and ascites (see Fluid Volume Excess to follow).	Fluid/Electrolyte Management Hypervolemia Management	Increases lung capacity.

Evaluation: Within a day after paracentesis or shunting surgery, the client will have decreased volume of ascitic fluid, tolerate activity better, perform more ADL, and experience less dyspnea and tachycardia. If ascitic fluid recollects after paracentesis, the activity intolerance will return. Blood transfusions will immediately improve hemoglobin and hematocrit levels, whereas iron replacement therapy will take longer to be effective. Activity therapy and treatment of anemia will result in an increase in activity endurance.

Nursing Diagnosis: Imbalanced Nutrition: Less than Body Requirements (NANDA) related to impaired utilization and storage of nutrients, increased pressure on stomach and intestines, feeling full, anorexia, nausea, loss of nutrients from vomiting.

Outcomes: Appetite, Nutritional Status, Weight: Body Mass (NOC). Client will maintain or increase body weight to ideal weight and will consume adequate nutrients.

Interventions	(NIC)	Rationales
1. Weigh daily.	Nutrition Management Nutritional Monitoring	Monitors weight gain or loss.
2. Monitor nutritional intake.	Nutrition Management Nutrition Therapy Nutritional Monitoring	Monitors intake of nutrients.
3. Monitor hemoglobin, hematocrit, albumin, total protein values.	Nutritional Management Nutritional Monitoring	Monitors intake of nutrients, presence of anemia, and colloidal osmotic pressure.
4. Provide oral hygiene before meals.	Nausea Management	Improves taste of food.
5. Administer antiemetics as ordered.	Nausea Management	Relieves nausea and vomiting.
6. Provide small, frequent meals.	Nausea Management Nutrition Therapy	Prevents feeling of fullness and ensures adequate nutritional intake.
7. Determine food preferences and assist in selection of those that contain low or no protein and low salt, as ordered.	Nausea Management Nutrition Management Nutrition Therapy	Allows preferred foods, when possible, to encourage nutrition.
8. Prevent constipation.	Nutrition Management Nutrition Therapy Constipation Management	Reduces abdominal pressure and fullness.

Evaluation: With interventions, the client will maintain weight and body mass (not fluid) or begin to gain weight by consuming adequate nutrients and following diet restrictions.

Nursing Diagnosis: Ineffective Protection (NANDA) related to decreased filtering of bacteria by liver, impaired synthesis of clotting factors.

Outcomes: Blood Coagulation, Immune Status (NOC). Client will remain free of infection and will have no bruising or hemorrhage.

Interventions	(NIC)	Rationales
1. Monitor for hemorrhage.	Bleeding Precautions	Decreased synthesis of clotting factors can lead to hemorrhage.
2. Provide assistance with ambulation and ADL.	Bleeding Precautions	Minimizes risk of trauma, injury, and bleeding.
3. Use small gauge needles for injections and apply prolonged pressure after injection.	Bleeding Precautions	Minimizes risk of bleeding into tissues.
4. Recommend soft-bristle toothbrush.	Bleeding Precautions	Reduces injury and bleeding of oral tissues.

5. Avoid vigorous blowing of nose or straining at stool.   Bleeding Precautions   Reduces risk of hemorrhage.

6. Administer vitamin K as ordered   Bleeding Precautions   Necessary for synthesis of clotting factors.

7. Monitor for infection (fever, leukopenia).   Infection Protection   Promotes identification and treatment of infection.

Evaluation: If interventions are successful, the client will not experience hemorrhage or infection.

Nursing Diagnosis: Acute Confusion (NANDA) related to portal systemic encephalopathy occurring in conjunction with gastrointestinal bleeding, accumulation of ammonia in the bloodstream.

Outcomes: Cognitive Orientation, Distorted Thought Self-Control, Information Processing, Neurological Status (NOC). Client will be oriented to person, place, and time. Serum ammonia levels will not increase and level of consciousness will not decrease.

Interventions	(NIC)	Rationales
1. Monitor for encephalopathy such as disorientation, changes in handwriting or speech, or coma.	Neurologic Monitoring	Liver is unable to convert ammonia to urea for excretion.
2. Encourage fluids unless restricted.	Cerebral Perfusion Promotion	Promotes excretion of ammonia and urea.
3. Give laxatives and enemas.	Medication Administration	Decreases serum ammonia.
4. Provide low-protein diet.	Nutrition Therapy	Reduces generation of ammonia, which is a by-product of protein metabolism.
5. Limit activity.	Environmental Management	Reduces generation of ammonia, a by-product of metabolism.
6. Treat gastrointestinal bleeding as ordered.	Medication Administration	Reduces generation of ammonia, a by-product of bacterial action on blood in the gut.

Evaluation: Within 1 or 2 days of treatment, the client's serum ammonia levels will decrease and the client will become oriented to person, place, and time.

Nursing Diagnosis: Disturbed Body Image (NANDA) related to yellowing of skin and sclera (jaundice), ascites, edema.

Outcomes: Adaptation to Physical Disability, Body Image, Psychosocial Adjustment: Life Change, Self-Esteem (NOC). Client will cope with body image disturbance, avoid isolation, and initiate or reestablish support systems.

Interventions	(NIC)	Rationales
1. Assess the client's response to body changes.	Body Image Enhancement	Determines the extent of body image disturbance.
2. Promote accepting and nonjudgmental attitude.	Active Listening Emotional Support	Respects the client's sensitivity to body image changes.
3. Listen and encourage ventilation of feelings.	Active Listening Emotional Support	Helps the client feel valued.
4. Suggest clothing colors and options and offer make-up tips.	Body Image Enhancement Self-Esteem Enhancement	Enhances self-esteem.

Evaluation: Within 1-2 days of beginning treatment, some of the body changes will be corrected. Jaundice usually resolves in about 3 weeks. The volume of ascitic and edematous fluid can be reduced in a few days. Some degree of ascites and muscle wasting is irreversible, and the client will learn to accept the altered body image. In addition, it is expected that the client will maintain or establish new interpersonal relationships and activities.

Nursing Diagnosis: Excess Fluid Volume (NANDA) related to retention of fluids secondary to decreased serum albumin, increased sodium and water, portal hypertension, possible shunting procedures causing hemodilution of blood.

Outcomes: Electrolyte/Acid-Base Balance, Fluid Balance, Fluid Overload Severity, Kidney Function (NOC). Client will maintain a normovolemic state and adequate respirations and will have a decreased abdominal girth.

Interventions	(NIC)	Rationales
1. Follow sodium and fluid restrictions.	Fluid/Electrolyte Management Hypervolemia Management	Help to decrease ascites and edema.
2. Administer diuretics as ordered.	Fluid Management Hypervolemia Management	Promotes excretion of fluid.
3. Weigh daily.	Fluid Monitoring	Evaluates treatment measures and determines if fluid is being retained.
4. Measure abdominal girth every day or shift.	Fluid Monitoring	Evaluates treatment measures.
5. Monitor intake and output.	Fluid Monitoring	Evaluates treatment measures and determines if fluid is being retained.
6. Monitor electrolytes, hemoglobin, and hematocrit.	Electrolyte Management Laboratory Data Interpretation	Diuretics may cause electrolyte imbalances; shunting may cause hemodilution.
7. Implement measures to prevent skin breakdown (see Impaired Skin Integrity).		Edema causes skin to break down faster.

(Continued)

C A R E   P L A N   *evolve*

Management of the Client with Hepatic Failure—Cont'd

8. Administer albumin as ordered.	Laboratory Data Interpretation Fluid Management	Albumin pulls fluid into blood vessels, where the action of diuretics can remove the excess fluid.
9. Assist with paracentesis procedure.	Fluid Management	Paracentesis may be used to remove 1 L or more of fluid from peritoneum.

Evaluation: If some liver function is restored, the client will produce more albumin to promote the return of fluid into the blood vessels. Administration of albumin and diuretics will promote diuresis within hours, but repeated administration may be necessary because their effect is temporary. Paracentesis is a temporary solution; ascitic fluid will accumulate again if albumin levels remain low and portal hypertension is untreated.

Nursing Diagnosis: Ineffective Breathing Pattern (NANDA) related to pressure on diaphragm, reduced lung capacity secondary to ascites, possible anemia.

Outcomes: Respiratory Status: Ventilation, Vital Signs (NOC). Client will breathe with minimal difficulty; no manifestations of hypoxia will be seen.

Interventions	(NIC)	Rationales
1. Place the client in the semi-Fowler or Fowler position with arms supported with pillows.	Positioning	Relieves pressure on diaphragm.
2. Assess for crackles and increased respirations.	Respiratory Monitoring Vital Signs Monitoring	Identifies fluid in lungs.
3. Administer oxygen and blood products as ordered.	Oxygen Therapy Intravenous Therapy	Improves gas exchange.

Evaluation: Treatment of ascites and anemia will enable the client to breath with minimal difficulty.

Nursing Diagnosis: Impaired Skin Integrity (NANDA) related to pruritus (itching), edema, ascites, decreased mobility.

Outcomes: Tissue Integrity: Skin and Mucous Membranes (NOC). Client will maintain skin integrity and obtain relief from pruritus.

Interventions	(NIC)	Rationales
1. Limit bathing to every 2-3 days, with sponge baths in between.	Pruritus Management	Keeps skin moist and minimizes itching.
2. Use warm (95°-100° F) rather than hot water.	Pruritus Management	Cooler water minimizes vasodilation and itching.
3. Avoid alkaline soaps.	Pruritus Management	Alkaline soap dries skin.
4. Apply emollients (mineral oil, baby oil, lanolin).	Pruritus Management	Emollients reduce evaporation and keep skin moist.
5. Use cool, light cotton clothing, which promotes evaporation.	Pruritus Management	Minimizes irritation and itching.
6. Keep clothing and bedding dry.	Pruritus Management	Minimizes itching.
7. Keep the environment cool (65°-70° F.)	Pruritus Management	Minimizes itching and vasodilation.
8. Avoid activities that promote sweating.	Pruritus Management	Minimizes itching and vasodilation.
9. Keep nails short and smooth.	Pruritus Management	Prevents breaking skin integrity when scratching.
10. Administer cholestyramine as ordered.	Medication Administration	Combines with bile salts and promotes intestinal elimination to decrease itching.
11. Administer diphenhydramine HCl (Benadryl).	Medication Administration	Antihistamine that has antipruritic and sedative effect; itching is worse at night.
12. Encourage diversional activities	Pruritus Management	Decreases perception of itching and improves coping.
13. Restrict sodium and fluid intake.	Fluid/Electrolyte Management	Prevents additional fluid retention.
14. Administer prescribed diuretics.	Fluid/Electrolyte Management	Reduces fluid retention and promotes diuresis.
15. Monitor intake and output and weigh daily.	Fluid Monitoring	Assesses renal function and fluid retention.
16. Reposition every 2 hours.	Pressure Management	Relieves pressure over bony prominences.
17. Use special mattress such as alternating air mattress.	Pressure Management	Reduces the likelihood of skin breakdown.

Evaluation: After jaundice resolves in about 3 weeks, the client will have relief from pruritus, will be able to sleep without interruption, and will maintain skin integrity. Prevention and treatment of edema will minimize risk of skin integrity breakdown.

Outcomes. The client will maintain skin integrity.

Interventions Turn the client frequently, providing adequate support for the distended abdomen. If the client has been prescribed bed rest, recommend a specialty mattress used to prevent skin breakdown. To prevent skin breakdown, inspect the client's skin daily, apply lotions and creams, keep the skin cool, and change soiled bed linens as soon as possible.

Evaluation. The client's ascites may be controlled to some extent, but once cirrhosis is advanced, it is difficult to control. The optimal outcome is that the client will stop drinking, thereby preventing further liver damage.

Surgical Management

Peritoneovenous Shunt
The client with refractory and disabling chronic ascites may obtain relief from the insertion of a peritoneovenous (LeVeen or Denver) shunt.

Indications. Insertion of a peritoneovenous shunt may be indicated for clients whose ascites is not responding to medical management. As Figure 47-5 shows, a properly functioning shunt moves fluid from the peritoneal (abdominal) cavity into the superior vena cava. Resolution of ascites may be dramatic after implantation of a peritoneovenous shunt. The shunt contains a one-way valve that prevents back-flow of ascitic fluid.

Contraindications. The main contraindication to placement of a peritoneovenous shunt is that the client's state of health is too poor to withstand the trauma of surgery.

Complications. Complications of shunt implantation include infection, hemodilution, DIC, heart failure, and shunt clotting. For additional information, see the earlier discussion of surgical management of portal hypertension.

Nursing Management of the Surgical Client

Preoperative and postoperative management of a client with ascites is similar to that of a client who has undergone surgery for portal hypertension and esophageal varices. See the discussion of nursing care of the client with surgical treatment of a hepatic problem.

HEPATIC ENCEPHALOPATHY

Etiology and Risk Factors
Hepatic encephalopathy constitutes a spectrum of CNS disturbances. These disturbances may appear in conjunction with severe liver injury or liver failure or after portosystemic shunt surgery. The cause of this disorder is the liver's inability to metabolize ammonia to form urea so that it can be excreted. Ammonia is a CNS depressant. Changes during the initial stages of hepatic encephalopathy include reduced mental alertness, confusion, and restlessness. Loss of consciousness, seizures, and irreversible coma occur in the terminal stage.

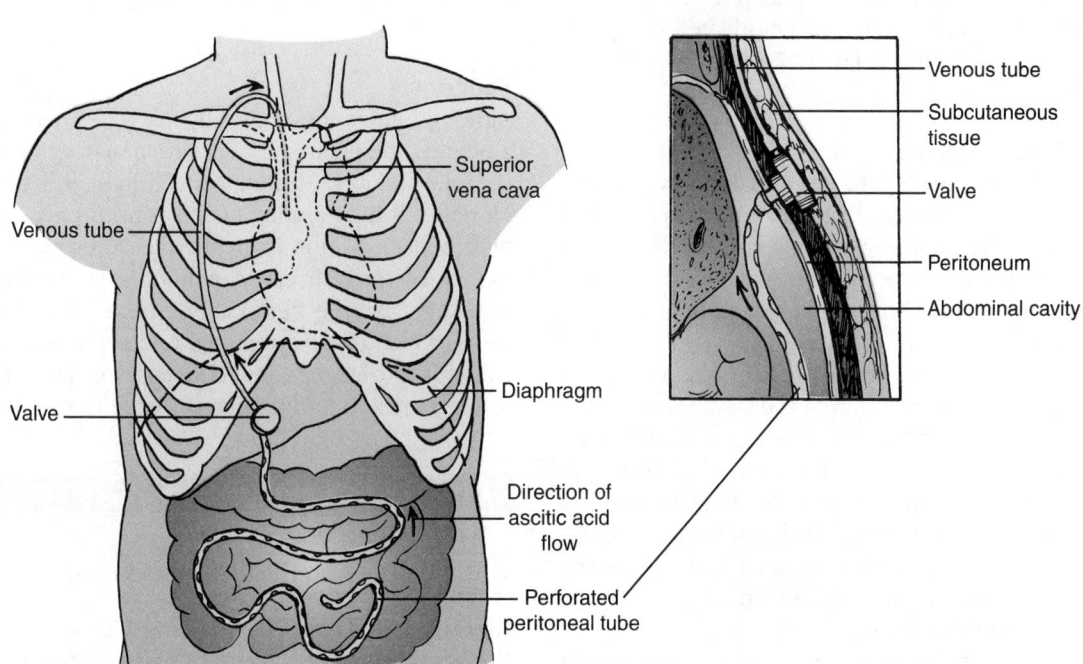

■ **FIGURE 47–5**   LeVeen peritoneovenous shunt for chronic ascites moves fluid from the peritoneal (abdominal) cavity into the superior vena cava.

Pathophysiology

The specific cause of hepatic encephalopathy is unknown, but it is characterized by elevations of ammonia levels in the blood and cerebrospinal fluid (CSF). Ammonia is produced in the gastrointestinal tract when protein is broken down by bacteria, by the liver, and, in lesser amounts, by gastric juices and peripheral tissue metabolism. The kidneys are another source of ammonia in the presence of hypokalemia. More recently implicated as a cause of encephalopathy are false neurotransmitters, elevated levels of mercaptans (organic chemicals that contain the sulfhydryl radical, formed when the oxygen of an alcohol molecule is replaced by sulfur), phenol, and short-chain fatty acids.

Normally the liver converts ammonia into glutamine, which is stored in the liver and is later converted to urea and excreted through the kidneys. Blood ammonia levels rise when the liver cells are unable to perform this conversion. Failure of the liver to perform this function may be due to liver cell damage and necrosis. It also may result from the shunting of blood from the portal venous system directly into the systemic venous circulation (bypassing the liver). In either case, as blood ammonia levels rise, many unusual compounds begin to form.

Some of these compounds (e.g., octopamine) apparently act as false neurotransmitters in the CNS. Ammonia also is a CNS toxin, affecting glial and nerve cells; it leads to altered CNS metabolism and function.

Any process that increases protein in the intestine, such as increased dietary protein or gastrointestinal bleeding, causes elevated blood ammonia levels and possible manifestations of hepatic encephalopathy in clients with hepatocellular failure or who have undergone portosystemic shunt surgery (Box 47-3).

Clinical Manifestations

The manifestations of hepatic encephalopathy are primarily neurologic and range from mild mental confusion to deep coma. The neurologic changes occur with cerebral accumulation of ammonia or gastrointestinal bleeding. Hepatic encephalopathy impairs memory, attention, concentration, and rate of response.

Sleep pattern reversal often occurs, with the client awake at night and sleepy during the day. Handwriting and speech show significant changes as intellectual deterioration occurs. Asterixis may be present. In some clients with hepatic encephalopathy, hyperventilation with respiratory alkalosis develops because high ammonia levels stimulate the respiratory center. The presence of methylmercaptan causes a characteristic odor on the breath called fetor hepaticus.

As the client's condition deteriorates, characteristic delta waves appear on the electroencephalogram (EEG). As the syndrome progresses, the client's level of consciousness

---

BOX 47-3   Hepatic Encephalopathy: Causes or Precipitating Factors

- Decrease in hepatocellular function
- Hypoxia
- Infection
- Diuretics (produce hypokalemia, alkalosis, and hypovolemia)
- Depressants: phenobarbital, narcotics, tranquilizers, and sedatives
- Gastrointestinal bleeding
- Medications containing ammonium or amino compounds
- Paracentesis
- Increased protein intake
- Constipation
- Dehydration
- Hypokalemia
- Portosystemic and portacaval shunts

---

slowly diminishes, and confusion becomes more severe; however, the level of CNS depression commonly fluctuates. Coma may eventually ensue, which deepens until there is no pain response and the reflexes, including the corneal reflex, are completely absent. Box 47-4 lists the stages of hepatic encephalopathy.

Laboratory results show elevated blood ammonia and CSF glutamine levels. Although these findings help to confirm the diagnosis of encephalopathy, they are not specific to it. Monitor serum ammonia levels, electrolyte levels, blood gases, and hepatic function test results (bilirubin, albumin, prothrombin, and enzymes) throughout the course. These findings help to determine the degree of imbalance and the extent of hepatic injury (see Chapter 42).

Prognosis

Although intervention usually alleviates hepatic encephalopathy, the client may die of circulatory or respiratory complications, infection, or delirium and convulsions. Mortality is high among clients who progress into coma with hepatic failure. Dramatic measures may be needed to reduce toxic levels of ammonia in the blood. Such measures include hemodialysis and exchange transfusions, which involve removal and replacement of about 80% of the client's blood. A liver transplant may be performed in cases of fulminant liver failure.

OUTCOME MANAGEMENT

Medical Management

Identify and Treat Precipitating Causes

Factors that may precipitate or severely aggravate hepatic encephalopathy in clients with severe liver disease include gastrointestinal bleeding, increased dietary

| BOX 47-4 | **Stages of Hepatic Encephalopathy** |

STAGE 1

- Fatigue
- Restlessness
- Irritability
- Decreased intellectual performance
- Decreased attention span
- Diminished short-term memory
- Personality changes
- Sleep pattern reversal

STAGE 2

- Deterioration in handwriting
- Asterixis
- Drowsiness
- Confusion
- Lethargy
- Fetor hepaticus

STAGE 3

- Severe confusion
- Inability to follow commands
- Deep somnolence, but arousable

STAGE 4

- Coma
- Unresponsive to painful stimuli
- Possible decorticate or decerebrate posturing

protein, constipation, infection, CNS-depressant drugs (e.g., opiates, benzodiazepines), and dehydration. Gastrointestinal bleeding and increased protein intake may lead to increased bacterial formation of nitrogenous compounds that induce encephalopathy. The use of CNS-depressant drugs should be avoided in these clients.

Protein may be totally eliminated from the diet, with an intake of only fruit juices and IV fluids, although this radical restriction leads to catabolism of the client's own protein stores. The usual protein restriction is 20 to 40 g daily. The client with chronic hepatic encephalopathy may need to adjust to a long-term, low-protein diet (50 to 60 g/day). Vegetable and dairy protein may be better tolerated than meats. These proteins contain fewer ammonia-forming amino acids than those in meat. A diet high in vegetables and dairy products also helps to prevent constipation, thus further reducing ammonia production.

Reduce Nitrogenous Waste (Ammonia) in Blood and Bacteria in Colon

Neomycin and lactulose are given to reduce bacteria in the intestinal tract. Because it is not absorbed into the circulation, neomycin exerts a powerful effect on the intestinal bacteria that are responsible for ammonia production. Undesirable side effects result from the

depletion of intestinal flora (e.g., diarrhea, vitamin K deficiency). Also, because neomycin is nephrotoxic, its use must be avoided in clients with renal insufficiency. Lactulose, which helps decrease blood ammonia levels by reducing absorption of ammonia, is given to clients to produce two to four stools a day. Antibiotics are administered to inhibit growth of gastrointestinal bacteria, and oral magnesium sulfate or enemas are given after hemorrhage to clean out the intestines.

Maintain Fluid Volume Balance

With the accumulation of fluid in the abdominal area (ascites), bleeding, and decreased fluid intake, the client may experience a fluid volume deficit. This deficit, along with electrolyte imbalances that may occur, should be corrected. IV fluids are administered, carefully monitoring the quantity and rate of administration.

Nursing Management of the Medical Client

Assessment. When working with a client susceptible to hepatic encephalopathy, use interviewing and assessment techniques to evaluate psychophysiologic status. For example, has the client's normally neat handwriting become sloppy and difficult to read? Is speech slow and slurred? Observe the client for personality changes with labile feeling states, and elicit liver flap or flapping tremor (asterixis) by asking the client to dorsiflex the hand with the rest of the arm resting on the bed. (In asterixis, the hand cannot be held steady.) The nurse is often the best person to assess a change in the level of mental functioning.

Early detection of a depressed or confused level of consciousness greatly improves the client's chances of recovery.

 SAFETY ALERT

Nursing progress notes should describe the client's behavior vividly and objectively, as in "States pigeons are pecking at his bedclothes," rather than offering interpretations that may have a different meaning for each reader, such as "Seems more confused." Make ongoing neurologic checks to determine the level of consciousness and/or progression to coma. See Unit 16 for neurologic assessment of comatose clients.

Diagnosis, Outcomes, Interventions
Diagnosis: Ineffective Therapeutic Regimen Management and Ineffective Family Therapeutic Regimen Management. The client and family members are vital players in the control of encephalopathy. Thus the nursing diagnoses *Ineffective Therapeutic Regimen Management* and *Ineffective Family Therapeutic Regimen Management related to reduction in protein in the diet and long-term pharmacologic intervention with neomycin* are common with hepatic encephalopathy.

Outcomes. The client will understand and comply with the reduction of protein in the diet and long-term pharmacologic intervention with neomycin as evidenced by the client's following a low-protein diet and stating reasons why neomycin should be taken.

Interventions

Promote Low-Protein Diet. It is important that the client understand the importance of the reduced protein diet to have the motivation to remain on this diet.

Monitor for Gastrointestinal Hemorrhage. In addition to ensuring a low-protein diet, assess for manifestations of gastrointestinal bleeding, checking for bright red blood in the stool or for black, tarry stools. To reverse the progression of manifestations, constipation must be prevented. Administer cathartics and enemas to hasten the exit of protein material from the intestines.

Encourage Bowel Cleansing. The client may need to learn to manage diarrhea, a possible side effect related to the laxative action of lactulose or neomycin sulfate. Intervention in severe hepatic encephalopathy commonly combines neomycin therapy with protein restriction and bowel cleansing. Administer the prescribed maintenance doses of neomycin and provide a low-protein diet for clients with chronic hepatic encephalopathy. In addition, administer oral lactulose, a combination of galactose and fructose that passes through the intestine unchanged, to decrease ammonia by trapping ammonium ions and allowing their evacuation from the bowel. As noted earlier, the appropriate lactulose dosage causes two to four soft stool evacuations daily. If severe diarrhea occurs, the dosage is reduced to prevent further electrolyte imbalance.

Diagnosis: Deficient Fluid Volume. The client often has difficulties with fluid volume, leading to the nursing diagnosis *Deficient Fluid Volume related to bleeding, decreased intake, and ascites.*

Outcomes. The client will maintain a balanced fluid volume, as evidenced by normal blood pressure, absence of edema, absence of ascites, and balanced intake and output.

Interventions. Hypovolemia often precipitates hepatic encephalopathy by reducing hepatocellular perfusion. Fluid balance must be achieved, maintained, and monitored to prevent further hepatic injury and reduced renal perfusion. Deliver IV fluids evenly over time. Monitor vital signs frequently. If necessary, measure urine output hourly.

Electrolyte and acid-base disturbances such as hypokalemia and alkalosis may precipitate hepatic encephalopathy or may develop during its course. Laboratory tests indicate which replacement therapy is necessary.

Diagnosis: Risk for Injury. Because of the multitude of problems faced by the client with encephalopathy, the nursing diagnosis *Risk for Injury related to loss of protective mechanisms secondary to hepatic coma* is common.

Outcomes. Injury or complications of immobility will be prevented or will be identified early as evidenced by the absence of problems related to immobility.

Interventions. Hepatic coma may create a multitude of problems for the client with encephalopathy.

Prevent Hypoxemia. Hypoxemia may precipitate hepatic encephalopathy by damaging the hepatic cell.

To prevent and treat hypoxemia, attend to respiratory interventions (e.g., maintain a patent airway).

Prevent Infection. Concurrent infection, with accumulation of protein from tissue catabolism, necessitates rapid intervention.

The client is particularly vulnerable to nosocomial (hospital-acquired) infections. Wash your hands thoroughly, and take other measures to prevent cross-contamination.

Prevent Ammonia Toxicity and Hypokalemia

Be alert to possible harmful accumulations of ammonia as a result of diuretic therapy. Hypokalemia from the use of diuretics contributes to hepatic encephalopathy by increasing ammonia production in the kidney.

Avoid Sedation

Agents with CNS-depressant effects may precipitate coma, and their use should thus be avoided. If agitation occurs in early encephalopathy, administer agents that are excreted partially through the kidney, instead of the liver (e.g., phenobarbital). Administer phenobarbital with caution. Know which opioids, tranquilizers, and sedatives are biotransformed by the liver; they are often contraindicated in clients with decreased hepatic function.

Prevent Complications of Immobility. The immobile client who lacks protective reflexes (blink or gag reflex) is vulnerable to numerous complications. Preventing complications requires intensive nursing intervention.

Prevent pneumonia and skin breakdown by turning the client frequently and promoting lung aeration.

As the body accumulates metabolic substances, physiologic disturbances develop that may produce a state of agitation.

Therefore protect the client from self-injury, for example, by lowering the bed and padding the side rails.

See Chapter 68 for further discussion of the comatose client and the client with neurologic disturbances.

Evaluation. The prognosis for the client with hepatic encephalopathy is poor. Generally the best outcome that can be hoped for is maintenance with slowed deterioration.

Self-Care

As the acute stages of cirrhosis subside, ongoing care of the client continues. If the care plan includes discharge from the hospital, provide extensive discharge teaching for the client with cirrhosis who has experienced complications. Family members and significant others need to know how to reduce the incidence of complications from cirrhosis. Review the potential complications with the caregivers as well as how to prevent and treat them.

Medications
Review all medications along with scheduled times of administration and their intended and adverse side effects. Potential medications include lactulose, diuretics, and vitamin supplements.

Diet Modifications
Explain the importance of a well-balanced, nutritional diet to the client, with specific information about limitations on dietary protein, sodium, and water. Teach family members and significant others about the need to encourage eating and still maintain food intake within prescribed limits.

Home Modifications
Teach that the client's home may need to be altered to adjust for limitations in mobility. Safety precautions should be taken to help prevent injury to the client. The client's bedroom should be near the bathroom if the client is receiving diuretics.

Follow-Up Assessments
The client's status should be followed closely. Be sure that the client's caregivers are aware of any changes that require immediate medical attention. They should also know that diagnostic testing at regular intervals is continued to monitor the status of the liver.

FATTY LIVER (HEPATIC STENOSIS)

Lipid infiltration may lead to hepatic stenosis, or "fatty liver," one of the most common metabolic diseases of the liver. This pathologic process causes liver enlargement and increased firmness and may result in decreased function.

Liver biopsy establishes the diagnosis. Laboratory studies disclose that triglycerides are the major type of lipid involved, but small amounts of cholesterol and phospholipid also may have infiltrated the liver.

Major causes of lipid infiltration include chronic alcoholism, protein malnutrition in early life, diabetes mellitus, obesity, Cushing's syndrome (natural or induced), jejunoileal bypass, prolonged IV hyperalimentation, chronic illnesses that involve impaired nutrition or malabsorption, some hepatotoxins (carbon tetrachloride and DDT [dichlorodiphenyltrichloroethane]), and Reye's syndrome in children.

The manifestations of fatty liver are related to the degree of fat infiltration, the amount of time fat has been accumulating, and the underlying cause. Clients with moderate to severe lipid infiltration are frequently asymptomatic; however, clients with massive infiltration experience anorexia, abdominal pain, and sometimes jaundice. Laboratory studies demonstrate elevated serum alkaline phosphatase and bilirubin levels.

Recovery begins after the source of the problem is removed and metabolic balance and adequate nutrition are restored. Residual damage, if it occurs, usually follows persistent fatty infiltration and chronic alcoholism. Fat embolization may occur and can cause death.

Nursing intervention for clients with fatty infiltration of the liver includes the following:

- Directing attention to correction of the cause (abstinence from alcohol, control of diabetes mellitus, weight loss, or correction of the intestinal absorptive defect)
- Preparing the client for diagnostic procedures
- Giving emotional support by allowing verbalization of concerns and fears
- Giving supportive physical care including adequate nutritional intake
- Designing teaching guidelines that promote proper diet and prevent recurrence

LIVER CANCERS

Tumors of the liver are either primary or metastatic. Primary liver tumors may arise from hepatocytes, connective tissue, blood vessels, or bile ducts. These tumors are either benign or malignant (Figure 47-6). Figure 47-7 presents a classification of the primary liver cancers. Metastatic malignant tumors arise from the gastrointestinal tract (particularly the colon), the breasts, and the lungs.

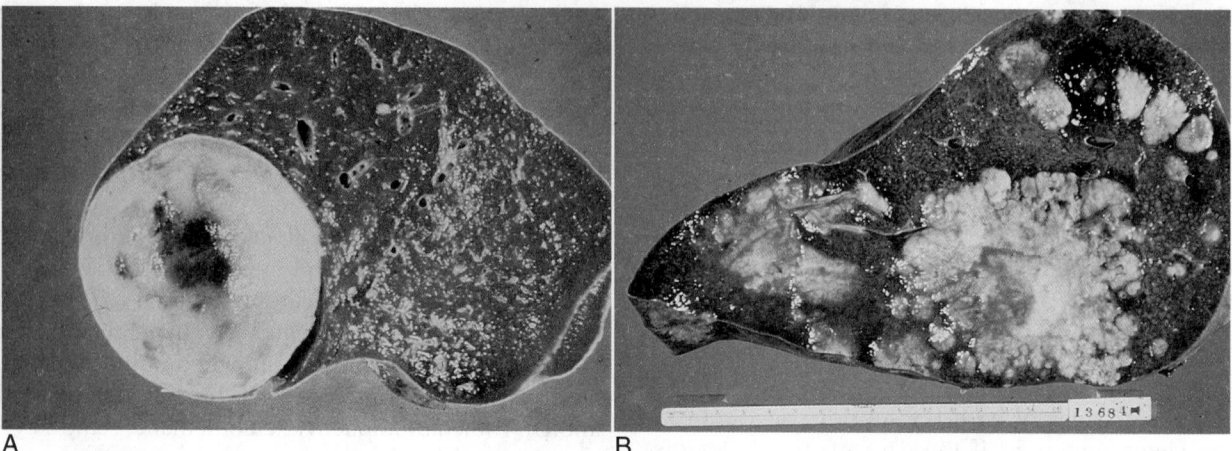

■ **FIGURE 47–6**   Benign liver tumor **(A)** and metastatic malignant liver tumor **(B)**. Note the encapsulated tumor in the benign lesion and the invasiveness of malignant lesion. Satellite lesions are also present with the malignant lesion.

ORIGIN	BENIGN	MALIGNANT
Hepatocytes	Adenoma	Hepatocellular carcinoma
Connective tissue	Fibroma	Sarcoma
Blood vessels	Hemangioma	Hemangioendothelioma
Bile ducts	Cholangioma	Carcinoma

■ **FIGURE 47–7**   Classification of primary liver cancers.

BENIGN HEPATIC TUMORS

Hepatic adenomas are benign tumors of the liver that occur most commonly in women in their 30s and 40s. Nearly 90% of cases are associated with oral contraceptive use. The fact that the tumors occur more commonly in women, especially women who take oral contraceptives, suggests a hormonal influence in their pathogenesis.

Although these tumors are classified as benign, they are nevertheless dangerous because of their vascularity. A benign adenoma may rupture, with consequent hemorrhage. Diagnosis is made by a combination of tests including sonography, CT scanning, selective hepatic arteriography, and radionuclide scanning. Liver biopsy is not warranted because the tumors are hypervascular. Intervention for benign adenoma depends on its cause. Discontinuation of oral contraceptives or androgens, when a tumor appears to be hormone dependent, may correct the condition. Otherwise treatment may include surgical excision of the involved liver segment. If acute hemorrhage calls for surgery, the surgeon may perform a hepatic lobectomy. Benign hepatic tumors are associated with an excellent prognosis if they are removed surgically before they rupture and cause death from hemorrhage.

MALIGNANT HEPATIC TUMORS

PRIMARY HEPATOCELLULAR CANCER

The rate of primary hepatocellular cancer is rising in the United States and other Western countries, presumably because of the high prevalence of hepatitis B and hepatitis C during the last 20 to 30 years.[1,7] The American Cancer Society estimates for 2007 were for more than 19,000 new cases and approximately 16,800 deaths of hepatocellular cancer in the United States.[1] Other etiologic factors that may contribute to hepatoma are hepatitis B, cirrhosis, chronic liver disease, hemochromatosis, ingestion of certain mycotoxins (aflatoxins), anabolic steroid use, and long-term androgen therapy. Primary hepatocellular carcinoma is the main cause of death from cancer in many areas of the world, including sub-Saharan Africa and parts of Asia.

After the diagnosis of liver cancer and if intervention fails to terminate the neoplastic process, the client usually dies of hepatic failure within 3 to 6 months. Surgical resection of the tumor is the only method of cure and may be attempted if the tumor is confined to one lobe. Many clients, however, do not have a resectable tumor because of underlying cirrhosis, involvement of both lobes, and distant metastases.

METASTATIC HEPATIC CANCERS

The liver is one of the common sites of metastasis for all cancers. In the United States, metastatic cancers of the liver are 20 times more common than primary liver tumors.[7]

Etiology and Risk Factors

The liver is a common site of metastasis because of the liver's high rate of blood flow, its size, and portal venous drainage from the major abdominal organs. Tumors of the gastrointestinal tract, lung, and breast metastasize to the liver more frequently than do tumors of the prostate or thyroid.

Pathophysiology

Metastatic cancers spread to the liver in three ways: by direct extension from adjacent organs (stomach and gallbladder), via the hepatic arterial system, or via the portal venous system. Also, as a result of cell migration, the surface of the liver may become seeded with metastatic cells.

Clinical Manifestations

Clients with primary (benign and malignant) and secondary (metastatic) tumors often show similar manifestations. Early indicators of liver cancer are usually vague. Many clients with metastatic malignancy of the liver have the following three types of manifestations:

- Manifestations that are specific only to the primary tumor, hepatic involvement being discovered incidentally in the course of a diagnostic evaluation
- Nonspecific manifestations of anorexia, diaphoresis, fever, weight loss, and weakness
- Manifestations of active liver disease, such as abdominal pain, ascites, and hepatomegaly

Diagnostic studies and physical examination may reveal the following: elevated alkaline phosphatase level, hepatomegaly, a liver mass, a friction rub or bruit over the liver, angiographic evidence of cancer hypoproteinemia, blood-tinged ascitic fluid, decreased liver function, and reversal of the albumin-globulin (A:G) ratio. The A:G ratio is a calculation of the distribution of two major protein fractions: albumin and globulin. The value of the A:G ratio is usually greater than 1. A high ratio is considered insignificant; however, a low ratio occurs in liver and renal diseases.

Some clients also may have metabolic derangements, such as in polycythemia, blood glucose disorders, and high levels of calcium. Other clients may present with marked leukocytosis and anemia. Jaundice occurs more often when a bile duct is the site of a primary tumor or when the tumor mass obstructs a major outflow duct. Other manifestations may be present, depending on the concurrent pathologic condition. At times the tumor process causes elevation of the diaphragm and some respiratory problems.

Although cancers of the liver create numerous clinical manifestations, many pathologic features may not appear until the tumors have grown quite large. Malignant tumor cells may have replaced as much as 90% of normal liver tissue before liver insufficiency becomes clinically evident.

In primary hepatocellular cancers, diagnostic tests often reveal high levels of alpha-fetoprotein (AFP). This substance is sometimes present in clients who have metastatic tumors, but levels rarely reach those found in clients with primary tumors.

A diagnosis of liver cancer is suggested by an elevated serum alkaline phosphatase level and by abnormal findings on ultrasonography, CT, liver scanning, or magnetic resonance imaging (MRI). Cytologic examination of aspirated fluid can also be used to establish the diagnosis.

Performing a liver biopsy is helpful in establishing the diagnosis. The route of access may be percutaneous, direct via laparotomy, or through a peritoneoscope. Each method has its limitations. Percutaneous procedures may cause seeding of tumor cells along the biopsy needle pathway as it is withdrawn. Laparotomy requires anesthesia, which may be too dangerous. Peritoneoscopy may be impossible if there are extensive adhesions. Because all these biopsy procedures require internal membrane puncture, be sure the client has an acceptable PT because of the risk of hemorrhage if the time is too prolonged.

Prognosis

Because hepatic tumors may be far advanced before clinical manifestations or laboratory data indicate their presence, and because severe liver disease (e.g., cirrhosis) frequently coexists, liver cancer carries a poor prognosis. In the United States, median survival from the time of diagnosis is about 6 months.

OUTCOME MANAGEMENT

Medical Management

Relief of Manifestations and Promotion of Palliation

As noted previously, treatment of liver cancer is aimed at relieving manifestations and supporting the client physically and emotionally. The treatment options for medical management include chemotherapy, radiation therapy, and other approaches, such as cryoablation.

Chemotherapy. Regional perfusion of the liver with infusions given directly into the hepatic artery may reduce pain or slow tumor growth and may produce fewer side effects than those incurred with systemic chemotherapy, which is not known to prolong life. Various chemotherapeutic agents have been used singly or in combination with other agents infused into the hepatic artery or have been given by regional infusion with other agents given systemically.

During surgery, the surgeon may implant a chemotherapy infusion pump. Such pumps, filled percutaneously, deliver medication continuously into the hepatic artery. With metastatic growths, the oncologist may prescribe systemic chemotherapy to reduce tumor size and pain.

Chemotherapeutic agents used to induce the regression of primary and metastatic tumors of the liver include 5-fluorouracil (5-FU) and doxorubicin (Adriamycin) for single-dose therapy and 5-FU with carmustine (BCNU), semustine (methyl CCNU), or streptozocin for combination therapy.

Radiation Therapy. Radiation therapy has produced disappointing results. Irradiation of liver tumors may provide temporary pain reduction but does not promote survival.

Other Approaches. Some other approaches that have been used for the treatment of primary hepatic tumor include hepatic artery embolization and chemotherapy (chemoembolization), alcohol ablation via ultrasound-guided percutaneous injection, ultrasound-guided cryoablation, and gene therapy with retroviral vectors containing genes that express cytotoxic agents. Biliary drainage achieved percutaneously or through an internal stent placed surgically helps to increase the passage of bile into the duodenum, thereby decreasing jaundice and discomfort.

The Food and Drug Administration (FDA) has approved a device called SIR-Spheres, which consists of biocompatible microspheres containing yttrium-90 that are 20 to 40 μm in diameter. It is implanted into a hepatic tumor by injection either into the common hepatic artery or into the right or left hepatic artery using a chemotherapy catheter port. Liver transplantation may be an option to prolong life if the client has cirrhosis but may be impractical because of the donor organ shortage.

Nursing Management of the Medical Client

Nursing diagnoses and interventions for clients with liver cancers vary according to the amount of liver dysfunction and the treatment modalities. Plan to assess the client for metabolic malfunctions, pain, bleeding problems, ascites, edema, an inability to biotransform endogenous and exogenous (drug) wastes, hypoproteinemia, jaundice, and endocrine complications.

Take time to prepare the client in the diagnostic stage for the various procedures, and assess carefully for postprocedure complications. If pain is a problem, administer medication at the prescribed time and dosage. In addition, assist the client and family members to gain knowledge about the condition and to offer support necessary for them to cope with the uncertainty and fear associated with cancer. See Chapters 16 and 17 for detailed discussions of nursing care of clients with malignant tumors. See also the Care Plan feature on Management of the Client with Hepatic Failure on pp. 1162 to 1164.

Surgical Management

Indications
Resection is indicated for tumors that are small and confined to one liver segment or lobe. The affected segment or lobe is removed surgically. Resection is curative if the remaining unaffected liver is normal. Liver transplantation may be considered as the therapeutic option for small unresectable tumors in a client with advanced cirrhosis; however, it may be curative in only a minority of clients. Recurrence of tumor or metastasis after transplantation has limited its usefulness.

Contraindications
The client may not be able to withstand the stress of surgery. An additional contraindication to surgery is the presence of liver disease too extensive for surgery to be beneficial.

Complications
Tumor rupture, gastrointestinal hemorrhage from varices, progressive cachexia, and hepatic failure are the primary complications of hepatic tumors. Management of the client with these complications is supportive and palliative and will vary according to the client's overall condition, degree of liver impairment, and extent of surgery.

Outcomes
Prognosis is poor. Most clients with hepatic carcinoma have a median survival time of 3 to 6 months.

Nursing Management of the Surgical Client

Nursing management of the client preoperatively and postoperatively includes many responsibilities. See the discussion of nursing management of the client who has undergone surgery for complications of portal hypertension, described earlier in this chapter.

LIVER TRANSPLANTATION

Surgical Management

Liver transplantation is now considered a feasible form of intervention for a variety of end-stage liver diseases. The number of liver transplants has continued to grow each year. From 2000 to 2002, more than 4500 people in the United States received liver transplants.[4] The demand for livers for transplantation continues to outpace availability. More than 6000 clients in the United States remain on a donor liver waiting list.

The duration of the surgical procedure is generally 8 hours but can be from 6 to 18 hours. The surgery may be orthotopic, involving removal of the diseased liver and insertion of the donor liver. Anastomoses of the vena cava, portal vein, hepatic artery, and bile duct are performed. In the heterotopic approach, the diseased liver is left in and the transplanted liver is inserted alongside it.

Orthotopic surgery is by far the more common of the two. Because excessive bleeding may occur, large amounts of blood, blood products, and volume expanders are needed.

Indications

The most appropriate candidates for liver transplantation are people who, in the absence of contraindications, have severe, irreversible liver disease for which alternative medical or surgical treatments have not been successful or are not available. Ideally transplantation should be considered in clients with end-stage liver disease who are experiencing life-threatening complications of liver dysfunction, whose quality of life has increasingly deteriorated, or who are predicted to experience neurologic effects of liver damage. If the surgery is performed sufficiently early, contraindications and extrahepatic deterioration are less likely.[4]

Some of the most common conditions warranting transplantation are as follows:

- Primary and secondary biliary cirrhosis (adult)
- Hepatitis—chronic with cirrhosis, chronic viral or fulminant (usually adult)
- Primary sclerosing cholangitis (adult)
- Biliary atresia (pediatric)
- Alpha$_1$-antitrypsin deficiency (usually pediatric)
- Confined hepatic malignancy (adult or pediatric)
- Wilson's disease
- Budd-Chiari syndrome (hepatic vein thrombosis)
- Alcoholic cirrhosis

Choosing clients with alcoholic cirrhosis, chronic viral hepatitis, and primary hepatocellular malignancies as liver transplant recipients may be questionable. Clients with any one of these conditions are considered high-risk surgical candidates, but liver transplantation may be offered to carefully selected individuals. The alcoholic client, for example, must be willing to adhere to certain guidelines, such as abstinence from alcohol and participation in a substance-abuse treatment program, to be eligible for the procedure. The client must be psychologically stable and have good support systems for the complex postoperative course.

Contraindications

Absolute contraindications include (1) life-threatening systemic diseases; (2) uncontrolled extrahepatic bacterial or fungal infections; (3) pre-existing advanced cardiovascular or pulmonary disease; (4) multiple uncorrectable, life-threatening congenital anomalies; (5) metastatic malignancy to the liver; (6) active alcoholism or drug abuse; (7) cholangiocarcinoma; and (8) human immunodeficiency virus (HIV) infection. See Chapter 80 for other contraindications to transplantation.

Complications

Postoperative complications can be hepatic or nonhepatic. They may include cardiovascular and pulmonary problems as well as infection, rejection, hemorrhage, atelectasis, failure of anastomosis, and acute renal failure. Rejection occurs most commonly between postoperative days 4 and 10.

Manifestations of acute rejection include fever, tachycardia, right upper quadrant or flank pain, and increasing jaundice. Drugs used to stop or prevent rejection include azathioprine, cyclosporine, FK506, OKT3, and steroids such as prednisone and methylprednisolone; otherwise, liver function rapidly deteriorates. Chapter 80 describes management of clients undergoing transplantation.

Outcomes

It is expected that the client will recover from the liver transplant surgery, be discharged from the hospital in 1 week, and within 3 to 4 months be able to resume a normal life as long as medication and health care regimens are followed closely. Complications such as rejection and infection will slow the progress of affected clients.

The survival rate after liver transplantation has improved steadily since the early 1980s from approximately 30% in the 1970s to greater than 85% today.

The survival rate is higher and the quality of life better after transplantation in people who had less hepatic damage before surgery and in those who had fewer extrahepatic manifestations.

Nursing Management of the Surgical Client

Preoperative Care

Once the client has chosen transplantation as an alternative to care and is placed on the recipient waiting list, an extensive physical and psychological evaluation is required (see Chapter 80). The client must undergo a variety of tests, including blood analysis, hepatic angiogram, abdominal CT scan, chest and hip x-ray studies, electrocardiogram (ECG), bone density studies, and nutritional assessment. The client may also have the opportunity to meet the transplant team. Matching donor and recipient organ size and blood and tissue type are important considerations in donor selection.

Focus on assessing the client's needs in relation to the client's level of knowledge and information. Ascertain how the client and the client's family members are coping with the situation. In addition, the needs dictated by the extent of organ failure will guide care. The specific nursing care needs of clients during the waiting period for a liver transplant depend on the degree of end-stage liver disease.

Postoperative Care

The major focus of care is to monitor for rejection, infection, and occlusion of vessels. Immunosuppressive therapy, which is started before surgery, must be continued on a regular schedule postoperatively to prevent rejection of the new liver. The client requires constant monitoring of respiratory, cardiovascular, neurologic, and hemodynamic status. Liver function is monitored through assessment of serum transaminases (ALT, AST), bilirubin, albumin, and clotting factors. Monitor fluid and electrolyte status, blood glucose levels, and pH.

Clients are always somewhat fluid overloaded from receiving extensive volumes of blood products during the long surgical procedure. This overload can lead to pulmonary edema and heart failure. Serum potassium level will be decreased as a result of transplantation, and blood glucose level will be increased. The serum pH will be normal to acidic.

Monitor wound drains and bile drains for patency, and note bile characteristics (amount, color, consistency). Obstruction of wound drains causes increased intra-abdominal pressure from the accumulation of ascitic fluid and blood. Obstruction of bile flow can cause damage to the liver and biliary system.

Assess the needs of family members and significant others, who may have traveled long distances from home and may be feeling powerless, stressed, and anxious.

Much of the care and many of the nursing diagnoses for a client who undergoes liver transplantation are the same as for a client after any other type of surgery. See Chapter 80 for care of the client after transplantation.

LIVER ABSCESS

A liver abscess is a localized collection of pus and organisms within the parenchyma of the liver. Liver abscess usually develops in association with one of the following three conditions:

- Bacterial cholangitis, which results from obstruction of the bile ducts by stone or stricture
- Portal vein bacteremia, which may develop following bowel inflammation or organ perforation
- Amebiasis (infestation with amebae from tropical or subtropical areas)

Other predisposing factors are diabetes mellitus, infected hepatic cysts, metastatic liver tumors with secondary infection, and diverticulitis.

The client commonly reports right upper quadrant pain and abdominal and right shoulder pain. Assessment may also reveal liver enlargement, tenderness, nausea, vomiting, weight loss, anorexia, fever, and diaphoresis. Sometimes a right pleural effusion develops. The liver's proximity to the base of the right lung contributes to this process.

Liver scanning is extremely valuable in diagnosis. Other useful diagnostic modalities include ultrasonography, CT, and arteriography. Laboratory data reflect slight to marked elevations of aminotransferases, alkaline phosphatase, and bilirubin. High levels indicate the presence of concurrent obstruction. Blood culture yields positive results in some cases.

Intervention in hepatic abscess consists of (1) percutaneous drainage of the abscess with antimicrobial therapy, (2) surgical drainage of large abscesses with postoperative antimicrobial therapy, or (3) antimicrobial therapy without drainage for a few months. Abscesses resulting from amebic infestation (such as by *Entamoeba histolytica*) require treatment with metronidazole (Flagyl) or chloroquine phosphate (Aralen phosphate) instead of broad-spectrum antibiotics. Early diagnosis and therapy for uncomplicated amebic liver abscess result in a death rate of less than 1%.

When caring for the client with liver abscess, assess vital signs regularly. High temperature and rapid pulse rate may indicate the presence of general sepsis, a likely complication. Encourage movement, coughing, and deep breathing to prevent or limit pulmonary complications related to hepatic abscess. Increase the client's fluid intake and provide skin care in the event of hyperpyrexia. Dispose of feces carefully, and wash your hands to prevent transmission of amebic infestations.

RARE DISORDERS

Hemochromatosis (an uncommon disorder of iron metabolism often associated with portal hypertension and hepatomegaly) and amyloidosis (a proteinaceous, starch-like substance that can infiltrate the liver and other organs) are two rare disorders that can occur. Hereditary hemochromatosis is addressed in the Genetics Links feature on p. 1175. Table 47-6 briefly describes these two disorders.

CONGENITAL CONDITIONS

Three congenital conditions affecting the liver are Wilson's disease, Caroli's disease, and congenital hepatic fibrosis. Table 47-7 briefly describes these three conditions.

LIVER TRAUMA

Liver injury usually results from a penetrating injury or blunt trauma. Either can lead to laceration and hemorrhage. Penetrating injuries are usually knife or missile (gunshot) wounds. A knife wound generally is superficial and leaves a sharp clear edge, whereas missile

GENETIC LINKS

Hereditary Hemochromatosis

DESCRIPTION

Hereditary hemochromatosis is an autosomal-recessive disorder of iron metabolism in which excessive iron accumulates in multiple organs such as the liver, heart, pancreas, joints, and skin. Common early clinical manifestations include abdominal pain, arthralgia, fatigue, weight loss, and lethargy. Manifestations tend to occur in men between 40 and 60 years of age and in women after menopause. Hepatic fibrosis or cirrhosis is common in untreated individuals after age 40. Other findings may include arthritis, diabetes mellitus, cardiac abnormalities, and increased skin pigmentation. Hereditary hemochromatosis (HHC) most often affects Caucasians of Northern European descent, although other ethnic groups are also affected.

GENETICS

About one in nine people in the general population is a carrier of the hemochromatosis gene. Hemochromatosis is associated mainly with mutations in a gene called *HFE*, located on chromosome 6. The two known common mutations in *HFE* are named *C282Y* (the most common mutation) and

H63D. HFE is inherited in an autosomal-recessive manner. Two copies of a mutant gene inherited from unaffected carrier parents are necessary to cause the disorder. Offspring of carrier parents have a 25% risk of having hemochromatosis.

DIAGNOSIS/TESTING

Diagnosis of individuals with clinical manifestations is typically based on screening tests such as serum transferrin-iron saturation and serum ferritin concentration and confirmatory tests such as histologic assessment of hepatic iron stores on liver biopsy or molecular genetic testing for the *C282Y* and *H63D* mutations in the *HFE* gene.

MANAGEMENT

Usual therapy is removal of excess iron by phlebotomy (i.e., removal of blood). Early diagnosis and treatment to normalize serum iron levels before manifestations of organ damage develop can prevent all the potential complications of HHC. People with HHC should avoid taking iron supplements. Because HHC is common and early detection and treatment are effective, widespread screening for this disorder has been proposed and is an area of current research.

TABLE 47–6   **Rare Disorders**

Factor	Hemochromatosis	Amyloidosis
Description/etiology	Disorder of iron storage. Excessive amounts of iron are deposited in parenchymal cells, causing eventual damage and impaired function of organs, especially liver, pancreas, heart, joints, and pituitary. Primary hemochromatosis is a recessive inherited metabolic defect that causes increased iron absorption from gastrointestinal tract. Secondary hemochromatosis is caused by alcoholism, excessive intake of iron, or conditions requiring repeated blood transfusions. Common problems associated with hemochromatosis include diabetes mellitus, enlarged liver, cirrhosis, cardiac disease, increased skin pigmentation, and arthritis.	Results from deposition of insoluble proteins in extracellular spaces of organs and tissues, causing them to cease functioning; is classified according to type of protein that forms amyloid deposits. Primary amyloidosis (AL) is formed from deposition of immunoglobulins and causes damage to tissues of cardiac, smooth muscle, skin, kidney, and liver origin. Primary amyloidosis is often associated with multiple myeloma. Amyloidosis caused by deposition of protein A (AA) occurs most often in chronic inflammations such as tuberculosis, rheumatoid arthritis, osteomyelitis, and bronchiectasis. Another type of amyloidosis is genetic and passed down through families (FAP). The tissues most affected by this type of amyloidosis include spleen, kidney, and liver.
Diagnosis	Elevated levels of plasma iron (>150 mg/ml; normal 2-5 g), more than 60% saturation of iron-binding protein (transferrin), manifestations of specific organ dysfunction, and liver biopsy.	Liver biopsy provides best data, but there is a high incidence of postbiopsy hemorrhage or liver rupture.
Clinical manifestations	Clinical manifestations are varied and depend on area of body involved. Often arthritis prompts clients to seek medical attention.	Clinical manifestations are varied and depend on area of body involved.
Interventions	Phlebotomy (surgical opening of a vein to withdraw blood) biweekly or weekly over a 1- or 2-year period (2 ml of blood = 1 mg of iron). Desferrioxamine mesylate, a chelating agent, facilitates removal of iron from body.	Treatment depends on type of amyloidosis present. Genetic counseling is important for heredofamilial types, and liver transplantation has been done for FAP. In AL, stem cell transplantation and immunosuppressive drugs (melphalan) have been effective.

Data from Sipe, J.D., & Cohen, A.S. (2005). Amyloidosis. In D. Kasper, et al. (Eds.), *Harrison's principles of internal medicine* (16th ed., pp. 2024-2029). New York: McGraw-Hill; and Powell, L.W. (2005). Hemochromatosis. In D. Kasper, et al. (Eds.), *Harrison's principles of internal medicine* (16th ed., pp. 2298-2303). New York: McGraw-Hill.

TABLE 47–7 Congenital Conditions

Condition	Description/Diagnosis	Symptoms	Intervention
Wilson's disease	Accumulation of copper in tissues of liver, brain, and kidney Is usually chronic but may be acute; acute form may be fatal Hallmark of disease is presence of Kayser-Fleischer rings encircling corneas (from copper deposits) Copper deposits also seen in liver biopsy	Abnormal liver function and neurologic changes Manifests itself from early childhood to adulthood	Penicillamine Liver transplantation may be performed for acute disease
Caroli's disease	Characterized by dilated bile ducts and cyst formations May be localized or widespread	Fever and bacterial cholangitis, right upper quadrant pain, and jaundice (from obstruction of biliary tract by one or more cysts or stones) Usually presents soon after birth, but may not be diagnosed until early adulthood	Antibiotics, external biliary drainage, or liver transplantation
Congenital hepatic fibrosis	Characterized by portal hypertension caused by portal vein fibrosis	Upper gastrointestinal bleeding from gastric or esophageal varices	Ranges from blood transfusions to sclerotherapy to portacaval shunting

wounds cause perforations through the liver tissue, that is, the entrance and exit points. The greater the velocity of the missile, the greater the damage. Often, a close-range missile injury is fatal because of the large amount of damage. Blunt trauma (e.g., from a steering wheel or a fall) can have various effects, ranging from small hematomas that remain under the liver capsule to large, star-like lacerations from severe impact forces.

Management of liver injuries consists of control of the hemorrhage, debridement, and drainage. Surgical resection of liver lobes may be necessary, but more often the major goal of surgical intervention is to control hemorrhage. Monitor victims of trauma carefully for falling blood pressure and tachycardia, which may indicate hemorrhage. The problem is more difficult when the liver's blood vessels or bile ducts are damaged as well. Later complications include bile peritonitis and abscess formation.

CONCLUSIONS

Hepatic disorders are complex and difficult for all involved. You should have a thorough understanding of the liver and its functions to care for these clients. Many hepatic disorders are the result of the client's lifestyle, further complicating an already difficult problem. The nurse must therefore consider both the physiologic and the psychosocial problems associated with many hepatic disorders. Helping the client make appropriate lifestyle changes is an important nursing function.

 THINKING CRITICALLY

1. A 37-year-old man is admitted to the hospital with a 10-day history of anorexia, fatigue, malaise, low-grade fever, dark urine, and upper abdominal discomfort. There is no history of jaundice, IV drug use, or blood transfusions. He is homosexual. Alcohol intake consists of several mixed drinks nightly and wine with dinner. Findings on physical examination include temperature of 99.6° F, jaundice, blood pressure of 150/80 mm Hg, and no spider nevi. The liver measures 12 cm in the midclavicular line and is moderately tender. The spleen is not palpable. Initial laboratory data were as follows: total bilirubin, 6.8 mg/dl (normal, 0.2 to 1.2 mg/dl); alkaline phosphatase, 240 units/L (normal, 20 to 90 units/L); AST, 980 units/L (normal, 5 to 40 units/L); ALT, 1200 units/L (normal, 5 to 35 units/L). The WBC count is 5600/mm³, with a normal differential count. What are the priorities for care in this situation? What interventions might be used?

Factors to Consider. Without further data, what would appear to be the major organ systems involved? What additional information do you, as his nurse, think is necessary to obtain? If you are caring for this client and you inadvertently sustain a needlestick from a syringe used to give an injection to this client, what action would you take?

2. A 48-year-old man arrives in the emergency department. He felt well until 2 hours ago, when he became nauseated and subsequently vomited a large amount of red blood and clots. He reports a long history of heavy alcohol use and cigarette smoking. He takes no medications. Laboratory data were the following: hemoglobin, 9.6 g/dl; hematocrit, 28.4%; platelet count, 92,000/mm³; PT, 16.5 seconds (normal, 11 to 15 seconds); alkaline phosphatase, 120 units/L (normal, 20 to 90 units/L); AST, 265 units/L; ALT,

112 units/L. What is likely to be a major underlying cause of this client's problem? Is it reversible? Can further damage be stopped? With the client vomiting blood, what should be your priority interventions?

Factors to Consider. What gastrointestinal disorders can be manifested in people who consume large quantities of alcohol? What risks does the client face in the present situation?

3. Your client is a 68-year-old man with cirrhosis. He is admitted for treatment of ascites and acute upper right abdominal pain. His abdomen is very large, and the ascitic fluid shifts from side to side whenever he moves. Diagnostic studies reveal that the cause of the pain is cholelithiasis, and surgery is scheduled. What are the client's priority needs on admission? What complications might he face following surgery?

Factors to Consider. What are the clinical manifestations of cirrhosis? Is the client with cirrhosis a good candidate for abdominal surgery?

Discussions for these questions can be found on the website.

BIBLIOGRAPHY

Citations appearing in red refer to primary research.

Citations appearing in blue refer to evidence-based practice guidelines and protocols.

1. American Cancer Society. (2007). *Cancer facts and figures 2007*. Atlanta: Author.
2. Arguedas, M.R., & Fallon, M.B. (2004). Cirrhosis of the liver and its complications. In T.E. Andreoli, et al. (Eds.), *Cecil essentials of medicine* (6th ed., pp. 411-417). Philadelphia: Saunders.
3. Chung, R.T., & Podolsky, D.K. (2005). Cirrhosis and its complications. In D. Kasper, et al. (Eds.), *Harrison's principles of internal medicine* (16th ed., pp. 1858-1869). New York: McGraw-Hill.
4. Dienstag, J.L. (2005). Liver transplantation. In D. Kasper, et al. (Eds.), *Harrison's principles of internal medicine* (16th ed., pp. 1873-1880). New York: McGraw-Hill.
5. Dienstag, J.L., & Isselbacher, K.J. (2005). Acute viral hepatitis. In D. Kasper, et al. (Eds.), *Harrison's principles of internal medicine* (16th ed., pp. 1822-1838). New York: McGraw-Hill.
6. Dienstag, J.L., & Isselbacher, K.J. (2005). Chronic hepatitis. In D. Kasper, et al. (Eds.), *Harrison's principles of internal medicine* (16th ed., pp. 1844-1855). New York: McGraw-Hill.
7. Dienstag, J.L., & Isselbacher, K.J. (2005). Tumors of the liver and biliary tract. In D. Kasper, et al. (Eds.), *Harrison's principles of internal medicine* (16th ed., pp. 533-536). New York: McGraw-Hill.
8. Dienstag, J.L., & Isselbacher, K.J. (2005). Toxic and drug-induced hepatitis. In D. Kasper, et al. (Eds.), *Harrison's principles of internal medicine* (16th ed., pp. 1838-1844). New York: McGraw-Hill.
9. Friedman, L.S. (2004). Liver, biliary tract, and pancreas. In L.M. Tierney, S.J. McPhee, & M.A. Papadakis (Eds.), *Current medical diagnosis and treatment 2004* (43rd ed., pp. 626-668). New York: Lange Medical.
10. Greenwald, B. (2004). The Minnesota tube: Its use and care in bleeding esophageal and gastric varices. *Gastroenterology Nursing*, *27*(15), 212-217.
11. Hench, C., & Simpkins, S. (2002, July). Hepatitis C: Risk factors, assessment and diagnosis. (Part 1 of 2). *Nurse Week*, 20-21.
12. Hench, C., & Simpkins, S. (2002, Aug). Hepatitis C: Treatment, prevention, and nursing interventions. (Part 2 of 2). *Nurse Week*, 17-18.
13. Holloway, M., & D'Acunto, K. (2006). An update on the ABCs of viral hepatitis. *The Clinical Advisor*, *9*(6), 26-39.
14. Krumberger, J. (2002). When the liver fails. *RN*, *65*(2), 26-29.
15. Lindseth, G. (2003). Disorders of the liver, gallbladder and pancreas. In S. Price & L. Wilson (Eds.), *Pathophysiology: Clinical concepts of disease processes* (6th ed., pp. 368-401). St. Louis: Mosby.
16. Monkemuller, K.E., & Fallon, M.B. (2004). Jaundice. In T.E. Andreoli, et al. (Eds.), *Cecil essentials of medicine* (5th ed., pp. 371-376). Philadelphia: Saunders.
17. Ostapowica, G., Fontana, R.J., Schiodt, F.V., et al. (2002). Results of a prospective study of acute liver failure at 17 tertiary care centers in the United States. *Annals Internal Medicine, 137*, 947-954. Synoptic article in Greenberger, N.J., & Sharma, P. (2004). Update in gastroenterology and hepatology. *Annals of Internal Medicine, 141*(5), 374-380.
18. Powell, L.W. (2005). Hemochromatosis. In D. Kasper, et al. (Eds.), *Harrison's principles of internal medicine* (16th ed., pp. 2298-2303). New York: McGraw-Hill.
19. Poynard, T., McHutchison, J., Manns, M., et al. (2002). Impact of pegylated interferon alfa-2b and ribavirin on liver fibrosis in patients with chronic hepatitis C. *Gastroenterology, 122*, 1303-1313. Synoptic article in Greenberger, N.J., & Sharma, P. (2004). Update in gastroenterology and hepatology. *Annals of Internal Medicine, 141*(5), 374-380.
20. Saunders, J.C. (2004). Living with hepatitis. *Gastroenterology Nursing, 27*(5), 239-241.
21. Sheikh, A.M., Fallon, M.B., et al. (2004). Acute and chronic hepatitis. In T.E. Andreoli, et al. (Eds.), *Cecil essentials of medicine* (6th ed., pp. 399-407). Philadelphia: Saunders.
22. Sip, J.D., & Cohen, A.S. (2005). Amyloidosis. In D. Kasper, et al. (Eds.), *Harrison's principles of internal medicine* (16th ed., pp. 2024-2029). New York: McGraw-Hill.
23. Sommers, M.S., & Johnson, S.A. (2002). Cirrhosis. In M.S. Sommers & S.A. Johnson (Eds.), *Diseases and disorders: A nursing therapeutics manual* (2nd ed., pp. 253-257). Philadelphia: F.A. Davis.

UNIT 11

INTEGUMENTARY DISORDERS

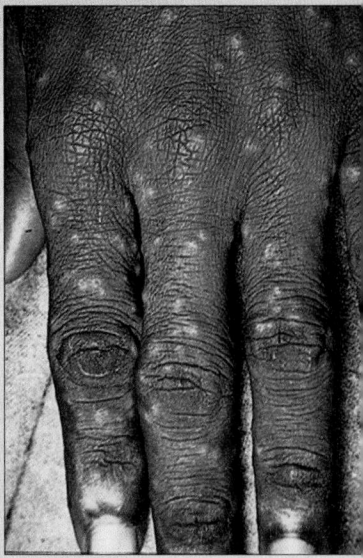

ANATOMY AND PHYSIOLOGY REVIEW:

The Integumentary System

Robert G. Carroll

The integument, or skin, makes up 15% to 20% of the body's weight. Intact skin is the body's primary defense system. It protects us from invasion by organisms, helps to regulate body temperature, manufactures vitamins, and provides our external appearance. Skin has three primary layers (i.e., *epidermis,* or outer layer; the *dermis,* or inner layer; and the *hypodermis,* or subcutaneous layer) as well as epidermal appendages (i.e., eccrine glands, apocrine glands, sebaceous glands, hair follicles, and nails).

The skin's *epithelium* is composed of cells that provide a continuous barrier between the body contents and the outside environment. Epithelial cells also cover the gastrointestinal (GI) tract, pulmonary airways and alveoli, renal tubules and the urinary system, and the ducts that empty onto the surface of the skin (lumen) of the GI and respiratory systems. Epithelial cells allow the selective transport of ions, nutrients, and metabolic wastes and have a permeability to water that is partially regulated. Epithelial cells are joined to each other through tight junctions and express different populations of protein transporters on the apical side (generally facing a lumen) and the basolateral (facing the blood, or serosal) side. The functional significance of epithelial transport is covered in the GI and renal chapters (see the Anatomy and Physiology Review for Units 7 and 8).

STRUCTURE OF THE INTEGUMENTARY SYSTEM

EPIDERMIS

The epidermis is the thin, stratified outer skin layer that is in direct contact with the external environment (Figure A&P11-1). The thickness of the epidermis ranges from 0.04 mm on the eyelids to 1.6 mm on the palms and soles. *Desmosomes* (points of intercellular attachment that are vital for cell-to-cell adhesion) are found in the epidermis.

Keratinocytes, the principal cells of the epidermis, produce *keratin* in a complex process. The cells begin in the basal cell layer and change constantly, moving upward through the epidermis. On the surface, they are sloughed off or lost by abrasion. Thus the epidermis constantly regenerates itself, providing a tough keratinized barrier.

Skin color reflects both the production of pigment granules *(melanin)* by melanocytes and, in light-skinned people, the presence of blood *(hemoglobin).* Skin color reflects a combination of four basic colors:

- Exogenously formed carotenoids (yellow)
- Melanin (brown)
- Oxygenated hemoglobin in arterioles and capillaries (red)
- Reduced hemoglobin in venules (blue or purple)

Melanin plays the largest role in skin color; it is produced in the epidermis and in corresponding layers of the hair follicle. Although melanin is not produced in the dermis, it can be deposited in the dermis from the epidermis through various processes (such as inflammation).

Melanosomes are granules in melanocytes that synthesize melanin. Skin color differences result from the size and quantity of melanosomes as well as from the rate of melanin production. In natives of equatorial Africa, there is an increase in the size and number of melanosomes (not melanocytes) as well as increased melanin production. The melanosomes are large, discrete, and dispersed. In natives of northern Europe, the melanosomes are small and aggregated, producing less melanin. Sun exposure initially increases the size and functional activity of both melanocytes and melanosomes. With chronic sun exposure, there is an increase in the concentration of melanocytes as well as in size and functional activity. The presence of melanin limits the penetration of sun rays into the skin and protects against sunburn and the development of ultraviolet light–induced skin carcinomas.

Epidermal Appendages

Epidermal appendages are down-growths of epidermis into the dermis. They consist of eccrine glands, apocrine units, sebaceous glands, hair, and nails.

Glands

Eccrine glands produce sweat and play an important role in thermoregulation. They are found throughout the skin except on the vermilion border (junction of the pink area of the lip with the surrounding skin), the ears, nail bed, glans penis, and labia minora. They are more numerous on the palms, soles, forehead, and

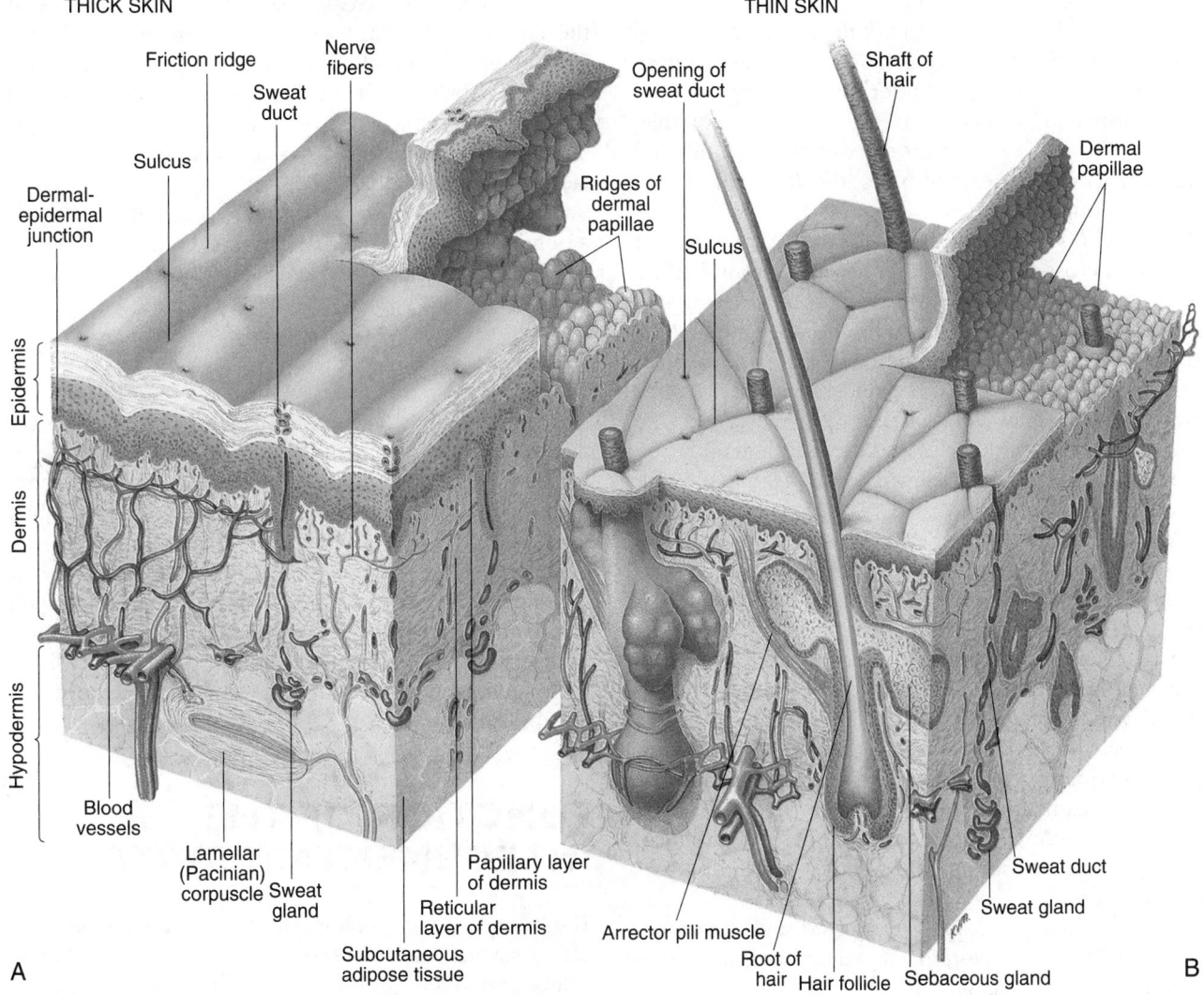

THICK SKIN

THIN SKIN

Friction ridge

Nerve fibers

Sweat duct

Sulcus

Dermal-epidermal junction

Epidermis

Dermis

Hypodermis

Blood vessels

Lamellar (Pacinian) corpuscle

Sweat gland

Reticular layer of dermis

Papillary layer of dermis

Subcutaneous adipose tissue

A

Opening of sweat duct

Shaft of hair

Ridges of dermal papillae

Dermal papillae

Sulcus

Arrector pili muscle

Root of hair

Hair follicle

Sebaceous gland

Sweat duct

Sweat gland

B

■ **FIGURE A&P11-1** Structure of the skin. **A,** Thick skin is found on the palms and on the soles of the feet. **B,** Thin skin is found on most other body surfaces.

axillae. Sweat is similar to plasma but sweat is more dilute. Eccrine gland secretion is stimulated by heat and emotional stress. Eccrine glands exit the body independently of the hair shaft (see Figure A&P11-1).

Apocrine glands occur primarily in the axillae, breast areolae, anogenital area, ear canals, and eyelids. In lower-order animals, apocrine secretions function as sexual attractants *(pheromones),* and the apocrine secretion musk is used as a perfume base. The role, if any, in humans is not established. Mediated by adrenergic innervation, apocrine glands secrete a milky substance that becomes odoriferous when altered by skin surface bacteria. These glands do not function until puberty, and they require a high output of sex hormone for activity.

Sebaceous glands are found throughout the skin except on the palms and soles and are most abundant

on the face, scalp, upper back, and chest. They are associated with hair follicles that open onto the skin surface, where *sebum* (a mixture of sebaceous gland–produced lipids and epidermal cell–derived lipids) is released. Sebum has a lubricating function and bactericidal activity. Androgen is responsible for sebaceous gland development. In utero androgen causes neonatal acne; after puberty sebum production can cause acne in adolescents.

Hair and Nails

Hair is a nonviable protein end product found on all skin surfaces except the palms and soles. Each hair follicle functions as an independent unit and goes through intermittent stages of development. Hair develops from the mitotic activity of the hair bulb. The rate of hair growth varies in different parts of the body. In a typical adult scalp, 85% to 90% of hairs are in an *anagen* (growth) phase. The remainder is in a *telogen* (rest) phase. About 50 to 100 hairs are lost each day. As a rule, the growing phase of hair on the eyebrows, trunk, and extremities does not exceed 6 months. Its resting phase is 3 to 4 months.

Hair form (straight or curly) depends on the shape of the hair in cross-section. Straight hair has a round cross-section; curly hair has an oval or ribbon-like cross-section. Curved follicles also affect the curliness of hair. Melanocytes in the bulb determine hair color. Hair follicles usually occur with sebaceous glands, and together they form a *pilosebaceous unit. Arrector pili* muscles of the dermis attach to hair follicles and elevate the hairs when body temperature falls or strong emotions are present, producing "goose bumps."

Nails are horny scales of epidermis. The nail matrix is the source of specialized, nonkeratinized cells. They differentiate into keratinized cells, which make up the nail protein. The matrix for nail formation is located in the proximal nail bed. It grows forward from the nailfold to cover the nail bed. Fingernails grow about 0.1 mm each day; complete reproduction takes 100 to 150 days. Toenails grow one third as fast as fingernails do. A damaged nail matrix, which may result from trauma or aggressive manicuring, produces a distorted nail. Nails are also sensitive to physiologic changes; for instance, they grow more slowly in cold weather and during periods of illness.

Nails and hair consist of keratinized and, therefore, "dead" cells. The ingestion of gelatin has not been shown to increase nail growth or strength.

DERMIS

The dermis, a dense layer of tissue beneath the epidermis, gives the skin most of its substance and structure. It varies from 1 to 4 mm in thickness and is thickest over the back. The dermis contains fibroblasts, macrophages, mast cells, and lymphocytes, which promote wound healing. The skin's lymphatic, vascular, and nerve supplies, which maintain equilibrium in the skin, are in the dermis.

The dermis is divided into two parts: papillary and reticular. The papillary dermis, which contains increased amounts of collagen, blood vessels, sweat glands, and elastin, is in contact with the epidermis. The *reticular* dermis also contains collagen but with increased amounts of mature elastic tissue. The dermis houses many specialized cells, blood vessels, and nerves.

The epidermis and dermis meet at the *dermoepidermal junction.* This area contains wave-like projections from the dermis called *papillae* (or rete pegs), which correspond to reciprocal structures in the epidermis.

These projections increase the area of contact between the layers of skin, and help to prevent the epidermis from being sheared off. They are not present in the skins of unborn babies but rapidly develop after birth, and are very noticeable in a young person's skin when it is examined under the microscope. As skin ages, the papillae get smaller and flatter.

The *subepidermal basement membrane zone* is a semipermeable filter that permits fluid exchange of components such as nutrients, metabolites, and waste products.

HYPODERMIS

The *subcutaneous layer* is a specialized layer of connective tissue. It is sometimes called the *adipose layer* because of its fat content. This layer is absent in some sites, such as the eyelids, scrotum, areola, and tibia. Age, heredity, and many other factors influence the thickness of the subcutaneous layer. Subcutaneous fat is generally thickest on the back and buttocks, giving shape and contour over the bone. This layer functions as insulation from extremes of hot and cold, as a cushion to trauma, and as a source of energy and hormone metabolism.

FUNCTION OF THE INTEGUMENTARY SYSTEM

The skin is a morphologically complex structure that serves several functions essential to life. The skin differs anatomically and physiologically in various areas of the body. Functions of the skin include protection, maintenance of homeostasis, thermoregulation, sensory reception, vitamin synthesis, and processing of antigenic substances.

PROTECTION

The skin protects the body against many forms of trauma (e.g., mechanical, thermal, chemical, radiant). The intact tough epidermal layer is a mechanical barrier. Bacteria, foreign matter, other organisms, and chemicals can penetrate it with difficulty. The oily and slightly acid secretions of its sebaceous glands protect the body further by limiting the growth of many organisms. The thickened skin of the palms and soles provides additional covering to absorb the constant use of or trauma to these areas.

Cells in both the epidermis and the dermis of the skin are important in immune function. Skin is now recognized not only as a physical barrier but also as a participant in immunologically mediated defense against various antigens. *Langerhans cells* are scattered among the keratinocytes located primarily in the epidermis; however, they can also be seen in the dermis. These cells originate in the bone marrow and migrate to the epidermis. Langerhans cells play a role in the cell-mediated immune responses of the skin through antigen presentation. An antigen entering immunologically competent skin is likely to encounter a coordinated response of Langerhans and T cells to neutralize its effect. An antigen entering diseased skin can induce and elicit immune responses. These reactions may be involved in the pathogenesis of many inflammatory skin diseases.

HOMEOSTASIS

Skin forms a barrier that prevents excessive loss of water and electrolytes from the internal environment. Intact skin also prevents the subcutaneous tissues from drying out. The effectiveness of this impermeable membrane is readily recognized when one observes the extreme loss of fluids that occurs with damage to the skin, as with burns and other injuries. Insensible loss of water and electrolytes occurs only through pores in this effective barrier.

THERMOREGULATION

Body temperature represents the balance between heat generation and heat loss processes. The skin, with its ability to alter the rate of heat loss, is the major point of regulation of body temperature. The rate of heat loss depends primarily on the surface temperature of the skin, which is in turn a function of the skin's blood flow. The blood flow of the skin varies in response to changes in the body's core temperature and to changes in temperature of the external environment.

The flow of blood to the skin is derived in two processes. Direct perfusion is from capillary beds entering in lateral directions. Skin is also perfused vertically from vessels that enter from the muscle and fascia supporting it.

In general, the vessels dilate during warm temperatures and constrict in cold temperatures. The hypothalamus is partly responsible for regulating skin blood flow, particularly to the extremities, the face, ears, and the tip of the nose. Maintenance of the thermal balance allows the internal temperature of the body to remain at approximately 37° C (98.6° F).

Under severe heat stress, increased cutaneous blood flow is inadequate to dissipate the thermal load. Eccrine glands produce sweat, and cooling is enhanced by fluid evaporation from the skin. Eccrine gland innervation is unique in that these sympathetic cholinergic nerves use acetylcholine (rather than norepinephrine) as the neurotransmitter. Sweating significantly enhances the body's capacity for thermoregulation.

SENSORY RECEPTION

Apart from sight and hearing, the major human sensory apparatus is in the skin. Sensory fibers responsible for pain, touch, and temperature form a complex network in the dermis. This information is transmitted in compartments to the spinal cord and is relayed to the somatosensory cortex, where the information is integrated into a somatotopic representation of the body.

The skin contains specialized receptors to detect discriminative touch and pressure. *Touch* (flutter) is sensed by Meissner's corpuscles; *pressure,* by Merkel cells and Ruffini endings; *vibration and pressure,* by Pacinian corpuscles; and *hair movement,* by hair follicle endings. Together these receptors communicate information to the somatosensory cortex via the dorsal column spinal pathways.

A second grouping of nerves communicates information about temperature and pain to the somatosensory cortex via the anterolateral spinal pathways. *Temperature* is sensed by specific thermoreceptors in the epidermis, and *pain* is sensed by free nerve endings throughout the epidermal, dermal, and hypodermal layers. The speed of conduction of pain information to the cortex results in a functional division. "Fast" pain is well localized and has a short latency. "Slow" pain is more diffuse, has a longer latency, and is more difficult to endure.

The density of receptors determines the sensitivity of the skin. For example, two-point discrimination is most accurate on the skin of the fingers and face, where the highest density of touch receptors occurs. In contrast, the skin on the back has a low density of touch receptors, and the ability to localize touch is therefore reduced.

VITAMIN D PRODUCTION

The epidermis is involved in synthesis of vitamin D. In the presence of sunlight or ultraviolet radiation, a sterol found on the malpighian cells is converted to form cholecalciferol (vitamin D_3) in the liver to its active form. Vitamin D_3 assists in the absorption of calcium and phosphate from ingested foods.

DERMATOLOGIC CARE

As the largest and most visible organ of the body, the skin plays a major role in our physical and mental health and protects us from an array of natural and man-made attacks. Yet the skin is rarely taken as seriously as other organ systems, such as the heart and the lung. In both outpatient and inpatient practice settings, as a nurse you have a unique opportunity to affect a client's dermatologic care. You can teach clients to appreciate the skin's important role and to recognize that some skin conditions are indeed life-threatening. For example, skin cancers and especially malignant melanoma are rising at rapid rates. Malignant melanoma is an aggressive form of skin cancer, and often fatal. In the United States today, one person dies every hour from skin cancer. Also, burn injuries continue despite advances in fireproofing homes and clothes. Pressure ulcers, a serious alteration in skin integrity, pose a growing concern as the older population increases, and may result in 60,000 deaths per year.

APPEARANCE AND SELF-ESTEEM

Skin is integral to self-image and self-esteem. Each client's unique appearance is established through the skin. The skin was once thought to reflect the normal "aging process" and how that aging process affected the genetic skin types we inherit. We now know that skin type more likely reflects the cumulative amount of sun exposure over a lifetime. It is hoped that with education, people will once again view untanned skin as attractive and healthy. Cosmetic surgery should not be considered a procedure for vanity but a procedure to enhance self-esteem.

Today's society has a long-standing prejudice that needs to be dispelled regarding impaired skin. Historically, skin diseases were perceived as divine punishment for being spiritually and physically "unclean." Subtle punishment for skin diseases still exists because of ignorance. For example, a woman with atopic dermatitis may sit isolated and shunned in a waiting room because others view eczematous lesions as contagious. A server at a restaurant may be encouraged to work in the back of the kitchen so that customers will not notice the healed burn scars on his or her hands and body. Vitiligo, loss of pigment in the skin, is sometimes mislabeled "white leprosy," and so on. Clients who have visible chronic skin problems often withdraw from social situations and have altered interpersonal relationships and increased social isolation. When these clients seek professional care for skin problems, psychosocial as well as physical concerns need to be met.

Another function of skin, hair, and nails is to provide an outward appearance or *cosmetic adornment*. The appearance of our skin, hair, and nails is crucial to our psychosocial well-being and can affect our experiences positively or negatively. Skin disorders are often a major cause of morbidity because we live in a beauty-conscious society. Health care providers must be acutely aware of the role of the skin in a person's self-esteem and ability to function in relationships.

EFFECTS OF AGING

The skin undergoes numerous changes that can be seen and felt throughout the life span. Many of these changes are natural, unchangeable, and harmless. Some may be bothersome or painful and are treated until there is an acceptable resolution or acceptance of the condition. Other skin changes may go unnoticed or might not be bothersome because they are slow growing, such as senile keratosis. Table A&P11-1 lists some age-associated changes.

Adolescence

During puberty, hormone secretion stimulates the maturation of hair follicles, sebaceous glands, and apocrine and eccrine units in certain body areas. Hair follicles on the face (males), pubic region, and axillae activate to produce coarse terminal hairs. Normal changes may bother teenagers, but adolescents must be cautioned about the potential for irritating the skin with excessive use of over-the-counter products.

New nevi can appear after adolescence. At any age, raised, pigmented lesions that bleed or change in color or size should be assessed by a physician to determine whether they require only minor care or removal because of early malignant changes.

Adulthood

Temporary *hormonal changes* account for some adult skin changes. Pregnancy and birth control pills may alter

TABLE A&P11-1	Common Skin Changes Associated with Aging
Skin Change	**Description**
Adolescence	
Folliculitis	Hair follicle inflammation
Acne	Inflammation of pilosebaceous follicle
Increased perspiration	Response to heat, emotional stress, exercise
Apocrine secretion	Related to sex hormone activity
Skin irritation	Often caused by overuse of over-the-counter skin products
Pigmented nevi	Benign cluster melanocyte-like cells
Adulthood	
Melasma	Blotchy hyperpigmentation
Alopecia	Baldness (hormonal and genetic factors)
Excessive facial or body hair	Androgen-related problem in women
Actinic keratosis	Slightly raised, red papules (premalignant)
Sebaceous cyst	Enclosed cyst in dermis (potentially infectious)
Acrochordon	Small, flesh-colored papule
Older Adulthood	
Xerosis	Dry skin (decreased natural oils and sweat)
Wrinkling	Natural change affected by many factors (e.g., loss of elasticity and subcutaneous fat, sun exposure, gravity, cigarette smoking)
Skin tears	Epidermal thinning; seen most in clients using oral corticosteroids
Senile lentigenes	Black or brown flat lesions ("liver spots")
Seborrheic keratosis	Harmless raised black or brown spots or wart-like growths
Cherry angiomas	Dilated blood vessels that form loops

hormonal status and thus change skin structures that are hormonally linked. Pregnancy may cause changes in hair growth patterns and a temporary thinning of hair after pregnancy. Pregnancy also leads to darkening skin of the areola and a linea nigra (dark line on the abdomen).

Heredity and exposure to environmental factors, such as sun, tobacco, alcohol, and chemicals, play a major role in many of the skin changes that occur in adults. Some lesions (i.e., seborrheic keratosis and acrochordons) may be removed for cosmetic reasons, if desired, or if physically irritating. Actinic keratoses (because of their premalignant status) and sebaceous cysts (because of their infectious potential) need to be assessed and may be removed. Basal and squamous cell cancers develop from sunlight exposure.

Older Adulthood

The skin of older people reflects the cumulative influence of environmental insults, decreased circulation, and diminished function of various skin structures. As the stratum corneum becomes thinner, the skin reacts more readily to minor changes in humidity, temperature, and other irritants. The skin also becomes more transparent. Hair loss is often noticeable on the trunk, pubic area, axillae, and limbs. Loss of pigment causes gray hair. Nails become brittle and may yellow or thicken. Skin may be leathery from overexposure to ultraviolet light.

There is no known treatment for past overexposure; protection from ultraviolet light is the only preventive measure. Wrinkles develop because of loss of tensile strength and elasticity in the skin.

CONCLUSIONS

The skin is the largest and most visible organ of the body. Anatomically, the skin is divided into (1) the epidermis (outer layer), (2) the dermis (inner layer), and (3) the hypodermis (subcutaneous layer). The skin serves many functions. It is the first line of defense against many forms of trauma. Skin maintains body temperature, prevents water loss, and provides sensations of touch, temperature, and pain. Skin also produces vitamin D and recognizes antigens. Finally, healthy skin is aesthetically pleasing.

BIBLIOGRAPHY

1. Berne, R., et al. (2004). *Physiology* (5th ed.). St. Louis: Mosby.
2. Carroll, R.G. (2007). *Elsevier's integrated physiology.* Philadelphia: Saunders.
3. Kierszenbaum, A.L. (2007). *Histology and cell biology: An introduction to pathology* (2nd ed.). St. Louis: Mosby.
4. Guyton, A., & Hall, J. (2006). *Textbook of medical physiology* (11th ed.). Philadelphia: Saunders.
5. Silverthorn, D. (2006). *Human physiology* (4th ed.). San Francisco, Calif: Pearson Benjamin Cummings.

CHAPTER 48

Assessment of the Integumentary System

NOREEN HEER NICOL

Assessment of skin disorders is a complex process because many skin disorders undergo a characteristic evolution. Observation is often required on more than one occasion for diagnosis. Additionally, diagnosis may require the information provided by a complete history, physical examination, laboratory tests, and histopathologic analysis. A complete health history assists in the diagnosis of integumentary disorders, such as occupationally related contact dermatitis, or in revealing psychosocial aspects of skin disorders. The medication history is important because side effects of certain medications can cause skin changes. The physical examination can confirm integumentary disorders as well as disclose disorders that the client may have omitted during the history.

HISTORY

The history includes questions about the chief complaint and current manifestations, a review of systems, past health history, past surgical history, allergies, medications, psychosocial history, and family health history.

Current Health
Chief Complaint

The most common problems related to the integument are itching (pruritus), dryness, rashes, lesions, ecchymoses (small hemorrhagic patches), lumps, masses, and cosmetic appearance. The onset, duration, and suspected trigger of each manifestation should be discussed. Ask about changes in the skin, hair, and nails that may be related to the chief complaint. Sample questions that elicit pertinent information related to the presenting dermatologic problem are listed in the website table Dermatologic Assessment History: Sample *evolve* Questions.

Clinical Manifestations

Conduct an analysis of clinical manifestations including the questions located in the Dermatology Assessment: Sample Questions located on the website. The sexual history may be significant if the differential diagnosis includes a sexually transmitted infection (STI) (see Chapter 41). Figure 48-1 demonstrates assessment information for clinical manifestations specific to skin complaints.

Pruritus. Persistent itching or pruritus is a manifestation that frequently brings clients to a health care provider. Note whether the itching is associated with skin lesions and whether it is localized or generalized. Persistent itching without associated lesions could suggest significant systemic disease such as biliary obstruction, diabetes mellitus, uremia, lymphoma, or hyperthyroidism. If pruritus is associated with skin lesions, consider scabies, many types of dermatitis, psoriasis, xerosis, and dermatophytosis in the diagnostic process.

Lesions. A change or new skin lesion will often prompt a client to seek evaluation. When assessing any lesion, it is important to inquire about the time the lesion has been present, any color changes, any exudate, and any other changes that have occurred. The lesion may have been altered because of scratching, trauma, or infection and scarring. It is also necessary to establish if the

---

evolve **Web Enhancements**

Appendix B A Health History Format That Integrates the Assessment of Functional Health Patterns

Tables Dermatologic Assessment History: Sample Questions

Glossary of Dermatologic Terms

Be sure to check out the bonus material on the Evolve website and the CD-ROM, including free self-assessment exercises. **http://evolve.elsevier. com/Black/medsurg**

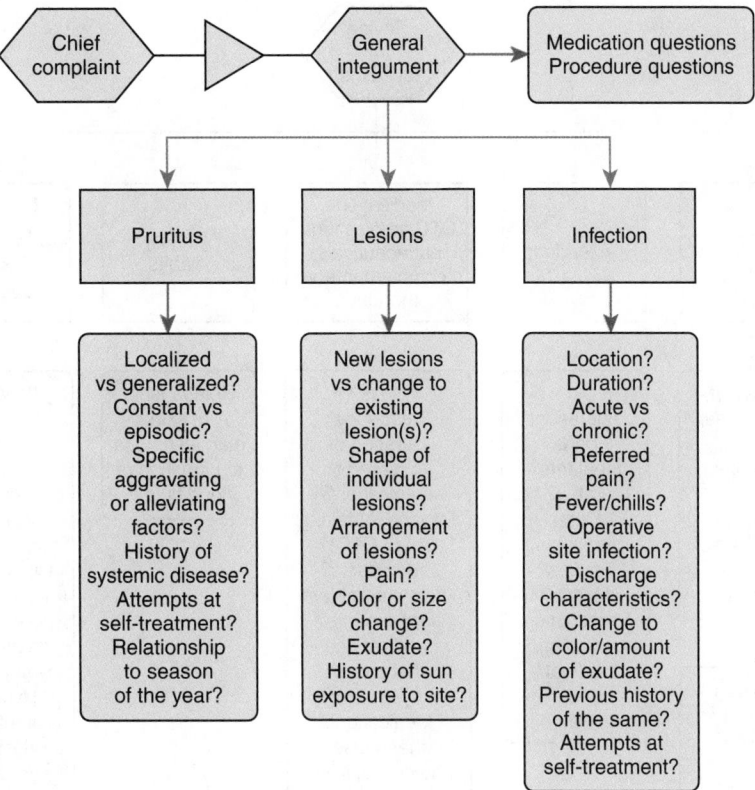

■ **FIGURE 48–1** Expanded integumentary assessment.

lesion is in an area of skin that has received significant sun exposure.

Infection. Skin infections will prompt clients to seek further evaluation, especially if there is a history of failure at attempts at self-treatment. As with any infection, establish if there has been fever, chills, the amount and type of exudate, and the presence of pain at the suspected site of infection.

Review of Systems
Obtain a complete history of the skin. Specifically, ask about past problems with unusual itching, dryness, lesions, rashes, lumps, ecchymoses, and masses. Determine if the client has problems with moles or other lesions, especially if they have undergone changes in size, shape, or color. Refer to Figure 48-2 for a guide to compiling an expanded integument history.

Past Medical History
Recent past medical history may be significant. For example, a recent acute or unresolved *Streptococcus* infection might explain diffuse hair loss or an unresolved rash. Ask about childhood diseases, and find out about the vaccination status.

Various systemic diseases are characterized by cutaneous manifestations. Does the client have other systemic disorders relevant to the skin (immunologic, endocrine, collagen, vascular, renal, or hepatic conditions)? Ask about childhood diseases, and find out about the vaccination status.

Surgical History
Evaluating previous trauma, procedure sites, and surgical interventions may explain unusual lesions and/or scars or their location.

Allergies
An *allergy* is an immunologic response that happens consistently with exposure. *Irritation* can occur unpredictably. Inquire about substances that may cause local skin irritation or lesions on direct contact, such as textiles or metals. Wool is irritating to most people. Jewelry that contains nickel can cause skin discoloration, irritation, rash, or other problems in people who are sensitive to this metal.

Ask the client about allergies to medications, foods, inhalants, latex, and other chemicals. Does the ingestion of certain foods cause itching, burning, or eruption of rashes? Does contact with pollens, inhalants, or animals result in hives? A history of past allergic reactions to foods or medications is important for avoiding inadvertent reaction through readministration. A history of contact with and discussion of compounds in the work environment, hobbies, and recent travel is

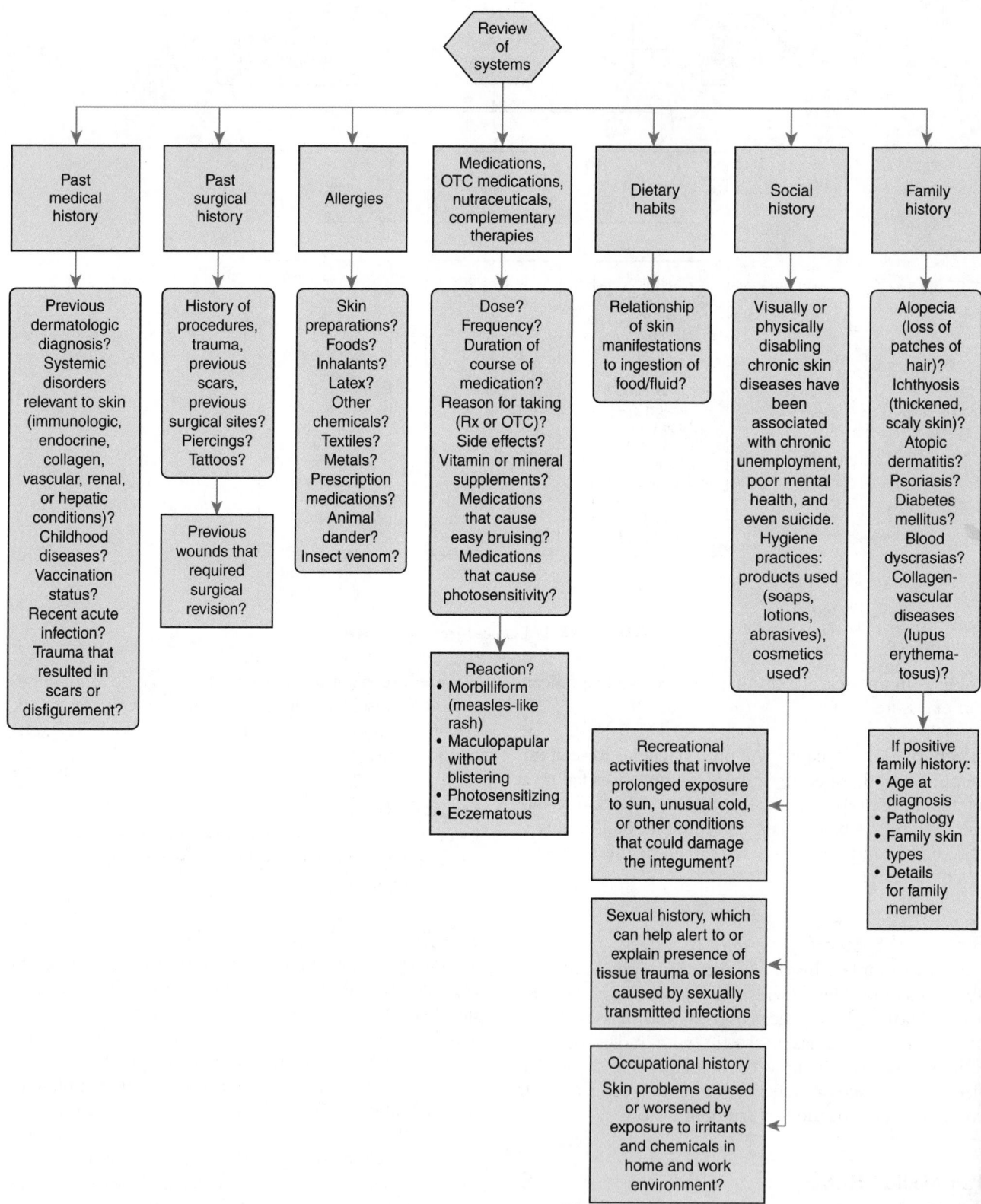

■ **FIGURE 48–2** Expanded integumentary history.

particularly useful when evaluating conditions such as suspected occupational or contact dermatitis or urticaria, which are very common reasons for dermatology consultation.

Medications

Note prescription and over-the-counter medications that the client is currently taking or has recently finished. Complications from these products can range from nuisance skin rashes to rare or life-threatening events. Medication reactions can be limited to the skin or may be part of a systemic process.

The most common type of allergic drug reactions is cutaneous. Most of these skin reactions are *morbilliform* (measles-like rash) or maculopapular without blistering or pustulation. These eruptions can be caused by many drugs, including penicillins, sulfonamides, nevirapine, and antiseizure medications. Sensitivity to antibiotics or other drugs that is manifested in the form of a skin rash may not occur until the end of a routine course of therapy or with subsequent exposures. Photosensitizing drugs (phenothiazines, tetracycline, diuretics, sulfonamides) may cause a sunburn-like rash in areas of sun exposure.[8] Topical preparations may include preservatives or active ingredients that are known sensitizers that frequently produce an eczematous rash. The most commonly encountered are neomycin, benzocaine, and diphenhydramine hydrochloride. Oral corticosteroids (prednisone), if used at high doses or routinely, can cause acne breakouts, thinning of skin, stretch marks, and many other systemic side effects.

Complementary and alternative medicine has grown in the United States, and providers at all levels realize that clients may be anxious to try these products, especially if they suffer from chronic skin disorders such as atopic dermatitis, psoriasis, or wounds. Some components of these medications are beneficial, but for others scientific evidence is lacking and is actually detrimental. When possible, clients need to be educated about these modalities and their possible adverse physiologic and immunologic side effects. Aloe vera *(Aloe barbadensis, Aloe ferox, Aloe africana, Aloe spicata)* is promoted for the relief of eczema and psoriasis and to aid in wound healing. Chamomile *(Matricaria recutita, Chamaemelum nobile)*, comfrey *(Symphytum officinale)*, evening primrose *(Oenothera biennis)*, gotu kola *(Centella asiatica)*, and Oregon grape *(Mahonia aquifolium)* have similar uses. Although these products in pure forms or in high quantities may have pharmacologic activities such as antiseptic, diaphoretic, diuretic, or analgesic effects, the effect of diluted topical formulas is not known.[1] Care must also be taken to watch how clients administer products. The answer to future use of these products is the need for more high-quality evidence-based studies.

Dietary Habits

The benefit of balanced nutrition in the areas of wound healing and general skin health continues to be common knowledge. However, discussions of other supplemental nutrition, such as megavitamins taken orally, continue to be causes of concern especially with fat-soluble vitamins. Another myth is the one associated with water and fluid intake for the correlation to xerosis or dry skin conditions. One needs to have almost clinical dehydration before turgor changes become apparent on clinical examination. And while good routine intake of water is a healthy practice for the genitourinary and other systems, there is no scientific evidence that it plays a role in routine hydration of the skin. Suspected food allergy can play a role in specific dermatologic conditions such as atopic dermatitis and urticaria. In these situations, true food allergy needs to be evaluated and established to avoid unnecessary elimination of food types or groups.

Social History

Psychosocial factors that influence dermatologic disorders often play a large role, particularly in long-term and chronic processes. Skin disease can greatly affect lifestyle and self-image. Cultural and familial influences in caring for a particular disorder may conflict with prescribed therapies. Misconceptions about skin problems (e.g., that acne lesions can be scrubbed away) need to be determined and corrected. Visually or physically disabling chronic skin diseases have been associated with chronic unemployment, poor mental health, and even suicide. Assess the client's sexual history, which can help to explain the presence of tissue trauma or lesions caused by STIs (see Chapter 41).

Socioeconomic factors may influence an individual's compliance with outlined therapies and return for follow-up care. When recommending therapies or medications, consider the impact on the client's day-to-day routine as well as the type of prescription insurance plan. Many topical therapies—whether or not they are covered by insurance—are expensive, and expense affects compliance.

Occupational history is important because a large number of skin problems are caused or worsened by exposure to irritants and chemicals in the home and work environment. The travel history can be helpful as well, especially if it includes hiking or exposure to outdoor agents that result in dermatologic disorders, such as poison ivy, poison sumac, poison oak, or Lyme disease. Ask about recent exposure to ticks, other insects, or infections.

Inquire about the client's habits, such as the frequency of hygiene practices, the products used (soaps, lotions, abrasives), and whether cosmetics are used. Record the products used, including brand names. Inquire whether there have been any changes in clothing or bedding, and discuss how these items are cleaned.

Does the client engage in recreational activities that involve prolonged exposure to the sun, unusual cold, or other conditions that could damage the integument? For example, does the client visit tanning salons? Advise clients that exposure to sun and tanning beds leads to premature aging, increased risk of skin cancer, risk of corneal burns if eye guards are not worn, exacerbation of photosensitivity disorders, and increased development of lentigines (age spots) and other types of photodamage.

Family Health History

A personal or family health history helps to determine genetic predisposition to skin disorders as well as a predisposition to parasitic or other conditions related to the family's lifestyle and living environment. Many dermatologic disorders or systemic disorders with a dermatologic presentation have a genetic or familial component. Genetically transmitted dermatologic conditions include *alopecia* (loss of patches of hair), *ichthyosis* (thickened, scaly skin), atopic dermatitis, and psoriasis. Systemic diseases with dermatologic manifestations include diabetes mellitus, blood dyscrasia, and collagen-vascular diseases (lupus erythematosus). Other diseases, such as scabies, are likely to be passed on to family members because of close and frequent exposure.

PHYSICAL EXAMINATION

Examine the skin as thoroughly as any other body organ. This procedure cannot be done properly in the hall or at a quick glance, which the health care provider is often requested to do. Use inspection, palpation, and olfaction to assess hair, nails, and skin. Effective assessment requires knowledge, awareness, and practice in describing the skin of people of all ages, ethnicities, and different lifestyles and in recognizing normal and abnormal skin changes. A description of normal conditions of the integumentary system is given in the Physical Assessment Findings in the Healthy Adult feature above, right.

Terminology

The terms routinely used in dermatology have been referred to as a "foreign language" and have been known to inhibit use of the correct terminology for skin disorders by health care providers. Use of standardized terminology often leads to differential diagnosis. This section clarifies some commonly used dermatologic terms and should assist the reader in recognizing and *evolve* describing skin disorders. See the Glossary of Dermatologic Terms on the website.

Types of Lesions

Examining and making the correct diagnosis of skin disorders depend on identifying skin lesions or changes. Two major types of lesions are distinguished: *primary* and *secondary* lesions.

The primary lesion is the first lesion to appear on the skin and has a visually recognizable structure. Figure 48-3, *A* depicts nine primary lesions: macule, papule, plaque, nodule, wheal, vesicle, bulla, cyst, and

---

Physical Assessment Findings in the Healthy Adult

The Integumentary System

INSPECTION

Skin. Even skin tones, darker on exposed areas of face, neck, arms, and lower legs; lighter on trunk and back. Small tan freckles scattered over face and arms. Scars, striae absent.

Hair and Scalp. Hair evenly distributed over scalp. Clean, without nits or lice. No dandruff, scaling, or scalp lesions. Axillae and legs probably shaved; pubic hair distributed as inverted triangle from symphysis pubis to perineum (female). Pubic hair distributed in diamond pattern from below umbilicus to perineum (male).

Nails. Regular, smooth, oval shape. Pink nail beds. Cuticles manicured, clean. Nail bed angle 160 degrees (no clubbing).

PALPATION

Skin. Warm, well hydrated, smooth, elastic, nontender. No lesions, masses, or lumps.

Hair and Scalp. Hair non-oily, even textured, resilient. Scalp smooth, intact, nontender.

Nails. Firm without tenderness or bogginess. Rapid blanch response.

---

pustule. Frequently, the health care provider does not see a primary lesion but sees only secondary lesions; the health care provider then must depend on the client's description of "how it looked when it first appeared." An in-depth look should be made to find a primary lesion because these are often key to clarifying the diagnosis.

When a primary lesion undergoes changes, it becomes a secondary lesion. These alterations, brought about by the client or by the client's environment, often occur in the epidermal layer. The changes may result from many factors, including scratching, rubbing, medication, natural disease progression over time, or processes of involution and healing. Figure 48-3, *B* presents eight secondary lesions: scale, crust, erosion, deep ulcer, scar, lichenification, excoriation, fissure, and atrophy.

Examination Environment

The best setting for conducting a dermatologic assessment is a well-lighted, private room with moderate temperature and neutral, white, or cream-colored walls. Excessive warmth can produce changes in skin color (redness) by causing vasodilation. Colored walls can affect normal skin hue (color). For a complete examination, ask the client to undress and provide a gown. Explain that all skin surfaces will be examined. Having a second health care provider in the room during a total body examination is frequently recommended. Avoid unnecessary exposure during the examination. Have

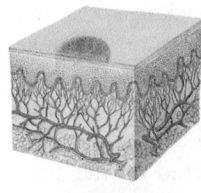

MACULE: Skin color change without elevation, i.e., flat (freckles or petechia). Described as a "patch" if greater than 1 cm (vitiligo).

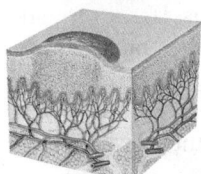

PAPULE: Elevated, solid lesion of less than 1 cm, varying in color (warts or elevated nevus).

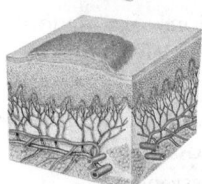

PLAQUE: Raised, flat lesion formed from merging papules or nodules.

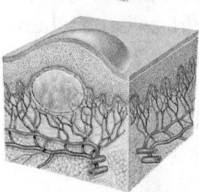

NODULE: Larger than a papule. Raised solid lesion extending deeper into the dermis. A large nodule is referred to as a tumor.

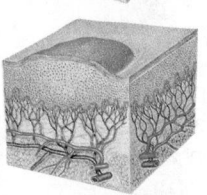

WHEAL (hive): Fleeting skin elevation that is irregularly shaped because of edema (mosquito bite or urticaria).

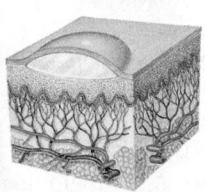

VESICLE (blister): Elevated, sharply defined lesion containing serous fluid. Usually less than 1 cm (blister, chickenpo, or herpes simplex).

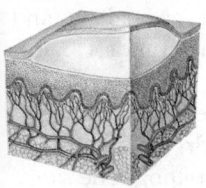

BULLA (plural, bullae): Large, elevated, fluid-filled lesion greater than 1 cm (partial-thickness burn).

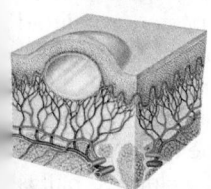

CYST: Elevated, thick-walled lesion containing fluid or semisolid matter.

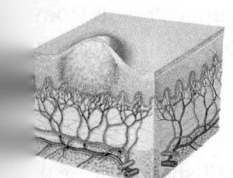

PUSTULE: Elevated lesion less than 1 cm containing purulent material. Lesions larger than 1 cm are described as boils, abscesses, or furuncles (acne or impetigo).

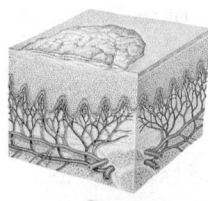

SCALE: Dried fragments of sloughed epidermal cells, irregular in shape and size and white, tan, yellow, or silver in color (dandruff, dry skin, or psoriasis).

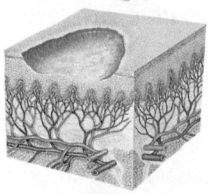

EROSION: A moist, demarcated, depressed area due to loss of partial- or full-thickness epidermis. Basal layer of epidermis remains intact (ruptured chickenpox vesicle).

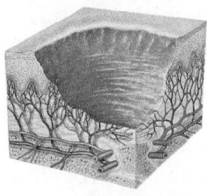

DEEP ULCER: Irregularly shaped, exudative, depressed lesion in which entire epidermis and all or part of dermis are lost. Results from trauma and tissue destruction (pressure ulcer).

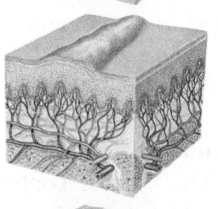

SCAR: Mark left on skin after healing. Replacement of destroyed tissue by scar tissue.

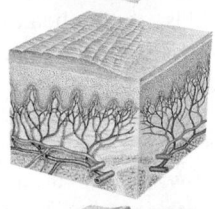

LICHENIFICATION: Epidermal thickening resulting in elevated plaque with accentuated skin markings. Usually results from repeated injury through rubbing or scratching (chronic atopic dermatitis).

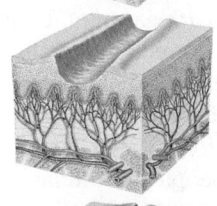

EXCORIATION: Superficial, linear abrasion of epidermis. Visible sign of itching caused by rubbing or scratching (atopic dermatitis).

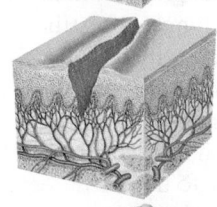

FISSURE: Deep linear split through epidermis into dermis (tinea pedis).

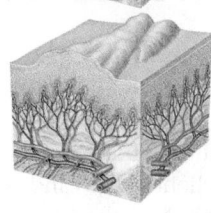

KELOID: Irregularly shaped, elevated, progressively enlarging scar; extends beyond the boundaries of the wound; caused by excessive collagen formation during post-surgical healing.

FIGURE 48–3 **A,** Primary lesions: visually recognizable structural changes in the skin that have specific characteristics. **B,** Secondary lesions: primary lesions that have changed because of the natural progression of the lesion or because of physical change (scratching, irritation, or secondary infection).

warm hands to avoid stimulation of the skin and to add to the client's overall comfort.

Depth of Examination

The examination is systematic and as complete as appropriate. A total-body skin examination involves assessment of the hair, scalp, nails, mucous membranes, and skin, including the axillae, areas in skinfolds, external genitalia, webs between toes and fingers, palms of hands, and soles of feet. Begin at the head, and proceed to the toes. General changes can alter total-body skin color (jaundice, cyanosis, pallor), thickness, turgor, temperature, and vascularity (purpura, petechiae). General findings can suggest systemic disease and may require complete physical examination and appropriate evaluation. The diagnosis of skin disorders is accomplished by careful observation and evaluation of individual lesions. This discussion is limited to assessment of hair, scalp, nails, and skin lesions.

Considerations in Ethnic Populations

As the demographics of the United States continue to change, the background and skills of the health care providers must continue to expand. Providers must learn to distinguish between normal and pathologic dermatologic variations in all ethnic populations, including Asians, African Americans, and Hispanics, as well as Caucasians (e.g., recognizing how inflammation, erythema, or follicular reactivity can appear in different skin pigments). Inflammation is underrecognized in dark-skinned people because erythema is difficult to assess. In diseases such as atopic dermatitis, nummular eczema, pityriasis rosea, or sarcoidosis, follicular accentuation is clearly visible in darker-skinned people. Post-inflammatory hyperpigmentation may persist longer after the disease has cleared in dark-pigmented skin than in fair-skinned people. In addition to appreciating physical differences in the skin of various ethnic populations, one must learn to value the social customs, traditional beliefs, mistrust, and fear that may influence adherence to treatment regimens.

Inspection and Palpation
Hair and Scalp

Examine the hair distribution patterns for symmetry and distribution according to the client's age and sexual development. Fine hair covers much of the body and is the same color as scalp hair. Increased distribution occurs normally in the axillae and pubic area. Having excess body hair is known as *hirsutism*.

Inspect the hair and scalp under good light, and always wear protective gloves while examining open lesions or if you suspect infestation with lice. Inspect and palpate the hair for distribution, thickness, texture, lubrication, and signs of infestation or infection. Because natural hair color varies greatly, ask the client whether hair dye is used because it alters the hair's texture. Hair should be resilient and distributed evenly over the scalp. Texture and lubrication are affected by the type of hair care products used as well as by a protein-deficient diet or severe health problems, which tend to leave hair dry and brittle. Hair loss or thinning *(alopecia)* can result from genetic predisposition to baldness or a health problem, such as recent chemotherapy or a thyroid disorder.

Inspect and palpate the scalp for lesions, excoriations (from scratching), lumps, or bruises, which should be absent. Examine hair shafts for the presence of nits, which are the eggs of the human head louse. Adult lice often bite the scalp behind the ears and along the back of the neck, which results in pustular lesions.

If you see lesions, describe them and ask the client about recent trauma or injury to the head. If the client has not already provided information during the health history interview, conduct an analysis of clinical manifestations.

Nails

Inspect the client's nails for color, shape, texture, integrity, and thickness (Table 48-1). The nails reflect the client's overall health, indicating nutrition and respiratory status.

Color and Shape. The nail plate is usually transparent and colorless and, when viewed from the side, has a convex shape. The vascular bed underlying the nail plate gives the nail its color. The color is pink in white clients and darker in dark-skinned clients. A hemoglobin deficiency is seen in the nail bed as pallor, and decreased arterial circulation appears as cyanosis.

Texture. Texture should be smooth; healthy nails are of uniform thickness with no signs of dryness, softness, brittleness, splitting, peeling, ridges, or pitting. The *angle* formed between the nail plate and the posterior nailfold is about 160 degrees without separation (see Table 48-1). Changes in nail shape and nail bed angle can indicate health problems. Clubbing of the nails refers to an increase of more than 160 degrees in the angle between the nail plate and nail base. The base of a clubbed nail is spongy and soft on palpation. These changes result from hypoxia (diminished tissue oxygenation). Nail clubbing commonly occurs in clients with congenital heart defects or chronic lung disease.

Integrity. The tissue surrounding the nail should appear intact without signs of inflammation, jagged edges

TABLE 48-1 Assessing the Nails

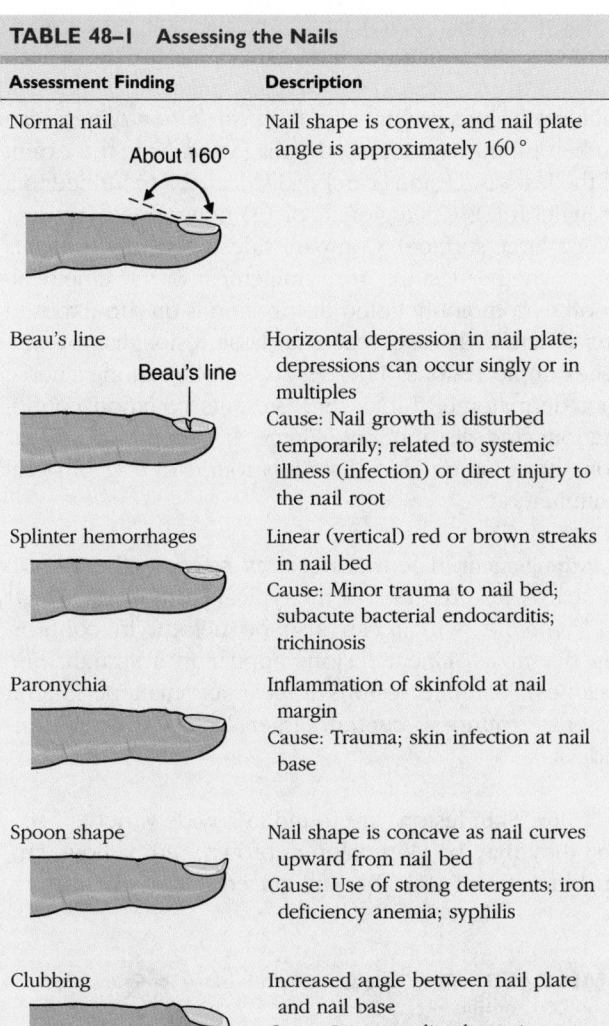

Assessment Finding	Description
Normal nail About 160°	Nail shape is convex, and nail plate angle is approximately 160°
Beau's line Beau's line	Horizontal depression in nail plate; depressions can occur singly or in multiples Cause: Nail growth is disturbed temporarily; related to systemic illness (infection) or direct injury to the nail root
Splinter hemorrhages	Linear (vertical) red or brown streaks in nail bed Cause: Minor trauma to nail bed; subacute bacterial endocarditis; trichinosis
Paronychia	Inflammation of skinfold at nail margin Cause: Trauma; skin infection at nail base
Spoon shape	Nail shape is concave as nail curves upward from nail bed Cause: Use of strong detergents; iron deficiency anemia; syphilis
Clubbing	Increased angle between nail plate and nail base Cause: Long-standing hypoxia

(hangnail), or dryness. Inferior or lateral nailfold inflammation is a sign of paronychia (nailfold infection). If these abnormalities are noted, ask the client about nail care habits such as biting or cutting cuticles.

Thickness. While examining the fingers and toes, you may note common abnormalities such as calluses or corns. A *callus* is a flat, painless thickening of a circumscribed area of skin. Calluses usually occur on the hands and feet. A *corn* is a horny induration and thickening of the skin caused by friction and pressure and is often painful.

Skin

Color. Assess overall skin color during the health history interview. Observe the client's face and visible skin surfaces for color tones, which should be congruent with the stated race. Abnormal findings include pallor

(paleness), a flushed or ruddy complexion, cyanosis (blue cast), jaundice (yellow cast), and areas of irregular pigmentation. Normal variation occurs from one region of the body to another, particularly in areas protected from the sun and exposure by clothing; these areas are lighter. Overall color should be uniform, but may range over a variety of colors.

Examine local areas of color change closely. *Hyperpigmentation* describes areas of increased pigmentation; *hypopigmentation* describes areas of decreased pigmentation. Skin color also results from the circulation; an increased blood supply may lead to the redness of inflammation *(rubor),* whereas extreme pallor may be a result of anemia or impeded arterial circulation to the area. Areas that are less pigmented reveal abnormal findings more readily than more heavily pigmented surfaces. *Pallor* is best seen in the buccal (mouth) mucosa, especially in clients with dark skin. *Cyanosis* is evident more readily in less pigmented areas, such as the nail beds, lips, and palms. *Jaundice* sharply contrasts with the white of the sclera, especially in dark-skinned clients who have more carotene deposits. Jaundice is best assessed in dark-skinned clients by inspecting color changes in the hard palate.

Moisture. Moisture refers to the skin's hydration level. Overall skin moisture in healthy individuals can be described as well hydrated. Skin moisture often reflects ambient temperature and humidity levels. Moistness usually occurs in intertriginous areas (where skin touches skin), such as the axillae and groin. Skin that feels overly moist and cool (clammy) or overly dry, scaling, or cracked is abnormal.

Temperature. Assess temperature with the dorsum of the hand. The skin should feel uniformly warm because it reflects circulation. Compare areas of hypothermia or hyperthermia with the same areas on the opposite side (Figure 48-4).

Texture. Palpate *texture* by stroking the skin lightly with the fingertips. The skin should feel smooth, soft, and resilient. There should be no areas of lumps or unusual thickening or thinning *(atrophy).*

Turgor. Turgor, a reflection of the skin's elasticity and hydration status, is measured by the time needed for the skin and underlying tissue to return to their original contour after being "pinched up." Lightly pinch the skin over the forearm between the thumb and index finger, and then release it. Skin with normal turgor is mobile and elastic and should return to baseline contour within 3 seconds. If the skin remains elevated (tented) for more than 3 seconds, turgor is decreased. Turgor decreases with age as the skin loses elasticity.

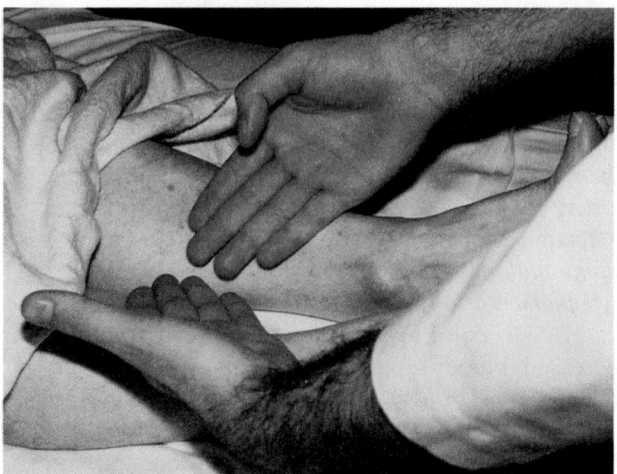

■ FIGURE 48–4 Assessing skin temperature uses the backs of the hands for the most accurate assessment.

Edema. Palpate for *edema* (fluid retention), particularly if areas of taut, shiny skin are noted. Edema refers to a collection of fluid in underlying tissues that separate the skin's surface from pigmented and vascular layers, resulting in a blanched appearance. It is an abnormal finding. Palpate edematous areas for consistency, temperature, shape (extent), tenderness, and mobility. Assess and describe edematous areas using the technique described in Chapter 51. Areas examined for edema include those over the sacrum (especially in bedridden clients), the feet, the ankles, and over the tibia.

Tenderness. Tenderness is an abnormal finding and is elicited with palpation. No areas of tenderness should be found in a healthy, uninjured client.

Odor. The skin should be free of pungent odors. Odors, when noted, are usually present in the axillae and skinfolds or in open wounds and are related to the presence of bacteria on the skin, inadequate hygiene, or infection. Assess odor in open wounds after cleansing the wound because odor can be related to the drainage itself or to the type of dressing used (hydrocolloid).

Lesions. Inspect the skin for detectable lesions. Assess and describe lesions in an orderly fashion: location, distribution, size, arrangement, color, configuration, secondary changes, and presence of drainage. Palpate skin lesions to determine the characteristics of contour (flat, raised, or depressed), size (using a measuring device), consistency (firm, soft), mobility, and tenderness. Lesions can be mobile or immobile (fixed to underlying tissue). Photographing lesions of concern is an excellent way to document changes over time.

Location, Distribution, and Size. Location is described in reference to anatomic landmarks. Measure the lesions for *size* to help classify their type (macule, papule). If multiple lesions are present, the *distribution pattern* can be helpful in determining the diagnosis. Note the extent of the lesions. Lesions can be (1) localized (confined to a specific area), (2) regional, or (3) generalized (present over a large surface). Compare sides bilaterally to determine whether lesions are symmetrical or asymmetrical. Another commonly noted distribution is on sun-exposed areas. Certain diseases feature a classic lesion distribution; for example, lesions of herpes zoster follow along a nerve root dermatome. Table 48-2 presents common configurations and distributions. Figure 48-5 depicts the locations of common skin disorders found during physical examination.

Arrangement. The *arrangement* refers to the pattern of nearby lesions. Two of the typical patterns are *linear* and *satellite,* which can also be helpful in confirming diagnosis. Linear lesions appear in a straight line (scabies). Satellite lesions appear as small peripheral lesions around a central larger lesion (diaper candidiasis).

Color. Skin lesions are found in a wide variety of colors; they may be skin-colored, brown, red, yellow, tan, or blue. Color can be influenced by many factors,

TABLE 48–2   Terminology for Skin Lesion Configuration and Distribution

Configuration*	Description
Annular	Ring-shaped
Iris	Concentric rings, "bull's eyes"
Gyrate	Spiral-shaped
Linear	Forming a line
Nummular	Coin-like
Polymorphous	Occurring in several forms
Punctate	Marked by points or dots
Serpiginous	Snake-like
Distribution†	**Description**
Solitary	Single lesion
Satellite	Single lesion occurring in close proximity to but separate from a large group of lesions
Grouped	Clustered
Confluent	Merged together
Diffuse	Widely distributed
Discrete	Separate from other lesions
Generalized	Diffusely distributed
Localized	Limited, clearly defined
Symmetrical	Bilaterally distributed
Asymmetrical	Unilaterally distributed
Zosteriform	Band-like distribution of lesions along a dermatome

* Position of lesions relative to other lesions.
† Grouping, or pattern, of lesions over entire skin surface.

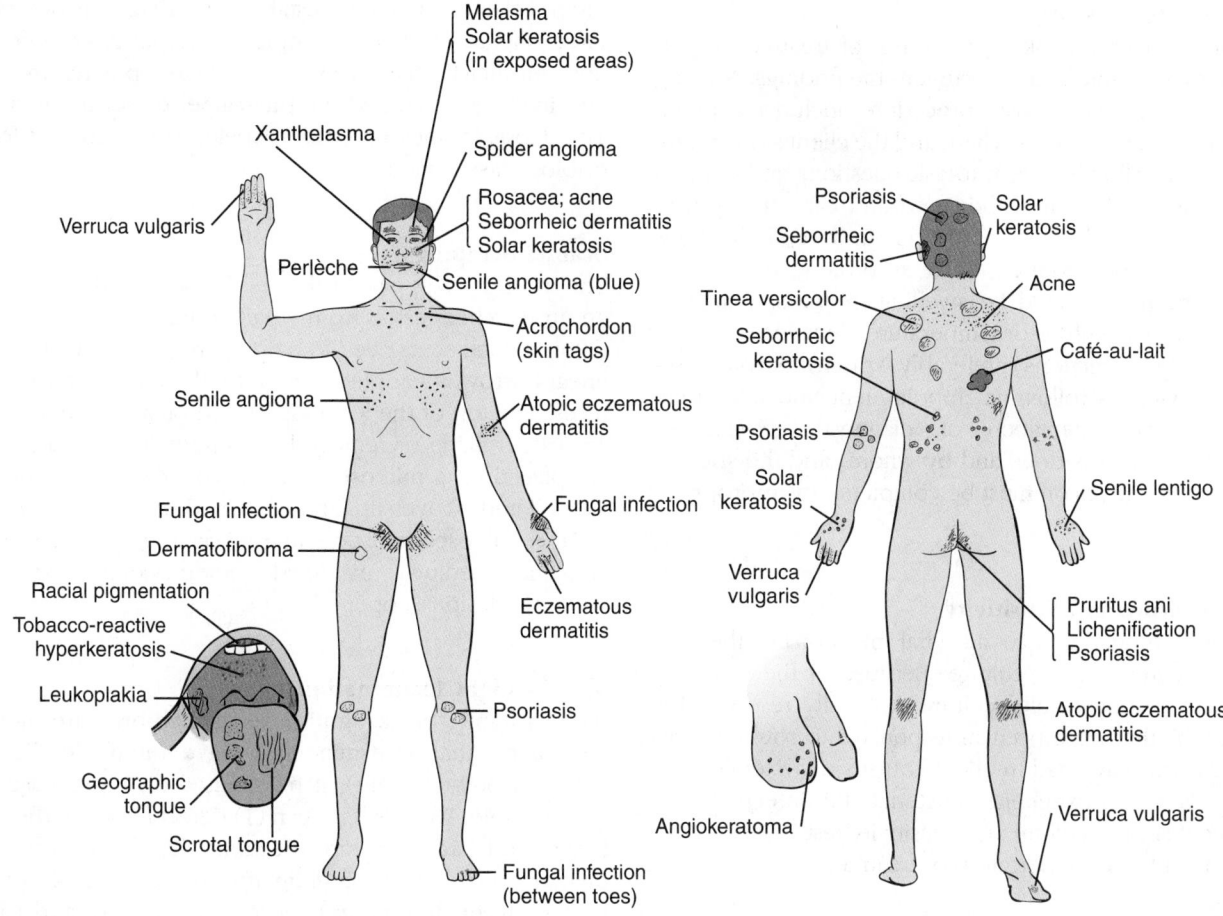

■ **FIGURE 48–5** Common disorders encountered during physical examination of the skin.

including the client's normal skin hue, which may make accurate description difficult. Slight color changes can best be assessed in areas having the least amount of natural pigmentation and those with superficial capillary beds (buccal membrane of the mouth, mucosa, lips, nail beds, ocular conjunctiva, palms, and soles). These areas are especially important in assessing darkly pigmented skin.

Configuration. The term *configuration* refers to the shape or the outline of the lesion. Most lesions are circular. The term *nummular* is used for a circular lesion that is the size of a large coin (nummular eczema). *Annular* describes lesions with an active ring-shaped border and some central clearing (granuloma annulare). Table 48-2 describes other configurations that may be found during assessment.

Skin Self-Examination

Although it is crucial that all health care providers learn to perform an accurate and complete assessment of the skin, it is more important to teach every individual how to perform a skin self-examination. Routine self-examination promotes skin health and awareness and greatly lowers individual risk for severe skin disorders, such as skin cancer. Teach clients to examine their entire bodies to look for any changes in the skin or in their moles or skin lesions. See the Client Education Guide feature on Skin Self-Examination in Chapter 49. Encourage clients to visit their health care provider for further evaluation of any suspicious-looking lesions.

Danger signals to look for are the *ABCDEs* of melanoma:

A, *Asymmetry:* one half is unlike the other half
B, *Border:* irregular, scalloped, or poorly circumscribed border
C, *Color:* varied from one area to another, shades of two colors, or changing colors
D, *Diameter:* larger than 6 mm as a rule (diameter of a Number 2 pencil eraser)
E, *Evolving:* any change (e.g., in size, shape, color, elevation), or another trait, or a new manifestation (such as bleeding, itching, or crusting)

Diagnostic Testing

Before a diagnostic skin procedure (or treatment), perform an assessment and document the findings. Nursing intervention for diagnostic procedures includes explaining the procedure to the client and the client's significant others and allowing them to ask questions and express concerns. Explain appropriate wound care and indications of possible side effects and complications that should be reported, such as prolonged bleeding or infection (indicated by swelling, redness, drainage, increased discomfort, or temperature elevation).

Provide instructions (preferably written) for follow-up care as well as follow-up appointment and telephone number. Documentation of diagnostic procedures (exactly what was done and by whom) and the specific location of the lesion must be completed by appropriate personnel.

Skin Culture and Sensitivity

Bacterial, fungal, and certain viral infections of the skin can be confirmed by culture. Because of the cost and delay in getting results, culture is usually reserved for infections that have been unresponsive to routine care. Clients who have had frequent courses of systemic antibiotics and still experience bacterial skin infections are candidates for a culture and sensitivity test to determine which antibiotic is indicated for treatment.

Potassium Hydroxide Examination and Fungal Culture

Fungal infection of skin, hair, or nails can be confirmed by microscopic identification or culture of scrapings from the area, or both. Any area of scaly dermatitis may be scraped for this test. Typical sites are the scalp, intertriginous areas (between the toes, axillae, groin, under or between the breasts, abdominal folds), and the nailfold.

Fine scales from the edge of the site are scraped with a number 15 scalpel blade or the edge of a glass slide onto a second glass slide. A drop of 10% to 20% potassium hydroxide is added to the scale, and a coverslip is placed over the specimen. Gentle pressure is applied to the coverslip to flatten the scales. The slide may be gently heated to dissolve the keratin or the cells more quickly. The scrapings are examined under the microscope. For a culture, scrapings from a suspicious lesion are implanted in the appropriate culture medium. For a nail culture, an altered, dystrophic nail is snipped and implanted in the medium. Debris from the nail's subungual area is less suitable for culture.

Tzanck's Smear

Tzanck's smear is used for microscopic assessment of fluids and cells from vesicles or bullae. The presence of multinucleated giant cells establishes a diagnosis of viral infection, such as herpes simplex or herpes zoster infection. An intact, recently evolved vesicle top is removed, and its base is scraped with a scalpel or small curette. The debris is smeared onto a labeled slide and sent for cytologic assessment.

Scabies Scraping

The most difficult part of the test for scabies is selecting an unscratched lesion from which to take the specimen. Often several areas need to be prepared. When visible, a linear burrow is sampled to look for the mite, its eggs, or feces. The top of the lesion is shaved off with a number 15 scalpel blade or removed by curette. The specimens are placed on a microscope slide, covered with immersion oil and a coverslip, and examined under low power on the microscope. Local anesthesia is not necessary, and fine bleeding is expected. Some discomfort occurs when the lesion is opened.

Wood's Light Examination

Wood's light ("black light") uses a high-pressure mercury lamp that transmits long-wave ultraviolet light (UVA, or 360-nm light); it has limited diagnostic uses. For example, Wood's light can (1) detect few superficial fungal and bacterial skin infections, (2) delineate pigmentary disorders by highlighting the degree of contrast between lesions and normal skin color, and (3) accentuate the contrast between hypopigmented and totally amelanotic areas. It is important to recognize that the most common types of fungi do not fluoresce, and for years this test has been of questionable use in diagnosing fungus.[11] Wood's light examination is done in a darkened room.

Patch Testing

Patch testing is done to attempt to identify substances that produce allergic skin responses.[4,13] It is a painless procedure, and a skilled evaluator must be on hand to read and interpret the results. Patch testing is often done to differentiate between an *irritant* contact dermatitis and an *allergic* contact dermatitis. Small amounts of various substances or allergens are applied to the skin using a commercially prepared tape containing the allergens, or allergens are placed on aluminum disks on a special tape. The client and the client's significant others need to understand that whereas potential allergic substances (allergens) can produce inflammatory skin reactions, compounds of low concentration are used to prevent possible excessive irritation.

Patch testing should not be performed if acute dermatitis is present or if the client is taking substantial amounts of oral steroids; the potential allergen might worsen the dermatitis.

TABLE 48–3 Methods of Lesion Biopsy

Biopsy Type	Details
Punch	Obtains skin specimen with full thickness (epidermal, dermal, and subcutaneous tissue) using circular sharp instrument of varying cutting diameters (2-8 mm) for diagnosis
Shave	Obtains tissue sample of epidermis and generally upper portion of dermis using blade-type instrument to remove lesions/specimen around the plane of surrounding skin for diagnosis or treatment
Snip excision	Used to remove lesion/specimen that can be cut off with blade-type instrument or scissor at base of pedunculated lesion for diagnosis or treatment
Curettage	Used to remove/obtain tissue/specimen using an oval or round scalpel-type instrument for diagnosis or treatment
Excision	Obtains a larger full-thickness specimen than is attainable by punch; usually used on large irregular lesion for diagnosis or treatment of a recurrent or aggressive lesion
Surgical excision	Used (1) when it is necessary to excise lesion completely (when full skin thickness is needed), (2) when lesion's borders are indistinct from surrounding skin, or (3) when there is recurrent or aggressive cancer. Lesion is excised with scalpel by means of a variety of surgical techniques

The tape must be worn for 48 hours without disturbing the patches; then it is removed. Interpretations are made at 48, 72, and 96 hours and sometimes at 1 week. A specific eczematous response at the test site with erythema, papules, or small vesicles indicates a positive reaction and confirms an allergic contact sensitivity to the substance on the disk. Counseling regarding allergen avoidance in a positive test or the meaning of the negative result is a critical part of the test.[4]

Biopsy

Skin biopsy refers to the removal of a skin tissue specimen for histologic (cellular microscopic) assessment and/or immunofluorescence (special media before special microscopic evaluation). In all procedures, local anesthesia is generally used. Small-gauge (26- to 30-gauge) needles are recommended to limit trauma to the skin. Refer to Table 48-3 for specifics regarding the types of biopsy.

Depending on the size and location of the biopsy specimen and the skill of the practitioner, the procedure is usually quick and almost painless. The most common source of pain is the initial administration of local anesthetic. The specimen is placed in a preservative such as formalin solution, properly identified, and sent for pathologic assessment. Clean or sterile technique is used as appropriate to dress or cover the biopsy site.

Preprocedure Care. Depending on the procedure, instruct the client to avoid the use of aspirin and products containing aspirin for 48 hours before the biopsy to avoid a prolonged postprocedure bleeding time. If the client is taking anticoagulants (heparin or warfarin), notify the physician. Review the client's medical history for systemic disorders such as liver malfunction, which affects clotting time. If the client has a history of cardiac valve replacement, be sure that prophylactic antibiotics are prescribed. Obtain an informed consent. The client may eat a light meal before the procedure to avoid syncope (fainting).

Postprocedure Care. After the procedure, cover most biopsy sites with an antibiotic ointment and a clean bandage or dry dressing unless ordered otherwise. Many nonadhesive types of dressings are available and may be preferable for clients who have fragile or sensitive skin. The client should be reminded that a follow-up assessment is necessary, and a follow-up appointment should be scheduled if needed for suture removal. Tell the client how and when biopsy results will be reported; individuals have different levels of anxiety about biopsy results.

CONCLUSIONS

The skin is the largest organ in the body, and it presents many health care challenges. The key to assessment of the skin or to the assessment of a rash or lesion is use of a comprehensive, systematic approach. Remember, the current view does not tell the whole story; multiple assessments over time or anticipating the changes that came before or those that will occur next will be important.

BIBLIOGRAPHY

Citations appearing in red refer to primary research.

Citations appearing in blue refer to evidence-based practice guidelines and protocols.

1. Boguniewicz, M. (2002). *Immunology and allergy clinics of North America: Atopic dermatitis.* Philadelphia: Saunders.
2. Callen, J.P. (2000). *Color atlas of dermatology* (2nd ed.). Philadelphia: Saunders.
3. Deleo, V.A., Elsner, P., & Marks, J.G. (2002). *Contact & occupational dermatology* (3rd ed.). St. Louis: Mosby.
4. Fitzpatrick, T.B., Johnson, R.A., & Wolff, K. (2001). *Color atlas and synopsis of clinical dermatology: Common and serious diseases* (4th ed.). New York: McGraw-Hill.
5. Freedberg, I.M., Eisen, A.Z., Wolff, K., et al (2003). *Fitzpatrick's dermatology in general medicine* (6th ed.). New York: McGraw-Hill.
6. Gilchrest, B.A. (2002). *Geriatric dermatology part II.* Philadelphia: Saunders.
7. Greaves, M.W., & Leung, D.Y.M. (2000). *Allergic skin disease: A multidisciplinary approach.* New York: Marcel Dekker.
8. Hill, M.J. (2003). *Dermatologic nursing essentials: A core curriculum* (2nd ed.). Pitman, NJ: Dermatology Nurses' Association.

9. Huether, S., & McCance, K. (2004). *Understanding pathophysiology* (3rd ed.). St. Louis: Mosby.

10. Lane, A.T., Morelli, J.G., & Weston, W.L. (2002). *Color textbook of pediatric dermatology* (3rd ed.). St. Louis: Mosby.

11. Lookingbill, D.P., & Marks J.G. (2006). *Principles of dermatology* (4th ed.). Philadelphia: Saunders.

12. McCance, K., & Huether, S.E. (2006). *Pathophysiology: The biological basis for disease in adults and children* (5th ed.). St. Louis: Mosby.

13. Williams, J.D., Berger, T.G., & Elston, D.M. (2006). *Andrews' diseases of the skin: Clinical dermatology* (10th ed.). Philadelphia: Saunders.

evolve **Did you remember to check out the bonus material on the Evolve website and the CD-ROM, including NCLEX®-Examination Style Review Questions, Open-Book Quizzes, and Chapter Review Audio Podcasts?**

http://evolve.elsevier.com/Black/medsurg

CHAPTER 49

Management of Clients with Integumentary Disorders

NOREEN HEER NICOL AND JOYCE M. BLACK

The skin is the largest and most visible organ of the body. Disorders of the skin offer the nurse an opportunity to provide care that makes a noticeable difference to clients. Anger, frustration, depression, and anxiety are commonly experienced by clients with skin disorders, particularly those with chronic dermatoses. Clients can become embarrassed about their appearance and shun socializing.

The educational needs of people affected by skin disease are vast. Health care providers need to consistently provide information that includes detailed skin care plans, general disease information, and availability of client-oriented support organizations as well as updates on encouraging research results. It behooves health care providers to stay current with new therapies to assist clients in obtaining information and treatment advances. Clients tend to forget or confuse important skin care treatment programs without written instructions. Clearly outlining the skin care recommendations orally and in writing is essential for increased compliance and good outcomes.

COMMON SKIN DISORDERS

PRURITUS

Pruritus (itching), one of the most common manifestations of skin problems, is a symptom, not a disease. Pruritus can lead to damage if scratching injures the skin, increasing risk for infection and scarring. Pruritus can be seen in conditions ranging from dry skin to severe systemic disease. Systemic diseases that can cause generalized and severe pruritus include chickenpox, liver and renal failure, diabetes mellitus, drug hypersensitivity reaction, immunodeficiency disorders, intestinal parasites, leukemia, and lymphoma. Relieving itching, especially for chronically ill clients, is challenging because of its common occurrence, detrimental effect on skin health, and the major effect it may have on quality of life.

Itching can begin by irritation from almost any chemical or physical substance, or allergic reaction, especially if skin is damaged. Once the itch sensation starts, the client has an almost uncontrollable urge to scratch; and scratching leads to further skin damage and increased inflammation. Thus the itch-scratch-itch cycle develops. To minimize skin trauma caused by scratching, fingernails should be short, smooth, and clean.

Appropriate management of itching requires a complete assessment that attempts to discover the underlying cause and knowledge of appropriate therapeutic modalities for treatment. Dry skin may be either the source of pruritus or a contributing factor, and good hydration is often helpful (see Xerotic Eczema), in addition to any other topical therapy. The Integrating Pharmacology feature on Common Topical Preparations describes medications used to treat dermatologic conditions (see p. 1200).

One bath or shower per day for 15 to 20 minutes with warm water and a gentle cleanser is recommended, immediately followed by the application of a sealing

evolve **Web Enhancements**

Care Plan The Client with Atopic Dermatitis

Case Management The Client with Impaired Skin Integrity

Client Education Guide Skin Self-Examination (Spanish Translation)

Topical Corticosteroids (Spanish Translation)

Simple Guidelines to Help Protect You from the Damaging Rays of the Sun (English Version and Spanish Translation)

Postoperative Care After Rhinoplasty (English Version and Spanish Translation)

Be sure to check out the bonus material on the Evolve website and the CD-ROM, including free self-assessment exercises. **http://evolve.elsevier.com/Black/medsurg**

INTEGRATING PHARMACOLOGY

Common Topical Preparations

The skin's large surface area allows the absorption, penetration, and permeation of topically applied preparations. The factors that determine how well these processes occur in the skin's layers include the client's age, the size of the affected region of skin, the condition of the stratum corneum, the cutaneous blood supply, the molecular weight of the drug, and the medication vehicle (the word *vehicle* is used here to mean the substance containing the medication or the form in which the medication is delivered).

Topical medications are chosen both for the action of the active ingredients (which are delivered directly to the skin surface) and for the vehicle. Topical medications have many different actions and cover a large spectrum of drug categories, including anti-infective, antipruritic, and anti-inflammatory.

Examples of various topical medication vehicles are ointments, creams, gels, lotions, solutions, and powders. Ointments are more occlusive, providing better delivery of the medication by preventing water loss from the skin. Use ointments cautiously with excessive heat or humidity because occlusion may result in increased itching or skin infection. When the weather is hot and humid, creams may be better tolerated. Although creams spread more easily than ointments, they are less occlusive, leading to increased skin drying in some people because of the evaporative property of the water. Creams also can be water based with ethyl alcohol and not be as drying as creams have been in the past. Sprays and lotions are available for use on the scalp and other hairy areas. The various ingredients used to formulate the different bases may be irritating to the skin, and care must be taken when recommending any product.

Both the active ingredient and the vehicle must be appropriate for the condition being treated. For acute dermatoses (i.e., weeping, blistering lesions), an aqueous (water-based) compound provides a drying effect. A greasy vehicle has the opposite effect; it promotes lubrication and occlusion and helps treat the dryness and scaling caused by chronic dermatosis. Differences in skin permeability also influence the effectiveness of topical medications. For example, absorption is increased in inflamed skin. Depending on the medication and the specific condition, topical medication may be applied to localized lesions or to larger skin surfaces. When increased absorption of the medication is needed, topical medication may be prescribed for application under an occlusive dressing. Be aware that some topical medication drug package-insert information states that they should or should *not* be used with or under occlusion. Ointments, creams, and gels have greatly increased absorption if they are applied to skin that is wet.

emollient, with or without other topical medications, to prevent evaporation of water from the hydrated epidermis. Other topical medications often added to emollients to help alleviate itching include menthol (0.25% to 0.5%), camphor (0.25% to 0.5%), urea (10% to 20%),

and lactic acid (12%). Camphor and menthol produce a cooling effect. Urea and lactic acid moisturize scaly skin by drawing moisture into the cell structure of the stratum corneum. Topically applied antihistamines and anesthetics are relatively ineffective and are best avoided because they can be potent allergic sensitizers. The sensitizing effect is especially pronounced if these products are used on inflamed skin. Use of topical corticosteroids should be reserved for the treatment of specific steroid-responsive dermatoses, not pruritus of unknown origin. Long-term application of topical steroids, especially on skin not affected with an eczematous condition, may result in thinning of the skin, striae, telangiectases, and easy bruising.

Systemic antihistaminic agents are most helpful in disorders in which histamine is the principal mediator but may be of benefit through a sedative or even placebo effect. A trial of a histamine$_1$ (H$_1$) blocker (hydroxyzine, diphenhydramine, cetirizine) is appropriate either on a regular schedule or as indicated for itching. Tricyclic antidepressants have a high binding capacity for H$_1$ receptors and may be helpful in clients who would benefit from their antidepressant as well as antipruritic effect. Mild analgesia can also be effective.

Older clients may have difficulty applying the needed topical agents properly, and assistive personnel may be required to ensure proper therapy. Oral sedating antihistamines should be administered carefully, with use of small doses initially, because many older people have a very low tolerance of these agents and may experience severe drowsiness, especially at the initiation of therapy.

ECZEMATOUS DISORDERS

Eczema is not a specific disease. *Dermatitis* and *eczema* are terms that may be used interchangeably to describe a group of disorders with a characteristic clinical appearance. Types of dermatitis are listed in Box 49-1.

BOX 49-1   Types of Dermatitis

- *Allergic contact dermatitis:* eruptions from allergy to poison ivy, sumac, or oak or another proven allergen
- *Irritant dermatitis:* eruptions from direct contact with irritating substances, which can be almost anything including cosmetics, chemicals, dyes, or detergents
- *Nummular eczema:* appearance of coin-shaped, oozing, crusting patches
- *Seborrheic dermatitis:* yellowish pink scaling of the scalp, face, and trunk
- *Stasis dermatitis:* eruptions resulting from peripheral venous disorders
- *Atopic dermatitis:* characteristic distribution of eczema in people with a family history of asthma, hay fever, or eczema

Eczema/dermatitis has three primary stages; the condition may be limited to any one of the three stages, or the three stages may coexist.

- *Acute dermatitis* is characterized by extensive erosions with serous exudate or by intensely pruritic, erythematous papules and vesicles on a background of erythema.
- *Subacute dermatitis* is characterized by erythematous, excoriated, scaling papules or plaques that are either grouped or scattered over erythematous skin; the scaling may be so fine and diffuse that the skin acquires a silvery sheen.
- *Chronic dermatitis* is characterized by thickened skin and increased skin marking secondary to rubbing and scratching (lichenification); excoriated papules, fibrotic papules, and nodules (prurigo nodularis); and postinflammatory hyperpigmentation and hypopigmentation.

ATOPIC DERMATITIS

Atopic dermatitis is a common, chronic, relapsing, pruritic type of eczema that begins in childhood. Clients with atopic dermatitis have familial hay fever, asthma, sensitive skin, and/or a history of atopic dermatitis.

Etiology

Atopic dermatitis (AD) is due to a combination of heredity and environmental factors. Genetic aspects are clear; most clients with atopic dermatitis report a family history of atopic diseases. The Genetic Links feature below lists other genetic disorders involving the skin. Atopic dermatitis is becoming increasingly prevalent in northern, industrialized, temperate countries. Many factors have been implicated in the increased prevalence of this disorder. Researchers point to environmental pollutants, food additives, a decrease in breast-feeding, and lifestyles involving primarily indoor dwelling, which increase exposure to house dust mites and indoor air pollution. Some theories suggest that an overly sterile, modern lifestyle, with its lack of exposure to immune-stimulating parasites, infections, and bacteria, creates an imbalance and immaturity of the immune system that predisposes to atopic disorders.

Pathophysiology

The pathophysiology of AD is poorly understood. Atopic dermatitis appears to be caused by dysfunction of skin T cells. A complex chain of events leads to T-cell activation and proliferation, resulting in the release of cytokines and inflammatory mediators, leading to the clinical manifestation of atopic dermatitis. Compared with normal skin, the dry skin of atopic dermatitis has reduced water-binding capacity, higher rate of transepidermal water loss, and decreased water content. Water loss leads to further drying and cracking of the skin, which leads to more itching. Rubbing and scratching of itchy skin are responsible for many of the changes seen in the skin.

GENETIC LINKS

Examples of Genetic Disorders Involving the Skin

Disorder	Skin Features	Inheritance	Metabolic/Gene Defect	Genetic Testing Available
Neurofibromatosis, type 1	Dermal neurofibromas, multiple café-au-lait spots, axillary and inguinal freckling	AD	Mutation in *NF1* gene on chromosome 17	Yes
Tuberous sclerosis	Hypomelanotic macules, facial angiofibromas, shagreen patches, fibrous facial plaques	AD	Mutation in *TSC1* gene on chromosome 9; *TSC2* gene on chromosome 16	Yes
Oculocutaneous albinism, type 1	Hypopigmentation of skin, hair, and eyes	AR	Mutation in tyrosinase gene, *TYR*, on chromosome 11	Yes
Waardenburg's syndrome	Hypopigmentation of skin and hair; white forelock; premature gray hair	AD	Mutation in *PAX3* gene on chromosome 2	Yes
Fabry's disease	Vascular cutaneous lesions (angiokeratomas)	XR	Mutation in *GLA* gene on chromosome X; deficient activity of enzyme alpha-galactosidase (α-Gal A)	Yes
Bloom syndrome	Sun-sensitive, telangiectatic, hypo- and hyperpigmented skin; predisposition to cancer	AR	Mutation in *BLM* gene on chromosome 15	Yes

AD, Autosomal dominant; *AR,* autosomal recessive; *XR,* X-linked recessive.

Clinical Manifestations

Atopic dermatitis begins in many clients during infancy. The dermatitis is usually of acute onset, with a red, oozing, crusting rash. Over time, the skin tends to show the chronic form of dermatitis, with thickened dry texture, brownish-gray color, and scales. The rash tends to become localized to the large folds of the extremities as the client becomes older (Figure 49-1). In older children and adults, it is found mainly on elbow bends, the backs of the knees, the neck, the eyelids, and the backs of the hands and feet. Hand and foot dermatitis becomes a significant problem in some adults.

Pruritus is the major clinical manifestation of atopic dermatitis and causes the greatest morbidity. The condition may be mild and self-limiting, or it may be intense, provoking scratching that results in severely excoriated lesions, infection, and scarring.

Clients with atopic dermatitis tend to experience viral, bacterial, and fungal skin infections. It is not clear whether these cutaneous infections arise secondary to a disruption of normal barrier function or are due to reduced local immunity. Honey-colored crusting, extensive serous weeping, folliculitis, pyoderma, and furunculosis indicate bacterial infection, usually secondary to *Staphylococcus aureus* colonization in clients with atopic dermatitis. Clients with atopic dermatitis are frequently heavily colonized with *S. aureus*. Superficial fungal infections may also appear more frequently. The most common viral infection is herpes simplex, which tends to spread locally or become generalized.

OUTCOME MANAGEMENT

The goal of therapy is to break the inflammatory cycle that causes excess drying and cracking as well as the itching and scratching.

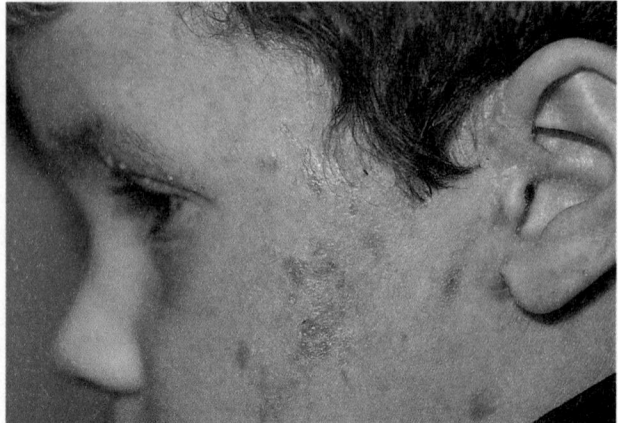

■ **FIGURE 49–1** Atopic dermatitis. Intense pruritus leads to scratching and open lesions.

Medical Management

Hydrate the Skin

Hydration is the key to management but is often difficult to achieve. Management begins with daily skin care that hydrates and lubricates the skin. Soaks followed by application of occlusive substances are usually prescribed.

Remove Allergens

Understanding each client's disease pattern and the discovery and reduction of exacerbating factors are crucial to effective management of this chronic disorder. Allergens, food, aeroallergens, and emotional stresses may be inciting factors. Many of these triggering factors are the same irritants or allergens that contribute to generalized pruritus (see Pruritus). Clients should avoid exposure to substances for which there is a positive result on allergy testing that correlates with history of precipitating dermatitis. Stringent restrictions on lifestyle and activities do not change the outcome.

Dietary management of atopic dermatitis has continued to be controversial. Food allergies in the causation of atopic dermatitis seem to be more significant in certain populations of young children and infants. The most common allergens appear to be eggs, cow's milk, soy, wheat, nuts, and fish. Proven allergens are avoided. People with food allergies must be taught to read labels. Care must be taken to avoid malnutrition when any type of restrictive diet is used.

Reduce Inflammation

Systemic medications may include antibiotics and antihistaminics (see Pruritus). The use of a systemic corticosteroid is rarely warranted in atopic dermatitis. Although systemic steroids can be a "quick and easy cure," they should be avoided in this chronic, non–life-threatening disorder. Although there may be dramatic improvement with their use, the recurrence of dermatitis after their discontinuation is equally dramatic. The side effects of long-term systemic steroid use are both unpleasant (moon face and buffalo hump) and dangerous (adrenal suppression, delayed healing).

Nursing Management of the Medical Client

Assess the client with atopic dermatitis for bathing habits, use of moisturizers, medication regimen, exposure to known allergens, environmental exposure, and history of skin eruptions. The Integrating Pharmacology feature on p. 1203 describes interventions for client with atopic dermatitis. See also the Care Plan on The Client with Atopic Dermatitis on the website.

Soaks and Wet Wraps

Soaks serve several purposes. Moisture softens dry epidermis, which aids in removal of crusts. Removal of cellular skin debris promotes healing and improves absorption of topical medication. The risk of infection is reduced by removal of necrotic tissue and occlusive crusts. Cooling also results from the gradual evaporation of water and has an anti-inflammatory effect, thus relieving itching (pruritus).

Soaks can be accomplished by either soaking the affected area or bathing for 15 to 20 minutes in warm water. The agent added to the soaks is the least important aspect of this therapy. Addition of substances such as colloidal oatmeal (Aveeno) or starch to the bath water may be soothing for some people but does nothing to increase water absorption. Coal tar preparations (Balnetar, T/Derm) have an anti-inflammatory effect and can be helpful in some eczematous and psoriatic conditions. Aluminum acetate (Burow's solution), aluminum sulfate and calcium acetate (Domeboro), povidone-iodine (Betadine), and diluted bleach in appropriate quantities are also effective antibacterial substances; however, they have drying effects and may cause increased stinging and noncompliance. Bath oils are usually not recommended because they give the client a false sense of lubrication and make the soaking area very slippery.

After soaking, clients should remove excess water by gently patting the skin with a soft towel. Then they should immediately apply the recommended topical substance. Immediate application of this substance to damp skin is the most important detail, because if the occlusive barrier is not provided within 3 to 5 minutes, evaporation begins to occur.

For moisturization and to seal in the water, use occlusives such as white petrolatum (Vaseline) or petrolatum with mineral oil and wool wax alcohol (Aquaphor ointment). Occlusives can be greasy and may be cosmetically unacceptable to some people. Clients may prefer creams or lotions because they are cosmetically pleasing products. Lotions and even creams may be irritating and drying because of the evaporative property of the water and the substances used as preservatives, solubilizers, and fragrances.

Wet wraps used immediately after soaking and occlusion can optimize hydration and topical therapy; this also promotes cooling of the skin. Wet wraps and occlusion can be applied in various ways and should not be confused with wet-to-dry dressings used for debridement. The location and severity of lesions often determine the choices. Total-body wet wraps can be accomplished by putting on wet pajamas or wet long underwear followed by dry pajamas or a dry or plastic sweat suit. The hands and feet can be covered with wet tube socks or wet cotton gloves followed by dry tube socks. Any extremity or the trunk can be covered with wet rolled (e.g., Kerlix) gauze and occluded with elastic bandages or by pieces of tube sock, wet followed by dry. The face can be wrapped with two layers of wet Kerlix gauze, followed by two layers of dry Kerlix gauze held in place with elasticized netting or other tubular dressings; holes are cut out for the eyes, nose, and mouth. If the dressing becomes dry, it should be rewetted before removal because debridement by the wet-to-dry method produces tissue damage and pain. Gentle debridement usually still occurs if dressings are removed when damp.[19]

Modifications for Older Clients

Dermatitis is a common skin disorder in the older population. It may be caused by venous insufficiency, allergens, irritants, or underlying malignancy such as leukemia or lymphoma. Because older adults often take many medications, the potential for dermatitis from drug-drug interactions is increased. The fragility of the skin as a result of the flattened epidermal-dermal junction and loss of dermis should be considered in planning any form of treatment.

XEROTIC ECZEMA

Xerotic (dry) skin lacks moisture in the top layer of the skin. Xerotic eczema may present as erythematous, scaling, and finely cracked skin. Xerosis occurs in patches and may involve any skin surface. It is common in the older population. If xerosis is severe, the skin is tight, itchy, and painful. Water loss causes xerotic chapping and fissures. The problem may be accentuated by use of drying skin cleansers, soaps, disinfectants, and solvents and infrequent use of moisturizers. Environmental factors play a large role, especially those that increase water loss in the stratum corneum. Any factors that decrease the relative humidity exacerbate this condition, such as cold or dry winter air, especially in artificially heated rooms.

Management includes hydration and moisturizing the skin plus avoiding irritating factors. Teaching the client correct daily skin care is essential to treating this condition (see Integrating Pharmacology feature on Soaks and Wet Wraps). Clients known to have xerosis every winter are advised to increase skin moisturizing before severe weather starts.

CONTACT DERMATITIS

Contact dermatitis is an inflammatory response of the skin. There are two types based on the etiology: irritant or allergic. Irritant contact dermatitis (ICD) is most common and is from exposure to anything that produces a chemical or physical irritant response. Allergic contact dermatitis (ACD) is a delayed hypersensitivity reaction resulting from contact with an allergen. This hypersensitivity reaction is an immune-mediated response by previously sensitized lymphocytes to a specific allergen. Common allergens are poison ivy, nickel, bacitracin, and formaldehyde.

The two conditions are difficult to distinguish. Clinical manifestations begin at the site of exposure with itching, stinging, erythema, and edema, which may extend to involve more distant sites. Manifestations may develop within an hour of contact or as late as 7 to 14 days after contact and may range from mild erythema to vesicles to ulceration (Figure 49-2). With even brief contact of the substance with the skin, an allergic response is possible. For example, contact with poison ivy may have happened quickly and the allergen washed off. However, areas of dermatitis may continue to appear for many days following the initial exposure.

Management begins with identification of the causative agent. First, question the client about recent exposure to substances such as plants, chemicals, and metals. Pain and itching may be controlled with topical medication or wet dressings (see Integrating Pharmacology on Soaks and Wet Wraps). Oral antihistaminic agents and topical or systemic steroids may be required. The Client Education Guide at right provides teaching information on topical corticosteroids. Patch testing is a test done to attempt to determine the specific agent. Each patch in a standardized test panel (TRUE test [thin-layer, rapid-use epicutaneous test]) contains a substance that is known to be one of the most common causes of allergic contact dermatitis. When these tests elicit a positive reaction, much can be done to teach the client about what to avoid (see Chapter 48).

INTERTRIGINOUS DERMATITIS

Intertriginous areas are between folds of skin. When the skin lays one fold on top of another, a superficial inflammatory dermatitis occurs. Inadequate ventilation

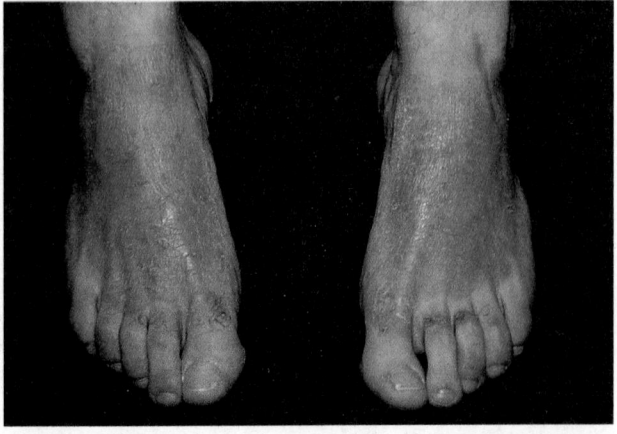

■ **FIGURE 49–2** Contact dermatitis. Note the distinct line of erythema.

Topical Corticosteroids

Corticosteroids are still among the most commonly used medications for treatment of a variety of dermatologic conditions. Corticosteroids can also be injected directly into the lesion, applied topically, or given systemically. Diagnosing the condition before any corticosteroid use is important because the effects of the medication can mask or change the clinical manifestations. Topical corticosteroids work through broad mechanisms, including anti-inflammatory, antimitotic, immunosuppressant, and vasoconstrictive actions. The effectiveness of these agents largely depends on the potency of the agent used and the degree of absorption through the skin. The greater the potency of a steroid, however, the greater the safety concerns. Skin hydration just before application increases absorption and effectiveness.

Topical steroids range in potency from low to high. Low-potency topical steroids are now available in over-the-counter (OTC) formulations (e.g., hydrocortisone, 0.5% or 1%) and in prescription strength (e.g., desonide, alclometasone). Generally, low-potency steroids are safe to use for longer periods of time and even on thin-skinned areas like the face, groin, or axilla. Prolonged use should still be monitored. Medium-potency (e.g., triamcinolone, fluocinolone) to high-potency (e.g., halcinonide, fluocinonide) corticosteroids should be used with caution and for short periods of time and not on the face, groin, or axilla. High-potency or super high-potency (e.g., betamethasone dipropionate, clobetasol) steroids should be reserved for use on acute or resistant dermatoses (e.g., contact dermatitis) or areas with thick plaque such as in psoriasis.

Clients should know the strength of the topical steroid they are using and its potential side effects. The lowest potency corticosteroid that is effective should be used. Side effects are more likely with prolonged use of medium-potency to high-potency topical corticosteroids. The most common side effect is skin atrophy, which presents as thin or shiny skin with increased prominence of blood vessels, telangiectases, and easy bruising. Other possible side effects include acne-like conditions, folliculitis, hypopigmentation, delayed wound healing, and striae.

Clients must clearly understand how, when, and where to use topical steroids. Properly applying the medication evenly and sparingly once or twice daily to the affected areas can eliminate many potential problems. More frequent application increases the chance of side effects, makes the therapy more costly, and does not usually increase effectiveness. The condition can recur if treatment is stopped abruptly. When the skin disease disappears or is under good control, a tar preparation, moisturizer, or other topical preparation may be substituted for the topical steroid.

especially in hot or humid weather, friction, heat, and moisture buildup result in maceration, erosions, fissures, itching, and burning. Skin folds prone to intertrigo are in the neck, axillae, antecubital fossae, the perineum finger and toe webs, abdomen, and beneath the breasts, particularly in obese clients. One of the most common causes of intertrigo is contamination with body fluids, as occurs in urinary incontinence. Secondary bacterial (*Pseudomonas* or *Staphylococcus*) or *Candida albicans* infection may occur. Whenever candidiasis is present, a careful evaluation is indicated. In an otherwise healthy person, candidiasis is a self-limiting disease that responds well to topical antifungal therapy; however, it can be the presenting manifestation of underlying systemic disease affecting the endocrine system (e.g., diabetes) or the immune system (e.g., immunodeficiency syndromes).

Treatment of intertrigo is to eliminate maceration by promoting drying and to aerate the body skinfolds. For mobile clients, review environmental changes that promote drying of the body folds, such as wearing loose-fitting cotton-blend clothing or periodic removal of clothing to dry off. Instruct clients to avoid tight-fitting clothing such as jeans as well as activities that promote sweating. Care recommendations depend on the degree of involvement and the overall condition of the skin. If the skin is still intact, recommendations include washing the area gently with tap water twice daily and then rinsing and drying the area, followed by sprinkling of a talc-containing powder or a cellulose-containing powder (e.g., Zeasorb) for extra absorption. Avoid using cornstarch in pure form because it encourages *C. albicans* overgrowth. Applying folded gauze or clean cotton handkerchiefs in skinfolds promotes healing by keeping skin surfaces apart. Wash cloths and paper towels should not be used; they do not wick drainage from the skin. Silver-impregnated dressings (e.g., InterDry), have been shown to work well for these skin folds. Apply cool, wet soaks with tap water or Burow's solution (an antiseptic) three to four times daily for removal of exudate if secondary infection is present.

If inflammation is present, a low-potency topical corticosteroid in a nonocclusive vehicle (e.g., hydrocortisone 1.0% or 2.5% cream or lotion) or a combination steroid-antibiotic-antifungal agent (Vytone 1%) may initially be helpful, but long-term use should be avoided (see the Client Education Guide on topical corticosteroids on p. 1204).

STASIS DERMATITIS

Stasis dermatitis is characterized by the development of areas of very dry, dark skin and sometimes shallow ulcers on the lower legs, primarily as a result of venous insufficiency. The dermatitis is treated with moisturizing agents and antihistamines; antifungal preparations may also be helpful. When fragile skin ulcerations are present, the wound is called a *venous stasis ulcer*. The treatment of these wounds is discussed in Chapter 53.

INCONTINENCE ASSOCIATED DERMATITIS

Dermatitis from exposure to urine or stool is called incontinence associated dermatitis (IAD). Risk factors include frequent exposure to urine or diarrheal stool and use of absorptive containment device. Secondary cutaneous infection (usually fungal) is common. When skin is exposed to urine, the urea is absorbed by the keratinocytes and once they are swollen, they cannot provide a barrier. The skin also develops an odor of ammonia. Diarrhea contains digestive enzymes that denude the skin.

These skin ulcers can be confused with pressure ulcers and may coexist with pressure ulcers. IAD ulcers are diffuse, often occurring as multiple areas of open skin in the perineum and perineal skin folds. They are partial thickness ulcers and do not develop necrotic tissue.

Treatment of IAD begins by determining the reason for the incontinence, for example, urinary tract infection. Skin must be kept clean by quickly cleansing incontinent clients. Reduce exposure of the skin to irritants. Keep the skin moisturized and provide a barrier on the skin by using wipes that contain dimethicone. It is most efficient and effective to keep the skin care products at the beside.

PSORIASIS VULGARIS

Psoriasis vulgaris is a chronic, recurrent, erythematous, inflammatory disorder with a worldwide distribution. The prevalence varies according to race and geographic location. Psoriasis occurs equally in both genders, usually starting in the early 20s to 40s. The Latin *vulgaris* (from *vulgus,* or "the public") means "common" and does not refer to "vulgar." Psoriasis is a genetic systemic disease with an immunologic basis that frequently manifests in the skin and joints.

Pathophysiology

T cells are one of the immune cells. In psoriasis, hordes of activated T cells are found in psoriatic skin and almost none in healthy skin. These activated T cells secrete interleukin-6, which has as one of its effects the ability to stimulate skin cell growth. A normal skin cell matures and is shed in 28 to 30 days, but a psoriatic skin cell takes only 3 to 4 days to mature and move to the surface. Instead of shedding, the cells pile up and form lesions.

Clinical Manifestations

The epidermis thickens with extra skin cells, and blood vessels dilate with increased blood supply to nourish those cells. At the surface, skin cells pile up. Dead cells create a white, flaky layer of silvery white scales over the patch of inflamed skin.

The eruptions (usually in a symmetrical distribution) commonly occur on the scalp, elbows, knees, genital,

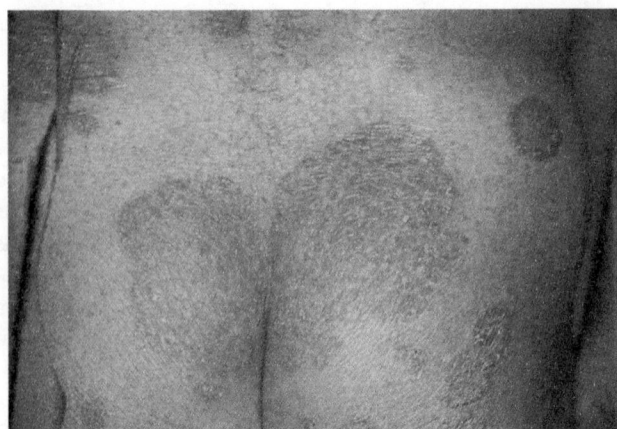

■ **FIGURE 49–3** Plaque psoriasis of the buttocks.

and sacral regions (Figure 49-3). Lesions may develop at the site of an injury, which is known as *Koebner's phenomenon.* A generalized eruption may occur with severe psoriasis vulgaris. Another type is palmar plantar psoriasis, which can be pustular or of a plaque type and only affects the palms and soles. In a rare form of psoriasis, known as *pustular psoriasis,* generalized, sterile cutaneous pustules are produced. Severe systemic involvement can be fatal. Up to one third of clients with moderate to severe psoriasis have psoriatic arthritis, which primarily affects the distal joints and may be deforming. Nail dystrophies and pitting occur frequently.

OUTCOME MANAGEMENT

The course of psoriasis vulgaris is unpredictable. It can be controlled with aggressive therapies but cannot be cured. Exacerbations and remissions are common. As with other chronic diseases, changes in physical and emotional health can precede flares. The goals of medical management of psoriasis are to decrease the T-cell counts in the epidermis, control the rate of epidermal cell turnover, and monitor for complications of therapy. Some individuals also may have associated psoriatic arthritis. In this group, selecting the appropriate treatment option is necessary to provide adequate pain relief and possibly reduce or prevent joint destruction.

Medical Management

Suppress T-Cell Activation

Steroids can be used to suppress the immune system (see the Client Education Guide Topical Corticosteroids on p. 1204). Injecting small, dilute amounts of corticosteroids (e.g., triamcinolone acetonide) into or just beneath a lesion gives a high drug concentration at the injection site. Systemic steroids are contraindicated in psoriasis. Tazarotene is a retinoid derivative that very commonly causes irritation and as such is typically used in conjunction with a topical steroid. Retinoid derivatives

alter the delayed hypersensitivity response and increase the number of Langerhans cells in the psoriatic lesion. For plaque psoriasis, retinoids can be used in combination with ultraviolet phototherapy to minimize the dose of each. Keratolytic agents (e.g., salicylic acid) may remove scales and allow greater penetration of topical agents. Anthralin reduces mitotic action in the cell and is an effective topical agent for treatment of psoriasis with widespread discrete lesions consisting primarily of thick plaques, but it is rarely used in the United States because of its complicated protocol. Calcipotriene is a synthetic vitamin D_3 analog that regulates skin cell production; however, it is not in widespread use.

Promote Desquamation

Artificial forms of ultraviolet light (UVL) are used therapeutically with topical or systemic photosensitizing drugs to cause desquamation (shedding or peeling of the epidermis). Ultraviolet A (UVA) light and ultraviolet B (UVB) light are used to treat diseases responsive to UVL, such as psoriasis, vitiligo, cutaneous T-cell lymphoma, uremic pruritus, and chronic eczematous eruptions. At present, two treatment modalities involve UVL: (1) broadband and narrowband UVB and (2) photochemotherapy, or PUVA (psoralen plus UVA). Initially, many of these regimens are given two or three times a week with the frequency decreased to two to four times per month for maintenance.

Obtaining a complete history and physical examination in every client before initiation of any UVL therapy is very important. One must take care to include the complete medication history, because the client may be taking one or more of the many photosensitizing drugs (e.g., thiazide diuretics, tetracycline). Ask clients specifically about previous herpes simplex infections, which can be reactivated by UVL. Pretreatment assessment includes identifying solar energy–induced skin malignancies, premalignant lesions, cataracts, or lupus erythematosus and any additional photodamage. Potential benefit must be weighed against potential risk. The skin changes of lupus erythematosus (LE) are worsened by sun exposure, and phototherapy is thus contraindicated. If LE is suspected, an antinuclear antibody (ANA) test should be obtained to rule out this condition before therapy is initiated.

A complete ophthalmologic examination before full body box treatment begins is important and should be performed yearly during long-term treatment. A history of cataract formation is a potential contraindication to PUVA therapy. Clients who exhibit early cataract changes need extra photoprotective measures (e.g., the complete occlusion provided by goggles or PUVA glasses) and more frequent ophthalmologic assessments (every 3 to 6 months).

Because UVL treatments add to the cumulative effects of natural and artificial UVL, minimize exposure by shielding the head, face, and male genitalia to reduce the risk of skin cancers. Periodic assessments must be done throughout the course of therapy for manifestations of actinic damage (e.g., severe wrinkling, "tissue paper" transparency) or cutaneous malignancy. All phototherapy should be administered by qualified and well-trained dermatologic personnel. Use of home UVL equipment and tanning salons should be considered only when the client has no access to qualified dermatologic personnel. Numerous risks and significantly diminished responses are associated with home and salon therapy.

Ultraviolet Light B Therapy

UVB therapy requires no oral medications and is usually the first-line UVL therapy used before progression to PUVA. Types of UVB therapy include (1) broadband or narrowband UVB treatment as monotherapy and (2) broadband or narrowband UVB in combination with topicals (tar, anthralin, calcipotriene, corticosteroids, or tazarotene). Topical anthralin and tar used with UVB are mainly of historical interest because they have generally been replaced by newer developments that are reimbursable and that are not as time-consuming.

Photochemotherapy

Photochemotherapy (PUVA) combines oral or topical 8-methoxypsoralen with UVA. PUVA is used to treat severe, unresponsive forms of psoriasis, atopic dermatitis, cutaneous T-cell lymphoma, graft-versus-host disease, and alopecia areata or vitiligo. The potent systemic photosensitizing medications (psoralens) used in PUVA increase skin sensitivity to long-wave UVL (UVA). In conjunction with exposure to artificially reproduced forms of UVA light, these medications induce repigmentation (melanin production) in vitiligo and have an antimitotic effect and reduce T-cell population in psoriasis and cutaneous T-cell lymphoma.

The skin and eyes must be protected from ambient UVL irradiation from the time psoralens are ingested until 8 hours after taking the photosensitizing medication. The client should (1) wear protective clothing, such as long sleeves, (2) apply sunscreen to exposed skin, (3) minimize natural skin exposure with topical psoralen, and (4) wear both UVA and UVB protective eyewear for 24 hours after taking the medication when outside or in an automobile.

Areas that are difficult to treat, such as the scalp and nails, remain a challenge. Scalp care in psoriasis consists of reducing scales and treating inflammation. Clients are instructed to avoid picking and scratching. Use of steroids and oil vehicles under occlusion is often necessary to enhance percutaneous absorption; on the scalp, a plastic shower cap can be used for this purpose. Other products such as tars, medicated shampoos, and

nonsteroidal treatments also play an important role in scalp care. There is no consistently effective treatment of psoriatic involvement of the nails. Tazarotene is showing promising results in reducing nail dystrophy. However, the scalp and nails do improve with clearing of psoriasis on the body surface.

Systemic treatments are being increasingly prescribed for psoriasis affecting 10% or more of the body surface area. Systemic agents are used to block the activation of T cells and prevent the migration of T cells into the skin. Agents include acitretin, methotrexate, and cyclosporine. Methotrexate and cyclosporine are potentially toxic to the renal, hepatic, and hematopoietic systems. Thus baseline assessment (e.g., blood chemistry, complete blood count, liver biopsy) is important before this medication is started. During treatment, periodic assessments are needed, including biopsy of the liver. If any serious side effects develop, such as bone marrow depression or gastrointestinal tract bleeding, treatment is discontinued. To limit potential liver damage, advise the client not to consume alcohol throughout therapy. Because methotrexate may cause chromosomal abnormalities, effective birth control methods are important for both women and men before and during treatment and for 3 months after completing methotrexate. Nausea, the most common side effect, can be limited by taking methotrexate with food, using prophylactic antiemetics, and adding supplemental folic acid.

Biologic drugs are the newest drugs in managing psoriasis and psoriatic arthritis and include etanercept, alefacept, efalizumab, and infliximab. This class of drugs is injected or infused and require specific monitoring.

Self-Care

Assist the client in coping with an altered self-concept. Psoriatic disease can have enormously negative effect on client quality of life, causing depression, disrupting work, and producing economic hardships. The appearance of skin lesions may make the client feel "dirty" or untouchable. Because open lesions are at high risk for secondary infection, the client should be taught to keep the creams or ointments on and to keep the area clean and dry. To keep psoriasis in remission, the client needs to control the causative factors. Stress should be minimized, and illness and infection should be treated early.

ACNE VULGARIS

Acne vulgaris is a common, multifactorial follicular disorder that affects pilosebaceous follicles, primarily of the face, neck, and upper trunk. It is characterized by both noninflammatory and inflammatory lesions. Acne is the most common chronic skin disease, affecting up to 85% of the population between the ages of 12 and 25. Genetic influences may determine client's susceptibility and severity of disease. Numerous topical and systemic drugs are available for the treatment of acne vulgaris; see a pediatric nursing textbook for further discussion.

ACNE ROSACEA

Acne rosacea is a chronic inflammatory skin eruption characterized by erythema, papules, pustules, and telangiectases. It occurs on the face, especially the cheeks and over the bridge of the nose. The onset is insidious, usually occurring between 30 and 50 years of age, and women are affected more frequently than men. It is more common in fair-skinned people with a history of easy facial flushing. Precipitating factors that appear to make the flushing worse include tea, coffee, alcohol (especially wine), caffeine-containing products, sunlight, extremes of hot and cold, spicy foods, and emotional stress.

Sebaceous hyperplasia of the nose (rhinophyma) often develops after many years of chronic acne rosacea. This condition results from chronic inflammation with an increase in the amount of connective tissue and may be mistaken for an indication of excessive alcohol consumption. Ocular changes such as eyelid inflammation and conjunctivitis may occur.

Avoidance of the stimuli that trigger acne rosacea may be sufficient for management of mild forms of the disorder. Treatment of rosacea is sometimes difficult. The topical agents generally used include antibiotics, metronidazole (MetroGel), and retinoids. Systemic drugs include antibiotics, isotretinoin, and metronidazole, but the pros and cons of using these must be weighed.

SKIN TEARS

Skin tears are wounds resulting from separation of the epidermis from the underlying connective tissue. The most common sites for skin tears, in order of frequency, are the forearm, hand, elbow, and upper arm. Skin tears are most common in older adults as a result of a thinning of the epidermis, a flattening of the dermal-epidermal junction, and a reduced adhesion of the dermis to the epidermis. They are very common in clients who have taken long-term oral steroids for conditions such as emphysema. Skin tears often result from trauma, such as falls and injury from wheelchair handles or brakes or injury that incurred during transfer to a chair. Even though the actual skin damage is minor, families and residents are disturbed by the presence of skin tears, often perceiving the injury as resulting from abuse.

OUTCOME MANAGEMENT

For tears with small to moderate losses of epidermal tissue, irrigate the wound with normal saline to remove blood or debris. Replace any flaps of epidermis and secure with strips of paper tape. Cover the open

wound with nonocclusive, moisture-retentive dressing such as petrolatum-impregnated gauze or opaque foam dressing. Do not use adherent clear dressings; when these dressings are removed, the skin can tear again. Table 49-1 shows how to select an appropriate dressing.

Prevention is important. Use protective gloves on the client's hands and soft armrests on wheelchairs, and train caregivers in proper transfer techniques (e.g., use of transfer belts). Daily assessment by unlicensed assistive personnel is critical to identify lesions early. The Management and Delegation feature on p. 1209 describes reportable skin abnormalities.

PRESSURE ULCERS

A pressure ulcer is localized injury to the skin and/or underlying tissue, usually over a bony prominence, as a result of pressure or pressure in combination with

TABLE 49-1 Choosing a Dressing for a Wound

Desired Purpose	Dressing Options
Prevent contamination of puncture sites	Transparent dressings
Prevent contamination from stool/urine	Skin protection with dimethicone
	Topical pastes and creams (dressing often lift up at the edges)
Prevent injury periulcer skin from frequent dressing changes	Hydrocolloids for window frame around wound
	Tubular gauze to hold dressing in place
Prevent injury to intact skin	Transparent dressings
Prevent injury to intact blisters	Lightly adhesive foams if removed often
Absorb drainage from incisions	Gauze and combination dressings
Absorb exudate from deep wounds	Alginate rope or dressings
	Foams
	Gauze packing
Control infection	Products with silver or iodine
	Dressings soaked with antibiotic solutions
Control odor	Products with iodine, silver, activated charcoal, or diluted Dakin's solution
	Crushed metronidazole
Control pain	Hydrogels
	Adaptic gauze
	Mepitel
Promote tissue hydration	Transparent dressings and films
	Hydrocolloids
	Gels
Promote autolytic debridement	Gels
	Transparent dressings and films
Conform to irregular body areas	Extra thin types of hydrocolloids
	Extra thin layers of foams
	Transparent films
Conform to depth for packing	Gels
	Rope alginate
	Gauze strips (do not pack deep wounds with single dressings)

Skin Inspection

Unlicensed assistive personnel frequently are in the position to observe the skin of clients as they assist with various activities of daily living and provide assistance with personal hygiene. Be sure to fully delineate their role in identifying and reporting skin abnormalities. Reportable findings are listed as follows.

Bruising or a change in skin color. Ecchymosis, erythema, jaundice, and pallor may indicate a serious disease process or acute deep tissue injury. Identification of these changes in skin color by unlicensed assistive personnel should be immediately reported to you for thorough assessment and intervention. Redness overlying bony structures may indicate prolonged or undue pressure. Purple areas over bony prominences or pressure prone areas may indicate deep tissue injury. Unlicensed assistive personnel should ensure pressure relief by assisting the client with frequent position changes.

Lumps. Assess any skin lesion or growth in further detail.

Dry, scaling, or cracked skin. Dry skin may indicate dehydration or other integumentary disorders. You may delegate the application of over-the-counter lotions to unlicensed assistive personnel if the skin is not broken. Some clients may need specific lubricants or medications prescribed by a physician; therefore have any findings of dry skin reported to you.

Skin that feels excessively moist and cool or excessively warm. It is appropriate for unlicensed assistive personnel to cover clients with extra bedding if they feel cool or to offer cool compresses for warm skin (see Chapter 27). Be certain that the client is not febrile. Localized areas of warmth may indicate underlying processes that need prompt attention. Clearly communicate that any of these findings should be immediately reported to you for prompt assessment and intervention.

Any break in the skin with drainage or bleeding. You may delegate the application of sterile gauze to the surface of the skin to unlicensed assistive personnel for the purpose of containing drainage (see Chapter 14). Skin tears should be treated with nonstick dressings. Assess such skin abnormalities promptly after identification by unlicensed assistive personnel.

Taut or shiny skin. This finding may indicate fluid shifting from the intravascular space. Such skin is susceptible to breakdown and infection. Employ proactive measures to prevent any undue pressure or damage to the skin. Assess the area carefully, and report any unknown disorders or significant change to a physician. Elevate the area to decrease swelling if present.

Client complaints of itching or tenderness. Instruct unlicensed assistive personnel identifying such client complaints to communicate these findings to you promptly. Assess the client for potential allergic reaction, an underlying tissue pathologic process, or the need for additional analgesics.

Rashes. New rashes or other skin eruptions sometimes suggest allergic reactions. Instruct that such findings be reported to you promptly.

You are ultimately responsible for thorough, ongoing assessment and evaluation of integument.

shear and/or friction. Although pressure ulcers are most common over bony prominences, they can be located in any area of the body that is subjected to pressure, shear, or friction. Pressure ulcers have also been called "bed sores" and "decubitus ulcers." The word *decubitus* comes from the Latin *decumbere,* which means to lie down. The ulcers were so named because they are common in bedridden clients.

Etiology and Risk Factors

Classically, pressure ulcers develop when soft tissues (skin, subcutaneous tissue, and muscle) are compressed between a bony prominence and a firm surface for a prolonged period. Recently, deep tissue injury pressure ulcers have been identified. These pressure ulcers develop during shorter periods of intense pressure, with the major site of injury initially being in the muscle. Therefore immobility and inactivity are major risk factors. In bedridden clients, infrequent turning and repositioning or lack of padding between surfaces that touch (e.g., knees) may lead to tissue damage. In addition, clients in bed are often positioned in semi-Fowler position to facilitate breathing or eating. This position increases the risk of ulcers on the sacrum and heels. The ischia are common sites of pressure ulcers in chairbound clients, especially if they sit erect in the chair. The length of time of exposure to pressure before skin breakdown varies among clients; in very debilitated clients, permanent tissue damage can result in less than 2 hours. Cognitive or sensory impairments also increase risk because the client cannot recognize the need to turn or move.

Protein-calorie malnutrition is another major risk factor. Malnourished clients have poor skin integrity, and their skin is damaged easily. In addition, incontinence, friction, and skin shearing can also lead to breakdown. These factors reduce the tolerance the skin has for pressure.

The reported incidence (number of new cases per year) of pressure ulcers in acute care facilities ranges from 2.7% to 29.5%. The prevalence (number of cases at one point in time) in acute care settings ranges from 3.5% to 29.5%. Several populations are at increased risk. Quadriplegic clients, older adults with femoral fractures, and clients in critical care units have the highest risk. Prevention of pressure ulcers begins with identifying the client at risk. Risk factors can be determined by assessing sensory perception, moisture, activity, mobility, nutrition, friction, and shear. Risk for pressure ulcers can be expressed numerically by using an instrument to appraise risk such as the Braden or Norton tool (see later discussion).

Pathophysiology

Pressure on soft tissues between bony prominences and external surfaces (mattress, chair) compresses capillaries and occludes blood flow. If the pressure is relieved, a brief period of rebound capillary dilation (called *reactive hyperemia*) occurs, and there is no tissue damage. If pressure is not relieved, microthrombi form in capillaries and completely occlude blood flow. A blister may form initially. When the blister breaks, an open wound is present. The open wound is rapidly colonized with surface bacteria. These bacteria can proliferate and cause a biofilm to develop. Today, slough in the wound is known to be a biofilm of bacteria covered by a surface that is not easily penetrated by antibiotics.

During periods of intense pressure it is hypothesized that the muscle becomes ischemic, resulting in necrosis of the injured muscle. The leakage of old blood causes the overlying skin to become purple. The necrotic tissue develops into eschar.

Healing occurs through secondary intention. Granulation tissue fills the base of full-thickness ulcers. Contraction of the ulcer edges closes the wound. Eventually, epithelial cells cover the wound. Stage III and IV pressure ulcers often require debridement and surgery to close the wound. Scar tissue predominates in ulcers that close without surgery.

Clinical Manifestations

The clinical manifestations of pressure ulcers have been described in four stages (Figure 49-4). Stage I is characterized by intact skin with nonblanchable redness of a localized area, usually over a bony prominence. Darkly pigmented skin may not have visible blanching, but its color may differ from the surrounding area. The area may be painful, firm or soft, and warmer or cooler compared with adjacent tissue. Stage I may be difficult to detect in clients with dark skin tones. This stage, considered a heralding sign, may indicate the client is at risk for pressure ulcers.

A stage II pressure ulcer is characterized by partial-thickness loss of dermis presenting as a shallow, open ulcer with a reddish-pink wound bed without slough. An ulcer at this stage may also present as an intact (serum-filled) or open (ruptured) blister. The wound is shiny or dry and shallow, without slough or bruising. (Bruising suggests a likelihood of deep tissue injury.) This stage should not be used to describe skin tears, tape burns, perineal dermatitis, maceration, or excoriation.

Ulcers classified as stage III are wounds that have full-thickness tissue loss. Subcutaneous fat may be visible, but bone, tendon, and muscle are not exposed. Slough may be present but does not obscure the depth of tissue loss. These ulcers may include undermining and tunneling. The depth of a stage III pressure ulcer varies by anatomic location. Ulcers most commonly occur on the sacrum, heel, greater trochanter, and ischial tuberosities. The bridge of the nose, ear, occiput, and malleolus do not have subcutaneous tissue, so stage III ulcers can be shallow. In contrast, areas of significant adiposity can

---

Stage I

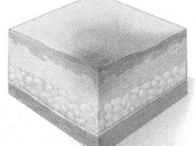

Intact skin with non-blanchable redness of a localized area usually over a bony prominence. Darkly pigmented skin may not have visible blanching; its color may differ from the surrounding area

The area may be painful, firm, soft, warmer, or cooler as compared to adjacent tissue. Stage I may be difficult to detect in individuals with dark skin. May indicate "at risk" persons (a heralding sign of risk)

Stage II

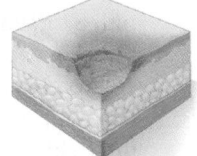

Partial-thickness loss of dermis presenting as a shallow open ulcer with a red pink wound bed, without slough. May also present as an intact or open/ruptured serum-filled blister

Presents as a shiny or dry shallow ulcer without slough or bruising.* This stage should not be used to describe skin tears, tape burns, perineal dermatitis, maceration, or excoriation

*Bruising indicates suspected deep-tissue injury

Stage III

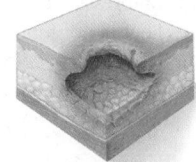

Full-thickness tissue loss. Subcutaneous fat may be visible but bone, tendon, or muscle are not exposed. Slough may be present but does not obscure the depth of tissue loss. May include undermining and tunneling

The depth of a stage III pressure ulcer varies by anatomical location. The bridge of the nose, ear, occiput, and malleolus do not have subcutaneous tissue, and stage III ulcers can be shallow. In contrast, areas of significant adiposity can develop extremely deep stage III pressure ulcers. Bone/tendon is not visible or directly palpable

Stage IV

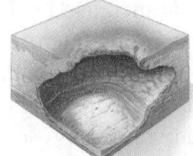

Full-thickness tissue loss with exposed bone, tendon, or muscle. Slough or eschar may be present on some parts of the wound bed. Often includes undermining and tunneling

The depth of a stage IV pressure ulcer varies by anatomical location. The bridge of the nose, ear, occiput, and malleolus do not have subcutaneous tissue and these ulcers can be shallow. Stage IV ulcers can extend into muscle and/or supporting structures (e.g., fascia, tendon, or joint capsule), making osteomyelitis possible. Exposed bone/tendon is visible or directly palpable

Unstageable

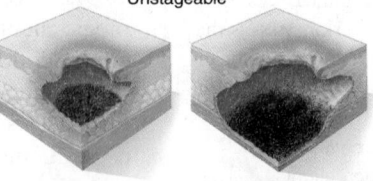

Full-thickness tissue loss in which the base of the ulcer is covered by slough (yellow, tan, gray, green, or brown) and/or eschar (tan, brown, or black) in the wound bed

Until enough slough and/or eschar is removed to expose the base of the wound, the true depth, and therefore stage, cannot be determined. Stable (dry, adherent, intact without erythema or fluctuance) eschar on the heels serves as the body's natural (biological) cover and should not be removed

Deep tissue injury

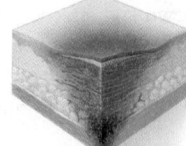

Purple or maroon localized area of discolored intact skin or blood-filled blister due to damage of underlying soft tissue from pressure and/or shear. The area may be preceded by tissue that is painful, firm, mushy, boggy, warmer, or cooler as compared to adjacent tissue

Deep-tissue injury may be difficult to detect in individuals with dark skin. Evolution may include thin blister over a dark wound bed. The wound may further evolve and become covered by thin eschar. Evolution may be rapid, exposing additional layers of tissue even with optimal treatment

■ **FIGURE 49–4** Stages of pressure ulcers.

develop extremely deep stage III pressure ulcers. Bone and tendon are neither visible nor directly palpable.

Stage IV ulcers show full-thickness tissue loss with exposed bone, tendon, or muscle. Slough or eschar may be present on some parts of the wound bed, and undermining and tunneling are often evident. The depth of a stage IV pressure ulcer varies by anatomic location. The bridge of the nose, ear, occiput, and malleolus do not have subcutaneous tissue, so these ulcers can be shallow. Stage IV ulcers can extend into muscle or supporting structures, such as fascia, tendon, and joint capsules, making osteomyelitis possible. Exposed bone or tendon is visible or directly palpable.

Some pressure ulcers cannot be staged because the bottom of the ulcer cannot be seen. These unstageable ulcers are characterized by full-thickness tissue loss in which the base of the ulcer is covered by slough (yellow, tan, gray, green, or brown) and/or eschar (tan, brown, or black) in the wound bed. Until enough slough or eschar is removed to expose the base of the wound, the true depth, and therefore the stage, cannot be determined. Some pressure ulcers will be "unstageable" for a long time, because the eschar provides a "biologic dressing." This is seen in stable (dry, adherent, and intact, without erythema or fluctuation ("buoyant") eschar on the heels, which serves as the body's natural (biological) cover and should not be removed.

Deep tissue injury is a new stage of pressure ulcers. Deep tissue injury is a purple or maroon localized area of discolored intact skin or blood-filled blister due to damage of underlying soft tissue from pressure and/or shear. This ulcer may be preceded by tissue that is painful, firm, mushy, boggy, and warmer or cooler as compared with adjacent tissue. Deep tissue injury may be difficult to detect in individuals with dark skin tones. Evolution may include a thin blister over a dark wound bed. The wound may further evolve and become covered by thin eschar. Evolution may be rapid, exposing additional layers of tissue even with optimal treatment.

Terminal ulcers, sometimes referred to as "Kennedy terminal ulcers," are pressure ulcers seen near the time of death. They are due to pressure in very poorly perfused skin and may represent "skin failure," especially because they are noted in conjunction with failure of other organs, such as the heart and lungs.

With pressure ulcers, few additional diagnostic assessments are required. Nurses can stage pressure ulcers based on their appearance. Sometimes osteomyelitis is present in deep wounds. Bone scans are used for confirming this problem. If malnutrition is suspected as a cause, serum protein, albumin, or prealbumin levels may be monitored. It is important to distinguish pressure ulcers from other wounds, such as arterial or venous ulcers. See Chapter 53 for a discussion of these wounds.

Medical Management

Management of the client with a pressure ulcer begins with a complete history and physical examination. There are many causes of delayed wound healing, and delayed healing of pressure ulcers may be the result of other health problems. The goal of medical management is to heal the ulcer by redistributing pressure over the ulcer (sometimes called decreasing tissue load), cleaning and dressing the wound, and improving nutrition. In addition, the ulcer is monitored for healing, and the client is monitored for complications.

Decrease Tissue Load

The term *tissue load* refers to the distribution of pressure, friction, and shear on the tissues. Interventions are designed to decrease tissue load and thereby decrease pressure. Increasing the frequency of turning helps disperse pressure over time. Clients should not lie on a pressure ulcer. Restricting blood flow to the ulcer delays healing. If the ulcer is on the sacrum, sitting should be reduced to 1 to 2 hours at a time and only for meals. If the client can turn or be repositioned so as not to lie on a pressure ulcer, a pressure-redistributing overlay may be placed on the mattress. However, these overlay devices can be compressed by the client's weight, and rendered ineffective. Check for bottoming out when using overlay mattresses (Figure 49-5). Special low-pressure beds may be required for clients with pressure ulcers on two or more turning surfaces (Figure 49-6). Heels should be floated from the bed by placing pillows under the calf or using pressure reduction boots. Chair cushions should be used if the client is sitting in a chair or getting up to a chair; 4 inches of foam is effective. In addition, clients who sit in chairs need to be repositioned hourly. Specialty cushions also exist for wheelchair-dependent clients.

Provide Ulcer Care

Moist, devitalized tissue supports bacterial growth. Therefore devitalized tissue must be removed from the ulcer. Several forms of debridement can be used depending on the client's goals and the type of wound. *Sharp debridement* is the use of a scalpel to excise devitalized thick, adherent eschar; this form of debridement is completed in the operating room by the physician. *Conservative sharp* debridement is carried out at the bedside using a scalpel and forceps to remove loose necrotic tissue. This form of debridement is done by trained personnel. *Mechanical debridement* is the use of wet-to-dry dressings, hydrotherapy, and high-pressure

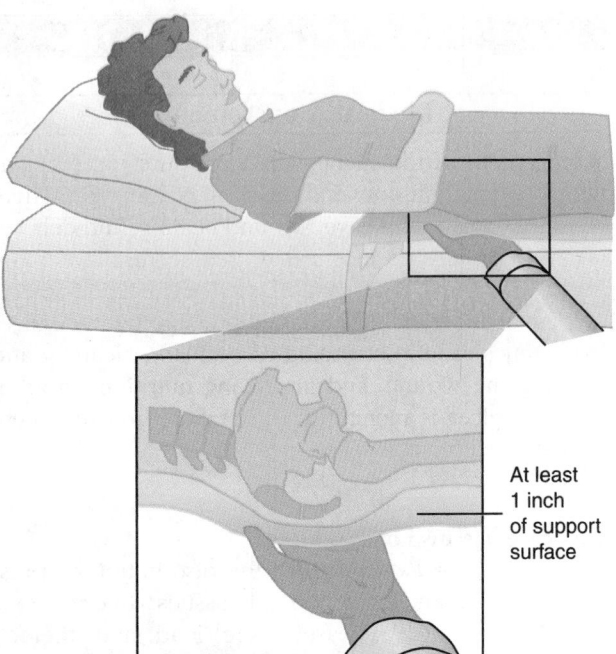

At least
1 inch
of support
surface

■ **FIGURE 49–5**   Assessment of pressure relief ("bottoming out"). Slide your hand (palm up and fingers flat) under the support surface, just under the pressure point. Do not flex your fingers. With adequate support, there will be at least 1 inch of uncompressed support surface between your hand and the client's body. *(Modified from Gaymar Industries, Inc., Orchard Park, NY.)*

wound irrigation to soften and remove devitalized tissues. *Enzymatic debridement* is the use of topical debriding agents to dissolve the collagen anchors that hold the necrotic slough tissue to the wound bed. *Biodebridement* is the use of sterile larvae (maggots), which secrete enzymes that digest wound tissue. Honey may also be used as a biodebriding agent. Finally, *autolytic debridement* involves the use of synthetic dressings to cover an ulcer, allowing enzymes in the wound bed to digest the devitalized tissues. This form of debridement is the slowest and is usually reserved for clients who cannot tolerate the other forms. Some ulcers should not be debrided, for example, ulcers on limbs where perfusion is insufficient to support healing and dry, stable eschar on heels. Stable eschar is hard and intact. If the eschar becomes soft, cracks, or exposes underlying open skin, it should be removed. Sharp, conservative debridement is painful; the client should be given analgesics before debridement begins. Some clients report burning pain with the enzymatic debriding agents.

Improve Nutrition

The association of malnutrition with pressure ulcer formation and delayed healing is clear. In fact, many clinicians believe that pressure ulcers are a specific indicator of malnutrition. If the client's serum albumin or prealbumin concentration is low, if the client is not eating, or if the client's body weight is less than 80% of ideal, consider nutritional supplementation. If the client has no gastrointestinal disorders and can swallow, provide oral supplements. Some clinicians use the phrase "if the gut works, use it" to summarize this recommendation. If the client cannot swallow without aspiration, tube-feeding may be required. If the client has digestive problems, consider total parenteral nutrition. These more aggressive forms of feeding must be compatible with the client's wishes, but in many cases a few weeks

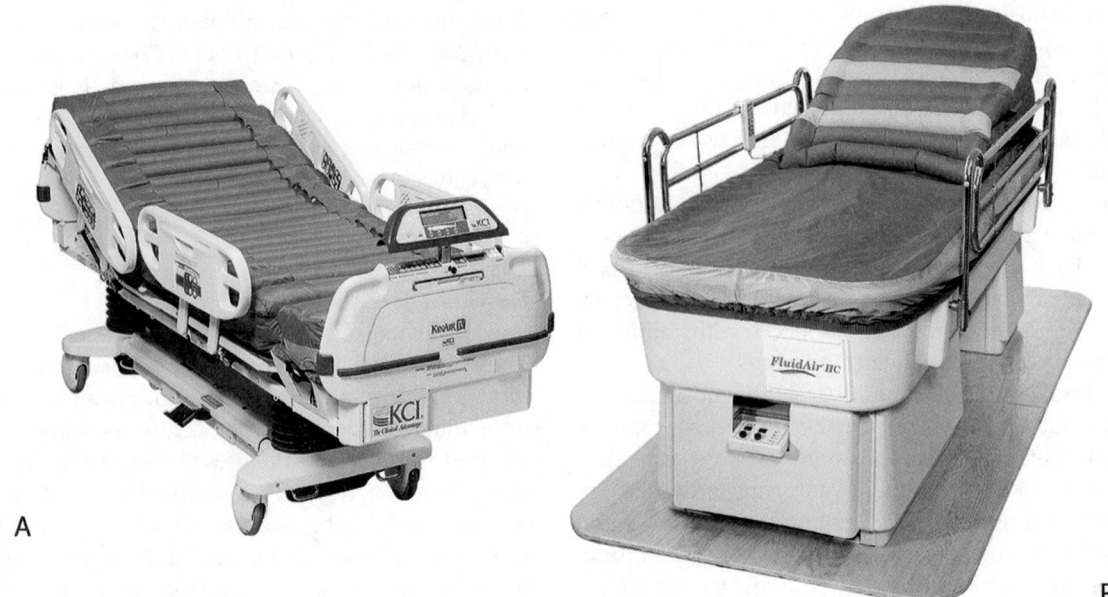

A

B

■ **FIGURE 49–6**   Pressure redistribution surfaces. **A,** KinAir beds provide controlled air suspension to redistribute body weight away from bony prominences. **B,** FluidAir beds use air flow and bead fluidization. Both of these beds are covered with Gore-Tex fabric, which resists tearing. This fabric is also water-proof and acts as a barrier against bacteria. *(Courtesy KCI Licensing, Inc., 2008.)*

of improved nutrition can "jump start" healing. Monitor nutritional status with repeated measurement of prealbumin, weight monitoring, or calorie counts. If tube-feeding must be stopped several times a day for medications or treatments, consider increasing the rate during the nighttime.

Monitor Healing

If the ulcer does not heal within 2 weeks despite adequate nutrition, pressure redistribution, daily cleaning, and use of appropriate dressings, the ulcer may be infected. An infected pressure ulcer looks like any other infected wound, with foul-smelling drainage, increasing size, increasing pain in the wound, and fever or elevation in white blood cell count. Older clients do not invariably demonstrate all of the manifestations of infection and are at risk for development of confusion; therefore vigilance in assessing the ulcer for changes is critical. If infection is suspected, a 2-week trial of topical antibiotics is considered. Swab cultures are not appropriate for diagnosis of infection in the ulcer, but can be used to diagnose heavy colonization or the presence of antibiotic resistance bacteria. Use a quantitative culture for suspected infection. Systemic antibiotics are used when the infection cannot be controlled locally or for systemic infection (manifested by fever or positive blood cultures).

Many conditions are associated with delays in healing. Diabetes, paralysis, and arterial diseases require close assessment because of increased risk of infection as a result of reduced blood flow to the wound. Urine and bowel incontinence lead to dermatitis and can contaminate open wounds.

Monitor for Complications

Many complications have been associated with pressure ulcers, including osteomyelitis, bacteremia and sepsis, and cellulitis. Wounds with osteomyelitis usually do not heal; if they do heal, they soon open again. The wound may become increasingly painful and drainage may be foul, often infected with *S. aureus, Enterobacter* species, and *Pseudomonas* species. Sepsis can follow osteomyelitis; confusion, reduced levels of consciousness, fever, hypotension, elevated white blood cell count, and other manifestations of septic shock may develop. The word *cellulitis* literally means "inflammation of the cells." It generally indicates an acute spreading infection of the dermis and subcutaneous tissues, resulting in pain, erythema, edema, and warmth. Associated red streaking visible in skin proximal to the area of cellulitis is characteristic of ascending lymphangitis. Cellulitis characterized by violaceous color and bullae suggests infection with *Streptococcus pneumoniae* (pneumococcus).

Nursing Management of the Medical Client

Assessment. All clients should be assessed for risk of pressure ulcers on admission and then daily, depending upon the client's condition. Less frequent assessment may be done if the client's condition is stable. The assessment of the client at high risk for development of pressure ulcers should identify any specific risk factors. The Braden scale (Figure 49-7) is an assessment tool that assists the nurse in predicting which clients are at greatest risk. Assess laboratory values on hemoglobin, hematocrit, albumin, prealbumin, total protein, and lymphocytes to further identify risks related to protein calorie malnutrition.

Skin should be fully assessed on admission and on each shift. To fully assess skin, look between folds of skin, remove anti-embolic stockings or devices, and use a mirror to see the heels. Also assess under oxygen tubing, especially on the ears and the cheeks, beneath splints and other medical devices. Pressure ulcers beneath medical devices are commonly overlooked! If the bath has been delegated to an unlicensed assistive person, arrange a time when the skin can be fully assessed. Sometimes helping with the bath is a convenient means to do a full skin assessment.

If the client has a pressure ulcer on admission to the facility, it must be recorded. Note objective data about the pressure ulcer (i.e., stage, length, width, depth, wound bed appearance, drainage, and condition of periulcer tissue). Reassessment of the ulcer is completed each time dressings are changed or sooner if the ulcer shows manifestations of deterioration. Analyses of the trends in healing are an important step in assessment. Consider whether the ulcer is increasing in size or depth or is developing more purulent drainage or odor, or whether the periulcer tissue is showing manifestations of deterioration. These changes in the pressure ulcer indicate that it is deteriorating and a change in treatment is needed. The physician or wound nurse should be notified, unless the agency protocol allows independent changes in treatment.

Diagnosis, Outcomes, Intervention
Diagnosis: Risk for Impaired Skin Integrity. Traditionally, clients who score between 12 and 16 on the Braden risk assessment scale are considered at risk for pressure ulcers. Scores below 12 indicate a high risk. A newer approach to reduce risk is to examine each risk factor independently and not rely on the total risk score, but rather the subscale score. This nursing diagnosis is written as *Risk for Impaired Skin Integrity related to malnutrition, unrelieved pressure, and/or incontinence as evidenced by Braden total risk score or subscale score.*

Outcomes. The client will have reduced risk of impairment of skin integrity, as evidenced by no actual tissue breakdown and no persistent reddened areas.

RISK PREDICTORS FOR SKIN BREAKDOWN

Patient's Name _____

Evaluator's Name _____

	1	2	3	4
SENSORY PERCEPTION ability to respond to discomfort	**1. Completely limited:** Unresponsive to painful stimuli, either because of state of unconsciousness or severe sensory impairment, which limits ability to feel pain over most of body surface	**2. Very limited:** Responds only to painful stimuli (but not verbal commands) by opening eyes or flexing extremities. Cannot communicate discomfort verbally, OR has a sensory impairment which limits the ability to feel pain or discomfort over one half of body surface	**3. Slightly limited:** Responds to verbal commands by opening eyes and obeying some commands, but cannot always communicate discomfort or need to be turned, OR has some sensory impairment which limits ability to feel pain or discomfort in one or two extremities.	**4. No impairment:** Responds to verbal commands by obeying. Can communicate needs accurately. Has no sensory deficit which would limit ability to feel pain or discomfort
MOISTURE degree to which skin is exposed to moisture	**1. Very Moist:** Skin is kept moist almost constantly by perspiration and urine. Dampness is detected every time patient is moved or turned. Linen must be changed more than one time each shift	**2. Occasionally Moist:** Skin is frequently, but not always kept moist, linen must be changed two to three times every 24 hours	**3. Rarely Moist:** Skin is rarely moist more than three to four times a week, but linen does require changing at that time	**4. Never Moist:** Perspiration and incontinence are never a problem; linen changed at routine intervals only
ACTIVITY degree of physical activity	**1. Bedfast:** Confined to bed	**2. Chairfast:** Ability to walk severely impaired or nonexistent and must be assisted into chair or wheelchair. Is confined to chair or wheelchair when not in bed	**3. Walks occasionally:** Walks occasionally during day, but for very short distances, with or without assistance. Spends majority of each shift in bed or chair	**4. Walks frequently:** Walks a moderate distance at least once every 1 to 2 hours during waking hours
MOBILITY ability to change and control body position	**1. Completely Immobile:** Unable to make even slight changes in position without assistance	**2. Very limited:** Makes occasional slight changes in position without help but unable to make frequent or significant changes in position independently	**3. Slightly limited:** Makes frequent though slight changes in position without assistance but unable to make or maintain major changes in position independently	**4. No limitations:** Makes major and frequent changes in position without assistance
NUTRITION usual food intake pattern	**1. Very Poor:** Never eats a complete meal. Rarely eats more than 1/3 of any food offered. Intake of protein is negligible. Takes even fluids poorly. Does not take a liquid dietary supplement, OR is NPO and/or maintained on clear liquids or IV for more than 5 days	**2. Probably Inadequate:** Rarely eats a complete meal and generally eats only about one half of any food offered. Protein intake is poor. Occasionally will take a liquid dietary supplement, OR receiving less than optimum amount of liquid diet or tube feeding	**3. Adequate:** Eats over half of most meals. Eats moderate amount of protein source one to two times daily. Occasionally will refuse a meal. Will usually take a dietary supplement if offered OR is on a tube feeding or TPN regimen which probably meets most of nutritional needs	**4. Excellent:** Eats most of every meal. Never refuses a meal. Frequently eats between meals. Does not require a dietary supplementation
FRICTION AND SHEAR	**1. Problem:** Requires moderate to maximum assistance in moving. Complete lifting without sliding against sheets is impossible. Frequently slides down in bed or chair, requiring frequent repositioning with maximum assistance. Either spasticity, contractures or agitation leads to almost constant friction	**2. Potential Problem:** Moves feebly Independently or requires minimum assistance. Skin probably slides against bedsheets or chair to some extent when movement occurs. Maintains relatively good position in chair or bed most of time but occasionally slides down	**3. No Apparent Problem:** Moves in bed and in chair independently and has sufficient muscle strength to lift up completely during move. Maintains good position in bed or chair at all times	

Key: 16, minimum risk; 13–14, moderate risk; 12 or less, high risk; NPO, nothing by mouth; IV, intravenously; TPN, total parenteral nutrition.

FIGURE 49–7 The Braden Scale for evaluation of risk of pressure ulcers. (Courtesy Barbara Braden and Nancy Bergstrom, © 1988.)

Interventions. Preventive measures to reduce the risk of pressure ulcers cannot be overemphasized (Box 49-2). Interventions are chosen to match the specific risk factors present (Table 49-2). Shearing injury can happen quickly in clients who are in semi-Fowler position. These clients should be repositioned often to reduce the risk of shear injury to the sacral area. Flexing the knee gatch of the bed will also prevent shearing when the head is elevated. It is also important to float heels from the bed by placing pillows under the calves.

Clients who have been placed on pressure-redistribution surfaces cannot be considered to be free from pressure ulcer risk. These clients must still be turned side to side and the skin inspected during turning. If the skin manifests stage I pressure ulcers, the turning frequency must be increased. If the client has been turned every 2 hours and is still showing stage I pressure ulcers, a higher level of pressure-redistribution device (e.g., mattress replacement) should be applied to the bed or a bed replacement should be used (e.g., low-air-loss bed).

Adequate hydration and nutrition are also important aspects of pressure ulcer prevention. Ask the unlicensed assistive personnel to offer food and fluids often and to accurately record what food and fluids are consumed. Skin should be lubricated when dry, and skin vulnerable to damage from incontinence should be protected with skin barriers. Indwelling catheters are commonly used in acute care settings; however, the continued use of catheters increases the risk of urinary tract infection.

Evaluation. Outcomes should be met in 24 to 48 hours. Recall that skin integrity can be impaired in just 2 hours. Therefore several hours are needed to determine whether skin injury occurred before risk reduction measures are implemented. If so, a more aggressive prevention plan is needed.

Diagnosis: Impaired Skin Integrity. If the client has a pressure ulcer, state the nursing diagnosis as *Impaired Skin Integrity related to pressure ulcer secondary to prolonged immobility, malnutrition, and unrelieved pressure as evidenced by (add description of the ulcer).*

BOX 49-2 Interventions for Treatment of Pressure Ulcers

- Continue to reduce risk of pressure ulcers using appropriate interventions.
- Assess and manage pain associated with the ulcer and its care. Even though clients cannot report pain, they still may be able to feel pain.
- Position the client to stay off the ulcer. If there is no turning surface without a pressure ulcer, use a pressure-redistribution bed and continue to turn the client. Do not rely on the bed exclusively to move the client. The client still needs to be repositioned and turned. Establish a written turning schedule.
- Elevate heels off the bed by using pillows or heel elevation boots. Fleece heel covers do not relieve pressure, but they can reduce friction.
- Maintain the head of the bed at the lowest elevation consistent with the client's medical condition. If the client must have the head elevated to prevent aspiration, reposition into a 30-degree lateral position. Use a seat cushion in the chair, and assess for sacral ulcers daily. For dyspneic clients, position erect and assess for sacral and ischial ulcers daily.
- Use support cushions (4 inches of foam, gels, flotation cushions) for the wheelchair-bound client or for any client who prefers to sit. Teach wheelchair-bound clients to reposition themselves every 15 minutes.
- Use support surfaces for clients with multiple ulcers or when there is no position for the client that does not place the client on an ulcer. Consider upgrading the support surface for those who are not able to keep off the ulcer surface. Begin with a reactive or active surface or mattress overlay. Progress to low-air-loss beds or air-fluidized beds if the ulcer does not heal. Check for bottoming out beneath the mattress. Place your hand between the mattress and the bed. If you feel less than an inch between the client's body and the mattress surface, the support is not adequate.

- Ensure adequate dietary intake to prevent malnutrition and delayed healing. Review the dietitian's recommendations for caloric and protein needs. Communicate these recommendations to the physician as needed.
- Provide oral supplementation, tube-feeding, or hyperalimentation to achieve positive nitrogen balance. For many clients, the decision not to eat is an important one that can give a sense of control over some aspect of existence. However, pressure ulcers cannot heal in clients with severe malnutrition.
- Supplement the diet with vitamins and minerals. Vitamin C and zinc are commonly prescribed to support wound healing in clients who are not consuming adequate calories.
- Remove devitalized tissue from the wound bed, except in avascular tissue or on the heels. Begin by cleansing the ulcer bed with normal saline; then use the appropriate technique for debridement. Once the ulcer is free of devitalized tissue, apply dressings that keep the wound bed moist and the surrounding skin dry. Do not use occlusive dressings on ulcers that may be infected.
- Prevent the ulcer from being exposed to urine and feces. Use indwelling catheters, bowel containment systems, and topical creams or dressings to prevent contamination.
- Follow body substance isolation precautions; use clean gloves and clean dressings for wound care.
- Monitor healing.

If the ulcer does not show signs of healing in 2 weeks or if manifestations of infection develop, the treatments must change to reduce the risk of sepsis and osteomyelitis.

SAFETY

ALERT

TABLE 49–2   Interventions to Reduce Pressure Ulcer Risk Based on Braden Subscale Scores

	Score 3	Score 2	Score 1
Sensory perceptual	Remind client to turn self and remain in off-loaded positions. Examine position of paralyzed limbs to be certain they are not trapped or pinned and do not rest on each other. Float heels from bed.	Inspect skin every shift. Protect client from self-injury on side rails, opposite limb, tubing, devices/monitors.	Assess all bony prominences (occiput, scapulae, elbows, heels). If positioned with head of bed elevated for tube-feeding, position in 30-degree lateral position rather than always supine. Examine skin beneath medical devices every shift
Activity	Place bed setting on prevention mode. Consider physical therapy consult.	Use padding of at least 4 inches of foam or a wheelchair cushion in wheelchair. Reposition wheelchair-bound clients every hour. Teach clients who are able to shift their weight every 15 min.	Depending on other factors (e.g., whether this client can turn at all), consider an upscaled bed. Float heels from bed.
Mobility	Use side rails and trapeze to facilitate self-movement.	Turn every 2 hr or more often and inspect bony prominences for skin breakdown. Do not massage red areas. Use pillows to keep bony prominences apart.	Turn every 2 hr using a written schedule for consistency. Consider an upscaled bed if other risk factors are present.
Moisture	Keep clean and dry between episodes of incontinence. Use skin protectant sprays, wipes, or lotions to protect skin. Treat dry skin with moisturizers. Keep skin care products at the bedside	Consider urinary tract infection as cause of incontinence. Consider infectious forms of diarrhea. Consider side effects of medications or tube-feeding as cause of diarrhea. Obtain order for antifungal powder or dressings if rash between skinfolds appears fungal.	Consider placing an indwelling catheter if denudement is severe. Consider a rectal bag if fecal incontinence is frequent. Monitor for dehydration from fluid loss. Avoid using plastic incontinence pads on specialty beds.
Nutrition	Offer oral supplements to diet. Monitor weight weekly.	Provide dietary consultation. Assess condition of mouth and ability to swallow. Monitor oral intake; consider calorie count.	Offer tube-feeding or hyperalimentation if within the goals of client or family.
Friction/shear	N/A	Apply lotions and creams to abraded areas. Apply cotton sleeves, socks, or heel and elbow protectors. Consider treatment for agitation or spasms.	Keep head of bed as low as possible. Use a lifting device to move client in bed. Apply adhesive dressings to abraded areas. If head of bed is elevated, monitor sacrum and heels closely for shear injury. Treat early manifestations of shear with protective dressings.

Outcomes. The client will experience healing of the ulcer, as evidenced by development of granulation tissue and decreasing ulcer size. Do not use lower stages of pressure ulcers to describe healing. For example, do not state a stage IV will heal to a stage III. The body does not heal by regeneration of tissue but, rather, by scar tissue. For clients who are terminally ill, outcomes such as healing may not be appropriate. For these clients, outcomes of pain management, comfort, or reducing risk of infection may be more appropriate.

Interventions. Consistency in the nursing care provided is an important aspect of interventions directed at achieving wound healing. It is important to develop scientific protocols in ulcer care and to use them consistently. It is also important to give one protocol time to work before changing to another. See Box 49-2 and Chapter 18 for information on wound healing.

Reducing the risk of pressure ulcer development and identifying early manifestations of pressure ulcers are frequently delegated to unlicensed assistive personnel. The Management and Delegation feature on p. 121 highlights important nursing instructions to give to unlicensed personnel caring for clients with pressure ulcers. Case managers often assist in managing care between facilities. When preparing for discharge to home, case managers assist with advocating and preventing readmission (see the Case Management feature on The Client with Impaired Skin Integrity on the website).

Care of Clients with Pressure Ulcers

When working with unlicensed assistive personnel (UAP) in the care of clients with pressure ulcers, help them to keep the following points in mind:

- Report any areas of skin redness that do not disappear after pressure relief.
- Report any new areas of purple or bruised skin.
- Report any development of foul odor or drainage from pressure ulcers.
- Reposition the client *at least* every 2 hours. Sometimes small shifts in the client's body weight may be sufficient, but the client must not be consistently positioned on the same tissue
- *Do not position the client on the ulcer.* If an ulcer is on the client's trunk, use a reactive mattress or an overlay mattress. However, the use of these support surfaces does not eliminate the need for turning.
- If the client is wheelchair-bound, instruct the UAP to reposition the client hourly. Ensure that the padding provides adequate pressure relief by checking for "bottoming out."
- Keep all pressure off the client's heels. Instruct the UAP how to float the heels using pillows for short term leg immobility. Be certain that any boots are applied properly. Instruct UAPs to remove boots and other devices on the legs to inspect the skin every shift.
- Keep the head of the bed at the lowest elevation to reduce shear and friction on the skin of the client's lower back.
- Keep the client's skin dry; clean any episodes of incontinence immediately.

Even though you have delegated the skin care of these clients, you are still accountable for their skin condition. Assess the entire skin surface every day. Ask for help in turning the client so that you can see the client's heels and sacrum. Use an assessment guide such as the Braden scale to determine the risk of further ulceration.

Evaluation. As the ulcer heals, assess the degree of outcome attainment every 3 to 4 days. Allow 2 weeks before changing the plan of care, unless the ulcer is deteriorating.

Self-Care

Clients at high risk for development of pressure ulcers who are going home should be referred to a home health agency before discharge from the acute care facility so that devices to reduce pressure can be obtained for home use. The family and the client need to understand the importance of frequent turning. A client who is wheelchair-bound and has arm function should be taught to lift the body, using the arms, off the chair twice every hour for repositioning. "Tilt in space" wheel chairs can be used for long-term wheelchair-dependent clients to assist with pressure redistribution. A client who is incontinent needs to wear protective pads to absorb the urine or stool and should be assessed often.

If the client is going home with an unhealed ulcer, the client and one or more family members must be taught wound care, wound assessment, and in some cases the administration of intravenous (IV) antibiotics. Teach these interventions before the day of discharge, so that return demonstrations can be used to evaluate learning. In addition, procurement of equipment is often necessary, which takes time. Community nurses need to be involved early in the planning for the discharge of the client with an ulcer. The Bridge to Home Health Care feature on p. 1218 describes ways to help the client and family manage pressure ulcers.

Surgical Management

Surgical repair is frequently performed on stage III and stage IV ulcers, on ulcers greater than 2 cm in diameter, and in clients who can tolerate surgery. In stage III ulcers, undamaged tissue near the wound is rotated to cover the ulcer. In stage IV ulcers, musculocutaneous flaps are often used (see later discussion).

PRECANCEROUS CHANGES IN THE SKIN

Precursors to cancer of the skin include damage from recurrent skin trauma and various skin lesions. To understand the role of prevention of skin cancer, these precursor conditions are discussed first. *Photodamage* refers to a spectrum of medical conditions caused by the sun. The spectrum includes sunburn; spider veins (telangiectasias); rough, thick skin; fine and deep wrinkling; actinic keratoses; and carcinomas. Sun protection at every age is the key to preventing short-term damage (sunburn and acute events), as well as the long-term damaging effects of sunlight such as photodamage and skin cancer. Tips for sun protection include daily use of sunscreen with SPF 15 or higher with broad-spectrum protection, wearing a T-shirt, broad-brimmed hat, and sunglasses, and staying out of the sun in the middle of the day. Use extra caution near water, snow, and sand because they reflect the damaging rays of the sun. Tanning beds should be avoided, and clients should be taught to check their skin regularly and consult a health-care provider if they see any skin lesions that are changing. Recall that "a change in a wart or mole" is one of the signs of cancer.

BRIDGE TO HOME HEALTH CARE

Managing Pressure Ulcers

For the client with pressure ulcers, a smooth transition from hospital to home care requires planning, preparation, and communication. For example, it may take a home health nurse several days to obtain special wound care supplies or pressure redistribution devices not ordinarily stocked by the home health agency. If a pressure redistribution bed or mattress overlay is required, the agency then contacts a durable medical equipment company and arranges delivery at a predetermined time. To facilitate the transition from hospital care, the home health agency should be notified of the referral before the client's discharge from the hospital and should receive specific instructions per physician orders for wound cleansing, dressing materials, and frequency of dressing changes. In addition, sending a day's supply home with the client minimizes disruption in the wound treatment regimen.

Clients who have stage IV or draining, infected pressure ulcers may initially require daily skilled nursing visits. However, as the infection is treated and drainage subsides, the frequency of skilled nursing visits is usually decreased and the family member or informal caregiver is taught to perform the dressing change. Caregivers should participate in or at least observe dressing change procedures in the hospital, and should receive information about turning and other aspects of care. The earlier the caregiver is introduced to prevention and treatment goals, the faster the client can reach the desired clinical outcome. Hospital nurses can significantly enhance the continuity of care by coordinating educational efforts with the home health agency. The home health nurse should obtain copies of any teaching materials distributed in the hospital. Older adults are often fearful of leaving the security of an inpatient setting; therefore reinforcing familiar teaching materials and wound care procedures helps to ensure a more seamless transition from inpatient to outpatient management.

Maintaining equipment and supplies is more difficult in the home than in inpatient settings. Estimate the needed amount of skin and wound care supplies, and arrange for delivery in a timely manner. Establish an intercommunication sheet in the home that flags a change in wound care orders for other members of the health care team. Leave specific directions for product use, especially when more than one product is being used. *Normal saline* can be made by using the following recipe: mix 8 teaspoons of salt in 1 gallon of bottled or boiled water. Do not use water from an outdoor well or an unknown water source.

Adapting the home environment to meet the needs of the client and family members or other caregivers requires creativity and skill. Note the conditions under which the client spends prolonged periods of time. Any firm, unyielding surface can contribute to development of a pressure ulcer in unusual body areas. Sitting on ridged, corded edges of chairs or stools or a firm toilet seat for extended periods can restrict blood flow, leading to pressure ulcer development.

The limitations of older clients and their older caregivers pose additional changes. For example, it may not be possible for a debilitated client to be turned as often as needed during the night to relieve pressure over bony prominences. Frequent turning schedules usually result in increased anxiety and sleep deprivation for older caregivers. Accurately assessing the client's risk category and using an effective pressure-relieving mattress overlay can help to reduce the physical demands for caregivers and increase the possibility that the client can receive needed care and remain at home.

SUNBURN

Sunburn is an acute inflammatory skin response that occurs as a reaction to excessive exposure to sunlight. Pathologic changes in the skin include the production of epidermal cells that exhibit cytoplasmic and nuclear changes. These changes are cumulative over the life span and lead to an increased incidence of skin cancer with aging.

A first-degree sunburn produces mild, tender erythema followed by desquamation (peeling), which heals without scarring. Second-degree sunburn causes more extreme erythema and edema, and blistering results from damage to the epidermal cells. Deep sunburn is uncommon unless it is induced by artificial sources such as tanning lamps or booths. Deep sunburn produces burns (see Chapter 50).

Prevention is the best approach to management of sunburn. Client teaching emphasizing sun protection should never be omitted when caring for the sunburned client. For a list of specific precautions, see the Client Education Guide feature on Simple Guidelines to Help Protect You from the Damaging Rays of the Sun on the website.

Treating sunburn involves decreasing inflammation and rehydrating the damaged skin. For localized, *superficial, partial-thickness* sunburn, use cool tap water soaks for 20 minutes or until the skin is cool. This measure limits skin destruction, prevents edema, and potentially reduces blisters. Tepid tap water baths are indicated for large sunburned areas. After a bath or soak, apply water-based emollients, lotions, foams, gels, or sprays, preferably refrigerated for an additional cooling effect. Emollients should also be applied throughout the day to soothe the skin and relieve dryness. Lotions, foams, or sprays containing camphor and menthol (e.g. Sarna) can also be beneficial. Avoid the use of OTC remedies containing local anesthetics—such as benzocaine dibucaine (Nupercaine), or lidocaine (Xylocaine)—because they are rarely effective and have the potential to induce contact sensitivity.

For *partial-thickness* sunburn, apply continuous cool, normal saline soaks or soaking baths to reduce oozing and edema. Very large blisters may be aspirated and dressed with sterile dressings. Avoid debridement unless there is evidence of secondary bacterial infection. Silver sulfadiazine may be prescribed.

Prostaglandin inhibitors (nonsteroidal anti-inflammatory drugs [NSAIDs]) may be used to reduce erythema and inflammation in adults. Topical corticosteroids may be prescribed to be used sparingly in nonocclusive vehicles (lotion, spray, gel) for their vasoconstrictive effects. Systemic corticosteroids are prescribed only for clients with extensive, painful burns, but their use has declined because they seem to offer little efficacy when given in a reasonable dose range.

ACTINIC KERATOSIS

Actinic keratosis, the most common epithelial precancerous lesion in Caucasians, is primarily caused by sun exposure. It affects nearly 100% of older Caucasian adults. There is a small but definite risk of malignant degeneration and subsequent metastatic potential in neglected lesions.

Actinic keratosis most frequently occurs in areas of chronic, usually high-intensity sun exposure, including the face, the tops of the ears, the back of the neck, the forearms, the backs of the hands, and the chest. The clinical appearance of actinic keratoses is varied. The typical lesion is an irregularly shaped, flat, slightly erythematous macule or papule with indistinct borders and an overlying hard keratotic scale or horn that feels rough or sharp to palpation. In some cases, the erythema or the horn may be absent. This scale can be periodically shed or peeled off, but then it regrows. The lesion varies in size from the size of a pinhead to several centimeters across and is often more easily palpated than observed. Single lesions may be seen, but more often they appear in groups on a background of sun-damaged skin.

OUTCOME MANAGEMENT

Medical Management

Topical application of fluorouracil (Carac, Efudex, and Fluoroplex), a topical antineoplastic, is currently one of the best approaches to treatment of widespread actinic damage with multiple lesions. The advantage is that large areas of widespread disease can be treated at the same time. Use not only removes the majority of premalignant and superficial malignant lesions that can be seen but also uncovers and destroys clinically undetectable lesions of this type. However, the major disadvantage is the inflammatory response that often accompanies successful treatment. This response sequence is erythema usually followed by vesiculation, erosion, ulcerations, necrosis, and epithelialization.

The medication should be applied twice daily with a gloved hand, carefully avoiding the eyes, folds around the nose, the mouth, and the scrotum. Medication should be continued until the inflammatory response reaches the erosion, necrosis, and ulceration stage, at which time the medication should be stopped. The usual duration of therapy is 2 to 4 weeks; by then, the client may experience extreme discomfort requiring pain medication. At the time these products are stopped, topical corticosteroid creams may be applied to reduce inflammation and provide the client with additional pain reduction. Complete healing of the lesions may not be evident for 1 to 2 months after cessation of therapy.

Surgical Management

Cryotherapy
Cryotherapy using liquid nitrogen is a common treatment for single lesions or for small numbers of actinic keratoses. Liquid nitrogen is usually applied with a cotton-tipped applicator or spraying device. No local anesthetic is required but the freezing process is associated with a small amount of discomfort, which may linger afterward. Intermittent application of a warm, damp wash cloth to the site may bring relief. Freezing frequently results in inflammation with blister formation, and blister care should be reviewed with the client.

Electrodesiccation and Curettage
Electrodesiccation produces superficial destruction. The procedure may be done using local anesthetics. The tissue is destroyed by mechanical disruption of cells and heat. The tissue is removed by scraping or scooping with a loop-shaped instrument called a curet. This method can provide tissue for histologic diagnosis if needed. The curetted areas usually heal quickly, with adequate wound care resulting in a small white permanent scar. The wound site should be kept moist with a less sensitizing topical antibiotic ointment such as bacitracin.

Laser Excision
Laser uses light energy to vaporize lesions. Depending upon the wavelength of the light, various portions of the cell are heated. Tissue is not available for histologic examination. Local anesthesia is used.

Punch or Excisional Biopsy
Punch or excisional biopsy is indicated for lesions that are large or have other characteristics of cancer. It is often difficult to distinguish a large actinic keratosis from a squamous cell carcinoma without histologic diagnosis. Biopsy should also be done on lesions that persist after

adequate treatment. Local anesthesia is used for the biopsy procedure and allows electrodesiccation to be done painlessly after biopsy. Excisional biopsy requires primary closure of the site and may be a more extensive procedure than the lesion warrants; however, it ensures more complete removal of the growth (see Chapter 48).

SKIN CANCER

Skin cancer is the most common cancer in the United States, and the number of new skin cancers and the number of skin cancer deaths are increasing at alarming rates. Skin cancer is a malignant condition caused by uncontrolled growth and spread of abnormal cells in a specific layer of the skin. The several different kinds of skin cancer are distinguished by the types of cells involved. The three most common types are (1) basal cell carcinoma, (2) squamous cell carcinoma, and (3) malignant melanoma. More than 90% of all skin cancers fall into the first two classifications. Both basal cell carcinoma and squamous cell carcinoma are slow-growing tumors with a cure rate of 95% or greater after early treatment

Etiology and Risk Factors

The cause of skin cancer is well known. Prolonged or intermittent, repeated exposure to UVL radiation from the sun, especially when it results in sunburn and blistering, plays a key role in the induction of skin cancer, especially malignant melanoma. Most non-melanoma skin cancers occur on parts of the body unprotected by clothing (face, neck, forearms, and backs of hands) and in people who have received considerable exposure to sunlight. All people are at risk of skin cancer regardless of skin tone and hair color, although some are at much greater risk than others. In general, people with red, blond, or light brown hair with light complexions or freckles, many of Celtic or Scandinavian origin, are most susceptible; blacks and Asians are least susceptible. The Genetic Links feature at right describes skin care for clients with reduced melanin synthesis.

Due to the rising numbers of skin cancers, all clients should be encouraged to use sunscreen. Clients should be taught to examine their own skin regularly and have someone examine their back looking for new moles or lesions. Danger signals in moles (pigmented nevi) are presented in Box 49-3. Suspicious lesions should be examined by a physician.

The pattern of reaction to acute sun exposure can be correlated with the development of actinic keratosis and skin cancer. People who never tan and always burn after 1 to 2 hours of midday summer sun are most susceptible. People who burn once or twice at the beginning of

GENETIC LINKS

Oculocutaneous Albinism Type I (OCA1)

DESCRIPTION

OCA1 is an autosomal recessive disorder characterized by reduced synthesis of melanin in the skin, hair, and eyes, and associated characteristic ocular findings. Ocular findings include nystagmus, reduced iris and retinal pigment, foveal hypoplasia with reduced visual acuity, and misrouting of the optic nerves, producing alternating strabismus and reduced stereoscopic vision. There are two categories of OCA1: OCA1A (most common), associated with absent melanin synthesis in all tissue; and OCA1B, associated with varying amounts of melanin synthesis in the skin, hair, and eyes. Clients with OCA1A have white hair, white skin that does not tan, and blue, fully translucent irises. Clients with OCA1B have white or light yellow hair that darkens with age, white skin that gradually develops some generalized pigment, and blue irises that may change color with age to green/hazel or brown/tan.

GENETICS

OCA1 is caused by mutations in the tyrosinase gene, *TYR*, located on chromosome 11. Molecular genetic testing of the *TYR* gene is clinically available. The carrier rate for OCA1 is approximately 1 in 100 in most populations throughout the world. OCA1 is an autosomal recessive disorder, and offspring of carrier parents have a 25% chance of being affected with OCA1, a 50% chance of being a carrier, and a 25% chance of being unaffected and not a carrier.

DIAGNOSIS AND TESTING

Diagnosis of OCA1 is established by clinical features of hypopigmentation of the skin and hair and eye findings. Genetic testing is rarely used in diagnosis and is most commonly used for carrier detection in genetic counseling.

MANAGEMENT

A critical aspect of the ongoing care of clients with OCA1 is ophthalmologic care, including, for example, correction of refractive errors (e.g., myopia, hyperopia, astigmatism) to improve visual acuity and annual eye examination. Skin care is dictated by the amount of skin pigment and cutaneous response to sunlight. Clients with OCA1A need to be protected from sun exposure with clothing and sunscreens.

summer and then tan are somewhat less susceptible. Those who never burn and always tan are the least susceptible. The most severely affected people usually have a history of long-term occupational (farmers, construction workers, surveyors, sailors) or recreational (swimmers, skiers, surfers, sunbathers) sun exposure. It is imperative that all people at risk of skin cancer examine their skin systematically. The Client Education Guide on p. 1222 summarizes teaching instructions recommended by The Skin Cancer Foundation.

- *Change in color,* especially red, white, and blue; sudden darkening; mottled shades of brown or black
- *Change in diameter,* especially sudden increase
- *Change in outline,* especially development of irregular margins
- *Change in surface characteristics,* especially scaliness, erosion, oozing, crusting, bleeding, ulceration, development of a mushrooming mass on the surface of the lesion
- *Change in consistency,* especially softening or friability
- *Change in symptoms,* especially pruritus
- *Change in shape,* especially irregular elevation from a previously flat condition
- *Change in surrounding skin,* especially "leaking" of pigment from the lesion into surrounding skin or pigmented "satellite" lesions

BASAL CELL CARCINOMA

Basal cell carcinoma (BCC), the most common form of skin cancer, is a malignant epithelial tumor of the skin that arises from the basal cells in the epidermis. The tumor is usually painless and slow growing, generally appearing on sun-exposed skin of the face, ears, head, neck, or hands. Occasionally, basal cell carcinoma may appear on the trunk, especially the upper back and chest. The majority of cases are caused by chronic overexposure to UVL radiation, and only a few cases can be linked to arsenic, burns, scars, exposure to radiation, or genetic predisposition. Clinical and histologic findings are used to identify the tumor.

The most common clinical presentation of basal cell carcinoma is the nodular lesion (Figure 49-8, *A*). This is a dome-shaped papule with a well-defined border having a classic "pearly" texture. Basal cell carcinoma has this flesh-colored "pearly" or shiny appearance because it does not keratinize. Telangiectatic (small spider-like) vessels frequently overlie the lesion. As the lesion enlarges, the center may flatten or ulcerate, but the border is still raised, giving a "rolled-edge" appearance.

Although basal cell carcinomas almost never metastasize, they can be locally destructive and invasive through tissue. This is particularly true on the face, where a lesion can invade deep structures with resultant loss of an eye or ear or the nose. If untreated, the tumor can invade bone and brain. If the tumor is identified and treated early, local excision or even nonexcisional destruction is usually curative.

Clients who have had one basal cell carcinoma are at risk for development of another. Recurrences of previously treated basal cell carcinomas are also possible but more unusual; recurrence is generally noted within the first 2 years after removal or therapy.

SQUAMOUS CELL CARCINOMA

Squamous cell carcinoma (SCC) (Figure 49-8, *B*) is the second most common skin cancer in Caucasians. It is a tumor of the epidermal keratinocytes and rarely occurs in dark-skinned people. It is found on areas often exposed to the sun, typically the rim of the ear, the face, the lips and mouth, and the backs of the hands.

Squamous cell carcinoma is more difficult to characterize than basal cell carcinoma. The tumor is poorly marginated; the edge often blends into surrounding sun-damaged skin. Squamous cell carcinoma may present as an ulcer, a flat red area, a cutaneous horn, an indurated plaque, or a hyperkeratotic papule or nodule. Often it presents as a red- to skin-colored papule surmounted by varying amounts of scale.

The lesions grow more rapidly than does basal cell carcinoma. These tumors are potentially dangerous because they may infiltrate surrounding structures and metastasize to lymph nodes, with a fatal outcome.

MALIGNANT MELANOMA

Malignant melanoma (Figure 49-8, *C* and *D*) is a cancer of melanocytes; it is the deadliest form of skin cancer. The incidence of melanoma is increasing, such that currently about 1 in 100 people in the United States can expect to develop this cancer in a lifetime. The incidence of and death rate from melanoma are increasing worldwide. In countries populated with fair-skinned Caucasian people, the incidence of melanoma and the death rate have increased 7% to 15% per year, more than doubling during the 1990s.

Exposure to UVL continues to be one of the most important causes of malignant melanoma. What causes melanocytes to transform to melanoma cells is poorly understood. Primary cutaneous melanoma may develop in precursor melanocytic nevi (common acquired, congenital, and atypical or dysplastic types), although more than 50% of cases are believed to arise without a preexisting pigmented lesion. Melanoma is multifactorial and appears to be related to multiple risk factors including (1) fair complexion, (2) excessive childhood sun exposure and blistering childhood sunburns, (3) increased number of common and dysplastic moles, (4) family history of melanoma, and (5) presence of a changing mole on the skin. The suspicion of melanoma is based on history as well as the clinical appearance.

Clinical Manifestations

The cardinal clinical manifestation of melanoma is a change in a skin lesion observed over a period of months. If a lesion grows so fast that it doubles in size in 10 days, it is usually an inflammation. If a lesion changes so slowly that neither the client nor the family

CLIENT EDUCATION GUIDE

Skin Self-Examination

You will need a bright light, a full-length mirror, a hand mirror, two chairs or stools, a blow dryer, body maps, and a pencil.

A. Examine your face—especially the nose, lips, mouth, and ears—front and back. Use one or both mirrors to get a clear view.

B. Thoroughly inspect your scalp, using a blow dryer and mirror to expose each section to view. Get a friend or family member to help, if you can.

C. Check your hands carefully: palms and backs, between the fingers, and under the fingernails. Continue up the wrists to examine both the front and back of your forearms.

D. Standing in front of the full-length mirror, begin at the elbows and scan all sides of your upper arms. Do not forget the underarms.

E. Next, focus on the neck, chest, and torso. Women should lift breasts to view the underside.

F. With your back to the full-length mirror, use the hand mirror to inspect the back of your neck, shoulders, upper back, and any part of the back of your upper arms you could not view previously.

G. Still using both mirrors, scan your lower back, buttocks, and backs of both legs.

H. Sit down; prop each leg in turn on the other stool or chair. Use the hand mirror to examine the genitals. Check front and sides of both legs, thigh to shin; ankles; and tops of feet, between toes, and under toenails. Examine soles of the feet and the heels.

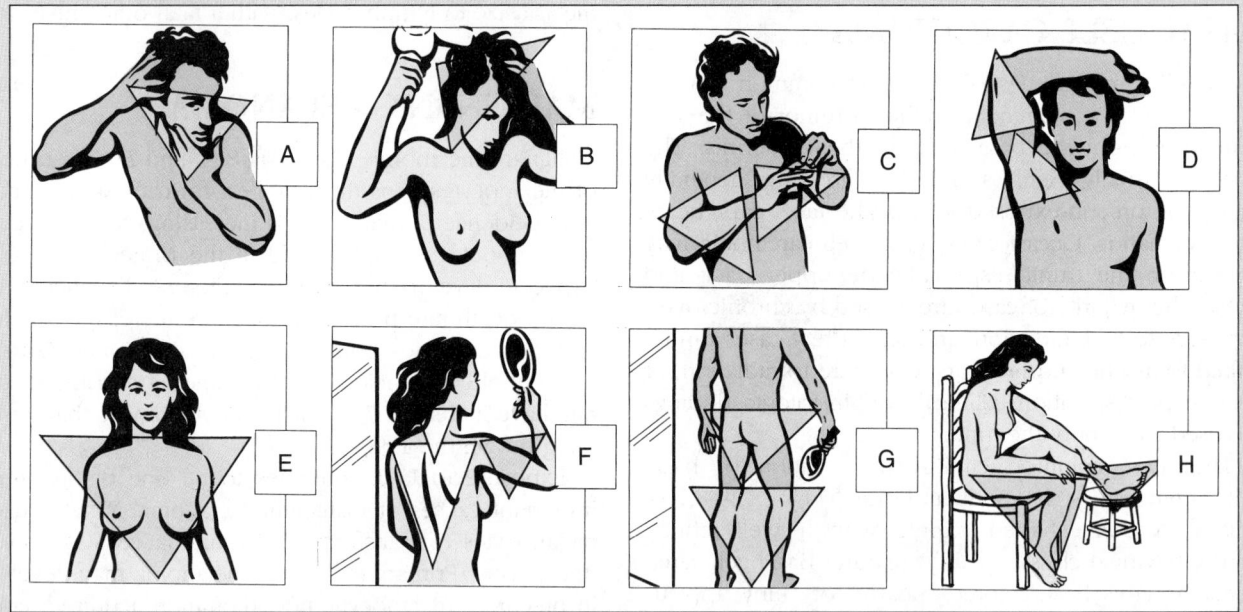

From The Skin Cancer Foundation (1992). *Skin cancer. If you can spot it, you can stop it.* New York: Author.

is sure of a change, it is usually benign. Changes that may signal melanoma are called the *A, B, C, D* changes in moles:

- Asymmetry
- Border notching
- Color variegation with black, brown, red, or white hue
- Diameter greater than 6 mm

Other changes include doubling size in 3 to 8 months, bleeding, itching, ulceration, a change in color, or development of a palpable lymph node. Four types of melanoma are presented in Table 49-3. The tumor can metastasize, usually to the brain, lungs, bones, liver, and skin, and is ultimately fatal.

OUTCOME MANAGEMENT

Management is directed at removing the tumor, if possible. Survival is directly related to the depth of tumor invasion: 10-year survival is greater than 90% if the tumor is less than 1 mm in depth, but if the tumor is larger than 4 mm in depth, 10-year survival decreases to only 40%. Microscopic ulceration is the next most

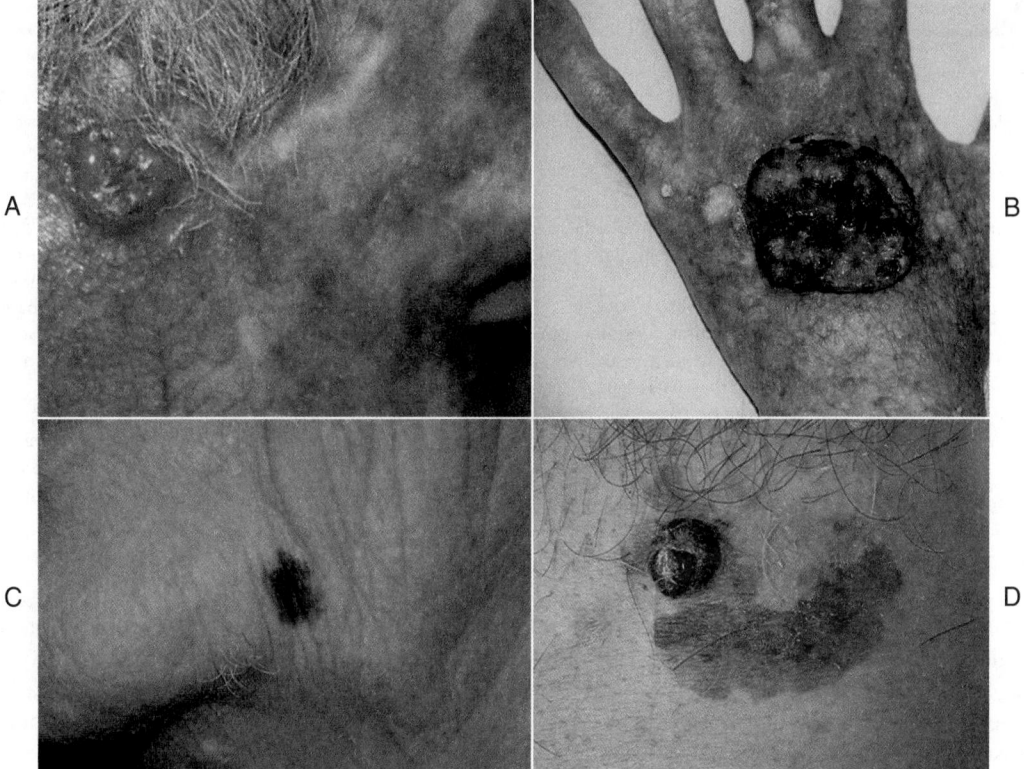

■ **FIGURE 49–8** **A,** Basal cell carcinoma characterized by rolled edges and a crater in the center of the lesion. Scars are from previous destruction of skin cancers. **B,** Squamous cell carcinoma on the hand. **C,** Superficial spreading melanoma. **D,** Nodular melanoma with satellite lesions.

important adverse prognostic pathologic feature. Metastatic melanoma is universally fatal. It is therefore extremely important for a malignant melanoma to be diagnosed early according to the ABCD rules.

Medical Management

Medical management begins with a high level of suspicion for any type of skin cancer but specifically for melanoma. The need for early detection cannot be overemphasized. Any indication, whether it is a confirmed risk factor or a suspicious lesion, is adequate reason for referral. Clients with localized cutaneous disease have been treated with adjuvant chemotherapy, nonspecific passive immunotherapy, radiation therapy, and biologic therapy. No increase in survival has been reported with these adjunctive therapies. Adjuvant interferon (IFN) alfa-2b and various experimental melanoma vaccines show promise in individuals with high-risk primary cutaneous melanoma and those with regional nodal disease. Melanoma vaccines are being investigated for therapeutic use. A variety of vaccines targeting melanoma cell antigens are in the clinical trial phase. The Complementary and Alternative Therapy feature on p. 1224 lists interventions that could reduce the risk or recurrence of melanoma.

Surgical Management

Treatment of all skin cancers requires removal of the lesion. The margins of the resected specimen must be free of tumor to a specified distance (depending on the type of skin cancer) to guarantee full removal.

A special surgical technique primarily used for the removal of skin malignancies such as basal cell carcinoma and squamous cell carcinoma is *Mohs' surgery,* which is also indicated for primary lesions in areas in which preservation of normal skin is necessary (e.g., eyelids, pinna, nasolabial folds). The technique involves a series of excisions with careful microscopic tissue assessment to "map" the presence or absence of malignant cells within each specimen. The procedure may be lengthy. After all tumor tissue is removed, the wound is closed with sutures or a flap, or is allowed to close by secondary intention.

Basal cell carcinomas and squamous cell carcinomas can also be excised and the surgical wound closed primarily (with skin edges sewn together) or with a skin flap. The advantage of this technique is that it requires much less time, and a fine line scar is produced. The tumor is completely excised with adequate margins of tumor-free tissue. If there is doubt about adequacy of margins, the specimen is sent for pathologic diagnosis (by permanent section technique).

TABLE 49–3 Types of Melanoma

Tumor Type	General Information	Clinical Manifestations
Superficial spreading melanoma (SSM)	Most common form of melanoma; slowly changing lesion with more rapid growth just before diagnosis	Deeply pigmented area contained within a brown nevus (freckle); usually flat and asymmetrical; as lesion grows, color changes may occur, ranging from jet black to dark blue to pale gray or white; looks lacy; lesions may have areas of no color; usually 2 cm wide
Nodular melanoma (NM)	Second most common form of melanoma; more aggressive tumor than SSM, with shorter clinical onset time	Common on trunk, head, and neck; usually 1-2 cm in diameter; often begins in normal skin, rather than in a pre-existing lesion; dark and more uniform in color; may resemble a blood blister or hemangioma; dome-shaped with sharp borders
Lentigo maligna melanoma (LMM)	Fairly uncommon tumor; typically appears on face of Caucasian women; usually has been present for long time (5-15 yr)	Generally a large, flat lesion that looks like a stain on the skin; typically tan with various shades of brown; metastasis less common
Acral-lentiginous melanoma (ALM)	Commonly occurs on palms and soles; more common in dark-skinned people; usually occurs in older adults; may evolve over a few months to years	Large lesion, about 3 cm in diameter; resembles LMM (a tan or brown flat lesion on palm or sole); can be misdiagnosed as a corn; ulceration is common; likely to metastasize

The treatment of malignant melanoma is wide local excision. Surgical excision begins with biopsy to determine the stage of the cancer. Excisional biopsy is the removal of the lesion and a narrow margin of normal-appearing tissue. The tumor is excised with a 1- to 2-cm margin of normal-appearing tissue. The margin width is based on the type of melanoma. The surgical wound is closed either primarily or with grafts or flaps.

Surgeons differ on the timing of the definitive surgery. Some surgeons excise the lesion after frozen section examination while the client is still on the operating table. Other surgeons wait for the results of permanent section pathologic diagnosis and then proceed with definitive treatment. The final excision is usually completed within 1 week of biopsy. Although there is a theoretical risk of tumor spread during biopsy, there is no convincing evidence that waiting 1 to even 6 weeks after biopsy jeopardizes the outcome. In fact, sometimes the delay gives the client time to prepare for surgery, both physically and psychologically.

Most clients with metastatic melanoma live less than 1 year. Currently, there is no cure for metastatic melanoma, but some of the new developments in clinical trials may change currently accepted treatments. A treatment plan is formulated on the basis of several factors: site of the tumor, number of metastases, rate of tumor growth, previous treatments, response to treatment, and the age, general health, and desires of the client. Some treatments include surgery to remove metastatic lesions, radiation therapy, chemotherapy, and local hyperthermia. Alternatively, the client can opt for no further treatment.

CUTANEOUS T-CELL LYMPHOMA (MYCOSIS FUNGOIDES)

Cutaneous T-cell lymphoma (CTCL), or mycosis fungoides, is a malignant disease involving the T helper cells. Malignant T cells in the blood migrate to the skin, where they have an affinity for the epidermis. The malignant cells continue to grow and change, eventually moving into the dermis. The cause is not known, and the course is unpredictable, varying with the type of presentation.

The three distinct clinical presentations are patch, plaque, and tumor. Clinical manifestations include eversion of the eyelids and hyperkeratosis of the palms and soles, often with fissuring. Finally, the plaques form tumors that ultimately ulcerate. Tumors can also develop spontaneously in previously unaffected areas, and eventual visceral or organ involvement ensues. This disease is often described as a slow-growing but highly disfiguring debilitating cancer. Clients often feel desperate by the time diagnosis is confirmed, which adds to the psychological difficulties. The tumor presentation

---

COMPLEMENTARY AND ALTERNATIVE THERAPY

Chemoprevention of Melanoma

A recent review of chemoprevention studies for melanoma found that several interventions could reduce the risk or the recurrence of melanoma. These include higher intakes of polyunsaturated fatty acids (such as fish oil), vitamin E from food, normal levels of selenium, green tea, soy, and nonsteroidal anti-inflammatory drugs (NSAIDs). More research is needed, but these are interesting initial data.

REFERENCE
Demierre M.-F., Nathanson L. (2003) Chemoprevention of melanoma: An unexplored strategy. *Journal of Clinical Oncology,* 21:158-165.

carries the worst prognosis, with a survival period of 3 years or less.

CTCL is extremely difficult to diagnose and is often misdiagnosed. In its early stages, CTCL can clinically mimic eczematous processes. The initial erythematous papules resemble those in other eczematous conditions, including psoriasis and atopic dermatitis. The original eruptions of CTCL may be either transitory or of prolonged duration and sometimes are pruritic.

OUTCOME MANAGEMENT

Control of pruritus is essential at all stages and is accomplished by rehydration of the skin, various dry skin therapies (see Xerotic Eczema), topical corticosteroids, and PUVA therapy (see Ultraviolet Light B Therapy). Prevention of secondary infections is important. Nitrogen mustard and other chemotherapy agents are administered topically. Daily application of chemotherapeutic agents often constitutes the initial treatment. Photophoresis, a treatment involving the removal of small amounts of blood that is irradiated and then returned to the body, is used frequently in more advanced stages. Total-body electron beam therapy with or without adjuvant chemotherapy is an aggressive approach often used.

The primary systemic drug used for treatment of CTCL was formerly intravenous methotrexate. With advances in treatment, newer drugs have replaced methotrexate: one is denileukin diftitox (Ontak), used primarily in the treatment of persistent or recurrent CTCL. This agent has produced sustained regression of the tumors, in some cases for longer than 2 years. Fatalities remain extremely high in this disease as a result of progression to systemic involvement.

BULLOUS DISORDERS: PEMPHIGUS

Pemphigus is a chronic disorder that results in the development of blisters *(bullae)*. It is fairly uncommon in the general population, but the incidence is increased in Jewish and Mediterranean people. There are several types: pemphigus vulgaris, pemphigus foliaceus, and pemphigus erythematosus. This discussion focuses on pemphigus vulgaris, the most common type.

Pemphigus is an autoimmune disease caused by circulating immunoglobulin G (IgG) autoantibodies. These autoantibodies react with the intracellular cement—the substance that holds epidermal cells together. The reaction causes intraepidermal bulla (blister) formation and acantholysis (loss of cohesion between epidermal cells).

Clinical manifestations include flaccid bullae that rupture easily, emitting a foul-smelling drainage and leaving crusted, denuded skin. Nikolsky's sign is the result when the epidermis can be rubbed off by slight friction or injury; this sign is a hallmark of pemphigus. Even slight pressure on an intact blister may cause it to spread to adjacent skin. The lesions are common on the face, back, chest, groin, and umbilicus.

OUTCOME MANAGEMENT

Management includes large doses of steroids and immunosuppressives. Plasmapheresis has been of some benefit in the treatment of pemphigus. If a large proportion of the skin is denuded, management is similar to that for a burn-injured client. The client is at increased risk for infection, fluid and electrolyte imbalance, and stress response complications (i.e., stress ulcers, body system failure). In addition, nursing management focuses on self-concept and pain management. Potassium permanganate baths may be used to reduce the risk of infection, control the odor of the drainage, and ease the pain.

INFECTIOUS DISORDERS

Several organisms lead to skin infections and infestations. Common skin infections are described in Table 49-4. The Terrorism Alert feature on p. 1227 describes smallpox, a serious viral infection. A few others are discussed in detail here.

ERYSIPELAS AND CELLULITIS

Cellulitis is a skin infection that extends into the deeper dermis and subcutaneous tissues and causes deep, red erythema without sharp borders that spreads widely through tissue spaces (Figure 49-9 on p. 1228). The skin is erythematous, edematous, tender, and sometimes nodular. *Streptococcus pyogenes* is the usual cause of this infection, although other pathogens may be responsible. Lymphangitis may occur; if cellulitis is untreated, gangrene, metastatic abscesses, and sepsis result.

Older clients are at increased risk for cellulitis due to lowered resistance from diabetes, malnutrition, steroid therapy, or the presence of wounds or ulcers. Other predisposing factors include the presence of edema and other cutaneous inflammation or wounds (e.g., tinea, eczema, burns, trauma). There is a tendency for recurrence, especially at sites of lymphatic obstruction.

Oral or IV antibiotics are used that are effective against both streptococci and *S. aureus*. Before antibiotics are administered, a wound specimen for culture and sensitivity testing should be obtained, although culture rarely yields the causative organism. Soaks may reduce edema and inflammation. The enzymes that facilitate a rapid spread of infection also seem to produce other significant manifestations such as high fever, tachycardia, confusion, and hypotension; appropriate interventions should be undertaken if these occur. Monitor

TABLE 49–4 Common Skin Infections and Infestations

Disease with Causative Organism	Clinical Manifestations	Management
Parasitic		
Scabies: *Sarcoptes scabiei*	Multiple straight or wavy thread-like lines beneath skin, itching	Application of a scabicide with retreatment in 1 wk to kill residual eggs. All clothing and linen should be washed and dried in hot cycles or dry-cleaned.
Lice: *Pediculus humanus, Phthirus pubis*	Intense itching; scratch marks may be evident	Application of pediculicides. For *head lice*, shampoo should be worked into dry hair until it is saturated. A fine-toothed comb should be used to remove dead lice and nits. Brushes and combs should be washed in pediculicide also. For *body lice*, pediculicide lotion is applied to involved body areas. Clothing should be washed and dried in hot cycles or dry-cleaned. Other items can be stored in plastic bags for 30-35 days. Family members, close contacts, and sexual partners should also be treated.
Bacterial		
Impetigo: group A streptococci, staphylococci	Pruritic vesicle or pustule that breaks and leaves a thick honey-colored crust	Antibiotics given until culture results available include erythromycin or dicloxacillin. Mupirocin is preferable to oral antibiotics when lesions are limited to small, localized area. **Teach control of contagion; infection is contagious as long as skin lesions are present. Use thorough hand-washing, separate laundry for client's linens, and separate washing of client's dishes.**
Folliculitis, furuncles, carbuncles: *Staphylococcus aureus*	White pustules on forehead, chest, upper back, neck, thighs, groin, and axillae; furuncles are deeper inflamed nodules; carbuncles are interconnected furuncles and often rupture, expelling purulent, foul-smelling thick drainage	Localized folliculitis is treated with warm compresses, gentle washing, and topical antibiotics. Furuncles are treated as for folliculitis with incision and drainage (I&D) to avoid rupture. Carbuncles are treated with systemic antibiotics and I&D. Instruct client to use disposable razors to avoid reinfection. **Reduce spread of infection by careful hand-washing and separate laundry of linens.**
Fungal		
Candidiasis: *Candida albicans*	Appearance depends on location; in *mouth*, infection is called thrush and appears as white plaques with an underlying red base with fissures on corners of mouth; *skin* lesions are pruritic, red, and moist with eroded scales, commonly found in axilla and gluteal, perianal, and interdigital folds; *vaginal* thrush causes intense itching and cheesy drainage	Eliminate or control predisposing factors such as antibiotics (which alter flora), malnutrition, diabetes, immunosuppression, pregnancy, or birth control pills. Use topical antifungal powders and creams. Keep skin dry and environment cool.
Tinea: variety of dermatophytes (tinea corporis, on body; tinea capitis, on scalp; tinea cruris, jock itch; tinea pedis, athlete's foot)	*Tinea corporis:* round red macules and papules with scales—lesions have advancing borders and healing centers; *tinea capitis:* patchy hair loss, inflammation, scales, and folliculitis; *tinea cruris:* red lesions with raised borders; *tinea pedis:* scaling, maceration, pain, and vesicles	Infection is controlled with antifungal solutions and creams. Acute lesions may require wet dressings, keratolytic agents, or both to remove scales. Client is taught to reduce risk by thoroughly drying after a bath or shower, wearing absorbent underwear and socks, applying talc to intertriginous areas, and wearing open shoes during warm weather.
Viral		
Herpes simplex: herpes simplex virus	Vesicles preceded by sensation of itching or burning; clear exudate from vesicles, followed by crusting; common to nose, lips, cheeks, ears, and genitalia	No cure is available. Treatment includes pain relief and topical anesthetics. Acyclovir, an antiviral drug, may decrease viral shedding and hasten healing. Avoiding sun and using sunscreens reduce recurrent lesions on lips. Reduce contagiousness by using frequent hand-washing, not picking at lesions, avoiding sexual intercourse and kissing while lesions are active, and not sharing lipsticks. Try to identify (and avoid or control) personal triggers for lesions.
Warts: human papillomavirus	Rough, fresh, or gray-colored skin protrusion	Numerous therapies, some with over-the-counter medication. May require electrodesiccation or cryosurgery. Intralesional injections of cytotoxic drugs may also be used. No treatment is also an acceptable option.

Smallpox

Smallpox is a serious, contagious, and sometimes fatal infectious disease caused by the variola virus. Smallpox outbreaks have occurred from time to time for thousands of years, but the disease has been eradicated after a successful worldwide vaccination program. The last case of smallpox in the United States was in 1949 and the last naturally occurring case in the world was in Somalia in 1977. After the disease was eliminated from the world, routine vaccination against smallpox among the general public was stopped because it was no longer necessary for prevention. Except for laboratory stockpiles, the variola virus has been eliminated. However, there is heightened concern that the variola virus might be used as an agent of bioterrorism.

Smallpox normally spreads from contact with infected people. Generally, direct and fairly prolonged face-to-face contact is required to spread smallpox from one person to another. Smallpox also can be spread through direct contact with infected body fluids or contaminated objects such as bedding or clothing. Indirect spread is less common. Rarely, smallpox has been spread by virus carried in the air in enclosed settings such as buildings, buses, and trains. Smallpox is not known to be transmitted by insects or animals.

There are two clinical forms of smallpox. *Variola major* is the severe and most common form of smallpox, with a more extensive rash and higher fever. *Variola minor* is a less common presentation of smallpox, and a much less severe disease, with death rates historically of 1% or less. There is no specific treatment for smallpox disease, although some medications are in laboratory trials; currently, the only prevention is vaccination.

The first phase of smallpox is an incubation period of 7 to 17 days after exposure to the virus. The person is not contagious and does not feel ill. The first manifestations of smallpox include fever, headache, muscle pain, and malaise (weakness, tiredness) over a 2- to 4-day time frame. A person with smallpox becomes most contagious with the onset of rash on the tongue and mouth. As the lesions open, the virus enters the mouth and airway, and the person is highly contagious. The rash spreads throughout the body over the next 2 to 3 days. The pox areas become pustular,

eventually form a crust, and then a scab. A person is contagious until the last smallpox scab falls off.

It is important to distinguish smallpox from other diseases that have skin eruptions, such as chickenpox. People with smallpox report a fever 1 to 4 days before the skin eruptions, all skin eruptions are at the small stage of development, and the skin lesions are deep-seated, round, and pustular that may be draining purulent, thick fluid. The person may recall that the first lesions were in the mouth and that they evolved over 2 to 3 days. Suspicious cases should be isolated and reported to the Centers for Disease Control and Prevention (CDC).

There is a detailed nationwide smallpox preparedness program to protect Americans against smallpox used as a biologic weapon. This program includes the creation of preparedness teams that are ready to respond to a smallpox attack on the United States. Members of these teams—health care and public health workers—are being vaccinated so that they might safely protect others in the event of a smallpox outbreak.

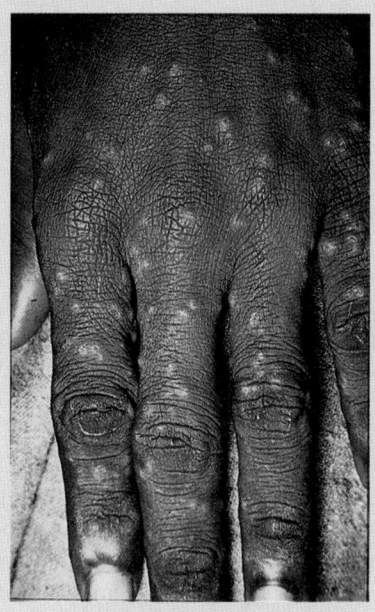

Data from Henderson, D.A. (1999). Smallpox as a biological weapon: Medical and public health management. *Journal of the American Medical Association, 281,* 2127-2137.

the client's temperature and administer prescribed antipyretic medication. Prevent cross-contamination by teaching the client proper hand-washing technique and careful handling of soiled linen, clothing, and dressings. Standard precautions should be used as appropriate. Close follow-up evaluation is necessary.

HERPES ZOSTER (SHINGLES)

Herpes zoster, or shingles, is an infection caused by the reactivation of the varicella zoster virus in clients who

have had chickenpox. Although zoster is much less communicable than varicella, people who have not had chickenpox are at risk after exposure to a person with herpes zoster. An increased incidence of herpes zoster is seen in clients with lymphoma, leukemia, or acquired immunodeficiency syndrome, probably because of their decreased immunologic response. Diagnostic tests may not be necessary because of the specific characteristics of herpes zoster; however, a Tzanck test demonstrates multinucleated giant cells (see Chapter 48), and a viral culture is also helpful.

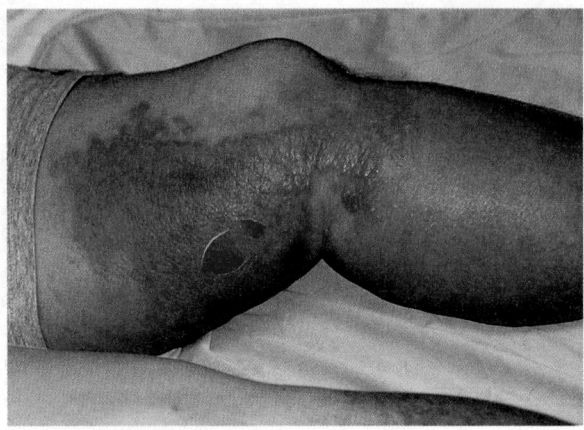

■ **FIGURE 49–9** Cellulitis in a client with long-standing diabetes and stasis dermatitis.

The primary lesion of zoster is a vesicle. The classic presentation is grouped vesicles on an erythematous base along a dermatome. The vesicles appear 1 to 2 days after onset of pain and itching at the site. Occasionally, only papules appear and not vesicles. Because they follow nerve pathways, the lesions do not cross the body's midline; however, rarely, the nerves of both sides may be involved. Herpes zoster lesions evolve into ulcers on the superficial mucous membrane.

The eruption generally clears in about 2 weeks, unless the period between the pain and the eruption is longer than 2 days. In such cases, a prolonged convalescence may be expected. Residual pain, called *postherpetic neuralgia,* and itching are the major complications with herpes zoster. The pain may be constant or intermittent and may range from light burning to a deep visceral sensation. The duration of the pain can be weeks or months to years. In older clients, the pain generally lasts months to years. Another potential complication is loss of sight when herpes zoster involves the facial or acoustic nerve. Involvement of the ophthalmic branch of the facial nerve requires close medical attention to avoid ocular damage.

OUTCOME MANAGEMENT

The primary goals of therapy are to limit extent, duration, and severity of pain and rash in the primary dermatome, prevent spread of the disease, and prevent postherpetic neuralgia. Treatment for herpes zoster is administration of antiviral medications. Antivirals, when started early in the course of the disease, reduce acute pain and accelerate healing of the lesions. Studies suggest that early oral antiviral therapy may assist in reducing postherpetic neuralgia. Analgesics and sedatives are prescribed for pain reduction.

Topical therapy is primarily symptomatic: applications of cool compresses; use of cooling antipruritic preparations, cornstarch, or baking soda; and measures to prevent secondary infection. If pain is present, the client's normal pain tolerance and current pain level must be assessed. Systemic analgesics are usually required and occasionally opioids; however, in chronic pain, use of these agents raises the possibility of addiction. Assess the effectiveness and side effects of prescribed analgesics. Because postherpetic neuralgia can last a long time, the client and significant others need continued intervention and support. Chronic pain management may include the use of tricyclic antidepressants, phenothiazines, and other local physical modalities such as electrical stimulating units.

PLASTIC SURGERY AND OTHER COSMETIC/ RESTORATIVE PROCEDURES

Plastic surgery is the surgical subspecialty that concentrates on the restoration of function and form to body structures damaged by trauma, transformed by the aging process, changed by disease processes (such as skin cancer), or malformed as a result of congenital defect. Plastic surgery can be divided into two major areas: (1) aesthetic (cosmetic) and (2) reconstructive.

Aesthetic plastic surgery improves physical features that are already within "normal" range. It is performed for changes that result from aging, to alter inherited features, or because of a client's personal desire. Because aesthetic surgery is considered "cosmetic," it is not covered by insurance; clients pay out of pocket. Most clients are enthusiastic and happy because the surgery is a culmination of a personal desire that they may have held for a long time. In contrast, other clients may or may not have social support for their decision. The client may feel vain, embarrassed, or guilty about taking health care away from "people who really need it." Become sensitive to these feelings in the client, and be comfortable with a person's normal desires to feel good about the way he or she looks.

Reconstructive surgery attempts to restore a more normal appearance or function in a person who has an abnormal body part or in whom a body part is missing. The abnormality may be a result of injury or disease, may be congenital, or it may be the cause of other medical problems. People undergoing reconstructive surgery are typically motivated to try to gain increased function of body parts and to improve their appearance. Although they may hope that plastic surgery will make them "normal," they usually know this may be unrealistic. Such clients are often struggling with diverse emotions: hope for a future without disease recurrence, eagerness to see final surgical results, anxiety over the surgery itself and impending postoperative pain, and weariness of the illness. The client having reconstructive surgery does have the advantage of social approval. Inasmuch as such a client is seen as a victim, society, as represented by either individuals or institutions, often provides treatment or makes appeals for payment of the operations.

Because of the significant impact of plastic surgery procedures on body image and self-esteem, psychological care is imperative. Plastic surgery not only is an operation on the skin but also reaches into the psyche of the person undergoing the surgery.

Minimal postoperative scarring is the hallmark of successful plastic surgery. It is important to understand that no surgery can be done without creating a scar. Plastic surgery is conducted to minimize scars, so at times it seems that surgery can be done without scars. The quality of scarring is affected by many variables, such as the client's age, general health, skin type, and healing ability. Surgical technique and the quality of wound care also affect the healing process.

Blacks, people of Mediterranean origin, and other people with dark skin tend to have more noticeable scars. Wounds located in areas in which the tissue moves as it heals (e.g., over joints) are also more susceptible to scarring. The skin of malnourished clients heals slowly, and those wounds may also develop more obvious scars.

BODY IMAGE AND SURGERY

The desire to be attractive or beautiful is present in people of all cultures, but the perception of what is attractive varies. The importance of physical appearance varies from person to person; however, it is an integral part of the sense of self. The desire to want to physically resemble one's peers reasonably closely—for instance, to have acceptably "normal" facial features—is a normal desire. A significant portion of any deformity rests in the client's perception of the abnormality. Perceptions develop in part from body image. Body image describes a person's perception of his or her body—how the person *thinks* he or she looks, rather than an objective assessment of the person's characteristics. Body image is a factor in determining self-image, self-concept, and self-esteem. People with a positive body image display more confidence and interact more easily with others. Body image changes continually, depending on individual expectations and feedback from others.

A person with a physical deformity, real or perceived, can have a severely damaged body image. Even the usual processes of aging can be detrimental to body image. A self-perception of "getting old" can impair self-confidence, affect behavior, and interfere with interactions in society. Body image is an important factor in the nursing assessment of the client having plastic surgery.

The client's ability to cope with a temporary or permanent or a perceived or actual disfigurement is also assessed. Assess the client's coping mechanisms. Some coping mechanisms may be effective; others may be ineffective. Men may have more difficulty expressing their feelings about their appearance than that typically noted in women. Listen to the client, be alert for positive and negative self-statements, and note the degree of anxiety and fear. Evaluate the client's willingness or unwillingness to touch or look at involved body areas and the client's comfort with being near other people.

Techniques for working with clients who have alterations in body image are presented in Box 49-4.

FACIAL REJUVENATING PROCEDURES

In childhood, skin is very elastic and is fully supported by adipose tissue ("baby fat"). During aging, the skin loses elasticity and the subcutaneous fat diminishes and changes character. Skinfolds and wrinkles become increasingly noticeable. Tissue around the eyes and jaw line sags, producing a drooping, tired, weary, or worried expression. The rate of skin change varies among people. Weight loss, habitual sun exposure, genetic tendencies, and alcohol and tobacco use affect the speed and character of the changes.

Facial Resurfacing
Skin Peels

Various products (alpha-hydroxy acid, glycolic acid, trichloroacetic acid) can be used to lift superficial layers of skin and remove fine wrinkles from the skin. These products are usually applied in an office setting with the client awake. The best candidates are those clients with fair skin and fine wrinkles. Trained nurses perform the peel procedure. Most skin peel procedures require a regimen of skin care before treatment. Care after the peel includes application of skin moisturizers, use of hydrocortisone to reduce edema and erythema, gentle cleansing, and use of sunscreen. The client often resumes the pre-peel skin regimen after the peel. Hyperpigmentation is the most common complication.

Laser Resurfacing

Laser treatment creates a shallow burn injury to the skin. Dormant herpes can be reactivated; therefore antiviral agents are used before treatments. Clients are sedated, or topical anesthetics such as eutectic mixture of local anesthetic (EMLA) are used. Postoperative edema can be reduced somewhat with ice packs and oral corticosteroids for 48 hours. Some clients also experience a burning sensation for 12 to 18 hours after treatment. The skin reepithelializes in about 5 to 10 days, depending on the depth of the injury. Sun-blocking agents are a must, in that hyperpigmentation can develop.

BOX 49-4 Supporting the Client Who Has a Changed Body Image

Many clients undergoing plastic surgery experience some form of body image alteration. Clients may experience body image changes before surgery because of disease or injury. They may also have problems after surgery from edema, bruising, or less than desired results. Try to anticipate these problems and work with the client as soon as possible to facilitate needed adjustments. You may want to work with the nursing diagnosis of *Risk for Disturbed Body Image* or *Situational Low Self-Esteem related to perceived or actual disfigurement and changes in self-concept.* The expected outcome must be tailored to the client but may include improved self-image with incorporation of the changed body part into the body image, as evidenced by effective coping and appropriate use of defense mechanisms; verbalizing feelings comfortably and appropriately; expressing satisfaction with the changed body image; having the ability to openly verbalize feelings; making positive statements about self; having a normal level of anxiety and normal fears; comfortably looking at self in mirror and/or touching the deformed body area, healed surgical site, or other scars; being able to be with others comfortably; and having no indications of depression.

Some interventions that you may find effective with clients who are experiencing body image disturbances include the following:

- Continue to assess apparent self-concept, coping methods, defense mechanisms, degree of anxiety, and fears frequently.
- Assist the client to explore and express feelings; do not use phrases such as "I know how you feel." These empty phrases create barriers to communication, whereas

statements such as "you are angry" or "you seem depressed," for example, identify the feeling.

- Be sensitive to and acknowledge the client's feelings and needs.
- Present reality; building false hope is detrimental (reality need not be brutal, however).
- Healing is unpredictable; refer questions about healing to the surgeon.
- Do not force the client to view or touch himself or herself; gently assist the client to look at and touch the deformity or healed surgical site (help incorporate it into the client's self-concept and body image).
- Encourage the client to begin meeting in public to begin desensitization to the reactions of others, such as by taking walks in halls; desensitization begins in safe environments and proceeds to new situations; prepare the client for stares and remarks.
- Discuss others' reaction to the client; support grief reactions.
- If the client has a facial deformity, prepare visitors and family members before they see the client.
- Look for vocal expressions or hand gestures in cases of facial disfigurement; facial expression may be limited in clients with extensive facial scars or skin grafts.
- Refer the client and family to local support groups, such as About Face.
- Assist the client with techniques to camouflage scars; licensed aestheticians can assist with make-up choices and techniques.

Dermabrasion

Dermabrasion is a process of sanding the surface layers of skin on cheeks and forehead with an electric rotating brush to smooth out pitting and surface blemishes. This operation is the preferred treatment for depressed acne scars and other deep scars. Local anesthesia with sedation is used. The abraded surfaces are covered with antibiotic ointment and gauze. After removal of the gauze, the facial skin weeps serous fluid for 5 to 7 days. Once the weeping stops and new skin has appeared, the client can apply make-up to camouflage the redness. The redness fades over the following 6 weeks.

Dermal Fillers

Soft tissue augmentation has become a popular means of addressing contour defects that result from aging, photodamage, trauma or scarification, or disease. Several products can be used (e.g., autologous fat, collagen, hyaluronic acid, Hylaform, Restylane to fill in small wrinkles or depressed blemishes in the skin. The client's reaction to collagen is tested before treatment, because some people experience induration (hard, raised area) and swelling at the injection site. Clients with autoimmune disorders

are not candidates for collagen injection. Restylane can also be used to fill medium to deep creases and folds.

Botulinum Injections

Botulinum toxin type A (Botox) can be injected to temporarily improve the appearance of moderate to severe frown lines between the eyebrows (glabellar lines). Botox is a protein produced by the bacterium *Clostridium botulinum*. Small doses of the toxin are injected into the affected muscles and block the release of the chemical acetylcholine that would otherwise signal the muscle to contract. The toxin thus paralyzes or weakens the injected muscle for up to 120 days. Following injection, some clients report headache, respiratory tract infection, flu syndrome, blepharoptosis (droopy eyelids), and nausea. Less frequent adverse reactions include pain in the face, redness at the injection site, and muscle weakness.

Rhytidectomy (Face Lift)

A rhytidectomy *(face lift)* may restore a more youthful appearance to the face (perhaps from 5 to 10 years younger) by removing wrinkled skin from the forehead and around the eyes and mouth (Figure 49-10).

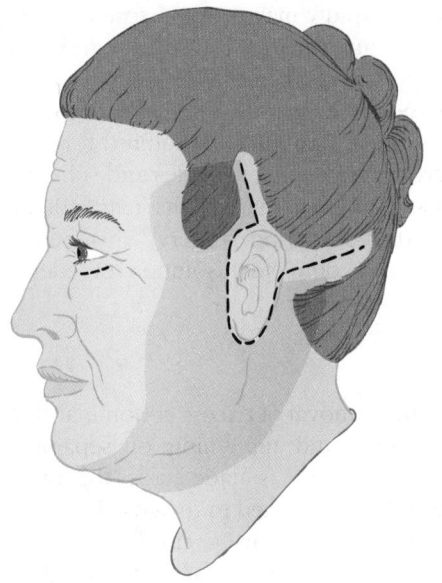

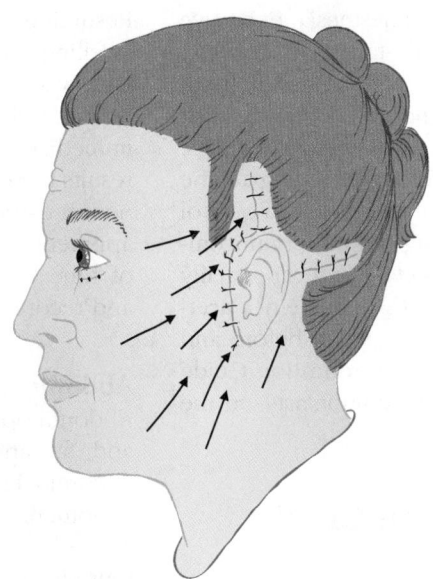

A Before face lift and blepharoplasty

B After face lift and blepharoplasty

■ **FIGURE 49-10** Face lift (rhytidectomy) and blepharoplasty. Face lifts enable removal of large wrinkles and folds of skin from the face and neck. **A,** Area in pink shows amount of tissue that is undermined (lifted from the fascial connection) and moved during a face lift. For the face lift, the incision lines go around the ear and into the hair-bearing scalp; other incisions may also be used. Note also the incision line beneath the eyelid for the blepharoplasty, which enables removal of excess eyelid tissue. **B,** The postoperative near-final result, with tightened facial skin and neck folds.

Rhytidectomy is usually performed on an outpatient basis with the client under general anesthesia, or using local anesthesia with IV sedation. Incisions are made from the temple along the ear and out into the hair-bearing scalp behind the ear. Through the incisions, excess facial skin is undermined and pulled back toward the ear. *Undermining* is a surgical technique in which the skin is separated from underlying structures.

Postoperatively, the client is placed in the Fowler position to reduce the risk of edema. Cold compresses can also be used to reduce swelling and bleeding. Suction drains are used to eliminate dead space and remove wound drainage. Drains are removed in 24 to 48 hours, when drainage has subsided. Facial movement (talking and chewing) should be limited. Increases in blood pressure should be avoided by keeping the head elevated; any prescribed antihypertensive medications should also be resumed. Coughing also increases blood pressure and should be avoided (by not operating on clients with colds) or treated if it manifests after surgery.

Complications include hematomas, which can cause tissue necrosis and must be surgically removed. Hematoma formation occurs most often in people who smoke or have pre-existing hypertension. Postoperative nausea and vomiting can also increase bleeding and hematoma formation. Hematoma development is first noted as increasing facial asymmetry associated with pain or tightness on one side of the face. Increasing drainage and changes in facial sensation should also be reported.

Blepharoplasty

Blepharoplasty is the surgical removal of excess skin and periorbital fat from the upper or lower eyelid.

Blepharoplasty is usually performed on an outpatient basis. General or local anesthesia with sedation can be used. Wide elliptical incisions are made on the upper eyelids. The excised wedge of excess tissue is lifted off, and herniated fat is removed. A lower-lid blepharoplasty incision is placed ⅛ inch below the edge of the eyelid.

Assess preoperative near and distant vision in each eye by asking the client to read from a book and from something in the distance while one eye is covered. These baseline data are crucial to assess postoperative visual changes. An ophthalmologic examination is indicated before surgery if vision problems are noted.

After blepharoplasty, the head is elevated to reduce edema. Iced normal saline compresses or patches are applied to the eyes as prescribed. Activity is limited for 1 week to reduce blood pressure elevations that often lead to increased edema and ecchymosis (bruising). Normally, severe pain is not experienced after blepharoplasty. An itching sensation, similar to that associated with dry eyes, is usually experienced as a result of slight corneal swelling. This can be prevented with cold wet dressings.

Rhinoplasty

Rhinoplasty is the surgical correction of nasal deformities. This procedure is frequently performed as an outpatient procedure using either local anesthesia and sedation or general anesthesia. Incisions are made inside the nose to reshape the dorsum, ala, or internal cartilage. After surgery, the inside of the nose may be packed and an external splint applied.

Preoperative nursing care focuses on teaching the client to breathe through the mouth after surgery and to not touch the nose. Postoperatively, assess for bleeding.

While the client is sleepy from the anesthesia, excessive swallowing may be the only manifestation of bleeding. Examine the back of the throat with a flashlight to look for blood. Some bleeding is normal down the back of the throat and on the nasal packs and dressings. The nurse promptly reports excessive bleeding to the surgeon. The head of the bed is kept elevated to control postoperative edema. Nasal packing can be very uncomfortable. Pain management is important and can usually be achieved with oral analgesics (e.g., codeine, acetaminophen). Aspirin is avoided for 1 week before and 3 weeks after surgery. (See the Client Education Guide feature on Postoperative Care After Rhinoplasty on the *evolve* website.)

BODY-CONTOURING SURGERY (LIPECTOMY)

Body-contouring surgical procedures (lipectomy) remove excess fatty tissue, skinfolds, or subcutaneous fat from various body parts, including the abdomen, thighs, arms, and buttocks.

Liposuction

Liposuction is a technique used (1) to aspirate fatty tissue from areas of the body resistant to diet and exercise (lipodystrophy), (2) to contour flaps, and (3) to remove lipomas (benign fatty tumors). A blunt, hollow cannula is inserted through very small incisions and then attached to a powerful suction machine that vacuums out adipose tissue. After surgery, compression garments are used to prevent fluid collection (hematoma and seroma), to maintain the desired body contour, and to promote healing. Tumescent technique involves the additional use of large volumes of dilute lidocaine and epinephrine. These medications promote vasoconstriction to minimize bleeding and provide postoperative analgesia. Ultrasonic lipectomy is the use of ultrasound to ease the removal of fat.

Complications of liposuction include hematoma, skin necrosis, infection, and undesirable scars or skin dimpling. If large volumes of fat are removed, hypovolemia may develop. Pulmonary embolism has also been reported.

After liposuction, assess the client for hypovolemia and electrolyte imbalance (manifested by syncope, dizziness, and abnormal blood values). If drains are used, monitor the quantity and quality of drainage. Ice and oral analgesics are effective in managing postoperative pain. Dressings usually remain in place for at least 24 hours. Nurses must ensure that dressings remain smooth and uniform; otherwise, contour irregularities can result. Sometimes the client wears a compression garment for several weeks postoperatively.

Clients may gradually resume normal activity except for strenuous exercise. It may be 4 to 6 weeks before the client works up to the preoperative level of exercise.

Resuming activity too rapidly may result in soreness and swelling. Bruising is common after liposuction and may take weeks to disappear completely.

Many clients expect the results of liposuction to be immediate. Usually up to 6 months is required for final results to be apparent after edema subsides and subcutaneous tissue heals. Reinforce that results may not be apparent for 6 months following surgery. This period of time is required for complete resolution of edema and reconnection of soft tissues.

Abdominoplasty

Abdominoplasty is the removal of excess abdominal skin and fat and the repair and tightening of separated abdominal muscles. An incision is made across the lower abdomen, and tissue is undermined to the costal margin. The excess skin and fatty tissue are excised and recontoured. The umbilical stalk is detached and reattached once the overlying skin is in its proper position.

After surgery, inspect the incision line for manifestations of pallor or lack of capillary refill. The operative site can swell, with resulting impairment of capillary blood supply. Smoking is prohibited, because nicotine further restricts blood flow to the skin. Tension on the suture line must be minimized; therefore the client must lie in semi-Fowler position with the knees flexed (a contouring position). The client also needs to walk in a "hunched-over" position until the swelling decreases and abdominal skin relaxes. Teach the client postoperative pain management techniques. Abdominoplasty is an abdominal operation and produces significant postoperative discomfort. Adequate analgesia and other pain-relieving measures are essential. As suggested in the Management and Delegation feature below, reinforce to unlicensed personnel that these plastic surgery clients require usual postoperative care.

MANAGEMENT AND DELEGATION

Care of Clients Recovering from Plastic Surgery

When unlicensed assistive personnel are caring for clients after plastic surgery, reinforce the need for adequate pain management and routine postoperative care. It is not uncommon for these clients to feel uncomfortable about asking for pain medications and for nursing assistance. Some people have the notion that surgery "for vanity" should hurt a little. This is a dangerous philosophy and should not be condoned. Any incision hurts, and these clients do not differ in their need for pain control. Likewise, measuring routine vital signs, providing pulmonary care, monitoring intake and output, and encouraging ambulation are routine aspects of postoperative nursing care. Withholding care is not acceptable.

Panniculectomy

In people who have experienced major weight loss, excess loose skin and subcutaneous tissue may remain over the abdomen, thighs, and arms, hanging in large folds. The folds of tissue are called *pannus,* and panniculectomy is the surgical removal of these tissue folds. As much as 10 pounds of redundant tissue has been surgically removed during one of these operations. Clearly, this operation is not for the cure of the client's obesity, but it can offer some positive gains in self-esteem and reduction in health-related problems.

Postoperative care is usually focused on reducing stress on the long suture lines. For example, place the client in the Fowler position after abdominal panniculectomy. Monitor the suture lines closely for manifestations of nonhealing. Fatty tissue is poorly perfused, and the client may have pre-existing diet-induced malnutrition. During the healing phase, the client needs to consume adequate amounts of protein and carbohydrate to heal. Other tissue folds must be treated for intertriginous dermatitis (see earlier discussion on intertrigo).

RECONSTRUCTIVE PLASTIC SURGERY

One of the greatest challenges in plastic surgery is the reconstruction of deformities. Skin grafting is discussed in Chapter 50. This section discusses flap surgery.

Flaps are areas of tissue raised from one area of the body without being completely detached, so that the blood supply is intact; the flap is transferred (e.g., by rotation) to adjacent areas. Flaps of tissue can also be transferred to distant areas, where a blood supply is reestablished; these are called *free flaps* and are discussed later. Local flaps are rotated or advanced to reconstruct an adjacent defect (Figure 49-11).

Preservation of the nutrient blood vessels is paramount to flap survival. The tissue attachment containing these vessels is sometimes called the *pedicle,* because in the past flaps were moved from site to site with a visible portion of tissue that "carried" the flap to the recipient site. This style of flap can be seen in the deltopectoral flaps used to repair neck resection tissue loss. Flaps are also used to cover extensive wounds from pressure ulcers and long-standing defects from osteomyelitis.

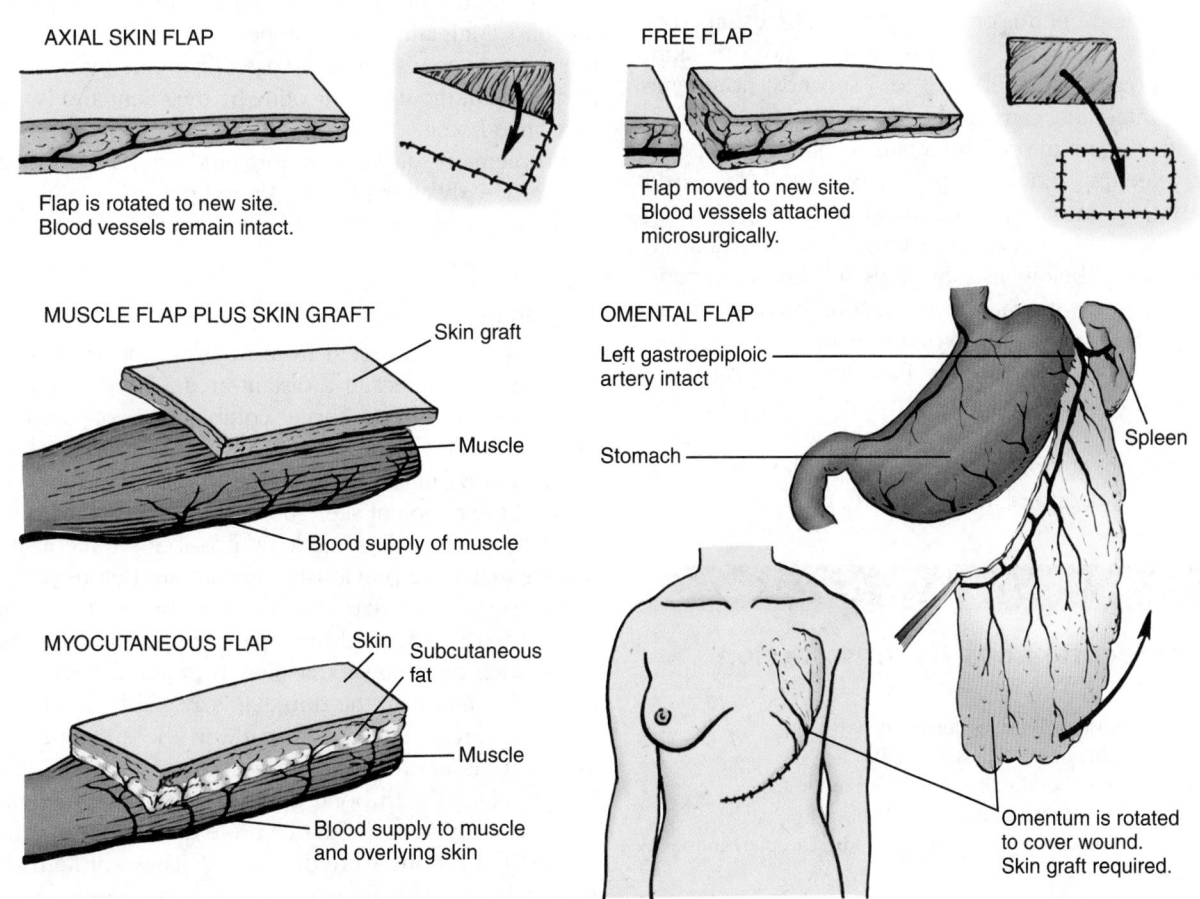

AXIAL SKIN FLAP

Flap is rotated to new site.
Blood vessels remain intact.

FREE FLAP

Flap moved to new site.
Blood vessels attached
microsurgically.

MUSCLE FLAP PLUS SKIN GRAFT
Skin graft
Muscle
Blood supply of muscle

OMENTAL FLAP
Left gastroepiploic artery intact
Stomach
Spleen

MYOCUTANEOUS FLAP
Skin Subcutaneous fat
Muscle
Blood supply to muscle and overlying skin

Omentum is rotated
to cover wound.
Skin graft required.

■ **FIGURE 49-11** Common flaps.

Skin Flaps

Skin flaps are sections of skin rotated from their origin to cover a defect. Common uses of skin flaps are to reconstruct a neck after excision of cancer (deltopectoral flap) or the face (rotation flap). Occasionally skin flaps are used to close pressure ulcers on the pelvis. Blood flow to the flap must be protected. Avoid securing dressings or tracheotomy ties across the flap.

Musculocutaneous Flaps

Flaps comprising both muscle and skin are called *musculocutaneous flaps.* They are commonly used to fill in defects where muscle is missing or where muscle can provide ample blood flow to heal osteomyelitis. These flaps are named by the muscle of origin. For example, large trochanteric pressure ulcers can be repaired with tensor fasciae latae flaps, named for the tensor fasciae latae muscle of the lateral thigh. Intrathoracic muscle flaps used for chest wall reconstruction include serratus anterior, latissimus dorsi, and pectoralis muscles.

Nursing care centers on maintaining perfusion and reducing tissue injury to the flap. You may choose to design your nursing care under the nursing diagnosis of *Risk for Ineffective Tissue Perfusion related to tissue transfer.*

The outcome is that the client will maintain effective peripheral tissue perfusion, as evidenced by usual color of skin, no pallor or cyanosis, warm and dry skin, blanching (capillary refill) in 3 to 5 seconds, no edema or blebs, intact incisions, and controllable pain.

The flap is monitored for color, capillary refill, and dermal bleeding. Look for pallor, coolness, decreased capillary refill, or dark dermal blood on lancing (lancing may not be allowed in some settings). The Critical Monitoring feature below lists findings to report immediately in clients with musculocutaneous reconstruction. It takes a fair amount of experience in clinical assessment of flaps to predict early flap demise using these subjective methods. Findings can vary because of oxygen content of the blood, capillary dilation, blood flow, and skin pigmentation. Therefore in complex flaps, temperature and Doppler monitors are used to monitor

circulation. The extremity is usually elevated to improve venous return as long as elevation does not interfere with arterial flow.

Protecting the blood supply to a flap is a primary nursing responsibility. Nursing interventions are designed to avoid factors that can jeopardize blood flow. Position the client so that the flap is relaxed and elevated. Gravity promotes edema and venous congestion, both of which impede blood flow. Interventions to increase venous return include elevating the involved body part and applying elastic stockings or wraps as prescribed. Tension on the flap can stretch or kink the feeding blood vessels, reducing the flow of blood to the tissues. A blood clot can restrict blood flow. The first manifestation of compromised blood flow is pallor.

Know the location of the pedicle that carries blood vessels to the flap. Most of the time the pedicle is buried, and little can be done to harm it. Some exceptions exist, though. When skin flaps are used, such as the deltopectoral flap, the pedicle is visible. Tracheostomy ties should not be tied tightly around the flap; otherwise, circulation to the distal portions will be compromised. When the breast is reconstructed after mastectomy with a latissimus dorsi flap, the pedicle is located in the ipsilateral axilla. The client cannot lie on the ipsilateral side or blood flow to the flap will be impaired.

Hydrate the client well, if prescribed, to help perfuse the flap. Maintain any postoperative splints to prevent tension on vessels. Limit the use of caffeine by the client and prohibit the use of nicotine by the client and by visitors once home.

Problems resulting from impaired arterial supply are apparent early after surgery. Altered perfusion caused by venous obstruction may not be evident for a few hours.

Free Flaps

Free flaps are harvested from one area of the body to reconstruct a defect in a distant area. The donor tissue (skin, muscle, bone, or a combination of these) is detached from its blood supply at the donor site and reattached by microvascular anastomosis to arteries and veins at the recipient site. The development of microvascular techniques has made it possible to reconstruct defects that were previously untreatable. Before surgical reconstruction, a flap can be prefabricated to build exactly what is needed for repair. Supplemental techniques, such as tissue expansion (discussed later), may be used to augment the skin that is available for closure. Other advances have been made in the areas of bone and soft tissue reconstruction. Bone has traditionally been replaced with bone grafts or alloplastic materials. More recently, osteoinductive proteins capable of differentiating into bone were discovered. These proteins can be combined with muscle flaps, and the tissue then is transformed into useful bone.

CRITICAL MONITORING

Musculocutaneous Reconstruction

Report the following findings immediately:
- Development of coolness in the flap
- Development of duskiness or pallor in the flap
- Slowing of capillary refill in the flap
- Loss of pulses (palpable or detected by Doppler) in the flap
- Increasing pain in the flap

Preoperative client characteristics to consider include health status and condition of potential donor tissue. Diabetes and cardiovascular, renal, and pulmonary disease do not present absolute contraindications, but these diseases do increase risk of flap failure. The vessels used for a flap must not be in proximity to sites of previous trauma or irradiation. After trauma, widespread changes occur in the walls and perivascular tissues of the major vascular bundles. These changes have been labeled as *post-traumatic vessel disease* (PTVD). Vessels with PTVD are more difficult to dissect, are easily damaged, and have little resistance against clots. Donor sites are chosen according to guidelines presented previously. The donor site pedicle is deliberately planned so that the flap can comfortably reach the recipient site.

Free Flap Failure

When all goes well, the advantages of free flaps are obvious. Nevertheless, the phantom called *free flap failure* looms large, limiting use of the procedure. Thrombosis is the most common cause of failure. After surgery, the free flap site is seldom dressed, so that clinical assessments can be performed. Several techniques have been developed in large clinical trials, but no consensus exists as to which is the best technique. The ideal monitoring system would provide a continuous recording of flap perfusion or flap metabolism. It should monitor both visible and buried tissues. Finally, the data should be easily interpreted by nursing personnel and junior medical staff.

Assess for trends in color, texture, and temperature of the flap, as well as Doppler pulses and drainage from wound drains. Other postoperative care includes maintaining adequate hydration, keeping the client warm, managing pain, and allowing only appropriate activities. Clients may express some concern with the decision to salvage a body part or may fear that the flap will fail

and amputation will be required. The nurse needs to be supportive of the decision for surgery and allow time for expression of fears.

SKIN EXPANSION

Skin expansion is a technique used to increase the amount of local tissue available to reconstruct a defect. An inflatable silicone balloon is placed under the skin or muscle flap adjacent to a defect. The expander is inflated sequentially over several weeks or months to stretch the overlying tissue. When tissue is sufficient to resurface the adjacent defect, the balloon is removed and the flap is contoured (shaped) and advanced to cover the defect.

REPAIR OF TRAUMATIC INJURIES

Facial Fractures

Fractures can occur in the individual bones of the face: the nasal bones, orbit, malar prominence, mandible, or maxilla (Figure 49-12). The client with facial fractures has often been involved in an automobile accident or an assault or has suffered a sports injury. Pain, improper bite (malocclusion), swelling, bruising, diplopia (double vision), facial asymmetry, enophthalmos (sunken eye), and exophthalmos (bulging eye) are clinical manifestations of facial fractures. Diagnostic assessment includes x-ray studies.

Life-threatening problems (e.g., airway obstruction, hemorrhage, or cervical spine injury) that may accompany facial trauma must be managed immediately. Because of the proximity of the injury to the airway, assess airway patency and breath sounds every 2 hours (more often if bleeding is present). Place suction equipment at the bedside. Teach the client to breathe through the nose. Trying to open the mouth may dislocate the fracture.

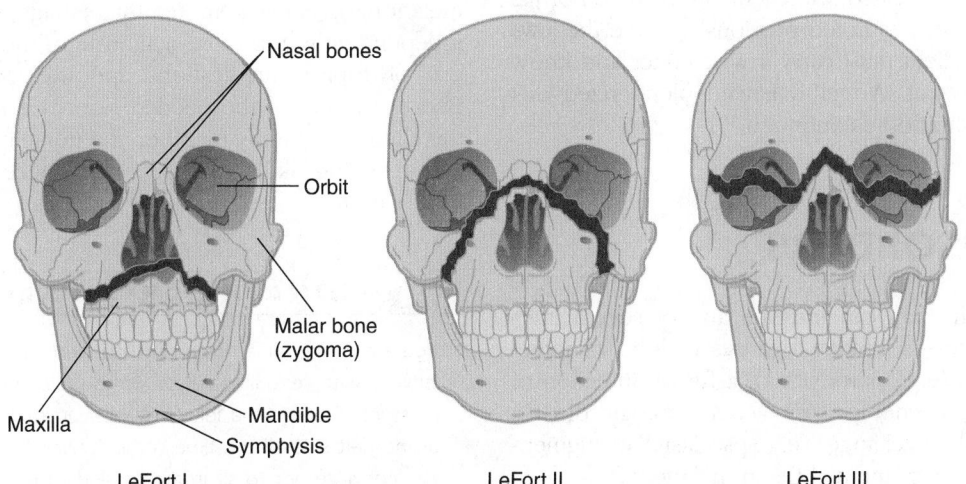

Nasal bones
Orbit
Malar bone (zygoma)
Maxilla
Mandible
Symphysis

LeFort I   LeFort II   LeFort III

■ **FIGURE 49-12** LeFort fractures. *LeFort I:* transverse fracture of the alveolar process separating the upper dental arch from the maxilla; *LeFort II:* fracture of the mid face, maxilla, and orbits; *LeFort III:* fracture of the orbit that creates craniofacial dissociation.

Repair of facial fractures can be delayed for up to 3 weeks and still achieve good results. Like all fractures, facial fractures must be reduced, stabilized, and immobilized to ensure proper healing. Methods vary according to the location of the fractures.

 When the client has intermaxillary wiring, wire cutters should be in the client's possession at all times. If airway problems develop that cannot be managed with suction, the wires that secure the upper and lower jaws should be cut. The nurse and the client need to be informed about which wires should be cut. These are the only wires that attach the top and bottom teeth. Do not try to cut off the bands attached to the teeth.

A liquefied diet is used until the wires are removed. Without adequate nutrition, clients can lose 10 to 20 pounds during convalescence. Instruct the client how to "blenderize" food and to maintain an adequate balance of carbohydrates, fat, protein, and calories. Milkshakes can be made with a wide variety of foods. High-calorie food supplements can augment the regular diet, and liquid multivitamins may be useful. Alcoholic and carbonated beverages can cause nausea and can fizz and foam in the back of the throat, leading to airway problems; they are to be avoided.

Oral hygiene aids in healing of oral wounds, prevents infection and destruction of teeth and gums, increases comfort, and enhances self-esteem. Rinsing the mouth with water or a mouthwash followed by use of an oral irrigation device on low pressure removes particles from the front of the mouth while the tissues are still tender. Once the initial swelling and tenderness subside, the teeth must be brushed and the mouth rinsed after every meal and at bedtime. Pieces of dental wax can be placed on the open ends of the wires if they irritate buccal surfaces.

Before discharge, the client and family members need to be taught about the wires, diet, and oral care. Once the incisions have healed, the client can resume normal activities. However, as noted previously, while the jaws are wired, the client must carry a wire cutter and know which wires to cut. A well-balanced blenderized diet and oral care should be continued.

NAIL DISORDERS

Disorders of the nail can indicate any of several dermatologic processes. Potential causes include an infection of the nail (e.g., paronychia), a fungal infection of the nail (e.g., onychomycosis), a dermatologic disease with prominent nail changes (e.g., psoriasis), or pigmentary abnormalities of the nail (as in melanoma).

Unguis incarnatus (ingrown nail) is one of the most common nail conditions and is caused by improper nail trimming and by wearing tight or ill-fitting shoes. It primarily involves the nail of the great toe that acts as a foreign body, leading to inflammation. A painful, warm inflammatory reaction results from excessive lateral growth of the nail into the nailfold. Decrease inflammation with warm soaks for 20 minutes several times a day. If the problem is minor, lifting the lateral portion of the nail by inserting a cotton wick prevents contact with the nailfold. Sometimes, the involved segment of the nailfold needs to be excised.

Paronychia, or infection around the nail, is characterized by red, shiny skin often associated with painful swelling. These infections frequently result from trauma, picking at the nail, or disorders such as dermatitis. Often these sites become secondarily infected with bacteria or fungi, which later involve the nail. As with ingrown toenail, warm soaks three or more times a day may reduce pressure and pain; however, incision and drainage of inflamed sites is frequently required. Samples for appropriate cultures of the purulent material and the nail should be obtained.

Onychomycosis refers to any fungal infection of the nail, whether caused by dermatophytes or candidiasis. Topical or systemic antibiotic or antifungal therapy is prescribed, with emphasis on medication regimen compliance. Unfortunately, even with good compliance, recurrence of fungal infections in nails is frequent.

Clients should understand the importance of reducing trauma and irritation to involved nails by (1) trimming nails straight across to reduce further trauma, (2) avoiding overmanicuring or self-induced trauma, (3) limiting harsh chemical irritants such as abrasive cleansers and drying nail products, and (4) keeping the nails dry.

CONCLUSIONS

Skin disorders range from those that are a mere nuisance (such as dry skin) to life-threatening disorders (such as melanoma). Nurses frequently manage skin disorders independently; therefore a thorough knowledge of the use of topical medications and therapies is crucial. Because much of the needed skin care is provided by the client or a family member, the nurse must use excellent teaching skills to convey the necessary self-care information.

THINKING CRITICALLY

1. You are caring for an older woman who has had a stroke that left her with residual paralysis on the left side. She also has a pressure ulcer on the left trochanter, in part because she lies on her left side all the time. While caring for her on Monday, you convince her to sit in a chair and to lie on her right side. When you care for her again on Thursday, the ulcer is twice as large and deeper. She refuses to turn to the right and says "I like lying on my left side." What can you do to help this client?

Factors to Consider. What pressure-redistribution methods should be instituted? Is there any harm in lying on a pressure ulcer? Why might she be at increased risk because of malnutrition?

2. The client is a 72-year-old Caucasian man who had undergone a wide excisional biopsy on his forearm to rule out squamous cell carcinoma. The next day the client calls the office complaining of pain at the surgery site. What additional questions need to be asked? What potential interventions might be necessary?

Factors to Consider. What clinical manifestations would indicate an infection is present? Is age a factor in wound healing?

3. The client is an otherwise healthy 41-year-old woman who presented to the clinic with a week-long history of intensely itchy, erythematous red lesions under her breasts. The rash appears to be spreading, and the centers of some of the lesions are seen to contain tiny pustules. In addition, the woman complains of a 12-pound weight loss over the past 6 months despite always feeling hungry and thirsty. She denies any medical problems and reports that she does not currently take systemic or topical medications.

Factors to Consider. What is the common cause of intertriginous dermatitis? What diagnostic study can determine the cause of the problem? What endocrine disorder is suggested by the history of skin rash, thirst, and weight loss?

Discussions for these questions can be found on the website.

BIBLIOGRAPHY

🔴 Citations appearing in red refer to primary research.

🔵 Citations appearing in blue refer to evidence-based practice guidelines and protocols.

1. Aly, R., Bayles, C., & Forney, R. (2001). Treatments for common superficial fungal infections. *Dermatology Nursing, 13*(2), 91-101.
2. American Society of Plastic Surgical Nurses. (2007). *Core curriculum for plastic and reconstructive surgical nurses* (3rd ed.). Pensacola, Fla: Author.
3. Ankrom, M., Bennett, R., Sprigle, S., & the National Pressure Ulcer Advisory Panel. (2005). Pressure-related deep tissue injury under intact skin and the current pressure ulcer staging systems. *Advances in Skin and Wound Care, 18*(1), 35-42.
4. Ayello, E.A., & Franz, R.A. (2003). Pressure ulcer prevention and treatment: Competency-based nursing curricula. *Dermatology Nursing, 15*(1), 44-55.
5. Berger, T.G., James, W.D., & Odom, R.B. (2000). *Andrews' diseases of the skin: Clinical dermatology* (9th ed.). Philadelphia: Saunders.
6. Bergstrom, N., & Braden, B. (1987). The Braden Scale for predicting pressure sore risk. *Nursing Research, 36*(4), 205-210.
7. Bergstrom, N., et al. (1994). *Treatment of pressure ulcers: Clinical practice guideline No. 15* (AHCPR Pub No. 95-0652). Rockville, Md: U.S. Department of Health and Human Services, Public Health Service, Agency for Health Care Policy and Research.
8. Bergstrom, N., et al. (1992). *Pressure ulcers in adults: Prediction and prevention* (AHCPR Pub No. 95-0050). Rockville, Md: U.S. Department of Health and Human Services, Public Health Service, Agency for Health Care Policy and Research.
9. Bielory, L., & Kanuga, M. (2002). Complementary and alternative interventions in atopic dermatitis. In M. Boguniewicz (Ed.), *Immunology and Allergy Clinics of North America: Atopic Dermatitis, 22*(1), 153-173.
10. Black, J., Baharestani, M., Cuddigan, J., et al. (2007). National Pressure Ulcer Advisory Panel's updated pressure ulcer staging system. *Advances in Skin and Wound Care, 20*(5), 269-274.
11. Black, J. (2006). Saving the skin during kinetic bed therapy. *Nursing 2006, 36*, 17.
12. Black, J., & National Pressure Ulcer Advisory Panel. (2005). Moving toward consensus on deep tissue injury and pressure ulcer staging. *Advances in Skin and Wound Care, 18*(8), 415-421.
13. Black, J. (2005). Treating heel pressure ulcers. *Nursing 2005, 35*(1), 68.
14. Black, J. (2004). Preventing heel pressure ulcers. *Nursing 2004, 34*(11), 17.
15. Black, J., & Black, S. (2003). Deep tissue injury. *Wounds: A Compendium of Clinical Research and Practice, 16*(11), 380.
16. Black, J. (2000). Improving outcomes in the elderly after pressure ulcer repair. *Plastic Surgical Nursing, 20*(3), 139-143, 170.
17. Boguniewicz, M., et al. (2003). Evolution in the treatment of atopic dermatitis: New approaches to managing a chronic skin disease. *Dermatology Nursing* (Suppl), *15*(4), 3-19.
18. Boguniewicz, M., & Leung, D.Y.M. (2001). Pathophysiologic mechanisms in atopic dermatitis. *Seminars in Cutaneous Medicine and Surgery, 20*(4), 217-225.
19. Boguniewicz, M., & Nicol, N.H. (2002). Conventional therapy for atopic dermatitis. In M. Boguniewicz (Ed.), *Immunology and allergy clinics of North America, atopic dermatitis* (pp. 107-124). Philadelphia: Saunders.
20. Bratcher, C., & Stover, B. (2001). Varicella-zoster virus: Infection, control, and prevention. *American Journal of Infection Control, 26*(3), 369-381.
21. Callen, J.P. (2000). *Color atlas of dermatology* (2nd ed.). Philadelphia: Saunders.
22. Camisa, C., & Warner, M. (1998). Treatment of pemphigus. *Dermatology Nursing, 10*(2), 115-118, 123-131.
23. Cohen, P.R., Schulze, K.E., Tolz, R., et al. (2006). Allergic contact dermatitis. *Dermatology Nursing, 18*(1), 48-49.
24. Christos, P.J., Oliveria, S.A., Masse, L.C., et al. (2004). Skin cancer prevention and detection by nurses: Attitudes, perceptions and barriers. *Journal of Cancer Education, 19*(1), 50-57.
25. Coolum, N., McInnes, E., Bell-Syer, S.E., et al. (2004). Support surfaces for pressure ulcer prevention. *Cochrane Database of Systematic Reviews* (electronic resource), CD001735.
26. Cullum, N., Deeks, J., Sheldon, T., et al. (2002). Beds, mattresses and cushions for pressure sore prevention and treatment. *The Cochrane Library,* 1.
27. DeLeo, V.A., Elsner, P., & Marks, J.G., Jr. (2002). *Contact & occupational dermatology* (3rd ed.). St. Louis: Mosby.
28. Duvic, M., et al. (2003). Analysis of long-term outcomes of combined modality therapy for cutaneous T-cell lymphoma. *Journal of the American Academy of Dermatology, 51*(1), 35-54.
29. Freedberg, I.M., Eisen, A.Z., & Wolff, K. (2003). *Fitzpatrick's dermatology in general medicine* (6th ed.). New York: McGraw-Hill, Health Professions Division.
30. Gilchrest, B.A. (2002). *Geriatric dermatology part II.* Philadelphia: Saunders.
31. Greaves, M.W., & Leung, D.Y.M. (2000). *Allergic skin disease: A multidisciplinary approach.* New York: Marcel Dekker.
32. Guile, K., & Nicholson, S. (2004). Does knowledge influence melanoma-prone behavior? Awareness, exposure, and sun protection among five social groups. *Oncology Nursing Forum, 31*(3), 641-646.
33. Heddens, C. (2001). Belt lipectomy: Procedure and outcomes. *Plastic Surgical Nursing, 21*(4), 185-189, 199.
34. Hill, M.J. (2003). *Dermatology nursing essentials: A core curriculum—Dermatology Nurses' Association* (2nd ed.). Pitman, NJ: Anthony J. Jannetti.
35. Kanzler, M.H., & Swetter, S.M. (2003). Malignant melanoma. *Journal of the American Academy of Dermatology, 48*(5), 781-783.
36. Leone, G., Rolston, K., & Spaulding, G. (2003). Alefacept for chronic plaque psoriasis: A selective therapy with long-lasting disease remissions and an encouraging safety profile. *Dermatology Nursing, 15*(3), 216-220.
37. Madison, L.K. (2001). Shingles update: Common questions in caring for a patient with shingles. *Dermatology Nursing, 13*(1), 51-55.
38. Memierre, M.F., Allten, S., & Brown, R. (2005). New treatments for melanoma. *Dermatology Nursing, 17*(4), 287-295.

39. Menter, M.A. (Ed.) (2003). Psoriasis for the clinician: A new therapeutics era ("the biologics") beckons. *Journal of the American Academy of Dermatology, 51*(Suppl), 39-142.

40. Naeyaert, J.M., & Brochez, L. (2003). Dysplastic nevi. *New England Journal of Medicine, 349*(23), 2233-2240.

41. Nicol, N.H. (2003). Dermatitis/eczemas. In M.J. Hill (Ed.), *Dermatologic nursing essentials: A core curriculum* (2nd ed., pp. 103-116). Pitman, NJ: Anthony J. Jannetti.

42. Nicol, N.H. (2000). Managing atopic dermatitis in children and adults. *Nurse Practitioner, 25*, 58-79.

43. Nicol, N.H., & Baumeister, L. (1997). Topical corticosteroid therapy: Considerations for prescribing and use. *Lippincott's Primary Care Practice, 1*(1), 62-69.

44. Nicol, N.H., & Boguniewicz, M. (1999). Understanding and treating atopic dermatitis. *Nurse Practitioner Forum, 10*(2), 48-55.

45. Noel, S., & Strohl, R. (2002). The management of high-risk melanoma: Staging, treatment, and nursing issues. *Dermatology Nursing, 14*(6), 363-371.

46. Nunley, J.R. (2000). Cutaneous manifestations of HIV and HCV. *Dermatology Nursing, 12*(3), 163-173.

47. Oliveria, S.A., Dusza, S.W., Phelan, S.L., et al. (2004). Patient adherence to skin self-examination. Effect of nurse intervention with photographs. *American Journal of Preventive Medicine, 26*(2), 152-155.

48. Pinnell, S.R. (2003). Cutaneous photodamage, oxidative stress, and topical antioxidant protection. *Journal of the American Academy of Dermatology, 48*(1), 1-22.

49. Smith, P., Black, J., & Black, S. (1999). Infected pressure ulcers in the long-term care facility. *Infection Control and Hospital Epidemiology, 20*(5), 358-361.

50. Spilsbury, K., Nelson, A., Cullum, N., et al. (2007). Pressure ulcers and their treatment and effects on quality of life: Hospital inpatient perspectives. *Journal of Advanced Nursing, 57*(5), 494-504.

51. Stulberg, D.L., Penrod, M.A., & Blatny, R.A. (2002). Common bacterial skin infections. *American Family Physician, 66*(1), 119-124.

52. Trioa, C. (2002). Promoting positive outcomes in obese patients. *Plastic Surgical Nursing, 22*(1), 10-17, 28.

53. Wheeler, T. (2006). Psychological consequences of malignant melanoma: Patients' experiences and preferences. *Nursing Standard, 21*(10), 42-46.

54. Wound Ostomy and Continence Nurses Society. (2003). *Guideline for prevention and management of pressure ulcers.* Glenview, Ill: Author.

55. Wound Ostomy and Continence Nurses Society. (2003). *Guideline for prevention and management of incontinence.* Glenview, Ill: Author.

evolve *Did you remember to check out the bonus material on the Evolve website and the CD-ROM, including NCLEX®-Examination Style Review Questions, Open-Book Quizzes, and Chapter Review Audio Podcasts?*

http://evolve.elsevier.com/Black/medsurg

CHAPTER **50**

Management of Clients with Burn Injury

GRETCHEN J. CARROUGHER AND CHARLES SANDIDGE

Injuries that result from direct contact with or exposure to any thermal, chemical, electrical, or radiation source are termed *burns*. Burn injuries occur when energy from a heat source is transferred to the tissues of the body. The depth of injury is related to the temperature and the duration of exposure or contact.

Burn care has improved in recent decades, resulting in a lower mortality for victims of burn injuries. Dedicated burn centers have been established in which multidisciplinary burn team members work together to care for the burn client and family. Advances in pre-hospital and inpatient care have contributed to survival. However, despite these advances, many people are still injured and die each year from burns. In the United States, it is estimated that 500,000 people are treated every year for a burn injury. Of these, approximately 40,000 will require hospitalization.[2]

Etiology

Burns can be caused from a number of substances or items that come into direct contact with the skin or lungs. To facilitate treatment, burn injuries are categorized according to the mechanism of injury.

Thermal Burns

Thermal burns are caused by exposure to or contact with flame, hot liquids, semiliquids (e.g., steam), semisolids (e.g., tar), or hot objects. Specific examples of thermal burns are those sustained in residential fires, explosive automobile accidents, cooking accidents, or with ignition of poorly stored flammable liquids.

Chemical Burns

Chemical burns are caused by contact with strong acids, alkalis, or organic compounds. The concentration, volume, and type of chemical, as well as the duration of contact, determine the severity of a chemical injury.

Chemical burns can result from contact with certain household cleaning agents and various chemicals used in industry, agriculture, and the military. Chemical injuries to the eyes and inhalation of chemical fumes can be very serious.

Electrical Burns

Electrical burn injuries are caused by heat that is generated by the electrical energy as it passes through the body. Electrical injuries can result from contact with exposed or faulty electrical wiring or high-voltage power lines. People struck by lightning also sustain electrical injury.

The extent of injury is influenced by the duration of contact, the intensity of the current (voltage), the type of current (direct or alternating), the pathway of the current, and the resistance of the tissues as the electrical current passes through the body. Contact with electrical current greater than 40 volts (V) is potentially dangerous because of cardiac dysrhythmias; current greater than 1000 V is considered to be high-voltage current and is associated with extensive tissue damage.

Radiation Burns

Radiation burns are the least common type of burn injury and are caused by exposure to a radioactive source. These types of injuries have been associated with nuclear radiation accidents, the use of ionizing radiation in industry, and therapeutic irradiation. Sunburn,

> **evolve** **Web Enhancements**
>
> **Ethical Issues in Nursing** Should the Severely Burned Client Be Allowed to Refuse Treatment?
>
> Be sure to check out the bonus material on the Evolve website and the CD-ROM, including free self-assessment exercises. **http://evolve.elsevier.com/Black/medsurg**

from prolonged exposure to ultraviolet rays (solar radiation), is also considered to be a radiation burn.

The amount of radioactive energy received after exposure depends on the distance the person is from the source of the radiation, the strength of the radiation source, the duration of exposure, the extent of body surface area exposed, and the amount of shielding between the source and the person. An acute, localized radiation injury appears similar to a cutaneous thermal injury. The injury is characterized by skin erythema, edema, and pain. In contrast, whole-body radiation exposure manifestations may begin with nausea, vomiting, diarrhea, and fatigue, continuing with a headache and fever within hours of exposure. As time proceeds, hematopoietic and gastrointestinal complications are seen. The severity of manifestations is dose-dependent.

Inhalation Injury

Exposure to asphyxiants (e.g., carbon monoxide) and smoke commonly occurs with flame injuries, particularly if the victim was trapped in an enclosed, smoke-filled space (e.g., in a residential fire). Victims who die at the scene of a fire usually do so as a result of hypoxia and carbon monoxide poisoning. The pulmonary pathophysiologic changes that occur with inhalation injury are multifactorial and relate to the severity and type of smoke or gases inhaled. Exposure to asphyxiants, smoke poisoning, and direct thermal (heat) injury to lung tissue constitute the three facets of an inhalation injury. However, not all of these injury components may be present in the client suffering from an inhalation injury. An inhalation injury increases the risk of mortality 7 times after controlling for the size of the cutaneous burn injury and other clinical and demographic factors.

Risk Factors and Injury Prevention

Adults with burn injuries are more likely to be male and in the 20 to 40 age group. Contact with fire/flame occurs in more than 60% of injuries. Structural fires account for approximately 5% of burn-related hospital admissions; however, they are responsible for the greatest number of burn-related deaths. Approximately 30% of all burn-related deaths are a result of structural fires, seemingly from the associated smoke inhalation. Ignition from cigarettes is the nation's largest single cause of all fire deaths. Alcohol and drug intoxication, which contributes to careless smoking, has been reported as a factor in 40% of residential fire deaths. In approximately 10% of cases of residential fire deaths, the fires were caused by children playing with matches or other ignition sources. Additionally, faulty chimneys, flue vents, fixed heating units, fireplaces, central heating systems, wood-burning stoves, ignition of wood-shingled roofs, as well as

human error have all been implicated as causes of residential fires that have resulted in deaths.

Clothing ignition during routine meal preparation has been cited as a leading cause of burn injury, particularly in the older population. Synthetic fabrics are especially dangerous, because they melt and adhere to the skin, causing prolonged contact with heat. Another age group at risk for clothing ignition is the pediatric population. During the early 1970s, the fatality rate among young children burned from ignition of sleepwear was significant. In 1975 it was mandated that children's sleepwear, sizes 0 to 6X, pass a standard flame test. This action significantly lowered mortality associated with children's clothing ignition. The mandate for sleepwear to pass a flame test has since been repealed, and testing is no longer required. Since the repeal, some have reported an increase in clothing-related flame burns occurring in 2- to 11-year-old girls.[19]

Scald burns occur in approximately 10% of adults, but 30% in children. Toddlers (children 2 to 4 years of age) suffer more scald injuries than people in any other age group. Scald injuries are frequently the result of mishaps in the performance of everyday tasks such as bathing and cooking. Overturned coffeepots, cooking pans spilling hot liquid and grease, overheated foods, liquids cooked in microwave ovens, and hot tap water have been identified as specific causes.

Of primary importance in reducing injuries and deaths from residential fires is the presence of a working smoke detector and fire extinguisher. It has been estimated that the risk of dying in a residential fire is reduced 50% when an operating smoke detector is in place.[5] One national burn prevention activity is the "Change Your Clock, Change Your Battery" campaign. This program is designed to remind people in the United States that when they set their clocks back in the fall, they should change the batteries in their smoke detector as well. Prevention efforts have also focused on passing legislation mandating the commercial production and sale of fire-safe cigarettes that are designed with a reduced propensity for ignition. To date, these efforts have been unsuccessful in achieving legislation in all states.

To reduce the incidence of scald injuries, the Consumer Products Safety Commission and Underwriters Laboratory has recommended that the maximum temperature on the thermostats of hot water heaters be lowered and that a warning label identifying the potential for injury be affixed to hot water heaters. Legislation requiring public buildings to lower water temperature to 120° F (48.8° C) has been successful in reducing scald injuries. In addition, a thermostatic control system (anti-scald device) has been developed that, when installed at the faucet or shower head, shuts off the flow of water when the temperature rises above a predetermined temperature, typically 119° F (48.3° C). Box 50-1 summarizes burn injury prevention recommendations.

In the kitchen:

- Turn pot handles toward the back of the stove.
- Purchase a stove with controls on the front or side to reduce the likelihood of clothing ignition as one reaches across hot elements.
- Use a cooking timer with an audible alarm.
- The use of turkey fryers to prepare holiday meals carries a high risk of severe injury and fire—consumers are encouraged to seek out commercial professionals to prepare the turkey or order the turkey from a supermarket or restaurant.

In the home:

- Store all matches and lighters securely so they are inaccessible to children.
- Infants and young children should wear flame-resistant sleepwear and costumes.
- Teach children to STOP, DROP, and ROLL on the ground if their clothing were to catch fire.
- Install smoke detectors on each level of the house and outside all sleeping areas. Test the batteries once a month and change the batteries twice a year.
- Install carbon monoxide detectors on each level of the house.
- Check the temperature on the hot water heater; the recommended setting is 120° F (48.8° C).
- Install water temperature-regulating valves (anti-scald device) that obstruct the flow of water when the water temperature exceeds a preset level.

In the community:

- Attend public fireworks displays conducted by professionals.
- Support fire-safe cigarette legislation in your state.

Pathophysiology

The pathophysiologic changes that occur following a cutaneous burn injury depend on the extent or size of the burn. For smaller burns, the body's response to injury is localized to the burned area. However, with more extensive burns (i.e., involving 25% or more of the total body surface area [TBSA]), the body's response to injury is systemic and proportional to the extent of the injury. The clinical manifestations of an extensive burn injury evolve in dramatic fashion over the post-injury clinical course. Extensive burn injuries affect all major systems of the body. The systemic response to burn injury is typically biphasic, characterized by early hypofunction followed later by hyperfunction of each of the organ systems.

Direct Injury to the Skin

With direct injury to the skin, heat from an external source is conducted to the skin, where it destroys tissue. The amount of damage depends on the length of exposure to

the heat and the temperature. At sustained temperatures of 40° to 44° C (104° to 111.2° F), various cellular enzyme systems and cellular systems fail. The sodium-potassium pump fails, which leads to cellular edema. As the temperature rises to 44° C, cell necrosis occurs. In addition, free radicals are produced, which leads to further cellular damage. These destructive processes continue until the heat source is withdrawn and the mechanisms for cooling return the cell temperature to a tolerable range.

Some types of burn create unique patterns of injury. In electrical injuries, heat is generated by electricity as it travels through the body, resulting in internal tissue damage. The concept of the "tip of the iceberg," where the true extent of the injury is not visually apparent, is helpful to understand these injuries. For instance, the cutaneous burn injury may appear negligible in size, but underlying muscle and soft tissue damage may be extensive, particularly with high-voltage electrical injuries. The voltage, type of current (direct or alternating), moisture content at the contact site, composition of the skin at the contact site, and duration of contact are important considerations affecting mortality and morbidity. Once the electrical current enters the body, it seeks to go to ground; en route, it creates heat and may damage vital organs as it passes through them. Alternating current (AC) is more dangerous than direct current (DC). AC produces more heat-related injury and, related to its rapid intermittent flow of electricity, is often associated with cardiopulmonary arrest, ventricular fibrillation, tetanic muscle contractions, and long bone or vertebral compression fractures. The risk of acute renal failure is noteworthy in clients following an electrical injury. Hemoglobin (released from heat-damaged erythrocytes) and myoglobin (the protein that supplies muscles with oxygen) are released in significant quantities into the bloodstream after deep burn injuries involving muscle damage. These substances pass through the glomeruli and are excreted in the urine. However, released in larger than normal quantities as a result of the muscle damage, they may precipitate and obstruct the renal tubules, causing renal damage. This damage can be minimized with the maintenance of a brisk urine output. In addition, victims of electrical injuries may have fallen from the point of electrical contact and sustained associated trauma-related injuries. Cataract formation is also associated with high-voltage electrical injury, especially when contact points are on the head or neck.

In chemical burns, systemic toxic effects may result from cutaneous absorption of the offending agent. Organ failure and even death have resulted from prolonged contact with and absorption of different chemicals.

Fluid Shifts

Immediately following a burn injury, vasoactive substances (catecholamines, histamine, serotonin, leukotrienes, kinins, and prostaglandins) are released from the injured tissues. These substances initiate changes in capillary integrity, allowing plasma to seep into surrounding tissues (Figure 50-1). Direct damage to vessels from heat further increases capillary permeability, which permits sodium ions to enter the cell and potassium ions to exit. The overall effect of these changes is creation of an osmotic gradient, which leads to increases in intercellular and interstitial fluid that further deplete intravascular fluid volumes. These vasoactive substances exert their effects both locally (in the area of injury) and systemically (throughout the body) with extensive injuries. The burn-injured client's hemodynamic balance, metabolism, and immune status are altered.

The body responds initially by shunting blood toward the brain and heart and away from all other body organs. Prolonged lack of blood flow to these other organs is detrimental. The resulting damage depends on the basal needs of the body organ. Some organs can survive for only a few hours without nutrient blood supply. For example, the lack of renal blood flow decreases

glomerular filtration rate, leading to oliguria (low urine output). If fluid resuscitation is delayed or inadequate, hypovolemia progresses, and acute renal failure may occur. However, with adequate fluid resuscitation and an increase in cardiac output, renal blood flow returns to normal. After resuscitation, the body begins to reabsorb the edema fluid and eliminate it through diuresis.

Blood flow to the mesenteric bed is also diminished initially, leading to the development of intestinal ileus and gastrointestinal dysfunction in clients with burns greater than 25% TBSA. With the reduction in blood flow to the gastric mucosa, ischemic changes to the upper gastrointestinal tract occur, which slows production of the protective mucous lining, resulting in small, superficial erosions to the stomach and duodenum. If the gastrointestinal tract is left untreated and unprotected by antacids or histamine H_2-receptor antagonists, the erosions can progress to ulcerations—called *Curling's ulcers* in burn-injured clients—and gastrointestinal bleeding.

Pulmonary System

Minute ventilation is often normal or slightly decreased early after an extensive burn injury. Following fluid resuscitation, an increase in minute ventilation—manifested by hyperventilation—may occur, especially if the client is fearful, anxious, or in pain. This hyperventilation is the result of an increase in both respiratory rate and tidal volume and appears to be the result of the hypermetabolism that is seen after burn injury. It typically peaks in the second post-injury week and then gradually returns to normal as the burn wound heals or is closed by grafting.

Pulmonary vascular resistance may increase slightly, and lung compliance may decrease. The changes in lung compliance cause a proportionate increase in the work of breathing. However, these changes are typically small, and in the absence of any pulmonary parenchymal (tissue) damage, they require no specialized treatment.

Inhalation Injury. Exposure to asphyxiants is the most common cause of early mortality from inhalation injury. Carbon monoxide (CO), a common asphyxiant, is produced when organic substances (e.g., wood or coal) burn. It is a colorless, odorless, and tasteless gas that has an affinity for the body's hemoglobin that is 200 times greater than that of oxygen. With inhalation of CO, the oxygen molecules are displaced, and CO binds to hemoglobin to form carboxyhemoglobin (COHb). Tissue hypoxia occurs from an overall decrease in the blood's oxygen-delivering capability.

Direct heat injury to the upper airway results from inhalation of the air heated by fire. The heat immediately produces injury to the airway, which results in edema, erythema, and ulceration. Thermal burns to the lower airways of the pulmonary system are rare because of

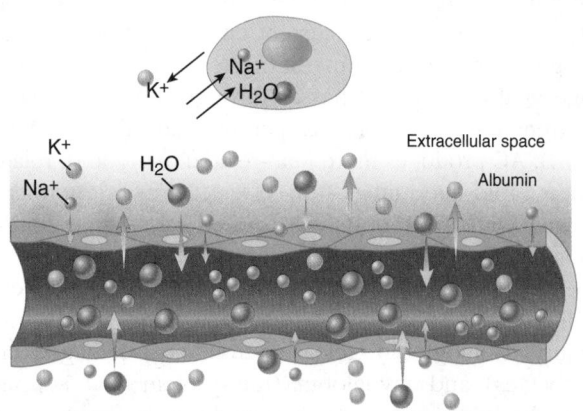

Fluid and electrolyte shift during burn shock

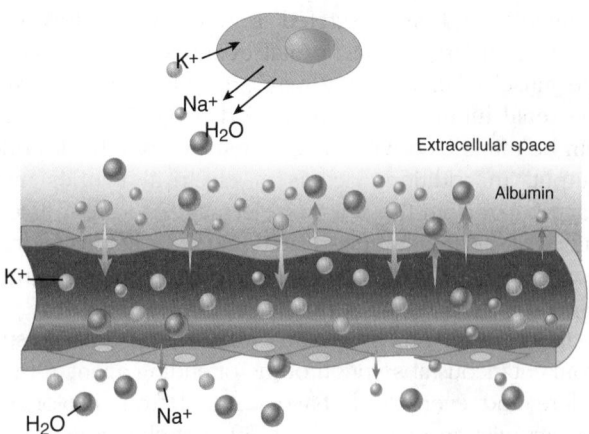

Fluid and electrolyte shift after burn shock

■ **FIGURE 50–1** Changes in capillary permeability allow plasma to seep into interstitial spaces. In addition, the sodium pump fails and sodium remains in the cell. There is a corresponding increase in serum potassium concentration.

the protective reflex closure of the glottis and the ability of the respiratory tract to exchange heat effectively. However, thermal burns to the lower airways can occur with the inhalation of steam or explosive gases or with aspiration of scalding liquids, especially in the unconscious victim.

Smoke poisoning results from the inhalation of the by-products of combustion: noxious chemicals (e.g., carbon monoxide, hydrogen cyanide, acrolein, ammonia) and particulate matter. The pulmonary response includes a localized inflammatory reaction, a decrease in bronchial ciliary action, and a decrease in alveolar surfactant. Mucosal edema occurs in the smaller airways. After several hours, sloughing of the tracheobronchial epithelium may occur, and hemorrhagic tracheobronchitis may develop. Adult (acute) respiratory distress syndrome may follow.

Myocardial Depression
Some research investigators have suggested that a myocardial depressant factor exists with more extensive injuries and circulates in the early post-injury period. A significant and immediate depression in cardiac output (CO) occurs, even before circulating plasma volumes decrease, suggesting a neurogenic response to some circulating agent. This depression in CO often continues for several days even after plasma volumes have been restored and urinary output normalizes. More recently, a combination of inflammatory mediators and hormones has been suggested as the cause of myocardial depression occurring after the injury.

Altered Skin Integrity
The burn wound itself exhibits pathophysiologic changes caused by disruption of the skin and alterations to the tissue beneath the surface. The skin, nerve endings, sweat glands, and hair follicles injured by the burn lose normal functioning. Most important, the skin's barrier function is lost. Intact skin normally keeps bacteria from entering the body and body fluids from seeping out, controls evaporation, and maintains body warmth. With destruction of the skin, mechanisms for maintaining normal body temperature can be altered, the risk of infection from invasion of bacteria increases, and evaporative water loss increases. Depending on the depth of the injury, nerve endings either become exposed, resulting in pain and discomfort until wound closure, or are damaged, leaving the innervated area insensate, with potential for permanent impairment of the ability to sense touch, pressure, and pain.

Individuals with severe burn injuries are at risk for developing hypertrophic scarring. This type of scar is best described as reddened, raised (above adjacent uninjured skin), rigid, and uncomfortable. Clients often suffer from pruritus (itch) and increased sensitivity. Hypertrophic scars can result in skin and tissue contractures, especially when the scar crosses over a joint The incidence of hypertrophic scarring varies; however, it is thought that the depth of burn and age and ethnic background of the survivor are key factors in whether or not this type of scar develops.

Immunosuppression
Immune system function is depressed following burn injury. Depression of lymphocyte activity, a decrease in immunoglobulin production, suppression of complement activity, and an alteration in neutrophil and macrophage functioning are evident following extensive burn injuries. In addition, the burn injury disrupts the body's primary barrier to infection—the skin. Together these changes result in an increased risk of infection and life-threatening sepsis.

Psychological Response
Numerous psychological and emotional responses to burn injuries have been identified, ranging from fear to psychosis. A victim's response is influenced by age, personality, cultural and ethnic background, the extent and location of the injury, impact on body image, and pre-injury coping abilities. In addition, separation from family and friends during hospitalization and the change in the client's normal role and responsibilities affect the reaction to burn trauma.[1]

Clinical Manifestations
Degree of Injury
Depending on the skin layers damaged, burn wounds are termed either *partial-thickness* burns or *full-thickness* burns. Burn wounds are also classified as first-, second-, third-, or fourth-degree burns. Partial-thickness burns involve injury to the epidermis and portions of the dermis. *First-degree* partial-thickness burns are superficial and painful and appear red. They heal on their own by epidermal cell regeneration within about 3 to 7 days. Sunburn is a good example of a first-degree partial-thickness burn. *Second-degree* partial-thickness burns appear wet or blistered and are extremely painful. They heal on their own (that is, without skin grafting) as long as they are fairly small and they do not become infected (Figure 50-2).

Third-degree full-thickness burns are characterized by damage through the entire epidermis and dermis (Figure 50-3). A full-thickness burn appears dry and may be mottled and colored black, brown, white, or red. The denatured skin is called *eschar* (pronounced "ES-car"). The burned tissue is most often painless as a result of damage to the nerve endings; however, the surrounding skin may be painful. Upon palpation, individuals with a full-thickness burn may feel pressure. Full-thickness injuries heal by formation of granulation tissue to fill the wound defect and contracture of the epithelium, also known as scarring, to close the wound. Unless the area is very small (the size of a half-dollar or less), the full-thickness burn will not heal adequately and must be skin-grafted to close the wound. *Fourth-degree* full-thickness burns involve skin, subcutaneous (fat) tissue, muscle, and sometimes bone. The skin appears charred or may be completely burned away. Fourth-degree burns require extensive surgical debridement and skin grafting. Amputations are common in these extensive injuries (Figure 50-4). The appearance of the burn relative to the depth of injury is described in Figure 50-5.

Hypothermia

In addition to altered physical appearance, the loss of skin leads to other problems. Hypothermia results from loss of body heat through the burn wound and is characterized by a core body temperature below 98.6° F (37° C). Hypothermia is extremely harmful because it leads to shivering, which in turn increases oxygen consumption and caloric demands as well as vasoconstriction in the periphery. Hypothermia is most common in extensive injuries during the early hours following injury, evacuation, and transport to a burn facility.

Fluid and Electrolyte Imbalance

The evaporative water loss through the burn contributes to the client's diminished fluid volume and compromised hydration status. Evaporative losses not compensated for by fluid replacement are evidenced by a low blood pressure, decreased urine output, dry mucous membranes, and poor skin turgor.

Hyponatremia, hypernatremia, and hyperkalemia are common electrolyte abnormalities that affect the burn-injured client at different points in the recovery process. Extensive burns (greater than 25% TBSA) result in generalized body edema affecting both burned and non-burned tissues and in a decrease in circulating intravascular blood volume. Hematocrit levels are elevated in the first 24 hours after injury, demonstrating hemoconcentration from the loss of intravascular fluid. In addition, evaporative fluid losses through the burn wound are 4 to 20 times greater than normal and remain elevated until complete wound closure is obtained. The result is a decrease in organ perfusion. If the intravascular space is not replenished with intravenous (IV) fluids, hypovolemic (burn) shock and, ultimately, death ensue for the victim of an extensive burn.

Urine output for the adult client receiving insufficient fluid replacement following a major burn injury diminishes to less than 30 ml/hour. Physical findings of the urine sample demonstrate dehydration, characterized by dark amber, concentrated urine and elevated specific gravity. Laboratory tests reveal elevated blood urea nitrogen (BUN) levels until the client is adequately hydrated.

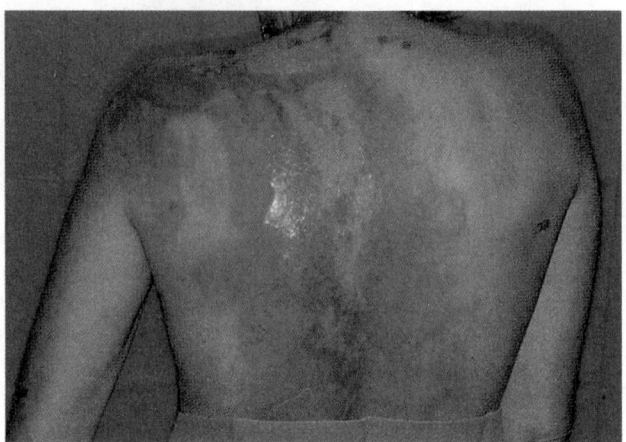

■ **FIGURE 50–2** Partial-thickness burn injury (second-degree burn).

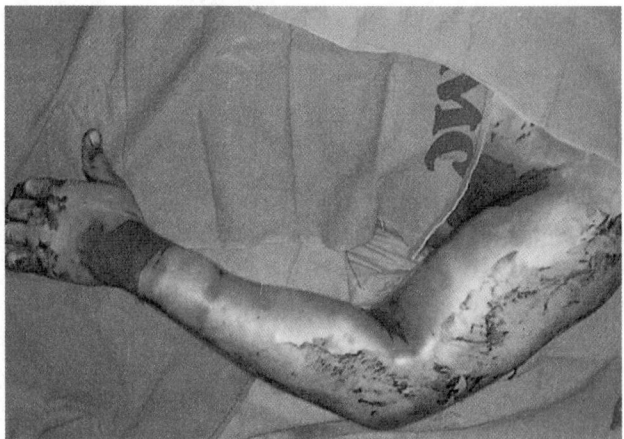

■ **FIGURE 50–3** Full-thickness burn injury (third-degree burn).

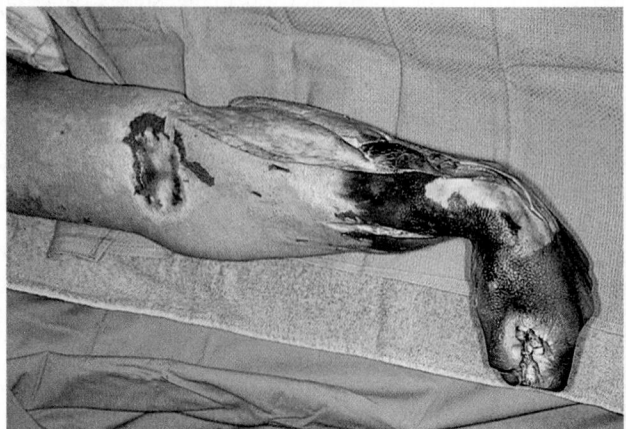

■ **FIGURE 50–4** Full-thickness burn injury of the forearm and hand caused by high-voltage electrical current. Injury extends into the muscle and bone of the hand and forearm (fourth-degree burn).

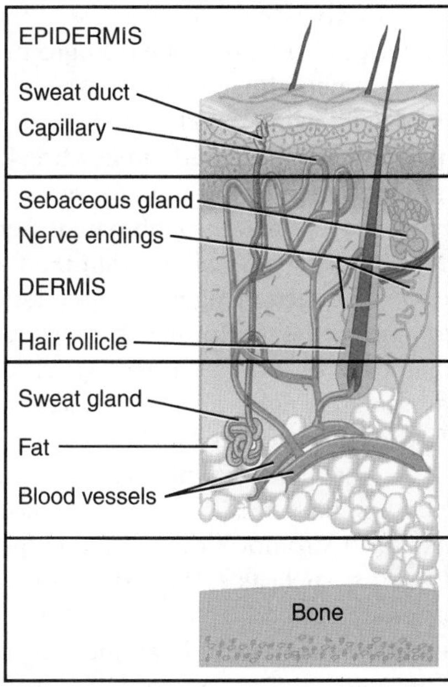

		WOUND APPEARANCE	WOUND SENSATION	COURSE OF HEALING
PARTIAL-THICKNESS BURN	1st-degree	Epidermis remains intact and without blisters Erythema; skin blanches with pressure	Painful	Discomfort lasts 48-72 hours. Desquamation occurs in 3-7 days.
PARTIAL-THICKNESS BURN	2nd-degree	Wet, shiny, weeping surface Blisters Wound blanches with pressure	Painful Very sensitive to touch, air currents	Superficial partial-thickness burn heals in <21 days. Deep partial-thickness burn requires >21 days for healing. Healing rates vary with burn depth and presence/absence of infection.
FULL-THICKNESS BURN	3rd-degree	Color variable (i.e., deep red, white, black, brown) Surface dry Thrombosed vessels visible No blanching	Insensate (↓ pinprick sensation)	Autografting is required for healing.
FULL-THICKNESS BURN	4th-degree	Color variable Charring visible in deepest areas Extremity movement limited	Insensate	Amputation of extremities is likely. Autografting is required for healing.

EPIDERMIS
Sweat duct
Capillary
Sebaceous gland
Nerve endings
DERMIS
Hair follicle
Sweat gland
Fat
Blood vessels
Bone

■ **FIGURE 50–5**   Burn injury classification according to depth of injury.

Manifestations of decreased gastrointestinal motility following major burn injuries include the absence of bowel sounds, stool, or flatus; nausea and vomiting; and abdominal distention. After adequate fluid resuscitation, gastrointestinal motility returns, signaled by a return of hunger and appetite, bowel sounds, flatus, and stool production.

At approximately 18 to 36 hours after burn injury, capillary membrane integrity begins to be restored. The initial increase in hematocrit, seen early after injury, falls to below normal by the third or fourth day after injury. The fall in hematocrit occurs as a result of red blood cell loss and damage incurred at the time of injury. Over the ensuing days and weeks, the body begins to reabsorb the edema fluid, and the excess fluid is excreted via diuresis.

Alterations in Respiration

Initially, the client may exhibit tachypnea following the burn injury. Arterial blood gas analysis may demonstrate a relatively normal arterial partial pressure of oxygen (Pa_{O_2}), with oxygen saturation lower than expected relative to the P_{O_2}. In those with an inhalation injury, respiratory insufficiency may develop during the resuscitative phase when fluid shifts are greatest and the injured lung parenchyma is particularly susceptible to edema formation. Later on in the course of recovery, respiratory failure may occur because of infection (often 10 days to 2 weeks following injury).

Diagnosis of CO poisoning is made by measuring the COHb level in the blood. The clinical manifestations of acute CO poisoning, shown in the Bridge to Critical Care

feature below, are directly related to the level of COHb saturation and relative degree of tissue hypoxia. The onset of clinical manifestations typically does not occur until COHb levels reach 15%. Initial manifestations are related to decreased cerebral tissue oxygenation and are neurologic in nature. The neurologic problems caused by CO exposure can lead to progressive and permanent cerebral dysfunction.

Thermal burns to the upper airways (mouth, nasopharynx, and larynx) characteristically appear erythematous and edematous, with mucosal blisters or ulcerations. Increasing mucosal edema can lead to upper airway obstruction, typically within the first 24 to 48 hours after

BRIDGE TO CRITICAL CARE

Clinical Manifestations of Carbon Monoxide (CO) Poisoning

CO Level (%)	Clinical Manifestations
5-10	Impaired visual acuity
11-20	Flushing, headache
21-30	Nausea, impaired dexterity
31-40	Vomiting, dizziness, syncope
41-50	Tachypnea, tachycardia
>50	Coma, death

From Cioffi, W.G. (1998). Inhalation injury. In G.J. Carrougher (Ed.), *Burn care and therapy* (p. 42). St. Louis: Mosby.

injury. Clinical manifestations observed in critical narrowing of the airway include stridor, dyspnea, increased work of breathing, use of respiratory accessory muscles, and eventually cyanosis.

Admission physical findings indicative of smoke exposure include soot on the face and nares, facial burns, soot in the sputum, coughing, and wheezing. The manifestations of tracheobronchitis typically do not present until 24 to 48 hours after injury. Early manifestations consist of bronchospasm evidenced as wheezing and bronchorrhea. Lung compliance is decreased, causing an increased work of breathing. Impaired clearance of secretions accentuates the problem. Normally, ventilation and perfusion are matched by equal volumes of air and blood at the alveolar-capillary level. The client with smoke inhalation exhibits pathophysiologic changes that reduce alveolar ventilation, causing a ventilation-perfusion ($\dot{V}/\dot{Q}$) mismatch, which impairs gas exchange.[8]

Decreased Cardiac Output

Following an extensive burn injury, heart rate and peripheral vascular resistance increase in response to the release of catecholamines and to the relative hypovolemia, but initial cardiac output decreases (hypofunction). At approximately 24 hours after burn injury in clients receiving adequate fluid resuscitation, cardiac output returns to normal and then increases (2 to 2.5 times normal) to meet the hypermetabolic needs of the body (hyperfunction). This change in cardiac output occurs even before circulating intravascular volume levels are restored to normal. Arterial blood pressure is normal or slightly elevated unless severe hypovolemia exists. The decreased cardiac output seen initially after burn injury is evidenced by decreased blood pressure, decreased urine output, weak peripheral pulses, and, if monitored via a pulmonary artery catheter, a cardiac output of less than 4 L/min, cardiac index of less than 2.5 L/min, and systemic vascular resistance of less than 900 dynes.

Pain Responses

The client experiences substantial pain as a result of the burn wound and exposed nerve endings from lack of skin integrity. Burn survivors typically describe three types of pain resulting from their injury: background, breakthrough, and procedural pain. Background pain is experienced when the client is at rest or engages in non–procedure-related activities, such as shifting position in bed, or with chest or abdominal wall movements that occur with deep breathing or coughing. Background pain is described as continuous in nature and low in intensity, typically lasting the duration of recovery. Management of background pain is often with the use of long-acting analgesic agents using such modalities as

patient-controlled analgesia (PCA), continuous infusion, or sustained-release oral agents. Breakthrough pain is an increase in the pain experienced that exceeds the low intensity level of background pain. Like background pain, it is experienced when the client is at rest or engages in activities of daily living or other minor activities that require movement of injured areas. Breakthrough pain occurs intermittently throughout the day. The intensity and frequency of breakthrough pain lessen as the burn heals. Management of breakthrough pain is often with the use of short-acting agents. Procedural pain is experienced during the performance of therapeutic measures commonly used in burn care, such as wound cleansing, dressing changes, and physical/occupational therapy. Procedural pain is described as acute and high in intensity. Management depends on the phase of recovery and includes short-acting opioids (e.g., morphine sulfate, fentanyl, hydromorphone, oxycodone, ketamine). Inhaled agents, such as nitrous oxide, may also be used to treat procedural pain.[11]

Clinical responses to pain may include an increase in blood pressure, heart rate, and respiratory rate with dilated pupils, rigid muscle tone, and guarded positioning. To assess pain, several different pain measurement tools are available for use in adults; they include numerical scales (e.g., 1 to 5, or 1 to 10), verbal descriptive scales (e.g., none, mild, moderate, or severe), and visual analog scales (e.g., 0 to 10 rating scale with verbal descriptors of none at the 0 mark to worst pain possible at the 10 mark).[16]

Altered Level of Consciousness

Rarely do burn-injured clients suffer neurologic damage unless prolonged exposure to smoke has occurred. The client with a major burn injury is most often awake and alert on admission to the hospital. If agitation develops in the immediate post-injury period, the client may be suffering from hypoxemia or hypovolemia and needs further assessment for identifying the origin of these changes. When an alteration in level of consciousness is present on admission to the hospital, it is most often related to neurologic trauma (e.g., fall, motor vehicle accident), impaired perfusion to the brain, hypoxemia (as from a closed-space fire), inhalation injury (as from exposure to asphyxiates or other toxic materials from the fire), electrical burn injury, or the effects of drugs present in the body at the time of injury.

Clients with associated head trauma may have scalp lacerations, swelling, tenderness, or ecchymosis. Level of consciousness may fluctuate between intervals of lucidity followed by rapid deterioration. Pupils may be of unequal size. Neurologic manifestations may include headache, dizziness, memory loss, confusion or loss of consciousness, disorientation, visual changes, hallucinations, combativeness, and coma.

Psychological Alterations

Immediately after injury, those with a major injury may respond with psychological shock, disbelief, anxiety, and feelings of being overwhelmed. The client and family members may be aware of what is happening but may be coping with the situation poorly. Because the client will have a limited ability to process new information, the familiar presence of family and friends can help alleviate anxiety. Simple preparatory instructions and information, especially before procedures, is important. Families of critically ill clients have a need for assurance, proximity to the injured person, and information. Specifically, families want to know how the client is being treated, specific facts about the client's progress, and why certain procedures are being done.

Once stabilized, the client may cope psychologically in many ways. The most common problems during the acute phase of recovery include grief, depression, anxiety, and acute stress disorder (i.e., persistent re-experiencing of the trauma, avoidance of stimuli associated with the trauma, and manifestations of increased arousal). Clients may experience nightmares or flashbacks of the injury, sleep problems, and behavioral regression. A combination of pharmacologic and psychological treatments is often used during this phase. Brief supportive therapy and behavior modification are psychological treatments often used, as is group therapy (e.g., inpatient support groups for burn survivors).

Following hospital discharge, clients may continue to suffer from anxiety and depression. They may report difficulties as they relate to vocational and emotional adjustment. However, the intensity of emotional difficulties often decreases significantly after a year post-burn.[1]

OUTCOME MANAGEMENT

The burn client undergoes a wide range of physiologic and metabolic changes in response to the burn injury. To accomplish the best outcomes, it is essential to have a clear understanding of the pathophysiologic process and the necessary treatment modifications needed over the entire recovery continuum. Three distinct periods or phases of treatment can be defined in the care of clients with major burns: the resuscitative, the acute, and the rehabilitation phases of recovery.

Resuscitative Phase

The resuscitative phase of burn injury consists of the time between the initial injury and 36 to 48 hours after injury. This phase ends when fluid resuscitation is complete. During this phase, life-threatening airway and breathing problems are of major concern. It is also characterized by the development of hypovolemia, which results as

capillaries leak fluid from the intravascular spaces into the interstitial spaces, causing edema. Although the fluid remains in the body, it is unable to contribute to maintaining adequate circulation, because it is no longer in the vascular space. The burn itself, except for initial assessment of severity and depth, is of less immediate concern; in certain cases, however, escharotomy may be performed to restore perfusion to areas exhibiting circulatory compromise. The adequacy of initial treatment of pulmonary and circulatory abnormalities sets the stage for subsequent management. Management of the burn client begins at the scene of the accident. The first step should be to remove the victim from the area of immediate danger, followed by stopping the burning process. Basic life support measures should be implemented during transport of the client to the hospital.

Medical Management in the Resuscitative Phase of Burn Injury

Assess Burn Severity

The American Burn Association has published a severity classification schedule for burn injuries, shown in the Bridge to Critical Care feature on p. 1248.[3] These guidelines are intended to assist the clinician in determining injury severity for the burn client. This classification schedule separates injuries into major, moderate, and minor categories. Clients with major burns are usually transferred to a specialized burn care facility after local emergency treatment has been provided. Clients with moderate burns can usually be managed on an inpatient basis at the receiving hospital. Clients with minor burns usually receive initial care in the emergency department and are then discharged for follow-up care on an outpatient basis.

The severity of a burn injury is classified according to the risk of mortality and the risk of cosmetic or functional disability. Several factors influence injury severity.

Burn Depth. The deeper the burn wound, the more serious the injury. Deep partial-thickness and full-thickness burns are more likely to become infected, have more profound systemic effects, and are more frequently associated with scarring and development of skin contractures.

Burn Size. The size of a burn (percentage of injured skin, excluding first-degree burns) is determined by one of three techniques: (1) the rule of nines; (2) the palm method; and (3) an age-specific burn diagram or chart. Burn size is expressed as a percentage of TBSA. The *rule of nines* was introduced in the late 1940s as a quick assessment tool for estimating burn size in the adult. The basis of the rule is that the body is divided into

American Burn Association Severity Classification for Burn Injuries

MAJOR BURN INJURY

- 25% TBSA* burn in adults <40 yr of age
- 20% TBSA burn in adults >40 yr of age
- 20% TBSA burn in children <10 yr of age

or

   Burns involving the face, eyes, ears, hands, feet, and perineum likely to result in functional or cosmetic disability

or

   High-voltage electrical burn injury

or

   All burn injuries with concomitant inhalation injury or major trauma

MODERATE BURN INJURY

- 15-25% TBSA burn in adults <40 yr of age
- 10-20% TBSA burn in adults >40 yr of age
- 10-20% TBSA burn in children <10 yr of age

   with

   Less than 10% TBSA full-thickness burn without cosmetic or functional risk to the face, eyes, ears, hands, feet, or perineum

MINOR BURN INJURY

- <15% TBSA burn in adults <40 yr of age
- <10% TBSA burn in adults >40 yr of age
- <10% TBSA burn in children <10 yr of age

   with

     <2% TBSA full-thickness burn and no cosmetic or functional risk to the face, eyes, ears, hands, feet, or perineum

*TBSA, Total body surface area.
Modified from American Burn Association. (1984). Guidelines for service standards and severity classification in the treatment of burn injury. *American College of Surgeons Bulletin, 69*(10), 24-28.

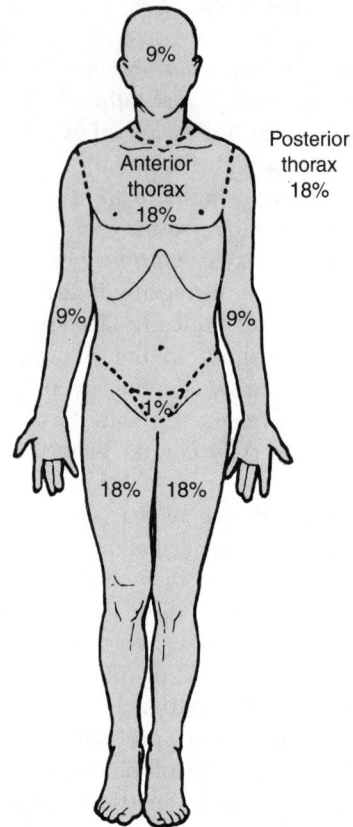

■ FIGURE 50–6 The rule of nines provides a quick method for estimating the extent of a burn injury in the adult.

anatomic sections, each of which represents 9%, or a multiple of 9%, of the TBSA (Figure 50-6). This method is easy and requires no diagrams to determine the percentage of TBSA injured. Therefore it is frequently used in emergency departments, where initial triage occurs. A second method for estimating the size of a burn is the *palm method*. The client's palm and digits make up approximately 1% of the total body surface area. The percent burn is derived by visualizing the number of client hands it would take to cover the burn area. This method is useful when the burned area or areas is small, less than 5%. Lastly, a *burn diagram* charts the percentages for body segments according to age and provides a more accurate estimate of burn size (Figure 50-7). It should be noted that the extent of burn injury is most accurate after initial debridement and should therefore be verified again at that time.

Burn Location. The location of injury on the body can affect outcome. Pulmonary complications are frequent with burns of the head, neck, and chest. When burns involve the face, associated injuries often include corneal abrasions. Burns of the ears are susceptible to auricular chondritis, infection, and further loss of tissue. Management of burns of the hands and joints often requires intense physical and occupational therapy, with the potential for major loss of work time and for permanent physical and vocational disability. Burns involving the perineal area are susceptible to infection because of auto-contamination by urine and feces. Circumferential burns of extremities may produce a tourniquet-like effect, leading to distal vascular compromise. Circumferential thorax burns may lead to inadequate chest wall expansion and pulmonary insufficiency.

Age. The client's age affects the severity and outcome of the burn. Death rates are higher for children younger than 4 years, particularly in newborns and infants up to 1 year of age, and for clients older than 65 years. High mortality and morbidity rates in the older burn-injured client are from the combination of age-related functional impairments (slower reaction time, impaired judgment, and decreased mobility), living alone, environmental

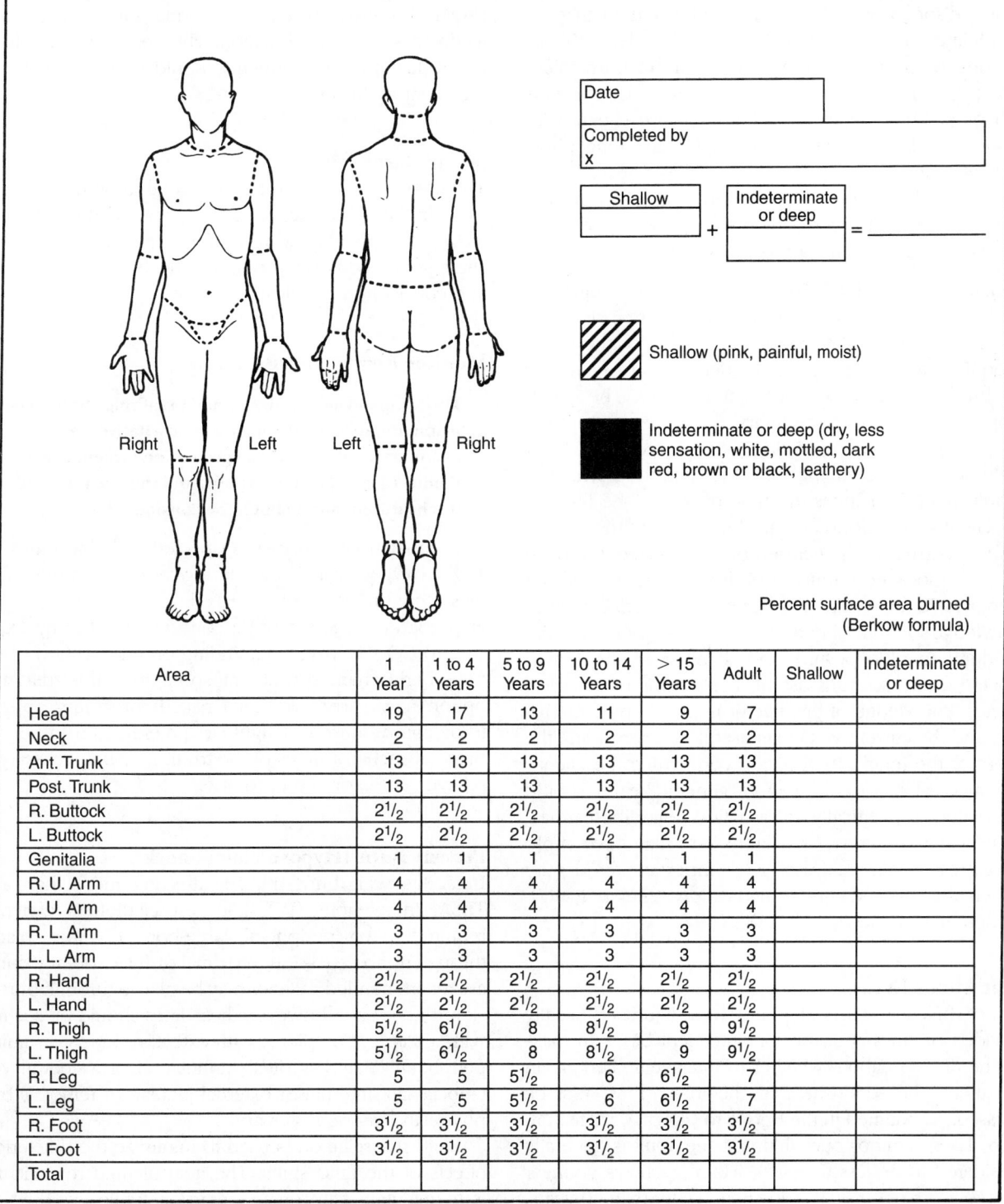

Area	1 Year	1 to 4 Years	5 to 9 Years	10 to 14 Years	> 15 Years	Adult	Shallow	Indeterminate or deep
Head	19	17	13	11	9	7		
Neck	2	2	2	2	2	2		
Ant. Trunk	13	13	13	13	13	13		
Post. Trunk	13	13	13	13	13	13		
R. Buttock	$2^1/_2$	$2^1/_2$	$2^1/_2$	$2^1/_2$	$2^1/_2$	$2^1/_2$		
L. Buttock	$2^1/_2$	$2^1/_2$	$2^1/_2$	$2^1/_2$	$2^1/_2$	$2^1/_2$		
Genitalia	1	1	1	1	1	1		
R. U. Arm	4	4	4	4	4	4		
L. U. Arm	4	4	4	4	4	4		
R. L. Arm	3	3	3	3	3	3		
L. L. Arm	3	3	3	3	3	3		
R. Hand	$2^1/_2$	$2^1/_2$	$2^1/_2$	$2^1/_2$	$2^1/_2$	$2^1/_2$		
L. Hand	$2^1/_2$	$2^1/_2$	$2^1/_2$	$2^1/_2$	$2^1/_2$	$2^1/_2$		
R. Thigh	$5^1/_2$	$6^1/_2$	8	$8^1/_2$	9	$9^1/_2$		
L. Thigh	$5^1/_2$	$6^1/_2$	8	$8^1/_2$	9	$9^1/_2$		
R. Leg	5	5	$5^1/_2$	6	$6^1/_2$	7		
L. Leg	5	5	$5^1/_2$	6	$6^1/_2$	7		
R. Foot	$3^1/_2$	$3^1/_2$	$3^1/_2$	$3^1/_2$	$3^1/_2$	$3^1/_2$		
L. Foot	$3^1/_2$	$3^1/_2$	$3^1/_2$	$3^1/_2$	$3^1/_2$	$3^1/_2$		
Total								

■ **FIGURE 50–7** A sample chart for recording the extent and depth of a burn injury using the Berkow formula. To estimate burn extent using this chart, the nurse outlines the injured areas, excluding first-degree burns. Shallow (second-degree) burns are designated by parallel lines, and deeper (third-degree and fourth-degree) burns are designated by shading in the appropriate areas. The percentage of each injured anatomic area is then estimated using the age-specific table. Total body surface area (TBSA) burn is then calculated.

hazards, and significant pre-injury morbidity. Compounding this vulnerability to burn injury is the thinning of the skin and atrophy of skin appendages that occur with aging.

General Health. Debilitating cardiac, pulmonary, endocrine, and renal disease—specifically, cardiopulmonary insufficiency, diabetes, alcoholism-related disease, and renal failure—can influence the client's response to injury and treatment. The death rate for clients with pre-existing cardiac disorders is 3.5 to 4 times higher than that for burn-injured clients without cardiac disorders. Clients suffering from alcoholism and a significant burn injury have a three-fold increase in mortality over that of clients with only a burn injury. In addition, those clients with alcoholism who survive their burn injury have longer hospital stays and more complications. The increased morbidity may be related to impaired immune function. Obese clients with burn injury are at increased risk because of cardiopulmonary complications.

Mechanism of Injury. The mechanism of injury is another factor used to determine the severity of injury. In general, special attention to this aspect of the injury is required for any electrical or chemical burn injury or any burn associated with inhalation injury. The client, people at the scene of the injury, and emergency medical personnel may have important information that could help in determining the severity of the burn. Useful information includes the time of injury, the level of the client's consciousness at the scene, whether the injury occurred in an enclosed or open space, the presence of associated trauma, and the specific mechanism of injury. If the victim has suffered a chemical burn, knowledge of the offending agent, its concentration, the duration of exposure, and whether irrigation was initiated at the scene is useful. For victims of electrical injuries, knowledge of the electrical source, type of current, and the current voltage is useful in determining the extent of the injury. Information concerning the client's past medical history as well as general health should be obtained. Specifically, information regarding cardiac, pulmonary, endocrine, or renal disease may have implications for treatment. Also, it is important to identify known allergies and current medication regimen, including herbal remedies.

Treat Minor Burns

Care of the client with only minor burn injuries is usually provided on an ambulatory or outpatient basis. In making the decision about whether to manage a client as an outpatient, the seriousness of the injury must first be assessed. As outlined in the Bridge to Critical Care feature on p. 1248, a minor burn injury in the adult is generally considered to be less than 15% TBSA in clients younger than 40 years or 10% TBSA in clients older than 40 years, without a risk of cosmetic or functional impairment or disability. In addition, the client or caregiver's ability to perform wound care in the home environment must be considered. Medical care of the minor burn includes wound evaluation and initial care, tetanus immunization, and pain management. While providing initial wound care, the nurse is responsible for teaching home wound care and the clinical manifestations of infection that necessitate further medical care. Other teaching needs

include the need to perform active range-of-motion (ROM) exercises to maintain normal joint function and to decrease edema formation. The need for any follow-up evaluations or treatments should be confirmed with the client at this time.

Major Burns 🪔

The medical goals for burn care depend on the phase of care. Initial goals are saving life, maintaining and protecting the airway, and restoring hemodynamic stability. Later goals focus on promoting healing, and assessing and correcting complications.

Monitor Airway and Breathing

The adequacy of the airway and breathing should take prime importance during the resuscitative phase. The oropharynx should be inspected for evidence of erythema, blisters, or ulcerations, and the need for endotracheal intubation should be considered.

If inhalation injury is suspected, administration of 100% oxygen via a tight-fitting non-rebreathing face mask continues until COHb levels fall below 15%. Hyperbaric oxygen may be considered with any exposure to CO. However, depending on the location of the hyperbaric chamber and transport time, this treatment option may carry additional risk. If breathing appears to be compromised by tight circumferential trunk burns, bilateral escharotomies of the trunk may be necessary to relieve ventilatory compromise.

Prevent Burn (Hypovolemic) Shock

In adults with burn injuries affecting more than 15% TBSA, intravenous (IV) fluid resuscitation is generally required. Two peripheral large-bore IV lines placed through nonburned skin, proximal to any extremity burns, are recommended. IV lines may be placed through burned skin if necessary; however, these lines should be secured with a suture. For clients with extensive burns or limited peripheral IV access sites, cannulation of a central vein (subclavian, internal or external jugular, or femoral) by a physician may be necessary.

Fluid resuscitation is used to minimize the deleterious effects of the fluid shifts. The goal of fluid resuscitation is to maintain vital organ perfusion while avoiding the complications related to either inadequate or excessive fluid administration. Several different formulas exist that are used to calculate fluid requirements. The formula currently recommended by the American Burn Life Support (ABLS) course, outlined in the Critical Monitoring feature on p. 1251, is 2 to 4 ml/kg/24 hours of lactated Ringer's solution. In the calculation of fluid infusion rates, the time of injury, not the time at which fluid resuscitation was initiated, serves as time zero. Thus if a burned client is delayed 2 hours in reaching an emergency department, those 2 hours must be considered in any calculation of needed fluid. However, adjustment to the fluid infusion rate is based on the client's physiologic response (e.g., urine production, vital signs, and lung sounds) and not missed resuscitation fluid.

It is important to remember that this resuscitation formula is only a guide and that fluid resuscitation volumes should be adjusted according to the client's physiologic response. Adequacy of fluid resuscitation is based on urine output and hemodynamic monitoring (if necessary and available). An indwelling urethral catheter connected to a closed drainage system should be placed to measure hourly urine production in order to guide IV fluid replacement in those with extensive or major burn injuries.

The exact amount of fluid is based on the client's weight and the extent of injury. Other factors to be considered include the presence of an inhalation injury or a high-voltage electrical injury, delay in initiation of resuscitation, history of excessive alcohol intake, associated trauma, and deep tissue damage. These factors tend to increase the amount of IV fluid required for adequate resuscitation above the calculated amount. Colloid-containing solutions are not given during this period because of the changes in capillary integrity that allow leakage of protein-rich fluid (e.g., albumin) into the interstitial space, resulting in the formation of additional edematous fluid. During the second 24 hours after burn injury, colloid-containing solutions may be administered, along with 5% dextrose and water in varying amounts.

Vital signs are used to provide a baseline of information as well as additional data for determining the adequacy of fluid resuscitation. Baseline laboratory studies should include blood glucose, BUN, serum creatinine, serum electrolytes, and hematocrit levels. Arterial blood gas and COHb levels should be obtained, particularly if an inhalation injury is suspected. A chest x-ray film should be obtained for all clients with extensive burns or inhalation injury. Other laboratory tests in addition to the radiographic study should be performed in all clients with associated trauma, as indicated. Depending on the circumstance of the injury, an alcohol or drug screen may be appropriate. Continuous electrocardiographic (ECG) monitoring should be initiated in all clients with major burn injuries, particularly those who have suffered a high-voltage electrical injury or who have a history of cardiac ischemia. ECG leads should be placed on nonburned skin, therefore interpretation of the rhythm must be interpreted in light of where the leads are placed.

Prevent Aspiration

Many burn centers advocate the placement of a nasogastric tube for management of unresponsive clients and clients with burns of 20% to 25% TBSA or more, to prevent emesis and reduce the risk of aspiration. Gastrointestinal dysfunction results from the intestinal ileus that develops almost universally in clients during the early post–burn injury period. All oral fluids should be restricted at this time.

Minimize Pain and Anxiety

During the resuscitative phase, pain management for the client with a major burn is achieved through the administration of IV opioids, typically morphine sulfate or fentanyl. In the adult, small doses are given and repeated in 5- to 10-minute intervals until pain is under control.

The intramuscular and subcutaneous routes are *not* used during the resuscitative phase because absorption from the soft tissues is unreliable when peripheral perfusion is sporadic. The oral route for pain medication administration is not used because of the likelihood of gastrointestinal dysfunction.

SAFETY

⚠

ALERT

Clients presenting to emergency departments with minor or moderate burn injuries often are initially given small doses of IV opioids (e.g., morphine sulfate). Oral analgesic agents are then prescribed.

To minimize anxiety, simple explanations concerning the hospital environment (e.g., cardiac monitoring devices, pumps used to administer intravenous fluids) and preparatory information before all procedures should be provided.[6,16]

Wound Care

Stop the Burning Process. All burn wound care begins at the scene of the injury. Clothing that continues to smolder should be carefully removed. In the case of a scald injury, all hot, wet clothing (includes diapers) should be removed immediately. Once the clothing is removed, the client should be covered with a dry sheet and blanket to preserve body heat.

Treatment of chemical burn injuries also begins at the scene of the injury. All clothing should be promptly removed, and any chemical powder brushed off the skin. Chemical burns should be irrigated continuously with copious amounts of water for at least 20 minutes and until the burning sensation stops. Neutralizing agents are not recommended because the neutralizing reaction causes heat, which results in further tissue damage.

For chemical eye injuries, irrigate the eyes with a gentle stream of normal saline, flushing both the injured eye and the conjunctiva. The recommended method is to irrigate the eyes from the inner canthus outward, to avoid washing any chemicals down the tear duct or toward the other eye.

Electrical burn care includes stopping the burning process.

It is important to remember, for your safety and the client's, to shut off any power source before approaching the victim.

Early care is directed at assessment of the entire person, because of the potential path of the electricity through the body (e.g., dysrhythmias, fractures).

Immediate Care. When transfer to a burn center will be accomplished within 12 hours of injury, wound care should consist of covering the wound with sterile towels and placing clean, dry sheets and blankets over the client. Initiation of debridement and application of topical antimicrobial agents are unnecessary. Definitive wound care begins following inpatient admission to the hospital.

Definitive wound care for burns consists of cleansing, debridement of devitalized tissue, removal of any damaging agents (e.g., chemicals, tar), and application of an appropriate topical agent and a dressing. Burn wounds should be washed with a mild soap and rinsed thoroughly with warm water. Loose, devitalized tissue should be carefully trimmed away, and any hair should be shaved to within a 1-inch margin around the burn wound (exception: do not shave eyebrows or eyelashes as they may not grow back in a normal pattern) to minimize surface organisms.

The removal of tar or asphalt is more easily accomplished with the use of a citrus-petroleum product such as Medisol (Orange-Sol, Inc., Chandler, Ariz) or with mineral oil and a petroleum-based antibiotic ointment such as bacitracin or polymyxin-neomycin-bacitracin (Neosporin ointment, Pfizer Inc., New York, NY).

Clients with minor burns are generally taught wound care and discharged home with instructions to continue wound care once to twice daily and return to the outpatient clinic or their private physician for follow-up assessment and care.

Prevent Tetanus. Burns, even minor ones, are susceptible to tetanus. The current protocol for tetanus immunization in clients with any burn injury is the same as those with other types of trauma. Clients who have not received immunization against tetanus within the past 5 years should receive a tetanus toxoid booster. For clients who have not been immunized, tetanus immunoglobulin (a passive immunizing agent) and the first of a series of active immunizations with tetanus toxoid should be administered.[4]

Prevent Tissue Ischemia. Circumferential burns of the extremities may compromise circulation in the affected limb. Elevating injured extremities 15 degrees above the level of the heart and performing active exercises help to reduce dependent edema formation. However, circulatory compromise may still occur. Therefore frequent assessment of distal extremity perfusion is necessary. Doppler flowmeter assessment of the palmar arch vessels (for the upper extremity) and the posterior tibial artery (for the lower extremity) provides the most precise indication of peripheral perfusion and should be performed regularly during the resuscitation period. The absence of flow or the progressive diminution of the Doppler flowmeter signal intensity is an indication that perfusion is impaired.

An escharotomy is the appropriate treatment for circulatory compromise caused by constricting, circumferential burns (Figure 50-8). A midlateral or midmedial incision of the involved extremity is made from the most proximal to the most distal extent of the full-thickness burn. The depth of the incision is limited to the eschar. It is generally performed at the bedside without local or general anesthesia, because full-thickness burns are insensate. However, viable tissue beneath the escharotomy may bleed if cut, and then the client may feel pain. Bleeding can be controlled with pressure, a topical clotting agent, suture ligation, or electrocautery. Pain control is achieved with IV opioid administration. After escharotomy, the burn wound can be dressed with topical antimicrobial creams and gauze dressings.

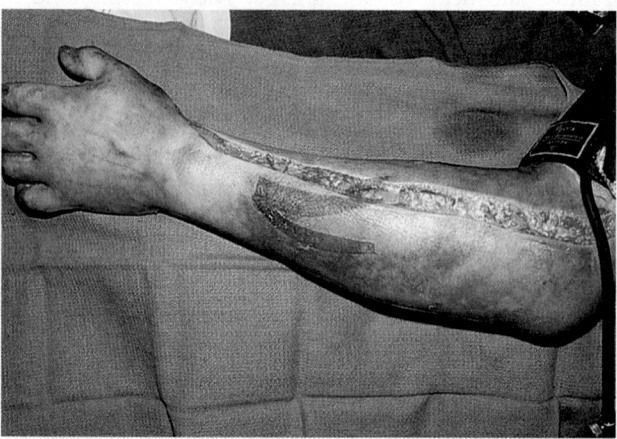

■ **FIGURE 50–8** Escharotomy. Incision is made through the constricting burn eschar to permit expansion of the underlying subcutaneous tissues as edema forms. *(Courtesy University of Washington Burn Center at Harborview Medical Center, Seattle, Wash).*

If adequate tissue perfusion does not return following escharotomy, a fasciotomy may be necessary. This procedure, in which the fascia is incised, is performed in the operating room with the client under general anesthesia. A fasciotomy is usually necessary only in injuries caused by high-voltage electricity or those with concomitant crush injury.

Transport to a Burn Facility. Consideration of transfer to a specialized burn care facility is appropriate for all clients with major burn injuries (see the Bridge to Critical Care feature on p. 1248 for burn classifications). Prompt contact with the receiving burn center is important to facilitate a smooth transfer. All copies of medical records, including administered fluids and medications, hourly urine output values, and vital signs, must accompany the client. The client's burn wounds should simply be covered with a dry sheet and blankets. Burn center personnel will perform a complete assessment of the wound; therefore it is best if topical wound care has not been initiated.

Nursing Management of the Medical Client in the Resuscitative Phase of Burn Care

Assessment. Because the body's immediate physiologic responses to burn injury can either be life-threatening or lead to significant morbidity, prudent nursing assessment during the resuscitative phase of burn injury is crucial.

Diagnosis, Outcomes, Interventions
Diagnosis: Impaired Gas Exchange. Effective gas exchange may become impaired when clients have experienced smoke inhalation because of tracheobronchial swelling, the presence of carbonaceous debris in the airway, or CO poisoning.

Outcomes. The client will have adequate gas exchange evidenced by a Pao_2 greater than 90 mm Hg, oxygen saturation (Sao_2) greater than 95%, arterial partial pressure of carbon dioxide ($Paco_2$) 35 to 45 mm Hg, respiratory rate 16 to 24 breaths/min with a normal pattern and depth, and clear bilateral breath sounds.

Interventions. The client must be frequently assessed for manifestations of respiratory distress such as restlessness, confusion, labored breathing, tachypnea, dyspnea, diminished or adventitious breath sounds, tachycardia, decrease in Pao_2 and Sao_2, and cyanosis. Monitor Sao_2 continuously in clients with major burns during the resuscitative phase of burn injury. Monitor arterial blood gas and COHb levels per physician order. Report changes in the client's condition immediately.

Instruct the client on the use of the incentive spirometer to encourage deep breathing every 2 hours. Elevate the head of the bed to facilitate lung expansion and to reduce facial and neck edema.

Diagnosis: Ineffective Airway Clearance. Because of the occurrence of airway epidermal sloughing, increase in secretions, inflammation and swelling of the nasopharyngeal mucous membranes from smoke irritation, and depressed ciliary action from inhalation injury, the client becomes at risk for *Ineffective Airway Clearance*.

Outcomes. Clients will have an effective airway clearance, as evidenced by clear bilateral breath sounds, clear to white pulmonary secretions, effective mobilization of pulmonary secretions, and unlabored respiration with a respiratory rate of 16 to 24 breaths/min.

Interventions. A thorough pulmonary assessment should be performed every 1 to 2 hours during the first 24 hours after injury, and every 2 to 4 hours the second 24 hours after injury, evaluating breath sounds, rate and depth of respirations, and level of consciousness.

> **Be alert to a declining respiratory status as evidenced by crackles, rhonchi, stridor, labored breathing, dyspnea, tachypnea, restlessness, or a decreasing level of consciousness. Report significant findings promptly.**

SAFETY ALERT

Have the client turn, cough, and deep breathe every 1 to 2 hours for 24 hours and then every 2 to 4 hours. Place an oral suctioning device within the client's reach for independent use. Perform endotracheal or nasotracheal suction as needed. Assess and document the character and amount of secretions.

Diagnosis: Deficient Fluid Volume. The client with an extensive burn injury is at risk for hypovolemia, most significantly during the first 36 hours after burn injury. The *Deficient Fluid Volume* is directly related to the increased capillary leakage and fluid shift from the intravascular to the interstitial space after the burn insult.

Outcomes. The client will have improved fluid balance, as evidenced by a urine output of 30 ml/hour, clear sensorium, pulse rate less than 120 beats/min, absence of dysrhythmias, adequate amplitude of peripheral pulses (2+ or better), and blood pressure within the expected range for age and medical history.

Interventions. Assess the client for manifestations of hypovolemia every hour for 36 hours, including tachycardia, decreased blood pressure, decreased amplitude of peripheral pulses, urine output of less than 30 ml/hour, thirst, and dry mucous membranes. Report significant findings.

> **Carefully monitor and document intake and output, administering fluid therapy as prescribed; titrate the infusion to maintain a urine output of 30 ml/hour. Early in the resuscitative phase, nurses should not wait for the full hour to adjust infusion of fluids; if little to no urine is present, fluid rates should be adjusted.**

SAFETY ALERT

Monitor serum electrolyte and hematocrit values. Hyponatremia, hyperkalemia, and elevated hematocrit levels are common findings during the resuscitative phase. As the circulation is restored, levels should return to normal values.

Diagnosis: Ineffective Tissue Perfusion: Renal. Clients who have suffered deep burn tissue injury, such as in electrical injury or crush injuries, and those in who adequate fluid resuscitation has not been achieved are at risk for renal failure. Myoglobin and hemoglobin are released from the damaged muscles and red blood cells and precipitate in the renal tubules, where they can create acute tubular necrosis.

Outcomes. The client with evidence of deep burn tissue injury will maintain a urine output of 75 to 100 ml/hour until the pigment load has decreased.

Interventions. Monitor and document hourly output and urine color. A dark brown or red color is indicative of the presence of hemochromogens. Send urine samples for myoglobin or hemoglobin assay per physician order to provide quantitative information for documentation of the client's condition. Ensure that the catheter is patent, because the tubing may become plugged with hemochromogens. Administer IV fluids per physician orders. Hemochromogens must be flushed from the body; therefore the rate of fluid administration is based on maintaining an hourly urine output of 75 to 100 ml/hour.

Diagnosis: Ineffective Tissue Perfusion: Peripheral. The client may exhibit *Ineffective Peripheral Tissue Perfusion* as a result of constricting circumferential burns and/or edema of peripheral tissues.

Outcomes. The client will have adequate peripheral perfusion, as evidenced by the presence of pulses on palpation or Doppler flowmeter assessment, capillary refill time for unburned skin of less than 2 seconds, absence of numbness or tingling, and absence of increased pain with active range-of-motion (ROM) exercises.

Interventions. Remove all constricting jewelry and clothing as early as possible, because constricting items may compromise circulation as edema formation ensues. Limit the use of the blood pressure cuff on the affected extremity, because the cuff can reduce arterial inflow and venous return. Elevate the burned extremity above the level of the heart to promote venous return and to prevent excessive dependent edema formation.

Monitor arterial pulses by palpation or with the use of an ultrasonic flow detector (Doppler flowmeter) hourly for up to 72 hours after burn injury. Pulses will diminish with circulation impairment. Assess capillary refill of unburned skin on the affected extremity; capillary refill will be prolonged with impaired circulation. Encourage ROM exercises, and assess the level of pain associated with efforts. Increasing pain with movement is a result of tissue ischemia. When pain is not present, increased movement of the affected area will promote venous return and assist in decreasing edema.

If tissue perfusion is threatened, anticipate and prepare the client for an escharotomy. Once the underlying tissue edema has exceeded the expansion ability of the burned skin, an escharotomy will be needed to restore perfusion. After the procedure is complete, recheck for restoration of circulation by assessing pulses, color, movement, and sensation of the affected extremity. Anticipate some bleeding after escharotomy, because the tissue beneath the eschar may bleed. Bleeding can be controlled by pressure, electrocautery, or suturing by the physician. Continue to observe and assess the extremity after the procedure.

Diagnosis: Acute Pain. The client can be expected to experience a significant amount of pain during the resuscitative phase of recovery. The pain experienced is associated with the burn wound and wound-related procedures.

Outcomes. The client will verbalize a level of acceptable pain control.

Interventions. Assess for pain, and administer appropriate opioids. Time the administration of medications so that the client receives the benefit of the drug's peak performance during painful procedures, and evaluate the effectiveness of interventions. Explain all procedures and allow adequate time for preparation. Assess the need for an anxiolytic medication, as anxiety can be a major contributor to pain. Document findings, including the client's response to pain interventions.

Diagnosis: Anxiety. The client can be expected to experience a significant amount of anxiety. The anxiety experienced is associated with the critical nature of the injury, wound- and care-related procedures, and pain.

Outcomes. The client will verbalize a level of acceptable anxiety control.

Interventions. Assess for anxiety. Explain all procedures and allow adequate time for preparation. Provide adequate pain medications to reduce pain-related anxiety. Assess the need for anxiolytic agents. Document findings.

Diagnosis: Risk for Infection. The burn-injured client faces an increased *Risk for Infection* related to inadequate primary and secondary defenses resulting from traumatized tissue, bacterial proliferation in burn wounds, and an immunocompromised status.

Outcomes. The client will remain free from significant burn wound microbial invasion, as evidenced by quantitative wound cultures containing less than 100,000 colony-forming units (CFUs)/g. In addition, core body temperature will be maintained between 99.6° and 101°F (37.5° C to 38.3° C); there will be no swelling, redness, or purulence present at IV line insertion sites; and results of blood, urine, and sputum cultures will be negative.

Interventions. Tetanus prophylaxis should be administered per physician order because the anaerobic environment beneath eschar is ideal for tetanus organism growth. Topical antimicrobial agents are used to deter the growth of bacteria on the surface of the wound.

It is essential to maintain infection control techniques at all times during the client's hospitalization to prevent cross-contamination. Ensure aseptic technique when administering care to burned areas and performing invasive techniques. Enforce strict hand-washing, and instruct family members or significant others on infection control measures.

When wound care is performed, it is important to debride the wound of loose, devitalized tissue, which serves as a medium for bacterial growth. Hair within and around a wound should be shaved (with the exception of eyebrows and eyelashes), because hair is contaminated and prevents adherence of the burn cream. Apply a topical antimicrobial agent or skin substitute per physician order.

Diagnosis: Impaired Physical Mobility. The client's mobility during the resuscitative phase of burn injury is impaired by tissue edema, pain, and dressings.

Outcomes. The outcomes related to physical mobility are measured throughout the hospitalization and recovery process. The long-term outcome goal is return of the client to maximum independence in performance of activities of daily living (ADL) with minimum disability and disfigurement. Although this outcome is demonstrated long after the resuscitative phase, it is important to initiate care on the day of admission and to follow through continually throughout hospitalization.

Interventions. Encourage the client to participate in self-care and ROM exercises at the earliest time possible. During the early postinjury fluid shifts, physical movement helps to improve circulation and decrease edema. Consult with occupational and physical therapists for initial assessment and follow-up care throughout the hospitalization.

Diagnosis: Disabled Family Coping. Because of the urgent and critical nature of the injury, the client and family are at risk for ineffective coping skills.

Outcomes. Family members and significant others will have accurate information about the immediate status of the client, as evidenced by their ability to verbalize an understanding of the client's injury and treatment goals. Support services will be provided as needed.

Interventions. It is important to prepare family members or significant others for their first visit with the client after injury. Provide a simple explanation of procedures and equipment, communicate the extent of the burn, and describe changes in the client's appearance. When client transfer is impending, provide family members or significant others with support services to assist with travel arrangements. Providing support at this time will help to reduce their anxiety during the client's transfer. Families of clients remaining in the facility should be provided with information that meets their basic needs (e.g., information about lodging, location of cafeteria, parking).

Acute Phase

The acute phase of recovery following a major burn begins when the client is hemodynamically stable, capillary integrity is restored, and diuresis has begun. This time-point begins at approximately 48 to 72 hours after the time of injury. Many of the same principles of care outlined for the resuscitative phase apply to the acute phase; however, more emphasis is placed on restorative therapies. For clients with either a minor or a moderate burn, the acute phase essentially begins at the time of injury. The acute phase continues until wound closure is achieved.

Medical Management in the Acute Phase of Burn Injury

Prevent Infection

Infection control is a major component of burn management. An infection control policy is necessary for managing burn-injured clients to control the transmission of microorganisms that can lead to infection. Standard precautions should be followed in caring for all clients with burn injuries; however, specific infection control practices and isolation techniques exist for all burn centers. These practices include the use of gloves, caps, masks, shoe covers, scrub clothes, and plastic aprons. Strict hand-washing is stressed to reduce the incidence of cross-contamination between clients and is the single most important means of preventing the spread of infection. Staff and visitors are generally prevented from client contact if they have any skin, gastrointestinal, or respiratory tract infections. See Box 50-2 for basic infection control strategies. All visitors as well as health care providers from other departments should be educated concerning established infection control practices before their first contact with the burn-injured client. Some burn centers limit the number of visitors in burn units.

SAFETY
ALERT

Provide Metabolic Support

Maintenance of adequate nutrition during the acute phase of burn care is essential in promoting wound healing and preventing infection. Basal metabolic rates may be 40% to 100% higher than normal levels, depending on the extent of the burn. This response is thought to be the result of a resetting of the homeostatic "thermostat" of the hypothalamic-pituitary-adrenal axis, leading

BOX 50-2 Basic Requirements of Infection Control

1. Hands should be washed before and after each client contact with antimicrobial agent and water or an alcohol hand rinse.
2. Appropriate garb, including clean aprons or gowns and clean gloves, should be donned before each client contact and discarded immediately after leaving the bedside or room.
3. Gloves should be changed when contaminated with secretions or excretions from one body site before contact with another site on the client.
4. Sterile gloves, hats, and masks should be worn when caring for an open burn wound and when preparing for and performing other sterile procedures.
5. Equipment, materials, and surfaces should be considered contaminated with organisms from the client and should be appropriately decontaminated before use on other clients.
6. Appropriate garb should be worn when handling or touching equipment, materials, and surfaces contaminated by clients.

Personal communication with Joan M. Weber, RN, BSN, CIC, Infection Control Coordinator, Shriners Burn Hospital, 51 Blossom St., Boston, Mass.

to an increase in heat production. Metabolic rates decrease as wound coverage and healing are achieved.

Aggressive nutritional support is required to meet the increased energy requirements necessary to promote healing and to prevent the untoward effects of catabolism. Several different formulas, shown in the Critical Monitoring feature below, are currently used to estimate energy requirements by factoring different indices: weight, gender, age, extent of burn, and amount of activity. Additional support is generally indicated for the burn-injured client with any of the following: 30% or greater TBSA burn, clinical course requiring multiple

CRITICAL MONITORING

Energy Calculation Formulas Used for the Adult with a Burn Injury

Formula/Author Name	Formula for Daily Caloric Expenditure Estimate
Curreri	(25 kcal/kg body weight) + (40 kcal × % TBSA burn)
Modified Harris-Benedict	RMR × Activity factor × Injury factor
U.S. Army Institute of Surgical Research	(Age- and gender-specific BMR) × (0.89142 + 0.01335 × % TBSA burn) × (m^2 × 24 × Activity factor)

BMR, Basal metabolic rate; *RMR,* resting metabolic rate; *TBSA,* total body surface area.
From Weber, J.M., & Tompkins, D.M. (1993). Improving survival: Infection control and burns. *AACN Clinical Issues in Critical Care Nursing, 4*(2), 418-419.

operations, need for mechanical ventilatory support, compromised mental status, and poor pre-injury nutritional state. Methods for delivering nutritional support include oral intake, enteral tube feedings, peripheral parenteral nutrition, and total parenteral nutrition, which may be used alone or in combination. The preferred feeding route is oral or enteral; however, the decision of how to best meet the client's nutritional needs should be individualized. Typically, parenteral nutrition is reserved for clients with a prolonged ileus or for those in whom enteral feedings fail to meet nutritional needs.

Minimize Pain

Procedural, background, and breakthrough pain continue to be important issues during this part of the recovery. During the acute phase of injury, an attempt is made to find the right combination of medications and interventions to minimize the discomfort and pain.

As in the resuscitative phase, the most common approach to pain control is with the use of pharmacologic agents. However, in addition to the opioids used during the resuscitative phase, other modalities may be used during the acute phase of burn injury to help alleviate the client's pain. Patient-controlled analgesia devices, inhalation analgesics such as nitrous oxide, oral analgesic "pain cocktails," and opioid agonist-antagonist agents may be beneficial during the acute phase of burn injury. Nonsteroidal anti-inflammatory drugs (NSAIDs) can be prescribed for the treatment of mild to moderate pain. When NSAIDs are used, extra precautions must be taken to prevent gastric ulceration.[11]

Nonpharmacologic modalities used to treat burn-related pain include hypnosis, guided imagery, art and play therapy, relaxation techniques, distraction, biofeedback, and music therapy. These modalities have been found to be effective in decreasing anxiety, thereby decreasing the perception of pain. They are often used as adjunctive therapies to the pharmacologic treatment of burn pain.[9]

Provide Wound Care

Care of the burn wound is ultimately aimed at promoting wound healing. Daily wound care involves cleansing, debridement of devitalized tissue, and dressing of the wound.

Wound Cleansing. The practice of hydrotherapy remains a mainstay of burn treatment plans for cleansing the wounds. This is accomplished by immersion, showering, or spraying (Figure 50-9). A hydrotherapy session of 30 minutes or less is optimal for clients with acute burns. Longer time periods may increase sodium loss (water is hypotonic) through the burn wound and may promote heat loss, pain, and stress. During hydrotherapy, the wounds are gently washed using any one of a variety of solutions.

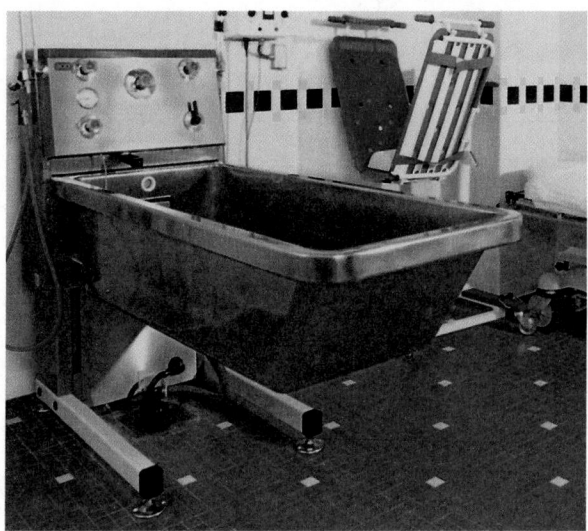

■ **FIGURE 50-9** A low-boy whirlpool tank is used for immersion hydrotherapy treatment of burn wounds. *(Courtesy of Shriners Hospitals for Children of Northern California.)*

Care should be taken to minimize bleeding and to maintain body temperature during this procedure. To prevent cross-contamination, single-use plastic hydrotherapy tub liners are available, with tub cleansing performed between clients. Clients excluded from hydrotherapy are generally those who are hemodynamically unstable and those with new skin grafts. If hydrotherapy is not used, wounds are washed and rinsed while the client is in bed, before the application of topical antimicrobial agents.

Debridement. Burn wound debridement involves the removal of eschar, exudate, and crusts. This promotes wound healing by preventing bacterial proliferation in and under the devitalized tissue. Debridement of the burn wound is accomplished through mechanical, enzymatic, or surgical means.

Mechanical debridement can be accomplished with careful use of scissors and forceps to lift and trim away loose devitalized tissue. Hydrotherapy softens and loosens devitalized tissue so that it is more easily removed. Wet-to-dry dressing changes are another effective means of mechanical debridement. Coarse gauze dressings are saturated with a prescribed solution, wrung out until the dressing is slightly moist, and applied to the wound. The dressing is left in place to dry. Typically 6 to 8 hours later the gauze is carefully removed from the wound, mechanically lifting drainage, exudate, and loose necrotic tissue that have dried onto the gauze. However, this method of wound debridement must be used cautiously, as it will also debride viable tissue. Mechanical debridement of the burn wound can be extremely painful; therefore effective pain management is paramount.

Enzymatic debridement involves the application of commercially prepared proteolytic and fibrinolytic topical enzymes (Accuzyme, Healthpoint Ltd., Ft. Worth, Tex;

Santyl, Abbott Laboratories, Columbus, Ohio) to the burn wound, which facilitates devitalized tissue removal. These agents require a moist environment to be effective and are applied directly to the burn wound.

> **Caution must be used when enzymes are used as pain and bleeding are common side effects. As the enzyme digests necrotic tissue, it may open up thrombosed blood vessels. This causes some oozing of blood from the vessels and creates a site for bacteria to enter the bloodstream. Bacteremia, pain, and bleeding can occur; therefore if enzymatic debridement is used, the client should be assessed for complications continuously throughout the course of treatment. The use of enzymatic debridement agents is contraindicated for wounds communicating with major body cavities and for wounds with exposed nerves or nervous tissue.**

SAFETY

ALERT

Surgical debridement of the burn wound involves excision of the devitalized tissue and coverage of the wound. Early surgical excision begins during the first week after injury, once the client is hemodynamically stable. Advantages of early excision include early mobilization, early wound closure (which reduces the potential for wound infection), and reduced length of hospitalization. A disadvantage of early excision is the risk of excising viable tissue that may heal with time.

Two techniques of surgical debridement are currently used. In *tangential* excision, very thin layers of devitalized tissue are sequentially shaved until viable tissue is reached. *Fascial* excision involves removing the burn tissue and underlying fat down to fascia. This technique is frequently used for debridement of very deep burns.

Topical Antimicrobial Treatment. Deep partial-thickness or full-thickness burn wounds are treated initially with topical antimicrobial agents. These agents are applied once or twice daily following cleansing, debridement, and inspection of the wound. The nurse assesses for separation of devitalized tissue, the presence of granulation tissue or reepithelialization, and manifestations of infection. The most commonly used topical antimicrobial agents are listed in Table 50-1. Although no single agent is used universally, many burn centers choose silver sulfadiazine cream as the initial topical agent.[7,14]

Burn wounds are treated using either an open or a closed dressing technique. For the *open method,* the antimicrobial cream is applied with a gloved hand and the wound is left open to the air without gauze dressings. The cream is reapplied as needed, although formal reapplication is common every 12 to 24 hours. The advantages of the open method include increased visualization of the wound, greater freedom for mobility and joint motion, and simplicity in wound care. The disadvantages include an increased chance of hypothermia and pain from exposure.

TABLE 50–1 Topical Antimicrobial Agents Used in Burn Care

Agent	Antimicrobial Spectrum	Application	Side Effects	Nursing Considerations
Water-Based Creams				
1% Silver sulfadiazine	Broad spectrum; effective against some fungi and yeast	1-2 times daily, 1/16-inch thickness	Transient leukopenia typically appearing after 2 or 3 days of treatment Macular rash	Do not store in warm environment (e.g., warm client room)
Mafenide acetate	Broad spectrum; little antifungal activity	Gauze dressing not required	Hyperchloremic metabolic acidosis from bicarbonate diuresis because of inhibition of carbonic anhydrase Pain/burning sensation on application to superficial burns Maculopapular rash	Assess for side effects Assess adequacy of pain management; if pain and discomfort continue, consider other topical treatments Use cautiously in clients with acute renal failure
Solutions				
5% Mafenide acetate	Broad spectrum	2 times daily, 1/16-inch thickness	Pain on application Pruritus Rash Fungal colonization	Assess for side effects Assess adequacy of pain management
0.5% Silver nitrate	Broad spectrum; effective against *Candida* species	Gauze dressing not required	Hyponatremia Hypochloremia Hypokalemia Hypocalcemia	Check serum electrolyte levels daily Penetrates eschar poorly Remoisten dressings every 2 hr to avoid wound desiccation Protect environment; stains everything blackish-brown color
Petroleum-Based Ointments				
Polymyxin B	Gram-negative organisms	Gauze dressing required, moistened with solution for application to wound	Hypersensitivity (rash)	Assess for side effects
Neomycin sulfate	Predominantly gram-negative organisms	Multiple layers of gauze dressing required, moistened with solution for application to wound	Overgrowth of nonsusceptible organisms including fungi	
Bacitracin	Predominantly gram-positive organisms	Apply as needed in a thin layer; gauze dressing not used unless clothing protection is needed		

In the *closed method* of wound care, gauze dressing is impregnated with antimicrobial cream and applied to the wound. To prevent circulatory compromise in extremity burns, the gauze should be wrapped from the most distal portion of the extremity in a proximal direction. The advantages of the closed method are decreases in evaporative fluid and heat loss from the wound surface. In addition, gauze dressings may aid in debridement. The disadvantages of gauze dressings are mobility limitations and a potential decrease in effectiveness of range-of-motion (ROM) exercises. Wound assessment is also limited to the times at which dressing changes are performed.

Temporary wound coverings (skin substitutes) are frequently used as a kind of wound "dressing." Table 50-2 outlines the most common biologic, biosynthetic, and synthetic wound coverings available. These products are temporary wound coverings, and each has specific

indications. The character of the wound (depth of injury, amount of exudate, location of the wound on the body, and phase of recovery) and treatment goals are considered in choosing the most appropriate wound covering.

Maximize Function
Maintenance of optimal physical functioning in the client with a burn injury is a challenge for the entire team. Nurses work closely with occupational and physical therapists to identify the rehabilitative needs of the burn-injured client. An individualized program of splinting, positioning, exercise, ambulation, performance of ADL, and pressure therapy should be implemented in the acute phase of recovery to maximize functional recovery and cosmetic outcome. Therapeutic goals at

TABLE 50–2 Wound Coverings Used in Burn Care

Category/Examples	Description/Indications	Nursing Considerations
Biologic		
Allograft (homograft/cadaver)	Donated human cadaver skin used to: Debride exudative wounds Protect excised wounds and test for receptivity before autograft placement Cover and protect meshed autografts	Gauze cover dressing is applied over allograft to protect from shearing forces and, with meshed allograft, used to absorb drainage. Staples may be used to hold allograft in place. Staples are placed intraoperatively. Negative pressure therapy may be used over allograft to increase vascularization of wound bed.
Xenograft (heterograft/pigskin)	Harvested porcine (pig) skin used to: Promote healing of clean, superficial partial-thickness burn wounds Debride exudative wounds	Gauze cover dressing applied over xenograft for first 24 hr until adhered (for clean partial-thickness wounds). Once xenograft is adhered, it may be left open to air. Gauze cover dressing applied over xenograft to protect from shearing forces and, with meshed xenograft, to absorb wound drainage. Xenograft is changed daily when used to promote debridement.
Biosynthetic		
Biobrane (Bertek Pharmaceuticals, Morgantown, WV)	Nylon fabric bonded to a silicone membrane containing collagenous porcine peptides used to: Cover donor sites Protect and facilitate healing of clean, superficial partial-thickness burn wounds	Secure to surrounding intact skin with tape, skin closure strips, or staples. Wrap Biobrane with coarse mesh roller gauze dressing. For donor sites, gauze wrap is secured with an outer dressing. Once Biobrane is adhered (usually at 48 hr postoperative), outer dressings can be removed and Biobrane left exposed to air. New and healing donor sites of legs require support during ambulation; figure-eight elastic (Ace) bandage wrapping technique is recommended to minimize trauma to newly formed capillaries. For superficial partial-thickness wounds, Biobrane is applied and secured with tape or skin closure strips. Assess for purulent drainage beneath fabric and at wound periphery (indicative of infection).
Integra (Integra Life Sciences, Plainsboro, NJ)	Bilayer matrix of bovine collagen and glycosaminoglycan covered by silicone layer used to: Provide a dermal layer to excised burn wounds	Applied in OR to excised wounds and secured with staples or securing devices. Silastic (outer) layer is removed approximately 2 weeks following application and covered with very thin split-thickness skin graft. Assess for infection; may appear as pockets of purulent fluid beneath Integra. If indicated, these areas may require debridement and topical antimicrobial coverage. Protect from shearing forces.
Calcium alginate (Kaltostat, ConvaTec/Bristol-Myers & Squibb Co., New York, NY; SeaSorb Ag, Coloplast Corp, Marietta, Ga; Silver Cel, Johnson & Johnson/Ethicon, Inc., Somerville, NJ) Hydrofiber (Aquacel/Aquacel Ag—ConvaTec/Bristol-Myers & Squibb Co., New York, NY)	Dressing produced from alginates found in brown seaweed or synthetically produced to create hydrofibers that are used to: Absorb exudate from moderate to heavily draining wounds Cover donor sites Reduce wound bioburden (those with silver (Ag) added to them)	Applied to wounds and donor sites following irrigation with physiologic solution, such as saline. Absorptive dressing covers calcium alginate or Hydrofiber dressing. Entire dressing should be changed when outer dressing is saturated with drainage.
Non-adhering fine mesh gauze (Aquaphor gauze, Beiersdorf Inc., Norwalk, Conn; Adaptic, Johnson & Johnson/Ethicon, Inc., Somerville, NJ; Xeroform gauze, Sherwood Medical, St. Louis, Mo)	Gauze impregnated with ointment used to: Cover meshed autograft Cover donor sites Cover and protect fragile, newly healed skin	Gauze dressing over healing autograft is often changed daily. Gauze dressing over donor sites should remain in place until healed (10-14 days; may be longer in older adults). Healing donor sites on legs require vascular support when out of bed; figure-eight (Ace) wrapping technique is recommended to minimize trauma to newly formed capillaries.

this stage in recovery are to prevent early contracture formation and to maintain soft tissue length.

Wound contracture and hypertrophic scarring are two major problems for the burn-injured client. Wound contractures are typically more severe with extensive burns. Areas seemingly predisposed to contracture are the hands, head and neck, and axilla. Measures used to prevent and treat wound contractures include therapeutic positioning, ROM exercises, splinting, and client and family education.

Table 50-3 lists corrective and therapeutic techniques for positioning clients with specific areas of burn injury during periods of inactivity or immobilization. Allowing the burn-injured client to assume a position of comfort most often contributes to contracture formation. Therefore proper positioning, both in and out of bed, should be maintained for the burn-injured client. These techniques place affected body parts in positions that are in opposition to positions of potential contracture or deformity. The natural tendency with healing and immobility is for muscles and joints to contract into a shortened, flexed position. For example, to reduce the risk of neck contractures, the use of pillows—which place the neck in flexion—is not allowed.

Active ROM exercises are prescribed early in the acute phase of recovery to promote resolution of edema and to maintain strength and joint function. In addition, ADL can be effective in maintaining function and ROM. Ambulation maintains strength and ROM of the lower extremities. They should begin as soon as the client is physiologically stable. Passive ROM and stretching exercises should be included as part of the daily treatment plan when the client is unable to perform active ROM exercises.

Splints are used to maintain proper joint position and to prevent or correct contractures. Two types of splints are frequently used. A *static splint* immobilizes the joint. Static splints do not replace exercise and are frequently applied for periods of immobilization or during sleeping hours or are used for clients who cannot maintain proper positioning. In contrast, *dynamic splints* exercise the affected joint. Care must be taken to ensure that all splints fit properly and do not apply excessive pressure, which may lead to further tissue or nerve damage.

🐚 Provide Psychological Support

The longest period of adjustment occurs during the acute phase. The burn-injured adult may demonstrate a variety of emotional and psychological responses. Anxiety and fearfulness related to potential disfigurement and perceived changes in role and identity plague the client during this time period. Depression, withdrawal, and regression may result.

The client may begin discussing the burn injury or accident, recounting significant events and searching for the meaning of what has happened. Allowing the expression of these worries and validating that they are "normal" are essential in providing support. Staff members need to actively listen and to allow the client to talk about the accident. Detailed and repetitious recounting of the injury is useful in desensitizing clients to the horror of what has happened and in decreasing nightmares.

Clients who have little information about specific treatment procedures, potential associated discomfort or pain, and available resources or options for pain management typically react with anxiety and a heightened pain response. Providing the client with information about what will occur during a particular procedure or what is expected over the course of recovery is a concept known as *providing preparatory information*. This technique is a psychologically based method that has proved successful in reducing pain and anxiety during certain procedures. To enhance the client's sense of personal control, teaching should include education about various coping mechanisms and the use of nonpharmacologic methods for pain control.

Involving clients in their own care helps them to feel some control over the situation at hand. Clients can be encouraged to participate in wound care (e.g., bathing, simple debridement, dressing application) and physical therapy (e.g., active versus passive ROM exercises, application of splints and pressure garments). These interventions have been found to be effective in supporting the client's psychological needs.

Nursing Management of the Medical Client in the Acute Phase of Burn Injury

Assessment. Once fluid balance is achieved, the client moves into the acute phase of burn care. During this phase, closure of the wounds is a major focus of care. Wounds are assessed daily with every dressing change for evidence of healing and infection. Other areas of assessment include respiratory condition; pain control, nutritional status, and stress ulceration; mobility and contractures; and psychological adjustments by both the client and the family.

Diagnosis, Outcomes, Interventions

Diagnosis: Impaired Gas Exchange. Note that the consequences of smoke inhalation may not be fully appreciated until the acute phase of burn care. The decreased ciliary action in the airways leads to a high risk for pulmonary infection (which usually is not manifested until day 3 or 4 after the burn injury), which is demonstrated first by tracheobronchitis and is followed by bronchopneumonia.

Outcomes. The client will have improved gas exchange, as evidenced by unlabored respirations, a respiratory rate

TABLE 50–3   Anticontracture Positioning for the Client with a Burn Injury

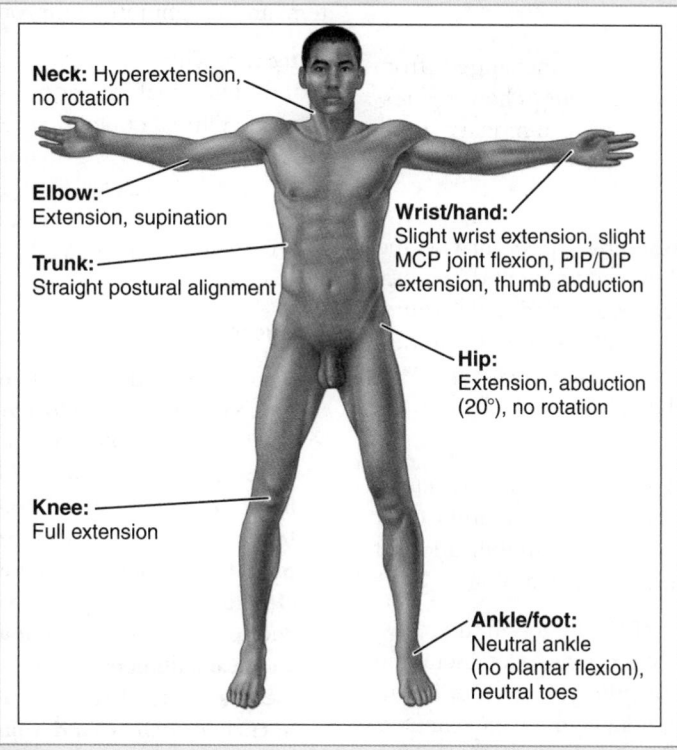

Neck: Hyperextension, no rotation

Elbow: Extension, supination

Trunk: Straight postural alignment

Wrist/hand: Slight wrist extension, slight MCP joint flexion, PIP/DIP extension, thumb abduction

Hip: Extension, abduction (20°), no rotation

Knee: Full extension

Ankle/foot: Neutral ankle (no plantar flexion), neutral toes

Burned Area	Therapeutic Position	Positioning Techniques
Neck		
Anterior	Extension	No pillow
		Small towel roll beneath shoulders to promote neck extension
Circumferential	Neutral toward extension	No pillow
Posterior or asymmetrical	Neutral	No pillow
Shoulder/axilla	Arm abduction to 90-110 degrees	Splinting
		Arms positioned away from body and supported on arm troughs
Elbow	Arm extension	Elbow splint
		Elbows positioned in extension with slight bend at elbow (no more than 10 degrees of elbow flexion)
		Arms supported on arm troughs with forearm in slight pronation
Hand		
Wrist	Wrist extension	Hand splint
MCP	MCP flexion at 90 degrees	Hand splint
PIP/DIP	PIP/DIP extension	Hand splint
Thumb	Thumb abduction	Hand splint with thumb abduction
Finger web spaces	Finger abduction	Web spacers of foam, silicone products, or custom-fitted pressure garments to decrease webbing formation
Hip	Hip extension	Supine with head of bed flat and legs extended
		Trochanter roll to maintain neutral hip rotation (toes should be pointing toward ceiling)
		Prone positioning
Knee	Knee extension	Supine with knees extended (toes should be pointing toward the ceiling)
		Prone positioning with feet extended over end of mattress
		Sitting in chair with legs extended and elevated
		Knee splint
Ankle	Neutral	Padded footboard
		Ankle positioning devices (avoid heel cord tightening)— provide heel protection to prevent pressure sore development

MCP, Metacarpal interphalangeal joint(s); *PIP/DIP,* proximal/distal interphalangeal joint(s).

of 16 to 24 breaths/min, Pao_2 greater than 90 mm Hg, $Paco_2$ of 35 to 45 mm Hg, Sao_2 greater than 95%, and clear bilateral breath sounds.

Interventions. Interventions continue unchanged from the resuscitative phase of injury. Comprehensive respiratory assessment and preventive pulmonary toilet should be performed every 2 hours while the client is awake.

Diagnosis: Ineffective Airway Clearance. Upper airway and facial edema caused by heat-induced tissue and mucosal damage begins to resolve between 2 and 4 days after injury with superficial burns. Full-thickness injuries, however, resolve more slowly, making *Ineffective Airway Clearance* a problem that may last well into the acute phase of treatment.

Outcomes. The client will have effective airway clearance, as evidenced by clear bilateral breath sounds, clear to white pulmonary secretions, effective mobilization of pulmonary secretions, and unlabored breathing.

Interventions. Continue interventions begun in the resuscitative phase of treatment. Pulmonary toilet including turning, coughing, and deep breathing; use of an incentive spirometer every 2 to 4 hours while the client is awake; and endotracheal suctioning as needed facilitates clearance of secretions and sputum. Leave an oral suctioning device within the client's reach for independent use.

Diagnosis: Hypothermia. Clients remain at risk for loss of body heat through burn injuries until wound closure is complete. During hydrotherapy, dressing changes, and lengthy operative procedures, clients are at increased risk for hypothermia.

Outcomes. The client will maintain a core body temperature between 99.6° and 101° F (between 37.5° and 38.3° C).

Interventions. To help prevent the loss of heat from open wounds that occurs as a result of evaporation, limit hydrotherapy treatment sessions to 30 minutes or less with water temperatures of 98° to 102° F (36.6° to 38.8° C). Cover the client with warm blankets after the hydrotherapy session, exposing only limited areas of body surface during topical agent and dressing application. Provide heat lamps or heat shields and increase the ambient temperature in the treatment room or in the client's room if the client exhibits subnormal temperatures. Intravenous fluids and warming blankets may be used in the operating room to maintain body temperature.

Diagnosis: Risk for Infection. During the acute phase of injury, infection remains an ongoing risk because of inadequate primary and secondary defenses resulting from traumatized tissue, bacterial proliferation in the burn wound, presence of invasive lines or urinary catheters, and an immunocompromised status.

Outcomes. The client will have no significant burn wound microbial invasion, as evidenced by quantitative wound cultures containing less than 100,000 CFUs/g. In addition, the client will maintain core body temperature at 99.6° to 101° F; will demonstrate evidence of no swelling, redness, or purulence at invasive line insertion sites; and will have negative results on blood, urine, and sputum cultures.

Interventions

Continue to follow infection control policy for burn-injured clients in an effort to prevent cross-contamination. Assess for clinical manifestations of infection in the burn wound: discoloration of wounds (e.g., brown, black, or hemorrhagic), drainage, odor, delayed healing, or spongy eschar. As in the resuscitative phase, provide meticulous wound care in an aseptic fashion, cleaning and rinsing the wound, and debriding loose devitalized tissue to discourage bacterial growth. Apply a topical antimicrobial agent to the wound to decrease the risk for local wound infection. Continue to shave or cut body hair around wound margins until complete wound closure (exception: do not shave eyebrows or eyelashes).

Observe for clinical indicators of sepsis: headache, chills, anorexia, nausea, changes in vital signs, hyperglycemia and glycosuria, paralytic ileus, and confusion, restlessness, or hallucinations. Assess for manifestations of infection at catheter insertion sites and wounds. Obtain cultures per physician order, and administer antibiotics and antipyretics as prescribed.

Collaborative Problem: Risk for Stress Ulceration. Stress ulcers can occur at any time after a burn injury. The assessment and preventive treatment started in the resuscitative phase of injury should continue until wound coverage is complete.

Outcomes. The nurse will monitor for manifestations of gastrointestinal bleeding and will maintain gastric pH greater than 5.

Interventions. Monitor and document gastric pH values and heme content every 2 hours while the client's nasogastric tube is in place. Administer antacids, H_2 blockers, or proton pump inhibitors per physician order to reduce the gastric acid content, because high acid levels may lead to bleeding. Monitor stools for occult blood.

Diagnosis: Imbalanced Nutrition: Less Than Body Requirements. The burn-injured client must maintain adequate protein and caloric intake to meet metabolic demands for wound healing.

Outcomes. The client will have adequate nutrition, as evidenced by maintenance of 85% to 90% of pre-burn weight and healing of burn wounds, donor sites, and skin grafts.

Interventions. Caloric needs are based on pre-injury weight. For clients with a major burn, obtain a daily weight to assess whether caloric needs are being met and to provide documentation for staff to follow trends. Weekly weight assessments are adequate for the client who is stable and has less than 25% TBSA burn wound. Assess eating habits and patterns, and identify food preferences and food allergies. Order meals high in calories and proteins. Encourage family members or significant others to bring favorite nutritional foods from home. Provide supplements between meals.

Document daily caloric intake, and consult with the dietitian to perform a nutritional assessment. Consider other methods to meet caloric needs such as tube-feeding or total parenteral feeding, because oral feeding may not provide adequate calories for healing.

Performing oral hygiene during each nursing shift and as needed helps to prevent stomatitis and enhance appetite. Provide an aesthetically pleasing environment that is conducive to eating. Treatments are scheduled to provide for uninterrupted meal times. Allow a period of rest before meal times if the client has endured a painful procedure or treatment, because pain will decrease appetite.

Diagnosis: Acute Pain. The client can be expected to experience a significant amount of pain during the acute burn phase. The pain experienced during this phase of recovery is associated with the burn wound, donor sites, wound care procedures, and ROM exercises.

Outcomes. The client will verbalize a level of acceptable pain control.

Interventions. Continue to assess for pain frequently, and administer appropriate opioids. Time the administration of medications so that the client receives the benefit of the drug's peak performance during painful procedures, and evaluate the effectiveness of interventions.

During the acute phase, nonpharmacologic interventions should be initiated to enhance medication effects and to assist in controlling pain. Explore the benefits of relaxation techniques, guided imagery, music therapy, distraction, and biofeedback. Explain all procedures and allow adequate time for preparation. Assess the need for anxiolytic agents, as anxiety can be a major contributor to pain. Document findings including response to pain interventions.

Diagnosis: Anxiety. The client can be expected to experience a significant amount of anxiety. The anxiety experienced is associated with wound- and care-related procedures, and pain.

Outcomes. The client will verbalize a level of acceptable anxiety control.

Interventions. Assess for anxiety. Explain all procedures and allow adequate time for preparation. Provide adequate pain medications to reduce pain-related anxiety. Provide a consistent treatment schedule (e.g., wound care and physical therapy times are prescheduled with the client on a daily basis). Assess the need for anxiolytic agents. Document findings.

Diagnosis: Impaired Physical Mobility. *Impaired Physical Mobility* during the acute phase of burn treatment is related to pain, the presence of dressings and splints, surgical procedures, and wound contractures.

Outcomes. The client will maintain soft tissue length, as evidenced by maintaining ROM without manifestations of early contracture formation.

Interventions. The main interventions during the acute phase of injury are splinting, positioning, and ROM exercises. Collaboration with physical and occupational therapists is essential for guidance in an individualized program for each client.

Optimal positioning of the client involves continuing use of anticontracture positions. Maintaining burned areas in a position of physiologic function by either splinting or positioning will help to prevent or reduce contracture development.

Encourage the client to participate in ADL, to ambulate, and to spend time sitting up in a chair. These activities will not only improve mobility but also assist in moving the client toward independence.

Diagnosis: Disturbed Personal Identity. During the acute burn phase, the client recognizes the extent of injury and realizes that his or her body is changed. Depression, grief, fear, and anxiety confront the client.

Outcomes. The client will acknowledge body changes and demonstrate movement toward incorporating these changes into the self-concept. The client will not exhibit maladaptive responses such as severe depression.

Interventions. The client can be expected to experience emotional lability while progressing through recovery. Staff members should provide an accepting atmosphere for the client, although the client should be assisted to exercise control over any destructive behaviors. Family members or significant others should be involved in care as much as possible to demonstrate continued support for the client. Staff members should be available to provide information about the appearance of burns and grafts and to explain changes that can be expected over time (healed burn wounds, graft sites, and donor sites may change in appearance for up to 1 year after injury). Providing information helps to reduce misconceptions and can give hope that the painful procedures can produce good cosmetic results.

Diagnosis: Disabled Family Coping. Recognize that families often imagine that the survival of the family unit is threatened following a member's injury. Normal coping mechanisms become overwhelmed.

Outcomes. Family members will demonstrate coping strategies, as evidenced by verbalizing realistic expectations for client outcomes, expressing knowledge of the goals of the treatment regimen, interacting appropriately with the client, and demonstrating decreased emotional stress.

Interventions. Once beyond the resuscitative phase, it is important to provide the family members or significant others with information about what to expect for the burn-injured client in the future. It is helpful to provide families with daily updates regarding changes in the client's condition. This assists in maintaining realistic perceptions of the client's progress. Assist the family in finding ways to nurture the client and to participate in some aspects of care. These measures not only assure the client of the family's love and acceptance but also allow family members or significant others to regain some feelings of control. It may also be useful to introduce the family members to the local burn support group. Burn survivors and their families can provide emotional support and validation and can reinforce the concept that it is possible to survive and live happily and productively after a burn injury.

Surgical Management in the Acute Phase of Burn Injury

Definitive wound care for full-thickness burns is accomplished by *autografting,* the surgical removal of a superficial layer of the client's own unburned skin, which is subsequently grafted to the excised or granulating burn wound. Because the epidermis is split (in layers) rather than taken in full, these grafts are referred to as *split-thickness grafts.* This procedure is performed in the operating room while the client is under general anesthesia. Autografts can be applied either as a sheet *(sheet graft)* or in a meshed form *(meshed graft).*

A sheet autograft is applied to the excised wound bed without alteration in its integrity (Figure 50-10). Sheet autografts are frequently used to graft burns in visible areas (e.g., face, neck, hands).

In contrast, a meshed autograft contains many little slits that allow for expansion of the donor skin (Figure 50-11). Meshing permits coverage of larger areas of irregularly shaped wounds and allows for drainage from a bleeding wound bed. When healed, the meshed pattern of the autograft remains visible. Therefore meshed grafts are often used on hidden body areas. When a thicker layer of skin is removed, consisting of the epidermis and the dermis, this is referred to as a *full-thickness graft.* For all autografts, the area of the body from which the skin was removed is referred to as the *donor site* (Figure 50-12).

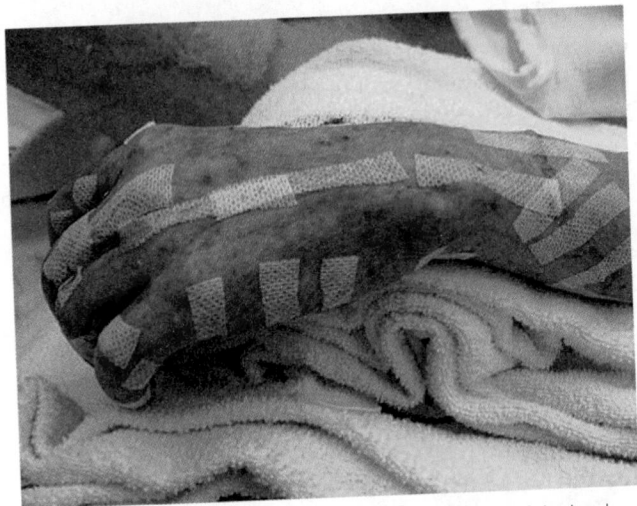

■ **FIGURE 50–10** Split-thickness sheet autograft of the hand on postoperative day 3. Note the use of medical adhesive tape (white coloring) that has been used at the junctions between grafts and graft and intact skin to help affix the graft to the wound bed. Tape is removed at postoperative day 7-10.

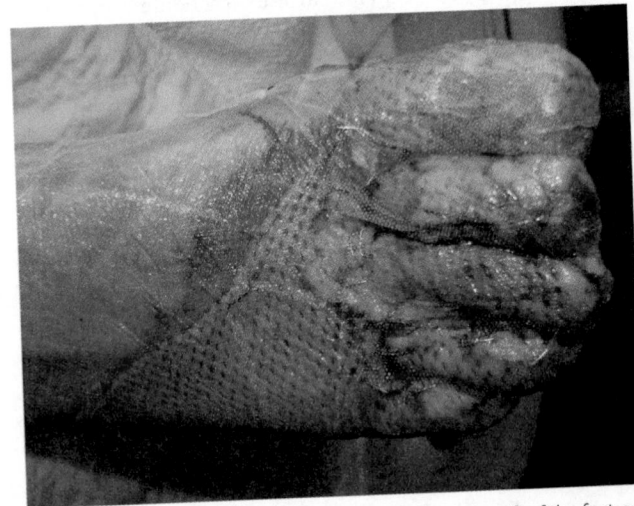

■ **FIGURE 50–11** Split-thickness meshed autograft of the foot on postoperative day 5. Note the thin layer of dressing material covering the meshed graft. This dressing provides protection while not preventing wound drainage.

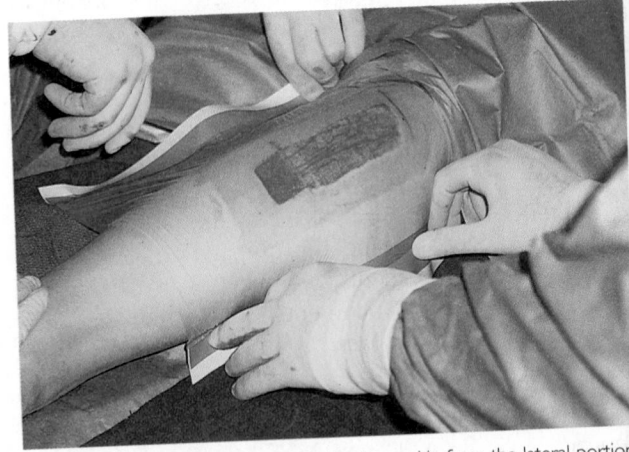

■ **FIGURE 50–12** Harvesting donor skin from the lateral portion of the client's thigh.

Graft adherence is dependent on the formation of a fibrin bond between the recipient bed and the graft. There are no vascular connections between the graft and the wound bed immediately after surgery. The graft is held in place only by weak fibrin bonds and is nourished by the diffusion of serum from the wound bed. The graft begins to stabilize after 3 days as a fibrovascular and collagen network form and provide durability to the graft.

A bleeding wound bed, hematoma formation, or shearing of the graft disrupts formation of this bond between graft and bed. Care must be taken during the postoperative period to assess for bleeding, remove accumulated serum beneath sheet grafts (as described next in the discussion on nursing management of the surgical client), and prevent unwanted movement and shearing of autografts.

Various types of dressings are used to cover donor sites, depending on the size, location, and condition of adjacent skin or tissue (see Table 50-2).

However, despite the differences in dressings, the donor site wound requires the same meticulous care as for other partial-thickness wounds, to expedite healing and prevent infection. If the donor site becomes infected, the dressing should be gently removed or soaked off. The wound can then be thoroughly cleansed and an antimicrobial agent applied.

Once the donor site has healed, lubricating lotions can be applied to soften the area and reduce itching. Donor sites can be reused after they are healed.

Cultured *epithelial autografting* is a technique for closure of massive burn wounds. The process of autologous epithelial cell growth begins with taking a full-thickness skin specimen from an uninjured body site. This specimen is sent to a specialized laboratory for culture and growth. Typically, in 3 to 4 weeks, several sheets of cultured epithelial autografts are ready for application. In the operating room, the cultured epithelial autograft sheets are carefully applied to an excised and nonbleeding wound bed and are secured in place with staples. Dressings are applied and moistened with an antibiotic solution shown to be nontoxic to the cultured epithelial autografts.

Reports demonstrating the success of cultured epithelial autografts in the treatment of massive burn wounds have been limited. Both early and late cultured epithelial autograft loss resulting from mechanical shearing, nutritional imbalance, infection, or an autoimmune response has been reported.

Nursing Management of the Surgical Client in the Acute Phase of Burn Injury

Preoperative Care

Routine care of clients undergoing surgery is discussed in Chapter 14. Specific preoperative care of the client scheduled for burn surgery includes providing information about areas to be excised and plans for pain control. Specific orders for medications to be given or withheld and the time to begin *nil per os* (NPO) (i.e., nothing by mouth) status should be obtained.

Before skin grafting, clients need information on the type of skin graft to be placed (e.g., sheet graft, meshed graft, cultured epithelial autografts), the location of the donor site, the postoperative plans for pain control, and the need for immobility and elevation of the graft site postoperatively. Fears over scarring should be addressed; in general, scarring cannot be predicted because scar tissue requires a full year to mature. Both debridement and grafting can require multiple procedures, and clients may become anxious over repeated surgical procedures. Severe anxiety should be communicated to the surgeon and anesthesia personnel.

Postoperative Care

Routine postoperative care is discussed in Chapter 14. Care specific to excised wounds includes assessment of bleeding and pain control. Many clients report more pain in donor sites (because of exposed nerve endings) than in recipient sites. Donor sites are dressed with occlusive dressings. Skin-grafted sites must be immobilized to promote adherence of the graft to the wound bed. Various techniques are used, including suture, staples, tape, splints and dressings. Because blebs (pockets) of serum or hematomas may develop beneath the sheet graft, postoperative dressings are often removed within 24 hours for an assessment. If blebs or hematomas are evident, they must be removed or the risk of graft loss is high. A small needle (e.g., 25 gauge) is used to aspirate fluid beneath the graft, or a small slit in the graft is made with a scalpel and the fluid is rolled out with a cotton-tipped applicator. Skin-grafted sites are elevated to prevent edema. Swelling of edematous tissue can lift the graft off of the wound bed. Bed rest may be prescribed. When the graft is on the lower legs, the client should typically not walk until postoperative day 3 to 7 to be certain the graft has appropriately adhered.

Rehabilitation Phase

The rehabilitation phase of recovery represents the final phase of burn recovery and encompasses the time from wound closure to discharge and beyond. In order for the best outcomes to be achieved, caregivers must understand the consequences of burn injury, and treatment for rehabilitation must begin from the day of injury. Rehabilitation should overlap the acute care phase and last well beyond the acute inpatient hospitalization. Ultimately, a burn rehabilitation program is designed for maximal functional and emotional recovery. Measures to promote wound healing, to prevent or minimize deformities and hypertrophic scarring, to increase physical strength and function, to promote emotional support, and to provide education are a part of the ongoing rehabilitation phase.

The Bridge to Home Health Care feature below describes rehabilitative care for the client after discharge from the hospital.

Medical Management in the Rehabilitation Phase of Burn Injury

Minimize Functional Loss

Early wound excision helps minimize short-term and long-term functional loss by closing the wound, minimizing infection, and eliminating wound pain. A skin graft, although more elastic than eschar, still does not have normal elasticity. The resultant wound stiffness must be counterbalanced with aggressive therapy and splinting.

Exercise, splinting, and positioning continue through all phases of burn injury; however, it is during this phase that the importance of these efforts becomes paramount. These measures are crucial to the client's progression to optimal functional independence.

Hypertrophic scarring, which results from an overabundant deposition of collagen in the healed burn wound, can be minimized with the use of massage and pressure therapy. Constant pressure applied to healing burn wounds through the use of custom-fit pressure garments has been found to reduce scarring in some individuals. Several commercially available products provide the constant, even pressure that is required. Although hypertrophic scarring usually does not peak until several months after the injury, it is important to plan ahead before the onset of loss of function. If custom-fit pressure garments are to be prescribed, the client should have been measured for the garments by the time of hospital discharge or by their first outpatient visit (Figure 50-13). It is important that these garments fit properly and are checked often during the early post-discharge phase of recovery.

Provide Psychosocial Support

In this last phase of recovery, during which the wounds are almost healed and specific plans are made for hospital discharge, the client will face numerous issues and concerns. Self-image issues, pain, physical limitations,

---

BRIDGE TO HOME HEALTH CARE

Managing After Burns

When admitting the burn-injured client to home health services, remember that each client is unique and involves detailed treatment instructions. In the nursing assessment, include the responses of both the client and the family members to hospital discharge and return home. If clients require assistance with wound care and activities of daily living (ADL), they will need a primary caregiver to provide both emotional support and direct care. This person is a critical member of the home health care delivery team.

Work with the client and the primary caregiver to set up a place in the home for dressing changes and storage of needed dressing materials. This area should be clean, comfortable, relaxing, and off-limits to family pets. If possible, select a room that clients do not use for other activities, especially sleeping, so that they do not associate these activities with painful dressing changes. The dressing materials and a current wound care plan can be neatly organized and stored in a sealed plastic box or plastic bag. Dressing supplies should be ordered in quantities that allow for single dressing changes, thus reducing wastage. In some agencies, prepackaged wound care kits provide an excellent method of infection control and significantly reduce the amount of waste.

Although dressing changes and physical therapy can be painful experiences for the client, both are essential for recovery. Identify ways to decrease the pain or the length of time during which pain is experienced. Work with the physical therapist, the client, and the family to determine the best schedule for these activities. Consider scheduling joint visits if this would improve

the care given to the client. Instruct a family member on when to give prescribed pain medications in order to provide the best relief for the client. Timing of medication administration depends on the dose and route of pain medication. Typically, at this stage in the recovery, the client is receiving only oral medications. While changing dressings, consider the use of music or relaxation techniques, and involve the client and family as much as possible. These strategies offer a sense of control and can decrease anxiety and the perception of pain.

Unless mechanical debridement of the wound is necessary, the dressings should not stick to the wound bed. Avoid removing dried-on, adhered dressings because they cause unnecessary pain. If the dressings are adhered to the wound, soak them off with normal saline or water. Collaborate with the primary physician or a wound care nurse to obtain an appropriate moisture-retentive dressing to reduce or eliminate pain with dressing changes.

Rehabilitation of clients who have suffered burn injury involves more than dressing changes and physical therapy. It is also important to consider the psychological stress of the initial injury, scarring, and surgical procedures and other treatments as well as the financial burden from loss of work time and the lengthy recovery period.[12] Evaluate the need of the client and family members for referrals to local agencies that offer social, counseling, financial, and spiritual services as well as support groups. Such services may be essential in order for clients and their families to cope with the traumatic life event that a major burn injury with its sequelae represents.

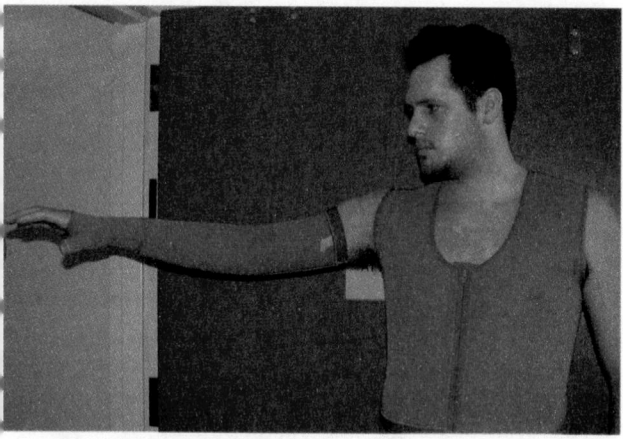

■ **FIGURE 50–13** Custom-fit pressure garments. Pressure therapy helps to minimize the development of hypertrophic (raised, reddened) scars.

reintegration into society, and fear of rejection represent only a few of the issues the client must handle as discharge nears. During this time, it is important to maintain good communication with the client. It is beneficial to the client for the staff to encourage independence and convey the message that survivors can find ways to achieve whatever goals they set for themselves. Pain control and anxiety prevention continue to require assessment and medical management as needed. Psychosocial assistance for the client and family members or significant others should carry through to hospital discharge. Providing information on local community resources that will be of assistance after hospital discharge is important for continued support and assistance. Additionally, national survivor organizations such as the Phoenix Society for Burn Survivors (www. phoenix-society.org) can be of great benefit and support. Providing clients with the names and telephone numbers of burn clinic staff and rehabilitation staff for urgent questions has also been found to be helpful during this transition period from hospital to home. Vocational rehabilitation may also be required if the burns involved the hands and arms.

Nursing Management of the Medical Client in the Rehabilitation Phase of Burn Injury

Assessment. Once the client and family are able to manage the care of the client, the focus becomes preparing them for discharge to a home setting (for some clients, other settings will be necessary). Nurses will assess the client and family's comprehension of teaching and ability to perform needed care. Nurses will also determine the best methods to teach the client and family. The client's psychological status and need for vocational rehabilitation will be addressed during this final phase.

Diagnosis, Outcomes, Interventions
Diagnosis: Impaired Physical Mobility. During the rehabilitation phase of burn injury, the client's physical mobility

and ability to provide self-care are impaired by the presence of dressings, pain, scarring, contracture, and muscle atrophy.

Outcomes. The client will have improved physical mobility, as evidenced by maximum independence in performance of ADL, with minimum disability and disfigurement.

Interventions. The physical and occupational therapy consultations initiated in the early phases of burn injury are especially important for continued treatment in the rehabilitation phase as the client works toward functional independence. Typically, the therapist provides an individualized rehabilitation schedule as well as needed assistive devices for the client.

Motivate the client to participate in self-care activities such as brushing teeth and self-feeding, because this increased activity will not only improve mobility but also lessen dependence. Provide assistive devices furnished by therapy consultants to assist the client with any limitations. Expect tasks to take longer when the client works independently. Allow adequate time for the client to complete the undertaking. Self-confidence will be gained with independent functioning regardless of the time spent.

Encourage active ROM every 2 to 4 hours while the client is awake unless contraindicated because of a recent grafting procedure. Increased activity prevents muscle atrophy, tendon adherence, joint stiffness, and capsular tightness. Help the client to ambulate to promote muscle strength and cardiopulmonary reserve. Provide passive exercise and stretching if the client is unable to actively participate.

Wrap donor sites on both burned and unburned legs with elastic bandage wraps (Ace bandages), using a figure-eight technique at the feet and a spiral up the legs, before placing the limbs in a dependent position. The support will decrease capillary venous stasis, which impairs wound healing.

Explain the rationale for activities to the client and family members, because understanding improves compliance. Avoid the position of comfort, and maintain burned areas in the position of physiologic function, within the client's limit of endurance. Continue to follow the splinting and positioning regimen recommended in the therapy consultation.

Diagnosis: Acute Pain and Chronic Pain. Pain experienced during the rehabilitation phase of burn injury is typically associated with wound care and therapeutic activity, particularly ROM exercises.

Outcomes. The client will have an acceptable level of comfort, as evidenced by verbalizing relief or control of pain or discomfort and actively participating in care.

Interventions. Formulate a plan for controlling the client's pain based on an assessment of the client's response to pain and documentation of previous successful treatment regimens. As in the earlier phases of injury, allow adequate time for the onset of the medication for maximum benefits of the medication. Nonpharmacologic methods of pain control, such as relaxation techniques, music therapy, guided imagery, distraction, and hypnosis, may improve the client's comfort, even if such methods were not successful in the earlier phases of injury. In preparation for impending discharge, the client should at some point during the rehabilitation phase progress to analgesia given only by the oral route. Again, document pain scores before and after analgesia.

Diagnosis: Disturbed Personal Identity. The client is at risk for self-esteem disturbances related to threatened or actual change in body image, physical loss, and loss of role responsibilities.

Outcomes. The client will develop improved self-esteem, as evidenced by making social contact with others outside the immediate family, developing effective coping mechanisms throughout the stages of recovery, and verbalizing feelings about self-concept.

Interventions. Allowing time for two-way communication with the client is especially important during this phase of injury. Provide an atmosphere of acceptance as the client tries various coping strategies to deal with the injury. Provide honest and accurate information about the client's projected appearance to reduce misconceptions that he or she may have.

Assess the need for limit setting for maladaptive behavior. Consult with burn team members to establish such limits and to formulate a treatment plan for such behaviors; explain limit setting to family members or significant others and assist them to maintain the same limits. Promote the client's self-confidence by providing information about the progress made, and support the client's role in care and treatment, providing encouragement and positive reinforcement.

Encourage family members to interact with the client, because this encouragement facilitates societal reintegration. During this phase of recovery, encourage the client to interact with others outside the facility. Use of a family day pass during this time is useful. Help to prepare the client for social interaction after discharge by discussing potential situations and how the client might deal with them. Such preparation provides rehearsal of events and reduces anxiety.

Diagnosis: Impaired Skin Integrity. The expectation is that by the time the client reaches the rehabilitation phase of burn injury, the majority of wounds will be healed (either by reepithelialization or autograft). The new skin over areas of donor site, graft, and healed burn is characteristically very thin, with disrupted oil glands. The

healed skin is fragile; it can be very dry and shears or cracks easily.

Outcomes. The client will have intact skin with no evidence of infection, breakdown, or blistering.

Interventions. Daily wound and skin care should continue throughout hospitalization. Clean burned areas, grafts, and donor sites daily with a mild soap (without fragrance) and water. Rinse thoroughly to remove the soap. After cleaning, the healed skin should be lubricated with a nonirritating, alcohol-free moisturizer. Itching associated with dry skin can be minimized with application of the moisturizer at least three times a day. Avoid any shearing of skin with dressings, clothing, or splints.

Diagnosis: Deficient Knowledge. The burn-injured client or a family member or significant other must have knowledge of important treatment modalities that need continuation after discharge from the hospital.

Outcomes. The client or a family member or significant other will verbalize knowledge and demonstrate techniques that facilitate continued wound healing and limb mobility.

Interventions. Demonstrate and discuss the following skin care interventions with the client and appropriate family member or significant other: daily skin and wound care and dressing instructions if any; lubrication of grafts, donor sites, and healed burn wounds using an alcohol-free skin moisturizer; wearing pressure dressings or garments for 23 hours daily; and avoidance of direct sunlight for 1 year after injury because of increased sensitivity to ultraviolet rays.

Review current medications and the dosage, precautions, and potential side effects. Discuss nutritional needs and the benefits of diets with adequate protein and calories.

Provide information on support groups of peers and/or counseling as needed for adjustment to life outside the hospital setting. Stress the need for follow-up care and provide appointment dates and times if these have been established.

CONCLUSIONS

Nursing care of the burn-injured client is both complex and challenging. The psychological and physical trauma sustained following a burn injury can be devastating for both the survivor and the family members or significant others. Having a thorough understanding of the pathophysiologic changes that occur after a burn, knowing what to expect clinically as a result of the injury, and becoming familiar with the standards of care will guide nursing care. As a key member of the burn team, you are responsible for an individualized plan of care that reflects the client's changing needs during progression through the different phases of recovery. Priority issues and care change as the client moves from the critical resuscitative phase into and, ultimately, through the rehabilitation period.

THINKING CRITICALLY

1. You are working on the night shift in your hospital's burn center and receive a call that a client is in transport via ambulance to your unit. He will be a direct admission and bypass the emergency department. The telephone report describes that the client was found unconscious on the floor of the bedroom. He is covered with soot and has obvious burns on his face, arms, and torso. An intravenous line of lactated Ringer's solution is started and is running wide open. Oxygen is being administered via face mask. On admission, the client is received lying in the supine position on a gurney. He is restless, confused, and combative. He appears anxious and in pain. The eyebrows, eyelashes, and hair are singed. There is soot in the nares and mouth and on the tongue. His voice is raspy, and he is coughing up thick black sputum. Breath sounds are scattered crackles; oxygen saturation is 75%. A face mask is in place but was disconnected from the oxygen tank while the client was being moved onto the burn center gurney.

Heart rate is 142 beats/min, with sinus tachycardia. Respiratory rate is 40 breaths/min and labored. Blood pressure is 144/88 mm Hg; temperature is 35° C. Bowel sounds are absent. There is thick, white leathery eschar on the chest, neck, left and right arms, and hands. The skin of the face and back are pink, moist, and blistered. The body from the waist to the feet is unburned. An IV line is infusing lactated Ringer's solution through the right antecubital vein. Weight is 85 kg. What priorities should be set for the client's care? What interventions should be undertaken?

Factors to Consider. What is the client's respiratory status? Do the physical examination and history provided by the ambulance crew give any clues to his respiratory status? What should you consider when administering analgesia or anxiolytics to this client? What is the client's fluid volume status? How will you monitor fluid resuscitation?

2. It is now 7 days after the injury and the client has just returned to the burn intensive care unit after receiving autografts on his chest, neck, bilateral arms, hands, and axillae. Donor skin was taken circumferentially from both thighs. What assessments should you perform? What interventions should be undertaken?

Factors to Consider. What factors disrupt graft adherence? What can you do to help prevent contracture formation?

3. It is now 2 months since the client was injured and discharge plans are being finalized. The client tells you that he is concerned about his ability to manage at home. What can you do to help the client?

Factors to Consider. What concerns might a burn survivor face upon discharge from the hospital? What professional resources might be helpful? What lay resources might be helpful?

Discussions for these questions can be found on the website.

BIBLIOGRAPHY

Citations appearing in red refer to primary research.

Citations appearing in blue refer to evidence-based practice guidelines and protocols.

1. Adcock, R., Boeve, S., & Patterson, D. (1998). Psychological and emotional recovery. In G.J. Carrougher (Ed.), *Burn care and therapy* (pp. 329-347). St. Louis: Mosby.
2. American Burn Association. (2006). *Burn incidence and treatment in the US: 2007 fact sheet* [online]. Available at www.ameriburn.org/resources_factsheetphp.
3. American Burn Association. (1984). Guidelines for service standards and severity classification in the treatment of burn injuries. *Bulletin of the American College of Surgeons, 69*, 24-28.
4. American College of Surgeons: Committee on Trauma. (1987). *A guide to prophylaxis against tetanus in wound management.* Chicago: American College of Surgeons.
5. Barillo, D.J., & Goode, R. (1996). Fire fatality study: Demographics of fire victims. *Burns, 22*, 85-88.
6. Carrougher, G.J., Ptacek, J.T., Honari, S., et al. (2006). Self-reports of anxiety in burn injured hospitalized adults during routine wound care. *Journal of Burn Care and Research, 27*, 676-681.
7. Carrougher, G.J. (1998). Burn wound assessment and topical treatment. In G.J. Carrougher (Ed.), *Burn care and therapy* (pp. 133-159). St. Louis: Mosby.
8. Cioffi, W.G. (1998). Inhalation injury. In G.J. Carrougher (Ed.), *Burn care and therapy* (pp. 35-59). St. Louis: Mosby.
9. deJong, A.E.E., Middelkoop, E., Faber, A.W., VanLoey, N.E.E. (2007). Non-pharmacological nursing interventions for procedural pain relief in adults with burns: A systematic literature review. *Burns, 33*, 811-827.
10. Esselman, P.C., Thombs, B.D., Magyar-Russell, G., et al. (2006). Burn rehabilitation: State of the science. *American Journal of Physical Medicine and Rehabilitation, 85*, 383-413.
11. Faucher, L., & Furukawa, K. (2006). Practice guidelines for the management of pain. *Journal of Burn Care and Research, 27*, 659-668.
12. Fauerbach, J.A., Engrav, L., & Kowalske, K. (2001). Barriers to employment among working-aged patients with major burn injury. *Journal of Burn Care and Rehabilitation, 22*, 26-34.
13. Hall, B. (2005). Wound care for burn patients in acute rehabilitation settings. *Rehabilitation Nursing, 30*, 114-119.
14. Honari, S. (2004). Topical therapies and antimicrobials in the management of burn wounds. *Critical Care Nursing Clinics of North America, 16*, 1-11.
15. Kramer, G., Lund, T., & Herndon, D.N. (2002). Pathophysiology of burn shock and burn edema. In D.N. Herndon (Ed.), *Total burn care* (pp. 78-87). London: Saunders.
16. Marvin, J.A. (1998). Management of pain and anxiety. In G.J. Carrougher (Ed.), *Burn care and therapy* (pp. 167-183). St. Louis: Mosby.
17. Pruitt, B., Goodwin, C., & Mason, A. (2002). Epidemiological, demographic and outcome characteristics of burn injury. In D.N. Herndon (Ed.), *Total burn care* (pp. 16-20). London: Saunders.
18. Runyon, C.W., Bangdiwala, S.I., & Linzar, M.A. (1992). Risk factors for fatal residential fires. *New England Journal of Medicine, 327*, 859-863.
19. Wilson, D., & Bailie, F. (1999). Night attire burns in young girls: The return of an old adversary. *Burns, 25*, 269-271.

evolve *Did you remember to check out the bonus material on the Evolve website and the CD-ROM, including NCLEX®-Examination Style Review Questions, Open-Book Quizzes, and Chapter Review Audio Podcasts?*

http://evolve.elsevier.com/Black/medsurg

UNIT 12

VASCULAR DISORDERS

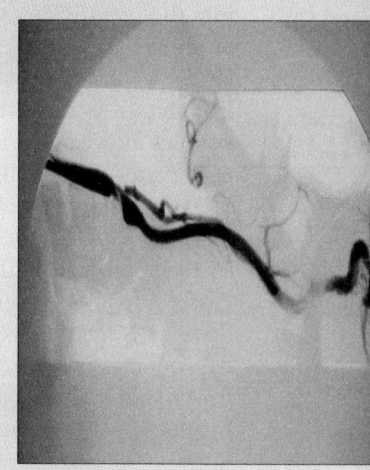

ANATOMY AND PHYSIOLOGY REVIEW:

The Vascular System

Robert G. Carroll

The vascular system is a vast network of vessels through which blood circulates in the body. The major functions of the cardiovascular system—delivery of nutrients to tissues and removal of metabolic wastes—are accomplished in the capillaries. Blood leaving the ventricles is distributed through arteries and arterioles, in progressively smaller branches to the capillaries (a *divergent* pattern, like a river to a delta). Blood leaving the capillaries follows progressively larger venules and veins on its way back to the atria (a *convergent* pattern, like tributaries flowing into a river).

The anatomic arrangement of blood vessels allows regulation of blood flow at the individual tissue level so that blood flow delivery can be proportional to the tissue's metabolic needs. Because the volume of blood flowing from the arteries to the capillaries is a major determinant of blood pressure, the blood pressure control systems also include control of arteriolar diameter by the sympathetic nervous system and circulating hormones.

STRUCTURES OF THE VASCULAR SYSTEM

Two series of blood vessels—the systemic and the pulmonary circulations—distribute blood to the capillaries and return blood to the heart. Blood exiting the left ventricle enters the *systemic circulation,* passing progressively through the aorta, arteries, arterioles, capillaries, venules, veins, and finally the vena cava before entering the right atrium (Figure A&P12-1). For the *pulmonary circulation,* blood flows from the right ventricle into the pulmonary artery, and then passes through arterioles, pulmonary capillaries, and venules before returning to the pulmonary vein and the left atrium.

GENERAL BLOOD VESSEL STRUCTURE

The anatomic division of blood vessels into arteries, arterioles, capillaries, venules, and veins is based on the presence of up to three histologic layers (Figure A&P12-2):

1. The *tunica intima* (innermost layer) consists of endothelial cells that separate the blood from the extravascular spaces. The tightness of the junctions between the endothelial cells varies among tissues. For example, the very tight junctions of cerebral capillaries restrict movement of some drugs to brain cells (the blood-brain barrier). In contrast, the endothelial cell holes and relatively loose junctions in the liver and spleen allow easy transit between the blood and tissue spaces in those organs. The endothelium has surface proteins, or *adhesion molecules,* that facilitate the attachment of white blood cells and their movement from the circulation to the tissues. The endothelium generates substances such as endothelial-derived relaxing factor (EDRF, or nitric oxide), allowing nitroglycerin, friction, and stress to cause vasodilation. Damage to the endothelium may allow blood to enter the middle layer of a blood vessel, creating an aneurysm.

2. The *tunica media* (middle layer) consists of elastic connective tissue and smooth muscle cells. Particularly in the aorta and large arteries, the elastic tissue contributes to the shape of the arterial pressure pulse. Smooth muscle contraction regulates the diameter of the vessel and causes a change in blood flow and blood pressure. Smooth muscle is normally partially contracted because of sympathetic nerve activity (also known as sympathetic tone). Smooth muscle contraction can also be regulated by circulating hormones and (in the smaller vessels) by tissue metabolic factors.

3. The *tunica adventitia* (outermost layer) consists of a relatively thin layer of connective tissue that provides shape for the blood vessels. This layer also houses the *vasa vasorum,* the small arteries and veins that provide nutrients to the cells of the blood vessel.

VASCULAR SEGMENTS

Arteries and Arterioles

Arteries, particularly the aorta, have an extensive elastic tissue layer that accounts for the difference between arterial pressure (120/80 mm Hg) and left ventricular pressure (120/10 mm Hg). The elastic tissue stretches during ventricular ejection, storing energy. When the aortic valve closes and ventricular ejection stops, recoil of the elastic tissue slows the fall of arterial pressure during the interval until the next period of ventricular ejection. The efficiency of the elastic tissue decreases with age and with

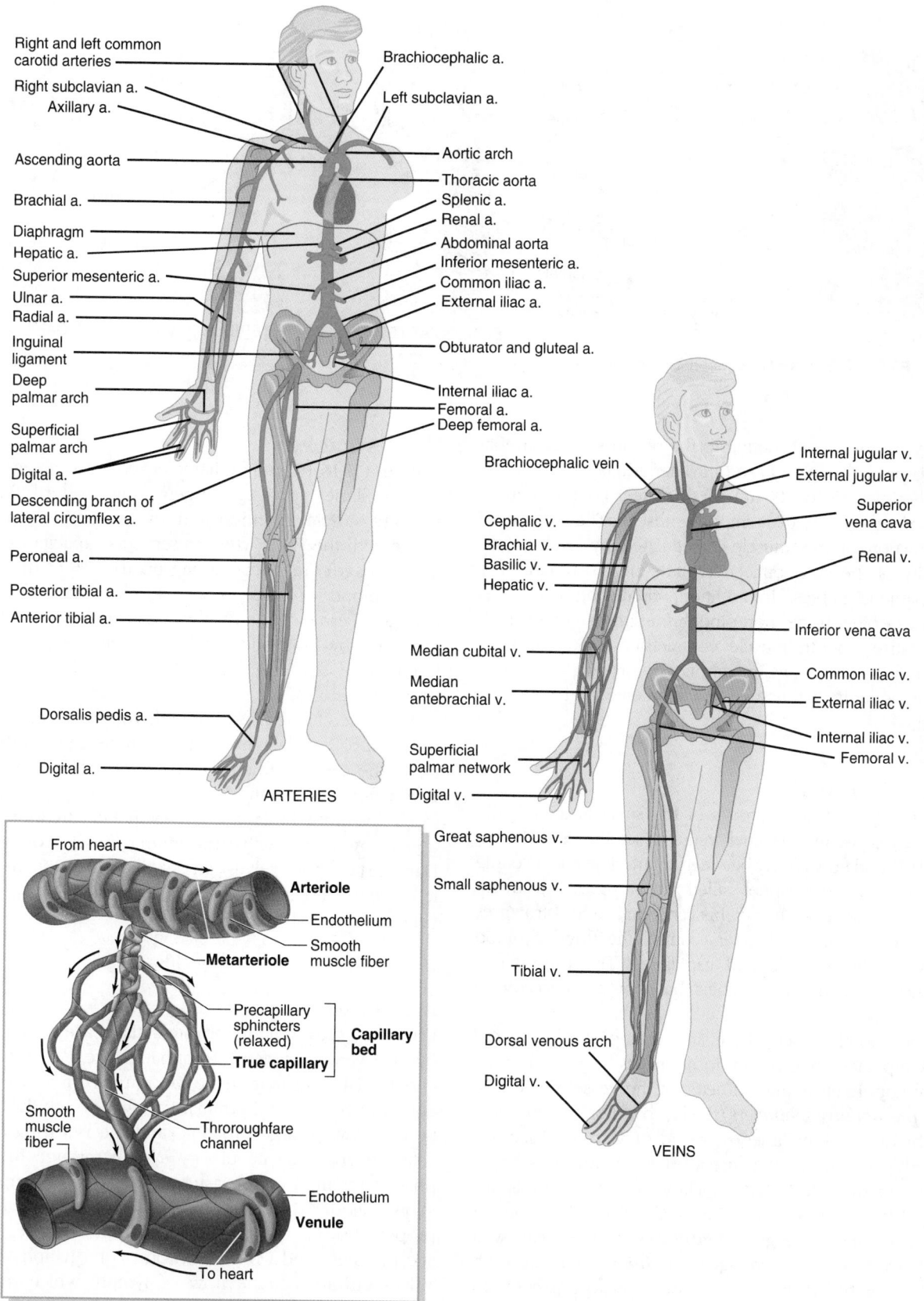

Right and left common carotid arteries

Brachiocephalic a.

Right subclavian a.

Left subclavian a.

Axillary a.

Ascending aorta

Aortic arch

Thoracic aorta

Brachial a.

Splenic a.

Diaphragm

Renal a.

Hepatic a.

Abdominal aorta

Superior mesenteric a.

Inferior mesenteric a.

Ulnar a.

Common iliac a.

Radial a.

External iliac a.

Inguinal ligament

Obturator and gluteal a.

Deep palmar arch

Internal iliac a.

Femoral a.

Superficial palmar arch

Deep femoral a.

Digital a.

Brachiocephalic vein

Internal jugular v.

External jugular v.

Descending branch of lateral circumflex a.

Cephalic v.

Superior vena cava

Peroneal a.

Brachial v.

Basilic v.

Renal v.

Posterior tibial a.

Hepatic v.

Anterior tibial a.

Inferior vena cava

Median cubital v.

Common iliac v.

Median antebrachial v.

External iliac v.

Internal iliac v.

Femoral v.

Dorsalis pedis a.

Superficial palmar network

Digital a.

Digital v.

ARTERIES

Great saphenous v.

Small saphenous v.

From heart

Arteriole

Endothelium

Smooth muscle fiber

Metarteriole

Tibial v.

Precapillary sphincters (relaxed)

Capillary bed

True capillary

Dorsal venous arch

Smooth muscle fiber

Throroughfare channel

Digital v.

Endothelium

Venule

VEINS

To heart

■ **FIGURE A&P12–1**   Major systemic arteries and veins. *Inset,* Capillary network.

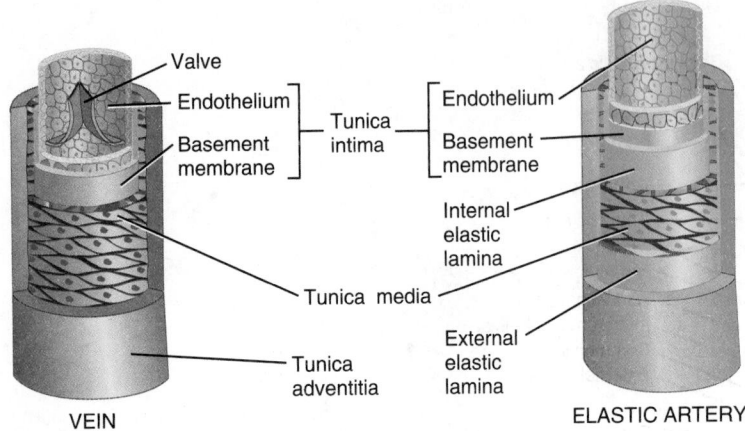
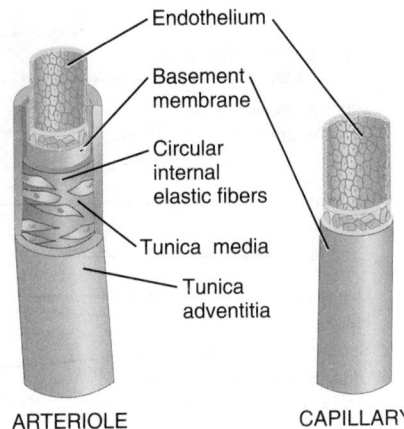

■ **FIGURE A&P12–2** Structure of blood vessels.

atherosclerosis, contributing to the rise in systolic arterial blood pressure usually seen in older adults.

Arterioles (5 to 100 μm in diameter) contain a high proportion of vascular smooth muscle. The degree of contraction of this muscle is regulated by background activity of the autonomic nervous system, primarily the sympathetic nerves. In addition, circulating hormones such as epinephrine, norepinephrine, and angiotensin II can cause smooth muscle contraction. These substances are produced as metabolic by-products, so they allow the individual tissue beds to receive the blood they need.

Microcirculation

The microcirculation consists of the small arterioles, the capillary beds, and the small venules (see Figure A&P12-1, *inset*). Blood flows freely between an arteriole and a venule through a vessel channel called a thoroughfare channel. Capillaries extend from this channel, and structures called precapillary sphincters control the flow of blood between the arteriole and capillaries. The precapillary sphincters contain muscle fibers that allow them to control blood flow.

The smooth muscle of the small arterioles is contracted by sympathetic nerves, but local factors become increasingly important as the diameter of the vessel decreases. The *precapillary sphincters* (the last band of smooth muscle before the capillaries) respond only to local factors. Blood passes from the arterioles into capillaries (5 to 10 μm in diameter). The capillary diameter approaches that of the red blood cell (7 μm). Capillaries have only a tunica intima (see Figure A&P12-2), and the small wall thickness facilitates exchange by diffusion. In tissues such as the skin, blood also passes through *metarterioles* (10 to 100 μm in diameter). Metarterioles are not exchange vessels but serve a separate role. Decreased blood flow through cutaneous metarterioles helps the body conserve heat; increased flow enhances heat loss.

Venules and Veins

Venules (10 to 100 μm in diameter) collect drainage from the capillaries in a convergent flow pattern. Venule smooth muscle is innervated by sympathetic nerves. Along with the veins, venules serve as capacitance (volume storage) areas, containing up to 75% of the circulating blood volume as a result of their ability to expand. Permeability of the postcapillary venules is regulated by hormones such as histamine and bradykinin. Note that angiogenesis is initiated in the postcapillary venules.

Veins are characterized by high volume and low pressure. Sympathetic nerve activity constricts the smooth muscle of the veins and helps move blood toward the heart. Blood flow toward the heart is also assisted by gravity (for veins in the head) and valves that ensure a unidirectional flow along with surrounding muscle contraction. Damage to venous valves can cause swellings, such as varicose veins, and lack of leg muscle movement can lead to venous stasis and clotting.

Lymphatics

Lymph is excess fluid in the interstitial space not removed by the venous system. Lymphatics are a network of endothelial tubes that merge to form two large ducts that enter the vena cava. Terminal lymphatics lack tight junctions, allowing large proteins (and metastasizing cancer cells) to enter the circulatory system through the lymphatic system. In the gastrointestinal tract, lymphatics allow digested fats to enter the circulation. Lymph is propelled by (1) massaging from adjacent muscle, (2) tissue pressure, and (3) contraction of the lymph vessels. Valves ensure that the flow of lymph, which over 24 hours is a volume equal to the total blood volume, is toward the vena cava. Lymph is filtered in lymph nodes before progressing back to the circulation (Figure A&P12-3).

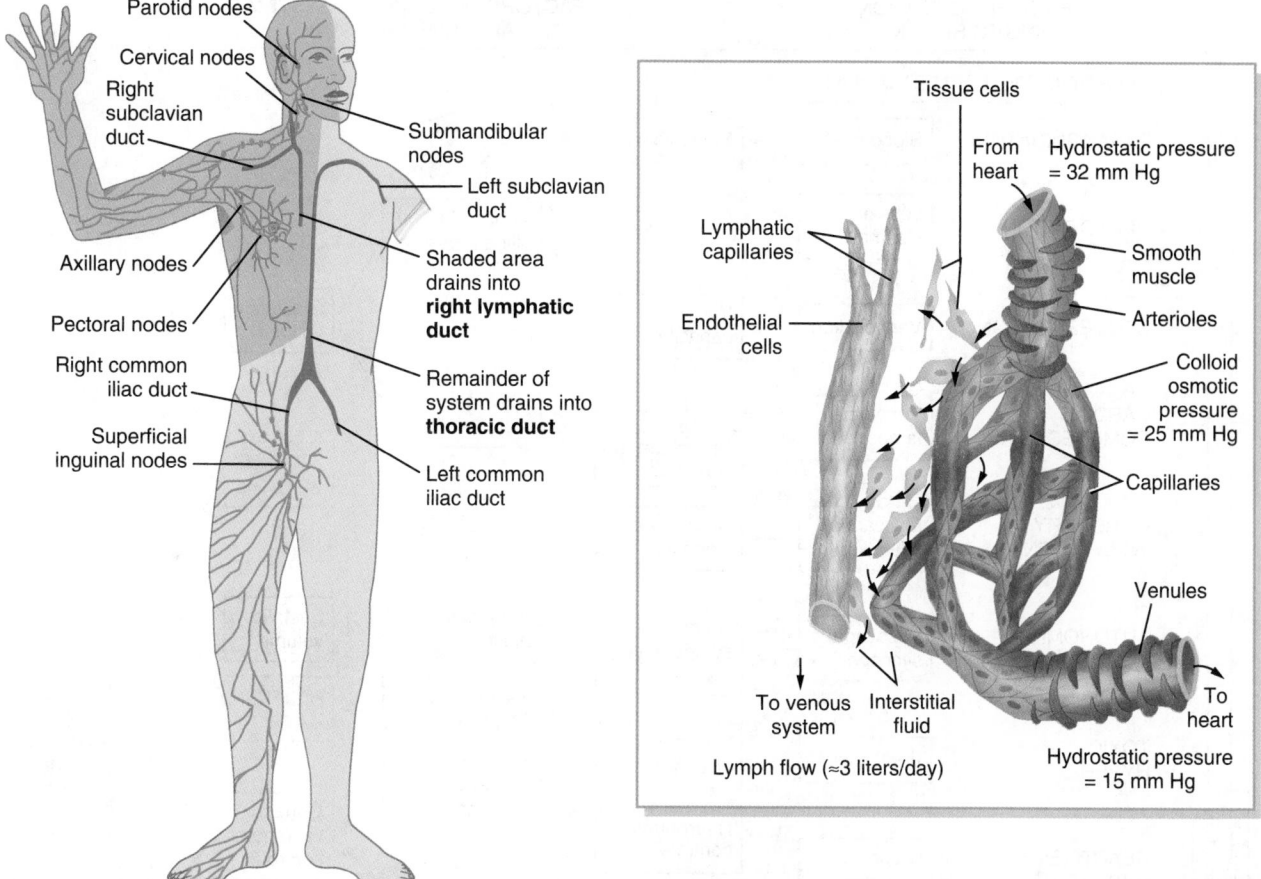

■ **FIGURE A&P12–3** Major lymphatic vessels and drainage. *Inset,* Fluid exchange at the capillary bed. The primary driving force to move fluids from the capillary is *hydrostatic pressure.* The primary pulling force to bring fluids back into the vessel is *colloid osmotic pressure* from the proteins in the capillary fluids (e.g., albumin). The hydrostatic pressure at the arterial end of the capillary is 32 mm Hg. As the fluid moves through the capillary, the pressure falls. Because proteins do not move across the capillary endothelium, colloid osmotic pressure is constant at 25 mm Hg. Thus at the arterial end the hydrostatic pressure is greater than the colloid osmotic pressure, and fluids then move into interstitial spaces. The opposite is true at the venous end where pressure falls to 15 mm Hg. The hydrostatic pressure is lower than the colloid osmotic pressure, and fluids thus return to the capillary. There is a net loss of fluids out of the capillary (approximately 3 L/day). This fluid is absorbed by the lymphatic system and is returned to circulation at the lymphatic duct.

FUNCTION OF THE VASCULAR SYSTEM

PRESSURE, FLOW, AND RESISTANCE

The relationship of arterial pressure, cardiac output, and total peripheral resistance is shown by the following equation:

$$Q = \frac{\Delta P}{R}$$

Or

$$\text{Flow} = \frac{\text{Pressure Gradient}}{\text{Resistance}}$$

Resistance

In the body, arterial *pressure* is regulated. A decrease in arterial pressure is corrected by a reflex increase in cardiac output and an increase in total peripheral resistance, both mediated by an increase in sympathetic nervous system activity. For a capillary bed, however, *flow* is regulated. If flow is too low, the arteriole dilates and the decrease in resistance allows flow to increase.

Resistance affects blood flow according to the (1) radius of the vessel, (2) fluid viscosity, and (3) length of the vessel. Of these factors, vessel radius is the most powerful mechanism for controlling resistance and the one that is physiologically most important. If the radius of the vessel decreases to one half the starting value, resistance to flow increases 16-fold. The body utilizes vascular smooth muscle to alter the diameter of arteries and arterioles and therefore to regulate both pressure and flow. Occasionally, changes in blood viscosity can alter resistance, particularly when the hematocrit is increased (*polycythemia*) or decreased (*anemia*). Resistance increases as viscosity increases and decreases as viscosity decreases.

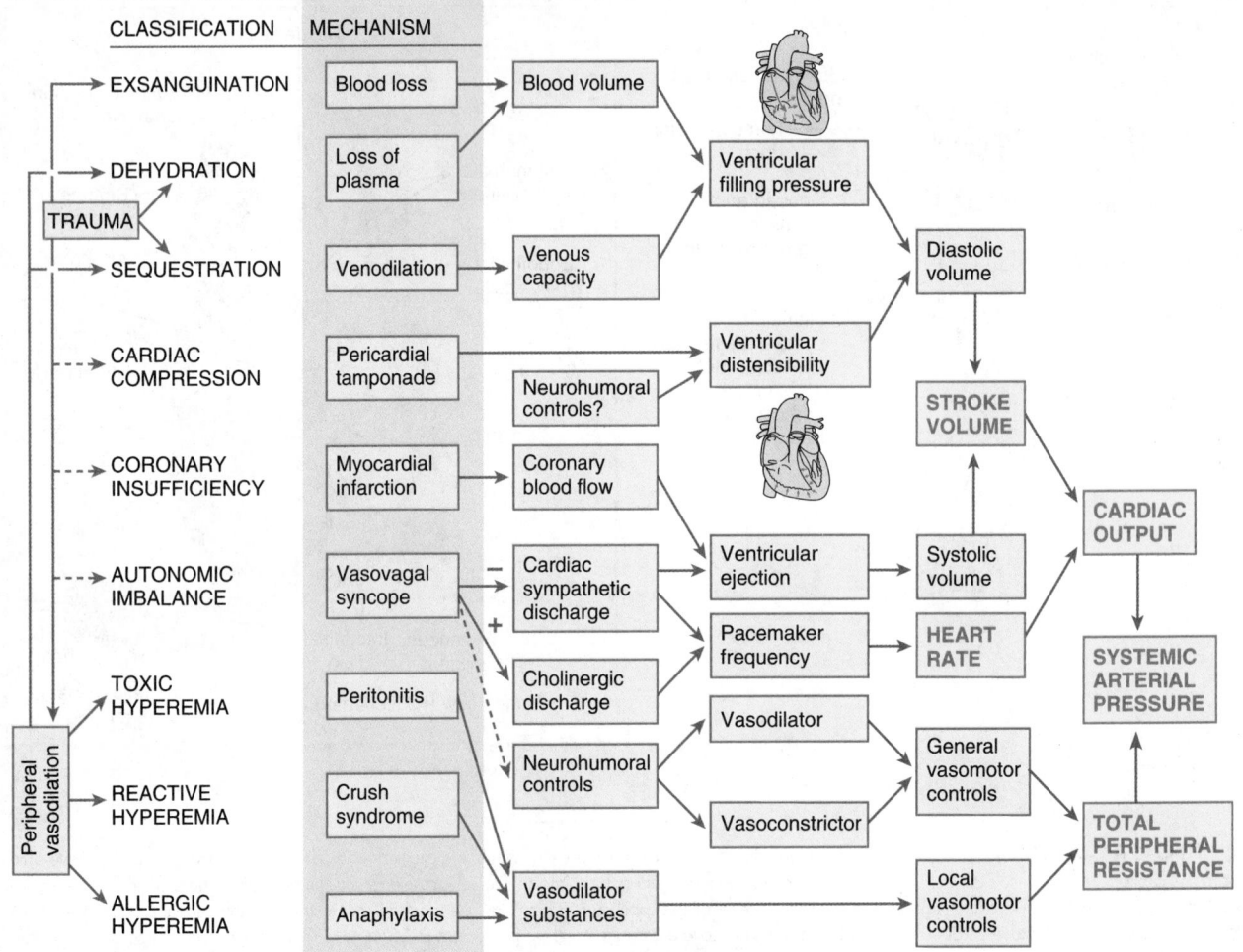

FIGURE A&P12–4 Control of arterial pressure. Arterial blood pressure is determined by several factors. *Right,* Systemic arterial blood pressure is controlled by two major factors: cardiac output and total peripheral vascular resistance. Cardiac output is also a function of two factors: stroke volume and heart rate. Reading the diagram from the right, you will find the factors that govern each step. Each bifurcation represents possible compensatory mechanisms. *Far left,* Disorders that can lead to shock. *(Modified from Rushmer, R.F. [1976]. Cardiovascular dynamics [p. 207]. Philadelphia: Saunders.)*

CAPILLARY EXCHANGE

Exchange of nutrients and wastes between the blood and the tissues is the primary purpose of the cardiovascular system. The movement of nutrients from the blood to the tissue and removal of metabolic wastes are driven by diffusion, filtration, and pinocytosis.

Diffusion

Diffusion is quantitatively the most important process. The rate of diffusion is enhanced by (1) increasing the surface area available for exchange, (2) increasing the concentration gradient, and (3) decreasing the distance that a substance must travel. In tissues such as exercising skeletal muscle, an increase in the number of perfused capillaries enhances the delivery of nutrients to the tissues. Altering arteriole flow to individual tissue beds is used to meet metabolic need.

Filtration

Fluid movement across the capillary depends on the balance of the hydrostatic pressure gradient (which favors filtration) and the oncotic pressure gradient from plasma proteins (which favors reabsorption) (Figure A&P12-4). In normal situations, the net force favors filtration at the arteriolar end of the capillary bed, and reabsorption at the venular end of the capillary bed. In most capillary beds, the volume filtered is slightly greater than the volume absorbed and the excess fluid is removed from the tissue spaces by the lymph vessels. *Edema* (accumulation of fluid in the tissue spaces) occurs because of (1) increased filtration (2) decreased reabsorption, or (3) impaired lymph drainage.

Pinocytosis

Pinocytosis is the movement of vesicles, especially from outside the cell to inside the cell. Pinocytosis is though to be important only as a route for large proteins to cross the capillary wall.

CARDIOVASCULAR CONTROL

Much like the power and water supply systems in a city, the distribution of blood flow in the body depends on a sufficient driving pressure (arterial pressure), allowing the end users (capillary beds) to determine how much of the resource to utilize. Cardiovascular control is best described in terms of (1) regulation of arterial pressure and (2) local regulation of tissue blood flow.

Regulation of Arterial Pressure
The normal arterial pressure is maintained by a negative feedback mechanism called the *baroreceptor reflex* (Figure A&P12-5). A decrease in blood pressure immediately activates the sympathetic nervous system, increasing cardiac output (heart rate, venoconstriction for venous return, and cardiac contractility) and increasing peripheral resistance to trap blood within the arteries, and restores arterial blood pressure.

Longer term management of blood pressure is through baroreceptor control by volume-sensitive receptors in the low-pressure atria and veins. The volume of circulating blood is controlled by renal fluid balance and by endocrine vasoconstrictor agents such as angiotensin II, antidiuretic hormone (ADH), and norepinephrine. Chronic regulation of blood pressure depends on the volume of blood in the system and, ultimately, is tied to renal regulation of body fluid balance.

Chemoreceptors in the carotid body and aortic body are associated primarily with respiratory control but can elicit cardiovascular responses. A decrease in arterial O_2 concentration, an increase in arterial CO_2 concentration, or a drop in arterial pH can elicit a sympathetic response similar to that caused by a drop in arterial blood pressure.

Local Regulation of Blood Flow
If arterial pressure is sufficient, tissues can regulate their blood flow to match their metabolic needs. If blood flow is inadequate, metabolites such as carbon dioxide, adenosine, potassium, and acids accumulate, acting as vasodilators of the arteriolar smooth muscle to promote blood flow only in that local area. The resulting increase in blood flow washes out the metabolites and diminishes the vasodilator stimulus. This control system allows tissue blood flow to increase as tissue metabolic activity

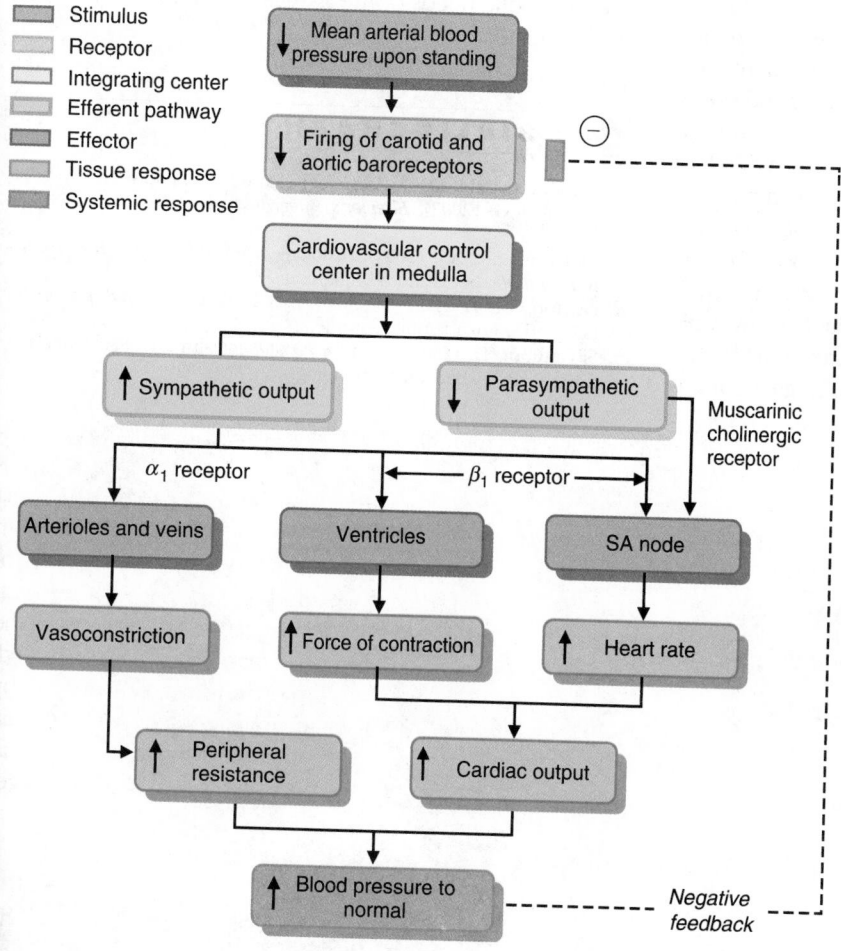

■ **FIGURE A&P12–5** Baroreceptor control of blood pressure. When baroreceptors sense a drop in blood pressure, they elicit an increase in sympathetic nervous system activity and a decrease in parasympathetic activity. The resultant vasoconstriction, increase in heart rate, and increase in ventricular contractility help to restore blood pressure to the starting point. *SA,* Sinoatrial. *(Modified from Silverthorn, D. [2001]. Human physiology [2nd ed.]. Upper Saddle River, NJ: Prentice Hall.)*

increases and accounts for the period of increased blood flow that follows a period of occlusion (called reactive hyperemia). In the long term, inadequate blood flow to a tissue can cause the growth of new capillaries (called collateral circulation), again matching blood flow to the tissue's metabolic needs. Blood flow to tissues such as the brain and myocardium is dominated by local control. The brain is exceptional at altering local flow, and in brain edema the systolic pressure rises in an attempt to provide the edematous brain with blood.

At the other extreme of regulation, cutaneous blood flow responds primarily to neural control. Because skin blood flow is tied to thermoregulation rather than nutrition, metabolic control is poorly developed. Other vascular beds, such as the kidney and the splanchnic circulation, respond both to sympathetic control and to local control. During increased sympathetic activity, blood flow to these tissues is decreased and is shunted to the brain and the myocardium.

CARDIOVASCULAR ADJUSTMENT TO EXERCISE

Cardiovascular control must balance the need for a steady arterial blood pressure against the ability to respond to a physiologic challenge. Exercise, which increases skeletal muscle consumption of oxygen and other nutrients, requires a marked increase in both cardiac output and skeletal muscle blood flow. The increase in cardiac output results from a cerebral cortical stimulation of the medullary cardiovascular center and activation of the sympathetic nervous system. The increased cardiac output requires an increased venous return, accomplished both by the arteriolar dilation of the skeletal muscle beds and by a sympathetic-mediated venous constriction. In rhythmic activity such as running, compression of the veins by the contracting skeletal muscle along with the negative intra-thoracic pressure from breathing assists the flow of venous blood toward the heart. In low cardiac output states, the brain and heart preferentially receive blood flow.

The increased cardiac output is preferentially directed to the exercising muscles (including the heart). Local factors in the exercising muscles cause a vasodilation of those vascular beds. The sympathetic activity constricts the arteriolar smooth muscle of the nonexercising vascular beds, such as the gastrointestinal tract, the kidney, and the nonworking muscles. Cerebral blood flow remains unchanged because that vascular bed is regulated primarily by local control. Cutaneous blood flow may be diminished initially but increases as the heat generated by the exercising muscles raises body core temperature, and cutaneous vasodilation helps to cool the body.

CONCLUSIONS

The vascular system is a series of vessels that transport blood to the capillary exchange vessels. In the capillaries, nutrients pass to the tissues and wastes pass into the blood for transport to excretory organs. Blood pressure regulation by the baroreceptor reflex ensures that arterial pressure remains sufficient to propel blood toward the tissues. Tissue blood flow is controlled by the metabolic needs of the tissues, and it increases when tissue metabolism increases.

BIBLIOGRAPHY

1. Berne, R., et al. (2004). *Physiology* (5th ed.). St. Louis: Mosby.
2. Carroll, R.G. (2007). *Elsevier's integrated physiology.* Philadelphia: Saunders.
3. Kierszenbaum, A.L. (2007). *Histology and cell biology: An introduction to pathology* (2nd ed.). St. Louis: Mosby.
4. Guyton, A., & Hall, J. (2006). *Textbook of medical physiology* (11th ed.). Philadelphia: Saunders.
5. Silverthorn, D. (2006). *Human physiology* (4th ed). San Francisco, Calif: Pearson Benjamin Cummings.

CHAPTER 51

Assessment of the Vascular System

MARY SIEGGREEN AND SUSANNE A. QUALLICH

There are several well-established risk factors for the development of atherosclerosis, including smoking, hyperlipidemia, hypertension, and diabetes. Several other conditions are contributors as well, such as obesity, a sedentary lifestyle, stress, hypertriglyceridemia, and family history.

Peripheral vascular disease is common among older clients and diabetic clients. It is characterized by disturbances of blood flow through the peripheral vessels. These disturbances eventually damage tissues as a result of ischemia, excessive accumulation of waste and fluid, or both. Damage can be a result of any disorder that narrows, obstructs, or injures blood vessels, thus impeding blood flow. Without intervention, damage may progress to the point of tissue or organ death.

HISTORY

When assessing the client, note risk factors for atherosclerosis and vascular disease (see Chapter 53), hypertension (see Chapter 52), diabetes mellitus (see Chapter 45), and cardiac (see Chapters 55 to 58) as well as lymphatic disorders. Some clients are reluctant to mention what they believe to be minor manifestations (swelling, intermittent discomfort). Consequently, perform a careful assessment, ask specific questions skillfully, and be alert for information that may indicate early manifestations of insidious conditions.

Studies have found that the effects of peripheral arterial disease (PAD) have significant psychosocial and emotional consequences. Assessment of quality of life as well as functional changes and symptom manifestations is needed to establish effective interventions. Seven themes emerged from one study[8] designed to evaluate the effects of PAD from clients' perspectives. The themes are (1) PAD diagnosis and management, (2) clinical manifestation (symptom) experience, (3) limitations in physical functioning, (4) limitations in social functioning, (5) compromise

of self, (6) uncertainty and fear, and (7) adaptation (see the website for a table with more information on these themes—Themes, Definitions, and Characteristics of Peripheral Arterial Disease).

Biographical and Demographic Data

Biographical data that are particularly relevant to the vascular system include the client's age. Atherosclerosis (hardening of the arteries) is more prevalent in older people. Venous disease, although also more prevalent in older clients, may be identified in younger people. Ask about occupation, and clarify whether the occupation increases the risk for vascular disease.

Current Health

Ask about the onset, precipitating factors, frequency, duration, and persistence of clinical manifestations that may indicate a vascular disorder. The following section describes the typical complaints of clients who have arterial and venous disorders.

Chief Complaint

Arterial Disorders. Arterial manifestations may occur in the head, upper extremities, abdomen, chest, or lower

---

evolve Web Enhancements

Assessment Terms English and Spanish

Appendix B A Health History Format That Integrates the Assessment of Functional Health Patterns

Figure Head-to-Toe Bilateral Pulse Assessment

Table Themes, Definitions, and Characteristics of Peripheral Arterial Disease

Be sure to check out the bonus material on the Evolve website and the CD-ROM, including free self-assessment exercises. **http://evolve.elsevier. com/Black/medsurg**

extremities. Clinical manifestations related to the head include visual disturbances, orientation, movement of extremities, facial symmetry, speech, and swallowing. These manifestations may be found in neurologic disorders as well as vascular disorders. ⚱ Document the activity required to cause pain when it is present. In lower extremity arterial disorders the extent of disease involvement can be gauged by the distance the client is able to walk without pain, or claudication distance.

Venous Disorders. Chronic venous disease has an insidious onset. Many clients do not recall a precipitating event. A positive family history, a job history involving standing in one place, multiple pregnancies, varicose veins, or a history of phlebitis or obesity may be factors. Acute venous disorders usually present as sudden swelling in a localized area. Upper extremity superficial venous occlusion causes discomfort along the course of the affected vein. Suspect deep vein thrombosis in the upper extremity if there is significant edema in the affected arm. Pain in chronic venous disease has a slow onset. Heaviness in the legs or nighttime cramping may be reported. Exercise and elevation improve venous return to the heart and generally relieve the discomfort and swelling.

Clinical Manifestations

Vascular disease may be arterial, venous, or lymphatic, but there are also neurologic conditions that cause similar manifestations. Table 51-1 compares arterial and venous clinical manifestations in the lower extremities. Figure 51-1 provides a guide for the evaluation of clinical manifestations related to vascular disease.

Pain. In arterial insufficiency of the lower extremities, the client may complain of cramping leg pain in the calf muscles that occurs during ambulation but disappears with 1 to 2 minutes of rest. The pain is called intermittent claudication. The pain occurs in the muscle group distal to the diseased artery and is a pathologic process similar to angina pectoris (chest pain). As an artery becomes more stenosed, the pain may become more severe. The Integrating Diagnostic Testing feature on p. 1283 demonstrates the evaluation of a claudication complaint.

Pain in chronic venous disease has a slow onset and is not associated with exercise or rest. The client who has venous disease may report chronic aching pain in the legs when they are in a dependent position.

Skin Changes. Skin changes noted with chronic venous disorders may include erythema (redness), followed in the late stages by lipodermatosclerosis (brawny, thick, darkly pigmented skin). The skin becomes dry and flaky, which leads to itching and scratching. With chronic

arterial insufficiency, the skin is pale when the legs are elevated above heart level and dusky red after they are placed in a dependent position.

Sensory Changes. Clients may report distal forefoot burning, numbness or tingling, pain at rest, or pain that awakens them during the night (rest pain). ⚱ These complaints may indicate that urgent attention is needed. This pain is related to arterial disease and exacerbated by decreased cardiac output during sleep.

Edema. In more severe forms of chronic venous disorders, lower extremity edema may be the initial complaint. Edema worsens toward the end of the day and diminishes after nighttime leg elevation. Skin temperature remains normal or slightly elevated and pulses are present, although they may be difficult to palpate through the edema. Pitting edema (see later discussion of edema) may be seen at first, but as the edema becomes more chronic, tissue sclerosis develops and the tissue becomes more difficult to compress. Lymphatic disorders also lead to edema. If the lymphatic obstruction is prolonged, edematous tissue becomes fibrotic and almost impossible to compress.

Lower Extremity Ulcers. With chronic venous disorders, the continued fluid leakage results in stasis dermatitis and the skin eventually ulcerates. Ulcers develop in the lower third of the leg, most commonly above the medial malleolus, where venous pressure is highest and there are more perforator veins than elsewhere in the leg.

Review of Systems

Review each body system as it relates to peripheral vascular disorders. Inquire about headaches, dizziness, pulmonary emboli, phlebitis, and leg or foot ulcers. Refer to Figure 51-2 on p. 1284 for vascular system-specific information to gather for the health history and review of systems.

Past Medical History

Note any history of vascular impairment. Inquire about changes that indicate vasospastic disorders, such as changes in color or temperature of digits. Ask specifically whether the client has a history of hypertension, diabetes, stroke, transient ischemic attacks (TIAs) changes in vision, pain in legs during activity, leg cramps, phlebitis, venous or arterial blood clots, pulmonary emboli, edema, varicose veins, or extremities that are cold, pale, or blue. Question any previous history of frostbite, which increases risk of vasospasm. Visual changes and TIAs may indicate carotid artery disease. Ask about previous treatment for diabetes mellitus, collagen disorders, or hypertension.

TABLE 51-1 Manifestations of Lower Extremity Arterial and Venous Disorders

	Arterial	Venous	Differentiating Neuropathic Disorder (Spinal Stenosis or Disc Disease)
Location of manifestation	Distal to arterial stenosis, buttocks, thigh, calf muscles, feet	Around ankle, over course of veins, often on medial side, may be entire leg	May radiate down lower back, legs, and buttocks after ambulation
Pain	Claudication, cramping pain occurs predictable distance Rest pain Continuous pain worsens with elevation	Aching, throbbing, burning, heaviness at end of day, nocturnal cramping	Burning, sharp, or aching pain
Relief of manifestation	Claudication—cessation of muscle use Rest pain—dependent position	Leg elevation	Must sit or flex lower back for relief May be able to walk only if bent over
Infection	May be present if open ulcer Thick toenails often indicate fungal infection but may also indicate arterial insufficiency	May be present if open ulcer	No
Skin	Pale Cooler than other skin areas In long-standing disease, skin is thin with absence of hair	Darkened brown color in gaiter area (area above the ankle to the knee) Dependent cyanosis Temperature may be higher than other skin areas Brawny edema Skin also may be thick and fibrotic (woody) May be oozing and crusted Pruritus may be present	No change
Sensation	Decreased Tingling, numbness may be present		Numbness, tingling, or other paresthesias in affected limb
Edema	Minimal unless leg kept dependent	May be severe	Not present
Pulses	Absent or diminished Often disappears with exercise	Usually present with only venous etiology but may be difficult to palpate if edema is present	Present
Muscle mass	Reduced in chronic disease	Unaffected in pure venous disease	Muscle wasting possible with long-term disease
Ankle-brachial index (ABI)	Decreased, 0.50 to 0.75	Not affected	Normal, 1.0 or greater
Ulcer description	Dry, pale gray or yellow May be necrotic Small, painful ulcers on pressure points, points of trauma, between toes, or distal points, especially lateral malleolus and toes	Broad, shallow, but may be deep pink or beefy red base with granulation tissue Ulcer bed moist; may have copious drainage Surrounding skin is brown, fibrotic	No ulcer
Operative procedures	Arterial bypass Angioplasty Stent placement	Vein ligation/stripping Valve grafts Sclerotherapy Laser or radiofrequency ablation	May require nerve decompression

Past Surgical History

Detail any previous operations that the client has endured, particularly vascular bypass surgery. Note if there has been any previous angiography, endovascular graft or stent placement, or harvesting of arteries or veins from the lower extremities. These are discussed in more detail in the following chapters on vascular and cardiac disorders.

Allergies

Note allergies, especially to iodine. Iodine is found in contrast agents used in diagnostic testing for vascular disorders.

Medications

Note specific medications that the client takes, including over-the-counter drugs and herbal remedies. Some

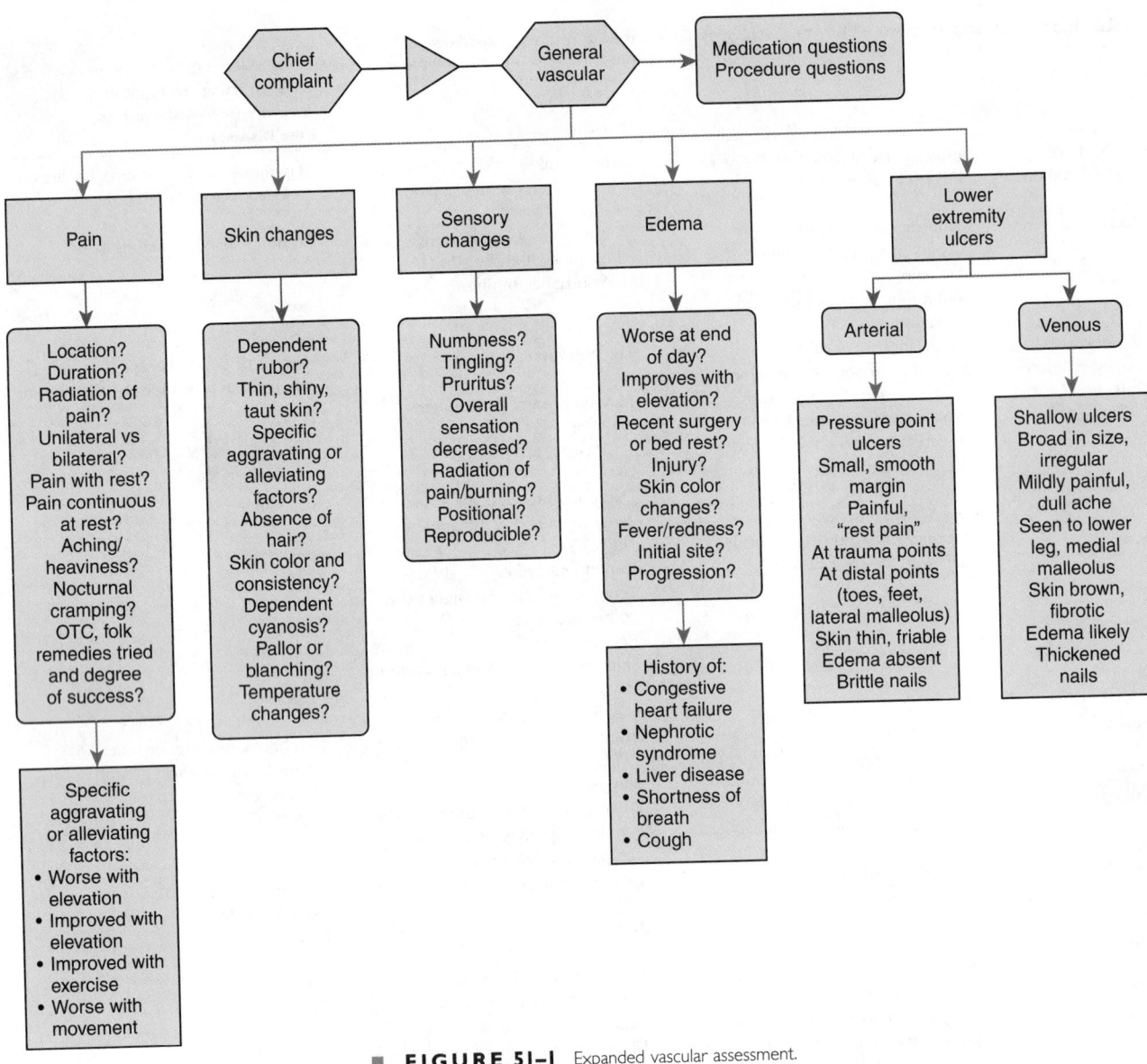

FIGURE 51-1 Expanded vascular assessment.

medications increase the risk for vascular disorders (such as birth control pills). Ask specifically about the use of prescription and over-the-counter nicotine products. Ask about use of illegal or street drugs.

Herbal remedies used to self-treat peripheral vascular disorders include those for hypertension, varicose veins, atherosclerosis, and vascular spasm. Herbs with antihypertensive action include garlic (*Allium sativum*), hawthorn (*Crataegus oxyacantha*), kudzu (*Pueraria lobata*), nettle (*Urtica dioica*), onion (*Allium cepa*), purslane (*Portulaca oleracea*), reishi mushroom (*Ganoderma lucidum*), and valerian (*Valeriana officinalis*). Garlic is thought to be preventive for atherosclerosis. Ginkgo biloba is used for varicose veins, obliterative arterial disease of the lower extremities, and intermittent claudication. Horse chestnut

(*Aesculus hippocastanum*) and butcher's broom (*Ruscus aculeatus*) are used for varicose veins and phlebitis, and valerian is used as an antispasmodic. Spices with possible antihypertensive effects include basil, black pepper, fennel, and tarragon.

Dietary Habits

Determine the client's nutrient and fluid intake (see Chapter 28). Ask about the usual intake of protein and calories. Also ask about sodium, cholesterol, and fat intake. The client who is underweight or overweight can be at risk for compromised healing and progression of vascular ulcers. Does the client report shortness of breath or fatigue when eating? Overall dietary intake

INTEGRATING DIAGNOSTIC TESTING

Claudication Pain

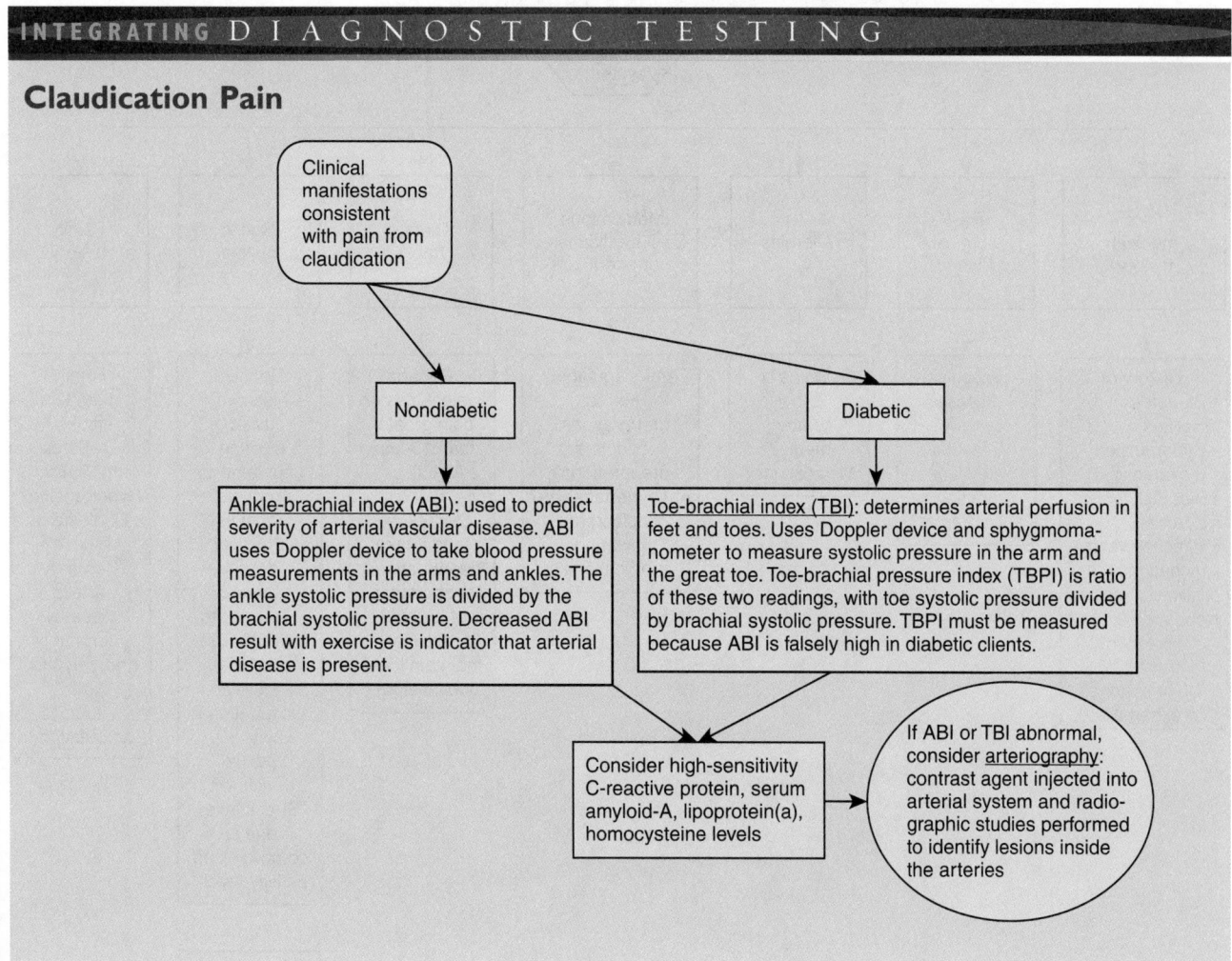

Clinical manifestations consistent with pain from claudication

Nondiabetic

Diabetic

Ankle-brachial index (ABI): used to predict severity of arterial vascular disease. ABI uses Doppler device to take blood pressure measurements in the arms and ankles. The ankle systolic pressure is divided by the brachial systolic pressure. Decreased ABI result with exercise is indicator that arterial disease is present.

Toe-brachial index (TBI): determines arterial perfusion in feet and toes. Uses Doppler device and sphygmomanometer to measure systolic pressure in the arm and the great toe. Toe-brachial pressure index (TBPI) is ratio of these two readings, with toe systolic pressure divided by brachial systolic pressure. TBPI must be measured because ABI is falsely high in diabetic clients.

Consider high-sensitivity C-reactive protein, serum amyloid-A, lipoprotein(a), homocysteine levels

If ABI or TBI abnormal, consider <u>arteriography</u>: contrast agent injected into arterial system and radiographic studies performed to identify lesions inside the arteries

should support maintenance of ideal body weight. Ask about recent weight loss or pain in the abdomen within 20 minutes of eating. This may indicate mesenteric artery ischemia.

Social History

Record the occupational history, including the number of hours spent in various positions or activities (standing, prolonged sitting, walking, using vibrating machinery). Some occupations involve contact with chemicals or are associated with cold or wet environments; these should be noted as well.

Nicotine in any form is a potent vasoconstrictor. A complete smoking history is necessary as part of the vascular assessment. Discuss previous and current use of chewing tobacco, cigarettes, cigars, and pipe tobacco.

Assess the client's activity, rest, and sleep habits. Assess the extent to which the clinical manifestations illustrated in Figure 51-1 interfere with activities of daily living. Obtaining information about the frequency and duration of manifestations, precipitating activities, and their influence on daily life enables determination of disease severity.

Disorders of the aorta and iliac vessels can lead to impotence. If a male client has aortoiliac disease, ask about problems with erectile function. Assessment of the client's stress level, emotional state, and coping mechanisms is important. Remain sensitive to the emotional effect of peripheral vascular disorders. Clients who have visible lesions may be embarrassed. Clients may have concern about the inability to perform self-care and about changes in role and sexual performance. Fear of amputation or functional loss may be significant.[2]

Family History

The family health history helps determine risk factors and provides clues about reported and observed manifestations. Note any family history of diabetes, hypertension, coronary artery disease, collagen diseases, and peripheral vascular disease.

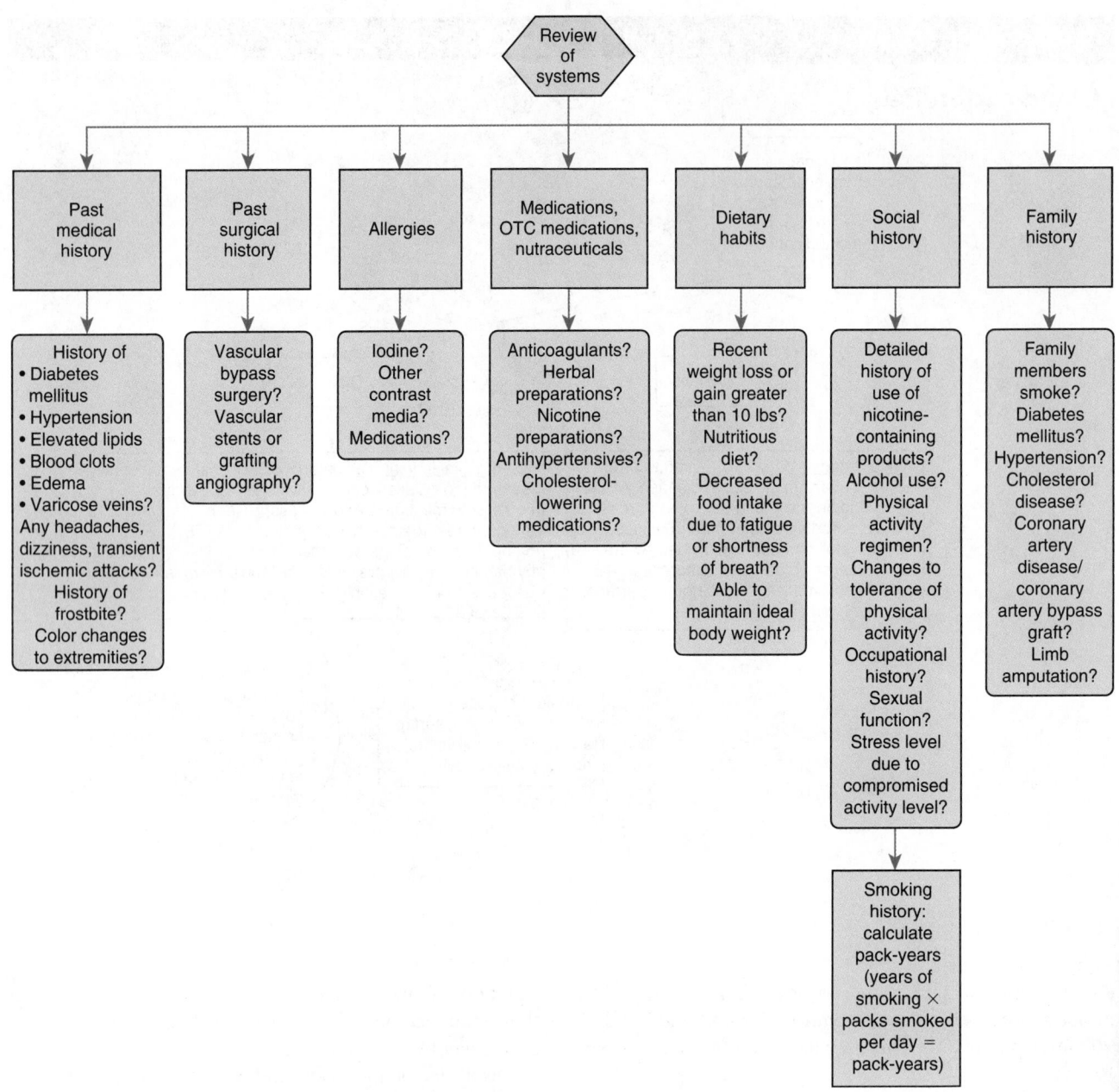

■ **FIGURE 51–2** Expanded vascular history.

PHYSICAL EXAMINATION

Assessment of the vascular system allows for the comparison of one side to the other. Blood pressure, pulse examination, color, and temperature assessment are bilateral. Differences between bilateral measurements may signify vascular disorders. Refer to the normal findings described in the Physical Assessment Findings in the Healthy Adult feature on p. 1285.

Inspection

Observe the extremities, noting skin color, hair distribution, nail beds and capillary refill time, presence of muscle atrophy or edema, venous pattern, and ulcers. Compare one side with the other. Begin with the head and upper extremities, and proceed toward the legs and feet.

Skin Color

There is a range of normal skin color. Localized areas of cyanosis, rubor, or pallor are easily noticed in a person with fair skin (Figure 51-3) but are more difficult to see in a person with darker skin tones (Figure 51-4). For all clients, changes in skin color are best assessed by comparison with the contralateral limb. Ischemic pallor may be detected by comparing the palms of the hands, the soles of the feet, or the nail beds. Clients with

The Peripheral Vascular System

INSPECTION

Extremities of even contour, without edema. Even hair distribution; symmetrical venous pattern. Varicosities, skin lesions, and ulcers absent. Capillaries refill in less than 3 seconds on blanching.

PALPATION

Extremities warm and dry without areas of localized heat or tenderness. Pulses (temporal, carotid, brachial, radial, ulnar, femoral, popliteal, posterior tibial, dorsalis pedis) are bilaterally equal and regular. No aneurysmal dilation of aorta.

AUSCULTATION

Blood pressures equal in contralateral extremities. Orthostatic hypotension absent. No bruits.

arterial disorders may have pale extremities and cyanotic (blue-tinged) or red extremities with venous disorders.

Hair Distribution

Lack of hair growth may indicate chronically inadequate circulation to an area. It is not a valid indicator of acute arterial insufficiency.

Capillary Refill Time

Capillary refill time is an evaluation of peripheral perfusion and cardiac output. This assessment is usually completed while pulses are assessed. Depress the nail bed or the pad of the toe or finger until it blanches or becomes pale. Release pressure on the blanched area, and note the length of time for usual skin color to return. Capillaries usually refill in a fraction of a second, but "normal" times range up to 3 seconds for color return.

Muscle Atrophy

There can be many reasons for muscle atrophy in an extremity. If atrophy is suspected, compare it with the muscle on the opposite side.

Edema

To assess edema of the leg, push with your thumb on the skin over the client's foot or tibia for 5 seconds. If the skin is edematous, an indentation or pit will remain (thus the term *pitting edema*) (Figure 51-5). Edema is often graded; however, scales used to grade edema are not universal. Clinicians should use their institution's approved scale. This may include documentation as basic as noting if edema is present or absent and, if present, whether it is pitting or non-pitting.

Edema resulting from cardiac disease is bilateral and occurs in dependent areas (in the legs of a client who is ambulatory and the sacrum of a client who is bedridden). Unilateral edema indicates venous or lymphatic obstruction. Long-standing edema destroys the structure of the skin and the subcutaneous tissue and is easily recognized from its fibrotic appearance and firm texture.

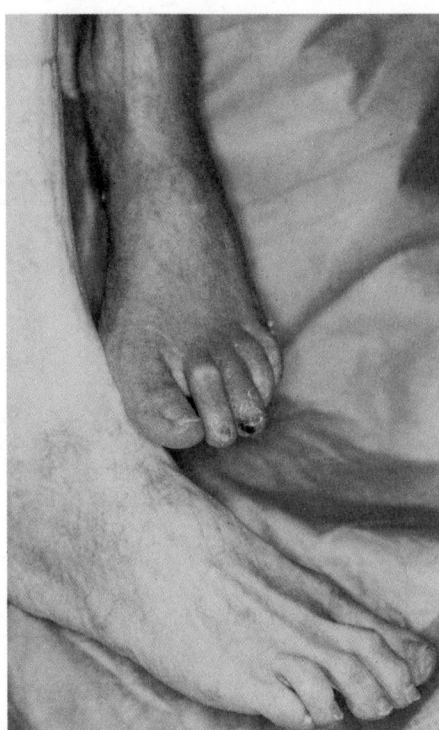

■ **FIGURE 51–3** Dependent rubor is noted as a ruddy color in severe arterial insufficiency in this white client's left leg just minutes before amputation. (Note area of ulceration and necrosis on the third toe.)

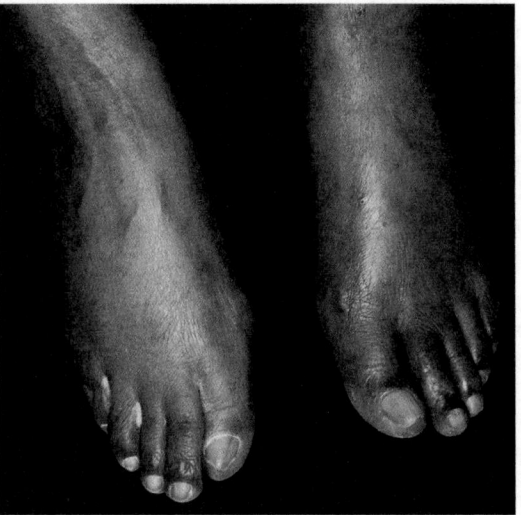

■ **FIGURE 51–4** Dependent rubor in dark skin (which can be difficult to see) in the client's left foot has a reddish hue when compared with the unaffected right foot.

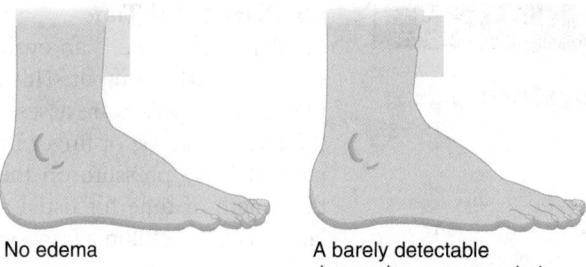

No edema

A barely detectable
depression accompanied
by normal foot and leg contours

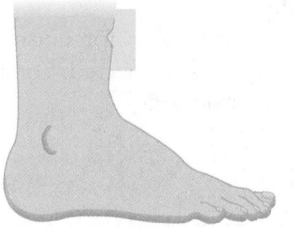

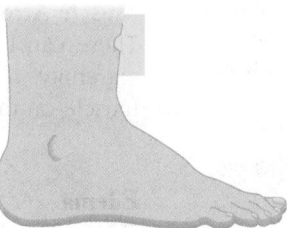

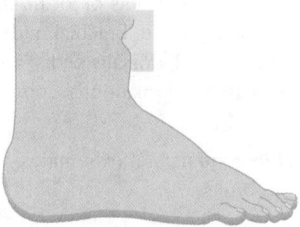

A deeper depression
(less than 5 mm) accompanied
by normal foot and leg contours

A deep depression
(5 to 10 mm) accompanied
by foot and leg swelling

An even deeper depression
(more than 1 cm) accompanied by
severe foot and leg swelling

■ **FIGURE 51–5**   To assess peripheral edema, press a finger into the skin over the client's tibia. Note the presence, depth, and persistence of any resulting depression. Use descriptive terms to record your findings.

Ulcers

Note the presence of skin lesions or scar tissue (indicating healed ulcers); fissures of the feet and ulcers of the ankles and heels may be signs of arterial insufficiency. Tissue necrosis (see Figure 51-4) and gangrene may be present with severe arterial disease. Examine between the toes for moist ulcers penetrating into the web spaces.

Palpation
Temperature

Palpate the arms and legs with the dorsal surface of your hand, and note the temperature (see Chapter 48). Temperature should be similar in contralateral limbs. Vasoconstriction produces cold, pale skin. Bilateral vasoconstriction may be caused by smoking, environmental temperature, anxiety, or generalized arterial disease. Unilateral or localized arterial vasoconstriction indicates arterial disease. Venous disorders may cause an increase in local skin temperature.

Pulses

Palpate pulses by placing the first three fingers of your dominant hand along the length of the selected artery. Apply gentle pressure against the artery, followed by a gradual release. Palpate temporal, carotid, brachial, radial, and ulnar pulses (upper extremities), and femoral, popliteal, posterior tibial, and dorsalis pedis pulses (lower extremities), as shown in the website *evolve* figure Head-to-Toe Bilateral Pulse Assessment. Palpate

pulses bilaterally and simultaneously, except for the carotid pulse. Palpate carotid pulses separately to avoid stimulation of the carotid sinus, which may produce bradycardia or sinus arrest. Assess the ulnar pulse during Allen's test (Box 51-1). Homans' test, which was used in the past to assess for deep venous thrombosis, is no longer used because the test itself

---

BOX 51-1

ALLEN'S TEST

Blood flow to the hand is supplied by both the ulnar and the radial arteries, which join at the volar arch in the palm. Allen's test is used to assess the patency of the radial and ulnar arteries distal to the wrist. It is commonly performed before arterial blood samples are drawn for analysis or before an arterial line is inserted. Perform Allen's test as follows:

1. Ask the client to make a tight fist while you compress the radial and ulnar arteries.
2. Have the client open the hand, which should be pale and mottled.
3. Release the pressure on the radial artery while continuing to compress the ulnar artery. If the client's hand regains full color within about 6 seconds, the radial artery has normal patency.
4. Repeat steps 1 to 3, this time releasing the pressure on the ulnar artery to assess its patency.

If the client's hand remains pale during either portion of the test, the artery being tested may be occluded. Allen's test is shown in Figure 59-13 on p. 1539.

may cause a clot to dislodge and become an embolus (Box 51-2).

Always note the rhythm, amplitude, and symmetry of pulses. Compare peripheral pulses on both sides for rate, rhythm, and quality. There are no standard numerical grades or rating scales for pulses although some systems use a numerical scale. It is most accurate to describe the pulse as palpable (or present), diminished (weak), absent, or aneurysmal (easily palpable, bounding).

Note whether a pulse feels unequal bilaterally. The dorsalis pedis pulse is congenitally absent in approximately 10% to 17% of the normal adult population.[1] The posterior tibial pulse is absent congenitally in 9% of the black adult population of the United States.[1] In older clients, dorsalis pedis and posterior tibial pulses may be more difficult to palpate. If they are found, mark the site with a pen to facilitate later examinations. Clients who have arterial grafts may have palpable pulses along the length of the graft. The aorta can easily be palpated on a thin person by placing the hand on the upper abdomen just below the xyphoid process.

Auscultation
Limb Blood Pressure

The measurement of arterial blood pressure is the most commonly performed noninvasive test of cardiac and vascular function. It may be the best single indicator of arterial perfusion. Arterial stenosis or occlusion produces regional hypotension. Auscultate the blood pressure in both arms. 🪔 A difference of 20 mm Hg between extremity readings may indicate aortic dissection or subclavian artery stenosis. Document asymmetrical readings. All subsequent blood pressure measurements should be performed on the arm with the higher reading. Measure blood pressure with the client in supine, sitting, and standing positions on the first assessment, and document the position of the client and the site used for each reading. Note orthostatic (positional) changes in blood pressure.

Auscultate over the carotid artery, the aorta, and the renal, femoral, and popliteal arteries to assess for the presence of bruits. A bruit is a "whooshing" sound that may be soft or loud; it results from turbulent blood flow from vessel wall irregularities. The presence of a bruit

indicates arterial narrowing. These arterial sounds are best heard with the bell of the stethoscope.

DIAGNOSTIC TESTING

The following is a summary of tests used to assess the extent of a client's vascular disease. For specifics on the nursing role with and pre- and postprocedure care with each test, consult a diagnostic testing textbook.

Noninvasive Tests

Noninvasive diagnostic techniques have assumed an increasingly important role in the management of vascular disorders. Noninvasive diagnostic tests provide reliable, objective data that can be used to evaluate the extent of vascular disease. Variables include blood flow velocity, blood flow abnormality, and some measure of functional limitations.

Ankle-Brachial Index

The ankle-brachial index (ABI) is a commonly used parameter for overall evaluation of extremity status. This test measures blood pressure at the ankle and in the arm while a person is at rest. Measurements are repeated at both sites after 5 minutes of walking on a treadmill. This ABI result is used to document the severity of lower extremity arterial disease. A decrease in the ABI measurement with exercise is an indicator that arterial disease is present.

Doppler Ultrasonography

Hand-held Doppler ultrasonographic instruments permit assessment of arterial disease through evaluation of audible arterial signals or measurement of limb blood pressures. Doppler ultrasonography is simple and inexpensive, but the technique may not detect minor disease, and it is less accurate than duplex scanning (see later discussion).

Brightness-mode (B-mode) ultrasound refers to the creation of a two-dimensional image from ultrasound waves. It can be used to assess the size and compressibility of a vessel, flow patterns, the presence or absence of thrombus, and valve function.

Ultrasonic Duplex Scan

Ultrasonic duplex scanners are used to localize vascular obstruction, evaluate the degree of stenosis, and determine the presence or absence of vascular reflux (backward flow). This anatomic and physiologic test evaluates the hemodynamic effects of arterial lesions. 🪔 It is also the most sensitive and specific noninvasive modality for detecting DVT. Both an ultrasound image of the vessel and a Doppler audible signal and waveform are provided. The visual ultrasound data allow more specific localization of stenosis than simple pressure or waveform techniques. No special client preparation is required.

Air Plethysmography

Air plethysmography (APG) uses a pneumatic plethysmograph to measure volume changes in the legs. Venous reflux, venous obstruction, calf muscle pump function, and venous volume can be measured. A large cuff is applied to the client's calf, and a known volume of air is instilled to calibrate the cuff. Venous volume, ejection fraction, and residual volume fractions are then measured.

Impedance Plethysmography

Impedance plethysmography (IPG) and photoplethysmography (PPG) are also used to measure venous blood volume changes in the extremities. During the procedure, electrodes from a plethysmograph are applied to a limb along with a pressure cuff. As pressure is increased, electrical resistance is increased; thus the quality of venous blood flow is demonstrated.

Exercise Testing

Exercise or stress testing provides an objective measurement of the severity of intermittent claudication. The most commonly used 🪔 method for stress testing is the treadmill exercise test. This test is similar to that used for clients who have cardiac stress testing, except that walking speed is usually 1.5 to 2 miles per hour (mph) with a grade elevation of 10% to 20% and a time limit of 5 minutes. A client who can walk 5 minutes is considered mildly symptomatic; a walking time of 1 minute represents severe disease.

Performance on the treadmill test is also gauged by measurement of ankle systolic pressure. In asymptomatic clients, the time required for return to pre-exercise ankle pressure is usually less than 3 minutes with a decline from baseline of 20% or less. In clients with intermittent claudication, recovery time is longer; ankle pressure is usually less than 50 mm Hg and may be unrecordable during recovery.

Computed Tomography

Computed tomography (CT) provides a cross-section of vessel walls and other structures. CT scans can be used to diagnose abdominal aortic aneurysms and postoperative complications, such as graft infection, graft occlusion, hemorrhage, and abscess.

Magnetic Resonance Imaging

Magnetic resonance imaging (MRI) is used to detect tissue changes, such as tumors, aneurysms, and DVT, in the pelvic iliac veins and leg veins. Blood flow in an extremity is evaluated, with the limb to be examined placed in a cradle-like support in a flow cylinder.

In the future, MRI techniques likely will supply much of the information that currently is available only with invasive angiography. Although MRI does not require ionizing radiation or injection into the arterial system, the expense and time necessary limit its use for routine screening and follow-up.

Invasive Tests
Arteriography

Contrast arteriography is performed if the client is willing to undergo a surgical or percutaneous intervention. It is used to identify lesions inside the arteries and intraoperatively to evaluate the results of an operation. The procedure involves injecting a contrast agent into the arterial system and performing radiographic studies.

Venography

Venography, performed in a manner similar to that for arteriography, is used to examine the venous system. Venograms can be used to detect DVT and other abnormalities, such as incompetent valves. This diagnostic test is performed less frequently than in the past. Newer, noninvasive vascular laboratory studies pose less risk, are more accurate, and provide functional information as well.

Magnetic Resonance Angiography

Magnetic resonance angiography (MRA) uses magnetic imaging techniques to access blood vessels. The advantage of this technique is that the images are not obscured by bone, bowel gas, fat, or vascular calcification. The vessel anatomy is displayed as a three-dimensional angiogram. MRA can be used to measure blood flow volume and blood viscosity. It is a noninvasive modality. The disadvantages are its limited availability, its cost, and the need for the client to hold still during the procedure. MRA cannot be used for people who have cardiac pacemakers or intracranial aneurysm clips.

Vascular Endoscopy (Angioscopy)

Vascular endoscopy permits imaging of intra-arterial disease with the use of fiberoptic technology. Images are in color and in three dimensions. The major advantage of angioscopy is the internal visualization of the vessel lumen. This enables identification of thrombus (blood clot), plaque, hemorrhage, ulceration, or embolus (clot that has broken off from a thrombus and lodged in a more distal artery). Angioscopes can be used to remove debris from vessels and to check the integrity of an anastomosis (suture line that connects a vessel grafted to a native vessel) from within a vessel. They may also be used to remove venous valves in preparation for use of the vein as a bypass graft.

Complications of vascular endoscopy are rare but may include intimal damage, vessel spasm, thrombosis or embolism, perforation, fluid overload, and infection. Postprocedure care is similar to that for clients who have undergone angiography.

Intravascular Ultrasonography

Intravascular ultrasonography provides information about the atherosclerotic intima beneath the luminal surface. It can thus determine the thickness of the arterial wall and can distinguish thrombus and calcified vessel walls from vascular tissue, allowing more exact removal of lesions. Specialized interpretation of the scan is necessary.

Laboratory Tests

Elevations in the total lipid profile, or specific portions of it, are a major risk factor in the development of atherosclerosis, and measures of the coagulation properties of a client's blood are part of the evaluation of the severity of cardiovascular disease. Refer to the discussion of the relevance of these laboratory values in the chapter about vascular disorders (Chapter 53) and functional cardiac disorders (Chapter 56).

CONCLUSIONS

Vascular assessment requires inspection, palpation, and auscultation skills. Knowledge of anatomy is critical for correct performance of assessments. Diagnostic modalities can range from simple, noninvasive tests to complex, sophisticated, invasive technology. A clear understanding of the indications for diagnostic tests and interpretation of the findings assists the clinical decision making.

BIBLIOGRAPHY

 Citations appearing in red refer to primary research.

Citations appearing in blue refer to evidence-based practice guidelines and protocols.

1. Fahey, V. (2004). Clinical assessment of the vascular system. In V.A. Fahey (Ed.), *Vascular nursing* (4th ed.). Philadelphia: Elsevier Saunders.
2. Hirsch, A., Haskal, Z., Hertzer, N., et al. (2006). ACC/AHA guidelines for the management of patients with peripheral arterial disease (lower extremity, renal, mesenteric, and abdominal aortic). *Journal of the American College of Cardiology, 147*, 1239-1312.
3. Hirsch, A.T. (Ed.) (2001). Primary care series: Peripheral arterial disease and intermittent claudication: A compilation of the American Journal of Medicine Continuing Education Series. An office based approach to the diagnosis and treatment of peripheral arterial disease. *Excerpta Medica*. Philadelphia: Elsevier.
4. Hirsch, A.T., et al. (2001). Peripheral arterial disease detection, awareness, and treatment in primary care. *Journal of the American Medical Association, 11*(286), 1317-1324.
5. Jaff, M.R., & Hiatt, W.R. (2001). Clinical and vascular laboratory evaluation of peripheral arterial disease. In W.R. Hiatt, A.T. Hirsch, & J.G. Regensteiner (Eds.), *Peripheral arterial disease handbook* (pp. 81-94). Boca Raton, Fla: CRC Press.
6. Moore, W.S. (Ed.) (2005). *Vascular and endovascular surgery: A comprehensive review* (7th ed.). Philadelphia: Saunders.
7. Negus, D. (2005). Diagnosis: History and examination. In D. Negus, P. Coleridge Smith, & J. Bergan (Eds.), *Leg ulcers: Diagnosis and management* (3rd ed., pp. 75-83). London: Hodder Arnold.
8. Treat-Jacobson, D., et al. (2002). A patient-derived perspective of health-related quality of life with peripheral arterial disease. *Journal of Nursing Scholarship, 34*(1), 55-60.

evolve Did you remember to check out the bonus material on the Evolve website and the CD-ROM, including NCLEX®-Examination Style Review Questions, Open-Book Quizzes, and Chapter Review Audio Podcasts?

http://evolve.elsevier.com/Black/medsurg

CHAPTER 52

Management of Clients with Hypertensive Disorders

JEAN ELIZABETH DEMARTINIS

HYPERTENSION

Arterial hypertension, simply stated, is high blood pressure. It is defined as a persistent elevation of the systolic blood pressure (SBP) at a level of 140 mm Hg or higher and diastolic blood pressure (DBP) at a level of 90 mm Hg or higher. The National Institutes of Health's report titled *The Seventh Report of the Joint National Committee on Detection, Evaluation, and Treatment of High Blood Pressure (JNC VII)* and the Centers for Disease Control and Prevention (CDC) publications *Healthy People 2000* and *2010* have documented the advances made over the last few decades in the prevention, detection, and treatment of hypertension. Members of the public have become more knowledgeable about high blood pressure, are more likely to visit a health care provider for hypertension, and are more likely to comply with medical advice. The use of increasingly effective antihypertensive agents has also dramatically reduced the death rate associated with hypertension. The percentage of people has increased significantly who receive treatment for hypertension and keep their blood pressure controlled. The combined effects from increased access to treatment and better control of existing hypertension have contributed to a greater than 60% decline in stroke and greater than 50% decline in the death rate from coronary artery disease. These impressive gains have been seen across all age groups, in both men and women, and in special populations.

The *JNC VII* and *Healthy People 2010,* however, also document some disturbing current trends. After years of decline, the death rates for coronary heart disease and stroke leveled off and have begun to rise again. The prevalence of hypertension is on the rise, and control rates are variable, with the majority of people with hypertension undercontrolled. Arterial hypertension affects more than 50 million people—1 in 4—in the United States, with the highest rates of occurrence among older adults, blacks, less educated people, and lower socio-economic groups. Estimates are that only about 25% of all people with hypertension have blood pressure controlled at a target level. Lack of client compliance and providers' continued ignorance of the need to prescribe and manage complex holistic treatment protocols are cited as the two major factors that have contributed to this abysmal decline in improved client outcomes.

Acute coronary syndrome events such as a "heart attack" are still the most common result of hypertension. Hypertension is also related to increased severity of atherosclerosis, stroke, nephropathy, peripheral vascular disease, aortic aneurysms, and heart failure. Nearly all people with heart failure have antecedent hypertension. If hypertension is left untreated, nearly half of hypertensive clients will die of heart disease, one third will die of stroke, and the remaining 10% to 15% will die of renal failure. Hypertension is also a "silent factor" leading to many deaths attributed to stroke or heart attacks.

These disturbing trends indicate the need for increased vigilance in the battle against hypertension. Hypertension-related morbidity and mortality rates will not significantly decrease until providers appreciate the need for adjustments or refinements in their existing treatment protocols that are based on current practice guidelines that suggest options for evidence-based practice that produce

---

evolve **Web Enhancements**

Client Education Guide Low-Sodium Diet (English Version and Spanish Translation)

Low-Fat, Low-Cholesterol Diet (English Version and Spanish Translation)

Calorie-Restriction Diet (English Version and Spanish Translation)

Concept Map Understanding Hypertension and Its Treatment

Be sure to check out the bonus material on the Evolve website and the CD-ROM, including free self-assessment exercises. **http://evolve.elsevier.com/Black/medsurg**

quantifiable client outcomes. For example, there are readily available non-invasive assessment devices that indirectly measure a client's internal hemodynamics; these measurements can be used to guide a provider's choices for appropriate medications and dosages for each individual client.

The *Healthy People 2010* guidelines are prevention focused, and the *JNC VII* guidelines are also now primarily prevention focused and strongly recommend the use of nonpharmaceutical as well as pharmaceutical measures to prevent and treat hypertension. The Translating Evidence into Practice feature at right examines new guidelines for preventing and managing hypertension. Nurses are faced with a profound urgency to enhance public and professional education toward this end and to translate the results of research into improved practice. An ambitious, but nevertheless feasible, goal is the diagnosis and treatment of hypertension in all affected people in the United States.

Types of Hypertensive Disease, Etiology, and Severity

Hypertension is characterized by type, cause, and severity. Most clients with a combination of systolic and diastolic blood pressure elevation are diagnosed with *primary hypertension,* also known as *essential* or idiopathic hypertension. The etiology is multifactoral, with no identifiable cause, but several interacting homeostatic forces are generally involved. The blood pressure remains elevated and continues to rise over time because of a persistent, progressive increase in peripheral arterial resistance. The persistent rise in arterial resistance is due to inappropriate renal retention of salt and water or abnormalities of or within the vessel wall. The severity of the condition directly relates to the number and magnitude of risk factors present, the length of time for which these risk factors have been present, and the presence of accompanying disease states. The severity of complications from hypertension increase as the blood pressure, both systolic and diastolic, increases.

Clients who develop hypertension from an identifiable cause—a specific disease state or problem—are diagnosed with *secondary hypertension,* and in many cases the underlying cause is correctable (Box 52-1 on p. 1294). Therefore it is important to isolate the root of the problem so that the most appropriate treatment regimen can be prescribed. Severity depends on underlying causes, personal and environmental factors, and duration of concurrent disease states.

When the systolic blood pressure is 140 mm Hg or higher but the diastolic blood pressure remains less than 90 mm Hg, the client is diagnosed with *isolated systolic hypertension* (ISH). ISH can result from increased cardiac output or atherosclerosis-induced changes in blood vessel compliance or both. Regardless of cause, this form of hypertension is treated in the same manner as

---

⛭ TRANSLATING EVIDENCE INTO PRACTICE

Guidelines for Hypertension Prevention and Management

The Seventh Report of the Joint National Committee on Prevention, Detection, Evaluation, and Treatment of High Blood Pressure provides a new guideline for hypertension prevention and management. The following are the report's key messages:

- In people older than 50 years, systolic blood pressure greater than 140 mm Hg is a much more important cardiovascular disease (CVD) risk factor than diastolic blood pressure.
- The risk of CVD beginning at 115/75 mm Hg doubles with each increment of 20/10 mm Hg; individuals who are normotensive at age 55 have a 90% lifetime risk for developing hypertension.
- Individuals with a systolic blood pressure of 120 to 139 mm Hg or a diastolic blood pressure of 80 to 89 mm Hg should be considered as prehypertensive and require health-promoting lifestyle modifications to prevent CVD.
- Thiazide-type diuretics should be used in drug treatment for most clients with uncomplicated hypertension, either alone or combined with drugs from other classes. Certain high-risk conditions are compelling indications for the initial use of other antihypertensive drug classes (such as angiotensin-converting enzyme inhibitors, angiotensin receptor blockers, beta-blockers, calcium channel blockers).
- Most clients with hypertension will require two or more antihypertensive medications to achieve goal blood pressure (<140/90 mm Hg, or <130/80 mm Hg for clients with diabetes or chronic kidney disease).
- If blood pressure is >20/10 mm Hg above goal blood pressure, consideration should be given to initiating therapy with two agents, one of which usually should be a thiazide-type diuretic.
- The most effective therapy prescribed by the most careful clinician will control hypertension only if clients are motivated. Motivation improves when clients have positive experiences with, and trust in, the clinician. Empathy builds trust and is a potent motivator.
- In presenting these guidelines, the committee recognizes that the responsible physician's judgment remains paramount.

From National High Blood Pressure Education Program, National Institutes of Health, National Heart, Lung and Blood Institute. (2003). *The Seventh Report of the Joint National Committee on Detection, Evaluation, and Treatment of High Blood Pressure.* Bethesda, Md: U.S. Government Printing Office.

---

primary hypertension. The likelihood of the development of ISH increases with advancing age, as does the severity of ISH.

Clients who develop refractory hypertension with persistent systolic or diastolic elevation and/or if diastolic blood pressure is protracted above 110 to 120 mm Hg are diagnosed with *resistant hypertension.* It results when hypertension is left untreated or is unresponsive to treatment and becomes a truly severe emergency condition as the pressure continues to rise unchecked. The unrelenting rise in arterial resistance is due to inappropriate renal retention of salt and water or abnormalities of or within the vessel wall. The severity of the condition directly relates to the number and magnitude of risk factors present, the length of time for which these risk factors have been present, and the presence of accompanying disease states.

Epidemiology and Risk Factors

Primary hypertension constitutes more than 90% of all cases of hypertension. Fewer than 5% to 8% of adult hypertensive clients have secondary hypertension; however, hypertension, regardless of type, results from an array of genetic and environmental factors. These risk factors are grouped into those that are modifiable and those which are not. Education for lifestyle change is directed at the modifiable risk factors.

Nonmodifiable Risk Factors

Family History

Hypertension is thought to be polygenic and multifactorial—that is, in any person with a family history of hypertension, several genes may interact with each other and the environment to cause the blood pressure to elevate over time. The genetic predisposition that makes certain families more susceptible to hypertension may be related to an elevation in intracellular sodium levels and to lowered potassium-to-sodium ratios, which are found more often in blacks than in other groups. Clients with parents who have hypertension are at greater risk for hypertension at a younger age.

Age

Primary hypertension typically appears between the ages of 30 and 50 years. The incidence of hypertension increases with age; 50% to 60% of clients older than 60 years have a blood pressure over 140/90 mm Hg. Epidemiologic studies, however, have shown a poorer prognosis in clients whose hypertension began at a young age. Isolated systolic hypertension occurs primarily in people older than 50 years, with almost 24% of all people affected by age 80 years. Among older adults, SBP readings are a better predictor of possible future events such as coronary heart disease, stroke, heart failure, and renal disease than are DBP readings.

Gender

The overall incidence of hypertension is higher in men than in women until about age 55 years. Between the ages of 55 and 74 years, the risk in men and that in women are almost equal; then, after age 74 years, women are at greater risk.

Ethnicity

Mortality statistics indicate that the death rate for adults with hypertension is lowest for white women at 4.7%; white men have the next lowest rate at 6.3%, and black men have the next lowest at 22.5%; the death rate is highest for black women at 29.3%. The reason for the increased prevalence of hypertension among blacks is unclear, but the increase has been attributed to lower renin levels, greater sensitivity to vasopressin, higher salt intake, and greater environmental stress.

Modifiable Risk Factors

Diabetes

Hypertension has been shown to be more than twice as prevalent in diabetic clients according to several recent research studies. Diabetes accelerates atherosclerosis and leads to hypertension from damage to the large vessels. Therefore hypertension *will* become a prevalent diagnosis in diabetics, even if diabetes is well controlled. When a diabetic client is diagnosed with hypertension, treatment decisions and follow-up care must be totally individualized and aggressive.

Stress

Stress increases peripheral vascular resistance and cardiac output and stimulates sympathetic nervous system activity. Over time hypertension can develop. Stressors can be many things, and noise, infection, inflammation, pain, decreased oxygen supply, heat, cold, trauma, prolonged exertion, responses to life events, obesity, old age, drugs, disease, surgery, and medical treatment can elicit the stress response. These noxious stimuli are perceived by a person as a threat or as capable of causing harm; subsequently, a psychophysiologic "fight-or-flight" response is initiated in the body. If stress responses become excessive or prolonged, target organ dysfunction or disease will result. A report from the American Institute of Stress estimates that 60% to 90% of all primary care visits involve stress-related complaints. Because stress is a matter of perception, people's interpretations of events are what create most stressors and stress responses.

Obesity

Obesity, especially in the upper body (giving an "apple" shape), with increased amounts of fat about the midriff, waist, and abdomen, is associated with subsequent development of hypertension. People who are overweight but carry most of the excess weight in the buttocks, hips, and thighs (giving them a "pear" shape) are at far less risk for development of hypertension secondary to increased weight alone. The combination of obesity with other factors can be labeled as metabolic syndrome, which also increases the risk of hypertension.

Nutrients

Sodium consumption can be an important factor in the development of essential hypertension. At least 40% of clients who eventually develop hypertension are salt-sensitive and the excess salt may be the precipitating cause of the hypertension in these individuals. A high-salt diet may induce excessive release of natriuretic hormone, which may indirectly increase blood pressure. Sodium loading also stimulates vasopressor mechanisms within the central nervous system (CNS). Studies also show that low dietary intake of calcium, potassium, and magnesium can contribute to the development of hypertension.

Substance Abuse

Cigarette smoking, heavy alcohol consumption, and some illicit drug use all are risk factors for hypertension. The nicotine in cigarette smoke and drugs such as cocaine cause an immediate rise in blood pressure that is dose dependent; however, *habitual* use of these substances has been implicated in an increased incidence of hypertension over time. The incidence of hypertension is also higher among people who drink more than 3 ounces of ethanol per day. The impact of caffeine is controversial. Caffeine raises blood pressure acutely but does not produce sustained effects.

Pathophysiology

Primary (Essential) Hypertension

The exact pathologic underpinnings of primary hypertension remain to be established. Any factor that produces an alteration in peripheral vascular resistance, heart rate, or stroke volume affects systemic arterial blood pressure (see Figure A&P12-4 in the Anatomy and Physiology Review on p. 1276). Four control systems play a major role in maintaining blood pressure: (1) the arterial baroreceptor and chemoreceptors' system; (2) regulation of body fluid volume; (3) the renin-angiotensin system; and (4) vascular autoregulation. Primary hypertension most likely occurs from a defect or malfunction in some or all of these systems. Probably no single defect causes essential hypertension in all affected people.

Arterial baroreceptors and chemoreceptors work reflexively to control blood pressure (see Figure A&P12-5 in Anatomy and Physiology Review on p. 1277). Baroreceptors, major stretch receptors, are found in the carotid sinus, aorta, and wall of the left ventricle. They monitor the level of arterial pressure and counteract increases through vasodilation and slowing of the heart rate via the vagus nerve. Chemoreceptors, located in the medulla and carotid and aortic bodies, are sensitive to changes in concentrations of oxygen, carbon dioxide, and hydrogen ions (pH) in the blood. A decrease in arterial oxygen concentration or pH causes a reflexive rise in pressure,

whereas an increase in carbon dioxide concentration causes a decrease in blood pressure. Changes in fluid volume affect systemic arterial pressure. Thus an abnormality in the transport of sodium in the renal tubules may cause essential hypertension. When sodium and water levels are excessive, total blood volume increases, thereby increasing blood pressure. Pathologic changes that alter the pressure threshold at which kidneys excrete salt and water alter systemic blood pressure. In addition, the overproduction of sodium-retaining hormones has been implicated in hypertension.

Renin and angiotensin play a role in blood pressure regulation. *Renin* is an enzyme produced by the kidney that catalyzes a plasma protein substrate to split off angiotensin I, which is removed by a converting enzyme to the lung to form angiotensin II and then angiotensin III. Angiotensins II and III act as vasoconstrictors and also stimulate aldosterone release. With increased sympathetic nervous system activity, angiotensins II and III also seem to inhibit sodium excretion, which results in elevated blood pressure. Increased renin secretion has been investigated as a cause of increased peripheral vascular resistance in primary hypertension.

Vascular endothelial cells are being shown to be important in hypertension. The cells of the endothelium produce nitric oxide that dilates the arteriole and endothelium that constricts it. Dysfunction of the endothelium has been implicated in human essential hypertension.

Secondary Hypertension

Many renal, vascular, neurologic, endocrine, and drug- and food-induced problems that directly or indirectly negatively affect the kidneys can result in serious insult to these organs that interferes with sodium excretion, renal perfusion, or the renin-angiotensin-aldosterone mechanism, leading to an elevation in blood pressure over time (Box 52-1).

Chronic glomerulonephritis and renal artery stenosis are the most common cause of secondary hypertension. Also, the adrenal glands can cause secondary hypertension if they produce excessive aldosterone, cortisol, and catecholamines. Excess aldosterone causes renal retention of sodium and water, expands blood volume, and elevates blood pressure. *Pheochromocytoma,* a small tumor of the adrenal medulla, can cause dramatic hypertension because of the release of excessive amounts of epinephrine and norepinephrine (called catecholamines). Other adrenocortical problems can result in excess production of cortisol (Cushing's syndrome). Clients with Cushing's syndrome have an 80% risk for development of hypertension. Cortisol increases blood pressure by increasing renal sodium retention, angiotensin II levels, and vascular reactivity to norepinephrine. Chronic stress elevates blood levels of catecholamines, aldosterone, and cortisol.

BOX 52-1   **Causes of Secondary Hypertension**

ACUTE STRESS
- Alcoholism
- Acute alcohol withdrawal
- Burns
- Chronic intermittent vasovagal response
- Hyperventilation
- Hypoglycemia
- Psychogenic

VASCULAR DISORDERS
- Arteriosclerosis
- Coarctation of the aorta
- Increased intravascular volume
- Sickle cell crisis
- Dissecting aortic aneurysm

ENDOCRINE DISORDERS
- Acromegaly
- Adrenal disorders
  - Cortical
    - Cushing's syndrome
    - Primary aldosteronism
  - Medullary
    - Pancreatitis
    - Pheochromocytoma
- Hypothyroidism
- Hyperthyroidism

NEUROLOGIC DISORDERS
- Autonomic dysreflexia
- Increased intracranial pressure
  - Brain tumor
  - Encephalitis
  - Respiratory acidosis
- Sleep apnea

MEDICATIONS
- Abrupt medication withdrawal
- Amphetamine use
- Anabolic and adrenogenic steroids
- Antihistamines/decongestants
- Cocaine use
- Cyclosporine
- Ergot alkaloids
- Erythropoietin
- Glucocorticoids
- Heavy metal poisons (lead, arsenic)
- Mineralocorticoids
- Monoamine oxidase inhibitors
- NSAIDs
- Oral contraceptives
- Sympathomimetics
  - Ephedrine
  - Phenylephrine
- Tricyclic antidepressants

PROBLEMS WITH PREGNANCY
- Pregnancy-induced hypertension
- Eclampsia

RENAL DISORDERS
- Renal artery stenosis
- Renal parenchymal disease
  - Acute glomerulonephritis
  - Chronic pyelonephritis
  - Connective tissue diseases
  - Diabetic nephropathy
  - Hydronephrosis
  - Polycystic disease
- Renin-producing tumors
- Renovascular diseases
- Atherosclerosis
- Vasculitis

SEVERE ANEMIA

TYRAMINE-CONTAINING FOODS
- Aged cheeses (especially cheddar)
- Beer, wine
- Chicken liver
- Yeast extract

From National High Blood Pressure Education Program, National Institutes of Health, and National Heart, Lung and Blood Institute. (2003). *The Seventh Report of the Joint National Committee on Detection, Evaluation, and Treatment of High Blood Pressure*. Bethesda, MD: U.S. Government Printing Office.

Vessel Changes

Early in the course of development of hypertension, no obvious pathologic changes in the blood vessels and organs may be seen other than intermittent elevations of blood pressure *(labile hypertension)*. Slowly, widespread pathologic changes take place both in the large and small blood vessels and in the heart, kidneys, and brain.

The large vessels, such as the aorta, coronary arteries, basilar artery to the brain, and peripheral vessels in the limbs, become sclerotic, tortuous, and weak. Their lumina narrow, with resultant decreased blood flow to the heart, brain, and lower extremities. As the damage continues, large vessels may become occluded or may hemorrhage, causing infarction of the tissue supplied by the vessel that has suddenly been robbed of its blood supply.

Small vessel damage, equally dangerous, causes structural changes in the heart, kidneys, and brain. Elevated DBP damages the intimal lining of the small vessels. Because of intimal damage, fibrin accumulates in the vessels, local edema develops, and intravascular clotting may occur. The net results of these changes are (1) a decreased blood supply to the tissues of the heart, brain, kidneys, and retina; (2) progressive functional impairment of these organs; and (3) finally, as a consequence of the chronic ischemia, infarction of the tissue

supplied by these vessels, originating in much the same way as with occlusion of the large vessels.

Clinical Manifestations

In the early stages of development of hypertension, no clinical manifestations are noted by clients or practitioners. Eventually the blood pressure will rise, and if it is not "found" during routine screening, clients will remain unaware that their blood pressure is elevated. If the condition is left undiagnosed, the blood pressure will continue to rise, clinical manifestations will become apparent, and clients will eventually report to a provider's office with complaints of persistent headaches, fatigue, dizziness, palpitations, flushing, blurred or double vision, or epistaxis.

Assessment of the client with hypertension involves the following three main objectives:

- To assess lifestyle and determine the presence of other cardiovascular risk factors or concomitant disorders that can affect prognosis and guide treatment
- To identify the type of hypertension (primary or secondary) and identifiable causes
- To verify the presence or absence of target organ involvement

Clinicians can obtain information relevant to these areas from the history, physical examination, and laboratory studies (Box 52-2). The diagnosis of hypertension is made after the seated client has been allowed to rest for at least 5 minutes and the average of two or more readings separated by at least 2 minutes is 140 mm Hg or higher for the SBP and 90 mm Hg or higher for the DBP. Follow-up examinations are scheduled to diagnose or rule out the presence of hypertension, unless first-visit measurement averages fall into either stage 2 or stage 3. In such cases, the client is diagnosed with hypertension on the basis of the first-visit measurements, and a

temporary management plan is implemented to bring the blood pressure down quickly (see Hypertensive Crises: Urgency Versus Emergency later in this chapter). Careful differentiation of primary from secondary causes of the high blood pressure must precede any long-term management plan.

Hypertension is classified into a prehypertension category and two stages according to blood pressure readings (Table 52-1). It is important to identify "prehypertensive" values because this range of blood pressures is associated with twice the risk of developing hypertension. Clients who are classified as prehypertensive,

---

BOX 52-2   Assessment of the Client with Hypertension

HISTORY

Note the following points when interviewing the hypertensive client:

- Family history of hypertension, diabetes mellitus, cardiovascular disease, hyperlipidemia, or renal disease; smoking; stress; obesity; or sedentary lifestyle.
- Previous documentation of high blood pressure, including age at onset, level of elevation, and currently prescribed medical regimen.
- History of all prescribed and over-the-counter medications and the client's exact compliance with taking the medications. **Note:** Medications that may either raise blood pressure or interfere with the effectiveness of antihypertensive medications include oral contraceptives, steroids, nonsteroidal anti-inflammatory drugs, nasal decongestants, appetite suppressants, cyclosporine, tricyclic antidepressants, monoamine oxidase inhibitors, and erythropoietin.
- History of any disease or trauma to target organs.
- Results and side effects of previous antihypertensive therapy.
- Clinical manifestations of cardiovascular disorders, such as angina, dyspnea, or claudication.
- History of or recent weight gain, exercise activities, sodium intake, fat intake, alcohol use, and smoking.
- Psychosocial and environmental factors (e.g., emotional stress, cultural food practices, economic status) that may influence blood pressure control.

PHYSICAL EXAMINATION

Physical assessment should include an accurate determination of blood pressure as well as an evaluation of target organs:
- Vital signs and weight.
- Blood pressure—because blood pressure is variable and can be affected by multiple factors, it should be measured so that readings are representative of the client's usual level; the following techniques are strongly recommended:
  - The client should be seated with the arm bare, supported, and positioned at heart level. The client should not have smoked tobacco or ingested caffeine within the previous 30 minutes.
  - Measurement should begin after at least 5 minutes of quiet rest. The client's back should be supported, and both feet should be flat on the floor with the legs uncrossed. The client should not speak while the blood pressure is being monitored.

- Use of the appropriate cuff size will ensure an accurate measurement. The rubber bladder should encircle at least 80% of the limb being measured. The bladder's width should be one third to one half the circumference of the limb. Several sizes of cuffs (e.g., child, adult, large adult) should be available.
- Measurements should be taken with a mercury sphygmomanometer, a recently calibrated aneroid manometer, or a validated electronic device.
- Postural blood pressures should be measured and recorded according to position and arm used, including lying, sitting, and standing measurements from both arms.
  - Both systolic and diastolic blood pressures should be recorded. The disappearance of sound (phase V) should be used for the diastolic reading.
  - Two or more readings should be averaged. If the first two readings differ by more than 5 mm Hg, additional readings should be obtained.
- Funduscopic examination for retinal arteriolar narrowing, hemorrhages, exudates, and papilledema.
- Examination of the neck for distended veins, carotid bruits, and enlarged thyroid.
- Auscultation of the heart for increased heart rate, dysrhythmias, enlargement, precordial impulses, murmurs, and S_3 and S_4 heart sounds.
- Examination of the abdomen for bruits, aortic dilation, and enlarged kidneys.
- Examination of extremities for diminished or absent peripheral pulses, edema, and bilateral inequality of pulses.
- Neurologic evaluation for signs of cerebral thrombosis or hemorrhage.

LABORATORY STUDIES

Studies used in the routine evaluation of hypertension include a complete blood cell count, urinalysis, determinations of serum potassium and sodium levels, fasting blood glucose level, serum cholesterol level, blood urea nitrogen and serum creatinine levels, electrocardiogram, and chest radiography. These tests provide useful information in determining the severity of vascular disease, the extent of target organ damage, and the possible causes of hypertension. Clients with the potential for secondary hypertension may need more extensive studies.

TABLE 52–1 Classification and Management of Blood Pressure for Adults*

BP Classification	SBP* (mm Hg)	DBP* (mm Hg)	Lifestyle Modification	Initial Drug Therapy Without Compelling Indication	Initial Drug Therapy With Compelling Indications
Normal	<120	and <80	Encourage		
Prehypertension	120-139	or 80-89	Yes	No antihypertensive drug indicated	Drug(s) for compelling indications‡
Stage 1 hypertension	140-159	or 90-99	Yes	Thiazide-type diuretics for most May consider ACEI, ARB, BB, CCB, or combination§	Drug(s) for compelling indications‡
Stage 2 hypertension	≥160	or ≥100	Yes	Two-drug combination for most† (usually thiazide-type diuretic and ACEI or ARB or BB or CCB)	Other antihypertensive drugs (diuretics, ACEI, ARB, BB, CCB) as needed

*Treatment determined by highest BP category.
†Initial combined therapy should be used cautiously in those at risk for orthostatic hypotension.
‡Treat clients with chronic kidney disease or diabetes to BP goal of <130/80 mm Hg.
§ACEI, Angiotensin-converting enzyme inhibitor; ARB, angiotensin receptor blocker; BB, beta-blocker; CCB, calcium channel blocker; DBP, diastolic blood pressure; SBP, systolic blood pressure.
From National High Blood Pressure Education Program, National Institutes of Health, National Heart, Lung and Blood Institute. (2003). *The Seventh Report of the Joint National Committee on Detection, Evaluation, and Treatment of High Blood Pressure.* Bethesda, Md: U.S. Government Printing Office.

particularly those who have additional risk factors, should be informed that they are at risk of developing hypertension and that they should institute appropriate lifestyle modifications.

Risk Stratification

Risk stratification (Box 52-3) of clients with hypertension is accomplished after assessing each individual for the type and number of major risk factors and the presence or absence of target organ damage (TOD) or clinical cardiovascular disease (CCD). Target organs, sometimes called *end organs,* are the body organs likely to be damaged by untreated disease (e.g., brain, eyes, kidneys).

OUTCOME MANAGEMENT

The goal of management is to normalize blood pressure and reduce risk factors in order to control the progression of the hypertension. The goal is to lower SBP below 140 mm Hg (goal of ≤120 mm Hg) and DBP below 90 mm Hg (goal of ≤80 mm Hg) while modifying and controlling risk factors. For clients with diabetes or progressive renal disease, the goal is <130/80 mm Hg (or 125/75 mm Hg for clients with renal disease and proteinuria >1 g/24 hour).

Long-term compliance and adherence has emerged as the most essential element in reducing morbidity and mortality rates associated with hypertension. The most pronounced positive client outcomes have resulted from a systematic, multifactorial, multidisciplinary team approach for primary and secondary prevention and management of hypertension using diverse qualified health care professionals. Multidisciplinary teams can provide the most comprehensive, cost-effective care of clients with a multitude of prevention and management

needs, including those related to the prevention, diagnosis, and management of hypertension.

Unfortunately, poor compliance with or adherence to antihypertensive therapy persists as one of the most frustrating blocks to effective therapeutic management

BOX 52-3 Cardiovascular Risk Stratification

MAJOR RISK FACTORS
- Hypertension*
- Smoking
- Age (>55 for men; >65 for women)
- Diabetes mellitus*
- Physical inactivity
- Dyslipidemia*
- Gender (men and postmenopausal women)
- Obesity (BMI ≥30)*
- Family history of cardiovascular disease: women <65 years or men <55 years
- Microalbuminuria or estimated GFR <60 ml/min

TARGET ORGAN DAMAGE/CLINICAL CARDIOVASCULAR DISEASE (TOD/CCD)
- Heart diseases
  - Left ventricular hypertrophy
  - Angina/prior myocardial infarction
  - Prior coronary revascularization
  - Heart failure
- Stroke or transient ischemic attack
- Nephropathy
- Peripheral arterial disease
- Retinopathy

*Components of metabolic syndrome.
Modified from National High Blood Pressure Education Program, National Institutes of Health, National Heart, Lung and Blood Institute. (2003). *The Seventh Report of the Joint National Committee on Detection, Evaluation, and Treatment of High Blood Pressure.* Bethesda, Md: U.S. Government Printing Office.

and is often due to clients' belief systems and values. Poor compliance or adherence is the reason that more than two thirds of clients with hypertension do not have adequate control of their blood pressure. For example, clients may choose not to have the initial prescription filled; successfully initiate therapy only to abandon it after a few weeks or months; or comply with only part of the regimen, thus failing to achieve optimal control.

Normalizing Arterial Pressure

The ultimate factors in evaluating whether the correct choice of treatment regimen has been made are as follows: the desired "control" blood pressure is reached, treatment choices are tolerated and safe, and the client is willing to *commit* to the regimen over the long term.

Lifestyle Modifications

Strong research evidence has illustrated conclusively that lifestyle modifications are effective in lowering blood pressure and reducing cardiovascular risk factors at little overall cost and with minimal risk. According to the *JNC VII* (Figure 52-1), lifestyle modifications are suggested as definitive first-line therapy for some clients, at least for the first 6 to 12 months after the initial diagnosis.

Lifestyle modification is also strongly encouraged as adjunctive therapy for all clients with hypertension who are receiving pharmacologic therapy. Continued healthy lifestyle practices, along with pharmacologic therapy, can reduce the number and dosage of antihypertensive medications needed to manage the condition.

Weight Reduction

Excess body weight, exhibited by a body mass index (BMI)—weight in kilograms divided by height in meters squared—of 27 or greater, correlates closely with elevated blood pressure. Also, excess body fat accumulated in the torso with a waist circumference of 35 inches or greater for women and 40 inches or greater for men has been associated with an increased risk for hypertension (waist/hip ratio). For many people with hypertension whose body weight is more than 10% greater than ideal, weight reduction of as little as 10 pounds can lower blood pressure up to 10 mm Hg. Weight reduction also enhances the effectiveness of antihypertensive medications. Therefore reassess the client's blood pressure during weight loss, and make appropriate changes in pharmacologic interventions as needed.

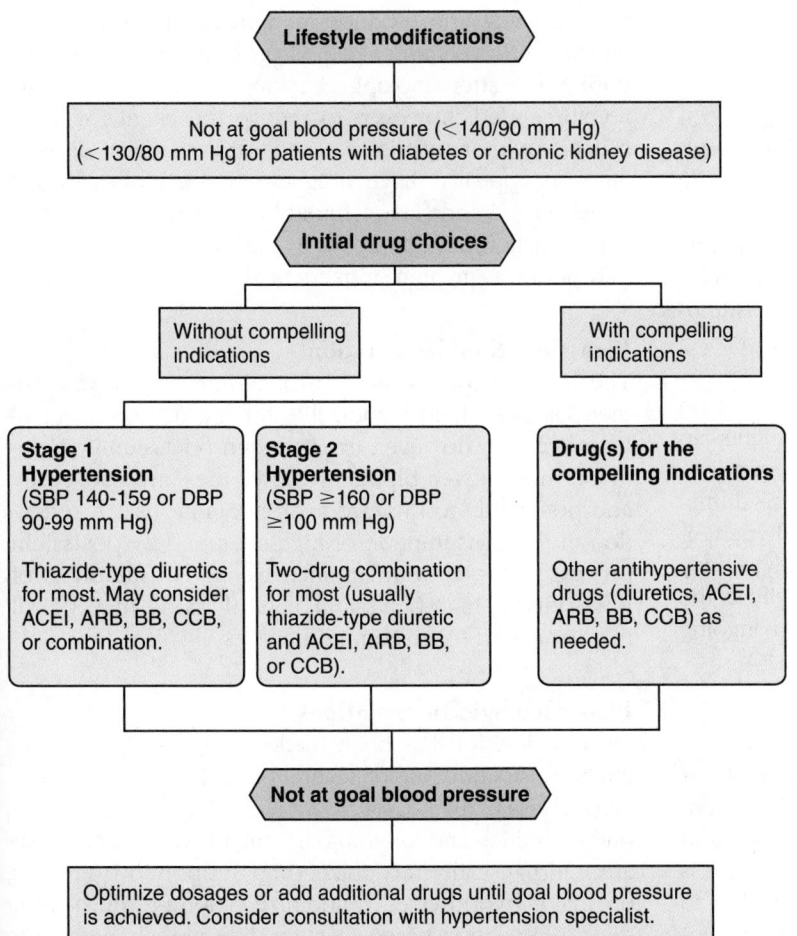

■ **FIGURE 52–1** Algorithm for treatment of hypertension. *ACEI*, Angiotensin-converting enzyme inhibitor; *ARB*, angiotensin receptor blocker; *BB*, beta-blocker; *CCB*, calcium channel blocker; *DBP*, diastolic blood pressure; *SBP*, systolic blood pressure. *(From National High Blood Pressure Education Program, National Institutes of Health, National Heart, Lung and Blood Institute. [2003]. The Seventh Report of the Joint National Committee on Detection, Evaluation, and Treatment of High Blood Pressure. Bethesda, Md: U.S. Government Printing Office.)*

Sodium Restriction

Most hypertensive people are sensitive to sodium, showing rises in BP after sodium intake. Therefore, a moderate restriction of sodium intake to 2 or 3 g of sodium can be used to lower blood pressure. The amount of medication otherwise needed may be decreased if sodium intake is lowered. In addition, this moderate sodium restriction may reduce the degree of potassium depletion that often accompanies diuretic therapy.

Dietary Fat Modification

Modification of dietary intake of fat by decreasing the fraction of saturated fat and increasing that of polyunsaturated fat has little, if any, effect on decreasing blood pressure but can decrease the cholesterol level significantly. Because dyslipidemia is a major risk factor in the development of atherosclerosis, diet therapy aimed at reducing lipids is an important adjunct to any total dietary regimen. In addition to the usual recommendations for sensible eating following the food pyramid (see Chapter 1), the Dietary Approaches to Stop Hypertension (DASH) diet (Table 52-2), which is rich in fruits, vegetables, nuts, and low-fat dairy foods with reduced saturated and total fats, should be recommended for clients who need a more structured, fat-limited dietary intervention.

Exercise

A regular program of aerobic exercise adequate to achieve at least a moderate level of physical fitness facilitates cardiovascular conditioning and can aid the obese hypertensive client in weight reduction and reduce the risk for cardiovascular disease and all-cause mortality. Blood pressure can be reduced with moderate-intensity (as low as 40% to 60% of maximum oxygen consumption) physical activity, such as a brisk walk (about 2.5 to 3 mph) for 30 to 45 minutes most days of the week.

Weight training using *light* weights is a positive addition to any exercise regimen; however, lifting *heavy* weights can be harmful because blood pressure rises, sometimes to high levels, with the vasovagal response that occurs during an intense isometric muscle contraction. Advise hypertensive clients to initiate exercise programs gradually, slowly increasing the intensity and the duration of activity as the body adjusts and becomes more conditioned with ongoing professional surveillance.

Alcohol Restriction

The consumption of more than 1 ounce of alcohol per day is associated with a higher prevalence of hypertension, poor adherence to antihypertensive therapy, and occasionally refractory hypertension. Carefully assess alcohol intake. Advise clients who do drink alcohol to do so in moderation (i.e., no more than 1 ounce of ethanol per day for men and 0.5 ounce for women). There is 1 ounce (30 ml) of ethanol in 2 ounces (60 ml) of 100-proof whiskey, in 10 ounces (300 ml) of wine, or in 24 ounces (720 ml) of beer.

Caffeine Restriction

Although acute ingestion of caffeine may raise blood pressure, chronic moderate caffeine ingestion appears to have no significant effect on blood pressure. Therefore caffeine restriction is not necessary unless cardiac response or other excessive sensitivity to caffeine is present.

Relaxation Techniques

A variety of relaxation therapies, including transcendental meditation, yoga, biofeedback, progressive muscle relaxation, and psychotherapy, can reduce blood pressure in hypertensive clients, at least transiently. Although each modality has its advocates, none has been conclusively shown to be either practical for the majority of hypertensive clients or effective in maintaining a significant long-term effect.

Smoking Cessation

Although smoking has not been statistically linked to the development of hypertension, nicotine definitely increases the heart rate and produces peripheral vasoconstriction, which does raise arterial blood pressure for a short time during and after smoking. Smoking cessation is strongly recommended, however, to reduce the client's risk for cancer, pulmonary disease, and cardiovascular disease. Smokers appear to have a higher frequency of malignant hypertension and subarachnoid hemorrhage. In addition, risk reduction brought about by antihypertensive therapy may not be as great in smokers as in nonsmokers.

Potassium Supplementation

The high ratio of sodium to potassium in the modern diet has been held responsible for the development of hypertension; however, even though potassium supplements may lower blood pressure, they are too costly and potentially too hazardous for routine use. A reduction in the consumption of high-sodium, low-potassium processed foods with an increase in consumption of low-sodium, high-potassium natural foods may be all that is needed for maximum benefits.

Pharmacologic Interventions

Once a decision has been made to use pharmacologic intervention, any one of several drugs from seven major drug classes can be used. Table 52-1 and Figure 52-1 outline initial and ongoing treatment suggestions that are internationally recognized and supported by results of major worldwide, randomized, long-term clinical trials. Prevention-based healthy lifestyle change with

TABLE 52-2 Dietary Approaches to Stop Hypertension (DASH) Diet

The DASH eating plan shown below is based on 2000 calories per day. Depending on your caloric needs, your number of daily servings in a food group may vary from those listed. This eating plan is from the Dietary Approaches to Stop Hypertension (DASH) clinical study supported by the National Institutes of Health. The DASH combination diet lowered blood pressure and so may help prevent and control high blood pressure.

Food Group	Daily Servings (Number)	Serving Size	Examples	Significance of Each Food Group to DASH Diet Pattern
Grains and grain products	7-8	1 slice bread; ½ cup dry cereal; ½ cup cooked rice, pasta, or cereal*	Whole wheat breads, English muffin, pita bread, bagel, cereals and fiber, grits, oatmeal	Major source of energy and fiber
Vegetables	4-5	1 cup raw, leafy vegetable; ½ cup cooked vegetable; 6 oz vegetable juice	Tomatoes, potatoes, carrots, peas, squash, broccoli, turnip greens, collards, kale, spinach, artichokes, beans, sweet potatoes	Rich sources of potassium, magnesium, and fiber
Fruits	4-5	6 oz fruit juice; 1 medium fruit; ¼ cup dried fruit; ½ cup fresh, frozen, or canned fruit	Apricots, bananas, dates, grapes, oranges, orange juice, grapefruit, grapefruit juice, mangoes, melons, peaches, pineapples, prunes, raisins, strawberries, tangerines	Important sources of potassium, magnesium, and fiber
Low-fat or nonfat dairy foods	2-3	8 oz milk; 1 cup yogurt; 1.5 oz cheese	Fat-free or 1% milk, skim or low-fat buttermilk, nonfat or low-fat yogurt, part skim mozzarella cheese, nonfat cheese	Major sources of calcium and protein
Meats, poultry, fish	2 or less	3 oz cooked meats, poultry, or fish	Select only lean; trim away visible fats; broil, roast, or boil, instead of frying; remove skin from poultry	Rich sources of protein and magnesium
Nuts, seeds, and legumes	4-5/wk	1.5 oz or ⅓ cup nuts; ½ oz or 2 tbsp seeds; ½ cup cooked dry beans	Almonds, filberts, mixed nuts, peanuts, walnuts, sunflower seeds, kidney beans, lentils, and peas	Rich sources of energy, magnesium, potassium, protein, and fiber
Fats and oils[†]	2-3	1 tsp soft margarine; 1 tbsp low-fat mayonnaise; 2 tbsp light salad dressing; 1 tsp vegetable oil	Soft margarine, low-fat mayonnaise, light salad dressing Vegetable oil (such as olive, corn, canola, or safflower)	Besides considering the fats added to foods, choose foods that contain less fat
Sweets	5/wk	1 tbsp sugar; 1 tbsp jelly or jam; ½ oz jelly beans; 8 oz lemonade	Maple syrup, sugar, jelly, jam, fruit-flavored gelatin, jelly beans, hard candy, fruit punch, sorbet ices	Sweets should be low in fat

*Serving sizes vary between ½ and 1½ cups. Check the nutrition label.
[†]Fat content changes per serving size of fats and oil. For example, 1 tbsp regular salad dressing equals 1 serving, 1 tbsp low-fat dressing equals ½ serving, and 1 tbsp fat-free dressing equals zero servings.
Modified from Kolasa, K.M. (1999). Dietary Approaches to Stop Hypertension (DASH) in clinical practice: A primary care experience. *Clinical Cardiology, 22*(7 Suppl), III-16-22.

the addition of pharmacologic therapy as indicated is the preferred treatment regimen for those clients in stages 1 and 2. If therapy is chosen carefully, more than half of mild hypertension cases can be controlled with one or two drugs. Most clients, however, will require two or more drugs to achieve goal blood pressure.

Antihypertensive medications can be classified into the following categories: diuretics, alpha- and beta-adrenergic antagonists [beta-blocker (BB)], vasodilators, calcium antagonists [calcium channel blocker (CCB)], angiotensin-converting enzyme (ACE) inhibitors, and angiotensin receptor blockers (ARBs). Diuretics, particularly thiazide-type diuretics, will continue to be the first line drug of choice for newly diagnosed, low level, uncomplicated hypertension, and BBs will continue to be first-line choices in other selected cases. However, there are compelling and specific indications for two- and three-drug initial and/or subsequent treatment regimes for various conditions.

Provider Responsibilities

The goal of antihypertensive therapy is to control blood pressure with a minimum of side effects (see the Integrating Pharmacology feature on Antihypertensive Medications at right). Clinicians must be currently knowledgeable regarding drug choices and must be able to extrapolate potential side effects or negative effects quickly and effectively to manage clients' blood pressures most successfully, especially if concomitant conditions exist. See a pharmacologic text for detailed descriptions of each drug or drug combination and its actions and side effects. See the Client Education Guide at right and the Concept Map feature on p. 1301.

If more than one drug is necessary, several combination therapies have proved effective. For example, the combination of a diuretic with a beta-adrenergic blocker or other adrenergic inhibitor has been effective in both blacks and whites, in contrast to the responses to the individual drugs, whereas blacks respond less well to beta-adrenergic blockers alone or as first-line treatment. The combination of a diuretic with an ACE inhibitor or a CCB has additive effects on blood pressure. Finally, combination drugs can be less expensive than the individual drugs, and the need for only one drug may improve compliance in a client who does not like "taking so many pills."

Reducing the number and amounts of antihypertensive medications should be considered once a client's blood pressure has been controlled effectively for at least 1 year. Medication dosages must be decreased slowly and progressively until the lowest effective dosages are reached and maintained. Regular follow-up evaluation is essential if drug therapy has been completely stopped secondary to success of weight loss or other lifestyle change practices because blood pressure can rise again over time.

INTEGRATING PHARMACOLOGY

Antihypertensive Medications

It is common to administer more than one antihypertensive along with diuretics for blood pressure control. Usually the use of more than one medication is designed to lower the dose of any single medication and reduce the side effects. However, when administering these medications, it is important to consider their synergistic effects.

Before administering antihypertensives, be certain that you are aware of the most recent blood pressure (BP). Many events during a hospitalization can lower BP, such as blood loss with surgery and pain control with analgesics. Conversely, fluid overload and stress or anxiety can raise BP. It is common to withhold antihypertensives following surgery during times when BP is low. If the BP is high, administer the antihypertensive medications ahead of schedule (e.g., at 0800 rather than waiting until 0900). Also note the pulse rate; beta-adrenergic blockers can lead to bradycardia.

Also make note of the most recent potassium level. Loop diuretics quickly reduce potassium levels, and potassium-sparing diuretics can lead to elevations in potassium levels. Further, aldosterone blocking agents, such as ACE inhibitors and angiotensin receptor blockers, can also lead to hyperkalemia. ACE inhibitors and calcium channel blockers can lead to orthostatic hypotension, and positional BP measurement may be warranted to reduce the risk of falls.

Recent data have shown that the use of beta-adrenergic blockers before surgery has reduced mortality. Therefore you may be asked to administer these medications before surgery even in clients with no history of hypertension or who do not routinely take beta blockers.

CLIENT EDUCATION GUIDE

Ten Ways to Control Your High Blood Pressure

- Know your blood pressure. Have it checked regularly.
- Know what your weight should be. Keep it at that level or below.
- Do not use too much salt in cooking or at meals. Avoid salty foods.
- Eat a low-fat diet according to American Heart Association recommendations.
- Do not smoke cigarettes or use tobacco products.
- Take your medicine exactly as prescribed. Do not run out of pills even for a single day.
- Keep appointments with the doctor.
- Follow your doctor's advice about exercise.
- Make certain that your parents, brothers, sisters, and children have their blood pressure checked regularly.
- Live a normal life in every other way.

From the American Heart Association. (2004). Retrieved 03/18/04 from http://americanheart.org/presenter.jhtml?identifier=578.

CONCEPT MAP

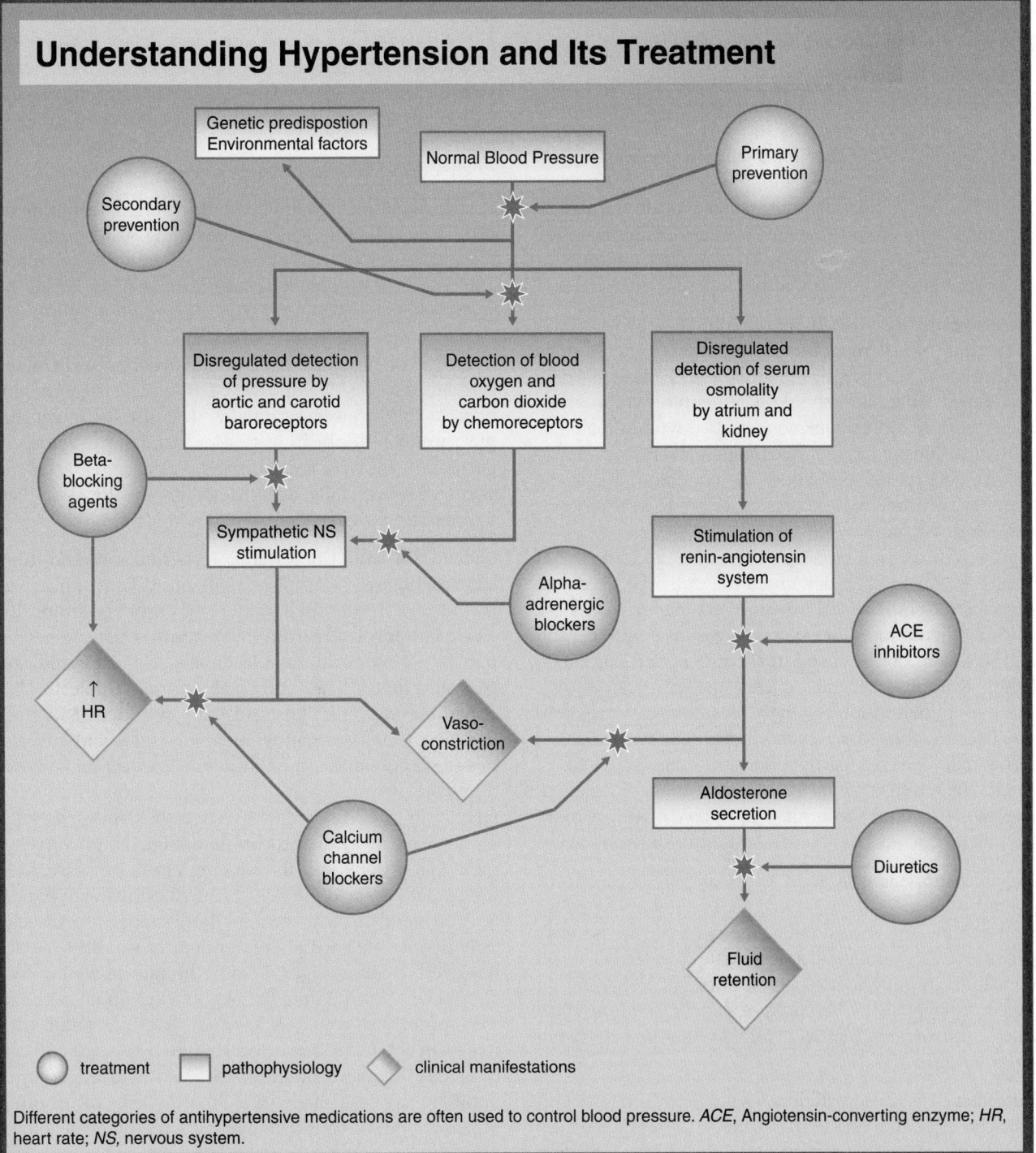

Understanding Hypertension and Its Treatment

Different categories of antihypertensive medications are often used to control blood pressure. *ACE,* Angiotensin-converting enzyme; *HR,* heart rate; *NS,* nervous system.

Nursing Management

Assessment. The many sequelae of untreated hypertension can be prevented, or the severity of such problems reduced, if hypertension is well managed. Client education and understanding are crucial to successful management.

Diagnosis, Outcomes, and Interventions

Diagnosis: Ineffective Therapeutic Regimen Management (Individual). Use the nursing diagnosis *Ineffective Therapeutic Regimen Management (Individual)* to identify the learning needs of the newly diagnosed hypertensive client. The nursing diagnosis can be written *Risk for*

Ineffective Therapeutic Regimen Management (Individual) related to a new diagnosis, no previous learning about the disease process, potential consequences, the rationale for life-long intervention and follow-up, and proper administration of prescribed medications.

Outcomes. The client and significant others will demonstrate knowledge required for self-care as evidenced by (1) describing hypertension and its associated risk factors; (2) discussing the importance of lifelong medical follow-up; (3) listing the prescribed medications, including drug name, rationale for use, dose, frequency, potential side effects, and measures to minimize side effects; and (4) demonstrating the proper technique for blood pressure monitoring at home.

Interventions. Because hypertension is a lifelong disease and has dangerous complications, clients with hypertension need clear, practical, and realistic learning guidelines. Guidelines should include information about hypertension and its management. Use written materials with clear illustrations for teaching the client with newly diagnosed hypertension about the condition. Teach the client to measure blood pressure at home at least once a week and to record the findings in a diary.

When measuring blood pressure, use the correct cuff size. For consistency, document the cuff size used and on which arm the blood pressure reading was assessed. Inform clients of their blood pressure reading, and advise them of the need for periodic measurement. When working with most clients, the examiner should refer to hypertension as *high blood pressure* to help avoid confusion. Many clients unfamiliar with medical terms may believe that hypertension denotes a state of being "hypertense"—that is, being worried or agitated. For these clients, the term *high blood pressure* more accurately conveys the nature of the health problem.

Diagnosis: Imbalanced Nutrition: More Than Body Requirements. Dietary adjustments can reduce the severity of hypertension and in some cases reduce the need for medication. Client teaching about and assessment of needed changes constitute an important aspect of nursing care. Write the nursing diagnosis as *Imbalanced Nutrition: More Than Body Requirements related to high sodium, fat, and total calorie intake.*

Outcomes. The client will demonstrate knowledge of and adherence to the nutritional regimen as evidenced by describing specific dietary modifications (including sodium, fat, and calorie restrictions) and explaining their rationales (reduction in levels of urine sodium and blood cholesterol, weight loss). (See the Client Education Guide features on Low-Sodium Diet, on Low-Fat, Low-Cholesterol Diet, and on Calorie-Restriction Diet on the website.)

Interventions. The two most important aspects of dietary intervention for hypertension are weight reduction (for overweight clients) and mild to moderate sodium restriction. Therefore advise the client with hypertension to eat a diet low in salt, calories, cholesterol, and saturated fat. Discuss the prescribed diet with the household members who prepare food. If possible, enlist the aid of a dietitian to provide detailed dietary instructions. Before dietary intervention begins, assess the client's patterns of food intake; lifestyle; food preferences; and ethnic, social, cultural, and financial influences. A highly individualized approach to dietary counseling is crucial to client compliance and adherence.

Restrict Sodium. Sodium is a hidden ingredient in many processed foods, beverages (including water from certain sources), and over-the-counter drugs (particularly antacids, cough remedies, and laxatives). It cannot be seen and often is not tasted. The average adult daily intake of salt is 5 to 15 g, but the therapeutic effects of sodium reduction on blood pressure do not occur until salt intake is reduced to 6 g/day or lower. Low-salt diets can be difficult to follow, at least initially. Reassure the client that dietary adherence becomes easier as the palate adjusts to decreased salt over several weeks to months. After the client becomes fully accustomed to the low-salt diet, unsalted foods usually cease to taste bland.

Reduce Fat and Cholesterol. Hypertension and high serum cholesterol levels (>250 mg/dl) are linked as risk factors in the development of coronary artery disease. The level of serum cholesterol is determined in part by the consumption of cholesterol, saturated and polyunsaturated fats, and total calories. Cholesterol is contained in animal fats and dairy products. Saturated fats occur predominantly in animal fats and tropical oils (e.g., coconut and palm oils). Unsaturated fats predominate in most plant-derived fats. Polyunsaturated fats occur predominantly in vegetable and seed oils. A diet low in saturated fats and high in polyunsaturated fats is beneficial in reducing blood pressure. (See the DASH diet in Table 52-2.) Not all clients with hypertension need to lose weight. As discussed previously, only people with a BMI greater than 27 should consider the need to lose weight. Ideally the rate of weight loss should be no more than 0.25 kg -0.5 kg (about one-half to 1 pound) a week. Advise the average adult with hypertension to reduce caloric intake by at least 250 calories/day. Caution the client to avoid over-the-counter appetite suppressants because these preparations often contain sympathomimetic agents, which elevate blood pressure.

Diagnosis: Ineffective Health Maintenance. Exercise is like dietary management: A regular exercise program can lower blood pressure in hypertensive clients. This nursing diagnosis can be written as *Ineffective Health Maintenance related to a lack of regular exercise regimen.*

Outcomes. The client will begin and maintain an appropriate exercise program as evidenced by self-report, demonstration of the ability to monitor heart rate during exercise, sensation of reduced physical and emotional stress, and reduced blood pressure.

Interventions. Exercise programs can heighten the client's sense of well-being, provide an outlet for emotional tension, produce relaxation of blood vessels, and raise the levels of high-density lipoproteins (HDLs) relative to total blood cholesterol. Elevated HDL levels are associated with a decreased risk of cardiovascular morbidity and mortality. Instruct the client, however, to avoid heavy weight-lifting, isometric exercises, and other activities inappropriate to the client's physical limitations. A modest but consistent exercise program provides greater benefits than those obtainable with spurts of strenuous activity mixed with periods of inactivity. A gradually increasing program of aerobic activity such as walking, jogging, or swimming can thus be recommended.

Maximum heart rate is calculated by subtracting the client's age from 220. Most clients without diagnosed heart disease or other concomitant conditions can safely exercise to 75% to 85% of the maximal heart rate. Clients with known cardiopulmonary disease and hypertension must be prescreened; a cardio-respiratory exercise stress test is most predictive of cardiopulmonary and exercise functional capacity. An *individualized* target heart rate can be designated from objective data obtained from this test that will allow the client to maximize his or her aerobic exercise. Ultimately, before an exercise prescription is advised and initiated for a hypertensive client, a qualified specialist must conduct a careful performance evaluation.

Diagnosis: Risk for Nonadherence. The greatest problem in the management of chronic hypertension involves the client's lack of adherence to nonpharmacologic and pharmacologic interventions. An estimated 40% to 60% of clients with hypertension fail to comply with prescribed therapy. There are several reasons why hypertensive clients do not follow prescribed regimens:

- The asymptomatic nature of the disease tends to minimize the perceived seriousness of the problem and importance of intervention.
- Therapeutic regimens often demand difficult lifestyle changes, such as low-sodium diets, weight loss, and smoking cessation.
- Many hypertensive agents produce annoying side effects, and clients who require antihypertensive medication may consider the intervention worse than the disease.
- The high cost of medications and the inconvenience of obtaining health care also contribute to noncompliance.

Assess the reasons for possible nonadherence, and then state the nursing diagnosis as *Risk for Nonadherence related to a lack of understanding about the seriousness of high blood pressure, cost of therapy, side effects of* *medications, complexity of management,* or *multiple changes in lifestyle.*

Outcomes. The client will actively participate in creating a treatment plan, describing the underlying causes of hypertension and self-care strategies, adhering to scheduled follow-up appointments, describing the actions and side effects of current medications, and expressing commitment to and self-responsibility for controlling hypertension.

Interventions. Nursing interventions for promoting adherence to the antihypertensive treatment regimen include individualizing care, ensuring adequate follow-up, communicating often with the client, and teaching the client and the client's family. Adherence usually improves dramatically when the client understands the causative factors underlying hypertension as well as the consequences of inadequate intervention and health maintenance.

Evaluation. Medications can lower blood pressure quickly. The remainder of the interventions, such as stress management, exercise, and smoking cessation, are more difficult to implement and maintain. Expect the client to struggle with compliance with any and all of the necessary changes in medications and/or lifestyle. Ask specific questions in a nonjudgmental manner. As needed, recommend involvement in various self-help groups, such as smoking cessation groups.

Modifications for Older Clients

Hypertension is one of the most prevalent cardiovascular diseases among older adults, and because of their advanced age, these clients are more likely to suffer from end-organ damage secondary to chronically elevated pressure.[7,14] Blood pressure readings in older adults show greater variability from one measurement to the next compared to younger clients; therefore the diagnosis is made after several readings. Recent research findings indicate a need to treat hypertension in older people, regardless of whether both the SBP *and* DBP are involved or there is evidence of only isolated systolic hypertension. Older adults are more likely to experience adverse reactions to antihypertensive drugs and are monitored closely for evidence of such reactions; they are given detailed advice on the specifics of their medication regimens; and the clinical course of the disease is carefully followed.

The ultimate goal of antihypertensive therapy in older adults is not to try to lower the pressure to "normal" values immediately but rather to lower the pressure gradually to a level sufficient to eliminate target organ damage and to minimize the risk of hypoperfusion. "Start low and go slow" is the principle followed for prescribing medications to the older adult. Too rapid a reduction in blood pressure in older clients, particularly those with chronic hypertension, may produce cerebral hypoperfusion that manifests by decreased mental status, weakness, and dizziness.

HYPERTENSIVE CRISES: URGENCY VERSUS EMERGENCY

Elevated blood pressure alone, in the absence of clinical manifestations or new or progressive target organ damage, rarely requires *emergency* therapy. In most cases the hypertensive crisis really constitutes a hypertensive *urgency* in which a severe elevation in blood pressure has been reached but there is mild or no acute target organ damage. Hypertensive urgencies include cases in which it is desirable to reduce blood pressure within a few hours to 24 hours. Clinicians treat urgent situations primarily with oral medications in an outpatient setting with close follow-up.

Because many clients have chronically elevated blood pressure that has not been diagnosed, the seriousness of any crisis correlates not so much with the level of blood pressure elevation as with the extent of target organ damage secondary to length of time the blood pressure has remained significantly high. Clients who qualify for emergent care are hospitalized, given intravenous medications, and monitored closely for at least 12 to 24 hours.

Without treatment persistent severe hypertension results in a 90% death rate within 1 year secondary to renal or heart failure, stroke, myocardial infarction, or aortic dissection. The most common cause of persistent severe hypertension is untreated hypertension. Other causes include eclampsia, dissecting aortic aneurysm, pyelonephritis, sudden catecholamine release (as from a pheochromocytoma), drug or toxic substance ingestion or exposure, and food and drug interactions (e.g., between a monoamine oxidase inhibitor [MAO] and aged cheese).

Clinical manifestations include those of hypertensive encephalopathy evidenced by restlessness, changes in level of consciousness (e.g., confusion, somnolence, lethargy, memory defects, coma), seizures, blurred vision, dizziness, headache, nausea, and vomiting. Assessment may also reveal renal insufficiency, proteinuria, hematuria, urinary sediment casts, hemolytic anemia, left ventricular failure, and pulmonary edema. Severe headache may be occipital or anterior in location, is steady and throbbing, and is often worse in the morning. Visual blurring, reduced visual acuity, and even blindness can occur. Acute renal failure, rapid vascular deterioration, and stroke can also develop.

OUTCOME MANAGEMENT

The initial goal of therapy in hypertensive crisis is to reduce mean arterial pressure by no more than 25% within the first minutes to 2 hours. Then a reduction in blood pressure toward 160/100 mm Hg is accomplished over the next 2 to 6 hours.

SAFETY

⚠

ALERT

Blood pressure is monitored frequently (every 5 to 15 minutes, depending on the drug and the route of administration used), and medications are titrated to manage the course of blood pressure reduction. It is essential to avoid excessive falls in blood pressure, which can precipitate renal, cerebral, or coronary ischemia.

Consequently restoration of normal blood pressure must be done slowly and with care. Once the client is out of immediate danger, oral medications are adjusted while vital signs are monitored continuously, and changes in drug therapy regimens are made if necessary. NOTE: Although sublingual administration of nifedipine had been widely used to reduce blood pressure in an urgent situation, it is no longer considered appropriate therapy because of several reports of severe adverse effects from its use.

COMMUNITY SCREENING AND SELF-CARE

Public Health Initiative

Research showing the importance of normalized blood pressure for clients' optimum health led to the introduction by the National Heart, Lung and Blood Institute (NHLBI) of the National High Blood Pressure Education Program (NHBPEP) in 1972. The NHBPEP is the first large-scale public outreach and education campaign to reduce high blood pressure. Its promotion of the detection, treatment, and control of high blood pressure has been credited with influencing the dramatic increase in the public's understanding of hypertension and its role in heart attacks and strokes.

The prevention and treatment of hypertension continue to be a major public health concern in the United States. Prevention of hypertension and early discovery of new cases depend on a broader national public health effort. With guidance from the *Healthy People/2010* initiatives, this national effort has begun. In addition to the diligent work of the NHBPEP, government support is increasing, and nationwide attention and assistance from business and industry, labor organizations, health care institutions, voluntary associations, and local communities are also on the rise. For example, the *JNC VII* guideline endorses the American Public Health Association (APHA) resolution challenging food manufacturers and restaurants to reduce sodium in foods by 50% over the next decade.

The following are the revised goals of the national public health plan:

- To prevent the rise of blood pressure with age
- To decrease the existing prevalence of hypertension
- To increase hypertension awareness and detection
- To improve control of hypertension
- To reduce cardiovascular risks
- To increase recognition of the importance of controlled isolated systolic hypertension
- To improve recognition of the importance of the persistence and damage from high-normal blood pressures
- To reduce ethnic, socioeconomic, and regional variations in hypertension
- To improve opportunities for treatment
- To enhance community programs

Managed Care and Community Screening

Because high blood pressure is so common, its management requires a major commitment from clinicians and managed care organizations. Managed care programs offer the opportunity for a coordinated systematic, multi-factorial, multidisciplinary approach to care. Nurse-managed clinics offer attractive opportunities to improve adherence and outcomes.

Hypertensive clients usually learn of their condition through incidental screening in health care facilities or through organized community screening in public settings (e.g., shopping malls, schools, and the workplace). Nurses are actively involved in both approaches. About 80% of Americans come into contact with some aspect of the health care system at least once a year (e.g., in a health care provider's office, clinic, or hospital). Each encounter with the health care system presents an opportunity for incidental blood pressure screening. Blood pressure measurement should be a routine procedure at every initial encounter with a health care practitioner and annually thereafter.

Organized community screening programs help to assess the remaining 20% of Americans not in contact with any part of the health care system. Such programs identify not only clients with untreated hypertension but also those who have discontinued intervention or whose hypertension is not adequately controlled by current intervention. In addition, screening programs provide an opportunity to educate the public. It is particularly important to screen members of high-risk "target groups," such as black and older populations. Community services need to keep target groups in mind when choosing the setting for blood pressure screenings. Practitioners who take blood pressure readings need to inform clients in writing of their blood pressure and its significance and, if necessary, the importance of follow-up evaluation. Culturally and linguistically appropriate counseling by health care providers is important to those efforts.

Self-Measurement of Blood Pressure

Measurement of blood pressure outside a health care provider's office can provide valuable information for initial evaluation and subsequent follow-up of people with hypertension. Most drug, medical supply, and grocery stores provide standardized blood pressure monitors that their customers can use at no cost. These monitoring stations are generally located near the pharmacy or medical supplies department. Such stores also usually carry a variety of self-measurement blood pressure devices for home use. Choosing a monitoring device may be confusing for some people; however, several models of accurate and appropriate electronic or aneroid-type sphygmomanometers are available. Most insurance packages cover the cost of a home blood pressure unit, and these devices are generally easy to use.

Manual and electronic arm cuffs are the most accurate. Finger and wrist monitors are available but have proved inaccurate in standardized testing. Periodically, the accuracy of the instrument used in the home should be checked by comparing home readings with those obtained in the health care provider's office, at a "health fair," or in a community nursing clinic. It is helpful if the client keeps a record of BP values; these findings will help with follow-up care.

SYNCOPE

Syncope (fainting) is defined as generalized muscle weakness and an inability to stand erect accompanied by loss of consciousness. It is a good measure of cardiovascular status because it may indicate decreased cardiac output, fluid volume deficits, or defects in cerebral tissue perfusion.

Syncope is a common occurrence when a person tries to stand after being bedridden for a while. This form of syncope, called *postural hypotension,* can be seen in clients attempting to ambulate the first few times after surgery, in clients who have been on prolonged bed rest, and in clients who have dysrhythmias. When a person moves quickly to a standing position, blood normally pools in the lower legs. The arterial pressure receptors in the aortic arch detect the fall in cardiac output that occurs with the lack of venous return, and they increase sympathetic tone to compress arterioles to improve venous return. If the sympathetic response is not adequate or is blocked by medication, the person becomes dizzy because of the decreased cerebral perfusion. All medications taken to reduce blood pressure have the potential to cause orthostatic hypotension or postural hypotension—some more than others, such as potent diuretics, alpha$_1$-receptor blockers, and vasodilators.

> **When a client reports dizziness or is at risk of syncope because of medication use or prolonged bed rest, assess fluid volume status and check the pulse for irregularities.**

 SAFETY ALERT

If syncope develops, it usually can be managed by having the client move slowly to a sitting position and rest a moment before standing. If the client becomes dizzy, instruct the client to breathe deeply and to keep both eyes open. Syncope should resolve within moments. If it is prolonged, place the client supine, use leg exercises to improve venous return, and wait until the blood pressure returns to a normotensive state.

> **Confused clients who do not wait for syncope to resolve before walking are at risk for falls. Bed alarms may be needed.**

 SAFETY ALERT

CONCLUSIONS

New coalitions between health care providers and individual communities are forming to focus on the prevention and management of hypertension throughout all stages of life. Support from the community and greater use of technology such as the Internet will play an increasingly greater role in promoting long-term adherence to lifestyle and pharmacologic regimens. Achieving long-term control of blood pressure risk factors requires that the same interest and attention given to initial evaluation and treatment decisions also be given to long-term lifestyle management issues. In addition, *JNC VII* has taken a strong stance toward mandating better pharmacologic control of high blood pressure. In their report, *JNC VII* stated that clinicians' failure to titrate or combine medications, despite knowing that a client's blood pressure is not at goal, represents clinical inertia and must be overcome.

THINKING CRITICALLY

1. A 50-year-old obese black man arrives at your clinic with persistent elevated blood pressure. He has had hypertension for 7 months. Despite attempts at lifestyle management, his blood pressure has continued to rise. He was started on a regimen of antihypertensive medication 1 month ago and has returned to the clinic today for a follow-up visit. His blood pressure is higher than it was initially. What might explain his continued elevated blood pressure?

Factors to Consider. What other history and physical examination data should you obtain to analyze this case more effectively? When and how long should lifestyle modifications alone be encouraged? How long does it take for various medications to be effective? What diseases worsen hypertension? What psychosocial factors affect compliance with or adherence to a treatment regimen? What modifications in the pharmacologic treatment plan, if any, would be most appropriate at this time?

Discussions for these questions can be found on the website.

BIBLIOGRAPHY

 Citations appearing in red refer to primary research.

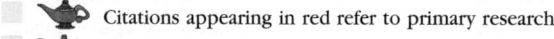 Citations appearing in blue refer to evidence-based practice guidelines and protocols.

1. Ades, P.A. (2001). Cardiac rehabilitation and secondary prevention of coronary heart disease. *New England Journal of Medicine, 345,* 892-902.
2. Agodoa, L.Y., et al. (2001). Effect of ramipril vs amlodipine on renal outcomes in hypertensive nephrosclerosis: A randomized control trial (AASK). *Journal of the American Medical Association, 285,* 2719-2728.
2a. American Heart Association. (2006, December). *Controlling blood pressure: Hypertension among United States adults 1999-2004.* Retrieved November 19, 2007, from www.heart.org/print_presenter.jhtml?identifier=3044518.
2b. Barlow, C.E., LaMonte, M.J., FitzGerald, S.J., et al. (2006). Cardiorespiratory fitness is an independent predictor of hypertension incidence among initially normotensive healthy women. *American Journal of Epidemiology, 163*(2),142-150.
3. Brenner, B.M., et al. (2001). Effects of losartan on renal and cardiovascular outcomes in patients with type 2 diabetes and nephropathy. *New England Journal of Medicine, 345,* 861-869.
4. Cardiac Rehabilitation Guideline Panel. (1995). *Cardiac rehabilitation* (AHCPR Pub. No. 96-0672). Rockville, Md: Agency for Health Care Policy and Research, Public Health Services, U.S. Department of Health and Human Services.

5. Davidson, M.H. (2002). Strategies to improve adult treatment panel III guideline adherence and patient compliance. *The American Journal of Cardiology 89*(Suppl), 8C-22C.
6. DeMartinis, J. (2001). Relaxation and stress management. In D. Robinson & C.P. Kish (Eds.), *Core concepts in advanced practice nursing.* St. Louis: Mosby.
7. DeMartinis, J. (2003). Principles and methods of the basic physical examination. In R. Jones & R. Rospond (Eds.), *Patient assessment in pharmacy practice.* Baltimore, Md: Lippincott Williams & Wilkins.
8. DeMartinis, J.E., Uphold, C.R., & Graham, M.V. (2003). Cardiovascular problems. In C.R. Uphold & M.V. Graham (Eds.), *Clinical guidelines in adult health* (3rd ed.). Gainesville, Fla: Barmarrae Books.
8a. Dengel, D.R., Brown, M.D., Reynolds, T.H. IV, Supiano, M.A. (2006). Effect of aerobic exercise training on renal responses to sodium in hypertensives. *American College of Sports Medicine, 217-222.* Retrieved November 19, 2007, from www.acsm-msse.org.
9. Epperly, T.D., & Fogarty, J.P. (2001). Syncope. In M.B. Mengel & L.P. Schwiebert (Eds.), *Ambulatory medicine: The primary care of families* (3rd ed.). New York: Lange Medical Books/McGraw-Hill.
10. Furberg, C.D., et al. (2001). Clinical implications of recent findings from the Antihypertensive and Lipid-Lowering Treatment to Prevent Heart Attack Trial (ALLHAT) and other studies of hypertension. *Annals of Internal Medicine, 135,* 1074-1078.
11. Isaacsohn, J., et al. (2002). The impact of the national cholesterol education program adult treatment panel III guidelines on drug development. *The American Journal of Cardiology, 89*(Suppl), 45C-49C.
11a. Margolis, K.L., Piller, L.B., Ford, C.E., et al. (2007). Blood pressure control in Hispanics in the Antihypertensive and Lipid-Lowering Treatment to Prevent Heart Attack Trial. *American Heart Association, 50,* 854-861.
12. McGowan, M.P. (2002). Lipid-lowering therapy in women: New treatment options. *Cardiology Review, December,* 1-12.
13. National Cholesterol Education Program (NCEP), National Institutes of Health, National Heart, Lung and Blood Institute. (2001). *Executive summary of the third report of the National Cholesterol Education Program (NCEP) Expert Panel on detection, evaluation, and treatment of high blood cholesterol in adults (Adult Treatment Panel III)* (NIH Publ. No. 01-3305). Bethesda, Md: U.S. Government Printing Office.
14. National High Blood Pressure Education Program, National Institutes of Health, National Heart, Lung and Blood Institute. (2003). *The Seventh Report of the Joint National Committee on Detection, Evaluation, and Treatment of High Blood Pressure.* Bethesda, Md: U.S. Government Printing Office.
15. Nutrition Committee of the AHA. (2000). AHA dietary guidelines: Revision 2000: A statement for healthcare professionals from the nutrition committee of the American Heart Association. *Circulation, 102,* 2284-2299.
15a. Ong, K.L., Cheung, B.M., Man, Y.B., et al. (2007). Prevalence, awareness, treatment, and control of hypertension among United States adults 1999-2004. *American Heart Association, 49,* 69-75.
16. Opie, L. (1991). *Drugs for the heart* (3rd ed.). Philadelphia, Saunders.
17. Pasternak, R. (2002). Adult treatment panel II versus adult treatment panel III: What has changed and why? *American Journal of Cardiology, 89*(Suppl), 3C-7C.
18. Rader, D. (2002). Lipid disorders. In E.J. Topol (Ed.), *Textbook of cardiovascular medicine* (2nd ed.). Philadelphia: Lippincott Williams & Wilkins.
19. U.S. Department of Health and Human Services. (2000). *Healthy People 2010: National health promotion and disease prevention objectives.* Washington, DC: U.S. Public Health Service.

evolve **Did you remember to check out the bonus material on the Evolve website and the CD-ROM, including NCLEX®-Examination Style Review Questions, Open-Book Quizzes, and Chapter Review Audio Podcasts?**

CHAPTER 53

Management of Clients with Vascular Disorders

JOYCE M. BLACK

PERIPHERAL ARTERY DISORDERS

Peripheral vascular disease (PVD) includes disorders of the arterial, venous, and lymphatic systems. In clinical settings, the term *PVD* is usually used to describe peripheral arterial disease. PVD is increasingly common and has the potential to cause loss of limb or, occasionally, life.

Etiology and Risk Factors

Peripheral arterial occlusive diseases are primarily caused by atherosclerosis, a complex and chronic inflammatory process that slowly occludes the elastic and muscular arteries. The atherosclerotic process gradually may progress to complete occlusion of medium and large arteries.

Primary risk factors for atherosclerosis include diabetes, smoking, hypertension, obesity, and elevated blood lipid levels. Phlebitis, surgery, and autoimmune disease are other risk factors. Clients with PVD often have other forms of atherosclerosis, such as coronary artery disease, myocardial infarction, atrial fibrillation, carotid stenosis, stroke, or renal disease.

Arteries can be occluded acutely from embolism, thrombosis, trauma, vasospasm, or edema. Multiple factors increase risk of thromboses including obesity, sepsis, hypotension, low cardiac output, aneurysms, aortic dissection, bypass grafts, and underlying atherosclerotic narrowing of the arterial lumen. Emboli, the most common cause of sudden ischemia, usually are of cardiac origin during periods of atrial fibrillation, but they also can originate from proximal atheroma, tumor, or foreign objects. Emboli tend to lodge at artery bifurcations or in areas where vessels abruptly narrow such as the femoral artery bifurcation.

Pathophysiology

The progressive nature of atherosclerosis slowly starves the tissues of oxygenated blood. Collateral arterioles develop to attempt to compensate for the occluded arterial supply. However, collateral vessels develop slowly. During the interim, vasodilation and anaerobic pathways are used to meet oxygen and nutrient demands. Vasodilation has a limited effect because arteries that become oxygen-deprived quickly become maximally dilated. Cellular anaerobic metabolism tries to meet the basic requirements, but the waste products of lactic acid and pyruvic acid build up quickly, are extremely toxic, and are excreted slowly.

Stenosis, the narrowing of a vessel, is progressive. The physiologic effect of any given stenosis is variable because it is determined not only by the degree of narrowing but also by the amount of collateral vessels that have developed. However, continued lack of arterial flow eventually results in pain. The pain is called *intermittent claudication* and is analogous to anginal pain. Intermittent claudication occurs when a muscle is forced to work without an adequate blood supply to meet its metabolic demands. Remember, muscles are metabolically active and use aerobic metabolism; therefore without blood they resort to anaerobic metabolism.

Clinical Manifestations

The process of atherosclerosis is insidious and the clinical manifestations of chronic arterial occlusion may not appear for 20 to 40 years.

evolve **Web Enhancements**

Client Education Guide   Foot Care (Spanish Translation)

Stump and Prosthesis Care (Spanish Translation)

Be sure to check out the bonus material on the Evolve website and the CD-ROM, including free self-assessment exercises. **http://evolve.elsevier.com/Black/medsurg**

Intermittent Claudication

The most important subjective manifestations of chronic arterial occlusive disease are *intermittent claudication* and *rest pain*. The client typically reports pain described as tightening pressure in the calves or buttocks or a sharp cramp or burning sensation that occurs during walking and disappears with rest. Claudication also may present as the hip or leg "giving out" after a certain period of exertion. The pain of claudication usually does not occur with sitting or standing. Claudication generally occurs in men, although there is an increased incidence in women after menopause. Usually, claudication strikes men in their sixth or seventh decade. Nearly half of clients who experience claudication also have associated severe coronary artery disease (Table 53-1).

Intermittent claudication is worsened by the speed or incline of the walk, conditions that increase the demand for oxygen by muscles of the legs. The more rapid the speed or the greater the incline, the faster claudication occurs. The client's exercise tolerance generally decreases over time; episodes of claudication occur with less exertion. Claudication response is constant, reproducible, and not positional. Reproducible means that the client who walks the same distance at the same speed and incline has manifestations at the same distance each time. The client who cannot walk the length of a house because of leg pain one day but can walk indefinitely the next day does not have intermittent claudication.

PVD can occur along any portion of the arterial system. Aortoiliac stenosis and occlusion result in hip, thigh, and buttock claudication with absent or diminished femoral and distal pulses (Figure 53-1). In males, impotence is also part of the syndrome, known as *Leriche syndrome*. A superficial femoral artery and popliteal occlusion leads to calf claudication, which may improve, stay the same, or potentially progress to rest pain. Popliteal artery disease and stenosis in the anterior or posterior tibial artery result in claudication in the distal leg and foot.

Rest Pain

As the disease progresses, clinical manifestations become more severe. The development of pain at rest, usually occurring at night when the client lies supine, indicates limb-threatening disease. Usually described as a dull, deep pain in the toes or forefoot, this sensation awakens the client from sleep and may cause the client to hang the foot over the side of the bed or get up and walk around for relief. The client may start to sleep in a chair with legs dependent. Placing the leg in a dependent position provides increased gravitational supply of blood. This often results in a moderate degree of lower extremity edema. The affected foot usually demonstrates dependent rubor. Ischemic rest pain often is exacerbated by poor cardiac output. PVD may also be acutely compounded by either emboli or thrombi. Many people live daily with PVD; however, in situations such as acute limb ischemia, the disease can be life-threatening and can require emergency intervention to minimize morbidity and mortality.

Lower extremity pain may also occur in several other disorders unrelated to arterial disease. Other conditions that cause a similar type of pain include arthritis, lumbar disk protrusion, neuritis, and muscle cramps. However, the pain of other conditions is not consistent, reproducible, or positional.

Paresthesias with exertion indicate ischemia of the peripheral nerves because of the phenomenon of *arterial steal*. This phenomenon occurs as arterioles of the muscles are maximally dilated because of hypoxia. To meet muscular metabolic needs, these arterioles steal from cutaneous and peripheral nerve vessels, which results in coldness and a "pins and needles" sensation.

Decreased Pulses

Objective data associated with arterial insufficiency include weak or absent peripheral pulses, low ankle-brachial index (ABI) scores (see p. 1287), dependent rubor and pallor with elevation, hypertrophied toenails, coolness of the skin, hairlessness of the extremity, tissue atrophy, ulceration, and gangrene (Figure 53-2). Dependent rubor is a dusky, purplish discoloration of the foot and leg when the foot is placed in a dependent position. This *dependent rubor* changes to white pallor when the leg is elevated. Dependent rubor is common when aortoiliac and femoropopliteal disorders are combined. Mottling, paralysis, and paresthesias tend to occur in limb-threatening conditions and prompt care to restore blood flow is required.

TABLE 53-1	Manifestations of Arterial Insufficiency
Type of Data	**Manifestations**
Subjective	Exertional pain
	Nocturnal pain
	Ischemic rest pain
	Claudication manifestations
	Foot, calf, thigh, or buttock pain
	Pain worse with exertion
	Pain relieved with several minutes rest
	Pain relieved with dependent position
Objective	Decreased skin temperature
	Shiny skin
	Skin hairless over lower extremity (e.g., shin)
	Dystrophic toenails
	Distal extremity color change with position
	Skin pallor when leg elevated
	Skin rubor when leg dependent
	Bilateral leg diminished pulses throughout
	Slow wound healing in legs
	Impotence

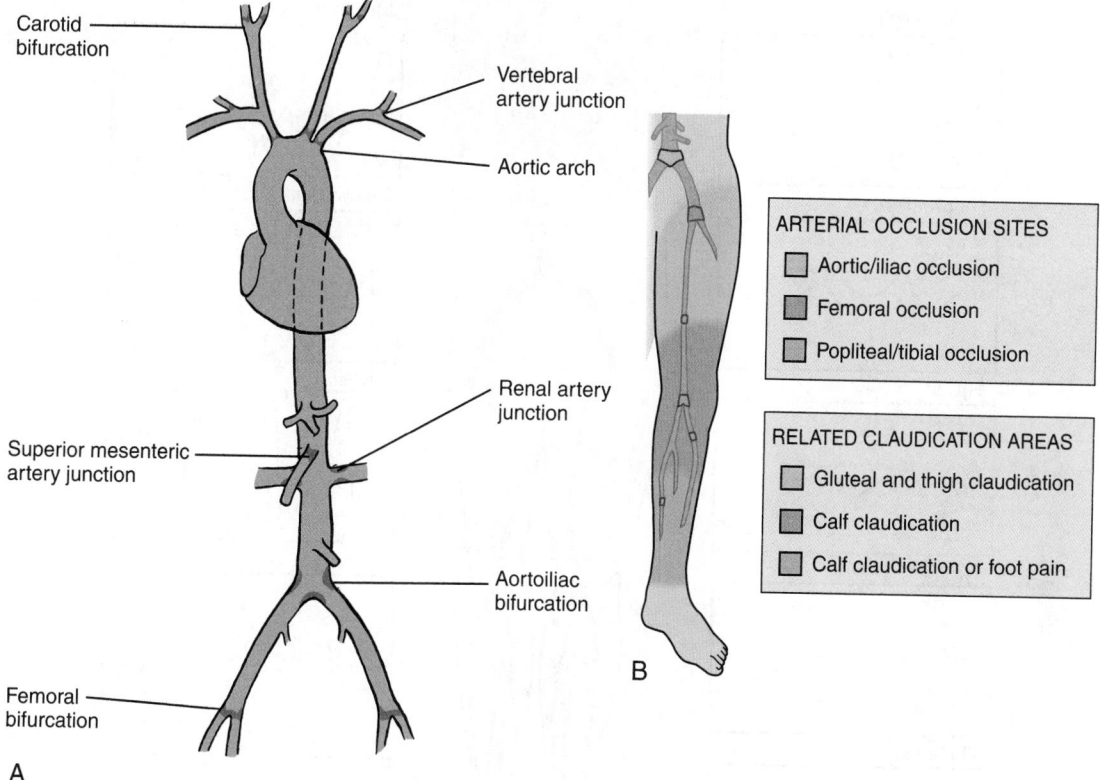

Carotid bifurcation

Vertebral artery junction

Aortic arch

Renal artery junction

Superior mesenteric artery junction

Aortoiliac bifurcation

Femoral bifurcation

A

B

ARTERIAL OCCLUSION SITES
- ☐ Aortic/iliac occlusion
- ☐ Femoral occlusion
- ☐ Popliteal/tibial occlusion

RELATED CLAUDICATION AREAS
- ☐ Gluteal and thigh claudication
- ☐ Calf claudication
- ☐ Calf claudication or foot pain

■ **FIGURE 53–1   A,** Major sites of peripheral atherosclerotic occlusive disease. **B,** Specific patterns of claudication in distal tissues.

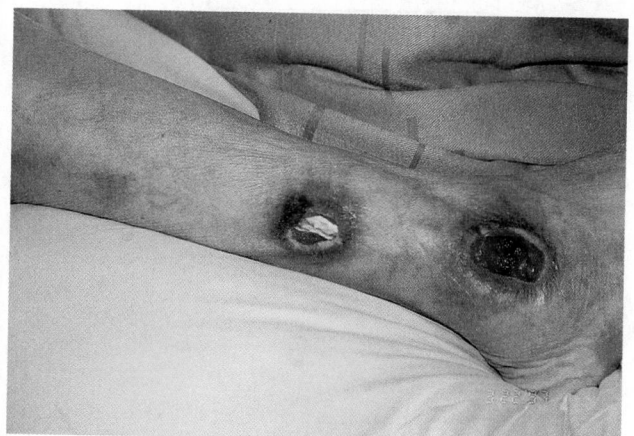

■ **FIGURE 53–2**   Arterial ulcers of the foot. Note the pale, hairless appearance of the leg and the smooth, round shape of the ulcers.

Delayed Wound Healing

Even small or shallow wounds do not heal because of the lack of arterial blood flow. The physician should be made aware of the presence of wounds.

Laboratory findings may reveal abnormal lipid profiles. If the renal arteries are involved, elevated levels of urea nitrogen and creatinine may be noted. An elevated level of total homocysteine (tHcy) in blood is emerging as a prevalent and strong risk factor for atherosclerotic vascular disease in the coronary, cerebral, and peripheral vessels, and for arterial and venous thromboembolism.

Diagnostic Evaluation

Diagnostic evaluation of the lower extremity includes both noninvasive and invasive techniques. ABI can be measured at the bedside. Using Doppler ultrasonography, the systolic pressure both at the brachial artery and at the posterior tibialis artery is measured. The ankle systolic pressure is divided by the brachial pressure, with both measured in the supine position. Normally, the ratio is more than 1. Comparison with ABI in the opposite extremity is helpful to determine the degree of ischemia. ABI is not accurate in diabetic clients using the ankle pulsation; pulsation in the great toe can be used instead.

Doppler ultrasound studies can determine the quality of blood flow (Figure 53-3). The femoral, popliteal, dorsalis pedis, and posterior tibial arteries are evaluated in the lower extremities. The axillary, brachial, ulnar, and radial arteries are evaluated in the arms. The shape of the waveform (i.e., monophasic, biphasic, triphasic) provides data on the presence of disease. A monophasic waveform can indicate proximal stenosis or occlusion in the iliac vessels. The biphasic or triphasic waveform is normal and occurs when the main blood vessels in the leg are elastic and dilated by the increased pressure during systole.

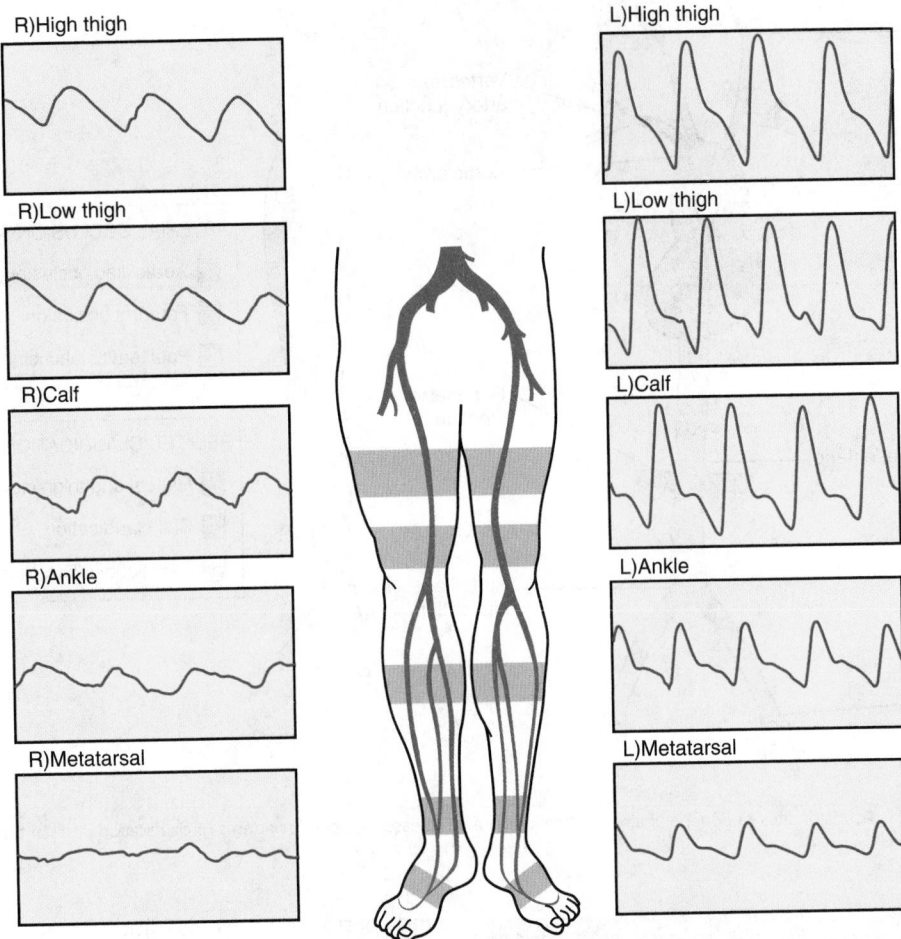

R)High thigh

L)High thigh

R)Low thigh

L)Low thigh

R)Calf

L)Calf

R)Ankle

L)Ankle

R)Metatarsal

L)Metatarsal

■ **FIGURE 53–3** Duplex ultrasound of a normal lower extremity (left leg) and one from a client with rest pain (right leg). *(From Townsend, C.M., Jr., Beauchamp, R.D., Evers, B.M., Mattox, K.L. [2004]. Sabiston textbook of surgery [17th ed.]. Philadelphia: Saunders.)*

Transcutaneous oximetry measures tissue levels of oxygen and carbon dioxide, providing data on impairments of flow in both large and small vessels.

Treadmill examination, a form of lower extremity stress testing, measures the decrease of arterial pressure with ambulation and the rapidity with which it returns to baseline. Color flow imaging visualizes the blood flow in the vessels and records pressures within the vessel.

Arteriography is the definitive examination when surgery is being considered. Arteriography shows the lumen of the blood vessels. It is not a measurement of actual blood flow like the noninvasive assessment, but instead shows the outline of the contrast media within the lumen. Use of contrast media, however, contributes to risk of many potential complications especially renal insufficiency.

OUTCOME MANAGEMENT

Medical Management

The goals of medical management are to reduce the risk of progressive arterial disease, to promote arterial flow,

and to save the limb for clients with intermittent claudication and non–limb-threatening ischemia. Additionally, medical management may be the only course of action in the client with multiple morbidities and who is a poor surgical risk.

Promote Arterial Flow

Pentoxifylline (Trental) has been reported to decrease blood viscosity and increase red cell flexibility, thereby increasing peripheral blood flow. Several studies have shown that pentoxifylline increases the duration of exercise in clients with claudication. Cilostazol has also been shown to increase walking distance. It works as a vasodilator and has antiplatelet properties. Platelet inhibitors, such as aspirin and clopidogrel, are used to reduce the risk of embolism in clients with PVD. New medications including L-arginine, which is the precursor of the endothelium-dependent vasodilator nitric oxide, and vasodilator prostaglandins are being studied.

In severe cases of arterial insufficiency, the physician may order reverse Trendelenburg position; this can be achieved by placing the head of the client's bed on 6-inch blocks (or heavy books such as encyclopedias) so that blood from the heart flows more easily to the extremities whenever the client sleeps or rests. Fleece boots may also be used to keep the feet warm and protected from injury. Float the heels from the bed to prevent pressure ulcers.

Reduce Risk

Because of the chronic nature of PAD, all clients are provided with information to reduce their risk of continued ischemia and injury to the peripheral leg and foot.

Smoking Cessation

The importance of stopping cigarette smoking cannot be overemphasized. Cigarette smoke is a potent vasoconstrictor, further impairing blood flow to the extremities. Clients who are able to stop smoking successfully improve their treadmill walking distance. Smoking cessation is extremely difficult, because nicotine is a highly addictive chemical. Social support, especially of friends and family members, seems to be an important factor in assisting smokers to quit their habit. Pharmacologic measures may be instituted by the primary care provider, if necessary. Educate clients about the dangers of cigarette smoke, encourage them to stop smoking, act as role models for nonsmoking, and support policies to prohibit smoking in the workplace. Primary care providers should question clients each time they visit about their desire to quit and the need to quit. (See Chapter 62 for techniques to help with smoking cessation.)

Control of Comorbid Diseases

Diabetes, obesity, hypertension, and lipid abnormalities should all be well controlled to slow the progression of the disease. Clients are advised and counseled to reduce body weight by following a low-fat, low-cholesterol diet containing more fruits and vegetables. Interventions for lowering blood lipid levels are recommended for clients with hyperlipidemia. The initial step for lowering cholesterol level is to reduce calorie intake to achieve ideal body weight. If weight loss is seen as improbable, the client should try to maintain current weight.

The next major step is to reduce the total fat intake in the diet to 30% or less of total calories. Saturated fat intake should be reduced. The most common sources of saturated fat in the American diet are red meat, fried foods, and dairy products, especially whole milk and cheese. Increasing the quantity of fish and poultry and changing to skim milk and nonfat cheese may be sufficient to meet saturated fat recommendations.

The third major goal is to reduce intake of cholesterol, which is found in egg yolks, organ meats, shellfish, and animal meats. Increasing dietary fiber, especially soluble fiber, such as that found in oats, lentils, and beans, has a beneficial effect on lipid levels. Fast foods, snack foods, and restaurant dining account for a large amount of the increased fat intake in the United States. Dietary counseling by a registered dietitian is a helpful intervention for clients and families who are attempting to change eating habits. See other chapters for treatment of diabetes (Chapter 45) and hypertension (Chapter 52).

Exercise

A prescribed moderate program of exercise and rest reduces claudication. Supervised exercise for 30 to 45 minutes 3 times a week for 12 weeks on a treadmill or track improves claudication by changing the metabolism in muscles, altering the endothelium of the vessels, and improving the gait. Improvements are not due to increased collateral circulation as once thought. The exercise program should begin slowly with the client stopping at the onset of pain and progress gradually until the client has substantially lengthened walking distances. For obese and chronically ill clients, it is important that an exercise program (1) be individually tailored to the client's abilities, goals, interests, and resources and (2) be written with specific instructions. Most clients can significantly increase their walking distance, and many can avoid surgery if they exercise regularly and stop smoking.

Prevention of Injury

As a result of poor blood flow to the feet, supportive measures include meticulous care of the skin. Feet should be kept clean and protected against excessive drying with moisturizing creams. Well-fitting and protective shoes are advised to reduce trauma. Sandals and shoes made of synthetic materials that do not "breathe" should be avoided. Elastic support hose should be avoided, because they reduce blood flow to the skin. In clients with ischemia at rest, "shock blocks" under the head of the bed together with a canopy over the feet may improve perfusion pressure and ameliorate some of the rest pain.

Nursing Management of the Medical Client

Assessment. The history should include questions regarding arterial disease, surgery, medications, and ulcerations. Some clients are not aware of chest pain, shortness of breath, or fatigue because their attention is focused on leg discomfort. Question them carefully about these discomforts. Because of the chronic nature of the problem, perform a psychosocial assessment. Clients may have feelings of powerlessness.

The physical examination should include peripheral pulses (begin with dorsalis pedis, then proceed proximally to the posterior tibial, popliteal, and femoral until a pulse is found); ABI; quality of arterial flow assessed with a hand-held Doppler instrument; notations of skin color, skin temperature, and level of hair on the leg; and assessment of skin integrity (including the presence of ulcers, darkened areas of skin, tinea pedis, or thickened nails), capillary refill time, and the presence of venous filling when the foot is dependent.

The Management and Delegation feature below provides additional information for ongoing assessment of clients with vascular disorders.

Diagnosis, Outcomes, Interventions

Diagnosis: Ineffective Peripheral Tissue Perfusion. The ideal nursing diagnosis for clients with arterial disorders is *Ineffective Peripheral Tissue Perfusion.* Write the diagnosis as *Ineffective Tissue Perfusion related to interruption of blood flow secondary to arterial occlusion.*

Outcomes. The client will maintain adequate peripheral tissue perfusion to affected extremities as evidenced by improvement from baseline of skin color, skin temperature, pulse rate measurements, and level of pain.

Interventions

Promote Arterial Flow. Position clients with arterial disease so that blood flows toward the legs and feet.

MANAGEMENT AND DELEGATION

Management of Clients with Vascular Disorders

Clients with peripheral vascular disorders require frequent monitoring and observation of the neurovascular status (NV) of their affected extremities. Likewise, you will implement interventions to minimize pressure and swelling to the affected extremity. Following your initial assessment and implementation of protective measures in an affected extremity, you may deem it appropriate to delegate the routine monitoring and recording of NV status to an unlicensed assistant.

Your baseline assessment establishes the NV status, including skin temperature, skin color, presence and location of pulses, sensation, and skin integrity. Skin integrity, especially overlying bony prominences like the heels, ankles, and elbows, is at especially high risk for compromise and breakdown and deserves close assessment. Pulses are best noted by marking their location with a waterproof marker, noting whether they are palpable or audible by Doppler.

Inform your assistants of the initial findings and instruct them to notify you of any changes in skin color or temperature, quality or detection of pulses, altered sensation (e.g., "pins and needles"), or client report of pain in the extremity. Assistants can help ensure protective measures are maintained by providing heel protectors, using pillows to elevate the heels from the bed, and implementing other pressure-reducing devices.

Perform ongoing assessment of your client as your institution and the client's clinical condition dictates. Changes in assessment may necessitate a change in delegation considerations. Vascular clients may have postoperative dressings on their affected extremities. Delegation considerations in the care of postoperative clients are described in Chapter 14 and apply in this population as well.

In milder cases, clients can benefit from simply sitting for periods of time with their feet flat on the floor. If reverse Trendelenburg position is used, assess for dependent edema. Remind clients with arterial insufficiency to avoid raising their feet above heart level unless the physician has specifically prescribed this as an exercise.

Explain the dangers of smoking to the client who uses tobacco. Encourage the client to stop smoking completely. The client who realizes that smoking literally threatens life and limbs may develop sufficient motivation to abstain permanently. Help the client locate therapy groups or biofeedback training. Do not advise the use of nicotine patches. Patches provide continuous administration of nicotine and thereby can cause continuous vasospasm.

Encourage the client to avoid stressful situations and to relax, both mentally and physically. Counseling services may be indicated for nervous, "high-strung" clients. Offer information regarding stress reduction classes. Involve significant others.

Prevent the client from becoming chilled. Stockings should be worn to keep the legs warm. Clients should wear protective clothing in layers during cold weather, warm their cars before entering them, and follow winter driving precautions (e.g., not running out of gas).

Be certain that the client understands how to take antiplatelet medications. The effect of these drugs is augmented by other anticoagulants including self-prescribed medications. Side effects often include gastrointestinal upset or bleeding when using aspirin.

Reduce Risk. Nurses should encourage the client to follow all risk reduction programs. These changes are prescribed for life and should be incorporated into daily living. This amount of change can be stressful and clients should be allowed to express their frustration at the changes prescribed, but also strongly encouraged to continue with them.

Diagnosis: Acute Pain. Intermittent claudication is caused by ischemia. The nursing diagnosis can be written *Acute Pain related to inadequate arterial blood supply to the legs.*

Outcomes. The client will experience increased comfort, as evidenced by self-report and demonstrated knowledge of pain reduction measures, both pharmacologic and nonpharmacologic.

Interventions. The pain of ischemia is usually chronic, continuous, and difficult to relieve. Arterial leg ulcers are exquisitely painful. Because of pain, clients with arterial disorders are often depressed and irritable. Pain limits their activities, disturbs their sleep, saps their energy, and has a demoralizing emotional effect. Thus pain must be reduced if the client is to rest and improve.

Help clients assess and plan ways of correcting the position of their beds at home. The head of the bed can be elevated to promote blood flow to the legs. Remind the client with arterial insufficiency of the following points:

- Avoid standing in one position for more than a few minutes.
- Avoid crossing the legs at the knees.
- In general, seek the most comfortable position.
- Watch for and report edema.

Any measure that increases circulation to the extremities helps alleviate ischemic pain. Although pain also can be subdued by analgesics, interventions that augment circulation are best. When strong analgesics, such as morphine, are necessary around the clock, the client may require amputation. Amputation can improve the quality of life by diminishing pain and improving mobility with a prosthesis.

Diagnosis: Risk for Impaired Skin Integrity. Because of altered peripheral tissue perfusion, the client is at risk of arterial ulceration and skin infection. Write the diagnosis as *Risk for Impaired Skin Integrity related to decreased peripheral circulation.* If the client has an arterial ulcer, this diagnosis can still be used for the remaining intact skin.

Outcomes. The client will reduce risk of skin impairment as evidenced by maintaining soft skin, protecting skin from trauma, and showing no signs of skin injury. If the client has an open wound, see later information in this chapter.

Interventions. Prevent injury to the extremities, particularly the feet. Excellent foot care should be an integral part of the daily routine of clients with peripheral vascular disorders, because prevention is easier to initiate and maintain than is correction. For bedridden clients, use fleece leg wraps or cotton stockings to keep the feet warm and reduce friction injury. The Client Education Guide below summarizes client instructions.

CLIENT EDUCATION GUIDE

Foot Care

CLIENT INSTRUCTIONS

Daily Hygiene

- Do not soak your feet; use mild soap and a washcloth to clean them.
- Dry well between your toes.
- Check water temperature with a bath thermometer or your elbow, not your toes, to prevent burns; 32.2° to 35° C (90° to 95° F) is safe.
- Gently rub corns or calluses. Avoid cutting, digging, or using harsh commercial products.

Daily Inspection and Lubrication

- Use good lighting.
- Put on your glasses or contacts, if you wear them.
- Promptly report ulcerations, redness, calluses, blisters, or cracking of the skin on the feet or thickening of the nails to the physician.
- Rub soothing lotions or lanolin on your hands, feet, legs, and arms to prevent dryness.
- Do not use lotion on sores or between your toes.
- Do not use perfumed lotions.
- Dust your feet lightly with cornstarch if they sweat.

Care of Toenails

- Use clippers, not scissors or razor blades.
- Cut straight across the nail.
- Do not perform "bathroom surgery."
- If your eyesight is poor or if you are unable to reach your toes, find qualified assistance.
- Place lamb's wool between overlapping toes.

Proper Footwear

- Never go barefoot, not even at the beach or at home.
- Avoid high heels and shoes with pointed toes.

- Make sure nothing is in your shoes before putting them on your feet.
- Avoid tight socks and shoes.
- Wear cotton socks for absorbency. Change your socks daily.
- Alternate several pairs of comfortable, firm, well-made shoes during the week.
- Avoid shoes that cause your feet to perspire (for example, canvas shoes and rubber boots).
- Make sure that your shoes and slippers fit well and are sturdy enough to prevent foot injury.

Safety

- Avoid sunburn.
- Avoid scratching insect bites on your legs to prevent creating open lesions.
- Do not use heating pads.
- Wear adequate foot protection on cold days.
- Turn on the lights before entering a dark hallway or room.
- Avoid sitting with your legs crossed.
- Use a cane or walker, if indicated.
- When in doubt, ask for help. Have telephone numbers of people who can assist you at hand.

Activity

- Walking is good, but get your physician's permission before beginning a regular program.
- Do not walk if you have open ulcerations.
- Walk until pain begins, stop and rest, and then begin again.
- Elevate your feet if they swell.
- Find a nurse and a physician who will get to know you and your foot problems and will take the time to talk with you when you need help.

Diagnosis: Risk for Activity Intolerance. Intermittent claudication may greatly deter activity. This common nursing diagnosis is written as *Risk for Activity Intolerance related to leg pain after walking.*

Outcomes. The client will develop appropriate levels of activity free from pain and excess fatigue, as evidenced by normal vital signs, absence of pain, and verbalized understanding of the benefits of gradual increase in activity and exercise.

Interventions. When assisting the client with a walking program, assert that *pain* should be the guide to the amount of activity to be undertaken. Intermittent claudication signals that the muscles and tissues of the legs are not receiving enough oxygen.

SAFETY ⚠ ALERT

Before the client begins a walking program, take a careful history and perform a physical assessment. Establish a cardiopulmonary profile and carefully examine the client's feet and legs to locate open ulcerations or anatomic deformities. The client should have sturdy shoes to prevent foot trauma.

Although exercise helps most clients with vascular disorders, some clients must not exercise. These clients have leg ulcers, pain at rest, cellulitis, deep vein thrombosis, or gangrene. Exercise and activity increase the metabolic needs of tissues and, consequently, tissue requirements for oxygenated blood. Thus clients with tissue breakdown or necrosis must remain for a period of time on complete bed rest. Even minimal activity raises the oxygen requirements of the tissues above that which damaged arteries can provide.

Diagnosis: Deficient Knowledge. The nursing diagnosis *Deficient Knowledge* can be used as a guide to teaching the client about a walking program. State the nursing diagnosis as *Deficient Knowledge related to walking program as evidenced by no previous experience.*

Outcomes. The client will develop and follow a progressive walking program.

Interventions. Remind clients that at first it may be painful to walk any distance and that they may need to stop frequently to rest. Walking on a track or treadmill is the best way to start exercising. Encourage them to walk in enclosed shopping malls in the winter for safety from falls on icy pavement and to avoid vasoconstriction from the environment. In the summer, walking in the malls helps avoid heat exhaustion or stress on other conditions such as heart disease. Clients should walk through the pain as much as possible without causing undue distress. It is important to stress that small increments of exercise increase are not dramatic, but rather are evidence of improvement. Even improvement to the point of being able to shop in the grocery store is a cause for celebration.

Diagnosis: Health-Seeking Behaviors. Health-conscious clients may request information about self-improvement and interventions to reduce the severity of manifestations. Write the nursing diagnosis as *Health-Seeking Behaviors related to lack of knowledge about the role of exercise, weight reduction, and smoking cessation in management of arterial disease.*

Outcomes. The client will begin and maintain the chosen health promotion program, as evidenced by demonstrated knowledge of the specific activities of the program, regular evaluation of goals against performance, and verbalized feelings of increased well-being.

Interventions. Instruct the client in areas of concern or interest. Refer to the nonpharmacologic intervention methods described earlier. Also refer to the Complementary and Alternative Therapy features below and on p. 1315. Refer the client to groups in the community if available. The client with intermittent claudication caused by arterial disease should be routinely reexamined at least every 3 months for progression of disease.

Evaluation. Arterial disorders are chronic, so do not expect to see reversal of the problems. Write outcomes that allow for time and client adjustments.

Modifications for Older Clients

Age-related changes and impairments of physiologic function along with arterial disease affect the nursing diagnoses of *Activity Intolerance* (possibly increased), *Altered Peripheral Tissue Perfusion* (possibly reduced),

COMPLEMENTARY AND ALTERNATIVE THERAPY

Vitamin E Supplements and Peripheral Vascular Disease

Recent data on the ability of vitamin E supplements to reduce the risk of cardiovascular disease have not shown a positive effect. For example, the Heart Outcomes Prevention Evaluation (HOPE) trial was a 4.5-year randomized controlled clinical trial of vitamin E or placebo in 9541 clients ages 55 years or older with a history of coronary artery disease (CAD), stroke, peripheral vascular disease, or diabetes and other cardiovascular disease risk factors. No difference was noted between vitamin E (400 international units/day) and placebo for the outcomes of stroke, death, or other cardiac outcomes for these high-risk clients.

REFERENCE

Yusuf, S., et al. (2000). Vitamin E supplementation and cardiovascular events in high-risk patients. The Heart Outcomes Prevention Evaluation (HOPE) study investigators. *New England Journal of Medicine, 342,* 154-160.

Antioxidant Vitamins to Reduce Cardiovascular Disease

Researchers attempted to determine whether dietary supplements reduce death, vascular events, and cancer in clients with a high 5-year risk for death. In a randomized, blinded, placebo-controlled trial with a mean follow-up of 5 years in the setting of 69 United Kingdom hospitals, 20,536 clients ages 40 to 80 years (28% were 70 years of age or older, and 75% were men) were studied. A total of 10,269 clients received antioxidant supplements (synthetic 600 mg/day of vitamin E, plus 250 mg/day of vitamin C, plus 20 mg/day of beta-carotene) and 10,267 received placebo. There was no difference in outcome between the group taking antioxidant supplements and those taking placebo. In clients with a high 5-year risk for death, antioxidant supplements did not reduce mortality or the occurrence of coronary events, stroke, vascular events, or cancer.

REFERENCE

MRC/BHF Heart Protection Study Group. (2002). MRC/BHF Heart Protection Study of antioxidant vitamin supplementation in 20,536 high-risk individuals: A randomized placebo-controlled trial. *Lancet, 360*, 23-33.

and *Pain* (acute or chronic). Recognition of pain may be complicated by physical or cognitive impairments, ongoing drug therapy, and psychosocial factors (e.g., depression or social isolation). Additionally, sight reduction and flexibility limitations may prevent or decrease self-care. Sight reduction may increase risk for falls or other injury, which may be disastrous in the client with impaired circulation.

Surgical Management

Surgical management of PAD is called *revascularization* and is reserved for clients with progressive, severe, or disabling manifestations, including ischemia at rest. Angiography is commonly used before surgery to mark the level of inflow or areas of obstruction. Revascularization can be done through endovascular techniques or surgical reconstruction with grafting.

Endovascular Interventions

Endovascular procedures include angioplasty, atherectomy, and stent placement. The goal is to operate from within the artery to remove partial or total blockages. Most of the procedures can be done in the radiology department or in cardiac catheterization laboratories. Using local anesthetics for sedation, many of these procedures can be performed through small puncture wounds. The client recovers quickly and costs are

reduced. Preprocedural and postprocedural care is discussed in Chapter 51.

Arterial Bypass

Arterial bypass operations are used to revascularize limbs. Selecting the client for surgery begins with a careful history and physical and diagnostic assessments, including arteriography. Arteriography provides a necessary road map to indicate the level of obstruction, because it is essential to reconstruct the arterial inflow to the legs before correcting the outflow. This process prevents newly placed bypass grafts from thrombosing because of inadequate blood supply to the graft. During the operation, the surgeon assesses inflow, and after it is ascertained that inflow to the femoral system is adequate, a distal site is chosen for outflow.

Improvements in vascular surgery have provided outstanding examples of long-term limb salvage in clients who in the past would have required amputation. Current data indicate that revascularization should be the first option considered in clients with critical limb ischemia. This recommendation is based on the following observations: (1) previous revascularization does not raise the level of amputation, (2) mortality rates for amputation are at least as high as for arterial bypass, and (3) there is no difference in cost between amputation and successful bypass.

Various locations along the arterial system can be reconstructed. The femoral artery can be bypassed with grafts anastomosed (surgically connected) to any one of three lower leg arteries (posterior tibial, anterior tibial, or peroneal artery) (Figure 53-4). The success of bypass grafts of the legs depends largely on what material is used for grafting. The client's own saphenous vein is the most successful grafting material. Up to 80% of saphenous vein grafts are patent after 5 years; in contrast, only 30% of synthetic material (polytetrafluoroethylene [PTFE]) is patent after the same length of time. (Gore-Tex is a common brand name for PTFE.) The client's own saphenous vein is not always large enough or long enough for the surgery, however, or it may have been removed during another operation. In these cases, PTFE is used. In situ grafts can also be used for reconstruction. In situ grafting uses the client's own vein for a bypass of the artery. A section of vein is anastomosed proximally and distally and then the valves are disabled. The vein then acts as an artery.

Axillofemoral grafting is reserved for clients who have increased operative risk, usually because of their cardiopulmonary status or the presence of intra-abdominal infection. The graft begins at the axillary artery and travels subcutaneously along the lateral chest wall to the femoral artery. It may then be combined with a femorofemoral graft to revascularize both extremities. Axillofemoral grafts have a higher incidence of occlusion than aortofemoral grafts. The patency rates are 60% to 70%

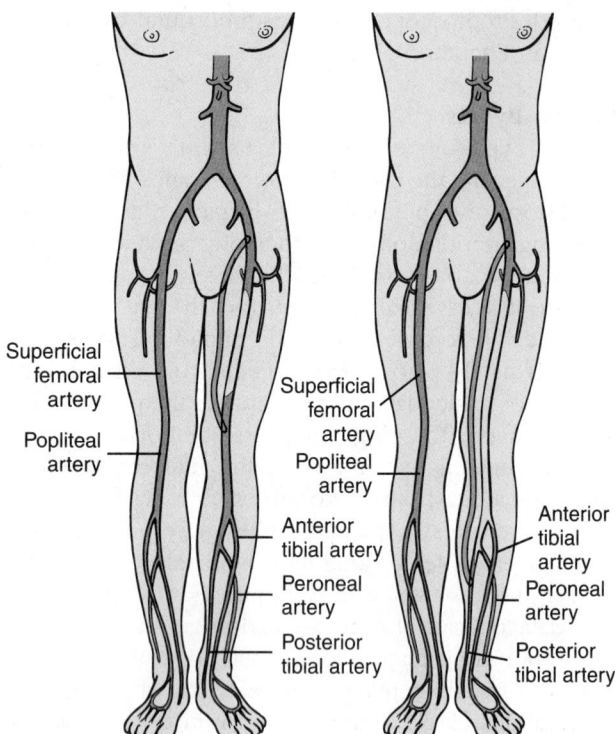

■ **FIGURE 53–4** The occluded femoral artery can be bypassed into the arteries supplying the lower leg.

at 5 years, in part because thrombi are easily removed from axillofemoral grafts.

Clots in the graft are a major complication after surgery. Clots cause immediate impairment in blood flow and the limb becomes cool, pale, painful, and pulseless. Anticoagulant medications (e.g., low-molecular-weight heparin, heparin sodium) or antiplatelet aggregates (e.g., aspirin and Plavix) can be used prophylactically. If the graft becomes occluded, fibrinolytics may be used depending on the amount of time that has lapsed since surgery (because of marked risk of bleeding) (see Chapter 56).

When an ischemic leg is revascularized and the ischemic muscle is reperfused, a variety of ions, structural proteins, and enzymes that accumulated in the ischemic tissue return to central circulation. This process is called reperfusion syndrome and can lead to renal failure when the myoglobin is trapped in the renal tubules. Lactic acid can lead to myocardial depression, and debris can impair blood flow in the limb as it enters smaller blood vessels. Edema can develop and create compartment syndrome.

Nursing Management of the Surgical Client

Preoperative Care

Preoperatively, obtain baseline vital signs and document the character of peripheral pulses, comparing one side to the other. Know exactly which pulses are palpable and which pulses can be assessed only with the Doppler. To assist with postoperative assessment, mark with ink the sites where peripheral pulses can be palpated. A lack of pulses postoperatively can be considered an occlusion if the quality of the pulses before surgery was not recorded.

As with any preoperative assessment, perform careful cardiac and pulmonary evaluation. Even though the incision for a femoral artery bypass is peripheral and major complications are infrequent, the client probably has other manifestations of atherosclerosis (such as heart and kidney disease) that may complicate the surgery. If the operation is not an emergency, malnutrition can be reversed and open wounds cleaned. The client should have a complete medical evaluation and hypertension should be controlled. Report to the surgeon or anesthesia department any blood pressure reading outside of normal parameters or well above the client's normal. All infections (e.g., tooth abscesses, urinary tract infections, respiratory tract infections) must be resolved, especially if the synthetic graft is planned.

Before the client goes to surgery, it is common to begin administration of intravenous fluids, insert a urinary catheter, and weigh the client. In addition, broad-spectrum antibiotics normally are administered.

The client and family are taught the various procedures involved and are offered psychological support. First assess the client's readiness and desire to learn about the surgery. The importance of maintaining the medication routine is to be stressed with appropriate guidance from the physician or anesthesia department.

Postoperative Care

The client is placed on bed rest for the evening after surgery, with the leg flat in bed. The leg is wrapped with light dressings or a fleece vascular boot. The Care Plan feature on Postoperative Care of the Client Who Has Had Arterial Bypass Surgery of the Lower Extremity on pp. 1318-1319 describes additional nursing care of the client.

Complications

Bleeding may develop along the suture line and can indicate a disruption in the suture line, pseudoaneurysm formation, or a slipped ligature (suture). These problems require additional surgery. Reclotting of the graft is also possible. Peripheral tissue perfusion is monitored and noninvasive follow-up studies are performed to assess patency.

Infection is not a common complication after bypass surgery, but it can occur, especially when synthetic grafting material is used. Because infection in a synthetic graft necessitates its removal, infection often results in the loss of a limb. Poorly nourished clients appear to be at highest risk of infection and delayed healing.

Reperfusion syndrome can lead to several problems. Compartment syndrome may also develop from swelling around the fascial compartments of the leg. The manifestations of compartment syndrome include pain out of proportion to the surgery, a tense swollen leg and pain with muscle stretching, and decreased sensation. In addition to loss of sensation and function, muscle cells can die and release myoglobin, which can cause acute tubular necrosis in the kidney. A change involving any of these manifestations or a change in the color of the urine to rusty brown should be reported immediately.

Self-Care

Most clients are discharged to home. Because activity was limited by claudication before surgery, the client needs to begin regular permissible exercise, including climbing stairs and going out of doors. The client is taught that swelling of the operative leg is normal and can last for 2 to 3 months. Elastic wraps can be used when the client is ambulating, but they should not be worn continuously. Smoking must stop; it can jeopardize the results of the operation.

CRITICAL LIMB ISCHEMIA

Critical limb ischemia differs from claudication. These clients have rest pain in the forefoot and toes that interferes with sleep as well as ischemic ulcers or gangrene of the forefoot or toes. There may be calf muscle atrophy, loss of hair on the dorsum or the foot, and shiny, scaly skin attributable to loss of subcutaneous tissues. Treatment includes antiplatelet medications and revascularization. The outcomes may not be as predictable, however.

AMPUTATION

Amputation is the oldest operation known to man, existing before recorded history. Early amputations were done as punishment for crime. Today's amputations are used to treat injuries, cancers, overwhelming limb gangrene, and limb-threatening arterial disease or rest pain. Amputation is common; nearly 2 million people in the United States have undergone amputations. Even though prosthetic devices can restore a reasonable degree of function after amputation, the visible loss engenders an additional emotional component that may not occur with other surgeries.

For many years, amputation was performed with an apology and often a sense of failure. Recently there has been increasing media publicity featuring amputees who have "overcome their handicap" and returned to mainstream society. There are organizations of amputee skiers, golfers, and runners. Publicity has removed much of the old stigma.

Clients with peripheral vascular disease are the most frequent candidates for amputation of the lower extremities. Diabetes mellitus is a major cause of arterial occlusion and has been associated with more than 55% of major amputations in clients with lower extremity occlusive disease. Traumatic injuries are also a common cause of amputation.

Preoperative Assessment

Usual preoperative assessment is performed (see Chapter 14). In addition, a rehabilitation team designs an individualized care plan focusing on the whole client rather than on a diseased or missing limb. Before amputation, the surgeon and rehabilitative team consider the following:

- *The client's physical condition.* The following physical conditions may predicate the rehabilitation potential: the age of the client, the ability to become ambulatory or remain ambulatory, the comprehension level of the client, the willingness of the client to participate in a rehabilitation program, and the condition of pre-existing conditions (e.g., chronic and progressive mental deterioration, advancing neurologic problems, chronic obstructive pulmonary disease, or cardiac disease with heart failure or angina). Ideally, clients should attain independent function with the use of a prosthesis.
- *The type of amputation to be performed.* There are two types of amputation procedures: the open, or guillotine, amputation and the closed, or "flap," amputation. The major indication for guillotine amputation is infection. In open amputation, the surgeon does not close the stump with a skin flap immediately but leaves the end open, allowing the wound to drain freely. Antibiotics are used. Once the infection is completely eradicated, the client undergoes another operation for stump closure.
- During a "flap" amputation, the surgeon closes or covers the stump with a flap of skin sutured over the end of the stump. This type of amputation is the most common and performed when there is no evidence of infection and, consequently, no need for open drainage. However, the surgeon may insert small drains to promote wound healing.
- *The level of amputation required.* The level of amputation for any extremity should be as distal as possible (Figure 53-5 on p. 1320). Arteriography is used to guide the decision about the level of amputation. Clients with below-knee amputations (even bilateral) more successfully achieve independent function with a prosthesis than do those with above-knee amputations (see Figure 53-5).
- *The client's general attitude toward amputation.* Attitude toward amputation depends to a large degree on the client's age and maturity. Young clients may resist amputation even though it would greatly improve their function. For some, the thought of amputation dramatically conflicts with their ideal

Postoperative Care of the Client Who Has Had Arterial Bypass Surgery of the Lower Extremity

Nursing Diagnosis: *Risk for Deficient Fluid Volume related to hemorrhage, hematoma, third-spacing of fluid, or diuresis from contrast given during angiography.*

NOC OUTCOMES	Fluid Balance, Hydration, Kidney Function, Bleeding Reduction (NOC).

Interventions	NIC INTERVENTIONS	Rationales
1. Observe the client for an increase in pulse rate, decrease in blood pressure, anxiety, restlessness, pallor, cyanosis, thirst, oliguria, clammy skin, venous collapse, and decreasing level of consciousness.	Bleeding Reduction	1. Hemorrhagic shock can develop from surgical or postoperative blood loss. Blood is shunted from peripheral stores because of the effect of sympathetic nervous system stimulation.
2. Check the client's dressings for excessive drainage. Also check under the leg.	Bleeding Reduction	2. Bleeding may appear on dressings and may also be found beneath the leg because of gravity.
3. Assess the client's pulmonary artery pressures and cardiac output if parameters are available.	Hemodynamic Regulation Invasive Hemodynamic Monitoring	3. Pulmonary artery pressures and cardiac output parameters are reliable indicators of hemodynamic stability.
4. Check the client's daily weights; monitor intake and output closely.	Fluid Monitoring	4. Intake should equal output. Weight is a reliable indicator of fluid balance.
5. Check hematocrit and hemoglobin values and notify the physician if they are abnormal.	Hypovolemia Management	5. Hematocrit and hemoglobin levels normally fall slightly because of surgical blood loss. Transfusion may be required.
6. Check the client's creatinine level after angiography.	Risk Identification	6. Contrast is excreted by the kidneys.

Evaluation: This outcome should be attainable within 24 hours. Bleeding usually occurs within the first few hours after the operation, and if bleeding develops it is usually visible on the dressings. Intravenous fluids are required until the client is drinking without nausea and producing adequate urine volumes.

Nursing Diagnosis: *Acute Pain related to surgical incision.*

NOC OUTCOMES	Pain Level, Pain Control, Comfort Level.

Interventions	NIC INTERVENTIONS	Rationales
1. Assess the client's level of pain: type, duration, and location.	Pain Management	1. Baseline data are used to evaluate the effectiveness of treatment and act as a guide to determine type of analgesia needed.
2. Medicate with prescribed analgesics based on current level of pain and prior effectiveness.	Medication Administration: IV, Oral Analgesic Administration	2. Analgesia is provided to obtain comfort, using the previous pain response to analgesia and current level of pain to guide the decision.
3. Evaluate the effectiveness of pain medication after each administration.	Pain Management	3. This helps determine the adequacy of analgesia.
4. Teach the client how pain will be controlled.	Patient-Controlled Analgesia Assistance	4. Clients can participate in pain management by notifying the nurse before intense pain and by using patient-controlled analgesia (PCA) devices.
5. Position the leg to promote blood flow and keep the leg warm.	Circulatory Care: Arterial Insufficiency	5. Arterial inflow and warmth are aided by supine position.

Evaluation: Acute pain should subside over 48 to 72 hours. The client should report less severe pain on a 1 to 10 scale, use less analgesia, and ambulate increasing distances. The client will likely require intravenous opioids for the first 24 hours and then should be able to remain comfortable on oral opioids, tapering to nonsteroidal medications in a few days. Pain that does not follow such a pattern should be investigated.

Nursing Diagnosis: *Impaired Physical Mobility related to a surgical procedure, pain, preoperative deconditioning, or nerve injury secondary to ischemia.*

NOC OUTCOMES	Ambulation, Balance, Coordinated Movement, Mobility.

Interventions	NIC INTERVENTIONS	Rationales
1. Assess the causative factors for immobility and the client's range of motion and ability to ambulate.	Exercise Promotion: Ambulation Exercise Promotion: Strength Training	1. Mobility can be facilitated once the cause of immobility is known.
2. Encourage range of motion while the client is in bed.	Exercise Promotion: Strength Training Body Mechanics Promotion	2. These activities promote venous return and muscle strength.

Interventions	NIC INTERVENTIONS	Rationales
3. Ambulate increasing distances daily. Monitor tolerance of ambulation. Monitor for balance, stamina, and unsteady gait if muscle atrophy is present.	Exercise Promotion: Strength Training Exercise Promotion: Balance Fall Prevention Exercise Therapy: Muscle Control	3. Ambulation increases muscle strength and endurance. Clients who have not ambulated for some time need to be monitored for safety (balance and gait) and stamina.
4. Request a physical therapy consult when appropriate.	Exercise Promotion: Strength Training Body Mechanics Promotion	4. Assistive devices may be necessary for ambulation.
5. Encourage independence in the client's activities of daily living.	Exercise Promotion: Strength Training	5. Independence improves both physical and psychological recovery.

Evaluation: Outcomes related to mobility may require several days, depending on initial physical status. Begin transferring to the bedside chair as soon as possible and proceed with ambulation as tolerated.

Nursing Diagnosis: *Risk for Impaired Skin Integrity related to altered circulation, altered nutritional state, infection, and surgical procedures.*

NOC OUTCOMES   Immobility Consequences: Physiologic, Wound Healing: Primary Intention.

Interventions	NIC INTERVENTIONS	Rationales
1. Inspect the client's lower extremities on a daily basis, including footdrop.	Skin Surveillance	1. Early detection of ulceration will allow early treatment of lesions.
2. Monitor the client for low-grade fever, elevated white blood cell count, any drainage from the wound, and graft exposure at each shift.	Incision Site Care	2. These are clinical manifestations of wound infection.
3. Monitor the client's nutritional status, oral intake, weight, and prealbumin and albumin levels. Obtain a dietitian's consultation, if necessary.	Nutritional Therapy	3. Malnutrition is the most common cause of delayed healing.
4. Provide proper skin care using lanolin-based creams.	Skin Care: Topical Treatments	4. Soft skin does not excoriate.
5. Protect the client's lower extremities from trauma.	Pressure Management	5. Tissue perfusion is decreased and injured sites heal poorly.
6. Use fleece vascular boots when appropriate.	Circulatory Precautions	6. Boots protect the skin from breakdown and keep the legs warm.
7. Elevate heels from the bed.	Pressure Ulcer Prevention	7. Pressure ulcers on the heels may be slow to heal because of poor circulation.
8. Avoid using tape on the skin below the client's knee.	Skin Care; Topical Treatments	8. Tape burns from tape removal may be slow to heal.
9. Observe strict aseptic technique during dressing changes.	Infection Control	9. Aseptic technique reduces the risk of infection.
10. Instruct the client to inspect feet and incisions daily. (See Client Education Guide on Foot Care.)	Teaching: Disease Process	10. Circulation to the legs and feet is impaired from arteriosclerosis. Daily assessment and proper care can lead to early intervention.

Evaluation: Expect the wound to heal slowly over 10 days if arteriosclerosis is extensive. Because of delays in wound healing, the client will remain at risk of infection.

Nursing Diagnosis: *Risk for Ineffective Tissue Perfusion related to graft thrombosis, compartment syndrome, progressive arterial disease, or inadequate anticoagulation.*

NOC OUTCOMES   Circulation Status, Tissue Perfusion; Peripheral, Kidney Function.

Interventions	NIC INTERVENTIONS	Rationales
1. Assess the client's pedal pulses every hour for 24 hours, then every shift, unless otherwise ordered. Obtain Doppler pressures per doctor's orders. Compare to baseline values.	Lower Extremity Monitoring	1. Pedal pulses indicate graft patency.
2. Assess the sensory and motor function of the client's extremities.	Neurologic Monitoring	2. Compartment syndrome may develop because of bleeding.
3. Assess the client's leg for hematoma or severe swelling.	Circulatory Precautions	3. Severe swelling may impede the flow through the graft.
4. Monitor creatine phosphokinase levels when appropriate.	Laboratory Value Interpretation	4. Enzymes are released from ischemic muscle.
5. Report dark red or brown urine and the presence of red blood cells in the client's urine.	Emergency Management	5. These manifestations may be caused by a release of myoglobin secondary to muscle ischemia.
6. Report any unexpected deviation in perfusion to the physician.	Circulatory Precautions	6. Early reporting allows early intervention.
7. Avoid raising the knee section of the Gatch bed and placing pillows under the client's knees.	Positioning	7. Pressure may increase the risk of thrombosis.

Evaluation: Outcomes related to tissue perfusion should be met within 48 hours. Preoperative decreases in pedal pulse measurements should be restored when the client returns from surgery. Some edema is common but should not become so severe that it impairs blood flow or nerve conduction.

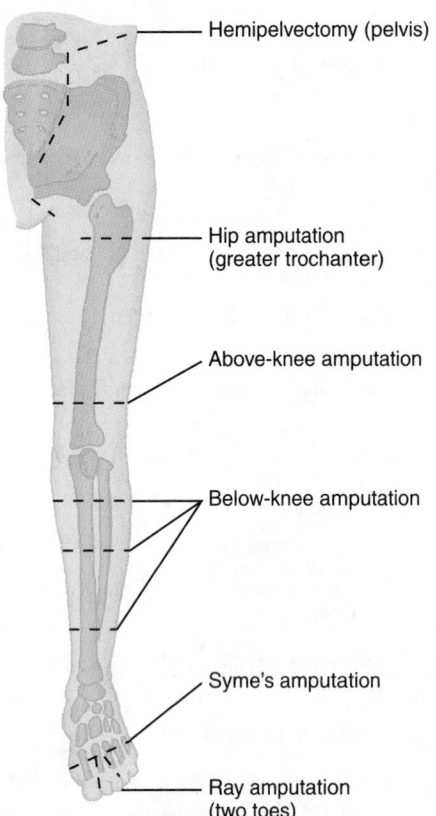

Hemipelvectomy (pelvis)

Hip amputation
(greater trochanter)

Above-knee amputation

Below-knee amputation

Syme's amputation

Ray amputation
(two toes)

■ **FIGURE 53–5** Common sites of lower extremity amputation.

self-image. Conversely, some clients who suffer from the pain of chronic ischemia may welcome amputation. These clients are often more concerned with removing the source of their pain than they are with altering their body image or function.

Diagnostic assessments include the usual preoperative blood studies and radiographs. In addition, the client may have arteriography to determine the level of blood flow in the extremity. Doppler studies are used to measure blood flow velocity, and transcutaneous tissue oxygen levels may also be measured (see Chapter 51). These studies assist with determining the level of amputation that is most likely to heal.

Phantom Limb Sensation

Phantom sensations are feelings that the amputated part is still present. Although these sensations are often referred to as phantom pain, not all of the sensations are painful. The client may describe sensations of warmth, cold, itching, or pain, especially in amputated fingers or toes. *Phantom sensations* are caused by intact peripheral nerves proximal to the amputation site that carried messages between the brain and the now amputated part. These sensations are normal, and the client should be prepared for them. Phantom sensations often are felt immediately after surgery and their frequency gradually decreases over the next 2 years.

Another condition called *phantom pain* is a form of central pain. The client reports actual pain. The pain is usually burning, cramping, squeezing, or shooting in nature. Phantom pain is less well understood and may occur in a large percentage of clients. It is thought to be caused by a combination of physiologic and psychological components. However, no research has identified a link between phantom pain and any clinical psychological disorder. Phantom pain occurs most often in clients who had pain in the limb before the amputation. Interventions that may reduce phantom pain include range-of-motion exercises, visual imaging, nerve-stabilizing medications, and other interventions for chronic pain (see Chapter 20).

Preoperative Care

Nursing Assessment of the Surgical Client

Assessment. Perform the usual preoperative assessments (see Chapter 14). In addition, support the client and family through their pain, suffering, and decision making as the client is prepared physically and psychologically for amputation. If the amputation is being done for an infectious process, administer antibiotics and monitor for sepsis (changes in mental status, fever and chills, increasing pain or odor from the wound, elevated white blood cell count). If the client has an infection in the leg to be amputated, it is important that the remaining leg is not wounded and also infected. Ulcers on the heel are hazardous, and the legs should be elevated to remove all pressure from the heel. Diabetic clients need close monitoring of blood glucose levels because infection makes blood glucose regulation erratic. Maintaining or promoting strength in the upper arms facilitates rehabilitation. Teach the client to use the trapeze and side rails for independent movement in bed. Maintain or promote nutrition to aid in healing. Older adults may have several problems that can lead to malnutrition. Ask the dietitian to evaluate the nutrient intake and offer suggestions to meet caloric and protein needs.

Diagnosis, Outcomes, Interventions
Diagnosis: Risk for Delayed Surgical Recovery. Some clients require amputation on an emergent basis; for those clients the usual preoperative care to stabilize health conditions cannot occur. The need for emergent surgery can create a risk for delayed recovery. State this nursing diagnosis as *Risk for Delayed Surgical Recovery related to pre-existing health conditions.*

Outcomes. The risk for delayed surgical recovery will be minimized.

Interventions. Clients with diabetes mellitus are a high-risk surgical group and require frequent assessment of their blood glucose level. Blood glucose level is normalized using frequent (e.g., four times daily) blood testing and sliding scale insulin. Clients with ulcerated legs or osteomyelitis may be treated with wound packing, antibiotics, and leg elevation with bed rest. Malnourished clients are nourished with foods high in protein or are administered tube feedings. They also may benefit from vitamin and mineral supplements. Severely anemic clients may require iron preparations and blood transfusions. Dehydrated clients should receive preoperative intravenous fluids to restore fluid balance.

Diagnosis: Anxiety. Clients may fear amputation because it destroys a familiar body image, imposes physical and social limitations, and temporarily upsets personal lifestyle. Such fears and anxiety must be resolved during the preoperative period to ensure successful postoperative recovery. Depending on the reason for the amputation, fear may lead the client to experience anticipatory grief. State this nursing diagnosis as *Anxiety related to impending loss of limb, change in mobility, loss of independence, pain, changes in body image, fear about feelings after amputation.* Other nursing diagnoses may also be appropriate, such as ineffective individual coping, self-esteem disturbance, or body image disturbance.

Outcomes. The client will have reduced anxiety as evidenced by openly discussing feelings and expressing reduced anxiety before surgery.

Interventions. Establish open, honest communication. Allow free expression of fears and negative feelings about the loss of a limb. Ask significant others how they feel about the amputation and how they perceive the client to be responding. The social worker or psychologist may need to be involved if the client is responding poorly.

The client may also be anxious about unknown consequences and sensations after the amputation. Provide and reinforce information. Most clients feel less anxious when they know what to expect on awakening from surgery. Prepare the client for *phantom limb sensation.* Most clients with new amputations experience the peculiar sensation that their missing limb is still present. This phantom limb sensation may or may not be painful. Also, it may either disappear within hours after surgery or persist for years. To avoid misunderstandings, inform clients that phantom limb sensations occur and are normal.

Diagnosis: Acute Pain. The client may experience severe to moderate pain before surgery. The nursing diagnosis of *Acute Pain related to ischemia of the limb* is used.

Outcomes. The client will have improved comfort as evidenced by statements of reduced pain, use of reduced doses of opioids (e.g., pain is controlled without increasing dosage), ability to move about comfortably, and ability to sleep or rest.

Interventions. Administer prescribed analgesics as necessary to reduce pain. Intervene with supportive measures. For example, use footboards and cradles to avoid pressure on injured or ischemic limbs. Keep ischemic limbs warm with wraps or fleece vascular boots.

Diagnosis: Deficient Knowledge. A common nursing diagnosis for clients having surgery is *Deficient Knowledge related to expectations after surgery.*

Outcomes. The client will express an understanding of the usual postoperative regimens.

Interventions. Clients want to know what to expect after surgery and what will be expected of them by health care professionals. Emphasize that the client is the most important member of the rehabilitation team. To achieve independence, teach the client about the following:

- Exercising legs and arms several times a day
- Strictly limiting weight-bearing (for leg amputations) until instructed otherwise
- Learning the intricacies of stump and prosthesis care
- Mastering the use of the prosthesis

Postoperative Care

After the operation is completed, the surgeon applies a small amount of fluffed gauze over the end of the stump. A rigid dressing (usually a cast) is applied, distributing pressure evenly over the end of the stump. The cast protects the stump from injury and reduces swelling by gently compressing the tissues. The socket of the distal end of the cast connects to a pylon. A pylon is an adjustable rigid support, the proximal end of which attaches to the below-knee socket or to the knee unit of an above-knee prosthesis. The distal end connects to a foot-ankle assembly. The rigid dressing is usually changed three to four times before application of a permanent prosthesis. Cast changes are necessary because the stump tends to shrink as it heals and, consequently, is no longer adequately compressed by the original cast.

Edema is controlled by elevating the stump for the first 24 hours after surgery. Then, the stump is placed flat on the bed to reduce hip contracture. Edema is also controlled by stump wrapping techniques. In below-knee amputations, the knee is immobilized to eliminate joint flexion. A trapeze is attached to the bed to assist the client to develop upper arm and shoulder strength.

Nursing Assessment of the Surgical Client

Assessment. Following an amputation, the usual postoperative care is given. Look for bleeding or oozing. If present, outline the drainage, including the time on the temporary prosthesis or soft dressing. If drains were placed in the wound, carefully monitor the amount and type of drainage.

Postoperative management of acute pain is essential. Acute surgical pain assessment and management is like those techniques used for other postoperative clients. To prevent increased pain, the nurse handles the stump carefully when assessing the site or drainage beneath the stump or dressings.

Because of pre-existent conditions such as diabetes, open infected wounds, and decreased perfusion, the client remains at high risk for infection. The nurse monitors the client and the wound for manifestations of wound infection, which usually develops about 72 hours after surgery. Broad-spectrum antibiotics are usually prescribed for several days after surgery, until there is indication that the wound is healing.

Diagnosis, Outcomes, Interventions

Diagnosis: Acute Pain. Following amputation, acute pain from the operation is present and phantom limb sensation can also be present. State this nursing diagnosis as either *Acute Pain related to traumatized tissues and phantom sensation in amputated limb* or *Anxiety related to phantom sensation in amputated limb.*

Outcomes. The client will have comfort and express an understanding of the sensations present and will recognize that they are normal and usually diminish in time.

Interventions. Provide pain control with ordered analgesics. Ischemia in the limb before surgery can sensitize the nerves, making pain somewhat more difficult to control after the amputation. If phantom sensations are present, empathetically reinforce the idea that this sensation is usual and, more importantly, subsides in time. It is not helpful to correct the client, telling the client that the limb cannot be hurting because it is absent.

Diagnosis: Ineffective Coping. For clients with some chronic disorders, such as diabetes, the amputation may signal further losses in their battle. These clients may express anger openly or covertly. Many clients express depression after amputation. The client may cry easily, eat little, sleep poorly or sleep more, or avoid interactions with others. Many times depression is a reaction to the fear of never walking again, and therefore early ambulation is therapeutic. State the nursing diagnosis as *Ineffective Coping related to reaction/response to change in body image, fear over loss of independence.*

Outcomes. The client will openly verbalize fears about changes in body image and loss of independence, and will begin to speak optimistically and realistically about the future.

Interventions. The nurse listens to the client and confronts misconceptions about the rehabilitation. If it is

possible, the nurse arranges for the client to meet with another amputee. The client may express concerns that it will be impossible to return to a previous lifestyle, including job, leisure activities, or intimate relationships. With advancements in prosthetic devices, many clients can have both functional and aesthetic prosthetic devices.

Some clients feel the use of the word "stump" to be distasteful and report feeling like they are part of a tree. Use of other terms may be controversial, however, if they encourage or support denial of the problem. Some rehabilitation specialists use the phrase "residual limb" instead.

Diagnosis: Deficient Knowledge. Clients require information and time to learn all the new information about the care of the stump and the prosthesis. Use the nursing diagnosis *Deficient Knowledge related to gait training, care of the stump, care of the prosthesis.*

Outcomes. The client will express an understanding of stump and prosthesis care.

Interventions. *The Prosthesis.* The most common prosthesis for clients with a below-the-knee amputation is a patellar tendon–bearing limb prosthesis. The interior of the prosthesis contacts all surfaces of the stump and weight-bearing is on several areas. Clients with above-the-knee amputation are fitted with either a quadrilateral socket or an ischial containment prosthesis. Weight is borne on the ischial tuberosity or the soft tissues of the proximal stump, respectively.

Prostheses for the upper extremity consist of a hook or hand device, a harness to supply force to the hand, and a socket for attachment. The client coping with an upper extremity amputation must be highly motivated to master the prosthesis and achieve independence. For successful rehabilitation, the client must integrate the prosthetic arm and hand into the total body image.

Cosmetic prostheses are primarily used to enhance self-esteem and make reentry into society minus a limb more tolerable for clients who are not candidates for a functioning prosthesis. Because the construction of cosmetic prostheses does not allow weight-bearing, caution the client never to attempt transfers or ambulation with a cosmetic prosthesis.

Immediate prosthetic fitting is not always possible. However, anyone with a new amputation who is capable of ambulating should receive a temporary prosthesis as soon as possible after surgery. When a conventional delayed prosthesis fitting is anticipated, the client returns from surgery with the stump dressed and covered with elastic bandages or stump socks. (See a fundamentals of nursing text on how to wrap these stumps.) When the sutures are removed 2 to 3 weeks after surgery, the surgeon or prosthetist fits the client with a provisional temporary prosthesis made of plaster of paris or plastic.

A permanent prosthesis is fitted once the stump is healed and molded (Figure 53-6).

Gait Training. Physical mobility will be compromised for the client who has just experienced an amputation. Amputating a limb displaces the center of gravity, normally located just below the umbilicus. A client coping with an amputation must relearn balance because the prosthesis, however similar, will not be an exact replica in weight and movement of the lost limb. Adapting to a change in the center of gravity occurs slowly but progressively until the conscious effort of maintaining balance comes under unconscious control. Physically, the client increases strength and endurance with regularly scheduled exercise, controls weight-bearing until the wound completely heals, and practices ambulating with the new prosthesis until a skillful, automatic gait is developed. Physical therapists usually work with the client twice daily for strengthening and gait training.

When the prosthesis is not worn (e.g., during the night), turning also requires a readaptation in body balance. Consequently, the client may need assistance while turning until awareness of the new center of gravity is present.

Self-Care

When making discharge plans for the client with a new amputation (and probably a prosthesis), consider the client's ambulatory level and the tasks with which the client may need help. Frequently, by the time amputees are aware of their changed circumstances, they are at home, alone, and without the informed and professional advice that can prepare them for their altered lives. Schedule home visits from community health care nurses until such clients have adjusted to their new situation and feel reasonably comfortable and confident in their ability to provide self-care.

The Client Education Guide feature below offers suggestions for care in the health care facility or at home for clients who have had lower limb amputation.

TRAUMATIC AMPUTATION

Not all amputations are planned. Some clients suffer traumatic loss of limb as a result of farm machinery

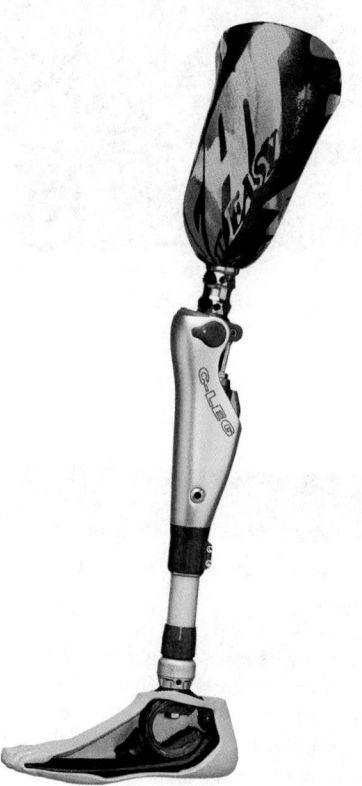

FIGURE 53–6 Permanent lower-extremity prosthesis. *(Courtesy Otto Bock Health Care, Minneapolis, Minn.)*

CLIENT EDUCATION GUIDE

Stump and Prosthesis Care

STUMP CARE

- Inspect the stump daily for redness, blistering, or abrasions.
- Use a mirror to examine all sides and aspects of the stump. Skin breakdown on the stump is extremely serious because it interferes with prosthesis training and may prolong hospitalization and recovery. If you have diabetes mellitus, you are particularly susceptible to skin complications, because changes in sensation may obliterate your awareness of stump pain.
- Perform meticulous daily hygiene. Wash the stump with a mild soap, and then carefully rinse and dry it. Apply nothing to the stump after it is bathed. Alcohol dries and cracks the skin, whereas oils and creams soften the skin too much for safe prosthesis use.
- Wear woolen stump socks over the stump for cleanliness and comfort. Wash woolen socks in cool water and mild soap to prevent shrinkage. To prevent stretching, wash socks gently. Dry stump socks flat on a towel. Replace torn socks; mending creates wrinkles that irritate the skin.
- Put on the prosthesis immediately when arising and keep it on all day (once the wound has healed completely) to reduce stump swelling.
- Continue prescribed exercises to prevent weakness.

PROSTHESIS CARE

- Remove sweat and dirt from the prosthesis socket daily by wiping the inside of the socket with a damp soapy cloth. To remove the soap, use a clean damp cloth. Dry the prosthesis socket thoroughly.
- Never attempt to adjust or mechanically alter the prosthesis. If problems develop, consult the prosthetist.
- Schedule a yearly appointment with the prosthetist.

accidents, chain saw accidents, or automobile accidents. Sometimes the amputated limb can be replanted because usually both the client and the limb were healthy up to the time of injury. It is important to properly store and transport the amputated limb before replantation. The limb should be wrapped in a cloth, placed in a plastic bag, and then placed on ice. The limb or digit itself should not come in contact with ice or water to prevent direct tissue damage. No promises should be made to the client about the ability to successfully replant an amputated limb before evaluation by the replantation surgery team. Individuals whose limbs were amputated because of trauma have had no time before surgery to grieve the loss or adjust to their perceived alterations in body image. They may express sadness or anger, or they may show a strong determination not to let the amputation alter their ability to function. Outcomes after replantation vary with the complexity of repair required and the amount of tissue replanted. Months of rehabilitation are required; the peripheral nerve repairs itself very slowly.

ACUTE ARTERIAL OCCLUSION

Acute occlusion of an artery may be caused by trauma, embolism, or thrombosis and may occur in a healthy or diseased artery. About 90% of acute occlusion occurs in the lower limbs. In arterial embolism, the wall of the artery is often healthy; the obstruction in the artery arises most frequently from a thrombus within the heart. Etiologies include atrial fibrillation, myocardial infarction, prosthetic heart valves, and rheumatic heart disease. Sometimes, portions of a blood clot, such as platelet emboli, which form at points of turbulence and then lodge at a bifurcation, can initiate a thrombus. Other noncardiac sources of emboli are clot in an abdominal aortic aneurysm or peripheral aneurysm, and up to 20% are from an unidentified source. Arterial thrombosis is usually superimposed on atherosclerosis and consequently develops in a damaged vessel; however, coagulopathy from heparin-induced thrombocytopenia, inherited coagulation disorders, disseminated intravascular coagulation, or polycythemia vera may also occur.

The circulatory changes that follow arterial occlusion and that predict the outcome are complex and depend on a variety of factors. Acute occlusion produces a decrease in mean and pulse pressures in the distal arteries and a decrease in tissue perfusion and oxygenation. In a normal artery, blood flow is restored by collateral channels, but with acute emboli, collateral vessels have not had time to develop.

It is important to differentiate between arterial thrombosis and arterial embolism. Acute arterial thrombosis is usually caused by arterial obstruction from a blood clot

that forms in an artery that has been damaged by atherosclerosis. Arterial thrombosis may also develop in an arterial aneurysm, especially aneurysms that form in the popliteal artery. Arterial emboli form in the terminal end of an artery and lead to distinct areas of necrotic tissue (Figure 53-7).

The classic manifestations of acute ischemia caused by peripheral thrombus or embolism, which are known as the *six P's*, are shown in Box 53-1. Muscle necrosis may start as early as 2 to 3 hours after occlusion. Paresthesias indicate advanced damage. Complete paralysis with stiffness of muscles and joints (rigor mortis) indicates irreversible damage. The leg must be amputated to prevent systemic reaction to the products of massive muscle destruction and systemic sepsis.

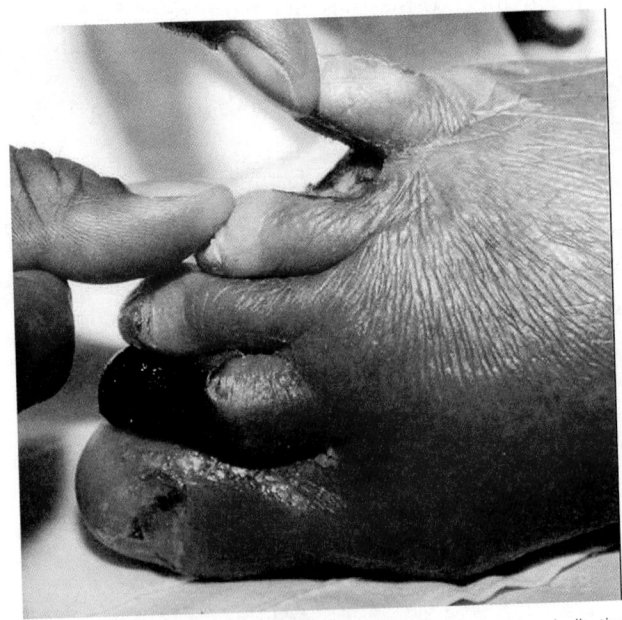

■ **FIGURE 53–7** Distal necrosis of toes from arterial embolization.

BOX 53-1 Clinical Manifestations of Acute Arterial Occlusion: The Six Ps

1. *Pain* or loss of sensory nerves secondary to ischemia
2. *Pulselessness*
3. *Poikilothermia* (coldness)
4. *Pallor* caused by empty superficial veins and no capillary filling; pallor can progress to a mottled, cyanotic, cadaverous, cold leg
5. *Paresthesias* and loss of position sense; the client cannot detect pressure or sense a pinprick; the client cannot tell whether toes are flexed or extended
6. *Paralysis*

OUTCOME MANAGEMENT

Surgery is required to correct arterial embolism. Arterial emboli can be removed by an embolectomy. Surgery for thrombosis usually involves an arterial reconstructive procedure for revascularization of the leg. If the decision is made to remove the occluding embolus or thrombus, surgery should be performed as quickly as possible, generally using local anesthetics. If hours have elapsed since the occlusion occurred, the viability of the limb determines whether embolectomy should be attempted.

If surgery is not performed immediately, anticoagulants are used to reduce the risk of further occlusion. Heparin is usually continued for a minimum of 2 to 7 days, after which a change to an oral anticoagulant may be made. The prevailing practice is to treat all clients who have a definite source of embolism and who have satisfactorily recovered from the acute episode of occlusion with long-term anticoagulant therapy. Fibrinolytic agents may also be used to dissolve a thrombus or embolus (see Chapter 56 for discussion of their use).

While decisions about surgery are being made, put the client to bed in a comfortable, warm room. Protect the limb from pressure and other trauma and keep it at room temperature, neither warm nor chilled. The best position for the limb is level or slightly dependent.

ARTERIAL ULCERS

Areas of an ischemic foot or leg subjected to pressure or minor trauma may have skin breakdown. The usual sites of arterial ulcers are the medial and lateral metatarsal heads and the tip of the toes. The ulcers are painful, which distinguishes them from the achy or "heavy" sensation of venous stasis ulcers. Arterial ulcers also have a sharp edge and pale base, and often are surrounded by atrophic tissue (see Figure 53-2). In contrast, venous stasis ulcers are irregular and have a red healthy base (see later discussion).

Once an ulcer develops, it tends to heal poorly, if at all (especially in diabetic clients). Without adequate blood flow, the damaged tissues fail to receive needed oxygen, nutrients, antibodies, and protective leukocytes, and the process of tissue damage continues. Eventually, the client may be forced to undergo limb amputation.

Although skin grafting may ultimately be required to cover the site of arterial ischemic leg ulcers (once the ulcerated area is free from infection and granulation tissue is evident), intervention for the skin lesion does not cure the underlying disease. Most ulcers require revascularization to heal. Arterial bypass surgery improves circulation when the client has an aortoiliac or femoral-popliteal occlusion. For this surgery to be successful, however, the arteries in the leg must be healthy enough to carry sufficient blood to the foot once the block has been removed or bypassed.

General intervention involves keeping the area of ulceration clean and free from pressure and irritation. Bed rest reduces the oxygen needs of the impaired tissues. Debridement is performed only when the client has reasonable blood flow to heal the wound. Dry, intact eschar should be left in place, that is not softened or removed. If surgical debridement is necessary, a qualified health care provider should perform this procedure. After revascularization, if the ulcer bed is clean and granulating, healing is enhanced with moist dressings.

ANEURYSMS

An aneurysm is a permanent localized dilation, stretching, or ballooning of an artery to around 50% increase in the size (Figure 53-8). The exact cause is unknown, but recent evidence includes atherosclerosis and hypertension. Abdominal aortic aneurysm may be caused by damage to the artery wall by metalloproteinase, infection, congenital weakening of the connective tissue component of the artery wall (e.g., Marfan syndrome or Ehlers-Danlos syndrome), mycotic (fungal) infections, or rarely by trauma. The most common locations for arteriosclerotic aneurysms are the thoracic and abdominal aorta, the iliac arteries, and the femoral and popliteal arteries.

Aneurysms are designated as being either *venous* or *arterial*. They are also described according to the specific vessel they affect (e.g., abdominal aortic aneurysm). Aneurysms are also labeled by their shape and size (see Figure 53-9). True aneurysms contain all three layers of the arterial wall (intima, media, and adventitia); saccular aneurysms have a neck or mouth. Fusiform aneurysms involve the entire circumference of the vessel. A dissecting aneurysm is not a true aneurysm, but rather is a hematoma in the arterial wall that separates the layers of the arterial wall. A *pseudoaneurysm,* or false aneurysm, results from the development of a sac around a hematoma that

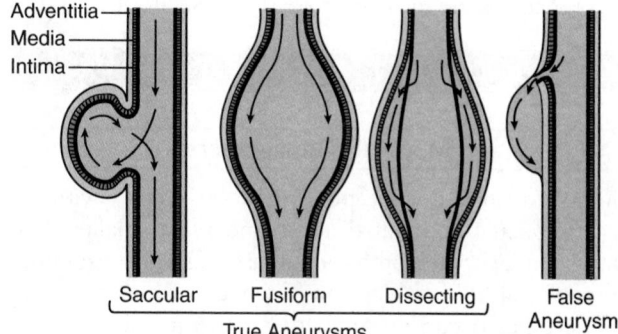

■ **FIGURE 53–8** Classification of aneurysms. In a true aneurysm, layers of the vessel wall dilate in one of the following ways: *saccular,* a unilateral outpouching; *fusiform,* a bilateral outpouching; or *dissecting,* a bilateral outpouching in which layers of the vessel wall separate, creating a cavity. In a false aneurysm, the wall ruptures, and a blood clot is retained in an outpouching of tissue, or there is a connection between a vein and an artery that does not close.

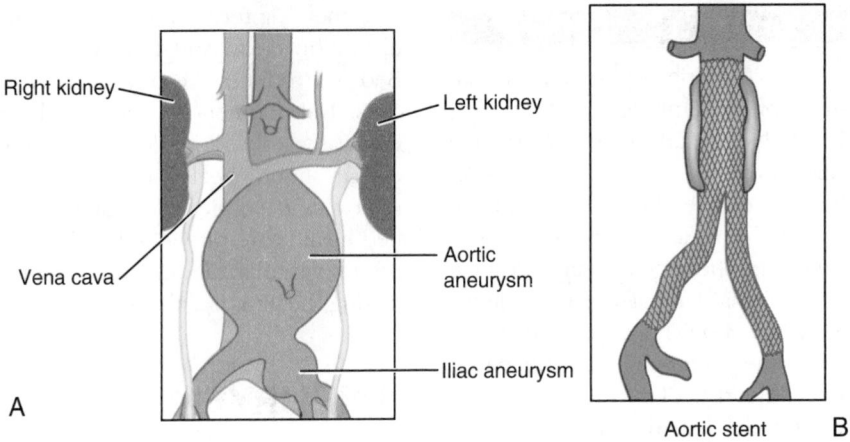

■ **FIGURE 53-9** **A,** An abdominal aortic aneurysm. **B,** A bifurcated synthetic graft in place.

maintains a communication with the lumen of an artery whose wall has been ruptured or penetrated.

ABDOMINAL AORTIC ANEURYSMS

Abdominal aortic aneurysms (Figure 53-9, *A*) are the most common type of aneurysm. They are seen most often in men 40 to 70 years of age. Most abdominal aneurysms are asymptomatic; discovery is usually made on physical or x-ray examination of the abdomen or lower spine for other reasons. When the aneurysm reaches about 5 cm in diameter, it can usually be palpated, except in obese clients. Smaller aneurysms and aneurysms in obese clients may be more difficult to confirm. The most common clinical manifestation is the client's awareness of a pulsating mass in the abdomen, with or without pain, followed by abdominal pain and back pain. Groin pain and flank pain may be experienced because of increasing pressure on other structures. Bruits can be heard over the aneurysm. Sometimes mottling of the extremities or distal emboli in the feet alert the clinician to a source in the abdomen. Ultrasonography and computed tomography (CT) scan are the most accurate diagnostic tools.

OUTCOME MANAGEMENT

Medical Management

Surgery is usually not performed on clients with an asymptomatic abdominal aortic aneurysm smaller than 4 to 5 cm. Every 6 months, an ultrasonographic examination is indicated to determine whether any change in the size has occurred. Antihypertensive medications are usually prescribed if indicated.

Surgical Management

Surgical resection of the aneurysm and creation of a new artery are the definitive treatments for aneurysm. There

are two types of surgery: endovascular surgery and traditional surgery through an abdominal incision.

Endovascular Procedures

Endovascular procedures are a newer method for non-emergency treatment to repair abdominal aortic aneurysm. Two small incisions are made in the groin, and a vascular graft is guided into the aorta (see Figure 53-9, *B*). At the tip of the catheter are a deflated balloon and a tightly wrapped polyester cloth graft. When properly positioned, the graft is secured in place by inflating the balloon and opening the graft to the diameter needed to prevent blood flow into the aneurysm. The balloon is then deflated and removed along with the catheter. At each end of the graft are hooks that help secure it to the inner walls of the aorta. The graft allows blood flow to continue through the aorta to the arteries in the pelvis and legs, without filling the aneurysm.

Postprocedure Care. The usual postoperative care is provided. Assess the surgical sites for swelling and pain (hematoma) and bleeding. Monitor peripheral perfusion closely, comparing findings to baseline. Ambulation is allowed the day after surgery. Clients may ask if they can "feel" the hooks in the aorta. They should be told that they will not be able to feel the hooks because the aorta cannot sense the hooks. Before dismissal, the location of the graft may be confirmed with CT scan, ultrasound, or x-ray study.

Aneurysm Repair

Surgical repair is usually recommended for all aneurysms greater than 6 cm wide. Elective repair is also generally recommended for aneurysms between 4 and 6 cm in clients who are good surgical risks. The more traditional surgical technique for aneurysm repair is done through a midline incision that extends from the xiphoid process to the symphysis pubis. The aneurysm is exposed, the aorta is clamped just above and below the aneurysm to stop the flow of blood, the aneurysm is opened, and a Dacron graft is placed within the aneurysm. The aneurysm sac is then wrapped around the graft to protect it (see Figure 53-9, *B*).

Complications. Abdominal aortic aneurysm repair is considered a major operation, and many specific postoperative complications can develop. Complications after abdominal aortic aneurysm repair are generally caused by underlying coronary artery disease and chronic obstructive pulmonary disease. These conditions decrease excretion of anesthetic, increase the risk of postoperative atelectasis, and decrease the client's tolerance of hemodynamic changes from blood loss and fluid shifts. To reduce the risk of acute myocardial infarction, one of the most serious complications, clients may undergo coronary artery bypass before aneurysm repair.

Prerenal failure can develop for several reasons. The kidney can sustain ischemia from decreased aortic blood flow, decreased cardiac output, emboli, inadequate hydration, or the need for clamps on the aorta above the renal arteries during surgery.

Emboli can also develop and lodge in the arteries of the lower extremities or mesentery. Clinical manifestations include those of acute occlusion in the leg. Bowel necrosis is exhibited as fever, leukocytosis, ileus, diarrhea, and abdominal pain.

The spinal cord can also become ischemic, resulting in paraplegia, rectal and urinary incontinence, or loss of pain and temperature sensation. Spinal cord ischemia tends to occur more commonly when an abdominal aortic aneurysm has ruptured.

Changes in sexual function may also develop following repair of an abdominal aortic aneurysm. Retrograde ejaculation occurs in about two thirds of male clients, and loss of potency occurs in one third of males who have undergone repair of abdominal aortic aneurysm.

Nursing Management of the Surgical Client

Preoperative Care

Abdominal aortic surgery is major surgery; it lasts approximately 4 hours. During the hours under anesthesia, the client faces a great risk of pulmonary and cardiac complications developing. Preoperative assessment must include detection of concurrent coronary artery disease and cerebrovascular disease. Also assess all peripheral pulses for baseline comparison postoperatively. For endovascular repair, the procedure is much shorter. Standard evaluation must occur because the potential for an open repair of the aneurysm still exists.

Postoperative Care

Assessment. Following surgery, clients usually return to an intensive care unit. A comprehensive postoperative assessment of the client after open surgical repair for abdominal aortic aneurysm repair is essential. Potential complications are many, because of the seriousness of the problem and the complexity of the repair. Even though extracorporeal perfusion (cardiopulmonary bypass) is not needed for the surgery, arterial flow to tissues distal to the aneurysm is reduced during the time required to perform the surgery because the aorta is clamped.

Diagnosis, Outcomes, Interventions

Collaborative Problem: Risk for Hemorrhage. Because of the risk of bleeding at the graft site, the client is at risk for hemorrhage. Use the collaborative problem *Risk for Hemorrhage.* You can also use the nursing diagnosis *Risk for Deficient Fluid Volume,* but recognize that the "fluid" that can be lost is blood.

Outcomes. The nurse will monitor for manifestations of hemorrhage and notify the physician if any manifestations occur.

Interventions. Assess for changes indicating hypovolemia.

> **Monitor the client for increase in pulse rate, decrease in blood pressure, clammy skin, anxiety, restlessness, decreasing levels of consciousness, pallor, cyanosis, thirst, oliguria (urine output less than 0.5 ml/kg/hour), increase in abdominal girth, increased chest tube output greater than 100 ml/hour for 3 hours, and back pain (from retroperitoneal bleeding). Monitor central venous pressure, left atrial pressure, pulmonary artery pressure, and pulmonary capillary wedge pressure continuously. Report any of these manifestations immediately.**

SAFETY ⚠ ALERT

Diagnosis: Risk for Impaired Gas Exchange. The large abdominal incision impairs deep inspiration and usually reduced effective coughing. Write the nursing diagnosis as *Risk for Impaired Gas Exchange related to ineffective cough secondary to pain from large incision.*

Outcomes. The client will have improved gas exchange as evidenced by oxygen saturation or Pao_2 greater than 95%, increasing effectiveness in coughing, and clearing of lung sounds.

Interventions. Monitor settings on the ventilator to ensure that the client is adequately oxygenated. Assess lung sounds every 1 to 2 hours. Report any adventitious sounds. Monitor oxygen saturation continuously. Report any desaturation. After extubation, assist with coughing by using incentive spirometry, provide splinting pillows before coughing, encouraging ambulation, and providing adequate analgesia.

Diagnosis: Risk for Ineffective Tissue Perfusion. During the operation, the aorta is clamped to stop bleeding while the graft is placed. During that time, distal peripheral tissues are not perfused. The graft site can also become occluded with thrombus. In addition, the client often has pre-existing arterial disease. Write the nursing diagnosis as *Risk for Ineffective Tissue Perfusion related to temporary decrease in blood supply*.

Outcomes. The client will maintain adequate tissue perfusion as evidenced by pedal pulses, warm feet, capillary refill of less than 5 seconds, absence of numbness or tingling, and ability to dorsiflex and plantiflex both feet equally.

Interventions. Assess dorsalis pedis and posterior tibial pulses every hour for 24 hours. Report changes in pulse quality or absent pulses (assess with Doppler if needed). Assess dorsiflexion and plantiflexion and sensation ("pins and needles" sensation) every hour for 24 hours. Inspect lower extremities for mottling, cyanosis, coolness, or numbness every 4 hours.

Diagnosis: Acute Pain. Abdominal aortic aneurysm repair necessitates a long incision. Write this common postoperative diagnosis as *Acute Pain related to surgical incision*.

Outcomes. The client will have increased comfort as evidenced by self-report of decreasing levels of pain, use of decreasing amounts of opioid analgesics for pain control, and ambulating or coughing without extreme pain.

Interventions. Opioids are usually provided via a patient-controlled analgesia system or through an epidural catheter. Assess the degree of pain often, and record the baseline level of pain and the degree to which pain is reduced by medications or other interventions. When changing to an oral route for pain management, plan to pretreat the pain with oral medications 30 minutes or more before discontinuing the infusion.

Collaborative Problem: Risk for Ischemia of the Bowel. If the client undergoes extensive aortic procedures that involve clamping the mesenteric vessels, ischemic colitis can develop. In addition, the inferior mesenteric artery can embolize. The lack of blood supply can lead to ischemia and ileus.

Outcomes. The nurse will monitor the client for abdominal distention, diarrhea, severe abdominal pain, sudden elevations in white blood cell count, and bowel sounds.

Interventions. Assess bowel sounds every 4 hours. Keep the client nothing by mouth (NPO) and provide oral care every 2 to 4 hours. Provide routine nasogastric (NG)

tube care and assess nares for tissue impairment. Perform guaiac tests of NG drainage every 4 hours or if bleeding is suspected (i.e., drainage has dark, coffee-ground appearance or is bright red).

Collaborative Problem: Risk for Spinal Cord Ischemia. A rare but devastating effect of aortic abdominal aneurysm repair is spinal cord ischemia leading to paralysis, with or without bowel and bladder involvement. It appears to be most common in clients who have suprarenal aortic reconstruction.

Outcomes. The nurse will monitor for manifestations of spinal cord damage and report any abnormal data.

Interventions

> **Monitor ability to move lower extremities (dorsiflexion and plantar flexion) and sensation in both legs every 1 to 2 hours. Report any changes from baseline.**

Self-Care

Most clients who require abdominal aortic aneurysm repair have significant degrees of arterial disease. Many of the postoperative instructions should address care of clients with arterial disorders, which is discussed earlier. Review all medications to be used by the client to be certain that the purpose, schedule, and side effects are understood.

> **Instruct the client about incision care and manifestations of infection.**

The client should ambulate as tolerated, including climbing stairs and walking outdoors. If leg swelling develops, the leg should be wrapped in elastic bandages or support stockings should be used. Activities that involve lifting heavy objects, usually more than 15 to 20 pounds, are not permitted for 6 to 12 weeks postoperatively. Activities that involve pushing, pulling, or straining may also be restricted. Driving may also be restricted because of postoperative weakness and decreased response time.

The client can resume sexual activity in about 4 to 6 weeks, when the client is able to walk without shortness of breath (e.g., two flights of stairs). The risk of impotence in male clients should be discussed before discharge. Causes vary from pre-existing aortoiliac disease or diabetes to side effects from aortic cross-clamping. Referral may be appropriate if the client is amenable.

RUPTURE OF AN ABDOMINAL AORTIC ANEURYSM

Rupture of an abdominal aortic aneurysm (AAA) is a catastrophe. Rupture occurs most often in aneurysm

5 cm or more in diameter; an abdominal aneurysm measuring 6 cm or more in diameter has a 20% chance of rupturing in 1 year. Less than 50% of people with a ruptured abdominal aortic aneurysm survive. Abdominal, back, or flank pain of sudden onset is characteristic of a rapidly expanding or ruptured AAA. The diagnosis should be entertained whenever a client older than 50 years presents with abdominal pain, particularly when pain is associated with syncope or signs of hemorrhagic shock.

The Critical Monitoring feature below lists clinical manifestations associated with ruptured abdominal aortic aneurysm.

Surgery is the only intervention for clients with ruptured abdominal aortic aneurysm. New surgical and grafting techniques and faster methods for transport (e.g., helicopters) permit rapid resection of ruptured abdominal aortic aneurysm. However, even with advances in surgery, the operative mortality rate for repair of ruptured abdominal aneurysm may be as high as 50%. Manage hemorrhagic shock with fluid resuscitation, and blood transfusion. If the client is hypertensive before surgery, there is greater risk of rupture. Treat the blood pressure to maintain a systolic pressure between 100 and 120 mm Hg. Care of the client following emergency repair of a ruptured AAA is the same as elective repair, except that the client has more hemodynamic instability because of preoperative blood loss and ischemic organ disease.

AORTIC DISSECTION

Aortic dissection is the longitudinal splitting of the medial (muscular) layer of the aorta by blood flowing through it. It is the most common catastrophe involving the aorta. Dissection occurs following a tear in the intima, or inner lining, of the aorta, which allows blood to dissect between it and the medial layer. As the dissection progresses, blood flow through the arterial branches of the aorta becomes blocked, and blood flow to the organs that are served by these branches is reduced. Aortic dissections occur more often in men between 50 and 70 years of age, most of whom are hypertensive. Aortic dissections differ from aneurysms in that a false lumen is formed by separation of the intima from the medial layers of the aorta. An aneurysm is a dilation of the entire aortic wall.

Etiology and Classification

The exact cause of dissection is not known. The medial layer of the aorta can become necrotic and thereby lose strength. Clients with Marfan syndrome (a hereditary condition of connective tissue that predisposes it to aneurysm formation) have a high incidence of dissection. Blunt trauma to the chest wall, such as impact on the steering wheel during a car accident, can also lead to tearing of the aorta.

Dissections are classified by the anatomic location using the Stanford classification system. There are two types of dissections: type A and type B. Type A involves the ascending aorta; type B does not. This system also helps delineate treatment. Usually, type A dissections require surgery, whereas type B dissections may be managed medically under most conditions.

Clinical Manifestations

Abrupt, excruciating pain is the most common presenting manifestation in clients with aortic dissection. Clients describe the pain as ripping or knife-like tearing sensations that radiate to the back, abdomen, extremities, or anterior part of the chest. Hypertension is a common finding, although the client looks "shocky," is sweating profusely, is severely apprehensive, and has diminished peripheral pulses. Other manifestations from decreased perfusion include unequal pulses, different blood pressures in the arms, paraplegia or hemiplegia, decreased urine output or hematuria, mental status changes, and chest pain. A murmur of aortic regurgitation can be heard if the dissection proceeds proximally.

Chest radiograph reveals a widened mediastinum and may show fractured ribs. Transesophageal echocardiogram can be used to determine the size, shape, and location of the tear. Laboratory tests during emergency settings are usually not helpful, except for hemoglobin and hematocrit assays to calculate blood loss and transfusion needs. If the client's condition is stable, helical CT or magnetic resonance imaging can be used to determine the extent of the dissection.

CRITICAL MONITORING

Ruptured Abdominal Aortic Aneurysm

- Pulsating sensation in the abdomen
- Severe, sudden, persistent or constant pain in the abdomen
  - Pain is not colicky or spasmodic
  - Pain radiates to groin, lower back, buttocks, or legs
- Abdominal rigidity
- Manifestations of shock
  - Pallor
  - Tachycardia with hypotension
  - Dry skin and mouth
  - Excessive thirst
  - Anxiety

Complications

Cardiac tamponade can develop when the client has dissection of the ascending aortic arch. This life-threatening complication occurs when blood escapes from the area of dissection into the pericardial sac. Clients have pulsus paradoxus, muffled heart sounds, narrowed pulse pressure, and distended neck veins. Pulsus paradoxus occurs when beats are weaker in amplitude during inspiration and stronger with expiration. Blood pressure readings decrease more than 10 mm Hg during inspiration and increase with expiration.

Because the dissection decreases blood supply to many vital organs, ischemic changes in many organs can develop. The spinal cord, kidneys, and abdominal organs are most commonly affected. Ischemia of the spinal cord can lead to manifestations ranging from weakness to paralysis. Renal ischemia can lead to oliguria. Ileus is the most common manifestation of decreased bowel perfusion.

OUTCOME MANAGEMENT

Emergency management is directed at lowering the blood pressure to decrease the force of the blood tearing the aorta. Potent vasodilators, such as nitroprusside, are used to quickly reduce blood pressure. Beta-blockers can also be used to decrease myocardial contractility.

If the client's condition is stable, management is directed at pain reduction, blood transfusion (as needed), and management of heart failure (as needed). Pain levels are used as a guide for needed treatment. Pain subsides when the dissection stabilizes.

Surgery is used for clients whose condition is unstable, in whom severe heart failure develops, who have leaking blood, or who have occlusion of arteries to major organs. During surgery, the torn area is resected and repaired with synthetic graft materials. The operation is similar to that for repair of AAA.

Nursing care is directed at reducing blood pressure. The client is maintained on bed rest in a semi-Fowler position. Unnecessary environmental stresses (e.g., noise) should be minimized. Use opioids to reduce pain; tranquilizers may also be needed. If the client is receiving potent antihypertensive agents, blood pressure should be monitored continuously with an arterial line. Usually the desired parameters for blood pressure are maintained by titrating the vasodilators. Observe the client often for manifestations of further tearing or rupture. Monitor peripheral pulses, level of anxiety, level of pain, and pulse pressure and check for pulsus paradoxus.

If the client is being managed medically, teach the client about the need for antihypertensive agents and beta-blocker drugs.

SAFETY ALERT **The client and family should understand that if pain returns they should immediately return to the emergency department.**

RAYNAUD'S SYNDROME

Raynaud's syndrome is a condition in which the small arteries and arterioles constrict in response to various stimuli. It is classified as either vasospastic or obstructive. Manifestations of vasospastic Raynaud's syndrome can be induced by cold, nicotine, caffeine, and stress. Obstructive Raynaud's syndrome is often found in association with autoimmune disorders such as systemic lupus erythematosus, scleroderma, or rheumatoid arthritis.

Raynaud's syndrome may be a benign primary disorder (previously called *Raynaud's disease*) or secondary to another disease or underlying cause (previously called *Raynaud's phenomenon*). Manifestations of both types are the same.

Clinical Manifestations

Raynaud's syndrome causes classic color changes in the hands. Exposure to causative stimuli leads to spasm of the digital arteries, which results in pallor. The resulting tissue hypoxia causes the arteries to dilate slightly. Because they carry mainly deoxygenated hemoglobin, the fingers look cyanotic. Finally, rubor develops when arterial spasms stop completely. Criteria for diagnosing primary Raynaud's disease include (1) manifestations for at least 2 years, (2) intermittent attacks of pallor or cyanosis of the digits by exposure to cold or from emotional stimuli, (3) bilateral or symmetrical involvement, (4) no evidence of occlusive disease in the digital arteries or of any systemic disease that might be the cause of the changes, and (5) gangrene, which (when it occurs) is limited to the skin of the tips of the digits.

Noninvasive blood flow studies to determine finger pressures both before and after cold challenge may be necessary. Occasionally, the presence of vasospasm during examination makes the use of cold challenge unnecessary.

OUTCOME MANAGEMENT

Conservative measures are essential. These measures include keeping hands and feet warm and dry, protecting all parts of the body from cold exposure to prevent reflex sympathetic vasoconstriction of the digits, and terminating tobacco use. Biofeedback has been of help to some clients.

Medication is used when the vasospastic attacks interfere with the client's ability to work or to perform activities of daily living. Medications are used to induce smooth muscle relaxation, to relieve spasm, and to increase arterial flow. Calcium antagonists, such as nifedipine, are the drugs of first choice because they have been shown to decrease the frequency, duration, and intensity of vasospastic attacks. Medications may be necessary only during the winter months. Individuals who rarely go out in the cold weather may take medications prophylactically 1 to 2 hours before exposure to the cold.

The manifestations of Raynaud's syndrome may be alarming, so reassure the client that the condition is not likely to lead to a serious disability. Advise the client to stay warm by wearing wool gloves and turtleneck sweaters, turning up the thermostat at home if necessary, and staying out of drafts. Teach the client to warm up a cold car before driving. Body core heating is important to prevent chilling and the shunting of blood from the extremities to the trunk. Encourage clients to limit their intake of caffeine or chocolate. They must stop smoking to control the disease. Stress can also trigger vasospasm, so stress management workshops and biofeedback programs may be beneficial. Also, teach the client about any prescribed medications.

BUERGER'S DISEASE (THROMBOANGIITIS OBLITERANS)

Buerger's disease (thromboangiitis obliterans) is an inflammatory disease of the small and medium-sized arteries and veins of the extremities. It is often seen in men and appears to be directly related to smoking. Many clients have a hypersensitivity reaction to intradermal injection of tobacco products, so there may also be an autoimmune element as well. Raynaud's phenomenon, ulcers, and pain are typically seen.

Pain is the outstanding clinical manifestation. Clients have digital ulcerations and pain from ischemia. The pain may be accompanied by manifestations of ischemia, such as color or temperature changes in the fingers. Cold sensitivity, with color changes and pain, may be another early manifestation. Various types of lower extremity paresthesias may occur. Claudication type pain is common, with pain in the arch of the foot. Pulsations in the posterior tibial and dorsalis pedis arteries are weak or absent. In advanced cases, the extremities may be abnormally red or cyanotic, particularly when dependent.

Ulceration and gangrene are frequent complications and may occur early in the course of the disease. These lesions can appear spontaneously from migratory superficial thrombophlebitis but can also follow trauma. Gangrene usually occurs in one extremity at a time. Edema of the legs is fairly common in advanced cases. Changes in the nails and skin appear, and segmental thrombophlebitis affects the smaller veins in about 40% of clients. The primary diagnostic study is leg arteriography. Biopsy may also be used; inflammatory lesions are usually noted.

OUTCOME MANAGEMENT

The goals for management include arresting progress of the disease, producing vasodilation, relieving pain, and providing emotional support. The need for smoking cessation must be clearly and unequivocally conveyed to the client and family. Information about programs to promote abstinence from tobacco should be provided. Because of vasoconstriction, the client should be taught to avoid exposure to cold. Work-related exposure to cold should be considered.

For clients with rest pain and ischemic lesions, adequate pain control is essential. Vasodilation by calcium-channel blockers may be used. Ulcerations need wound care to facilitate healing. Amputation should be deferred until conservative interventions have failed. Thromboangiitis is usually not life-threatening. It does, however, result in disability from pain and amputation.

VENOUS DISORDERS

Venous disorders can be separated into acute and chronic conditions. Chronic venous disorders can be further separated into varicose vein formation and chronic venous insufficiency. Acute venous disorders include thromboembolism. Acute venous disorders are discussed first.

ACUTE VENOUS DISORDERS

Acute venous disorders are caused by thrombus (clot) formation that obstructs venous flow. Blockage may occur in either the superficial or the deep veins.

THROMBOPHLEBITIS

Superficial thrombophlebitis is usually an easily diagnosed condition; it may iatrogenic, resulting from intravenous catheters or infusion of caustic solutions. Deep vein thrombosis (DVT) is thrombophlebitis of the deep veins. DVT is a common disorder, more so in women than in men, and among hospitalized clients. DVT develops in approximately one third of clients older than 40 years who have had major surgery, orthopedic surgery, or an acute myocardial infarction. In addition, clients with cancer or a family history of clotting disorders are at high risk.

Etiology and Risk Factors

There are many risk factors for the development of venous thrombosis (Box 53-2). Thrombus formation is usually attributed to Virchow's triad: (1) venous stasis, (2) hypercoagulability, and (3) injury to the venous wall. At least two of the three conditions must be present for thrombi to form.

Venous stasis is usually caused by immobilization or lack of use of the calf muscle pump. Other conditions that may cause stasis are age older than 40 years, surgery, immobility, prolonged travel, stroke, obesity, pregnancy, paralysis, and heart disease such as heart failure, myocardial infarction, and cardiomyopathy. Some of the highest risk clients are those having orthopedic surgery.

> **BOX 53-2 Common Conditions Associated with Venous Thrombosis and Thromboembolism**
>
> - Age >40 years
> - Surgery requiring more than 30 minutes of general, spinal, or epidural anesthesia
> - Postoperative edema in the pelvis
> - Prolonged position of hip flexion
> - Venous stasis (bed rest, prolonged travel, stroke)
> - Previous deep vein thrombosis
> - Cardiac disease (heart failure, myocardial infarction, cardiomyopathy)
> - Pregnancy
> - Trauma, especially of the lower extremities
> - Estrogen therapy or oral contraceptives
> - Malignancy
> - Obesity
> - Family history of clotting disorders

Hypercoagulability often accompanies malignant cancers (especially visceral and ovarian tumors). Dehydration and blood dyscrasias may raise the platelet count, decrease fibrinolysis, increase the clotting factors, or increase the viscosity of the blood. Oral contraceptives and hematologic disorders may also increase the coagulability of the blood.

SAFETY ⚠ ALERT

Conditions that may cause vein wall trauma are intravenous injections; fractures and dislocations; severe blows to an area; chemical injury from sclerosing agents, contrast x-ray studies, or certain antibiotics (such as chlortetracycline); and thromboangiitis obliterans (Buerger's disease). The resulting damage to the vein wall attracts platelets, and blood debris accumulates. Platelets do not stick to an intact endothelium. This injury, in combination with low blood flow and a hypercoagulable state, results in thrombus formation.

Pathophysiology

Usually, venous return is aided by the calf muscle pump. When the legs are inactive or the pump is ineffective, blood pools by gravity in the veins (Figure 53-10). Thrombus development is a local process. It begins by platelet adherence to the endothelium. Several factors promote platelet aggregation, including thrombin, fibrin, activated factor X, and catecholamines. In addition, where the platelets adhere to collagen, adenosine diphosphate (ADP) is released. ADP is also released from the damaged tissues and disrupted platelets. ADP produces platelet aggregation that results in a platelet plug. Approximately 24 to 48 hours after formation, thrombi undergo lysis or become organized and adhere to the vessel wall, a process that diminishes the risk of embolization.

Deep vein thrombi vary from 1 mm in diameter to long tubular masses filling main veins. Small thrombi are found commonly in the pocket of deep vein valves. As thrombi become larger in diameter and length, they obstruct the

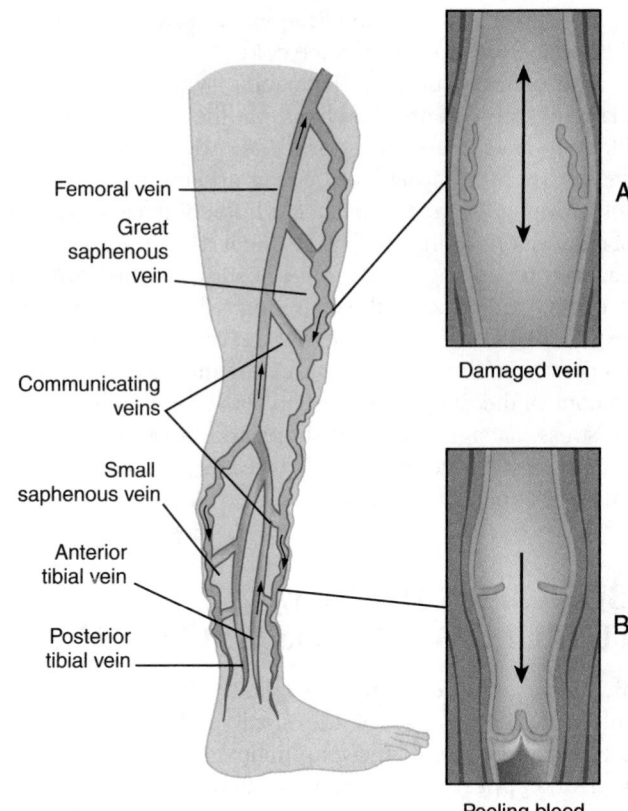

Femoral vein
Great saphenous vein
Communicating veins
Small saphenous vein
Anterior tibial vein
Posterior tibial vein

Damaged vein

A

Pooling blood

B

■ **FIGURE 53-10** Venous return from the legs. **A,** Normal flow **B,** Varicosities and retrograde venous flow.

veins. If a thrombus occludes a major vein (e.g., femoral, vena cava, axillary), the venous pressure and volume increase distally. Conversely, if a thrombus occludes a deep small vein (e.g., tibial, popliteal), collateral venous channels usually relieve the increased venous pressure and volume. The resulting inflammatory process can destroy the valves of the veins; thus venous insufficiency and postphlebitic syndrome are initiated.

Newly formed thrombi may embolize and travel. Pulmonary emboli, most of which start as thrombi in the large deep veins of the legs, are an acute and potentially lethal complication of DVT. Pulmonary embolism (PE) is discussed in Chapter 61.

Prevention

Because of the frequency of DVT and the risk of PE, prevention is imperative. Prevention is geared toward reversing the three risk factors by promoting venous return, treating hypercoagulability, and reducing risk of injury to the venous wall.

Venous stasis is improved by any activity that causes the leg muscles to contract; passive or active contraction promotes venous return. Leg exercises and ambulation promote venous return. Passive leg muscle contraction occurs by using intermittent sequential compression devices (SCDs) (Figure 53-11). These devices are applied

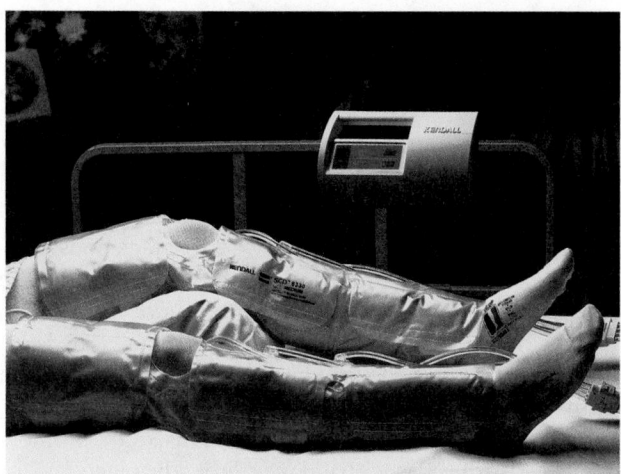

■ **FIGURE 53-11** Pneumatic compression devices, such as the Kendall sequential compression device, are commonly used to prevent deep vein thrombosis in high-risk clients. *(Courtesy Kendall Company, Mansfield, Mass.)*

after surgery and carefully used until the client is ambulatory. Research has shown that SCDs are clinically effective in reducing the incidence of DVT. It is also a good alternative for clients who cannot tolerate anticoagulation. These devices should *not* be used in clients with known DVT. Other methods of promoting venous return include elevating the foot of the bed, applying compression stockings, using motorized foot compressive devices, and providing passive range-of-motion exercises. Encouraging postoperative deep-breathing exercises promotes thoracic pull as a result of the negative thoracic pressure on venous stores in the legs.

Pharmacologic prevention directed at reducing the hypercoagulability includes warfarin, platelet antiaggregation agents (aspirin being the most common), heparin, and low-molecular-weight heparin. Other methods to reduce coagulation include preventing the venous blood from pooling.

> **Avoid using pillows under the client's knees postoperatively. Teach the client to avoid sitting or standing in one position for prolonged periods.**
>
> **Measures to prevent injury to the vein wall include avoidance of (1) infiltration during intravenous therapy, (2) pressure on the calf veins during prolonged surgery, and (3) trauma to veins in procedures requiring prolonged positioning (e.g., childbirth, colonoscopy). In addition, access ports should be used in clients requiring multiple intravenous punctures.**

Clinical Manifestations and Diagnostic Findings

Clinical manifestations of superficial thrombophlebitis include redness (rubor), induration, warmth (calor), and tenderness (dolor) along a vein. Discomfort may be relieved by applying heat. Activity should be encouraged, and a supportive wrap or stocking should be applied.

The clinical manifestations of DVT are less distinctive; about half of clients are asymptomatic. The most common clinical manifestation is unilateral leg swelling. Other clinical manifestations include pain, redness or warmth of the leg, dilated veins, and low-grade fever. The first clinical manifestation may be PE. Clients may have thrombi in both legs even though the manifestations are unilateral, but this is more common in the client with malignancy.

Homans' sign—discomfort in the upper calf during forced dorsiflexion of the foot—is commonly assessed during physical examination, but findings are insensitive and nonspecific. Homans' sign is present in less than one third of clients with documented DVT. In addition, more than 50% of clients with a positive Homans' sign do not have venous thrombosis. For example, shin splints from running create a positive Homans' sign without DVT.

Venous duplex scanning has become the primary diagnostic test for DVT because it allows visualization of the vein, which provides a reliable diagnosis of venous thrombus. Venography, the previous gold standard of diagnosis, results in exposure to contrast medium and is seldom used. The D-dimer blood test is being used more frequently in evaluation of DVT. The D-dimer is a product of fibrin degradation and is indicative of fibrinolysis, which occurs with thrombosis. Recent studies seem to indicate that the use of the D-dimer test, a risk assessment score, and duplex imaging are excellent at predicting and diagnosing DVT in an asymptomatic population. Plethysmographic examination of the venous system is seldom used, although results of these studies may be found in client records.

OUTCOME MANAGEMENT

Medical Management

The goals of medical management are to reduce risk of DVT, detect the thrombus early, prevent extension or embolization of the thrombus, and prevent further thrombus formation.

Superficial thrombophlebitis can be managed with local measures, such as warm packs and elevation of the extremity. Ambulation is encouraged. Sometimes anti-inflammatory medications are required. Clients are encouraged to be seen in follow-up, because an extension of a superficial phlebitis can result in a DVT.

Anticoagulation

Anticoagulant therapy is designed to prevent initiation or extension of thrombi by inhibiting the synthesis of clotting factors or by accelerating their inactivation. Anticoagulant agents do not break up or dissolve clots; they prevent new clots from forming. Various agents that can be used for anticoagulation are discussed in the Integrating Pharmacology feature on p. 1334.

Nursing Management of the Medical Client

Goals of nursing management are to prevent DVT in high-risk clients, prevent existing thrombi from becoming emboli, and prevent new thrombi from forming. Nurses also closely monitor the effect of anticoagulant medications.

Prevent DVT

All clients prescribed bed rest should be encouraged to move their legs because blood stasis leads to clotting. Sequential compression devices (SCDs) should be used for those clients expected to be prescribed bed rest for longer than 24 hours. SCDs are removed twice daily to inspect the skin and allow perspiration to evaporate. High-risk clients may also be prescribed anticoagulants.

Promote Venous Return

Elevation of the legs above the level of the heart facilitates blood flow by the force of gravity. The increase of blood flow prevents venous stasis and the formation of new thrombi. Elevation of the legs also decreases venous pressure, which in turn reduces edema and pain. Elevate the foot of the bed 6 inches (Trendelenburg's position), with a slight knee bend to prevent popliteal pressure. The veins of the legs should be level with the right atrium. The head of the bed may be raised to facilitate eating and bathing. Various forms of elastic support are used to promote venous return. Elastic bandages are advantageous for

---

INTEGRATING PHARMACOLOGY

Anticoagulant Therapy for the Prevention and Treatment of Deep Vein Thrombosis

Anticoagulation prevents the extension of the original thrombus and the development of new thrombi while the existing thrombus is lysed naturally by fibrinolysis. Oral warfarin (Coumadin) and parenterally administered heparin have been the mainstays of anticoagulant therapy since the 1940s. Even though it is well-known that these medications are effective, they have several undesirable characteristics, such as unpredictability in dosage required for therapeutic effect, the need for careful laboratory monitoring, and the potential for life-threatening toxicity.

Acute deep vein thrombosis (DVT) is treated with continuous intravenous heparin or injected low-molecular-weight heparin (LMWH). Heparin is normally administered according to the client's weight and blood levels of activated partial thromboplastin time (aPPT or PTT), which is maintained either at more than 60 seconds or at a level 1.5 to 2.5 times a baseline established before the beginning of therapy. Heparin is usually infused in the range of 700 to 1400 units/hour. When the client has marked elevated PTT levels, frequent assessment of bleeding or bruising and institution of bleeding precautions are important. Bleeding precautions include avoidance of injections, brushing teeth with a soft sponge device, supervision with ambulation to prevent falls, and increasing intake of fiber and fluids to prevent straining and constipation. Heparin has a short half-life of 4 hours and can be quickly reversed with protamine. Heparin has increased effects when simultaneously administered with other anticoagulants. Therefore a full list of prescribed and over-the-counter medications must be reviewed for potential drug-drug interactions.

LMWH has been available for the past decade. LMWHs are longer acting, homogeneous molecules, with a reliable dose-response curve requiring little or no monitoring, but they are much more expensive than heparin. The actions of heparin and LMWHs are similar. Both bind to antithrombin III, increasing its activity and inhibiting thrombin and other factors. Whereas the anticoagulant function of heparin can be measured through PTT, no such blood test is available for LMWH. This may seem like a drawback for LMWHs, but the reason that standard heparin therapy must be monitored is because heparin has an unpredictable bioavailability and pharmacokinetics, particularly when administered subcutaneously. LMWHs, however, have extremely high bioavailability. The same bleeding precautions and drug-drug interactions apply with LMWH.

Coumadin (warfarin or coumarin) is an oral anticoagulant. It is often used as a long-term anticoagulant after the acute DVT has been treated with injectable forms of heparin. Coumadin has a long half-life (3 to 5 days). Therefore the drug must be stopped for 3 days before any invasive procedure is done. Coumadin is prescribed based on International Normalized Ratio (INR) levels; the recommended therapeutic range is 2 to 3.5. Coumadin can also be prescribed based on prothrombin (ProTime) levels, but there is variation from one laboratory to another, so INR levels are becoming more common, especially with long-term use of warfarin (Coumadin). For hospitalized clients, warfarin (Coumadin) is administered in the afternoon or early evening. This schedule allows for dose adjustments based on daily INR or ProTime results. Warfarin (Coumadin) can be reversed with injections of vitamin K (phytonadione). The therapeutic effect of warfarin (Coumadin) is altered by a host of medications and foods, and in clients with liver disease. Potential drug-drug and drug-food interactions should be reviewed by a pharmacist if the intended response (e.g., changes in INR) is not seen as predicted.

PREVENTION OF DEEP VEIN THROMBOSIS

Several medications can be used to prevent DVT. Standard heparin is increased by adjusting the dose to maintain the aPTT ratio in the upper normal range. An average dose is 5000 units given subcutaneously in the abdomen twice daily. LMWH is also given subcutaneously. Subcutaneous injection of anticoagulants can lead to bruising at the injection sites. Clients and families should be taught that this is an expected response and does not indicate active bleeding. The development of painful masses in the abdomen should be reported and may indicate more active bleeding.

The use of antiplatelet drugs, aspirin, and nonsteroidal anti-inflammatory drugs may have a place in the prevention of DVT postoperatively or once conventional anticoagulant therapy for DVT has been concluded, although there is still debate on this topic.

clients with large or misshapen legs. Apply elastic wraps snugly from toe to groin. Use a narrower elastic wrap for the foot and a wider one for the leg. Rewrap them every 4 to 8 hours. If compression stockings are prescribed, they must be fitted correctly and removed for a short time every day. Bathe the legs and inspect them closely for manifestations of skin breakdown while the stockings are off.

Reduce Discomfort

Elevation of the extremity and application of warm packs usually reduce discomfort. Some clients need a mild analgesic.

Monitor Anticoagulant Therapy

Most physicians use an algorithm to adjust the dose of heparin based on the client's body weight and partial thromboplastin time (PTT) results. Blood is sampled every 4 to 8 hours for measurement of PTT or International Normalized Ratio (INR), and the dose is adjusted accordingly. Warfarin therapy requires the prothrombin time (PT) or INR be determined on a regular basis. Low-molecular-weight heparin requires no testing.

> **Bleeding can occur in any client receiving anticoagulation. The client should also be observed for frank bleeding in the urine, tarry or frank blood in the stool, bleeding with brushing the teeth, easy subcutaneous bruising, and flank pain. When invasive studies are necessary (e.g., arterial blood gas analyses), apply pressure for 30 minutes to the puncture site.**

Monitor for Pulmonary Embolism

PE is an acute and potentially lethal complication of DVT. Tachypnea and anxiety are the most common manifestations of PE. Pleuritic chest pain can also occur. It is often sudden and aggravated by breathing. Pleuritic pain is caused by an inflammatory reaction of the lung parenchyma or by pulmonary infarction or ischemia caused by obstruction of small pulmonary arterial branches.

Other clinical manifestations may include cough without hemoptysis, diaphoresis, dyspnea, crackles, and wheezing. Hemoptysis can occur as a result of pulmonary infarction, or atelectasis may produce alveolar hemorrhage. Because of the seriousness of PE, promptly notify the physician of these clinical manifestations. Document the lack of manifestations or PE in clients with DVT to provide evidence of monitoring for the condition. PE is fully discussed in Chapter 61.

Surgical Management

Surgical treatment of thrombophlebitis is aimed at reducing PE by inserting a filter into the vena cava to filter the blood before it reaches the lungs (see Chapter 61).

Thrombectomy can also be performed, but it is not common.

Self-Care

Prevention is the key to managing DVT. Therefore teach the client about risk factors of DVT and how to avoid them. Continue teaching with explanations of medications being taken, actions, doses, timing, adverse effects, and importance of monitoring coagulation status. Begin teaching on the first day of heparinization, discussing reasons for anticoagulants. Clients need to know who to contact and how to reach a health care provider in case problems develop. Inform the client about the monitoring required while receiving anticoagulation therapy.

After thrombosis of a deep calf vein, clients should wear elastic support for at least 3 to 6 months and probably for life. Elastic support compresses the superficial veins when the client walks, and blood flow in the larger veins is increased while venous pressure is kept to a minimum. Standing and sitting are not allowed for long periods during the acute phase so as not to increase the hydrostatic pressure in the capillaries, which promotes edema. Encourage walking and exercises in bed to decrease venous pressure and promote blood flow.

CHRONIC VENOUS DISORDERS

VARICOSE VEINS

Varicose veins are permanently distended veins that develop from the loss of valvular competence. Faulty valves elevate venous pressure, causing distention and tortuosity of the superficial veins. The greater and lesser saphenous veins and perforator veins in the ankle are common sites of varicosities.

Varicose veins may be either primary or secondary. Primary varicose veins often result from a congenital or familial predisposition that leads to loss of elasticity of the vein wall. Secondary varicosities occur when trauma, obstruction, DVT, or inflammation causes damage to valves.

Varicose veins affect a large percentage of the adult population. An estimated 24 million Americans have varicose veins. The prevalence increases with age and peaks between the fifth and sixth decades of life. Varicose veins are more common in women; however, the gender ratio decreases with advancing age and almost disappears in clients older than 70 years. Prolonged standing has been implicated as a cause of varicose veins, but epidemiologic studies have not demonstrated an association between standing at work and an increased incidence of varicose veins.

Clients with varicose veins often complain of aching, a feeling of heaviness in the legs, itching, moderate swelling, and, frequently, the unsightly appearance of their legs. Severity of discomfort is difficult to assess and does not seem related to the size of varicosities. A superficial inflammation may occasionally develop along the path of the varicose vein. To assess for varicose veins, carefully examine both of the client's legs in good lighting. Varicosities appear as dilated, tortuous skin veins (Figure 53-12).

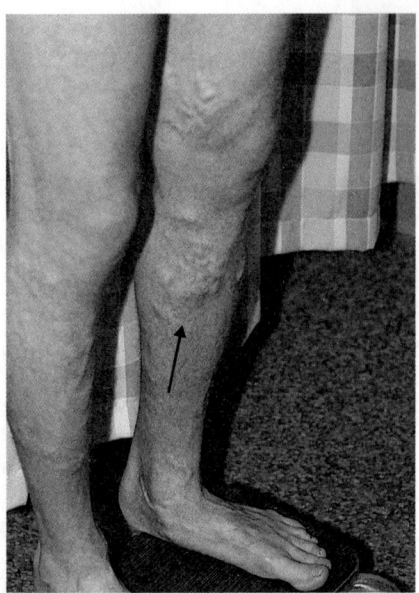

■ **FIGURE 53–12** Varicose veins on the surface of the leg (arrow). Note the tortuous pattern.

 OUTCOME MANAGEMENT

Medical Management

In early stages of varicose veins, the goal is to reduce venous pooling, prevent complications, and improve comfort levels. The simplest form of treatment is the application of below-the-knee compression stockings or elastic wraps. These stockings are designed to apply the greatest amount of pressure over the ankle.

Nursing Management of the Medical Client

The client should be taught that varicose veins are a chronic problem. Even though they do not subside, various activities can help prevent ulceration or new varicosities. The client should avoid standing still in one position for extended periods of time. Legs should be elevated when seated and, if swelling is present, legs should be elevated higher than the heart. Elastic stockings or support hose should be worn to help with venous blood return. Fit of elastic stockings is important. Many clients with venous disease have misshapen legs and standard stockings do not fit them well, being too tight in the ankle. Custom stockings may be needed. Elastic wraps need to be wrapped twice daily so that greatest pressure is at the ankle, with lesser pressure gradually applied to the level of the knee.

Surgical Management

Sclerotherapy

Sclerotherapy is the injection of a sclerosing agent into varicose veins. The agent damages the vein and endothelium,

causing an aseptic thrombosis that closes the vein. Application of pressure causes the vein walls to grow together. Sclerotherapy is usually performed for cosmetic reasons, but it may relieve the discomfort of both short segments of varicosities and spider veins. It is most effective in closing small, residual varicosities after surgical intervention for varicose veins. (Sclerotherapy is contraindicated before such surgery, because it makes vein stripping more difficult.) Within minutes after injection of the sclerosing agent, elastic compression and active walking should commence. Elastic bandages are worn for 1 to 3 weeks, from morning to night (but not 24 hours a day).

Vein Ligation and Stripping

Surgical management of varicose veins consists of ligation (tying off) of the greater saphenous vein with its tributaries at the saphenofemoral junction, combined with removal of the saphenous vein (stripping) and ligation of incompetent perforator veins. Removal of the vein is performed through multiple, short incisions. An incision is made at the ankle over the saphenous vein and a nylon wire is threaded up the vein to the groin. The wire is brought out through the groin, capped, and then the wire and vein are pulled out through the ankle incision. If the perforator veins alone are ligated, it may be done through multiple small endoscopic incisions.

Elastic compression bandages are applied from foot to groin. The client is rarely hospitalized overnight. Complications are infrequent and include bleeding, infection, and nerve damage. Hemorrhage most commonly occurs at the surgical wound site in the groin. Bleeding comes primarily from the stripped canal. The risk of serious bleeding can be decreased by carefully wrapping the leg from foot to groin and by applying compression, especially to the upper thigh and groin. Some discoloration and bruising along the stripped tract are normal.

Saphenous nerve damage may occur with surgery. In the distal third of the leg, the saphenous nerve runs close to the saphenous vein. Thus risk of nerve injury increases when the distal part of the vein is involved. DVT, embolism, and infection are rare following varicose vein surgery, especially if postoperative precautions (e.g., bandaging, movement, exercise) are taken.

Saphenofemoral Ligation

Some clients require only tying off of the junction of the saphenous and the femoral vein at the groin. This involves one short incision, often local anesthesia, and no hospital stay. Postoperative care is the same.

Nursing Management of the Surgical Client

Routine postoperative assessment and care are provided. Specific care includes maintaining firm elastic pressure over the whole limb, reducing the risk of thrombophlebitis by promoting regular movement and exercise of the legs, and improving venous return by elevating the foot of the bed 6 to 9 inches so that the legs are above the heart level when the client is in bed. The client ambulates for short periods, starting immediately after surgery. Clients should walk rather than stand or sit. After ambulation, elevate the client's legs again.

CHRONIC VENOUS INSUFFICIENCY

Chronic venous insufficiency is also known as *postphlebitic syndrome* and follows most severe cases of DVT. Chronic venous insufficiency results from dysfunctional valves that reduce venous return, which thus increases venous pressure and causes venous stasis. Because existing valves are destroyed, venous blood flow is bidirectional, resulting in inefficient venous outflow. The net effect of this change is that the weight of the venous blood column from the right atrium is transmitted along the full length of the veins. Very high venous pressure is exerted at the ankle and the venules become the final pathway for the highest venous pressure. The current theory is that the abnormal capillaries lead to extravasation of red blood cells, activation of endothelial cells, and trapping of white blood cells. The end result is capillary thrombosis. Skin ulcerations also occur.

Chronic venous insufficiency is marked by the following characteristics:

- Chronically swollen legs
- Thick, coarse, brownish skin around the ankles (referred to as the "gaiter" area)
- Venous stasis ulceration (Figure 53-13)
- Itchy, scaly skin

OUTCOME MANAGEMENT

Goals of management are to increase venous blood return and to decrease venous pressure. Antigravity measures increase blood return to the heart. They include elevating the client's legs above the heart level and avoiding prolonged standing or sitting. Encourage the client to sleep with the foot of the bed elevated 6 inches. At least one third of every 24 hours should be spent with the feet and legs elevated above the heart. The client should also be taught *not* to cross the legs, sit in chairs that are too high to allow the feet to touch the floor or that are too deep (and press on the popliteal area), or wear garters, rolled stockings or tight girdles.

The Bridge to Home Health Care feature on p. 1338 describes how increased venous pressure on the tissues of the leg can be counteracted by the compression of elastic support hose. Ideally, this support should just balance the increased venous pressure. Thus hose should be fitted individually to the client's legs. Measurements of the ankle and calf circumference and from 1 inch below the knee or 1 inch below the groin to the bottom of the foot are usually taken. Measure after the client has

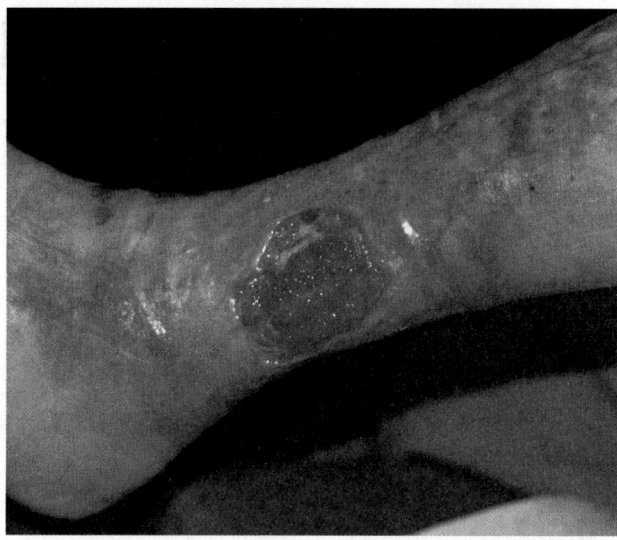

■ **FIGURE 53–13** Venous stasis ulcers usually develop in the lower outer leg, appear irregular, and have a beefy red base. Note the dark-stained skin from venous disease.

been recumbent and leg edema is minimal. Stockings that extend above the knee often bind the popliteal space and act as a tourniquet, especially when the knee is bent. Knee-length elastic stockings are preferable. Elastic wraps are often preferable for clients who have periods of leg swelling. Apply the elastic wrap using a graded technique, placing more tension on the lower leg. The problem with elastic wraps is that they only maintain their elastic properties for a few washings (with a few exceptions), and clients tend to use them long past their effective compression. Additionally, wraps often are not used properly and do not exert adequate compression.

VENOUS STASIS ULCERATION

Venous stasis ulceration is the end stage of chronic venous insufficiency. Prolonged venous pressure slows nutrient blood flow, which deprives cells of needed oxygen, glucose, and other substances. Skin of the lower legs ulcerates, causing a stasis ulcer, which occurs as a result of stasis of blood. It is characteristically located in the malleolar or gaiter (lower third of the leg) area (see Figure 53-13). It is important to determine the cause of the ulcer before beginning treatment. Determining whether arterial disease is present is imperative; compression devices are contraindicated in arterial disease because they can restrict arterial inflow of blood.

Management of venous stasis ulceration includes leg elevation, wound care, moist dressings, and support stockings. Gravity is the major enemy of venous stasis disease. The client should rest with his or her legs elevated 6 inches. Regular walking is encouraged.

When ulcers are present, cultures are often obtained of painful, odorous, or weeping wounds to rule out infection.

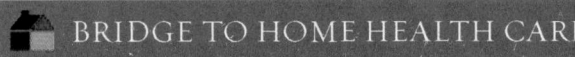

Managing Peripheral Vascular Disease

Many clients who are referred to home health agencies or clinics that serve older people have peripheral vascular disease. Consider what you can do to help clients prevent further complications through assessment and evaluation, blood pressure monitoring, health education, and reporting changes in your clients' status to their physicians.

ASSESSMENT

Inspect clients for temperature variations; color changes in the skin; dorsal and ankle foot pulses; extremity size comparisons; shiny, taunt, hairless, or blistered skin; diminished toenail growth and color change; pain with palpation, dependent position, or weight-bearing; and skin breakdown and ulcerations. As part of the assessment, measure the calves, ankles, and feet correctly, as the involved areas of edema indicate. Use a monofilament (thin plastic filament) test for sensation and dorsiflexion and plantar flexion of the great toe (proprioception), especially for diabetic clients. The loss of touch sensation may require special foot protection. The loss of proprioception of the foot (position perception) indicates the need to discourage or stop driving. For many clients, this news is very traumatic. You may want to discuss this safety recommendation with a family member or significant other. Be prepared to problem-solve transportation alternatives.

EDUCATION

Health education is an essential component of the care you provide. It is important for clients to avoid smoking, wearing constrictive clothing, and applying excessive heat to their extremities. Clients need information about elevating their legs and performing daily foot hygiene. They may be able to reduce lower extremity edema by wearing properly fitted anti-embolic hose or compression socks (Sigvaris or TEDS); home health clients need physicians' orders. Before ready-made compression socks are bought, measure the heel to knee or the heel to thigh distance and the largest calf circumference; the cost ranges from $8 to $15. Before purchasing custom-ordered anti-embolic socks, clients need a prescription and are measured by a supply company; these socks cost up to several hundred dollars. Clients need to exercise caution when using compression socks. Most ready-made ones lose significant compression after 6 to 12 months and need to be replaced. When possible, use the "open toe" design to prevent excess pressure on the toes, especially with diabetic clients. The nylon content in these socks causes moisture retention and leads to skin maceration in clients who have poor circulation. The socks should not be worn around-the-clock.

Antibiotics may be required to treat infection or cellulitis. Local wound care is essential and should be provided by a health care provider familiar with the disease process. Some ulcers require debridement of eschar (see Chapter 14).

To clean the ulcer, use normal saline. Clean the dry, scaly skin around the ulcer and on the leg with saline or mild soaps. Gently clean the area and apply a lanolin-containing lotion every day to keep skin moist and supple. Avoid lotions containing alcohol and perfumes because they dry and irritate the skin. Protect granulation tissue with saline gel dressings or antibiotic ointments. Cover with a nonadherent dressing that does not accumulate heat or humidity at the wound bed. Monitor for sensitivity to topical agents, seen as blistering, itching, and erythema on the treated areas. If the ulcer is large and heavily exuding, more frequent dressing changes, with absorptive dressings, are required.

No topical treatment is adequate without compression. Graduated compression systems, with adequate padding, capable of sustaining compression for at least a week, should be the first line of treatment for uncomplicated venous leg ulcers with an ABI ≥ 0.8. Stockings are the easiest to apply, although soiling may be a problem. In addition, stockings do not fit abnormally shaped legs or those clients with dressings over the ulcer. Elastic wraps can be adjusted for size. Elastic wraps must be wrapped with the most tension at the foot and ankle and rewrapped twice daily.

An Unna boot is a popular form of bandage impregnated with calamine, zinc oxide, and glycerin. When wrapped snugly around the leg, it provides excellent compression during ambulation and applies minimal pressure during limb elevation. An Unna boot is a permeable dressing that can be applied directly over skin ulcers, thereby allowing drainage of exudate. It creates a moist and warm interface between the ulcerated skin and the bandage. It can be changed on a weekly or biweekly basis; the client wears the boot without interruption and thereby improves compliance. Disadvantages of the Unna boot include allergy, skin irritation, discomfort, difficulty in bathing, and pain while changing the boot. The Unna boot has been shown to achieve healing rates of 70%.

Skin grafting is rarely necessary to achieve healing. Surgery to remove incompetent varicose veins or incompetent perforator veins may also be necessary.

LYMPHATIC DISORDERS

LYMPHEDEMA

Lymphedema is an accumulation of lymphatic fluid in the interstitial tissue that causes swelling, most often in the arms or legs, and occasionally in other parts of the body. Lymphedema can develop when lymphatic vessels are missing or impaired (primary), or when lymph vessels are damaged or lymph nodes removed (secondary). Lymphedema should not be confused with edema resulting from venous insufficiency, which is not lymphedema.

When the impairment becomes so great that the lymphatic fluid exceeds the lymphatic transport capacity, an abnormal amount of protein-rich fluid collects in the tissues of the affected area. Left untreated, this stagnant protein-rich fluid not only causes tissue channels to increase in size and number, but also reduces oxygen availability in the transport system, interferes with wound healing, and provides a culture medium for bacteria that can result in lymphangitis (infection).

Primary lymphedema may be classified according to age at onset: congenital (present at birth), praecox (before age 35 years), or tarda (after age 35 years). Congenital and familial lymphedema is also called *Milroy disease*. It is inherited as an autosomal dominant trait. The edema usually appears spontaneously and without known cause.

Secondary lymphedema occurs because of some damage or obstruction to the lymph system by another disease process or by a procedure: trauma, cancers (primary or metastatic), filariasis, inflammation, surgical excision, or high doses of radiation. Postoperative lymphedema is usually seen after surgical excision of axillary, inguinal, or iliac nodes. These operations are usually performed as a prophylactic or therapeutic treatment for metastatic tumor. For example, lymphedema of the arm is encountered after mastectomy (Figure 53-14, *A*). Radiation in moderate amounts does not appear to damage the lymph vessels. However, heavy radiation for a particularly resistant tumor usually leads to lymphatic obstruction.

Filariasis, caused by the filarial nematode *Wuchereria bancrofti* (and others), is one of the most common diseases in undeveloped nations; it is transmitted by mosquitoes from human to human. The living embryos (microfilariae) of the adult worms are found in the bloodstream. The larvae migrate to the lymphatics, where they mature into adult worms. Adult worms in the lymph nodes and lymphatics lead to obstruction, lymphedema, and elephantiasis.

Lymphedema secondary to cancer in the lymph nodes is common. The malignant disease may be primary (lymphoma or Hodgkin's disease) or metastatic from another site.

Clinical Manifestations

Primary lymphedema presents as bilateral mild edema of ankles and legs in women at puberty or shortly after puberty, unilateral edema of the entire leg in men and women, or bilateral edema present at birth or early age. The skin of clients with congenital lymphedema contains vesicles (blisters) filled with lymph. A dull, heavy sensation is present, but actual pain is absent. Elevation of the limb and rest in bed cause a reduction but not disappearance of the sensation. Smooth skin becomes roughened; the edema is nonpitting. Acute lymphangitis and cellulitis are infrequent. Ulceration of the skin does not occur. However, the limb becomes greatly enlarged, uncomfortable, and unsightly (see Figure 53-14, *B*). Lymphedema can be diagnosed with isotopic lymphography, lymphangiography, and phlebography.

OUTCOME MANAGEMENT

There is no known cure for lymphedema once the swelling appears. The goal of treatment is to remove as much fluid as possible from the affected extremity and to maintain as normal-appearing an extremity as possible.

Physical therapy for arm or leg lymphedema involves mechanical or manual squeezing of the tissue in order to

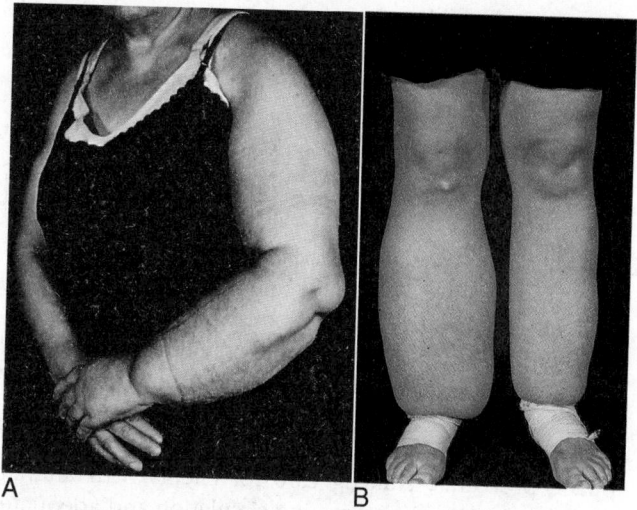

■ FIGURE 53–14 Types of lymphedema. **A,** Secondary lymphedema of the arm following mastectomy. **B,** Severe lymphedema. The client's feet were bandaged so that shoes could be worn.

press the stagnant lymphatic fluid to the proximal part of the limb. This is followed by specific active and passive exercises to transport the lymph farther into the lymphatic system and finally into the bloodstream. Many pneumatic pumping devices for intermittent compression are available. Diuretics may also be prescribed. Elastic stockings or sleeves are used to maintain the effects of the pneumatic pump.

To reduce the swelling, the extremity is elevated above the right atrium. Pneumatic pumps may be used to reduce the extremity size. If pumps are used, teach the client how to apply the device, the frequency of application, and the reasons for its use. When stockings or sleeves are used, ascertain that they fit and do not gather at the knee or elbow. Activity such as walking, rather than sitting or standing, should be promoted. For bedridden clients, teach bed exercises to promote venous and lymphatic return and to maintain muscle strength.

The client with lymphedema is at high risk for infection. The affected extremity is monitored for clinical manifestations of infection such as redness, warmth, and pain. Meticulous skin care is given to the extremity using mild soaps and lotions. Skin should be gently dried, especially between creases of skin. Nails are kept trimmed. Skin should be lubricated to maintain its suppleness; avoid using products with alcohol, dyes, lanolin, mineral oil, petroleum products, talc, or perfumes. Chemical hair removers and regular razors are not used. If shaving is desired, a well-maintained electric razor should be used. Hot water should be avoided. SAFETY ALERT

Clients with lymphedema may suffer from disturbances in self-concept because of the visibility of their deformity. Encourage the client to discuss these feelings and help the client understand that such feelings are normal. Variations in clothing style may be suggested to disguise the deformity. When caring for clients with lymph disorders, remember that these clients must cope with difficult, chronic diseases. Take time to give emotional support to the client and the family. Emphasize the possible need for lifelong follow-up.

CONCLUSIONS

Clients with vascular diseases can challenge a broad range of the nurse's capability and skill, from monitoring a client with rupture of an abdominal aortic aneurysm in an intensive care unit, to performing and teaching meticulous foot care, to educating and counseling a client to make significant lifestyle changes. Vascular diseases involve a broad spectrum of arterial, venous, and lymphatic problems. Nursing care for clients with arterial disorders centers on promoting circulation and adequate tissue perfusion, protecting against skin breakdown and injury, managing pain, and encouraging positive lifestyle changes. Limb amputation requires particularly sensitive assessment, teaching, and counseling skills. Nursing care for clients with venous disorders focuses on monitoring therapeutic regimens such as thrombolytic therapy, controlling and preventing thrombus formation, and promoting circulation by increasing venous blood return and decreasing venous pressure. Nursing care for lymphedema is palliative.

THINKING CRITICALLY

1. The client is admitted to the hospital for the care of leg ulcers. He is homeless and usually wanders the streets, sleeping on external heating grates in the sidewalk. He has large, irregularly shaped ulcers covered with thick, yellow, devitalized tissue. The ulcers are weeping and his stockings have adhered to the ulcers. What types of ulcers are present? What type of wound care will he need? How can he continue to do wound care after discharge?

Factors to Consider. How are arterial and venous ulcers distinguished? Is it important to remove the devitalized tissue? If so, how? How does his lifestyle influence his recovery?

2. A middle-age man enters the emergency department with complaints of a painful leg. The pain began about 3 hours before he noted a very rapid heartbeat. You note that his leg and foot are cold and white. What may have happened? What other factors need to be addressed in relation to his leg? What are the possible treatments available? What might his post-hospital instructions include?

Factors to Consider. How do you determine the acuteness of the tissue insult? What are the potential outcomes if you delay treatment? What might be the source of emboli, and how can this be assessed?

 Discussions for these questions can be found on the website.

BIBLIOGRAPHY

 Citations appearing in red refer to primary research.

1. Aquila, A.M. (2001). Deep venous thrombosis. *Journal of Cardiovascular Nursing, 15*(4), 25-44.
2. Belkin, M., et al. (2004). Peripheral arterial occlusive disease In C.M. Townsend, et al. (Eds.), *Sabiston textbook of surgery* (17th ed.). Philadelphia: Saunders.
3. Bryant, C., et al. (2002). Abdominal aortic aneurysm repair: A look at the first 24 hours. *Journal of Perianesthesia Nursing, 17*(3), 164-169.
4. Cosmi, B., Conti, E., & Coccheri, S. (2001). Anticoagulants (heparin, low molecular weight heparin, and oral anticoagulants) for intermittent claudication. *Cochrane Database of Systematic Reviews,* Issue 2, Article CD001999, DOI 10.1002/14651858.CD001999.
5. Cumming, J.C.O., Barr, S., & Howe, T.E. (2006). Prosthetic rehabilitation for older dysvascular people following a unilateral transfemoral amputation. *Cochrane Database of Systematic Reviews,* Issue 4, Article CD005260, DOI 10.1002/14651858.CD005260.pub2.
6. Dörffler-Melly, J., Koopman, M.M.W., Prins, M.H., et al. (2005). Antiplatelet and anticoagulant drugs for prevention of restenosis/reocclusion following peripheral endovascular treatment. *Cochrane Database of Systematic Reviews,* Issue 1, Article CD002071, DOI 10.1002/14651858.CD002071.pub2.
7. Doughty, D., & Holbrook, R. (2006). Lower extremity ulcers of vascular etiology. In R. Bryant & D. Nix (Eds.), *Acute and chronic wounds* (3rd ed., pp. 258-306). St. Louis: Mosby.
8. Ennis, W.J., & Meneses, P. (2003). Standard, appropriate and advanced care and medical-legal considerations: Venous ulcerations. *Wounds, 15*(4), 107-122.
9. Eskandari, M., Matsumura, J., & Anderson, L. (2004). Surgery on the aorta. In V. Fahey (Ed.), *Vascular nursing* (4th ed., pp. 215-236). Philadelphia: Saunders.
10. Frost-Rude, J.A., et al. (2000). Buerger's disease. *Journal of Vascular Nursing, 18*(4), 128-130.
11. Hafner, J., et al. (2000). Leg ulcers in peripheral arterial disease: Impaired wound healing above the threshold of chronic critical limb ischemia. *Journal of the American Academy of Dermatology, 43*(6), 1001-1008.
12. Hayes, J.M. (2002). Graduated compression stockings: Updating practice, improving compliance. *MEDSURG Nursing, 11*(4), 163-166.
13. Keeling, W.B., et al. (2007). Plaque excision with the Silverhawk catheter: Early results in patients with claudication or critical limb ischemia. *Journal of Vascular Surgery, 45*(1), 25-31.
14. Juynh, T., et al. (2004). Thoracic vasculature. In C.M. Townsend, et al. (Eds.), *Sabiston textbook of surgery* (17th ed.). Philadelphia: Saunders.
15. Leng, G.C., Davis, M., & Baker, D. (2000). Bypass surgery for chronic lower limb ischemia. *Cochrane Database of Systematic Reviews,* Issue 3, Article CD002000, DOI 10.1002/14651858.CD002000.
16. Lewis, C.D. (2001). Peripheral arterial disease of the lower extremity. *Journal of Cardiovascular Nursing, 15*(4), 45-63.
17. Jones, M.A., et al. (2000). Endovascular grafting for repair of abdominal aortic aneurysm. *Critical Care Nurse, 20*(4), 38-48.
18. Nelson, E.A., et al. (2003). Compression for preventing recurrence of venous ulcers. *Cochrane Review The Cochrane Library,* (2) Oxford: Update Software.
19. Rudolph, D. (2001). Standards of care for venous leg ulcers: Compression therapy and moist wound healing. *Journal of Vascular Nursing, 19*(1), 20-27.
20. Treat-Jacobson, D. (2003). Treating patients with peripheral arterial disease and claudication. *Journal of Vascular Nursing, 21*(1), 5-14.

evolve *Did you remember to check out the bonus material on the Evolve website and the CD-ROM, including NCLEX®-Examination Style Review Questions, Open-Book Quizzes, and Chapter Review Audio Podcasts?*

http://evolve.elsevier.com/Black/medsurg

UNIT 13

CARDIAC DISORDERS

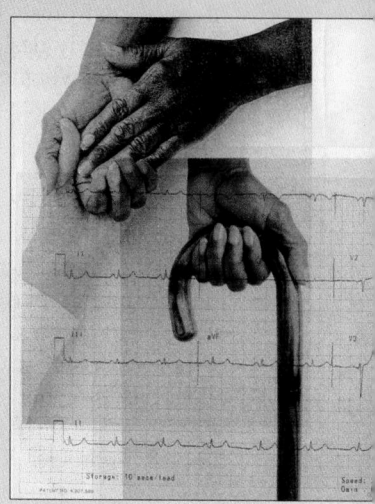

ANATOMY AND PHYSIOLOGY REVIEW:

The Heart

Robert G. Carroll

The human heart, through rhythmic contraction, provides the pressure necessary to propel blood through the body. Blood flow is essential to deliver nutrients to the tissues of the body and to transport metabolic wastes, including heat, to removal sites. The presence of an arterial pulse, caused by the beating of the heart, is appropriately designated as a vital sign.

The heart weighs about 300 g and is located within the mediastinum; it is cone-shaped and tilted forward and to the left. Because of a rotation in orientation during fetal development, the apex of the heart (tip of the cone) is at its bottom and lies left of the midline. The base is at the top, where the great vessels enter the heart, and lies posterior to the sternum. The heart consists of four chambers: two smaller atria at the top (the base) of the heart and two larger ventricles at the apex. A band of fibrous tissue separates the atria from the ventricles and seats the four cardiac valves. A muscular septum separates the right from the left atrium and the right from the left ventricle. Table A&P13-1 describes the basic structures and their functions.

Functionally, the heart is actually two pumps working simultaneously (Figure A&P13-1). The right atrium and right ventricle generate the pressure to propel the oxygen-poor blood through the pulmonic circulation; the left atrium and left ventricle propel oxygen-rich blood to the remainder of the body through the systemic circulation. At rest, each side of the heart pumps approximately 5000 ml (5 L) of blood per minute *(cardiac output)*. This is accomplished by a contraction frequency *(heart rate)* of 72 beats/min, with each contraction ejecting a volume of 70 ml *(stroke volume)* into the arterial system. Cardiac output can increase five-fold during exercise as a result of increases in both heart rate and stroke volume.

STRUCTURE OF THE HEART

LAYERS OF THE HEART

The heart consists of three distinct layers of tissue: endocardium, myocardium, and epicardium (Figure A&P13-2, inset). The *endocardium* (innermost layer) consists of thin endothelial tissue lining the inner chambers and the heart valves. The *myocardium* (middle layer) consists of striated muscle fibers forming interlaced bundles and is the actual contracting muscle of the heart. The *epicardium* or *visceral pericardium* covers the outer surface of the heart. It closely adheres to the heart and to the first several centimeters of the pulmonary artery and aorta.

The visceral pericardium is encased by the *parietal pericardium,* a tough, loose-fitting, fibrous outer membrane that is attached anteriorly to the lower half of the sternum, posteriorly to the thoracic vertebrae, and inferiorly to the diaphragm. Between the visceral pericardium and the parietal pericardium is the *pericardial space,* which holds 5 to 20 ml of pericardial fluid. This fluid lubricates the pericardial surfaces as they slide over each other when the heart beats. Excessive fluid accumulation in the pericardial space can diminish the filling of the ventricles *(cardiac tamponade).*

CHAMBERS OF THE HEART

The heart consists of four chambers: two upper collecting chambers *(atria)* and two lower pumping chambers *(ventricles)* (see Figure A&P13-2). A muscular wall *(septum)* separates the chambers of the right side from those of the left side. The *right atrium* receives deoxygenated blood from the body. The blood moves to the *right ventricle,* which pumps it to the lungs against low resistance. The *left atrium* receives oxygenated blood from the lungs. The blood flows into the *left ventricle* (the heart's largest, most muscular chamber), which pumps it against high resistance into the systemic circulation.

CARDIAC VALVES

The cardiac valves are delicate, flexible structures that consist of fibrous tissue covered by endothelium. They permit only unidirectional blood flow through the heart. The valves open and close passively, determined by pressure gradients between the cardiac chambers (Figure A&P13-3). "Leaky" valves that do not seal when closed are called *regurgitant* or *insufficient.* "Stiff" valves that cannot open completely are called *stenotic.*

Cardiac valves are of two types: (1) atrioventricular (AV) and (2) semilunar (see Table A&P13-1). *Atrioventricular valves* lie between the atria and ventricles. The *tricuspid valve,* on the right side, is composed of three leaflets. The *mitral (bicuspid)* valve, on the left, is composed of two. Attached to the edges of the AV valves are strong, fibrous filaments called *chorda*

TABLE A&P13–1 **The Heart:** *Its Structure and Functions*

Structure	Function
Pericardium	Two-layered case that encases and protects heart
Atrium	Upper, receiving chambers of heart
Right atrium	Receives deoxygenated systemic blood via superior and inferior vena cava; blood passes to right ventricle
Left atrium	Receives oxygenated blood from lungs; blood passes to left ventricle
Ventricles	Lower, pumping chambers of heart
Right ventricle	Receives blood from atrium via tricuspid valve; pumps it to pulmonary circulation
Left ventricle	Receives blood from atrium via tricuspid (mitral) valve; pumps it to systemic circulation
Cardiac valves	Prevent backflow of blood
Tricuspid and bicuspid (mitral) valves	Prevent backflow from right ventricle to right atrium and from left ventricle to left atrium, respectively
Semilunar valves	Prevent backflow from pulmonary artery to right ventricle (*pulmonary semilunar*) and from aorta to left ventricle (*aortic semilunar*)
Coronary arteries (common pattern)	Supply blood to heart
Right coronary artery	Perfuses right atrium, right ventricle, inferior portion of left ventricle and posterior septal wall, SA node, and AV node
Left coronary artery	Supplies blood to anterior wall of left ventricle, anterior ventricular septum, and apex of left ventricle
Left anterior descending artery	Supplies blood to left atrium, lateral and posterior surfaces of left ventricle, occasionally posterior interventricular septum; sometimes supplies SA and AV nodes
Circumflex artery	
SA node	"Pacemaker" node; initiates heartbeat by generating an electrical impulse
AV node	Normal pathway for impulses originating in atria to be conducted to ventricles; can be a secondary pacemaker
Bundle of His, bundle branches, Purkinje's fibers	Rapidly transmit cardiac action potentials to enable synchronous contraction of ventricles

tendineae, which arise from papillary muscles on the ventricular walls. The papillary muscles and chordae tendineae work together to prevent the AV valves from bulging back into the atria during ventricular contraction *(systole).*

The *semilunar valves* consist of three cup-like cusps that open during ventricular contraction and close to prevent backflow of blood into the ventricles during relaxation *(diastole).* Unlike the AV valves, the semilunar valves open during ventricular contraction. The *pulmonic semilunar valve* (right ventricle to pulmonary artery) and the *aortic semilunar valve* (left ventricle to aorta) do not have papillary muscles.

CARDIAC BLOOD SUPPLY

The heart muscle requires a rich oxygen supply to meet its own metabolic needs. The *coronary arteries* (right and left) branch off the aorta just above the aortic valve, encircle the heart, and penetrate the myocardium (Figure A&P13-4). Coronary vessel distribution can vary greatly, but the pattern described in Table A&P13-1 is the most common.

Contraction of the muscle of the left ventricle generates enough extravascular pressure to occlude the coronary blood vessels and prevent blood flow to the muscle of the heart during ventricular systole. Thus 75% of the

coronary artery blood flow occurs during diastole, when the heart is relaxed and resistance is low. For adequate blood flow through the coronary arteries, the diastolic blood pressure must be at least 60 mm Hg. Coronary blood flow increases with increased heart workload (e.g., exercise). The coronary veins return blood from most of the myocardium to the coronary sinus of the right atrium. Some areas, particularly on the right side of the heart, drain directly into the cardiac chambers.

FUNCTIONS OF THE HEART

ELECTROPHYSIOLOGIC PROPERTIES

The electrophysiologic properties of cardiac muscle regulate the heart rate and rhythm. These properties include excitability, automaticity, contractility, refractoriness, and conductivity.

Excitability

The ability of cardiac muscle cells to depolarize in response to a stimulus—*excitability*—is influenced by hormones, electrolytes, nutrition, oxygen supply, medications, infection, and autonomic nerve activity.

PULMONIC
CIRCULATION

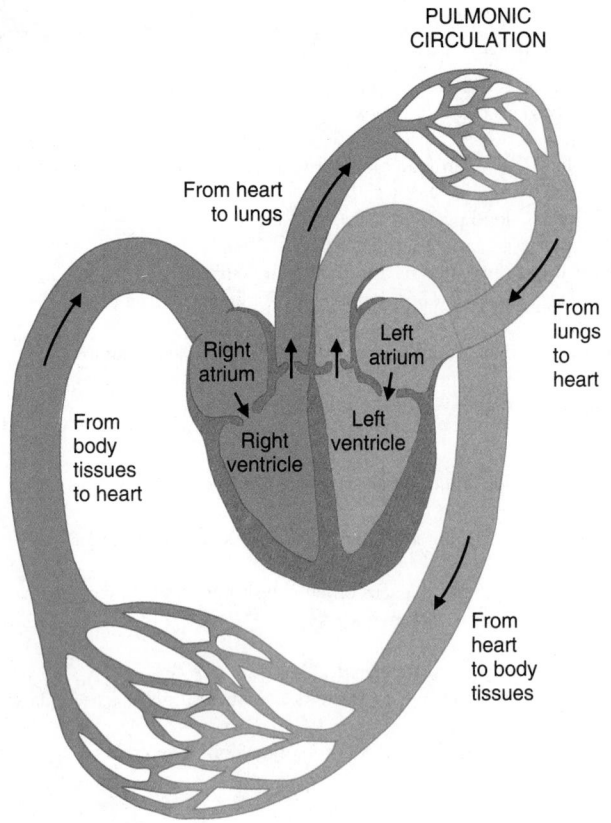

SYSTEMIC CIRCULATION

■ **FIGURE A&P13–1** Functions of the heart. In the peripheral capillaries in systemic circulation, blood oxygen is exchanged for carbon dioxide. The oxygen-poor blood returns to the right atrium and right ventricle to be pumped into the lungs, where carbon dioxide is exchanged for oxygen. Oxygen-rich blood from the lungs enters the left atrium and left ventricle of the heart to be pumped once again into the systemic circulation.

In myocardial cells, as in other types of muscle and neurons, differences in intracellular and extracellular ion concentrations create electrical and concentration gradients for ionic movement across the semipermeable cell membrane. At rest, the inside of a myocardial cell is more negative than the outside. This *resting membrane potential* results primarily from the differences in concentrations of potassium (K^+) and sodium (Na^+) ions. Although both ions are present on either side of the cell membrane, potassium has a greater intracellular concentration and sodium has a greater extracellular concentration. Selective channels can increase membrane permeability for specific ions, allowing the ion to move down the electrochemical gradient and to alter the resting membrane potential.

When the cardiac cell is stimulated to a certain threshold, a sequence of ion permeability changes cause a dramatic change in the transmembrane potential; this is known as an *action potential* (Figure A&P13-5, *A*). The action potential consists of depolarization and repolarization phases. The electrocardiogram (ECG) reflects

currents generated during the depolarization and repolarization of regions of the heart.

Depolarization is caused by an increase in cell membrane permeability to sodium. The cell returns to its resting (relaxed) state during *repolarization*. Sodium permeability drops sharply, and potassium permeability increases, returning the membrane to the negative resting potential. In the process of depolarization and repolarization, small amounts of sodium leak into the cell and potassium leaks outward. The cell compensates for this by actively pumping sodium back out and potassium inward (using the enzyme Na, K-ATPase).

Other ions, such as calcium and chloride, also play a role in the action potential and the contraction it causes. For the heart, calcium is especially important because it initiates contraction. During depolarization, myocardial cell membrane permeability to calcium increases and calcium moves into the cell. This inward Ca^{++} flux triggers the release of more calcium stored in the sarcoplasmic reticulum (see Contractility). As the intracellular concentration of calcium increases, calcium reacts with contractile proteins and myocardial muscle fibers contract.

Automaticity (Rhythmicity)

The ability of cardiac pacemaker cells to initiate an impulse spontaneously and repetitively, without external neurohormonal control, is known as *automaticity*, or *rhythmicity*. Given the proper conditions, the heart can continue to beat outside the body. In contrast, skeletal muscle must be stimulated by a nerve to depolarize and contract. The sinoatrial (SA) node pacemaker cells have the highest rate of automaticity of all cardiac cells, and thus govern the heart rate. The conduction tissue area with the highest automaticity, or rate of spontaneous depolarization, assumes the role of pacemaker (see Chapter 57). SA node cell automaticity is due to changes in ionic permeability of the membrane. Even at rest, a decreasing potassium permeability and increasing slow channel permeability (for Na^+ and Ca^{++} ions) move the cell membrane potential more positively toward threshold voltage. When threshold is reached, the cell initiates an "all-or-none" action potential. Norepinephrine and acetylcholine cause heart rate to increase and decrease, respectively (Figure A&P13-5, *B*). The rate of spontaneous depolarization can also be affected by other hormones, body temperature, drugs, and disease.

Contractility

The heart muscle is composed of long, narrow cells or fibers. Cardiac muscle fibers, like striated skeletal muscle, contain myofibrils, Z bands, sarcomeres, sarcolemmas, sarcoplasm, and sarcoplasmic reticulum. Contraction results from the same sliding filament mechanism

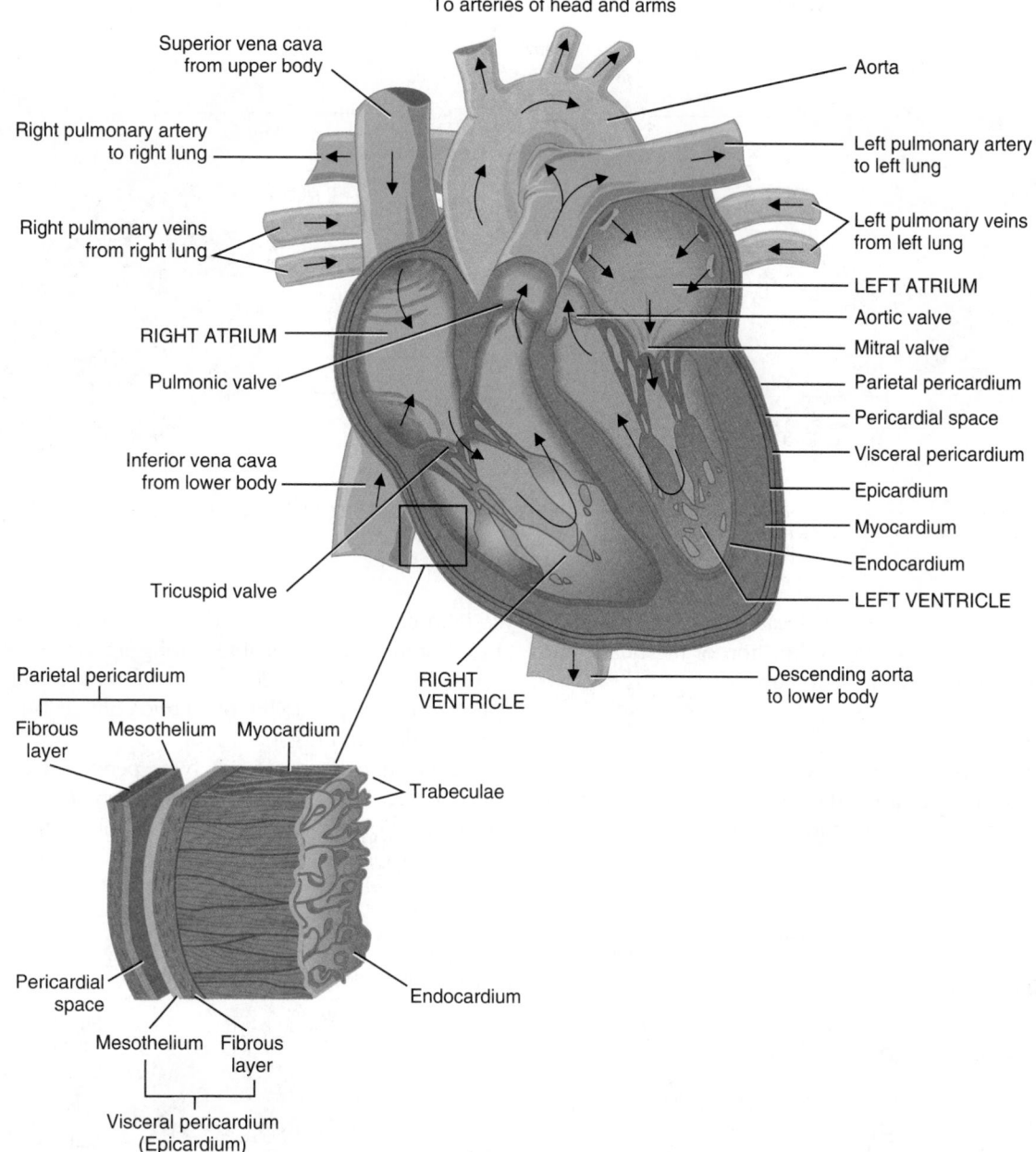

To arteries of head and arms

Superior vena cava
from upper body

Aorta

Right pulmonary artery
to right lung

Left pulmonary artery
to left lung

Right pulmonary veins
from right lung

Left pulmonary veins
from left lung

LEFT ATRIUM

RIGHT ATRIUM

Aortic valve

Pulmonic valve

Mitral valve

Parietal pericardium

Pericardial space

Visceral pericardium

Inferior vena cava
from lower body

Epicardium

Myocardium

Endocardium

LEFT VENTRICLE

Tricuspid valve

Descending aorta
to lower body

RIGHT
VENTRICLE

Parietal pericardium

Fibrous
layer

Mesothelium   Myocardium

Trabeculae

Pericardial
space

Endocardium

Mesothelium   Fibrous
layer

Visceral pericardium
(Epicardium)

■ **FIGURE A&PI3–2**   Structure of the heart and circulation of blood through the heart. Blood entering the left atrium from the right and left pulmonary veins flows into the left ventricle. The left ventricle pumps blood into the systemic circulation through the aorta. From the systemic circulation, blood returns to the right atrium through the superior and inferior venae cavae. From there, the right ventricle pumps blood into the lungs through the right and left pulmonary arteries. *Inset,* The pericardium and layers of the heart.

described for skeletal muscle (see the Unit 6 Anatomy and Physiology Review).

The action potential initiates the muscle contraction by releasing calcium through the T tubules of the cell membrane. The calcium reaches the sarcoplasmic reticulum, causing additional calcium release. The intracellular calcium diffuses to myofibrils, where it binds with troponin. When the actin filaments become activated by calcium, the heads of the cross-bridges from the myosin filaments immediately become attracted to

the active sites of the actin. Contraction then occurs by power stroke repetition. After contraction, free calcium ions are actively pumped back into the sarcoplasmic reticulum, and muscle relaxation begins.

One important difference between cardiac and skeletal muscle is that cardiac muscle needs extracellular calcium. All the calcium involved in skeletal muscle comes from the sarcoplasmic reticulum. In cardiac muscle, however, extracellular calcium enters through the T tubules and triggers the release of more calcium from

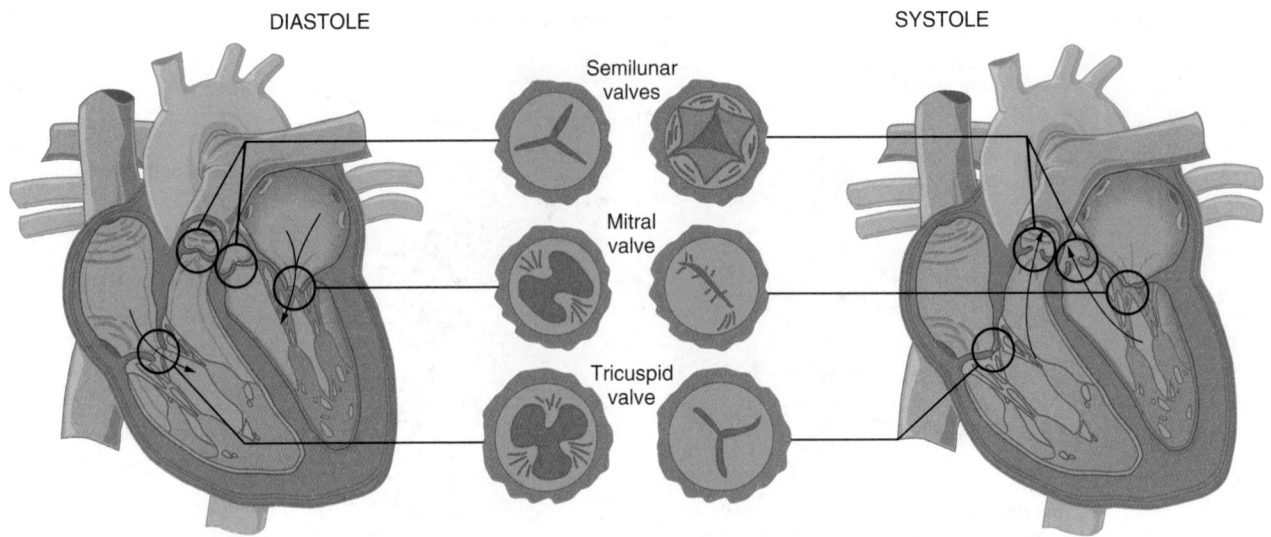

DIASTOLE   SYSTOLE

Semilunar valves

Mitral valve

Tricuspid valve

■ **FIGURE A&PI3–3** Valves of the heart. The semilunar, mitral, and tricuspid valves are shown as they appear during diastole, or ventricular filling *(left)*, and during systole, or ventricular emptying *(right)*.

the sarcoplasmic reticulum. Because of this, calcium-channel blockers can alter contraction of the heart, but not the contraction of skeletal muscle.

Refractoriness

Refractoriness is the heart's inability to respond to a new stimulus while still in a state of depolarization from an earlier stimulus. Refractoriness develops when the

sodium channels of the cardiac cell membrane become inactivated and unexcitable during an action potential. Thus the heart muscle does not respond to restimulation, preventing the possibility of tetanic contractions that are seen in skeletal muscle.

Refractoriness occurs in two periods (see Figure A&P13-5, *A*). The *absolute refractory period* occurs during depolarization and the first part of repolarization. During

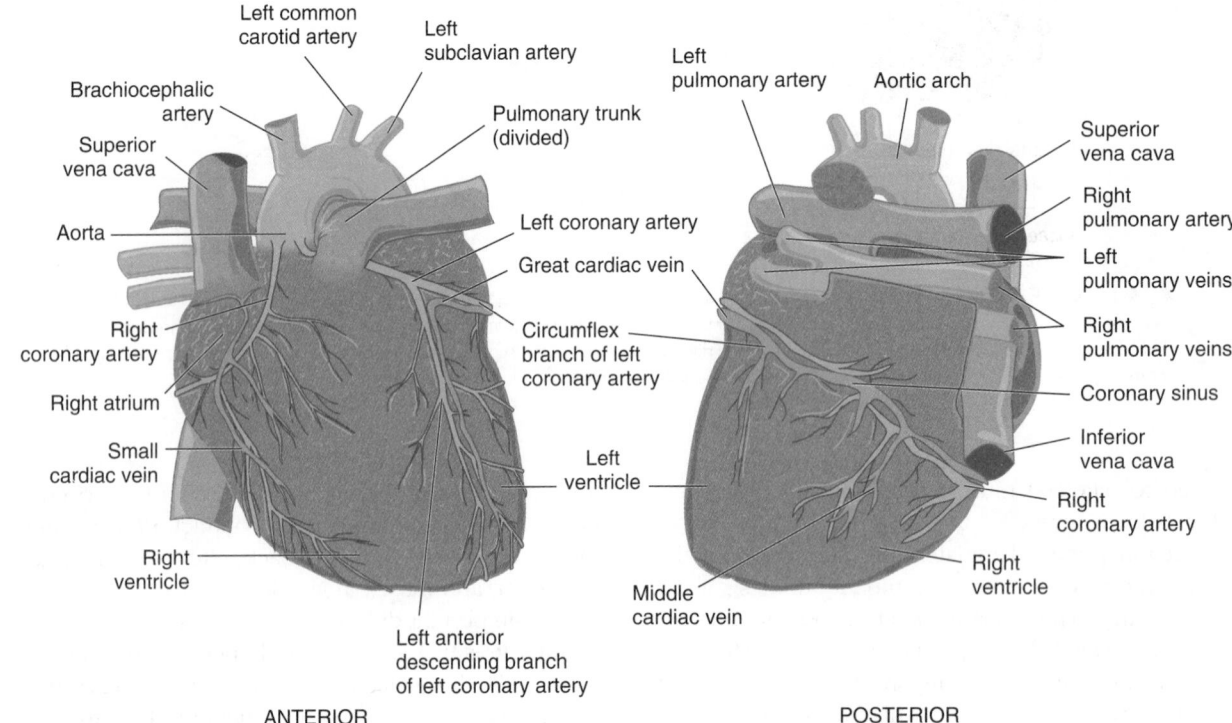

Left common carotid artery
Left subclavian artery
Brachiocephalic artery
Pulmonary trunk (divided)
Superior vena cava
Aorta
Left coronary artery
Right coronary artery
Great cardiac vein
Right atrium
Circumflex branch of left coronary artery
Small cardiac vein
Left ventricle
Right ventricle
Left anterior descending branch of left coronary artery

ANTERIOR

Left pulmonary artery
Aortic arch
Superior vena cava
Right pulmonary artery
Left pulmonary veins
Right pulmonary veins
Coronary sinus
Inferior vena cava
Right coronary artery
Right ventricle
Middle cardiac vein

POSTERIOR

■ **FIGURE A&PI3–4** The coronary arteries. The right and left coronary arteries branch off the aorta just above the aortic valve; they normally supply the myocardium with oxygenated blood.

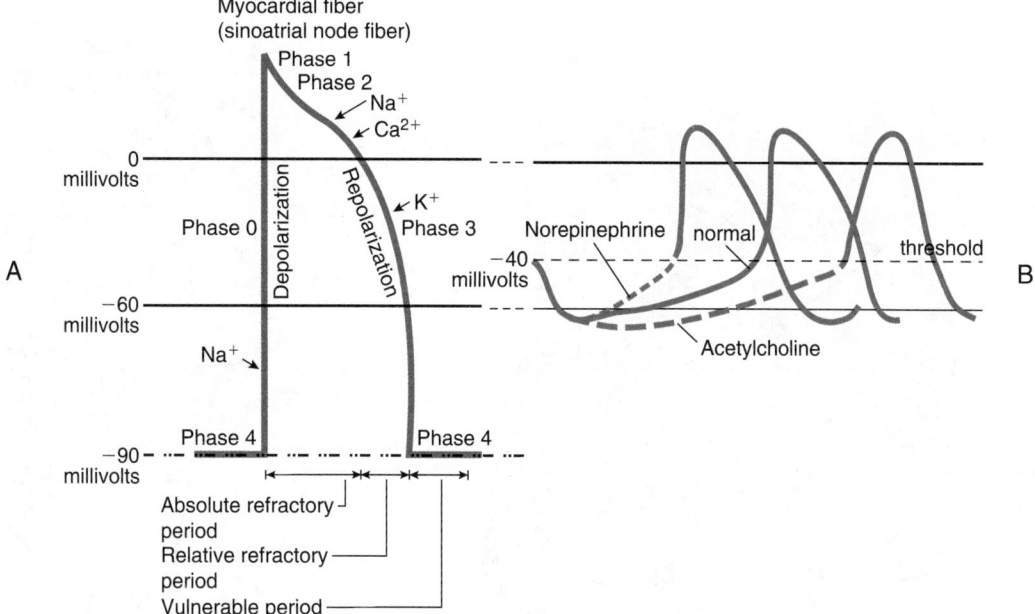

■ FIGURE A&P13–5 Action potential. **A,** The action potential of cardiac cells has five phases: *Phase 0:* Sodium permeability increases through fast sodium channels, and cell depolarization (contraction) begins. *Phase 1:* The fast sodium channels close. *Phase 2:* Some sodium and calcium permeability remains through slow Na+/Ca++ channels. *Phase 3:* Potassium permeability increases in the cell. *Phase 4:* The cell returns to its resting potential, sodium is pumped out of the cell, and potassium is pumped into the cell through the cell's sodium-potassium pump. In all cardiac cells, a period occurs during which the cells cannot be stimulated to fire another action potential. During the end of the action potential, the membrane is relatively refractory and can be reexcited only by a larger than usual stimulus. Immediately after the action potential, the membrane has transitory hyperexcitability and is said to be in a vulnerable state. **B,** The sympathetic neurotransmitter norepinephrine increases slow channel activity, allowing cells to reach threshold more rapidly (increased heart rate). Conversely, the parasympathetic neurotransmitter acetylcholine *(dashed line)* increases potassium permeability, moving the cell membrane potential away from threshold, and causes the cell to reach threshold more slowly (decreased heart rate). Calcium-channel blockers slow the heart rate by decreasing slow channel activity.

this period, cardiac cells do not respond to any stimuli, however strong. The *relative refractory period* occurs in the final stages of repolarization; refractoriness diminishes and a stronger-than-normal stimulus can excite the heart muscle to contract. At the end of the refractory period, there is a transient hyperexcitability *(vulnerable period)*. The sodium channels are reset and the cardiac cells can again conduct action potentials. The refractory period is the time when the heart chambers are filling with blood for the next beat.

Normally, the ventricles have an absolute refractory period of 0.25 to 0.3 second, which approximates the duration of the action potential. The relative refractory period for the ventricles lasts about 0.05 second. The atria have a refractory period of about 0.15 second, and they can therefore contract rhythmically much more quickly than the ventricles. The durations of the action potential and the refractory period are not fixed, however; both can shorten as heart rate increases.

Conductivity

Conductivity is the ability of heart muscle fibers to propagate electrical impulses along and across cell membranes.

The heart muscle must conduct the action potential from its origin throughout the heart both rapidly and smoothly so that the atria and ventricles contract as a unit. Intercalated disks join adjacent myocardial cells, allowing the action potential to travel over the entire muscle mass (Figure A&P13-6) through gap junctions. The fibrous band of tissue that separates the atria and ventricles lacks intercalated disks. Therefore the atria are isolated electrically from the ventricles except for the only normal conduction pathway, including the atrioventricular node. Cardiac conduction is a sequential depolarization of the following:

■ Sinoatrial (SA) node
■ AV node
■ Bundle of His and bundle branches
■ Purkinje fibers
■ Ventricular myocardium

The *SA node,* or *pacemaker,* is located at the junction of the superior vena cava and right atrium. Under normal circumstances, the SA node initiates electrical impulses (heartbeats) approximately 60 to 100 times per minute, but it can adjust its rate. Three internodal and one interatrial tract carry the wave of depolarization through the right atrium to the AV node and to the left

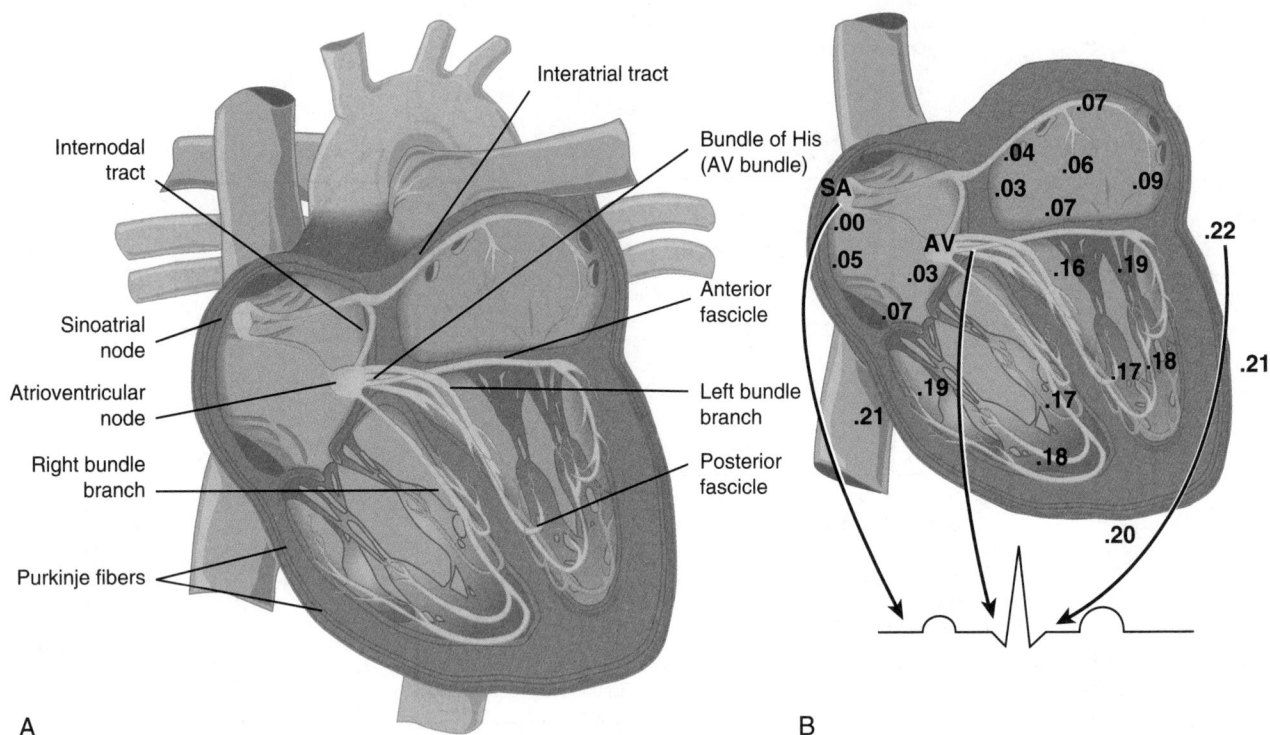

■ **FIGURE A&P13–6 A,** The cardiac conduction system. **B,** Transmission of the cardiac impulse through the heart, showing the time of appearance (in fractions of a second) of the impulse in different parts of the heart. (**B,** *Modified from Guyton, A.C., & Hall, J.E. [2001]. Textbook of medical physiology [10th ed.]. Philadelphia: Saunders.)*

atrium, respectively. The sympathetic and parasympathetic nervous systems regulate the SA node. Any myocardial tissue that generates impulses at a higher rate than the SA node can become an abnormal, or *ectopic,* pacemaker.

The (AV) node, or *AV junction,* is located in the lower aspect of the atrial septum. The AV node can be a secondary cardiac pacemaker, but it normally receives electrical impulses from the SA node and is the only pathway for conducting impulses from the atria to the ventricles. Within the AV node, the impulse is delayed 0.07 second while the atria contract. This delay enables atrial contraction to be completed before the ventricles contract.

The common *bundle of His* in the interventricular septum is relatively short, branching into right and left segments. The *right bundle branch* (RBB) courses down the right side of the interventricular septum. The *left bundle branch* (LBB) bifurcates into anterior and posterior fascicles, both of which extend into the left ventricle. The right and left bundle branches terminate in Purkinje fibers.

Purkinje fibers are a diffuse network of conducting strands beneath the ventricular endocardium; they rapidly spread the wave of depolarization through the ventricles. Activation of the ventricles begins in the septum and then moves from the apex of the heart upward. Within the ventricular walls, depolarization proceeds

from endocardium to epicardium. Repolarization occurs in each cell and does not involve the conduction system. Repolarization occurs in reverse order, so that the last cells to depolarize are the first to repolarize. The action potentials of Purkinje fibers have the longest duration, and their repolarization is occasionally seen as a U wave of the electrocardiogram (ECG).

CARDIAC CYCLE

One cardiac cycle (Figure A&P13-7) is equivalent to one complete heartbeat. The sequence of events in the cardiac cycle is divided into two parts: ventricular *systole* (contraction) and ventricular *diastole* (relaxation). The cardiac cycle normally begins with the spontaneous depolarization of the pacemaker cells of the SA node and ends following the filling of the relaxed ventricles.

Atrial Systole

Depolarization of the SA node spreads through the atria both in a cell-to-cell manner and by using the internodal and interatrial pathways. Depolarization of the atrial cells (P wave of the ECG) allows calcium entry, followed by contraction and pressure generation (a wave of the venous pressure tracing). Contraction of the atria propels a small amount of blood into the ventricles, called the "atrial kick."

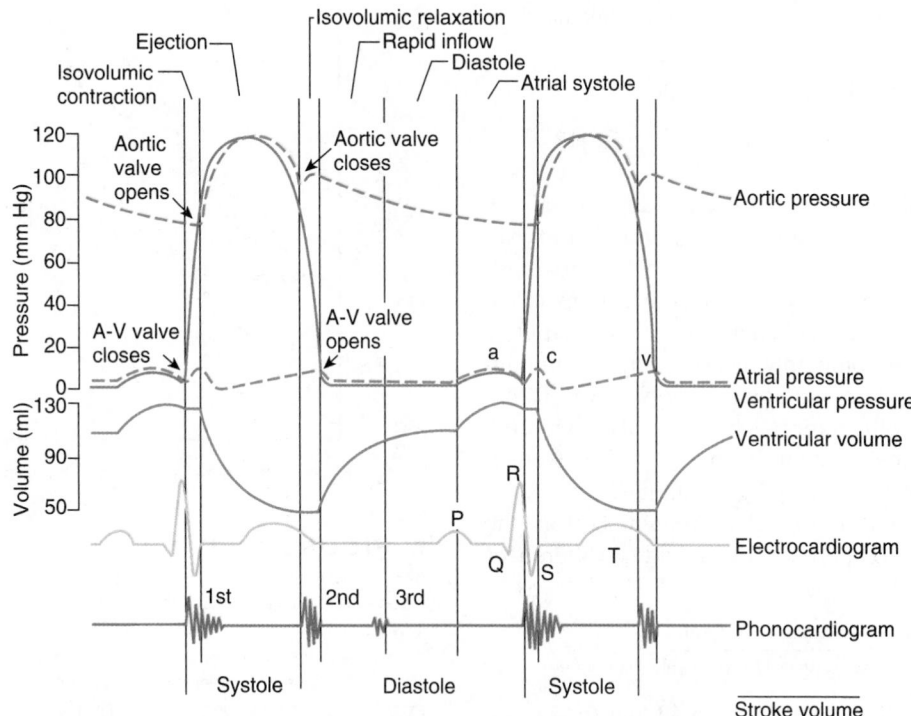

FIGURE A&P13–7 Changes that occur during the cardiac cycle in left atrial pressure, left ventricular pressure, aortic pressure, ventricular volume, the electrocardiogram, and the phonocardiogram. *(From Guyton, A.C., & Hall, J.E. [2001]. Textbook of medical physiology [10th ed.]. Philadelphia: Saunders.)*

Ventricular Systole

Following a delay at the AV node, the wave of depolarization enters the ventricles, where it is spread rapidly by the bundle branches and Purkinje fibers (QRS complex of the ECG). Following depolarization, calcium enters, initiating contraction of the ventricle. In the *isovolumic contraction phase,* the ventricles begin to contract, closing the AV valves and building up pressure within the ventricles. As the AV valves close, the first heart sound (S_1) is heard. Because the aortic and pulmonic valves remain closed at this point, no blood leaves the ventricle. The *ejection phase* begins when pressure in the ventricles exceeds the aortic and pulmonic pressures. The semilunar valves open, and the ventricles pump blood into the systemic and pulmonary circulations.

Ventricular Diastole

In early diastole, as the ventricles begin to relax, aortic and pulmonary artery pressures exceed ventricular pressures, and the semilunar valves close. The valve closure causes the second heart sound (S_2). The AV valves remain closed, and no blood moves in or out of the ventricles. This is called *isovolumic relaxation.* As the ventricles continue to relax, pressure in the ventricles falls below that of the atria, and the AV valves open, allowing blood that has been pooling in the atria to flow into the ventricles *(ventricular filling).* When the ventricles have filled passively, the cardiac cycle is ready to begin again.

Extra Heart Sounds

The ventricular wall must expand to accommodate rapid ventricular filling. If ventricular wall compliance is decreased (as in heart failure or valvular regurgitation), blood and structures within the ventricular wall vibrate and a third heart sound (S_3) may be heard. Because of increased filling, an S_3 heart sound may be a normal finding in people younger than age 30 years. During the last phase of ventricular diastole, atrial contraction (atrial systole or atrial kick) occurs, contributing 5% to 30% more blood volume to the ventricles.

A fourth heart sound (S_4) may be heard on atrial systole if resistance to active ventricular filling is present. This is not a normal finding and is commonly caused by a stiff ventricle from hypertrophy, disease, or injury of the ventricular wall.

CARDIAC OUTPUT AND CARDIAC INDEX

Cardiac output (CO) is the volume of blood ejected per minute by rhythmic ventricular contraction. At the end of ventricular diastole, each ventricle contains approximately 140 ml of blood (end-diastolic volume [EDV]). Normally, during systole, the heart ejects approximately half of this volume. The volume ejected with each contraction (heartbeat) of the ventricle is the stroke volume and ejection fraction. Cardiac output can be calculated as follows:

$$CO = [EDV - ESV] \times HR$$

where ESV is the end-systolic volume and HR is the heart rate.

Cardiac output averages between 4 and 8 L/min in adults. For a normal 150-pound (70-kg) adult at rest, cardiac output is 5 to 6 L/min. Adjustments in either stroke volume or heart rate can compensate for fluctuations in the other, or both can rise or fall to maintain cardiac output.

Cardiac output is commonly measured by thermodilution with the use of a pulmonary artery (Swan-Ganz) catheter. Several other approaches can also be used, such as obtaining heart rate from an ECG and stroke volume through ventricular imaging techniques.

Clinicians compute the *cardiac index* (CI) from the cardiac output to compensate for individual differences in body size:

$$CI = \frac{Cardiac\ output}{Body\ surface\ area}$$

The normal cardiac index is 2.5 to 4 L/min/m^2.

Stroke volume has a major influence on cardiac output and is determined by (1) preload, (2) afterload, and (3) the contractile state of the heart (reviewed in Figure A&P12-4).

Preload

Preload is the myocardial fiber length of the left ventricle at end diastole. It is determined by the EDV. The Frank-Starling law of the heart states that the greater the resting myocardial fiber length, or stretch, the greater its force of contraction. Preload therefore increases when increased EDV (e.g., from increased venous return) subjects myocardial fibers to greater stretch. The ventricles respond with a greater force of contraction, producing a larger stroke volume and increased cardiac output. This phenomenon, however, has limits (Figure A&P13-8), such as the greatly distended ventricles characteristic of heart failure.

Afterload

Afterload is the resistance to left ventricular ejection. More specifically, it is the amount of pressure required by the left ventricle to open the aortic valve during systole and to eject blood. Afterload directly relates to arterial blood pressure and the characteristics of the valve. If arterial blood pressure is high, the heart must work harder to pump blood into the circulation. Stroke volume is inversely related to afterload. For example, if afterload increases because of peripheral vasoconstriction (which increases arterial blood pressure), myocardial fiber shortening is reduced and ejections are less effective. Then the ventricles cannot eject a normal stroke volume.

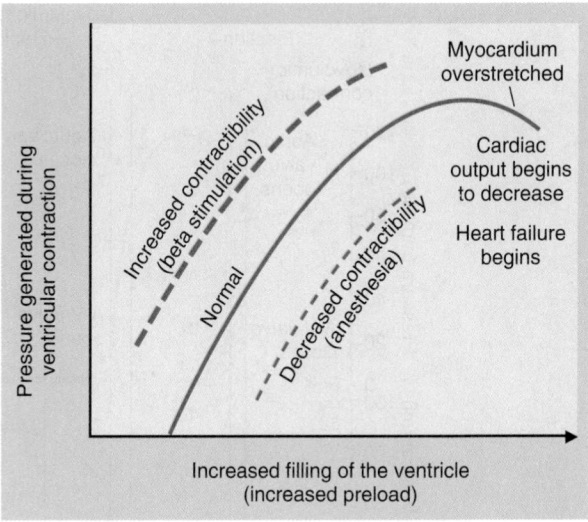

■ **FIGURE A&P13–8** According to the Frank-Starling law, the more the left ventricle fills with blood (preload), the greater the quantity of blood ejected into the aorta. If the left ventricle fills to such an extent that it overdistends the myocardium *(arrow)*, however, cardiac output begins to decrease and the heart begins to fail. Agents that change contractility can shift this relationship. Norepinephrine increases contractility (positive inotrope) and improves cardiac performance; anesthesia decreases contractility (negative inotrope) and impairs cardiac performance.

Contractile State

The contractile *(inotropic)* state refers to the vigor of contraction generated by the myocardium regardless of its blood volume (preload). Unlike skeletal muscle, the myocardium can alter contractile velocity and therefore force. The rate of cross-bridge cycling in the myocardium is calcium dependent, and agents that increase intracellular calcium level thus increase contractile force. For example, sympathetic stimulation increases myocardial contractility and ventricular pressure, thereby ejecting blood more rapidly and increasing stroke volume. Metabolic abnormalities (e.g., hypoxemia) and metabolic acidosis decrease myocardial contractility, therefore reducing stroke volume (see Figure A&P13-8).

Cardiac Pressures

With the use of a pulmonary artery pressure (Swan-Ganz) catheter, pressures in the right atrium, right ventricle, and pulmonary artery can be measured. Inflation of a balloon at the catheter tip allows measurement of pulmonary capillary wedge pressure (PCWP), an estimate of left atrial pressure. Assuming normal aortic valve function, arterial systolic pressure reflects left ventricular systolic pressure. These pressures are useful in determining factors that characterize cardiac performance, such as preload, afterload, volume, filling pressures, and resistance. Normal cardiac pressures are shown in Figure A&P13-9.

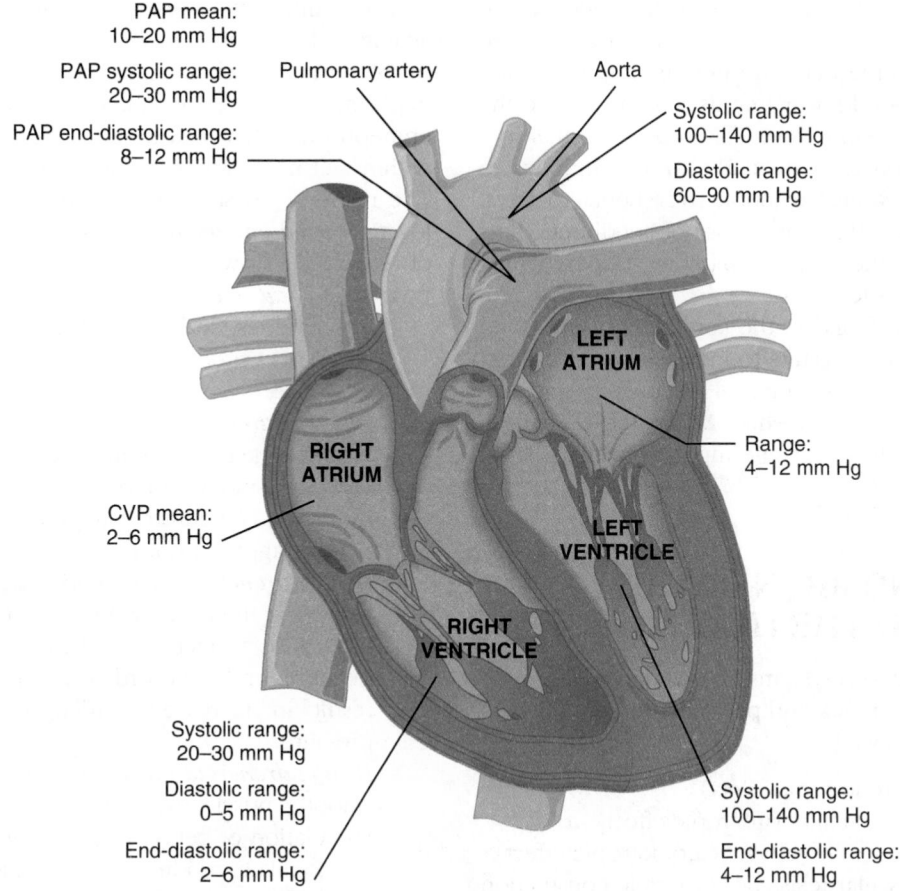

PAP mean:
10–20 mm Hg

PAP systolic range:
20–30 mm Hg

PAP end-diastolic range:
8–12 mm Hg

Pulmonary artery

Aorta

Systolic range:
100–140 mm Hg

Diastolic range:
60–90 mm Hg

LEFT ATRIUM

RIGHT ATRIUM

Range:
4–12 mm Hg

CVP mean:
2–6 mm Hg

LEFT VENTRICLE

RIGHT VENTRICLE

Systolic range:
20–30 mm Hg

Diastolic range:
0–5 mm Hg

End-diastolic range:
2–6 mm Hg

Systolic range:
100–140 mm Hg

End-diastolic range:
4–12 mm Hg

■ **FIGURE A&PI3–9** Normal pressures in the cardiac chambers and associated major blood vessels. *CVP,* Central venous pressure; *PAP,* pulmonary artery pressure.

HEART RATE

The normal heart rate is 60 to 100 beats/min. *Sinus tachycardia* is a rate of more than 100 beats/min; *sinus bradycardia* is a rate of fewer than 60 beats/min. (The *sinus* in these terms indicates that the impulse arose in the sinoatrial node, the normal pacemaker region of the heart.) The intrinsic heart rate is 90 beats/min. At rest, the heart rate of 70 beats/min reflects the dominant control by the parasympathetic nervous system. Variations in heartbeat can be caused by exercise, the size of the client, age, hormones, temperature, blood pressure, anxiety, stress, and pain.

ARTERIAL PRESSURE

Arterial pressure (see the Unit 12 Anatomy and Physiology Review) is the pressure of blood against arterial walls. *Systolic pressure* is the maximum pressure of the blood exerted against the artery walls when the heart contracts (normally 100 to 140 mm Hg). *Diastolic pressure* is the force of blood exerted against the artery walls during the heart's relaxation (or filling) phase (normally 60 to 90 mm Hg). *Blood pressure* is expressed as systolic pressure/diastolic pressure (e.g., 120/80 mm Hg). Cardiac

output is a key determinant of arterial pressure (see Figure A&P12-4).

Baroreceptors, Stretch Receptors, and Chemoreceptors

Changes in sympathetic and parasympathetic activity occur in response to messages sent from sensory receptors in various parts of the body. Important receptors in cardiovascular reflexes include (1) arterial baroreceptors, (2) stretch-sensitive cardiopulmonary receptors of the atria and veins, and (3) chemoreceptors.

Baroreceptors (pressoreceptors) are stretch-sensitive nerve endings affected by changes in arterial blood pressure. They are located in the walls of the aortic arch and carotid sinuses. Increases in arterial pressure stimulate baroreceptors, which send impulses to the medulla, resulting in heart rate and arterial pressure decreases (the *vagal response*). When arterial pressure decreases, baroreceptors receive less stretch and thus send fewer impulses to the medulla (see Figure A&P12-5). Then sympathetic-mediated increase in heart rate and vasoconstriction occurs.

Cardiopulmonary stretch receptors are located in terminal sections of the vena cava and the atria. These receptors respond to length changes, which reflect circulatory volume status. When blood pressure decreases in the vena cava and the right atrium (e.g., hypovolemia), stretch receptors send fewer impulses than usual to the central nervous system (CNS). This process results in a sympathetic response, particularly to the kidney, to enhance salt and water retention over hours to days. These changes also stimulate release of antidiuretic hormone (ADH) from the posterior pituitary. Hypervolemia produces the opposite effects.

Chemoreceptors, found in the aortic arch and carotid bodies, are primarily sensitive to increased carbon dioxide levels and decreased arterial pH (acidemia) and secondarily sensitive to hypoxemia. When these changes occur, chemoreceptors transmit impulses to the CNS to increase heart rate.

THE AUTONOMIC NERVOUS SYSTEM AND THE HEART

The autonomic nervous system (ANS) is the effector limb of the baroreceptor reflex and plays an important role in regulating the following:

- Heart rate (chronotropic effect)
- Myocardial contractility (inotropic effect)
- AV node conduction velocity (dromotropic effect)
- Peripheral vascular resistance (arteriole constriction and dilation)
- Venous return (venule and vein constriction and dilation)

The two subdivisions of the ANS (sympathetic and parasympathetic) generally exert opposing influences and balance their activities to promote cardiovascular adaptation to internal and external demands. ANS responses are involuntary.

Parasympathetic nerves arise from the dorsal motor nucleus of the vagus nerve, located in the medulla oblongata. They innervate the SA node atria, AV node, and to a lesser extent the ventricles and Purkinje system. When stimulated, parasympathetic nerve endings release the neurotransmitter acetylcholine, which produces inhibitory effects by binding to muscarinic receptors. Parasympathetic stimulation decreases the rate of SA node firing, thus lowering heart rate; atrial conductivity lessens as well.

Sympathetic nerve fibers originate between the first and fifth thoracic vertebrae and terminate in all areas of the heart. With stimulation, the nerve endings release the neurotransmitter norepinephrine and produce the following effects: (1) increased heart rate, (2) increased conduction speed through the AV node, (3) increased atrial and ventricular contractility, and (4) peripheral vasoconstriction, by binding to adrenergic receptors, activating G proteins, and opening ionic channels.

The sympathetic nervous system influences adrenal activity. The adrenal medulla responds to stimulation by secreting catecholamines (norepinephrine and epinephrine) into the circulation. Norepinephrine and epinephrine interact with adrenergic receptors found within cell membranes of the heart and blood vessels. The response to stimulation depends on the type and location of adrenergic receptors involved. The five types of receptors follow:

1. *Alpha$_1$-adrenergic* receptors are located in peripheral arteries and veins. When stimulated, alpha receptors produce a dramatic vasoconstrictive response.
2. *Alpha$_2$-adrenergic* receptors are located in several tissues. Their actions include contraction of some vascular smooth muscle, inhibition of lipolysis, inhibition of neurotransmission, and promotion of platelet aggregation.
3. *Beta$_1$-adrenergic* receptors are predominantly located in the heart. When stimulated, beta$_1$ receptors cause an increase in heart rate, AV node conduction, and myocardial contractility. This may result in increased cardiac output and blood pressure.
4. *Beta$_2$-adrenergic* receptors are found in the smooth muscle of arteriolar and bronchial walls. Stimulation of beta$_2$ receptors causes smooth muscles to dilate, producing vasodilation of arterial vessels and bronchodilation.
5. *Beta$_3$-adrenergic* receptors are found in adipose tissue, where they promote lipolysis. Indirectly, this may assist cardiac performance because the myocardium can utilize fatty acids as metabolic fuels. Currently, no direct cardiac role for beta$_3$ adrenoreceptors has been identified.

Hormonal and Other Influences

In addition to epinephrine and norepinephrine from the adrenal medulla, several other hormones regulate cardiac output indirectly by controlling body fluid volume (and thus venous pressure and venous return). The most important hormones include ADH and the renin-angiotensin-aldosterone mechanism.

Other factors also influence cardiac activity and blood pressure. For example, cerebral cortical input from anger, fear, pain, or excitement can augment the effects of the sympathetic nervous system.

EFFECTS OF AGING

At birth, the neonate ventricles are of equal size; however, the vascular changes associated with birth lead to a decrease in pulmonary vascular resistance and pressure and an increase in systemic vascular resistance and pressure. During childhood, the greater work o the left ventricle to eject its cardiac output into the high-pressure systemic circulation causes a hypertrophy of the left ventricular muscle, which is characteristic of the adult heart. The heart muscle also undergoes changes with further aging that lead to dilation of the cardiac chambers and lessening of contractility. This has little effect on stroke volume, but it reduces cardiac reserve. Coronary arteries become thickened and rigid. These changes decrease the ability of the heart to respond to additional demands and increase the likelihood of coronary artery disease. Heart valves may thicken and become incompetent, resulting in a systolic ejection murmur.

CONCLUSIONS

Although the heart can be viewed simply as a pump, this remarkable, durable organ is much more than that. The heart is a continuously beating organ that never rests. It moves blood throughout the body to oxygenate cells for energy. It propels blood through its four chambers in one direction, from right to left. Left ventricular contraction moves blood into the arteries under high pressure. This pressure propels blood through the systemic circulation.

Heart disease remains the major cause of death and involves disorders both of structure and of function of the heart. These disorders are studied in the following chapters.

BIBLIOGRAPHY

1. Berne, R., et al. (2004). *Physiology* (5th ed.). St. Louis: Mosby.
2. Carroll, R.G. (2007). *Elsevier's integrated physiology*. Philadelphia: Saunders.
3. Kierszenbaum, A.L. (2007). *Histology and cell biology: An introduction to pathology* (2nd ed.). St. Louis: Mosby.
4. Guyton, A., & Hall, J. (2006). *Textbook of medical physiology* (11th ed.). Philadelphia: Saunders.
5. Silverthorn, D. (2006). *Human physiology* (4th ed.). San Francisco, Calif: Pearson Benjamin Cummings.

CHAPTER 54

Assessment of the Cardiac System

BETH F. CROWDER

Since 1918 cardiovascular disease (CVD) has been the number one cause of death in the United States. In 2003 CVD accounted for 37.3% of all deaths, or 1 in every 2.7 deaths, in the United States. In fact, CVD claimed more lives than the next four leading causes of death combined (cancer, chronic lower respiratory tract diseases, accidents, and diabetes mellitus).[3] The 2006 estimated direct and indirect cost of CVD is $403.1 billion. According to the Social Security Administration, CVD is the leading cause of premature, permanent disability in the U.S. labor force today.[3] For those age 60 years and older, CVD is the number one killer worldwide. Of those who die from CVD, 80% to 90% have one or more risk factors. The worldwide incidence and prevalence of CVD are on the rise and CVD is a pandemic that knows no boundaries.[32]

According to World Health Organization estimates for 2003, deaths from CVD totaled 16.7 million. Approximately 80% of CVD deaths occurred in countries with low- and middle-income populations. By 2010 CVD is estimated to be the leading cause of death in developing countries.[32] Heart disease has no geographical, gender, or socioeconomic boundaries; at least 20 million people survive CVD attacks every year. Cardiovascular disease affects individuals in their peak midlife years, disrupting the future of the families dependent on them and undermining the development of nations by depriving them of workers in their most productive years.[32]

It is estimated that more than 50% of CVD deaths and disability can be eliminated by a combination of cost-effective national and individual efforts to reduce risk factors.[3] The goal of *Healthy People 2010* is to improve overall cardiovascular health and quality of life through prevention, assessment, detection, risk factor management, and early diagnosis and treatment.[7,24] The prevalence and complications of CVD have significant implications for nurses, requiring them to use holistic assessment and treatment skills. Assessment of the cardiovascular system involves incorporating data from history-taking, relating the information to the physical examination and diagnostic tests, and correlating the data with the underlying pathophysiology to institute a plan of care.

HISTORY

The history encompasses all of the subjective information gathered from the client and his/her present family members and/or friends. If the client is stable, a detailed history can and should be obtained. A careful history allows a care provider to evaluate the impact the presenting illness has on the client's personal and social life, personality, occupation, and responsibilities.[6]

Biographical and Demographic Data
Biographical and demographic data include name, age, gender, place of birth, race, marital status, occupation, and ethnic background. Alterations in health may have caused changes in the main provider's occupation and

---

evolve Web Enhancements

Client Education Guide Stress Testing (English and Spanish)

Assessment Terms Assessment Terms (English and Spanish)

Appendix A Religious Beliefs and Practices Affecting Health Care

Appendix B Health History Format That Integrates the Assessment of Functional Health Patterns

Tables Common Electrocardiographic Tests

Common Radiographic Cardiac Tests

Common Cardiac Ultrasonographic Tests

Common Cardiac Invasive Procedures

Common Cardiac Laboratory Tests

Be sure to check out the bonus material on the Evolve website and the CD-ROM, including free self-assessment exercises. **http://evolve.elsevier.com/Black/medsurg**

status within the family. There are known transcultural considerations regarding heart disease and stroke among culturally diverse individuals. 🪔 Economic transition, urbanization, industrialization, and globalization bring about lifestyle changes that promote heart disease.

🪔 Prevalence, incidence, and mortality of CVD vary among differing races and by gender. The average incidence of a first major cardiovascular event rises from 7/1000 men ages 35 to 44 to 68/1000 at ages 85 to 94.[3] For women, comparable rates occur a decade later in life. The prevalence of CVD is highest among native Hawaiians (16.6%) followed by American Indians (13.8%), whites (11.4%), and blacks (9.9%).[3] Black and Hispanic women have a higher prevalence of CVD risk factors than white women of comparable socioeconomic status. The age-adjusted death rates for CVD are 17% for Hispanics, 15% for whites, 14% for Asians, 11% for blacks, and 8% for American Indians.[3] The death rates for CVD in men and women were higher compared to the death rates from cancer in the two groups. Among minority women, the CVD death rate is higher in black women compared to white women. For many unaware women, CVD caused greater mortality than the next five leading causes of death combined (cancer, chronic obstructive pulmonary disease [COPD], Alzheimer's disease, diabetes mellitus, and accidents), resulting in about one death every minute.[3]

Current Health

Documenting the progression of the first manifestation to the current complaints or problems helps organize the history and reveals the sequence of events that led the client to seek help.

Chief Complaint

There can be a tendency to rely on objective testing (laboratory values, x-rays, scans, angiography) to diagnose a client's illness. However, the client's history remains the richest source of information concerning the presenting illness or chief complaint.[28] Eliciting a client's history not only assists with individualizing the plan of care but also helps to establish a bond with that client.[6] The history begins with an open-ended question that allows the client to provide his/her own account of clinical manifestations leading up to the illness presentation. Upon completion of the client's clinical manifestations, "probe" questions are asked in order to analyze the manifestations and gather specific information regarding the *o*nset, *l*ocation, *d*uration, *c*haracteristics, *a*ssociated manifestations, *a*ggravating factors, and *r*elieving factors. The mnemonic "OLD CAAR" can help you remember what to ask each client.[11] There are many common cardiac manifestations, however; many disorders can cause chest pain. Table 54-1 differentiates between the various chest pain conditions and clinical manifestations.

Table 54-1 will aid in comparing and contrasting conditions as the mnemonic OLD CAAR assessment skills are reinforced. Some conditions are life-threatening that require immediate attention. As a medical-surgical nurse standing at that client's bedside, you may be the first one to (1) see the client and obtain the history, (2) witness the sudden development of clinical manifestations, or (3) alert the attending health care provider of important information you obtained during assessment of the client. In caring for adults (or children, as they may have congenital anomalies) you will encounter a client with a history of CVD or clinical manifestations that could be due to CVD. What you learn in this chapter may help you diagnose, treat, and save your client's life.

Clinical Manifestations

Conduct an analysis of the client's clinical manifestations to evaluate and clarify the chief complaint. This will help you deduce, or narrow, the possible cause of the presenting illness. While evaluating and caring for any client, keep these three rules foremost in mind: (1) the initial or admitting diagnosis may be incorrect or inconclusive; (2) do not bias the severity of the client's presenting illness based on the client's bed/unit assignment; and (3) keep an open mind to alternative diagnoses.[11] Figure 54-1 on p. 1358 provides questions and manifestations to guide your assessment for cardiac clinical manifestations. The cardinal manifestations of CVD are located in Box 54-1. There may be more than one major manifestation. When this occurs, assess them in the order of importance.

Chest pain. Chest pain is one of the most common manifestations of cardiac disease; however, almost 30% of clients with confirmed myocardial infarction (MI) may not report chest pain at all.[11] Many women and long-standing diabetic clients with neuropathy do not experience chest pain resulting in undiagnosed or unknown cardiac ischemia and a silent MI. Chest pain may also result from pulmonary, gastrointestinal, musculoskeletal, neurologic, and anxiety-related conditions. *Angina pectoris* is the true manifestation, or typical chest pain, of coronary artery disease (CAD). Angina is caused by myocardial ischemia (hypoxia), an imbalance of oxygen supply and demand as the coronary arteries support myocardial tissue. Because chest pain is caused by a number of conditions, it is highly variable.

Chest pain not caused by myocardial ischemia is termed atypical chest pain. Evaluate chest pain and its cause with careful analysis. Table 54-1 compares selected cardiac, pulmonary, gastrointestinal, musculoskeletal, neurologic, and anxiety-related conditions in relation to chest pain. Chest pain manifestations may appear to overlap with the various body systems. A thorough analysis of clinical manifestations will assist in

TABLE 54–1 Differential Assessment of Chest Pain

Conditions	Location	Characteristics	Quantity	Onset/Duration	Aggravating and Relieving Factors	Associated Manifestations
Angina pectoris	Substernal or retrosternal region; radiates to neck, jaw, epigastrium, shoulders, arms (especially left)	Pressure, burning, squeezing, tight heaviness, indigestion	Moderate to severe	<10 min	Aggravated by exertion, cold, stress, or after meals; relieved by rest or nitroglycerin; atypical (Prinzmetal's) angina may be unrelated to activity and caused by coronary artery spasm	Sinus tachycardia, bradycardia, S_4, paradoxical split S_2 during pain episode
Coronary insufficiency	Same as angina	Same as angina	Increasingly severe	>10 min	Same as angina, with gradually decreasing tolerance for exertion	Same as angina
Myocardial infarction	Precordial, substernal; may radiate like angina	Heaviness, crushing pressure, burning, constriction	Severe, sometimes mild (in 30% of clients)	Sudden onset; lasts longer than 15 min	Unrelieved	Dyspnea, sweating, weakness, nausea, vomiting, severe anxiety
Pericarditis	Usually begins over sternum and may radiate to neck and down left upper extremity	Sharp, stabbing, knife-like	Moderate to severe	Lasts many hours to days	Aggravated by deep breathing, rotating chest or supine position; relieved by sitting up and leaning forward	Fever, infection, pericardial friction rub, syncope, dyspnea, orthopnea
Dissecting aortic aneurysm	Anterior chest; radiates to thoracic area of back; may be abdominal; pain shifts in chest	Tearing	Excruciating, tearing, knife-like	Sudden onset, lasts for hours	Unrelated to anything	Lower blood pressure in one arm, absent pulses, stroke, dyspnea, murmur of aortic insufficiency, pulsus paradoxus, stridor; myocardial infarction can occur
Mitral valve prolapse syndrome	Usually not substernal; sometimes radiates to left arm, back, jaw	Stabbing, sharp, sticky quality, "kick"	Variable; generally mild but can become severe	Sudden, recurrent	Not related to exertion, not relieved by nitroglycerin or rest	Variable palpitations, dysrhythmias, dizziness, syncope, dyspnea, late systolic or pansystolic murmur

Condition	Location	Quality	Severity	Onset/Duration	Aggravating factors	Associated findings
Pulmonary embolism (many pulmonary emboli do not produce chest pain)	Substernal, "anginal"	Deep, crushing; if pulmonary infection, may be pleuritic	Can be absent, mild, or severe	Sudden onset; lasts minutes to <1 hr	May be aggravated by breathing	Fever, tachypnea, tachycardia, hypotension, elevated jugular venous pressure, right ventricular lift, accentuated pulmonary valve (P_2) sound during S_2, occasional murmur of tricuspid insufficiency and right ventricular S_4; with infarction usually in presence of heart failure; crackles, pleural rub, hemoptysis, clinical phlebitis present in minority of cases
Spontaneous pneumothorax	Unilateral	Sharp, well localized, stabbing	Moderate, severe	Sudden onset; lasts many hours	Painful breathing	Dyspnea, shock, tension pneumothorax
Pneumonia with pleurisy	Localized over area of consolidation	Sharp, grabbing, aching	Variable	Sudden	Painful breathing	Dyspnea, cough, fever, hemoptysis, crackles, occasional pleural rub
Gastrointestinal disorders (esophageal reflux)	Lower substernal area, epigastric, right or left upper quadrant	Burning, colic-like aching, tightness, pressure	Moderate to severe	Waves, continuous radiation	Precipitated by recumbency, large meals, alcohol ingestion	Nausea, regurgitation, food intolerance, melena, hematemesis, jaundice
Musculoskeletal disorders	Variable	Aching	Variable	Short or long duration	History of muscle exertion, viral illness	Tender to pressure or movement
Neurologic disorders (herpes zoster)	Dermatomal in distribution	Aching, constant burning, pins and needles, sharp	Moderate, severe	Prolonged period of time	Aggravated by systemic stress	Pain before rash, vesicles
Psychogenic states (depression, self-gain, or attention-seeking)	Usually localized to a point	Vague, burning, diffuse	Mild to moderate, disabling	Unassociated with external events	Situational anger, depression, anxiety	Sighing, chest wall tenderness, fatigue, dyspnea, anorexia

CVA, Cerebrovascular accident; P_2, pulmonic second sound; S_2, second heart sound; S_4, fourth heart sound.
Modified from Andreoli, K., et al. (1987). *Comprehensive cardiac care* (6th ed., pp. 54-55). St. Louis: Mosby; Seller, R.H. (1996). *Differential diagnosis of common complaints* (3rd ed., pp. 57-68). Philadelphia: Saunders; and Hill, B., & Geraci, S.A. (1998). A diagnostic approach to chest pain based on history and ancillary evaluation. *Nurse Practitioner, 23*(2), 20-45.

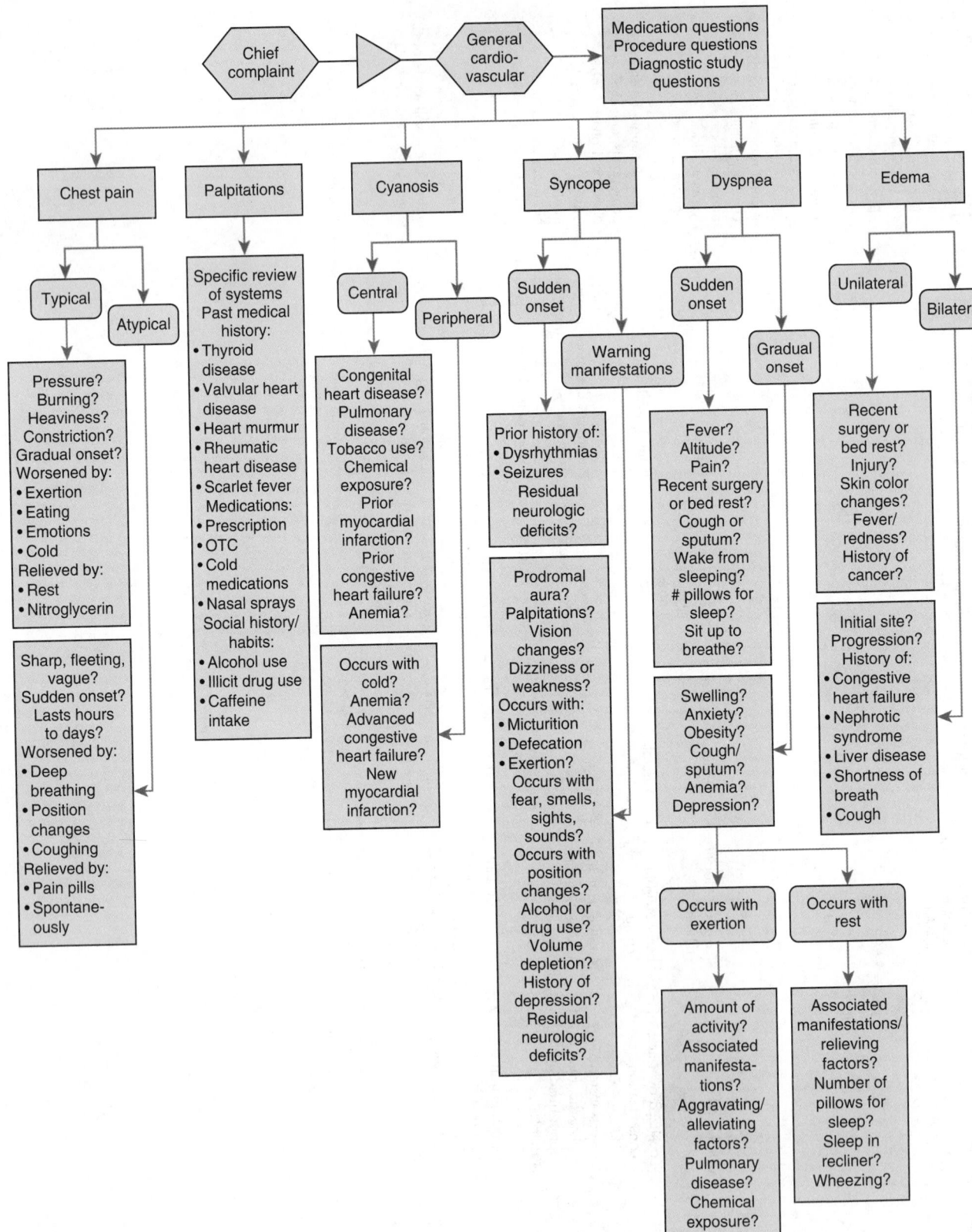

■ **FIGURE 54–1** Expanded cardiac assessment.

BOX 54-1 Common Clinical Manifestations of CVD

- Chest pain
- Dyspnea
- Cyanosis
- Syncope
- Palpitations
- Edema
- Epigastric discomfort
- Fatigue*

*Women often have several weeks of fatigue before a myocardial infarction, so this is often a warning sign for women.

prioritizing treatment and testing strategies.[6,11,16,30] Gender-specific knowledge of CVD is also needed, as research indicates women present with differing (frequently termed "atypical") manifestations, such as fatigue, caused by CVD.[19,20] Although some women may experience chest pain, many women present with dyspnea, nausea, vomiting, fatigue, neck pain, jaw pain, back pain, dizziness, palpitations.[19]

Onset. The onset of chest pain provides not only the time line between when the manifestations began and when the client presented for further evaluation, but also a description of the beginning of pain. Angina pain has a gradual onset that intensifies, especially with continued activities. Pain described as sudden in its onset is atypical for angina.

Location. The site of discomfort provides additional information for determining its cause. Angina pain is ordinarily retrosternal, felt slightly to the left of the midline or partly under the sternum. Angina pain tends to radiate bilaterally across the chest into the arms, left greater than right, and into the neck and lower jaw. Occasionally, radiation to the back or occiput is noted. Chest pain may be diffuse, localized, or so minor that clients dismiss true ischemic pain or possible infarction. Painless or atypical presentation of myocardial infarction occurs in up to 30% of clients, particularly in diabetic and older clients. Diabetic clients in particular have a two-fold to four-fold increase in developing CVD.*

Duration. Note the time the pain begins and ends to determine the duration of discomfort. Several intermittent small episodes of chest pain are not considered as one long period of pain. Generally, angina pain has an increasing pattern that reaches maximum intensity after several minutes and is usually relieved within 10 minutes by rest, with or without the use of vasodilator drugs such as nitroglycerin. Angina pectoris rarely lasts less than 1 minute or longer than 15 minutes. Unstable angina usually lasts less than 20 minutes, and pain from myocardial infarction usually lasts 30 minutes or longer. Pain that is "constant" or "prolonged" is atypical for angina.[‡]

Characteristics. Angina pain may be described as a "strange feeling" in the chest, a "dull heavy pressure, burning, crushing, constricting, squeezing, aching, or tightness." Some clients present with complaints of "gas" or "indigestion" that is caused by angina. Angina pectoris characteristically has a crescendo (gradually increasing) pattern at onset. Pain described as "shooting, stabbing, sudden onset, pleuritic, sharp, or fleeting" is often caused by pulmonary, gastrointestinal, musculoskeletal, neurologic, and anxiety-related conditions.**

To better quantify chest pain, ask the client to use a scale of 1 (least severe) to 10 (most severe). This recorded scale can then be used to compare future episodes of chest pain. For example, the client may report 10/10 for pain on admission and then report 3/10 for pain after administration of a vasodilating medication. Please refer to Chapter 20 for a further discussion of pain and its assessment.

Associated Manifestations. Radiation of pain to the arms (especially the left), throat, jaw, ear, shoulders, or back is typical of angina. Epigastric, unilateral, or right upper quadrant is atypical for angina. Clinical manifestations of dyspnea, nausea, vomiting, diaphoresis, palpitations, or syncope are commonly associated with angina. Fatigue for several weeks before a cardiac episode is common in women and is becoming a well-known warning sign. Tachycardia, coughing, or an associated rash is atypical for angina.[‡]

Aggravating Factors. Angina pain may be associated with certain factors or conditions. Chest pain resulting from stable angina pectoris develops after exertion, eating a heavy meal, or emotional excitement (the three Es), but may also occur with sexual excitement, temperature extremes, or straining to have a bowel movement. Rest or sublingual nitroglycerin will relieve the pain promptly. Chest pain caused by acute coronary syndrome or myocardial infarction occurs at rest or awakens the client from sleep, requiring sublingual nitroglycerin or medical attention for relief. Pain that worsens with position changes, palpation, coughing, deep breathing, or eating is atypical for angina.[6,11,16,17,30]

Relieving Factors. Angina pain is usually relieved by rest, vasodilator drugs such as nitroglycerin, oxygen, and relaxation. Chest pain that is not reduced by these interventions and lasts 20 minutes or longer is suggestive

---

* References 2,6,11,16,17,30.

** References 2,6,8,11,14,16,17,28,30.

‡ References 2, 6, 11, 16, 17, 30.

of an acute coronary syndrome (ACS). Chest pain that is relieved with position changes, eating, antacids, or movement is atypical for angina.[6,11,16,30] The Integrating Diagnostic Testing feature below outlines the steps necessary to integrate the chief complaint of chest pain with clinical manifestations and appropriate tests in order to diagnose the presenting illness.

Palpitations. The word *palpitation* is derived from the Latin *palpitare,* which means "to throb." *Palpitations* are uncomfortable sensations in the chest associated with a wide range of dysrhythmias.[6] Box 54-2 provides common causes of palpitations. Palpitations are commonly caused by extra atrial or ventricular systoles and do not necessarily indicate serious heart disease. The Integrating Diagnostic Testing feature on p. 1361 outlines the assessment of palpitations and the steps necessary to integrate the chief complaint of palpitations with other clinical manifestations and appropriate tests in order to diagnose the presenting illness.

A palpitation is a sensation of rapid heartbeats, skipping, irregularity, thumping, or pounding and may be accompanied by anxiousness. The onset and termination of palpitations are often abrupt. Some also report manifestations similar to syncopal episodes (vision changes, weakness, dizziness, nausea, or diaphoresis) with the aura they thought they were going to pass out, but do not lose consciousness. This is known as presyncope. Presyncope with palpitations is a more serious occurrence and warrants evaluation consistent with a syncopal evaluation.[6,11,16]

Ask the client about (1) medications, especially the use of over-the-counter cold medications or nasal sprays

INTEGRATING DIAGNOSTIC TESTING

Chest Pain

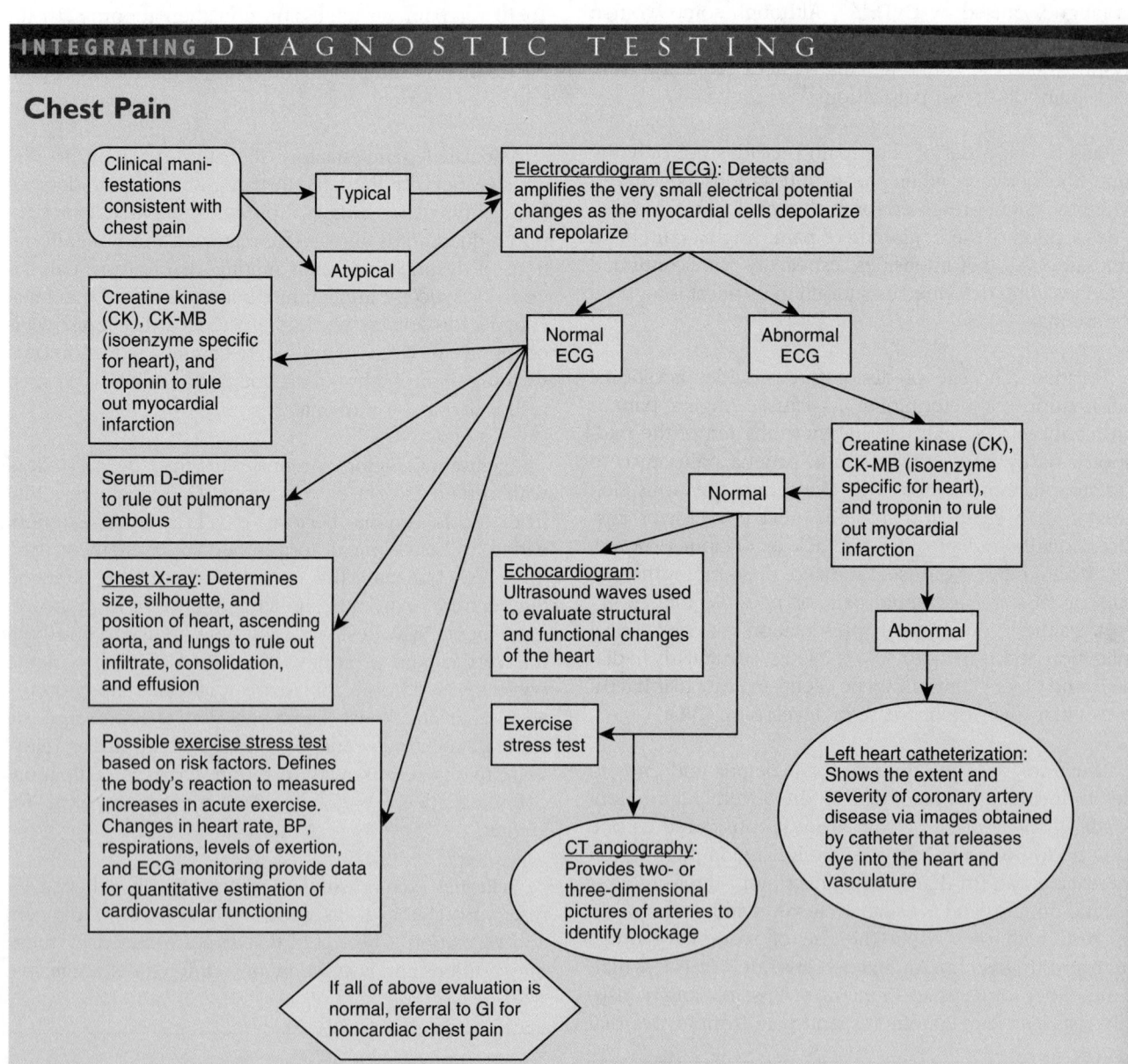

BOX 54-2   *Common Causes of Palpitations*

DYSRHYTHMIAS

1. Bradydysrhythmias
   a. Heart block
   b. Sinus arrest
2. Extrasystoles
   a. Premature atrial contractions (PACs)
   b. Premature nodal contractions
   c. Premature ventricular contractions (PVCs)
3. Tachydysrhythmias
   a. Atrial fibrillation
   b. Atrial flutter
   c. Multifocal atrial tachycardia
   d. Paroxysmal supraventricular tachycardia
   e. Ventricular tachycardia

OTHER

1. Anemia
2. Anxiety states
3. Caffeine
4. Drugs
   a. Antidepressants
   b. Bronchodilators
   c. Digitalis
5. Fever
6. Hyperthyroidism
7. Hypoglycemia
8. Perimenopausal
9. Pheochromocytoma
10. Smoking
11. Thyrotoxicosis

with decongestants; (2) caffeine intake; (3) history of thyroid disease; (4) the frequency or pattern (if any) of palpitations; (5) the duration of the palpitations; and (6) any manifestations such as dizziness, shortness of breath, or chest pain associated with the onset of the palpitations. Is there a family history of dysrhythmia or pacemakers?

Cyanosis. Cyanosis is a bluish discoloration of the mucous membranes or skin caused by decreased hemoglobin level or decreased blood perfusion. The two forms of cyanosis are central and peripheral. *Central cyanosis* is a result of decreased arterial oxygen saturation caused by impaired pulmonary function (either a reduced inspired oxygen concentration or an inability to oxygenate blood in the lungs). Causes include advanced pulmonary disease, right-to-left shunting within the heart, or pulmonary edema. Central cyanosis does not occur early in the disease process; it is often a later sign that may indicate advanced disease. *Peripheral cyanosis* is a result of decreased blood flow to the extremities caused by cutaneous vasoconstriction (from exposure to the cold) or low cardiac output (from shock or heart failure).[6,11,16]

Ask clients about any congenital heart disease or history of blood disorder. Inquire about underlying lung or heart disease including chronic obstructive pulmonary disease, emphysema, tobacco use, chemical or asbestos exposure, prior myocardial infarction, or congestive heart failure.

Syncope. Syncope, or fainting, is a transient loss of consciousness related to inadequate cerebral perfusion. The

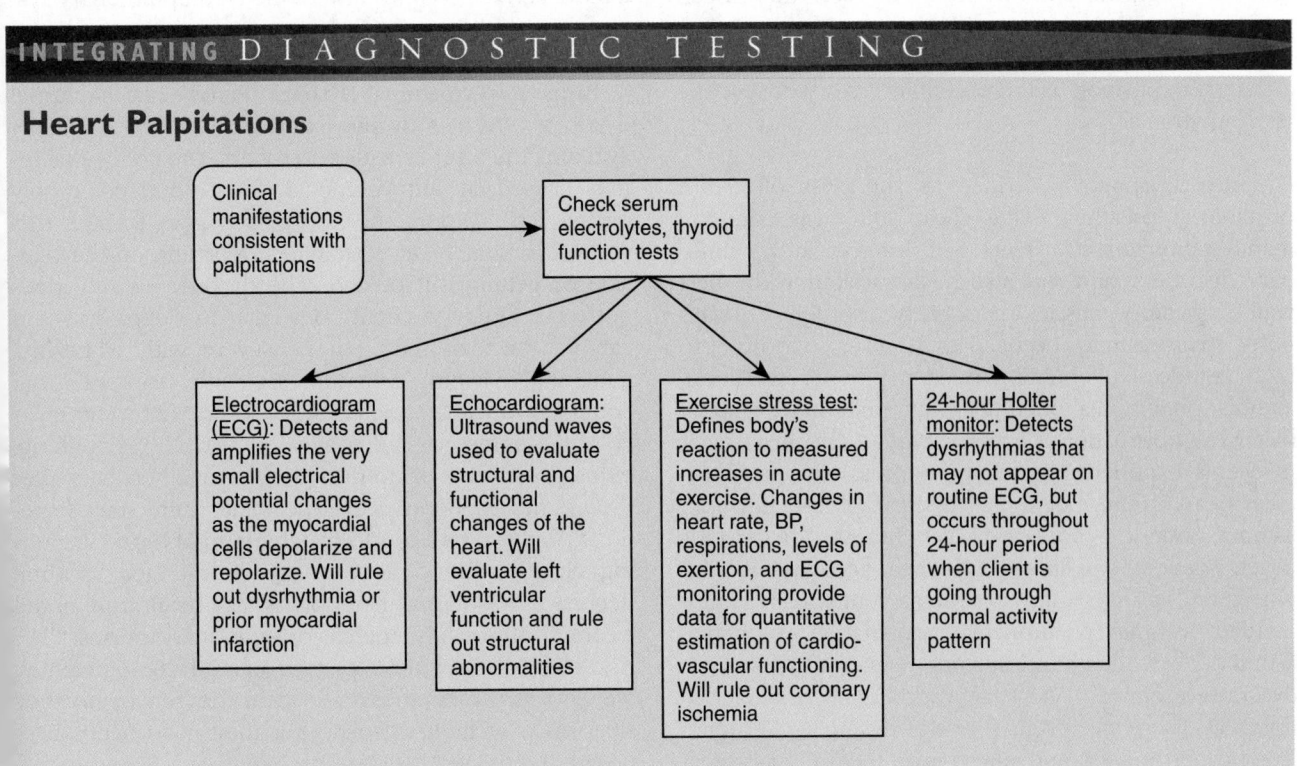

INTEGRATING DIAGNOSTIC TESTING

Heart Palpitations

Clinical manifestations consistent with palpitations → Check serum electrolytes, thyroid function tests

Electrocardiogram (ECG): Detects and amplifies the very small electrical potential changes as the myocardial cells depolarize and repolarize. Will rule out dysrhythmia or prior myocardial infarction

Echocardiogram: Ultrasound waves used to evaluate structural and functional changes of the heart. Will evaluate left ventricular function and rule out structural abnormalities

Exercise stress test: Defines body's reaction to measured increases in acute exercise. Changes in heart rate, BP, respirations, levels of exertion, and ECG monitoring provide data for quantitative estimation of cardiovascular functioning. Will rule out coronary ischemia

24-hour Holter monitor: Detects dysrhythmias that may not appear on routine ECG, but occurs throughout 24-hour period when client is going through normal activity pattern

most important tool in the evaluation of syncope is the medical history, which usually uncovers the likely cause. If the syncopal episode was witnessed, it is essential to speak directly to those witnesses in order to obtain a complete history.

Most syncopal episodes have a cardiac origin including either dysrhythmias, vasovagal, or neurocardiogenic syncope. Many syncopal episodes are preceded by warning manifestations such as rapid heart action, vision changes, weakness, dizziness, nausea, or diaphoresis. However, cardiac dysrhythmias (irregular heart rhythms) can precipitate a sudden decrease in cardiac output, causing syncope without warning. Certain medications (antidysrhythmics, antibiotics) can prolong the QT interval in the cardiac cycle, resulting in syncope. Valvular disorders, especially aortic stenosis, may also lead to an adverse change in circulatory hemodynamics precipitated by exertion and cause syncope or vertigo. Micturition, defecation, transient ischemic attacks, or volume depletion (from diuretics, nausea, vomiting, diarrhea, severe anemia) can cause syncope. Seizures often have a prodromal aura (warning manifestations) preceding the seizure, as well as urinary incontinence and a postictal state of confusion.

Vasovagal syncope (caused by heightened vagus nerve tone) occurs after sudden or unexpected pain, fear, or unpleasant sight, smell, or sound. Neurocardiogenic syncope is often preceded by position changes from lying or sitting to standing, or by prolonged standing. Psychiatric disorders (anxiety or major depression), pain disorder, or alcohol or drug dependence can also cause syncope.[6,10,11,16] Ask the client if anyone was with him/her when the episode occurred. Have there been previous episodes of syncope? Were any preceding manifestations noted? Was the syncopal episode preceded by a change in position? Is there a family history of syncope or dysrhythmia?[16]

Dyspnea. Dyspnea is defined as shortness of breath or labored breathing. Like chest pain, this common manifestation affects clients with cardiac and pulmonary disorders, and can also be associated with chest wall, respiratory muscle, and anxiety disorders. *Sudden-onset dyspnea* may occur with a fever, exposure to high altitude, acute pulmonary edema, hyperventilation, anemia, pneumonia, pneumothorax, pulmonary emboli, or airway obstruction. *Chronic dyspnea* also may occur in clients experiencing anxiety, depression, left ventricular heart failure, pulmonary disease, pleural effusion, asthma, obesity, poor physical fitness, or various psychosomatic conditions. Dyspnea accompanied by wheezing is secondary to left ventricular failure (cardiac asthma) or bronchial constriction (bronchial asthma).[6,11,16] Identification and treatment of obstructive sleep apnea (OSA) are additional risk factors for CVD. There are several forms of dyspnea: exertional dyspnea, orthopnea, and paroxysmal nocturnal dyspnea.

Exertional Dyspnea. This is the most common form of cardiac-related dyspnea. Also known as *dyspnea on exertion,* or dyspnea of angina equivalent, this occurs during mild to moderate exercise or activity and disappears with rest. If severe, exertional dyspnea can greatly limit activity tolerance. Ask the client to describe the degree of activity that typically precipitates the onset of dyspnea, for example, walking up one flight of stairs, or walking to the mailbox. How long does the shortness of breath last? Are there any accompanying manifestations with the shortness of breath? What relieves the shortness of breath? Noncardiac conditions such as obesity, poor physical conditioning, anemia, asthma, and obstructions of the nasal passages may also lead to dyspnea after mild exercise.

Orthopnea. Orthopnea (difficult breathing except when sitting erect or standing) results from an increase in pulmonary venous and capillary pressure in the lungs when the person is lying flat, and is relieved when the person sits upright or in a semivertical position. It consists of a cough and dyspnea in clients with left ventricular failure or mitral valve disease, and may also occur with severe chronic obstructive lung disease or asthma. Clients with orthopnea have learned to use two or more pillows when lying down in order to avoid dyspnea.

Ask clients what actions they take to facilitate breathing. In what position do they sleep? On how many pillows do they sleep? Do they sit up in a chair, dangle their feet at the bedside? Record the degree of head elevation required to breathe. Orthopnea usually indicates a more serious compromise of the cardiopulmonary system than does exertional dyspnea.[5,7,8]

Paroxysmal Nocturnal Dyspnea. Paroxysmal nocturnal dyspnea (PND) is dyspnea during sleep that suddenly awakens the sleeper with a "terrifying breathing attack." It is caused by left ventricular failure and commonly occurs 2 to 4 hours after the person goes to bed. It is relieved within 15 to 30 minutes by sitting on the bedside or getting out of bed. The dyspnea usually does not recur after the client goes back to sleep. Episodes can be mild, or they can be severe with wheezing, coughing, gasping, diaphoresis, and apprehension. Some episodes associated with severe left ventricular failure progress to pulmonary edema.[6,11,16] Coughing, either productive or nonproductive, usually occurs after PND as the sleeper tries to expectorate pulmonary secretions. *Hemoptysis* refers to coughing up of blood, including clots of blood as well as blood-tinged sputum. Recurrent episodes of hemoptysis may result from mitral stenosis, pulmonary edema, or pulmonary causes.[6,11,16] Ask clients about their pattern of PND (e.g., nightly, weekly). Are they able to sleep in the bed or do they sleep in a recliner? Also note if they have been diagnosed and treated for OSA.

Fatigue. Fatigue can accompany complaints of dyspnea. Fatigue is weariness or exhaustion with exertion. Women may report experiencing fatigue (rather than chest pain) for several weeks before or during a cardiac episode. Complaints of fatigue in women should be considered a warning sign of an impending cardiac event. Easy fatigability on mild exertion is a frequent problem for clients experiencing cardiac disease; it is a common manifestation of decreased cardiac output. Progressive deterioration of activity tolerance results from the heart's inability to pump an effective volume of blood to meet the varying metabolic demands of the body. Fatigue, however, is not specific for cardiac problems. Other causes of fatigue include anemia, anxiety, chronic diseases, depression, and thyroid dysfunction.[6,11,16]

Edema. Edema, or swelling, is an excess accumulation of fluid in the tissues. The location of the edema aids in clarifying the cause of the edema. For instance, unilateral edema is most commonly caused by deep vein thrombosis, cellulitis, or lymphatic blockage of that extremity. Cardiac edema is generally symmetrical and progresses. It will often start in the feet or ankles and ascend to the thighs, genitalia, and abdomen. In those clients confined to bed, fluid also accumulates in the sacral area. Edema that is diffuse or generalized (anasarca) is usually associated with nephrotic syndrome, severe heart failure, or hepatic cirrhosis. Edema that is localized around the eyes and face is characteristic of nephrotic syndrome, myxedema, angioneurotic edema, acute glomerulonephritis, or hypoproteinemia. Edema evident in the evening that is not present in the mornings is generally caused by heart failure or venous insufficiency.[6,11,16]

Along with locating the edematous area(s), ask the client if there are any associated manifestations such as dyspnea, orthopnea, PND, pain, color changes of the skin, or jaundice. Daily weight measurement is important for clients with cardiac problems. Changes in weight should be reported to the health care provider.[16]

Review of Systems

Following the history of the presenting illness and clinical manifestations, a detailed past medical history follows, including CVD risk factor analysis, past health history and hospitalizations, surgical history, allergies, medications, dietary habits, social habits (tobacco, alcohol, street drugs, exercise), and family history. After all subjective information has been obtained from the client, the physical examination (which began through observation when you walked into the client's room) is completed. Figure 54-2 provides questions to aid with completing an expanded cardiac history.

Past Medical History and Hospitalizations

Ask the client about the following areas: childhood and infectious diseases, immunizations, hospitalizations, obstetric history, major illnesses and hospitalizations. Has CVD been a recurrent or pre-existing illness? Has the client been denied admittance into the armed services or sports, failed an insurance examination, or received a high rating on an insurance examination? Specifically ask about prior history, including rheumatic fever, scarlet fever, severe streptococcal infections, or enlarged heart or heart murmur. These conditions are associated with structural mitral valve disease. Investigate known or corrected congenital anomalies (atrial or ventricular septal defect, persistent patent ductus arteriosus, tetralogy of Fallot, Eisenmenger's syndrome).[6,11,16] Clients with chronic conditions, such as cardiovascular disorders, should be vaccinated yearly against influenza and at least once against pneumococcal pneumonia with additional immunizations every 5 years for high-risk clients. Cardiovascular problems also affect the renal and neurologic systems. Ask about decreased urination, dark or concentrated urine, edema of the legs, dizzy spells, and memory loss.[6,11,16]

Risk Factor Analysis. The Framingham Heart Study of 1961 provided us with today's "risk factor" term. This benchmark cohort study described the natural history and epidemiology of CVD, outlining certain factors that increase the risk of developing CVD.[15] A risk factor assessment not only identifies clients at risk for having manifestations caused by CVD, but also identifies areas to target for nursing intervention. Risk factors are divided into four categories, which are outlined and defined in Table 54-2.[6] Risk factor modification in those with known CVD is referred to as secondary prevention. Risk factor modification in those without CVD is primary prevention.[6] Because of the CVD epidemic, INTER-HEART, a worldwide case-control study on acute myocardial infarctions, was conducted to assess the modifiable CVD risk factors.[25] Results revealed that nine modifiable risk factors accounted for greater than 90% of acute myocardial infarction risk in both males and females: smoking, abnormal lipid levels, hypertension, diabetes mellitus, abdominal obesity, psychosocial factors, poor fruit and vegetable consumption, alcohol consumption, and physical activity level. Obstructive sleep apnea (OSA) is also a risk factor for development of CVD and stroke.[1,4]

According to the American Heart Association, for people who are free of CVD at age 50 years, more than 50% of men and 40% of women will develop CVD during their remaining years. The more risk factors that are present, the greater the lifetime risk. Those with known vascular disease in one part of the body, either coronary, cerebrovascular, or peripheral arteries (which includes erectile dysfunction in men), are at higher risk of having

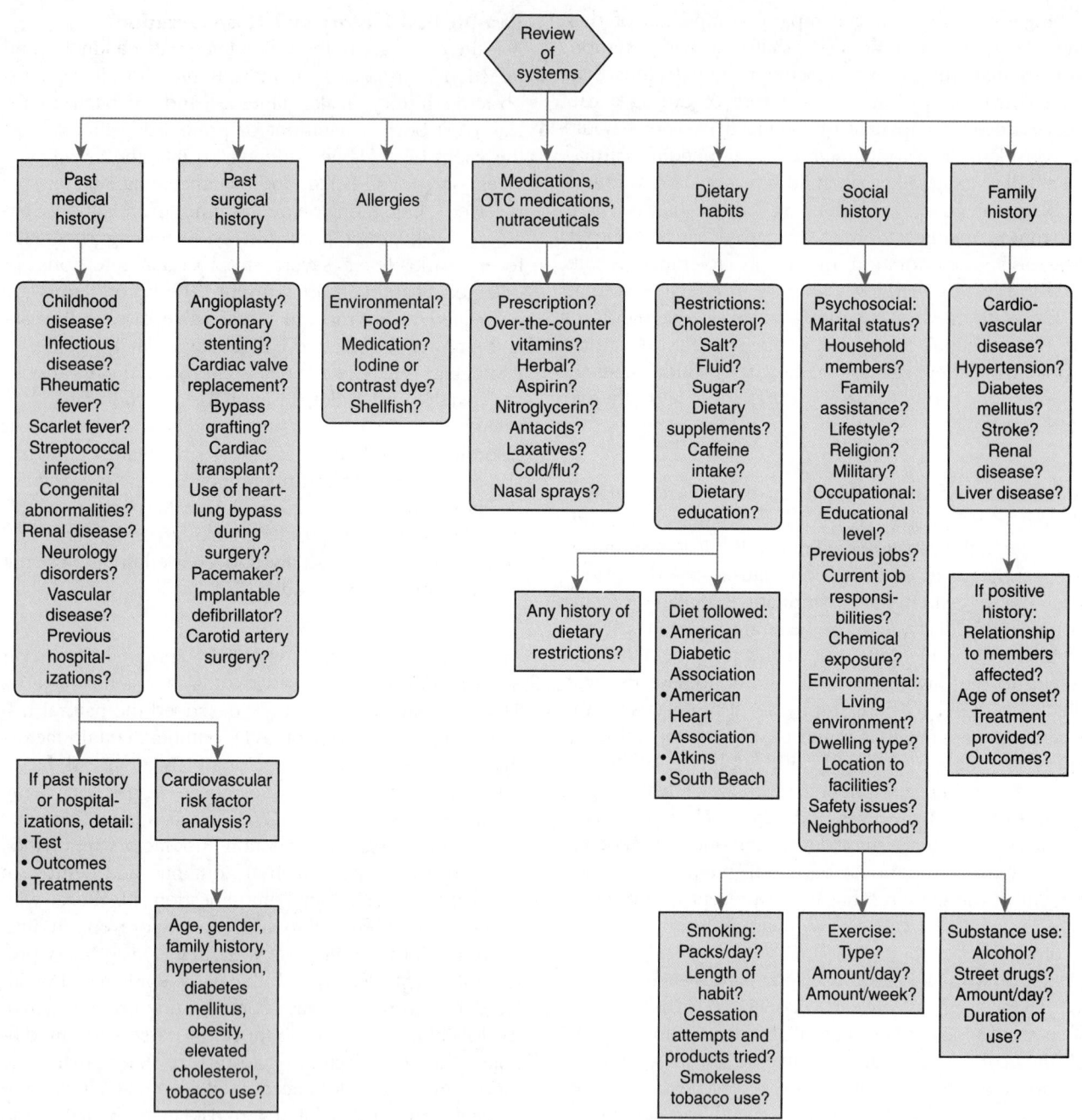

■ **FIGURE 54–2** Expanded cardiac history.

TABLE 54–2 Four Categories of Risk Factors

Category	Risk Factor
Predisposing factors	Age, gender, family history
Modifiable risk factors	Smoking, diet, alcohol intake, inactivity, obstructive sleep apnea
Metabolic risk factors	Dyslipidemia, hypertension, obesity, diabetes mellitus, metabolic syndrome
Identified disease markers	Abnormalities on CT scanning, cardiac catheterization, stress testing, echocardiography, and laboratory results

vascular disease in other areas.[6] Ask if the client experiences muscle cramping in the leg(s) with walking, called claudication, occurring because of arterial blockage supplying blood to those muscles. Ask the client about sleepiness during the day, wakefulness during the night, a dry throat in the morning, and other manifestations of OSA. Table 54-3 summarizes common risk factors for CVD.

Hypertension (defined as systolic pressure of 140 mm Hg or higher, or diastolic pressure of 90 mm Hg or higher) is an important independent risk factor for CVD and requires both primary and secondary prevention.

TABLE 54–3 Risk Factor Analysis for Cardiovascular Disease

Risk Factor	High Risk	Highest Risk
Gender and age	Women after menopause	Men older than 60
Family history of high blood pressure	Two blood relatives	Three or more blood relatives
Family history of heart attack	One relative, before age 60	Two relatives, before age 60
Family history of diabetes mellitus	One or more relatives with type 1 diabetes mellitus	One or more relatives with type 2 diabetes mellitus
Blood pressure[†] (degree of control somewhat modifiable)	Systolic: 160-200 mm Hg	Systolic: >200 mm Hg
	Diastolic: 90-110 mm Hg	Diastolic: >110 mm Hg
Diabetes mellitus[†] (degree of control somewhat modifiable), $HbA_{1C} <7\%$	Type 1 diabetes mellitus uncontrolled or type 2 diabetes mellitus controlled	Type 2 diabetes mellitus uncontrolled
Weight* BMI 18.5-24.9 kg/m^2 Normal weight	30%-40% overweight Overweight = BMI 25-29.9	50% or more overweight Obesity = BMI of 30 or greater
Waist circumference <40 inches (no increased risk for men) <35 inches (no increased risk for women)	>40 inches (men) >35 inches (women)	
Cholesterol level[†] HDL-C >40 mg/dl	240-280 mg/dl	>280 mg/dl
LDL-C <100 mg/dl	100-129 mg/dl	130 mg/dl
Serum triglycerides, fasting[†] <150 mg/dl	200-499 mg/dl	>500 mg/dl
Percentage of fat in diet[†]	30%-50%	>50%
Frequency of recreational exercise*	Minimal	No activity
Frequency of occupational exercise*	Minimal	Sedentary occupation
Cigarette smoking*	20-40 per day	>40 per day
Stress at home*	High	Extremely high
Stress at work[†]	High	Extremely high
Behavior pattern (especially men)[†]	Type A	Type A
Use of oral contraceptives (women)[†]	Younger than 40 and use oral contraceptives	Older than 40 and use oral contraceptives
Air pollution[†]	Moderate	High
Sleep patterns*	More than 8 hr sleep a night	4-6 hr sleep a night Sleep disrupted by obstructive sleep apnea (OSA)

* Modifable risk factors.
[†] Possibly modifiable risk factors.

According to the American Heart Association, blood pressure (BP) levels to prevent heart attack and/or stroke are as follows: BP maintained below 140/90 mm Hg; below 130/85 mm Hg for people with kidney damage or heart failure; or below 130/80 mm Hg for people with diabetes mellitus.[4] More recent data recommend lower BP values as treatment goals because the risk of CVD, beginning at 115/75 mm Hg, doubles with each increment of 20/10 mm Hg.[23] The report concluded that a systolic BP of more than 140 mm Hg in persons older than 50 years is a much more important CVD risk factor than elevated diastolic BP and that individuals with a systolic BP of 120 to 139 mm Hg or a diastolic BP of 80 to 89 mm Hg should be considered prehypertensive and require health-promoting lifestyle modifications to prevent CVD.[23]

Diabetes mellitus is another important independent risk factor for CVD. The total number of people with diabetes mellitus is projected to increase from 171 million in 2000 to 366 million in 2030.[31] It is estimated that at least 65% of people with diabetes mellitus will die of some form of heart or blood vessel disease, making heart disease the leading cause of diabetes-related death. With the prevalence of obesity, metabolic syndrome and diabetes mellitus have escalated.[3,22,23] See Chapter 45 for information related to diabetes mellitus and metabolic syndrome and their role for development of CVD.

The National Center for Health Statistics began tracking obesity in 1960 through the National Health and Nutrition Examination Survey (NHANES). This continued survey revealed an unanticipated jump in the prevalence of obesity. Obesity is becoming a global epidemic and is now an independent risk factor for CVD. Weight loss therapies (dietary intervention, physical activity, pharmacotherapy, and surgery) can improve or prevent many of the CVD risk factors caused by obesity.[3,22,23] For adults, overweight is a body mass index (BMI) of 25.0 to 29.9 kg/m^2; while obesity is defined as a BMI greater than 30.0 kg/m.[23]

The 2001 National Cholesterol Education Program Adult Treatment Panel III (ATP III) guidelines highlighted several modifiable and nonmodifiable major risk factors for CVD. Serum lipid levels are among the most important modifiable risk factors, and the cardiovascular benefit of lowering lipid levels is well-defined.[13,16,33]

The recently published Multi-Ethnic Study of Atherosclerosis (MESA) findings reveal that ATP III guidelines are not being fully implemented.[5] This coupled with increasing worldwide obesity is increasing the prevalence not only of CVD but also of other comorbidities such as type 2 diabetes mellitus, hypertension, certain cancers, and sleep apnea.[4]

Those with known CVD or who have two or more risk factors are considered high risk, while those without a CVD history or who have only one risk factor are considered low risk.[6] Data from the Behavioral Risk Factor Surveillance System revealed the reporting of two or more risk factors for CVD increased among successive age groups. The prevalence of having two or more risk factors was highest among blacks (48.7%) and American Indians (46.7%), and lowest among Asians (25.9%). The prevalence of two or more risk factors was similar in men (37.8%) and women (36.4%).[6,7]

The American Heart Association recommends that health care providers routinely assess a client's general risk of CVD beginning at age 20. The AHA guidelines also recommend that providers calculate the risk of developing CVD in the next 10 years for people age 40 and older or for anyone who has multiple risk factors. Risk factor screening includes measuring blood pressure, body mass index, waist circumference, and pulse rate at least every 2 years; obtaining a cholesterol profile and performing glucose testing at least every 5 years beginning at age 20; and obtaining a smoking history.[1]

Past Surgical History

Explore previous cardiac-related outpatient procedures, interventions, or surgery. This includes relatively minor procedures such as a diagnostic cardiac catheterization to major surgery such as a heart transplant. Inquire about the details of each procedure, including any adverse events or prolonged recovery.

Allergies

Note and describe any environmental, food, or drug allergies. Particularly inquire about allergies to Betadine, iodine, shrimp, shellfish, contrast, or dye (in case CT scanning or angiography is warranted). Clearly document the manifestations of an allergic reaction, such as rashes, itching, or anaphylaxis (a sudden severe allergic reaction).[6,16]

Medications

Evaluate the use of prescription medications, over-the-counter medications, herbals, and recreational drugs. Whenever possible, use brand names or simple descriptors instead of generic names. For example, ask clients whether they are currently taking "water pills," "heart pills," or "blood pressure" medications.[6,16]

Numerous medications can affect the cardiovascular system. Ask specifically about the use of antihypertensives, diuretics, vasodilators (nitroglycerin), cardiotonic drugs (digoxin), anticoagulants, bronchodilators, contraceptives, hormones, and steroids. Noncardiac medications can have profound secondary effects on cardiovascular performance. For example, tricyclic antidepressants and other psychotropic medications can potentiate dysrhythmias. Oral contraceptives increase the incidence of thrombophlebitis.[6,27] Steroid use increases fluid retention and may cause hypertension. Various antineoplastic agents may be cardiotoxic, causing dysrhythmias and cardiomyopathy. Elevated levels of thyroid hormones can result in thyrotoxicosis and a resultant hyperdynamic cardiovascular state (bounding pulses, palpitations, tachycardia). Decreased levels of thyroid hormone (hypothyroidism) may explain a client's dyspnea on exertion, fatigue, decreased cardiac output, and heart failure.[6,16,27]

Finally, discuss the use of over-the-counter drugs such as aspirin, cold remedies, and vitamins. Note the dose and times of administration. Inquire about the use of antioxidants (folic acid, vitamin B_6 or B_{12}, nuts, ginger, purslane, or rosemary) or cholesterol-lowering agents (omega 3 fatty acids, niacin, pigweed). Ask about use of herbal remedies. Herbs are used for cardiac disorders such as angina, dysrhythmias, and heart disease and for related disorders such as high blood pressure (BP) and peripheral vascular disease.[27] See Box 54-3 for a list of commonly used antianginal herbs and Box 54-4 for antidysrhythmic herbs.

In addition to the types and names of the medications the client takes, ask how many pills and how often they are taken. Is the client currently taking these medications as prescribed? Clients with cardiac disease occasionally stop taking prescribed medications because they (1) are taking too many pills, (2) are experiencing unwanted

---

BOX 54-3 Antianginal Herbs

- Angelica (*Angelica archangelica*)
- Bilberry (*Vaccinium myrtillus*)
- Evening primrose (*Oenothera biennis*)
- Flaxseed (*Linum usitatissimum*)
- Garlic (*Allium sativum*)
- Ginger (*Zingiber officinale*)
- Hawthorn (*Crataegus laevigata*)
- Khella (*Ammi majus*)
- Kudzu (*Pueraria lobata*)
- Onion (*Allium cepa*)
- Purslane (*Portulaca oleracea*)
- Sichuan lovage (*Ligusticum chuanxiong*)
- Willow (*Salix*)

BOX 54-4 Antidysrhythmic Herbs

- Angelica
- Astragalus (*Astragalus*)
- Barberry (*Berberis vulgaris*)
- Canola (*Brassica*)
- Cinchona (*Cinchona*)
- Gingko (*Gingko biloba*)
- Hawthorn
- Horehound (*Marrubium vulgare*)
- Khella
- Motherwort (*Leonurus cardiaca*)
- Purslane
- Reishi (*Ganoderma lucidum*)
- Scotch broom (*Cytisus scoparius*)
- Valerian (*Valeriana officinalis*)

side effects, (3) believe that the problem has resolved, (4) worry about the cost, or (5) some combination of these factors. A client may neglect to take prescribed diuretics because "it makes me go to the bathroom all the time." Clients who take antihypertensives or lipid-lowering medications may stop taking them when their BP or cholesterol level reaches a normal range because they perceive that the problem has resolved. Careful questioning can identify areas for client teaching.

Dietary Habits

Assess excess or deficit caloric intake and the client's approximate intake of foods high in sodium, cholesterol, saturated fat, and caffeine. Although these are common components of the average American diet, they have been linked to the development of atherosclerosis and hypertensive disease. Elevated serum cholesterol levels are associated with coronary artery disease. The Translating Evidence into Practice feature below details how nurses can help clients make the connection between diet and cardiovascular health.

Caffeine is a stimulant that, in excessive amounts, can increase heart rate and provoke palpitations. For clients with tachycardia or palpitations, caution regarding more than two 8-ounce cups of a caffeinated beverage is

TRANSLATING EVIDENCE INTO PRACTICE

Diet and Heart Disease

Being in the medical field, we all know the importance of dieting. Diets have been studied for decades and the choice of diets plans spans from A to Z. In spite of this vast knowledge, disease mortality and morbidity are escalating as a result of both national and international obesity, which not only is a risk factor for CVD but also is now considered a worldwide pandemic.[1]

The importance of dieting, from a medical standpoint, focuses on risk factor modification for disease prevention or control. The DASH (Dietary Approaches to Stop Hypertension) diet showed reduced weight and improved physical fitness with a decreased prevalence of hypertension at 6 months after implementation of the diet.[7] Diabetes mellitus has also been positively impacted through dietary restriction and statin therapy.[2,7]

IMPLICATIONS

Although outcomes are positive regarding dietary restrictions, many people either have not read or do not understand the literature. Implications for nurses include ensuring that every client is made aware of these research findings and is encouraged to follow a heart-healthy diet. Nutrition counseling is recommended, including written literature providing examples of heart-healthy foods. Too often clients have heard of a low-fat or low-cholesterol diet, but do not fully understand their benefits regarding risk factor modification.

For those clients who will not adhere to dietary restrictions, multiple trials using statin medications have replicated previous findings that statin therapy helps to lower LDL-C levels and may actually decrease some of the plaque burden in the artery lumen, thereby decreasing CVD

morbidity and mortality.[3-6] Future research is needed to evaluate effective methods for providing dietary information to clients, follow-up on those methods, and client responses to those methods in hopes of better understanding the dietary actions and views of the client.

REFERENCES

1. American Heart Association. (2006). Obesity and cardiovascular disease: Pathophysiology, evaluation, and effect of weight loss: An update of the 1997 American Heart Association Scientific Statement on Obesity and Heart Disease from the Obesity Committee of the Council on Nutrition, Physical Activity, and Metabolism. *Circulation, 113*(6), 898-918.
2. Davidson, M.H. (2006). Statin/fibrate combination in patients with metabolic syndrome or diabetes: Evaluating the risks of pharmacokinetic drug interactions. *Expert Opinions on Drug Safety, 5*, 145-156.
3. Diabetes Prevention Program Research Group. (2002). Reduction in the incidence of type 2 diabetes with lifestyle intervention or metformin. *New England Journal of Medicine, 346*, 393-403.
4. Dierkes, J., Westphal, S., & Luley, C. (2004). The effect of fibrates and other lipid-lowering drugs on plasma homocysteine levels. *Expert Opinions on Drug Safety, 3*, 101-111.
5. Nissen, S.E., Tuzcu, E.M., Schoenhagen, P., et al. (2004). Effect of intensive compared with moderate lipid-lowering on progression of coronary atherosclerosis: A randomized controlled trial. *JAMA, 291*, 1071-1080.
6. Taylor, A.J., Sullenberger, L.E., Lee, H.J., et al. (2004). Arterial Biology for the Investigation of the Treatment Effects or Reducing Cholesterol (ARBITER) 2: A double-blind, placebo-controlled study of extended-release niacin on atherosclerosis progression in secondary prevention patients treated with statins. *Circulation, 110*, 3512-3517.
7. Writing group of the PREMIER Collaborative Research Group. (2003). Effects of comprehensive lifestyle modification on blood pressure control. Main results of the PREMIER clinical trial. *JAMA, 289*, 2083-2093.

recommended. Regarding caffeine and blood pressure or coronary artery disease, restriction of caffeine is no longer indicated.[23,29]

Examine not only daily food habits but also attitudes toward food and resistance to therapeutic alterations in diet. Cultural beliefs and economic status greatly affect food choices. Consider these factors before recommending dietary changes. Identify and include the primary food purchaser and preparer in dietary instruction.

Social History/Social Habits

Psychosocial History. The psychosocial history includes data on lifestyle, household members, marital status, children, relationships with significant others, military service, religious beliefs (in relation to perceptions of health and treatment), and hobbies. Note data that help identify support systems and coping mechanisms. Psychosocial data provide information about risk factors for the development of CVD. Background information can be used to formulate a plan to assist the client in making necessary lifestyle adaptations to promote health and lessen disease.

Occupation. Inquire about the client's educational level and all occupations of the client as well as the duration of each job. The present occupation may be relevant to the significance of the disease; that is, coronary artery disease or dysrhythmias may be incompatible with continuing a career as an airline pilot or truck driver. The amount of perceived job-related stress may need to be evaluated; stress is a modifiable risk factor for CVD. Ask about possible occupational exposure to agents or chemicals (asbestos).

Environment.

> **SAFETY** ⚠ **ALERT**
>
> **After a stroke or with deteriorating cardiac function and output, a client may need assistance or environmental adjustments to live safely and fully and meet daily needs. Inquire about the following: (1) the home, such as safety issues, type of dwelling (number of steps), state of repair, exits for fire, heating and cooling adequacy; (2) mode of transportation; (3) the neighborhood, in regard to noise, pollution, and violence; and (4) access to family and friends, grocery store, a pharmacy, laundry, church, and health care facilities.**

Smoking. If the client smokes, inquire about the duration of the smoking habit and the number of cigarettes smoked daily. If the client is not smoking currently, does the client use a nicotine inhalation system or a nicotine transdermal product or chew nicotine gum or smokeless tobacco? Determine the pack-year history (number of cigarette packs smoked per day multiplied by the number of years smoked). All nicotine products have a vasoconstrictive effect on the heart and vessels. Cigarette smoking increases the risk of coronary artery disease and worsens hypertension. Nicotine, a major ingredient in cigarettes, causes peripheral vasoconstriction, increasing resistance to left ventricular emptying and thus increasing the myocardial workload. Cigarette smokers are three to four times more likely to develop CVD than nonsmokers, smoking doubles the risk for stroke, and smokers are 10 times more likely to develop peripheral vascular disease.[3] At 5 to 15 years after tobacco cessation, clients have a death rate from CVD similar to that of nonsmokers.[7]

Substance Abuse. Review for daily substance abuse, including alcohol or street drugs along with the amount(s) ingested. Evidence that alcohol ingestion increases the risk of atherosclerosis is inconclusive. Researchers state that only excessive alcohol intake has deleterious effects on the cardiovascular system and its performance. An intake of 100 g of pure (100%) alcohol may slightly increase BP and heart rate; this amount is approximately equal to three beers or one mixed drink. Alcoholism, in contrast, has been associated with the development of hypertension and damage to the heart muscle, leading to cardiomyopathy.[6] Ask about the client's approximate daily and weekly alcohol consumption. Keep in mind that the alcoholic client may lie about the type and amount consumed.

Discuss the use of recreational drugs. Cocaine toxicity is a major threat to the cardiovascular system. The systemic sympathomimetic effects of cocaine result in a "fight-or-flight" reaction that increases heart rate, contractility, blood glucose levels, and peripheral vasoconstriction. Cocaine can potentiate the effects of circulating catecholamines (epinephrine and norepinephrine), resulting in sudden death.[6,27]

Exercise. Ask about the type and amount of exercise routinely engaged in during an average week before and after the onset of current manifestations. Research confirms that a sedentary lifestyle potentiates the lethality of myocardial infarction or stroke, and it is considered a significant risk factor in the development of coronary artery disease. Effective, routine aerobic exercise is thought to lower the likelihood of a coronary event. Aerobic exercise includes such activities as swimming, jogging, brisk walking, bicycling, and rowing.[3,4,6]

 To be beneficial, aerobic exercise should raise the heart rate from 50% to 100% of baseline (depending on age and prior physical conditioning) for at least 30 minutes three to five times a week. Along with general body conditioning, this form of exercise increases the heart's efficiency in using oxygen. Advise clients who are older than 40 years or who have a history of CVD to consult their physician before beginning an exercise program.[1,4]

Ask about current activities and limitations. Do any activities trigger the clinical manifestations discussed in Figure 54-1? How far can the client walk, run, or climb steps? Can the client complete housework, mow the lawn, participate in sports, shop, do a full day's work, or have sexual intercourse?

Family History

Ask about prolonged contact with a communicable disease or the effect of a family member's illness on the client. Specifically, inquire about a family history of heart disease, high BP, stroke, diabetes mellitus, or kidney disease. A detailed health history of the client's family can provide insight into possible genetic, environmental, and lifestyle conditions contributing to a cardiac condition.

PHYSICAL EXAMINATION

The cardiac physical examination begins with a general inspection, followed by assessment of the vital signs, palpation, auscultation, and percussion. The examination logically proceeds from head to toe with the client in supine position (the head of the bed or examination table may be elevated for comfort). Stand at the client's right side. Cardiac examination abnormalities are noted in Table 54-4. Necessary equipment includes a stethoscope with diaphragm and bell, a ruler, and a sphygmomanometer.[6] Please refer to the normal cardiovascular findings described in the Physical Assessment Findings in the Healthy Adult feature on p. 1371.

General Appearance and Level of Consciousness

Begin with inspection. Assessment of *general appearance* and *level of consciousness* provides an initial composite picture of the client and indicates the level of comfort and distress. Look at the client and consider the following: (1) Does the client lie quietly, or is there restlessness or continual moving about? (2) Can the client lie flat, or is only an upright, erect position tolerated? (3) Does the facial expression reflect pain or obvious manifestations of respiratory distress? (4) Are there manifestations of significant cyanosis or pallor? (5) Can the client answer questions without dyspnea during the interview?

Note the client's general *level of consciousness* (LOC). The LOC reflects the adequacy of cerebral perfusion and oxygenation. Also assess whether the client manifests appropriate behavior for the surroundings: (1) What is the client's affect? (2) Are there obvious manifestations of anxiety, fear, depression, or anger? (3) How does the client react to those in the immediate vicinity, including significant others?

Vital Signs

Vital signs include bilateral arm blood pressures, heart and respiratory rates, and temperature. A weight should also be obtained to aid in body mass index calculation and risk factor assessment.

Blood Pressure

Blood pressure measurements should be made with the appropriate cuff size and with the client lying, sitting, and standing, as shown in Figure 54-3. Blood pressure readings normally may vary 5 to 15 mm Hg with postural changes. *Orthostatic hypotension* is a blood pressure drop of more than 15 mm Hg with position changes. Blood pressure readings may also vary with inspiration from 5 to 10 mm Hg. *Pulsus paradoxus* is an abnormal decrease in systolic BP of more than 10 mm Hg during inspiration. If the arms are inaccessible, obtain pressures from the thighs and popliteal arteries or the calves and posterior tibial arteries. When pressures are difficult to auscultate, systolic pressures can be determined through palpation or by Doppler ultrasonography.[6,16]

Pulse

Pulse characteristics can vary. If the pulse is irregular, assess for a pulse deficit by taking apical and radial pulses simultaneously, noting differences in rate. Pulse volume can be described as bounding, thready, or absent. Peripheral pulse assessment is discussed in Chapter 51.

Respiratory Rate

Note the rate, rhythm, depth, and quality of the breathing pattern. Look for accessory muscle use. Does the client have to sit up to breathe easily, or is the client able to lie flat comfortably? (See Chapter 59 for respiratory assessment information.)

Head and Neck

When examining the head, pay particular attention to the eyes, ear lobes, lips, and buccal mucosa. Examine the eyes for *arcus senilis* (a light gray ring around the iris, possibly caused by cholesterol deposits) and *xanthelasma* (yellow raised plaques around the eyelids resulting from lipid deposits).[6,16]

Neck Vein Assessment

Neck vein distention can be used to estimate *central venous pressure* (CVP). The amount of distention reflects pressure and volume changes in the right atrium. The internal jugular veins, although more difficult to detect than the external jugular veins, are more reliable indicators of CVP. The external jugular vein engorges easily with only slight provocation, for example, by holding

TABLE 54–4 **Cardiac Examination Abnormalities**

Findings	Possible Etiology
Vital Signs	
Unequal arm blood pressures	Aortic dissection, coarctation of the aorta, vascular obstruction, vascular outlet syndrome, measurement error
Pulsus paradoxus	Cardiac tamponade, pericarditis
Tachycardia (>100 beats/min)	Anxiety, hypovolemia, shock, hyperthyroidism
Bradycardia (<60 beats/min)	Medication side effect, SA or AV node abnormality, physical conditioning, hypothyroidism
Irregular pulse	Dysrhythmia, myocardial ischemia, medication side effect
Bounding pulse	Bradycardia, anemia, aortic valve insufficiency
Thready pulse	Hypovolemia, mitral valve stenosis
Absent pulse	Atherosclerosis, embolus, thrombus, trauma
Tachypnea	Anxiety, pain, pulmonary edema, COPD exacerbation
Head	
Arcus senilis	Hyperlipidemia, atherosclerosis
Xanthelasma	Hyperlipidemia, atherosclerosis
Neck	
Neck vein distention	Right ventricular failure, tricuspid failure, cardiac tamponade
Flat jugular veins	Extracellular volume depletion
Carotid bruit	Atherosclerosis, aortic stenosis
Thorax	
Displaced PMI	Left ventricular enlargement, left ventricular aneurysm
Heaves	Valvular heart disease, pulmonary hypertension
Thrills	Valvular heart disease, partially obstructed blood vessels
Crackles	Pulmonary edema
Heart Sounds	
S_3 gallop	Pulmonary edema, myocardial infarction, valvular insufficiency
S_4 gallop	Ventricular hypertrophy, hypertension, cardiomyopathy, cor pulmonale, aortic stenosis, pulmonic stenosis, pulmonary fibrosis
Pericardial rub	Pericarditis
Systolic murmur	Aortic or pulmonic stenosis, anemia, tachycardia
Diastolic murmur	Mitral or tricuspid stenosis, aortic or pulmonic insufficiency
Abdomen	
Ascites	Chronic right ventricular failure; liver failure
Hyperactive bowel sounds	Laxative use, antidysrhythmic medication side effect
Hypoactive bowel sounds	Hyperkalemia
Bruits	Atherosclerosis
Pronounced and widened aortic pulsation	Abdominal aortic aneurysm
Skin	
Central cyanosis	Advanced pulmonary disease, right-to-left shunting within heart, pulmonary edema
Peripheral cyanosis	Cutaneous vasoconstriction, exposure to cold, shock, heart failure
Decreased turgor	Dehydration, volume depletion, rapid weight loss, advanced age
Warm to touch	Thyrotoxicosis
Cool to touch	Vascular disease
Edema	Right ventricular failure, venous insufficiency, medication side effect
Nail	
Clubbing	Advanced pulmonary or cardiovascular disease
Splinter hemorrhages	Subacute bacterial endocarditis

the breath, twisting the neck, and being constricted by clothing (except in weight lifters, football players, and professional speakers and singers, who have overdeveloped neck muscle tendons). The vessels are prominent and visible but soft and compressible.[6,16]

A relaxed supine position with the head of the bed inclined between 15 and 30 degrees maximizes jugular vein prominence. Clients who have greatly increased right atrial pressure may require head elevation from 45 to 90 degrees. Support the client's head with a small

The Cardiovascular System

INSPECTION

Skin color even; capillary refill less than 3 seconds. Thorax symmetrical, without visible lifts or point of maximal impulse (PMI). Jugular venous distention absent with client at 45-degree angle. Lower extremity superficial vessels without tortuosity upon standing.

PALPATION

Skin warm. PMI palpable in fifth intercostal space at left midclavicular line, approximately 1 cm in diameter. Forceful thrusts, heaves, and pulsations absent. No palpable thrills. Abdominal aorta pulsations slightly palpable over epigastrium without lateral radiation. Carotid and peripheral pulses equal and readily palpable bilaterally. Evidence of unimpeded arterial flow and venous return to upper and lower extremities. No edema evident.

PERCUSSION

Right heart border not discerned.

AUSCULTATION

S_1 and S_2 heard without splitting. Apical rate, 72 beats/min, regular. Murmurs and extra heart sounds absent.

pillow and avoid sharp neck flexion. Turn the client's head slightly away from you and loosen or remove clothing that compresses the neck or upper thorax. Tangential (oblique) lighting enhances the appearance of the vein. Observe both sides of the neck. The internal jugular vein lies deep to the sternocleidomastoid muscle and runs parallel along its length to the jaw and ear lobe. Identify the pulsations of the internal jugular. Use the external jugular vein if the internal jugular is not visible.[6]

Note the highest point at which the internal jugular pulses can be seen (the *meniscus*). The *sternal angle* (manubrial joint) is a reference point to measure the height of venous pulsation, approximately 4 to 5 cm above the center of the right atrium. Use a centimeter ruler to measure the vertical distance between the sternal angle and the point of highest venous pulsations (Figure 54-4). The value is usually less than 3 or 4 cm above the sternal angle when the head of the bed is elevated 30 to 40 degrees.[6,16]

Carotid Artery Assessment

Carotid artery examination indicates the adequacy of stroke volume and the patency of the arteries. Using your finger tips, gently palpate the carotid arteries one side at a time in order to avoid vagal stimulation. Check and compare the rate, rhythm, and amplitude of the pulses. Note whether a *bruit* (a blowing sound) is present by listening with the diaphragm of a stethoscope over the arteries while the client holds the breath. Tracheal breath sounds are heard while respiration is ongoing.[6,16]

Thorax
Inspection

Perform inspection and palpation of the precordium together to determine the presence of normal and abnormal pulsations. Ideally, the client should be supine with the chest exposed. The left lateral position allows the heart to move closer to the chest wall, accentuating precordial movements and certain heart sounds. Good lighting and a warm, quiet environment are essential. Stand at the client's right side and observe the anterior chest for size, shape, symmetry of movement, and any evident pulsations. Record the location of pulsation in relation to the intercostal space and the midclavicular line. Confirm your observation with palpation.

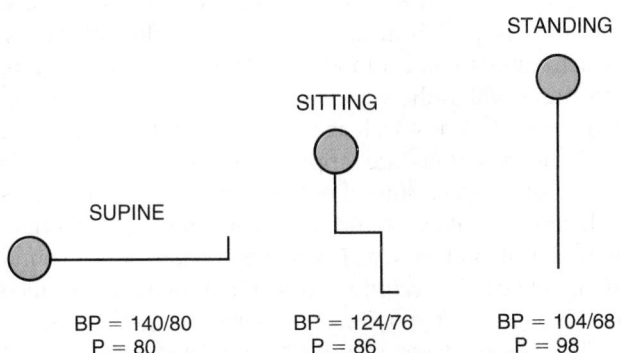

■ **FIGURE 54-3** Recording postural blood pressure (BP). After measuring the client's BP and pulse in the supine position, leave the BP cuff in place and help the client sit. Then measure the BP within 15 to 30 seconds. Help the client stand, and measure again. Postural hypotension is indicated by a BP decrease of more than 10 to 15 mm Hg systolic pressure and more than 10 mm Hg diastolic pressure. Postural hypotension is typically accompanied by a 10% to 20% increase in heart rate (pulse rate).

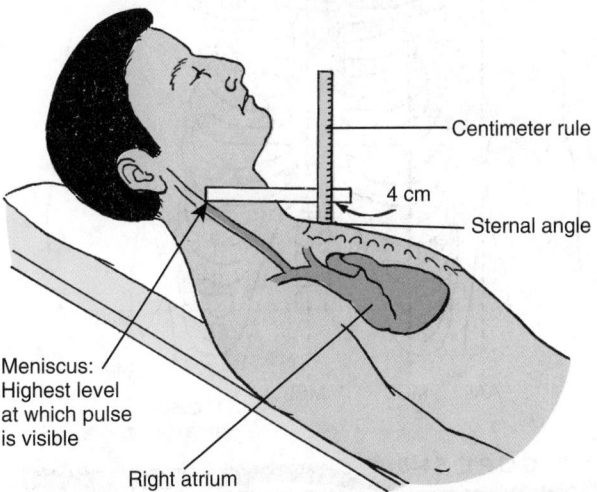

■ **FIGURE 54-4** Estimation of jugular vein measurement to assess central venous pressure.

Palpation

When palpating, use the fingers and palm of the hand. The *point of maximum intensity* (PMI), or apical impulse, is usually seen at the fifth intercostal space medial to the left midclavicular line. It may be prominent in thin people and obscured in those who are obese or have large breasts. When palpated, the PMI is a single, faint, instantaneous tap beneath the fingers, no more than 2 cm in diameter. The left lateral recumbent position may enhance locating the PMI, but its position is displaced. With left ventricular enlargement and aneurysm, the PMI is more diffuse, sustained, and displaced downward and to the left of the midclavicular line.[6,11]

Right ventricular enlargement can produce an abnormal pulsation, called *"heaves"* or *"lifts,"* that may be seen as a sustained thrust along the left sternal border. *Thrills* represent turbulent blood flow through the heart, especially across abnormal heart valves. Use the heel or ulnar surface of the hand to palpate over each of the five cardiac landmarks (Figure 54-5). Thrills are perceived as a rushing vibration, much like feeling the throat of a purring cat.[6,11,16]

Auscultation of the Posterior Chest

With the client sitting forward, auscultate both sides of the lungs. Crackles (high-pitched, noncontinuous sounds) frequently signal left ventricular failure. As the left ventricle fails, crackles occur because of increasing pulmonary capillary pressure that forces fluid to shift into the intra-alveolar spaces. Crackles are best heard at the lung bases (because of gravitational effects on the fluid) during late inspiration.[6,11,16]

Auscultation of the Precordium

With the client in a supine position, auscultation of the precordium yields valuable information about normal or abnormal heart rate and rhythm, ventricular filling, and blood flow across heart valves. Use the bell to hear low-pitched sounds and the diaphragm to hear high-pitched sounds. Always warm the chestpiece before placing it on the client's skin. A quiet environment is key to successful auscultation. The left lateral position may facilitate auscultation. An upright position, leaning forward and holding the breath after exhalation, helps when assessing early diastolic murmurs and pericardial friction rubs.

Examine heart sounds from the base (right second intercostal space) of the heart to the apex (left fifth intercostal space). Figure 54-5 diagrams specific cardiac areas to auscultate. Use the mnemonic "APE To Man" to remember the areas (aortic, pulmonic, Erb's point, tricuspid, and mitral). Each area corresponds to a specific valvular outflow tract. Concentrate on one component of the cardiac cycle at a time, that is, the first heart sound (S_1), then the second heart sound (S_2), and so on. Listen to several complete cardiac cycles at each of the five precordial areas. Listen carefully, noting the quality (crisp or muffled), intensity (loud or soft), rhythm (irregular or regular), and presence of extra sounds (murmurs, gallops, rubs, or clicks). Repeat this process using the bell over each of the precordial areas.[6,11,16]

Normal Heart Sounds

The *first heart sound* (S_1) is linked to closure of the mitral and tricuspid valves (atrioventricular [AV] valves). It marks the onset of systole (ventricular contraction). It is heard best with the diaphragm at the apex (the mitral valve area) and left lower sternal border (the tricuspid valve area). S_1 results from abrupt closure of the AV valves, which causes some blood turbulence and vibration of structures within the ventricles. This vibration is transmitted across the chest wall as a heart sound. Phonetically, if both heart sounds are appreciated as "lub-dub," S_1 is "lub." Although closure of both mitral and tricuspid valves is heard as a single sound, the mitral valve closes a fraction of a second earlier.[6] If you are not sure which sound is S_1, check the carotid artery for a pulsation (which occurs with S_1 or systole), as outlined in Figure 54-6.

The *second heart sound* (S_2) is related to closure of the pulmonic and aortic (semilunar) valves and is heard best with the diaphragm at the aortic area. Phonetically, it is the "dub" of the heart sounds. It signifies the end of systole and the onset of diastole (ventricular filling). At the base of the heart, normal S_2 is always louder than S_1, whereas both sounds are usually of nearly equal

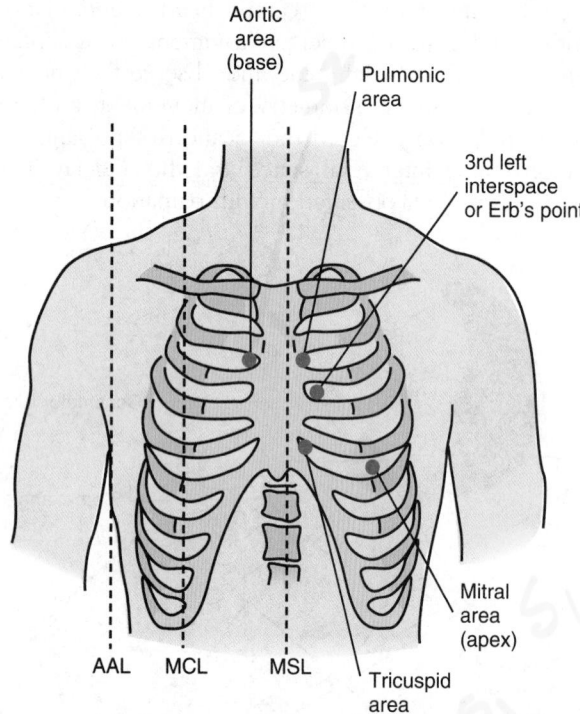

Aortic area (base)
Pulmonic area
3rd left interspace or Erb's point
Mitral area (apex)
Tricuspid area
AAL   MCL   MSL

■ **FIGURE 54–5** Cardiac auscultatory sites. S_1 is heard loudest at mitral and tricuspid areas. S_2 is heard loudest at aortic and pulmonic areas. S_3 and S_4 are heard best at the mitral area. *AAL,* Anterior axillary line; *MCL,* midclavicular line; *MSL,* midsternal line.

intensity at the left sternal border over Erb's point. Usually, S_1 is the louder of the two sounds at the apex and occurs just after or along with the carotid pulse.[6] Figure 54-6 shows the relationship of heart sounds to events during the cardiac cycle.

Abnormal Heart Sounds

Many abnormal heart sounds may indicate a serious heart disorder or change in cardiac function. You may not be able to label each abnormality, but with a thorough understanding of the normal sounds, you should be able to recognize various abnormal sounds and refer the problem to the physician or primary health care provider.

Gallops. Diastolic filling sounds or *gallops* (S_3 and S_4) occur during the two phases of ventricular filling. Sudden changes of inflow volume cause vibrations of the valves and ventricular supporting structures, producing low-pitched sounds that occur either early (S_3) or late (S_4) in diastole. Such sounds can originate in either side of the heart. These extra heart sounds create a triplet rhythm, acoustically mimicking a horse's gallop. For that reason, the term "gallop" is often used to denote these heart sounds. Figure 54-6 shows the timing of S_3 and S_4 during the cardiac cycle.[6,11,16]

A gallop sound that occurs in early diastole, during passive, rapid filling of the ventricles, is known as the *third heart sound* (S_3). It is heard best with the bell at the apex and with the client in the left lateral recumbent position. An S_3 immediately follows S_2 and is a dull, low-pitched sound. An S_3 gallop is considered a normal finding in children and young adults. In adults older than 30 years of age, an S_3 is considered characteristic of left ventricular dysfunction.[6,11,16]

A *fourth heart sound,* or S_4 gallop, occurs in the later stage of diastole, during atrial contraction and active filling of the ventricles. This soft, low-pitched sound is heard immediately before S_1 and is also referred to as an *atrial gallop.* S_4 is heard best with the bell of the stethoscope at the apex, with the client in the supine, left lateral position.[6,11,16] An atrial gallop is found most commonly in disorders involving increased stiffness of the ventricle. The ventricles become resistant to filling, and the structures within the ventricles vibrate in response to the added blood input during the "atrial kick." S_4 is never heard in the absence of atrial contraction (atrial fibrillation).

Pericardial Friction Rub. A pericardial friction rub is produced by inflammation of the pericardial sac. The roughened parietal and visceral layers of the pericardium rub

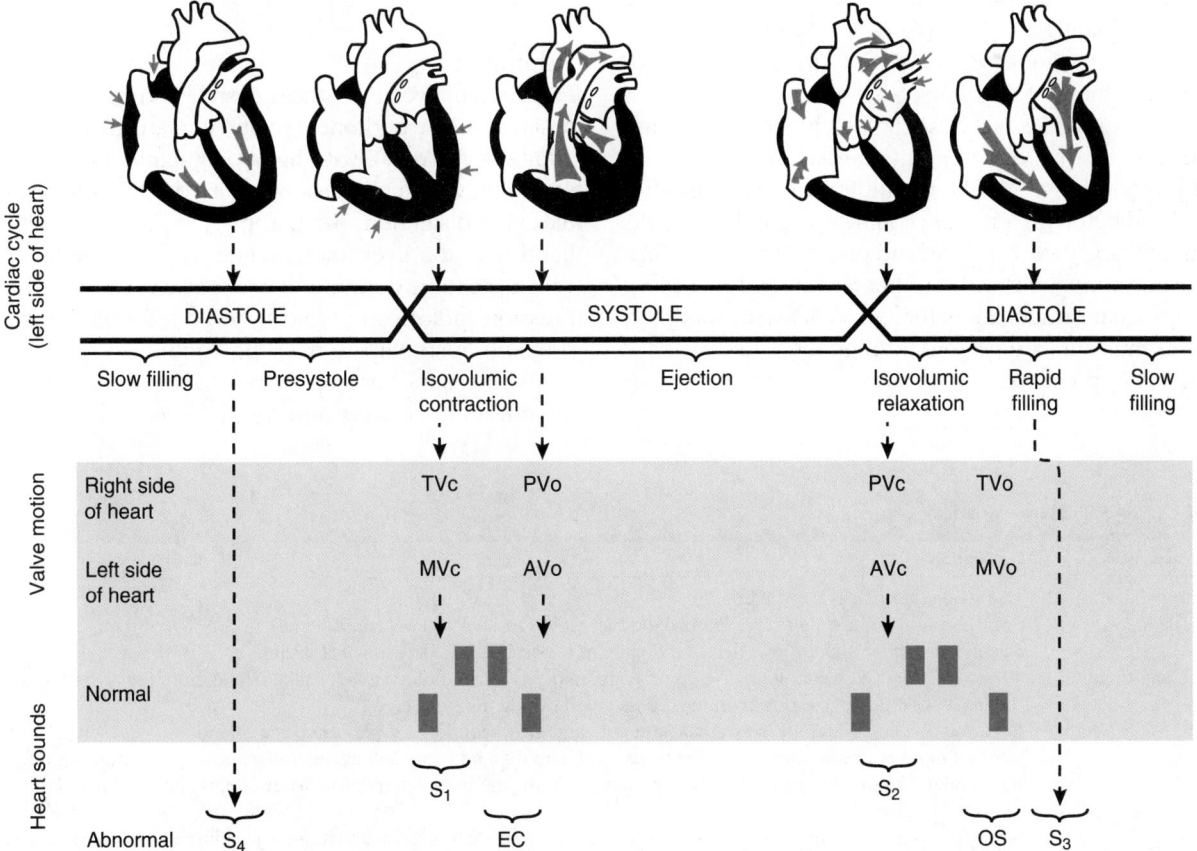

■ **FIGURE 54–6** Relationship of heart sounds to events during the cardiac cycle. Understanding heart sounds is facilitated when they are correlated with cardiac cycle events and valvular movements. *EC,* Ejection click; *MVc,* mitral valve closing; *MVo,* mitral valve opening; *OS,* opening snap; *PVc,* pulmonic valve closing; *TVc,* tricuspid valve closing; *TVo,* tricuspid valve opening.

against each other during cardiac motion. A pericardial friction rub is best detected with the diaphragm at the apex and along the left sternal border. It may be accentuated when a person leans forward or lies prone and exhales. Friction rubs produce a sound that is described as "to and fro," scratchy, and much like the sound made when rubbing your hair between your thumb and forefinger. Friction rubs may be present during the first week after myocardial infarction or after open heart surgery. Differentiate a pericardial friction rub from a pleural friction rub by noting the timing of the rub in relation to breathing. Pleural friction rubs are heard during inspiration; pericardial friction rubs are heard throughout the respiratory cycle.[6,16]

Murmurs. Murmurs are heard as a consequence of turbulent blood flow through the heart and large vessels. Turbulent blood flow produces vibrations in the heart and great vessels that can be detected as a blowing or swooshing sound. Murmurs are caused by (1) increased rate or velocity of blood flow, (2) abnormal forward or backward flow across stenosed or incompetent valves, (3) flow into a dilated chamber, or (4) flow through an abnormal passage between heart chambers. Murmurs are best heard with the bell of the stethoscope when the client is in the left lateral recumbent position. Certain maneuvers (Valsalva, deep inspiration, sudden postural changes, squatting, isometric exercise) can change the murmur's qualities.[6,11,16] Table 54-5 describes the characteristics of murmurs. Box 54-5 gives the scale for grading the loudness of murmurs.

Systolic murmurs, also called "benign" murmurs, are often caused by vigorous myocardial contraction or strong blood flow. Systolic murmurs begin with or after S_1 and end before S_2. They are common in children, adults younger than 50 years of age, and pregnant women. *Diastolic* murmurs begin with or after S_2 and end before S_1. All diastolic murmurs are pathologic. *Holosystolic* or *continuous* murmurs are present throughout S_1 and S_2.[6,11,16] Table 54-6 presents a comparison of selected heart murmurs.

BOX 54-5	Grading of Heart Murmurs*
Grade I	Faint; heard after listener has "tuned in"
Grade II	Faint murmur heard immediately
Grade III	Moderately loud, with accompanying thrill
Grade IV	Loud
Grade V	Very loud; heard only with the stethoscope
Grade VI	Very loud; heard without the stethoscope

*Heart murmurs are graded on a scale of 1 to 6 (I to VI).

Abdomen
Inspection
Examination of the abdomen provides information regarding cardiac competence. Abdominal assessment is described in Chapter 28, 32 and 42. Inspection may reveal abdominal distention.

Auscultation
Auscultation can yield clues about cardiovascular function including electrolyte imbalance, or atherosclerosis. Aortic bruits are heart just over or above the umbilicus. Renal bruits are heard over the upper midclavicular line laterally from the umbilicus.[6]

Palpitation
Palpation may confirm the presence of *ascites* (fluid accumulation in the peritoneal cavity) and an enlarged liver. In addition, you may elicit a hepatojugular reflex in the client with right ventricular distention. To do this, assess for jugular vein distention. Next, apply mild pressure with one hand over the liver for 1 minute. An increase in jugular vein distention during and immediately after liver compression indicates chronically elevated right ventricular pressure. Also palpate over the abdominal aorta located at midline, superior and inferior to the umbilicus. Assess the pulsation intensity and width.[6,11,16]

TABLE 54–5	Characteristics of Murmurs	

Characteristic	Description
Location	Area where murmur is best heard
Loudness	Graded on a 6-point scale from I (barely audible) to VI (audible without stethoscope)
Pitch	Classified as either high or low; describe quality as musical, harsh, blowing, or buzzing
Place and duration	When murmur occurs during cardiac cycle: early, middle, or late; holosystolic or pansystolic murmurs are heard during entire systolic phase; ejection murmur is best heard during midsystole
Quality	A murmur's sound pattern; a *crescendo* starts low and grows louder; a *decrescendo* starts loud and gets softer; a *crescendo-decrescendo* starts softly, becomes loud, and then becomes soft again; a *plateau* is a consistent sound
Radiation	Sound migration to other parts of body; for example, aortic murmurs often radiate to carotid arteries, and mitral murmurs radiate to axillae
Timing	Refers to whether murmur occurs in systole or diastole; systolic murmurs, unlike diastolic murmurs, are harmless
Variations	Changes that occur with movement or interruption of normal respirations

Modified from Alexander, R.W., et al. (Eds.) (1998). *Hurst's the heart* (9th ed.). New York: McGraw-Hill; and O'Hanlon-Nickols, T. (1997). The adult cardiovascular system. *American Journal of Nursing*, 97(12), 34-40.

TABLE 54–6 Heart Murmurs

Type of Heart Sound	Origin	Preferred Method of Auscultation
Systolic Murmurs		
Ejection type 	Systolic ejection murmurs are associated with forward blood flow during ventricular contraction across stenotic aortic or pulmonic valves.	Use the stethoscope diaphragm. Ejection murmurs are typically of medium pitch and harsh quality and may be associated with early ejection click. Aortic ejection murmurs are best heard over aortic valve and radiate into neck, down left sternal border, and occasionally to apex. May be accompanied by decreased S_2. Pulmonic ejection murmurs are heard best over pulmonic valve, and they radiate toward left shoulder and left neck vessels. May be accompanied by a wide split S_2.
Pansystolic regurgitant murmurs 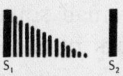	Pansystolic murmurs occur when blood regurgitates through incompetent mitral and tricuspid valves (AV valves) or ventricular septal defect as pressures rise during systole and blood seeks chambers of lower pressure. Damage to valve leaflets, papillary muscles, and chordae tendineae results in mitral valve insufficiency (blood regurgitates from left ventricle to left atrium) and tricuspid valve insufficiency (blood regurgitates from right ventricle to right atrium). Ventricular septal defect results in blood regurgitation from left ventricle to right ventricle.	All regurgitant murmurs are high-pitched, and those of AV valve incompetence have blowing quality. Mitral regurgitant murmurs are heard at apex, radiate into left axilla, and may be accompanied by ejection click and signs of left ventricular failure. Tricuspid regurgitant murmurs are heard loudest over tricuspid area and radiate into sternum. Ventricular septal defects are usually loud, harsh, and heard best over left sternal border in fourth, fifth, and sixth intercostal spaces and radiate over precordium but not axilla.
Early systolic murmurs 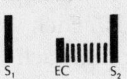	Early systolic (innocent) murmurs are associated with high cardiac outputs, as blood flow velocity is increased across normal semilunar valves. Causes include anemia, tachycardia, thyrotoxicosis, and fever. Murmur disappears with correction of underlying condition. Normal variant in children.	These are best heard with bell over base of heart or along lower left sternal border. Are usually no greater than grade II, are of medium pitch, and have a blowing quality. Intensity may increase during inspiration with client in left recumbent position or with increased heart rates.
Late systolic murmurs 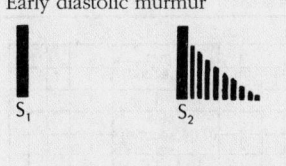	These imply mild mitral regurgitation as mitral valve balloons into left atrium late in ventricular systole.	Best heard with diaphragm of stethoscope over apex and are often preceded by midsystolic or late systolic ejection click.
Diastolic Murmurs		
Early diastolic murmur 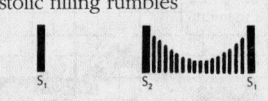	These (decrescendo murmurs) are usually caused by semilunar valve insufficiency, with regurgitation resulting from valvular deformity or dilation of valvular ring. Are heard immediately after S_2 and then diminish in intensity as pressure in aorta or pulmonary artery falls and ventricles fill.	Heard best with diaphragm at base of heart while client leans forward in deep expiration. Are high-pitched and blowing and radiate down left sternal border, perhaps to apex or down right sternal border. Accompanying signs of heart failure may be present.
Diastolic filling rumbles	Caused by blood flow across stenotic AV valves (more often mitral). May also occur during augmented blood flow across normal AV valves. Murmur has two phases, becoming louder as blood flows from atrium to ventricle and increases with passive ventricular filling just after AV valve opening and again during atrial contraction (presystole).	Using bell, this murmur is heard over only a small area at and just medial to apex. Exercise and a left lateral position of the client increase intensity of sound. It is a low-pitched, rumbling sound often accompanied by an augmented S_1 and an opening snap.

AV, Atrioventricular.
Modified from Huang, S.L., et al. (1989). *Coronary care nursing* (2nd ed., p. 19). Philadelphia: Saunders; and Alexander, R.W., et al. (Eds.) (1998). *Hurst's the heart* (9th ed.). New York: McGraw-Hill.

Extremities
Skin

Observe the skin and mucous membranes for abnormalities such as central or peripheral *cyanosis*. The presence of a bluish tinge or duskiness is indicative of central cyanosis. Peripheral cyanosis is seen in lips, ear lobes, and nail beds.[6] Assess *capillary refill* (circulation) by putting slight pressure on a nail bed until it blanches (see

Chapter 51). Quickly release the pressure. When circulation is adequate, nail color returns to baseline in less than 3 seconds. Always check capillary refill before using pulse oximetry; if capillary refill is abnormal, pulse oximetry findings are inaccurate.

Skin Turgor

Assess skin turgor (elasticity) by lifting a fold of skin over the sternum or lower arms and releasing it (see Chapter 48). Normal skin immediately returns to the baseline position, but skin with decreased turgor stays pinched (tenting) for up to 30 seconds. Decreased skin turgor occurs with dehydration, volume depletion, rapid weight loss, and advanced age.

Temperature

The temperature of the skin may reflect cardiac disease. Along with the locations of warm or cold skin areas, the location of temperature changes assists in differentiating underlying pathology.[6,11,16]

Clubbing

Check fingers for clubbing, in which the distal tips of the fingers become bulbous and the angle between the base of the nail and the skin next to the cuticle increases from the normal 160 to 180 degrees or more (see Chapter 48). Also look for splinter hemorrhages of the nails.

Edema

Inspect dependent areas for edema. In the mobile client, edema is best seen in the feet, ankles, and lower legs. In the chair-ridden or bedridden client, edema may be palpated over the sacrum, abdomen, or scapula. Assess the severity of edema by pressing a thumb or finger carefully into the area. A depression that does not rapidly resume its original contour is noted as orthostatic, or pitting, edema.[6,11,16] Record whether edema is present or absent, and, if present, whether it is pitting or non-pitting.

DIAGNOSTIC TESTING

Diagnostic tests add objective findings that when added to the client's subjective information help to diagnose the presenting illness. Cardiac diagnostic procedures are both noninvasive (laboratory, electrocardiograms, Holter monitors, ultrasounds, x-rays, CT scans, stress tests, MRIs, tilt-table tests) and invasive (arteriography, hemodynamic studies, electrophysiologic studies). Nursing responsibilities for these various tests include (1) scheduling the procedure, (2) explaining the purpose and the procedure and answering any questions, (3) witnessing signing of the consent form, (4) providing any necessary preliminary care (adjustments in medications and special diets), (5) promoting maximal emotional and physical comfort, and (6) providing postprocedure care and instructions for home care, returning to work, and general

aftercare.[6,11,16,21] Please refer to a diagnostic and laboratory testing textbook for more specific information for the tests described in the following paragraphs.

Noninvasive Tests
Electrocardiographic Tests

Electrocardiographic tests are noninvasive tests in which patches are placed on the chest wall to obtain the electrical activity of the heart. The table Common Electrocardiographic Tests on the website describes the common electrographic tests and the clinical manifestations that may indicate the need for these tests.

Electrocardiogram. The electrocardiogram (ECG) is an essential tool in evaluating the heart's rhythm and signs of ischemia. The impulse waves, recorded by the ECG machine on graph paper, are designated by the letters P, QRS, and T. Figure 54-7 below depicts the typical ECG pattern formed by these waves. The P wave represents depolarization of the atria. The QRS complex represents depolarization of the ventricles. The T wave represents repolarization of the ventricles.[6]

An ECG tracing also shows the voltage of the waves and the duration of both the waves and the intervals. ECG graph paper is divided into horizontal lines and vertical lines, large squares and small squares. Voltage is represented on the vertical axis of the ECG paper. Each small square is 1 mm in height. Five small squares are equivalent to 5 mm, which is equivalent to 0.5 mV. Voltage yields information about the presence and degree of atrial or ventricular hypertrophy. Time is measured on the horizontal axis. Each small square signifies the passage of 0.04 second. Each large square indicates the passage of 0.20 second. By studying the

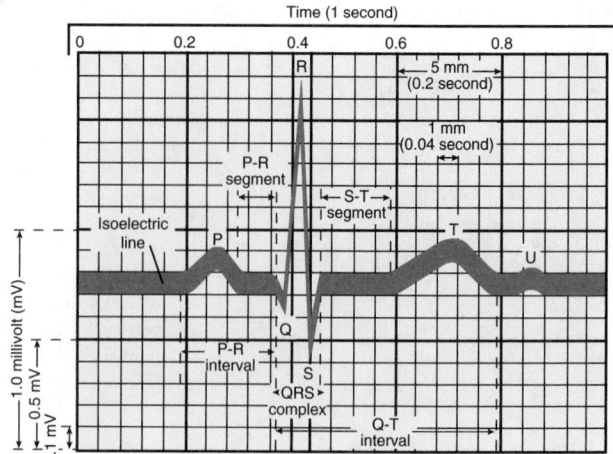

■ **FIGURE 54–7** Normal electrocardiographic (ECG) patterns. The P wave represents depolarization of the atria to the ventricles. The QRS complex represents depolarization of the ventricles, and the T wave represents repolarization of the ventricles. The small U wave is sometimes seen following the T wave. Time and voltage lines of ECG paper: *vertically*, 1 mm = 0.1 mV; 5 mm = 0.5 mV; 10 mm = 1 mV; *horizontally*, one small box = 0.04 second; five small boxes = 0.20 second; 25 small boxes = 1 second.

duration of the waves and intervals, the examiner can diagnose abnormal impulse formation and conduction.[6]

Normal time durations for waves and intervals are as follows:

- *P wave:* less than 0.11 second
- *PR interval:* 0.12 to 0.20 second
- *QRS complex:* 0.04 to 0.11 second
- *QT interval:* in women, up to 0.43 second; in men, up to 0.42 second

The standard ECG has a 12-lead system, offering 12 points of reference for recording the electrical activity of the heart, looking in both horizontal and vertical planes. The placement of 12-lead electrodes is shown in Figure 54-8. The standard 12-lead ECG has 6 *limb* leads (used to view the heart in a frontal or vertical plane) and 6 *precordial* leads (used to view the heart in a horizontal plane). Together, the 12 leads permit multidirectional examination of the electrical events in the heart. The location of pathologic change within the heart, which alters electrical activity (usually ST-segment elevation or depression), can be pinpointed.[6] Table 54-7 correlates the area of infarct with expected ECG changes and coronary artery lesion location.

Holter Monitoring. When the client wears a portable Holter monitor, an ECG tracing is recorded continuously, usually for 24 hours, on an outpatient basis. The Holter monitor may be used to detect dysrhythmias that may not appear on a routine ECG or evaluate the effectiveness of antidysrhythmics or pacemaker therapy. Clients may be asked to record manifestations that develop during the time they are wearing the monitor. A standard ECG records only seconds of cardiac activity.[6]

TABLE 54–7 Coronary Artery Lesion Location, Area of Infarct, and Electrocardiographic Changes

Coronary Artery	Area of Infarct	ECG Leads	Dysrhythmias
LAD	Anterior	V_{2-4}	RBBB, LAH, Mobitz type II, CHB
	Septal	V_{1-2}	
	Anteroseptal	V_{1-4}	
Circumflex	Lateral	I, aV_L	Ventricular and possibly SA and AV node conduction disturbances
	Anterolateral	I, aV_L, V_{5-6}	
	Inferolateral	aV_F, II, III, V_{5-6}	
	Posterior	Reciprocal, V_{1-3}	
RCA	Inferior	II, III, aV_F	SA node, AV node, and His bundle conduction disturbances
	Right ventricle	II, III, aV_F, V_{4-6_R}	

AV, Atrioventricular; *CHB,* complete heart block; *LAD,* left anterior descending; *LAH,* left anterior hemiblock; *RBBB,* right bundle branch block; *RCA,* right coronary artery; *SA,* sinoatrial.
From Alspach, J.G. (Ed.) (1992). *Instructor's resource manual for the AACN core curriculum for critical care nursing.* Philadelphia: Saunders.

Exercise Tests

Exercise testing provides physiologic information regarding the heart's functional capacity to meet the metabolic demands caused by increasing exertion. Exercise testing is most often used in conjunction with nuclear scanning, and sometimes echocardiography, using a radionuclide tracer (thallium, dipyridamole, Cardiolite) to provide additional information regarding left ventricular wall motion

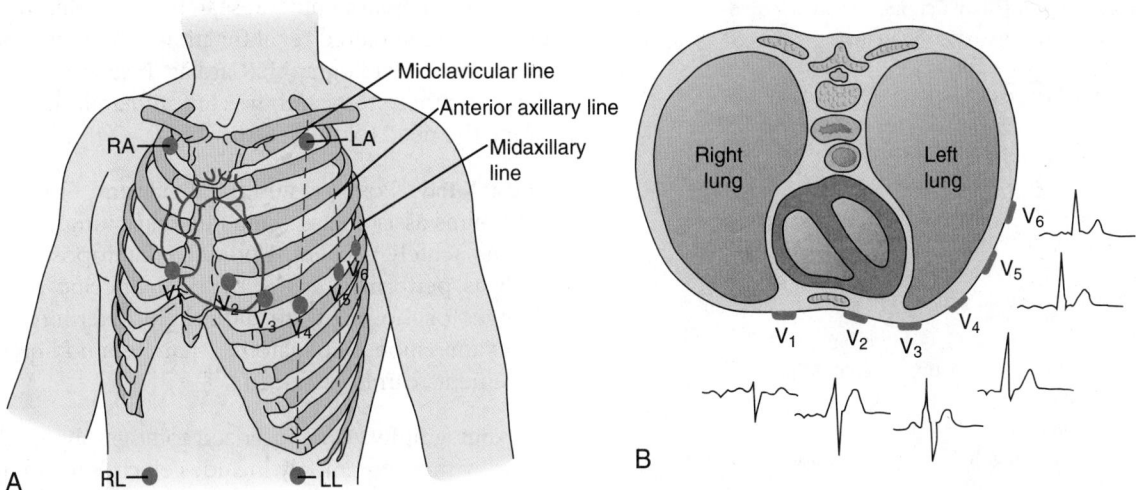

■ FIGURE 54–8 Common positions for continuous monitoring lead placement. **A,** Five-lead system: RA electrode, below right clavicle at MCL; LA electrode, below left clavicle at MCL; RL electrode, right abdomen at MCL; LL electrode, left abdomen at MCL. V_1 to V_6 are the precordial or chest leads: V_1, fourth ICS at right sternal border; V_2, fourth ICS at left sternal border; V_3, fourth ICS, midway between left sternal border and MCL; V_4, fifth ICS at left MCL; V_5, fifth ICS, midway between left MCL and AAL; V_6, fifth ICS at left AAL. **B,** Normal electrocardiographic findings with corresponding chest leads to cross-section at the fourth rib level. *AAL,* Anterior axillary line; *ICS,* intercostal space; *LA,* left arm; *LL,* left leg; *MAL,* midaxillary line; *MCL,* midclavicular line; *RA,* right arm; *RL,* right leg.

during stress. Echocardiography also aids in revealing any wall motion abnormalities post stress. The perfusion scanning is performed with a special camera that is capable of showing the source of emitted low-energy photons on a screen. Each photon detected by the camera is recorded on film and a computer screen. The computer refines and enhances the images and then provides quantitative perfusion information about the myocardial walls.[21]

Exercise testing helps evaluate the presence, absence, or severity of coronary artery disease, both in clients with known CVD and in those initially seen with chest pain of unknown origin.[6,21] Exercise testing is usually indicated in low-risk clients only but may be indicated in post–open heart clients before beginning cardiac rehabilitation. Box 54-6 lists contraindications to exercise testing. Clients are instructed not to eat or smoke for 2 to 3 hours before the test and to dress appropriately for exercise. Most clients are allowed to take their usual medications unless the clinician orders otherwise.

Exercise testing may include bicycle ergometry or treadmill testing. Clients are exercised in stages in order to increase their heart rates to a value based on their age. Achieving their age-adjusted heart rate increases the reliability of test results. For those who cannot walk on the treadmill, or have underlying left bundle branch block on ECG (which may alter test results), nuclear scanning with intravenous Persantine provides reliable results. Persantine dilates coronary arteries to increase blood flow; however, arteries with plaque and blockage are unable to significantly dilate to allow increased perfusion. Intravenous dobutamine is an option for clients who cannot exercise.

BOX 54-6 Contraindications to Exercise Testing

ACUTE CARDIOVASCULAR DISEASE
- Acute myocardial infarction (usually avoided in clients less than 2 weeks after infarction)
- Unstable angina pectoris
- Heart failure
- Pericarditis
- Myocarditis
- Endocarditis
- Life-threatening dysrhythmias
- Thrombophlebitis
- Recent systemic embolism
- Dissecting or enlarging aneurysm

OTHERS
- Severe diseases restricting mobility
- Renal failure
- Severe pulmonary disruptions
- Orthopedic disorders affecting the spine or lower extremities
- Neurologic impairment (stroke or paralysis)
- Systemic infection
- Left ventricular outflow obstruction (aortic stenosis, hypertension, or hypertrophic cardiomyopathy)

A positive exercise test is indicated by one of the following results: (a) It must be terminated before the predicted maximal (or submaximal) limits have been achieved because of manifestations of cardiovascular intolerance. (b) ST-segment changes have occurred (horizontal ST-segment depression, ST-segment downsloping, or ST-segment upsloping is indicative of abnormal tracings). (c) Echocardiography or nuclear scanning will reveal wall motion abnormalities or reversible perfusion defects. In some people, ST-segment alterations may occur during exercise even though coronary artery disease is not present. Hyperventilation, certain drugs, and electrolyte imbalances can produce false-positive readings. On the other hand, false-negative findings also occur, although with less frequency. Medications such as beta-blocking agents and nitrates can produce false-negative results.[6,21] These medications may be held before the stress test to avoid inaccurate results.

Upright Tilt-Table Tests
Clients are tilted upright to a maximum of 60 to 80 degrees for 20 to 45 minutes while their heart rate and blood pressure are continuously monitored. Tests are positive for vasopressor syncope if both the heart rate and the blood pressure fall in unison. This procedure, when positive, reproduces the client's presenting manifestations.[6] Three to five electrodes are placed on the chest and connected to a monitor (with rhythm recording capabilities) at the client's side.

Radiographic Cardiac Tests
Renal functioning must be obtained before CT scanning or CT angiography because of contrast use. Because of the tracer used with MRI or MRA (which is not cleared through the kidneys), renal function is not a contraindication. This makes these tests especially useful for those clients with renal impairment.[34] Research reassessing the effect of tracer on impaired renal function continues. The table on Common Radiographic Cardiac Tests on the website describes these tests and the clinical manifestations indicating the need for these tests.

Chest X-Ray. Posteroanterior, lateral, and oblique chest x-ray films assist in assessing the heart, lungs, and aorta. For the acutely ill client, a portable anteroposterior x-ray study is performed at the bedside. Specific pathologic changes of the heart are difficult to determine with x-ray examination, but anatomic changes, and line or tube placements can be assessed.[6,16]

CT Angiography. Computerized tomography (CT) angiography most commonly includes electron beam tomography (EBT) or modern multivector computerized tomography (MVCT). This scan allows a noninvasive way to evaluate the coronary arteries, great vessels, aorta, renal arteries, and lower extremity arteries through two- or three-dimensional images.[6,16]

CT Scan per Pulmonary Embolus Protocol. In a CT scan with pulmonary embolus protocol, extra contrast is used to enhance the pulmonary arteries. This is an alternative to ventilation-perfusion lung scans, and is now used as the principal diagnostic test to rule out pulmonary emboli.[6,16]

Magnetic Resonance Imaging. Although MRI is one of the most expensive noninvasive diagnostic options, a variety of data may be obtained in a single image. MRI can show the heart beating and the blood flowing in any direction. All standard quantitative functional indices, except transstenotic gradients, can be obtained from an MRI study.[6,16]

Magnetic Resonance Angiography. MRA is similar to MRI, but it uses gadolinium as intravenous contrast medium to evaluate arterial disease. Gadolinium differs from other contrast media because it is not nephrotoxic; thus clients with renal insufficiency can safely undergo this procedure. Research regarding the safety of Gadolinium on impaired renal function is in progress. Along with coronary MRA, pulmonary, renal, and peripheral arteries can also be studied.[6,16]

Viability Scan. Positron emission tomography (PET) allows visualization of regional physiologic function and biochemical changes that often separate normal from diseased myocardium. Cellular metabolic information is obtained by mapping regional myocardial glucose metabolism while a tracer is used to obtain left ventricular perfusion. Combining information from the perfusion and metabolism images provides a thorough assessment of regional cardiac viability. Clients with decreased perfusion but preserved glucose uptake have viable, or hibernating, myocardium. This information is critical regarding the need for coronary artery revascularization, which is indicated if viable myocardium is detected.[21]

Echocardiogram

Echocardiography, a noninvasive diagnostic procedure based on the principles of ultrasonography, provides another way to look at the heart's structure. An echocardiogram is obtained by placing a transducer on several areas of the chest wall. Bursts of ultrasound waves are directed at the part of the heart under investigation. The echocardiogram records the structure and motion of that area in relation to its distance from the anterior chest wall. An ECG is recorded simultaneously on the graph. Two-dimensional echocardiography generates a continuous picture of the beating heart. The images are recorded on videotape for analysis.[6] The table Common Cardiac Ultrasonographic Tests on the website describes these tests and the clinical manifestations that may indicate the need for these tests.

Invasive Cardiac Tests

Transesophageal Echocardiography

Transesophageal echocardiography (TEE) yields a higher quality picture of the heart than does regular echocardiography. It is especially useful for clients who have thickened lung tissue or thick chest walls or who are obese. Transesophageal echocardiography eliminates the interference of the thoracic structures and provides an excellent image of the heart and great vessels from a posterior view. Because the probe is placed behind the heart, it allows the left atrium to be viewed easily. The procedure may also be used intraoperatively, where conventional echocardiography is ineffective.[6]

Cardiac Catheterization

This complex procedure involves insertion of a catheter into the heart, coronary arteries, and surrounding vessels to obtain detailed information about the structure and performance of the heart, the valves, and the circulatory system. Cardiac catheterization includes both left and right heart catheterization and is performed in a special cardiac catheterization laboratory.[6] Please refer to a diagnostic procedures handbook for discussion of the preprocedure and postprocedure nursing care and possible complications after cardiac catheterization. The table Common Cardiac Invasive Procedures on the website describes the evolve common invasive cardiac procedures and the clinical manifestations that may indicate the need for these tests.

Left Heart Catheterization. Catheters are inserted through the femoral artery or radial artery leading to the aorta and coronary arteries. Each coronary artery is selectively cannulated and contrast is injected into the artery as cineangiography is obtained. Cineangiography provides moving pictures of contrast flow through the coronary arteries or as the left ventricle contracts. These pictures can be viewed at both rapid and slow speeds, permitting detailed and unlimited review of the study. Plaque, or blockage, manifests itself by narrowing of the artery lumen. This information is critical to optimize treatment of atherosclerotic heart disease. There is less that 1% risk of major complication and less than 0.08% mortality risk with this procedure.[6]

Right Heart Catheterization. Although right heart catheterization is conducted in the cardiac catheterization laboratory, hemodynamic monitoring can be conducted at the bedside. A Swan-Ganz catheter is inserted via the brachial vein or femoral vein and progressed through the vena cava into the right atrium, right ventricle, and finally the pulmonary artery. The catheter has several end or side holes that allow blood withdrawal for oxygen analysis from the various cardiac chambers. Hemodynamic pressure monitoring provides information about blood volume, fluid balance, how well the heart is pumping, valvular structures, or shunting.

Current technology allows measurement of right atrial pressure or central venous pressure (CVP); pulmonary artery (PA) pressures during systole and diastole, which reflects right and left ventricular pressures; and pulmonary capillary wedge pressure (PCWP), which is an indirect indicator of left ventricular pressure and cardiac output (CO), reflecting the heart's output in liters per minute, cardiac index (CI), systemic vascular resistance (SVR), pulmonary vascular resistances (PVR) and various stroke volumes. These pressures are obtained by attaching the catheter to a transducer with its connecting amplifier and recording device. Critical care nurses perform all of these studies routinely at the bedside. Hemodynamic studies provide a wealth of information reflecting the earliest changes in the circulatory system that are not yet clinically detectable.[6,11,16] The Bridge to Critical Care feature below and on p. 1381 illustrates Swan-Ganz monitoring.

BRIDGE TO CRITICAL CARE

Swan-Ganz Monitoring (PA Catheter)

POSITIONING THE SWAN-GANZ CATHETER

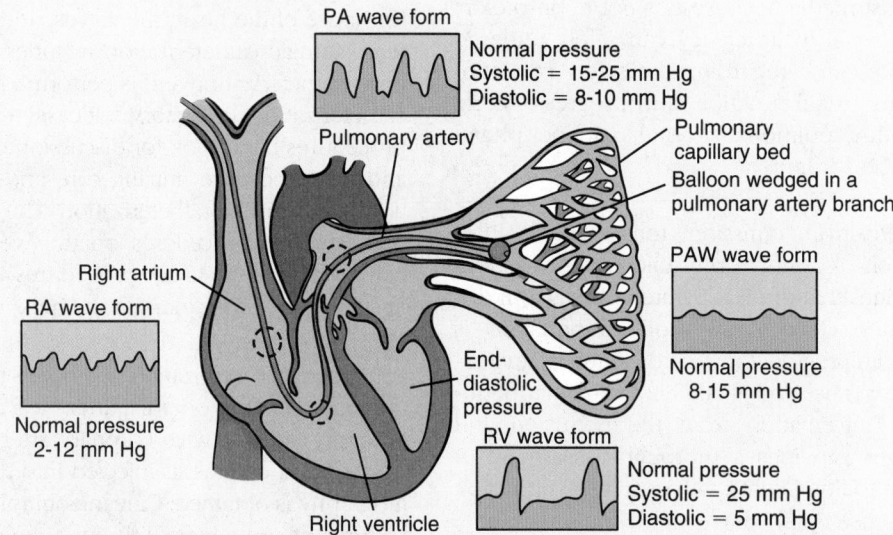

PA wave form
Normal pressure
Systolic = 15-25 mm Hg
Diastolic = 8-10 mm Hg

Pulmonary artery

Pulmonary capillary bed
Balloon wedged in a pulmonary artery branch

PAW wave form
Normal pressure
8-15 mm Hg

Right atrium

RA wave form
Normal pressure
2-12 mm Hg

End-diastolic pressure

RV wave form
Normal pressure
Systolic = 25 mm Hg
Diastolic = 5 mm Hg

Right ventricle

The Quadruple-Lumen Swan-Ganz Catheter

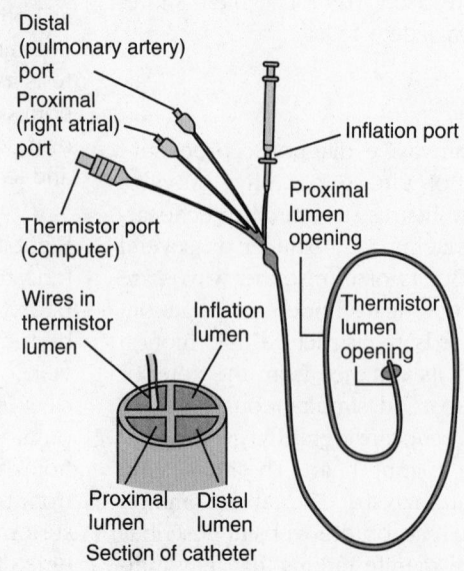

Distal (pulmonary artery) port
Proximal (right atrial) port
Inflation port
Proximal lumen opening
Thermistor port (computer)
Wires in thermistor lumen
Inflation lumen
Thermistor lumen opening
Proximal lumen
Distal lumen
Section of catheter

Electrophysiologic Studies

The electrophysiologic study is an invasive method of recording intracardiac electrical activity. It is used to (1) shed light on the mechanisms of dysrhythmias, (2) differentiate between supraventricular and ventricular dysrhythmias, (3) evaluate sinoatrial (SA) or AV node dysfunction, (4) determine the need for a pacemaker, and (5) evaluate the effect of antidysrhythmic agents used to prevent the occurrence of tachycardias. These studies, like cardiac catheterization, are conducted in a specialized laboratory where equipment and monitors are readily available.[6]

The purpose of the procedure is to reproduce any dysrhythmia so that its origin may be isolated. If a dysrhythmia is induced, the client's BP and hemodynamic responses are observed. It is possible to record simultaneously arterial pressure, surface ECGs, and ECGs from intracavitary catheters. The morphology and rate of any induced dysrhythmias are compared with those of the client's spontaneous dysrhythmia.

BRIDGE TO CRITICAL CARE

Swan-Ganz Monitoring (PA Catheter)—Cont'd

MEASURING CARDIAC OUTPUT BY THERMODILUTION

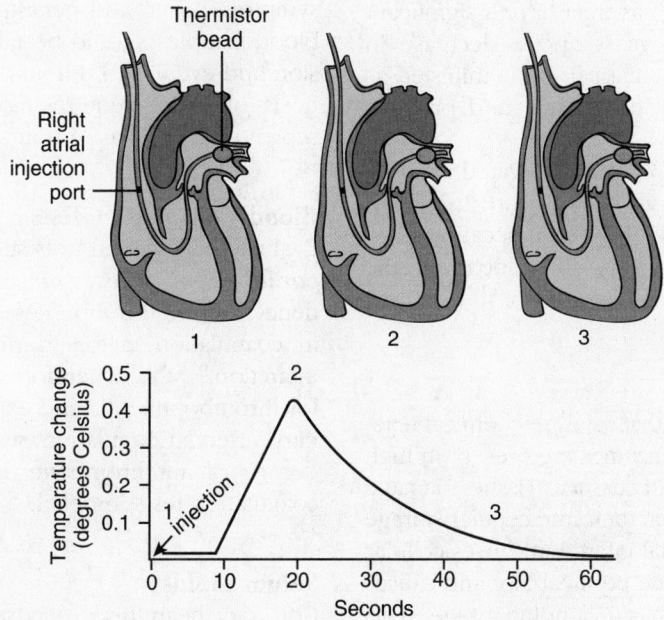

Conditions with Expected Pressure Changes

	Pressure Changes			
Condition	**RAP**	**RVP**	**PAP**	**PAWP**
Heart failure (volume overload)	↑	↑	↑	↑
Hypovolemia	↓	↓	↓	↓
Cardiogenic shock*	none or ↑	none or ↑	none or ↑	none or ↑ (diastolic)
Pulmonary hypertension	↑	↑	↑	none or ↑
Cardiac tamponade	↑	↑	↑	↑ (diastolic)
Pulmonary emboli	↑	↑	↑	↑ (systolic)
Mitral valve stenosis/insufficiency†	↑	↑	↑	↑

PAP, Pulmonary artery pressure; *PAWP*, pulmonary artery wedge pressure; *RAP*, right atrial pressure; *RVP*, right ventricular pressure.
*Pressure readings depend on the heart's ability to handle circulating volume. Chronic lung disease elevates all readings.
†Mitral valve disease produces unreliable pressure readings.

Laboratory Tests

Laboratory test data are used to (1) diagnose a variety of cardiovascular ailments (myocardial infarction), (2) screen people considered at risk for CVD, (3) determine baseline values, (4) identify concurrent disorders (anemia, diabetes mellitus, electrolyte imbalance, renal or liver abnormalities) that may affect treatment, and (5) evaluate the effectiveness of intervention. Tests that are more commonly used to determine cardiovascular function and disease are discussed here. The table Common Cardiac Laboratory Tests on the website provides a description of the tests and possible etiologies for abnormal findings. Please refer to a laboratory tests textbook for the specifics of collecting and handling these blood samples.

Complete Blood Cell Count

Measuring the packed cell volume, or *hematocrit,* is the easiest way to ascertain the concentration of red blood cells in the blood. Clients with anemia have a significant reduction in red blood cell mass and a decrease in oxygen-carrying capacity. Anemia can be manifested as angina or it can exacerbate heart failure and produce heart murmurs.[6,12]

The *white blood cell (WBC) count* is elevated in infectious and inflammatory diseases of the heart. It is commonly seen after myocardial infarction because large numbers of WBCs are necessary to dispose of the necrotic tissue resulting from the infarction.[6,12]

Cardiac Enzymes

Enzymes are special proteins that catalyze chemical reactions in living cells. Cardiac enzymes are present in high concentrations in myocardial tissue. Tissue damage causes release of enzymes from their intracellular storage areas. For example, myocardial infarction causes cellular anoxia, which alters membrane permeability and causes spillage of enzymes into the surrounding tissue. This leakage of enzymes can be detected by rising plasma levels. Cardiac enzyme levels reflect myocardial infarction (cellular death).[6,12]

Myoglobin is a useful marker of myocardial necrosis; it is rapidly released from the circulation within 1 to 2 hours of infarction. Its release allows very early detection of myocardial infarction, but its short half-life makes it less useful in clients who present several hours after onset. This enzyme is not cardiac specific and although it increases early, it is not the most reliable indicator of an MI. Measurement of myoglobin levels is not recommended if there is evidence of muscle damage, trauma, or renal failure because of the greater potential for false-positive test results in these circumstances.[6,12]

The enzymes most commonly used to detect myocardial infarction because of their excellent sensitivity are *creatine kinase* (CK) and *troponin.* There are three CK isoenzymes: CK-MM (skeletal muscle), CK-MB (myocardial muscle), and CK-BB (brain). Troponin has three components: I, C, and T. Troponin I modulates the contractile state, troponin C binds calcium, and troponin T binds troponins I and C. Although troponin is present in all striated muscle, troponin components in cardiac muscle have different amino acid sequences. Therefore antibodies against cardiac troponins I and T are very specific. Elevated levels of troponin I are as sensitive as CK-MB for the detection of myocardial injury. Because of their higher specificity for myocardial injury, troponins can be used to exclude myocardial infarction when CK-MB may be falsely positive.[6,12,16] Troponin I is the definitive laboratory test for diagnosis of an MI.

Plasma CK-MB can be initially seen within 2 hours of symptom onset, is significantly elevated within 6 to 8 hours of symptom onset, and returns to normal after 48 to 72 hours. Troponin can also be seen in 2 hours after symptom onset, peaks within 6 to 10 hours of symptom onset, and persists for 4 to 7 days. Therefore blood samples should be taken immediately on admission and every 6 to 8 hours for the first 24 hours. Diagnosis of injury requires no fewer than two samples separated by at least 4 hours.[6,10,12,16]

Blood Coagulation Tests

Evaluate coagulation tests such as *prothrombin time* and *partial thromboplastin time* in people with a greater tendency to form thrombi. Research has shown an increase in coagulation factors during and after a myocardial infarction.[6] Therefore the client is at greater risk for thrombophlebitis and extension of clots in the coronary artery. Coagulation studies are ordered to guide dosage of antithrombotic drugs. Chapter 74 discusses coagulation tests in detail.

Serum Lipids

Coronary heart disease is secondary to atherosclerosis and accumulation of lipids within the arterial wall, which is associated with inflammation and vascular remodeling. The cholesterol-containing lipid fraction most closely associated with atherogenesis is low-density-lipoprotein cholesterol (LDL-C). Coronary heart disease risk increases as blood levels of LDL-C increase. The recommended goal for LDL-C is <100 mg/dL, but when the client's risk is very high as with a previous event, the LDL-C goal is <70 mg/dL.[13] A second lipid fraction that plays a major role in determining CVD risk is high-density-lipoprotein cholesterol (HDL-C). Coronary heart disease risk decreases as blood levels of HDL-C increase. These lipids are composed of fatty substances that are insoluble in water. They are derived from fats in the diet or synthesized in the liver.[3,5,12] Serum lipids are discussed in Chapter 56.

C-Reactive Protein

Atherosclerosis is in part a chronic low-grade inflammatory condition. Elevation of levels of C-reactive protein (CRP), an acute-phase protein that measures the presence and degree of inflammation within the arterial walls, has been linked to future cardiovascular risks, including stroke, myocardial infarction, and cardiovascular death.[6,12]

D-Dimer

Plasma D-dimer level is determined by enzyme-linked immunosorbent assay; levels reflect plasmin's breakdown of fibrin (indicating thrombolysis). D-dimer levels are elevated in greater than 90% of clients with pulmonary embolus. If positive, and pulmonary embolus is a suspicion, lung scanning or ventilation-perfusion scanning is recommended.[6,12]

Serum Electrolytes

Fluid and electrolyte regulation may be affected by cardiovascular disorders or medications. In addition, electrolyte levels can alter cardiac muscle contraction.[6,12] Chapters 11 and 12 describe fluids and electrolytes in more detail.

Potassium. *Hypokalemia* (abnormally low potassium level) increases cardiac electrical instability, the occurrence of ventricular dysrhythmias, and the risk of digitalis toxicity. A characteristic change on the ECG is a U wave but this finding alone is not considered diagnostic for hypokalemia. *Hyperkalemia* (elevated potassium level) can lead to a tall T wave on the ECG, asystole, and ventricular dysrhythmias.[6,11,12,16]

Sodium. The serum sodium level reflects water balance. Hyponatremia indicates water excess. Hypernatremia indicates sodium excess.[12]

Calcium. Calcium is considered an important mediator of many cardiovascular functions because of its effect on cardiac excitability, contractility, and vascular tone. Hypocalcemia (low calcium level) can lead to serious ventricular dysrhythmias, a prolonged QT interval, and cardiac arrest. Hypercalcemia (elevated calcium level) shortens the QT interval and causes AV block, tachycardia, bradycardia, digitalis hypersensitivity, and cardiac arrest.[6,12]

Magnesium. Magnesium helps regulate intracellular metabolism, activates essential enzymes, and aids transport of sodium and potassium across the cell membrane. It plays a vital role in neuromuscular excitability. Low magnesium levels (hypomagnesemia) may cause mental apathy, facial tics, leg cramps, respiratory depression, and severe cardiac dysrhythmias, including ventricular tachycardia and fibrillation. Elevated magnesium levels (hypermagnesemia) may cause profound muscle weakness, hyporeflexia, hypotension, and bradycardia with a prolonged PR interval and wide QRS complex.[6,12]

Phosphorus. Most extracellular phosphorus is present in the bone with calcium (85% of the body's total phosphorus). A small amount of phosphorus is found in intracellular fluid. There, it helps regulate energy formation (adenosine triphosphate [ATP]) and maintain acid-base balance and neuromuscular excitability. Phosphate levels are inversely related to calcium levels as the kidneys retain or excrete one or the other. Interpret the two levels together. Low phosphorus levels (hypophosphatemia) may cause bleeding, decreased WBC levels, muscular weakness (including respiratory muscles), and nausea and vomiting. Elevated levels (hyperphosphatemia) may cause manifestations similar to those of hypocalcemia, with muscle tetany being the most common finding.[6,12]

Urea Nitrogen, Creatinine, and GFR. Urea nitrogen, also known as blood urea nitrogen (BUN), serum creatinine, and glomerular filtration rate (GFR) are indicators of renal function, specifically the ability of the kidney to excrete urea and protein. Renal function must be assessed before any procedures using contrast (CT scans, angiography, or angiograms). Contrast is cleared through the kidneys and clients may be at risk for acute renal failure when undergoing those procedures.[6,12]

Serum Glucose. Diabetes mellitus is a major risk factor for the development of atherosclerosis. In addition, the stress of an acute cardiac event can greatly elevate blood glucose level, causing unstable hyperglycemia in clients with latent diabetes mellitus. For these reasons, blood glucose level is routinely assessed in all clients with acute cardiovascular disorders.[6,12,16]

CONCLUSIONS

With the rising incidence and prevalence of CVD, the role of nurses is more important than ever regarding client assessment, treatment, and education. Especially important is education regarding risk factor modification, as it is estimated that more than 50% of CVD deaths and disability can be eliminated by a combination of cost-effective national and individual efforts to reduce risk factors.[3] Learning to obtain a thorough history and conduct a comprehensive physical examination requires repetition and perseverance. These data are just as important as the results of noninvasive and invasive studies if the nurse is to continue to assess the client effectively, provide primary preventive care, and monitor treatment. Assessment skills and nursing interventions can make a significant difference in the client's quality of life by preventing complications and improving outcomes. By helping the client you also impact that client's family and support system, who in turn may by compelled to modify risk factors and seek preventive care. Through these efforts, the goal of *Healthy People 2010* (to improve overall cardiovascular health and quality of life through prevention, assessment, detection, risk factor management, and early diagnosis and treatment) may be attained.

BIBLIOGRAPHY

Citations appearing in red refer to primary research.

Citations appearing in blue refer to evidence-based practice guidelines and protocols.

1. American Heart Association. (2005). *American Heart Association guidelines for primary prevention of cardiovascular disease and stroke.* Accessed 03/28/06 at www.americanheart.org/presenter. jhtml?identifier=4704.
2. American Heart Association. (2003). Case definitions for acute coronary heart disease in epidemiology and clinical research studies: A statement from the AHA Council on Epidemiology and Prevention; AHA Statistics Committee; World Heart Federation Council on Epidemiology and Prevention; the European Society of Cardiology Working Group on National Heart, Lung, and Blood Institute. *Circulation, 108*(20), 2543-2549.
3. American Heart Association. (2006). Heart disease and stroke statistics—2006 update: A report from the American Heart Association Statistics Committee and Stroke Statistics Subcommittee. *Circulation, 113*(6), 85-151.
4. American Heart Association. (2006). Obesity and cardiovascular disease: Pathophysiology, evaluation, and effect of weight loss: An update of the 1997 American Heart Association Scientific Statement on Obesity and Heart Disease from the Obesity Committee of the Council on Nutrition, Physical Activity, and Metabolism. *Circulation, 113*(6), 898-918.
5. American Heart Association. (2006). Prevention of coronary heart disease and the National Cholesterol Education Program. *Circulation, 113*(5), 598-600.
6. Braunwald, E., Zipes, D.P., Libby, P., et al. (2005). *Braunwald's heart disease: A textbook of cardiovascular medicine* (7th ed.). Philadelphia: Saunders.
7. Centers for Disease Control and Prevention. (2004). *Smoking among adults: Coronary heart disease and stroke.* Accessed 8/6/06 at www. cdc.gov.tobacco/sgr/sgr_2004/Factsheets/3.htm.
7a. Centers for Disease Control and Prevention. (2008). Healthy People 2010. Accessed 1/2/08 at www.cdc.gov/nchs/hphome.htm#Healthy %20People%202010.
8. Chahal, P.S., & Rao, S.S. (2005). Functional chest pain: Nociception and visceral hyperalgesia. *Journal of Clinical Gastroenterology, 39* (4, Suppl 3), 204-209.
9. Chen, W., Woods, S.L., & Puntillo, K.A. (2005). Gender differences in symptoms associated with acute myocardial infarction: A review of the research. *Heart & Lung, 34*(4), 240-247.
10. Ferri, F.F. (2006). *Ferri's clinical advisor: Instant diagnosis and treatment.* Philadelphia: Mosby.
11. Fink, M.P., Abraham, E., Vincent, J., et al. (2005). *Textbook of critical care* (5th ed.). Philadelphia: Saunders.
12. Fishbach, F.T. (2004). *A manual of laboratory & diagnostic tests* (7th ed.). Philadelphia: Lippincott.
13. Grundy, S.M., Cleeman, J.L., & Merz, C.N., et al. (2004). Implications of recent clinical trials for the National Cholesterol Education Program Adult Treatment Panel III Guidelines. *Circulation, 110,* 227-239.
14. Habib, P.A., Huang, G., Mendiola, J.A., et al. (2004). Anterior chest pain: Musculoskeletal considerations. *Emergency Radiology, 11,* 37-45.

15. Kannel, W.B. (1961). The Framingham study. *Annals of Internal Medicine, 55,* 33-50.
16. Kasper, D.L., Braunwald, E., Fauci, A.S., et al. (2005). *Harrison's principles of internal medicine* (16th ed.). New York: McGraw-Hill.
17. Kris-Etherton, P.M. (1999). American Heart Association Science Advisory: Monounsaturated fatty acids and risk of cardiovascular disease. American Heart Association Nutrition Committee. *Circulation, 100,* 1253-1258.
18. Kuczmarski, R.J., Flegal, K.M., Campbell, S.M., et al. (1994). Increasing prevalence of overweight among United States adults: The National Health and Nutrition Examination Surveys, 1960 to 1991. *Journal of the American Medical Association, 272,* 205-211.
19. McSweeney, J.C., Cody, M., O'Sullivan, P., et al. (2003). Women's early warning symptoms of acute myocardial infarction. *Circulation, 108,* 2619-2623.
20. McSweeney, J.C., Lefler, L.L., & Crowder, B.F. (2005). What's wrong with me? Women's coronary heart disease diagnostic experiences. *Progress in Cardiovascular Nursing, 20*(2), 48-57.
21. Meltler, F.A., & Guiberteau, M.J. (2006). *Essentials of nuclear medicine imaging* (5th ed.). Philadelphia: Saunders.
22. Mokdad, A.H., Serdula, M.K., Dietz, W.H., et al. (1999). The spread of the obesity epidemic in the United States, 1991-1998. *Journal of the American Medical Association, 282,* 1519-1522.
23. National Heart, Lung, and Blood Institute Joint National Committee on Prevention, Detection, Evaluation, and Treatment of High Blood Pressure. (2003). The seventh report of the Joint National Committee on Prevention, Detection, Evaluation, and Treatment of High Blood Pressure: The JNC-7 report. *Journal of the American Medical Association, 289*(19), 2560-2572.
24. National Institutes of Health. (2005). *Heart and circulation.* Accessed 03/28/06 at www.nih.gov.
25. Ounpuus, S., Negassa, A., & Yusuf, S. (2001). INTER-HEART: A global study of risk factors for acute myocardial infarction. *American Heart Journal, 141,* 711-721.
26. Postgraduate Institute for Medicine. (2006). *New insights in efficacy and safety of combination therapy with statins and fibrates. [Brochure].* New York: Jobson Publishing Group.
27. *Remington: The science and practice of pharmacy* (21st ed.). (2005). Philadelphia: Lippincott Wilkins & Wilkins.
28. Sapira, J.D. (1990). *Science of bedside diagnosis.* Baltimore: Urban & Schwatzneberg.
29. Sudano, I., Binggeli, C., Spieker, L., et al. (2005). Cardiovascular effects of coffee: Is it a risk factor? *PCVN, 20*(2), 65-69.
30. Swap, C.J., & Nagurney, J.T. (2005). Value and limitations of chest pain history in the evaluation of patients with suspected acute coronary syndromes. *Journal of the American Medical Association, 294*(20), 2623-2630.
31. Wild, S., Roglic, G., Sicree, et al. (2004). Global prevalence of diabetes: Estimates for the year 2000 and projections for 2030. *Diabetes Care, 27,* 1047-1053.
32. World Health Organization. (2005). *Cardiovascular disease.* Accessed 03/28/06 at www.who.int/.
33. World Health Organization Expert Panel on Detection, Evaluation, and Treatment of High Blood Cholesterol in Adults. (May 2001). *Third report of the National Cholesterol Education Program (NCEP)* (NIH Pub No. 01-3670.) Washington, DC: National Heart, Lung, and Blood Institute.

evolve **Did you remember to check out the bonus material on the Evolve website and the CD-ROM, including NCLEX®-Examination Style Review Questions, Open-Book Quizzes, and Chapter Review Audio Podcasts?**

http://evolve.elsevier.com/Black/medsurg

CHAPTER 55

Management of Clients with Structural Cardiac Disorders

BARBARA B. OTT AND MARIE A. DEFRANCESCO-LOUKAS

The movement of blood through the heart is crucial for human life. But in addition to perfusion, blood must flow through the heart in an efficient and orderly manner. This chapter focuses on the cardiac disorders that affect the structure of the heart and impair the efficiency of the heart as a pump.

VALVULAR HEART DISEASE

When heart valves that normally move blood efficiently through the heart chambers cannot fully open or fully close, perfusion of the heart and distal tissues is impaired and the heart muscle is strained. A stenosed valve may impede the flow of blood from one chamber to the next; an insufficient (incompetent) valve may allow blood to regurgitate (flow backward) (Table 55-1). The aortic and mitral valves become dysfunctional more often than do the pulmonary and tricuspid valves. This change occurs because the left side of the heart is a system of higher pressures compared with the lower pressures in the pulmonary circulation.

Valvular heart disease remains fairly common in the United States even though the incidence is steadily decreasing as the incidence of rheumatic fever decreases. Mitral valve prolapse syndrome is one of the most common cardiac abnormalities; as much as 5% of the population is affected, and women are affected more often than men.

MITRAL VALVE DISEASE

The mitral valve separates the left atrium from the left ventricle. Therefore problems with blood flow through the mitral valve affect left ventricular output and hence activity tolerance.

Etiology and Risk Factors

The predominant cause of mitral valve disease is rheumatic fever. Acute rheumatic fever leads to inflammation of the endocardium. The inflammation causes the valve leaflets and chordae tendineae to become fibrous. The chordae tendineae shorten, which narrows the outflow tract (see Table 55-1).

Mitral regurgitation develops from problems with the leaflets, chordae tendineae, papillary muscles, or mitral opening. The major causes of mitral regurgitation are mitral valve prolapse, myocardial ischemia, rheumatic heart disease, cardiomyopathy, and calcification of the opening. Rheumatic heart disease is preventable with early detection of beta-hemolytic streptococcal infections (the precursor to rheumatic heart disease).

Myocardial ischemia from coronary artery disease affects the mitral valve in many ways. Ischemia leads to loss of contractility, which affects mitral valve performance. Portions of the papillary muscle are fed by the coronary vessels, and when the vessels cannot provide blood flow to the myocardium, the leaflets may also not be supplied.

Mitral valve prolapse is the bulging of one or both of the valve leaflets into the left atrium during ventricular systole. Usually it occurs as a primary condition that is not associated with other diseases. However, it can occur in genetic diseases of connective tissues—such as

TABLE 55–1 Mitral and Aortic Valve Stenosis and Regurgitation

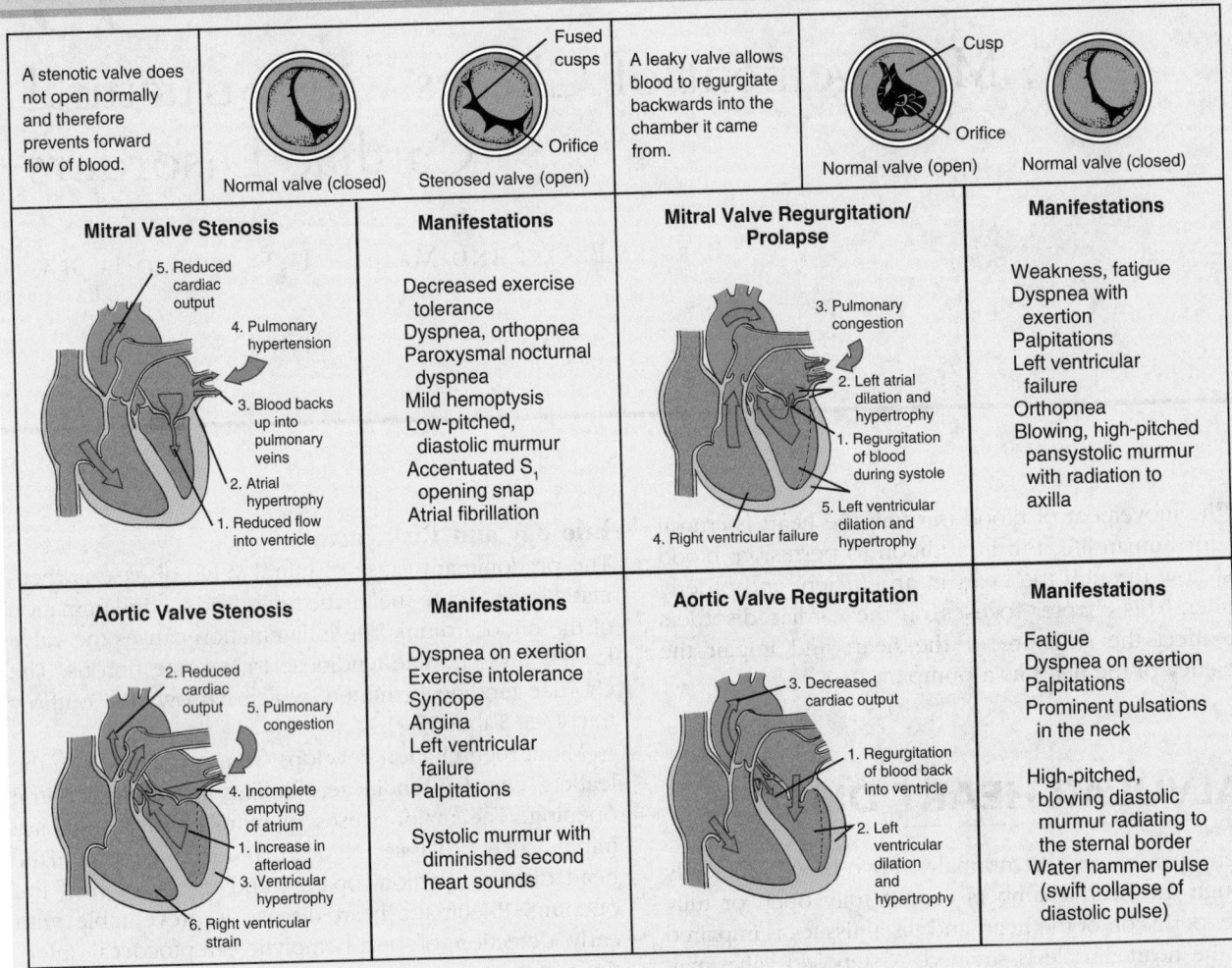

Mitral Valve Stenosis	Manifestations
5. Reduced cardiac output 4. Pulmonary hypertension 3. Blood backs up into pulmonary veins 2. Atrial hypertrophy 1. Reduced flow into ventricle	Decreased exercise tolerance Dyspnea, orthopnea Paroxysmal nocturnal dyspnea Mild hemoptysis Low-pitched, diastolic murmur Accentuated S_1 opening snap Atrial fibrillation

A stenotic valve does not open normally and therefore prevents forward flow of blood.

Normal valve (closed) — Fused cusps — Stenosed valve (open) — Orifice

A leaky valve allows blood to regurgitate backwards into the chamber it came from.

Cusp — Normal valve (open) — Orifice — Normal valve (closed)

Mitral Valve Regurgitation/ Prolapse	Manifestations
3. Pulmonary congestion 2. Left atrial dilation and hypertrophy 1. Regurgitation of blood during systole 5. Left ventricular dilation and hypertrophy 4. Right ventricular failure	Weakness, fatigue Dyspnea with exertion Palpitations Left ventricular failure Orthopnea Blowing, high-pitched pansystolic murmur with radiation to axilla

Aortic Valve Stenosis	Manifestations
2. Reduced cardiac output 5. Pulmonary congestion 4. Incomplete emptying of atrium 1. Increase in afterload 3. Ventricular hypertrophy 6. Right ventricular strain	Dyspnea on exertion Exercise intolerance Syncope Angina Left ventricular failure Palpitations Systolic murmur with diminished second heart sounds

Aortic Valve Regurgitation	Manifestations
3. Decreased cardiac output 1. Regurgitation of blood back into ventricle 2. Left ventricular dilation and hypertrophy	Fatigue Dyspnea on exertion Palpitations Prominent pulsations in the neck High-pitched, blowing diastolic murmur radiating to the sternal border Water hammer pulse (swift collapse of diastolic pulse)

Marfan syndrome and osteogenesis imperfecta—and after the ingestion of appetite suppressant drugs.

Pathophysiology

Mitral stenosis (MS) is a narrowing of the inlet valve into the left ventricle that prevents proper opening during diastolic filling. Clients with mitral stenosis typically have mitral valve leaflets that are thickened, openings that are fused, and/or chordae tendineae that are thickened and shortened. As the opening gets smaller, the left atrial pressure (LAP) rises to maintain a normal cardiac output. The increase in LAP also enlarges the left atrium and raises pulmonary venous and capillary pressures. The resulting pulmonary congestion and reduced cardiac output can mimic primary left ventricular failure, but left ventricular contractility is normal in most cases of mitral stenosis. As the disease evolves, chronic elevation of LAP

eventually leads to pulmonary hypertension, tricuspid and pulmonary valve incompetence, and secondary right heart failure. Eventually, there is loss of blood flow into the left ventricle and cardiac output falls.

Mitral insufficiency and regurgitation is due to scarring and retraction of the valve leaflets, resulting in incomplete closure. Mitral regurgitation occurs during systole, when much pressure is generated within the left ventricle to eject it forward into the aorta. When the mitral valve does not close, blood flows backward into the left atrium. The backward flow of blood causes left atrial and left ventricular enlargement. The left atrium dilates and hypertrophies in response to the large volume of blood it is receiving during systole. In response to the large amount of blood lost to the left atrium, the left ventricle must pump harder to preserve cardiac output and also hypertrophies. This hypertrophy of the left ventricle eventually leads to left ventricular failure (see Table 55-1). Over time the increase in blood flow to the left atrium causes a rise in left atrial pressure. This pressure is reflected backward into the pulmonary venous and arterial system. With continued high pressures, right-sided heart failure can develop.

Mitral valve prolapse occurs when the anterior and posterior cusps of the mitral valve billow upward into the atrium during systolic contraction. The chordae tendineae lengthen, allowing the valve cusps to stretch upward. The cusps may be enlarged and thickened. Mitral valve prolapse is often accompanied by mitral regurgitation, causing backward flow of blood into the atrium during systole.

Clinical Manifestations

The clinical manifestations of mitral valvular heart disease may appear gradually or suddenly. Auscultation will reveal a typical pattern of murmur. It is important to note where on the chest wall the murmur is heard best and during what phase of the cardiac cycle it occurs. Asking the client to hold his or her breath may help to distinguish the murmur from respiratory sounds.

Mitral Stenosis

Manifestations of mitral stenosis are usually insidious, occurring over several years after the infection. Clients often report decreased exercise tolerance, dyspnea, orthopnea, and paroxysmal nocturnal dyspnea. On auscultation a loud first heart sound is heard and then an opening "snap" that ushers in a low-pitched, rumbling diastolic murmur. The opening snap is best heard at the apex with the diaphragm of the stethoscope. The diastolic murmur is best heard at the apex using the bell of the stethoscope while the client is in a left lateral recumbent position. Manifestations of right-sided heart failure may also be present.

Atrial fibrillation is a common finding in clients with mitral stenosis. During episodes of atrial fibrillation, the pulse becomes irregular and faint and the blood pressure often drops. Hemoptysis is also seen frequently. Ineffective atrial contractions allow some stagnation of blood in the left atrium and encourage the formation of mural thrombi. These thrombi easily break away and travel as emboli throughout the arterial system, causing tissue infarction. These areas appear as dark areas or areas of necrotic tissue, especially on the toes, where vessels are small.

Mitral Regurgitation

Clients with mitral regurgitation may be asymptomatic until cardiac output falls. Reduced cardiac output first leads to fatigue and dyspnea. Clinical manifestations gradually increase to include orthopnea, paroxysmal nocturnal dyspnea, and peripheral edema. Pulmonary manifestations are less severe than in mitral stenosis because changes in the mean pulmonary capillary pressure are less exaggerated. When the right side of the heart is affected, the manifestations are the same as in mitral stenosis.

Auscultation reveals a blowing, high-pitched systolic murmur with radiation to the left axilla, heard best at the apex. The first heart sound may be diminished, and often a splitting of the second sound is heard. Severe regurgitation is associated with a third heart sound (S_3). Vital signs are usually normal unless mitral regurgitation is severe. Atrial fibrillation is common in clients with this condition; however, emboli and hemoptysis occur far less often than in mitral stenosis.

Mitral Valve Prolapse

It is not uncommon for clients with mitral valve prolapse to be completely asymptomatic. In a healthy client, physical examination may disclose a regurgitant murmur or a midsystolic click on auscultation. Manifestations may be vague; if present, they include tachycardia, light-headedness, syncope, fatigue, weakness, dyspnea, chest discomfort, anxiety, and palpitations related to dysrhythmias. Minimal morbidity and mortality are associated with mitral valve prolapse, and clinically clients have no physical limitations.

Various diagnostic assessments are used to detect valvular lesions or structural heart changes. These studies include echocardiography, chest radiography, stress tests, and cardiac catheterization.

OUTCOME MANAGEMENT

The goals of treatment for the asymptomatic client are to prevent beta-hemolytic streptococcal infection, which could lead to infective endocarditis, as discussed in the Translating Evidence into Practice feature on p. 1388. The prognosis is good for this group of clients. The goals of medical management of the symptomatic clients are to maintain cardiac output and activity tolerance. When cardiac output falls or the client is unable to tolerate simple activities, the valve can be surgically replaced.

Mitral Stenosis

Clients with mitral stenosis resulting from rheumatic heart disease should receive penicillin prophylaxis for beta-hemolytic streptococcal infections as well as for infective endocarditis. Prompt aggressive treatment of anemia and infections is also warranted. Adolescents and young adults with severe mitral stenosis should avoid entering professions and occupations that may require strenuous physical exertion. For clients that have experienced one or more previous pulmonary embolic episodes, anticoagulant therapy is helpful in preventing venous thrombosis and pulmonary embolism.

TRANSLATING EVIDENCE INTO PRACTICE

Preventing Infective Endocarditis

The number of cases of infective endocarditis is rising and the types of clients are changing. It remains a life-threatening infection responsible for substantial morbidity and mortality. The American Heart Association (AHA) has established guidelines for antibiotic prophylaxis to prevent bacterial endocarditis in high-risk clients.[1,2] Prophylactic antibiotics are administered according to the risk associated with various procedures. Risk for bacteremia is highest with dental extractions and oral surgical procedures, moderate for procedures affecting the genitourinary tract, and lowest for gastrointestinal diagnostic procedures.

Successful prophylaxis depends on client adherence. If clients do not understand the reason for prophylaxis and implications for their health, they may not adhere to the regimen. Nurses can play a key role in preventing bacterial endocarditis in high-risk clients by teaching them and their families the significance of prophylactic antibiotic treatment. Stucki and colleagues found that even after an educational program on the need for prophylaxis, 15% did not remember receiving such education and only 21% had not informed their dentist of their risk for IE.[6] Lynch states that these findings are not surprising considering the volume of information given when a heart lesion is diagnosed.[5] It is understandable that clients' recall of bacterial endocarditis prophylaxis might be poor.

Nurses are often in the ideal position to convey appropriate information to clients about their disease process and available prevention measures. Lynch and Estlow offer examples of teaching modules for promoting awareness of effective bacterial endocarditis prophylaxis in children.[4,5] The teaching package must be understandable, concise, and logical. Nurses possess the education necessary to provide teaching in the most effective manner with content based on the most current medical recommendations. This intervention can result in favorable outcomes such as decreased incidence of bacterial endocarditis, decreased cost for treatment through disease prevention, and decreased morbidity and mortality associated with the disease.

Further research is needed to compare client outcomes and prophylaxis compliance in clients who have received intense nursing instruction compared to those clients who have not had the benefit of such intervention. With the present cost constraints on health care services, research is also needed to quantify the cost-benefit for improved outcomes in preventing bacterial endocarditis when extensive teaching is provided to clients and their families.

Implications for nursing practice include the need to develop a structured program for education. Strong client teaching skills, allocation of adequate nursing hours to provide client teaching, and evaluation methods to measure client outcomes will validate the need for client education provided by qualified nurses.

REFERENCES

1. Taubert, K.A., & Dajani, A.S. (1998). Preventing bacterial endocarditis: American Heart Association guidelines. *American Family Physician, 57*(3), 457-469.
2. Dajani, A.S., et al. (1997). Prevention of bacterial endocarditis: Recommendations by the American Heart Association. *Journal of the American Medical Association, 277*(22), 1794-1801.
3. Durack, D.T. (1995). Prevention of infective endocarditis. *New England Journal of Medicine, 332*(1), 38-44.
4. Estlow, M.M. (1998). Prevention of infective endocarditis in the pediatric congenital heart population. *Pediatric Nursing, 24*(3), 205-212.
5. Lynch, L.I. (1999). A teaching module: Promoting awareness of effective bacterial endocarditis prophylaxis in children. *Pediatric Nursing, 25*(6), 621-626.
6. Stucki, C., Mury, R., & Bertel, O. (2003). Insufficient awareness of endocarditis prophylaxis in clients at risk. *Swiss Medicine Weekly, 133*(9-10), 155-159.
7. Moons, P., De Volder, E., Budts, W., et al. (2001). What do adult patients with congenital heart disease know about their disease, treatment and prevention of complications? A call for structured patient education. *Heart, 86*(1), 74-80.

Heart failure is treated with oral diuretics and a sodium-restricted diet. Digitalis is useful in clients with atrial fibrillation for slowing the ventricular heart rate. Beta-blockers may also decrease the heart rate and therefore increase exercise tolerance. Clients with premature atrial contractions (PACs) should be treated because PACs often precede atrial fibrillation. A client with untreated mitral stenosis can progress from having mild disability to severe disability in less than 10 years.

Mitral Regurgitation

The client should restrict physical activities that produce fatigue and dyspnea. Reducing sodium intake and promoting sodium excretion with diuretics can lessen the work of the heart. Nitrates, digitalis, and angiotensin-converting enzyme (ACE) inhibitors have brought about hemodynamic improvement and symptomatic relief in clients with chronic mitral regurgitation.

Mitral Valve Prolapse

Treatment of mitral valve prolapse depends on the manifestations. Beta-blockers are helpful in relieving syncope, palpitations, and chest pain. Aspirin can also help to prevent transient ischemic attacks. For preventing infective endocarditis, the client may receive antibiotics prophylactically before any invasive procedures are performed.

AORTIC VALVE DISEASE

The aortic valve is the last valve through which blood flows before entering systemic circulation. In aortic stenosis the orifice of the aortic valve becomes narrowed, which causes a decrease in the blood flow from the left ventricle into the aorta and systemic circulation. This obstruction to flow creates a resistance to ejection and increased pressure in the left ventricle. Aortic regurgitation (aortic insufficiency) allows blood to leak back from the aorta into the left ventricle. During systole blood that is ejected into the aorta reenters the left ventricle. To maintain normal pressures, the left ventricle hypertrophies. Both aortic stenosis and aortic regurgitation overwork the left ventricle. Aortic valve disease is far less common than mitral valve disease but often occurs in conjunction with mitral valve disease. A dilation of the ascending aorta, or aortic root disease, is also quite common.

Etiology and Risk Factors

Aortic stenosis can be caused by several congenital defects of the aortic valve and by two degenerative processes: (1) calcification of the valve in older adults and (2) retraction and stiffening of the valve from rheumatic fever. As the population in the United States ages, the incidence of aortic stenosis from calcification has been rising.

Aortic regurgitation is most often a result of infectious disorders such as rheumatic fever, syphilis, and infective endocarditis. Connective tissue disorders can also lead to aortic regurgitation. Acute aortic regurgitation is usually due to aortic dissection, bacterial endocarditis, or trauma, which may be either penetrating or blunt.

Pathophysiology

When aortic stenosis is present, the pressure within the left ventricle rises as the blood is ejected through the narrowed opening. A pressure gradient develops between the left ventricle and the aorta. The elevated pressure in the left ventricle during systole causes the ventricle to hypertrophy. Dilation of the left ventricle occurs over time when the contractility of the hypertrophied muscle deteriorates. Eventually dilation and hypertrophy of the left ventricle are unable to maintain adequate cardiac output, resulting in elevated left ventricular end-diastolic pressure, decreased cardiac output, and increased pulmonary hypertension (see Table 55-1).

Aortic regurgitation is a diastolic event in which blood that is propelled forward into the aorta regurgitates back into the left ventricle through an incompetent valve. The backward flow of blood causes abnormal filling and a volume overload of the left ventricle. The magnitude of the overload depends on the severity of the incompetence; however, a small incompetent area can result in significant aortic regurgitation over time.

Because the left ventricle receives blood from both the atrium and the systemic circulation, aortic regurgitation gradually increases left ventricular end-diastolic volume. Left ventricular stroke volume is increased to produce an effective forward-moving volume into the systemic circulation. Compensatory dilation of the left ventricle occurs, but the increase in left ventricular end-diastolic pressure is minimal.[1] The compensatory mechanisms of dilation and hypertrophy help to maintain an adequate cardiac output. As the condition progresses and the contractile state of the myocardium declines, however, cardiac output declines (see Table 55-1).

Clinical Manifestations
Aortic Stenosis

Clinical manifestations of aortic stenosis tend to occur gradually and late in the course of the disease. Usually a long latent period in which the client is asymptomatic occurs. Manifestations begin to appear as the obstruction and ventricular pressure increase to critical levels. Angina pectoris (chest pain) is a frequent finding in about 66% of clients. The character of the angina is similar to that in clients with coronary artery disease, and pain is commonly brought on by exertion and relieved by rest. Myocardial oxygen consumption is higher in clients with aortic stenosis because of the hypertrophy of the left ventricle, and this probably accounts for the angina.

Syncope, another common clinical manifestation, also occurs during exertion because of a fixed cardiac output during a period of increased demand. Syncope at rest may be due to dysrhythmias. Exertional dyspnea, paroxysmal nocturnal dyspnea, and pulmonary edema occur with increasing pulmonary venous hypertension attributable to left ventricular failure. In severe aortic stenosis, additional manifestations may include palpitations, fatigue, and visual disturbances. On auscultation the systolic murmur may be associated with a diminished second heart sound and an early ejection click. A systolic thrill is present over the aortic areas.

Aortic Regurgitation

Clients with chronic severe aortic regurgitation may be asymptomatic for a long time. During this time the left ventricle gradually enlarges. Clients may complain of an uncomfortable awareness of the heartbeat and palpitations because of the large left ventricular stroke volume with rapid diastolic runoff. Clients may also have prominent pulsations in the neck and even head-bobbing with each heartbeat. Sinus tachycardia or premature ventricular contractions may make palpitations more pronounced.

On physical examination, low systolic blood pressure may be due to the large stroke volume and a decreased diastolic blood pressure resulting from the regurgitation and distal runoff. Carotid artery pulsations may be exaggerated. The arterial pulse pressure widens, and palpable pulse amplitude increases, often noted as a sudden sharp pulse, followed by a swift collapse of the diastolic pulse (Corrigan's or water-hammer pulse). Auscultation reveals a soft, high-pitched, blowing decrescendo diastolic murmur heard best at the second right intercostal space and radiating to the left sternal border. Noninvasive assessment of clients with Doppler echocardiography should be performed at intervals.[1]

Medical Management

The goals of medical management are to maintain or improve cardiac function and activity tolerance. When the client reaches the maximum benefit from medications, surgery may be warranted. Aortic valve surgery may be necessary if angina or heart failure develops even though the client has been on medications.

Aortic Stenosis

Prophylactic antibiotics may be given on an individual basis for invasive medical or dental procedures for the prevention of infective endocarditis (see the Translating Evidence into Practice feature on Preventing Infective Endocarditis on p. 1388). Digitalis and diuretics usually used for ventricular failure must be used with caution because dehydration can reduce the cardiac output. Beta-blockers are not usually ordered because they can depress myocardial function and induce left ventricular failure. Cardiac dysrhythmias should be treated pharmacologically. With aortic stenosis, there is an associated gradual increase in the severity of obstruction that should be monitored with Doppler echocardiography. Advise clients with known or suspected critical obstruction of the aortic valve to avoid vigorous physical activity. Clients with mild obstruction may continue exercise if it is tolerated. For symptomatic clients, it is recommended that exercise stress-testing be avoided. The prognosis for clients with symptomatic aortic stenosis is poor without surgical intervention. The incidence of sudden death rises once myocardial failure develops.

Aortic Regurgitation

Medical intervention for aortic regurgitation is the same as that for aortic stenosis: relief of manifestations of heart failure and prevention of infection in the already deformed aortic cusps. Prompt surgical treatment is indicated when there is left ventricular failure. Death from pulmonary edema, ventricular dysrhythmias, electromechanical dissociation, or circulatory collapse is common in acute severe AR, even with intensive medical management. Early surgical intervention is recommended. Nitroprusside and possibly inotropic agents such as dopamine or dobutamine to augment forward flow and reduce LV end-diastolic pressure may be used temporarily before surgery. Intra-aortic balloon counterpulsation is contraindicated.

TRICUSPID AND PULMONIC VALVE DISEASE

Tricuspid stenosis, or regurgitation, usually develops from rheumatic fever or in combination with other structural disorders of the heart. Because the tricuspid valve is on the right side of the heart, the major hemodynamic alterations are decreased cardiac output and increased right atrial pressure. The inability of the right atrium to propel blood across the stenosed valve may account for these changes. With tricuspid regurgitation, the pressure in the right atrium is also elevated because of regurgitation of the blood volume in the right ventricle back into the right atrium during systole.

Clinical manifestations of tricuspid stenosis are dyspnea and fatigue, pulsations in the neck, and peripheral edema and weight loss. Physical assessment reveals prominent waves in the neck veins as the atrium vigorously contracts against the stenotic valve. A diastolic murmur is heard best along the left lower sternal border. The murmur increases with inspiration. The ECG reveals tall, tented P waves. Tricuspid insufficiency causes hepatic congestion and peripheral edema. Often atrial fibrillation is present, and jugular waves are evident. The murmur is holosystolic along the left sternal border.

Tricuspid stenosis usually responds well to diuretics and digitalis therapy. If the leaflets are severely stenotic, surgery may be required. Surgery for tricuspid regurgitation, however, may not be necessary unless pulmonary hypertension is present.

Abnormalities of the pulmonic valve are usually congenital defects. Few lesions develop after birth. Pulmonary hypertension, caused by mitral stenosis, pulmonary emboli, or chronic lung disease, can precipitate functional pulmonary regurgitation. Pulmonic stenosis and regurgitation lead to a decrease in cardiac output because blood does not reach the left side of the heart in adequate supply for metabolic demands. Pulmonic regurgitation may lead to dyspnea and fatigue. The murmur is a high-pitched diastolic blow along the left sternal border. No significant changes in the ECG are noted. Pulmonic stenosis causes similar clinical manifestations, but the murmur is often a crescendo-decrescendo type. Right-sided heart failure can also develop. Intervention focuses on treating the underlying cause and treating right-sided heart failure.

Nursing Management of the Medical Client

Nursing assessment should address the type, severity, and progress of the valvular disorder; the presence of fatigue; clinical manifestations of heart failure; heart rhythm (including ECG); vital signs; auscultation and palpation of the heart; the client's support systems; and the degree of knowledge that the client and the client's family have concerning the nature of and intervention in the disorder.

The main focus of nursing intervention in valvular heart disease is to help the client maintain a normal cardiac output, thereby preventing manifestations of heart failure, venous or pulmonary congestion, and inadequate tissue perfusion. To evaluate the effectiveness of therapeutic interventions, perform ongoing hemodynamic assessment. Monitor vital signs closely every 1 to 4 hours. A decrease in cardiac output is manifested in a compensatory rise in the heart rate, a drop in blood pressure, and/or a decrease in urine output. Carefully auscultate the chest every 4 hours to identify the presence of abnormal breath sounds (crackles, rhonchi), heart gallops (S_3, S_4) or new heart murmurs.

Self-Care

Clients with valvular heart disease require lifelong management. With a sincere desire to understand and accept each client's response to chronic illness, you can help these clients adapt to difficult lifestyle changes and achieve a positive sense of well-being.

Clients may find it difficult to cope physically and psychosocially after hospital discharge. The chronicity of valvular heart disease and its potential complications can create an atmosphere of uncertainty, fear, and frustration. Take time to help the client identify support people, personal strengths, and coping strategies. Assess how the client handles frustration or anger and which activities are particularly relaxing. Address the client's fears and misconceptions. In some cases counseling referrals may help. Stress the importance of follow-up physical examinations and intervention.

Before discharge prepare detailed teaching materials for the client and family concerning the therapeutic regimen, the disease process, factors contributing to manifestations, and the rationale for intervention. Give information about the prescribed medications. Frequently prescribed medications include digoxin, diuretics, beta-blockers, potassium supplements, anticoagulants, and sometimes prophylactic antibiotics. Explain their rationale, dosages, side effects, and special considerations in their use.

Review the exercise prescriptions with the client. Clients with aortic stenosis often require activity restrictions. The client should demonstrate ability to pace activity, verbalize improvement in fatigue, and accept activity restrictions.

Address dietary restrictions, and plan interdisciplinary follow-up. Make sure the client knows whom to call when questions arise.

Surgical Management

Valves can be reconstructed or replaced. Valve reconstruction can be accomplished if the preoperative assessment indicates that the valve is pliable. If the valve is not pliable, valve replacement is necessary. Indications for valve replacement include the following symptomatic clients:

1. Clients with progressive impairment of cardiac function caused by scarring and thickening of the valve with either impaired narrowing of the valvular opening (stenosis) or incomplete closure (insufficiency, regurgitation)
2. Clients with gradual enlargement of the heart with manifestations of decreased activity, shortness of breath, and heart failure.

Valve Repair Procedures

In clients with mitral regurgitation, valve reconstruction or annuloplasty may be done, which may include the use of a flexible ring that is sewn into the valve for stabilization. Aortic stenosis may be surgically treated with valve replacement or balloon aortic valvuloplasty. In the valvuloplasty procedure, a catheter with a balloon is used to dilate the valve orifice. Commissurotomy is used to repair the leaflets of a valve that have become fused at the base (or annulus).

Balloon Valvuloplasty

Sometimes it is possible to open the valves without resorting to open heart surgery. Balloon valvuloplasty is a procedure in which a narrowed heart valve is stretched open (Figure 55-1). The procedure is performed in a cardiac catheterization laboratory. The client is usually awake but given local anesthesia and sedation. A catheter is placed in the groin and threaded into the heart to measure pressures in the chambers and to gauge the disease in the valve. The first catheter is then withdrawn, and a second catheter which contains a guidewire is threaded into one of the branch pulmonary arteries.

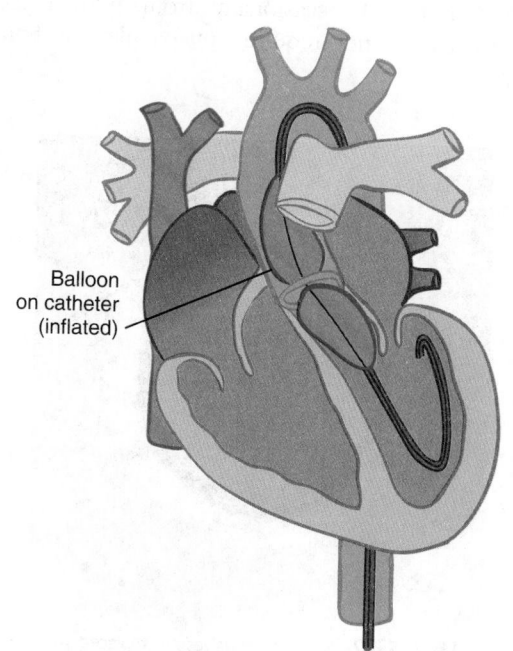

Balloon on catheter (inflated)

■ **FIGURE 55-1** Balloon valvuloplasty is a procedure used to stretch stenotic valves.

The purpose of the wire is to steady the catheter. The balloon catheter is then advanced into the heart and across the narrowed valve. The deflated balloon is positioned in the valve opening and then is inflated repeatedly. The inflated balloon widens the valve's opening by splitting the valve leaflets apart.

The main risk of stretching a mitral valve is for the valve to become severely leaky. A mild increase in the amount of leakage *(regurgitation)* is common with the procedure. In about 5% of clients, however, the valve becomes significantly leaky and will require replacement in 6 months. In about 2% of clients this is necessary as an emergency procedure during the valvuloplasty procedure.

Valve Replacement

Artificial heart valves are continuing to show improvements in design, safety, function, and durability. Mechanical and tissue prosthetic valves are available. The overall advantages and disadvantages of tissue and mechanical valves are almost equal. Mechanical valves are durable, but blood tends to clot on them, and anticoagulant therapy is therefore necessary. Fortunately, some of the newer artificial valves have reduced rates of thrombus formation. Some physicians recommend mechanical valves in clients younger than 65 or 70 years of age and tissue valves in clients 70 years or older. An artificial valve is shown in Figure 55-2. The type of valve prosthesis used is based on a number of considerations. The surgeon primarily considers (1) the durability of the valve and (2) the client's tolerance of anticoagulation. Therefore if the client has a preoperative history of bleeding or noncompliance with pharmacologic regimens, a tissue valve may be preferable.

Tissue valves are commonly from porcine (pig) or bovine (cow) and occasionally from human tissue. These valves do not require anticoagulation therapy, which makes them valuable for older clients, for women of childbearing age, and for clients who live in areas where anticoagulation monitoring is difficult. However, they are less durable. Tissue valves may degenerate or calcify or develop structural abnormalities. The rate of the tissue valve failure is 30% in 10 years, with the rate accelerating over the following 10 years.

Techniques for valve replacement can include the usual sternotomy approach. Advances in valvular surgery include the use of robotic techniques and minimally invasive surgery. Aortic valve replacement incisions are performed through a mini-sternotomy, in which an incision is made from the sternal notch to the third intercostal space. Mitral valve replacement/repair incisions are performed through a right parasternal incision in which small portions of the third and fourth costal cartilages are excised, a limited thoracotomy, or a partial sternotomy. These techniques reduce the size of the incisions and length of recovery. Nursing management of the client after heart surgery is discussed in Chapter 56.

CARDIOMYOPATHY

Cardiomyopathy is a broad term that includes subacute or chronic disorders of the myocardium. It is also used to refer to a group of systemic diseases and processes that are toxic to or alter the myocardium. There are three major types: dilated (congestive), hypertrophic, and restrictive (Figure 55-3). Although there have been several attempts to standardize the classification of the cardiomyopathies,

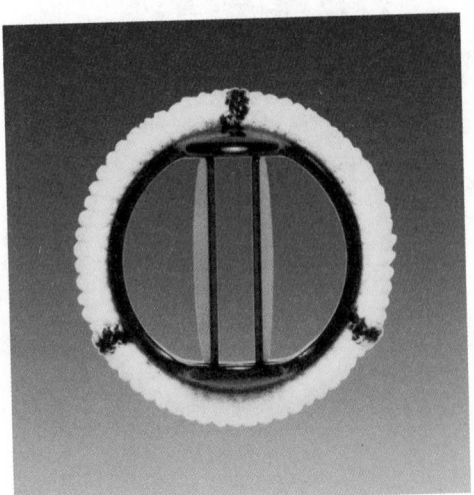

■ **FIGURE 55-2** Some heart valves are replaced with prosthetic ones. This is a St. Jude bileaflet mechanical valve. *(Courtesy St. Jude Medical, Inc., St. Paul, Minn.).*

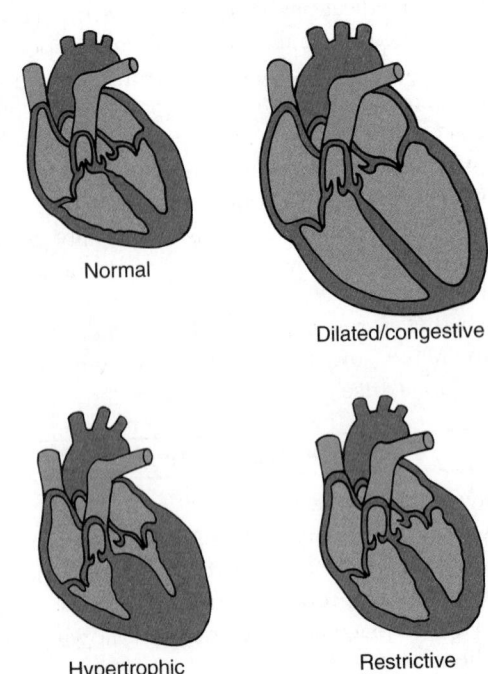

Normal

Dilated/congestive

Hypertrophic

Restrictive

■ **FIGURE 55-3** The three types of cardiomyopathy. The ventricle is enlarged and significantly reduces cardiac output.

the most widely recognized method was devised through a joint effort by the World Health Organization (WHO) and the International Society and Federation of Cardiology. Early research in animal models is being conducted in cardiac stem cell therapy for these clients.

The risk of cardiomyopathy increases in clients who chronically ingest excessive amounts of alcohol, are pregnant, have systemic hypertension, and have had some forms of infections. Table 55-2 compares the diagnostic data for the three types of cardiomyopathy. These forms of cardiomyopathy are described separately.

DILATED CARDIOMYOPATHY

Dilated cardiomyopathy is characterized by ventricular dilation, contractile dysfunction, and heart failure. It is the most common form, seen in about 60% of all cases. This form of cardiomyopathy has also been called hypertrophic subaortic stenosis, idiopathic hypertrophic subaortic stenosis, and asymmetrical septal hypertrophy. Some forms of dilated cardiomyopathy are idiopathic. Other causes include viral myocarditis, infections, metabolic problems, toxins, pregnancy, neuromuscular disorders, connective tissue disorders, and genetic predisposition (20% of cases).

In dilated cardiomyopathy usually both the left and right ventricles dilate, the myocardial fibers degenerate, and fibrotic tissue replaces viable tissue. Fibrotic tissue is not pliable, which leads to reduced contractility and decreased stroke volume and low cardiac output, with a compensatory increase in heart rate. These changes eventually lead to heart failure accompanied by lethal ventricular dysrhythmias. The combination of ventricular dilation and ineffective myocardial contractility also increases the risk of blood pooling within the heart and subsequent clot formation. Many clients (75%) with idiopathic dilated cardiomyopathy die within 5 years after the onset of manifestations. Spontaneous rapid improvement occurs in some women and early fatality in others. The clinical manifestations of dilated cardiomyopathy are presented in Table 55-2.

OUTCOME MANAGEMENT

Treatment is similar to that for heart failure, including diuretics and sodium-restricted diets, angiotensin-converting enzyme inhibition, and beta-adrenergic blocking agents. Digoxin is also used and because of its narrow window of therapeutic index, the serum level must be closely monitored, keeping the range between 0.5 and 0.8 ng/ml. Inotropic agents are used to enhance myocardial contractility and to unload the heart. Nitroglycerin as a vasodilator can be used to decrease preload and afterload. Anticoagulants may help to prevent clots and emboli. Antidysrhythmic agents may help suppress ventricular irritability. In appropriate candidates implantation of the automatic internal cardiac defibrillator may be used to prevent sudden cardiac death.

Rest improves cardiac function. During the early stages, most clients find it difficult to accept rigidly imposed restrictions on activity. Clients should avoid poorly

TABLE 55–2 Findings in the Three Types of Cardiomyopathy		
Dilated	**Restrictive**	**Hypertrophic**
Manifestations		
Heart failure, particularly left sided Fatigue and weakness Systemic or pulmonary emboli	Dyspnea, fatigue Right-sided heart failure manifestations of systemic disease (e.g., amyloidosis, iron storage disease)	Dyspnea, angina pectoris Fatigue, syncope, palpitations
Physical Examination		
Moderate to severe cardiomegaly: S_3 and S_4 Atrioventricular valve regurgitation, especially mitral	Mild to moderate cardiomegaly: S_3 or S_4 Atrioventricular valve regurgitation; inspiratory increase in venous pressure (Kussmaul's sign)	Mild cardiomegaly Apical systolic thrill and heave; brisk carotid upstroke; S_4 common Systolic murmur that increases with Valsalva maneuver
Chest X-ray Study		
Moderate to marked cardiac enlargement, especially left ventricle Pulmonary venous hypertension	Mild cardiac enlargement Pulmonary venous hypertension	Mild to moderate cardiac enlargement Paroxysmal nocturnal dyspnea Left atrial enlargement
Electrocardiogram		
Sinus tachycardia Atrial and ventricular dysrhythmias ST-segment and T-wave abnormalities Intraventricular conduction defects	Low voltage Intraventricular conduction defects Atrioventricular conduction defects	Left ventricular hypertrophy ST-segment and T-wave abnormalities Abnormal Q waves Atrial and ventricular dysrhythmias

Modified from Zipes, D. (2005). *Braunwald's heart disease: A textbook of cardiovascular medicine* (7th ed.). Philadelphia: Saunders.

tolerated activities. Advise clients that physical and emotional stress exacerbate the disease. Most clients experience severe activity intolerance during the later stages of the disease, which automatically limits their activities. Because alcohol depresses myocardial contractility, the client should abstain from drinking alcoholic beverages.

Only transplantation and specific vasodilator therapy (hydralazine plus nitrates) have resulted in prolonged life. Heart transplantation shows a 5-year survival of greater than 70% in appropriately selected clients.

HYPERTROPHIC CARDIOMYOPATHY

The disproportionate thickening of the interventricular septum in hypertrophic cardiomyopathy leads to wall rigidity and thereby increases resistance to blood flow from the left atrium. There is also obstruction of left ventricular outflow. In its severest form, the left ventricular wall reaches tremendous dimensions and encroaches on the left ventricular chamber, which becomes small and elongated. Septal hypertrophy may obstruct the left ventricular outflow tract during systole. Frequently diastolic dysfunction in the form of stiffness of the left ventricle occurs during diastolic filling. This stiffness raises left ventricular end-diastolic pressure, which eventually results in elevation of left atrial, pulmonary venous, and pulmonary capillary pressures.

Hypertrophic cardiomyopathy appears to be a genetically transmitted disease (approximately 50% of cases).[10] It can also be idiopathic, caused by hypertension or hypoparathyroidism. It appears most often in young adults, both men and women.

The clinical manifestations most commonly manifest in late adolescence or early adulthood but may appear at any age. Many clients with hypertrophic cardiomyopathy are asymptomatic and can lead long lives. They often have relatives with incapacitating manifestations of the disease. Sadly, sudden death is frequently the first clinical manifestation of the disease in asymptomatic clients. Sudden death appears more often in younger clients (i.e., less than 30 years of age, family history of sudden death, genetic abnormalities, and syncope, especially in children) and, if the presence of the disease is known, may be avoided by elimination of strenuous exercise. Clients who carry a high risk for sudden death should be considered and evaluated to receive an implantable cardioverter defibrillator (ICD).

The most common manifestation is dyspnea, which occurs in up to 90% of clients.[8] Dyspnea is due to the high pulmonary pressures produced by the elevated left ventricular end-diastolic pressure. Table 55-1 presents the remainder of clinical manifestations.

OUTCOME MANAGEMENT

The goals of intervention for hypertrophic cardiomyopathy are to alleviate manifestations, prevent complications, and reduce the risk of sudden death. Clients with hypertrophic cardiomyopathy should be evaluated using a full history and physical examination, a two-dimensional echocardiography, a 24- to 48-hour ambulatory Holter monitor evaluation, and treadmill or bicycle exercise testing.[11] These goals can be accomplished by reducing ventricular contractility and relieving left ventricular outflow obstruction. Beta-adrenergic blocking agents and calcium channel blocking medications reduce the heart rate, which lowers the myocardial contractility and oxygen consumption and prevents dysrhythmias. With decreased vigor of ventricular contraction, outflow obstruction diminishes. Beta-adrenergic blockade also reduces the heart rate (which further reduces myocardial workload) and prevents dysrhythmias.

Medications that decrease preload (e.g., nitrates, diuretics, morphine) and that increase contractility (e.g., isoproterenol, dopamine, digitalis) should be avoided. Currently, it has not been established whether asymptomatic clients should receive drug therapy because adequate controlled studies are not available.[12-14] Anticoagulants are used if the client is in atrial fibrillation. The client is at risk for endocarditis and should follow the prophylactic care for that condition. Alcohol should be avoided because its vasodilation properties can exacerbate an outflow problem.

RESTRICTIVE CARDIOMYOPATHY

Restrictive cardiomyopathy is the least common of the three clinically recognized and described cardiomyopathies. Its principal abnormality is diastolic dysfunction. Differentiation from constrictive pericarditis, a clinically similar entity, is difficult but important because the treatment options and prognosis differ drastically. Any infiltrative process of the heart that results in fibrosis and thickening can cause restrictive cardiomyopathy. The most frequently associated disease is amyloidosis (deposition of eosinophilic fibrous protein in the heart). Other disorders include glycogen storage disease, hemochromatosis, and sarcoidosis. Fibrotic infiltrations into the myocardium, endocardium, and subendocardium cause the ventricles to lose their ability to stretch. The excessively rigid ventricular walls impair filling during diastole; however, contractility with systole is usually normal. Filling pressures increase, and cardiac output falls. Eventually cardiac failure and mild ventricular hypertrophy occur. As cardiac output falls and intraventricular pressures rise, manifestations of heart failure appear. Table 55-1 presents the clinical manifestations. In severe or end-stage restrictive cardiomyopathy, the clinical manifestations are almost indistinguishable from those for chronic constrictive pericarditis. It is important to distinguish between the two problems because surgery can be used to treat cardiomyopathy.

OUTCOME MANAGEMENT

At present no specific interventions have been established for restrictive cardiomyopathy. Intervention aims at diminishing heart failure using pacemakers, diuretics, vasodilators, and salt restrictions to accomplish this goal. Digitalis may also help in some forms of restrictive cardiomyopathy. Clients with restrictive cardiomyopathy often have dysrhythmias that are refractory to antidysrhythmic drugs. These clients may benefit from a permanent pacemaker. Clients who carry a high risk for sudden death should be considered and evaluated to receive an implantable cardioverter defibrillator (ICD). Death attributable to dysrhythmia may occur suddenly, or a more progressive course may be followed by eventual, intractable heart failure. Candidates with intractable heart failure have been selected to undergo heart or heart-lung transplantation; unfortunately, however, recurrent sarcoid involvement can occur in the transplanted heart. The prognosis depends largely on the underlying cause. Unfortunately, intervention rarely results in long-term improvement.

Nursing management of the client with dilated cardiomyopathy is outlined in the Care Plan feature on The Client with Dilated Cardiomyopathy on the website. In addition, clients who are acutely or chronically ill with cardiomyopathy require strong psychosocial support. The uncertain and serious consequences of the disease create fear and anxiety. The chronic nature of the disorder can deplete coping resources, leaving clients with feelings of helplessness and hopelessness. As physical capabilities diminish, feelings of inadequacy, frustration, and poor self-esteem grow. Clients may become irritable, angry, withdrawn, or dependent.

Even though the prognosis is often poor, you can help clients who suffer from this debilitating disorder to maintain hope and dignity. Encouragement, a caring touch, a listening ear, and attainable goals can promote a high quality of life. Create an environment in which clients can openly express concerns and acknowledge fears. Acceptance, empathy, and kindness can help clients with cardiomyopathies to adopt more successful coping strategies.

Self-Care

With hypertrophic cardiomyopathy, syncope or sudden death may follow physical exertion. Therefore warn the client with hypertrophic cardiomyopathy to avoid strenuous physical exercise such as running or active competitive sports. In addition, encourage household members to learn cardiopulmonary resuscitation (CPR). Although chest pain often accompanies this disease, nitroglycerin can worsen the obstruction; clinicians can therefore treat chest pain with reduced activity and beta-blocking agents.

Hypertrophic cardiomyopathy predisposes the client to the risk of infective endocarditis. Advise clients **with this cardiomyopathy to check with their physician about taking prophylactic antibiotics before and after dental and surgical procedures because American Heart Association guidelines have changed.[19]**

All clients with cardiomyopathy need clear, honest education concerning the disease and its cause and intervention. Both you and the client must be watchful for adverse effects of therapy. Clients with restrictive cardiomyopathy are especially vulnerable to the toxic effects of digitalis (see Chapter 56).

Surgical Management

Surgical procedures have been developed for hypertrophic cardiomyopathy procedures to reduce the outflow gradient. Myotomy is the surgical incision into or resection of a portion of the ventricular septum. The excision of fibrotic endocardium is successful in a limited number of clients with restrictive cardiomyopathy. Surgical ablation can reduce some dysrhythmias.

Heart Transplantation

Cardiac transplantation is now a standard and effective treatment for clients with end-stage cardiac disease.
In 2005, 2125 hearts were transplanted in the United States. About 80% of clients with heart transplants are still living 2 years after the operation. While the benefits are obvious to the recipient, finding a donor can be difficult because the healthy heart must come from a fresh cadaver. Outcomes of heart transplantation depend on how quickly the transplant can be performed once a donor is found. There is a 10% to 20% death rate for clients on the waiting list. As of 2006, 84% to 86% of heart transplant clients survived 1 year and 74% to 78% survived 3 years. (Survival differs by gender; woman have lower survival rates.) Heart transplant recipients who die after the procedure usually do so within the first 30 days postoperatively.

Potential candidates must be evaluated and screened. Their cardiac status is evaluated to determine the need for the heart transplant. The candidates are also evaluated for underlying conditions that predispose to an unfavorable outcome. Box 55-1 shows the selection criteria for heart transplantation

The current orthotopic technique retains a large portion of the right and left atrium in the recipient and implants the donor heart to the atria (Figure 55-4). Cardiopulmonary bypass is used during the operation (see Chapter 56). Temporary pacemaker wires and chest drainage catheters are inserted.

The newly transplanted heart does not have a vagus nerve or sympathetic nerve fibers. Increases or decreases in cardiac output are due to changes in the venous return causing changes in the stretch of the heart muscle. Therefore the client has a subnormal capacity for exercise. The clients can usually perform

SAFETY

⚠

ALERT

BOX 55-1   **Indications and Contraindications for Heart Transplant**

INDICATIONS

- New York Heart Association (NYHA) class III or IV symptoms
- Dilated cardiomyopathy
- Ischemic cardiomyopathy
- Ejection fraction of less than 25%
- Intractable angina or malignant cardiac dysrhythmias for which conventional therapy has been exhausted
- Age younger than 65 years
- Pulmonary vascular resistance less than 2 Wood's units
- Ability to comply with medical follow-up care

CONTRAINDICATIONS

- Lack of indications
- Active systemic infection
- Active systemic disease such as collagen vascular disease or sickle cell disease
- Active malignancies; clients with malignancies who have been tumor free for 3 to 5 years may be considered depending upon the type of cancer
- An ongoing history of substance abuse (e.g., alcohol, drugs, tobacco)
- Psychosocial instability

---

activities of daily living and at least moderate exercise and probably most importantly enjoy an excellent quality of life. Without nerves, the client cannot experience angina in response to cardiac ischemia or infarction. Instead they will experience dyspnea or dysrhythmias. Treatment of dysrhythmias does not include medications in these clients.

Assisted Circulation and Mechanical Hearts

About 2600 clients in the United States are waiting to receive a heart transplant, but only about 2100 donated hearts are received each year. Clients who are waiting for a heart donor and transplant are at great risk of dying before a heart becomes available. During this waiting period, a ventricular assist device (VAD) may be inserted to keep these clients alive, as explained in the Bridge to Critical Care feature on p. 1397. These high-tech machines help the failing heart to pump blood throughout the body, bridging the time until a donor heart becomes available. In some cases the machine allows the heart to rest and recover so that the VAD can be removed and the client no longer needs a transplant.

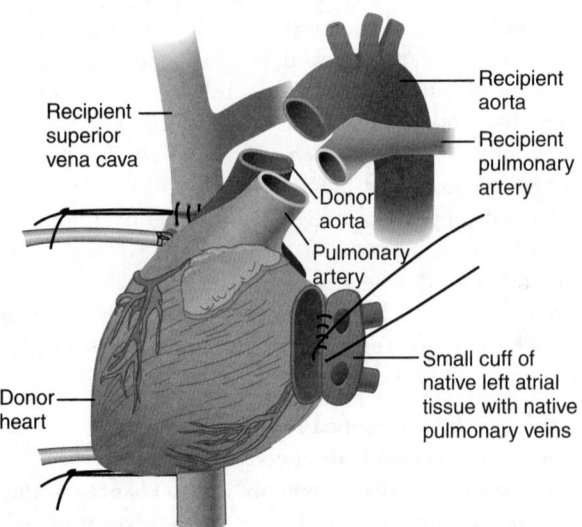

■ **FIGURE 55–4**   During heart transplantation, all but the posterior walls of the atrium are removed. The donor heart is sewn into place.

Recipient superior vena cava

Recipient aorta

Recipient pulmonary artery

Donor aorta

Pulmonary artery

Donor heart

Small cuff of native left atrial tissue with native pulmonary veins

Management of the Surgical Client

Management of the postoperative client is discussed in Chapter 56. The client will receive immunosuppressant medications, commonly cyclosporine, prednisone, and tacrolimus. Drug therapy is adjusted to give the maximum amount of immunosuppression with the minimum amount of side effects using an individualistic regimen. The risk of acute rejection is highest soon after transplantation and decreases dramatically after 3 months. Even with this intensive regimen, almost all heart transplant recipients experience some acute rejection during the first postoperative year. The most reliable technique for assessing organ rejection is the endomyocardial biopsy, which enables identification of the diffuse interstitial infiltrate associated with rejection.

INFECTIOUS DISORDERS

Bacteria and other microbes are found in abundance in our environment. Because the heart valves do not actually receive any blood supply of their own, which may be surprising given their location, defense mechanisms (such as leukocytes) cannot enter. Therefore if an organism infiltrates the valves, the body cannot combat it. Normally, blood flows smoothly through these valves but if they have been damaged, bacteria have a chance to thrive.

RHEUMATIC FEVER

Rheumatic fever (RF) is a diffuse inflammatory disease characterized by a delayed response to an infection by group A beta-hemolytic streptococci (GAS) in the tonsillopharyngeal area. RF is classified as a collagen-vascular disease or connective tissue disease. Many organs are involved through these rheumatic processes, including the heart, the joints, and the central nervous system. This process is caused by an inflammatory reaction. Although

BRIDGE TO CRITICAL CARE

Left Ventricular Assist Devices

INDICATIONS

- Transplant-ready clients who are in danger of dying before a donor heart is available
- Heart failure not responsive to standard cardiac treatments
- Heart failure following various forms of heart surgery

DEVICES

Consist of a pump, which is implanted in the abdominal wall and connected to the left ventricle of the heart. Although the ventricle may be too weak to pump blood to the entire body, the pump draws blood from the ventricle and, in turn, propels it out to the rest of the body.

Pneumatic: External pulsatile pump that propels blood.

Electric: An electrical line attached to the device connects to a portable, external controller, which fits onto the client's belt and operates and monitors the pump. Clients carry reserve battery packs on their belt or shoulder bag so they can change the batteries every 3 to 4 hours, a procedure like changing the batteries in a cell phone.

PLACEMENT

The surgeon connects the VAD to the bottom of the heart and the main heart artery (aorta). Blood then flows into the heart and out of the aorta by means of a small electrically or pneumatically driven motor that is part of the VAD. A tube is passed through the client's skin. The tube connects to a controller and a battery pack that the client wears or carries. This allows the client to be fully mobile with the device in place.

COMPLICATIONS

- Infection, especially pneumonia related to immobility
- Bleeding from anticoagulant use
- Right-sided heart failure
- Thromboembolism
- Device malfunction

NURSING PRECAUTIONS

- Monitor cardiac output and hemodynamic status.
- Perform range-of-motion exercises to maintain muscle strength and joint flexibility.
- Monitor lung sounds; suction secretions from airway or assist client to deep breathe and cough.
- Monitor level of anticoagulation, especially during weaning.
- Monitor for specific device-related problems.
- Educate about how to change batteries, reportable problems if client is ambulatory.

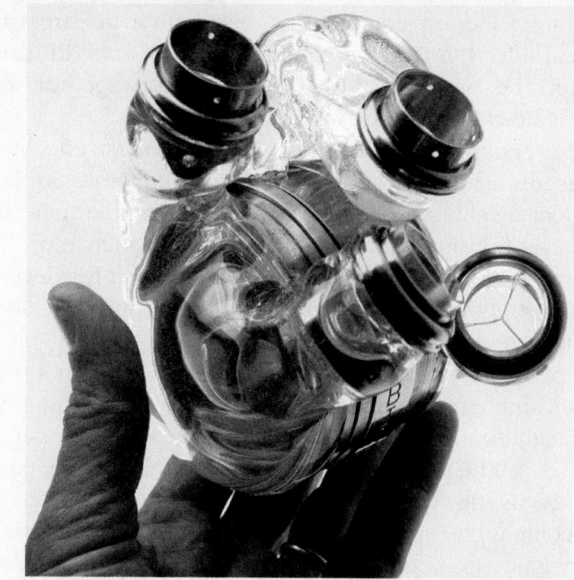

AbioCor pump.

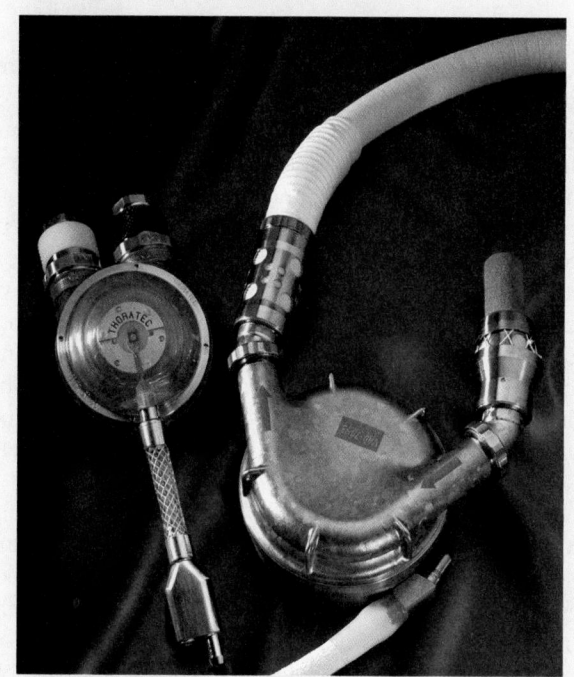

HeartMate left ventricular assist device.

Data from Mahmood, A.K., et al. (2000). Critical review of current left ventricular assist devices. *Perfusion, 15*(399), 420-432.

this infection remains common, the incidence of RF has declined dramatically to about 2 per 100,000 people in the United States. This decline is due to an emphasis on prevention. The incidence in developing countries is about 100 per 100,000 people.

Etiology and Risk Factors

Rheumatic fever develops in only a relatively small percentage of people (3%), even after a virulent bout of streptococcal infection; there is therefore some evidence of host predisposition. There is also a familial predisposition to the disease. Once RF is acquired, the client becomes more susceptible than the general population to recurrent infection. Poor hygiene, crowding, and poverty are risk factors for acute RF. If appropriate antibiotic therapy for group A beta-hemolytic streptococcal infection is given within the first 9 days, RF can usually be prevented. The most common age for an initial attack of RF is between 6 and 15 years.

Prevention is the best treatment. The most effective measures against RF are probably socioeconomic. In the affluent neighborhoods of Western cities, where there is spacious housing with no crowding, the incidence of RF is low. Certain populations are at a higher risk for developing streptococcal pharyngitis. These groups include military recruits, people living in crowded conditions, and people in close contact with school-age children. Both males and females have the same incidence for acquiring RF. Identification of high-risk people is also important. Nurses can help to identify mitral valve prolapse (see earlier discussion) early to prevent valvular disease. Nurses in community settings can identify those with beta-hemolytic streptococcal infections and refer clients for appropriate diagnosis and medical management.

Pathophysiology

Rheumatic fever initiates a diffuse, proliferative, and exudative inflammatory process involving all layers of the heart, joints, subcutaneous tissue, central nervous system (CNS), and skin. Although the cellular disease process is not clear, the mechanism is probably an abnormal humoral and cell-mediated response to streptococcal cell membrane antigens. There is a positive correlation that links group A streptococci as the causative agent for initial and recurrent attacks of RF. These antigens bind to receptors on the heart, other tissues, and joints, which begins the autoimmune response. The inflammatory process often produces permanent and severe heart damage. Complications of RF include valvular disorders, cardiomegaly, and heart failure.

All layers of the heart swell, a condition called carditis. Necrosis develops in areas of inflamed myocardium, called Aschoff's bodies. These areas are minuscule nodules with localized fibrin deposits surrounded by areas of necrosis in the myocardium. Endocardial inflammation causes swelling of the valve leaflets, which leads to valve dysfunction and murmurs. Small bacterial vegetations form on the valve tissues. Rough eroded areas of the valves attract platelets, which adhere and form platelet-fibrin clumps that eventually scar and shorten the valve. The valves lose their elasticity, and cardiac function is impaired. After a latent period of about 3 weeks following a group A streptococcal infection, the clinical manifestations of acute rheumatic fever are evident.

First, the damaged valve may become scarred and stenosed, increasing the cardiac workload because higher pressure must be generated to propel blood through the narrow valve. Second, the valve leaflets may become so short that they cannot close securely. As a result blood regurgitates backwards from the damaged valve. Both valvular stenosis and regurgitation eventually cause heart failure from the high workload.

Clinical Manifestations

The clinical manifestations of rheumatic fever are related to the inflammatory response and can last about 3 months.

Major manifestations include the following:

- Carditis is the most destructive consequence of RF. It is present in at least 50% of clients with acute RF and is the most specific manifestation of RF. Characteristics include a significant murmur, cardiomegaly, pericarditis that produces a significant friction rub, and heart failure. Chest pain resulting from pericardial inflammation may be present. Sometimes myocardial involvement produces atrioventricular (AV) conduction defects (first-degree AV block) or atrial fibrillation.
- Arthritis, the most common finding of RF, is painful and migratory. It most often affects the larger joints, such as the ankles, knees, elbows, shoulders, and wrists. The arthritis may or may not be symmetrical. If the client takes aspirin early in the course of the disease, arthritis manifestations may not be as apparent. Joint manifestations may last hours or days. Arthritis that is not treated usually lasts 2 to 3 weeks. RF-associated arthritis has a good response to salicylates.
- Chorea, a disorder of the basal ganglia and caudate nuclei, is a late manifestation of RF, usually appearing 3 months or longer after the streptococcal infection. Chorea, which is from the Greek word for movement and the origin of the word choreography, is manifested by sudden, irregular, aimless involuntary movements. The client may also have emotional lability. Chorea disappears without treatment and produces no permanent sequelae. Chorea may disappear during sleep and be more prevalent when the client is awake and/or under stress.
- Erythema marginatum is an unusual rash that is seen primarily on the trunk. The application of heat may induce this rash. The lesions are crescent-shaped and have clear centers. The rash is transitory and its appearance may change in minutes or hours. This rash is a distinctive feature of RF; however, it is rare.
- Subcutaneous nodules are small, painless, firm yet freely mobile nodules that adhere loosely to the tendon sheaths, especially in knees, knuckles, and elbows. They are usually evident only during the first week or two and generally only in children.

Minor manifestations include the following:

- Fever, with a temperature of 38° C (100.4° F) or higher, alternates with normal temperature. Weakness, malaise, weight loss, and anorexia probably develop as a result of fever, pain, and the general debilitation associated with serious illness. When only a single major manifestation is present, fever is used to support the diagnosis of RF. There is no distinguishing pattern to these fevers in the acute phase of RF.

■ A positive throat culture for group A beta-hemolytic streptococci can help to confirm the diagnosis. An elevated white blood cell (WBC) count, erythrocyte sedimentation rate (ESR), and C-reactive protein level may indicate inflammation. An ECG or echocardiogram can help to confirm rhythm problems and structural changes.

The diagnosis is made by the presence of major manifestations; the Jones criteria (Box 55-2) and abnormal laboratory findings are used to make the diagnosis. Not many clients with acute RF have a positive throat culture for group A streptococci. Therefore anti-streptococcal antibody titers are drawn to determine if a recent streptococcal infection has been present.

OUTCOME MANAGEMENT

Medical Management

The goals of medical management include (1) eradicating infection, (2) maximizing cardiac output, and (3) promoting comfort.

BOX 55-2 Jones' Criteria for the Diagnosis of Rheumatic Fever*

MAJOR MANIFESTATIONS
1. Carditis
2. Polyarthritis
3. Chorea
4. Erythema marginatum
5. Subcutaneous nodules

MINOR MANIFESTATIONS
1. Clinical findings
   a. Previous rheumatic fever or rheumatic heart disease
   b. Arthralgia
   c. Fever
2. Laboratory findings
   a. Elevated acute phase reactants
      (1) Erythrocyte sedimentation rate
      (2) C-reactive protein
      (3) Leukocytosis
   b. Prolonged P-R interval

EVIDENCE OF GROUP A STREPTOCOCCAL INFECTION
1. Positive throat culture for Strep A
2. Elevated or rising anti-streptococcal antibody titer
3. Recent scarlet fever

In some instances, rheumatic fever can be diagnosed without fulfillment of Jones' criteria.
Modified from Special Writing Group of the American Heart Association. (1992). Guidelines for the diagnosis of rheumatic fever: Jones criteria. 1992 update. *Journal of the American Heart Association, 268*(15), 2069-2072.

Eradicate Infection

The first priority is to eradicate the streptococcal infection. At the time of diagnosis of RF, only a few clients will still have throat cultures positive for streptococcal infection. This is because of the elimination of the organism by the host before manifestations of RF appear. Penicillin or erythromycin is usually prescribed for 10 days even if the cultures are negative. The client typically takes prophylactic agents for rheumatic fever for 5 years after the initial attack. After 5 years, recurrences are rare and prophylaxis continues only in high-risk clients. Clients who have had rheumatic fever remain vulnerable to bacterial endocarditis. Therefore in addition to the antibiotics they take to prevent rheumatic fever recurrence, they must be referred for evaluation for possible prophylactic medications before and after any surgical procedure or dental work. Specific evaluation for prophylaxis medication must be individualized according to recommendations by the American Heart Association. (See the Translating Evidence into Practice feature on Preventing Infective Endocarditis on p. 1388.)

Maximize Cardiac Output

Corticosteroids are used to treat carditis, especially if heart failure is evident. If heart failure develops, treatment, including ACE inhibitors, beta blockers, and diuretics, is effective.

Promote Comfort

Clients with arthritic manifestations obtain clinical relief with salicylates; however, because these drugs can result in a misdiagnosis, a firm diagnosis should be in place before salicylates are given. Bed rest is usually prescribed to reduce cardiac effort until evidence of inflammation has subsided. For clients with rheumatic valvular heart disease, bacterial endocarditis prophylaxis may be necessary (see Infective Endocarditis).

Nursing Management of the Medical Client

Assessment. Nursing assessment involves gathering baseline and ongoing subjective and objective data. Obtain baseline vital signs, assess the heart for a friction rub and the lungs for crackles, and palpate peripheral pulses. A baseline ECG is used to determine whether heart block is present. Assess baseline nutritional and hydration data. Continue to reassess vital signs to determine the patterns of fever and the stability of blood pressure. Vital signs are also used as a measure of activity tolerance.

Assess psychosocial data about the client's feelings regarding restrictions of activity, support systems, coping strategies, level of discomfort, and knowledge (both the client and the client's family) concerning the nature of, and intervention for, rheumatic fever.

Diagnosis, Outcomes, Interventions

Diagnosis: Activity Intolerance. A reduced cardiac reserve and enforced bed rest can quickly lead to activity intolerance. The nursing diagnosis statement would be *Activity Intolerance related to reduced cardiac reserve and enforced bed rest.*

Outcomes. The client will have improved tolerance of activity and progress toward an optimal level of physical activity tolerance based on underlying cardiovascular status and psychosocial readiness as evidenced by the ability to (1) steadily increase activity level to include climbing one flight of stairs without chest pain or without ECG changes, while the heart rate remains under 90 beats/min; (2) verbalize improvement in fatigue; (3) express acceptance of any imposed activity restrictions; and (4) pace activities.

Interventions. Bed rest is important in the acute phase because it reduces myocardial oxygen demand and usually continues until the following criteria are met:

- Temperature remains normal without use of salicylates.
- Resting pulse rate remains less than 100 beats/min.
- ECG tracings show no manifestations of myocardial damage.
- ESR returns to normal.
- Pericardial friction rub is not present.

Once ambulatory, the client must still refrain from overexertion. Assess the client's stamina and response to exercise to gauge the degree of gradual activity progression.

SAFETY ⚠ **ALERT**
Assess vital signs before and after exercise. After 3 to 5 minutes of rest, reassess vital signs. They should have returned to baseline within 3 minutes of cessation of exercise. The client should reduce or discontinue activity if chest pain, vertigo, dyspnea, confusion, a drop in blood pressure, an irregular pulse or abnormal heart rate develops.

The length of activity restriction depends on whether carditis develops and on the extent of permanent heart damage. Restrictions may extend for months. In severe cases of rheumatic carditis, clients may be forced to undergo restrictions on a permanent basis. Encourage a gradual increase in activity within the limits of the client's condition.

The client experiencing chorea requires sedatives, bed rest, and protection from self-injury. A carefully planned and supervised activity schedule should be maintained and evaluated.

Diagnosis: Chronic Pain. The inflammatory response in the joints can lead to pain. The nursing diagnosis statement would be *Chronic Pain related to the inflammatory response in the joints.*

Outcomes. The client will experience increased comfort as evidenced by (1) reports of reduced discomfort, (2) expression of joint pain reduction, (3) reduced use of pain medications, (4) a relaxed body posture and a calm facial expression, and (5) ability to sleep.

Interventions. Obtain a clear description of the pain or discomfort. Identify the source of greatest discomfort as a focus for intervention. Administer analgesics as needed and use salicylates around the clock. Balance rest and activity according to the degree of pain and activity tolerance. Other pain interventions are discussed in Chapter 20.

Diagnosis: Imbalanced Nutrition: Less Than Body Requirements. Hypermetabolism seen with fever and inflammation and other factors in rheumatic fever can lead to protein-calorie malnutrition. This nursing diagnosis is stated as *Imbalanced Nutrition: Less Than Body Requirements, related to fever, inflammation, anorexia, and fatigue.*

Outcomes. The client will maintain or restore adequate nutritional balance as evidenced by (1) the resumption of pre-illness body weight or no further weight loss, (2) consumption of 75% or more of each meal served, (3) normal serum albumin or prealbumin levels, and (4) increasing energy and stamina.

Interventions. A high-protein, high-carbohydrate diet helps maintain adequate nutrition in the presence of fever and infection. Hypermetabolic states (fever and infection) can induce a catabolic state, thus delaying healing. Vitamin and mineral supplements may also benefit the client. Oral hygiene every 4 hours; small, attractive meal servings; and foods that are not overly rich, sweet, or greasy stimulate the appetite. Adequate fluid intake prevents dehydration resulting from fever. If the client shows manifestations of severe carditis or heart failure, sodium and fluids must be restricted. Daily weights can serve as an indication of nutritional and fluid status.

Diagnosis: Risk for Ineffective Therapeutic Regimen Management (Individuals). Following rheumatic fever, the client must follow a lifelong regimen to reduce the risk of rheumatic heart disease. This nursing diagnosis is stated as *Risk for Ineffective Therapeutic Regimen Management (Individuals) related to a need for lifelong therapy.*

Outcomes. The client and the client's family will demonstrate adequate knowledge of rheumatic fever and its ability to lead to rheumatic heart disease including the need to complete the entire course of antibiotics; consuming adequate calories, protein, and fluids; and the rationale for lifelong prevention.

Interventions. Today streptococcal infections do not have to develop into rheumatic fever if the client seeks immediate assessment and begins antibiotics. Clients who have recovered from an episode of rheumatic fever can avoid subsequent attacks by taking prophylactic doses of antibiotics and observing good health practices. Because repeated attacks may lead to serious heart disease and permanent cardiac disability, it is important to emphasize means of avoiding subsequent attacks.

Instruct the client about how to reduce exposure to streptococcal infection as follows:

1. Take good care of the teeth and gums, and obtain prompt dental care for cavities and gingivitis. Prophylactic medication may be needed before invasive dental procedures, and individualized evaluation for prophylaxis medication is needed.
2. Avoid people who have an upper respiratory tract infection or who have had a recent streptococcal infection.
3. Notify the physician if any manifestations of streptococcal sore throat *(pharyngitis)* develop. It is extremely important to begin antibiotic therapy promptly for any infection. The clinical manifestations include fever (102° to 104° F, 38.8° to 40° C), chills, sore throat, and enlarged, painful lymph nodes. Advise clients who have had rheumatic fever that they must guard against infections for the rest of their lives to avoid development of heart disease.

Evaluation. Rheumatic fever is treated over 10 days. Expect activity tolerance to improve once fever and pain are controlled. Altered nutrition may require more than 2 weeks to show improvement, depending on the severity of anorexia and fever.

INFECTIVE ENDOCARDITIS

Endocarditis is an inflammatory process of the endocardium, especially the valves. This disorder carries high morbidity and death rates, but outcomes can be improved greatly with rapid diagnosis and effective treatment.

Many different terms and classifications are used to describe infective endocarditis. Some are defined in the following list:

- Subacute bacterial endocarditis (SBE): develops gradually over several weeks or months; usually caused by organisms of low virulence, such as *Streptococcus viridans,* which has a limited ability to infect other tissues
- Acute bacterial endocarditis: develops over days or weeks with an erratic course and earlier development of complications; commonly caused by *Staphylococcus aureus,* which is capable of infecting other body tissues
- Native valve endocarditis: an infection of a previously normal or damaged valve
- Prosthetic valve endocarditis: an infection of a prosthetic valve
- Nonbacterial thrombotic endocarditis: caused by sterile thrombotic lesions (often aggregates of platelets) that may develop in people with cancer or other chronic diseases

Changes in the population at risk are altering the classic picture of infective endocarditis (IE). The incidence is continuing to rise. Each year 15,000 to 20,000 new cases are diagnosed and IE is now the fourth leading cause of life-threatening infectious disease syndromes. The changes are traced to several notable alterations in the population. The increased incidence of endocarditis caused by yeasts and fungi is attributable to the increased number of people with valve prostheses, to the increased number of people using intravenous (IV) drugs, and to the rising use of long-term antimicrobial therapy or immunosuppression. Nosocomial infections are now the cause of up to 29% of all cases.

The decreased incidence of rheumatic fever results in a lower incidence of endocarditis, whereas the number of children surviving congenital heart disease results in an increased incidence. The growing population of older adults also leads to an increase in the number of endocarditis episodes.

Etiology and Risk Factors

Common infecting organisms include staphylococci *(S. aureus, S. faecalis, S. epidermidis),* streptococci, *Escherichia coli,* gram-negative organisms *(Klebsiella, Pseudomonas, Serratia marcescens),* fungi *(Candida, Aspergillus),* and HACEK organisms *(Haemophilus parainfluenzae, Haemophilus aphrophilus, Actinobacillus actinomycetemcomitans, Cardiobacterium hominis, Eikenella* species, and *Kingella* species). These organisms enter the body through the oral cavity after dental procedures, mouth or tooth abscesses, oral irrigations, or oral irritations from dental floss or bridgework. The upper respiratory tract is another port of entry following surgery, intubations, or infections. Direct exposure of the bloodstream to organisms can occur with prolonged IV catheters, hemodialysis catheters, and IV drug use. Procedures involving the gastrointestinal and genitourinary tracts (e.g., barium enemas, sigmoidoscopy, colonoscopy, percutaneous liver biopsy, catheterization, urethrotomy, prostatectomy, cystoscopy) have been associated with infective endocarditis.

Reproductive conditions have also been linked (e.g., delivery of a newborn, abortion, intrauterine devices, pelvic inflammatory diseases). Defective heart valves causing changes in blood flow and pressures encourage the proliferation of vegetations. Open heart surgery to replace damaged valves increases the risk of endocarditis. Fortunately, coronary artery bypass grafting (CABG), one of the most frequently performed surgical procedures in the United States, carries a low risk of infective endocarditis because the endocardium is not invaded during the operation.

Circulating microorganisms in the bloodstream attach to the endocardial surface and multiply. Usually multiplication of these organisms requires a rough or abnormal endocardium. IV drug abusers may be injecting particulate matter into the bloodstream, causing damage to the previously normal right heart endocardium that allows the organism to adhere, thereby initiating acute bacterial endocarditis.

Pathophysiology

Microorganisms enter the bloodstream in many ways. Once the colonization process begins on the endothelium, replication occurs and bacterial colonies form within layers of platelets and fibrin. As the colonies become entangled within the tight layers of fibrin and platelets, the colony becomes less and less vulnerable to the body's defense mechanisms. The bacteria stimulate the humoral immune system to produce nonspecific antibodies, but the bacteria are protected by the fibrin-platelet aggregation. It is not uncommon for these vegetations to form clots that travel to other organs, forming abscesses. The vegetations can severely damage heart valves by perforating and deforming the valve leaflets (Figure 55-5). Extensions of the bacteria may invade the aorta or pericardium. The amount of damage depends on the type and virulence of the organisms causing the infection.

Many complications are possible. Heart failure may develop as a result of structural valvular damage. Arterial emboli can occur from the vegetation. Systemic embolization occurs in 30% to 40% of clients with left-sided infective endocarditis. Common infarction sites are the kidney, spleen, and brain. Pulmonary embolus is associated with right-sided infective endocarditis. Emboli can also travel to the brain and produce a myriad of manifestations. Occasionally immune complex glomerulonephritis will develop. Renal function usually returns to normal after the infection has been controlled.

Clinical Manifestations

Clinical manifestations of infective endocarditis include those related to the infectious process, heart murmurs, embolization, and the immune response.

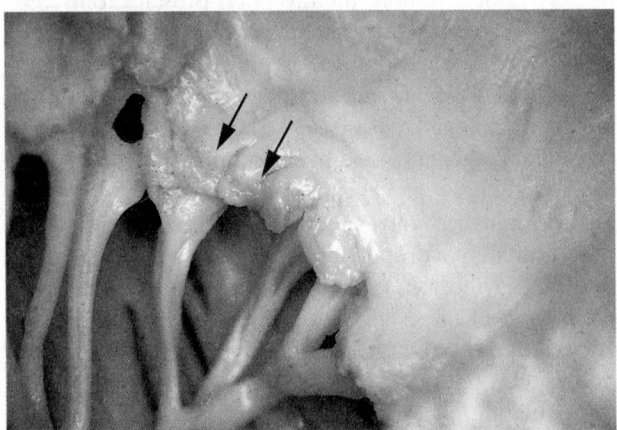

■ **FIGURE 55-5** Vegetations of the heart valves resulting from infective endocarditis. *(From Kumar, V.A., Abbas, A.K., & Fausto, N. [2004]. Robbins and Cotran pathologic basis of disease [7th ed.]. Philadelphia: Saunders.)*

Clinical manifestations related to the infection include fever, chills alternating with sweats, malaise, weakness, anorexia, weight loss, pallor, backache, and splenomegaly. Clients may report feeling as though they have the flu, with headaches and musculoskeletal aching. In acute infection, clients appear very ill. Fever, chills, and prostration are so severe that hospital admission is usually necessary within a few days.

Cardiac murmurs eventually develop, but they may be absent in the early stages of infection. In clients with pre-existing valvular disease, new murmurs may be heard. Heart failure may develop suddenly in either acute or subacute endocarditis. Mechanical complications include perforation of a valve leaflet, rupture of one of the chordae tendineae, or development of a functional stenosis from the obstruction of blood flow by large vegetations.

Clinical manifestations related to embolization can occur in any part of the body. They are presented in the following list in order from head to toe:

- Stroke, transient ischemic attacks, aphasia, or ataxia
- Loss of vision from embolization to the brain or retinal artery
- Petechiae on the neck, conjunctiva, chest, abdomen, and mouth
- Roth's spots—a white or yellow center surrounded by a bright red, irregular halo seen by ophthalmoscope
- Myocardial infarction, which may develop as a result of coronary artery embolism
- Pulmonary embolus
- Splinter hemorrhages, which look like tiny splinters under the nail
- Osler's nodes—painful, erythematous, pea-sized nodules on tips of the fingers and toes resulting from inflammation around a small, infected embolus
- Finger clubbing, although less common today, may occur in clients with long-standing infective endocarditis; pathogenesis remains unclear
- Janeway's lesions—flat, small, nontender red spots on the palms of the hands and the soles of the feet
- Evidence of an immunologic reaction to infection, including arthralgia, proteinuria, hematuria, casts, and acidosis

Because the clinical manifestations of endocarditis are numerous and often nonspecific, several modalities are used for the differential medical diagnosis. Blood cultures for bacteria, fungus, and yeast are the most important diagnostic tests. Blood cultures should be obtained for all clients with both fever and heart murmur. ECGs and echocardiograms should be done on admission to the hospital and repeated during the hospital stay.[25] A chest x-ray study is useful in identifying early heart failure. A complete blood count (CBC) and other routine diagnostic procedures are also helpful. Diagnosis is confirmed by clinical manifestations, blood cultures, and echocardiography.

OUTCOME MANAGEMENT

Medical Management

The chief goals of management are to eradicate the infecting organism in the vegetation and to treat the complications. Because the bacteria reside inside the vegetation, getting antibiotics to them is difficult. Antibiotics cannot reach the organism directly, because the valves do not receive a blood supply; therefore antibiotics have to reach the vegetation passively. Penicillin plus ceftriaxone and gentamicin or vancomycin is commonly used. Because of resistive strains of bacteria, other antibiotics might be needed. Therapy is usually administered by the IV route and continued for 4 to 6 weeks. Antibiotics are usually begun in the hospital and continued as an outpatient at the client's home if the living situation is appropriate. Risk for IE will continue for the client's lifetime and prophylaxis against infection will remain important.

IE can lead to valve disease, and surgery may be required once the infection is under control (negative blood cultures, absence of fever, and normal WBC count). Severe valve disease with heart failure can require surgical eradication of the infection.

Nursing Management of the Medical Client

Nursing assessment focuses on gathering data about the client's hemodynamic stability (particularly the presence of a new heart murmur and embolic complications), level of comfort, coping ability, support from significant others, and potential for self-care. Auscultate the heart every 8 hours for murmurs. Assess for rapid pulse rate, easy fatigability, dyspnea, restlessness, manifestations of heart failure, and embolic manifestations. Document these manifestations if they occur, and report them to the physician.

Administer IV antibiotics as prescribed. Antibiotics relieve much discomfort within a few days. Treat fever, when present, with rest, cooling measures, forced fluids, and sometimes salicylates. As with most infectious processes, encourage the client to eat a nutritious diet, drink sufficient fluids, and rest mentally and physically.

The client may need to be hospitalized or transferred to a setting that can provide IV medications for 2 to 6 weeks if home care is not an option. Do not enforce complete bed rest unless fever or manifestations of heart damage develop.

When the client's condition improves, plan and implement a progressive activity schedule and a teaching plan (see the Client Education Guide feature on Infective Endocarditis on the website). As activity increases, monitor the client's physical response to exercise. For example, assess blood pressure, heart rate, diaphoresis, vertigo, and weakness.

Self-Care

The trend toward early hospital discharge has changed the course of treatment for clients with infective endocarditis. IV therapy may now be routinely given in the home. Clients who are alert, cooperative, and reasonably stable and who want to return home may be allowed to do so. Typically the nurse, pharmacist, and physician teach the techniques of self-administered IV antibiotics. Before discharge, the client must demonstrate the knowledge and technique required. The physician's office or home health care nurses often monitor the client's progress.

Home IV antibiotic therapy offers many benefits. It is less costly than hospital care, motivates clients to become active participants in their own care, reestablishes a more normal lifestyle, and promotes a sense of control that aids in psychosocial and physiologic recovery. To be effective, this program calls for exceptional communication and cooperation between members of the health care team and the client.

Invasive procedures, especially dental work, increase the risk of endocarditis. Oral antibiotics are advised before most dental procedures are performed (Box 55-3). Other invasive diagnostic and surgical procedures also require antibiotics.

MYOCARDITIS

Myocarditis is an inflammation of the myocardial wall. Frequently, the inflammation is not limited to the myocardium but extends to the pericardium, with production of an associated pericarditis.

In the United States, most cases of myocarditis are due to viral infections, Coxsackie virus being the most common. Other viral causes include mumps, influenza, rubella, measles, adenoviruses, echoviruses, cytomegalovirus, and Epstein-Barr virus. Bacterial, fungal, rickettsial, spirochetal, helminthic, and protozoal infections can also cause myocarditis. Hypersensitivity immune reactions seen with acute rheumatic fever and postcardiotomy syndrome, toxins and chemicals such as alcohol, and large doses of radiation therapy to the chest for the treatment of malignancy are other causes.

Most viral pathogens enter the body through the upper respiratory or gastrointestinal tract. The virus enters the myocyte, replicates, and destroys the cell. The body's immune system responds. Over the next days to weeks, the cells that survive do not appear normal and are also destroyed by the immune system. If myocardial contractility is impaired, ventricular diastolic pressures and volumes may be elevated to maintain stroke volume. Disruptions leading to cardiac dysrhythmias can decrease cardiac output. Unfortunately, the outcome is commonly dilated cardiomyopathy and heart failure.

BOX 55-3 Dental Procedures and Endocarditis Prophylaxis in Adults

ENDOCARDITIS PROPHYLAXIS RECOMMENDED*

- Dental extractions
- Periodontal procedures, including surgery, scaling and root planing, probing, and recall maintenance
- Dental implant placement and reimplantation of avulsed teeth
- Endodontic (root canal) instrumentation or surgery only beyond the apex
- Subgingival placement of antibiotic fibers or strips
- Initial placement of orthodontic bands but not brackets
- Intraligamentary local anesthetic injections
- Prophylactic cleaning of teeth or implants where bleeding is anticipated
- Restoration of decayed teeth (filling cavities) and replacement of missing teeth
- Selected circumstances that may create significant bleeding

ENDOCARDITIS PROPHYLAXIS NOT RECOMMENDED

- Restorative dentistry (operative and prosthodontic) with or without retraction cord
- Local anesthetic injections (non-intraligamentary)
- Intracanal endodontic treatment; post placement and buildup
- Placement of rubber dams
- Postoperative suture removal
- Placement of removable prosthodontic or orthodontic appliances
- Taking of oral impressions
- Fluoride treatments
- Taking of oral radiographs
- Orthodontic appliance adjustment
- Shedding of primary teeth

*Standard general prophylaxis for adults is amoxicillin 3 g orally 1 hour before procedure, half the dose 6 hours later. If client is allergic to penicillin, erythromycin 800 mg or clindamycin 300 mg 1 hour before procedure, then half the dose 6 hours later.

From Dajani, A.S., et al. (1997). Prevention of bacterial endocarditis. *Journal of the American Medical Association, 277,* 1794-1801.

Clinical Manifestations

Clients who have viral myocarditis will present with a history of recent upper respiratory or gastrointestinal tract infection. After the viral illness is over, there is a delay of days to weeks before cardiac manifestations appear. Cardiac problems include heart failure, lethal dysrhythmias, and embolic problems. The most frequent manifestations are fatigue, dyspnea, palpitations, and chest pain. The client often experiences chest pain as a sharp, stabbing precordial pain, which can then be distinguished from the pressure sensation of angina pectoris. The client also has sinus tachycardia and abnormal heart sounds of murmurs, gallops, and rarely a pericardial friction rub.

ECG abnormalities and elevated serum levels of cardiac enzymes are helpful in the diagnosis. The ECG may show a bundle branch block or complete AV heart block, ST-segment elevation, or T-wave flattening. The chest x-ray may show an enlarged cardiac silhouette resulting from ventricular enlargement or pericardial effusion. Blood tests may show a moderate leukocytosis and elevated cardiac enzymes. Echocardiograms show impairments in the left ventricle and heart wall abnormalities. Ventricular thrombus is not uncommon. Cardiac MRI can reveal abnormal signal intensity in the heart muscle. Endomyocardial biopsies are used in diagnosis of the viral infection.

OUTCOME MANAGEMENT

Clients with acute myocarditis are usually admitted to the hospital for observation. Clients with pericardial effusion, dysrhythmias, heart failure, or hypotension are usually admitted to the intensive care unit (ICU) and may be in cardiogenic shock. Medical management begins with specific therapy for the underlying infection. Bed rest is suggested to decrease cardiac workload. Supplemental oxygen may be prescribed for clients with low cardiac output or dysrhythmias. Immunosuppressive therapy is being investigated. Antipyretic agents are helpful for the fever and its hemodynamic effects, which result in increased myocardial workload. Clients who remain at home may use Holter monitoring, which provides continuous surveillance of the client's heart rhythm. In most cases myocarditis is self-limiting and uncomplicated. Although most clients recover rapidly, some have recurrent or chronic myocarditis and some become very ill and die.

Nursing management for the client experiencing myocarditis is essentially the same as that provided to clients with infective endocarditis and rheumatic fever. Review those sections in this chapter.

Teaching begins when acute manifestations have subsided and the client has demonstrated physical and emotional readiness. Teach clients how to monitor their pulse rate and rhythm. Instruct them to report any sudden changes in heart rate, rhythm, or palpitations immediately. Encourage family members to take CPR training, which can be obtained from such groups as the local fire department, the American Red Cross, or the American Heart Association. Educating family members about CPR can enhance their sense of preparedness for an emergency.

Because the myocardial infectious process resolves slowly and late complications can occur, advise clients to continue self-monitoring and to schedule clinical follow-up appointments, even after apparent recovery.

The potential of lethal dysrhythmias may frighten the client and the client's significant others. The client who is experiencing extreme anxiety, fear, and ineffective coping may manifest insomnia, tearfulness, somatic complaints, an inability to problem-solve, and agitation. Determine with the client (and family) the specific focus of anxiety. Clarify any misconceptions. Speak slowly and calmly, and focus on the present situation, giving feedback about current reality. Encourage the use of relaxation techniques to help allay stress. Schedule activities around periods of undisturbed sleep.

PERICARDITIS

Pericarditis is inflammation of the pericardium and it may be either acute or chronic (recurrent). It is not known why pericarditis may be an acute illness in some clients and recurrent in others.

ACUTE PERICARDITIS

Acute pericarditis is a syndrome resulting from inflammation of the parietal and visceral pericardium. Because of the proximity of the pericardium to the pleura, lungs, sternum, diaphragm, and myocardium, pericarditis may be a consequence of a number of inflammatory or infectious processes (Box 55-4). Acute pericarditis is usually viral (idiopathic) in origin.

Agents or processes causing pericardial inflammation create an exudate of fibrin, WBCs, and endothelial cells. The exudate covers the pericardium and causes further inflammation of the surrounding pleura and tissues. The fibrinous exudate may localize to one region of the heart, or it may be generalized. Acute pericarditis may be either

---

BOX 55-4   Causes of Pericarditis

INFECTIONS
- Viral: Coxsackie, influenza
- Bacterial: tuberculosis, staphylococcus, streptococcus, meningococcus, pneumococcus
- Parasitic
- Fungal

MYOCARDIAL INJURY
- Myocardial infarction (Dressler's syndrome)
- Cardiac trauma: blunt or penetrating
- Post cardiac surgery
- Hypersensitivity

COLLAGEN DISEASES
- Rheumatic fever
- Scleroderma
- Systemic lupus erythematosus
- Rheumatoid arthritis

DRUG REACTION
- Procainamide
- Methysergide
- Hydralazine

RADIATION THERAPY

COBALT THERAPY

METABOLIC DISORDERS
- Uremia
- Myxedema

CHRONIC ANEMIA

NEOPLASM: LYMPHOMA

AORTIC DISSECTION

---

dry (fibrinous) or exudative. Under normal conditions the pericardial sac contains about 50 ml of clear, serous-like fluid. Volumes from 100 to 3000 ml of serofibrinous exudate can accumulate with pericarditis. The exudate accumulates in the pericardial sac, causing cardiac tamponade that restricts cardiac filling and emptying (see below). Without prompt treatment, shock and death can result from decreased cardiac output.

Dry pericarditis can occur after a common viral infection, myocardial infarction, tuberculosis, bacteremia, or renal failure. Delicate adhesions form within the pericardial space along with serous fibrin deposition, hemorrhage, and calcification. Adhesions may eventually obliterate the pericardial sac. Inflammation of the pericardium frequently penetrates the myocardium to some degree, which produces myopericarditis.

Although chest pain is common, the nature of this pain varies. Sometimes the pain is similar to that of myocardial infarction; at other times it mimics the pain of pleurisy. The pain is exacerbated with respiration and rotating the trunk but usually does not radiate to the arms. Sitting up and bending forward often relieves the pain.

Pericardial friction rub is a classic objective manifestation of acute pericarditis. The rub is produced by inflamed, roughened pericardial layers that create friction as their surfaces rub together during heart movement. Auscultation over the precordium reveals a scratchy, leathery, or creaky sound that is heard anywhere over the precordium but most frequently at the third intercostal space left of the sternal border. The rub is best heard with the diaphragm of the stethoscope and with the client holding his or her breath (to eliminate the breath sounds). In some clients the sound is best heard with the client sitting up. Pericardial friction rubs vary in intensity from hour to hour and from day to day.

Fever is another common finding in clients with pericarditis. The temperature may rise to 39.4° C (103° F). Chills, malaise, joint pain, anorexia, nausea, and weight loss accompany the fever. Dyspnea and chest pain can potentiate anxiety. An increase in heart rate usually corresponds to the degree of fever and anxiety.

The ECG may indicate tachycardia, but with underlying heart disease or uremia, bradycardia can occur. Laboratory studies show an elevated ESR and may show an elevated WBC count. Cardiac enzymes are usually normal but may be elevated.

OUTCOME MANAGEMENT

When the cause of acute pericarditis is known, treatment of the cause can be planned accordingly. If no causal agent is known, symptomatic intervention for acute dry pericarditis is provided. Clients may be hospitalized for diagnosis and for the treatment of complications. Pain and fever, usually self-limited, may be eased by aspirin given in the maximally tolerated doses.

Nonsteroidal anti-inflammatory drugs (NSAIDs) may also be prescribed. Stronger analgesia, such as morphine sulfate, may be necessary if chest pain becomes severe.

If acute pericarditis is present after a myocardial infarction (called Dressler's syndrome), reassure the client that the pain experienced with pericarditis does not mean that another infarction is occurring. If the client becomes anxious, worrying about the cause of the pain, oxygen demand increases and myocardial ischemia may develop.

The focus of nursing care related to pericarditis is the same as that described for the other inflammatory cardiac diseases discussed in this chapter. Nursing assessment of the client with pericarditis also includes scrutiny for the presence of pericardial tamponade (pulsus paradoxus, distended neck veins). Vigilant assessment is necessary. Provide reassurance about the temporary nature of the disease.

ACUTE PERICARDITIS WITH EFFUSION

Acute pericarditis with effusion results when fluid accumulates rapidly within the pericardial sac. The fluid may compress the heart and reduce ventricular filling and cardiac output. When fluid accumulates slowly, the fibrous pericardium is better able to stretch and accommodate its presence. Clients can tolerate 1 to 2 L of fluid without an increase in intrapericardial pressure if accumulation is slow and may show no manifestations. The heart sounds are often distant or muffled. The friction rub may disappear. Fever may develop.

Rapid accumulation of only 80 to 200 ml of fluid in the pericardial space can create a decrease in cardiac output. The client usually appears uncomfortable, with varying degrees of reduced cardiac output or even obvious shock. The client may have tachycardia, diaphoresis, cool or cyanotic extremities, and anxiety or confusion. A paradoxical pulse is often present. Carefully assess for an exaggeration of the normal variation in the pulse or a change in blood pressure by 10 mm Hg during the inspiratory phase of respiration, in which the pulse becomes weaker as one inhales and stronger as the client exhales. Echocardiography is the most accurate technique for evaluating pericardial effusion and pericardiocentesis. The fluid withdrawn is sent for analysis. Care of the client with pericardial effusion is similar to the plan of intervention for dry pericarditis. Bed rest, analgesia, and proper positioning can help to alleviate manifestations. Psychological support is important.

CHRONIC CONSTRICTIVE PERICARDITIS

Chronic constrictive pericarditis is a chronic inflammatory condition in which the pericardium changes into a thick, fibrous band of tissue. This tissue encircles, encases, and compresses the heart, preventing proper ventricular filling and emptying. Cardiac failure eventually results from this slow compression. This condition usually begins with an episode of acute pericarditis characterized by fibrin deposition, often with pericardial effusion. In most cases the visceral and parietal layers become completely fused.

Clinical manifestations include right ventricular failure first, followed by decreased cardiac output manifesting as fatigue on exertion, dyspnea, leg edema, ascites, low pulse pressure, distended neck veins, and delayed capillary refill time. Constrictive pericarditis is a progressive disease without spontaneous reversal of manifestations.

Medical treatment includes digitalis, diuretics, and sodium restriction to relieve manifestations of right ventricular failure. Excision of the damaged pericardium (pericardiectomy) may be required.

CARDIAC TAMPONADE

Cardiac tamponade is a life-threatening complication caused by accumulation of fluid in the pericardium. This fluid, which can be blood, pus, or air in the pericardial sac, accumulates fast enough and in sufficient quantity to compress the heart and restrict blood flow in and out of the ventricles. This is a cardiac emergency.

Large or rapidly accumulating effusions raise the intrapericardial pressure to a point at which venous blood cannot flow into the heart, which decreases ventricular filling. As a result, venous pressure rises and cardiac output and arterial blood pressure fall. A narrowing pulse pressure signals cardiac tamponade. The heart attempts to compensate by beating rapidly (tachycardia), but tachycardia cannot sustain cardiac output for long. Prompt intervention is necessary to prevent shock and death.

Hypotension, tachycardia, jugular venous distention, cyanosis of lips and nails, dyspnea, muffled heart sounds, diaphoresis, and paradoxical pulse (a decrease in systolic arterial pulsation exceeding 10 mm Hg, during inspiration) are present. The client may be comfortable and quiet one minute and then restless with a feeling of impending doom. Clients may panic when fluid accumulates rapidly as a result of seriously reduced cardiac output. Slowly developing tamponade is characterized by manifestations that resemble those of heart failure: nonspecific ECG changes, decreased voltage, and visualization of fluid in the pericardial sac on echocardiogram. These clinical manifestations and related interventions are outlined in the Critical Monitoring feature on p. 1407.

Immediate intervention is required. The emergency intervention of choice is pericardiocentesis, a procedure in which fluid or air is aspirated from the pericardial sac (Figure 55-6). This procedure relieves pressure on the heart, thereby improving cardiac function and perhaps saving the client's life. Pericardiocentesis is performed with a soft catheter to reduce the risk of cardiac lacerations.

Cardiac Tamponade

Report the following manifestations of cardiac tamponade immediately!

- Elevated venous pressure (increased central venous pressure)
- Distended neck veins
- Kussmaul's sign (distended neck veins on inspiration)
- Hypotension
- Narrowed pulse pressure
- Tachycardia
- Dyspnea
- Restlessness, anxiety
- Cyanosis of lips and nails
- Diaphoresis
- Muffled heart sounds
- Pulsus paradoxus
- Decreased friction rub
- Decreased QRS voltage and electrical alternans

CONGENITAL DISORDERS

Congenital heart disorders result from faulty development of cardiac structures in utero. With today's available treatments, about 85% of children with congenital heart disease will survive to adulthood. Therefore we can expect to see more adults with congenital defects in the future. Many people with a congenital heart defect have remained asymptomatic; others have had varying levels of functional ability. Clients may have both residual problems and sequelae. Common lifelong problems include the risk of infective endocarditis in clients with artificial valves or with suture repair of an atrial septal defect. It is not uncommon for a client with a repaired coarctation of the aorta to find that the aorta has gradually become narrowed again. In such cases hypertension may develop. Clients who as children underwent repair for cyanotic defects tend to experience sequelae and complications in adulthood. Some degree of exercise intolerance may be present that can be better managed after proper stress testing.

Dysrhythmias frequently present a lifelong complication. Clients who have had intraventricular repairs may present with ventricular dysrhythmias or complete heart block. A 24-hour Holter monitor and stress testing may help to evaluate the client's tolerance for activity.

Many people who have had surgical procedures as infants and children had to have repeated operations as they "outgrew" their repairs or prosthetic devices. Our growing geriatric population also may be experiencing unknown late consequences of congenital heart disease or surgical repair. It is important to encourage these people to participate in long-term follow-up.

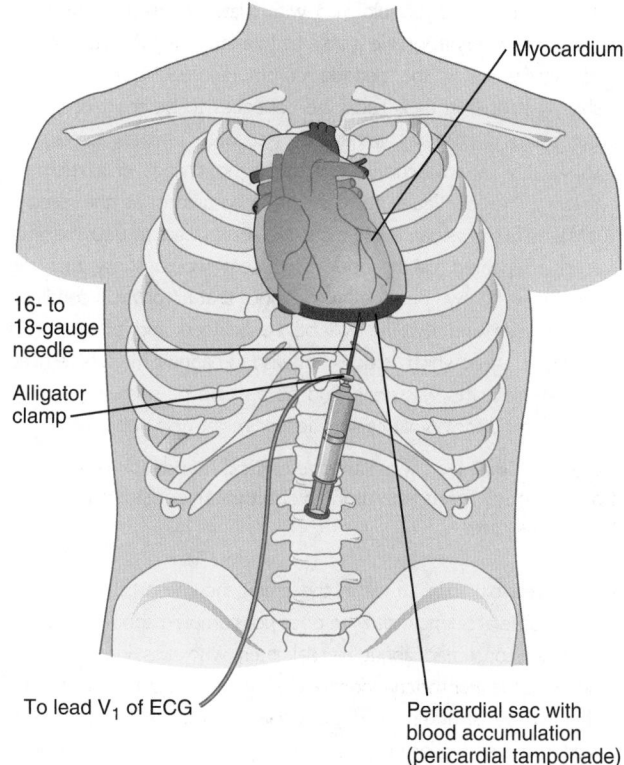

■ **FIGURE 55–6** Pericardiocentesis to remove blood from the pericardial sac during tamponade. *ECG*, Electrocardiogram.

Your role as a nurse who is caring for the adult with congenital heart disease varies with the setting; however, you play an integral role in helping these clients to achieve optimal health and functioning. Nursing assessment, intervention, education, and follow-up are directed toward improving functional levels, managing medications, assisting in psychosocial adjustment, and preventing complications.

CONCLUSIONS

The client with a cardiac disorder frequently has activity intolerance, decreased cardiac output, and ineffective coping because of the seriousness of the disorder. Nurses must be skilled in the physical and psychosocial aspects of disease when providing care.

THINKING CRITICALLY

1. A 52-year-old man with a lengthy history of mitral valve prolapse is recovering from kidney transplantation surgery. This is his fourth postoperative day, and he and his spouse are asking questions about care at home. What priorities for client education should be established?

Factors to Consider. What complication is associated with mitral valve prolapse? How does the medication regimen following transplantation surgery further place the client at risk?

2. The client is a 60-year-old man with dilated cardiomyopathy. His prognosis is very poor. He is able to tolerate only minimal amounts of activity—using the bedside commode, feeding himself, and shaving himself in bed. Today he continues to be short of breath but seems particularly withdrawn. Repeated physical assessment to identify cardiovascular status shows no change in assessment findings. He continues to take his medications at the proper dosages. His physician thinks these medications are at their maximal levels. Repeated psychosocial assessment would show that the client is withdrawn because he is anxious that his physical condition will worsen and that he will be hospitalized and placed on a ventilator again, which he does not wish to happen. He was terrified the last time this was done, and he sees no purpose in just prolonging his dying. What nursing actions might help your client?

Factors to Consider. What are the clinical manifestations of cardiomyopathy? What are the psychological considerations for the client's care?

3. A 45-year-old man arrives in the emergency department after an automobile accident. Initially he does not complain about himself; he is more concerned about his daughter, who was injured in the accident. Neither the child nor the client was wearing a seat belt when their car was struck from behind. While sitting at his daughter's bedside in the emergency department, the client becomes increasingly anxious; his respiratory rate increases, and he becomes restless. The vital signs show a blood pressure of 88/72 mm Hg, pulse rate of 118 beats/min, and respirations of 28 breaths/min. What other assessments are needed to rule out cardiac tamponade? What intervention will relieve pressure on the heart and improve cardiac function?

Factors to Consider. What are the clinical manifestations of cardiac tamponade? How is cardiac output affected by cardiac tamponade?

evolve   *Discussions for these questions can be found on the website.*

BIBLIOGRAPHY

🪔 Citations appearing in red refer to primary research.

🪔 Citations appearing in blue refer to evidence-based practice guidelines and protocols.

1. American Health Association. (2002). *2002 Heart and stroke statistical update.* Dallas, Tex: American Heart Association.
2. Autore, C., Conte, M.R., Piccininno, M., et al. (2002). Risk associated with pregnancy in hypertrophic cardiomyopathy. *Journal of the American College of Cardiology, 40*(10), 1864-1869.
3. Baddour, L., Wilson, W., Bayer, A., et al. (2005). Infective Endocarditis: American Heart Association Scientific Statement. *Circulation 111*, 3167-3184.
4. Baughman, K.L., & Braunwald, E. (2005). Myocarditis. In E. Braunwald (Ed.), *Heart disease* (7th ed., pp. 1697-1717). Philadelphia: Saunders.
5. Bayer, A.S., et al. (1998). AHA Scientific statement: Diagnosis and management of infective endocarditis and its complications. *Circulation, 98*, 2936-2948.
6. Bond, A.E., Bolton, B., & Nelson, K. (2004). Nursing education and implications for left ventricular assist device destination therapy. *Progress in Cardiovascular Nursing, 19*(3), 85-91.
7. Bonow, R.O., & Braunwald, E. (2005). Valvular heart disease. In E. Braunwald (Ed.), *Heart disease* (7th ed., pp. 1553-1632). Philadelphia: Saunders.
8. Bonow, R.O., Carabello, B., Chatterjee, K., et al. (2006). ACC/AHA 2006 practice guidelines for the management of patients with valvular heart disease: Executive summary: A report of the American College of Cardiology/American Heart Association Task Force on Practice Guidelines. *Journal of American College of Cardiology, 48*(3), 598-675.
9. Bonow, R.O., Carabello, B.A., Chatterjee, K., et al. (2006). ACC/AHA 2006 guidelines for the management of patients with valvular heart disease: A report of the American College of Cardiology/American Heart Association Task force on Practice Guidelines. *Journal of American College of Cardiology, 48*(3), e1-148.
10. Dajani, A.S. (2005). Rheumatic fever. In E. Braunwald (Ed.), *Heart disease* (7th ed., pp. 2093-2099). Philadelphia: Saunders.
11. Dajani, A.S., et al. (1997). Prevention of bacterial endocarditis: Recommendations by the American Heart Association. *Journal of the American Medical Association, 277*(22), 1794-1801.
12. Durack, D.T. (1995). Prevention of infective endocarditis. *New England Journal of Medicine, 332*(1), 38-44.
13. Greffe, G., Chalabreysse, L., Mouly-Bertin, C., et al. (2007). Valvular heart disease associated with fenfluramine detected 7 years after discontinuation of treatment. *Annals of Thoracic Surgery, 83*(4), 1541-1543.
14. Karchmer, A.W. (2005). Infective endocarditis. In E. Braunwald (Ed.), *Heart disease* (7th ed., pp. 1633-1658). Philadelphia: Saunders.
15. LeWinter, M.M., & Kabbani, S. (2005). Pericardial diseases. In E. Braunwald (Ed.), *Heart disease* (7th ed., pp. 1757-1780). Philadelphia: Saunders.
16. Maron, B.J. (2002). Hypertrophic cardiomyopathy: A systematic review. *Journal of the American Medical Association, 287*(10), 1308-1320.
17. McRae, M.E. (2005). Repaired tetralogy of Fallot in the adult. *Progress in Cardiovascular Nursing, 20*(3), 104-110.
18. Mogensen, J., Klausen, I.C., Pedersen, K., et al. (1999). Alpha-cardiac actin is a novel disease gene in familial hypertrophic cardiomyopathy. *The Journal of Clinical Investigation, 103*(10), R39-43.
19. Myers, R.B., & Spodick, D.H. (1999). Constrictive pericarditis: Clinical and pathophysiologic characteristics. *American Heart Journal, 138*, 219-232.
20. Otto, C.M., Burwash, I.G., Legget, M.E., et al. (1997). A prospective study of asymptomatic valvular aortic stenosis: Clinical, echocardiographic, and exercise predictors of outcome. *Circulation, 95*(9), 2262-2270.
21. Rahimtoola, S.H., Durairaj, A., Mehra, A., et al. (2002). Current evaluation and management of patients with mitral stenosis. *Circulation, 106*(10), 1183-1188.
22. Rathore, S.S., Curtis, J.P., Wang, Y., et al. (2003). Association of serum digoxin concentration and outcomes in patients with heart failure. *Journal of the American Medical Association, 289*(7), 871-878.
23. Richardson, P., McKenna, W., Bristow, M., et al. (1996). Report of the 1995 World Health Organization/International Society and Federation of Cardiology Task Force on the Definition and Classification of Cardiomyopathies. *Circulation, 93*(5), 841-842.
24. Shabetai, R. (2000). Sarcoidosis and the heart. *Current Treatment Options in Cardiovascular Medicine, 2*(5), 385-398.
25. Shepler, S.A., & Patel, A.N. (2007). Cardiac cell therapy: A treatment option for cardiomyopathy. *Critical Care Nursing Quarterly, 30*(1), 74-80.
26. Shimada, T., Shimada, K., Sakane, T., et al. (2001). Diagnosis of cardiac sarcoidosis and evaluation of the effects of steroid therapy by gadolinium-DTPA-enhanced magnetic resonance imaging. *American Journal of Medicine, 110*(7), 520-527.
27. Spirito, P., Seidman, C.E., McKenna, W.J., et al. (1997). The management of hypertrophic cardiomyopathy. *New England Journal of Medicine, 336*(11), 775-785.
28. Supino, P.G., Borer, J.S., Preibisz, J., et al. (2006). The epidemiology of valvular heart disease: A growing public health problem. *Heart Failure Clinics, 2*(4), 379-393.

29. Wang, A., Athan, E., Pappas, P., et al. (2007). Contemporary clinical profile and outcome of prosthetic valve endocarditis. *Journal of the American Medical Association, 297,* 1354-1361.

30. Winters, M., & Obriot, P. (2007). Mitral valve repair. *AORN Journal, 85*(1), 152-170.

31. Wynne, J., & Braunwald, E. (2005). The cardiomyopathies. In E. Braunwald (Ed.), *Heart disease* (7th ed., pp. 1659-1696). Philadelphia: Saunders.

32. Yazaki, Y., Isobe, M., Hiroe, M., et al. (2001). Prognostic determinants of long-term survival in Japanese patients with cardiac sarcoidosis treated with prednisone. *American Journal of Cardiology, 88*(9), 1006-1010.

evolve **Did you remember to check out the bonus material on the Evolve website and the CD-ROM, including NCLEX®-Examination Style Review Questions, Open-Book Quizzes, and Chapter Review Audio Podcasts?**

http://evolve.elsevier.com/Black/medsurg

CHAPTER 56

Management of Clients with Functional Cardiac Disorders

PATRICIA A. KERESZTES AND MARY WCISEL

Normal functioning of the heart is based on a balance between oxygen supply and oxygen demand. To function as an effective pump, the heart muscle must be adequately supplied with blood from the coronary arteries. In *coronary heart disease* (CHD), atherosclerosis develops in the coronary arteries, causing them to become narrowed or blocked. When a coronary artery is narrowed or blocked, blood flow to the area of the heart supplied by that artery is reduced. If the remaining blood flow is inadequate to meet the oxygen demands of the heart, the area may become ischemic and injured and myocardial infarction (MI) may result. In addition, the heart may fail to pump sufficient blood supply to the other organs and tissues in the body. Over time, changes resulting from CHD may lead to the development of chronic heart failure.

The terms *coronary heart disease, coronary artery disease,* and *ischemic heart disease* all refer to diseases of the heart that result from a decrease in blood supply to the heart muscle. This chapter reviews the risk factors, etiology, pathophysiology, clinical manifestations, and medical and nursing interventions for two major disorders of cardiac function: CHD and heart failure. The related conditions of angina pectoris and myocardial infarction (MI) are discussed in Chapter 58.

CORONARY HEART DISEASE

CHD is the single largest killer of both men and women in the United States, with nearly 2500 deaths per day. Although these numbers seem high, the death rate from CHD decreased by 30% from 1993 to 2003. Contributing to this decline in the death rate are factors such as improved technology for diagnosis and treatment, the use of thrombolytic drugs in acute MI, improved interventional therapies and surgical techniques, and modification of risk factors in populations at risk.

Etiology and Risk Factors

Although several mechanisms and many risk factors for CHD are present, it appears that the primary cause of CAD is inflammation and lipid deposition in the wall of the artery. Risk factors that precipitate CHD can be presented in two categories: modifiable and nonmodifiable risk factors (Box 56-1). The more risk factors a person has, the greater the risk of CHD. Although risk factors influence the development of CHD in all people, the importance of selected risk factors may vary by gender and race. African-American and Mexican-American women have a higher prevalence of CHD risk factors than white women. The prevalence of having two or more risk factors for CHD has been shown to be higher in African Americans and American Indians/Alaska Natives. There is a lower prevalence of risk factors seen in Asians. Reduction of risk is based on control of the modifiable risk factors.

Nonmodifiable Risk Factors

Heredity (Including Race)

Children whose parents had heart disease are at higher risk for CHD. This increased risk is related to genetic

---

BOX 56-1	Risk Factors for Coronary Heart Disease

NONMODIFIABLE MAJOR RISK FACTORS
- Heredity, including race
- Age
- Gender

MODIFIABLE MAJOR RISK FACTORS
- Cigarette smoking
- Hypertension
- Elevated serum cholesterol level
- Diabetes mellitus
- Physical inactivity
- Obesity

CONTRIBUTING RISK FACTORS
- Stress
- Homocysteine level

predisposition to hypertension, elevated lipid levels, diabetes, and obesity, all of which increase the risk of CHD.

For people 35 to 74 years of age, the age-adjusted death rate from CHD for African-American women is 72% higher than that for white women and Native Americans. The prevalence of CHD is lowest among Mexican Americans.

Increasing Age

Age influences both the risk and the severity of CHD. Symptomatic CHD appears predominantly in people older than 40 years of age, and 4 of 5 people who die of CHD are age 65 years or older. Angina and MI, however, can occur in a person's 30s and even in one's 20s. At older ages, women who have heart attacks are twice as likely as men to die from the heart attack.

Gender

Coronary heart disease is the number one killer of both men and women. In 1999 mortality from CHD was almost equal for men and women. Although men are at higher risk for heart attacks at younger ages, the risk for women increases significantly at menopause, so that CHD rates in women after menopause are two to three times that of women the same age before menopause. Women who take oral contraceptives and who smoke or have high blood pressure are at greater risk for CHD. Women with an early menopause are also at higher risk than are women with a normal or late menopause.

Two lifestyle changes during the past 2 decades may be responsible for the increased incidence of CHD among women. More women (many with full responsibility for the household and children) have entered the work force, and more women have begun to smoke tobacco at an earlier age.

Modifiable Risk Factors

Smoking, hypertension, elevated serum cholesterol levels, physical inactivity, obesity, and diabetes mellitus constitute the modifiable risk factors for CHD. These factors can be modified or reduced by lifestyle changes and treatment.

Smoking

Both active smoking and passive smoking have been strongly implicated as a risk factor in the development of CHD. Currently 23% of men and 18% of women are smokers. The prevalence of smoking is higher in people with 11 years of education or less. Smoking triples the risk of heart attack in women and doubles the risk of heart attack in men. It also doubles the risk of dying from a heart attack and may quadruple the risk of sudden death. Nonsmokers who are exposed to second-hand tobacco smoke at home or work may also have a higher death rate from CHD. The risk of CHD is decreased by 50% 1 year after smokers quit. The risk is further reduced to that of nonsmokers within 5 to 10 years after smoking cessation.

Tar, nicotine, and carbon monoxide contribute to the damage. Tar contains hydrocarbons and other carcinogenic substances. Nicotine increases the release of epinephrine and norepinephrine, which results in peripheral vasoconstriction, elevated blood pressure and heart rate, greater oxygen consumption, and increased likelihood of dysrhythmias. In addition, nicotine activates platelets and stimulates smooth muscle cell proliferation in the arterial walls. Carbon monoxide reduces the amount of blood available to the intima of the vessel wall and increases the permeability of the endothelium.

Hypertension

High blood pressure afflicts nearly 1 in 3 adults in the United States. It increases the workload of the heart by increasing afterload, enlarging and weakening the left ventricle over time. As blood pressure increases, the risk of a serious cardiovascular event also escalates. When clients have hypertension, obesity, tobacco use, high cholesterol levels, and diabetes, the risk of heart attack increases significantly.

More men than women have hypertension until the age of 45, when it is more prevalent in women. The prevalence of hypertension in African Americans is among the highest in the world. In addition, African Americans have hypertension at an earlier age and it is more severe at any age. Consequently, the rate of heart disease in African Americans is 1.5 times greater than that of white Americans. Although hypertension cannot always be prevented, it should be treated to lower the risk of CHD and premature death.

Elevated Serum Cholesterol Levels

The risk of CHD increases as blood cholesterol levels increase. This risk increases further when other risk factors are present. In adults total cholesterol levels of 240 mg/dl are classified as "high" and levels ranging from 200 to 239 mg/dl are classified as "borderline high." At young and middle ages, men have higher cholesterol levels. In women cholesterol levels continue to increase up to about age 70.

Cholesterol circulates in the blood in combination with triglycerides and protein-bound phospholipids. This complex is called a *lipoprotein*. There are four basic groups of lipoproteins, all produced in the intestinal wall. Elevation of lipoproteins is called *hyperlipoproteinemia*. Elevation of lipids, a component of lipoproteins, is called *hyperlipidemia*. Lipoproteins and their functions are as follows:

- Chylomicrons primarily transport dietary triglycerides and cholesterol.
- Very-low-density lipoproteins (VLDLs) mainly transport triglycerides synthesized by the liver.
- Low-density lipoproteins (LDLs) have the highest concentration of cholesterol and transport endogenous cholesterol to body cells.
- High-density lipoproteins (HDLs) have the lowest concentration of cholesterol and transport endogenous cholesterol to body cells.

People with high levels of HDL in proportion to LDL are at lower risk for CHD than people with a low HDL-LDL ratio. High concentrations of HDL seem to protect against the development of CHD. Experts believe that the cholesterol in HDL, in contrast to that in LDL, does not become incorporated into the fatty plaques that develop in the lining of the artery wall. The ratio of total cholesterol to HDL or of LDL to HDL is the best test for predicting the risk of CHD. Exercise and low-fat, low-cholesterol diets increase the amount of HDL in the blood. The following are the current recommendations for cholesterol and lipoproteins:

- Total blood cholesterol <200 mg/dl
- LDL <160 mg/dl if fewer than two other risk factors (<130 mg/dl if two or more risk factors)
- HDL >40 mg/dl

Triglycerides are not an independent risk factor in men, but their significance in women is unknown; however, the combination of a high triglyceride level and a low HDL level seems to be a more important predictor of CHD in women than in men. The Consensus Panel Statement from the American Heart Association (AHA) recommends that triglyceride levels be below 150 mg/dl.

In the average American diet, about 45% of the total calories come from fat. This level exceeds that recommended in the AHA Step 1 Diet. Dietary fat comes in many forms and "disguises." A high intake of cholesterol and saturated fats is associated with the development of CHD, whereas a proportional intake of polyunsaturated and monounsaturated fats is linked with lower risk. Following a Mediterranean diet, described in the Complementary and Alternative Therapy feature below, may lower the risk of CHD. The AHA Step 1 Diet contains no more than 30% of calories from fat, 55% from carbohydrate (at least half of which should be complex), and 15% from protein. When fat intake does not exceed 30% of total calories, the expected rise in triglyceride levels from a high-carbohydrate diet is minimal. Saturated fats should account for no more than 10% of caloric intake.

COMPLEMENTARY AND ALTERNATIVE THERAPY

Mediterranean Diets and Cardiovascular Disease

A traditional Mediterranean diet may reduce the risk of dying from cardiovascular disease and cancer. Researchers evaluated more than 22,000 apparently healthy individuals ages 22 to 86 in Greece. Participants were rated on how closely they followed a Mediterranean diet. This type of diet is traditionally high in fruits and vegetables, legumes, nuts, cereal grains, and olive oil (monounsaturated fat); contains moderate amounts of fish, dairy (mostly cheese and yogurt), and alcohol; and is low in saturated fat. Adherence to the diet was measured on a scale of 0 (did not follow the diet closely) to 9 (strictly followed the diet). After about 4 years of follow-up, the researchers found that the more closely individuals adhered to the diet, the lower their risk of death, including death from cardiovascular disease and cancer (about a 25% decrease for every 2-point increase on the scale). Thus a greater adherence to the traditional Mediterranean diet was associated with a significant reduction in total mortality.[2]

The first clinical-trial evidence in support of the health benefits of the Mediterranean diet came from the Lyon Diet Heart Study, in which 605 clients with a previous MI were randomly assigned to a Mediterranean diet or a control diet similar to the AHA Step 1 Diet. Clients in the Mediterranean diet arm were encouraged to eat more fruits, vegetables, and fish; to eat less red meat; and to replace butter and cream with margarine high in alpha-linolenic acid (canola oil based margarine). After a mean follow-up of 27 months, the trial was stopped because of a 73% reduction in coronary events and a 70% reduction in all-cause or total mortality in the Mediterranean diet arm of the study.[1]

REFERENCES

1. de Lorgeril, M., et al. (1994). Mediterranean alpha-linolenic acid–rich diet in secondary prevention of coronary heart disease. *Lancet, 343,* 1454-1459.
2. Trichopoulou, A., et al. (2003). Adherence to a Mediterranean diet and survival in a Greek population. *New England Journal of Medicine, 348,* 2599-2608.

See the Complementary and Alternative Therapy features Eggs and Heart Disease, Do All Fish Products Prevent Heart Disease?, and Nuts and the Risk of Sudden Cardiac Death on the website.

Physical Inactivity

In the United States about 25% of adults report no leisure-time physical activity, even though regular aerobic exercise is important in preventing heart and blood vessel disease. There is an inverse relationship between exercise and the risk of CHD. Those who exercise reduce their risk of CHD because they have (1) higher HDL levels; (2) lower LDL cholesterol, triglyceride, and blood glucose levels; (3) greater insulin sensitivity; (4) lower blood pressure; and (5) lower body mass index. The AHA recommends 30 to 60 minutes of physical activity on most days of the week.

Obesity

Obesity places an extra burden on the heart, requiring the muscle to work harder to pump enough blood to support added tissue mass. In addition obesity increases the risk for CHD because it is often associated with elevated serum cholesterol and triglyceride levels, high blood pressure, and diabetes. The prevalence of obesity has increased to 30% in the years 1999 to 2002 compared to 22% from 1988 to 1994. Since 1993 the prevalence of those who are obese increased to 61%.

Distribution of body fat is also important. A waist measurement is a way to estimate fat. For men a high-risk waistline measurement is more than 40 inches, and for women a high-risk waist measurement is more than 35 inches. Body mass index (BMI) is another measure to estimate body fat. A BMI from 18.5 to 24.9 is considered healthy. Extreme obesity, or a BMI greater than 40, is estimated to occur in 4.9% of the population. People can lower their heart disease risk by losing as little as 10 to 20 pounds. An alternating pattern of weight gain and weight loss, however, is associated with an increased risk for CHD.

Diabetes

Since 1990 the prevalence of people diagnosed with diabetes increased by 61%. In addition, the prevalence of diabetes has increased by 8% since 2000 to 2001. Contributing to these statistics is the increased frequency of obesity and sedentary lifestyles. A fasting blood glucose level of more than 126 mg/dl or a routine blood glucose level of 180 mg/dl and glucosuria signals the presence of diabetes and represents an increased risk for CHD. Clients with diabetes have a two- to four-fold higher prevalence, incidence, and mortality from all forms of CHD.

Contributing Risk Factors

Response to Stress

A person's response to stress may contribute to the development of CHD. Some researchers have reported a relationship between CHD risk and stress levels, health behaviors, and socioeconomic status. Stress response appears to increase CHD risk through its effect on major risk factors. For example, some people respond to stress by overeating or by starting or increasing smoking. Stress is also associated with elevated blood pressure. Although stress is unavoidable in modern life, an excessive response to stress can be a health hazard. Significant stressors include major changes in residence, occupation, or socioeconomic status.

Homocysteine Levels

Researchers have reported that elevated levels of plasma homocysteine (an amino acid produced by the body) are associated with an increased risk of CHD (see the Complementary and Alternative Therapy feature on Elevated Homocysteine Levels and Heart Disease on the website). Scientists do not know whether homocysteine directly or indirectly increases CHD risk, however, because homocysteine levels are related to renal function, smoking, fibrinogen, and C-reactive protein (CRP). Elevated homocysteine levels can be reduced by treatment with folic acid, vitamin B_6, and vitamin B_{12}. Experts currently recommend that homocysteine levels be measured in people with a history of premature CHD, stroke, or both in the absence of other risk factors.

Inflammatory Responses

A newly identified risk factor currently being researched is the presence of any chronic inflammatory state that leads to an increase in the body's production of C-reactive protein (CRP). Too much CRP tends to destabilize plaque inside artery walls. When plaque lesions crack or break, a clot is formed and this may lead to a heart attack. Researchers have discovered that a high CRP level is a marker for coronary disease. This means that clients with chronic inflammatory diseases, such as arthritis, lupus, and autoimmune deficiency, may be at higher risk for heart attack.

Menopause

The incidence of CHD markedly increases among women after menopause. Before menopause estrogen is thought to protect against CHD risk by raising HDL and lowering LDL levels. Epidemiologic studies have shown that the loss of natural estrogen as women age may be associated with increases in total and LDL cholesterol and a gradually increasing CHD risk. If menopause is caused by surgical removal of the uterus and ovaries, the risks of CHD and MI increase.

Multiple research studies on the potential benefits of estrogen replacement therapy (ERT) and hormone replacement therapy (HRT) have yielded inconsistent results. Recent recommendations by the AHA outline the potential benefits and risks associated with HRT.

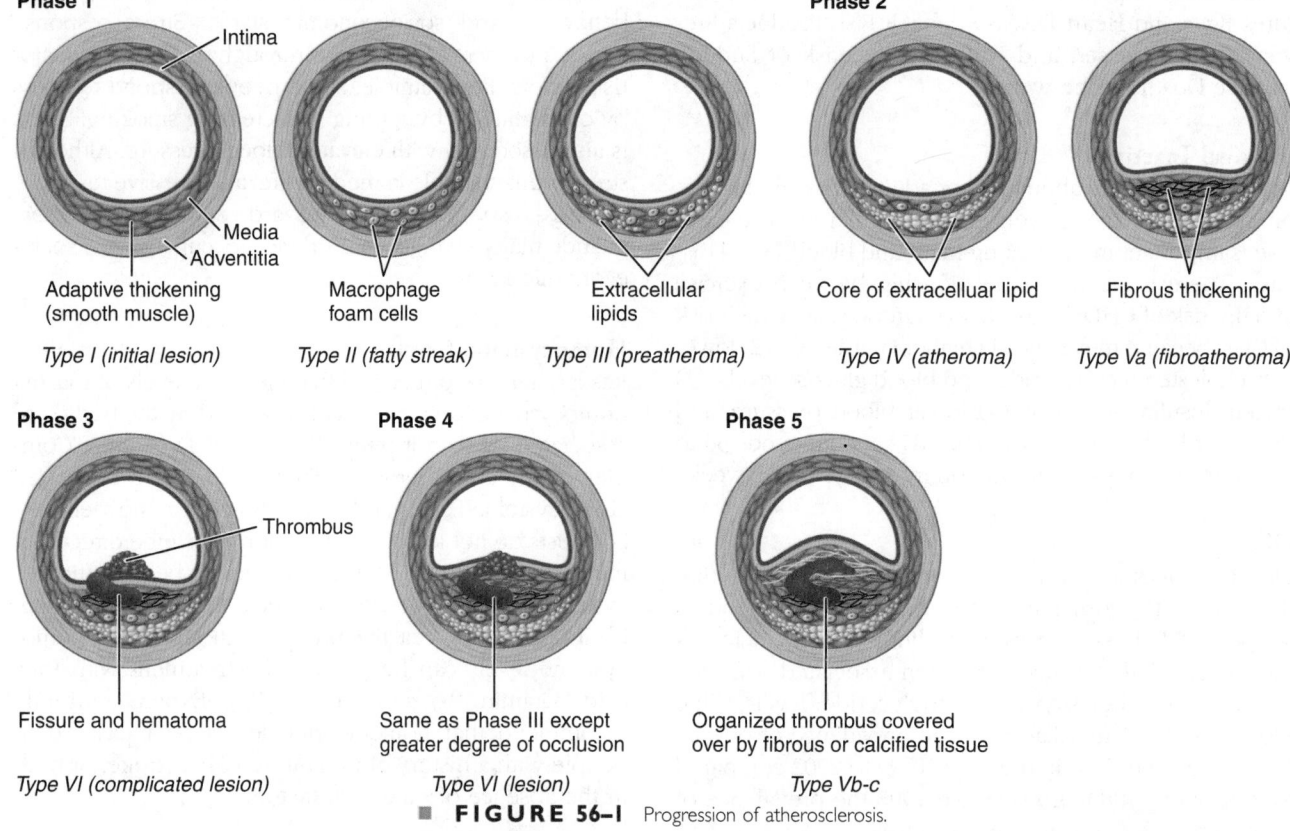

■ **FIGURE 56–1** Progression of atherosclerosis.

The recommendations advise against the use of HRT for the secondary prevention of CHD. There continues to be research to investigate the use of HRT for the primary prevention of CHD.

Pathophysiology

Coronary artery atherosclerosis is a progressive disease that begins early in life. Although several risk factors are present, endothelial injury is caused by an inflammatory response in the intimal layer of the wall and the deposition of lipids into the wall. This process has been shown to occur in five phases that include six progressive types of lesions (Figure 56-1).

Phase 1 is present in most people 30 years of age and younger and is characterized by clinically silent lesions of types I through III that do not appreciably thicken the arterial wall or narrow the arterial lumen. *Type I* lesions are microscopic adaptations of smooth muscle and occur most often near branches in the arteries. Type I lesions progress and mature into *type II* lesions. *Type III* lesions, known as *intermediate* lesions, develop during one's 20s. These lesions surround the smooth muscle cells. Type III lesions are also referred to as *pre-atheromas* because they form the bridge between early and advanced lesions. In phase 1, the progression of lesions is predictable, characteristic, and uniform.

Phase 2, characterized by type IV and V lesions, represents the development of vulnerable plaques. The *type IV* lesion, also called an *atheroma,* is characterized by further changes in the intimal structure caused by the accumulation of large amounts of extracellular lipids and fibrous tissue localized into a lipid core. The lipid core thickens the artery wall but often does not narrow the lumen of the artery. The periphery of type IV lesions is vulnerable to rupture, which may lead to rapid progression to more severe lesions.

When new fibrous connective tissue forms a thin protective cap over the atheroma, the lesion is classified as *type V.* These lesions are further subdivided into types Va, Vb, and Vc. *Type Va* lesions contain irregularly stacked multiple layers of lipid cores separated by thick layers of fibrous connective tissue. These lesions may rapidly progress to a *type VI* lesion or continue to develop into stenotic plaques that eventually occlude the entire lumen of the artery. A type V lesion that contains calcium in the lipid core and other parts of the lesion is referred to as *type Vb.* The absence of a lipid core, with minimal lipid deposition in other parts of the lesion, is characteristic of a *type Vc* lesion. *Type Vc* lesions are often seen in arteries in the legs.

Phase 3 is marked by the acute disruption of type IV and V lesions that causes thrombus formation and the development of a type VI lesion *(complicated).* If thrombus formation during phase 3 does not limit the flow of blood through the artery, these events are often asymptomatic. The net result of phase 3 is a rapid increase in plaque size that may result in stable angina. If the thrombus reduces or significantly blocks flow through the artery *(phase IV)*, an acute coronary syndrome such as unstable angina, MI, or sudden cardiac death often results (see Chapter 58). Type VI lesions are characterized by a core that contains extracellular lipids, tissue factor, collagen, platelets, thrombin, and fibrin. These lesions may also be associated with disruption of the plaque surface, hematoma or hemorrhage into the plaque, and thrombosis.

Phase 5 follows a phase 3 or 4 event and occurs when the thrombus over the disrupted plaque begins to calcify (type Vb lesion) or fibrose (type Vc lesion), forming a chronic stenotic lesion. The phase 5 lesion often contains organizing thrombi from several earlier episodes of plaque disruption, ulceration, hemorrhage, and organization. As the phase 5 lesion progresses, it occludes a greater portion of the arterial lumen and eventually may lead to total occlusion. Phase 5 lesions are associated with chronic stable angina and are often accompanied by the development of collateral circulation.

Collateral circulation is the presence of more than one artery supplying a muscle (Figure 56-2). Normally some collateral circulation is present in the coronary arteries, especially in older people. Collateral vessels develop when the blood flow through an artery progressively decreases and causes ischemia to the muscle. Extra blood vessels develop to meet the metabolic demands of the muscle. The development of collateral circulation takes time. Therefore an occlusion of a coronary artery in a younger person is more likely to be lethal because there are no collateral arteries present to supply the myocardium with blood.

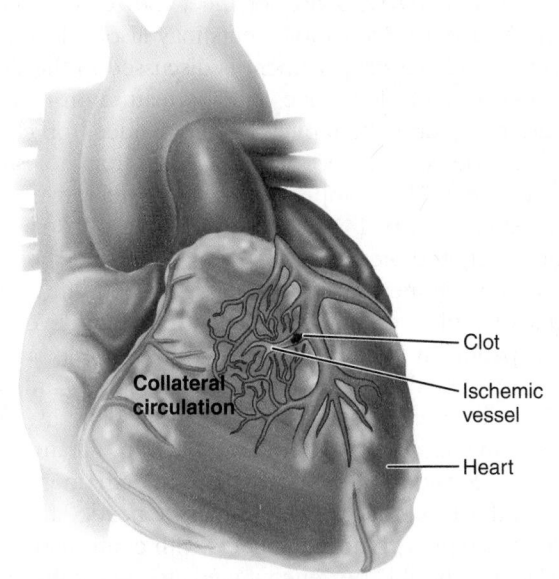

FIGURE 56–2 Collateral circulation develops when new vessels form during ischemic periods.

For many years researchers thought that the more obstructive lesions (types Vb and Vc) were responsible for most occlusions of the coronary arteries and acute coronary events. In contrast, more recent studies suggest that lesions that produce mild stenosis (types IV and Va) are more frequently associated with rapid progression to coronary occlusion. In fact nearly 60% to 70% of all acute coronary syndromes occur in arteries with mild (<50% stenosis) or moderate (50% to 70% stenosis) occlusion. It is thought that this occurs because less occlusive lesions are more vulnerable to plaque rupture and thrombosis. Plaque disruption is thought to result from external stresses on the vessel and internal changes that increase plaque fragility. Physical forces that exert external pressure on the atherosclerotic plaques, such as blood and pulse pressures, heart contraction, vasospasm, and shear stress, may trigger plaque rupture. Internal factors, such as inflammation, may increase plaque vulnerability.

Clinical Manifestations

Atherosclerosis by itself does not necessarily produce subjective clinical manifestations. For manifestations to develop, there must be a critical deficit in the blood supply to the heart in proportion to the demands for oxygen and nutrients; in other words, a supply-and-demand imbalance must exist. When atherosclerosis progresses slowly, the collateral circulation that develops generally can meet the heart's demands. Thus whether manifestations of CHD develop depends on the total blood supply to the myocardium (by way of the coronary arteries and collateral circulation) and not solely on the condition of the coronary arteries.

Rapid progression of atherosclerotic lesions (type VI) may cause ischemia and may result in the development of acute coronary syndromes of unstable angina, MI, and sudden cardiac death. Slow progression of atherosclerotic lesions (types Vb and Vc) is associated with stable coronary artery disease and the clinical manifestation of chronic stable angina. These lesions usually cause ischemia during periods when myocardial oxygen demand increases. Angina, MI, and sudden cardiac death are discussed in Chapter 58.

Techniques to determine the extent of CHD and identify the affected vessels include the electrocardiogram (ECG); B-mode ultrasonography; Doppler flow studies; intravascular ultrasound; electron-beam computed tomography; and thallium, sestamibi, or echocardiographic stress tests (see Chapter 58).

OUTCOME MANAGEMENT

Medical Management

The primary goals that guide the medical management of a client with CHD are reducing and controlling risk factors and restoring blood supply to the myocardium.

Reduce Risk Factors

Prevention, rather than treatment, is the goal with regard to CHD. Modification of risk factors can significantly improve prognosis even after an acute coronary event. Recent findings indicate reducing risk factors may limit and even prevent the progression of CHD by increasing the stability of atherosclerotic plaques, decreasing thrombogenicity, and limiting external stress on the vessel. For people without diagnosed CHD, the goal of medical treatment is to prevent the development of risk factors and clinical disease. Cessation of cigarette smoking; participating in regular exercise; and controlling blood pressure, diabetes, cholesterol levels, and weight can reduce the risk of CHD.

Primary and secondary prevention goals are in place for all the major risk factors. Ideally primary prevention should begin with promoting healthy lifestyles in children. Primary care should include family-oriented education about the risk factors, review of the family history, and modification of risk factors. For clients with diagnosed CHD, the goals of prevention are to (1) reduce the incidence of subsequent coronary events, (2) decrease the need for treatments such as angioplasty and coronary artery bypass graft (CABG) surgery, (3) extend overall survival, and (4) improve the quality of life.

Blood pressure should be measured at least every 2 years in adults, and clients should be encouraged to control blood pressure by maintaining ideal weight, exercising regularly, moderating alcohol intake, and following a moderately low sodium diet (alcohol intake is discussed in the Complementary and Alternative Therapy feature at right). Blood pressure should be below 140/90 mm Hg (<130/85 mm Hg for those with heart failure, diabetes, or renal insufficiency). Antihypertensive therapy should begin if blood pressure exceeds 140/90 mm Hg after 6 months of lifestyle modification or if the initial blood pressure exceeds 160/100 mm Hg (130/85 mm Hg for those with heart failure, diabetes, or renal insufficiency). Clients should stop smoking and avoid contact with secondary smoke. Health professionals should provide counseling, nicotine replacement, and referrals to smoking-cessation programs for clients who smoke.

Total, LDL, and HDL cholesterol should be measured annually for adults older than 20 years. The following are the primary prevention goals for cholesterol management:

- LDL <160 mg/dl if no risk factors or only one risk factor
- LDL <130 mg/dl if two or more risk factors
- HDL >40 mg/dl
- Triglycerides <150 mg/dl

The following are the secondary prevention goals for cholesterol management:

- LDL <100 mg/dl
- HDL >40 mg/dl
- Triglycerides <150 mg/dl

COMPLEMENTARY AND ALTERNATIVE THERAPY

Which Type of Alcohol Reduces the Risk of Heart Disease?

Researchers studied the association of alcohol ingestion with the risk of MI among more than 38,000 male health professionals who were free of cardiovascular disease and cancer at baseline. Alcohol consumption and type of alcohol were documented every 4 years using a food-frequency questionnaire. After 12 years of follow-up, the total number of MIs was 1418. Compared with men who consumed alcohol less than once a week, men who consumed alcohol 3 or 4 or 5-7 days per week had a 32% and 37% reduction of MI, respectively. The risk was similar in men who consumed less than 10 g of alcohol per drinking day and those who consumed 30 g or more (a single alcoholic drink contains 11 to 14 g of alcohol). No single type of alcoholic beverage provided an additional benefit. In other words, red wine, white wine, beer, and liquor were similar in their effect. Therefore moderate drinking was associated with a reduced risk of MI. The problem with this large study is that although alcohol in moderation seems to reduce the risk of dying from a MI, researchers are not sure whether or not it reduces the risk of all-cause mortality (this needs to be studied). Regardless, for now moderate consumption reduces the risk of death from cardiovascular disease.

REFERENCE

Mukamal, K., et al. (2003). Roles of drinking pattern and type of alcohol consumed in coronary heart disease in men. *New England Journal of Medicine, 348,* 109-118.

The AHA Step 1 Diet should be recommended for clients who are unable to meet the primary prevention goals, and the Step 2 Diet should be recommended for those with CHD who do not meet the recommended goals. Red-yeast rice supplements may also reduce cholesterol level. This supplement is discussed in the Complementary and Alternative Therapy feature on p. 1417. In addition, drug therapy is recommended for clients who do not meet the recommended goals for cholesterol management. The Complementary and Alternative Therapy features on p. 1417 consider the interplay of statin drugs, diet, and dietary supplements.

During routine physical examinations, health professionals should determine the client's activity level and participation in exercise. Clients should be encouraged to exercise at least five times weekly for 30 minutes and to increase their physical activity in daily life. The Complementary and Alternative Therapy feature on p. 1417 considers the benefits of strength training in men with CHD. An exercise test may be needed to guide an exercise prescription for clients with confirmed CHD.

Clients should be encouraged to maintain ideal body weight as indicated by a BMI between 18.5 and

Red Yeast Rice Supplements to Reduce Cholesterol

Chinese red yeast rice supplements have been available on the U.S. market for several years, and currently they have been involved in litigation because some companies argue that this natural supplement has a similar structure to cholesterol-lowering drugs (statins). This supplement was tested against a placebo in 83 individuals (46 men, 37 women). A total of 2.4 g of red yeast rice or placebo was given daily for 3 months. Levels of total cholesterol, LDL, and triglycerides decreased compared with the placebo arm of the study. Total cholesterol level had the largest reduction, with an average decrease of 45 mg/dl. This supplement showed no effect on HDL (good cholesterol) levels. No apparent adverse effects were seen with this supplement, but this study was of short duration.

REFERENCE

Ashley, J., et al. (1999). Cholesterol-lowering effects of a proprietary Chinese red-yeast-rice dietary supplement. *American Journal of Clinical Nutrition, 69,*231-236.

Statin Drugs and Dietary Supplements

The largest randomized trial of statin drugs in combination with supplements included 160 individuals studied over 3 years. The supplement combination included 800 international units of vitamin E plus 100 mcg of selenium plus 1000 mg of vitamin C and 25 mg of beta-carotene with or without a statin drug plus niacin. Simvastatin plus niacin provided a marked clinical angiographically measurable benefit in clients with coronary disease and low HDL levels. The group taking the supplement combination plus the statin drug experienced a significant reduction in HDL (or "good cholesterol") compared with the group that took the statin drug alone. Further study is needed to determine whether the desired effects of statin drugs are diminished when taken in combination with antioxidant vitamin supplements.

REFERENCE

Brown, B.G., et al. (2001). Simvastatin and niacin, antioxidant vitamins, or the combination for the prevention of coronary disease. *New England Journal of Medicine, 345,*1583-1592.

Diet Versus Statin Therapy for High Cholesterol

A preliminary recent study randomly assigned 55 healthy hyperlipidemic men and women to receive 1 of 3 treatments: a very low saturated fat diet based on low-fat dairy foods and whole-grain cereals (control arm); the same diet plus 20 mg daily of lovastatin (statin group); or a diet with a high intake of plant sterols, soy protein, soluble fibers, and almonds (dietary portfolio group). The data were based on 46 clients who completed the 4-week study. The researchers reported that the statin and dietary portfolio treatment arms had about a 30% decrease in LDL ("bad cholesterol") versus an 8% reduction in the control group. Although a longer and larger trial is needed, this unique study suggests that over a short period, individuals willing to try a more directed dietary change could potentially reduce their cholesterol as much as some cholesterol-lowering drugs; however, cholesterol-lowering drugs are still the treatment of choice for clients who cannot significantly reduce their cholesterol levels with diet and physical activity over a period of 3 to 6 months.

REFERENCE

Jenkins, D., et al. (2003). Effects of a dietary portfolio of cholesterol-lowering foods vs lovastatin on serum lipids and C-reactive protein. *Journal of the American Medical Association, 290,* 502-510.

Lifting Weights and Coronary Heart Disease in Men

A cohort of 44,452 men enrolled in the Health Professionals' Follow-up Study were followed up at 2-year intervals from 1986 to 1998. Men who trained with weights for 30 minutes or more per week had a 23% risk reduction in coronary heart disease compared with men who did not train with weights ($P = 0.03$ for trend). In summary, researchers found that total physical activity, running, weight training, and walking were each associated with a reduced risk of coronary heart disease.

REFERENCE

Tanasescu, M., et al. (2002). Exercise type and intensity in relation to coronary heart disease in men. *Journal of the American Medical Association, 288,* 1994-2000.

24.9 kg/m^2 and a waist circumference less than 40 inches in men and 35 inches in women. Height, weight, BMI, and waist-to-hip ratio should be measured at each visit. People with BMI and waist circumferences higher than those recommended should be counseled regarding weight management and physical activity.

Fasting blood glucose concentration should be maintained near normal levels in clients with diabetes mellitus. Hypoglycemic therapy should be used to achieve normal fasting blood glucose as indicated by hemoglobin A_{1C} (HbA$_{1C}$) value. The recommended goal for HbA$_{1C}$ is <7%. Other risk factors should be treated aggressively.

Hormone replacement therapy should be considered for all postmenopausal women without diagnosed CHD, particularly if they have multiple risk factors. The decision about HRT, however, should be made by considering the risks for breast cancer, gallbladder disease, thromboembolic disease, and endometrial cancer. Estrogen-progesterone therapy reportedly increases cardiovascular events in women with diagnosed CHD during the first year of treatment but decreases events in the fourth and fifth years. Consequently, initiating estrogen-progesterone therapy for women with confirmed CHD is not recommended. For women with CHD who have already been receiving HRT for more than 1 year, continuing therapy is recommended until the results of additional research are known.

Additional management strategies are recommended for clients with diagnosed CHD. These include the use of antiplatelet therapies such as acetylsalicylic acid (aspirin), heparin, and low-molecular-weight heparin if it is not contraindicated. Aspirin reduces the risk of fatal or nonfatal MI by 71% during the acute phase, by 60% at 3 months, and by 52% at 2 years[14] (see the website Complementary and Alternative Therapy feature Aspirin to Reduce the Risk of Coronary Artery Disease). Adjunctive therapies, such as angiotensin-converting enzyme (ACE) inhibitors, beta-blockers, and nitrates, are also recommended.

Glycoprotein IIb/IIIa (GPIIb/IIIa) receptor antagonists are the most recent pharmacologic treatment for secondary prevention of CHD. These drugs prevent platelet aggregation in acute coronary syndromes, and when combined with aspirin they decrease the incidence of recurrent cardiac events. The therapeutic effects, adverse responses, and nursing implications of pharmacologic agents used in the primary prevention of CHD are outlined in the Integrating Pharmacology feature below.

Restore Blood Supply

For some clients even aggressive management of risk factors fails to prevent coronary occlusion. Various techniques have been developed to open the vessels and restore blood flow through the coronary arteries. Percutaneous coronary intervention (PCI) includes percutaneous luminal coronary angioplasty, rotational atherectomy, directional atherectomy, laser angioplasty, and implantation of intracoronary stents. The American College of Cardiology, along with the AHA, issues guidelines for the use of PCI and reports on all procedures collectively. More than 500,000 PCI procedures are performed yearly. The use of percutaneous transluminal coronary angioplasty (PTCA) alone has decreased dramatically, whereas the use of PCTA with placement of intracoronary stents has dramatically increased. Stents have been shown to reduce late restenosis in coronary arteries. The use of GPIIb/IIIa platelet receptor antagonists has also improved outcomes of PCI. PCI is recommended for clients with mild angina, single or multivessel coronary artery disease, unstable angina, and acute MI and following thrombolytic therapy. These procedures are performed in a "catheterization laboratory," which is outfitted with high-resolution fluoroscopy and x-ray.

INTEGRATING PHARMACOLOGY

Preventive Pharmacology for Coronary Heart Disease

Several medications can be prescribed to prevent the development or progression of coronary heart disease. They include statins to reduce elevated LDL levels and antiplatelet aggregates to reduce the risk of clotting in narrowed vessels.

STATINS

A reduction in elevated LDL levels can significantly reduce coronary events in individuals without CHD. Lipid-lowering drug therapy for primary CHD prevention is most clearly indicated when two or more CHD risk factors are present and the LDL level remains higher than 160 mg/dl after an adequate dietary trial. In addition, clients with LDL levels higher than 160 mg/dl and with one other strong risk factor (diabetes, smoking, or a family history of early CHD) may also be candidates for drug therapy. For clients with elevated risk attributable to sudden cardiac death in family members and elevated LDL levels, drug treatment may be beneficial.

Educating the client about the need to take this medication for a lifetime is important. Noticeable effects will not be seen and may lead clients to discontinue the medication without informing their care provider. If cost is an issue, consider prescribing half-pill doses or recommending ingestion of grapefruit juice when the drug is taken to increase drug absorption. Follow-up assessment of serum lipid levels is important to monitor progress.

Clients should be taught that the medication must be taken every day indefinitely to maximize benefit, noting that the LDL level returns to the pretreatment level soon after the medication is discontinued. Dietary adjustments must also be continued.

ANTIPLATELET AGGREGATING AGENTS

Aspirin in low doses is the best known agent for the prevention of coronary heart disease. Aspirin's benefits include reducing the coagulability of blood so that it can flow more freely through tight, narrow vessels. Aspirin is also an anti-inflammatory agent and can reduce the inflammatory process, which destabilizes plaque inside artery walls. A risk factor with the consumption of aspirin is that clients may take the medication because it is readily available without prescription believing it could not harm them. Aspirin should not be used by clients with allergy to aspirin or other salicylates, asthma, uncontrolled high blood pressure, severe liver or kidney disease, excess alcohol consumption, or bleeding disorders. Clients taking other medications that affect bleeding or clotting also should not take aspirin.

Percutaneous Transluminal Coronary Angioplasty. Percutaneous transluminal coronary angioplasty (PTCA) is a technique in which a balloon-tipped catheter is usually inserted into the femoral artery (although the brachial or radial artery can be used) and threaded under x-ray guidance into a blocked coronary artery. The balloon is inflated several times to reshape the lumen by stretching it and flattening the atherosclerotic plaque against the arterial wall (analogous to making footprints in the snow), thus opening the artery (Figure 56-3). PTCA is less invasive and less expensive than open heart surgery and therefore is an attractive alternative.

Directional Coronary Atherectomy. Directional coronary atherectomy (DCA) reduces coronary stenosis by excising and removing atheromatous plaque. The DCA cutter consists of a catheter that contains a rigid cylindrical housing with a central rotating blade (Figure 56-3, *E*). The blade shaves off the atherosclerotic material and deposits it in the nose cone of the housing for later histopathologic study. DCA is appropriate for lesions in medium to large coronary arteries located in the proximal or middle portions of the vessel. It is not recommended for use with tortuous vessels, distal lesions, or heavily calcified lesions.

Intracoronary Stents. Intracoronary stents were originally designed to reduce restenosis and abrupt closure of coronary vessels resulting from complications of coronary angioplasty. They are now used instead of PTCA to eliminate the risk of acute closure and to improve long-term patency. Several different stent designs are available, but most are balloon-expandable or self-expandable tubes that, when placed in a coronary artery, act as a mechanical scaffold to reopen the blocked artery (Figure 56-3, *C*). Coronary stents are made of numerous materials, ranging from stainless steel to bioabsorbable compounds. The procedure for placing a stent is similar to that for PTCA. Once the coronary lesion is identified by angiography, the balloon catheter bearing the stent is inserted into the coronary artery and the stent is positioned at the site of the occlusion. A major concern related to stent placement is the prevention of acute thrombosis, especially during the first several weeks after the procedure. The use of

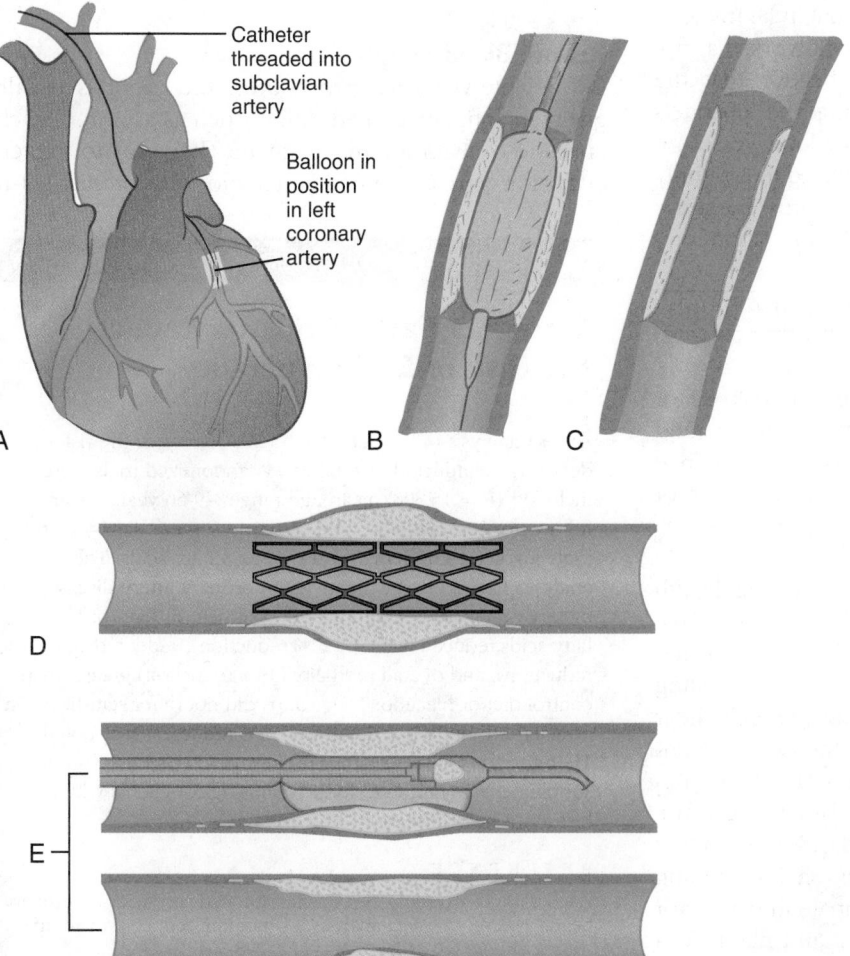

Catheter threaded into subclavian artery

Balloon in position in left coronary artery

A

B

C

D

E

■ **FIGURE 56–3** Interventional cardiology can be performed to open occluded coronary arteries. **A,** Percutaneous transluminal coronary angioplasty (PTCA). **B,** The balloon-tipped catheter is centered in the lesion and expanded to compress the blockage. **C,** The artery is restored to its original diameter. **D,** Placement of a coronary artery stent at the site of the lesion. **E,** Atherectomy. If the plaque has hardened and become calcified, atherectomy can be used to pulverize the material. Some catheters are fitted with a laser that dissolves the lesions.

GPIIb/IIIa platelet receptor antagonists has decreased the risk of thrombus formation following stent placement. New technology, including the use of intracoronary gamma and beta radiation with stent placement, has reduced restenosis rates by 3% to 50%. The use of stents coated with antiplatelet drugs has been shown to decrease rates of restenosis.

Laser Ablation. Lasers are used with balloon angioplasty to vaporize atherosclerotic plaque. After the initial balloon angioplasty, a brief burst of laser radiation is administered and additional remaining plaque is removed. Results of clinical trials indicate that laser ablation combined with balloon angioplasty is more effective in treating lesions that typically respond poorly to angioplasty alone. Complications include coronary dissection, acute occlusion, perforation, and embolism.

Transmyocardial Revascularization. A new type of laser catheter, used in a procedure called transmyocardial revascularization (TMR), may be able to help clients who are not candidates for surgery or angioplasty because of ill health or degree of disease. The high-powered laser is guided into the left ventricle between heartbeats when the ventricle is filling with blood. The laser creates from 15 to 40 1-mm channels through the myocardium. The exact mechanism by which TMR works has not been established; however, scientists believe that the "controlled trauma" caused by creating the channels may promote the growth of small new blood vessels, a process called *angiogenesis*. TMR is estimated to cost only slightly more than PTCA, and sustained improvement has been seen up to 27 months following the operation.

Nursing Management of the Medical Client

Reduce Risk Factors

Nursing management for CHD focuses on risk factor modification through risk assessment, screening, and education. The client's level of motivation to reduce cardiovascular risk factors is the primary predictor of success. Nursing researchers are studying methods to improve motivation.

Primary prevention efforts include providing health education about reducing the risk factors for CHD. Encourage clients to reduce their risk by lowering dietary intake of fats and cholesterol, exercising, controlling diabetes and hypertension, keeping body weight near ideal levels, and ceasing smoking (see the Complementary and Alternative Therapy feature on Moderate Lifestyle Change and Coronary Artery Disease on the *evolve* website). The risk and incidence of CHD are so high that many clients are doing these activities on an ongoing basis. Reinforce these behaviors. Participate in risk factor screening for both children and adults, and maintain a high index of suspicion for clients at increased risk for

CHD. Teach stress-reduction techniques, such as progressive muscle relaxation and guided imagery. Instruct postmenopausal women to discuss the need for estrogen HRT with their physician. Monitor blood pressure control in clients with diagnosed hypertension, and monitor HbA_{1C} levels in diabetic clients.

Nursing interventions for clients with diagnosed CHD include assessing their CHD risk and explaining diagnostic tests, when to seek treatment, clinical manifestations of complications, and the actions, dosages, and side effects of prescribed medications. Assess cardiovascular risk factors, and provide individualized education on risk reduction. Emphasize the importance of adopting risk-reduction behaviors and participating in cardiac rehabilitation to prevent recurrence or progression of CHD. Teach clients the clinical manifestations of angina and MI. Monitor therapeutic drug levels as appropriate. Emphasize the importance of keeping follow-up appointments with health care practitioners. Most important, instruct clients to seek prompt medical attention if manifestations of CHD return.

Many clients use forms of alternative therapies for self-treatment of heart disease. The Complementary and Alternative Therapy feature below examines one commonly used therapy.

Restore Blood Supply

Before interventional procedures, the client is usually given an antiplatelet medication, such as aspirin. The client is also given an anticoagulant (heparin) to prevent occlusion and calcium-channel blockers or nitrates to

---

COMPLEMENTARY AND ALTERNATIVE THERAPY

Omega-3 Fatty Acids to Reduce the Risk of Early Mortality

A meta-analysis of omega-3 fatty acids to reduce the risk of death was conducted. A total of 11 randomized trials were included ($n = 15,806$; mean age range, 49-66 years; mean follow-up, 20 months). Of the 11 trials, 2 were dietary, and 9 trials involved supplements of omega-3 fatty acids. The meta-analyses found that in clients with coronary artery disease, dietary or supplemental intake (1 g of fish oil/day) of omega-3 fatty acids reduced fatal MI (27% reduction), sudden death (31% reduction), and overall mortality (19% reduction) greater than a control diet or placebo. The groups did not differ statistically in nonfatal MI, but a nonsignificant 20% reduction was noted. Therefore diets high in omega-3 fatty acids (fish) or fish oil supplements continue to look promising for clients with a history of heart disease.

REFERENCE

Bucher, H., et al. (2002). N-3 polyunsaturated fatty acids in coronary heart disease: A meta-analysis of randomized controlled trials. *American Journal of Medicine, 112*, 298-304.

reduce coronary spasm during the procedure. After the procedure, the client may continue with this drug regimen to prevent reocclusion or arterial spasms.

The client's blood is also typed and crossmatched in the event emergency CABG surgery is needed. A consent form is signed for the interventional procedure and surgery, if required, for spasm, perforation of the artery, or acute occlusion. Following interventional procedures, monitor the vital signs for changes, especially the quality and rhythm of the pulse and in the ECG. Report any indication of coronary ischemia to the physician. ST-segment monitoring is frequently used to detect ischemia.

Complications include bleeding and hematoma formation at the puncture site, acute MI resulting from perforation of an artery, refractory spasm, or occlusion. If the client complains of chest pain, obtain a 12-lead ECG immediately. Force fluids, orally or intravenously, to assist the body in excreting contrast medium, which causes diuresis and may cause acute renal tubular necrosis. Monitor the puncture site for hematoma, and palpate pulses to assess peripheral perfusion.

The physician may order bed rest for longer periods for clients undergoing stent placement and DCA because of the larger sheaths used to dilate the vessels in these procedures.

Nursing considerations specific to the care of the client with a coronary stent include close monitoring of anticoagulation status and ongoing assessment for bleeding. Until the sheath is removed, instruct the client to limit movement of the sheathed leg and keep the head of the bed below 30 degrees to prevent bleeding and hematoma formation at the site. Clients with coronary stents usually have longer hospital stays than clients undergoing other interventional procedures because their antithrombin therapy must be monitored closely.

Surgical Management

Cardiac Surgery
There are three types of cardiac surgery:
1. *Reparative* procedures are likely to produce a cure or excellent and prolonged improvement. Examples are closure of a patent ductus arteriosus, atrial septal defect, and ventricular septal defect; repair of mitral stenosis; and simple repair of tetralogy of Fallot.
2. *Reconstructive* procedures are more complex. They are not always curative, and reoperation may be needed. Examples are CABG and reconstruction of an incompetent mitral, tricuspid, or aortic valve.
3. *Substitutional* procedures are not usually curative because of the preoperative condition of the client. Examples are valve replacement, cardiac replacement by transplantation, ventricular replacement or assistance, and cardiac replacement by mechanical devices.

Open Heart Surgery
Cardiopulmonary bypass is used during cardiac surgery to divert the client's unoxygenated blood to a machine in which oxygenation and circulation occur. Reoxygenated blood is then returned to the client's circulation. This technique, called extracorporeal circulation (ECC, also called the heart-lung machine), allows the surgeon to stop the heart during the time of surgery. The heart-lung machine does the following:

- Diverts circulation from the heart and lungs, providing the surgeon with a bloodless operative field
- Performs all gas exchange functions
- Filters, rewarms, or cools the blood
- Circulates oxygenated, filtered blood back into the arterial system

The three components of cardiopulmonary bypass are hemodilution, hypothermia, and anticoagulation. Hemodilution occurs as the client's blood becomes diluted with the isotonic crystalloid solution used to prime the bypass machine. Hypothermia (28° to 36° C) is used to reduce tissue oxygen requirements by approximately 50% to protect the organs from ischemic injury. Anticoagulation is necessary to prevent coagulation in the bypass machine once the client's blood comes into contact with the surfaces in the machine. These three components contribute to the clinical sequelae and the complications associated with cardiopulmonary bypass, including coagulopathies. Excessive bleeding after cardiac surgery is related to the hemodilution and excessive activation of the hemostatic system because blood cells are injured as they contact the bypass machine. The risk of complications is high when the duration of cardiopulmonary bypass exceeds 2 hours and dramatically increases whenever bypass persists beyond 3 to 4 hours. This proportional increase in complications is attributed to the increase in blood trauma, altered capillary membrane permeability, and subsequent tissue hypoxia.

Coronary Artery Bypass Graft
Coronary artery bypass graft (CABG) surgery involves the bypass of a blockage in one or more of the coronary arteries using the saphenous veins, mammary artery, or radial artery as conduits or replacement vessels. Before surgery, coronary angiography precisely locates lesions and points of narrowing within the coronary arteries.

During traditional CABG surgery, a median sternotomy incision is made so that the heart and aorta can be seen. The client is placed on cardiopulmonary bypass (CPB) and the heart is stopped (*cardioplegia*) using a solution of iced saline containing potassium. After the bypasses have been performed, the client is taken off of the machine, and the heart takes over again. Three different types of "less invasive" CABG surgery are also performed: (1) off-bypass CABG performed through a median sternotomy with a smaller incision; (2) minimally

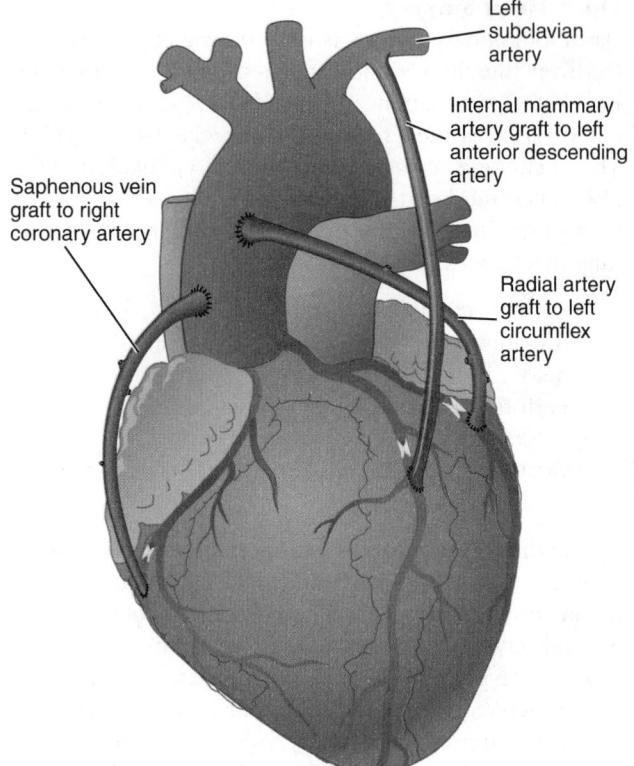

■ **FIGURE 56–4** Coronary artery bypass grafting (CABG). **A,** A section of saphenous vein is harvested from the leg and anastomosed (upside down, because of its directional valves) to a coronary artery to bypass an area of occlusion on the right coronary artery. **B,** Bypass of the left coronary artery with the internal mammary artery.

invasive direct CABG (MIDCABG) performed through a left anterior thoracotomy without cardiopulmonary bypass; and port-access CABG with femoral-to-femoral bypass and cardioplegia with a limited incision. Many institutions are performing MIDCABG surgery. In off-bypass CABG, the surgery is performed on a beating heart after a reduction in cardiac motion with several different medications and devices. The benefit of this type of CABG surgery is the avoidance of the use of CPB because of the many potential complications of CPB.

Saphenous veins can be used as the new coronary artery. The distal end of the vein is sutured to the aorta, and the proximal end is sewn to the coronary vessel distal to the blockage (Figure 56-4). The veins are reversed so that their valves do not interfere with blood flow. The internal mammary artery (IMA) can also be grafted to a coronary artery. It is more routinely used to revascularize the portion of the myocardium supplied by the left anterior descending (LAD) artery. The disadvantage of the IMA is that more time is required to remove it and the mammary artery is shorter. An advantage is that IMA grafts have a greater chance of remaining patent. Radial arteries have also been used in repeat CABG and when radiation therapy to the chest makes it impossible to use the IMA. The radial artery has had excellent patency rates.

For clients who need revascularization of the anterior coronary arteries, MIDCABG is a less invasive approach. The IMAs are used as conduits, and the client does not need to be placed on CPB. MIDCABG surgery is less costly than traditional CABG surgery and is associated with fewer postoperative complications. A small study comparing outcomes in CABG to minimally invasive bypass procedures found that fewer cardiac and pulmonary complications were reported in the minimally invasive group.

Outcomes. The use of calcium-channel blockers, PTCA, atherectomy, and stents has reduced the number of CABG surgical procedures being performed. Survival rates using CABG have not been significantly better than those of medically treated clients. CABG nevertheless remains a common procedure; and, because it can reduce angina in 80% to 90% of clients who do not respond to medical management, it will continue to be an important intervention in the management of CHD. Benefits from CABG surgery also include prolongation of life, increased exercise tolerance, reduced need for medication, and ability to resume former activities.

In studies comparing CABG with and without CPB, the advantages of surgery on a beating heart have been documented. These advantages include a decrease in mortality, in postoperative need for mechanical ventilation, in pulmonary complications, and in the incidence of stroke and atrial fibrillation. Clients who benefit from this type of CABG include those who refuse transfusions of blood and blood products and those with advanced respiratory disease, impaired renal function, and heavily calcified aortas.

Regardless of the type of operation, surgical methods only ease the manifestations. Surgery cannot halt the process of atherosclerosis, although it may prolong life in some cases. Recent studies documented an improvement in perceived quality of life following CABG, including improvements in physical functioning, social functioning, and mood states. Data on the outcomes of surgery for CHD in women continue to have conflicting results. Smaller body size in women along with smaller coronary arteries seems to be a consistent finding to explain poorer outcomes for women following CABG. Scientists are continuing to conduct research in this area.

Complications. Possible complications of CABG surgery occur in 6 areas:

Cardiovascular complications include dysrhythmias, decreased cardiac output, and persistent hypotension. While the heart's metabolic demands are reduced during surgery, the myocardium still needs nutrient blood and oxygen supply. Following surgery, the heart can be ischemic and not fully contracting. Dysrhythmias may develop from electrolyte imbalances, surgery near the conduction system, and ischemia. Inotropic medications are used to maintain cardiac output, and antidysrhythmics are used to control dysrhythmias.

When cardiac output is low, other organs can become impaired, including the brain and kidneys. In the absence of treatment, shock can develop. To improve cardiac output, the surgeon may use a mechanical device to support the failing heart if inotropic medications are unsuccessful.

The intra-aortic balloon pump (IABP) is a counterpulsation device that supports the failing heart by increasing coronary artery perfusion during diastole and reducing afterload. It consists of a sausage-shaped balloon catheter that is passed through the femoral artery and positioned in the descending thoracic aorta just distal to the subclavian artery. The catheter is attached to a power console that inflates and deflates the balloon in time with the heart.

The balloon is inflated during diastole; blood is pushed back into the aorta, and coronary artery perfusion is improved. The balloon is deflated during systole; resistance is decreased, and the workload of the heart is thus reduced. This procedure is described in the Bridge to Critical Care feature below. The timing of the balloon inflations and deflations is critical. A nurse educated in the use of the balloon pump is assigned to care for the client. Monitoring the effects of the pumping on the client's vital signs requires special skills.

Hematologic complications include bleeding and clotting. The bypass machine leads to clot formation, so the blood is anticoagulated, but this can lead to persistent

---

BRIDGE TO CRITICAL CARE

Intra-Aortic Balloon Pumping— Counterpulsation Device

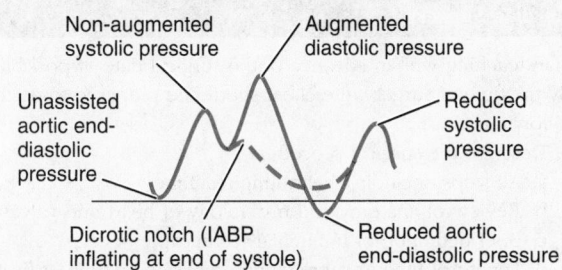

Red line represents an actual pressure tracing. An initial systolic waveform is followed by a pump-generated waveform. Then the systolic waveform is seen following a balloon waveform when systolic pressure is reduced.

When the left ventricle fails to support adequate circulation and perfusion, an intra-aortic balloon pumping (IABP) device can be used to augment coronary artery filling and decrease left ventricular workload. A polyethylene balloon is inserted via the femoral artery into the descending thoracic aorta distal to the left subclavian artery and connected to an external pneumatic pumping system. The pump inflates the balloon with helium or carbon dioxide during diastole and deflates it during systole. The inflation-deflation cycle is triggered by the client's ECG, specifically by the R wave, which signals the beginning of systole. Balloon inflation during diastole augments coronary artery filling. Systolic balloon deflation decreases afterload.

The IABP device is used in clients with cardiogenic shock, septic shock, acute anterior myocardial infarction (MI), complications following MI, angioplasty with MI, ventricular dysrhythmias with ischemia, left ventricular failure, unstable angina refractory to medications, and low cardiac output after surgery.

GUIDELINES FOR MANAGEMENT

1. Select an ECG lead that optimizes the R wave.
2. Time the IABP device using an arterial waveform.
3. Monitor perfusion in the extremity with IABP.
4. Monitor perfusion in arms (catheter can occlude subclavian artery).

5. Monitor arterial pressures (which should improve).
6. Monitor urine output (the catheter can occlude the renal artery).
7. Keep the affected limb straight to prevent dislodgment of the catheter.
8. Monitor for balloon rupture and misplacement (loss of augmentation, wrinkled appearance in safety chamber, blood in tubing).
9. Monitor for bleeding resulting from anticoagulant use.
10. Monitor for aortic dissection (acute back, retroperitoneal, testicular, or chest pain; decreased pulses; variations in blood pressure between arms; decreased cardiac output; tachycardia; decreased filling pressures; decreased hemoglobin and hematocrit levels).
11. Monitor skin integrity on the sacrum, the coccyx, and the heels.
12. Do not elevate the head of the bed above 15 degrees.
13. Clarify or reinforce the client's and family's understanding of the IABP device.

COMPLICATIONS

- Dissection of the femoral or iliac artery or aorta
- Bleeding
- Plaque dislodgment, which can cause embolization
- Balloon rupture
- Arterial occlusion with limb ischemia or neuropathy
- Mechanical destruction of red blood cells
- Inability to wean from the IABP device
- Hematoma at the insertion site
- Mesenteric/renal ischemia (catheter too low)
- Arm ischemia (catheter too high)

WEANING

The ratio of IABP-assisted beats to unassisted beats is decreased from 1:1 to 1:2 based on the following parameters:

- Heart rate <110 beats/min
- No dysrhythmias
- Mean arterial pressure >70 mm Hg without vasopressors
- Pulmonary arterial wedge pressure <18 mm Hg
- Cardiac index >2.5 L/min/m^2
- Capillary refill >3 sec
- Urine output >0.5 ml/kg/min
- SVO_2 between 70% and 80%

bleeding. In addition, the inflammatory response is triggered and leads to edema from increased capillary permeability. Edema is common after surgery; some clients gain 10 kg of fluid.

Renal complications including renal failure can develop if cardiac output is low. Prerenal renal failure can be prevented by managing fluids closely and avoiding medications that further impair renal blood flow, such as nonsteroidal anti-inflammatory drugs.

Pulmonary complications include atelectasis. Because the lungs are not ventilated during bypass surgery, the alveoli collapse. In addition, surfactant may not be produced normally. Both changes make ventilation more difficult, because each breath has to open collapsed lung tissue. Clients also have incisional pain with deep breathing and coughing and guard the chest wall to prevent pain. Early extubation and ambulation have reduced pulmonary complications.

Neurologic complications can be devastating and include stroke and encephalopathy. Stroke can be embolic or thrombotic; embolic from disrupted plaques or air in the bypass machinery. Thrombotic stroke is usually from the walls of the atria or the carotid arteries. Encephalopathy can develop from mild stroke, cerebral edema, or cerebral ischemia.

SAFETY ALERT

Wound infection and sternal dehiscence can occur following surgery. Mupirocin nasal ointment has been shown to reduce the risk of mediastinitis. Sternal dehiscence risk can be reduced by preventing strain on the incision line, for example by placing a bra on large-breasted women.

Nursing Management Before Cardiac Surgery

Clients may have experienced cardiopulmonary clinical manifestations for varying amounts of time. Some clients will have had cardiac disease for months or years. Others may have had their first manifestations of heart disease today and already be on their way to surgery.

Note the client's psychological readiness for surgery and his or her reaction to the need for heart surgery. The client may initially experience shock and grief over the impending surgery. Chief concerns may be helplessness and fear of disability or death.

The psychological preparation of the cardiac surgery client is very important. Many hospitals throughout the United States have extensive preoperative education programs that greatly reduce client and family anxiety. Such a program should include a thorough explanation of the preoperative, intraoperative, and postoperative procedures. Also helpful is the introduction of the client to involved health care team members and the health care facility environment. Box 56-2 provides a list of topics for education. Your institution probably has written material for you to use.

Allow clients to tell you in their own words about their heart problem and the surgery. Correct any misconceptions, using pictures and a model of the heart. Clients tend to ask the greatest number of questions about what will happen to them in the recovery room and intensive care unit (ICU).

Explain that they will awaken from the anesthetic with a chest tube in place. Discuss the ventilator that will assist the client's breathing for the first few to 24 hours. Remind clients that during this time they will be unable to talk. Explain that an IV line for fluid or blood will be inserted in an arm, chest and/or neck and that various equipment needed to continuously monitor vital signs will be attached to their skin.

Answer questions concerning the necessity of using blood products. Use these facts to respond to concerns about transfusion. Postoperative blood transfusions are used only as needed; blood is screened carefully, and there is little risk of contracting blood-borne illnesses.

BOX 56–2 Guidelines to Prepare the Client Undergoing Cardiac Surgery

Plan teaching well in advance of the surgical date, if possible. By the time of surgery, the client should be prepared to do the following:

1. Describe the surgical procedure:
   a. All steps, including heart-lung machine
   b. Review of anatomy and physiology of heart and valves
   c. Brief definition of unfamiliar technical terms
   d. Length of time in surgery and approximate time of first visit by family
   e. Give the client pictures of the heart and involved valve for future reference
2. Describe the intensive care unit (ICU) environment and monitoring equipment:
   a. Cardiac monitor and alarm
   b. Endotracheal (ET) tube and projected length of time with ET tube in place
   c. Mechanical ventilator and alarm
   d. Suctioning procedure
   e. Arterial line and automatic blood pressure cuff
   f. Any limitation on visits from family
   g. Chest tubes or mediastinal tubes
   h. Nasogastric tube and length of NPO (nothing by mouth) status
   i. Urinary catheter
   j. High noise level in ICU
   k. Multiple intravenous lines and fluids
3. Describe preoperative preparation:
   a. Showering with antimicrobial soap
   b. Shaving of chest, abdomen, neck, and groin
   c. Special cardiac studies: echocardiogram, electrocardiogram, cardiac catheterization
4. Describe comfort measures:
   a. Pain reduction
   b. Turning, range-of-motion exercises
   c. Out of bed next morning
   d. Medication for sleep, if needed

Emphasize that although the client will experience pain, the pain will be swiftly reduced by medication and comfort measures.

Finally, explain that the client will be awakened frequently following surgery for vital nursing assessments and interventions. Give examples of scheduled activities: vital signs every 15 minutes; temperature every 2 hours; frequent turning, coughing, and deep breathing; blood drawn for tests every morning.

Clients also need information concerning discharge from the ICU and health care facility. Explain the average length of stay in the ICU, the room to which the client will return from the ICU, the average length of stay in the health care facility, and the diet and activities permitted once the client returns home. Be general in the discussion. Remember, many unforeseen events can arise and greatly alter the postoperative course.

Give verbal and written information concerning health care facility services, rules, and regulations; visiting hours; the chaplain's name and visiting hours (if appropriate); and the names of the clinical nurse specialists and other health care professionals who can be contacted for information. Most clients benefit from a tour of the recovery room and ICU. If they are not physically able to participate in a tour, audiovisual material is helpful.

Familiarize the client with the equipment that will be used in the ICU (e.g., chest drainage tubes, oxygen apparatus, ventilators, cardiac monitors, IV setups). Reassure the client that lights and alarm noises are part of the critical care environment and are not indicators that something is wrong.

Nursing Management of the Surgical Client

Clients are usually initially cared for in the intensive care unit (ICU). Initial assessment is focused on the level of consciousness, lung sounds, peripheral pulses and vital signs including heart rhythm, cardiac output/index, and temperature. Clients have continuous blood pressure readings via an arterial line, central venous pressure lines, and occasionally monitors for cardiac output and pulmonary artery pressures. The clients remain intubated and ventilated via a respirator. Mediastinal tube drainage should be measured hourly; surgeons differ on their orders about milking the tubes, but blood should not be allowed to clot in the tube because it would prohibit drainage and lead to tamponade. Urine output is also measured hourly. Laboratory studies are drawn including hemoglobin, hematocrit, platelet count, blood glucose, electrolytes, blood urea nitrogen, creatinine, prothrombin time, partial thromboplastin time, and arterial blood gases. A chest x-ray is taken to verify placement of the endotracheal tube and identify any chest abnormalities (e.g., pneumothorax). Within 4 to 8 hours, if the client is hemodynamically stable, as they awaken and are able to sustain breathing independently, they may be extubated according to physician's orders. Oxygen will need to be used to maintain desired oxygen saturations.

The goals for the first 24 hours after surgery are to maintain adequate blood pressure and cardiac output, to correct problems with coagulation and calcium levels, and to stabilize intravascular volume. Medications to maintain cardiac output include inotropic agents, calcium, and vasoconstrictors. Vasodilators may also be used to improve flow through the coronary arteries and reduce peripheral vascular resistance and preload.

> **It is imperative that the target parameters (e.g., cardiac output, cardiac index, blood pressure, heart rate) be known and which medications are titrated to achieve these goals. The increments of titration should also be known, along with the side effects and ceiling limits for each drug.**

SAFETY ⚠ ALERT

Many hospitals have initiated rapid recovery programs for cardiac surgery clients that reduce the hospital stay to 4 days. With rapid recovery programs, most of the client's recovery takes place in the home, with the client and family assuming primary responsibility for many aspects of care. Discharge planning begins at the time of admission, activity progression in the postoperative period is accelerated, and client and family education continues on a daily basis throughout hospitalization.

Many hospitals have developed clinical pathways for CABG. See the Clinical Pathway feature on Coronary Bypass Grafting on the website. Immediate care of the *evolve* client after CABG is shown in the Care Plan on pp. 1426 to 1429. In addition, a three-phase program of activity is implemented.

Phase 1 (In-Hospital) Rehabilitation Programs

Most CABG clients participate in cardiac rehabilitation following surgery. Phase 1 begins immediately after the client returns from surgery. The following are the goals of phase 1 inpatient rehabilitation:

- To prevent the negative effects of prolonged bed rest
- To assess the client's physiologic response to exercise
- To manage the psychosocial issues related to recovery from CABG surgery
- To educate the client and family concerning recovery and the adoption of risk reduction behaviors

While in ICU the client is turned every 2 hours during the first several hours after surgery. Once extubated, the client gets up in a chair and ambulates in the room. After transfer to the intermediate care unit, the client continues to walk three or four times a day, increasing the distance walked each time.

Assess the client's blood pressure, heart rate, ECG, and oxygen saturation before, during, and after activity. Systolic blood pressure should not increase more than 20 mm Hg or decrease more than 10 to 15 mm Hg after exercise. Heart rate should not increase more than 20 beats/min

C A R E   P L A N   *evolve*

Coronary Bypass Surgical Clients

Nursing Diagnosis: Decreased Cardiac Output related to alterations in preload/afterload/contractility/heart rate.
Outcomes: The client will have improved cardiac output as evidenced by stable blood pressure (and/or cardiac output/cardiac index) with decreasing need for vasoactive medications, normal sinus rhythm without pacing, clear lung sounds, warm and dry skin, preoperative mental status, urine output greater than 0.5 ml/kg without diuretics, and palpable pedal pulses.

NOC OUTCOMES   Cardiac Pump Effectiveness (NOC)

Interventions	NIC INTERVENTIONS	Rationales
1. Monitor cardiac output and/or cardiac index, SVR, PAP, CVP, PCWP as appropriate or according to protocol.	Hemodynamic Regulation	1. Monitoring allows for early intervention.
2. Monitor heart rhythm continuously. Treat dysrhythmias per protocol	Dysrhythmia Management	2. Dysrhythmias can include atrial fibrillation or ventricular dysrhythmias. They must be identified and treated early.
3. Monitor weight daily and compare to previous weights	Fluid Management	3. Body weight is a reliable indicator of fluid volume.
4. Monitor for peripheral edema every 4 hours.	Hemodynamic Regulation	4. Peripheral edema may develop with dilutional hypoproteinemia or heart failure.
5. Auscultate heart sounds every 4 hours.	Hemodynamic Regulation	5. A ventricular gallop (S_3) is an early sign of heart failure. S_4 may indicate decreased ventricular compliance.
6. Auscultate lung sounds for crackles every 4 hours.	Fluid Management	6. Crackles may indicate left ventricular failure.
7. Monitor intake/output, urine output hourly.	Fluid Management	7. Hourly assessment allows for rapid adjustments in fluids to prevent hypotension and maintain renal perfusion.
8. Monitor potassium and calcium levels	Electrolyte Management	8. Hypokalemia and hypocalcemia can lead to ventricular dysrhythmias.
9. Maintain fluid balance by administering IV fluids, packed red blood cells, or colloids.	Shock Management: Cardiac	9. Hypovolemia is a common cause of low cardiac output.
10. Administer prescribed vasodilators (specify).	Cardiac Care: Acute	10. Reducing afterload reduces stress on the left ventricle.
11. Administer positive inotropic/contractility medications as prescribed (specify).	Cardiac Care: Acute	11. Inotropic medications enhance myocardial contractility, leading to improved cardiac output by more complete emptying of the ventricles.
12. Monitor the ECG and arterial blood pressure to verify timing and effect of balloon counterpulsations (IABP). (See also the Bridge to Critical Care feature on IABP.)	Circulatory Care: Mechanical Assist Device	12. IABP must receive a signal to identify the beginning of a new cardiac cycle. Dysrhythmias may affect the timing of balloon deflation and inflation. MAP should remain approximately 80 mm Hg on IABP.
13. Protect external pacemaker wires from water and accidental exposure to electricity by placing them in a rubber glove.	Injury Prevention	13. Static electricity and water can cause the pacer wires to conduct electricity.

Evaluation: The goal for this diagnosis can be written for 24 hours; most clients who were fairly healthy before surgery usually are awake and up in a chair by the day after surgery.

Nursing Diagnosis: Impaired Gas Exchange related to ventilation/perfusion mismatch or intrapulmonary shunting.
Outcomes: The client will have adequate gas exchange as evidence by Pao_2 >90 mm Hg, $Paco_2$ <35 mm Hg, pH between 7.35 and 7.45, and oxygen saturation >90%.

NOC OUTCOMES   Respiratory Status: Gas Exchange

Interventions	NIC INTERVENTIONS	Rationales
1. Monitor oxygen saturation continuously. If the levels fall below 90%, either encourage the client to deep breathe, or consider if the endotracheal tube needs suctioning.	Mechanical Ventilation	1. Continuous monitoring allows for early intervention

2. Monitor results of ABGs; report abnormal or unexpected findings to the surgeon.	Mechanical Ventilation	2. Hypoxemia or acidosis may require modification in ventilation parameters.
3. Monitor settings on ventilator, position of ET tube, lung sounds, and response to mechanical ventilation.	Artificial Airway Management Mechanical Ventilation	3. Mechanical ventilation is used with positive pressure to facilitate alveolar ventilation. The ET tube must remain at the carina; its position within the airway is monitored by confirming placement. Lung sounds should be present in each lung.
4. Securely tape or hold the ET tube in place; move the tube in the mouth every 12 hours.	Mechanical Ventilation	4. Securing the ET tube allows the client to be moved in bed without dislodgement. Moving the tube prevents pressure ulcers on the lips.
5. Use an oral bite block prn.	Mechanical Ventilation	5. Bite blocks prevent obstruction of the tube from biting.
6. Collaborate with respiratory therapists to assess weaning parameters per protocol.	Mechanical Ventilation	6. Weaning parameters help determine if the client is ready for extubation.

Evaluation: The goal for this care plan can be fairly short term; early extubation (within 4-8 hours after surgery) is becoming more common in clients undergoing elective CABG.

Nursing Diagnosis: Ineffective Airway Clearance related to retained secretions and excess secretions.
Outcomes: The client will have improved airway clearance as evidenced by deep breathing and coughing productively.

NOC OUTCOMES   Respiratory Status: Ventilation

Interventions	NIC INTERVENTIONS	Rationales
1. Monitor lung sounds q 2 hr.	Respiratory Monitoring	1. Fluids in the alveoli accumulate as a result of atelectasis and dilutional hypoproteinemia.
2. Monitor coughing effort.	Respiratory Monitoring	2. After extubation, coughing is used to clear the airways. Because of incisional pain, many clients cough poorly.
3. Administer supplemental oxygen to maintain oxygen saturation levels >93%.	Oxygen Therapy	3. Oxygen saturation levels >93% equate to 90% arterial blood saturation, which is adequate in most clients.
4. Maintain comfort using prescribed opioids.	Cough Enhancement	4. Pain control can facilitate adequate coughing.
5. Splint the incision with "heart pillows" or pillows.	Cough Enhancement	5. Splinting the incision before coughing promotes more intense coughing efforts.
6. Ambulate when tolerated.	Ventilation Assistance	6. Respiratory effort is increased with ambulation; therefore deep breathing occurs.
7. Teach proper use of the incentive spirometer (ICS) once extubated. Demonstrate as needed.	Cough Enhancement	7. Correct use of ICS encourages sustained inspiration to open alveoli.

Evaluation: Expect this outcome to be met after 4 to 5 days; clearing the chest of secretions requires time and client effort.

Collaborative Problem: Risk of Hemorrhage related to inadequate hemostasis, disruption of suture lines, or coagulopathy.
Outcomes: The nurse will monitor for bleeding in excess of expectations (should be less than 70 ml/hr), visible blood loss, decreased blood pressure, and increased heart rate.

NOC OUTCOMES   Blood Loss Severity

Interventions	NIC INTERVENTIONS	Rationales
1. Monitor mediastinal chest tubes for output hourly.	Bleeding Reduction	1. Hourly assessment of output and total output is analyzed. Clients with IMA grafts are at increased risk of bleeding because of the surgical resection needed.
2. Report excess volumes and/or institute prescribed treatments for blood loss.	Bleeding Reduction	2. Agents such as protamine (to reverse heparin), aminocaproic acid (inhibits lysis of clots by blocking the conversion of plasminogen to plasmin), fresh-frozen plasma, platelets, and fluids may be used to restore volume.
3. Retransfuse blood from mediastinum as ordered.	Blood Products Administration	3. Autotransfusion is one mechanism of using the client's own blood for transfusion.

(Continued)

C A R E   P L A N   *evolve*

Coronary Bypass Surgical Clients—Cont'd

4. Keep chest tubes positioned without kinks and/or strip them (per agency or physician protocol).	Tube Care: Chest	4. Maintain patency of the tube. Aggressive chest tube stripping can lead to bleeding by dislodging small clots.
5. Monitor for manifestations of cardiac tamponade: Elevated CVP, PADP, PAP Decreased CO, BP Pulsus paradoxus Muffled heart sounds Sudden cessation of chest tube drainage	Cardiac Care: Acute	5. Cardiac tamponade, which is the collection of blood/fluid in the pericardial sac, can severely restrict ventricular filling.

Evaluation: The risk of bleeding is highest in the first 24 hours after surgery.

Nursing Diagnosis: Acute Pain related to tissue trauma secondary to sternotomy and leg incision.

Outcomes: The client will have improved comfort as evidenced by reporting pain at tolerable levels, using less potent analgesia.

NOC OUTCOMES   Pain Level, Analgesic Administration

Interventions	NIC INTERVENTIONS	Rationales
1. Monitor reported level of pain.	Pain Management	1. Reported pain levels are the most accurate method of describing the intensity of pain.
2. Assess the nature of the pain.	Pain Management	2. Angina must be differentiated from incisional pain. Clients with IMA grafts will often have chest wall pain. Saphenous vein graft harvest incisions are often quite painful.
3. Administer ordered opioids for surgical pain by prescribed route management to meet client goal.	Analgesic Administration	3. Treatment of acute pain reduces sympathetic stimulation and thereby cardiac workload. Pain control also enhances recovery.
4. Premedicate before activities such as ambulation and coughing.	Medication Management	4. Premedication assists the client to fully participate.

Evaluation: Expect pain levels to be highest for the first 48 hours after surgery. Clients often require IV analgesia for 24-48 hours, and then the pain should be controllable with oral analgesia.

Collaborative Problem: Risk of Postcardiotomy Delirium or Stroke.

Outcomes: The nurse will monitor for the return to baseline levels of consciousness and mental acuity.

NOC OUTCOMES   Cognitive Ability: Cranial Sensory/Motor Function

Interventions	NIC INTERVENTIONS	Rationales
1. Monitor for return of consciousness when off of sedating medications.	Neurologic Monitoring	1. Neurologic examination is accurate only if the client is awake and able to participate.
2. Assess neurologic status every shift. Compare current level of mental acuity to baseline levels. Report any deviations to surgeon.	Neurologic Monitoring	2. Baseline levels of mental acuity provide a comparison. Early intervention for stroke may limit permanent damage.
3. Reorient frequently to setting, timing, and procedures being performed.	Reality Orientation	3. Delirium is short-term, and reorientation is helpful to assist the client in restructuring thoughts.
4. Explain all procedures, using a calm and clear voice.	Reality Orientation	4. The environment of an ICU may threaten the confused client. Explanations also build trust and gain cooperation.
5. Secure all invasive lines and tubes.	Environmental Management: Safety	5. Disoriented clients may accidentally pull or remove lines. Accidental dislodgement may injure the client and/or require replacement of the device.
6. Administer sedative medications cautiously.	Medication Management	6. Mild sedation may help prevent injury. However, the use of sedation in older adults may increase agitation.
7. Avoid restraints in lieu of other methods to prevent self-injury.	Physical Restraint	7. Physical restraints may increase agitation.

Interventions	NIC INTERVENTIONS	Rationales
8. Explain that changes in mental acuity, agitation, confusion, and/or hallucinations are temporary (as applies).	Reality Orientation	8. Transient changes in acuity are usually caused by decreased cerebral perfusion and microemboli during the cardiac bypass pump run. Discussion of permanent changes is left to the neurologist.
9. Organize nursing care to provide time for sleep. Limit environmental noise as much as possible.	Sleep Enhancement	9. Sleep deprivation may increase confusion.
10. Liberalize visitation time with family.	Reality Orientation	10. Familiar voices and faces will help with reorientation.

Evaluation: Once the sedative effects of the medications and anesthetics wear off, mental acuity of baseline levels should return.

Nursing Diagnosis: Risk for Infection related to sternotomy incision, diabetes, and obesity.
Outcomes: The client will have decreased risk of infection as evidenced by primary healing of the sternotomy and leg incisions.

NOC OUTCOMES   Wound Healing: Primary Intention

Interventions	NIC INTERVENTIONS	Rationales
1. Initially monitor temperature every hour, and every 4 hr once stable.	Incision Site Care	1. Temperature >38.3° C (101° F) may indicate atelectasis early in recovery. Later fever may indicate sternal wound infection or infective endocarditis.
2. Monitor incision for signs of delayed primary healing.	Incision Site Care	2. Erythema, pain, drainage, or opening of the sternal margin are signs of delayed healing.
3. Administer insulin drip as ordered to control blood glucose levels to desired values as ordered.	Infection Protection	3. Blood glucose levels >200 mg/dl create ineffective phagocytosis and increase the risk of infection.
4. Apply a front-closing brassiere or other supportive dressings for obese female clients.	Incision Site Care	4. Pendulous breasts can create tension on the suture lines and impair sternotomy healing.
5. Collaborate with the dietitian to ensure that a diet of adequate calories and protein is delivered.	Infection Protection	5. Protein and calorie needs increase after major stress and are needed for wound healing.
6. Administer antibiotics as prescribed (specify), including nasal ointments.	Infection Protection	6. Antibiotics reduce the risk of surgical site infection. Nasal application of mupirocin has been shown to reduce the risk of MRSA infections in the sternal incision.

Evaluation: Incisions should heal by primary intention in 7 to 10 days.

BP, Blood pressure; *CI,* cardiac index; *CO,* cardiac output; *CVP,* central venous pressure; *IABP,* intra-aortic balloon pump; *MAP,* mean arterial pressure; *PADP,* pulmonary artery diastolic pressure; *PAP,* pulmonary artery pressure; *PAWP,* pulmonary artery wedge pressure; *PCWP,* pulmonary capillary wedge pressure; *RAP,* right atrial pressure; *SVR,* systemic vascular resistance.

above resting, and no significant dysrhythmias should occur. Activity levels will be reduced if clients have adverse physiologic responses (e.g., tachycardia, dysrhythmias, pain) to exercise. Clients are seated for all meals. Research has demonstrated that early mobilization improves cardiac function and benefits the client psychologically.

Education for a healthier lifestyle is an important part of each phase of cardiac rehabilitation. The emphasis in phase 1 is on the identification and modification of reversible risk factors to prevent further deleterious cardiac events.

Deep breathing and coughing must continue to reduce the risk of pneumonia. The client is taught and encouraged to cough, not just clear the throat, using a pillow to splint the sternum.

Self-Care

Before hospital discharge, instruct the client and family (or significant other) about medication actions and side effects, dietary restrictions, physical activity restrictions and progression, and incisional care. Because it is not always possible to anticipate all the problems clients may encounter the first few days at home, instruct the client whom to call when there is an emergency or when there are questions or concerns. If possible, introduce the client to the home health nurse who will be supervising home care. Following discharge, the home health care nurse provides additional education and counseling and assesses the client for complications.[36] In addition, instruct the client on how to assess response to exercise and activity.[5]

Before discharge, a low-level symptom-limited exercise test may be performed to evaluate the client's ability to perform activities of daily living (ADL) and exercise. The test results are used to prescribe a safe and effective exercise program for the first few weeks at home and serve as a basis for the initial exercise prescription in phase 2.

Phase 2 (Outpatient Exercise Training) Rehabilitation Programs
Outpatient (phase 2) exercise training usually takes place in a facility that provides continuous ECG monitoring, emergency equipment, and medically supervised

exercise. Outpatient treatment usually begins 10 to 14 days after discharge and requires physician referral. The following are the goals of phase 2:

- To restore clients to a desirable exercise capacity appropriate to their health status, lifestyle, and occupation
- To provide additional education and support to the client and family for adoption of risk-reduction behaviors
- To meet the psychosocial needs of clients and families, restore confidence, and minimize anxiety and depression
- To promote early identification of medical problems through close observation and monitoring of clients during exercise
- To assist clients in returning to occupational and leisure activities

Exercise therapy is conducted three times weekly for 2 to 3 months. The duration of the aerobic exercise session ranges from 20 to 40 minutes at an intensity of 70% to 85% of the baseline exercise heart rate. During each exercise session, blood pressure, heart rate, respiratory rate, and ECG are monitored before, during, and after exercise. Activity levels are increased gradually, based on the client's response. A nutritionist may counsel clients about proper diet, and a psychologist or social worker may counsel clients about stress management and adoption of other risk prevention behaviors.

At the end of the program, clients are given a symptom-limited exercise test and are reevaluated. Decisions regarding progression to a phase 3 or home program are based on the client's results of the stress test, the client's ability to self-monitor the response to exercise, the client's stability, and the client's psychological or emotional status. Periodic evaluations are scheduled so that activity progression and cardiopulmonary function can be assessed.[5]

Phase 3 (Community) Rehabilitation Programs

Phase 3 programs are conducted in community settings, such as a "Y" or a health club. The following are the goals of phase 3:

- To maintain and, if possible, increase exercise capacity
- To institute long-term follow-up of risk-reduction behavior change
- To encourage clients to take responsibility for continuing lifestyle changes

Exercise consists of walking, jogging, weight training, and recreational games. Clients are usually not monitored while exercising, although some facilities obtain exercise ECGs on a monthly basis. Clients are responsible for monitoring their own heart rate response to exercise, although blood pressure can be taken by program personnel if indicated.[5]

Home Exercise Rehabilitation Programs

For CABG clients, a home exercise program is usually prescribed in conjunction with or in place of the outpatient program. Clients are given detailed exercise instructions and are told to keep a log of heart rates, perceived exertion rates, exercise parameters, and any problems that occur during the home program. Cardiac rehabilitation staff members or the client's physician should analyze the data and adjust the home exercise program if necessary. Once clients reach their optimal level of functional capacity, they are instructed to continue to exercise at least three times weekly so that cardiopulmonary exercise capacity can be maintained.

Modifications for Older Clients

More than half of all CABG procedures are performed on people older than 65 years, and 71% of them are performed on men. Older clients have a postoperative recovery similar to that for younger clients, but the pace is slower and they typically remain hospitalized an average of 2 to 4 days longer. They also have a higher death rate.

Postoperative complications that are more prevalent in older clients include dysrhythmias related to aged sinoatrial node cells, drug toxicity associated with impaired hepatic and renal perfusion, multiple drug interactions, and decreased physical stamina. These complications contribute to a 15-day mean length of hospital stay for clients older than 80 years.

During the first and second weeks after discharge, depression, fatigue, incisional chest discomfort, dyspnea, and anorexia are common. By the fourth to fifth weeks, older clients report improved mood, comfort, and appetite. At 1 year, almost all (93%) clients are pleased with the outcome and improved quality of life.

HEART FAILURE

Despite aggressive medical and surgical treatment, CHD may eventually lead to the development of heart failure. Heart failure is a physiologic state in which the heart cannot pump enough blood to meet the metabolic needs of the body (determined as oxygen consumption). Heart failure results from changes in systolic or diastolic function of the left ventricle. The heart fails when, because of intrinsic disease or structural defects, it cannot handle a normal blood volume or, in the absence of disease, cannot tolerate a sudden expansion in blood volume (e.g., during exercise). Heart failure is not a disease itself; instead, the term refers to a clinical syndrome characterized by manifestations of volume overload, inadequate tissue perfusion, and poor exercise tolerance. Whatever the cause, pump failure results in hypoperfusion of tissue, followed by pulmonary and systemic venous congestion. Because heart failure causes vascular congestion, it is often called *congestive heart failure,* although most cardiac specialists no longer use this term. Other terms used to denote heart failure include *chronic heart failure, cardiac decompensation, cardiac insufficiency,* and *ventricular failure.*

Heart failure affects about 5 million people in the United States, with 500,000 new cases diagnosed each year. In contrast to decreases in mortality associated with other cardiovascular diseases, the incidence of heart failure and the mortality associated with it have increased steadily since 1975. Annually about 300,000 clients die from direct or indirect consequences of heart failure, and the number of deaths attributed to heart failure has increased six-fold over the past 40 years.

Heart failure can affect both women and men, although the mortality is higher among women. There are also racial differences; at all ages death rates are higher in African Americans than in non-Hispanic whites. Heart failure is primarily a disease of older adults, affecting 6% to 10% of those older than 65. It is also the leading cause of hospitalization in older people.

Etiology and Risk Factors

Heart failure is caused by conditions that weaken or damage the myocardium. Heart failure can be caused by factors originating from the heart (i.e., intrinsic disease or pathology) or from external factors that place excessive demands upon the heart. Etiologies of heart failure are shown in Table 56-1.

Intrinsic Factors

The most common cause of heart failure is coronary artery disease. CAD reduces blood flow through the coronary arteries and therefore reduces oxygen delivery to the myocardium. Without oxygen, the muscle cells cannot function. Another common cause of heart failure is myocardial infarction (MI). During MI, myocardium is starved of blood, and the tissue dies and therefore cannot contract. The remaining myocardium must compensate for the loss of tissue. Other intrinsic causes of heart failure include valve disease, cardiomyopathy, and dysrhythmias.

Certain conditions externally compress the heart, thereby limiting ventricular filling and myocardial contractility. Disorders that greatly restrict cardiac chamber filling and myocardial fiber stretch include *constrictive pericarditis,* an inflammatory and fibrotic process of the pericardial sac; and *cardiac tamponade,* which involves the accumulation of fluid or blood within the pericardial sac. Because the pericardium encloses all four heart chambers, compression of the heart both decreases diastolic relaxation, thereby elevating diastolic pressure, and hampers forward blood flow through the heart.

Extrinsic Factors

Factors external to the heart include increased afterload (e.g., hypertension), increased stroke volume from hypervolemia or increased preload, and increased body demands (high output failure; e.g., thyrotoxicosis, pregnancy). The weakened myocardium cannot tolerate the usual changes in the volume of blood entering the left ventricle. These conditions include abnormal volumes of blood reaching the left ventricle (called a load), abnormal muscle in the ventricle from scarring after injury, and problems that reduce the contractility of the heart muscle. They will be examined in more detail.

Abnormal loading occurs when either the pressure or the volume of blood in the ventricle increases. The effect of increasing volume on the ventricle can be explained by the analogy that the heart muscle is like a stretched rubber band. When the rubber band is stretched, it contracts with more force. The heart muscle does the same. Venous return stretches the heart and improves contractility. When the rubber band is overstretched, however, it becomes limp and cannot contract. Likewise, when the heart is overloaded with blood, excessive stretch and decreased contraction occur. Overload develops because blood does not leave the ventricles during contraction. Therefore the workload on the heart increases in an effort to move blood. Loading, called preload and afterload, can occur in normal or abnormal conditions.

TABLE 56-I   Etiology of Heart Failure

Abnormal Loading Conditions	Abnormal Muscle Function	Limited Ventricular Filling
Conditions That Increase Preload		
Regurgitation of mitral or tricuspid valve	Myocardial infarction	Mitral or tricuspid stenosis
Hypervolemia	Myocarditis	Cardiac tamponade
Congenital defects (left-to-right shunts)	Cardiomyopathy	Constrictive pericarditis
Ventricular septal defect	Ventricular aneurysm	Hypertrophic obstructive cardiomyopathy
Atrial septal defect	Long-term alcohol consumption	
Patent ductus arteriosus	Coronary heart disease	
	Metabolic heart disease	
	Endocrine heart disease	
Conditions That Increase Afterload		
Hypertension, pulmonary or systemic		
Aortic or pulmonic stenosis		
High peripheral vascular resistance		

Preload can be defined as the initial stretching of the cardiac muscle fiber length before contraction. Changes in ventricular preload dramatically affect ventricular stroke volume by what is called the Frank-Starling mechanism. Increased preload increases stroke volume, whereas decreased preload decreases stroke volume by altering the force of contraction of the cardiac muscle. Preload, therefore, is related to the sarcomere length, but since sarcomere length cannot be determined in the intact heart, other indices of preload are used such as ventricular end-diastolic volume or pressure. For example, when venous return is increased, the end-diastolic pressure and volume of the ventricle are increased, which stretches the sarcomeres (increases their preload). As another example, hypovolemia resulting from a loss of blood by hemorrhage leads to less ventricular filling and therefore shorter sarcomere lengths (reduced preload). Increased pressure load in the ventricle is related to *afterload,* the amount of tension the heart must generate to overcome systemic pressure and to allow adequate ventricular emptying. Thus afterload indicates how hard the heart must pump to force blood into circulation. The tone of systemic arterioles, the elasticity of the aorta and large arteries, the size and thickness of the ventricle, the presence of aortic stenosis, and the viscosity of the blood all determine afterload. High peripheral vascular resistance and high blood pressure force the ventricle to work harder to eject blood. Subjected to prolonged high pressures, the ventricle eventually fails.

Pathophysiology

The healthy heart can meet the demands for oxygen delivery through the use of cardiac reserve. *Cardiac reserve* is the heart's ability to increase output in response to stress. The normal heart can increase its output up to five times the resting level. The failing heart, even at rest, however, is pumping near its capacity and thus has lost much of its reserve. The compromised heart has a limited ability to respond to the body's needs for increased output in situations of stress.

When cardiac output is not sufficient to meet the metabolic needs of the body, compensatory mechanisms, including neurohormonal responses, become activated. These mechanisms initially help to improve contraction and maintain integrity of the circulation, but if continued lead to abnormal cardiac muscle growth and reconfiguration (remodeling) of the heart. The compensatory responses to a decrease in cardiac output are ventricular dilation, increased sympathetic nervous system stimulation, and activation of the renin-angiotensin system. Figure 56-5 depicts the pathophysiology of heart failure in an algorithm.

Ventricular Dilation

Ventricular dilation refers to lengthening of the muscle fibers that increases the volume in the heart chambers.

Dilation causes an increase in preload, and thus cardiac output, because a stretched muscle contracts more forcefully (Starling's law); however, dilation has limits as a compensatory mechanism. Muscle fibers, if stretched beyond a certain point, become ineffective. Second, a dilated heart requires more oxygen. Thus the dilated heart with a normal coronary blood flow can suffer from a lack of oxygen. Hypoxia of the heart further decreases the muscle's ability to contract.

Increased Sympathetic Nervous System Stimulation

Sympathetic adrenergic stimulation produces arteriolar constriction, tachycardia, and increased myocardial contractility, all of which work to increase cardiac output and improve delivery of oxygen and nutrients to tissues. Arterial baroreceptors are important components of this response. This compensatory effect occurs at the cost of increasing peripheral vascular resistance (afterload) and myocardial workload, however. In addition, sympathetic stimulation reduces renal blood flow and stimulates the renin-angiotensin system.

Stimulation of the Renin-Angiotensin System

When blood flow through the renal artery is decreased, the baroreceptor reflex is stimulated and renin is released into the bloodstream. Renin interacts with angiotensinogen to produce angiotensin I. When angiotensin I contacts ACE, it is converted to angiotensin II, a potent vasoconstrictor. Angiotensin II increases arterial vasoconstriction, promotes the release of norepinephrine from sympathetic nerve endings, and stimulates the adrenal medulla to secrete aldosterone, which enhances sodium and water absorption. Stimulation of the renin-angiotensin system causes plasma volume to expand and preload to increase.

Cardiac compensation exists when the initial compensatory mechanisms of ventricular dilation, sympathetic nervous system stimulation, and renin-angiotensin system stimulation succeed in maintaining an adequate cardiac output and oxygen delivery to the tissues in the presence of pathologic changes. Once cardiac output is restored, the body produces counter-regulatory substances that restore cardiovascular homeostasis. If underlying pathologic changes are not corrected, prolonged activation of the compensatory mechanisms eventually leads to changes in the function of the myocardial cell and excess production of the neurohormones. These processes are responsible for the transition from compensated to decompensated heart failure. At this point manifestations of heart failure develop because the heart cannot maintain adequate circulation.

When compensatory mechanisms fail, the amount of blood remaining in the left ventricle at the end of diastole increases. This increase in residual blood in turn decreases the ventricle's capacity to receive blood from the left atrium.

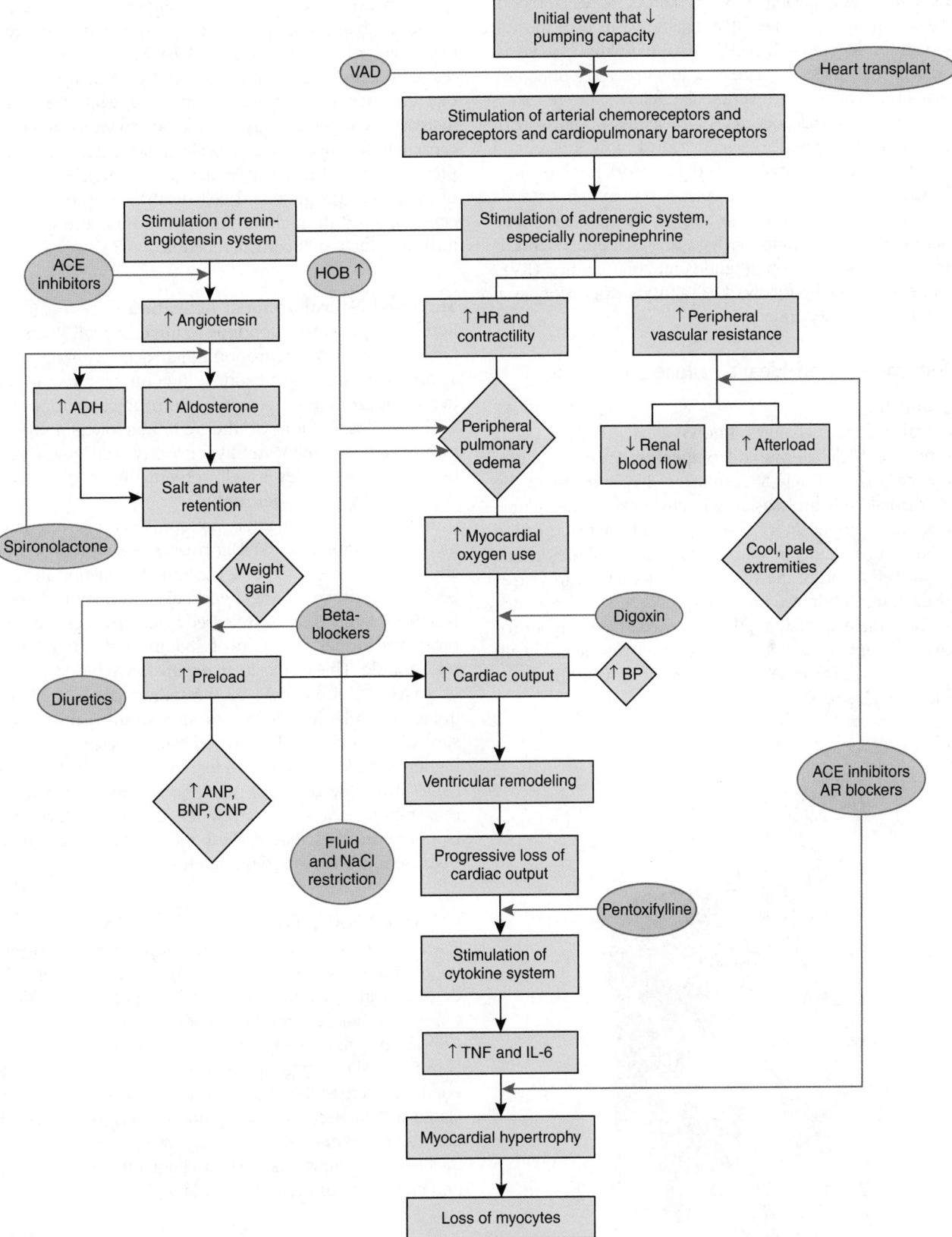

■ **FIGURE 56–5** Pathophysiology of heart failure. *ACE,* Angiotensin-converting enzyme; *ADH,* antidiuretic hormone; *ANP,* atrial natriuretic peptide; *AR,* aldosterone receptor; *BNP,* brain natriuretic peptide; *BP,* blood pressure; *BUN,* blood urea nitrogen; *CNP,* C-natriuretic peptide; *HOB,* head of bed; *HR,* heart rate; *VAD,* ventricular assist device.

The left atrium, having to work harder to eject blood, dilates and hypertrophies. It is unable to receive the full amount of incoming blood from the pulmonary veins, and left atrial pressure increases; this leads to pulmonary edema (Figure 56-6). Left ventricular failure (LVF) results.

The right ventricle, because of the increased pressure in the pulmonary vascular system, must now dilate and hypertrophy to meet its increased workload. It too eventually fails. Engorgement of the venous system then extends backward to produce congestion in the gastrointestinal tract, liver, viscera, kidneys, legs, and sacrum; edema is the main manifestation. Right ventricular failure (RVF) results. RVF usually follows LVF, although occasionally it may develop independently.

Decompensated Heart Failure

Remodeling

Several structural changes, known as *remodeling,* occur in the ventricle during decompensated heart failure. Remodeling is thought to result from hypertrophy of the myocardial cells and sustained activation of the neurohormonal compensatory systems. Recall that one of the initial compensatory responses to a decrease in cardiac output is dilation of the ventricle. This dilation increases cardiac output but also increases wall stress in the ventricle. To reduce wall stress, the myocardial cells hypertrophy, resulting in a thickening of the ventricular wall. According to Laplace's law, an increase in wall thickness reduces wall stress.

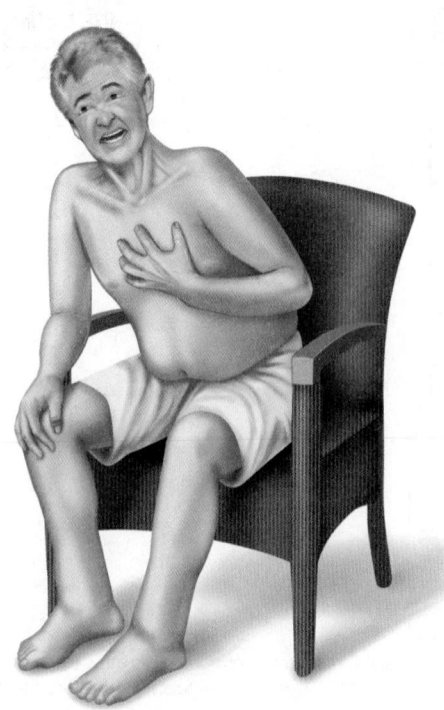

■ **FIGURE 56–6** Appearance of a client with both right-sided and left-sided heart failure.

When used over time, these compensatory responses produce changes in the structure, function, and gene expression of the myocardial cell. Changes in the myocardial cells eventually increase failure by reducing myocardial contractility, increasing ventricular wall stress, and increasing oxygen demand. In addition to increasing myocardial dysfunction, the genetically abnormal myocytes die prematurely and at an accelerated rate through the process of *apoptosis* (programmed cell death). Apoptosis affects cells scattered throughout the myocardium and causes a further reduction in cardiac function.

Sustained Neurohormonal Activation

Remodeling changes continue to increase wall stress and further stimulate neurohormonal activity. Long-term sympathetic activation exerts a direct toxic effect on the heart that promotes myocyte hypertrophy and apoptosis. Prolonged activation of the renin-angiotensin system also stimulates myocyte hypertrophy and myocardial fibrosis. This creates a self-perpetuating cycle of cell death and further hypertrophy.

In addition, if renal artery pressure falls, a lowered glomerular filtration rate (GFR) increases retention of sodium and water. In response to a continued reduction in renal blood flow, the renin-angiotensin-aldosterone mechanism is activated. Aldosterone, released from the adrenal cortex, promotes further retention of sodium and water by the renal tubule. This results in an expansion in blood volume of up to 30% and edema. As the sodium concentration in the extracellular fluid increases, so does the osmotic pressure of the plasma. The hypothalamus responds to the higher osmotic pressure by releasing antidiuretic hormone (ADH) from the posterior pituitary. This in turn promotes renal tubular reabsorption of water. Aldosterone, however, is more important than ADH in the production of edema because it promotes sodium retention.

Clinical Manifestations

The manifestations of heart failure depend on the specific ventricle involved, the precipitating causes of failure, the degree of impairment, the rate of progression, the duration of the failure, and the client's underlying condition. Conditions that precipitate heart failure are listed in Box 56-3. Manifestations of pulmonary congestion and edema dominate the clinical picture of LVF; RVF is associated with manifestations of abdominal organ distention and peripheral edema. Heart failure has been classified into several stages based on a client's functional ability and clinical manifestations (Table 56-2).

Types of Heart Failure

Heart failure may be categorized as (1) LVF versus RVF, (2) backward versus forward, and (3) high output versus low output.

BOX 56-3	Conditions That Precipitate Heart Failure

- Dysrhythmias, especially tachycardia
- Systemic infections (sepsis)
- Anemia
- Thyroid disorders
- Pulmonary embolism
- Thiamine deficiency
- Chronic pulmonary diseases
- Medication dose changes
- Physical or emotional stress
- Endocarditis, myocarditis, or pericarditis
- Fluid retention from medication or salt intake
- A new cardiac condition

Left Ventricular Versus Right Ventricular Failure

The theory of LVF versus RVF is based on the fact that fluid accumulates behind the chamber that fails first. Because the circulatory system is a closed circuit, however, impairments of one ventricle commonly progress to failure of the other. This is referred to as *ventricular interdependence*. Figure 56-7 depicts clinical manifestations that differentiate LVF from RVF.

Left Ventricular Failure. Left ventricular failure causes either pulmonary congestion or a disturbance in the respiratory control mechanisms. These problems in turn precipitate respiratory distress. The degree of distress varies with the client's position, activity, and level of stress.

Dyspnea (difficult breathing) is a subjective problem, and it does not always correlate with the extent of heart failure. Because breathing is usually effortless at rest, the feeling of breathlessness can mean anything from an awareness of breathing to extreme distress. An apprehensive client with only moderate ventricular failure may be more aware of dyspnea than a client with advanced disease. To some degree, exertional dyspnea

occurs in all clients. Therefore elicit from the client a description of the degree of exertion that results in the sensation of breathlessness. The mechanism of dyspnea may be related to the decrease in the lung's air volume *(vital capacity)* as air is displaced by blood or interstitial fluid. Pulmonary congestion can eventually reduce the vital capacity of the lungs to 1500 ml or less.

Orthopnea is a more advanced stage of dyspnea. The client often assumes a "three-point position," sitting up with both hands on the knees and leaning forward. Orthopnea develops because the supine position increases the amount of blood returning from the lower extremities to the heart and lungs (preload). The client learns to avoid respiratory distress at night by supporting the head and thorax on pillows. In severe heart failure, the client may resort to sleeping upright in a chair.

Paroxysmal nocturnal dyspnea (PND) resembles the frightening sensation of suffocation. The client suddenly awakens with the feeling of severe suffocation and seeks relief by sitting upright or opening a window for a "breath of fresh air." Respirations may be labored and wheezing *(cardiac asthma)*. PND represents an acute exacerbation of pulmonary congestion. It stems from a combination of increased venous return to the lungs during recumbency and suppression of the respiratory center to sensory input from the lungs during sleep. Once the client is upright, relief from the attack of PND may not occur for 30 minutes or longer.

Cheyne-Stokes respirations sometimes occur in clients with severe forms of heart failure. Cheyne-Stokes respirations probably result from the prolonged circulation time between the pulmonary circulation and the central nervous system (CNS).

Cough is a common manifestation of LVF. The cough, often hacking, may produce large amounts of frothy, blood-tinged sputum. The client coughs because a large amount of fluid is trapped in the pulmonary tree,

TABLE 56–2   Stages of Heart Failure and Treatments

Stage	Extent of Disease	NYHA Class	Outcomes and Goals in Order of Importance	Treatments
1	Asymptomatic myocardial dysfunction with mild heart failure	I/II	Reverse or prevent remodeling Prevent overt heart failure	ACE inhibitors or ARBs Beta-adrenergic blockers
2	Mild to moderate heart failure	II/III	Reverse or prevent remodeling Improve symptoms and functional capacity Reduce disability and hospitalizations Reduce mortality	ACE inhibitors or ARBs/beta-adrenergic blockers Diuretics, digoxin
3	Advanced heart failure	III/IV	Reduce mortality Reduce disability and hospitalizations Improve symptoms and functional capacity	ACE inhibitors, spironolactone, beta-adrenergic blockers Positive inotropic agents, including digoxin
4	Severe heart failure with frequent or sustained decompensation	III/IV	Reduce disability and hospitalizations Improve symptoms and functional capacity Reduce mortality	Diuretics, ACE inhibitors Positive inotropic agents for periods of decompensation Beta-adrenergic blockers

ACE, Angiotensin-converting enzyme; ARB, angiotensin receptor blocker; NYHA, New York Heart Association.

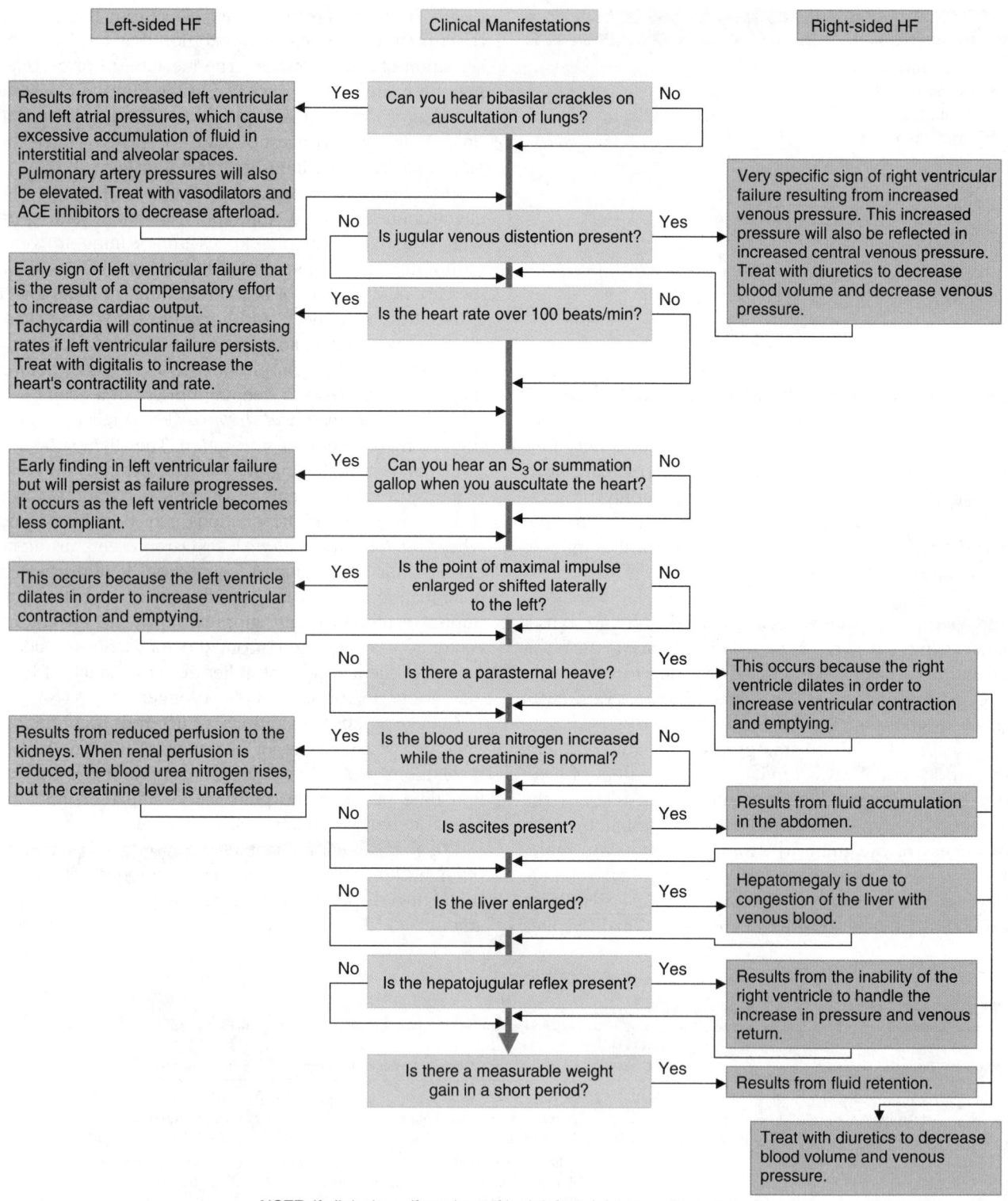

NOTE: If clinical manifestations of both left and right ventricular failure are present, the client is experiencing biventricular failure.

■ **FIGURE 56–7** Clinical manifestations of left-sided and right-sided heart failure. *HF*, Heart failure.

irritating the lung mucosa. On auscultation bilateral crackles may be heard.

Cardiovascular manifestations also denote LVF. Inspecting and palpating the precordium may reveal an enlarged or left laterally displaced apical pulse. This occurs because the left ventricle dilates in an effort to supplement ventricular contraction and emptying. Heart gallop (S_3 or S_4) sounds may be an early finding in heart failure as the left ventricle becomes less compliant and its walls vibrate in response to filling during diastole. The appearance of pulsus alternans (alternating strong and weak heartbeats) may also herald the onset of LVF.

Cerebral hypoxia may occur as a result of a decrease in cardiac output, causing inadequate brain perfusion. Depressed cerebral function can cause anxiety, irritability, restlessness, confusion, impaired memory, bad dreams, and insomnia. Impaired ventilation with resultant hypercapnia may also be a precipitant.

Fatigue and muscular weakness are often associated with LVF. Inadequate cardiac output leads to hypoxic tissue and slowed removal of metabolic wastes, which in turn cause the client to tire easily. Disturbances in sleep and rest patterns may worsen fatigue.

Renal changes can occur in both RVF and LVF but are more striking in LVF. Nocturia occurs early in heart failure. During the day the client is upright, blood flow is away from the kidneys, and the formation of urine is reduced. At night urine formation increases as blood flow to the kidneys improves. Nocturia may interfere with effective sleep patterns, which may contribute to fatigue. As cardiac output declines, decreased renal blood flow may result in oliguria, a late manifestation of heart failure.

Complications of Left Ventricular Failure. Acute pulmonary edema, a medical emergency, usually results from LVF. In clients with severe cardiac decompensation, the capillary pressure within the lungs becomes so elevated that fluid is pushed from the circulating blood into the interstitium and then into the alveoli, bronchioles, and bronchi. The resulting pulmonary edema, if untreated, may cause death from suffocation. Clients with pulmonary edema literally drown in their own fluids. The dramatic manifestations of acute pulmonary edema, listed in the Critical Monitoring feature above, right, terrify the client and the client's significant others.

Right Ventricular Failure. When right ventricle functioning decreases, peripheral edema and venous congestion of the organs develop. Liver enlargement (*hepatomegaly*) and abdominal pain occur as the liver becomes congested with venous blood. If this occurs rapidly, stretching of the capsule surrounding the liver causes severe discomfort. The client may notice either a constant aching or a sharp pain in the right upper quadrant. In chronic heart failure, abdominal tenderness generally disappears.

In severe RVF, the lobules of the liver may become so congested with venous blood that they become anoxic. Anoxia leads to necrosis of the lobules. In long-standing heart failure, these necrotic areas may become fibrotic and then sclerotic. As a result, a condition called *cardiac cirrhosis* develops, manifested by ascites and jaundice.

In chronic heart failure, the increased workload of the heart and the extreme work of breathing increase the metabolic demands of the body. Anorexia, nausea, and

---

CRITICAL MONITORING

Acute Pulmonary Edema

- Severe dyspnea
- Orthopnea
- Pallor
- Tachycardia
- Expectoration of large amounts of frothy, blood-tinged sputum
- Fear
- Wheezing
- Sweating
- Bubbling respirations
- Cyanosis
- Nasal flaring
- Use of accessory breathing muscles
- Tachypnea
- Vasoconstriction
- Hypoxia in ABG findings

bloating develop secondary to venous congestion of the gastrointestinal tract. The combination of increased metabolic needs and decreased caloric intake results in a marked wasting of tissue mass, called *cardiac cachexia*. Anorexia and nausea may also result from digitalis toxicity.

Dependent edema is one of the early manifestations of RVF. Venous congestion in the peripheral vascular beds causes increased hydrostatic capillary pressure. Capillary hydrostatic pressure overwhelms the opposing pressure of plasma proteins, and fluid shifts out of the capillary beds and into the interstitial spaces, with resultant pitting edema. Edema is usually symmetrical and occurs in the dependent parts of the body, where venous pressure is highest. In ambulatory clients edema begins in the feet and ankles and moves up the lower legs. It is most noticeable at the end of the day and often subsides after a night's rest. In the recumbent client, pitting edema may develop in the presacral area and, as it worsens, progress to the genital region and medial thighs. Concurrent jugular vein distention differentiates the edema of heart failure from that of lymphatic obstruction, cirrhosis, and hypoproteinemia.

Anasarca, a late manifestation in heart failure, is substantial and generalized edema. It can involve the upper extremities, genital area, and thoracic and abdominal walls. Cyanosis of the nail beds appears as venous congestion reduces peripheral blood flow.

Clients with heart failure often feel anxious, frightened, and depressed. Almost all clients realize that the heart is a vital organ and that when the heart begins to fail, health also fails. As the course of the disease progresses and manifestations worsen, the client may have an overwhelming fear of permanent disability and death. Clients express their fears in varying ways: nightmares, insomnia, acute anxiety, depression, or withdrawal from reality.

Backward Versus Forward Failure

The clinical presentation of heart failure arises from inadequate cardiac output, the pooling of blood behind the failing chamber, or both. *Backward* failure focuses on the ventricle's inability to eject completely, which increases ventricular filling pressures, causing venous and pulmonary congestion. *Forward* failure is a problem of inadequate perfusion. It results when reduced contractility produces a decrease in stroke volume and cardiac output. As cardiac output falls, blood flow to vital organs and peripheral tissues diminishes. This causes mental confusion, muscular weakness, and renal retention of sodium and water. Each of these types of failure is usually present to some degree in the client with heart failure.

High-Output Versus Low-Output Failure

High-output failure occurs when the heart, despite normal-output to high-output levels, is simply not able to meet the accelerated needs of the body. Causes include sepsis, Paget's disease, beriberi, anemia, thyrotoxicosis, arteriovenous fistula, and pregnancy.

Low-output failure occurs in most forms of heart disease, resulting in hypoperfusion of tissue cells. The underlying disorder is related not to increased metabolic needs of the tissues but to poor ventricular pumping action and a low cardiac output.

Decompensated Versus Chronic Heart Failure

The onset of heart failure may be *acute,* leading to decompensation, or stable, called *chronic* heart failure.

Diagnostic Findings

The diagnosis of heart failure rests primarily on presenting manifestations and pertinent data from the client's health history. Diagnostic studies assist in determining the underlying cause and the degree of heart failure. B-type natriuretic peptide (BNP) is a protein secreted from the ventricles in response to overload, such as occurs in heart failure. As the degree of heart failure worsens, the level of BNP secreted into the blood increases. Liver enzymes may reflect the degree of liver failure. Elevated blood urea nitrogen (BUN) and creatinine levels reflect decreased renal perfusion.

Additional studies include an echocardiogram, chest x-ray, and ECG. A two-dimensional (2-D) echocardiogram, coupled with Doppler flow studies, provides information about cardiac chamber size and ventricular function. These tests aid in assessing myocardial, valvular, congenital, endocardial, and pericardial heart disease, allowing the clinician to determine whether the dysfunction is systolic or diastolic. In LVF, chest x-ray often depicts an enlarged cardiac silhouette, pulmonary and venous congestion, and interstitial edema. On x-ray interstitial edema produces images called Kerley's B lines. Pleural effusions

may develop and generally reflect biventricular failure. An ECG may give clues to the cause of LVF. Abnormalities in the ECG arise from the underlying cardiac disorder and from therapeutic agents. It may demonstrate evidence of a prior MI, dysrhythmias, or left ventricular dysfunction.

Arterial blood gas analysis may be performed. Early heart failure with pulmonary edema may lead to respiratory alkalosis that is due to hyperventilation. As the disorder progresses and oxygenation becomes more impaired, acidosis develops. Pulse oximetry values show decreased oxygen levels.

OUTCOME MANAGEMENT OF DECOMPENSATED HEART FAILURE

Medical Management

The management of heart failure is divided into two situations: the treatment of decompensated heart failure and the treatment of stable chronic heart failure. Diuretics, nitrates, analgesics, and inotropic agents are indicated for the treatment of decompensated heart failure and pulmonary edema. The goals of the management are to reduce myocardial workload, improve ventricular pump performance, perfuse essential organs, and prevent further heart failure by affecting the process of cardiac remodeling.

Reduce Myocardial Workload

Diuretics are an important aspect of treatment because of the central role of the kidney as the target organ of many of the neurohormonal changes in response to the failing heart. First-line therapy generally includes a loop diuretic such as furosemide, which will inhibit sodium chloride reabsorption in the ascending loop of Henle. Diuretics reduce circulating blood volume, diminish preload, and lessen systemic and pulmonary congestion. Loop diuretics can also produce mild to severe electrolyte imbalance. Hypokalemia, a particularly dangerous side effect, can cause myocardial weakness and cardiac dysrhythmias. Hypokalemia also potentiates digitalis toxicity. Moreover, vigorous diuresis may produce hypovolemia and hypotension, jeopardizing cardiac output.

Vasodilators also reduce myocardial workload by reducing both preload and afterload. Nitroglycerin reduces myocardial oxygen demand by lowering preload and afterload. It is often given intravenously. Morphine IV is often used for clients with acute heart failure. In addition to being both an anxiolytic and an analgesic, its most important effect is venodilation, which reduces preload. Morphine also causes arterial dilation, which reduces systemic vascular resistance (SVR) and increases cardiac output. Medications can be direct vasodilators acting through nitric oxide on the vessel walls. Nesiritide is a newer medication and also works by dilating arteries and veins.

Beta-adrenergic antagonists (beta-blockers) are used to inhibit the effects of the sympathetic nervous system and reduce the oxygen needs of the myocardium. They increase clinical improvement and decrease mortality. These findings are apparent when clients are concurrently receiving ACE inhibitory therapy, suggesting that the combination of two agents that have inhibitory effects on two neurohormonal systems may have an additive effect. Beta-blockers, possibly by restoring beta$_1$-receptor activity or via prevention of catecholamine activity, appear to be cardioprotective in clients with depressed left ventricular function.

Elevate the Client's Head

The client is placed in a high Fowler position or chair to reduce pulmonary venous congestion and to relieve the dyspnea. The legs are maintained in a dependent position as much as possible. Even though the legs are edematous, they should not be elevated. Elevating the legs rapidly increases venous return.

Reduce Fluid Retention

Controlling sodium and water retention improves cardiac performance. Sodium restrictions are placed on the diet to prevent, control, or eliminate edema. Diets with 2 to 4 g of sodium are usually prescribed (Table 56-3).

From the use of some loop diuretics, potassium is lost via the kidneys, which can lead to dysrhythmias and electrolyte imbalances. Hypokalemia sensitizes the myocardium to digitalis and therefore predisposes the client to digitalis toxicity. Potassium supplements and adequate dietary potassium are important.

It is usually not necessary to restrict fluid intake in clients with mild or moderate heart failure. In more advanced cases, however, it is beneficial to limit water to 1000 ml/day (1 L/day). The reason is that excessive water intake tends to dilute the amount of sodium in body fluids and may produce a low-salt syndrome *(hyponatremia)*. Hyponatremia is characterized by lethargy and weakness; it results more often from the combination of a restricted sodium diet, increased sodium loss during diuresis, and excessive water intake.

Improve Ventricular Pump Performance

The most powerful way to increase contractility of the heart is to use adrenergic agonist, or inotropic medications. Angiotensin-converting enzyme (ACE) inhibitors also commonly yield pronounced improvement in hemodynamics, and are discussed below.

Inotropes. Principal inotropic agents include dobutamine, milrinone, dopexamine, and digoxin. In the hypotensive client with heart failure, dopamine and

TABLE 56-3 Sodium Content of Selected Foods	
Foods Low in Sodium	
Dairy products	Skim milk, eggs, cottage cheese, cream cheese, ice cream
Meats*	Turkey, chicken, veal, lamb, liver, fresh fish, tuna packed in water (meats should be unprocessed)
Fruits and vegetables*	Any fresh or frozen food in this group
Beverages	Any juice (except tomato or V8 brand vegetable), coffee, tea, bottled water
Breads	Some breads and cereals
Seasonings	Garlic, onion, bay leaf, pepper, dill, nutmeg, rosemary, allspice, thyme, sage, caraway, cinnamon, almond and vanilla extract, fresh dried herbs
Fats	Margarine, oils, shortening, unsalted salad dressings
Desserts	Sherbet, fruit ice, gelatin, fruit drinks
Miscellaneous	Unbuttered, unsalted popcorn; unsalted nuts; vinegar
Foods High in Sodium	
Milk and dairy products	Aged, hard cheese; pasteurized, processed cheese; buttermilk
Meats	Sausage, frankfurters, ham, bacon, corned beef; all smoked, pickled, or cured meats; canned meats, salami, most luncheon meats, beef jerky; frozen dinners
Fruits and vegetables	Pickled or canned fruits and vegetables, olives, sauerkraut, pickles
Breads and cereals	Salted crackers, macaroni and cheese, pretzels, rye rolls, pizza, commercial pancake mixes
Beverages	Tomato juice, V8 vegetable juice, beef broth, bouillon
Fats	Commercial salad dressings, dips and party spreads, peanut butter
Seasonings	Garlic, celery, or onion salt; Accent, monosodium glutamate (MSG), meat tenderizer, soy sauce, ketchup, steak sauce, mustard, canned soup
Desserts	Fruit pies, doughnuts, cakes, commercial puddings
Miscellaneous	Baking soda, baking powder, salted popcorn, salted nuts, potato chips

*Food sources high in potassium.

dobutamine are agents usually used. These medications facilitate myocardial contractility and enhance stroke volume. They also can lead to dysrhythmias.

Dobutamine is a very useful medication for heart failure because it produces strong beta-stimulatory effects within the myocardium; it increases heart rate, atrioventricular (AV) conduction, and myocardial contractility. Dobutamine is capable of increasing cardiac output without increasing myocardial oxygen demands or reducing coronary blood flow.

Dopamine is a naturally occurring catecholamine with alpha-adrenergic, beta-adrenergic, and dopaminergic activity. Dopamine, given in small doses

(<4 mcg/kg/min), opens the kidney's vascular beds. Vasodilation in the kidney is especially advantageous, leading to improved GFR, urine output, and excretion of sodium. When dopamine is given in higher doses it produces tachycardia and dysrhythmias; therefore it is not commonly used in decompensated heart failure.

Milrinone is another inotropic medication and also dilates the pulmonary vascular beds. Amrinone, the first of the phosphodiesterase inhibitors, is seldom used because it leads to thrombocytopenia. Dopexamine has been used in some clients, and is still being investigated. Digoxin is used less and less in the emergency management of heart failure. Digoxin is discussed with chronic heart failure; it has little to no role in the treatment of decompensated heart failure.

Supplement Oxygen

High concentrations of oxygen by mask or cannula are provided to relieve hypoxia and dyspnea and to improve oxygen–carbon dioxide exchange. For hypoxemia, partial rebreather masks with a flow rate of 8 to 10 L/min can be used to deliver oxygen concentrations of 40% to 70%. A non-rebreathing mask can achieve even higher oxygen concentrations. If these methods do not raise the arterial oxygen tension (Pao_2) above 60 mm Hg, the client may need intubation and ventilatory management. Intubation also provides a route for removing secretions from the bronchi. If severe bronchospasm or bronchoconstriction occurs, bronchodilators are given. The heart rhythm is monitored because some bronchodilators may lead to dysrhythmias.

Control Dysrhythmias

Atrial fibrillation with a rapid ventricular response is the most common dysrhythmia seen in heart failure clients. Atrial fibrillation can lead to embolic stroke, so clients are given anticoagulants. The rhythm is often controlled with medications such as amiodarone.

Reduce Myocardial Remodeling

Angiotensin-converting enzyme inhibitors are now considered first-choice treatment and are the cornerstone of heart failure drug therapy. ACE inhibitors have proved to slow the progression of heart failure by reducing remodeling changes in the heart. ACE inhibitors reduce afterload by blocking the production of angiotensin, a potent vasoconstrictor. They also increase renal blood flow and decrease renal vascular resistance, which enhances diuresis. Side effects include orthostatic hypotension, persistent hacky cough and kidney problems, skin rashes, an altered sense of taste, and hyperkalemia. Potassium levels should be monitored, especially if diuretics or potassium supplements are being used.

Reduce Stress and Risk of Injury

In addition to improving ventricular pump performance and reducing myocardial workload, the client also needs to reduce physical and emotional stress. Sometimes clinicians overlook rest as an intervention to diminish the workload of the heart. The proper use of rest as the initial step in management offers many benefits. Rest can promote diuresis, slow the heart rate, and relieve dyspnea, all of which allow more conservative use of pharmacologic agents (e.g., ACE inhibitors, diuretics, beta-blockers).

Whether the physician prescribes complete, modified bed rest depends on the seriousness of the client's condition. The physician may prescribe a mild sedative or small doses of barbiturates and tranquilizers to promote rest and overcome problems of restlessness, insomnia, and anxiety.

The client may also be at risk for injury because of immobility. The client should be confined to bed only long enough to regain cardiac reserve but not so long as to promote complications of immobility. Give the client confined to bed rest specific guidelines to prevent the harmful effects of immobility. Clients should perform passive leg exercises several times daily to prevent venous stasis, which may lead to the formation of venous thrombi and pulmonary emboli. Anticoagulant therapy prevents these potentially deadly complications.

Nursing Management of the Medical Client

The following are the goals of nursing management for the client with heart failure:

- To monitor for reduced cardiac output
- To maintain adequate fluid balance
- To reduce myocardial workload
- To monitor for pulmonary edema
- To assess response to medical therapies

Consider the psychosocial effect of heart failure on the client and family. Nursing diagnoses that may apply to the client with heart failure are discussed in the Care Plan on pp. 1441-1445.

Surgical Management for Heart Failure

Ventricular Assist Devices

Advances continue to be made in perfecting methods of mechanical ventricular support. The goal of mechanical circulatory support is to decompress the hypokinetic ventricle, decrease myocardial workload, reduce oxygen demands, and maintain adequate systemic perfusion to sustain end-organ function. In the client with heart failure, the two most common options are ventricular assist

CARE PLAN *evolve*

The Client with Decompensated Heart Failure

Nursing Diagnosis: Decreased Cardiac Output related to heart failure or dysrhythmias or both.
Outcomes: The client will have an increase in cardiac output as evidenced by regular cardiac rhythm, heart rate, blood pressure, respirations, and urine output within normal limits.

NOC OUTCOMES Cardiac Pump Effectiveness

Interventions	NIC INTERVENTIONS	Rationale
1. Assess blood pressure for hypotension or hypertension and respiratory rate for tachypnea q 1 hr (more or less frequently, depending on the client's stability).	Vital Signs Monitoring	1. Hypotension may indicate decreased cardiac output and may lead to a decrease in coronary artery perfusion. Hypertension may be caused by chronic vasoconstriction or may indicate fear or anxiety, and increased respiratory rate may indicate fatigue or increased pulmonary congestion.
2. Assess heart rate and rhythm q 1 hr for tachycardia. Continuously monitor for dysrhythmias.	Vital Signs Monitoring	2. Tachycardia can increase myocardial and oxygen demands and may be a compensatory mechanism related to the decreased cardiac output (increased heart rate to compensate for decrease in stroke volume). Ventricular enlargement decreases conduction of cardiac impulses and may lead to dysrhythmias. Dysrhythmias further compromise cardiac output by reducing ventricular filling time and myocardial contractility and by increasing myocardial oxygen demands.
3. Document rhythm strips q 8 hr and if dysrhythmias occur. Measure and note rate; QRS, PR, and QT intervals; and ST segment with each strip and note any deviations from baseline.	Acute Cardiac Care	3. Common dysrhythmias include premature atrial contractions (PACs), premature ventricular contractions (PVCs), and paroxysmal atrial tachycardia (PAT). Changes in the ST segment may indicate myocardial ischemia, which may be present because of decreased coronary artery perfusion.
4. Report dysrhythmias to the physician, or follow protocol for emergency treatment.	Acute Cardiac Care	4. Dysrhythmias can decrease cardiac output. Particular attention must be paid to ventricular dysrhythmias because they can increase the chance of sudden death.
5. Monitor lab values for isoenzymes, atrial peptide, CK, LDH, AST, BUN, creatinine, liver function tests, CBC, electrolytes, glucose, thyroid function, blood lipids.	Acute Cardiac Care	5. These lab values may indicate myocardial infarction, severe heart failure, renal failure, or liver failure. Thyroid disease can precipitate heart failure.
6. Auscultate heart rate q 2 hr for changes in heart sounds such as murmurs, S_3, or S_4.	Vital Signs Monitoring	6. Delayed filling time, incomplete ejection, and structural changes within the heart and fluid overload may cause abnormal heart sounds detected by auscultation. S_3 may indicate a noncompliant or stiff ventricle, and S_4 may indicate a weak, overdistended ventricle.
7. Monitor lung sounds q 2 hr for adventitious sounds such as crackles and for the presence of coughing.	Vital Signs Monitoring	7. Increased ventricular pressures are transmitted back to the pulmonary circulation, increasing pulmonary capillary hydrostatic pressure and exceeding oncotic pressure fluid moving within the alveolar septum; evidenced by auscultation of crackles, increased shortness of breath, and sputum production. This indicates a further decrease in cardiac output and the possibility of the development of pulmonary edema. Coughing can be caused by the increased fluid in the lungs or by angiotensin-converting enzyme (ACE) inhibitors.

(Continued)

C A R E   P L A N   *evolve*

The Client with Decompensated Heart Failure—Cont'd

8. Monitor intake and output (I&O) and analyze findings q 8 hr and as required (prn). Note color and amount of urine q 2 hr and prn.	Acute Cardiac Care	8. If intake exceeds output, the client is at risk for fluid overload and may not be excreting fluids because of a decompensating heart. Dark, concentrated urine and oliguria may reflect a decrease in renal perfusion. Diuresis is expected in clients receiving diuretic therapy.
9. Assess for changes in mental status.	Acute Cardiac Care	9. Change in mental status may indicate decreased cerebral perfusion or hypoxia.
10. Assess peripheral pulses for strength and quality and for pulsus alternans.	Acute Cardiac Care	10. Decreased strength of peripheral pulses is often found in clients with decreased cardiac output, and a further decrease in pulses from baseline may indicate further cardiac failure. Pulsus alternans may be detected and indicates severe heart failure.
11. Administer prescribed medications and evaluate responses by the client for the intended effect (specify).	Acute Cardiac Care	11. Prescribed medications are used to increase contractility responses and decrease preload or afterload, and their effects must be evaluated. Therapeutic levels and side effects must be monitored.
12. Encourage physical and psychological rest.	Cardiac Precautions	12. Increased physical or mental strain can increase myocardial oxygen demands.
13. Avoid rectal temperatures, rectal meds, enemas, and rectal examinations.	Cardiac Precautions	13. Stimulation of the rectum causes a Valsalva response, which can trigger bradycardia.
14. Encourage clients to eat small meals and rest afterward.	Cardiac Precautions	14. Larger meals increase myocardial workload and may cause vagal stimulation, which may lead to bradycardia.

Evaluation: Following the administration of ACE inhibitors and diuretics, dyspnea should improve. Heart failure is a chronic disorder and complete resolution is not possible; expect small gains in cardiac output in the days that follow.

Nursing Diagnosis: Excess Fluid Volume related to reduced glomerular filtration, decreased cardiac output, increased antidiuretic hormone (ADH) and aldosterone production, and sodium and water retention.

Outcomes: The client will demonstrate adequate fluid balance as evidenced by output equal to or exceeding intake, clearing breath sounds, and decreasing edema.

NOC OUTCOMES   Fluid Balance

Interventions	NIC INTERVENTIONS	Rationales
1. Monitor I&O q 4 hr (more or less frequently).	Fluid Monitoring	1. I&O balance reflects fluid status (depending on client's status).
2. Weigh clients daily and compare to previous weights.	Fluid Monitoring	2. Body weight is a sensitive indicator of fluid balance and an increase indicates fluid volume excess.
3. Auscultate breath sounds q 2 hr and prn for the presence of crackles and monitor for frothy sputum production.	Fluid Monitoring	3. When increased pulmonary capillary hydrostatic pressure exceeds oncotic pressure, fluid moves within the alveolar septum and is evidenced by the auscultation of crackles. Frothy, pink-tinged sputum is an indicator that the client is developing pulmonary edema.
4. Assess for presence of peripheral edema. Do not elevate the legs if the client is dyspneic.	Fluid Monitoring	4. Heart failure causes venous congestion, resulting in increased capillary pressure. When hydrostatic pressure exceeds interstitial pressure, fluids leak out of the capillaries and present as edema in the legs, sacrum, and scrotum. Elevation of the legs increases venous return to the heart.
5. Assess for jugular vein distention, hepatomegaly, and abdominal pain.	Fluid Monitoring	5. Elevated volumes in the venae cavae occur from inadequate emptying of the right atrium. The excess fluid is transmitted to the jugular vein, liver, and abdomen and manifests as distention.

6. Follow low-sodium diet and/or fluid restriction.

Hypervolemia Management

6. Decreased systemic blood pressure can lead to stimulation of aldosterone, which causes increased renal tubular absorption of sodium. Low-sodium diet helps prevent increased sodium retention, which decreases water retention. Fluid restriction may be used to decrease fluid intake, hence decreasing fluid volume excess.

7. Administer diuretic therapy as ordered and evaluate effectiveness of therapy. Empty indwelling catheter bags before administration of diuretics to record volume diuresed.

Hypervolemia Management

7. Diuretics are commonly prescribed to promote the diuresis of accumulated fluid. The nurse should expect an increase in urine output, improved breathing, and weight loss after the client receives diuretic therapy.

8. Encourage or provide oral care q 2 hr.

Oral Health Maintenance

8. The client senses thirst because the body senses dehydration. Oral care can alleviate the sensation without an increase in fluid intake.

Evaluation: After administration of diuretics, expect profound urine output if the client has reasonable cardiac output. Weight loss and output should stabilize in 2 to 3 days. Expect fairly rapid improvement in peripheral edema.

Nursing Diagnosis: Impaired Gas Exchange related to fluid in alveoli.
Outcomes: The client will have improved gas exchange as evidenced by decreased dyspnea, no cyanosis, normal arterial blood gases, and a decrease in pulmonary congestion on auscultation.

| NOC OUTCOMES | Respiratory Status: Gas Exchange |

Interventions	NIC INTERVENTIONS	Rationales
1. Auscultate breath sounds q 2 hr.	Vital Sign Monitoring	1. Auscultation of crackles may indicate pulmonary congestion.
2. Encourage the client to turn, cough, and deep breathe and use the incentive spirometer q 2 hr.	Cough Enhancement	2. This will help facilitate oxygen delivery and clear the airways.
3. Administer oxygen as ordered. Monitor for the development of dry nasal mucous membranes and skin injury from the oxygen tubing.	Oxygen Therapy	3. Oxygen therapy will improve oxygenation by increasing the amount of oxygen available for delivery. Administration of nonhumidified oxygen can dry and injure nasal membranes. Tubing pulled tightly can lead to pressure ulcers on the face and ears.
4. Assess respiratory rate and rhythm q 2 hr and prn.	Vital Sign Monitoring	4. Increased respiratory rate indicates difficulty with oxygenation, and a decreased respiratory rate may indicate impending respiratory failure.
5. Assess for cyanosis q 4 hr and prn.	Respiratory Monitoring	5. Circumoral cyanosis or cyanosis to the finger tips or end of nose indicates hypoxia from lack of oxygen in peripheral tissues. Cyanosis is a late sign of poor oxygenation.
6. Position the client to facilitate breathing and observe for paroxysmal nocturnal dyspnea.	Airway Management	6. Fowler position and orthopneic positioning facilitate diaphragmatic excursion. Paroxysmal nocturnal dyspnea may occur because as the client assumes a supine position, venous return to the heart is increased. This increase in return increases preload and will increase pulmonary capillary hydrostatic pressure and lead to pulmonary edema.
7. Monitor pulse oximetry. Move the probe to ensure good contact with the skin or ear.	Vital Sign Monitoring	7. A low Sao_2 reflects hypoxia.
8. Obtain arterial blood gases if ordered.	Acid-Base Management	8. Arterial blood gases indicate whether the client has hypoxia, acidosis, or both.
9. Administer diuretic therapy as ordered, and monitor for effectiveness.	Hypervolemia Management	9. Diuretics promote fluid loss in the alveoli as well as systemically.

Evaluation: Expect dyspnea to improve rapidly once the diuresis has occurred unless the client has significant lung disease from other problems. Because the lung is a low-pressure area, the redevelopment of edema in the lung can occur quickly and continued monitoring is important.

(Continued)

C A R E   P L A N   *evolve*

The Client with Decompensated Heart Failure—Cont'd

Nursing Diagnosis: Ineffective Tissue Perfusion related to decreased cardiac output.
Outcomes: The client will have adequate tissue perfusion as evidenced by warm, dry skin, peripheral pulses, and adequate urine output.

NOC OUTCOMES   Tissue Perfusion

Interventions	NIC INTERVENTIONS	Rationales
1. Note color and temperature of the skin q 4 hr.	Acute Cardiac Care	1. Cool, pale skin is indicative of decreased peripheral tissue perfusion.
2. Monitor peripheral pulses q 4 hr.	Acute Cardiac Care	2. Decreased pulses are indicative of decreased tissue perfusion from vasoconstriction of the vessels.
3. Provide a warm environment.	Temperature Regulation	3. A warm environment promotes vasodilation, which decreases preload and promotes tissue perfusion.
4. Encourage active range of motion.	Circulatory Precautions	4. Range of motion helps decrease venous pooling and promotes tissue perfusion.
5. Monitor urine output q 4 hr.	Fluid Monitoring	5. Decreased perfusion to the kidneys may result in oliguria.
6. Protect the skin from trauma by applying cotton socks or fleece boots.	Circulatory Precautions	6. Poorly perfused skin heals slowly, if at all, once injured.

Evaluation: Once cardiac output is improved, expect peripheral blood flow to improve slightly. Pre-existing atherosclerosis will prevent the skin from making dramatic improvement, but the client should return to baseline condition.

Nursing Diagnosis: Risk for Activity Intolerance related to decreased cardiac output.
Outcomes: The client will have improved levels of activity without dyspnea.

NOC OUTCOMES   Activity Tolerance

Interventions	NIC INTERVENTIONS	Rationales
1. Space nursing activities.	Energy Management	1. Clustering activities increases myocardial demand and may cause extreme fatigue.
2. Schedule rest periods.	Energy Management	2. Rest periods help alleviate fatigue and decrease myocardial workload.
3. Monitor the client's response to activities. Assess vital signs before and after an activity.	Vital Sign Monitoring	3. Dyspnea, tachycardia, angina, diaphoresis, dysrhythmias, and hypotension are all indicative that the activity required more myocardial demand than the heart was able to supply. The time it requires for the vital signs to return to baseline indicates the degree of cardiac deconditioning.
4. Increase activity as ordered or according to the rehabilitation nurse's directions.	Exercise Promotion: Ambulation	4. Gradually and appropriately increasing physical activity may help the client gain cardiac conditioning and improve activity tolerance.
5. Instruct the client to avoid activities that increase cardiac workload.	Counseling	5. Activities such as stair climbing, working with arms above the head, or sustained arm movement may cause extreme fatigue and demand more cardiac output than the body can supply.

Evaluation: The client will perform spaced activities without dyspnea and will gradually increase activity tolerance. This goal will require time; deconditioning caused by marked dyspnea often prevents rapid improvement.

Nursing Diagnosis: Risk for Impaired Skin Integrity related to decreased tissue perfusion and activities.
Outcomes: The client will have reduced risk of skin impairment.

NOC OUTCOMES   Tissue Integrity: Skin

Interventions	NIC INTERVENTIONS	Rationales
1. Reposition the client q 2 hr if client moving self. Turn side to side q 2 hr if client unable to turn self.	Pressure Ulcer Prevention	1. Changing position frequently deters the formation of pressure ulcers by decreasing the amount of time there is pressure on any given area.
2. Provide a therapeutic mattress or bed while the client is in bed.	Pressure Ulcer Prevention	2. Pressure-redistribution mattresses and beds are available to decrease the pressure on the sacrum when the client is sitting up in bed.

3. Assess the skin, especially bony prominences, for redness each shift and as needed. Use protective devices if redness is noted. Inspect between skinfolds in obese clients.	Skin Surveillance	3. Redness is indicative of increased pressure to an area and is the first sign of breakdown. Risk areas include the sacrum, coccyx, heels, elbows, and back of the head.
4. Float the heels from the bed if the client has little spontaneous leg movement.	Pressure Ulcer Prevention	4. The posterior prominence of the heels makes them high risk for breakdown in clients in Fowler position.
5. Assist the client with morning care and lubricate the skin.	Pressure Ulcer Prevention	5. Clients may have difficulty providing themselves with adequate skin care, and the nurse must ensure the skin is clean and has proper moisture to prevent cracking.

Evaluation: Intact skin should remain intact.

Nursing Diagnosis: Risk for Anxiety related to decreased cardiac output, hypoxia, diagnosis of heart failure, and fear of death or debilitation.

Outcomes: The client will not exhibit manifestations of anxiety and will be able to express concerns.

| NOC OUTCOMES   Anxiety Control |

Interventions	NIC INTERVENTIONS	Rationales
1. Provide a calm environment.	Anxiety Reduction	1. A calm environment decreases additional anxiety.
2. Explain in advance all procedures and routine regimens.	Anticipatory Guidance	2. By providing information in advance, the client should not feel anxious about the routine care being provided.
3. Encourage the client to ask questions.	Anxiety Reduction	3. By encouraging the client to ask questions, the nurse is providing an open forum for discussion with the client.
4. Provide emotional support to clients and their significant others.	Anxiety Reduction	4. By allowing clients and their support systems to vent fears and anxiety, the nurse assists them in decreasing anxiety.
5. Encourage the client to use additional support systems.	Coping Enhancement	5. Additional support people such as religious leaders, social workers, counselors, and clinical nurse specialists may increase the client's support system and decrease anxiety.

Evaluation: Anxiety should improve once dyspnea improves. Concerns over deteriorations in health will require additional time for discussion and may require changes in living arrangements.

---

devices (VADs) as a bridge to transplantation and as permanent support.[28] VADs have the capability to support circulation, either partially or totally, until the heart recovers or is replaced. Devices may be right ventricular, left ventricular, or biventricular VADs. Complications of any VAD include bleeding, hemolysis, thromboembolism, infection, and multiorgan failure. Intra-aortic balloon pumping as a treatment for VAD is discussed in the Bridge to Critical Care feature on p. 1423.

Traditionally nonpulsatile pumps have been used as VADs. Difficulties with these devices include end-organ dysfunction, thromboembolic complications, and the need for full anticoagulation. Their use in clients with heart failure is diminishing because better technology has become available. These pumps can be used for a relatively short period of about 10 days.

Total artificial hearts provide complete control of the cardiovascular system and allow total mobility. Their use is limited in smaller people because the device may not fit the client's small body. Complications include infection, thromboembolism, and the possibility of mechanical failure. Initially, total artificial hearts were limited to people awaiting transplantation. Currently,

these devices are being used when there are contraindications to transplantation, such as advanced age.

Extracorporeal membrane oxygenation (ECMO) systems are widely used for short-term hemodynamic stabilization. These devices remove blood from the inferior vena cava to a centrifugal pump that pumps the blood to an oxygenator. The oxygenated blood is returned to the client via the femoral artery. Long-term use (<48 hours) does not promote recovery. In addition, bleeding is a concern because anticoagulation therapy is needed.

Heart Transplantation

When the heart is irreversibly damaged and no longer functions adequately and when the client is at risk of dying, cardiac transplantation and the use of an artificial heart to assist or replace the failing heart are measures of last resort. With the development of cyclosporine, and more recently FK-506 and mycophenolate mofetil, and with improvements in the procurement and preservation of donor hearts, cardiac transplantation has become an accepted therapeutic procedure. One-year survival rates after transplantation are greater than 85%. Although transplantation may not be appropriate for all clients, it may be the only option available to some. Heart transplantation is discussed in Chapter 55.

Cardiomyoplasty

For clients with low cardiac output who are not candidates for cardiac transplantation, a procedure called *cardiomyoplasty* may support the failing heart. This procedure involves wrapping the latissimus dorsi muscle around the heart and electrostimulating it in synchrony with ventricular systole.

Immediate postoperative care is similar to that of any cardiac surgery client. Continuous cardiac and hemodynamic monitoring is initiated. Inotropic and vasopressor agents are administered to maintain cardiac output until the pulse generator is activated (within 2 to 3 weeks). Because the muscle flap obliterates the left upper lobe of the lung and can reduce vital capacity by as much as 20%, aggressive pulmonary hygiene and judicious pain management are essential to prevent atelectasis or pneumonia. In addition an upper-extremity exercise regimen is prescribed.

OUTCOME MANAGEMENT OF CHRONIC HEART FAILURE

Chronic heart failure has been classified according to severity (see Table 56-2). Outcome management for clients with chronic heart failure usually follows guidelines based on the degree of severity. This form of heart failure is treated by the client at home, as described in the Bridge to Home Health Care feature below. Interventions must be tailored to the client and taught to improve adherence. Specific instructions should include the following guidelines:

- Adhere to dietary restrictions. Sodium in the diet should be limited to 4 g per day initially until fluid and weight gain are controlled. Fluid restrictions may also be needed. Clients should be shown how to weigh themselves daily and how to adjust sodium and fluid intake if their weight fluctuates from day to day.
- Monitor blood pressure. Clients or family members should be taught how to measure BP daily, especially if the client has diastolic heart failure.
- Modify activity. During severe stages of heart failure, the client should remain on bed rest with the head

---

BRIDGE TO HOME HEALTH CARE

Managing Heart Failure

One third of all clients hospitalized for heart failure are readmitted within 90 days of discharge. Problems with self-monitoring techniques, medication, and diet are the primary reasons. Home health and outpatient care nurses can make a positive difference in readmission rates through nursing interventions.

Review clients' cardiovascular history, disease etiology, and medical management plan to guide your assessment. Auscultate the heart and lungs during each visit, and look for manifestations of fluid accumulation. Measure blood pressure with the client both sitting and standing. If blood pressure decreases significantly and the client experiences lightheadedness or dizziness upon standing, it may be necessary to adjust diuretic or vasoactive medications. Worsening cardiac status or drug toxicities can cause changes in pulse rate or rhythm.

Clients may experience unique manifestations such as fullness in their ears, increased urination at night, and chest heaviness. The client, family members, and informal caregivers need to be educated about the correlation between manifestations and clinical status. Evaluate changes in the prevalence and severity of manifestations. The assessment can include measuring food and fluid intake, abdominal girth and lower extremities, and weight. Instruct clients to call you or their physicians if they lose or gain 2 to 3 pounds in 1 day or 5 to 7 pounds in 1 week. When manifestations are noted and cardiac decompensation is detected early, heart failure can be managed successfully in non-institutional outpatient settings.

Use various techniques to help clients manage their medications. Write the medication schedule clearly, and suggest reminder systems such as pill boxes. Examine all pill bottles for the

drug name, strength, expiration date, and available refills. Review brand versus generic labeling to minimize confusion and prevent drug administration errors. Simplify dosing frequencies; by limiting doses to twice a day (bid), three times a day (tid), or four times a day (qid), medication administration can be associated with daily routines such as meals and bedtime. Flexible dose times can promote drug tolerance and increase accurate administration. Discourage the use of over-the-counter medications because of the potential for drug interactions.

Limiting sodium intake to 2000 mg a day can help prevent fluid retention. Rarely do clients need to restrict fluid intake to less than 2000 ml/day. Evaluate the client's appetite, meal frequency, portion sizes, and food preferences, and provide appropriate health education. If possible, open cupboards and the refrigerator to gain insight into the client's eating patterns. Suggest a food diary to assess intake accurately. Teach clients, family members, and informal caregivers how to distinguish the sodium content of foods by reading food labels.

Because a client's functional status is often severely impaired, explain energy-conservation techniques before initiating limited mobility and aerobic routines. Even the most severely affected client may benefit from chair exercises done in a sitting position. Instruct clients to keep an activity log to demonstrate their progress toward activity goals. Clients should perceive their activities as only somewhat hard to do and should not participate in activities that worsen their manifestations or produce fatigue.

Clients who have chronic illnesses, including heart failure, often have feelings of depression. Consider whether clients need psychosocial and financial assistance. Antidepressant medications benefit some clients and improve their sense of well-being.

of the bed elevated and elastic stockings or wraps worn to mobilize edema. Once the client can breathe comfortably during activity, activity should be increased gradually to help increase strength.

- Adhere to medications. The multiple medications will require some type of system to prevent missed or duplicate doses. Be certain that the client knows how to monitor for side effects. Many people find it best to take diuretics in the morning so that trips to the bathroom to urinate happen during the day. Taking diuretics in the evening or at night often results in interrupted sleep because the urge to empty the bladder continues for hours.

Digoxin

Digoxin is often added to the medication regimen in chronic heart failure. Digoxin is a positive inotrope, often taught to clients as a medication that "slows and strengthens the heart beat." Improved cardiac output enhances kidney perfusion, which may create a mild diuresis of sodium and water. Digoxin does not appear to have an effect on long-term mortality in clients with heart failure. Digoxin therapy may also be initiated to control the ventricular response in atrial fibrillation, the most common dysrhythmia in heart failure.

Digoxin has a narrow therapeutic index, and toxicity occurs in about one in five clients. Clients at risk for the toxic effects of digoxin are older adults; those with advanced heart disease, severe dysrhythmias, or acute MI; and those concurrently using quinidine, verapamil, and amiodarone. Digoxin dosage may need to be reduced if the client is taking any of these medications. Digoxin toxicity is more prevalent when the serum concentration is equal to or greater than 2 mcg/L, serum potassium level is less than 3 mEq/L, or serum magnesium level is low. Digoxin toxicity, described in the Critical Monitoring feature below, may be a life-threatening condition.

CRITICAL MONITORING

Digoxin Toxicity

Digoxin remains a common medication for clients in heart failure because it increases ventricular contractility and emptying by slowing the heart rate, which promotes ventricular filling. Digoxin preparations, however, have a narrow window of therapeutic efficacy, and toxicity from digitalis is not uncommon. Nurses play a significant role in early detection of the subtle manifestations of digoxin toxicity. The diagnosis of digoxin toxicity remains a clinical challenge, in part because therapeutic and toxic digoxin concentrations overlap from one individual to another.

Several causes are known:

- Deteriorating renal function, especially in clients with hyperthyroid conditions
- Dehydration
- Electrolyte imbalances, especially potassium and magnesium imbalances
- Myocardial ischemia
- Acidosis
- Medication interactions:
  - Amiloride
  - Amiodarone
  - Calcium-channel blockers
  - Hydrochlorothiazide and other loop diuretics
  - Indomethacin
  - Propafenone
  - Quinidine
  - Quinine
  - Spironolactone
  - Triamterene

CLINICAL MANIFESTATIONS

- Nausea, vomiting, diarrhea
- Anorexia
- Palpitations
- Irregular heart block, bradycardia and junctional tachycardia

- Confusion
- Lethargy, ataxia
- Visual changes (unusual)
  - Halos or rings of light around objects
  - Seeing lights or bright spots
  - Changes in color perception, especially yellow-green
  - Blind spots in vision
  - Diagnosis

Serum levels of digoxin are used to determine whether toxicity is present. A key factor in determining digoxin toxicity is whether or not blood is drawn at least 6 hours after the last digoxin dose, which ensures that adequate distribution of the drug has been achieved before blood sampling. Blood levels would not be elevated in acute forms of toxicity, such as overdose. Toxic plasma levels are greater than 2.4 ng/ml.

TREATMENT

Because of its long half-life of 38 to 48 hours, treatment is directed at removing the drug. Acute toxicity can be treated with gastric lavage, activated charcoal to limit absorption, or digoxin-Fab fragments (Digibind), which is an antidote. Digibind is composed of digoxin-specific antibody fragments prepared from the immunoglobulin G (IgG) of sheep immunized with digoxin. The smaller Fab fragment avidly binds digoxin but is minimally immunogenic in humans and is excreted renally. Clients are admitted for cardiac monitoring. Factors that led to the toxicity are addressed.

PREVENTION

- Assess potential drug-drug interactions.
- Assess for manifestations of toxicity.
- Assess electrolyte levels (potassium, magnesium).
- Hold the medication if the heart rate is below 60 beats/min or if a new dysrhythmia has developed.
- Push IV digoxin slowly over 5 minutes.
- Schedule serum digoxin levels to be drawn at least 4 hours after an intravenous (IV) dose and 6 hours after an oral dose.

Modifications for Older Clients

Heart failure is becoming increasingly a disorder of the very old. Decompensated heart failure can be triggered by seemingly minor illnesses and dietary indiscretions. Medications commonly used by older people may have an impact on heart performance even though they pose little risk of interaction with cardiovascular medications. Nonsteroidal anti-inflammatory drugs (NSAIDs) tend to worsen heart disease because they promote sodium retention; tricyclic antidepressants (TCAs) and neuroleptic agents lead to orthostatic hypotension. Conversely, cardiac performance can affect the medication's action. The development of RVF can markedly increase the prothrombin time and thereby increase the action of anticoagulants. See the Case Management feature on Heart Failure on the website. Continuous monitoring of homebound clients with heart failure can be facilitated by computer-assisted programs. Nurse researchers are studying the effect of daily interaction via the computer with heart failure clients.

CONCLUSIONS

Disorders of cardiac function are the leading causes of death in the industrialized world. It is imperative that you fully understand the care of clients with heart disease to improve the outcomes and quality of life and to reduce morbidity and mortality. CHD is the precursor to several problems. Your role is to educate the client about risk reduction. Heart failure is a frequent endpoint of cardiac disease. It is important to maximize cardiac output and reduce system demands on the heart.

THINKING CRITICALLY

1. Your client is a 67-year-old man with newly diagnosed insulin-dependent diabetes in end-stage heart failure. The client was recently released from the hospital. You are to begin intravenous dobutamine therapy during this initial home visit. What assessment should be made before initiating dobutamine therapy? What other assessment interventions might be done?

Factors to Consider. How does heart failure respond to the administration of dobutamine? What teaching or learning needs might be assessed in the client?

2. A 70-year-old man is scheduled for a coronary artery bypass graft. What postoperative complications are most prevalent in older adults?

Factors to Consider. How is CABG surgery accomplished? Why is the CABG surgery a popular option?

 Discussions for these questions can be found on the website.

BIBLIOGRAPHY

 Citations appearing in red refer to primary research.

Citations appearing in blue refer to evidence-based practice guidelines and protocols.

1. Ades, P. (2001). Cardiac rehabilitation and secondary prevention of coronary heart disease. *New England Journal of Medicine, 345*(12), 892-900.
2. Albert, N. (1999). Heart failure: The physiologic basis for current therapeutic concepts. *Critical Care Nurse, 19*(Suppl 6), 2-13.
3. Allen, B., et al. (1999). Comparison of transmyocardial revascularization with medical therapy in patients with refractory angina. *New England Journal of Medicine, 341*, 1029-1036.
4. American Heart Association. (2002). *2002 Heart and stroke facts statistical update.* Dallas: Author.
5. Baig, M.K., et al. (1998). The pathophysiology of advanced heart failure. *Heart and Lung, 28*, 87-97.
6. Balady, G., et al. (2000). Core components of cardiac rehabilitation/secondary prevention programs. *Circulation, 102*, 1069-1073.
7. Chen-Scarabelli, C. (2002). Beating heart coronary artery bypass graft surgery: Indications, advantages, and limitations. *Critical Care Nurse, 22*(5), 44-58.
8. Coffey, M., Crowder, G., & Cheek, D. (2003). Reducing coronary artery disease by decreasing homocysteine levels. *Critical Care Nursing, 23*(1), 25-30.
9. Colbert, K., & Greene, M. (2003). Nesiritide (Natrecor): A new treatment for acutely decompensated congestive heart failure. *Critical Care Nursing Quarterly, 26*(1), 40-44.
10. Collins, A. (2001). More than a pump: The endocrine functions of the heart. *American Journal of Critical Care, 10*(2), 94-96.
11. Cosgrove, J., et al. (2006). Drug-eluting stent restenosis. *Journal of the American College of Cardiology, 47*, 2399-2409.
12. Doering, L.V. (1999). Pathophysiology of acute coronary syndromes leading to acute myocardial infarction. *Journal of Cardiovascular Nursing, 13*(3), 1-20.
13. Eagle, K., et al. (2004). ACC/AHA 2004 guideline update for coronary artery bypass graft surgery. Available at www.acc.org.
14. Epstein, F. (1999). Hormones and hemodynamics in heart failure. *New England Journal of Medicine, 341*(8), 577-585.
15. Fischer, A., et al. (1999). Thrombosis and coagulation abnormalities in the acute coronary syndromes. *Cardiology Clinics, 17*, 283-294.
16. Hunt, S., et al. (2005). ACC/AHA 2005 guideline update for the diagnosis and management of chronic heart failure in the adult: Summary article. *Circulation, 112*, 1825-1852.
17. Kherea, A., et al. (2006). Relationship between C-reactive protein and subclinical atherosclerosis. *Circulation, 113*, 38-43.
18. Kim, W., et al. (2006). The clinical results of a platelet glycoprotein IIb/IIa receptor blocker (abciximab-ReoPro)-coated stent in acute myocardial infarction. *Journal of the American College of Cardiology, 47*, 933-938.
19. LaFramboise, L., et al. (2003). Comparison of health buddy with traditional approaches to heart failure management. *Family and Community Health, 26*(4), 275-288.
20. Lorenz, B., & Coyle, K. (2002). Coronary artery bypass graft surgery without cardiopulmonary bypass: A review and nursing implications. *Critical Care Nurse, 22*(1), 51-60.
21. MacKlin, M. (2001). Managing heart failure: A case study approach. *Critical Care Nurse, 21*(2), 36-51.
22. Maglish, B.L., et al. (1999). Outcomes improvement following minimally invasive direct coronary artery bypass surgery. *Critical Care Nursing Clinics of North America, 11*(2), 177-208.
23. Mosca, L., et al. (2001). Hormone replacement therapy and cardiovascular diseases. *Circulation, 104*, 499-503.
24. National Institutes of Health. (2001). *Detection, evaluation, and treatment of high blood cholesterol in adults (Adult Treatment Panel III)* (NIH Pub No. 01-3670). Bethesda, Md: NIH.
25. Packer, M., & Cohn, J.N. (1999). Consensus recommendation for the management of chronic heart failure. *American Journal of Cardiology, 83*, 1A-38A.

26. Parson, C. (1999). Evidence based clinical outcome management in interventional cardiology. *Critical Care Nursing Clinics of North America*, 11(2), 143-157.

27. Pasternak, R., et al. (2002). ACC/HA/NHLBI clinical advisory on the use and safety of statins. *Circulation, 106*, 1024-1028.

28. Piano, M., Bondmass, M., & Schwertz, D. (1998). The molecular and cellular pathophysiology of heart failure. *Heart and Lung, 27*, 3-19.

29. Poirier, V. (1997). The HeartMate left ventricular assist system: Worldwide clinical results. *European Journal of Cardio-Thoracic Surgery, 11*, 539-544.

30. Puskas, J. (2004). Off-pump versus conventional coronary artery bypass grafting. Early and 1-year graft patency, cost and quality of life outcomes. *Journal of the American Medical Association, 291*, 1841-1849.

31. Reger, T., & Vargas, G. (1999). The return of the radial artery in CABG. *American Journal of Nursing, 99*(9), 26-32.

32. Ross, A., & Ostrow, L. (2001). Subjectively perceived quality of life after coronary artery bypass surgery. *American Journal of Critical Care, 10*(1), 11-16.

33. Scherr, K., Jensen, L., & Koshal, A. (1999). Mechanical circulation as a bridge to cardiac transplantation: Toward the 21st century. *American Journal of Critical Care, 8*, 324-335.

34. Shah, P.K. (1996). Pathophysiology of plaque rupture and the concept of plaque stabilization. *Cardiology Clinics, 14*(1), 17-28.

35. Shekar, P. (2006). On-pump and off-pump coronary artery bypass grafting. *Circulation, 113*, e51-e52.

36. Smith, A., & Brown, C. (2003). New advances and novel treatments in heart failure. *Critical Care Nurse Supplement*, 11-20.

37. Smith, S., et al. (2001). ACC-AHA guidelines for percutaneous coronary intervention (revision of the 1993 PTCA guidelines)—Executive summary. *Circulation, 103*, 3019-3041.

38. Smith, S., et al. (2006). AHA/ACC guidelines for secondary prevention for patients with coronary and other atherosclerotic vascular disease—2006 update. *Journal of the American College of Cardiology, 47*, 2130-2139.

39. St. Joer, S., et al. (2001). Dietary protein and weight reduction: A statement for healthcare professionals from the nutrition committee on nutrition, physical activity, and metabolism of the American Heart Association. *Circulation, 104*, 1869-1874.

40. Stary, H.C., et al. (1995). A definition of advanced types of atherosclerotic lesions and a histological classification of atherosclerosis. *Circulation, 92*, 1355-1374.

41. Stevenson, L., & Kormos, R. (2001). Mechanical Cardiac Support 2000: Current applications and future trial design. *Journal of Thoracic and Cardiovascular Surgery.* 121(3),418-24.

42. Taccetta-Chapnick, M. (2002). Using carvedilol to treat heart failure. *Critical Care Nurse, 22*(2), 36-58.

43. Teirsteine, P., et al. (2000). Three-year clinical and angiographic follow-up after intracoronary radiation. *Circulation, 101*, 360-370.

44. Wenger, N.K. (1999). Women, myocardial infarction, and coronary revascularization. *Cardiology in Review, 7*, 117-120.

45. Zhou, J., et al. (1999). Plaque pathology and coronary thrombosis in the pathogenesis of acute coronary syndromes. *Scandinavian Journal of Clinical and Laboratory Investigation, 59*(Suppl 230), 3-11.

46. Zimmerman, L., et al. (2002). Comparison of recovery patterns for patients undergoing coronary artery bypass grafting and minimally invasive direct coronary artery bypass in the early discharge period. *Progress in Cardiovascular Nursing, 17*(3), 132-141.

evolve *Did you remember to check out the bonus material on the Evolve website and the CD-ROM, including NCLEX®-Examination Style Review Questions, Open-Book Quizzes, and Chapter Review Audio Podcasts?*

http://evolve.elsevier.com/Black/medsurg

CHAPTER 57

Management of Clients with Dysrhythmias

BETH F. CROWDER*

The heart is endowed with a specialized conduction system for generating rhythmic electrical impulses and for moving these impulses rapidly throughout the heart to cause coordinated contraction of the myocardium. When this system functions normally, the atria contract about one sixth of a second ahead of the ventricles. This orderly electrical activity must precede contraction to provide adequate cardiac output for perfusion of all body organs and tissues.

The rhythmic and conduction systems of the heart are susceptible to damage by heart disease, especially by ischemia of the heart tissues resulting from decreased coronary artery blood flow. The consequence is often a bizarre heart rhythm or abnormal sequence of contraction through the heart chambers. The abnormal rhythms, called *dysrhythmias* (or *arrhythmias*), can severely decrease the heart's ability to pump effectively, even causing death.

In 2003 dysrhythmias caused or contributed to 479,000 of more than 2,400,000 deaths in the United States.[1] Dysrhythmias are historically linked to human awareness of the strength and rhythm of the palpable pulse.[14] As early as the 6th century BC, the irregularity of the pulse was observed in China, and then later by the Greeks. Many irregularities were discovered before the availability of electrocardiography. In 1895 Willem Einthoven published a paper on the electrical system of the heart noting five distinct electrical patterns, labeled P, Q, R, S, and T. In 1903 Einthoven modified his string galvanometer, enabling him to record more extensive electrocardiograms (ECGs). In 1912 Einthoven and Thomas Lewis separately published works representing decades of research, observations, and findings regarding cardiac dysrhythmias. Through their discoveries and publications of the heart's electrical system and irregularities, Einthoven and Lewis are considered the pioneers of electrocardiography.[14] Before reading about dysrhythmias, you may want to review the electrical conduction system of the heart in the Unit 13 Anatomy and Physiology Review and the electrocardiogram (ECG) in Chapter 54.

NORMAL SINUS RHYTHM

A *normal sinus rhythm* is the usual heart rhythm that begins in the sinoatrial (SA) node, is between 60 and 100 beats/min, and has normal intervals and no aberrant or ectopic beats (Figure 57-1). Characteristics of normal sinus rhythm are shown in Table 57-1 and discussed in Chapter 54.

DYSRHYTHMIAS

Dysrhythmias are disorders of the heart rhythm. Dysrhythmias are common in people with cardiac disorders but also occur in people with normal hearts. Dysrhythmias are often detected because of associated manifestations of dizziness, palpitations, and syncope. Abnormalities in conduction are dangerous because of reduced cardiac output, which can lead to impaired cerebral perfusion. The most serious complication of a dysrhythmia is sudden death.[5] Because seconds can literally make the difference between life and death for the person who is experiencing

*The author would like to thank Andrea R. Cain and Sheila Melander for their contribution to this chapter in the seventh edition of *Medical-Surgical Nursing*.

---

evolve **Web Enhancements**

Client Education Guide The Client with a Permanent Pacemaker (Spanish Translation)

Ethical Issues in Nursing What Is Your Role in a "Do Not Resuscitate" Decision?

Be sure to check out the bonus material on the Evolve website and the CD-ROM, including free self-assessment exercises. **http://evolve.elsevier.com/Black/medsurg**

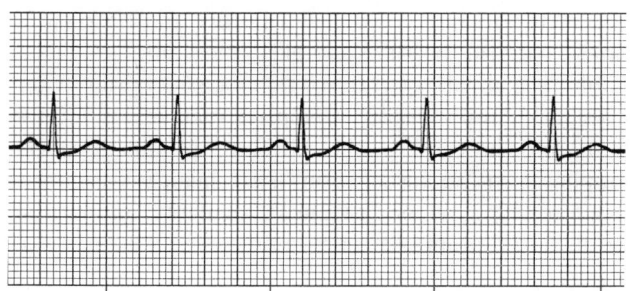

■ **FIGURE 57–1** Normal sinus rhythm as seen on an electrocardiogram (ECG) strip. Note the regular R-R interval, a rate of 80 beats/min, and a P-R interval of 0.16 second.

a serious dysrhythmia, evaluating responsiveness, quickly activating the emergency medical service (EMS), and initiating cardiopulmonary resuscitation (CPR) can determine the outcome.[2]

Etiology and Risk Factors

Dysrhythmias result from disturbances in three major mechanisms: (1) automaticity, (2) conduction, and (3) reentry of impulses.[3,6]

Disturbances in Automaticity

Automaticity is used here to describe the normal processes of generating a heart rhythm. This process of automatically initiating an impulse can be altered if the normal pacemaker cells are firing too rapidly or if an impulse is generated by a cell that normally does not initiate heartbeats, called an ectopic pacemaker. Enhanced normal automaticity occurs when cells conduct an impulse because they were not suppressed. An ectopic pacemaker occurs when cardiac muscle cells that normally do not exhibit pacemaker potential or activity (latent cells) fire to originate an impulse.

Recall that the SA node is the pacemaker of the heart because it possesses the highest level of automaticity. It normally produces a rhythm of 60 to 100 beats every minute. The SA node is regulated by the nervous system through the vagus nerve. Sympathetic stimulation increases the rate of firing, while lack of sympathetic stimulation or vagal stimulation (which is parasympathetic) decreases the rate. If the SA node fails to fire, other latent sites in the atria can fire (60 to 100 beats/min). If the atria

do not initiate a beat, it can begin in the atrioventricular (AV) node; if the AV node does not initiate a beat, one can start in the ventricles. This fail-safe mechanism is crucial during heart disease. Latent pacemaker cells in the AV junction usually assume the role of pacemaker of the heart but at a slower rate (40 to 60 beats/min). Such a pacemaker is called an *escape* pacemaker. If the AV junction cannot take over as the pacemaker because of disease, an escape pacemaker in the electrical conduction system below the AV junction (i.e., in the bundle branches or Purkinje fibers) can take over, but at a still lower rate (less than 40 beats/min). In general, the further the escape pacemaker is from the SA node, the slower the impulse rate generated.

Risk Factors. Abnormal automaticity is commonly caused by myocardial ischemia, decreased left ventricular function, valvular heart disease, electrolyte imbalance, hypoxia, adrenergic (sympathetic nervous system) stimulation, impaired cellular metabolism, use of antidysrhythmic medications, digitalis toxicity, and administration of atropine (which blocks vagal stimulation).

Disturbances in Conduction

Conduction is the speed the impulse travels through the sinus node, AV node, and Purkinje fibers. Latent pacemaker cells can also fire at rates above or below their inherent rate. A rhythm slower than the intrinsic rate is called *bradycardia*. A rhythm faster than the intrinsic rate is called *accelerated* or *tachycardia*. For example, sinus bradycardia is identified as a heart rate below 60 beats/min and sinus tachycardia is defined as a heart rate above 100 beats/min. An accelerated junctional tachycardia can develop with a rate higher than 60 beats/min (the inherent AV node rate).

Impulses can also occur prematurely or may be blocked anywhere between the SA node and the Purkinje fibers. Premature beats are ones that occur before the expected impulse. Premature beats can develop from any of the latent pacemaker cells. Blocks are impulses that are generated normally, but do not reach their destination. Blocks need more time to travel to their destination; the ECG wave is wider than normal. Disturbances in conduction can also lead to decreased cardiac output and life-threatening dysrhythmias.

Risk Factors. Conduction disturbances can result from myocardial ischemia, scarring and compression of conduction pathways, valvular heart disease or valvular surgery, inflammation of the AV node, extreme vagal stimulation of the heart, electrolyte imbalances, increased atrial preload, digitalis toxicity, beta-blocking agents, non-dihydropyridine calcium-channel blockers, impaired cellular metabolism, and myocardial infarction (MI) (especially inferior).

TABLE 57–1	Characteristics of Normal Sinus Rhythms
Rhythm	Regular, P-P intervals and R-R intervals may vary as much as 3 mm and still be considered regular
Rate	60-100 beats/min
P waves	One P wave preceding each QRS complex
P-R interval	0.12-0.20 sec, consistent with each complex
QRS complex	0.04-0.10 sec, consistent with each complex
Q-T interval	<0.40 sec

Reentry of Impulses

Reentry of impulses occurs when cardiac tissue is depolarized multiple times by the same impulse. Normally the impulse enters into the tissue, excites the tissue (causing depolarization), and leaves the tissue after the refractory period is over (repolarization). It occurs along one pathway with a constant conduction velocity. Reentry of impulses occurs when two pathways are present (a "slow" pathway and a "fast" pathway). Two pathways can develop from anatomic abnormalities (accessory pathway, fibrosis) or functional defects (ischemia, drug interactions). The two pathways are separated by an area of unexcitable tissue. As the impulse enters both pathways, the "fast" pathway exhibits a resistance that will not allow the impulse to travel forward but the impulse is able to travel down the slow pathway. When the impulse reaches the distal end of the slow pathway, it travels backwards into the fast pathway, causing the impulse to repeat itself.[3] Reentry of impulses creates problems because some cells have been repolarized sufficiently so that they can prematurely depolarize again, producing ectopic beats and rhythm disturbances.

Risk Factors. Reentry can result from myocardial ischemia, the action of antidysrhythmic medications, myocardial fibrosis, existence of an accessory pathway, or bundle-branch block.

Pathophysiology

The significance of all dysrhythmias is their effect on cardiac output and therefore cerebral and vascular perfusion. Recall that cardiac output is the result of stroke volume times the heart rate. During normal sinus rhythm, the atria contract to fill and stretch the ventricles with about 30% more blood. This process, called the *atrial kick,* increases the amount of blood (stroke volume) in the ventricles before contractility, thereby increasing cardiac output by 30%. When the impulse originates below the SA node, or more than one area fires in the atria to originate a beat (such as with atrial fibrillation or atrial flutter), the atrial kick is lost and cardiac output falls that 30%.[3]

Clinical Manifestations

The reduced cardiac output leads to clinical manifestations of palpitations, dizziness, presyncope or syncope, pallor, diaphoresis, altered mentation (restlessness and agitation to lethargy and coma), shortness of breath, chest pain, orthopnea, paroxysmal nocturnal dyspnea, hypotension, sluggish capillary refill, swelling of the extremities, and decreased urine output.

The initial assessment includes a careful history regarding the onset, duration, associated manifestations, aggravating factors, and relieving factors. Following the history and symptom analysis, a detailed past medical history follows including cardiovascular disease (CVD) risk factor analysis, past health history and hospitalizations, surgical history, allergies, medications, dietary habits, social habits (tobacco, alcohol, street drugs, exercise), and family history. Complete your review of systems and proceed to the physical examination with emphasis on the auscultation of the heart for abnormal heart tones, slow or fast rate, irregularity, murmur(s), or displaced point of maximum intensity.

Diagnostic Assessment
Noninvasive Recording

Electrocardiography. Electrocardiography remains the most important and definitive noninvasive diagnostic test for dysrhythmias. Each rhythm strip or ECG must be approached in a systematic manner for analysis (Box 57-1). The key to dysrhythmia interpretation is the analysis of the form and interrelations of the P wave, the P-R interval, and the QRS complex. Are P waves present? Is there a P wave preceding every QRS complex? What is the duration of the P-R interval? Is the P-R interval constant? What is the duration of the QRS complex? What are the atrial and ventricular rates? Are the P-P and R-R intervals regular? Are all P waves and QRS complexes identical? The ECG should also be analyzed with respect to its rate, rhythm, and site of the dominant pacemaker as well as the configuration of the P and QRS waves (Table 57-2). Remember, any ECG findings should be correlated with clinical observations of the client; that is, treat the client, not the monitor.

Holter Monitors. Holter monitors continuously record the cardiac rhythm for 24 hours. This method of prolonged ECG monitoring, with clients engaged in their usual daily activities, is one of the most useful noninvasive methods for capturing and documenting the type, frequency, and complexity of the dysrhythmia. Holter monitors also allow correlation between the dysrhythmia and the client's manifestations. The Holter tape is timed and clients keep a diary noting the clinical manifestation and the time the manifestation was noted.

Event Monitors. For those clients who do not experience dysrhythmia within that 24-hour period of recording, event monitors are available. This monitor is smaller with fewer electrodes placed on the client. Unlike the 24-hour Holter monitor (which records continuously), the event monitor is client activated. When a dysrhythmia is noted, the client pushes a small button to activate the recorder. Multiple episodes can be recorded and downloaded over the telephone. Clients usually keep event monitors for 2 weeks (or longer) in order to capture their dysrhythmia.

Invasive Electrophysiologic Studies

An electrophysiologic (EP) study involves the positioning of a multipolar catheter electrode into the venous

BOX 57-1 Electrocardiographic Interpretation of Dysrhythmias

There are seven basic steps to assist you in the identification of dysrhythmias. The electrocardiogram (ECG) should be studied in an *orderly* fashion as follows:

Step 1. Calculate the heart rate. The simplest method for obtaining the rate is to count the number of R waves in a 6-inch strip of the ECG tracing (which equals 6 seconds). Multiply this sum by 10 to get the rate per minute (beats/min). Because the ECG paper is marked into 3-inch intervals (at the top margin), the approximate heart rate can be rapidly calculated.

Another method is to count the number of large squares between R waves. Find an R wave crossing a large square. Count the number of large squares until the next R wave. The approximate heart rate is as follows:

- 1 large square = 300 beats/min
- 2 large squares = 150 beats/min
- 3 large squares = 100 beats/min
- 4 large squares = 75 beats/min
- 5 large squares = 60 beats/min
- 6 large squares = 50 beats/min
- 7 large squares = 43 beats/min
- 8 large squares = 37 beats/min
- 9 large squares = 33 beats/min
- 10 large squares = 30 beats/min

Step 2. Measure the regularity (rhythm) of the R waves (ventricular rhythm). This can be done by gross observation or actual measurement of the intervals (R-R).

If the R waves occur at regular intervals (variance <0.12 second between beats), the ventricular rhythm is normal. When there are differences in R-R intervals (>0.12 second), the ventricular rhythm is said to be irregular. The division of

ventricular rhythm into regular and irregular categories assists in identifying the mechanism of many dysrhythmias.

Note atrial regularity and measure the atrial rate. Measure the regularity (rhythm) of the P waves (P-P). Use the previously described method, but calculate the distance between the same point on two consecutive P waves.

Step 3. Examine the P waves. If P waves are present and precede each QRS complex, the heartbeat originates in the sinus node and a sinus rhythm exists. The absence of P waves or an abnormality in their position with respect to the QRS complex indicates that the impulse started outside the sinoatrial node and that an ectopic pacemaker is in command.

Step 4. Measure the P-R interval. Normally this interval should be between 0.12 and 0.20 second. Prolongation or reduction of this interval beyond these limits indicates a defect in the conduction system between the atria and the ventricles.

Step 5. Measure the duration of the QRS complex. If the width between the onset of the Q wave and the completion of the S wave is greater than 0.12 second (three fine lines on the paper), an intraventricular conduction defect exists.

Step 6. Examine the ST segment. Normally this segment is isoelectric, meaning it is neither elevated nor depressed because the positive and negative forces are equally balanced during this period. Elevation or depression of the ST segment indicates an abnormality in the onset of recovery of the ventricular muscle, usually because of injury (e.g., acute myocardial infarction).

Step 7. Examine the T wave. Normally the T wave is upright and one third the height of the QRS complex. Any condition that interferes with normal repolarization (e.g., myocardial ischemia) may cause the T waves to invert. An abnormally high serum potassium level causes the T wave to become very tall, sometimes the height of the QRS complex.

---

system, placing the electrode at various sites along the atria, ventricles, His bundle, bundle branches, accessory pathways, and other structures to record electrical activity. These areas can also be stimulated through the catheter tip to assess for function or rhythm disturbances. Electrophysiologic studies are performed for three primary reasons:

(1) diagnostically (to provide information on the dysrhythmia type and its origin), (2) therapeutically (to evaluate the effects of antidysrhythmic drugs or function of an automatic internal cardioverter-defibrillator), and (3) prognostically (to identify clients at risk for sudden death).[3]

TABLE 57–2 Cardiac Dysrhythmia Characteristics

Type of Dysrhythmia	Atrial Rate (beats/min)	P-Wave Rhythm/Contour	Ventricular Rate (beats/min)	QRS Complex Rhythm/Contour
Sinus rhythm	60-100	Regular/normal	60-100	Regular/normal
Sinus tachycardia	>100	Regular/normal	>100	Regular/normal
Sinus bradycardia	<60	Regular/normal	<60	Regular/normal
Atrial fibrillation	350-600	Irregular/undulations	100-180	Irregular/normal
Atrial flutter	220-350	Regular/sawtooth	75-175	Regular/normal
1° AV block	60-100	Regular/normal	60-100	Regular/normal
2° AV block type I	60-100	Regular/normal	30-100	Regular/normal
2° AV block type II	60-100	Regular/normal	30-100	Regular/normal
3° (complete) AV block	60-100	Regular/normal	40-60	Regular/normal
Ventricular tachycardia	Cannot calculate	Absent	70-250	Fairly regular to irregular/wide
Ventricular fibrillation	Cannot calculate	Absent	150-300	Grossly irregular/wide

The goal of management is to control or ablate the dysrhythmia and reduce potential complications. The specific management of dysrhythmias depends on the type and on the client's response to the dysrhythmia. All dysrhythmias can reduce cardiac output, which can cause a client to have no manifestations or to have many. Rhythm disturbances resulting in syncope, near-syncope, or near sudden death warrant further evaluation. Ventricular dysrhythmias can be life-threatening, demanding immediate treatment. This chapter reviews dysrhythmias and their management, including rhythm disturbances arising (1) in the sinoatrial node, (2) in the atria, (3) in the AV junction, (4) in an accessory pathway, (5) in the ventricles, and (6) with impulse conduction.

SINOATRIAL NODE DYSRHYTHMIAS

DISTURBANCES IN AUTOMATICITY

Sinus Tachycardia

Sinus tachycardia in an adult is defined as a heart rate faster than 100 beats/min. Sinus tachycardia begins in the sinus node, with a regular rhythm between 100 and 180 beats/min. The P wave and QRS complex are normal duration (Figure 57-2, *A*). It often occurs in response to an increase in sympathetic stimulation or decreased vagal (parasympathetic) stimulation.

Causes include the following:

- Fever
- Emotional and physical stress
- Heart failure
- Fluid volume loss
- Hyperthyroidism
- Hypercalcemia
- Medications, including atropine, nitrates, epinephrine, isoproterenol, and over-the-counter cold medications containing decongestants (pseudoephedrine dextromethorphan)
- Caffeine
- Nicotine
- Exercise

Sinus tachycardia usually does not produce noticeable clinical manifestations except for occasional palpitations; however, if the heart rate is very rapid it will reduce cardiac output. Between these quick beats, there is little time for atrial contraction and ventricular filling. Clients with underlying heart disease may not tolerate the increased myocardial workload and reduced coronary artery filling time that accompany the increased heart rate. These clients may experience hypotension and *angina pectoris* (chest pain).

Management

Management focuses on alleviating the underlying cause and reducing further demands on the heart. Medications such as digitalis, beta-blocking agents (e.g., propranolol), and calcium-channel blockers (e.g., verapamil) may be prescribed, or intravenous fluids may be given

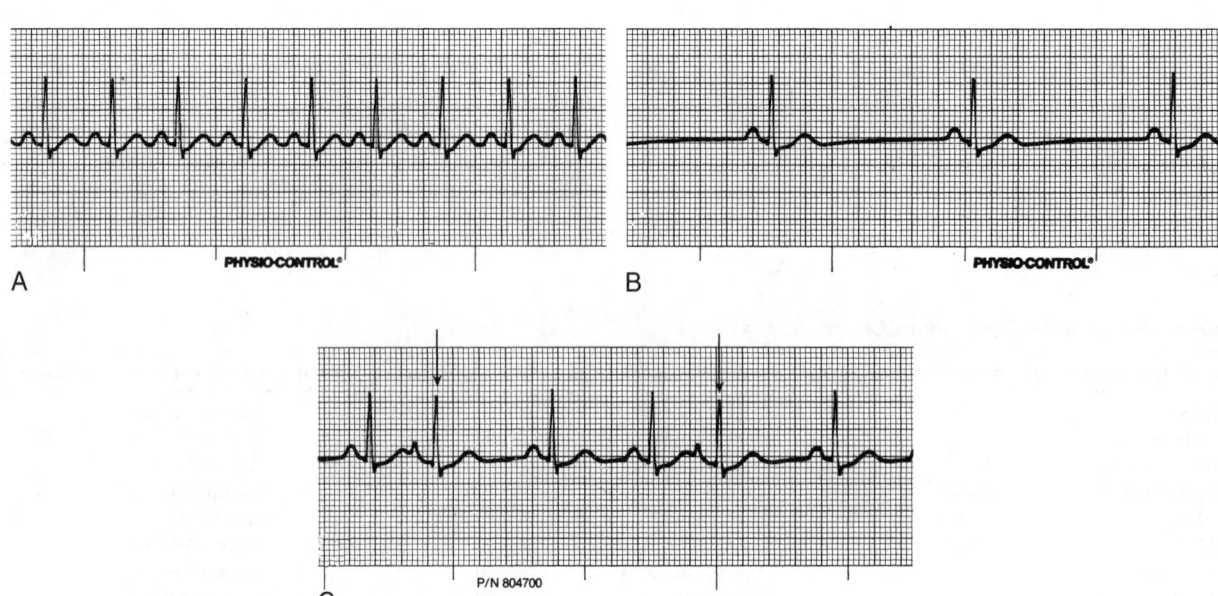

■ **FIGURE 57–2** Atrial dysrhythmias. **A,** Sinus tachycardia—regular R-R interval, rate 125 beats/min; P-R interval, 0.16 second. **B,** Sinus bradycardia— regular R-R interval, rate 40 beats/min; P-R interval, 0.16. **C,** Premature atrial contractions. The second and fifth beats are premature atrial contractions (PACs). Note the difference in the appearance of the P wave and the shortened R-R interval.

if hypovolemia is suspected.[5,6] Bed rest or decreased physical activity reduces metabolic demand. Oxygen may be prescribed to supply the myocardium adequately. Elimination of tobacco, alcohol, caffeine, and other stimulants is recommended.

Sinus Bradycardia

Sinus bradycardia in an adult occurs when the SA node fires at a rate of less than 60 beats/min. The P wave and QRS complex are normal (Figure 57-2, B). Sinus bradycardia may result from the following:

- Increased vagal (parasympathetic) tone, as with vomiting or Valsalva's maneuver (straining with bowel movements)
- Drugs (especially digitalis, propranolol, or verapamil)
- MI (most often inferior MI)
- Hyperkalemia
- Various diseases, such as hypothyroidism, myxedema, and obstructive jaundice
- Severe hypoxia
- Increased intracranial pressure

Asymptomatic sinus bradycardia frequently occurs in young, healthy adults or athletes because of conditioning and a greater than normal stroke volume. In adolescents and young adults during sleep, the normal heart rate may fall to 40 beats/min.

Manifestations develop when cardiac output is decreased and can include fatigue, hypotension, lightheadedness, dizziness, presyncope, syncope, shortness of breath, decreased level of consciousness, pulmonary congestion, or heart failure. The slowed rate of SA discharge may allow junctional or ventricular pacemakers to take over, thereby producing ectopic beats sensed as palpitations.

Management

The goal of management is to correct the underlying cause of sinus bradycardia, and the goal of intervention is to increase the heart rate just enough to relieve manifestations but not enough to cause tachycardia. The intervention sequence for treating hospitalized symptomatic bradycardia is atropine; transcutaneous pacing if available; dopamine, epinephrine, and isoproterenol; or insertion of a temporary transvenous pacemaker.[5,6] Permanent transvenous pacemakers can also be inserted if warranted. Medications to increase the heart rate safely and reliably over long periods without side effects are not available.

Sinus Dysrhythmia

Sinus dysrhythmia is characterized by phasic changes in the automaticity of the SA node, causing it to fire at varying speeds. The heart rate generally ranges between 60 and 100 beats/min. The ECG shows a normal P wave, P-R interval, and QRS complex, with the only abnormality being an irregular P-P interval. Sinus dysrhythmia may develop from alterations in vagal tone and in response to delayed atrial filling with inspiration. During inspiration, venous return to the right atrium is delayed because of increased intrathoracic pressure. In quiet respiration, the heart rate can decrease about 5%; with deep inspiration, the rate can decrease up to 30%.[3] Clients with sinus dysrhythmia do not usually require intervention unless blood pressure is affected, particularly with orthostatic position changes. If dizziness, presyncope, or syncope occur, elastic support stockings and/or sodium-retaining drugs (to expand the vascular volume) are helpful.

Sick Sinus Syndrome

Sick sinus syndrome encompasses different abnormalities of the sinus node including (1) persistent sinus bradycardia (not caused by medications or physiologic disturbances), (2) sinus arrest or pauses, (3) combinations of SA and AV nodal conduction disturbances, and (4) alternating paroxysms of rapid atrial tachycardias. Manifestations are intermittent and unpredictable, and affect client lifestyles. Causes are also similar to those for tachycardia and bradycardia.[3]

Management

Often, clients are found to have tachycardia and are prescribed digitalis, propranolol, verapamil, or other medications that slow the SA node impulse. The drugs then affect the impulse conduction and can lead to bradycardia. Decreasing the drug dose usually leads to recurrence of tachycardia. For clients with sick sinus syndrome, treatment is two-fold including drugs to slow the automaticity and heart rate, along with insertion of a permanent transvenous pacemaker to prevent symptomatic bradycardia.

DISTURBANCES IN CONDUCTION

SINOATRIAL NODE CONDUCTION DISTURBANCES

Under certain circumstances, the impulse from the SA node is either (1) not generated in the SA node (*SA arrest*) or (2) not conducted from the SA node (*sinus exit block*). Causes of SA node conduction abnormalities include the following:

- Conditions that increase vagal tone
- Coronary artery disease
- MI
- Digitalis and calcium-channel blocker toxicity
- Hypertensive disease
- Tissue hypoxia
- Scarring of intra-atrial pathways
- Electrolyte imbalances

SA Arrest

During *SA arrest,* neither the atria nor the ventricles are stimulated, resulting in a pause in the rhythm. An entire

PQRST complex will be missing for one or more cycles. After the pause of sinus arrest, a new pacemaker focus assumes the pacing responsibility. The new pacemaker paces the heart at its inherent rate, which is usually slower than the original SA node rate. The new pacemaker site is often another atrial focus, but the AV junction or ventricle can also assume pacing responsibility.

Management

Intervention may include administration of a vagolytic (atropine) or a sympathomimetic (isoproterenol) agent to increase the rate of SA node firing. If pharmacologic measures fail, a temporary transvenous pacemaker may be required. A permanent transvenous pacemaker may also be warranted depending on the underlying cause of the dysrhythmia.[3,5]

Sinus Exit Block

During *sinus exit block,* a conduction delay occurs between the sinus node and the atrial muscle. Unlike the rhythm in SA arrest, the rhythm of SA node discharge in sinus exit block remains constant and uninterrupted. The ECG characteristically displays a normal sinus rhythm interrupted intermittently by pauses. This creates a pattern of pauses that, when measured, comprises multiples of the underlying P-P interval. Sinus arrest differs from SA exit block in that the SA node at times does not fire at all. The result is the occurrence of pauses that are longer and not a multiple of the underlying P-P interval. These pauses are also frequently terminated by escape ectopic beats. Sinus arrest often is associated with a more serious prognosis.[3] The client usually remains asymptomatic, depending on the duration and frequency of the pauses; however, lengthy pauses can cause lightheadedness, dizziness, presyncope, or syncope. Intervention is unnecessary unless the client becomes symptomatic and exhibits manifestations of decreased cardiac output.

Management

Management is similar to SA arrest and is based on symptoms or alterations in vital signs.

ATRIAL DYSRHYTHMIAS

DISTURBANCES IN AUTOMATICITY

Premature Atrial Contractions

Premature atrial contractions (PACs) are early beats arising from ectopic atrial foci, interrupting the normal rhythm. They commonly result from enhanced automaticity of the atrial muscle and can occur in both normal and diseased hearts. PACs are associated with valvular disease and atrial chamber enlargement; they may also be seen with stress, fatigue, alcohol or caffeine ingestion, smoking, coronary artery disease (CAD), cardiac ischemia, heart failure, cardioactive medications (digitalis, quinidine, procainamide), pulmonary congestion, and pulmonary hypertension. Frequent PACs may mark the onset of atrial fibrillation or heart failure or may reflect electrolyte imbalances.[3]

In clients with PACs, P waves are premature and often differ from the normal sinus P wave in appearance, size, or shape (Figure 57-2, *C*). When a PAC occurs, conduction may not be normal as the AV node may still be refractory from the preceding beat. Thus the impulse may be blocked or slowed, prolonging the P-R interval. Premature beats from any ectopic focus can be palpated as skipped or irregular beats. The client who experiences numerous PACs may note palpitations, or "missed beats." PACs are usually benign; however, if the client has increasing numbers of "skipped beats" or feels palpitations often, the problem should be evaluated.

Management

PACs generally do not require treatment. Intervention usually focuses on correcting the underlying cause and may include administration of digitalis, a beta-blocker, or a calcium-channel blocker.

REENTRY OF IMPULSES

Paroxysmal Atrial Tachycardia

Paroxysmal atrial tachycardia (PAT) is the sudden onset and sudden termination of a rapid firing from an ectopic atrial pacemaker (Figure 57-3, *A*). Atrial tachycardias are referred to as *supraventricular* because the dysrhythmia source is above the ventricles and often P waves are difficult to detect, which leads to difficulty in trying to name the dysrhythmia. The atrial rate is 150 to 200 beats/min with change in P-wave contour from the sinus P wave. At faster atrial rates, the P waves may become lost in the preceding T wave. Rapid atrial rates may overcome the conduction limits of the AV node, causing varying degrees of AV block [2:1 block (i.e., two P waves for every QRS complex)]. If the atrial rate is not excessive, then conduction through the AV node is usually 1:1. If the atrial rate is excessive, the AV node blocks some of the impulses from further conduction. The QRS complexes are usually normal, although aberrant ventricular conduction may occur at very rapid atrial rates or when a conduction defect exists within the ventricle.[3]

Occasionally PAT appears in clients with a normal heart but most commonly develops in clients with cardiac disease. Common cardiac problems precipitating PAT include the following:

- Coronary artery disease
- MI
- Cardiomyopathy
- Extreme emotions
- Caffeine ingestion

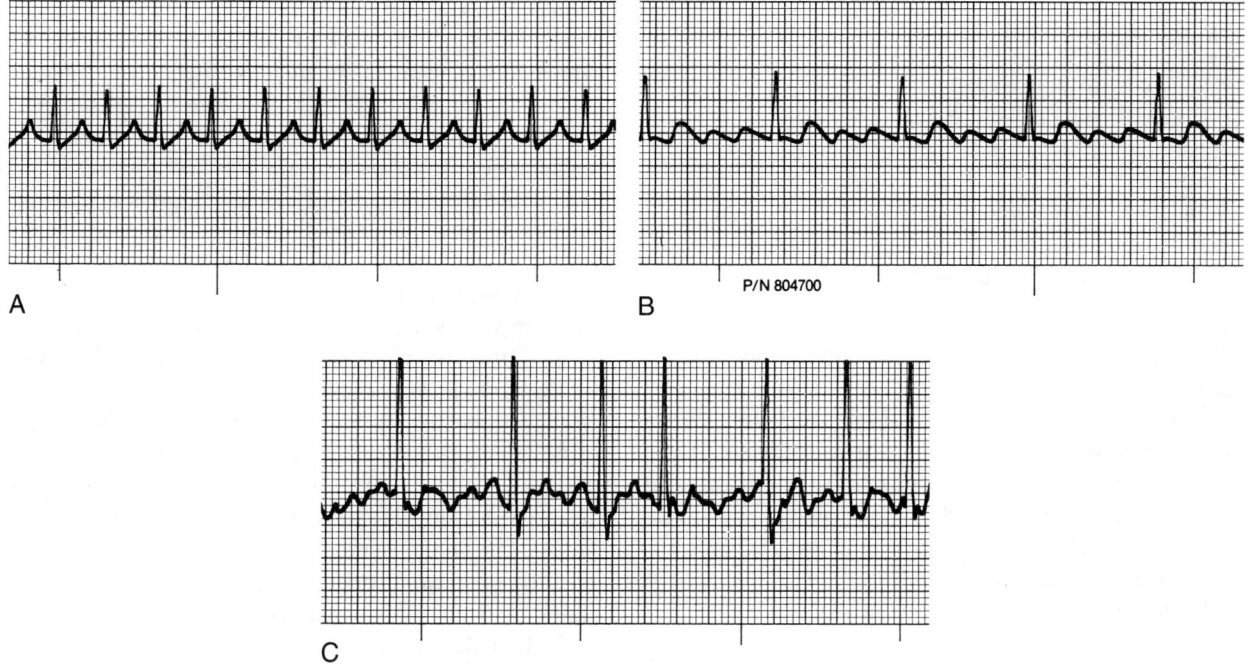

■ FIGURE 57–3 A, Paroxysmal atrial tachycardia (PAT). The rate is rapid, about 175 beats/min. The P wave is not distinguishable, but the QRS complex is narrow, indicating that the impulse began above the atrioventricular node. **B,** Atrial flutter. Note the saw-toothed appearance of the P waves. There are three P waves for every QRS complex, indicating a 3:1 block. Atrial rate is 75 beats/min. **C,** Atrial fibrillation is identifiable by a chaotic P wave, not one clear P wave, and an irregular R-R interval.

■ Cor pulmonale (heart failure from lung disease)
■ Digitalis toxicity
■ Hypokalemia

Less common causes include rheumatic heart disease, valvular disease, pulmonary emboli, thyrotoxicosis, and cardiac surgery. Paroxysmal atrial tachycardia decreases ventricular filling time and mean arterial pressure and also increases myocardial oxygen demand. Clients may report palpitations, heart racing, dizziness, and lightheadedness.

Management

Management varies with the severity of manifestations. Clients with extremely rapid heart rates or significant underlying cardiovascular disease may experience syncope and heart failure. In such instances, heart rate must be immediately slowed. Any maneuver that stimulates the vagus nerve can successfully terminate PAT or increase AV block. The vagus nerve can be stimulated by carotid sinus massage and/or Valsalva's maneuver. Useful pharmacologic agents include adenosine, verapamil, and beta-blockers. Sedatives may also be used to reduce sympathetic stimulation. If medications and vagal stimulation are not effective, cardioversion (discussed later in this chapter) is an effective means of terminating PAT. Ablation procedures that block a part of the reentrant path are being more widely used (discussed later in this chapter). Such procedures can result in a long-term cure in selected clients.[3–11]

ATRIAL FIBRILLATION

Atrial fibrillation (A Fib) is the most common supraventricular dysrhythmia encountered in the emergency department, affecting 1% to 2% of the general population, especially older adults.[3,6] Atrial fibrillation is characterized by rapid, chaotic atrial depolarization from a reentrant pathway. Ectopic atrial foci produce impulses between 350 and 600 beats/min. At extremely rapid rates, however, the entire atrium may not be able to recover from one depolarization wave before the next begins, resulting in mechanical and electrical disorganization of the atria without effective atrial contraction. Small irregular baseline undulations that vary in size and shape, called *f* waves, are identified, which differ from the formed "saw-toothed" waves of atrial flutter. Similar to atrial flutter, the AV node is bombarded with more impulses than it can conduct so a rapid ventricular response comparable to the atrial rate cannot occur. Most of these impulses are blocked; however, as a result of the erratic atrial impulses, the ventricular rhythm is very irregular. The ventricular rate ranges from 100 to 180 beats/min.

Examination of the ECG reveals erratic unidentifiable P waves and underlying ventricular rhythm that appears to be irregular (Figure 57-3, *C*). Because of atrial disorganization, "atrial kick" is lost, thereby decreasing cardiac output by as much as 30%. With increasing ventricular rates allowing less filling time, cardiac output declines even further and may result in dyspnea, angina pectoris, heart failure, and shock. The client may have a pulse deficit between apical and radial pulses.

Atrial fibrillation most commonly occurs because of the following:

- Coronary artery disease
- Congestive heart failure
- Valvular heart disease (particularly mitral and aortic)
- Sick sinus syndrome
- Advanced age
- Longstanding hypertension
- Pericarditis

During atrial fibrillation, blood pools in the "quivering" atria because of lack of adequate contraction of atrial appendages. Pooling blood is prone to clot, forming a mural thrombus, which increases the risk of cerebral and peripheral vascular emboli. Most clients with sudden onset of atrial fibrillation are given anticoagulants to reduce risk of thrombus formation and embolic events. Approximately 20% to 25% of cerebral vascular accidents are due to cardiogenic emboli.[11]

OUTCOME MANAGEMENT

The initial treatment goal is to reduce the risk of thromboembolism and to convert the rhythm to sinus rhythm or control the ventricular response. Anticoagulation in the form of heparin or a low-molecular-weight heparin is started. Oral anticoagulation in the form of Coumadin or warfarin should be started on any reliable client. The dose of Coumadin or warfarin should achieve an international normalized ratio (INR) of 2.0 to 3.0 for stroke prevention. Clients with contraindications to anticoagulation (previous cerebral hemorrhage, history of hemorrhage or gastrointestinal bleeding while taking Coumadin, prone to falls, or cannot reliably follow dosing regimen) can be treated with aspirin therapy. Anticoagulation therapy is 50% more effective than aspirin for stroke prevention.[3,11] Conversion of the atrial fibrillation back to sinus rhythm can be accomplished with medications or cardioversion. Diltiazem, verapamil, beta-blockers, or digoxin is used to control the ventricular heart rate. Chemical cardioversion, usually after 4- to 6- week period of anticoagulation therapy, can then be attempted with procainamide, quinidine, sotalol, propafenone, amiodarone, or other antidysrhythmic agent. Electrical cardioversion is another therapeutic option. The risk of stroke following cardioversion, whether chemical or electrical, in clients not treated with anticoagulation is up to 7%. An alternative option to 4 to 6 weeks of anticoagulation therapy, especially in symptomatic clients, is transesophageal echocardiogram to exclude the presence of atrial thrombus. Please see Chapter 54 for a review of transesophageal echocardiography. After return to sinus rhythm, anticoagulation therapy is continued for an additional 4 to 6 weeks.[3]

Electrical Cardioversion

Cardioversion, most often an elective procedure for dysrhythmias caused by reentry, involves the use of a synchronized biphasic direct current (DC) electrical countershock that depolarizes all the myocardial cells simultaneously, allowing the SA node to resume the pacemaker role. The electrical discharge is synchronized with or triggered by the client's QRS complex for avoidance of accidental discharge during the repolarization phase when the ventricle is vulnerable to the development of ventricular fibrillation. A QRS complex must be present for successful conversion of the dysrhythmia.

Biphasic defibrillators have replaced monophasic defibrillators because biphasic energy requires about half the joules for successful cardioversion. Low voltages (50 to 100 J) are tried initially. If the attempt is unsuccessful, cardioversion using larger voltages can be repeated. Only specially trained physicians can perform this procedure.[3]

Cardioversion is used to treat atrial fibrillation, atrial flutter, and supraventricular tachycardia (see later discussion) that is resistant to medication, and is also used in ventricular tachycardia in an unstable client. The unstable client may be hypotensive or dyspneic, may be experiencing chest pain, or may have evidence of heart failure, MI, or ischemia. Analgesia or sedation may be provided before the electrical shock.[11]

Care Before Cardioversion

The physician evaluates the ECG to identify the type of dysrhythmia present. The client must sign an informed consent, after which the intervention is scheduled. The client and family must receive a full explanation of the cardioversion procedure. The client should be in a fasting state with normal electrolyte balance. For those clients receiving digoxin, a therapeutic drug level must be present. Digitalis toxicity may predispose the client to ventricular dysrhythmias during cardioversion. An INR should between 2.0 and 3.0 after 4 to 6 weeks of receiving anticoagulation therapy (or may be normal if transesophageal echocardiography precedes the cardioversion).[3]

Cardioversion is typically performed at the client's bedside in the critical care unit, or similar specialized area, along with the physician, nurses, and respiratory therapist. If a life-threatening dysrhythmia develops after cardioversion, emergency equipment and trained clinicians are immediately at hand. Start an intravenous (IV) line for medication delivery. Self-adhesive pads (instead of paddles) are used and placed in the standard apex-anterior or apex-posterior positions.

The client is premedicated with a rapid, short-acting sedative. Anesthesia personnel may be present to sedate the client. Oxygen is administered before cardioversion and discontinued if oxygenation saturation is within normal limits.

Care During Cardioversion

The physician performs the following steps and they are repeated with each increase in joules:

1. Sets the biphasic machine within a range of 50 to 200 joules (more or less, depending on the underlying impedances)
2. Turns the synchronizer switch to "on" to deliver the shock during the QRS complex, not on the downslope of the T wave
3. Calls for all health care personnel to stand back from the bed
4. While standing back from the bed, depresses and holds the buttons on the paddles until the shock is delivered
5. Reassess the cardiac rhythm, rate, blood pressure, and pulse oximetry and client's airway after every shock delivered.

Care After Cardioversion

Clinicians immediately assess the ECG, pulse, blood pressure, and respiratory status after the procedure. In some cases ventricular fibrillation or ventricular tachycardia occurs, demanding emergency action. Monitor the client's ECG rhythm and vital signs continuously for at least 2 hours, and carefully assess for rhythm changes and complications. A successful response to cardioversion resolves the dysrhythmia and restores normal sinus rhythm. The client's airway is protected until sedation lightens. With a good response and no complications, the client may be discharged later that day when fully awake and able to eat.

Surgical Management

The Cox-Maze procedure (typically called the MAZE procedure) is an open heart operation for clients with lone atrial fibrillation and no other structural heart disease. The operation involves making a series of incisions that encircle abnormal foci usually near the pulmonary veins. The client requires the usual care of anyone having open-heart surgery (see Chapter 54).

ATRIAL FLUTTER

Atrial flutter is a dysrhythmia from an ectopic pacemaker or the site of a rapid reentry circuit in the atria, characterized by rapid "saw-toothed" atrial wave formations that are usually followed by a slower, regular ventricular response. Atrial flutter differs from PAT in that it produces a much more rapid atrial rate. The P waves are actually inverted or bidirectional because of the clockwise or counterclockwise reentrant pathway, producing a "saw-toothed" pattern of "flutter waves" (Figure 57-3, *B*). The atrial rate generally ranges from 220 to 350 beats/min. The AV node cannot conduct all the atrial impulses that bombard it; therefore the ventricular rate is

always slower than the atrial rate. Thus the pulse, which reflects the ventricular rate, may be normal even though the atrial rate may be quite rapid. The ratio of atrial to ventricular beats may be constant (2:1, 3:1, 4:1, and 5:1, for example), or it may vary. A variable degree of block produces an irregular ventricular rhythm.[3,6]

Atrial flutter most commonly occurs in association with the following:

- Coronary artery disease
- Mitral valve disease
- Atrial enlargement caused by septal defects
- Pulmonary embolus
- Thyrotoxicosis
- Alcoholism
- Pericarditis

In addition, it may occur after cardiac surgery. The client may sense palpitations, shortness of breath, and chest pain, especially when rapid ventricular rates exist. The use of carotid massage helps to slow the ventricular response temporarily so that flutter waves can be identified.

Medical Management

Intervention is based on manifestations and aims at controlling rapid ventricular rates. Anticoagulation is imperative, initially with heparin or a low-molecular-weight heparin, followed by Coumadin or warfarin therapy with an international normalized ratio (INR) of 2.0 to 3.0. Intravenous ibutilide, a short-acting antidysrhythmic medication, has a 60% to 90% success rate for converting atrial flutter. Cardioversion also promptly restores sinus rhythm, usually at energy levels as low as 25 to 100 J. Other medications used include digitalis, diltiazem, flecainide, propafenone, amiodarone, procainamide, and sotalol. Clients with atrial flutter should be referred for electrophysiologic evaluation/study in hopes of dysrhythmia ablation.[3,5,6]

ATRIOVENTRICULAR JUNCTIONAL DYSRHYTHMIAS

If the SA node fails to fire and an impulse is not initiated in other ectopic sites in the atria, the AV junction is the next pacemaker for the heart. An impulse begins in the AV junction and simultaneously spreads up to the atria and down into the ventricles. During junctional rhythms, cardiac output decreases because there is no atrial kick to the ventricles. A junctional rhythm is not dependable as the long-term cardiac pacemaker because its intrinsic rate is slow and more irritable ectopic foci may fire, such as from the ventricles. Consider junctional rhythms to be a warning or forerunner of more serious dysrhythmias.[6]

Two major types of dysrhythmias arise in the AV junction:

- Disturbances in automaticity, with the AV junctional tissue assuming the role of the pacemaker
- Disturbances in conduction, with the AV junction blocking impulses journeying from the atria to the ventricles

Both types of dysrhythmias can result from ischemia, MI, congenital heart disease, valvular heart disease, hyperkalemia, thyrotoxicosis, infectious or inflammatory diseases, or with the use of digoxin, beta-blockers, certain calcium-channel blockers, or certain antidysrhythmics.

Junctional rhythms produce abnormal upward direction of impulse (e.g., in lead II the P waves are inverted) because the impulse is traveling through the atria in a direction opposite that found in normal sinus rhythm. Also, the P-R interval shortens to less than 0.12 second. The impulse may spread through the atria at the same time that the ventricles are being activated by the AV junction. In this instance, the P wave would be buried in the QRS complex and not observed on the ECG. Also, the atria may contract after the ventricles. In this case the P wave would follow the QRS complex. The QRS complex is normal if ventricular conduction is normal.

DISTURBANCES IN AUTOMATICITY

The major junctional dysrhythmias caused by changes in automaticity are (1) premature junctional contractions (PJCs), (2) junctional escape rhythm, and (3) junctional tachycardias. As with PACs, an ectopic focus in the AV junctional tissue may develop increased automaticity and discharge prematurely, initiating depolarization of the heart.[3]

Premature Junctional Contractions

A PJC is the single, early firing of a junctional ectopic focus (Figure 57-4). PJCs are slower as a result of lower intrinsic rates. Usually clients can tolerate junctional rhythms without significant loss of cardiac output; however, clients with underlying cardiac disease may become symptomatic depending upon the amount and frequency

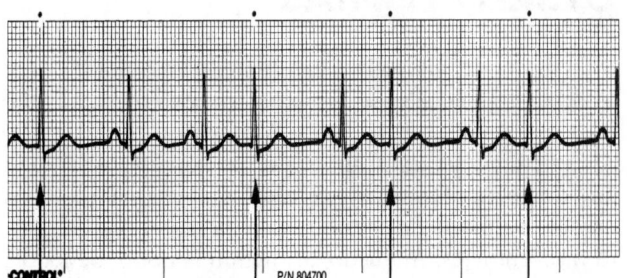

■ **FIGURE 57-4** A premature junctional contraction. The beats marked with *arrows* are premature junctional contractions. Note the absence of a P wave but otherwise normal deflection, indicating that the impulse was initiated above the ventricles.

of ectopic beats. Clients are usually asymptomatic and no interventions are warranted.

Paroxysmal Junctional Tachycardia

A junctional rhythm with a rate that exceeds 60 beats/min is termed a *junctional tachycardia*. It usually stops and starts abruptly, thereby acquiring the name *paroxysmal junctional tachycardia*, or PJT. The usual rate is 140 to 220 beats/min. Causes of PJT include metabolic imbalances and increased sympathetic stimulation. Rapid ventricular rates can lead to left ventricular failure resulting from increased myocardial oxygen demand and decreased myocardial blood supply. PJT that cannot be distinguished from PAT on the ECG is called *supraventricular tachycardia* (SVT).

Medical Management

Management of rapid junctional rhythms begins with vagal stimulation, such as carotid sinus massage. If clinical manifestations develop, treatment consists of pharmacologic agents and cardioversion. Common medications include propranolol, quinidine, and digitalis. Assessment of serum electrolytes and digitalis levels is indicated.[3,6]

DISTURBANCES IN IMPULSE CONDUCTION

The second group of dysrhythmias arising in the area of the AV junction is the AV block. Impulses passing through the AV junction are blocked to varying degrees. Therefore the conduction of impulses from the atria to the ventricles slows or stops entirely, depending on the degree of the AV block. Normally the impulse coming from the SA node is delayed at the AV junction for less than 0.20 second before traveling on to the bundle of His. If the AV junction has been damaged (by one or more of the above etiologies), impulses are delayed or completely blocked at the AV junction for abnormally long periods. Impulse conduction disturbances are classified by the severity of block: first-degree, second-degree, or third-degree AV block.

FIRST-DEGREE ATRIOVENTRICULAR BLOCK

First-degree AV block is a delay in passage of the impulse from atria to ventricles creating a prolonged P-R interval that is greater than the normal 0.20 second. This delay usually occurs at the level of the AV node. Although conduction time is prolonged, all impulses are conducted. The rhythm is regular and each P wave is followed by a QRS complex. The P-R interval usually remains constant (Figure 57-5, *A*). This characteristic is an important differentiation between first-degree AV block and other AV blocks. This block is often associated with structural abnormalities such as right atrial enlargement or atrial septal defect

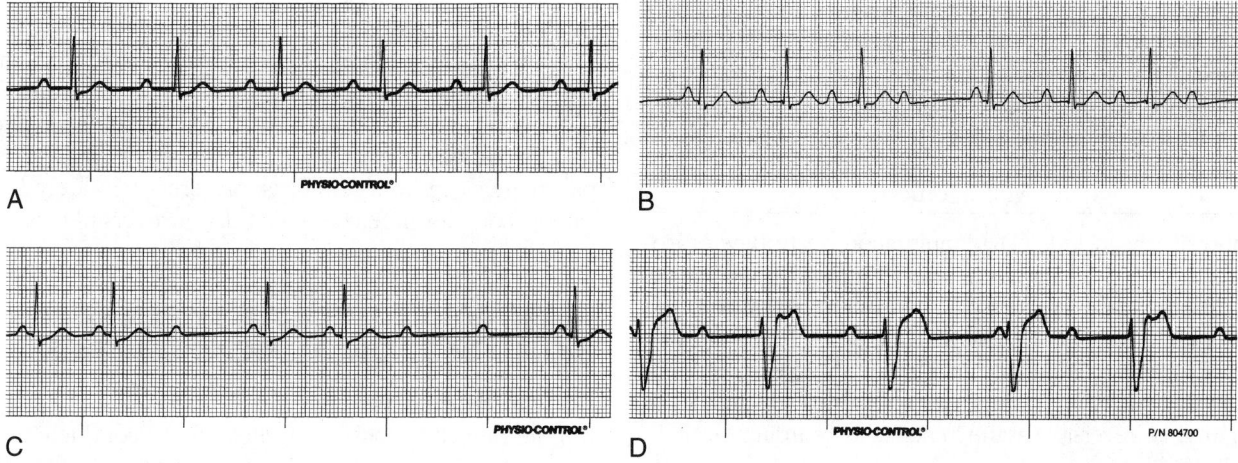

■ **FIGURE 57–5** Junctional dysrhythmias. **A,** First-degree atrioventricular (AV) block. **B,** Second-degree AV block (Mobitz type I, Wenckebach phenomenon; note the regularly occurring P waves and the increasing P-R intervals). **C,** Second-degree AV block (Mobitz type II). **D,** Third-degree AV block (note variable P-R interval and lack of association of the P wave with the QRS complex).

It occurs in 0.5% of young adults without heart disease; however, in the older population it is often seen with idiopathic degenerative disease of the conduction system.[3,6]

Management

First-degree AV block, existing alone as the only abnormal feature of a client's ECG, produces no clinical manifestations and requires no intervention. If the block is a result of digitalis, the medication may be discontinued. Because first-degree AV block can progress to a higher-degree AV block, the client requires routine evaluation including ECG monitoring.[3]

SECOND-DEGREE ATRIOVENTRICULAR BLOCK

Second-degree AV block is a more serious form of conduction delay in the heart; some impulses are conducted and others are blocked. Second-degree block results in intermittently dropped QRS complexes. Atrial depolarization continues producing normal-appearing P waves at regular intervals. Second-degree AV block does not usually affect conduction through the ventricles, and QRS complexes appear normal in configuration. Second-degree AV block develops from coronary artery disease (CAD), digitalis toxicity, rheumatic fever, viral infections, and inferior wall MI.[3,6]

Second-degree AV block is subdivided into two additional types: Mobitz type I (Wenckebach phenomenon) and Mobitz type II.

Mobitz Type I Block (Wenckebach Phenomenon)

The Mobitz type I form of second-degree block is an abnormally long refractory period at the AV node. This delay causes the P-R interval to progressively lengthen until the P wave fails to conduct to the ventricles and a QRS complex is dropped (Figure 57-5, *B*). As the P-R interval lengthens, the R-R interval becomes shorter. With

Wenckebach phenomenon, the QRS complexes are typically "grouped" into twos, threes, fours, and so on. Because of this characteristic grouping, the rhythm is described by recording the number of P waves compared to the number of QRS complexes (e.g., 3:2 or 4:3).[3,6]

Mobitz type I is the mildest form of second-degree heart block and carries a better prognosis compared to type II. The etiology is similar to first-degree AV block, except that Mobitz type I is caused by a block in the AV node. Mobitz type I is a stable rhythm that usually does not result in clinical manifestations because the ventricular rate is adequate; however, the client may have an irregular pulse rate. Vertigo, weakness, or other manifestations of low cardiac output may be experienced if the ventricular rate drops precipitously.

Management

Intervention is not required as long as the ventricular rate remains adequate for perfusion. The client is assessed for progression to a higher (more serious) degree of block. Clinicians focus primarily on managing the underlying cause. Intervention, if needed, is similar to that described for Mobitz type II block.[3]

Mobitz Type II Block

Mobitz type II block occurs when a P wave is not conducted, resulting in a dropped QRS complex. Although a QRS complex is dropped in type I, in type II the P-R interval remains constant without prolongation. In type II the P waves are normal and are followed by normal QRS complexes at regular intervals until suddenly a QRS complex is dropped (Figure 57-5, *C*). The block is described by the ratio of the number of P waves to QRS complexes (e.g., 2:1, 3:1, 4:1). This is considered an unstable rhythm that is usually caused by an infranodal conduction disturbance. Mobitz type II blocks result from ischemia, MI, drug toxicity, idiopathic fibrosis of the conduction system, congenital or valvular heart disease, or hyperkalemia.[3,6]

Mobitz type II is a more serious condition than Mobitz type I because it may progress to third-degree AV block, especially in clients with an anterior wall MI. Clients with second-degree AV block require close ECG monitoring for possible progression to complete heart block.

Management

Interventions include (1) administration of atropine or isoproterenol (which speed the rate of impulse conduction), (2) insertion of a temporary or permanent pacemaker, and (3) withholding cardiac depressant drugs (e.g., digitalis, beta-blockers, certain calcium-channel blockers). Second-degree block, which occurs after MI, particularly an inferior MI, may be reversible as the ischemic myocardium heals.[3]

THIRD-DEGREE ATRIOVENTRICULAR BLOCK

Third-degree AV block is the complete dissociation of the impulse between the atria and ventricles. The atria are regularly paced by the SA node, but because the message is completely blocked, the ventricles are being regularly paced by a ventricular ectopic pacemaker (Figure 57-5, *D*). Third-degree heart block is sometimes called *AV dissociation* or complete heart block because upper and lower chambers of the heart are working independently of each other. The atrial rate is always equal to or faster than the ventricular rate in complete heart block. The ventricular rate is typically 40 to 60 beats/min.[3,6]

Other features of the ECG in third-degree heart block include (1) regular P-P intervals, (2) regular R-R intervals, (3) an absence of meaningful or consistent P-R intervals, and (4) normal-appearing P waves. The greatest danger inherent in third-degree AV block is ventricular standstill or asystole. If an ectopic focus in the ventricles does not initiate a heartbeat, asystole will lead to immediate loss of consciousness and in some cases even death.

Third-degree AV block results from a variety of causes, including the following:

- Fibrotic or degenerative changes in the conduction system
- MI (especially inferior wall MI)
- Congenital anomalies
- Cardiac surgery
- Myocarditis
- Viral infections of the conduction system
- Drug toxicity (digitalis, beta-blockers, calcium-channel blockers)
- Trauma
- Cardiomyopathy
- Lyme disease

The slow ventricular rate leads to decreased cardiac output and circulatory impairment. Clients may experience hypotension, angina pectoris, heart failure, dyspnea, dizziness, presyncope, or syncope.

Management

The major interventions for complete heart block are atropine, transcutaneous pacing, catecholamine infusions (dopamine or epinephrine), and transvenous pacemaker. If asystole develops, CPR is used until a transvenous pacemaker can be inserted. Isoproterenol is rarely indicated. Long-term management for irreversible causes includes permanent pacemaker implantation.[3,5]

INTRAVENTRICULAR IMPULSE CONDUCTION ABNORMALITIES

Bundle-Branch Block

Bundle-branch block indicates that conduction is impaired in one of the bundle branches (distal to the bundle of His), and thus the ventricles do not depolarize simultaneously. The abnormal conduction pathway through the ventricles is causing a wide (greater than 0.20 second) or notched QRS complex.

The defect may result from the following:

- Myocardial fibrosis
- Chronic CAD
- MI
- Cardiomyopathy
- Inflammation
- Pulmonary embolism
- Severe left ventricular hypertrophy
- Congenital anomalies

These disturbances of conduction through the ventricles result in either a right bundle-branch block (RBBB) or a left bundle-branch block (LBBB). A 12-lead electrocardiogram is needed to distinguish left and right BBB. In LBBB the QRS complex in V_1 is described as rS or QS (Figure 57-6, *B*). In RBBB the QRS complex in V_1 is described as rsR (Figure 57-6, *C*). Because of its association with left ventricular disease, LBBB carries a worse prognosis. The left bundle branch is composed of anterior and posterior fascicles (small bundles), and one or both fascicles may be involved. No specific intervention for this conduction defect has been established; however, if RBBB exists along with block in one of the fascicles of the left bundle, the one remaining fascicle represents the only conduction pathway to the ventricles. Therefore in this situation, a pacemaker is required.[3]

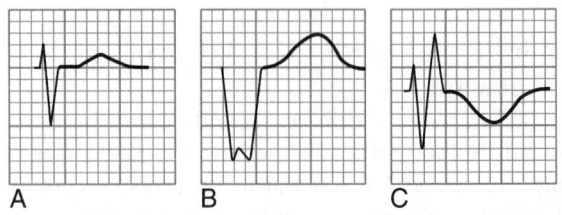

■ **FIGURE 57–6** Bundle-branch block. **A,** Normal QRS in V **B,** Left bundle-branch block in V_1. **C,** Right bundle-branch block in V_1.

VENTRICULAR DYSRHYTHMIAS

Ventricular dysrhythmias arise below the level of the AV junction. Like dysrhythmias in the atria or junction, dysrhythmias in the ventricles are caused by abnormalities of automaticity or conduction. Ventricular dysrhythmias are generally more serious and life-threatening than atrial or junctional dysrhythmias because ventricular dysrhythmias more commonly develop in association with intrinsic heart disease. Also, ventricular dysrhythmias usually cause greater hemodynamic compromise (e.g., hypotension, heart failure, shock). The independent contraction of the ventricles results in a reduced stroke volume and therefore a reduced cardiac output. Rapid ventricular rates prevent optimal filling of the ventricular chambers and reduce stroke volume even further. At rates of less than 40 contractions per minute, cardiac output is simply not sufficient to support the body's vital functions.[13]

The ECG tracing of a client with ventricular dysrhythmias reveals wide and bizarre QRS complexes. Normally impulses traverse the ventricles via the shortest, most efficient route. This normal pathway results in a narrow QRS complex. When an impulse originates in the ventricles, however, the impulse follows an abnormal pathway through the ventricular muscle tissue. This abnormality appears as a wide (greater than 0.12 second) complex on the ECG.

DISTURBANCES IN AUTOMATICITY

Dysrhythmias resulting from problems in automaticity are characterized by ectopic impulses, which result from either myocardial irritability or the phenomenon of reentry. Ventricular dysrhythmias caused by problems with automaticity are premature ventricular contractions (PVCs), ventricular tachycardia (VT), and torsades de pointes.

Premature Ventricular Contractions

Premature ventricular contractions are the most common of all dysrhythmias other than those of the sinus node. They are usually caused by firing of an irritable pacemaker in the ventricle and result from enhanced ventricular automaticity or reentry. Factors promoting PVCs are listed in Box 57-2.[3,6] Premature ventricular contractions

BOX 57-2 **Causes of Premature Ventricular Contractions**	
■ Myocardial hypoxia	■ Heart failure
■ Hypokalemia	■ Toxic agents (e.g.,
■ Hypocalcemia	digitalis, tricyclic
■ Acidosis	antidepressants)
■ Alcohol	■ Exercise
■ Caffeine	■ Hypermetabolic states
■ Nicotine	■ Intracardiac catheters
■ Coronary artery disease	

produce easily recognized ECG changes. They occur earlier than the expected beat of the underlying rhythm and are not preceded by a P wave. The QRS complex is wide (greater than 0.12 second) and bizarre. The T wave is commonly large and in the opposite direction of the QRS deflection (Figure 57-7, *A*).

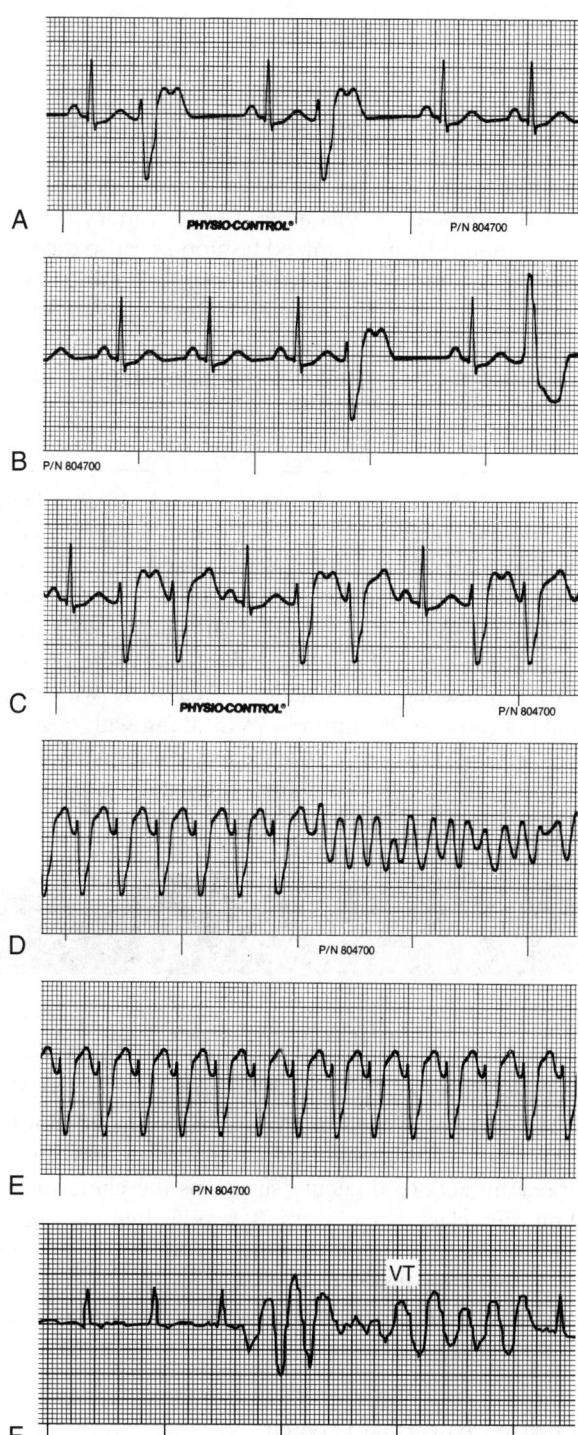

■ **FIGURE 57–7** Ventricular dysrhythmias. **A,** Beats 2 and 4 are unifocal premature ventricular contractions (PVCs). **B,** Multifocal PVCs. **C,** Paired PVCs. **D,** R-on-T phenomenon, leading to ventricular fibrillation. **E,** Ventricular tachycardia. **F,** Polymorphic ventricular tachycardia.

In the following situations PVCs are considered dangerous:

- Frequent (greater than 6 per minute)
- Coupled with normal beats (bigeminy)
- Multiform (Figure 57-7, *B*)
- In pairs after every third beat (trigeminy) (Figure 57-7, *C*)
- A result of acute MI
- On the T wave (Figure 57-7, *D*)

Clinicians refer to "falling on the T wave" as the R-on-T phenomenon. The downward slope of the T wave is the most vulnerable period of the cardiac cycle. If the heart is stimulated at this time, it often cannot respond to the stimulus in an organized fashion because the muscle fibers are in various stages of repolarization. Therefore PVCs that occur during this vulnerable period can precipitate the more life-threatening dysrhythmias of VT (Figure 57-7, *E*) and ventricular fibrillation.

Management

Isolated PVCs are usually not treated. If the client becomes symptomatic because of decreased cardiac output, lidocaine or any of the other class I, II, or III antidysrhythmics can be given to treat PVCs. Intravenous magnesium may also be useful. In clients with acute MI, the development of PVCs indicates that the myocardium is ischemic and irritated. Treatment with beta-blockers can help to suppress PVCs along with restoring myocardial blood flow. In the ischemic setting, PVCs can progress to VT or ventricular fibrillation quickly, so prompt attention and treatment is warranted.[3,6]

OUTCOME MANAGEMENT OF NONTHREATENING DYSRHYTHMIAS

Medical Management

Suppress Irritable Foci

Management of dangerous PVCs involves the administration of antidysrhythmic agents that have myocardial depressant actions. In acute situations the clinician may administer class I and class II antidysrhythmic agents intravenously (IV), followed by a continuous IV drip. The Integrating Pharmacology feature on Toxicity and Antidysrhythmic Agents on p. 1465 describes a variety of antidysrhythmic agents.[3]

Improve Myocardial Oxygen

Oxygen is an essential component of dysrhythmia management, especially for dysrhythmias that result from irritable foci in an ischemic myocardium. These include PVCs and other ventricular dysrhythmias. Oxygen should be given to all clients at risk of ventricular dysrhythmias, such as those with chest pain or hypoxemia or during cardiac arrest.

Nursing Management of the Medical Client

Assessment. Assess the client for clinical manifestations of decreased cardiac output. Monitor the ECG continuously for patterns of dysrhythmias that indicate further deterioration (e.g., sudden onset of atrial fibrillation, PVCs increasing in number; PVCs from different foci, moving closer to the preceding T wave).

Diagnosis, Outcomes, Interventions
Diagnosis: Decreased Cardiac Output. Dysrhythmias often lead to decreased ventricular filling as a result of the rapid rate or from not being coordinated to allow for atrial kick. Express this common nursing diagnosis as *Decreased Cardiac Output related to decreased ventricular filling time secondary to (name the rhythm).*

Outcomes. The client will have an adequate cardiac output as evidenced by (1) return of normal heart rate, rhythm, palpable pulse, and blood pressure to baseline levels; (2) return of level of consciousness to baseline value; (3) warm, dry skin; (4) clear lung sounds; (5) the absence of S_3 or S_4; (6) the absence of dysrhythmias; and (7) adequate urine output.

Interventions. Monitor heart rate and rhythm and vital signs continuously, aided by the computer as needed. Assess skin temperature, lung sounds, heart sounds, and peripheral pulses every 2 to 4 hours. Monitor laboratory studies, especially if a myocardial infarction is suspected. Give antidysrhythmic medications according to orders. Use blood levels as a guide to dosage. Many medications, especially antidysrhythmics, can rise to toxic levels, especially if the client has a pre-existing liver, renal, or electrolyte disorder. Do not attempt to memorize the Integrating Pharmacology box; rather, commit a few drugs to memory (amiodarone, lidocaine, verapamil, and sotalol). Some of these medications can be administered orally or by continuous IV infusion. You must be diligent in monitoring for the intended effect and side effects of the medication.

Assess for manifestations of stroke in clients with atrial fibrillation or flutter. Teach the client to report to the nursing staff any unusual manifestations, especially changes in speech or ability to move.

Administer anticoagulant medications to maintain target partial thromboplastin time (PTT) or INR. If the client is discharged on Coumadin, be certain that the need for follow-up monitoring of INR and the effect of diet on anticoagulation are understood.

Maintain a quiet atmosphere, and administer analgesic to control pain. Stimulation can lead to increased levels of catecholamine release and may trigger tachycardias an

INTEGRATING PHARMACOLOGY

Toxicity and Antidysrhythmic Agents

Numerous antidysrhythmic agents are used to treat and prevent disturbances in cardiac rhythms. Antidysrhythmic drugs have and will continue to have a significant role in decreasing the incidence of sudden cardiac death. Unfortunately, antidysrhythmic drugs also can lead to dysrhythmias at both therapeutic and toxic drug concentrations. See Chapter 56 for a discussion of digoxin toxicity.

CLASS I: SODIUM CHANNEL BLOCKERS

All class I agents block fast sodium channels and reduce the rate of increase of the action potential (phase 0) in certain cells. They inhibit depolarization of neuronal cells, thereby producing local anesthesia. They inhibit depolarization in atrial, ventricular, and Purkinje myocytes, thereby decreasing conduction velocity and automaticity. Class I agents are further categorized as A, B, or C subclasses based on the degree of sodium channel blockade and effects on repolarization. Class IA agents prolong action potential duration and produce moderate slowing of cardiac conduction; prolongation of action potential duration occurs from blockade of outward-rectifying potassium channels. Class IB agents shorten the duration of action potentials and selectively depress cardiac conduction in ischemic cells. Class IC agents have little effect on the potential duration of action potentials but markedly depress cardiac conduction (potent sodium channel blockers).

Procainamide is a commonly used class IA medication used to treat sustained ventricular dysrhythmias. At toxic levels it leads to prolongation of the Q-T interval and QRS complex. Other toxic manifestations include gastrointestinal disturbances, headache, mild hypotension, rash, insomnia, dizziness, ataxia, hallucinations, and weakness.

Lidocaine is a class IB agent used for suppression of VTach or dysrhythmias associated with cardiac surgery. Evidence supporting the efficacy of lidocaine is lacking at this time. ACLS protocol recommends other antidysrhythmics, such as amiodarone, as a better choice. Lidocaine blocks sodium channels and shortens the action potential. Side effects are blurred vision, tinnitus, drowsiness, nausea or vomiting, lightheadedness, confusion, hypotension, and atrioventricular block.

CLASS II: BETA-ADRENERGIC BLOCKERS

Class II beta-adrenergic blockers indirectly block calcium-channel opening and block the ability of catecholamines to cause dysrhythmias. Beta-blockers are used to treat hypertension and myocardial infarction. They are also used to treat migraine headaches, essential tremors, thyrotoxicosis, glaucoma, anxiety, and various other disorders. As a result of their expanded use, the incidence of overdose with these agents has also increased. Manifestations of beta-blocker overdose are related to blocking sympathetic beta-adrenergic receptors. Seizures have been reported.

CLASS III: POTASSIUM CHANNEL BLOCKERS

Class III potassium channel blockers prolong refractoriness and delay repolarization by blocking potassium channels; they have little direct effect on sodium channels. Amiodarone is commonly used to suppress dysrhythmias. Toxic effects include photosensitivity, neurotoxicity, hyperthyroidism, heart failure, complete heart block, pulmonary fibrosis, skin pigmentation (blue nail coloration), and corneal deposits. It may induce Q-T prolongation.

CLASS IV: CALCIUM-CHANNEL BLOCKERS

Class IV calcium-channel blockers slow sinoatrial node pacemaker cell and atrioventricular conduction by direct blockade of L-type voltage-gated calcium channels. Calcium-channel blocker overdose is rapidly emerging as the most lethal prescription drug ingestion. Overdose by short-acting agents is characterized by rapid progression to cardiac arrest. Overdose by extended-relief formulations results in delayed onset of dysrhythmias, shock, sudden cardiac collapse, and bowel ischemia.

As in the case of any client with suspected or known acute poisoning, attempt to obtain the original medication containers, pill counts, the quantity that may have been ingested, approximate time of ingestion, and a report of any potential co-ingestants. To clarify the role of the antidysrhythmic agent, ask the client the following:

- What were the indications for starting the drug?
- How long has the client used this medication?
- How do the manifestations correlate with the initiation of drug therapy?
- Is the client compliant with the drug regimen? Does the client take any extra doses?
- What other medications has the client begun recently? Include nonprescription and herbal medications as well.

From Cummings, R. (2001). *ACLS provider manual.* Dallas, Tex: American Heart Association; Asselin, M.E., & Cullen, H.A. (2002). A new beat for BLS and ACLS guidelines. *Nursing Management, 33*(2), 31-38; Ophie, L.H., & Marcus, F.I. (2001). Antiarrhythmic drugs. In L.H. Ophie (Ed.), *Drugs for the heart* (5th ed.). Philadelphia: Saunders; and Miller, J.M., & Zipes, D.P. (2001). Management of the patient with cardiac arrhythmias. In E. Braunwald (Ed.), *Heart disease* (6th ed.). Philadelphia: Saunders.

ncreased oxygen demand. Apply oxygen with nasal prongs to supplement serum levels. Hypoxia can lead to urther myocardial ischemia and dysrhythmias.

If life-threatening dysrhythmias develop, many nurses re trained to use defibrillation for the client. Other emergency interventions include CPR, various medica-ions, and preparation of the client for a transcutaneous r permanent pacemaker (see the Bridge to Critical Care eature on Defibrillation on p. 1466).

Diagnosis: Anxiety. The risk of death from sudden onset of life-threatening dysrhythmias, fear of the unknown, or fear of defibrillation weighs heavily on most clients.

Outcomes. The client will experience a reduced level of anxiety as evidenced by (1) reporting less anxiety or fewer feelings of helplessness or hopelessness, (2) an increased ability to sleep and rest, (3) a return of the heart rate to baseline level, and (4) a reduction of dyspnea.

BRIDGE TO CRITICAL CARE

Defibrillation

When a client is in ventricular fibrillation or pulseless ventricular tachycardia, the nurse must be able to safely and effectively use an automatic external defibrillator (AED) or conventional (manual) defibrillator (monophasic or biphasic).

GUIDELINES FOR USE OF AN AUTOMATIC EXTERNAL DEFIBRILLATOR (AED)

1. Turn the power on the AED device.
2. Attach cables to the adhesive defibrillator pads.
3. Peel paper from pads and attach pads to the client's chest at the upper right sternal border and the cardiac apex.
4. Place the AED in analyze mode.
5. Announce loudly, "Analyzing rhythm, stand clear!"
6. If VF/VT is present, the AED will charge to the appropriate joules and signal that a shock is indicated.
7. Announce, "Shock is indicated, stand clear!"
8. Confirm that no one is touching the client.
9. Press the shock button when indicated.
10. Repeat the analyze and shock steps until VF/VT is no longer present. The device will signal "No shock indicated."
11. For each set of three shocks, provide 1 minute of CPR.

GUIDELINES FOR THE USE OF CONVENTIONAL DEFIBRILLATORS (MONOPHASIC AND BIPHASIC)

1. Turn on the defibrillator.
2. Select energy level at 200 J for monophasic defibrillation.
3. Set the lead switch to paddles.
4. Apply gel on the paddles or use conductor pads, and place on the client's chest (at second right intercostal space and at the anterior axillary line in fifth left intercostal space).
5. Look at the monitor display, and assess the cardiac rhythm. If VF/VT is present, proceed to the next step.
6. Press the charge button on the apex paddle (the right hand).
7. When the defibrillator is fully charged, state loudly, "Shocking on three, all clear!"
8. Chant "Shocking on three. One, I'm clear. Two, you're clear. Three, all clear!"
9. Apply 25 pounds of pressure with both paddles, and press the discharge button on both paddles simultaneously.
10. Look at the monitor display. If VF/VT is still present, immediately recharge the defibrillator.
11. Shock at 200 to 300 J, then at 360 J. Always remember to make sure the client's surroundings are clear, repeating the chant and assessing for safety each time before shocking.

From Cummings, R. (2001). *ACLS provider manual.* Dallas, Tex: American Heart Association.

Interventions. Identify the client's anxiety and assist the client in discussing sources of fear. Clarify misconceptions. Commonly the client or a member of the family has had a heart condition, and the client's ability to cope may be directly influenced by that experience.

Explain the equipment present in the room. Most rooms are stocked with several types of equipment, and its presence does not always indicate the severity of the client's condition. Remain with the client, and tell the client and family what is happening now and what will be happening (e.g., blood will be drawn soon, an ECG will be obtained).

Finally, explore the usual coping methods with the client. Positive coping methods are usually supported; discuss maladaptive coping mechanisms, and suggest substitutions. For example, smoking may be a common coping mechanism, but it is not permitted in hospitals. Therefore if smoking is the client's coping mechanism when stressed, a substitute would need to be found, such as nicotine patches or chewing gum. Be aware that these patches can lead to chest pain because of vasoconstriction from the nicotine. Adjust the dose of the patch appropriately, beginning with the lowest levels.

Ventricular Tachycardia

Ventricular tachycardia is a life-threatening dysrhythmia that occurs when an irritable ectopic focus in the ventricles takes over as the pacemaker. It occurs in the presence of significant cardiac disease, such as in clients with CAD,

cardiomyopathy, mitral valve prolapse, heart failure, acut MI with hypoxia and acidosis, and digitalis toxicity.[13]

Ventricular tachycardia is characterized by a rapidl occurring series of PVCs (three or more) with no norma beats in between (Figure 57-7, *E*). P waves are absen and the P-R interval is absent. The QRS complex is wid (greater than 0.12 second) and bizarre. The ventricula rate ranges between 70 and 250 beats/min, usually 13 to 170 beats/min. The ventricular rhythm is slightly irregu lar. VT produces a very low cardiac output that can quickl lead to cerebral and myocardial ischemia. At any time VT can develop into ventricular fibrillation. Clients wit VT commonly express feelings of impending death.[3,6]

Ventricular tachycardia can be described as mono morphic or polymorphic. Monomorphic VT originate from one focal site in the ventricle, producing VT tha has a similar contour throughout the run. Polymorphi VT, on the other hand, results from discharges from mu tiple foci in the ventricle, producing differing contou throughout the run (Figure 57-7, *E*). Polymorphic V usually occurs because of a prolonged Q-T interval (sim ilar to torsades de pointes discussed later in this section or as a result of underlying cardiac ischemia.[3]

Management

Manifestations of VT depend on underlying structura cardiac disease, the ventricular rate, and the duration o the VT. Sustained but hemodynamically stable VT is initial eated with antidysrhythmics (i.e., lidocaine, procainamide, r amiodarone). If the dysrhythmia does not respond to antiysrhythmics, cardioversion may be required for conversion ɔ sinus rhythm (see earlier discussion). When the client is in T and unconscious, defibrillation is indicated. Striking the lient's sternum, called a precordial thump or thumpversion, ay interrupt the dysrhythmia. The physician may also rder IV antidysrhythmic agents, usually lidocaine or amioarone. Another drug gaining favor is magnesium sulfate, articularly if the client has low magnesium levels.[3,5,9] The ɔal of long-term therapy includes class IC antidysrhythmics r implantation of an automatic internal cardiodefibrillator y an electrophysiologist.

ifferentiating VT from SVT

can be difficult to differentiate VT from SVT when ventriclar rates are rapid and the QRS complex is not wide. Some ues to help distinguish SVT follow: (1) onset of dysrhythia included a premature P wave, (2) slowing of the venicular rate or termination of the dysrhythmia by vagal imulation, (3) a very short R to P interval (less than 100 illiseconds or 0.1 second), (4) a QRS configuration similar ɔ previously documented supraventricular ectopy, and (5) noted P wave or notch before every QRS complex signalg that ventricular activation is linked to atrial activity.[3]

orsades de Pointes

ɔrsades de pointes is a form of VT in which the QRS ɔmplexes appear to be constantly changing or twisting ɔund an isoelectric line. Delayed repolarization of the entricle is revealed as a prolonged Q-T interval and a ɔad flat T wave in the preceding sinus rhythm. The ythm is regular or irregular with a ventricular rate of ɔ0 to 250 beats/min (Figure 57-8, A). The QRS complex wide and bizarre.[3,6]

Torsades de pointes is usually a result of drug toxicity ɔrocainamide, quinidine, disopyramide) or electrolyte imbalances (hypokalemia or hypomagnesemia), which can lengthen the Q-T interval (see the Genetic Links feature on Long Q-T Syndrome, p. 1468). Clinical manifestations begin with palpitations and syncope. This rhythm often precedes ventricular fibrillation and sudden death.[13]

Management

Torsades de pointes is treated only if the Q-T interval is prolonged. Intravenous magnesium is the initial treatment of choice, along with intravenous potassium if indicated, followed by temporary ventricular or atrial pacing. Discontinuation of offending agents is also crucial.[3,6,9]

REENTRY OF IMPULSES

Two rhythms occur in the ventricles as a result of the reentry phenomenon: ventricular fibrillation and preexcitation syndromes. The usual pathway through the ventricles is not used and the wave of depolarization must spread from cell to cell. As a result the complex is wide and prolonged.

Ventricular Fibrillation

Ventricular fibrillation (VF) is a life-threatening dysrhythmia characterized by extremely rapid, erratic impulse formation and conduction (Figure 57-8, B). Ventricular fibrillation (VF) leads to inadequate myocardial contractions. The heart consequently immediately loses its ability to function as a pump. As the initial reentry pattern of excitation breaks up into multiple smaller wavelets, the level of disorganization increases. Sudden loss of cardiac output with subsequent tissue hypoperfusion creates global tissue ischemia; brain and myocardium are most susceptible. VF is the primary cause of sudden cardiac death (SCD).

This lethal dysrhythmia usually results from severe myocardial damage (such as MI), hypothermia, R-on-T phenomenon, hypoxia, contact with high-voltage electricity,

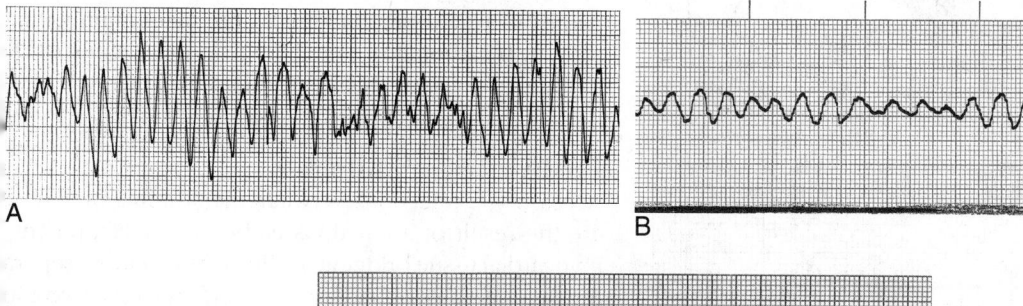

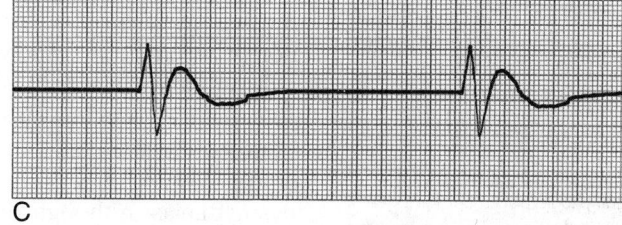

FIGURE 57–8 A, Torsades de pointes. **B,** Coarse ventricular fibrillation. **C,** Ventricular asystole in a dying heart. **(B** from Phillips, R.E., Feeney, M.K. 90]. *The cardiac rhythms: A systematic approach to interpretation* [3rd ed., p. 393]. Philadelphia: Saunders.)

GENETIC LINKS

Long Q-T Syndrome*

DESCRIPTION

Long Q-T syndrome (LQT) produces episodic tachydysrhythmias including *torsades de pointes* (TdP), which may eventually lead to ventricular fibrillation. The most common manifestation of LQT is syncope typically occurring without warning. Undetected or untreated ventricular fibrillation may result in premature sudden death.

GENETICS

LQT is inherited in an autosomal-dominant pattern of inheritance with most individuals (90%) inheriting the gene from an affected parent. Offspring of an affected parent have a 50% chance of inheriting the disease-causing mutation. LQT is caused by mutations in one of five known genes associated with this disorder: *KCNQ1, KCNH2, SCN5A, KCNE1,*

and *KCNE2.* A family history of syncope, sudden death, or successful reversal of cardiac arrest may be suspicious of LQT syndrome.

DIAGNOSIS/GENETIC TESTING

LQT syndrome produces a prolongation of the Q-T interval and T-wave abnormalities, which can be determined clinically by electrocardiography. Clinical molecular genetic testing of the five genes associated with LQT may also make the diagnosis of LQT. About 30% of clinically affected families do not have a detectable mutation in one of these five genes. It is thought that one or more genes not yet identified may be responsible.

MANAGEMENT

Most affected individuals live normal lifestyles. Management is focused on client education, avoidance of triggering events, administration of beta-blockers, insertion of pacemakers, and ready availability of external defibrillators.

*Also known as Romano-Ward syndrome (RWS).

electrolyte imbalance, antidysrhythmic drug side effect, or toxicity from quinidine, procainamide, or digitalis.[13]

The ECG tracing displays bizarre fibrillatory wave patterns, and it is impossible to identify P waves, QRS complexes, or T waves (Figure 57-9, *A*). VF may be either coarse or fine with ventricular rates between 150 and 300 beats/min. Untreated, the deflections become smaller,

and eventually all ventricular activity ceases. Death results within minutes without immediate intervention (i.e., CPR, defibrillation, and medications).[3,6]

Management

When VF appears, the clinician must immediately initiate CPR until the defibrillator is engaged. Defibrillate up to three times if needed. Defibrillation can be performed by nurses who have advanced training (see Defibrillation). A standard monophasic pattern of energy and current can be used. Defibrillation begins with 200 joules (J); if not successful, it is advanced to 300 J, and then to 360 J. With persistent VF, epinephrine is given and the clinician defibrillates at 360 J. Most defibrillators now are biphasic and each manufacturer has it's own recommendations, but the energy used is significantly less than with an old monophasic defibrillator. Other medications are alternated with defibrillation (lidocaine, magnesium sulfate, sodium bicarbonate), depending on the client's cardiac rhythm and electrolyte and acid-base balance.[3,5,6]

Pre-Excitation Syndromes

Accessory connections between the atrium and ventricle are the result of anomalous embryonic development of myocardial tissue bridging the fibrous tissues that separate the two chambers. This tissue allows for electrical conduction between the atria and ventricles at sites other than the atrioventricular node (AVN). Passage through this accessory pathway circumvents the usual conduction delay between the atria and ventricles, which normally occurs at the AVN and predisposes the client to develop tachydysrhythmias. Although dozens of locations for bypass tracts can exist in pre-excitation, including atriofascicular, fasciculoventricular, intranodal, or nodoventricular, the

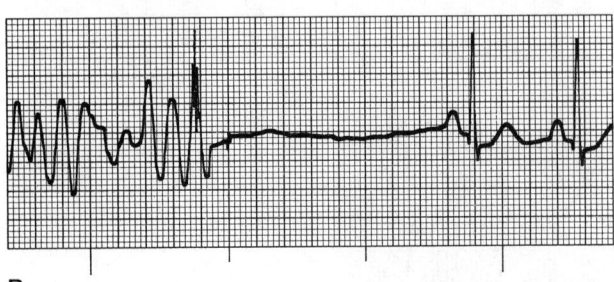

A

B

■ **FIGURE 57–9 A,** Anterolateral paddle placement for external countershock. External paddles are placed at the second right intercostal space and at the anterior axillary line in the fifth left intercostal space. **B,** Ventricular fibrillation converted to normal sinus rhythm.

most common bypass tract is an accessory atrioventricular (AV) pathway otherwise known as a Kent bundle. This is the anomaly seen in *Wolff-Parkinson-White syndrome* (WPW).

Three basic ECG abnormalities are seen as a result of pre-excitation syndromes: (1) a P-R interval less than 120 milliseconds during sinus rhythm; (2) a QRS complex duration exceeding 120 milliseconds with a slurred, slowly rising QRS complex (delta wave) with the remainder of the QRS complex being normal; (3) secondary ST segment and T-wave changes that are usually directed in the opposite direction of the delta wave and QRS complex vectors.[3] Of the several types of disorders in this category, *Wolff-Parkinson-White syndrome* (WPW) appears most frequently. In clients with WPW, attacks of very rapid supraventricular dysrhythmias suddenly develop. Most adults with WPW have normal hearts, but if the tachydysrhythmias occur persistently, myocardial fatigue and ventricular failure may result.

Management

Clients with WPW do not require intervention unless they experience recurring tachydysrhythmias. In this instance, the physician may elect to use vagotonic maneuvers; cardioversion, adenosine, propranolol, amiodarone, and sotalol can affect both the AV node and the accessory pathway. The use of lidocaine or verapamil can increase the ventricular rate and can precipitate ventricular fibrillation. Electrophysiologic evaluation is recommended for appropriate drug therapy and possible accessory pathway radiofrequency ablation (an interventional procedure that destroys the accessory pathway).[3,6]

DISTURBANCES IN CONDUCTION

VENTRICULAR ASYSTOLE

Ventricular asystole (cardiac standstill) represents the total absence of ventricular electrical activity (Figure 57-8, *C*). The client has no palpable pulse (no cardiac output), and a rhythm is absent if the client is monitored. The occurrence of sudden ventricular asystole in a conscious person results in dizziness followed within seconds by loss of consciousness, seizures, and apnea. If the dysrhythmia remains untreated, death ensues. Ventricular asystole must be treated immediately.[3,6]

Cardiac standstill can occur as a primary event, or it may follow VF or pulseless electrical activity. Asystole can occur also in clients with complete heart block (CHB) in whom there is no escape pacemaker. Possible causes include the following:

- Hypoxia
- Hyperkalemia and hypokalemia

- Pre-existing acidosis
- Drug overdose
- Hypothermia

Management

The treatment of choice consists of CPR, epinephrine, atropine, transcutaneous pacing, and correction of the cause.[3,5,6]

PULSELESS ELECTRICAL ACTIVITY

Pulseless electrical activity (PEA), formerly called electromechanical dissociation (EMD), represents the presence of electrical activity in the heart, as seen on the monitor; however, a pulse cannot be detected by palpation of any artery. Thus the ventricles fail to produce an effective contraction despite continued electrical activity. Common causes include end-stage cardiac disease, cardiac tamponade, massive pulmonary embolus, tension pneumothorax, severe hypovolemia, prolonged cardiac resuscitation, exsanguination, or acute malfunction of a prosthetic valve.[3]

Management

Rapid searching for the cause is imperative. Until the cause is located, CPR is initiated in conjunction with advanced cardiac life support measures.

SUDDEN CARDIAC DEATH

Sudden cardiac death is defined as death resulting from an abrupt loss of heart function (cardiac arrest). The victim may or may not have known heart disease. The time and mode of death are unexpected, and death occurs within minutes after the manifestations appear. More than 163,000 deaths occur annually because of sudden cardiac death, with an annual incidence of 0.55 per 1000.[1]

OUTCOME MANAGEMENT OF LIFE-THREATENING DYSRHYTHMIAS

Medical Management

The goal of management is to stop the dysrhythmia immediately and to restore normal sinus rhythm. Remember, because there is inadequate or no perfusion of blood during these dysrhythmias, CPR with advanced cardiac life support measures are performed. Finally, the cause of the dysrhythmia is identified and treated.

Life-threatening dysrhythmias can often be effectively controlled by defibrillation. The most crucial element for survival after cardiac arrest is the time interval from collapse to care, especially defibrillation. With each passing minute, the chances of survival decline as much as 10%.

Electrical intervention can (1) abruptly stop the heart's erratic electrical discharge or (2) restore the flow of electrical current where there is none. Methods of electrical therapy include defibrillation and cardioversion.[3,6]

Defibrillation

The use of defibrillation delivers an electrical biphasic current (shock) of preset voltage to the heart through paddles or special patches placed on the chest wall (closed chest procedure). This current causes the entire myocardium to depolarize completely at the moment of shock, thus producing transient asystole and allowing the heart's intrinsic pacemaker to regain control. The amount of energy required to produce this effect is determined largely by the client's *transthoracic impedance,* or resistance to current flow. Because of this factor, the amount of energy that reaches the heart is less than the amount that the defibrillator is charged to deliver.[10]

The procedure is associated with potential hazards, particularly myocardial damage. The higher the amount of energy or frequency of the shocks, the greater the risk of injury. Advances in the equipment now allow measurement of transthoracic impedance. Once impedance is determined, the defibrillator automatically selects the amount of biphasic current needed that can restore rhythm and cardiac output. It is expected this mode of defibrillation will reduce the risk of complications.[3,6]

The degree of transthoracic resistance depends on several variables:

1. *Energy level.* The higher the energy level that is selected, the more current will follow.
2. *Number and frequency of shocks.* The more shocks administered and the shorter the time between them, the lower the transthoracic resistance.
3. *Ventilation phase.* Resistance is lower when shocks are delivered during exhalation, when there is less air (and therefore smaller diameter) in the lungs.
4. *Paddle or patch size.* The larger the paddle, the lower the resistance.
5. *Chest size.* The smaller the distance between the defibrillator electrodes once they are in place, the lower the resistance.
6. *Paddle-skin or patch-skin interface material.* Conductive material between the skin and paddles/patches reduces transthoracic impedance.
7. *Paddle or patch pressure.* Applying firm pressure increases contact between the skin and the paddles/patches, helping to overcome transthoracic resistance. Exert about 25 pounds of pressure on each paddle.
8. *Paddle or patch placement.* Place one paddle on the upper chest, to the right of the sternum; place the other paddle on the lower left chest, to the left of the nipple, with the center of the paddle in the midaxillary line. If patches are used, they can be placed in a similar fashion or in an anterior-posterior fashion.

If the client has a permanent pacemaker or an internal cardiac defibrillator, place the paddles or patches at least 5 inches away from the generator to avoid damaging it. If a temporary pacing system is in use, disconnect the pacing lead from the pulse generator immediately before defibrillation and reconnect it after the shock.[4,10]

Most defibrillators can be used to perform either *synchronized* cardioversion or *unsynchronized* cardioversion (commonly called *defibrillation*). Defibrillation (unsynchronized) is always indicated in VF and is also used in VT when the client is unconscious and pulseless. Specially trained nurses, emergency medical technicians, and physicians perform this procedure in acute settings.[3]

Care Before Defibrillation

Immediately before defibrillation, assess the client's responsiveness and do the following:
1. **If the client is not responsive, call for immediate assistance (or activate the EMS system).**
2. **Call for the defibrillator and crash cart.**
3. **Assess the client's airway, breathing, and circulation (ABCs). Open the airway. Look, listen, and feel.**
4. **If the client is not breathing, give two slow breaths.**
5. **Assess the client's circulation; if no pulse is present, start CPR.**
6. **Perform CPR until the defibrillator is in place.**
7. **Check the ECG to verify the presence of VF or pulseless VT; confirm in two leads.**
8. **Check leads for any loose connections.**
9. **Remove any nitroglycerin patch.**

On confirmation of the emergency, the code is announced overhead so that the physician and ancillary and support staff can be present to assist with advanced cardiac life support measures. Continue CPR measures and ensure that intravenous access is available. Once the physician arrives, he/she will take charge of the situation and guide further management.

Care During Defibrillation. When VF develops, clinicians must attempt defibrillation at the earliest opportunity. The paddles are lubricated with electrode gel or conducting pads to enhance conduction and prevent burning of the skin. The gel should not extend beyond the paddles and the paddles must lie flat against the body to avoid current arching or burns. The clinician places the paddles firmly against the chest. A transverse (anterolateral) position for paddle placement is used. One paddle is placed at the second intercostal space, at the right of the sternum, and the other paddle is positioned at the fifth intercostal space on the anterior axillary line (see Figure 57-9, *A*).

To ensure safe defibrillation, people who perform defibrillation must always announce when they are about to shock. The phrase "One. I'm clear. Two. You're clear. Three. All clear" is recommended. Because electricity is

carried along metal devices and the client, all personnel, including the clinician administering the shock, must stand back from the bed. Open chest defibrillation occurs when electrical current is applied directly to the heart.

Care After Defibrillation. The clinician immediately assesses the ECG and pulse after defibrillation. If the first countershock is unsuccessful, immediate defibrillation must be performed again at a higher energy level (300 and 360 J). Monophasic defibrillation may be applied up to three times (200, 300, 360 J) if needed for persistent VF or pulseless VT. Defibrillators are frequently equipped with paddles that can monitor the ECG, even immediately after defibrillation. Therefore if the paddles are left in place after the shock has been delivered, the cardiac response can be quickly evaluated.

If the three defibrillations have not been successful, CPR should be continued. A successful response is indicated by cessation of fibrillation, restoration of sinus rhythm, and palpation of a regular pulse (see Figure 57-9, *B*). After successful defibrillation, continuous ECG monitoring is required. The client's vital signs and neurologic status must also be continuously assessed.

For clients with a pacemaker or an automatic implantable cardioverter-defibrillator (AICD), a programmer-analyzer should be available to examine the system for damage and erroneous reprogramming after defibrillation. Continue to monitor for pacemaker or AICD malfunction for at least the next 24 hours.

In documenting the outcome of defibrillation, record the following points:

- Preprocedure rhythm
- Times and voltage of shocks delivered
- Post-defibrillation rhythm pattern
- Names, times of administration, and doses of administered medications
- Other hemodynamic data available before, during, and after defibrillation

Automated External Defibrillator. An automated external defibrillator (AED) delivers biphasic electrical shocks to a client after it "auto-analyzes" VT or VF through an internal microprocessor-based detection system that analyzes the rhythm for the characteristics of VF or VT. The device is attached to the client with adhesive sternal-apex pads on flexible cables, which allows "hands-free" defibrillation, a feature available with conventional defibrillation as well. When VF or VT is present, the AED "advises" the operator to deliver a shock. This device was a milestone development in the fight against sudden cardiac death, and was designed for use by non-medical personnel with little or no medical training.[3]

The most common cause of unconsciousness in an adult is VF. Defibrillation is the only effective treatment.

AEDs are present in emergency response units and have been placed in many public settings because of the ease in using them and their impact on sudden cardiac death.

Termination of Resuscitation

In general, if an organized rhythm and pulse have not returned, the advanced cardiac life support team leader can cease efforts to resuscitate clients from confirmed and persistent asystole when the client has received successful endotracheal intubation, successful IV access, suitable CPR and advanced cardiac life support measures, and all rhythm-appropriate medications. Always consider any pre-existing problems that may make the client less responsive to defibrillation (acidosis, hypokalemia, hyperkalemia, hypoxia, hypovolemia), and treat them appropriately. In many cases clients may have other, noncardiac, disorders that make resuscitation attempts futile.

The American Heart Association guidelines for emergency cardiac care do not state a specific time limit beyond which rescuers cannot have a successful resuscitation. Cardiac arrests in special situations such as hypothermia, electrocution, and drug overdose present exceptions to any rules. Special situations call for common sense and clinical judgment.[5]

Interventional Medical Management

Ablating Conduction Pathways

A variety of procedures can be used to treat dysrhythmias when medications are not successful in bringing about conversion of the abnormal rhythm to a normal rhythm. Interventions include (1) chemical and mechanical ablation and (2) radiofrequency ablation of the abnormal pathway. These procedures involve risk to normal conduction tissue, and a pacemaker may be needed either temporarily or permanently.[3]

Chemical Ablation. Alcohol or phenol is inserted into involved areas of the myocardium through an angioplasty catheter leading to myocardial necrosis. Recurrences of tachycardia after successful chemical ablation are common. Chemical ablation is used only when other ablative approaches have failed and no other options are available. Postprocedural care is the same as that for angioplasty, with the exception of expected cardiac enzyme elevation following chemical ablation.[3]

Mechanical Ablation. The abnormal pathway is surgically removed or treated with a cryoprobe to interrupt its effect on heart rhythms. SVT, atrial fibrillation, atrial flutter, and WPW syndrome may be treated with this method when the client does not respond to medication. Before the procedure the myocardium is mapped to determine whether other forms of surgery (e.g., coronary bypass grafting, valve replacement) might correct the dysrhythmia. Mapping also isolates the area to be treated. The procedure may be performed through open-heart or closed-heart methods.[3] Postprocedure care and recovery are similar to those following cardiac catheterization.

Radiofrequency Ablation. Radiofrequency catheter ablation (RFA) is used primarily for SVT associated with WPW or AV nodal reentry, although it has also been used successfully to treat refractory VT. A steerable pacing catheter directs low-power, high-frequency current to a localized accessory pathway and necroses a small portion of myocardium along that pathway. When radiofrequency current is applied, the temperature of the contact tissue rises, water is driven out, and coagulation necrosis results. The amount of tissue injury depends on the amount of energy delivered (5 to 50 W), the length of time it is delivered (10 to 90 seconds), and the resistance at the end of the catheter. RFA produces lesions that are smaller and more controllable than DC catheter ablation lesions.[3]

The major advantage of RFA is the high rate of success, especially with SVT, and low morbidity. RFA can be more successful with AV node reentry or AV reentry tachycardia than conventional drug therapies.

Although RFA is a relatively safe procedure, the following complications can occur:

- Cardiac tamponade (1%)
- Deep vein thrombosis (1%)
- Trauma to vessel (1%)
- Transient ischemic attack or stroke (0.5%)
- Perforation of AV leaflet (extremely rare)
- Hematoma at introducer site (common)
- Unintentional AV block requiring pacemaker implantation (up to 10%)

Postprocedure nursing care and recovery are similar to those following cardiac catheterization. Specific nursing responsibilities include (1) preprocedure education of client and family, (2) interventions to reduce anxiety before and during the RFA procedure, (3) monitoring of vital signs and lower-extremity perfusion during and after the procedure, and (4) discharge instructions. Clients are usually discharged within 24 hours after RFA and are instructed to resume normal activities gradually but to avoid strenuous activities for 7 to 10 days. ECGs are obtained routinely at 1, 3, 6, and 9 months after RFA.[3]

Surgical Management

Clients with persistent heart rhythm problems may benefit from implanted devices to control their rhythm to control abnormal impulses or generate an impulse.

Controlling Impulses

Automatic Implantable Cardioverter-Defibrillator

Abnormal impulses can be controlled with an implanted device to cardiovert or defibrillate the heart. Before the development of the automatic implantable cardioverter-defibrillator (AICD), antidysrhythmic drugs were the standard of treatment for recurrent VT and VF; however, these drugs had dangerous side effects including a propensity to cause dysrhythmias. Antidysrhythmic drug therapy is now primarily used for clients with a low risk of sudden cardiac death or for clients with supraventricular dysrhythmias, while AICDs are the standard of treatment for clients at high risk for sudden cardiac death. Therefore the primary purpose of the AICD is detection and termination of VT and VF. The MADIT II trial outlines inclusion criteria for clients needing AICD implantation, including (1) post-myocardial infarction, (2) ejection fraction of equal to or less than 30%, (3) greater than 10 PVCs per hour.[11]

The AICD consists of a pulse generator and lead (Figure 57-10). The generator consists of electronic circuits that monitor the cardiac rhythm, analyze

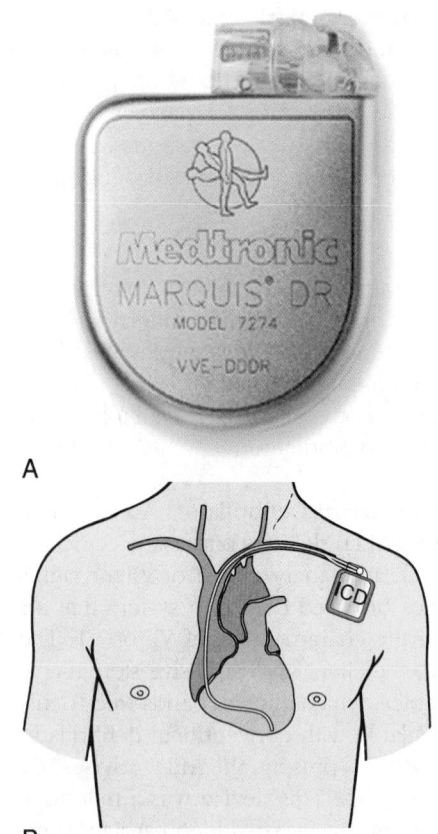

A

B

■ FIGURE 57–10 A, An automatic implanted cardioverter-defibrillator (ICD) from Medtronic. **B,** The device can be implanted in the upper chest or in the abdomen. It detects dysrhythmias and delivers an electric shock to the heart muscle.

dysrhythmias, and begin appropriate treatment; a capacitor that charges and discharges; batteries; and information storage so that the device can be interrogated and its history obtained. The device also has a "back-up" pacemaker as postshock bradycardia is common. Compared with external defibrillation, this implanted system does not require as much energy because less energy is lost when the impulse is applied directly to the heart. Interrogation of the AICD provides information regarding manufacturer, model, settings, recorded events, battery life, and lead parameters.[3]

The AICD is usually implanted surgically into a pouch below the left clavicle (similar to implantation of a permanent pacemaker) for two types of conditions.[3,11]

1. Survival of one or more episodes of sudden cardiac death resulting from VT or VF
2. Recurrent, refractory, life-threatening ventricular dysrhythmias that can develop into VT or VF, or both, despite antidysrhythmic therapy

Clients who require AICDs have a great deal of anxiety. Anxiety can develop from past episodes of near death as well as from feelings of not ever being able to die. Other clients may fear that the AICD will not be able to reverse the dysrhythmia. Be sensitive to these thoughts, and facilitate their discussion.[4,10]

Restoring Impulse Generation

Pacemakers

Pacemakers provide an artificial SA node and/or Purkinje system. A pacemaker is indicated if the conduction system fails to transmit impulses from the sinus node to the ventricles, to generate an impulse spontaneously, or to maintain primary control of the pacing function of the heart. Many conditions can affect the ability of the heart's conduction system to function normally, creating circumstances that warrant pacing (Box 57-3). Pacemakers can be *permanent* or *temporary*. Pacemakers can be used temporarily or prophylactically until the condition underlying the disturbance resolves. Pacemakers also can be used on a permanent basis if the client's condition persists despite adequate therapy.

BOX 57-3 Conditions That May Necessitate a Pacemaker

- Ablation
- Acute myocardial infarction
- Autonomic nervous system failure
- Cardiac surgery
- Drug toxicity (antidysrhythmics)
- Electrolyte imbalance
- Myocardial ischemia

Pacemaker Design. A pacemaker provides an external energy source for impulse formation and delivery. Whereas numerous pacemaker models are available, each with unique capabilities, every pacemaker consists of a pulse generator with circuitry, the lead(s), and the electrode system. *Single-chamber* pacemakers pace either the atria or the ventricles; *dual-chamber* pacemakers pace both the atria and the ventricles.

The pulse generator is essentially the pacemaker's power source. It houses the electronic circuitry responsible for sending out appropriately timed signals and for sensing the client's cardiac activity. The pulse generator can be external or internal. The external unit is designed for temporary pacing, primarily for support of transient dysrhythmias that impair cardiac output. The unit is the size of a small transistor radio and operates by dry-cell batteries (Figure 57-11). It has dials for the adjustment of power, rate of discharge, and mode. A pulse generator can also be permanently implanted. The surgeon places the permanent pulse generator into a small tunnel burrowed within the subcutaneous tissue below the right or left clavicle. The pulse generator is small (about the size of a vanilla wafer) and contains a sealed lithium battery. Pacemaker generators can be reprogrammed after insertion as

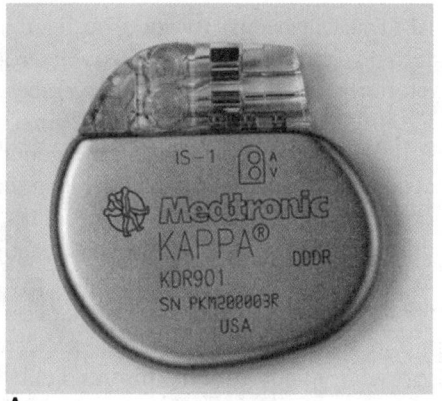

A

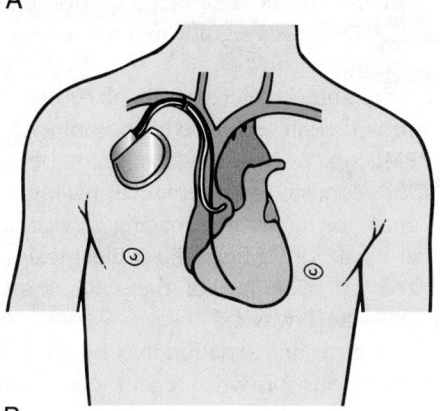

B

■ **FIGURE 57-11**   A permanent pacemaker. The pulse generator is placed under the pectoralis muscle (but above the breast). This is a dual-chamber pacemaker with leads in both the right atria and the ventricle.

needed. The output circuit controls the current pulse delivery rate, pulse duration, and refractory period. The sensing circuit is responsible for identifying and analyzing any spontaneous intrinsic electrical activity and responding appropriately.

The lead delivers the electrical impulse from the pulse generator to the myocardium. The lead(s) consist(s) of flexible conductive wires enclosed by insulating material. The electrode is the end of the lead that delivers the impulse directly to the myocardial wall. It is usually made of platinum-iridium, a highly conductive material that also deters the adherence of platelets. This system not only delivers electrical impulses but also relays information about spontaneous impulses back to the sensing circuit within the pulse generator.

Electrodes can be *unipolar* or *bipolar*. Unipolar designs incorporate the cardiac electrode as the negative terminal of the electrical circuit; the metallic shell or second wire of the impulse generator is the positive electrode. Bipolar systems use two wires, each ending in an electrode a short distance apart.

Pacemaker Methods. Impulses can be delivered to myocardial tissue by three major modes of artificial pacing: external, epicardial, and endocardial.

External (Transcutaneous) Pacing. The heart is stimulated externally through large, gelled electrode pads placed anteriorly and posteriorly and connected to an external transcutaneous pacemaker. Transcutaneous pacing is the treatment of choice in emergency cardiac care because it can be started quickly while a temporary transvenous pacemaker is being inserted or as prophylaxis against dysrhythmias. It is also the least invasive pacing technique. Because no vascular puncture is needed for electrode placement, transcutaneous pacing is preferred in clients who are receiving anticoagulation therapy or who might require thrombolytic therapy. However, many clients feel extreme discomfort with each paced beat; this is a significant limitation to transcutaneous pacing.

Because the anterior electrode is placed to the left of the sternum and centered close to the point of maximal impulse (PMI), excessive chest hair must be shaved to ensure good contact, or alternative pacing electrode positions must be used. The pacing device is usually activated at a rate of 70 beats/min. Electrical capture is characterized by widening of the QRS complex and broadening of the T wave.

Opioid analgesia and sedation may be given to clients who are conscious or who regain consciousness to reduce discomfort and anxiety. Additional complications of external transcutaneous pacing can include skin burns, muscle twitching, psychological reactions, failure to "capture" (inability of the impulse to initiate a contraction), and failure to "sense" (inability of the pacemaker to sense intrinsic electrical activity) (Table 57-3).

Epicardial (Transthoracic) Pacing. With this method of artificial pacing, the electrical energy travels through lead wires from an external pulse generator through the thoracic muscles directly to the epicardium. Epicardial pacing is most commonly used during and immediately after open-heart surgery because there is direct access to the epicardium at this time.

> **Some occasional complications include lead dislodgment, microshock, cardiac tamponade, infection, psychological reactions, failure to capture, and failure to sense.**

Endocardial (Transvenous) Pacing. Endocardial pacing is the most common mode of pacing the heart in emergency situations. The cardiologist inserts the pacing electrode via the transvenous route (the antecubital, femoral, jugular, or subclavian vein) and then threads the electrode into the right atrium or right ventricle so that it comes into direct contact with the endocardium (Figure 57-12). This procedure can be done at the bedside under fluoroscopic control or in a cardiovascular laboratory.

> **Major drawbacks include thrombophlebitis, infection at the insertion site, sepsis from nonsterile technique, increased chance of lead displacement as the client changes position, and the discomfort of having the extremity nearest the insertion site immobilized.**

Other additional complications occasionally seen are pacer-induced dysrhythmias, hiccups, abdominal twitching, myocardial irritability, perforation of chamber or septum, failure to capture, and failure to sense.

Temporary Pacing. Temporary pacing can be used in emergent or elective situations that require limited, short-term pacing (less than 1 week). The pulse generator is external. Temporary pacemakers are most commonly inserted transvenously, but they can be applied transcutaneously and can be inserted transthoracically.

Nursing Management

Although the principles of cardiac pacing are the same for temporary and permanent pacemakers, each type presents distinct issues for nurses to assess and to teach to the client and family. Clients with a temporary pacemaker need the following:

- An explanation about the pacemaker
- Monitoring for response to the pacemaker
- Maintenance of electrical safety
- Monitoring for pacing parameters (sensing, capturing, threshold)
- Protection against injury and infection

TABLE 57-3 Pacemaker Malfunctions and Nursing Interventions

Problem	Possible Cause	Nursing Interventions*
Failure to Pace Properly		
Intermittent or complete absence of pacing artifact	Battery failure A break or loose connection anywhere along system	Replace pulse generator. Replace battery unit.
Rapid, inappropriate firing of pacemaker (pacemaker-mediated tachycardia)	Pulse generator failure Circuitry failure "Oversensing" or "undersensing" by pacemaker	Check and tighten all connections between pulse generator and leads. Reduce or increase sensitivity threshold of pacemaker unit. Assess client's tolerance of pacemaker failure; have emergency drugs on hand; perform CPR[†] as indicated.
Failure to Capture		
Pacing artifact present but not followed by QRS complex or P wave	Increased pacing threshold; can be related to electrolyte imbalance, ischemia, drug toxicity, perforation, or excessive fibrosis of tissue at electrode site	Increase voltage by 1-2 mA (temporary pacemaker). Increase amplitude of pacemaker output/pulse width. Reposition client to either side in attempt to improve contact of electrode with endocardium; in temporary pacemaker, try moving arm if lead wire is inserted in antecubital area.
	Lead displacement caused by migration, or idle manipulation of pulse generator ("twiddler's syndrome")	Obtain chest film to determine pacemaker position. Have emergency drugs on hand; initiate CPR if necessary.
Failure to Sense		
Pacing artifact present despite presence of QRS complexes and P waves A competitive rhythm may develop	Sensitivity threshold set too low Intrinsic beats are of too-low voltage and go undetected by pacemaker's sensing mechanism	Increase sensitivity threshold on pulse generator. Reposition client.
		If client's intrinsic rhythm or rate is adequate, turn off pacemaker. Increase pacing rate to overdrive client's intrinsic heart rate.
	Dislodged or fractured lead Circuitry failure Electromagnetic interference	Give antidysrhythmics to decrease ectopy. Notify physician. Obtain chest x-ray to determine electrode placement.
Oversensing		
Results from inappropriate sensing of extraneous electrical signals or myopotentials (which should be ignored)	Sensitivity threshold set too high T wave sensing myopotentials Electromagnetic interference Two leads touching	Decrease sensitivity threshold. Correct conditions that produce large T waves.

*For all problems document malfunction by an electrocardiogram. If the pacemaker is programmable, have the reprogramming machine available. Monitor the client's tolerance to pacemaker malfunction (vital signs, chest pain).

[†]CPR, Cardiopulmonary resuscitation.

From Urden, L.D., Stacy, K.M., Lough, M.E. (Eds.), (2007) *Thelan's critical care nursing: Diagnosis and management* (4th ed.). St. Louis: Mosby.

Before the procedure, explain the purpose of the temporary pacemaker to the client and family. Ensure that a permit for the procedure has been signed and that all questions have been answered. Necessary equipment is gathered, and the external generator is checked (battery and sense and pace modes). Assess the client's vital signs and oxygen saturation; obtain a rhythm strip. Assess the need for sedation or analgesics, the client's level of anxiety, and the risk for bleeding.

During the procedure, monitor the client's ECG and vital signs continuously. Large P waves are seen as the catheter passes through the atrium, and larger QRS complexes are seen in the ventricles. Set and maintain the stimulus and sensitivity settings according to the physician's orders. Tape or suture the electrode at the insertion site.

After the procedure assess vital signs and peripheral pulses routinely along with emotional reactions to the procedure and pacing. Clients with temporary pacemakers must be placed on a cardiac monitor. Document the location and type of pacing lead. Note the pacing mode, stimulus threshold, sensitivity setting, pacing rate and intervals, and intrinsic rhythm. Pacing intervals are shown in Figure 57-13. Secure and check all

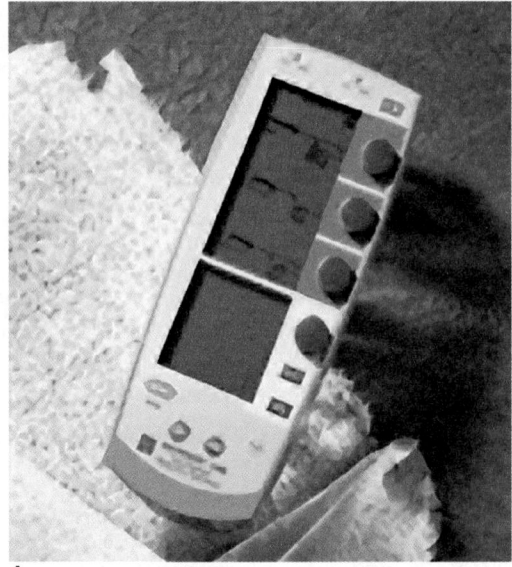

A

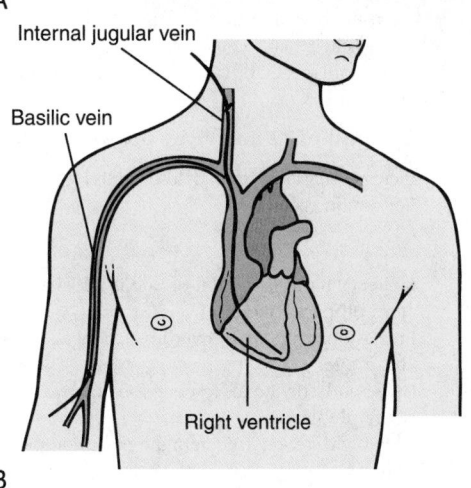

Internal jugular vein

Basilic vein

Right ventricle

B

■ **FIGURE 57–12** Transvenous temporary endocardial pacing is routine for most cardiac surgical procedures. This can be established by insertion of electrode wires through a vein (subclavian or internal jugular) and into the right atrium or right ventricle. Temporary pacing wires can also be advanced through pulmonary artery catheters.

connections. Monitor battery and control settings. Clean and dress the incision site according to protocols.

SAFETY ⚠ ALERT **Keep the generator dry and protect the controls from mishandling. The client must be protected from electrical microshocks and electromagnetic interference. Wear rubber gloves when exposed wires are handled. Check electrical equipment for adequate grounding.**

Limit the motion of the extremity at the insertion site. Stabilize the arm, catheter, and pacemaker to an arm board and avoid movement of the arm above shoulder level. Do not lift the client from under the arm. If the leg is the insertion site, limit its motion, especially hip flexion by limiting elevation of the head of the bed.

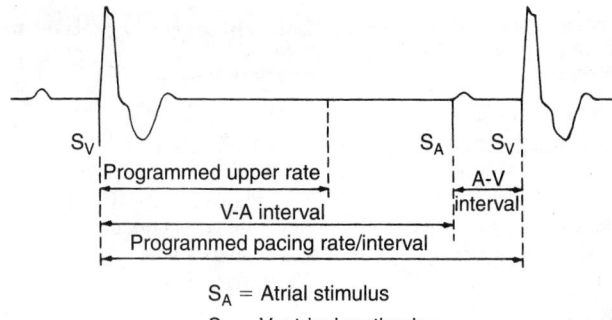

S_A = Atrial stimulus
S_V = Ventricular stimulus

■ **FIGURE 57–13** Pacing intervals. The atrioventricular (A-V, del interval can be thought of as an artificial P-R interval. The programmed pac rate, or *interval*, is also called the ventriculoventricular (V-V) interval. Ventricu pacing occurs if intrinsic ventricular activity does not occur within the V-V int val. *(From Symbiotics series: Selecting the DDD patient [1984]. Minneapo Medtronic.)*

PERMANENT PACING

Permanent pacing is indicated for chronic or recurren dysrhythmias that are severe, unresponsive to antidys rhythmic medication, and caused by AV block or sinu node malfunction. The need for permanent pacemaker is confirmed through ECGs, Holter monitoring, and elec trophysiology studies. Indications for permanent pace makers have been grouped into three classes. Class criteria are identified in Box 57-4.[8] 🪔

Clinical manifestations that are directly attributable t the slow heart rate include transient dizziness, lighthead edness, near syncope or frank syncope as manifestation of transient cerebral ischemia, and more generalized manifestations such as marked exercise intolerance o frank heart failure.[3,5,6]

Pacemaker Modes

There are two basic types of pacemakers:

1. *Fixed-rate* (non-demand or asynchronous). Fixed rate pacemakers are designed to fire constantly a a preset rate without regard to the electrical activit of the client's heart. This mode of pacing is appro priate in the absence of any electrical activity *(asys tole)* but is dangerous in the presence of a intrinsic rhythm because of the potential of th pacemaker to fire during the vulnerable perio of repolarization and initiate lethal ventricula dysrhythmias.

2. *Demand* pacemakers contain a device that sense the heart's electrical activity and fires at a prese rate only when the heart's electrical activity drop below a predetermined rate (Figure 57-14).

In addition to a variety of capabilities, permanen pacemakers now have special programmable and ant tachydysrhythmic functions that are quite comple. To communicate all the functions of the individu;

pacemakers, international codes were developed. Pacemakers are identified with a five-digit letter code. Although the last two letters contain pertinent information, commonly a pacemaker is referred to only by its first three letters (Box 57-5).

Pacemaker Function

Because there are many types of pacemakers with more than 250 programs, the general functions are discussed first. A simple demand pacing system works in the following manner. The cardiac cycle normally begins with the client's own beat. The pacemaker's sensor senses whether the intrinsic beat has occurred; if not, the pacer sends out an impulse to begin myocardial depolarization through a pulse generator. The impulse generator is said to "capture" the myocardium and thereby maintain heart rhythm.

ELECTRONIC PACEMAKER SPIKES

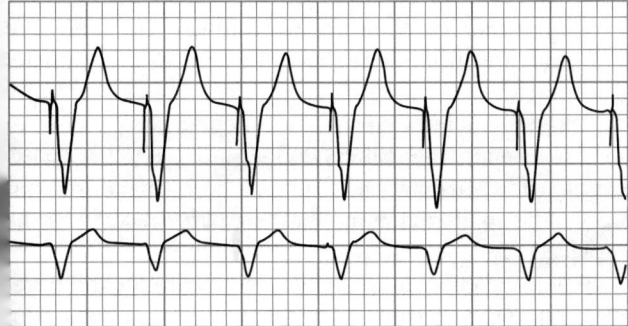

■ **FIGURE 57-14** Demand pacing. The pacemaker initiates an electrical impulse when the sinus node fails to pace the heart.

For a predetermined amount of time after the pacemaker impulse, the pacemaker cannot sense incoming signals. This feature prevents the pacer from sensing its own generated electrical current and from acting again. The *refractory period* is followed by the *noise-sampling period*. If any electromagnetic interference is sensed during this phase, the pacemaker goes into a fixed-rate mode of operation and remains in this mode until the source of interference is removed. At the end of the noise-sampling period, the *alert period* begins and the cycle starts again. If a PVC or PAC occurs during the alert period, the pacemaker can sense it and start its cycle again without emitting any impulse.

Electrocardiography of Paced Beats

In order to "turn on" a pacemaker and record its impulse generation and conduction, place a magnet over the pacemaker. The magnet disables the sensing mechanism, causing the pacemaker to fire at its programmed rate, regardless of the underlying cardiac rhythm.

Never place a magnet over an AICD as the magnet will suspend detection of VT and VF by the AICD, thus preventing the AICD from firing when VT or VF is present.

SAFETY

⚠

ALERT

The ECG appearance of a paced rhythm differs from that of a normal sinus rhythm. A pacing artifact is seen. With atrial pacing, a P wave follows the artifact but is hidden in some leads. Examination of leads II and V_1 is best for deciding whether a P wave follows a pacer spike. The QRS complex appears normal with atrial pacing; the impulse travels through the usual conduction system.[3]

The ECG with ventricular pacing shows an abnormal QRS complex because the impulse begins in the ventricle. With right ventricular endocardial pacing, a pseudo-LBBB wave is created on ECG. If the left ventricle is paced, a pseudo-RBBB is created.

Assess the ECG strip for pacer spikes followed by the expected appearance of a P wave or QRS complex. Spikes not followed by depolarization waves or paced beats that appear too early or too late may signal pacemaker failure.

Pacemaker Failure

Malfunctions can occur in the pacemaker's sensor or pulse generator. Complications associated with the components of the pacemaker system itself (see Table 57-3) may include the following:
1. *Failure to sense*—an inability of the sensor to detect the client's intrinsic beats; as a result, the pacemaker sends out impulses too early (Figure 57-15, *A*). The failure may be due to improper position of the catheter, tip or lead dislodgment, battery failure, the sensitivity being set too low, or a fractured wire in the catheter.

BOX 57-5 Classification System for Pacemakers

FIRST LETTER: CHAMBER PACED

Indicates which chamber(s) of the heart will be stimulated:

- V = Ventricle
- A = Atrium
- D = Dual-chamber (both atria and ventricles stimulated)

SECOND LETTER: CHAMBER SENSED

Indicates the chamber(s) of the heart in which the lead is capable of recognizing intrinsic electrical activity:

- V = Ventricle
- A = Atrium
- D = Dual-chamber (sensing capabilities in atria and ventricles)
- O = No sensing capability

THIRD LETTER: MODE OF RESPONSE

Indicates how the pacemaker will act based on the information it senses:

- T = Triggered (may have energy output triggered)
- I = Inhibited (pacing output inhibited by intrinsic activity)
- D = Dual-chamber (may be either inhibiting or triggering of both chambers)

FOURTH LETTER: PROGRAMMABLE FUNCTIONS

Indicates ability to change function once the pacemaker has been implanted:

- P = Programmable for one or two functions
- M = Multiprogrammable ability to change functions other than the rate or output

FIFTH LETTER: TACHYDYSRHYTHMIC FUNCTIONS

Indicates specific methods of interrupting tachydysrhythmias:

- B = Bursts of pacing
- N = Normal rate competition
- S = Scanning

EXAMPLES

Pacing Modes Within Single-Chamber Pacemakers

- *Atrial demand pacemaker (AAI).* A pacemaker that senses spontaneously occurring P waves and paces the atria when they do not appear.

- *Atrial fixed-rate pacemaker (AOO).* A pacemaker that paces the atria and does not sense.
- *Ventricular demand pacemaker (VVI).* A pacemaker that senses spontaneously occurring QRS complexes and paces the ventricles when they do not appear.
- *Ventricular fixed-rate pacemaker (VOO).* A pacemaker that paces the ventricles and does not sense.

Pacing Modes Within Dual-Chamber Pacemakers

- *Atrial synchronous ventricular pacemaker (VDD).* A pacemaker that senses spontaneously occurring P waves and QRS complexes and paces the ventricles when QRS complexes fail to appear after spontaneously occurring P waves, as in complete atrioventricular (AV) block. In this type of pacemaker, the pacing of ventricles is synchronized with the P waves so that the ventricular contractions follow the atrial contractions in a normal sequence. A major benefit is that it permits the heart rate to vary, and AV synchrony occurs, depending on the physiologic demands of the body. A built-in safety mechanism causes ventricular depolarizations to occur at a fixed rate should atrial rates become too fast.
- *AV synchronous pacemaker (VAT).* A pacemaker that has ventricular pacing, atrial sensing, and triggered response to sensing. The ventricular pacing stimulus will fire at a set time after sensing a spontaneous atrial depolarization.
- *AV sequential pacemaker (DVI).* A pacemaker that senses spontaneously occurring QRS complexes and paces both the atria and ventricles (the atria first, followed by the ventricles after a short delay) when QRS complexes do not appear.
- *AV sequential fixed-rate pacemaker (DOO).* A pacemaker that paces both the atria and ventricles but does not sense.
- *Optimal sequential pacemaker (DDD).* A pacemaker that senses spontaneously occurring P waves and QRS complexes and (1) paces the atria when P waves fail to appear, as in sick sinus syndrome; and (2) paces the ventricles when QRS complexes fail to appear after spontaneously occurring or paced P waves. In this type of pacemaker, like the VDD pacemaker, the pacing of ventricles is synchronized with the P waves so that the ventricular contractions follow the atrial contractions in a normal sequence.

---

2. *Failure to pace*—a malfunction of the pulse generator. The ECG shows an absence of any impulse (Figure 57-15, *B*). Component failure to discharge (pace) can be due to battery failure, lead dislodgment, fracture of the lead wire inside the catheter, disconnections between catheter and generator, or a sensing malfunction.

3. *Failure to capture*—a disorder in the pacemaker electrodes; the impulse does not generate depolarization (Figure 57-15, *C*). This complication can result from low voltage, battery failure, faulty connections between the pulse generator and catheter,

improper position of the catheter, catheter wire fracture, fibrosis at the catheter tip, or a catheter fracture.

Clinical manifestations associated with pacemaker malfunctioning include syncope, bradycardia or tachycardia, and palpitations. When these manifestations occur, the malfunctioning leads or pacemaker must be replaced.

Teach the client and family how to care for the pacemaker and the precautions to follow (see the Client Education Guide feature on the Client with a Permanent Pacemaker, p. 1480).[12]

FAILURE TO SENSE

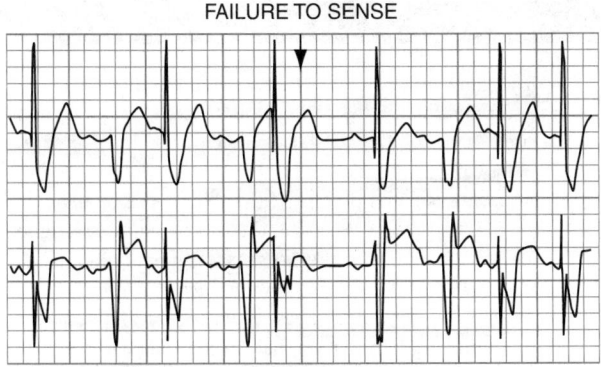

A The pacemaker fails to recognize normal beats and generates an unnecessary pacemaker spike.

FAILURE TO PACE

The pacemaker fails to generate a pacemaker spike when needed. **B**

FAILURE TO CAPTURE

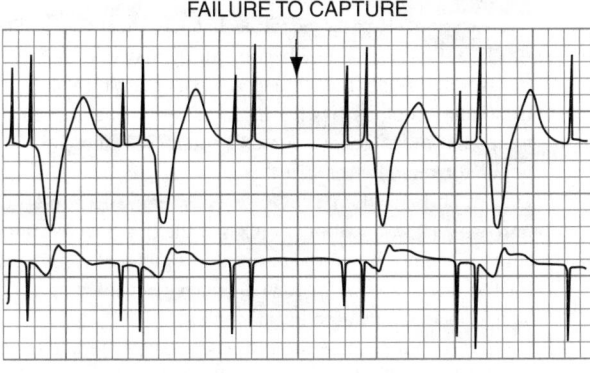

C The pacemaker generates a pacemaker spike but fails to produce a QRS.

FUSION BEAT

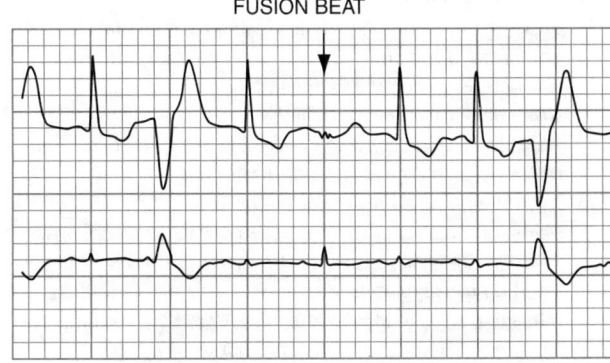

D

■ **FIGURE 57–15** Pacemaker failures. **A,** Failure to sense. **B,** Failure to pace. **C,** Failure to capture. **D,** Fusion beat.

Nursing Management of Clients with Pacemakers

Assessment. Assess the client for *subjective* clinical manifestations of dysrhythmias and alterations in cardiac output: palpitations, syncope, fatigue, shortness of breath, chest pain, or skipped beats felt in the chest. The client may also feel anxiety about the heart disorder and may manifest nervousness, fear, sleeplessness, uncertainty, or hopelessness. *Objective* clinical manifestations may include diaphoresis, pallor or cyanosis, variations in radial and apical pulse rates such as bradycardia or tachycardia, rhythm changes, hypotension, crackles, and decreased mental acuity. The client may be fearful of being left alone. Monitoring is begun, and the heart rhythm is observed continuously by a nurse, a computer, and an ECG technician. Rhythm strips are examined at least every shift.

Explain the purpose of the pacemaker and the experience of having a pacemaker inserted to the client and family. Most permanent pacemakers are inserted transvenously. Try to keep the ECG leads off the possible insertion site. The insertion site is prepared according to hospital policy.

A preoperative ECG is obtained, and a patent IV line is maintained. Prophylactic antibiotics may be given.

After insertion, monitor vital signs and pacemaker function. Pain can usually be managed with oral analgesics if the transvenous approach has been used. Initially instruct the client to avoid excessive extension or abduction of the arm on the operative side. Perform passive range-of-motion exercises on the arm.

Obtain paced and nonpaced ECGs. A magnet can be placed over the pulse generator, converting it to a fixed-rate pacing mode, so that the client's intrinsic rhythm can be determined. The location of the pacemaker electrodes is determined by x-ray. The model and serial numbers of the pulse generator and leads, along with the date of implantation and programmed functions of the initial implant, are recorded.

Transtelephonic Pacemaker Monitoring. Special telephone monitoring of the client's pacemaker can be done on a routine outpatient basis. Telephone ECG systems are designed for follow-up monitoring of clients with pacemakers. Via finger tip, wrist, or ankle electrodes, the transmitter detects, amplifies, and converts a client's

CLIENT EDUCATION GUIDE

Client With a Permanent Pacemaker

WOUND CARE

1. Assess your wound daily, and keep the incision clean and dry until it heals.
2. Report any fever, redness, drainage, warmth, discoloration, or swelling to the physician.
3. Avoid constrictive clothing (e.g., tight brassiere straps), which puts excessive pressure on the wound and the pulse generator.
4. Avoid extensive "toying" with the pulse generator because this may cause pacemaker malfunction and local skin inflammation.

PACEMAKER MANAGEMENT

1. Measure your pulse rate as instructed by your physician in your wrist or on your neck. You will be taught how to do this before leaving the hospital.
2. Notify the physician if your pulse rate is slower than the set rate; also report sensations of feeling your heart "racing," beating irregularly, fatigue, or dizziness.
3. Avoid being near areas with high voltage, magnetic force fields, or radiation; this can cause pacemaker problems.
4. Avoid being near large running motors (gas or electric) and standing near high-tension wires, power plants, radio transmitters, large industrial magnets, and arc welding machines. Riding in a car is safe, but do not bring the pacemaker to within 6 to 12 inches of the distributor coil of a running engine.
5. You can continue to operate safely most appliances and tools that are properly grounded and in good repair, including microwave ovens, televisions, video recorders, AM and FM radios, electric blankets, lawn mowers, leaf blowers, and cars.
6. You can safely operate office and light industrial equipment that is properly grounded and in good repair, such as electric typewriters, copying machines, and personal computers.
7. An airport's metal detector can be triggered by the pacemaker's metal casing and the programming magnet. Mention your pacemaker to security guards. The metal detector itself does not harm the pacemaker.
8. At all times carry a pacemaker identity card (including programming information, pacemaker manufacturer, emergency phone numbers). Wear a medical alert bracelet.
9. Avoid activity that might damage the pulse generator, such as playing football or firing a rifle with the butt end against the affected shoulder.
10. Some stores sell antitheft devices that may affect pacemaker function. If you suddenly become dizzy, move away from the area and notify the store clerk about the pacemaker.
11. If radiation therapy has been prescribed to the area in which the pulse generator was implanted, the pulse generator must be relocated.
12. Do not lift more than 5 to 10 pounds (equivalent to a full grocery sack or a gallon of milk) for the first 6 weeks after surgery. Do not move your arms and shoulders vigorously for the first 6 weeks. Normal activities (including sexual activity) can be resumed in 6 weeks.
13. Discuss with the nurse the purpose, dose, schedule, and possible side effects of prescribed medications. Consult your written information sheets to reinforce learning.
14. Plan to see your physician to test your pacemaker. Your cardiologist periodically will reevaluate pacemaker function and can reprogram it if needed. You may also be able to check your pacemaker by telephone. If this is possible, you will receive instructions.

---

electrical activity and pacemaker artifacts to frequency-modulated audio tones for transmission, via the telephone, to an ECG receiver. From the transmitted signals, the ECG receiver provides an ECG strip recording and printout of the rate and pulse width of a client's implanted pacemaker.

Self-Care

It may be necessary to teach about the nature of the dysrhythmia several times because the client's attention span may be shorter than normal as a result of severe anxiety.

SAFETY ⚠ **ALERT** **Before discharge, make certain that clients appreciate the importance of taking antidysrhythmic agents as prescribed. Include details about medication administration, dosage, and side effects in the discharge plan. If discharged too early and in an unstable condition, many clients risk further exacerbations or additional complications. Make sure that nursing discharge criteria are met and documented.**

Clients who have experienced cardiac dysrhythmias while at a health care facility may be apprehensive about leaving the facility. Those who have experienced innocuous dysrhythmias may need only calm reassurance and an explanation of the cause of the disorder. Clients with recurring life-threatening dysrhythmias, such as VT, require comprehensive and specialized attention. These clients may have experienced frightening events in the course of their hospitalization.

When a client is at risk for development of a life-threatening dysrhythmia, ascertain whether the client's housemates and significant others know how to perform CPR. Refer them to community agencies that provide CPR training (e.g., the American Heart Association, the American Red Cross, local fire department, local hospital).

Sometimes clients with serious, chronic, or potential dysrhythmias use portable telemetry units for self-monitoring at home after discharge. This allows resumption of daily activities while providing continuous 24-hour surveillance of cardiac rhythm. Nurses are often responsible for instructing clients in the use of these units

Ask the client to keep a diary of daily activities so that clinicians can correlate factors in the client's life that are contributing to the development of dysrhythmias.

Finally, instruct clients about the importance of regular medical follow-up. Advise them to keep regular appointments with their physician after discharge. Explain to the client and his or her significant others about how to obtain emergency medical attention if it becomes necessary.

Living under the constant threat of sudden death provokes anxiety, depression, and occasionally dependent behavior. In some cases psychological counseling can bolster coping resources. Recommend community and private counseling services for the client and the client's significant others.

CONCLUSIONS

Cardiac dysrhythmias can vary from benign to life-threatening, and the cardiac rhythm can change as quickly as a heartbeat and without warning. It is imperative to be aware of life-threatening dysrhythmias and immediate nursing interventions, including client assessment, CPR, and activation of colleagues or the EMS. Treatment methods may include temporary pacemaker insertion or application, permanent pacemaker implantation, a prescribed medical regimen, ablation therapy, or AICD implantation. Client education regarding taking medications as directed, reporting any manifestations or side effects, caring for the device wound, and following up with the cardiologist is necessary before discharge to complete client care regarding dysrhythmias.

THINKING CRITICALLY

1. You are walking with a client in the hospital. He is recovering from an MI. A dysrhythmia develops. What assessments should you perform? What care does the client need?

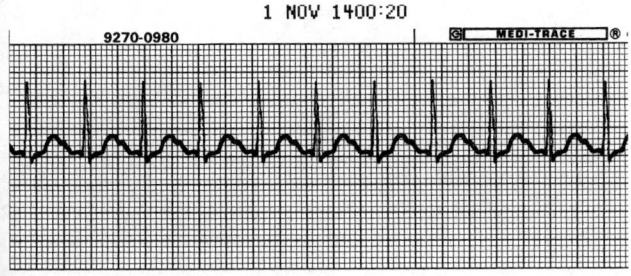

Factors to Consider. What is the usual heart rhythm response to activity? How can you assess if your client is tolerating this rhythm? How should the client be returned to his room?

2. An 82-year-old woman is brought to the emergency department by her son after losing consciousness and hitting her head after falling. She is now awake and states that she has been having periods of dizziness and blackouts for the past few weeks. During your physical examination, you notice what appears to be a pacemaker device implanted under her left clavicle. What additional assessments should you make? What information should you obtain about the pacemaker?

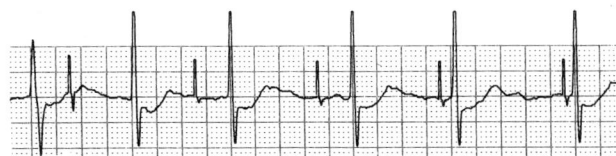

Factors to Consider. What might have happened to the pacemaker during the fall? Could a faulty pacemaker be responsible for the loss of consciousness?

Discussions for these questions can be found on the website. **evolve**

BIBLIOGRAPHY

 Citations appearing in red refer to primary research.

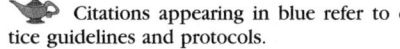 Citations appearing in blue refer to evidence-based practice guidelines and protocols.

1. American Heart Association. (2006). Heart disease and stroke statistics—2006 update: A report from the American Heart Association statistics committee and stroke statistics subcommittee. *Circulation, 113*(6), 85-151.
2. AHA scientific statement: Practice standards for electrocardiographic monitoring in hospital settings: An AHA scientific statement from disease in the young: Endorsed by the International Society of Computerized Electrocardiology and the American Association of Critical-Care Nurses. (2005). *Journal of Cardiovascular Nursing, 20*(2), 76-106.
3. Braunwald, E., Zipes, D.P., Libby, P., et al.. (2005). *Braunwald's heart disease: A textbook of cardiovascular medicine* (7th ed.). Philadelphia: Elsevier Saunders.
4. Conover, M.B. (2003). *Understanding electrocardiography* (8th ed.). St. Louis: Mosby.
5. Cummings, R. (2001). *ACLS provider manual*. Dallas, Tex: American Heart Association.
6. Fink, M.P., Abraham, E., Vincent, J., et al. (2005). *Textbook of critical care* (5th ed.). Philadelphia: Elsevier Saunders.
7. Greenberg, H., Case, R.B., Moss, A.J., et al. (2004). Analysis of mortality events in the Multicenter Automatic Defibrillator Implantation Trial (MADIT-II). *Journal of the American College of Cardiology, 43*, 1459-1465.
8. Gregoratos, G., Abrams, J., Epstein, A.E., et al. (2002). ACC/AHA/NASPE 2002 Guideline update for implantation of cardiac pacemakers and antiarrhythmia devices: Summary article: A report of the American College of Cardiology/American Heart Association task force on practice guidelines (ACC/AHA/NASPE Committee to update the 1998 pacemaker guidelines). *Circulation, 106*(16), 2145-2165.
9. Massie, B.M., & Amidon, T.A. (2004). Conduction disturbances. In L.M. Tierney, et al.. (Eds.), *Current medical diagnosis and treatment* (43rd ed.). Stamford, Conn: Appleton and Lange.
10. Massie, B.M., & Amidon, T.A. (2004). Disturbances in rate and rhythm. In L.M. Tierney, et al. (Eds.), *Current medical diagnosis and treatment* (43rd ed.). Stamford, Conn: Appleton and Lange.
11. McCabe, P.J. (2005). Spheres of clinical nurse specialist practice influence evidence-based care for patients with atrial fibrillation. *Clinical Nurse Specialist, 19*(6), 308-317.

12. Morton, P.G., Fontaine, D., Hudak, C., et al.. (2003). *Critical care nursing: A holistic approach* (8th ed.). Philadelphia: Lippincott Williams & Wilkins.
13. Shah, M., Akar, F.G., Tomaselli, G.F., et al. (2005). Molecular basis of arrhythmias. *Circulation, 12*(16), 2517-2529.
14. Surawicz, B. (2003). Brief history of cardiac arrhythmias since the end of the nineteenth century: Part 1. *Journal of Cardiovascular Electrophysiology, 14*, 1365-1371.

evolve **Did you remember to check out the bonus material on the Evolve website and the CD-ROM, including NCLEX®-Examination Style Review Questions, Open-Book Quizzes, and Chapter Review Audio Podcasts?**

http://evolve.elsevier.com/Black/medsurg

CHAPTER 58

Management of Clients with Myocardial Infarction

PATRICIA A. KERESZTES AND MARY WCISEL

The heart requires a balance between oxygen supply and oxygen demand in order to function properly. The integrity of the coronary arteries is an important determinant of oxygen supply to the heart muscle. Any disorder that reduces the lumen of one of the coronary arteries may cause a decrease in blood flow and oxygen delivery to the area of the myocardium supplied by that vessel and lead to acute coronary syndromes of angina, acute myocardial infarction (AMI), and sudden cardiac death.

Coronary heart disease (CHD) is the primary underlying cause of these syndromes and is the single largest killer of American men and women. The clinical syndromes associated with CHD are familiar to most Americans. Almost every day, the news media cover a story on a celebrity who has suffered from or was treated for chest pain, heart attack, or cardiac arrest. Turn on any television hospital drama and you will see someone seeking treatment for an episode of chest pain. Many of us also have had personal experience with CHD through the illness of a relative or close friend.

It is estimated that 1 million Americans will have a new or recurrent acute coronary syndrome this year. Acute coronary syndromes are responsible for more than 250,000 deaths annually and result from a progressive atherosclerotic process that culminates in rupture of atherosclerotic plaques and thrombus formation. This chapter reviews the risk factors, pathophysiology, clinical manifestations, and medical and nursing interventions for the acute coronary syndromes of angina pectoris (a type of chest pain) and AMI.

ANGINA PECTORIS

Angina pectoris is chest pain resulting from myocardial ischemia (inadequate blood supply to the myocardium). It is a common manifestation of CHD and affects about 6,400,000 Americans—2,400,000 men and 4,000,000 women. According to the Framingham Heart Study, approximately 400,000 new cases of angina occur each year. Angina can also occur in clients with normal coronary arteries, but it is less common. Clients with aortic stenosis, hypertension, and hypertrophic cardiomyopathy can also have angina pectoris.

Etiology and Risk Factors

Angina pectoris is associated with atherosclerotic lesions and is a manifestation of CHD (see Chapter 56). Angina can be caused either by chronic or acute blockage of a coronary artery or by coronary artery spasm. Chronic blockages are associated with fixed calcified (type Vb) or fibrotic (type Vc) atherosclerotic lesions that occlude more than 75% of the vessel lumen.

When fixed blockages are present in the coronary arteries, conditions that increase myocardial oxygen demand (e.g., physical exertion, emotion, exposure to cold) may precipitate episodes of angina. Because the severely stenosed arteries cannot dilate to deliver enough oxygen to meet the increased demand, ischemia results. In contrast, acute blockage of a coronary artery results from rupture or disruption of vulnerable atherosclerotic plaques that cause platelet aggregation and thrombus formation (see Etiology and Risk Factors under Acute Myocardial Infarction). Acute blockages are associated with unstable angina and AMI.

---

evolve **Web Enhancements**

Case Management Acute Myocardial Infarction

Case Study Cardiogenic Shock, Tachycardia, and Heart Failure

Concept Map Understanding Myocardial Infarction and Its Treatment

Tables Differential Diagnosis of Chest Pain

Be sure to check out the bonus material on the Evolve website and the CD-ROM, including free self-assessment exercises. **http://evolve.elsevier. com/Black/medsurg**

Primary prevention is through the lifelong commitment to reducing the risk factors of CHD (see Chapter 56). Secondary prevention is through recognition and early treatment of anginal attacks (see the Critical Monitoring feature below). Tertiary prevention consists of resolution of angina before myocardial damage occurs.

Pathophysiology

Three coronary arteries normally supply the myocardium with blood to meet its metabolic needs during varying workloads. The right coronary artery supplies arterial blood to the right side of the heart; the left coronary artery divides into the left circumflex artery, which feeds the posterior heart muscle, and the anterior descending artery, which supplies the anterior myocardium, especially the left ventricle. The coronary vessels are usually efficient and perfuse the myocardium during diastole. When the heart needs more blood, the vessels dilate. As the vessels become lined and eventually occluded with atherosclerotic plaques and thrombi, the vessels can no longer dilate properly.

If the coronary vessels slowly become occluded, collateral vessels develop to provide the myocardium with needed arterial blood. Collateral vessels are more common in clients with long-term coronary artery disease.

Myocardial ischemia develops if the blood supply through the coronary vessels or oxygen content of the blood is not adequate to meet metabolic demands. Disorders of the coronary vessels, the circulation, or the blood may lead to deficits in supply.

Disorders of the coronary vessels include atherosclerosis, arterial spasm, and coronary arteritis. Atherosclerosis increases resistance to flow. Arterial spasm also increases resistance. Coronary *arteritis* is inflammation of the coronary arteries caused by infection or autoimmune disease.

Disorders of circulation include hypotension and aortic stenosis and insufficiency. Hypotension may be a result of spinal anesthesia, potent antihypertensive drugs, blood loss, or other factors that result in decreased blood return to the heart. Aortic valve stenosis or insufficiency results in decreased filling pressure of the coronary arteries.

Blood disorders include anemia, hypoxemia, and polycythemia. Anemia and hypoxemia result in decreased oxygen flow to the myocardium. Polycythemia increases blood viscosity, which slows blood flow through the coronary arteries.

The opposite of supply is demand, and increased demands can be placed on the heart. Conditions that increase demands on the myocardium are those that increase cardiac output or increase myocardial need for oxygen (Box 58-1).

Myocardial ischemia occurs when either supply or demand is altered. In some people, the coronary arteries can supply adequate blood when the person is at rest

---

BOX 58-1 Factors Influencing Myocardial Supply and Demand

FACTORS THAT DECREASE SUPPLY

Coronary Vessel Disorders

- Atherosclerosis
- Arterial spasm
- Coronary arteritis

Circulation Disorders

- Hypotension
- Aortic stenosis
- Aortic insufficiency

Blood Disorders

- Anemia
- Hypoxemia
- Polycythemia

FACTORS THAT INCREASE DEMAND

Increased Cardiac Output

- Exercise
- Emotion
- Digestion of a large meal
- Anemia
- Hyperthyroidism

Increased Myocardial Need for Oxygen

- Damaged myocardium
- Myocardial hypertrophy
- Aortic stenosis
- Aortic insufficiency
- Diastolic hypertension
- Thyrotoxicosis
- Strong emotions
- Heavy exertion

CRITICAL MONITORING

Angina from Impending Myocardial Infarction

- Continuous, enduring, severe chest pain lasts more than 20 minutes.
- Pain is usually felt in the retrosternal area, possibly radiating to the arms (the pain is most common in the left shoulder and arm), back, neck, or lower jaw.
- Pain is described as squeezing, pressing, or a sensation of heaviness.
- Deep breathing or changing posture does not change the severity of the pain.
- Pain may occur in the upper abdomen, accompanied by nausea and vomiting.
- Pain is relieved by nitroglycerin; pain is not relieved by antacids or food.
- ECG often shows ischemic changes.
- Chest radiograph is normal for client.

when the person attempts activity or is taxed in some other manner, however, angina develops. Myocardial cells become ischemic within 10 seconds of coronary artery occlusion. After several minutes of ischemia, the pumping function of the heart is reduced. The reduction in pumping deprives the ischemic cells of needed oxygen and glucose. The cells convert to anaerobic metabolism, which leaves lactic acid as a waste product. As lactic acid accumulates, pain develops. Angina pectoris is transient, lasting for only 3 to 5 minutes.[3,13] If blood flow is restored, no permanent myocardial damage occurs.

Clinical Manifestations
Characteristics of Angina

Angina is a clinical syndrome characterized by discomfort in the chest, jaw, shoulder, back, or arm. Angina pectoris produces transient paroxysmal attacks of substernal or precordial pain with the following characteristics:

- *Onset.* Angina can develop quickly or slowly. Some clients ignore the chest pain, thinking that it will go away or that it is indigestion. Ask what the client was doing when the pain began.
- *Location.* Nearly 90% of clients experience the pain as retrosternal or slightly to the left of the sternum.
- *Radiation.* The pain usually radiates to the left shoulder and upper arm and may then travel down the inner aspect of the left arm to the elbow, wrist, and fourth and fifth fingers. The pain may also radiate to the right shoulder, neck, jaw, or epigastric region. On occasion, the pain may be felt only in the area of radiation and not in the chest. Rarely is the pain localized to any one single small area over the precordium.
- *Duration.* Angina usually lasts less than 5 minutes. However, attacks precipitated by a heavy meal or extreme anger may last 15 to 20 minutes.
- *Sensation.* Clients describe the pain of angina as squeezing, burning, pressing, choking, aching, or bursting pressure. The client often says the pain feels like gas, heartburn, or indigestion. Clients do not describe anginal pain as sharp or knife-like.
- *Severity.* The pain of angina is usually mild or moderate in severity. It is often called "discomfort," not "pain." Rarely is the pain described as "severe."
- *Associated characteristics.* Other manifestations that may accompany the pain include dyspnea, pallor, sweating, faintness, palpitations, dizziness, and digestive disturbances.
- *Atypical presentation.* Women, older adults, and clients with diabetes may have atypical presentations of CHD that are equivalent to angina. In women, CHD may be manifested as epigastric pain, dyspnea, or back pain, whereas older adults frequently experience dyspnea, fatigue, or syncope.
- *Relieving and aggravating factors.* Angina is aggravated by continued activity, and most anginal attacks

quickly subside with the administration of nitroglycerin and rest. The typical "exertion-pain, rest-relief" pattern is the major clue to the diagnosis of angina pectoris.

- *Treatment.* Treatments to reduce the demand on the heart, such as rest, or treatments that dilate the coronary arteries will commonly reduce the pain. The client may have used nitroglycerin and the client should be asked if the angina subsided.

An important aspect of assessing angina is to determine quickly and accurately if the pain is indeed angina. Other conditions also lead to chest pain, such as pulmonary embolism, pleurisy, and pneumonia (see the table on Differential Diagnosis of Chest Pain on the website).

SAFETY

⚠️

ALERT

evolve

As vessels become lined with atherosclerotic plaques, plaques may be disrupted and thrombi may form, leading to clinical manifestations of inadequate blood supply in the tissues supplied by these vessels. Problems such as stroke, claudication, and angina develop. Stroke is described in Chapter 70 and claudication is discussed in Chapter 53.

Patterns of Angina

Classic angina pectoris can be subdivided into the following basic patterns:

- *Stable angina.* Stable angina is paroxysmal chest pain or discomfort triggered by a *predictable* degree of exertion (e.g., walking 20 feet) or emotion. Characteristically, a stable pattern of onset, duration, severity, and relieving factors is present. Normally, stable angina is relieved with rest or nitroglycerin, or both.
- *Unstable angina.* Unstable angina (preinfarction angina, crescendo angina, or intermittent coronary syndrome) is paroxysmal chest pain triggered by an *unpredictable* degree of exertion or emotion, which may occur at night. Unstable angina attacks characteristically increase in number, duration, and severity over time. If unstable angina occurs, it must be treated as a medical emergency with the client receiving immediate medical attention.
- *Variant angina.* Variant angina (*Prinzmetal's angina*) is chest discomfort similar to classic angina but of longer duration; it may occur while the client is at rest. These attacks tend to happen between midnight and 8 AM. Variant angina results from coronary artery spasm and may be associated with elevation of the ST segment on the electrocardiogram (ECG).
- *Nocturnal angina.* Nocturnal angina is possibly associated with rapid eye movement (REM) sleep during dreaming.
- *Angina decubitus.* Angina decubitus is paroxysmal chest pain that occurs when the client reclines and lessens when the client sits or stands up.

- *Intractable angina.* Intractable angina is chronic incapacitating angina that is unresponsive to intervention.
- *Postinfarction angina.* Pain occurs after MI, when residual ischemia may cause episodes of angina.

Diagnostic Tests

Initial laboratory testing and noninvasive testing of clients with suspected angina include resting ECG, chest radiography, hemoglobin, fasting glucose, and fasting lipid profile. Enzymes may be drawn for the more severe forms of angina in order to rule out myocardial infarction. Further testing is based on initial results of these and individual risk factors for CHD. The following modalities are described in Chapter 54.

Electrocardiography

The ECG tracings remain normal in more than 50% of clients with angina pectoris at rest. An ECG recorded in the presence of pain may document transient ischemic attacks with ST-segment elevation or depression. An ECG recorded during an episode of pain also suggests coronary artery involvement and the extent of cardiac muscle affected by the ischemic event.

Exercise Electrocardiography

During a *stress test,* the client exercises on a treadmill or stationary bicycle until reaching 85% of maximal heart rate. ECG or vital sign changes may indicate ischemia. Exercise electrocardiography is less sensitive in women and older adults.

Radioisotope Imaging

Various nuclear imaging techniques are used to evaluate myocardial muscle. Regions of poor perfusion or ischemia appear as areas of diminished or absent activity (cold spots).

Electron-Beam (Ultrafast) Computed Tomography (EBCT)

This noninvasive method enables detection of the amount of calcium in coronary arteries. Because calcification occurs with atherosclerotic plaque formation, measurement of coronary calcium may reflect the extent of coronary atherosclerosis. High coronary calcium values have been associated with obstructive coronary disease.

Coronary Angiography

Angiography remains the most accurate test to diagnose the percentage of blockage in coronary arteries because of atherosclerosis.

Chest X-Ray

Chest x-rays are an inexpensive technique that allow detection of cardiomegaly and noncardiac causes of chest pain (e.g., pleuritis or pneumonia).

OUTCOME MANAGEMENT

The aims of therapy in the treatment of chronic stable angina are to reduce manifestations and ultimately to reduce the risk of mortality and morbid events. These goals are accomplished through (1) antianginal pharmacologic intervention, (2) education and risk factor modification to control or eliminate known cardiovascular risk factors, and (3) in some instances, revascularization through interventional cardiology or coronary artery bypass graft (CABG) surgery. Smoking cessation after 1 year decreases the risk of CHD by 50%, a 10% reduction in cholesterol level lowers the risk of CHD by 20%, and 6 mm Hg reduction in diastolic blood pressure lowers the risk of CHD by 10%. The American Heart Association (AHA) recommends that people with angina control their modifiable risk factors and seek prompt treatment for episodes of chest pain. The mnemonic "A, B, C, D, E" is promoted for health care professionals and clients alike in aiding to reduce manifestations and control risk factors:

- *A* for aspirin and antianginal therapy
- *B* for beta-blocker therapy and blood pressure control
- *C* for cigarettes and cholesterol
- *D* for diet and diabetes
- *E* for education and exercise

Clients with chronic stable angina (CSA) are usually managed effectively with risk factor reduction and pharmacologic therapy. Revascularization through interventional cardiology procedures or CABG surgery is reserved for those clients with triple-vessel (all three coronary arteries) or left main coronary artery disease, with left ventricular dysfunction, or whose manifestations are not adequately controlled by pharmacologic therapy. Revascularization is used most often for clients with unstable angina or AMI. Interventional cardiology procedures and CABG are discussed in Chapter 56.

Medical Management

Medical management of clients with angina pectoris focuses on three goals: (1) relieve the acute pain, (2) restore coronary blood flow, and (3) prevent further attacks to reduce the risk of AMI.[13]

The diagnosis of angina pectoris is confirmed by history and various tests. A complete history of the pain and its pattern is collected to discriminate angina from other causes of chest pain. Clients are encouraged to describe the pain in their own words. Record a complete analysis of manifestations. This description provides a baseline that can be used in ongoing care.

Most physical findings are transient. The client exhibits pallor or has cold, clammy skin. Tachycardia and hypertension may be recorded. Pulsus alternans (the force of each beat varies) may be present at the onset of ischemic attacks. On auscultation, an S_3 or S_4 gallop or a paradoxical split of S_2 may be noted. If mitral regurgitation is present because of ischemia of the papillary muscle, a murmur can be heard.

Relieve Acute Pain and Restore Coronary Blood Flow

The primary goal of pharmacologic treatment of angina is to balance myocardial oxygen supply and demand by altering the various components of the process, thereby increasing oxygen supply to the myocardium or reducing myocardial oxygen demand. The components of myocardial oxygen consumption that can be pharmacologically treated are (1) blood pressure, (2) heart rate, (3) contractility, and (4) left ventricular volume. Drugs used in the treatment of angina and associated nursing implications are listed in the Integrating Pharmacology feature below.

The major types of medications used to treat the acute attack in angina pectoris are as follows:

- *Opiate analgesics* are used to relieve or reduce acute pain. By reducing pain, the heart rate often lowers and the need for oxygen by the myocardium also is reduced.
- *Vasodilators* help reduce acute pain and prevent further attacks by widening the diameter of coronary arteries and increasing the supply of oxygen to the myocardium. *Nitroglycerin,* a *short-acting* nitrate, has been the treatment of choice against anginal attacks since 1867. Administered sublingually, per tablet, or via translingual spray, nitroglycerin helps relieve or reduce anginal pain within 1 to 2 minutes. *Long-acting* nitrates, given orally or transdermally, help maintain coronary artery vasodilation, thereby promoting greater flow of blood and oxygen to the heart muscle.
- *Beta-adrenergic blockers* help reduce the workload of the heart, decrease myocardial oxygen demand, and may decrease the number of anginal attacks.
- *Calcium-channel blockers* are used to dilate coronary arteries, thereby increasing oxygen supply to the myocardium.
- *Antiplatelet* agents inhibit platelet aggregation and reduce coagulability, thus preventing clot formation.

Prevent Further Attacks

Education and counseling regarding modification of risk factors are necessary to reduce the progression of CHD and to prevent further attacks. Recommendations

---

INTEGRATING PHARMACOLOGY

Treatment of Angina

Angina is ischemic pain in the myocardium. The medications used to treat acute angina episodes are vasodilators designed to restore arterial flow (supply) or reduce oxygen consumption (demand).

Nitroglycerin is the most common medication used and should be given to clients with known ischemic heart disease who report manifestations of angina. Because of its potent vasodilatory effect, assess the blood pressure before beginning treatment and 5 minutes after each dose. The most common practice is to give three doses of sublingual nitroglycerin 5 minutes apart as long as the client does not become severely hypotensive. If the pain is not relieved, notify the physician immediately; morphine may be required. If the client does not have a history of ischemic heart disease, collect a thorough assessment of the pain and notify the physician immediately if there are any indications of serious forms of chest pain. Some physicians order simultaneous liquid antacids and nitroglycerin to reduce both cardiac and gastrointestinal pain. If the medications are given 5 minutes apart, it may help with clinical decision making about the cause of the pain. Concurrent use of sildenafil (Viagra) may cause severe hypotension and death.

Clients with long-standing angina may also use topical nitroglycerin of extended-release forms. These forms of nitroglycerin provide continuous vasodilation. Tolerance to the medication can develop, especially in doses with longer half-lives; hence topical nitroglycerin is removed during the night to restore efficacy. Assessment of nocturnal angina, especially during REM sleep, is needed.

A second method of controlling pain is to reduce the myocardial need for oxygen. Beta-blocking agents reduce myocardial oxygen consumption by controlling the high-oxygen demands from the effects of the sympathetic nervous system. Original forms of beta-blocking agents contained both $beta_1$ and $beta_2$ antagonists and therefore could prompt bronchoconstriction. Newer forms are selective $beta_1$ antagonists only.

Aspirin is commonly used in acute events and to promote blood flow through narrowed and tortuous coronary arteries, where slowed blood is likely to clot and prevent forward flow of blood. Aspirin prevents platelets from aggregating (collecting) by blocking prostaglandin synthesis. Aspirin is irritating to the gastrointestinal tract and should be given with food. It also leads to increased bleeding risk from all invasive procedures. Concurrent use of other medications that also slow clotting must be carefully monitored.

Other medications for the treatment of angina are the same as the medications used for the treatment of coronary artery disease (see Chapter 56).

should follow the guidelines established by the AHA for primary and secondary prevention of CHD. Specific recommendations for risk factor modification are described in Chapter 56.

Nursing Management of the Medical Client

Relieve Acute Pain and Restore Coronary Blood Flow

In addition to documenting the clinical manifestations of angina, ascertain how long the client has had angina, whether risk factors for CHD are present, and the client's emotional reaction to chest pain. Start cardiac monitoring, obtain a 12-lead ECG, and control ongoing angina. Until the angina is controlled and coronary blood flow is reestablished, the client is at risk for myocardial damage from myocardial ischemia. If the client reports angina, assess the pain and ask the client whether the pain is the same as that experienced in the past. Note new characteristics or increased pain. The phrase "all clients with chest pain get MONA" is used to guide treatment of clients with chest pain:

- *M,* morphine sulfate
- *O,* oxygen therapy
- *N,* nitrates
- *A,* aspirin

Give sublingual nitroglycerin tablets or spray as prescribed. Nitroglycerin dilates coronary arteries, reducing pain and restoring coronary blood flow. Because nitroglycerin causes vasodilation and hypotension, monitor blood pressure. If the pain is not relieved after three nitroglycerin tablets, each taken 5 minutes apart, or after morphine, notify the physician. In addition, an environment that provides rest and security as well as allays fear and anxiety helps reduce pain. Oxygen therapy is used to ensure adequate oxygenation. Aspirin is given for its antiplatelet activities.

Self-Care

The client must be knowledgeable about the care of episodes of angina and how to reduce the risk factors that exacerbate the process. Use the following information to help clients control risk factors for angina pectoris:

- Educate the client to avoid activities or habits that precipitate angina (eating large meals, drinking coffee, smoking, exercising too strenuously, going out in cold weather, becoming anxious and stressed). If an attack begins, the client should stop the activity and sit down. An antianginal medication (e.g., nitroglycerin) should be taken. Three pills can be taken sublingually 5 minutes apart. If the pain does not subside, worsens, or radiates, the client should take an aspirin. The client should call "911" and explain that he or she is experiencing chest pain;

the client would then be taken promptly to the emergency department. Emphasize this point because if the client is experiencing an AMI, the sooner treatment is initiated, the lower the death rate. Family members should not drive the client to the hospital because of the risk for sudden death precipitated by ventricular fibrillation. If the client is taken by ambulance, defibrillators are available in case of ventricular fibrillation.

- Explain the importance of daily management of hypertension. Advise the client to take daily medication even if no clinical manifestations are evident (see Chapter 52).
- Encourage and help plan a regular program of daily exercise to promote improved coronary circulation and weight management.
- Instruct clients who smoke to quit smoking at once. Smoking cigarettes raises carboxyhemoglobin levels in the blood, which reduces the amount of oxygen available to the myocardium. Clients with angina pectoris exposed for 2 hours to cigarette smoke have elevations in carboxyhemoglobin concentration, decreased exercise tolerance, increased heart rate, and elevated blood pressure. Advise clients to avoid "passive smoking" (i.e., being with a smoker or in a smoke-filled room).
- Urge overweight clients to lose excess weight. Explain that weight reduction may also reduce blood pressure, cholesterol level, and the incidence of adult-onset diabetes. Encourage them to eat small meals, avoid high-calorie and high-cholesterol diets, abstain from gas-forming foods, and rest for short periods after meals. In addition, recommend a high-fiber diet, which not only may prevent constipation and other intestinal tract ailments but also may decrease the number and severity of angina attacks. Diets high in fiber may also help lower serum cholesterol and triglyceride levels. CHD is less common among clients with a high intake of dietary fiber than in those with a low intake. High fiber diets can also decrease hypertension.
- Help the client who leads an active, hectic life to adjust activities to a level below that which precipitates anginal attacks. Encourage brief rest periods throughout the working day, an early bedtime, and longer or more frequent vacations. Advise clients who are anxious and nervous to consider counseling. Relaxation techniques may also be used.

ACUTE MYOCARDIAL INFARCTION

Acute coronary syndrome refers to the clinical manifestations that are compatible with AMI. An AMI is also known as a heart attack, coronary occlusion, or simply a "coronary," which is a life-threatening condition characterized by the formation of localized necrotic areas within the myocardium. AMI usually follows the sudden occlusion of a coronary artery and the abrupt cessation of blood and oxygen flow to the heart muscle. Because the heart muscle must function continuously, blockage of blood to the muscle and the development of necrotic areas can be lethal.

AMI is the leading cause of death in America and is responsible for an estimated 529,000 deaths each year. Every year about 1.1 million Americans have AMIs. Every 29 seconds an American suffers a coronary event and approximately every 1 minute someone dies of a coronary event. About 250,000 people a year die before they reach the hospital. Studies indicate that half of all AMI victims wait more than 2 hours before getting help. On the basis of data from the Framingham study, about 45% of all AMIs occur in people younger than age 65 years and 5% occur in those younger than age 40. Eighty-five percent of people who die of AMI are 65 years of age or older. Women have higher in-hospital mortality than men. The difference may result from differences in treatment for men and women. In studies of women with AMI, aspirin, beta-blocking drugs, coronary thrombolysis, acute cardiac catheterization, percutaneous transluminal coronary angioplasty (PTCA), and CABG surgery were used less often than in men with AMI. Death rates for CHD are higher for African Americans, Hispanics, and American Indians than for Caucasians.

Etiology and Risk Factors

The most common cause of AMI is complete or nearly complete occlusion of a coronary artery, usually precipitated by rupture of a vulnerable atherosclerotic plaque and subsequent thrombus formation. Plaque rupture can be precipitated by both internal and external factors.

Internal factors include plaque characteristics, such as the size and consistency of the lipid core and the thickness of the fibrous cap, as well as conditions to which it is exposed, such as coagulation status and degree of arterial vasoconstriction. Vulnerable plaques most frequently occur in areas with less than 70% stenosis and are characterized by an eccentric shape with an irregular border; a large, thin lipid core; and a thin, fibrous cap.

External factors result from actions of the client or from external conditions that affect the client. Strenuous physical activity and severe emotional stress, such as anger, increase sympathetic nervous system responses, that may lead to plaque rupture. At the same time, sympathetic nervous system responses increase myocardial oxygen demand. Scientists have reported that external factors, such as exposure to cold and time of day, also affect plaque rupture. Acute coronary events occur more frequently with exposure to cold and during the morning hours. Researchers hypothesize that the sudden increases in sympathetic nervous system responses associated with these factors may contribute to plaque

rupture. The role of inflammation in triggering plaque rupture is currently being studied.

Regardless of the cause, rupture of the atherosclerotic plaque results in (1) exposure of the plaque's lipid-rich core to flowing blood, (2) seepage of blood into the plaque, causing it to expand, (3) triggering of thrombus formation, and (4) partial or complete occlusion of the coronary artery.

Unstable angina is associated with short-term partial occlusion of a coronary artery, whereas AMI results from significant or complete occlusion of a coronary artery that lasts more than 1 hour. When blood flow ceases abruptly, the myocardial tissue supplied by that artery dies. Coronary artery spasm can also cause acute occlusion. The risk factors that predispose a client to a heart attack are the same as for all forms of CHD (see Chapter 56).

Pathophysiology

AMI can be considered the end-point of CHD. Unlike the temporary ischemia that occurs with angina, prolonged unrelieved ischemia causes irreversible damage to the myocardium. Cardiac cells can withstand ischemia for about 15 minutes before they die. Because the myocardium is metabolically active, manifestations of ischemia can be seen within 8 to 10 seconds of decreased blood flow. When the heart does not receive blood and oxygen, it converts to *anaerobic metabolism,* creating less adenosine triphosphate (ATP) and more lactic acid as a by-product. Myocardial cells are very sensitive to changes in pH and become less functional. Acidosis causes the myocardium to become more vulnerable to the effects of the lysosomal enzymes within the cell. Acidosis leads to conduction system disorders, and dysrhythmias develop. Contractility is also reduced, decreasing the heart's ability to pump. As the myocardial cells necrose, intracellular enzymes are introduced into the bloodstream, where they can be detected by laboratory tests.

Figure 58-1 illustrates the depth of various types of infarctions in the wall of the ventricle. Cellular necrosis

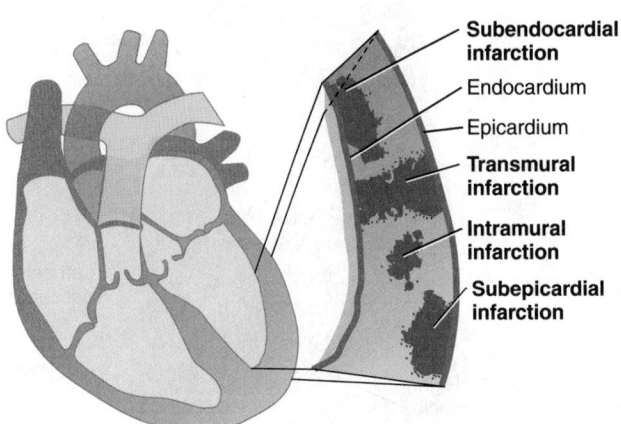

■ **FIGURE 58–1** Depth of infarction in the wall of the ventricle. Subendocardial, intramural, and subepicardial injuries are only in one layer. Transmural infarction extends through all three layers.

occurs in one layer of myocardial tissue in subendocardial, intramural, and subepicardial infarctions. In a transmural infarction, cellular necrosis is present in all three layers of myocardial tissue. The infarct site is called the *zone of infarction and necrosis*. Around it is a zone of hypoxic injury, also called a penumbra. This zone can return to normal but may also become necrotic if blood flow is not restored. The outermost zone is called the *zone of ischemia;* damage to this area is reversible.

Within the first few hours of AMI, the necrotic area stretches in a process called *infarct expansion*. This expansion is furthered by the neurohormonal activation that occurs with AMI. Increased heart rate, ventricular dilation, and activation of the renin-angiotensin system increase preload during AMI in order to maintain cardiac output. Transmural infarctions heal by scar formation of the left ventricle, called *remodeling*. Expansion may continue for up to 6 weeks after an AMI and is accompanied by progressive thinning and lengthening of infarcted and noninfarcted areas. The gene expression of remodeled cardiac cells changes, causing permanent structural changes to the heart. Remodeled tissue does not function normally and can result in acute or chronic heart failure with left ventricular dysfunction and increases in ventricular volumes and pressures. Remodeling may continue for years after an AMI (see Chapter 56).

The most common site of an AMI is the *anterior wall* of the left ventricle near the apex, resulting from thrombosis of the descending branch of the left coronary artery (Figure 58-2). Other common sites are (1) the *posterior wall* of the left ventricle near the base and behind the posterior cusp of the mitral valve and (2) the *inferior (diaphragmatic) surface* of the heart. Infarction of the posterior left ventricle results from occlusion of the right coronary artery or circumflex branch of the left coronary artery. An inferior infarction occurs when the right coronary artery is occluded. In nearly 25% of inferior wall AMIs, the right ventricle is the site of infarction. Atrial infarctions develop less than 5% of the time. The Concept Map on p. 1491 further outlines the cellular effects that occur during an MI.

Clinical Manifestations

The clinical manifestations associated with AMI result from ischemia of the heart muscle and the decrease in function and acidosis associated with it. The major clinical manifestation of AMI is chest pain (Figure 58-3), which is similar to angina pectoris but more severe and unrelieved by nitroglycerin. The pain may radiate to the neck, jaw, shoulder, back, or left arm. The pain also may present near the epigastrium, simulating indigestion. AMI may also be associated with less common clinical manifestations, including the following:[3]

- **Atypical chest, stomach, back, or abdominal pain**
- **Nausea or dizziness**
- **Shortness of breath and difficulty breathing**
- **Unexplained anxiety, weakness, or fatigue**
- **Palpitations, cold sweat, or paleness**

Women experiencing AMI frequently present with one or more of the less common clinical manifestations.

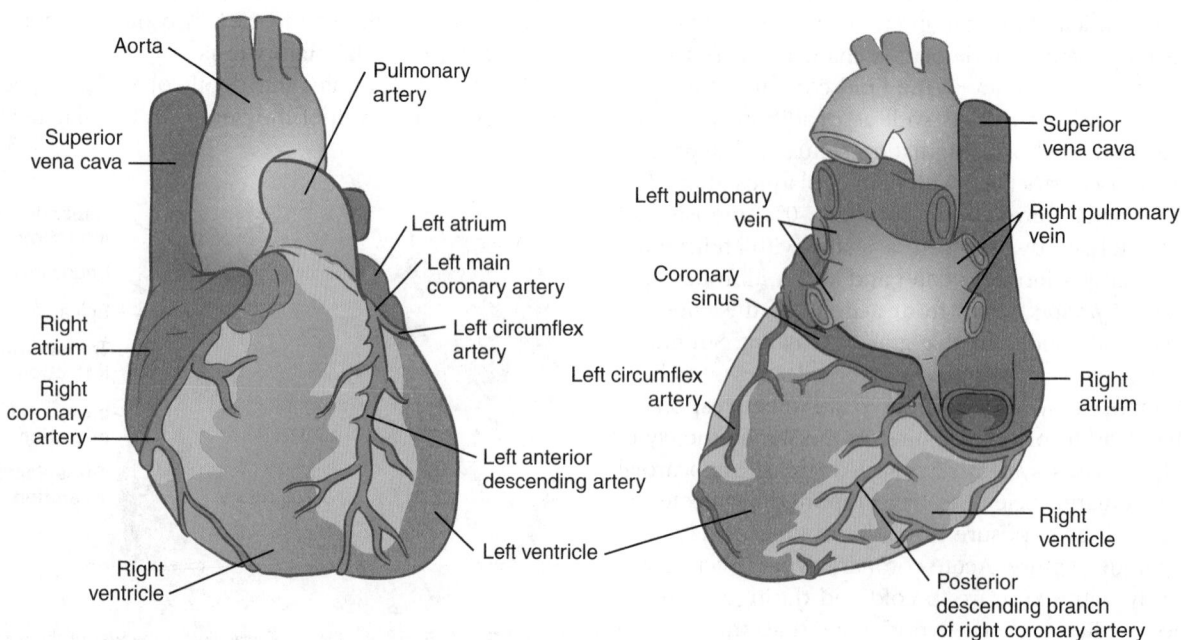

■ **FIGURE 58–2** There are three coronary arteries. The right coronary artery supplies arterial blood to the right side of the heart; the left coronary artery divides into the left circumflex artery, which feeds the posterior heart muscle, and left anterior descending artery, which supplies the anterior myocardium

Understanding Myocardial Infarction and Its Treatment

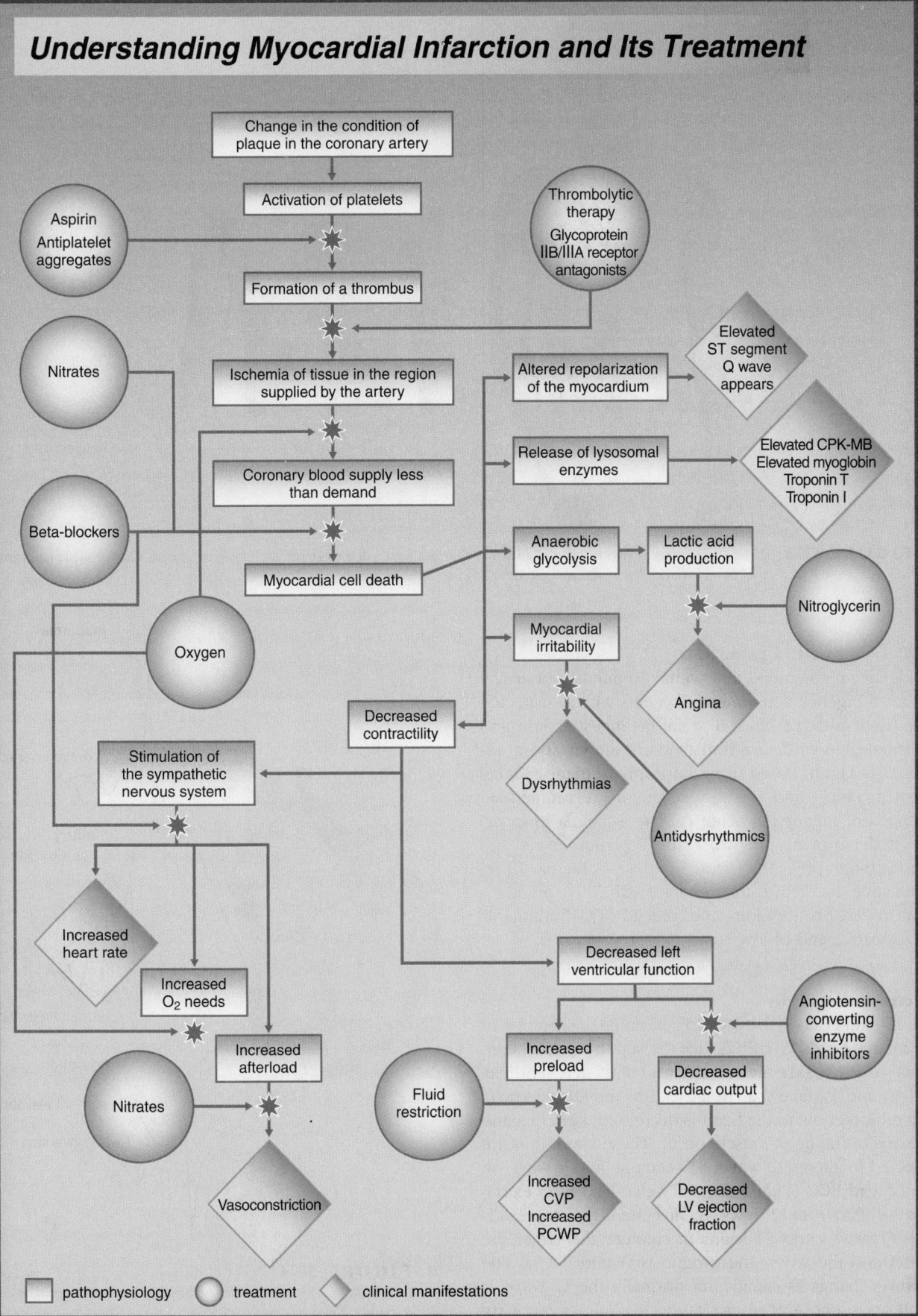

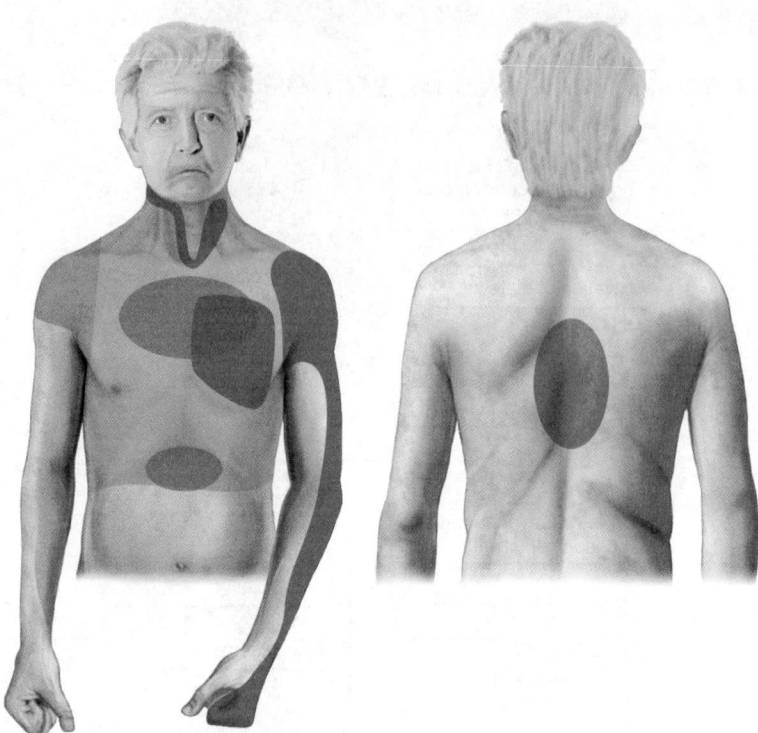

■ **FIGURE 58–3** Possible pain patterns with myocardial infarction. The red area is the most common location of pain. Orange areas are areas of referred pain and the location of pain in women. However, pain can develop in any area of the chest (yellow).

🪔 Diagnostic Evaluation

Guidelines recommend that within 10 minutes of arrival in the emergency department all clients with a suspected AMI (ischemic-type chest discomfort) ingest aspirin and have baseline cardiac serum markers drawn and a 12-lead ECG taken. Based upon appropriate triage, 30-day survival rates, and cost-effectiveness, recommended methods of identifying acute cardiac ischemia in emergency departments are troponin T serum levels and echocardiography. The Acute Cardiac Ischemia Time-Insensitive Predictive Instrument (ACI-TIPI), an algorithm based on questions and 12-lead ECG findings, is also accurate and of low cost.

Electrocardiography

The 12-lead ECG can be used to determine the location of the infarct. Leads V_1 and V_2 face the septum of the heart, leads V_3 and V_4 face the anterior wall of the left ventricle, and V_5 and V_6 face the lateral wall of the left ventricle. When blood flow to the heart is decreased, ischemia and necrosis of the heart muscle occur. These conditions are reflected in altered Q wave, ST segment, and T wave on the 12-lead ECG (Figure 58-4). Twelve-lead ECG examines the heart from 12 views, and in general the more leads with Q waves and ST segment changes the larger the infarct and the worse the prognosis (Figure 58-5). The Q-wave change is significant; normally the Q wave is small or absent. AMI from total occlusion of a coronary

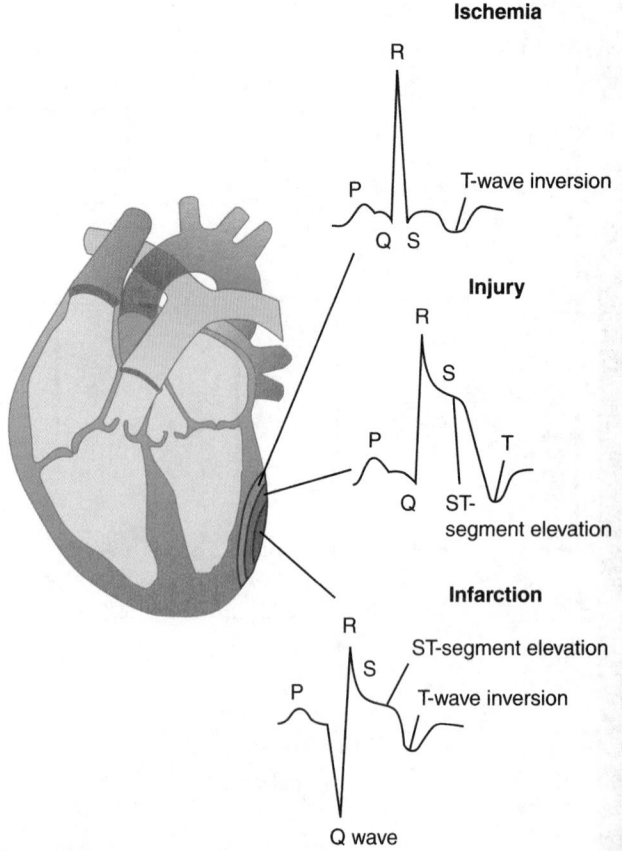

■ **FIGURE 58–4** Zones of hypoxic injury, zone of infarction, zone of necrosis, and the electrocardiographic patterns accompanying these changes during myocardial infarction.

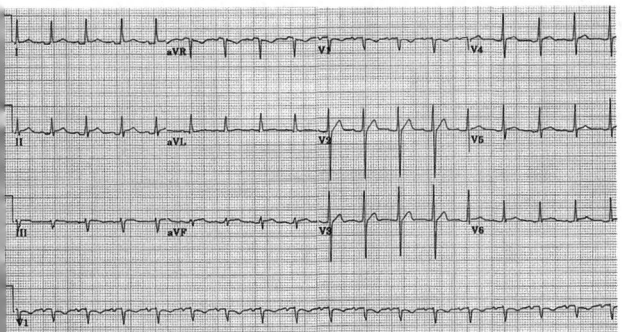

■ **FIGURE 58–5** A 12-lead ECG showing sinus tachycardia and ST elevation consistent with acute myocardial infarction.

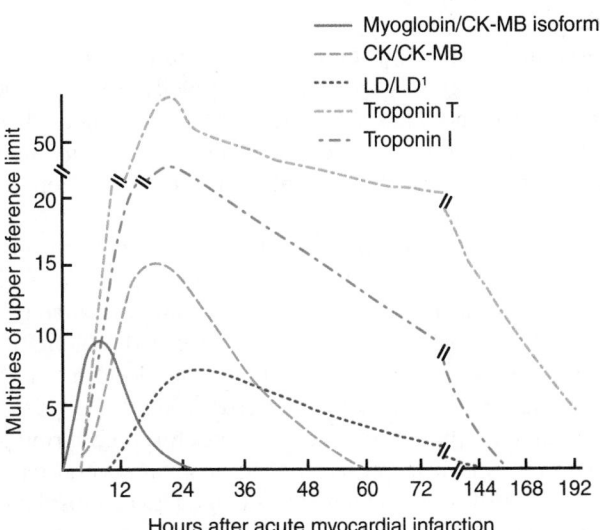

■ **FIGURE 58–6** Isoenzyme alterations in acute myocardial infarction. *(From Wong, S.S. [1996]. Strategic utilization of cardiac markers for the diagnosis of acute myocardial infarction. Annals of Clinical Laboratory Science, 26, 301-312. Copyright 1996 by the Institute for Clinical Science, Inc.)*

artery causes a visible Q wave on the ECG; AMI with less than total occlusion does not lead to Q wave changes. Ischemic tissue produces an elevation in the ST segment and a peaked T wave or inversion of the T wave. ST-segment elevation is considered significant if greater than 1 mm. Through the course of an MI, changes occur first in the ST segment, then the T wave, and finally the Q wave. As the myocardium heals, the ST segment and T wave return to normal, but the Q-wave changes persist. However, an ECG can be completely normal in a client with AMI, especially in the early hours following infarct.

Laboratory Tests

Laboratory findings include elevated levels of serum creatine kinase (CK)-MB isoenzyme, myoglobin, cardiac troponin T, and cardiac troponin I. Historically, elevations in lactate dehydrogenase (LDH) M1 isoenzyme, serum aspartate transaminase (AST), leukocytes (leukocytosis), and erythrocyte sedimentation rate (ESR) have aided in the diagnosis of AMI. Although serum levels of these substances can be drawn, isoenzymes are used today to diagnose AMI. Isoenzyme changes in AMI follow a typical pattern (see Figure 58-6). Knowing the typical pattern allows an estimation of the time of the actual injury.

Troponin. The cardiac troponin complex is a basic component of the myocardium that is involved in the contraction of the myocardial muscle. Positive levels of troponin are considered virtually diagnostic of AMI.

Cardiac *troponin T* is similar to CK-MB with regard to sensitivity, and levels increase within 3 to 6 hours after pain has started. Levels remain elevated for 14 to 21 days. This is useful (and more accurate than LDH) in confirmation of distant AMI.[15,21]

Cardiac *troponin I* levels increase 7 to 14 hours after AMI. This is a very specific and sensitive indicator of AMI and is not affected by any other disease or injury to any other muscle except cardiac muscle. Elevation persists for 5 to 7 days.

Myoglobin. Myoglobin is a heme protein found in striated muscle fibers. Myoglobin is rapidly released when myocardial muscle tissue is damaged. Because of the rapid release, it can be detected within 2 hours after AMI. Although many other factors can raise the serum myoglobin level (e.g., strenuous exercise, heavy ethanol use), myoglobin is a highly sensitive indicator of AMI if serum levels double when a second sample is drawn within 2 hours of the first. Conversely, it is reliable to exclude the diagnosis of AMI if the levels do not increase every 2 hours. The diagnostic window ends 24 hours after an AMI.[21]

CK-MB. Serum levels of CK-MB (an isoenzyme of CK found primarily in cardiac muscle) increase 3 to 6 hours after the onset of chest pain, peak in 12 to 18 hours, and return to normal levels in 3 to 4 days.

LDH. The LDH_1 subunit is plentiful in heart muscle and is released into the serum when myocardial damage occurs. Serum levels of LDH elevate 14 to 24 hours after onset of myocardial damage, peak within 48 to 72 hours, and slowly return to normal over the next 7 to 14 days. Figure 58-6 illustrates the pattern of enzyme changes after AMI.

AST. Serum levels of AST increase within several hours after the onset of chest pain, peak within 12 to 18 hours, and return to normal within 3 to 4 days.

Leukocytosis. Leukocytosis ($10,000/mm^3$ to $20,000/mm^3$) appears on the second day after AMI and disappears in 1 week. Myeloperoxidase, a leukocyte enzyme, was recently shown to be predictive of AMI even in clients without elevations in troponin T level.

Imaging Studies

Radionuclide imaging studies provide information on the presence of coronary artery disease as well as the location of ischemic and infarcted tissue. Cardiac imaging studies have been used to provide information for management decisions of clients who present to the emergency department with acute chest pain.

When a client experiences acute chest pain, perfusion imaging with agents such as thallium, sestamibi, and teboroxime can be used to identify ischemic and infarcted tissue. Perfusion imaging is sometimes called "cold spot" imaging because the radioisotope in the bloodstream is not taken up by ischemic or infarcted tissue.

Infarct, or "hot spot" imaging, is useful in confirming AMI in clients who present to the hospital several days after an AMI. Technetium 99 m–tagged pyrophosphate binds with calcium in areas of myocardial necrosis. Areas of uptake (hot spots) seen on nuclear imaging indicate areas of infarction. Because this test does not give positive results for 24 hours, however, it cannot be used to identify an acute, early-stage MI. Radiolabeled antimyosin is also used for hot spot imaging, but its diagnostic value is limited because it cannot differentiate between a new infarct and a scar from an earlier infarct.

Positron Emission Tomography. Positron emission tomography (PET) is used to evaluate cardiac metabolism and to assess tissue perfusion. It can also be used to detect CHD, assess coronary artery flow reserve, measure absolute myocardial blood flow, detect AMI, and differentiate ischemic from nonischemic cardiomyopathy. It may also be used to assess myocardial viability to determine which clients can benefit from CABG.

Magnetic Resonance Imaging. Magnetic resonance imaging (MRI) helps identify the site and extent of an MI, assess the effects of reperfusion therapy, and differentiate reversible and irreversible tissue injury. Its use as a diagnostic tool for coronary artery disease is increasing, although MRI cannot be used in clients with implanted metallic devices, such as pacemakers or defibrillators.

Echocardiography. Echocardiography is useful in assessing the ability of the heart walls to contract and relax. The transducer is placed on the chest, and images are relayed to a monitor screen. Wall motion is abnormal in ischemic or infarcted areas. Complications such as mitral regurgitation, rupture of the left ventricle, and pericardial effusion can be detected.

Transesophageal Echocardiography. Transesophageal echocardiography (TEE) is an imaging technique in which the transducer is placed against the wall of the esophagus. The image of the myocardium is clearer when the esophageal site is used because no air and no ribs are between the transducer and the heart. This technique is particularly useful for viewing the posterior wall of the heart.

OUTCOME MANAGEMENT

Since the advent of coronary care units and devices that aid in promptly recognizing and treating life-threatening dysrhythmias, 70% to 80% of people experiencing an AMI survive the initial attack. Chances for survival greatly diminish with the presence of the following:

- Older age (clients 80 years or older have a 60% death rate)
- Manifestations of heart failure
- ST-segment elevation
- Elevation of cardiac markers
- Hypotension (systolic blood pressure less than 55 mm Hg on admission has a 60% death rate)
- More than three coronary risk factors
- More than two anginal events within 24 hours

Deaths generally result from severe dysrhythmias, cardiogenic shock, heart failure, rupture of the heart, and recurrent AMI. Clients who avoid complications after AMI still require 6 to 12 weeks for complete recovery. However, 25% of men and 38% of women die within 1 year after having AMI and 22% of men and 46% of women are disabled with heart failure within 6 years of an AMI.

Medical Management

Major goals of care for clients with AMI include the following:

- Initiating prompt care
- Determining the type of AMI (STEMI vs. NSTEMI)
- Reducing pain
- Delivering successful treatment for the acute pain and reperfusion of the myocardium
- Preventing complications
- Preventing remodeling and heart failure
- Rehabilitating and educating the client and significant others

Treat the Acute Attack Immediately

Clients with manifestations of AMI must receive immediate treatment. Delays may increase damage to the heart and reduce the chance of survival. The goal for treatment of AMI is "door to needle" in less than 30 minutes, or specifically from onset of pain till thrombolytic therapy within 30 minutes or percutaneous angioplasty within 1 hour.

Most communities have an emergency medical system (EMS) that responds quickly (call "911"). Until EMS personnel arrive, keep the client quiet and calm. It is recommended that, if conscious, a client chew an aspirin at the onset of manifestations, because mortality is reduced 23% with this action alone.[1]

Many people who experience manifestations of AMI delay calling for help because they misinterpret what they are sensing. Their expectations of what AMI should feel like and their experience are not the same. In women, this delay may even be longer. Community education to "call first, call fast" is important.

While waiting for EMS to arrive, elevate the client's head and loosen any tight clothing around the neck. Once EMS workers arrive, the client is assessed and transported quickly to an emergency department. EMS workers are trained to respond to possible AMI clients with protocols to ensure quick and proper treatment. Sudden death from AMI caused by ventricular tachycardia degenerating first to ventricular fibrillation and later to asystole is the most common cause of sudden cardiac death. The client is given oxygen; an intravenous (IV) line is inserted, and the client is connected to a heart monitor. Portable automatic external defibrillators (AEDs) are becoming standard in public places. These devices can guide amateurs on how to resuscitate a person with chest pain who is having a dysrhythmia. Clients who become unconscious before reaching the emergency department may require defibrillation or cardiopulmonary resuscitation (CPR).

The client experiencing AMI needs immediate admission to a hospital with a coronary care unit if possible. The first 24 hours after AMI is the time of highest risk for sudden death. There is a significant benefit if treatment is administered within the first hour of onset of manifestations. The first hour after the onset of pain is the crucial time frame for salvage of the myocardium. Therefore efforts have been made to decrease the time for initial treatment. All emergency departments treat AMI clients within 30 minutes of presenting to the hospital. The mnemonic *4D's* (*d*oor, *d*ata, *d*ecision, and *d*rug), along with treatment algorithms, has been adopted by many emergency departments to treat those with AMI and remains current. Equally important is for everyone to have 911 access for EMS personnel who are trained in triage of chest pain and defibrillation.

Determining the Type of AMI

For purposes of determining appropriate treatment, AMI is viewed as part of a spectrum of coronary syndromes, which includes (1) ST-segment elevation myocardial infarction (STEMI), (2) non–ST-segment elevation myocardial infarction (NSTEMI), and (3) unstable angina. Clients with persistent ST elevation should be considered for reperfusion therapy (thrombolysis or primary percutaneous coronary interventions [PCIs]). Those without ST elevation will be diagnosed either with NSTEMI if cardiac markers are elevated or with unstable angina if serum cardiac markers provide no evidence of myocardial injury. Clients with no ST-segment elevation are not candidates for immediate thrombolytics but should receive anti-ischemic therapy and may be candidates for PCI urgently or during admission. Confirmation of

the diagnosis of NSTEMI requires waiting for the results of cardiac markers. In the case of unstable angina, diagnosis may await further diagnostic studies such as coronary angiography or imaging studies to confirm the diagnosis and to distinguish it from noncoronary causes of chest pain.

The initial focus should be on identifying clients with STEMI. An ECG should be performed and read within 10 minutes of ED arrival. If STEMI is present, the decision as to whether the client will be treated with thrombolysis or primary PCI should be made within the next 10 minutes. The goal for clients with STEMI should be to achieve a door-to-drug time of within 30 minutes and a door-to-balloon time of within 90 minutes. If STEMI is not present, then the workup proceeds looking for unstable angina or NSTEMI and for other causes of chest pain.

Reduce Pain

Upon admission, the client who complains of chest pain is admitted to the emergency department, given oxygen therapy, and placed on ECG monitoring. An IV line is placed, serum cardiac markers are drawn, and a 12-lead ECG is undertaken within 10 minutes. Pain control is a priority, and pain is usually treated with IV morphine. Continued pain is a manifestation of myocardial ischemia. Pain also stimulates the autonomic nervous system and increases preload, which in turn increases myocardial oxygen demand. Oxygen is used to treat tissue hypoxia.

Monitor Heart Rhythm

Because dysrhythmias are common, ECG monitoring is essential and antidysrhythmic medications should be on hand. A two-dimensional echocardiogram and test may be performed in the emergency department to aid in ruling in or ruling out AMI.

Improve Perfusion

The general principles of pharmacologic treatment of AMI consist of anti-ischemic and antithrombotic therapies, which are outlined in the Integrating Pharmacology feature on p. 1496.[1] Anti-ischemic therapy usually consists of beta-blockade and IV nitroglycerin. Antithrombotic therapy and the combination of different antithrombotic agents are being studied widely. Antithrombotic therapy is usually initiated with the administration of an aspirin if the client has not taken one before reaching the emergency department. Heparin therapy is the next step.

Antithrombotic therapy continues with medications that lyse (dissolve) the clot that forms part of the blockage of the coronary artery. Thrombolytic therapy includes streptokinase, urokinase, tissue-type plasminogen activator (t-PA), anisoylated plasminogen-streptokinase activator complex (anistreplase, APSAC), alteplase,

INTEGRATING PHARMACOLOGY

Medications for Myocardial Infarction

The portion of the coronary artery occluded by a thrombus can be opened by using various medications that dissolve the clot or prevent new clots from forming or extending. Non–clot-specific thrombolytic agents (streptokinase, urokinase) can be infused over 60 minutes after the client is premedicated with a steroid and diphenhydramine to prevent allergic responses. For large or anterior infarcts, clot-specific agents are more common forms of plasminogen activator. This medication is given in a bolus followed by an infusion. Several relative and absolute contraindications exist for thrombolytic therapy (see Box 58-2).

Heparin is also used in combination with the thrombolytic to prevent new clot formation. The dose of heparin is based on lean body weight and adjusted to the partial thromboplastin time. Heparin is contraindicated in clients with known bleeding conditions or recent stroke. Low-molecular-weight heparin is more commonly used because of ease of administration.

Preventing platelet aggregation is an important component of therapy. Aspirin continues to be used routinely in coronary angioplasty and to treat clients with myocardial infarction or unstable angina. The advantages of early aspirin administration are clear; it is strongly advised that aspirin be consumed early in care. Glycoprotein (GP) IIb/IIIa serves as the receptor on platelets that permits platelet aggregation. Agents that block this final common pathway by blocking the binding of adhesive proteins to GP IIb/IIIa, termed *GP IIb/IIIa antagonists,* are currently considered the most powerful specific inhibitors of platelet participation in acute thrombosis.

Pain is managed with morphine or intravenous nitroglycerin. Nitroglycerin is a coronary vasodilator used to reduce preload and afterload. Other medications, beta-blockers, ACE inhibitors, and statins are discussed in Chapter 56.

BOX 58-2 Absolute and Relative Contraindications for Thrombolytic Therapy

ABSOLUTE CONTRAINDICATIONS

- Any prior intracranial hemorrhage
- Ischemic stroke within 3 months *except* acute ischemic stroke within 3 hours
- Known structural cerebral vascular lesion (i.e., AVM)
- Known malignant intracranial neoplasm (primary or metastatic)
- Active bleeding or bleeding diathesis excluding menses
- Suspected aortic dissection
- Significant closed head trauma or facial trauma within past 3 months

RELATIVE CONTRAINDICATIONS

- History of chronic, severe, poorly controlled hypertension
- Severe uncontrolled hypertension on presentation (SBP >180 or DBP >100 mm Hg)
- History of prior ischemic stroke >3 months
- Dementia
- Known intracranial pathology not covered in contraindications
- Traumatic or prolonged CPR or major surgery in last 3 weeks
- Noncompressible vascular punctures
- Pregnancy
- Active peptic ulcer
- Current use of anticoagulants, the higher the INR the greater the risk
- Prior exposure (>5 days ago) to streptokinase/anistreplase
- Allergic reaction to streptokinase or anistreplase

---

urokinase plasminogen activator, and reteplase. For best efficacy, thrombolytic agents should be given within an hour after the onset of chest pain. However, new AHA guidelines advise that thrombolytic agents can still be given for up to 12 hours after the onset of chest pain. The choice of thrombolytic agent is not as important as the speed with which it is given. After the thrombolytic agent is administered, IV heparin or a glycoprotein IIb/IIIa is usually continued. All of these thrombolytic agents can be given intravenously.

Not all clients with AMI are suitable candidates for thrombolytic therapy (Box 58-2). History of recent cerebral vascular accident, surgery, pregnancy, and use of anticoagulants are contraindications for thrombolytic therapy. Complications of thrombolytics include bleeding, allergic reactions, and stroke. Successful reperfusion of the coronary arteries is evidenced by (1) return of ECG changes to normal, (2) relief of chest pain, (3) presence of reperfusion dysrhythmias, usually sudden onset of frequent premature ventricular contractions (PVCs) or short runs of PVCs, and (4) a rapid, early peak of the CK-MB isoenzyme ("washout"). If reperfusion is not attained or if the client is not a candidate for thrombolytic therapy, then primary angioplasty, stenting, or CABG may be performed. Interventional cardiology procedures and bypass surgery are discussed in Chapter 56. If ST elevation is present, reperfusion strategies are to be promptly initiated.[1] Guidelines suggest that thrombolytic therapy should be initiated within 30 minutes or PTCA should be initiated within 60 minutes. PTCA may be considered before thrombolytic therapy in institutions that have cardiac surgery capabilities, that have skilled physicians in PCTA, and that perform more than 200 PTCA procedures per year.

Antidysrhythmic agents are initiated. Clinicians begin beta-blockade and angiotensin-converting enzyme (ACE) inhibitors within 72 hours of onset to reduce ventricular remodeling and reduce mortality. Stool softeners are used to relieve constipation and to lower the risk of bradycardia from straining that stimulates the vagus nerve.

Determine the Location of the Myocardial Infarction

Determining the exact coronary vessel that has infarcted is done through analysis of the 12-lead ECG and is validated with coronary angiography to determine the degree of occlusion (expressed in percentage of blockage of each coronary artery). Determining the exact artery that is involved is important so potential complications can be assessed and minimized (Table 58-1). Knowledge of the area of the heart with infarct can prevent complications and allow diagnosis of AMI when ECG changes are not present.

Monitor for Complications

The possibility of death from complications always accompanies an AMI. Thus prime collaborative goals include the prevention of life-threatening complications or at least recognition of them.

Dysrhythmias. Dysrhythmias are the cause of 40% to 50% of deaths after AMI. Ectopic rhythms arise in or near the borders of intensely ischemic and damaged myocardial tissues. Damaged myocardium may also interfere with

the conduction system, causing dissociation of the atria and ventricles *(heart block).* Supraventricular tachycardia (SVT) sometimes occurs as a result of heart failure. Spontaneous or pharmacologic reperfusion of a previously ischemic area may also precipitate ventricular dysrhythmias.

Provide continuous cardiac monitoring and frequent counts of PVCs (many monitoring systems count continuously). Notify the physician if more than six PVCs occur per minute and the client is symptomatic (e.g., hypotension, chest pain). For *dysrhythmias,* provide prompt intervention per protocol or orders. For new-onset, symptomatic *ventricular ectopy* (runs, couplets), administer amiodarone or lidocaine per order or protocol. For *ventricular tachycardia,* administer amiodarone or lidocaine; if pulseless ventricular tachycardia occurs, provide synchronized cardioversion. For *ventricular fibrillation,* provide immediate defibrillation coupled with CPR and administration of epinephrine or vasopressin. For *supraventricular tachycardia (SVT),* administer a vagal maneuver, adenosine, diltiazem, or amiodarone,

---

TABLE 58–1 Clinical Manifestations Based on Location of Acute Myocardial Infarction

Area	ST-Segment Elevation and Q Waves on 12-Lead ECG	Common Dysrhythmias	Other Manifestations	Complications
Left anterior descending (LAD)	V_1-V_6 depending on branch	Ventricular tachycardia Bundle branch blocks (BBBs) Premature ventricular contractions (PVCs) Atrial fibrillation or flutter	Severe heart failure Low CO, BP Elevated pulmonary artery diastolic pressure (PAD), pulmonary capillary wedge pressure	Cardiogenic shock Myocardial rupture High mortality with this location
Circumflex/V_5	I, aV_L, V_5, V_6 ST depression of V_1-V_4 (reciprocal)	AV nodal blocks (especially Mobitz 1)	Heart failure and left ventricular dysfunction Bradycardia	Papillary muscle dysfunction Aneurysms
Right circumflex artery (RCA)	II, III, and aV_F	Premature atrial contractions (PACs) and atrial fibrillation Atrioventricular (AV) block (all types)	Hypotension resulting from decreased right ventricle ejection, especially when client is given nitroglycerin or morphine sulfate Requires large volumes of fluids to maintain BP	Ventricular tachycardia/ventricular fibrillation
Inferior wall	II, III, aV_F	Atrial dysrhythmias	Hiccups, nausea, vomiting	Papillary muscle rupture Septal rupture
Anterior wall	V_3, V_4	Second-degree AV block Sinus tachycardia		Cardiogenic shock Extension of infarct to lateral wall
Septal wall	V_1, V_2	Infranodal BBB and second- and third-degree heart block		Septal rupture
Lateral wall	I, aV_L, V_5, V_6	AV nodal blocks		Cardiogenic shock and heart failure
Posterior wall	ST-segment depression V_1-V_4	Bradycardia	Nausea	Papillary muscle dysfunction Aneurysms

The classic pattern of ECG changes with AMI begins with an abnormal T wave that is prolonged and peaked. This is followed within minutes by ST-segment elevation in the leads facing the area of injury with reciprocal changes of ST-segment depression in the opposite leads. Q-wave formation follows, and the Q-wave changes only disappear over months. The classic evolution of ST-segment elevation and Q-wave formation is often diagnostic of AMI. Knowledge of the area of the heart with infarct can prevent complications and allow diagnosis of AMI when ECG changes are not present.

BP, Blood pressure; *CO,* cardiac output.

and prepare for possible elective cardioversion. For *heart block or symptomatic bradycardia,* administer atropine and prepare for use a temporary pacemaker. Dysrhythmias are discussed in Chapter 57.

Cardiogenic Shock. Cardiogenic shock accounts for only 9% of deaths from AMI, but more than 70% of clients in shock die of it.[2] Causes include (1) decreased myocardial contraction with diminished cardiac output, (2) undetected dysrhythmias, and (3) sepsis. Clinical manifestations include systolic blood pressure significantly below the client's normal range, diaphoresis, rapid pulse, restlessness, cold and clammy skin, and grayish skin color. Shock can be prevented with sufficient IV fluids to prevent circulatory collapse and the identification of dysrhythmias.

Vasopressors are administered (dopamine, dobutamine) to raise blood pressure by increasing peripheral resistance. In other cases, vasodilators (nitroprusside, nitroglycerin) promote better blood flow in the microcirculation and reduce afterload. Positive inotropic agents (dobutamine, epinephrine, milrinone) increase cardiac contractility and cardiac output and improve tissue perfusion. Administer oxygen therapy and antidysrhythmic agents as prescribed, and continuously monitor arterial and pulmonary artery pressures. Analgesics such as morphine sulfate should be given to ensure client comfort. Chapter 81 explains shock in detail.

Heart Failure and Pulmonary Edema. The most common cause of in-hospital death in clients with cardiac disorders is heart failure. Heart failure disables 22% of male clients and 46% of female clients who experience an AMI and is responsible for one third of deaths after an AMI.

Heart failure may develop at the onset of the infarction or may occur weeks later. Clinical manifestations include dyspnea, orthopnea, weight gain, edema, enlarged tender liver, distended neck veins, and crackles. It is managed by correcting the underlying cause, relieving clinical manifestations, and enhancing cardiac pump performance.[22,24,27] Heart failure is discussed in Chapter 56, in the Case Study feature above, right, and on the website.

Pulmonary Embolism. Pulmonary embolism (PE) may develop secondary to phlebitis of the leg or pelvic veins (venous thrombosis) or from atrial flutter or fibrillation. PE occurs in 10% to 20% of clients at some point, during either the acute attack or convalescence. PE is discussed in Chapter 61.

Recurrent Myocardial Infarction. Within 6 years after an initial AMI, 18% of men and 35% of women may experience recurrent MI. Possible causes include overexertion, embolization, and further thrombotic occlusion of a

CASE STUDY

Cardiogenic Shock, Tachycardia, and Heart Failure

Mr. Borg is a 70-year-old retired African-American man who was admitted to the emergency department (ED) after arriving by rescue squad. According to his wife, he had been vomiting and experiencing progressive weakness earlier in the day. When the rescue squad arrived at his home, he was in supraventricular tachycardia with a heart rate more than 180 beats/min. The squad administered adenosine (Adenocard) 6 mg IV, followed by an additional 12 mg 3 minutes later. En route he denied chest pain or shortness of breath, but he was becoming cyanotic and his heart rhythm was again becoming tachycardic. . . . *Case Study continued on the website and the CD-ROM with discussions, multiple-choice questions, and a nursing care plan.*

coronary artery by an atheroma. The clinical manifestation is the return of angina. Management is the same as that for AMI.

Complications Caused by Myocardial Necrosis. Complications that are due to necrosis of the myocardium include ventricular aneurysm, rupture of the heart *(myocardial rupture),* ventricular septal defect (VSD), and ruptured papillary muscle. These complications are infrequent but serious, usually occurring about 5 to 7 days after MI. Weak, friable necrotic myocardial tissue increases vulnerability to these complications (Figure 58-7).

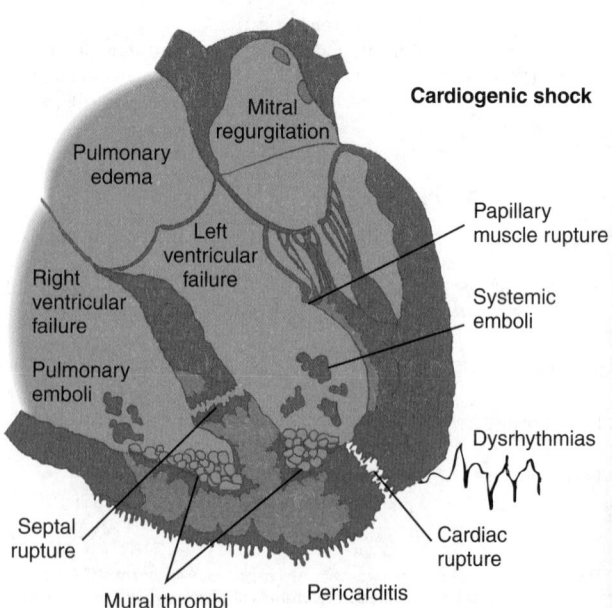

FIGURE 58–7 Major complications of acute myocardial infarction.

Manifestations of heart failure develop with ventricular aneurysm, rupture of the ventricular septum, and rupture of the papillary muscle. Manifestations of severe mitral insufficiency often develop when the papillary muscle of the left ventricle ruptures. Ventricular dysrhythmias (e.g., frequent PVCs and ventricular tachycardia) occur often in the presence of a ventricular aneurysm (the necrotic tissue is very irritable). Manifestations of cardiac tamponade develop with rupture of the heart.

The goal of treatment is to decrease the workload of the heart and increase the oxygen supply to keep the area of infarction and necrotic tissue as small as possible. Surgery is performed to (1) excise the ventricular aneurysm, (2) replace the mitral valve if the papillary muscle is ruptured, or (3) repair the VSD. Pericardiocentesis and immediate surgery help relieve cardiac tamponade that occurs after rupture of the heart.

Pericarditis. In up to 28% of clients with an acute transmural MI, early pericarditis develops (within 2 to 4 days). The inflamed area of the infarction rubs against the pericardial surface and causes it to lose its lubricating fluid. A pericardial friction rub can be auscultated across the precordium. The client complains that chest pain is worse with movement, deep inspiration, and cough. The pain of pericarditis is relieved by sitting up and leaning forward.

Frequent assessment may lead to early identification and intervention. Relieve pain with analgesics, such as acetaminophen, nonsteroidal anti-inflammatory drugs (NSAIDs), or other anti-inflammatory agents. Reduce the client's anxiety by differentiating the pain of pericarditis from the pain of AMI.

Dressler's Syndrome (Late Pericarditis). Dressler's syndrome, a form of pericarditis, can occur as late as 6 weeks to months after AMI. Although the etiologic agent is unknown, an autoimmune cause is suggested. The client usually presents with a fever lasting 1 week or longer, pericardial chest pain, pericardial friction rub, and occasionally pleuritis with pleural effusions. This is a self-limiting phenomenon, and no prevention is known. Treatment includes aspirin, prednisone, and opioid analgesics for pain. Anticoagulation therapy may precipitate cardiac tamponade and should be avoided in these clients.

Nursing Management of the Medical Client

The goals of nursing management after AMI are as follows:

- Recognize and treat cardiac ischemia.
- Administer thrombolytic therapy as ordered, or ready client for PTCA and observe for complications.
- Recognize and treat potentially life-threatening dysrhythmias.

- Monitor for complications of reduced cardiac output.
- Maintain a therapeutic critical care environment.
- Identify the psychosocial impact of AMI on the client and family.
- Educate the client in lifestyle changes and rehabilitation.
- A care plan on care of the client with AMI lists specific nursing diagnoses, interventions with rationale and evaluation outcomes.

Rehabilitation and Education

Cardiac rehabilitation following AMI is an essential component of professional and personal management. The following are recommendations for managing rehabilitation of clients who have suffered an AMI:

- All clients with cardiovascular disease should adopt a cardioprotective dietary pattern.
- Intensive dietary advice, compliance checks, and long-term follow-up should be given, preferably by a dietitian.
- There is insufficient evidence to recommend nutritional supplements of antioxidant vitamins, minerals, or trace elements for the prevention of cardiovascular disease.
- Fish and fish oil supplements may reduce the risk of sudden cardiac death.
- For overweight and obese clients with CHD, the combination of reduced-carbohydrate diet and increased physical activity is recommended.
- Initial goal of weight loss therapy should be to reduce the client's weight by 10%.
- All clients with cardiovascular disease should be advised to quit smoking and should be supported to stop smoking as a priority measure.
- All clients with CHD should consider having standard pharmacotherapy with aspirin, beta-blocker, ACE inhibitor, and a statin unless contraindicated.
- Comprehensive cardiac rehabilitation should embrace a case management approach.

Strengthen the Myocardium. A successful rehabilitation program begins the moment the client enters the coronary care unit for emergency care and continues for months and even years after discharge from the health care facility. The overall goal of rehabilitation is to help the client live as full, vital, and productive a life as possible while remaining within the limits of the heart's ability to respond to increases in activity and stress. Six important subgoals of the rehabilitation process are as follows:

- Developing a program of progressive physical activity
- Educating the client and significant others about the cause, prevention, and treatment of CHD
- Helping the client accept the limitations imposed by illness

- Aiding the client in adjusting to changes in occupational goals
- Lessening the exposure to risk factors
- Changing the psychosocial factors adversely affecting recovery from CHD

Cardiac rehabilitation is a comprehensive, long-term program that involves periodic medical evaluation, prescribed exercises, and education and counseling about cardiac risk factor modification. Cardiac rehabilitation is a multifactorial program that begins when the client is still hospitalized and continues throughout recovery. Cardiac rehabilitation consists of four phases: phase I (inpatient), phase II (immediate outpatient), phase III (intermediate outpatient), and phase IV (maintenance outpatient).

Phase I (Inpatient). Phase I begins with admission to the coronary care unit. After AMI, clients usually remain on bed rest for less than 24 hours unless complications such as heart failure or dysrhythmias develop. Although the myocardium must rest, bed rest puts the client at risk for hypovolemia, hypoxemia, muscle atrophy, and pulmonary embolus. Thus the client must avoid both invalidism and reckless overexertion. These considerations are outlined in the Care Plan on pp. 1502-1509. Case managers may be assigned to coordinate care. See the Case Management feature on Acute Myocardial Infarction on the website.

Provide complete bed rest for the first day or two with use of a bedside commode for bowel movements. Most clients receive a 2-g sodium diet. If the client is nauseated, provide a clear liquid diet until nausea subsides. A coronary care nurse or physiotherapist should start passive exercises. As the client regains strength, have the client sit for brief periods on the side of the bed and dangle the feet. Allow the client to ambulate to a bedside chair for 15 to 20 minutes after the first day if dangling has been tolerated without development of chest pain, dysrhythmias, or hypotension. When the client is transferred from the coronary care unit to an intermediate or regular unit, bathroom privileges and self-care activities are encouraged. Wireless heart monitoring (telemetry) may continue. Allow brief walks in the hall with supervision. The length and duration of these walks are increased progressively, working up to 5 to 10 minutes according to the client's endurance. The client loses 10% to 15% of skeletal muscle and contractile strength within the first week of bed rest and 20% to 25% after 3 weeks of bed rest. The client must increase activities gradually to avoid overtaxing the heart as it pumps oxygenated blood to the muscles. The metabolic equivalent test (MET) provides one way of measuring the amount of oxygen needed to perform an activity:

$$1 \text{ MET} = 3.5 \text{ ml of } O_2/\text{kg/min}$$

One MET is about equivalent to the oxygen uptake a client requires when resting. Early mobilization activities after AMI should not exceed 1 to 2 METs, as from shaving, washing, and self-feeding. (Later activities can increase to 10 or 11 METs, such as cycling or running.)

With each activity level increase, monitor the heart rate, blood pressure, and fatigue level, adjusting the client's activity level accordingly. During early activities, the heart rate should not increase more than 25% above resting level. Blood pressure must not increase more than 25 mm Hg above normal.

Help the client avoid fatigue. Dyspnea, chest pain, tachycardia, and a sense of exhaustion warn that the client is attempting to do too much. Instruct the client regarding these warning signs of overexertion. Include family members in these discussions; family members may fear that allowing the client to become active again will precipitate another AMI and while attempting to help, they may discourage autonomy.

During phase I, client education should include cardiac anatomy and physiology risk factors and management of CHD, behavioral counseling, and home activities.

Phase II (Immediate Outpatient). If no complications arise, the physician discharges the client to the home after a week. Nearly 50% of clients after AMI have an uncomplicated hospital course without evidence of angina, heart failure, or major dysrhythmias. There is a growing trend toward early discharge of clients with uncomplicated AMI. A team at one health care facility discharges post-AMI clients at the end of the fourth day but allows clients to go home early only if the household has adequate help and is conducive to rest. Such clients are followed up carefully by trained nurse-clinicians who visit the home and supervise physiologic status, exercise, and diet every other day. The Bridge to Home Health Care feature on p. 1501 discusses how to promote heart-healthy living after an AMI. Researchers believe that earlier discharge after AMI reduces depression as well as hospital expenses.

Resuming sexual activity may be one of the most difficult aspects of returning to normal life after AMI. Sexual intercourse usually may resume 4 to 8 weeks after an AMI. The client should be able to climb two flights of stairs before resuming sexual activity. Caution clients not to eat or drink alcoholic beverages immediately before intercourse. Taking nitroglycerin before intercourse may help prevent exertional angina. However, clients cannot take sildenafil (Viagra) while taking nitroglycerin; both medications are vasodilators.

Advise the client to stop smoking. Encourage frequent walks, but warn against strenuous activities, such as shoveling snow. The walking program aims for a goal of 2 miles in less than 60 minutes.

Heart-Healthy Living After an Acute Myocardial Infarction

The role of the home health nurse is to teach heart-healthy living to clients who had an AMI so that they can adjust their lifestyle. Focus your teaching on areas that will help clients become responsible for self-care. Assume that you need to repeat health education that was provided in the hospital during the AMI episode. When stress is high, clients usually recall little of what was taught.

Instruct the client and significant other or family member to monitor for clinical manifestations that may indicate extensions and recurrences of the AMI. Clients need to report indigestion, shortness of breath, increased edema, and palpitations. Learning when to call the physician or nurse for these physical problems is important.

Determine what your clients know about their medications. Knowing what the medication is called, its function, the schedule for taking it, and its side effects is required for client safety. Generally, multiple medications are prescribed, and you need to give the client written instructions and information about each medication. Many pharmacists provide a computer printout of medications and interactions for the client to keep. Medication planners that have compartments for various times of day allow the client to prefill medications for a week at a time and may prevent errors.

The convalescence period for the client and family creates anxiety about daily activities. Instruct the client to avoid prolonged baths or showers to prevent vasodilation. Use tepid water and a stool or bath chair in the shower. Encourage the use of energy-conservation techniques, such as keeping the arms at waist level and getting enough rest to prevent fatigue. Routine household activities and mild recreational activities, such as playing golf, are usually permitted.

Climbing more than two flights of stairs and lifting more than 20 pounds are restricted. If clients do not ask about resuming sexual relations, consider introducing the topic. They may be too timid to consult their physicians about this subject.

An appropriate unsupervised exercise is a prescribed indoor walking program. Exercising after a heavy meal or during mild illness is contraindicated. Instruct the client to begin each exercise session with a warm-up period that may last as long as 15 minutes and to end the session with a cool-down period. Walking should be constant and should last long enough to increase blood flow to the muscles.

The client or caregiver should have an emergency plan that includes having someone available to drive if a ride is needed and someone in the home who knows basic cardiopulmonary resuscitation (CPR). A personal emergency response system may be appropriate for clients who live alone. Some emergency response systems are worn around the neck, and the push of a button summons medical assistance. Caregiver stress, communication problems, and fear of the unknown are valid concerns. Community resources and additional information can be obtained by calling the American Heart Association's toll-free number: 1-800-242-8721.

A monitored group program may help the client achieve the best possible physical conditioning. These programs typically last from 10 to 12 weeks and are implemented in a supervised setting. They offer various training devices, such as treadmills, stationary bicycles, and rowing machines. During phase II, the client performs large-muscle exercises for at least 20 to 30 minutes three or four times a week. In addition, clients are trained in warm-up and stretching exercises. During the sessions, cardiac rehabilitation staff monitors cardiac rhythm, heart rate, and blood pressure before exercise, at peak exercise, and during recovery. Clients also report their level of perceived exertion several times during the exercise session.

Some clients may be able to return to work at the end of 8 or 9 weeks if they remain asymptomatic. Clients with less physically strenuous jobs can sometimes resume a full-time schedule, but manual laborers may have to work part time or find less taxing work. Occupational evaluations can be done to assess cardiac impairment in relation to job requirements and client skills.

Between the eighth and tenth weeks, the client requires a complete physical examination, including ECG, exercise stress tests, lipid analysis, and chest x-ray study. Clinicians must correct pre-existing health problems that might have contributed to the development of CHD (e.g., hypertension, anemia, hyperthyroidism).

Recovery after AMI may be lengthy and difficult. The client may have undergone surgery or may have been managed medically. In either case, a serious threat to integrity has occurred. Initially after AMI, clients may attempt to prove that they are not seriously ill. Coping strategies include denial and minimization. Some clients conceal the recurrence of chest pain. As recovery continues, clients begin to comprehend that a heart attack has really occurred, to understand why it happened, and to consider its impact on the future. Clients begin the process of life adjustment to find a lifestyle that can be tolerated and maintained while preserving a sense of self-worth. Several strategies are used to regain self-control, such as gauging progress, seeking reassurance, learning about health, and being cautious. Eventually, most clients come to terms with the fact that they will not be living life to the fullest. Clients learn to accept limitations and to refocus on other aspects of life. Some clients are unable to adjust. Sometimes clients find that they have had too many setbacks and are powerless to make changes or gain control. The education and counseling that accompany a structured cardiac rehabilitation program can help improve psychological well-being, social adjustment, and functioning.

Phase III (Intermediate Outpatient). The extended outpatient phase of cardiac rehabilitation lasts from 4 to 6 months. Exercise sessions continue to be supervised, and clients are taught how to monitor their exercise intensity by measuring their pulse rate or, if in a walking

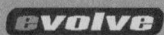
The Client with Acute Myocardial Infarction

Nursing Diagnosis: Acute Pain related to myocardial ischemia resulting from coronary artery occlusion with loss or restriction of blood flow to an area of the myocardium and necrosis of the myocardium.

Outcomes: The client will experience improved comfort in the chest, as evidenced by a decrease in the pain rating, the ability to rest and sleep comfortably, have less need for analgesia or nitroglycerin, and have reduced anxiety.

NOC OUTCOMES	Comfort Level, Pain Control, Pain: Disruptive Effects, Pain Level

Interventions	NIC INTERVENTIONS	Rationales
1. Assess the characteristics of chest pain, including location, duration, quality, intensity, presence of radiation, precipitating and alleviating factors, and associated manifestations. Have the client rate pain on a scale of 0 to 10, and document findings in nurses' notes.	Pain Management Cardiac Care: Acute	1. Pain is an indication of myocardial ischemia. Assisting the client in quantifying pain may differentiate pre-existing and current pain patterns as well as identify complications. Usually a scale of 0 to 10 is used, with 10 being the worst pain and 0 being none.
2. Assess respirations, blood pressure, and heart rate with each episode of chest pain.	Cardiac Care: Acute	2. Respirations may be increased as a result of pain and associated anxiety. Release of stress-induced catecholamines increases heart rate and blood pressure.
3. Obtain a 12-lead electrocardiogram (ECG) on admission and then each time chest pain recurs for evidence of further infarction.	Cardiac Care: Acute	3. Serial ECGs and stat ECGs record changes that can give evidence of further cardiac damage and location of myocardial ischemia.
4. Monitor the response to drug therapy. Notify the physician if pain does not abate within 15-20 minutes.	Pain Management Analgesic Administration	4. Pain control is a priority because it indicates ischemia.
5. Provide care in a calm, efficient manner that reassures the client and minimizes anxiety. Stay with the client until discomfort is relieved.	Cardiac Care: Acute Anxiety Reduction	5. External stimuli may worsen anxiety and increase cardiac workload as well as limit coping abilities.
6. Limit visitors as the client requests.	Cardiac Care: Acute Anxiety Reduction	6. Limiting visitors prevents overstimulation and promotes rest.
7. Administer morphine as ordered.	Pain Management Analgesic Administration	7. Morphine is an opiate analgesic and alters the client's perception of pain and reduces preload time vasoconstriction.
8. Administer nitrates as ordered.	Cardiac Care: Acute Medication Administration	8. Nitrates relax the smooth muscles of coronary blood vessels, decreasing ischemia and hence decreasing pain.

Evaluation: The client should be pain-free within 15 to 20 minutes after administration of drug therapy. The client will verbalize relief of pain and will not exhibit associated manifestations of pain.

Nursing Diagnosis: Ineffective Tissue Perfusion (Cardiopulmonary) related to thrombus in coronary artery, resulting in altered blood flow to myocardial tissue.

Outcomes: The client will demonstrate improved cardiac tissue perfusion, as evidenced by a decrease in the rating of pain and resolving ST segments.

NOC OUTCOMES	Cardiac Pump Effectiveness, Circulation Status

Interventions	NIC INTERVENTIONS	Rationales
1. Keep the client on bed rest with a quiet environment.	Cardiac Care: Acute Hemodynamic Regulation, Circulatory Care: Arterial Insufficiency	1. Stress activates the sympathetic nervous system and increases myocardial oxygen needs.
2. Administer oxygen as ordered.	Cardiac Care: Acute Hemodynamic Regulation, Circulatory Care: Arterial Insufficiency	2. Oxygen increases myocardial supply of oxygen.
3. Administer thrombolytics or send the client for angioplasty as ordered.	Cardiac Care: Acute Circulatory Care: Arterial Insufficiency Medication Administration	3. Thrombolytic therapy or angioplasty can break apart the thrombus and increase myocardial tissue perfusion.
4. Monitor ST segments.	Cardiac Care: Acute Dysrhythmia Management	4. ST-segment elevation indicates myocardial tissue injury; ST-segment depression indicates decreased myocardial perfusion.

Evaluation: The return of ST segments to baseline is dependent on the degree of ischemia and rapidity of treatment.

Collaborative Problem: Dysrhythmias related to electrical instability or irritability secondary to ischemia or infarcted tissue, as evidenced by an increase or decrease in heart rate, change in rhythm, and atrial or ventricular dysrhythmias.

Outcomes: The client will have no dysrhythmias, as evidenced by normal sinus rhythm or return to the client's own baseline rhythm.

| NOC OUTCOMES | Cardiac Pump Effectiveness, Circulation Status (NOC) |

Interventions	NIC INTERVENTIONS	Rationales
1. Teach the client and family about the need for continuous monitoring. Keep alarms on and limits set at all times.	Dysrhythmia Management Cardiac Care: Acute Anxiety Management	1. Continued monitoring keeps staff aware of rhythm changes. Family anxiety is decreased when explanations are provided.
2. Assess the apical heart rate. Auscultate for change in heart sounds (murmurs, rub, S_3, and S_4).	Dysrhythmia Management Cardiac Care: Acute Circulatory Care: Arterial Insufficiency	2. The apical heart rate suggests early cardiac decompensation and potential loss of cardiac output.
3. Document the rhythm strip every shift and prn (as needed) if dysrhythmias occur. Measure the pulse rate, QRS, PR, and QT segments with each strip. Note and report any deviations from the client's baseline values.	Dysrhythmia Management Cardiac Care: Acute Circulatory Care: Arterial Insufficiency	3. Dysrhythmias are the most common complication after AMI.
4. Report six or more multifocal premature ventricular contractions (PVCs) per minute to the physician.	Dysrhythmia Management Cardiac Care: Acute Circulatory Care: Arterial Insufficiency	4. Multifocal PVCs indicate ventricular irritability, which decreases cardiac output and may lead to life-threatening dysrhythmias.
5. Give antidysrhythmic agents as ordered.	Dysrhythmia Management Cardiac Care: Acute Medication Administration	5. Antidysrhythmic drugs reduce myocardial irritability.
6. Monitor the effects of antidysrhythmic agents.	Dysrhythmia Management Cardiac Care: Acute Medication Administration	6. The desired results are increased diastolic threshold potential and decreased action potential duration.
7. Monitor serum potassium levels.	Dysrhythmia Management Cardiac Care: Acute	7. Altered potassium levels can affect cardiac rhythms.
8. Maintain a patent intravenous (IV) line or heparin lock at all times.	Dysrhythmia Management Cardiac Care: Acute Medication Administration	8. This measure is for emergency administration of IV cardiac medications.
9. Monitor ST segments, and document changes.	Dysrhythmia Management Cardiac Care: Acute	9. ST depression indicates myocardial ischemia, and ST elevation indicates injury; either may precipitate dysrhythmias.

Evaluation: Within 24 hours of admission, the client's cardiac rhythm will remain stable and the client will exhibit no manifestations of rhythm disturbance.

Nursing Diagnosis: Decreased Cardiac Output related to negative inotropic changes in the heart secondary to myocardial ischemia, injury, or infarction, as evidenced by change in the level of consciousness, weakness, dizziness, loss of peripheral pulses, abnormal heart sounds, hemodynamic compromise, and cardiopulmonary arrest.

Outcomes: The client will have improved cardiac output as evidenced by normal cardiac rate, rhythm, and hemodynamic parameters; dysrhythmias controlled or absent; and absence of angina.

| NOC OUTCOMES | Cardiac Pump Effectiveness, Circulation Status |

Interventions	NIC INTERVENTIONS	Rationales

Assess for and document the following as evidence of myocardial dysfunction with decreasing cardiac output:

Interventions	NIC INTERVENTIONS	Rationales
1. Mental status—be alert to restlessness and decreased responsiveness.	Cardiac Care: Acute, Hemodynamic Regulation Acid-Base Management Shock Management: Cardiac	1. Cerebral perfusion is directly related to cardiac output and aortic perfusion pressure and is influenced by hypoxia and electrolyte and acid-base variations.
2. Lung sounds—monitor for crackles and rhonchi.	Shock Management: Cardiac Cardiac Care: Acute, Hemodynamic Regulation Airway Management	2. Crackles may develop, reflecting pulmonary congestion related to alterations in myocardial function.
3. Blood pressure—monitor for hypertension or hypotension.	Shock Management: Cardiac Cardiac Care: Acute, Hemodynamic Regulation	3. Hypotension related to hypoperfusion, vagal stimulation, dysrhythmias, or ventricular dysfunction may occur; it may be related to pain, anxiety, catecholamine release, or pre-existing vascular problems.
4. Heart sounds—note the presence of gallop, murmur, and increased or decreased heart rate.	Shock Management: Cardiac Cardiac Care: Hemodynamic Regulation	4. Bradycardia may be present because of vagal stimulation or conduction disturbances related to the area of myocardial injury. Tachycardia may be a compensatory mechanism related to decreased cardiac output. A gallop may be related to fluid volume overload or heart failure, and a murmur may be present if ruptured chordae tendineae occurred.

(Continued)

C A R E P L A N *evolve*

The Client with Acute Myocardial Infarction—Cont'd

5. Urine output—be alert to output less than 0.5 ml/kg/hr.	Shock Management: Cardiac, Hemodynamic Regulation Circulatory Care: Arterial Insufficiency	5. Urine output less than 0.5 ml/kg/hr may reflect reduced renal perfusion and glomerular filtration as a result of reduced cardiac output.
6. Peripheral perfusion— monitor for pallor, mottling, cyanosis, coolness, diaphoresis, and peripheral pulses.	Shock Management: Cardiac, Hemodynamic Regulation Circulatory Care: Arterial Insufficiency	6. Decreased peripheral pulses may indicate a decrease in cardiac output.
7. Monitor arterial blood gas (ABG) levels.	Shock Management: Cardiac, Hemodynamic Regulation, Acid-Base Management	7. Acidosis may cause dysrhythmias and depressed cardiac function and some cardiac medications increase oxygen demand and may cause hypoxia.
8. If a pulmonary artery catheter is used, record hemodynamic parameters every 2 to 4 hours and as required (prn). Be alert to pulmonary capillary wedge pressure (PCWP) greater than 18 mm Hg, cardiac output less than 4 L/min, and cardiac index less than 2.5 L/min.	Shock Management: Cardiac, Hemodynamic Regulation	8. A PCWP greater than 18 mm Hg may indicate fluid volume overload or heart failure. A cardiac output less than 4 L/min and a cardiac index less than 2.5 L/min indicate heart failure or decrease in cardiac output. Use hemodynamic monitoring to assess drug therapy and for prevention or early detection of complications of AMI (i.e., extension, heart failure, cardiogenic shock).
9. Maintain hemodynamic stability by monitoring the effects of beta-blockers and inotropic agents.	Shock Management: Cardiac, Hemodynamic Regulation, Medication Management	9. Assess the effect of drug therapy on myocardial contractility and function.
10. Monitor and assess angina for type, severity, and duration.	Shock Management: Cardiac, Hemodynamic Regulation	10. Angina indicates myocardial ischemia, which may decrease cardiac output.

Evaluation: Within 2 to 3 days of admission, the client should have normal hemodynamic pressures, normal vital signs, clear breath sounds, no shortness of breath, normal ABG values, and normal sinus rhythm with rate between 60 and 100 beats/min.

Nursing Diagnosis: Impaired Gas Exchange related to decreased cardiac output, as evidenced by cyanosis, impaired capillary refill, reduced arterial oxygen tension (Pao_2), and dyspnea.

Outcomes: Tissue Perfusion: The client will demonstrate improved gas exchange, as evidenced by absence of cyanosis, brisk capillary refill, absence of dyspnea, and ABG levels within normal limits.

NOC OUTCOMES Pulmonary

Interventions	NIC INTERVENTIONS	Rationales
1. Administer oxygen as ordered; maintain continuous oximetry.	Oxygen Therapy Respiratory Monitoring	1. Increases amount of oxygen available for myocardial uptake; measures peripheral oxygen saturation.
2. Monitor ABGs as ordered.	Oxygen Therapy Respiratory Monitoring Acid-Base Management	2. The presence of hypoxia indicates a need for supplemental oxygen. Monitoring provides data on the adequacy of tissue perfusion and oxygenation.
3. Continue to assess the client's skin, capillary refill, and level of consciousness every 2-4 hours and prn.	Respiratory Monitoring Cardiac Care	3. Cyanosis (circumoral or in extremities) indicates hypoxia. Capillary refill greater than 3 seconds indicates poor perfusion and possibly hypoxia.
4. Assess respiratory status for dyspnea and crackles.	Oxygen Therapy Respiratory Monitoring	4. Dyspnea may indicate inadequate oxygenation, and the presence of crackles may impair gas exchange because of decreased exchange of oxygen and carbon dioxide through fluid in alveoli.
5. Prepare for intubation and mechanical ventilation if hypoxia increases.	Oxygen Therapy Respiratory Monitoring Airway Management	5. With increasing hypoxia, mechanical ventilation may be necessary to oxygenate the client adequately.

Evaluation: Within 2 to 3 days of admission, client's breath sounds will be clear, and ABG values will be within normal limits.

Collaborative Problem: Risk for Bleeding related to coagulopathies associated with thrombolytic therapy or arterial puncture after angioplasty.

Outcomes: The nurse will monitor for bleeding and reduce bleeding risk. If bleeding does occur, it will be recognized and treated at once.

NOC OUTCOMES   Blood Loss Severity

Interventions	NIC INTERVENTIONS	Rationales
1. Obtain coagulation studies as ordered. Follow protocols for adjustments of anticoagulants	Bleeding Precautions	1. Coagulation studies can help determine the tendency to bleed and if adjustments in anticoagulant medications are needed.
2. Monitor invasive line sites for active bleeding.	Bleeding Precautions	2. Thrombolytic therapy disrupts the normal coagulation process, and bleeding may occur at any invasive site.
3. Inspect all body fluids for presence of blood.	Bleeding Precautions	3. Internal bleeding may be manifested in urine, sputum, and gastrointestinal drainage.
4. Hold pressure on any discontinued lines for 15 minutes; if arterial, hold for 30 minutes.	Bleeding Precautions, Bleeding Reduction	4. Pressure is used to achieve hemostasis at catheter sites.
5. If the client has had an angioplasty, monitor puncture site frequently for hemorrhage.	Bleeding Precautions	5. Active bleeding may occur after angioplasty.
6. Observe neurologic status.	Bleeding Precautions	6. A change in neurologic status may indicate intracranial bleeding.
7. Avoid intramuscular (IM) injections.	Bleeding Precautions, Bleeding Reduction	7. IM injections may cause bleeding.
8. Assess for back or flank pain.	Bleeding Precautions	8. Flank or back pain may suggest retroperitoneal bleeding.
9. Keep IV line patent.	Bleeding Precautions, Bleeding Reduction Fluid Management Hypovolemia Management	9. In case of active bleeding, a patent line must be maintained to transfuse blood products.
10. Maintain an active type and crossmatch on the client.	Bleeding Precautions, Bleeding Reduction Fluid Management Hypovolemia Management	10. If the client requires blood or blood products, an active type and crossmatch helps eliminate any delay in treatment.

Evaluation: The nurse will monitor for and prevent bleeding.

Nursing Diagnosis: Powerlessness related to a near-death experience and anticipated lifestyle changes, as evidenced by verbalized "feelings of doom," crying, and anger.

Outcomes: The client will regain a sense of "control," as evidenced by feeling able to express feelings of powerlessness over the present situation and future outcomes.

NOC OUTCOMES   Fear Level

Interventions	NIC INTERVENTIONS	Rationales
1. Provide opportunities for the client to express feelings about oneself and the illness.	Coping Enhancement	1. These opportunities create a supportive climate and send the message that caregivers are willing to help.
2. Explore reality perceptions, and clarify if necessary.	Coping Enhancement	2. Listening to the client's feelings and words can help the client acquire a more hopeful outlook.
3. Eliminate the unpredictability of events by allowing adequate preparation for tests and procedures.	Coping Enhancement Anxiety Reduction	3. Information helps the client and family feel more hopeful and be more willing to participate in care.
4. Reinforce the client's right to ask questions.	Coping Enhancement	4. Maintain a supportive climate to let the client feel free to ask questions or have information repeated.
5. Allow choices when possible.	Coping Enhancement Decision-Making Support	5. Self-care allows the client to feel independent.
6. Provide positive reinforcement for increased involvement in self-care.	Coping Enhancement	6. When clients participate in planning for care, they are more likely to feel a sense of control and to follow through with actions.
7. Help the client identify strengths and areas of control.	Coping Enhancement	7. Self-confidence and security come with a sense of control; foster full client participation.

Evaluation: Within 24 hours of admission, client will verbalize a feeling of control over the situation and will actively participate in decisions regarding care.

(Continued)

CARE PLAN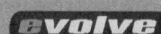

The Client with Acute Myocardial Infarction—Cont'd

Nursing Diagnosis: Anxiety and Fear related to hospital admission and fear of death, as evidenced by client and family appearing restless, hostile, or withdrawn; client and family verbalize fatalism or act extremely emotional as if in the grieving process.

Outcomes: The client will have reduced feelings of anxiety and fear, as evidenced by demonstrating appropriate range of feelings and initial manifestations of effective coping (participating in the treatment regimen), being able to rest, and asking fewer questions.

NOC OUTCOMES Anxiety Level

Interventions	NIC INTERVENTIONS	Rationales
1. Limit nursing personnel; provide continuity of care.	Anxiety Reduction Coping Enhancement	1. Continuity of care promotes security and development of rapport with and trust of health care providers.
2. Allow and encourage the client and family to ask questions; do not avoid questions. Bring up common concerns.	Anxiety Reduction Coping Enhancement Decision-Making Support	2. Accurate information about the situation reduces fear, strengthens the client-nurse relationship, and assists the client and family to face the situation realistically.
3. Allow the client and family to verbalize fears.	Anxiety Reduction Coping Enhancement Decision-Making Support	3. Sharing information elicits support and comfort and can relieve tension and unexpressed worries.
4. Stress that frequent assessments are routine and do not necessarily imply a deteriorating condition.	Anxiety Reduction	4. The client may feel reassured after learning that frequent assessments may prevent development of more serious complications.
5. Repeat information as necessary because of the reduced attention span of the client and family.	Anxiety Reduction	5. The client's attention span is short, and time perception may be altered. Anxiety decreases learning and attention.
6. Provide a comfortable, quiet environment for the client and family.	Anxiety Reduction Coping Enhancement	6. A comfortable environment enhances coping mechanisms and reduces myocardial workload and oxygen consumption.

Evaluation: Coping is very individualized. Base the timing of outcomes on the client's demonstrated behaviors and statements.

Nursing Diagnosis: Risk for Constipation related to bed rest, pain medications, and NPO (nothing by mouth) or soft diet, as evidenced by subjective feeling of fullness, abdominal cramping, painful defecation, and palpable impaction.

Outcomes: The client will have improved bowel elimination, as evidenced by eliminating a stool without straining or having a vasovagal response (bradycardia).

NOC OUTCOMES Bowel Elimination

Interventions	NIC INTERVENTIONS	Rationales
1. Ensure that the client has adequate bulk in diet and adequate fluid intake (without violating fluid restrictions).	Constipation/Impaction Management	1. Bulk and fluid within the colon prevent straining.
2. Monitor the effectiveness of softeners or laxatives. Instruct the client on prevention of straining and avoiding Valsalva (vasovagal) maneuver.	Constipation/Impaction Management Medication Management	2. Stool softeners decrease the myocardial workload of straining. The Valsalva maneuver causes bradycardia, decreasing the cardiac output.
3. Encourage the client to use a bedside commode rather than a bedpan.	Constipation/Impaction Management	3. Use of bedpans necessitates more straining and increases the vasovagal response.

Evaluation: Within 2 to 3 days of admission, client should have normal bowel function.

Nursing Diagnosis: Ineffective Health Maintenance related to AMI and implications for lifestyle changes.

Outcomes: The client and family will learn about the medical regimen and lifestyle changes, as evidenced by verbalizing an understanding of a heart attack and the necessary lifestyle changes regarding diet, medications, stress reduction, quitting smoking, and cholesterol, weight, and blood pressure reduction.

NOC OUTCOMES Knowledge: Treatment Regimen

Interventions	NIC INTERVENTIONS	Rationales
1. Explain the following, providing both oral and written instructions: anatomy and functions of heart muscle and atherosclerotic process; definition of a "heart attack"; healing process of the heart; and role of collateral circulation.	Teaching: Disease Process, Coping Enhancement	1. Use of multiple learning methods enhances retention of material; information helps the client understand the underlying coronary arteries, problems of overall heart functions.

2. Assist the client with identifying personal risk factors.	Teaching: Disease Process, Coping Enhancement	2. Risk factor identification is the first step before changes can be implemented.
3. Assist the client in devising a plan for risk factor modification (e.g., diet; smoking cessation; cholesterol, stress, and blood pressure reduction).	Teaching: Disease Process, Coping Enhancement Decision-Making Support	3. This information is helpful in providing opportunity for the client to identify risk factors, assume control, and participate in treatment regimen.
4. Provide guidelines for a diet low in cholesterol and saturated fat. Arrange for dietary consultation before hospital discharge.	Teaching: Prescribed Diet, Coping Enhancement	4. Consultation with other health professionals enhances client learning from others. Guidelines developed with the client and family before discharge help once they are home.
5. Teach the client and family about medications that will be taken after hospital discharge (name, purpose, dosage, schedule, precautions, potential side effects).	Teaching: Prescribed Medications, Coping Enhancement	5. The more clients understand the medical regimen and potential side effects, the more adept they will be in monitoring for them.
6. Discuss post-AMI activity progression; arrange for a cardiac rehabilitation consultation.	Teaching: Prescribed Activity/Exercise, Coping Enhancement	6. Continued follow-up will let clients know how they are doing; outpatient cardiac rehabilitation supports and assists clients in the lifestyle changes necessary for a healthy recovery and life.
7. Use other professionals to collaborate in the care of the client.	Teaching: Disease Process Teaching: Prescribed Activity/Exercise Teaching: Prescribed Diet, Coping Enhancement	7. Dietitians can assist in diet education; social services can identify assistance in the area of finances and home help; cardiac rehabilitation personnel can assist in exercise regimens; clergy can assist in coping strategies; and support groups can assist in social support.

Evaluation: Adaptation to new self-care strategies is very individualized. Plan the projected time frame once the client's learning style is known.

Nursing Diagnosis: Risk for Activity Intolerance related to an imbalance between oxygen supply and demand, as evidenced by weakness, fatigue, change in vital signs, dysrhythmias, dyspnea, pallor, and diaphoresis.

Outcomes: The client will have improved activity tolerance, as evidenced by participating in desired activities, meeting activities of daily living (ADL), reduced fatigue and weakness, vital signs within normal limits during activity, and absence of cyanosis, diaphoresis, and pain.

NOC OUTCOMES Activity Intolerance

Interventions	NIC INTERVENTIONS	Rationales
1. Monitor vital signs before and immediately after activity and 3 minutes later. If blood pressure decreases and heart rate increases, cardiac decompensation is suggested and activity should be decreased.	Cardiac Care: Rehabilitative	1. Vital signs should return to baseline levels in 3 minutes. The development of cardiac decompensation chest pain or dyspnea may indicate a need for an alteration in exercise regimen or medication.
2. Monitor for tachycardia, dysrhythmias, dyspnea, diaphoresis, weakness, fatigue, or pallor after activity.	Cardiac Care: Rehabilitative Oxygen Therapy Respiratory Monitoring	2. These indicators of myocardial oxygen deprivation may call for decreased activity, changes in medications, or use of supplemental oxygen.
3. Encourage verbalization of feelings or concerns regarding fatigue or limitations.	Cardiac Care: Rehabilitative Coping Enhancement	3. Knowing limitations prevents exertion and increasing myocardial workload.
4. Provide assistance with self-care activities, and provide frequent rest periods, especially after meals.	Cardiac Care: Rehabilitative	4. Large meals may increase myocardial workload and cause vagal stimulation, with resultant bradycardia or ectopic beats; caffeine, a cardiac stimulant, increases heart rate.
5. Increase activity per cardiac rehabilitation nurse and physician orders.	Cardiac Care: Rehabilitative	5. Gradual increase in activity increases strength and prevents overexertion, enhances collateral circulation, and restores a normal lifestyle as far as possible.

Evaluation: With stable acute myocardial infarction, the client should progress normally through steps of phase I cardiac rehabilitation without manifestations of exercise intolerance in 3 to 4 days.

(Continued)

The Client with Acute Myocardial Infarction—Cont'd

Collaborative Problem: Risk for Heart Failure related to disease process, as evidenced by tachycardia, hypotension or hypertension, S_3 or S_4 heart sounds, dysrhythmias, ECG changes, decreased urine output, decreased peripheral pulses, peripheral edema, cool ashen skin, diaphoresis, crackles, jugular vein distention, edema, and chest pain.

Outcomes: The nurse will monitor for clinical manifestations of heart failure by assessing cardiac rate, rhythm, hemodynamic parameters, skin perfusion, and CNS perfusion.

NOC OUTCOMES   Cardiac Pump Effectiveness

Interventions	NIC INTERVENTIONS	Rationales
1. Auscultate the apical pulse.	Cardiac Care: Acute Shock Management: Cardiac, Hemodynamic Regulation	1. Atrial (S_3) or ventricular (S_4) gallop rhythms are common and reflect tissue noncompliance or distention of chambers.
2. Assess heart rate and rhythm.	Cardiac Care: Acute Shock Management: Cardiac, Hemodynamic Regulation Dysrhythmia Management	2. Sinus tachycardia, paroxysmal atrial contractions, paroxysmal atrial tachycardia, multifocal atrial tachycardia, and PVCs are commonly seen with heart failure.
3. Document dysrhythmias, if present, as necessary.	Dysrhythmia Management Cardiac Care: Acute	3. Dysrhythmias reduce ventricular filling time, decrease myocardial contractility, and increase myocardial oxygen demands, which further compromises cardiac output.
4. Note lung sounds every 2 to 4 hours and as needed.	Cardiac Care: Acute, Respiratory Monitoring	4. Crackles may develop; ineffective cardiac output causes pulmonary venous congestion that leaks into the alveolar tissue, resulting in congestion.
5. Palpate peripheral pulses every 2 to 4 hours and as necessary.	Cardiac Care: Acute Circulatory Care: Arterial Insufficiency	5. Pulses may be weak, thready, or difficult to obtain when cardiac output is decreased.
6. Monitor blood pressure every 2 to 4 hours and as needed.	Cardiac Care: Acute	6. Hypotension related to hypoperfusion, vagal stimulation, or ventricular dysfunction may occur. Hypertension may be related to pain, anxiety, catecholamine release, or pre-existing vascular problems.
7. Inspect skin for pallor, cyanosis, and diaphoresis every 2 to 4 hours and as needed.	Cardiac Care: Acute Circulatory Care: Arterial Insufficiency	7. Pallor is associated with vasoconstriction, reduced cardiac output, and anemia. Cyanosis may develop during severe episodes of pulmonary edema. Dependent areas are often blue or mottled with increased venous congestion.
8. Monitor urine output, noting changes or decreasing output and dark or concentrated urine, every 2 to 4 hours and as needed.	Fluid Management Cardiac Care: Acute	8. Urine output less than 0.5 ml/kg/hr may reflect reduced renal perfusion and glomerular filtration as a result of reduced cardiac output.
9. Assess for chest pain.	Cardiac Care: Acute Pain Management	9. Chest pain may indicate inadequate cardiac perfusion related to the hypertrophied myocardium.
10. Assess for peripheral edema.	Cardiac Care: Acute	10. In heart failure, especially right-sided, the inability to pump blood forward results in venous pooling and increased pressure in the vascular space that leaks in the interstitium, presenting as peripheral edema.
11. Assess changes in sensorium.	Cardiac Care: Acute Circulatory Care: Arterial Insufficiency	11. Cerebral perfusion is directly related to cardiac output, and mentation may be a sensitive indicator of deterioration.
12. Provide frequent rest periods.	Cardiac Care: Acute	12. Physical rest decreases the production of catecholamines, which increases heart rate, myocardial oxygen demand, and blood pressure.
13. Instruct the client on avoidance of activities that increase cardiac workload.	Teaching: Disease Process Teaching: Prescribed Activity/Exercise	13. Avoidance of activities provides an opportunity for myocardial recovery and decreases workload and myocardial oxygen consumption.
14. Provide a bedside commode. Avoid the Valsalva maneuver.	Cardiac Care Teaching: Disease Process	14. The Valsalva maneuver stimulates the vagus nerve and causes bradycardia that temporarily decreases cardiac output.
15. Elevate the client's legs and avoid pressure under the knees. Permit increase in activity as tolerated and observe for breathing difficulty.	Teaching: Disease Process Teaching: Prescribed Activity/Exercise Cardiac Care	15. This position enhances venous return, reduces dependent swelling, decreases venous stasis, and may reduce the incidence of thrombus and embolus formation. If the left heart cannot pump blood forward, it may become trapped in the lungs/
16. Administer medications as ordered.	Medication Administration Cardiac Care	16. ACE inhibitors and beta-blockade were shown to help reduce the incidence of heart failure after AMI in clinical trials.[21]

Evaluation: The nurse will monitor for heart failure and report manifestations promptly.

Nursing Diagnosis: Excess Fluid Volume related to reduced glomerular filtration rate (GFR), decreased cardiac output, increased antidiuretic hormone (ADH) production, and sodium and water retention, as evidenced by orthopnea, S_3 heart sound, oliguria, edema, jugular neck vein distention, increased weight, increased blood pressure, respiratory distress, and abnormal breath sounds.

Outcomes: The client's fluid volume balance will be adequate, as evidenced by balanced intake and output (I&O), clear or clearing breath sounds, vital signs within normal limits, stable weight, and minimal edema.

| NOC OUTCOMES | Fluid Overload Severity |

Interventions	NIC INTERVENTIONS	Rationales
1. Monitor I&O (especially note color, specific gravity, and amount) every 2 to 4 hours, and as needed, and 24-hour totals.	Fluid Management	1. Intake greater than output may indicate fluid volume excess. If client receives diuretic therapy, an increase in output is expected.
2. Maintain chair or bed rest in the semi-Fowler position.	Cardiac Care Fluid Management	2. This position promotes diuresis by recumbency-induced increased GFR and reduced ADH production.
3. Involve the client and family in fluid schedules, especially if there are restrictions, and provide frequent oral care.	Coping Enhancement Teaching: Disease Process Fluid Management	3. Involving the client in the therapy regimen may enhance a sense of control and fosters cooperation with restrictions. Fluid restrictions dry the oral mucous membranes.
4. Weigh the client daily.	Fluid Management	4. Daily weights can show the increase or decrease in congestion and edema in response to therapy. A gain of 5 pounds represents about 2 L of fluid.
5. Assess for jugular neck vein distention, edema, peripheral pulses, and presence of anasarca.	Cardiac Care, Fluid Management	5. Excessive fluid retention may be demonstrated by venous engorgement and edema formation. Peripheral edema often begins in the feet and ascends upward as heart failure worsens.
6. Auscultate breath sounds. Note adventitious sounds, increased vascular volume, and pulmonary hypertension or worsening of heart failure.	Respiratory Monitoring Cardiac Care	6. These manifestations of pulmonary congestion reflect and monitor for dyspnea or tachypnea.
7. Monitor for sudden extreme shortness of breath, and feelings of panic.	Respiratory Monitoring Cardiac Care	7. These are manifestations of pulmonary edema.
8. Palpate for hepatomegaly. Note complaints of right upper quadrant pain or tenderness.	Cardiac Care	8. Advancing heart failure leads to venous congestion, which results in liver engorgement and altered liver function (i.e., impaired drug metabolism, prolonged drug half-life).
9. Evaluate the effectiveness of diuretics and potassium.	Fluid Management Medication Management Cardiac Care	9. Fluid shifts and use of diuretics can alter electrolytes, especially potassium and chloride supplements, which affects cardiac rhythm and contractility.
10. Note increased lethargy, hypotension, and muscle cramping.	Cardiac Care	10. These are manifestations of hypokalemia and hyponatremia that may occur because of fluid shifts and diuretic therapy.
11. Assess the need for dietary consultation as needed.	Cardiac Care Teaching: Prescribed Diet	11. Restrictions of foods high in sodium may be necessary. The client may need to eat foods enriched with potassium when taking loop diuretics.

Evaluation: Depending on the degree of heart failure, fluid volume excess may be slow to resolve. Initially, there may be a resolution of manifestations after diuresis. Fluid balance adjustments may then be made daily.

Nursing Diagnosis: Risk for Impaired Skin Integrity related to bed rest, edema, and decreased tissue perfusion, as evidenced by reddened areas and the presence of areas of breakdown.

Outcomes: The client will have intact skin integrity, as evidenced by an absence of reddened areas and no areas of breakdown.

| NOC OUTCOMES | Tissue Integrity: Skin and Mucous Membranes |

Interventions	NIC INTERVENTIONS	Rationales
1. Inspect the client's skin; note bony prominences, edema, altered circulation, pigmentation, obesity, and emaciation.	Pressure Ulcer Prevention	1. Altered skin color in isolated areas suggests damage caused by pressure or decreased circulation.
2. Assist with active or passive range-of-motion (ROM) exercises.	Pressure Ulcer Prevention	2. ROM exercises enhance venous return. Isometric exercises may adversely affect cardiac output by increasing myocardial work and oxygen consumption.
3. Reposition the client every 2 hours in a bed or chair.	Pressure Ulcer Prevention	3. Repositioning increases circulation and reduces the time that weight deprives any one area of blood flow.
4. Provide pressure-reducing devices, sheepskin, elbow protectors, and heel elevation if needed.	Pressure Ulcer Prevention	4. These devices reduce pressure to bone prominences and maintain skin integrity.
5. Assess and provide special air or flotation beds for clients at high risk for pressure ulcers.	Pressure Ulcer Prevention	5. These beds reduce pressure to skin and may improve circulation.
6. Pad the chair with a pressure reduction pad or 4 inches of foam.	Pressure Ulcer Prevention	6. Weak clients do not move spontaneously. Pressure reduction surfaces can prevent pressures in excess of capillary filling pressures.

Evaluation: Skin impairment may be evident within 48 hours of admission or a significant change in condition.

program, by counting the number of steps they take in a 15-second interval. Clients with dysrhythmias are monitored more closely, and intermittent rhythm strips may be taken. For clients who prefer to exercise at home, clinicians trained in cardiac rehabilitation can provide detailed, written instructions for a long-term exercise program. Various methods are used to determine the appropriate exercise routines. Periodic evaluation is necessary to assess the client's endurance and tolerance to the prescribed exercise program.

Phase IV (Maintenance Outpatient). Phase IV, the final phase of cardiac rehabilitation, usually takes place in the home or community and is unsupervised. The client maintains a program of regular exercise and other lifestyle modifications to modify cardiac risk. Clients should undergo an exercise testing and risk factor assessment annually.

CONCLUSIONS

CHD is a progressive occlusive disorder that commonly results in reduced coronary blood flow. This reduction in blood flow is manifested clinically by angina and AMI. AMI, permanent damage to the myocardium, may be the first indicator of the seriousness of the heart disease. Your responsibilities in the care of these clients are to educate them about the warning signs of AMI, to monitor their response to therapy, to prevent complications, and to promote rehabilitation.

THINKING CRITICALLY

1. Mrs. Polk, a 62-year-old housewife who cares for her two grandchildren, is admitted to the emergency department with complaints of chest pain. She is diaphoretic and pale and complains of pain "under my left breast that pushes to my back." She rates the pain as an 8 on a scale of 1 to 10. Her ECG shows an elevated ST segment. She is placed on oxygen therapy, and an IV line is inserted. Cardiac serum markers are drawn and sent to the laboratory. Her vital signs are temperature 36.9° C, apical pulse rate 110 beats/min, and blood pressure 108/68 mm Hg.

Factors to Consider. What additional testing is necessary to rule in or rule out an acute MI? What other information from Mrs. Polk's history might aid in the diagnosis?

2. The physician immediately orders reteplase, a thrombolytic agent, for Mrs. Polk.

Factors to Consider. What information must be obtained from Mrs. Polk to safely initiate thrombolytic therapy?

3. You administer the thrombolytic therapy as ordered. Mrs. Polk states her pain is now a 1 on a scale of 1 to 10. ST segments are resolving, and she is no longer diaphoretic.

Factors to Consider. What effects from the thrombolytic therapy appear to be occurring? Which side effects of the therapy should you anticipate?

4. A client with long-standing coronary artery disease experiences severe chest pain unrelieved by nitroglycerin. He is admitted with an acute MI to the coronary care unit. What are the priorities on admission? What medical treatment may be instituted in the first hours following the infarction?

Factors to Consider. What time frame is considered most crucial to the salvage of myocardial muscle? What care is given to the newly admitted client?

Discussions for these questions can be found on the website.

BIBLIOGRAPHY

 Citations appearing in red refer to primary research.

 Citations appearing in blue refer to evidence-based practice guidelines and protocols.

1. American Heart Association. (2005). 2005 American Heart Association guidelines for cardiopulmonary resuscitation and emergency cardiovascular care. Part 8: Stabilization of the patient with acute coronary syndrome. *Circulation, 112*(Suppl IV), IV89-111.
2. American Heart Association (2006). *2006 Heart disease and stroke statistics: 2006 Update.* Dallas, Tex: American Heart Association. Available at www.americanheart.org/.
3. American Heart Association. (2002). *Heart attack, stroke & cardiac arrest warning signs.* Available at www.americanheart.org/.
4. Antman, E., et al. (2000). The TIMI risk score for unstable angina/non-ST elevation MI: A method for prognostication and therapeutic decision making. *Journal of the American Medical Association, 284*(7), 876-878.
5. Antman, E., et al. (2006). ACC/AHA guidelines for the management of patients with ST-segment elevation myocardial infarction: Executive summary. *Circulation, 110*(5), 588-636.
6. *Best practice evidence-based guideline—Cardiac rehabilitation.* (2002)The New Zealand Guideline Group. Available at www.nzgg.org.nz/library/gl-complete/Cardiac-Rehab/index.cfm.
7. Beattie, S. (1999). Management of chronic stable angina. *Nurse Practitioner, 24*(5), 44, 49, 53, 56, 59-61.
8. Braunwald, E., et al. (2002). ACC/AHA 2002 guideline update for the management of patients with unstable angina and non-ST-segment elevation myocardial infarction: A report of the American College of Cardiology/American Heart Association Task Force on Practice Guidelines. Available at www.acc.org/clinical/guidelines/unstable/unstable.pdf.
9. Brennen, M.L., et al. (2003). Prognostic value of myeloperoxidase in patients with chest pain. *New England Journal of Medicine, 349*(17), 1595-1604.
10. Cummings, R. (2001). *ACLS provider manual.* Dallas, Tex: American Heart Association.
11. Doering, L.V. (1999). Pathophysiology of acute coronary syndromes leading to acute myocardial infarction. *Journal of Cardiovascular Nursing, 13*(3), 1-20.
12. Dracup, K., & Cannon, C. (1999, April). Combination treatment strategies for management of acute myocardial infarction. *Critical Care Nurse Supplement,* 1-17.
13. Gibbons, R.J., et al. (2003). ACC/AHA 2002 guideline update for the management of patients with chronic stable angina: A summary article. *Circulation, 107,* 149-158.
14. Gibbons, R., et al. (2002). ACC/AHA 2002 guideline update for exercise testing: Summary article. *Circulation, 106,* 1883-1890.
15. Hudson, M., et al. (1999). Cardiac markers: Point of care testing. *Clinica Chimica Acta, 28*(4), 223-237.

16. Huikuri, H., et al. (2001). Sudden death due to cardiac arrhythmias. *New England Journal of Medicine, 345*(20), 1473-1482.

17. Lau, J., et al. (2001). Evaluation of technologies for identifying acute cardiac ischemia in emergency departments. *AHRQ Publication Evidence Report/Technology Assessment Number 26.* Available at www.ahrq.gov/.

18. Lee, T.H., & Goldman, L. (2000). Evaluation of the patient with acute chest pain. *New England Journal of Medicine, 342*(16), 1187-1193.

19. Libby, P., Ridker, P., & Maseri, A. (2002). Inflammation and atherosclerosis. *Circulation, 105,* 1135-1143.

20. McAvoy, J. (2004). Case studies of ST-segment elevation before and after percutaneous coronary intervention in patients with acute myocardial infarction. *Critical Care Nurse, 21*(6), 32-39.

21. Murphy, M., & Berding, C. (1999). Use of myoglobins and cardiac troponins in the diagnosis of acute myocardial infarction. *Critical Care Nurse, 19*(1), 58-65.

22. O'Connor, C.M., Gattis, W.A., & Swedberg, K. (1999). Current and novel pharmacologic approaches in advanced heart failure. *Heart and Lung, 28,* 227-239.

23. Peeters, A., et al. (2002). A cardiovascular life history—A life course analysis of the original Framingham Heart Study cohort. *European Heart Journal, 23*(6), 795-799.

24. Rich, M.W. (1999). Heart failure disease management: A critical review. *Journal of Cardiac Failure, 5*(1), 64-75.

25. Rosenfeld, A. (2006). State of the heart: Building science to improve women's cardiovascular health. *American Journal of Critical Care, 15,* 556-567.

26. Smith, S., et al. (2006). ACC/AHA guidelines for secondary prevention for patients with coronary and other atherosclerotic vascular diseases: 2006 update. *Journal of American College of Cardiology, 47,* 2130-2139.

27. Soran, O., Schneider, V.M., & Feldman, A.M. (1999). Basic therapy for congestive heart failure: Current practice, new prospects. *Journal of Critical Illness, 14*(2), 78-89.

28. Thygesen, K., et al. (2000). Myocardial infarction redefined. A consensus document of the Joint European Society of Cardiology/American College of Cardiology Committee for the Redefinition of Myocardial Infarction. *Journal of American College of Cardiology, 36*(3), 959-969.

evolve *Did you remember to check out the bonus material on the Evolve website and the CD-ROM, including NCLEX®-Examination Style Review Questions, Open-Book Quizzes, and Chapter Review Audio Podcasts?*

http://evolve.elsevier.com/Black/medsurg

UNIT 14

OXYGENATION DISORDERS

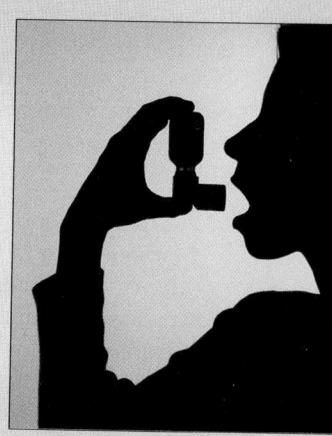

ANATOMY AND PHYSIOLOGY REVIEW:

The Respiratory System

Robert G. Carroll

Our body needs a constant supply of oxygen to support metabolism. The respiratory system brings oxygen through the airways of the lung into the alveoli, where it diffuses into the blood for transport to the tissues. This process is so vital that difficulty in breathing is experienced as a threat to life itself. Whether death is a real possibility or not, people with respiratory disorders are often anxious and fearful that they may die, perhaps agonizingly.

The respiratory system also has other essential functions:

- Expels carbon dioxide (CO_2), a metabolic waste product that is transported from the tissues to the lungs for elimination
- Filters and humidifies air that enters the lungs
- Traps particulate matter in the mucus of the airways and propels it toward the mouth for elimination by coughing or swallowing
- Prevents the entry of inhaled pathogens by activating the immune system

Respiratory control is tied most closely to arterial blood and brain CO_2 levels as well as to arterial blood oxygen levels. Respiration is also controlled by higher cortical centers. For example, an increase in ventilation accompanies exercise and keeps arterial blood gases within the normal range.

Respiratory problems are widespread. Acute disorders range from minor inconveniences (colds or flu) to more life-threatening problems (asthma, some types of pneumonia, and chest trauma). Chronic disabling conditions include *chronic airflow limitation* (also called chronic obstructive pulmonary disease) and certain restrictive lung diseases. Chronic respiratory problems affect many people, often causing them to make radical lifestyle changes, such as retiring from work earlier than they wish.

Respiratory problems are associated with many causes: allergies, occupational factors, genetic factors, smoking and tobacco use, infection, neuromuscular disorders, chest abnormalities, trauma, pleural conditions, and pulmonary vascular abnormalities. The most significant factor in chronic respiratory illness and lung cancer is cigarette smoking.

STRUCTURE OF THE RESPIRATORY SYSTEM

UPPER AIRWAYS

The airways are the regions through which air passes on its way to the exchange areas of the lungs. The upper airways consist of the nasal cavities, pharynx, and larynx.

Nasal Cavity

The nose is formed from both bone and cartilage. The nasal bone forms the bridge, and the remainder of the nose is composed of cartilage and connective tissue (Figure A&P14-1). Each opening of the nose on the face (*nostrils* or *nares*) leads to a cavity (*vestibule*). The vestibule is lined anteriorly with skin and hair that filter foreign objects and prevent them from being inhaled. The posterior vestibule is lined with a mucous membrane, composed of columnar epithelial cells, and goblet cells that secrete mucus. The mucous membrane extends throughout the airways, and cilia (hair-like projections) propel mucus to the pharynx for elimination by swallowing or coughing. The portion of the mucous membrane that is located at the top of the nasal cavity, just beneath the cribriform plate of the ethmoid bone, is specialized (*olfactory*) epithelium, which provides the sense of smell. Because the olfactory epithelium does not lie along the usual path of air movement, smell is enhanced by sniffing.

Along the sides of the vestibule are *turbinates,* mucous membrane–covered projections that contain a rich blood supply from the internal and external carotid arteries. They warm and humidify inspired air.

Paranasal sinuses, open areas within the skull, are named for the bones in which they lie: frontal, ethmoid, sphenoid, and maxillary. Passageways from the paranasal sinuses drain into the nasal cavities. The nasolacrimal ducts, which drain tears from the surface of the eyes, also drain into the nasal cavity.

The mouth is considered part of the upper airway but only because it can be used to deliver air to the lungs

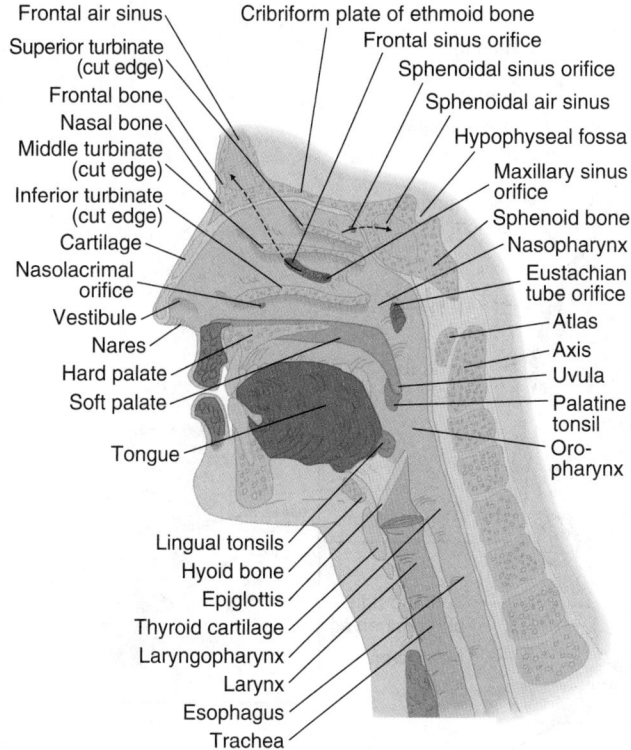

Frontal air sinus
Superior turbinate (cut edge)
Frontal bone
Nasal bone
Middle turbinate (cut edge)
Inferior turbinate (cut edge)
Cartilage
Nasolacrimal orifice
Vestibule
Nares
Hard palate
Soft palate
Tongue

Cribriform plate of ethmoid bone
Frontal sinus orifice
Sphenoidal sinus orifice
Sphenoidal air sinus
Hypophyseal fossa
Maxillary sinus orifice
Sphenoid bone
Nasopharynx
Eustachian tube orifice
Atlas
Axis
Uvula
Palatine tonsil
Oro-pharynx

Lingual tonsils
Hyoid bone
Epiglottis
Thyroid cartilage
Laryngopharynx
Larynx
Esophagus
Trachea

■ **FIGURE A&PI4–I** Structures of the upper airway. Air enters the body through the nares or mouth and is filtered and humidified while passing toward the alveoli. The epiglottis directs air into the trachea during respiration and directs food into the esophagus during swallowing. Dashed arrows indicate passage of air into sinuses.

when the nose is obstructed or when high volumes of air are needed, such as during exercise. The mouth does not perform the nasal functions efficiently, especially those of warming, humidifying, and filtering air.

Pharynx

The pharynx is a funnel-shaped tube that extends from the nose to the larynx. It can be divided into three sections.

The *nasopharynx* is located above the margin of the soft palate and receives air from the nasal cavity. From the ear, the eustachian tubes open into the nasopharynx. The pharyngeal tonsils (called *adenoids* when enlarged) are located on the posterior wall of the nasopharynx.

The *oropharynx* serves both respiration and digestion. It receives air from the nasopharynx and food from the oral cavity. Palatine (faucial) tonsils are located along the sides of the posterior mouth, and the lingual tonsils are located at the base of the tongue.

The *laryngopharynx (hypopharynx),* located below the base of the tongue, is the most inferior portion of the pharynx. It connects to the larynx and serves both respiration and digestion.

Larynx

The larynx is commonly called the *voice box.* It connects the upper (pharynx) and lower (trachea) airways. The larynx lies just anterior to the upper esophagus. Nine cartilages form the larynx: three large unpaired cartilages (epiglottis, thyroid, cricoid) and three smaller paired cartilages (arytenoid, corniculate, cuneiform). The cartilages are attached to the hyoid bone above and below the trachea by muscles and ligaments, all of which prevent the larynx from collapse during inspiration and swallowing.

The larynx consists of the endolarynx and a surrounding triangle-shaped bone and cartilage. The endolarynx is formed by two paired folds of tissue, forming the false and the true vocal cords. The slit between the vocal cords forms the *glottis.* The *epiglottis,* a leaf-shaped structure immediately posterior to the base of the tongue, lies above the larynx. When food or liquids are swallowed, the epiglottis closes over the larynx, protecting the lower airways from aspiration.

The thyroid cartilage protrudes in front of the larynx, forming the "Adam's apple." The cricoid cartilage lies just below the thyroid cartilage and is the anatomic site for an artificial opening into the trachea (tracheostomy, or cricothyroidotomy). The internal portion of the larynx is composed of muscles that assist with swallowing, speaking, and respiration and that contribute to the pitch of the voice. The blood supply to the larynx is through the branches of the thyroid arteries. The nerve supply is through the recurrent laryngeal and superior laryngeal nerves.

LOWER AIRWAYS

The lower airway, or tracheobronchial tree, is composed of the trachea, right and left mainstem bronchi, segmental bronchi, subsegmental bronchi, and terminal bronchioles (Figure A&P14-2). Smooth muscle, wound in overlapping clockwise and counterclockwise helical bands, is found in all of these structures. This arrangement allows contraction of the smooth muscle to decrease the diameter of the airways, increasing the resistance to air flow. This muscle is subject to spasm in many airway disorders. The lower airways continue to warm, humidify, and filter inspired air as it flows toward the lungs.

Trachea

The trachea (windpipe) extends from the larynx to the level of the seventh thoracic vertebra, where it divides into two main *(primary)* bronchi. The point at which the trachea divides is called the *carina.* The trachea is a flexible, muscular, 12-cm-long air passage with C-shaped cartilaginous rings. Along with all other regions

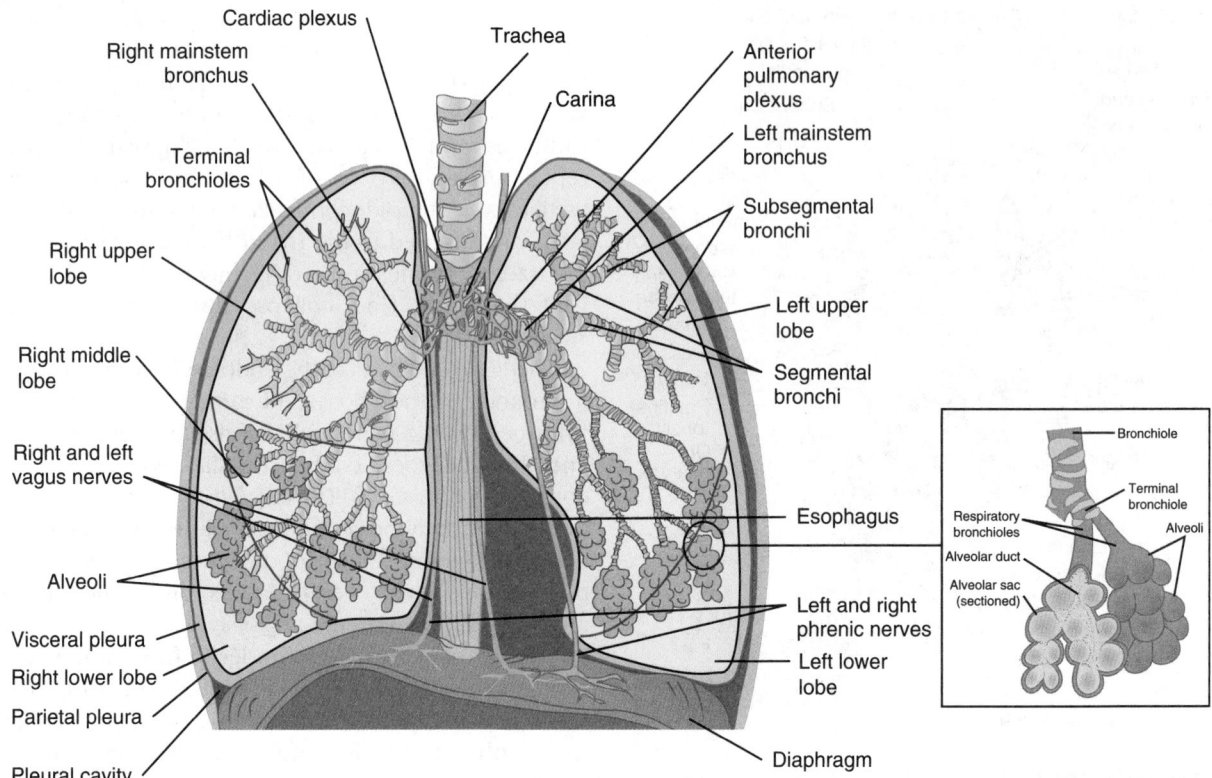

■ **FIGURE A&P14–2** Structures of the lower airways. Air passes from the trachea through bronchi and bronchioles before reaching the alveoli. Cartilage in the bronchi and trachea prevents airway collapse during forced expiration. *Inset:* Gas exchange occurs in the respiratory zone, which consists of the respiratory bronchioles, alveolar ducts, and alveolar sacs.

of the lower airways it is lined with pseudostratified columnar epithelium that contains goblet (mucus-secreting) cells and cilia (Figure A&P14-3). Because the cilia beat upward, they tend to propel foreign particles and excessive mucus away from the lungs to the pharynx. No cilia are present in the alveoli.

Bronchi and Bronchioles

The right mainstem bronchus is shorter and wider, extending more vertically downward, than the left mainstem bronchus. Thus foreign bodies are more likely to lodge there than in the left mainstem bronchus. The *segmental* and *subsegmental bronchi* are subdivisions of the main bronchi and spread in an inverted, tree-like formation through each lung. Cartilage surrounds the airway in the bronchi, but the bronchioles (the final pathway to the alveoli) contain no cartilage and thus can collapse and trap air during active exhalation.

The *terminal bronchioles* are the last airways of the conducting system. The area from the nose to the terminal bronchioles does not exchange gas and functions as *anatomic dead space*. The lack of gas exchange means that the first air out of the mouth during exhalation resembles room air, but the last air out (end-tidal air) resembles alveolar air.

LUNGS AND ALVEOLI

Lungs

The lungs lie within the thoracic cavity on either side of the heart (see Figure A&P14-2). They are cone-shaped, with the apex above the first rib and the base resting on the diaphragm. Each lung is divided into superior and inferior lobes by an oblique fissure. The right lung is further divided by a horizontal fissure, which creates a middle lobe. The right lung, therefore, has three lobes; the left lobe has only two. In addition to these 5 lobes, which are visible externally, each lung can be subdivided into about 10 smaller units *(bronchopulmonary segments)*. Each segment represents the portion of the lung that is supplied by a specific tertiary bronchus. These segments are important surgically, because a diseased segment can be resected without the need to remove the entire lobe or lung. The two lungs are separated by a space (the *mediastinum*) where the heart, aorta, vena cava, pulmonary vessels, esophagus, part of the trachea and bronchi, and the thymus gland are located.

The lungs contain gas, blood, thin alveolar walls, and support structures. The alveolar walls contain elastic and collagen fibers; these form a three-dimensional, basket-like structure that allows the lung to inflate in all directions. These fibers are capable of stretching when

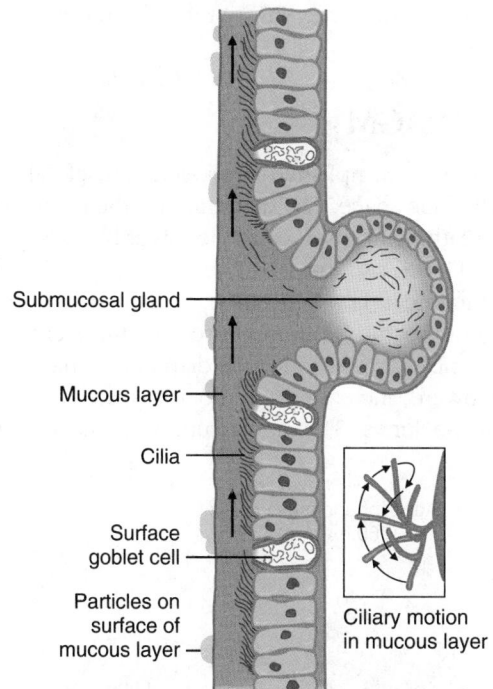

Submucosal gland

Mucous layer

Cilia

Surface goblet cell

Particles on surface of mucous layer

Ciliary motion in mucous layer

■ **FIGURE A&P14–3** The mucociliary blanket is an important respiratory defense mechanism. Mucus is secreted by surface goblet cells. About 100 ml of mucus is normally secreted each day by the submucosal glands. Mucus covers the epithelial lining of the tracheobronchial tree in two layers: the watery solution layer close to the mucosal surface and the thicker gel layer. The cilia (hair-like projections) beat in an upward direction toward the upper airway. Particulate matter is trapped on the mucous layer and moved upward by the cilia. Debris-laden mucus is then either swallowed or expectorated as sputum.

pulling force is exerted on them from outside of the body or when they are inflated from within. The elastic recoil helps return the lungs to their resting volume.

Branches of the pulmonary artery provide most of the blood supply to the lungs. The blood is oxygen-poor, but oxygen is supplied by inspired air. The trachea and bronchioles, which are not part of the oxygen exchange surface, receive oxygen-rich blood from branches of the aorta.

Lung Volumes

The lungs of an average 19-year-old man have a total capacity of about 5900 ml. However, a person cannot exhale all the air from the lungs, and about 1200 ml of air always remains, no matter how forceful the expiration. This remaining volume *(residual volume)* prevents the collapse of the lung structures during expiration. The volume of air that moves in and out with each breath is called the *tidal volume.* During quiet breathing, tidal volume is about 500 ml. When a person takes a deep breath, the lung is more fully expanded. The amount of extra air inhaled, beyond the tidal volume, is called the *inspiratory reserve volume;* the extra air that can be exhaled after a forced breath is called the *expiratory reserve volume.*

Lung volumes are often combined into capacities:

- ■ *Total lung capacity:* all four volumes
- ■ *Vital capacity:* all volumes except residual volume, which is the amount a person can ventilate
- ■ *Functional reserve capacity:* expiratory reserve plus residual volumes
- ■ *Inspiratory capacity:* tidal volume plus inspiratory reserve volume

The rate at which air can be expelled from the lungs also provides diagnostic information. The "timed" forced expiratory volume (FEV) is obtained by having the client perform a maximum inspiration (to total lung capacity) followed by a maximal exhalation (to residual volume). The total amount of air exhaled is the vital capacity. FEV_1 indicates the volume of air exhaled during the first second, usually about 80% of vital capacity, and FEV_3 indicates the volume of air exhaled during 3 seconds, usually about 95% of vital capacity.

These volumes and capacities are frequently altered by disease. The pattern and severity of the change correlate with the severity of the disease processes. Lung volumes as measured by spirometry are shown in Figure A&P14-4. Pulmonary function tests are described in Chapter 59.

Alveoli

The lung parenchyma, which consists of millions of alveolar units, is the working area of the lung tissue. At birth, a person has approximately 24 million alveoli; by age 8 years, a person has 300 million. The total working alveolar surface area is approximately 750 to 860 square feet. The blood supply flowing toward the alveoli comes from the right ventricle of the heart.

The entire alveolar unit (respiratory zone) is made up of respiratory bronchioles, alveolar ducts, and alveolar

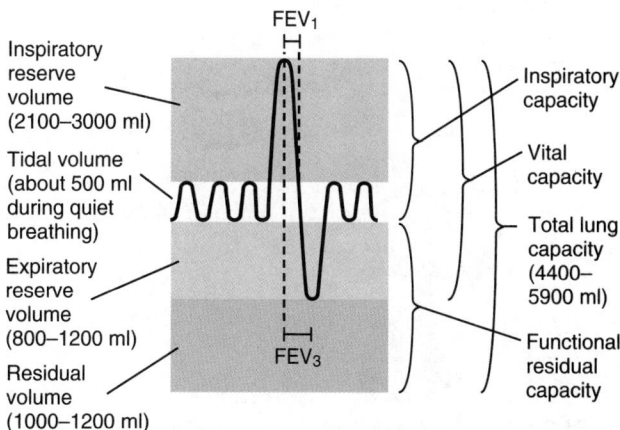

FEV_1

Inspiratory reserve volume (2100–3000 ml)

Tidal volume (about 500 ml during quiet breathing)

Expiratory reserve volume (800–1200 ml)

Residual volume (1000–1200 ml)

FEV_3

Inspiratory capacity

Vital capacity

Total lung capacity (4400–5900 ml)

Functional residual capacity

■ **FIGURE A&P14–4** Lung volumes and capacities as measured by spirometry. The four volumes of the lungs (identified on the left) are combined to form four capacities (identified on the right).

sacs (see Figure A&P14-2). The alveolar walls are extremely thin, with an almost solid network of interconnecting capillaries. Because of the extensiveness of the capillary system, the flow of blood in the alveolar wall has been described as a "sheet" of flowing blood.

Oxygen and CO_2 are exchanged through a respiratory membrane, about 0.2 mm thick (Figure A&P14-5). The average diameter of the pulmonary capillary is only about 5 μm, but red blood cells (7 μm in diameter) must squeeze through, actually touching the capillary wall. Thus the distance across which oxygen and CO_2 must diffuse is greatly reduced. Thickening of the respiratory membrane (e.g., with pulmonary edema or fibrosis) may interfere with normal exchange of gases.

The alveolus comprises two cell types: *type I pneumocytes,* which line the alveolus, are thin and incapable of reproduction but are effective in gas exchange. *Type II pneumocytes* are cuboidal and do not exchange oxygen and CO_2 well. They produce surfactant and are important in lung injury and repair because they differentiate into alveolar macrophages. They differentiate into type I cells; oxygenation is impaired during the transition from type II to type I cells.

THORAX

The bony thorax provides protection for the lungs, heart, and great vessels. The outer shell of the thorax is made up of 12 pairs of ribs. The ribs connect posteriorly to the transverse processes of the thoracic vertebrae of the spine. Anteriorly, the first seven pairs of ribs are attached to the sternum by cartilage. The 8th, 9th, and 10th ribs *(false ribs)* are attached to each other by costal cartilage. The 11th and 12th ribs *(floating ribs)* allow full chest expansion because they are not attached in any way to the sternum.

DIAPHRAGM

Breathing is accomplished by skeletal muscle alteration of the thoracic space. The diaphragm is the primary muscle of breathing and serves as the lower boundary of the thorax (Figure A&P14-6). The diaphragm is dome-shaped in the relaxed position, with central muscular attachments to the xiphoid process of the sternum and the lower ribs. Contraction of the diaphragm pulls the muscle downward, increasing the thoracic space and actively inflating the lungs. The nerve supply of the diaphragm

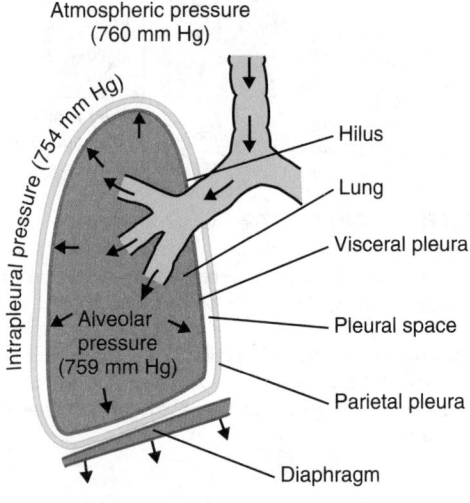

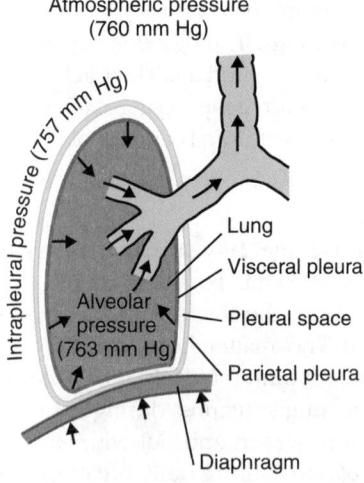

■ **FIGURE A&P14-6** Normal inspiration and expiration. Contraction of the diaphragm increases the size of the thoracic cavity, and reduces alveolar pressure to below atmospheric pressure. Relaxation of the diaphragm allows the elastic recoil of the lungs to diminish the size of the thoracic cavity, increasing alveolar pressure to greater than atmospheric pressure.

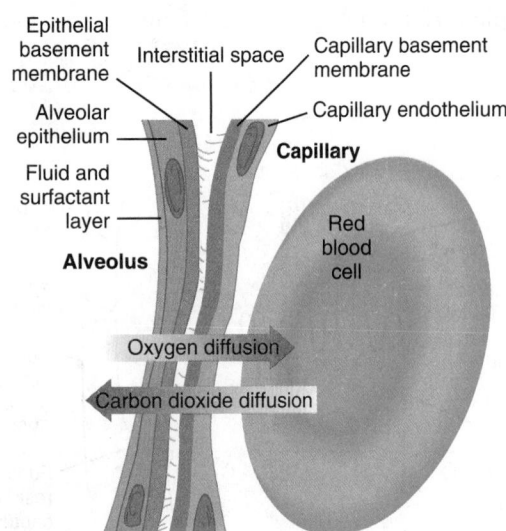

■ **FIGURE A&P14-5** The ultrastructure of the respiratory membrane where oxygen is exchanged. Accumulation of fluid in the interstitial space (pulmonary edema) diminishes the diffusion of oxygen into the pulmonary capillary.

(phrenic nerve) comes through the spinal cord at the level of the third cervical vertebra. Thus spinal injuries at C3 or above can impair ventilation.

PLEURAE

The pleurae are serous membranes that enclose the lung in a double-walled sac. The *visceral* pleura covers the lung and the fissures between the lobes of the lung. The *parietal* pleura covers the inside of each hemithorax, the mediastinum, and the top of the diaphragm; it joins the visceral pleura at the *hilus* (a notch in the medial surface of the lung, where the mainstem bronchi, pulmonary blood vessels, and nerves enter the lung).

Normally, no space exists between the pleurae; the *pleural space* is a potential space between the two layers of pleura. A thin film (only a few milliliters) of serous fluid acts as a lubricant in the potential space. The fluid also causes the moist pleural membranes to adhere, creating a pulling force that helps to hold the lungs in an expanded position because the parietal pleura is attached to the rib cage. The action of the pleurae is analogous to coupling two sheets of glass with a thin film of water. It is extremely difficult to separate the sheets of glass at right angles, yet they readily slide along each other. Because of the nature of this coupling, the movement of the lungs closely follows the movement of the thorax. If air or increased amounts of serous fluid, blood, or pus accumulate in the thoracic space, the lungs are compressed and respiratory difficulties follow. These conditions constitute *pneumothorax* (air in the pleural space) or *hemothorax* (blood in the pleural space) and pleural effusion (fluid in the pleural space).

FUNCTION OF THE RESPIRATORY SYSTEM

The respiratory system enhances gas exchange. Inspiration brings oxygen-rich air into the alveoli. The upper and lower airways filter and humidify inspired air. Gas exchange between the air and the blood occurs in the alveolus. Oxygen diffuses into the blood, and CO_2 diffuses from the blood into the alveolar air. The CO_2-enriched air is removed from the body during expiration. The large number and large surface area of alveoli are necessary to meet both resting and exercise gas exchange requirements.

The thorax and diaphragm alter pressures in the thorax to drive air movement. The movement of air depends on pressure gradients between the atmosphere and the air in the lungs, with air flowing from regions of higher pressure to regions of lower pressure. On inspiration, the dome of the diaphragm flattens and the rib cage lifts. As thoracic and lung volumes increase, alveolar pressure decreases and air is drawn into the lungs.

Airway resistance also affects air movement and is affected primarily by the diameter of the airways. Decreasing the diameter by half results in a 16-fold increase in airway resistance. Thus a decreased diameter of the airways caused by bronchial muscle contraction or by secretions in the airways increases resistance and decreases the rate of air flow. This is a common finding in obstructive airway diseases such as asthma.

During quiet breathing, expiration is usually passive, that is, does not require the use of muscles. The chest wall, in contrast to the lungs, tends to recoil outward. The opposing forces of lung and chest wall create a subatmospheric (negative) force of about −5 cm of water in the intrapleural space at the end of quiet exhalation. Exhalation is also a result of elastic recoil of the lungs.

VENTILATION

Ventilation, the movement of air in and out of the lungs (especially the removal of carbon dioxide from the lungs), involves three forces: (1) compliance properties of the lung and the thorax (chest wall), (2) surface tension, and (3) the muscular efforts of inspiratory muscles.

Compliance

Compliance refers to the ease with which the lung expands and indicates the relationship between the volume and the pressure of the lungs. The lungs are elastic structures that tend to recoil to a volume slightly less than *residual volume* (the volume of gas remaining in the lungs after a full exhalation). The force required to distend the lungs is the difference between the alveolar pressure and the intrapleural pressure. Diseases that cause fibrosis of the lungs result in "stiff" lungs with low compliance; stiff lungs require high inspiratory pressures to achieve a set volume of gas. In contrast, diseases such as emphysema that damage the elastic structure of the alveolar walls result in "floppy" lungs with greater compliance but poor recoil. Relatively low pressures can achieve the same volume of air during inspiration. Passive exhalation, normally a function of elastic recoil, is impaired.

Surface Tension

Changes in the surface tension of the liquid film lining the alveoli also affect compliance by changing resistance. *Surface tension,* the result of the air-liquid interface at each alveolus, restricts alveolar expansion on inspiration and aids alveolar collapse on expiration. Surfactant produced by type II cells in the alveolar lining lowers surface tension and thus increases compliance and aids ventilation and oxygenation. A deficiency of surfactant results in stiff lungs. Premature babies lacking surfactant may suffer infant respiratory distress syndrome, formerly called hyaline membrane disease.

Muscular Effort

Ventilation also requires muscular effort. For inspiration to occur, the pressure within the alveoli must be less than atmospheric pressure. Contraction of the diaphragm and the external intercostal muscles enlarges the size of the thorax. The external intercostal muscles pull the ribs upward and forward, thus increasing the transverse and anteroposterior diameter. Two accessory muscles of inspiration—the scalene and sternocleidomastoid muscles—elevate the first and second ribs during inspiration to enlarge the upper thorax and stabilize the chest wall. The sternocleidomastoid muscle elevates the sternum. The expanding thorax creates a more negative intrapleural pressure, which expands the lungs. When the alveolar pressure becomes lower than the atmospheric pressure, air flows into the lungs.

During exhalation, the inspiratory muscles relax. The elastic recoil of the lung tissue increases alveolar pressure above atmospheric pressure and causes air to move out of the lungs. Air flow stops when the recoil pressure of the lungs balances the muscular and elastic forces of the chest (see Figure A&P14-6).

Although expiration is usually passive, forced expiration and coughing employ accessory muscles to decrease the size of the thoracic space and cause expiration. Contraction of the abdominal muscles forces the diaphragm upward to its dome-shaped position. Contraction of the internal intercostal muscles pulls the ribs inward, thus decreasing the anteroposterior diameter of the chest wall.

Work of Breathing

Respiratory muscle contraction represents a significant metabolic load. Tidal volume and respiratory rate are adjusted to minimize the workload on the body. For example, clients with obstructive lung disease use slower but deeper breaths to maintain appropriate alveolar ventilation. Clients with restrictive lung disease use frequent, shallow breaths to maintain alveolar ventilation.

RESPIRATORY CONTROL

Human metabolism is not one of steady state. The oxygen needs of the tissues change with changing metabolic demands. Respiratory control mechanisms match the elimination of CO_2 and supply of oxygen to the metabolic needs. The lungs have no intrinsic control of themselves; instead, they are controlled by the central nervous system.

Central Nervous System Control

The medulla has several levels of respiratory centers. The dorsal respiratory group primarily provides for inspiration. The ventral respiratory group is normally quiet unless increased ventilation is needed or if active exhalation is performed. The pons has an apneustic center, which contains both expiratory and inspiratory neurons. The upper pons contains the pneumotaxic center, which fine-tunes breathing. For example, the pneumotaxic center allows for talking and breathing.

Output from the respiratory neurons, located in the medulla, descends via the ventral and lateral columns of the spinal cord to phrenic motor neurons of the diaphragm and intercostal motor neurons of the intercostal muscles. The result is rhythmic respiratory movements.

The cortex also allows voluntary control of breathing (holding our breath or altering the rate or depth of breathing).

Reflex Control

The cough reflex is a neural reflex stimulated by mechanical stimuli (Table A&P14-1). Inhaled irritants and mucus (mechanical stimuli) excite rapidly adapting pulmonary stretch receptors concentrated in the region of the carina and the large bronchi. The stimulation of the receptors results in high-velocity expiratory gas flow (cough).

Peripheral Control

Peripheral control of respiration is due to the sensing of the partial pressure of oxygen (Po_2) and the partial pressure of CO_2 (Pco_2) in the blood. In the blood, CO_2 is an acid. An increase in Pco_2 causes acidosis, and a decrease in pH. Receptors that are responsive to changes in oxygen, CO_2, and pH are located in the brain and in structures adjacent to blood vessels. Arterial blood oxygen and CO_2 pressures are sensed by receptors in the carotid body and the aortic body. The carotid body receptors are located close to the carotid sinus, and the aortic

TABLE A&P14-1	Physiologic Elements of a Cough
Deep inspiration	Inhaled volume of air must be sufficient to increase lung volume, to increase diameter of bronchi and bronchioles, and to move mucus up and out of airways
Inspiratory pause	Allows a buildup and distribution of air and pressure distal to mucus
Closed glottis	Intact muscles and nerves supplying larynx required; allows development of high intrapleural pressures, resulting in a high air flow velocity to propel mucus out of airway
Abdominal muscles	Increase intra-abdominal pressure, which forces diaphragm upward to increase intrapleural pressure against closed glottis
Open glottis	After intrapleural pressures increase, glottis opens suddenly to allow a high velocity of air to leave lungs; flow rates may be as high as 300 L/min
Mucus is expelled	Expulsion caused by high velocity of air leaving airway

bodies are located near the aortic arch. Chemoreceptors are also located on the brain side of the blood-brain barrier. These receptors respond only to Pco_2 (or pH). An elevated Pco_2 in arterial blood is the normal stimulus to increase ventilation. Low levels of partial pressure of oxygen in arterial blood (Pao_2) can stimulate ventilation, but only when Po_2 drops below 70 mm Hg. There is a powerful synergism between these respiratory stimuli, with the greatest ventilatory drive caused by a simultaneous increase in Pco_2 and decrease in Po_2.

GAS EXCHANGE AND TRANSPORT

The exchange of gases occurs between air and blood in the respiratory membrane. Respiration is the exchange of oxygen and CO_2 at the alveolar-capillary level *(external respiration)* and at the tissue-cellular level *(internal respiration)*. During respiration, body tissues are supplied with oxygen for metabolism and CO_2 is released.

In the earth's atmosphere, air contains 20.84% oxygen, 78.62% nitrogen, 0.04% CO_2, and 0.50% water vapor. Each gas exerts a pressure *(partial pressure)* as

if it were the only gas present. The sum of the partial pressures is the *barometric pressure*. When a liquid is exposed to a gas, gas enters the liquid in proportion to the individual pressures. Po_2 in the alveoli is about 104 mm Hg, and Pco_2 is about 40 mm Hg. Venous blood has a Po_2 of 40 mm Hg and a Pco_2 of about 45 mm Hg. These differences in concentration result in the movement of oxygen into the pulmonary capillary bloodstream and of CO_2 out of the pulmonary capillary bed into the alveoli (Figure A&P14-7).

The high Po_2 gradient between the alveolar air and blood is necessary because oxygen is less soluble than CO_2. Diseases that decrease gas diffusion generally alter oxygen exchange before altering carbon dioxide exchange.

Oxygen Transport

After diffusing into the pulmonary capillaries, oxygen is transported throughout the body by the circulatory system. The oxygen is dissolved in the plasma (3%) or bound in the ferrous iron–containing protein hemoglobin (97%). The combination of hemoglobin and oxygen forms *oxyhemoglobin,* which greatly increases the

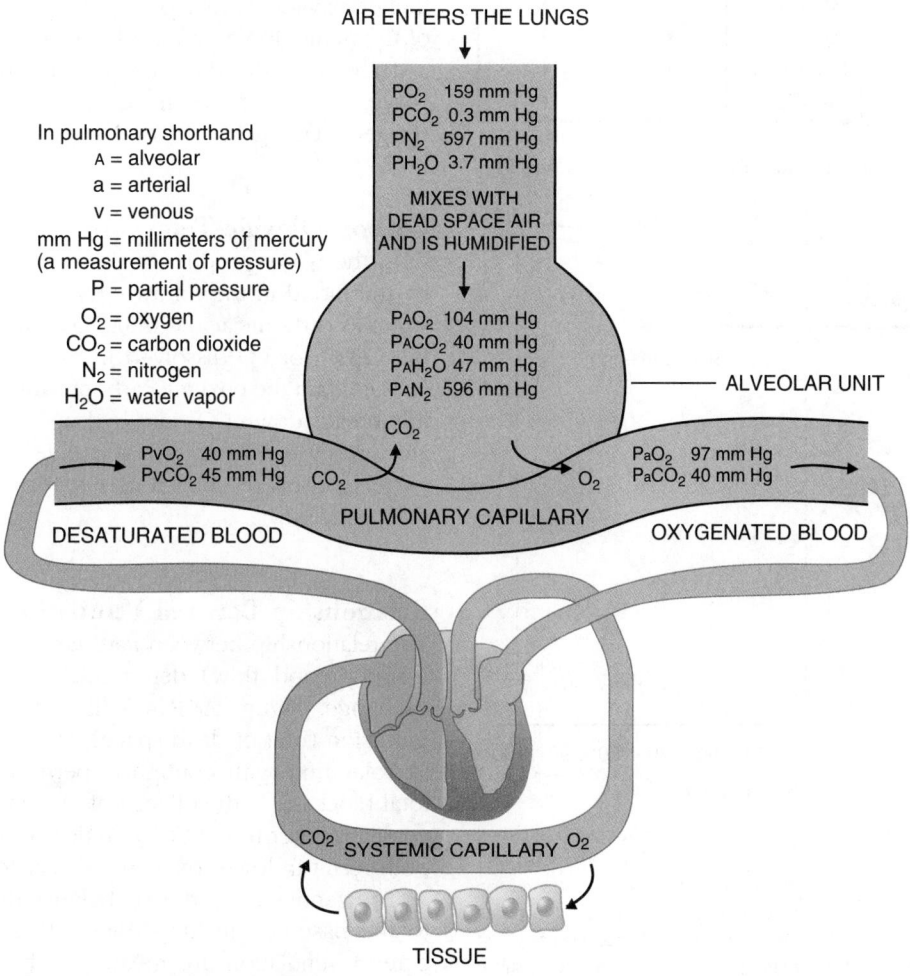

■ **FIGURE A&P14–7** Partial pressures of gases during normal respiration.

oxygen content of the blood above that dissolved in plasma. Tissues take up oxygen at varying rates; the rate of oxygen consumption creates an oxygen pressure gradient between the blood and the mitochondria. Carbon monoxide (CO) and other chemicals impair the ability of hemoglobin to transport oxygen in the blood.

The *oxyhemoglobin dissociation curve* represents the relationship between Pao$_2$ and the saturation of hemoglobin. This saturation reflects the amount of oxygen available to the tissues. For a normal curve, it is assumed that the client's temperature is 37° C, pH is 7.40, and Pco$_2$ is 40 mm Hg. The oxyhemoglobin dissociation curve is affected by a number of factors, including (1) temperature, (2) pH, (3) Pco$_2$, (4) substances in the red blood cell (2,3-diphosphoglycerate [2,3-DPG]), (5) presence of CO, and (6) abnormal hemoglobin. Changes in the affinity of oxygen for hemoglobin cause the oxyhemoglobin curve to move from its normal contour, or to *shift* (Figure A&P14-8).

A *shift to the left* of the oxyhemoglobin dissociation curve increases the affinity of the hemoglobin molecule for oxygen. It is easier for oxygen to bind to hemoglobin, but oxygen is not easily released at the tissues. Thus at any Po$_2$ level, oxygen saturation is greater than normal but tissue hypoxia is present. Clinical situations that diminish the tissue delivery of oxygen include alkalosis, hypocapnia, hypothermia, decreased 2,3-DPG levels, and CO poisoning.

A *shift to the right* indicates an easier release of oxygen at the tissue level but more difficulty in binding in the lungs. This shift protects the body by allowing oxygen attached to hemoglobin to be released in the tissues to maintain adequate tissue oxygenation. Exercise improves the delivery of oxygen to the tissues, as do a number of clinical situations, including acidosis, hypercapnia, hyperthermia, hyperthyroidism (which increases 2,3-DPG levels), anemia, and chronic hypoxia.

Alternatively, shifts in the oxyhemoglobin dissociation curve can be expressed by a single numerical value—the P$_{50}$. The P$_{50}$ represents that oxygen partial pressure at which 50% of the hemoglobin is bound to oxygen, that is, the 50% saturation point. If the affinity of hemoglobin for oxygen is decreased (shifted to the right), then a higher oxygen partial pressure is needed to bind 50% of the hemoglobin and the P$_{50}$ is increased. Conversely, a decrease in the P$_{50}$ represents a leftward shift in the curve, or an increase in the affinity of hemoglobin for oxygen (see Figure A&P14-8).

Carbon Dioxide Transport

CO$_2$, the waste product of tissue metabolism, is carried by the blood in the following ways: (1) combined with water as carbonic acid (70%), (2) coupled with hemoglobin (23%), or (3) dissolved in plasma (7%). Red blood cells contain the enzyme carbonic anhydrase, which rapidly breaks down CO$_2$ into hydrogen ions and bicarbonate ions. When venous blood enters the lungs for gas exchange, this reaction reverses, forming CO$_2$, which is then exhaled.

Relationship Between Ventilation and Perfusion

The relationship between *ventilation* (air flow) and *perfusion* (blood flow) determines the efficiency of gas exchange. Figure A&P14-9 illustrates ventilation with perfusion (unit of dead space), lack of ventilation of an alveolar unit with continued perfusion (a shunt), and total blockage with collapse of alveoli (atelectasis). Low ventilation-perfusion ($\dot{V}/\dot{Q}$) ratios and high $\dot{V}/\dot{Q}$ ratio both result in lower oxygen delivery to the body.

The ventilation-perfusion balance differs from the top to the base of the lung. Blood flow and (to a lesser extent) ventilation are greater in the more dependent lung segments at the base of the lung. Consequently

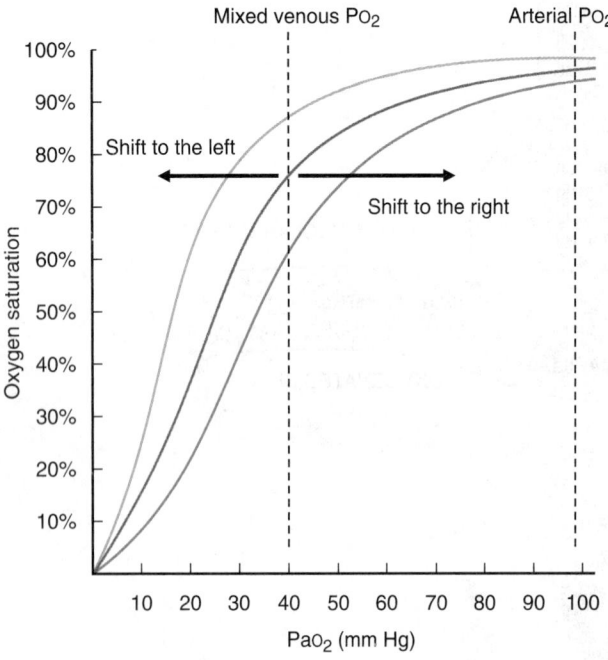

	Factors shifting curve...	
	To the left	To the right
[H⁺], pH	↑	↓
Pco$_2$	↓	↑
Temperature	↓	↑
2,3-DPG	↓	↑

■ **FIGURE A&P14–8** The normal oxyhemoglobin dissociation curve, showing how changes in the affinity of oxygen for hemoglobin shift the curve to the right or the left. Changes in the Pao$_2$ at the flattened top portion of the curve result in small changes in oxygen saturation. The opposite is true as the slope of the curve becomes steeper. At the steepest portion of the curve, with the Pao$_2$ below 60 mm Hg, small changes in the Pao$_2$ result in large decreases in oxygen saturation.

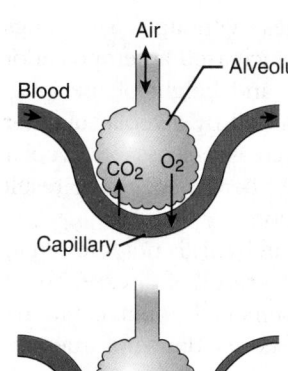

NORMAL
A normally functioning alveolus and normal pulmonary capillary flow. Ventilation and perfusion match.

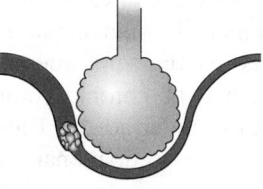

DEAD SPACE UNIT
When there is ventilation without perfusion, a dead space unit exists. Example: Pulmonary embolus preventing blood flow through the pulmonary capillary.

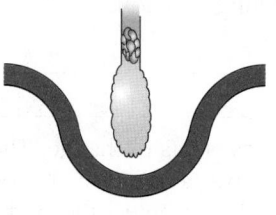

SHUNT UNIT
When there is no ventilation to an alveolar unit but perfusion continues, a shunt unit exists, and unoxygenated blood continues to circulate. Examples: atelectasis, pneumonia. The alveoli collapse.

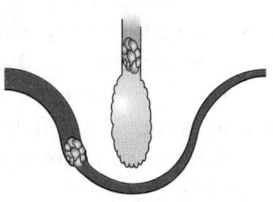

SILENT UNIT
When there is neither ventilation nor perfusion, a silent unit develops. Example: Pulmonary embolus combined with ARDS (adult respiratory distress syndrome). The alveoli collapse.

■ **FIGURE A&P14–9** Relationships between ventilation (air flow) and perfusion (blood flow).

the base of the lung has the lowest $\dot{V}/\dot{Q}$ ratio, and the apex of the lung has the highest $\dot{V}/\dot{Q}$ ratio.

The $\dot{V}/\dot{Q}$ balance is controlled at both the airway and vascular levels. Hypoxia, resulting from underventilation of an alveolar region, causes vasoconstriction, which redirects blood to well-ventilated alveoli. CO_2 in the airways dilates the airway smooth muscle. Poorly perfused alveoli have low CO_2 levels, and the resultant airway constriction directs ventilation to better perfused alveoli.

REGULATION OF ACID-BASE BALANCE

The lungs, through gas exchange, have a key role in regulating the acid-base balance of the body. Pulmonary disorders that change the CO_2 level in the blood cause either respiratory acidemia or respiratory alkalemia. Insufficient ventilation causes *hypercapnia,* a respiratory acidemia caused by retention of excessive amounts of CO_2. Hyperventilation, conversely, causes *hypocapnia,* a respiratory alkalemia caused by the low amounts of CO_2 in the blood.

The effectiveness of ventilation is best measured by the P_{CO_2} in the arterial blood (Pa_{CO_2}). Because the respiratory system normally maintains a Pa_{CO_2} between 35 and 45 mm Hg at sea level, a Pa_{CO_2} above this range represents *hypoventilation.* Anesthetic agents, sedatives, and opioids all tend to increase the resting Pa_{CO_2}. (Acid-base balance is detailed in Chapter 13.)

REACTION TO INJURY

The elaborate defense mechanisms of the lungs involve clearance mechanisms, defense by the respiratory epithelium, and immunologic responses in the lungs. Any injury to the lung affects the barrier between the atmosphere and the bloodstream. This barrier, which lies within the alveolar septum, is made up of epithelial (types I and II pneumocytes) and vascular endothelial cells. Injury resulting from airborne or blood-borne agents may increase vascular permeability and cause pulmonary edema. Inflammatory cells (e.g., neutrophils) arrive soon after acute injury. Then the proportion of lymphocytes, monocytes, and macrophages increases following a typical inflammatory process.

The basic lung repair processes include lymphatic drainage of excess fluid and phagocytic removal of protein and debris. This action generally restores lung function and structure. More severe injury requires endothelial and epithelial cell regeneration and proliferation of interstitial cells (fibroblasts). Type II cells that are generated for defense eventually differentiate into thin type I cells, which permit gas exchange. The lung's ability to recreate alveolar septa determines the degree to which normal lung function and structure are restored.

Defense by Clearance Mechanisms

The *upper airways* filter particles. Because the nose has a larger surface-volume ratio and a much more tortuous pathway for airflow than the mouth, particle deposition and conditioning of the air are more efficient when a person breathes through the nose. Larger particles (>10 mm) are generally trapped; smaller particles (<1 mm) may readily enter the lower airways.

There are four clearance mechanisms of the lower airways and alveoli:

- Cough (first five to eight bronchial generations)
- Mucociliary system (to terminal bronchioles)
- Macrophages (alveoli and respiratory bronchioles)
- Lymphatics (alveoli and interstitium)

The cough, an automatic protective reflex used to clear the trachea, occurs most rapidly in the clearing process (see Table A&P14-1). If the swallowing reflex is delayed or absent, a cough may be stimulated to avoid aspiration of particles into the lower airways.

Defense by the Respiratory Epithelium

Unlike the upper and lower airways, the alveoli lack a mucous layer to trap foreign particles and cilia to propel them to the pharynx for elimination. The alveolar lining is made up of flat, membranous pneumocytes (type I cells) and rounded granular (type II) cells. The type II cells are resistant to injury and cover most of the alveolar surface after exposure to infectious agents. Alveolar macrophages, derived from type II pneumocytes, are also found over the surface of the alveoli. Alveolar macrophages are active phagocytes that remove dead cells and protein and that synthesize and secrete substances that regulate the immune system. They leave the lung by the mucociliary system or the lymphatic system.

Defense by Immunologic Mechanisms

The systemic immune system responds to the lung during inflammatory processes by mobilizing blood neutrophils and monocytes. Recruited thymus-dependent (T) and thymus-independent (B) lymphocytes contribute to local cell-mediated immune reactions and the production of specific antibodies within the alveoli. Cell-mediated immunity is a key determinant in resistance to organisms such as *Mycobacterium tuberculosis* and *Pneumocystis (carinii) jiroveci*. Immune mechanisms are generally a host defense function. However, hypersensitivity immune reactions lead to tissue injury and are responsible for clinical conditions such as asthma, granuloma formation, and lung transplant rejection. (Chapter 76 describes types I, II, III, and IV hypersensitivity reactions.)

EFFECTS OF AGING

Most of the changes that occur with aging affect the lower airway. Movement of cilia in the upper airway slows and becomes less effective. This change predisposes older clients to a greater number of respiratory tract infections.

Lung structure also changes with age. The lungs become rounder as a result of increased anteroposterior diameter, circumference, area, and height of the lung. The proportion of the lung formed by alveolar duct air increases, and alveolar air decreases. Loss of alveolar wall tissue and its elastic tissue fibers is seen. The result is a deterioration of lung function.

The air spaces enlarge, although this is not referred to as emphysema because it is not a result of disease. These changes may be due to environmental pollutants rather than to aging alone. An increased incidence of true emphysema and a greater prevalence of chronic cough and sputum production are seen in older adults. These findings suggest that environmental or occupational pollutants, in addition to the normal aging process, may be a component in the decline of lung function.

CONCLUSIONS

The primary function of the lungs is gas exchange. The physical structure of the airways allows air to be warmed, filtered, and humidified as it enters the body. In the alveolar sacs, oxygen is exchanged for CO_2. The mechanics of breathing are coordinated by the ribs, diaphragm, pleural space, elastic recoil of the lungs, and the nervous system. The respiratory system also helps regulate acid-base balance. Alterations in structure and function can result in various disorders.

BIBLIOGRAPHY

1. Berne, R., et al. (2004). *Physiology* (5th ed.). St. Louis: Mosby.
2. Carroll, R.G. (2007). *Elsevier's integrated physiology*. Philadelphia: Saunders.
3. Kierszenbaum, A.L. (2007). *Histology and cell biology: An introduction to pathology* (2nd ed.). St. Louis: Mosby.
4. Guyton, A., & Hall, J. (2006). *Textbook of medical physiology* (11th ed.). Philadelphia: Saunders.
5. Silverthorn, D. (2006). *Human physiology* (4th ed.). San Francisco: Pearson Benjamin Cummings.

CHAPTER 59

Assessment of the Respiratory System

DIANA MOXNESS AND SUSANNE A. QUALLICH

Nurses who care for clients experiencing respiratory disorders perform and interpret a variety of assessment procedures. This chapter discusses history and physical assessment as well as diagnostic procedures used to plan care for clients with respiratory disorders.

HISTORY

Biographical Data

Note the client's biological age and compare it with the client's appearance. Does the client look his/her stated age? Chronic respiratory disorders such as lung cancer or chronic obstructive pulmonary disease often make the client appear older.

Current Health
Chief Complaint

The client's clinical manifestations, sometimes described as the chief complaint, help to establish priorities for medical and nursing intervention. In emergency or acute situations, brief and simple questions regarding the chief complaint(s) are asked until the client's condition is stabilized.

Clinical Manifestations

Common clinical manifestations related to the respiratory system include noncardiac chest pain, dyspnea (difficulty breathing), cough, hemoptysis (bloody sputum), wheezing, stridor, and complaints related to the nose and sinuses. Figure 59-1 summarizes the assessment data that should be collected regarding common respiratory clinical manifestations. Note the onset, location, duration, characteristics, aggravating and relieving factors, associated manifestations, timing, setting, and severity of the problem. Some students use the mnemonic OLD CARTS to remember assessment data to collect from the client.

Noncardiac Chest Pain. Chest pain may be associated with pulmonary, cardiac, or gastrointestinal problems, and being able to distinguish between the three is important. Determine the location, duration, and intensity of the chest pain to provide early clues to the cause. Ask the client what instigates the pain (e.g., activity, coughing, movement) and what relieves the pain (e.g., nitroglycerin, splinting the chest wall, heat).

Pleuritic chest pain is commonly a sharp, stabbing pain that occurs at one site on the chest wall and increases with chest wall movement or deep breathing. Retrosternal (behind the sternum) pain is usually burning, constant, and aching. Pain can also originate in the bony and cartilaginous parts of the thorax.

Angina pectoris (pain of the chest) is cardiac in origin and may be associated with decreased blood flow to the heart and is a potentially life-threatening problem. Cardiac chest pain is usually described as an aching, heavy, squeezing sensation with pressure or tightness in the substernal area and can radiate into the neck or arms

---

evolve Web Enhancements

Assessment Terms English and Spanish

Appendix B Expanded Health History Format That Integrates the Assessment of Functional Health Patterns

Web Tables Modified Borg Scale

Pulmonary Function Test (PFT) Components

Categorization of Obstructive and Restrictive Pulmonary Disorders and Pulmonary Function Test (PFT) Findings

Figures Thoracic Landmarks and Underlying Structures

Assessing Respiratory Patterns

Assessment of Thoracic Excursion

Be sure to check out the bonus material on the Evolve website and the CD-ROM, including free self-assessment exercises. **http://evolve.elsevier.com/Black/medsurg**

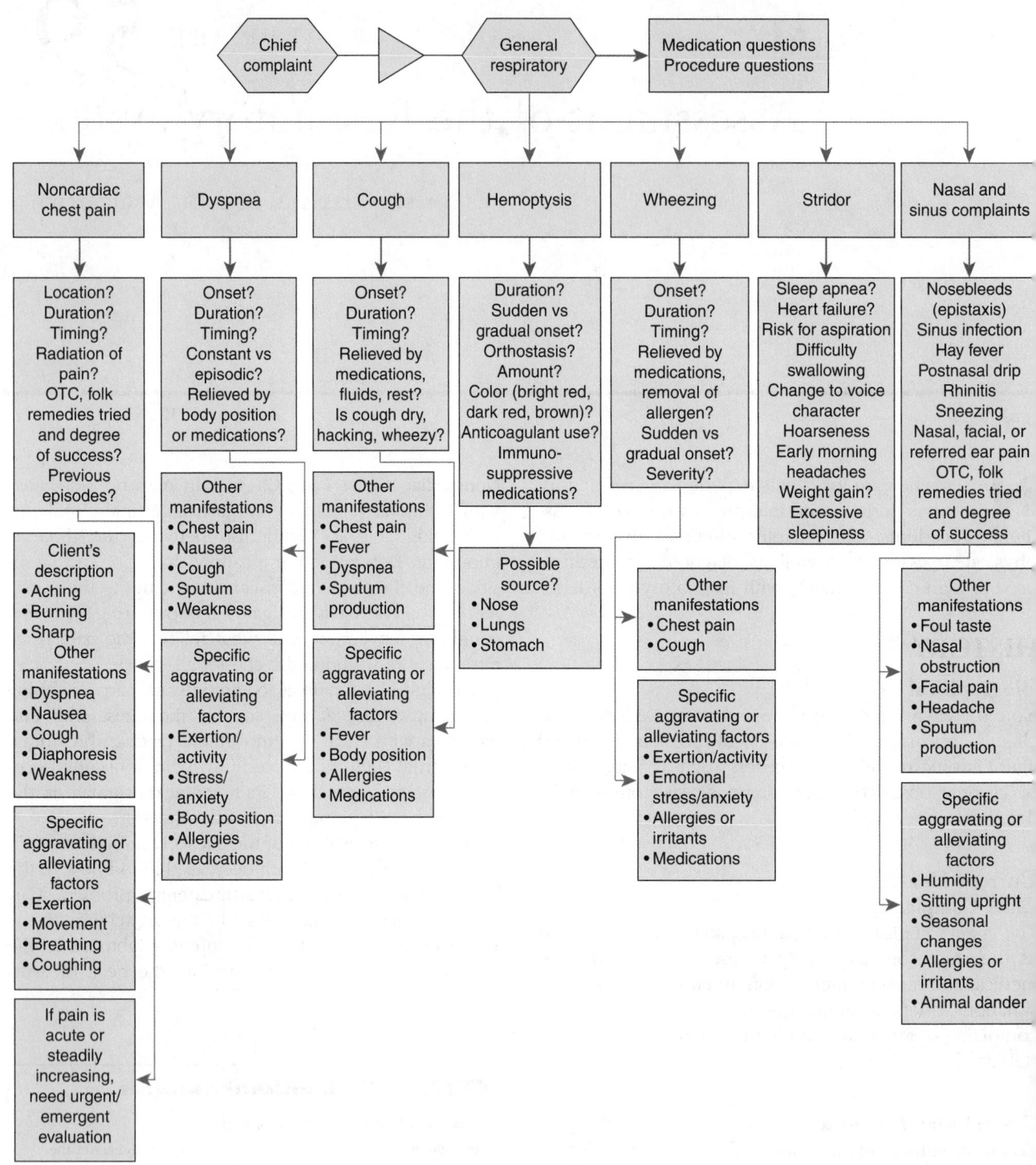

■ **FIGURE 59–1** Expanded respiratory assessment.

(see Chapters 54 and 56 for more information related to cardiac chest pain).

Clients with esophageal problems such as esophagitis, gastrointestinal reflux disease (GERD), and hiatal hernias may complain of chest pain. See Chapter 28 for more information related to assessment of these disorders.

Dyspnea. Dyspnea (difficulty breathing) is a common manifestation experienced by clients with pulmonary

and cardiac disorders. It is a client's subjective assessment of the degree of work of breathing exerted for given task or effort. Clients may define dyspnea as shortness of breath, suffocation, tightness, being winded, c being breathless. The subjective nature of dyspne makes it difficult to quantify objectively.

Several methods are used to assess accurately the leve of dyspnea experienced by a client. The Visual Analogu Scale (Figure 59-2) is used to quantify breathlessness l

How short of breath are you right now?

None

Extremely
severe

■ **FIGURE 59–2** The Visual Analogue Scale of dyspnea. Although the scale can be in the form of either a vertical or a horizontal line, the most commonly used scale consists of a 100-mm horizontal line, like the one shown here.

using the client's response to particular questions. It is easy to understand, and the amount of dyspnea during various activities can be assessed. The modified Borg Category Ratio Scale for assessment of dyspnea (found on the website) is used to rate the intensity of dyspnea. The scale is simple, and results have been reproduced in several populations.

In addition to a subjective assessment, document the characteristics of the dyspnea. Assess all the characteristics because many respiratory and nonrespiratory causes can result in dyspnea. The Integrating Diagnostic Testing feature below further details the evaluation of dyspnea.

Cough. Note when and how the cough began (suddenly or gradually) and how long it has been present. Determine the frequency of the cough and the time of day when the cough is better or worse (early morning, late afternoon, nighttime). The client may describe the cough as hacking, dry, hoarse, congested, barking, wheezy, or bubbling. The Integrating Diagnostic Testing feature on p. 1528 further details the evaluation of a client with a cough.

Determine which medications or treatments the client has used for the cough (antitussives, codeine, inhalers, nebulizers, rest, sitting up).

Find out what precautions are used to prevent the spread of infection (if it is present).

SAFETY

ALERT

Sputum is the substance expelled by coughing or clearing the throat, but sputum production with coughing is not normal. The tracheobronchial tree normally produces about 3 ounces of mucus a day as part of the normal cleaning mechanism. Question the client about sputum color (clear, yellow, green, rusty, bloody), odor, quality (watery, stringy, frothy, thick), and quantity (teaspoon, tablespoon, cup) and document any changes. Ascertain whether sputum is produced only after the client is lying in a certain position. Sputum may also be a

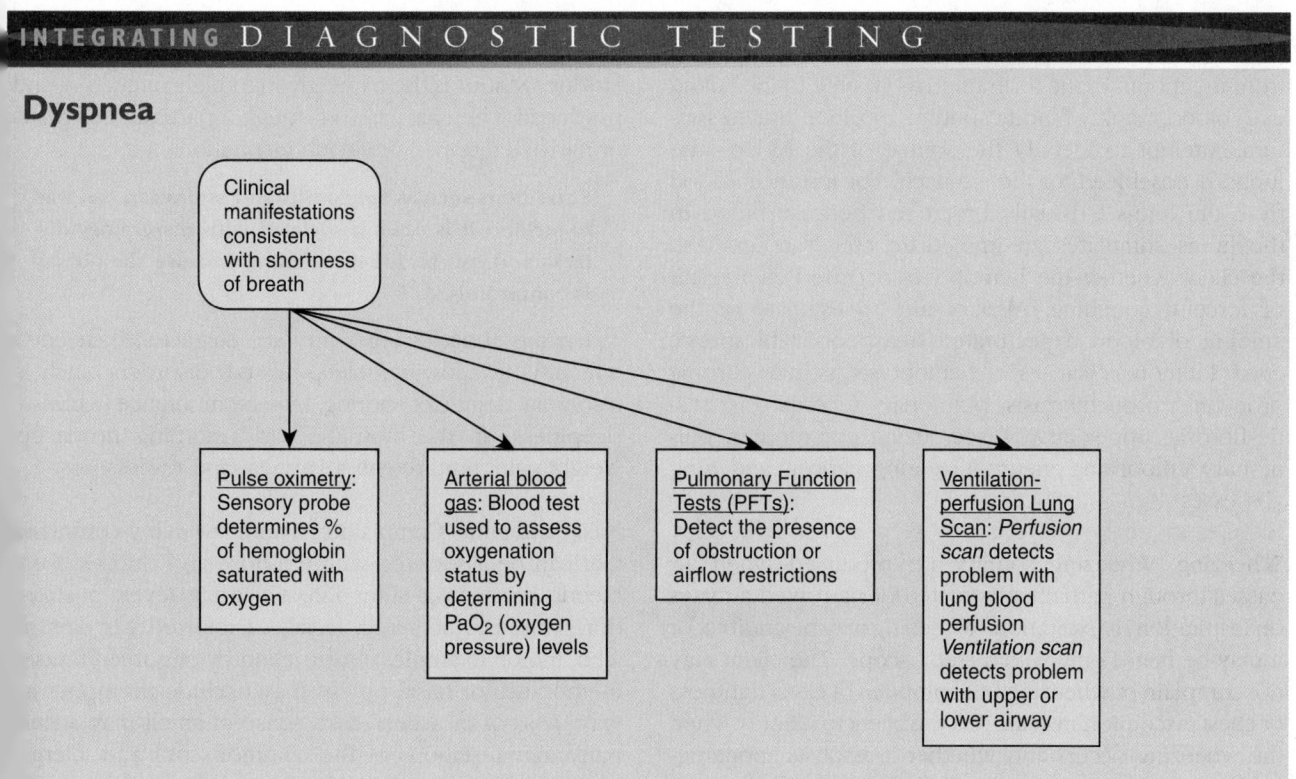

INTEGRATING DIAGNOSTIC TESTING

Dyspnea

Clinical manifestations consistent with shortness of breath

Pulse oximetry: Sensory probe determines % of hemoglobin saturated with oxygen

Arterial blood gas: Blood test used to assess oxygenation status by determining PaO_2 (oxygen pressure) levels

Pulmonary Function Tests (PFTs): Detect the presence of obstruction or airflow restrictions

Ventilation-perfusion Lung Scan: *Perfusion scan* detects problem with lung blood perfusion *Ventilation scan* detects problem with upper or lower airway

INTEGRATING DIAGNOSTIC TESTING

Cough

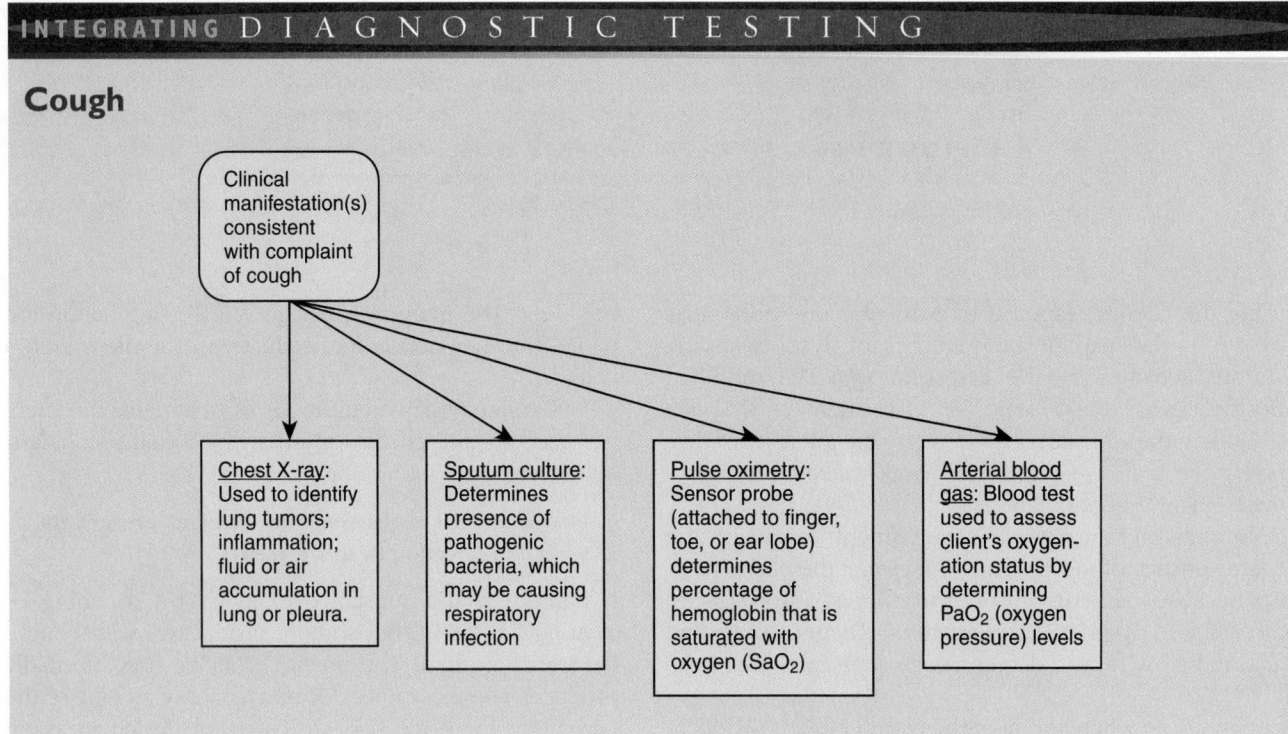

secretion from the oral or nasopharyngeal area or sinuses rather than from the tracheobronchial tree. For example, draining sinuses may provoke a productive cough.

Hemoptysis. Hemoptysis refers to blood expectorated from the mouth in the form of gross (visible to the naked eye) blood, frankly bloody sputum, or blood-tinged sputum. Attempt to identify the source of the blood—the lungs, a nosebleed, or the stomach. For instance, blood from the lungs is usually bright red because blood in the lungs stimulates an immediate cough reflex. Ask the client whether the hemoptysis occurred as a result of forceful coughing. Also obtain an estimate of the amount of blood expectorated (teaspoon, tablespoon, cup). Pulmonary causes of hemoptysis include chronic bronchitis, bronchiectasis, pulmonary tuberculosis, cystic fibrosis, upper airway necrotizing granulomas, pulmonary embolism, pneumonia, lung cancer, and lung abscesses.

Wheezing. Wheezing sounds are produced when air passes through partially obstructed or narrowed airways on inspiration or expiration. Wheezing may be audible, or it may be heard only with a stethoscope. The client may not complain of wheezing but complain of chest tightness or chest discomfort instead. Ask the client to identify when the wheezing occurs and whether it resolves spontaneously or medication is required for relief. Not all wheezing

is caused by asthma; wheezing can be caused by mucosal edema, airway secretions, collapsed airways resulting from loss of elastic tissue, and foreign objects or tumors partially obstructing air flow.

Stridor. Stridor is the name given to high-pitched sounds produced when air passes through a partially obstructed or narrowed upper airway on inspiration.

> Conditions such as epiglottitis and aspiration can lead to stridor; it is often associated with respiratory distress and can be life-threatening because the airway is compromised.

Inquire about changes in voice character, hoarseness, difficulty swallowing, sleep-related disorders such as insomnia, degree of snoring, hypersomnolence (excessive sleepiness) in the morning, early morning headache, weight gain, fluid retention, apnea, and restlessness.

Nasal and Sinus Complaints. There are many complaints that can be associated with the nose and sinuses. Nose bleeds (epistaxis), sinus infection, hay fever, postnasal drip, rhinitis, and nasal, facial, or referred ear pain are all common examples. Obstruction by engorged mucous membranes or nasal polyps may occlude the upper airway. Loss of or a decreased sense of smell may accompany manifestations of the common cold and allergy or may signal a more serious neurologic problem.

Inquire whether the client has experienced these manifestations previously and, if so, under what conditions. Ask the client about attempts at self-treatment, such as nasal sprays, decongestants, antihistamines, and other over-the-counter and herbal cold and allergy medications.

Ask the client about factors that alleviate or worsen the manifestations and any other conditions that seem to be related. This includes increased humidity, sitting upright, lying supine, weather and seasonal changes, or allergies. Nasal and sinus problems may be allergy related and provoked by pollen, fumes, smoke, animal dander, or dust particles. A foul taste in the mouth, unpleasant breath odor (halitosis), nasal obstruction, and facial pain (particularly over the frontal and maxillary sinuses) may accompany sinusitis. Chronic sinusitis may be accompanied by headache or facial pain present on awakening and diminishing during the day as the sinuses drain.

Review of Systems

In addition to the common clinical manifestations, the client may report other complaints that may be directly or indirectly related to a respiratory condition. These symptoms include fever, hoarseness, night sweats, anorexia, weight loss, dependent edema, recent or frequent colds, nasal discharge, sinus pain or pressure, and epistaxis (nosebleed). In addition, coughing may result in stress incontinence; you may want to ask female clients about this problem. Figure 59-3 provides a summary of specific history data that should be collected for a client with respiratory complaints.

Past Medical History

Review the past health history of the client and family members for data related to the upper and lower respiratory systems, which are common sources of both acute and chronic health problems. Assess clients with chronic conditions for changes in their ongoing respiratory manifestations as these changes provide clues to the cause of the new problem.

In addition to obtaining data regarding common childhood diseases and vaccinations, ask the client about the occurrence of tuberculosis, bronchitis, influenza, asthma, and pneumonia and the frequency of lower respiratory tract infections after upper respiratory tract infection. Determine the existence of congenital problems, such as cystic fibrosis and premature birth history, which can be associated with respiratory complications in the adult client. Inquire about vaccination against pneumonia and influenza. A one-time administration of the polyvalent pneumococcal vaccine Pneumovax provides lifelong immunity against pneumococcal pneumonia in most clients. However, revaccination has been a topic of discussion in recent years and may be necessary with some clients. Influenza or "flu" shots must be received annually in the fall of the year.

Ask about the date and results of the client's most recent chest x-ray or other pulmonary diagnostic tests. These test results can provide baseline data for the evaluation of the current problem. Inquire about previous injuries to the mouth, nose, throat, or chest (e.g., blunt trauma, fractured ribs, or pneumothorax).

Surgical History

Discuss the client's history of any procedure or surgery that pertains to the upper or lower respiratory system, such as biopsies or procedures to directly visualize the structures.

Allergies

Question the client about a history of allergies and timing of manifestations to help identify a possible allergic basis for the condition. Has the client been tested for allergies? When? Are medications (including allergy shots) taken prophylactically or on an as-needed basis to provide relief from manifestations?

Ask about precipitating and aggravating factors, such as foods, medications, pollens, smoke, fumes, dust, and animal dander. Ask the client to describe the allergic manifestations experienced (chest tightness, wheezing, cough, rhinitis, watery eyes, scratchy throat) and their severity. Determine the age at which allergies first occurred and whether they have become progressively more severe.

Medications

Obtain detailed information regarding both prescribed and over-the-counter medications, including herbal remedies, because many products affect the respiratory system. The client may routinely require antibiotics, bronchodilators, or steroids for respiratory tract infections. Specify the route of administration (pill, liquid, or inhalation). Many respiratory medications are inhaled through a metered-dose inhaler (MDI) or mini-nebulizer. Some medications can affect smell and taste; these include metronidazole, local anesthetics, clofibrate, some antibiotics, some antineoplastics, allopurinol, phenylbutazone, levodopa, codeine, morphine, carbamazepine, lithium, and trifluoperazine.

Herbal medicines for respiratory problems include remedies for nasal discharge and congestion, cough, sore throat, fever and headache, and possible immunostimulants. Expectorants include anise (*Pimpinella anisum*), coltsfoot (*Tussilago farfara*), and horehound (*Marrubium vulgare*). Coltsfoot and horehound are also believed to have antitussive action. Sore throat remedies include mint (*Mentha piperita* [peppermint], *Mentha spicata* [spearmint]) and slippery elm (*Ulmus rubra*). Remedies for the fever and headache that may accompany colds and influenza include boneset (*Eupatorium perfoliatum*), feverfew (*Tanacetum parthenium*), and white

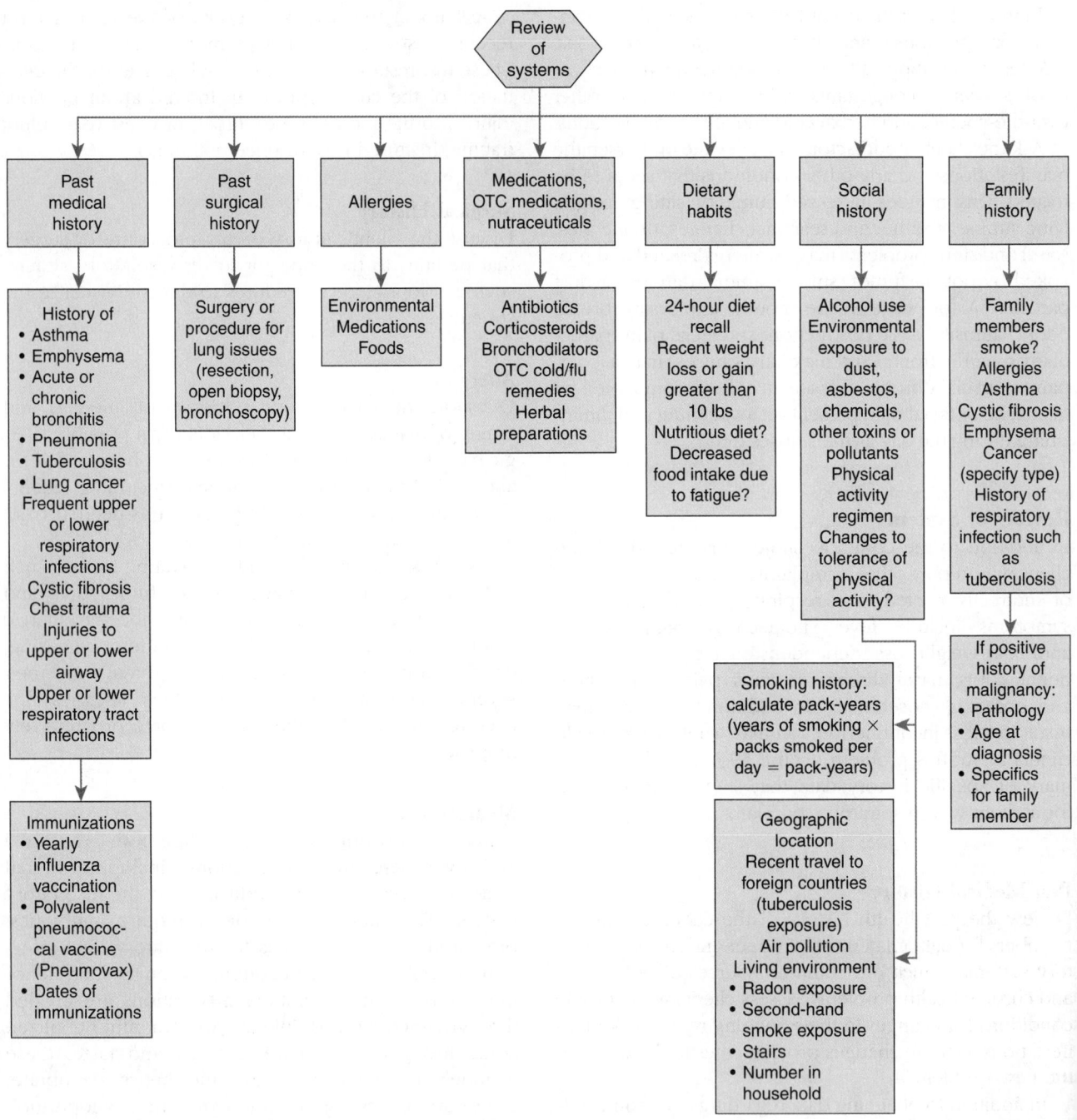

■ FIGURE 59–3 Expanded respiratory history.

willow *(Salix purpurea, Salix fragilis).* Stimulants of the immune system, believed to help ward off colds and flu, include *Echinacea (E. angustifolia, E. pallida, E. purpurea)* and goldenseal *(Hydrastis canadensis).* Refer to Chapter 4 for further discussion.

Dietary Habits

Maintaining a nutritious diet is important for clients with chronic respiratory disease, which can result in decreased lung capacity and greater workload for the lungs and cardiovascular system. The added workload increases caloric expenditure, and weight loss may occur. Clients may

become anorectic because of the effects of medications and fatigue. The client may not have enough energy to consume the needed calories to maintain body weight. Ask the client to recall intake for the last 24 hours. Assess the amount of protein, kilocalories, and sodium intake (see Chapter 28).

Social History

Respiratory status is affected by numerous factors that may lead to acute problems or that may affect the client's coping with chronic respiratory problems. Identify any environmental agents that might be contributing to the lient's condition. Ask specifically about the work envi-onment and hobbies. Focus on exposure to dust, asbes-os, beryllium, silica, and other toxins or pollutants. armers are exposed to airborne particles such as grain ust, fertilizers, and animal dander. Hobbies may involve nemicals, heat, dust, and airborne particles from grind-ig, soldering, or welding.

Ask about recent travel to areas where respiratory dis-ases are prevalent, such as Asia (tuberculosis), the Ohio iver valley (histoplasmosis), or the San Joaquin valley valley fever). Polluted city air has also been related) increasing incidence and severity of asthma.

Ask about the client's living conditions. Assess for nvironmental hazards such as stairs or poor air cir-ulation. A client with a chronic respiratory condition lay have difficulty climbing stairs or breathing unfil-red air. How many people are in the household? rowded living conditions increase risk of exposure to nfectious respiratory diseases such as tuberculosis and old viruses. Recent exposure to continuous air condi-oning in a hotel or motel setting may be related to egionnaires' disease.

Inquire about any history of smoking tobacco pro-ucts and of drinking alcohol. Smoking has been asso-ated with decreased ciliary function of the lungs, creased mucus production, and the development of ng cancer and chronic lung problems. Ask the ient about the use of smokeless tobacco (snuff, chew-g tobacco) and smoking non-tobacco substances (mar-ıana and clove cigarettes). The pack-year history, hich helps quantify the smoking history, is determined / using the following equation:

$$\text{Years of Smoking} \times \text{Packs Smoked per Day} = \text{Pack-Years}$$

Ciliary action is slowed by alcohol, which reduces ucus clearance from the lungs. Heavy alcohol inges-on depresses the cough reflex and increases risk of piration.

Clients who are active may describe the onset of >ughing and wheezing during exercise. These clients ed to be further evaluated for exercise-induced thma before continuing workouts. Clients with chronic spiratory conditions often do not have the lung capac-/ to sustain even mild forms of exercise and subse-ıently become dyspneic. Has tolerance for activity :creased or remained stable? Ask the client to describe pical activities, such as walking, light housekeeping iores, or grocery shopping, that are tolerated or, con-rsely, that result in shortness of breath.

ımily Health History

uestion the client about the family history of respira-ry diseases. Identify blood relatives (in regard to genet-ılly transmitted diseases) and family members (in gard to infectious conditions) who have had asthma,

cystic fibrosis, emphysema, chronic obstructive pulmo-nary disease (COPD), lung cancer, respiratory tract infec-tions, tuberculosis, or allergies. List the age and cause of death of each deceased family member. Do any house-hold members smoke cigarettes, pipes, or cigars? Second-ary inhalation of smoke often precipitates or worsens respiratory manifestations.

PHYSICAL EXAMINATION

Hypoxia as a result of respiratory conditions may precip-itate subtle neurologic alterations, such as restlessness, fatigue, disorientation, and personality changes. Tachy-cardia usually accompanies respiratory problems as the body attempts to compensate for decreased oxygen deliv-ery. Anorexia and weight loss are seen in many chronic respiratory conditions. Please refer to the normal findings as described in the Physical Assessment Findings in the Healthy Adult feature below. Refer to a physical assess-ment text for the details of a complete respiratory system assessment.

Physical Assessment Findings in the Healthy Adult

The Respiratory System

INSPECTION
Nose. Nose straight, without flaring or discharge; nares patent; mucosa pink and moist; septum midline, without masses or perforation.
Sinuses. Transilluminate.
Thorax. Even color; regular, even contour; respirations quiet, unlabored, of even depth, and without retractions, bulges, masses, or use of accessory muscles; anteroposterior-transverse diameter ratio 1:2.
Digits. Clubbing absent; nail beds pink; immediate capillary refill on blanching.

PALPATION
Nose. Nontender, without masses or lesions.
Sinuses. Nontender, without swelling or bogginess.
Trachea. Midline and mobile without crepitus.
Thorax. Chest wall symmetrical, smooth, without lumps, masses, tenderness, or crepitus; thoracic excursion symmetrical; tactile fremitus present.

PERCUSSION
Sinuses. Nontender.
Thorax and Lungs. Resonant throughout peripheral lung fields; cardiac dullness; diaphragmatic excursion ranges from 3 to 6 cm for each hemidiaphragm, with the right side slightly higher than the left.

AUSCULTATION
Thorax and Lungs. Vesicular sounds throughout peripheral lung fields; bronchovesicular sounds over the area of tracheal bifurcation, both anteriorly and posteriorly; bronchial sounds over the trachea anteriorly; adventitious sounds absent; vocal resonance absent.

General Assessment

Assess the client's level of consciousness and orientation. Note the skin and lip color. Assess the nail beds for color and the presence of clubbing, which occurs as a compensatory measure for chronic hypoxia. The Shamroth technique is a useful assessment for the presence of clubbing (Figure 59-4).

Nose and Paranasal Sinuses
External Nose

Inspect and palpate the external nose for deviations from normal alignment, symmetry, color, discharge, nasal flaring, lesions, and tenderness. The client should be able to breathe quietly through the nose rather than breathe through the mouth. Check the nasal canals for patency by asking the client to occlude one naris with a finger and to breathe through the open naris while closing the mouth. Ask the client to tip the head back, and inspect the outer nares for crusting, bleeding, or dryness, which should be absent.

Internal Nose

Next inspect the vestibules with a penlight while the client's head is tipped back. Normal findings include coarse hairs, dark red nasal mucosa, a clear passage without discharge, and a midline septum. Further examination of the internal nose requires the use of a nasal speculum and is not conducted unless indicated. Inspection may be hampered by nasal congestion.

Paranasal Sinuses

Palpate and percuss the frontal and maxillary sinuses to assess for swelling and tenderness, which are normally

absent. Palpate the frontal sinuses simultaneously b placing the thumbs above the eyes, just under the bor ridge of the eye orbits, and apply gentle pressure. Pa pate the maxillary sinuses by using either the inde and third fingers or the thumbs to press gently on eac side of the nose just under the zygomatic bones. Us direct percussion over the eyebrows for the front sinuses and on either side of the nose below the ey in line with the pupils for the maxillary sinuses.

Smell

The senses of taste and smell are closely related. Smell perceived mainly via the olfactory nerves, although som smell is perceived through the trigeminal nerves. Mar conditions affect taste and smell, such as viral infectior normal aging, head injuries, and local obstruction. Sme impairment may be (1) hyposmia (a decrease in sme sensitivity) or (2) anosmia (bilateral and comple absence of smell sensitivity). Assess smell by having th client identify various odors by testing each nostr separately.

Thorax and Lungs

Accurate physical examination of the thorax and lun requires being familiar with the anatomic landmarks the posterior, anterior, and lateral thorax (see the figu of Thoracic Landmarks and Underlying Structures c the website). Use these landmarks to identify the unde lying structures, particularly the lobes of the lung and t heart. When performing inspection, palpation, percu sion, and auscultation of the respiratory system, th examiner should compare one side of the thorax to th other side to help determine the presence or absen of abnormalities (Figure 59-5).

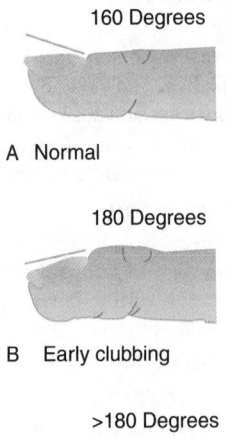
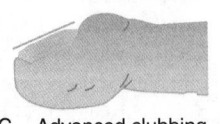
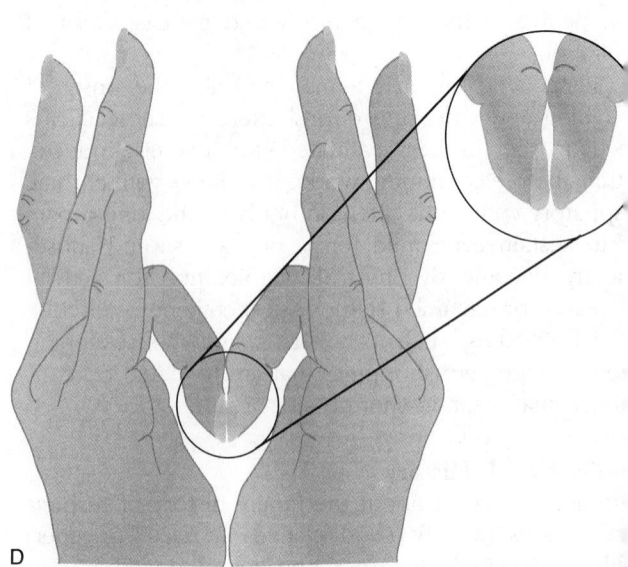

■ **FIGURE 59–4** Clubbing. **A,** A normal digit, with an angle of 160 degrees. **B,** A flattened angle between the nail and the skin, exceeding 180 degrees. **C,** Advanced clubbing with a rounded nail. **D,** Assess clubbing with the use of the Shamroth technique. Instruct the client to place the nails of the fourth (ring) fingers together while extending the other fingers and to hold the hands up. A diamond-shaped space between the nails is a normal finding and indicates the absence of clubbing.

160 Degrees

A Normal

180 Degrees

B Early clubbing

>180 Degrees

C Advanced clubbing

D

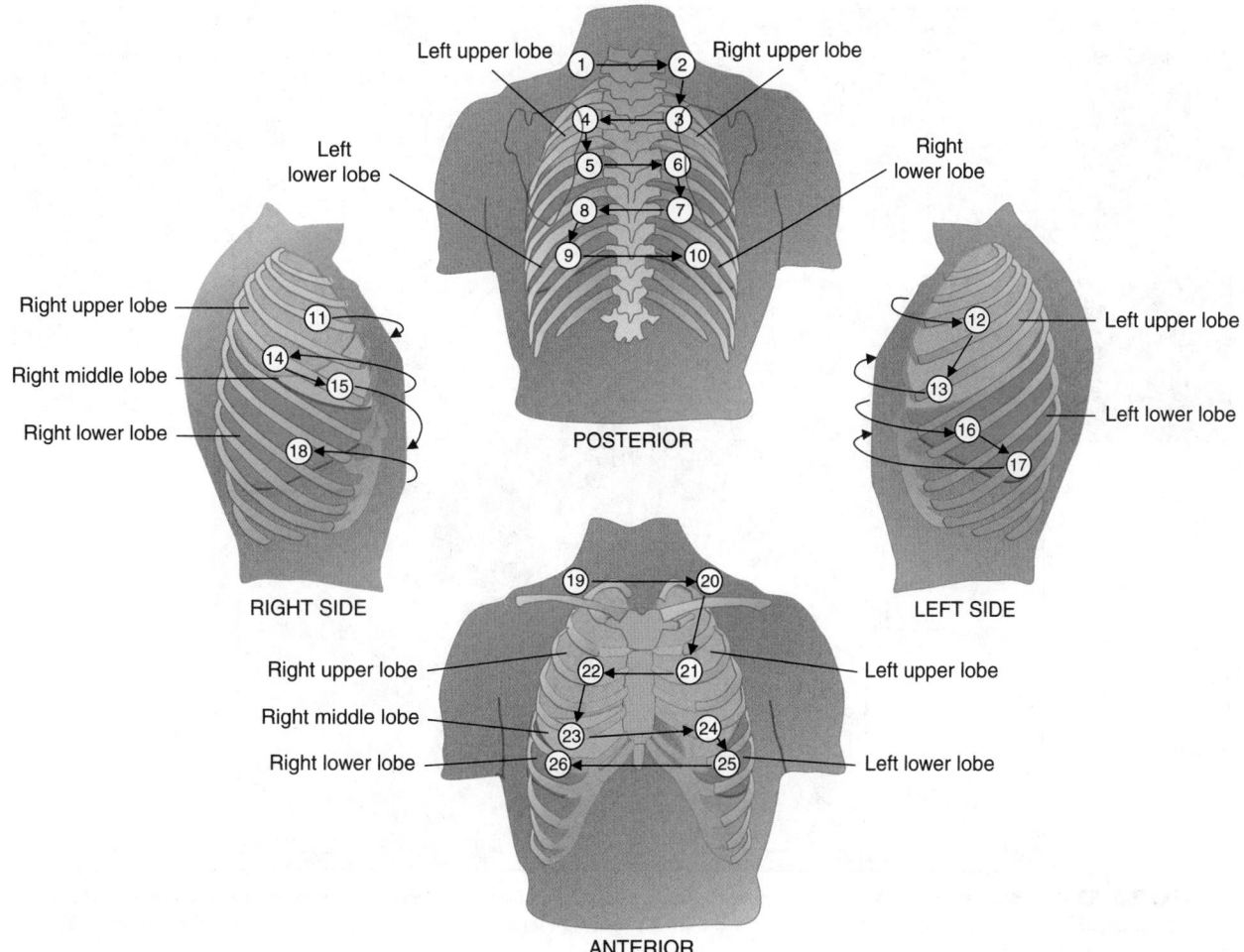

■ **FIGURE 59–5** Sequence for palpation, percussion, and auscultation of the thorax (posterior, lateral, and anterior).

Inspection

Note the client's rate, rhythm, and depth of respirations. The normal respiratory rate for an adult is 14 to 20 breaths per minute. The Assessing Respiratory Patterns figure on the website describes examples of normal and abnormal respiratory patterns. Observe for signs of respiratory distress, such as nasal flaring or retractions, and bulging of intercostal or sternocleidomastoid muscles to facilitate breathing. Inspect the chest wall configuration by comparing the anteroposterior (AP) diameter to the transverse (lateral) diameter; the lateral diameter is normally twice the AP diameter. Figure 59-6 provides information about chest deformities.

Palpation

Palpate the trachea for midline position and slight movability. Palpate the chest wall for symmetrical thoracic excursion during inspiration and expiration (see Assessment of Thoracic Excursion figure on the website). Palpate costal angle (angle at the base of the rib cage); the costal angle should be less than 90 degrees. A costal angle greater than 90 degrees with an AP/lateral

diameter ratio of 1:1 indicates an abnormal barrel chest wall shape, as seen in clients with chronic obstructive pulmonary disease. Additionally, palpate for tactile fremitus, which involves palpating the posterior chest wall while the client says "ninety-nine"; compare the intensity of the vibrations on both sides for symmetry.

Percussion

Percussion over healthy lung tissue produces a resonant (low-pitched, hollow) sound. The pitch and qualities of other percussion sounds can be summarized as follows: (1) tympany (high-pitched, hollow, drum-like); (2) flat (high-pitched, soft); (3) dull (medium-pitched, thud-like). Figure 59-7 illustrates the location of various thoracic percussion sounds and the associated anatomic structures that produce the various sounds.

Auscultation

Lung auscultation provides critical assessment data in terms of a client's respiratory health. Auscultate in a pattern that compares the right side of the thorax to the left side. Auscultate all areas of the lungs over a bare chest in order to

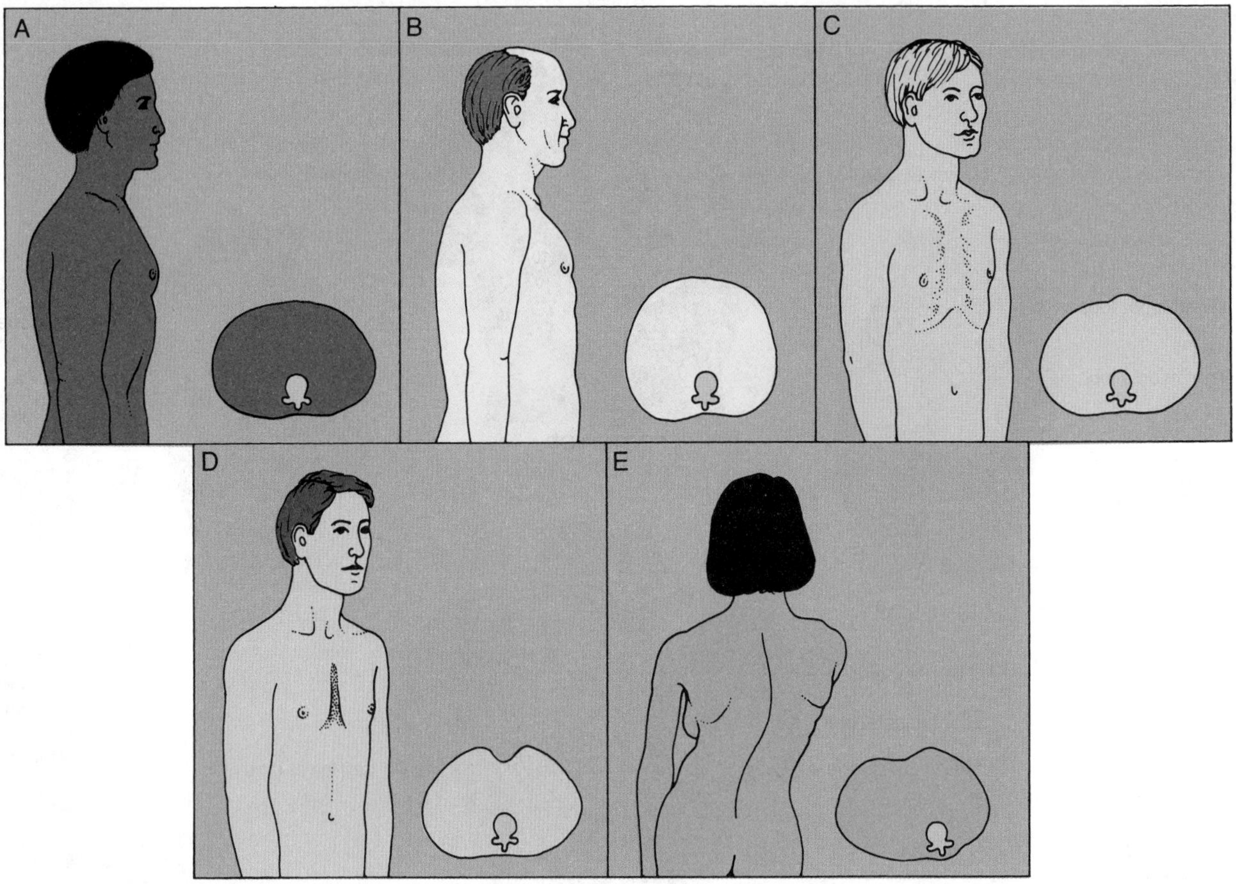

■ **FIGURE 59–6** Chest deformities. **A,** Normal adult, for comparison. The ratio of anteroposterior diameter to transverse diameter can be seen here as 1:2. **B,** Barrel chest. The anteroposterior-transverse diameter ratio is 1:1. **C,** Pigeon chest (pectus carinatum). **D,** Funnel chest (pectus excavatum). **E,** Thoracic kyphoscoliosis.

achieve accurate findings. At each auscultation location, listen for a full respiration cycle of inspiration and expiration as the client breathes through the mouth. Auscultate for the type or character of the breath sounds and the presence of adventitious (extra) sounds. Table 59-1 describes the characteristics of normal breath sounds, and Figure 59-8 illustrates the normal anatomic location of these sounds. Bronchovesicular or bronchial breath sounds heard in the peripheral lung fields can indicate consolidation of the lung resulting from inflammation and infection. Absent

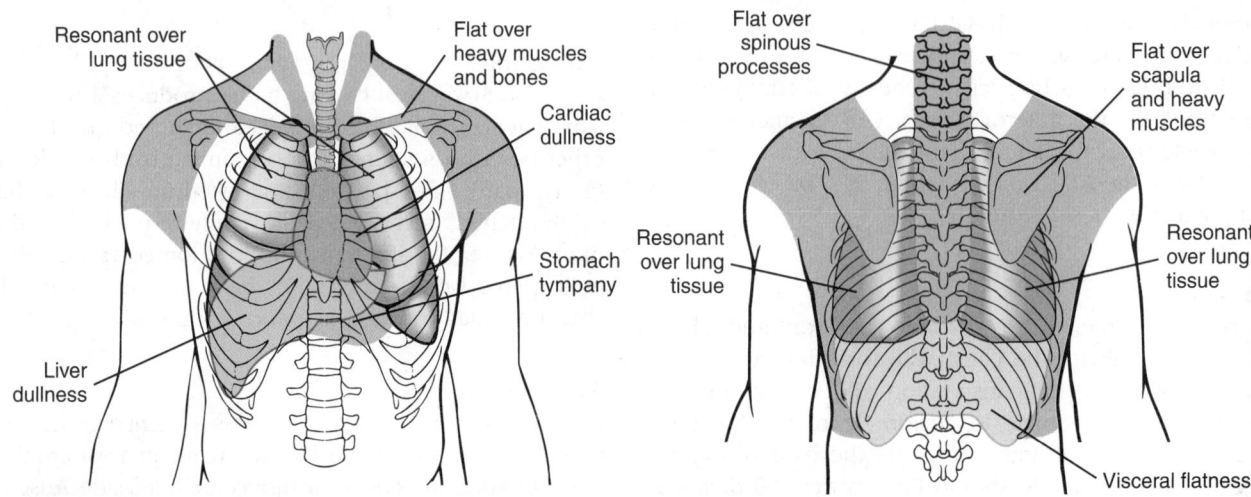

■ **FIGURE 59–7** Location of thoracic percussion sounds and their associated structures.

TABLE 59-1   Characteristics of Normal Breath Sounds

	Pitch	Amplitude	Duration	Quality	Normal Location
Bronchial (tracheal)	High	Loud	Inspiration < expiration	Harsh, hollow, tubular	Trachea and larynx
Bronchovesicular	Moderate	Moderate	Inspiration = expiration	Mixed	Over major bronchi where fewer alveoli are located: posterior, between scapulae, especially on right; anterior, around upper sternum in first and second intercostal spaces
Vesicular	Low	Soft	Inspiration > expiration	Rustling, like sound of wind in trees	Over peripheral lung fields where air flows through smaller bronchioles and alveoli

From Jarvis, C. (2006). *Physical examination and health assessment* (4th ed.). Philadelphia: Saunders.

or diminished breath sounds can also indicate lung disease. Table 59-2 provides a summary of adventitious lung sounds and the associated abnormal client conditions. Refer to a physical assessment textbook for additional details.

DIAGNOSTIC TESTING

Noninvasive Tests

Diagnostic procedures facilitate the assessment and diagnosis of client respiratory disorders. Commonly available diagnostic tests include pulmonary function tests, arterial blood gas analysis, pulse oximetry, ventilation-perfusion scan, chest x-ray, and sputum cultures.

Pulse Oximetry

The pulse oximeter passes a beam of light through the tissue, and a sensor attached to the finger tip, toe, or ear lobe measures the amount of light absorbed by the oxygen-saturated hemoglobin. The oximeter then gives a reading of the percentage of hemoglobin that is saturated with oxygen (SaO_2). SaO_2 is closely correlated with the saturations obtained from the pulse oximeter if it is greater than 70% (Table 59-3).

Pulmonary Function Testing

Pulmonary function tests (PFTs) provide information about respiratory function by measuring lung volumes, lung mechanics, and diffusion capabilities of the lungs. PFTs performed in a pulmonary function laboratory can measure respiratory volumes and capacities. PFTs done outside a laboratory are modified to include ventilation tests of forced expiratory volume, vital capacity, and maximal voluntary ventilation measures. Refer to the table Pulmonary Function Test (PFT) Components and the table Categorization of Obstructive and Restrictive Pulmonary Disorders and Pulmonary Function Test (PFT) Findings on the website for an explanation of *evolve* the PFT recordings and results that indicate obstructive and restrictive lung disease.

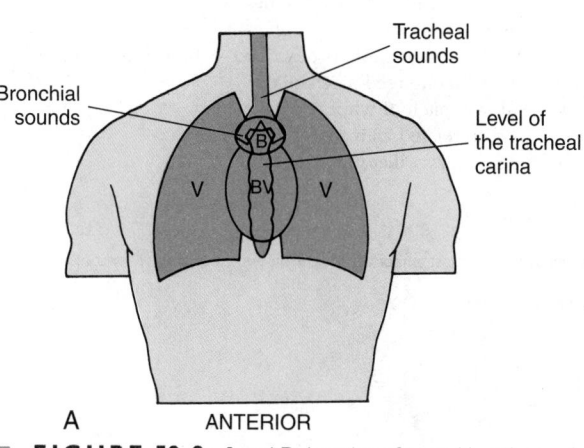

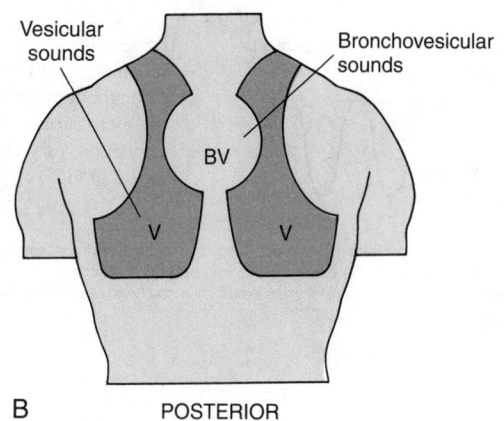

■ **FIGURE 59-8   A** and **B,** Location of normal breath sounds.

TABLE 59–2 Adventitious Breath Sounds

Sound*	Description	Mechanism	Clinical Example
Discontinuous Sounds			
Crackles—fine (rales, crepitations)	Discontinuous, high-pitched, short crackling, popping sounds heard during inspiration that are not cleared by coughing; this sound can be simulated by rolling a strand of hair between fingers near the ear or by moistening thumb and index finger and separating them near the ear	Inhaled air collides with previously deflated airways; airways suddenly pop open, creating a crackling sound as gas pressures between two compartments equalize	*Late inspiratory crackles* occur with restrictive disease: pneumonia, heart failure, and interstitial fibrosis *Early inspiratory crackles* occur with obstructive disease: chronic bronchitis, asthma, and emphysema
Crackles—coarse (coarse rales)	Loud, low-pitched, bubbling, and gurgling sounds that start in early inspiration and may be present in expiration; may decrease somewhat by suctioning or coughing but will reappear shortly; sound like opening a self-fastening tape (Velcro) fastener	Inhaled air collides with secretions in trachea and large bronchi	Pulmonary edema, pneumonia, pulmonary fibrosis, and in terminally ill who have a depressed cough reflex
Atelectatic crackles (atelectatic rales)	Sound like fine crackles but do not last and are not pathologic; disappear after first few breaths; heard in axillae and bases (usually dependent) of lungs	When sections of alveoli are not fully aerated, they deflate and accumulate secretions; crackles are heard when these sections reexpand with a few deep breaths	In aging adults, bedridden people, or in people just aroused from sleep
Pleural friction rub	Very superficial sound that is coarse and low-pitched; it has a grating quality as if two pieces of leather are being rubbed together; sounds just like crackles, but *close* to the ear; sounds louder if stethoscope is pushed harder onto chest wall; sound is inspiratory and expiratory	Caused when pleurae become inflamed and lose their normal lubricating fluid; their opposing roughened pleural surfaces rub together during respiration; heard best in anterolateral wall where there is greatest lung mobility	Pleuritis, accompanied by pain with breathing (rub disappears after a few days if pleural fluid accumulates and separates pleurae)
Continuous Sounds			
Wheeze—high-pitched (sibilant rhonchi)	High-pitched, musical squeaking sounds that predominate in expiration but may occur in both expiration and inspiration	Air squeezed or compressed through passageways narrowed almost to closure by collapsing, swelling, secretions, or tumors; passageway walls oscillate in apposition between closed and barely open positions; resulting sound is similar to a vibrating reed	Obstructive lung disease such as asthma or emphysema
Wheeze—low-pitched (sonorous rhonchi)	Low-pitched, musical, snoring, moaning sounds; they are heard throughout cycle, although they are more prominent on expiration; may clear somewhat by coughing	Air flow obstruction as described by vibrating reed mechanism above; pitch of wheeze cannot be correlated with size of passageway that generates it	Bronchitis

*Although nothing in clinical practice seems to differ more than the nomenclature of adventitious sounds, most authorities concur on two categories: (1) discontinuous, discrete crackling sounds and (2) continuous, coarse, or musical sounds.

Modified from Jarvis, C. (2006). *Physical examination and health assessment* (4th ed.). Philadelphia: Saunders.

TABLE 59–3 Comparing Oxygen Saturation to Partial Pressure of Arterial Oxygen (Pao$_2$)

Oxygen Saturation (%)	Pao$_2$ (mm Hg)	Client Status
50	25	Life-threatening hypoxemia
75	40	Moderate hypoxemia
90	55	Mild hypoxemia

Chest X-Ray

Chest x-rays (Figure 59-9) provide information about the chest that may not be available through other assessment means and may be able to illustrate graphically the cause of respiratory dysfunction. Chest films may reveal abnormalities when there are no physical manifestations of pulmonary disease. Chest x-ray studies may be performed for a variety of reasons, including the following: as part of a routine screening procedure; when pulmonary disease is suspected; to monitor the status of respiratory disorders and abnormalities (pleural effusion, atelectasis, tubercular lesions); and to confirm endotracheal or tracheostomy tube placement.

Ventilation-Perfusion Scan

Ventilation-perfusion ($\dot{V}/\dot{Q}$) scans are used to assess lung ventilation and lung perfusion. $\dot{V}/\dot{Q}$ scans are used to confirm pulmonary embolism, pulmonary infarction, emphysema, fibrosis, and bronchiectasis. Although pulmonary angiography is the most specific diagnostic tool for pulmonary emboli, it is invasive; the $\dot{V}/\dot{Q}$ scan is less invasive and less dangerous. Quantitative perfusion scans may be helpful in preoperative assessment of clients undergoing surgical resection of thoracic malignancy.

Computed Tomography and Magnetic Resonance Imaging

Computed tomography (CT) provides more sophisticated tomography than is possible with conventional x-ray equipment. The CT scan is particularly helpful in identifying peripheral (pleural) or mediastinal disorders. Special techniques can be used to view pulmonary nodules. Thin cuts of CT scans are used in diagnosing interstitial lung disorders such as pulmonary fibrosis and bronchiectasis. Spiral or helical CT scan of the chest is an alternative to the lung scan for identifying pulmonary emboli.

Magnetic resonance imaging (MRI) employs magnetic fields rather than radiation to create images of body structures. MRI is used in much the same way as CT, although MRI is more definitive than CT because it creates more detailed images of anatomic structures.

Invasive Tests

The following paragraphs briefly describe other diagnostic tests used to detect pulmonary disorders. For a complete description of tests used to aid in the diagnosis of pulmonary disease, consult a diagnostic and laboratory tests textbook for more information related to pre- and postprocedure nursing care.

Laryngoscopy

Laryngoscopy is visual examination of the larynx and is used to diagnose laryngeal papillomas, nodules, polyps, or cancer. Laryngoscopy can be performed during bronchoscopy or as a separate procedure. Figure 59-10 shows a tumor on the vocal cord as seen via laryngoscopy.

Bronchoscopy

Bronchoscopy (Figure 59-11) is a test used for diagnostic and therapeutic uses. A flexible fiberoptic bronchoscope or a rigid bronchoscope permits visualization of the larynx, trachea, and bronchi. A bronchoscopy is useful for the diagnostic detection of tumors, inflammation, or strictures as well as to obtain tissue biopsies. Therapeutic uses of bronchoscopy include the removal of retained secretions or foreign bodies blocking air passages and to control bleeding within the bronchus.

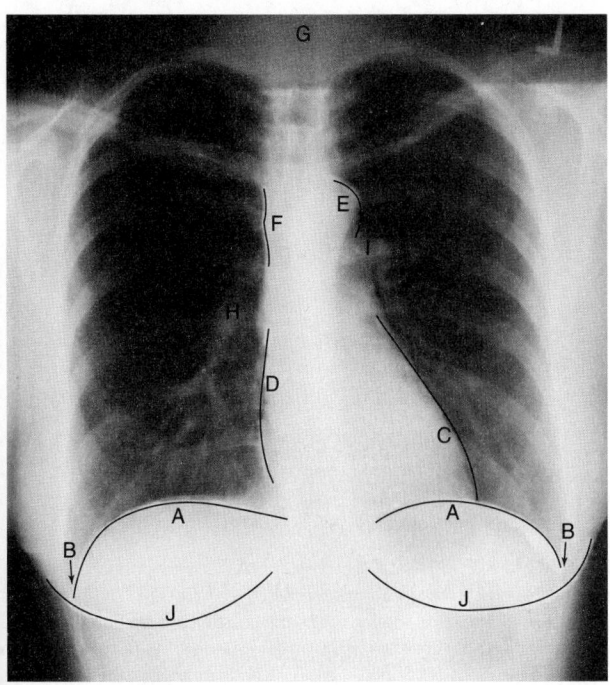

FIGURE 59–9 A normal chest x-ray film taken from the posteroanterior view. The backward L in the upper right corner is placed on the film to indicate the left side of the client's chest. **A,** Diaphragm; **B,** costophrenic angle; **C,** left ventricle; **D,** right atrium; **E,** aortic arch; **F,** superior vena cava; **G,** trachea; **H,** right bronchus; **I,** left bronchus; **J,** breast shadows.

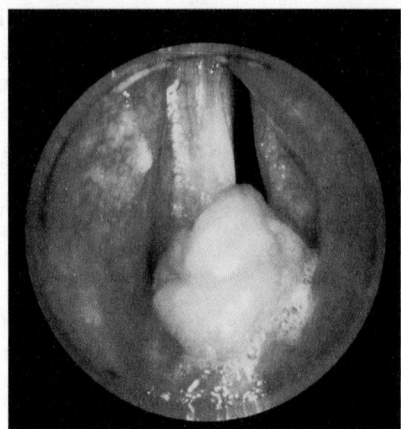

■ **FIGURE 59–10** Large granular cell tumor of the true vocal cord, as seen during laryngoscopy. *(From Fu, Y.S., et al. [2001]. Head and neck pathology—With clinical correlations. New York: Churchill Livingstone.)*

Thoracentesis and Pleural Fluid Analysis

Thoracentesis is an invasive procedure that involves insertion of a needle into the pleural space for removal of pleural fluid or air (Figure 59-12). Pleural fluid is removed to therapeutically relieve pain or shortness of breath caused by excessive pleural pressure. A thoracentesis and pleural fluid analysis can also be a diagnostic tool to detect various disorders, such as inflammatory, infectious, or cancerous conditions.

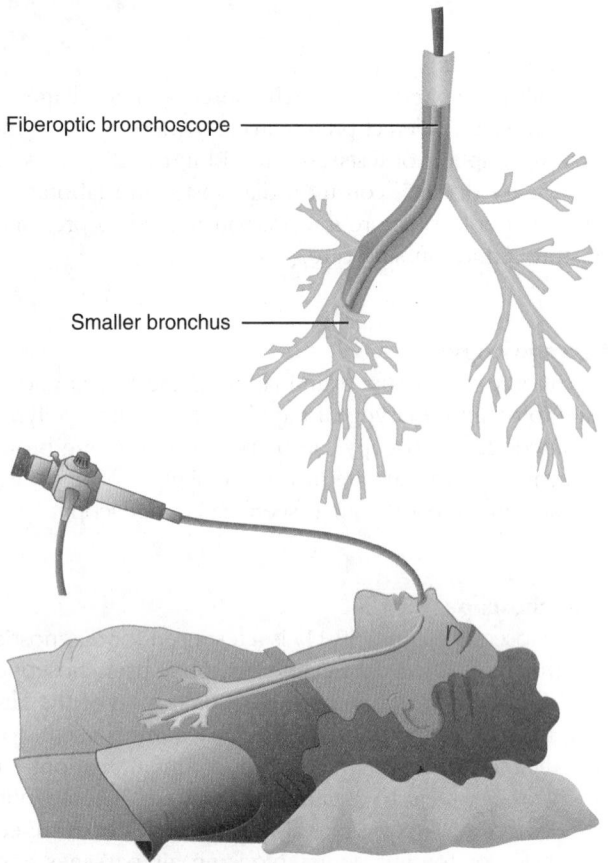

■ **FIGURE 59–11** Bronchoscopy.

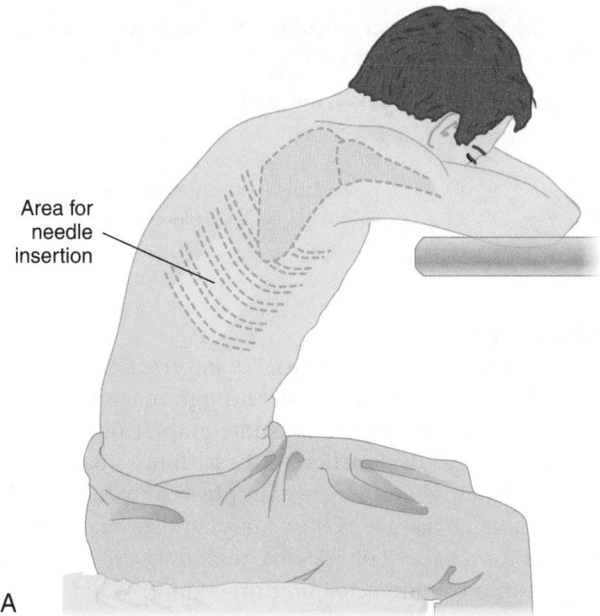

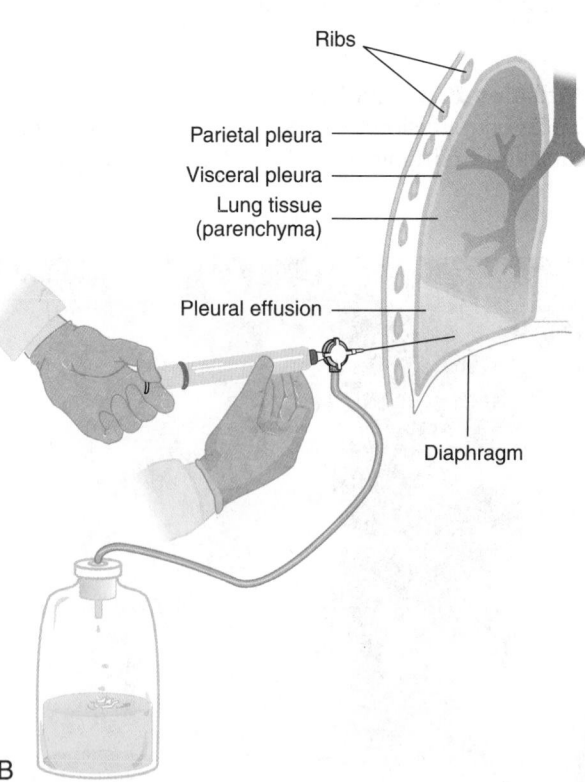

■ **FIGURE 59–12** Thoracentesis. **A,** Correct position of the client for the procedure. The arms are raised and crossed. The head rests on the folded arm. This position allows the chest wall to be pulled outward in an expanded position. If an institutional over-bed table is not available, you may leave the client's arms down, but position them toward the client's hips or cross them in front of the chest. **B,** Usual site for insertion of a thoracentesis needle for a right-sided effusion. The actual site varies, depending on the location and volume of the effusion. The needle is kept as far away from the diaphragm as possible but is inserted close to the base of the effusion so that gravity can help with drainage.

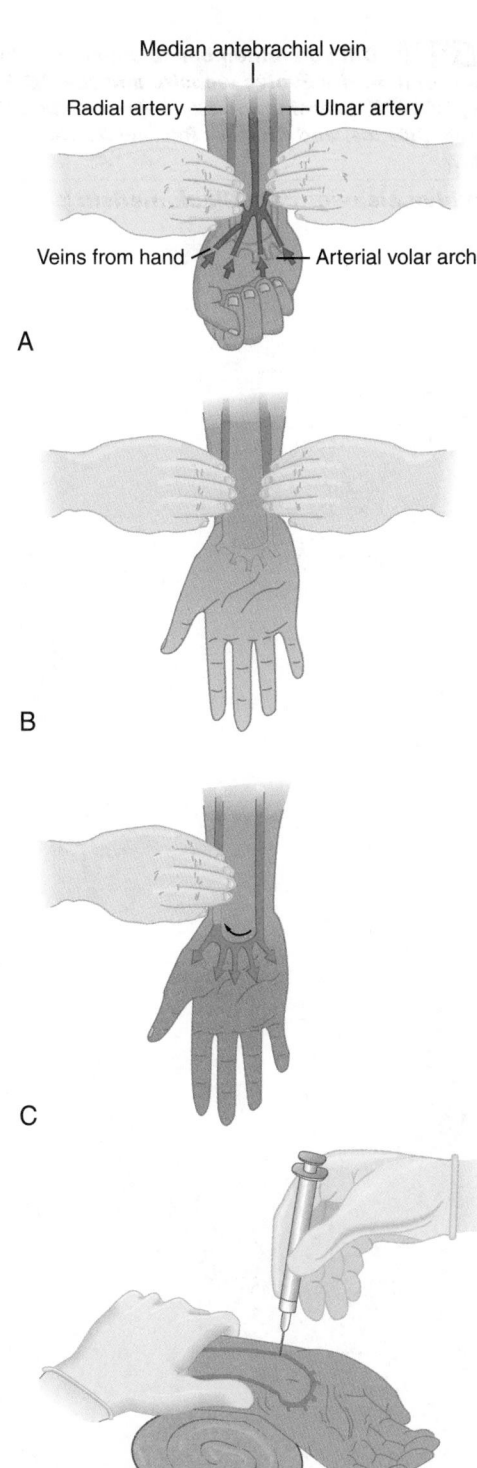

A

B

C

D

FIGURE 59–13 Obtaining a sample of arterial blood by arterial puncture. First, perform Allen's test, a quick assessment of collateral circulation the hand. This test is essential before radial artery puncture. **A,** Occlude oth the radial and the ulnar arteries with your fingers. Ask the client to close e hand into a fist. **B,** When the client opens the hand with the arteries still ccluded, the hand is pale. **C,** When you release either the radial or the ulnar tery, the client's hand should become pink because of collateral circulation. ssess the patency of each of the two arteries in this way, one at a time. **D,** If llateral circulation is adequate, you can draw arterial blood from the radial tery with a heparinized needle and syringe as shown.

Biopsy

Biopsy of the lung or pleura requires a surgical excision of tissue. The tissue is examined for abnormal cellular structure (cancer cells) or infection.

Laboratory Tests
Sputum Culture

An infectious process can lead to excessive production of mucus (commonly called sputum). Assessment of sputum for bacteria, fungi, or cellular elements guides the treatment of an underlying infection. If possible, sputum should be collected before antimicrobial treatment is begun.

Nose and Throat Cultures

The throat and nose normally contain many organisms. Using a flexible sterile cotton swab, cultures of these areas are taken to identify certain pathogens, such as *Streptococcus* species, *Bordetella pertussis, Corynebacterium diphtheria, Haemophilus influenzae,* or respiratory syncytial virus (RSV). Bacteria in the nose and throat can be identified by culture during assessment of the upper airway. Some bacteria are normally present (streptococci, staphylococci, pneumococci, *Haemophilus influenzae,* and *Klebsiella pneumoniae*). Other organisms are abnormal (those causing diphtheria or tuberculosis). The culture should be collected before antimicrobial treatment is begun.

Arterial Blood Gases (ABGs)

The ABG analysis involves the use of arterial, rather than venous, blood to measure PaO_2, $PaCO_2$, and pH directly (Figure 59-13). Bicarbonate concentration (HCO_3^-) and SaO_2 are calculated as well. PaO_2 reflects the efficiency of gas exchange, whereas $PaCO_2$ reflects the effectiveness of alveolar ventilation. The acid-base status of the body (see Chapter 13) is indicated by the pH of arterial blood. ABG analysis is helpful in the assessment of clients who are acutely ill with either pulmonary or nonpulmonary disorders, who require an artificial airway, who are dependent on mechanical ventilation, or who are experiencing chronic respiratory disease.

CONCLUSIONS

The nurse's involvement in a general respiratory assessment includes a variety of interventions. The nurse must obtain specific history data, including information about smoking history and other environmental hazards. The physical examination includes the assessment techniques of inspection, palpation, percussion, and auscultation. In addition, the nurse also monitors and reports the results of various diagnostic tests used to evaluate the client's respiratory status.

BIBLIOGRAPHY

1. Bickley, L.S. (2003). *Bates' guide to physical examination and history taking* (8th ed.). Philadelphia: Lippincott Williams & Wilkins.
2. Hardin, K.A., Tharratt, R.S., & Louie, S. (2005). Asthma in adulthood: different and complex. *The Clinical Advisor, 8*(10), 34-40.
3. Infectious Disease Leadership Council. (2005). Management of respiratory tract infections: Practical approaches. *Clinical Advisor Supplement, 8*(4).
4. Jarvis, C. (2004). *Physical examination and health assessment* (4th ed.). Philadelphia: Saunders.
5. Pagana, K.D., & Pagana, T.J. (2005). *Mosby's diagnostic and laboratory test reference* (7th ed.). St. Louis: Mosby.
6. Regueiro, C.R. (2004). The latest approaches to managing pneumonia. *The Clinical Advisor, 7*(11), 25-31.

evolve *Did you remember to check out the bonus material on the Evolve website and the CD-ROM, including NCLEX®-Examination Style Review Questions, Open-Book Quizzes, and Chapter Review Audio Podcasts?*

http://evolve.elsevier.com/Black/medsurg

CHAPTER 60

Management of Clients with Upper Airway Disorders

MARGARET M. ECKLUND

The upper airway is considered to be the nasal passages, sinuses, and trachea. The initial complaint for clients with disorders of the upper airway is a problem with breathing. Obstructions to nasal breathing are observed in clients with nasal polyps, deviated nasal septum, or nasal fractures. Sinus infections create inflammation and congestion. Laryngeal disorders may also result in breathing problems. Tumors of the larynx create obstruction to air entering the trachea, as well as to air being exhaled. Vocal cord paralysis and laryngospasm may also affect the passage of air through the larynx and vocal cords. Because of the priority need to have a patent airway, the chapter will begin with maintaining the airway.

METHODS OF CONTROLLING THE AIRWAY

Airway obstruction can be prevented or treated with many modalities, depending on the underlying cause. Antihistamine treatment is discussed in Chapter 76. Intubation to support ventilation and oxygenation is discussed in Chapter 63. This chapter begins with a discussion of tracheostomy because it is a strategy of airway management in hospitalized clients, creating a portal to manage secretions, relieve obstruction, or provide ongoing mechanical ventilation.

Tracheostomy

A *tracheotomy* is a surgical incision into the trachea through overlying skin and muscles for airway management. A *tracheostomy* is the surgical creation of a stoma, or opening, into the trachea through the overlying skin (Figure 60-1). These terms are often used interchangeably. For simplicity, the term *tracheostomy* is used here.

Tracheostomy can be performed as an emergency procedure or as an elective procedure, depending on the indication. A competent provider can perform a percutaneous tracheostomy at the bedside in critical care

units. This method is cost-effective as it avoids the operating room cost, saves time, and avoids transporting critically ill clients to the operating room. The surgical approach, done as an open procedure in the operating room, includes removal of a portion of the tracheal ring to facilitate creation of a stoma for the tube placement. Surgically created tracheostomies may have sutures holding the tube in place for the first few postoperative days. A tracheostomy provides the best route for long-term airway maintenance. There are many indications for this procedure, including the following:

- Relief of acute or chronic upper airway obstruction, such as obstructive sleep apnea, trauma, bleeding, tumors, tissue swelling, infections, or burns (chemical or inhalation)
- Access for continuous mechanical ventilation, with the inability to wean (broadly defined as greater than 2 weeks of ventilation)
- Promotion of pulmonary hygiene by accessing airway for secretion removal
- Bilateral vocal cord paralysis
- Inability to protect own airway

---

evolve Web Enhancements

Bridge to Home Health Care Living with a Tracheostomy

Client Education Guide Swallowing Technique After a Partial Laryngectomy (Spanish Translation)

Care of a Tracheoesophageal Puncture Wound (English Version and Spanish Translation)

Exercises After Radical Neck Surgery (English Version and Spanish Translation)

Ethical Issues in Nursing What Type of Client Education Is Needed for Informed Consent to Radical Procedures?

Be sure to check out the bonus material on the Evolve website and the CD-ROM, including free self-assessment exercises. **http://evolve.elsevier. com/Black/medsurg**

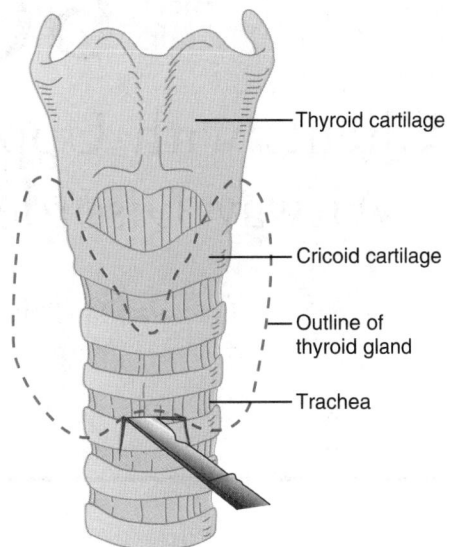

Thyroid cartilage

Cricoid cartilage

Outline of
thyroid gland

Trachea

■ **FIGURE 60–1** Incision for a tracheostomy is made through the fibrous tissue above the third tracheal cartilage. Two small vertical incisions create a flap that can be closed later.

A tracheostomy is by far the most satisfactory artificial airway. It bypasses the upper airway and glottis, making stabilization, suction, and the attachment of respiratory equipment much easier than with other types of artificial airways. The client has the potential to eat and, depending on the type of tube placed, talk, which can improve quality of life. Advantages to placement of tracheostomy tubes in critically ill clients include the need for less sedation, increased mobility, and reduced complications from immobility.

Tracheostomy Tubes

The tracheostomy opening is fitted with a tube to maintain airway patency. Tracheostomy tubes vary in their composition, number of separate parts, shape, and size. Tracheostomy tubes are chosen specifically for each client. Incorrectly fitted tubes can precipitate permanent or life-threatening damage.

The diameter of a tracheostomy tube must be smaller than the trachea so that it lies comfortably within the tracheal lumen. Air should be able to pass between the outer wall of the tracheostomy tube and the tracheal mucosa, and allow adequate perfusion to tracheal tissue. Although there is no standard tracheostomy tube sizing system, all packages indicate the inner and outer diameters in millimeters. Common size range for adult tracheostomy tubes is 6 to 8 mm. Tracheostomy tubes are made of various substances, such as nonreactive plastic, stainless steel, sterling silver, or silicone. Plastic tubes are disposable and used for only one person. Metal tubes may be reused after being sterilized. A tube must have a 15-mm hub for attachment to mechanical ventilation circuits, or manual resuscitation bags.

The length and curve of a tracheostomy tube are important to note. Tracheostomy tubes may be long or short. They may be angled, with the angle ranging from 50 to 90 degrees. Short to moderately short tubes with an angle of about 60 degrees are most often used. A tube must be long enough to avoid dislodgment into paratracheal tissue when the client coughs or turns his or her head. The lower end of a tracheostomy tube should be located above the carina. The curve of the tube must allow the tip to be in a straight line with the trachea, rather than pressing on the anterior or posterior tracheal wall. Tubes vary in material, and manufacturers produce standard as well as custom-made tubes to meet clients' needs. The ear, nose, and throat (ENT) surgeon selects the tube based on need, but as time progresses, it may be the bedside caregiver team of nurse, respiratory therapist (RT), and provider who determines the tube best suited for a client's needs. Tubes may have a single cannula, or may have an inner cannula. Inner cannulas will need to be removed periodically for cleaning; they may be reusable or disposable.

Tracheostomy tubes may be cuffed or uncuffed. An inflated cuff permits mechanical ventilation. Inflated cuffs deter secretions from the upper airway leaking into the lower airway, but do not create an absolute barrier. (Box 60-1). Tracheostomy cuffs do not hold the tube in place. Cuffs may be inflated with air, sterile water, or foam.

Standard Tracheostomy Tube. A standard tracheostomy tube (Figure 60-2) has (1) an outer cannula with cuff, flange, and pilot balloon and (2) an obturator. The parts fit together as one unit and may not be interchanged with other units. The tube fits in the tracheostomy stoma to keep it open. The tracheostomy tube has a flange or neckplate that fits flush with the neck and has holes on each side to attach the securing tapes or ties. A tracheostomy tube must be secured in place to prevent accidental extubation, excessive motion, or misalignment. Cloth tape or commercially available self-fastening (Velcro) ties may be used.

The obturator is placed into the outer tube before insertion. Its rounded tip smooths the end of the cannula and facilitates nontraumatic insertion of the tube into the stoma, with the aid of sterile lubricating jelly. The obturator is removed immediately after insertion to open the tube. Place the obturator in a plastic bag and tape it to the head of the client's bed in a conspicuous place. If the tracheostomy tube is accidentally displaced, the obturator can be immediately placed into the outer cannula for quick reinsertion.

A spare tube of the same type kept at the bedside is an important safety strategy. Accidental decannulation in the initial postoperative period may be considered an airway emergency. If the tube cannot be placed back in the stoma, the client may need urgent reintubation with an endotracheal tube. As the stoma matures postoperatively, the tube can be placed with greater ease.

BOX 60-1   **Inflation and Deflation of Tracheostomy Tube Cuff***

INFLATION (MINIMAL LEAK TECHNIQUE)
Objective
Inflate the cuff with the minimum volume of air required to adequately seal the trachea during positive-pressure ventilation and to prevent aspiration of foreign material while exerting the lowest possible cuff-to-tracheal wall pressure.

Intervention
1. Withdraw all residual air from the cuff.
2. Place 6 ml of air in a syringe.
3. Place the diaphragm of a stethoscope over the client's neck in the area of the tracheostomy tube cuff.
4. On inhalation, slowly inject air through the one-way valve into the pilot line in 1-ml increments.
5. Auscultate the neck area over the cuff.
6. Apply positive pressure to the tracheostomy tube with a manual self-inflating bag. An audible air leak can be heard via the stethoscope unless the cuff is inflated.
7. Continue slowly injecting air until the air leak is no longer present during inhalation.
8. When a leak is no longer auscultated, withdraw a small amount of air from the cuff until a very small leak is heard. This is called a *minimal leak*.
9. Note the amount of air necessary to achieve the minimal leak. This is the *minimal occluding volume* (MOV).
10. Once minimal leak is attained, measure the cuff pressure with a manometer.
11. Routinely measure and document cuff pressures.

DEFLATION
Objective
Allow air to flow around the tracheostomy tube to permit phonation and to provide an opportunity to blow secretions above the cuff into the oropharynx, where they can be removed by suctioning.

Intervention
Routinely deflating the cuff is not necessary provided that safe cuff inflation and cuff pressure measurements are performed.
1. Remove the ventilator assembly (if present) and attach a self-inflating bag to the 15-mm adapter on the inner cannula.
2. Hyperoxygenate, hyperinflate, and suction the trachea to remove secretions below the cuff. Remove secretions above the cuff by gently applying suction deep into the oropharynx.
3. Insert an empty syringe into the one-way valve, and pull back on the plunger to remove the air in the cuff. At the same time, apply positive pressure with the manual self-inflating bag. This maneuver blows secretions lying directly above the cuff into the mouth, which prevents secretions accumulated above the cuff from draining into the trachea and lower airway.
4. Suction the oropharynx again.
5. If the person is ventilator-dependent, remember that with the cuff "down" or deflated, a portion of ventilation volume will not reach the lungs. Air will escape through the upper airway, which may compromise the person's respiratory status. This volume loss creates an audible leak. Phonation is possible during the exhalation phase of ventilation.

*The same procedure is used for inflation and deflation of endotracheal tube cuffs.

Once the obturator is removed, the inner cannula is placed into the outer cannula. Lock it into place to prevent accidental removal (e.g., when the client coughs). Frequent removal and cleaning of the inner cannula are necessary to maintain airway patency. At the distal end, most inner cannulas have a standard 15-mm adapter that fits respiratory therapy and anesthesiology equipment.

Single-Cannula Tracheostomy Tube. A single-cannula tracheostomy tube is slightly longer than the standard tube and does not have an inner cannula. The longer single-cannula tube is used in the client with a thick neck or with an altered airway in whom a standard tracheostomy tube would be too short. Single-cannula tubes may have cuffs of variable types, or no cuff. Air-cuffed tubes may not be safely plugged because of the bulk of cuff within the airway. Silicone tubes with "tight to shaft" cuffs that inflate with sterile water offer safe options for plugging if the client has adequate air flow. Clients in whom a single-cannula tube is used must have continuous supplemental humidification to prevent obstruction by accumulated secretions.

Double-Cannula Tracheostomy Tube. Tubes with inner cannulas may be cuffed or uncuffed. Inner cannulas can be used when intermittent manual cleaning is desired. Inner cannulas are removed, inspected, cleaned, and put back in place or, if disposable, exchanged. Both inner and outer cannulas may have fenestrations.

Fenestrated Tracheostomy Tube. A fenestrated tracheostomy tube has one large opening (Latin, *fenestra*), or several small ones, on the curvature of the posterior wall of the outer cannula. Fenestrated tubes have an inner cannula and may be cuffed or cuffless. When the inner cannula is removed, the fenestration permits air to flow through both the upper airway and the tracheostomy opening. This may facilitate speech and more effective coughing. This tube may be used while a client is being weaned from a tracheostomy and for a client in whom use of the tracheostomy is expected to be prolonged. When the inner cannula is in place, the fenestration may be closed.

Foam Cuff Tracheostomy Tube. Tubes with a single cannula are for specialized needs. The cuff on the tube is

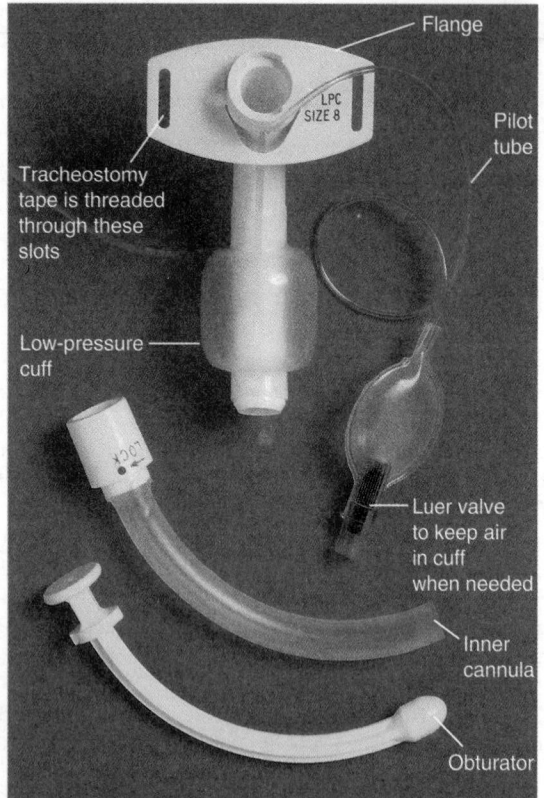

■ FIGURE 60–2 Parts of a tracheostomy tube. *(Courtesy of Shiley, Inc., Irvine, Calif.)*

made of foam, so the cuff passively inflates to the desired size at atmospheric pressure. This design is intended to prevent injury to the trachea from over-inflated cuffs and used for clients who may have erosion of the airway or tracheomalacia.

Tracheostomy Speaking Valves. A speaking valve is a one-way plastic valve attached to the 15-mm end of a tracheostomy tube. This modification permits talking without the need to plug the tracheostomy tube. The one-way valve allows air (and the aerosol of supplemental humidification and oxygen) to flow into the tube during inspiration. On exhalation, the one-way valve closes, directing air from the lungs up through the vocal cords and upper airway. Phonation and effective coughing are facilitated by this normal passage of air.

SAFETY ALERT

A talking tracheostomy is never used unless there is enough room around the tracheostomy tube to permit sufficient air flow for breathing. Always deflate a cuffed tracheostomy tube before the client uses the talking tracheostomy adapter. Cuff inflation prevents exhalation, potentially causing suffocation.

An important first step is assessment of the air flow initially with cuff deflation while monitoring the client with oximetry. Speech therapists are important team members to collaborate with respiratory care nurses

and providers to ensure safety and quality for speakin[g] valve use. Individuals may eat with valves on, and ma[y] have improved intake with better ability to sme[ll]. Because of the risk of airway occlusion, individua[ls] should not sleep with speaking valves in place.

Talking Tracheostomy Tube. This tracheostomy tub[e] allows speech by coordination of phonation efforts. Ve[n]tilation and phonation are separated because of differe[nt] air sources. With this device, an air flow tube (that look[s] like a second pilot tube) runs outside the pilot (main[)] tube and opens just above the cuff. There is a port [at] the distal end of the air flow tube. When the port [is] occluded by a finger and compressed air or oxygen [is] directed through the air flow tube, a current of air is gen[]erated up through the vocal cords. With practice, the cl[i]ent learns to use this air flow for speech, although th[e] "voice" produced in this way does not sound norma[l.] Mucosal irritation may develop from the forced flow [of] air or oxygen into the upper airway. The portal can clo[g] with mucus, creating less effective air flow and n[o] vocalization.

Tracheostomy Button. Use of a tracheostomy button [is] sometimes indicated during weaning as an intermediat[e] measure between using a standard tracheostomy tub[e] and extubation. A button is a short, straight, plastic cylin[]der secured by a flange to the anterior tracheal wall bu[t] is not deep enough to enter the tracheal lumen. It has [a] removable cap with a one-way flap inside that permit[s] inhalation but not exhalation. Exhalation occurs throug[h] the normal upper airway. When the cap is on, the clie[nt] can talk. Without a 15-mm hub, the button cannot b[e] used for ventilation.

It can replace a standard tracheostomy tube for clien[ts] with retained secretions who do not require ventilator[y] assistance. A button creates less airway resistance tha[n] that produced by a plugged standard tracheostomy tub[e;] hence, breathing is easier. Artificial humidification [of] inspired air is necessary with a button (as with an[y] tracheostomy tube), because the natural airway [is] bypassed.

Metal Tracheostomy Tube. Metal tracheostomy tube[s] are made of sterling silver or stainless steel. The mo[st] popular type is the Jackson tracheostomy tube. Met[al] tubes are cuffless and most often used in clients wh[o] have a permanent tracheostomy or laryngectomy. Th[e] inner cannula locks together with the outer cannul[a.] Because metal tubes do not have a standard 15-m[m] adapter, rapid adaptation to respiratory or anesthes[ia] equipment is impossible unless a specific adapter [is] available. The Hollinger tube is also made of metal an[d] is similar to the Jackson tube. A plastic decannulatio[n] stopper, or plug, allows communication and upper ai[r]way breathing.

Permanent Tracheostomy. Most clients with a permanent tracheostomy use a cuffless tracheostomy tube. For appearance's sake, many clients prefer a low-profile inner cannula. This design does not incorporate a 15-mm adapter. Instead, the inner cannula fits into the outer cannula and lies flush with the neck. If the client has had a total laryngectomy, the cut end of the trachea is sutured to the skin, creating a permanent stoma. Once the stoma is healed, most laryngectomy clients do not need a tube.

🜂 Potential Problems Associated with Tracheostomy Tubes and Cuffs

The presence of an artificial airway bypasses the normal mechanism for protection against infection. Breathing that bypasses the upper airway does not permit the nose and mouth to warm or moisten inspired air. To prevent complications, caregivers must provide attention to aseptic technique and adequate humidification.

The oral cavity becomes colonized with nosocomial bacteria within 48 hours of admission. Oral care, including plaque removal from teeth, even in clients who are nothing by mouth (NPO), helps prevent hospital-acquired pneumonia. Clients with artificial airways are at highest risk for this complication.

Airway Obstruction. The flow of air through a tracheostomy tube may become occluded for several reasons. The tracheostomy tube may be misaligned so that its opening lies against the tracheal wall, preventing air flow. Cuff overinflation causes the cuff to herniate over the tip of the tube, obstructing air flow. Without adequate airway care, the inner cannula can become occluded with dried secretions or excessive bronchial secretions. Collaborate with respiratory care therapists to ensure adequate humidification is delivered to the airway. Heating and humidifying the inspired air will help keep mucus thin.

Infection. Tracheostomies increase the risk of bronchopulmonary infection because they (1) bypass upper airway protective mechanisms (i.e., filtering, warming, and humidifying) and (2) decrease mucociliary transport and coughing, thus increasing retained secretions. Stoma site infection may occur as well.

Nosocomial infection is also a potential problem. The lower airway (below the larynx) is normally sterile. Therefore all solutions and equipment entering the trachea must be sterile. Organisms (e.g., *Pseudomonas aeruginosa* and other gram-negative bacteria) grow readily in respiratory equipment, which can then contaminate the lower airway. In addition, some bacteria may colonize a tracheostomy without causing infection.

Ventilator-associated pneumonia (VAP) prevention strategies are implemented, including head-of-bed positioning greater than 45 degrees and frequent oral care for all clients with mechanical ventilation or artificial airways. Nurses need to be aggressive when performing oral care and clean the entire mouth, not just the lips and in front of the teeth.

Stoma care, including cleaning and skin care, should begin at its creation. Stoma maintenance promotes adequate skin integrity and provides a barrier to infection.

Changing Tracheostomy Tubes. Recommendations for changing tracheostomy tubes vary and therefore most physicians and health care facilities have established protocols. No standards exist in the literature. Each client has a unique set of circumstances that dictate the frequency of tracheostomy tube changes. Change of the tube based on need may be the best strategy to minimize risk and discomfort for the client. Tracheostomy care is discussed in a fundamentals of nursing textbook.

Accidental Decannulation. A tracheostomy tube that is not properly secured may be accidentally dislodged from the stoma. Because most new tracheostomy tubes are sutured in place, decannulation is rare, but it is serious nonetheless. Decannulation may occur while the ties are being changed. Manipulation of a tracheostomy tube or suctioning often produces vigorous coughing, which can expel the tube from the stoma unless the tube is held firmly. A stoma less than 4 days old may also close because a tract is not yet formed. If extubation occurs, call for help immediately and follow the steps in Box 60-2.

Maintain ventilation and oxygenation by bag and mask. If ventilation is impossible, you must reinsert the tube. To do so, deflate the cuff, remove the inner cannula of the tube, insert the obturator in the outer cannula, elevate the client's shoulders with a pillow, and gently hyperextend the neck. If accidental decannulation occurs once a tract has formed following a tracheostomy, the same procedure is used, but reinsertion of the tube is generally easier. If bleeding occurs or the airway is obstructed, use emergency measures as indicated earlier. If the tube cannot be reinserted, it should be considered an airway emergency and preparation for reintubation begun.

SAFETY ALERT

Tracheal Wall Necrosis. Necrosis of the tracheal wall can lead to the formation of an opening between the posterior trachea and the esophagus, called a *tracheoesophageal fistula*. The fistula allows air to escape into the stomach, causing distention. It also promotes aspiration of gastric contents. Fistulae most often develop when a

---

BOX 60-2 Accidental Decannulation of Tracheostomy Tube

PREPARE FOR POTENTIAL DECANNULATION

Keep the following equipment at the client's bedside:
- Extra tracheostomy tubes of the same size and one size smaller
- Obturator belonging to the existing tube
- Tracheal dilator (spreader)
- Oxygen source
- Suction catheters and suction source
- Resuscitation bag

IF DECANNULATION OCCURS
- Call for help.
- Hyperextend the client's neck to facilitate tube reinsertion.
- Assess the presence of tracheal retention sutures and use them to maintain an airway:
  - Pull top suture upward and outward.
  - Pull lower suture downward and outward.
- If retention sutures are not present, insert the tracheal dilator into the tracheostoma to open the airway.
- Place the obturator into the outer cannula and reinsert the tracheostomy tube into the tracheostoma. If the replacement tube is cuffed, deflate the cuff before insertion.
- Secure the tube with ties or Velcro strap.
- Assess tube placement by auscultating for breath sounds. Insert the inner cannula and reconnect oxygen/ventilation equipment.
- If the tracheostomy tube cannot be reinserted in 1 minute, call a code.

---

cuffed tube is used in conjunction with a standard nasogastric (NG) tube. Use of small-lumen NG tubes can decrease the risk of fistula formation. Necrosis of the anterior trachea can lead to the rare but life-threatening complication of hemorrhage resulting from erosion into the innominate artery. This complication is manifested by bleeding in and around the tracheostomy or by pulsation of the tracheostomy tube. Immediate intervention is mandatory because exsanguination can occur.

Most tracheostomy tube cuffs are designed to exert a low pressure against the tracheal wall. These cuffs are easily distensible, so that they accept a high volume of air without generating excessive force (i.e., high-volume, low-pressure cuffs). Low cuff pressure is necessary to prevent damage to the tracheal mucosa. The volume of air in the cuff determines the pressure exerted on the tracheal mucosa. Cuff pressures should not exceed 20 cm H_2O. With pressures greater than 42 cm H_2O, circulation to the tracheal mucosa is impaired, resulting in ischemia and necrosis. This is because the normal pressure within tracheal arteries is 42 cm H_2O. In the veins and lymphatic vessels, the normal pressures are 24 and 7 cm H_2O, respectively. Tracheal damage from cuff pressure is a frequent complication of intubation. Cuffed tubes can cause tracheal damage in as few as 3 to 5 days.

Tracheal Dilation. Prolonged intubation can lead to dilation of the trachea from the cuff. This complication should be suspected when increasing amounts of air are needed to seal the cuff or when bulging of the tracheal wall is seen on x-ray films.

Tracheal Stenosis. Tracheal stenosis is narrowing of the trachea and may be noted 1 week to 2 years after intubation. It results from chronic inflammation, fibrosis, and necrosis, which cause scar formation in the inflamed trachea. It can also result from excessive movement of the tracheostomy tube from ventilator tubing. The severity of stenosis can be prevented by choosing the right size of tube, maintaining adequate cuff pressure, keeping intubation time short, preventing infection, and reducing movement of the tube. Tracheal stenosis is a potential complication of long-term tracheostomy and may require tracheal resection.

Tracheomalacia. Tracheomalacia is a softening of the trachea resulting from secretions pooling above the cuff and thinning the cartilage. This weakened area of the trachea collapses on deep inspiration, impeding air flow and making it difficult to achieve an adequate seal. This problem may be managed by using a foam cuff tracheostomy tube. This tube has a sponge-like consistency. The cuff is foam-filled and self-expands with air after insertion, conforming to the size and shape of the client's trachea, and reducing pressure on the tracheal wall.

Subcutaneous Emphysema. Subcutaneous emphysema develops when air escapes from the tracheostomy incision into the tissues, dissects fascial planes under the skin, and accumulates around the face, neck, and upper chest. These areas appear puffy, and slight finger pressure produces a crackling sound and sensation. Generally this is not a serious condition; the air is eventually absorbed. The underlying cause determines the serious nature of the treatment.

Weaning, Removal, and Rescue Breathing
Weaning from a Tracheostomy Tube

Clients can be weaned from mechanical ventilation if they can clear their secretions by mouth with an adequate cough, maintain oxygenation, and have a functional upper airway without obstruction. The multidisciplinary team collaborates for this assessment.

A tracheostomy tube is usually plugged by inserting a tracheostomy plug (decannulation stopper) into the opening of the outer cannula if the tube has a "tight to shaft" cuff, fenestration, or no cuff. This closes off the tracheostomy, allowing air flow and respiration to occur normally through the nose and mouth.

When a cuffed tracheostomy tube is plugged, the cuff must be deflated. If the cuff remains inflated, ventilation cannot occur, and respiratory arrest could result.

Air-cuffed tubes without fenestrations may not be safely capped.

Explain the process to the client and family. Most clients are anxious about weaning because they fear they may not be able to breathe. Constant, supportive observation during weaning is necessary. Encourage the client to begin to think about breathing through the nose again. This breathing is a strange sensation for people who have used a tracheostomy tube for a long time. Explain ways to facilitate optimal respiration and to maintain control of breathing (e.g., inhale slowly and completely through the nose; avoid holding the breath).

Arterial blood gas (ABG) analysis and measurement of spontaneous respiratory mechanics (respiratory rate, tidal volume, vital capacity, inspiratory effort, expiratory effort) are important assessments during the decannulation process. Oximetry and other noninvasive assessment modes may also be used once baseline ABG values are established. During weaning from tracheostomy, assess for indications of respiratory distress or ventilation impairment and suction frequency. Clinical manifestations of problems may include the following:

- Abnormal respiratory rate and pattern
- Use of accessory muscles to assist breathing
- Abnormal pulse and blood pressure measurements
- Abnormal skin and mucous membrane color
- Abnormal ABG levels or decreased oxygen saturation

Inability to Clear Mucus. Remove the tracheostomy plug immediately if any manifestation of respiratory distress or ventilation impairment appear. Also assess the client's quality of phonation and ability to deep-breathe and cough effectively. If oxygen has been administered via the tracheostomy, administer it at the prescribed rate of flow using nasal prongs. Prepare for possible return to mechanical ventilation, and have a manual resuscitation bag available at the bedside.

Removing a Tracheostomy Tube

A tracheostomy tube is removed after resumption of normal respirations as indicated by the client's ability to breathe comfortably with the tracheostomy plugged, to cough and expectorate secretions, and to maintain normal ABG values or oxygen saturation. Gradually increase the length of plugging sessions until the client is comfortable and confident with the tube plugged continuously for at least 24 hours.

After a tracheostomy tube is removed, place a petroleum gauze pad covered by a sterile dressing over the stoma. Providing an occlusive dressing minimizes air leak during the stoma healing process. Initially, every 8 hours, clean the skin around the stoma, remove mucus with hydrogen peroxide, rinse the area with normal saline, and apply a fresh, dry dressing over the healing stoma. Document the condition of the stoma and the surrounding skin. If either appears irritated or infected, notify the physician. Topical antibiotic ointment may be prescribed. A tracheostomy stoma closes gradually (over a period of several days). As long as the stoma is open, an air leak is present. Instruct the client to place clean fingers firmly over the dressing to facilitate normal speech and coughing.

After decannulation, ongoing assessment of respiratory function is necessary. Some complications of tracheostomy, such as tracheal stenosis, can appear months after tracheostomy tube removal.

Performing Rescue Breathing

Emergency rescue breathing in the bag-to-neck mode (i.e., mouth to tracheostomy or mouth to stoma) may be necessary if a client who has a tracheostomy or laryngectomy experiences respiratory depression or respiratory arrest. If a tracheostomy tube is in place, provide ventilation by attaching a manual self-inflating bag to the standard 15-mm adapter on the inner cannula. Some volume is lost from an uncuffed tube. Compensation of adequate ventilation can often be accomplished by altering the usual method of manual inflation (e.g., compress the bag more forcefully and quickly). If the tracheostomy tube is cuffed, inflate the cuff and maintain ventilation at the correct rate—that is, 12 to 16 breaths/min for an adult. If inflation of the cuff impedes ventilation, immediately deflate the cuff, and attempt to compensate for volume loss by compressing the bag more forcefully or quickly.

Nursing Management of the Client with a Tracheostomy

Preoperative Care

For clients who are to undergo elective tracheostomy, reinforce education provided by the physician. You may delegate some respiratory assistance tasks to other staff members, as discussed in the Management and Delegation feature on p. 1548. The client's understanding of the tracheostomy tube may be enhanced by looking at anatomic diagrams and by handling a tracheostomy tube. The postoperative changes in ability to speak and eat should be explained. If the tracheostomy is expected to be permanent, information about living a productive life with modifications in clothing can be provided. A visit by a client with a permanent tracheostomy may be desirable.

When an emergency tracheostomy is needed, precious seconds may be all the time available for teaching.

MANAGEMENT AND DELEGATION

Assisting with Respiratory Care

Assisting with respiratory care is one of the more controversial areas involving the use of assistive personnel. Opinions differ widely on the role of assistive personnel in caring for clients who need respiratory care. The performance of suctioning in particular is central to this debate. Your clinical facility should provide you with clear guidelines about the role of assistive personnel in this aspect of care.

The following aspects of respiratory care are commonly delegated to unlicensed assistive personnel:

- Setting up oxygen delivery equipment and suction equipment
- Stocking routine respiratory care supplies at the bedside
- Assisting clients with the use of an incentive spirometer (after client instruction from a nurse or respiratory care clinician)
- Assisting clients with coughing and deep-breathing (after client instruction from a nurse or a respiratory care clinician)
- Measuring and recording peripheral oxygen saturation (SpO$_2$)

Before the delegation of any aspect of respiratory care, consider the following:

- What is the client's respiratory status? Complete a thorough respiratory assessment.
- What is the indication for respiratory care? Is the client's condition stable? A client with acute respiratory compromise should receive your full attention and care; the care of such a client should not be delegated.
- Is your client receiving oxygen therapy? Oxygen is a type of medication for your client. All guidelines that pertain to medications also apply to oxygen. You may delegate the setup of oxygen delivery equipment to assistive personnel. However, you are responsible to verify that the ordered amount (dose) of oxygen is actually being delivered to the client.
- Does this client have a new or long-term tracheostomy? The tracheostomy tube that has been placed through a new surgical incision should be evaluated as for any other fresh postoperative site.
- Have the client and family members managed this tracheostomy at home? This is an opportunity to evaluate their sterile technique, to provide reinforcement, and to review instructions with the client and family. After doing so, you may choose to delegate suctioning for this client to assistive personnel.

Findings that are immediately reportable to you, the registered nurse, should be described for the assistive personnel. These include any change or difficulty that the caregiver or the client experiences during the provision of care, changes in the respiratory rate or pattern, and changes in the consistency, color, and quantity of respiratory secretions.

The client may be anxious or even unconscious. Education is often provided to the family to provide support to the individual.

Postoperative Care

Assessment. After tracheostomy, usual frequent assessment is required, including assessing amount, color, and consistency of secretions; and observing for indications of shock, hemorrhage, respiratory insufficiency, or complications related to the client's general condition or the surgical intervention.

Diagnosis, Outcomes, Interventions
Diagnosis: Ineffective Airway Clearance. Numerous factors can lead to ineffective airway clearance in clients with tracheostomy—for example, dehydration, fever, anesthesia, anticholinergic drugs, sedatives, and immobility.

Outcomes. The client will have effective airway clearance, as evidenced by no retained secretions, clear (or clearing) lung sounds, and no fever.

Interventions. Promote airway clearance and pulmonary aeration by changing the client's position frequently, providing humidification and hydration, using sedatives cautiously, and performing frequent hyperinflation and suctioning to promote lung expansion and reduce the risks of atelectasis, pulmonary infection, and ineffective gas exchange. Hyperinflation creates an "artificial sigh," improving lung aeration and facilitating removal of tracheobronchial secretions by enhancing the cough effort. When the client's condition is stabilized sufficiently, coughing may be enhanced by having the client place a finger over the tracheostomy tube opening while attempting to cough, if the tube is cuffless or the cuff is deflated. It is important that the client wash his or her hands before doing this. Have the client cough into clean gauze squares and dispose of them carefully. Paper tissues are not recommended for use with a tracheostomy.

Perform Suctioning. When a cuffed tracheostomy tube is used, secretions collect above the cuff. It is difficult to remove such secretions by oropharyngeal suctioning. Oral suction devices allow pharyngeal suctioning.

Suction clients' secretions based on assessment, not routinely, using sterile technique, preoxygenation, and hyperinflation, without routine instillation of normal saline. Routine suctioning increases airway trauma, and routine instillation of normal saline for suctioning increases the risk of pulmonary edema. Use proper technique to reduce mucosal trauma, which can lead to tracheal infection.

Mucosal trauma is indicated by tracheal irritation, tracheitis, and bloody tracheal secretions.

If the client is unable to cough, suction the airway through the tracheostomy tube. See the Management and Delegation feature on p. 1548 before delegating activities to unlicensed assistive personnel.

Provide Tracheostomy Care. Tracheostomy care is detailed elsewhere in fundamentals of nursing textbooks. Reinsertion of the clean inner cannula is shown in Figure 60-3.

Provide Adequate Hydration. The normal hydrating mechanisms of the upper airway are bypassed by a tracheostomy. Hydration can be provided by an oral, parenteral, or inhalation route. Inhalation techniques include increasing the humidity of room air with a room humidifier and administering oxygen with heated humidification via a ventilator circuit or aerosol device and sterile water.

If humidification is insufficient, the body tries to compensate for the deficit by using its own water stores. The result is tenacious (very thick) mucus, which can compromise airway patency and increases the risk of secretion pooling and subsequent infection. Dried mucus also occludes air passages and leads to atelectasis, pneumonia, and potentially severe gas exchange abnormalities.

Prevent Tube Movement. Secure a tracheostomy tube in midline tracheal alignment. Support ventilator and aerosol tubing to prevent pulling on the tracheostomy tube. Be careful not to disconnect tubing when turning the client. If cloth tape is used to secure the tube, tie a square knot, allowing room for two fingers to slide comfortably under the tape. Avoid placing the knot over the client's carotid artery or spine. Inspect the skin under the securing tape for skin irritation. When a tracheostomy is required for prolonged periods, the use of fastening devices such as padded straps with self-adhesive fasteners promotes comfort.

Diagnosis: Risk for Impaired Gas Exchange. After tracheostomy, impaired gas exchange may occur because of various factors. Factors affecting oxygen delivery include

(1) aspiration of blood, oral secretions, or gastric contents; (2) restricted lung expansion from immobility; (3) excessive tracheobronchial secretions; (4) inability to cough and deep-breathe; and (5) pre-existing medical conditions (e.g., obesity, fever, inadequate hydration, pneumonia, tracheal injury such as from burns).

Factors affecting the removal of carbon dioxide include (1) the use of sedatives or anesthetic agents, (2) deteriorating level of consciousness, and (3) any other condition potentially affecting ventilatory efficiency and leading to hypoventilation and retention of carbon dioxide.

Outcomes. The client will have adequate gas exchange, as evidenced by maintaining oxygen saturation at greater than 90% (or ABG values within normal limits) and having no manifestations of respiratory distress.

Interventions. Assessment of gas exchange by ABG analysis is important immediately after tracheostomy and whenever there is a change in the client's condition or a change in treatment. Continuous noninvasive monitoring with pulse oximetry is also used. If shock or hypotension exists, or if peripheral vasoconstrictive drugs are used, data obtained by transcutaneous monitoring may be incorrect because of vasoconstriction and probes should be placed on the ears if the fingers are cool.

> **Do not allow smoking in the room of a person who has a tracheostomy. Do not use aerosol spray cans (e.g., room deodorizers) near the person. Do not shake bedding or create dust clouds. Be careful when shaving or tending the person's hair that whiskers or hair does not fall into the trachea. Cover the tracheostomy with a thin cloth towel during shaving.**   SAFETY ⚠ ALERT

Diagnosis: Risk for Infection. The tracheostomy bypasses normal upper airway protective mechanisms. The client also has an incision. Both areas can become infected.

Outcomes. The client will exhibit no indications of infection, as evidenced by the absence of fever and by having a clean and dry tracheostomy site, healing incisions, and clear sputum.

Interventions

> **Use aseptic technique when working with the tracheostomy. This includes performing careful hand-washing; appropriately using gloves, sterile supplies, and solutions; and changing and decontaminating respiratory equipment per CDC standards. Create a "loop" in the aerosol or ventilator tubing assembly; that is, let the tube loop down to catch condensate. Drain water and condensate in the tubing away from the tracheostomy into a receptacle.**   SAFETY ⚠ ALERT
>
> **Clean and inspect the skin around the stoma and the stoma itself. Observe for indications of irritation, inflammation, skin breakdown, and purulent**

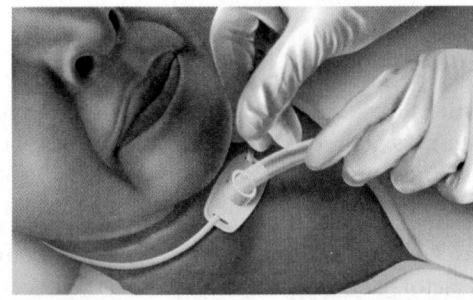

FIGURE 60–3 Reinserting a cleaned inner cannula.

drainage. Use a topical barrier to deter moisture, such as vitamin A and D ointment. If skin or stomal infection does occur, a topical antibacterial ointment may be prescribed.

Tracheostomy dressings (Figure 60-4) are often used, especially in the early postoperative stage. Damp blood and mucus-soaked dressings constitute a perfect medium for the growth of microorganisms. These conditions promote tissue irritation and breakdown. Change dressings whenever they are soiled or damp. Using normal saline and cotton-tipped applicators, carefully clean the skin each time the dressing is changed. Do not use plastic-backed or waterproof dressings. Moisture, secretions, and blood may seep behind the dressings, which retain warmth and moisture. Skin then becomes irritated and macerated.

Diagnosis: Risk for Aspiration. The presence of a tracheostomy increases the risk of aspiration because the tubes tether the larynx, preventing normal upward movement of the larynx and closure by the epiglottis on swallowing.

Outcomes. The client will exhibit no evidence of aspiration—that is, the client will have clear lung sounds, no fever, and no choking with swallowing.

Interventions. Intravenous fluids are usually given during the first 24 hours after tracheostomy. Then, if the client is alert and if swallowing and gag mechanisms are intact, oral intake of fluid and food may be attempted. Speech therapists can provide assessments and contributions to the plan of care. If a cuffed endotracheal tube was used before the tracheostomy, assess for the presence of tracheoesophageal fistula before permitting oral feedings. A client in whom normal swallowing is not

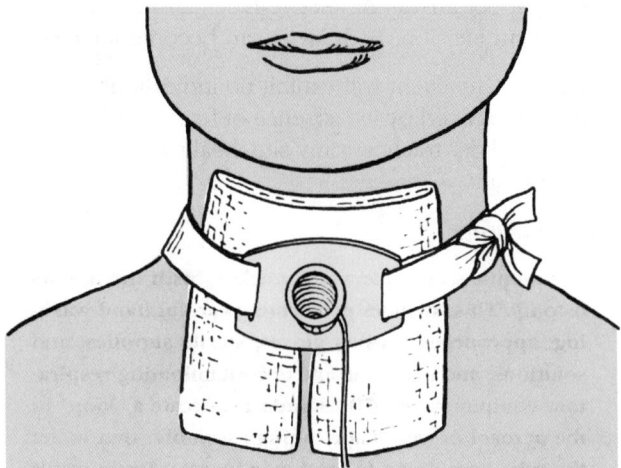

■ **FIGURE 60–4** Tracheostomy dressings. If there is significant bleeding or tracheal secretions, cleaning the skin and changing the dressing frequently may prevent infection and skin breakdown. Manufactured dressing with a precut slit has no fine threads that could unravel and enter the stoma. Place the dressing around the tracheostomy tube with the slit downward, as shown, or upward.

expected to return for some time, or in whom the swallowing mechanism is permanently impaired (e.g., after a stroke), requires gastrostomy feedings or a permanent feeding tube (see Chapter 30). Tube feedings may cause reflux, and the formula may be aspirated into the trachea. Before administering tube feedings, inflate the cuff of the tracheostomy tube. Leave it inflated for at least 1 hour after feeding. Suction above the cuff before deflating it to remove any tube-feeding material.

When feeding a client with a tracheostomy, have the client sit upright. Often, food and fluids with semi-solid consistency (e.g., pudding) are easier to swallow than water. Overinflation of the cuff causes swallowing difficulty. If oral fluid intake is limited, continue intravenous fluids or enteral feedings.

Diagnosis: Impaired Verbal Communication. Because the vocal cords are bypassed by the tracheostomy tube, the client cannot talk. The nursing diagnosis of *Impaired Verbal Communication* may need to be combined with the nursing diagnosis of *Fear* or *Anxiety* if the client feels afraid of not being able to summon help.

Outcomes. The client will have a satisfactory method of communicating with the nursing staff, as evidenced by being able to summon help and have needs met.

Interventions. Make sure the client can always reach an emergency call system to summon help. Be sure all staff members who may be answering the call system are aware that the client is unable to talk. Make a written list of common needs, words, and phrases that the client can point to (e.g., "I want to pass urine," "I am thirsty," or "I have pain") to communicate needs. Provide paper and pencil or a picture communication board to facilitate communication. Clients can seldom write clearly and it may be difficult to comprehend their written messages. When possible, assess the client's reading ability preoperatively and select appropriate communication tools to be used postoperatively. Other options include using a speaking valve, plugging of an appropriate tube, or using an electrolarynx.

Diagnosis: Risk for Constipation. When the glottis and vocal cords are bypassed (as with tracheostomy), the client cannot perform a Valsalva maneuver. This deficit impairs the person's ability to defecate.

Outcomes. The client will have regular bowel movements (according to a usual schedule).

Interventions. Assess for most recent bowel movement Elimination is a frequently overlooked area of client care. Use prescribed stool softeners, laxatives, and even enemas or suppositories as necessary.

Diagnosis: Anxiety and Fear. Anxiety and fear are caused b' various factors affecting the client with a tracheostomy— for example, inability to talk, fear of suffocating, anxiet' about diagnosis, or fear that the tracheostomy tube will come out.

Outcomes. The client will have decreasing manifestations of anxiety and fear, as evidenced by a pulse rate within normal limits, a calm facial expression, the ability to communicate, and no expressed fears.

Interventions. Frequent observation is essential. Your presence and skilled nursing care are reassuring. Be certain to allow the client adequate time to communicate needs and concerns. Assist the family in reassuring the client that nurses are present and that the client is not alone.

Diagnosis: Risk for Ineffective Therapeutic Regimen Management (Individuals) and Risk for Ineffective Family Therapeutic Regimen Management. The client and family members need a lot of new information about permanent or long-term tracheostomy care.

Outcomes. Before discharge from the health care facility, the client and significant others will be confident in performing tracheostomy care, suctioning, and preoxygenation and will demonstrate proper use of safety measures, emergency airway management, aerosol therapy, and other aspects of the client's airway maintenance regimen.

Interventions. Learning self-care is important for the client with a permanent tracheostomy. It provides a sense of self-control and reduces dependency on others. The client and significant others should begin performing self-care procedures as soon as possible postoperatively in order to allow sufficient time for learning. Multimedia resources, videotape, and booklets should be used to supplement the demonstrations and teaching. Follow-up telephone calls, contact through the physician's office, and home health nursing care (see the Bridge to Home Health Care website feature on Living with a Tracheostomy) are necessary to identify the effectiveness of the teaching.

Significant others must also be able to provide tracheostomy care and other components of airway management. Teach family members how to provide rescue breathing using the information presented previously.

The client and significant others are often anxious about home management. Send home a duplicate tracheostomy tube for use in changing the tube or in the event of accidental decannulation. Close follow-up is essential. Arrange for home equipment and follow-up visits by a home health agency or community health nurse with expertise in caring for people with complex airway needs. Involve a tracheostomy nurse specialist in client teaching when available. Order home health care equipment from medical suppliers who employ respiratory therapists or nurses. Ideally, have the equipment initially delivered to the hospital, so that the client and significant others can learn its use under the supervision of professionals.

Evaluation. Nursing diagnoses related to airway management should be resolvable within a few days. Problems with communication, infection, constipation, and eating remain areas of concern and require long-term planning.

NEOPLASTIC DISORDERS

BENIGN TUMORS OF THE LARYNX

Papillomas are one type of benign tumor of the larynx. They are small, wart-like growths believed to be viral in origin. Papillomas may be removed by surgical excision or laser. Surgery must be exact, because the nondiseased portion of the vocal cords needs to be retained for function. Other benign tumors of the larynx are *nodules* and *polyps*. Nodules and polyps frequently occur in people who abuse or overuse their voice.

CANCER OF THE LARYNX

Cancer of the larynx accounts for 2% to 3% of all malignancies. Care of the client with cancer of the larynx presents a unique challenge to the nurse because of the cosmetic and functional deformities commonly resulting from the disorder and its treatment. Benign and early malignant tumors may be treated with limited surgery, and the client recovers with little functional loss. Advanced tumors require extensive treatment, including surgery, radiation treatments, and chemotherapy. When a total laryngectomy is required, postoperatively the client is unable to speak, breathe through the nose or mouth, or eat normally. In addition, the creation of a permanent tracheostoma resulting from surgery has a tremendous impact on the client's functional ability and quality of life.

Laryngeal cancer is classified and treated by its anatomic site. Cancer of the larynx (voice box) may occur on the glottis (true vocal cords), the supraglottic structures (above the vocal cords), or the subglottic structures (below the vocal cords) (Box 60-3).

The American Cancer Society estimates 8900 new cases of laryngeal cancer each year, most occurring in men. However, the incidence of cancer of the larynx in women is increasing. If untreated, cancer of the larynx is inevitably fatal; 90% of untreated people die within 3 years. It is potentially curable if diagnosed and treated early.

Etiology and Risk Factors

The primary etiologic agent in laryngeal cancer is cigarette smoking. Three of four clients in whom laryngeal cancer develops have smoked or currently smoke. Alcohol appears to act synergistically with tobacco to increase the risk of development of a malignant tumor in the upper airway. Additional risk factors include occupational exposure to asbestos, wood dust, mustard gas,

BOX 60-3 Clinical Manifestations of Laryngeal Cancer

GLOTTIC TUMOR

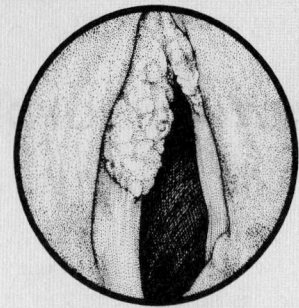

True glottic tumors interfere with normal closure and vibration of the vocal cords

Manifestations

- *Early:* Voice change, hoarseness, hemoptysis
- Dyspnea, respiratory obstruction, dysphagia, weight loss, pain
- *Metastasize:* Through regional lymph nodes (rare except in superior or inferior tumors)

SUPRAGLOTTIC TUMOR

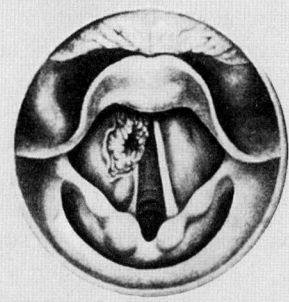

Carcinoma of the false cord partially hiding the true cord

Manifestations

- *Early:* Aspiration on swallowing (especially liquids), persistent unilateral sore throat, foreign-body sensation, dysphagia, weight loss, neck mass, hemoptysis (expectoration of blood)
- *Late:* Dyspnea, pain in the throat or referred to the ear

SUBGLOTTIC TUMOR

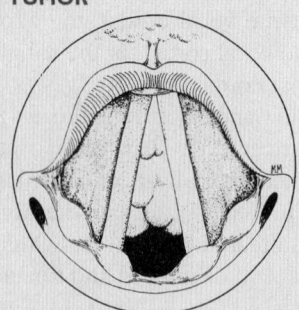

Subglottic polyp; this type of polyp can be single and smooth or lobulated as shown

Manifestations

- *Early:* None
- *Late:* Dyspnea, airway obstruction, dysphagia, weight loss, hemoptysis

Top and bottom figures from DeWeese, D.F., & Saunders, W.H. (1982). *Textbook of otolaryngology* (6th ed.). St. Louis: Mosby; middle figure from Del Regato, J.A., et al. (1985). *Ackerman and Del Regato's cancer* (6th ed.). St. Louis: Mosby.

and petroleum products and the inhalation of other noxious fumes. Chronic laryngitis and voice abuse may also contribute to the disorder. Research points to a link between tobacco exposure and mutation of the *p53* gene in squamous cell carcinoma of the head and neck.

Pathophysiology

Squamous cell carcinoma is the most common malignant tumor of the larynx, arising from the membrane lining the respiratory tract. Metastasis from cancer of the glottis is unusual because of the sparse lymphatic drainage from the vocal cords. Cancer elsewhere in the larynx spreads more quickly because there are abundant lymphatic vessels. Metastatic disease often may be palpated as neck masses. Distant metastasis may occur in the lungs. Patterns of spread of head and neck cancer are shown in Figure 60-5.

Clinical Manifestations

The earliest clinical warning signs of laryngeal cancer are dependent on the location of the tumor. In general, hoarseness that lasts longer than 2 weeks should be evaluated. Hoarseness occurs when the tumor invades muscle and cartilage surrounding the larynx, causing fixation of the vocal cords. Most clients wait before seeking a diagnosis for chronic hoarseness.

Tumors on the glottis prevent glottic closure during speech, which causes hoarseness or a voice change. Supraglottic tumors may cause pain in the throat (especially with swallowing), aspiration during swallowing, a sensation of a foreign body in the throat, neck masses, or pain radiating to the ear by way of the glossopharyngeal and vagus nerves. Subglottic tumors have no early

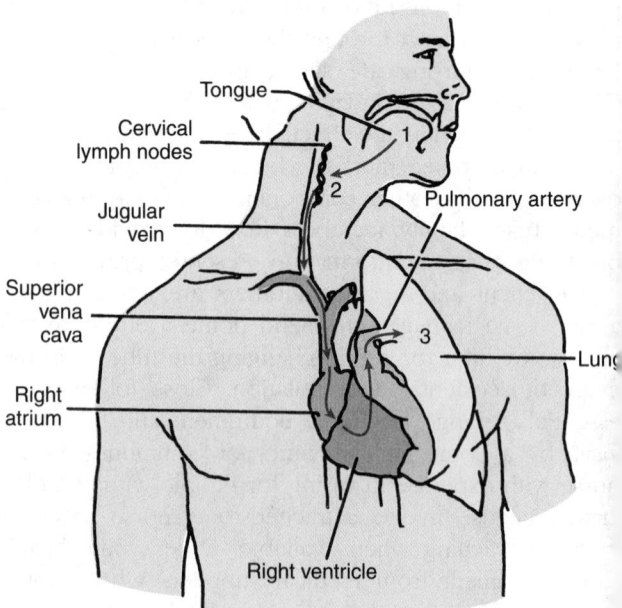

■ FIGURE 60–5 Pattern of spread of head and neck cancer *(From Black, J. [1991]. Reconstructive surgery in the elderly. Plastic Surgic Nursing, 11, 157.)*

manifestations; clinical evidence does not appear until the lesion grows to obstruct the airway.

Diagnostic Findings

The diagnosis of laryngeal cancer is made by visual examination of the larynx using direct or indirect laryngoscopy. The nasopharynx and posterior soft palate are inspected indirectly with a small mirror or an instrument resembling a telescope. While the mirror is inserted, slight pressure is applied to the tongue, and the client is instructed to say "a" and then "e," which elevates the soft palate. The instrument should not touch the tongue, or the client will gag. The nasopharynx is then inspected for drainage, bleeding, ulceration, or masses. Direct visualization of the larynx may be accomplished with use of several different instruments; most devices used are lighted endoscopes. The client is instructed to protrude the tongue, and the examiner *gently* holds the tongue with a gauze sponge and pulls it forward. A laryngeal mirror or telescopic endoscope is inserted into the oropharynx; again, contact with the tongue is avoided. The client is instructed to breathe in and out rapidly through the mouth, or to "pant like a puppy." Panting decreases the gagging sensation caused by the examination. During quiet respiration, the base of the tongue, epiglottis, and vocal cords are examined for manifestations of infection or tumor. The client is instructed to vocalize a high-pitched *eee* to approximate (close) the vocal cords. The examiner observes the movement of the cords, the color of the mucous membranes, and the presence of any lesions. If the client is unable to cooperate as described, the examination may be performed with a fiberoptic endoscope inserted through the nose.

Before any definitive treatment for tumor is initiated, a panendoscopy and biopsy are performed to determine the exact location, size, and extent of the primary tumor. Computed tomography (CT) or magnetic resonance imaging (MRI) is used to assist with this process. Laboratory analysis includes a complete blood count, determination of serum electrolytes including calcium, and kidney and liver function tests. These data help determine the physiologic readiness of the client for surgery. Because the airway will be altered after surgery, the client requires a thorough pulmonary assessment with ABG analysis for identification of any pre-existing pulmonary disorders that would interfere with breathing. Clients who are to undergo partial laryngectomy must have an adequate pulmonary reserve in order to produce an effective cough postoperatively. The operation is associated with an increased risk of aspiration, and the client must be able to cough to rid the airway of aspirated secretions. Finally, for ascertaining possible tumor spread or other primary tumors, a chest radiography and barium swallow study or esophagography are performed.

Once the tumor has been identified and a biopsy performed, the tumor can be staged. Staging has important implications for treatment choice and outcome. It is essential to determine the extent of the primary tumor in order to select the most appropriate intervention. Staging is accomplished by (1) measuring the size of the primary tumor, (2) determining the presence of enlarged lymphatic nodes, and (3) determining the presence of distant metastasis. This system of staging is called the TNM (tumor-node-metastasis) classification system (see Chapter 17).

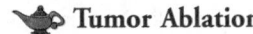 **OUTCOME MANAGEMENT**

Medical Management

Tumor Ablation

The goal of client care is ablation of the tumor, with sparing of undiseased tissue when possible. The choice of treatment for glottic cancer depends on the degree of tumor involvement. If the tumor is limited to the true vocal cord, without causing limitation of the cord's movement, radiation therapy is usually the best treatment, with cure rates of 85% to 95%. The radiation dose depends on the size and location of the tumor; it is usually a minimum dose of 5500 to 6000 centigray (cGy; *gray* is a more accurate unit than *rad*) over 5 to 7 weeks. Hyperfractionation (delivery of radiation twice a day) may be done to improve tumor control. During radiation therapy, the client needs to be assessed for manifestations of destruction of normal tissue, ability to eat, airway distress, and other side effects. The complications of radiation therapy to the larynx include skin irritation, xerostomia, mucositis, laryngeal edema, and delayed healing. Radiation therapy is discussed in Chapter 17.

Supraglottic tumors may be treated with radiation therapy or a partial laryngectomy, with or without lymph node dissection. Subglottic tumors are usually more advanced carcinomas in which the tumor has spread to surrounding tissues. Metastasis is common. Treatment requires a total laryngectomy with or without radical neck dissection on the same or both sides of the tumor (see later discussion). The operative site may require reconstruction with pectoralis myocutaneous flaps (see Chapter 49).

Chemotherapy alone is not considered to be curative in treating head and neck cancers but it is now integrated into standard therapy for head and neck cancer. It may be administered preoperatively to reduce tumor size, concurrently with radiation therapy, postoperatively to reduce the risk of metastasis, or as palliative treatment. Larynx preservation may be possible with induction chemotherapy followed by radiation. Chemotherapy is generally not effective in advanced laryngeal cancer, but it may control the development of new primary tumors through a process called *chemoprevention.*

Clients with laryngeal tumors often present in a compromised nutritional state because of dysphagia and weight loss. In addition, surgery, radiation therapy, and chemotherapy can directly affect oropharyngeal structures and impair swallowing. Nutritional intervention should begin before treatment to prevent malnutrition, thereby improving the overall prognosis.

Nursing Management of the Medical Client

The client undergoing radiation therapy for laryngeal cancer should be taught about the procedure and how to assess for and manage any expected problems at home. Written material is usually best, so that the client and family can refer to it as needed. Skin care for the irradiated site should include using prescribed creams and sunscreens, which are "patted" onto the skin; avoiding extremes of temperature; avoiding rough or tight garments; and avoiding rubbing or scratching the area.

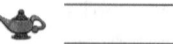

Surgical Management

The goals of surgical intervention for laryngeal cancer are to (1) remove the cancer, (2) maintain adequate physiologic function of the airway, and (3) achieve a personally acceptable physical appearance. Many clients require tracheostomy for airway management (see earlier discussion). Most clients with advanced laryngeal cancer also have malnutrition from obstruction to swallowing by the tumor, as well as from the effects of the cancer. Before surgery, supplemental nutrition may be provided by NG tube feedings or gastrostomy feedings. If long-term difficulty in swallowing is anticipated, a gastrostomy tube may be inserted at the time of surgery.

Laser Surgery

Small tumors can often be eradicated with the use of laser. Laser surgery for vocal cord tumors can preserve much of the normal glottis, leaving the client with a usable voice. Sometimes laser surgery is combined with radiation therapy.

Partial Laryngectomy

For cancer involving one true vocal cord, or one cord plus a portion of the other, a partial laryngectomy is feasible. This procedure is also called a vertical partial laryngectomy and involves the removal of half or more of the larynx (Figure 60-6). A horizontal neck incision is made, and the diseased portion of the vocal cord is removed. Sometimes up to one third of the contralateral cord is also removed. This operation is generally well tolerated, and the client has only mild difficulty swallowing and an altered but adequate voice.

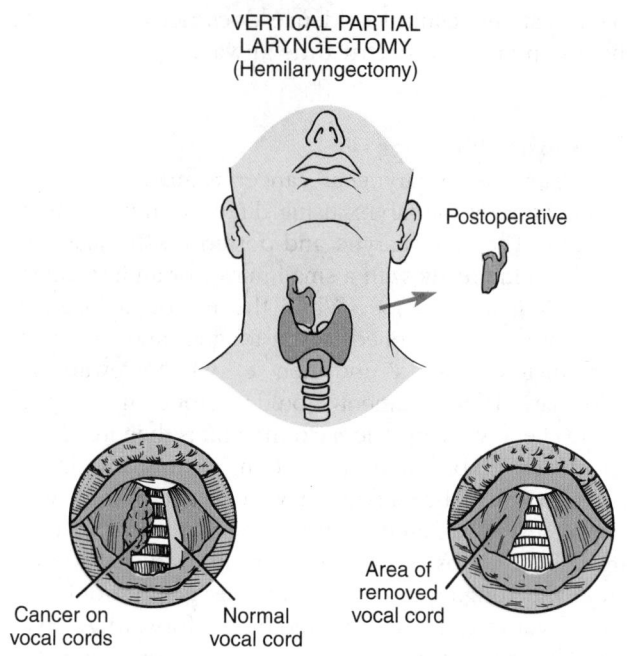

FIGURE 60–6 Technique of partial laryngectomy.

Another form of partial laryngectomy is the supraglottic laryngectomy. This procedure is performed for cancer of the supraglottis. The surgeon removes the superior portion of the larynx from the false vocal cords to the epiglottis and may also remove a portion of the base of the tongue. Lymph node dissection also may be performed. Because the true vocal cords are preserved, voice quality is maintained. The major postoperative problem is risk of aspiration, because the epiglottis, which normally closes over and protects the larynx, has been removed. The airway is managed with a tracheostomy after surgery; when the edema subsides in surrounding tissues, the tracheostomy tube can usually be removed and the stoma allowed to heal. The client then needs to be taught how to swallow to avoid aspiration.

For selected confined transglottic carcinomas, a supracricoid partial laryngectomy may be indicated. This conservative procedure preserves functional speech and swallowing without a permanent tracheostomy.

Total Laryngectomy

For large glottic tumors with fixation of the vocal cords, a total laryngectomy is required. The larynx is the connection of the pharynx (upper airway) and the trachea (lower airway) (Figure 60-7, *A*). When the larynx is removed, a permanent opening is made by suturing the trachea to the neck. The esophagus remains attached to the pharynx (Figure 60-7, *B*). Because no air can enter the nose, the client loses the sense of smell. The biggest problem for the client after laryngectomy is loss of voice

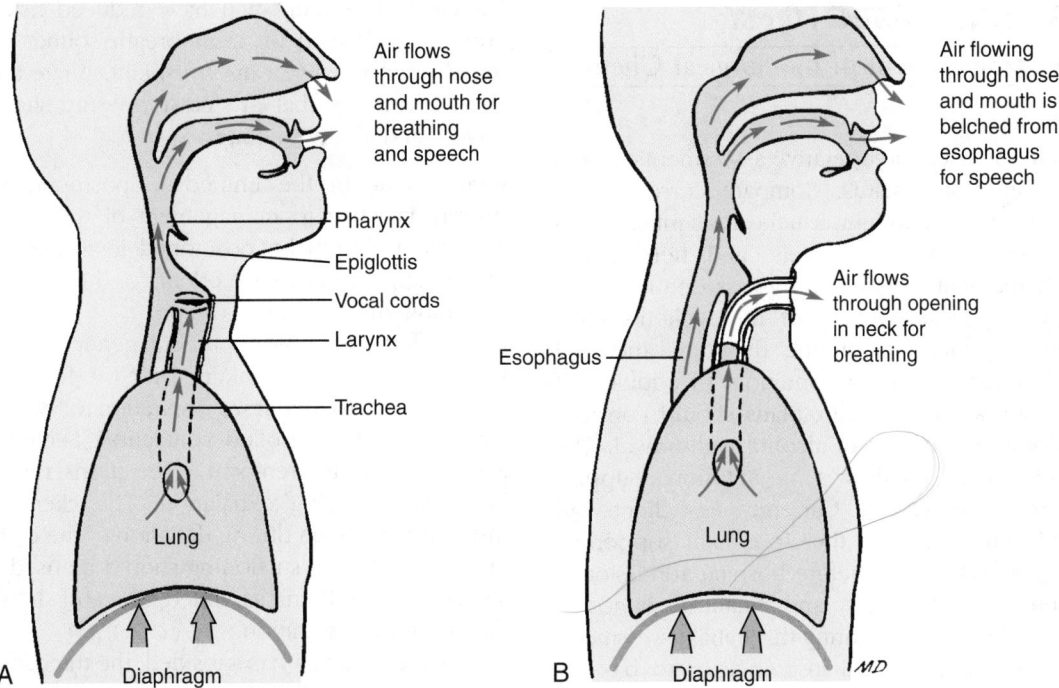

■ FIGURE 60–7   A, Before laryngectomy, air flow is through the nose and mouth. **B,** After surgical removal of the larynx, a new opening must be made for air passage. The trachea and esophagus are separated.

The client should be made aware that without surgery, the voice quality worsens as the tumor enlarges, but in any case the loss of voice constitutes a serious psychological issue. Because the trachea and esophagus are permanently separated by surgery, there is no risk of aspiration unless a fistula forms from the trachea to the esophagus. Besides this, the potential complications of the total laryngectomy are the same as those for the partial laryngectomy (see earlier discussion).

Cervical Lymph Node Dissection

Metastasis to the cervical lymph nodes is common with tumors of the upper aerodigestive tract. Surgical management of laryngeal tumors often includes neck dissection. Radical neck dissection (also called en bloc) involves the removal of lymphatic drainage channels and nodes, the sternocleidomastoid muscle, the spinal accessory nerve, the jugular vein, and tissue in the submandibular area. A modified radical neck dissection spares the spinal accessory nerve, and a selective neck dissection removes only the lymph nodes within the area of anticipated spread.

Complications

Possible complications after laryngeal surgery are airway obstruction, hemorrhage, carotid artery rupture, and fistula formation. Airway obstruction is due to edema in the surgical site, bleeding into the airway, or loss of airway from a plugged tracheostomy tube. Airway obstruction constitutes an emergency and requires immediate intervention for restoration of the airway.

Hemorrhage is usually the result of inadequate hemostasis during surgery. Some blood-tinged sputum is expected in the tracheal secretions for the first 48 hours, but frank bleeding from the tracheotomy site or tube is a manifestation of hemorrhage and must be reported to the physician immediately. Also assess the client for other manifestations of bleeding such as evident hematoma or unilateral swelling, tachycardia, hypotension, and changes in respiratory patterns.

Carotid artery rupture is usually a late complication and is related to poor condition of the neck tissue. It may be the result of previous radiation therapy to the area, pharyngocutaneous fistula, recurrent tumor, or infection. This condition is also a life-threatening emergency and carries an extremely high mortality. Mild bleeding from the oral cavity, neck, or trachea may precede impending rupture by 24 to 48 hours. A pulsating tracheostomy tube may indicate that the tip of the tube is resting on the innominate artery, which may cause injury to the artery and result in hemorrhage.

Fistulae between the hypopharynx and the skin may also develop. Many fistulae heal on their own, but treatment may require surgery, depending on the location and size.

PARTIAL LARYNGECTOMY

Nursing Management of the Surgical Client

Preoperative Care

In addition to the usual preoperative assessments, assess the client's nutritional status. Compare current body weight with ideal body weight, usual caloric intake, total lymphocyte count, albumin levels, and hemoglobin value and hematocrit. In addition, assess dentition and the oral cavity. Because many of these clients have abused tobacco and alcohol, the dentition and oral cavity are frequently in poor condition. In addition, if the client is an active alcoholic, plans should consider support through the period of alcohol withdrawal. The ideal plan of care would allow some nutritional support and oral care before surgery. Currently, few clients can be admitted before surgery; therefore such supportive care must be accomplished before hospital admission.

The client's work history and financial concerns should also be investigated during this initial assessment. Inability to purchase medical insurance or to pay for health care services may account for the client's lack of personal and medical care.

The client's usual coping strategies and family support should also be evaluated. Some degree of cosmetic (aesthetic) change will result after surgery, and the client will be unable to speak for some time. Preoperative plans should consider alternative methods of communication and family support networks. Preoperative education by rehabilitated laryngectomees is important for these clients.

Because of the multiple problems common in these clients, a team approach to their care is used. Members of the team usually include the primary physician or surgeon, nurses, a social worker, a dietitian, a speech or swallowing therapist, a physical therapist, a respiratory therapist, and home health care nurses. If extensive surgery is required, a plastic surgeon and a maxillofacial prosthodontist may also care for the client during reconstruction.

Postoperative Care

Assessment. In addition to the routine postoperative assessments, after a partial laryngectomy the client needs to undergo careful assessment of the airway, lung sounds, and position of the tracheostomy tube, as well as checking for potential complications related to the surgical procedure and the tracheostomy tube (see earlier discussion).

Diagnosis, Outcomes, Interventions

Diagnosis: Risk for Aspiration. Because of the removal of the epiglottis (which normally acts as a trap door to close the airway and prevent aspiration) and because secretions are excessive after surgery, the client is at very high risk for aspiration. This is a priority diagnosis.

Outcomes. The client will have reduced risk of aspiration, as evidenced by clear breath sounds throughout the chest, normal (for age) respiratory rate and rhythm, chest secretions that are clear or only slightly blood-tinged, and ability to cough.

Interventions. In the immediate postoperative period, priority is given to management of the upper airway. The client should be positioned in a greater than 45-degree angle to decrease edema of the airway, facilitate breathing, and improve comfort.

A cuffed tracheostomy tube is generally inserted during surgery and is maintained for the first several days after surgery to minimize aspiration of secretions and for assisted or controlled ventilation. Secretions collect above the cuff. For removal of secretions, the cuff should be deflated during exhalation. The client should be instructed to cough during deflation of the cuff. If the client cannot cough, suctioning should be used to prevent secretions from being aspirated. The cuff should be reinflated during inspiration.

When the edema has subsided, the tracheostomy tube may be removed. The decannulation process is slow and begins with observation of the client for aspiration, as follows. The cuff of the tube is deflated, and the client is observed for the ability to swallow saliva and other secretions without coughing or requiring additional suctioning. If increased secretions are present through and around the tracheostomy tube, aspiration is occurring and the cuff should be reinflated. If no aspiration is occurring, the tracheostomy tube can be replaced with a smaller, uncuffed tube. If the uncuffed tube is tolerated without aspiration, the tube is capped (plugged) to determine the client's ability to breathe through the upper airway. If the client can breathe through the upper airway for 24 hours, the tracheostomy tube is removed, and the stoma is taped closed and covered with an occlusive dressing.

Diagnosis: Ineffective Airway Clearance. The physical alteration in the airway and the presence of a tracheostomy tube interfere with normal movement of mucus up and out of the bronchial tree. In addition, as a result of prior smoking, the cilia have become ineffective. *Ineffective Airway Clearance* is also a priority nursing diagnosis for several days.

Outcomes. The client will have improved airway clearance, as evidenced by effortless, quiet respirations at baseline rate and clear breath sounds.

Interventions. The client may have copious secretions because of the presence of the tracheostomy tube, a history of chronic obstructive lung disease, and aspiration. There may also be oral secretions that cannot be swallowed. Oral secretions accumulate because of the disruption of normal air flow, and swallowing may be impaired as a result of surgery. In the alert and conscious client, coughing and deep-breathing mobilize and eliminate many of these secretions. However, in the client who has undergone head and neck surgery and is just emerging from anesthesia, these measures may not be possible. Suctioning of the trachea is needed for the first 24 to 48 hours after surgery. The frequency of suctioning depends on the client's needs, but suctioning every hour or more often is common for the first 24 hours. Suctioning techniques can be found in fundamentals of nursing textbooks.

Sterile technique must be used to avoid introducing microorganisms into the tracheobronchial tree in a client with impaired immune defenses resulting from malignancy and surgery.

If present, the inner cannula of the tracheostomy tube should be cleaned as often as necessary to provide a clear airway. In the immediate postoperative phase, the inner cannula is cleaned after suctioning. Once the client is ambulatory and can handle secretions safely, the cannula can be cleaned three times a day and as necessary.

Aerosol administration of bronchodilators into deeper parts of the respiratory tract is recommended to prevent pulmonary complications. These treatments are performed every 4 hours for the first few days after surgery and then usually decreased to four times a day once the client can ambulate.

Diagnosis: Risk for Impaired Gas Exchange. Like other postoperative clients, clients with neck surgery have a high risk for atelectasis related to low tidal volume breathing secondary to pain, sedation, and increased mucus production.

Outcomes. The client will have adequate oxygenation, as evidenced by pulse oximetry values above 90%, ABG values within normal limits (that take into consideration any pre-existing lung disorders, such as emphysema), no air hunger, and clear lung sounds.

Interventions. Oxygenation is assessed through ABG analysis or pulse oximetry and the fraction of inspired oxygen (Fio_2) may be adjusted. If the client has pre-existent chronic air flow limitations, oxygen may have to be delivered at lower percentages or not at all. Compressed air with high humidity may be substituted in such cases.

Diagnosis: Impaired Nutrition: Less Than Body Requirements. A combination of the pre-existing malignancy and swallowing difficulties sets the stage for malnutrition. In addition, concomitant lung disorders and alcoholism, which are common in this population, increase the tendency for malnutrition.

Outcomes. The client will have an improved nutritional status, as evidenced by maintaining baseline body weight or losing less than 5 pounds; consuming adequate fluid, protein, fat, and carbohydrate each 24 hours; swallowing without aspirating or choking; and maintaining hemoglobin, hematocrit, albumin, and total lymphocyte values within normal limits.

Interventions. Immediately after surgery, typically an NG tube is inserted for removal of gastric secretions until postoperative ileus subsides. If long-term difficulty in swallowing is anticipated, a gastrostomy tube may be inserted at the time of surgery. Assess for hunger and passage of flatus as manifestations of returning gastrointestinal function; bowel sounds may or may not be present In some clients, tube-feeding with commercial supplements is indicated. Continually ascertain the correct position of the tube before each feeding. (Techniques for checking feeding tube placement can be found in fundamentals of nursing textbooks.) The tube-feeding can be administered by pump, slow drip, or bolus feeding, depending on the client's tolerance. Aspiration remains a high risk with partial laryngectomy, and precautions to guard the client from this event with its untoward results are critical.

When the epiglottis has been removed, the timing for resumption of oral feeding after a partial laryngectomy is controversial. One approach is to begin oral feedings with the tracheostomy tube in place when edema has subsided and the client is able to swallow secretions. The advantage of this technique is that aspirated liquid can be suctioned. A second technique is to delay oral feeding until the client has been decannulated and the stoma has healed. The advantage of this technique is that with a closed stoma, the client is able to increase intrathoracic pressure and remove any aspirated material through an effective cough.

Whenever the client eats, eating should be evaluated with a speech therapist. The Client Education Guide on p. 1558 lists precautions to teach clients undergoing a partial laryngectomy. Once swallowing can be accomplished without aspiration, carbonated beverages may be added. Thin liquids should be withheld until the risk of aspiration is minimal.

Diagnosis: Risk for Infection. The loss of primary defenses of the skin and delayed healing attributable to pre-existing malignancy and malnutrition make *Risk for Infection* a common nursing diagnosis.

Outcomes. The client will have no clinical manifestations of wound infection, as evidenced by continued approximation of incisional edges; decrease in the amount of wound drainage; absence of purulent drainage; absence of redness, swelling, tenderness, or warmth beyond the suture lines; absence of fever; and a white blood cell count within normal limits.

CLIENT EDUCATION GUIDE

Swallowing Technique After a Partial Laryngectomy

- Begin with soft or semi-solid foods.
- Stay with a nurse or swallowing therapist during meals until you master the technique of swallowing without choking.
- Be patient; learning to swallow again is frustrating.
- Follow these steps in sequence:
  1. Take a deep breath.
  2. Bear down to close the vocal cords.
  3. Place food into your mouth.
  4. Swallow.
  5. Cough to rid the closed cord of accumulated food particles.
  6. Swallow.
  7. Cough.
  8. Breathe.

Interventions. During surgery, a wound drain is placed into the surrounding tissues of the neck and attached to constant suction. A closed wound drainage system is attached to the client's gown to prevent accidental dislodgment. Using standard precautions, assess the amount and color of the drainage every 4 hours for the first 24 hours. Assess the wound for manifestations of hematoma or seroma formation by noting whether the amount of drainage is increasing or whether there is a change in the color or consistency of the drainage. Also assess the color of the surgical incisions. If the amount of drainage is decreasing, the drain may be removed by the physician. Dressings are placed over the drain puncture sites on the skin. Small to moderate amounts of serosanguineous drainage should be expected for another 48 to 72 hours.

The suture lines should be cleaned at least twice daily with saline rinse. A thin film of a protective barrier ointment may be applied to the suture line to prevent crusting of secretions and to promote healing.

Evaluation. Expect the problems with airway management to resolve within a few days. Infection, apart from atelectasis, does not arise for about 72 hours. Nutritional problems and problems with healing may require several weeks to resolve.

Self-Care

The client who has undergone partial laryngectomy may be discharged from the hospital before completion of wound healing. If upper airway edema has not subsided, the client is discharged with a temporary tracheostomy. The client and significant others should understand and demonstrate proper care of the tube, including inner cannula care, technique for insertion of the entire tube in case

of accidental decannulation, suctioning, humidification techniques, and emergency resuscitation measures.

Once decannulation has been performed, the stoma must be cleansed and an occlusive dressing applied at least once a day. Additional wound care includes cleaning the incision area with hydrogen peroxide and water and applying an antibiotic ointment. All instructions given to the client should be in writing, with additional teaching materials used as available. Ongoing assessment for healing, recurrent tumor, or a new tumor is required.

TOTAL LARYNGECTOMY

Nursing Management of the Surgical Client

The nursing management of the client after a total laryngectomy is the same as the care given to a client with a partial laryngectomy, except for feeding and teaching about permanent stoma care. Clients who have a total laryngectomy have a permanent tracheostomy and need to learn how to speak using alternative methods.

Nutrition

Immediately after surgery, the client's nutrition is supplemented with tube feedings. The client continues to receive tube feedings until edema has subsided and suture line healing has occurred. When the client can swallow saliva, oral feedings can begin. The diet usually begins with liquid or semi-soft foods and progresses as healing occurs.

Communication

For the first few days after surgery, the client should communicate by writing. If the client is very fatigued, requests such as "I need something for pain" may be expressed by using a communication board so that the client can just point to the statement. Even though the client cannot speak, conversation should still include the client's input through nodding and pointing and not be directed only to others, such as the family. Avoiding conversation with the client because of difficulty in communication is demeaning to the client and leads to frustration.

Artificial Larynx

An artificial larynx may be used as early as 3 to 4 days after surgery. These battery-operated speech devices are held alongside the neck or can be adapted with a plastic tube that is inserted in the mouth. The air inside the mouth is vibrated, and the client articulates as usual (Figure 60-8). The speech quality is monotone and mechanical-sounding but intelligible.

Esophageal Speech

Esophageal speech is a technique that requires the client to swallow and hold air in the upper esophagus. By

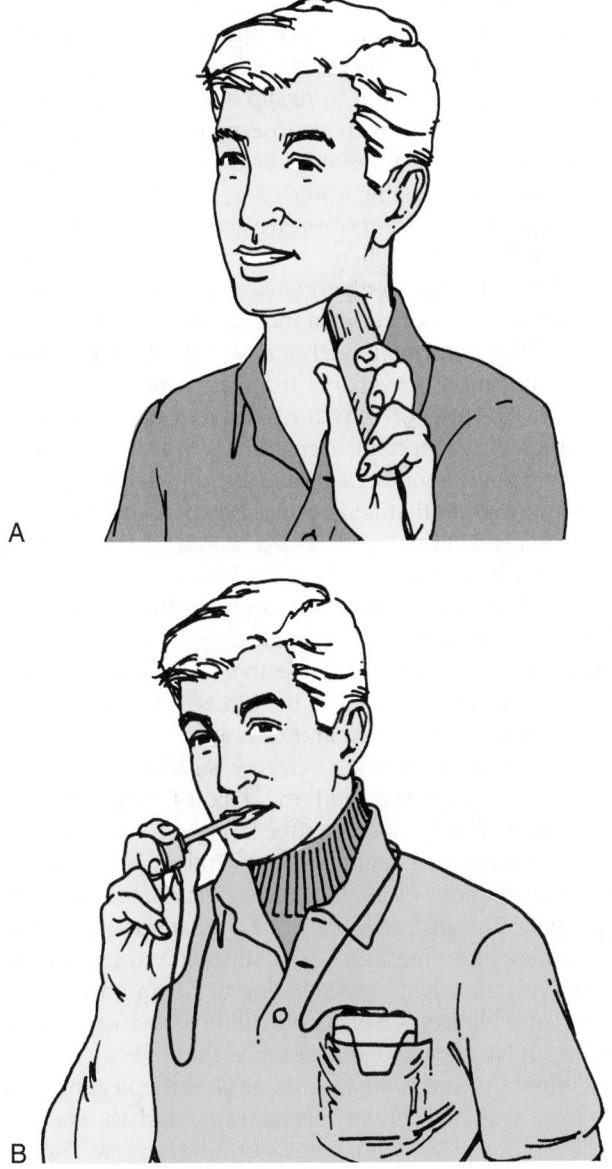

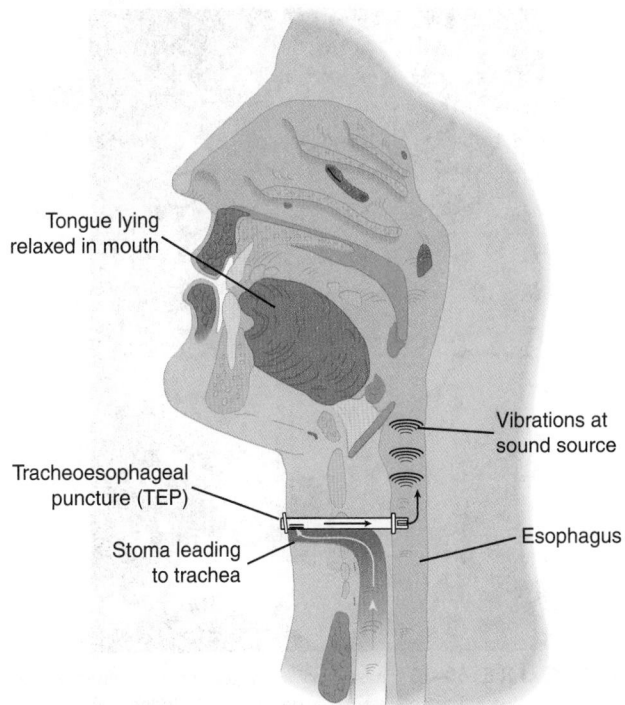

- **FIGURE 60–9** Tracheoesophageal puncture for voice rehabilitation after laryngectomy. A prosthesis is inserted into a fistula created in the neck. The prosthesis has a one-way valve that permits air to pass into the esophagus but prevents accidental aspiration. To speak, the client occludes the prosthesis with a finger or attachment. Exhaled air is then shunted through the prosthesis, where it vibrates, and exits the mouth as a spoken word.

- **FIGURE 60–8** Artificial larynx. This hand-held, battery-powered speech aid is placed against the neck. **A,** When the artificial larynx is activated, it creates a vibration that is transmitted to the neck and into the mouth. Words silently formed by the mouth become sounds from the vibrations emitted by the device. Any type of artificial larynx requires muscle and tongue control and hand strength; usually, such a device is not used until immediate postoperative neck tenderness has subsided. **B,** Electronic speech aid allows the client to adjust tone, pitch, and volume. An oral connector permits speech without the necessity of placing the device against the neck. This is an advantage immediately after surgery, when the neck is too sensitive for a neck-vibrating device.

puncture is made into the upper tracheostoma to the cervical esophagus for creation of a fistula. After the fistula tract has healed, a small one-way valve, or voice prosthesis, is inserted. By occlusion of the prosthesis, air can be shunted into the esophagus and used to produce speech. The TEP may be done concurrently with a total laryngectomy or as a secondary procedure after healing and radiation therapy. These devices require maintenance; therefore only clients who are highly motivated, who are able to perform self-care, and who have good manual dexterity are eligible for this procedure. Care of the TEP surgical wound is presented in the Client Education Guide feature on the website.

controlling the flow of air, the client can pronounce as many as 6 to 10 words before stopping to swallow more air. The voice is deep but is loud and effective once the technique is mastered.

Tracheoesophageal Puncture

Tracheoesophageal puncture (TEP) is a surgical technique that also restores speech (Figure 60-9). A small

Self-Care

Clients should be discharged with an extra tracheostomy tube to allow tube changes at home (Figure 60-10). To provide supplemental humidification, normal saline may be instilled into the stoma several times each day to stimulate coughing, moisten the mucosa, and loosen dried secretions and crusts. Use of a bedside humidifier or vaporizer also aids in humidifying the inspired air. A stoma bib or covering should be worn to warm and filter inspired air and to prevent foreign bodies from entering the stoma.

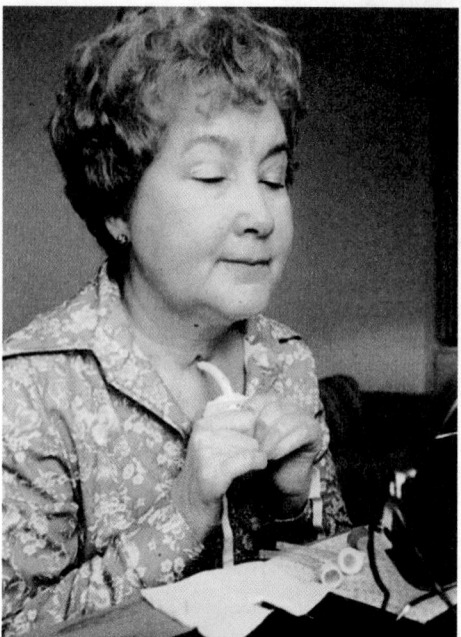

■ **FIGURE 60-10** Insertion of a laryngectomy tube into a permanent tracheostoma. The obturator or guide is inserted into the outer cannula. After the tube is lubricated with water-soluble ointment, the client takes a deep breath and the lubricated tube is inserted. The obturator is removed, and the tube is tied in place.

These coverings can be purchased, or the client may improvise by using a scarf, necktie, or turtleneck shirt.

The client must be encouraged to continue speech therapy as begun in the hospital. The techniques to restore speech require much time for mastery; the client is seen by a speech therapist after dismissal from the hospital. Community support groups for clients after laryngectomy such as the Lost Cord Club and the International Association of Laryngectomees offer needed reassurance. Much patience is required by the client and family while the client is relearning to speak. The process is time-consuming and frustrating, and progress may sometimes be slow. Encourage the family to give the client enough time to formulate the words and not speak for the client.

Once the incision has completely healed, the tracheostomy tube is no longer required (Figure 60-11). This process varies but usually takes about 6 to 8 weeks. Occasionally, the tube may be required at night, if the

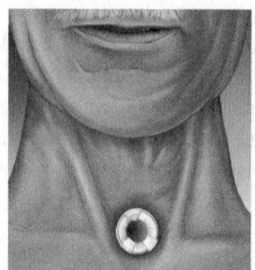

■ **FIGURE 60-11** Healed tracheostomy incision.

stoma is small or the client does not get adequate air exchange during sleep. Once the tracheostomy tube has been removed, the client can disguise the stoma with clothing and begin to regain a sense of normalcy.

Tub baths or showers are permitted, but the client must use caution to prevent introduction of water into the stoma, aiming the water spray at midchest. Commercial stoma shower covers are available. Water sports are prohibited. The client should wear a medical alert bracelet and carry an emergency wallet card to identify the fact that resuscitation cannot be performed through the mouth. Information about obtaining these forms of identification is available from the American Cancer Society. The use of mouth-to-stoma rescue breathing is imperative when resuscitation is needed in these clients. Family members should be directed to a community program that teaches mouth-to-stoma resuscitation. For additional security, a wireless "beeper" or automatic response monitoring device can be useful.

The client may require a nutritional plan for the first few weeks at home. The dietitian should work with the client and family to determine the consistency of food easiest to swallow as well as the kinds of foods required to obtain needed protein and calories.

It is essential that the client not smoke so that lung function is preserved and the risk of other cancers reduced. For some clients after laryngectomy, the process of smoking cessation seems pointless. Some clients continue to smoke by inhaling the cigarette smoke through the stoma. The attitude is one of "Why quit now? What else could happen to me?" Use extra support and encouragement with the client, remembering to be an advocate of the client's choice as well as providing assurance that the quality of life after smoking cessation improves.

Follow-up care is important to assess the healing process, to evaluate coping mechanisms, and to examine the client for possible metastasis or new tumors. The client should be taught to report any of the following manifestations to the physician:

- A lump anywhere in the neck or body
- Persistent cough, sore throat, or earache
- Hemoptysis
- Sores around the stoma or within the trachea that do not heal
- Difficulty swallowing or breathing

NECK DISSECTION

Nursing Management of the Surgical Client

Preoperative Care

Before surgery, the client's understanding of the plans for surgery should be assessed. Determine what the surgeon has told the client and how much information has been retained or lost because of anxiety. In addition, ldress the fears the client has about the diagnosis of ncer and fears of deformity after surgery. Assist the cli- nt to understand the anatomic and physiologic altera- ons that will occur as a result of radical surgery. xplain to the client and family what to expect after sur- ery (e.g., placement in the intensive care unit, tracheos- my, drainage tubes) and review postoperative care .g., communication techniques to be used if a trache- stomy is to be placed).

The client's support systems and degree of coping lould be assessed. If the client is an alcoholic, alcohol ay be the usual coping tool. Because alcohol will not e available, assess the other coping mechanisms avail- le to the client, and encourage the client to use them. urces may include friends and family. Identify new lpport systems, if needed, such as interaction with peo- e who have had the same surgery or diagnosis.

ostoperative Care

fter surgery, the usual postoperative assessments are erformed, with special attention given to the airway. irway patency can be lost as a result of edema of the eck or bleeding within the area. Assess the client for anifestations of airway edema or bleeding. Auscultate ng sounds every 2 hours for the first 24 hours. Report anifestations of airway obstruction immediately.

Position the client with the head of bed elevated greater an 45 degrees to minimize postoperative edema. Monitor eck drainage for volume and color. Sanguineous or rosanguineous drainage is expected for the first 72 hours ter surgery. Once drainage has stopped, the wound ains are removed.

Pressure dressings may be used in the immediate ostoperative period, depending on physician prefer- ice. If a dressing is used, it should be reinforced as eeded and observed for any drainage. If musculocuta- eous flaps were needed for coverage, pressure dres- ngs are not used, and special flap care is required. ee Chapter 49 for specific care of flaps.)

If the surgical defect was repaired with musculocuta- eous flaps, the flap should be assessed for arterial inflow nd venous outflow. Flap temperature, color, and blanch- g should be noted every hour for the first 24 hours and very 4 hours after that time. Other means of monitoring ap perfusion (Doppler signals) may be used.

Because of the disruption of the sensory nerve fibers om the incisions used, most clients report only minimal ain at the surgical site. If an en bloc radical neck dissec- on has been performed, postoperative shoulder dys- inction is the rule, with forward rotation and ropping of the shoulder. Sectioning of the spinal acces- ory nerve during neck dissection also interrupts inner- ation to the upper trapezius muscle.

Exercises to increase range of motion and muscle rength, shown in the Client Education Guide website

feature on Exercises After Radical Neck Surgery, are encouraged to prevent a "frozen shoulder" and to restore full movement. If a selective or modified neck dissection has been performed, minimal alterations in range of motion and muscle strength are anticipated. Encourage use of exercise to prevent permanent disability.

Self-Care

After neck dissection, caution clients about the potential for injury to neck tissue because of lack of sensation. The use of a heating pad or exposure to temperature extremes may result in tissue injury (burns, frostbite) in a client who cannot feel these temperatures. Clients who have a tracheostomy need specific instructions for its man- agement. Explain ongoing evaluations and follow-up.

INFECTIOUS, INFLAMMATORY, AND HEMORRHAGIC DISORDERS

SINUSITIS

Sinusitis is a common infection that may occur in any of the paranasal sinuses. *Pansinusitis* is infection of more than one sinus. The term *rhinosinusitis* is thought to more accurately describe respiratory manifestations referable to an inflammatory disease of the nose or sinuses. However, the terms *rhinitis* and *sinusitis* may still be used.

Sinusitis is a common medical condition that affects an estimated 35 million people a year. The sinuses are protected against infection by mucociliary action. The normal mucus produced by the sinuses is removed through small openings in the nose called *ostia*. When the ciliary action is impaired or the ostia are obstructed, mucus can accumulate in the sinus, which may then become infected. Blockage of the ostia may be due to a deviated nasal septum, bony abnormalities, congenital malformations, infections, or allergy.

A medical diagnosis of sinusitis is suggested by the cli- ent's clinical manifestations and confirmed by x-ray find- ings. Fever and chills along with headaches and facial pain exacerbated with bending, pain or numbness in the upper teeth, and a purulent or discolored nasal dis- charge may be present. Sinus radiographs or CT scans may show opacification of the sinus, thickened mucous membranes, and an air-fluid level (attributable to accumu- lation of secretions in the sinus), all indicative of sinusitis.

OUTCOME MANAGEMENT

Medical Management

Medical management of sinusitis includes (1) use of the appropriate antibiotic to manage the bacterial infection,

(2) decongestants to reduce nasal edema, (3) corticosteroid nasal sprays to reduce mucosal inflammation, and (4) humidification by use of normal saline solution irrigations or a vaporizer or humidifier to prevent nasal crusting and to moisten secretions.

Antibiotics are not prescribed routinely, because many cases of sinusitis are viral. Initial selection of antibiotics is based on the likely causative organisms indicated by the manifestations and the probability of resistant strains within a community. First-line therapy at most centers is amoxicillin for 14 days.

Medical means of providing drainage include topical and systemic vasoconstrictors. Oral alpha-adrenergic vasoconstrictors, including pseudoephedrine and phenylephrine, can be used for 10 to 14 days, allowing for restoration of normal mucociliary function and drainage. They may be contraindicated in clients with cardiovascular disease because they may cause hypertension and tachycardia. They also may be contraindicated in competitive athletes because of rules of competition.

Mucolytic agents, such as guaifenesin and saline lavage, have been shown to decrease the duration of sinus infections and can be performed by the client at home. Intranasal steroids are also commonly prescribed.

Antihistamines are beneficial for reducing osteomeatal obstruction in clients with allergies and acute sinusitis.

Antral irrigation or sinus lavage may be performed in clients who are not responding to treatment or who have increased purulent exudate in the maxillary sinus. Antral irrigation is performed with the use of a local anesthetic. A trocar (a sharp metal instrument) is inserted through the ostium in the lateral wall of the nose into the sinus. Prepare the client for the procedure with thorough explanations of the anesthetic procedure, the sensation of passage of the trocar through the ostium, and feelings of pressure. Normal saline solution is then injected through the cannula to rinse the sinus of purulent exudate. The client is placed in a sitting position, leaning slightly forward with the mouth open to allow drainage of the irrigating solution through the nose and mouth. A specimen of the exudate may be obtained for culture to determine the causative organism for prescription of an appropriate antibiotic. Sinus irrigations with normal saline can be performed by the client at home also.

Surgical Management

Functional Endoscopic Sinus Surgery

If nonoperative measures fail, functional endoscopic sinus surgery (FESS) may be necessary. The major objective of FESS is the reestablishment of sinus ventilation and mucociliary clearance. FESS is usually performed as an outpatient surgical procedure using local anesthesia (with or without conscious sedation) or with the client under general anesthesia. Small fiberoptic endoscopes are passed through the nasal cavity and into the

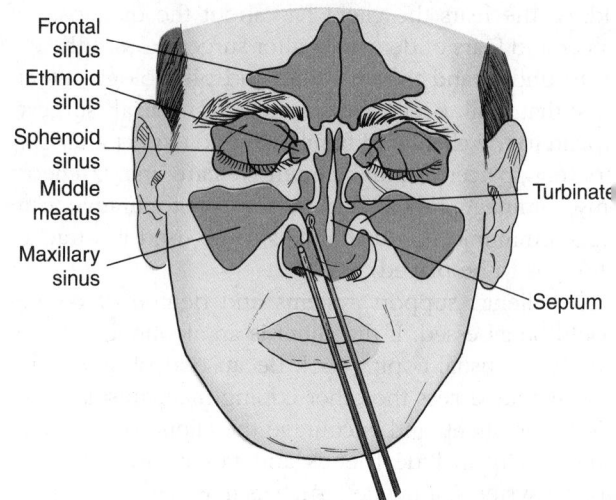

■ FIGURE 60–12 Functional endoscopic sinus surgery. The middle meatus is the site to which most of the sinuses drain; if it is plugged drainage is obstructed. With an endoscope, the sinuses can be seen and obstructions removed.

sinuses to allow direct visualization of the sinuses in order to remove diseased tissue and to enlarge sinus ostia (Figure 60-12).

Possible complications of FESS include nasal bleeding, pain, scar formation, and, rarely, cerebrospinal fluid leak and blindness resulting from intraorbital hematoma formation or direct injury to the optic nerve. After FESS, nasal packing may be inserted to minimize nasal bleeding. Packing is removed within a few hours of the surgical procedure.

External Sphenoethmoidectomy

External sphenoethmoidectomy is a surgical procedure performed to remove diseased mucosa from the sphenoidal or ethmoidal sinus. A small incision is made over the ethmoidal sinus on the lateral nasal bridge, and the diseased mucosa is removed. Nasal and ethmoidal packing is then inserted. An eye pressure patch is usually applied to decrease periorbital edema.

Nursing Management of the Surgical Client

For the first 24 hours after sinus surgery, observe the client for profuse nasal bleeding, respiratory distress, ecchymosis, and orbital and facial edema. Apply ice compresses to the nose and cheek to minimize edema and control bleeding. Place the client in a position with the head of the bed greater than 45 degrees for 24 to 48 hours after surgery to minimize postoperative edema. The nasal packing is generally removed the morning after surgery; however, antral packing may remain in place for 36 to 72 hours. Give mild analgesics to the client to minimize discomfort postoperatively and before removal of the packing.

Instruct clients to increase fluid intake, which maximizes the water content of secretions. Although there may be some pain, a mild analgesic is usually all that is required. Minor nasal bleeding is expected for 24 to 48 hours after surgery. Use of a drip pad under the nose may eliminate the need for constant wiping (Figure 60-13). Instruct clients to avoid blowing the nose for 7 to 10 days after surgery; tell them to sniff backward or spit, not blow. Teach the client to sneeze only with the mouth open. Nasal saline sprays may be started 3 to 5 days after surgery to moisten the nasal mucosa. Explain that the client is to engage in minimal physical exercise and to avoid strenuous activity, lifting, and straining for approximately 2 weeks. After FESS, the client needs to return to the physician's office for removal of crusts and debris and for examination of the nose.

PHARYNGITIS

Pharyngitis is inflammation of the pharynx (tonsils, palate, uvula) and may be viral, bacterial, or fungal in origin. Beta-hemolytic streptococci are the most common infecting organisms. Clients may complain of a sore throat, difficulty in swallowing, fever, malaise, and cough and have an elevated white blood cell count. A culture of the pharyngeal mucosa is sometimes indicated before treatment is started. Treatment of pharyngitis depends on the causative agent. Both viral pharyngitis and bacterial pharyngitis are contagious by droplet spread. Good hand-washing technique is essential, and the use of a mask may prevent spread. Antibiotics are used to treat the bacterial

pharyngitis, antifungal agents are used to treat fungal infections, and use of comfort measures is required for viral types. Bed rest, fluids, warm saline irrigations or gargles, analgesics, and antipyretics are recommended until the clinical manifestations are alleviated.

Chronic pharyngitis (chronic pharyngeal inflammation) is most common in people who habitually use tobacco and alcohol, have a chronic cough, are employed or live in dusty environments, or use their voices excessively. Clinical manifestations vary according to the degree of irritation and inflammation.

EPISTAXIS

Epistaxis (nosebleed) may result from irritation, trauma, infection, foreign bodies, or tumors. Epistaxis may also be the result of systemic disease (e.g., atherosclerosis, hypertension, blood dyscrasias) or systemic treatment (e.g., chemotherapy or anticoagulants), or it may be idiopathic.

OUTCOME MANAGEMENT

Medical Management

Anterior epistaxis is initially treated by assisting the client to a sitting position. Apply pressure by pinching the anterior portion of the nose for a minimum of 5 to 10 minutes. This maneuver is often successful because the most common source of epistaxis is the anterior part of the septum in an area known as Kiesselbach's plexus, a venous plexus vulnerable to trauma. In addition, the application of ice compresses to produce vasoconstriction may also reduce bleeding. If more definitive treatment is necessary, anterior epistaxis can usually be controlled by cauterization of the bleeding vessel with applications of silver nitrate. If these measures do not stop the bleeding, nasal packing may be inserted unilaterally or bilaterally. Antibacterial ointment is applied to 0.5-inch gauze, which is then gently but firmly inserted into the anterior nasal cavities to apply pressure to the bleeding vessels. The use of petrolatum gauze packing should be avoided, because it has no antimicrobial properties, and a malodorous discharge may develop within 1 to 2 days of insertion. Nasal packing should remain in place for a minimum of 48 to 72 hours.

Ten percent of nosebleeds are posterior, usually occurring in people older than 50 years. Posterior bleeding tends to cause increased swallowing of blood, which can be noted in the pharynx. For clients with posterior epistaxis, a *posterior plug* may be necessary in addition to the anterior nasal packing (Figure 60-14). Insertion of a posterior plug is very uncomfortable, and a mild analgesic may be required to reduce anxiety and discomfort. A small, red rubber catheter is passed through the nose into the oropharynx and mouth. A gauze pack

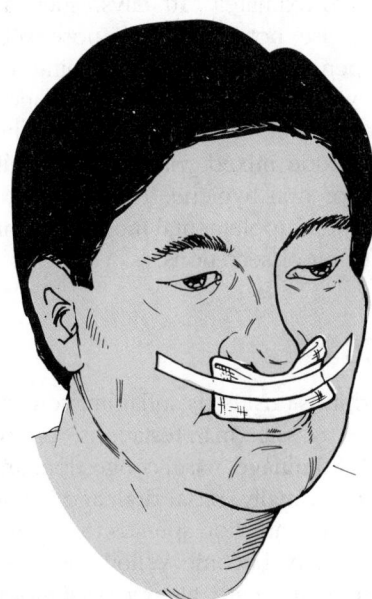

■ **FIGURE 60-13** A nasal drip pad is taped beneath the nares to absorb drainage after nasal or sinus surgery. The usual technique consists of folding 4 × 4 dressings into thirds and taping them in place. These dressings can be changed at the nurse's discretion.

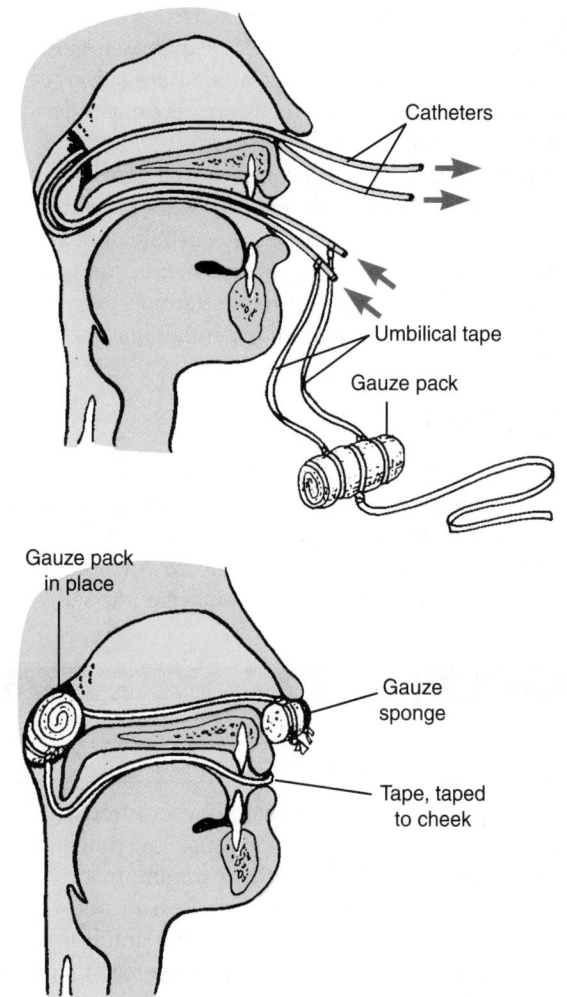

■ **FIGURE 60–14** Instillation of a posterior nasal pack (plug), typically used in an emergency. A catheter can also be used with the balloon placed to tamponade the bleeding.

is tied to the catheter, and the catheter is withdrawn; this moves the pack into proper placement in the nasopharynx and posterior nose to apply pressure. The nasal cavity is packed with 0.5-inch gauze, and the strings from the posterior pack are tied around a rolled gauze or bolus to maintain its position outside the nasal vestibule. The ties from the oral cavity are taped to the client's face to prevent loosening or dislodgment of the plug. A nasal balloon may be substituted for the traditional nasal pack. When the balloon is inflated with normal saline, pressure is applied to the lateral nasal wall.

Nursing Management of the Medical Client

Clients with a posterior plug and anterior nasal packing may be admitted to the hospital and monitored closely for hypoxia. The presence of posterior packing may alter consciousness and respiratory status, especially in older

adults. Because hypertension is frequently cited as a risk factor for epistaxis, monitor the client's blood pressure. General comfort measures, such as humidification, the use of a drip pad to collect bloody drainage and mucus, and application of water-soluble ointment around the nares to provide lubrication, help alleviate the discomfort. Monitor the client closely for any manifestations of airway obstruction and bleeding from the anterior or posterior nares. Inspect the oral cavity for the presence of blood, soft palate necrosis, and proper placement of the posterior plug. If the posterior plug is visible, notify the physician for readjustment of the packing. Posterior nasal packs remain in place for 5 days. Prophylactic antibiotics are used to prevent toxic shock syndrome and sinusitis.

Surgical Management

If anterior and posterior packs fail to control epistaxis, internal maxillary or ethmoidal surgical *artery ligation* may be required. An incision is made in the gum line above the incisor on the affected side, and the maxillary sinus is entered. The artery that supplies the area of bleeding is identified, and a metal clip or suture is used to ligate the artery.

Nursing Management of the Surgical Client

The nasal packing inserted to control epistaxis remains in place for a minimum of 24 hours, during which time the client must be observed for additional bleeding, evidence of hypertension or hypotension, and infection. Upon discharge, the client is instructed to minimize activity for approximately 10 days, such as avoiding strenuous exercise; not blowing the nose; sneezing with the mouth open; and not lifting, stooping, or straining. The use of water-soluble ointment around the nares may provide comfort, and mouth rinses of half-strength hydrogen peroxide mixed with water or saline should be provided for oral hygiene. The use of a humidifier or vaporizer adds supplemental moisture to prevent dryness and crusting of secretions.

RHINITIS

Rhinitis, or rhinosinusitis, is inflammation of the nasal mucosa. The classic manifestations of rhinitis are increased nasal drainage, nasal congestion, and paroxysmal sneezing. Normally, nasal drainage is composed of clear mucus. If the infection spreads to the sinuses, however, drainage may become yellow or green. Rhinitis may be classified as acute, allergic, vasomotor, or drug-related (rhinitis medicamentosa).

Acute rhinitis is also known as the common cold, or coryza. Acute rhinitis may be bacterial or viral in origin; it is treated symptomatically. Acute rhinitis usually lasts

5 to 7 days, with or without treatment. Common interventions for acute rhinitis are symptomatic and include supplemental humidification, decongestants to reduce the edema of the nasal mucosa, increased fluids to prevent dehydration, and analgesics to relieve the generalized myalgia. Sometimes antibiotics are given to prevent a secondary infection by bacteria.

Allergic rhinitis affects between 15% and 20% of the American population and occurs most often as a seasonal disorder. In addition to obstruction to nasal breathing, the client may also experience irritation of other mucous membranes (e.g., the conjunctiva, causing tearing and edema of the eyelids). There is a broad association between allergic rhinitis and disease affecting other body systems. Treatment is symptomatic. A complete allergy evaluation may be required to determine the offending allergen. Most clients are placed on a desensitization program and instructed to avoid the antigen (substance that causes the allergic reaction); treatment is with antihistamines, steroids, or mast cell–stabilizing sprays.

Vasomotor rhinitis causes the same manifestations as those of acute and allergic rhinitis but has no known cause. Clients with vasomotor rhinitis in whom results of bacterial culture and allergy evaluation are negative are given symptomatic treatment. If medications have been prescribed for the treatment of rhinitis (especially nasal sprays), the client must be taught the use of medications, including side effects and possible interactions with other medications.

Rhinitis medicamentosa is caused by abuse or overuse of topical nasal decongestant sprays or intranasal cocaine. These substances initially cause vasoconstriction. When used frequently, however, the initial decongestion is followed by severe mucosal edema. The edema is self-treated with more medication, and the rhinitis becomes cyclic. Management of rhinitis medicamentosa consists of avoidance of the causative agent and evaluation and treatment of the original problem.

LARYNGITIS

Laryngitis may be caused by an inflammatory process or vocal abuse. The laryngeal membrane is continuous with the lining of the upper respiratory tract, and infections in other areas of the nose and throat may include the larynx. Edema of the vocal cords caused by the chronic irritation of an upper respiratory tract infection inhibits the normal mobility of the vocal cords, which causes an abnormal sound.

Laryngitis may also be the result of gastroesophageal reflux disorder (GERD). In this syndrome, the cardiac sphincter between the stomach and the esophagus relaxes, and gastric acid is allowed to enter the esophagus. Reflux of gastric secretions, especially during sleep, may result in the aspiration of gastric secretions into the larynx, causing a chemical irritation or burning of the mucous membrane lining the larynx. Clients with gastroesophageal reflux may complain of hoarseness from the chemical irritation of the gastric acid on the vocal cords, increased mucus production from the body's natural tendency to protect the irritated membrane, foreign body sensation, or sore throat. Chronic cough and asthma may also be associated manifestations of GERD.

Hoarseness is a common manifestation of disorders of the larynx and may be caused by inflammation of the vocal cords, abnormal movements of the vocal cords, or a benign or malignant tumor of the vocal cords. All of these problems interfere with normal mobility of the vocal cords, which produces a change in sound. Abnormal voice may also be the result of vocal abuse. Screaming, shouting, and loud speaking over a period of time may produce edema of the vocal cords and the formation of nodules or polyps—outpouchings of inflamed mucous membranes.

The treatment of laryngitis is aimed at the causative factors. If inflammatory laryngitis is suspected, the inflammation should be treated. Antibiotics may be used if a bacterial infection is suspected. In severe cases, systemic steroids (e.g., methylprednisolone [Medrol]) may be prescribed to reduce inflammation and edema. Supplemental humidification may add increased moisture to liquefy secretions, and mucolytic agents may be prescribed to thin and mobilize mucus. The client with laryngitis may also be placed on voice rest to allow the edema of the vocal cords to subside without added strain. Caution the client to avoid whispering, which also causes excessive vocal cord strain.

Gastroesophageal reflux is initially treated symptomatically. The client is instructed to elevate the head of the bed 6 to 10 inches to minimize reflux; to avoid lying on the right side; to avoid eating or drinking for 2 to 3 hours before going to sleep; to avoid caffeine, alcohol, and tobacco, which are known to increase gastric secretions; and to use antacids and histamine-2-receptor blockers (famotidine [Pepcid], ranitidine [Zantac], omeprazole [Prilosec]) to neutralize and decrease acid production.

Chronic laryngitis may stem from repeated infections, allergy, chronic irritant exposure, long-term voice abuse, or reflux esophagitis of acidic gastric contents. Chronic laryngitis is manifested as a tickling sensation in the throat, voice huskiness, and painful or difficult phonation. Management involves correction or removal of the irritation, in addition to measures to increase comfort. Long-term voice retraining may be necessary if improper use or overuse of the voice is the main cause of chronic laryngitis. This retraining includes (1) learning to use the voice without straining and (2) forming and projecting words to use the diaphragm without shouting.

OBSTRUCTIONS OF THE UPPER AIRWAY

ACUTE LARYNGEAL EDEMA

Acute laryngeal edema may be associated with inflammation, injury, or anaphylaxis. This condition is manifested by hoarseness and dramatic shortness of breath of acute onset. Dyspnea progresses rapidly, and unless a patent airway is established, respiratory arrest occurs. Endotracheal intubation may be very difficult because the larynx is edematous and is likely to bleed. Emergency tracheostomy may be required. If anaphylaxis is the precipitating cause, subcutaneous epinephrine 1:1000 is given. Intravenous corticosteroids are also used.

CHRONIC LARYNGEAL EDEMA

Chronic laryngeal edema may occur when lymph drainage is obstructed, as with infection or tumor or after radiation therapy. If the edema is significant, an artificial airway may be required (either a tracheostomy or an endotracheal tube). The choice of route depends on the severity of the edema.

LARYNGOSPASM

Laryngospasm (spasm of the laryngeal muscles) may occur (1) after administration of some general anesthetic agents, (2) after repeated and traumatic attempts at endotracheal intubation, (3) as a response to some inhaled agents and foreign material, such as industrial fumes, dusts, and chemicals, and (4) from hypocalcemia.

Management is directed at reestablishing the airway as quickly and efficiently as possible. Administer 100% oxygen until the airway is fully reestablished and the larynx relaxes and spasms stop. Titrate Fio_2 according to ABG or pulse oximetry values. If the laryngospasm persists, paralysis with neuromuscular blocking agents, such as succinylcholine, may be required to allow intubation until the spasm subsides. Manual or mechanical ventilation is then necessary until the effects of the paralyzing agent have worn off. Occasionally, emergency cricothyroidotomy or tracheotomy may be necessary and should not be delayed.

LARYNGEAL PARALYSIS

Laryngeal paralysis may be the result of neck surgery, peripheral disorders, central nervous system (CNS) disorders, tumor, or viral infections; or it may be of unknown cause. One of the most common causes of laryngeal paralysis is trauma to the recurrent laryngeal nerve during thyroidectomy. Other causes of laryngeal paralysis are aortic aneurysm; mitral stenosis; thoracic surgery; thyroid gland carcinoma; neck injuries; tuberculosis; tumors of the bronchi, lungs, and mediastinum; metallic poisons (e.g., lead); and infection (e.g., diphtheria). CNS disorders that may lead to laryngeal paralysis include stroke and myasthenia gravis. Bilateral laryngeal paralysis is rare, and when it occurs, the client usually exhibits difficulty in breathing or stridor.

With unilateral vocal cord paralysis (in which only one vocal cord is affected), the airway is usually not impaired and the primary manifestation is hoarseness. The client may have a breathy quality of the voice. Aspiration of food or saliva may occur until the normal, moving cord compensates by approximating the paralyzed cord (bringing the cords together). The client must be observed for manifestations of aspiration such as coughing upon swallowing, ineffective cough, decreased breath sounds, and crackles, rhonchi, or wheezes. The client with bilateral vocal cord paralysis can have a near-normal voice if the vocal cords are paralyzed in the adducted position. However, the major concern is airway compromise, especially on exertion. Dyspnea, intercostal muscle retraction, and stridor may occur with activity or upper airway infections.

If the paralyzed cords are bilaterally adducted, an emergency tracheotomy may be required. Surgery, such as arytenoidectomy, in which one or both arytenoid cartilages are removed and the vocal cords are held in an open position, may be used to open the glottis.

Injection of absorbable sponge (Gelfoam), as a temporary measure, or of polytetrafluoroethylene (Teflon), for permanent correction, may be used if the client with unilateral vocal cord paralysis exhibits manifestations of aspiration or requires strength or projection of the voice. The injected material is placed into the paralyzed cord to add bulk and to allow better approximation with the functioning cord.

Type I thyroplasty is recommended for permanent unilateral vocal cord paralysis. For this procedure, a window is made in the thyroid cartilage through an external incision, and a stent is inserted to move the paralyzed vocal cord into a midline position. The client may show manifestations of airway edema from both the injection and the thyroplasty and should be observed for respiratory distress.

LARYNGEAL INJURY

Laryngeal injury most often results from trauma during a motor-vehicle accident, when the driver's neck strikes the steering wheel. Other causes include inhalation of hot gases and aspiration of caustic liquids. If complete airway obstruction does not occur, carefully assess for post-traumatic edema, which may lead to complete obstruction. Few outward manifestations may be present. It is often easy to overlook potential problems in the neck structures while focusing on other, possibly more dramatic injuries. Observe for increased dyspnea, intercostal muscle retraction, neck swelling, laryngeal tenderness, dysphagia, stridor, inability to speak, and change in respiration patterns.

The thyroid cartilage may be fractured. This problem leads to soft tissue and laryngeal edema as well as hematoma formation. If airway obstruction occurs, tracheostomy may be necessary. Indications of a fractured thyroid cartilage include (1) a tender, swollen ecchymotic neck, (2) stridor, (3) cyanosis in some cases, and (4) subcutaneous emphysema in some cases.

Damage to the larynx above the cricoid cartilage may lead to tracheal stenosis. The cricoid cartilage forms the only complete circle of cartilage in the upper airway, and it maintains the open lumen of the upper end of the airway.

CHRONIC AIRWAY OBSTRUCTION

NASAL POLYPS

Nasal polyps are outpouchings of mucous membrane lining the nose or paranasal sinuses and may occur as solitary or multiple lesions. Polyps may be exacerbated by allergic manifestations, although they are not caused by allergies. Most people who have symptomatic polyps seek medical attention for obstruction to nasal breathing.

The medical management of clients with nasal polyps is symptomatic. Attempts are made to reduce the size of the polyps by eliminating or treating the causative factor (i.e., allergy). In many clients, surgery is needed to remove nasal polyps in order to restore nasal breathing before allergy treatment. Nasal polypectomy (removal of nasal polyps) can be done in the physician's office or in the operating room. Nasal polypectomy is usually performed with use of a local anesthetic. The anesthetic (commonly lidocaine with epinephrine) eliminates discomfort while also producing vasoconstriction to minimize bleeding during the procedure. A snare-like instrument is used to remove the polyps. The bleeding sites are cauterized, and intranasal packing is inserted. Intranasal splints can be used to prevent formation of adhesions. The nasal packing is maintained for several hours to minimize the possibility of postoperative bleeding and is generally removed before discharge of the client from the health care facility.

Because of the presence of nasal packing and edema, clients need to breathe through their mouth for the first 24 to 48 hours. The use of humidification, frequent mouth care, and increasing oral fluids minimize the dryness and oropharyngeal discomfort. Inspect the oral cavity frequently to evaluate the effectiveness of these measures. Clients with polyps frequently also have asthma (when combined with aspirin allergy, this is called *triad disease*). Asthmatic manifestations may be exacerbated after surgery.

The client is positioned with the head of the bed greater than 45 degrees after surgery to minimize edema. In addition, continuous use of ice compresses is recommended for the first 48 hours to reduce edema and to control bleeding. With the proper application of nasal packing at the time of surgery and the use of ice compresses in the immediate postoperative period, nasal bleeding should be minimal. However, the client should be assessed for changes in vital signs and the oropharynx should be inspected for the presence of blood. Because the nasal packing absorbs anterior bleeding, it is essential to observe the client for posterior nasal bleeding. Manifestations of active posterior bleeding include frequent swallowing and the presence of blood in the throat.

Most clients experience only minimal discomfort after a nasal polypectomy. Mild analgesics may be given for any postoperative discomfort. The use of aspirin and aspirin-containing products should be avoided because of their anticoagulant effects. Instruct the client not to blow his or her nose and to refrain from sneezing if possible. When the stimulus to sneeze cannot be overcome, the client should sneeze through an open mouth.

DEVIATED NASAL SEPTUM AND NASAL FRACTURE

The nasal septum (the dividing structure of the nose) is usually straight and separates the nose into two equal chambers. After trauma, the septum may become deviated, creating asymmetrical breathing passages. For some clients, the deviation may cause an obstruction to nasal breathing, dryness of the nasal mucosa leading to bleeding, and occasionally a cosmetic deformity. A deviated nasal septum changes the velocity of air, altering normal nasal activity and resulting in dryness, crusting, nasal bleeding, and changes in the membranes lining the nose.

If a nasal fracture occurs, immediate medical management is advised. Within several hours of nasal injury, severe edema may occur, which causes difficulty in reducing the fracture. Immediately after the injury, ice should be applied. A simple nasal fracture may be reduced in an emergency facility with use of local anesthesia. If immediate reduction of the nasal fracture is not possible, it is advisable to wait several days until edema subsides but before healing begins.

For correction of a deviated nasal septum, reconstruction of a cosmetic deformity of the nose, and reduction of a nasal fracture, the principles of surgical management are similar. All three procedures are usually performed with use of local anesthesia combined with mild sedation. Because of the vasoconstrictor properties of local anesthetics, these agents reduce bleeding during and immediately after surgery. Surgery to correct a deviated nasal septum is known as a nasal septoplasty and consists of making an incision on either side of the septum, elevating the mucous membrane, and straightening or removing the offending portion of the cartilage. If a cosmetic deformity is also of concern or if the deformity interferes with septal reconstruction, a rhinoplasty (reconstruction of the external nose) may be done in conjunction with the nasal septoplasty or as a separate procedure. (See also Chapter 49.)

After these three procedures, intranasal packing and internal splints may be used to maintain the position of the septum, to control bleeding, and to prevent hematoma formation. If the client has undergone rhinoplasty or reduction of a nasal fracture, an external splint and a small dressing may also be applied. Postoperative care is directed at airway management, control of edema and hemorrhage, pain reduction, client education, and emotional support. Because of the presence of bilateral nasal packing, clients require the same care as discussed for the client who has undergone nasal polypectomy.

CONCLUSIONS

Disorders of the upper airway range from the common cold to cancer of the larynx. This chapter presents care of clients most commonly hospitalized with upper airway disorders. Nursing management ranges from assessment of life-threatening airway obstruction to teaching techniques that reduce the spread of infection.

THINKING CRITICALLY

1. The client has a temporary tracheostomy after undergoing a supraglottic laryngectomy. On the second postoperative day, the client indicates to you that he is having trouble breathing. How should you evaluate the client and eliminate the problem?

Factors to Consider. What principles are used as the basis of tracheostomy care? How does evaluation of pulse oximetry contribute to decision making for care?

2. You walk into the room of a client who underwent total laryngectomy 12 hours ago. The client is complaining of severe nausea but has not vomited. What are the client's risks following this type of surgery? How should you respond to the present problem?

Factors to Consider. What risks are inherent in the occurrence of tracheal interruption? How well can the client communicate with you at this time?

3. You enter the room of a client in whom a nosebleed has developed. Bright red blood is seeping continuously from the nares, and the client states that it feels like some blood is going down the back of his throat. What is the priority intervention? What are the implications if the bleeding continues?

Factors to Consider. What are the causes of epistaxis? What are the psychological effects of a nosebleed?

Discussions for these questions can be found on the website.

BIBLIOGRAPHY

 Citations appearing in red refer to primary research.

 Citations appearing in blue refer to evidence-based practice guidelines and protocols.

1. AACN Practice Alert: Ventilator-associated pneumonia. (2005). *AACN Clinical Issues, 16,* 105-109. Accessed 08/04/06 at www.aacn.org />clinical practice>practice alerts.
2. American Cancer Society. (2002). *Cancer facts and figures 2002.* Atlanta, Ga: Author.
3. Branson, R.D., Campbell, R.S., Chatburn, R.L., et al. (1992). AARC Clinical Practice Guideline: Humidification during mechanical ventilation. *Respiratory Care, 37,* 887-890. Accessed 08/03/06 at www.rcjournal.com/online_resources/cpgs/hdmvcpg.html.
4. Britton, D., Jones-Redmond, J., & Kasper, C. (2001). The use of speaking valves with ventilator dependent and tracheostomy patients. *Current Opinions in Otolaryngology and Head and Neck Surgery, 9,* 147-152.
5. Cady, J. (2002). Laryngectomy: Beyond loss of voice: Caring for the patient as a whole. *Clinical Journal of Oncology Nursing, 6*(6), 347-351.
6. Ch'ien, A.P.Y., et al. (2002). Managing gastroesophageal reflux disease. *The Nurse Practitioner: The American Journal of Primary Health Care, 27*(5), 36-53.
7. Chulay, M. (2005). Suctioning: Endotracheal or tracheostomy tube. In D.L.M. Wiegand, & K. Carlson (Eds.), *AACN procedure manual for critical care* (4th ed., pp. 62-70). Aliso Viejo, Calif: American Association of Critical-Care Nurses.
8. Coltart, L., Elder, F., & Grant, F. (2003). Caring for the patient with a tracheostomy: Best practice statement. *2003 NHS Quality Improvement Scotland.* Accessed 05/19/06 at www.nahshealthquality.org.
9. Cutler, C.J., & Davis, N. (2005). Improving oral care in patients receiving mechanical ventilation. *American Journal of Critical Care, 14,* 389-394.
10. Devine, P., & Doyle, T. (2001). Brachytherapy for head and neck cancer: A case study. *Clinical Journal of Oncology Nursing, 5*(2), 55-57.
11. Dropkin, M.J. (1999). Body image and quality of life after head and neck cancer surgery. *Cancer Practice, 7*(6), 309-313.
12. Gaziano, J.E. (2002). Evaluation and management of oropharyngeal dysphagia in head and neck cancer. *Cancer Control, 9*(5), 400-409.
13. Gosselin, T.K., & Pavilonis, H. (2002). Head and neck cancer: Managing xerostomia and other treatment induced side effects. *ORL—Head and Neck Nursing, 20*(4), 15-22.
14. Hahn, M.J., & Jones, A. (2000). *Head and neck nursing.* London: Churchill Livingstone-Harcourt Publishers.
15. Heffner, J.E. (2001). The role of tracheotomy in weaning. *Chest, 120,* 477-481.
16. Higgins, T.S., et al. (1998). Nasal cavity, paranasal sinuses, nasopharynx conditions and care. In L.L. Harris & M.B. Huntoon (Eds.), *Core curriculum for otorhinolaryngology and head-neck nursing* (pp. 169-206). New Smyrna Beach, Fla: Society of Otorhinolaryngology and Head-Neck Nurses.
17. Jemal, A., et al. (2002). Cancer statistics, 2002. *CA: A Cancer Journal for Clinicians, 52*(1), 23-45.
18. Kearney, K. (2001). Epiglottitis. *American Journal of Nursing, 101* (8), 37-38.
19. Koch, W.M., et al. (1999). Head and neck cancer in nonsmokers: A distinct clinical and molecular entity. *Laryngoscope, 109,* 1544-1551.
20. Krouse, J.H. (1999). Introduction to sinus disease: I. Anatomy and physiology. *ORL—Head and Neck Nursing, 17*(2), 7-12.
21. Krouse, J.H., & Krouse, H.J. (1999). Introduction to sinus disease: II. Diagnosis and treatment. *ORL—Head and Neck Nursing, 17*(3), 6-16.

22. Krouse, J.H., & Krouse, H.J. (2002). Allergic disease and associated concurrent medical illnesses. *ORL—Head and Neck Nursing, 20*(4), 10-14.

23. McKenna, M. (1999). Postoperative tonsillectomy/adenoidectomy hemorrhage: A retrospective chart review. *ORL—Head and Neck Nursing, 17*(3), 18-21.

24. St. John, R.E., & Seckel, M.A. (2007). Airway management. In S.M. Burns (Ed.), *AACN protocols for practice: Care of mechanically ventilated patients* (2nd ed., pp. 1-57). Sudbury, Mass: Jones and Bartlett.

25. Scott, J.M., & Vollman, K.M. (2005). Endotracheal tube and oral care. In Lynn-McHale, D. Wiegand, & K. Carlson (Eds.), *AACN procedure manual for critical care* (4th ed., pp. 28-33). Aliso Viejo, Calif: American Association of Critical-Care Nurses.

26. Skillings, K.N., & Curtis, B.L. (2005). Tracheal tube care. In D.L.M. Wiegand, & K. Carlson (Eds.), *AACN procedure manual for critical care* (4th ed., pp. 79-86). Aliso Viejo, Calif: American Association of Critical-Care Nurses.

27. Skillings, K.N., & Curtis, B.L. (2005). Tracheal tube cuff care. In D.L.M. Wiegand, & K. Carlson (Eds.), *AACN procedure manual for critical care* (4th ed., pp. 71-78). Aliso Viejo, Calif: American Association of Critical-Care Nurses.

28. Skillings, K.N., & Curtis, B.L. (2005). Extubation/decannulation. In D.L.M. Wiegand, & K. Carlson (Eds.), *AACN procedure manual for critical care* (4th ed., pp. 34-37). Aliso Viejo, Calif: American Association of Critical-Care Nurses.

29. Sparacino, L.L. (2000). Epistaxis management: What's new and what's noteworthy. *Lippincott's Primary Care Practice, 4*(5), 498-507.

30. Spaulding, M.B. (2002). Recent advances in the treatment of head and neck cancer: A patient care perspective. *ORL—Head and Neck Nursing, 20*(1), 9-18.

31. Stapleton, E.R., et al. (Eds.) (2001). *BLS for healthcare providers.* Dallas: American Heart Association.

32. Steyer, T.E. (2002). Peritonsillar abscess: Diagnosis and treatment. *American Family Physician, 65*(1), 93-96.

33. Sue, R.D., & Susanto, I. (2003). Long-term complications of artificial airways. *Clinics in Chest Medicine, 24*, 457-471.

34. Wilkinson, J.M. (2000). *Nursing diagnosis handbook with NIC interventions and NOC outcomes.* Upper Saddle River, NJ: Prentice Hall.

evolve *Did you remember to check out the bonus material on the Evolve website and the CD-ROM, including NCLEX®-Examination Style Review Questions, Open-Book Quizzes, and Chapter Review Audio Podcasts?*

http://evolve.elsevier.com/Black/medsurg

CHAPTER 61

Management of Clients with Lower Airway and Pulmonary Vessel Disorders

SHERILL NONES CRONIN AND KIM MIRACLE

A distinguishing feature of lower airway and pulmonary vessel disorders is the presence of dyspnea. *Dyspnea* (shortness of breath) is a subjective experience that results when air flow, oxygen exchange, or both are impaired. The sensation of uncomfortable breathing can be as distressing as pain and can lead to severe functional disability. The intensity and frequency of dyspnea as well as its association with specific activities must be assessed to develop realistic expectations of treatment outcomes. Because the experience of dyspnea is associated with much anxiety, nursing interventions to relieve this manifestation are essential to the care of clients with conditions of the lower airways and pulmonary vessels.

DISORDERS OF THE LOWER AIRWAYS

ASTHMA

Asthma is a disorder of the bronchial airways characterized by periods of reversible bronchospasm (spasms of prolonged contraction of the bronchial airways). Asthma is often called *reactive airway disease*. This complex disorder involves biochemical, immunologic, endocrine, infectious, autonomic, and psychological factors. In 2005 approximately 22.2 million Americans were diagnosed with asthma, with 12.2 million having an asthma attack. The annual financial impact of this disease is approximately $16.1 billion in direct care and lost productivity.

Etiology and Risk Factors

Asthma occurs in families, which suggests that it is an inherited disorder. Apparently, environmental factors (e.g., viral infection, allergens, pollutants) interact with inherited factors to produce disease. Other inciting factors can include excitatory states (stress, laughing, crying), exercise, changes in temperature, and strong odors. Asthma also is a component of *triad* disease: asthma, nasal polyps, and allergy to aspirin.

Pathophysiology

Asthma involves a chronic inflammatory process that produces mucosal edema, mucus secretion, and airway inflammation (Figure 61-1). When people with asthma are exposed to extrinsic allergens and irritants (e.g., dust, pollen, smoke, mold, medications, foods, respiratory tract infections), their airways become inflamed, producing shortness of breath, chest tightness, and wheezing. Initial clinical manifestations, termed *early-phase reaction,* develop immediately and last about an hour.

When a client is exposed to an allergen, immunoglobulin E (IgE) is produced by B lymphocytes. IgE antibodies attach to mast cells and basophils in the bronchial walls. As shown in the Concept Map feature on p. 1572, the mast cell empties, releasing chemical mediators of inflammation, such as histamine, bradykinin, prostaglandins, and slow-reacting substance of anaphylaxis (SRS-A). These substances induce capillary dilation,

---

evolve Web Enhancements

Case Management Chronic Obstructive Pulmonary Disease
The Older Adult
Case Study COPD with Nutritional Concerns
Client Education Guide Asthma (Spanish Translation)
Clinical Pathway Chronic Obstructive Pulmonary Disease
Concept Map Understanding Asthma and Its Treatment

Be sure to check out the bonus material on the Evolve website and the CD-ROM, including free self-assessment exercises. **http://evolve.elsevier.com/Black/medsurg**

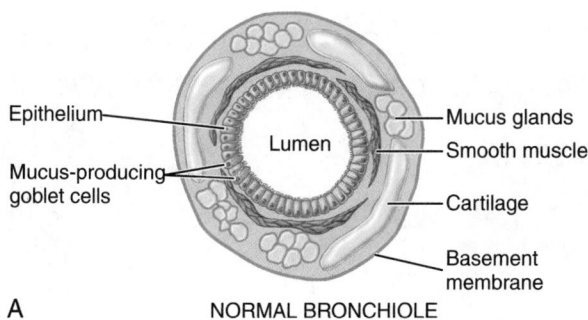

Epithelium
Lumen
Mucus-producing goblet cells
Mucus glands
Smooth muscle
Cartilage
Basement membrane

A   NORMAL BRONCHIOLE

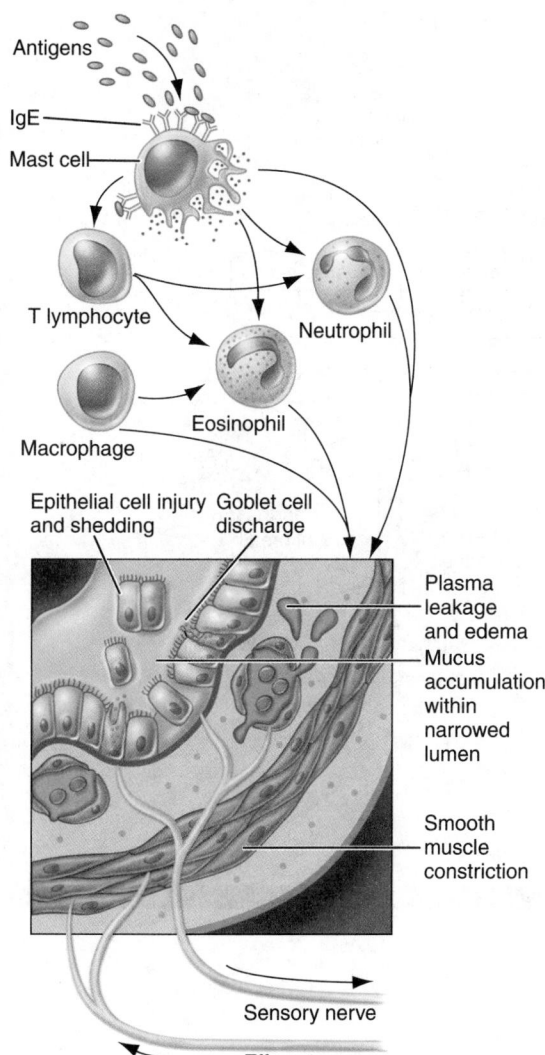

Antigens

IgE

Mast cell

T lymphocyte

Neutrophil

Macrophage

Eosinophil

Epithelial cell injury and shedding   Goblet cell discharge

Plasma leakage and edema

Mucus accumulation within narrowed lumen

Smooth muscle constriction

Sensory nerve

Efferent nerve

B   MECHANISM OF AIRWAY OBSTRUCTION IN ASTHMA

■ **FIGURE 61–1** Common bronchial wall changes in asthma are hypertrophied smooth muscle, edema, mucus gland hypertrophy, and mucus in the lumen. *(From Copstead, L.C., & Banasik, J.L. [2000]. Pathophysiology: Biological and behavioral perspectives. Philadelphia: Saunders.)*

leading to edema of the airway in an attempt to dilute the allergen and wash it away. They also induce airway constriction in an attempt to close the airway to prevent inhalation of more allergen.

About half of all asthma clients also experience a *delayed (late-phase) reaction*. Although clinical manifestations are the same as those in the early phase, they do not begin until 4 to 8 hours after exposure and may last for hours or days.

In both phases, the release of chemical mediators produces the airway response. In the late-phase response, however, the mediators attract other inflammatory cells and create a self-sustaining cycle of obstruction and inflammation. This chronic inflammation produces hyperresponsiveness of the airways. This hyperresponsiveness causes subsequent episodes in response not only to specific antigens but also to stimuli such as physical exertion and breathing cold air. Clinical manifestations may occur with increasing frequency and severity.

Both alpha-adrenergic and beta-adrenergic receptors of the sympathetic nervous system are found in the bronchi. Stimulation of alpha-adrenergic receptors causes bronchoconstriction; conversely, stimulation of beta-adrenergic receptors causes bronchodilation. Cyclic adenosine monophosphate (cAMP) balances the two receptors. Some theories suggest that asthma may be a result of lack of beta-adrenergic stimulation.

Clinical Manifestations

During asthma attacks, clients are dyspneic and have marked respiratory effort. Manifestations of marked respiratory effort include nasal flaring, pursed-lip breathing, and use of accessory muscles. Cyanosis is a late development.

Auscultation of breath sounds usually reveals wheezing, especially during expiration. The inability to auscultate wheezing in an asthmatic client with acute respiratory distress may be an ominous sign. It may indicate that the small airways are too constricted to allow any air flow. The client may require immediate, aggressive medical intervention. In addition, bronchospasm may lead to almost continuous coughing in an attempt to exhale and clear the airway.

The diagnosis of asthma is based on clinical manifestations, spirometry results, and response to treatment. Spirometry reveals decreased peak expiratory flow rate (PEFR), timed forced expiratory volume (FEV), and forced vital capacity (FVC). Functional residual capacity (FRC), total lung capacity (TLC), and residual volume (RV) are increased because air is trapped within the lungs. A 12% improvement in forced expiratory volume in 1 second (FEV_1) after inhaled administration of a beta-agonist bronchodilator implies a reversible air flow obstruction, that is, by definition, asthma. Figure 61-2 shows a peak flowmeter for monitoring air flow.

Baseline assessment of pulmonary status also may include pulse oximetry and arterial blood gas (ABG) analysis. Pulse oximetry usually reveals low oxygen

CONCEPT MAP

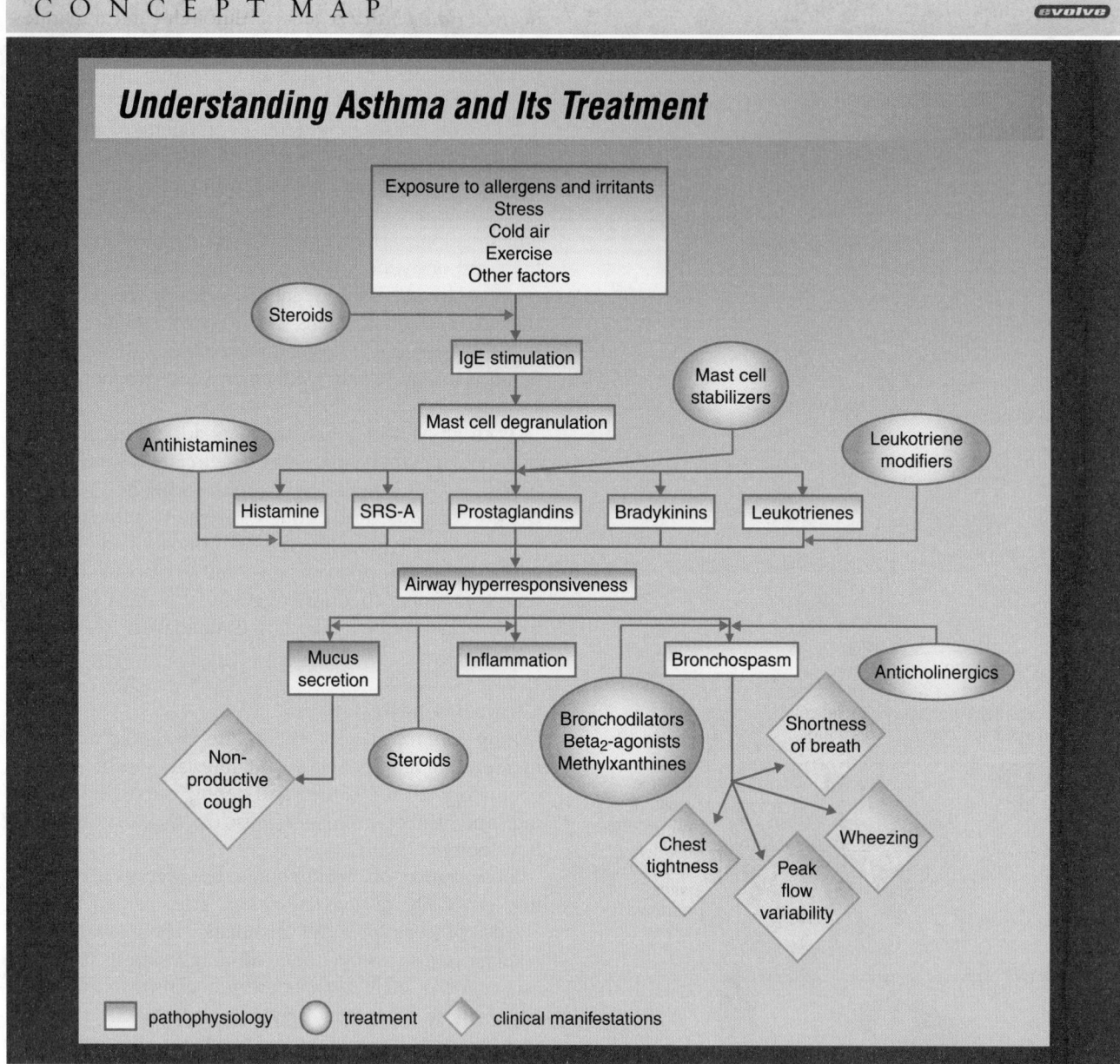

Understanding Asthma and Its Treatment

saturation. ABG results often show some degree of hypoxemia, with elevated partial pressures of arterial carbon dioxide ($Paco_2$) in severe cases.

Status asthmaticus is a severe, life-threatening complication of asthma. It is an acute episode of bronchospasm that tends to intensify. With severe bronchospasm, the workload of breathing increases 5 to 10 times, which can lead to acute cor pulmonale (right-sided heart failure resulting from lung disease). When air is trapped, a severe paradoxical pulse (i.e., drop in blood pressure >10 mm Hg during inspiration) develops as venous return is obstructed. Pneumothorax commonly develops. If status asthmaticus continues, hypoxemia worsens and acidosis begins. If the condition is untreated or not reversed, respiratory or cardiac arrest ensues.

OUTCOME MANAGEMENT

Medical Management

Many disorders can cause wheezing, such as sinusitis, gastroesophageal reflux disease (GERD), heart failure, bronchitis, and lung tumors. These conditions are ruled out before an asthma diagnosis is given.

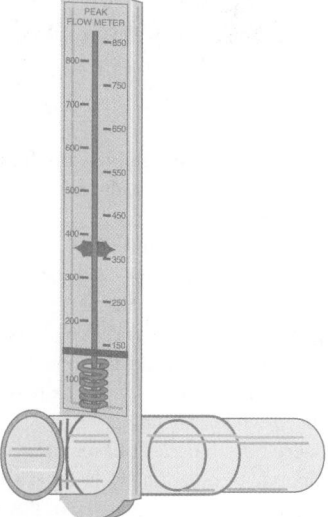

■ **FIGURE 61-2** Peak flowmeters. Several types of portable meters are available for self-monitoring of air flow.

Management of asthma is based on the severity of the disease (Table 61-1) and is directed at reversing airway spasm. The general goals of asthma therapy include the following:

- Prevention of chronic asthma and asthma exacerbations
- Maintenance of normal activity levels
- Maintenance of normal or near-normal lung function
- Minimal or no side effects while receiving optimal medications
- Client satisfaction with asthma care

Emphasis has moved away from episodic treatment of manifestations after they occur to long-term control through inhaled corticosteroids to prevent asthma whenever possible.

Reverse Airway Spasm

A severe asthma episode may constitute a medical emergency. Medical intervention for such episodes is aimed primarily at the following:

- Maintaining a patent airway by relieving bronchospasm and clearing excess or retained secretions
- Maintaining effective gas exchange
- Preventing complications, such as acute respiratory failure and status asthmaticus

Emergency management of the client begins with inhaled beta$_2$ agonists. Beta$_2$ agonists stimulate the beta-adrenergic receptors and dilate the airways. If the spasm does not abate (i.e., if FEV$_1$ remains <50% of predicted), nebulized atropine sulfate or intravenous (IV) steroids may be given. Atropine is an anticholinergic that blocks the effect of the parasympathetic system. When the vagus nerve is stimulated, bronchial smooth muscle tone increases. If these treatments do not reverse the clinical manifestations, the client usually is admitted to the hospital for further treatment.

If the client has an acute asthma attack and no medications are nearby, the attack sometimes can be lessened by *pursed-lip breathing*, which increases pressure in the airways so that they remain open and trapped air can be exhaled more easily.

SAFETY ALERT

Supplemental oxygen is indicated if Pao$_2$ levels decrease to less than 60 mm Hg. Monitor the client closely for clinical manifestations of increasing anxiety, increased work of breathing, and indications of tiring. Endotracheal intubation and mechanical ventilation may be necessary. Sedation, and in rare cases administration of paralytic agents, may be necessary to blunt the client's respiratory effort and to prevent further air trapping and pressure increases. Status asthmaticus is treated

TABLE 61-1 Classifying Asthma Severity

	Symptoms	Nighttime Symptoms	Lung Function
Step 4 Severe persistent	Continual symptoms Limited physical activity Frequent exacerbations	Frequent	FEV$_1$ or PEF ≤60% predicted* PEF variability >30%
Step 3 Moderate persistent	Daily symptoms Daily use of inhaled short-acting beta$_2$ agonist Exacerbations affect activity Exacerbations ≥2 times a week; may last days	>1 time a week	FEV$_1$ or PEF >60% to <80% predicted PEF variability >30%
Step 2 Mild persistent	Symptoms >2 times a week but <1 time a day Exacerbations may affect activity	>2 times a month	FEV$_1$ or PEF ≥80% predicted PEF variability 20%-30%
Step 1 Mild intermittent	Symptoms ≤2 times a week Asymptomatic and normal PEF between exacerbations Exacerbations brief (from a few hours to a few days); intensity may vary	≤2 times a month	FEV$_1$ or PEF ≥80% predicted PEF variability <20%

FEV$_1$, Forced expiratory volume in 1 second; *PEF*, peak expiratory flow.
Data from National Institutes of Health. (1997). *Guidelines for the diagnosis and management of asthma* (NIH Pub No. 97-4051). Washington, DC: Author; and National Institutes of Health. (2002). *The NAEPP Expert Panel report: Guidelines for the diagnosis and management of asthma—Update on selected topics 2002* (NIH Pub No. 02-5075). Washington, DC: Author.

with aggressive use of IV corticosteroids and frequent administration of inhaled beta-adrenergic medications to avoid intubation and mechanical ventilation.

Control Inflammation

Mucosal inflammation is controlled through the use of inhaled corticosteroids. Steroids prevent the mast cell from emptying, reducing the edema and spasm.

Mast cell stabilizers and leukotriene modifiers are included in special circumstances. Mast cell stabilizers, such as cromolyn (Nasalcrom, Intal) and nedocromil (Tilade), suppress the release of bronchoconstrictive substances during antigen-antibody reactions. Leukotriene modifiers are used in the treatment of both acute and chronic asthma. The release of leukotrienes into the asthmatic airways causes smooth muscle constriction, increased vascular permeability, edema of the airway mucosa, mucus release, and inhibited mucus clearance. Leukotrienes also attract eosinophils to the airway mucosa, which subsequently promote inflammation. Drugs that block leukotriene receptors mediate the actions of leukotrienes and serve as a useful addition to other therapies during an exacerbation. Leukotriene modifiers have also become an important component of therapy for chronic asthma, offering another class of medications for long-term asthma control. A growing body of evidence indicates that leukotriene modifiers are effective, are well tolerated, and have a low risk of adverse effects. Clinical trials have addressed the effectiveness of these drugs in clients with asthma. These medications have shown improvement in the FEV_1, a decreased need for rescue inhalers, and improvement in asthma symptoms. Leukotriene modifiers are not listed as preferred first-line treatment, yet they do have a potential role in the treatment of asthmatics of all severities. The concept of anti-IgE therapies is continuing to be explored as another therapy since there is a significant association between asthma and atopy, and since IgE plays a central role in the pathogenesis of atopy. However, no formal recommendations have been made thus far.

Nursing Management

Assessment

SAFETY ALERT

Initially, assess the client for clinical manifestations of airway distress. If present, they constitute an emergency that must be managed before a detailed history of the disease or other health problems is obtained. The Critical Monitoring feature above, right, lists manifestations of acute airway distress caused by asthma.

Asking clients to rate dyspnea on a scale of 0 to 10 is an easy and effective measure of present dyspnea and may help to monitor and evaluate dyspnea in clinic and home care settings: "On a scale of 0 to 10, indicate

Asthma

Notify the physician if the client still has the following manifestations after treatment for asthma:

- Increased anxiety
- Increased respiratory rate and effort
- Feelings of not being able to "catch one's breath"
- Continued low oxygen saturation
- Wheezing, both inspiratory and expiratory
- Almost continuous nonproductive cough
- Nasal flaring as respiratory distress increases
  - Lips pursed while exhaling
  - Use of accessory muscles of breathing
  - Increasing tachycardia (tachycardia is a normal response to beta-adrenergic drugs)
  - Paradoxical pulse as bronchospasm worsens
  - Cyanosis and central nervous system depression as late findings

how much shortness of breath you are having right now, with 0 meaning no shortness of breath and 10 meaning shortness of breath as bad as can be."[18]

Determine any known medication allergies so that they can be avoided during treatment. Ascertain whether the client has a history of cardiac disease because nonselective $beta_2$ agonists can produce tachycardia and stress a diseased heart.

Once the acute episode is controlled, explore the history of the client's asthma. Assist the client to determine whether there is a pattern to the manifestations in order to help identify a trigger that precipitates the asthma. If an extrinsic trigger can be identified, it may be possible to reduce or eliminate it. For example, if the client is allergic to mold, common sources of mold can be avoided. Ask about current medications. Some clients are inadvertently given medications that may induce bronchospasms. For example, a noncardioselective beta-blocker, such as propranolol (Inderal), prescribed for hypertension may cause bronchospasm.

Within the psychosocial domain, ask about the client's ability to manage the asthma as well as the client's general adaptation to the illness. Denial of the illness can interfere with early treatment. Determine whether the client feels control over the illness and feels capable of managing it. Clients who have this feeling of control show better compliance with treatments. Determine whether the client is experiencing an increased number of stressors. A stressful lifestyle may exacerbate asthma.

Assess the attitude of the family. The family can be a great source of support and can assist the client in recognizing early manifestations. In contrast, an unsupportive family may contribute to denial or may be an additional source of stress to the client. Involve the case manager (see the Case Management website feature on Chronic Obstructive Pulmonary Disease).

The client with a new diagnosis of asthma may be asked to assess the home and work environment for likely triggers of the clinical manifestations. In addition, skin testing for allergy may be performed.

Diagnosis, Outcomes, Interventions

Diagnosis: Ineffective Breathing Pattern. Because of airway spasm and edema, the client cannot move air in and out of the lungs as needed to maintain adequate tissue oxygenation. The correct nursing diagnosis would be *Ineffective Breathing Pattern related to impaired exhalation and anxiety.* Anxiety with dyspnea is another cause of breathing pattern problems.

Outcomes. The client will have improved breathing patterns, as evidenced by (1) a decreasing respiratory rate to within normal limits; (2) decreased dyspnea, less nasal flaring, and reduced use of accessory muscles; (3) decreased manifestations of anxiety; (4) a return of ABG levels to normal limits; (5) oxygen saturation greater than 95%; and (6) vital capacity measurements within normal limits or greater than 40% of those predicted.

Interventions. Assess the client frequently, observing respiratory rate and depth. Assess the breathing pattern for shortness of breath, pursed-lip breathing, nasal flaring, sternal and intercostal retractions, or a prolonged expiratory phase. During an acute asthma attack, these assessments can be conducted continuously.

Place the client in the Fowler position, and give oxygen as ordered. Monitor ABGs and oxygen saturation levels to determine the effectiveness of treatments. Compare pulmonary function test results with normal levels. The degree of dysfunction assists in planning client activity.

Diagnosis: Ineffective Airway Clearance. The excessive production of mucus and spasm in the airway makes it difficult to keep the airway patent. The nursing diagnosis *Ineffective Airway Clearance related to increased production of secretions and bronchospasm* is appropriate.

Outcomes. The client will have effective airway clearance, as evidenced by (1) decreased inspiratory and expiratory wheezing; (2) decreased rhonchi; and (3) decreasing dry, nonproductive cough.

Interventions. If the airway is compromised, the client's secretions may require suctioning. Some clients experience asthma episodes as a result of pulmonary infection. Monitor the color and consistency of the sputum, and assist the client to cough effectively. Encourage oral fluids to thin the secretions and to replace fluids lost through rapid respiration. The humidity in the room may be increased slightly. If chest secretions are thick

and difficult to expectorate, the client may benefit from postural drainage, lung percussion and vibration, expectorants, and frequent position changes. Give frequent oral care, every 2 to 4 hours, to remove the taste of the secretions and remoisten the oral mucous membranes that have dried from mouth breathing.

The approach to pharmacologic therapy often is referred to as *step care,* meaning that the medications ordered and the frequency of administration are adjusted according to the severity of the client's asthma. Asthma medications are categorized into two major classes: (1) *long-term–control* medications, used to achieve and maintain control of persistent asthma; and (2) *quick-relief* medications, used to treat acute air flow obstruction and its accompanying manifestations. The most effective long-term–control medications are those that reduce inflammation, with inhaled steroids being the most potent. Quick-relief medications include short-acting inhaled beta$_2$ agonists and oral steroids.

For clients who respond poorly to inhaled agents, theophylline and aminophylline are still used at times. These medications are regarded as weak bronchodilators. Wide variations exist in their rates of metabolism, and these medications have a high potential for toxicity; for these reasons, their use is declining. Theophylline levels must be monitored to evaluate effectiveness and possible toxicity.

Figure 61-3 depicts a stepwise approach for managing asthma in adults. All clients with asthma require a short-acting inhaled beta$_2$ agonist as needed for acute manifestations. Clients with mild, moderate, or severe persistent asthma require daily long-term–control medications. The preferred treatment strategy is to start with more intensive therapy to achieve rapid control and then "step down" to the minimum therapy needed for maintenance.

Diagnosis: Impaired Gas Exchange. When air is trapped within alveoli, the alveoli are eventually drained of oxygen and the client can become hypoxic. The nursing diagnosis is *Impaired Gas Exchange related to air trapping.*

Outcomes. The client will have adequate gas exchange, as evidenced by (1) decreased inspiratory and expiratory wheezing; (2) decreased rhonchi; (3) oxygen saturation >90%; (4) Pao$_2$ greater than 60 mm Hg; (5) Paco$_2$ equal to or less than 45 mm Hg; (6) pH of 7.35 to 7.45; (7) usual skin color (no cyanosis); and (8) decreasing dry, nonproductive cough.

Interventions. Assess lung sounds every hour during acute episodes to determine the adequacy of gas exchange. Assess skin and mucous membrane color for cyanosis. Cyanosis is a late manifestation of hypoxia and an indication of serious gas-exchange problems. Monitor pulse oximetry for oxygen saturation levels. Administer oxygen as ordered to maintain optimal oxygen saturation.

Stepwise Approach for Managing Asthma in Adults and Children Older Than 5 Years of Age: Treatment

Classify Severity: Clinical Features Before Treatment or Adequate Control			Medications Required to Maintain Long-Term Control
	Symptoms/Day Symptoms/Night	PEF or FEV₁ PEF Variability	Daily Medications

Step 4
 	
Severe Persistent
	Continual
	Frequent
		≤60%
		>30%
			■ Preferred treatment:
			– High-dose inhaled corticosteroids
			  AND
			– Long-acting inhaled beta₂-agonists
			  AND, if needed,
			– Corticosteroid tablets or syrup long term (2 mg/kg/day, generally do not exceed 60 mg/day). (Make repeat attempts to reduce systemic corticosteroids and maintain control with high-dose inhaled corticosteroids.)

Step 3 **Moderate Persistent**	Daily >1 night/week	>60% – <80% >30%	■ Preferred treatment: – Low-to-medium dose inhaled corticosteroids and long-acting inhaled beta₂-agonists. ■ Alternative treatment (listed alphabetically): – Increase inhaled corticosteroids within medium-dose range OR – Low-to-medium dose inhaled corticosteroids and either leukotriene modifier or theophylline. If needed (particularly in patients with recurring severe exacerbations): ■ Preferred treatment: – Increase inhaled corticosteroids within medium-dose range and add long-acting inhaled beta₂-agonists. ■ Alternative treatment: – Increase inhaled corticosteroids within medium-dose range and add either leukotriene modifier or theophylline.
Step 2 **Mild Persistent**	>2/week but <1 time/day >2 nights/month	≥80% 20%-30%	■ Preferred treatment: – Low-dose inhaled corticosteroids. ■ Alternative treatment (listed alphabetically): cromolyn, leukotriene modifier, nedocromil, OR sustained-release theophylline to serum concentration of 5-15 mcg/ml.
Step 1 **Mild Intermittent**	≤2 days/week ≤2 nights/month	≥80% <20%	■ No daily medication needed. ■ Severe exacerbations may occur, separated by long periods of normal lung function and no symptoms. A course of systemic corticosteroids is recommended.

Quick Relief

All Patients

- ■ Short-acting bronchodilator: 2-4 puffs short-acting inhaled beta₂-agonists as needed for symptoms.
- ■ Intensity of treatment will depend on severity of exacerbation; up to 3 treatments at 20-minute intervals or a single nebulizer treatment as needed. Course of systemic corticosteroids may be needed.
- ■ Use of short-acting beta₂-agonists >2 times a week in intermittent asthma (daily, or increasing use in persistent asthma) may indicate the need to initiate (increase) long-term control therapy.

 Step down
Review treatment every 1 to 6 months; a gradual stepwise reduction in treatment may be possible.

 Step up
If control is not maintained, consider step up. First, review patient medication technique, adherence, and environmental control.

Goals of Therapy: Asthma Control

- ■ Minimal or no chronic symptoms day or night
- ■ Minimal or no exacerbations
- ■ No limitations on activities; no school/work missed
- ■ Maintain (near) normal pulmonary function
- ■ Minimal use of short-acting inhaled beta₂-agonist (<1 time/day, <1 canister/month)
- ■ Minimal or no adverse effects from medications

Note
- ■ The stepwise approach is meant to assist, not replace, the clinical decision making required to meet individual patient needs.
- ■ Classify severity: assign patient to most severe step in which any feature occurs (PEF is % of personal best; FEV₁ is % predicted).
- ■ Gain control as quickly as possible (consider a short course of systemic corticosteroids); then step down to the least medication necessary to maintain control.
- ■ Provide education on self-management and controlling environmental factors that make asthma worse (e.g., allergens and irritants).
- ■ Refer to an asthma specialist if there are difficulties controlling asthma or if step 4 care is required. Referral may be considered if step 3 care is required.

■ **FIGURE 61-3** Stepwise approach for managing asthma in adults and children older than 5 years of age. *(From National Institutes of Health. [2002]. The National Asthma Education and Prevention Program Expert Panel report: Guidelines for the diagnosis and management of asthma—Update on selected topics [NIH Pub No. 02-5075]. Washington, DC: Author.)*

Nursing Diagnosis: Knowledge Deficit. If the client has just been diagnosed with asthma, the diagnosis of *Knowledge Deficit* may be used to identify specific topics needing education. State the diagnosis as *Knowledge Deficit related to use of inhaled and nebulized medications.*

Outcomes. The client will have increased knowledge about how and when to use nebulized medications as evidenced by explaining the manifestations to be treated with nebulized medications and the outcomes expected as well as how to hold the devices.

Interventions. Nebulized medications can be difficult to learn to use. The client must coordinate inhalation with compression of the metered-dose inhaler canister (Figure 61-4). The Client Education Guide on p. 1578 provides directions for using an inhaler. Observe the client's use of the nebulizer to ascertain whether the medication is entering the airway. Be certain the client knows what manifestations require the use of the nebulizer; also see the Self-Care section on this page.

Nursing Diagnosis: Risk for Decisional Conflict. This nursing diagnosis is related to allergens present in the environment and fits the client who must change a previous lifestyle or make an environmental change to reduce the risk of asthma.

Outcomes. The client will express an understanding of the conflict involved with maintaining the present lifestyle and its effect on asthma.

Interventions. The presence of pets that shed hair or dander, cigarette smoke, or occupational exposure to other allergens may require some lifestyle changes. In many cases, the pets can remain in the house but cannot sleep with the asthmatic client. Encourage clients to stop smoking, and teach clients and others about the dangers of second-hand smoke. Elimination of irritants is generally

performed in a reasonable fashion, such as removing exposure to one allergen at a time. Potential improvements in a client's manifestations that might result from a major lifestyle change, such as job change or loss of a pet, may be offset quickly by the stress felt from such a change.

See the Care Plan feature on pp. 1582-1585 when working with COPD clients who have diagnoses of *Activity Intolerance, Anxiety, Imbalanced Nutrition,* or *Disturbed Sleep Pattern.*

Evaluation. Generally, asthma episodes can be reversed quickly if there is no underlying problem, such as infection. Expect the client to be hospitalized only briefly; plan a coordinated approach to assessment and follow-up.

Self-Care

Through appropriate use of the peak flowmeter and medications, clients with asthma should be able to anticipate most exacerbations and enhance their quality of life. Peak flow values fall about 24 hours before manifestations develop. Clients should be taught to increase their routine medications in anticipation of asthma exacerbations. Many clients can manage their asthma effectively with a thorough action plan to guide their decisions. An action plan for asthma is presented in Figure 61-5. It is recommended that a written plan be used as part of the overall effort to educate the client in self-management.

Changes in the treatment plan may be needed as asthma severity and control vary over time. Follow-up visits every 1 to 6 months are recommended to monitor the disease and to maintain control. The presence of one or more indicators of poor control (i.e., awakening at night with dyspnea or coughing, increased use of short-acting inhaled beta$_2$ agonists, increased urgent care visits) may suggest a need to "step up" therapy. Before increasing medications, however, consider other possible reasons for poor control (Table 61-2).

CHRONIC OBSTRUCTIVE PULMONARY DISEASE

Also known as *chronic obstructive lung disease,* chronic obstructive pulmonary disease (COPD) refers to several disorders that affect the movement of air in and out of the lungs. Although the most important of these—obstructive bronchitis, emphysema, and asthma—may occur in a pure form, they most commonly coexist with overlapping clinical manifestations. COPD can occur as a result of increased airway resistance secondary to bronchial mucosal edema or smooth muscle contraction. It may also be a result of decreased elastic recoil, as seen in emphysema. Elastic recoil, similar to the recoil of a stretched rubber band, is the force used to passively

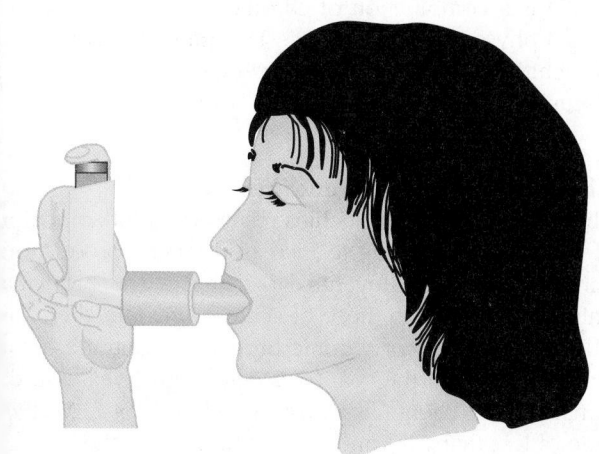

■ **FIGURE 61-4** A client using a metered-dose inhaler with a spacer.

CLIENT EDUCATION GUIDE

Asthma

CLIENT INSTRUCTIONS

Asthma may be triggered by pollen, dust, animal dander, molds, smoke, or other allergens. Learn what triggers your asthma and minimize your exposure to it.

Monitor the pollution index and pollen counts. Limit outdoor activities when these indicators are high.

Take all medications as prescribed by your physician. If you are taking both a bronchodilator and a steroid via inhaler, take the bronchodilator first to open the airways.

Use your peak flowmeter daily.

Follow these directions on how to use a peak flowmeter:

- Attach the mouthpiece and set the pointer to zero (0).
- Stand up and take a deep breath.
- Put the mouthpiece in your mouth, and close your lips tightly around it.
- Blow into the mouthpiece as hard and as fast as you can.
- Record the value and reset the meter.
- Repeat the procedure for a total of three readings.
- Record the highest value on your record sheet.
- Monitor peak flow daily; know your "green zone," when air flow is normal; the "yellow zone," when values have fallen and you need to increase your routine medications; and the "red zone," when you need to increase your rescue medications and notify your doctor.

Use these directions for using an inhaler:

- Remove the cap and shake the inhaler well.
- Hold the canister upright with your index finger on the top and your thumb on the bottom.

- Breathe out through your mouth.
- Place the mouthpiece 1 to 2 inches away from your opened mouth (unless using a spacer).
- Begin with a slow, deep breath. As you breathe in, press the canister down with your finger to give yourself one puff of medication.
- Hold your breath in for at least 5 to 10 seconds.
- Slowly breathe out, holding your lips tight (pursed).

If your physician has prescribed more than one puff, wait 1 minute between puffs to let the medication open up the upper airway. That way, the next puff can reach lower into your lungs.

Pursed-lip breathing, progressive muscle relaxation, and tripod positioning (i.e., leaning on your arms positioned in front of you) may improve your breathing during asthma episodes.

Unless your physician has told you to limit fluids, drink 8 to 10 glasses of water every day. Water helps to thin your sputum so that you can cough it up more easily.

Some forms of asthma may be triggered by exercise. Before starting an exercise program, discuss the exercise plan with your physician.

Call your physician if you experience any of the following manifestations:

- Wheezing and shortness of breath, even though you are taking your medications as prescribed
- Fever, muscle aches, chest pain, or thickening of sputum
- Sputum color changes to yellow, green, gray, or red (bloody)
- Problems that may be related to your medications (e.g., rash, itching, swelling, or trouble breathing)

---

deflate the lung and exhale. Decreased elastic recoil, analogous to an overstreched and weak rubber band, results in a decreased driving force to empty the lung.

COPD is a widespread disorder, 11.4 million U.S. adults (age 18 and over) are estimated to have the disease. However, close to 24 million have evidence of impaired lung function, suggesting an under-diagnosis of the condition. It is the fourth leading cause of death in America, claiming the lives of 122,283 Americans in 2003. Caring for clients with COPD has been estimated at $20.9 billion annually in direct care costs alone; however, the burden of COPD is even greater from a global perspective, where it is projected to rank fifth in 2020 in burden of disease caused worldwide.

Etiology and Risk Factors

Smoking is the primary risk factor for COPD. The numerous irritants found in cigarette smoke stimulate excess mucus production and coughing, destroy ciliary function, and lead to inflammation and damage of bronchiolar and alveolar walls. Other risk factors include air pollution,

second-hand smoke, a history of childhood respiratory tract infections, and heredity. Occupational exposure certain industrial pollutants may also increase risk.

Pathophysiology

COPD is a combination of chronic obstructive bronchitis, emphysema, and asthma. The pathophysiology bronchitis and emphysema is presented here (see earlier discussion of pathophysiology of asthma).

Chronic Obstructive Bronchitis

Chronic obstructive bronchitis results from inflammation of the bronchi, leading to increased mucus production, chronic cough, and eventual scarring of the bronchi lining. In contrast to those of acute bronchitis, the clinical manifestations of chronic bronchitis continue for least 3 months of the year for 2 consecutive years. Additionally, if the client has a post-bronchodilator FEV_1/FV ratio of less than 70% and chronic bronchitis, the client said to have chronic *obstructive* bronchitis, indicating that the client has obstructive lung disease combined

ASTHMA ACTION PLAN FOR _____

Doctor's Phone Number _____ Doctor's Name _____ Date _____

Hospital/Emergency Room Phone Number _____

Take These Long-Term-Control Medicines Each Day (include an anti-inflammatory)

Medicine	How much to take	When to take it

GREEN ZONE: Doing Well

- No cough, wheeze, chest tightness, or shortness of breath during the day or night
- Can do usual activities

And, if a peak flow meter is used,
Peak flow: more than _____
(80% or more of my best peak flow)

My best peak flow is: _____

Before exercise   ☐ _____   ☐ 2 or ☐ 4 puffs   5 to 60 minutes before exercise

YELLOW ZONE: Asthma Is Getting Worse

FIRST — Add: **Quick-Relief Medicine – and keep taking your GREEN ZONE medicine**

- Cough, wheeze, chest tightness, or shortness of breath, or
- Waking at night due to asthma, or
- Can do some, but not all, usual activities

-Or-

Peak flow: _____ to _____
(50% - 80% of my best peak flow)

_____ (short-acting beta₂-agonist) ☐ 2 or ☐ 4 puffs, every 20 minutes for up to 1 hour   ☐ Nebulizer, once

SECOND — If your symptoms (and peak flow, if used) *return to GREEN ZONE* after 1 hour of above treatment:
- ☐ Take the quick-relief medicine every 4 hours for 1 to 2 days.
- ☐ Double the dose of your inhaled steroid for _____ (7-10) days.

-Or-

If your symptoms (and peak flow, if used) *do not return to GREEN ZONE* after 1 hour of above treatment:

- ☐ Take: _____ (short-acting beta₂-agonist)   ☐ 2 or ☐ 4 puffs or ☐ Nebulizer
- ☐ Add: _____ (oral steroid)   _____ mg per day For _____ (3-10) days
- ☐ Call the doctor ☐ before/ ☐ within _____ hours after taking the oral steroid.

RED ZONE: Medical Alert!

- Very short of breath, or
- Quick-relief medicines have not helped, or
- Cannot do usual activities, or
- Symptoms are same or get worse after 24 hours in Yellow Zone

-Or-

Peak flow: less than _____
(50% of my best peak flow)

Take this medicine:

- ☐ _____ (short-acting beta₂-agonist)   ☐ 4 or ☐ 6 puffs or ☐ Nebulizer
- ☐ _____ (oral steroid)   _____ mg

Then call your doctor NOW.   Go to the hospital or call for an ambulance if:
- You are still in the red zone after 15 minutes AND
- You have not reached your doctor.

DANGER SIGNS

- Trouble walking and talking due to shortness of breath
- Lips or fingernails are blue

→ ■ Take ☐ 4 or ☐ 6 puffs of your quick-relief medicine *AND*
■ Go to the hospital or call for an ambulance (_____) *NOW!*

■ **FIGURE 61–5** Asthma action plan. *(From National Institutes of Health. [1997]. Practical guide for the diagnosis and management of asthma [NIH Pub No. 97-4053]. Washington, DC: Author.)*

TABLE 61–2   Possible Reasons for Poor Asthma Control—"ICE"

Possible Reasons	Interventions
*In*haler technique	Check client's technique
*C*ompliance	Ask when and how much medication the client is taking
*E*nvironment	Ask client whether something in the environment has changed
Also consider Alternative diagnosis	Assess client for the presence of concomitant upper respiratory disease or alternative diagnosis

From National Institutes of Health. (1997). *Practical guide for the diagnosis and management of asthma* (NIH Pub No. 97-4051). Washington, DC: Author.

with chronic cough. Chronic bronchitis is characterized by the following:

- An increase in the size and number of submucous glands in the large bronchi, which increases mucus production
- An increased number of goblet cells, which also secrete mucus
- Impaired ciliary function, which reduces mucus clearance

The lung's mucociliary defenses are impaired, and there is increased susceptibility to infection. When infection occurs, mucus production is greater, and the bronchial walls become inflamed and thickened. Chronic bronchitis initially affects only the larger bronchi, but eventually all the airways are involved. The thick mucus and inflamed bronchi obstruct the airways, especially during expiration. The airways collapse, and air is trapped in the distal portion of the lung. This obstruction leads to reduced alveolar ventilation. An abnormal ventilation-perfusion $\dot{V}/\dot{Q}$ ratio develops, with a corresponding fall in Pa_{O_2}. Impaired ventilation may also result in increased levels of Pa_{CO_2}. As compensation for the hypoxemia, polycythemia (overproduction of erythrocytes) occurs.

Emphysema

Emphysema is a disorder in which the alveolar walls are destroyed. This destruction leads to permanent overdistention of the air spaces. Air passages are obstructed as a result of these changes, rather than from mucus production as in chronic bronchitis. Some forms of emphysema may result from a breakdown in the lung's normal defense mechanisms (alpha₁-antitrypsin [AAT]) against certain enzymes. Research has shown that the enzymes protease and elastase can attack and destroy the connective tissue of the lungs. Difficult expiration in emphysema is the result of destruction of the walls (septa) between the alveoli, partial airway collapse, and loss of elastic recoil. As the alveoli and septa collapse, pockets

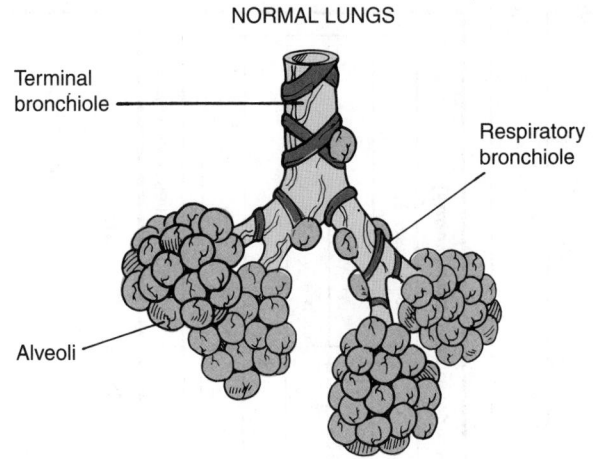

NORMAL LUNGS

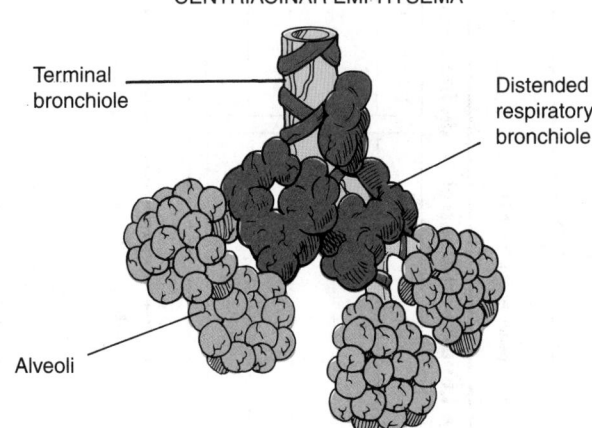

CENTRIACINAR EMPHYSEMA

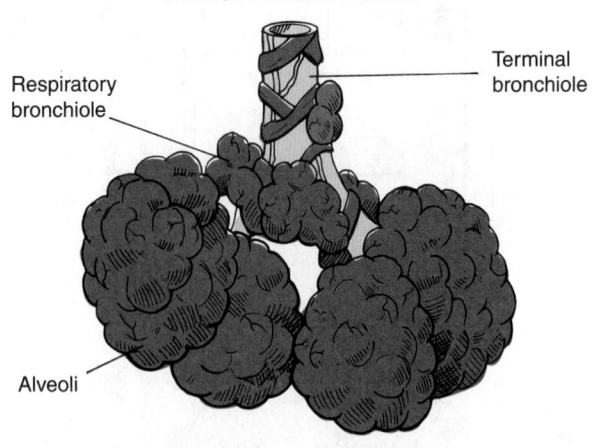

PANACINAR EMPHYSEMA

■ **FIGURE 61–6** Types of emphysema.

of air form between the alveolar spaces (blebs) and within the lung parenchyma (bullae). This process leads to increased ventilatory dead space from areas that do not participate in gas or blood exchange. The work of breathing is increased because there is less functional

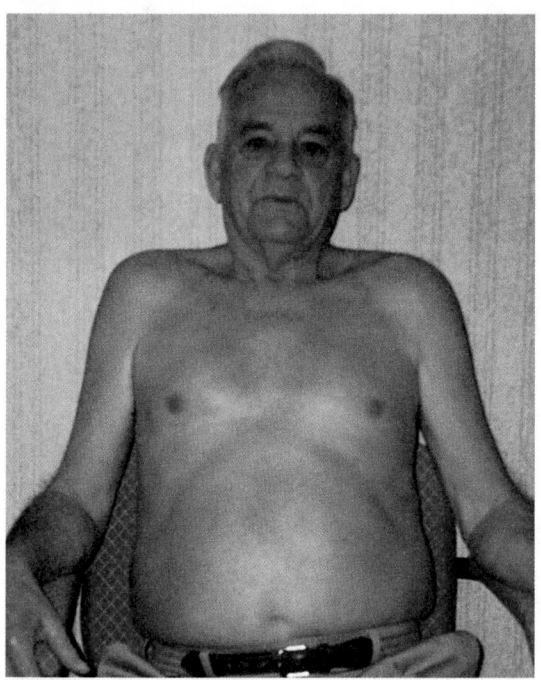

■ **FIGURE 61-7** A client with chronic obstructive bronchitis. Note the stocky build and the presence of pursed-lip breathing. The slight gynecomastia is a side effect of corticosteroid therapy. The client's shoulders are raised because of shortness of breath and increased work of breathing.

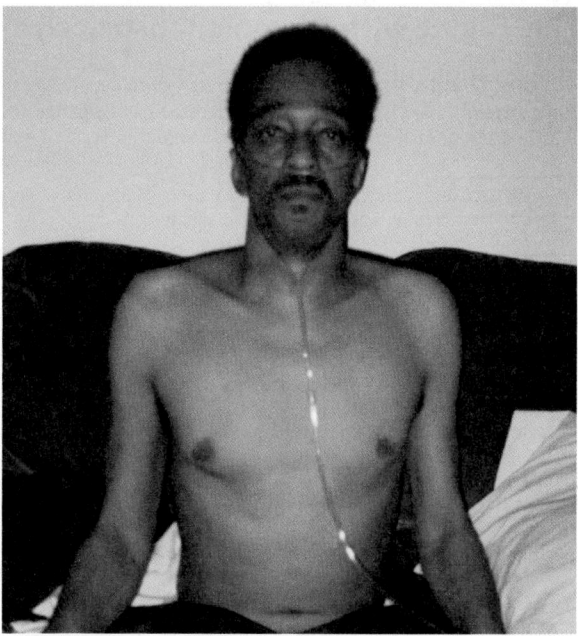

■ **FIGURE 61-8** A client with emphysema. Note the thin appearance and the presence of continuous oxygen therapy. The use of accessory muscles of respiration (neck and shoulder muscles) reflects the client's shortness of breath and increased work of breathing necessary to increase minute ventilation and to maintain adequate arterial blood gas values.

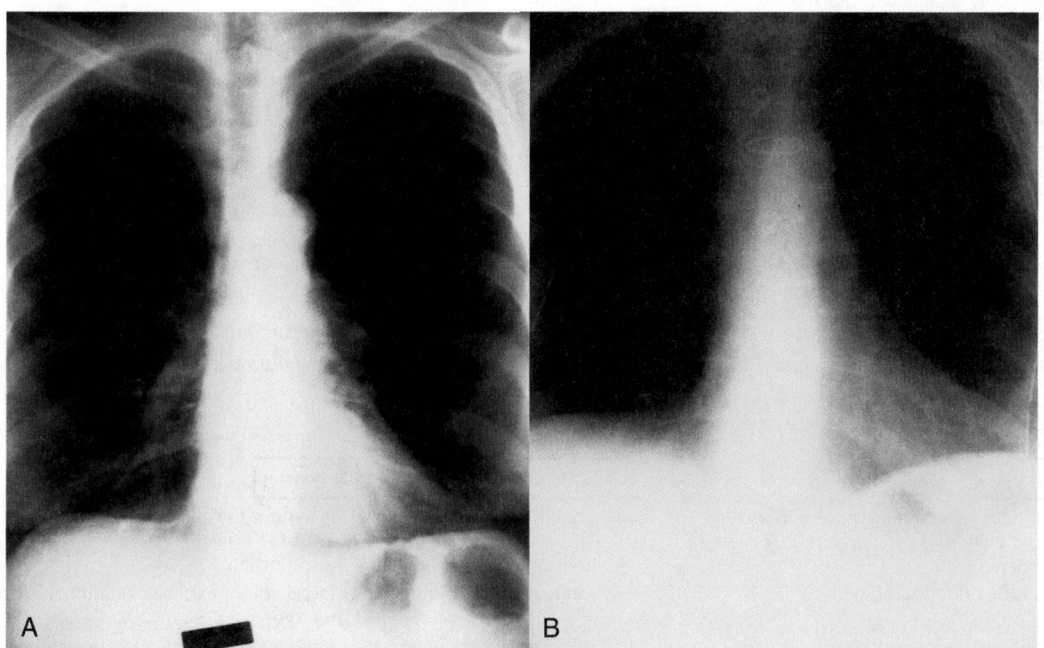

■ **FIGURE 61-9 A,** Preoperative chest x-ray of a client with emphysema. Note the flattened diaphragm and the laterally hyperexpanded chest walls. **B,** Postoperative chest x-ray after lung volume reduction surgery. The right side of the diaphragm is rounded and no longer flattened by emphysematous lung tissue. *(From Allen, G. [1996]. Surgical treatment of emphysema using bovine pericardium strips. AORN Journal, 63[2], 373-388.)*

The Client with Chronic Obstructive Pulmonary Disease

Nursing Diagnosis: Impaired Gas Exchange related to decreased ventilation and mucus plugs.
Outcomes: The client will maintain adequate gas exchange as evidenced by arterial blood gas (ABG) values (i.e., Pao_2 of at least 60 mm Hg, pH within normal limits, and $Paco_2$ at baseline) or oxygen saturation greater than 90%, mental status at baseline, minimal anxiety.

NOC OUTCOMES	Electrolyte and Acid-Base Balance, Respiratory Status: Gas Exchange, Respiratory Status: Ventilation, Tissue Perfusion: Pulmonary, Vital Signs Status

Interventions	NIC INTERVENTIONS	Rationales
1. Regularly monitor the client's respiratory rate and pattern, pulse oximetry, ABG results, and manifestations of hypoxia or hypercapnia. Report significant changes or a lack of response promptly.	Respiratory Monitoring	1. Prompt recognition of deteriorating respiratory function can reduce potentially lethal outcomes.
2. Administer low-flow oxygen therapy (1 to 3 L/min on 24% to 31% Fio_2) as needed via nasal prongs or a high-flow Venturi mask.	Oxygen Therapy	2. Oxygen corrects existing hypoxemia.
3. Assist the client into the high-Fowler position.	Positioning	3. The upright position allows full lung excursion and enhances air exchange.
4. Administer bronchodilators if ordered. Monitor for side effects.	Medication Administration: Inhalation	4. Bronchodilators relax bronchial smooth muscle, facilitating air flow. Common side effects include tremor, tachycardia, and other cardiac dysrhythmias.
5. Use caution when administering opioids, sedatives, and tranquilizers.	Medication Management	5. These medications are respiratory depressants and can further impair ventilation.

Evaluation: Bronchospasm is fairly quickly reversible with inhaled bronchodilators and steroids, but until the underlying trigger is controlled, it may quickly recur.

Nursing Diagnosis: Ineffective Airway Clearance related to excessive secretions and ineffective coughing.
Outcomes: The client will have improved airway clearance as evidenced by effective coughing techniques and a patent airway.

NOC OUTCOMES	Respiratory Status: Airway Patency, Respiratory Status: Ventilation, Vital Signs Status

Interventions	NIC INTERVENTIONS	Rationales
1. Monitor lung sounds every 4 to 8 hours and before and after coughing episodes.	Respiratory Monitoring	1. Rhonchi present in the large airways may impair airway patency.
2. Teach the client to maintain adequate hydration by drinking at least 8 to 10 glasses of fluid per day (if not contraindicated) and increasing the humidity of the ambient air.	Fluid Management	2. Hydration helps to thin secretions.
3. Teach and supervise effective coughing techniques.	Airway Management	3. Proper coughing techniques conserve energy, reduce airway collapse, and lessen client frustration.
4. Teach and supervise incentive spirometer techniques 10 times per hour while awake.	Ventilation Assistance	4. Incentive spirometer is an objective measure of the depth of inhalation to promote lung expansion.
5. Perform chest physical therapy, if needed, and instruct the client and significant others in these techniques.	Airway Management	5. Chest physical therapy techniques use forces of gravity and motion to facilitate secretion removal.
6. Assess the condition of the oral mucous membranes and perform or offer oral care every 2 hours.	Oral Health Maintenance	6. Thick secretions line the mouth when the client coughs; oral care removes them.

Evaluation: The client will often require 48 or more hours to clear severely congested lungs.

Nursing Diagnosis: Anxiety related to acute breathing difficulties and fear of suffocation.
Outcomes: The client will express an increase in psychological comfort and demonstrate the use of effective coping mechanisms.

NOC OUTCOMES	Aggression Control, Anxiety Reduction, Coping, Impulse Control

Interventions	NIC INTERVENTIONS	Rationales
1. Remain with the client during acute episodes of breathing difficulty, and provide care in a calm, reassuring manner.	Anxiety Reduction	1. Reassures the client that competent help is available if needed. Anxiety can be contagious; remain calm.
2. Provide a quiet, calm environment.	Environmental Management	2. Reduction of external stimuli helps promote relaxation.
3. During acute episodes, open doors and curtains and limit the number of people and unnecessary equipment in the room. Provide a fan if the client perceives a benefit from the moving air.	Environmental Management	3. Environmental changes may lessen the client's perceptions of suffocation.

4. Encourage the use of breathing retraining and relaxation techniques.	Calming Technique	4. A feeling of self-control and success in facilitating breathing helps reduce anxiety.
5. Give sedatives and tranquilizers with extreme caution. Nonpharmaceutical methods of anxiety reduction are more useful.	Medication Management	5. Oversedation may cause respiratory depression.

Evaluation: Anxiety can usually be controlled quickly but may recur with each episode of dyspnea and requires both short-term and long-term interventions.

Nursing Diagnosis: Activity Intolerance related to inadequate oxygenation and dyspnea.

Outcomes: The client will have improved activity tolerance as evidenced by maintaining a realistic activity level (specify based on underlying condition and baseline activity) and demonstrating energy conservation techniques.

NOC OUTCOMES   Activity Tolerance, Endurance, Energy Conservation

Interventions	NIC INTERVENTIONS	Rationales
1. Monitor the severity of dyspnea and oxygen saturation with and following activity	Respiratory Monitoring	1. Activity increases the demand for oxygen, and the inability to meet the demand may result in dyspnea and desaturation.
2. Stop or slow any activity that leads to a significant change in respiratory rate, failure of pulse to return to near resting rate within 3 minutes of activity, and/or changes in mental status.	Energy Management	2. Significant changes in respiratory, cardiac, or circulatory status signal activity intolerance.
3. Maintain supplemental oxygen therapy as needed during activity.	Oxygen Therapy	3. Supplemental oxygen helps alleviate exercise-induced hypoxemia, thus improving activity tolerance.
4. Schedule active exercise after respiratory therapy or treatment (e.g., bronchodilator in metered-dose inhaler).	Exercise Promotion	4. Lung function is maximized during peak periods of medication and drug effect.
5. Assist the client in scheduling a gradual increase in daily activities and exercise.	Activity Therapy	5. Gradual increases in physical activity improve respiratory and cardiac conditioning, thus improving activity tolerance.
6. Advise the client to avoid conditions that increase oxygen demand, such as smoking, temperature extremes, excess weight, and stress.	Teaching: Disease Process	6. These factors increase peripheral vascular resistance, which increases cardiac workload and oxygen requirements.
7. Instruct the client in energy conservation techniques, such as pacing activities throughout the day, interspersed with adequate rest periods, and alternating high-energy and low-energy tasks.	Energy Management	7. Conservation techniques allow the client to accomplish more tasks with a limited energy supply.
8. Teach the client to use pursed-lip and diaphragmatic breathing techniques during activities.	Teaching: Prescribed Activity/Exercise	8. Breathing retraining ensures maximal use of available respiratory function. Pursed-lip breathing leaves positive end-expiratory pressure in the lungs and helps keep airways open.

Evaluation: Depending on the degree of underlying lung disease, activity intolerance may be slow to be correctable, and this goal should be long term for complete resolution.

Nursing Diagnosis: Imbalanced Nutrition: Less Than Body Requirements related to reduced appetite, decreased energy level, and dyspnea.

Outcomes: The client will eat 75% of served foods during the acute phase and maintain body weight within normal limits for gender and body build, and hemoglobin, prealbumin, and albumin levels will be within normal ranges.

NOC OUTCOMES   Nutritional Status, Nutritional Status: Food and Fluid Intake, Nutritional Status: Nutrient Intake, Weight Control

Interventions	NIC INTERVENTIONS	Rationales
1. Assist the client with mouth care before meals and as needed.	Oral Health Maintenance	1. Coughing and sputum production may impair appetite. Mouth-breathing dries mucous membranes.
2. Advise the client to eat small, frequent meals (e.g., six meals a day) that are high in protein and low in carbohydrates.	Nutrition Therapy	2. Large meals may create an excessive feeling of fullness that may make breathing uncomfortable and difficult. Protein is needed to maintain nutritional status because of the increased work of breathing. Carbohydrate intake should be reduced because they produce carbon dioxide.
3. Advise the client to avoid gas-producing foods, such as beans and cabbage.	Teaching: Prescribed Diet	3. Gas-forming foods may cause abdominal bloating and distention and thus impair ventilation.
4. Instruct the client in the use of high-calorie liquid supplements if indicated.	Teaching: Prescribed Diet	4. Liquid supplements provide high-calorie concentrations in a relatively small volume.
5. Advise hypoxemic clients to use oxygen via nasal cannula during meals.	Oxygen Therapy	5. Adequate oxygenation increases the energy available for eating.
6. Suggest methods to make meal preparation more convenient (e.g., Meals on Wheels program).	Nutritional Counseling	6. Reducing the energy expenditure of preparation maximizes the energy available for eating.

(Continued)

C A R E   P L A N   *evolve*

The Client with Chronic Obstructive Pulmonary Disease—Cont'd

7. Consult with the dietitian to assist with food choices that reduce the production of carbon dioxide.	Consultation Teaching: Disease Process	7. Clients with carbon dioxide retention benefit from foods that do not produce excess CO_2.
8. Monitor the client's food intake, weight, and serum hemoglobin, prealbumin, and albumin levels.	Nutritional Monitoring	8. Changes in body weight reflect the degree of nutrition or malnutrition. Hemoglobin, prealbumin, and albumin levels reflect protein intake.

Evaluation: Improving nutrition, lab values, and body weight are long-term goals. During an acute exacerbation of dyspnea, short-term goals such as the amount of dietary intake may be accomplishable.

Nursing Diagnosis: Disturbed Sleep Pattern related to dyspnea and external stimuli.
Outcomes: The client will report feeling adequately rested.

NOC OUTCOMES   Rest, Sleep, Well-Being

Interventions	NIC INTERVENTIONS	Rationales
1. Promote relaxation by providing a darkened, quiet environment; ensuring adequate room ventilation; and following bedtime routines.	Sleep Enhancement	1. The hospital environment can interfere with relaxation and sleep. Using established bedtime rituals increases relaxation.
2. Schedule care activities to allow periods of uninterrupted sleep.	Sleep Enhancement	2. For most people, completing four to five complete sleep cycles (60 to 90 minutes) per night promotes a feeling of being rested.
3. Avoid the use of "sleeping pills."	Sleep Enhancement	3. Many forms of hypnotics, sedatives, and barbiturates impair sleep cycles.

4. Instruct the client in measures to promote sleep:
  a. Plan physical exercise during the day and passive, nonstimulating activities in the evening.
  b. Avoid stimulants, such as caffeine.
  c. Maintain a consistent bedtime and a regular bedtime routine.
  d. Eat a high-protein snack before bedtime.
  e. Use relaxation techniques (e.g., meditation, warm bath, massage, warm beverage).
  f. If the client awakens during the night, suggest a quiet, diverting activity, such as reading, in another room.
  g. If dyspnea is severe, a recliner chair or hospital bed may be more comfortable than a regular bed.
	Sleep Enhancement	4.
		  a. Activity increases the need for sleep and contributes to a feeling of tiredness.
		  b. Stimulants increase metabolism and inhibit relaxation.
		  c. Consistency promotes relaxation and prevents disruptions of the biologic clock.
		  d. Protein digestion produces tryptophan, an amino acid that may have a sedative effect.
		  e. Sleep is difficult unless the client is relaxed.
		  f. Frustration over being awake deters sleep efforts further. The bedroom should be associated mentally with sleep to enhance future sleep promotion.
		  g. The upright position facilitates ventilation.

Evaluation: During acute respiratory problems, sleep may be difficult because of interruptions and dyspnea. Short-term outcomes such as napping may be accomplishable. Long-term plans for sleep may have to be deferred until dyspnea is controlled.

Nursing Diagnosis: Interrupted Family Processes related to chronic illness of a family member.
Outcomes: The family will verbalize their feelings, participate in the care of the ill family member, and seek external resources as needed.

NOC OUTCOMES   Caregiver Emotional Health, Caregiver Well-Being, Family Coping, Family Normalization

Interventions	NIC INTERVENTIONS	Rationales
1. Plan interventions considering the client and significant other as the unit of care. Encourage participation in the planning process.	Family Involvement Promotion	1. COPD affects the client and the client's significant others.
2. Assess family communication patterns, and intervene if they are ineffective. Family counseling may be needed.	Family Process Maintenance	2. Effective communication helps each member to understand his or her own and others' feelings. Counseling may facilitate healthy interaction.
3. Encourage as wide a social support network as feasible.	Family Support	3. The use of a wide support group prevents a few family members from being overloaded with responsibility.
4. Encourage the client and family to seek support from other sources (e.g., self-help groups and support groups, such as the Better Breathers clubs sponsored by the American Lung Association).	Support System Enhancement	4. Clients may benefit from opportunities to share common experiences and to learn from others in similar situations.
5. Provide the family with anticipatory guidance as the client's COPD progresses.	Teaching: Disease Process	5. Knowing what to expect facilitates family adjustment.

Evaluation: Coping with a family member's illness may require weeks or months to accomplish as the family learns to recognize and treat various exacerbations and live through various family events and activities with the disease (e.g., travel).

Nursing Diagnosis: Sexual Dysfunction related to dyspnea, reduced energy, and changes in relationships.

Outcomes: The client will report increased satisfaction with sexual function.

| NOC OUTCOMES | Sexual Functioning, Endurance |

Interventions	NIC INTERVENTIONS	Rationales
1. Provide an opportunity for the client to discuss concerns.	Sexual Counseling	1. Many people are embarrassed or reluctant to talk about sexual concerns.
2. Suggest measures that may facilitate sexual activity (e.g., alternative positions, use of bronchodilator therapy before beginning sexual activity, choosing a time of day when dyspnea is minimal).	Sexual Counseling	2. Such measures can reduce physical exertion and maximize available oxygen levels.
3. Encourage the client and partner to consider alternative forms of sexual expression (e.g., hugging, cuddling, stroking, kissing).	Sexual Counseling	3. Alternative methods require less energy expenditure compared with intercourse.
4. Recommend a professional sex therapist if appropriate.	Sexual Counseling	4. Talking with a skilled professional may assist the client with constructive problem-solving.

Evaluation: During an acute flare-up of dyspnea, the discussion of sexual activity should be introduced when appropriate. Resolution of the problems and issues is a long-term goal.

Nursing Diagnosis: Risk for Infection related to ineffective pulmonary clearance.

Outcomes: Client will have a decreased risk of infection as evidenced by health promotion behaviors and awareness of manifestations of pulmonary infection.

| NOC OUTCOMES | Knowledge: Infection Control, Tissue Integrity: Skin and Mucous Membranes |

Interventions	NIC INTERVENTIONS	Rationales
1. Teach the client to wash his or her hands after contact with potentially infectious material.	Infection Control	1. Hand-washing is the primary defense against the spread of infection.
2. Encourage the client to obtain a flu vaccination yearly and a pneumococcal vaccination every 5 years.	Infection Protection	2. Vaccination provides immunity for infections.
3. Teach the client and family how to care for and clean respiratory equipment used at home.	Infection Protection	3. Water in respiratory equipment is a common source of bacterial growth.
4. Teach the client and family the manifestations of pulmonary infections (change in color or volume of sputum, fever, chills, malaise, productive cough, confusion, increased dyspnea), and when to call the physician.	Infection Protection	4. Early recognition of manifestations can lead to a rapid diagnosis. Self-care with preplanned interventions (e.g., antibiotics) should be understood.

Evaluation: Risk reduction cannot be measured in a short period of time. Verbal statements of comprehension and plans to follow the instructions should be noted. Sometimes a reduction in the number of acute pulmonary infections or hospitalizations can be measured.

Nursing Diagnosis: Decisional Conflict related to smoking cessation.

Outcomes: The client and family will seriously consider the value of smoking cessation and develop a plan to stop smoking.

| NOC OUTCOMES | Decision Making, Participation: Health Care Decisions |

Interventions	NIC INTERVENTIONS	Rationales
1. Ask the client if he or she was smoking before hospitalization.	Smoking Cessation Assistance	1. Validates the frequency of smoking.
2. Advise the client and family on the benefit of smoking cessation.	Smoking Cessation Assistance	2. Many clients believe there is no benefit to stopping smoking now because lung damage is already present. Even though it is difficult to stop, most clients experience less dyspnea within a few weeks.
3. Assess if the client is ready to stop smoking now (or at dismissal).	Smoking Cessation Assistance	3. It is important for the client to determine if he or she is willing to try. Family may be helpful by discarding all remaining cigarettes.
4. Assist with plans for counseling and pharmacotherapy.	Smoking Cessation Assistance	4. Both cognitive and behavioral strategies are needed and can be provided by therapists.
5. Arrange follow-up care.	Smoking Cessation Assistance	5. Many clients benefit from nicotine patches or antidepressant medications to assist with smoking cessation.

Evaluation: Smoking cessation is a difficult problem. A short-term goal would be for the client to value the need to stop. The long-term goal would be the cessation of tobacco use.

lung tissue to exchange oxygen and carbon dioxide. Emphysema causes destruction of the pulmonary capillaries, further decreasing oxygen perfusion and ventilation.

The three types of emphysema are centriacinar, panacinar, and paraseptal (Figure 61-6). *Centriacinar* (or *centrilobular*) *emphysema,* the most common type, produces destruction in the bronchioles, usually in the upper lung regions. Inflammation begins in the bronchioles and spreads peripherally, but usually the alveolar sac remains intact. This form of emphysema occurs most often in smokers.

Panacinar emphysema destroys the entire alveolus and most commonly involves the lower portions of the lung. This form of the disease is generally observed in individuals with AAT deficiencies. Focal panacinar emphysema may also be seen at the lung bases in smokers with the centriacinar form.

Paraseptal (or *distal acinar*) *emphysema* primarily involves the distal airway structures, alveolar ducts, and alveolar sacs. The process is localized around the septa of the lungs or pleura, resulting in isolated blebs along the lung periphery. It is believed to be the likely cause of spontaneous pneumothorax. Giant bullae occasionally cause severe compression of adjacent lung tissue. The diagnosis of the disease, along with severity determination, is primarily accomplished through spirometry.

While all three disorders—asthma, chronic bronchitis, and emphysema—are present to some degree in clients with COPD, those individuals with chronic obstructive bronchitis as the major disease typically demonstrate a productive cough, decreased exercise tolerance, wheezing, shortness of breath, and prolonged expiration. As the chronic bronchitis progresses, copious amounts of sputum are produced and pulmonary infection is common. The client suffers from chronic hypoxemia and hypercapnia (Figure 61-7). The characteristic sitting position is leaning over a table with the shoulder girdle raised. Gait and walking pace correspond to the client's breathing with frequent rest periods to breathe.

Clients who have primary emphysema have progressive dyspnea on exertion that eventually becomes dyspnea at rest (Figure 61-8). The anteroposterior diameter of the chest is enlarged, and the chest has hyperresonant sounds to percussion. Chest films show overinflation and flattened diaphragms (Figure 61-9, *A*). ABG values are usually normal until later stages, when compensated respiratory acidosis is often evident. The client may have an enlarged heart and right ventricular lift. The electrocardiogram (ECG) shows right heart strain pattern and right axis deviation. Other manifestations may be cyanosis around the lips, neck vein distention, and pitting peripheral edema.

Complications

Respiratory tract infections commonly develop in clients with COPD. This situation is a result of alterations in the normal respiratory defense mechanisms and decreased immune resistance. Because respiratory status already is compromised, infection frequently leads to acute respiratory failure and is a common reason for hospitalization (see Chapter 63).

Spontaneous pneumothorax may develop from rupture of an emphysematous bleb. This rupture results in a closed pneumothorax and requires insertion of a chest tube for reexpansion of the lung (see Chapter 63).

Similar to asthma, chronic obstructive bronchitis and emphysema may worsen at night. Clients often report sleep-onset dyspnea and frequent or early-morning awakenings. During sleep, there is a decrease in the muscle tone and activity of the respiratory muscles. This decreased tone leads to hypoventilation, an increase in resistance of the airways, and $\dot{V}/\dot{Q}$ mismatch. Eventually, the client becomes hypoxemic.

OUTCOME MANAGEMENT

Medical Management

The treatment goals for the client with COPD are to improve ventilation, to facilitate the removal of bronchial secretions, to reduce complications, to slow the progression of clinical manifestations, and to promote health maintenance and client management of the disease. As in asthma, a step-care approach is used to guide medical intervention (Figure 61-10). The use of inspiratory muscle training may also be recommended in selected clients with COPD (see the Translating Evidence into Practice box on p. 1588).

Improve Ventilation

Bronchodilators remain the mainstay in the symptomatic management of COPD. These drugs reduce airway obstruction and are given on an as-needed basis or on a regular basis to prevent or reduce manifestations and exacerbations. They are usually administered via the inhalation route but in rare occasions may be given orally or administered intravenously. Regular treatment with long-acting bronchodilators is more effective and convenient than treatment with short-acting forms.

The principal bronchodilator treatments are beta$_2$ agonists, anticholinergics, and methylxanthines used singly or in combination. Beta$_2$ agonists are sympathomimetic drugs that act on the beta$_2$-adrenoceptors in the smooth muscles of the airways and cause bronchodilation. These drugs may also enhance mucus clearance and improve the endurance of respiratory muscles. Short-acting beta$_2$ agonists (e.g., albuterol) have minimal adverse effects, with rapid onset of action, a peak effect in 60 to 90 minutes, and duration of 4 to 6 hours. Side effects that may develop with the use of these drugs are tachycardia, tremor, nervousness, and nausea.

Summary of the GOLD guidelines

Therapy at each stage of COPD

Old	0: At risk	I: Mild	II: Moderate IIA IIB	III: Severe	
New	0: At risk	I: Mild	II: Moderate	III: Severe	IV: Very severe
Characteristics	Chronic symptoms Exposure to risk factors Normal spirometry	FEV_1/FVC <70% FEV_1 ≥80% With or without symptoms	FEV_1/FVC <70% 50% ≤FEV_1 <80% With or without symptoms	FEV_1/FVC <70% 30% ≤FEV_1 <50% With or without symptoms	FEV_1/FVC <70% FEV_1 <30% OR FEV_1 <50% predicted Plus chronic respiratory failure

Avoidance of risk factor(s); influenza vaccination

Add short-acting bronchodilator when needed

Add regular treatment with one or more long-acting bronchodilators

Add rehabilitation

Add inhaled glucocorticosteroids if repeated exacerbations

Add long-term oxygen if chronic respiratory failure

Consider surgical treatments

■ **FIGURE 61-10** Step-care approach to COPD care. *(From Global Initiative for Chronic Obstructive Lung Disease [GOLD]. [2006]. Global strategy for the diagnosis, management and prevention of COPD. Available at www.goldcopd.org.)*

Anticholinergic agents offer greater bronchodilator effect and fewer side effects than short-acting inhaled beta₂ agonists. These drugs work by blocking the cholinergic receptors located in the larger airways, resulting in bronchodilation. Ipratropium bromide (Atrovent) is the most commonly used drug in this category. When given by metered-dose inhaler, two puffs achieve maximal bronchodilation in 1.5 to 2 hours and last 6 to 8 hours. Adverse reactions from these drugs include dry mouth, nervousness, dizziness, fatigue, and headache.

Methylxanthines (e.g., theophylline, aminophylline), in both parenteral and oral forms, are also used to treat acute exacerbations. In addition to their bronchodilatory properties, methylxanthines enhance mucociliary clearance, stimulate the central respiratory drive, reduce pulmonary vascular resistance, and improve lung function during sleep. The level of benefit achieved with these agents is dose related, but there is no uniform relationship between the drug's effectiveness and serum blood levels. Age, smoking status, circulatory status, and hepatic function are factors that affect metabolism. Toxicity with methylxanthines may occur even at therapeutic levels, so blood levels of these agents need to be monitored closely. Several drugs also interfere with these agents even when administered in therapeutic levels. Side effects may include gastric upset, tachycardia, nausea and vomiting (possible toxicity), tremors, and nervousness.

Systemic glucocorticosteroids are used in the management of exacerbations of COPD. The exact mechanisms of action of these drugs in obstructive airway disease are poorly understood, but they shorten recovery time, improve lung function, and decrease hypoxemia. If used, corticosteroids should be administered either orally or parenterally, depending on the severity of the exacerbation. They should be used early in the course of treatment because their effect is not apparent for several hours. Clients who show a rapid response to parenteral steroids can be switched to oral forms on the third or fourth day of treatment, followed by a tapering course. The most common adverse effects are hypertension, peptic ulcer, dysphoria, hyperglycemia, cough, oral thrush, and fragile skin. A short course of corticosteroids may result in few adverse effects, but prolonged use does not result in greater efficacy and increases the risk of side effects.

Long-term oxygen therapy (>15 hours per day) has been shown to improve survival and quality of life in hypoxemic clients. Oxygen by nasal cannula should be provided at a flow rate sufficient to produce a resting Pao_2 of at least 60 mm Hg, or an Sao_2 greater than 89%. It

TRANSLATING EVIDENCE INTO PRACTICE

Inspiratory Muscle Training in COPD

COPD is characterized by progressive deterioration of inspiratory muscle strength. A number of factors are suspected of contributing to this deterioration, including chronic hyperinflation of the lungs, loss of muscle mass, decline in nutritional status, effects of corticosteroid use, and aging.[2] Decreased inspiratory muscle strength worsens the sensation of dyspnea and places clients at risk for respiratory muscle fatigue and declines in functional status.[1]

General interventions, such as pulmonary rehabilitation, nutritional counseling, and client education to prevent acute exacerbations, help to improve overall muscle strength and reduce dyspnea. However, targeted training of the inspiratory muscles has been proposed as an approach for directly improving their strength and endurance. Inspiratory muscle training (IMT) is accomplished through resistance training techniques. These involve the use of commercially available hand-held devices that require the user to generate an increased inspiratory effort to allow inspiratory flow.

Although a significant amount of research has been done on IMT, its benefits have been debated.[4] This is largely due to methodological limitations of many of the studies.[3] In general, the evidence supports the effectiveness of the intervention when training is adequate in duration and frequency (for example, 20 to 30 minutes per day, 4 to 6 days per week) as well as intensity (40% to 70% maximal inspiratory pressure).[5] Current evidence-based guidelines for pulmonary rehabilitation issued by the American College of Chest Physicians and the American Association of Cardiovascular and Pulmonary Rehabilitation recommend the use of IMT in selected clients with COPD who have decreased inspiratory muscle strength and breathlessness despite receiving optimal medical therapy.[6] Supervision and monitoring during training are recommended to ensure that adequate training loads are generated and to evaluate client tolerance.

REFERENCES

1. Hill, K., Jenkins, S.C., Hillman, D.R., et al. (2004). Dyspnea in COPD: Can inspiratory muscle training help? *Australian Journal of Physiotherapy, 50*(3), 169-180.
2. Larson, J.L., Covey, M.K., & Corbridge, S. (2002). Inspiratory muscle strength in chronic obstructive pulmonary disease. *AACN Clinical Issues, 13*(2), 320-332.
3. Padula, C.A. (2006). Inspiratory muscle training: Integrative review. *Research and Theory for Nursing Practice, 20*(4), 291-304.
4. Ram, F.S.F., Wellington, S.R., & Barnes, N.C. (2006). Inspiratory muscle training for asthma. *Cochrane Library, 1*, CD003792.
5. Reid, W.D., Geddes, E.L., Brooks, D., et al. (2004). Inspiratory muscle training in chronic obstructive pulmonary disease. *Physiotherapy Canada, 56*(3), 128-142.
6. Reis, A.L., Bauldoff, G.S., Carlin, B.W., et al. (2007). Pulmonary rehabilitation: Joint ACCP/AACVPR evidence-based clinical practice guidelines. *Chest, 131*, 4-42.

is important to note that some clients with chronic hypercapnia (elevated $Paco_2$ level) may be oxygen sensitive; that is, their $Paco_2$ levels may rise when given supplemental oxygen, leading to suppression of the central nervous system and significant lethargy. This phenomenon is commonly known as *CO_2 narcosis*. There are several theories as to why supplemental oxygen increases hypercapnia in some CO_2 retainers and, in all likelihood, there are probably multiple factors involved. However, the key point is that clients with high $Paco_2$ levels who are receiving oxygen should be closely monitored to determine their response to therapy.

At times, the client may require mechanical ventilatory support for adequate oxygenation during exacerbations. Ventilatory support includes both noninvasive intermittent ventilation, using either negative- or positive-pressure devices, and invasive continuous ventilation via endotracheal tube or tracheostomy.

Remove Bronchial Secretions

Pulmonary hygiene is needed to rid the lungs of secretions and to reduce the risk of infection. In the hospital, the client may be treated with nebulized bronchodilators and positive-pressure air flow or positive end-expiratory pressure devices to increase the caliber of the airways. Postural drainage and chest physiotherapy may be prescribed to move the secretions from the small to the large airways, from which they can be expelled.

Reduce Complications

Deep venous thrombosis prophylaxis may be needed in clients who are immobilized, polycythemic, or dehydrated. Influenza vaccines can reduce serious illness. Pneumococcal polysaccharide vaccine is also recommended for clients 65 years and older and for those clients younger than age 65 with an FEV_1 <40% predicted.

Promote Exercise

All clients with COPD benefit from exercise programs, showing improvement in exercise tolerance and decreased dyspnea and fatigue. Aerobic exercise is used to enhance cardiovascular fitness and to train respiratory muscles to function more effectively. Exercise does not improve lung function, but respiratory muscles can be strengthened even when the lungs are diseased. Progressively increased walking is the most common form of exercise. Before a walking program is begun, ABGs should be assessed and compared with resting levels. Supplemental oxygen should be used during exercise if the client becomes severely hypoxemic.

Breathing exercises may also be prescribed. Encourage diaphragmatic breathing and pursed-lip breathing and discourage rapid, shallow *panic* breathing.

Improve General Health

The most effective way to slow disease progression is for the client to stop smoking. Exposure to second-hand smoke, occupational dusts and chemicals, air pollution, and known allergens should also be minimized. All clients with COPD should avoid high altitudes, and supplemental oxygen may be required for air travel. No specific climate has been shown to alter the course of the disorder.

Adequate nutrition is essential to maintain respiratory muscle strength. Malnutrition is common and contributes to decreased respiratory muscle strength and reduced diaphragmatic mass. Consult a clinical dietitian to assist clients in modifying their diet to meet their caloric needs. Clients with COPD often have difficulty eating because of dyspnea. Offer the client frequent small meals rather than large meals. When the client must be tube-fed, substrate metabolism also may affect lung function. Normal carbohydrate metabolism produces carbon dioxide and water. Excess carbohydrate leads to increased production of carbon dioxide and can lead to respiratory distress. Enteral formulas are designed for pulmonary disease and provide more calories from fat, as discussed in the Case Study below. Adjust oxygen delivery devices so that the mouth is not obstructed but oxygen is delivered through the nose during eating.

Nursing Management of the Medical Client

Assessment. The nursing assessment should include a thorough exploration of the client's clinical manifestations. Determine the client's ability to recognize manifestations that require further care. For example, if a client says, "I knew I was developing an infection and went to the doctor," this statement indicates an understanding of the disorder. In contrast, if a client does not fully understand the reasons for hospitalization, educate the client about COPD. A review of past medical history helps to determine whether the client has other disorders, such as heart disease, that might affect treatment.

Complete a physical examination with an emphasis on the respiratory and cardiac systems. Note the degree of dyspnea, the presence of orthopnea, decreased breath sounds, and clinical manifestations of heart failure.

Evaluate mental status because confusion and restlessness may be early indicators of increasing hypoxia and hypercapnia. Record the client's baseline oximetry and the level of inspired oxygen. Ask if the client smokes and, if so, if he or she has interest in smoking cessation. Infection is a common cause of exacerbation of COPD. Note the presence of a productive cough, pain with coughing, fever, and the color and consistency of sputum.

Consider the impact of stressors that may have led to exacerbations of COPD. Possible factors include the progressive illness itself, marital or other family problems, and financial concerns. Review the client's usual coping strategies and determine effectiveness. Support systems, such as friends and family, also are important components of psychosocial stability. Determine the reliability of the client's support system.

The psychosocial impact of COPD is significant. Clients commonly have feelings of loss of control over their bodies and their social environment. These responses leave the client socially isolated and depressed and can severely affect quality of life. Psychosocial intervention is important.

A thorough history may need to be delayed until the client is able to breathe comfortably, or it may be taken over short periods of time or obtained through the family. Likewise, the physical examination should not tire the client. Protein-calorie malnutrition may be evident. Consult the dietitian for methods to improve the client's intake.

Evaluation. Dyspnea will be slow to improve. Expect several days for the client to return to baseline levels. Clients with COPD often continue to deteriorate despite medical care. It is difficult to cope with failing health that limits activity and employment. As much as possible, encourage the client to live an active life with daily exercise. The support of significant others is essential.

Diagnosis, Outcomes, Interventions. Common nursing diagnoses and interventions for the client with COPD are listed in the Care Plan for the client with COPD. Because COPD is common, many institutions use clinical paths or care maps to guide care. (See the Care Plan feature on pp. 1582-1585 and the Clinical Pathway on Chronic Obstructive Pulmonary Disease on the website.)

Surgical Management

In some clients, bullectomy (removal of large bullae, which compress the lung and add to dead space) may be of benefit. Lung transplantation may be used to provide relief of disabling manifestations and improve quality of life for clients with end-stage COPD, although its effect on survival remains unclear.

Lung volume–reduction surgery (LVRS) may improve work capacity and health-related quality of life for a select group of COPD clients. In this operation, portions

---

CASE STUDY   *evolve*

COPD with Nutritional Concerns

Bill Smith is a 55-year-old disabled car salesman who is cared for at home by his wife of 36 years. Bill is being seen in the office today for a routine visit. He reports that he has been coughing up more sputum than normal and that sometimes he feels as if he is choking. Bill's wife also reports that she is afraid he is not getting enough to eat, because she has noticed he has put three more holes in his leather belt to hold up his pants . . . .
Case Study continued on the website and the CD-ROM with discussions, multiple-choice questions, and a nursing care plan.

of diffusely emphysematous lungs are removed to help restore more normal chest-wall configuration and to improve respiratory mechanics and functional capacity (see Figure 61-9, *B*). The ideal candidates for LVRS are individuals with severe upper-lobe emphysema and markedly reduced exercise capacity. In this group, the surgery may also improve survival.

Nursing Management of the Surgical Client

After surgery, monitor closely the client's ABG values. Chest assessment and radiographs help to determine whether the lungs are expanding. Assess the chest tubes for air leaks and drainage. Intensive pulmonary toilet is essential. Repeated coughing and deep breathing help to prevent pulmonary complications. Many clients have chest physiotherapy every 4 hours and nebulized aerosol treatments. Manage pain aggressively to promote activity and pulmonary hygiene.

After discharge, the client is assessed for adequate ventilation and tissue oxygenation (with pulse oximetry) and progressive wound healing. Pulmonary treatments may continue until lung sounds are clear. The client is weaned from oxygen and placed into a formal pulmonary rehabilitation program.

Modifications for Older Clients

The prevalence of COPD rises significantly in people in the middle to late adult years and is a leading cause of hospitalizations in older clients. The older client frequently has other problems that influence the treatment of COPD. For example, the client may have decreased exercise tolerance, impaired nutrition, or multiple comorbid conditions. Also consider the possibility of drug interactions in older clients. Remember, too, that the older adult has special requirements when chronic conditions are exacerbated (see the Case Management feature on the Older Adult on the website).

Self-Care

Pulmonary rehabilitation is designed to reduce the toll of pulmonary disease for the client and the health care system. The goals of pulmonary rehabilitation are to reduce clinical manifestations, to improve quality of life, and to increase physical and emotional participation in everyday activities. Clients are taught how to administer medications, what side effects to look for and how to manage them, and the safe and correct use of oxygen. Lower-body exercise (walking, cycling) is commonly prescribed. Upper-body exercise is also used in some cases.

To facilitate self-care and adherence, the client and significant others need thorough information about the disease process. Review the manifestations of impending respiratory problems (e.g., increased confusion or drowsiness), respiratory tract infection, and right-sided

heart failure (e.g., peripheral edema, distended neck veins) so that prompt intervention can be obtained if these complications develop. The need for routine respiratory follow-up should also be discussed. In your teaching, include a discussion of the hazards of infection and ways to decrease personal risk (i.e., avoid crowds during the flu and colds season, clean respiratory equipment well, obtain flu vaccines yearly). Review the need for lifestyle modifications, especially smoking cessation.

Clients with end-stage lung disease experience significant, intensely distressing manifestations, especially dyspnea. Whether care is provided in the home or in an extended-care facility, the focus is on minimizing dyspnea and making the client as comfortable as possible. The Bridge to Home Health Care feature on p. 1591 details client teaching and nursing interventions for the home setting.

BRONCHIECTASIS

Bronchiectasis, an extreme form of obstructive bronchitis, causes permanent, abnormal dilation and distortion of bronchi and bronchioles. It develops when bronchial walls are weakened by chronic inflammatory changes in the bronchial mucosa and occurs most often after recurrent inflammatory conditions. Any condition producing a narrowing of the lumen of the bronchioles, however, may result in bronchiectasis, including tuberculosis, adenoviral infections, and pneumonia.

Some forms of bronchiectasis are congenital and are associated with cystic fibrosis, sinusitis, dextrocardia (heart located on right side), and alterations in ciliary activity (Kartagener's syndrome). Bronchiectasis is usually localized to a lung lobe or segment rather than generalized throughout the lungs. At times, however, persistent, nonresolving infection may cause the disorder to spread to other parts of the same lung. Diagnosis may be confirmed by chest radiograph, bronchogram, or computed tomography (CT) scan.

Manifestations vary according to the etiologic agent. The main manifestations are cough and purulent sputum production in large quantities. Fever, hemoptysis, nasal stuffiness, and drainage from sinusitis also are common. The client may complain of fatigue and weakness. Clubbing of the fingers may be present.

OUTCOME MANAGEMENT

Management of bronchiectasis is the same as that for COPD. Most clients are managed medically to prevent progression of the disorder and to control clinical manifestations. Antibiotics, chest physical therapy, hydration, bronchodilators, and oxygen commonly are prescribed. Severe cases may be treated by surgical resection if the pathologic process is well localized in one lobe or two adjacent lobes and when no contraindications to surgery exist

Conserving Oxygen with Chronic Obstructive Pulmonary Disease

Clients with chronic obstructive pulmonary disease (COPD) are challenged to make the most of their lives, given their available oxygen.

Usually, home health nurses are primarily responsible for monitoring manifestations; reviewing and reinforcing previously taught oxygen-conservation techniques; giving further instructions; and determining whether referrals to registered dietitians and occupational, physical, or respiratory therapists are needed. Evaluate what your clients already know, and proceed from there. Be certain that your clients understand the importance of using pursed-lip breathing, abdominal breathing, and metered-dose inhalers consistently and correctly. Have them demonstrate their technique.

Help your clients develop an oxygen-conservation plan that allows them to participate in activities that are most important to them. Ask them to keep a simple diary and to record their usual behavior during a 1- or 2-day period that includes all waking hours. When you analyze the diary, identify your clients' priorities. Help them relate specific activity to feelings of dyspnea during the day. In this way, you can teach specific oxygen-conservation techniques and pacing of activities to meet their priorities. To increase comfort, have your clients schedule the use of inhalers before activities and keep them within easy reach.

Encourage clients who are concerned about adequate oxygen for sexual activity to assume passive positions and to allow their partners to be more active. If winded, clients should use massage and other relaxation techniques as part of foreplay.

Adequate nutrition is essential to clients who have COPD; they may be malnourished because of respiratory muscle wasting. The diet should be high in protein and fat and low in carbohydrates. Answer your clients' questions, and determine whether they are willing or able to purchase, prepare, and eat the foods that were suggested. Encourage easy food preparation to prevent fatigue. Use foods that are prepackaged or can be heated in the microwave. Consider home-delivered meals. Use liquid food supplements to increase protein; many brands are available, including some that are specially formulated for people who have pulmonary problems.

Encourage clients to rest just before eating and to follow these suggestions. Eat in a relaxed and quiet area. Small, frequent meals are best. Schedule meals early in the day if fatigue increases as the day continues. Snack frequently. Schedule inhalers after meals because inhaler medications can taint the taste of food and make it more difficult to achieve adequate nutrition.

Clients who have COPD often feel isolated because of their decreased ability to leave their homes. Suggest that they and their families join local support groups where they can share their experiences and feelings about the disease and learn new techniques to improve their quality of life. Many hospitals sponsor groups. Another valuable resource is the American Lung Association, which has local offices throughout the United States; call for information about prevention and the latest developments in treatment.

DISORDERS OF THE PULMONARY VASCULATURE

PULMONARY EMBOLISM

Pulmonary embolism (PE) is an occlusion of a portion of the pulmonary blood vessels by an embolus. An embolus is a clot or other plug (thrombus) that is carried by the bloodstream from its point of origin to a smaller blood vessel, where it obstructs circulation. Depending on its size, an embolus can be lethal. It is estimated that in the United States more than 650,000 cases of pulmonary embolism are diagnosed annually.

Etiology and Risk Factors
Virtually all PEs develop from thrombi (clots), most of which originate in the deep calf, femoral, popliteal, or iliac veins. Other sources of emboli include tumors, air, fat, bone marrow, amniotic fluid, septic thrombi, and vegetations on heart valves that develop with endocarditis.

Major operations, especially hip, knee, abdominal, and extensive pelvic procedures, predispose the client to thrombus formation because of the reduced flow of blood through the pelvis. Traveling in cramped quarters for a long time or sitting for long periods is also associated with stasis and clotting of blood. Preventive measures, such as early ambulation, frequent leg exercises, sequential compression stockings, and anticoagulant prophylaxis, are essential.

Pathophysiology
When emboli travel to the lungs, they lodge in the pulmonary vasculature. The size and number of emboli determine the location. Blood flow is obstructed, leading to decreased perfusion of the section of lung supplied by the vessel. The client continues to ventilate the lung portion, but because the tissue is not perfused, a $\dot{V}/\dot{Q}$ mismatch occurs, resulting in hypoxemia (Figure 61-11).

If an embolus lodges in a large pulmonary vessel, it increases proximal pulmonary vascular resistance, causes atelectasis, and eventually reduces cardiac output. If the embolus is in a smaller vessel, less dramatic clinical manifestations follow but perfusion is still altered.

The arterioles constrict because of platelet degranulation, accompanied by a release of histamine, serotonin, catecholamines, and prostaglandins. These chemical agents result in bronchial and pulmonary artery

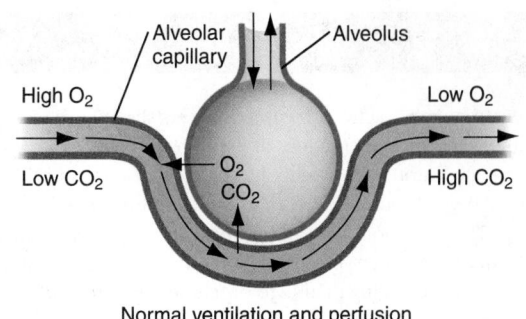

Normal ventilation and perfusion

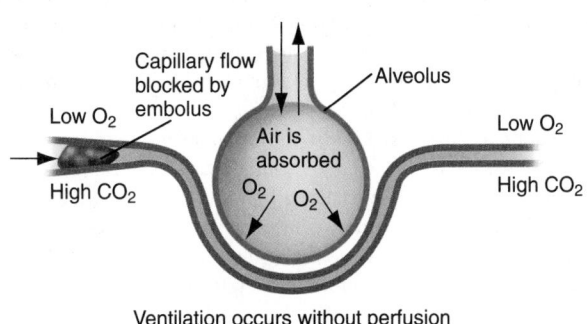

Ventilation occurs without perfusion
(dead space ventilation)

■ **FIGURE 61-11** V̇/Q̇ mismatch occurs when the blood flow to a pulmonary arteriole is halted by a blood clot, but for a while air is still exchanged in the alveolus it serves. Because there is no blood to exchange oxygen for carbon dioxide, eventually the alveolus collapses.

constriction. This vasoconstriction probably plays a major role in the hemodynamic instability that follows PE.

Pulmonary embolism can lead to right-sided heart failure. Once the clot lodges, affected blood vessels in the lung collapse. This collapse increases the pressure in the pulmonary vasculature. The increased pressure increases the workload of the right side of the heart, leading to failure. Massive PE of the pulmonary artery can also result in cardiopulmonary collapse from lack of perfusion and resulting hypoxia and acidosis.

Clinical Manifestations

The clinical manifestations of PE are nonspecific and, in some clients, may not appear until late in the event. The most common manifestations of PE are tachypnea, dyspnea, anxiety or fretfulness, and chest pain. Hypoxemia may be present depending on the size of the embolism. Because these clinical manifestations are similar to those seen with myocardial infarction and other cardiovascular illnesses, overdiagnosis is as likely as underdiagnosis. Extensive differential diagnosis often is required. The pain usually experienced with PE is pleuritic in nature, caused by an inflammatory reaction of the lung parenchyma or by pulmonary infarction or ischemia, resulting from obstruction of small pulmonary arterial branches. Typical pleuritic chest pain is sudden in onset and exacerbated by breathing. The client is usually dyspneic, especially if the embolus has occluded major arteries or

major portions of lung tissue. Apprehension, cough, diaphoresis, syncope, and hemoptysis may occur. The presence of hemoptysis indicates that the infarction or areas of atelectasis have produced alveolar damage.

Respirations typically increase. Crackles, an accentuated second heart sound, tachycardia, and fever may also develop. Less common findings include heart gallops, edema, heart murmur, and cyanosis.

Diagnostic Findings

When PE is suspected, the optimal strategy for diagnosis is an integrated approach that includes a thorough history and physical examination, supplemented by selective diagnostic tests. Pulse oximetry will be low and may be unresponsive to inhaled oxygen. ABG analysis indicates arterial hypoxemia (low Pao_2) and hypocapnia (low $Paco_2$) in massive PE. Severe respiratory alkalosis may occur. Lactate dehydrogenase (LDH) isoenzymes show an increase in LDH_3 if there is lung tissue injury. A chest radiograph may help to rule out other pulmonary diagnoses.

A noninvasive diagnostic test for PE is the V̇/Q̇ lung scan. A radioisotope lung scan is performed by IV injection of particles of human serum albumin that have been labeled with iodine 131 or technetium 99m. These particles are trapped in the pulmonary microvasculature and are distributed according to pulmonary flow. Both lungs are scanned with a scintillation counter, and the amount of radioactivity counted gives an indication of obstruction to flow. An alternative to lung scanning that is being used more frequently is spiral CT scan of the chest. This approach is particularly effective for identifying PE in the proximal pulmonary vascular tree and for clients who are unstable or have limited cardiopulmonary reserve.

Pulmonary angiography remains the definitive means of diagnosis of PE (Figure 61-12). A radiopaque contrast agent is injected into the right atrium and pulmonary artery via a catheter threaded through a peripheral vein. Visualization of any filling defects of the heart and right pulmonary artery is achieved by taking sequential radiographs. Because of the invasive nature of the test pulmonary angiography typically is reserved for cases in which the index of clinical suspicion is high despite nondiagnostic findings on other tests.

The D-dimer plasma test helps exclude PE when the value is below 500 ng/L. It does not always help predict PE, however, because it is elevated from myocardial infarction, sepsis, and other systemic illnesses.

OUTCOME MANAGEMENT

Medical Management

Successful management of PE depends on having a high index of suspicion for manifestations such as dyspnea

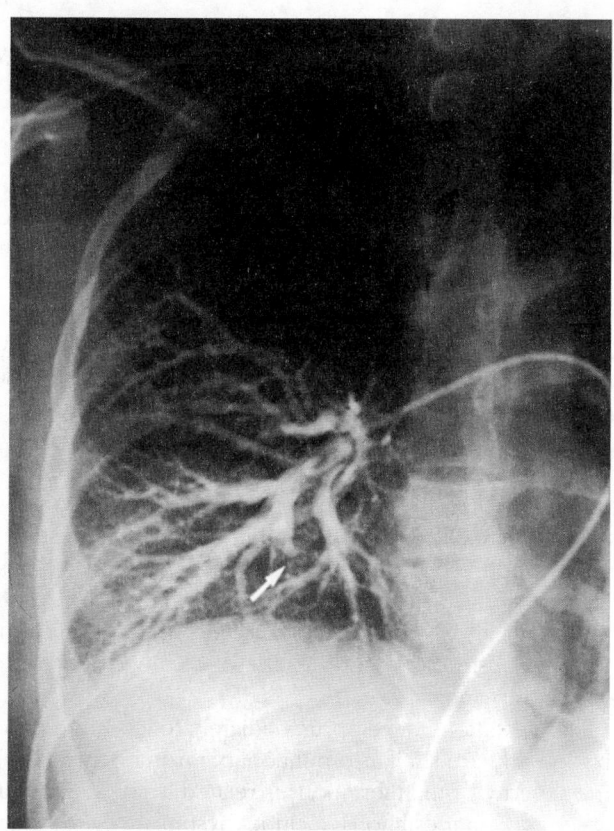

■ **FIGURE 61-12** Angiogram showing a pulmonary embolus (arrow).

and anxiety in high-risk clients such as those who are immobile or have a malignancy. Prompt recognition of the condition and immediate treatment are essential. Goals are to stabilize the cardiopulmonary system and reduce the threat of a further PE with anticoagulation therapy or trapping with an umbrella in the vena cava. For some clients, the clot can be lysed.

Stabilizing the Cardiopulmonary System

Maintenance of cardiopulmonary stability is the first priority. Sometimes hypoxemia can be reversed with low-flow oxygen by nasal cannula. Other clients may require endotracheal intubation to maintain Pao_2 greater than 60 mm Hg. Hypotension is treated with fluids. If fluids do not raise the preload (right ventricular end-diastolic pressure) enough to raise blood pressure, inotropic agents may be required. Acidosis, which has a powerful vasoconstricting effect, is corrected with bicarbonate.

Anticoagulant Therapy

Typically, anticoagulation begins with IV standard (unfractionated) heparin sodium based initially on body weight and current level of anticoagulation to reduce the risk of further clots and to prevent extension of existing clots. *Anticoagulants do not break up existing clots*, but they do prevent extensions of existing clots. Clinical trials have shown that subcutaneously administered low-molecular-weight heparin is as safe and effective as standard heparin in the treatment of hemodynamically stable clients with PE. Anticoagulants are administered until a therapeutic partial thromboplastin time (PTT) is achieved. In general, the initial target International Normalized Ratio should be 2.5 to 3.0. Administration of sodium warfarin is begun about 3 to 5 days before heparin is stopped to provide a transition to oral anticoagulation. Because the half-life of warfarin is long, about 2 to 3 days is required to achieve adequate anticoagulation. Clients are maintained on warfarin for 3 to 6 months.

Fibrinolytic Therapy

The effectiveness of fibrinolytic therapy in the management of a massive PE is not clear, but it may be useful in clients who are hemodynamically unstable. Thrombolytic agents lyse the clots and restore right-sided heart function; however, some clinicians have found that although the clot dissolves, the death rate is not improved.

Nursing Management of the Medical Client

Monitor the client closely for hypoxemia and respiratory compromise, and assess vital signs and lung sounds frequently. Monitor ABG or oximetry values, and monitor the client for manifestations of right-sided heart failure. Auscultate heart sounds frequently, assessing for murmurs or extra heart sounds. Check for peripheral edema, distended neck veins, and liver engorgement.

To facilitate breathing, elevate the head of the bed and apply oxygen per physician's orders. Because the usual cause of a PE is thrombus from the lower legs, elevate the legs with caution to avoid severe flexure of the hips. Such flexure would slow blood flow and increase the risk of new thrombi.

The client typically experiences fear with the sudden onset of severe chest pain and inability to breathe. Anxiety, restlessness, and apprehension are common. Emotional support can reduce anxiety and lessen dyspnea. Stay with the client and give calm, yet efficient, nursing care.

Analgesics are given as needed to reduce pain and anxiety. Morphine is the most common agent. Anxiety and pain increase oxygen demand and dyspnea. Administer oral care with soft brushes or rinses while oxygen is in use, especially if the client breathes through the mouth.

Follow the anticoagulation protocols to achieve desired blood levels. Expect variations in PTT or INR during a 24 hour period with higher levels during the night and lower levels in the morning. Once

SAFETY

ALERT

anticoagulation is achieved, watch for manifestations of excess anticoagulation, such as blood in the urine, in the stool, or along the gums or teeth; subcutaneous bruising; or flank pain. When invasive studies, such as ABGs, are necessary, apply pressure to the puncture site for at least 10 minutes.

The client is discharged with oral anticoagulation therapy. Instruct the client about side effects, the importance of follow-up to monitor prothrombin times, the effect of diet on anticoagulation, and precautions to prevent bleeding. Review methods to reduce thrombophlebitis if that was the likely cause of the embolus (see Chapter 53).

Surgical Management

Surgical interventions that may be used in the treatment of PE include (1) vena caval interruption with the insertion of a filter (Figure 61-13) and (2) pulmonary embolectomy. The Greenfield filter, a basket-like cone of wires bent to look like an umbrella, is the most commonly used filter. The filter is inserted by threading it up the veins in the leg or neck until it reaches the vena cava at the level of the renal arteries. The filter allows blood flow while trapping emboli; however, vena cava filters are less effective than anticoagulation and may lead to deep vein thrombosis, and so these generally are used only when anticoagulants are contraindicated or ineffective.

Embolectomy is used in clients with significant hemodynamic instability caused by the embolus, especially those with unstable circulation and contraindications to thrombolytic therapy. An embolectomy involves surgical removal of emboli from the pulmonary arteries by either a thoracotomy or an embolectomy catheter.

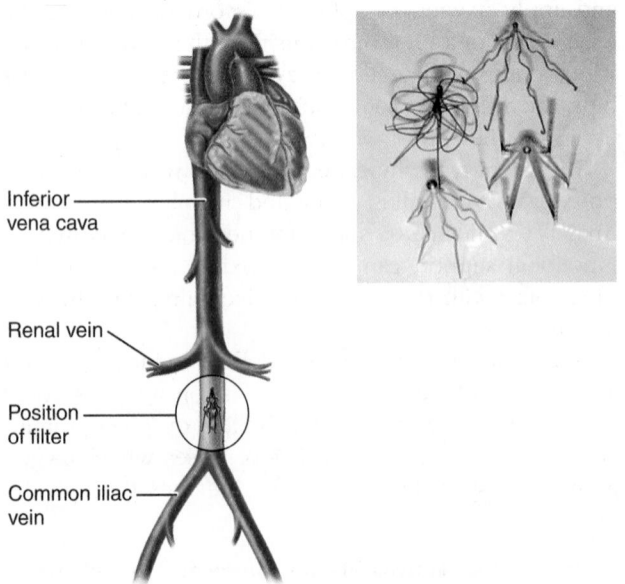

Inferior
vena cava

Renal vein

Position
of filter

Common iliac
vein

■ **FIGURE 61-13** Inferior vena cava filters inserted into the vena cava through the iliac vein, such as the Greenfield filter, prevent emboli from traveling to the lung.

Newly developed catheters use high-velocity jets of saline to draw the thrombus toward the catheter tip and pulverize it.

VENOUS AIR EMBOLISM

Venous air embolism (VAE) is the entry of air into the venous system. VAE may occur in any condition in which an open vein above the right atrium level is exposed to the atmosphere (e.g., trauma to a vein, insertion or removal of central venous catheters or pulmonary artery catheters, surgical procedures on the head and neck [e.g., craniotomy], pelvic operations in Trendelenburg position, and during gas insufflation in laparoscopy.

Entry of air into the venous system produces manifestations in the right ventricle, pulmonary circulation, or systemic circulation (if right-to-left shunts are present). Small amounts of air do not produce manifestations because air is removed from the circulation. Large boluses of air (3 to 8 ml/kg) can cause right ventricular outflow obstruction and result in cardiogenic shock and circulatory arrest.

Manifestations develop immediately following embolization and are similar to pulmonary thromboembolism. The severity of manifestations is related to the degree of air entry. Manifestations include dyspnea, chest pain, "mill wheel" murmur (a loud, churning, machinery-like murmur heard over the precordium), tachycardia, hypotension, decreased consciousness, circulatory shock, or sudden death (with severe VAE).

Reduce the risk of air embolus by carefully priming all intravenous tubing. Secure all connections in central lines and protect them from becoming dislodged when the client moves in bed or from the bed.

If VAE is suspected, any central line procedure in progress is immediately terminated and the line is clamped. Promptly place the client in Trendelenburg position and rotate toward the left lateral decubitus position. This maneuver helps trap air in the apex of the ventricle, prevents its ejection into the pulmonary arterial system, and maintains right ventricular output. The client is given 100% oxygen, and mechanical ventilation may be needed for significant respiratory distress or refractory hypoxemia. If a central venous catheter is present, aspirate from the distal port and attempt to remove air.

PULMONARY HYPERTENSION

Pulmonary hypertension is defined as a prolonged elevation of the mean pulmonary artery pressure (PAP) at or above 25 mm Hg (normal, 10 to 20 mm Hg) with a pulmonary capillary wedge pressure of 15 mm Hg or higher, both measured at rest. Forms of pulmonary hypertension are categorized according to the exact nature of the disease mechanism; i.e., those conditions that directly affect the pulmonary arterial tree (termed pulmonary arterial hypertension [PAH]), those that predominantly affect the venous circulation (pulmonary venous hypertension), and those conditions that affect the pulmonary circulation by altering respiratory structure or function (pulmonary hypertension associated with hypoxemia or chronic thromboembolic disease). PAH is further classified as either *idiopathic* or *familial* when supported by genetic investigation. The idiopathic form occurs in the absence of known causes. It occurs most often in young adults between the ages of 30 and 40 years, with women affected more often than men. A relationship with sleep-disordered breathing has also been found. The familial form is associated with an identified genetic mutation, increasing the risk among family members. The condition is relatively rare. However, increasing numbers of pulmonary hypertension–related hospitalizations and deaths seen among adults ages 65 and older suggest that as the U.S. population ages, pulmonary hypertension might become a more frequent diagnosis, particularly with accompanying chronic heart failure.

The pulmonary circulation is generally a low-pressure, low-resistance system. Increased cardiac output in a healthy person, as with exercise, causes minimal elevations in PAP because of the large pulmonary vascular reserve. When pulmonary vasoconstriction is present, however, pressure elevation occurs because the pulmonary vasculature cannot accommodate increased blood flow.

Milder forms of pulmonary hypertension are generally caused by pulmonary vasoconstriction resulting from chronic hypoxia, acidosis, or both. Administration of oxygen, correction of acid-base imbalance, and use of vasodilating medications in selected cases generally return PAP to normal, either completely or partially.

Clients with mild pulmonary hypertension may be relatively asymptomatic. In moderate to severe forms, the main (and occasionally only) manifestation is dyspnea. Fatigue, syncope, angina-like chest pain, palpitations, and muscular weakness also may occur.

A chest x-ray study shows right ventricular hypertrophy, enlarged pulmonary arteries, prominent hilar vessels, and normal or reduced intrapulmonary vascular markings. Right-heart cardiac catheterization is required to confirm the diagnosis and determine severity. Typical findings include elevated PAP and increased arteriovenous oxygen differences accompanied by normal systemic blood pressure and normal to low cardiac output.

OUTCOME MANAGEMENT

The overall prognosis in severe pulmonary arterial hypertension is poor, although treatment options are improving and survival rates are increasing. Supportive intervention with supplemental oxygen helps to reduce

hypoxemia, whereas anticoagulants may be used to prevent thromboembolic events. Other conventional non-specific therapy includes digoxin, diuretics, and high-dose calcium-channel blockade in those clients with acute vasoreactivity.

Vasodilator therapy is the cornerstone of pharmacologic management. Long-term prostacyclin (epoprostenol) therapy has been found to improve hemodynamic status and physical manifestations. Prostacyclin is a potent pulmonary vasodilator that also reduces right ventricular dilation, prevents tricuspid regurgitation from worsening, and has antithrombotic properties related to its effects on platelets. However, treatment with prostacyclin is expensive and difficult to manage because, among other drawbacks, it requires long-term, continuous central infusion. An oral endothelin-receptor antagonist, Bosentan, has been found to be just as effective in some clients. In addition, subcutaneous treprostinil and inhaled iloprost are prostacyclin analogs that have also shown some promising results.

Pulmonary thromboendarterectomy may provide a potential surgical cure in cases resulting from chronic thromboembolic disease. Some clients with severe pulmonary hypertension may undergo heart-lung or bilateral-lung transplantation. In addition, atrial septostomy may be performed in clients with severe PAH in whom other therapies either are unavailable or have failed, and who find themselves in need of palliative or bridging maneuvers. This procedure involves the creation of an intra-atrial right-to-left shunt to decompress the right atrium and right ventricle and augment left ventricle filling and cardiac output. This helps to increase tissue oxygenation delivery.

CONCLUSIONS

Lower-airway disorders include asthma, chronic air flow limitations, and inflammations of the airways. Nursing care centers on reversal of any airway spasms and education of the client about how to live with the disorder and how to reduce the risk of future problems. PE is a potentially life-threatening disorder that usually can be managed effectively with prompt recognition. Pulmonary hypertension is a disorder that is often difficult to diagnose and challenging to treat, although remarkable improvements in therapy have been made.

THINKING CRITICALLY

1. A 52-year-old woman is being treated at the neighborhood health clinic for chronic bronchitis. Her husband of 30 years smoked two to three packs of cigarettes a day. The client never smoked. During this exacerbation, she presents with shortness of breath; wheezing; a deep, throaty, productive cough when she tries to talk; and fatigue. Her blood pressure is 180/90 mm Hg, pulse is 90 beats/min, respirations are 28 breaths/min and labored, and

temperature is 99.4 ° F. She tells you that she tried to shovel the driveway on this cold winter day and did not wear a scarf over her mouth as she usually does. She further states that her inhalers did not seem to help her. She is taking a diuretic for hypertension, with blood pressure controlled at about 160/86 mm Hg. What is your priority nursing action? What teaching is appropriate at this time?

Factors to Consider. What are the clinical manifestations of chronic obstructive emphysema? What nursing assessments are in order?

2. An older client is recovering from pelvic surgery. Because of a previous stroke, she is hemiplegic. She has been on bed rest since the surgery. While the nursing assistant is giving her a bath, she notices the client grimacing as if in pain. The client responds to her question by pointing to her chest and nodding when asked if the pain is severe. The nursing assistant notifies you that the client is in distress. What is the priority assessment?

Factors to Consider. What complications of surgery and resulting bed rest might pose a risk for this client? How would you compare and contrast the clinical manifestations for pneumonia and pulmonary embolus?

3. You enter the room of the client from question 2 and discover that she is apprehensive. She is trying to hold her breath because it hurts to breathe. She is sweating, and there is frothy sputum on her lips. What nursing interventions are appropriate? What treatment might be ordered?

Factors to Consider. What are the clinical manifestations of pulmonary embolus? What diagnostic studies may be ordered?

evolve *Discussions for these questions can be found on the website.*

BIBLIOGRAPHY

🪔 Citations appearing in red refer to primary research.

🪔 Citations appearing in blue refer to evidence-based practice guidelines and protocols.

1. American Lung Association. (2006). *Asthma in adults fact sheet.* Available at www.lungusa.org.
2. American Lung Association. (2006). *Chronic obstructive pulmonary disease fact sheet.* Available at www.lungusa.org.
3. Benditt, J.O. (2006). Surgical options for patients with COPD: Sorting out the choices. *Respiratory Care, 51,* 173-178.
4. Brown, M.D., Rowe, B.H., & Reeves, M.J. (2004). The accuracy of the enzyme-linked immunosorbent assay D-dimer test in the diagnosis of pulmonary embolism: A meta-analysis. *Annals of Emergency Medicine, 40,* 133-144.
5. Burkstein, D., et al. (2005). Discussing the costs of asthma: Controlling outcomes, symptoms, and treatment strategies. *American Journal of Managed Care, 11*(11), s318-s328.
6. Capriotti, T. (2005). Changes in inhaler devices for asthma and COPD. *MEDSURG Nursing, 14*(3), 185-194.
7. Chu, E., & Drazen, J. (2005). Asthma: One hundred years of treatment and onward. *American Journal of Respiratory and Critical Care Medicine, 171*(11), 1202-1208.
8. Crompton, G.K. (2004). How to achieve good compliance with inhaled asthma therapy. *Respiratory Medicine, 98* (Suppl B), s35-s40.
9. Decramer, M., & Selroos, O. (2005). Asthma and COPD: Differences and similarities. *International Journal of Clinical Practice, 59*(4), 385-398.
10. Dolovich, M., et al. (2005). Device selection and outcomes of aerosol therapy: Evidence-based guidelines. *Chest, 127*(1), 335-371.
11. Doyle, R.L., McCrory, D., Channick, R.N., et al (2004). Surgical treatments/interventions for pulmonary arterial hypertension: ACCP evidence-based clinical practice guidelines. *Chest, 126* (Suppl 1), 63S-72S.
12. Geller, D. (2005). Comparing clinical features of the nebulizer, metered-dose inhaler, and dry powder inhaler. *Respiratory Care, 50*(10), 1313-1322.
13. Gift, A.G., & Narsavage, G. (1998). Validity of the numeric rating scale as a measure of dyspnea. *American Journal of Critical Care, 7*(3), 200-204.
14. Global Initiative for Chronic Obstructive Lung Disease (GOLD). (2006). *Global strategy for the diagnosis, management and prevention of COPD.* Available at www.goldcopd.org.
15. Hayashino, Y., Goto, M., et al (2005). Ventilation perfusion scanning and helical CT in asuspected pulmonary embolism: Meta analysis of diagnostic performance. *Radiology, 234,* 740-748.
16. Koschel, M. (2004). Pulmonary embolism. *American Journal of Nursing, 104*(6), 46-57.
17. National Heart, Lung, and Blood Institute. (2004). *Morbidity and mortality: 2004 chart book on cardiovascular, lung, and blood diseases.* Available at www.nhlbi.nih.gov/resources/docs/04_chtbk.pdf.
18. MacIntyre, N.R. (2006). Corticosteroid therapy and chronic obstructive pulmonary disease. *Respiratory Care, 51,* 289-296.
19. Mahler, D.A. (2005). Measurement of dyspnea: Clinical ratings. In D.A. Mahler & D.E. O'Donnell (Eds.), *Dyspnea: Mechanisms, measurement, and management* (pp. 147-165). Boca Raton, Fla: Taylor & Francis.
20. Mather, S., & Busse, W. (2006). Asthma: Diagnosis and management. *Medical Clinics of North America, 90*(1), 39-60.
21. Naunheim, K.S., Wood, D.E., Mohsenifar, Z., et al. (2006). Long-term follow-up of patients receiving lung-volume reduction surgery versus medical therapy for severe emphysema by the National Emphysema Treatment Trial Research Group. *Annals of Thoracic Surgery, 82,* 431-443.
22. O'Neill, B., Bradley, J.M., Macmahon, J., et al. (2004). Subjective benefit of inhaled therapies in patients with bronchiectasis: A questionnaire study. *International Journal of Clinical Practice, 58,* 441-443.
23. Rubin, L.J. (2004). Diagnosis and management of pulmonary arterial hypertension: ACCP evidence-based clinical practice guidelines. *Chest, 126*(Suppl 1), 4S-6S.
24. Simmons, P., & Simmons, M. (2004). Informed nursing practice: The administration of oxygen to patients with COPD. *MEDSURG Nursing, 13,* 82-85.
25. Tran, H., McRae, S., & Ginsberg, J. (2006). Anticoagulant treatment of deep vein thrombosis and pulmonary embolism. *Clinics in Geriatric Medicine, 22*(1), 113-134.
26. Wezel, S. (2005). Severe asthma in adults. *American Journal of Respiratory and Critical Care Medicine, 172*(2), 149-160.
27. Wick, J. (2006). Beyond the basics: Special issues in venous thromboembolism prevention. *Annals of Long-Term Care, 14*(1), 17-22.
28. Widlitz, A.C., McDevitt, S., Ward, G.R., et al. (2007). Practical aspects of continuous intravenous treprostinil therapy. *Critical Care Nurse, 27*(2), 41-50.
29. Young, B., & Flynn, T. (2005). Pulmonary emboli: The differential diagnosis dilemma. *Journal of Orthopedic & Sports Physical Therapy, 35*(10), 637-644.

evolve **Did you remember to check out the bonus material on the Evolve website and the CD-ROM, including NCLEX®-Examination Style Review Questions, Open-Book Quizzes, and Chapter Review Audio Podcasts?**

CHAPTER 62

Management of Clients with Parenchymal and Pleural Disorders

NANCY L. YORK

The parenchyma of any organ, in this case the lung, is the tissue essential for the function of the organ. This chapter reviews disorders of the lung parenchyma, such as pneumonia, tuberculosis, cystic fibrosis, and cancer.

ATELECTASIS

Atelectasis is the collapse of alveoli or lung tissue. It develops when the alveoli become airless from absorption of their air without replacement of the air with breathing. Common causes of atelectasis include inhalation of irritating anesthetics, localized airway obstruction, insufficient pulmonary surfactant, or increased elastic recoil. Examples of each of these causes are given in Box 62-1. Atelectasis is particularly common after surgery, especially upper abdominal or thoracic procedures. Clients who are older, obese, or bedridden or who have a history of smoking are also more susceptible to atelectasis.

Atelectasis may be diagnosed through physical examination, although generally it is detected on chest radiograph. Some clients are asymptomatic. If significant hypoxemia is present, however, dyspnea, tachypnea, tachycardia, and cyanosis may occur. Chest auscultation may reveal bronchial or diminished breath sounds and crackles over the involved area. Temperature of less than 101° F (38.3° C) is common. However, older adults with atelectasis typically do not exhibit a fever.

If atelectasis is severe, physical assessment findings include the following:

- A dull percussion note over the affected lung area
- A decrease in tactile fremitus over the affected lung area
- Decreased chest movement on the involved side
- A tracheal shift toward the side of the atelectasis

None of these manifestations is specific for atelectasis, and the entire clinical picture must always be considered.

One of the primary goals of nursing intervention is to prevent atelectasis in the high-risk client. Frequent position changes and early ambulation help promote drainage of all lung segments. Deep-breathing and effective coughing enhances lung expansion and prevents airway obstruction. Incentive spirometry is an excellent means of encouraging a client to deep-breathe. Administration of pain medications may assist the client in taking deeper breaths; however, they should be used with caution to prevent respiratory depression from occurring.

If atelectasis develops, treatment is directed toward the underlying cause. If the client becomes hypoxic, oxygen should be administered as prescribed (e.g., per nasal cannula, 1 to 4 L/min). More aggressive measures to maintain airway patency, such as postural drainage, chest physiotherapy, and tracheal suctioning, may also be ordered. If an airway obstruction is causing atelectasis, bronchoscopy may be used to remove the material.

BOX 62-1   **Causes of Atelectasis**

REDUCTION IN LUNG DISTENTION FORCES
- Pleural space encroachment (e.g., pneumothorax, pleural effusion, pleural tumor)
- Chest wall disorders (e.g., scoliosis, flail chest)
- Impaired diaphragmatic movement (e.g., ascites, obesity)
- Central nervous system dysfunction (e.g., coma, neuromuscular disorders, oversedation)

LOCALIZED AIRWAY OBSTRUCTION
- Mucus plugging
- Foreign body aspiration
- Bronchiectasis

INSUFFICIENT PULMONARY SURFACTANT
- Respiratory distress syndrome
- Inhalation anesthesia
- High concentrations of oxygen (oxygen toxicity)
- Lung contusion
- Aspiration of gastric contents
- Smoke inhalation

INCREASED ELASTIC RECOIL
- Interstitial fibrosis (e.g., silicosis, radiation pneumonitis)

INFECTIOUS DISORDERS

INFLUENZA

The term *flu* is often used inappropriately to describe many clinical manifestations and disorders. *Influenza* refers to an acute viral infection of the respiratory tract. Influenza usually occurs seasonally in epidemic form. People most at risk are very young children, older adults, people living in institutional settings, people with chronic diseases, and health care personnel. Influenza viruses have been identified as types A, B, and C. Type A is the most prevalent and is associated with the most serious epidemics. Type B outbreaks also can reach epidemic levels, but the disease produced is generally milder than that caused by type A. Type C viruses have never been connected with a large epidemic.

Clinical manifestations of influenza include fever, myalgias (muscular pain), and cough. Influenza predisposes to complications such as viral bronchitis or pneumonia, bacterial pneumonia, and superinfections (infections that occur during the course of antimicrobial therapy). Influenza differs from a common cold primarily in its sudden onset and widespread occurrence within the population. Conversely, colds have a slow onset of manifestations, usually do not cause fever, have malaise as a major manifestation, and commonly cause nasal manifestations.

In 2003 a large outbreak of influenza A (H5N1) or avian flu spread among poultry in Asia. By 2004 humans had become infected in nine countries; however, to date, no infection has been identified in the United States.

Spread of the avian influenza virus from an ill person to another person has been rarely reported. The majority of avian influenza infections in humans have resulted from direct or close contact with infected poultry or surfaces contaminated with secretions and excretions from infected birds. Symptoms can be mild but are more often severe and include cough, fever, acute respiratory failure, leukopenia, and thrombocytopenia. Death rates have been reported between 50% and 75%.

OUTCOME MANAGEMENT

Interventions for influenza are based on manifestations as they arise (i.e., supportive measures to relieve fever, myalgia, and cough). The Complementary and Alternative Therapy feature below summarizes research findings for certain supplements commonly used for respiratory tract infections. Antiviral medications can be prescribed for very early stages of influenza and may reduce the severity of the symptoms and shorten the duration of illness by 1 to 2 days. These drugs do not, however, replace the need for immunization.

COMPLEMENTARY AND ALTERNATIVE THERAPY

Vitamin E Supplements and Acute Respiratory Tract Infections in Older Adults

Older adults have a potentially increased risk of infectious diseases and related conditions because of reduced immune function. Therefore a randomized controlled trial was conducted to examine the effect of two capsules daily of one of the following: a multivitamin and mineral complex, vitamin E (200 mg/day), a multivitamin-mineral complex plus vitamin E, or a placebo for a maximum of 15 months. The primary outcomes measured were incidence and severity of acute respiratory tract infections. After a median study duration of 441 days, 1024 episodes of acute respiratory tract infections were reported by 68% of the participants. When the treatment groups were compared with the placebo group, results were similar for all aspects of incidence and severity of acute respiratory tract infection, except more clients in the multivitamin-mineral treatment arm experienced a significant reduction in activity restriction (34.8% versus 48.5%; $p = .04$, number needed to treat = 8). Individuals taking either multivitamin-mineral or vitamin E supplementation did not have a reduced incidence rate of acute respiratory tract infections. Interestingly, multivitamin-mineral supplementation had no effect on the severity of infection, whereas vitamin E supplementation was associated with illnesses of significantly greater severity.

REFERENCE

Gratt, J., Schouten, E., & Kok F. (2002). Effect of daily vitamin E and multivitamin-mineral supplementation on acute respiratory tract infections in elderly persons: A randomized controlled trial. *Journal of the American Medical Association, 288,* 715-721.

Influenza is a communicable disease spread by droplet infection.

Prevent the spread of this infection by encouraging clients with influenza to remain at home, practice frequent hand-washing, and cover the nose and mouth when sneezing or coughing.

Encourage clients at risk for influenza to obtain an annual immunization before the start of "flu season" each winter. Vaccination prevents influenza for many high-risk clients. Vaccination with the nasal-spray flu vaccine is now available for healthy people between the ages of 5 and 49 and who are not pregnant. However, clients who are severely allergic to eggs, have a history of Guillain-Barré syndrome, or are less than 6 months of age should not receive any type of influenza immunization.

PNEUMONIA

Pneumonia (pneumonitis) is an inflammatory process in lung parenchyma usually associated with a marked increase in interstitial and alveolar fluid. Advances in antibiotic therapy have led to the perception that pneumonia is no longer a major health problem in the United States. Among all nosocomial infections (hospital acquired), pneumonia is the second most common, but has the highest mortality.

Etiology and Risk Factors

There are many causes of pneumonia, including bacteria, viruses, mycoplasmas, fungal agents, and protozoa. Pneumonia may also result from aspiration of food, fluids, or vomitus or from inhalation of toxic or caustic chemicals, smoke, dusts, or gases. Pneumonia may complicate immobility and chronic illnesses. Pneumonia often follows influenza and together they rank as the seventh leading cause of death in the United States, and are the fifth leading cause in people older than 65.

Major risk factors for pneumonia include the following:

- Advanced age
- History of smoking
- Upper respiratory tract infection
- Tracheal intubation
- Prolonged immobility
- Immunosuppressive therapy
- A nonfunctional immune system
- Malnutrition
- Dehydration
- Homelessness
- Chronic disease states (such as diabetes, heart disease, chronic lung disease, renal disease, and cancer)

Additional risk factors are dysphagia; exposure to air pollution; altered consciousness (from alcoholism, drug overdose, general anesthesia, or a seizure disorder); inhalation of noxious substances; aspiration of food, liquid, or foreign or gastric material; and residence in institutional settings, where transmission of the disease is more likely. The Terrorism Alert feature on p. 1600 discusses the pneumonic plague.

Pathophysiology

Streptococcus pneumoniae, a major cause of bacterial pneumonia, generally resides in the nasopharynx and is carried asymptomatically in approximately 20%-50% of healthy individuals. It is the most common type of community-acquired pneumonia. Viral infections increase attachment of *S. pneumoniae* to the receptors on respiratory epithelium. Once inhaled into the alveolus, pneumococci infect type II alveolar cells. They multiply in the alveolus and invade alveolar epithelium. Pneumococci spread from alveolus to alveolus through the pores of Kohn, thereby producing inflammation and consolidation along lobar compartments. Inflamed and fluid-filled alveolar sacs cannot exchange oxygen and carbon dioxide effectively. Alveolar exudate tends to consolidate, so it is increasingly difficult to expectorate. Bacterial pneumonia may be associated with significant ventilation-perfusion mismatch as the infection grows.

Clinical Manifestations

The onset of all pneumonias is marked by any or all of the following manifestations: fever, chills, sweats, fatigue, cough, sputum production, and dyspnea. Less common symptoms include hemoptysis, pleuritic chest pain, and headache. Older clients may present not with fever or respiratory manifestations but with altered mental status and dehydration.

Chest auscultation reveals bronchial breath sounds over areas of *consolidation* (seen as dense white areas on the chest radiograph). Consolidated lung tissue transmits bronchial sound waves to outer lung fields. Crackling sounds (from fluid in interstitial and alveolar areas) and whispered *pectoriloquy* (transmission of the sound of whispered words through the chest wall) may be heard over affected areas. Tactile fremitus is usually increased over areas of pneumonia, whereas percussion sounds are dulled. Unequal chest wall expansion may occur during inspiration if a large area of lung tissue is involved; this is due to decreased distensibility in the affected area. Table 62-1 lists the most common types of pneumonia and their clinical manifestations.

A chest radiograph provides information about the location and extent of the pneumonia consolidation. Definitive diagnosis is usually determined through sputum culture analysis and sensitivity or serologic testing. Fiberoptic bronchoscopy or transcutaneous needle

Pneumonic Plague

Plague is a life-threatening infectious disease caused by the *Yersinia pestis* bacteria. These bacteria are found in rodents, notably rats, and the fleas that feed on them. However, the bacteria can also be found in wild animals such as prairie dogs. Plague-causing bacteria exist in the environment today and intentional transmission through aerosol distribution is considered a potential bioterrorism tactic.

Yersinia pestis—also called the bubonic plague—leads to skin masses and necrosis and has been responsible for the deaths of thousands of people over time. A variant of plague is the pulmonary form, which is quickly fatal. Clinical manifestations occur anytime from 1 to 6 days after becoming infected. Bubonic plague should be suspected when a person develops flu-like symptoms including swollen glands, fever, chills, headache, and extreme exhaustion, and has a history of possible exposure to infected rodents, rabbits, or fleas. Once a person has the disease, he or she can spread the bacteria to others in close contact through droplets in the air during talking, coughing, or sneezing. The bacteria can be spread before the person even shows manifestations of the disease. Because of the delay between being exposed to the bacteria and becoming ill, people could travel over a large area—possibly infecting others—before showing manifestations of the disease.

When bubonic plague is left untreated, plague bacteria invade the bloodstream and can lead to pneumonic plague. Clinical manifestations of pneumonic plague include fever, weakness, and rapidly developing pneumonia with shortness of breath, chest pain, cough, and sometimes bloody or watery sputum. Nausea, vomiting, and abdominal pain may also occur. Without early treatment, pneumonic plague usually leads to respiratory failure, shock, and rapid death. The development of these severe respiration infection manifestations in a group of people should lead to the consideration of pneumonic plague. The bacterium used in an aerosol terrorism attack could cause the pneumonic form of plague.

Pneumonic plague is typically treated with the antibiotics gentamicin and streptomycin, which should be given within 24 hours of the first manifestations. People in direct and close contact with someone with pneumonic plague should wear tight-fitting disposable surgical masks. Clients with the disease should be immediately placed in isolation and medically supervised for at least the first 48 hours of antibiotic treatment. People who have been exposed to a contagious person can be protected from developing plague by receiving prompt antibiotic treatment.

REFERENCES

1. Snow, M. (2005). Preparing for a plague outbreak. *Nursing 2005, 35,* 14.
2. Weir, E. (2005). Plague: A continuing threat. *Canadian Medical Association Journal, 172,* 155.

aspiration/biopsy may be necessary for confirmation. Additional evaluation may consist of (1) transcutaneous oxygen level analysis or arterial blood gas (ABG) measurements to assess the need for supplemental oxygen, (2) skin tests, if tuberculosis or coccidioidomycosis is suspected, and (3) blood and urine cultures to assess systemic spread.

Pneumonia may involve one or more lobe segments of the lungs *(segmental pneumonia),* one or more entire lobes *(lobar pneumonia)* (Figure 62-1, *A*), or lobes in both lungs *(bilateral pneumonia).* On the basis of location and radiologic appearance, pneumonias may be classified as bronchopneumonia, interstitial pneumonia, alveolar pneumonia, or necrotizing pneumonia. *Bronchopneumonia* (bronchial pneumonia) (see Figure 62-1, *B*) involves the terminal bronchioles and alveoli. *Interstitial (reticular) pneumonia* involves inflammatory responses within lung tissue surrounding the air spaces or vascular structures rather than the air passages themselves. In *alveolar* (or *acinar*) *pneumonia,* there is fluid accumulation in a lung's distal air spaces. *Necrotizing pneumonia* causes the death of a portion of lung tissue surrounded by viable tissue; x-ray examination may reveal cavity formation at the site of necrosis. Necrotic lung tissue, which does not heal, constitutes a permanent loss of functioning parenchyma.

OUTCOME MANAGEMENT

Medical Management

Treatment of pneumonia should include organism-specific antibiotic therapy, respiratory support as needed, nutritional support, and fluid and electrolyte management. Initial drug therapy should consist of empirical broad-spectrum antibiotics until the specific organism has been identified through sputum culture analysis. Oxygen should be administered as ordered, and bronchodilator medications, postural drainage, chest physiotherapy, and nasotracheal suctioning may be used to maintain airway patency. See the Clinical Pathway feature on Pneumonia on the website for a Care Map and clinical guide to treating pneumonia.

Nursing Management of the Medical Client

Assessment. The nursing history should explore the following areas with the client in whom pneumonia is suspected or confirmed:

- Contact with other clients experiencing similar manifestations (suggests viral or mycoplasmal pneumonia)
- Factors suggesting the presence of noninfectious diseases that produce manifestations similar to those of pneumonia (e.g., pulmonary embolism, allergic reaction to drugs or other substances, cancer)
- Lowered levels of consciousness, which increase the risk of aspiration

TABLE 62–1   Assessment and Treatment of Pneumonia

Common Name	Clinical Manifestations
Pneumococcal pneumonia (caused by *Streptococcus pneumoniae*)	Sudden onset with a single shaking chill, high fever, stabbing pleuritic chest pain, malaise, weakness, occasional vomiting, tachypnea, dyspnea, and elevated WBC count Single or multiple lobar consolidation on chest x-ray film Cough productive of rusty brown or blood-streaked purulent sputum that turns yellow and mucoid
Staphylococcal pneumonia (caused by *Staphylococcus aureus*)	Sudden onset with fever, multiple chills, pleuritic pain, dyspnea, rales, decreased breath sounds, elevated WBC count, and exaggerated cough productive of purulent golden-yellow or blood-streaked sputum Chest x-ray film may show patchy infiltrates, empyema, abscesses, and pneumothorax Disease may start with headache, cough, and myalgia
Influenzal pneumonia (caused by *Haemophilus influenzae*)	Similar to those of pneumococcal pneumonia Cough productive of apple- or lime-green purulent sputum, which may be blood-tinged
Gram-negative bacterial pneumonia (most commonly caused by *Klebsiella pneumoniae*)	Sudden onset with high fever, multiple chills, pleuritic pain, dyspnea, cyanosis, and elevated WBC count Lobar consolidation and cavitation on chest x-ray film Cough productive of red sputum resembling currant jelly (mucoid, sticky, and difficult to expectorate)
Anaerobic bacterial pneumonia, hypostatic pneumonia (caused by normal oral flora)	Insidious onset with low-grade fever, dyspnea, crackles, cyanosis, hypertension, tachycardia, and elevated WBC count Patchy infiltrates in dependent lung segments on chest x-ray film Cough productive of purulent, greenish-yellow, foul-smelling sputum
Legionnaires' disease (caused by *Legionella pneumophila*)	Prodrome of 24-48 hours with fever, headache, and malaise followed by high fever with pulse-temperature dissociation, dyspnea, hypoxia, pleuritic pain, nausea, vomiting, diarrhea, confusion, and elevated WBC count Single or multilobar consolidation and small pleural effusions on chest x-ray film Dry cough productive of scant mucoid or blood-tinged sputum
Mycoplasma pneumonia (caused by *Mycoplasma* microorganisms)	Insidious onset with slowly rising fever, headache, myalgia, malaise, and normal WBC count Pulmonary infiltrate—sometimes extensive—on chest x-ray film Cough productive of scant mucoid sputum Client may show only minimal signs and symptoms
Viral pneumonia (caused by influenza A virus)	Prodrome with headache and myalgia followed by high fever, dyspnea, normal breath sounds with occasional wheezing and crackles, and normal or slightly elevated WBC count Diffuse, patchy infiltrates on chest x-ray film Dry cough with initial mucoid sputum that later turns purulent Cough may be unproductive
Fungal pneumonia (caused by histoplasmosis, blastomycosis, coccidioidomycosis, aspergillosis, candidiasis)	Usually asymptomatic When manifestations occur; they range from brief periods of malaise to severe, life-threatening illness Typical illness resembles influenza
Parasitic pneumonia (caused by protozoa, nematodes, platyhelminths); common organism is *Pneumocystis (carinii) jiroveci*	Clients who have *P. (carinii) jiroveci* pneumonia are invariably immunocompromised (HIV) Nonproductive cough, dyspnea, pleuritic chest pain, fever and night sweats, crackles
Aspiration pneumonia (caused by aspiration of gastric contents, food, or oropharyngeal secretions)	Often asymptomatic with minor aspiration Major aspiration may lead to tachypnea, apnea, cyanosis, hypotension, fever, adventitious lung sounds (crackles, rhonchi, wheezing), hypoxemia, respiratory failure, leukocytosis

HIV, Human immunodeficiency virus; *WBC*, white blood cell.

- Presence of tuberculosis or contact with others who have active tuberculosis
- Presence and character of any chest pain
- Presence and character of cough and sputum production

Perform respiratory assessments every 4 hours, including determination of the rate and character of respirations, auscultation of breath sounds, and assessment of skin and nail beds to determine the severity of hypoxia. In addition to the physical examination, transcutaneous oxygen level analysis or ABG measurements may be used to evaluate the need for oxygen support.

Diagnosis, Outcomes, Interventions. Nursing diagnoses common to pneumonia are described here. Other applicable nursing diagnoses are *Anxiety related to shortness of air; Deficient Fluid Volume related to fever, diaphoresis, and mouth breathing; Imbalanced Nutrition: Less Than Body Requirements related to dyspnea; Pain related to frequent coughing;* and *Impaired Oral Mucous Membranes related to mouth breathing and frequent*

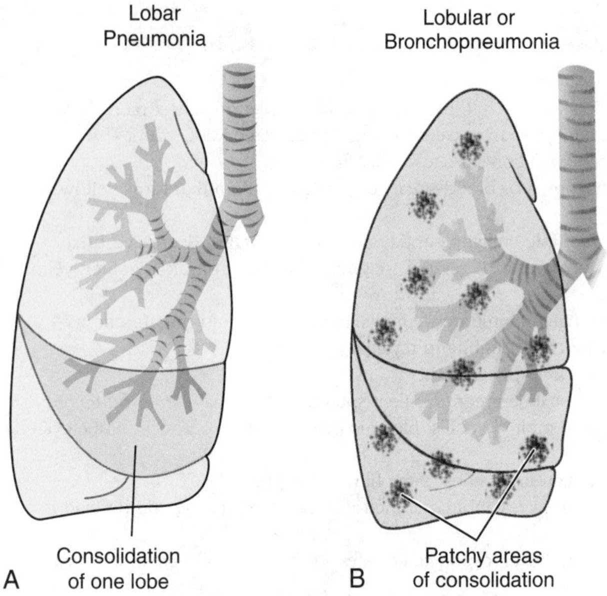

Lobar
Pneumonia

Lobular or
Bronchopneumonia

A — Consolidation
of one lobe

B — Patchy areas
of consolidation

■ **FIGURE 62–1** Two types of pneumonia. **A,** Lobar pneumonia with consolidation of one lobe of one lung. **B,** Lobular or bronchopneumonia with patchy consolidation throughout.

cough. Collaborative problems include risk of hypoxemia, respiratory failure, and sepsis.

Diagnosis: Impaired Gas Exchange. The nursing diagnosis is written as Impaired Gas Exchange related to retained secretions and inflammatory pulmonary infection.

Outcomes. The client will have improved gas exchange, as evidenced by maintaining oxygen saturations over 92% on decreasing amounts of inspired oxygen, having no manifestations of pallor or cyanosis, and retaining or improving baseline mental status.

Interventions. Titrate oxygen delivery rates to maintain oxygen saturations above 92% (or as ordered).

SAFETY
ALERT

If oxygen is administered, use needed safety precautions with oxygen and monitor oral mucous membranes.

Assess the nares for signs of drying from oxygen use and assess the skin underneath the oxygen tubing for signs of pressure ulcers. Compare ongoing assessments of skin color and mental status; improvements in oxygen saturation should improve pallor and/or cyanosis and mental status to baseline.

Diagnosis: Ineffective Airway Clearance. Ineffective airway clearance is a common diagnosis and is related to excessive secretions and weak cough. The inflammation and increased secretions seen with pneumonia make it difficult to maintain a patent airway.

Outcomes. The client will maintain effective airway clearance, as evidenced by keeping a patent airway and effectively clearing secretions.

Interventions. Take measures to promote airway patency, such as increasing fluid intake, teaching and encouraging effective coughing and deep-breathing techniques, and frequent turning. Encourage clients to use their incentive spirometer every 2 hours while awake. Clients with an altered level of consciousness should be turned at least every 2 hours and should be placed in side-lying positions, unless contraindicated, to prevent aspiration. Only thickened liquids should be given to clients with dysphagia. Administer bronchodilating medications, if prescribed. If indicated, more aggressive measures to maintain airway patency may be required (e.g., chest physiotherapy, suctioning, artificial airway).

Diagnosis: Ineffective Breathing Pattern. This diagnosis is related to tachypnea. Many clients experience compensatory tachypnea because of an inability to meet metabolic demands. This occurs because affected alveoli cannot effectively exchange oxygen and carbon dioxide. Higher respiratory rates can also develop as a result of chest pain and increased body temperature.

Outcomes. The client will have improved breathing patterns, as evidenced by (1) a respiratory rate within normal limits, (2) adequate chest expansion, (3) clear breath sounds, and (4) decreased dyspnea.

Interventions. Position the client for comfort and to facilitate breathing (e.g., raise the head of the bed 45 degrees). Teach the client how to splint the chest wall with a pillow for comfort during coughing and about the use of incentive spirometry.

Administer prescribed cough suppressants and analgesics cautiously because opioids may depress respirations more than desired. Routinely monitor respiratory rate/depth and transcutaneous oxygen levels, auscultate the chest, and document findings. Monitor ABG values, and observe for manifestations of hypoxemia, hypercapnia, and acid-base imbalance.

Diagnosis: Activity Intolerance. This diagnosis is related to decreased oxygen levels for metabolic demands. Depleted energy reserves, resulting from not eating during periods of dyspnea, and impairment of oxygen and carbon dioxide transport leave little oxygen to meet metabolic demands.

Outcomes. The client will have improved activity tolerance, as evidenced by an ability to perform activities of daily living and a progressive increase in physical activity without excessive dyspnea and fatigue.

Interventions. Assess the client's baseline activity level and response to activity. Note how well the client tolerates activity by assessing for changes in respiratory and pulse rates, marked dyspnea, fatigue, pallor or cyanosis, and dysrhythmias. Schedule activities after treatments or medications. Provide psychological support and a quiet environment to reduce anxiety and promote rest. Regulate nursing care and visitors as warranted by the client's condition. Gradually increase activity on the basis of tolerance. Balance activity with adequate rest periods.

Teach the client to avoid conditions that increase oxygen demand, such as smoking, temperature extremes, weight gain, and stress. Pursed-lip and diaphragmatic breathing, which improve air flow, as well as techniques to lower energy use, should be reinforced. Activities that are tiring should be interspersed with rest

Diagnosis: Impaired Oral Mucous Membranes. The nursing diagnosis *Impaired Oral Mucous Membranes* may be indicated and is related to breathing through the mouth

Outcomes. The client will have improved oral mucous membranes as evidenced by improved oral assessment scores.

Interventions. Assess the oral mucous membranes every shift. If the client can swab the mouth, leave swabs and water on the over-bed table. If the client cannot moisten the mouth, swab the mouth for the client. Moisten the mouth and lips before meals.

Evaluation. Pneumonia should resolve quickly once the client is receiving organism-specific antibiotics, and as long as there are no immune disorders or malnutrition. Older clients may require additional time to fully recover.

ASPIRATION PNEUMONIA

Aspiration can lead to pneumonia. Healthy people aspirate during sleep, and an even higher proportion of severely ill clients aspirate routinely, which can lead to pneumonia. Tube-feeding and thin liquids can be aspirated, especially in clients with dysphagia. Reduce the risk of aspiration in clients with dysphagia by sitting them up to 90 degrees during eating. Tube-fed clients also need the head of bed elevated, at least 30 degrees. Furthermore, hold tube feedings when residual volume is high, and stop feeding 1 hour before treatments that require lowering the head of the bed (e.g., x-ray examination, chest physical therapy [CPT]). Recognize that when holding tube-feeding often, the client is not getting the needed calories, and the volumes administered at other times may need to be increased.

Self-Care

Clients with pneumonia who are ambulatory but have an ongoing health problem may require hospitalization. For clients with intact defense mechanisms and good general health, recuperation can often take place at home with rest and supportive treatment; the term *walking pneumonia* is sometimes used to describe this situation. Walking pneumonia is generally caused by the *Mycoplasma pneumoniae* organism.

LUNG ABSCESS

Lung abscess is a collection of pus within lung tissue. Single lung abscesses usually occur distal to a bronchial obstruction, commonly from aspirated foreign material (vomitus) or tumors. Multiple lung abscesses can follow pneumonia caused by necrotizing bacteria (such as *Staphylococcus aureus,* which creates necrotic lung tissue). Bacteria may also arise from septic emboli from infected foci, such as septic phlebitis. The body attempts to wall off the abscess with fibrous tissue. If the attempt is unsuccessful, the abscess ruptures into a bronchus, causing a cough that produces copious amounts of sputum.

Early clinical manifestations are similar to pneumonia (i.e., chills, fever, pleuritic pain, cough with abundant sputum). The sputum is purulent, foul-smelling, and foul-tasting. After bronchial rupture, hemoptysis often occurs. Chest auscultation reveals decreased breath sounds and dullness to percussion over the affected area. Crackles may be present when the abscess drains. The diagnosis is commonly confirmed by chest radiography or computed tomography (CT) scan. Sputum cultures assist with identification of the organism.

OUTCOME MANAGEMENT

Antibiotics are prescribed on the basis of culture results. The client's response to antibiotics is monitored. Caring for a client with a lung abscess is similar to caring for a client experiencing pneumonia (e.g., promoting hydration, teaching effective cough techniques, and administering postural drainage).

Lung abscesses produce copious volumes of sputum. Note the color, quantity, quality, and smell of the expectorated material, including the presence of blood. Use gloves when handling articles contaminated with sputum. The sputum may have a foul taste. Provide frequent opportunities for the client to use mouthwash, brush the teeth, and floss. Because long-term antibiotic administration is usually necessary, observe oral mucous membranes for indications of *Candida albicans* overgrowth (i.e., white patches). Encourage long-term dental care. Oral nystatin (which the client swishes around the mouth and swallows or spits) may be ordered.

Antibiotic therapy for a lung abscess may be needed for 8 weeks or longer. Clients with lung abscesses must understand the importance of compliance with the medication schedule. The entire course of antibiotics must be taken. Teaching about medications should cover (1) the reasons for taking them, (2) specific directions, such as time of day, frequency, and when to take in relation to food, (3) potential side effects, and (4) what to do if side effects occur. Reassessment after the antibiotic course is completed (e.g., with culture of sputum or chest films) is essential to evaluate the effectiveness of treatment.

PULMONARY TUBERCULOSIS

Tuberculosis (TB) is one of the two most prominent mycobacterial diseases known to humankind; the other is leprosy. The Centers for Disease Control and Prevention reports an estimated 2 billion people, or one third of the world's population, are infected with the bacterium that causes tuberculosis. Before the development of anti-TB drugs in the late 1940s, TB was the leading cause of all deaths in the United States. Drug therapy, along with improvements in public health and general living standards, resulted in a marked decline in incidence over the next 3 decades. However, between 1985 and 1992, the number of reported TB cases increased by 20%. This increase was attributed to the emergence of the human immunodeficiency virus (HIV) epidemic, drug misuse, influx of immigrants from developing countries, and deterioration of the nation's health care infrastructure.

In 2005 there were 14,093 reported cases of TB in the United States, a 3.8% decline from the previous year. However, two prevalent public health concerns remain about TB. First is the increase in the number of TB cases attributable to multi-drug-resistant organisms (MDR-TB) and extensive drug-resistant organisms (XDR-TB). These forms of TB have been found worldwide and are a threat to public health as a potential epidemic that is considered practically untreatable. Resistance to drugs has developed because of the long treatment course; and clients either stop taking their medication once they begin to feel well or are noncompliant with treatment as a result of other health problems, such as substance abuse.

The second public health concern is that clients with HIV infection are particularly susceptible to TB because *Mycobacterium tuberculosis,* the organism causing TB, is an extremely opportunistic pathogen. In some HIV-seropositive populations, the TB infection rate is 1000-fold higher than the annual rate in the United States. Clients infected with HIV are at greater risk for acquiring a new infection with rapid progression to active disease or for experiencing reinfection from dormant lesions.

Etiology and Risk Factors

TB is a communicable disease caused by *M. tuberculosis,* an aerobic, acid-fast bacillus (AFB). TB is an airborne infection and generally acquired by inhalation of a particle small enough (1 to 5 mm in diameter) to reach the alveolus. Droplets are emitted during talking, coughing, laughing, sneezing, or singing. Infected droplet nuclei may then be inhaled by a susceptible person (host). Before pulmonary infection can occur, the inhaled organisms must overcome the lung's defense mechanisms and penetrate lung tissue.

Brief exposure to TB does not usually cause infection. People most commonly infected are those who have repeated close contact with an infected person whose disease is not yet diagnosed. Such people may include anyone who has repeated contacts with medically underserved clients, low-income populations, foreign-born people, or residents of long-term care facilities or institutional settings. Other high-risk populations are intravenous drug users, homeless people, and people who are occupationally exposed to active TB (health care workers).

In countries that do not have public health programs and those in which TB commonly occurs in cattle, humans may experience bovine TB after drinking raw milk from infected cattle. This form of TB can be prevented by pasteurizing milk and maintaining tuberculin skin-testing programs for cattle.

Pathophysiology
Primary (First) Infection

The first time a client is infected with TB, the disease is said to be a *primary infection.* Primary TB infections are usually located in the apices of the lungs or near the pleurae of the lower lobes. Although a primary infection may be only microscopic (and hence may not appear on chest radiograph), the following sequence of events is typically observed.

A small area of bronchopneumonia develops in the lung tissue. Many of the infecting tubercle bacilli are phagocytosed (ingested) by wandering macrophages. However, before the development of hypersensitivity and immunity, many of the bacilli may survive within these blood cells and may be carried into regional bronchopulmonary (hilar) lymph nodes via the lymphatic system. The bacilli may even spread throughout the body. Thus the infection, although small, spreads rapidly.

The primary infection site may or may not undergo a process of necrotic degeneration, called caseation because it produces cavities filled with a cheese-like mass of tubercle bacilli, dead white blood cells (WBCs), and necrotic lung tissue. In time, this material liquefies, may drain into the tracheobronchial tree, and may be coughed up. Most primary tubercles heal over a period of months by forming scars and then calcified lesions, also known as Ghon's complex. These lesions may contain living bacilli that can be reactivated, especially if the client becomes immunocompromised, even after many years, and cause secondary infection.

Primary TB infections cause the body to develop an allergic reaction to tubercle bacilli or their proteins. This cell-mediated immune response appears in the form of sensitized T cells and is detectable as a positive reaction to a tuberculin skin test. The development of this tuberculin sensitivity occurs in all body cells 2 to 6 weeks after the primary infection. It is maintained as long as living bacilli remain in the body. This acquired immunity usually inhibits further growth of the bacilli and the development of active infection.

Approximately 10% of people infected with TB will eventually develop active disease within their lifetime. The reason active TB disease develops in some clients (instead of being controlled by the acquired immune response and thereby remaining dormant) is poorly understood. However, factors that seem to play a role in the progression from a dormant TB infection to active disease include the following:

- Repeated close contact with a person who has active TB
- Advanced age
- HIV infection
- Immunosuppression
- Prolonged corticosteroid therapy
- Living or working in a high-risk congregate areas (prison, long-term care facilities)
- Low body weight (10% or more below ideal weight)
- Substance abuse
- Presence of other diseases (e.g., diabetes mellitus, end-stage renal disease, or malignancy)

Secondary Infection

In addition to progressive primary disease, reinfection may also lead to a clinical form of active TB, or secondary infection. Primary sites of infection containing TB bacilli may remain latent for years and then may be reactivated if the client's resistance is lowered. Because reinfection is possible and because dormant lesions may be reactivated, it is extremely important for clients who have had a TB infection to be reassessed periodically for new evidence of active disease.

Clinical Manifestations

The detection and diagnosis of TB are achieved through subjective assessment findings and objective test results. The diagnosis can be difficult because TB mimics many other diseases and may occur concurrently with other pulmonary diseases. Nurses and other health care providers should maintain a high index of suspicion for TB in high-risk clients.

The history includes assessing the probability of recent or past exposure to TB as well as the client's occupation, other usual activities, and travel to or residence in countries with a high incidence of TB. A history of TB exposure is important, but most clients are unaware of exposure. It is advisable to determine whether the client has been previously tested for TB and to obtain the results of that testing. Typical findings in pulmonary TB are found in Box 62-2.

Primary TB infections may remain unrecognized because they are relatively asymptomatic. Calcified lesions

BOX 62-2 Symptoms of Active Tuberculosis
PULMONARY SYMPTOMS
■ Dyspnea
■ Nonproductive or productive cough
■ Hemoptysis
■ Chest pain that may be pleuritic or dull
■ Chest tightness
■ Crackles may be present on auscultation
GENERAL SYMPTOMS
■ Fatigue
■ Anorexia (loss of appetite)
■ Weight loss
■ Low-grade fever with chills and sweats (often at night)

on chest radiograph and a positive skin test reaction are frequently the only indications that a primary TB infection has occurred. Most clients harbor tubercle bacilli for life and never experience active disease because their body defenses are adequate to arrest primary infection. The tubercles heal through fibrosis and calcification. When an infected person develops the active disease, the following may occur: (1) the primary complex sites progress and worsen, (2) cavitation within the lung occurs, (3) active infection is spread, and (4) the client becomes clinically ill.

Diagnostic Findings

Tuberculin Skin Testing. Tuberculin skin testing, typically the Mantoux test, is performed on a routine basis in high-risk groups when active TB is suspected. Mantoux testing uses purified protein derivative (PPD) tuberculin to identify TB infection. A small amount (0.1 ml) of the derivative is administered intradermally to form a 6- to 10-mm wheal. The wheal must be examined ("read") in 48 to 72 hours by a trained professional. The presence of induration (a palpable, hard, raised formation), not erythema, indicates a positive test result. Table 62-2 shows how to interpret the TB skin test.

False-positive reactions to tuberculin skin testing can occur in clients who have other mycobacterial infections or who have received the bacille Calmette-Guérin (BCG) vaccination. False-negative reactions are also possible, especially in people who are immunosuppressed or anergic (impaired ability to react to antigens). For these clients, and for anyone who has a positive skin test reaction, the AFB sputum smear examination and chest radiograph are used to identify active disease. It is critical to initiate respiratory isolation of such clients until AFB sputum results are known.

The term tuberculin converter refers to a client who does not show radiologic or bacteriologic evidence of pulmonary TB but whose tuberculin skin test "converts" from a known negative reaction to a known positive

TABLE 62–2 Classifying Positive Tuberculosis Skin Test Reactions

Reaction ≥5-mm induration is considered positive in:	Reaction ≥10-mm induration is considered positive in:	Reaction ≥15-mm induration is considered positive in:
People suspected of having TB disease	Recent immigrants from high prevalence countries	People with no known risk factors for TB
HIV-infected people	IV drug users	
Recent contacts of infectious TB	Residents or employees of high-risk congregate areas	
People with fibrotic changes on chest x-ray consistent with prior TB	Mycobacteriology lab personnel	
Organ transplant recipients	Children <4 years, or children or adolescents exposed to adults at high risk	
People taking immunosuppressive therapy		

From Centers for Disease Control and Prevention. (2006) Prevention and control of tuberculosis in correctional and detention facilities: Recommendations from the CDC. *Morbidity and Mortality Weekly Report,* 55, 1-62.

reaction. The absence of a positive (reactive) tuberculin test result does not always mean that TB is absent.

QuantiFERON-TB Gold Test. The QuantiFERON-TB Gold Test is a newer diagnostic exam that was introduced in 2005. It is a blood test used to determine how a client's immune system reacts to *M. tuberculosis*. A positive QuantiFERON-TB Gold Test only tells that a person has been infected, and like the Mantoux skin test, does not confirm if a client has progressed to the active TB disease.

Acid-Fast Bacillus Smear and Culture. A more definitive diagnosis of TB is made from the AFB smear and culture. Three different sputum specimens are collected on three consecutive mornings. Sputum AFB smears are not extremely sensitive, but the positive result of a sputum AFB smear confirms active disease. A more reliable indicator is a positive culture for *M. tuberculosis,* which does confirm active TB; however, final culture results may not be available for 2 to 12 weeks. Although newer detection tests can generate faster results and show clinical promise, the increasing prevalence of MDR-TB and XDR-TB still mandates the use of traditional culture methods for diagnosis.

OUTCOME MANAGEMENT

Medical Management

Most people with newly diagnosed active TB are not hospitalized. If pulmonary TB is diagnosed in the hospitalized client, the client may be kept in the hospital until therapeutic drug levels are established. Some clients with active TB may be hospitalized for the following reasons:

- They are acutely ill.
- Concomitant diseases are present and acute.
- Their living situation is considered a high risk.
- They are thought to be noncompliant with therapy.

- They have a history of previous TB and noncompliance, and the disease has been reactivated.
- Improvement does not occur after treatment.
- The organisms are highly resistant, requiring second-line or third-line drugs, and brief hospitalization is required to monitor the effects and side effects of therapy.

Treatment of TB is a long-term process that should be initiated immediately upon suspicion of infection. Clients with a diagnosis of active TB are usually started on a minimum of four medications to ensure elimination of resistant organisms. The dose of some drugs may initially be large because the bacilli are difficult to kill. Treatment continues long enough to eliminate or substantially reduce the number of dormant or semidormant bacilli.

Medications used for TB may include *first-line* and *second-line* agents. *First-line* agents are almost always initially prescribed until results of culture and sensitivity tests are available. In clients with a previous history of incomplete TB treatment, resistant organisms may have developed and secondary agents are used.

The CDC currently recommends a two-phase approach for treatment, consisting of (1) an *induction* phase, using four drugs aimed at destroying large numbers of rapidly multiplying organisms, and (2) a *continuation* phase, usually using two drugs directed at eliminating remaining bacilli.

The recommended treatment regimen for previously untreated clients is 2 months of isoniazid (INH), rifampin (RIF), pyrazinamide, and ethambutol. This treatment, outlined in the Integrating Pharmacology feature on p. 1607, is followed by 4 or 7 months of a combination of INH with either rifampin or rifapentine. The length of time a client remains infectious varies. Sputum cultures and clinical responses (absence of fever and dyspnea, reduction in cough) are used to evaluate the effectiveness of the therapy.

If compliance with daily dosing is a problem, TB protocols call for administration of medications two or three

Tuberculosis Medications

Four medications are considered *first-line* for the treatment of tuberculosis: isoniazid, rifampin, pyrazinamide, and ethambutol. There are four different medication regimen choices using these drugs. Each regimen choice has an initial 2-month *induction* phase, followed by a *continuation* phase of either 4 or 7 months, depending upon laboratory findings.[1]

Isoniazid (INH) is the single most important drug used in treating TB. It is most frequently administered orally; however, other routes include intramuscular and intravenous administration. INH is low cost and can be given daily or two or three times weekly. It is metabolized by the liver and should be temporarily discontinued if liver enzymes are elevated to three times the normal range or if manifestations of hepatic toxicity (such as nausea, vomiting, anorexia, fatigue, or jaundice) occur. Typically INH is well tolerated by clients; however, the risk of developing hepatitis increases with age, alcohol consumption, and underlying liver disease.

Rifampin (RIF) is also a potent antituberculosis medication that can be given either orally or intravenously and is metabolized by the liver. Both INH and RIF are bactericidal and the combination of the two drugs allows action against active, slow, and intermittently growing organisms. A common side effect of RIF is that it colors the body fluids such as urine, sweat, saliva, sputum, and tears orange. Gastrointestinal upset is also a common side effect that can be decreased by dividing the dose in half and taking it twice a day with meals instead of once a day. Hepatotoxicity is rare but can occur.

Pyrazinamide and ethambutol provide adjunct effects that reduce the risk of acquired drug resistance while accelerating the client's response to treatment. Pyrazinamide is given to clients because of its effects of eliminating bacteria that are resistant to INH and RIF. Ethambutol is also given to clients until susceptibility to INH and RIF is demonstrated, at which time the drug can be discontinued.

Because of the duration of treatment, medication side effects, and lack of awareness of the severity of TB, noncompliance remains a serious problem. Local and national health initiatives, including providing medications at no cost, have been used to address these issues.

REFERENCES

1. Driver, C.R., Matus, S.P., Bayuga, S., et al. (2005). Factors associated with tuberculosis treatment interruption in New York City. *Journal of Public Health Management Practice, 11*, 361-368.
2. Sheff, B., & Hayes, D.D. (2005). Connecting the DOTS to treat pulmonary TB. *Nursing 2005, 35*, 24-25.

times a week rather than daily. If intermittent dosing is being used, clients should be assigned to receive *directly observed therapy* (DOT). Fixed-dose combinations of drugs are also available as a means to reduce clients' noncompliance to medical therapy. Rifamate (a combination of INH and RIF) and Rifater (a combination of

INH, RIF, and pyrazinamide) combine drugs into one pill to decrease the risk of acquired drug resistance and medication errors because clients are required to take only a single daily dose. The Translating Evidence into Practice feature on p. 1608 describes how to assist with medication compliance among tuberculosis patients.

If the medication regimen does not seem effective (e.g., worsening manifestations, continued presence of AFB in sputum, increasing infiltrates or cavity formation on radiograph), then the treatment program needs reevaluation and the client's compliance should be assessed. At least two medications (never just one) are added to a failing TB treatment program.

Because medications used to treat TB have potentially serious side effects, baseline studies (depending on the specific drugs prescribed) are performed first. Drug toxicity can limit the treatment of TB. Drug tolerance, drug effect, and drug toxicity depend on factors such as the medication dosage, the time since last dosage, the medication's chemical formula, and the client's age, renal and intestinal function, and compliance with treatment.

Nursing Management of the Medical Client

Nursing management of the client with TB includes many interventions already discussed for the client with pneumonia, depending on the specific nursing diagnoses identified. Possible nursing diagnoses for the client with TB are as follows: *Anxiety; Ineffective Airway Clearance; Impaired Gas Exchange; Pain; Imbalanced Nutrition: Less Than Body Requirements; Ineffective Coping; Compromised Family Coping; Ineffective Health Maintenance; Deficient Knowledge related to treatment; Noncompliance;* and *Disturbed Sleep Pattern*.

Prevention of Transmission

During hospitalization, appropriate infection control and hospital employee health practices are essential. First, early identification of clients with TB is crucial. High-risk clients and clients with clinical manifestations of pneumonia should be placed immediately in airborne isolation until results of AFB smears and cultures are obtained. Private airborne isolation rooms should be maintained with negative pressure relative to the hallway; negative pressure keeps room air from flowing out into the hallway when the door is opened, thereby avoiding the spread of infectious particles outside the room. Negative-pressure ventilation sends room air directly to the outside, with at least six air exchanges per hour. Additional equipment, such as ultraviolet lamps (proven to kill mycobacteria) and high-efficiency particulate air (HEPA) filters, should also be used.

Personal protective equipment, called *particulate respirators,* is required for all health care workers entering a TB isolation room. When fitted properly,

SAFETY

ALERT

these respirators filter droplet nuclei; the fit of a particulate respirator should be reassessed if there is a change in the wearer's facial shape.

Monitoring health care workers' TB status is essential. Skin testing should be performed yearly in all health care workers who may be exposed to TB. Semi-annual testing should be completed in high-risk areas or where high rates of TB skin test conversion are occurring.

When a client is found to have TB, public health officials (often nurses) talk with the client and develop a contact list. Everyone with whom the client has had contact is then assessed with a tuberculin skin test and chest radiograph to evaluate for TB infection.

Preventive Therapy

Clients infected with *M. tuberculosis*, without the active TB disease, are considered to have a latent TB infection. These clients usually have a positive reaction to the tuberculin skin test; however, they are asymptomatic. Those with latent TB infection are not infectious and cannot spread TB infection to others, but approximately 10% will develop active TB disease in the future. Chemoprophylaxis may assist clients in avoiding active TB, as well as preventing initial infection in people recently exposed. Current recommendations for clients with latent TB infection include taking either isoniazid for 6 or 9 months or rifampin for 4 months.[15]

Self-Care

TB treatment is a long process. Nurses in clinics and public health facilities are often responsible for follow-up assessment and monitoring, including (1) determining medication compliance, (2) understanding the pharmacologic actions of medications, (3) monitoring unwanted side effects, (4) collecting follow-up sputum specimens, (5) obtaining serial chest radiographs, and (6) observing for reversal or worsening of initial assessment findings, all of which are part of the ongoing follow-up. It is essential that clients with TB, and their significant others, receive the information summarized in the Client Education Guide feature on Tuberculosis on the website. Providing complete information and ongoing support helps clients understand the long-term recovery process. The more information clients have and the more personal control they feel they have, the more likely they are to comply with treatment.

EXTRAPULMONARY TUBERCULOSIS

Extrapulmonary tuberculosis (XPTB) is TB that occurs anywhere outside the lungs. Pulmonary TB is the most common form of the disease, but after initial invasion, tubercle bacilli can spread throughout the body via the

---

TRANSLATING EVIDENCE INTO PRACTICE

Directly Observed Therapy for Tuberculosis

Directly observed therapy (DOT) for tuberculosis (TB) is the practice of health care personnel observing or assisting clients as they take their prescribed medications. In addition, DOT allows health care personnel to provide immediate information and support to clients who require it. Directly observed therapy may be given in a variety of settings including a clinic, hospital, client's home, school, or workplace.

Directly observed therapy is the result of increasing nonadherence to the long-term treatment plan for TB. Nonadherence is a major problem facing health care providers and clients, and was a major contributing factor in the resurgence of TB in the 1990s. Clients who do not complete their drug regimen face an increased chance of spreading the disease to others, treatment failure, relapse of disease, emergence of drug-resistant forms of the disease, increased costs of therapy, disability, and even death.

Reasons for nonadherence are many. Factors relating to nonadherence include duration of treatment, medication side effects, homelessness, and cost. Additionally, lack of awareness of the severity of their TB disease has led to interruptions in clients completing their medication therapy.

Studies have documented the positive outcomes of DOT. Clients who participate in a DOT program demonstrate higher completion rates of therapy, lower relapse rates, less acquired drug resistance, and faster sputum conversion rates (from positive to negative). These outcomes ultimately lead to lower costs of treating TB for the client and society.

IMPLICATIONS

DOT is recommended by the CDC and is currently the basis for treating tuberculosis in the United States. If properly implemented, DOT can lead to successful cure rates, decrease spreading of the disease, decrease drug-resistant forms of the disease, and decrease costs to society. Nurses need to be aware of the positive outcomes of DOT and be able to educate clients on its purpose and results. Nurses need to conduct careful assessments to identify clients who are at risk or who do not adhere to their prescribed therapy. These clients need to be introduced immediately to DOT therapy until a cure is obtained.

REFERENCES

1. Driver, C.R., Matus, S.P., Bayuga, S., et al. (2005). Factors associated with tuberculosis treatment interruption in New York City. *Journal of Public Health Management Practice, 11*, 361-368.
2. Lobato, M.N., Wang, Y., Becerra, J.E., et al. (2006). Improved program activities are associated with decreasing tuberculosis incidence in the United States. *Public Health Reports, 121*, 108-115.
3. Sheff, B., & Hayes, D.D. (2005). Connecting the DOTS to treat pulmonary TB. *Nursing 2005, 35*, 24-25.

blood and lymph. *M. tuberculosis* thrives in oxygen-rich areas such as the cervical lymph nodes, pleura, renal cortex, bone growth plates, and meninges. It may also occur in the genitourinary tract, pericardium, abdomen, and endocrine glands.

Widespread dissemination throughout the body *(miliary tuberculosis)* involves the lungs and many other organs. It is more common in clients who are HIV-seropositive or are 50 years or older. Miliary TB may develop from delayed or late dissemination after immune system compromise in older people who were infected with TB many years earlier.

Despite the severity of the disease, XPTB is often difficult to detect. Weight loss, fatigue, malaise, fever, lymphadenopathy, and night sweats may or may not be present. The only physical finding that is specific for disseminated TB is a granuloma in the choroid of the retina. Clinical manifestations may precede changes in the chest radiograph.

The diagnosis and treatment of XPTB proceed similarly to those of pulmonary TB. However, the treatment period may be longer, and more medications may be used. Treatment depends on the extent, severity, course, and complications of the disease.

NONTUBERCULOUS MYCOBACTERIAL INFECTION

Nontuberculous mycobacteria (NTM), also known as MOTT (mycobacteria other than tubercle [bacilli]), are responsible for growing numbers of mycobacterial infections. Although NTM infection is still relatively uncommon, the following changes in disease patterns have appeared: (1) more cases, (2) wider geographical distribution, and (3) new groups of vulnerable hosts, most notably clients with HIV infection.

NTM are widely distributed in nature (i.e., in food, standing fresh water, saltwater, animal bedding, soil, animals, and birds), and most clients acquire their infections from environmental sources rather than from other diseased clients. Infection is common in the southeastern part of the United States and more prevalent in rural areas. The most commonly occurring NTM diseases are caused by *Mycobacterium avium* complex, *Mycobacterium kansasii,* and *Mycobacterium fortuitum.* The primary site of NTM disease is the lungs, although extrapulmonary sites (e.g., liver, spleen, lymph nodes, skin, joints) may occur. Disseminated disease with multiple organ involvement is also possible, most commonly in immunosuppressed clients.

Pulmonary NTM disease is similar to TB, although the clinical manifestations may be less severe. Clinical manifestations of the disease include (1) fever, (2) anorexia, (3) night sweats, (4) diarrhea, (5) abdominal pain, and (6) weight loss. Clients with pre-existing bronchopulmonary disease (e.g., bronchiectasis, chronic obstructive pulmonary disease [COPD], or healed pulmonary TB) are at highest risk of pulmonary involvement.

Diagnosis of NTM disease is often difficult because of the widespread distribution of the organisms in the environment. Definitive diagnosis of disease is possible only if NTM are isolated from specimens collected from normally sterile sites (e.g., blood, cerebrospinal fluid, bone marrow, lymph nodes) or through biopsy. However, NTM disease is strongly suspected when (1) a client presents with a clinical syndrome that is compatible with NTM, (2) no other pathogens can be identified, and (3) repeated sputum cultures reveal large numbers of NTM.

OUTCOME MANAGEMENT

The same medications used to treat TB are prescribed for NTM disease. However, NTM are considerably more resistant to drugs than *M. tuberculosis.* Consequently, combined drug regimens and treatment periods up to 24 months in duration are necessary. The more clients understand about the condition and its management, the more likely they will be to complete the full course of medication.

Other aspects of the nursing management of NTM disease are the same as for pulmonary TB (see earlier discussion). Because these diseases are not transmitted from person to person, isolation and measures to control infection, other than good hygiene, are not necessary.

SEVERE ACUTE RESPIRATORY SYNDROME

Severe acute respiratory syndrome (SARS), a coronavirus respiratory illness, was initially identified in 2003 in a unique risk group—previously healthy people. However, no new cases have been reported since late 2004. The incubation period for SARS is typically 2 to 7 days. The illness typically begins with a prodrome of fever (temperature >100.4° F [>38° C]) that is sometimes associated with chills, rigors, headache, diarrhea, malaise, and myalgia. Occasional mild respiratory manifestations are noted.

After 3 to 7 days, a lower respiratory phase begins with the onset of a dry, nonproductive cough or dyspnea, which can progress to hypoxemia requiring mechanical ventilation. As the condition progresses, chest radiograph shows focal interstitial infiltrates progressing to more generalized, patchy, interstitial infiltrates. In the late stages, chest radiograph shows areas of consolidation. Laboratory tests reveal leukopenia and thrombocytopenia or low-normal platelet counts. Early in the respiratory phase, elevated levels of both creatine phosphokinase (as high as 3000 international units/L) and hepatic transaminases (two to six times the upper limits of normal) have been noted. In most clients, renal function remains normal.

The virus is transmitted by close person-to-person contact, either when an infected person talks, coughs, or sneezes, exposing a non-infected person to respiratory droplets; or when a non-infected person touches a surface contaminated with infectious droplets and then touches their own mucous membranes. The majority of non-infected people who have close contact with a SARS-infected client remain well, while some people have reported a mild febrile illness without the severe respiratory manifestations. This suggests the illness does not always progress to the severe respiratory phase.

SAFETY ⚠️ **ALERT** **However, because of the critical nature of the illness, SARS clients should be placed in airborne isolation rooms and health care workers should wear masks and gloves when in the client's room.**

Treatment regimens currently are supportive and include antipyretics, oxygen, and ventilation. Antibiotics known to treat bacterial agents of atypical pneumonia have been found to be ineffectual. Initially, steroids were administered; however, no studies have supported their efficacy.

FUNGAL PULMONARY INFECTIONS

Most fungi that are pathogenic to humans limit their activities to the skin. However, the spores of some fungi become airborne and can be inhaled into the respiratory tract, causing pulmonary diseases that, in their chronic forms, produce granulomas similar to TB. The most common of these are coccidioidomycosis and histoplasmosis. Opportunistic fungal infections occur in clients with impaired immunity, including those who require long-term high-dose immunosuppressant therapy, have hematologic malignancies, or have undiagnosed HIV.

Coccidioidomycosis
Coccidioidomycosis is found in the Western hemisphere, primarily in the San Joaquin Valley of California, Utah, Nevada, New Mexico, Arizona, western Texas, and northern Mexico and South America. The disease is most likely to develop in people engaging in desert recreational activities or working in construction or other occupations that involve digging (e.g., archaeology, mining). The disease is mild and self-limiting in 60% of those affected. Such clients either are asymptomatic or have only mild upper respiratory tract assessment findings. The remaining 40% experience a syndrome similar to influenza, with cough, fever, pleuritic chest pain, myalgias, and arthralgias. *Erythema multiforme,* a flat, red rash that erupts with dark red papules, occurs in some people.

Histoplasma capsulatum
The causative organism of *histoplasmosis,* the fungus *Histoplasma capsulatum,* is endemic to the central and eastern portions of North America, most notably the Ohio River, Missouri River, and Mississippi River valleys.

It is also found in South and Central America, India, and Cyprus. This fungus lives in moist soil of appropriate chemical composition, in mushroom cellars, on the floors of chicken houses and bat caves, and in bird droppings, especially those from starlings, pigeons, and blackbirds.

H. capsulatum infections are usually asymptomatic or mild. Clinical manifestations include fever, fatigue, cough, dyspnea, and weight loss of 1 to 2 months' duration. A few clients may demonstrate disseminated or chronic forms of pulmonary fungal disease and have central nervous system, liver, spleen, gastrointestinal tract, or musculoskeletal involvement. Chronic disease may result in progressive changes similar to those seen with TB, including emphysema-like pulmonary structural changes.

OUTCOME MANAGEMENT

The diagnosis of fungal pulmonary diseases is usually based on history and clinical assessment findings. Skin testing is also used for coccidioidomycosis and can indicate exposure but not active infection. Chest radiographs may show hilar adenopathy (lymph gland enlargement), small areas of infiltrates, or manifestations of pneumonia. Sometimes, cavities and calcified nodules may form, usually remaining in the lungs as permanent indicators of previous infection. In addition to the pathogenic fungi, common fungal spores may cause serious, potentially fatal pulmonary disease in immunocompromised people. These fungi include *Aspergillus, Blastomyces dermatitidis, Candida,* and *Cryptococcus neoformans.*

Mild primary forms of fungal pulmonary disease usually do not require treatment. Progressive, disseminated, or chronic forms are usually treated with intravenous itraconazole or amphotericin B until the client is asymptomatic for 7 to 10 days. Initial treatment of clients diagnosed with HIV includes either itraconazole or amphotericin B. Amphotericin B is toxic and frequently causes acute reactions (e.g., chills, fever, vomiting, headache, decreased renal function) during infusion. Antiemetics, antihistamines, antipyretics, or hydrocortisone may be prescribed as premedications. To reduce the common problem of thrombophlebitis at the intravenous site, a small amount of heparin may be added to the infusion. If the disorder is not responsive to drug therapy, surgical removal of affected areas (e.g., lung cavities) may be necessary.

Nursing management in relation to fungal pulmonary infection consists of (1) providing preventive education to minimize exposure of clients to infectious fungi (i.e., learning to avoid high-risk situations and to recognize early indications of infection) and (2) offering appropriate support and education for infected clients and their significant others, along with symptomatic management of the disease. Education involves teaching not only about the disease and intervention measures but also about reportable indications of complications.

NEOPLASTIC LUNG DISORDERS

MALIGNANT LUNG TUMORS

Lung cancer is the malignant transformation and expansion of lung tissue, and is the most lethal of all cancers worldwide, responsible for 1.2 million deaths. Though declining, lung cancer remains the leading cause of cancer deaths in the United States, killing approximately 173,000 Americans annually.

There are three types of lung cancer based on the size and appearance of the cancer cells:

1. Non-small cell lung cancer (NSCLC) includes squamous cell carcinoma and adenocarcinoma. Squamous cell cancers start in the large bronchi and adenocarcinomas begin in the alveolus. Recently, specific oncogenes and inactivation of tumor suppressor genes have been found. The most important abnormalities detected are mutations involving the *ras* family of oncogenes.

2. Small cell carcinoma, also called "oat cell carcinoma," begins in the larger airways and becomes sizeable. It is linked to an oncogene called L-*myc*. The "oat" cell contains dense neurosecretory granules that often cause an endocrine/paraneoplastic syndrome. It is initially more sensitive to chemotherapy, but ultimately carries a worse prognosis and has often metastasized when initially found. This type of lung cancer is strongly associated with smoking.

3. Metastatic lung cancer is another common form of lung cancer. Tumors of the breast, colon, prostate, and bladder commonly metastasize to the lungs; however, any cancer has the capacity to spread to the lungs. Table 62-3 compares the types of lung cancer.

Etiology and Risk Factors

Cigarette smoking is by far the leading risk factor for lung cancer. People who smoke are 10 times more likely to develop lung cancer than nonsmokers. Approximately 90% of males and 80% of females who develop lung cancer are, or have been, smokers. The risk of lung cancer increases as the duration of smoking and the number of cigarettes smoked per day increases. The lung cancer death rate is directly related to the total amount (often expressed in "cigarette pack-years") of cigarettes smoked.

Second-hand smoke (SHS) is also a risk factor and has been classified by the Environmental Protection Agency as a group A carcinogen. Second-hand smoke is known

TABLE 62–3   Overview of Malignant Pulmonary Cancers

Cell Type	Approximate Incidence	Specific Characteristics	Growth Rate
Epidermoid (squamous cell)	30%	Arises from bronchial epithelium As growth occurs, cavitation may develop in lung distal to tumor; Pancoast's tumor arises in apex and upper lung zones Secondary infections distal to obstructive tumor in bronchioles commonly occur	Slow growth, with metastasis not common If metastasis occurs, usually to lymph, adrenals, and liver
Adenocarcinoma	45%	Majority arise from bronchial mucous gland Often subpleural; rarely cavitates; often arises in previously scarred lung tissue Incidence strongly linked to cigarette smoking Increasing incidence in women Bronchioloalveolar cell carcinoma is a subtype	Slow growth Can metastasize throughout lung or to other organs of body
Large cell	20%	More often peripheral mass, either single or multiple masses Cavitation common May be located centrally, midlung, or peripherally Rare hilar involvement Often grows to large tumor mass before diagnosis	Slow growth Metastasis may occur to kidney, liver, and adrenals
Small cell (oat cell)	15%	65%-75% manifest as hilar or central mass May compress bronchi Involvement of diaphragm through paralysis of phrenic nerve and hoarseness through paralysis of recurrent laryngeal nerve Pleural and pericardial effusions and tamponade often seen Does not form cavities	Rapid growth Metastasis to mediastinum and to thoracic and extrathoracic structures occurs early

to contain more than 60 cancer-causing compounds. There are no safe levels of SHS exposure for nonsmokers. Approximately 3000 lung cancer deaths are attributable to SHS annually in the United States.

People who develop lung cancer may also have a genetic predisposition. First-degree relatives of people with lung cancer have a two- to three-fold excess risk of lung cancer or other cancers, many of which are not smoking related. Age also has a role because lung cancer rarely occurs in people younger than 45 years. Tuberculosis and low levels of radiation, radon, and asbestos exposure also increase the risk of developing lung cancer. Recent studies have also suggested that smoking marijuana may increase the risk of developing lung cancer because of the high levels of tar and smokers' prolonged and deep inhalations.

Pathophysiology

Normal lung tissue is made up of cells that are programmed by genes to create lung cells of a certain size and shape that perform certain functions. Lung cancer develops when these cells mutate and reproduce excessively. The cancerous lung tissue cannot exchange oxygen and carbon dioxide and therefore performs no biological function. Furthermore, tumor cells grow and invade surrounding lung tissue. This will limit expansion of the affected lobes of the lung and interfere with gas exchange of oxygen and carbon dioxide. Airways are invaded, obstructing the flow of air. Cancerous cells invade local lymph nodes and the thoracic duct. Significant growth of the tumor and invasion may occur before diagnosis.

Clinical Manifestations

The warning signals of lung cancer are presented in Box 62-3. In many instances, lung cancer may mimic other pulmonary conditions. Extrapulmonary manifestations may occur before pulmonary manifestations. Specific clinical assessment findings vary according to tumor type, location, and extent as well as pre-existing pulmonary health.

BOX 62-3 Warning Signals of Lung Cancer

- Hoarseness
- Any change in respiratory patterns
- Persistent cough
- Sputum streaked with blood
- Frank hemoptysis
  - Rust-colored or purulent sputum
  - Fatigue
  - Chest, shoulder, back, or arm pain
  - Recurring episodes of pleural effusion, pneumonia, or bronchitis
  - Unexplained dyspnea, fever, or weight loss

Centrally located pulmonary tumors usually obstruct air flow, producing clinical manifestations such as coughing, wheezing, stridor, and dyspnea. As obstruction increases, bronchopulmonary infection often occurs distal to the obstruction. Chest, shoulder, arm, and back pain may develop as the tumor invades the perivascular nerves. Squamous and small cell tumors often cause hemoptysis. Small cell tumors may also extend into the pericardium, causing pericardial effusion and, possibly, tamponade. Cardiac dysrhythmias are also likely.

Peripheral pulmonary tumors often do not produce early assessment findings. In time, pleural pain develops that increases on inspiration, is sharp and severe, and is usually localized. Pleural effusion (see later) also occurs and, along with the pain, limits lung expansion.

Pancoast's tumor occurs in the apices of the lungs in both squamous cell and adenocarcinomatous cancers. The tumor is asymptomatic until it extends into surrounding structures. Clinical manifestations are caused by compression of the brachial plexus in the distribution from the eighth cervical nerve to the first two thoracic nerves. This results in arm and shoulder pain on the affected side along with atrophy of the arm and hand muscles. With continuing tumor growth, the ribs over the tumor (usually the first and second ribs) may be invaded, resulting in bone pain. Later, involvement of the cervical sympathetic nerve ganglia may lead to *Horner syndrome*. This syndrome consists of miosis (contraction of the pupil), partial ptosis (drooping upper eyelid), and anhidrosis (absence of sweating) on the affected side of the face.

Diagnostic Findings

Numerous diagnostic tests may be used to determine the presence and extent of lung cancer. Sputum cytologic study and chest radiograph may be initially used. Bronchoscopy may be used to biopsy a tumor located in the bronchial tree. Low-dose spiral CT scans detect involved lymph nodes and small (less than 1 cm) lung tumors in their early and treatable stages. A promising development in diagnosing lung cancer combines spiral CT screening with positron emission tomography (PET) scanning. Physiologic images show areas of accumulation in areas of the cancer. PET scans obtain images of the entire body and are used to determine whether lung cancer is isolated in one area or has metastasized.

Mediastinoscopy and thoracotomy are considered the "gold standard" for staging of lung cancer. Percutaneous transthoracic needle biopsy, esophageal endoscopic ultrasound, and endobronchial ultrasound for aspiration of involved nodes have also been used successfully to confirm the diagnosis of certain lung cancers. Radionuclide scans may be used to detect metastasis to the bone, liver, or brain. Central pulmonary tumors are easiest to locate and identify with fiberoptic bronchoscopy and sputum cytologic study. During bronchoscopy bronchial washings or brushings are performed to obtain tumor cells for cytologic and pathologic study.

The appropriate staging of lung cancer is critical because treatment and prognostic information is based on both the type and stage of cancer. Table 62-4 explains the tumor-node-metastasis (TNM) classification scheme used for lung cancer staging, which is based on the anatomic extent of the disease (Figure 62-2). Staging information is valuable in helping clients and their families make treatment decisions and set appropriate short-term and long-term goals. Staging is primarily for non-small cell lung cancer only.

Metastasis

If tumors spread, by either direct extension or metastasis, further clinical manifestations may result. Direct extension to the recurrent laryngeal nerve produces hoarseness. Compression of the esophagus may cause dysphagia. Invasion or compression of the superior vena cava produces superior vena cava syndrome, a potentially life-threatening emergency. Obstruction of venous blood flow leads to clinical manifestations, including (1) shortness of breath, (2) facial, arm, and trunk swelling, (3) distended neck veins, (4) chest pain, and (5) venous stasis. Immediate palliative surgical treatment may be necessary.

Regional lymph node involvement may produce manifestations caused by impaired lymph drainage. Involvement of the mediastinal lymph nodes may result in vocal cord paralysis, dysphagia, diaphragmatic paralysis on the affected side (resulting from phrenic nerve compression), vena cava compression, and malignant pleural effusion (see later discussion). Usually, when mediastinal lymph nodes are involved, surgical excision of the pulmonary tumor is no longer possible.

OUTCOME MANAGEMENT

Early detection is the key to improving survival rates for clients with lung cancer. When premalignant changes begin, dysplastic cells are identifiable with fiberoptic bronchoscopy and sputum cytologic studies. At this stage, lesions are potentially curable. Unfortunately, a tumor must be at least 1 cm in diameter before it is detectable on a chest radiograph and typically invasion to surrounding tissues and metastasis have usually already occurred once the tumor reaches this size.

TABLE 62–4 Staging of Lung Cancer

Stage	Tumors	Node Involvement	Distant Metastasis Present
Occult carcinoma	TX	N0	M0
Stage 0	Tis	Carcinoma in situ	
Stage IA	T1	N0	M0
Stage IB	T2	N0	M0
Stage IIA	T1	N1	M0
Stage IIB	T2	N1	M0
Stage IIIA	T3	N0	M0
	T3	N1	M0
	T1-T3	N2	M0
Stage IIIB	Any T	N3	M0
	T4	Any N	M0
Stage IV	Any T	Any N	M1

T = extent of the size and location of the primary tumor; N = regional lymph node involvement; M = presence or absence of distant metastasis. Higher numbers indicate more advanced stages and/or spread of the disease. X indicates tumor cells are present; however, no tumor is visible on radiologic exam or bronchoscopy washings.

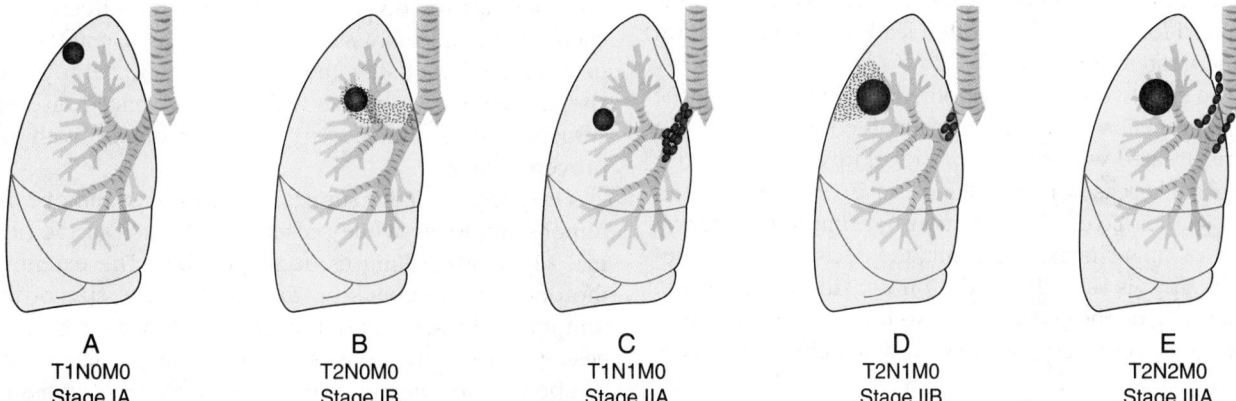

A	B	C	D	E
T1N0M0	T2N0M0	T1N1M0	T2N1M0	T2N2M0
Stage IA	Stage IB	Stage IIA	Stage IIB	Stage IIIA

■ **FIGURE 62–2** Examples of stages of lung cancer by the tumor-node-metastasis (TNM) classification system. **A,** Stage IA—T1N0M0: tumor is 3 cm or less in diameter with no metastases to regional lymph nodes and no distant metastasis. **B,** Stage IB—T2N0M0: tumor is greater than 3 cm in diameter or is any size that either invades the visceral pleura or has associated atelectasis or obstructive pneumonitis extending to the hilar region; however, there are no metastases to lymph nodes or distant metastasis. **C,** Stage IIA—T1N1M0: tumor is 3 cm or less in diameter with metastasis to lymph nodes in the peribronchial or ipsilateral hilar region, or both, without distant metastasis. **D,** Stage IIB—T2N1M0: tumor is greater than 3 cm in diameter or is any size that either invades the visceral pleura or has associated atelectasis or obstructive pneumonitis extending to the hilar region, with metastasis to lymph nodes in the peribronchial or ipsilateral hilar region, or both, without distant metastasis. **E,** Stage IIIA—T2N2M0: tumor is greater than 3 cm in diameter or is any size that either invades the visceral pleura or has associated atelectasis or obstructive pneumonitis extending to the hilar region, with metastasis to ipsilateral mediastinal or subcarinal nodes, without distant metastasis.

Medical Management

Management of the client with lung cancer depends on tumor type and stage as well as the client's underlying health status. Following diagnosis, primary treatment modalities are surgery, radiation therapy, and chemotherapy.

Radiation Therapy

Radiation therapy (radiotherapy) may potentially cure clients with locally advanced disease (1) for whom surgery poses an unacceptably high risk, (2) who have technically inoperable tumors, or (3) who refuse a thoracotomy. Radiotherapy may also be used in combination with surgery or chemotherapy to improve outcomes.

Radiation doses are limited by the presence of other structures in the treatment area and by normal tissue tolerance. Irreversible fibrotic changes and other pulmonary side effects may occur. To delineate precisely the area to be irradiated, CT scanning is often performed before treatment begins. This method also minimizes tissue damage to surrounding areas.

Radiotherapy may also be used in advanced cancers for palliation of manifestations such as chest pain, shortness of breath, cough, hemoptysis, and obstruction or compression of bronchi, blood vessels, or esophagus.

Chemotherapy

The response of lung cancer to chemotherapy depends on the tumor's cell type. SCLC responds to chemotherapeutic agents because of its rapid growth rate. Studies have demonstrated that survival in clients with SCLC can be improved with an intensive combination chemotherapy and radiotherapy to the mediastinum. However, because of the required escalating chemotherapy doses required for SCLC, toxicity often leads to discontinuation of the treatment course.

The effectiveness of chemotherapy in the treatment of NSCLC remains poor. This modality is commonly used in clients treated with surgery or radiation who experience recurrent disease or distant metastasis. However, large-scale studies have failed to demonstrate improved survival rates for such clients. As a result, the decision to use chemotherapy is usually made on an individual basis, depending on the client's previous history, current condition, and acceptance of the risks and side effects involved.

Nursing Management of the Medical Client

Diagnostic Phase

The client who is undergoing diagnostic tests for lung cancer faces an uncertain future. If the diagnosis is confirmed, the client can anticipate a variety of physical difficulties, potentially extensive medical treatment, and many emotional changes. The nursing assessment plays a critical role in developing a plan of care that will provide needed support.

The nursing history should include an exploration of the client's chief complaints, particularly cough (productive or nonproductive), fatigue, dyspnea, pain, weight loss, and recurrent infections. Ask the client about the presence of risk factors, such as a smoking history, exposure to occupational respiratory carcinogens, or a family history of the disease. Assess the client's socioeconomic situation and available social support because these factors affect subsequent management options.

Nursing management during the diagnostic phase focuses on emotional support and client education along with required physical care. Help clients maintain a sense of control by keeping them informed about all scheduled tests. Once a diagnosis of lung cancer is confirmed, nursing care must incorporate measures designed to help the client cope with anxiety and fear, family responses, financial considerations, absence from work and social activities, and possible changes in life goals.

Treatment Phase

Nursing care of the client receiving radiation and chemotherapy is detailed in Chapters 16 and 17.

Surgical Management

Surgical intervention is the treatment of choice in early-stage NSCLC. Cure is possible if the disease is still localized to the thoracic cavity and no distant metastases are present. However, few clients with NSCLC meet these criteria at the time of diagnosis. For clients who successfully undergo surgical resection, 15% will survive 5 years.

The role of surgical resection in the treatment of SCLC is limited because small cell cancer of the lung grows and metastasizes quickly. Surgery may be effective for clients with the early stages of SCLC, as a component of combined modality therapy with radiotherapy and chemotherapy. For clients with more advanced disease, surgery causes unnecessary risk and stress, with no proven benefits.

The primary aim of surgical resection is to remove the tumor completely while preserving as much of the normal surrounding lung tissue as possible. The extent of the operation depends on the location and size of the tumor and the severity of the underlying pathologic process. Clients with pre-existing pulmonary disease may not be able to tolerate extensive removal of lung tissue, anesthesia, or the risks of surgery.

Preoperative Management

Extensive pulmonary function testing may be performed before surgery to determine the client's ability to tolerate the proposed surgical intervention. Clients with impaired pulmonary function may be treated with antibiotics, bronchodilating medications, intermittent positive-pressure breathing procedures, and supervised breathing exercises to improve respiratory efficiency. Clients are encouraged to refrain from smoking during the preoperative period because smoking increases pulmonary secretions and diminishes blood oxygen saturation.

Surgical Procedures

Laser Surgery

Laser therapy is used as a palliative measure for relief of endobronchial obstructions that are not surgically resectable. However, the tumor must be accessible by bronchoscopy. Therefore tumors pressing on bronchial tissue from outside the bronchus are not amenable to laser therapy. Laser procedures do not produce systemic or cumulative toxic effects and are well tolerated. Laser therapy may be provided in an outpatient setting.

Pulmonary Resection

Complete resection of tumor remains the best chance of cure. Common pulmonary resection procedures are shown in Figure 62-3 and are discussed here.

Wedge Resection. In a wedge resection, a small, localized area of tumor near the surface of the lung is removed using special stapling devices. This operation can be performed either through a thoracotomy or by video-assisted thoracoscopic surgery (VATS). Because the resected area is small, pulmonary structure and function are relatively unchanged after healing. It is generally tolerated by most clients even if they have poor lung function.

Segmental Resection. Segmental resection is removal of one or more lung segments (a bronchiole and its alveoli). The remaining lung tissue overexpands to fill the previously occupied space.

Lobectomy. A lobectomy is the removal of an entire lobe of the lung. Postoperatively, the remaining lung overexpands to fill the open portion of the thoracic space. Clients with better lung function can tolerate removal of an entire lobe. A lobectomy is believed to be a better cancer operation since more surrounding normal lung tissue is removed. Therefore if there are microscopic cancer cells present, removal of more tissue is beneficial. A lobectomy is usually performed via a thoracotomy, but in some instances VATS can be used.

Pneumonectomy. Pneumonectomy is removal of an entire lung. Once the lung is removed, the involved side of the thoracic cavity is an empty space. To reduce the size of the cavity, the surgeon severs the phrenic nerve on the affected side to paralyze the diaphragm in an elevated position. A thoracoplasty, which is the removal of several ribs or portions of ribs to further reduce the thoracic space, may also be performed.

Closed-chest drainage is not used after pneumonectomy because there is no lung to reexpand. The empty chest can be filled with various products, such as balloons and implants to prevent shifting of the mediastinum, heart, and remaining lung.

Chest Tubes

Chest surgery causes a pneumothorax on the operated side. During a thoracotomy the parietal pleura is incised and the pleural space is entered. Atmospheric air enters the pleural space, changing the normally negative pressure in that pleural space to a positive pressure. As a result, the lung recoils to its unexpanded size and remains collapsed. Chest tubes are usually inserted in an operating room during chest surgery. However, in some emergencies, a chest tube may be inserted in a treatment room or at the bedside.

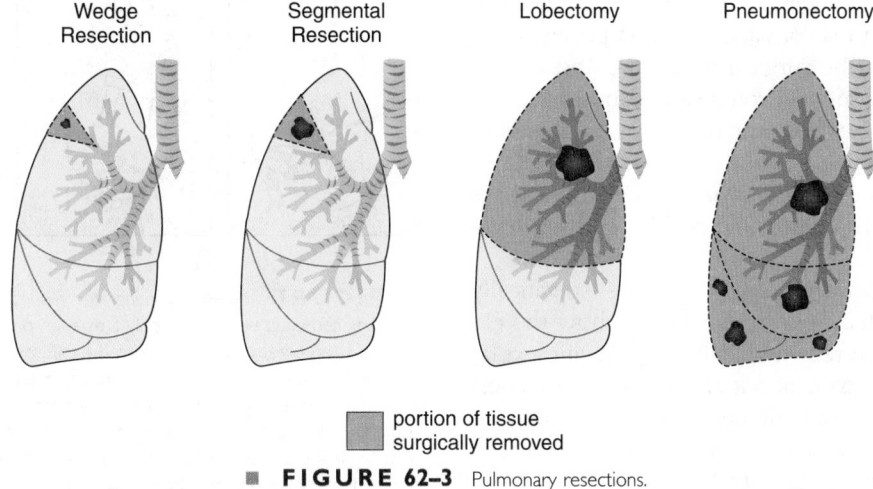

Wedge Resection · Segmental Resection · Lobectomy · Pneumonectomy

□ portion of tissue surgically removed

■ **FIGURE 62–3** Pulmonary resections.

Two catheters are usually placed in the chest following resectional surgery (except pneumonectomy). One catheter (the upper [or anterior] tube) is placed anteriorly through the second intercostal space to permit the escape of air rising in the pleural space. The second catheter (the lower [or posterior] tube) is placed posteriorly between the sixth to ninth intercostal spaces in the midaxillary line to drain serosanguineous fluid accumulating in the lower portion of the pleural space. The lower tube may have a larger diameter than the upper tube, to enhance fluid drainage. Chest tubes are brought out of the chest wall through stab wounds made by the surgeon. The catheters are secured to the client's skin with sutures.

The two chest tubes may be joined to each other with a plastic Y-junction and then attached to one closed-chest drainage system. However, it is preferable to leave them separate and to attach them to separate drainage systems. This arrangement makes it possible to monitor air and fluid drainage from each tube separately and later to remove a non-draining tube without disrupting the rest of the system. Flexible drainage tubing connects the chest tube to the drainage collection apparatus. Usually, chest tubes are connected to a closed-chest drainage apparatus before the client leaves the operating room.

Nursing Management of the Surgical Client

Preoperative Assessment
Preoperative preparation of the client with lung cancer who is to undergo surgery is the same as for any surgical client but with greater emphasis on assessment and preparation of the respiratory system (see Chapter 14 for discussion of preoperative nursing care).

Preoperative Care
Nursing interventions during the preoperative period are aimed primarily at reducing the client's anxiety level. Anxiety results from fear of cancer and its prognosis as well as from fear of the surgical procedure and insufficient knowledge of surgical routines and postoperative self-care activities. The client and family are taught about the following issues:

The anticipated surgical procedure: Assess the client's (and family's) understanding, and provide further information as needed.

The early postoperative period: Discuss specifically what can be expected postoperatively and how the client can participate in recovery activities. Specific explanations should be given about the presence of chest tubes (except with pneumonectomy) and drainage tubes, intubation and mechanical ventilation, oxygen therapy, and available pain reduction measures.

Postoperative exercises: These include (1) respiratory exercises, such as the use of incentive spirometry (IS) to maintain effective pulmonary function, (2) splinting techniques to promote effective coughing and deep breathing (Figure 62-4), and (3) leg exercises to prevent thrombophlebitis. All of these exercises should be demonstrated preoperatively, and opportunity should be given for practice and return demonstration. Document the client's preoperative inspiratory capacity using the IS and use that volume as a target goal postoperatively.

Postoperative Assessment
During the immediate postoperative period a thorough assessment is essential. Make observations as often as the client's condition warrants. Frequency of observations is determined by the following factors:

- Amount of anesthesia received and the client's reaction to it
- Amount of intraoperative blood loss
- The client's preoperative condition (e.g., presence of pre-existing medical conditions, such as COPD, diabetes, and heart disorders)
- The client's response to pain
- Facility protocols

Postoperative Care
Nursing interventions are based on careful assessment and appropriate nursing diagnoses. General postoperative nursing measures are applicable (see Chapter 14). The Care Plan feature on pp. 1618-1621 discusses nursing management of the client undergoing thoracic surgery.

Maintain Closed-Chest Drainage. Clients have closed-chest drainage after all forms of chest surgery (except pneumonectomy) and some forms of chest trauma. The chest drainage system is airtight, or closed, to prevent

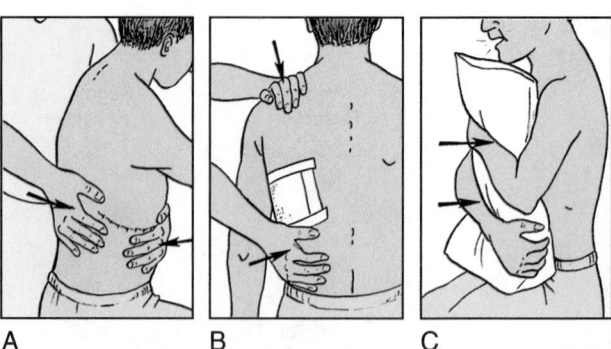

A   B   C

■ **FIGURE 62–4** Splinting techniques to promote effective coughing and deep breathing. Apply firm, even pressure after the client has taken a deep breath and during forced expiratory cough. Do not squeeze the chest or interfere with chest inspiratory expansion. **A,** Place one hand around the client's back and the other around the incisional area. **B,** Support the area below the incision with one hand while exerting downward pressure on the shoulder on the affected side with the other. **C,** Have the person hug a pillow during forced expiratory coughing.

the inflow of atmospheric pressure. Closed-chest drainage after a thoracotomy or chest trauma is used to do the following:

- Promote evacuation of air and serosanguineous fluid from the pleural space
- Prevent the reflux of atmospheric air into the pleural space
- Help reexpand the remaining lung tissue by reestablishing normal negative pressure in the pleural space
- Prevent mediastinal shift and pneumothorax by equalizing pressures on the two sides of the thoracic cavity

Two types of closed-chest drainage systems are available. The *wet suction control* systems have three main compartments (Figure 62-5, *A*):

- The *collection chamber* collects drainage and allows monitoring of the volume, rate, and nature of drainage from the pleural space.
- The *water-seal chamber* is used as a one-way valve so that air or fluids can drain from the client's chest but not return.
- The *suction-control chamber* uses suction to promote drainage from the pleural space (at a greater rate than achieved by gravity alone) and assist in reexpanding the lung.

The *dry suction control* systems have two main compartments (Figure 62-5, *B*). Regulating the level of suction is not performed through a column of water, but controlled with a self-compensating regulator using a spring or dial mechanism. Advantages of the dry system include ease in setup, no noise of bubbling water in the suction-control chamber, no evaporation of water over time, and provision of higher and more precise levels of suction. The collection chamber and water-seal chamber of a dry system are the same as for the wet systems.

Assess Chest Drainage. Measure and document the amount of drainage coming from the pleural space in the collection chamber. This record helps determine the amount of blood loss and the flow rate of drainage from the pleural space. Disposable systems are manufactured with a marked write-on surface on which to record the amount of drainage. Drainage rates and amounts are used in planning blood replacement therapy and assessing the client's status. As much as 500 to 1000 ml of drainage may occur in the first 24 hours after chest surgery. Between 100 and 300 ml of drainage may accumulate during the first 2 hours; after this time, the drainage should lessen. Excessive drainage or a sudden large increase may require further surgery to determine its cause.

Normally, chest drainage is grossly bloody immediately following surgery, but it should not continue to be so for more than several hours. Assess blood loss by monitoring the rising fluid level in the collection chamber. Suspect hemorrhage if the pulse rate becomes rapid and the blood pressure drops. Check fluid in the drainage collection chamber. If the fluid level has not risen, check the tubes for patency. Notify the surgeon if (1) the drainage remains frankly bloody for longer than the first few postoperative hours, (2) bleeding recurs after it has slowed, or (3) there are any other manifestations of hemorrhage.

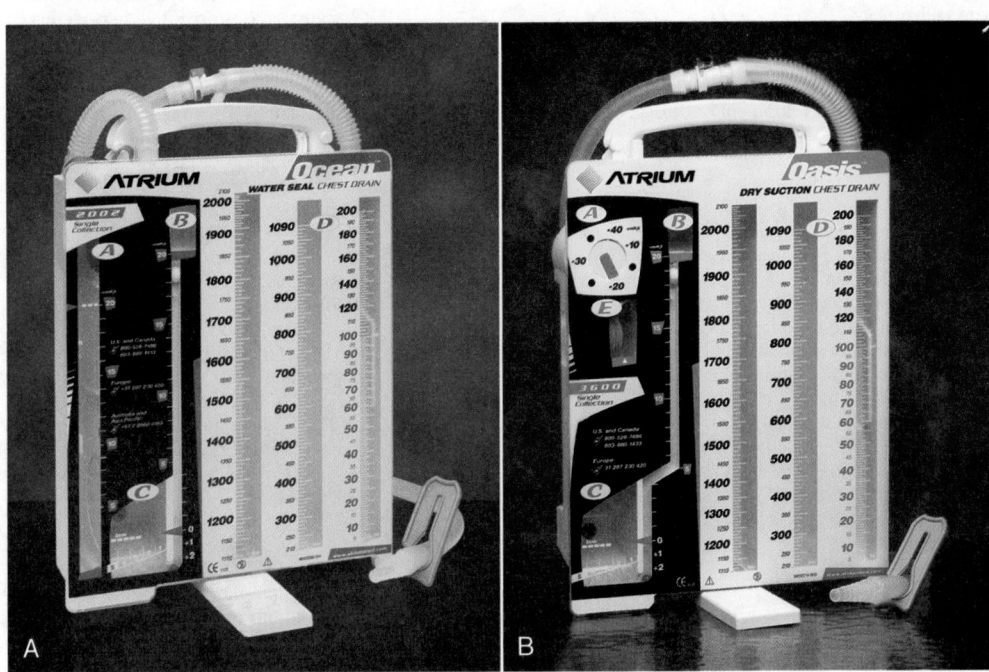

■ **FIGURE 62–5** Closed chest tube drainage systems. **A,** Three-chamber chest tube drainage system—wet suction control. **B,** Two-chamber chest tube drainage system—dry suction control.

C A R E   P L A N   *evolve*

The Client Undergoing Thoracic Surgery

Collaborative Problems: Potential complications of thoracic surgery: pulmonary edema; pneumothorax and mediastinal shift; subcutaneous emphysema; pulmonary embolism; cardiac dysrhythmias; hemorrhage, hemothorax, and hypovolemic shock; and thrombophlebitis.

Outcomes: The nurse will monitor for respiratory, cardiac, and vascular complications.

Interventions	NIC INTERVENTIONS	Rationales

1. Monitor for manifestations of acute pulmonary edema:
  a. Dyspnea
  b. Crackles
  c. Persistent cough
  d. Frothy sputum
  e. Cyanosis
  f. Decreased Sao_2 values
	Monitoring	1. Circulatory overload may result from the reduced size of the pulmonary vascular bed because of surgical removal of pulmonary tissue and delayed reexpansion of the affected lung. Additionally, hypoxia increases capillary permeability, causing fluid to enter pulmonary tissue.

2. Monitor chest tube drainage system:
  a. Amount and color of drainage
  b. Water-seal chamber for tidaling and bubbling
  c. Suction-control chamber filled to appropriate level and bubbling
  d. Intact and occlusive dressing at insertion site
	Monitoring	2. Chest tube drainage systems promote evacuation of air and drainage from the pleural space and assist in the reexpansion of lung tissue by reestablishing negative pressure in the pleural space after surgery.

3. Monitor for manifestations of tension pneumothorax:
  a. Severe dyspnea
  b. Tachypnea and tachycardia
  c. Extreme restlessness and agitation
  d. Progressive cyanosis
  e. Laryngeal and tracheal deviation to unaffected side
  f. Lateral or medial PMI shift
	Monitoring	3. Postoperative tension pneumothorax can result from air leaking through pleural incision lines if closed-chest drainage fails to function properly.

4. Observe for subcutaneous emphysema around incision and in the chest and neck:
  a. Assess progression by periodically marking the chest with a skin-marking pencil at the outer periphery of emphysematous tissue; if neck involvement occurs, measure neck circumference at least every 1-2 hours
  b. Keep emergency tracheostomy tray at bedside
	Monitoring	4. Subcutaneous emphysema may result from air leakage at the pulmonary incision site.
		  a. Rapid progression (i.e., an increase of more than a hand's width in 1 hour) may indicate leakage through the bronchial stump
		  b. Severe subcutaneous emphysema in the neck may compress the trachea and may require tracheostomy

5. Monitor for manifestations of pulmonary embolus:
  a. Chest pain
  b. Dyspnea and tachypnea
  c. Fever
  d. Hemoptysis
  e. Indications of right-sided heart failure
	Monitoring	5. Pulmonary embolism is a serious potential complication after chest surgery and a significant cause of postoperative hypoxemia.

6. Assess cardiac monitor for the development of cardiac dysrhythmias, particularly atrial fibrillation, atrial flutter, and paroxysmal atrial tachycardia.	Monitoring	6. Cardiac dysrhythmias are fairly common after chest surgery. Rhythm disturbances result from a combination of factors, including increased vagal tone, hypoxia, mediastinal shift, and abnormal blood pH.
7. Monitor intravenous flow rates. Consult physician if fluid amounts (maintenance plus intermittent medications) exceed 125 ml/hr.	Monitoring	7. After chest surgery, intravenous fluids should not exceed 125 ml/hr because of possible circulatory overload (e.g., antibiotics).
8. Assess dressing and incisional area every 4 hours for evidence of bleeding (increase to every 1 to 2 hours if any bleeding develops). Assess drainage in closed-chest drainage system for manifestations of bleeding per hospital protocol.	Monitoring	8. Blood loss may be great with major thoracic surgery because blood vessels in the thorax are of large diameter and the incision is often large and produces considerable capillary oozing.

9. Monitor for manifestations of hypovolemic shock:
  a. Increased pulse rate
  b. Decreased blood pressure measurement
  c. Restlessness and decreased level of consciousness
  d. Decreased urine output (<0.5 ml/kg/hr)
  e. Cool, pale, clammy skin
  f. Increased respirations
	Monitoring	9. The body compensates for lost blood volume by increasing blood flow (through increased heart rate) to vital organs and decreasing peripheral circulation.

10. Monitor for thrombophlebitis:
  a. Unilateral leg edema
  b. Calf tenderness, redness, unusual warmth
	Monitoring	10. Anesthesia and immobility reduce vasomotor tone, leading to decreased venous return and peripheral pooling of blood.

11. Encourage client to perform leg exercises. Discourage placing pillows under knees, crossing the legs, or prolonged sitting. Apply elastic hose or pneumatic compression stockings, if ordered.	Monitoring	11. These measures prevent venous stasis, thus reducing the risk of thrombophlebitis.

Evaluation: Most complications occur early after surgery, except for pulmonary embolus.

Nursing Diagnosis: Ineffective Airway Clearance related to increased secretions and to decreased coughing effectiveness due to pain.
Outcomes: The client will demonstrate effective airway clearance, as evidenced by clear breath sounds, effective coughing, and adequate air exchange in the lungs.

NOC OUTCOMES	Airway Patency

Interventions	NIC INTERVENTIONS	Rationales
1. Once vital signs are stable, place the client in semi- or high-Fowler's position.	Airway Management	1. The upright position enhances lung expansion and facilitates ventilation with minimal effort.
2. Help the client cough and deep breathe every 1 or 2 hours (while awake) during the first 24 to 48 postoperative hours.	Cough Enhancement	2. Increasing the volume of air in the lungs promotes expulsion of secretions.
3. Instruct the client to take a deep breath slowly and to hold it for 3 to 5 seconds, then exhale; to take a second breath and then, while exhaling, to cough forcefully twice.	Cough Enhancement	3. Coughing helps move tracheobronchial secretions out of the lung. Deep breathing dilates the airways, stimulates surfactant production, and expands lung tissue.
4. When possible, schedule coughing and deep-breathing sessions at times when pain medication is maximally effective.	Cough Enhancement	4. The less postoperative pain a client experiences, the more effective are coughing and deep breathing.
5. Assess breath sounds before and after coughing. Provide support and reassurance: a. Explain that breathing exercises will not damage the lungs or the suture line b. Manually splint the incision area during coughing and deep breathing c. Offer sips of warm water d. Maintain adequate level of hydration and adequate humidity of inspired air e. Monitor results of chest radiographs f. Evaluate the need for suctioning	Cough Enhancement	5. This helps in evaluation of coughing effectiveness. a. Client's fear of "splitting open" the incision may hamper coughing efforts b. Physical support of the incision is both comforting and reassuring c. Warm water can aid relaxation and produce more effective coughing d. Fluids and moisture help thin secretions, making them easier to expectorate e. Frequent chest films help detect atelectasis and infection f. If coughing is ineffective, suctioning may be required to remove pulmonary secretions; suctioning should be performed cautiously so that disruption of pulmonary suture lines is avoided

Evaluation: The client will maintain clear and open airways, as evidenced by clear breath sounds, a normal rate and depth of respirations, and effective coughing. Outcomes on effective airway clearance may require days to achieve.

Nursing Diagnosis: Ineffective Breathing Pattern related to hypoventilation, pain, and decreased energy.
Outcomes: Effective breathing pattern as evidenced by a normal rate and depth of respirations, absence of dyspnea, and Sao_2 levels greater than 92%.

NOC OUTCOMES	Respiratory Status: Airway Patency, Respiratory Status: Ventilation

Interventions	NIC INTERVENTIONS	Rationales
1. Monitor for manifestations of ineffective breathing pattern: a. Tachypnea and tachycardia b. Dyspnea c. Use of accessory muscles or retractions d. Cyanosis e. Restlessness f. Decreased level of consciousness	Respiratory Monitoring	1. Postoperatively, ineffective breathing patterns may result from an altered level of consciousness because of anesthesia or decreased respiratory effort because of chest pain.
2. Monitor for and report a significant decrease in Sao_2 and Pao_2 levels and/or increased $Paco_2$ levels.	Respiratory Monitoring	2. Measuring Sao_2, Pao_2, and $Paco_2$ levels will assist in evaluating a client's respiratory status.
3. Provide interventions to reduce chest pain if present: a. Splint incisions b. Provide prescribed analgesics	Pain Control	3. A client with chest pain may take shallow breaths to prevent additional discomfort.
4. Maintain semi- to high-Fowler's positioning unless contraindicated.	Positioning	4. Fowler's positioning maximizes ventilation-perfusion

(Continued)

The Client Undergoing Thoracic Surgery—Cont'd

5. Implement measures to reduce client anxiety and fear: a. Provide reassurance b. Answer questions c. Maintain calm and supportive interactions with client and family d. Provide calm and restful environment e. Instruct client on relaxation techniques	Anxiety Reduction	5. Anxiety and fear may cause a client to breathe shallow or to hyperventilate

Evaluation: If interventions are successful, the client will demonstrate an effective breathing pattern with a normal rate and depth of respirations, absence of dyspnea, and Sao_2 levels greater than 92% within the first day postoperatively.

Nursing Diagnosis: Acute Pain related to surgical procedure.

Outcomes: The client will be more comfortable, as evidenced by verbalizing that discomfort is reduced, using less opioid medication, and increased participation in activities.

NOC OUTCOMES	Comfort Level

Interventions	NIC INTERVENTIONS	Rationales
1. Assess pain intensity using a self-report measurement tool.	Pain Management	1. Use of a consistent, valid tool promotes communication and evaluation of pain intervention effectiveness.
2. Administer pain medication as ordered.	Medication Management	2. Use of opioids is a common method of postoperative pain control. Opioids bind to opiate receptors, decreasing sensations of pain.
3. Observe for side effects of medication used.	Medication Management	3. Side effects are monitored.
4. Offer and instruct clients to ask for pain medication before pain becomes severe.	Medication Management	4. A preventive approach to pain control provides a more consistent level of relief and reduces client anxiety.
5. Assess medication effectiveness and avoid overmedication.	Pain Management	5. Adequate pain reduction must be obtained. However, overmedication can depress respirations and the cough reflex.
6. Use nonpharmacologic pain reduction measures concurrently.	Pain Management	6. Proper positioning and relaxation techniques and similar measures can augment effects of medications.

Evaluation: Pain will be most acute for the first 48 to 72 hours postoperatively, requiring opioids for pain control. Expect pain to subside after that time, and offer less potent opioids or analgesics.

Nursing Diagnosis: Impaired Physical Mobility related to pain, muscle dissection, restricted positioning, and chest tubes.

Outcomes: The client will maintain physical mobility in the arm and shoulder, as evidenced by regaining of preoperative arm and shoulder function.

NOC OUTCOMES	Joint Motion: Active

Interventions	NIC INTERVENTIONS	Rationales
1. Position client as indicated by phase of recovery and surgical procedure: a. Nonoperative side-lying position may be used until consciousness is regained b. Semi-Fowler's position (head of bed elevated 30 to 45 degrees) is recommended once vital signs are stable c. Avoid positioning client on operative side if a wedge resection or segmentectomy has been performed d. Avoid complete lateral positioning after pneumonectomy e. Avoid traction on chest tubes while changing client position; check for kinking or compression of tubing	Positioning	1. Repositioning maximizes lung expansion and drainage of secretions, promotes ventilation and oxygenation, and enhances comfort: a. This position prevents aspiration b. The upright position enhances lung expansion and facilitates chest tube drainage c. Lying on the operative side hinders expansion of remaining lung tissue and may accentuate perfusion of poorly ventilated tissue, thus further impeding normal gas exchange d. Because the mediastinum is no longer held in place on both sides by lung tissue, extreme turning may cause mediastinal shift and compression of the remaining lung e. Traction may dislodge the chest tubes; kinking or compression inhibits drainage and reestablishment of negative intrapleural pressure
2. Gently turn the client every 1 to 2 hours, unless contraindicated.	Positioning	2. Frequent turning promotes mobilization and drainage of air and fluid from the pleural space. Turning also improves circulation, promotes lung aeration, and enhances comfort.
3. Encourage regular ambulation, once the client's condition is stable. Maintain supplemental oxygen, if ordered.	Exercise Therapy: Ambulation	3. Early ambulation improves ventilation, circulation, and morale. Oxygen therapy is used to avoid hypoxia.

4. Begin passive ROM exercises of the arm and shoulder on the affected side 4 hours after recovery from anesthesia. Exercises should be performed two times every 4 to 6 hours through the first 24 postoperative hours, with progression to 10 to 20 times every 2 hours. — Exercise Promotion: Joint Mobility — 4. ROM exercises help prevent adhesion formation in the operative area, which can lead to dysfunction syndrome (i.e., "frozen shoulder").

5. Active ROM exercises are begun once the client's condition permits. — Exercise Promotion — 5. Active ROM exercises prevent adhesions of the incised muscle layers.

6. Encourage the client to use the arm on the affected side in daily activities (e.g., eating, reaching, grooming). Keep bedside stand on the operative side to encourage reaching. Teach the importance of continued use of the arm after discharge. — Exercise Promotion: Joint Mobility — 6. Regular use of the affected arm and shoulder reduces the possibility of contractures.

Evaluation: Expect the client to be able to turn independently after 24 hours. Improvement in ROM requires a few days, until pain subsides and the chest tube is removed.

Nursing Diagnosis: Activity Intolerance related to difficulty in maintaining oxygenation secondary to pain and reduced lung volume.

NOC OUTCOMES Activity Intolerance, Endurance

Interventions	NIC INTERVENTIONS	Rationales
1. Carefully assess client's response to activity and exercise. Observe for manifestations of dyspnea, fatigue, tachycardia, and tachypnea that do not subside in 3 minutes.	Monitoring	1. It may take time for the client's activity tolerance to increase, because the body must adjust to reduced respiratory capacity after resectional surgery.
2. Allow adequate rest periods between activities.	Energy Management	2. Adequate rest enables the client to cooperate more fully with activities.

Evaluation: The client's ability to tolerate activity is based on underlying lung disease, level of conditioning before surgery, and pain control. Expect the client to require several days to return to baseline.

Nursing Diagnosis: Risk for Ineffective Coping related to temporary dependence and loss of full respiratory function.
Outcomes: The client will use adaptive coping mechanisms, as evidenced by verbalizing feelings related to emotional state and taking appropriate actions to regain self-care capabilities.

NOC OUTCOMES Coping, Information Processing, Role Performance, Social Support

Interventions	NIC INTERVENTIONS	Rationales
1. Provide opportunity for client to express feelings.	Emotional Support	1. Loss of normal body function and self-care capabilities can lead to feelings of powerlessness, anger, and grief. Open expression of these feelings can help client begin coping.
2. Encourage use of positive coping strategies that have been successful in the past.	Coping Enhancement	2. The use of effective coping actions can decrease feelings of hopelessness and helplessness.
3. Allow client to have as much control over daily activities and decision making as is possible.	Coping Enhancement	3. Active involvement in the plan of care gives the client a sense of control and promotes return to independence.
4. Support and praise all independent activities that promote recovery.	Emotional Support	4. Emotional support and encouragement help motivate the client to continue progress toward independence.

Evaluation: The use of effective coping mechanisms depends on prior coping strategies. This outcome may be met quickly if the client is able to cope with a diagnosis of cancer and has hope for recovery and a support system. On the contrary, coping in the face of a dreaded diagnosis, fear of pain, little hope for recovery, and limited support systems taxes the client's coping mechanisms.

Nursing Diagnosis: Knowledge Deficit related to self-care after discharge.
Outcomes: Client will be able to state or demonstrate discharge plans.

NOC OUTCOMES Knowledge: Disease Process, Health Behaviors, Medication, Treatment Regimen

Interventions	NIC INTERVENTIONS	Rationales
1. Provide thorough instruction and preparation for hospital discharge: a. Surgical wound and chest tube insertion site care b. Continuation of exercise program c. Precautions regarding activity and environmental irritants d. Clinical manifestations to be reported to health care professionals e. Importance of regular follow-up care f. Community agencies that can provide resources, as needed	Teaching: Procedure/Treatment	1. Thorough understanding promotes compliance and enhances self-care capabilities. a. Wound care varies according to condition of incision and client b. Continued exercise increases activity tolerance and prevents complications c. Heavy lifting should be avoided; return to work depends on the client's condition and type of job; however, it is usually possible to return to work within 4 to 6 weeks; environmental irritants can cause severe coughing episodes d. Evidence of infection, deteriorating respiratory status, or other complications should be reported promptly e. The client should be monitored closely for manifestations of surgical complications, recurrence of malignancy, and metastasis f. Community resources can facilitate home management

Evaluation: Client and family must demonstrate understanding of discharge teaching before leaving the hospital.

Assess Water-Seal Function. A water seal provides a one-way valve between atmospheric pressure and subatmospheric (negative) intrapleural pressure. It allows air and fluid to leave the intrapleural space but prevents the back-flow of atmospheric air into the chest.

On expiration, air and fluid in the pleural space travel through the drainage tubing. This air bubbles up through the water seal and enters atmospheric air. On inspiration, the water seal prevents atmospheric air from being sucked back into the pleural space (which would collapse the lung). The fluid in the water-seal compartment is not drawn into the chest cavity because the negative pressures generated during inspiration in the intrapleural space are not high enough to pull the fluid through the drainage tubing. However, fluctuation of the fluid occurs during respiration; this fluctuation is called *tidaling* (tidal movement) or *vacillation*.

A closed-chest drainage system must be airtight between the pleural space and the water-seal compartment. Any air leak allows the entry of atmospheric air into the pleural space during inspiration, creating a positive pressure that collapses the lung. All connections within the drainage system must be tight and secure. Securing of tubing connections should be done with waterproof tape. The water-seal chamber itself must have an air vent to provide an escape route for air passing through the water seal from the pleural space.

Observe the Water Seal. Fluid in the water-seal compartment should rise with inspiration and fall with expiration (tidaling). When tidaling occurs, the drainage tubes are patent and the apparatus is functioning properly. Tidaling stops when the lung has reexpanded or if the chest drainage tubes are kinked or obstructed. If tidaling does not occur:

1. Check to make sure the tubing is not kinked or compressed.
2. Change the client's position.
3. Have the client deep breathe and cough.
4. If these measures do not restore tidaling, notify the surgeon. (*Note:* Tidaling may not occur or may be minimal in systems not using suction.)

Observe for Bubbling in the Water-Seal Compartment. Bubbling in the water-seal compartment is caused by air passing out of the pleural space into the fluid in the chamber. *Intermittent* bubbling is normal on expiration and indicates that the system is accomplishing one of its purposes, that is, removing air from the pleural space.

Continuous bubbling during both inspiration and expiration, however, indicates that air is leaking into the drainage system or pleural cavity. Because air entering the system also enters the pleural space, this situation must be corrected in the following manner:

1. Locate the source of the air leak, and repair it if you can. Begin by inspecting the chest wall where the catheters are inserted.
2. If a chest catheter is loose or has been partially removed, gently squeeze the skin up around the catheter or apply sterile petrolatum gauze around the insertion site. Determine whether this measure stops the continuous bubbling in the chamber.
3. If the air leak continues, check the tubing, inch by inch, and all the connections. A break in the tubing or a loose connection may be found that can be sealed with tape.
4. If the leak still cannot be located, it may be necessary to replace the drainage system.

Rapid bubbling in the absence of an air leak indicates considerable loss of air, as from an incision or tear in the pulmonary pleura. When this occurs, notify the physician *immediately* so that appropriate measures can be taken to prevent collapse of the lung or mediastinal shift, such as (1) application of suction, (2) increase in the amount of suction, or (3) thoracotomy.

When caring for a client with water-seal drainage, find out whether this particular client's water-seal chamber should be bubbling. Having this knowledge facilitates accurate assessment of the drainage pattern (e.g., if intermittent bubbling changes to constant bubbling or if an apparatus that has not been bubbling begins to bubble).

Suction. Most clients who require a chest tube postoperatively need suction for 24 to 72 hours. Suction may be applied to a closed-chest drainage system for the following reasons:

- Gravity drainage is not adequate to pull air and fluid out of the pleural space through the chest catheters.
- The client's cough and respirations are too weak to force air and fluid out of the pleural space through the chest catheters.
- Air is leaking into the pleural space faster than it can be removed by a water-seal apparatus.
- The removal of air from the pleural space must be accelerated.

The amount of suction is typically 10 to 20 cm H_2O for a *wet suction control* system. This suction is regulated by the height of the water column in the suction chamber. The more water in the chamber, the more suction (subatmospheric pressure) is created. If there was no water in the chamber, atmospheric air would go straight from the air vent into the suction source as fast as the suction was applied. Passage of the air through water slows it, and the suction force is evenly controlled. Increasing the source of suction only causes more air to travel through the air vent. The suction applied to the client remains stable. An occluded atmospheric air vent is dangerous because it causes the suction to be applied directly to the pleural cavity.

For *dry suction control* systems, up to 40 cm H_2O of suction may be applied. Conditions requiring higher amounts of suction include a large air leak from the lung parenchyma, empyema, thick pleural effusions, or hemothorax. A suction force greater than 50 cm H_2O may cause parenchymal damage and should not be applied by any type of system.

Assess Suction Apparatus Function. Because most suction regulators can create potentially damaging amounts of suction, the amount of suction in the system must be controlled. Proper functioning of a wet suction control compartment is indicated by continuous bubbling in the suction-control chamber. Vigorous bubbling does not increase the amount of suction; rather, it causes the water in the bottle to evaporate more rapidly.

Absence of bubbling in a suction-control chamber means that the system is not functioning properly and that the correct level of suction is not being maintained. Possible reasons for malfunction of a mechanical suction apparatus include (1) large amounts of air leaking into the pleural space or into the drainage apparatus and (2) mechanical problems in the regulator (suction power source). The most serious problem is air leaking into the pleural space. Check for air leaks by briefly clamping the chest drainage tube close to the client's body and observing the chamber.

If bubbling begins in the suction-control chamber, there is nothing wrong with either the drainage apparatus or the regulator. The problem is therefore an air leak into the pleural space around the chest tubes. If the air leak cannot be sealed off (e.g., with petrolatum gauze), notify the surgeon immediately.

If bubbling does not begin in the suction-control chamber when the chest catheter is clamped, the problem is in the drainage connections or the regulator. Check the system carefully, looking for loose connections and for air leaks around compartment tops and in the tubing (e.g., split tubing). Make sure that the tubing is not kinked, is correctly positioned, and has no dependent loops. If the suction power source appears to be causing the problem, obtain another suction canister and regulator.

Because the chest catheter remains clamped during this inspection, observe the client closely for indications of tension pneumothorax (e.g., dyspnea, tachycardia, hypotension, tracheal shift). As soon as the problem is corrected, the fluid in the suction-control chamber begins to bubble. Immediately remove the clamps on the chest catheter.

Promote Chest Drainage. Closed-chest drainage systems must always be placed lower (preferably 1 to 2 feet) than the client's chest. Drainage by gravity is thus maintained, and fluid is not forced back into the pleural space. Chest drainage systems must be placed upright on the floor or hung from the foot of the bed.

If the drainage apparatus is on the floor, be careful not to lower a high-low bed or side rails onto it. If a client with closed-chest drainage is to be moved, always keep the chest drainage system below the level of the client's chest.

If the apparatus is placed above the level of the client's chest, even for a moment, fluid from the drainage chamber is siphoned back into the pleural cavity. If absolutely necessary, chest tubes may be clamped briefly during momentary movement of the apparatus above the level of the person's chest (e.g., when moving drainage apparatus from one side of the bed to the other if the tubing is not long enough to allow movement around an end of the bed).

Follow positioning orders carefully. If a client can be positioned on the side that has chest tubes, be sure the client is not lying on (compressing or kinking) the catheters or tubing. This may impair drainage, cause retrograde pressure (forcing drainage back into the pleural cavity), and increase the client's discomfort. Coil the drainage tubing (connecting the chest tube to the drainage apparatus) on the client's mattress so that it falls straight to the drainage apparatus, with no dependent loops. Dependent loops of tubing that contain fluid obstruct fluid flow and create back-pressure, thus impairing air or fluid drainage.

Drainage tubing should be neither too short nor too long. Excessive tubing length causes tangling and kinking. However, make sure the tubing is long enough to allow the person to turn and sit up without pulling on the chest tubes. Each time the client is turned or moved, check the chest tubes to make sure they are not being pulled or displaced. Check the drainage tubing to be certain it is properly positioned.

Tube patency is unlikely to be a problem when chest tubes are evacuating only air or when fluid or blood is draining well by gravity. However, if fragments of a blood clot or lung tissue are visible in the tube, *milking* a chest tube may be indicated. *Milking* entails compressing the tube intermittently using a twisting or squeezing motion. Theoretically, this technique will dislodge clot material from the tube lumen and propel it toward the drainage collection chamber.

Encourage Activity. Encourage a client with closed-chest drainage to cough and deep breathe frequently. In addition to clearing the bronchi of secretions, these activities promote lung expansion and the expulsion of air and fluid from the pleural space by increasing intrapulmonary and intrapleural pressures.

A client with a chest drainage system can sit up in bed, get in and out of bed, and ambulate without clamping of the chest tubes as long as the apparatus stays upright and below the level of the chest. Do not exert traction (pull) on the tubing. Various arrangements are used to hold a chest drainage system during ambulation. The device may be placed in a wheelchair in front of the client. Many disposable units have handles to allow for carrying. If the client's condition warrants, removal of suction during ambulation may be ordered, allowing gravity drainage.

Mobile Chest Tube Drainage Systems. Mobile chest drains (Heimlich valve, Tru-Close Thoracic Vent, Pneumostat Chest Drain Valve) are smaller chest tubes that use a mechanical one-way valve instead of a water-seal chamber; and do not have a suction-control chamber. Air is allowed to leave the chest on exhalation through the one-way collapsible flutter-type valve, which then prevents air from reentering on inhalation. Mobile chest drains are used for clients who require a chest tube but do not require suction to reinflate the lung and are not draining large amounts of fluid from the pleural cavity. They are used for clients who require long-term treatment for pleural effusions or persistent air leaks. Because of their small size and lack of large drainage collection system, clients are allowed to be more mobile earlier in their recovery.

Clamp Chest Drainage Tubing. In most situations, clamping of chest tubes is contraindicated. When the client has a residual air leak or pneumothorax, clamping the chest tube may precipitate a tension pneumothorax because the air has no escape route. If the tube becomes disconnected, it is best to immediately reattach it to the drainage system or to submerge the end in a bottle of sterile water or saline to reestablish a water seal; therefore one of these sterile solutions should be at the bedside at all times. If fluid is not readily available, it is preferable to leave the tube open because the risk of tension pneumothorax outweighs the consequences of an open tube.

There are occasions, however, when clamping is appropriate, such as the following:

- Assessing a persistent air leak
- Evaluating the client's readiness for removal of the drainage system
- Changing the drainage system

Except when clamping is clearly indicated, *never* clamp chest drainage tubes without an order to do so. If clamps must be used, the best time to apply them is after an exhalation. Then remove the clamps as soon as possible.

Remove Chest Tubes. The physician determines when to remove chest tubes and closed-chest drainage. One indication that the lung has reexpanded is the cessation of tidaling in the water-seal chamber (if suction is not applied). Chest auscultation, chest percussion, and chest radiographs confirm lung reexpansion.

Usually, a lung is fully reexpanded after 2 or 3 postoperative days of chest drainage. Chest tubes are generally left in place and connected to drainage systems for an additional 24 hours after all air and significant fluid drainage have stopped. The tubes may be temporarily clamped to determine how the client will tolerate their removal. Chest tubes may not be removed if the chest is draining more than 50 to 70 ml of fluid daily. The sooner the chest tubes can be removed, the better. Their presence often contributes to postoperative pain and inactivity. The longer the tubes are in place, the greater the risk of infection. Chest tubes used for treatment of empyema (see later discussion) may be in place longer than tubes placed after chest surgery.

Clients report removal of chest tubes is moderately to severely painful. The prescribed premedication for pain reduction should be administered approximately 30 minutes before the procedure. Assemble equipment as necessary, such as sterile scissors or a suture removal kit to cut sutures securing the tubes, sterile petrolatum gauze, 4-inch × 4-inch gauze to cover the wound, and occlusive waterproof tape.

> If chest tubes are accidentally removed, cover the insertion site with sterile petrolatum gauze and notify the surgeon. Do not apply an occlusive dressing because it increases the client's risk of developing a tension pneumothorax. Observe the client closely and remove the petrolatum gauze to allow air to escape if respiratory distress develops.

BENIGN LUNG TUMORS

Benign pulmonary cancers account for approximately 2% to 5% of all primary pulmonary tumors. The term *benign* may be misleading because these tumors can mechanically interfere with lung function (e.g., obstruction of a major bronchus may occur), depending on the tumor's location. The most common benign lung tumor is the hamartoma, which usually arises in peripheral lung parenchyma. This tumor is more common in older men. Other benign tumor types are fibroma, hemangioma, lipoma, and papilloma.

Benign lung tumors are often difficult to diagnose because clients are generally asymptomatic. Unless there is pre-existing lung disease or major airway obstruction, pulmonary function study results and ABG values are usually within normal limits. The tumor may be first detected on chest radiograph or autopsy. Confirmatory diagnosis usually requires bronchoscopy or thoracotomy. Until the diagnosis is confirmed, most clients are anxious and fearful of the possibility of cancer. Emotional support is an important adjunct to the physical preparation required for diagnostic procedures.

Surgical intervention is the treatment of choice for all benign cancers. Tumor removal promptly alleviates any respiratory manifestations that may have resulted from pressure on lung structures. Postoperative management is the same as that after surgical treatment of malignant lung disease.

OCCUPATIONAL LUNG DISEASES

Occupational lung diseases are the leading cause of work-related illnesses in the United States. They are caused by the inhalation of various chemicals, dusts, and other particulate matter that are present in certain settings. Clients who are smokers or who have underlying lung disease are at a much greater risk of developing occupational lung diseases. The most commonly encountered occupational lung diseases are described in Table 62-5.

Acute respiratory irritation results from the inhalation of chemicals such as ammonia, chlorine, and nitrogen oxides in the form of gases, aerosols, or particulate matter. If such irritants reach the lower airways, alveolar damage and pulmonary edema can result. Although the effects of acute irritants are usually short-lived, some may cause chronic alveolar damage or airway obstruction.

Occupational asthma is often attributed to workplace exposure to allergens, such as plant and animal proteins (e.g., wheat flour, cotton, flax, and grain mites). In most cases, the asthma resolves after exposure is terminated. However, hyperactivity of the airways may persist for years.

Hypersensitivity pneumonitis, or allergic alveolitis, is most commonly due to the inhalation of organic antigens of fungal, bacterial, or animal origin. The nature of the exposure and the client's immunologic reactivity determine the pulmonary response. Nonatopic people (i.e., those with no history of allergies) demonstrate a pulmonary response to organic dusts more often than atopic people, although atopic people, too, may exhibit pulmonary reactions.

Pneumoconioses, or the "dust diseases," result from inhalation of minerals, notably silica, coal dust, or asbestos. These diseases are most commonly seen in miners, construction workers, sandblasters, potters, and foundry and quarry workers. Pneumoconioses usually develop gradually over a period of years, eventually leading to diffuse pulmonary fibrosis that diminishes lung capacity and produces restrictive lung disease. Early clinical manifestations are cough and dyspnea on exertion. Chest pain, productive cough, and dyspnea at rest develop as the condition progresses.

OUTCOME MANAGEMENT

Early detection is vital in preventing progression of occupational lung disease. The respiratory history should consist of (1) a complete occupational history and questions about the actual job performed rather than title or job description, (2) past as well as current occupations, (3) exposure to organic and inorganic substances in each job, and (4) smoking history. The physical examination should include assessment of respiratory pattern and effort, presence of cough, lung sounds, and other manifestations indicating potential lung disease. Some employers support ongoing assessment programs (e.g., routine pulmonary function studies or chest radiographs) for workers at risk for occupational lung disorders. Diagnosis

TABLE 62–5 Characteristics of Occupational Lung Disease

Disease	Onset of Symptoms	Diagnosis	Treatment	Clinical Course
Acute respiratory irritation	Immediate—within minutes of exposure Pulmonary edema may be delayed for hours	Consistent history Physical findings of respiratory tract irritation	Avoidance of exposure Respiratory support as needed	Resolves in hours to days Pulmonary edema may last days to weeks
Occupational asthma	Immediate—within minutes of exposure Can be delayed up to 6 hours	PFTs demonstrate reduced rates of FEV_1 to FVC Chest x-ray usually normal	Avoidance of exposure Asthma medication Steroids Bronchodilators	Resolves within hours Permanent loss of physiologic lung function may occur
Hypersensitivity pneumonitis	Within a few hours of exposure	Chest x-ray findings range from normal to fine or diffuse infiltrates PFTs demonstrate a reduction in vital capacity	Avoidance of exposure Steroids	Symptoms typically lessen in 48 hours Chest x-ray and PFT findings may last for weeks to months or may be permanent
Pneumoconiosis	Requires long-term exposure First manifestation is often cough progressing to dyspnea	Restrictive pattern on PFTs Chest x-ray with asbestosis shows interstitial markings in lower lobes and with silicosis shows opacities in upper lobes	Avoidance of exposure Cessation of smoking	Gradual worsening with fatigue, loss of appetite, chest pain, respiratory failure, and death

FEV₁, Forced expiratory volume in 1 second; *FVC,* forced vital capacity; *PFTs,* pulmonary function tests.

of occupational asthma allergens includes the nonspecific challenge test or skin-prick testing.

SAFETY

⚠

ALERT

Exposure precautions are essential for avoiding permanent pulmonary disability. Safety measures include adequate ventilation, the wearing of masks, and care in the handling of garments worn in dusty environments.

If occupational lung disease is significant, the client may qualify for a disability allowance. Refer clients to community resources, such as federal or state departments of labor, if they have questions about their eligibility for such allowances.

Nursing interventions for clients experiencing occupational lung diseases are similar to those for clients with other restrictive lung disorders (see the following discussion). Supportive measures can help clients adjust their lifestyles to their conditions.

RESTRICTIVE LUNG DISORDERS

Restrictive lung disorders constitute a major category of pulmonary problems. The category includes any disorder that limits lung expansion and produces a pattern of abnormal function on pulmonary function tests characterized by a decrease in total lung capacity (TLC). Restrictive lung diseases may result from conditions affecting lung tissues (intrapulmonary) or from extrapulmonary causes. Extrapulmonary causes include neurologic and neuromuscular disorders and disorders affecting the thoracic cage, pleura, and movement of the diaphragm. Obesity may also lead to restrictive lung disorders. Box 62-4 lists restrictive lung disorders.

Manifestations vary according to the cause of the restrictive disorder. For example, kyphosis, scoliosis, and kyphoscoliosis result in changes in the thoracic cage (Figure 62-6). Generally, clients with restrictive lung disease exhibit a rapid, shallow respiratory pattern. Chronic hyperventilation occurs in an effort to overcome the effects of reduced lung volume and compliance. Shortness of breath is experienced, at first only with exertion, but later at rest. As the disease progresses, respiratory muscle fatigue may occur, leading to inadequate alveolar ventilation and carbon dioxide retention. Hypoxemia is a common finding, especially in the later stages of restrictive lung disease.

Pulmonary function tests demonstrate impairment of the bellows' action of the lungs. Reduced total lung capacity (TLC) of less than 80% of expected value is the primary indicator of the restrictive lung disease. In addition, the ratio of forced expiratory volume in 1 second (FEV_1) to forced vital capacity (FVC), or FEV_1/FVC ratio, is normal or increased (i.e., 75% or more of expected values).

BOX 62-4   Restrictive Lung Diseases

Restrictive lung diseases are disorders affecting lung volumes and compliance of either chest wall or lung tissue. Their causes are classified as intrapulmonary or extrapulmonary.

INTRAPULMONARY
- Pulmonary fibrosis
- Sarcoidosis and other interstitial lung diseases
- Pneumonia
- Atelectasis
- Pneumoconiosis
- Surgical lung resection
- Neoplastic disease

EXTRAPULMONARY
- Head or spinal cord injury
- Amyotrophic lateral sclerosis
- Myasthenia gravis
- Muscular dystrophy
- Congenital chest wall deformity
- Acquired chest wall changes (e.g., kyphosis or scoliosis)
- Abdominal distention restricting diaphragmatic movement
- Sleep disorders
- Poliomyelitis
- Pleural effusion
- Pleurisy
- Excessive obesity

Often a specific diagnosis of restrictive lung disease is made only after extensive testing, including chest radiography, biopsy, immunologic testing, and testing to differentiate neurologic dysfunction, such as electromyography and cerebrospinal fluid analysis.

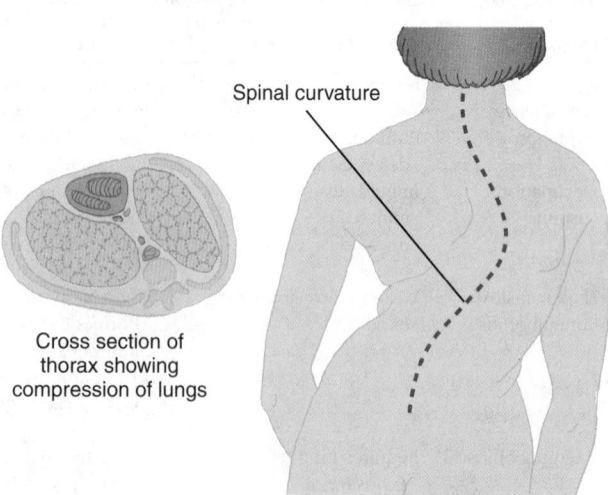

Spinal curvature

Cross section of thorax showing compression of lungs

■ **FIGURE 62–6** Thoracic scoliosis. Note the S shape of the spine. These thoracic deformities alter the chest cage space. Lung tissue may be compressed, producing altered lung function (restrictive lung disease).

Management is based on the severity of impairment and the ability to reverse the condition. Clients with spinal deformities may be helped by corrective spinal surgery. Likewise, obese clients breathe better after weight loss. Selected clients may benefit from the use of transtracheal oxygen administration or nighttime mechanical ventilation with a mask or cuirass respirator (a device that covers the chest and moves the chest wall out and back through changes in pressure), especially clients who have postpoliomyelitis syndrome.

The primary goals of nursing management of the client with restrictive lung disease are (1) promotion of adequate oxygenation, (2) maintenance of a patent airway, and (3) achievement of the highest possible functional level. Interventions to attain these goals are similar to those used in the treatment of COPD (see Chapter 61). ABG analysis is important for monitoring oxygen needs, acid-base balance, and the effects of physical activity. $Paco_2$ values should be monitored because rising carbon dioxide level is an indicator of impending respiratory failure.

Most restrictive lung disorders are not reversible. End-stage disease is characterized by the development of pulmonary hypertension, cor pulmonale, severe hypoxemia, and eventual respiratory failure. Efforts should be made to maintain the client's functional status and quality of life at as high a level as possible.

CYSTIC FIBROSIS

Cystic fibrosis (CF) is a congenital restrictive lung disorder in which the secretions of the exocrine (mucus-producing) glands are abnormal. This disorder affects the sweat glands, respiratory system, digestive tract (particularly the pancreas), and reproductive tract. CF is the most common inherited genetic disease in the Caucasian population. There are approximately 30,000 people with CF in the United States, with almost 1000 new cases diagnosed each year. CF is an autosomal recessive trait, resulting from mutations at a single gene locus on the long arm of chromosome 7. CF used to be considered a "pediatric problem" because it was fatal in childhood. However, advances in early diagnosis and treatment, including antibiotics, chest physiotherapy, and nutrition programs, have extended the median life expectancy into the mid-30s.

Pathophysiology

A gene found on chromosome 7 is responsible for the function of the CF transmembrane conductance regulator (CFTR). When the CFTR is defective, both the rate of active ion transport and the resistance to ion flow across the superficial epithelium are altered. CF airway epithelia exhibit both raised transport rates (Na^+) and decreased Cl^- permeabilities. These abnormalities in the sodium and chloride transport alter water movement across the membrane, leading to thick secretions of mucoproteins that plug the airway. Furthermore, the mucociliary transport is slowed, which decreases the ability to clear the airways of mucus and leads to stasis of mucus and a medium for infection. Lung infections often develop from *Staphylococcus aureus* and *Pseudomonas aeruginosa* organisms, which seldom infect the lungs of healthy people.

The thick mucus also plugs the glands and ducts of the pancreatic acini, intestinal glands, intrahepatic bile ducts, and the gallbladder, causing dilation and fibrosis. These changes result in decreased production of pancreatic enzymes needed for digestion of carbohydrates, fats, and proteins. Sweat glands, salivary glands, and lacrimal glands are also affected, leading to high concentrations of sodium and chloride in these secretions.

Clinical Manifestations

The most common clinical manifestation is a persistent cough that is worse at night and upon arising. As CF progresses, the cough becomes productive and then paroxysmal, with gagging and emesis. Recurrent lung infections lead to tenacious purulent, often green sputum. Asthmatic wheezing is common. Because of the pancreatic involvement, clients may have steatorrhea.

Chest radiography shows hyperinflation, and pulmonary function tests reveal increased airway resistance. The airways are hyperreactive and clients often complain of dyspnea with cold air, smoke, and exercise. CF is diagnosed by elevated chloride levels in the sweat. Distal intestinal obstruction can occur, which presents as right lower quadrant pain, loss of appetite, occasional emesis, and often a palpable mass. The syndrome can be confused with appendicitis, which occurs frequently in clients with CF.

Delayed puberty is common in both males and females with CF. The delayed maturational pattern is likely secondary to the effects of chronic lung disease and inadequate nutrition on reproductive endocrine function. Most male clients with CF are azoospermic, reflecting obliteration of the vas deferens. Twenty percent of women with CF are infertile as a result of effects of chronic lung disease on the menstrual cycle. Thick, tenacious cervical mucus blocks sperm migration, and there are possible fallopian tube and uterine wall abnormalities in liquid transport. However, more than 90% of completed pregnancies produce viable infants, and women with CF are generally able to breast-feed infants normally.

OUTCOME MANAGEMENT

The goals of CF are to ensure a reasonable quality of life for as long as possible and to prevent or slow the decline in pulmonary functioning. Goals are achieved by removing secretions, improving aeration, promoting optimal nutrition, suppressing inflammation, and administering antibiotic agents.

Clearing tracheobronchial secretions is promoted by the following measures:

- Adequate hydration
- Bronchodilators and mucolytic aerosols
- Synthetic DNase—an enzyme that breaks down deoxyribonucleic acid (DNA) released from neutrophils and causes the "stickiness" of mucus
- Twice daily inhalation of hypertonic saline solution
- Effective coughing techniques

Additional interventions to assist clients with aeration and secretion removal include noninvasive ventilation such as positive expiratory pressure devices, postural drainage, and chest physiotherapy, percussion, and exercise. Oxygen is used if hypoxemia is present. Sitting erect also facilitates breathing.

Anti-inflammatory agents decrease inflammatory responses in the respiratory tract epithelium and improve pulmonary function. Short-term systemic corticosteroids are used during acute exacerbations and nonsteroidal anti-inflammatory drugs are often given long term.

Antibiotic therapy has played an important role in extending the life expectancy of clients with CF. Administration of intravenous antibiotics is essential during acute infections. Inhaled antibiotics provide a high concentration of drugs directly into the pulmonary system while minimizing systemic side effects. The choice of antibiotic should be determined by results of sputum culture and sensitivity testing. Sputum should be assessed for color, quality, and quantity.

SAFETY
ALERT

All respiratory equipment should be thoroughly cleaned on a routine basis to prevent reinfection from contaminated equipment.

Persistent pulmonary infection with *Pseudomonas* organisms is common in the end stages of CF. Prolonged course of treatment with larger than normal doses of intravenous antibiotics is usually indicated. Moderate to severe hemoptysis can occur if the infection causes erosion of pulmonary blood vessels. Blood replacement and temporary cessation of postural drainage may be required.

Maintenance of adequate nutrition is critical. The majority of CF clients benefit from pancreatic enzyme replacement. The dose of enzymes is adjusted on the basis of weight gain, abdominal manifestations, and character of stools. Replacement of fat-soluble vitamins, particularly vitamins A, D, E, and K, is usually required.

Treatment of end-stage disease is primarily concerned with the management of severe complications. Obstruction of the airways leads to hyperinflation. In time, restrictive lung disease is superimposed on the obstructive disease. Pneumothorax (air in the chest cavity) develops in 20% of all adult clients, requiring lung reexpansion with chest tubes.

Over time, pulmonary obstruction leads to chronic hypoxemia, hypercapnia, and acidosis. Pulmonary hypertension and, eventually, cor pulmonale may result. Treatment consists of digitalis, diuretics, and oxygen therapy. Clients with severely reduced lung function (FEV_1 <30% of predicted) whose disease no longer responds to maximal therapy and who are experiencing a decline in quality of life are often considered candidates for bilateral lung transplantation.

Attention to psychosocial concerns is a nursing priority throughout the course of the disease. In the adult client with CF, psychosocial concerns center on the following three major areas:

- Disease management (e.g., treatment compliance, sleep disturbance, hemoptysis, nutrition, and hospitalizations)
- Growth and development (e.g., daily activities, work, and sex and reproduction)
- Family relations (e.g., substance abuse, depression, anxiety, and marital problems)

Nursing intervention involves helping clients cope with these problem areas as well as providing emotional support to both clients and their families.

LUNG TRANSPLANTATION

Lung transplantation is the definitive therapy for many end-stage lung diseases that are unresponsive to medical therapy. Transplantation can involve replacement of one or both of the diseased lungs with lungs from a cadaver donor or lobar transplantation from a live donor. Lung transplantation is an accepted treatment modality for end-stage pulmonary diseases such as emphysema, cystic fibrosis, alpha$_1$-antitrypsin deficiency, drug-induced pulmonary fibrosis, sarcoidosis, and primary pulmonary hypertension. Although long-term survival after lung transplantation has improved, it still lags behind other solid organ transplants.

Preoperative Care
Preoperative assessment consists of both medical and psychosocial evaluation. After the severity of lung disease is established, a battery of tests is performed to rule out active infection and to evaluate cardiac, hepatic, hematopoietic, and renal functions. The client who smokes or has an active non-pulmonary infection, significant disease in other organ systems, or poor nutritional status will be ruled out as a transplant candidate. Psychosocial evaluation focuses on assessing the client's history of compliance with medical therapy, history of substance abuse, and ability to cope with stress.

Postoperative Care

Postoperatively, the client is observed for excessive bleeding. Vital signs, hemodynamic pressures, electrocardiograms (ECGs), ABG values, urine output, transcutaneous oxygen level analysis, and chest tube drainage are monitored hourly, or more frequently as the client's condition warrants. Pulmonary edema may develop in the denervated transplanted lung. Therefore the client will be placed on mechanical ventilation with positive end-expiratory pressure (PEEP) for 24 to 48 hours.

Serum electrolytes, complete blood counts, and chest radiographs are obtained at least daily. Fluids are restricted, lung sounds are auscultated, and the severity of peripheral edema is monitored. Pain control is important to allow deep breathing and coughing in addition to chest physiotherapy. Many clients benefit from epidural analgesia. Following extubation, maintain good pain control and help the client cough, deep breathe, and use incentive spirometry to expand the lung.

The client who has received a lung transplant is at risk for infection, organ rejection, pneumothorax, pleural effusions, pulmonary embolism, venous thromboembolism, lung hyperinflation, and phrenic nerve injury. Isolation is used to decrease inadvertent exposure to pathogens. Laboratory values are monitored frequently, especially the WBC and absolute neutrophil counts. Evaluate the client for clinical manifestations of infection, such as (1) changes in vital signs (especially fever), (2) local infections at intravenous access sites and incision lines, and (3) changes in respiratory status (excessive secretions, tachypnea, dyspnea, fatigue).

Rejection of the transplanted lung may manifest as dyspnea, development of infiltrates on chest radiograph, need for ventilatory support, and fatigue. Cyclosporin A is the most important immunosuppressive agent for lung transplant clients to prevent rejection. It is initially given IV and then converted to an oral route before the client's discharge.

Following the initial procedure, the client may experience alterations in self-concept related to changes in (1) appearance, from the side effects of medications such as steroids and immunosuppressants, (2) lifestyle, or (3) work ability and role performance. Be sensitive to these issues, and encourage the client and family to discuss their feelings and explore options.

Self-Care

Before discharge from the facility, teach the client about the medication regimen, and stress the need for daily medications despite a lack of any rejection manifestations. The client should report fever, dyspnea, cough, new or increased productive sputum, chest pain, reduced exercise tolerance, excessive weight gain, and fatigue to the physician. In addition, the client should begin a pulmonary rehabilitation program.

During follow-up visits, the client is monitored for manifestations of rejection, compliance with immunosuppressive therapy, and progress in functional status.

Lung transplantation offers some hope for extended life to clients with previously fatal conditions. However, it is a frightening and stressful surgery. Clients receiving lung transplants are always critically ill before surgery. In addition, they must undergo a radical, major surgical procedure and endure prolonged intensive care and isolation procedures. Clients with transplants also must adapt to an altered self-concept. The client and significant others need constant emotional support for achievement of a successful outcome.

Successful transplant outcomes can include markedly improved ABG levels 3 months after transplantation. Unilateral lung recipients may continue to have mild hypoxemia but rarely require supplemental oxygen. Pulmonary function studies have shown that some unilateral graft recipients can reach 60% to 65% of their predicted FVC and FEV_1 values. The values for bilateral lung recipients often approach normal predicted values, but these clients can have mild restrictive physiology.

Improved exercise capacity is also observed in recipients of both unilateral and bilateral lung transplants. Typically, transplant recipients can walk 100 to 120 m/min within 6 months of transplantation and are generally able to sustain this rate over time. Any limitations in exercise capacity appear to be related to muscle deconditioning and abnormalities in skeletal muscle oxidative capacity.

SARCOIDOSIS

Sarcoidosis is an inflammatory condition that affects many body systems. While the onset of sarcoidosis typically occurs between 20 and 40 years of age, it can be present in children and older adults. The disease is characterized by the formation of widespread granulomatous lesions. In addition to lung involvement, which occurs in more than 90% of cases, clients may present with clinical manifestations involving the peripheral lymphatic system, eyes, skin, liver, spleen, bones, salivary glands, joints, nervous system, and heart.

The cause of sarcoidosis remains unknown; it is suggested that a triggering agent (which may be genetic, infectious, immunologic, or toxic) stimulates enhanced cell-mediated immune processes at the site of involvement. A series of interactions between T lymphocytes and monocyte-macrophages leads to the formation of noncaseating (i.e., having no cheesy necrotic degeneration) granulomas, which are characteristic of the disease. Granuloma formation may regress with therapy or as a result of the disorder's natural course, but it may also progress to fibrosis and restrictive lung disease. In chronic cases, approximately 10% of clients die of the disease.

As many as half of clients are asymptomatic, and the diagnosis is confirmed by chest radiography. Clients with pulmonary manifestations usually present with a dry cough and shortness of breath. Chest pain, hemoptysis, or pneumothorax may also be present. Systemic manifestations include fatigue, weakness, malaise, weight loss, and fever. A definitive diagnosis of sarcoidosis is made from tissue biopsy. When lung involvement is suspected, bronchoscopy, bronchoalveolar lavage, mediastinoscopy, or open lung biopsy may be performed.

OUTCOME MANAGEMENT

Medical management is primarily determined by the extent to which the client's life is disturbed by the manifestations experienced. If the client with sarcoidosis is asymptomatic, management involves ongoing assessment for further disease progression, such as obtaining a chest radiograph every 6 months. When manifestations are present, medical treatment usually consists of systemic corticosteroids to suppress the immune process and often leads to dramatic improvement.

Nursing intervention in clients with sarcoidosis is the same as that in clients with other restrictive lung diseases and hypoxemia. Assess for drug side effects, especially adverse responses to corticosteroids (such as weight gain, change in mood, and development of diabetes mellitus). Also assess for manifestations of improvement, such as increased exercise tolerance, disappearance of initial assessment findings, improved pulmonary function studies, and better oxygenation. If assessment findings worsen, document them and notify the physician.

INTERSTITIAL LUNG DISEASE

Interstitial lung diseases (ILDs) comprise a group of chronic and diffuse inflammatory lower respiratory tract disorders. The term *interstitial* is used to indicate that the interstitium of the alveolar walls is thickened and has become fibrotic. The alveolar walls thicken as a result of the accumulation of inflammatory cells. The thickened alveolus becomes nonfunctional.

The cause of ILD is not clearly defined. It most commonly develops from idiopathic pulmonary fibrosis, sarcoidosis, and collagen-vascular disorders. ILD can also result from the inhalation of inorganic dust (such as crystalline silica, asbestos, and coal dust) or of organic dust from organisms encountered in farming, use of air conditioning, and animal husbandry. Other possible causes are radiation damage and infectious agents.

Manifestations of ILD are insidious and nonspecific, such as fatigue, progressive dyspnea, dyspnea at rest, and nonproductive cough. Because the clinical manifestations are nonspecific, ILD may remain undiagnosed for years.

The client's history plays a major part in diagnosis because it is important to determine the agents to which the client has been exposed. Physical examination may reveal reduced chest expansion, which is reflected as a decrease in TLC. Inspiratory and expiratory crackles are frequently heard. The crackles have a characteristic sound, like the sound of hook-and-loop tape (Velcro) being pulled apart. Clubbing of the finger tips may be present.

Diagnostic assessment includes gallium ventilation-perfusion scans. These scans usually reveal impaired perfusion in the lower lobes and multiple areas of impaired ventilation. The ventilation-perfusion mismatch results in hypoxemia and carbon dioxide retention. Bronchoscopy and biopsy may also be used to confirm ILD.

OUTCOME MANAGEMENT

Management of a client with ILD is based on the level of respiratory impairment. Inflammation is controlled with corticosteroids. Explain to the client that corticosteroids reduce further impairment but previously injured alveolar-capillary units are permanently damaged. Clients often show subjective improvement while taking steroids, the dosage of which can eventually be tapered and stopped. If the offending agent is known, the initial treatment is to remove the client from exposure to the agent. As the disorder progresses, inhaled corticosteroids and bronchodilators help mobilize secretions and provide oxygen during periods of exercise. Nursing management is the same as that for clients with restrictive lung disorders.

DISORDERS OF THE PLEURA AND PLEURAL SPACE

PLEURAL PAIN

Pleural pain is a common pulmonary manifestation arising from the parietal pleura, which is richly supplied with sensory nerve endings. Pleuritic pain indicates the presence of pleural inflammation (*pleurisy*) caused by pneumonia, pulmonary infarction, pleural effusion (see the following discussion), or pneumothorax, among others. It is often accompanied by a pleural friction rub that is discovered during chest auscultation.

Pleuritic chest pain often develops abruptly and is usually severe enough that the client seeks medical attention. It commonly occurs on only one side of the chest, usually in the lower lateral portions of the chest wall, and is aggravated by deep breathing or coughing. Often the client can point directly to the exact location of the pain. However, pleural pain may also be referred to the neck, shoulder, or abdomen. Because other types of chest pain (e.g., cardiac pain, chest wall pain) may be misinterpreted as pleuritic pain, careful assessment is necessary.

Pleuritic pain may restrict normal respiratory efforts, leading to problems with gas exchange and airway clearance. If pain-relieving measures, including administration of prescribed analgesics, do not relieve the pain, the physician may perform an intercostal nerve block (see Chapter 20).

PLEURAL EFFUSION

Pleural effusion is an accumulation of fluid in the pleural space. Pleural fluid normally seeps continually into the pleural space from the capillaries lining the parietal pleura and is reabsorbed by the visceral pleural capillaries and lymphatic system. Any condition that interferes with either secretion or drainage of this fluid leads to pleural effusion.

Causes of pleural effusion can be grouped into four major categories:

- Increased systemic hydrostatic pressure (e.g., heart failure)
- Reduced capillary oncotic pressure (e.g., liver or renal failure)
- Increased capillary permeability (e.g., infections or trauma)
- Impaired lymphatic function (e.g., lymphatic obstruction caused by tumor)

Clinical manifestations depend on the amount of fluid present and the severity of lung compression. If the effusion is small (i.e., 250 ml), its presence may be discovered only on a chest radiograph. With larger effusions, lung expansion may be restricted, and the client may experience dyspnea, primarily on exertion, and a dry, nonproductive cough caused by bronchial irritation or mediastinal shift. Tactile fremitus may be decreased or absent, and percussion notes dull or flat.

Thoracentesis (see Chapter 59) is used to remove excess pleural fluid. The removed fluid is analyzed to determine whether it is transudate or exudate. Transudates are substances that have passed through a membrane or tissue surface. They occur primarily in conditions in which there is protein loss and low protein content (e.g., hypoalbuminemia, cirrhosis, nephrosis) or increased hydrostatic pressure (e.g., heart failure). Exudates are substances that have escaped from blood vessels. They contain an accumulation of cells, have a high specific gravity and a high lactate dehydrogenase (LDH) level, and occur in response to malignancies, infections, or inflammatory processes. Exudates occur when there is an increase in capillary permeability. Differentiating between transudates and exudates helps establish a specific diagnosis. Diagnosis may also require analysis of the fluid for white and red blood cells, malignant cells, bacteria, glucose content, pH, and LDH.

Pleural fluid may be (1) hemorrhagic (or bloody), such as when a tumor is present or after trauma or pulmonary embolus with infarction; (2) chylous (or thick and white), such as after lymphatic obstruction or trauma to the thoracic duct; or (3) rich in cholesterol, such as in chronic, recurrent effusions caused by tuberculosis or rheumatoid arthritis. If there is a high WBC count and the pleural fluid is purulent, the effusion is called an empyema. An empyema of any volume requires drainage and treatment of the infection.

If the pus is not drained, it may become thick and almost solidified or loculated (containing cavities), a condition called fibrothorax. Fibrothorax may significantly restrict lung expansion and may require surgical intervention. The procedure, known as decortication, involves removal of the restrictive mass of fibrin and inflammatory cells. Decortication is usually not performed until the fibrothorax is relatively solid, so it can be easily removed.

After the thoracentesis, closed-chest drainage with suction is used to reexpand the lung rapidly and fill the pleural space. If the fibrous material has restricted the lung for some time, the lung may not reexpand effectively and further intervention (usually thoracoplasty) may be needed.

RECURRENT PLEURAL EFFUSIONS

In some cases, pleural effusions may recur despite repeated thoracenteses (e.g., malignancy-induced effusions), with resultant compromise of lung function or persistent pleural pain. Treatment of recurrent effusions is accomplished through obliteration of the pleural space. Methods of obliterating the pleural space are as follows:

- **Pleurectomy (pleural stripping):** Surgical stripping of the parietal pleura away from the visceral pleura, which produces an intense inflammatory reaction that promotes adhesion formation between the two layers during healing.
- **Pleurodesis:** Instillation of a sclerosing substance (e.g., unbuffered tetracycline, bleomycin) into the pleural space via a chest tube to create an inflammatory response that causes the pleura to adhere and sclerose to each other. During the instillation, the client is rolled side to side to spread the substance throughout the pleural space.

Because pleural space obliteration creates permanent changes, the client's existing and predicted postprocedure respiratory status must be carefully evaluated. If a large area is involved, significant alterations in ventilatory mechanics (e.g., deep breathing, coughing) may occur, leading to compromised respiratory function.

After the procedure, closely monitor lung function, including respiratory rate and ventilation pattern. Document alleviation or persistence of pleural pain and watch for indications of a return of the pleural effusion.

Pulmonary function studies (see Chapter 59) and ABG measurements should also be performed.

BRONCHOPLEURAL FISTULA

A bronchopleural fistula is a communication between the pleural space and a bronchus. It may occur when an undrained empyema erodes into a bronchus or when the pleural space does not heal spontaneously after removal of a chest tube. A bronchopleural fistula raises the risk of pleural infection and may compromise ventilation and oxygenation.

The management of clients with bronchopleural fistulas is complex because they are often slow to heal. The client may be discharged home with a chest tube still in place and connected to a collection drainage system. Teach the client and family how to care for the chest tube and collection system and to recognize both manifestations of irritation at the chest puncture site and changes in chest drainage (e.g., blood) that require the physician to be notified.

METASTATIC PLEURAL TUMORS

Primary tumors in the lungs and other organs often metastasize to the pleura. The primary tumor is usually in a lung but may occur in the breast, ovaries, liver, kidneys, uterus, testicles, or larynx or may result from leukemia or lymphoma. Metastatic pleural disease frequently causes pleural effusions. Assessment findings in malignant pleural effusion are the same as those in pleural effusion from other causes. Diagnosis of pleural effusion is by chest radiograph. The source of the effusion is determined from cytologic examination of pleural fluid obtained by thoracentesis. Intervention is the same as for any pleural effusion, along with treatment of the primary malignancy.

DISORDERS OF THE DIAPHRAGM

SUBDIAPHRAGMATIC ABSCESS

A subdiaphragmatic abscess can compromise a client's respiratory status or erode and perforate the client's diaphragm. Clinical manifestations include pleuritic pain or pain referred to the shoulder on the affected side. Dyspnea and poor or no diaphragmatic movement are common. Flank pain or tenderness and a palpable abdominal mass in the region of the abscess are noted. The client has fever, anorexia, weight loss, and vomiting. Chest radiograph shows the diaphragm is generally elevated on the affected side. Fluoroscopic studies of diaphragmatic movement reveal limitation or absence of diaphragmatic movement on the affected side. Pleural effusion also commonly occurs. Thoracentesis and analysis of the pleural fluid reveal an exudate.

Subdiaphragmatic abscesses are drained and treated with antibiotics. Supportive measures are used to maintain ventilation and respiratory status. An untreated subdiaphragmatic abscess is nearly always fatal. With treatment, the death rate is still high but drops to approximately 25%.

DIAPHRAGMATIC PARALYSIS

Diaphragmatic paralysis can involve either the entire diaphragm (bilateral) or one side (unilateral). The most common causes of bilateral paralysis include high spinal cord injury, thoracic trauma (including cardiac surgery), multiple sclerosis, tumor nerve compression, anterior horn disease, and muscular dystrophy. Unilateral paralysis of the diaphragm is much more common than is bilateral paralysis. The most common cause is nerve invasion from malignancy or trauma.

Although the diaphragm is the primary muscle of respiration, its role can be assumed in part by the accessory and abdominal muscles. As a result, unilateral diaphragmatic paralysis is often difficult to detect. The diagnosis is suggested by finding an elevated hemidiaphragm on the chest radiograph and is confirmed by fluoroscopy. During the fluoroscopic procedure, the client is asked to "sniff." If paralysis is present, the nonparalyzed side of the diaphragm descends during inspiration (the sniff), and the paralyzed side paradoxically rises. Clients with unilateral diaphragmatic paralysis usually experience dyspnea when lying on the affected side. Dyspnea on exertion is not usual unless there is underlying lung disease. Both TLC and vital capacity (VC) are reduced by about 20%. There is also less ventilation to the affected side, and mild hypoxemia occurs because of shifts of ventilation and blood flow. Pre-existing lung disease combined with unilateral diaphragmatic paralysis may be disabling, depending on the extent of the lung disease.

The effects of bilateral diaphragmatic paralysis are potentially much more severe. However, the problem is often subtle and overlooked, especially if the client has a neuromuscular disorder. Fatigue, disturbed sleep, and morning headache are frequently the only manifestations. Classic manifestations of bilateral paralysis of the diaphragm are increased dyspnea, paradoxical inward abdominal movement, and active use of accessory muscles when the client is lying supine. Functional residual capacity (FRC) is also decreased, as is lung compliance. In the side-lying position, ventilation is preferentially distributed to the uppermost lung tissue and away from blood flow, leading to a significant mismatch of ventilation and perfusion. Severe hypoxemia results. Reduced tidal volume leads to retention of carbon dioxide and respiratory acidosis.

Little can be done to treat diaphragmatic paralysis. Management is aimed at supporting ventilatory function as needed. If the phrenic nerve is intact, a phrenic nerve pacer may be surgically inserted. Use of a phrenic nerve pacer is useful primarily for clients with spinal cord injuries.

Nursing management focuses on maintenance of a patent airway and detection of deteriorating gas exchange. Because inspiration is impaired, the client may need assistance to cough and deep breathe effectively. Position the client on the unaffected side in the semi-sitting or sitting position. Suction secretions as necessary. Increase hydration to liquefy secretions. Administer oxygen as prescribed. If respiratory function declines significantly, the physician and client (or possibly significant others) must decide whether a permanent tracheostomy should be placed and whether mechanical ventilation or other assistance devices should be used.

CONCLUSIONS

Clients with lung disorders are a challenge to the nurse providing care. In addition to common nursing diagnoses centering on *Impaired Gas Exchange* and *Ineffective Airway Clearance,* the client is often anxious because of the feelings of dyspnea and air hunger. Management of lung disorders consists of methods to open the airway (bronchodilators), clear infection (antibiotics), and improve oxygenation (position, coughing and deep breathing, oxygen).

THINKING CRITICALLY

1. Your client, who has undergone a thoracotomy, has a pleural chest tube connected to water-seal drainage. While your client is being positioned for a bedside chest radiograph, the drainage tubing is inadvertently disconnected from the chest drainage apparatus. What actions should you take?

Factors to Consider. What happens to the normally negative pressure in the pleural space when it is exposed to room air? Is this a dangerous problem?

2. A client with exertional dyspnea is admitted to the unit with a diagnosis of pleural effusion. He has difficulty breathing during the transfer from the cart to bed. You are asked to prepare the client for a thoracentesis. How would you prioritize care? What preparations are necessary for a thoracentesis?

Factors to Consider. What is the purpose of a thoracentesis? How are complications avoided? What clients are at risk for pleural effusion?

Discussion for these questions can be found on the website.

BIBLIOGRAPHY

 Citations appearing in red refer to primary research.

 Citations appearing in blue refer to evidence-based practice guidelines and protocols.

1. Ahluwalia, G., Ahluwalia, A., Gupta, K., et al. (2005). Extrapulmonary tuberculosis, part 1: Pleura and lymph node disease. *Journal of Respiratory Diseases, 26*, 326-332.
2. Alberg, A.J., & Samet, J.M. (2003). Epidemiology of lung cancer. *Chest, 123*, 21S-49S.
3. American Cancer Society. (2006). *What are the key statistics about lung cancer?* Retrieved 12/01/06 from www.cancer.org/docroot/CRI/content/CRI_2_4_1x_What_Are_the_Key_Statistics_About_Lung_Cancer_15.asp?sitearea=.
4. American Lung Association. (2006). *Lung disease data at a glance: Influenza and pneumonia.* Retrieved 12/10/06 from www.lungusa.org/site/pp.asp?c=dvLUK9O0E&b=316591.
4a. American Thoracic Society, Centers for Disease Control and Infectious Diseases Society of America. (2003). Treatment of tuberculosis. *Mortality and Morbidity Weekly Report, 52(RR11),* 1-77.
5. Anstead, G.M., & Graybill, J.R. (2006). Coccidioidomycosis. *Infectious Disease Clinics of North America, 20,* 621-623.
6. Arcasoy, S.M., & Wilt, J. (2006). Medical complications after lung transplantation. *Seminars in Respiratory and Critical Care Medicine, 27,* 508-520.
7. Barron, A., Brassell, S.A., & Shulman, L.P. (2005). Early cancer diagnosis: Present and future. *Patient Care, 39,* 27-30.
8. Bruce, E.A., Howard, R.F., & Franck, L.S. (2006). Chest drain removal pain and its management: A literature review. *Journal of Clinical Nursing, 15,* 145-154.
9. Centers for Disease Control and Prevention. (2006). Emergence of *Mycobacterium tuberculosis* with extensive resistance to second-line drugs—worldwide, 2000-2004. *Morbidity and Mortality Weekly Report, 55,* 301-328.
10. Centers for Disease Control and Prevention. (2006). Update: Influenza activity—United States, April 2-8, 2006. *Morbidity and Mortality Weekly Report, 55,* 421-448.
11. Centers for Disease Control and Prevention. (2006). *Testing for TB disease and infection—Tuberculin skin testing.* Core Curriculum on Tuberculosis. Retrieved 12/10/06 from www.cdc.gov/nchstp/tb/pubs/corecurr/Chapter4/Chapter_4_Skin_Testing.htm.
12. Centers for Disease Control and Prevention. (2006). Trends in tuberculosis—United States, 2005. *Morbidity and Mortality Weekly Report, 55,* 301-328.
13. Couppie, P., Aznar, C., Carme, B., et al. (2006). American histoplasmosis in developing countries with a special focus on patients with HIV: Diagnosis, treatment, and prognosis. *Current Opinion in Infectious Diseases, 19,* 443-449.
14. Cystic Fibrosis Foundation. (2005). *Patient registry—Annual data report 2004.* Retrieved 12/05/06 from www.cff.org/ID=4573/TYPE=2676/2004%20Patient%20Registry%20Report.pdf.
15. Davis, P.B. (2006). Cystic fibrosis since 1938. *American Journal of Respiratory and Critical Care Medicine, 173,* 475-482.
15a. Diagnosis and management of lung cancer: ACCP evidence-based guidelines. *Chest, 123* (15), 337S.
16. Driver, C.R., Matus, S.P., Bayuga, S., et al.. (2005). Factors associated with tuberculosis treatment interruption in New York City. *Journal of Public Health Management Practice, 11,* 361-368.
17. Dunn, L. (2005). Pneumonia: Classification, diagnosis, and nursing management. *Nursing Standard, 19,* 50-54.
18. Elkins, M.R., Robinson, M., Rose, B.R., et al.. (2006). A controlled trial of long-term inhaled hypertonic saline in patients with cystic fibrosis. *New England Journal of Medicine, 354,* 229-240.
19. Flanders, S.A., Collard, H.R., & Saint, S. (2006). Nosocomial pneumonia: State of the science. *American Journal of Infection Control, 34,* 84-93.
20. Gift, A.G., Jablonski, A., Stommel, M., et al. (2004). Symptom clusters in elderly patients with lung cancer. *Oncology Nursing Forum, 31,* 203-210.
21. Jett, J.R., & Miller, Y.E. (2006). Update in lung cancer 2005. *American Journal of Respiratory and Critical Care Medicine, 173,* 695-697.

22. Lawrence, V.A., Cornell, J.E., & Smetana, G.W. (2006). Strategies to reduce postoperative pulmonary complications after noncardiothoracic surgery: Systematic review for the American College of Physicians. *Annals of Internal Medicine, 144,* 596-608.

23. Leonard, M.K., Egan, K.B., Kourbatova, E., et al. (2006). Increased efficiency in evaluating patients with suspected tuberculosis by use of a dedicated airborne infection isolation unit. *American Journal of Infection Control, 34,* 69-72.

24. Lobato, M.N., Want, Y.C., Becerra, J.E., et al. (2006). Improved program activities are associated with decreasing tuberculosis incidence in the United States. *Public Health Reports, 121,* 108-115.

25. Mandell, L.A. (2005). Symposium on community-acquired pneumonia. Update on community-acquired pneumonia: New pathogens and new concepts in treatment. *Postgraduate Medicine, 118*(4), 35-46.

25a. Mandell, L.A., Bartlett, J.G., Dowell, S.F., et al. (2006). Update of guidelines for the management of community-acquired pneumonia in immunocompetent adults. *Clinics in Infectious Disease, 37,* 1405-1433.

26. Mapp, C.E., Miotto, D., & Boschetto, P. (2006). Occupational asthma. *La Medicina del Lavoro, 97,* 404-409.

27. Mehra, R., Moore, B.A., Crothers, K., et al. (2006). The association between marijuana smoking and lung cancer: A systematic review. *Archives of Internal Medicine, 166,* 1359-1367.

28. Moran, F., & Bradley, J. (2006). Non-invasive ventilation for cystic fibrosis. *Cochrane Library, 4,* 1-30.

29. O'Meara, E.S., White, M., Siscovick, D.S., et al. (2005). Hospitalization for pneumonia in the cardiovascular health study: Incidence, mortality, and influence on longer-term survival. *Journal of the American Geriatrics Society, 53,* 1108-1116.

30. Page, K.R., Sifakis, F., Montes de Oca, R., et al. (2006). Improved adherence and less toxicity with rifampin vs isoniazid for treatment of latent tuberculosis: A retrospective study. *Archives of Internal Medicine, 166,* 1863-1870.

31. Pirozynski, M. (2006). 100 years of lung cancer. *Respiratory Medicine, 100,* 2073-2084.

32. Trow, T.K. (2006). Clinical year in review: Occupational lung disease, pulmonary vascular disease, bronchiectasis, and chronic obstructive pulmonary disease. *Proceedings of the American Thoracic Society, 3,* 557-560.

33. United States National Institutes of Health. (2006). *Small cell lung cancer: Treatment.* National Cancer Institute. Retrieved 12/01/06 from www.cancer.gov/cancertopics/pdq/treatment/small-cell-lung/HealthProfessional/page1/print.

34. United States Department of Health and Human Services. (2006). *The health consequences of involuntary exposure to tobacco smoke: A report of the Surgeon General.* Atlanta, Ga: Department of Health and Human Services, Public Health Service, Centers for Disease Control and Prevention, National Center for Chronic Disease and Prevention and Promotion, Office of Smoking and Health.

35. Valdivia, L., Nix, D., Wright, M., et al. (2006). Coccidioidomycosis as a common cause of community-acquired pneumonia. *Emerging Infectious Diseases, 12,* 958-962.

36. van der Schans, C., Prasad, A., & Main, E. (2006). Chest physiotherapy compared to no chest physiotherapy for cystic fibrosis. *Cochrane Library, 4,* 1-21.

37. Vivek, N.A., & Kawut, S.M. (2005). Noninfectious pulmonary complications after lung transplantation. *Clinics in Chest Medicine, 26,* 613-622.

38. Westerdahl, E., Lindmark, B., Eriksson, T., et al. (2003). The immediate effects of deep breathing exercises on atelectasis and oxygenation after cardiac surgery. *Scandinavian Cardiovascular Journal, 37,* 363-367.

39. Williams, V.G. (2006). Tuberculosis: Clinical features, diagnosis and management. *Nursing Management, 20,* 49-53.

40. Yen, M.Y., Lin, Y.E., Su, I.J., et al. (2006). Using an integrated infection control strategy during outbreak control to minimize nosocomial infection of severe acute respiratory syndrome among healthcare workers. *Journal of Hospital Infection, 64,* 195-199.

evolve *Did you remember to check out the bonus material on the Evolve website and the CD-ROM, including NCLEX®-Examination Style Review Questions, Open-Book Quizzes, and Chapter Review Audio Podcasts?*

http://evolve.elsevier.com/Black/medsurg

CHAPTER 63

Management of Clients with Acute Pulmonary Disorders

LYNN WHITE

RESPIRATORY FAILURE

The most important function of the respiratory system is to provide the body tissues with oxygen and to remove carbon dioxide. The body relies primarily on the central nervous system (CNS), the pulmonary system, the heart, and the vascular system to accomplish effective respiration. Respiratory failure develops when one or more of these systems or organs fail to maintain optimal functioning. If the respiratory failure occurs so rapidly that the compensatory mechanisms cannot accommodate or if the compensatory mechanisms are overwhelmed, acute respiratory failure develops.

Respiratory failure is a broad, nonspecific clinical diagnosis indicating that the respiratory system is unable to supply the oxygen necessary to maintain metabolism or cannot eliminate sufficient carbon dioxide (CO_2). *Acute respiratory failure* is defined as a partial pressure of arterial oxygen (Pao_2) of 50 mm Hg or less on room air or a partial pressure of arterial CO_2 ($Paco_2$) of 50 mm Hg or more with a pH ≤ 7.25, along with clinical presentation. Some experts will also identify a pH of ≤ 7.35 as another indication of acute respiratory failure. In clients with chronic hypercapnia, $Paco_2$ elevations of 5 mm Hg or more from their previously stable levels indicate that acute respiratory failure has been superimposed on chronic respiratory failure.

Acute respiratory failure may be classified as hypoxemic or ventilatory failure with a rapid onset over minutes to hours or gradually over days. Clients with acute *hypoxemic* respiratory failure have severe arterial hypoxemia and are minimally responsive to supplemental oxygen despite adequate ventilation. Hypoxemic respiratory failure may be caused by diffuse problems such as pulmonary edema; near-drowning; adult (acute) respiratory distress syndrome (ARDS); or localized problems such as pneumonia, bleeding into the chest, or lung tumors.

Ventilatory or hypercapnic respiratory failure is when the client is unable to support adequate gas exchange leading to elevated $Paco_2$ levels that can result from CNS depression, inadequate neuromuscular ability to sustain breathing, or respiratory system overload. Conditions such as acute deterioration of chronic obstructive pulmonary disease (COPD), and status asthmaticus are other causes of ventilatory failure. Clients may have a combination of hypoxemic and hypercapnic respiratory failure.

HYPOXEMIC RESPIRATORY FAILURE
PULMONARY EDEMA

Pulmonary edema is the abnormal accumulation of fluid in the alveolar sacs and in the interstitial spaces surrounding the alveoli. Pulmonary edema is classified by its underlying causes: *Cardiogenic* causes include left ventricular failure, mitral valve stenosis, cardiogenic shock, hypertension, and cardiomyopathy. *Noncardiogenic* causes are shown in Box 63-1. Pulmonary edema can also develop after catastrophic injury to the CNS, such as head injury; this form of pulmonary edema is called *neurogenic* pulmonary edema.

Etiology
Normally, fluid moves into the interstitial space at the arterial end of the capillary as a result of hydrostatic pressure in the vessel and returns to the venous end of the capillary because of oncotic pressure and increases in interstitial hydrostatic pressure (see the Anatomy and

---

evolve Web Enhancements

Bridge to Home Health Care Living with a Ventilator
Concept Map Understanding ARDS and Its Treatment

Be sure to check out the bonus material on the Evolve website and the CD-ROM, including free self-assessment exercises. **http://evolve.elsevier. com/Black/medsurg**

BOX 63-1 Causes of Noncardiogenic Pulmonary Edema

- Aspiration of gastric contents, especially if a large amount of HCl is present
- Barotrauma (e.g., with PEEP with mechanical ventilation)
- Drugs (e.g., after administration of narcotics)
- Fluid overload from IV fluids or renal failure
- Hypoalbuminemia (e.g., nephrotic syndrome, hepatic disease, malnutrition)
- Sepsis
- Inhalation of toxic chemicals (e.g., sulfur dioxide, paraquat, phosgene, chlorine, nitrogen oxides)
- High altitudes (>8000 ft)
- Neurogenic stimulus (e.g., increased intracranial pressure, epileptic seizures, head trauma)
- Near-drowning syndrome
- Mechanical ventilation, oxygen toxicity, ARDS
- Malignancies blocking outflow of lymph within the lungs
- Pancreatitis
- Pneumonia
- Smoke inhalation (e.g., trapped in a burning building)
- Unilaterally, after reexpansion of collapsed lung (pneumothorax)

ARDS, Adult (acute) respiratory distress syndrome; *HCl,* hydrochloric acid; *IV,* intravenous; *PEEP,* positive end-expiratory pressure.

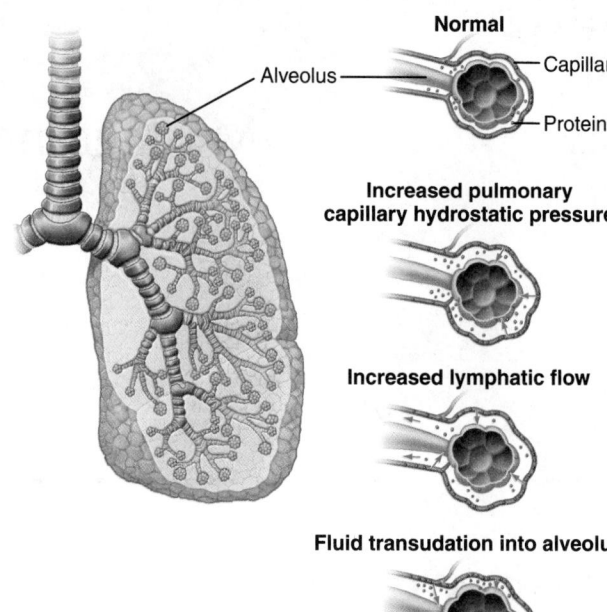

■ **FIGURE 63–1** Progression of pulmonary edema. Pulmonary edema occurs when capillary hydrostatic pressure is increased, promoting movement of fluid into the interstitial space of the alveolar-capillary membrane. Initially, increased lymphatic flow removes the excess fluids, but continued leakage eventually overwhelms this mechanism. Gas exchange becomes impaired by the thick membrane. Increasing interstitial fluid pressure ultimately causes leaks into the alveolar sacs, impairing ventilation and gas exchange.

Physiology Review for Unit 3). Fluid movement through the lung is no different; in fact, fluid in the interstitial spaces of the lungs is not uncommon. It normally escapes from the microcirculation and enters the interstitium, providing nutrients for the cells. The residual fluid is returned via the lymphatic system. Increased volume of fluid in the pulmonary arteries from obstruction of forward flow is the most common cause of pulmonary edema, and heart failure is the most common example of the obstruction of forward flow. Lung tumors can obstruct lymphatic flow and lead to pulmonary edema.

Pathophysiology

Increased hydrostatic pressure in the pulmonary vessels creates an imbalance in the Starling forces, resulting in an increase of fluid filtration into the interstitial spaces of the lung that exceeds the lymphatic capacity to drain the fluid away. Increasing volumes of fluid leak into the alveolar spaces (Figure 63-1). The lymphatic system attempts to compensate by draining excess interstitial fluid volume through the hilar lymph nodes and back into the vascular system. If this pathway becomes overwhelmed, fluid moves from the pleural interstitium into the alveolar walls. If the alveolar epithelium is damaged, the fluid begins to accumulate in the alveoli. Alveolar edema is a serious late manifestation in the progression of fluid imbalance.

Hypoxemia develops when the alveolar membrane is thickened by fluid hindering the exchange of oxygen and CO_2. As fluid fills the interstitium and alveolar spaces, lung compliance decreases and oxygen diffusion is impaired. If pulmonary edema has developed because of left ventricular failure, right ventricular failure may occur because the pulmonary artery pressure is elevated. This elevation increases afterload for the right ventricle, resulting in increased workload of the heart and manifestations of right ventricular failure.

Clinical Manifestations

The manifestations of pulmonary edema are due to failure of the regulatory factors guiding fluid movement. Most manifestations are seen in the respiratory system and include marked dyspnea, tachypnea, weak and thready tachycardia, hypertension (if cardiogenic), orthopnea at less than 90 degrees, and the use of accessory muscles to aid breathing. The client's frequent coughing is an attempt to rid the chest of fluid. The sputum is thin and frothy because it is combined with water. If the hydrostatic pressure is very high, small capillaries break and sputum becomes pink tinged. The client may be anxious from dyspnea and restless from hypoxemia. Chest auscultation reveals crackles, wheezes, and the presence of an S_3 heart sound. A heart murmur may be noted if the cause is mitral valve disease. Pulse oximetry readings are commonly less than 85% and arterial blood gas (ABG) determinations may reveal an arterial Pao$_2$ of less than 50 mm Hg. Respiratory alkalosis is common because of the tachypnea. Pressure in the pulmonary artery and pulmonary artery wedge pressure (PAWP) are elevated. The chest x-ray shows areas of "whiteout" where fluid has replaced air-filled lung tissue, which normally appears black. Right ventricular failure may also be noted, with manifestations of hepatomegaly, jugular venous distention, and peripheral edema.

OUTCOME MANAGEMENT

Medical Management

Medical management concentrates on the following four areas: (1) correction of hypoxemia, (2) reduction in preload, (3) reduction of afterload, and (4) support of perfusion.

Correct Hypoxemia

It is imperative to maintain adequate oxygenation. Clients with severe pulmonary edema commonly require oxygen therapy at high Fio$_2$ levels and may require noninvasive positive- pressure ventilation (NPPV) such as continuous positive airway pressure (CPAP) or mechanical ventilation if they cannot meet the work of breathing. NPPV is any type of respiratory support that does not require endotracheal tube (ET) intubation.

Reduce Preload

The client is placed in an upright position. Usually, the client does not want to lie down because of orthopnea and a feeling of choking when supine. Diuretics are prescribed to promote fluid excretion. Nitrates, such as nitroglycerin, are used for their vasodilating properties, decreasing the workload of the heart muscle. Other management strategies consist of treating the underlying condition.

Reduce Afterload

Afterload is reduced to diminish workload on the left ventricle. Antihypertensive agents, including potent agents such as nitroprusside, are prescribed. Angiotensin-converting enzyme (ACE) inhibitors are considered essential in the treatment of pulmonary edema from congestive heart failure. ACE inhibitors reduce afterload and improve stroke volume and cardiac output. There is also a slight reduction in preload when renal perfusion is improved and diuresis begins. Morphine is prescribed to reduce the sympathetic nervous system response and to reduce anxiety from the dyspnea.

Support Perfusion

The left ventricle is supported by using inotropic medications such as dobutamine, dopamine, and norepinephrine. Nesiritide is also used to decrease PCWP, pulmonary artery

pressure, right atrial pressure, and systemic vascular resistance while increasing cardiac output. Urine output is monitored closely to determine whether renal perfusion is adequate. An intra-aortic balloon pump (IABP) may be required with severe heart failure and pulmonary edema (see Chapter 55).

Nursing Management

Assessment. The client with pulmonary edema is assessed quickly on admission, concentrating on only the information and assessment findings essential to begin treatment. The client is typically anxious and having significant shortness of breath. Managing the client's anxiety and reducing the dyspnea are imperative. A complete assessment is carried out over the following hours, when the client can breathe more comfortably and answer questions. A baseline weight and lung assessment is essential, because these parameters will assist in determining the effectiveness of treatments.

Diagnosis, Outcomes, Interventions

Diagnosis: Impaired Gas Exchange. The fluid-filled alveoli block the exchange of gases. Use the nursing diagnosis *Impaired Gas Exchange related to capillary membrane obstruction from fluid* to plan care. This is the priority diagnosis.

Outcomes. The client will demonstrate improved gas exchange, as evidenced by rising Pao$_2$ to 55 or 60 mm Hg, oxygen saturation above 90%, normalizing pH, decreasing anxiety and dyspnea, and fewer crackles and wheezing within 12 hours.

Interventions. Monitor vital signs every 15 minutes initially, until the client is stable. Administer oxygen as ordered using a high-flow rebreather bag to maintain oxygenation. Titrate the actual liter flow of oxygen to maintain saturation above 90%.

> **Continuous assessment is needed because the client may not be able to tolerate the work of breathing and may quickly require NPPV or endotracheal (ET) intubation with mechanical ventilation. NPPV, mechanical ventilation, and intubation equipment should be readily available.**

SAFETY ALERT

To reduce preload, position the client with the legs in a dependent position. Raising edematous legs increases venous return and will stress the overtaxed left ventricle. Preload is reduced with morphine and nitroglycerin. Because perfusion to the skin is often compromised, repositioning is important.

Air hunger can lead to panic and feelings of suffocation. Administering opioids (morphine) and anxiolytics to control both dyspnea and anxiety will relax the client and improve breathing. Stay with the client and use breathing techniques to support the client.

Diagnosis: Excess Fluid Volume. Accumulation of fluid from several causes leads to fluid overload. Use the nursing diagnosis *Excess Fluid Volume related to excess preload.*

Outcomes. The client will demonstrate improved fluid balance, as evidenced by diuresis (input less than output), decreased number of crackles and wheezes, eupnea, weight loss, resolving peripheral edema, decreased anxiety, and normalizing blood urea nitrogen levels.

Interventions. Administer a diuretic (furosemide is the most common) as prescribed to promote diuresis. Place an indwelling catheter to monitor response to diuretics. Monitor urine output hourly, weight, and potassium levels (potassium loss is a side effect of furosemide). Monitor blood pressure to determine whether the client can maintain perfusion without inotropic support. Because oral fluids are restricted, oral hygiene is completed every 2 hours.

Evaluation. If the previously described interventions are implemented immediately, a fairly rapid response to diuresis and oxygen therapy should be seen. It is not uncommon to diurese several liters of fluid, resulting in dramatic weight loss and reduction of dyspnea.

Self-Care

Consider the reasons for development of pulmonary edema when developing a plan for self-care. Clients may need further education on daily weights, dietary choices, and scheduling of medications. Instruct the client and family members on the early manifestations of fluid overload so that early intervention is possible.

ACUTE VENTILATORY FAILURE

Ventilatory failure is the inability of the body to sustain respiratory drive or the inability of the chest wall and muscles to mechanically move air in and out of the lungs. The hallmark of ventilatory failure is an elevated CO_2 level.

Etiology and Risk Factors

In acute ventilatory failure, the respiratory load placed on the lung to exchange oxygen and CO_2 is impaired by (1) problems of resistance to moving air in and out of the lung, (2) the ability of the lung to expand and contract (elastic recoil), and (3) conditions that increase the production of CO_2 or decrease the surface available for exchange of gases. The competence of the nerves and muscles coordinating the movement of the chest can also be impaired by loss of drive to breathe, impaired transmission of signals to the chest and diaphragm, and muscle fatigue.

Pathophysiology

Alveolar ventilation is maintained by the CNS acting through nerves and the muscles of respiration to drive breathing. Failure of alveolar ventilation leads to a ventilation-perfusion (expressed as $\dot{V}/\dot{Q}$) mismatch resulting in hypercapnia (rising CO_2 levels) and eventually acidosis develops. Left untreated, acute ventilatory failure leads to death.

Functional residual capacity (FRC) is the volume of air remaining in the lung after normal expiration. In obstructive forms of ventilatory failure, the residual pressure in the chest impairs inhalation and increases the workload of breathing. When end-expiratory alveolar volumes remain above their critical closing point, the alveoli remain open and functioning, allowing oxygen to diffuse into the bloodstream. If alveolar volumes fall below the closing point, the alveoli tend to collapse. When alveoli collapse, no oxygenation or blood flow to the alveoli occurs (Figure 63-2). In acute ventilatory failure, the residual volume and FRC are decreased, resulting in a true intrapulmonary shunt (perfusion without oxygenation) and decreased lung compliance.

Once alveolar collapse occurs, reinflation necessitates very high opening pressures, the generation of which significantly increases the work of breathing. The hypoxemia resulting from alveolar collapse and the increased oxygen consumption caused by the increased work of breathing may severely compromise the client.

Clinical Manifestations

To avoid frank apnea, recognizing impending ventilatory failure is critical. Continuous monitoring of high-risk clients concentrating on changes in respiratory rate and depth, mental status, and patterns of breathing is essential. The hallmark manifestations of hypercapnia are headache and dyspnea. The client may also verbalize that dyspnea is increasing despite treatment. Altered respiratory patterns can herald impending ventilatory failure. The client's respiratory rate can rise to 50 to 60 breaths/min, but the breaths are shallow and impaired by spasm of the airway. The rate can also fall to 4 to 6 breaths/min. Clients become confused and less conversant, and

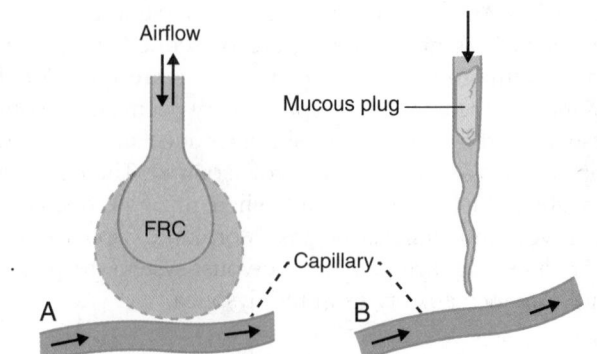

■ **FIGURE 63-2** Effects of positive airway pressure on the alveolus. **A,** The collapsed alveolus continues to be perfused with blood, but cannot exchange oxygen for carbon dioxide. **B,** The alveolus is opened by positive pressure.

are difficult to arouse. Electrolyte abnormalities, caused by a falling pH level, may cause cardiac dysrhythmias. If the cause of ventilatory failure is obstruction of the airway, the systolic blood pressure falls during inspiration as a result of intrathoracic resistance. This change, called *pulsus paradoxus,* is present when systolic blood pressure falls more than 10 mm Hg during inspiration. Pulse oximetry indicates steadily decreasing oxygen saturation values, and ABG analysis shows falling Pao_2 and rising $Paco_2$ values.

OUTCOME MANAGEMENT

Medical Management

Medical management is directed at reversing bronchospasm, maintaining oxygenation, treating the underlying problem, and providing ventilatory assistance. Mechanical ventilation is not used until other methods of maintaining ventilation have been tried.

Reverse Bronchospasm
Several forms of bronchodilators are used to treat obstructions to airflow in clients with COPD and asthma. These agents include inhaled $beta_2$-selective agonists (albuterol), ipratropium, corticosteroids, and rarely theophylline. If infection is the underlying cause, broad-spectrum antibiotics are given.

Maintain Oxygenation
Oxygen by mask may be adequate to support oxygenation. Using forms of NPPV such as CPAP reduces the workload of breathing by decreasing the force needed to overcome the pressure in the chest. Outcomes after mechanical ventilation with lower tidal volumes may be better than the traditional formula (10 to 15 ml of body weight per kilogram), which sometimes lead to stretch-induced lung injury.

Manage the Underlying Problem
There are many causes of ventilatory failure. Some of these causes can be quickly managed, such as reversing opiate overdose with naloxone, but others require more aggressive treatment. Supportive therapies are used to reverse or control the underlying problem.

Maintain Ventilation
Initially, NPPV should be used if the client is alert and can maintain the mask over the nose or mouth without becoming claustrophobic. NPPV keeps small airways open and improves gas exchange with the goal being to keep oxygen saturation above 90%. Frequent ABG readings may need to be taken to ensure that adequate oxygenation is being achieved. If NPPV is not successful, mechanical ventilation is required and helps to minimize the work of breathing while effectively promoting gas exchange (oxygenation and ventilation). The client requires an artificial airway, usually by ET intubation and the use of positive-pressure ventilation (PPV). If prolonged intubation is required, the ET tube is replaced with a tracheostomy.

Endotracheal Intubation

Intubation
The ET tube is a long, slender, hollow tube usually made of polyvinyl chloride and is inserted into the trachea via the mouth or nose. In addition to providing a connection for ventilators, the ET tube provides a stable airway and facilitates removal of secretions. However, it allows the normal respiratory defenses to be bypassed and may reduce cough effectiveness. The ET tube also prevents verbal communication. It passes through the vocal cords, and the distal tip is positioned just above the bifurcation of the main stem of the bronchus (carina). Oral intubation is usually used for short-term airway management. Nasal intubation, a more secure method, is believed to be more comfortable because the tube does not move as much in the airway. However, nasal intubation is not being used much because of the risk of sinusitis. Before intubation, the client is supine, and all dental bridgework and plates and loose teeth are removed because these items can be jarred loose and aspirated during the procedure. The client's head is hyperextended, the lower aspect of the neck is flexed, and the mouth is opened (Figure 63-3). This position brings the mouth, pharynx, and larynx into a straight line. A laryngoscope is used to hold the airway open, expose the vocal cords, and serve as a guide for the tube into the trachea. ET tubes are inserted only by fully trained health care team members.

Intubation should not cause or exacerbate hypoxia. If the client's neck and mandible are mobile, the procedure usually takes about 30 seconds. Certain pre-existing conditions such as obesity with a stocky neck, a possible spinal cord injury, or rheumatoid arthritis of the neck can make intubation difficult. For clients with expected difficulty of intubation, an oxygen mask can be used to provide oxygen through the mouth. An oxygen saturation monitor may also be used to warn of hypoxemia.

A good practice to remember during difficult intubation is to hold your breath while intubation is attempted. If you must stop to breathe before the client is intubated, the intubation is taking too long. Stop the intubation, reoxygenate the client by mask, and reattempt intubation.

Immediately after ET tube insertion, tube placement is verified by auscultation and chest x-ray to ensure aeration of both sides of the chest. An end-tidal CO_2 monitor and assessment of oxygen saturation levels are also indications of correct ET tube placement. Record in the nurses' notes and on the respiratory flow sheet the point

■ **FIGURE 63–3** **A,** A laryngoscope is used to visualize the vocal cords. **B,** The endotracheal tube is inserted with the client's head extended to align the airway.

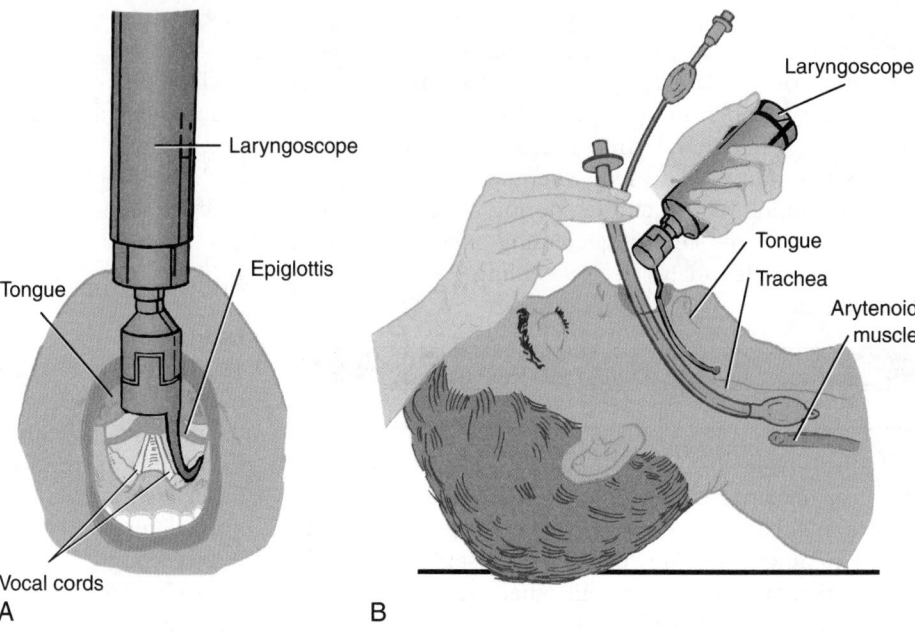

Laryngoscope

Tongue

Epiglottis

Vocal cords

A

Laryngoscope

Tongue

Trachea

Arytenoid muscle

B

at which the tube meets the lips or nostrils by using the numbers listed on the side of the ET tube. If the tube slips, its correct position can be reestablished quickly. Secure the ET tube immediately after intubation with adhesive tape, twill tape, or specially designed ET tube holders (Figure 63-4). Current recommendations favor the use of commercial ET tube holders to minimize the

Irrigation port for saline lavage

Removable plug

Catheter

Thumb control for suction

Modified T piece for ventilator circuit

Ventilator circuit

Catheter sheath

To vacuum source

■ **FIGURE 63–4** Secured cuffed endotracheal tube with closed tracheal suction system. *(From Sill, J.R. [1991]. Respiratory care certification guide. St. Louis: Mosby.)*

risk of unplanned extubations. Retaping is required only if the tape becomes loose or soiled.

Cuff Inflation

The cuff of an ET tube seals the tube against the tracheal wall to facilitate PPV and protects the respiratory tract from aspiration of foreign material. The amount of air required to seal an ET tube cuff is reflected by the cuff pressure, which is usually maintained at less than 20 mm Hg. Most ET tubes are designed with soft plastic cuffs for use with high volumes of air at low pressures. Cuffs are inflated with a volume of air high enough to seal the trachea while exerting the lowest possible pressure on the tracheal wall. Low cuff pressure is necessary to prevent damage to the tracheal mucosa. Arterial pressures in the tracheal wall are approximately 20 to 25 mm Hg; venous pressures are 18 to 20 mm Hg. Therefore cuff pressures greater than 18 to 20 mm Hg impair circulation to the tracheal mucosa and necrosis may develop. Assess cuff pressures every 8 hours or as institutional policy dictates.

The most common method of cuff inflation *(minimal occlusion volume technique)* aims to provide an adequate seal in the trachea at the lowest possible cuff pressure. Slowly inject air into the cuff while auscultating with a stethoscope placed over the larynx (over the cuff) during a positive-pressure breath. At the point when sounds (from air movement) cease, inflation is stopped, indicating that the cuff is sealed against the tracheal wall.

Cuff Deflation

Generally, ET cuffs should remain inflated at all times. If cuff deflation is required for any reason, suction the trachea (with the client being hyperventilated and hyperoxygenated before and during this procedure) and clean the area above the cuff of secretions by gently suctioning deep into the oropharynx. Advance the suction catheter to the end of the ET tube and deflate the cuff while applying suction to the suction catheter so that any secretions lying above the cuff can be removed. If necessary, repeat pharyngeal suctioning.

Cuff Leaks

Cuff leaks can be a major problem. They may be caused by a rupture or tear in the cuff or pilot system or by a change in ET tube position in the trachea. There are several signs of a leak in or around the ET tube cuff, including the pilot balloon not filling when air is injected, the client can talk when the cuff is inflated, or air is heard leaking during positive-pressure breathing.

If the system is not functional, the ET tube may need to be replaced. Before replacement, increasing tidal volume may help maintain ventilation by compensating for the escaping gas. The client is at high risk for aspiration while the cuff is leaking.

Continuous Mechanical Ventilation

Normal respiration begins with the contraction of the diaphragm and respiratory muscles to create negative pressure in the chest: A vacuum is created and air flows in. When a ventilator is used, positive pressure (rather than negative pressure) forces air into the lungs. The positive pressure is necessary for gas exchange and to keep alveoli open. Unfortunately, positive-pressure forces can also damage the alveoli and may retard venous return and cardiac output. Trauma from high pressures in a ventilator is called barotrauma; the prefix "baro" means pressure. The high-risk groups for barotrauma include those clients with underlying lung disease.

The goals of continuous mechanical ventilation (CMV) are the following:

- To maintain adequate ventilation
- To deliver precise concentrations of Fio_2
- To deliver adequate tidal volumes to obtain an adequate minute ventilation and oxygenation
- To lessen the work of breathing in those clients who cannot sustain adequate ventilation on their own
- To prevent complications from the underlying problems

Modes of Ventilation

The ventilation mode refers to the way the client receives breaths from the ventilator. A control panel of one ventilator system is shown in Figure 63-5. Two common types of mechanical ventilation include volume-cycled and pressure-cycled. When selecting a mode of

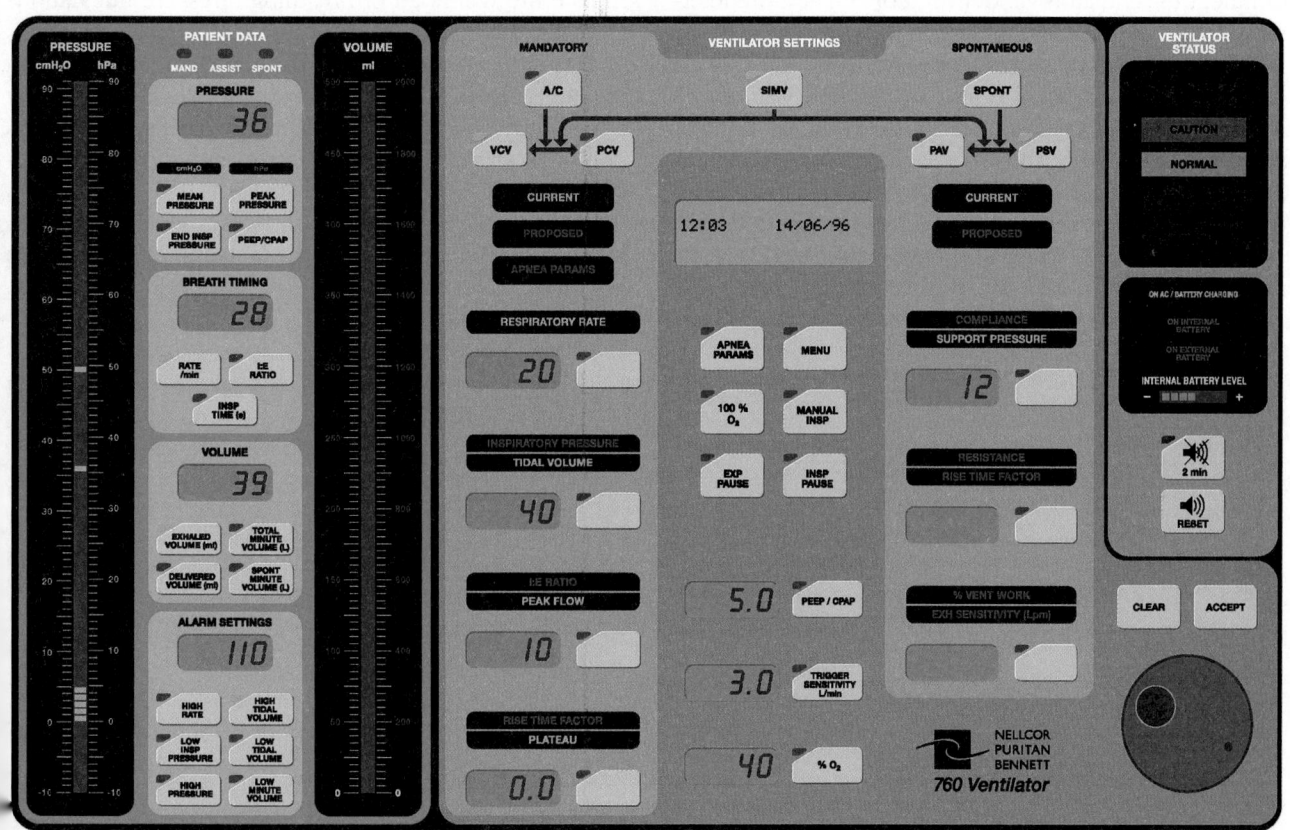

■ **FIGURE 63-5** Nellcor Puritan Bennett 760 Ventilator. *(Courtesy Mallinckrodt, Inc., Nellcor Puritan Bennett Ventilator Division.)*

ventilation, it is important to consider which mode will provide for adequate gas exchange while synchronizing with the clients own respiratory efforts, while decreasing the potential for barotrauma.

Pressure-cycled ventilation delivers a volume of gas to the airway using positive pressure during inspiration. This positive pressure is delivered until the preselected pressure has been reached. When the preset pressure is reached, the ventilator will cycle into passive exhalation. A disadvantage to this type of ventilation is that the volume delivered may not be sufficient depending on the compliance of the lung and the integrity of the ventilatory circuit (e.g., kinked tubing).

Volume-cycled (volume-controlled or *volume-limited) ventilation* delivers a preset tidal volume of inspired gas. The tidal volume has been preselected based on the ideal body weight, and is delivered to the client regardless of the pressure required to deliver this volume. The ventilator will automatically adjust the pressure needed to deliver the preset volume. If the client's breathing has become shallow, the ventilator will increase pressure to continue delivering the preset volume. A pressure limit can be set to prevent the occurrence of dangerously high airway pressures.

Table 63-1 describes several conventional modes of CMV. *Assist-control (A/C) ventilation* will deliver a preset volume of gas each time the client initiates a breath. If the client fails to initiate a breath within a preset amount of time, the ventilator will deliver a breath at a predetermined volume and rate. Each breath, whether client or ventilator generated, is delivered to a preset tidal volume or pressure limit. *Synchronous intermittent mandatory ventilation (SIMV)* delivers the preset volume or pressure breath for only those breaths that are ventilator initiated. Additional breaths are the result of the client's own efforts. The ventilator-delivered breaths are synchronized with the client's spontaneous breaths. This mode is often used for ventilator weaning.

When clients have special ventilation or oxygenation needs, a high-frequency ventilation mode may be indicated. High-frequency ventilation allows the delivery of smaller tidal volumes using a high-speed ventilation rate, up to as high as 360 breaths/min. The advantage of this mode is a decreased risk for alveolar trauma. Clients must be sedated to tolerate this type of ventilation. There are three types of high-frequency ventilation: high-frequency jet ventilation, high-frequency positive-pressure ventilation, and high-frequency oscillation. The most common indication for use is adult respiratory distress syndrome. It is also used in neonatal or pediatric clients.

Triggering Mechanisms

All breaths given to the client must be initiated or triggered. Triggering mechanisms can be based on (1) time, (2) negative pressure, (3) flow, or (4) volume.

Time-triggered inhalation is used to manage clients who cannot breathe on their own. The ventilator will trigger a breath after a preset time, serving as a backup in case a client's own breathing rate falls below a preset value.

Negative pressure inhalation is triggered by the initial negative pressure that begins inspiration. As soon as the client initiates a breath, the ventilator is triggered to produce inhalation. The sensitivity of the system is set to reduce the workload of breathing. Pressure fluctuations (e.g., hiccoughs, leaks) can cause premature triggering.

Flow-triggered inhalation occurs when the client can initiate a breath. The ventilator completes the breath by sensing the flow of air into the chest. This system works well in combination with positive end-expiratory pressure (PEEP).

Volume-triggered ventilation occurs when the ventilator completes the breath to maximize inhaled gas volumes.

TABLE 63–1 Modes of Mechanical Ventilation		
Mode of Ventilation	**Clinical Application**	**Nursing Implications**
Continuous mandatory ventilation (CMV), also known as assist control A/C, delivers gas at preset tidal volumes	Primary ventilatory mode in clients who are apneic or have weak respiratory efforts	May hyperventilate Sedation may be needed to control spontaneous breaths
Pressure controlled ventilation delivers gas at preset pressures over a set inspiratory time	Primary ventilatory mode for clients with changing pulmonary mechanics, such as airway resistance or lung compliance (e.g., ARDS)	Increased thoracic pressure may lead to decreased cardiac output for impaired venous return Requires sedation and/or paralysis
Pressure support ventilation	Primary ventilatory mode for clients with stable respiratory drive to overcome airway resistance from ET tube Primary weaning mode	Client should have less work to breathe Monitor for hypercapnia
Intermittent mandatory ventilation	Primary ventilatory mode for clients with decreased lung compliance or increased airway resistance Occasionally used for weaning	Monitor for hypercapnia

Safety and Alarms

Ventilators have several alarms to assist with their safe use.

> **Alarms should be ON at all times to alert the caregiver to changes in the client's condition and hazardous situations such as unplanned extubation. Emergency equipment such as a hand-held resuscitation bag should be readily available. *High-pressure* alarms are triggered when there is increased airway resistance or decreased lung compliance. Increased airway resistance may be caused by secretions, bronchospasm, ET tube dislodgement or biting, coughing, or kinked ventilatory circuit tubing. Decreased lung compliance may be caused by pulmonary edema, pneumothorax, atelectasis, or acute respiratory distress syndrome. *Low-pressure* or *low-minute* volume alarms are caused by disconnected tubing, ET tube cuff leak, or apnea. An alarm should never be silenced until the cause has been investigated and corrected. If the source of the alarm cannot be determined, disconnect the client from the ventilator and use a hand-held resuscitation bag for manual ventilation with 100% oxygen until the problem can be resolved.**

The Bridge to Critical Care feature on p. 1644 provides additional discussion of the alarm systems most commonly seen with ventilators.

Client-Ventilator Dyssynchrony

Ventilators breathe into the client through positive pressure (normal inhalation is through negative pressure), and this change in inhalation can lead to uncoordinated breathing. Ideally, the client should inhale and exhale when the ventilator inhales and exhales. When the client is not "in sync" with the ventilator, it appears that the client is "fighting" or "bucking" the ventilator. To avoid this problem, the ventilator is set to sense the client's own inhalation efforts and to support any spontaneous breathing. Also the patency of the ET tube should be confirmed by suctioning. If adjusting the ventilator settings does not help, the client may need to be sedated.

Positive End-Expiratory Pressure/Continuous Positive Airway Pressure

The techniques PEEP and CPAP are applied during expiration to prevent intrathoracic pressures from returning to ambient atmospheric pressure. CPAP is applied to a client with spontaneous respiration; PEEP is applied during mechanical ventilation. CPAP and PEEP are used to apply positive airway pressure that keeps the alveoli open and reduces the amount of shunting with the goal that the FiO_2 may be reduced to the lowest possible level to maintain gas exchange and to prevent oxygen toxicity. This increased pressure also increases functional residual capacity (FRC) and enhances oxygenation as a result of the enlarged surface area that is available for diffusion. In normal conditions, 10 cm H_2O is needed to keep the alveoli open. High tidal volumes and continuous cyclic expansion and collapse of the alveoli deplete surfactant in the alveoli and create the need for higher PEEP. Positive pressures of 10 to 25 cm H_2O are typically used in adults. Pressures may be adjusted until the level is found that produces the best PaO_2 without producing adverse effects. This level is called "best PEEP."

Risks of PEEP include overdistention of the alveoli, $\dot{V}/\dot{Q}$ mismatch, subcutaneous emphysema, and decreased cardiac output from increased intrathoracic pressure.

Physiologic Changes After Mechanical Ventilation

Many physiologic changes occur when a client is placed on mechanical ventilation. Decreased cardiac output is the most common of these. Normal unassisted respiration begins with subatmospheric pressure. Negative pressure increases during inhalation and decreases during exhalation. Positive pressure applied to the airway has the opposite effect. As positive pressure inflates the lungs, the pressure in the thorax builds, decreasing the flow of blood to the vena cava and to the right atrium of the heart. Exhalation is passive and pressures return to the normal resting subatmospheric level. Blood flow to and from the right ventricle is also decreased if PPV is continued for more than a few minutes. This, in turn, decreases the filling of the left ventricle, leading to a lowered cardiac output. The lowered cardiac output is reflected in the hypotension that clients commonly exhibit immediately after initiating mechanical ventilation. It is imperative that blood pressures be monitored closely.

Positive pressure may also briefly affect the left side of the heart by increased filling and output. This increase is due to the displacement of blood from the pulmonary system into the left ventricle. However, this effect is noted only immediately after institution of PPV.

PPV may lead to stretch injury in the alveoli and the release of inflammatory mediators. To minimize stretch injury, the lowest possible tidal volume and PEEP should be used.

Other body systems are also affected by PPV. During the inspiratory phase, the diaphragm descends into the abdomen, resulting in decreased blood flow to the splanchnic area, leading to ischemia of the gastric mucosa. Ischemia of the gastric mucosa may be one of the reasons that clients receiving PPV for an extended period have a high incidence of gastrointestinal bleeding and stress ulcerations. Decreasing blood flow to the splanchnic region also results in decreased blood flow to the kidneys. Decreased blood flow signals the posterior pituitary gland to increase secretion of vasopressin (antidiuretic hormone [ADH]). Elevated vasopressin levels lead to reabsorption of free water in the renal tubular cells, thereby increasing water retention. Lymphatic flow also decreases.

BRIDGE TO CRITICAL CARE

Troubleshooting Alarms

Display Message	Possible Cause	Remedy
High continuous pressure	Airway pressure higher than set PEEP plus 15 cm H_2O for more than 15 sec	Check client Check circuit Check ventilator settings and alarm limits
Check tubings	Disconnected pressure transducer (expiratory) Blocked pressure transducer (expiratory) Water in expiratory limb of ventilator Wet bacterial filter Clogged bacterial filter	Check ventilator internals on expiratory side Refer to service Replace filter Remove water from tubing and check humidifier settings (i.e., relative humidity) Check heater wires in humidifier (if present)
Airway pressure too high *Note:* If airway pressure rises 6 cm H_2O above set upper pressure limit, the safety valve opens Safety valve also opens if system pressure exceeds 120 cm H_2O	Kinked or blocked client tubing Mucus or secretion plug in endotracheal tube or in airways Client coughing or fighting ventilator Inspiratory flow rate too high Improper alarm setting	Check client Check ventilator settings and alarm limits
Limited pressure *Note:* Alarm is active only in PRVC and VS modes	Kinked or blocked client tubing Mucus or secretion plug in endotracheal tube or in airways Client coughing or fighting ventilator Improper alarm setting Client's lung/thorax compliance decreasing Client's airway resistance increasing	Check ventilator settings and alarm limits
Expired minute volume too high	Increased client activity Ventilator self-triggering (autocycling) Improper alarm limit setting Wet flow transducer	Check client Check trigger sensitivity setting Check alarm limit settings Dry the flow transducer
Expired minute volume too low	Low spontaneous client breathing activity Leakage in cuff Leakage in client circuit Improper alarm limit setting	Check client Check cuff pressure Check client circuit (perform leakage test if necessary) Check pause time and graphics to verify Consider more ventilatory support for client
Expired minute volume display reads 0	Flow transducer faulty Circuit disconnected from client	Replace flow transducer Connect Y-piece to client
Apnea alarm *Note:* If in VS, ventilator will revert to PRVC; back-up rate and time must be set	Time between two consecutive inspiratory efforts exceeds: Adult: 20 sec Pediatric: 15 sec Neonate: 10 sec	Check client Check ventilator settings
PEEP/CPAP and/or plateau pressure fails to be maintained	Leakage in cuff Leakage in client circuit Improper alarm limit setting	Check cuff pressure Check client circuit (perform leakage test if necessary) Check pause time and graphics to verify Consider more ventilatory support for client

Modified from *Servo Ventilator 300 operating manual 8.0* (1996). Solna, Sweden: Siemens-Elema AB. *CPAP,* Continuous positive airway pressure; *PEEP,* positive end-expiratory pressure; *PRVC,* pressure-regulated volume control; *VS,* volume support.

In addition, PPV can cause neurophysiologic changes. When the oxygenation levels improve in a client with respiratory failure, cerebral oxygenation also improves. A client with compensated *respiratory acidosis* (chronic CO_2 retention) may be adversely affected by positive-pressure breathing because too much CO_2 is exhaled, or "blown off." If acute respiratory alkalosis occurs, the client may exhibit dizziness, lightheadedness, and anxiety. If severe alkalosis persists, convulsions, cardiac dysrhythmias, and cerebral edema may occur. Cerebral edema may also contribute to intensive care unit (ICU) psychosis.

Oxygen toxicity can develop in clients who receive oxygen at concentrations greater than 70% for as little as 16 to 24 hours. Oxygen free radicals are produced in excess of their normal consumption by antioxidants; oxygen free radicals damage cell membranes, which increases the risk of pulmonary fibrosis. Manifestations of oxygen toxicity include fatigue, lethargy, weakness, restlessness, and nausea and vomiting. Later manifestations include severe dyspnea, coughing, tachycardia, tachypnea, crackles, and cyanosis. Because these manifestations are vague, oxygen concentration is limited to the minimal percentage and amount of time needed to maintain oxygenation.

Nursing Management

The nurse coordinates efforts of the health care team, teaches and supports the client and family, monitors the client's response to ventilation, intervenes to maintain oxygenation and ventilation, and ensures that the client's complex needs are met. The Care Plan feature on pp. 1646-1649 describes this coordinated care.

Neuromuscular Blocking Agents

Sedation with paralysis is often necessary to maintain ventilation by creating a synchronous respiratory pattern and reducing oxygen demand. In some clients, paralysis with neuromuscular blocking agents is also needed. The most common agents given are vecuronium (Norcuron) and pancuronium (Pavulon). Because neuromuscular blocking agents do not inhibit pain or awareness, they are combined with a sedative or an anxiolytic agent. Unfortunately, the use of paralytics has been linked to prolonged paralysis from either overdose of the medication or accumulation of active metabolites. Sedation assessment scales and/or bispectral index monitoring are techniques used to determine adequate sedation levels. Peripheral nerve stimulation, using a train-of-four (TOF) peripheral nerve stimulator, is commonly used to guide sustained paralysis. TOF delivers four low-energy impulses over a nerve; usually the ulnar nerve is used. When the ulnar nerve is stimulated, the response of the thumb is observed. The ideal response is two twitches of the thumb with four impulses. If no twitching is noted, the client is too paralyzed; if four twitches are noted, there is no

paralysis. There is some evidence that clients recall unusual dreams while under paralysis and sedation.

> **While necessary to provide comfort and facilitate treatment, careful monitoring to determine the minimum amount of sedation to meet treatment goals is important. Pain medication may also be required if the client has pain. If the client is awake, be aware of the anxiety or fear related to inability to breathe independently. Several nursing precautions are needed while these neuromuscular blocking agents are administered. Reorient the client often, and explain all procedures because the client can still hear but cannot move or see.**
>
> **Safety is a major concern because the client cannot verbalize or identify problems. Specific attention should be given to the eyes to prevent corneal abrasions and other eye injuries. Eye care with lubricating ointment is important.**   SAFETY ALERT

Suctioning

Because the client loses the ability to cough while on mechanical ventilation and secretions tend to pool and obstruct the airways, suctioning is often required.

> **The client should be suctioned through the ET tube only when needed to prevent hypoxemia and to prevent injury to bronchial and lung tissue. Priorities when suctioning a client include hyperoxygenation before suctioning and maintaining sterile technique including the use of the closed tracheal suction system (see Figure 63-4).**   SAFETY ALERT

See the nursing Care Plan on pp. 1646-1649 for additional guidelines for suctioning a client.

Complications of Mechanical Ventilation

There are several potential complications of mechanical ventilation. Ventilator-associated pneumonia (VAP) is a potentially avoidable nosocomial infection that occurs greater than 48 hours after mechanical ventilation. Clients that develop VAP are at increased risk of mortality as well as prolonged intubation times and increased ICU stays. The endotracheal tube provides a pathway for bacteria to enter the lower respiratory tract.

> **A major cause of VAP is colonization and aspiration of oropharyngeal secretions. Measures to prevent VAP include keeping the client's head of bed elevated at 30 degrees or higher and changing ventilator circuits only when visibly contaminated, providing frequent and thorough oral hygiene and meticulous suctioning techniques can prevent VAP.**   SAFETY ALERT

Other interventions found to be helpful in the prevention of VAP include stress ulcer and deep venous thrombosis prophylaxis. The Translating Evidence into Practice feature on p. 1650 describes additional nursing interventions to prevent or reduce this complication.

CARE PLAN *evolve*

The Mechanically Ventilated Client

Nursing Diagnosis: Impaired Spontaneous Ventilation related to imbalance between ventilatory capacity and ventilatory demand.
Outcomes: The client will have a normal respiratory rate and pattern, return of arterial blood gases (ABGs) and pulse oximetry to normal, decreased dyspnea, absence of air trapping, and no complications after continuous mechanical ventilation (CMV).

NOC OUTCOMES   Mechanical Ventilation Response

Interventions	NIC INTERVENTIONS	Rationales
1. Check ventilator settings, Fio_2, alarms, connections, and endotracheal (ET) tube placement (use cm markings) at beginning of each shift, hourly thereafter, and after any changes. Ensure that alarms are functional.	Mechanical Ventilation	1. Determine baseline values, and validate that settings are accurate.
2. Assess lung sounds every 1-2 hours as indicated.	Mechanical Ventilation	2. Lung sounds should be present bilaterally (unless a previous change in lung sounds is known).
3. Check placement of the ET tube, and secure the tube. Check previous records for a mark that is visible (in cm).	Mechanical Ventilation	3. The visible portion of the ET tube should not change. Securing prevents dislodgment.
4. Use a bite block.	Mechanical Ventilation	4. A bite block prevents the client from chewing on the tube and ET tube compression.
5. Assess for pressure ulcers of skin or mucous membrane irritation every shift.	Skin Surveillance	5. Devices can cause pressure on the skin. ET tubes can place pressure on the lips and oral mucosa at the ET tube site.
6. Assess for agitation, distress, and "fighting" the ventilator.	Mechanical Ventilation	6. An incorrect ventilator setup may be providing less air than the client requires.
7. Assess for an obstructed airway. If it is obstructed, manually inflate lungs with a resuscitation bag and 100% oxygen and suction the airway.	Emergency Care	7. Airway obstruction with mucus may prevent oxygenation. Providing air to the client is imperative. A common cause of obstruction is retained secretions.
8. Sedate and paralyze the client if ventilator settings and oxygenation are adequate.	Mechanical Ventilation	8. Sedation and paralysis may be required to prevent mismatch.
9. Medicate the client if pain is present.	Comfort Care	9. Pain can lead to agitation.
10. Perform passive range-of-motion (ROM) or assisted ROM exercises and transfer the client to a chair when feasible.	Body Mechanics Promotion	10. Immobility leads to decreased respiratory muscle strength.

Evaluation: The timing of goal attainment will vary greatly because of underlying co-morbid conditions. Expect postoperative clients to require CMV for 24 hours or less. Clients with end-stage pulmonary disease may require prolonged ventilatory support.

Nursing Diagnosis: Impaired Gas Exchange and Ineffective Breathing Pattern related to underlying disease process and artificial airway and ventilator system.
Outcomes: The client will have improved gas exchange and breathing pattern, ventilation of both lungs, no manifestations of hypoxemia (O_2 saturation >90%, respiratory rate <24 breaths/min, no restlessness); arterial blood gases (ABGs) and acid-base balance will return to preintubation level or normal values.

NOC OUTCOMES   Respiratory Status: Gas Exchange

Interventions	NIC INTERVENTIONS	Rationales
1. Auscultate lung sounds and respiratory rate and pattern every 1 to 2 hours as needed.	Oxygen Therapy	1. Auscultation reveals the amount of fluid and secretion in the lungs, validates that the ET tube is placed correctly so that both lungs can be ventilated, and determines ventilatory effectiveness.
2. Provide adequate humidity via the ventilator or nebulizer.	Mechanical Ventilation	2. Replaces the function of the upper airway to warm and humidify the inspired air; thins secretions to facilitate their removal.
3. Turn and reposition the client every 2 hours.	Skin Integrity	3. Turning promotes the ventilation of both lungs and mobilization of secretions.
4. Monitor ABG values and pulse oximetry.	Oxygen Therapy	4. Degree of oxygenation can be indicated; lack of improvement in ABGs or falling oximetry may require a change in interventions.

Evaluation: If the client's underlying problem has been corrected by mechanical ventilation, these outcomes will be met quickly. If the client has a pre-existing pulmonary disease or is acutely ill, it may take several days for attainment of outcomes.

Nursing Diagnosis: Ineffective Airway Clearance related to inability to cough and stimulation of increased secretion formation in the lower tracheobronchial tree from the ET tube.

Outcomes: The client will have improved airway clearance, as evidenced by fewer crackles, fewer wheezes, and an absence of fever.

| NOC OUTCOMES | Respiratory Status: Airway Patency |

Interventions	NIC INTERVENTIONS	Rationales
1. Assess the need for suctioning: noisy, wet respirations; restlessness; increased pulse and respirations; visible mucus bubbling into the ET tube; and an increase in peak airway pressure.	Airway Suctioning	1. Detecting the need for suctioning early can prevent desaturation.
2. Thoroughly explain the procedure before starting, and provide reassurance to the client throughout.	Airway Suctioning	2. Suctioning can be an uncomfortable and frightening experience.
3. Airway suctioning is performed on an "as-needed" basis, not at regularly scheduled intervals.	Airway Suctioning	3. Suctioning can traumatize the airway and mucosa.
4. Select a catheter of appropriate size. The most common sizes for adults are 12F and 14F.	Airway Suctioning	4. The suction catheter should never exceed half the diameter of an artificial airway or the natural airway it is to enter.
5. Avoid excessive vacuum pressures that may traumatize the airway.	Airway Suctioning	5. The safe range of pressure for adults is 80 to 120 mm Hg.
6. Maintain sterility throughout the procedure. Use closed system for suctioning. Clean gloves can be used for closed suctioning; sterile gloves are needed for open suctioning.	Airway Suctioning	6. Usual cilia clearance and cough are suppressed. Closed systems avoid opening the ET tube and exposing the airway to the environment.
7. Hyperoxygenate before and after each suctioning attempt and after the procedure. Increase the Fio$_2$ on ventilator (remember to return to previous setting upon completion) or manually ventilate the client.	Airway Suctioning	7. Providing extra oxygen prevents desaturation from suctioning.
8. Instill saline infrequently and only when secretions are tenacious.	Airway Suctioning	8. Excess saline instillation before suctioning has been associated with pulmonary edema.

Evaluation: The ability to maintain a clear airway will require several days until the underlying problem (e.g., pneumonia) is stabilized and the client's strength returns.

Nursing Diagnosis: Anxiety related to dependence on CMV for breathing.

Outcomes: The client will exhibit decreased anxiety as evidenced by reduction in the level of stress or anxiety and decreased feelings of powerlessness.

| NOC OUTCOMES | Anxiety |

Interventions	NIC INTERVENTIONS	Rationales
1. Develop a means of communication.	Anxiety Reduction	1. Communication allows the client to have needs met.
2. Place a nurse-call device within the client's reach.	Anxiety Reduction	2. Anxiety is increased when fear of being alone is present.
3. Be available and visible.	Presence	3. The client's anxiety is alleviated when not alone.
4. Provide distractions (e.g., television, radio).	Calming Techniques	4. Anxiety is reduced because the client does not focus on the ventilator and noises.
5. Explain all procedures.	Anxiety Reduction	5. The client feels respected and fears are alleviated.
6. Medicate as necessary for anxiety.	Medication Administration	6. Antianxiety medications and opioids may be needed, but use them with caution during weaning because these drugs suppress respiratory drive.
7. Provide privacy.	Anxiety Reduction	7. Providing privacy demonstrates respect for the client.
8. Respect the client's rights and opinions.	Anxiety Reduction	8. The client feels respected and maintains dignity when included in discussion.
9. Provide a calm environment.	Calming Techniques	9. A frenzied environment engenders anxiety; if the client becomes anxious, ventilation is more difficult and oxygen needs increase.
10. Explain to the client and family that the client's vocal cords have been bypassed, which prevents talking; encourage them to use other modes of communication.	Emotional Support	10. Clients can hear and respond even though they cannot talk.

Evaluation: Expect the client to remain moderately anxious while receiving CMV.

(Continued)

The Mechanically Ventilated Client—Cont'd

Collaborative Problem. High Risk for Complications of CMV and Positive-Pressure Ventilation (PPV).
Outcomes: The nurse will monitor the client for pulmonary barotrauma, cardiovascular depression, inadvertent extubation, and improper positioning of the ET tube.

Interventions	NIC INTERVENTIONS	Rationales
1. Assess for acute, increasing, or severe dyspnea; agitation; panic; decreased or absent breath sounds; localized hyperresonance; increased breathing effort; tracheal deviation away from the side with abnormal findings; subcutaneous emphysema; and decreasing Pao_2 levels.	Mechanical Ventilation	1. Barotrauma can lead to pneumothorax or tension pneumothorax.
2. Assess for an acute or gradual fall in blood pressure, tachycardia (early manifestation), bradycardia (late manifestation), dysrhythmias, weak peripheral pulses, acute or gradual increase in pulmonary capillary wedge pressure (PCWP), and respiratory "swing" (depression) in arterial or pulmonary artery wave forms during inspiration.	Mechanical Ventilation	2. Cardiovascular depression can occur after an increase in tidal volume, positive end-expiratory pressure (PEEP), continuous positive airway pressure (CPAP), or with hyperinflation; positive pressure decreases venous return and cardiac output because of an increase in intrathoracic pressure.
3. Monitor for manifestations of inadvertent extubation: vocalization, low-pressure alarm, bilateral decrease in upper lobe airway sounds, gastric distention, clinical manifestations of inadequate ventilation; change in length of portion of ET tube that extends beyond the lip. If inadvertent extubation occurs, notify the physician, because reintubation may be necessary; manage ventilation and oxygenation with a self-inflating resuscitation bag.	Mechanical Ventilation	3. Inadvertent extubation can be obvious, as when the tube is found in the client's hand; it can also be obscure, as when the tube slips into the hypopharynx or esophagus.
4. Keep an intubation tray readily available.	Mechanical Ventilation	4. Intubation supplies may be needed quickly

Evaluation: Most complications of PPV occur within 48 hours after intubation. Inadvertent extubation can occur at any time.

Nursing Diagnosis: Risk for Infection related to impaired primary defenses in respiratory tract.
Outcomes: The client will remain free of infection, as evidenced by clear sputum, no fever, clear lung sounds, no increased difficulty with ventilation (e.g., increased peak inspiratory pressure), white blood cell (WBC) count within normal limits, and respiratory rate less than 24 breaths/min.

NOC OUTCOMES   Infection Severity

Interventions	NIC INTERVENTIONS	Rationales
1. Wash your hands thoroughly.	Infection Control	1. Hand-washing reduces spread of infection.
2. Use sterile technique for open suctioning.	Infection Control	2. The respiratory tract is considered sterile.
3. Monitor the client for increased breathing effort, localized changes on auscultation, and changes in Pao_2.	Respiratory Monitoring	3. Infected lung segments transmit sound differently (more solid) and do not permit gas exchange.
4. Provide oral care every 2 hours.	Infection Protection	4. The client's mouth becomes dry, and stomatitis may develop from lack of oral secretions.
5. Drain water from ventilator tubing; do not drain water back into the humidifier.	Infection Control	5. Water may become a source of contamination, especially from *Pseudomonas*.
6. Monitor laboratory values, WBC count, and differential.	Respiratory Monitoring	6. WBC count increases may indicate pulmonary infection.
7. Monitor sputum for changes in color, consistency, amount, and odor.	Respiratory Monitoring	7. Infection may cause sputum to increase, darken, thicken, and become malodorous.

Evaluation: Infection usually develops after 72 hours of intubation unless the client is immunosuppressed; then infection develops more rapidly.

Nursing Diagnosis: Imbalanced Nutrition: Less Than Body Requirements related to lack of ability to eat while on a ventilator and to increased metabolic needs.

Outcomes: The client will exhibit adequate nutritional intake, as evidenced by (1) stable weight or weight appropriate to height, (2) intake of adequate calorie levels, (3) no manifestations of catabolism, (4) wound healing, (5) absence of infection, (6) laboratory values within normal limits (prealbumin, total protein, transferrin), and (7) adequate muscle strength to breathe spontaneously.

NOC OUTCOMES   Nutritional Status

Interventions	NIC INTERVENTIONS	Rationales
1. Provide adequate nutrition (high calorie intake, protein, vitamins, and minerals); provide a nutrition consult as needed.	Nutritional Therapy	1. Inadequate nutrition decreases diaphragmatic muscle mass, decreases pulmonary function, and increases mechanical ventilation requirements. Calorie and protein needs are calculated by a dietitian.
2. Begin tube-feeding as soon as it is evident that the client will remain on CMV for a length of time (usually 2-3 days).	Nutritional Therapy	2. The client should not be allowed to go into a catabolic state.
3. Avoid excessive carbohydrate loads.	Nutritional Therapy	3. Carbohydrate loads may increase carbon dioxide production to the point of producing hypercapnia.
4. Weigh the client daily.	Nutritional Monitoring	4. Changes in body weight are a reliable indicator of nutritional balance.
5. Monitor intake and output.	Nutritional Monitoring	5. Fluids are still required, and output should match intake.
6. Assess for complications of tube-feeding: aspiration, diarrhea, constipation. Position the client sitting upright for feeding, with the cuff inflated. Check for residual tube-feeding every 4 hours (continuous feeding) or before beginning another feeding (intermittent feeding).	Nutritional Therapy	6. Diarrhea is often caused by osmotic changes from an excessive concentration of tube-feeding or the use of sorbitol-based elixirs; consider reducing the concentration or changing to crushed pills. Constipation is caused by a lack of free water within the feeding; add 100 ml of water every 4 to 6 hours if allowable.
7. If the client cannot tolerate enteral feeding, consider parenteral nutrition to meet metabolic needs.	Nutritional Monitoring	7. Clients with decreased gastrointestinal function may require total parenteral feeding (TPN).
8. Monitor bowel sounds.	Nutritional Monitoring	8. Bowel obstruction and ileus present as changes in bowel sounds.
9. Before tube-feeding or between bolus feedings, obtain gastric pH and Hemoccult test every 8 hours.	Nutritional Therapy	9. A change in pH may indicate an increased risk of stress ulcer. A positive Hemoccult test indicates bleeding.

Evaluation: Malnutrition is preventable. Expect the client's weight to stabilize (unless there is fluid imbalance).

Nursing Diagnosis: Impaired Verbal Communication related to mute state when the ET tube is in place.

Outcomes: The client will be able to communicate with health care providers in order to have basic needs met.

NOC OUTCOMES   Communication

Interventions	NIC INTERVENTIONS	Rationales
1. Help the client develop a means of communication. Keep a pencil and paper pad or a picture board readily available.	Communication Enhancement: Speech Deficit	1. With an ET tube passing through the vocal cords, the client cannot cough effectively or speak.
2. Be patient and willing to spend time communicating.	Communication Enhancement: Speech Deficit	2. Prevents feelings of frustration, and reduces anxiety.

Evaluation: Depending on pre-existing problems (language), disease-related problems (confusion), or treatment-related problems (restraints) affecting communication, the timing to develop effective communication may be long or short.

Nursing Diagnosis: Impaired Oral Mucous Membrane related to nothing by mouth (NPO) status.

Outcomes: The client's gums and mouth will remain moist and ulcer-free.

NOC OUTCOMES   Oral Hygiene

Interventions	NIC INTERVENTIONS	Rationales
1. Provide oral hygiene every 2 hours, moistening the entire mouth and tongue.	Oral Health Restoration	1. Oral mucous membranes dry in 2 hours.
2. Moisten the mouth with solutions that do not contain alcohol or lemon.	Oral Health Restoration	2. Alcohol and lemon solutions dry mucous membranes.
3. Moisten lips with lubricant.	Oral Health Restoration	3. Lubricants prevent drying, cracking, and excoriation.
4. Brush the client's teeth twice daily.	Oral Health Restoration	4. Dental caries are prevented by saliva.
5. Suction oral secretions from mouth.	Oral Health Restoration	5. Secretions pool in the oropharynx because of the inflated tracheal cuff.
6. Assess for pressure areas from the ET tube and reposition daily.	Oral Health Restoration	6. ET tubes can lead to pressure ulcers on lips.

Evaluation: Oral mucous membranes can be restored to pink and moist within 24 hours. Oral care, however, is an ongoing need.

❦ TRANSLATING EVIDENCE INTO PRACTICE

Ventilator-Associated Pneumonia

Ventilator-associated pneumonia (VAP) is a nosocomial pneumonia that is a common problem in clients with ARDS, compared to other respiratory problems requiring mechanical ventilation. Bacteria may enter the respiratory tract from aspiration of oral-pharyngeal secretions or inhalation of aerosols containing bacteria. Aspiration is especially common in those clients who have decreased levels of consciousness, had devices or instruments in the lungs or gastrointestinal (GI) tract, or had surgery on the lungs or abdomen.

PREVENT GASTRIC REFLUX

Gram-negative bacillus infections from organisms originating in the GI tract are the most common. Usually bacteria are destroyed by acidic gastric pH, but when the pH is greater than 4 the bacteria can thrive. Tube feedings, histamines, and proton pump blockers contribute to lowering the gastric pH and have been associated with increased risk of pneumonias. Many ventilated clients have nasogastric tubes that predispose them to gastric reflux, which increases the risk of aspiration.[1] The most important intervention to prevent gastric reflux is elevation of the head of the bed. Unless medically contraindicated, the bed of a client on mechanical ventilation should remain elevated 30 to 45 degrees at all times.[2] Two studies have shown that head of bed elevation significantly decreases the incidence of VAP.[3,4]

PREVENT ASPIRATION

ET tubes prevent the glottis from closing, which leaves the airway exposed and allows oropharyngeal secretions that accumulate above the tube cuff to leak into the lungs. Mucus can accumulate on the top of the cuff of the ET tube and along the tube, where neither antibiotics nor white blood cells can reach the organisms to destroy them. Suctioning secretions from the ET tube cannot reach mucus on the top of the cuff. The CDC suggests using a particular type of ET tube, sometimes referred to as a continuous aspiration of subglottic secretions (CASS) tube.[5] It features an additional lumen that ends with an evacuation port just above the cuff, making it possible to remove secretions from above the cuff by applying continuous or intermittent suction through the extra lumen. Studies have found that the use of a CASS tube can significantly reduce the incidence of VAP.[2,6] Use only sterile fluid to clear a catheter that you are using to suction secretions from the client's lower respiratory tract if you are planning to reinsert it into the ET tube.[6]

Suction catheters are used to remove secretions in the ET tube. Two types exist: a closed system and an open system. Open suction systems are single use, and the frequency of changing closed systems is not clear. Studies have not shown significant differences in VAP and one study showed a significant reduction in days in the ICU.[7,8]

PROVIDE ORAL CARE

Although oral care has been linked to reduced VAP cases,[9] the frequency of oral care has not been described. Toothettes are the most common device used.

HAND-WASHING

Prevention of VAP is best accomplished through adequate hand-washing and wearing gloves when suctioning or manipulating the ET tube. Compliance with hand-washing is far from ideal and the use of alcohol gels may help increase compliance.[10,11]

IMPLICATIONS

VAP is a common complication in clients on ventilators because of changes in their risk profile for aspiration and lowered immune status. Nursing care can prevent or reduce the number of VAP cases.

REFERENCES

1. Kollef, M.H. (1999). The prevention of ventilator-associated pneumonia. *New England Journal of Medicine, 340*(8), 627.
2. Smulders, K., van der Hoeven, H., et al. (2002). A randomized clinical trial of intermittent subglottic secretion drainage in patients receiving mechanical ventilation. *Chest, 121*(3), 858.
3. Drakulovic, M.B., Torres, A., et al. (1999). Supine body position as a risk factor for nosocomial pneumonia in mechanically ventilated patients: A randomized trial. *Lancet, 354*(9193), 1851.
4. Ibanez, J., Penafiel, A., et al. (1992). Gastroesophageal reflux in intubated patients receiving enteral nutrition: Effect of supine and semirecumbent positions. *Journal of Parenteral and Enteral Nutrition, 16*(5), 419.
5. Centers for Disease Control and Prevention. (2004). *Guidelines for preventing health-care-associated pneumonia, 2003: Recommendations of CDC and the Healthcare Infection Control Practices Advisory Committee (HICPAC).* Retrieved 05/22/07 from www.cdc.gov/ncidod/hip/pneumonia/default.htm.
6. Valles, J., Artigas, A., et al. (1995). Continuous aspiration of subglottic secretions in preventing ventilator-associated pneumonia. *Annals of Internal Medicine, 122*(3), 179.
7. Johnson, K.L., Kearney, P.A., Johnson, S.B., et al. (1994). Closed versus open suctioning: Costs and physiologic consequences. *Critical Care Medicine, 22*(4), 658-666.
8. Cook, D., De Jonghe, B., Brochard, E., et al. (1998). Influence of airway management on ventilator associated pneumonia: Evidence from an randomized trial. *Journal of the American Medical Association, 279*(10), 781-787.
9. Mori, H., Hirasawa, H., Oda, S., et al. (2006). Oral care reduces incidence of ventilator-associated pneumonia in ICU populations. *Critical Care Medicine, 32*(2), 230-236.
10. Kim, P.W., Roghmann, M.C., et al. (2003). Rates of hand disinfection associated with glove use, patient isolation, and changes between exposure to various body sites. *American Journal of Infection Control, 31*(2), 97.
11. Sharir, R., Teitler, N., et al. (2001). High-level handwashing compliance in a community teaching hospital: A challenge that can be met!. *Journal of Hospital Infection, 49*(1), 55.

Dental or vocal cord trauma and tracheal mucosa damage from prolonged ET tube placement are a risk. Therefore tracheostomy may be used in clients who need long-term ventilation. Barotrauma may occur from excessive intra-alveolar pressure and is prevented by careful PEEP adjustment and avoiding high tidal volumes if possible. Gastric complications include distention from air entering the gastrointestinal tract and stress ulcers from hyperacidity and inadequate nutrition. Aspiration of oral secretions or gastric contents can be prevented by maintaining head of bead elevation at >45 degrees, careful monitoring of gastric residuals, meticulous suctioning, and maintaining adequate cuff inflation. Medications that block production of gastric acids are often prescribed.

Self-extubation often occurs during times of agitation or turning and repositioning the client. Because the cuff is inflated, the tracheal wall can be damaged and bleeding can ensue. In most cases, the client requires reintubation, which must be done swiftly to prevent hypoxemia and to avoid inserting the ET tube through swollen tissues. Sometimes, the client can be monitored and not reintubated, especially if the time for extubation was approaching. Unplanned extubation often leads to increased duration of mechanical ventilation and longer ICU stays. Nursing interventions to prevent unplanned extubation are shown in Box 63-2.

Other complications that arise from extended mechanical ventilation include problems from limited mobility such as deep venous thromboembolism, skin breakdown, malnutrition, and stress and anxiety.

Weaning from a Ventilator

Weaning is the gradual withdrawal of mechanical ventilation. The criteria for weaning are shown in Box 63-3. The client's ability to breathe independently is the most important criterion for successful weaning. Minute ventilation and tidal volume are indicators that the client is meeting adequate tidal volume requirements; creating negative inspiratory force, which indicates inspiratory muscle strength; and generating positive expiratory pressure, which indicates respiratory muscle strength and ability to cough. The length of time required for successful weaning generally relates to the underlying disease process and to the client's state of health before the ventilator was used. For example, a young client who is recovering from an overdose of drugs can usually be weaned rapidly, but a client with COPD and acute

---

BOX 63-3 Criteria for a Ventilator Weaning Trial

- Reversal of underlying cause of respiratory failure
- Adequate oxygenation, indicated by the following:
  - $Pao_2 \geq 60$ mm Hg on $Fio_2 \leq 40\text{-}50\%$
  - PEEP requirement $\leq 5\text{-}8$ cm H_2O
  - pH ≥ 7.25
  - $Pao_2/Fio_2 > 150\text{-}300$
- Heart rate ≤ 140 beats/min
- Stable BP with no or minimal vasopressive medications, such as dopamine or norepinephrine ≤ 5 mcg/kg/min
- No myocardial ischemia
- Temperature $\leq 100.4°$ F ($38°$ C)
- Hemoglobin $\geq 8\text{-}10$ g/dl
- Acceptable electrolyte values
- Adequate cough
- Capability to initiate inspiration/maximum inspiratory pressure less than or equal to -20 cm H_2O
- Adequate mentation without continuous IV sedation

From MacIntyre, N.R., Cook, D.J., et al. (2001). Evidenced based guidelines for weaning and discontinuing ventilatory support. A collective task force facilitated by the American College of Chest Physicians, the American Association for Respiratory Care and the American College of Critical Care Medicine. *Chest, 120*(6 Suppl), 375S.

---

respiratory failure with little or no pulmonary reserve often takes longer and requires much professional patience and skill. Weaning should be instituted after paralytics are discontinued, and sedation is tapered off. During the weaning process, the client should be observed for increased respiratory rate, shallow breathing, and decreased tidal volume, which may indicate muscle fatigue.

Techniques for Weaning

Spontaneous Breathing Trial. With the client still connected to the ventilator, the head of the bed is elevated and the client's ability to breathe on his or her own is measured. Most clients will be excited about coming off of the ventilator but at the same time concerned about being able to breathe on their own. Explain the weaning plan and assure the client you will remain at the bedside to monitor progress and problems with the trial.

Pressure Support Ventilation (PSV). Using this form of weaning, the ventilator delivers a set amount of positive pressure into the lungs with each breath initiated by the client. With PSV, the client controls both the length and the depth of each breath. This form of weaning is used for clients who have been on mechanical ventilation for longer periods of time.

Synchronized Intermittent Mandatory Ventilation (SIMV). With this mode of ventilation, the ventilator provides a set amount of breaths and tidal volumes in coordination

---

BOX 63-2 Strategies to Prevent Unplanned or Accidental Extubation

- Provide adequate sedation and pain control.
- Use wrist restraints according to hospital protocol.
- Secure the ET tube with tape or other commercial devices.
- Record the centimeter reference number at the lips.
- Assess the position of the ET tube routinely and after each position change.
- Support the ventilator tubes and suction tubing and keep them out of the client's reach.
- Use two staff members to reposition the ET tube.
- Explain the purpose of the tube and the need for restraints to the client and family.

*, Endotracheal.

with the client's efforts. As the client breathes more independently, the number of breaths by the ventilator decreases eventually to zero. This form of weaning is also used when more time is needed for weaning.

Difficulties in Weaning

A first weaning attempt may not be successful for several reasons, including decreased muscular strength caused by protein-carbohydrate malnutrition, underlying disease processes, or inability of respiratory muscles to sustain respiratory efforts as a result of disuse after prolonged CMV. Increased work of breathing caused by increased airway resistance, abdominal distention, a small-diameter artificial airway, upper airway obstruction, or unresolved acute lung diseases may also affect the success of the first weaning attempt. Other reasons include increased ventilation requirements, difficulty managing secretions, and psychological factors, such as fear and anxiety.

If the first attempt at weaning is not successful, determine the reasons and try to eliminate them in subsequent attempts. Clients who require prolonged ventilatory support and extended periods of weaning often do best in a setting that promotes rehabilitation concepts. These clients can usually be transferred to subacute or long-term acute care facilities.

Extubation

Extubation is the removal of the ET tube. Once the client has been weaned successfully, has demonstrated adequate ventilatory effort, and has maintained an acceptable level of consciousness to sustain spontaneous respiration, the ET tube may be removed. ET tubes are removed on physician's orders and only by health care team members qualified to reintubate if necessary. The occurrence of laryngospasm and tracheal edema after extubation may occlude the airway, requiring immediate reintubation.

The ET tube is suctioned, the cuff deflated, and the tube removed. Immediately after extubation, the client is usually placed on an oxygen mask. Assess the client for manifestations of respiratory distress and hypoxemia, as evidenced by restlessness, irritability, tachycardia, use of accessory muscles, and tachypnea. ABGs are obtained and monitored for decreased Pao_2 or increased $Paco_2$ levels, which indicate an inability to sustain ventilation. If these manifestations are noted, notify the physician and prepare for reintubation.

Dysfunctional Ventilatory Weaning Response

Some clients cannot adjust to lowered levels of mechanical ventilation, and the process of weaning them from the ventilator is delayed. The nursing diagnosis *Dysfunctional Ventilatory Weaning Response related to respiratory muscle fatigue or anxiety* was developed for these situations. Manifestations of respiratory muscle fatigue include a respiratory rate more than 30 breaths/min, increased $Paco_2$ level, abnormal patterns of breathing, hemodynamic changes such as dysrhythmias, diaphoresis, anxiety, and dyspnea.

An unsuccessful attempt to wean the client may have taken place, resulting in reintubation. When the client cannot sustain ventilation independently, the ventilator is set at full ventilation; the client has no spontaneous breaths and therefore can rest. Once the client has rested, attempts at weaning should begin again. Some clients can never be weaned from mechanical ventilation. Those clients can be managed in less acute care units or at home for many years.

Ventilator-Dependent Clients

Some clients become stable and can be discharged from acute care and return home (see the website Bridge to Home Health Care feature titled Living with a Ventilator for ways to assist the ventilator-dependent client).

ADULT (ACUTE) RESPIRATORY DISTRESS SYNDROME

Adult (acute) respiratory distress syndrome (ARDS) is a sudden, progressive form of respiratory failure characterized by severe dyspnea, refractory hypoxemia, and diffuse bilateral infiltrates. It follows acute and massive lung injury that results from a variety of clinical states, often occurring in previously healthy people. The syndrome was first described in 1967 and has been referred to by several terms, including shock lung, wet lung, post-traumatic lung, congestive atelectasis, capillary leak syndrome, and adult hyaline membrane disease. Tremendous advances in the treatment of this condition have occurred over the last 2 decades.

Etiology and Risk Factors

ARDS develops as a result of ischemia in the alveolar capillary membrane during shock, oxygen toxicity, inhalation of noxious fumes or fluids (e.g., gastric acid), or inflammation from pneumonia or sepsis. There may be a direct insult to lung tissue or indirect injuries occurring in other body areas, with inflammatory mediators sent to the lung through the vascular system. Conditions leading to ARDS are listed in Box 63-4. Early recognition and treatment of these conditions may reduce the risk of ARDS.

Pathophysiology

The hallmark of ARDS is a massive inflammatory response by the lungs that increases permeability of the alveolar membrane, with resultant fluid movement into the interstitial and alveolar spaces. This leads to th

---

BOX 63-4 **Risk Factors for Adult (Acute) Respiratory Distress Syndrome**

DIRECT PULMONARY TRAUMA

- Viral, bacterial, or fungal pneumonias
- Lung contusion
- Fat embolus
- Aspiration (e.g., foreign material, drowning, vomitus)
- Massive smoke inhalation
- Inhaled toxins
- Prolonged exposure to high concentrations of oxygen

INDIRECT PULMONARY TRAUMA

- Sepsis
- Shock
- Multisystem trauma
- Disseminated intravascular coagulation
- Pancreatitis
- Uremia
- Drug overdose
- Anaphylaxis
- Idiopathic
- Prolonged heart bypass surgery
- Massive blood transfusions
- Pregnancy-induced hypertension
- Increased intracranial pressure
- Radiation therapy

---

development of noncardiogenic pulmonary edema, which decreases lung compliance and impairs oxygen transport. Three phases of ARDS have been described:[27]

1. *Phase 1 (exudative)* is seen approximately 24 hours after the initial insult and consists of damage to the capillary endothelium and leakage of fluid into the pulmonary interstitium. Microemboli also develop and cause a further increase in pulmonary artery pressures. Inflammatory responses accompany the pulmonary parenchymal damage, leading to the release of toxic mediators, the activation of complement, the mobilization of macrophages, and the release of vasoactive substances from mast cells. There is further damage to the basement membrane, interstitial space, and alveolar epithelium. Fibrin, blood, fluid, and protein exude into the interstitial spaces around the alveoli and increase the distance across the capillary membrane.

2. *Phase 2 (proliferative)* begins about 7 to 10 days later. Type I and type II alveolar cells are ultimately damaged, resulting in decreased surfactant production, alveolar collapse, and atelectasis, leading to further impairment in gas exchange. Significant hypoxemia is present because of decreased surfactant production, intrapulmonary shunting, and $\dot{V}/\dot{Q}$ mismatch.

3. *Phase 3 (fibrotic)* occurs in about 2 to 3 weeks. There is irreversible deposition of fibrin into the lung, resulting in pulmonary fibrosis, further decreasing lung compliance and worsening hypoxemia. The end result is a significant $\dot{V}/\dot{Q}$ imbalance and profound arterial hypoxemia. (The Concept Map feature on Understanding ARDS and Its Treatment, p. 1654, illustrates these concepts.)

Clinical Manifestations

The initial insult of ARDS is followed by a period of apparently normal lung function that may last from 1 to 24 hours. Then hypoxemia rapidly develops and progresses along with decreasing lung compliance and development of diffuse lung infiltrates.

The earliest clinical manifestation of ARDS is usually an increased respiratory rate and profound dyspnea 12 to 24 hours after the initial injury. Breathing becomes increasingly labored; the client may exhibit air hunger and retractions. Chest auscultation may or may not reveal the presence of adventitious sounds. If present, abnormal sounds may range from fine inspiratory crackles to widespread coarse crackles. ABG analysis discloses increasing hypoxemia (Pao_2 <60 mm Hg) that does not respond to increased fractions of inspired oxygen levels (Fio_2 <40%) and compensatory hypocapnia. In the early stages, respiratory alkalosis is present because of hyperventilation. Later, metabolic acidosis develops from increased work of breathing and hypoxemia. The chest x-ray usually demonstrates diffuse, bilateral, and rapidly progressing interstitial or alveolar infiltrates (Figure 63-6).

Recommended diagnostic criteria include bilateral infiltrates seen on chest x-rays in the absence of fluid overload, ratio of Pao_2 (partial pressure of oxygen) to Fio_2 (fraction of inspired oxygen) less than or equal to 200 mm Hg (regardless of PEEP levels), and PAWP less than or equal to 18 mm Hg.[27] Additional diagnostic tests may be needed based on the underlying cause and include bronchial washing and biopsy to determine whether infection is present.

OUTCOME MANAGEMENT

The keys to successful management of ARDS are early detection and initiation of treatment. The goals of medical management are (1) respiratory and ventilatory support, (2) maintenance of hemodynamic stability, (3) treatment of the underlying cause, when possible, and (4) prevention of complications.

Medical Management

Support Respiration and Ventilation

Mechanical ventilation, ET intubation, and PEEP are usually required to maintain adequate blood oxygen levels. The goal of ventilatory support is to use the least amount of Fio_2 and PEEP possible to maintain oxygen saturation at or above 90% while decreasing the potential of

CONCEPT MAP

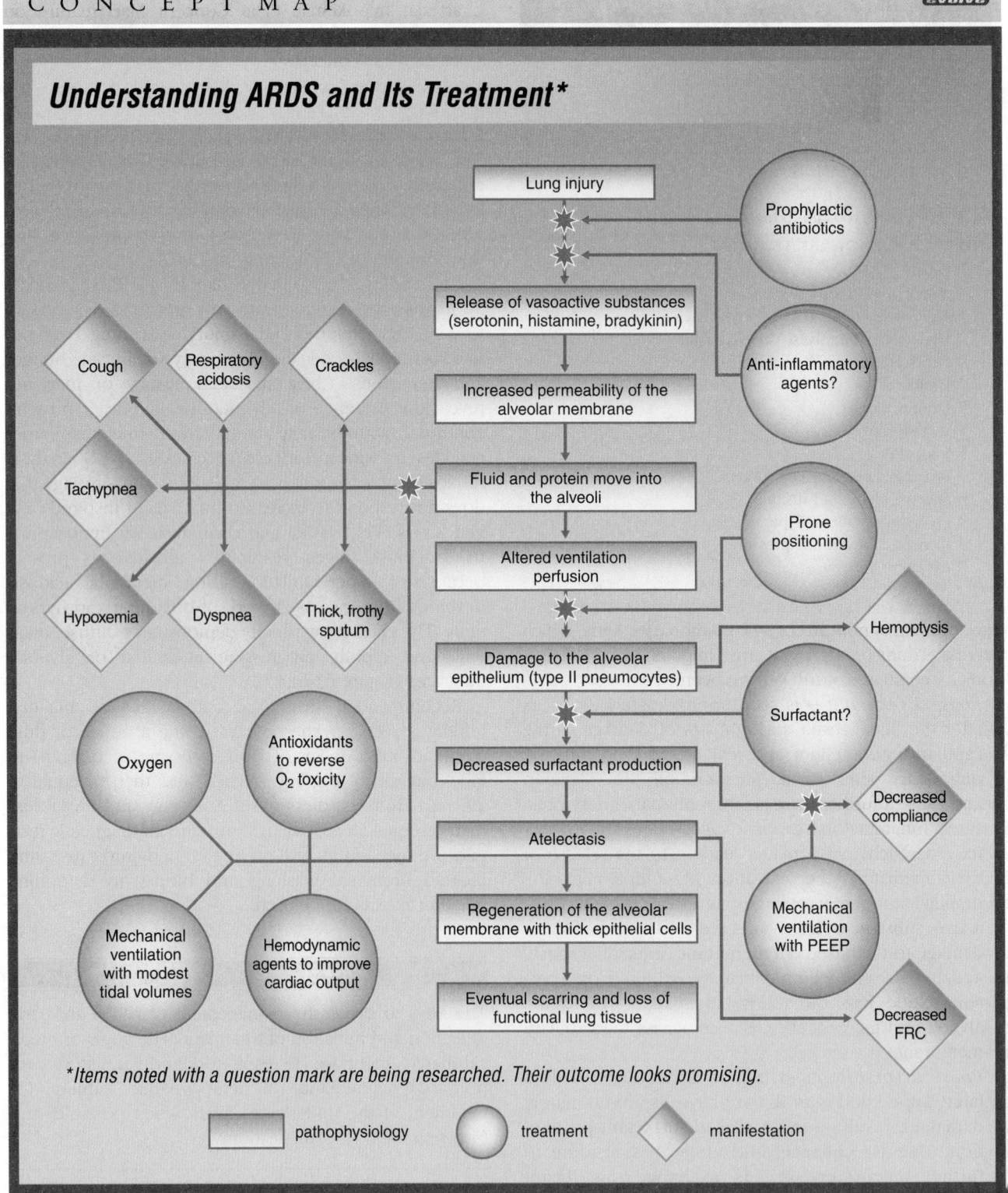

Understanding ARDS and Its Treatment*

*Items noted with a question mark are being researched. Their outcome looks promising.

□ pathophysiology   ○ treatment   ◇ manifestation

oxygen toxicity. PEEP will also be used to decrease intra-pulmonary shunting and to recruit collapsed alveoli. Studies have shown that using smaller tidal volumes (permissive hypercapnia) and the least amount of PEEP possible can reduce the risk of lung injury (low levels of CO_2 [hypocapnia] have been shown to decrease lung compliance).[16,22] Additional studies have encouraged the use of inverse ratio ventilation (IRV) as one method of increasing mean airway pressure without creating further peak pressures in the alveolus from PEEP.[6] IRV

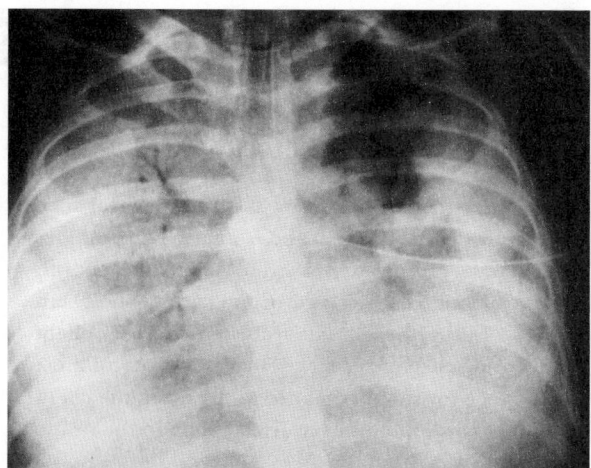

■ **FIGURE 63–6** Adult (acute) respiratory distress syndrome (ARDS). This chest x-ray study shows massive consolidation from pulmonary edema following multisystem trauma. *(From Fraser, R.G., et al. [1990]. Diagnosis of diseases of the chest [3rd ed., p. 493]. Philadelphia: Saunders.)*

increases the inspiratory portion of each breath to more than half the respiratory cycle. Because IRV maintains a prolonged positive pressure through the ventilatory cycle, alveoli stay open and gas exchange is improved. Other alternative modes of ventilation (e.g., extracorporeal membrane oxygenation [ECMO] and partial liquid ventilation) may be used in some situations but are still considered investigational therapies. Surfactant therapy has been successful for neonates but to date has not had the same results in adults with ARDS.

Nitric oxide (NO) is now being used more often in the treatment of ARDS. NO causes selective vasodilation in the pulmonary vascular system and is a powerful bronchodilator. Inhaled NO dilates the capillary bed of the lungs, which in turn reduces the pressure in the pulmonary arteries without lowering systemic blood pressure.

Antioxidants, scavengers of oxygen free radicals, are also being used. *N*-Acetylcysteine and procysteine have been effective in reducing the degradative effect of the proteases. Pharmacologic efforts to inhibit the substances released by the endotoxins, neutrophils, and macrophages are also being explored. Prostaglandins are also being investigated as a possible treatment therapy for ARDS clients, especially those with sepsis and multiple organ failure. Steroids have been used with improvement in pulmonary function.

The prone position has been used to improve oxygenation by changing the distribution of perfusion. The belief is that ARDS does the greatest damage in the gravity-dependent parts of the lungs. By placing the client in a prone position, there is a change in the dependent portions of the lung, resulting in increased perfusion to the less damaged portions of the lungs and decreased pulmonary shunting. Prone positioning is also thought to

reduce compression of the lung by the heart, improve chest wall compliance, and result in better draining of bronchial secretions. Placing a client in a prone position requires coordination by many health care professionals to turn the client while maintaining equipment patency (e.g., ET tube) and decreasing client anxiety. Side effects include hypotension, desaturation, and dysrhythmias, although these appear to be short term. A plan for immediate repositioning in the event of deteriorating condition or cardiac or respiratory arrest should be in place before placing the client in the prone position. The prone position is shown in Figure 63-7 and is further discussed in the Translating Evidence into Practice feature on p. 1656.

Kinetic therapy via continuously rotating beds can also be used to improve ventilation. The constant postural drainage assists in removing airway plugs. To be effective, the movement must be at least 45 degrees from side to side, which is best accomplished by a rotation bed.

Shearing of the sacrum may develop, and therefore the client's skin should be completely assessed twice daily. Beds set to rotate at less than 40 degrees do not provide adequate pressure relief; if used at that degree, manual turning must also be completed. The nurse needs to stop the motion of the bed and inspect the skin to examine for shear and offload the sacrum for periods of time.

SAFETY ALERT

Maintain Hemodynamic Stability

Hemodynamic monitoring is used to observe the effect of fluids and degree of pulmonary edema. The use of pharmacologic agents in the treatment of ARDS varies according to the client's underlying disease process. Inotropic agents (e.g., dobutamine or dopamine) may be indicated to improve cardiac output and to increase systemic blood pressure. Fluids are carefully monitored to prevent systemic fluid overload.

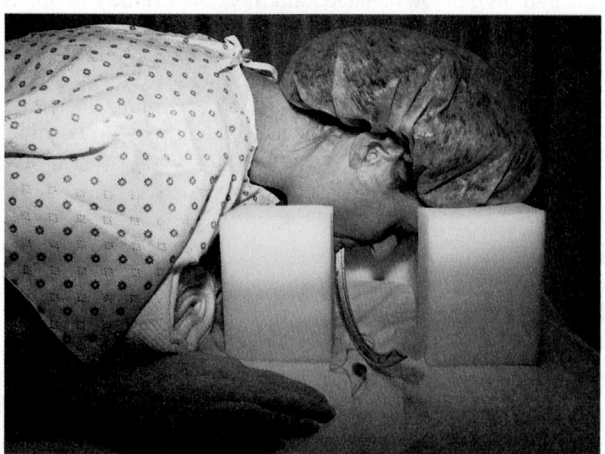

■ **FIGURE 63–7** Use of the prone position to improve ventilation-perfusion. *(Courtesy H.E.A.D. Prone, Inc., Cambridge, Mass.)*

Prone Positioning and Adult (Acute) Respiratory Distress Syndrome

Adequate perfusion and ventilation of lung tissue are important to provide adequate oxygenation to tissues and maintain life. Adult (acute) respiratory distress syndrome (ARDS) is typically characterized by decreased lung compliance and severe hypoxia. Using mechanical ventilation has long been accepted as a means to overcome the decreased compliance and to correct the life-threatening hypoxia. Additional studies are beginning to investigate the use of prone positioning with mechanical ventilation as another means to improve oxygenation while decreasing some of the complications associated with mechanical ventilation.

A meta-analysis completed by Curley identified 17 primary research studies that investigated the use of prone positioning.[3] Ryan and Pelosi presented findings from 11 studies investigating the use of prone positioning.[4] Although the studies all had different methodologies, each study met the criteria for scientific rigor and investigated the use of prone positioning to improve oxygenation. When combining the results of all 17 studies in the Curley meta-analysis, 69% of the clients (169 of 213 clients) responded positively to being placed in a prone position as demonstrated by an increase in the oxygenation saturation and Fio_2 ratio of 20% or more.[3] The studies reviewed by Ryan and Pelosi identified that 70% of the clients demonstrated improvement in oxygenation.[4] Various reasons were given for the improvements noted, including reexpansion of dependent portions of the lungs leading to atelectasis, changes in the $\dot{V}/\dot{Q}$ ratio, increase in functional residual capacity, and reduction in the amount of venous stasis.[4] As a result, the percentage of oxygen for mechanical ventilation could be decreased, thereby also decreasing the possibility of oxygen toxicity.

Several contraindications to the use of prone positioning included shock, hemorrhage, multiple trauma, spinal injury or instability, pregnancy, increased intracranial pressure, and recent abdominal surgery.[2,4] Both studies also identified complications associated with placing a client in a prone position, including the potential for impaired skin integrity, development of dependent edema in the face and anterior chest wall, damage to the eyes (corneal abrasions and ulcerations), nerve damage, and most importantly potential to dislodge extraneous tubes such as the endotracheal tube, venous and arterial lines, and Foley catheter. Care must be taken to prevent any of these complications. Strategies identified to prevent skin breakdown, eye injury, facial edema, and nerve damage included using padded cushions for bony prominences, repositioning the head every

2 hours, placing extremities in a functional position, inspecting the eyes and skin every 2 hours, and using pressure reduction devices.

To prevent loss of a line or the endotracheal tube when turning the client to and from a prone position, the nursing, respiratory therapy, and other health care professionals involved in the care of the client must work together in a coordinated effort for client safety and sense of security. Finally, a protocol must be in place for rapid response in the event the client goes into cardiopulmonary arrest while in the prone position.

Another concern identified by the researchers was the use of tube feedings while the client is in the prone position. The increased potential for regurgitation and possible aspiration of feedings or stomach contents into the lungs was mentioned.[1] The need for caloric intake was recognized as important for the critically ill client. If the gastrointestinal function is confirmed, enteral feedings can be used with a client in the prone position with careful monitoring for potential aspiration.

None of the studies reported aspiration as a noted complication.

IMPLICATIONS

Additional studies need to be conducted on the effects of prone positioning for clients with adult (acute) respiratory distress syndrome. All the studies reviewed in the meta-analyses had small sample sizes (fewer than 30 clients in any one study). Consistent results of all the studies demonstrated the improved oxygenation of a majority of the clients. Prone positioning has been found to be an effective means to improve oxygenation in clients with adult (acute) respiratory distress syndrome, especially in the early stages of the adult (acute) respiratory distress syndrome when edema in the lungs and atelectasis are apparent.

REFERENCES

1. Balas, M. (2000). Prone positioning of patients with acute respiratory distress syndrome: Applying research to practice. *Critical Care Nurse, 20*(1), 24-36.
2. Breiburg, A., et al. (2000). Efficacy and safety of prone positioning for patients with acute respiratory distress syndrome. *Journal of Advanced Nursing, 32*(4), 922-929.
3. Curley, M. (1999). Prone positioning of patients with acute respiratory distress syndrome: A systematic review. *American Journal of Critical Care, 8*(6), 397-405.
4. Ryan, D., & Pelosi, P. (1996). Prone positioning in acute respiratory distress syndrome. *British Medical Journal, 312*, 860-861.

Treat the Underlying Condition

Antibiotics are administered if suspected or confirmed infection is present. Although controversial, the use of large doses of corticosteroids is also common. The rationale for steroid administration is to reduce inflammatory response and to promote pulmonary membrane stability; however, controlled clinical trials have not demonstrated

their effectiveness in ARDS. Indiscriminate use should be avoided.[6]

Monitor for Complications

In addition to lung fibrosis, other complications may arise during supportive management of the client with ARDS, such as cardiac dysrhythmias caused by hypoxemia, oxygen toxicity, renal failure, thrombocytopenia, gastrointestinal bleeding secondary to stress ulcers, sepsis from invasive lines, and disseminated intravascular coagulation (DIC) (see Chapter 75).

Prognosis

The outcome for any one client is difficult to predict. For most of the 1970s and 1980s, death rates seemed to be constant at 60% to 70%. In the 1990s, however, rates improved, and current rates are about 40%; however, a 90% death rate remains for clients with sepsis or multiple organ failure who develop ARDS.[8]

Nursing Management

The principles of nursing management of clients with pulmonary edema and care of the client requiring mechanical ventilation are appropriate in the care of the client with ARDS. Placing a client in prone position clearly is within the realm of nursing. Evaluation of the client's response to treatment as well as careful monitoring for potential complications is essential. Emotional support for the client's family and significant others is also important. The disease can progress very rapidly, leaving family members unprepared for the severity of the client's condition. Clear communications and frequent condition updates are essential to keeping the family adequately informed.

CHEST TRAUMA

The chest is a large, exposed portion of the body that is vulnerable to impact injuries. Because the chest houses the heart, lungs, and great vessels, chest trauma is frequently life-threatening. Injury to the thoracic cage and its contents can restrict the heart's ability to pump blood or the lungs' ability to exchange air and oxygenate blood. Major dangers associated with chest injuries are internal bleeding and punctured organs.

Chest injuries can range from relatively minor bumps and scrapes to severe crushing or penetrating trauma. Chest injuries may be *penetrating* or *blunt*.[30] Penetrating chest injuries may cause an open chest wound, permitting atmospheric air into the pleural space and disrupting the normal vacuum ventilation mechanism. Penetrating chest injuries may seriously damage the lungs, heart, and other thoracic structures. Blunt injuries are most commonly deceleration injuries associated with motor-vehicle crashes. Blunt chest trauma may also result from falls or blows to the chest.

Initial assessment is directed toward identifying and treating immediate life-threatening conditions. Any client with chest trauma should be considered to have a serious injury until proven otherwise. Airway patency, adequacy of breathing, and circulatory sufficiency (i.e., presence of shock), or ABCs, are always of primary concern.

Immobilization of a potential spinal cord injury should also be initiated.

Once initial emergencies have been addressed, assess the client more thoroughly (Box 63-5). A medical history helps to identify any pre-existing conditions that could further complicate the injury. A thorough physical examination should be performed, with care being taken not to focus only on obvious injuries. Information about the accident (obtained from the injured client or witnesses) assists in the diagnosis of regional as well as anatomic injuries. A chest x-ray and electrocardiogram (ECG) are obtained for detection of possible pulmonary or cardiac impairment.

OUTCOME MANAGEMENT

Initial management should focus on airway patency, ventilation, hemorrhage control, stabilization of any thoracic fractures, and immobilization of the spinal column. Clients are typically divided into two categories: stable

---

BOX 63-5 Chest Trauma: Assessment and Interventions

1. Assess "ABCs":
   a. Maintain *a*irway, *b*reathing, and *c*irculation.
   b. Ensure adequate air movement.
2. Obtain a quick history:
   a. What happened?
   b. What was the mechanism of injury?
   c. How long ago did it happen?
   d. Where is the pain? Does it radiate?
   e. Is there anything that makes the pain better or worse?
   f. What does the pain feel like?
   g. How severe is the pain on a scale of 1 to 10?
   h. Is there a significant medical history?
3. Perform a quick (1-minute) assessment for:
   a. Shortness of breath and cyanosis
   b. Vital signs
   c. Skin color and temperature
   d. Wound size and location
   e. Paradoxical chest movement
   f. Distended neck veins
   g. Tracheal deviation
   h. Respiratory stridor
   i. Bilateral breath sounds
   j. Use of accessory muscles
   k. Estimated tidal volume
   l. Subcutaneous emphysema
   m. Sucking chest wounds
   n. Heart sounds
   o. Dysrhythmias
4. Quickly intervene:
   a. Administer oxygen.
   b. Cover any open chest wound.
   c. Control flail segment.
   d. Prepare to insert a chest tube.
   e. Initiate a large-bore intravenous line.

and unstable. The stable client needs careful and continuous monitoring, and the unstable client requires immediate management of ventilation-perfusion imbalances, shock, and pain.

Ventilation-perfusion imbalances may result from atelectasis, hemopneumothorax, flail chest, aspiration, or pulmonary contusion. Oxygen or mechanical ventilation may be required. General respiratory status (e.g., rate and depth of respirations, chest movement, spontaneous vital volumes) and ABG values should be monitored closely. Deterioration of any of these parameters may indicate previously undetected injury or late-developing complications.

Therapeutic measures such as thoracentesis, chest tube insertion, bronchoscopic aspiration, video-assisted thoracic surgery (VATS), and thoracotomy (see Chapter 62) may be indicated. Management should focus on maintaining effective functioning of any equipment used (e.g., chest drainage system) and supporting the client and significant others to understand the procedures and the rationale for their use.

Monitor continually for clinical manifestations of shock. Shock often results from hypovolemia, but in the chest-injured client it may also be caused by cardiac tamponade, cardiac contusion, flail chest, or tension pneumothorax. Central vascular pressure readings (central venous pressure or pulmonary artery pressure) require careful interpretation. Once the cause of shock is determined, rapid treatment is crucial (see Chapter 81).

Excessive blood loss may further compromise oxygenation. Assess external bleeding carefully, and estimate blood loss. Internal bleeding may result from injuries to the thoracic or abdominal viscera, torn muscles, or fractures. Considerable bleeding (2 L or more) into the pleural space may occur. This is usually detected quickly as hypovolemic shock. Bleeding into areas such as the chest wall (e.g., from torn intercostal muscles) is more difficult to assess. A liter of blood can accumulate between the chest wall muscles without producing much swelling.

Fluid replacement is with blood and blood products, if indicated, or with crystalloid intravenous solutions (e.g., lactated Ringer's solution, normal saline). A chest-injured person may require large quantities of blood replacement. Until the results of typing and crossmatching are available, the client is given O-negative blood. The volume of blood replacement is determined through assessment of clinical findings, hemodynamic measurements, and laboratory results (e.g., hemoglobin and hematocrit). When possible, surgery is delayed until blood volume is restored.

Pain associated with chest injuries may cause the client to breathe rapidly and shallowly, which leads to atelectasis and pooling of tracheobronchial secretions. Analgesics minimize pain, permit periods of rest and relaxation, and allow the client to cough and to take deeper breaths.

Opioids are most effective if given via the intravenous route. Intercostal nerve blocks or epidural analgesia may be used in clients with underlying health problems. Splinting the chest may also be helpful.

SPECIFIC CHEST INJURIES

FRACTURED RIBS

Etiology and Risk Factors

Rib fractures are common chest injuries, particularly in older adults. Such fractures are usually associated with a blunt injury, such as a fall, a blow to the chest, coughing or sneezing, the impact of the chest against a steering wheel during rapid deceleration, or less obvious traumas, such as pushing furniture when osteoporosis is present. The fifth through the ninth ribs are most commonly affected.

Clinical Manifestations

Clinical manifestations include (1) localized pain and tenderness over the fracture area on inspiration and palpation, (2) shallow respirations, (3) the client's tendency to hold the chest protectively or to breathe shallowly to minimize chest movements, (4) sometimes bruising or surface markings from the trauma at the site of injury, (5) protruding bone splinters if the fracture is compound, and (6) a clicking sensation during inspiration when costochondral separation or dislocation is present.

Fractured ribs compromise ventilation by three mechanisms. Pain from the injury causes splinting, shallow breathing, and ineffective cough, which predisposes to atelectasis and pneumonia. Secretions accumulate and obstruct the bronchi, becoming a site of infection; shallow breathing reduces lung compliance.

> **Rib fractures can result in a flail chest, which interferes with the normal physiology of breathing, and bone splinters from fractured ribs may penetrate the lung or pleura, resulting in a pneumothorax or hemothorax.**

Chest x-rays are carefully reviewed for 24 to 48 hours after injury for indications of these complications. Bright-red sputum may be coughed up if the lung has been penetrated. Continuously assess the client for manifestations of pneumothorax or hemothorax, and report such findings promptly.[10]

OUTCOME MANAGEMENT

Fractured ribs are generally treated conservatively with good pulmonary physiotherapy, rapid mobilization and proper pain management. Strapping the ribs with tape is no longer recommended because it restricts deep breathing and can increase the incidence of atelectasis and pneumonia.

Adequate pain control and splinting of the chest during coughing and deep breathing help the client with rib fractures to carry out painful but vital mobilization activities more comfortably. If pain is severe enough to impair ventilation significantly, a local anesthetic solution may be injected at the fracture site itself. Intercostal nerve blocks may also be used.[12] A client with an underlying chest or heart disease (e.g., COPD, heart failure) may benefit particularly from this type of pain management. A chest x-ray should be taken after this procedure to ensure that pneumothorax has not occurred. Hospitalization may be required, especially in older adults, whose vital capacity may be significantly compromised. The pain from fractured ribs usually lasts 5 to 7 days. Complete healing occurs in approximately 6 to 8 weeks.

FRACTURED STERNUM

Sternal fractures usually result from blunt deceleration injuries, such as impact from a steering wheel. About 40% to 60% of the clients with fractured sternums have other major injuries, such as flail chest; pulmonary and myocardial contusions; ruptured aorta, trachea, bronchus, or esophagus; and hemothorax or pneumothorax.[12]

Clinical manifestations include sharp, stabbing pain; swelling and discoloration over the fracture site; and crepitus. The main priority is to control associated injuries. A client with a nondisplaced fracture may need analgesics or intercostal nerve blocks for pain reduction. Surgical fixation may be required for severe sternal fractures.

FLAIL CHEST

Etiology and Risk Factors

Severe blunt injury to the chest often fractures multiple ribs and crushes the ribs onto lung tissue. By definition, a flail chest is one that has paradoxical movement of a segment of chest wall caused by fractures of 3 or more ribs anteriorly and posteriorly within each rib (Figure 63-8). The flail segment most commonly involves the lateral side of the chest. It is common for the end of a fractured rib to tear the pleura and lung surface (thereby producing *hemopneumothorax*) and for a crushed chest to have a flail segment. Pulmonary edema, pneumonitis, and atelectasis often develop rapidly with a crushed chest when fluids increase and collect at the injured site.

The "flail" segment no longer has bony or cartilaginous connections with the rest of the rib cage. Lacking attachment to the thoracic skeleton, the flail section "floats," moving independently of the chest wall during ventilation. This abnormality disrupts the normal bellows action of the thorax by causing *paradoxical motion,* during which the flail portion of the chest and its underlying lung tissue are (1) "sucked in" with inspiration (instead of expanding outward as normal) and (2) "blown out" with expiration (instead of collapsing normally inward).[12] This alteration in normal chest wall mechanics diminishes the client's ability to achieve an adequate tidal volume and to produce an adequate cough. Hypoventilation and hypoxia may result, leading to respiratory failure. Furthermore, mediastinal structures tend to swing back and forth (mediastinal flutter) with significant paradoxical

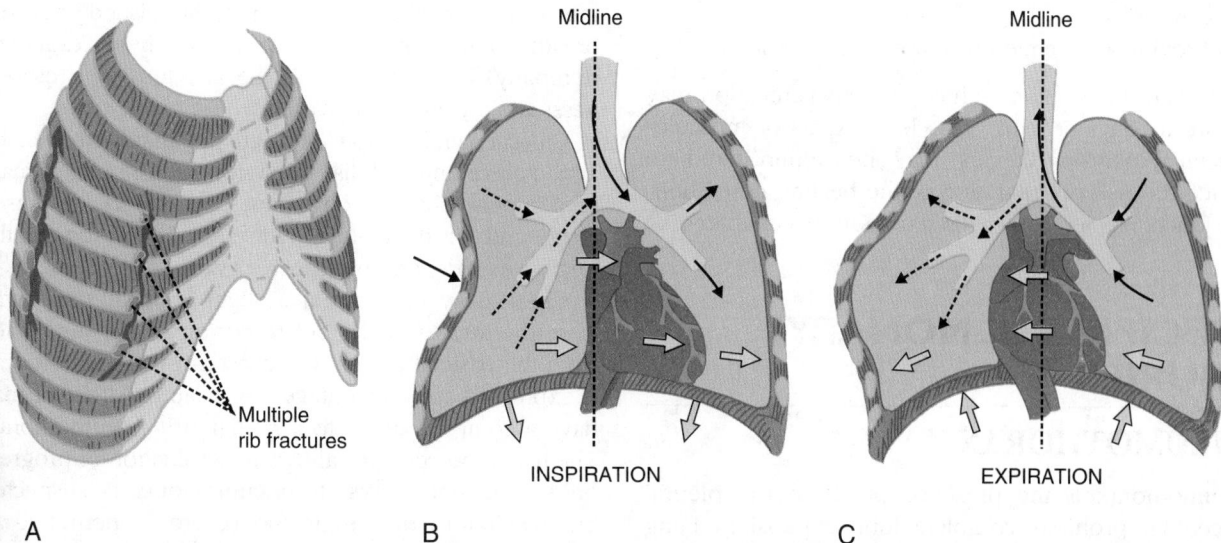

■ **FIGURE 63–8** Flail chest. *Solid and dashed arrows* indicate air movement; *open arrows* indicate structural movement. **A,** A flail chest consists of fractured rib segments that are unattached (free-floating) to the rest of the chest wall. **B,** On inspiration, the flail segment of ribs is sucked inward. The affected lung and mediastinal structures shift to the unaffected side. This compromises the amount of inspired air in the unaffected lung. **C,** On expiration, the flail segment of ribs bellows outward. The affected lung and mediastinal structures shift to the affected side. Some air within the lungs is shunted back and forth between the lungs instead of passing through the upper airway.

motion. These swings may seriously affect circulatory dynamics, producing elevated venous pressure, impaired filling of the right side of the heart, and decreased arterial pressure.

In addition, pulmonary contusion occurs, resulting in an accumulation of fluid in the affected alveoli, which leads to intrapulmonary shunting and further hypoxia. The full effects of pulmonary contusion may not be manifested until the height of the body's inflammatory response in 24 to 48 hours.

The client with a flail chest commonly experiences emotional and physical distress while trying to breathe despite excruciating pain. Respirations are usually rapid, shallow, and labored. Paradoxical movement of the chest wall is usually obvious if the client's bare chest is inspected. Breath sounds are absent or decreased on the affected side and crepitus may be heard or felt at the fracture site. Hypercapnia and hypoxia worsen as the effort necessary to breathe further depletes the already diminished oxygen supply. Frequent assessment of ABGs is needed to monitor respiratory effectiveness and to detect acidosis. Various factors produce metabolic and respiratory acidosis in chest-injured clients.

OUTCOME MANAGEMENT

Treatment is usually with intubation and mechanical ventilation, which can accomplish the following:

- Restore adequate ventilation, thus reducing hypoxia and hypercapnia
- Decrease paradoxical motion by using positive pressure to stabilize the chest wall internally
- Reduce pain by decreasing movement of the fractured ribs
- Provide an avenue for removal of secretions

Internal stabilization with continuous ventilation may require 21 days or more. Muscle relaxants or musculoskeletal paralyzing agents may be administered to reduce the risk of separation of the healing costochondral junctions. See earlier discussion in this chapter.

SPECIFIC PULMONARY INJURIES

PNEUMOTHORAX

Pneumothorax is the presence of air in the pleural space that prohibits complete lung expansion. Lung expansion occurs when the pleural lining of the chest wall and the visceral lining of the lung maintain negative pressure in the pleural space. When the continuity of this system is lost, the lung collapses, resulting in a pneumothorax.[24]

Pathophysiology

A pneumothorax may be closed or open. In a closed pneumothorax, air may escape into the pleural space from a puncture or tear in an internal respiratory structure such as the bronchus, bronchioles, or alveoli (Figure 63-9, *A*). Fractured ribs may also lead to closed pneumothorax. In an open pneumothorax, air may enter the pleural space directly through a hole in the chest wall or diaphragm (Figure 63-9, *B*).

A pneumothorax may be classified as spontaneous or traumatic, and either classification may result in a tension pneumothorax. A spontaneous pneumothorax may be idiopathic in that no cause can be found (primary) or as a result of another lung illness such as COPD, tuberculosis, or cancer (secondary). Whereas the chest wall remains intact, a bleb or bulla ruptures, leading to a collapsed lung. A traumatic pneumothorax results in a collapsed lung caused either by blunt force trauma to the chest wall or by the creation of an open sucking chest wound caused by a motor-vehicle accident, gun or knife wound, or a diagnostic procedure such as a thoracentesis. Additional risk factors for developing a pneumothorax are listed in Table 63-2.

A tension pneumothorax develops when air is trapped in the pleural space during inspiration and cannot escape during expiration. The intrapleural pressure becomes greater than the lung tissue pressure, resulting in compression of the lung and surrounding structures.

Clinical Manifestations

Clinical manifestations of *moderate* pneumothorax include tachypnea; dyspnea; sudden sharp pain on the affected side with chest movement, breathing, or coughing; asymmetrical chest expansion; diminished or absent breath sounds on the affected side; hyperresonance (tympany) to percussion on the affected side; restlessness; anxiety; and tachycardia.

Clinical manifestations of *severe* pneumothorax include all the preceding and distended neck veins; point of maximal impulse shift; subcutaneous emphysema; decreased tactile and vocal fremitus; tracheal deviation toward the unaffected side; and progressive cyanosis.

Chest x-ray may reveal a slight tracheal shift away from the affected side and retraction of the lung back from the parietal pleura. On chest x-ray, pneumothorax is expressed as a percentage. For example, a client may have a complete 100% to a partial 10% pneumothorax. The use of percentages allows for evaluation of progress on subsequent x-rays. If pneumothorax is suspected but respiratory distress is too severe to permit x-ray confirmation, the physician may insert an 18-gauge needle (emergency thoracentesis) into the second or third intercostal space in the midclavicular line. Aspiration demonstrates whether free air is present in the pleural space.

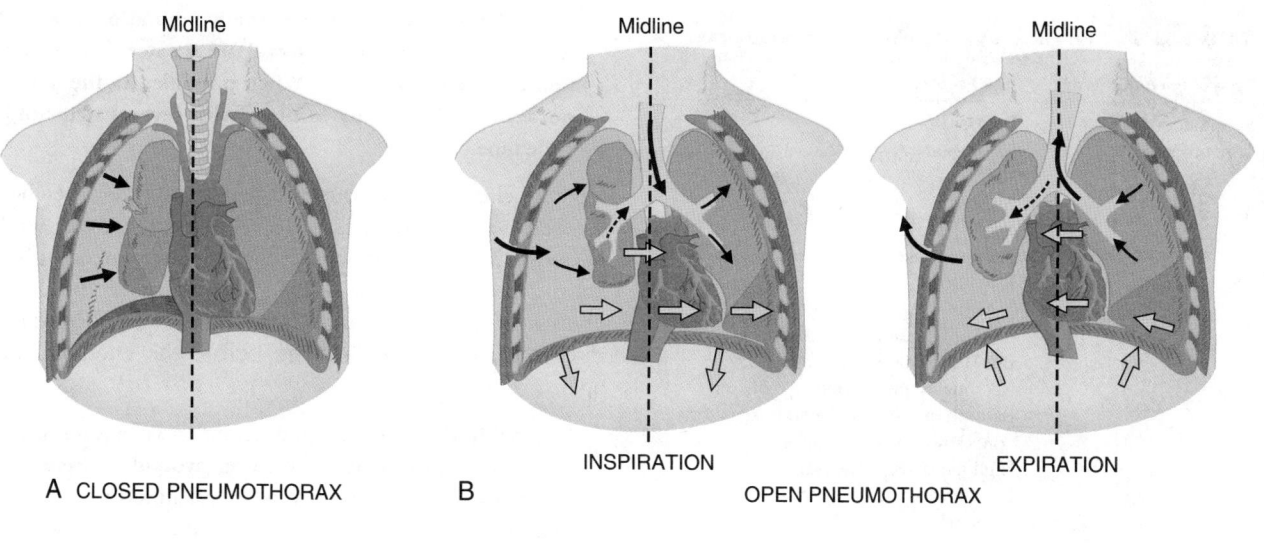

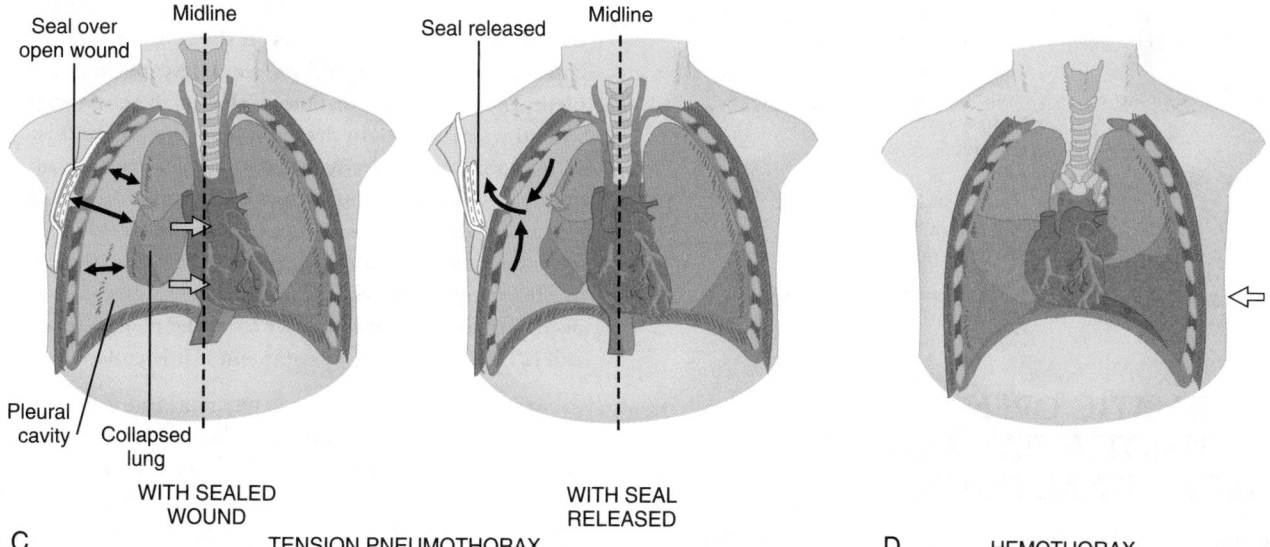

■ **FIGURE 63–9** Pneumothorax. **A,** Closed pneumothorax. The lung collapses as air gathers in the pleural space. **B,** Open pneumothorax (sucking chest wound). *Solid and dashed arrows* indicate air movement; *open arrows* indicate structural movement. A chest wall wound connects the pleural space with atmospheric air. During inspiration, atmospheric air is sucked into the pleural space through the chest wall wound. Positive pressure in the pleural space collapses the lung on the affected side and pushes the mediastinal contents toward the unaffected side. This reduces the volume of air in the unaffected side considerably. During expiration, air escapes through the chest wall wound, lessening positive pressure in the affected side and allowing the mediastinal contents to swing back toward the affected side. Movement of mediastinal structures from side to side is called mediastinal flutter. **C,** Tension pneumothorax. *Left,* If an open pneumothorax is covered (e.g., with a dressing), it forms a seal, resulting in tension pneumothorax with a mediastinal shift. A tear in lung structure continues to allow air into the pleural space. As positive pressure builds in the pleural space, the affected lung collapses, and the mediastinal contents shift to the unaffected side. *Right,* Tension pneumothorax is corrected by removing the seal (e.g., dressing), allowing air trapped in the pleural space to escape. **D,** Massive hemothorax (*arrow*) below the left lung, causing collapse of lung tissue.

OUTCOME MANAGEMENT

Most physicians prefer to insert a chest tube immediately into the pleural space via the fourth intercostal space at the midaxillary or anterior axillary line. The chest catheter is connected to closed-chest drainage (see Chapter 62). The catheter permits the continuous escape of air and blood from the pleural space, thus helping the lung expand by reestablishing negative subatmospheric pressure in the pleural space. Sometimes a thoracotomy is done to explore the chest surgically and to repair the site of origin of the pneumothorax or hemothorax. Surgical treatment may also be accomplished through VATS.[24] A thoracoscopy is completed with direct visualization of the defect in the chest that needs to be repaired. Because the VATS is less invasive than a thoracotomy, the client experiences less pain, has a smaller chest wound, and recovers faster and with fewer side effects, compared with a thoracotomy where the chest is opened.

TABLE 63–2 Risk Factors for Developing Pneumothorax

Type of Pneumothorax	Risk Factors
Spontaneous pneumothorax	Bleb or bulla
	Emphysema
	AIDS
	Asthma
	Cystic fibrosis
	Tuberculosis
	Sarcoidosis
	Malignancy
	Idiopathic pulmonary fibrosis
	Birt-Hogg-Dubé syndrome
	Necrotizing pneumonia
	Barotrauma or positive end-expiratory pressure
	High altitudes
	Decompression diving injuries
	Smoking
	Marfan syndrome
	Cocaine use
Traumatic pneumothorax	Chest surgery
	Insertion of central line
	Thoracentesis
	Gunshot wound
	Knife wound
	Penetrating foreign object
	Falls
	Motor-vehicle accidents
	Blunt chest trauma
	Fractured rib

Revised from Bucher, L., & Melander, S. (1999). *Critical care nursing.* Philadelphia: Saunders.

TRAUMATIC OPEN PNEUMOTHORAX AND MEDIASTINAL FLUTTER

A traumatic open pneumothorax occurs with sucking chest wounds. With this type of wound, a traumatic opening in the chest wall is large enough for air to move freely in and out of the chest cavity during ventilation (Figure 63-9, *B*). This abnormal movement of air through the chest wound produces a sucking noise that is audible in a quiet environment. Open sucking chest wounds may result from accidental injuries or surgical trauma. For example, if a chest drainage catheter is accidentally pulled out of a chest, the remaining puncture incision in the chest wall may become a sucking wound.

OUTCOME MANAGEMENT

SAFETY

ALERT

When an open sucking chest wound is detected, emergency intervention includes immediately covering the wound securely with anything available. An airtight covering usually prevents tension pneumothorax and preserves ventilation of the opposite lung. Do not waste time looking for a sterile gauze petrolatum dressing (the ideal covering for such a wound) if it is not immediately available. Cover the wound at once with whatever is at hand (e.g., a towel) until a sterile petrolatum dressing is available. When possible, fix the temporary dressing firmly in place with several strips of wide tape.

If the client is conscious and cooperative, ask the client to take a deep breath and to try to blow it out while keeping the mouth and nose closed. This pushing effort against a closed glottis helps push air out through the chest wound and reexpand the lung. When the client does this, apply the dressing before the client inhales again.

Stay with the chest-injured client after a dressing has been applied to a sucking wound. Carefully assess for indications of tension pneumothorax and *mediastinal shift* (contents of mediastinum [heart, great vessels, trachea, esophagus] are pushed to the unaffected side of the chest). These complications may develop if the air leak is in the lung or a bronchus; such a situation allows air to escape into the pleural space. In such instances, closing the chest wall wound with an airtight dressing prevents the outflow of escaping air, thereby accidentally converting an open pneumothorax into a tension pneumothorax. If a tension pneumothorax appears to be developing after the wound is sealed, immediately unplug the seal to allow the air to escape. Closed-chest drainage is necessary to (1) remove the air from the pleural space and (2) allow the lung to reexpand if it is collapsed.

In addition to experiencing dyspnea and collapse of the lung on the affected side, the client with a traumatic open pneumothorax may experience *mediastinal flutter.* This complication results from air rushing in and out of the thoracic cavity on the affected side. With inspiration, the mediastinal structures (heart, trachea, esophagus) and collapsed lung are pushed toward the unaffected side. With expiration, these structures then move back toward the affected side. Fluttering back-and-forth movements of these vital mediastinal structures produce severe cardiopulmonary compromise, which is fatal if not treated promptly.

Chest tubes are inserted on the affected side away from the open wound. Surgical closure of the wound may follow. Supplemental high-flow oxygen should be administered.

TENSION PNEUMOTHORAX AND MEDIASTINAL SHIFT

Although it is dangerous to have air moving in and out of the pleural space with each respiration, the client is at even greater risk when air moves only into the pleural space and cannot move back out (tension pneumothorax). Tension pneumothorax (Figure 63-9, *C*) is a tru emergency. Air enters the pleural space with each inspiration, becomes trapped there, and is not expelled during expiration (i.e., one-way valve effect). Pressure builds in the chest as the accumulation of air in the pleural space increases. Tension pneumothorax most commonly occurs with blunt traumatic injuries and is frequently associated with flail chest injuries.

If untreated, tension pneumothorax collapses the lung on the affected side as intrapleural pressure or tension increases, causing a mediastinal shift (mediastinal contents—heart, trachea, esophagus, great vessels—pushed or "shifted" toward the chest's unaffected side). Mediastinal shift may cause (1) compression of the lung in the direction of the shift (i.e., the lung opposite the pneumothorax) and (2) compression, traction, torsion, or kinking of the great vessels; thus blood return to the heart is dangerously impaired. The latter situation causes a subsequent decrease in cardiac output and blood pressure. Tension pneumothorax produces serious circulatory and pulmonary impairment that can be rapidly fatal. This is a high-priority emergency requiring prompt assessment and intervention.

Clinical Manifestations

Clinical manifestations of tension pneumothorax may include (1) marked, severe dyspnea; (2) tachypnea; (3) subcutaneous emphysema in the neck and upper chest; (4) progressive cyanosis; (5) acute chest pain on the affected side; (6) hyperresonance (tympany) upon percussion of the affected side; (7) tachycardia; (8) asymmetrical chest wall movement; (9) diminished or absent breath sounds on the affected side; and (10) extreme restlessness and agitation. Other manifestations include (1) neck vein distention; (2) laryngeal and tracheal deviation or shift to the unaffected side; (3) a feeling of tightness or pressure within the chest; (4) a point of maximal impulse (PMI) shift laterally or medially; (5) severe hypotension leading to shock; and (6) muffled heart sounds.

A suspected mediastinal shift may be confirmed by x-ray. Laryngeal and tracheal deviation toward the unaffected side can be detected by gentle palpation and with x-ray study. ABG analysis demonstrates hypoxia and respiratory alkalosis. When mediastinal shift is severe and not immediately corrected, respiratory acidosis may ensue.

OUTCOME MANAGEMENT

The immediate intervention is to convert a *tension* pneumothorax into an *open* pneumothorax, a less serious disorder. Large-bore chest tubes (36F to 40F) are inserted on the affected side at the fifth intercostal space anterior to the midaxillary line. Once tubes are inserted, suction drainage should be established. If a delay in the chest tube insertion is anticipated, a 14- to 18-gauge needle may be inserted into the pleural space of the affected side at the level of the second intercostal space at the midclavicular line. Prompt thoracentesis to remove air may be life-saving. As trapped air rushes from a tension pneumothorax, the tension is relieved and the lung should reexpand; and if mediastinal shift is present, it corrects itself. Supplemental oxygen is administered.

HEMOTHORAX

Hemothorax may be present in clients with chest injuries. A small amount of blood (<300 ml) in the pleural space may cause no clinical manifestations and may require no intervention, with the blood being reabsorbed spontaneously. Severe hemothorax (1400 to 2500 ml) may be life-threatening because of resultant hypovolemia and tension (Figure 63-9, *D*). Massive hemothorax is associated with 50% to 75% mortality.

Clinical manifestations include respiratory distress, shock, and mediastinal shift. There is dullness upon percussion of the affected side. A chest film confirms a diagnosis of hemothorax. If the client is in severe distress, the physician may aspirate blood from the pleural space by inserting a 16-gauge needle into the fifth or sixth intercostal space at the midaxillary line. To drain intrathoracic accumulations of blood, the physician inserts a large-caliber (36F or larger) chest catheter, which is then connected to a drainage system. An initial drainage of 500 to 1000 ml is considered moderate, and additional treatment may not be required. An initial drainage of more than 1500 ml or continued large amounts of drainage (200 ml/hr) warrants immediate exploratory thoracotomy or the use of VATS to repair the site of active bleeding. Fluid replacement with O-negative blood or autotransfusion of blood should be used.

OTHER TRAUMATIC LUNG EVENTS

NEAR-DROWNING

Clients who initially survive suffocation after submersion in a water or fluid medium are said to have experienced a near-drowning or *immersion syndrome*. Immersion syndrome is the immersion into cold water that leads to cardiac dysrhythmias. Freshwater drowning (i.e., in a swimming pool) is more common than saltwater drowning. Risk factors that increase the potential for near-drowning are alcohol or drug ingestion, overestimation of swimming skills, hypothermia, hyperventilation, extreme fatigue, sudden acute illness (seizure or acute myocardial infarction), head or spinal cord injury from a diving mishap, and hypoglycemia.

Pathophysiology

Regardless of the fluid aspirated, the ultimate result is pulmonary edema. Both freshwater and saltwater wash out alveolar surfactant. Freshwater also changes the surface tension of surfactant. The loss of surfactant leads to alveolar collapse, intrapulmonary shunting, decreased lung compliance, and hypoxemia. Poor perfusion and hypoxemia result in acidosis and eventual pulmonary edema. Near-drowning also compromises the respiratory system and leads to hypoxia, hypercapnia, cardiac arrest, and severe alterations in fluid-electrolyte balance.

Clinical Manifestations

The client may be unconscious or awake but restless and complaining of chest pain or a headache. Vomiting often occurs. Hypothermia may also be present. Cardiac manifestations include tachycardia, hypotension, and dysrhythmias. Pink frothy sputum indicates that pulmonary edema is already present. Auscultation may reveal crackles, rhonchi, and wheezes. Hemoglobin, hematocrit, and electrolyte levels may be abnormal. White blood cell count may be elevated, especially if the water aspirated contained impurities.

OUTCOME MANAGEMENT

Begin assessment and interventions with the ABCs. If there is a possibility of spinal cord injury (such as with a diving injury), the spinal column should be immobilized. Basic cardiopulmonary resuscitation (CPR) should be initiated if necessary and continued, especially with hypothermic clients. Resuscitation efforts for clients with hypothermia have been successful long after typical CPR time guidelines would indicate to discontinue resuscitation efforts. Attempting to drain the fluid from the lungs is not advised.

Obtain a history of the submersion from the client or someone who has the information needed. Include the length of submersion, temperature of the water, any associated injuries, and type of water. Assess the level of consciousness. Note any respiratory efforts and adventitious sounds. Open the airway while maintaining spinal immobility. Look for manifestations of hypoxia, such as confusion, irritability, lethargy, or unconsciousness. Obtain a complete set of vital signs and assess for any additional injuries that may be present, including associated trauma, spinal cord injury from diving, air embolism from scuba diving, and seizures.

For respiratory insufficiency, intubate and ventilate with 100% oxygen and 5 to 10 cm of PEEP to prevent the alveoli from collapsing. If PEEP is used, slow and cautious removal of PEEP is required. Surfactant levels may remain low for up to 48 to 72 hours, especially after freshwater aspiration. If the client is breathing, provide respiratory support with a non-rebreather mask. Oxygen saturation should be maintained above 90%.[9]

Remove the client's wet clothing, and wrap the client in a warm blanket. Core rewarming may be indicated if the client is hypothermic. Rewarm the client slowly to avoid a rapid influx of anaerobic metabolites (lactic acid) that may be trapped in the cold extremities.

Once the vital functions are stabilized, correct any acid-base or electrolyte abnormalities. Diagnostic studies include ABG analysis, complete blood count, electrolytes, appropriate toxicology studies if alcohol or drug ingestion is suspected, and a chest film. Clients are at high risk for pulmonary edema even several hours after a near-drowning incident. Monitor neurologic status carefully. A deteriorating level of consciousness may indicate cerebral edema, severe acidosis, or increased hypoxia. Table 63-3 identifies factors associated with near-drowning outcomes.

CARBON MONOXIDE POISONING

Carbon monoxide (CO) is a colorless, odorless, tasteless gas that is formed by the incomplete combustion of any carbon fuel. Intoxication by CO is the leading cause of death by poisoning. CO preferentially binds to hemoglobin, with an affinity for hemoglobin 200 to 230 times greater than that of oxygen. CO displaces oxygen, leading to reduced supplies of oxygen in the arterial blood and development of tissue hypoxia. CO also shifts the oxygen-hemoglobin dissociation curve to the left, which further reduces the oxygen levels by decreasing the release of oxygen into the tissues.

Generally, there is a history of exposure to CO after being found in an enclosed space in the presence of gases or fire. Faulty furnaces are also associated with CO poisoning. If CO poisoning is due to smoke inhalation, manifestations such as hoarseness, stridor, burns, or soot on the mouth or nose may be present. Sputum may be black because of inhalation of soot.

TABLE 63-3 Factors Associated with Prediction of Outcome in Near-Drowning

Factors Suggestive of Favorable Outcome	Factors Suggestive of Poor Outcome
Submersion time <5 minutes	Submersion time >10 minutes
Immediate resuscitation	No resuscitation within first 10 minutes
CPR given <10 minutes	CPR given >25 minutes
Spontaneous cardiac rhythm in ED	Use of cardiotonic medications in field or ED
GCS score >6 on arrival at ED	GCS score <5
Spontaneous purposeful movement and intact brain stem function at 24 hours	No spontaneous purposeful movements 24 hours after submersion

CPR, Cardiopulmonary resuscitation; *ED,* emergency department; *GCS,* Glasgow Coma Scale.
From Shoemaker, W.C., et al. (2007). *Textbook of critical care* (5th ed.). Philadelphia: Saunders.

Clinical Manifestations

Clinical manifestations are vague until levels of CO bound to hemoglobin (carboxyhemoglobin, or COHb) are around 40%. With levels below 20%, manifestations include headache, vertigo, dizziness, nausea, and dyspnea on exertion. Above 20%, the client may have impaired concentration, clumsiness, and throbbing headache. Only when levels exceed 30% are manifestations more evident, including irritability, visual changes, impaired thought, and vomiting. At 40% vital signs change, and eventually seizures and coma ensue when levels are greater than 50%. The diagnosis is confirmed by measurement of carboxyhemoglobin levels in the blood. Pulse oximetry should not be used because the readings are unreliable because of the detection of carboxyhemoglobin as oxyhemoglobin.

OUTCOME MANAGEMENT

Removal of the CO from the body is imperative. When the client is breathing room air, the CO will be removed from the body in about 320 minutes. Administering 100% oxygen will shorten the half-life of CO to 80 minutes. Hyperbaric oxygen may be required to reduce the half-life of CO to minutes by forcing it off of the hemoglobin molecule for clients with severe CO poisoning. Hyperbaric oxygen will decrease the half-life of CO to 23 minutes.

Reasons for CO poisoning must be explored and interventions directed at correcting those problems should begin before hospital discharge. If the client's home furnace is faulty, it must be repaired. If the CO poisoning was a suicide attempt, crisis counselors should be used. Long-term neurologic and psychiatric consequences may develop, and the client should be observed and followed up by their usual health care provider.

CONCLUSIONS

Two forms of respiratory failure exist: hypoxemic and ventilatory. Hypoxemic failure includes problems that lead to failure to transport oxygen and CO_2 across the capillary. Ventilatory failure includes disorders that impair neurologic triggers to breathe and neuromuscular movement with respiration. Mechanical ventilation is a common method of treatment for both problems. Chest trauma involves life-threatening problems that demand prompt recognition and treatment.

THINKING CRITICALLY

1. You are caring for a client who is receiving mechanical ventilation. You have just suctioned the client's airway and begin to leave the room when the high-pressure alarm sounds. What should you do?

Factors to Consider. What changes in the client can trigger the high-pressure alarm? What changes in the ventilator can cause high pressure?

2. You are going to position the client prone to improve ventilation and perfusion. What considerations should be made before, during, and after the prone position is used?

Factors to Consider. How can the tubes be moved safely with the client? What complications might occur in a prone position? What procedures cannot be done while the client is prone?

Discussions for these questions can be found on the website.

BIBLIOGRAPHY

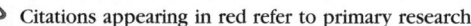 Citations appearing in red refer to primary research.

Citations appearing in blue refer to evidence-based practice guidelines and protocols.

1. Anas, N., & Lewis, K. (2000). Drowning and near-drowning. In A. Grenvik, et al. (Eds.), *The textbook of critical care* (4th ed., pp. 200-211). Philadelphia: Saunders.
2. Austan, F., & Polise, M. (2002). Management of respiratory failure with noninvasive positive pressure ventilation and heliox adjunct. *Heart and Lung, 31*(3), 214-218.
3. Balas, M. (2000). Prone positioning of patients with acute respiratory distress syndrome: Applying research to practice. *Critical Care Nurse, 20*(1), 24-36.
4. Ballard, N. (2006). Patients' recollections of therapeutic paralysis in the intensive care unit. *American Journal of Critical Care, 15*(1), 86-94.
5. Berenholtz, S., et al. (2004). Improving Care for the Ventilated Patient. *Joint Commission Journal on Quality and Safety, 30*(4), 195-204.
6. Brochard, L. (2000). Noninvasive ventilation. In A. Grenvik, et al. (Eds.), *The textbook of critical care* (4th ed., pp. 1302-1306). Philadelphia: Saunders.
7. Brower, R., et al. (2001). Treatment for ARDS [Electronic version]. *Chest, 120*(4), 1347-1367.
8. Burns, S. (1999). Making weaning easier: Pathways and protocols that work. *Nursing Clinics of North America, 11*(4), 465-479.
9. Burton, S., & Alexander, E. (2006). Avoiding the pitfalls and ensuring the safety of sustained neuromuscular blockade. *AACN Advanced Critical Care, 17*(3), 239-243.
9a. Centers for Disease Control and Prevention. (2004). *Guidelines for preventing health-care associated pneumonia.* Atlanta: CDC.
10. Chesnutt, M., & Prendergast, T. (2003). Lung. In L. Tierney, S. McPhee, & M. Papadakis (Eds.), *Current medical diagnosis and treatment* (pp. 306-311). New York: Lange Medical Books.
11. Cohen, R., & Moelleken, B. (2003). Disorders due to physical agents. In L. Tierney, S. McPhee, & M. Papadakis (Eds.), *Current medical diagnosis and treatment* (pp. 1549-1551). New York: Lange Medical Books.
12. Combes, A. (2007). Early predictors for infection recurrence and death in patients with ventilator-associated pneumonia. *Critical Care Medicine, 35*(1), 146-154.
13. Easter, A. (2001). Management of patients with multiple rib fractures [Electronic version]. *American Journal of Critical Care, 10*(5), 320-329.
14. Eutereuer, D. (2006). Health related quality of life in patients with chronic respiratory failure after long-term mechanical ventilation. *Respiratory Medicine, 100*(3), 477-486.
15. Fenstermacher, D., & Hong, D. (2004). Mechanical ventilation: What have we learned? *Critical Care Nursing Quarterly, 27*(3), 258-294.
16. Golden, P. (2000). Thoracic trauma [Electronic version]. *Orthopedic Nursing, 19*(5), 37-47.
17. Goll, C. (2001). Near drowning. In P. Swearingen & J. Hicks Keen (Eds.), *Manual of critical care nursing* (4th ed., pp. 136-140). St. Louis: Mosby.
18. Goll, C. (2001). Acute respiratory failure. In P. Swearingen & J. Hicks Keen (Eds.), *Manual of critical care nursing* (4th ed., pp. 243-246). St. Louis: Mosby.

19. Guerin, C. (2004). Effects of systematic prone positioning in hypoxemic acute respiratory failure. *Journal of the American Medical Association, 292*(17), 2379-2387.

20. Hardin, K.A. (2006). Sleep in critically ill chemically paralyzed patients requiring mechanical ventilation. *Chest, 129*(6), 1468-1477.

21. Hogarth, D.K., & Hall, J. (2004). Management of sedation in mechanically ventilated patients. *Current Opinion in Critical Care, 10*(1), 40-46.

22. Klein, D. (1999). Prone positioning in patients with acute respiratory distress syndrome: The Vollman Prone Positioner. *Critical Care Nurse, 19*(4), 66-71.

23. Lafferty, J., & Kavanagh, B. (2002). Hypocapnia. *New England Journal of Medicine, 347*(1), 43-53.

24. Lenart, S., & Garrity, J. (2000). Eye care for patients receiving neuromuscular blocking agents or propofol during mechanical ventilation. *American Journal of Critical Care, 9*(3), 188-191.

25. MacIntyre, N., et al. (2001). Evidence-based guidelines for weaning and discontinuing ventilatory support. *Chest, 120*(6), 375S-389S.

26. Markou, N., Myrianthefs, P., & Baltopoulos, G. (2004). Respiratory failure: An overview. *Critical Care Nursing Quarterly, 27*(4), 353-379.

27. Meade, M., & Herridge, M. (2001). An evidence-based approach to acute respiratory distress syndrome [Electronic version]. *Respiratory Care, 46*(12), 1368-1376.

28. Meduri, G.U. (2007). Methylprednisolone infusion in early severe ARDS: Results of a randomized controlled trial. *Chest, 131*(4), 954-963.

29. Moon, R., Dear, G., & Stolp, B. (2000). Hyperbaric oxygen in critical care. In A. Grenvik, et al. (Eds.), *The textbook of critical care* (4th ed., pp. 1534-1535). Philadelphia: Saunders.

30. Mortelli, M., & Manning, H. (2002). Acute respiratory distress syndrome [Electronic version]. *American Family Physician, 65*(9), 1823-1830.

31. Pierson, D. (2001). The future of respiratory care. *Respiratory Care, 46*(7), 705-718.

32. Rodger, M. (1999). Common respiratory problems: Pulmonary embolism, pneumothorax, and thoracic pulmonary surgery. In L. Bucher & S. Melander (Eds.), *Critical care nursing* (pp. 486-496). Philadelphia: Saunders.

33. Sakallaris, B. (1999). Acute respiratory failure. In L. Bucher & S. Melander (Eds.), *Critical care nursing* (pp. 411-445). Philadelphia: Saunders.

34. Sassoon, C., & McGovern, J. (2000). Oxygenation strategy. In A. Grenvik, et al. (Eds.), *The textbook of critical care* (4th ed., pp. 1308-1323). Philadelphia: Saunders.

35. Sole, M.L., Byers, J.F., Ludy, J.E., et al. (2003). A multi-site survey of suctioning techniques and airway management practices. *American Journal of Critical Care, 12*, 220-230.

36. Stacy, K. (2006). Pulmonary disorders. In L. Urden, K. Stacy, & M. Lough (Eds.), *Thelan's critical care nursing: Diagnosis and management* (5th ed., pp. 551-560, 570-573). St. Louis: Mosby.

37. Stacy, K. (2006). Pulmonary therapeutic management. In L. Urden, K. Stacy, & M. Lough (Eds.), *Thelan's critical care nursing: Diagnosis and management* (5th ed., pp. 587-613). St. Louis: Mosby.

38. Staudinger, T., et al. (2001). Comparison of prone positioning and continuous rotation of patients with adult respiratory distress syndrome: Results of a pilot study. *Critical Care Medicine, 29*(1), 51-56.

39. Tarizan, A.J. (2000). Caring for dying patients who have air hunger. *Journal of Nursing Scholarship, 32*(2), 137-143.

40. Taylor, R., & Trottier, S. (2000). Pathophysiology of acute lung injury. In A. Grenvik, et al. (Eds.), *The textbook of critical care* (4th ed., pp. 1382-1390). Philadelphia: Saunders.

41. The Acute Respiratory Distress Syndrome Network. (2000). Ventilation with lower tidal volumes as compared to traditional tidal volumes for acute lung injury and the acute respiratory distress syndrome. *New England Journal of Medicine, 342*(18), 1301-1308.

42. Voggenreiter, G., et al. (1999). Intermittent prone positioning in the treatment of severe and moderate posttraumatic lung injury. *Critical Care Medicine, 27*(11), 2375-2382.

evolve   *Did you remember to check out the bonus material on the Evolve website and the CD-ROM, including NCLEX®-Examination Style Review Questions, Open-Book Quizzes, and Chapter Review Audio Podcasts?*

http://evolve.elsevier.com/Black/medsurg

UNIT 15

SENSORY DISORDERS

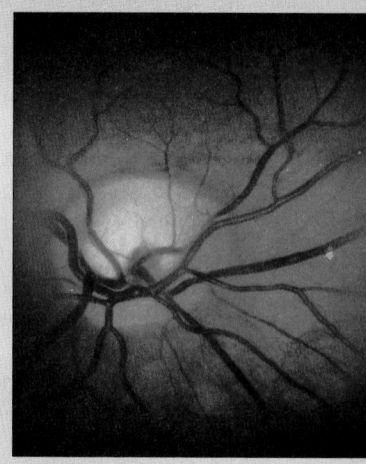

ANATOMY AND PHYSIOLOGY REVIEW:

The Eyes and Ears

Robert G. Carroll

OVERVIEW

The visual, auditory, and olfactory systems are "distance" senses, bringing information about our environment to our perception. Each system detects the intensity and quality of stimuli, encodes and processes this information, and transmits it to various areas of the cerebral cortex. Together these senses provide much of the available information about our environment. This review covers vision and hearing; smell is described in Unit 7.

The *visual apparatus* is specialized to detect light. Light passes through the cornea, aqueous humor, lens, and vitreous humor before striking the retina. The visual receptors—rods and cones—encode data about the intensity and wavelength of light. This information is processed and transmitted through nerve cells of the retina, the optic nerve, and the thalamus before arriving at the visual cortex. The information is constructed in the primary and associated visual cortex into a conscious perception.

The *auditory apparatus* is specialized to detect sound. Sound waves pass through the pinna, through the auditory canal to the eardrum (tympanic membrane), through the bones of the middle ear, and then to the receptors in the cochlea. The auditory hair cells are arranged on the organ of Corti (the end organ for hearing) and are coded to detect the intensity and frequency of sound. This information passes through the auditory nerve through the lateral lemniscus and, finally, to the auditory cortex. Within the primary and secondary auditory cortex, auditory discrimination occurs.

VISUAL SYSTEM

STRUCTURE OF THE VISUAL SYSTEM

External Structures

The visual system is a complex group of structures that includes the eyeballs, muscles, nerves, fat, and bones. The *ocular adnexa* (Figure A&P15-1, *A*) are the accessory structures of the eye (muscles, fat, and bone) that support and protect it. The bony orbit (eye socket) surrounds and protects most of the eye so that only a small portion is visible. The orbit is formed from portions of the frontal, lacrimal, ethmoid, maxillary, zygomaticus,

sphenoid, and palatine bones. These bones are thin and fragile and break easily when pressure is applied to the eye (as in a fist fight). In addition to bone, the orbit also contains fat, various connective tissues, blood vessels, and nerves.

The *eyeball* is moved by six ocular muscles that are attached to the surface of the globe (Figure A&P15-2) and move the eye through six cardinal gazes. The four rectus muscles (the medial, lateral, superior, and inferior) move the eyes horizontally and vertically. The two oblique muscles (superior and inferior) rotate the eye in circular movements to allow vision at all angles.

The upper and lower *eyelids* are folds of skin that close to protect the anterior eyeball. When the eyelids close, they distribute tear film, which prevents evaporation and drying of the surface epithelium. The elliptic space between the two open lids is the *palpebral fissure*. The corners of the fissure are called the *canthi*. The medial, or inner, canthus is next to the nose; the lateral, or outer, canthus is the outside corner. Oil-secreting *meibomian glands* are embedded in both upper and lower lids (see Figure A&P15-1, *B*).

The *lacrimal gland,* in the upper lid over the outer canthus, produces tears that reach the eyeball through secretory ducts. Tiny openings *(puncti)* in both the upper and lower lids at the inner canthus direct tears to the lacrimal sac. The *nasolacrimal duct* directs the flow of tears into the nose. The tear film is composed of lipids secreted by the meibomian glands and dissolved salts, glucose, urea, protein, and lysozyme secreted by the lacrimal glands. The tear film lubricates, cleans, and protects the ocular surface. Mucus, secreted by goblet cells located in the lids, assists these processes.

Internal Structures

The *conjunctiva* is a thin transparent layer of mucous membrane that lines the eyelids and covers the eyeball (see Figure A&P15-1, *C*). The *cornea* is a transparent avascular structure with a brilliant, shiny surface. It is convex in shape, is about 0.5 mm thick, and acts as a powerful lens to bend and direct (refract) rays of light to the retina. The cornea is composed of five layers. It derives oxygen from the atmosphere. A rich network of nerve fibers in the outer layer (epithelium) produces a sensation of pain whenever the fibers are exposed or stimulated.

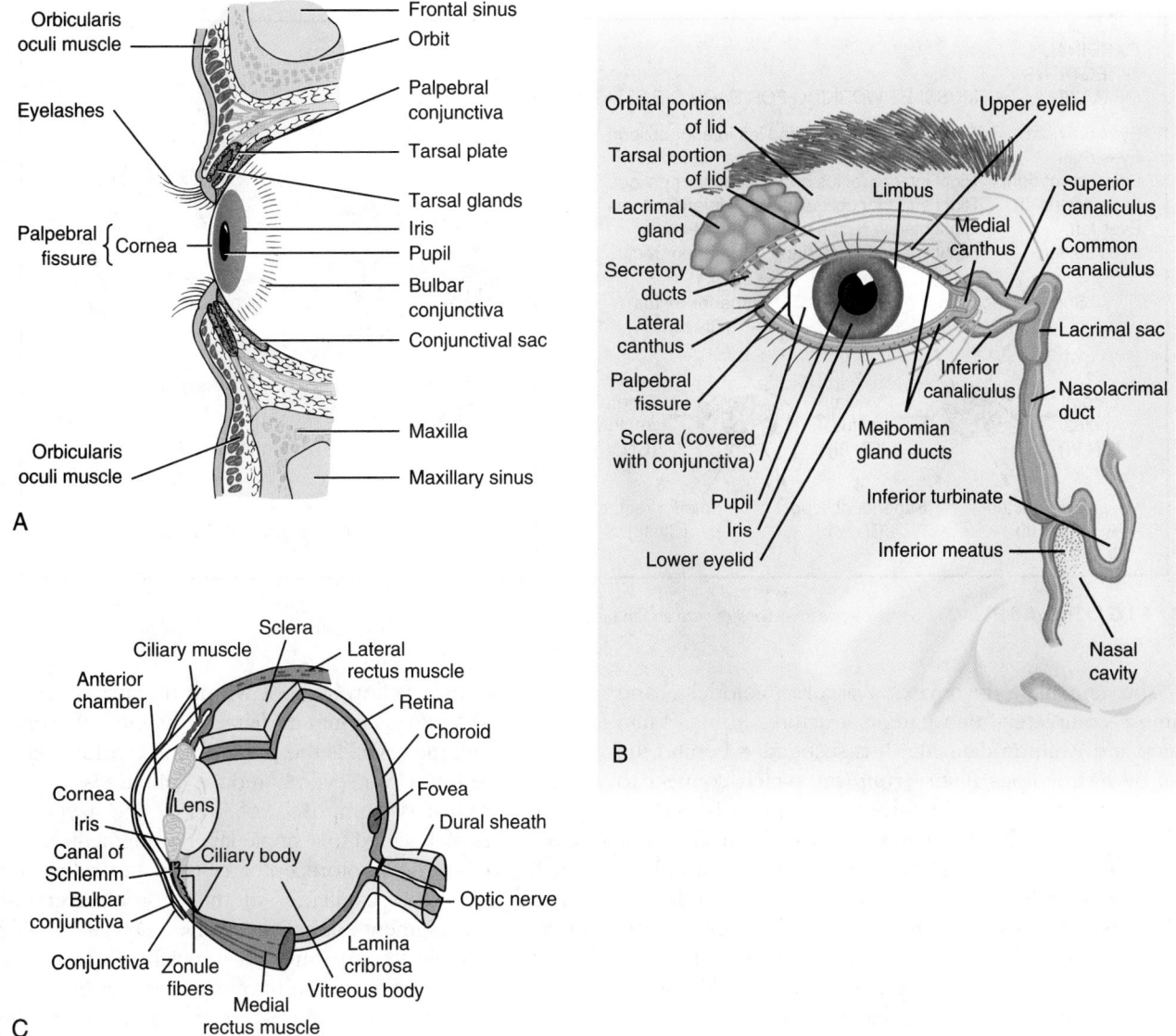

■ FIGURE A&P15–1 Surface anatomy of the eye. **A,** Ocular adnexa. **B,** Frontal view of the lacrimal drainage system. **C,** Horizontal section of the eye.

The *sclera* is the fibrous protective coating of the eye. It is white, dense, and continuous with the cornea. In children, the sclera is thin and appears bluish because of the underlying pigmented structures. In old age, it may become yellowish from degeneration.

The *uveal tract,* the middle vascular layer of the eye that furnishes the blood supply to the retina, consists of three structures:

1. The *iris* is a thin, pigmented diaphragm with a central aperture, the pupil. Iris color is determined by the degree of pigmentation in the stromal melanocytes. The interaction of the two iris muscles (sphincter and dilator) determines pupil diameter. Expansion and contraction of the iris regulate the amount of light entering the eye.

2. The *ciliary body* produces and secretes *aqueous humor,* a clear alkaline fluid composed mainly of water that occupies the space between the iris and the cornea (the anterior chamber of the eye). The ciliary body is in direct continuity with the iris and is circular, surrounding the lens. Aqueous humor circulates from the posterior chamber through the pupil into the anterior chamber. The flow continues into the anterior chamber angle and is filtered out through the trabecular meshwork into Schlemm's canal. From there, the aqueous humor is channeled into a capillary network and into episcleral veins. Normal intraocular pressure is maintained as long as there is a balance between aqueous production and aqueous humor outflow.

3. The *choroid* is the posterior segment of the uveal tract between the retina and the sclera. It is composed of three layers of vessels and is attached to both the ciliary body and the optic nerve.

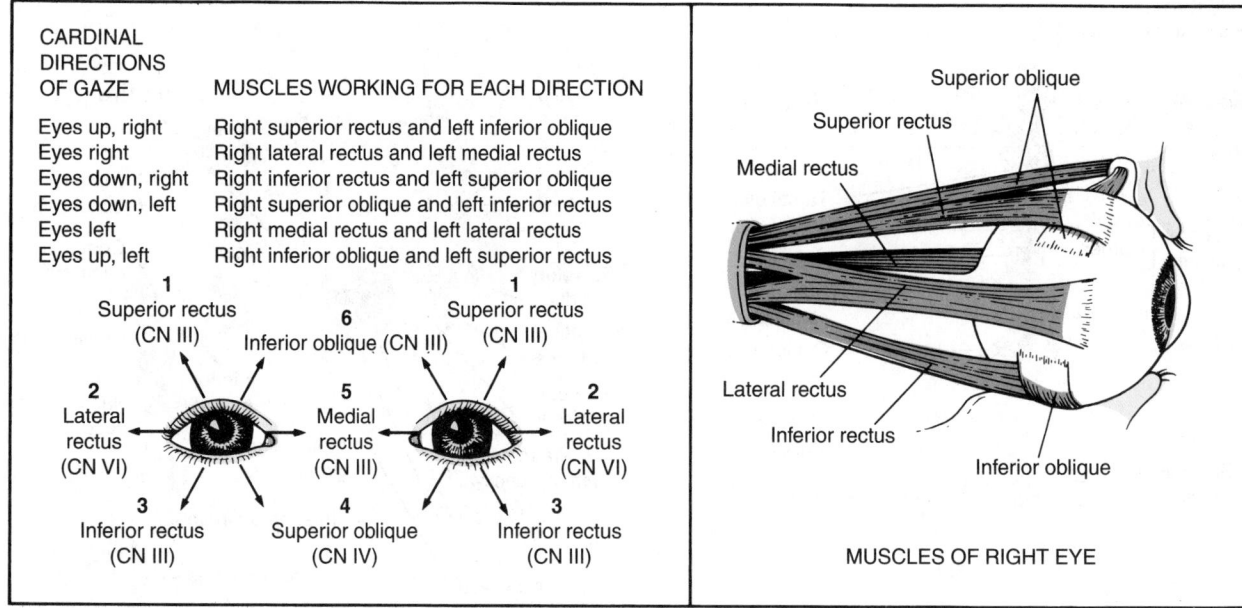

■ **FIGURE A&P15–2** The six cardinal directions of gaze and the muscles responsible for each.

The *lens* is a biconvex, avascular, colorless, and almost completely transparent structure, about 4 mm thick and 9 mm in diameter. It is suspended behind the iris by ligamentous fibers *(zonules),* which connect to the ciliary body. The sole purpose of the lens is to focus light on the retina. The change of focus from distant to near is called *accommodation.* There are no pain fibers or blood vessels in the lens. The lens is surrounded by a transparent envelope (the capsule). The lens of the eye consists of about 65% water and 35% protein.

The *vitreous body* is a clear, avascular, jelly-like structure. Vitreous fluid is thick and viscous, and occupies a space called the *vitreous chamber.* It fills the largest cavity of the eye, accounting for two thirds of its volume. It helps maintain the shape and transparency of the eye.

Retina

The retina is a thin, semitransparent layer of nerve tissue that forms the innermost lining of the eye. It consists of 10 distinct layers of highly organized, delicate tissue. The retina contains all the sensory receptors for the transmission of light and is actually part of the brain.

There are two types of retinal receptors: rods and cones. About 125 million *rods* are distributed in the periphery of the retina; they function best in dim light. Damage to these structures results in night blindness. The *cones,* numbering about 6 million and concentrated in the center of the retina, provide resolution of small visual angles, resulting in perception of fine details. They are also responsible for color vision.

The center of the retina *(macula)* is an area about 5 mm in diameter. In an ophthalmoscopic examination,

it appears as a yellowish spot with a depressed center, the *fovea.* An area 1.5 mm in diameter where only cones are present, the fovea is the point of finest vision. Damage to the fovea can severely reduce central vision.

The retina is composed of many fine layers of neural tissue attached to a single layer of pigmented epithelial cells. The photoreceptor cells in the retina are nourished by the capillaries of the choroid layer just beneath the pigment epithelial cell layer. Oxygen supply to these delicate structures is crucial, because the conversion of visual stimuli into impulses that the brain records as images requires very active metabolic processes.

Optic Nerve and Neural Pathways

The optic nerve is located at the posterior portion of the eye and transmits visual impulses from the retina to the brain. The head of the optic nerve *(optic disc)* can be seen by ophthalmoscopic examination. The optic nerve contains no sensory receptors (rods or cones) and represents a blind spot in the eye. The nerve emerges from the back of the eye and extends for 25 to 30 mm, traveling through the muscle cone to enter the bony optic foramen, eventually joining the other optic nerve to form the optic chiasm. The optic nerve neurons synapse in the thalamus, and thalamic nerves then transmit the visual information to the occipital lobe of the cortex.

FUNCTION OF THE VISUAL SYSTEM

Vision requires accurate transmission of light to the photoreceptors of the retina, encoding of the wavelength and intensity by the retinal receptors, and interpretation of the coded signals by the visual cortex.

Transmission of Light

Light passes through the cornea, aqueous humor, lens, and vitreous humor before striking the retina. Blood vessels are opaque, and the cornea, lens, and fovea are sparsely vascularized, which enhances light transmission. The cornea and lens refract light, allowing it to converge to a focal point on the fovea of the retina. Refraction at the lens is regulated by contraction of the ciliary muscles.

Near vision is accomplished by contraction of the ciliary muscles, which increases curvature of the lens and brings near objects into focus on the retina. *Far vision* is accomplished by relaxing the ciliary muscles and flattening the lens. With age, lens elasticity decreases because of protein degeneration, reducing the ability to accommodate for near vision. Visual abnormalities are corrected by placing an appropriate refractor (eyeglasses or contact lens) in the light pathway.

Visual Receptors of the Retina: Cones and Rods

Three types of cones are sensitive to specific wavelengths of light, with peak sensitivities in the red, green, and blue wavelengths. Density of the cone receptors is highest in the fovea (the area of highest visual acuity). Bright light causes contraction of the iris, limiting the light entering the eye and focusing the light on the fovea. Exposure to light bleaches retinal photopigments, reducing the receptor responsiveness to subsequent exposure (light adaptation). However, prolonged exposure to dark allows the receptors to recover; cones recover completely in about 10 minutes.

Rods are sensitive to light in the green and yellow wavelengths and impart night *(scotopic)* vision. Rods are distributed throughout the retina, but few rods are in the fovea. In the dark, the iris dilates, admitting light to large portions of the retina. Consequently, night vision is enhanced by looking just to the side of the object of interest. After light exposure, rods recover slowly, taking about 20 minutes to return to peak sensitivity (dark adaptation). Because the rod photopigments are not sensitive to red light, exposure to red light does not interfere with dark adaptation.

Image Processing and the Visual Cortex

Interneurons in the retina process the receptor output and transmit information via the optic nerve to the thalamus. The thalamus processes information about the wavelength and intensity of the light and relays the information to the visual cortex. Visual space in the cortex is completely crossed; objects appearing on the left side of the body are represented on the right visual

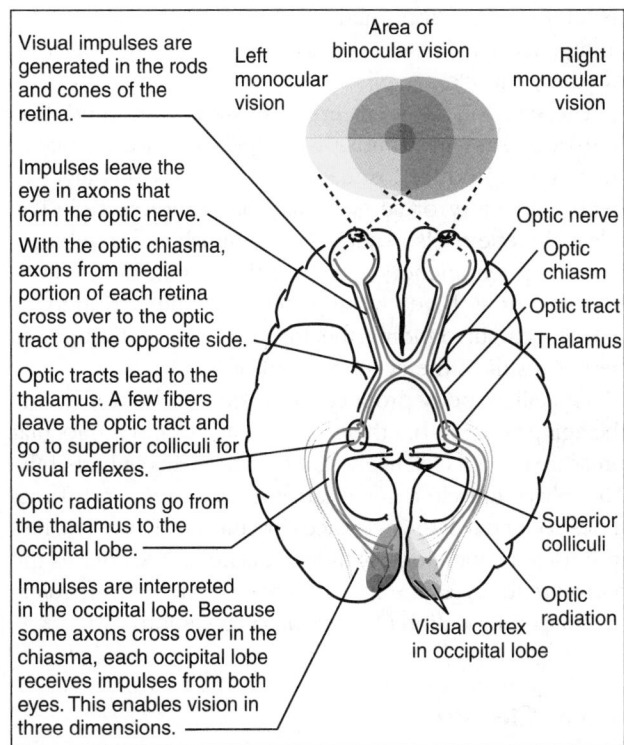

■ FIGURE A&P15–3 Visual pathways from the retina to the occipital lobe. The pathway is partially crossed, so that objects in the visual space of one side are interpreted in the contralateral visual cortex.

cortex and vice versa (Figure A&P15-3). The two eyes work together as one, focusing on the same point in space and fusing their images so that a single mental impression is obtained. The ability of the eyes to fuse two images into a single image is called *binocular vision,* accounting for one aspect of depth perception.

EFFECTS OF AGING ON VISION

Structural Changes

Several age-related changes occur in the structures of the eye and surrounding tissue. Eyebrows and eyelashes turn gray, and skin around the eyelids becomes wrinkled and loose because of loss of muscle tone and elasticity. Loss of orbital fat causes the eyes to sink deeper into the orbit and sometimes limits the upward gaze. Tear secretions may also diminish, resulting in the condition of dry eyes.

The most frequent and significant age-related change in the eye is the formation of a *cataract.* With age, the thickness and density of the lens increase and the lens becomes progressively yellowed and opaque. Throughout the life span, the lens continues to grow by forming new fiber cells. Although the rate of growth gradually diminishes, the accumulation of cells over time contributes to lens density. Loss of transparency also results from protein deterioration from absorption of ultraviolet radiation. The yellow material is associated with the development of abnormal fluorescent substances in the aging lens. The lens accommodation diminishes because of ciliary muscle atrophy.

The cells of the inner layer of the cornea (endothelium) decrease in number with age. Because this layer does not reproduce lost cells, the ability of this layer to heal after injury or surgery may be compromised. The corneal reflex also may be diminished or absent. Another phenomenon characteristic of aging is the *arcus senilis,* a grayish yellow ring found on the periphery of the cornea surrounding the iris. This ring is thought to be the result of the accumulation of lipids.

The ciliary body produces less aqueous humor during the aging process, but there is less outflow and intraocular pressure remains relatively stable or increases only slightly. The ciliary muscle tends to atrophy with age, and sometimes connective tissue replaces lost muscle tissue. The loss in muscle action along with lens thickening decreases the focusing ability of the lens. Decreasing ability to focus at near accommodation *(presbyopia)* is common.

Visual Changes

The major visual changes with aging include decreases in (1) visual acuity, (2) tolerance of glare, (3) ability to adapt to dark and light, and (4) peripheral vision. Each of these decreases is related to changes in the eye structure and each affects the quality and intensity of the light able to reach the retina.

Glare is a particular problem for older people. In combination with difficulty adjusting to dark and light, it is often the reason older adults stop driving at night. The lights from oncoming vehicles produce a glare when passing through both cornea and lens, which may make it very difficult to discern objects. Bright sunlight, either indoors or outdoors, causes an equally blinding glare. Indoor rooms should be lighted with soft incandescent lights, and sheer curtains can be used to diffuse bright sunlight.

Because the eye takes longer to adapt to changes from dark to light and vice versa, older people are at a greater risk for falls and injuries. Any place subject to sudden changes in lighting (e.g., inside a theater) can be dangerous. Getting up at night can be particularly hazardous for older adults. However, because red wavelengths are longer and are perceived by the cones, a red light in the bathroom at night allows enough vision to function without interfering with dark vision.

Peripheral vision decreases with age and may interfere with social interactions and physical activities. Older adults suffering from loss of peripheral vision may not notice someone sitting next to them. They may also have difficulty finding objects out of their range of vision.

The iris loses pigment with age, and older people may thus appear to have grayish or light blue eyes. The pupil becomes gradually smaller with age. A decrease in pupil size results in a smaller amount of light reaching the retina, meaning that the light must pass through the densest, most opaque area of the lens.

AUDITORY SYSTEM

STRUCTURE OF THE AUDITORY SYSTEM

The ear is housed in the *temporal bone* of the skull. The temporal bones are two of the eight cranial bones that form part of the base and lateral wall of the skull. The petrous portion of the temporal bone houses the otic capsule, the densest bone in the body. The temporal bone articulates with the sphenoid, parietal, and occipital bones.

External Ear

The ears are located on each side of the head at approximately eye level. The external ear is divided into the auricle *(pinna)* and the external auditory canal *(ear canal).* The tympanic membrane *(eardrum)* separates the external ear from the middle ear.

Auricle (Pinna)

The *auricle* (pinna), the conspicuous part of the ear, is attached to the side of the head by skin at approximately a 20- to 30-degree angle. Except for the fat and subcutaneous tissue in the lobule, it is composed mostly of cartilage. The cartilage is held to the skull by small muscles (the posterior, anterior, and superior auricular muscles), which are innervated by the posterior auricular branch of the facial nerve.

The parts of the pinna are illustrated in Figure A&P15-4. The *helix,* the outer rim of the pinna, leads inferiorly to the

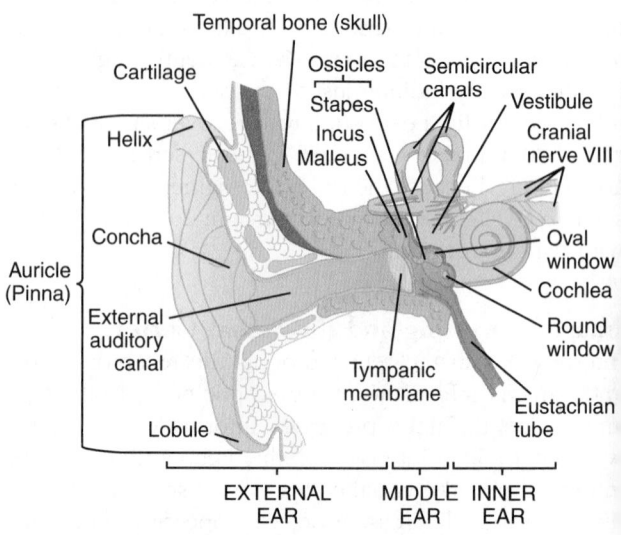

■ **FIGURE A&P15–4** Anatomy of the ear.

lobule. The *concha* is the deepest part, leading to the ear canal. The tragus and antitragus are triangular folds of cartilage that project over the entrance to the ear canal. Hair covers most of the ear, but it is usually rudimentary, except in the region of the tragus and antitragus.

In front of the external opening of the ear is the temporomandibular joint (TMJ). Often, TMJ problems produce referred pain to the ear (otalgia) because of their shared sensory nerve supply.

External Auditory Canal (Ear Canal)
The ear canal extends from the concha of the pinna to the tympanic membrane (see Figure A&P15-4). In adults, this slightly S-shaped canal is approximately 2.5 cm (1 inch) in length and follows an inward, forward, and downward path. The skeleton of cartilage in the outer third is continuous with the cartilage of the pinna. The inner two thirds is a bony canal entering the skull. The lumen of the ear canal is irregularly shaped and is narrowest where the transition from cartilage to bone occurs. The skin covering the cartilage portion is thick, containing sebaceous and ceruminous glands and hair follicles. The sebaceous and ceruminous glands secrete a golden to black substance called *cerumen* (wax). The skin covering the bony portion is very thin.

Tympanic Membrane
The tympanic membrane (eardrum) is an oval disk (approximately 1 cm in diameter); it covers the end of the auditory canal and separates the canal from the middle ear (see Figure A&P15-4). The eardrum is a thin, translucent, pearly gray membrane obliquely directed downward and inward, so that the posterior part is more accessible than the anterior part.

Middle Ear
The middle ear consists of the middle ear cleft and contents: ossicles, oval and round windows, eustachian tube, and facial nerve (see Figure A&P15-4). The middle ear lies between the ear canal and the *labyrinth* (inner ear). The middle ear cavity has a mucosal lining.

Ossicles
The middle ear contains the three smallest bones *(ossicles)* of the body, named according to their appearance. The outermost and largest ossicle is the *malleus* (hammer), which is firmly attached to the tympanic membrane. The innermost and smallest ossicle is the *stapes* (stirrup); its footplate occupies the oval window, in direct contact with the perilymph of the inner ear. The *incus* (anvil) lies between the other two and is shaped like a tooth with two roots (see Figure A&P15-4).

Windows
The middle ear contains two windows, whose names reflect their shape. The *round window* is an opening in the inner ear from which sound vibrations exit. The *oval window* is an opening in the inner ear into which sound vibrations enter. The oval window is not a true window because the footplate of the stapes bone covers it.

Eustachian Tube
The eustachian tube is a narrow channel approximately 35 mm (1½ inches) long and only 1 mm wide at its narrowest end. This tube connects the middle ear to the nasopharynx (see Figure A&P15-4). The structure consists mostly of fibrous tissue, cartilage, and bone; it extends downward, forward, and inward from each middle ear. The eustachian tube is lined with a mucous membrane that is continuous with the lining of the middle ear at one end and with the nasopharynx at the other end. A small section of this tube, originating in the middle ear, remains permanently open. Otherwise, the walls of the tube lightly oppose or touch each other, closing the tube to both the throat and ear and preventing the sound of normal nasal respiration and of one's own voice from passing up the eustachian tube.

Mastoid Bone
The mastoid section of the temporal bone includes the cone-shaped *mastoid process;* the *mastoid antrum,* a large cavity posteriorly continuous with the middle ear; and the *mastoid air cells,* which extend from the antrum and fill the temporal bone with air pockets.

The mastoid bone is a bony protuberance behind the lower portion of the pinna. The mastoid cavity is close to several important cranial structures: the dura of the temporal lobe, the cerebellar dura, the sigmoid sinus, and the jugular bulb. The middle ear is also bounded by the internal carotid artery. Therefore infection of the middle ear and mastoid cavities can also involve these structures.

Inner Ear (Labyrinth)
The inner ear or labyrinth is located deep within the petrous section of the temporal bone; it contains the sense organs for hearing and balance, which form the eighth cranial nerve (Figure A&P15-5). The inner ear is a complicated system of intercommunicating chambers and connecting tubes composed of two structures:
1. The *bony labyrinth* is the rigid capsule (otic capsule) that surrounds and protects the delicate membranous labyrinth. The *vestibule* connects the cochlea (for hearing) to the three semicircular canals (for balance). The *cochlea,* which looks like a snail shell with 2½ turns, is approximately 7 mm in diameter at the widest part and is structurally

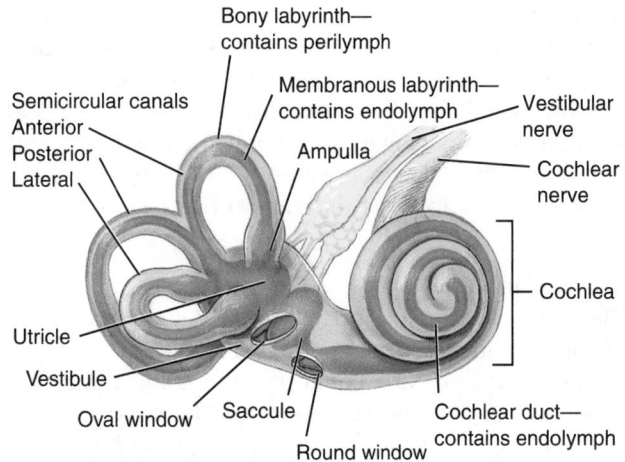

■ **FIGURE A&P15–5** The labyrinths of the inner ear. *(From Applegate, E.J. [2000]. The anatomy and physiology learning system [2nd ed.]. Philadelphia: Saunders.)*

divided into 3 compartments (Figure A&P15-6). The upper compartment *(scala vestibuli)* leads from the oval window to the apex of the cochlear spiral. The lower compartment *(scala tympani)* leads from the apex of the cochlear spiral to the round window. The *scala media,* which contains the organ of Corti, lies between the scala vestibuli and scala tympani.

2. The *membranous labyrinth,* lying within but not completely filling the bony labyrinth, is bathed in a fluid called *perilymph,* which communicates with the cerebrospinal fluid (CSF) via the cochlear duct. The membranous labyrinth consists of the utricle, the saccule, the semicircular canals, the cochlear duct, and the *organ of Corti* (the end organ for

hearing). The membranous labyrinth contains a different fluid *(endolymph).* This fluid also protects the end organ because it acts as a cushion against abrupt movements of the head.

The three *semicircular canals* are at right angles to each other and are named the anterior (superior), posterior (inferior), and lateral (horizontal) canals. The horizontal canal lies closest to the middle ear. This arrangement allows detection of movement in all three dimensions.

FUNCTION OF THE AUDITORY SYSTEM

External Ear

The ears are a pair of complex sensory organs for both hearing and balance. Their location on either side of the head produces binaural hearing, allows the detection of sound direction, and aids in maintaining equilibrium. The temporal bone provides protection for the organs of hearing and balance. It houses (1) the external and internal auditory canals; (2) the mastoid air cells, which provide an air reservoir for the middle ear; (3) the blood vessels; (4) the facial, vestibular, and cochlear nerves; (5) the labyrinth; and (6) the cochlea.

Sound Wave Conduction

The head, pinna, and ear canal act as an integrated system to transmit sound vibrations to the eardrum. Sound is transmitted from the external ear through the middle ear (which amplifies the sound) to the inner ear (see

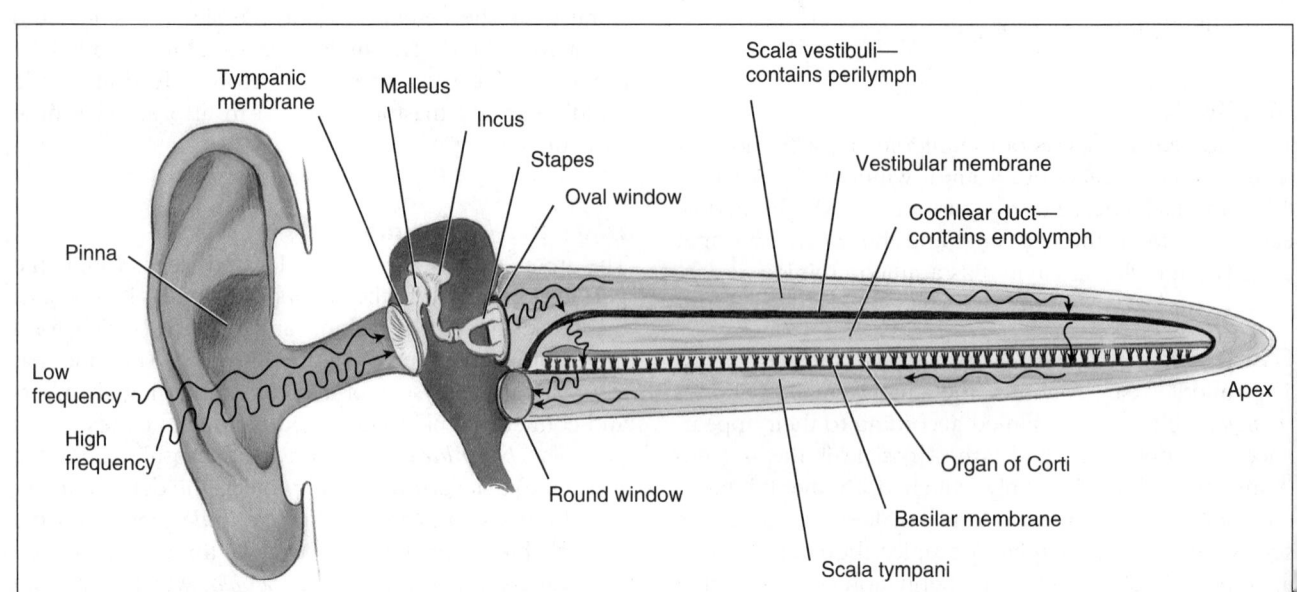

■ **FIGURE A&P15–6** The uncoiled cochlea, showing the pathway of pressure waves. *(From Applegate, E.J. [2000]. The anatomy and physiology learning system [2nd ed.]. Philadelphia: Saunders.)*

Figure A&P15-6). The funnel shape of the pinna collects and directs sound to the eardrum.

The tympanic membrane, a common membrane between the external ear canal and the middle ear space, protects the middle ear and conducts sound vibrations from the external ear to the ossicles. The tympanic membrane changes its tension to muffle sound. The sound pressure applied to the stapes (the smallest ossicle) in the oval window is 22 times greater than the sound pressure exerted on the eardrum. The pressure of the sound vibrations is increased as a result of transmission from a larger area to a smaller area, and the lever effect of the ossicular chain. The sound energy, after transformation, is carried by neural elements to the brain for decoding and, thus, hearing.

Wax Production

Cerumen (wax) protects the ear. Wax is to the ear what tears are to the eyes. The sticky consistency of the wax and the fine hairs of the ear canal help clean the ear canal of foreign matter and protect it from water damage. Impacted cerumen can cause hearing losses in clients of all ages. At times, wax must be mechanically removed.

Middle Ear
Sound Wave Conduction

The ossicles transmit sound vibrations mechanically (see Figure A&P15-6). The ossicles are held in place by joints, muscles, and ligaments, which also offer some protection from loud sounds. The light weight and the configuration of the ossicles provide an efficient means of transmitting sound vibrations from the air molecules of the external ear to the fluid molecules of the inner ear. Fluids offer more resistance than air and need more force to transmit movement. The ossicular chain produces and magnifies this force in order to move the inner ear fluids.

Ventilation and Pressure Regulation

The eustachian tube provides an air passage from the nasopharynx to the middle ear to equalize pressure on both sides of the eardrum. This tube regulates ventilation and pressure, both of which are necessary for normal hearing. During yawning, swallowing, and sneezing, the eustachian tube is opened by the *tensor veli palatini* muscle. The natural opening and closing of the eustachian tube also allows drainage of exudate from the middle ear mucosa. The tube can be forcibly opened by increasing nasopharyngeal pressure. This act is accomplished by attempting to blow air through the nose while holding the nose closed.

Inner Ear
Hearing

Sound waves are transmitted by the ossicles to the delicate membrane of the oval window (see Figure A&P15-6).

These vibrations move the perilymph in the scala vestibuli. The perilymph of the scala vestibuli is continuous with that of the scala tympani at the extreme tip of the "snail shell," called the *helicotrema*. The sound energy vibrations enter through the oval window and exit through the round window.

Vibrations in the perilymph of the scala vestibuli are transmitted through the vestibular membrane (*Reissner's membrane*) to the endolymph that fills the cochlear duct. The cochlear duct is located between the scala vestibuli and the scala tympani. The *organ of Corti,* which is bathed in the endolymph, lies on the basilar membrane in a spiral strip from the basal turn near the round window to the apex at the helicotrema. This organ transforms mechanical sound vibrations into neural activity and separates sound into different frequencies. The electrochemical impulse travels via the acoustic nerve to the brain stem. Auditory nerve input from both ears joins at the lateral lemniscus, reducing the possibility of unilateral deafness from central nervous system damage. The auditory nerves ascend through the thalamus to the cortex by a variety of pathways, reaching both the primary and secondary auditory regions of the temporal cortex of the brain. Efferent innervation via the acoustic nerve (eighth cranial nerve) reaches the cochlea and vestibule via the internal auditory canal, which also carries the facial nerve (seventh cranial nerve).

Sound is filtered by the ear components. Human auditory sensitivity ranges from 15 to 20,000 Hz. The auditory canal diminishes the passage of sounds with frequencies greater than 3500 Hz, the higher end of the human voice frequency. The middle ear diminishes passage of sounds with frequencies less than 1000 Hz, the lower end of human voice frequency. The muscles of the middle ear decrease sound transmission by uncoupling the ossicles. For example, contraction of the tensor tympani allows reflex adaptation to a noisy environment. Contraction of the stapedius decreases sound transmission while speaking.

Balance

The *utricle* and *saccule* are vestibular receptors that position the head as it relates to the pull of gravity. The utricle and saccule contain hair cells arranged in sheets (maculae). These hair cells detect changes in linear acceleration, including the force of gravity. The *semicircular canals* are arranged to sense rotational movements, such as movements or changes in position. Each of the semicircular canals connects with the utricle. Where the canals connect with the utricle is an enlarged portion (*ampulla*). The ampulla contains a cluster of hair cells (*crista*) concerned with dynamic balance. For example, when head position is changed, movement of the endolymph stimulates the hair cells, initiating increased impulses that travel over the vestibular division of the acoustic nerve to the brain. Balance functions in the vestibular system, along with visual cues and musculoskeletal cues, combine to maintain balance. Hearing and balance are partially maintained with the loss of function of one ear.

EFFECTS OF AGING ON HEARING

Many physiologic changes lead to changes in hearing in older people. The hairs become coarser during the aging process; thus retention of wax is more of a problem. *Presbycusis,* a gradual sensorineural loss caused by nerve degeneration in the inner ear or auditory nerve, is a type of hearing loss that occurs with aging, even in people living in a quiet environment. Loss of auditory neurons in the organ of Corti and cochlear hair cell degeneration create an inability to hear high-frequency sounds. There may also be degeneration of the cochlear conductive membrane and decreased blood supply to the cochlea, leading to inability to hear at all (but especially higher) frequencies. Finally, a loss of cortical auditory neurons leads to diminished hearing and speech comprehension.

CONCLUSIONS

Vision and hearing are two senses that allow distance perception of the environment. Because we rely on these senses for communication with those around us, alterations in either sense can have a profound social and emotional impact. Some reductions in the ability to see or to hear are a normal part of age-related changes.

BIBLIOGRAPHY

1. Applegate, E.J. (2000). *The anatomy and physiology learning system* (2nd ed.). Philadelphia: Saunders.
2. Guyton, A.C., & Hall, J. (2007). *Textbook of medical physiology* (11th ed.). Philadelphia: Saunders.
3. Kandel, E.R., Schwartz, J.H., & Jessel, T.M. (2000). *Principles of neural science* (4th ed.). New York: McGraw-Hill.
4. McPhee, S.J., et al. (1999). *Pathophysiology of disease.* New York, McGraw-Hill.
5. Nolte, J. (2002). *The human brain* (5th ed.). St. Louis: Mosby.
6. Silverthorn, D. (2001). *Human physiology* (2nd ed.). Upper Saddle River, NJ: Prentice Hall.

CHAPTER 64

Assessment of the Eyes and Ears

Sharon Lanzetta and Lianne F. Herbruck

ASSESSMENT OF THE EYE

The eye is a unique organ because its external anatomy can be assessed easily. Internal eye structures, including blood vessels and central nervous system (CNS) tissue (the retina and optic nerve), are also easily visualized through the cornea without invasive procedures. The effects of many systemic problems, such as infections, cancer, and vascular and autoimmune disorders, can be detected during an internal eye examination. Clients may voice misconceptions about vision and the eyes (Box 64-1). If you encounter such misconceptions while conducting a physical examination, be prepared to address them.

HISTORY

A complete ophthalmic history includes demographic data, exploration of chief complaint and related manifestations, review of systems, past medical history, past surgical history, allergies and medications, dietary habits, psychosocial history and lifestyle, and family health history.

Biographical and Demographic Data

Demographic data relevant to ocular assessment include age and gender. The incidence of cataracts, dry eye, retinal detachment, glaucoma, esotropia (eyes turning inward), and exotropia (eyes turning outward) increases with age. Hereditary color vision deficits are more common in men than in women.

Current Health

As with many body systems, care must be taken when assessing ocular manifestations. Of the five senses, vision is the system that provides the most information. There may be a fear of vision loss or uncorrectable visual

manifestations. Many disease processes, or their treatments, have potential to negatively impact visual health. Some eye issues, like wide-angle glaucoma, are usually found during routine eye examinations.

The four most common preventable causes of permanent vision loss in developed nations are (1) *amblyopia* (reduced visual acuity that is not correctable with glasses in the absence of anatomic defects in the eye or visual pathways), (2) diabetic retinopathy, (3) age-related maculopathy, and (4) glaucoma. Many of these ophthalmic disorders are asymptomatic, so routine eye examinations are therefore imperative.

Chief Complaint

The most common chief complaint is a change or loss of vision. The complaint may also be less specific, such as headache or eyestrain. Sometimes the client may be unable to verbalize a specific complaint, and the chief complaint could be as vague as "something is wrong with my eyes."

---

evolve Web Enhancements

Assessment Terms English and Spanish

Appendix B A Health History Format That Integrates the Assessment of Functional Health Patterns

Web Figures Snellen's Chart

An Otoscope

Weber and Rinne Tests for Hearing Impairment

Web Tables Constriction and Accommodation Tests for the Pupil

Tonometry and Slit-Lamp Examinations

Web Box Guidelines for Using an Ophthalmoscope

Be sure to check out the bonus material on the Evolve website and the CD-ROM, including free self-assessment exercises. **http://evolve.elsevier.com/Black/medsurg**

BOX 64-1 Common Misconceptions About Vision and the Eyes

The following statements are often passed along as "advice." All of the following are false:

- Reading in the dark is harmful to the eyes.
- Children will outgrow crossed eyes.
- A cataract is a film growing over the surface of the eye.
- Cataracts must "ripen" before they are removed.
- The surgeon takes out the eye to operate on it.
- A person with failing eyesight should avoid reading to save the eyes.
- Children must be cautioned not to sit too close to the television.
- Wearing someone else's glasses may damage your eyes.
- Misuse of the eyes in childhood results in the need for glasses later in life.
- Cataracts can be removed by a laser.
- Emotional stress increases intraocular pressure.

Clinical Manifestations

Ocular manifestations can be divided into three basic categories: (1) vision, (2) appearance, and (3) sensations of pain and discomfort. Whenever possible, characterize clinical manifestations according to onset, location, duration, and characteristics, such as frequency and severity. The circumstances surrounding onset as well as the client's response to treatment are important. Refer to Figure 64-1 for details on the initial assessment of the client with eye complaints.

Pain (Ophthalmalgia). Eye pain is often poorly localized. Nonspecific complaints include eyestrain, pulling, pressure, fullness, or generalized headache. The pain may be periocular, ocular, or retrobulbar (behind the globe). Foreign-body sensation produces a sharp superficial pain that can be relieved by topical anesthesia. Deeper internal aching may indicate glaucoma, inflammation, muscle spasm, or infection. The Integrating Diagnostic Testing feature on p. 1680 provides further cues for evaluation of the client with eye pain.

Abnormal Vision. Visual changes or loss of vision can be caused by abnormalities in the eye or anywhere along the visual pathway. Considerations may include refractive (focusing) error; lid ptosis (drooping eyelid); clouding or interference in the cornea, lens, or aqueous or vitreous space; and malfunction of the retina, optic nerve, or intracranial visual pathway. Refer to the Integrating Diagnostic Testing feature on p. 1681 for further details on the evaluation of the client with a visual changes complaint.

Abnormal Appearance. External changes in appearance include growths or lesions, edema, ptosis, and abnormal position. The most common abnormal appearance is a red eye (Box 64-2). Refer to the Integrating Diagnostic Testing feature on p. 1682 for further details on the evaluation of the client with a possible eye infection.

Abnormal Sensation. Adequate description of ocular sensation can help guide an appropriate diagnosis (Table 64-1 on p. 1683). Reflex spasm of the ciliary muscle and iris sphincter that occurs with inflammation may produce brow ache and *photophobia* (sensitivity to light) or a constricted pupil *(miosis)*. Itching is usually a sign of an allergic response. Dryness, burning, grittiness, and mild foreign-body sensation can occur with dry eyes or mild corneal irritation.

Review of Systems

The review of systems (ROS) information in Figure 64-2 on p. 1684 can be used as a guide to help determine underlying etiology of potential and realized visual issues. Many disease processes can affect vision. Vascular problems, such as hypertension, can impact blood flow to the eyes, causing changes in vision. Headaches with visual changes may indicate a tumor in the brain or be a cue to migraines. Obtaining the family visual history can alert the client to potential visual risks, and can assist the practitioner in helping the client to reduce these risks.

ROS relevant to ocular assessment includes asking about manifestations such as headaches and problems with sinusitis. Determine whether manifestations occur in association with pain or discomfort, visual changes, swelling, redness, or drainage from the eye. Record time of day and the season of year during which manifestations occur as well as any sensitivity to light.

Past Medical History

The past medical history focuses on systemic disorders commonly associated with ocular manifestations. Some of these illnesses, such as diabetes mellitus, rheumatoid arthritis, and thyroid disorders, may be recently acquired by adults, or may have occurred in the client's childhood. Inquire about childhood vaccinations, particularly for measles (rubella).

In addition to childhood and systemic diseases, ask about hypertension, multiple sclerosis, and myasthenia gravis. If the client wears eyeglasses or contact lenses, ask when the last eye examination took place and when the prescription was last changed. Hospitalizations related to the eyes or brain, including a history of head or eye trauma, must be assessed.

Surgical History

Record the client's surgical history. This may include corrective vision surgery such as laser-assisted in-situ keratomileusis (LASIK), radial keratotomy (RK), cataract removal, glaucoma treatment, or eye muscle correction. Some eye surgeries, such as those for glaucoma, car

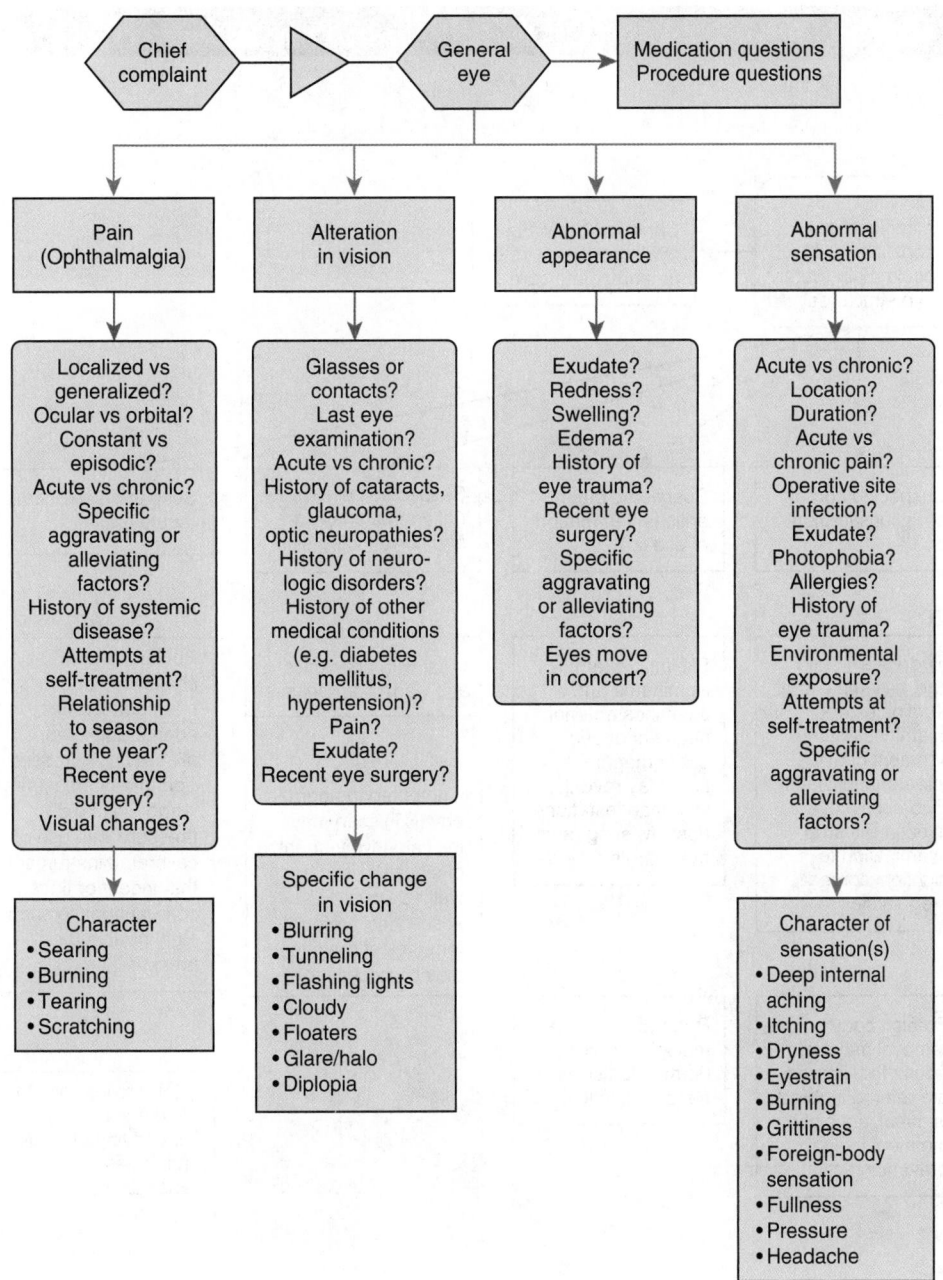

■ **FIGURE 64-1** Expanded eye assessment.

precipitate other eye issues (cataracts). History of brain or facial surgeries should also be assessed as these have the potential to affect vision.

Allergies

Note any allergies to medications (eye drops) and other substances, such as inhalants (dust, chemicals, or pollens) and environmental contacts (cosmetics or pollens). Allergic manifestations include eye redness, tearing, and itching.

Medications

Many medications, including prescription drugs, affect the eyes. Note the name, dose, and frequency the

medication is taken. Specifically ask about use of over-the-counter (OTC) eye drops, as those with antihistamines and decongestants can dry the ocular surface. Record current eye and systemic medications being used, and all other current and past ocular disorders.

Dietary Habits

Inquire about the use of herbal remedies and dietary supplements (vitamins). Some clients may consume large doses of vitamins, believing these substances will prevent the development of vision problems such as cataracts and macular degeneration. Studies have shown that diets rich in fruits, vegetables, and fish, or

INTEGRATING D I A G N O S T I C   T E S T I N G

Eye Pain

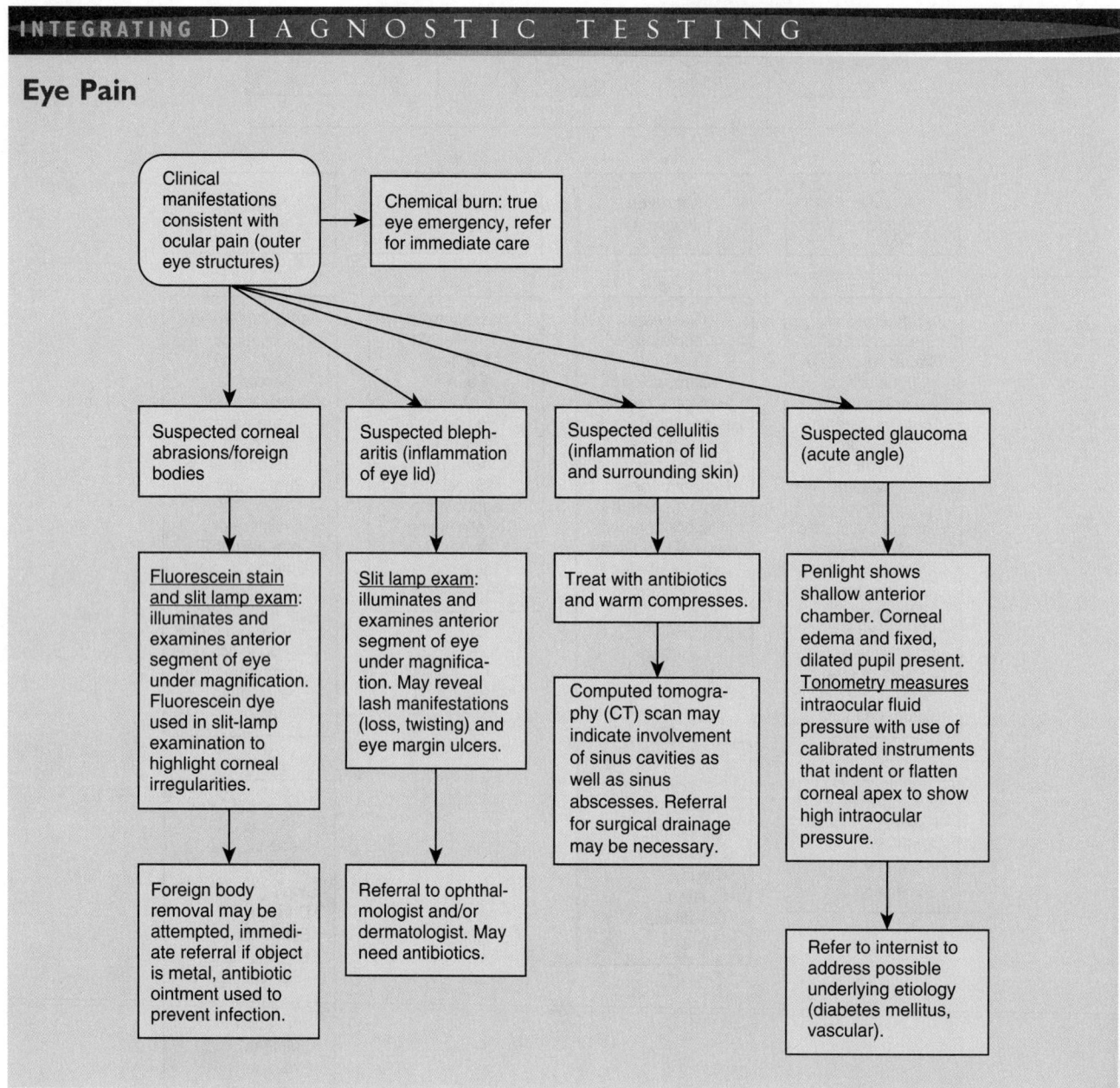

supplements of antioxidants C, E, and beta-carotene, have potential to reduce the incidence of visual problems like macular degeneration. However, many OTC preparations taken in too large a quantity can be harmful. Clients need to be aware of the risks and should be encouraged to be truthful about supplement ingestion.

Social History
Psychosocial history and lifestyle data significant to the ocular health history include occupational hazards, leisure activities and hobbies, and health management behaviors. Assess the client's work and/or hobbies that may include exposure to irritating fumes, smoke, or airborne particles. Also assess participation in activities that

increase the risk for eye or head trauma (such as football, racquetball, or baseball), as well as those that increase the risk of foreign-body injury or abrasion (e.g., hiking or gardening). Address client use of protective eye gear (such as safety goggles or sunglasses) when engaging in these activities.

Health management behaviors related to the eyes include self-care measures as mismanagement can negatively impact eye health. For example, is the diabetic client aggressively managing his/her disease? Is the client with contact lenses cleaning and storing them as recommended? Sunglasses are important as the ultraviolet rays of the sun can damage the eyes. Smoking is associated with increased risk of macula

INTEGRATING DIAGNOSTIC TESTING

Visual Changes

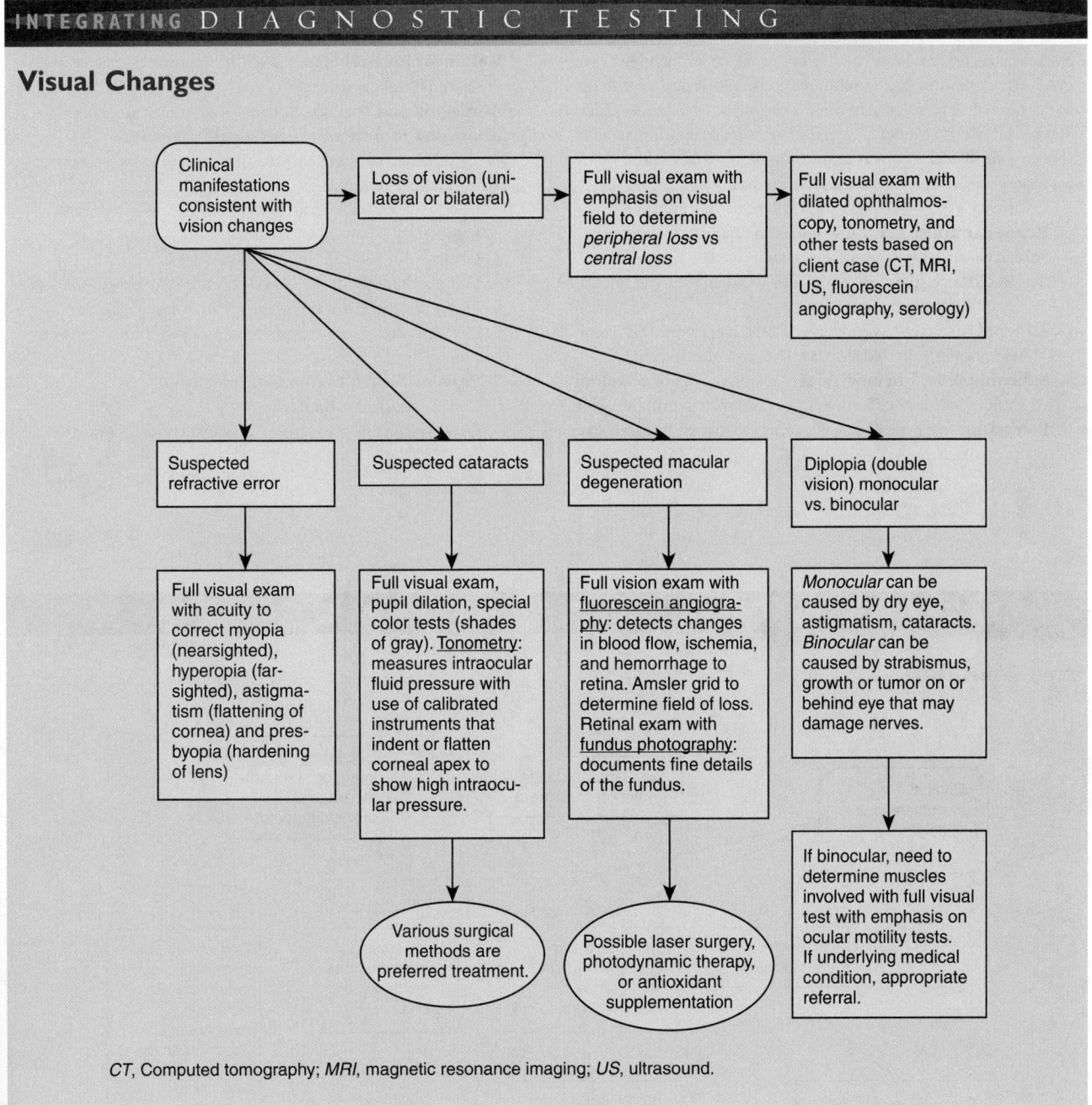

CT, Computed tomography; MRI, magnetic resonance imaging; US, ultrasound.

degeneration. Also, eating a healthy diet and getting adequate exercise can positively impact other disease processes, such as hypertension, which increases the odds of good visual health.

Visual ability is one of several capabilities necessary for a person to operate a motor vehicle. Use tact when reviewing a driving history for a client who may have impaired vision. Clients may not answer truthfully if they feel driving privileges may be lost.

The social stigma of blindness underlies the anxiety that clients experience with actual or potential vision loss. Loss of control in personal, family, and work

situations can be devastating. Total loss of vision isolates a person within a different reality. Clients with actual or potential vision loss may be faced with barriers in their vocations that force an unwanted change, as not all work environments can be adapted for someone who is visually impaired. Issues of dependence versus independence are often a factor in the client's ability to cope with the stressors of vision loss.

Family Health History

Many ocular disorders tend to be familial (strabismus, glaucoma, myopia, hyperopia). Other conditions such as

---

BOX 64-2   Red Eye

Nurses often encounter a client whose chief complaint is a "red eye." The condition causing the eye to be red (engorgement of the conjunctival vessels) may be a subconjunctival hemorrhage that requires no treatment, or it may be a manifestation of a serious eye disorder, which requires immediate attention. Disorders involving red eye include the following:

Conjunctivitis—bacterial, viral, allergic, and irritative
Herpes simplex keratitis—inflammation of the cornea
Scleritis—inflammation of the sclera
Angle-closure glaucoma—sudden occlusion of the anterior chamber angle by iris tissue
Adnexal disease—stye, dacryocystitis, blepharitis, lid lesions (carcinoma), thyroid disease, and vascular lesions
Subconjunctival hemorrhage—accumulation of blood in the potential space between the conjunctiva and the sclera
Pterygium—abnormal growth of tissue that progresses over the cornea

Keratoconjunctivitis sicca—inflammation associated with lacrimal deficiency
Abrasions and foreign bodies—hyperemic response
Abnormal lid function—Bell's palsy, thyroid ophthalmopathy, or lesions that cause ocular exposure

To evaluate a red eye:

1. Check the client's visual acuity with a Snellen chart.
2. Inspect for a pattern of redness.
3. Observe for the presence of discharge.
4. Using a penlight or slit lamp, observe for corneal opacities.
5. Using fluorescein stain, observe for corneal defects.
6. Examine the anterior chamber for depth, blood cells, or pus.
7. Examine the pupils for irregularity.
8. Check intraocular pressure.
9. Observe for the pressure of proptosis or a lid disorder.

INTEGRATING DIAGNOSTIC TESTING

Eye Infection

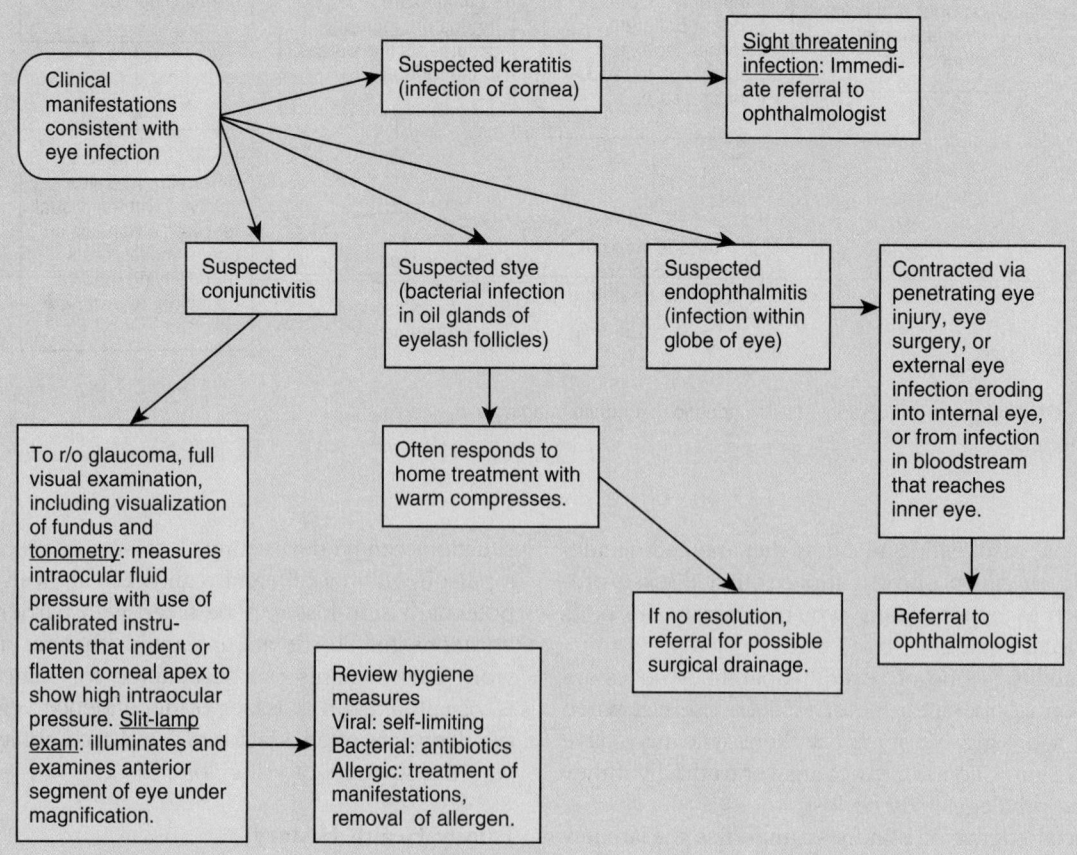

TABLE 64–1 Ocular Manifestations and Common Causes

Clinical Manifestation	Potential Cause
Blurring	Cataracts, iritis, macular degeneration, refractive error, eye fatigue, myopia, diabetes mellitus, corneal edema, optic neuritis or neuropathy
Eye numbness	Diabetes mellitus, peripheral neuropathy, conjunctivitis, stroke
Eye pain	Injury, infection, inflammation, glaucoma, foreign body, eye strain, sinusitis, corneal abrasions, hypertension, migraine, multiple sclerosis, tumor
Flashes	Retinal detachment, blow to the head, ocular migraine
Floaters	Red and white blood cells or gel-like clumps in the vitreous, retinal tear or detachment, normal part of aging
Foreign body	Object in eye, corneal scratches, abrasions or erosion, dry eye, conjunctivitis, contact lens issue, keratitis
Headache	Eyestrain, migraine headache, cluster headache, sinusitis, shingles, conjunctivitis, corneal abrasion or ulcer
Itching	Blepharitis (eyelid infection), conjunctivitis, contact lens issues, ocular allergy
Light sensitivity	Acute glaucoma, iritis, scleritis, corneal ulcer, thyroid disease, ectropion/entropion
Tearing	Blocked tear duct, dry eye, infection of lacrimal sac, ectropion (everted lid) or entropion (inverted lid)

diabetes mellitus, retinoblastoma, retinitis pigmentosa, and macular degeneration also tend to appear in families. Lack of a family health history does not rule out the possibility of a genetic disorder. Some clients do not know the ocular history of family members, and some may be embarrassed or hesitant to share the information. Accurate reporting of the family history can alert both client and caregiver to potential issues in the future.

PHYSICAL EXAMINATION

Basic physical examination of the eyes includes assessment of external structures via inspection and palpation. Other important assessments include testing of corneal reflexes, ocular motility (see the Snellen chart for assessment of visual acuity on the web and see Table 64-2 on p. 1685), visual acuity, and visual fields (Table 64-3 on p. 1686). It also includes examination of the internal eye structures with an ophthalmoscope. For an example of an assessment recording, see the Physical Assessment Findings in the Healthy Adult feature on p. 1687. For more in-depth physical examination explanations and techniques, please refer to a physical examination textbook.

External Eye

External eye structures include the eyebrows, eyelashes, eyelids, the lacrimal apparatus, anterior portion of the eyeballs, conjunctivae, sclerae, corneas, anterior chambers, pupils, and irides. Inspect and palpate these structures while the client sits at eye level. Table 64-4 on p. 1687 presents abnormal physical examination findings of the external eye.

Eye Position

Assess eye position for symmetry and alignment.

Eyebrows

Inspect the eyebrows for symmetry, hair distribution, skin conditions, and movement. The eyebrows normally move up and down smoothly under control of the facial nerves.

Eyelids and Eyelashes

Examine the eyelids and eyelashes for placement and symmetry. Normally, the sclerae are not visible above or below the irides when the eyelids are open. Elevate the eyebrows to inspect the upper lids for lesions. Inspect the lower lids by asking the client to open the eyes. Examine the skin of the eyelids and orbit by palpating for texture, firmness, mobility, and integrity of the underlying tissues. Assess the blink response. Blinking is an involuntary reflex that occurs bilaterally up to 20 times a minute.

Eyeballs and Lacrimal Apparatus

To palpate the eyeballs, instruct the client to close the eyes and look down. Place the tip of the index fingers on the upper eyelids, over the sclerae, and palpate gently. Normally, the eyeballs feel firm and symmetrical. Visualize the lacrimal apparatus by retracting the upper lid and having the client look down. The area should be free of swelling, edema, and excessive moisture, and there should be no regurgitation of fluid from the sac or puncta.

Conjunctivae and Sclerae

Inspect the conjunctivae and sclerae for color changes, texture, vascularity, lesions, thickness, secretions, and foreign bodies. The bulbar conjunctivae are colorless and transparent, allowing the sclerae to be seen. Small blood vessels may be visible. In Caucasians, the sclerae are white; in people with darker skin, they may appear light yellow. Retract the lower eyelids to expose the conjunctivae without applying pressure to the eyeballs. You (or the client) should gently push the lower lids down against the bony orbit while the client looks up. Healthy conjunctivae are pink to light red. If the lower palpebral conjunctivae are normal, the upper palpebral conjunctivae usually are not inspected. Wear gloves to inspect the palpebral conjunctivae, and wash your hands both before and after this portion of the examination.

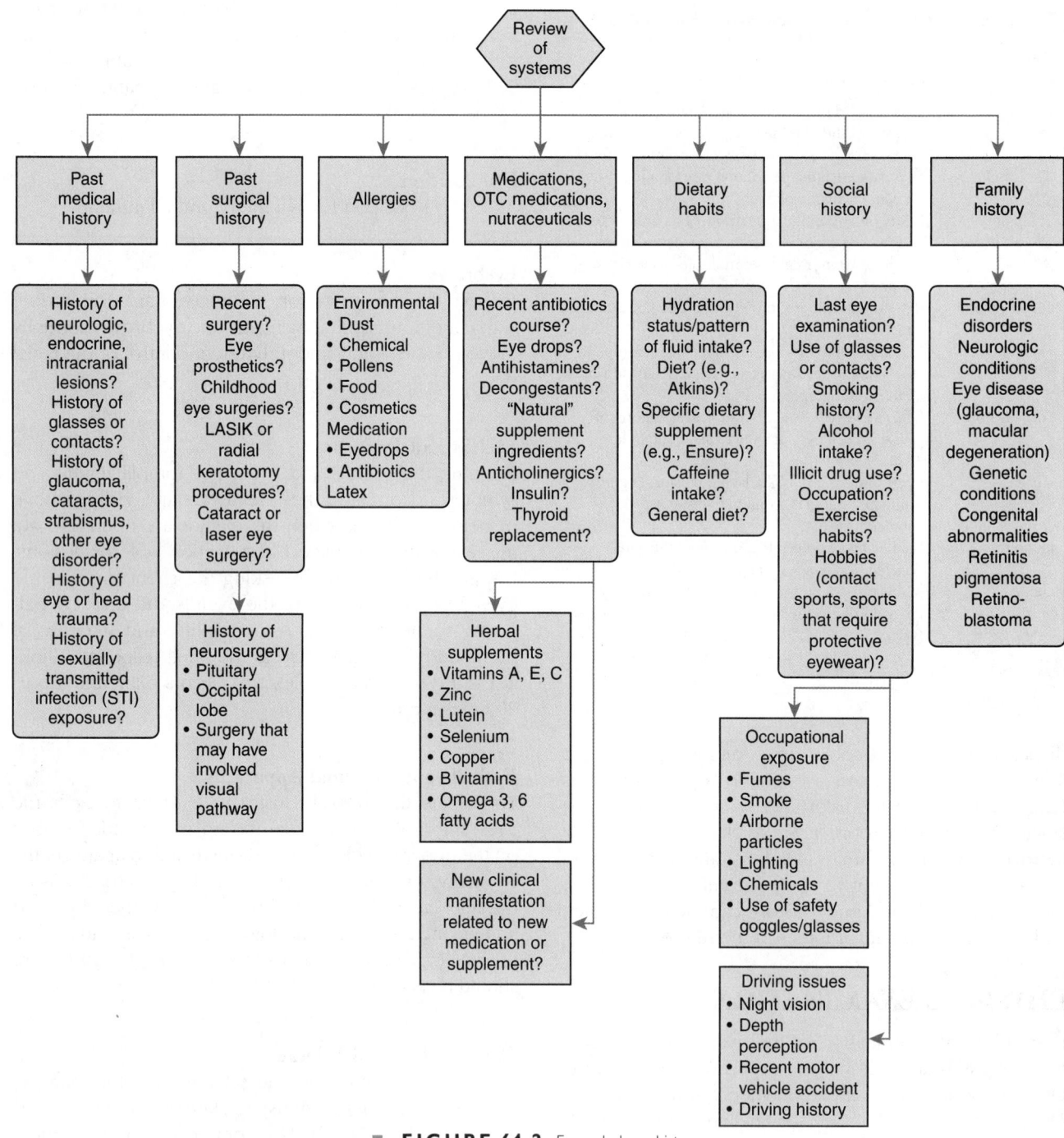

■ **FIGURE 64-2** Expanded eye history.

Cornea and Anterior Chamber

Inspect the cornea and anterior chamber from an oblique angle while shining a penlight on the corneal surface. The irides are easily visible. In older adults, a thin, grayish white ring around the edge of the cornea *(arcus senilis)* may be seen. The anterior chambers should appear clear and transparent with no cloudiness or shadows cast on the irides. The depth of the chamber between the cornea and iris is normally about 3 mm.

Iris and Pupil

Inspect the iris and the pupil with the same oblique lighting from the penlight. The iris should light up and have a consistent color. The light should also cause the iris to constrict as the optic nerves are stimulated, causing the pupil to become smaller. Dim lighting causes the pupil to dilate. Pupils are normally black and round, have smooth borders, and are equal in size. Inspect the pupils for size, equality, shape, and ability to react to

TABLE 64–2 **Physical Examination Tests of the Eye:** *Reflexes and Motility*

Test	Purpose	Procedure	Results
Corneal reflex	Assesses function of fifth cranial nerve (trigeminal)	Client looks straight ahead; bring sterile cotton wisp from behind and lightly touch cornea; may also use syringe to puff air gently across cornea	Blinking and tearing indicate intact nerves
Corneal light reflex test (Hirschberg's test)	Determines eye alignment	Shine penlight 12-15 inches from bridge of nose with client staring straight ahead; observe light reflection from both corneas	Symmetrical reflection is normal Asymmetrical reflection can indicate strabismus, esotropia (deviates to nose), exotropia (deviates away from nose), hyperopia (vertical up), or hypotropia (vertical down)
Ocular motility	Gathers information about extraocular muscles; orbit; oculomotor, trochlear, and abducens nerves; brain stem connections; and cerebral cortex	Client tracks target with both eyes as it is moved through the 6 cardinal directions of gaze (see Fig. A&P15-2 in the Anatomy & Physiology Review). Nerve function testing: stand directly in front of client with penlight 12 inches from eyes; keeping head still, client follows light with eyes only; move in orderly fashion from center to outer edge of each of 6 cardinal directions	Eyes normally move parallel to each other in smooth unison Involuntary, rapid oscillating movement of eyeball (nystagmus) abnormal Eyes not parallel or eyelid covering more than a tiny portion of iris also abnormal
Cover-uncover test	Assesses eye muscle function and alignment for tropia (deviation of ocular alignment) and phoria (latent deviations with one eye covered)	Client stares at fixed point 20 inches away; cover one eye with opaque card and observe uncovered eye for lateral or medial movement as it focuses on fixed point; remove cover and observe that eye for movement as it focuses on fixed point Repeat for other eye	No movement is a normal finding Test may need to be repeated several times to confirm abnormal findings

light and accommodation. (See the table on the website titled Constriction and Accommodation Tests for the Pupil.) Pupil abnormalities may be caused by neurologic disease, intraocular inflammation, iris adhesions, systemic or ocular medication side effects, or surgical alteration.

Internal Eye

Internal eye structures are visible only with illumination such as that provided by a direct, or indirect, ophthalmoscope. These instruments are used to inspect the structures posterior to the iris, including the lens and fundus (which includes the retina, retinal vessels, choroid, optic disc, macula, and fovea). Using the ophthalmoscope requires considerable skill and practice. This section presents a brief overview of basic internal eye assessment. Please refer to a physical examination textbook for more in-depth discussion.

Direct Ophthalmoscopy

The direct ophthalmoscope uses a light source and reflective mirrors to provide a magnified (×15) image of the fundus (posterior portion of the eye) and a detailed view of the disc and retinal vascular bed. In a

darkened room, the instrument is held 1 to 2 inches away from the client's eye for examination (see the box on the website titled Guidelines for Using an Ophthalmoscope) (Figures 64-3 and 64-4). Retinal veins radiate from the disc and are darker, and slightly thicker, than arteries. They should not be pulsating, although as a normal variation you may see an occasional spontaneous pulsation. The retinal background is pink in Caucasian people and heavily pigmented in people with a dark complexion. Choroidal vessels may appear as linear orange streaks. The presence of a cataract, or cloudy cornea, may impair examination.

The fundus is the only site in the body where the vascular bed may be observed directly. Thus funduscopic examination yields information about many systemic diseases. Abnormal findings include an altered arteriovenous ratio, narrowed arteries, widened veins, pinched-off vessels, abnormal arterial light reflex, excessive tortuosity, numerous arteriovenous nicks, exudates, white patches, and focal hemorrhage.

Indirect Ophthalmoscopy

Indirect ophthalmoscopy provides a stereoscopic picture over a large area of the retina. The light source comes from a head-mounted light. The examiner holds a convex

TABLE 64–3 Vision Testing

Test	Purpose	Procedure	Results
Visual acuity	Determines clarity of cornea, lens, and vitreous; determines function of visual pathway from retina to brain. *For best corrected vision, allow client to wear glasses or contact lenses during exam.	1. Position client 20 ft in front of Snellen chart* (see website). 2. Client sits with one eye covered. 3. Ask client to read smallest line of print seen. 4. Credit client with line read with >50% accuracy; record results according to standardized numbers. 5. Assess with and without corrective lenses for both eyes.	Abnormal acuity implies uncorrected refractive error or pathology. *Normal is 20/20. *Myopia (nearsighted) is 20/30 or more. *Farsighted is 20/15 or less, but may be greater than average acuity. *20/200 with corrected vision is legal blindness.
Visual fields	To evaluate peripheral vision, you can use *confrontational method* (at right) or a computerized instrument. Computerized equipment permits more accurate detection and quantification of scotoma (area of decreased visual function).	1. Client sits 2 ft away from you, looking into your eyes. 2. Cover your right eye and client's left eye. 3. Hold a penlight equidistant between you and client, just out of view of peripheral visual field. Starting with superior field, bring object down until client states it is visible (you should also be able to see it). Repeat at 45-degree angles, through superior, temporal, inferior, and nasal fields. 4. Repeat for other eye.	Gross visual field abnormalities can be detected. If found, refer for further exam. Visual field alteration may be caused by CNS disorders (lesions, syphilis) or ocular disorders (glaucoma, retinal detachment).

Special Tests

Color Vision

Problems are genetic and more often seen in men (7%) than women (0.5%); also affected by nutrition, optic nerve disorder, fovea centralis problems	Not always common screening test. Detects those with altered color perception.	Common test involves use of color plates with numbers outlined in primary colors and surrounded by "confusion" colors.	Clients with color vision problems are unable to recognize figure presented.

Central Area of Blindness

	Used to detect and follow development of central area blindness (scotoma), such as seen with macular degeneration.	Amsler grid: 20-cm square divided into 5-mm squares with dot in center. Holding the grid 12 inches from face, client fixes gaze on central dot and describes any areas of distortion or absence in grid.	If distortion or grid absence noted, refer for further exam.

Examples: 20/20 is normal; client reads at 20 ft what person with normal vision reads at 20 ft.
  20/60 means client reads at 20 ft what person with normal vision reads at 60 ft.
  20/15 means client reads at 20 ft what person with normal vision reads at 15 ft.
* Snellen chart: Generally placed at a distance of 20 feet, the distance at which rays of light from an object are practically parallel and little accommodation effort is needed. Sizes of symbols are identified according to the distances at which they are normally visible. For example, the largest symbols can be read 200 feet away by people with unimpaired vision.

lens in front of the client's eye and, through a viewing device attached to the headband, sees an inverted reversed image. The indirect ophthalmoscope provides for binocular visual inspection with depth perception and permits a wider field of view compared with the direct method.

Advanced Eye Assessment
Some common, but advanced, skills in internal assessment of the eye include tonometry, which is a method of measuring intraocular fluid pressure, and slit-lamp examination, which examines the anterior segment of the eye under magnification (see the Tonometry and Slit-Lamp Examinations table on the website).

DIAGNOSTIC TESTING

There are many diagnostic tests to help determine the etiology of vision difficulties. A brief overview of some of these tests is presented in Table 64-5 on p. 1688. Please refer to diagnostic testing and physical examination textbooks for a more in-depth discussion of these tests.

Physical Assessment Findings in the Healthy Adult

The Eye

INSPECTION

Visual acuity 20/20. Eyebrows full, mobile. Eyelashes curve out and away from eyelids. Ptosis absent. Eyelids without lesions or inflammation. Eyes moist. Palpebral conjunctivae pink; bulbar conjunctivae clear. Scleral color even, without redness. Corneal light reflection symmetrical. PERRLA, directly and consensually. Cornea smooth; lens and anterior chamber clear. Irides evenly colored. EOMs full, without nystagmus. Conjugate movement. No strabismus. Visual fields full to confrontation.

PALPATION

Eyeballs firm. Orbits without edema. No regurgitation from puncta. Tenderness absent over lacrimal apparatus.

FUNDUSCOPIC EXAMINATION

Red reflexes visualized. AV ratio approximately 2:3. Vessels without tortuosity, narrowing, pulsation, or nicking. Disc margins clear, no cupping, cup-to-disc ratio 1:3. No evidence of retinal hemorrhage, patches, spots.

AV, Artery-to-vein; *EOM,* extraocular movement;
PERRLA, pupils equal, round, reactive to light and accommodation.

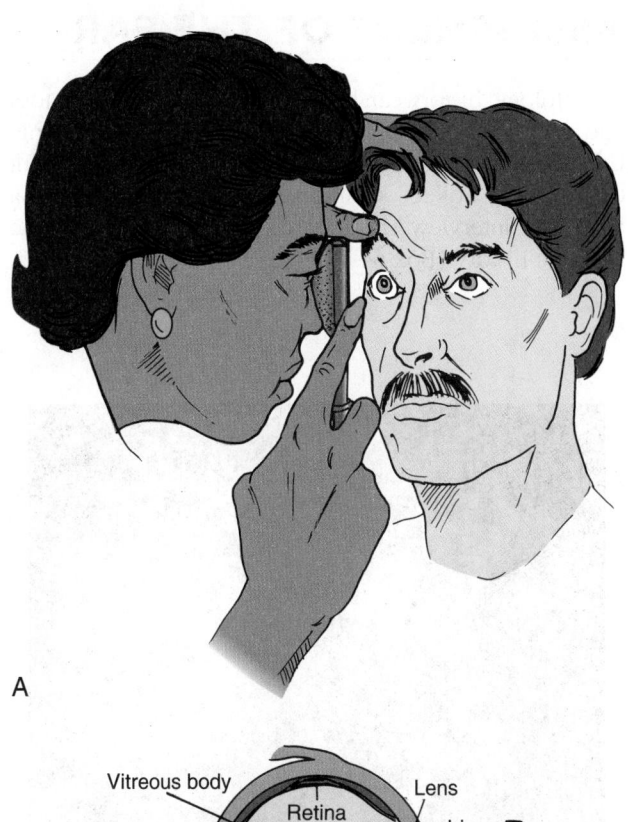

A

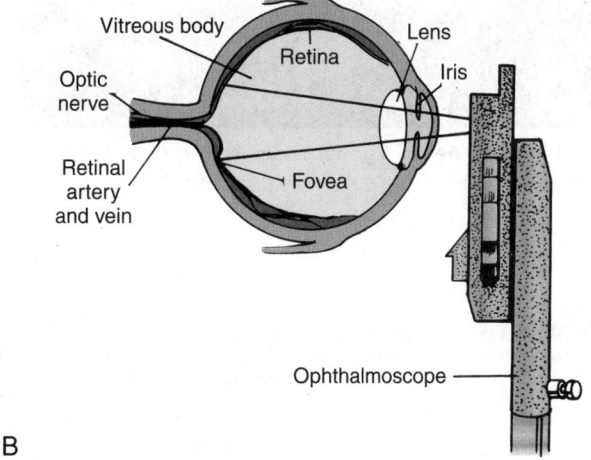

B

TABLE 64–4   Abnormal Physical Examination Findings of the External Eye

Eye Structure	Abnormal Findings
Eye position	Sunken or protruding eyes, such as protrusion of one eye or both eyes (exophthalmos)
Lids	Sagging of upper lids that covers part of pupil (ptosis)
	Eyelids that turn inward (entropion) or outward (ectropion)
	Lid eversion and inversion
Blink	Rapid, infrequent, or asymmetrical blinking
Eyeball	Asymmetrical, hard, or soft
Lacrimal apparatus	Swelling, edema, excessive moisture, and regurgitation of fluid
Conjunctiva	Paleness or a bright red color
Cornea	Surface irregularity and cloudiness (opacity)
Anterior chamber	Shallow or deep chambers (3 mm is normal) are abnormal
	Cloudy or nontransparent
Iris	Bulging or uneven coloring
Pupil	Light intolerance *(photophobia)*
	Irregular or unequal pupils
	Pupils that do not react to light or accommodation

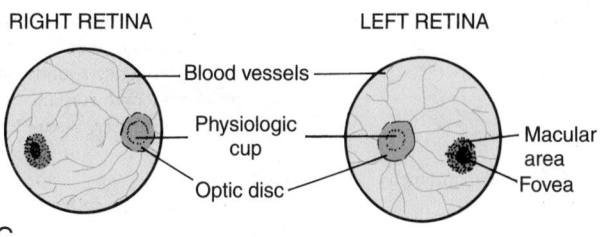

C

■ **FIGURE 64–3   A,** The examiner uses the right hand to hold the ophthalmoscope to the right eye to examine the client's right eye. The examiner uses the left hand when examining the client's left eye. Note the positioning of the examiner's free hand, which is placed to steady the client's head and to slightly retract the eyebrow. **B,** The examiner sees what appears in the angle of light through the viewing aperture. **C,** The actual area of retina visualized depends on the dilation of the pupil. Note the structures that may be examined.

ASSESSMENT OF THE EAR

The otologic history can be an important assessment tool and should be obtained before audiometric testing. Certain behavioral cues can indicate hearing impairment (Box 64-3). Collect significant data by conducting a thorough interview. Include the specific items in the otologic history (Box 64-4).

HISTORY

An otologic history includes demographic data, current clinical manifestations, past health history, family health history, psychosocial history, and review of systems. Ear problems often result from childhood illnesses or abnormalities associated with adjacent structures. The history interview is essential for determining current problems related to the ear.

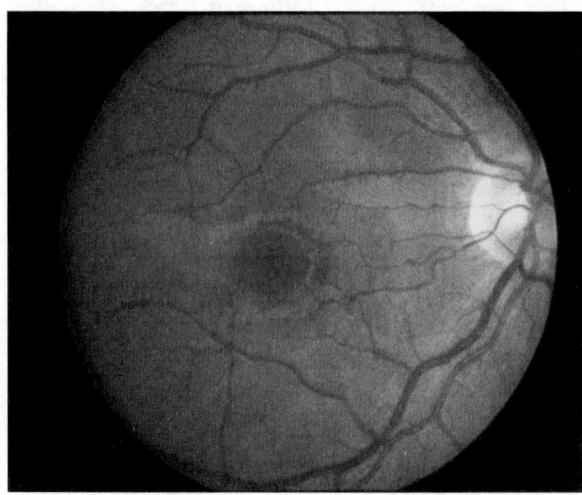

■ **FIGURE 64–4**   A normal fundus. (*Courtesy Ophthalmic Photography at the University of Michigan W.K. Kellogg Eye Center, Ann Arbor, Mich.*)

BOX 64-3   Clues Suggesting Hearing Impairment

Any adult who exhibits one or more of the following traits may be experiencing hearing impairment:

- Is irritable, hostile, hypersensitive in interpersonal relations
- Has difficulty hearing upper frequency consonants (such as "sl" or "sh")
- Complains about people mumbling
- Turns up volume on television
- Asks for frequent repetition and answers questions inappropriately
- Loses sense of humor, becomes grim
- Leans forward to hear better or turns head to preferred side
- Shuns large-group and small-group audience situations
- Shuns areas with increased background noise
- Might appear aloof and "stuck up"
- Complains of ringing in the ears
- Has an unusually soft or loud voice

TABLE 64–5 Diagnostic Tests for the Eye	
Test	**Description**
Fundus photography	Special retinal cameras are used to document fine details of the fundus for study and future comparison. Photographs are compared over time to identify subtle changes in disc shape and color (see Figure 64-4).
Exophthalmometry	Exophthalmometer is designed to measure forward protrusion of the eye. It provides a method of evaluation and record of progression/regression of the prominence.
Ophthalmic radiography	X-ray study, tomography, and computed tomography (CT) are useful in evaluation of orbital and intracranial conditions, as well as detection of foreign bodies.
Magnetic resonance imaging (MRI)	MRI allows multidimensional views to be obtained without repositioning client. MRI is used to image edema, areas of demyelination, and vascular lesions.
Ultrasonography (US)	US uses high-frequency sound waves transmitted through a probe placed directly on the eyeball. A-scan US measures axial length (distance from cornea to retina) to determine the refractive power of an intraocular lens in cataract surgery. B-scan US is used to evaluate lesions and their growth over time, or the presence of a foreign body.
Ophthalmodynamometry	Ophthalmodynamometry is a test that exerts pressure on the sclera with a spring plunger while the central retinal vessels emerging from the disc are observed. This instrument gives an approximate measurement of the relative pressures in the central retinal arteries and indirectly assesses carotid arterial flow on either side.
Electroretinography (ERG)	ERG measures the change in electrical potential of the eye caused by a diffuse flash of light through electrodes incorporated onto a contact lens that is placed directly on the eye.
Visual evoked response (VER)	VER is similar to ERG in that it also measures the electrical potential resulting from a visual stimulus. The entire visual pathway from the retina to the cortex can be evaluated through placement of electrodes on the scalp.
Fluorescein angiography (FA)	FA enhances fundus photography. The client receives an intravenous fluorescein dye injection, and the dye passes through the retinal and choroidal circulation, allowing those spaces to be visualized and photographed. A rapid sequence of photos captures perfusion of vessels and helps locate abnormalities, changes in flow, and hemorrhage.

BOX 64-4   Otologic History Assessment Guide

CURRENT PROBLEM

- What changes are you having in your hearing?
- Do you have any of the following manifestations?

Distortion of hearing	Yes	No
Differences in the pitch of sound	Yes	No
Noise in your ear	Yes	No
Fullness or pressure in your ear	Yes	No
Pain in your ear	Yes	No
Drainage from your ear	Yes	No

- Have you ever had a hearing examination?
  - If yes, why?
  - What were the results?

USE OF HEARING AIDS

Are you wearing hearing aids now?	Yes	No
Are your hearing aids effective?	Yes	No
How old are your hearing aids?	L _____ yr	R _____ yr

ASSOCIATED PROBLEMS

- Do you have any of the following manifestations?

Head noise or ringing	Yes	No
Feeling dizzy or unsteady	Yes	No
Blurred vision	Yes	No
Double vision	Yes	No
Numbness in the hands or feet	Yes	No
Weakness in the arms or legs	Yes	No
Tingling around the mouth or face	Yes	No
Loss of consciousness or blackouts	Yes	No
Fainting	Yes	No
Convulsions or seizures	Yes	No

RISK FACTORS

Have you ever worked around loud noises?	Yes	No
How long?	_____ yr	
Do you still work around loud noise?	Yes	No
Do you wear ear protection?	Yes	No

PAST HEALTH HISTORY

Did you have hearing problems as a child?	Yes	No
Did you have frequent ear infections as a child?	Yes	No
Did you ever have a perforation in your eardrum?	Yes	No
Did you ever get hit in the ear?	Yes	No
Have you had ear surgery?	Yes	No

- If yes,

	Date	Operation	Surgeon
Right ear	_____	_____	_____
Left ear	_____	_____	_____

- Do you have any food or medication allergies?
- Please list and describe your reaction.

FAMILY HISTORY

- Do you have family members who had difficulty hearing before 50 years of age?
  - If yes, explain.

- Have any members of your family ever had ear surgery?
  - If yes, explain.

Biographical and Demographic Data

Demographic data relevant to otologic assessment include the client's age. Hearing impairment may occur as a consequence of the aging process (Table 64-6).

Current Health

Hearing problems can affect a client's ability to communicate as well as limit their social activities and job opportunities. A reduction in their physical, functional, and social activities, attributable to ear problems or hearing loss, can interfere with the client's independence, which can lead to isolation and depression. Hearing loss can result in feelings of frustration, embarrassment, and loneliness. It is important to assess both verbal and nonverbal feedback and to listen attentively. The nurse's communication style is adapted to the client. The nurse should face the client as directly as possible when speaking, speak slowly, and enunciate distinctly. This individualized approach will assist with the development of trust between the nurse and client that will provide a valid database.

Chief Complaint

When discussing ear complaints, ask about common clinical manifestations of the ear (Figure 64-5). The client may also complain of associated nausea or vomiting. Complete an analysis of clinical manifestations to determine the onset, duration, frequency, and precipitating and relieving factors. Explore the client's past health history to determine the chronicity of the problem and the probable cause (see Box 64-4).

Clinical Manifestations

The most common clinical manifestations of ear disorders are pain, hearing loss, vertigo, tinnitus, drainage, and infection. Systemic manifestations will also be described.

Pain (Otalgia). Pain may be perceived as a feeling of fullness in the ear. It may be intensified by movement and relieved by holding the head still or by applying heat. Ear pain may occur as a result of related problems of the nose, sinuses, oral cavity, pharynx, or temporomandibular joint (TMJ). Pain may occur in and around the ear and it may be intense. Fever, headache, nausea,

and vomiting may also be present. The Integrating Diagnostic Testing feature on p. 1692 describes the evaluation of a client with ear pain.

Hearing Loss. Hearing loss may occur suddenly or gradually and can accompany the normal aging process. The loss may be conductive, a result of damage to the middle ear or otosclerosis; sensory neural, a result of disease of the inner ear, nerve pathways or a result of loss of hair cells; or related to a CNS disorder. Central hearing loss may be due to brain tumors and lesions of the auditory pathway in the central nervous system. The client may report an inability to hear certain words or sounds or that sounds are muffled.

Vertigo. Vertigo is a sensation of motion while the person is not moving. A client may feel that either he or she or the room is moving. Sudden movement of the head may precipitate vomiting. Vertigo may last for hours or all day. *Dizziness* is a sensation of unsteadiness and a feeling of movement within the head or lightheadedness.

Tinnitus. Tinnitus (ringing in the ears) may be reported as high-pitched or low-pitched, roaring, humming, hissing, or loud and persistent. Tinnitus may occur more commonly at certain times of the day and may involve one or both ears. This sensory neural form of auditory disorder occurs even in the absence of sound waves.

Ear Drainage (Otorrhea). Ear drainage can be bloody (sanguineous), clear (serous), mixed (serosanguineous), or it may contain pus (purulent). Drainage may also be accompanied by odor and pain.

Infection. Ear infections in infants can impair their ability to hear spoken words and impede the development of the auditory nerve used for hearing and speech. The assessment of an adult client should also include a careful review of frequent ear infections as a child.

Systemic Manifestations

Hearing is essential in interacting with the environment. The ear is a special sensory receptor that is connected to specific areas of the cerebral cortex through the afferent pathways of the central nervous system (CNS). Clinical manifestations of the disease and treatment of the

---

TABLE 64-6 Changes in Auditory Acuity Caused by Aging

Anatomic Changes	Physiologic Changes
Degeneration of basilar conductive membrane of cochlea	Decreased ability to hear at all frequencies, with higher frequencies being most affected
Degeneration of cochlear hair cells	Decreased ability to hear high-frequency sounds
Decreased vascularity of cochlea	Loss of hearing equal at all frequencies
Loss of auditory neurons in spiral ganglia of organ of Corti	Loss of ability to hear high-frequency sounds
Loss of cortical auditory neurons	Diminished hearing and speech comprehension

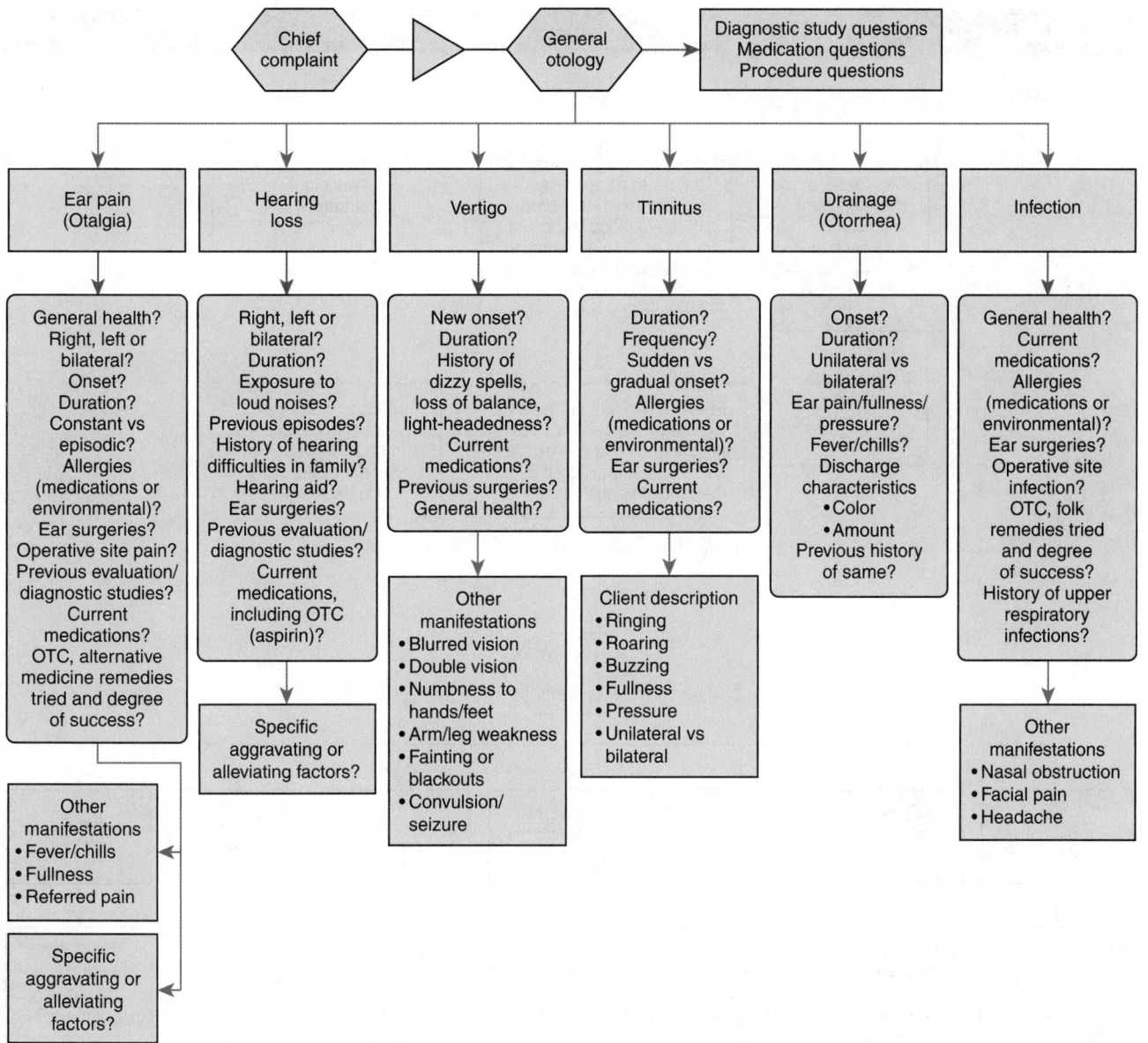

FIGURE 64–5 Expanded ear assessment.

underlying problem are important. Hearing loss, pain, infection, vertigo, tinnitus, and ear drainage are all principal manifestations attributed to the ears. Not all clients will present with the textbook common manifestations that are only related to the ears. Special consideration with emphasis on the nose, nasopharynx, and paranasal sinuses should also be included with the history and physical examination. Referred pain may also be from the teeth, tongue, tonsils, hypopharynx, larynx, salivary glands, and temporomandibular joint and should also be considered in the assessment.

Review of Systems
The past health history, family health history, and psychosocial history are integrated with the otologic history

assessment (Figure 64-6). The nurse conducts a review of systems to provide focus for the physical examination. The review of systems related to the ear includes gaining information about problems or concerns that the client reports. Focus areas include asking about the location, quality, quantity, timing, precipitating factors, and aggravating or relieving factors.

Past Medical History
Common childhood diseases involving the ears include the following: acute middle ear infections (otitis media); eardrum perforations resulting from otitis media; complications of ear infections such as chronic otitis media, frequent upper respiratory tract infections, and acute and chronic sinus infections.

INTEGRATING D I A G N O S T I C   T E S T I N G

Ear Pain

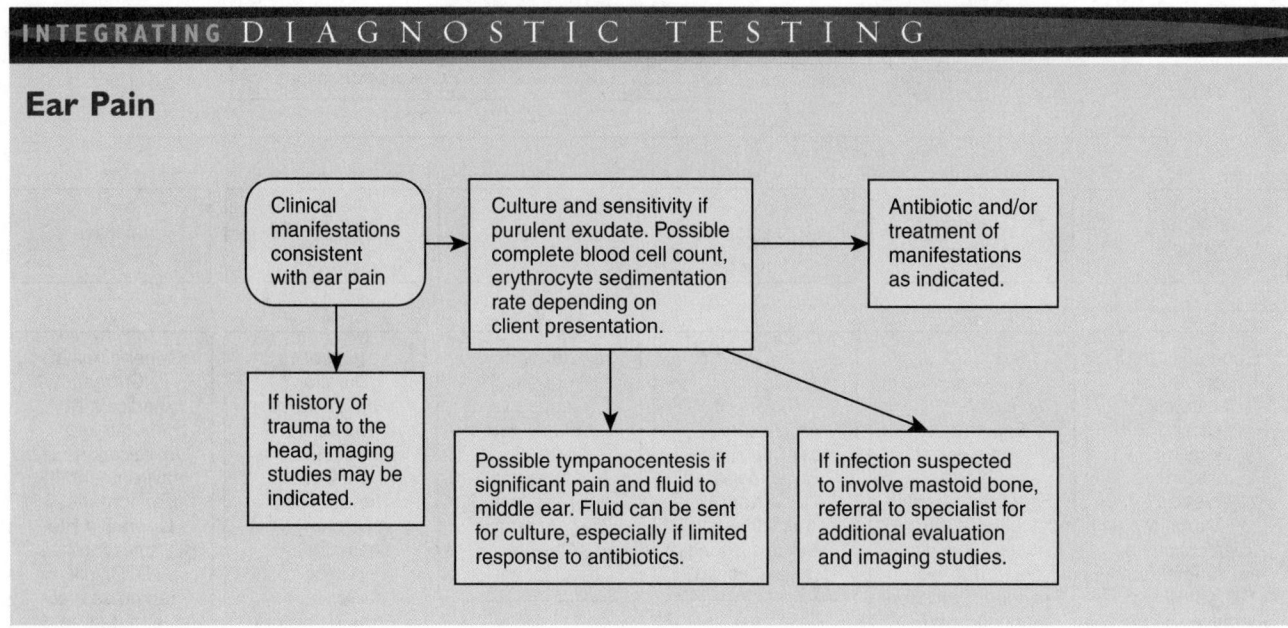

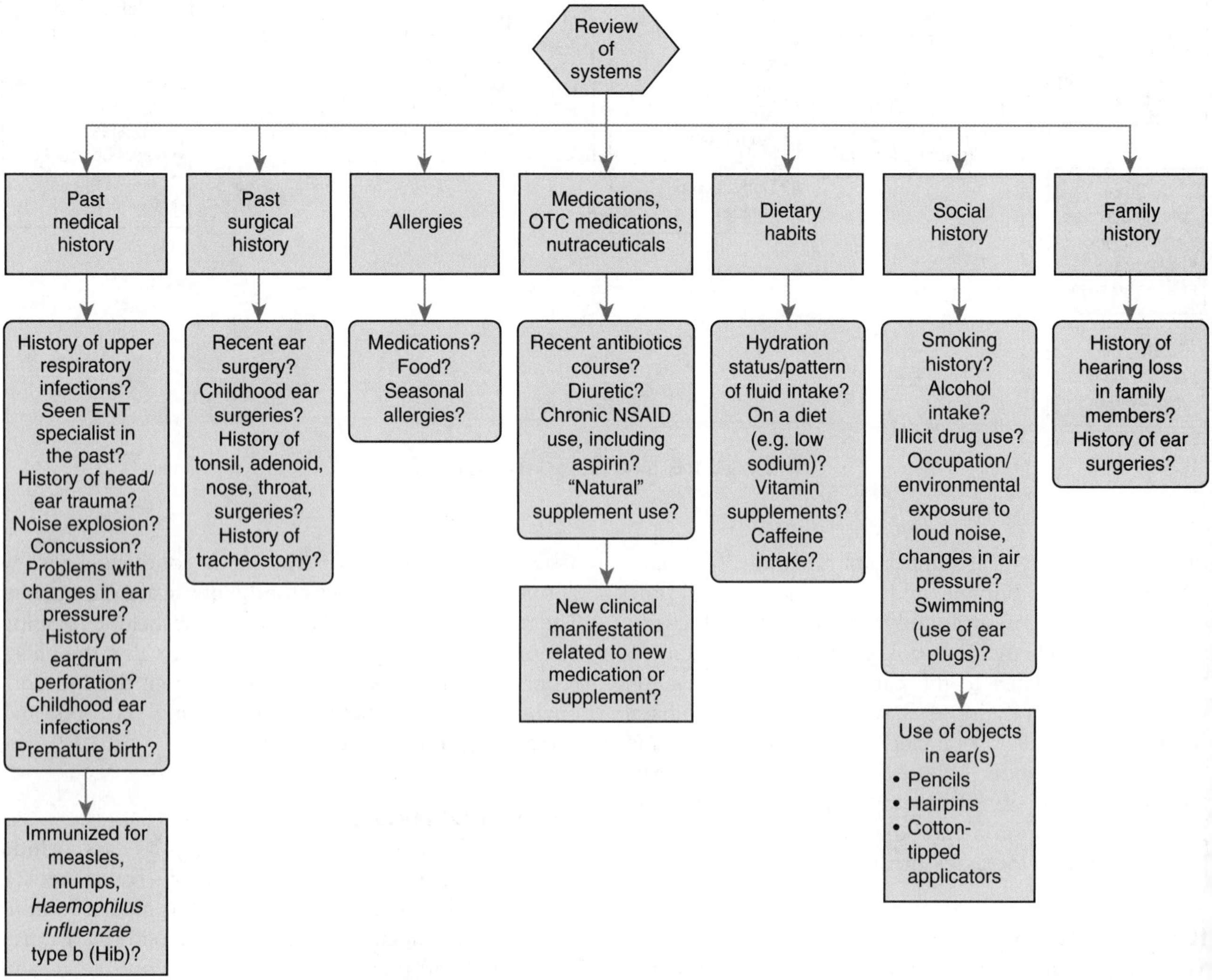

```
┌─────────────┐     ┌──────────────────────┐     ┌──────────────────┐
│ Clinical    │     │ Culture and          │     │ Antibiotic and/or│
│ manifesta-  │────▶│ sensitivity if       │────▶│ treatment of     │
│ tions       │     │ purulent exudate.    │     │ manifestations   │
│ consistent  │     │ Possible complete    │     │ as indicated.    │
│ with ear    │     │ blood cell count,    │     └──────────────────┘
│ pain        │     │ erythrocyte          │
└─────────────┘     │ sedimentation rate   │
       │            │ depending on client  │
       ▼            │ presentation.        │
┌─────────────┐     └──────────────────────┘
│ If history  │          │           │
│ of trauma   │          ▼           ▼
│ to the head,│   ┌──────────────┐ ┌──────────────┐
│ imaging     │   │ Possible     │ │ If infection │
│ studies may │   │ tympano-     │ │ suspected to │
│ be indicated│   │ centesis if  │ │ involve      │
└─────────────┘   │ significant  │ │ mastoid bone,│
                  │ pain and     │ │ referral to  │
                  │ fluid to     │ │ specialist   │
                  │ middle ear.  │ │ for          │
                  │ Fluid can be │ │ additional   │
                  │ sent for     │ │ evaluation   │
                  │ culture,     │ │ and imaging  │
                  │ especially   │ │ studies.     │
                  │ if limited   │ └──────────────┘
                  │ response to  │
                  │ antibiotics. │
                  └──────────────┘
```

```
                    ⬡ Review
                      of
                      systems ⬡
```

Past medical history	Past surgical history	Allergies	Medications, OTC medications, nutraceuticals	Dietary habits	Social history	Family history
History of upper respiratory infections? Seen ENT specialist in the past? History of head/ ear trauma? Noise explosion? Concussion? Problems with changes in ear pressure? History of eardrum perforation? Childhood ear infections? Premature birth?	Recent ear surgery? Childhood ear surgeries? History of tonsil, adenoid, nose, throat, surgeries? History of tracheostomy?	Medications? Food? Seasonal allergies?	Recent antibiotics course? Diuretic? Chronic NSAID use, including aspirin? "Natural" supplement use?	Hydration status/pattern of fluid intake? On a diet (e.g. low sodium)? Vitamin supplements? Caffeine intake?	Smoking history? Alcohol intake? Illicit drug use? Occupation/ environmental exposure to loud noise, changes in air pressure? Swimming (use of ear plugs)?	History of hearing loss in family members? History of ear surgeries?

Immunized for measles, mumps, *Haemophilus influenzae* type b (Hib)?

New clinical manifestation related to new medication or supplement?

Use of objects in ear(s)
• Pencils
• Hairpins
• Cotton-tipped applicators

■ **FIGURE 64–6** Expanded ear history.

Infectious diseases with ear sequelae include mumps, measles, and meningitis. Specifically inquire whether the client has been immunized for mumps, measles, and *Haemophilus influenzae* type b (Hib). In utero exposure to maternal influenza or rubella may result in congenital hearing loss in the child. Premature birth is also associated with hearing problems.

Inquire about a history of upper respiratory tract infections. Has the client had tonsil, adenoid, or other nose or throat surgery? Has the client ever consulted an ear specialist? Has the client suffered trauma to the head or ear, such as a severe blow or sustained loud noise exposure or concussion from sudden changes in air pressure (such as may occur in an explosion)? Does the history include chronic eardrum perforation?

Surgical History

A thorough surgical history is vital to the assessment of ear complaints. If the client has a history of ear diagnoses, inquire about any surgical procedures that may have been performed. This may include a mastoidectomy, tympanoplasty, stapedectomy, or a labyrinthectomy. Whenever possible, the date and the precise procedure should be documented, as there are various methods for performing a specific procedure, such as a myringoplasty for repair of perforation of the eardrum.

Allergies

In addition to asking about allergies to medications and other substances, inquire about allergies resulting in nasal stuffiness and congestion. Close proximity of the eustachian tubes to the nasal mucosa may result in edema, which obstructs the flow of air between the middle ear and nose so that air pressure cannot be equalized.

Medications

Obtain a complete medication history for prescription and over-the-counter drugs and herbal remedies. Determine the medication or supplement, and establish the dose, route, recent dosage changes, and length of time taken to ascertain if there is any relationship to the onset of the chief complaint.

Certain medications can damage the vestibulocochlear nerve (eighth cranial nerve), with resultant hearing loss, tinnitus, or disturbances in equilibrium. Aspirin is a common cause of tinnitus. Other drugs include aminoglycosides, analgesics, salicylates, quinine, chemotherapeutic agents, and antiprotozoal agents (Box 64-5).

Review the use of herbal remedies. Ginger *(Zingiber officinale)* is known for its antinausea effect and can be used for the relief of motion sickness. *Ginkgo biloba* has been used for tinnitus and vertigo.

Dietary Habits

Nutritional factors that describe the client's food and fluid consumption in relationship to the body's metabolic needs are important to assess. Adequacy of nutrient supply to local tissues should be considered. Inquire about dietary restrictions, use of food supplements (e.g., vitamins), ability to swallow and chew, and a history of any feeding problems. Ménière's disease may present with attacks of vertigo and tinnitus. Recent findings have indicated the use of a low-salt diet may be involved with the initial treatment of the disease.

Psychosocial History

Psychosocial and lifestyle factors that influence the incidence of hearing impairment include occupational hazards, environmental exposure, and leisure activities and hobbies. Leisure activities should include questions

---

BOX 64-5 Selected Ototoxic* Drugs

AMINOGLYCOSIDE ANTIBIOTICS
- Streptomycin
- Neomycin
- Gentamicin
- Tobramycin
- Amikacin
- Kanamycin
- Netilmicin

OTHER ANTIBIOTICS
- Vancomycin
- Viomycin
- Polymyxin B
- Polymyxin E
- Erythromycin
- Capreomycin
- Chloramphenicol
- Minocycline

OTHER DRUGS
- Chemotherapeutic agents (bleomycin, cisplatin, nitrogen mustard)
- Salicylates
- Quinine drugs
- Quinidine
- Chloroquine

DIURETICS
- Furosemide
- Ethacrynic acid
- Acetazolamide
- Bumetanide
- Mannitol

CHEMICALS
- Metals (lead, mercury, gold, arsenic)
- Alcohol
- Aniline dyes
- Caffeine
- Carbon monoxide
- Nicotine
- Potassium bromate
- Povidone-iodine

*Substances toxic to the ear.

about swimming. Contaminated water can provoke an external ear infection and, if the tympanic membrane is perforated, may lead to infection in the middle ear. Also, explore the client's ear hygiene habits to see if objects are used or inserted into the ear canal. Inserting objects into the ear canal to clean the ear may traumatize the ear canal and damage or perforate the tympanic membrane.

Ask about exposure to loud noises (Table 64-7), including the type, frequency, and duration. Sound intensity is measured in units known as *decibels (dB)*. Ordinary speech level measures about 50 dB; heavy traffic is about 70 dB; at above 80 dB noise becomes uncomfortable to the human ear. Exposure to levels greater than 85 to 90 dB for months or years causes cochlear damage.

Family Health History
Ask about a history of hearing loss or ear surgery among family members. Determine the age at onset for hearing loss or changes in hearing acuity.

PHYSICAL EXAMINATION

Physical examination of the ear includes assessment of hearing acuity, balance, and equilibrium. Because the external ear is completely visible, it is easy to identify anatomic landmarks and to assess abnormalities. Most of the middle ear and the entire inner ear, however, are inaccessible to direct examination; testing of auditory and vestibular function should be completed to help assess these structures. Refer to the Physical Assessment Findings in the Healthy Adult feature at right.

Inspection and Palpation
External Ear
Inflammation and infection are the most frequent conditions of the external ear seen by the nurse. In assessing the external ear, manipulation of the ear is important. Care must be exercised not to cause unnecessary pain.

Gross examination of both ears should precede individual examination of either ear. Use inspection and palpation to assess the external ear. Note the size, configuration, and angle of attachment to the head. Observe the configuration of the pinna for gross deformity. Note whether the ears protrude and, if so, the degree of protrusion; note the color of the skin of the ears; and determine whether additional skin tags are present. The skin of the ear should be smooth and without breaks or inflammation, especially in the crevice behind the ear. Note any lumps, skin lesions, or cysts, and record approximate size and location.

Perform palpation and manipulation of the pinna to detect tenderness, nodules, or *tophi* (small, hard nodules in the helix that are deposits of uric acid crystals characteristic of gout). During palpation, move the pinna, feel

---

Physical Assessment Findings in the Healthy Adult

The Ear

INSPECTION
Auricles symmetrical, superior portion level with outer canthus of eye. Outer canals clear. Preauricular and postauricular areas without swelling, masses, or lesions. AC > BC, bilaterally. No lateralization. Whisper heard at 3 feet.

PALPATION
Tenderness over tragus and mastoid absent. No masses.

OTOSCOPIC EXAMINATION
Soft cerumen present in canals. No discharge. TMs intact, gray. Cone of light at 4:00 in right ear and at 7:00 in left ear. Landmarks visualized. No retraction or bulging. TM freely movable with pneumatic pressure.

AC, Air conduction; *BC,* bone conduction; *TM,* tympanic membrane.

TABLE 64–7 Decibel (dB) Ratings and Hazardous Time Exposure of Common Noises

Typical Level* (dB)	Example	Dangerous Time Exposure
0	Lowest sound audible to human ear	
30	Quiet library, soft whisper	
40	Quiet office, living room, bedroom away from traffic	
50	Light traffic at a distance, refrigerator, gentle breeze	
60	Air conditioner at 20 ft, conversation, sewing machine	
70	Busy traffic, noisy restaurant (constant exposure)	Critical level begins
80	Subway, heavy city traffic, alarm clock at 2 ft, factory noise	More than 8 hr
90	Truck traffic, noisy home appliances, shop tools, lawnmower	Less than 8 hr
100	Chain saw, boiler shop, pneumatic drill	2 hr
120	Rock concert in front of speakers, sandblasting, thunderclap	Immediate danger
140	Gunshot blast, jet plane	Any length of exposure time is dangerous
180	Rocket launching pad	Hearing loss is inevitable

* Sound levels refer to intensity experienced at typical working distances. Intensity drops 6 dB with every doubling of distance from noise source.
Courtesy American Academy of Otolaryngology—Head and Neck Surgery, Washington, DC.

the mastoid area, and press on the tragus, noting any pain or discomfort, which may indicate inflammation or infection (see the Physical Assessment Findings in the Healthy Adult feature, p. 1694).

Ear Canal

Direct Observation. Inspection of the ear canal is carried out by direct observation, otoscopy, or microscopic examination. The extent and depth of the otology examination are determined by the nurse's skill level, training, and the health care setting. A basic understanding of the anatomy and physiology of the ear, and additional training by a health care professional, are required for the nurse to appreciate the wide range of normal findings. A physical examination text provides detailed instructions to perform direct observation of the ear canal.

Otoscopy. The eardrum is located at the end of the only skin-lined canal in the body. Proper visualization requires illumination and magnification for accurate assessment. An otoscope is portable, and otoscopic examination is the most commonly used method. An otoscope is a device (see the otoscope figure on the website and see Figure 64-7) that consists of a handle, a light source, a magnifying lens, and an attachment for visualizing the ear canal and eardrum. A pneumatic device attached to the otoscope is used for injecting air into the ear canal to test the mobility and integrity of the eardrum. Figure 64-8 shows a normal right eardrum.

Tests for Auditory Acuity

Assessment of the middle and inner ear for hearing is accomplished by sophisticated methods of indirect testing (audiometry and vestibular testing). A gross assessment of hearing can be made simply through conversation, by evaluating the logical sequence of replies, and the appropriateness of the responses. Gross assessments can be made at the bedside or in the office.

Test each ear separately to estimate hearing ability. Begin by occluding one of the client's ears with a finger. Then, standing 1 foot away, whisper two-syllable numbers softly toward the unoccluded ear and ask the client to repeat the numbers. Increase the intensity of your voice from a soft, medium, or loud whisper to a soft, medium, or loud voice. If you suspect that the client is lip-reading, turn the client's face to one side. Ask the client whether hearing is better in one ear than in the other ear. If auditory acuity between the two ears is different, test the ear that hears better first. Next produce noise in the better-hearing ear by rapidly but gently moving the finger in the client's ear canal while the other ear is tested.

Although the ticking of a watch can also be used to test hearing, it produces a higher-pitched sound, which is less relevant to functional hearing compared with the voice test.

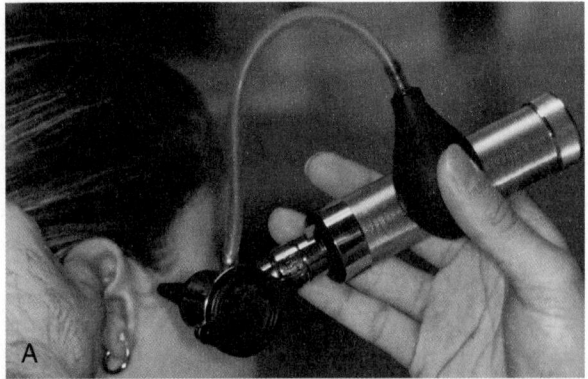
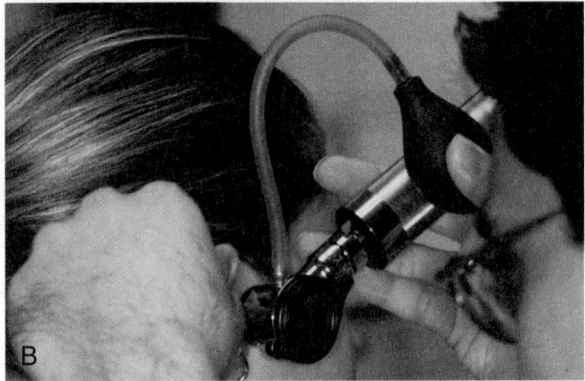

■ **FIGURE 64–7** Use of the otoscope. **A,** Hold the otoscope handle between the thumb and fingers. Pull the pinna backward and upward in the adult to straighten the auditory canal. **B,** Carefully insert the speculum into the ear canal while allowing the back of the fingers that hold the otoscope handle to rest against the client's head. If a pneumatic bulb attachment will be used, position the bulb between thumb and otoscope handle to facilitate compression of the pneumatic bulb.

The tuning fork also provides a general estimate of hearing loss. A frequency of 512 Hz is recommended. The two major tuning fork tests date from the 19th century and are named after their originators: Weber and Rinne (see Table 64-8 and the figure of Weber and Rinne tests on the website).

Tests for Vestibular Acuity

Romberg Test. Assess the inner ear for balance by performing a Romberg test. The client stands with the

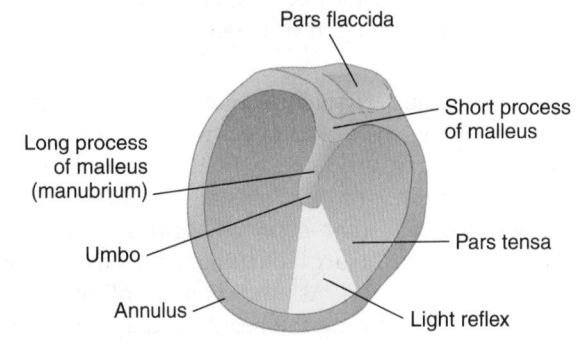

■ **FIGURE 64–8** Normal right eardrum (tympanic membrane).

TABLE 64–8 Auditory Acuity Tests

Auditory Acuity Test	Purpose	Procedure	Interpretation
Weber	To assess conduction of sound through bone	Strike tuning fork on hand	Normal: sound is heard equally in both ears by bone conduction
		Place rounded tip of handle on center of client's forehead or nasal bone	Sensorineural (nerve) hearing loss: sound is heard in unaffected ear
		Placement on teeth, even false teeth, is reliable	Conductive (air conduction) hearing loss: sound is heard better in affected ear
		Ask if client can hear the tone in the center of the head, right ear, or left ear	
Rinne	Compares air conduction to bone conduction to help differentiate conductive from sensorineural hearing loss	Shift tuning fork between 2 positions: first against the mastoid bone (bone conduction) and second 2 inches from opening of ear canal (air conduction)	Normal: sound is heard twice as long or as loud by air conduction than by bone conduction
		Move tuning fork when client can no longer hear sound by bone conduction	Normal hearing: air conduction is greater than bone conduction = positive test
		Ask client to indicate if tone is louder in front or behind the ear	Conductive hearing loss: bone conduction sounds louder or longer than air conduction sound = negative test
		Ask client to state when tone is no longer heard by air conduction	Sensorineural hearing loss: client hears better by air conduction = positive test

feet together, arms by the sides, and eyes closed. Note the ability to maintain an upright posture with only a minimal amount of sway. Stand close to the client to offer balance support if it is needed. If the client loses his or her balance, this is a positive Romberg sign, suggesting a vestibular ear problem or cerebellar ataxia.

A *tandem* Romberg test should also be performed. Instruct the client to walk forward and backward, heel to toe. A peripheral vestibular lesion can cause marked swaying or falling. A client without pathologic vestibular change can usually maintain balance, depending on his or her age.

A *past-pointing test* can also indicate a labyrinthine disorder. While the client is seated, facing you with eyes open, hold out your index finger at the client's shoulder level. Instruct the client to touch your finger with the right index finger. Ask the client to lower the arm, close the eyes, and touch your finger again. Repeat the procedure, testing the client's left index finger. Observe and record the presence or absence as well as the degree and direction, of past-pointing. A labyrinthine disorder can lead to past-pointing when the eyes are closed. Cerebral lesions are indicated when past-pointing occurs whether the eyes are open or closed.

Test for Nystagmus. Nystagmus is involuntary, rhythmic oscillation of the eyes associated with vestibular dysfunction. Nystagmus occurs normally when a client watches a rapidly moving object or looks beyond 30 degrees laterally *(end-point nystagmus)*. To assess for *gaze nystagmus,* place your finger directly in front of the client at eye level. Ask the client to follow (track) the finger without moving the head. Starting at the midline, slowly move your finger toward the client's right

ear and then the left ear, but not more than 30 degrees laterally, superiorly, or inferiorly. Observe the client's eyes for any jerking movements. For example, if the eyes jerk quickly to the left, and drift slowly back to the right, the client has left spontaneous *(horizontal)* nystagmus. Nystagmus is named for the direction of the fast phase. Nystagmus can be horizontal, vertical, or rotary.

DIAGNOSTIC TESTING

Noninvasive Tests
Tests for Aural Structure
The temporal bone and its structures can be examined easily by radiography (x-ray study). The oldest, but not necessarily most useful, study is x-ray examination of the mastoid bone. Radiographic techniques have largely been replaced by imaging studies, such as CT and MRI.

Computed Tomography
Computed tomography without contrast medium is the most commonly ordered CT scan for imaging of the temporal bone. Contrast is not generally needed because most bony structures are seen well. Contrast may be used to delineate vascular or soft tissue structures.

Magnetic Resonance Imaging
Magnetic resonance imaging reveals membranous organs as well as nerves and blood vessels of the temporal bone. MRI is the test of choice for tumors of the temporal bone. Contrast can be used for enhancement. For certain diagnostic assessments, both MRI and CT scans are obtained.

Invasive Tests
Arteriography

Arteriography is used to assess vascular abnormalities in the temporal bone.

Tests for Auditory Function
Audiometric Tests

Audiology may be broadly called the science of hearing. Audiometric tests are performed to measure hearing and comprehension. A hearing test is performed in a sound-proof booth by an *audiologist*. An *audiometer* is an electronic instrument used to test hearing by producing sounds of varying pure-tone frequencies. The client is asked to signal the audiologist by raising a hand or pressing a button when a tone is heard; the responses are plotted on a graph called an *audiogram*. Earphones are used for the audiogram.

Normal hearing is a range established nationally by testing the hearing levels of people of all ages. A client with normal hearing ability has 80% or more hearing, depending on the client's age.

Some audiometric tests are performed by computer-assisted instruments. The objective of these special tests is to reveal whether a disorder is in the cochlea, acoustic nerve, or brain stem (see Table 64-9).

Tests for Vestibular Function
Electronystagmography

The vestibular system can be tested by electrophysiologic means. Although the physical assessment of balance is important, the most common objective measurement of balance is accomplished by electronystagmography (ENG). The ENG instrument was developed to measure nystagmus (involuntary, rapid eye movement) in response to stimulation of the vestibular system. This stimulation includes testing the client at rest in different positions for both the eyes and the head and with different temperatures of air or water in the ear canals, thus stimulating the semicircular canals. The different test results give a recording (electronystagmogram) that reflects the status of each labyrinth and can indicate CNS disorders.

Platform Posturography

Platform posturography is another balance test that helps to identify, quantify, and localize the source of balance disorders. The client stands in a tall box-like device

---

TABLE 64–9 **Auditory Function Tests**

Tests for Auditory Function	Purpose	Procedure	Interpretation
Audiography	Components of hearing are tested through air conduction, bone conduction, and speech	Air conduction: tones presented through earphones Bone conduction: tones presented through bone conduction oscillator placed behind ear on mastoid bone	Difference between air and bone conduction signifies conductive hearing loss; if air and bone conduction are the same, either normal hearing or sensorineural (nerve) hearing loss exists
Tympanometry	Differentiates problems in middle ear Measures compliance (mobility) and impedance (opposition to movement) of tympanic membrane and ossicles of middle ear Also used to measure stapedius muscle reflex and its decay Also indicates function of acoustic nerve	Positive, normal, and negative air pressure is applied into external meatus and measures resultant sound energy flow; then traced on graph (tympanogram)	Abnormalities reveal dysfunction of middle ear, eustachian tube, and ossicles
Brain stem response	Assessment of auditory nervous system	Determined by presenting sound to ear and measuring response (computer averaging) in brain stem	Examiner obtains specific diagnostic information; imaging tests of the head are usually ordered to confirm abnormality
Electrocochleography	Measures response of cochlea and eighth cranial nerve to acoustic stimulation	Electrodes are placed through tympanic membrane onto promontory near round window or in ear canal, and acoustic stimulation is applied	Evaluates presence of Ménière's disease or perilymphatic fistula
Otoacoustic emissions (OAEs)	Low-level sounds produced by cochlea are involved in modulation of hearing mechanism	Can be measured quickly and are generally easier to obtain than test, especially in uncooperative and crying infants	Evoked OAEs can be observed in nearly all normal-hearing people; therefore serve as a useful screen for hearing acuity

while the floor moves. No visual cues are provided, and the response to correcting balance is recorded. Most people correct posture changes with adjustments in muscles (of the feet and ankles).

SAFETY ⚠ ALERT **The client is strapped in for safety in case he or she loses balance.**

This test can help to isolate the etiologic basis of balance disorders as vestibular, visual, or proprioceptive.

Rotary Chair Assessment

Rotary chair or harmonic acceleration can also be used. Rotation of the client in a chair in darkness provides information about vestibular dysfunction and the level of central compensation.

Laboratory Tests
Blood Tests

Blood tests that are diagnostic for systemic abnormalities are only secondarily significant for ear disease. For example, an elevated white blood cell (WBC) count suggests an infection but is not diagnostic of ear disease. In the presence of clinical manifestations of ear infection, and in the absence of other manifestations of infection, however, an elevated WBC count does suggest acute ear infection. Other blood tests are useful for diagnosis of autoimmune diseases and other systemic illnesses that can affect hearing and balance.

Cultures

Drainage samples from the ear canal are sometimes obtained for culture to identify an infecting organism. When long-term drainage is present, such as in chronic otitis media, cultures are more helpful because multiple pathogenic organisms can be present.

Tests for the Presence of Cerebrospinal Fluid

Clear drainage found in the ear presents a dilemma. Is this cerebrospinal fluid (CSF) or serous drainage? A fistula from the inner ear to the middle ear can drain CSF. This pathway can also lead to meningitis by retrograde contamination. Therefore an analysis of clear fluid drainage from the ear or nose is often helpful in the diagnosis.

Tissue Specimens

Biopsy specimens of abnormal tissue from the ear canal or from other tissue harvested during surgery are necessary to rule out a malignancy and to identify unusual problems. In an infected ear, abnormal tissue is readily identified by visual assessment.

CONCLUSIONS

Understanding the complexity of ocular structures and the physiology of vision is essential to providing comprehensive nursing care for clients with ocular disorders.

Hearing and balance are vital to a person's safety and independence. Understanding the physiology of hearing and balance is essential to providing comprehensive nursing care for clients with ear disorders.

Ophthalmic and otolaryngology registered nurses perform the roles of educator, technician, counselor, and coordinator in the diagnostic setting.

BIBLIOGRAPHY

🪔 Citations appearing in red refer to primary research.

🪔 Citations appearing in blue refer to evidence-based practice guidelines and protocols.

1. Eagle, R. (1999). *Eye pathology: An atlas and basic text.* Philadelphia: Saunders.
1a. Eskola, J., et al. (2001). Efficacy of a pneumococcal conjugate vaccine against acute otitis media. *New England Journal of Medicine, 344*(6), 403-409.
2. Folmer, R., Martin, W., & Shi, Y. (2004). Tinnitus: Questions to reveal the cause, answers to provide relief. *Journal of Family Practice, 53*(7), 532-540.
3. Goldblum, K. (Ed.) (2002). *Ophthalmic nursing core curriculum.* Dubuque, Iowa: Kendall.
4. Harris, L.L., & Huntoon, M.B. (Eds.) (1998). *Core curriculum for otorhinolaryngology and head-neck nursing.* New Smyrna Beach, Fla: Society of Otorhinolaryngology and Head-Neck Nurses.
5. Henry, J., Dennis, K., & Schechter, M. (2005). General review of tinnitus: Prevalence, mechanisms, effects, and management. *Journal of Speech, Language, and Hearing Research, 48*(5), 1204-1235.
6. Jarvis, C. (2004). *Physical examination and health assessment* (4th ed.). Philadelphia: Saunders.
7. Kanski, J. (2003). *Clinical ophthalmology* (5th ed.). Oxford: Butterworth Heinemann.
8. Rados, C. (2005). Sound advice about age-related hearing loss. *FDA Consumer, 39*(3), 20-27.
9. Scudder, S., et al. (2003). Predictive validity and reliability of adult hearing screening techniques. *Journal of the American Academy of Audiology, 14*(1), 9-19.
10. Vaughan, D., Asbury, T., & Riordan-Eva, P. (1999). *General ophthalmology* (15th ed.). Norwalk, Conn: Appleton & Lange.
11. Wilson, S., Giddens, J., & Thompson, J. (2004). *Health assessment for nursing practice* (3rd ed.). St. Louis: Mosby.
12. Woodson, G. (2001). *Ear, nose and throat disorders in primary care.* Philadelphia: Saunders.

evolve *Did you remember to check out the bonus material on the Evolve website and the CD-ROM, including NCLEX®-Examination Style Review Questions, Open-Book Quizzes, and Chapter Review Audio Podcasts?*

http://evolve.elsevier.com/Black/medsurg

CHAPTER 65

Management of Clients with Visual Disorders

SARAH C. SMITH

The role that vision plays in our lives is difficult to define because it is so deeply personal and intimate. It is the connection between the mind and the body and the rest of the world. The visual pathway is a multidimensional system with many structures and processes subject to trauma or disorders. When there is a failure of any part along the visual pathway, the result is loss of vision.

Loss of vision is closely associated with loss of independence. Even simple tasks become difficult to perform without assistance. Seeing what food is being served at the table; selecting clothes for color and design; avoiding objects while walking; and reading books, magazines, or personal mail are no longer possible. The visually impaired person must adapt to this loss to maintain control in the daily affairs of life.

The nursing diagnosis *Disturbed Sensory Perception (Visual)* is commonly identified for clients with visual problems or impairment. Nursing interventions focus on providing a safe environment and education for self-care. The most important assessment you can make, however, is to address your client's grieving process. Visual impairment is more than a physiologic deficit. It is a loss that has physical, emotional, and spiritual effects on the person afflicted. Even minor changes in vision can provoke feelings of anger and frustration in people who must rely on clear and sharp vision in their work (e.g., airline pilots, artists, photographers, architects). Permanent and profound loss of vision can result in morbid grieving in which an individual is unable to cope with or adapt to life changes.

Surveys have shown that most people are more afraid of going blind than dying of cancer. Although we have made some improvements in the way our society views and provides for people who are physically challenged, blind people are frequently regarded with pity. Loss of vision is a threat to a person's independence, self-esteem, and self-control.

GLAUCOMA

Glaucoma comprises a group of ocular disorders characterized by increased intraocular pressure, optic nerve atrophy, and visual field loss. It is estimated that more than 80,000 people in the United States are blind as a result of glaucoma. The incidence of glaucoma is about 1.5%, and in blacks between ages 45 and 65 years, the prevalence is at least five times that of whites in the same age group. In most cases blindness can be prevented if treatment is begun early.

Classification

Many terms are used to describe the various types of glaucoma:

- *Primary* and *secondary glaucoma* refer to whether the cause is the disease alone or another condition.
- *Acute* and *chronic* refer to the onset and duration of the disorder.
- *Open* (wide) and *closed* (narrow) describe the width of the angle between the cornea and the iris (Figure 65-1, *A*). Anatomically narrow anterior-chamber angles predispose people to an acute onset of *angle-closure glaucoma*.

Primary Open-Angle Glaucoma

Primary open-angle glaucoma, the most common form, is a multifactorial disorder that is often genetically

---

evolve **Web Enhancements**

Client Education Guide   Care After Cataract Removal (Spanish Translation)

Be sure to check out the bonus material on the Evolve website and the CD-ROM, including free self-assessment exercises. **http://evolve.elsevier. com/Black/medsurg**

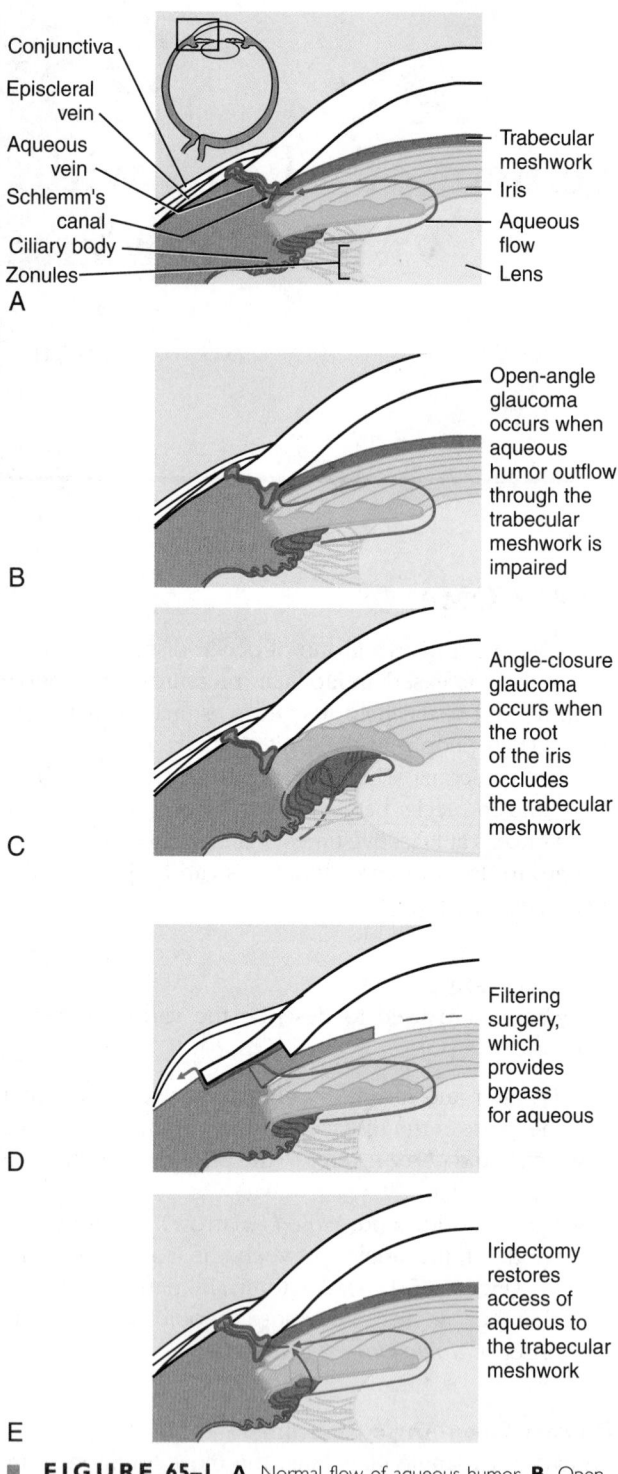

Conjunctiva
Episcleral vein
Aqueous vein
Schlemm's canal
Ciliary body
Zonules

A

Trabecular meshwork
Iris
Aqueous flow
Lens

B

Open-angle glaucoma occurs when aqueous humor outflow through the trabecular meshwork is impaired

C

Angle-closure glaucoma occurs when the root of the iris occludes the trabecular meshwork

D

Filtering surgery, which provides bypass for aqueous

E

Iridectomy restores access of aqueous to the trabecular meshwork

■ **FIGURE 65–1** **A,** Normal flow of aqueous humor. **B,** Open-angle glaucoma occurs when aqueous humor outflow is impaired by the trabecular meshwork. **C,** Angle-closure glaucoma occurs when the root of the iris occludes the trabecular meshwork. Filtering surgery (**D**) and iridectomy (**E**) restore the flow of aqueous humor through the trabecular meshwork.

determined, bilateral, insidious in onset, and slow to progress. This type of glaucoma is often referred to as the "thief in the night" because no early clinical manifestations are present to alert the client that vision is

being lost. Aqueous humor flow is slowed or stopped because of obstruction by the trabecular meshwork (see Figure 65-1, *B*).

Angle-Closure Glaucoma

An acute attack of angle-closure glaucoma can develop only in an eye in which the anterior chamber angle is anatomically narrow. The attack occurs because of a sudden blockage of the anterior angle by the base of the iris (see Figure 65-1, *C*).

Other Forms of Glaucoma

Normal-tension glaucoma resembles primary open-angle glaucoma. In this type of glaucoma, the optic nerve is damaged even though intraocular pressure (IOP) is not high. *Secondary glaucoma* may occur as a result of trauma that can disrupt the flow pattern of aqueous humor.

Etiology and Risk Factors

About 90% of primary glaucoma occurs in people with open angles. Because there are no early warning clinical manifestations, it is imperative that regular ophthalmic examinations include tonometry and assessment of the optic nerve head (disc). The most common cause of chronic open-angle glaucoma is degenerative change in the trabecular meshwork, resulting in decreased outflow of aqueous humor. Hypertension, cardiovascular disease, diabetes, and obesity are associated with the development of glaucoma. Increased IOP also results from *uveitis* (inflammation of filtering structures). Encroachment by a rapidly growing tumor and chronic use of topical corticosteroids may also produce manifestations of open-angle glaucoma. Neither the causes of *low-tension glaucoma* nor the reasons optic nerves are damaged even though the IOP is "normal" (i.e., between 12 and 22 mm Hg) are known. People at higher risk for this form of low-tension glaucoma are those with a family history of normal-tension glaucoma, people of Japanese ancestry, and people with a history of systemic heart disease, such as irregular heart rhythm.

Secondary glaucoma develops from edema, eye injury (*hyphema*), inflammation, tumor, or advanced cases of cataract or diabetes. Edematous tissue may inhibit the outflow of aqueous humor through the trabecular meshwork. Delayed healing of corneal wound edges may result in epithelial cell growth into the anterior chamber.

Pathophysiology

Intraocular pressure is determined by the rate of aqueous humor production in the ciliary body and the resistance to outflow of aqueous humor from the eye. IOP varies with diurnal cycles (the highest pressure is usually on awakening) and body position (increased when lying down). Normal variations do not usually exceed 2 to 3 mm Hg. IOP and blood pressures are independent of each other, but variations in systemic blood pressure may be associated with corresponding variations in IOP. Increased IOP may result from hyperproduction of aqueous humor or obstruction of outflow. As aqueous fluid accumulates in the eye, the increased pressure inhibits blood supply to the optic nerve and the retina. These delicate tissues become ischemic and gradually lose function.

Clinical Manifestations

Acute angle-closure glaucoma causes severe pain and blurred vision or vision loss. Some clients see rainbow halos around lights, and some experience nausea and vomiting. Secondary glaucoma has the same clinical manifestations as acute angle-closure glaucoma. Visual field defects are the result of the loss of blood supply to areas in the retina. The individual response to IOP varies; some clients sustain damage from relatively low pressures, whereas others sustain no damage from high pressure.

An ophthalmoscopic examination shows *atrophy* (pale color) and *cupping* (indentation) of the optic nerve head. The visual field examination is used to determine the extent of peripheral vision loss (see visual fields in Chapter 64). In chronic open-angle glaucoma, a small crescent-shaped *scotoma* (blind spot) appears early in the disease. In acute angle-closure glaucoma, the fields demonstrate larger areas of significant loss of vision.

In clients with angle-closure glaucoma, a slit-lamp examination may demonstrate an erythematous conjunctiva and corneal cloudiness. The aqueous humor in the anterior chamber may also appear *turbid* (hazy), and the pupil may be nonreactive. Increased IOP (>23 mm Hg) indicates the need for further evaluation. Gonioscopy is performed to determine the depth of the anterior chamber angle and to examine the entire circumference of the angle for any abnormal changes in the filtering meshwork.

OUTCOME MANAGEMENT

The goal of management is to facilitate the outflow of aqueous humor through remaining channels and to maintain IOP within a range that prevents further damage to the optic nerve. If the IOP is very high, it must be reduced to retain vision. If vision is lost, the goals are to restore independence for the client.

Medical Management

Reduce Intraocular Pressure (Promote Aqueous Flow)
Intraocular pressure can be reduced by increasing the outflow of aqueous fluids. In narrow-angle glaucoma

the pupil is constricted using topical miotics or epinephrine, which opens the canal of Schlemm and promotes drainage of aqueous humor. Further, the production of aqueous humor can be reduced by using topical beta-blocker or alpha-adrenergic agents or oral carbonic anhydrase inhibitors. Figure 65-2 shows the sites of action for various drugs.

Nursing Management of the Medical Client

Assessment. Nursing assessment includes establishing demographic data of age and race because open-angle glaucoma occurs most often in clients more than 40 years of age and in blacks. Determine whether there is a family history of glaucoma or other eye problems and whether the client has had ocular surgery, infections, or trauma. An accurate list of current medications is imperative because over-the-counter medications (such as antihistamines) may dilate the pupil, increasing the risk for angle-closure glaucoma. Always note a history of allergic reactions, particularly to medications or dyes.

Ask the client to describe any changes in vision. Although the manifestations of primary open-angle glaucoma are insidious, the client may describe blind spots in the periphery or an overall decreased visual acuity with loss of contrast sensitivity. Decreased, uncorrectable visual acuity usually occurs when there has been irreversible damage to the optic nerve.

If it has been previously established that the client has visual loss from glaucoma, assess how the client is coping with this loss. Although people adapt to the loss of vision

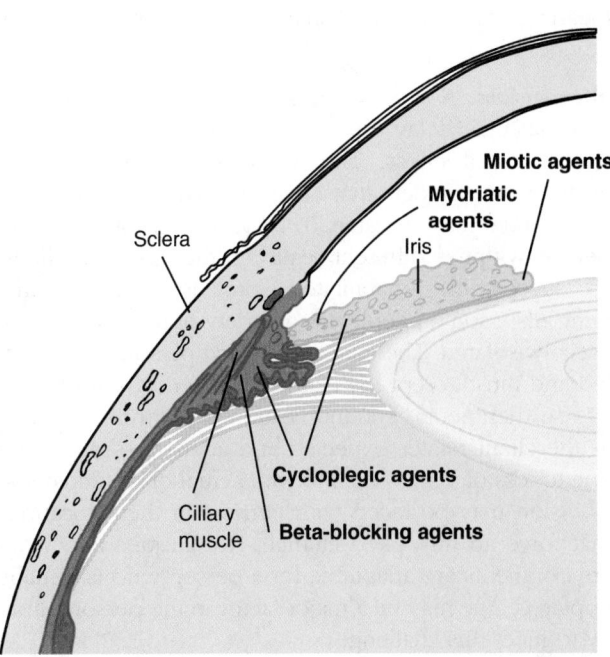

■ **FIGURE** **65–2** Sites of action of mydriatic, beta-blocking, cycloplegic, and miotic agents.

in different ways, they usually manifest grief and loss at any stage of the disease process. Clients may be understandably anxious during examinations because they may fear discovery that further vision loss has occurred. Assess the client's perception of glaucoma and the effect it has on quality of life. Help the client identify effective coping skills that may have been used in the past.

Diagnosis, Outcomes, Interventions

Diagnosis: Disturbed Sensory Perception (Visual). The increased IOP alters the function of the optic nerve, decreasing vision. The nursing diagnosis *Disturbed Sensory Perception (Visual) related to recent loss of vision* may be appropriate if the loss of vision is a new problem for the client.

Outcomes. The client will maintain as much functional vision as possible, report no further loss of vision, adapt to any visual loss, be able to perform activities of daily living (ADL), and recognize clinical manifestations of complications.

Interventions. Reassure the client that although some vision has been lost and cannot be restored, further loss may be prevented by adhering to the treatment plan.

Diagnosis: Grieving. Vision lost to glaucoma is irreparable. Even with the most aggressive medical and surgical management, vision loss may progress. A typical nursing diagnosis would therefore be *Grieving related to loss of vision.* Significant loss of vision represents the need for compromise and adaptation for both the client and the client's family.

Outcomes. The client will express grief, describe the meaning of the loss, and share the grief with significant others.

Interventions. Assess the causative and contributing factors that may delay the work of grieving and promote family cohesiveness. The social stigma of blindness underlies the anxiety that clients experience with actual or potential loss of vision. Total loss of vision isolates a person within a different reality. Although most clients are successfully rehabilitated, some losses are permanent. Also, some people, for a variety of reasons, remain socially isolated. The image of a blind person who is pitied and must accept the charity of others is disturbing.

Use therapeutic communication to express empathy as the client relates expected and actual losses that are due to loss of vision. People with actual or potential loss of vision may be faced with barriers in their vocations that force an unwanted change. Not all jobs and work environments are adaptable for a person who is visually impaired. Age may be a major factor in the person's ability to meet this challenge.

Self-esteem is closely related to the roles of people in their particular lifestyle. Loss of control in personal, family, and work situations can be devastating. The issue of dependence versus independence may also be a factor in the person's ability to cope with the stressors of vision loss.

Diagnosis: Risk for Ineffective Therapeutic Regimen Management (Individuals). The regimen for eyedrops and oral medications to control glaucoma ranges from simple to complex. This nursing diagnosis should be stated as *Risk for Ineffective Therapeutic Regimen Management (Individuals) related to complex medication schedule.*

Outcomes. The client will describe the disease process and the regimen for disease control and will relate how the medication routine will be incorporated into ADL.

Interventions. The client may need to instill as many as three or four different eyedrops from one to six times a day. Constricting eyedrops are usually prescribed four times a day, and beta-blockers are usually prescribed every 12 hours; however, the eyedrops may be needed every 4 to 6 hours. The schedule is designed to provide the best possible control of IOP around the clock.

Medications are an integral part of the treatment and care of a client with glaucoma, and nursing interventions must thus be directed at the client's ability to understand and comply with prescribed therapy. First, determine the client's current level of knowledge. Provide necessary information about glaucoma and its treatment in understandable terms. Diagrams may be helpful to the client and the client's significant others. Because treatment for glaucoma is often complex, involving both oral and topical ophthalmic medications, review a written plan of care in large print with the client and family. To maximize compliance, ensure that the plan of care fits into the client's lifestyle.

The administration of eyedrops is a critical component of self-care for the client with glaucoma. After instructing the client and family on the technique of instillation, validate the client's or the family's ability to instill eyedrops properly by asking for a return demonstration. Be sure to include discussion of medications and their side effects.

Evaluation. Independent self-care is the area for evaluation in the medically managed client. Evaluate the client's ability for self-care (a short-term outcome) and compliance with the medical regimen (a long-term outcome).

Modifications for Older Clients

Older clients with arthritic or shaking hands have difficulty instilling their own eyedrops. Instruct the client to lie down on a bed or sofa. Tilting the head back can lead to loss of balance. The eyedrop regimen for glaucoma requires accurate timing. Older clients may need visual reminders, such as a check-off list and may also need to use a timer or an alarm clock to help them remember

Surgical Management

When maximal medical therapy fails to halt the progression of visual field loss and optic nerve damage, surgical intervention is recommended. Many procedures are used to improve aqueous humor outflow; however, no operation has been uniformly successful.

Laser Trabeculoplasty

The use of the laser to create an opening in the trabecular meshwork is often indicated before filtering surgery is considered. The laser produces scars in the trabecular meshwork, causing tightening of meshwork fibers. The tightened fibers allow increased outflow of aqueous humor. IOP is reduced through improved outflow in about 80% of cases. The effect of the laser treatment decreases with time, and the procedure may need to be repeated. Medical treatment with topical eyedrops is usually continued.

Trabeculectomy

Trabeculectomy is the creation of an opening through which the aqueous fluid escapes. A half-thickness scleral flap is loosely sutured over the created opening through which the fluid escapes, again resulting in subconjunctival absorption of aqueous humor (see Figure 65-1, *C*).

Filtering Procedures

Operations such as trephination, thermal sclerostomy, and sclerectomy create an outflow channel from the anterior chamber into the subconjunctival space (see Figure 65-1, *D*). Aqueous humor is absorbed through the conjunctival vessels. In about 25% of cases, the opening closes because of scar tissue formation and reoperation is necessary. Such filtering procedures are less successful in young and black clients, who tend to have an increased ability to produce thicker scar tissue. Topical corticosteroids are used postoperatively because their anti-inflammatory action inhibits proliferation of fibroblasts at the surgical site.

Iridotomy

Iridotomy is the creation of a new route for the flow of aqueous humor to the trabecular meshwork. The laser is used to create the new opening in the iris (see Figure 65-1, *E*).

Other Techniques

5-Fluorouracil (5-FU), mitomycin, and other antimetabolites are sometimes injected subconjunctivally because they also inhibit fibroblast proliferation and thereby reduce postoperative scarring. Ocular implantation devices (e.g., Molteno implant, Baerveldt seton) are sometimes used to control the flow of aqueous humor in clients with complicated types of glaucoma. A device is sutured to the outer surface of the eyeball on the sclera between the ocular muscles. A tiny probe is inserted under the scleral flap directly into the anterior chamber that directs the flow of aqueous humor more posteriorly than in the more common filtering procedures.

Cyclodestructive Procedures

When other surgical procedures have failed, *cyclocryotherapy* (application of a freezing tip) or cyclophotocoagulation (applied with a laser) may be used to damage the ciliary body and decrease production of aqueous humor.

Nursing Management of the Surgical Client

Preoperative Care

Preoperative nursing care includes preparing the client for a surgical procedure that may be performed in either an outpatient or an inpatient setting (see Chapter 14).

Laser therapy is most commonly performed in a clinic or office, including the use of a topical anesthetic. Explain both the expected outcome of the procedure and the "popping" sounds and flashing lights that the client will experience. Explain that there will be a waiting period (usually 1 to 2 hours) after the procedure to evaluate a possible rise in IOP. Because of the instability of the IOP, the client should arrange for a friend or family member to accompany him or her and to provide transportation.

Postoperative Care

Following surgery, the eye is covered with a patch and a metal or plastic shield for protection to protect from light and trauma. Instruct the client not to lie on the operative side to avoid pressure on the surgical site. When the effects of perioperative sedation have diminished, the client may ambulate and eat as desired.

Frequent monitoring of IOP is necessary because the surgical site is microscopic. Assess the client for continued or increasing pain, nausea, and decreased vision. Follow-up care is needed to monitor for delayed healing. The anterior chamber may fail to heal, or the wound may seal too tightly. Both situations warrant further surgery.

Self-Care

The postoperative plan must include client education and evaluation of the home environment and available care. Because the level of independence varies with each client, use information supplied by the client and family or friends to assess how much support may be needed. Although many clients with glaucoma undergo repeated surgical procedures, it is necessary to carefully review the information each time. The Client Education Guide on p. 1704 summarizes this essential information.

CATARACTS

A *cataract* is opacity of the lens. Some degree of cataract formation is to be expected in most people more than 70 years of age. Worldwide, cataract is the primary cause of reduced vision and blindness. More than 1 million cataract operations are now being performed annually in the United States. A person with a normal life span is more likely to undergo a cataract operation than any other major surgical procedure.

The most common cataract is the age-related or senile type. Senile cataracts usually begin around the age of 50 years and consist of cortical, nuclear, or posterior subcapsular opacities, which may coexist in various combinations. In cortical cataracts, spoke-like opacifications are found in the periphery of the lens. They progress slowly, infrequently involve the visual axis, and often do not cause severe loss of vision. Nuclear sclerotic cataracts are a result of a progressive yellowing and hardening of the central lens (nucleus). Most people older than 70 have some degree of nuclear sclerosis. Posterior subcapsular opacities occur centrally on the posterior lens capsule and cause visual loss early in their development because they lie directly on the visual axis.

Etiology and Risk Factors

The cumulative exposure to ultraviolet light over a person's life span is the single most important risk factor in cataract development. People who live at high altitudes or who work in bright sunlight, such as commercial fishermen, appear to experience cataract formation earlier in life. Glassblowers and welders who do not wear eye protection are also at higher risk.

Cataracts may develop as a result of many other systemic, ocular, and congenital disorders. *Systemic* disorders include diabetes, tetany, myotonic dystrophy, neurodermatitis, galactosemia, Lowe syndrome, Werner's syndrome, and Down syndrome. *Intraocular* disorders include iridocyclitis, retinitis, retinal detachment, and onchocerciasis. Infections (German measles, mumps, hepatitis, poliomyelitis, chickenpox, infectious mononucleosis) during the first trimester of pregnancy may cause *congenital* cataracts. Blunt trauma, lacerations, foreign bodies, radiation, exposure to infrared light, and chronic use of corticosteroids may also result in cataracts.

Pathophysiology

Cataract formation is characterized chemically by a reduction in oxygen uptake and an initial increase in water content followed by dehydration of the lens. Sodium and calcium contents are increased; potassium, ascorbic acid, and protein contents are decreased. The protein in the lens undergoes numerous age-related changes, including yellowing from formation of fluorescent compounds and molecular changes. These changes, along with the photoabsorption of ultraviolet radiation throughout life, suggest that cataracts may be caused by a photochemical process.

Cataracts progress in a predictable pattern. They begin as immature cataracts that are not completely opaque, and some light is transmitted through them, allowing useful vision. Mature cataracts are completely opaque (the former term for this stage was *ripe*). Vision is significantly reduced. Hypermature cataracts are those in which the lens proteins break down into short-chain polypeptides that leak out through the lens capsule. The pieces of protein are engulfed by macrophages, which may obstruct the trabecular meshwork, causing phacolytic glaucoma.

Clinical Manifestations

Blurred vision, sometimes monocular diplopia (double vision), photophobia (light sensitivity), and glare occur because the opacity of the lens obstructs the reception of light and images by the retina. Clients usually see better in low light, when the pupil is dilated, which allows for vision around a central opacity. There is no complaint of pain. A cloudy lens can be observed (Figure 65-3).

A cataract should be suspected when the red reflex seen with the direct ophthalmoscope is distorted or absent. Although cataracts can usually be easily identified with the direct ophthalmoscope, an accurate determination of the type and extent of the lens change requires a slit-lamp examination.

OUTCOME MANAGEMENT

Surgical Management

There is no known treatment other than surgery that prevents or reduces cataract formation. The role of diet

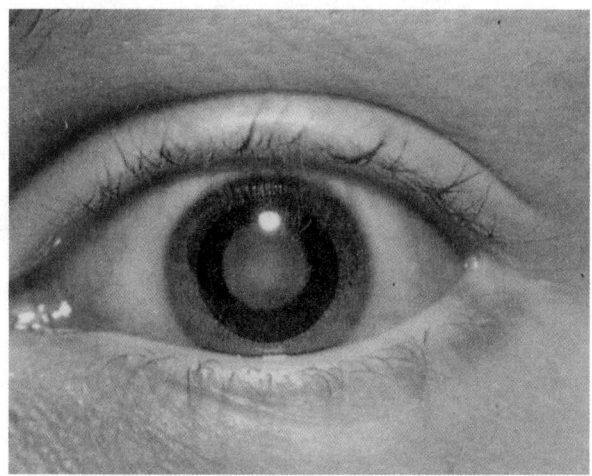

■ **FIGURE 65–3** The cloudy appearance of a lens affected by cataract. *(Courtesy Ophthalmic Photography at the University of Michigan W. K. Kellogg Eye Center, Ann Arbor, Mich.)*

is not clear. Some research, presented in the Complementary and Alternative Therapy feature below, suggests that egg yolks may improve vision. Unless other ocular complications or health factors exist, cataract surgery is performed on an outpatient basis. Preoperative eyedrops may include a dilating agent such as tropicamide (Mydriacyl) to facilitate the surgery. A cycloplegic cyclopentolate (Cyclogyl) may also be administered to paralyze the ciliary muscles. Cataract surgery is performed under topical anesthesia using eyedrops or regional anesthesia (retrobulbar injection of local anesthetic solution). The client is often given an intravenous sedative in addition.

The cataract is removed by making a small incision in the cornea. The cataract is broken into microscopic particles using an ultrasonic probe. The use of high-energy sound waves is called *phacoemulsification*. Then a folded intraocular lens (IOL) is inserted through the microincision, then unfolded, and locked into permanent position (Figure 65-4). The small incision is "self-sealing" and usually requires no stitches. It remains tightly closed by the natural outward pressure within the eye. This type of incision heals fast and provides a much more comfortable recuperation.

Complications

Postoperative infection, bleeding, macular edema, and wound leaks are possible; however, side effects after cataract surgery are rare. The incidence of retinal

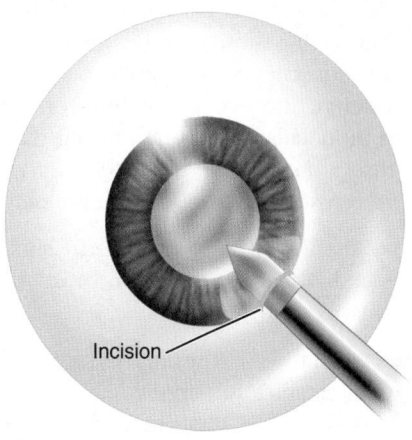

A

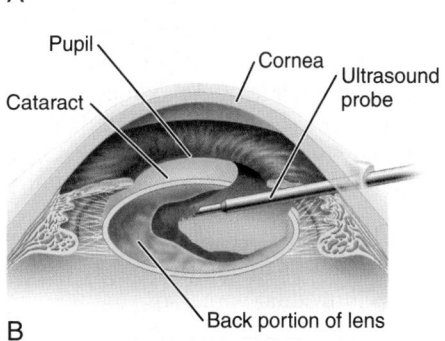

B

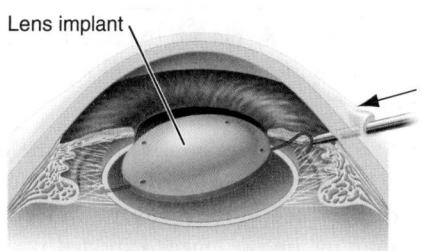

C

■ **FIGURE 65–4** **A,** A small incision is made into the cornea for the insertion of the phacoemulsification tip. **B,** Using ultrasound, the cataract is dissolved. **C,** An artificial lens is inserted into the eye, which unfolds into place.

COMPLEMENTARY AND ALTERNATIVE THERAPY

Egg Yolks and Better Vision

Two carotenoids may be deposited in the eye and prevent macular degeneration or cataracts (leading causes of blindness in older adults in the United States). These carotenoids are lutein and zeaxanthin, and they are found in large amounts in egg yolks. Researchers gave slightly more than 1 egg yolk per day to 11 individuals. About 1 month later, the researchers found significantly increased levels of the two carotenoids in the subjects' blood; however, the subjects' low-density lipoprotein (LDL, or bad cholesterol) levels also increased significantly. These carotenoids can also come from dark-green, leafy vegetables and corn; however, they are better absorbed when they come from egg yolks. In moderation (several times a week), egg yolks may prevent some eye problems, but clients must pay attention to cholesterol intake.

REFERENCE

Handelman, G., et al. (1999). Lutein and zeaxanthin concentrations in plasma after dietary supplementation with egg yolk. *American Journal of Clinical Nutrition, 70,* 247-251.

detachment is higher in the first 12 months after cataract surgery.

Nursing Management of the Surgical Client

Assessment. During the history and physical examination, ask the client about any predisposing factors (trauma, systemic diseases, medications such as corticosteroids, and other ocular problems). Visual acuity (both distant and near) in each eye is documented. Ask the client to describe visual disturbances. The client's visual acuity may be relatively close to normal ranges, and yet the client may experience difficulty in performing ADL. The client's individual perception of the quality of vision is an important factor in determining the need for surgery.

Diagnosis, Outcomes, Interventions
Diagnosis: Disturbed Sensory Perception (Visual). An IOL does not provide the same visual acuity as the natural lens of the eye. Although vision may be greatly improved, varying degrees of change in depth perception may remain. In addition, the eye is patched for protection, making vision monocular. Write the nursing diagnosis as *Disturbed Sensory Perception (Visual) related to lens extraction and replacement and use of eye patch.*

Outcomes. The client will have improved visual perception as evidenced by improved vision or adaptation to changes in visual acuity.

Interventions. Adaptation is the key issue in caring for the client having cataract surgery. Nursing interventions are based on assisting the client to gain or maintain as much independence as possible. Evaluate the client's lifestyle, abilities, and home environment. A 55-year-old client who is an architect and otherwise healthy may have an early cataract removed because it interferes with his work in areas where bright light is used. A 75-year-old diabetic client who is retired and mainly watches television has entirely different needs.

Evaluation. Adaptation to restored normal vision is usually rapid. Adaptation to limited vision requires more time based on individual variations.

Self-Care

After cataract surgery, clients are expected to return for a follow-up visit the next morning and again at 1 week and at 1 month.

SAFETY ALERT **Postoperative care includes observation of the ocular dressing, if present, and assessment of the client's ability to perform ADL at the preoperative level. Nausea and vomiting are no longer expected outcomes of the surgical procedure but, if present, should be reported immediately. The eye patch is usually removed the next morning but may be removed after a few hours if the client has limited vision in the other eye. Instruct the client to wear a metal or plastic shield to protect the eye from accidental injury and not to rub the eye.**

Glasses may be worn during the day. The Client Education Guide below provides instructions for clients to follow.

Restrictions on postoperative activity vary according to the practice of the ophthalmologist. Generally, the client should avoid heavy lifting (>15 pounds) or straining in the early postoperative period.

Eye care for the client after cataract surgery is the same as that for glaucoma clients (see Glaucoma). Postoperative eye medications may include antibiotics, corticosteroids, or both. Assess the client's or the family's ability to instill eyedrops appropriately. Review the rationale and schedule for the medications with the client and family. Postoperative discomfort should be minimal to moderate and is usually relieved by acetaminophen. Clients commonly experience an itching sensation after cataract surgery. Instruct the client to report any pain that is unrelieved. Review the clinical manifestations of infection and increased IOP with the client and family.

Depending on the client's age, ability, and availability of assistance, make a referral for home health care if indicated. Adjustment to changes in vision also varies with the individual client.

RETINAL DISORDERS

RETINAL DETACHMENT

Retinal detachment is the separation of the retina from the choroid, a membrane dense with blood vessels that

---

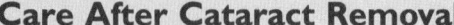

CLIENT EDUCATION GUIDE

Care After Cataract Removal

- Leave the eye patch in place.
- For 24 hours, limit your activity to sitting in a chair, resting in bed, and walking to the bathroom.
- Do not rub your eye.
- You can wear your glasses.
- Do not lift more than 5 pounds (the weight of a gallon of milk).
- Do not strain (or bear down).
- Do not sleep on the operative side of your body.
- Take your eyedrops.
- Take acetaminophen (e.g., Tylenol) as needed for pain or itching.
- DO NOT take aspirin or drugs containing aspirin.
- Report any pain that is unrelieved, redness around the eye, nausea, or vomiting.
- Wear an eye shield to protect your eye.

is located between the retina and the sclera ("white" of the eye). The retina is a thin layer of light-sensitive tissue that lines the back portion of the eye. When the retina detaches, it is deprived of its blood supply and source of nourishment and loses its ability to function. This can impair vision to the point of blindness.

Rhegmatogenous retinal detachment is the most common type and is due to a retinal hole. Liquid in the vitreous body seeps through the hole and separates the retina from its blood supply. Without intervention, the detachment continues to spread and the detached retina loses the ability to function. It may become increasingly detached over a period of hours to years.

Predisposing factors to retinal detachment include aging, cataract extraction, degeneration of the retina, trauma, severe myopia, previous retinal detachment in the other eye, and a family history of retinal detachment. Retinal holes and tears usually occur from spontaneous vitreous traction, but abnormal adhesions may be present between the retina and vitreous body secondary to diabetic retinopathy, injury, or other ocular disorders. Atrophy of the vitreous body may also result in a retinal tear.

Characteristic clinical manifestations of retinal detachment are described by clients as a shadow or curtain falling across the field of vision. Shadows or black areas in the field of vision are the result of separation of visual receptors from the neural pathway. No pain is associated with a detached retina. The onset is usually sudden and may be accompanied by a burst of black spots or floaters indicating that bleeding has occurred as a result of the detachment. The person may also see flashes of light caused by separation of the retina.

Visual field loss occurs in the opposite quadrant of the actual detachment. For example, a tear in the temporal region, which is affected more frequently, creates a visual defect in the nasal area. The extent of loss of vision is related to the portion of the retina involved. Giant retinal tears involving the entire retina may result in temporary blindness, whereas peripheral tears may not interfere with central vision at all.

The pupil must be widely dilated for a retinal examination. Tell clients that they will experience an extremely bright light and will be asked to change their gaze frequently to facilitate the ophthalmoscopic examination. A scleral depressor also may be used externally on the lid or conjunctiva to assist in rotating the eyeball and to indent the retina for increased viewing ability. Areas of detachment appear bluish gray as opposed to the normal red-pink color (Figure 65-5).

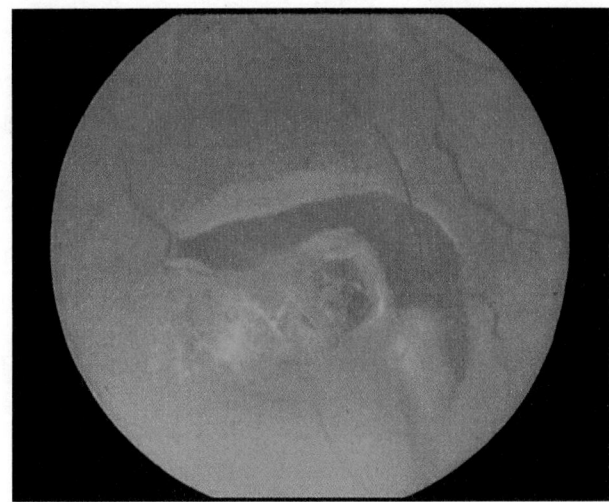

■ **FIGURE 65-5** Bluish gray appearance of areas of retinal detachment. *(Courtesy Ophthalmic Photography at the University of Michigan W. K. Kellogg Eye Center, Ann Arbor, Mich.)*

is to place the retina back in contact with the choroid and to seal the accompanying holes and breaks. Because retinal detachment repair may take several hours, general anesthesia is commonly used. The pupil must be widely dilated before the operation, and the client may be given a sedative.

Laser Photocoagulation

If the retina is torn or the detachment is slight, a laser can be used to burn the edges of the tear and halt progression. If the detachment is small, the laser can seal the retina against the choroid. Laser surgery is usually performed as an outpatient procedure under local anesthesia.

Cryopexy

Cryopexy uses nitrous oxide to freeze the tissue behind the retinal tear, stimulating scar tissue formation that will seal the edges of the tear. It is usually done as an outpatient procedure with the client under local anesthesia.

Pneumatic Retinopexy

Pneumatic retinopexy is most effective for detachments that occur in the upper portion of the eye. The eye is numbed with local anesthesia, and a small gas bubble is injected into the vitreous body. The bubble rises and presses against the retina, pushing it against the choroid. The gas bubble is slowly absorbed over the next 1 or 2 weeks. Cryopexy or laser is used to seal the retina into place.

Scleral Buckling

The surgical procedure to place the retina back in contact with the choroid is called *scleral buckling* (Figure 65-6). The sclera is actually depressed from the outside by

OUTCOME MANAGEMENT

Surgical Management

There is no known medical treatment for a detached retina. The goal of surgical repair of retinal detachment

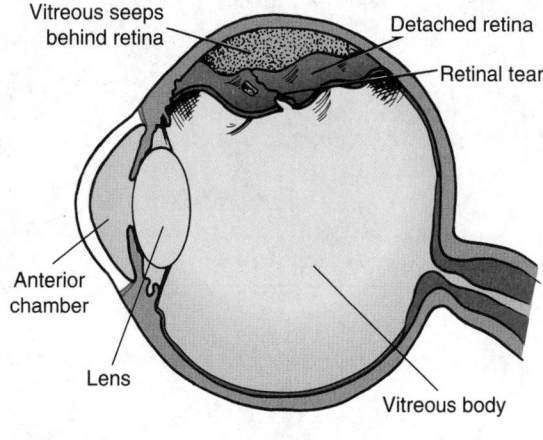

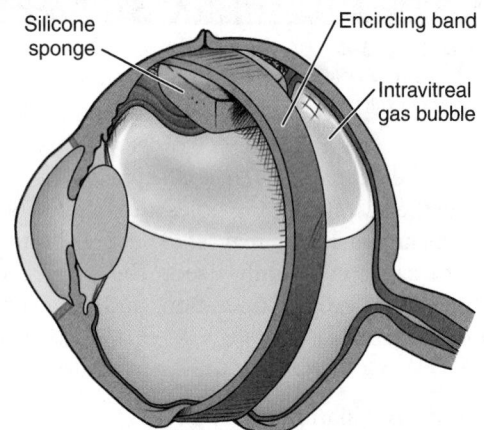

■ **FIGURE 65–6 A,** Detached retina. **B,** Scleral buckling to repair a detached retina. A silicone sponge implant is placed over the tear and held in place with an encircling band. An air or gas bubble may be used to apply pressure on the retina from the inside of the eye. When the buckle is tightened, the implant indents the sclera, holding the choroid and retina together.

rubber-like silicone (Silastic) sponges or bands that are sutured in place permanently. In addition to the buckling procedure, an intraocular injection of air or sulfur hexafluoride (SF6) gas bubble, or both, may be used to apply pressure on the retina from the inside of the eye. This holds the retina in place by gravitational force during the healing phase. Postoperative positioning of the client maximizes the tamponade effect of the air or gas bubble. The bubble is slowly absorbed.

Postoperative swelling of tissues and cells in the anterior chamber caused by the inflammatory process or compromise of the venous drainage system may result in increased IOP. Because of the fragility of the tissues involved in the repair, re-detachment of the retina may occur at any time. At times, the retina has been separated from its blood supply long enough that, even when reattached, it no longer has useful function and the client's vision does not improve significantly. Postoperative infection is also a risk.

The client should not expect immediate return of vision. Postoperative inflammation and the dilating drops interfere with vision. As healing takes place over weeks and months, vision may improve gradually.

Nursing Management

Nursing care focuses on helping the client cope with the fears and reality of loss of vision and to adapt to changes in vision. The client must be aware of the clinical manifestations of further loss of vision.

Following surgery, observe the eye patch for any drainage. Blood loss in retinal detachment surgery is minimal, and only serous drainage is expected on the postoperative dressing. Assess the level of pain and the presence of nausea.

Activity restrictions may be necessary if an air or gas bubble has been injected. The client needs to be positioned so that the bubble can apply maximal pressure on the retina by the force of gravity. This position, usually head down and to one side, is maintained for several days. Provide suggestions for comfort and support with the positioning (pillows under stomach, elbows, or ankles).

Encourage the client to resume a regular diet and fluids as tolerated. The eye patch and shield are removed the next morning. Redness and swelling of the lids and conjunctiva should be expected from the surgical manipulation. After several days, the swelling and ecchymosis of the lids subside, but the conjunctiva may remain red or pink for a few weeks.

Postoperative eye medications generally include an antibiotic-steroid combination eyedrop to prevent infection and reduce inflammation. Cycloplegic agents are prescribed to dilate the pupil and relax the ciliary muscles, which decreases discomfort and helps prevent the formation of iris adhesions to the corneal endothelium (*synechiae*). Either warm or cold compresses may be applied for comfort several times a day.

Self-Care

Because retinal detachment surgery is often performed on an urgent basis, the client rarely has an opportunity to plan for the surgery. Evaluate the home environment, and assist the client and family in preparing for any necessary support. You may need to find help at home for independent living until sight returns or the client adapts to changes in vision. Although the eye patch is usually removed early in the postoperative period, clients commonly have decreased functional vision in the eye. The Bridge to Home Health Care feature on p. 1709 suggests ways to help clients cope with failing vision.

Instruct the client to clean the eye with warm tap water using a clean washcloth. Warm compresses may be continued at home. Either an eye shield or glasses should be worn during the day, and the shield should be worn during naps and at night. Advise the client to avoid vigorous activities and heavy lifting during the

Coping with Failing Vision

Providing a safe home environment for the client with failing vision is essential. Promoting an autonomous lifestyle is desirable. Assessing the client's ability to remain safely at home is an important responsibility of home health care nurses.

Basic emergency procedures can be implemented by the use of nationwide services such as Lifeline. This service provides a portable electronic device usually worn around the client's neck or wrist. By simply pushing the button, immediate contact is made with emergency personnel. The toll-free phone number is 1-800-852-5433.

Local telephone companies can provide special adaptive equipment for 9-1-1 access. Telephones that can be programmed and have lighted or large numbers are available in most retail stores.

Home safety precautions can be simple. Burns can be prevented by color-coding water faucets. Use red for hot water and blue for cold water. Marking the "Off" dials on stoves and microwave ovens with colored tape or paint reduces the chance of injury.

Adequate lighting is essential. During the day, natural light is preferable. Open drapes or shades to provide ample light. Replace light bulbs with the highest wattage recommended.

Removal of hazards, such as throw rugs, clutter, and unnecessary furniture, can promote unrestricted ambulation. Handrails can be installed in hallways, in bathrooms, and on steps to prevent falls. Equipment such as canes, walkers, raised toilet seats, and bathtub rails promote safety. These items are available at medical supply stores.

Many commercial products are now marketed that can be of great assistance in the home. Pill organizers are clearly marked boxes with the day of the week and the times pills are to be taken. These can be filled by family members for a week at a time. Electronic lamp timers and voice-activated switches will allow the client to function more independently.

Access to a television and a radio is important. Large-print newspapers and reading materials help keep the client in touch with current events. The local library and the American Association for the Blind can provide assistance in obtaining needed items.

Creativity and planning can allow the client to remain at home in a safe environment for as long as possible.

immediate postoperative period. If an air or gas bubble has been injected, it may take several weeks to be totally absorbed. Clients are advised to avoid air travel during this time because the gas and air expand at high altitudes.

DIABETIC RETINOPATHY

Diabetic retinopathy is a progressive disorder of the retina characterized by microscopic damage to the retinal vessels, resulting in occlusion of the vessels. As a result of inadequate blood supply, sections of the retina deteriorate and vision is permanently lost. Diabetic retinopathy is one of the leading causes of blindness worldwide. All diabetic people are at risk for retinopathy, although there appears to be a strong correlation between incidence and severity of retinopathy and duration of the disease and blood glucose control. About 30% to 40% of the diabetic population has some degree of retinopathy. Clients who have had diabetes for 15 to 20 years have an 80% to 90% risk for development of retinopathy. Recently a genetic predisposition to retinopathy was found in the Asian Indian population with diabetes. People with allele 210 bp have increased risk.

The two types of diabetic retinopathy are (1) background (*nonproliferative*) and (2) *proliferative*. In background retinopathy, the retinal vessels are hyperpermeable and weak. The capillaries develop microaneurysms, and the retinal veins become dilated and tortuous. Multiple hemorrhages occur from these defective vessels. Retinal edema is caused by leaking capillaries, and after the serous fluid is absorbed, a yellowish precipitate ("hard exudate") remains. Hemorrhages, exudates, and ischemia contribute to impaired vision, particularly if these occur on or around the macula. Progressive retinal ischemia stimulates the growth of new but ineffective blood vessels. These new and fragile blood vessels proliferate and grow into the vitreous body. These vessels leak, hemorrhage, and undergo fibrous changes that may form bands that pull on the retina, causing detachment. This process is called *proliferative retinopathy* (Figure 65-7). With increasing ischemia, micro-infarcts of the nerve fiber layer, called "cotton-wool spots," appear.

Clinical manifestations are quite varied. Clients may report "spiders," "cobwebs," or tiny specks floating in their vision; dark streaks or a red film that blocks vision; vision loss, usually in both eyes, but more so in one eye; blurred vision that may fluctuate; a dark or empty spot in the center of the vision; poor night vision; or difficulty adjusting from bright light to dim light (Figure 65-8).

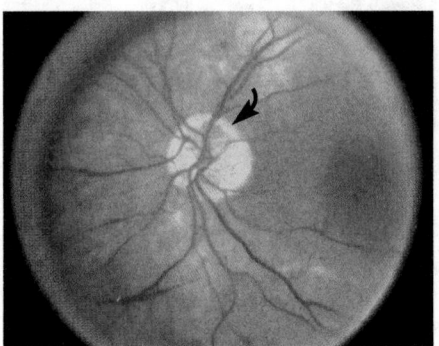

■ **FIGURE 65–7** Proliferative diabetic retinopathy. Neovascularization covers one fourth to one third of the optic disc *(arrow)*.

OUTCOME MANAGEMENT

The two main treatments for diabetic retinopathy are photocoagulation and vitrectomy. In most cases, these treatments are effective and slow or stop the progression of the disease for some time.

Photocoagulation

The goal of photocoagulation is to stop the leakage of blood and fluid in the retina and thus slow the progression of diabetic retinopathy. In photocoagulation a high-energy laser beam creates small burns in areas of the retina with abnormal blood vessels to seal any leaks. The procedure can be done as an outpatient using local anesthesia. A medical contact lens is placed on the cornea to help focus laser light on the sections of the retina to be treated. Fluorescein angiographic photographs may serve as maps to show where the laser burns should be placed. For proliferative diabetic retinopathy, panretinal or scatter photocoagulation can be used to treat the entire retina except the macula. The treatment causes the abnormal new blood vessels to shrink and disappear. Thus it reduces the chances of vitreous hemorrhage. Panretinal photocoagulation is usually done in two or more sessions. The treatment significantly reduces the risk of severe vision loss.

Vitrectomy

Vitrectomy is removal of the blood-filled vitreous. A vitreous cutter cuts the tissue and removes it, piece by piece, from the eye. The volume of removed tissue is replaced with saline to maintain the normal shape and pressure of the eye. During a vitrectomy the surgeon may also use a laser probe to perform a procedure called *panretinal photocoagulation* to prevent renewed growth of abnormal blood vessels and bleeding.

Nursing Management of the Surgical Client

Shortly after laser treatment, the client can usually return home driven by someone else. Vision will be blurry for about a day. Mild pain, headache, and sensitivity to light are expected and can be controlled with an eye patch and over-the-counter pain relievers. Immediately following laser surgery to treat macular edema, small spots caused by the laser burns may appear in the visual field. The spots generally fade and disappear with time. Follow-up care should be arranged before the client leaves; new areas of leakage may appear later and may require additional laser treatments.

RETINITIS PIGMENTOSA

Retinitis pigmentosa, described in the Genetic Links feature on p. 1711, is a genetic disorder that initially destroys the rods of the eye. Because the rods perceive black and white vision, the earliest manifestation is noticed during childhood as night blindness. Over the next several years, manifestations progress until a total loss of peripheral vision occurs. In time, central vision is also lost. No treatment is available to slow or stop this disorder. Genetic counseling is advised.

AGE-RELATED MACULAR DEGENERATION

Age-related macular degeneration (AMD) is a degenerative process that affects the macula and surrounding tissues, resulting in central visual deficits. AMD is found to some degree in most adults over 65 years of age. It is one of the most common causes of visual loss in older people. The exact cause is unknown, but the incidence increases with each decade in people over 50 years of age. It may be hereditary. It has been demonstrated that the blue rays of the spectrum (sunlight or its reflection in the ocean or desert) seem to accelerate macular degeneration more than other rays of the spectrum. There are two types of age-related macular degeneration: (1) nonexudative *(dry)* and (2) exudative *(wet)*. Both types are usually bilateral and progressive.

Nonexudative AMD is characterized by atrophy and degeneration of the outer retina and underlying structures. Seventy percent of clients have the dry form, which involves thinning of the macular tissues and disturbances in its pigmentation. Yellowish round spots *(drusen)* may be seen on the retina and macula with an ophthalmoscope. Drusen are deposits of amorphous material from the pigment epithelial cells of the retina. Over time, these spots increase, enlarge, and may calcify.

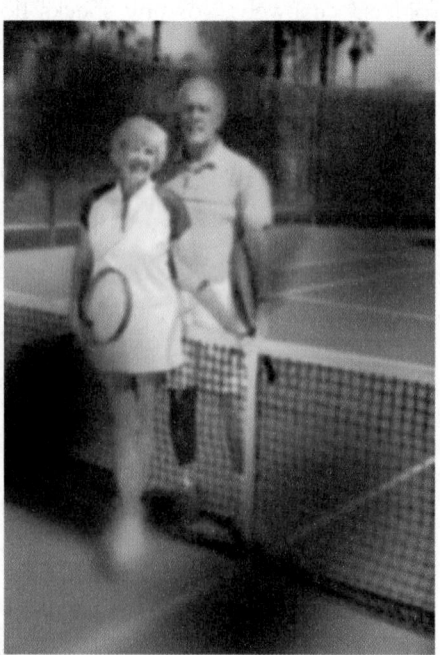

■ **FIGURE 65–8** Vision with diabetic retinopathy.

GENETIC LINKS

Retinitis Pigmentosa

DESCRIPTION

Retinitis pigmentosa (RP) describes a group of inherited disorders in which abnormalities of the photoreceptors (rods and cones) or the retinal pigment epithelium (RPE) of the retina lead to progressive visual loss. Clients initially experience "night blindness" (decreased night vision), followed by constriction of the peripheral visual field and eventually loss of central vision in the advanced stage of the disease. Most clients are legally blind by age 60. The prevalence of RP is approximately 1 in 3500 to 1 in 4000 individuals in the United States and Europe; it is considered the most common inherited cause of blindness.

GENETICS

RP can be inherited in an autosomal-dominant, autosomal-recessive, or X-linked recessive fashion. The molecular genetic causes of RP are unusually complicated. Many different genes may cause the same disease, and different mutations in the RP genes may cause different diseases. The mode of inheritance is determined by family history. To date, at least 34 different genes are known to cause RP; mutations in at least 12 genes cause autosomal-dominant RP, 16 genes cause autosomal-recessive RP, and 6 genes cause X-linked RP.

DIAGNOSIS/TESTING

The diagnosis of RP is based on documentation of progressive loss in photoreceptor function by electroretinography (ERG) and visual field testing. DNA testing is available for all the cloned genes causing RP on a research basis only. Routine genetic testing for RP is not available in clinical laboratories.

MANAGEMENT

RP is neither preventable nor curable, but therapy with high-dose vitamin A has been suggested to have a possible effect on slowing changes in retinal function. Various optical aids have been promoted for RP clients, and referral to agencies for the visually impaired can assist in providing vocational training, mobility training, and skills for independent living.

At the exudative stage of AMD, Bruch's membrane, which lies just beneath the pigment epithelial cell layer of the retina, becomes compromised. Thirty percent of clients have the wet form, which can involve bleeding within and beneath the retina, opaque deposits, and eventually scar tissue. The wet form accounts for 90% of all cases of legal blindness in clients with macular degeneration. It results in serous fluid leaks from the choroid, with accompanying proliferation of choroidal blood vessels. A dome-shaped retinal pigment epithelium may be seen when examining the fundus. These leaks produce a visual effect called metamorphopsia, which appears as distorted lines; the center of vision appears more distorted than the rest of the scene. A dark, blurry area or "whiteout" appears in the center

of vision. Color perception changes or diminishes. Fundus photography and angiography may be performed on a regular basis to document and evaluate changes.

OUTCOME MANAGEMENT

Recent research findings, reviewed in the Complementary and Alternative Therapy feature below, have shown that the use of high-dose antioxidant vitamins C and E, beta-carotene, and zinc supplements may delay progression of AMD and vision loss. Currently there are several drugs that are injected inside the eye to halt the angiogenesis that causes the distortion and loss of central vision. VEGF (vascular endothelial growth factor) drives the production of blood vessels, and there are new drugs that block the release of VEGF.

The client with AMD is threatened with the loss of central vision (see the Bridge to Home Health Care feature on Coping with Failing Vision on p. 1709). To evaluate changes in vision, teach the client to use the Amsler chart at home. You may assist the client to maximize remaining vision with low-vision aids and community referral to a low-vision specialist and low-vision support groups.

CORNEAL DISORDERS

CORNEAL INJURY

The cornea can be injured in many ways, such as with direct trauma, over-worn contact lens, chips of flying metal or glass fragments, or even dirt. A client with a

---

COMPLEMENTARY AND ALTERNATIVE THERAPY

Macular Degeneration and Dietary Supplements

The largest randomized trial ($n = 3640$) of a combination daily dietary supplement (500 mg of vitamin C, 400 international units of vitamin E, 15 mg of beta-carotene, 80 mg of zinc, plus 2 mg of copper) compared with placebo for macular degeneration found a significant reduction in the risk of disease progression over the 6-year study. The only individuals who benefited, however, were those with intermediate to advanced stages of already diagnosed macular degeneration. Individuals at risk or with early stage macular degeneration did not benefit from taking this supplement combination over the study period. In addition, the supplement combination did not have any effect on cataract development or risk.

REFERENCE

Age-Related Eye Disease Study Research Group. (2001). A randomized, placebo-controlled, clinical trial of high-dose supplementation with vitamins C and E, beta carotene, and zinc for age-related macular degeneration and vision loss: AREDS report no. 8. *Archives of Ophthalmology, 119,* 1417-1435.

corneal injury will typically have a dramatic, painful, profusely lacrimating eye. The bulbar conjunctiva blood vessels will be prominent (injected).

SAFETY ALERT **Treatment includes removing any imbedded items and then resting the eye (keeping it closed, using antibiotic ointments). Clients who are unconscious can also develop corneal dryness attributable to lack of blinking (Box 65-1).**

CORNEAL DYSTROPHIES

Corneal dystrophies comprise a group of hereditary and acquired disorders of unknown cause, characterized by deposits in the layers of the cornea and alteration of the corneal structure. Corneal dystrophies are associated with all five layers of the cornea. Although the disease usually originates in the inner layers (Descemet's membrane, the stroma, and Bowman's membrane), the degeneration, erosion, and deposits affect all layers. Corneal endothelium constantly removes fluids from the cornea to maintain its clarity. As the endothelial cells are gradually lost, the dystrophy progresses. Once lost, the endothelial cells do not grow back but instead spread out to fill the empty spaces. The pump system becomes less efficient, causing corneal clouding, swelling, and eventually reduced vision.

OUTCOME MANAGEMENT

The goal of treatment is to restore visual clarity for both safety and improved quality of life.

Medical Management

Dystrophies cannot be cured; however, with certain medications, blurred vision resulting from corneal swelling can be controlled. Saline eyedrops or ointments are often prescribed to draw fluid from the cornea and reduce swelling. Another simple technique that reduces moisture in the cornea is to hold a hair dryer at arm's length, blowing air into the face with the eyes closed. This technique draws moisture from the cornea, temporarily decreases swelling, and improves vision.

Surgical Management

Corneal Transplantation

Corneal transplantation *(keratoplasty)* is the use of donor corneas to improve the clarity of vision. Two depths of keratoplasty are performed. Penetrating keratoplasty indicates full-thickness corneal replacement; lamellar keratoplasty denotes a partial-thickness procedure. Because there is a direct relationship between age and health of the endothelial layer of the cornea, young donor tissue is preferred. Donor eyes are obtained from cadavers; donor eyes must be enucleated soon after death because of rapid endothelial cell death and must be stored in a preserving solution. Storage, handling, and coordination of donor tissue with surgeons are provided by a network of state eye-bank associations around the country.

Corneal transplantation surgery is usually performed with the client under local anesthesia. Figure 65-9, *A,* shows the eye after keratoplasty. Unlike cataract surgery, however, visual return after a corneal transplant is relatively slow and typically takes 6 to 12 months. The reason for the slow return of vision is that the sutures holding the new cornea in place tend to distort the vision, and they must be left in place for a considerable time before it is safe to remove them.

Rejection of donor tissue can occur following corneal transplantation from unsuitable storage of donor tissue, dystrophy of the donor's endothelium, surgical trauma, or immunologic rejection. Wound leakage, bleeding into the anterior chamber, glaucoma, cataract, and infection are other complications that may occur. At the first sign of graft rejection, when the cornea becomes cloudy and edematous and when there is an anterior chamber reaction (the presence of white blood cells or protein) (see Figure 65-9, *B*), topical steroids are prescribed in frequent doses to control the inflammatory response and to reverse the rejection reaction. In severe cases, a second transplantation may be necessary.

Nursing Management of the Postoperative Client

Corneal transplantation is usually performed as outpatient surgery. Postoperatively the client returns from the operating room with an eye patch and protective shield in place. Observe the patch for signs of drainage. No bleeding is expected with this procedure. The client should experience only mild to moderate discomfort, which should be relieved by acetaminophen. Unreduced

---

BOX 65-1   Eye Care for Unconscious Clients

Unconscious, sedated, or paralyzed clients are at high risk of corneal injury because they cannot maintain normal lid closure. Normal lid closure during sleep is provided by tonic contraction of the orbicularis oculi muscle. The use of muscle relaxants reduces the tonic contraction of the muscle and leads only to passive closure of the eyelids. Further, the client may have lost the blink reflex when sedatives are used. Tears quickly evaporate from the eye and increase the risk of injury. Corneal abrasion has been reported in as little as 48 hours.

Eye protection and lubrication are important to preserve sight. The use of eyedrops or ointments is effective in maintaining eye moisture. Films that preserve humidity in the eye can also be used; however, the family may be alarmed by the client's appearance with these products.

Data from Joyce, N. (2002). *Eye care for intensive care patients. A systematic review.* Adelaide, South Africa: The Joanna Briggs Institute for Evidence Based Nursing and Midwifery.

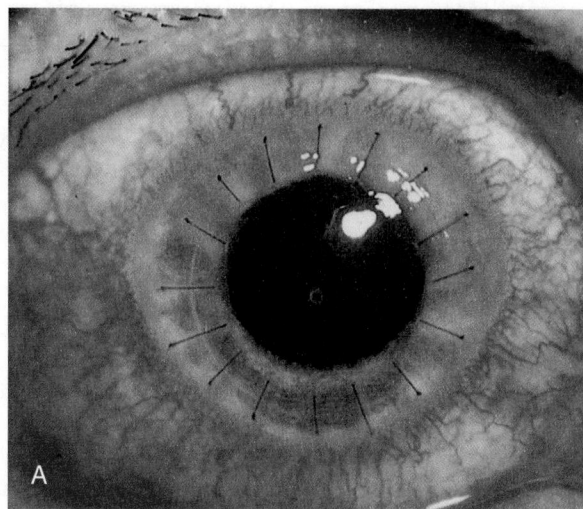

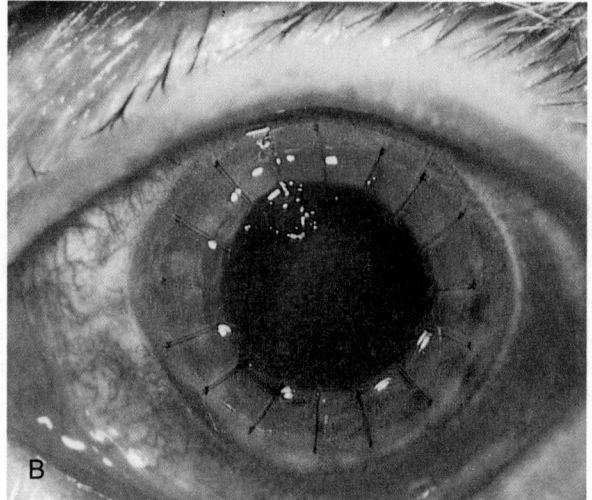

■ **FIGURE 65–9 A,** Clinical appearance of the eye after keratoplasty. **B,** Acute graft rejection. *(Courtesy Ophthalmic Photography at the University of Michigan W.K. Kellogg Eye Center, Ann Arbor, Mich.)*

pain may indicate a rise in IOP and should be reported to the surgeon. Because the eye patch is to be in place until the following morning, assess the client's ability for self-care and reinforce information on the hazards of monocular vision.

The eye is examined the next morning with the slit lamp. Depending on the extent of preoperative visual limitations, most clients experience improved vision immediately. Instruct clients, however, not to overestimate their expectations for full vision. Vision continues to improve gradually because the healing process may take up to a year or more. Glasses or contact lenses are usually needed to obtain the best result. Many months may be required for restoration of vision, and revisions in the care plan may be needed.

Self-Care

Postoperative eyedrops usually include an antibiotic and a corticosteroid. Topical corticosteroid therapy may

be needed indefinitely. Discharge instructions include the rationale for the medications and proper instillation technique.

> It is important for the client to wear eye protection in the form of regular glasses, sunglasses, or a protective shield to prevent injury to the eye. Advise the client never to rub the eye. The area around the eye may be cleaned with warm tap water using a clean washcloth.

SAFETY ALERT

Teach the client and family to recognize the clinical manifestations of increased IOP, infection, and graft rejection. A mnemonic tool may be useful in teaching the client to remember the signs of graft rejection (RSVP):

- R Redness
- S Swelling
- V Decreased vision
- P Pain

Advise the client to evaluate vision in the eye each day. A picture on the wall or some object in a well-lighted room should be selected as a point of reference. If a change in vision from the day before is noted, the client should reevaluate his or her vision in a few hours. If no improvement is noted or if vision is worse, the client should notify the physician. Because graft rejection may occur at any time (even years) after the surgery, advise the client to make the vision check a routine part of ADL for the rest of his or her life.

OCULAR MELANOMA

Although less than 1% of the people in the United States are affected by malignant ocular tumors, treatment of these tumors can be a challenge for both client and nurse. Choroidal melanomas are often detected during a routine ocular examination because there is no pain associated with the development of the tumor. By the time the tumor has grown large enough to obstruct vision, there may be involvement of the macula and metastasis.

OUTCOME MANAGEMENT

The goal of treatment is to care for the malignancy while preserving the eye.

Medical Management

When ocular melanoma is discovered early, radiation therapy alone may be the treatment of choice. Radiation therapy to the eye is accomplished through insertion of a tiny plate or plaque about the size of a dime that holds tiny seeds of radioactive iodine 125. The plaque is sutured to the sclera directly over the site of the tumor. It is left in place for several days, depending on the required dose, and then removed. Both insertion and removal are performed in the operating room. During treatment a lead shield is placed over the eye. Radiation exposure to the nurse who cares for the client is minimal—a small fraction of a chest x-ray study. Despite this extremely low exposure, the routine restrictions for hospital personnel and visitors are implemented for consistency. Hospitalization for treatment with radioactive iodine is required, depending on regulations.

SAFETY ALERT   **Follow the principles of radiation safety: reduce distance from the client, wear a lead shield and use a lead shield at the bedside, and limit time at the bedside by condensing assessments and interventions.**

During the client's hospitalization for this treatment, provide support and encouragement for the client. The plaque is only mildly to moderately uncomfortable, and discomfort should be relieved with acetaminophen. The difficult challenge for clients is confinement to their room with limitations on visitors at a time when support is essential. Eye medications include a cycloplegic agent and an antibiotic-steroid eyedrop.

Surgical Management

Enucleation

The goal of surgical removal is to preserve life by removing the tumor. Removal of the entire eyeball *(enucleation)* has been the traditional method of treatment and may be combined with radiation treatments. *Exenteration* (removal of the eyeball and surrounding tissues and bone) may also be necessary. The goal for clients following enucleation is adaptation to monocular vision and return to their former level of independence.

Enucleation is usually performed with the client under general anesthesia, but IV conscious sedation may also be used. The ocular muscles are dissected from the eyeball, which is removed by severing the optic nerve and vessels at the back. An acrylic sphere covered by donor scleral tissue is usually placed within the capsule of tissue that formerly held the eyeball. Scleral tissue encourages fibrovascular ingrowth, which prevents migration and extrusion of the implant. A soft plastic scleral shell is placed in the visible outer portion of the socket as a support until a permanent prosthesis can be made. A newer type of implant, hydroxyapatite, which is made of the same inorganic material present in human bone, is now being used.

Several weeks later a central hole is drilled into the sphere and covering tissues. A peg (which later fits into a depression on the posterior surface of the artificial eye) is then inserted into the hole. The movement of the implant by the muscle cone is transferred directly to the prosthesis. With the artificial eye being primarily supported by the peg instead of the lids and socket tissues, fewer cosmetic and structural complications occur.

Nursing Management

The client undergoing enucleation for a malignant tumor is stressed not only by the threat of cancer but also by disfigurement of the face. Assess the client's response, home, and family for support mechanisms. Nursing interventions are focused on assisting the client to grieve for the lost body part and lost vision and to identify coping mechanisms that will facilitate rehabilitation.

Preoperative Care

Assist the client in preparing for the surgical procedure. Most often the client is made aware of the tumor at a routine office visit. Surgery is usually scheduled within a few days. Recognizing that the client is most appropriately in a state of shock and denial, carefully explain the perioperative events. Although it is possible to have an enucleation as an outpatient procedure, the client may stay overnight in the hospital.

Postoperative Care

Provide routine postoperative care. The client returns from the operating room with a pressure dressing over the eye. Assess the dressing for bleeding using standard postoperative routines. Clients are understandably anxious about the removal of the dressing the next morning. Prepare the client by explaining how the eye and conformer will appear. The socket and lids will be swollen, and the white plastic conformer is visible.

Determine the client's or the family's ability to care for the wound postoperatively.

Some clients fear that their appearance will frighten others, especially children. In this case, an eye patch may be worn during the 4 to 6 weeks before the prosthesis is fitted but should not be worn continuously. Eventually the eye prosthesis can be worn and looks pleasingly normal (Figure 65-10). Refer to a fundamentals of nursing textbook for insertion and removal of the prosthesis.

The area around the lids may be cleaned with warm tap water with a clean washcloth. Soap and water should be kept away from the socket. If the plastic conformer accidentally comes out, it should be washed and replaced. Antibiotic ophthalmic ointment is usually ordered to be instilled in the socket once or twice a day.

Self-Care

Adjustment to monocular vision is a challenge the client begins to face immediately. Depth perception is altered, and the client needs to exercise caution in walking, crossing streets, and driving. Advise the client to practice ADLs until visual and body adjustments are made.

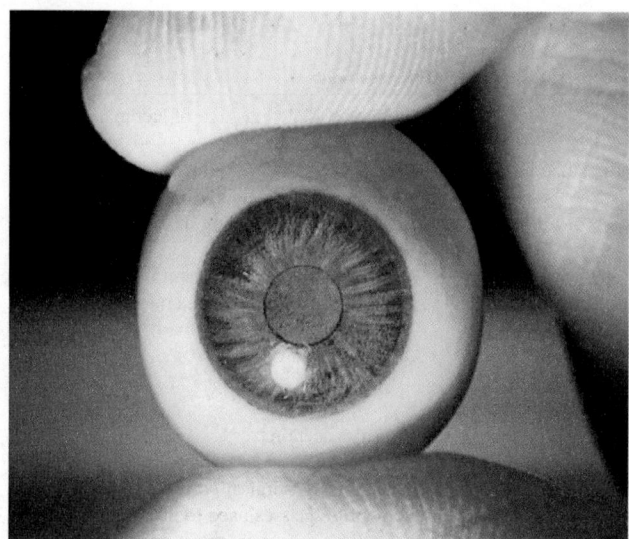

■ **FIGURE 65–10** An ocular prosthesis. *(Courtesy Ophthalmic Photography at the University of Michigan W.K. Kellogg Eye Center, Ann Arbor, Mich.)*

Emphasize the need for extra precaution with the remaining eye. Eye protection should be worn when engaging in any activity that might even remotely result in an injury. Many clients are advised to wear glasses even if no correction is needed.

EYELID, LACRIMAL, AND CONJUNCTIVAL DISORDERS

DRY EYE SYNDROME

Dry eye syndrome is a condition in which tear production is inadequate. It most commonly occurs in women between 50 and 60 years of age. Three primary causes are lacrimal gland malfunction, mucin deficiency, and mechanical abnormalities that prevent the spread of tears across the surface of the eye. The lacrimal gland can be genetically malformed or malformed because of injury or infection. Tear production is also decreased in Sjögren's syndrome, an autoimmune disorder that commonly accompanies rheumatoid arthritis. Facial nerve (seventh cranial nerve) palsy disrupts tear production. Mechanical abnormalities include problems with eyelid structure, eyeball extrusion, and misuse of contact lenses. Conjunctivitis and mumps can obstruct the gland. Some medications, such as antihistamines, atropine, and beta-adrenergic blocking agents, decrease tear production.

Manifestations include burning, itching eyes and a sensation of "something" in the eye. The term *keratoconjunctivitis sicca* is used to describe the problem.

Management includes determining the degree of injury to the cornea. Artificial tears (eyedrops and lubricants) can be used. In addition, some clients benefit from using airtight goggles at night to prevent tear evaporation. Postmenopausal women have found some relief from estrogen replacement therapy. Surgery can be used to open the lacrimal duct or to repair lid problems.

Other eyelid, lacrimal, and conjunctival disorders are discussed in Table 65-1.

REFRACTIVE DISORDERS

Light is bent (refracted) as it passes through the cornea and lens of the eye. Refractive errors exist when light rays are not focused appropriately on the retina of the eye. Three basic abnormalities of refraction occur in the eye: (1) myopia, (2) hyperopia, and (3) astigmatism. Optical correction is important to distinguish between visual loss caused by disease and visual loss caused by refractive error. *Refractometry* is the measurement of refractive error and should not be confused with *refraction,* the method used to determine which lens or lenses (if any) will most benefit the client.

MYOPIA

Myopia, or *nearsightedness,* is a condition in which the light rays come into focus in front of the retina (Figure 65-11, *A*). In this case the refractive power of the eye is too strong and a concave, or minus, lens is used to focus light rays on the eye. In most cases myopia is caused by an eyeball that is longer than normal, which may be a familial trait. Transient myopia may occur with the administration of a variety of medications (sulfonamides, acetazolamide, salicylates, and steroids) and has been associated with other disorders, such as influenza, typhoid fever, severe dehydration, and large intakes of antacids (for stomach ulcers). Correction is accomplished with eyeglasses or contact lenses.

HYPEROPIA

The hyperopic, or *farsighted,* eye focuses light rays behind the eye, and consequently the image that falls on the retina is blurred (see Figure 65-11, *B*). Vision may be brought into focus by placing a convex, or plus, lens in front of the eye. The lens supplies the magnifying power that the eye is lacking. Hyperopia may be caused by an eyeball that is shorter than normal or a cornea that has less curvature than normal. Because children have a greater ability to accommodate, they are less often affected than adults. Demands for close work and reading usually instigate manifestations of headache or eyestrain. Correction is based on a person's age and individual needs and complaints.

ASTIGMATISM

Astigmatism is a refractive condition in which rays of light are not bent equally by the cornea in all directions

TABLE 65-1 Eyelid, Lacrimal, and Conjunctival Disorders

Disorder	Definition	Appearance	Management
Dacryocystitis	Inflammation of tear drainage system	Pus-like drainage or raised, red lump near puncta	Antibiotics, daily massage of lacrimal system
Hordeolum (stye)	Infection of glands of eyelids	Redness and swelling of localized area of eyelid	Warm compresses and antibiotics; may need to be incised and drained
Chalazion	Chronic granuloma of meibomian gland	Painless, localized swelling of lid margin	If cosmetically distracting, may be surgically removed
Blepharitis	Chronic, bilateral inflammation of eyelids	Itching and burning of eyes; eyes appear red; scales noted on lashes	Wash eyelids with baby shampoo, water, and cotton-tipped applicators; antibiotic ointments may be prescribed
Conjunctivitis	Inflammation of conjunctiva from various microorganisms	Redness, tearing, and exudation of eyelid; may progress to eyelid drooping, abnormal tissue growth	Antibiotic eyedrops
Entropion	Turning in eyelid margin	Inversion of lower eyelid; dry and irritated eyes	Surgical resection
Ptosis	Drooping of eyelid from several causes	Irritation of eye caused by drying, loss of tears	Artificial tears; surgical correction needed; sometimes glasses used to lift redundant skin
Lagophthalmos	Inadequate closure of eyelids	Irritation of eye caused by drying	Artificial tears, eye shields at night; surgical correction
Absence of blinking	Lack of blinking seen with Parkinson's disease and hyperthyroidism	Blinking fewer than 20 times/min	Artificial tears; eye shields at night

so that a point of focus is not attained (see Figure 65-11, *C*). In most instances, astigmatism is caused because the curvature of the cornea is not perfectly spherical. This is the cause of poor vision for both distant and near objects. Astigmatism is corrected with cylindrical lenses.

Surgical Management

Refractive Surgery

Laser in situ keratomileusis (LASIK) is the most commonly used corrective surgery for nearsightedness in the United States. An extremely thin layer of the cornea is peeled back for laser reshaping on the middle layer of the cornea, and then the thin layer is put back in place. There is little postoperative discomfort, rapid recovery of clear vision, and quick stabilization of refractive change. LASIK is performed in a surgeon's office or same-day surgery center and does not require a hospital stay. It takes about 10 to 15 minutes per eye. It has a high success rate and low complication rate for low to moderate nearsightedness and may also be used to correct more severe nearsightedness.

LASEK (laser epithelial keratomileusis) is a relatively new procedure that is technically a variation of others. Also called epithelial LASIK or E-LASIK, LASEK is used mostly for people with corneas that are too thin or too flat for LASIK. It was developed to reduce the chance of complications that occur when the flap created during LASIK is not the ideal thickness or diameter.

Corneal ring implants (In-tacs) are clear pieces of acrylic that can be surgically implanted into the cornea. The implants flatten the cornea and thereby reduce

nearsightedness. The implants are shaped like crescents or half-circles. Two implants are used for each eye, and the implants are inserted along the sides of the cornea (*corneal periphery*). They do not cover the central

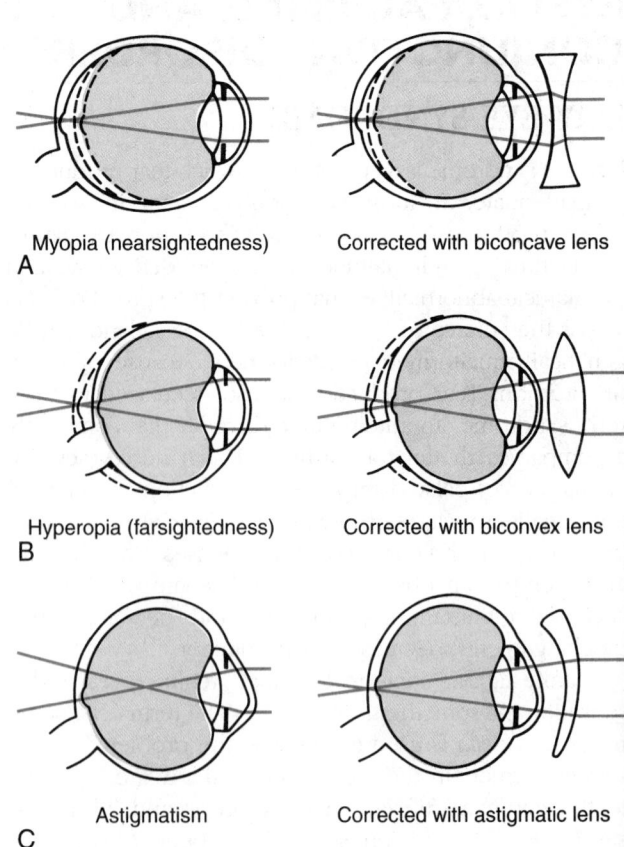

Myopia (nearsightedness)
A

Corrected with biconcave lens

Hyperopia (farsightedness)
B

Corrected with biconvex lens

Astigmatism
C

Corrected with astigmatic lens

■ **FIGURE 65-11 A-C,** Common refractive disorders and their correction. *Dashed lines* in **A** and **B** indicate normal eye contour.

portion of the cornea. Corneal ring implants appear to be very effective for correcting mild nearsightedness.

Nursing Management of the Surgical Client

Clients are assessed preoperatively for degree of myopia or astigmatism. Clients with severe refraction problems may not achieve full correction. Surgery is performed on an outpatient basis with local anesthesia. Eye protection is used, such as goggles to prevent dry eyes. Vigorous activities, activities that could get water in the eye, and eye makeup are to be avoided.

The eye is treated with steroid eyedrops, and most clients report watering of the eyes and minimal pain. Refraction slowly stabilizes after surgery. There is a period of adjustment during which visual acuity waxes and wanes. Reduced contrast sensitivity in night vision and daytime glare is common. Some clients require re-treatment for scarring that is unresponsive to topical steroids.

OCULAR MANIFESTATIONS OF SYSTEMIC DISORDERS

ENDOCRINE DISORDERS: GRAVES' DISEASE

Graves' disease may exist with or without any clinical evidence of thyroid dysfunction. Ocular manifestations include retraction of both upper and lower lids, resulting in a staring or frightened expression (Stellwag's sign); and lid lag (Graefe's sign), the retarded lowering of the upper lid when looking down (Figure 65-12). When the gaze is changed from down to up, the globe then lags behind the upper lid. Other signs are infrequent blinking, marked fine tremor with lid closure, and jerky movements on lid opening.

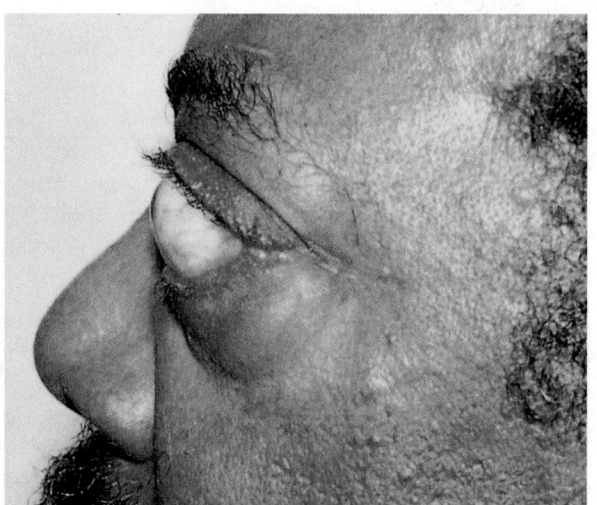

■ **FIGURE 65–12** Graves' exophthalmos. *(Courtesy Ophthalmic Photography at the University of Michigan W.K. Kellogg Eye Center, Ann Arbor, Mich.)*

The globes enlarge because of the increased size of extraocular muscles, edema of tissues, and excess orbital fat. The eye develops *proptosis* (forward protrusion of the eyeballs), which is called *exophthalmos*. Subsequent degeneration of muscle tissue leads to fibrosis, which restricts muscle movement, resulting in double vision.

As a primary measure, adequate control of thyroid abnormalities is essential. Diuretics as well as steroid therapy and radiotherapy may be indicated. Surgical interventions include corrective lid surgery and tarsorrhaphy for lid retraction to protect the cornea. Decompression of the orbit, which usually involves removal of the inferior and medial walls of the orbit, may be necessary to accommodate proliferative orbital fat and enlarged ocular muscles. Ocular muscle surgery may also be indicated. If the surgery is extensive, suction drains may be placed at the operative sites. Drainage is usually serosanguineous.

> **It is important that the client sleep with the head elevated to reduce postoperative swelling.**
> **Advise the client to expect redness, swelling, and ecchymoses around the eyes and lids. In the immediate postoperative period, check the client's visual acuity with a near-vision card every hour to monitor the possibility of pressure on the optic nerve (see Thinking Critically). Caution the client to modify normal activities for the first 2 weeks after surgery.**

SAFETY

ALERT

RHEUMATOID AND CONNECTIVE TISSUE DISORDERS

Sjögren's syndrome includes keratoconjunctivitis sicca, a common condition in which tear secretion is reduced in association with a systemic disorder such as rheumatoid arthritis, psoriatic arthritis, connective tissue disorders, sarcoidosis, or Crohn's disease. Manifestations include ocular irritation and foreign-body sensation. Frequent instillation of lubricating eyedrops or ointment is effective in most cases.

Several ocular problems may be associated with systemic lupus erythematosus (SLE), a connective tissue disorder. The eyelids may be involved, with the discoid lesions characteristic of the disease. Punctate epithelial keratopathy and secondary Sjögren's syndrome may also occur. Retinopathy of SLE produces cotton-wool spots and increased retinal vessel fragility, as in diabetes. Optic neuropathy can also occur.

NEUROLOGIC DISORDERS

About 90% of clients with myasthenia gravis have ocular involvement. In most cases it is the presenting manifestation. *Ptosis* (drooping of the eyelid) is bilateral but may be asymmetrical. Diplopia is frequently in the vertical plane. Nystagmus is also present. Ocular myopathy and cranial nerve palsy may develop later, as may ophthalmoplegia (paralysis of all extraocular muscles). Medical treatment is supportive and includes systemic steroids.

There is also a close association between optic neuritis and multiple sclerosis. About three fourths of women and one third of men with optic neuritis have multiple sclerosis at 15-year follow-up. Typically an attack of optic neuritis starts with acute onset of loss of vision in one eye, with periocular discomfort made worse by movement of the eye. Visual impairment is progressive over 2 weeks and usually resolves after 4 to 6 weeks. Recovery may take longer and may be incomplete. Medical treatment consists of oral, IV, and retrobulbar steroids.

CIRCULATORY DISORDERS

The primary response of retinal arterioles to hypertension is a narrowing. In clients with chronic hypertension, the blood-retina barrier is disrupted in small areas, resulting in increased vascular permeability. Funduscopic examination reveals vasoconstriction, leakage, and arteriosclerosis. Hypertensive retinopathy is graded for severity on a scale of 1 to 4, with 4 the most severe. Systemic hypertension is also associated with an increased risk of retinal vein occlusion. There is no known treatment for retinal vein occlusion.

LYME DISEASE

Lyme disease *(Borrelia burgdorferi),* transmitted by the bite of a tick, consists of three stages. The initial stage involves a lesion and erythema around the bite, accompanied by regional lymphadenopathy, malaise, fever, headache, myalgia, arthralgia, and frequently conjunctivitis. Several weeks to months later, the second phase is associated with neurologic and cardiac problems. Along with these problems, there may be cranial nerve palsies, uveitis, optic neuropathy, keratitis, choroiditis, and exudative retinal detachments. Rheumatologic complications may develop in the third stage, which may occur over several years. Tetracycline and penicillin are effective in treating the initial infection and in preventing late complications.

CONCLUSIONS

To provide comprehensive nursing care for clients, it is essential to understand the complexity of ocular structures and the physiology of vision. The specialty practice of ophthalmic nursing is devoted to caring for clients with eye disorders. Ophthalmic registered nurses perform the roles of caregiver, advocate, educator, counselor, technician, coordinator, and researcher. Ophthalmic nursing care not only is directed at those biologic systems that are affected by an actual or potential deficit but also is

an integration of how actual or potential visual deficits affect the individual as an entire being.

THINKING CRITICALLY

1. Your client is a 72-year-old retired carpenter who has undergone outpatient cataract surgery. He and his wife live an hour away from the surgery center, where they received instructions to call the emergency number if any unusual pain or nausea occurs. They have an appointment to return for a follow-up evaluation the next morning. After supper the client's wife calls to report that her husband has a headache. She says that her husband also has an upset stomach, but she thinks he feels queasy because he ate some spicy food. The client does not want his wife to drive him back at night and thinks she should not have bothered to call because they have an appointment in the morning. How would you proceed? What further assessment data are needed? What are the likely complications following cataract surgery, and what are their clinical manifestations?

Factors to Consider. Might the headache and upset stomach be related to the cataract surgery, or are they likely to be unrelated?

2. Your client, a 55-year-old woman with Graves' ophthalmopathy, has undergone surgery in the late afternoon today for a right orbital decompression. An incisional drain is in place at the right temple with a bulb attached for suction. The surgeon has ordered postoperative vision checks with a near-vision card every hour throughout the night. The surgery lasted more than 3 hours; general anesthesia was used, and the client is still sedated. Her right eye is extremely swollen; she is unable to open it to read the vision card. She winces and cries when her operative eye is touched, and she is so sleepy that she cannot respond by reading the vision card. What should you do to carry out the surgeon's postoperative orders?

Factors to Consider. Are such severe eye pain and swelling normal postoperative findings? How would you assess the eye? How would you rouse the client to perform these crucial eye assessments?

Discussions for these questions can be found on the website.

BIBLIOGRAPHY

Citations appearing in red refer to primary research.

Citations appearing in blue refer to evidence-based practice guidelines and protocols.

1. Age Related Eye Disease Study. (2001). Age-related eye disease study: A randomized, placebo-controlled clinical trial for high dose supplementation with vitamins C, E, and beta carotene for AMD and vision loss. *Archives of Ophthalmology*, 119(10), 1417-1436.
2. Banerjee, S. (2006). A review of developments in the management of retinal diseases. *Journal of the Royal Society of Medicine*, 99(3), 125-127.
3. Evans, J.R. (2006) Antioxidant vitamin and mineral supplements for slowing the progression of age-related macular degeneration. *Cochrane Database of Systematic Reviews* 2006, 19(2), CD000254 DOI: 10.1002/14651858.CD000254.pub2.

4. Garvican, L., Cloves, J., & Gillow, T. (2000). Preservation of sight in diabetes: Developing a national risk reduction program. *Diabetic Medicine, 17*(9), 627-634.

5. Goldblum, K. (Ed.) (2007). *Ophthalmic nursing core curriculum.* Dubuque, Iowa: Kendall Publishing.

6. Greenlee, E.C. (2005). Laser and surgical treatment for glaucoma: An overview. *Insight, 30*(4), 32-37.

7. Halle, C. (2002). Achieve new vision screening objectives. *Nurse Practitioner, 27*(3), 21-22, 25–26.

8. Kanski, J. (1999). *Clinical ophthalmology* (4th ed.). Oxford: Butterworth Heinemann.

9. Smith, S.C., Lamp, P., & Liu, J. (2005). Age-related macular degeneration: Answers to some common questions. *Insight, 30*(3), 17-21.

10. Smith, S. (2001). The dry eye: An introduction. *Plastic Surgical Nursing, 21*(3), 135-140.

11. Subramanian, M.L., & Topping, T.M. (2004). Controversies in the management of primary retinal detachments. *Ophthalmology Clinic 2004, 44*(4), 103-114.

12. Ticho, B.H., & Dreger, V. (2000). Enucleation: Indications, methods and prosthetic devices. *Insight, 25*(1), 23-27.

13. Vaughan, D., Asbury, T., & Riordan-Eva, P. (2004). *General ophthalmology* (16th ed.). Norwalk, Conn: Appleton & Lange.

14. Watkinson, S., & Chetram, N. (2005). A nurse-led approach to diabetic retinal screening. *Nursing Times, 101*(36), 32-34.

15. Whitaker, R., & Whitaker, V. (1999). Glaucoma: What the ophthalmic nurse should know. *Insight, 24*(3), 86.

evolve *Did you remember to check out the bonus material on the Evolve website and the CD-ROM, including NCLEX®-Examination Style Review Questions, Open-Book Quizzes, and Chapter Review Audio Podcasts?*

http://evolve.elsevier.com/Black/medsurg

CHAPTER 66

Management of Clients with Hearing and Balance Disorders

HELENE J. KROUSE

HEARING IMPAIRMENT

Hearing impairment ranges from minor difficulty in understanding words or hearing certain sounds to total deafness. Hearing impairment is the nation's primary disability: 1 in 15 Americans is affected. By the year 2050, about 1 in 5 people in the United States will be 55 years or older; of these estimated 58 million people, 26 million are expected to have hearing impairment. Of the 10 million people in the United States with a hearing loss who are now 65 years or older, more than 90% have a sensorineural hearing loss. Because of fear, misinformation, lack of information, and vanity, many people do not admit that they have a hearing problem. Up to 80% of all hearing impairments are caused by hearing nerve disorders, for which no cure is currently available. Hearing impairments diminish the quality of life for one third of adults between 65 and 75 years of age.

Etiology and Risk Factors

Many factors influence the type and amount of hearing loss. Hearing loss is not an actual disorder but is a clinical manifestation of many possible problems. Both common and uncommon causes of hearing impairment are examined in this chapter. Hearing loss can be classified into three main areas:

- Conductive hearing loss (i.e., otosclerosis, trauma)
- Sensorineural hearing loss (i.e., presbycusis, noise-induced, and sudden hearing loss)
- Mixed hearing loss

Conductive hearing loss results from interference of sound transmission through the external ear and middle ear. It may be caused by (1) anything that blocks the external ear, such as wax, infection, or a foreign body; (2) thickening, retraction, scarring, or perforation of the tympanic membrane; or (3) any pathophysiologic changes in the middle ear that affect or freeze one or more of the ossicles (Figure 66-1).

Sensorineural hearing loss is caused by impairment of the function of the inner ear, the eighth cranial nerve, or the brain. Causes are congenital and hereditary factors, noise injury, aging and degenerative processes, Ménière's disease, and ototoxicity. Systemic disorders, such as autoimmune disease, syphilis, certain collagen disorders, and diabetes, may cause sensorineural hearing losses. Cigarette smoking and exposure to environmental tobacco smoke have been associated with age-related hearing loss. Many medications can be ototoxic; see the Integrating Pharmacology feature, p. 1721.

In a *mixed hearing loss,* conductive and sensorineural hearing components are present simultaneously. A client with a perforated eardrum and presbycusis has both conductive and sensorineural hearing losses.

Conductive Hearing Loss

Ear Obstructions

Obstruction of the ear is most commonly caused by impacted cerumen (wax). Although the ear canal is self-cleaning, cerumen may become impacted from a disorder or from improper cleaning. Older people are more susceptible to cerumen impaction because hair in the ear becomes coarser with age and traps the wax. Some people produce more cerumen in the ear canal

---

evolve **Web Enhancements**

Care Plan   The Client with Vertigo

Client Education Guide   Infection of the Tympanic Membrane, Middle Ear, or Mastoid Cavity (English Version and Spanish Translation)

Precautions After Ear Surgery (Spanish Translation)

Be sure to check out the bonus material on the Evolve website and the CD-ROM, including free self-assessment exercises. **http://evolve.elsevier.com/Black/medsurg**

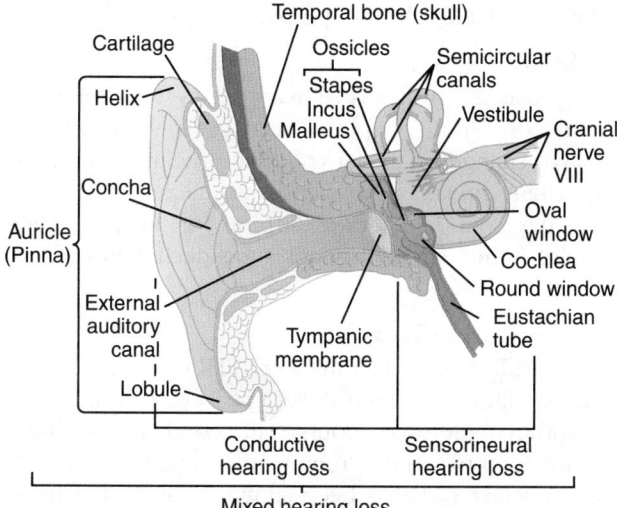

■ **FIGURE 66–1** Hearing loss can result from three causes. Conductive hearing loss occurs in areas of the outer ear when sound is conducted. Sensorineural hearing loss occurs in the inner ear where sound is transmitted by the nerves. In addition, both types can be present, called mixed hearing loss.

and require a regular routine for eliminating excessive buildup of wax in the ear canal. Insertion of cotton-tipped swabs into the ear canal can create further impaction of ear wax or can even traumatize the ear canal or perforate the eardrum.

Ear obstruction can also be caused by a wide array of foreign bodies that fit into the ear canal and impede conduction of sound waves. The most common foreign bodies found in the adult ear are pieces of cotton (such as cotton swabs) and insects. Foreign bodies commonly seen in children consist of small toys, beads, insects, and food, such as kernels of corn.

Infection

Many infections can lead to hearing loss. An infection of the inner ear, called *labyrinthitis,* can be either viral or bacterial in origin. Viral labyrinthitis can be associated with recent respiratory tract infections, measles, mumps, or rubella. Bacterial labyrinthitis, which is rare, is associated with otitis media or meningitis. Otitis media is a common disorder of the middle ear. Repeated infections or allergic inflammation can lead to fluid accumulation

---

INTEGRATING PHARMACOLOGY

Ototoxic Medications

Ototoxic medications are those drugs that have the potential to cause damage to the inner ear structures that may result in temporary or permanent loss of hearing or an aggravation of an existing sensorineural hearing loss. As a result of using ototoxic medications, the degree of hearing loss that occurs and the amount of recovery that follows depend upon the amount and duration of the use of that particular medication. A client receiving more than one ototoxic medication is even more vulnerable to developing a sensorineural hearing loss or aggravating an existing sensorineural hearing loss.

With high peak plasma concentrations, the aminoglycosides diffuse into the perilymph where their half-lives are five to six times longer than those in plasma. Diffusion out of the perilymph is enhanced when a low trough level occurs. Ototoxicity occurs because of hair cell destruction. They usually affect the sensory cells in the basal turn of the cochlea, first producing a high-frequency sensorineural hearing loss that can progress to involve the middle and lower frequencies. It is thought that aminoglycosides cause an imbalance in the ionic equilibrium of the inner ear by interfering with active transport systems. Damage can occur following a single administration of these drugs or after repeated doses. Clients who receive these medications must be monitored with peak and trough serum concentrations assessed for therapeutic and safe levels. The risk of ototoxicity is increased when more than one ototoxic medication is given.

Diuretics alter the electrolyte composition of the endolymph of the inner ear. Chemotherapeutic medications produce

permanent hearing loss. Cisplatin is a common cancer treatment and, unfortunately, it is cochleotoxic. The toxicity of cisplatin is synergistic with gentamicin, and high doses of cisplatin have been reported to cause total deafness. The other medications listed here produce transient hearing loss or tinnitus and some produce permanent hearing loss.

Ototoxic medications include these groups of medications.

Aminoglycoside antibiotics	Gentamicin, kanamycin, neomycin, streptomycin, tobramycin, amikacin
Antibiotics	Vancomycin, erythromycin, polymyxin B, polymyxin E, minocycline, chloramphenicol, Biaxin, Zithromax
Diuretics (loop)	Furosemide (Lasix), bumetanide (Bumex), ethacrynic acid (Edecrin)
Diuretics (osmotic)	Mannitol, acetazolamide
Analgesics/antipyretics/ NSAIDs and antimalarial drugs	Salicylates (aspirin compounds) Advil, Aleve, Anaprox, Clinoril, Feldene, Indocin, Lodine, Motrin, Nalfon, Naprosyn, Nuprin, Toradol, Voltaren, quinine, chloroquine
Antineoplastic drugs	Cisplatin, nitrogen mustard, vincristine, bleomycin
Miscellaneous	Alcohol, atropine, barbiturates, caffeine, ergot, gold, lidocaine, nicotine

behind the eardrum, causing dampening of the sound being conducted to the inner ear. In addition, drainage, perforation, or scarring of the tympanic membrane can result in a conductive hearing loss. Otitis media and other infectious ear processes are discussed later in the chapter under Otalgia.

Otosclerosis

Otosclerosis is a genetic disorder in which repeated resorption and redeposition of abnormal bone gradually leads to fixation of the footplate of the stapes in the oval window (Figure 66-2, *A*). The immobility of the footplate prevents transmission of sound vibration into the inner ear, leading to conductive hearing loss. This disorder occurs twice as often in women and is 10 times more prevalent in whites. The disorder is autosomally dominant with variable penetrance and therefore can be transmitted to offspring if only one parent has the disorder.

Tympanosclerosis

Tympanosclerosis is the result of repeated infection and trauma to the tympanic membrane. It consists of a deposit of collagen and calcium within the middle ear that can harden around the ossicles, causing a conductive hearing loss. Tympanosclerotic deposits can also be found mounded in the middle ear or as plaque on the tympanic membrane.

Trauma to the Tympanic Membrane

The tympanic membrane can be damaged by trauma. Increased pressure from a hand slap, falling in water, sports injuries, cleaning the ear with a sharp instrument, and industrial accidents involving welding sparks can rupture the thin membrane. Trauma to the tympanic membrane from a blast or blunt injury can involve the middle ear, causing a fracture or dislocation of the ossicles and tearing of the tympanic membrane. When the tympanic membrane is perforated, infection is a concern.

Sensorineural Hearing Loss

Presbycusis

Presbycusis is a progressive hearing loss found predominantly in older people. This degenerative process involves changes in the labyrinthine structures over time. The client initially experiences a decrease in high-frequency sound. At times, *tinnitus,* or the perception of noise in the ear, accompanies this decline in hearing.

Sudden Hearing Loss

Sudden (idiopathic) hearing loss (SHL) is a fairly common condition in which the client loses hearing in an ear within minutes or hours. This condition is almost exclusively unilateral. Prompt early intervention with oral corticosteroids has been shown to at least partially restore the lost hearing in many clients with sudden hearing loss.

Sensorineural hearing loss of abrupt onset can sometimes occur from discrete causes. Some of these specific causes are (1) rapid infectious processes, such as meningitis or mumps; (2) ototoxic agents; (3) trauma; (4) metabolic disturbances; and (5) immunologic disorders. In most cases of SHL, however, no specific cause is found.

Hearing Loss

Congenital episodes of sensorineural hearing loss are not uncommon. These losses can be severe and present at birth or can develop during childhood or early adulthood and gradually worsen with time. Congenital hearing loss often results in total deafness. It can occur either in a genetic pattern within families or spontaneously. Both autosomal-recessive and autosomal-dominant methods of transmission have been documented. In milder cases of congenital hearing loss, the individual may not be aware of a loss until hearing is screened for work or school. In families with a history of congenital hearing loss, infant screening is essential to allow early detection of the problem and rehabilitation of congenitally deaf infants.

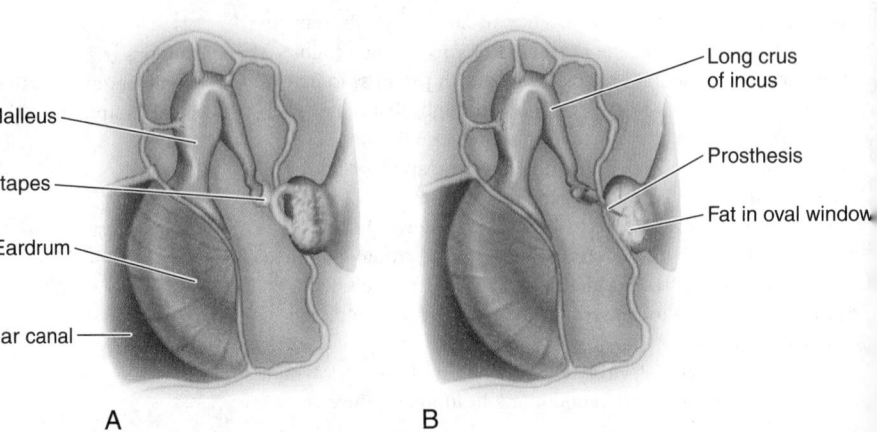

■ **FIGURE 66–2 A,** Stapedial otosclerosis. A chain of three ossicles connects the tympanic membrane to the oval window and cochlea. Otosclerosis knits the bone of the middle ear to the stapes, preventing sound transmission from the eardrum to the middle ear. **B,** Stapedectomy removes the ankylosed bone and replaces it.

Malleus

Stapes

Eardrum

Ear canal

Long crus of incus

Prosthesis

Fat in oval window

A

B

Noise-Induced Hearing Loss

Noise-induced hearing loss is a specific type of sensorineural hearing loss that most often occurs over time from repeated acoustic trauma from loud noise. The major causes are industrial noise, the use of firearms, and listening to loud music. Traumatic injury associated with a sudden loud noise, such as a blast, can also result in noise-induced hearing loss.

Benign and Malignant Tumors

Both benign and malignant tumors of the temporal bone can involve the inner ear and lead to sensorineural hearing loss. The most common benign tumor is an acoustic neuroma or schwannoma of the eighth cranial nerve. The tumor usually develops in the internal auditory canal, the bony channel through which the vestibular nerve passes as it leaves the inner ear. The tumor presses on the nerve, which then sends false signals to the brain. If the vestibular portion of the nerve is compressed, the client is unable to interpret stimuli about position and movement. If the cochlear branch is compressed, the client experiences tinnitus. The first clinical manifestation is often partial or complete sensorineural hearing loss followed by tinnitus. The client may also report dizziness.

Other tumors in the cerebellopontine angle likewise involve the seventh and eighth cranial nerves as they enter the internal acoustic meatus. Malignant tumors invade the entire inner ear, usually spreading from the middle ear and mastoid system.

Ménière's Disease

Ménière's disease is a disorder that affects both vestibular and auditory function. It is caused by excess endolymph (intracellular fluid in the membranous labyrinth of the inner ear) in the vestibular and semicircular canals. Hearing loss is fluctuant and usually subtle and reversible in the early stages. Later the hearing loss becomes permanent. Although Ménière's disease is associated with sensorineural hearing loss, the most prominent clinical manifestation is *vertigo* (feeling that the surroundings or one's own body is revolving). Therefore it is fully discussed in the section Balance Disorders.

Central Auditory Dysfunction

Central auditory dysfunction is a phenomenon whereby the central nervous system (CNS) cannot interpret normal auditory signals. Central auditory dysfunction, also known as *central deafness,* is a rare form of sensorineural hearing loss. Diseases that alter the CNS, such as strokes and tumors, can cause central deafness.

Mixed Hearing Loss

Some causes of hearing impairment can result in both sensorineural and conductive hearing losses. These types of losses are referred to as *mixed hearing loss.* Clients with mixed hearing loss present with clinical manifestations associated with both sensorineural and conductive hearing losses.

Pathophysiology

Conductive hearing loss is the result of interference of sound transmission into and through the external ear and middle ear. The inner ear is not affected in a pure conductive loss; therefore sound transmission from the inner ear to the brain is normal. Normal movement of sound vibrations through the ear canal, tympanic membrane, or ossicles is impeded because of the nature of the disease process involved in the conductive loss. Sound is perceived as faint or distant, but it remains relatively clear. Most conductive hearing losses are correctable by medical or surgical treatment.

Sensorineural hearing loss, however, results from disease or trauma to the organ of Corti or auditory nerve pathways of the inner ear leading to the brain stem. Normal reception and transmission of sound waves are disrupted. Sound is distorted and faint. Sensorineural hearing losses are usually permanent and are generally not correctable by medical or surgical treatment.

Clinical Manifestations

Most hearing loss is gradual and goes unnoticed by the client until several incidents of communication problems have occurred. Significant others and co-workers are usually aware of the client's hearing problem long before the client realizes or admits to the problem. Box 66-1 lists the manifestations of hearing loss.

The hearing impaired or "hard-of-hearing" client may repeat the information, even incorrectly, or may ask for clarification. Clients with a hearing loss can also experience distorted or abnormal sounds. Sometimes a sound is heard at different pitches for each ear; this is called *diplacusis.* A sound may cause a rapid increase in loudness; this is called *recruitment.* These abnormal sounds can cause discomfort.

BOX 66-1 Manifestations of Hearing Loss

- Failure to respond to oral communication
- Frequently asking others to repeat statements
- Inappropriate response to oral communication
- Failing to respond when not looking in the direction of the sound
- Excessively loud speech
- Abnormal awareness of sounds
- Strained facial expressions
- Tilting of head when listening
- Faulty speech articulation
- Listening to radio and television at increased volume
- Avoiding crowds and better understanding of speech when in small groups

The onset of a conductive hearing loss can be sudden or progressive. In cases of fluid in the middle ear, hearing loss is often bilateral but is usually restored with medical or surgical treatment. In other conductive processes, such as otosclerosis, clinical manifestations consist of slow progressive hearing loss with changes noted even in adolescence. Hearing loss is usually bilateral but may be asymmetrical. Other manifestations are mild tinnitus, recurrent vertigo, and postural imbalance. It is common for the client to speak in a soft voice.

If damage to the tympanic membrane is suspected, such as perforation, examination of the client may reveal a conductive hearing loss and serous drainage in the ear canal. The hearing loss found with a total perforation of the eardrum is approximately 35 dB (one third of the hearing range). With small perforations, no loss may be present. If a perforation is present, damage to the ossicles should be suspected. Diagnostic findings of conductive hearing loss include greater bone conduction than air conduction on the Rinne test. If hearing loss is greater in one ear, Weber's test shows lateralization to the more affected ear. Pure-tone audiometry confirms hearing loss. *Speech discrimination* (understanding of words) is usually maintained.

Noise-induced hearing loss is characterized by a greater loss in the higher frequencies. Sudden or fluctuating hearing losses are recognized as separate disorders from routine sensorineural hearing loss. Although fluctuating losses usually suggest syphilis or Ménière's disease, sudden sensorineural hearing losses are believed to be viral in origin. Recognition of these patterns is important because medical treatment of such disorders can result in significant improvements in hearing. A characteristic of a severe hearing loss is loss of discrimination. To some clients, a hearing loss feels like a blockage or fullness in the ear or an inability to distinguish the direction of sounds.

Tinnitus accompanies most sensorineural hearing losses and is annoying. *Tinnitus* literally means "ringing" but can actually sound like roaring, the chirping of crickets, or occasionally music. Tinnitus is not a disease but a distressing manifestation, and it is sometimes a warning sign of hearing loss or other, more serious problems. Ear noise that cannot be heard by an observer is classified as *subjective tinnitus,* which is the most common kind. Any ear noise that can be heard by someone other than the client is called *objective tinnitus.* In some clients the tinnitus becomes the problem, and the underlying cause may be forgotten.

The major nursing responsibility in a client with tinnitus is to perform a thorough history and assessment of the onset, frequency, constancy, and level of intensity of the tinnitus. Unilateral tinnitus merits a complete neuro-otologic evaluation with the goal of ruling out the possibility of a tumor, most likely an acoustic neuroma. The nurse must keep in mind that tinnitus is a manifestation of an underlying pathologic process that warrants further referral.

Table 66-1 presents the clinical manifestations of conductive and sensorineural hearing losses. Diagnostic measures include (1) testing for hearing of pure tones on audiometry, (2) speech reception and discrimination, (3) tympanometry, and sometimes (4) brain stem auditory evoked responses. Tones are presented using earphones (air conduction) and vibrators (bone conduction). The minimal level at which the client can hear is determined. The *speech reception threshold* is the lowest intensity at which the client can correctly repeat 50% of the words presented. The speech discrimination test is a measure of the client's ability to understand speech when it is presented at a volume that is easily heard.

OUTCOME MANAGEMENT

Medical Management

All health providers should teach clients how to prevent hearing loss and should screen for hearing loss in high-risk groups (Box 66-2). The goals for medical management of the client with hearing impairment are to (1) restore hearing, (2) assist hearing, (3) manage tinnitus, and (4) implement aural rehabilitation.

Restore Hearing

Hearing loss that results from blockage or fullness in the ear associated with an infectious process may be restored to normal with administration of antibiotics for bacterial infections. In the case of sudden hearing loss, prompt administration of oral corticosteroids is used in an attempt to lessen the progressive hearing loss or to reverse a sudden loss. Antiviral medications have been advocated for sudden sensorineural hearing loss, although they have not been shown in clinical trials to be of additional benefit. If ototoxicity is suspected, all ototoxic medications are discontinued.

TABLE 66–1 Clinical Manifestations of Conductive and Sensorineural Hearing Losses

	Conductive Hearing Loss	Sensorineural Hearing Loss
Voice quality	Soft voice	Loud voice
Effect of environmental noise on hearing	Hearing improved	Hearing made worse
Speech discrimination	Good	Poor
Ability to hear on telephone	Good	Poor
Lateralization on Weber's test	To diseased ear	To normal ear
Result of Rinne test	Negative, AC < BC	Positive, AC > BC

AC, Air conduction; *BC,* bone conduction.

BOX 66-2   Hearing Impairment: Prevention and Screening

Identification of clients at risk for hearing loss and adequate protection of the ears are important to maintain normal function.

PRIMARY PREVENTION

- Avoid ototoxic drugs.
- Recognize and treat infectious diseases such as meningitis, mumps, and measles.
- Wear protective headgear or helmets when participating in sports.
- Avoid insertion of hard instruments or objects into the ear canal.
- Wear earplugs and avoid prolonged exposure to noise levels in excess of 80 decibels (dB).

SECONDARY PREVENTION

- Perform hearing screenings in children and adults 65 years and older.
- Monitor blood levels of medications with ototoxic side effects, observing for vertigo, lessened hearing acuity, and tinnitus.

TERTIARY PREVENTION

- Encourage hearing-impaired clients to attend rehabilitation programs.
- Teach the proper use and care of hearing aids.
- Encourage family to continue to communicate with the hearing impaired.

Assist Hearing

Unfortunately, most hearing losses are permanent, and hearing cannot be restored. The use of hearing aids and assistive listening devices can greatly improve the client's ability to communicate and interact with others. Hearing aids amplify sound in a controlled manner. They are used by both *hearing-impaired* clients (those with slight or moderate hearing loss) and *deaf* clients (those with severe or profound hearing loss). Hearing aids make sound louder but do not improve the quality of sound. Therefore clients with decreased discrimination benefit less from a hearing aid. The hearing aid amplifies all background noises, such as hospital machinery, background conversation in restaurants, footsteps, and department store noises, as well as speech. These noises may mask conversation or confuse the hearing-impaired client, especially older adults.

A client should undergo a trial period before purchasing a hearing aid to see whether he or she can adapt to its use. In fact, in most states, such a trial period is mandatory. Bilateral (binaural) aids may be desirable. Hearing aids can be worn in the following locations: in the ear, in the ear canal, behind the ear (postauricular), in eyeglasses, and in the middle of the chest (body-worn aid).

Regardless of type, the hearing aid consists of four parts. The microphone receives sound waves from the air and changes sounds into electrical signals. The amplifier increases the strength of electrical signals. The receiver (loudspeaker) changes the electrical signals into sound waves, and the battery provides the electrical energy needed to operate the hearing aid. On all types of hearing aids except the body-worn type, all four components are housed in one small case. The louder sounds are then directed into the ear through a custom-molded earpiece.

The evolution in hearing aid design has led to smaller and more effective aids. Small hearing aids are available that fit into the ear canal. The latest advancements in hearing aids are digital processing and directional microphones, which enhance the voice of a speaker in front of the client and suppress background noise. Programmable hearing aids allow the selection of various amplification patterns by the user and may have some added benefit for clients. Hearing aid technology continues to advance in improving the person's quality of life.

Assistive listening devices help the hearing-impaired client hear the television or radio as well as use the telephone. Stationary devices called *teletypewriters* and a portable instrument called a *telecommunication device for the deaf* (TDD) are used for telephone communication by the profoundly deaf. A flashing light signals the presence of a dial tone, a busy signal, or a ring. When another teletypewriter or TDD is reached, messages are typed and displayed on a screen or printed. Other devices, such as flashing lights that alert a deaf person to a ringing doorbell, alarm clock, or smoke alarm, are available. Hearing dogs are trained to be sensitive to certain noises, such as the telephone, doorbells, and crying children. On hearing the sound, a hearing dog moves back and forth between the client and the sound to alert the client.

Manage Tinnitus

Tinnitus can be a distressing disorder associated with sensorineural hearing loss. Many approaches have been tried to alleviate this problem, including biofeedback, electrostimulation, hypnosis, medication, hearing aids, and tinnitus maskers. They have all met with minimal success. Tinnitus maskers appear similar to hearing aids except that they generate noise. The tinnitus masker is of benefit only while it is being used. Every approach for relief from tinnitus is only moderately successful, at best. Clients should be counseled to avoid unproved treatments for tinnitus. The nurse and the client's family must be alert to manifestations of depression if the tinnitus is chronic. The quality of the spouse's support of the client with tinnitus has been shown to be strongly correlated with role function. In addition, the nurse should be alert to spousal interaction and should facilitate problem-solving as needed.

Implement Aural Rehabilitation

Aural rehabilitation may improve communication if (1) hearing loss is irreversible or is not amenable to surgical intervention or (2) the client elects not to have surgery. The purpose of aural rehabilitation is to maximize the hearing-impaired client's communication skills.

Hearing is one of our primary modes of communication. Rehabilitation is directed toward teaching the client to use the other senses more effectively, those of vision, touch, and vibration, and to maximize the use of any remaining hearing ability. The outcome of rehabilitation is affected by all demographic variables and the severity of impairment. As with other forms of rehabilitation, success depends partly on the client's level of motivation.

Speech reading, the current term used for lip reading, is an important means of communication. Speech reading is the process of understanding vocal communication by the integration of lip movements with facial expressions, gestures, environmental clues, and conversation contexts. Speech reading is difficult without auditory cues for several reasons. Many movements for speech are rapid, many sounds are similar (*b, m, p*), and the production of certain sounds in any language is not visible. The hearing-impaired client must guess at a high percentage of words. Knowledge of this fact alone helps the nurse be more understanding of the client who is using this communication approach.

Because of reduced auditory feedback (the inability of hearing-impaired clients to monitor their own speech), the clearness, pitch quality, or rate of the client's speech may deteriorate. These changes may alter the efficiency of communication and reduce the intelligibility of speech. The goal of speech training is to conserve, develop, or prevent deterioration of speech skills.

Last, but still important, is sign language. Sign language allows communication by hand signals that represent different letters of the alphabet, words, and phrases.

Nursing Management of the Medical Client

Assessment. The client's ability to communicate may be informally assessed during the history. The nurse should assess the client's ability to follow conversation. During the interview, the nurse should look for answers to the following questions:

1. Does the client admit to having a hearing loss and difficulty communicating, or does the client blame other people for not speaking clearly?
2. In what settings does the client have more problems with hearing or communicating?
3. Are family members, co-workers, and friends aware of the hearing problem? Are they supportive of the client, making communication easier and including the client in conversation? Do others feel frustrated or angry when the client cannot hear correctly or

does not respond? Does the client feel left out or embarrassed?
4. Does the client try to understand spoken words? Or does the client withdraw or refuse to participate, letting others do the talking?
5. Does the client wear a hearing aid? Does it appear to work?

Occasionally, laboratory, radiologic, and vestibular examinations are used for assessment. In an otology office, the nurse may have the responsibility of performing the history, otologic examination, and screening audiometry. The history is often the most important part of the clinical assessment, as previously described (see Chapter 64, Box 64-4). The extent of assessment of the sensorineural hearing loss depends on the setting and the nurse's educational preparation and experience. Nurses should be able to inspect the outer ear and grossly assess auditory acuity.

Visualization of the ear canal and tympanic membrane is accomplished with the otoscope. Cerumen in the canal or on the eardrum can interfere with the examination and may need to be removed. The blind removal of ear wax with an ear syringe should be performed only if the ear is free of other abnormalities, such as an infection or perforation of the eardrum.

Impacted accumulations of ear wax may be softened and loosened for removal by alternating instillations of glycerin and hydrogen peroxide eardrops. The eardrops are warmed to body temperature and used daily as directed for 1 to 2 weeks. The ear is then irrigated gently with warm water for removal of the softened wax or cleaned under magnification with a cerumen spoon. Wax on the tympanic membrane should be removed by an otolaryngologist or an advanced-practice nurse in otorhinolaryngology.

Diagnosis, Outcomes, Interventions

Diagnosis: Impaired Verbal Communication. Clients who have lost their ability to hear are best described with the nursing diagnosis *Impaired Verbal Communication related to effects of hearing loss.*

Outcomes. The client will develop effective methods to communicate needs and will be included in conversation.

Interventions. When normal conversation is impossible, writing may be used successfully by clients who have good comprehension of English (or their primary language). Writing may cause frustration when the client's primary language is American Sign Language because it is grammatically different from standard English. Visual aids, such as pictures, diagrams, and models, may also improve the nurse's ability to explain medical terminology or procedures. An expert interpreter should be used when other attempts to communicate have failed or when speed and accuracy are critical. The National Registry of Interpreters for the Deaf (NRID) has loca-

chapters and offers certification for qualified individuals. Box 66-3 lists common nursing interventions to improve communication with hearing-impaired clients. They can apply to all clients, regardless of the type or severity of hearing loss.

Many hearing-impaired clients live in the community. Nurses may see these clients for their hearing problems or for many other problems. The Bridge to Home Health Care feature at right addresses approaches to home care of hearing-impaired clients.

Diagnosis: Ineffective Coping. The individual with a loss of hearing goes through the same stages of grieving as others experiencing a loss. Rehabilitation cannot begin until some acceptance of the hearing loss has taken place, leading to the nursing diagnosis *Ineffective Coping related to recent loss of hearing.*

BOX 66-3   Common Nursing Interventions for Hearing-Impaired Clients

- Get the client's attention by raising your arm or hand.
- Stand with a light on your face; this helps the client to speech-read.
- Talk directly to the client while facing him or her.
- Speak clearly, but do not overaccentuate words.
- Speak in a normal tone; do not shout. Shouting overuses normal speaking movements and so may cause distortion and may be too loud for the client with sensorineural damage. If the client has conductive loss only, it is sometimes helpful to make the voice louder without shouting.
- If the client does not seem to understand what is said, express it differently. Some words are difficult to "see" in speech reading, such as "white" and "red."
- Move closer to the client and toward the better-hearing ear.
- Write out proper names or any statement that you are not sure was understood.
- Do not smile, chew gum, or cover the mouth when talking.
- Remember that a client's inattention may indicate tiredness or lack of understanding.
- Use phrases rather than one-word answers to convey meaning. State the major topic of the discussion first, and then give details.
- Do not show annoyance by careless facial expressions. Clients who are hard of hearing depend more on visual clues for understanding.
- Encourage the use of a hearing aid if it is available; allow the client to adjust it before speaking.
- In a group, repeat important statements, and avoid making asides to others in the group.
- Avoid the use of the intercommunication system because this may distort sound and cause poor communication.
- Do not avoid conversation with a client who has hearing loss. It has been said that to live in a silent world is much more devastating than to live in darkness, and clients with hearing loss appear to have more emotional difficulties than do those who are blind.

 BRIDGE TO HOME HEALTH CARE

Living with a Severe Hearing Loss

People are often reluctant to admit that they have a hearing impairment. This reluctance results in difficulty with verbal communication, inability to follow instructions, and social isolation. To maximize communication, reduce background noise (turn off the television or radio), face the person, and speak clearly without shouting. Sometimes the only way to communicate is by writing. Develop written materials for repeated use. Include introduction materials (e.g., your name, your agency's name, the purpose of your visit), reportable problems, and treatment regimens.

In many cases, hearing loss is due to accumulation of cerumen. Use an otoscope to visualize the ear canal. If cerumen is present, a physician may need to remove it. If you are responsible for removing the cerumen, contact the physician to discuss a prescription for an ear irrigation solution, instill the solution, and evaluate the amount and color of drainage.

When people experience a hearing loss, they need a medical evaluation and a hearing aid evaluation. Many older adults are reluctant to wear a hearing aid for various reasons. It is a visual manifestation of an impairment, it is expensive, and it necessitates leaving home for evaluation, fitting, and follow-up appointments. If a client's reluctance is due to cosmetic reasons, show pictures of hearing aids and discuss individuals who wear hearing aids, such as former President George Bush. Newer hearing aids are available that are smaller, less noticeable, and more discreet.

If cost is a problem, consider a referral to a social worker to identify local resources. Currently Medicare pays for the cost of a hearing evaluation and little for the hearing aid; Medicaid usually pays for the hearing aid. Consider other financial resources, such as the American Association of Retired People and local hearing aid vendors. When leaving home is a problem, check whether a vendor will make a home visit. If this is not possible, suggest that the client use a head-set amplifier that can be purchased from a local electronics store.

Teaching is an important nursing intervention related to hearing impairment. It involves cleaning the devices and changing the batteries. Also, evaluate the client's ability to use the telephone and answer the door. Local telephone companies can equip the telephone with an adjustable volume control, hearing aid adapters, loud ringing signals, and a telecommunication device for the deaf (TDD). A TDD allows the hearing-impaired individual to communicate by typing information into a specially designed device. To receive information, the receiver must have a specific TDD telephone number. Teach the client with a TDD about TDD telephone numbers for an emergency response, and provide information about the home health agency and community resources.

It is important to involve informal caregivers, significant others, and family members in the management of a hearing impairment. Teach these people to maximize communication with a variety of techniques and adaptive equipment.

Outcomes. The client will discuss or will demonstrate problem-solving–based coping strategies, as evidenced by the following:

1. Taking the initiative to inform others of the hearing impairment and requesting that they assist with communication by using techniques that promote comprehension
2. Not experiencing feelings of embarrassment, frustration, or withdrawal
3. Not blaming others for failure to communicate effectively
4. Avoiding situations and environments, such as noisy areas, that impair hearing

Interventions. Work with the client and family on methods to enhance communication and thereby enhance coping. Encourage the client to role-play how he or she might tell people about the hearing impairment and indicate what techniques should be used to help hearing. Self-help groups, such as Self-help for Hard of Hearing People (SHHH), located in Bethesda, Maryland, can assist with resources, information, and support for clients and their families.

Diagnosis: Impaired Social Interaction. Clients with hearing losses can experience fears of inadequacy, feelings of inferiority, depression, and varying degrees of stress and isolation. The nursing diagnosis *Impaired Social Interaction related to perceived inability to interact with others secondary to hearing loss* can be used to guide interventions.

Outcomes. The client will exhibit a willingness to be involved in social situations as evidenced by (1) attempting to become a part of social events, (2) conversing with others, (3) indicating lessened feelings of inadequacy, and (4) responding appropriately to questions asked (not fabricating answers to cover hearing loss).

Interventions. The American Speech-Language Hearing Association (ASHA) urges that all clients with hearing impairments *not* be grouped into one category. Each client is unique and has an individual hearing problem. The nurse functions as a role model in accepting the client as an individual and demonstrating effective communication techniques.

Work with the client to enhance coping, encourage continued social involvement, and advocate the use of various organizations to their fullest extent. Many agencies and associations exist for the hearing-impaired client. Services are offered by audiology clinics and sponsored by universities, hospitals, community programs, state or local departments of health, the Department of Veterans Affairs (VA), and national organizations.

Diagnosis: Deficient Knowledge of Managing Hearing Loss. Clients with new hearing aids need information about their care and proper use. Therefore *Deficient Knowledge of managing hearing loss related to lack of previous exposure to a hearing aid* is an important nursing diagnosis.

Outcomes. The client will have greater knowledge about the hearing aid as evidenced by proper use and care of the aid.

Interventions. The hearing aid user should know how to care for the aid and what to do if the device does not work. Gain a basic knowledge of the hearing aid to help with insertion for clients who are ill. Encourage the client to use the hearing aid and to store it safely when not using it. Turn the device off before removal to prevent squealing feedback. The maintenance of a hearing aid is becoming less of a problem today. Usually the aid is returned to the dealer for factory repair while the client uses a "loaner" hearing aid. Unlicensed assistive personnel often care for clients with hearing aids. Delegation of care of the hearing aid and the hearing-impaired client is shown in the Management and Delegation feature on p. 1729.

Cost has been cited as a major factor in the non-use of hearing aids. Clients needing financial assistance should be referred to the state department of vocational rehabilitation, the local Lions Club, and, in some states, Medicaid.

Evaluation. A client with a new hearing loss or disorder needs frequent evaluation to determine the severity of hearing loss, coping strategies, and ability to communicate adequately. Because many forms of hearing loss are permanent or progressive, long-term evaluation should also be performed to be certain the client is adapting positively. Also determine whether the client has questions about the equipment used for hearing rehabilitation and the need for further education.

Surgical Management

Surgery is usually not warranted for sensorineural hearing loss; however, because mixed, conductive, and sensorineural hearing loss exists, surgery may be performed to (1) restore the conductive hearing loss, (2) remove a tumor, and (3) assist hearing in profoundly deaf people.

Restore Conductive Hearing Loss

The most common cause of conductive hearing loss is serous otitis media (see later discussion). Although most commonly seen in children, this disorder can occur at any age. In cases of serous otitis media and persistent conductive hearing loss that do not resolve after 2 to months of medical management, an incision into the tympanic membrane and evacuation of fluid can be performed with the client sedated using local or general anesthesia. This procedure, known as *myringotomy*, will restore hearing. It is discussed later in this chapter.

Hearing Aids

Caring for hearing aids and helping clients with maintenance of these devices may be delegated to unlicensed assistive personnel. Clients with new hearing aids need individualized teaching provided by you, the registered nurse. You are to evaluate the client's understanding of the instruction. Before delegating hearing aid care, consider the following issues:

The client's learning needs. Is this a new hearing aid? Does the client have a new hearing loss disorder? If so, you should instruct the client to care for these devices and provide consistent teaching.

The competency level of the unlicensed assistive personnel who will potentially perform hearing aid care. Unlicensed assistive personnel may not provide the initial instruction but may reinforce the instructions you have provided.

Instruct unlicensed assistive personnel caring for the client with a hearing aid to achieve the following:

- Encourage the use of hearing aids and independent care by clients without cognitive impairment.
- Provide safe storage of the hearing aids when not in use (in the client's personal case or another small storage device). If the client is hospitalized, ensure that the case is labeled with the client's name and location.
- Turn the device off when it is not in use. If the aid is to be off for a prolonged duration (such as during the night or sleeping hours), open the battery compartment to avoid additional drainage of battery power.
- Cleanse the ear mold with mild soap and water each day or as needed.
- Completely dry the ear mold before reconnecting it to the hearing aid.
- Help the client insert the ear mold into the ear. If the hearing aid makes a whistling noise, the device is not inserted properly into the ear. At this point, it may be necessary for you to assess more completely placement in the ear canal.
- Allow the client to adjust the volume before speaking.
- Speak clearly in a normal tone to the client. Do not shout.
- Turn off the device before removing it to prevent squealing "feedback."

If the hearing aid fails to work:

- Check the on-off switch.
- Inspect the ear mold for cleanliness.
- Examine the battery for correct insertion.
- Examine the cord plug for correct insertion.
- Examine the cord for breaks.
- Replace the battery, cord, or both, if necessary. The life of batteries varies according to the amount of use and power requirements of the aid. Batteries last 2 to 14 days.

Findings that are immediately reportable to you are (1) difficulty with placement in the ear, (2) redness or drainage in the ear, (3) mechanical failure of the device, and (4) other issues of concern to the client.

Another type of conductive hearing loss that can be treated medically or corrected surgically results from otosclerosis. Because speech discrimination is usually unimpaired, simple amplification of sound is quite effective. People who are at high risk of otosclerosis or who are not candidates for surgery can be given medications in an attempt to reduce the severity of the bony fusion. The clinical efficacy of medical therapy remains unsubstantiated.

Stapedectomy

Surgical intervention for otosclerosis has been very successful. *Stapedectomy* is a surgical procedure whereby the damaged stapes is removed and replaced with a stainless-steel, polytetrafluoroethylene (Teflon), or plastic prosthesis (see Figure 66-2, *B*). The oval window is grafted with absorbable gelatin sponge (Gelfoam) or tissue grafts. Stapedectomy was once a common middle ear procedure; however, the pool of clients with otosclerosis is dwindling, and today stapedectomy is performed less often.

The client must be free of otitis externa and otitis media before surgery. To reduce the risk of bleeding, the client should use no aspirin or products with aspirin for 1 week before surgery. Preoperative and postoperative audiograms and tympanograms are performed to test hearing acuity levels.

After surgery the client is often instructed to lie on the nonoperative ear with the head of the bed elevated. This position helps reduce edema and prevent dislodgment of the prosthesis. Antibiotics are prescribed. The packing in the ear canal should not be disturbed. On discharge from the hospital, the client is told to report the acute onset of vertigo. To reduce the risk of development of a perilymph fistula (rupture of the oval window, which permits leakage of perilymph fluid), the client should avoid excessive exercise, straining, and activities that might lead to head trauma. If the client needs to blow the nose, it should be done gently, one nostril at a time. The client should sneeze with the mouth open. No airplane travel is allowed for 1 month.

Hearing aids may still be required after stapedectomy, and the client's hearing will need to be reevaluated. Complications of the operation include granuloma formation and perilymph fistula. Either complication may result in profound deafness and persistent vertigo. Hearing loss may also develop after surgery from middle ear adhesions or shifting of the prosthesis.

Tumor Excision

Surgery and gamma knife radiotherapy are current treatments of acoustic neuroma. Current microsurgical techniques often allow preservation of hearing and usually enable resection of the tumor without injury to the facial nerve. In older clients, especially those with total deafness in the affected ear, a more conservative, non-surgical approach is sometimes taken because acoustic neuroma is benign and very slow growing.

Assist Hearing in Profound Deafness

Use of implantable hearing devices (IHDs) may be appropriate in certain clients. There are three types of IHDs: cochlear implants, temporal bone stimulators, and middle ear implants.

Cochlear Implants. Cochlear implants provide auditory sensation to clients with severe to profound sensorineural hearing loss who cannot benefit from a hearing aid (Figure 66-3). The cochlear implant contains a small computer that changes the spoken word to electrical impulses. The impulses are transmitted across the skin to an implanted coil that carries the impulse to the hearing nerve endings in the cochlea by means of an electrode introduced through the round window. The

most effective cochlear implants use multiple-frequency channels. In multichannel cochlear implants, up to 22 electrodes are inserted along the cochlear partition. The surgery for insertion of a cochlear implant is similar to mastoid surgery. The success of a cochlear implant varies widely, ranging from minimal improvement in auditory awareness to the ability to understand speech on the telephone. Preoperative vestibular testing is highly recommended for all clients in whom a cochlear implant is being considered.

Temporal Bone Stimulators (BAHA, Bone-Anchored Hearing Aid). In some cases of hearing loss, sound can be transmitted by applying stimulation directly to the temporal bone, thereby transmitting sound through the skull to the inner ear. For clients with a conductive hearing loss, a device is available in which the receiver is implanted under the skin into the skull. The external device transmits the sound through the skin. This device is worn above the ear rather than in the ear canal.

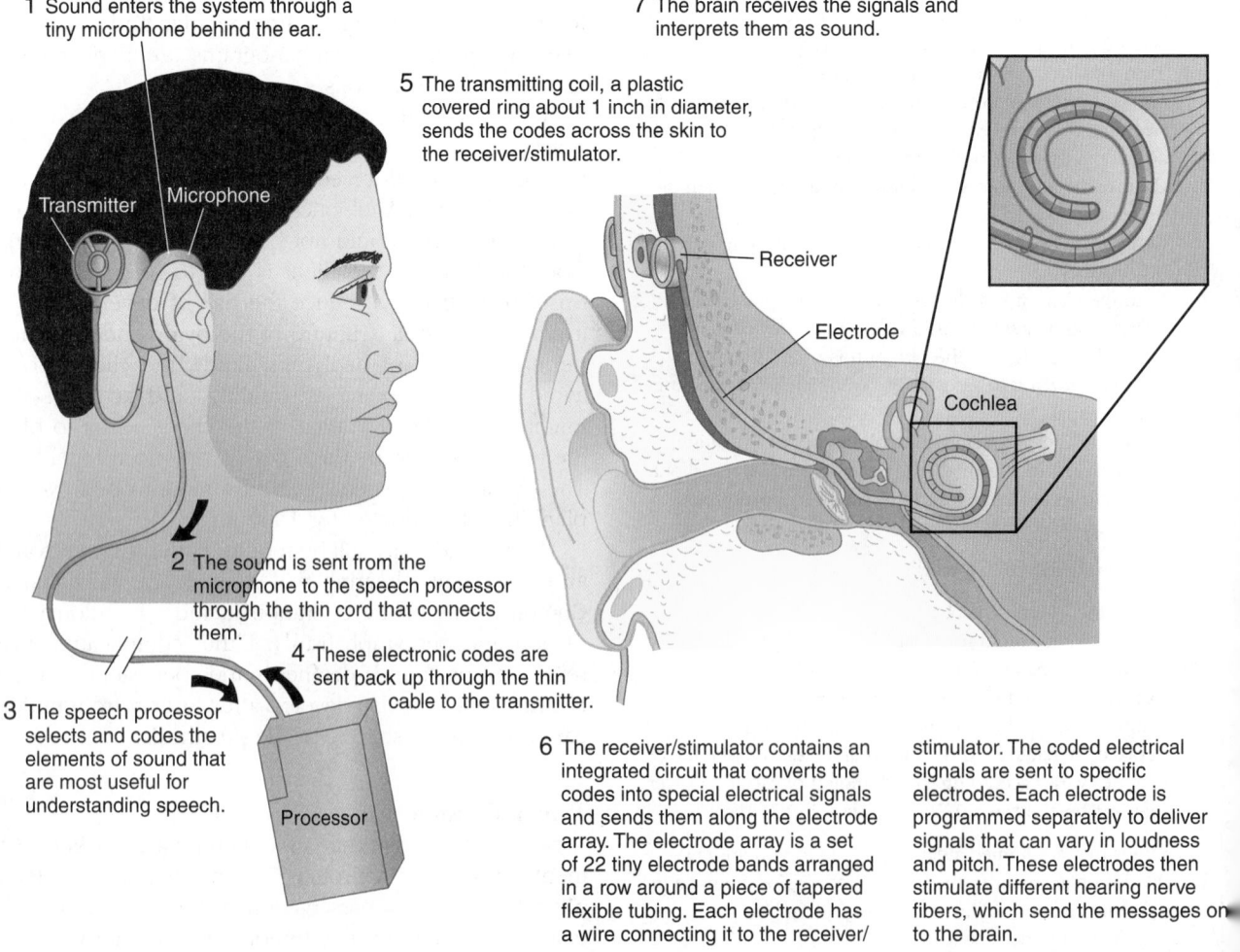

1 Sound enters the system through a tiny microphone behind the ear.

7 The brain receives the signals and interprets them as sound.

5 The transmitting coil, a plastic covered ring about 1 inch in diameter, sends the codes across the skin to the receiver/stimulator.

Transmitter Microphone

Receiver

Electrode

Cochlea

2 The sound is sent from the microphone to the speech processor through the thin cord that connects them.

4 These electronic codes are sent back up through the thin cable to the transmitter.

3 The speech processor selects and codes the elements of sound that are most useful for understanding speech.

Processor

6 The receiver/stimulator contains an integrated circuit that converts the codes into special electrical signals and sends them along the electrode array. The electrode array is a set of 22 tiny electrode bands arranged in a row around a piece of tapered flexible tubing. Each electrode has a wire connecting it to the receiver/

stimulator. The coded electrical signals are sent to specific electrodes. Each electrode is programmed separately to deliver signals that can vary in loudness and pitch. These electrodes then stimulate different hearing nerve fibers, which send the messages on to the brain.

■ **FIGURE 66–3** Cochlear implant to restore hearing.

Because some conductive hearing losses cannot be surgically repaired, the temporal bone stimulator may provide an alternative rehabilitative method to conventional hearing aids. It is not widely used at present.

Middle Ear Implants (Semi-Implantable Hearing Device). A variety of IHD devices are being evaluated for sound amplification and quality for individuals with moderate to moderately severe sensorineural hearing loss. However, many challenges have to be met before a workable device is available. This method of hearing aid technology is still in the research stage.

OTALGIA

Otalgia is defined as pain in the ear, or earache. Otalgia can be primary in origin (i.e., coming from a disorder in the ear), infectious, or referred (i.e., coming from a disorder outside the ear). Otalgia from ear pain can be the result of infection in the external or middle ear or of trauma to the ear and head. Referred otalgia can be caused by disorders in the temporomandibular joint (TMJ), cranial nerves, face, scalp, pharynx, tonsils, thyroid, trachea, teeth, or cervical muscles.

Etiology and Risk Factors

Otalgia can be related to infectious processes in the external ear and middle ear. Bacterial contaminants can enter the ear through insertion of unclean articles, such as fingers or toys. Insertion of any sharp object into the ear canal can traumatize the skin and provide an open medium for infection. Instillation of contaminated solutions into the ear or swimming in polluted water raises the risk for development of ear infection and inflammation. Clients with recent upper respiratory tract infections, eustachian tube dysfunction, and allergies are also at increased risk for ear infections.

Infectious and neoplastic processes of the pharynx can also cause referred otalgia. It is not uncommon for clients with acute tonsillitis to complain of significant ear pain, even though the ears may be normal on examination. Otalgia following tonsillectomy is universal and is not a manifestation of infection. In clients with unilateral otalgia and a history of smoking, consideration must be given to a neoplastic process of the lateral pharynx, especially if concurrent manifestations, such as hoarseness or dysphagia, are present. Examination of the lower pharynx by means of a fiberoptic endoscope is necessary in the smoker with persistent hoarseness, and referral to an otolaryngologist is indicated.

Trauma to the head, temporal bone, and ear can also result in ear pain. Engaging in contact sports without protective headgear can result in severe trauma to the head, injuring the hearing apparatus. A blow to the ear by an object such as a ball or hand can cause local or diffuse pain in the area. Noise trauma from a blast or loud noise may create a ringing sensation that is perceived as painful and uncomfortable. Nerve damage may be accompanied by intolerance to even soft sounds, resulting in severe pain. Exposure to extremely hot or cold temperatures can lead to burns or severe frostbite, respectively, of the external ear.

Blockage of the eustachian tube and otalgia can be the result of enlarged adenoid tissue and tonsils in children, middle ear infections often associated with upper respiratory tract infections, and *barotrauma* (pressure injury to the middle ear). Acute blockage from altitude changes caused by flying or underwater diving will cause middle ear problems. Hyperbaric oxygen treatments can also cause barotrauma. Hyperbaric oxygen treatment is common for carbon monoxide poisoning as well as other disorders. The incidence of barotrauma is increased when an upper respiratory tract infection is present. *Aerotitis media* is a form of serous otitis media in which fluid or air is trapped in the middle ear during descent in an airplane. Any long-term blockage of the eustachian tube leads to serous otitis media and a hearing loss.

Mouth and gum pain, TMJ pain, cervical muscle tenderness, and pain from dental work can cause referred pain to the ear. TMJ arthralgia may result from teeth grinding, gum chewing, excessive talking, or biting down on hard objects. The resultant inflammation to this joint can be perceived by the client as an earache. Similarly, stress on the neck muscles can be referred to the ear.

External Ear Trauma

Auricular trauma is common because ears are prominent and unprotected. The pinna is subject to lacerations, blunt injury, abrasions, burns, and frostbite. A special concern with ear trauma is that a hematoma can quickly develop between the skin and cartilage (called *perichondrial hematoma*). The hematoma exerts pressure on the cartilage, impairing its healing. Such hematomas are common after blunt injuries such as occur in wrestling, fighting, or boxing and are responsible for so-called "cauliflower ear."

People can often avoid ear trauma by wearing headgear for contact sports, wide-brimmed hats in the summer, and earmuffs or hats in the winter; heavy pierced earrings should not be worn because they can lacerate the lobule.

Foreign Bodies

Surprisingly a wide array of foreign bodies fit into the ear canal. The most common foreign body found in the adult ear is either a piece of cotton or, most annoying, an insect.

Ear pain from obstruction usually results from the buildup of matter in the ear canal, which leads to pressure and pain. Clients may also report decreased hearing, a sense of fullness, a throbbing sensation, and itching. The onset, duration, frequency, and intensity of manifestations should be noted.

Eustachian Tube Disorders

Because the eustachian tube connects the middle ear to the nasopharynx, pharyngeal disorders also cause eustachian tube dysfunction and thus secondary middle ear problems. For example, in children a common disorder is blockage of the eustachian tube by enlarged adenoid tissue. In adults swelling of the mucosa in the eustachian tube during an upper respiratory tract infection can lead to serous otitis media (see later discussion). For persistent unilateral blocked eustachian tube, a malignant tumor must be ruled out as the cause.

Ear Infections

Otitis Externa. The most common problems found in the external ear are infections, primarily bacterial or fungal. The most frequent infection, called *external otitis,* involves the external ear canal. Infection begins when the protective waxy coating has been damaged by dryness, moisture, or treatment. Infection can lead to edema, which can occlude the canal. External otitis occurs more frequently in the summer than in the winter. The most common form of external otitis is also called *swimmer's ear,* because it is prevalent in clients in whom water remains in the ear canal after swimming. In addition, opportunistic fungal infections are common. When a debilitating systemic disease such as diabetes is present, the external otitis can spread aggressively through cartilage and bone and is then named *malignant external otitis; Pseudomonas aeruginosa* is the usual offending pathogen.

Occasionally infection involves only the cartilage of the pinna (chondritis), with resultant necrosis of the cartilage and loss of the distinctive shape of the pinna if the infection is not treated quickly. Frostbite of the pinna has findings similar to those of infection. Another form of infection is seen as an ear canal furuncle or abscess.

Tympanic Membrane Infection. Infections of the external ear canal can involve the surface of the tympanic membrane. A specific infection of the tympanic membrane is *bullous myringitis*. This inflammatory disease forms blisters or bullae between the layers of the eardrum, which are extremely painful. It is usually caused by the bacterium *Mycoplasma pneumoniae.* Holes or perforations of the tympanic membrane can be caused by infection and also can be accompanied by drainage.

Tympanic membrane disorders can lead to perforation of the membrane. A perforation may be acute, as seen in trauma and acute infection, or chronic, as seen in repeated infection. An acute perforation has a better chance of healing spontaneously than does a chronic perforation.

Otitis Media. Otitis media is the most prevalent disorder of the middle ear. It is most common in children but does occur in adults. When an infection is sudden in onset and short in duration, the diagnosis is acute suppurative otitis media. When the infection is repeated, usually causing drainage and perforation, the problem is chronic otitis media. Chronic otitis media is often caused by organisms such as *Pseudomonas, Staphylococcus,* and *Klebsiella*. Anaerobes such as *Bacteroides* have also been identified in culture analysis of specimens from the ear. Infection can cause swelling of the mucosa throughout the middle ear and eustachian tube. At times *serous otitis media* is found in conjunction with upper respiratory tract infections or allergies.

Chronic otitis media can lead to tympanic membrane retraction, adhesive otitis media, or necrosis of the tympanic membrane (perforations) or of the ossicles. Both problems create a conductive hearing loss. Necrosis of the bone covering of the facial nerve may cause facial paralysis. Because of the anatomy of the temporal bone, middle ear infection can also lead to brain abscesses that are life-threatening if not treated properly. Cholesteatoma, another complication, is discussed on p. 1733.

Subsequent to infectious otitis media or allergic disease, fluid may form in the middle ear, known as *serous otitis media*. This fluid is formed when a vacuum develops in the middle ear, caused by a blocked eustachian tube. When the swelling subsides, the fluid may be too thick to drain. Tympanometry is a useful diagnostic assessment to distinguish a normal ear from one with a middle ear effusion.

Mastoiditis. The mastoid system is a series of air cells contained within the temporal bone that communicate with the middle ear. Before the discovery of antibiotics, a mastoid infection was a life-threatening event. Now acute mastoiditis is rare, although chronic mastoiditis does sometimes occur. With repeated middle ear infections, the mastoid cavity becomes a significant part of the problem, increasing the amount of drainage. A chronic infection also leads to the development of cholesteatoma (see following section).

Drainage from the mastoid cavity via the ear canal is the most likely manifestation to appear. The drainage courses through the middle ear and out the tympanic membrane through a perforation. Tenderness over the mastoid cavity behind the ear points to an infection but usually is caused by an acute exacerbation of chronic mastoiditis rather than an acute mastoiditis. The protrusion of the pinna as a result of swelling over the mastoid may be part of this process.

Cholesteatoma. *Cholesteatoma* is a cyst in the middle ear or mastoid system that is lined with squamous epithelium and filled with keratin debris. Often infection is present in the mass of the cholesteatoma. Although cholesterol granules can be present in the specimen, yielding the term *cholesteatoma,* they are not the primary pathologic process.

Cholesteatoma most often results from chronic otitis media or marginal perforation of the tympanic membrane. Clients have conductive hearing loss and foul-smelling discharge from the ears. Although it is a benign growth, the cholesteatoma causes erosion of the surrounding structures, leading to other problems, such as brain abscesses, vertigo, and facial paralysis. Fortunately, these complications are uncommon.

Other Masses. Benign masses of the external ear canal are usually cysts that arise from a sebaceous gland or, more rarely, from the cerumen glands. Cysts can also be congenital in nature. Bony protrusions seen in the bony portion of the ear canal are called *exostoses*. The skin covering an exostosis is normal. If the skin is red, the mass is usually an abscess. Infectious polyps found in the ear canal arise from either the tympanic membrane or, more commonly, the middle ear, through a hole in the tympanic membrane.

Malignant tumors are also found in the external ear. The cutaneous carcinomas are most often basal cell carcinoma on the pinna and squamous cell carcinoma in the ear canal. If not treated, the carcinomas can invade underlying structures; squamous cell carcinoma may spread throughout the temporal bone. Rare tumors of the cerumen glands are of the adenoma cell type. Masses of the external ear are diagnosed through physical examination and biopsy to rule out malignancy. Surgical excision may be required.

Both benign and malignant tumors can involve the tympanic membrane, but they seldom arise from it; however, an infectious glandular polyp can be isolated to the tympanic membrane. Tumors in the middle ear can be seen through or protrude through the tympanic membrane.

The same tumors that arise in the middle ear can be found in the mastoid cavity. Because the mastoid cavity is connected to other air cells throughout the temporal bone and is close to the brain, malignant tumors at this location carry a poor prognosis.

Pathophysiology

Otalgia related to a problem in the ear is usually the result of an inflammatory process that can be caused by trauma or infection. Inflammation causes chemical mediators to be released into the tissue and the chemotaxis of leukocytes to the damaged area, resulting in tissue edema, pain, heat, and redness. This inflammatory process results in swelling of tissue that impinges on nerve endings and surrounding areas, causing the otalgia. Masses such as tumors grow and press on nearby tissue and nerves, causing pain. Sometimes the infection or mass erodes into tissue and bone as in cholesteatoma and causes further inflammation and pain.

Otalgia can also be caused by referred pain to the ear. In conditions such as TMJ or cervical adenopathy, the pain does not originate in the ear; however, the neuronal pain pathways for these processes cross over and are perceived in the ear. Although the perception of pain in the ear is real, the cause of the pain is not related to a pathologic process in that area.

Clinical Manifestations

In the case of head trauma and damage to the tympanic membrane, clients often report an episode of brief but intense otalgia. If the tympanic membrane is ruptured from barotrauma or otitis media, the client often notes a sudden reduction of pressure and pain. Pain is not usually elicited on palpation of the external ear; this phenomenon usually provides a differential diagnosis between problems of the external ear and middle ear. Disorders involving the tympanic membrane are painful, perhaps the most painful of all middle ear disorders. Hearing loss may be noted but is often reversible. Vertigo may also be present.

Ear pain from obstruction usually results from the buildup of matter in the ear canal, which leads to pressure and pain. Clients may also report decreased hearing, a sense of fullness, a throbbing sensation, and itching. The onset, duration, frequency, and intensity of manifestations should be noted.

Pain in the external ear is the most common clinical manifestation of infection. Pain ranges from mild to severe and is generally unilateral. Pain is more intense when the ear canal is swollen. Painful sites are tender because of the close proximity of bone (a hard surface) when the ear is palpated. A clue to early external otitis is tenderness when the pinna is gently pulled, in contrast to otitis media, in which touching the ear does not cause pain. A forerunner of pain in external otitis is itching in the ear canal. Inflammation (redness) is easily identified with an otoscope. At different stages of infection, drainage will be found from the ear canal. In early infectious disorders, the drainage may be clear rather than discolored by pus.

Manifestations of otitis media include ear pain and an immobile tympanic membrane. Because the tympanic membrane is a semitransparent membrane, what lies beneath it is visible. It can also become discolored or displaced. Therefore both fluid and infection can be seen in the middle ear. The tympanic membrane may be dull or red instead of the normal pearly gray. The eardrum may be normal, perforated, infected, retracted, or bulging depending on the disease process involved. In addition, the client may report bubbling, crackling, or popping sensations in the ear, especially during swallowing. There is a sense of fullness in the ear and conductive hearing loss that fluctuates.

Suppurative otitis media is invasion of the middle ear by virulent organisms and formation of pus, often accompanied by purulent *otorrhea* (drainage). Clinical manifestations include intense ear pain, fever, mild to moderate conductive hearing loss, thickened and bulging tympanic membrane, and occasional dizziness.

OUTCOME MANAGEMENT

Medical Management

The goals of medical management are to (1) promote healing, (2) alleviate pain, and (3) restore normal function of the ears.

Promote Healing

Ear Irrigation. The ear is commonly irrigated to cleanse the external auditory canal or to remove impacted wax, debris, or foreign bodies to promote healing. Irrigation is not used in clients with a history or clinical suspicion of perforated eardrum. Ear irrigation is performed as follows.

Warm the irrigating solution (usually water) to body temperature, and place it in the irrigating syringe. Dizziness is a common side effect of irrigating with fluids that are colder or warmer than body temperature. Protect the client's clothes with a plastic drape, and place a kidney-shaped basin below the ear to catch the irrigating solution. Have the client sit with the ear to be irrigated toward you and downward to drain the material. In the adult, pull the external ear upward and backward (or in children pull the external ear directly back), and direct the tip of the syringe along the upper wall of the ear canal (Figure 66-4). The canal should not be completely obstructed by the syringe to allow the back-flow of solution. When charting the ear irrigation, include the type of irrigation solution used and the nature of returned solution regarding amount, texture, color of cerumen, and type of debris. In addition, instruct the client to report pain, vertigo, or nausea during the procedure.

Sometimes the client is instructed to use a medicinal ear irrigation solution. The most common solution for ear irrigation is boric acid and alcohol, which is obtained by prescription. This solution cleanses the ear of debris and infection and provides a drying agent. A 2- or 3-ounce ear syringe is needed for irrigation. A family member performs the irrigation for the client. Usually the ear irrigation is followed by the use of eardrops.

Candling is a folk remedy that has gained popularity in recent years. In this technique, a candle is placed in

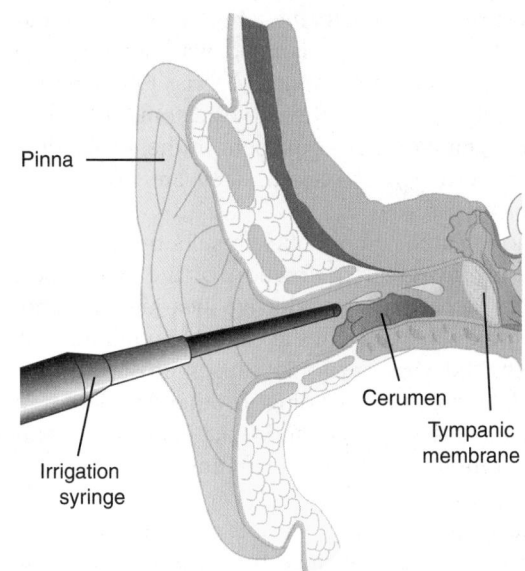

■ **FIGURE 66–4** Ear irrigation. The tip of the syringe is directed along the upper wall of the ear canal.

the ear canal. The wick is lighted and the candle is allowed to burn for a short period of time. Supposedly, the burning flame creates a vacuum at the other end of the candle, which can suck wax and other evil humors from the canal. When the candle is removed, the base of the candle typically will appear dark brown, leading the person to believe that their ear wax has been removed by candling. Candling has shown no benefit and, in fact, has been associated with harm. Hot wax can burn the external ear or tympanic membrane. It can also lead to perforation of the tympanic membrane.

Antibiotics. Local and systemic antibiotics are the cornerstone of preventing and managing infections of the ear canal; however, the first rule of treating infection is meticulous cleaning of the site so that the local antibiotic can reach the infected area. Suction, irrigation, or manual removal of matter with a cotton-tipped swab can be used. Regular application of antibiotic-steroid ear drops for a week is required.

If the ear canal is swollen shut, a wick may be inserted to allow the drops to penetrate the canal. Ear drops are placed directly on the wick. Commercially prepared wicks or single pieces of one-fourth-inch gauze can be used. The wick serves not only as a bandage but also as an excellent vehicle to medicate the ear canal. The wick is gently inserted into the ear canal by means of forceps while the external ear is gently pulled upward and backward. The wick is usually slightly less than 1 inch long (Figure 66-5). The client should lie on the unaffected side for 3 to 5 minutes to allow gravity to promote movement of the medication

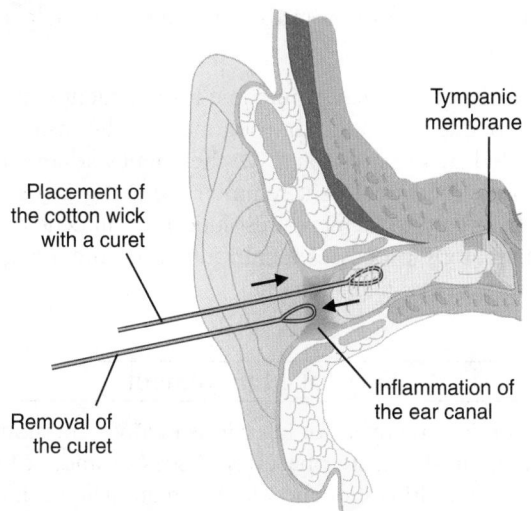

FIGURE 66-5 Administration of antibiotics for otitis externa. A curette with a cotton wick around it is placed in the ear canal. The wick is gently placed in the canal, and an antibiotic or treatment solution is added to the wick.

into the ear canal. If the infection is generalized or severe, systemic antibiotics are used. An infection that involves cartilage has to be treated aggressively and quickly with systemic antibiotics to avoid complications.

With any form of otitis media, appropriate antibiotic therapy may be necessary. If drainage is present, a specimen may be collected for culture analysis and sensitivity testing. Most episodes of acute otitis media, however, do not produce drainage, and the specific bacterial cause need not be identified. Otitis media is generally easily managed, but if it is not treated properly, it can lead to meningitis and brain abscess because of the proximity of the ear to these tissues.

Suppurative otitis media is managed with systemic antibiotics, topical antibiotic drops, and analgesics. If otitis media becomes chronic, myringotomy may be required to ventilate the middle ear and equalize pressure between the middle ear and external ear. Because infection starts in the middle ear, the problems in the mastoid cavity are avoided by early use of antibiotics with otitis media.

Alleviate Pain

Because external otitis is one of the most painful disorders of the ear, appropriate analgesics are required. Pain persists for 24 to 48 hours after treatment is initiated. Once the swelling and drainage are reduced by treatment, in about 48 hours the pain subsides.

Restore Normal Function and Remove Foreign Bodies

Removal of foreign bodies from the ear canal can be quite difficult. The nurse should not spend a long time attempting to remove an object from the ear without asking for help. The external auditory canal is an exquisitely sensitive, elliptical, cylinder-like structure. In adults, it is about 24 mm long and has two anatomic points of narrowing. Objects caught behind these narrow points create the greatest problems for removal. If perforation of the tympanic membrane is deemed unlikely and the object is not tightly wedged, you can irrigate the external canal with warm water. Direct the stream of water superiorly and anteriorly into the ear canal and around the object (see Figure 66-4). Water pressure builds up and forces the object outward. It often takes about 200 to 300 ml of water to remove an object. Do not irrigate vegetable foreign proteins, such as beans, because they swell and become even more difficult to remove.

For removal of a live insect, the ear canal is filled with mineral oil, lidocaine, or an ether-soaked cotton ball, *not water,* to kill or stupefy the insect. Water would cause the insect to swell and become more difficult to remove.

The least traumatic method of removing a foreign body is with the aid of an operating microscope. After removing the object, inspect the tympanic membrane and ear canal for manifestations of trauma. If trauma is noted, the client should be treated for external otitis and seen again in 4 to 5 days.

Nursing Management of the Medical Client

Assessment. When obtaining the history of the pain, ask the client about what events have triggered the ear pain, paying special attention to a recent history of upper respiratory tract infection, travel by airplane, exposure to loud noises, trauma to the head, and stressors that lead to teeth grinding or dental work.

The nurse first observes the external ear for redness, swelling, lumps, scaling, crusting, or drainage, either serous or purulent. During assessment of the external ear, manipulation of the ear is important. If the client complains of pain when any part of the ear is palpated, an abscess, a lesion, or some kind of inflammatory process of the ear canal is suspected. If an otoscopic examination is performed, care must be taken not to cause the client unnecessary pain. An abscess may be close to the opening of the canal, where the pressure of the speculum may cause greater pain.

During the physical examination, determine the presence of pain with swallowing, neck rotation, palpation of the face and head (over the sinuses), palpation of the mastoid process, and manipulation of the pinna. Assess the TMJ by inserting your index fingers into the external auditory canals and applying pressure anteriorly while the client opens and closes the mouth. TMJ syndrome may cause pain, clicking, or crepitation of the joint during movement.

Diagnosis, Outcomes, Interventions

Diagnosis: Risk for Infection. Because of tissue damage from trauma, foreign body, or pathogen, the nursing diagnosis *Risk for Infection related to tissue destruction* may be appropriate in the client with otalgia.

Outcomes. The client will have reduced risk of infection or will experience resolution of infection without complications.

Interventions. Monitor for clinical manifestations of infection, and administer antibiotics as prescribed. Other medications, such as antihistamines, decongestants, and steroid nasal sprays, may be ordered to reduce inflammation that can damage tissue. Teach the client to complete the entire prescription of the antibiotic even though manifestations may have cleared (see the Client Education Guide on Infection of the Tympanic Membrane, Middle Ear, or Mastoid Cavity on the website).

During an infectious process, instruct the client to avoid getting water in the ear while bathing or showering by using earplugs or placing cotton balls coated with petroleum jelly in the ear canal.

Eardrops may also be prescribed for bacterial or fungal infections, which are often seen in otitis externa. Various irrigations of the mastoid system and middle ear are used for chronic infections along with antibiotic eardrops or powders. In chronic otitis media with discharge, both broad-spectrum oral antibiotics and topical antibiotic drops are used.

Diagnosis: Acute Pain. Otalgia may be caused by a process in the ear or may be referred from a source outside the ear, resulting in the nursing diagnosis *Acute Pain related to inflammation in the external or middle ear or from referred pain in the head and neck area*.

Outcomes. The client will be able to reduce pain and achieve an acceptable comfort level.

Interventions. Otalgia is managed by treating the primary problem. Comfort can be promoted by using anesthetic ear solutions or systemic analgesics. After the physician has prescribed the analgesic therapy, instruct the client as to the amount, frequency, and duration. Other measures are the application of heat by warm compress, a soft diet, a quiet environment, and positioning of the client with the affected ear down.

The client with TMJ syndrome should avoid chewing and hyperextension of the jaw (e.g., during dental examination and care). The client should also try to stop grinding the teeth. A specially fitted mouth guard to be worn while sleeping can be helpful in preventing teeth grinding at night.

In the case of eustachian tube dysfunction or barotrauma, teach the client how to facilitate opening of the eustachian tube. Chewing gum, sucking hard candy and swallowing often, yawning, and blowing air out against closed nostrils (Valsalva maneuver) help open the tube.

Evaluation. The positive outcome for the client with otalgia depends on (1) the thoroughness of the instructions provided by the nurse and (2) the client's adherence to the prescribed treatment regimen. Ongoing assessment of the client to achieve resolution of infectious and inflammatory processes contributing to the otalgia is key to effective management.

Surgical Management

The surgical treatment of infections involves incision and drainage in the acute phase for abscesses and, at times, for perichondritis. Perichondrial hematomas are incised and drained and then dressed in large, bulky dressings. The most common surgical treatment is excision of cysts and cutaneous carcinomas. For conditions that occlude the ear canal, more extensive surgery that involves removal of bone and skin grafting, known as a *canaloplasty*, is performed.

Myringoplasty

Surgery can be performed on the tympanic membrane with use of an operating microscope for magnification. Closure of a simple perforation is called a *myringoplasty*.

Tympanoplasty

Tympanoplasty is the surgical correction of a perforated tympanic membrane. In tympanoplasty, a graft of temporalis fascia or other connective tissue is placed to restore the damaged tympanic membrane. The location of the graft depends on the original defect. Sometimes tympanostomy (ventilation) tubes are inserted.

Ossiculoplasty

The surgical procedure of ossicular reconstruction is called *ossiculoplasty*. Various methods of repositioning these tiny ear bones are now in use. In addition, various synthetic prostheses have been used to reconnect the ossicles to carry sound. In an attempt to prevent extrusion of the prostheses, tissue is combined with the prostheses to rebuild the ossicles (Figure 66-6).

Myringotomy

An incision into the tympanic membrane through which fluid is removed by suction is called *myringotomy*. To keep the incision open and to prevent a recurrence of fluid, various types of transtympanic tubes can be inserted into the incision. These tubes extrude by themselves in 3 to 12 months and rarely have to be removed. More permanent tubes (T tubes) with larger flanges may be used for clients who require repeated myringotomies.

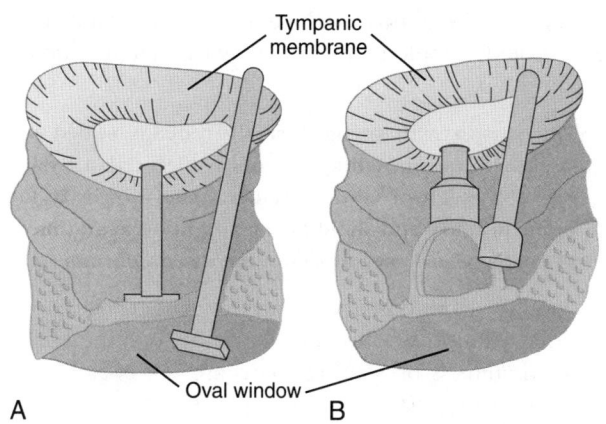

■ **FIGURE 66–6** Middle ear prostheses used for reconstruction. **A,** Ossicle columella prosthesis (total ossicular replacement). **B,** Ossicle cup prosthesis (partial ossicular replacement). *(Courtesy Arnold G. Shuring, MD.)*

Mastoidectomy

Radical mastoidectomy removes the contents of the mastoid bone for control of infection and cholesteatoma. Because the radical mastoidectomy sacrifices hearing, a modified radical mastoidectomy was developed to save the remaining middle ear structures. With the advent of antibiotics, simple mastoidectomy became possible, which maintained a normal-appearing ear canal. Because radical and modified mastoidectomies exteriorize the mastoid cavity to the external ear canal, they are known as *open* or *canal wall–down mastoidectomies. Closed* or *canal wall–up mastoidectomies* are simple mastoidectomies with modifications that are performed in conjunction with tympanoplasty and ossiculoplasty to retain or regain hearing. Today even the open mastoidectomy is performed with various tympanoplasties.

Nursing Management of the Surgical Client

Preoperative Care

The scope of nursing activities for the client undergoing ear surgery can be as broad as a preoperative assessment performed in an office or clinic or as limited as an assessment performed in the holding area of the surgical suite. Before surgery, an audiogram and tympanogram are obtained to assess preoperative hearing acuity. The client's level of knowledge about the procedure, expectations, and psychosocial readiness for surgery are evaluated along with the physiologic status.

The client undergoing ear surgery should be told what to expect during the procedure because local anesthesia with sedation is often used. Instructions should be given about the duration of the procedure, the estimated length of hospital stay, and immediate postoperative instructions.

Postoperative Care

Pain is not usually a major problem, but mild analgesia may be required. Vertigo or lightheadedness may occur when the client ambulates for the first time. Clients should be supervised when ambulating on the day of surgery to protect themselves from falling. Some clients who are quite vertiginous exhibit nystagmus (see Chapter 64) from stimulation of the inner ear. The vertigo usually passes very quickly and seldom requires medication.

Position the client as ordered; usually the client lies with operated ear up for several hours after surgery. The ear rarely bleeds after surgery. A small amount of serosanguineous drainage on a cotton ball is expected. The Client Education Guide below lists precautions for clients to take after ear surgery.

BALANCE DISORDERS

Vertigo is the perception that either oneself or one's surroundings are moving. Vertigo is often described as "dizziness." Dizziness, which can involve feelings of

---

CLIENT EDUCATION GUIDE

Precautions After Ear Surgery

To prevent injury and promote healing:
- Continue to blow your nose gently one side at a time and to sneeze or cough with your mouth open for 1 week after surgery.
- Avoid physical activity for 1 week and exercises or sports for 3 weeks after surgery.
- Return to work as recommended, usually 3 to 7 days after surgery (3 weeks if work is strenuous).
- Avoid heavy lifting, especially after stapedectomy.
- Change the cotton ball in your ear daily as prescribed.
- Keep your ear dry for 4 to 6 weeks after surgery.
- Do not shampoo for 1 week after surgery.
- Protect your ear when necessary with two pieces of cotton (outer piece saturated with petroleum jelly).
- Avoid airplane flights for the first week after surgery. For sensation of ear pressure, hold your nose, close your mouth, and swallow to equalize pressure.
- Wear noise defenders in loud environments.
- Report any drainage other than a slight amount of bleeding to the physician.
- Normal occurrences in the initial period after ear surgery may include the following:
  - Decreased hearing in operated ear from surgical packing (people may sound like they are talking in a barrel)
  - Noises in the ear, such as cracking or popping
  - Minor earache and discomfort in cheek and jaw
  - Ear swelling

disorientation in space or lightheadedness, is different, however. Vertigo results from imbalance of neural signals from the vestibular system in the ears. The imbalance of signals is interpreted by the brain as constant motion in space.

Disorders of balance and coordination result from problems of the vestibular system and "righting" reflexes. Balance can also be affected by problems outside the vestibular system. Few problems are more private than those involving one's sense of balance. Balance problems may be debilitating and may also cause embarrassing gait problems, which can jeopardize safety. More than 90 million Americans age 17 years or older have experienced vertigo or a balance problem. Vertigo is second only to chronic pain as the most common manifestation reported in America today.

Although vertigo and dizziness are not synonymous, they both relate to a sense of balance and equilibrium. Dizziness, vertigo, and syncope (fainting) are all manifestations of one of the following types of problems:

- Peripheral vestibular disorders (i.e., labyrinthine or inner ear)
- Central disorders (i.e., medullary, cerebellar, or cortical)
- Systemic disorders (i.e., cardiovascular or metabolic)

Peripheral vestibular disorders involve problems in the labyrinth or internal ear. Central disorders result from a problem in the brain or nerves, such as a tumor of the eighth cranial nerve (acoustic neuroma) or stroke. Systemic disorders begin in a nerve or organ outside the cranium (e.g., orthostatic hypotension, hypoglycemia). Examples of common causes of vertigo and dizziness, grouped by etiology, are presented in Box 66-4.

BOX 66-4   Disorders Associated with Vertigo and Dizziness

PERIPHERAL LABYRINTHINE (INNER EAR) DISORDERS
- Benign paroxysmal positional vertigo (BPPV)
- Labyrinthitis
- Ménière's disease
- Cholesteatoma

CENTRAL NERVOUS SYSTEM DISORDERS
- Cerebellar lesions
- Temporal lobe lesions
- Tumors of cranial nerve VIII (e.g., acoustic neuroma)
- Stroke
- Multiple sclerosis

SYSTEMIC DISORDERS
- Diabetes
- Postural hypotension
- Arthritis
- Hypoglycemia
- Allergies

Little can be done to reduce the risk of balance disorders. Clients should be treated early for manifestations of ear problems.

The person with vertigo usually remains seated or supine to prevent falling. Clients at high risk for falling as a result of vertigo should stand up slowly to prevent injury and should keep a light on at all times to enable visual cues to lessen the disequilibrium.

Finally, situations that lead to vertigo should be avoided. Motion sickness occurs normally if the provocative stimulus is present. Humans are not evolutionarily adapted to special environmental situations, such as deep-sea diving, high-speed flying, and space travel. Vertigo or dizziness may occur in these environments.

PERIPHERAL VESTIBULAR DISORDERS

Benign Paroxysmal Positional Vertigo

Benign paroxysmal positional vertigo (BPPV) is a common cause of vertigo. It tends to follow head injury and viral infections of the inner ear. BPPV is due to *cupulolithiasis*, the presence of calcium crystals in the semicircular canals. These crystals are normally deposited on small hair-like structures in the ear called *otoliths*, and they slow responses to head movement. When they are dislodged, head movement creates a hypersensitive response. BPPV is provoked when the head is placed in certain positions, usually hyperextended and to one side. Clinical manifestations usually consist of brief attacks of rotational vertigo, a rapid head tilt to the affected ear, and a lag time of 3 to 6 seconds between change of position and vertigo with nystagmus. It is usually self-limited and resolves spontaneously over weeks to months.

Labyrinthitis (Vestibular Neuronitis)

Labyrinthitis is infection or inflammation of the cochlear or vestibular portion of the inner ear or both. Causes are not fully understood, but the syndrome tends to occur in spring and early summer and to be preceded by an upper respiratory tract infection. A virus has therefore been implicated but has never been isolated. Three classic manifestations are reported: vertigo, nausea, and vomiting. There are no hearing changes. Vertigo is usually sudden in onset; it peaks in 24 to 48 hours and then gradually subsides over 1 to 2 weeks. Supportive treatment is usually given during the wait for the underlying problems to clear.

Ménière's Disease

Ménière's disease is caused by excess endolymph in the vestibular and semicircular canals. Normal vestibular activity depends on the stability of fluid pressure

Ménière's disease causes hearing changes and vertigo. Ménière's disease is an episodic illness that waxes and wanes, often remaining quiescent for many years and then reappearing. A cluster of manifestations develops consisting of (1) paroxysmal whirling vertigo, (2) fluctuating hearing loss, (3) tinnitus, and (4) aural fullness. Only one or two manifestations may be present initially. Vertigo is characterized by remission and relapses without apparent cause, although the manifestations become less severe in time. The initial attacks consist of approximately 30 minutes of intense vertigo, which commonly provokes nausea and vomiting. Remaining stationary reduces vertigo. A sensorineural hearing loss (see Hearing Impairment) that may be reversible in the early stages is a serious consequence of Ménière's disease.

CENTRAL DISORDERS OF BALANCE

Dizziness may be a manifestation of a transient ischemic attack (TIA) ("small stroke"). A temporary loss of blood flow to the brain leads to several manifestations, depending on the brain area that is not being perfused. Clients can experience momentary losses of consciousness; transient numbness, tingling, and weakness; and changes in speech. TIAs should be reported and treated aggressively to prevent true ischemic changes.

SYSTEMIC DISORDERS LEADING TO VERTIGO

Physiologic Vertigo
Physiologic vertigo is involved in common disorders such as motion sickness. In these conditions, vertigo is minimal or absent, but autonomic manifestations are present. Motion sickness leads to perspiration, nausea, vomiting, increased salivation, yawning, and malaise. Physiologic vertigo can usually be suppressed by supplying sensory cues that come from other stimuli. For example, motion sickness from reading in a car can be reduced by looking out the window at the moving environment.

Presbyastasis
A disorder that is recognized more and more is *presbyastasis,* or disequilibrium of aging. Because of the generalized degenerative changes that occur in aging, balance and stability are affected. In addition to the labyrinth, balance also depends on the visual system and the proprioceptive changes in the muscles. Because all three systems are involved in aging, older adults have difficulty with stability, which results in falls and subsequent trauma.

Orthostatic Hypotension
Orthostatic hypotension is a sudden drop in blood pressure and dizziness on sitting or standing. The manifestations noted are lightheadedness and faintness, not vertigo, which is due to inadequate cerebral blood flow. Older adults are at high risk of orthostatic hypotension because of atherosclerosis and the use of medications that lead to diuresis or hypotension (e.g., furosemide, calcium-channel blockers). Orthostasis is diagnosed through assessment of positional blood pressure changes. Clients should be taught to change position slowly, and medications may require adjustment if blood pressure is too low.

Pathophysiology
The body maintains balance and equilibrium by responding to an intricate network of information. The ability to maintain balance depends on the intactness of four systems:

- Vestibular system (the labyrinth or inner ear)
- Visual system (the eyes)
- Proprioceptive system (the somatosensory nerves of joints and muscles)
- Cerebellar system (the coordinator)

The sensations transmitted from the ears, the eyes, and the somatosensory nerves are integrated in the brain stem and cerebellum and perceived in the cerebral cortex. Gradual interference of vestibular input causes compensatory changes that allow the brain to adjust slowly. Quick changes demand more adjustments than can be made. Infections can destroy the nerve and alter transmission of messages. Ménière's disease is an increase in the volume of endolymph with distention of the entire endolymphatic system. This distention and increased fluid results in permanent damage to both the vestibular and the cochlear apparatuses. Overproduction of endolymph can slow transmission of messages and lead to the perception that the body is in constant motion. Head trauma can shake free calcium carbonate crystals on the utricular macule and alter endolymph movement.

Clinical Manifestations
Vertigo is the most common clinical manifestation in a client with a balance problem. The clinical manifestations of balance disorders vary widely depending on (1) the cause, (2) the location (one or both ears), (3) the client's age at onset, (4) the extent of the loss of vestibular function, and (5) the rapidity with which damage occurs. Disease in the external ear, middle ear, and inner ear usually leads to vertigo that is sudden, transient, and accompanied by vagal manifestations (e.g., nausea, vomiting, sweating, pallor). The vertigo associated with cerebrovascular lesions does not follow a pattern; however, tinnitus and hearing loss are usually not present.

An important differentiation is whether the vertigo is associated with hearing loss. The close anatomic relationship between the balance and hearing systems

TABLE 66–2   Vestibular and Nonvestibular Vertigo

	Vestibular	Nonvestibular
Common descriptions	Spinning (environment moves), on a merry-go-round	Lightheadedness, feeling of being dissociated from body, swimming, giddiness, spinning inside (environment stationary)
Clinical manifestations	Drunkenness, tilting, motion sickness, off balance	
Course of illness	Episodic	Constant
Precipitating factors	Head movement, position change	Stress, hyperventilation, cardiac dysrhythmia, orthostatic hypotension
Associated manifestations	Nausea, vomiting, tinnitus, hearing loss, impaired	Perspiration, pallor, paresthesias, palpitations, vision, unsteadiness, syncope, difficulty concentrating, tension headache; anxiety

sometimes causes the sensation of vertigo in conjunction with a hearing loss. In most instances, vertigo is present without a hearing loss. It is also important to distinguish between vertigo from vestibular problems and other forms of vertigo. Table 66-2 differentiates the two forms of vertigo.

Dizziness is described by clients in such varied terms that it is almost impossible to define. Not all the terms listed here suggest true vertigo. The nurse should record the terms or description the client uses to help find the actual cause. Clinical manifestations are listed in Box 66-5.

For the client with vertigo, the differential diagnosis may be accomplished by means of a thorough medical assessment, including audiometry, vestibular tests, imaging evaluation, and, sometimes, laboratory studies. Clients who have had vertigo may become quite anxious when they think about experiencing it again. Even after the vertigo has abated, anxiety tends to persist. Because vertigo is only a clinical manifestation, the diagnosis and treatment of the underlying disease are important. Unlike with vision or hearing problems, no single organ

is responsible for balance problems. Therefore the diagnosis, treatment, and rehabilitation of the client with a balance problem can be difficult as well as frustrating.

OUTCOME MANAGEMENT

Medical Management

Control of episodes of the disease is usually possible, although a cure is not yet available. Two main treatment goals guide the medical management of the client with vertigo. They are (1) suppression of the CNS and the vestibular system and (2) vestibular rehabilitation.

Suppress the Central Nervous System and Vestibular System

Treatment of acute vertigo involves several medicines, called *antivertigo agents*. These medicines tend to suppress the balance system or the CNS, allowing recovery over time. They should be used judiciously in clients with BPPV because they slow recovery of function.

A low-salt diet and a diuretic may reduce the frequency of attacks of Ménière's disease by decreasing the volume of endolymph. Other changes in lifestyle include avoiding caffeine, smoking, and alcohol. The client should try to reduce stress, get regular sleep, and remain physically active, but avoid excessive fatigue. If clients have had vertigo without warning, they should not drive. Safety may require they forego ladders, scaffolds, and swimming.

A recent treatment for manifestations associated with Ménière's disease is the application of low-pressure pulses through the ear canal to the middle ear. This airwave transmission passes through the external and middle ear structures to the fluids in the inner ear. The initial use of this device shows promise in relieving vertigo and improving hearing function during the early stages of Ménière's disease.

Promote Vestibular Rehabilitation

Vestibular rehabilitation is a recognized form of control for vertigo. Because the balance system can compensate,

BOX 66-5   Clinical Manifestations of Vertigo

- Staggering
- Giddiness
- Lightheadedness
- Disorientation
- Visual blurring
- Veering in one direction while walking
- Unsteadiness
- Reeling
- Faintness
- Wooziness
- Shakiness
- Instability
- Wobbliness
- Bewilderment
- Confusion
- Being dazed
- Clumsiness
- Sense of floating
- Sense of falling
- Weakness
- Vague feeling of uncertainty

head and total body exercises are performed by the client to hasten compensation. Vestibular rehabilitation consists of exercises that promote vestibular adaptation, habituation, and activities of daily living. Usually physical therapists are involved in structuring this treatment. Vestibular rehabilitation uses all three organ systems that provide balance.

The exercises included in vestibular rehabilitation are performed as follows:

1. While lying in bed, slowly and then quickly turn the eyes up, down, and from side to side, and the head forward, backward, and from side to side.
2. Perform the same exercises while sitting; in addition, bend forward and pick up objects from the ground.
3. While standing, perform the previously mentioned exercises; in addition, change from sitting to standing position with the eyes open and then closed, and turn around in between (i.e., change direction as well as position with eyes open and closed).
4. While moving about, walk up and down steps with the eyes open and then closed, or play games involving stooping and stretching, such as basketball.

It is believed that when vertigo is induced by these exercises, a tolerance for it is acquired. Clients should perform these exercises from the time of the acute attack and continue until they are free of manifestations for 2 consecutive days. Driving a car safely needs to be addressed with clients who have vertigo. Vestibular rehabilitation therapy has been found efficacious in treating vertigo associated with certain types of vestibular deficits. Several studies have found marked improvements in postural stability, walking, and symptom control in clients who have undergone vestibular rehabilitation therapy compared with those who have not participated in this treatment. Appropriateness of this therapy in treating vertigo in older clients has been evaluated in a few studies. As discussed in the Translating Evidence into Practice feature at right, initial findings indicate that vestibular rehabilitation is well tolerated and can be effective treatment for vertigo in the older person.

A specific intervention strategy that is currently being used involves a series of manipulative interventions known as the *Epley maneuvers*. These maneuvers, which are used specifically for BPPV, are designed to facilitate return of dislodged otoliths to their more normal position within the labyrinth. The Epley maneuvers are essentially a more direct, rapid method to restore normal function and are of variable efficacy.

Nursing Management of the Medical Client

Assessment. Nursing assessment of the client with a balance problem should consist of the following areas:

1. A client interview to obtain a health history and specific information about the onset and characteristics

---

 TRANSLATING EVIDENCE INTO PRACTICE

Vestibular Rehabilitation in Older Adults

Vestibular rehabilitation therapy (VRT) provides a comprehensive approach to management of the vertiginous client, which includes exercises that promote stability and alleviate manifestations while improving daily functioning. VRT is implemented in phases. Initially the person performs vestibular adaptation exercises to promote compensatory processes in the central nervous system. These adaptation exercises focus on improving stability in different postural positions (supine, sitting, and standing) and facilitating performance of activities of daily living. Habituation exercises are instituted later in the process during the maintenance phase of treatment.

Vestibular rehabilitation (VR) intervention is effective in reducing manifestations and improving balance and postural control in clients with dizziness and vertigo. Clients with chronic vestibular disorders accompanied by unsteadiness, imbalance, or motion intolerance often experience significant symptom improvement and reduction in falls after receiving weekly sessions of VR designed for daily home use.

The effectiveness of VR treatment is strongly related to the client's strict adherence to the regimen of activities during the rehabilitation period. This involves ongoing support, instruction, and evaluation to obtain benefits from VR in managing vertigo. While performing these exercises, individuals often experience manifestations of vertigo and dizziness and may become unsteady. Older people commonly experience dizziness and unsteadiness as a result of age-related deterioration of the vestibular system. Along with the physical consequences of gait alteration and disequilibrium, the older person may feel anxious and less confident in functioning independently. Inclusion of general precautions and protective adaptations to prevent falls, such as the use of walkers and handrails, is included in the rehabilitation program, especially with older clients.

Vestibular rehabilitation can be an effective treatment in managing vertigo in certain vestibular disorders. It is beneficial in alleviating manifestations and improving function and activities in older adults. VR is well tolerated by the older client, especially with the inclusion of specific protective measures to reduce the risk of falls and injury. Maintaining positive, ongoing support of the client throughout the rehabilitation period can increase adherence and improve treatment outcomes.

---

of the balance problem and associated hearing problems. Attempt to distinguish the type of vertigo reported, and note aggravating conditions (e.g., head movement)
2. Assessment of the effect of the vertigo on the client's performance of activities of daily living
3. An interview with a family member to determine the effects of the client's balance problem on others

The importance of the history and interview cannot be overemphasized. An adequate description of vertigo should include information about the onset, exacerbating and alleviating factors, associated clinical manifestations, and predisposing factors in the medical history, as previously described. All clients bring some degree of anxiety regarding this illness to the examination. Balance problems can have devastating effects on a client's behavior. The disruption of the client's routine, the severity of the "attacks," and the fear of the unknown can make the client agitated, anxious, or depressed. The nurse must be aware of these feelings and must demonstrate self-confidence, patience, courtesy, and gentleness.

A structured questionnaire such as the one shown in Box 66-6 should be completed by the client. These questions can also be used to facilitate the interview; however, the interview should be guided by client cues. A gross assessment of the client's balance can be made by watching the client's gait. Evidence of instability

---

BOX 66-6 Assessment Guide for Clients with Balance Disorders

A. When you are dizzy, do you experience any of the following sensations? Please read the entire list first. Then circle the numbers of those sensations that describe what you experience most accurately.
1. Lightheadedness
2. Tendency to lose balance or to fall
3. Objects spinning or turning around you
4. Sensation that you are turning
5. Headache
6. Nausea or vomiting
7. Pressure in the head

B. Please fill in the blank spaces.
1. When did the dizziness first occur? _____
2. Is your vertigo constant? _____
3. Does it come in attacks? _____
4. How often do attacks occur? _____
5. How long are the attacks? _____
6. Does vertigo occur only in certain positions?
   ▪ When upright?
   ▪ When lying flat?
   ▪ Turning to the right?
   ▪ Turning to the left?
7. Have you ever stumbled or fallen because of vertigo?
8. Do you know of anything that will stop the vertigo or make it better?
   Make your vertigo worse?
   Bring on an attack?
9. Did you ever injure your head?
10. Do you take any medications regularly (e.g., tranquilizers; oral contraceptives; barbiturates; a course of antibiotics, such as streptomycin, neomycin)?
11. Do you use tobacco in any form?
    Alcohol?
12. Have you worked for long in a noisy environment?
13. Do you suffer easily from motion sickness?

---

may be noted if the client touches the wall or walks with a wide-based, waddling gait.

The same inspection, palpation, and otoscopic examination should be performed for the client with a balance problem as was performed for the client with hearing loss (see earlier discussion). The client must be questioned about the loss of hearing and tinnitus, which can accompany a balance problem.

Diagnosis, Outcomes, Interventions. Nursing care is detailed in the Care Plan feature on The Client with Vertigo on the website.

Surgical Management

About 5% or less of all clients with vertigo undergo surgical intervention.

Endolymphatic Sac Surgery

The endolymphatic sac procedures include decompression and various forms of shunts to the CNS or mastoid cavity. The intent of these procedures is to lessen the fluid pressure within the labyrinth and control the vertigo of Ménière's disease. A collective review of the results of 1800 cases of various surgical approaches to the endolymphatic sac found that 22% of clients had improved hearing, 53% had no change in hearing acuity, and 25% had worsened hearing as determined by the established guidelines. Refinement of surgical approaches and outcomes research on these techniques continues to be important.[16a]

Labyrinthectomy

Labyrinthectomy is a form of surgery designed to destroy the labyrinth and eliminate its abnormal input. It is performed through the oval or round window (membranous limits of cochlear and inner ear). This is a destructive procedure that removes the membranous labyrinth, either subtotally through the oval window or totally through the mastoid bone. Any remaining hearing is sacrificed.

In a nonsurgical approach to labyrinthectomy, an ototoxic drug can be injected through the tympanic membrane into the middle ear to destroy the hair cells of the vestibular system. This procedure is carried out over a series of visits and is designed to decrease the abnormal vestibular signal in the affected ear. A secondary and sometimes unavoidable effect is concurrent cochlear toxicity. Clients are treated until their vestibular manifestations improve significantly, with the goal of preserving as much hearing as possible.

Vestibular Nerve Resection

Vestibular nerve resection is a highly effective procedure performed to alleviate vertigo. Vestibular nerve resection can be performed through the labyrinth (sacrificing hearing) or around the labyrinth (saving hearing). The retrolabyrinthine surgical approach is the most common form of surgical control for vertigo today. This method preserves the inner ear structures and approaches the vestibular nerve from behind the semicircular canal. Alleviation of the client's vertigo is usually immediate. Because of the compensation by all the other structures related to maintaining balance, a client can function with only one labyrinth.

CONCLUSIONS

Nurses caring for clients with hearing and balance problems need to focus on safety and on promoting independence. Many hearing-impaired clients live a normal life with hearing augmentation and aural rehabilitation.

Clients who have diminished hearing or balance disorders are at increased risk for injury because of lack of awareness of the risks or from losing balance.

Infections of the ears remain common, but excellent antibiotics have reduced the incidence of chronic problems caused by infections. Tumors of the ear are rare, but when they occur, they are quite destructive.

THINKING CRITICALLY

1. A middle-age man comes to the health clinic with ear pain and difficulty hearing. He had some serous drainage 1 day ago but does not recall any recent infection (throat or ear). The problem has persisted intermittently over the past 6 months and is getting progressively more painful and occurring more frequently. If surgery were deemed necessary for this client, how would you prepare him? What discharge teaching might need to be completed for this client after ear surgery?

Factors to Consider. What preoperative assessments are needed? How should equal pressures be maintained on the tympanic membrane? What normal occurrences might the client expect in the initial period following surgery?

2. An older woman reveals a 10-year history of ear infection. She is experiencing sensorineural hearing loss associated with presbycusis, which affects older people. During her clinic appointment, she tells the nurse that her right ear is painful and is keeping her awake at night. She explains that she can hear most sounds, although sounds on the right side seem to be coming through a filter. She has been using her eardrops as directed but has stopped taking her oral antibiotic because she felt better 2 days ago. She requests information about daily medication or a surgical procedure that might alleviate the problem. How should you respond to the client's request? How do age-related changes contribute to her problem?

Factors to Consider. What is the assessment focus for this client? What is the prognosis for the client with presbycusis? What type of teaching does the client require?

Discussions for these questions can be found on the website.

BIBLIOGRAPHY

 Citations appearing in red refer to primary research.

1. Barreire, S.O. (2005). Spin cycle: Evaluation and management of dizziness and vertigo. *Advance Nurse Practitioner, 13*(3), 22-27.
2. Brackmann, D.E., Shelton, C., & Arriaga, M.A. (Eds.) (2001). *Otologic surgery.* Philadelphia: Saunders.
3. Chawla, N., & Olshaker, J.S. (2006). Diagnosis and management of dizziness and vertigo. *Medical Clinics of North America, 90*(2), 291-304.
4. Copeland, B.J., & Pillsbury, H.C. (2004). Cochlear implantation for treatment of deafness. *Annual Review of Medicine, 55,* 157-167.
5. Cummings, C.W., Haughey, B.H., Thomas, J.R., et al. (2004). *Cummings otolaryngology: Head and neck surgery* (4th ed.). St. Louis: Mosby.
6. Das, S., & Buchman, C.A. (2005). Bilateral cochlear implantation: Current concepts. *Current Opinions in Otolaryngology—Head and Neck Surgery, 13*(5), 290-293.
7. Ferrite, S., & Santana, V. (2005). Joint effects of smoking, noise exposure and age on hearing loss. *Occupational Medicine, 55*(1), 48-53.
8. Gates, G.A. (2006). Ménière's disease review 2005. *Journal of the American Academia of Audiology, 17*(1), 16-26.
9. Gottshall, K.R., Hoffer, M.E., Moore, R.J., et al. (2005). The role of vestibular rehabilitation in the treatment of Meniere's disease. *Otolaryngology—Head and Neck Surgery, 133*(3), 326-328.
10. Halmagyi, G.M. (2005). Diagnosis and management of vertigo. *Clinical Medicine, 5*(2), 159-165.
11. Hannon, S.A., Sami, F., & Wareing, M.J. (2005). Tinnitus. *British Medical Journal, 330*(7485), 237.
12. Harris, L.L., & Huntoon, M.B. (Eds.) (2008). *Core curriculum for otorhinolaryngology and head-neck nursing* (2nd ed.). New Smyrna Beach, Fla: Society of Otorhinolaryngology—Head and Neck Nurses, Inc.
13. Hol, M.K., Bosman, A.J., Snik, A.F., et al. (2005). Bone-anchored hearing aids in unilateral inner ear deafness: An evaluation of audiometric and patient outcome measurements. *Otology and Neurotology, 26*(5), 999-1006.
14. Macias, J.D., Massingale, S., & Gerkin, R.D. (2005). Efficacy of vestibular rehabilitation therapy in reducing falls. *Otolaryngology—Head and Neck Surgery, 133*(3), 323-325.
15. Meli, A., Zimatore, G., Badaracco, C., et al. (2006). Vestibular rehabilitation and 6-month follow-up using objective and subjective measures. *Acta Otolaryngology, 126*(3), 259-266.
16. Rosenfeld, R.M., & Bluestone, C.D. (Ed.) (2003). *Evidence-based otitis media* (2nd ed.). New York: Marcel Dekker.
16a. Moffat, D.A. (1994). Endolymphatic sac surgery: Analysis of 100 operations. *Clinical Otolaryngology 19*(3), 261-266.
17. Rosenfeld, R.M., Singer, M., Wasserman, J.M., et al. (2006). Systematic review of topical antimicrobial therapy for acute otitis externa. *Otolaryngology—Head and Neck Surgery, 134*(4 Suppl), S24-48.
18. Roy, D., & Chopra, R. (2002). Tinnitus: An update. *Journal of the Royal Society of Health, 122*(1), 21-23.
19. Semaan, M.T., Alagramam, K.N., & Megerian, C.A. (2005). The basic science of Ménière's disease and endolymphatic hydrops. *Current Opinions in Otolaryngology—Head and Neck Surgery, 13* (5), 301-307.
20. Sen, P., Georgalas, C., & Papesch, M. (2005). Co-morbidity of migraine and Ménière's disease—Is allergy the link? *Journal of Laryngology and Otology, 119*(6), 455-460.

21. Snik, A.F., Mylanus, E.A., Proops, D.W., et al. (2005). Consensus statements on the BAHA system: Where do we stand at present? *Annals of Otology, Rhinology, and Laryngology, 195*(Dec Suppl), 2-12.
22. Waddell, A. (2004). Tinnitus. *Clinical Evidence, 12*, 798-807.
23. White, J., Savvides, P., Cherian, N., et al. (2005). Canalith repositioning for benign paroxysmal positional vertigo. *Otology and Neurotology, 26*(4), 704-710.

evolve *Did you remember to check out the bonus material on the Evolve website and the CD-ROM, including NCLEX®-Examination Style Review Questions, Open-Book Quizzes, and Chapter Review Audio Podcasts?*

http://evolve.elsevier.com/Black/medsurg

UNIT 16

COGNITIVE AND PERCEPTUAL DISORDERS

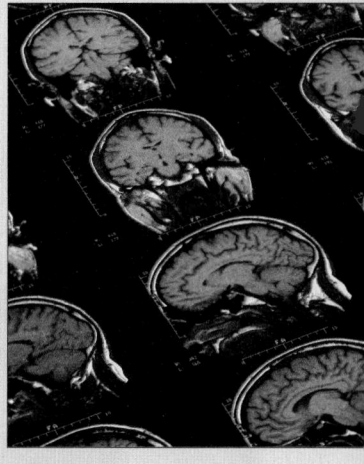

ANATOMY AND PHYSIOLOGY REVIEW:

The Neurologic System

Robert G. Carroll

The nervous system is the body's most organized and complex structural and functional system. It profoundly affects both psychological and physiologic functions. This unit discusses the importance of the nervous system to human functioning and the major consequences of neurologic disorders.

CENTRAL NERVOUS SYSTEM

The brain and spinal cord are known collectively as the *central nervous system* (CNS). The CNS is divided into three major functional divisions:
1. Higher-level brain, or cerebral cortex
2. Lower brain level (basal ganglia, thalamus, hypothalamus, midbrain, pons, medulla, cerebellum)
3. Spinal cord

These structures are protected by a rigid bony encasement, three layers of membranes, a fluid cushion, and a blood-brain or blood–spinal cord barrier.

BRAIN

The brain is the largest and most complex part of the nervous system. It is composed of more than 100 billion neurons and associated fibers. The brain tissues have a gelatin-like consistency. This semi-solid organ weighs about 1400 g (approximately 3 pounds) in the adult human.

Cerebrum

The cerebrum is divided by a deep groove *(longitudinal fissure)* into two sections called *cerebral hemispheres*. A transverse fissure separates the cerebrum from the cerebellum. The outermost layer of the cerebrum, the *cerebral cortex,* is only 2 to 5 mm thick. Directly beneath the cerebral cortex are varying thicknesses of association tracts above the commissural tracts, known as the *corpus callosum* (Figure A&P16-1).

The cerebral cortex is composed of gray matter (predominantly nerve cell bodies and dendrites) formed into raised convolutions, or *gyri*. About 75% of the neuronal cell bodies in the brain are found in the cortex. The shallow grooves between the gyri *(sulci)* divide the cerebral cortex into five lobes: frontal, parietal, occipital, temporal, and central (insula) (Figure A&P16-2).

The term *neocortex* is often used to refer to the cerebral cortex. The neocortex includes all the cerebral cortex except the olfactory portions and the hippocampal regions.

Both the left cortex and the right cortex interpret sensory data, store memories, learn, and form concepts; however, each hemisphere dominates the other in many functions. In most people, for example, the *left* cortex has dominance for systematic analysis, language and speech, mathematics, abstraction, and reasoning. The *right* cortex has dominance for assimilation of sensory experiences, such as visual-spatial information, and activities such as dancing, gymnastics, music, and art appreciation.

In the frontal lobes, the precentral gyrus *(motor cortex)* controls voluntary motor activity. Most of these fibers cross to the opposite side of the brain at the medulla and descend via the spinal cord as the *lateral corticospinal tracts*. The area anterior to the precentral gyrus *(premotor area)* is also associated with voluntary motor activities. *Broca's area,* which lies anterior to the primary motor cortex and superior to the lateral sulcus, coordinates the complex muscular activity of the mouth, tongue, and larynx and makes expressive *(motor)* speech possible. Damage to this area leaves the client unable to speak clearly, a disorder called *Broca's aphasia*.

The *prefrontal areas* control (1) attention over time (concentration); (2) motivation; (3) the ability to formulate or select goals; (4) the ability to plan; (5) the ability to initiate, maintain, or terminate actions; (6) the ability to self-monitor; and (7) the ability to use feedback (called *executive functions*). These same areas are thought to contribute to reasoning, problem-solving activities, and emotional stability by inhibiting the limbic areas of the cerebrum (see later discussion).

Each *parietal lobe* is located posterior to the central sulcus of Rolando and contains a primary somatic (tactile) receptive area and the somatic (tactile) association areas. The post-central gyrus and the anterior portion of the parietal lobe are the primary receptive (interpretation) areas for tactile sensations (e.g., temperature, touch, pressure). The association areas occupy the remainder of the parietal lobe. Concept formation and abstraction are carried out by the parietal association areas. The right parietal areas are also dominant for spatial orientation and awareness of size and shapes *(stereognosis)* and body position *(proprioception)*. The left parietal areas assist with right-left orientation and mathematics.

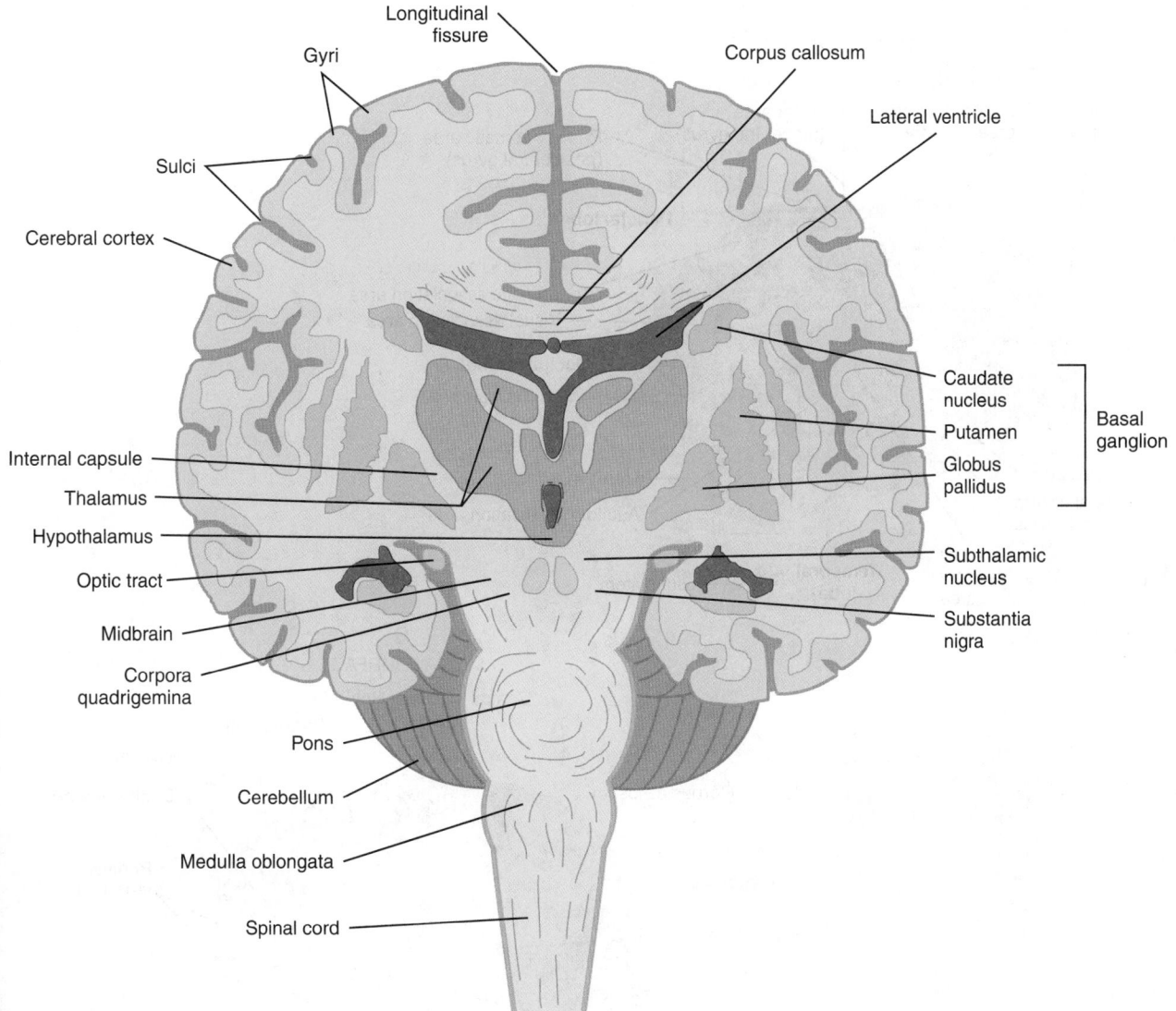

■ **FIGURE A&P16–1** Structures of the brain (coronal section).

Each *occipital lobe* contains a primary visual receptive interpretation) area and visual association areas. The primary visual cortex is on either side of the calcarine sulcus. The other areas of the occipital cortices are visual association areas. Visual memories are stored in these areas, which contribute to our ability to recognize visually and understand our environment.

Each *temporal lobe* is located under (inferior to) the lateral sulcus. The temporal lobe contains a primary auditory receptive area and secondary auditory association areas. Spoken language memories are stored in the left temporal auditory association areas. All other sound memories that are not language (e.g., music, various animal sounds, other noises) are stored in the right temporal lobe auditory areas. Damage to these areas would have one unable to understand spoken or written language or to recognize music or other environmental sounds. Cells that facilitate understanding language reside in *Wernicke's area.*

The *central (insula) lobe* is located deep within the lateral sulcus and is surrounded by the frontal, parietal, and temporal lobes. Nerve fibers for taste pass through the parietal lobe to the insular lobe. Many association fibers leading to other parts of the cerebral cortex pass through this lobe.

Hippocampus

The hippocampus, a part of the medial section of the temporal lobe, plays an essential role in the process of *memory,* a complex phenomenon. Three levels of memory have been identified:

1. *Short-term (recent) memory* is lost after seconds or minutes.
2. *Intermediate memory* lasts days to weeks and eventually is lost.
3. *Long-term (remote) memory* is stored and lasts a lifetime.

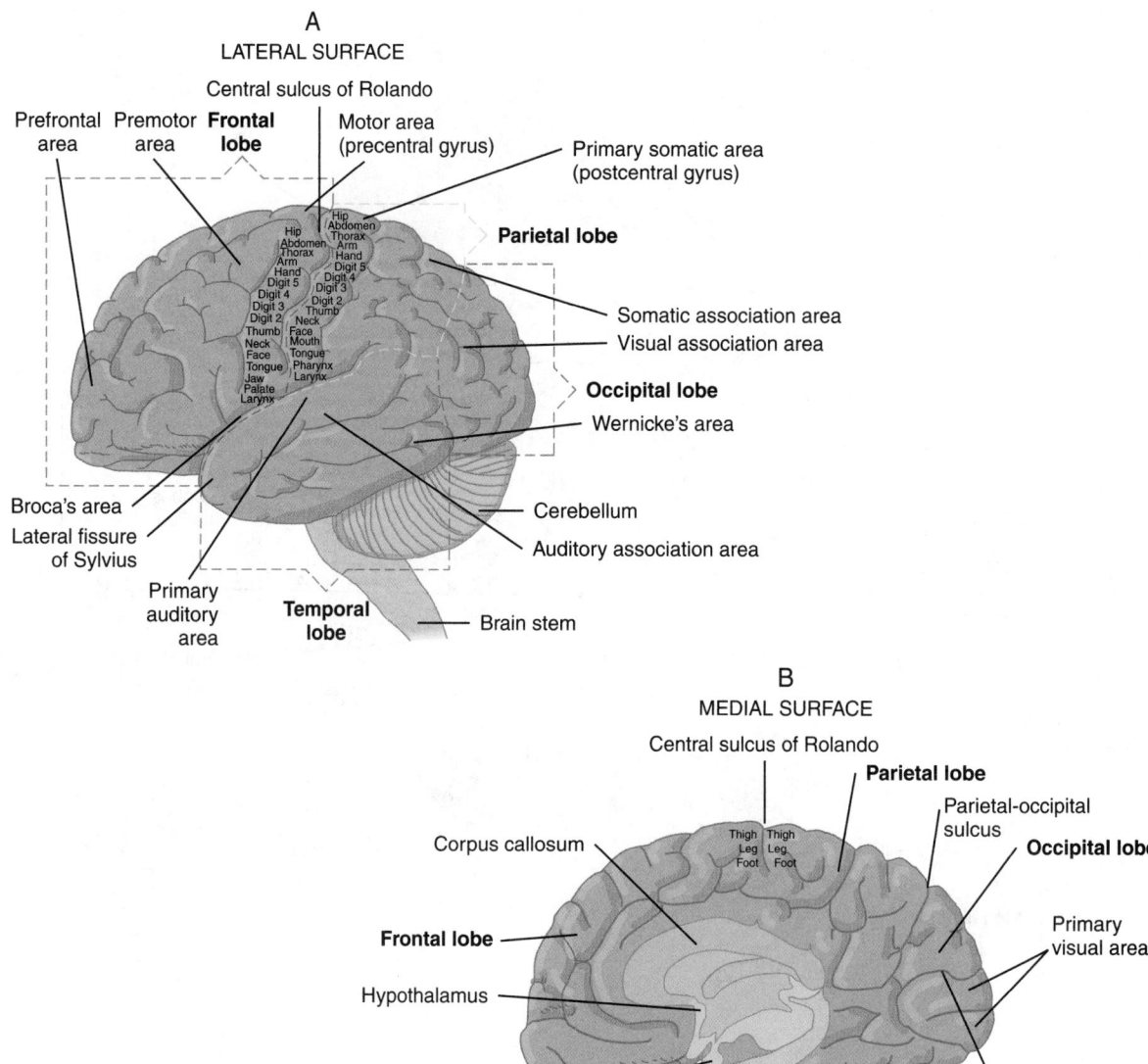

A
LATERAL SURFACE

Central sulcus of Rolando

Prefrontal area   Premotor area   **Frontal lobe**   Motor area (precentral gyrus)

Primary somatic area (postcentral gyrus)

Hip, Abdomen, Thorax, Arm, Hand, Digit 5, Digit 4, Digit 3, Digit 2, Thumb, Neck, Face, Tongue, Jaw, Palate, Larynx

Hip, Abdomen, Thorax, Arm, Hand, Digit 5, Digit 4, Digit 3, Digit 2, Thumb, Neck, Face, Mouth, Tongue, Pharynx, Larynx

Parietal lobe

Somatic association area
Visual association area

Occipital lobe

Wernicke's area

Broca's area
Lateral fissure of Sylvius

Cerebellum
Auditory association area

Primary auditory area   **Temporal lobe**   Brain stem

B
MEDIAL SURFACE

Central sulcus of Rolando

Parietal lobe

Parietal-occipital sulcus

Occipital lobe

Corpus callosum

Thigh, Leg, Foot   Thigh, Leg, Foot

Primary visual area

Frontal lobe

Hypothalamus

Hypophysis

Hippocampus

Calcarine sulcus

Temporal lobe

■ **FIGURE A&P16–2** The lateral **(A)** and medial **(B)** surfaces of the cerebral cortex. The central lobe is the fifth lobe.

Theories about the physiologic basis of memory suggest that reverberating neuronal messages cause short-term memory and that actual neuronal structural changes lead to long-term memory. The hippocampus assists in the conversion of short-term memory into intermediate and long-term memory in the thalamus. The association fibers of the frontal, parietal, temporal, and occipital lobes as well as the diencephalon are important in long-term memory.

Basal Ganglia

The basal ganglia consist of several structures of subcortical gray matter buried deep in the cerebral hemispheres. These structures include the caudate nucleus, putamen, globus pallidus, substantia nigra, and subthalamic nucleus. The basal ganglia serve as processing stations that link the

cerebral cortex to thalamic nuclei. Almost all the motor and sensory fibers connecting the cerebral cortex and the spinal cord travel through the white matter pathways near the caudate nucleus and putamen ganglia. These pathways are known as the *internal capsule*. The basal ganglia, along with the corticospinal tract, are important in controlling complex motor activity.

Diencephalon

The *diencephalon* is composed of the thalamus and the hypothalamus. The paired *thalami* lie between the cerebral hemispheres and superior to the brain stem. Its gray matter surrounds the lateral edges of the third ventricle. The *hypothalamus* forms the floor and portions of the wall of the third ventricle. Other important structures found in and near the diencephalon include (1) the optitracts and optic chiasm, (2) the pituitary gland on the floor of the diencephalon, and (3) the pineal gland on the roof of the diencephalon.

The thalamus channels all ascending (sensory) information, except smell, to the appropriate cortical cells. The hypothalamus regulates autonomic nervous system (ANS) functions, such as heart rate, blood pressure, water and electrolyte balance, stomach and intestinal motility, glandular activity, body temperature, hunger, body weight, and sleep-wakefulness. It also serves as the regulator of the pituitary gland by releasing factors that stimulate or inhibit pituitary gland output.

Limbic System

The limbic system comprises many nuclei, including parts of the medial portion of the frontal and temporal lobes (hippocampus), thalamus, hypothalamus, and the basal ganglia. It is considered the center for feelings and control of emotional expression (fear, anger, pleasure, sorrow). The limbic system (the temporal lobe component) also receives nerve fibers from the olfactory bulbs and thus plays an essential role in the interpretation of smells.

Brain Stem

The brain stem is composed of the midbrain, pons, and medulla oblongata (Table A&P16-1). They are composed of ascending pathways, the reticular formation, cranial nerves and their nuclei, and descending autonomic and motor pathways.

Reticular Formation

The reticular formation is composed of a complex network of gray matter (nuclei), ascending reticular pathways, and descending reticular pathways. Its nuclei extend from the superior part of the spinal cord to the diencephalon and communicate with the basal ganglia, cerebrum, and cerebellum.

The reticular formation assists in regulation of skeletal motor movement and spinal reflexes. It also filters incoming sensory information to the cerebral cortex. About 99% of sensory information is disregarded as unessential. One component of the reticular formation, the *reticular activating system,* controls the sleep-wake cycle (see Chapter 22) and consciousness.

Cerebellum

The cerebellum is composed of gray and white matter. The *cortex* of the cerebellum is a thin layer of gray matter arranged in parallel long and deep gyri, called *folia,* and separated by cerebellar sulci (Figure A&P16-3). Deep fissures divide the cerebellum into three lobes, but the functional division of the cerebellum consists of a right and left hemisphere separated by a narrow band of white matter called the *vermis.* An extension of dura mater, the *falx cerebelli,* partially separates the hemispheres.

TABLE A&P16–1 Brain Stem Structures and Their Functions

Structures	Functions
Midbrain	
Corpora quadrigemina	
Superior colliculi	Visual reflexes
Inferior colliculi	Auditory reflexes
Cerebral aqueduct	
Origin of CN III and IV	
Ascending sensory pathways	
Reticular formation	
Red nuclei	Motor pathways to spinal cord, cerebellum
Substantia nigra	Part of basal ganglia
Descending motor pathways	
Pons	
Fourth ventricle	
Nuclei of inferior colliculus	Auditory processing
Nuclei of CN V, VI, VII	
Locus ceruleus	Secretes norepinephrine
Raphe nuclei	Secrete serotonin
Ascending sensory pathways	
Medical lemniscus, auditory pathway	Discriminative touch
Descending motor pathways	
Medial longitudinal fasciculi	Efferent pathway to spinal cord
Reticular formation	
Respiratory centers	
Pontine nuclei; pontocerebellar fibers	
Medulla Oblongata	
Fourth ventricle	
Central canal	
Raphe nuclei	Secrete serotonin
Ascending sensory pathways	
Medial lemniscal pathways	Discriminative tactile pathways
Spinothalamic and trigeminothalamic tracts	Pain pathways / Tactile, temperature
Lateral lemnisci	Auditory pathways
Nuclei of CN VIII, IX, X, XI, XII	
Olive and vestibular-cerebellar systems	
Pyramids (corticospinal, corticobulbar, corticopontine)	Voluntary motor
Reflex centers: respiratory, vasomotor, cardiac, coughing, swallowing, sneezing, vomiting	
Reticular formation	
Descending motor pathways (pyramids)	Voluntary motor

CN, Cranial nerve.

The cerebellum integrates sensory information related to the position of body parts, coordinates skeletal muscle movement, and regulates muscle tension, which is necessary for balance and posture. Three pairs of nerve tracts (*cerebellar peduncles*) provide the communication pathways. The inferior peduncles are sensory (*afferent*)

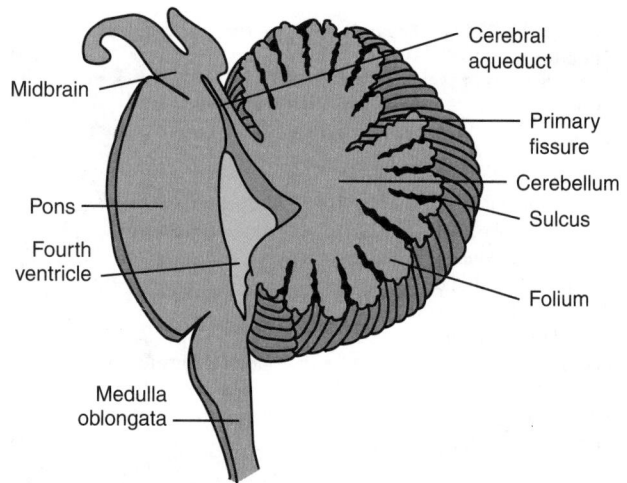

■ **FIGURE A&P16–3** Sagittal view of the brain stem, fourth ventricle, and cerebellum.

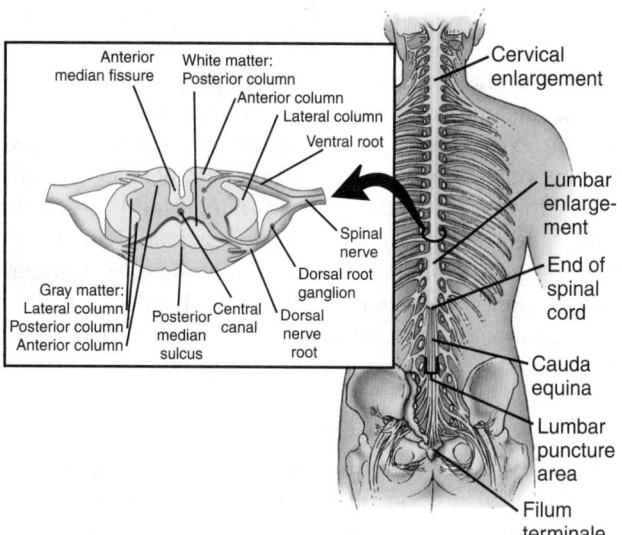

■ **FIGURE A&P16–4** The spinal cord ends at L-2. *Inset,* Transverse section *(left)* of the spinal cord. *(Modified from Thibodeau, G., & Patton, K. [2007]. Anatomy and physiology [6th ed.]. St. Louis: Mosby.)*

pathways from the spinal cord and medulla, which carry information related to the position of body parts to the cerebellum. The middle peduncles carry information about voluntary *(purposeful)* motor activities from the cerebral cortex to the cerebellum. The cerebellum also receives sensory input from the receptors in the muscles, tendons, joints, eyes, and inner ear. After this information is integrated and analyzed, the cerebellum sends impulses via the superior peduncles *(efferent pathways)* to the brain stem, thalamus, and cortex.

Most of the tracts in the cerebellum travel through various nuclei without crossing. Therefore the right cerebellar hemisphere predominantly affects the right (ipsilateral) side of the body and vice versa.

SPINAL CORD

The *spinal cord,* that portion of the CNS surrounded and protected by the vertebral column, is continuous with the medulla and lies within the upper two thirds of the *vertebral canal* (the cavity within the vertebral column). The lower spinal cord terminates caudally in a cone-shaped structure known as the *conus medullaris* at the level of the first (L1) and second (L2) lumbar vertebrae. The spinal cord is subdivided into four areas: (1) cervical cord, (2) thoracic cord, (3) lumbar cord, and (4) sacral cord (conus medullaris) (Figure A&P16-4).

Within the spinal cord, butterfly-shaped gray matter (mostly unmyelinated) is surrounded by mostly myelinated white matter. The white matter consists of *ascending tracts* and *descending tracts* that conduct nerve impulses between the brain and the cells outside the CNS. The cell bodies in the gray matter are grouped into clusters of nuclei and *laminae* (a defined group or column of cells). The tracts in the white matter are arranged into three paired columns: posterior, lateral, and anterior (Figure A&P16-4, *inset*).

Ascending and Descending Pathways

The *ascending (sensory) pathways* carry sensory information through the spinal cord to the brain. For example, the spinothalamic tract carries sensory information from the spinal cord to the thalamus. After synapsing in the thalamus, information is relayed to regions of the brain such as the parietal lobe. *Descending (motor) pathways* carry mostly efferent signals to the spinal cord. The corticospinal tract *(upper motor neuron)* is a descending tract passing from the frontal lobe of the cerebral cortex to the motor neurons of the spinal cord. *Lower motor neurons* are cells that begin in the anterior horn of the spinal cord and pass through the spinal nerves to the muscle cells. *Propriospinal tracts* remain within the cord.

Table A&P16-2 summarizes the specific functions of the major brain and spinal cord tracts.

Many of the tracts communicating with the cerebral cortex cross (decussate), but not all cross at the same place. The term *contralateral* refers to the opposite side of the body and is used to describe tracts that cross (often at the medulla) and ascend or descend; *ipsilateral* (same-sided) tracts do not cross. For example, sensory tracts (including the anterior spinothalamic, posterior, and anterior spinocerebellar tracts) cross in the medulla as they ascend to the cerebral cortex. Therefore the sensory neurons in the cerebral cortex interpret sensory stimuli from the contralateral side of the body.

The lateral corticospinal spinal tract *(pyramidal tract)* crosses at the medulla as it descends from the frontal lobe of the cerebral cortex to the spinal cord. The posterior spinocerebellar tracts are ipsilateral tracts and thus coordinate muscular function on the same side of the body. The crossing of the lateral spinothalamic tract is unique.

TABLE A&P16–2 Major Nerve Tracts of the Spinal Cord

Tract	Location	Function
Ascending Tracts		
Fasciculus gracilis	Posterior column	Touch, pressure, body movement, position
Fasciculus cuneatus	Posterior column	Pain, temperature
Spinothalamic	Lateral and anterior columns	Light (crude) touch
Spinocerebellar		
Posterior	Lateral column	Coordination of muscle movements
Anterior	Lateral column	
Descending Tracts		
Corticospinal		
Lateral	Lateral column	Voluntary motor
Ventral	Anterior column	Voluntary motor
Reticulospinal		
Anterior	Anterior column	Muscle tone, sweat glands
Medial	Anterior column	
Rubrospinal	Lateral column	Coordination of muscle movements
Lateral	Lateral column	Autonomic nervous system fibers

PROTECTIVE AND NUTRITIONAL STRUCTURES

Cranium and Vertebral Column

Eight bones that fuse early in childhood compose the cranium. The fused junctions are called *sutures*. The cranium encloses the brain structures and serves as a source of protection.

The floor, or *basilar plate*, of the cranial vault has three depressions, called *fossae*. The frontal lobes lie in the anterior fossa. The temporal lobes and the base of the diencephalon lie in the middle fossa. The cerebellum rests in the posterior fossa.

The vertebral column, a flexible series of vertebrae, surrounds and protects the spinal cord. It consists of 7 cervical vertebrae, 12 thoracic vertebrae, 5 lumbar vertebrae, 5 sacral vertebrae fused into a sacrum, and 4 coccygeal vertebrae fused into a coccyx. Ligaments hold the vertebrae together, and disks between the vertebrae prevent the bones from rubbing together.

Meninges

The *meninges,* three membranes that envelop the brain and spinal cord, are predominantly for protection (Figure A&P16-5). Each layer—the pia mater, arachnoid, and dura mater—is a separate membrane.

The *pia mater* is a vascular layer of connective tissue that is so closely connected to the brain and spinal cord that it follows every sulcus and fissure. This layer serves as a supporting structure for blood vessels passing through to the tissues of the brain and spinal cord. The

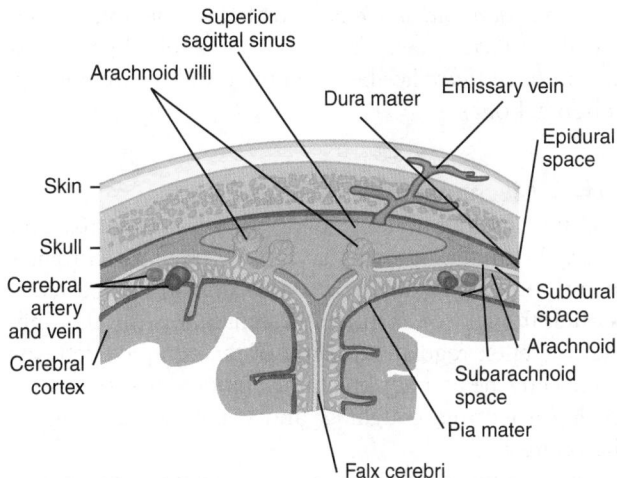

■ **FIGURE A&P16–5** The meninges (coronal section through the superior sagittal sinus).

pia mater and astrocytes together form the membrane part of the blood-brain barrier (see Blood-Brain Barrier).

The *arachnoid,* a thin layer of connective tissue, extends from the top of each gyrus to the top of the adjacent gyrus; it does not extend into the sulci and fissures. The space between this layer and the pia mater is known as the *subarachnoid space*. Cerebrospinal fluid (CSF) flows through this space.

The cranial *dura mater* is a tough, nonstretchable vascular membrane with two layers. The *outer* dura mater is actually the membrane *(periosteum)* of the cranial bones. The *inner* dura mater forms the plates that separate the two cerebral hemispheres *(falx cerebri),* the cerebrum and the brain stem and cerebellum *(tentorium cerebelli),* and the cerebellar hemispheres *(falx cerebelli).* The tentorium cerebelli is a landmark term that is often used by clinicians to separate parts of the brain; it is often referred to as *tentorium. Supratentorial* refers to the cerebrum and all the structures superior to the tentorium cerebelli; *infratentorial* refers to structures inferior to the tentorium cerebelli: the brain stem and the cerebellum.

Brain spaces that often fill with blood after head trauma include the potential space *(subdural space)* between the inner dura mater and the arachnoid and the *epidural space* between the dura mater and the periosteum.

The meninges anchor the spinal cord. The pia mater, which closely surrounds the spinal cord, continues from the tip of the conus as a thread-like structure *(filum terminale)* to the end of the vertebral column, where it is anchored into the ligament on the posterior side of the coccyx. The *denticulate ligaments* extend laterally from the pia mater to the dura mater to suspend the spinal cord from the dura mater.

Two common spaces that are commonly accessed by physicians are the subarachnoid space (for diagnostic studies) and the epidural space (for delivery of medications).

The *subarachnoid space* extends below the level of the spinal cord to the second sacral (S2) vertebral level, and the *epidural space* lies between the dural sheath and the vertebral bones.

Reflex Mechanisms

Our unconscious automatic responses to internal and external stimuli, known as *reflex responses,* provide many homeostatic functions. Although the spinal cord is often thought of as the reflex center, it is not the only site for reflex regulation. Many of the complex reflexes controlling heart rate, breathing, blood pressure, swallowing, sneezing, coughing, and vomiting are found in the brain stem.

Some intrinsic reflex circuits in the spinal cord create patterns of movement (flexion and extension) that are the basis for posture and forward progression. Other reflex circuits are the basis for spinal cord reflexes, which include the myotatic (deep tendon, stretch) reflex, the flexor withdrawal reflex, the crossed extension reflex, and the extensor thrust reflex. Visceral-somatic reflexes can also excite or inhibit the motor neurons, producing changes in muscle tone and even in movement.

Neuromuscular spindles monitor muscle stretch. As a muscle stretches, increased firing of spindles leads to contraction of the same muscle, commonly seen as the *knee-jerk reflex.* The Golgi tendon organs are sensory nerve endings that protect against excessive force developed during contraction.

Simple reflexes require only two or three neurons; for example, the *knee-jerk reflex* requires only a sensory neuron and a motor neuron. The *withdrawal reflex* helps prevent or decrease tissue injury when a body part touches a potentially harmful object. The harmful stimuli are sent via the sensory neuron to the interneuron in the spinal cord for interpretation, and the response message is sent via the motor neuron, resulting in the withdrawal response (Figure A&P16-6).

Cerebrospinal Fluid and the Ventricular System

The CSF is a clear, colorless fluid. About 100 to 160 ml of CSF circulates through the ventricles and within the subarachnoid space. When a person is lying in a horizontal position, the average CSF pressure is 100 to 180 mm Hg.

About two thirds of the CSF is made in the choroid plexus of the four ventricles, primarily in the lateral ventricles. Small amounts are produced by ependymal, arachnoid, and other brain cells. The *choroid plexus* is a network of blood vessels within the pia mater that is in direct contact with the lining of the ventricles. The choroid plexuses together produce about 500 ml of CSF per day. If CSF were allowed to accumulate, it would exert enough pressure to damage the brain. Normally, however, it is absorbed into the blood at the same rate at which it is formed.

The *ventricular system* is a series of cavities within the brain. CSF flows from each of the lateral ventricles via the foramen of Monro into the third ventricle (Figure A&P16-7). The third ventricle is midline just beneath the fornix. CSF drains from the third ventricle through the aqueduct of Sylvius into the fourth ventricle. The fourth ventricle is located in the brain stem just anterior to the cerebellum. From the fourth ventricle, CSF passes via one of three foramina (two foramina of Luschka and one foramen of Magendie) into a large

■ **FIGURE A&P16–6** Patellar reflex and neural pathway involved in the reflex response. *(From Thibodeau, G., & Patton, K. [2007]. Anatomy and physiology [6th ed.]. St. Louis: Mosby.)*

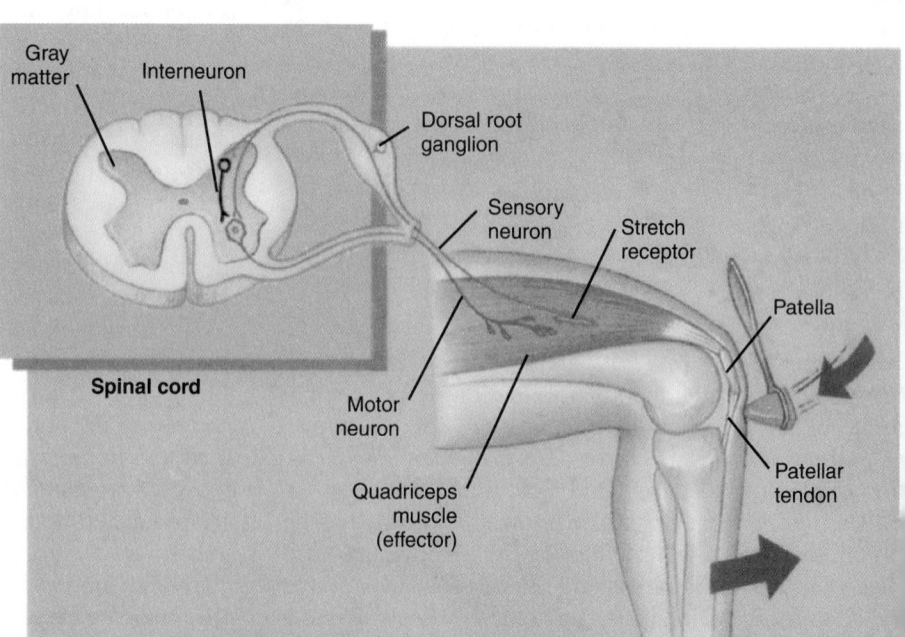

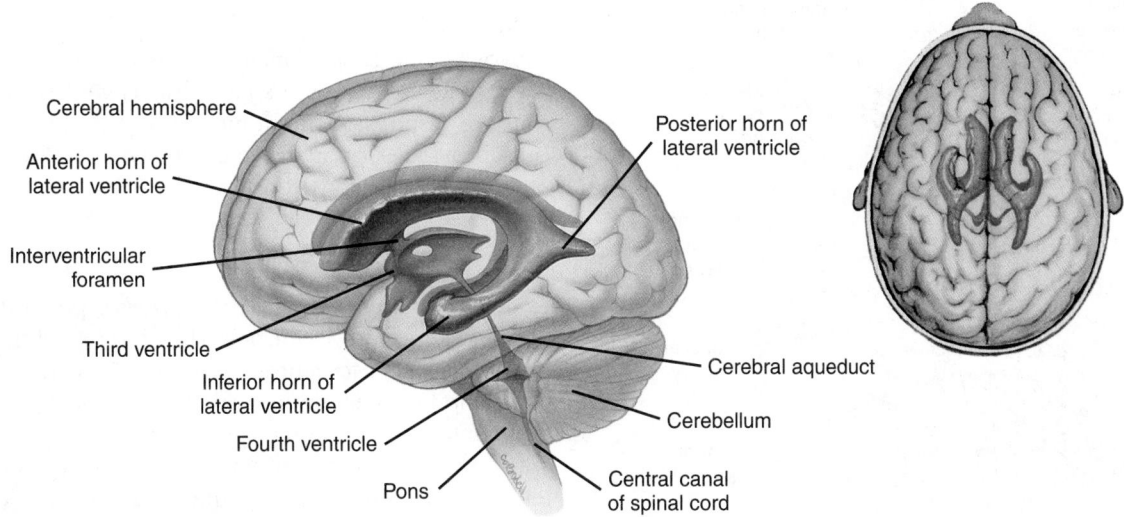

■ FIGURE A&P16–7 The ventricles of the brain produce and circulate cerebrospinal fluid. *(From Thibodeau, G., & Patton, K. [2007]. Anatomy and physiology [6th ed.]. St. Louis: Mosby.)*

subarachnoid space that lies behind the medulla and below the cerebellum, called the *cisterna magna*. The cisterna magna is continuous with the subarachnoid space, which surrounds the brain and spinal cord.

Eventually, the CSF circulates upward into the region of the superior sagittal sinus, where it is absorbed across the arachnoid villi. The arachnoid granulations are extensive tufts of pia-arachnoid that, along with the inner dura, extend into the superior sagittal sinus and permit one-way flow of CSF into the sinus.

Blood-Brain Barrier

Three brain barriers (blood-brain, blood-CSF, and brain-CSF) primarily regulate and maintain an optimal and stable chemical environment for neurons. Brain barriers are either physical barriers or physiologic processes (transport systems) that slow movement of certain substances from one CNS compartment to another by regulating ion movement between the compartments. Physical barriers include tight junctions of the endothelial cells lining the capillaries, pores of the capillaries of the choroid plexuses, the basement membrane (ependymal cells) next to the choroid plexuses, and the pial-glial membrane.

An intact blood-brain barrier may prevent some drugs from crossing into the brain, a fact that must be considered when medications are prescribed for nervous system disorders. Certain events, including dilutional hyponatremia, acute hypertension, high doses of some anesthetics, vasodilation, and hypercarbia, can increase the permeability of the blood-brain barrier.

BLOOD SUPPLY

The brain receives 20% of the cardiac output and uses 20% of the body's oxygen. Glucose is catabolized or burned for its energy. Gray matter has higher metabolic needs than white matter. Blood flow is regulated by levels of the metabolite carbon dioxide. An increase in neuronal metabolism produces an increase in carbon dioxide, leading to a local vasodilation. Local regulation of blood flow ensures that blood flow is proportional to neuronal metabolic needs.

The vertebral arteries and the internal carotid arteries (Figure A&P16-8) provide the arterial supply to the brain.

Arterial Supply

The *vertebral arteries* branch from the subclavian arteries, travel through the transverse foramina in the cervical vertebrae, and enter the cranial vault through the foramen magnum. The vertebral arteries are located on the anterolateral surface of the medulla. At the junction of the medulla and pons, the vertebral arteries join to form the basilar artery. The basilar artery bifurcates at the midbrain level to form two posterior cerebral arteries. The vertebral artery system supplies the brain stem, the cerebellum, the lower portion of the diencephalon, and the medial and inferior regions of the temporal and occipital lobes.

The *internal carotid arteries* branch from the common carotid arteries and enter through the carotid canals at the base of the skull. The internal carotid arteries bifurcate into the anterior and middle cerebral arteries.

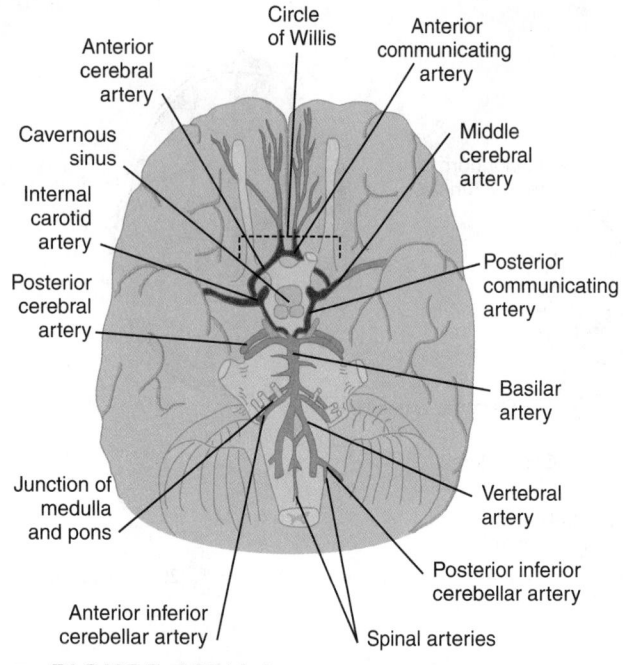

FIGURE A&P16–8 Inferior view of the cerebral circulation.

Labels:
- Anterior cerebral artery
- Circle of Willis
- Anterior communicating artery
- Cavernous sinus
- Middle cerebral artery
- Internal carotid artery
- Posterior communicating artery
- Posterior cerebral artery
- Basilar artery
- Junction of medulla and pons
- Vertebral artery
- Anterior inferior cerebellar artery
- Posterior inferior cerebellar artery
- Spinal arteries

CELLS OF THE NERVOUS SYSTEM

Structure

Nervous tissue consists mainly of *neuroglia* and *neurons* (as well as vascular and some connective tissues). Neurons are responsible for communication, and neuroglial cells provide support for the activity of neurons. The brain and spinal cord constitute the CNS.

Neuroglia

Glial cells, collectively called *neuroglia,* provide structure and support for neurons. They are plentiful, with a ratio of glial cells to neurons as high as 50 to 1. They also control ion concentrations within the extracellular space and contribute to the transport of nutrients, gases, and waste products between neurons and the vascular system and the CSF. Clinically, these cells are responsible for the development of many intracranial tumors. Four types of neuroglial cells exist (Figure A&P16-9).

In addition to these functions, each type of glial cell has specific functions.

1. *Astrocytes* supply nutrients to the neurons. They have specialized contacts with blood vessels in the pial-glial membrane and form part of the blood-brain barrier. Astrocytes appear to be the CNS cells that respond to brain trauma by forming scar tissue.
2. *Oligodendrocytes* are comparable to the Schwann cells in the peripheral nervous system (PNS). These cells wrap themselves around axons, and the spiraled part of their membrane is referred to as *myelin.* The outermost part of the Schwann cells also makes up the *neurilemma,* a sheath that surrounds the myelin sheath. The neurilemma is essential to nerve regeneration (see later discussion).
3. *Microglia* are phagocytic scavenger cells and are related to macrophages. They phagocytose products from injured neurons.
4. *Ependymal cells* line the ventricles, choroid plexuses, and the central canal that extends through the spinal cord. They create a one-cell-layered membrane that allows regulated diffusion of substances between the interstitial fluid and the CSF.

Neurons

A neuronal cell body *(soma)* is like other cells in that it contains most of the organelles seen in other cells. Unique structures in the neuron include *neurofibrils,* which are networks of thread-like structures supporting other structures. *Nissl bodies* are dark-staining sections of rough endoplasmic reticulum and are unique to the neuron.

Tree-like *dendrites* carry messages to the neuronal cell body; *axons* carry messages away from the cell body (Figure A&P16-10).

Near this bifurcation, the *circle of Willis* (a ring of blood vessels at the base of the brain) is formed by the posterior cerebral arteries, posterior communicating arteries, internal carotid arteries, anterior cerebral arteries, and anterior communicating branches. The internal carotid arteries supply the upper diencephalon, basal ganglia, lateral temporal and occipital lobes, and parietal and frontal lobes. The middle cerebral arteries supply large portions of the frontal, parietal, temporal, occipital, and insular lobes and the basal ganglia, internal capsule, and thalamus. The anterior cerebral arteries supply the medial portions of the frontal and parietal lobes and the upper basal ganglia and internal capsule (see Figure A&P16-8).

The spinal cord derives its arterial blood supply from small spinal arteries that branch off larger arteries, including the vertebral, ascending cervical, deep cervical, intercostal, lumbar, and sacral arteries. These arteries and their branches form the three main arteries of the spinal cord—the anterior spinal artery and a pair of posterior spinal arteries, which extend the length of the cord.

Venous Supply

Most of the venous blood from the head returns to the heart through the internal jugular veins, the external jugular veins, and the vertebral veins.

Venous distribution is similar to arterial distribution of the spinal cord. The venous system drains into the venous sinuses located between the dura mater and the periosteum of the vertebral column.

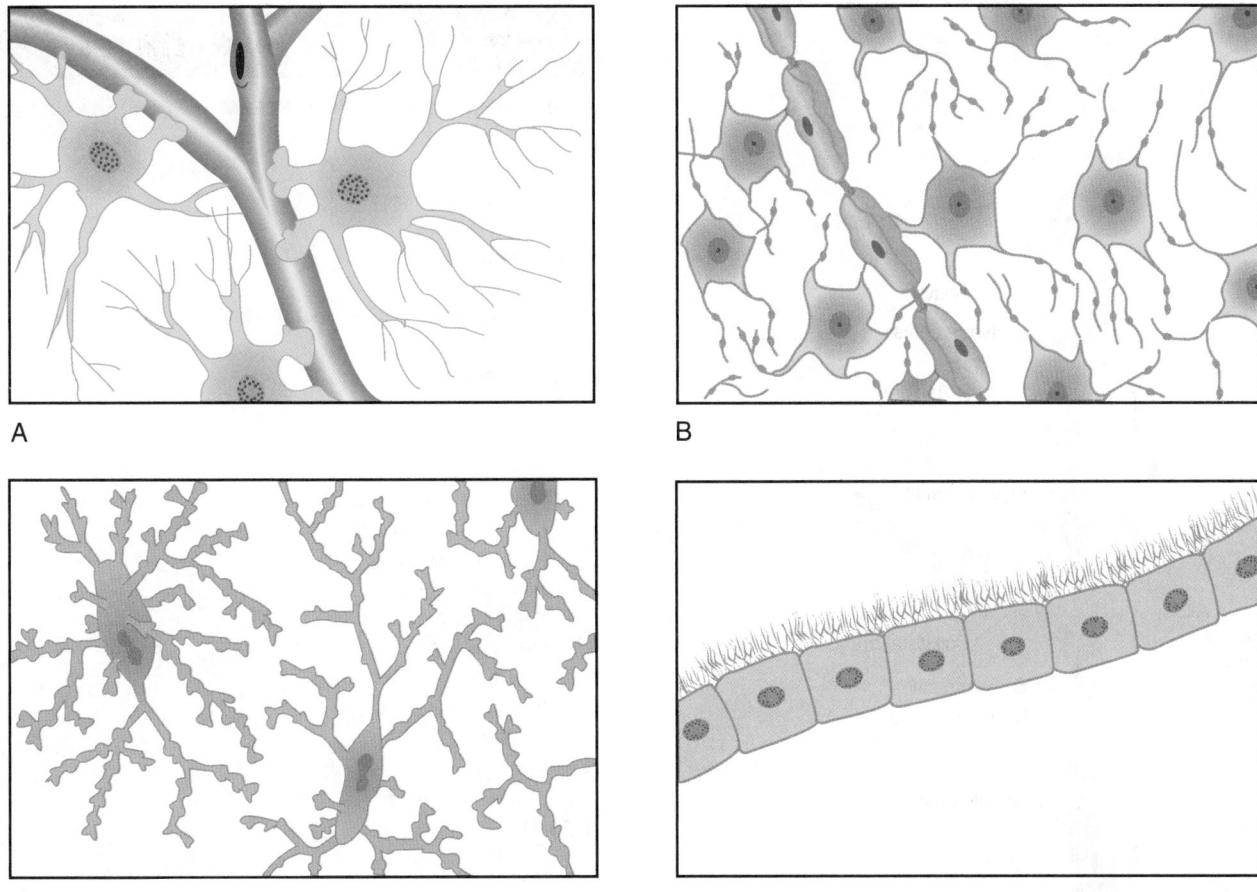

■ **FIGURE A&P16–9** Neuroglial cells. **A,** Astrocytes along the capillary. **B,** Oligodendrocytes along the nerves. **C,** Microglia (phagocytes). **D,** Ependymal cells form a sheet that lines fluid cavities in the brain.

Three types of neurons exist:

1. *Unipolar* neurons have only one nerve fiber leaving the cell body, but they branch to form a dendrite and axon. Unipolar neurons often send general sensory signals.
2. *Multipolar* neurons have numerous afferent synapses and axons that make multiple synapses.
3. *Bipolar* neurons are often utilized in the pathways of special sensory systems (eyes, nose, and ears).

Synapses, which are crucial to nerve function, are small spaces between neurons and their targets (other neurons, muscles, or glands). As a message travels down the neuron, it reaches a synapse that it must cross to "jump" to the next neuron. There are two types of synapses; *chemical* synapses dominate. In an *electrical synapse,* the electrical nerve impulses of two cells cross directly through a very small separation (called *gap junctions* or a *nexus*) from the presynaptic to the postsynaptic cell; this type of synapse is also found in smooth and cardiac muscle cells.

Chemical substances called *neurotransmitters* are discharged into the space *(cleft)* between two neurons and propel the message onto the next neuron. Transmitters are manufactured in the cell body and transported anterograde to the terminals *(boutons),* stored, and secreted from the vesicles in the first neuron *(presynaptic neuron)* into the synaptic cleft (see Figure A&P16-10). The neurotransmitter excites, inhibits, or modifies signals to the second neuron *(postsynaptic neuron)* by interacting with the receptors on its membrane. More than 100 neurotransmitters have been identified. Box A&P16-1 lists the more common transmitters.

IMPULSE CONDUCTION

Resting Potential

A neuron not conducting a nerve impulse is said to be "resting." Although it is resting, it remains charged and potentially ready to fire. The potential to fire is produced by a difference in electrical charge between the interstitial fluid outside the neuron and the intracellular fluid within (Figure A&P16-11). The inside of the nerve cell is electrically negative, and the interstitial fluid is electrically positive. A resulting membrane potential, measured in millivolts (mV), results from this difference in electrical potential between the two compartments. The *resting*

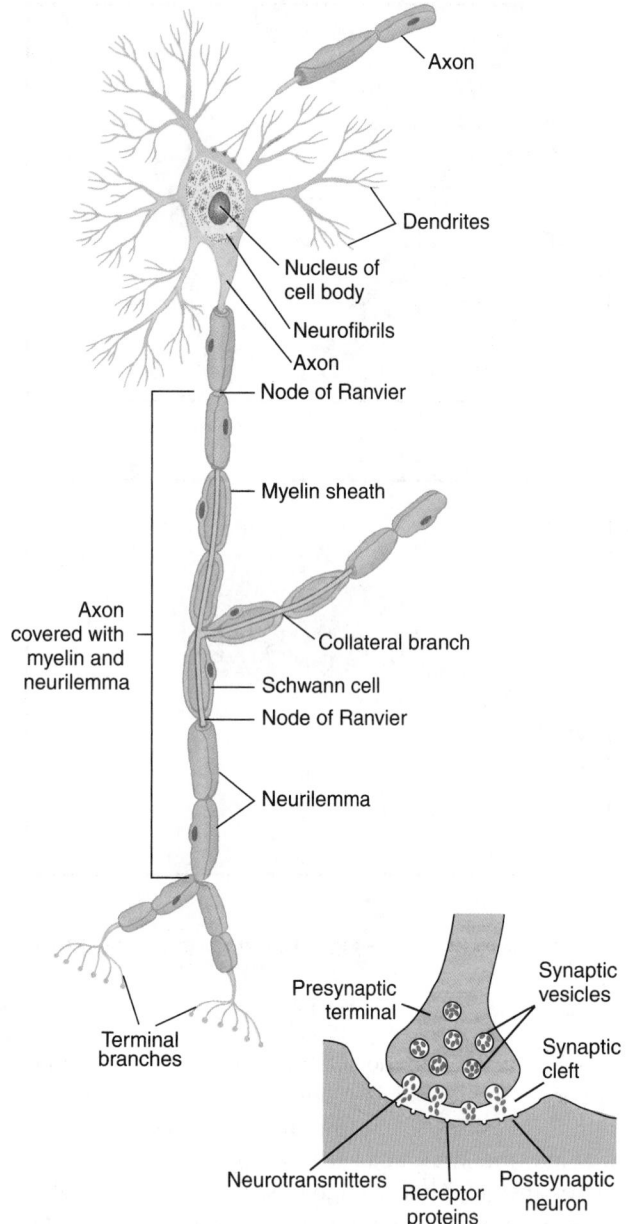

■ **FIGURE A&PI6–I0** A neuron (the basic element of the nervous system) and a chemical synapse.

BOX A&PI6-I   Common Neurotransmitters and Neuropeptides

SMALL-MOLECULE TRANSMITTERS
- Acetylcholine
- Dopamine
- Norepinephrine
- Epinephrine
- Histamine
- Serotonin
- Gamma-aminobutyric acid (GABA)
- Glycine
- Glutamate
- Aspartate
- Nitric oxide

NEUROPEPTIDES
- Hypothalamic-releasing hormones (thyrotropin, luteinizing, growth)
- Pituitary hormones
- Beta-endorphin
- Enkephalin
- Substance P
- Gastrin
- Insulin
- Glucagon
- Cholecystokinin
- Angiotensin II
- Bradykinin
- Calcitonin

Modified from Guyton, A.C., & Hall, J.E. (2007). *Textbook of medical physiology* (11th ed.). Philadelphia: Saunders.

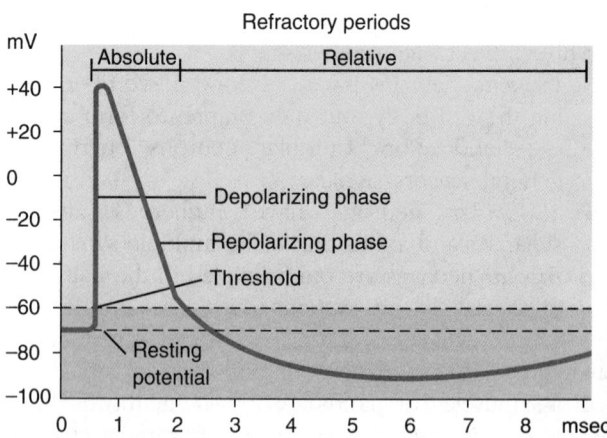

■ **FIGURE A&PI6–II** Generation of nerve impulses. The resting membrane potential is shown at −70 mV.

membrane potential (RMP) of neurons is between −45 and −75 mV, somewhat less polarized than the −90 mV RMP of cardiac and skeletal muscle cells.

The cell is *depolarized* when an influx of sodium makes the membrane potential more positive (i.e., rising to zero). In most cells, this is due to an electrical stimulus transmitted by an adjacent cell.

As the membrane potential rises during depolarization, it reaches a specified level *(threshold)*. When threshold is reached, the excited cell is committed to full action potential because the cell follows an all-or-none phenomenon.

Repolarization is the restoration of the membrane polarity, and sodium and potassium are returned to their usual places via the sodium-potassium pump.

After an action potential is generated, no segment of the nerve fiber can conduct another action potential for a brief period of time (<1 ms). This interval is called the *absolute refractory period.* Sodium and potassium are returning to their original locations during this period, and sodium cannot enter the nerve cell. During the next period, called the *relative refractory period,* only a stimulus stronger than the ordinary one can produce an action potential. On average, a return to a resting potential takes approximately 10 to 30 ms.

Nerve Impulses

Because neurons are arranged in chain-like pathways, impulses must travel quickly from one cell to another. In nerve cells the impulse begins at the axon. When the action potential reaches the presynaptic knob at the dendrite, the membrane's permeability to calcium increases, allowing increased calcium influx. Calcium promotes fusing of the vesicles with the membrane and release of the neurotransmitters inside. Some neurotransmitters are transported back into the vesicles *(reuptake).* Others are decomposed by an enzyme process. For example, acetylcholinesterase decomposes acetylcholine at the postsynaptic membrane.

Myelin

Myelin surrounds most large nerve fibers and is separated by nodes of Ranvier. Action potentials are generated only at the nodes, and thus they skip between them rather than depolarize the entire membrane. This jumping characteristic is known as *saltatory conduction.* Conduction using this process is rapid. Neurons with their axons covered by myelin are called *myelinated nerve fibers;* neurons with little or no myelin are called *unmyelinated nerve fibers.* Myelinated fibers in the CNS constitute the *white matter* in the brain and spinal cord. *Gray matter* consists of cell bodies. The speed of the nerve impulse conduction is also related to the diameter of the fiber; the greater the diameter, the faster the impulse.

Receptors

Receptors are biologic transducers that use the stimulus of one form of energy—mechanical, electrical, chemical, thermal, or light—to initiate the "electrical" energy of the nerve impulse. Although sensory receptors may be stimulated by more than one form of energy, each receptor is especially sensitive to a particular form of energy.

Receptors exhibit a phenomenon known as *adaptation,* a decreased receptor sensitivity in response to steady continuous stimuli. Slow-adapting receptors can maintain the lower rate of discharge for minutes to even hours. Fast-adapting receptor bursts of impulses terminate less than 1 second after initiation of the stimulus. The mechanism of adaptation is not known.

Receptors respond more effectively to change than to continuous stimulation. This characteristic of nerve "fatigue" is protective.

PERIPHERAL NERVOUS SYSTEM

The PNS includes all neurons other than those in the brain and spinal cord. It consists of pathways of nerve fibers between the CNS and all outlying structures in the body. Included in the PNS are 12 pairs of cranial nerves and 31 pairs of spinal nerves.

Nerves that conduct impulses to the brain and spinal cord are called *sensory (afferent) neurons.* Nerves that conduct impulses away from the brain and spinal cord are called *motor (efferent) neurons.* Most nerves are mixed, having both sensory and motor components.

SPINAL NERVES

The spinal nerves develop from a series of nerve rootlets that collect laterally as spinal roots. Each spinal nerve consists of a *dorsal (sensory) root* and a *ventral (motor) root,* which unite to form a spinal nerve. The dorsal root emerges from the posterolateral cord. The ventral root emerges from the anterolateral spinal cord. There are 31 pairs of spinal nerves: 8 pairs of cervical nerves, 12 pairs of thoracic nerves, 5 pairs of lumbar nerves, 5 pairs of sacral nerves, and usually 1 pair of coccygeal nerves (see Figure A&P16-4). The specific area of sensory reception for each dorsal root is called a *sensory dermatome* (Figure A&P16-12).

The peripheral nerves that are formed into plexuses have specific names. There are three major plexuses:

1. The *cervical plexus* supplies the muscles and skin of the neck and branches to form the phrenic nerve, which innervates the diaphragm.
2. The *brachial plexus* supplies the muscles and skin of the shoulder, axilla, arm, forearm, and hand. It branches to form the ulnar, median, and radial nerves.
3. The *lumbosacral plexus* supplies sensory and motor impulses to the muscles and skin of the perineum, gluteal region, thighs, legs, and feet. Its many branches include the pudendal, gluteal, femoral, sciatic, tibial, and common fibular nerves.

CRANIAL NERVES

Twelve pairs of cranial nerves arise from the brain. Most of the cranial nerves are composed of both motor and sensory neurons, although a few cranial nerves carry only sensory impulses (Figure A&P16-13). Except for the olfactory and optic nerves, whose nuclei lie just below the cerebrum, all other cranial nerve nuclei lie within the brain stem. Table A&P16-3 presents the 12 pairs of cranial nerves.

■ **FIGURE A&P16–12** Dermatomes (segments of the spinal cord) indicate distribution of spinal nerves. *Solid lines* divide the regions of the spinal cord (i.e., cervical, thoracic, lumbar, sacral). *Dotted lines* indicate dermatomes. **A,** Torso and limbs. **B,** Anterior chest. **C,** Perineum. **D,** Feet. Dermatomes are used during assessment to identify specific areas of sensory impairment (e.g., touch, pain, temperature).

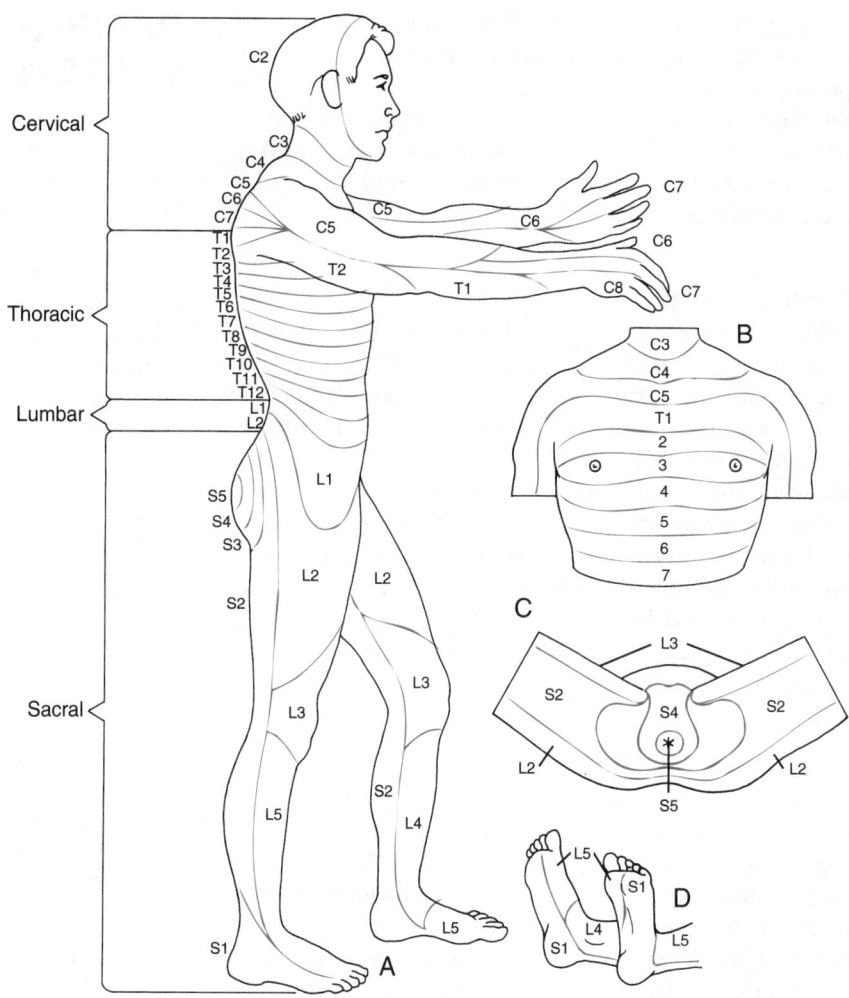

AUTONOMIC NERVOUS SYSTEM

The autonomic nervous system (ANS) is the part of the PNS that coordinates involuntary activities, such as visceral functions, smooth and cardiac muscle changes, and glandular responses. Although it can function independently, its primary control is from the brain and spinal cord. The ANS has two divisions: the *sympathetic* and *parasympathetic nervous systems*. The efferent ANS fibers travel within some cranial and spinal nerves. These two systems are highly integrated and interact with each other to maintain a stable internal environment.

Unlike the *somatic* neurons, which usually are single neurons linking the CNS to a muscle or gland, the ANS has a *two-neuron chain* leading to the effector organ. The terminal of the first neuron is located in the CNS and synapses with nerve fibers whose cell bodies are within an autonomic ganglion. The axon of the second neuron (*postganglionic fiber*) carries impulses to the target viscera. An exception is the adrenal medulla, which is innervated directly by preganglionic fibers.

The medulla is actually composed of postganglionic neurons that secrete epinephrine into the bloodstream during an "adrenaline rush."

The *sympathetic nervous system* coordinates activities used to handle stress and is geared for action as a whole for short periods. The preganglionic neurons of the sympathetic nervous system emerge from the spinal cord via the motor (ventral) roots of the thoracic and upper two lumbar spinal nerves (T1-L2) (Figure A&P16-14). Preganglionic axons are short; postganglionic axons are long.

The *parasympathetic nervous system* is associated with conservation and restoration of energy stores and is geared to act locally and discretely for a longer duration. The preganglionic fibers emerge from the brain stem via the cranial nerves and from the spinal cord via the sacral spinal nerves at S-4. These preganglionic fibers have long axons that synapse with the postganglionic neurons in ganglia close to or located within the organs to be innervated. Each postganglionic neuron has a relatively short axon. Most, but not all, organ systems have both parasympathetic and sympathetic innervation. About 75% of the parasympathetic fibers are in the vagus nerve.

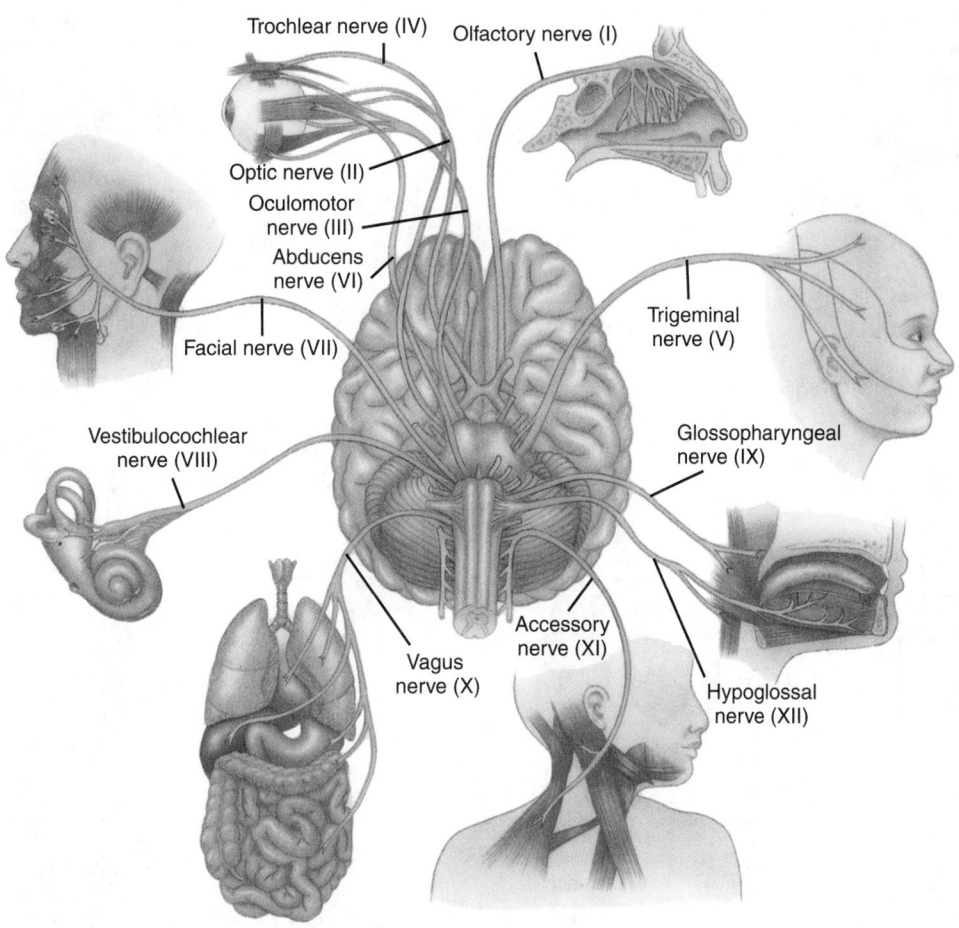

■ **FIGURE A&P16–13** Ventral surface of the brain showing the attachment of the cranial nerves. *(From Thibodeau, G., & Patton, K. [2007]. Anatomy and physiology [6th ed.]. St. Louis: Mosby.)*

TABLE A&P16–3   Functions and Types of Cranial Nerves

	Name	Function	Type
I	Olfactory	Olfaction (smell)	Sensory
II	Optic	Vision	Sensory
III	Oculomotor	Extraocular eye movement	Motor
		Elevation of eyelid	
		Pupil constriction	Parasympathetic
IV	Trochlear	Extraocular eye movement	Motor
V	Trigeminal		
	Ophthalmic division	Somatic sensations of cornea, nasal mucous membranes, face	Sensory
	Maxillary division	Somatic sensations of face, oral cavity, anterior two thirds of tongue, teeth	Sensory
	Mandibular division	Somatic sensation of lower face	Sensory
		Mastication (chewing)	Motor
VI	Abducens	Lateral eye movement	Motor
VII	Facial	Facial expression	Motor
		Taste, anterior two thirds of tongue	Sensory
		Salivation	Parasympathetic
VIII	Vestibulocochlear		
	Vestibular	Equilibrium	Sensory
	Cochlear	Hearing	Sensory
IX	Glossopharyngeal	Taste, posterior third of tongue; pharyngeal sensation	Sensory
		Swallowing	Motor
X	Vagus	Sensation in pharynx, larynx, external ear	Sensory
		Swallowing	Motor
		Thoracic and abdominal visceral parasympathetic nervous system activities	Parasympathetic
XI	Spinal accessory	Neck and shoulder movement	Motor
XII	Hypoglossal	Tongue movement	Motor

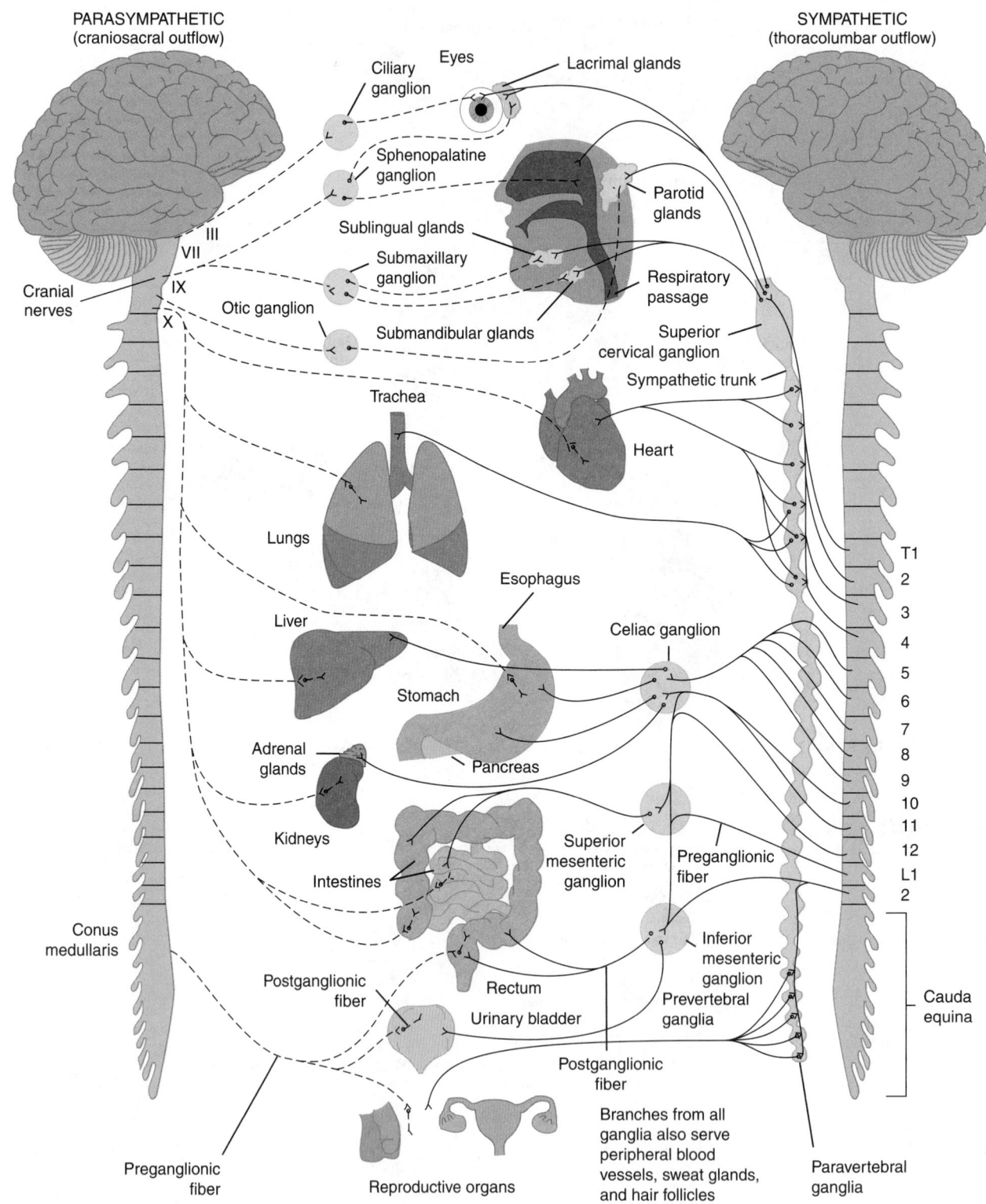

PARASYMPATHETIC
(craniosacral outflow)

SYMPATHETIC
(thoracolumbar outflow)

Eyes

Ciliary ganglion

Lacrimal glands

Sphenopalatine ganglion

Parotid glands

III
VII

Sublingual glands

Cranial nerves

Submaxillary ganglion

IX
X

Otic ganglion

Respiratory passage

Submandibular glands

Superior cervical ganglion

Sympathetic trunk

Trachea

Heart

Lungs

Esophagus

Liver

Celiac ganglion

Stomach

Adrenal glands

Pancreas

Kidneys

Intestines

Superior mesenteric ganglion

Preganglionic fiber

Conus medullaris

Inferior mesenteric ganglion

Postganglionic fiber

Prevertebral ganglia

Rectum

Cauda equina

Urinary bladder

Postganglionic fiber

Preganglionic fiber

Reproductive organs

Branches from all ganglia also serve peripheral blood vessels, sweat glands, and hair follicles

Paravertebral ganglia

T1
2
3
4
5
6
7
8
9
10
11
12
L1
2

■ **FIGURE A&P16–14** Autonomic nervous system.

Table A&P16-4 lists the effects of both the sympathetic and parasympathetic nervous systems on different organs. These functions and responses are related to the type of neurotransmitter released. The preganglionic fibers of the sympathetic and parasympathetic nerves and the postganglionic fibers of the parasympathetic nerves release acetylcholine. The postganglionic fibers of the sympathetic nerves release norepinephrine. Fibers that secrete

TABLE A&P16–4   Effects of the Sympathetic and Parasympathetic Nervous Systems on Organs

Organ	Effect of Sympathetic Stimulation	Effect of Parasympathetic Stimulation
Eye		
Pupil	Dilation (alpha)	Constriction
Ciliary muscle	Slight relaxation (far vision)	Constriction (near vision)
Glands	Vasoconstriction and slight secretion	Stimulation of copious secretion (containing many enzymes for enzyme-secreting glands)
Nasal		
Lacrimal		
Parotid		
Submandibular		
Gastric		
Pancreatic		
Sweat glands	Copious sweating (cholinergic)	Sweating on palms of hands
Apocrine glands	Thick, odoriferous secretion	None
Heart		
Muscle	Increased rate (beta$_1$)	Slowed rate
	Increased force of contraction (beta$_1$)	Decreased force of contraction (especially of atria)
Coronaries	Dilated (beta$_2$); constricted (alpha)	Dilation
Lungs		
Bronchi	Dilation (beta$_2$)	Constriction
Blood vessels	Mild constriction	? Dilation
Gut		
Lumen	Decreased peristalsis and tone (beta$_2$)	Increased peristalsis and tone
Sphincter	Increased tone (alpha)	Relaxation (most times)
Liver	Gluconeogenesis, glycogenolysis (beta$_2$)	Slight glycogen synthesis
Gallbladder and bile ducts	Relaxation	Contraction
Kidney	Decreased output and renin secretion	None
Bladder		
Detrusor	Relaxation (slight) (beta$_2$)	Contraction
Trigone	Contraction (alpha)	Relaxation
Penis	Ejaculation	Erection
Systemic arterioles		
Abdominal viscera	Constriction (alpha)	None
Muscle	Constriction (alpha)	None
	Dilation (beta$_2$)	
	Dilation (cholinergic)	
Skin	Constriction	None
Blood		
Coagulation	Increase	None
Glucose	Increase	None
Lipids	Increase	None
Basal metabolism	Increase up to 100%	None
Adrenal medullary secretion	Increase	None
Mental activity	Increase	None
Piloerector muscles	Contraction (alpha)	None
Skeletal muscle	Increased glycogenolysis (beta$_2$)	None
	Increased strength	
Fat cells	Lipolysis (beta$_3$)	None

Modified from Guyton, A.C., & Hall, J.E. (2007). *Textbook of medical physiology* (11th ed.). Philadelphia: Saunders.

acetylcholine are called *cholinergic fibers;* fibers that secrete norepinephrine are called *adrenergic fibers.*

The complexity of the sympathetic and parasympathetic response also depends on the type of receptor that combines with the neurotransmitter. The sympathetic nervous system has five types of receptors: alpha$_1$, alpha$_2$, beta$_1$, beta$_2$, and beta$_3$. The parasympathetic nervous system has two general classes of receptors, muscarinic and nicotinic.

EFFECTS OF INJURY ON THE NERVOUS SYSTEM

REGENERATION

For many years it was thought that nerve cell bodies were not able to regenerate; however, it appears that CNS cortical neurons do attempt to regenerate. PNS regeneration can occur if only the axon in the PNS is injured. Initially there is breakdown of the myelin sheath and axon. The axon swells and fragments while the myelin sheath disintegrates distal to the injury. The cell body takes up water. Macrophages phagocytose the breakdown products. Neurilemma cells migrate into the emerging space (Figure A&P16-15).

The injured axon tip forms a new plasma membrane. A few days after injury, sprouts emerge from the tip. Peripheral nerve sprouts enter the distal stump and often come in contact with a neurilemma cord, which serves as a guide. The regenerating axon grows along the cord at a rate of 4 mm daily. Later the neurilemma cells encapsulate the regenerating nerve fibers. With time the axon and myelin sheath both thicken. Axons within the CNS sprout and form growing tips but appear unable to sustain the metabolic responses necessary for extensive regeneration. It is believed that the axon tip is not able to penetrate the glial scar formed at the injury site, such as after spinal cord injury.

An uninjured axon may sprout a collateral branch at a node of Ranvier that may enter into an adjacent denervated neurilemma cord. Collateral nerve regeneration occurs in both the PNS and the CNS, for example, after peripheral nerve trauma or inflammation of a peripheral nerve, as in Bell's palsy.

EFFECTS OF AGING ON THE NERVOUS SYSTEM

Neurons undergo senescence. Intracellular, cellular, and biochemical changes occur. Lipofuscin accumulates in the cell. Neurofibrillary tangles and senile plaques develop. After we reach 30 years of age, neurons decrease in number and neuroglial cells increase in size and number. The number of dendrites decreases, but the intrinsic dendritic changes are quite variable in hippocampal areas of the brain on postmortem examination in the normal aging population. Variations in dendrite length, stability, and growth have been attributed to compensatory response to death of dendrites.

Aging has little effect on sensory and primary memory but causes a decrease in working memory, including longer retrieval times for short-term memory, categorization, and episodic memory. Dendritic changes are quite pronounced in pathologic conditions such as Alzheimer's disease (see Chapter 72). The axons also change in normal aging; their diameters thin, and the number of receptors decreases.

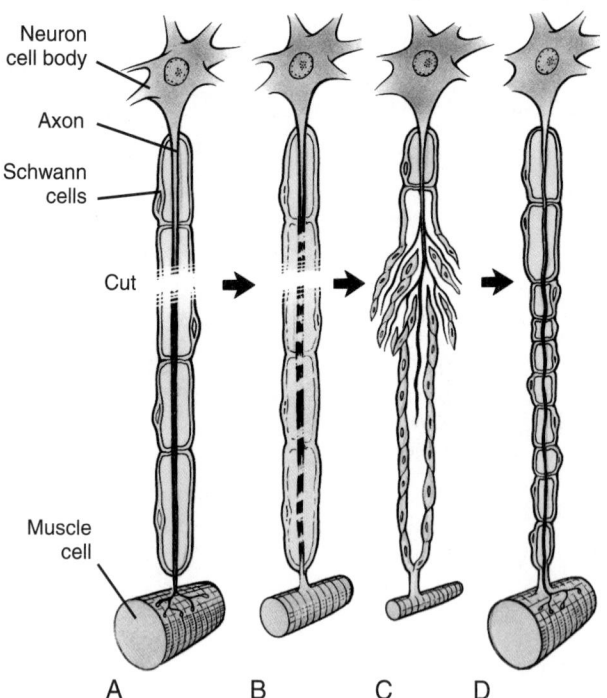

■ **FIGURE A&P16–15** Regeneration of peripheral nerve tissue. **A,** An injury results in a cut nerve. **B,** Immediately after the injury, the distal portion of the axon degenerates, as does its myelin sheath. **C,** The remaining neurilemma cells tunnel from the point of injury to the effector. New Schwann cells grow within this tunnel, maintaining a path for regrowth of the axon. Meanwhile, several growing fibers reach the tunnel. **D,** The neuron's attachment is reestablished. *(From Thibodeau, G., & Patton, K. [2007]. Anatomy and physiology [6th ed.]. St. Louis: Mosby.)*

 CONCLUSIONS

The nervous system has three major divisions:
1. The CNS regulates higher-level processes, such as thought and vital functions.
2. The PNS provides pathways to the CNS.
3. The ANS coordinates involuntary activities such as digestion.

The *neuron* is the structural and functional unit of the nervous system. The typical neuron is composed of a cell body, one axon, and several dendrites. The impulses along the nerve are carried through the action of several electrolytes. Neurotransmitters carry the impulse from neuron to neuron.

BIBLIOGRAPHY

1. Berne, R., et al. (2007). *Physiology* (5th ed.). St. Louis: Mosby.
2. Guyton, A.C., & Hall, J.E. (2007). *Textbook of medical physiology* (11th ed.). Philadelphia: Saunders.
3. Kandel, E.R., Schwartz, J.H., & Jessel, T.M. (2000). *Principles of neural science* (4th ed.). New York: McGraw-Hill.
4. Thibodeau, G., & Patton, K. (2007). *Anatomy and physiology* (6th ed.). St. Louis: Mosby.

CHAPTER 67

Assessment of the Neurologic System

CLARE M. SEKERAK

Assessment of a client experiencing a neurologic disorder is a challenge. Neurologic disorders range from simple to complex and can have profound consequences for activities of daily living (ADL) and survival. Neurologic assessment establishes baseline data that are used to compare ongoing assessments, diagnose actual and potential health problems, manage client care, and evaluate the outcome. Because of the complexity of the nervous system, neurologic assessment is both multifaceted and lengthy. A comprehensive history, a neurologic examination, and general or specific neurodiagnostic studies are the primary components of a neurologic assessment.

Neurologic assessment is both anatomic and functional. Continuous observations of the client are made and compared with baseline data. Astute observations are essential because many neurologic changes occur subtly. Nurses collect data on the client's ability to function physically (self-care deficit) and mentally (confusion and altered problem solving). Finally, because many neurologic disorders are serious, the nurse provides skillful, crisis-oriented support for the client and significant others.

This chapter presents basic neurologic assessment procedures. Additional assessment techniques for specific neurologic disorders are discussed throughout Unit 16. To avoid missing parts of a complex examination, novice practitioners should follow the assessment sequence described in this chapter. The sequence suggested in Table 67-1 integrates cranial nerve and reflex testing into motor and sensory examinations.

HISTORY

The history consists of biographical data, the chief complaint and clinical manifestation analysis, a review of systems, past medical history, surgical history, allergies, medications history, dietary habits, psychosocial history, and family health history.

The health history guides the physical examination. Some complaints require a complete neurologic examination while other complaints may require a more focused examination on a particular system or anatomic area. For example, a complaint of dizziness cues a focus on examination of the eyes, ears (vestibular nerve), and cerebellar function instead of motor and sensory functions. Detailed neurologic examination is indicated when the client reports behavioral changes, altered level of consciousness (LOC), growth and development problems, pain, changes in motor or sensory function, infection, or trauma.

Assess for neurologic problems that may be related to other problems, such as alcohol and recreational drug use, metabolic imbalances, and metastatic lesions.

Biographical and Demographic Data

Biographical data comprise demographic, administrative, and insurance information. Often included are (1) a personal profile or brief description of the client, (2) the source of the history (client or a significant other),

---

evolve **Web Enhancements**

Assessment Terms   English and Spanish

Appendix A   Religious Beliefs and Practices Affecting Health Care

Appendix B   A Health History Format That Integrates the Assessment of Functional Health Patterns

Web Figures   Cerebral Angiography

Electromyography

Web Tables   Normal Cerebrospinal Fluid (CSF) Values and Significance of Abnormal Values

Web Boxes   Terms Associated with Gait Disorders

Types of Electrical Brain Waves

Be sure to check out the bonus material on the Evolve website and the CD-ROM, including free self-assessment exercises. **http://evolve.elsevier. com/Black/medsurg**

TABLE 67–1 Neurologic Assessment Guidelines

Functional Category	Specific Category	Area of Nervous System Involved	Assessment Technique	Examples of Disorders
1. Consciousness (awareness of self and environment)	Arousal response to verbal, tactile, and visual stimuli	Reticular activating system (mesencephalon, diencephalon) Both hemispheres	Is client alert? What is attention span? Is there normal response to visual and auditory stimuli? Reaction to loud noises, shaking, deep pressure over eye orbits or sternum?	Elevation: insomnia, agitation, mania, delirium Depression: somnolence, lethargy, semicoma, coma
2. Mentation	Thinking	Cerebral hemispheres plus specific regional functions	Are vital signs, pupils, and reflexes normal? Is client oriented (time, place, person)?	Disorientation
	Insight, judgment, planning	Frontal lobe, with association fibers to other area of cerebrum	Does client recognize implication of illness? Are goals congruent with abilities? How would client respond to given situation (house on fire)?	Lack of judgment, inattention to grooming, appearance, and personal habits
	Fund of information	Basic biologic intellect (frontal lobe) integrated into other areas	Calculation ability, knowledge of current events consistent with educational level. Who is U.S. president?	Impairment—functioning not congruent with level of education
	Memory	Temporal lobe and association to most other areas of cortex		
	Recent	Hippocampus	What did client eat for breakfast? What happened yesterday?	Dementia
	Past	Frontal lobe	Recall past events during taking of history.	Lapses of memory for past events may coincide with past CNS problems (trauma, infection, psychic trauma)
	Feeling (affect) (congruence of response to stimulus)	Limbic system (usually involves both hemispheres)	Compare observed with expected reactions. Are emotions labile? Appropriate?	Blunted affect: hysteria, schizophrenia, bilateral frontal lobe lesions
	Perceptual distortions (illusions, hallucinations)	General and specific cortical areas in hallucinations	Observe for behavior indicating perceptual problems.	Irritative lesions of cortex may lead to hallucinations (occipital cortex → visual, postcentral gyrus → somatic sensation, uncus → smell)
3. Language and speech	Dysarthria (defects in articulation, enunciation, and rhythm in speech)	Impairment of muscles of tongue, palate, pharynx, or lips (may be due to impulses or incoordination) Brain stem, cerebellum, or extraneural causes; CN V, VII, IX, X, XII	Have client repeat a difficult phrase ("Susie sells seashells by the seashore").	Slurring, slowness, indistinctness, nasality, break in normal speech rhythm (speech of intoxication); amyotrophic lateral sclerosis; pseudobulbar palsy; myasthenia gravis; stroke
	Dysphonia (abnormal production of sounds from larynx)	Many extraneural causes Recurrent laryngeal nerve problems (part of vagus, CN X)	Is client's voice hoarse, strained, soft? Whispered voice is intact. Use indirect laryngoscopy findings.	Parkinsonism, dystonia Compression of recurrent laryngeal nerve by bronchogenic carcinoma of left mainstem bronchus Left atrial hypertrophy
		Medulla (area of nucleus of CN X)		Brain stem tumors, occlusion of posterior inferior cerebellar or vertebral artery

	Aphasia (inability to use and understand written and spoken words)	Fluent (receptive): left temporal and parietal lobes (Wernicke's area)	Observe vocal expression, written expression, comprehension of spoken and written language, and gesture communication.	Stroke of middle cerebral artery; Trauma, tumor, abscess in left temporal and parietal lobe areas
		Nonfluent (expressive): Broca's area (lateral) inferior portion of frontal lobe of dominant side		Damage to Broca's area or association fibers (stroke, tumor)
		Global (combined)		
	Agnosia (inability to recognize objects or symbols by means of senses)	Primarily in parietal, temporal, and occipital areas	Sense organs intact? Can the client recognize objects by sight, touch, hearing?	Stroke
4. Motor function	Expression (facial)	CN VII	Symmetry of smile, frown, raising of eyebrows	Central facial weakness (upper motor neuron dysfunction); weakness of lower half of face *Causes:* stroke, corticobulbar tract Peripheral facial weakness (lower motor dysfunction); weakness of entire half of face *Causes:* Bell's palsy, brain stem tumor, fracture of temporal bone
	Eating (chewing, swallowing)	CN V, VII, IX, X, XII	Strength of masticator muscles, gag reflexes, ability to swallow	Tetanus, peripheral spasm of muscle; amyotrophic lateral sclerosis, medullary tumor; pseudobulbar palsy may be associated with dysarthria
	Eye movements	CN III, IV, VI	Extraocular movement, pupil size, reactivity, pupils react equally to accommodation, diplopia, nystagmus	Cerebral peduncle pressure → CN III dysfunction, cavernous sinus thrombus → CN III, IV, VI problem Muscular problems (myasthenia gravis, hyperthyroid) Horner's syndrome (ptosis, constricted pupil), anisocoria
	Moving	Motor precentral gyrus (pyramidal) and cerebellar systems, basal ganglia, CN XI, spinal cord, upper motor neuron (brain → spinal cord via corticospinal tract)	Gait, heel-to-toe walking, presence or absence of involuntary movements, coordination, muscle tone, mass, strength, Romberg's test, ability to shrug shoulders and to rise from chair	*Upper motor neuron:* Brain and cord-sparing anterior horn cell Tone ↑↑ (spastic) Bulk ↓ because of atrophy of disuse Reflexes ↑↑ because of loss of central inhibition No fasciculations Frequent clonus *Lower motor neuron:* Segment anterior horn cell peripheral nerve Tone ↓↓ (flaccid) Bulk ↓ because of tone loss Reflexes ↓ or absent from loss of anterior horn cell Fasciculations No clonus
		Lower motor neuron (motor cells of cranial and spinal nerves and anterior horn cells → peripheral muscles)		
		Involves cerebellum		*Cerebellar problem* → loss of coordination and balance

(Continued)

TABLE 67-1   Neurologic Assessment Guidelines —Cont'd

Functional Category	Specific Category	Area of Nervous System Involved	Assessment Technique	Examples of Disorders
5. Sensory function	Seeing	CN II: optic, occipital lobe	Acuity, visual fields, funduscopy	Field test: loss in retina or optic nerve → loss in eye involved, optic chiasm → bitemporal hemianopsia Optic tract → homonymous hemianopsia, parietal lobe → quadrant problems (inferior), temporal lobe → superior quadrant problems ↑ Intracranial pressure → papilledema (raised disc → hemorrhage)
	Smelling	CN I: temporal lobe (uncus)	Ability to detect familiar odors	Usually ↓ smell from extraneural causes (upper respiratory tract infection, allergy, smoking); olfactory groove; meningioma, olfactory hallucinations
	Hearing	CN VIII: cochlear division, temporal lobe	Acuity of hearing, presence or absence of unusual sounds, Weber and Rinne tests	May have conductive (nerve OK) or neural hearing loss; Ménière's syndrome (tinnitus, hearing loss, vertigo, and nystagmus), basilar skull fracture → otorrhea Brain stem vascular dysfunction or tumors → ↓ hearing
	Taste	CN VII, IX: insular lobe	Ability to differentiate sweet, salt, sour, and bitter	Brain stem or insula lesions → ↓ taste; extraneural causes, smoking, poor oral hygiene
	Feeling (sensory)	Peripheral nerves → Dermatomes → Spinal cord → Tracts (leading to)	Pain: pinprick Touch: cotton touched to skin Proprioception: check where digit is in space	Polyneuropathy (diabetes mellitus, anemia) Spinal cord lesions → dermatome alterations Upper pons → thalamus, contralateral loss Thalamus → contralateral loss + paresthesias
		Pain-temperature–tactile, anterolateral system, proprioception, stereognosis, dorsal roots → thalamus leading to somasthetic area (postcentral gyrus, parietal lobe)	Vibration: place vibrating tuning fork on bony prominence Temperature: test tubes of cold and warm water laid against skin; person identifies whether hot or cold	Thalamus → cortex → cortical sensory loss
6. Bowel and bladder function	Bowel function	Afferent Spinal nerve S3-5 External sphincter (voluntary control) Internal sphincter	Check for fecal impaction or incontinence Check muscle tone	Fecal incontinence with lesions S3-5 Anal anesthesia—conus medullaris and tabes dorsalis
		Autonomic nervous system		May be extraneural causes
		Cerebral cortex		Loss of inhibitory control (stroke)
	Bladder function	Autonomic nervous system	Feels when bladder is full, complete emptying Does client have urgency, frequency?	Urinary incontinence
		Afferent Spinal nerve T9-L2, S2-4 Pudendal nerve Efferent Spinal nerve T11-L2 External sphincter (voluntary) Spinal nerve S2-4 Cerebral cortex		Flaccid bladder Spastic bladder Loss of inhibitory control (stroke) May be extraneural causes

CN, Cranial nerve; CNS, central nervous system; L, lumbar; S, sacral; T, thoracic; ↑, increased; ↑↑, significantly increased; ↓, decreased; ↓↓, significantly decreased; →, may affect or lead to.

and (3) the client's mental status (indicating the reliability of the data). Neurologic problems often affect mental status, sometimes making it difficult to obtain an accurate history directly from the client.

Current Health

Ask about the client's current state of health. Neurologic disorders often affect the client's lifestyle. The history should begin with an open-ended and non-direct inquiry to allow the client to describe the problem. Allow the client to describe how current conditions impact daily life. Explore areas of concern for the client.

Chief Complaint

Obtain a detailed description of the events that have led the client to seek care. Avoid suggesting manifestations to the client, and use open-ended questions. Allow clients to describe the problem in their own words and try not to interrupt. When given the opportunity, often clients will disclose their real concerns as the history-taking proceeds. A client with a complaint of headaches may only be concerned about headaches or may be fearful of a more serious problem such as brain tumor or aneurysm. If the client feels rushed or interrupted, these concerns may not be revealed. Elicit a detailed report from the client regarding the issues that relate to the chief complaint (Figure 67-1).

Clinical Manifestations

Determine the onset and sequence of manifestations and their progress. Ask the client to describe neurologic disease processes accurately to facilitate the diagnostic process. Allow the client to describe manifestations using his or her own words. Use a systematic analysis to elicit the characteristics and progression of manifestations (see Chapter 2). Inquire about the frequency, duration, and location of manifestations. Ask about related complaints. For example, urinary retention and bowel incontinence can occur in spinal injuries. Ask the client what improves or aggravates the condition. Common clinical manifestations of neurologic problems include pain, dizziness, sensory and/or motor function complaints, and LOC issues. The chief complaint guides the discussion of the clinical manifestations.

Pain. Pain is a common complaint of clients presenting with neurologic problems. Discussion should focus on the site (headache, back pain, pain in extremities), onset (sudden, gradual), frequency, duration, and character (throbbing, achy, dull, or sharp). Does the pain go anywhere else? What are the precipitating factors (headaches: aura, walking, neck movement) and relieving factors (medications, stretching, rest, applying cold/heat)? Ask about injury or trauma, including previous neurologic

injuries. Inquiry should also include related manifestations (headache: nausea, back pain: muscle spasms). Refer to the Integrating Diagnostic Testing feature on p. 1769 for details of further diagnostic evaluation of the client with complaints related to suspected nerve root compression, a possible cause for pain of neurologic origin.

Dizziness. Many clients present with a complaint of dizziness. Ask the client to describe what is meant by "dizziness" (lightheaded vs. room spinning). Ask if it is related to postural changes (orthostatic blood pressure drop, positional vertigo). What head movements cause problems? What happens when the client turns rapidly or rolls over in bed? Does the client have vision problems? Does the client have ear problems such as hearing loss, ringing, or buzzing (tinnitus)? Does the dizziness improve or worsen when eyes are closed? Does visual fixation help? Inquire about other causes of dizziness (cardiac dysrhythmias, anxiety [panic attacks], history of diabetes mellitus [decreased blood glucose level], ear infection).

Sensory Complaints. Common sensory complaints of the neurologic client include alterations in the ability to see, taste, hear, smell, and feel (pain, numbness, tingling). Ask the client to describe the sensation and its quality (shooting, stabbing, dull, sharp) and its severity. Ask about the site of the sensory abnormality as well as the distribution (stocking glove, extremity). Inquire about onset, frequency, and duration of manifestations. What are the precipitating factors (walking, neck movement, chewing, exposure to cold)? What relieves the manifestations (rest, change of position, medications)? Refer to the Integrating Diagnostic Testing feature on p. 1770 for details of the evaluation of a sensory complaint.

Motor Complaints. Motor complains include weakness, problems with coordination (balance, clumsiness, and gait disturbances), and involuntary movements (tremor, tics). Inquire about the site, onset, frequency, and duration of any manifestations. What precipitates and what improves these conditions?

Loss of Consciousness/Alterations in Mental Status. Impaired consciousness level is a common neurologic problem. Inquire about onset (gradual or sudden) and duration (transient or persistent). If the client's LOC remains diminished at the time of the interview, other sources of information such as family, friends, and the ambulance team may need to be questioned. Refer to the Integrating Diagnostic Testing feature on p. 1771 for details of the evaluation of the client who presents with alterations in level of consciousness.

Is there a history of head trauma (immediately leading to admission or recent: within 6 weeks)? If there is a history of trauma, what type of trauma occurred (fall, blunt force, motor vehicle accident, sports injury with head

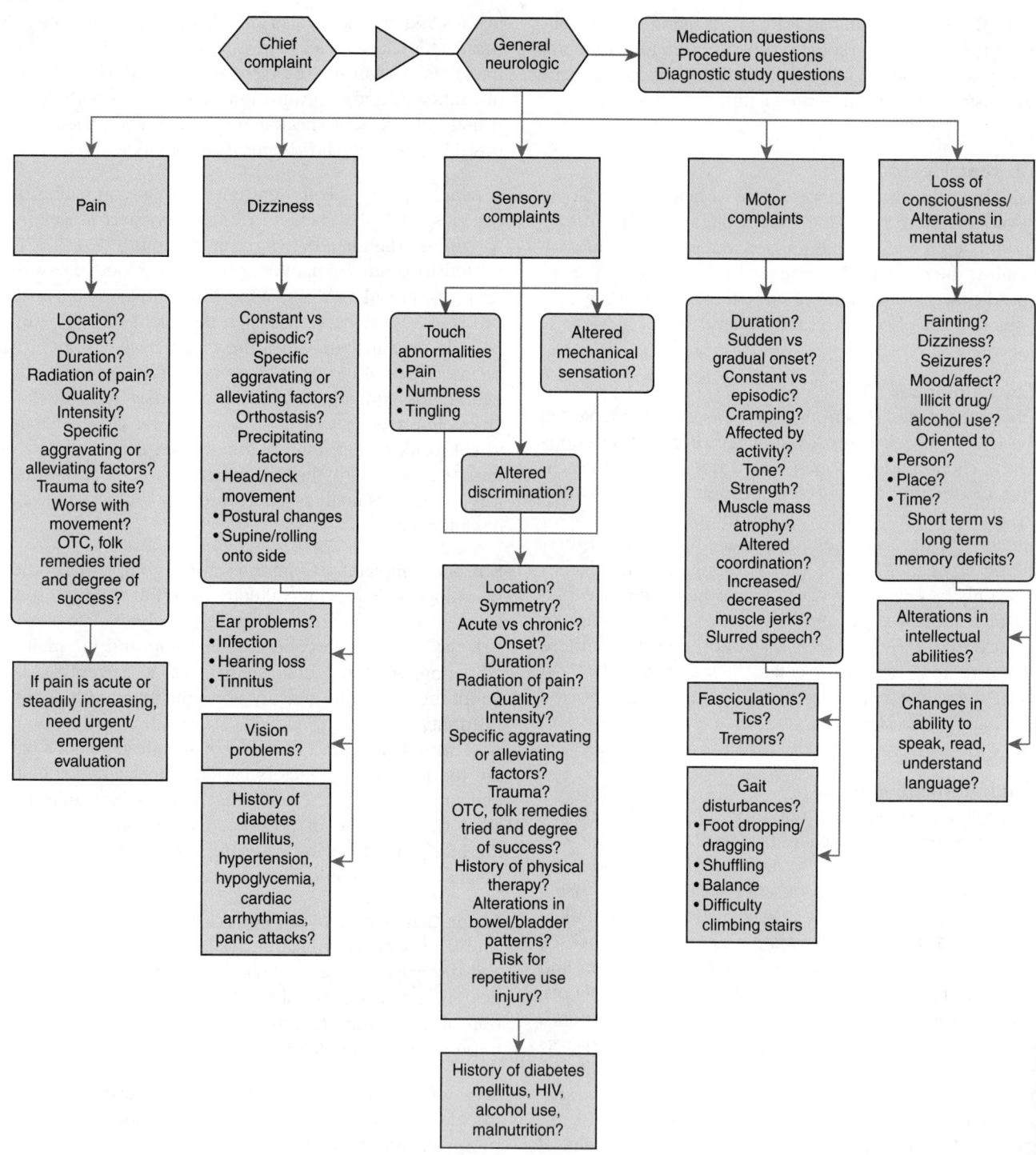

■ **FIGURE 67–1**   Expanded neurologic assessment.

impact)? Is there limb twitching and incontinence (seizure) associated with the episode of decreased level of consciousness? What precipitated the episode (injury, infection, fever, aura)? Does the client have a history of diabetes mellitus, alcoholism, drug abuse, psychiatric illness (drug overdose), or epilepsy?

Review of Systems

In contrast to the assessment of current health where the client is encouraged to give information through open-ended and general questions, the review of systems (ROS) uses direct questions. The purpose of the ROS is to gain more information about the client's presentation.

Nerve Root Compression

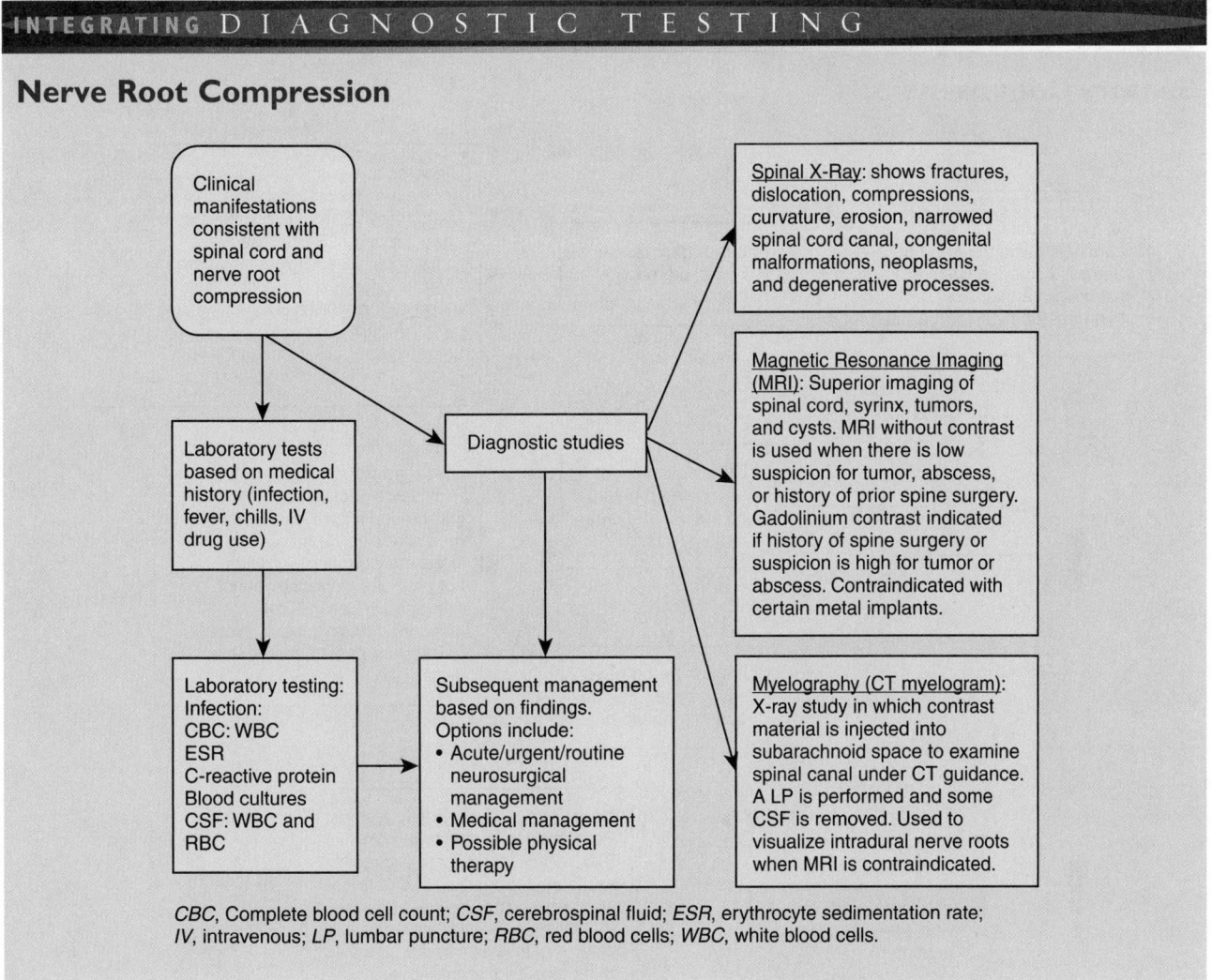

Clinical manifestations consistent with spinal cord and nerve root compression

Laboratory tests based on medical history (infection, fever, chills, IV drug use)

Diagnostic studies

Laboratory testing:
Infection:
CBC: WBC
ESR
C-reactive protein
Blood cultures
CSF: WBC and RBC

Subsequent management based on findings.
Options include:
• Acute/urgent/routine neurosurgical management
• Medical management
• Possible physical therapy

Spinal X-Ray: shows fractures, dislocation, compressions, curvature, erosion, narrowed spinal cord canal, congenital malformations, neoplasms, and degenerative processes.

Magnetic Resonance Imaging (MRI): Superior imaging of spinal cord, syrinx, tumors, and cysts. MRI without contrast is used when there is low suspicion for tumor, abscess, or history of prior spine surgery. Gadolinium contrast indicated if history of spine surgery or suspicion is high for tumor or abscess. Contraindicated with certain metal implants.

Myelography (CT myelogram): X-ray study in which contrast material is injected into subarachnoid space to examine spinal canal under CT guidance. A LP is performed and some CSF is removed. Used to visualize intradural nerve roots when MRI is contraindicated.

CBC, Complete blood cell count; *CSF*, cerebrospinal fluid; *ESR*, erythrocyte sedimentation rate; *IV*, intravenous; *LP*, lumbar puncture; *RBC*, red blood cells; *WBC*, white blood cells.

Do not repeat questions already asked earlier in the health history, but ask questions regarding topics not previously assessed (Figure 67-2 on p. 1772).

Neurologic disorders often subtly affect the ability to function in an integrated fashion. Ask the client to describe any neurologic manifestations, such as behavior changes, mood swings, loss of consciousness, seizures, headaches, dizziness, vertigo, memory deficits, speech or motor function problems (unstable balance or posture, gait changes, tics, tremors), and sensory function problems (vision changes, pain, paresthesia or tingling, paralysis). Has the client had any difficulty swallowing or a change in voice? Has the client experienced sexual difficulties such as erectile difficulties or loss of libido? Significant neurologic assessment data are listed in Box 67-1 on p. 1773. Detailed questions for the review of systems can be found on the website.

The client who has a neurologic problem may be unaware of its presence. Attempt to supplement and corroborate the history and review of systems by speaking with a family member or significant other who knows the client well. Ask specifically about mental or physical changes that have been noticed.

Past Medical History

Collect data regarding common childhood diseases and immunizations. Diseases associated with neurologic sequelae include rubella, rubeola, cytomegalovirus infection, herpes simplex, influenza, and meningitis. Ask whether the client has completed the recommended immunization schedule. Public health resources provide schedules for childhood immunizations as well as recommendations for travelers to foreign countries.

The growth and development history may help determine whether neurologic dysfunction was present at an early age. The perinatal history may contain data about maternal toxemia; neural tube defects; or in utero exposure to viruses (rubella), alcohol, tobacco, or other drugs, and radiation. Ask whether the client was born at full term. Premature birth increases the risk of neurologic damage from inadequate oxygenation and intracranial bleeding

INTEGRATING DIAGNOSTIC TESTING

Sensory Complaints

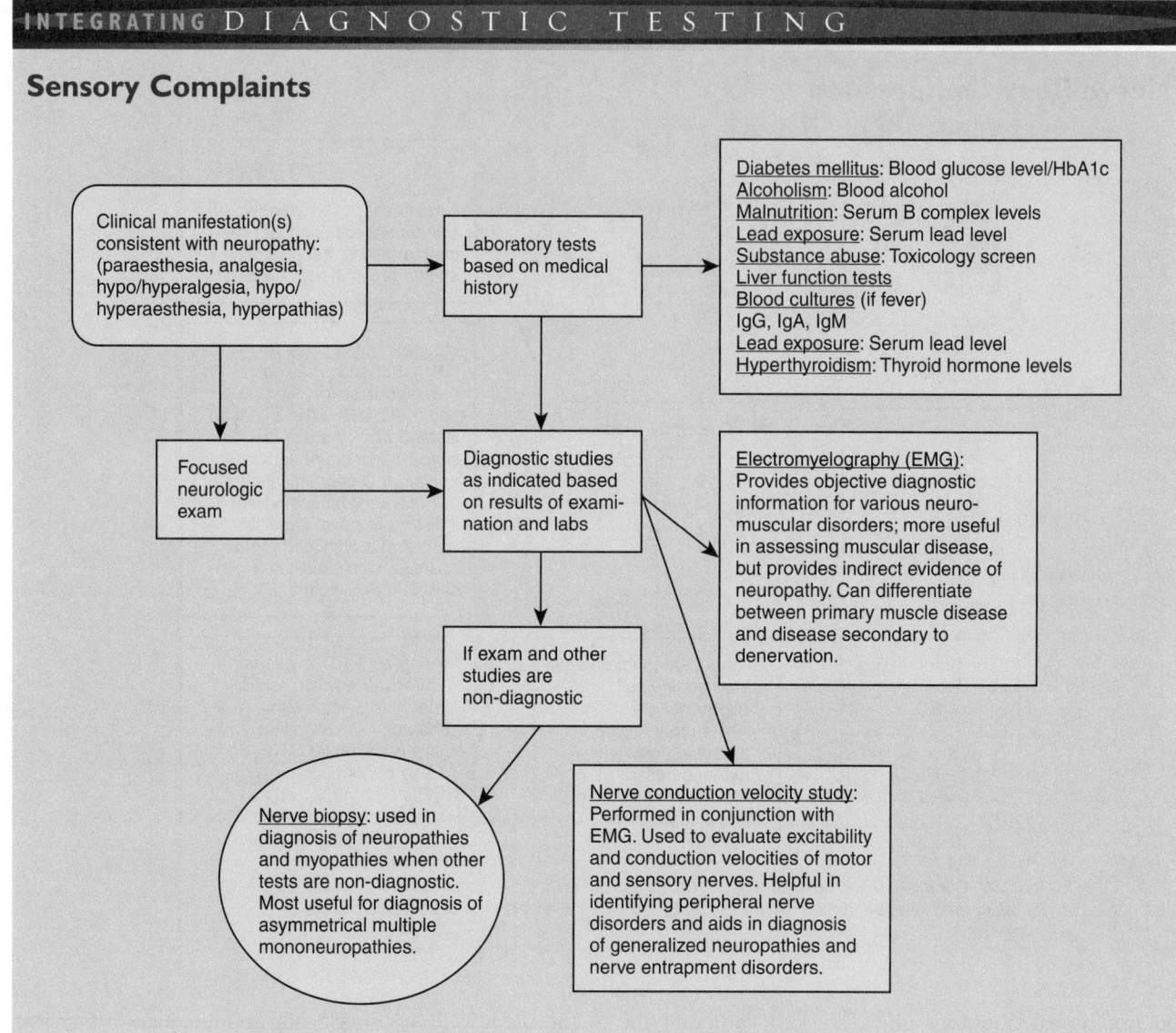

if ventilator support was used. A difficult or prolonged labor and delivery can result in hypoxia or use of forceps or vacuum extraction for delivery, with consequent central and peripheral neurologic damage.

At what age did the client accomplish major developmental tasks, such as walking and talking? Was the client able to participate in games, sports, and other childhood activities with peers? Did the client have any problems with coordination, balance, or agility?

A number of major illnesses are associated with neurologic changes, such as HIV, tuberculosis, diabetes mellitus, pernicious anemia, cancer, infections, shingles, and hypertension. Vascular disorders such as cardiac valve disease and atrial fibrillation are associated with transient ischemic attacks (TIAs) and stroke. Hypertension increases the risk of intracerebral bleeding. Systemic metabolic effects of advanced liver and renal diseases

can affect mental function. Inquire about injuries and hospitalizations for neurologic system problems such as head trauma, seizures, stroke, and crushing tissue injury.

Has the client undergone a neurologic diagnostic study, such as electroencephalography (EEG), electromyography (EMG), magnetic resolution imaging (MRI), or computed tomography (CT)? Results of such diagnostic studies provide valuable data for future comparison.

Past Surgical History

Inquire about the client's past surgeries, especially those related to neurologic problems such as spinal disorders, peripheral neuropathies, and cranial surgeries. Ask about surgical complications as some surgeries have a potential for nerve damage to surrounding tissue. Ask about past exposure to spinal and epidural anesthetics as well as any complications.

INTEGRATING DIAGNOSTIC TESTING

Altered Level of Consciousness

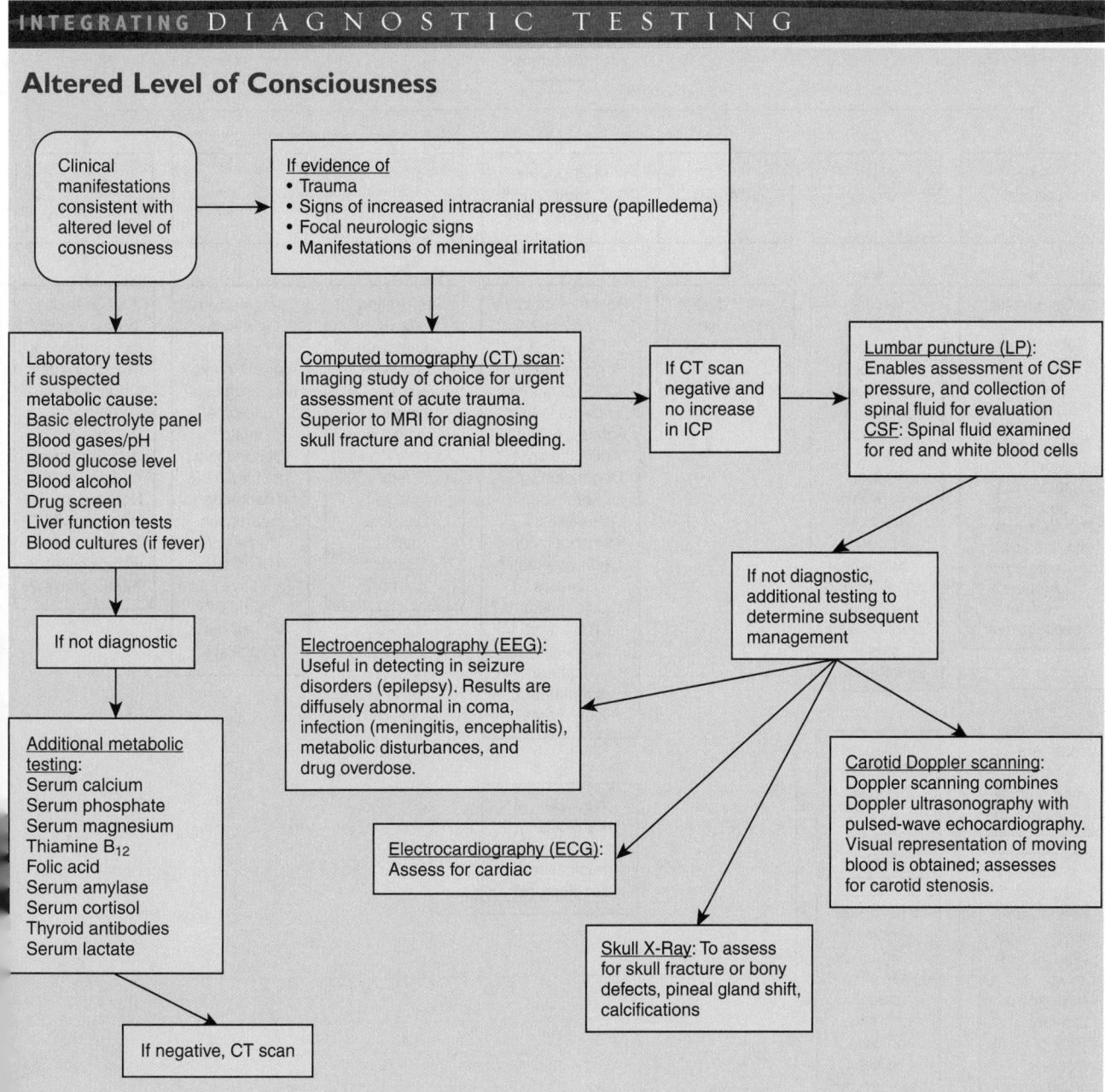

Allergies

Ask the client about food and drug allergies, especially to antibiotics, shellfish, and IV contrast dye.

Medications

The medication history includes all medicines that the client is taking or has taken, both prescription and over-the-counter, including herbal preparations. Specifically ask about aspirin and other anticoagulants, anticonvulsants, antidepressants, antihypertensives, oral contraceptive pills, central nervous system (CNS) stimulants such as diet pills, and CNS depressants such as opioids, antibiotics, antimicrobials, antirheumatics, tranquilizers, and sedatives.

Many medications have side effects involving the parasympathetic or sympathetic nervous system. Medications can have side effects involving the central nervous system, such as confusion, sedation, or agitation. Diet pills have been linked to stroke.[13] Many preparations for allergies and colds contain ingredients that can cause drowsiness. There are many types of medications that can cause peripheral nerve damage. Steroids can cause myopathies. Chemotherapy is associated with neuropathies.

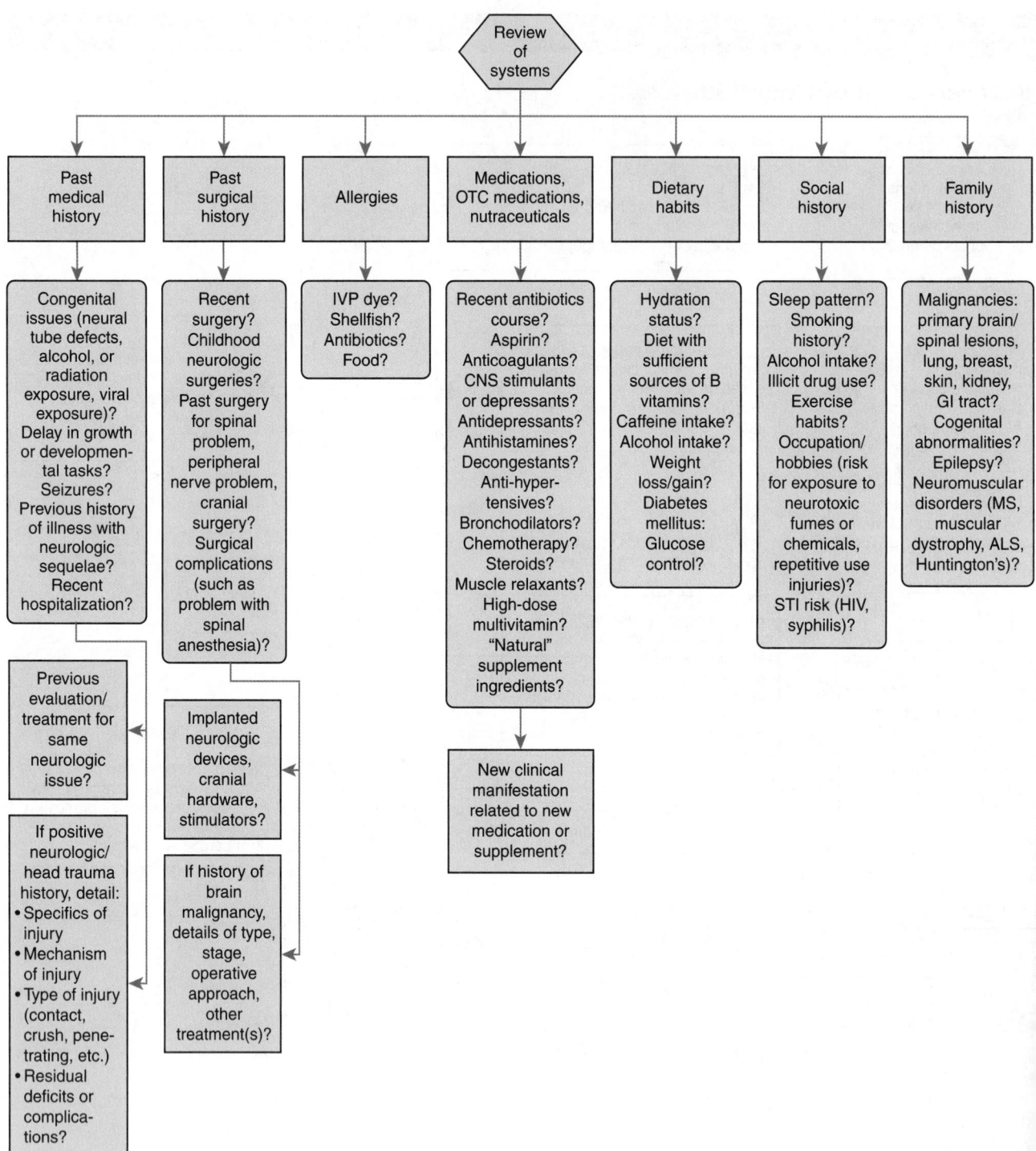

■ **FIGURE 67–2** Expanded neurologic history. *ALS,* amyotrophic lateral sclerosis; *CNS,* central nervous system; *IVP,* intravenous pyelogram; *MS,* multiple sclerosis; *STI,* sexually transmitted infection.

A number of medications may alter the sense of smell, such as antibiotics, antihistamines, decongestants, antihypertensives, bronchodilators, muscle relaxants, and psychiatric agents.

Clients are increasingly turning to herbal medications to treat neurologic problems, may not consider them to be medications, and fail to mention them unless specifically asked. Common herbal preparations used for neurologic problems are listed in Box 67-2.

Dietary Habits

Inquire about the client's dietary habits. Ask the client what was eaten in the previous 24 hours as an example of a typical day's diet. Specifically ask about intake of

---

BOX 67-1 Manifestations Related to Neurologic Assessment

EYE
- Vision and visual field loss
- Diplopia
- Ptosis
- Proptosis

EAR, NOSE, AND THROAT
- Infections
- Hearing loss
- Tinnitus
- Dizziness
- Vertigo
- Voice change
- Dysphagia
- Changes in taste or smell
- Experiences of unusual smells

CARDIOVASCULAR
- Syncope
- Palpitations
- Hypotension
- Hypertension
- Vertigo
- Transient ischemic attacks
- Stroke

NEUROLOGIC
- Weakness
- Numbness
- Paresthesias
- Headache
- Pain
- Altered thinking
- Speech difficulty
- Vomiting
- Vertigo
- Ataxia
- Fainting
- Seizures
- Any loss of consciousness
- Distortions of reality
- Use of consciousness-altering drugs
- Disorientation to time, place, or person
- Altered sleep patterns
- Changes in ability to speak, read, or understand language
- Changes in memory of recent or remote events
- Changes in ability to concentrate

SKIN
- Hair and nail changes

MUSCULOSKELETAL
- Tremor
- Weakness
- Altered coordination
- Staggering
- Difficulty climbing stairs

BOX 67-2 Common Herbal Preparations Used for Neurologic Problems

CNS stimulants: Betel nut *(Areca catechu)*; ephedra *(Ephedra sinica, E. vulgaris, E. nevadensis)*, also known as Ma Huang, and illegal in some areas; nutmeg *(Myristica fragrans)*

Sedatives/hypnotics: Chamomile *(Matricaria recutita, Chamaemelum nobile)*; gotu kola *(Centella asiatica)*; hops *(Humulus lupulus)*; kava kava *(Piper methysticum)*; St. John's wort *(Hypericum perforatum)*; valerian *(Valeriana officinalis)*

Antidepressives: Ginkgo biloba; sage *(Salvia officinalis)*; St. John's wort; sage can be used as an aid for dizziness, as can *G. biloba*; *G. biloba* has also been indicated for treating tinnitus, short-term memory loss, and headache

Analgesics: Cayenne *(Capsicum)*, taken internally for headache and toothache or applied externally for neuralgia; feverfew *(Tanacetum parthenium)*, used for prevention of migraine and cluster headaches; white willow *(Salix purpurea, S. fragilis, S. daphnoides)*, used as an analgesic and antipyretic

Antihypertensive or anti-stroke effects: Garlic *(Allium sativum)*; *G. biloba*; onion *(Allium cepa)*; reishi mushroom *(Ganoderma lucidum)*

---

whole grains and cereals. Deficiency of vitamin B_{12} causes central nervous system damage leading to polyneuritis and weakness. 🪔 Deficiencies of B complex vitamins [B_1 (thiamine), B_2 (riboflavin), B_3 (niacin), B_5 (pantothenic acid), or B_6 (pyridoxine)] lead to peripheral nerve damage. Inquire about folic acid supplementation in female clients of childbearing age. Ask about the client's pattern of fluid intake and caffeine consumption. Review diet and blood glucose control of clients with diabetes mellitus because neuropathies may be related to diabetes mellitus. Discuss weight loss and gain patterns.

Social History

An understanding of personal psychosocial factors (educational background, level of performance, and personality changes) enhances assessment. Inquire about changes that have occurred in daily routines. Ask about changes in sleep patterns, exercise routines, perceived stressors, and sexual interest and performance. Ask about sexual history. Has the client engaged in sexual behaviors that increase risk of infections? Inquire about alcohol and tobacco intake. Ask about the client's hobbies, recreational activities, and occupation. Is there risk of exposure to neurotoxic fumes or chemicals such as pesticides, paints, or bonding agents (glue)? Does the client spend time in an inadequately ventilated living area or workspace? Inquire about the current or past use of recreational drugs, the type of drug, and the duration of use.

Family Health History

Ask about a family history of neurologic disorders to determine the presence of genetic risk factors. Inquire about epilepsy, Huntington's disease, amyotrophic lateral sclerosis, muscular dystrophy, hypertension, stroke, mental retardation, and psychiatric disorders. Inquire about family history of cancer such as primary brain or spinal lesions as well as other cancers. Common sources of metastatic brain tumors are cancers of the lung, breast, skin, kidney, and gastrointestinal tract.

PHYSICAL EXAMINATION

The physical examination is intended to detect abnormalities in neurologic functioning. Variations in client age, physical condition, and LOC determine how detailed an examination can be. The neurologic examination is described here. Adapt the examination to the client's severity of illness and ability to cooperate. Box 67-3 presents a guide for adapting the assessment in various situations. A suggested sequence for the physical examination is as follows:

1. Vital signs
2. Mental status (including language and communication)
3. Head, neck, and back
4. Cranial nerves (including pupils)
5. Motor system (including coordination and gait)
6. Sensory function
7. Reflexes
8. Autonomic nervous system

Neurologic findings are summarized in the Physical Assessment Findings in the Healthy Adult feature on p. 1775. For a detailed guide to neurologic assessment, consult a physical examination textbook.

Vital Signs

Assess vital signs first because neurologic disorders can cause life-threatening changes. Clients who have cervical spinal cord injuries exhibit a classic triad of hypotension, bradycardia, and hypothermia related to the loss of sympathetic nervous system function. Changes in vital signs can accompany the late stages of increased intracranial pressure (ICP) in an attempt to preserve brain tissue. *Cushing's response* consists of elevated systolic blood pressure, widened pulse pressure, and bradycardia. Respiratory rate and rhythm can be altered by increased ICP on the brain stem.

Mental Status

Assess and document general data about the client's mental status. The mental status examination includes assessment of level of consciousness (LOC), orientation, memory, mood and affect, intellectual performance,

---

BOX 67-3 The Initial Neurologic Examination in the Clinical Setting

The sequence in which the neurologic examination is performed and the amount of time devoted to each step are dictated by the client's situation. For example, assessment of the head-injured client in the emergency department requires evaluation of vital signs, pupil reactivity, level of consciousness, and motor response. These clients may not be stable or cooperative enough to allow completion of the cranial nerve and sensory response assessment. Spinal cord–injured clients, however, are usually coherent and able to participate in the sensory examination. The sensory assessment information is essential for documenting changes in the status of spinal cord–injured clients.

As clients become more stable and cooperative, the examination can be performed in more depth and with less frequency. Remember that neurologically impaired clients frequently experience fluctuations in status. Alter the assessment schedule and technique to detect and report these fluctuations.

Following are suggested modifications in the screening neurologic examination that may be made on the basis of the client's initial presentation:

Initial examination for diagnosis and triage:
- Client history based on chief complaint
- Physical examination, including vital signs
- Level of consciousness
- Pupillary response
- Brain stem function (corneal reflex)
- Motor and sensory functions in all four extremities

If the client is conscious and stable:
- Complete baseline neurologic examination
- Focused examinations at prescribed intervals

If the client is conscious and unstable:
- Quick baseline physical assessment
- Frequent focused examinations until client is stable
- Vital signs
- Level of consciousness
- Pupillary response
- Brain stem function
- Motor and sensory functions in extremities
- Spinal cord function

If the client is unconscious but stable:
- Vital signs
- Level of consciousness and ability to arouse
- Cranial nerve function
- Motor and sensory functions
- Pathologic reflexes

If the client is unconscious and unstable:
- Vital signs
- Level of consciousness
- Cranial nerve function
- Motor and sensory functions relative to the ability to test for them
- Pathologic reflexes
- Frequent focused examinations on ongoing basis (hourly or more often)

If spinal cord involvement is suspected:
- Motor functions in detail with testing of specific muscle groups
- Sensory function
- Reflexes
- Bowel and bladder functions
- Vital signs

The Neurologic System

INSPECTION

Mental Status. Oriented to person, place, time, and situation. No difficulty recalling recent and past events. Serial 7's deferred. Mood and affect congruent, cooperative, and pleasant. Thought process clear and logical. Demonstrates effective problem solving. Speech articulate, clear, and fluent.

Head, Neck, and Back. Normocephalic without obvious lesions. Maintains head position. Spine in straight alignment with normal cervical, thoracic, and lumbar curves. Neck and back have full range of motion.

CRANIAL NERVES

CN I. Discerns smell of coffee, cinnamon, alcohol.

CN II. Visual acuity per Snellen chart is OU = 20/20. Visual fields full to confrontation. Optic disc margins sharp, no cupping; cup-to-disc ratio is 1:3. Retina-arteriovenous ratio is 2:3, without nicking. Fovea visualized.

CN III, CN IV, CN VI. PERRLA, direct and consensual. Accommodation present. EOMs intact without nystagmus or strabismus. Cover-uncover test negative. Corneal light reflections symmetrical.

CN V. Opens and closes mouth; chews, clenches teeth, and moves jaw side to side voluntarily. Sensation intact to forehead, cheeks, and chin. Corneal reflexes present.

CN VII. Face movements symmetrical with smiling, frowning, eyebrow raising, lip pursing, and cheek puffing. Discerns sweet, salty, sour, and bitter tastes (also CN IX).

CN VIII. Gross hearing intact. Whisper heard at 3 feet. Air conduction greater than bone conduction bilaterally.

CN IX and CN X. Tongue and uvula midline. Uvula and soft palate rise in midline with phonation. Gag reflex present bilaterally. Swallows, coughs, and speaks without difficulty.

CN XI. Performs shoulder shrugs. Turns head against resistance. Maintains head position against resistance.

CN XII. Tongue protrudes midline without deviation; pushes side to side with equal strength.

Motor Function. Muscle groups symmetrical. Gross and fine motor coordination intact. Moves all extremities through range of motion. Romberg's test negative. Pronator drift absent. Gait smooth, steady. Maintains balance walking on toes and heels. Rapid alternating movements and point-to-point maneuvers performed without difficulty.

Sensory Function. Sensation to light touch, pain, and vibration intact distally and over trunk, neck, and face. Position sense of fingers and toes intact. Stereognosis and graphesthesia present bilaterally. Two-point discrimination: 2 mm on index fingers. Discerns 2-point simultaneous stimulation.

PALPATION

Head, Neck, and Back. Skull without lesions or tenderness; smooth and firm. Neck and paravertebral muscles firm, relaxed, and nontender. No pain or tenderness over spinous processes.

Motor Function. Muscle bulk full and tone firm; strength rated as 5/5 bilaterally.

PERCUSSION

Reflexes. Deep tendon reflexes rated 2+ (on a scale of 0 to 4+) in triceps, biceps, wrists, knees, and ankles. Plantar reflexes present bilaterally. Abdominal reflexes present in all four quadrants.

AUSCULTATION

Vascular Flow. Absence of bruit over carotid arteries bilaterally.

---

judgment and insight, and language and communication. Cultural and educational background of the client must be considered when evaluating mental status. The mental status examination is summarized in Box 67-4.

Level of Consciousness

The level of consciousness (LOC) is the most sensitive indicator of changes in neurologic status. LOC refers to level of arousal and wakefulness and the ability to respond to the environment. Begin by observing spontaneous behavior before using stimuli. To be certain that you are assessing cerebral function, rather than spinal cord reflex, use central stimuli whenever possible. Noxious stimuli are discussed in Chapter 68. Document the location and type of stimuli applied along with the client's response.

The time between assessments should also be noted to assess how quickly changes occur. The *Glasgow Coma Scale* is an assessment tool designed to note trends in a client's response to stimuli in terms of eye opening, verbal response, and motor response (see Chapter 68). Many variations of this scale now exist for use with other client populations.

Orientation

Establish *orientation* to time, place, person (×3), and event or situation (×4). Orientation to time is usually lost first. Orientation to self (person) is usually maintained except in advanced dementia.

Memory

Identify gross deficits in long-term and short-term memory with simple tests. Test *long-term memory* when the client relates the past health history (of course, another source must be able to validate the data). Test *short-term memory* by asking the client to recall recent information.

BOX 67-4 Mental Status Examination

Level of consciousness (LOC): Most important part of assessment. (LOC is the most sensitive indicator of changes in neurologic status) Assess client's ability to respond to environment. Begin with least invasive stimuli; increase stimuli if no response. Document BEST response.

Types of stimuli: None, verbal, light touch, pain (use central stimuli: pressure on trapezius or pectoralis major muscle, sternal rub, supraorbital pressure).

Types of responses:
- Obeys simple commands.
- Localizes pain: Moves arm across the midline away from stimuli.
- Withdrawal: Movement to move away from stimuli but does not cross midline.
- Abnormal posturing: Only seen in coma, may be unilateral or bilateral.
  - (a) Flexion—arm abduction and elbow flexion, possibly with flexion of wrists, plantar flexion and extension of lower extremities
  - (b) Extension—arm adduction and elbow extension with flexion of wrists, rigid extension of lower extremities

Orientation:
- Person (usually not lost): What is your name?
- Time (usually lost first): What year is this?
- Place and event (or situation = orientation × 4): What kind of place is this? Where are you? What brought you to the hospital today?

Memory (must be able to verify information to evaluate for confabulation):
- Long-term memory (preserved except in advanced dementia): Past health history, historical dates such as date of high school graduation, birth date, names of family members.
- Short-term memory: Recent events: "What brings you here today?" "Tell me what you ate for breakfast."
- Ability to learn: Three words to remember (red, Broadway, three). Ask the client to say the words immediately, and then to repeat them after a few minutes.

Mood and affect: Ask the client to describe how he or she feels; observe facial expression. Is the client's affect appropriate to the situation?

Intellectual performance: Ability to identify commonly known people, places, current events, reversed *serial 7's* or *3's*, simple addition or subtraction problem.

Judgment and insight reasoning: Are the answers logical? Do they relate to the question? "What would you do if you lost your house keys?" Ask the client to explain a proverb such as "A rolling stone gathers no moss."

Language and communication:
- Expression: Evaluate speech for flow, choice of words, and completion of phrases or sentences. Assess speech quality. Assess speech for articulation problems (usually motor disorders) or comprehension or expression problems (aphasic disorders). Test comprehension in aphasic clients by asking *yes* or *no* questions or to follow simple verbal commands. Assess written expression by having the client write answers to simple questions on paper.
- Comprehension of spoken language: Ability to follow commands ("Stick out your tongue").
- Comprehension of written language: Ability to read several words or sentences and explain them. Have the client read a simple command and then perform the command.

Integrated sensory functions: Integration of cortical functioning (calculation) and visual recognition with expressive speech. Ask the client to identify common objects, such as a pen, a key, and a watch. Ask the client to write a sentence.

Mood and Affect

Facial expression may reveal emotions such as anxiety, distrust, and depression. Is the client's affect appropriate to the situation?

Intellectual Performance

Intellectual performance consists of the fund of knowledge and calculation ability. Ask the client to identify commonly known people, places, or current events.

Judgment and Insight

Judgment and insight include reasoning, abstract thinking, problem solving, and the client's perception of the situation. Assess reasoning, abstract thinking, and problem solving for indications of major problems with thought content. Listen to how the client answers questions. Can the client concentrate and remain focused, or is the client easily distracted?

Language and Communication

Language and communication assessment tests the ability to express and comprehend one's environment. Gross evaluation of *comprehension* and *expression* begins with the initial interview. Does the client initiate speech? Is speech fluent and appropriate? Assess speech quality. Assess speech for articulation problems (dysarthrias, usually motor disorders) or comprehension or expression problems (aphasic disorders).

Assess comprehension to both spoken and written language. If the client is expressively aphasic, test comprehension by asking *yes* or *no* questions or by having the client follow simple verbal commands.

Evaluate verbal expression as the client responds to questions that require more than a nod or a "yes" or "no" answer. Evaluate speech for flow, choice of words, and completion of phrases or sentences. Assess written expression by having the client write answers to simple questions on paper.

Integrated sensory functions involving language are often tested with this portion of the neurologic examination. Have the client perform simple addition or subtraction without writing or ask the client to orally identify common objects. These skills require integration of cortical functioning (calculation) and visual recognition with expressive speech.

Head, Neck, and Back

Examine the head, neck, and spine using inspection, palpation, percussion, and auscultation. Tumors, vascular disorders, traumatic disorders, and problems involving the vertebrae and surrounding muscles may be detected.

Inspection

Inspect the head for size, shape, contour, and symmetry. Note any ecchymosis (bruising) around the eyes or behind the ears. Anterior basilar skull fractures often result in "raccoon eyes," with periorbital ecchymosis and, occasionally, drainage of cerebrospinal fluid (CSF) from the nares. Middle fossa basilar skull fractures often result in ecchymosis over the mastoid process behind the ears (Battle's sign) and drainage of blood, CSF, or both from the ears. Assess the spine and back for symmetry. Look for skin tags, lipomas, hairy patch (hypertrichosis), or dermal sinus tract along the spine.

Palpation

Palpate the skull lightly for nodules or masses and to supplement inspection findings. The skull normally feels smooth and firm. Areas of bogginess or depressions are abnormal. Palpation of neck muscles may identify masses or tender areas. Ask the client to flex the neck with the chin touching the chest and look for nuchal (back of the neck) rigidity, which is a manifestation of meningeal irritation.

Inspect and palpate spine alignment. Note any deviation from the normal curvatures. Palpate the paravertebral muscles for masses, tenderness, and spasm (also see Chapter 25).

Percussion

Gentle percussion over the spinous processes may produce pain or tenderness, which are abnormal findings.

Auscultation

Auscultation of major neck and other vessels may reveal bruits or other sounds suggesting an abnormality. Use the bell of the stethoscope to auscultate the carotid arteries. Bruits result from turbulent flow, usually a manifestation of atherosclerotic disease.

Cranial Nerves

The cranial nerves are referred to by specific name or Roman numeral. Cranial nerve (CN) examination is important for two reasons. First, CN III through CN XII arise in the brain stem. Testing their function provides information about the brain stem and related pathways. Second, three reflexes involving cranial nerves are called *protective reflexes* (corneal, gag, and cough reflexes). The presence or absence of protective reflexes indicates the ability to protect the eye surfaces and airway. This is especially important in unconscious clients.

Normal cranial nerve reflexes require an appropriately received stimulus *(input)* that produces an appropriate response *(output)*. During testing of cranial nerves, the absence of a normal response may indicate (1) failure to receive stimuli (input failure), (2) failure to respond appropriately (output failure), or (3) a combination of input and output failure. Cranial nerves occur in pairs (right and left). Dysfunction may be unilateral or bilateral. The cranial nerves are part of the peripheral nervous system (PNS) and abnormalities may be a manifestation of a systemic neurologic disease (e.g., Guillain-Barré syndrome). Refer to Table 67-2 for details of cranial nerve testing.

Be aware that some abnormal findings are not clinically significant. Anosmia may develop in older people as a normal aging process. CN I cannot be accurately assessed in clients with upper respiratory infections (URI). In about 20% of the population, *anisocoria* (unequal pupils) is a normal finding. Older clients who have undergone cataract surgery with lens implants may have irregular, nonreactive pupils. This finding does not indicate neurologic damage.

Motor System

Assessing the motor system thoroughly involves numerous procedures. The following discussion focuses on the screening examinations and common abnormalities.

Muscle Size

Inspect all major muscle groups bilaterally for symmetry, hypertrophy, and atrophy.

Muscle Strength

Assess the power in major muscle groups against resistance (see Chapter 25). Assess and rate muscle strength on a 5-point scale in all four extremities, comparing one side with the other (Table 67-3 on p. 1781).

Next, test for subtle weakness in upper and lower extremities. For upper extremities, have the client hold the arms straight out in front with the palms up ("like holding a tray"). Ask the client to close the eyes and to maintain the position. A *pronator drift* is said to be present if one arm pronates and falls lower than the other. For the lower extremities, have the client walk on the heels and then on the toes to test dorsiflexion, plantiflexion, and balance.

Assessment of specific muscle groups evaluates deficits in certain areas, such as spinal cord disorders. Disorders of muscle strength may be exhibited as weakness

TABLE 67-2 Cranial Nerve Testing

Nerve	Function	Method for Assessment	Indication of Dysfunction	Causes of Dysfunction
Olfactory nerve (CN I)	Purely sensory Smell	Identify an aromatic, nonirritating odor (coffee, toothpaste) with each nostril separately and with eyes closed	Anosmia	Neurogenic: fracture of cribriform plate or ethmoid bone; tumor of frontal lobe or olfactory bulb/tract Nonneurogenic: sinus disorders or surgery; tobacco smoker, cocaine use, URI, advanced age
Optic nerve (CN II)	Purely sensory Vision: central and peripheral	Visual Acuity: Read Snellen chart or newspaper; or identify number and movement of fingers Visual fields: Confrontation: compare peripheral vision to examiner	Amaurosis (blindness): decreased or absent central vision Vision loss in one or more directions or in a portion of visual field (half of visual field, middle portion, or both sides)	Nonneurogenic: corneal defect or cataracts Neurogenic: trauma, stroke, occipital lobe lesion, diabetes mellitus, multiple sclerosis One eye: globe or anterior optic chiasm lesions Bilateral: optic chiasm or tract or occipital cortex Bitemporal: optic chiasm defect (pituitary tumor)
		Funduscopic and gross exam: inspect for trauma and cataracts Examine fundus with ophthalmoscope	Diabetic retinopathy; loss of venous pulsation; papilledema: optic disc swelling	Fracture of optic foramen; diabetes mellitus; laceration or blood clot in temporal, parietal, or occipital lobes; increased ICP
CN III, IV, VI assessed together: Oculomotor nerve (CN III)	Purely motor Eyelid elevation (III)		CN III: ptosis: upper eyelid droop	Horner's syndrome (unilateral ptosis and pupil constriction); myasthenia gravis (bilateral ptosis)
Trochlear nerve (CN IV) Abducens nerve (CN VI)	EOMs: nasally, up and temporal, up and nasally, down and temporal (III); downward and nasally (IV); far lateral gaze (VI)	EOMs: "six cardinal fields of gaze" (CN III, IV, VI) Nystagmus (involuntary eye movements), seen as fine, rhythmic eye movements that can be vertical, horizontal, or rotational	Inability of an eye to move nasally, up and nasally, up and temporally, or downward Double vision (diplopia)	Pressure on CN III, CN IV, or CN VI at brain stem because of fracture of orbit; increased ICP and tumor/trauma to base of brain, degenerative neurologic diseases such as multiple sclerosis, myasthenia gravis
		Inability to look down or to walk down steps because of visual disturbance		CN IV dysfunction
		Inability of an eye to move laterally outward		CN VI dysfunction
	Pupil size at rest and pupil constriction (III)	Pupil constriction: shine light at eye from side	Irregular shaped pupils Anisocoria: unequal pupils; no or sluggish response to light or accommodation	Cataract surgery; glaucoma; COPD: large sluggish pupils because of hypoxemia CN III dysfunction: nerve damage
		Direct response: connection in midbrain of CN II and ipsilateral CN III consensual response (other eye): connection in midbrain of CN II and contralateral CN III		Increased ICP or edema in uncus of temporal lobe Medications: opiates: small and sluggish; atropine: large and sluggish
		Accommodation: bring a pen or finger toward center of client's face		

Nerve	Type/Function	Assessment Technique	Abnormal Findings	Possible Causes
Trigeminal nerve (CN V)	Mixed Motor: masticator Innervates muscles for chewing	Clamp jaw shut, open mouth against resistance, open mouth widely, move jaw from side to side, and make chewing movements	Weakness (rare), aching, or spasm of masseter or temporal muscles	Jaw clenching; temporal arteritis, tetanus, parotitis, dystonic reaction to antipsychotic drugs
	Sensory: All sensations for entire face, scalp, cornea, and nasal and oral cavities	With client's eyes closed, test sensations on both sides of entire face: pain (sharp pin), touch (wisp of cotton), and temperature (hot and cold objects) Corneal reflexes: gently touch cornea with sterile wisp of cotton or gently stroke eyelash (CN V, sensory; CN VII, motor; eye blink)	Facial pain, paresthesias	Trigeminal neuralgia Medulla (loss of pain and temperature), pons (touch), and brain stem tumor or trauma, orbital fracture, and trigeminal neuralgia
Facial nerve (CN VII)	Mixed Motor: facial expression	Observe face for symmetry Assess facial muscles: smile, frown, raise forehead and eyebrows, tightly close eyes against resistance, whistle, show teeth, and puff out cheeks	Central deficits: affects lower half of face only; caused by CNS defect Peripheral deficit: deficit involving both upper face and lower face; caused by CN VII lesion Facial asymmetry loss of nasolabial fold, inability to close eye and blink reflexively, drooling, difficulty swallowing secretions, loss of tearing	Stroke (cerebral causes) Peripheral CN VII injury: facial weakness, Bell's palsy, temporal bone fracture, peripheral laceration or contusion of parotid region
	Sensory	Test taste on anterior part of tongue with eyes closed, eyes and tongue protruding Place taste substance on one side of anterior tongue Test taste on each side for sweet, salty, sour, and bitter	Loss of taste on anterior two thirds of tongue	
Vestibulocochlear or acoustic nerve (CN VIII)	Purely sensory Hearing (cochlear)	Auditory acuity: listen and respond to whispered words, fingers rubbing; test ears separately Air and bone conduction: Weber test: vibrating tuning fork placed midline on skull	Whispered words, fingers rubbing not heard correctly or equally Sound lateralized to one side (negative Weber); sound lateralizes toward side with hearing loss (conductive); sound lateralizes toward side without hearing loss (sensorineural)	Conductive hearing loss: tympanic membrane damage, ear wax, otitis media Sensorineural hearing loss: possibly caused by medications (gentamicin), acoustic nerve tumor
		Rinne test: vibrating tuning fork placed on mastoid process; when client indicates it is no longer heard, move tuning fork by ear and have client indicate when no longer heard	Bone conduction equal to or longer than air conduction (negative Rinne)	

(Continued)

TABLE 67-2 Cranial Nerve Testing —Cont'd

Nerve	Function	Method for Assessment	Indication of Dysfunction	Causes of Dysfunction
	Balance (vestibular)	Equilibrium tests Romberg: stands with feet together and eyes closed	Swaying, wide-based stance to maintain balance (positive Romberg)	Ménière's syndrome, acoustic neuroma
		Caloric tests: oculovestibular reflex (usually performed on comatose client only): inject cold or warm water into each ear and observe eye movement away from (cold) or toward (warm) stimulus	No response	Lesion in pons or lower brain stem: impending brain death
CN IX and X assessed together Glossopharyngeal nerve (CN IX) Vagus nerve (CN X)	Mixed *Motor:* swallow, gag, vocalization (IX, X); posterior pharynx muscles (IX); cough (X) *Sensory:* taste to posterior third of tongue, inner ear sensation (IX); decreases heart rate, increases GI motility (X)	Say "Ahhh": soft palate and pharynx rise symmetrically, uvula is midline Assess voice: stimulate back of throat with tongue blade to check gag Assess taste to back of tongue with sugar and salt, listen to heart rate and rhythm, bowel sounds	Uvula deviates, palate fails to rise Hoarse voice Nasal voice No gag Weak cough Loss of taste, tachycardia, ileus	Lower brain stem tumor or stroke, Guillain-Barré Vocal cord paralysis Palate paralysis Brain stem trauma or tumor, neck trauma, stroke
Spinal accessory nerve (CN XI)	Purely motor Shoulder elevation and lateral head rotation	Shoulders symmetrical, shrugs shoulders against resistance, turns head laterally against resistance toward midline, able to lift head off pillow	Drooping of a shoulder, muscle atrophy, weak shoulder shrug, or weak turn of head	Possible causes of abnormal findings include neck trauma, radical neck surgery, and torticollis
Hypoglossal nerve (CN XII)	Purely motor Tongue movement	Stick out tongue, move it side to side and against inside of each cheek; says "light, tight, dynamite"	Deviation of tongue to weak side, atrophy, fasciculations, slurred speech (dysarthria)	Stroke, ALS, neck trauma with major blood vessel damage, multiple CN lesions: V, VII, XII

TABLE 67–3   Neuromuscular Strength Assessment

Movement	Test Against Resistance	Muscle	Spinal Cord Level
Shoulder elevation	Shrug shoulders	Supraspinatus	C4-5
Elbow flexors	Flex elbow: pull forearm to face	Biceps	C5-6
Elbow extensors	Straighten elbow	Triceps	C7-8
Wrist extensors	Flex wrist up	Extensor carpi radialis	C6-7
		Extensor carpi ulnaris	C7-8
Hand intrinsics	Spread fingers apart	Interossei	C8-T1
Hip flexors	Raise knee to chest	Iliopsoas	L1-3
Knee extensors	Bend knee 90 degrees and straighten knee	Quadriceps	L3-4
Ankle dorsiflexors	Pull ankle up/toes toward head	Tibialis anterior	L4-5
Ankle plantiflexors	Push ankle/toes down (press gas pedal)	Gastrocnemius	S1-2

on one side of the body, in both lower extremities, or in both upper and lower extremities. If asymmetry is detected, ask the client or family whether it is long-standing or recent. Consider the client's age, handedness, and physical condition when interpreting the results of muscle-strength testing.

Muscle Tone

Assess muscle tone while moving each extremity through its range of passive motion. When tone is decreased *(hypotonicity)*, the muscles are soft, flabby, or flaccid; when tone is increased *(hypertonicity)*, the muscles are resistant to movement, rigid, or spastic. Note the presence of abnormal flexion or extension posture.

Muscle Coordination

Assessment of muscle coordination consists of testing rapid alternating movements, point-to-point maneuvers, and maintenance of truncal balance and head position. Test *rapid alternating movements* by asking the client to touch (approximate) each finger to the thumb quickly in succession. Alternatively, ask the client to pat the thighs first with the palms, then with the back of the hands, and to repeat the patting quickly.

For *point-to-point testing,* hold up an index finger approximately 18 inches from the client. Ask the client first to touch his or her nose with a finger, then touch your index finger, and then touch the nose again. Repeat this several times while you move your index finger to different locations. Perform the test for the client's right and left hands. Test lower-extremity coordination by asking the client to place the heel of the foot below the other knee and then slide the heel down the shin toward the great toe. Repeat for the other leg.

Assess *truncal balance* with the client sitting. Can the client remain upright without support? Gently push the client to a leaning position. Can the client return to an upright position? Note *head position* by observing the ability to move the head while following your movements.

Disorders related to coordination indicate cerebellar or posterior column lesions. The defining characteristics of cerebellar dysfunction are (1) ataxia, (2) intention tremor (tremor upon nearing the object), (3) nystagmus, (4) ocular dysmetria (inability to gaze on an object), and (5) dysdiadochokinesia (arresting one motor impulse and substituting an opposite one).

Gait and Station

Assess gait and station by having the client stand still, walk, and walk in tandem (one foot in front of the other in a straight line). Walking involves the functions of motor power, sensation, and coordination. The ability to stand quietly with the feet together requires coordination and intact *proprioception* (sense of body position).

> **If the client has difficulty standing, assess further to determine whether the client is weak or unsteady. If the client is weak, protect the client from falling.**

SAFETY

ALERT

The box Terms Associated with Gait Disorders on the website lists and describes terms used to describe gait disorders. *evolve*

Movement

Examine the muscles for fine and gross abnormal movements. Examples of fine abnormal movements are *fasciculations* (involuntary ripples or twitches that occur while the client is relaxed), which may indicate lower motor neuron disease. Examples of more grossly abnormal movements, often representing extrapyramidal disease, are described in Box 67-5.

Move all joints through a full range of passive motion. Abnormal findings include pain, joint contractures, and muscle resistance.

Test for *apraxia* (the inability to carry out a learned movement on command in the absence of weakness or paralysis). Ask the client to perform a common activity, such as tying shoes or combing hair. Apraxia is present if a client can follow other commands (indicating intact comprehension), has the motor strength to move the extremity involved, but cannot carry out the command.

Motor Testing of the Unconscious Client

An unresponsive client can be tested only for response to painful stimuli (reflex withdrawal of limbs, wincing,

---

BOX 67-5   Abnormal Movements Associated with Extrapyramidal Disease

Akinesia: Reduced body movement in the absence of weakness or paralysis; habitual movements (swinging arms) limited or absent

Athetosis: Gross, writhing, worm-like movements of body, face, or extremities

Ballismus: A form of chorea; involuntary dramatic movements of arms and legs (**hemiballismus** involves only one side)

Bradykinesia: Slow movement

Chorea: Discrete, jerky, purposeless movements in distal extremities and face

Dystonia: Prolonged twisting movements or postures

Myoclonus: Sudden muscle contractions of varying intensity that may involve a small part of one extremity or the entire body; may violently fling a client to the floor

Spasms: Involuntary contraction of large muscle groups (arms, legs, neck)

Tic: Involuntary movement of groups of muscles in stereotypic patterns; may be physical or psychogenic in origin; pathologic causes of tics include Tourette's syndrome

Tremors: Involuntary trembling or quivering; may vary in direction, amplitude, rhythmicity, parts involved, speed, and timing in relation to rest or activity; types include parkinsonian, essential, and cerebellar

---

grimacing). Although a pain stimulus is used, the response is usually recorded as a motor system response. These responses are often incorporated into the motor scale of the Glasgow Coma Scale. (See Chapter 68 for further information.) Box 67-6 describes the most common responses to painful stimuli.

Sensory Function

Sensory assessment involves testing for touch, pain, vibration, position (proprioception), and discrimination. Assessment of hearing, vision, smell, and taste is also

---

BOX 67-6   Responses to Painful Stimuli

Localization: Reaches for the source of the stimulus and attempts to push the examiner away

Flexion withdrawal: Moves without purpose and may exhibit minimal movement, grimacing, or wincing

Abnormal flexion (decorticate posturing): Flexes, adducts, and internally rotates the wrists and arms to the chest and rigidly extends the legs (indicates damage in the corticospinal tracts near the cerebral hemispheres that has left the rubrospinal tract intact)

Abnormal extension (decerebrate posturing): Extends and pronates the arms while rigidly extending the legs (indicates damage in the upper brain stem)

No response: No visible reaction to painful stimuli

---

sensory assessment. Sensory assessment may identify dermatomes as having normal, absent, reduced, exaggerated, or delayed sensation. A complete sensory examination is possible only on a conscious and cooperative client. Always test sensation with the client's eyes closed. Help the client relax and keep warm.

Conduct sensory assessment systematically. Test a particular area of the body, and then test the corresponding area on the other side. Begin testing a selection of dermatomes that represent cervical, thoracic, lumbar, and sacral segments of the spinal cord. If you note a sensory loss, you can perform a more detailed testing of surrounding dermatomes. Sensation assessment may be documented on a body chart of dermatomes.

Superficial Sensation

Test superficial sensations by stimulating the skin in symmetrical areas on each side of the body according to dermatome distribution.

Test *superficial pain* by alternating the sharp and dull ends of a broken cotton applicator. The wooden broken end is pointed enough for testing sharp sensation, yet dull enough not to break the skin. The cotton swab end serves as the dull stimulus. Ask the client to close the eyes. Explain that the client will feel a sharp or a dull stimulus. Alternate the two stimuli inconsistently (so that the client cannot predict which is being used), and ask the client to distinguish sharp from dull.

Use a cotton wisp to assess *light touch*. Follow the same guidelines as for testing superficial pain sensation, stimulating symmetrical areas of the dermatomes.

Temperature is not assessed routinely. Where there is a loss of the sense of pain, test for awareness of temperature. Pain and temperature sensations travel on related pathways. Use two test tubes, one filled with warm water and one with cold water.

Mechanical Sensation

Mechanical sensations are assessed with vibration and proprioception. Use a tuning fork to test for *vibration*. Place the end of a vibrating tuning fork on a distal bony prominence, such as a finger or great toe joint. Ask the client to indicate when the vibration is felt and when is no longer felt. Once the client indicates that the sensation has stopped, test your own joint to see whether you can feel vibration. You serve as the control. If the client reports that the sensation has stopped but you can still sense a clear vibration, the client has reduced vibratory sense.

Test *proprioception* by holding the side of the client's fingertips, then the great toes, between thumb and index finger. As each of the client's fingers and toes are gently flexed and extended, ask the client to state when movement is felt and in what direction. Test more proximal joints if impairment is detected.

Discrimination

Cortical discrimination depends on the ability to integrate and interpret sensory stimuli in the parietal lobe. Included are tests for stereognosis, graphesthesia, extinction phenomenon, and simultaneous two-point stimulation (Box 67-7).

Abnormalities of sensation are defined in Box 67-8, and Figure 67-3 summarizes patterns of sensory loss. Sensory changes are part of the normal aging process. Careful assessment of such changes is the basis of nursing intervention for older clients. Table 67-1 contains guidelines for assessment.

BOX 67-7   Tests for Cortical Discrimination

Stereognosis (discernment of the form and configuration of objects felt, or three-dimensional discrimination): Place three small, familiar objects (such as a coin, a key, and a paper clip) one at a time in the client's hands. Ask the client to identify each with the eyes closed.

Graphesthesia (recognition of the form and configuration of written symbols): Trace different separate letters and numbers on the client's palm with the blunt end of a pen. Ask the client to identify each with the eyes closed. Orient the figures so that they are right-side-up for the client.

Extinction phenomenon (simultaneous stimulation): Prick the client's skin at the same point on the two sides of the body at the same time. Ask the client to state whether one or two pricks are felt.

Two-point stimulation (two-point discrimination): Simultaneously prick the skin with two pins at varying distances apart to identify the smallest distance at which the client can perceive two pricks. Normal distances at which two-point discrimination is lost are as follows: upper arms, 75 mm; thighs, 75 mm; back, 40 to 70 mm; chest, 40 mm; forearms, 40 mm; palms, 8 to 12 mm; toes, 3 to 8 mm; fingertips, 2.8 mm; and tongue, 1 mm.

BOX 67-8   Abnormalities of Sensation

Dysesthesias: Well-localized, irritating sensations, such as warmth, cold, itching, tickling, crawling, prickling, and tingling

Paresthesias: Distortions of sensory stimuli (light touch may be experienced as burning or painful sensation)

Anesthesia: Absence of the sense of touch

Hypoesthesia: Reduced sense of touch

Hyperesthesia: Pathologic (abnormal) overperception of touch

Analgesia: Absence of the sense of pain

Hypalgesia: Reduced sense of pain

Hyperalgesia: Increased sense of pain

Agraphesthesia: Inability to identify symbols traced on the palm when the eyes are closed

Astereognosis: Loss of sense of three-dimensional discrimination

---

Reflex Activity

Reflex testing evaluates the integrity of specific sensory and motor pathways. Reflex activity assessment, always a part of neurologic assessment, provides information about the nature, location, and progression of neurologic disorders.

Normal Reflexes

Two types of reflexes are normally present: (1) superficial, or cutaneous, reflexes; and (2) deep tendon, or muscle-stretch, reflexes (Table 67-4).

Superficial (Cutaneous) Reflexes. Superficial (cutaneous) reflexes are elicited by stimulation of the skin or mucous membranes. The stimulus is produced by stroking a sensory zone with an object that will not cause damage. Superficial reflexes (abdominal, plantar, corneal, pharyngeal [gag], cremasteric, and anal) are absent in pyramidal tract disorders.

Deep Tendon (Muscle-Stretch) Reflexes. Deep tendon reflexes are also called muscle-stretch, or myotactic, reflexes because reflex muscle contraction normally results from rapid stretching of the muscle. This is produced by sharply striking a muscle tendon's point of insertion with a sudden, brief blow of a reflex hammer (Figure 67-4 and Box 67-9 on p. 1786). Reflexes commonly assessed include the biceps, triceps, brachioradialis, patella, and ankle jerk (Achilles tendon).

Other Normal Reflexes. Some normal reflexes involve structures other than skeletal muscles. For example, reflex mechanisms help maintain respiration and keep blood pressure within normal limits. Reflex salivation may follow the taste (or smell) of food. Flashing a light in an eye causes the pupils of both eyes to constrict *(light reflex* or *pupillary reflex)*.

Abnormal Reflexes

Pathologic reflexes indicate neurologic disorders, often related to the spinal cord or higher centers. These responses include Babinski's, jaw, palm-chin (palmomental), clonus, snout, rooting, sucking, glabella, grasp, and chewing reflexes. Babinski's reflex and clonus are discussed below. Box 67-10 on p. 1787 lists additional abnormal reflexes.

Babinski's Reflex. When exaggerated deep reflexes are present, superficial reflexes are usually diminished or absent and pathologic reflexes (Babinski's reflex) are observed. The presence of Babinski's reflex is indicative of an upper motor neuron lesion. Test for Babinski's reflex by gently scraping the sole of the foot with a blunt object. To elicit the reflex, start the stimulus at the

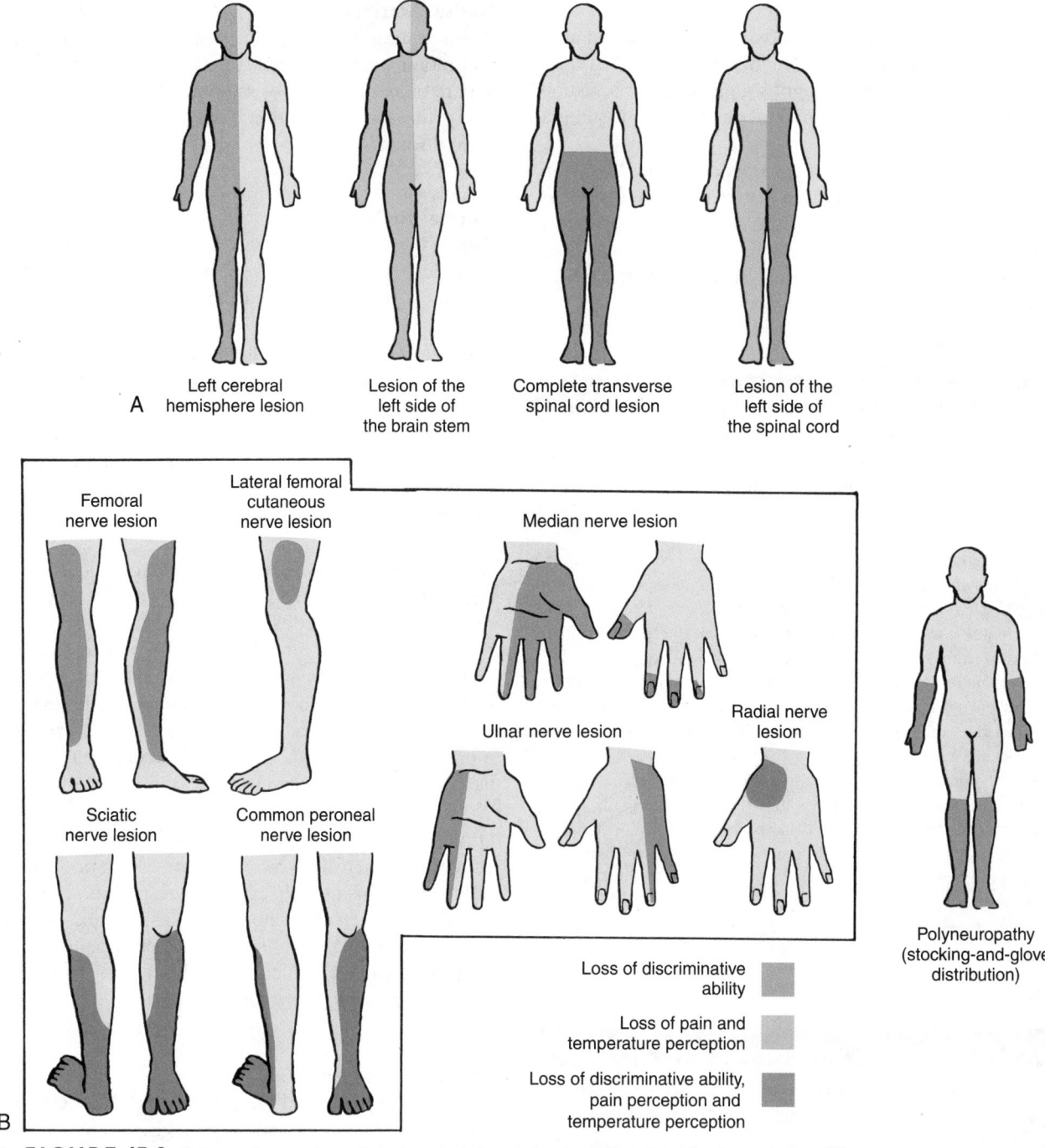

■ **FIGURE 67–3** Patterns of sensory loss with brain and spinal cord disorders **(A)** and peripheral nerve lesions **(B).**

midpoint of the heel, and move upward and laterally along the outer border of the sole to the ball of the foot. Continue the stimulus across the ball of the foot (without touching the toes) toward the medial side and off the foot. Alternatively, start the stimulus at the midlateral sole and carry it down toward the heel. A normal response is plantar flexion of the toes. An abnormal response (presence of Babinski's reflex) is dorsiflexion of the great toe and, often, fanning of the other toes (Figure 67-5). In extreme circumstances, a Babinski reflex may be accompanied

by dorsiflexion of the foot at the ankle and flexion at the knee and hip (called *triple flexion*).

Clonus. Clonus consists of rapidly alternating joint flexions and extensions resulting from continuous rhythmic contractions of a stretched muscle. This is not like a normal stretch reflex, which typically produces one reflex action. With clonus, the action continues. Support the leg at the knee, and help the client relax the leg. Rapidly flex the foot, and hold it in a flexed position. The flexion

TABLE 67–4 Important Reflexes

Reflex	Assessment Technique	Expected Response	Pathway Involved*
Tendon Reflexes			
Biceps reflex	A blow on examiner's thumb placed over biceps tendon	Flexion of elbow	C5-6
Brachioradialis reflex (supinator)	Styloid process of radius is tapped while forearm is in semiflexion and semipronation	Flexion of elbow, fingers, and hand with supination of forearm	C5-6
Triceps reflex	Strike on triceps tendon just above olecranon	Extension of elbow	C6-8 (C7 primarily)
Patellar reflex (knee jerk)	Tap on patellar tendon	Leg extends	L2-4
Achilles reflex (ankle jerk)	Tap on Achilles tendon	Plantiflexion of foot	S1-2
Superficial Reflexes			
Corneal reflex	Light touch at corneoscleral junction	Closure of eyelids	CN V, VII
Palatal and pharyngeal reflexes	Light touch to soft palate and pharynx	Elevation of palate; gagging	CN IX, X
Abdominal reflexes	Stroke skin of upper, middle, and lower abdomen toward umbilicus	Contraction of abdominal wall toward stimulus	Upper: T7-9 Middle: T9-11 Lower: T11-12
Cremasteric reflex	Stroke medial surface of upper thigh	Elevation of ipsilateral scrotum and testicle	T12-L2
Anal reflex	Stroke perianal region	Contraction of external anal sphincter	S3-5
Plantar reflex (normal)	Stroke sole of foot	Plantar flexion of toes	L4-S2
Plantar reflex (pathologic; Babinski's sign)	Stroke sole of foot	Dorsiflexion of great toe and fanning of other toes	L4-S2

* *C*, Cervical; *CN*, cranial nerve; *L*, lumbar; *S*, sacral; *T*, thoracic.
Modified from Bader, M., & Littlejohns, L. (Eds.) (2004). *AANN core curriculum for neuroscience nursing* (4th ed.). Philadelphia: Saunders.

stretches the calf muscles and causes repeated "beats" of clonus if this reflex is present.

Grading Reflex Activity

Figure 67-6 shows the grading and documentation of superficial reflexes. Although 1+ or 3+ responses are not considered normal, they may not be significant findings. Asymmetrical responses are more significant. Abnormal reflexes may be present in both neurologic and metabolic disorders. See Table 67-4 for a summary of important reflexes.

Autonomic Nervous System

The autonomic nervous system cannot be examined directly. The autonomic nervous system innervates many body organs through sympathetic and parasympathetic pathways; thus its function is evaluated by a full body systems assessment. Clinical manifestations of autonomic nervous system disorders occur in many body systems. Unit 16 focuses on neurologic disorders (heatstroke, autonomic dysreflexia). Disorders of other portions of the autonomic system are discussed in the cardiac, urinary, digestive, reproductive, and endocrine units of this book.

The following are examples of activity under autonomic nervous system influence:

- Increased or decreased heart rate
- Peripheral vasoconstriction or vasodilation
- Bronchoconstriction or bronchodilation
- Increased or decreased peristalsis
- Constriction or dilation of the pupil

Review medications the client is taking. Many medications have side effects involving the parasympathetic or sympathetic nervous system.

DIAGNOSTIC TESTING

Noninvasive Tests of Structure
Skull and Spinal X-Ray Studies

Skull x-ray studies reveal the size and shape of the skull bones, suture separation in infants, fractures or bony defects, erosion, calcification, sella turcica erosion, and pineal gland shift (>12 years of age). Spinal x-ray studies show fractures, dislocation, compressions, curvature, erosion, narrowed spinal cord canal, congenital malformations, cancers, and degenerative processes.

Computed Tomography

Computed tomography (CT) uses a computer to reconstruct a cross-sectional image from measurements of x-ray tissue penetration. The primary purpose of CT scanning is to detect intracranial bleeding, space-occupying lesions, cerebral edema, and shifts of brain structures (Figure 67-7). Infarctions, hydrocephalus, and cerebral atrophy can also be identified. It is especially useful in acute trauma not only because it can identify the extent

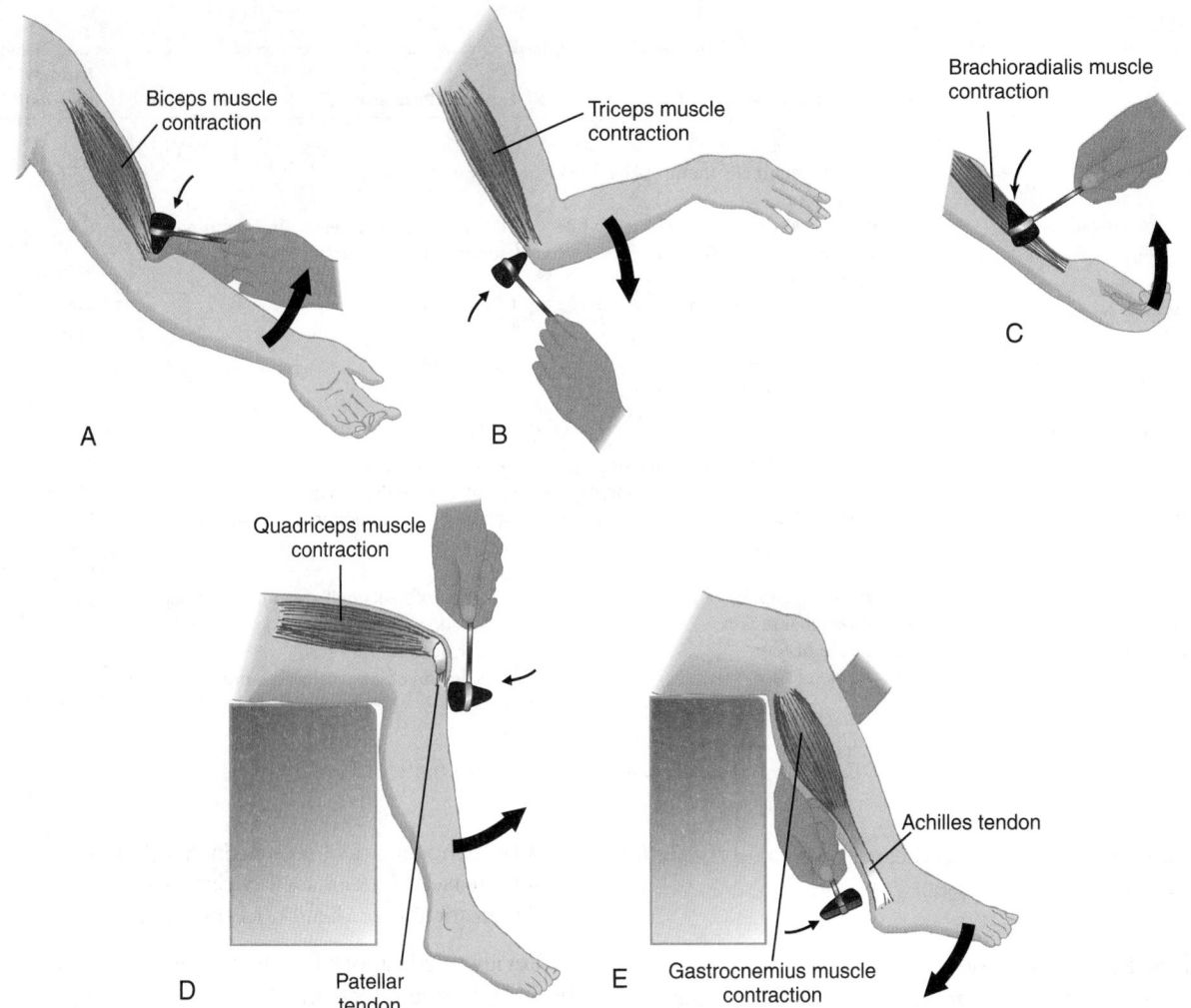

■ **FIGURE 67–4** Deep tendon (muscle-stretch) reflexes. **A,** Biceps jerk (C5-6). **B,** Triceps jerk (C7-8). **C,** Brachioradialis jerk (C5-6). **D,** Patellar reflexes (L2-4). **E,** Ankle jerk (S1-2).

BOX 67-9 Assessing Deep Tendon Reflexes

Use the following guidelines when assessing deep tendon reflexes:

1. Test deep tendon reflexes with the client either sitting or supine.
2. Support the joint where the tendon is being tested so that the attached muscle is relaxed.
3. Use the pointed end of a triangular reflex hammer to strike over small areas while you place your thumb over the biceps tendon. Use the flat end of the hammer to strike over larger areas, such as the Achilles tendon.
4. Hold the reflex hammer loosely between thumb and fingers so it can swing in an arc.
5. Swing the reflex hammer using only wrist motion, not the arm or elbow.
6. Tap the tendon briskly.
7. Note the speed, force, and amplitude of reflex responses.
8. Compare reflex responses on the two sides of the body.

9. Grade reflexes on a 0 to 4+ scale. Consider the strength of the reflex in relation to the bulk of the muscle mass.

   Repeat testing of reflexes graded 0 or 1+ by using the technique of reinforcement (see next phase). Note in the record that *reinforcement* was used. Reinforcement is a maneuver used to enhance deep tendon reflex responses when they are graded 0 or 1+. Reinforcement maneuvers for various deep tendon reflexes are as follows:

1. Ask the client to perform isometric contraction of other muscles, which may increase the generalized reflex response.
2. For the upper extremities, have the client either clench the teeth together or contract the quadriceps muscles (push the thighs against the table).
3. For the lower extremities, have the client lock the fingers together and try to pull them apart at the same time you test the tendon.

BOX 67-10 Abnormal Reflexes

Jaw reflex. The jaw reflex is also called the *mandibular reflex* or *jaw jerk*. Have the client relax the mouth, leaving it open slightly. Then tap gently on the lower jaw below the mouth. The jaw normally contracts and closes the mouth as a result of downward tapping. This reflex is absent in most people but may be present in clients who have lesions in the corticobulbar tract above the mid-pons.

Palm-chin (palmomental) reflex. The palm-chin reflex is produced by vigorous, rapid irritation on the mound of the palm at the thumb's base with a blunt instrument, which causes the chin muscles to pull up on the same side.

Snout reflex. A brisk midline tap above or below the mouth results in pursing of the lips. This reflex is normal in infants but is abnormal in adults.

Rooting reflex. Stroking the side of the face causes the mouth to open and the head to turn to the stimulated side. This reflex is normal in infants but is abnormal in adults.

Sucking reflex. Touching the lips with a blunt object results in movement of the tongue, lips, and jaws. This reflex is normal in infants but is abnormal in adults.

Glabella reflex. Tapping the forehead between the eyebrows results in sustained closure of the eyelids.

Grasp reflex. Placing an object in the palm of the hand causes the fingers to curl around it.

Chewing reflex. A tongue blade placed between the teeth results in the tight closing of the jaws.

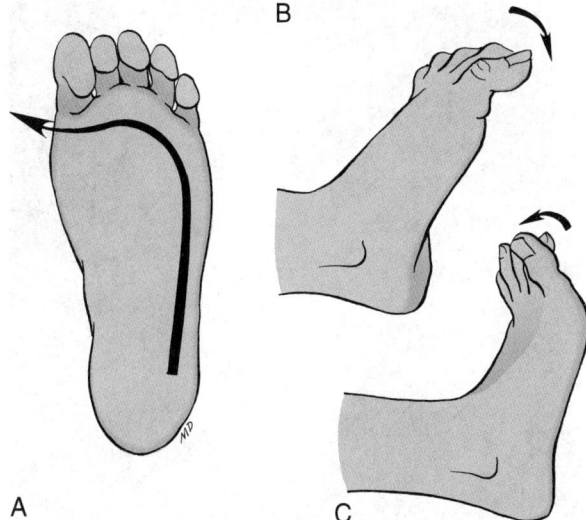

■ **FIGURE 67–5** Babinski's reflex. **A,** Test maneuver: Using a blunt point, scratch the sole of the foot as shown. **B,** Normal response (absence of Babinski's response) is plantiflexion of the toes. **C,** Abnormal response (presence of Babinski's response) is dorsiflexion of the big toe and often a fanning of the other toes.

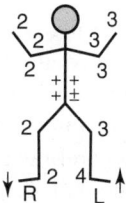

■ **FIGURE 67–6** Documentation of muscle-stretch and superficial reflexes in left hemiparesis. Muscle-stretch reflex grades: 0, absent; 1, diminished; 2, normal; 3, brisker than normal; 4, hyperactive (clonus). Superficial reflex grades: 0, absent, ±, equivocal or barely present; +, normally active.

of injuries quickly but also because it is readily available at lower cost than other types of scans. It is superior to MRI for diagnosing skull fractures and subarachnoid hemorrhage.

Advances in technology have expanded the uses of CT. CT fluoroscopy combines CT with real time imaging, which is useful during interventional procedures such as surgery and spinal injections. Spiral CT uses injection of contrast material followed by rapid image sequencing to study movement of the contrast material through the cerebral blood vessels. Xenon CT uses inhaled xenon gas, which is absorbed into the bloodstream, to enhance views that depict regional cerebral blood flow. CT angiography is a noninvasive alternative to conventional angiography for viewing intracranial blood vessels in two-dimensional and three-dimensional format. The image can be rotated 360 degrees.

CT scans can be used for stereotactic procedures. Before the scan, a frame is applied to the client's head with pins inserted into the skull. The scan is performed with the frame in place. The computer marks reference measurements on the scan to guide the location of treatment.

Magnetic Resonance Imaging

Magnetic resonance imaging (MRI) combines radiofrequency (RF) waves and magnetic fields to provide more

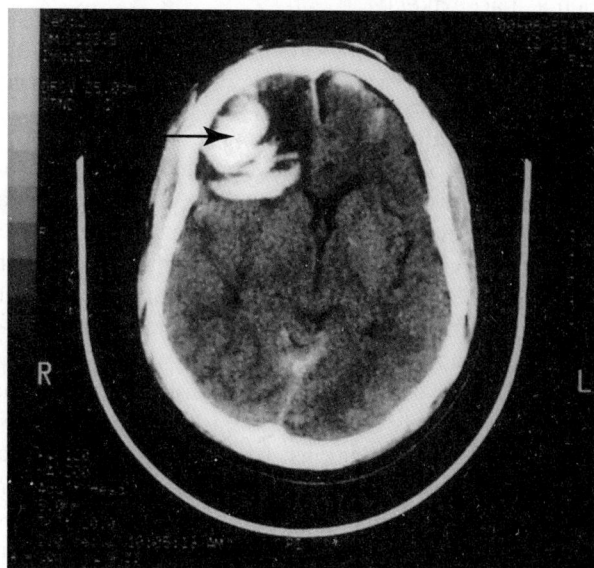

■ **FIGURE 67–7** A computed tomography scan of the head. The brain tissue is gray, and the skull is white. The mass in the left frontal lobe *(arrow)* is blood from a head injury.

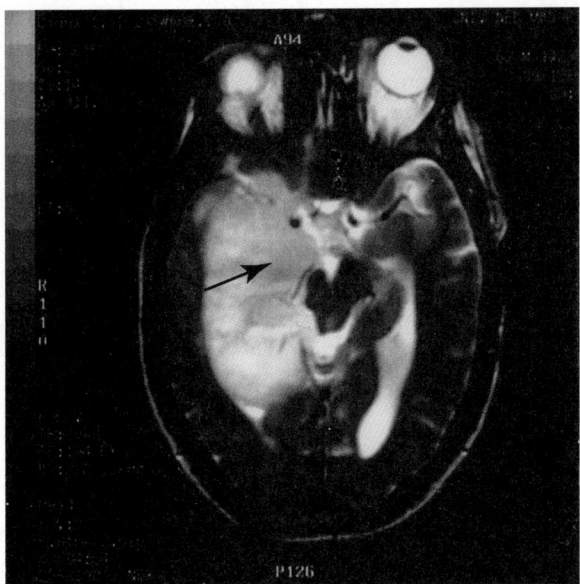

■ **FIGURE 67–8** Magnetic resonance imaging of the head. The eyes are evident at the top of the image. The client has a brain tumor (*arrow*).

anatomically detailed pictures than are available with CT (Figure 67-8). MRI has several advantages over CT. MRI can detect disorders in white matter pathways caused by loss of myelin, as in multiple sclerosis, better than CT. MRI can evaluate cerebral infarction within hours of the event; CT would not demonstrate the ischemic stroke for several days. MRI is the scan of choice for congenital brain malformations and spinal cord lesions. MRI with contrast material delineates blood flow through cerebral blood vessels in more detail than is possible with CT. MRI is contraindicated with certain metal implants, such as pacemakers.

Noninvasive Tests of Function
Electroencephalogram

An electroencephalogram (EEG) is a measurement of the electrical activity of the superficial layers of the cerebral cortex. The electrical potentials from neuron activity within the brain are recorded in the form of wave patterns. See the box Types of Electrical Brain Waves on the website for a description of the common types of brain wave patterns.

The EEG is used to assess seizure disorders. The results are diffusely abnormal in various metabolic disturbances, toxic conditions (drug overdose), coma, dementias, infections (meningitis and encephalitis), narcolepsy, and insomnia. The EEG may be used in the operating room to monitor cerebral activity during surgery on the blood vessels in the head or neck. Absence of waves on the recording ("flat lines") may be one of the criteria for defining brain death.

Evoked Potential Studies

Evoked potential (EP) studies measure evoked potentials or the brain's electrical response to various stimuli. EP studies assess the transit time of afferent pathways of the cerebral hemispheres and the brain stem. Typical stimuli are flashing lights, buzzing tones, and peripheral nerve stimulation. EP studies can be used to assess blindness, deafness, and brain stem injury. Evoked potential studies are carried out in the same fashion as EEG studies. EP studies can detect abnormalities in infants, children, and clients who are sedated or paralyzed with neuromuscular blocking agents.

Neuropsychological Testing

Neuropsychological testing involves a series of tests to evaluate cortical function by localizing the area and the extent of impairment and determining the rate of progression or recovery. The tests gauge many types of abilities, such as motor, perceptual, language, visuospatial, and cognitive. General measures of intelligence (Wechsler Adult Intelligence Scale) as well as tests of emotional and personal adjustment (the Minnesota Multiphasic Personality Inventory) are used. Test results can provide information regarding the extent of cognitive impairment and the effect it may have on functional ability and can aid in determining decision-making ability for legal and insurance matters. Test results may be used to make recommendations about treatment, including educational and vocational rehabilitation.

Magnetic Resonance Spectroscopy

Magnetic resonance spectroscopy (MRS) is a noninvasive MRI method of studying the distribution of chemicals or molecules in the body. MRS can detect abnormal amounts or those that are not normally present. The amount or presence of certain molecules or markers is associated with specific neurodegenerative diseases such as multiple sclerosis, Huntington's disease, dementia, and disorders of the mitochondria. Presently, MRS is mainly used in research.

Functional Magnetic Resonance Imaging

Similar to MRI, functional magnetic resonance imaging (fMRI) uses a strong magnet and radiofrequency waves to produce an image. Instead of lying still and quiet, the client performs cognitive, motor, or sensory tasks during the scan. The client may be asked to recite all the words they can remember that start with a certain letter or press a button at the sound of a noise. Certain areas of the brain are activated with each type of task. The fMRI detects changes in venous blood oxygenation and blood flow in activated areas. Blood flow increases in areas where neuronal activity increases. The fMRI is currently used more for experimental than diagnostic purposes. It increases understanding of the effects of stroke, hypoglycemia, and neurodegenerative diseases on specific areas of the brain. Clinically, it is useful for pre-surgical brain mapping to minimize damage to eloquent regions.

Positron Emission Tomography

Positron emission tomography (PET) enables visualization of physiologic function in body areas. Often the function of diseased tissue is different from that of normal tissues. PET has three primary uses: determining the amount of blood flow to specific body tissues; revealing how adequately tissues use blood or nutrients, such as oxygen; and mapping specific receptors, such as medications and neurotransmitters.

Cerebral blood flow, cerebral glucose metabolism, and oxygen extraction can be measured by PET. It is used in the diagnosis of stroke, brain tumors, and epilepsy and to chart the progress of Alzheimer's disease, Parkinson's disease, head injury, schizophrenia, and bipolar disorder.

A modification of the procedure, called single-photon emission computed tomography (SPECT), has been developed. SPECT uses less precise but more stable and more commercially available isotopes to measure cerebral blood flow rather than metabolic activity as measured with PET. SPECT is used to analyze blood flow in clients with ischemic stroke, subarachnoid hemorrhage, migraine, Alzheimer's disease, epilepsy, and other neurodegenerative diseases, such as Parkinson's disease.

Noninvasive Tests for Vascular Abnormalities

The noninvasive tests described here are useful in assessing cerebrovascular disorders.

Doppler Ultrasonography

Doppler ultrasonography may be used to measure blood flow (including direction and velocity) in the supraorbital region. In clients with occlusion or stenosis of the internal carotid artery, the direction of blood flow is altered (reversed) in the supraorbital artery, a change that may be detected by ultrasonography. Transcranial Doppler studies evaluate arterial flow in the circle of Willis and its major branches.

Doppler Scanning

Doppler scanning combines Doppler ultrasonography with pulsed-wave echocardiography. Visual representation of moving blood is obtained. Assessment of flow through carotid arteries is a common use of Doppler scanning.

Invasive Tests of Structure
Lumbar Puncture

In a lumbar puncture (LP), also known as a *spinal tap,* a needle is inserted into the subarachnoid space in the lumbar region of the spine below the level of the spinal cord. CSF can be withdrawn or substances can be injected into this space.

Lumbar puncture is performed for assessment and therapeutic purposes. LP enables assessment of CSF pressure and collection of CSF for evaluation. In adults, CSF can be assessed for WBCs, RBCs, chloride, glucose, protein, and lactate dehydrogenase (LDH) as well as pressure. Other tests that can be performed include serology for syphilis, glutamine, C-reactive protein, and a variety of cell stains. See the table Normal Cerebrospinal Fluid (CSF) Values and Significance of Abnormal Values on the website for common abnormalities seen on CSF analysis. *evolve*

Therapeutically, LP is used to administer spinal medications such as analgesics, antispasmodics, chemotherapy, and anesthetics. These medications can also be delivered via continuous infusion pump.

Myelography

A *myelogram* is an x-ray study in which contrast material is injected into the subarachnoid space to examine the spinal canal. A LP is performed and some CSF is removed. Myelography is used to visualize intradural nerve roots in selected clients in whom MRI cannot be performed.

Cerebral Angiography

Aneurysms and arteriovenous malformations (AVMs) are best detected by angiography. A *cerebral angiogram* consists of injection of contrast material into an artery to visualize intracranial circulation (see the Cerebral Angiography figure on the website). Angiography is the procedure used most often to visualize aneurysms, AVMs, major vessel displacement, vascular occlusion, and thrombi. *evolve*

Interventional Angiography

A polymer, glue, or small balloons are used to occlude feeding vessels in tumors or AVMs. Blocking the feeding vessels reduces the size and vascularity of the tumor or AVM, thus diminishing the need for, and the complications of, its surgical removal. Interventional angiography also enables balloon angioplasty to be performed to expand atherosclerotically narrowed cerebral vessels.

Digital Venous Angiography

Computerized digital video subtraction systems allow visualization of vascular structures. Much less contrast medium is required compared with that needed for cerebral angiography. A central venous line is necessary to inject the contrast medium. Indications for digital venous angiography include the following:

- Assessment for transient ischemic attacks
- Serial follow-up evaluations for known carotid stenosis
- Assessment of intracranial tumors
- Postoperative assessment of aneurysms
- Follow-up evaluations after extracranial or intracranial bypass procedures
- Assessment of dural venous sinuses

Invasive Tests of Function
Caloric Testing

The oculovestibular reflex, or *caloric test,* provides information about the function of the vestibular portion of CN VIII and pathways in the pons and midbrain. It aids in the differential diagnosis of brain stem lesions (see also Chapter 68).

The test is performed only in an unconscious client to determine the presence of brain stem function. Check that the ear canal is patent and that the tympanic membrane is intact. Ice-cold water is introduced into the auditory canal. If brain stem function is intact, the eyes move in a conjugate fashion away from the irrigated side and then quickly move back to midline. Irrigation with warm water results in the eyes moving toward the side where the ear is being irrigated. With brain stem death, this nystagmus pattern does not occur. Oculovestibular tests are contraindicated for clients with perforated eardrums or with acute labyrinthine disease.

Peripheral Nerve Studies

Electromyography. Electromyography (EMG) is used to measure and document electrical currents produced by skeletal muscles, called *muscle action potentials.* Small-needle electrodes are inserted into muscles. The electrical potentials of each muscle are amplified, transmitted to an oscilloscope, and displayed on a screen. The recording can be made audible and documented on *evolve* paper (see the figure Electromyography on the website).

EMG can differentiate between primary muscle disease and disease secondary to denervation. The results may indicate a transmission defect at the neuromuscular junction, such as myasthenia gravis. The procedure can be used to help to differentiate diseases of the anterior horn cells from those primarily of peripheral nerves.

Nerve Conduction Velocity Study. A nerve conduction velocity (NCV) study, often performed in conjunction with EMG, is used to evaluate the excitability and conduction velocities of motor and sensory nerves. It is helpful in identifying peripheral nerve disorders. A stimulating electrode and a recording electrode are placed to test specific nerves (usually on a limb). The time required for the passage of a nerve impulse from the point of stimulation to the point of recording is measured precisely.

Conduction velocity is calculated. Both motor and sensory modalities can be altered in peripheral nervous system disorders (carpal tunnel syndrome), whereas only motor fibers are affected in chronic disease of the anterior horn cell or motor nerve roots.

Muscle or Nerve Biopsy

When other tests are inconclusive, muscle and nerve biopsies are used in the diagnosis of myopathies and neuropathies. An EMG is helpful in locating those muscle areas that are most abnormal. It is important that areas that have been traumatized by needle electrodes be avoided when tissue is taken for biopsy. Different techniques are used to obtain the specimens, for example, open incision or needle biopsy.

Cellular Assessment

With analysis of the human genome, genetic testing has increased in importance in recent years. Chromosomes can be prepared for microscopic examination from tissue culture of cells obtained from peripheral blood, bone marrow, skin, chorionic villus, and autopsy specimens. Chromosome analysis assists diagnosis of some abnormal neurologic conditions and provides the basis for genetic counseling in families with evidence of congenital neurologic malformations and inherited neurologic diseases. Mental retardation and convulsive seizures may result from neurologic dysfunction associated with inborn errors of metabolism.

CONCLUSIONS

Neurologic assessment begins with the history of the disorder and proceeds to the physical examination. The physical examination can be lengthy because of the complexity of the CNS. The neurologic examination consists of assessments of cognition, sensation, motor function, and reflexes. The complexity and length of time required for the assessment may tempt you to omit portions to speed up the process. Before omitting portions, remember that the assessments provide baseline data for further evaluation and legal proof of a client's status. Diagnostic tests include LP, CT, MRI, and angiography. Understanding how a test is performed enables the nurse to provide adequate client preparation and to perform appropriate follow-up assessments.

BIBLIOGRAPHY

Citations appearing in red refer to primary research.

Citations appearing in blue refer to evidence-based practice guidelines and protocols.

1. Bader, M., & Littlejohns, L. (Eds.) (2004). *AANN core curriculum for neuroscience nursing* (4th ed.). Philadelphia: Saunders.
2. Blumenfeld, H. (2002). *Neuroanatomy through clinical cases.* Sunderland, Mass: Sinauer Associates.

3. Cipriano, J. (2003). *Photographic manual of regional orthopaedic and neurologic tests* (4th ed.). Atlanta: Lippincott Williams & Wilkins.

4. Estes, M. (2006). *Health assessment & physical examination* (3rd ed.). Australia: Delmar Thomson Learning.

5. Evans, R.W. (2003). *Saunders manual of neurologic practice*. Philadelphia: Saunders.

6. Goetz, C. (2003). *Textbook of clinical neurology* (2nd ed.). Philadelphia: Saunders.

7. Guyton, A., & Hall, J. (2006). *Textbook of medical physiology* (11th ed.). Philadelphia: Saunders.

8. Hickey, J.V. (2003). *Clinical practice of neurological and neuroscience nursing* (5th ed.). Philadelphia: Lippincott Williams & Wilkins.

9. Jarvis, C. (2004). *Physical examination and health assessment* (4th ed.). Philadelphia: Saunders.

10. Kernan, W., et al. (2000). Phenylpropanolamine and the risk of hemorrhagic stroke. *New England Journal of Medicine, 343*(25), 1826-1832.

11. Lindsay, K., & Bone, I. (2004). *Neurology and neurosurgery illustrated* (4th ed.). Edinburgh: Churchill Livingstone.

12. Lynn-McHale, D., & Carlson, K. (Eds.) (2005). *AACN procedure manual for critical care* (5th ed.). Philadelphia: Saunders.

13. Pagana, K., & Pagana, T. (2006). *Manual of diagnostic and laboratory tests* (3rd ed.). St. Louis: Mosby.

evolve Did you remember to check out the bonus material on the Evolve website and the CD-ROM, including NCLEX®-Examination Style Review Questions, Open-Book Quizzes, and Chapter Review Audio Podcasts?

http://evolve.elsevier.com/Black/medsurg

CHAPTER **68**

Management of Comatose or Confused Clients

CHRISTINA STEWART-AMIDEI

Perhaps more than any other clients we encounter, clients who are comatose or confused need to be cared for in a holistic manner. All aspects of physiologic and psychological function need to be addressed. Even if clients cannot interact with their surroundings the nurse must care for them in a respectful and dignified manner. It is important for family members to see that their loved ones are spoken to and cared for in a professional and caring way. The term *patient* is used in this chapter to describe the client who is comatose. It is assumed that such a client cannot be an active participant in care and that the *family* serves as the *client* in these circumstances.

DISORDERS OF CONSCIOUSNESS

Consciousness is a state of being with two important aspects: (1) wakefulness and (2) awareness of self, environment (including place), and time. Wakefulness is the ability to maintain an awake state or to be easily aroused from sleep. *Awareness of self* means that the client can identify himself or herself. *Awareness of place* indicates that the client can identify his or her present location and reason for being there. *Awareness of time* indicates that a client knows the date, month, and year and can identify common current facts, such as the season.

Unconsciousness can be brief, lasting for a few seconds to minutes, or sustained, lasting for an hour or longer. To produce unconsciousness, a disorder must (1) disrupt the ascending reticular activating system, which extends the length of the brain stem and up into the thalamus; (2) significantly disrupt the function of both cerebral hemispheres; or (3) metabolically depress overall brain function, as in a drug overdose.

Coma is a state of sustained unconsciousness in which the patient (1) does not respond to verbal stimuli, (2) may have varying responses to painful stimuli, (3) does not move voluntarily, (4) may have altered respiratory patterns, (5) may have altered pupillary responses to light, and (6) does not blink. In general the longer the coma lasts, the more likely it is irreversible. Duration of coma is also associated with mortality and outcome; the longer the coma, the higher the mortality, and the poorer the neurologic outcome.

Etiology and Risk Factors

Two types of disorders produce coma (Table 68-1):

1. Structural lesions in the brain that place pressure on the brain stem or the structures within the posterior cranial fossa, including the cerebellum, midbrain, pons, and medulla. These types of lesions affect the reticular activating system (RAS).
2. Metabolic disorders and diffuse lesions, which impair wakefulness and awareness by reducing the supply of oxygen and glucose, by allowing waste products to accumulate in the brain, or by altering other cerebral metabolic processes.

Structural causes of coma include head trauma, ischemic or hemorrhagic stroke, and brain tumors. Automobile and motorcycle accidents, physical assaults, gunshot wounds, and falls are common causes of head injury

TABLE 68–1	Causes of Altered Consciousness
Type of Lesion	**Causes**
Structural Brain Lesions	
Supratentorial lesions (cause upper brain stem dysfunction)	Cerebral edema
	Brain tumor
	Brain abscess
	Cerebral hemorrhage
	Cerebral infarction (large)
	Epidural hematoma
	Subdural hematoma
Infratentorial lesions (compress or destroy reticular formation)	Cerebellar abscess
	Brain stem or cerebellar hemorrhage
	Brain stem or cerebellar infarction
	Brain stem or cerebellar tumor
Metabolic disorders and diffuse lesions	Diseases of other organs (e.g., heart, liver, lungs, endocrine glands, kidney)
	Poisons, alcohol, and drugs
	Fluid, electrolyte, acid-base imbalances
	Seizures
	Infections (e.g., encephalitis, meningitis)
	Severe nutritional deficiencies
	Hypoglycemia
	Ischemia or anoxia
	Syncope
	Temperature regulation disorders

The impact of the initial injury causes damage, but further damage can occur as a result of ischemic consequences of injury. Ischemic stroke occurs with interruption of blood supply to the brain. Ischemia can directly affect structures involved in consciousness or cause swelling of the brain, leading to coma. Hemorrhagic stroke can occur as a consequence of hypertension or from rupture of a vascular anomaly. Hemorrhage causes coma by placing pressure on brain tissue. Tumors may metastasize from other organs or arise from the brain itself. Increased intracranial pressure caused by the tumor may lead to coma.

There are many metabolic causes of coma. The term *metabolic* is used to describe any problem that alters brain metabolism. *Hypoxia* is a common cause of metabolic coma. Blood loss, high altitudes, or carbon monoxide poisoning may deprive the brain of oxygen. *Ischemia,* inadequate tissue levels of oxygen, may occur with cardiac disorders in which cardiac output is decreased, such as cardiac arrest or even fainting.

Of note is that coma may be purposely induced as a means to treat neurologic and other serious illnesses. In this situation, medication such as propofol is given to produce coma to rest the brain and hopefully prevent further injury to the brain. Induced or therapeutic coma may be considered for clients with extreme brain swelling secondary to brain injury, stroke, or metabolic disease. Therapeutic coma may be continued for days to a few weeks. Care for patients in induced coma is largely the same as for those who are comatose from some disease process. Full life support in an intensive care setting is required.

Pathophysiology

Consciousness is a complex function controlled by the RAS and its integrated components. The RAS begins in the medulla as the reticular formation (RF) (Figure 68-1). The reticular formation connects to the RAS, located in the midbrain, which then connects to the hypothalamus and thalamus. Integrated pathways connect to the cortex via the thalamus and to the limbic system via the hypothalamus. Feedback systems also connect at the brain stem level. The reticular formation produces wakefulness, whereas the RAS and higher connections are responsible for awareness of self and the environment. Diffuse cortical connections allow maximum integration of all conscious-related activities.

Disorders that affect any part of the RAS can produce coma. To produce coma, a disorder must affect both cerebral hemispheres or the brain stem itself. Disorders affect these areas in one of three ways:

1. Direct compression or destruction of structures responsible for consciousness. A tumor or hemorrhage in the brain stem or swelling in the cerebral hemispheres can cause coma in this manner.
2. Decrease in availability of oxygen or glucose, both of which are needed for cerebral metabolism. Hypoxia and ischemia are the most common causes; without oxygen and glucose, the brain cannot form the chemicals necessary to carry out its functions.
3. Toxic effects of substances on structures of the RAS. Toxic wastes from liver or kidney disease, bacterial invasion from meningitis, and metabolites from drug overdose are examples of such substances.

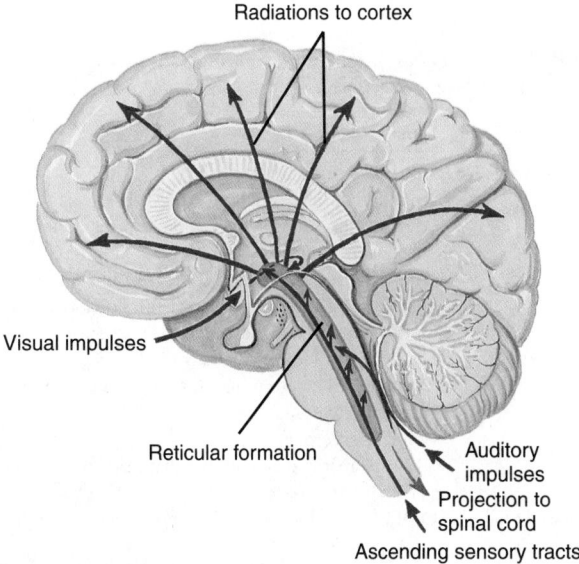

■ **FIGURE 68-1** The reticular activating system (RAS) consists of centers in the brain stem reticular formation along with fibers conducting to the centers from below and fibers conducting from the centers to widespread areas of the cerebral cortex. A functioning RAS is essential for consciousness. *(From Thibodeau, G., & Patton, K. [2003]. Anatomy and physiology [5th ed., p. 395]. St. Louis: Mosby.)*

The causes may overlap. The anatomic location and the severity of the problem determine the depth of coma.

Clinical Manifestations

Supratentorial lesions (located above the dura roofing the cerebellum) cause a fairly predictable set of clinical manifestations (Table 68-2). Such lesions can involve cortical or subcortical areas of the brain tissue, as with ischemia. The disorder may also be located in only one hemisphere, as with tumor or hemorrhage. These lesions produce manifestations such as headache, localized sensorimotor deficits, and seizures. The manifestations are related to the specific area of the brain affected.

For example, if the client has a mass in the frontal lobe, early clinical manifestations may consist of headaches, memory deficits and subtle motor deficits (unilateral arm drift), or partial seizures on the side of the body opposite the brain lesion. *Partial seizures* are seizures that occur in one area of the body, such as the hand. As the lesion expands, manifestations worsen because the lesion places pressure on nearby areas. This pressure may cause a more pronounced unilateral motor deficit (e.g., client cannot raise the right leg or arm), aphasia, or a deficit in the visual field (blind in one half of the visual field). The client usually has intact pupillary reflexes. The Critical Monitoring feature on p. 1795 describes these and other neurologic changes. If the lesion progresses, coma eventually develops. Coma indicates that the lesion has expanded and now compresses structures deep in the brain stem.

TABLE 68–2 Differential Manifestations of Structurally Induced and Metabolic Coma

Mechanism	Manifestations
Supratentorial coma	History of progressive onset; initiating manifestation is usually focal cerebral dysfunction; neurologic manifestations at any given time point to one anatomic area (e.g., frontal lobes, thalamus)
	Signs of dysfunction progress cephalocaudad
	Motor manifestations are often symmetrical
Infratentorial coma	History of sudden onset of coma
	Localizing brain stem manifestations precede or accompany coma onset
	Cranial nerve palsies
	"Bizarre" respiratory patterns that appear at coma onset
Metabolic coma	Confusion and stupor commonly precede motor manifestations
	Motor manifestations are usually symmetrical
	Pupillary reactions are usually preserved
	Asterixis, myoclonus, tremor, and seizures are common
	Acid-base imbalances with hyperventilation or hypoventilation are common

---

Disorders of the infratentorial area (located beneath the dura roofing the cerebellum) cause the client to lose consciousness suddenly either (1) by directly affecting the RAS or its pathways or (2) by invading the brain stem or reducing its blood supply. Infratentorial lesions may produce unusual respiratory patterns (Table 68-3). The brain stem houses the center for rhythmic breathing. This center's function is lost as consciousness decreases, and the lower brain stem begins to regulate breathing by responding to changes primarily in the carbon dioxide levels as well as in acid-base balance and oxygen levels. The result is a very irregular breathing depth and pattern. A lesion in the brain stem commonly compresses the cranial nerves, and various cranial nerve deficits can be seen. In particular, abnormal eye movements and loss of pupillary reactivity to light are noted. Specific patterns of pupil size and reactivity to light occur when pressure is exerted at various levels (see Table 68-3).

Coma caused by a metabolic disorder more often is manifested as the presence of bilateral or symmetrical findings because the disorder affects the entire brain. The client usually demonstrates confusion and stupor before any physical manifestations are noticed. Physical manifestations of coma caused by a metabolic disorder include tremor, asterixis (flapping tremors of the hands), *myoclonus* (a single, sudden jerking movement), and seizures. Pupillary response is usually normal unless the condition is related to drug overdose. Depending on the underlying cause, acid-base imbalances may be noted. For example, metabolic acidosis would be present in a patient with diabetic coma.

Level of consciousness is the single most important indicator of neurologic function. In the comatose patient, this indicator is lost and other indicators of neurologic function must be evaluated. Information about the time frame of onset, motor response, pupil size and reactivity to light, presence or absence of oculocephalic and oculovestibular responses and other cranial nerve functions, and breathing pattern can localize the level of involvement and determine the depth of coma. For further discussion about these indicators, see Chapter 73.

Diagnostic Findings

The neurologic examination is supplemented by diagnostic testing. Tests identify structural or physiologic abnormalities that affect brain function.

Computed Tomography and Magnetic Resonance Imaging

A computed tomography (CT) or magnetic resonance imaging (MRI) scan usually provides data that indicate a structural cause for the coma. In coma a CT scan is usually performed first because it is quicker. Tumors and areas of bleeding are evident on the scan. In metabolic

CRITICAL MONITORING

Manifestations of Changes in Neurologic Status

"Change" is the key word. Notify the physician whenever there is a change in the patient's neurologic status. The following manifestations are listed in the order that indicates a *worsening* in the patient's condition. Remember, a patient may display a "transient" deterioration in neurologic responses that does not warrant calling a physician. For example, after you have just performed suctioning of the patient's airway or have turned the patient, you would anticipate a possible change in neurologic status. If you hyperoxygenate the patient and ensure proper positioning for venous return from the jugular veins and airway maintenance, however, any manifestations of increased deficit should last only a few seconds or no more than a few minutes. Worsening deficit that lasts longer than this increases the risk for irreversible brain injury and requires immediate attention.

NORMAL

- Alert, oriented to person, place, time
- Responds appropriately to verbal commands
- Eyes open spontaneously with any stimulus, unless in a deep sleep

ABNORMAL; CHANGES CAUSED BY ALTERED PERFUSION OF THE CEREBRAL CORTEX

- Altered level of consciousness
- Altered perception of time, then place, and lastly person
- Motor deficits (e.g., hemiparesis, hemiplegia)
- Speech deficits (e.g., expressive or receptive speech or both)
- Memory deficits (e.g., recent, intermediate, remote)
- Hyperreflexia
- Babinski's sign
- Seizures
- Decorticate rigidity
- Emotional lability
- Altered sensory interpretation
- Cheyne-Stokes respiration
- Headache, nausea, vomiting, papilledema

ABNORMAL; CHANGES CAUSED BY ALTERED PERFUSION JUST INFERIOR TO THE CORTEX

- Pupillary changes: asymmetry of size, shape, or time-responsiveness
- Loss of reaction to direct light
- Visual field changes (e.g., homonymous hemianopsia; see Chapter 70)

ABNORMAL; CHANGES CAUSED BY ALTERED PERFUSION OF THE DIENCEPHALON

- Altered temperature; first high fevers, then hypothermia
- Cheyne-Stokes respiration

ABNORMAL; CHANGES CAUSED BY ALTERED PERFUSION OF THE POSTERIOR PITUITARY GLAND

- Diabetes insipidus (decreased antidiuretic hormone)

ABNORMAL; CHANGES CAUSED BY ALTERED PERFUSION OF THE MIDBRAIN

- Dysfunction of CN III (loss of reaction to indirect or consensual light, disconjugate eye movement)
- Dysfunction of CN IV (disconjugate eye movement)
- Central neurogenic hyperventilation

ABNORMAL; CHANGES CAUSED BY ALTERED PERFUSION OF THE UPPER PONS

- Dysfunction of CN V (altered sensory function to cornea, nasal membranes, face, oral cavity, tongue, teeth, or altered mastication)
- Dysfunction of CN VI (altered lateral eye movement)
- Dysfunction of CN VII (altered facial expression, taste, and salivation)
- Central neurogenic hyperventilation
- Abnormal extension posture
- Pinpoint pupils

ABNORMAL; CHANGES CAUSED BY ALTERED PERFUSION OF THE LOWER PONS

- Apneustic breathing
- Flaccidity

ABNORMAL; CHANGES CAUSED BY ALTERED PERFUSION OF THE MEDULLA

- Dysfunction of CN VIII (altered equilibrium and hearing)
- Dysfunction of CN IX (altered taste, pharyngeal sensations, and cough and swallowing)
- Dysfunction of CN X (altered sensations in pharynx, larynx, external ear, and altered cough and swallowing; altered parasympathetic nervous system functions in thoracic and abdominal viscera)
- Dysfunction of CN XI (altered neck and shoulder movement)
- Dysfunction of CN XII (altered tongue movement)
- Projectile vomiting
- Cushing's triad (increased systolic blood pressure, wide pulse pressure, bradycardia)
- Ataxic (Biot's respiration)

CN, Cranial nerve.

coma the structures may appear unremarkable, or edema or diffuse nonspecific changes may be seen.

Lumbar Puncture

A lumbar puncture can be performed when it is known, from data provided by the CT or MRI scans, that the patient does not have an expanding intracranial mass.

Obtaining this information before lumbar puncture is done avoids the risk of herniation caused by sudden changes in cerebrospinal fluid (CSF) pressures (low in the spinal column and high in the ventricles). A lumbar puncture can assist in the diagnosis of infection or bleeding as a cause of coma. The CSF may be cloudy when the client has an infection or bloody when there is bleeding into the ventricles or the subarachnoid space.

TABLE 68–3 Eye Manifestations and Respiratory Patterns by Level of Involvement in Coma

Level of Involvement	Eye Manifestations	Respiratory Pattern
Supratentorial	Small reactive pupils	Cheyne-Stokes: regular respirations with regular periods of apnea
Upper midbrain	Fixed, dilated pupils (unilateral or bilateral) or midposition fixed pupils	Central neurogenic hyperventilation: regular, deep respirations
Upper pons	Midposition fixed or pinpoint pupils	Apneustic breathing: regular but deep inspiration and expiration with regular periods of apnea
Lower pons	Pinpoint pupils	Cluster breathing: clusters of irregular inspiration and expiration between periods of apnea
Medulla	Pinpoint or midposition fixed pupils	Ataxic breathing: completely irregular respirations with apneic periods

Electroencephalography

Electroencephalography (EEG) can be used to determine whether the patient is comatose because of continuous seizures. EEG results are abnormal in many patients with coma and do not serve as a clear diagnostic tool. A portion of the general population may have abnormal EEG results as well.

Laboratory Tests

Liver, endocrine, and kidney function may be evaluated through blood tests. A urine or blood toxicology screen may be useful in distinguishing drug-induced coma. Blood oxygenation tests may be used to evaluate for hypoxia. Other laboratory tests specific to the patient's situation may be ordered. Chapter 67 covers specific neurologic diagnostic tests.

Tests for Abnormal Ocular Reflexes

Oculocephalic Response

The oculocephalic response (OCR), also known as *doll's eye reflex,* is movement of the eyes in the direction opposite that in which the head is moved. For example, the doll's eye reflex is present if the eyes move to the right when the head is rotated to the left, and vice versa. This test can be performed only in unconscious patients because conscious patients have voluntary control over eye movements. The absence of the doll's eye reflex indicates that brain stem function is preserved. The reflex is present in patients with brain stem problems. The doll's eye test should never be performed in comatose patients with suspected or known cervical spine injury because the head movement required may produce permanent spinal cord damage.

The brain stem in a comatose patient may be functioning even in the absence of the doll's eye reflex. Patients in metabolic coma, except that caused by barbiturate or phenytoin (Dilantin) poisoning, retain ocular reflexes. Other agents and disorders can block the eye's response. Neuromuscular drugs, such as succinylcholine, and Ménière's disease, which destroys the labyrinth in the ear, obliterate the oculocephalic response. In the patient without Ménière's disease or evidence of neuromuscular drugs,

however, absence of the oculocephalic response supports the diagnosis of brain death.[4]

Oculovestibular Response

If oculocephalic responses (OCRs) are absent, an oculovestibular response (OVR) (caloric) test can be performed to test cranial nerves III, IV, VI, and VIII (see Chapter 67). A normal response to instillation of iced water into one ear canal is seen as slow, smooth movement of both eyes toward the irrigated ear, followed by fast movement to the opposite side with nystagmus. Instillation of warm water results in slow eye movement away from the irrigated ear, followed by a fast movement to the same side with nystagmus. *Nystagmus* is the involuntary oscillation of the eyeballs; it may be horizontal, vertical, oblique, rotary, or mixed, with various rates of movement.

Failure to produce eye movement and nystagmus with the instillation of warm or cold water into the ear canal indicates an altered brain stem, with a few exceptions. The use of ototoxic drugs, barbiturates, sedatives, phenytoin, or tricyclic antidepressants or the presence of Ménière's disease may produce a false-negative caloric test result. In a patient without these conditions, the absence of an OVR supports the diagnosis of brain death.

Testing the OVR is contraindicated in a patient with a ruptured tympanic membrane (eardrum) or otorrhea (ear discharge). This test is usually performed only in comatose patients because awake patients may vomit in response to stimulation of cranial nerve VIII.

OUTCOME MANAGEMENT

Medical Management

The goals of medical management are to preserve brain function and to prevent additional brain injury. The primary focus is on maintaining the supply of oxygen and glucose to the brain.

The patient's airway, breathing, and circulation ("ABCs") must be maintained. A nasal or oral airway may be inserted for a short time. If the patient is breathing spontaneously, closely monitor the airway and respirations because the airway may become obstructed and aspiration may occur as consciousness decreases. If the patient is completely unresponsive or respiratory patterns become ineffective, an endotracheal tube is inserted, with care taken to avoid injury to the cervical spine (see also Chapter 63). Ventilation and supplemental oxygen are given.

Normal cerebral perfusion is promoted through monitoring blood pressure and maintenance of the systolic pressure between 100 and 160 mm Hg. Blood pressures lower or higher than these levels may alter cerebral perfusion pressure. Use of vasoactive agents may be required to keep the systolic pressure at 100 mm Hg or the *mean* systolic blood pressure above 80 mm Hg, or medications may be needed to lower the blood pressure. Blood pressure must be cautiously lowered, however, because high blood pressure may represent a compensatory mechanism to perfuse the brain.

Determine Level of Involvement

Once airway, breathing, and circulation are established, initial assessment of the comatose patient includes evaluation of the following factors:

1. Level of consciousness, through observation of response to stimuli.
2. Presence or absence of localizing neurologic manifestations, such as unilateral lack of movement or posturing, indicating focal intracranial disease.
3. Pupil size and reactivity to light.
4. Deep tendon and superficial reflexes (see Chapter 67). Superficial reflex assessment is particularly valuable in comatose patients because it provides objective information about brain stem function in the absence of consciousness. Assess the corneal reflex carefully to avoid corneal abrasion.
5. Response to noxious stimuli. First, loud verbal stimuli and then shaking are performed to produce a response. If none is noted, the examiner applies a painful stimulus, such as pressure to the sternum, nail beds, or supraorbital notch. Care must be taken not to damage skin underlying the areas where pressure is applied. Other aspects of sensory assessment are not possible or are unreliable in comatose patients.
6. Evidence of trauma. Trauma may be the result of coma rather than the cause of it (e.g., a tongue bite may result from a seizure). Examine the ears for ruptured eardrums and otorrhea.
7. Determination of serum oxygenation, blood alcohol, blood urea nitrogen, ammonia, and glucose levels if manifestations suggest a metabolic disorder.
8. History from significant others (or observers of what has happened), if possible.

Reverse Common Causes of Coma

Immediate interventions for the patient in a coma include treatment of common causes of coma while assessment of neurologic status and diagnostic testing continue. For example, after a blood specimen is drawn for testing, intravenous (IV) glucose is given to reverse potential insulin reactions. For comatose patients who appear malnourished and have a possible history of alcohol abuse, Wernicke's encephalopathy may occur. These patients are commonly given thiamine for prevention of Wernicke's encephalopathy, especially if they are given glucose.

If the patient is having repetitive seizures, coma and brain damage can follow. The patient is given IV diazepam or lorazepam to stop the seizures. If the patient is not intubated, closely monitor the airway because of the respiratory depressant effects of these medications.

Many metabolic causes of coma lead to acid-base, fluid, and electrolyte imbalances. The patient's acid-base balance should be restored quickly. Fluid imbalances should be restored slowly to prevent rebound fluid shifts into the brain (see Chapter 11). Isotonic saline is usually given if the patient is dehydrated, and fluids are withheld if the patient is fluid overloaded. If cerebral edema is present, osmotic diuretics may be used to promote shifting of extracellular brain fluid back into the plasma. Other medications, such as steroids, barbiturate therapy, and neuromuscular blocking agents, decrease intracranial pressure (ICP) through more indirect means. (Electrolyte imbalances are covered in Chapter 12.)

If infection is suspected, specimens for culture are obtained from the blood, urine, throat, and wounds (if present). Once such specimens have been collected, antibiotics are given. Body temperature should be normalized as much as possible by means of antipyretics, air circulation, and cooling blankets. Care must be taken to ensure that the patient does not shiver because shivering increases ICP.

Coma from drug overdose may be reversed by specific antidotes if the ingested drug can be identified. Often, however, the specific drug ingested is not known. A urine or blood specimen should be collected for a toxicity screen. Opioid overdose may be reversed with naloxone. Because the duration of action of naloxone is 2 to 3 hours shorter than that of most opioids, naloxone may need to be administered again. Seizures resulting from cocaine overdose can be treated with diazepam. Patients with cocaine overdose often have cardiac dysrhythmias and irregular respirations. Instillation of activated charcoal can be used to absorb medications. In rare circumstances, hemodialysis may be used to remove toxins from the blood.

Structural causes of coma may require surgery to decompress the cranial vault. Burr holes may be created to drain a subdural hematoma. A craniotomy may be performed to remove a tumor, abscess, or intracerebral hematoma. A ventricular catheter or shunt may be placed to relieve hydrocephalus.

To stimulate your thought process, see Thinking Critically at the end of this chapter for the description of a scenario involving a patient with coma from a hypertensive hemorrhage.

Prevent Complications

If the coma is prolonged, initiate enteral feeding to promote nutrition and prevent muscle wasting. Parenteral nutrition may be used if paralytic ileus is present. Take care to avoid hyperglycemia, which can exacerbate brain injury in the presence of ischemia. Brain cells have a high glucose need compared with other cells; however, supplying the necessary glucose without causing brain damage requires a delicate balance.

Prevent the complications of immobility, such as pneumonia and pressure ulcers, with frequent turning or the use of an oscillating bed. Continue to reposition the patient to relieve skin pressure unless the bed provides more than 40 degrees of rotation. The eyes may need to be taped closed to avoid corneal abrasion. Suctioning may be needed to keep the airway clear and prevent pneumonia. Passive range-of-motion exercises keep joints mobile and minimize muscle wasting. Position the extremities in correct alignment to prevent contractures. Use sequential compression stockings to prevent deep venous thrombosis (DVT); low-dose heparin may also be ordered. All these complications are continually assessed for and are treated promptly if they occur.

Outcomes. In the past, little information was available on which to base a prediction about the outcome for a patient in coma. Most of the time, a "wait-and-see" approach was taken. Today the family and the health care team should have some idea of the probable eventual outcome for the patient. It is discouraging and inappropriate to treat a patient vigorously who has no chance of recovery, but it is even more inappropriate to deny treatment to a patient with a reasonable chance of recovery.

Coma after head injury has a statistically better outcome than coma associated with medical illness. About 50% of patients in coma from head injury die, many instantly. Immediate treatment may improve the outcome somewhat for those who reach the hospital. Recovery in traumatic cases is closely linked to age; the younger the patient, the better the recovery. Severely abnormal neuro-ophthalmologic manifestations reflecting brain stem dysfunction imply a poor prognosis; about 90% of patients with such manifestations either die or remain in near-vegetative states.

The absence of pupillary, corneal, or oculovestibular responses during the early stages of coma is highly predictive of mortality or significant morbidity (e.g., persistent vegetative state). The recovery of these responses and a return to purposeful movement correlate with a better prognosis. Patients who lapse into coma as a result of metabolic disorders have an extremely poor prognosis if the coma lasts longer than 1 week.

Some patients in coma awaken slowly and begin to respond normally. They often require physical, occupational, and speech therapy to return to maximal levels of function. Persistent unresponsiveness is caused by damage to any area of the brain that destroys the patient's ability to respond to the environment. The brain stem and cerebellum remain intact, however, so that vital functions, such as heart, lung, and GI functions, continue. Patients can remain unresponsive for years. Significant ethical and legal debates have arisen regarding the maintenance of nutritional intake for such a patient, particularly when a patient's family questions the rationale for artificial feeding.

Coma stimulation—application of planned meaningful, multimodality sensory stimulation—has been suggested as a measure to enhance outcome from coma. Clinical validity of coma stimulation has not been clearly established. The type of stimulation, timing of application, and outcomes measures used vary among studies, making it difficult to determine whether coma stimulation is of benefit.[2] Nonetheless the nurse is encouraged to interact with comatose patients through all their sensory systems.

Nursing Management of the Medical Client

Assessment. Frequent, systematic, and objective nursing assessment of the comatose patient, including neurologic status, is essential. Serial observations are important for comparison and to facilitate prompt reporting of even subtle changes in status. Even if assessment findings seem insignificant for long periods, documentation provides an objective pattern and an important baseline for future observations. Assessment of consciousness is most effective when the assessments are performed by a consistent nurse. The neurologic assessment is performed as often as every 15 minutes during the first few hours of coma. Depending on the patient's condition, assessments may need to be continued hourly for several days.

See the Critical Monitoring feature on Manifestations of Changes in Neurologic Status on p. 1795, which lists the neurologic manifestations of a person who is unconscious. Presenting manifestations are ordered according to the degree of seriousness. Remembering these subtle changes in assessment helps in early identification of a patient's improvement or worsening. A decrease in the patient's Glasgow Coma Scale (GCS) score also indicates worsening. The GCS is the most common neurologic assessment tool used in clinical practice (see Chapter 73).

Although neurologic assessment is the priority evaluation, the entire body of a comatose patient must be periodically observed because the patient is unable to offer any specific complaints. Complications of the initial condition causing coma, injuries sustained from other causes, and/or immobility can arise at any time during the course of care. If surgery has been performed, post-operative assessments must be performed as well.

Diagnosis, Outcomes, Interventions. This section describes interventions appropriate for all comatose patients regardless of the cause of the coma. Interventions specific to particular forms of coma are described elsewhere (e.g., hepatic coma in Chapter 47, and uremic coma in Chapter 36).

Comatose patients are completely dependent on others because their protective reflexes are impaired. Nursing intervention provides the safety normally afforded by protective reflexes. Coma is often life-threatening and requires aggressive medical intervention. Physicians are concerned with establishing a medical diagnosis and prescribing appropriate treatment; nurses are responsible for meeting basic human needs and preventing the complications associated with coma. Nurses are also responsible for assessing and intervening to reduce ICP.

Altered cerebral tissue perfusion is one of the highest risks for a patient with an altered level of consciousness. This outcome is often seen as a direct consequence of increasing ICP. Nursing management of this problem is described in Chapter 73.

Diagnosis: Risk for Suffocation. Patients who are unconscious cannot swallow because of loss or suppression of the gag or coughing reflex and thus are at risk for suffocation. Airway obstruction is the most common source of harm to patients with decreased consciousness. Write the nursing diagnosis as *Risk for Suffocation related to loss of gag reflex.*

Outcomes. The patient will exhibit no manifestations of accidental suffocation or airway obstruction as evidenced by (1) clear lung sounds; (2) equal lung expansion; and (3) the absence of stridor, cyanosis, and pallor.

Interventions. For initial airway management, an oral airway can be inserted in an unconscious patient. Endotracheal intubation, with the use of a ventilator, may be required to maintain airway patency or improve ventilation.

For extended airway management, a tracheostomy may be required to (1) allow long-term continuous mechanical ventilation, (2) facilitate removal of tracheobronchial secretions, and (3) separate the upper and lower airways (see Chapter 63).

Diagnosis: Risk for Aspiration. The lack of effective airway clearance and gag reflex puts the comatose patient at **very** high risk for aspiration. Write the nursing diagnosis as *Risk for Aspiration related to lack of effective airway clearance and loss of gag reflex.*

Outcomes. The patient will exhibit no manifestations of aspiration as evidenced by (1) clear lung sounds, (2) no stridor, (3) absence of fever, (4) minimal amounts of clear mucus on suctioning, and (5) clear lungs as demonstrated by chest x-ray.

Interventions. Monitor the results of arterial blood gas (ABG) analysis and pulse oximetry to determine the level of oxygenation provided by ventilators or oxygen. Assess breath sounds every 1 to 2 hours in acutely ill patients. Keep suctioning equipment available.

Perform tracheobronchial suctioning only as needed to prevent or decrease the accumulation of secretions from immobility, the lack of a cough and sigh reflex, or pneumonia. Failure to suction secretions of a person who cannot expectorate can cause hypoxia and result in neurologic damage. Suctioning should be gentle, and the catheter should not remain in the airway for longer than 10 seconds. While suctioning, observe the cardiac monitor for bradycardia and dysrhythmias (e.g., premature ventricular contractions) secondary to hypoxia. Hyperoxygenating the patient before, during, and after suctioning decreases the risk of dysrhythmias and cerebral desaturation. Limiting the suctioning time to 10 seconds also minimizes increased ICP associated with suctioning. Never suction the nasal passages in any patient with facial or skull base fractures because the suction catheter can enter the cranial cavity.

A comatose patient may lack pharyngeal reflexes and be unable to swallow. Pneumonia secondary to aspiration is a common cause of death in unconscious patients.

> **To reduce the risk of aspiration, never give a comatose patient fluids to swallow.**   **SAFETY ⚠ ALERT**

Secretions also accumulate in the posterior pharynx and may be aspirated. If the patient is intubated or has a tracheostomy, make sure the cuff is inflated. Suction the upper trachea and posterior pharynx as often as necessary to remove secretions. After tracheal suctioning, the same suction catheter can be used for oral or pharyngeal suctioning, but not vice versa. Also, turn the patient from side to side every 2 hours to facilitate drainage of secretions and prevent pneumonia; position the patient upright or prone periodically if the patient's condition permits.

As consciousness returns and the patient begins to respond to verbal stimuli and has a gag reflex, test the patient's ability to suck and to swallow liquids. Before the test, position the patient in high Fowler's position, and have suction equipment nearby in case it is needed. Use a thick juice, nectar, or ice chips rather than water; liquid of a thick consistency is easier to swallow. Place about 1 teaspoon of liquid into the back of the mouth. Observe for swallowing, and suction as needed to prevent aspiration. If a patient cannot suck through a straw or drink from a glass because of facial paralysis, place fluids in the unaffected side of the mouth with an irrigation syringe. Watch for difficulty in swallowing. Suction as needed.

If there is any question about a patient's ability to swallow, a formal swallow evaluation should be performed by a speech therapist. Patients who cannot swallow for long periods may require placement of a gastrostomy tube. Many rehabilitation and extended-care facilities require the use of gastrostomy tubes rather than nasogastric (NG) tubes because there is less risk of aspiration with gastrostomy tube feedings.

Patients with impaired swallowing require special instruction. Swallowing can be stimulated by having the patient lean the head forward and, after taking fluid, quickly tip the head backward. Stroking the anterior neck may also promote swallowing.

Once a patient can safely swallow, begin oral nutrition with small liquid feedings, progressing to a soft diet. Discontinue tube feedings only when the patient can take adequate nutrition orally. Many patients are fed orally during the daytime and tube-fed at night to maintain adequate nutrition.

When changing from tube-feeding to oral feeding, turn off the tube-feeding several hours before the meal. This will stimulate the appetite. When a patient begins to eat independently, allow adequate time and be reassuring and encouraging. Remind the patient to eat slowly and to swallow after each bite. Position the patient sitting up as tolerated.

Diagnosis: Impaired Oral Mucous Membrane. Several factors can impair oral mucous membranes. The comatose patient usually has an NPO (nothing by mouth) order, is unable to swallow, and breathes through the mouth. A possible nursing diagnosis might be *Impaired Oral Mucous Membrane related to mouth breathing.*

Outcomes. The patient will maintain intact oral mucous membranes as evidenced by oral and nasal mucous membranes that are pink, moist, and without lesions, crusts, or bloody drainage.

Interventions. Using a flashlight and tongue depressor, inspect the patient's mouth every 8 hours. Keep the patient's lips coated with a water-soluble lubricant to prevent encrustation, drying, and cracking. Carefully inspect a paralyzed cheek for crusts or other conditions that require intervention.

At least twice a day, brush the patient's teeth with a small or sponge toothbrush, and rinse the mouth. Place a comatose patient in a lateral position to prevent aspiration. If facial paralysis is present, keep the affected side uppermost. Keep the patient's mouth open by placing an oral airway or bite block between the teeth. Clean the oral mucous membranes (especially the roof of the mouth), tongue, and gums. Pay close attention to the roof of the mouth in patients who breathe through the mouth

for long periods. Crusts of dried mucus may form, break off, and be aspirated. Use of artificial moisturizers may help prevent crust formation; however, frequent oral care is the best prevention. Avoid using agents that contain lemon or alcohol because they dry the membranes. Suction excess secretions to prevent aspiration. Toothbrushes with suction attachments are now available in many health care agencies.

Nasal passages may become occluded because an unconscious patient is unable to sniff, blow, sneeze, or otherwise clear the nose. To clear the nasal passages of mucus and crust formations, gently swab the nose with an applicator moistened with water or normal saline. Then apply a thin coat of water-soluble lubricant with a cotton-tipped applicator. Do *not* clean the nasal passages or ears of a patient with a skull base fracture. If bleeding occurs from the ears or nose or if CSF (a watery discharge) appears to be draining from these areas, notify the physician.

Diagnosis: Risk for Impaired Skin Integrity. Normal reflexes reduce the risk of skin ischemia by signaling conscious (even sleeping) people to shift their body weight. Comatose patients have lost these protective reflexes and are completely immobile. Sometimes patients are agitated and can shear the skin with frequent nonpurposeful movements; this diagnosis also applies to these patients. Write the nursing diagnosis as *Risk for Impaired Skin Integrity related to immobility.*

Outcomes. The patient will have reduced risk of skin impairment, as evidenced by no reddened areas over bony prominences and no areas or manifestations of skin irritation or dryness.

Interventions. Provide nursing intervention for all self-care needs, including bathing and care of the hair, skin, and nails. Patients often scratch themselves as the depth of unconsciousness lessens; therefore keep the nails trimmed. Patients who are comatose for long periods may be lifted occasionally into a bathtub half-filled with warm water. It may be helpful to apply solutions high in fatty acids (e.g., castile soap, baby oil, or cold cream) daily and to bathe the patient weekly to prevent loss of cutaneous oils as well as skin irritation and dryness.

Perineal care should be performed at least every 8 hours and after every episode of incontinence. If perineal care is not effective for a woman with vaginal discharge or odor, consult the physician about the use of cleansing douches.

When the patient cannot respond to local tissue hypoxia from being in one position for an extended time, the risk of pressure ulcers increases. Patients should be turned at least every 2 hours. If turning is impossible because of the patient's medical condition, place the patient on a special mattress or bed (Figure 68-2). The use of a special bed, however, does not eliminate the

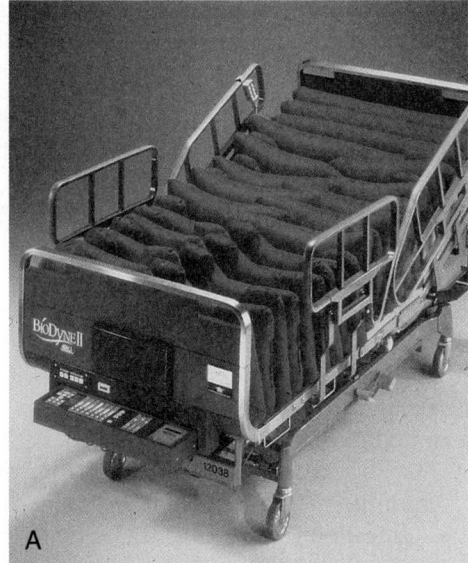

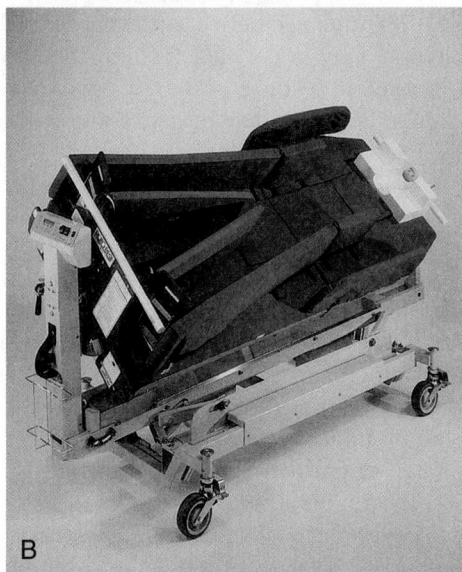

■ **FIGURE 68–2 A,** BioDyne, an oscillating-air support surface. **B,** Roto Rest, an oscillating bed. Both devices are used to prevent tissue hypoxemia and reduce the incidence of nosocomial pneumonia in patients that are unable to move or care for themselves. (*Courtesy Kinetic Concepts, Inc., San Antonio, Tex.*)

need to turn the patient and assess the skin. In addition, meet the nutritional needs of the patient to reduce the risk of pressure ulcers.

Diagnosis: Risk for Disuse Syndrome (Contractures). Normal movement and stretch are needed to prevent tightening of one group of muscles. When muscle groups are not used during periods of immobility, joint contractures can develop. Footdrop is of special concern. Write the nursing diagnosis as *Risk for Disuse Syndrome (Contractures) related to lack of voluntary movement.*

Outcomes. The patient will maintain full range of motion in any joint as evidenced by an absence of contractures.

Another outcome could be that the patient will have a reduced risk of contractures as evidenced by (1) a normal range of motion, (2) an absence of flexed arms and legs, and (3) no manifestations of footdrop.

Interventions. Prevent contractures by maintaining the patient's extremities in functional positions with proper support. Hand and forearm splints prevent flexion contracture of the fingers and wrists. Orthotic devices or high-top athletic shoes are used to support the feet. Remove the support devices every 4 hours to perform skin care and passive exercises. Assess the heel closely.

Diagnosis: Imbalanced Nutrition: Less Than Body Requirements. Comatose patients cannot eat and yet have normal or even increased metabolic needs; they can quickly become malnourished. Write the nursing diagnosis as *Imbalanced Nutrition: Less Than Body Requirements related to inability to eat and swallow.*

Outcomes. The patient will demonstrate the following manifestations of adequate nutrition: (1) stable weight; (2) adequate calories for age, height, and weight; (3) intake equaling output; (4) healing of incisions and wounds within 12 to 14 days; and (5) hemoglobin, blood urea nitrogen, total lymphocyte count, total protein, and serum albumin values within normal limits for age and gender.

Interventions. Intravenous fluids are begun on admission for comatose patients. Initially the IV site provides access to the circulatory system for the administration of medications. Because fluid intake is restricted and only limited amounts of glucose and few electrolytes are given by the IV route, an IV infusion cannot be considered nutritional support. Consider that 1 L of solution of 5% dextrose provides only 200 kilocalories!

Just because a patient is comatose, never assume that hunger is not present and that caloric needs are reduced. In fact, the opposite is true; such a patient's caloric needs are usually increased. Nutritional and fluid needs of comatose patients are usually met through enteral feedings because of the risk of aspiration with the oral route. If the patient does not have paralytic ileus or delayed gastric emptying and if bowel sounds are audible, start enteral feedings. The Management and Delegation feature on p. 1802 describes nursing considerations when administering or delegating enteral therapy.

The nutritional requirements of a patient in coma are complex; a complete nutritional assessment with comparison of height and weight charts, laboratory tests, and clinical examination is essential. Comatose patients may have a marked increase in metabolic needs. Malnutrition increases the morbidity and mortality of neurologically ill patients. Diarrhea and delayed gastric emptying may result from malabsorption. Healing cannot take place in the presence of a negative nitrogen state. Immunodeficiency, with increased risk of infection, sepsis, stress ulcers,

MANAGEMENT AND DELEGATION

Preparing Enteral Nutrition

Enteral nutrition may be delivered via oral, nasal, gastrostomy, or jejunostomy tubes. Gastrostomy or jejunostomy tubes are most commonly used because they pose a lower risk of aspiration. The delivery of enteral nutrition, including the verification of tube placement, is your responsibility. You may choose to delegate the reconstitution or preparation of enteral feedings to assistive personnel. Before delegating the preparation of tube-feeding or refilling the nutrition reservoir bag, consider the following:

- Your abdominal assessment does not reveal abdominal distention, pain, discomfort, or complaints of nausea. Your examination includes verification of tube placement and residual volume of less than 50% of the previous hour's intake. The presence of any of these findings would prompt you to delay the tube-feeding and notify the physician of your examination findings.
- You have checked the physician's order for the type and rate of tube-feeding to be delivered.
- Instruct assistive personnel in the proper dilution and handling of enteral feeding. (*Hint:* When mixing powdered enteral feedings, always place the powder in the mixing container before the water; this will ensure that the powder fully dissolves.)
- Instruct assistive personnel to place a 4-hour supply of feeding in the reservoir bag and to store the remaining mixture in a refrigerator for future use. Label the storage container with the patient's name, date on which mixture was prepared, and description of mixture.
- Although assistive personnel may prime the pump, you must set the pump and ensure that the flow rate matches the ordered flow rate.
- You are responsible for performing any irrigation of the tube.
- You may delegate care of gastrostomy and jejunostomy tube site to assistive personnel.
- You are responsible for monitoring fluid and nutritional balance via input and output and changes in weight.
- Describe findings that are immediately reportable to you for assistive personnel. They include any difficulty in preparing the enteral feeding and patient complaints of fullness, nausea, or vomiting.
- Verify the competence of assistive personnel in performing these tasks during orientation and annually thereafter.

weight loss, skeletal-muscle protein wasting, and lung tissue catabolism, leading to diaphragmatic weakness with respiratory reduction, results from prolonged calorie and protein deprivation. Starvation can lead to death.

Nursing responsibilities in tube-feeding of comatose patients are critical because these patients cannot communicate and may have lost protective cough and gag

reflexes. The possible complications from enteral feeding, and their prevention, are described in the following list:

- Vomiting and aspiration if the stomach is overfilled or the head of the patient is below the level of the stomach, such as during chest physiotherapy. When tube-feeding a patient, elevate the head of the bed at least 30 degrees to minimize possible aspiration.
- Delayed gastric emptying. Check residual volumes every 4 hours. If the residual volume is more than 100 ml, delay the feeding for 1 hour and then reassess. Assess bowel sounds, and check for gastric distention; if this complication persists after several hours, notify the physician. If there is a high suspicion that the patient has a bowel obstruction, do not return the gastric residue to the stomach.
- Tube dislocation into the trachea or lungs, causing aspiration. Comatose patients are often restless. Tape the tube securely to prevent dislodgment. Aspiration may occur if a feeding tube is pulled out during a feeding session or whenever it is unclamped. During feeding sessions, cloth "wristlets" or wrist restraints may be needed.
- Verify NG tube placement by aspirating for gastric contents. Some agency policies and some manufacturers of small-bore tubes require checking tube placement by listening with a stethoscope for "whooshing" while instilling air through the tube. Never tube-feed a patient in the supine position unless all other positions are impossible to use. Leave the head of the bed elevated 30 degrees for at least 30 minutes after bolus feedings.
- Ulcerated or crusted nares caused by local pressure from the feeding tube.
- Tracheoesophageal fistula, that is, breakdown of the anterior esophageal wall from prolonged contact between the NG tube and a tracheostomy tube. This complication is manifested by gastric contents in tracheal secretions. Stop the feeding and notify the physician immediately.
- Trauma to the gastric mucosa if the tube's distal end hardens, as may happen over time.
- Fluid volume deficit if hypertonic tube feedings are given. To prevent this problem, ensure that the patient receives approximately 1 ml of fluid for every kilocalorie of feeding. Depending on the agency's policy, this intervention may require consultation with the dietitian or the physician.
- Constipation or diarrhea, which may develop from the osmolarity of the feeding, the use of liquid medications with a sorbitol base, or a too rapid infusion
- Sacral pressure ulcers from continued positioning in the semi-Fowler position. Turn the patient 30 degrees lateral (to the side) with the head of the bed elevated to reduce pressure on the sacrum.

Diagnosis: Risk for Deficient Fluid Volume. The comatose patient cannot drink fluids or respond to normal thirst mechanisms. Such a patient is therefore at *Risk for Deficient Fluid Volume*. Recall that hypertonic tube feedings also increase this risk.

Outcomes. The patient will have reduced risk of deficient fluid volume as evidenced by (1) intake and output being equal for 24, 48, and 72 hours; (2) stable body weight; (3) absence of excessive perspiration, diarrhea, or vomiting; (4) serum glucose, hematocrit, BUN, creatinine, sodium, potassium, and chloride values within normal limits; and (5) moist oral mucous membranes with an absence of tongue furrows.

Interventions. Important aspects in maintaining fluid and electrolyte balance in unconscious patients are (1) accurate documentation of intake and output, (2) daily weights with comparison of trends, and (3) assessment and documentation of conditions that might increase fluid volume deficit (e.g., diaphoresis, polyuria, diarrhea, vomiting, hypertonic tube feedings).

Before fluid and electrolyte intervention is planned for a comatose patient, carefully assess the fluid-electrolyte status. The coma itself may have a fluid or electrolyte cause. Blood tests such as glucose, hematocrit, BUN, creatinine, sodium, potassium, chloride, and carbon dioxide measurements help determine fluid and electrolyte status (see Chapters 11 and 12). Dehydration and water intoxication (true hyponatremia) are common causes of electrolyte imbalance associated with coma.

Always avoid overhydration in a patient receiving IV fluids because of the risk of cerebral edema. Diuretics may be prescribed to correct fluid overload and reduce edema. Monitor the response to these medications. When evaluating the response to any diuretic, empty the indwelling catheter before administering the diuretic. Evaluation of the response should consider the diuretic given, the dose, and the patient's renal status.

Diagnosis: Risk for Injury. It may not be apparent that the comatose patient is at *Risk for Injury* because he or she does not move.

> If the coma starts to lighten, however, the patient can move and without protection could fall or be injured. Seizures may also occur, leading to injury. Although loss of the corneal blink reflex, which increases the risk of corneal abrasions, is also a type of injury, it is addressed as a collaborative problem.

Nursing interventions for a loss of the corneal blink reflex are discussed in Chapter 65.

Outcomes. The patient will not sustain injury as evidenced by an absence of abrasions or bruises and experiencing no falls from bed.

Interventions

> Keep the side rails up on the bed and the bed in the lowest position whenever the patient is not receiving direct care or is unattended. Observe seizure precautions for anyone who has a history of seizure or is at risk of seizure. Protect the patient from injury during seizures or periods of agitation (e.g., use padded side rails, keep the patient's nails short and filed). It is of utmost importance to protect the patient's head. Give the prescribed seizure medication on time to maintain a high seizure threshold. If a dose of the medication is missed for any reason (e.g., vomiting), notify the physician. Antiepileptic medication should not be withheld without a physician order.
>
> Use caution when moving the patient, who cannot voice pain. Give adequate support to the limbs and head when moving or turning the unconscious patient. Limbs without tone may dislocate if they are allowed to fall unsupported. Always turn an unconscious patient toward you or someone else to prevent falls. Protect an unconscious patient from external sources of heat (e.g., heating pads).
>
> Do not restrain the patient unless absolutely necessary because restraint is likely to worsen confused and combative behavior. If restraints are used, they must be released at least every 2 hours for range-of-motion exercises and skin checks. Do not leave unstable patients unattended. Attempt to manage the patient's behavior without restraints first. "Sitters," hospital volunteers, or family members or friends may be able to provide attendant services. Avoid oversedation because it may alter respirations, which increases ICP and masks changes in a patient's level of consciousness.

Diagnosis: Bowel Incontinence. Once a paralytic ileus is corrected, the patient will produce feces. Most patients are incontinent because voluntary control is required for the function of the external anal sphincter. Write the nursing diagnosis as *Bowel Incontinence related to inability to respond to normal cues about evacuation;* also consider *High Risk for Impaired Skin Integrity related to fecal incontinence.*

Outcomes. The patient will have reduced fecal incontinence, as evidenced by (1) a bowel movement every 2 to 3 days and (2) no manifestations of fecal impaction.

Interventions. Plan interventions to (1) control bowel movements, (2) maintain the patient's normal elimination schedule, and (3) prevent fecal impaction or constipation. As soon as the patient is able, begin a program of bowel retraining. Maintain a regular schedule, administering stool softeners and suppositories, and performing digital removal of stool at about the same times each day. Examine the abdomen frequently for distention.

Constipation and fecal impaction may occur. Small, frequent liquid stools may indicate impaction. If diarrhea or constipation persists, assess for possible causes, such as medications, enteral feedings, and intestinal bacterial infections.

SAFETY ALERT

Consult with the physician before performing digital removal of stool in a patient with an altered level of consciousness. This intervention has been known to induce seizures and may increase ICP. Rectal application of an anesthetic jelly before the stimulus decreases this risk.

Diagnosis: Interrupted Family Processes. Having a family member in a coma is a significant stressor. A possible nursing diagnosis is *Interrupted Family Processes related to uncertain future or impending death of a family member.* Individualize the etiology portion of the diagnosis to fit the specific patient and family.

Outcomes. Family members will exhibit positive coping behaviors as evidenced by (1) showing an ability to solve problems, (2) meeting the needs of other family members, and (3) asking questions about the patient that indicate understanding of previous teaching.

Interventions. The significant others of a comatose patient are often very distressed. It is difficult for family members when they cannot communicate with the patient. The uncertainty of not knowing whether the patient will recover is a major stressor. Include family members in the patient's care to the extent that they can and want to be involved. Family members need information and realistic hope.

It is important for the family to see the patient receiving high-quality, professional, and compassionate nursing care. For example, talk to the patient as though he or she can understand. Initially this behavior will seem awkward, but in time it will feel appropriate. Tell the patient that he or she will be turned to the side, bathed, and so on before performing the task. Depending on the depth of the coma, the patient's sense of hearing may still be intact. Therefore speak to the patient as if he or she can hear, and tell the family to do the same. Comatose patients have awakened and reported that they remember hearing specific voices.

The family is often in a state of shock, needing someone to recognize their needs and help them through this difficult situation. They may experience various conflicting feelings, such as guilt and anger. The Client Education Guide feature on When a Loved One Is in an Altered State of Consciousness on the website suggests ways for the patient's family members to cope with these feelings.

Allow significant others to stay with the patient when and where possible. At times family members may become zealous about attending and may stay at the patient's bedside continuously. Encourage family members to care for themselves also by eating regular meals and obtaining adequate sleep. Have them consider using external support systems (e.g., neighbors and church groups). Tell them they will be telephoned if any significant changes occur in their loved one's status, and ask them to leave a phone number where they can be reached. Encourage family members to phone if they have questions or concerns.

Social workers may be contacted to provide additional support. Some hospitals, especially tertiary care centers, have "family homes," where family members who must travel a long distance to the hospital may stay to be close to the hospital and the patient.

Evaluation. The patient may remain comatose for a few hours or even months. Some comatose patients (e.g., patients with diabetic coma) awaken and make a complete recovery while in the hospital. Therefore some expected outcomes have brief time frames (e.g., airway obstruction), whereas others are prolonged, requiring frequent reevaluation (e.g., family coping). Your evaluation may identify a need for revision of the care plan.

Modifications for Older Adults

The older patient in a coma requires the same quality of care as patients in other age groups; however, the older patient is at higher risk for all complications of immobility, especially pressure ulcers and pneumonia. Urinary retention is common in older men because of prostatic enlargement. Finally, fully assess the patient for the common disorders of aging (e.g., diabetes) that might be the cause of the coma.

Self-Care

The site to which a patient with coma is discharged from an acute care setting depends on (1) the condition of the patient, (2) the cause of the coma, and (3) the level of available family support. If the patient is recovering from coma, plan for placement in a rehabilitation center. Patients remaining in coma but showing slow recovery may be placed in an extended-care facility until they can participate in rehabilitation.[2,4] Coma stimulation programs, although not readily available, provide an alternative for the patient who is slow to recover.[2]

If the patient is in a coma and is not expected to awaken but may live for a time with nutritional support, placement in a skilled nursing center is common.[4] In these centers, supportive care is given. Family members usually specify how aggressively they wish the patient to be treated in the event of a deterioration in status. Your role in discharge of the comatose patient centers on communication with the receiving nurses and the family. If the patient is ventilator dependent or combative special consideration is required for transport to the new facility. Provide a complete plan of care.

CONFUSIONAL STATES

Confusion is a mental state marked by alterations in thought and attention deficit, followed by problems in comprehension. It is accompanied by a loss of short-term memory and, often, irritability alternating with drowsiness. Confusion is a common clinical manifestation in many neurologic and metabolic disorders, and increases in incidence with age. Since confusion has been shown to increase both morbidity and length of hospital stay, this is of major concern.

Etiology and Risk Factors

Confusion has many causes. Common causes of acute confusion are alcohol withdrawal and drug ingestion. Confusion can also follow fever, head injury, and use of anesthetics. Other causes of confusion are decreased cerebral perfusion, hypoxia, hypoglycemia, severe fluid and electrolyte disorders, sepsis, liver or renal failure, poisons, and drug overdose.

Types of confusion include delirium and dementia. Delirium is an acute reversible form of confusion. Three features are common to all types of *delirium:*

- A disturbance of consciousness with a reduced ability to focus, sustain, or shift attention
- A change in cognition (memory, language, disorientation) or development of a perceptual disturbance that is not better accounted for by a pre-existing, established, or evolving dementia
- A change that develops over a short time (hours to days) and may fluctuate during the course of the day

Several classifications of delirium have each of the three common features but specific causes. They are (1) delirium related to a general medical condition, (2) delirium resulting from substance intoxication (prescribed drugs, over-the-counter medications, or street drugs), (3) delirium caused by substance withdrawal, (4) delirium with multiple causes, and (5) delirium "not otherwise specified."[6]

Sundowning is defined as agitation, confusion, and restlessness that occur after the sun sets; however, diurnal variations may be responsible for these changes as well.[3]

Dementia is the chronic form of confusion. Common features in dementia are the following:

- The development of multiple memory impairments
- One or more of the following cognitive disturbances: *aphasia* (problems with expressing speech or understanding sounds), *apraxia* (inability to convert a thought to action), *agnosia* (inability to recognize objects), and impaired executive functioning
- Significant impairment and decline in social or occupational functioning
- A gradual onset and continuing cognitive decline

The classifications of dementia include the four common features with variable causes and characteristics. There are many subtypes of dementia of the Alzheimer's type. Other types of dementia are (1) vascular dementia (multi-infarct), (2) dementia secondary to other general medical conditions, (3) substance-induced persisting dementia, (4) dementia with multiple causes, and (5) dementia "not otherwise specified."[7]

An in-depth discussion of the care related to specific types of delirium and dementia, as well as the memory changes that occur in patients with amnesic disorders and other cognitive disorders not meeting the criteria for any of the preceding classifications, is beyond the scope of this book. The reader should see a psychiatric textbook for this information. This discussion focuses on the general care of a patient with confusion; however, because dementia of the Alzheimer's type is a growing problem, Chapter 72 details the pathologic processes and care related to this type of degenerative disease.

Risk factors that lead to confusion vary with the specific etiologic factors. In general, the proper management of various diseases, such as diabetes mellitus, would reduce the incidence of confusion. Disorders such as Alzheimer's disease have no known prevention at this time, although new drugs may slow disease progression. Avoid the use of any medications that contribute to confusion in people who are at risk for confusion.

Pathophysiology

Three mechanisms account for the development of *acute confusional states:* (1) damage to the brain with swelling or loss of oxygen, blood, or both (functional disorder); (2) impairment of the action of the nervous system by chemicals or other substances (metabolic disorder); and (3) the rebound overactivity of a previously depressed center in the brain. Chemicals that cross the blood-brain barrier, such as alcohol, impair the metabolism of neuronal cells. When the drug action wears off or the drug is withdrawn from the patient, the lower centers in the brain are overactive. This overactivity accounts for the development of acute confusion, combativeness, and other abnormal behaviors.

Chronic confusional states are due to disorders that cause brain tissue destruction, biochemical imbalances, or compression of the brain. For example, people with Alzheimer's disease lack acetylcholine, a neurotransmitter that is necessary for short-term memory. Other disorders that cause chronic confusion may be inherited; may be secondary to a transmissible agent, as with Creutzfeldt-Jakob disease; or may follow diseases such as encephalitis.

Clinical Manifestations

The earliest manifestation of a confusional brain disorder is a *disorder of attention*. The patient may report the loss of concentration or may appear preoccupied. At the same time, restlessness, emotional lability, insomnia or drowsiness, and vivid nightmares may begin. Patients may appear anxious and may fear that they are "going crazy." As the disorder progresses, stupor and coma develop. Behaviors seen in the patient are reflective not of personality but of the cause of the disorder. For example, barbiturate or alcohol abuse and withdrawal and liver disorders cause agitated delirium. In contrast, anoxia and kidney and lung disorders are associated with a quieter response. Disorders that develop rapidly are more likely to cause an agitated response than those that develop slowly.

Fluctuations in cognition (the ability to think and reason) are common in patients with metabolic brain disorders. Patients may be totally irrational one moment and lucid the next. Some of the fluctuations are caused by the environment. Delirious patients become more disoriented at night, in unfamiliar surroundings, when they hear unfamiliar noises or see unfamiliar people, or when restraints are used. The lack of a window in the room has caused many patients to become disoriented.

Loss of memory for recent events is a hallmark of metabolic brain disorders. The patient commonly has difficulty with both immediate recall and abstract thought. Patients who are delirious quickly lose orientation to time. Normal people can readily recall six or seven digits forward and five or six backward and identify the commonalities between an orange and an apple or a tree and a bush; delirious patients cannot do these things. The patient's general intelligence level can affect the behaviors observed, however. If possible, the patient's level of education should be known before the assessment.

Perceptual errors (e.g., mistaking the nurse for a daughter) as well as hallucinations, illusions, and delusions are common accompaniments of delirium.

Hallucinations are sensations occurring in the absence of external stimuli. A patient may hear, see, feel, smell, or taste something that is not present. The patient may or may not realize that the experience is "not real." Unfortunately, the most common hallucinations involve rodents and unfriendly animals (e.g., snakes, spiders). These visions are terribly frightening.

Illusions differ from hallucinations in that illusions are the misinterpretation of something actually in the environment. For example, if a patient sees a shadow on the drape and mistakes it for a real person, the patient is experiencing an illusion.

Delusions are thoughts or beliefs that have no basis in fact. For example, a patient may think that he or she has been robbed or poisoned when there is no basis for this belief.

No specific diagnostic tests for confusion exist. The patient may undergo CT or MRI scanning to determine whether there is a structural cause for the confusion, such as a tumor or stroke. In addition, a series of laboratory studies may be performed to look for a metabolic cause. Common studies include a complete blood count, electrolyte measurements, determination of vitamin B_{12} and folate levels, thyroid and liver function studies, drug toxicity screening tests, and an EEG. A lumbar puncture may be performed for CSF analysis.

OUTCOME MANAGEMENT

Medical Management

In all care settings, the medical management of the confused patient begins by determining the cause of the confusion and correcting it, if possible.[3] When no specific cause is found, the medical management focuses on controlling manifestations. Sometimes medications can be given to calm agitation. Nutritional needs also must be monitored.

Nursing Management of the Medical Client

Assessment. A thorough history is required for assessment of the confused patient. The history should include the onset of the confusion, past medical illnesses, work and occupational history, and past injuries. Disorders such as diabetes or liver failure may be out of control and responsible for the confusion. The patient may have been exposed to heavy metals or toxic wastes at work. Record past injuries, especially head injury. Depending on the level of confusion, the patient may not be able to answer each question, and you may need to rely on the family or others who have been with the patient. Review medications, including over-the-counter drugs and nutritional supplements.

Specific questions about the patient's ability to handle routine financial transactions or home safety with tasks such as cooking, dressing, and driving will help determine whether the patient can be safely returned home or is in need of an alternative arrangement. At times the family will report a change in personality, such as apathy, social isolation, disinterest in current events, and irritability. Record these observations because they may be clinical manifestations of Alzheimer's disease or frontal lobe lesions.

The confused patient requires ongoing assessment with the Mini-Mental State Examination (see Chapter 67). This examination is much more sensitive than other tools for serial evaluations of confused patients.[7] Analyze the data collected to determine whether the confusion is improving, worsening, or unchanged.

The confused patient is often combative and argumentative. Observe for factors in the patient's environment that might affect confusion. Assess whether the patient is able to refrain from self-injury or injury to others. If not bedridden, the patient may wander about and become lost or injured if harmful items are not secured (e.g., knives).

Confusion can occur in patients of any age or culture and from variable causes. The nurse's role as a patient advocate supersedes personal bias related to any of these variables.

Diagnosis, Outcomes, Interventions. This section describes interventions appropriate to the confused patient, regardless of the cause, with an emphasis on the issue of safety.

Diagnosis: Disturbed Thought Processes. Use the nursing diagnosis *Disturbed Thought Processes related to failure in memory and lack of self-protective behavior to address needs for safety*.

Outcomes. The patient will have improved thought processes as evidenced by (1) higher scores on the Mini-Mental State Examination and (2) decreased frequency of hallucinations, illusions, and delusions.

Interventions. The confused patient will benefit from consistency in the environment and care routine. Keep objects, such as the tray table and bedside chair, in the same place. If possible, the same staff member should care for the patient. Give the patient short explanations as events occur, such as "You need an x-ray" and "Please sit in the wheelchair." Saying to a confused patient, "In 2 hours, an x-ray tech will be coming to take you for a CT scan," is useless because such a patient will neither understand nor remember it. Response time may be slowed in confusion; allow the patient time to respond.

Reorient the patient as often as necessary, but use caution about the specific communication used. Patients with chronic untreatable confusion do not benefit from reorientation and may become more agitated when you attempt to reorient them. For example, in one study in which a 92-year-old patient was told repeatedly that her mother or father could not possibly be alive, the patient reacted each time as if it was the first time she had been told and grieved deeply. For these selected patients, avoid reorienting, redirect their thoughts and agitation, or "go along" with the confusion. Of course, when the patient is at risk of injury, safety precautions are foremost. Clocks and calendars in the room also help with reorientation. The use of familiar objects is helpful when a patient's remote memory is intact. For example, the use of a quilt from home on the bed may help the confused patient recognize the bed as his or her own.

Promote reduction of unfamiliar noise because it adds to confusion. The patient's room should be quiet and softly lighted without producing shadows.

Consistency in the care of a patient with confusion requires communication among caregivers. This communication occurs not only through the oral reporting method but also in the care plan and documentation records.

Diagnosis: Risk for Injury. Confusion greatly increases risk of harm. The patient cannot interpret, or may not be able to respond to, environmental stimuli that precede danger. Write the nursing diagnosis as *Risk for Injury related to the unpredictable behavior and inability to interpret environmental stimuli*.

Outcomes. The patient will have reduced risk of injury and will not injure others.

Interventions

> **Assess patients at risk of falling often and toilet them every 2 hours. Falls are commonly due to attempting to reach the toilet.**

SAFETY

ALERT

The patient must be protected from self-injury. The patient should be in a room near the nursing station so that assessments can be performed every 30 to 60 minutes. In addition, the bed should be in the low position. Structure the patient's environment to minimize injury; remove any extraneous equipment.

The routine use of physical restraints (e.g., side rails, cloth restraints) or chemical restraints (e.g., medication) is discouraged.[8] The use of side rails and restraints does not guarantee that patients will not fall and often either makes them more agitated or leads to more severe injury when they do fall. Alternatives to restraints include the use of sitters for ongoing observation and placement of the patient in an area permitting constant observation, such as the nursing station. Motion detection devices can be applied to the patient or the bed to signal the nursing staff when movement occurs. If all other alternatives have been unsuccessful and restraints are used, make frequent assessments and record the data. Cloth restraints must be removed every 2 hours to assess the skin beneath them and perform range-of-motion exercises. Chemical restraint (e.g., tranquilizers) can result in greater confusion and tremors (extrapyramidal symptoms). Net beds may be required for highly agitated clients. Follow manufacturer's recommendations and agency policy when using these beds.

The patient with brain alteration is not in control of his or her behavior. Behaviors may be unpredictable, irrational, or impulsive, or the patient may be frightened and suspicious. Never "punish" a confused patient for inappropriate behavior or remarks. Instead, remember that these personality changes are a result of brain lesions, and adjust the care plan accordingly. If a patient is agitated, provide reassurance and a calm environment. Redirect or distract the patient. Monitoring systems may be used for patients who wander.

SAFETY
⚠
ALERT

Confused older patients are at increased risk for falls. A formal assessment of the risk of falls should be completed. Some institutions have programs for patients who are at risk for falling or who have fallen. These programs include frequent assessments, identification of risk on the door or door frame, routine toilet trips, bed and wandering monitors, and environmental changes (mattress on the floor, use of a lap buddy). Trying to ambulate to the bathroom is a common time for falls, and toilet trips should be offered routinely (every 2 hours).

Diagnosis: Disturbed Sleep Pattern. A common problem seen in confused patients consists of daytime napping and nighttime hallucinations. This problem is stated as *Disturbed Sleep Pattern related to alterations in usual sleep habits.*

Outcomes. The patient will have improved sleep patterns as evidenced by (1) sleeping 4 to 6 hours continuously at night and (2) not sleeping as often during the day.

Interventions. Plan nighttime interventions to allow 4 to 6 hours of uninterrupted sleep. Recall that a sleep cycle requires 1.5 to 2 hours, and the loss of rapid eye movement (REM) sleep can increase confusion. When you enter the room at night, assess the patient for REM. If REM is present, the patient should be allowed to complete the REM portion of the sleep cycle. You should return later to care for the patient.

Keep the patient active during the day so that there is some fatigue by nighttime. Daytime sleeping is a difficult pattern to break, and the patient may have to be kept awake for this pattern to be reversed. Bedtime routines should be developed. Avoid the use of caffeinated beverages and alcohol, which may prevent sleep. For the older patient, the normal changes in sleep with aging need to be considered, such as the greater use of short naps and less sleep during the night. Sleeping medications are seldom given to the confused patient because they often alter sleep cycles and rob the patient of REM sleep. See Chapter 22 for further information about sleep disorders.

Diagnosis: Risk for Caregiver Role Strain. The unfamiliar behavior of the confused patient or the stress of providing continual care for the patient at home may increase stress in the family and alter their ability to cope. This nursing diagnosis is stated as *Risk for Caregiver Role Strain related to long-term, stressful, and complex care required by family member.*

Outcomes. The patient's family members will maintain their own physical and psychological health as evidenced by (1) improved use of support systems, (2) obtaining of adequate equipment to provide care, (3) limited use of addictive substances for coping, (4) interaction with friends and extended family (as desired), and (5) appropriate analysis of the patient's condition.

Interventions. Teach the family to monitor for the effects of confusion. When confusion is a new problem for the patient, the family will be distressed by the behavior. Explain to the family that the patient is not able to control behavior or speech at this time. Assess whether the patient becomes calm or agitated when the family is present, and advise visitations accordingly. If possible, the need for and use of restraints should be explained to the family before they see a patient in restraints. The family may become very upset when they see their loved one "tied" to a bed. Advance explanations can avert some of this reaction. In some instances, patients have suffered injury because the family did not understand the purpose for the restraints and untied them. The Management and Delegation feature on p. 1809 describes goals and assessments related to physical restraints.

Planning discharge from the hospital for the confused patient varies with the cause of confusion. If the confusion is acute and full recovery is expected, the patient may be able to go home under the care of family members. If the confusion is chronic, the patient needs either care or supervision at home or placement in an extended-care facility. Some communities offer adult day care and respite services that give family members relief from the constant care of the confused person. See Chapter 72 for care of the patient with Alzheimer's disease at home.

Advise the family to have legal counsel determine the patient's competence and the need for guardianship or durable power of attorney. The family may also need to grieve the loss of the patient's previous functional role, personality, companionship, and so on. Assess for evidence of violence in the caregiver and the patient. Caregiver violence is possible, especially if the patient was violent toward the caregiver in the past.

Help the caregiver find respite care and personal time to meet his or her own needs and to learn stress management techniques. Female caregivers are especially vulnerable to social isolation.

Evaluation. Most of the time, confusion will require many months to abate. The diagnosis of a chronic, progressive condition such as Alzheimer's disease or dementia of the Alzheimer's type may require an entire change in care plan prioritization. These conditions are discussed in Chapter 72.

Modifications for Older Patients

It is common but incorrect to believe that older people naturally undergo a marked deterioration in mental function. In general, older people have difficulty recalling

Physical Restraints

The use of physical restraints to protect a patient from self-harm or injury or to manage a patient at risk for disruption of medical therapies is a decision made collaboratively between you and the physician and may include consultation with other members of the interdisciplinary team. The serious decision to use physical restraints is made after your comprehensive assessment and evaluation of previous interventions and alternatives.

A clear goal is the use of the least restrictive device for the shortest interval possible. Regulatory agencies consider the use of restraints to be a high-risk intervention. Death and injury have been associated with restraint use in hospital environments. Your clinical site should provide you with clear guidelines regarding the use of restraints and the role of unlicensed assistive personnel in caring for restrained patients.

Before delegating care of the patient in physical restraints, consider the following:

- Have the patient and family been informed and educated regarding the need for restraints to protect the patient? Your education of the patient and family should include standards of care and discussion of what factors lead to discontinuation of restraints.
- Have you assessed the patient to determine the most appropriate type of restraint? The restraint must be the right size. Follow the manufacturer's recommendations for sizing. Never use anything other than a manufactured device that has been approved by the Food and Drug Administration.
- Have you obtained a physician's order for the use of restraints? In addition to the initiation order for restraints, there should be ongoing discussion of the need to continue restraint use with the interdisciplinary team and physician order updates every 24 hours.

Your assessment of the patient's safety and comfort needs must occur at regular intervals as defined by your institution. You are accountable for assessing and documenting the patient's condition, the patient's response to restraints, and the safety and comfort interventions provided.

Consider the following points when delegating components of care to assistive personnel:

- Be clear about the type of restraint being used. In addition to applying restraints according to the manufacturer's instructions, restraints are to be secured only to the bed frame or chair with slip knots.
- Explain that restraints are never used as a punishment.
- Patients with altered mental status experiencing unmet elimination needs may become agitated. Instruct assistive personnel to offer assistance with elimination at regular intervals.
- Provide specific expectations and a time schedule for observation of the patient.
- Provide instruction about how to remove restraints one at a time in agitated patients.
- Explain how to respond to patients who ask for the restraints to be "cut off" by re-explaining the need for them.

You may delegate these components of care to assistive personnel:

- Assistance with activities of daily living, such as bathing, grooming, and feeding.
- Active or passive range of motion.
- Turning and repositioning the patient. The assistive personnel should be instructed to resecure restraints after position changes.

Describe for the assistive personnel the findings that are immediately reportable to you. Such findings may include skin redness or irritation noted at points of contact with the restraint device, changes in color or movement of areas distal to the restraint, the patient's unplanned removal of a restraint, disruption of a medical therapy, and the patient's complaints of discomfort or distress. Verify the competency of assistive personnel in caring for restrained patients during orientation and in an ongoing manner thereafter.

---

new information, but their remote memory is intact. In addition, depression occurs in 20% to 30% of older people. Depression may follow the loss of friends, spouse, health, and independence and may lead to manifestations such as memory loss and confusion.

Older adults are particularly at risk for confusion during hospitalization.[3,6] They are dealing not only with the stress of being ill but also with the stress of an unfamiliar environment. Older patients may rely heavily on familiar landmarks and routines to help them maintain an independent lifestyle. These cues are often lost in the hospital or extended-care setting. A large percentage of the population in hospital and extended-care settings are older adults, who typically have other conditions that contribute to confusion. Confusion is best managed by using a team approach and teaching unlicensed assistive personnel to (1) introduce themselves at the beginning of a work shift; (2) use the same time for the patient's sleep, naps, and meals; (3) routinely place the patient on the toilet or commode; (4) talk to the patient about the past; (5) gently redirect lost or wandering patients; and (6) encourage self-care (eating, dressing, and so on).

CONCLUSIONS

Patients who are confused or comatose are vulnerable to many complications, including injury, aspiration, malnutrition, and skin breakdown. Nurses provide a lifeline for these patients, giving protection and promoting normal body functions. The families of these patients require therapeutic management because they face many difficult decisions.

THINKING CRITICALLY

1. A 48-year-old man is brought to the emergency department by ambulance. His wife states that he had been shaving in the bathroom when she heard a thud. She found him unresponsive on the floor. How do you intervene?

Factors to Consider. What was the patient's neurologic baseline when he was received in the emergency department? What other clinical manifestations did the patient display? Were there any physical manifestations of injury to his head or other parts of his body? Does he have any other significant medical history or allergies?

2. You are caring for a 72-year-old woman who recently underwent repair of a hip fracture. Her husband indicates that she had recently been confused, which led to her falling and fracturing her hip. How do you intervene?

Factors to Consider. What do you include in your assessment? What types of interventions do you need to consider? How do you involve her family?

evolve *Discussions for these questions can be found on the website.*

 BIBLIOGRAPHY

Citations appearing in red refer to primary research.

Citations appearing in blue refer to evidence-based practice guidelines and protocols.

1. Bateman, D.E. (2001). Neurologic assessment of coma. *Journal of Neurology, Neurosurgery, Psychiatry, 71*(1), 13-17.
2. Hansen, L., Archbold, P.G., Stewart, B. et al. (2005). Family caregivers making life-sustaining treatment decisions: factors associated with role strain and ease. *Journal of Gerontological Nursing, 31* (11), 28-35.
3. Hickey, J.V. (2002). Management of the unconscious patient. In *The clinical practice of neurological and neurosurgical nursing* (5th ed., pp. 288-299). Philadelphia: J.B. Lippincott.
4. Hilgers, J. (2003). Comforting a confused patient: Learn how simple interventions and diversions can help. *Nursing, 33,* 48-50.
5. Laplante, J., & Cole, M.G. (2001). Assessment. Detection of delirium using the Confusion Assessment Method. *Journal of Gerontological Nursing, 27*(9), 16-23.
6. Miller, J., Campbell, J., Moore, K., Schofield, A. (2004). Elder care supportive interventions protocol: Reducing discomfort in confused, hospitalized older adults. *Journal of Gerontological Nursing, 30*(8), 10-18.
7. Neri, M., Bonati, P.A., Pinelli, M. et al. (2007). Biological, psychological and clinical markers of caregiver's stress in impaired elderly with dementia and age-related disease. *Archives of Gerontology and Geriatrics, 44,* Suppl (1), 289-294.
8. Oh, S., & Seo, W. (2003). Sensory stimulation programme to improve recovery in comatose patients. *Journal of Clinical Nursing, 12*(3), 394-404.
9. Park, M., & Tang, J.H. (2007). Evidence-based guidelines changing the practice of physical restraint use in acute care. *Journal of Gerontological Nursing, 33*(2), 9-16.
10. Rapp, C.G. (2001). Acute confusion/delirium protocol. *Journal of Gerontological Nursing, 28*(4), 21-33.
11. Wijdicks, E.F. (2000). Coma in the critically ill: Using neurologic findings and clinical context as clues to diagnosis. *Journal of Critical Illness, 15*(11), 609-610, 615-618.

evolve **Did you remember to check out the bonus material on the Evolve website and the CD-ROM, including NCLEX®-Examination Style Review Questions, Open-Book Quizzes, and Chapter Review Audio Podcasts?**

http://evolve.elsevier.com/Black/medsurg

CHAPTER 69

Management of Clients with Cerebral Disorders

CHRISTINA STEWART-AMIDEI*

SEIZURE DISORDERS

Seizures are sudden, abnormal electrical discharges from the brain that result in changes in sensation, behavior, movements, perception, or consciousness. A seizure may occur in isolation or with low blood glucose level, drug or alcohol withdrawal, or traumatic brain injury. *Epilepsy* is a chronic disorder of recurrent seizures. An isolated, single seizure does not constitute epilepsy.

EPILEPSY

Epilepsy is derived from the Greek *epilepsia,* meaning "seizure." In early times, epilepsy was viewed as being of divine origin and was called the "sacred disease" because someone with epilepsy was thought to be "seized" or struck down by the gods. An epileptic syndrome consists of recurrent episodes of one or more of the following manifestations: loss of consciousness, convulsive movements or other motor activity, sensory phenomena, and behavioral abnormalities. About 2.3 million Americans are known to have seizures or epilepsy. About 181,000 new cases of seizures are documented annually.

Etiology and Risk Factors

Epilepsy can be caused by any process that disrupts the stability of the neuronal cell membrane. A variety of conditions are associated with an extremely high likelihood of onset of a chronic seizure disorder. For example, severe, penetrating head trauma is associated with up to a 50% risk of the development of epilepsy. This association suggests that the injury results in a long-lasting pathologic change in the central nervous system (CNS) that transforms a presumably normal neural network into one that is abnormally hyperexcitable.

The identified mechanisms responsible for neuronal malfunction are unknown. Possible theories include neuronal cell membrane impairment, abnormalities involving the sodium-potassium pump, and changes in various neurochemicals. The neuronal cell membrane appears to be more permeable and more sensitive to various offending factors than other cell walls. An epileptogenic focus may develop at an area of altered cell membrane permeability, be limited to a specific area, or encompass the entire cortical surface.

Most seizures have no identifiable cause and are termed idiopathic. Idiopathic epilepsy most often begins before the age of 20 years and rarely begins after age 30. Seizures beginning in newborns and infants are often caused by congenital brain defects, birth injuries, or metabolic problems such as anoxia, hypoglycemia, or hypocalcemia. Although the underlying cause may be perinatal, seizures may not begin for many years, often with onset during puberty. Seizures may be induced by high temperatures in children who are otherwise normal and who never develop other neurologic problems, including epilepsy. After the age of 20 years, generalized seizures usually have an identifiable cause. Primary causes include traumatic brain injury, brain tumor, and infection. Other than in children younger than age 5 years, the highest

---

The author thanks Melanie S. Minton for her contributions to this chapter in the seventh edition of *Medical-Surgical Nursing.*

> **evolve** **Web Enhancements**
>
> **Client Education Guide**   Epilepsy (Spanish Translation)
>
> **Migraine Headache** (Spanish Translation)
>
> Be sure to check out the bonus material on the Evolve website and the CD-ROM, including free self-assessment exercises. **http://evolve.elsevier.com/Black/medsurg**

incidence of new-onset seizures is in people older than 65 years. In this age group, the increased risk is attributed to the increase in conditions that cause neurologic changes. These include cerebrovascular disease, tumor, delirium, Alzheimer's disease, infection, brain trauma, and chronic alcoholism, as well as the aging process itself.

Simulated convulsive episodes may occur in clients with psychiatric disorders. These are called "pseudoseizures." One key to differentiating between pseudoseizures and actual seizures is to look for stereotypical movements and a paroxysmal nature of the episodes. Clients with recurrent seizures exhibit the same stereotypic movements with each seizure. Clients exhibiting pseudoseizure make different movements with each seizure.

Pathophysiology

When the integrity of the neuronal cell membrane is altered, the cell begins firing with increased frequency and amplitude. When the intensity of the discharges reaches the threshold, the neuronal firing spreads to adjacent neurons, ultimately resulting in a seizure. Normally, excitatory messages from a single hypersensitive neuron in the cerebral cortex are modulated by deeper structures (e.g., thalamus and brain stem) (Figure 69-1). In epilepsy, these bursts of electrical activity from the cortex are not modulated. Eventually, inhibitory neurons in the cortex, anterior thalamus, and basal ganglia slow neuronal firing. Once inhibitory processes develop or the epileptogenic neurons are exhausted, the seizure stops. These later events depress CNS activity and impair consciousness. This period of impaired consciousness after a seizure, called a *postictal state,* may be manifested as sleep, confusion, or fatigue.

Seizure activity increases cerebral oxygen consumption and the need for adenosine triphosphate (ATP). Supplies of oxygen and glucose are rapidly consumed. To meet these demands, cerebral blood flow increases during a seizure. If the seizure is ongoing (as in status epilepticus), severe hypoxia and lactic acidosis occur and may result in brain tissue destruction.

Clinical Manifestations

Epilepsy may be classified according to the age at onset, cause, area of origin, abnormalities on the electroencephalogram (EEG), and clinical manifestations of seizure. The International Classification of Epileptic Seizures, used here, is based on the clinical seizure type and on EEG findings during seizures (the ictal period) and between seizures (the interictal period). According to this classification, there are two major categories of seizures. The neurologic abnormality may be limited to a specific part or focus of the brain, hence the term *partial* seizures. Additionally, the seizure may involve the entire cortical surface, to produce a *generalized* seizure.

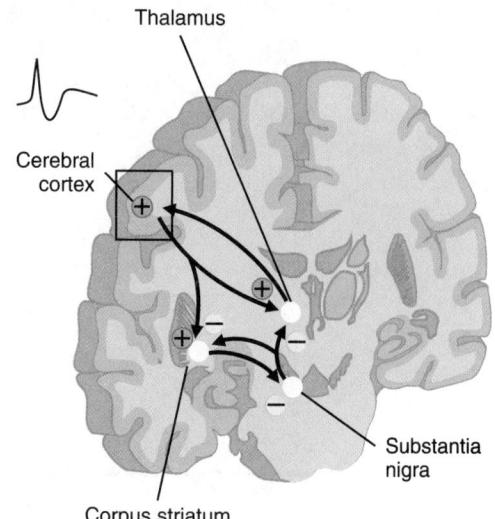

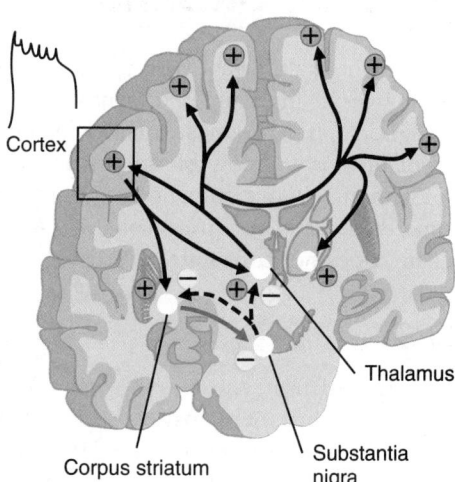

■ **FIGURE 69-1 A,** Normally, excitatory messages from the cerebral cortex are modulated by deeper structures. **B,** In clients with epilepsy, bursts of activity from the cortex are not modulated and these bursts spread. *(From Devinsky, O. [1994]. Seizure disorders. Clinical Symposia, 46[1], 1-54. Modified from an original illustration in Clinical Symposia, illustrated by John Craig, MD, copyright by Ciba-Geigy Corp.)*

Partial Seizures with No Loss of Consciousness

Partial seizures are the most common type of epilepsy. The first clinical and electroencephalographic changes indicate initial activation of neurons in one part of the cerebral hemisphere. They are further classified according to whether or not consciousness is impaired. There are four types of simple partial seizures that do not impair consciousness. These include seizures with motor manifestations, those with somatosensory or "special senses" manifestations, those with autonomic manifestations, and those with psychic manifestations.

Motor Manifestations. Partial seizures with motor manifestations arise from a focus in the motor cortex. The resulting motor activity (seizure) occurs in the part of the body innervated by motor neurons originating in the affected region of the cortex. Because the hand and fingers have the largest cortical representation, many focal motor seizures begin with convulsive movement in the upper extremity. Involuntary movements may spread centrally and involve the entire limb, including one side of the face and lower extremity. This progression or spread is known as the "Jacksonian march." The client also may exhibit changes in posture or spoken utterances.

Somatosensory Manifestations. If the epileptogenic focus is in the parietal region, the client experiences sensory phenomena such as numbness and tingling in the affected area. If the focus is in the occipital region, the client may experience bright, flashing lights in the field of vision opposite the side of the focus. Likewise, the client can have changes in speech or taste with involvement of the posterior temporal area of the dominant hemisphere.

Autonomic Manifestations. Seizures of the autonomic system produce epigastric sensations, pallor, sweating, flushing, piloerection (goose flesh), pupillary dilation, tachycardia, and tachypnea.

Psychic Manifestations. Seizures arising in the anterior temporal lobe can begin with psychic manifestations. These seizures frequently begin with an aura, a subjective sensation that helps localize the focus. An aura may be a strange smell, noise, or sensation preceding a seizure, or a sense of "rising" or "welling up" in the epigastric region. Visual distortions and feelings such as déjà vu are common.

Complex Partial Seizures

There are two types of complex partial seizures: complex partial seizures with automatisms and partial seizures evolving into generalized seizures.

Complex Partial Seizures with Automatisms. The most characteristic features of a complex partial seizure are the accompanying *automatisms*. These automatic behaviors include purposeless repetitive activities such as lip-smacking, chewing, patting a part of the body, or picking at clothes while in a dreamy state. Inappropriate or antisocial behavior may also occur during the seizure. This unusual behavior may cause the client to be viewed as psychotic or otherwise mentally disturbed. However, abnormalities may be subtle and detected only by a trained observer.

Complex partial seizures with automatisms usually last 2 to 3 minutes but can last up to 15 minutes. The client is usually unaware of any activity during the seizure and may be confused or drowsy postictally. Attempts to restrain the client during a seizure may induce combative and uncooperative behavior.

Partial Seizures Evolving to Secondary Generalized Seizures. These seizures start from a particular focus, and then the electrical discharges spread throughout the brain. Clinically, the client first shows focal manifestations; for example, one side of the face moves, and then the whole body becomes involved. Consciousness is lost if the discharges spread throughout the brain.[46]

Generalized Seizures

Generalized seizures lead to a loss of consciousness. They can be convulsive or nonconvulsive. Generalized seizures involve both hemispheres. About one third of seizures are generalized. Types of generalized seizures are absence, myoclonic, clonic, tonic, tonic-clonic, and atonic.

Absence Seizures. Absence seizures are abrupt periods of staring and lapses of awareness lasting a few seconds to a few minutes. They occur in childhood and early adolescence. Tonic-clonic or partial seizures may develop at any time in clients who have had absence seizures.

Myoclonic Seizures. Myoclonic seizures involve sudden uncontrollable jerking movements of either a single muscle group or multiple groups, sometimes causing the client to fall. The client loses consciousness for a moment and then is confused postictally. These seizures often occur in the morning; clients often report that they spill their coffee with their seizure.

Clonic Seizures. The clinical manifestations of clonic seizures include rhythmic muscular contraction and relaxation lasting several minutes. Distinct phases of clonic seizures are not easily observed.

Tonic Seizures. Tonic seizures include an abrupt increase in muscular tone and muscular contraction. In addition, with tonic seizures there is a loss of consciousness and the presence of autonomic manifestations. Tonic seizures may last from 30 seconds to several minutes.

Tonic-Clonic Seizures. Formerly known as "grand mal" seizures, tonic-clonic seizures are the type of seizures most closely associated with epilepsy. However, this type of generalized seizure comprises only 10% of all seizures. A tonic-clonic seizure typically proceeds as follows:

1. An aura may or may not be present.
2. Sudden loss of consciousness may occur.
3. In the tonic phase, the entire body becomes rigid (Figure 69-2, *A*). If standing or sitting, the client falls stiffly to the floor. A cry may be uttered. Respirations are interrupted temporarily, and the

client may become cyanotic. The jaw is fixed and the hands are clenched. The eyes may be opened wide; the pupils are dilated and fixed. The tonic phase lasts 30 to 60 seconds. At the end of this phase the client breathes deeply.

4. The clonic phase begins next, with rhythmic, jerky contraction and relaxation of all body muscles, especially those of the extremities (see Figure 69-2, *B*). The client is usually incontinent and may bite the lips, tongue, or inside of the mouth. Excessive saliva is blown from the mouth, which creates frothing at the lips.

5. An entire tonic-clonic seizure may last from 2 to 5 minutes, after which the client enters the postictal phase, during which the client relaxes and remains totally unresponsive for a time (see Figure 69-2, *C*). The client may rouse briefly and then go into a postictal sleep lasting 30 minutes to several hours. This sleep may be followed by general fatigue, depression, confusion, or headache, all of which gradually resolve. The client has complete amnesia for the seizure episode and may feel nauseated, stiff, and sore. Bruising may occur as the result of falls. Petechial hemorrhages may develop on the face and chest due to the vasovagal responses.

SAFETY ⚠ ALERT **Tongue biting or falling during the seizure may cause other injury.**

Tonic-clonic seizures vary in frequency from many times daily to once or twice a year. Tonic-only and clonic-only seizures may also occur.

Atonic Seizures. Atonic seizures are associated with a total loss of muscle tone. They may be mild, with the client briefly nodding the head, or the client may fall to the floor. Consciousness is impaired only briefly.

Diagnostic Tests

The major diagnostic tool for assessment of clients suspected of having epilepsy is the EEG (see Chapter 67). This test assists in (1) locating the focus of abnormal electrical discharges, if present, (2) establishing a diagnosis of epilepsy, and (3) identifying the specific type of seizures. The EEG records only the electrical activity of the cerebral cortex at the time it is taken. With this limitation, a normal EEG tracing does not always exclude a diagnosis of epilepsy, and EEG abnormalities do not always confirm the diagnosis. During a seizure, EEG abnormalities involve all parts of the cortex. Between seizures, clients with epilepsy may show EEG abnormalities not characteristic of seizure disorders. An ambulatory EEG study can be used to clarify suspected seizures that occur frequently. The monitor used is similar to a Holter monitor. Long-term video EEG monitoring may help classify seizures, and is also used to rule out pseudoseizures.

Occasionally, diagnostic tests such as computed tomography (CT) and magnetic resonance imaging (MRI) are used to rule out brain lesions that can trigger seizures. Positron emission tomography (PET) and single-photon emission computed tomography (SPECT) may be helpful to measure cerebral blood flow in clients undergoing surgery for epilepsy. A complete seizure profile and history is as important as the EEG and other diagnostic studies. The seizure profile includes a baseline neurologic examination

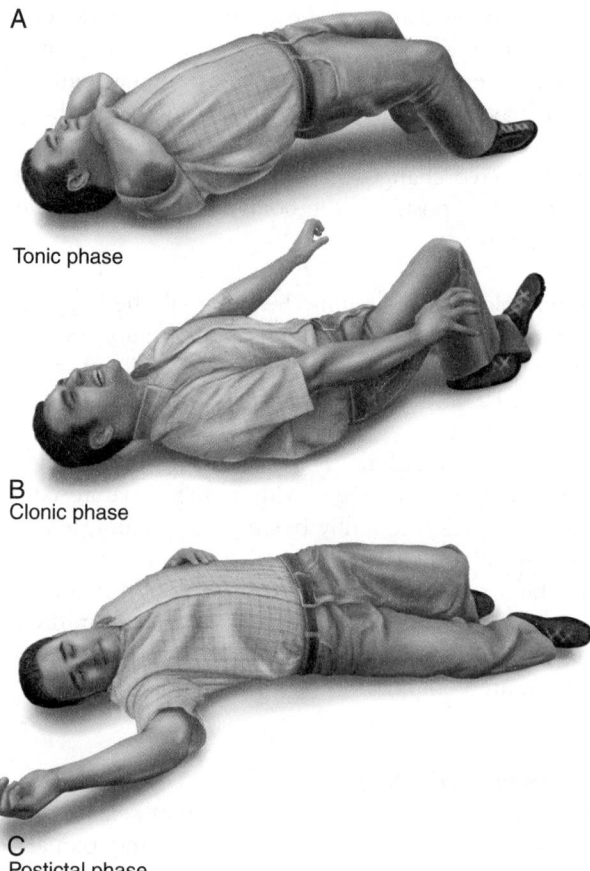

A

Tonic phase

B
Clonic phase

C
Postictal phase

■ **FIGURE 69–2 A,** Generalized convulsive seizures may begin with myoclonic jerks or, rarely, with absences. The tonic phase begins with flexion of the trunk and elevation and abduction of the elbows. Subsequent extension of the back and neck is followed by extension of arms and legs. This can be accompanied by apnea, which is secondary to laryngeal spasm. Autonomic signs are common during this phase and include increase in pulse rate and blood pressure, profuse sweating, and tracheobronchial hypersecretion. This stage lasts for 10 to 20 seconds. **B,** In the clonic phase, the tonic muscles relax intermittently, lasting for a variable period of time. During the clonic stage, a generalized tremor occurs at a rate of 8 tremors per second, which may slow down to about 4 tremors per second. The atonic periods gradually become longer until the last spasm. Voiding may occur at the end of the clonic phase as sphincter muscles relax. The atonic period lasts about 30 seconds. The client continues to be apneic during this phase. **C,** Postictal state includes a variable period of unconsciousness during which the client becomes quiet and breathing resumes. The client gradually awakens, often after a period of stupor or sleep, and often is confused, with some automatic behavior. Headache and muscular pain are common. The client does not recall the seizure itself.

and description of the seizure activity. Laboratory studies may rule out other causes for the seizure.

OUTCOME MANAGEMENT

Medical Management

The goals of management of clients with seizures and epilepsy are to prevent injury during seizures, eliminate factors that precipitate seizures, diagnose and treat the cause of the seizure, and control seizures to allow a desired lifestyle.

During a seizure, the major goals are to maintain the airway, prevent injury to the client, observe the seizure activity, and administer appropriate anticonvulsant medications. In a hospital setting, suction equipment should be readily available.

The person experiencing a seizure usually requires protection from the environment. Objects should be moved out of the way so that the client does not strike his or her head or extremities. Any tight clothing around the person's neck is loosened. Put a pillow or folded blanket under the affected person's head, but do not flex the neck sharply or close the airway. Turning the person to his or her side displaces the tongue and usually opens the airway once the tonic phase has ceased. Do not attempt to open the airway with your fingers or an oral airway. A jaw thrust will open the airway without the potential to harm the client or the caregiver.

Factors that precipitate seizures should be eliminated, if possible. Eating a balanced diet, restricting excessive caffeine and alcohol intake, sleeping well, avoiding seizure triggers (e.g., flashing lights), and minimizing emotional stress may be helpful in preventing seizures.

Observers' descriptions of a seizure can be helpful in making a diagnosis, especially if the descriptions include details such as the sequence in which phenomena occurred. Instruct the family and unlicensed assistive personnel to make the following observations:

- How long did the seizure last?
- Where in the body did the seizure begin and how did it progress?
- Did the client's eyes or head deviate?
- Were the respirations labored or frothy?
- Was the client incontinent?
- Did the client lose consciousness?
- What were the types of movements and what body parts moved?

Medications are used to control seizures. Currently available antiepileptic drugs appear to act primarily by blocking the initiation or spread of seizures. Phenytoin, fosphenytoin sodium (Cerebyx), carbamazepine, valproic acid, and lamotrigine inhibit sodium-dependent action potentials, blocking the burst and firing of neurons. Phenytoin also appears to suppress seizure spread through inhibition of specific voltage-gated calcium channels.

Benzodiazepines and barbiturates augment inhibition by interacting with gamma-aminobutyric acid (GABA) receptors (see the Unit 16 Anatomy and Physiology Review). Valproic acid elevates the concentration of GABA in the brain, perhaps through interaction with enzymes involved in the synthesis (glutamic acid decarboxylase) and catabolism (GABA transaminase) of GABA. Gabapentin and pregabalin, which are structural analogs of GABA, appear to increase GABA levels by enhancing GABA synthesis and release, and may also cause a decrease in glutamate synthesis. The two most effective drugs for absence seizures, ethosuximide and valproic acid, probably act by reducing calcium conduction in thalamic neurons. Topiramate enhances GABA activity to facilitate seizure control.

Initial treatment begins with a single drug until either seizure control is attained or unacceptable side effects appear. Large doses of a single antiepileptic drug (AED) are often more helpful than smaller doses of several drugs. If side effects become intolerable before seizures are controlled, a second drug is added. Combining medications does carry the potential risk of drug-drug interactions, which can decrease effectiveness, as described in the Integrating Pharmacology feature on p. 1816. Nondrug therapies may also contribute to seizure control. The Complementary and Alternative Therapy feature on p. 1817 outlines a non-drug alternative for seizure control.

The use of AEDs is not without adverse effects. Although myriad adverse effects can occur, for the most part they can be grouped into three categories: idiosyncratic, dose-related, and allergic reactions. It is the responsibility of the nurse, as well as other health care team members, to instruct the client about the action, dosing, and possible side effects of the various AEDs. Developing a program of correctly prescribed AEDs requires weeks to months of medication adjustment by trial and error. (The desired outcome of pharmacologic management is monotherapy [use of one AED].)

Nursing Management of the Medical Client

The management of epilepsy does not usually involve hospitalization. However, a client may be hospitalized for a new-onset seizure for assessment, diagnosis, and education. Hospitalization may also be required if seizures become uncontrolled, for seizure monitoring, or if status epilepticus develops. Nurses have a role in assessing for ineffective health maintenance related to knowledge deficit or other barriers, anticipating risk of injury, and providing support for clients and their families who experience life changes related to seizure disorders.

INTEGRATING PHARMACOLOGY

Antiseizure Drugs

Many seizure disorders are controlled by various types of antiseizure drugs (sometimes called antiepileptic drugs). As well, different types of seizures require different medications. Epilepsy medication may be prescribed alone or in combination. If a client has more than one type of seizure, he or she may have to take more than one type of drug to gain control. More than 20 different antiepileptic drugs are available, all with different benefits and side effects. The choice of which drug to prescribe, and at what dosage, depends on many different factors, including the type of seizures, the person's lifestyle and age, how frequently the seizures occur, and, for a woman, the likelihood that she will become pregnant. People with epilepsy should follow their physician's advice and share any concerns they may have regarding their medication.

The first line of drug therapy is often phenytoin, carbamazepine, valproate, or levetiracetam, unless the epilepsy is a type that is known to require a different kind of treatment. For absence seizures, ethosuximide is often the primary treatment. For the client with stereotyped recurrent severe seizures that can be easily recognized by the person's family, the drug diazepam is available as a gel that can be administered rectally by a family member. This method of drug delivery may stop prolonged seizures before they develop into status epilepticus.

Most side effects of antiepileptic drugs are relatively minor, such as fatigue, dizziness, or weight gain. However, severe and life-threatening side effects such as allergic reactions can occur. Epilepsy medication also may predispose people to developing depression or psychoses. Clients with epilepsy should consult a physician immediately if they develop any kind of rash while on medication, or if they find themselves depressed or otherwise unable to think in a rational manner. Other danger signs that should be discussed with a physician immediately are extreme fatigue, staggering or other movement problems, blurring of vision, and slurring of words. Clients with epilepsy should be aware that their epilepsy medication can interact with many other drugs in potentially harmful ways. For this reason, people with epilepsy should always tell their treating physicians which medications they are taking. Women also should know that some antiepileptic drugs can interfere with the effectiveness of oral contraceptives, and they should discuss this possibility with their physicians.

Because older adults are more sensitive to medications, blood levels of medication are checked occasionally to determine whether the dose needs to be adjusted. The effects of a particular medication also sometimes wear off over time, leading to an increase in seizures if the dose is not adjusted.

DISCONTINUING MEDICATION

Some physicians advise clients with epilepsy to discontinue their antiepileptic drugs after 2 years have passed without a seizure. Others believe it is better to wait for 4 to 5 years. Discontinuing medication should only be done with a physician's advice and supervision. It is very important to continue taking epilepsy medication for as long as it is prescribed. Clients should ask their physician or pharmacist ahead of time what they should do if they miss a dose. Discontinuing medication without a physician's advice is one of the major reasons people who have been seizure-free begin having new seizures. Seizures that result from suddenly stopping medication can be serious and can lead to status epilepticus. Furthermore, there is some evidence that uncontrolled seizures trigger changes in neurons that can make it more difficult to treat the seizures in the future.

The chance that a client will eventually be able to discontinue medication depends on the person's age and his or her type of epilepsy. More than half of children who go into remission with medication can eventually stop their medication without having new seizures. One study showed that 68% of adults who had been seizure-free for 2 years before stopping medication were able to do so without having more seizures and that 75% could successfully discontinue medication if they had been seizure-free for 3 years. However, the odds of successfully stopping medication are not as good for clients with a family history of epilepsy, those who need multiple medications, those with partial seizures, or those who continue to have abnormal EEG results while taking medication.

Assessment. Assessment of clients not actively experiencing seizures includes the following:

- History, including prenatal, birth, and developmental history; family history; age at seizure onset; history of all illnesses and trauma; previous brain surgery or stroke; complete description of seizures, including precipitating factors; and presence of an aura
- Medication use and postictal (period of time following a seizure) manifestations
- Psychosocial assessment, including mental status examination

- Complete physical examination, focusing on neurologic manifestations (usually physical examination between seizures is normal)

Diagnosis, Outcomes, Interventions
Diagnosis: Risk for Injury. The diagnosis *Risk for Injury* is related to uncontrolled movement and/or loss of airway patency during a seizure.

Outcomes. The client will have reduced risk of injury and maintain a patent airway during a seizure as evidenced by showing no bruises or bumps following a seizure and by being able to regain adequate oxygenation following the seizure.

Low-Carbohydrate or Ketogenic Diet for Seizures

The ketogenic diet (KD) is actually a non-drug therapy for children with epileptic seizures. It was developed in the 1920s and was based on the clinical observation that fasting suppresses seizures, probably through the induction of ketosis. Interestingly, the high-fat, low-carbohydrate KD tends to mimic the ketogenic effects of fasting and places the body into a constant state of ketosis. KD suppresses many different types of seizures, including those that do not respond to the conventional anticonvulsant drugs. The KD is given only after drug therapy has failed to provide adequate seizure control. KD is effective for tonic-clonic, absence, complex partial, and the multiple types of intractable seizures associated with Lennox-Gastaut syndrome.

REFERENCE

Likhodii, S., et al.. (2003). Anticonvulsant properties of acetone, a brain ketone elevated by the ketogenic diet. *Annals of Neurology, 54,* 219-226.

Interventions

Seizure precautions should be implemented in all clients with a history of epilepsy and seizures. No oral temperatures should be taken; use axillary or rectal routes. The bedrails should be padded and up when the client is in bed. Seizure precautions also include inserting an intravenous needle for medication administration, and keeping oxygen with a nasal cannula and suction equipment, including suction catheters, at the bedside. Fall risk precautions are also needed.

See earlier discussion about assessments and how to maintain the airway during a seizure. After the seizure is completed, place the client in a lateral position and assess oxygen status.

Diagnosis: Risk for Impaired Adjustment. A diagnosis of epilepsy requires major modifications in lifestyle, and these changes are long term. Based on the assessment of the client's adaptation to the diagnosis, the nursing diagnosis is *Risk for Impaired Adjustment* related to complex and long-term health management needs, inability to be involved in high-risk activities, feelings of embarrassment about risk of seizing in public areas, or cost of treatments.

Outcomes. The client and family will state that they understand the need for ongoing treatments, safety awareness during high-risk activities, potential feelings of embarrassment or loss of control and/or costs of treatment.

Interventions. The major problem for clients with epilepsy is the unpredictability of the next seizure. For any

activity, it is important to ask, "What would happen if I had a seizure while doing this?"

Five types of seizure precautions should be discussed with clients and their families. These lifestyle precautions are clearly more applicable to some clients than others.

1. Driving motorized vehicles: Generally no driving is allowed for 6 to 12 months following a seizure. However, state laws vary and also consider the pattern of seizures, for example, whether the client has seizures that occur exclusively during sleep. Consult current state and federal laws and regulations. For example, to resume commercial driving across state lines, a client must have a 5-year seizure-free period. The recommendation for driving cars and trucks extends to the operation of other motorized vehicles, such as boats, motorcycles, and others. Aircraft pilots are typically no longer permitted to fly.
2. Water precautions: Clients with seizures should ensure that they are in the presence of an adult lifeguard who can pull them out of the water if needed. Wearing a life jacket in a boat is important. Showers should be encouraged because taking a bath could lead to drowning with as little as 1 inch of water during the flaccid postictal phase.
3. Heights: Clients with seizures should not work at heights because they could fall and sustain injuries
4. Fire: Burns from injuries related to cooking are not uncommon. Teach clients to cook with other people present, and to avoid using the front burners.
5. Power tools: Caution with the use of power tools is required. In particular, supervision during their use is needed, and the use of safety devices, such as automatic shutoff switches, is recommended. Even the use of kitchen knives should be limited.

Diagnosis: Ineffective Health Maintenance. *Ineffective Health Maintenance* is the nursing diagnosis appropriate for clients who are having difficulty adjusting their life to their epileptic condition.

Outcomes. The client will have improved health maintenance as evidenced by maintaining routine dosing, consulting a physician whenever there is a problem, and wearing a medical alert identification tag or bracelet.

Interventions. Provide the client with verbal information and written reinforcement about (1) how AEDs prevent seizures, (2) the importance of taking prescribed medication regularly, and (3) care during seizures. Consult with the client to plan ways to make taking medication part of daily activities. Also, help the client to identify factors that precipitate seizures and ways of avoiding these factors. Such factors include increased stress, lack of sleep, emotional upset, and alcohol use. The Client Education Guide on p. 1818 lists other important client teaching information.

CLIENT EDUCATION GUIDE

Epilepsy

- Take prescribed dosages of medications to maintain your blood levels.
- Consult your physician if you are unable to take medication because of illness.
- Observe for side effects of antiepileptic drugs. Do not stop taking medications because of annoying side effects; this is very dangerous. Consult your physician first.
- Notify the physician if seizures are not controlled. Provide specific descriptions of the seizure activity.
- Do not take any over-the-counter medications without consulting your physician.
- Obtain a medical alert identification card (or bracelet or tag) with the name of the drug, dosage, and frequency; and your physician's name and phone number. Carry this identification with you at all times.

Evaluation. The short-term outcomes for the client who is experiencing a seizure are usually met within hours. An example is that the seizure stops and the client returns to the previous level of functioning. Nursing care of clients with confirmed epilepsy should focus on the long-term outcomes with self-care.

Modifications for Older Clients

With the increasing frequency of epilepsy in the older population, nurses need to be more aware of the changes in pharmacokinetics in this age group. Concurrent disease, foods, and drug-drug interactions affect absorption of anticonvulsant medication. A decrease in albumin, as is commonly seen in older adults, can increase the free plasma level of these drugs. Decreased metabolism can increase the half-life of these drugs, and decreased elimination can result in higher plasma levels.

Enteral feedings inhibit the absorption of phenytoin (Dilantin). Therefore the feeding should be turned off 2 hours before and after administration of phenytoin, or the dose should be adjusted based on plasma levels. Altered vitamin D metabolism with phenytoin increases the risk of osteoporosis. Carbamazepine (Tegretol) carries an increased risk of slowed cardiac conduction and heart failure; hyponatremia secondary to increased secretion of antidiuretic hormone, especially if the client is receiving a low-sodium diet; and altered cholesterol metabolism in the older population. Valproate (Depakene) carries an increased risk of causing hyperammonemia in older clients, leading to hepatic dysfunction, decrease in platelets, and toxicity related to its longer half-life in this population.

Surgical Management

For approximately 75% of clients with seizures, medical management with AEDs and follow-up evaluation suffices. The remaining 25% continue to have seizures. For about 5% of people with epilepsy, surgery is recommended to control the disease. A few years ago, the most common palliative surgery was anterior callosotomy. This surgery is still performed, but rarely. Several curative surgeries are possible, including lobectomy and lesionectomy.

Thorough assessment is necessary before surgery to determine the epileptogenic focus is located in the "dispensable" areas of the cerebral cortex. Dispensable areas are those for which there is a duplicative area in the cortex. A variety of neurologic tests are used, including video EEG, SPECT, or PET. Intelligence quotient (IQ) testing and psychological assessments are usually performed. Deep EEG electrodes may be surgically placed; this is done when surface electrodes are not sensitive enough to locate the seizure focus exactly. Electrodes are placed in the temporal and frontal lobes of the brain or in the subdural space. These techniques allow identification of deeper seizure foci. Intraoperative mapping may also be used to identify adjacent eloquent tissue that cannot be interrupted during seizure focus resection surgery. A *Wada test* simulates what may occur with surgery and may be used to determine hemispheric dominance, and the location of the speech and memory areas. An injection of amobarbital sodium (Amytal sodium) is given directly into the left internal carotid artery via a cerebral angiogram. If the left hemisphere is dominant, speech is arrested for 1 or 2 minutes, followed by misnaming and misreading for up to 8 to 9 minutes. After 30 minutes, the process is repeated in the right internal carotid artery. The physician looks for changes in sensation, abstract thought, and coordination. Postprocedural care is the same as that for cerebral angiography (see Chapter 67).

Operations for epilepsy include the following:

- Selective amygdalohippocampectomy: In this procedure the two structures within the temporal lobe that are commonly the genesis of seizure activity are removed.
- Temporal lobectomy: Focal resection of part of the temporal lobe, usually on the right side, is performed. If the dominant temporal lobe is removed, the client may experience language defects for a few weeks. Visual defects from loss of visual projection fibers are compensated for quickly. Other areas of the cortex (e.g., the frontal lobe) may also be resected, assuming there is either a defined structural abnormality or a highly localized seizure focus (Figure 69-3, *B*).
- Sub-pial resection: Fine cuts are made into the motor areas of the brain that do not control motor function, but do prevent the spread of the seizure.

- Resection: A cyst or lesion causing the seizures is removed.
- Hemispherectomy: An entire damaged side of the brain is removed; this procedure is performed to treat very severe epilepsy (see Figure 69-3, *C*).
- Corpus callosotomy: Fibers that connect the two halves of the brain are cut; this procedure is also done for treatment of severe epilepsy (see Figure 69-3, *A*).
- Vagal nerve stimulator implantation: The implantation of a vagal nerve stimulator (VNS) offers clients another treatment modality.

Although the underlying mechanism is not fully understood, the VNS is believed to provide a stimulus that desynchronizes the abnormal uncontrolled electrical discharge of the brain activity during a seizure. One study has reported that the benefits from VNS increase over time. For example, 40% to 45% of clients continue to experience a decrease in the frequency of seizures at 18 months after implantation of the VNS.

Nursing Management of the Surgical Client

Preoperative Care

The role of the nurse during the evaluation phase before surgery is to provide support and education. Clients who have epilepsy have been trying to control their seizures for most of their lives. Now, as part of the preoperative assessment, the health care team needs to observe the client during seizure activity. Therefore AEDs are stopped in the controlled hospital setting. This withdrawal period is often confusing and frightening. In addition, some clients are far from family and may be rethinking their decision to undergo surgery. Memory impairments are common because of both the side effects of medications and postictal states. Be certain to provide written material and reinforce education often.

Postoperative Care

Postoperative nursing care is the same as that for any client undergoing a craniotomy (see later discussion). The client is often placed in an intensive care unit (ICU) to facilitate frequent assessment. AEDs are continued after surgery and after leaving the hospital.

Self-Care

It is important for the client with epilepsy to live as normal a life as possible. The client and family members must learn to accept the condition and not exaggerate it or overprotect the client. The restriction on driving can be emotionally and economically devastating for clients of all ages and socioeconomic backgrounds.

A regular pattern of adequate diet, fluid intake, sleep, and moderate recreation and exercise is helpful. Many clients find that skipping meals or not getting enough sleep lowers the threshold for seizures. Alcoholic beverages are contraindicated for two reasons. First, alcohol lowers the seizure threshold; second, alcohol is detoxified by the liver. Most AEDs are also metabolized by

Corpus callosotomy

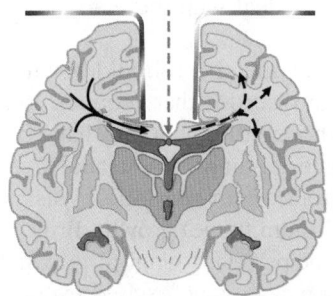

Division of the corpus callosum disrupts the interhemispheric pathway for secondary generalization of partial seizures (unilateral seizure focus)
A

Temporal lobectomy

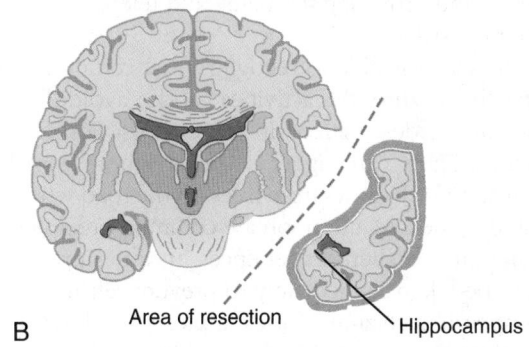

B   Area of resection   Hippocampus

Hemispherectomy

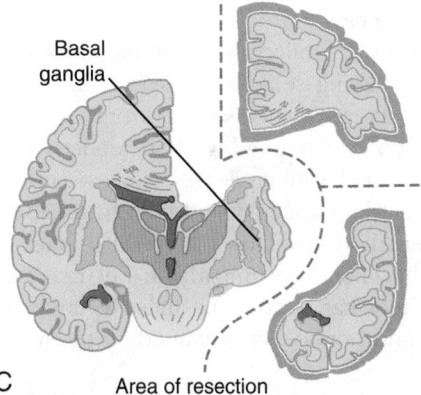

Basal ganglia

C   Area of resection

■ **FIGURE 69–3** Surgery for epilepsy can consist of corpus callosotomy **(A)**, temporal lobectomy **(B)**, or hemispherectomy **(C)**. *(From Devinsky, O. [1994]. Seizure disorders.* Clinical Symposia, *46[1], 1-54. Modified from an original illustration in* Clinical Symposia, *illustrated by John Craig, MD, copyright by Ciba-Geigy Corp.)*

the liver. Consuming alcohol while taking an anticonvulsant places an increased strain on the metabolizing functions of the liver.

For some clients, the psychosocial impact of epilepsy is overwhelming. Because most seizures occur without warning, many clients spend their lives anticipating inappropriate behavior, embarrassment, and self-injury. Clients with epilepsy often have a poor self-image, feelings of inferiority, self-consciousness, guilt, anger, depression, and other emotional problems. Education and support groups can help clients deal with the emotional impact of epilepsy.

The client and family members should be taught that epilepsy is a chronic disorder that requires long-term management. Even though the client may have been seizure-free for some time, it is important to take medication as prescribed. Phenytoin, a common anticonvulsant, leads to excessive gingival (gum tissue) growth. Brushing two to three times daily helps retard gingival growth. Some clients have excess gingival tissue excised every 6 to 12 months. Medications may also cause diplopia, ataxia, sedation, and bone marrow depression. Most AEDs require periodic monitoring of serum drug levels, liver function, and complete blood counts. Clients with epilepsy should always wear or carry identification stating that they have epilepsy and providing the name and telephone number of their physician.

If the client is able to recognize that certain activities trigger the seizure, the activities can be avoided, or the client can be desensitized in some cases. For example, flickering lights can trigger seizures. Fluorescent lights and flickering shadows from trees on the road while driving during the late afternoon are common precipitants of seizures. If the client experiences an aura, precautions should be taken immediately to prevent self-injury from the impending seizure—for example, lying down on the ground or floor or, if driving a vehicle, pulling over to the side of the road and lying on the seat. Instruct clients to carry a large pillow in the vehicle or to use their arms to protect their heads.

Some clients with epilepsy cannot find employment if they admit to having seizures. However, falsifying job applications can result in dismissal from employment. These factors contribute to a higher incidence of depression among clients with epilepsy. Nurses can educate the public regarding epilepsy and help to dissipate prejudices. When discussing the long-term impact of epilepsy with the client, be empathetic but realistic. It is hoped the client can accept the lifestyle limitations of the disorder and not be overwhelmed by them.

SAFETY
⚠️
ALERT

The client's family needs to know what to do in the event of a seizure. The affected person should be protected from self-injury. Clothing should be loosened, the head protected from impact, and sharp objects in the environment removed. The person should not be forcibly restrained during a seizure but protected from self-injury. Hard objects or fingers should not be inserted into the mouth. People experiencing a seizure do not swallow the tongue—a common misconception. However, the tongue can occlude the airway, and positioning the head is important to protect the airway. After the head is protected from injury, the person should be placed in a side-lying position to displace the tongue and allow oral secretions to drain from the airway. Someone should stay with the person until full consciousness has returned. An ambulance should be called if the seizure lasts for longer than 10 minutes, if another seizure occurs before consciousness returns, if there is respiratory difficulty or evidence of injury, or if the person is pregnant. Sleepiness is common in the postictal period.

Various organizations exist that try to educate the public, introduce appropriate legislation, and assist people with epilepsy. In the United States, these include the Epilepsy Foundation of America and Epilepsy Services. Similar organizations exist in other countries.

STATUS EPILEPTICUS

Status epilepticus, a medical emergency, is a state in which a client has continuous seizures or seizures in rapid succession, without regaining consciousness, lasting at least 30 minutes. The most common cause of status epilepticus is the sudden withdrawal of AEDs. During a seizure, the brain's metabolic needs increase dramatically. If these heightened requirements continue without opportunity for the body to recover, the supply of glucose and oxygen to the brain becomes depleted, and permanent brain damage may occur.

OUTCOME MANAGEMENT

The major goals in managing a client with status epilepticus are to establish and protect the airway, to control the seizure, and to monitor for adverse outcomes.

The airway is maintained and aspiration prevented by placing the client in a side-lying position, suctioning the airway, and providing oxygen. Oxygen offers nothing to a client who is apneic; therefore intubation may be necessary to ventilate and oxygenate the client.

AEDs are given to terminate seizures and to prevent exhaustion. Intravenous (IV) infusion is begun immediately and maintained during treatment. Status epilepticus is treated with diazepam in doses of 5 to 10 mg (0.2 mg/kg) given every 10 to 20 minutes, for a total dose of up to 30 mg in an 8-hour period. Lorazepam (0.1 mg/kg) can also be administered in 4-mg doses given over 2 to 5 minutes, repeated every 10 to 15 minutes to a maximum of 8 mg (0.2 mg/kg). In addition, phenytoin can be given to a total dose of 15 to 18 mg/kg by slow IV push (no more than 50 mg/min). Assess the client for bradycardia and heart block while phenytoin is given. If this agent is not effective, diazepam or lorazepam can be used. Because each of these medications can depress respiration, emergency ventilation equipment should be readily available.

If diazepam or lorazepam is not effective, pentobarbital or propofol can be used to suppress brain activity. Inducing coma is used only after attempts with AEDs have failed. The client in drug-induced coma is ventilator-dependent and requires nursing care in an ICU for ventilatory assistance, continuous EEG monitoring, and hemodynamic monitoring.

Once status epilepticus has been controlled, the client may be unresponsive for a period of time. Clients may be in a postictal state or experiencing subclinical seizures. After the seizures have been controlled, maintenance AEDs are prescribed.

It is especially difficult for significant others to watch clients experiencing status epilepticus. The family needs support and information. Always explain to family members the treatment being given.[21,26,35,48-50]

BRAIN TUMORS

The Central Brain Tumor Registry for the United States (CBTRUS) estimated that 190,600 brain tumors would be diagnosed in the United States in 2005. Of that total, 43,800 were estimated to be primary brain tumors and the remainder to be secondary or metastatic. The overall incidence for primary brain and CNS tumors is 14 cases per 100,000 person years. The incidence of brain tumors appears to be increasing, but this may reflect improved and earlier diagnosis. CBTRUS notes that, as of 2000, approximately 359,000 people in the United States were living with a primary brain tumor, with 75% having benign tumors and 23% having malignant tumors.

Etiology

No clear etiologic factor has been established for any of the primary brain tumors. Although the type of cell that develops into the tumor can often be identified, the mechanism causing the cells to act abnormally remains unknown. Familial tendencies, immunosuppression, and environmental factors are being considered. The peak time for brain tumor development is the fifth to seventh decades of life; men are affected more commonly than women.

Pathophysiology
Intracranial Tumors

Brain tumors are described as "space-occupying lesions." This description means that the tumor displaces normal tissue. When normal brain tissue is compressed, blood flow is altered and ischemia develops. If unchecked, necrosis may occur. Tumors may also irritate surrounding tissue, producing considerable cerebral edema. Because little room is available for expansion of any of the intracranial contents, edema as well as the tumor cause progressively increased intracranial pressure (ICP), which leads to herniation of the brain (see Chapter 73). Both of these mechanisms can contribute to nonspecific neurologic deficits. Tumor location may produce deficits specific to the area of involvement.

Brain tumors are identified as primary or secondary lesions. Tumors arising from the brain or its supporting structures are called *primary* brain tumors; those metastasizing from other areas in the body to the brain are *secondary* tumors. Brain tumors may also be referred to as *intra-axial* or *extra-axial*. Intra-axial tumors are those that arise from within the cerebrum, cerebellum, or brain stem. Extra-axial tumors have their origin in the skull, meninges, or cranial nerves. Primary intracranial tumors may arise from the support cells (the neuroglial cells [gliomas]), from neurons (neuromas), or from supporting structures.

Glial Tumors. Gliomas are the most common type of glial cell tumor and can be found throughout the brain or spinal cord. These tumors occur in adults and children. Depending on the exact location, clinical manifestations may result in increased ICP or focal compression. Gliomas are often further classified based on their specific cell or origin. Astrocytomas arise from astrocyte cells, oligodendroglioma tumors arise from oligodendroglial cells, and ependymomas arise from ependymal cells (Table 69-1). Much confusion exists about pathologic and histologic nomenclature. Historically, staging or grading scales identified glial tumors as grade I (benign) through grade IV (malignant). The grade is assigned according to the degree of tumor cell differentiation. Tumors that are well-differentiated are classified as a lower grade while high-grade tumors are poorly differentiated.

Astrocytomas. These are tumors arising from the cells that repair and maintain the nervous system These are the most common of all primary brain tumors and can be found anywhere in the cerebral hemispheres. Peak age for occurrence is 50 to 60 years, but these tumors can afflict younger and older age groups. Their location determines the exact clinical manifestations.

Oligodendrogliomas. Oligodendrogliomas arise from cells that produce myelin and specifically affect myelinated (white matter) brain. They tend to develop in the cortex of the frontal and parietal lobes. This tumor is fairly slow-growing and calcifies, which makes it recognizable on x-ray studies. The calcification may contribute to the development of seizures as a presenting clinical manifestation. Oligodendrogliomas peak in clients

TABLE 69–1 Schema for Classifying Brain Tumors*

Type of Tumor	Criteria
Astrocytoma	Increased number of astrocytes; mature astrocytes; normally developed astrocytes
Anaplastic astrocytoma	Increased number of less mature astrocytes; possibility of mitotic figures (mitotic figures represent increased cellular division and malignant changes)
Glioblastoma multiforme	Increased number of astrocyte cells; immature astrocytes; presence of mitotic figures; hemorrhage, necrosis, swelling, and obscure tumor margins

*This schema of astrocytoma, anaplastic tumor, and glioblastoma multiforme is also used for the astrocytoma, ependymoma, and oligodendroglioma.

between the ages of 30 and 50 years. Clinical manifestations in addition to seizures are headache, personality changes, and papilledema.

Ependymomas. These tumors arise from cells that line the ventricles and form the inner lining of the spinal cord. Although ependymomas may be found anywhere within the CNS, they are more commonly found adjacent to the fourth or lateral ventricles or within the spinal cord tissue. This tumor affects all age groups. Manifestations are caused by ventricular obstruction and include headache, vomiting, diplopia, dizziness, ataxia, vision changes, and motor and sensory abnormalities.

Neuromas. Neuromas can arise from any neuron but most commonly arise from the acoustic neurons. Neuromas account for only about 10% of all intracranial tumors.

Acoustic Neuromas. Acoustic neuromas are tumors of the Schwann cells of the eighth cranial nerve, the acoustic nerve. Manifestations are tinnitus, dizziness, and unilateral and permanent hearing loss. If the tumor is allowed to grow, it can displace the other cranial nerves—especially cranial nerves IV to X—and the brain stem. An excellent outcome can be expected with surgical resection or stereotactic radiosurgery, assuming the remaining cranial nerves are preserved. However, many clients experience at least temporary tinnitus, balance problems, and facial weakness after surgery or radiosurgery.

Pituitary Tumors. Pituitary tumors are usually slow-growing tumors that involve only the anterior lobe of the pituitary gland or extend into the floor of the third ventricle. Although histologically benign, they can reoccur after surgery. Manifestations can be related to hypofunctioning of the gland and include visual field defects, irregular or absent menstrual cycles, infertility, decreased libido, impotence, decreased body hair, and decreased production of pituitary-stimulating hormones; this decrease results

in decreased thyroid and adrenal function. Hypersecretion can also occur and is related to the hormones that are in excess. Combinations of hyposecretion and hypersecretion can also be seen. Manifestations of pituitary tumors are often overlooked for months because they are so diverse. Clients are usually diagnosed by MRI scan and blood testing for the presence of pituitary-stimulating hormones. Visual abnormalities may also occur because of the proximity of the pituitary to the optic nerve. Tumor growth in this area may cause optic nerve compression, manifested as loss of visual field.

Meningiomas. Meningiomas are common benign tumors that may involve all meningeal layers; however, these tumors are believed to originate in the arachnoid cells (Figure 69-4). Most meningiomas are benign, but some tumors may become malignant.[14] Meningiomas may be found in the brain or spinal cord. They are slow-growing and occur at any age, most commonly at midlife and in women. Manifestations depend on location of the tumor and can be diverse. Outcomes are related to the site of the tumor. Recurrence is a concern.

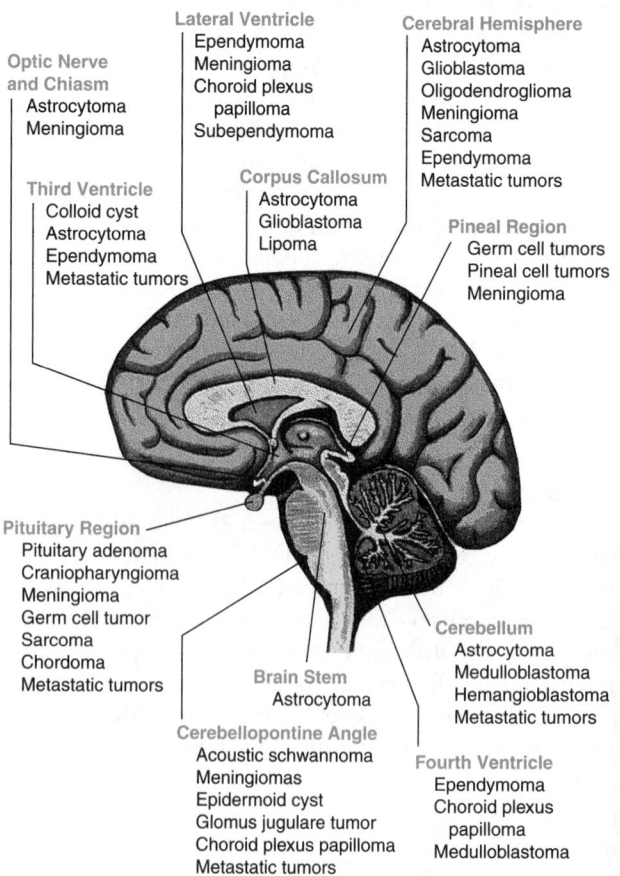

Optic Nerve and Chiasm
Astrocytoma
Meningioma

Third Ventricle
Colloid cyst
Astrocytoma
Ependymoma
Metastatic tumors

Lateral Ventricle
Ependymoma
Meningioma
Choroid plexus papilloma
Subependymoma

Corpus Callosum
Astrocytoma
Glioblastoma
Lipoma

Cerebral Hemisphere
Astrocytoma
Glioblastoma
Oligodendroglioma
Meningioma
Sarcoma
Ependymoma
Metastatic tumors

Pineal Region
Germ cell tumors
Pineal cell tumors
Meningioma

Pituitary Region
Pituitary adenoma
Craniopharyngioma
Meningioma
Germ cell tumor
Sarcoma
Chordoma
Metastatic tumors

Cerebellopontine Angle
Acoustic schwannoma
Meningiomas
Epidermoid cyst
Glomus jugulare tumor
Choroid plexus papilloma
Metastatic tumors

Brain Stem
Astrocytoma

Cerebellum
Astrocytoma
Medulloblastoma
Hemangioblastoma
Metastatic tumors

Fourth Ventricle
Ependymoma
Choroid plexus papilloma
Medulloblastoma

■ **FIGURE 69–4** Common intracranial tumors and their usual locations. *(Modified from Osteen, R.T., Gansler, T & Lenhard, R.E. [2001]. American Cancer Society textbook of clinical oncology [3rd ed., p. 381]. Atlanta: American Cancer Society.)*

Metastatic Brain Tumors

Metastatic brain tumors are those with primary sites outside of the brain. Cancers of the lung, breast, and kidney and malignant melanoma are the major sources of metastatic brain cancers. Metastatic tumors to the brain are more commonly multiple, making them less amenable to therapy. The tumor location may be in the brain itself or in the meninges lining the brain. The common locations of brain tumors are shown in Figure 69-4.

Clinical Manifestations

Clinical manifestations may be nonspecific, caused by edema and increased ICP, or specific and related to a particular anatomic location.

Mental Status Changes

As in any neurologic or neurosurgical disorder, a change in the level of consciousness (LOC) or sensorium is often noted. Mental and emotional status changes such as lethargy and drowsiness, confusion, disorientation, and personality changes may be found.

Headaches

Headaches may be localized or generalized. They are usually intermittent, are of increasing duration, and may be intensified by a change in position or straining. Recurrent, severe headaches in a client who was previously free of headaches, or recurrent headaches in the morning, increasing in frequency and severity, may indicate an intracranial tumor and indicate the need for further assessment.

Nausea and Vomiting

The clinical manifestations of nausea and vomiting are believed to occur because of pressure on the medulla, where the vomiting center is found. The client often complains of a severe headache after lying flat in bed. As the headache increases in severity, the client may also experience nausea or spontaneous vomiting. During the episode of emesis, the client may hyperventilate, which decreases brain swelling, and after the vomiting episode may note that the headache is less severe.

Papilledema

Compression of the second cranial nerve, the optic nerve, may result in papilledema. The underlying pathophysiologic mechanism of papilledema is not clearly understood. Increased intracranial pressure obstructs venous return from the eye and backs up blood in the central retinal vein. Also known as "choked disc," papilledema is common in clients with intracranial tumors and may be the first manifestation of increased ICP. Early papilledema does not cause visual acuity changes and can be detected only through an ophthalmologic examination. Severe papilledema may be manifest by decreased visual acuity.

Seizures

Seizures, focal or generalized, are common in clients with intracranial tumors, especially cerebral hemisphere tumors (see earlier discussion). Seizures may be partial or generalized; partial seizures usually help localize tumor location.

Localized Manifestations

Localized clinical manifestations are caused by destruction, irritation, or compression of the part of the brain where the tumor is located. Table 69-2 lists specific clinical manifestations based on tumor location. Localized manifestations include the following:

- Focal weaknesses (e.g., hemiparesis)
- Sensory disturbances, including absence of feeling (anesthesia) or abnormal sensation (paresthesia)
- Language disturbances
- Coordination disturbances (e.g., staggering gait)
- Visual disturbance such as diplopia (double vision) or visual field deficit (monopia)

Despite the availability of extremely sensitive and sophisticated equipment, brain tumor diagnosis is often delayed because of difficulty recognizing early manifestations. No two adults with the diagnosis of brain tumor present with the same clinical manifestations. Older clients especially fail to report such problems during regular examinations because they forget or think that the manifestations are "just part of growing old."

Diagnostic Findings

If an intracranial tumor is suspected, noninvasive studies such as CT and MRI are performed (Figure 69-5). Other disorders may be ruled out with EEG, radionuclide scans, angiogram, or lumbar puncture. A stereotactic biopsy may confirm the diagnosis of a brain tumor and help in planning appropriate therapy. Three-dimensional imaging techniques help further localize the tumor in the brain and can assist with plans for resection. PET scans can also be used to study the biochemical and physiologic effects of the tumor.

OUTCOME MANAGEMENT

Medical Management

For the adult client with a brain tumor, there are many options for treatment. Regardless of which treatment modality is selected, the initial goal is to establish a

TABLE 69–2 Clinical Manifestations of Brain Tumors by Location

Location	Clinical Manifestations
Frontal lobe	Disturbed mental state, apathy, inappropriate behavior, dementia, depression, emotional lability, inattentiveness, inability to concentrate, indifference, loss of self-restraint and social behavior, impaired long-term memory, difficulty with abstraction, quiet but flat affect, dominant hemisphere expressive speech disturbance, impaired sphincter control with bowel and bladder incontinence, motor disorders, gait disturbances, paralysis, "frontal release signs," seizures
Temporal lobe	Receptive aphasia, generalized psychomotor seizures, visual field changes, personality changes, ataxia, headache, manifestations of increased ICP, tinnitus, recent memory impairment
Parietal lobe	Sensory deficits, motor and sensory focal seizures, agnosias, hypoesthesias, paresthesias, dyslexia, visual field cut, diminished appreciation of side opposite the tumor, headache, apraxia, tactile inattention, right/left disorientation
Occipital lobe	Headache, manifestations of increased ICP, visual impairment (homonymous hemianopsia), visual agnosia, cortical blindness, hallucinations, seizures
Cerebellar	Unsteady gait, falling, ataxia, incoordination, tremors, head tilt, nystagmus, CSF obstruction/hydrocephalus, truncal ataxia if vermis is tumor site
Brain stem	Vertigo, dizziness, vomiting, CN III-XII palsies/dysfunction, nystagmus, decreased corneal reflex, headache, vomiting, gait disturbance, motor and sensory deficits, deafness, intranuclear ophthalmoplegia, sudden death from cardiac and respiratory failure
Pituitary and hypothalamus	Visual deficits, headache, hormonal dysfunction, sleep disturbances, water imbalance, temperature fluctuations, imbalance in fat and carbohydrate metabolism, Cushing's syndrome
Ventricle	Obstruction of CSF circulation, hydrocephalus, rapid increase in ICP, postural headache

CN, Cranial nerve; *CSF,* cerebrospinal fluid; *ICP,* intracranial pressure.

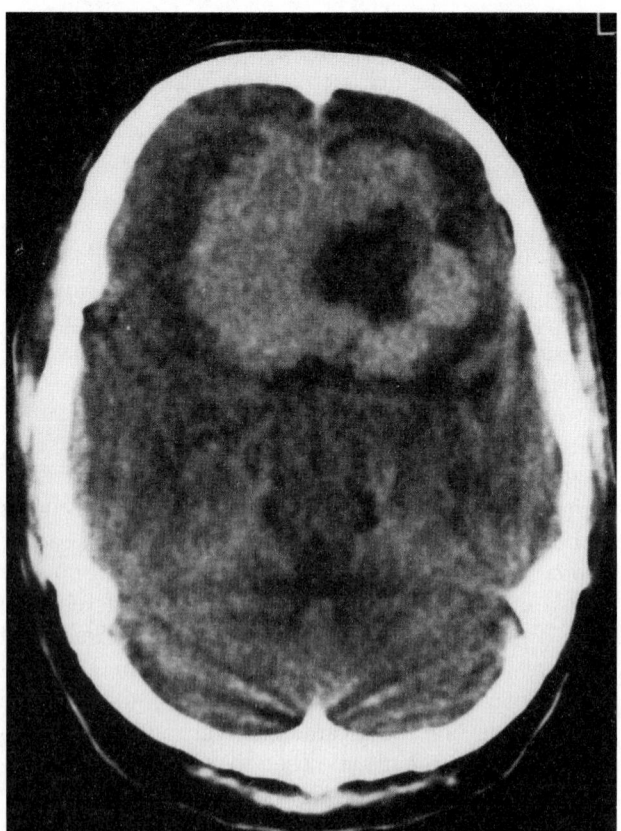

■ **FIGURE 69–5** Magnetic resonance image revealing a midline frontal meningioma.

diagnosis. Most often this is accomplished through surgery; therefore surgical management is discussed first. Additional goals include managing increased ICP, controlling or preventing seizures, and monitoring for motor or sensory deficits and cranial nerve deficits.

Intervention depends on the type and location of the intracranial tumor and the client's medical condition. Management is always interdisciplinary, with several members forming a clinical team to support the client through care.

Surgical Management

Surgical intervention may range from biopsy to total removal of the brain tumor by way of a craniotomy. Surgical biopsy or resection confirms the histologic or pathologic diagnosis. Surgical resection also decreases the tumor burden, making other treatments and adjunctive therapeutic treatments more effective, and helps control increased ICP. With only a few exceptions, all clients with brain tumors require a craniotomy for surgical intervention.

Craniotomy

The term *craniotomy* means to surgically create an opening into the skull. A craniectomy (removal of a portion of the cranium) may be performed for decompression. There are many methods of removing the tumor, regardless of the type of tumor and the extent of tumor removed (Table 69-3).

Intraoperatively the client may be positioned in various ways to facilitate exposure and visualization. Such positions and head-supporting frames have the potential to cause skin pressure on the head, edema of the face, and muscle soreness, especially in the neck. Preoperatively or postoperatively, a ventriculostomy, in which a catheter is inserted through a burr hole into the ventricle, may be needed to drain cerebrospinal fluid (CSF) or blood. Drains may be used if a large area of dead space remains after tumor removal.

TABLE 69–3 Surgical Options for Brain Tumor Diagnosis and Excision

Procedure	Description
Preoperative Procedures to Locate and Map the Tumor and Nearby Structures	
Brain-mapping technique	Uses viewing wand to precisely identify location of specific anatomic functions (i.e., motor, sensory, and/or speech); methods developed include localizing tumors with ultrasound techniques and various wand-like devices
Cortical mapping	Intraoperative cortical EEG recording and monitoring, facilitating areas for greater accuracy of resection without loss of eloquent motor and/or sensory functions
Direct cortical stimulation	Electrical current is directed to specific area in brain, causing visible movement of corresponding body part
Frameless stereotactic localization systems	External devices are placed preoperatively and client's body is scanned using CT or MRI; localization systems scanning data are transferred to operating room, allowing determination of boundaries of lesion by means of a surgical "wand"
Intraoperative ultrasonography	Uses a hand-held device to differentiate tumors with a cystic component; ultrasound techniques allow identification of tumor margins
Somatosensory evoked potentials (SSEPs)	Measurement of electrical response of specific areas (e.g., visual, auditory, brain stem); after functions of such critical areas have been determined, these areas can be avoided during surgical manipulation
Surgical Techniques Used for Precise Location of the Tumor	
Intraoperative imaging techniques	Real-time CT or MRI for improved visualization
Stereotactic surgery	Localization of a specific target within three-dimensional space; with client stabilized in a head frame, tumor is imaged using either CT or MRI; data from scans are analyzed by a computer and a trajectory location is identified; stereotactic procedures may be used for biopsy or craniotomy
Treatment Options for Tumor Excision	
Embolization	Decreases blood supply to tumor; may be used in conjunction with surgical procedures
Laser surgery	Destroys tumor tissue using heat from laser without causing adjacent edema or damage
Neuro-endoscopic techniques	For treatment of third and/or lateral ventricle lesions; provides access to lesions in areas otherwise difficult to locate
Polymer wafer implants	Chemotherapeutic wafers are placed in tumor bed; carmustine is currently available, and other agents are being tested
Ultrasonic aspirator	Suction-like device used in removing solid tumors

CT, Computed tomography; *EEG,* electroencephalography; *MRI,* magnetic resonance imaging.

Nursing Management of the Surgical Client

Preoperative Care

More than at any other time, the role of the nurse caring for the client with the diagnosis of a brain tumor is diverse. The nurse in the neurosurgeon's office begins preoperative teaching. During the perioperative and postoperative periods, the nurse prepares the client for various transitions in the continuum of care.

Preoperative assessment includes the routine assessment data (see Chapter 2). In addition, a detailed history and physical examination provides a baseline for comparison of neurologic data. The nurse will obtain and record data on the following:

- Presenting clinical manifestations such as headache, nausea and vomiting, or focal deficits
- Vital signs, level of consciousness, and orientation to person, place, and time; ability to follow instructions; pupil equality, size, reactivity, accommodation, and reaction to light; extraocular eye movements; and cranial nerve function
- Limb strength, movement, and sensation; note limited or exaggerated movements, pronator drift, hand grip, dorsiflexion/plantiflexion, any paresis or paralysis, or sensory abnormalities
- Mental status—note any difficulties in problem-solving, limited memory, or behavior change

Preoperative interventions are similar to those for the care of other clients before surgery (see Chapter 14). The suddenness of the diagnosis and possibility of a cancer diagnosis may produce anxiety for both the client and family. Offer explanations and clarification as needed especially about placement in an intensive care unit and initial appearance altered by dressings, edema, and bruising. Be certain not to offer empty promises about recovery.

Postoperative Care

General postoperative complications after intracranial surgery do not differ from those after other forms of surgery. Ecchymosis and periorbital edema may be present after intracranial surgery but are transient. These changes affecting the appearance of the eyes and the face overall can be frightening to the client as well as to the family members.

Postoperative care of the client after craniotomy is shown in the accompanying Care Plan feature on pp. 1826-1828. See also the information on care of clients with increased ICP in Chapter 73.

C A R E   P L A N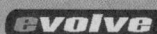

The Client Who Has Undergone Craniotomy

Nursing Diagnosis: Risk for Ineffective Tissue Perfusion: Cerebral related to edema or bleeding after craniotomy.
Outcomes: The client will have intracranial pressure (ICP) less than 15 mm Hg, mean arterial pressure (MAP) greater than 70 mm Hg, cerebral perfusion pressure (CPP) greater than 50 mm Hg, neurologic assessments and vital signs at baseline values or improved, no clinical manifestations of increased ICP and/or herniation, and body temperature less than 38.5 ° C.

NOC OUTCOMES	Cognitive Ability, Neurologic Status, Neurologic Status: Consciousness, Tissue Perfusion: Cerebral

Interventions	NIC INTERVENTIONS	Rationales
1. Assess neurologic status and vital signs frequently and compare with baseline values.	Neurologic Monitoring Vital Signs Monitoring	1. A change in level of consciousness is the first sign of increasing intracranial pressure (ICP).
2. Elevate head of bed to 30 degrees.	Cerebral Perfusion Promotion	2. Elevation facilitates venous drainage and reduces edema.
3. Maintain head and neck in neutral alignment.	Cerebral Perfusion Promotion	3. Neutral alignment facilitates venous drainage and reduces edema.
4. Change position slowly.	Cerebral Perfusion Promotion	4. Rapid changes in position increase cerebral blood flow and pressure.
5. Avoid Valsalva maneuver.	Cerebral Perfusion Promotion	5. Straining during coughing, movement in bed, or moving bowels increases ICP.
6. Monitor intake and output frequently.	Fluid Monitoring	6. Excess fluids can promote edema; dehydration can decrease cerebral arterial flow.
7. Monitor pulse oximetry and arterial blood gases.	Oxygen Therapy, Acid-Base Monitoring	7. The cerebrum is sensitive to lack of oxygen, and damage can occur within minutes after onset of hypoxia.
8. Reduce environmental stress by minimizing interruptions and stimuli.	Cerebral Perfusion Promotion Environmental Management	8. Noise and frequent interruptions may increase ICP.
9. Administer steroids as ordered.	Medication Administration	9. Steroids reduce cerebral edema.
10. Administer antiepileptic drugs as ordered.	Medication Administration Seizure Management	10. Seizures are common sequelae of brain surgery.

Evaluation: Depending on the etiology of edema or amount of bleeding, it may require hours to days to control ICP.

Nursing Diagnosis: Decreased Intracranial Adaptive Capacity related to neurologic changes from edema of surgical excision of sections of brain or tumor.
Outcomes: The client will have intracranial adaptive capacity as evidenced by controlled intracranial pressures.

NOC OUTCOMES	Electrolyte and Acid-Base Balance, Fluid Balance, Neurologic Status: Autonomic, Neurologic Status: Cranial Sensory/Motor Function

Interventions	NIC INTERVENTIONS	Rationales
1. Perform Glasgow Coma Scale and other neurologic assessments q 1 hr. Compare findings to baseline, and report changes.	Neurologic Monitoring	1. Hourly observations allow early intervention when changes occur.
2. Maintain patent airway with Po_2 values greater than 85 mm Hg and Pco_2 between 25 and 30 mm Hg.	Cerebral Perfusion Promotion	2. Prevent cerebral hypoxia; hypercapnia increases cerebral blood flow.
3. Maintain sterile and patent CSF drain, keeping stopcock at level of tragus (or as specified). Monitor CSF color.	Cerebral Perfusion Promotion	3. CSF drainage is normally sterile. A plugged CSF drain would increase ICP. The tragus is level with the ventricles and allows normal intracranial pressures when maintained at that level.

Evaluation: Stabilizing the brain in order to reach normal levels of adaptation to changes in intracranial volume and pressures will require at least 72 hours depending upon the initial amount of edema and tissue injury.

Nursing Diagnosis: Ineffective Coping related to fear of changes in body image, role performance, or life expectancy.
Outcomes: The client will have improved individual coping, as evidenced by statements indicating feelings of self-worth, behaviors demonstrating self-worth, and less use of dependent behaviors.

NOC OUTCOMES   Aggression Control, Coping, Decision-Making, Impulse Control, Role Performance

Interventions	NIC INTERVENTIONS	Rationales
1. Encourage family members/significant others to assist in meeting need for close contact.	Support System Enhancement, Anxiety Reduction, Coping Enhancement	1. Family members may also fear that they will injure the client.
2. Anticipate needs.	Support System Enhancement, Anxiety Reduction, Coping Enhancement	2. Anxiety increases feelings of loneliness.
3. Offer praise and encouragement during ongoing assessment of client's readiness to move toward more competent coping.	Self-Esteem Enhancement, Anxiety Reduction, Coping Enhancement	3. Positive reinforcement helps to guide future steps toward independence.
4. Provide opportunities for expression and ventilation of feelings and issues.	Anxiety Reduction, Coping Enhancement, Emotional Support	4. Problem-solving coping styles are initiated by talking about feelings.
5. Utilize consistent personnel.	Support System Enhancement, Anxiety Reduction, Coping Enhancement	5. A therapeutic relationship is easier to maintain than to build.
6. Establish trust relationship; follow through on promises.	Support System Enhancement, Anxiety Reduction, Coping Enhancement	6. Feelings of fear and anxiety are reduced.

Evaluation: Coping skills will wax and wane over time. Expect periods of coping and periods of failure to cope with changes in prognosis.

Nursing Diagnosis: Anxiety related to uncertain future and prognosis.
Outcomes: The client will have decreased anxiety and express fears and concerns openly.

NOC OUTCOMES   Aggression Control, Anxiety Control, Coping

Interventions	NIC INTERVENTIONS	Rationales
1. Repeat information; provide information in different forms; encourage the client and/or significant other to write down questions and/or concerns.	Support System Enhancement, Anxiety Reduction, Coping Enhancement, Teaching: Individual	1. Depending on the type of tumor, the location of the tumor, and/or motor or sensory deficits, the client may be faced with the loss of specific functions and the possibility of having a malignancy. Appropriate interventions may help the client better understand the prescribed plan of care.
2. Encourage open communication between the client, significant others, and members of the health care team.	Support System Enhancement, Anxiety Reduction, Coping Enhancement	2. Having a diagnosis of brain cancer may immobilize all of the normal coping mechanisms of the client and significant others.
3. Involve the client's clergy or hospital chaplain if desired.	Spiritual Support	3. Spiritual support is crucial at times of serious illness for the client, family members, and significant others. The client need not be "religious" to gain support from clergy.

Evaluation: Anxiety should be controllable in a short time. However, changes in response to therapy or other outcomes will increase anxiety.

Nursing Diagnosis: Risk for Disturbed Thought Processes related to neurologic changes from edema or surgical excision of sections of brain or tumor.
Outcomes: The client will make decisions and process information at expected levels, express and identify anger, exercise control over own behavior, make appropriate choices, and/or cease hostile behavior.

NOC OUTCOMES   Cognitive Ability, Cognitive Orientation, Decision-Making

Interventions	NIC INTERVENTIONS	Rationales
1. Allow client to verbalize concerns, and channel these concerns to the appropriate person.	Emotional Support, Anxiety Reduction	1. Problem-solving coping begins with verbalization of concerns.

(Continued)

CARE PLAN evolve

The Client Who Has Undergone Craniotomy—Cont'd

2. Offer reasonable choices to client.	Emotional Support, Anxiety Reduction	2. Feelings of control can be reestablished by offering choices to client. All options must be safe and implementable for the client.
3. Assist client to recognize alternatives and the implications of choices.	Emotional Support, Anxiety Reduction	3. This measure helps client with problem-solving abilities.
4. Report client's status to client, and allow for opportunity to make decisions about treatment or no treatment.	Client Rights' Protection	4. Do not keep facts from the client. The client has the right to know the diagnosis and to be a part of decisions about care.
5. Inform family about physiologic reasons for behavior, and teach them how to respond to client.	Family Support	5. The family needs to be informed about any abnormal behavior and how best to respond to it.
6. Use a consistent approach to inappropriate behavior; establish contracts if needed.	Anxiety Reduction, Behavior Management	6. Consistent approaches help the client relearn acceptable ways of personal expression.
7. Maintain nonjudgmental behavior.	Self-Esteem Enhancement, Emotional Support	7. The nurse realizes that the client's outbursts are not personal attacks but are due to the disease or feelings of loss of control.

Evaluation: Expect restoration of thought and behavior control to take weeks or months. Long-term coping by the family is important.

Nursing Diagnosis: Anticipatory Grieving related to potential loss of function, previous abilities, or life from brain cancer or surgery.

Outcomes: The client will have resolution of grief or progression through stages of grief, as evidenced by expressing feelings, maintaining hope, identifying problems with changes in body function, seeking help with anticipated problems, or developing realistic plans for the future.

NOC OUTCOMES   Aggression Control, Coping, Family Coping, Grief Resolution, Psychosocial Adjustment: Life Change

Interventions	NIC INTERVENTIONS	Rationales
1. Acknowledge reality, but do not force its acceptance.	Truth Telling, Active Listening, Emotional Support	1. Denial is a powerful defense mechanism; clients will examine reality when they are ready.
2. Establish regular time to spend with client, family members, and/or significant others for the exclusive purpose of discussing feelings and concerns.	Family Support, Active Listening, Emotional Support	2. Discussions about feelings can be difficult; giving the client time to plan and prepare facilitates the discussion.
3. If denial is beneficial, respond by listening with and reflecting statements by client.	Active Listening, Emotional Support	3. It is important to understand that not all clients reach acceptance of their disease; some remain in complete denial.
4. Accept emotions and assist client, family members, and/or significant others to clarify them.	Active Listening, Emotional Support, Family Support, Counseling	4. This measure reinforces the ideas that emotional response is normal and that family members should be accepting of the client at all stages of grief.
5. Assess perceptions about realistic goals and the future.	Truth Telling, Active Listening, Emotional Support	5. Inaccurate perceptions about the future can prevent or stall planning.
6. Have the client list those activities he or she wants to perform/resume.	Hope Instillation, Normalization Promotion	6. Plans for the future can be uplifting.

Evaluation: Expect each client and family to cope differently with grief over losses or impending death. Clients may go through the "typical" stages in order or go back and forth between them.

Transsphenoidal Approaches to the Pituitary

Clients with tumors of the pituitary gland have surgical options for excision of the tumor. The most direct approach is the transsphenoidal approach, across the sphenoid bone at the base of the skull. This may be accomplished endoscopically, through the nose, or through an incision at the junction of the inner aspect of the upper lip and gingiva above the teeth. The floor of the sella turcica in the sphenoid bone is opened and the tumor is removed (Figure 69-6). Fat or muscle grafts, using tissue from the inside cheek, abdomen, or upper thigh, may be implanted at the surgical site to assist in healing of the wound. Nasal packing may or may not be used. Pituitary tumors that are not able to be accessed through the transsphenoidal approaches may require a craniotomy to resect the tumor.

Postoperative Care Following Pituitary Surgery

Postoperative care after pituitary surgery using a transsphenoidal approach includes protection of the oral/gingival or incision site. Frequent oral hygiene is provided, and a cool vaporizer mist may be used to keep oral mucous membranes moist. The nasal drip pad ("moustache" dressing) is assessed frequently for blood or clear fluid (CSF). The donor site and dressings are also assessed, and dressings are changed as needed. The client must be instructed to avoid nose blowing or sneezing if possible.

A serious complication of pituitary surgery is the development of diabetes insipidus (DI). In most clients, the DI is temporary; however, in clients in whom the stalk of the pituitary is removed or damaged, DI is permanent. DI results from a decreased secretion of antidiuretic hormone (ADH). The clinical manifestations of DI are polyuria (large urine volumes) and polydipsia (increased thirst). Clients with DI produce large volumes

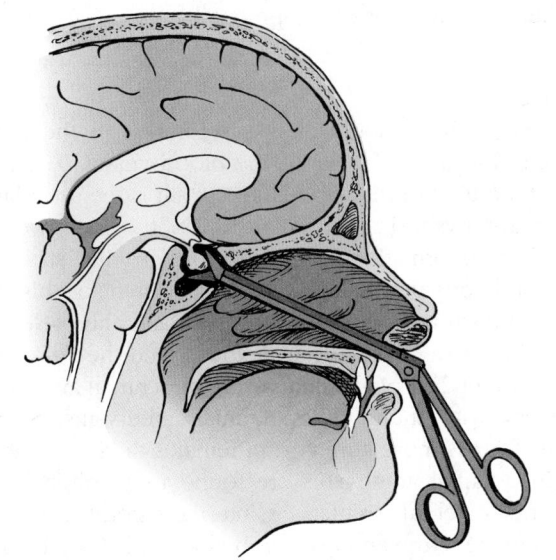

■ **FIGURE 69–6** Transsphenoidal approach to the excision of pituitary tumors.

(2 to 15 L/day) of dilute urine with a specific gravity of 1.005 or less. These clients require laboratory assessment of serum and urine sodium levels and serum osmolalities. If left untreated, dehydration quickly occurs. Circulatory collapse (hypovolemic shock) and hypertonic encephalopathy occur as a result of fluid shifts in the brain. Usual treatment is with fluid replacement first, and then IV vasopressin (Pitressin) or inhalation or oral desmopressin (DDAVP) if DI persists. Long-acting forms of these agents can be used to treat chronic DI.

Medical Management

After surgery, when an exact histologic diagnosis has been obtained, the client may be offered adjuvant therapy, including radiation therapy and chemotherapy. These modes of cancer treatment are discussed in Chapters 16 and 17; this material is also applicable to the care of clients with brain cancer.

Radiation Therapy

Conventional radiotherapy delivers radiation using a linear accelerator. The standard dose for primary brain tumors is approximately 6000 Gy given five times a week for 6 weeks. For clients with metastatic tumors, a standard dose of radiation is approximately 3000 Gy. The exact dose depends on tumor characteristics, volume of tissue to be irradiated, and the goals of radiation therapy. Radiation treatments are usually given over shorter periods of time to allow for protection of normal surrounding tissues. The cancer cells in CNS tumors tend to be more slowly dividing; therefore the tumor response often takes longer. This concept is important for clients to understand, because they may be disappointed when they do not see effects during or immediately following irradiation.

As in many areas of medicine, new methods of treatment and improved delivery devices are helping clients daily. This is also the case with radiation therapy. Newer methods of delivery and more sophisticated machines are available. Table 69-4 lists examples of advances made in the area of radiotherapy for clients with brain tumors. A recent development is an inflatable balloon-filled catheter with radioactive iodine 125 placed directly in the tumor bed (GliaSite Radiation Therapy System). Additional forms of radiation therapy, although not considered conventional and, more important, not readily available, are heavy particle radiation therapy, fast neutron radiotherapy, photodynamic therapy, and boron neutron capture therapy. Despite its wide use, radiation therapy is not without consequences. Effects may be acute, early, delayed, or late delayed (see Chapter 17).

Chemotherapy

As part of a multimodal approach, chemotherapy may be given before, during, or after other therapies. There

TABLE 69–4 Radiation Therapy Modalities for Treatment of Brain Tumors

Procedure	Description
Interstitial radiation (also called brachytherapy, tumor implants, tumor seeding, or radioactive pellets)	Temporary or permanent placement of radioactive substances in tumor bed Advantages: minimal effects to surrounding tissue Generally not advised in large tumors because of secondary swelling and edema Disadvantages: implantation requires a surgical procedure; because of radioactive substances, client must be protected and isolated to prevent exposure to family members and health care personnel
Stereotactic radiosurgery, stereotactic radiotherapy	Allows for a high dose of radiation beams to be directed precisely to a small brain tumor in a single session by localizing specific tumor site three dimensionally Gamma knife, Cyberknife, linear accelerator, or cyclotron is used to deliver radiation Best results when used on small, round, well-defined tumors Peacock technique incorporates stereotaxis, radiosurgery, and computers to deliver radiation exactly to tumor, skipping over vital areas that may be embedded in tumor such as nerves or blood vessels
Radiation sensitizing therapy	Use of various pharmacologic agents as "sensitizers" to make tumor more responsive to radiation therapy and other therapies
Intraoperative radiation	Direct irradiation of tumor while exposed in surgery; bypasses normal tissues
Conformal radiation	High or higher dose of external radiation "conformed" to match tumor's shape; goal is to deliver a uniform amount of radiation to entire tumor
Radioactive monoclonal antibodies	Antibodies that are cloned or mated to kill tumor cells

are several challenges in the use of chemotherapy in the treatment of brain tumors. The blood-brain barrier blocks chemotherapy from entering into the brain; however, some progress has been made. Recently, substances to open up the blood-brain barrier are being used. The osmotic diuretic mannitol may be used to disrupt the blood-brain barrier, allowing for greater drug concentration. There are also newer chemotherapeutic agents that cross the blood-brain barrier. Certain agents may enter and directly bind with the CSF or have a direct effect on the tumor. Brain tumor biology is still not well understood; hence it is difficult to find the optimal agent. Studies using newer agents have shown only minimal increase in survival, so research is ongoing.

Temozolomide is the most frequently used and effective chemotherapy agent for brain tumors. Nitrosoureas, for example, carmustine (BCNU) and lomustine (CCNU), are often used when temozolomide fails. Other agents are available. For the client with a brain tumor, the chemotherapy regimen may involve oral medication, IV solutions, intra-arterial routes, or intraventricular, intratumor, or epidural administration. Implanted devices, such as the Ommaya reservoir (see Chapter 17, Figure 17-3),[8] may also be used.

As with the treatment of any cancer invading the body and especially the brain, the hope lies in future research. Biologic response modifiers and modulation of the immune system are two of the keys that scientists hope may hold the answers.

The care of the client with a brain tumor is a challenging task for all involved. The client should not feel abandoned or uninformed during any portion of the care or treatment. To assist the client, family members, significant others, and the health care team, the American Cancer Society, the American Brain Tumor Association, and the National Brain Tumor Foundation are valuable resources.

SUBARACHNOID HEMORRHAGE

Subarachnoid hemorrhage (SAH) is bleeding into the subarachnoid space. Traumatic SAH develops from traumatic brain injury (TBI) (see Chapter 73). Spontaneous SAH is seen with intracranial aneurysms and arteriovenous malformations (AVMs). Other potential causes of spontaneous SAH include brain tumors (see earlier discussion), blood dyscrasias, and anticoagulant therapy.

Etiology
Spontaneous SAH occurs when an abnormal artery or vein ruptures and blood spills into the subarachnoid space or ventricles. In adults, aneurysms are the most common cause of SAH. Most intracranial aneurysms are either congenital or developmental.

Aneurysms
An intracranial aneurysm is a weakness in the tunica media, the middle layer of the blood vessel. The most common type of intracranial aneurysm is the saccular or berry aneurysm. The muscular walls of the artery weaken and lead to formation of a sac-like or berry-like structure.

Conditions that hasten the development of this type of aneurysm are smoking, hypertension, atherosclerosis, alcohol abuse, stimulant drug abuse, and the aging process. About 25% of all clients with intracranial aneurysms present with multiple intracranial aneurysms. Statistically, SAH is more common in females than in males.

Intracranial aneurysms are found more often in the anterior cerebral circulation (internal carotid artery and its branches—the anterior cerebral artery [ACA], the middle cerebral artery [MCA], and the posterior cerebral artery [PCA])—than in the posterior cerebral circulation, including the vertebral and basilar arteries. Intracranial aneurysms are found in locations where normal anatomic weaknesses occur—that is, in bifurcations and trifurcations.

Saccular aneurysms most commonly occur at the bifurcations of the large arteries at the base of the brain. Approximately 85% of aneurysms occur in the anterior circulation, mostly in the circle of Willis. The common sites include the junction of the anterior communicating artery with the ACA, the junction of the PCA with the internal carotid artery, and the bifurcation of the MCA. The top of the basilar artery, the junction of the basilar artery and the superior cerebellar artery or the anterior inferior cerebellar artery, and the junction of the vertebral artery and the posterior inferior cerebellar artery comprise most of the remaining sites of aneurysm formation.

Pathophysiology

As an aneurysm develops, it often forms a neck with a dome. The arterial internal elastic lamina disappears at the base of the neck. The media thins, and connective tissue replaces smooth muscle cells. At the site of rupture (most often the dome), the wall thins, and the tear that allows bleeding is often no more than 0.5 mm long. It is not possible to predict which aneurysms are likely to rupture, but limited data suggest that most ruptured aneurysms average 7 mm in diameter.

Blood byproducts from the SAH contribute to serious delayed effects. The most serious is vasospasm, defined as the constriction or narrowing of the cerebral vessels. In general, the more blood there is surrounding the arteries, the more likely there will be symptomatic vasospasm. Vasospasm causes ischemia and infarction and is the major cause of delayed morbidity or death following SAH.

Clinical Manifestations

Aneurysms found during incidental assessment, such as a work-up for headache, may be completely asymptomatic. More commonly, they are found after a SAH occurs. They may also produce symptoms without bleeding by placing pressure on adjacent structures as they enlarge. Once hemorrhage occurs, the symptoms are usually sudden and severe. The classic presentation is sudden onset of the "worst headache of my life." Hemorrhage is often accompanied by vomiting and generalized seizures may occur.

The client may lose consciousness immediately or may become confused and lethargic and gradually become comatose within hours, or the client may remain conscious and coherent. Manifestations of meningeal irritation (e.g., nuchal rigidity and pain, photophobia, back pain) are often present, caused by blood in the subarachnoid space. Depending on the location and size of the

aneurysm and the SAH, focal clinical manifestations may be noted (e.g., motor or sensory deficits, speech and cranial nerve deficits). Retinal hemorrhages may be present. Various grading scales have been developed. Table 69-5 presents criteria for the Hunt-Hess scale and the Fisher scale.

Manifestations of vasospasm appear 4 to 14 days after the hemorrhage, most frequently at about 7 days. The severity, duration, and distribution of vasospasm determine whether ischemia progresses to infarction. Manifestations of vasospasm vary according to the specific arterial territories involved. However, collateral blood flow may prevent the appearance of some expected manifestations. Spasm of the MCA typically causes contralateral hemiparesis and dysphasia (dominant hemisphere). Proximal ACA vasospasm causes bilateral leg weakness, abulia (faulty problem-solving), and incontinence, whereas severe vasospasm of the PCA causes hemianopia. Severe spasm of the basilar or vertebral arteries occasionally produces focal brain stem ischemia. All of these focal neurologic manifestations may develop over a few days, fluctuate, or present abruptly.

Diagnosis of SAH is usually based on history and physical examination. In about 80% to 90% of affected clients, enough blood is present to be visualized on a noncontrast CT scan. A small hemorrhage may not be seen on CT scan. If the scan fails to establish the diagnosis of SAH in the presence of symptoms, a lumbar puncture may be performed to look for the presence of subarachnoid blood. Lumbar puncture is contraindicated when ICP is elevated.

CT scan will also identify associated intracerebral clots, large clots surrounding an aneurysm, and the presence of hydrocephalus. Digital subtraction angiography or CT angiography is done to identify the presence,

TABLE 69–5 Grading Scales for Subarachnoid Hemorrhage	
Grade	**Clinical Criteria**
Hunt-Hess Clinical Grading Scale for Clients with Aneurysmal Subarachnoid Hemorrhage	
I	Alert, minimal headache
II	Alert, moderate to severe headache (cranial nerve palsy allowed)
III	Lethargic or confused, or mild focal deficit
IV	Stuporous, moderate to severe hemiparesis, possibly early decerebrate rigidity
V	Deep coma, decerebrate rigidity, moribund appearance
Fisher Scale for CT Grading of Clients with Aneurysmal Subarachnoid Hemorrhage	
1	No SAH on CT scan
2	Thin SAH (<1 mm)
3	Thick SAH (>1 mm)
4	Intracerebral or intraventricular hemorrhage, with no or thin SAH (<1 mm)

CT, Computed tomography; *SAH,* subarachnoid hemorrhage.

location, and configuration of an aneurysm; these same tests may be ordered during the peak time of vasospasm to identify the extent of vasospasm. Transcranial Doppler is a useful bedside tool to identify increased blood velocity indicative of vasospasm.

OUTCOME MANAGEMENT

Medical Management

The client with an SAH resulting from an intracranial aneurysm presents a multidisciplinary challenge. SAH constitutes a medical emergency, and clients with SAH are critically ill, cared for in an ICU. Definitive treatment is often instituted within 24 hours of onset of manifestations. Recovery is variable; one third of SAH survivors may succumb to the disease and another one third may have permanent sequelae.

The goals for the management of a client with SAH include preventing rebleeding, maintaining cerebral perfusion pressure, controlling ICP, minimizing effects of vasospasm, managing hydrocephalus, and managing cardiac dysrhythmias.

Prevent Rebleeding

Rebleeding is prevented by the neurosurgeon or interventional radiologist securing the aneurysm. While waiting for a securing procedure, the nurse must keep the client quiet and comfortable. Reducing hypertension may minimize rebleeding risk as well. Ongoing neurologic assessment is essential regardless of the setting in which care is provided. For the first 24 to 72 hours, the nurse examines the serial data to note trends in the neurologic assessments that suggest changes or deterioration. The LOC is the most sensitive and early indicator of neurologic change, usually evident before pupillary changes, new hemiparesis, or changes in respiratory patterns are noted. The onset of lethargy or restlessness may be the first clinical manifestation of increased ICP, hydrocephalus, or vasospasm.

Cardiac and respiratory function is also closely monitored, particularly because of the direct role in providing adequate cerebral perfusion pressure (CPP) and oxygen supply to the brain. Because cardiovascular disease is common in people with aneurysms, and since SAH can have cardiac complications, continuous electrocardiographic monitoring is necessary to identify life-threatening dysrhythmias. Pulse oximetry is imperative to monitor peripheral oxygen saturation. In the ICU setting, most clients have a central IV line or a pulmonary artery catheter in place to monitor hemodynamic status for prescription of fluids and vasoactive medications. Central venous pressure or pulmonary capillary wedge pressure measurements are used for targeted therapy to manage fluid administration.

Reduce Vasospasm

To prevent vasospasm, liberal isotonic fluids are used. If needed, volume expansion is added to promote cerebral perfusion. If vasospasm occurs, induced hypertension and hypervolemia are used. With the major goal of increasing cerebral blood flow and cerebral perfusion, the measures used have the potential to precipitate a cardiopulmonary crisis. Simply stated, if the client cannot tolerate an increase in fluid status or an increase in blood pressure, how can the vasospasm be relieved? Table 69-6 is a guide to various clinical interventions. The goal of

TABLE 69–6 Example Treatment Protocol for Vasospasm	
Interventions	**Rationales**
1. Glasgow Coma Scale and other neurologic assessments q 1 hr. Compare findings to baseline, and report changes.	1. Hourly observations allow early intervention when change occurs.
2. Maintain patent airway with Po_2 values >85 mm Hg and Pco_2 between 25 and 30 mm Hg.	2. Prevents cerebral hypoxia; hypercapnia increases cerebral blood flow.
3. Continuous hemodynamic monitoring of RAP, PAP, and PAWP. Perform CO/CI assessments as ordered. Titrate medications and fluids to maintain desired ranges. Usual ranges are as follows: ■ RAP: 1-7 mm Hg ■ PAWP (no congestion): 6-12 mm Hg ■ CI: >2.5 L/min ■ Target hematocrit is 33-38%. ■ Hypertensive goals are minimally hypertensive state (10 mm Hg above baseline), with SBP 110-160 mm Hg.	3. Hypervolemic, hemodilution, and hypertensive therapies are used to improve perfusion through cerebral vessels. Fluid balance must be monitored closely to prevent fluid volume overload.
4. Nimodipine (Nimotop) 60 mg q 4 hr for at least 3 weeks.	4. Calcium-channel blocker; promotes relaxation of blood vessels, decreasing vasospasm.
5. Morphine as required.	5. Sedative effect; allows for continuous monitoring.
6. Accurate I&O q 1 hr.	6. Fluid balance is crucial to maintaining CPP.

BP, Blood pressure; *CI*, cardiac index; *CO*, cardiac output; *CPP*, cerebral perfusion pressure; *I&O*, (fluid) input and output; *MAP*, mean arterial pressure; *PAP*, pulmonary artery pressur
PAWP, pulmonary artery wedge pressure; *RAP*, right atrial pressure; *SBP*, systolic blood pressure.

such therapies is to increase cerebral blood flow and cerebral perfusion pressure (CPP) without producing cerebral infarction or cardiopulmonary compromise. Angioplasty may be employed if medical measures fail; however, its success is limited.

Maintain Cerebral Perfusion Pressure

Medical and nursing management focuses on maintaining blood pressure to facilitate CPP. Once the aneurysm is secured, the blood pressure must be maintained to keep the systemic pressure at a level high enough to provide adequate CPP. Various medications and infusions are used to maintain the blood pressure approximately 10% above the client's normal pressure. In addition to medications supporting the blood pressure, blood products and albumin are used when indicated.

Surgical Management

Successful treatment of the aneurysm requires either a surgical procedure or an endovascular intervention (Figure 69-7). If surgery is the chosen treatment, several different procedures may be used; however, the one most commonly used is clipping of the intracranial aneurysm. Aneurysms not anatomically suited to clipping can be wrapped in a surgical gauze material and coated with an acrylic material.[49,67]

Aneurysm Clipping

Surgical obliteration of the aneurysm with a metal clip eliminates the risk of rebleeding. A craniotomy incision is used; the surgeon dissects down to the aneurysm and places a metal clip over the neck of the aneurysm. The craniotomy is then closed. Surgical obliteration of an aneurysm is usually performed within 24 hours of rupture. Medical instability, delay in transfer from one hospital to another, and client or family reluctance to seek medical care or consent to surgery may also delay prompt intervention.

Postoperatively, the client's neurologic status is carefully monitored. The usual postoperative care is given, including cardiac monitoring. As with any neurologic disorder, the physician must be promptly notified about any neurologic changes.

Endovascular Therapy and Embolization

An embolization procedure involves obliteration of the aneurysm by means of platinum coils. An interventional radiologist performs the procedure in an angiography suite. A cerebral angiogram is first performed to visualize the aneurysm. A small platinum coil is guided carefully into the aneurysm and then detached using a small current of electricity, leaving the coil to remain in the aneurysm. The process is repeated with as many coils as

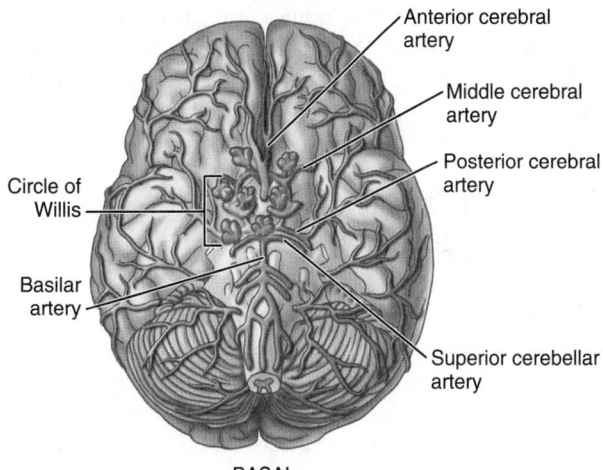

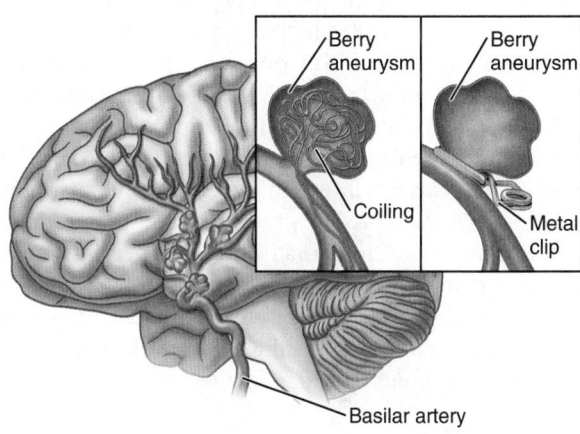

■ **FIGURE 69–7** Common locations of cerebral aneurysms are around the circle of Willis. Surgical resection of aneurysms includes clipping the neck of the aneurysm or inserting a coil into the sac to obliterate the aneurysm.

needed to block blood flow into the aneurysm but not through the adjacent vessel. As the aneurysm is embolized, it thromboses and closes off.

After embolization, the client is admitted to the ICU. The client may receive heparin for 12 to 24 hours after the procedure. The catheter sheath (from the angiogram site) remains in the femoral/groin area with a saline infusion to maintain patency of the artery. Care of the femoral/groin site includes assessing the puncture site for bleeding and hematoma formation, as well as frequent checking of peripheral pulses of the legs. The client remains flat in bed to avoid bending the leg at the groin. Nursing measures to maintain comfort are provided. Ongoing and frequent assessment of neurologic status is required.

Complications can result from the embolization procedure. If the aneurysm has not bled, there is a risk of rupture at the time of embolization. Ischemic stroke can occur if the coil does not stay in the aneurysm or if the parent vessel thromboses. Other problems may be related to the cerebral angiogram (see Chapter 67). Regardless of the treatment, the most important factor is the extent of SAH. Further details may be found in Chapter 70.

ARTERIOVENOUS MALFORMATIONS

Etiology and Pathophysiology

AVMs are vascular lesions in which there is a congenital lack of capillaries; a tangled array of arteries and veins form. Because of the lack of a capillary bed, the blood is shunted directly from the artery to the vein. At the core or center of the AVM is the major artery, referred to as the *nidus*. From the nidus are multiple feeding vessels. Blood flowing from the higher pressure arterial system after shunting to the lower pressure venous system can contribute to hemorrhage. AVMs range in size from small to those encompassing an entire hemisphere.

AVMs may be found in the brain or spinal cord. The majority of AVMs are found in the cerebral hemispheres. In the spinal cord, AVMs predominantly occur on the posterior aspect of the thoracic cord. Depending on the size of the malformation, the number of feeders, and the magnitude of circulatory steal, the AVM can bleed or undergo thrombosis, resulting in transient to permanent brain or spinal cord damage.

Clinical Manifestations

The onset of clinical manifestations may be seen at any age; however, increased incidence is noted in clients younger than 40 years of age. Manifestations are related to the anatomy of the malformation and the vessels involved, and occur as the result of the weakening of the vessels and of the shunting of blood in the tortuous mass. Manifestations may also be due to increasing size of the AVM. As the AVM expands, the anomalous vessels dilate and require more blood. The process of acquiring more blood flow is referred to as circulatory "steal." In this phenomenon, blood is diverted (stolen) from normal areas to maintain flow through the anomalous vessels. Consequently, localized hypoperfusion and hypoxia occur in the tissue adjacent to the AVM.

When the AVM bleeds, the client may present with any of the following: complaints of headache, seizures, or focal deficits. Bleeding may occur into the subarachnoid spaces or the brain tissue itself (intracerebral hemorrhage). Once an AVM has bled, there is a 25% chance of rebleeding.

OUTCOME MANAGEMENT

The management of an AVM is similar to that of an intracranial aneurysm. Nursing goals are comparable to those for aneurysm management, with limitation of activity,

seizure control, and blood pressure management. The goals of AVM treatment are complete and permanent obliteration of the lesion. This goal may be accomplished with surgery, endovascular embolizations, radiosurgery, or a combination of these methods. The client's condition and the characteristics of the AVM determine the course of treatment. For example, in a client who has had a large SAH, vasospasm may develop. In this case, treatment is delayed until the vasospasm is decreased or resolved. With an improvement in the clinical status of the client, a treatment plan can then be developed.[49,67]

Clients commonly require a combination of treatments. Surgical resection may be the preferred treatment. Depending on the size and location of the aneurysm, the client may undergo serial embolizations, and surgery is the final form of treatment. For the serial embolizations, a thrombosing agent, Histoacryl glue, may be used. The goal of the embolization is to place the glue as close to the nidus of the AVM as possible.

Another treatment option for cerebral AVMs is radiosurgery. This approach may constitute the main treatment or may be used in combination with other therapies. Radiosurgery consists of direction of a focused beam of radiation toward the nidus of the AVM. The dose delivered is determined by the size of the AVM. The use of radiotherapy is recommended with small AVMs.

The treatment and management of hemorrhagic cerebral disorders is an area of active research. For example, "liquid coils" (coils that take the shape within the vascular lesion), stent-assisted coils, and new coatings on currently used coils are being studied.

INFECTIONS

The brain and spinal cord are remarkably resistant to infection, but when they become infected, the consequences are usually very serious. Infections may be caused by bacteria, viruses, fungi, and occasionally protozoa or parasites. The most common types of brain infections are discussed here; others are presented in Table 69-7.

BACTERIAL MENINGITIS

Meningitis is characterized by inflammation of the meninges, the membranes lining the brain and spinal cord. Bacterial, viral, fungal, and parasitic organisms can all cause meningitis, but bacterial meningitis is by far the most common and this discussion will focus on bacterial meningitis.

Almost any bacteria entering the body can cause meningitis. The most common are meningococci (*Neisseria meningitidis*), pneumococci (*Streptococcus pneumoniae*), and *Haemophilus influenzae*. These organisms are often present in the nasopharynx. *S. pneumoniae*

TABLE 69–7 Central Nervous System Infections

Type of Infection	Organism	Clinical Manifestations	Management
Viral Infections			

Viral meningitis
Aseptic meningitis
	Mumps virus
	Picornaviruses
	Enteroviruses
	  (coxsackievirus,
	  echovirus)
		Drowsiness, headache, weakness, photophobia
		Nuchal rigidity (Brudzinski's sign)
		Spine stiffness with flexion (Kernig's sign)
		Blood in CSF
		Clinical manifestations usually resolve in 2 weeks
		Seizures may be present
			Symptomatic management to reduce
			  headache, control fever, and increase
			  general comfort
			Anticonvulsants for seizure
			Isolation

	Arthropod-borne
	virus (arbovirus)
		Unpredictable course of illness
		Acute fever, malaise, sore throat, vomiting, listlessness,
		  photophobia
		Later, mental deterioration, personality changes,
		  hemiparesis
		May develop coma or seizures
		Arbovirus encephalitis often leads to severe residual
		  disabilities including mental retardation, seizures,
		  blindness, deafness, speech disorders, and hemiplegia
			Symptomatic management with close
			  assessment for neurologic deterioration
			If antiviral medications, close
			  monitoring of vital signs, lungs, airway,
			  fluid balance, and serum electrolytes

	Herpes simplex 1	Similar to above, plus headache, fever, vomiting, and
		  seizures
		Permanent neurologic and mental disabilities are
		  common
		If not aggressively treated, will lead to brain herniation,
		  coma, and brain death
			Infectious agent confirmed with biopsy
			Symptomatic management with close
			  assessment for neurologic deterioration
			Acyclovir given early in course

Fungal Infections			

Granulomatous
  meningitis
	Cryptococcus	Concurrent diseases that reduce immune response
		Drowsiness, headache, weakness, photophobia, fever
		Nuchal rigidity
		Spine stiffness with flexion
		Cryptococci in CSF
			IV antifungal medications, such as
			  amphotericin B, flucytosine, and
			  fluconazole

Parasitic Infections			

Neurocysticercosis	Cysticercosis	Consumption of raw or undercooked pork by history
		May be asymptomatic unless near a vital portion of
		  brain, which leads to local manifestations
		CT or MRI shows cysts
			Praziquantel
			Surgical excision of cyst if medication
			  is ineffective

Toxoplasmosis	*Toxoplasma
	gondii*
		Most common opportunistic infection in clients with
		  AIDS
		Confusion, headache, lethargy, low-grade fever
		Focal manifestations of weakness, ataxia, speech
		  problems, apraxia, seizures, and sensory changes
		  (depending on location of mass)
		Multiple brain abscesses
			Pyrimethamine, sulfadiazine,
			  leucovorin, or clindamycin
			Symptomatic treatments

AIDS, Acquired immunodeficiency syndrome; *CSF,* cerebrospinal fluid; *CT,* computed tomography; *IV,* intravenous; *MRI,* magnetic resonance imaging.

and *N. meningitidis* are found most often in adults. Factors predisposing to bacterial meningitis include any circumstance where the dura has been compromised, such as open brain injury or brain surgery, systemic infection, anatomic defects of the skull, immunocompromise, and other systemic illnesses. Close quarters, poor hygiene, and malnutrition also place people at risk.

Pathophysiology

The route of entry into the intact CNS is uncertain. Invasion may occur through the choroid plexus (across the blood-brain barrier) or directly through an opening in the dura. Organisms colonize in the CSF, leading to inflammation of the meninges that contain it. Exudate forms, and the meninges become thickened, and adhesions form, leading to hydrocephalus. The arteries supplying the subarachnoid space may also become inflamed, leading to rupture or thrombosis of these vessels. If severe enough, underlying brain can become inflamed, leading to cerebral edema and increased ICP, as well as vasculitis and cerebral infarction. The CSF and meninges have no effective immune defense, so infections in this region can spread very quickly.

Clinical Manifestations

The classic manifestations of meningitis are nuchal rigidity (rigidity of the neck), Brudzinski's sign and Kernig's sign, and photophobia. To assess for *Kernig's sign,* begin

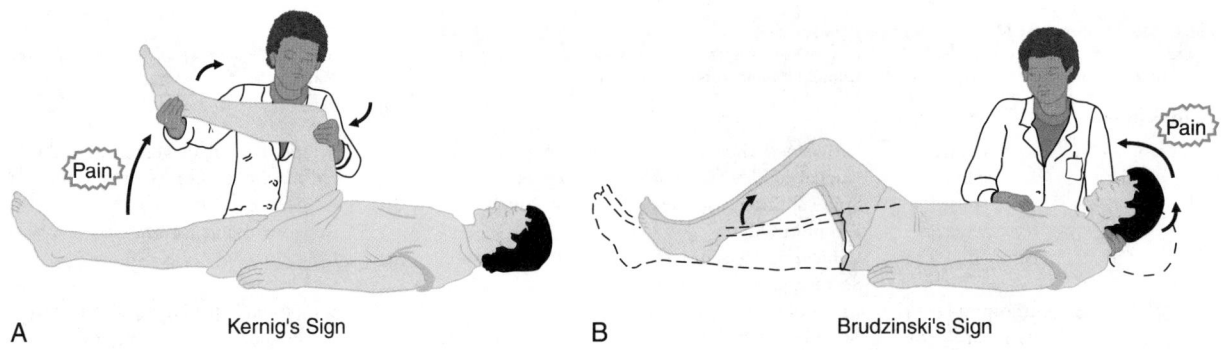

A   Kernig's Sign   B   Brudzinski's Sign

■ **FIGURE 69–8**   Assessment of meningeal irritation. Stretching the inflamed meninges by flexing the neck or legs causes pain. **A,** Kernig's sign. **B,** Brudzinski's sign.

with the client recumbent and the thigh flexed at a right angle to the abdomen, and with the knee flexed at a 90-degree angle to the thigh. Then extend the client's lower leg. In meningeal irritation, extending the leg upward causes pain, spasm of the hamstring muscles, and resistance to further leg extension at the knee (Figure 69-8, *A*). To assess for *Brudzinski's sign,* with the client supine lift the head rapidly up from the bed. If meningeal irritation is present, forward neck flexion produces flexion of both thighs at the hips and flexure movements of the ankles and knees (see Figure 69-8, *B*).

Other general manifestations related to infection may also be present, such as headache, fever, tachycardia, prostration, chills, fever, nausea, and vomiting. The client may be irritable at first, but, as the infection progresses, the client appears acutely ill and confused, stuporous, or comatose. Seizures may occur. A petechial or hemorrhagic rash may develop. Diagnosis is made by lumbar puncture. The CSF is cloudy. Gram stain of the CSF reveals organisms in 70% to 80% of cases. When the organism cannot be identified, bacterial antigens can be determined. *H. influenzae* is frequently detected with this technique. Clients with bacterial meningitis demonstrate the following:

- Moderately elevated CSF pressures
- Elevated CSF protein level (normal, 15 to 45 mg/dl)
- Decreased CSF glucose level (normal, 60 to 80 mg/dl, or two thirds of the serum glucose value)
- Elevated white blood cell count, usually increased (100 to 10,000/cm³), with predominantly polymorphonuclear leukocytes

OUTCOME MANAGEMENT

Bacterial meningitis constitutes a medical emergency. Prognosis varies according to the causative organism. The use of antibiotics has reduced the death rate to less than 5% for all types of bacterial meningitis. If untreated, it can be fatal within hours to days. Deaths most often occur in newborn infants and in older adults. Complications are rare

but may include septic shock, vasomotor collapse, seizures, and increased ICP attributable to hydrocephalus, brain swelling, and fluid overload. Residual neurologic deficits are rare in adults.

Medical diagnosis is made by assessment of clinical manifestations and is confirmed by isolating the causative organism from the CSF. Empirical therapy in bacterial meningitis includes cephalosporins, rifampin, and vancomycin. The empirical use of penicillin or ampicillin in the treatment of CNS infections is avoided because of the beta-lactamase–producing *H. influenzae* and *N. meningitidis*. It is believed that the cephalosporins are more potent against the beta-lactamase organisms. Chloramphenicol and trimethoprim-sulfamethoxazole are recommended for clients allergic to penicillin. Once the organism is known, antibiotics with greater sensitivity may be used. High doses of the appropriate antibiotic are usually prescribed for at least 10 days. Factors contributing to development of meningitis also need to be addressed.

A unique problem in treating CNS infection is that an intact blood-brain barrier prevents complete penetration of the antibiotic. However, inflammation inhibits the blood-brain barrier, so for a short time antibiotics penetrate the CNS. Antibiotics are given intravenously; the blood-brain barrier recovers as inflammation subsides, and high doses are required to reach the CSF.

If meningococcal meningitis is suspected, place the client in respiratory isolation and ensure that all personnel who had contact with the patient receive prophylaxis.

Adequate fluid and electrolyte balance must be maintained. Frequent assessment of the neurologic status is indicated to detect early manifestations of increasing ICP and seizures. Anticonvulsants may be prescribed for seizure prevention.

Outbreaks of meningitis can be a major health problem in the community, especially when they occur in schools. A vaccine is now available and is recommended for those living in tight quarters, such as dormitories or barracks.

ENCEPHALITIS

Encephalitis is an infection of the brain tissue that may be caused by a virus, bacterium, fungus, or parasite. Viral encephalitis is the most common and many different viruses can cause encephalitis. The disease course is extremely variable. Some viruses have a particular affinity for the nervous system, and the nervous system has a limited ability to mount a host response. Immunocompromised clients are at greatest risk for developing encephalitis, but the very young and very old are also at risk. Organisms can enter the body through oral or respiratory routes, or through animal or insect bites. Post-vaccine transmission can also occur.

Once the organisms invade the neuron, they replicate, and destroy the cell. The infection can be acute or the organism may remain latent and cause a more chronic type of infection years later. In acute encephalitis, the brain becomes inflamed, with a pathophysiology similar to that seen in brain involvement with bacterial meningitis. The exact pathophysiology varies and depends on the organism.

Clinical manifestations vary with the type of organism and the area of brain involved. Common manifestations include mild headache, low-grade fever, and mental status changes such as confusion. Hemiparesis, seizures, aphasia, and cranial nerve deficits may be seen. Diagnosis may be difficult. A comprehensive history must be obtained to include recent illnesses and immunizations, travel, and exposure to animals, birds, or insects. A lumbar puncture will show slight elevation in CSF protein with normal glucose level; lymphocytosis may be present. Enzyme-linked immunosorbent assay (ELISA) or other serologic assays may show elevated immunoglobulin M (IgM) (early) or IgG (late). Polymerase chain reaction (PCR) testing may be positive for specific antigens. It may take many days to weeks to get ELISA and PCR test results, so empirical care may be provided in the interim. Rarely, brain tissue biopsy is necessary to identify the organism.

OUTCOME MANAGEMENT

There is no specific treatment for encephalitis. Vaccines are available against eastern and western equine encephalitis. Prevention is an important factor; remaining indoors at dawn and dusk or, if outdoors, wearing long-sleeved clothing and using diethyltoluamide (DEET)-based insect repellants minimize the risk for insect and tick bites. Anti-inflammatory medications may be used for symptomatic relief while progressive cases of viral encephalitis may be treated with antiviral medications such as acyclovir. Complete supportive care is necessary during the time of acute illness; rehabilitation may be necessary for those with pre-existing neurologic deficits.

BRAIN ABSCESS

A brain abscess is a collection of pus within brain tissue arising from a primary focus elsewhere (e.g., ear, mastoid sinuses, nasal sinuses, heart, distal bones, lungs, or primary bacteremia). A brain abscess may occur after penetrating traumatic brain injuries or intracranial surgery. The frontal lobe is the most common site of a brain abscess. They vary in size; a large abscess may involve most of one cerebral hemisphere. Multiple abscesses are microscopic. Brain abscesses are relatively rare; when they do occur, they are most common in people younger than age 30. Morbidity and mortality increase greatly with multiple brain abscesses.

Staphylococci are the most common organisms in trauma-related cases; however, many organisms may be implicated. *Toxoplasma* is the usual agent found in clients with human immunodeficiency virus (HIV) infection.

In its early stages, the abscess produces inflammation, necrotic tissue, and surrounding edema. Within several days, the center of the abscess is purulent, and a wall of granulation tissue forms, encapsulating the abscess. Infection may spread through thin places in the wall of the capsule, resulting in development of additional abscesses.

Clinical manifestations of a brain abscess are essentially the same as those seen with any space-occupying brain lesion. Headache and lethargy are the most common manifestations. Manifestations of infection (e.g., fever, chills) are present about half the time. The client may experience drowsiness, confusion, and a depressed mental status as a result of the cerebral edema; increasing ICP; and intracranial effects of the brain abscess. Transient focal neurologic disorders (e.g., weakness on one side, loss of speech) occur when the abscess is located in a specific area such as the motor or speech area. Early manifestations may subside, and then within a few days or weeks, indications of increasing ICP may develop (e.g., recurrent headaches, changes in level of consciousness, focal or generalized seizures).

Medical diagnosis of a brain abscess is made by CT or MRI. However, the appearance is similar to a brain tumor and misdiagnosis is possible.

OUTCOME MANAGEMENT

Pyogenic brain abscess may be treated either with 6 to 12 weeks of antibiotic therapy or with antibiotics combined with surgical aspiration or craniotomy for excision. Needle aspiration may be performed stereotactically (guided by CT imaging) with the use of local anesthesia. Corticosteroids may also be given to reduce cerebral edema. Penicillin is the antibiotic of choice for this type of infection. When antibiotics are used to treat the abscess, follow-up CT or MRI scans are used to monitor progress.

HEADACHE

Headache, the most common of pains, may occur either in the absence of organic disease or as a manifestation of serious disease. Most headaches are transient and of only moderate or slight severity. However, a few types are chronic, intense, and recurrent over a period of months or years. Headache is a manifestation of an underlying disorder, rather than a disease itself. The cause of headache must be identified so that appropriate treatment can be given.

Clients often self-treat headaches with over-the-counter medications. Most headaches do not indicate serious disease. However, some headaches and headache patterns require more complete assessment, as shown in the Critical Monitoring feature below. Serious disorders that typically produce headache include intracranial tumors and hemorrhage, CNS infections, acute systemic infections, severe hypertension, and acute or chronic diseases of the eye, ear, or nose.

Assessment of headaches may include detailed history, psychosocial assessment, and physical examination. Neurologic assessment is particularly important. Possible neurologic diagnostic tests include CT, MRI, EEG, and lumbar puncture with CSF examination.

History should determine (1) location of the pain, intensity, and paths of radiation; (2) character of the headache (e.g., sharp, dull, throbbing); (3) mode of headache onset, duration, and frequency; (4) methods used to treat the headache; (5) presence of localized tenderness; (6) associated phenomena or precipitating factors; and (7) familial incidence.

Classification and Etiology
Tension Headaches
Tension headaches result from muscle contraction (Figure 69-9, *A*). This type of headache is described as a tight band-like discomfort that is unrelenting, with few headache-free intervals. The pain typically builds slowly, fluctuates in severity, and may persist more or less continuously for many days. Triggers include fatigue and stress. The diagnosis of tension headache is confirmed when the headaches occur more often than 15 days a month. Clients may report that the head feels as if it is in a vise or that the posterior neck muscles are tight. In some clients, anxiety or depression coexists with tension headache.

Cluster Headaches
Cluster headaches are classified as a form of migraine (see Figure 69-9, *B*). These headaches have a cyclical pattern of one to three short-lived attacks of periorbital pain lasting from 4 to 8 weeks, with an increased incidence in spring and fall. These headaches also have quiescent periods lasting months to years. Cluster headaches occur more often in men.

The headache lasts between 15 minutes and 3 hours. It may occur from every other day to eight times each day and may awaken the client from sleep. The pain is described as deep, boring, intense pain of such severity

CRITICAL MONITORING

Headache

Headaches are the most common form of pain and most headaches are due to primary causes, such as migraines or tension. However, headache requires further evaluation when any of the following exists:

- There is a significant change in the progression or pattern of the pain.
- The pain recurs in one particular area, such as over the eye or in the temple.
- The pain is described as "the worst headache" the client has ever had.
- The pain is severe and begins abruptly, waking the client from sleep.
- The client also has neck stiffness or fever.
- The client had a recent injury to the head.
- The client has neurologic changes lasting more than 1 hour, or loss of consciousness.
- There is a change in vision, such as light waves in the line of vision.
- The headache is present in clients with cancer, immunosuppression, or pregnancy.
- The headache is triggered by physical exertion, sexual activity, or the Valsalva maneuver.

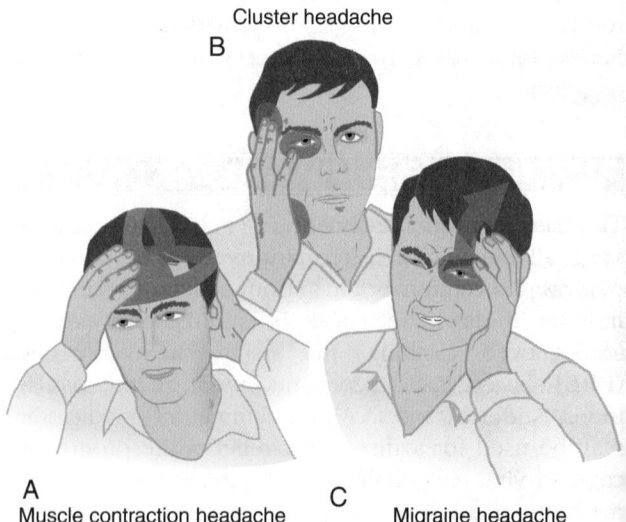

Cluster headache
B

A
Muscle contraction headache

C
Migraine headache

■ **FIGURE 69–9** Types of headaches. The red areas show the regions of greatest pain. **A,** Muscle contraction headache. **B,** Cluster headache. **C,** Migraine headache.

that the client has difficulty remaining still. The client may also develop Horner syndrome with constricted pupils, injected conjunctiva, unilateral lacrimation, and rhinorrhea during the headaches. Cluster headaches are triggered by consumption of alcohol.

The most satisfactory treatment is the administration of drugs to prevent cluster attacks until the bout is over. Effective prophylactic drugs are prednisone, lithium, methysergide, ergotamine, and verapamil. Lithium appears to be particularly useful for the chronic form of the disorder. A 10-day course of prednisone, followed by a rapid taper, may interrupt the pain bout for many clients.

For the attacks themselves, oxygen inhalation (9 L/min via a loose mask) is the most effective modality; inhalation of 100% oxygen for 15 minutes is often necessary. The self-administration of intranasal lidocaine, either 4% topical or 2% viscous, to the most caudal aspect of the inferior nasal turbinate can produce a ganglionic block that is usually remarkably effective in terminating an attack.

Migraine Headaches

Migraine headache is often considered to be a "vascular" headache, with vasospasm and ischemia of intracranial vessels being the cause of the pain (see Figure 69-9, *C*). These headaches usually begin in puberty and are more common in women, often associated with hormonal changes following the menstrual cycle. About 66% of cases of migraine are familial.

Migraine headaches last between 4 and 72 hours, with headache-free intervals between attacks. The headache is most often unilateral, but pain may occur on alternate sides with different attacks. Pain is described as throbbing and pulsatile. Photophobia, phonophobia, anorexia, nausea, vomiting, and focal neurologic manifestations are often present. Some clients have a visual aura that precedes the headache by 10 to 60 minutes (usually 20 minutes). The client sees a jagged edge of light in the visual fields. Other premonitory manifestations occur 12 to 24 hours before an attack and may include euphoria, fatigue, yawning, and craving for sweets. Migraine headache can be triggered by relief of intense stress, missing meals, or tyramine-rich foods. The Client Education Guide above, right lists additional triggers and stress-management interventions.

Typically, the client finds pain reduction in a quiet, dark environment. When aspirin and acetaminophen alone fail, the addition of butalbital, caffeine, ibuprofen (600 to 800 mg), and naproxen (375 to 750 mg) is often useful. Isometheptene compound, one to two capsules, is effective for mild to moderate "common migraine." When these measures fail, more aggressive therapy should be considered. Drug absorption is impaired during migrainous attacks because of reduced gastrointestinal motility. Delayed absorption occurs in the absence of nausea and is related to the severity of the attack and not

---

CLIENT EDUCATION GUIDE

Migraine Headache

- Many things can trigger a migraine headache. Find out what triggers your headaches and avoid those triggers. If this is not possible, consult your physician about adjusting the dosage of your medication.
- If menstruation and ovulation are triggers, consult your physician for adjustments to your medication dosage.
- Alcohol temporarily increases the diameter of your blood vessels (a process called vasodilation), which may trigger migraines.
- Some foods, such as chocolate, cheese, citrus fruits, coffee, pork, and dairy products, contain substances that may trigger migraines.
- Low food intake may lead to a low blood glucose (sugar) level (hypoglycemia), which can trigger migraines. Eat small, frequent meals to decrease this risk.
- Stress management is essential. Adjust your lifestyle to reduce fatigue and exposure to bright sunlight, heat, or humidity. Get enough sleep. If you are having trouble managing the stresses in your life, seek expert guidance.

---

its duration. Therefore when oral agents fail to cure, alternative therapies, including rectal ergotamine, subcutaneous or intranasal sumatriptan, sublingual zolmitriptan, parenteral dihydroergotamine, and IV chlorpromazine and prochlorperazine, should be tried. Narcotics should be avoided if possible. The Complementary and Alternative Therapy feature on p. 1840 presents one alternative therapy that is effective and inexpensive, with minimal side effects.

A number of drugs have the capacity to stabilize migraine. They must be taken daily. The decision to use daily medication as a prophylactic measure depends on the frequency of attacks and on how well acute treatment is working. The occurrence of at least two or three attacks per month may be an indication for this approach. There is usually a lag of 2 weeks before an effect is seen. The major drugs are propranolol, amitriptyline, valproate, verapamil, phenelzine, and methysergide.

Lumbar Puncture Headaches

Loss of CSF volume with lumbar puncture decreases the brain's supportive cushion. Headache after lumbar puncture usually begins within 48 hours but may be delayed for up to 12 days. Head pain is dramatically positional; it begins when the client sits or stands upright, and reduction is obtained upon reclining or with abdominal compression. The longer the client is upright, the longer the latency before head pain subsides. It is worsened by head shaking and jugular vein compression. The pain is usually a dull ache but may be throbbing; its location is occipitofrontal. Nausea and stiff neck often accompany

High-Dose Vitamin B₂ (Riboflavin) for Headaches

Because of the high cost and side effects of current migraine drug treatments, there is ongoing interest in alternative and cheaper options. For example, in a controlled trial, 55 clients were randomized to 3 months of vitamin B_2 (riboflavin) 400 mg once a day or placebo for 3 months. Clients were included who experienced 2 to 8 migraines a month. Responders were defined as those having a 50% reduction in manifestations. The two groups were similar in terms of age, co-morbidities, and severity of migraine at baseline. After 3 months of treatment, the number of migraines per month for clients taking riboflavin was reduced from 3.83 to less than 2 ($P = .0001$), with parallel reductions in the number of days ($P = .0001$) and the duration of migraines ($P = .018$). There were no changes in the placebo group. These changes were moderate but were also significant. Headache severity and medication use during headache did not change. Side effects were minimal; only one riboflavin recipient left the study, complaining of diarrhea after 2 weeks. Health professionals should keep in mind that riboflavin may work more slowly than other agents (taking 2 to 3 months to reach full effect). High doses of other B vitamins such as B_6 (pyridoxine) may cause peripheral neuropathy. Clients should be warned about the potential of this vitamin to create fluorescent yellow urine, as well as not attempting to obtain the 400 mg of B_2 with a multivitamin, which contains other toxic vitamins in excess. Thus clients should take B_2 as a separate individual supplement.

REFERENCE

Schoenen, J., Jacquy, J., & Lenaerts, M. (1998). Effectiveness of high-dose riboflavin in migraine prophylaxis: A randomized controlled trial. *Neurology, 50*, 466-470.

headache, and occasionally blurred vision, photophobia, tinnitus, and vertigo are reported. The pain usually resolves over a few days but may sometimes persist for weeks to months.

Treatment with IV caffeine sodium benzoate promptly terminates headache in most clients. An epidural blood patch accomplished by injection of 15 ml of autologous whole blood rarely fails for those who do not respond to caffeine. The mechanism for these treatment effects is not certain. The blood patch has an immediate effect, making it unlikely that sealing off a dural hole with a blood clot is its mechanism of action.

Postconcussion Headaches and Syndrome

After seemingly trivial head injuries and particularly after rear-end motor vehicle collisions, many clients report varying combinations of headache, dizziness, vertigo, and impaired memory. Anxiety, irritability, and difficulty with concentration are other hallmarks of *postconcussion syndrome*. Manifestations may remit after several weeks or persist for months and even years after the injury.

Postconcussion headaches may occur whether or not a client was rendered unconscious by head trauma. Typically, findings on neurologic examination are normal, with the exception of the behavioral abnormalities. Chronic subdural hematoma may on occasion mimic this disorder. Although the cause of postconcussive headache disorder is not known, it should not in general be viewed as a primary psychological disturbance. It often persists long after the settlement of pending lawsuits.

Treatment is symptomatic support. Repeated encouragement that the syndrome eventually remits is important.

Other Causes of Headache

Head pain may also develop from disorders of the eyes, ears, teeth, and paranasal structures. Headaches may result from errors of refraction, glaucoma (with increased intraocular pressure), inflammation, and ocular muscle disturbances (see Chapter 65). Pain associated with sinus infection is usually caused by irritation and inflammation of sinus openings. Sinus walls are less sensitive. The pain of a sinus headache may be reduced or eliminated by decongestants and analgesics. Sometimes antibiotics are needed. Surgery to drain the sinuses may also be required (see Chapter 60).

CONCLUSIONS

Because of the complexity of brain disorders and the emotional reactions of the client and family members to these problems, neurologic nursing is one of the most challenging areas of nursing practice. Common nursing problems center on cerebral perfusion and cognition as well as on those related to functional rehabilitation. Prevention and early intervention are key to optimal client outcome.

THINKING CRITICALLY

1. A client suffered a temporal lobe contusion from a motor vehicle accident 3 days ago. He is disoriented to time and place and has short-term memory deficits. During your assessment of the client, he stops answering questions and begins tonic movements of his extremities.

Factors to Consider. What are the highest priorities for this client? What are the interventions related to these priorities? What interventions come next? What significance does the site of injury have?

2. A client with a history of headaches, dizziness, and vertigo experienced a first-time seizure at age 27 years. Immediately after the episode, he noted the onset of blurred vision. Subsequent studies revealed the presence of a brain tumor, and cranial surgery was

scheduled. Two days after surgery, the client is transferred to the regular unit. What are your responsibilities regarding monitoring for an increase in intracranial pressure? What are the general interventions for the client after craniotomy?

Factors to Consider. What is the major complication following intracranial surgery? How do the general interventions prevent complications associated with this type of surgery?

3. You are caring for a client who had a malignant brain tumor resected 72 hours ago. During previous assessments, she was alert and oriented; her pupils were equal, round, reactive to light, and accommodative (PERRLA); her eyes opened spontaneously; and she was moving all four extremities equally and on command. Her Glasgow Coma Scale score was 15. Now, however, she is slow to respond although still oriented to person, place, and time. Her right pupil is equal in size to the left but exhibits a sluggish reaction to direct light. Her left pupil responds normally. She still responds to verbal commands appropriately, has equal motor strength, and opens her eyes spontaneously. Thus her score on the Glasgow Coma Scale is still 15. You decide to notify the physician. Why?

Factors to Consider. How sensitive is the Glasgow Coma Scale? What abnormality may be indicated by the decreased response time and the change in pupil reaction?

4. A 33-year-old woman, Miss Brown, arrives in the emergency department with a severe headache. She has vomited twice. She states, "This is the worst headache I have ever had." The headache has lasted for about 6 hours, and two doses of acetaminophen have given no relief. Miss Brown cannot lift her head off of the pillow or position herself for comfort. Her pupils are equal, and there is no diaphoresis. What further nursing history and assessments should be done? How soon can medication to alleviate the headache be administered?

Factors to Consider. How crucial is a thorough pain assessment? How can a migraine headache mimic manifestations of a cerebral disorder? Would it be advisable to delay giving an analgesic? Why? Why not?

Discussions for these questions can be found on the website.

BIBLIOGRAPHY

Citations appearing in red refer to primary research.

Citations appearing in blue refer to evidence-based practice guidelines and protocols.

1. American Brain Tumor Association. (2000). *A primer of brain tumors* (7th ed.). Chicago: Author.
2. Anderson, S.I., et al. (1999). Mood disorders in patients after treatment for primary intracranial tumors. *British Journal of Neurosurgery, 13*(5), 480-485.
3. Angelle, D. (2002). Brain attack. *Leading Medicine, 1*(Spring), 8-12.
4. Bader, M.K., & Littlejohns, L.R. (2004). *AANN core curriculum for neuroscience nursing* (4th ed.). Philadelphia: Elsevier.
5. Breslau, N., et al. (2000). Headache and major depression. *Neurology, 54*(2), 308-313.
6. Broderick, S., Connolly, E., Feldmann, D., et al. (2007). Guidelines for the management of spontaneous intracerebral hemorrhage in adults: 2007 update: A guideline from the American Heart Association/American Stroke Association Stroke Council, High Blood Pressure Research Council, and the Quality of Care and Outcomes in Research Interdisciplinary Working Group. *Stroke, 38*(6), 2001-2023.
7. Buffalo Neurosurgery Group. (2003). *Endoscopic endonasal removal of pituitary tumors.* Accessed July 2007 from www.buffaloneuro.com/cranial/brain%20tumors.htm.
8. Central Brain Tumor Registry for the United States (CBTRUS), Accessed December 2007 from www.cbtrus.org
9. Clinical Guideline 20. (2004). *The epilepsies: The diagnosis and management of the epilepsies in adults and children in primary and secondary care.* Accessed July 2007 from www.nice.org.uk/CG020NICEguideline.
10. Columbia-Presbyterian Department of Neurological Surgery. (2003). *Endoscopic neurosurgery.* Accessed July 2007 from www.cumc.columbia.edu/dept/nsg/NSGCPMC/specialties/endoscopy.html.
11. Dunleavy, K., Finck, A., Overstreet, W., et al. (2005). Doing it better: Putting research into practice. Improving care of patients with subarachnoid hemorrhage. *Nursing, 35*(11), 26-27.
12. Engle, J., & Pedley, T.A. (Eds.) (2007). *Epilepsy—A comprehensive textbook* (Vol. I, II, and III). Philadelphia: Lippincott, Williams and Wilkins.
13. Faylor, C.R. (1999). Using transcranial Doppler to augment the neurological examination after aneurysmal subarachnoid hemorrhage. *Journal of Neuroscience Nursing, 31*(5), 285-293.
14. Gahart, B., & Nazareno, A. (2008). *Intravenous medications* (24th ed., pp. 362-365). St. Louis: Mosby.
15. Gibson, P.A. (2005). Beyond pharmacologic therapy: Quality of life issues and counseling needs of the newly diagnosed patient. *Advanced Nursing Studies, 3*(3), 79-84, 91–93.
16. Gusa, D. (2004). Clinical updates. Aneurysmal subarachnoid hemorrhage. *Journal of Continuing Education in Nursing, 35*(4), 150-151.
17. Kaniecki, R. (2003). Headache assessment and management. *Journal of the American Medical Association, 289*(11), 1430-1433.
18. Krapohl, B.D., Keutinger, M., & Komurcu, F. (2007). Research for practice. Vagal nerve stimulation: Treatment modality for epilepsy. *MEDSURG Nursing, 16*(10), 39-44.
19. Laino, C. (2003). Changes in brain function associated with recovery identifiable two weeks after stroke. *Neurology Today*, September, 45-46.
20. Lawal, M. (2005). Epilepsy management. Management and treatment options for epilepsy. *British Journal of Nursing, 14*(16), 854-858.
21. Lech, J., Dungay, J., & Dowson, A. (2006). Headache management in primary care. *Primary Health Care, 16*(9), 25-31.
22. Longatti, P., Fiorindi, A., DiPaola, F., et al. (2006). Coiling and neuroendoscopy: A new perspective in the treatment of intraventricular hemorrhages due to bleeding aneurysms. *Journal of Neurology, Neurosurgery, and Psychiatry, 77*(12), 1354-1358.
23. Mayo Clinic. (2003). *Treatment options for brain tumors.* Accessed July 2007 from www.mayoclinic.org/braintumors.
24. McLendon, R.E., Bigner, D.D., & Rosenblum, M.K. (Eds.) (2006). *Russell and Rubinstein's pathology of tumors of the nervous system* (7th ed.). London: Hodder Arnold.
25. Minton, M. (1999). Primer of neuroanatomy and neurophysiology. *Nursing Clinics of North America, 34*(3), 555-572.
26. Moloney, M.F., et al. (2000). Caring for the woman with migraine headaches. *Nurse Practitioner, 25*(2), 17-41.
27. Morrison, S.R. (1997). Guglielmi detachable coils: An alternative therapy for surgically high-risk aneurysms. *Journal of Neuroscience Nursing, 29*(4), 232-237.
28. Mower-Wade, D., Cavanaugh, M.C., & Bush, D. (2001). Protecting the patient with a ruptured cerebral aneurysm. *Nursing, 31*(2), 52-58.
29. Myers, F. (2000). Meningitis: The fears, the facts. *RN, 63*(11), 52-58.
30. Rogers, G. (2003). Emerging guidance for epilepsy. *Primary Health Care, 13*(6), 39-41.
31. Rowan, J.A., & Tuchman, L. (2003). Management of seizures in the elderly. *Profiles in Seizure Management, 2*(4), 4-9.

32. Schiller, Y., et al. (2000). Discontinuation of antiepileptic drugs after successful epilepsy surgery. *Neurology, 54*(2), 346-349.

33. Schmidek, H.H., & Roberts, D.W. (2005). *Schmidek's and Sweet's operative neurosurgical techniques* (5th ed., Vol. I and II). Philadelphia: Saunders.

34. Shafer, P.O. (1999). Epilepsy and seizures—Advances in seizure assessment, treatment and self-management. *Nursing Clinics of North America, 34*(3), 743-759.

35. Shafer, P.O. (2005). Improving quality of life in adults with new-onset epilepsy. *Advanced Studies in Nursing, 3*(4), 120-125, 139-141.

36. Shah, S.M., & Kelly, K.M. (2007). *Emergency, neurology—Principles and practice.* Cambridge: Cambridge University Press.

37. Shuttleworth, A. (2004). Implementing new clinical guidelines on epilepsy management. *Nursing Times, 100*(45), 28-29.

38. Spencer, D.C., et al. (2000). The role of intracarotid amobarbital procedure in evaluation of patients for epilepsy. *Surgery, 42*(3), 302-325.

39. Snively, C., et al. (1998). Vagal nerve stimulator as a treatment for intractable epilepsy. *Journal of Neuroscience Nursing, 30*(5), 286-289.

40. Stewart-Amidei, C. (2005). Managing symptoms and side effects during brain tumor illness. *Expert Reviews in Neurotherapeutics, 5,* S71-S76.

41. Vitners, H.V. (1998). *Diagnostic neuropathology.* New York: Marcel Dekker.

42. Winn, H.R. (2004). *Youmans' neurological surgery: A comprehensive reference guide to the diagnosis and management of neurosurgical problems.* Philadelphia: Elsevier.

43. Wisniewski, A. (2203). Combating infection. Closing in on clues to encephalitis. *Nursing, 33*(4), 70-71.

evolve **Did you remember to check out the bonus material on the Evolve website and the CD-ROM, including NCLEX®-Examination Style Review Questions, Open-Book Quizzes, and Chapter Review Audio Podcasts?**

http://evolve.elsevier.com/Black/medsurg

CHAPTER 70

Management of Clients with Stroke

LISA BOWMAN

STROKE

Stroke is a term used to describe neurologic changes caused by an interruption in the blood supply to a part of the brain. The two major types of stroke are *ischemic* and *hemorrhagic*. Ischemic stroke is caused by a thrombotic or embolic blockage of blood flow to the brain. Bleeding into the brain tissue or the subarachnoid space causes a hemorrhagic stroke. Ischemic strokes account for about 83% of all strokes. The remaining 17% of strokes are hemorrhagic.

Cerebrovascular disorders are the third leading cause of death in the United States and account for about 150,000 mortalities annually. An estimated 550,000 people experience a stroke each year. When second strokes are considered in the estimates, the incidence increases to 700,000 per year in the United States alone. Stroke is a leading cause of adult disability and a leading primary diagnosis in long-term care. More than 4 million stroke survivors are living with varying degrees of disability in the United States. Along with a high death rate, strokes produce significant morbidity in people who survive them. Of stroke survivors, 31% require assistance with self-care, 20% require assistance with ambulation, 71% have some impairment in vocational ability up to 7 years following the stroke, and 16% are institutionalized.

Before 1995 health care professionals could offer only supportive measures and rehabilitation to stroke survivors. Thrombolytic therapies can prevent or limit the extent of damage to brain tissue caused by acute ischemic stroke. Thrombolytic therapy must be administered as soon as possible after onset of the stroke; a treatment window of 3 hours from the onset of manifestations has been established. To convey this sense of urgency regarding the evaluation and treatment of stroke, health care professionals now refer to stroke as a *brain attack*. Public education is focused on prevention, recognition of manifestations, and early treatment.

Etiology and Risk Factors

Blood flow to the brain can be decreased in several ways. Ischemia occurs when the blood supply to a part of the brain is interrupted or totally occluded. Ultimate survival of ischemic brain tissue depends on the length of time it is deprived plus the degree of altered brain metabolism. Ischemia is commonly due to thrombosis or embolism (Figure 70-1). Thrombotic strokes are more common than embolic strokes.

Strokes can also be "large vessel" and "small vessel." Large vessel strokes are caused by blockage of a major cerebral artery, such as the internal carotid, anterior cerebral, middle cerebral, posterior cerebral, vertebral, and basilar arteries. Small vessel strokes affect smaller vessels that branch off the larger vessels to penetrate deep into the brain.

Thrombosis

A thrombus starts with damage to the endothelial lining of the vessel. Atherosclerosis is the primary culprit. Atherosclerosis causes fatty material to deposit and form plaques on vessel walls. These plaques continue to enlarge and cause stenosis of the artery. Stenosis alters the usual smooth flow of blood through the artery. Blood swirls around the irregular surface of the plaques, causing platelets to adhere to the plaque. Eventually the

---

evolve **Web Enhancements**

Case Management Stroke

Case Study Meningioma, Fractured Hip, and Possible Stroke

Client Education Guide Transfer from Bed to Wheelchair by a Hemiplegic Client (Spanish Translation)

Clinical Pathway Stroke

Be sure to check out the bonus material on the Evolve website and the CD-ROM, including free self-assessment exercises. **http://evolve.elsevier.com/Black/medsurg**

■ **FIGURE 70–1** **A,** Events causing stroke. **B,** Hemorrhagic stroke caused by blood leaking into brain tissue and ischemic stroke caused by clot blocking the blood supply to area in brain.

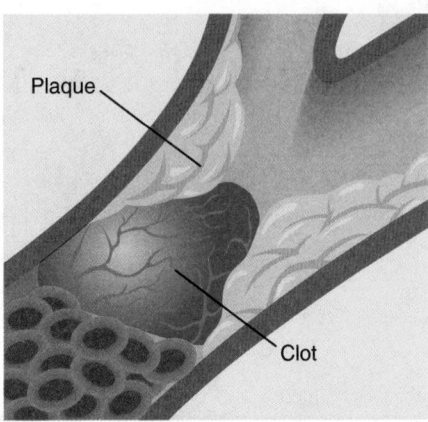

Thrombotic stroke. Cerebral thrombosis is a narrowing of the artery by fatty deposits called *plaque*. Plaque can cause a clot to form, which blocks the passage of blood through the artery.

A

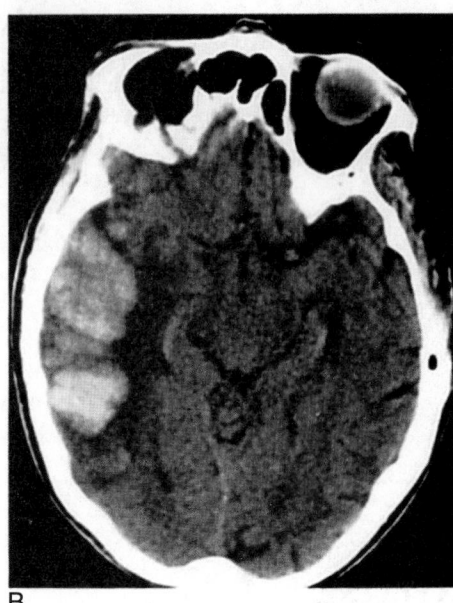

B

vessel lumen becomes obstructed. Rarely occlusion is due to inflammation of the arteries, called *arteritis* or *vasculitis*.

A thrombus can develop anywhere along a carotid artery or its branches. A common site is at the bifurcation of the common carotid into the internal and external carotid arteries. Thrombotic stroke is the most common type of stroke in people with diabetes.

Lacunar strokes are small vessel strokes. The endothelium of smaller vessels is affected primarily by hypertension, which causes a thickening of the vessel wall and stenosis. Lacunar infarctions are also common in people with diabetes mellitus.

Embolism

The occlusion of a cerebral artery by an embolus causes an embolic stroke. An embolus forms outside the brain, detaches, and travels through the cerebral circulation until it lodges in and occludes a cerebral artery. A common embolus is plaque. A thrombus can detach from the internal carotid artery at the site of an ulcerated plaque and travel into the cerebral circulation. Chronic atrial fibrillation is associated with a high incidence of embolic stroke. Blood pools in the poorly emptying atria. Tiny clots form in the left atrium and move through the heart and into the cerebral circulation. Mechanical prosthetic heart valves have a rougher surface than the normal endocardium and can also cause an increased risk of clots. Both bacterial and nonbacterial endocarditis can be sources of emboli. Other sources of emboli include tumor, fat, bacteria, and air. Any cerebrovascular territory may be affected. The incidence of cerebral embolism increases with age.

Hemorrhage

Most intracerebral hemorrhages are caused by the rupture of arteriosclerotic and hypertensive vessels, which causes bleeding into brain tissue. Intracerebral hemorrhage is most often secondary to hypertension and is most common after age 50 years. Aneurysms are another cause of hemorrhage. Aneurysms are weakened outpouchings in a vessel wall. Although cerebral aneurysms are usually small (2 to 6 mm in diameter), they can rupture. An estimated 6% of all strokes are caused by aneurysm rupture.

Stroke secondary to bleeding often produces spasm of cerebral vessels and cerebral ischemia because the blood outside of the vessels acts as an irritant to the tissues. Hemorrhagic stroke usually produces extensive residual functional loss and has the slowest recovery of all types of stroke. The overall mortality of intracerebral hemorrhage varies between 25% and 60%. The volume of the hemorrhage is the single most important predictor of client outcome. Therefore it is not surprising that hemorrhage into the brain causes the most fatalities of all strokes.

Other Causes

Cerebral arterial spasm, caused by irritation, reduces blood flow to the area of the brain supplied by the constricted vessel. Spasm of short duration does not necessarily cause permanent brain damage.

Hypercoagulable states, including protein C and protein S deficiencies and disorders of the clotting cascade, can cause thrombosis and ischemic stroke. Compression of cerebral vessels may result from a tumor, large blood clot, swollen brain tissue, brain abscess, or other disorders. These causes are fairly rare.

Risk Factors

The incidence of stroke and stroke mortalities has gradually declined in many industrialized countries in recent years as a result of increased recognition and treatment of risk factors. Modifiable risk factors can be reduced or eliminated through lifestyle changes. Hypertension is the most important modifiable risk factor for both ischemic and hemorrhagic stroke. Adequate blood pressure control is associated with a 38% reduction in stroke incidence.

Cardiovascular disease and atrial fibrillation are also associated with an increased risk of stroke. The Complementary and Alternative Therapy feature below discusses elevated homocysteine levels. Diabetes mellitus increases the risk of stroke and morbidity and mortality after stroke. The mechanism is related to macrovascular changes in people with diabetes mellitus. Prior stroke, carotid stenosis, and a history of transient ischemic attacks (TIAs) are considered modifiable risk factors for stroke. Reduction in the risk factors for initial stroke may prevent stroke recurrence. Early recognition and treatment of carotid stenosis and treatment of TIAs with antiplatelet agents reduce the risk of stroke.

Other modifiable risk factors for stroke include hyperlipidemia, cigarette smoking, heavy alcohol consumption, cocaine use, and obesity. Current research suggests that although heavy alcohol consumption increases one's risk of a stroke, light or moderate alcohol consumption may protect against ischemic stroke. Stroke is uncommon in women of childbearing age; however, high-dose estrogen oral contraceptives combined with hypertension, cigarette smoking, migraine headaches, and increasing age increase the risk of stroke in women. The Complementary and Alternative Therapy feature below examines whether vitamin E has any value in preventing stroke.

Client education is aimed at stroke prevention. *Primary* prevention of stroke includes the following:

- Maintaining an ideal body weight
- Maintaining safe cholesterol levels
- Smoking cessation
- Using low-dose estrogen contraceptives only in the absence of other risk factors
- Reducing heavy alcohol consumption
- Eliminating illicit drug use

Secondary prevention includes the following:

- Adequate blood pressure control
- Care of diabetes mellitus
- Treatment of cardiovascular disease, TIA, and atrial fibrillation

Nonmodifiable risk factors cannot be prevented or treated. Advancing age is one of the most significant risk factors for stroke. The incidence of stroke in men is

---

COMPLEMENTARY AND ALTERNATIVE THERAPY

Elevated Homocysteine Levels and Stroke

A recent meta-analysis of studies from 1966 to 1999 was conducted to evaluate the ability of homocysteine levels to predict heart disease or stroke. A total of 30 studies were found (12 prospective and 18 retrospective) that met the inclusion criteria. Researchers found that lower plasma homocysteine levels were associated with a modest reduction in cardiovascular disease (CVD) risk, but a true causal association cannot be concluded. None of the studies that were reviewed adjusted for the presence of renal impairment, a condition known to increase both plasma homocysteine levels and risk for CVD. Also, genetic studies and large intervention trials are required to establish causation. Interestingly, plasma homocysteine levels can be lowered in most clients using 1 mg/day oral folic acid, with or without vitamins B_{12} and B_6. Some researchers suggest that until ongoing primary and secondary prevention trials of homocysteine reduction and CVD are completed, the measurement of homocysteine levels should be done only in those with unexplained premature CVD.

REFERENCE

The Homocysteine Studies Collaboration. (2002). Homocysteine and risk of ischemic heart disease and stroke: A meta-analysis. *Journal of the American Medical Association, 288*, 2015-2022.

COMPLEMENTARY AND ALTERNATIVE THERAPY

Vitamin E and Stroke

In a randomized, controlled clinical trial of 29,133 Finnish male smokers, the overall net stroke morbidity and mortality with alpha-tocopherol (vitamin E) and beta-carotene was not significantly different from that of the placebo group. However, a trend toward higher rates of subarachnoid hemorrhages was found (relative risk [RR] = 1.5, number needed to harm = 833), but the cerebral infarction rate was decreased (RR = 0.86, number needed to treat = 239).[2] The Italian GISSI* study of 11,324 clients with a recent myocardial infarction showed no effect of vitamin E on the combined outcomes of death, myocardial infarction, and stroke.[1] Therefore recommending vitamin E supplements for cardiovascular disease reduction cannot be advocated at this time.

REFERENCES

1. GISSI Investigators. (1999). Dietary supplementation with n-3 polyunsaturated fatty acids and vitamin E after myocardial infarction: Results of the GISSI Prevenzione Trial. *Lancet, 354*, 447-455.
2. Leppala, J., et al. (2000). Controlled trial of alpha-tocopherol and beta-carotene supplements on stroke incidence and mortality in male smokers. *Arteriosclerosis, Thrombosis, and Vascular Biology, 20*, 230-235.

*Gruppo Italiano per lo Studio della Streptochinasi Nell'Infarto Miocardico (Italian Group for the Study of Streptokinase in Myocardial Infarction).

slightly higher than that in women. Stroke is also more prevalent in African Americans than in whites or Hispanics. This difference is probably related to the increased incidence of hypertension and diabetes mellitus in this group. Family history of stroke increases one's risk for stroke.

Pathophysiology

The brain is very sensitive to a loss of blood supply. Hypoxia can cause cerebral ischemia because unlike other body tissues, such as muscle, the brain cannot use anaerobic metabolism in the absence of oxygen and glucose. The brain is perfused at the expense of other less vital organs to preserve cerebral metabolism. Short-term ischemia leads to temporary neurologic deficits or a TIA. If blood flow is not restored, brain tissue sustains irreversible damage or infarction within minutes. The extent of infarction depends on the location and size of the occluded artery and the adequacy of collateral circulation to the area it supplies.

Ischemia quickly alters cerebral metabolism. Cell death and permanent changes can occur within 3 to 10 minutes. The client's baseline oxygen level and ability to compensate determine how quickly irreversible changes occur. Blood flow can be altered by localized perfusion problems, such as stroke, or by generalized perfusion problems, such as hypotension or cardiac arrest. Cerebral perfusion pressure must fall to two thirds of normal (a mean arterial pressure of 50 mm Hg or below assuming a normal baseline) before the brain does not receive adequate blood flow. A client who has lost compensatory autoregulation experiences manifestations of neurologic deficit sooner.

Decreased cerebral perfusion is usually caused by occlusion of a cerebral artery or intracerebral hemorrhage. Occlusion produces ischemia in the brain tissue supplied by the affected artery and edema in the surrounding tissue. Cells in the center of the stroke area, or the core, die almost immediately after stroke onset; this is referred to as *primary neuronal injury*. A zone of hypoperfusion also exists around the infarcted core; this zone is called the *penumbra*. The size of this zone depends on the amount of collateral circulation present. Collateral circulation describes the vessels that augment the major circulatory vessels of the brain. Differences in the size and number of collateral vessels help to explain variations in the severity of manifestations experienced by clients with strokes in the same anatomic area.

A cascade of biochemical processes occurs within minutes of cerebral ischemia. Neurotoxins, including oxygen free radicals, nitric oxide, and glutamate, are released. Local acidosis develops. Membrane depolarization occurs. This results in an influx of calcium and sodium. Cytotoxic edema and cell death are a result; this is secondary neuronal injury. Penumbral neurons are

highly susceptible to the effects of the ischemic cascade. The area of edema after ischemia may lead to temporary neurologic deficits. Edema may subside in a few hours or sometimes in several days, and the client may regain some function.

Clinical Manifestations
Early Warnings

Some strokes have early warning signs, called transient ischemic attacks (TIAs, see later discussion also). Manifestations of impending ischemic stroke include *transient* hemiparesis, loss of speech, and hemisensory loss. Manifestations of a thrombotic stroke develop over minutes to hours to days. The slow onset is because the thrombus is still increasing in size. First there is partial, and then complete, occlusion of the affected vessel. In contrast, manifestations of embolic strokes occur suddenly and without warning.

Hemorrhagic stroke also occurs rapidly, with manifestations developing over minutes to hours. Common manifestations include severe occipital or nuchal headaches, vertigo or syncope, paresthesias, transient paralysis, epistaxis, and retinal hemorrhages.

Manifestations of deficit must persist longer than 24 hours to be diagnostic of stroke. TIAs are focal neurologic deficits lasting less than 24 hours.

Generalized Findings

Most clients are hypertensive when arriving in the emergency department. General findings of stroke unrelated to specific vessel sites include headache, vomiting, seizures, changes in mental status, fever, and changes on the electrocardiogram (ECG). ECG changes may include atrial fibrillation, which can help indicate the cause of the stroke. Recent myocardial infarction can be seen with T-wave changes, shortened PR interval, prolonged QT interval, premature ventricular contractions, sinus bradycardia, and ventricular and supraventricular tachycardias. Subarachnoid hemorrhage (SAH) can lead to ST-segment and T-wave abnormalities also. Fever can indicate hypothalamic injury.

Specific Deficits After Stroke

Stroke manifestations can be correlated with the cause (Table 70-1) and with the area of the brain in which perfusion is impaired (Table 70-2). The middle cerebral artery is the most common site of ischemic stroke. The client's deficit also varies according to whether the dominant or the nondominant side of the brain is affected. The degree of deficit can also vary from little impairment to serious functional loss.

Hemiparesis and Hemiplegia. *Hemiparesis* (weakness) or *hemiplegia* (paralysis) of one side of the body may

TABLE 70–1 **Clinical Manifestations of the Various Causes of Stroke**

Cause	Clinical Manifestations
Thrombosis	Tends to develop during sleep or within 1 hour of arising
	Ischemia is produced gradually; therefore clinical manifestations develop more slowly than those caused by hemorrhage or emboli
	Relative preservation of consciousness
	Hypertension
Embolism	No discernible time pattern, unrelated to activity
	Clinical manifestations occur rapidly, within 10-30 seconds, and often without warning
	May have rapid improvement
	Relative preservation of consciousness
	Normotension
Hemorrhage	Typically occurs during active, waking hours
	Severe headache and nuchal rigidity occur (if client is able to report manifestations)
	Rapid onset of complete hemiplegia, occurs over minutes to 1 hour
	Usually results in extensive, permanent loss of function with slower, less complete recovery
	Rapid progression into coma

occur after a stroke. These deficits are usually caused by a stroke in the anterior or middle cerebral artery, leading to an infarction in the motor strip of the frontal cortex. Complete hemiplegia involves half of the face and tongue as well as the arm and leg of the ipsilateral side of the body. Infarction in the right side of the brain causes left-sided hemiplegia and vice versa because nerve fibers cross over in the pyramidal tract as they pass from the brain to the spinal cord. Strokes causing hemiparesis or hemiplegia usually affect other cortical areas in addition to the motor strip. As a result, hemiparesis and hemiplegia are often accompanied by other manifestations of stroke, including hemisensory loss, hemianopia, apraxia, agnosia, and aphasia. Muscles of the thorax and abdomen are usually not affected because they are innervated from both cerebral hemispheres.

Over time, when voluntary muscle control is lost, strong flexor muscles overbalance the extensors. This imbalance can cause serious contractures. For example, a hemiplegic client's affected arm tends to rotate internally and to adduct because adductor muscles are stronger than abductors. The elbow, wrist, and fingers also tend to flex. The affected leg tends to rotate externally at the hip joint, flex at the knee and plantar flex, and supinate at the ankle joint (Figure 70-2).

Aphasia. *Aphasia* is a deficit in the ability to communicate. Aphasia may involve any or all aspects of communication, including speaking, reading, writing, and understanding spoken language. The primary language center is usually located in the left cerebral hemisphere

and is affected by stroke in the left middle cerebral artery. Several different types of aphasia exist; the most common are described here.

Wernicke's (sensory or *receptive) aphasia* affects speech comprehension as a result of an infarction in the temporal lobe of the brain. *Broca's (expressive* or *motor) aphasia* affects speech production as a result of an infarction in the frontal lobe of the brain. Branches of the middle cerebral artery supply both areas. *Global aphasia* affects both speech comprehension and speech production.

Other methods of classifying aphasia are by fluency or by the degree of difficulty in articulation. Clients with fluent aphasia (Wernicke's) have speech that is well articulated and grammatically correct but lacks content. Clients with nonfluent aphasia (Broca's) have varying degrees of difficulty in producing speech, and what words are spoken are uttered slowly, with great effort and poor articulation. Clients with global aphasia typically repeat the same sounds they hear and have poor comprehension.

Sensory or fluent aphasias involve loss of the ability to comprehend written, printed, or spoken words. A client with acoustic aphasia can hear the sounds of speech, but the parts of the brain that give meaning to these sounds are damaged. Clients have difficulty understanding what is being said. They hear sound but cannot make sense of it because they cannot understand the symbolic communication associated with the sound. Visual aphasia is similar. Affected clients cannot read words but can see them. They cannot understand the symbolic content of printed or written symbols.

Motor or nonfluent aphasias include aphasias in which the ability to write, make signs, or speak is lost. For example, with motor aphasia, words may be recalled but the client cannot combine speech sounds into words and syllables. Pure motor or pure sensory aphasias are rare. Most aphasias are mixed, affecting both expressive and receptive elements.

Most aphasias are partial rather than complete. The severity of aphasia varies with the area involved and the extent of cerebral damage. Severe damage may deprive the client of any meaningful relationship with the environment and family. Global aphasia can be so extensive that neither expressive nor receptive language abilities are retained. Early determination of the client's yes-no reliability facilitates communication. Verbal skills are often the best. Reading and writing are usually more impaired. The use of gestures can aid in communication.

Aphasia is frequently associated with hemiplegia involving the dominant hemisphere. The speech center for a right-handed client is usually located in the left cerebral hemisphere; the speech center for a left-handed client may be in the brain's right or left side. Thus a right-handed client with right-sided hemiplegia usually has

TABLE 70–2 Clinical Manifestations of Stroke Associated with Area of Brain Affected

Location	Middle Cerebral Artery	Anterior Cerebral Artery	Posterior Cerebral Artery
Motor changes	Contralateral hemiparesis or hemiplegia, face and arm deficits greater than leg	Contralateral hemiparesis, foot and leg deficits greater than arm, footdrop, gait disturbances	Mild contralateral hemiparesis (with thalamic or subthalamic involvement) Intention tremor
Sensory changes	Contralateral hemisensory alterations Neglect of involved extremities	Contralateral hemisensory alterations	Diffuse sensory loss (thalamic)
Visual or ocular changes	Homonymous hemianopia Inability to turn eyes toward affected side	Deviation of eyes toward affected side	Pupillary dysfunction (brain stem) Loss of conjugate gaze, nystagmus Loss of depth perception Cortical blindness Homonymous hemianopia
Speech changes	Dyslexia, dysgraphia, aphasia	Expressive aphasia	Perseveration Dyslexia
Mental changes	Memory deficits	Confusion, amnesia Flat affect, apathy Shortened attention span Loss of mental acuity	Memory deficits
Other changes	Vomiting may occur	Apraxia (inability to carry out purposeful movements in unaffected areas) Incontinence	Visual hallucinations
Contralateral hemiparesis with facial asymmetry	Alternating motor weaknesses Ataxic gait, dysmetria (uncoordinated actions)	Ipsilateral ataxia Facial paralysis	Ataxia Paralysis of larynx and soft palate
Contralateral sensory alterations	Contralateral hemisensory impairments	Ipsilateral loss of sensation in face, sensation changes on trunk and limbs	Ipsilateral loss of sensation in face, contralateral on body
Homonymous hemianopia	Double vision Homonymous hemianopia	Nystagmus	Nystagmus
Ipsilateral periods of blindness (amaurosis fugax)	Nystagmus, conjugate gaze paralysis		
Aphasia if dominant hemisphere is involved	Dysarthria Memory loss Disorientation		Dysarthria
Mild Horner syndrome	Drop attacks	Horner syndrome	Horner syndrome
Carotid bruits	Tinnitus, hearing loss Vertigo Dysphagia Coma or locked-in syndrome	Tinnitus, hearing loss	Hiccups and coughing Vertigo Nausea, vomiting

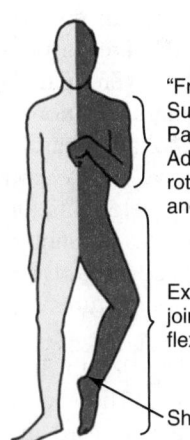

"Frozen" shoulder
Subluxation of the shoulder
Painful shoulder-hand dystrophy
Adduction of arm with internal rotation; flexion of elbow, wrist, and fingers

External rotation of leg at hip joint; flexion at knee; and plantar flexion and supination at ankle

Shortened heel cord

■ **FIGURE 70–2** Hemiplegic contractures. The elbow is bent, the wrist is flexed, and the fingers are curled into palmar flexion; the knee is bent and the heel cord is shortened.

aphasia because the speech center is in the damaged left hemisphere. Most people have left-sided speech dominance.

Dysarthria. *Dysarthria* is imperfect articulation that causes difficulty in speaking. It is important to differentiate between dysarthria and aphasia. With dysarthria the client understands language but has difficulty pronouncing words and may slur them, enunciating poorly. No disturbance is evident in grammar or in sentence construction. A dysarthric client can understand verbal speech and can read and write (unless the dominant hand is paralyzed, absent, or injured).

Dysarthria is caused by cranial nerve (CN) dysfunction from a stroke in the vertebrobasilar artery or its branches. It may result from weakness or paralysis of the muscles of the lips, tongue, and larynx or from a loss of sensation. In addition to speaking problems, clients with dysarthria often have difficulty chewing and swallowing because of poor muscle control.

Dysphagia. Swallowing is a complex process that requires the function of several cranial nerves. The mouth must open (CN V), the lips must close (CN VII), and the tongue must move (CN XII). The mouth must sense the quantity and quality of the food bolus (CN V and VII) and must send messages to the swallowing center (CN V and IX). During swallowing, the tongue moves the food bolus toward the oropharynx. The pharynx elevates and the glottis closes. Contraction of the pharyngeal muscles transports food from the pharynx to the esophagus. Peristalsis moves food to the stomach. A stroke in the territory of the vertebrobasilar system causes dysphagia.

Apraxia. *Apraxia* is a condition that affects complex motor integration and therefore can result from a stroke in several areas in the brain. Clients who have apraxia cannot carry out a skilled act such as dressing even when they are not paralyzed. A client with apraxia may be able to conceive or conceptualize the content of messages to send to muscles. The motor patterns or schema necessary to convey the impulse message cannot be reconstructed, however. Thus accurate "instructions" do not reach the limb from the brain, and the desired action or movement does not happen. Apraxia ranges from relatively simple to highly complex disorders. For example, a client may have less difficulty writing than speaking or vice versa.

Visual Changes. Vision is a complex process controlled by several areas in the brain. Parietal and temporal lobe strokes may interrupt visual fibers of the optic tract en route to the occipital cortex and impair visual acuity. Depth perception and visual perception of horizontal and vertical planes may also be impaired. In clients with hemiplegia, this causes motor performance problems in gait and posture (Figure 70-3). Clients may or may not be aware of a perceptual difficulty, but it may cause them to be accident prone, and their behavior may appear bizarre. Visual disorders can interfere with a client's ability to relearn motor skills. Infarcts affecting the function of CN III, IV, and VI may produce CN palsies and result in diplopia.

Homonymous Hemianopia. *Homonymous hemianopia* (Figure 70-4) is a visual loss in the same half of the visual field of each eye, so the client has only half of normal vision. For example, the client may see clearly on one side of the midline but see nothing on the other side. Clients with homonymous hemianopia cannot see past the midline without turning the head toward that side.

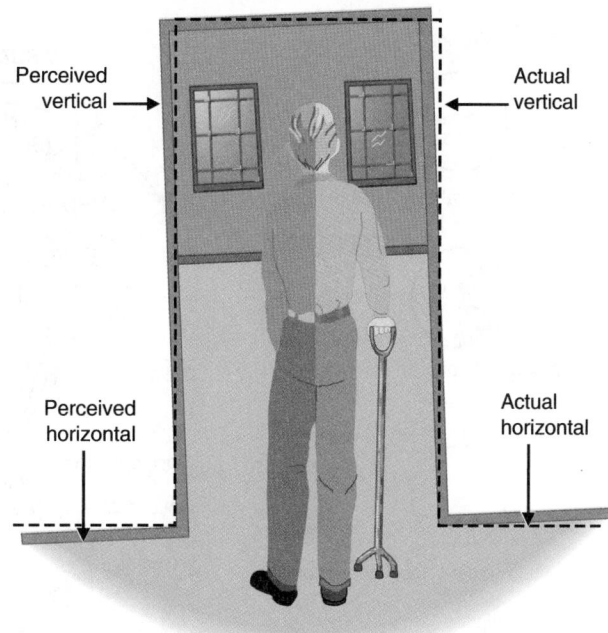

■ FIGURE 70–3 Perceptual disturbances in left-sided hemiplegia. Such disturbances can be both unpleasant and unsafe.

Horner Syndrome. *Horner syndrome* is paralysis of the sympathetic nerves to the eye, causing sinking of the eyeball, ptosis of the upper eyelid, slight elevation of the lower lid, constriction of the pupil, and lack of tearing in the eye.

Agnosia. *Agnosia* is a disturbance in the ability to recognize familiar objects through the senses. The most common types are visual and auditory. Agnosia may result from an occlusion of the middle or posterior cerebral arteries supplying the temporal or occipital lobes.

A client with visual agnosia sees objects but is unable to recognize or attach meaning to them. Disorientation occurs because of an inability to recognize environmental cues, familiar faces, or symbols. Such a client may examine objects curiously but might be unable to determine their function. This can cause considerable self-care deficit when common, necessary objects, such as silverware, clothing, or toilet articles, are unfamiliar. Visual agnosia greatly increases the risk for injury because the client cannot recognize danger or symbols that warn of danger. Extensive visual agnosia can produce such extreme behavioral effects that the client's condition may be inaccurately diagnosed as diffuse dementia.

A client with auditory agnosia cannot attach meaning to sounds in the absence of hearing loss or decreased level of consciousness. Some degree of aphasia is almost always present. Often these people are initially considered hysterical or psychotic.

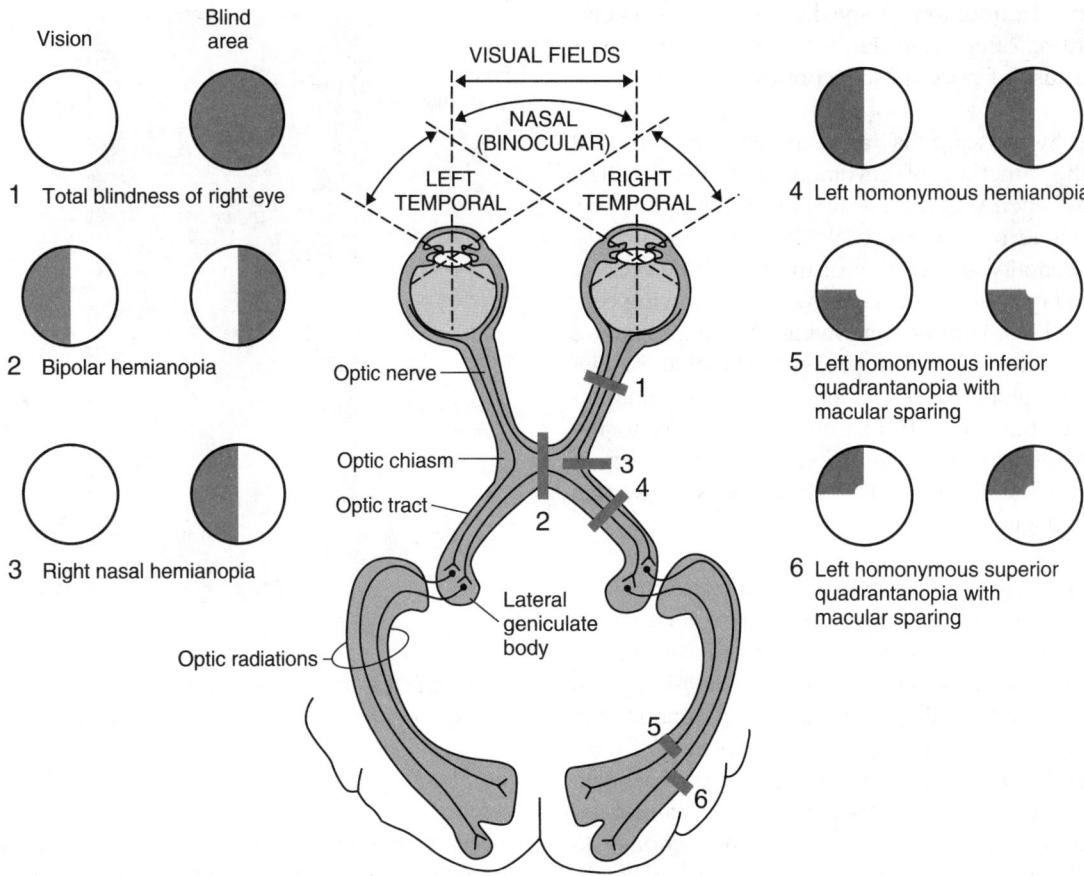

■ **FIGURE 70–4** Visual-field defects associated with optic nerve lesions.

Unilateral Neglect. *Unilateral neglect* is the inability of a person to respond to a stimulus on the contralateral side of a cerebral infarction. Clients with injury to the temporo-parietal lobe, inferior parietal lobe, lateral frontal lobe, cingulate gyrus, thalamus, and striatum as a result of a middle cerebral artery occlusion most commonly develop neglect. Because of the dominance of the right hemisphere in directing attention, neglect is most commonly seen in clients with right hemisphere damage.

Clinical manifestations of unilateral neglect include failure to (1) attend to one side of the body, (2) report or respond to stimuli on one side of the body, (3) use one extremity, and (4) orient the head and eyes to one side. Unilateral neglect may be accompanied by inaccurate beliefs about the position of a limb in space or its existence or ownership. For example, a man with unilateral neglect may not believe that his arm is part of his body, he may be unaware of his arm's position, or he may deny that a limb is paralyzed when it is.

Sensory Deficits. Several types of sensory changes can result from a stroke in the sensory strip of the parietal lobe supplied by the anterior or middle cerebral artery. The deficit is on the contralateral side of the body and is frequently accompanied by hemiplegia or hemiparesis. *Hemisensory loss* (a loss of sensation on one side

of the body) is generally incomplete and may not be noticed by the client. The superficial sensations of pain, touch, pressure, and temperature are affected in varying degrees. *Paresthesia* is described as persistent, burning pain; feelings of heaviness, numbness, tingling, or prickling; or heightened sensitivity. *Proprioception* (the ability to perceive the relationship of body parts to the external environment) and postural sense disturbances may occur with loss of muscle-joint sense. This may seriously interfere with the client's ability to ambulate because of a lack of balance control and inappropriate movements. The risk of falling is high because of the tendency to malposition the feet when walking.

Behavioral Changes. Various portions of the brain assist with control of behavior and emotions. The cerebral cortex interprets stimuli. The temporal and limbic areas modulate emotional responses to stimuli. The hypothalamus and pituitary glands coordinate the motor cortex and language areas. The brain can be seen as a modulator of emotions, and when the brain is not fully functional, emotional reactions and responses lack this modulation.

Behavioral changes after a stroke are common. People with stroke in the left cerebral, or dominant, hemisphere are frequently slow, cautious, and disorganized

People with stroke in the right cerebral, or nondominant, hemisphere are frequently impulsive, overestimate their abilities, and have a decreased attention span, which increases their risk of injury. Frontal lobe infarcts from a stroke in the anterior or middle cerebral arteries can lead to disturbances in memory, judgment, abstract thinking, insight, inhibition, and emotion. The client may exhibit a flat affect, a lack of spontaneity, distractibility, and forgetfulness. The client may have emotional lability and burst into tears or, less commonly, laughter without provocation. There is little or no relationship between the emotion and what is occurring in the person's environment. Significant clinical depression occurs in 25% to 60% of clients with strokes. Because depression can interfere with rehabilitation and functional recovery, it is important to identify it and initiate treatment.

Incontinence. Stroke may cause bowel and bladder dysfunction. One type of neurogenic bladder, an uninhibited bladder, sometimes occurs after stroke. Nerves send the message of bladder filling to the brain, but the brain does not correctly interpret the message and does not transmit the message not to urinate to the bladder. This results in frequency, urgency, and incontinence. Sometimes clients with a type of neurogenic bowel seem fixated on having a bowel movement. Other causes of incontinence may be memory lapses, inattention, emotional factors, inability to communicate, impaired physical mobility, and infection. The duration and severity of the dysfunction depend on the extent and location of the infarct.

Diagnostic Findings

With the advent of thrombolytic therapy in the treatment of acute ischemic stroke, accurate brain imaging plays an important role in the diagnosis and treatment of stroke. A noncontrast computed tomography (CT) scan of the head is performed to rule out hemorrhagic stroke as a cause of acute neurologic deficits. Cellular changes that are diagnostic of stroke do not appear on the head CT scan acutely. Standard magnetic resonance imaging (MRI) has limited value in diagnosing acute ischemic stroke because the infarct is usually not apparent until 8 to 12 hours after the onset of symptoms. New MRI techniques—diffusion-weighted imaging (DWI) and perfusion imaging (PI)—may improve the diagnosis and treatment of acute stroke. These techniques have greater sensitivity and anatomic resolution and the potential to allow earlier detection and characterization of acute ischemic stroke.

Further diagnostic studies include ECG to rule out atrial fibrillation and echocardiogram if atrial emboli are suspected. Carotid duplex scanning is used to identify carotid artery stenosis or occlusion.

OUTCOME MANAGEMENT

Medical Management

Medical management of the client with stroke is directed at early diagnosis and early identification of the client who can benefit from thrombolytic treatment. Preserving cerebral oxygenation, preventing complications and stroke recurrence, and rehabilitating the client are other goals.

Identify Stroke Early

A critical factor in the early intervention and treatment of stroke is the proper identification of stroke manifestations and establishing the onset of the manifestations. Because manifestations vary by the location and size of the infarct, standardized assessment tools, including the Acute Stroke Quick Screen and the National Institutes of Health Stroke Scale (NIHSS) (Table 70-3), can be used to identify rapidly which clients might benefit from thrombolytic therapy. The assessment must be complete and accurate to provide a baseline for ongoing assessments. A score of less than 5 on the 42-point scale indicates a minor stroke.

The initial assessment of the client who is thought to have had a stroke includes the level of consciousness, pupillary response to light, visual fields, movement of extremities, speech, sensation, reflexes, ataxia, and vital signs. These data are often recorded and scored in addition to the information assessed on the Glasgow Coma Scale (GCS). In addition, if intracranial pressure monitors are in place, baseline pressure values and waveforms should be noted.

A complete history of the presenting problem as well as past medical and social history can provide data about the cause of the stroke. This information also guides stroke treatment. The time of onset of manifestations must be determined because thrombolytic therapy must be administered within 3 hours of the onset of manifestations. A history of hypertension or cardiac valve disorders is commonly associated with stroke.

Maintain Cerebral Oxygenation

Emergency care of the client with stroke includes maintaining a patent airway. The unconscious client should be turned on the affected side to promote drainage of saliva from the airway. The collar of the shirt should be loosened to facilitate venous return. The head should be elevated, but the neck should not be flexed. The client should be kept quiet, and emergency help should be contacted.

Once the client is in the emergency department (ED), a patent airway is maintained and oxygen is supplied. If the client demonstrates poor ventilatory effort,

TABLE 70–3 National Institutes of Health (NIH) Stroke Scale

Administer stroke scale items in the order listed. Scores should reflect what the client does, not what the clinician thinks the client can do. Except where indicated, the client should not be coached (i.e., repeated requests to client to make a special effort). For the total score, 0 = normal examination, >4 often represents acute stroke, and >20 often represents profound neurologic deficit.

Instruction	Scale Definition
1a. Level of Consciousness The investigator must choose a response, even if a full evaluation is prevented by such obstacles as an endotracheal tube, language barrier, or orotracheal trauma or bandages. A 3 is scored only if the client makes no movement (other than reflexive posturing) in response to noxious stimulation.	0 = Alert, keenly responsive 1 = Not alert, but arousable by minor stimulation to obey, answer, or respond 2 = Not alert, requires repeated stimulation or painful stimulation to make movements (not stereotyped) 3 = Responds only with reflex motor or autonomic effects, or totally unresponsive, flaccid, areflexic
1b. LOC Questions The client is asked the month and his or her age. The answer must be correct—there is no partial credit for being close. Aphasic and stuporous clients who do not comprehend the questions will score 2. Clients unable to speak because of endotracheal intubation, orotracheal trauma, severe dysarthria from any cause, language barrier, or any other problem not secondary to aphasia are given a 1. It is important that only the initial answer be graded and that the examiner not "help" the client with verbal or nonverbal cues.	0 = Answers both questions correctly 1 = Answers one question correctly 2 = Answers neither question correctly
1c. LOC Commands The client is asked to open and close the eyes and then to grip and release the nonparetic hand. Substitute another one-step command if the hands cannot be used. Credit is given if an unequivocal attempt is made but not completed because of weakness. If clients do not respond to command, the task should be demonstrated to them (pantomime) and score the result (i.e., follows none, one, or two commands). Clients with trauma, amputation, or other physical impediments should be given suitable one-step commands. Only the first attempt is scored.	0 = Performs both tasks correctly 1 = Performs one task correctly 2 = Performs neither task correctly
2. Best Gaze Only horizontal eye movements will be tested. Voluntary or reflexive (oculocephalic) eye movements will be scored, but caloric testing is not done. If the client has a conjugate deviation of the eyes that can be overcome by voluntary or reflexive activity, the score will be 1. If a client has an isolated peripheral nerve paresis (CN III, IV, or VI), score a 1. Gaze is testable in all aphasic clients. Clients with ocular trauma, bandages, pre-existing blindness, or other disorder of visual acuity or fields should be tested with reflexive movements, and a choice made by the investigator. Establishing eye contact and then moving about the client from side to side will occasionally clarify the presence of a gaze palsy.	0 = Normal 1 = Partial gaze palsy; this score is given when gaze is abnormal in one or both eyes, but where forced deviation or total gaze paresis is not present 2 = Forced deviation or total gaze paresis not overcome by the oculocephalic maneuver
3. Visual Visual fields (upper and lower quadrants) are tested by confrontation, using finger counting or visual threat as appropriate. Client must be encouraged, but if he or she looks at the side of the moving fingers appropriately, this can be scored as normal. If there is unilateral blindness or enucleation, visual fields in the remaining eye are scored. Score 1 only if a clear-cut asymmetry, including quadrantanopia, is found. If client is blind from any cause, score 3. Double simultaneous stimulation is performed at this point. If there is extinction, client receives a 1 and the results are used to answer question 11.	0 = No visual loss 1 = Partial hemianopia 2 = Complete hemianopia 3 = Bilateral hemianopia (blind, including cortical blindness)
4. Facial Palsy Ask or use pantomime to encourage the client to show teeth or smile and close eyes. Score symmetry of grimace in response to noxious stimuli in the poorly responsive or noncomprehending client. If facial trauma or bandages, orotracheal tube, tape, or other physical barrier obscures the face, these should be removed to the extent possible.	0 = Normal symmetrical movement 1 = Minor paralysis (flattened nasolabial fold, asymmetry on smiling) 2 = Partial paralysis (total or near total paralysis of lower face) 3 = Complete paralysis (absence of facial movement in the upper and lower face)

TABLE 70–3   National Institutes of Health (NIH) Stroke Scale—Cont'd

Instruction	Scale Definition
5 and 6. Motor Arm and Leg The limb is placed in the appropriate position: extend the arms 90 degrees (if sitting) or 45 degrees (if supine) and the leg 30 degrees (always tested supine). Drift is scored if the arm falls before 10 seconds or the leg before 5 seconds. The aphasic client is encouraged using urgency in the voice and pantomime but not noxious stimulation. Each limb is tested in turn, beginning with the nonparetic arm. Only in the case of amputation or joint fusion at the shoulder or hip may the score be 9, and the examiner must clearly write the explanation for scoring as a 9.	0 = No drift; limb holds 90 degrees (or 45 degrees) for full 10 seconds 1 = Drift; limb holds 90 degrees (or 45 degrees) but drifts down before full 10 seconds; does not hit bed or other support 2 = Some effort against gravity; limb cannot get to or maintain (if cued) 90 degrees (or 45 degrees); drifts down to bed but has some effort against gravity 3 = No effort against gravity; limb falls 4 = No movement 9 = Amputation, joint fusion; explain: 5a = Left arm 5b = Right arm 0 = No drift; leg holds 30 degrees for full 5 seconds 1 = Drift; leg falls by the end of the 5-second period but does not hit bed 2 = Some effort against gravity; leg falls to bed by 5 seconds but has some effort against gravity 3 = No effort against gravity; leg falls to bed immediately 4 = No movement 9 = Amputation, joint fusion; explain: 6a = Left leg 6b = Right leg

7. Limb Ataxia
This item is aimed at finding evidence of a unilateral cerebellar lesion. Test with eyes open. In case of visual defect, ensure testing is done in intact visual field. The finger-nose-finger and heel-shin tests are performed on both sides, and ataxia is scored only if present out of proportion to weakness. Ataxia is absent in the client who cannot understand or is hemiplegic; only in the case of amputation or joint fusion may the item be scored 9, and the examiner must clearly write the explanation for not scoring. In case of blindness, test by touching nose from extended arm position.
	0 = Absent
	1 = Present in one limb
	2 = Present in two limbs
	If present, is ataxia in
	  Right arm: 1 = Yes 2 = No
	9 = Amputation or joint fusion; explain:
	  Left arm: 1 = Yes 2 = No
	9 = Amputation or joint fusion; explain:
	  Right leg: 1 = Yes 2 = No
	9 = Amputation or joint fusion; explain:
	  Left leg: 1 = Yes 2 = No
	9 = Amputation or joint fusion; explain:

8. Sensory Sensation or grimace to pinprick when tested or withdrawal from noxious stimulus in the obtunded or aphasic client. Only sensory loss attributed to stroke is scored as abnormal, and the examiner should test as many body areas (arms [not hands], legs, trunk, face) as needed to accurately check for hemisensory loss. A score of 2, "severe or total," should only be given when a severe or total loss of sensation can be clearly demonstrated. Stuporous and aphasic clients will therefore probably score 1 or 0. The client with brain stem stroke who has bilateral loss of sensation is scored 2. If the client does not respond and is quadriplegic, score 2. Clients in coma (question 1a = 3) are arbitrarily given a 2 on this item.	0 = Normal; no sensory loss 1 = Mild to moderate sensory loss; client feels pinprick is less sharp or is dull on the affected side, or there is a loss of superficial pain with pinprick but client is aware of being touched 2 = Severe to total sensory loss; client is not aware of being touched
9. Best Language A great deal of information about comprehension will be obtained during the preceding sections of the examination. The client is asked to describe what is happening in the attached picture, to name the items on the attached naming sheet, and to read from the attached list of sentences. Comprehension is judged from responses here as well as to all of the commands in the preceding general neurologic examination. If visual loss interferes with the tests, ask the client to identify objects placed in the hand, repeat, and produce speech. The intubated client should be asked to write a sentence. The client in coma (question 1a = 3) will arbitrarily score 3 on this item. The examiner must choose a score in the client with stupor or limited cooperation, but a score of 3 should be used only if the client is mute and follows no one-step commands.	0 = No aphasia; normal 1 = Mild to moderate aphasia; some obvious loss of fluency or facility of comprehension, without significant limitation on ideas expressed or form of expression. Reduction of speech and/or comprehension, however, makes conversation about provided material difficult or impossible. For example, in conversation about provided materials, examiner can identify picture or naming card from client's response. 2 = Severe aphasia; all communication is through fragmentary expression; great need for inference, questioning, and guessing by the listener. Range of information that can be exchanged is limited; listener carries burden of communication. Examiner cannot identify materials provided from client response. 3 = Mute, global aphasia; no usable speech or auditory comprehension

(Continued)

TABLE 70–3   National Institutes of Health (NIH) Stroke Scale—Cont'd

Instruction	Scale Definition
10. Dysarthria If the client is thought to be normal, an adequate sample of speech must be obtained by asking client to read or repeat words from the attached list. If the client has severe aphasia, the clarity of articulation of spontaneous speech can be rated. Only if the client is intubated or has other physical barriers to producing speech may the item be scored 9, and the examiner must clearly write an explanation for not scoring. Do not tell the client why he or she is being tested.	0 = Normal 1 = Mild to moderate; client slurs at least some words and, at worst, can be understood with some difficulty 2 = Severe; client's speech is so slurred as to be unintelligible in the absence of or out of proportion to any dysphasia, or is mute/anarthric 9 = Intubated or other physical barrier; explain:
11. Extinction and Inattention (formerly Neglect) Sufficient information to identify neglect may be obtained during the prior testing. If the client has severe visual loss preventing visual double simultaneous stimulation, and the cutaneous stimuli are normal, the score is normal. If the client has aphasia but does appear to attend to both sides, the score is normal. The presence of visual spatial neglect or anosognosia may also be taken as evidence of neglect. Because neglect is scored only if present, the item is never untestable. *Additional item, not part of the NIH Stroke Scale score.*	0 = No abnormality 1 = Visual, tactile, auditory, spatial, or personal inattention or extinction to bilateral simultaneous stimulation in one of the sensory modalities 2 = Profound hemi-inattention or hemi-inattention to more than one modality; does not recognize own hand or orients to only one side of space

12. Distal Motor Function
The client's hand is held up at the forearm by the examiner, and client is asked to extend his or her fingers as much as possible. If the client cannot or does not extend the fingers, the examiner places the fingers in full extension and observes for any flexion movement for 5 seconds. The client's first attempts only are scored. Repetition of the instructions or of the testing is prohibited.
	0 = Normal (no flexion after 5 seconds)
	1 = At least some extension after 5 seconds but not fully extended; any movement of the fingers that is not a command is not scored
	2 = No voluntary extension after 5 seconds; movement of the fingers at another time is not scored
	  a. Left arm
	  b. Right arm

CN, Cranial nerve; *LOC*, level of consciousness.
Modified from National Institutes of Health, Bethesda, Md.

intubation and mechanical ventilation may be required to prevent hypoxia and increased cerebral ischemia. An ECG is performed to assess for cardiac disorders, such as atrial fibrillation, that increase the risk for embolic stroke. Blood pressure is also evaluated, and hypertension may be reduced with vasodilators. Caution is exercised when treating blood pressure because lowering the blood pressure too far may lower cerebral perfusion pressure and increase cerebral ischemia. Laboratory tests for hematology, chemistry, and coagulation are obtained to rule out stroke-mimicking conditions and to detect bleeding disorders that would increase the risk of bleeding during thrombolytic therapy.

Restore Cerebral Blood Flow

The client is evaluated as a candidate for thrombolytic therapy once an intracerebral hemorrhage is ruled out. The goal of thrombolytic therapy is recanalization of the occluded vessel and reperfusion of ischemic brain tissue. Thrombolytic agents are exogenous plasminogen activators, which dissolve the thrombus or embolus blocking the cerebral blood flow. Clients who receive recombinant tissue plasminogen activator (rt-PA) within 3 hours of the onset of stroke are 30% more likely to have minimal or no disability from acute ischemic stroke without an increase in mortality. Several contraindications to thrombolytic therapy are shown in Box 70-1.

BOX 70-1   Inclusion Criteria for Intravenous rt-PA Therapy for Acute Ischemic Stroke

- Diagnosis of ischemic stroke with a measurable neurologic deficit
- Neurologic signs are not clearing spontaneously
- Neurologic signs should not be minor and isolated
- Caution should be used in treating clients with major deficits
- Symptoms should not be suggestive of subarachnoid hemorrhage
- Onset of manifestations <3 hours before the start of probable infusion
- No head trauma or prior stroke in past 3 months
- No myocardial infarction in prior 3 months
- No GI/GU hemorrhage in past 21 days
- No arterial puncture in a noncompressible site during prior 7 days
- No major surgery in prior 14 days
- No history of prior intracranial bleed
- Systolic BP <185, diastolic BP <110
- No evidence of acute trauma or bleeding
- Not taking an oral anticoagulant, or if so INR <1.7
- If taking heparin within 48 hours must have a normal aPTT
- Platelet count >100,000
- Blood glucose level >50 mg/dl (2.7 mmol)
- No seizure with residual postictal impairments
- CT does not show evidence of multilobar infarction

aPTT, Activated partial thromboplastin time; *CT*, computed tomography; *INR*, International Normalized Ratio.

Treatment should begin immediately after the client is deemed to be a candidate for rt-PA. The dose of rt-PA for acute ischemic stroke is 0.9 mg/kg administered intravenously over 1 hour. Ten percent of the total dose is given as a bolus over 1 minute before initiation of the intravenous dose. The pharmacologic half-life of rt-PA is approximately 5 to 7 minutes. After thrombolytic therapy, the client is sent to the intensive care unit (ICU) for careful monitoring of blood pressure, neurologic status, and bleeding.

The risk-benefit ratio for the use of thrombolytic therapy must be considered in certain client populations. The choice of whether to pursue aggressive treatment focuses on several factors, such as the client's age, the client's preference (if known), the presence and severity of other disorders, the severity of the stroke, and how much time has elapsed since the infarction. The risk of intracerebral hemorrhage after rt-PA is greater in clients with early signs of a major infarct on CT scan. Clients who have severe neurologic deficits at presentation (NIHSS >22) are at increased risk for intracerebral hemorrhage and poor outcome.

At present the treatment for most clients with large areas of infarction or large intracerebral hemorrhage is supportive care. It is hoped that future research can improve the treatment outcomes for these clients.

Prevent Complications

Bleeding. After administration of rt-PA, the client is monitored for potential complications of rt-PA, which may include intracranial hemorrhage and systemic bleeding. In the initial studies of rt-PA in acute ischemic stroke, symptomatic intracranial hemorrhage occurred in 6.4% of clients within the first 36 hours after treatment. Intracranial hemorrhage carries a death rate greater than 50%. All fatal intracranial hemorrhages occurred within the first 24 hours of treatment. The expanding clot of an intracranial hemorrhage destroys brain tissue. The pressure of the clot also disrupts blood flow and causes additional ischemia. Increased intracranial pressure (ICP) results from the space-occupying clot and surrounding edema of ischemic tissue and can lead to midline shift of intracranial contents, possible brain stem herniation, and death. To decrease the risk of intracranial or systemic bleeding, administration of anticoagulants and antiplatelet medications is not recommended until 24 hours after administration of rt-PA.

Stringent blood pressure management is the single most important measure to prevent intracranial hemorrhage after thrombolysis. Frequent vital signs and neurologic checks are necessary to prevent hypertension and detect manifestations of intracranial hemorrhage. Hypertension frequently accompanies acute ischemic stroke. Therefore blood pressure is usually not treated unless it increases to 185 mm Hg systolic or 105 mm Hg diastolic. In addition, the mean arterial pressure should be lowered by no more than 10% and in gradual increments. This is less likely to lead to hypoperfusion and worsening cerebral ischemia.

An intracranial hemorrhage should be suspected if the client has new complaints of headache, nausea, and vomiting, or a sudden change in level of consciousness. An intracranial hemorrhage should be assumed with any acute worsening of neurologic function until it can be ruled out by CT scan. If the rt-PA is still infusing, the infusion should be stopped. A complete blood count, coagulation studies, and type and crossmatch are done. If a head CT scan reveals intracranial hemorrhage, fresh frozen plasma with fibrinogen or cryoprecipitate is administered to correct coagulopathies.

Systemic bleeding may also occur as a complication of rt-PA. Clinical manifestations include change in level of consciousness (LOC), tachycardia, hypotension, and cool, clammy, and pale skin. Thrombolytic therapy may be stopped depending on the site and severity of the bleeding.

Cerebral Edema. Increased ICP is a potential complication of large ischemic strokes. Increased ICP is also a potential complication of intracerebral hemorrhage, either primary or secondary to thrombolytic therapy. Manifestations of increased ICP include change in LOC, reflex hypertension, and worsening neurologic status. Invasive monitoring of ICP is done for clients with decreased LOC who are at high risk for increased ICP. All clients are placed on bed rest with the head of the bed elevated to 30 degrees to decrease ICP and to facilitate venous drainage. Ideally the degree of head elevation is based on the response of the client's ICP for those clients on ICP monitoring.

External *ventriculostomy* drainage is sometimes used to reduce pressure from cerebrospinal fluid (CSF) accumulation. A burr hole is placed through the skull, and a catheter is passed into the lateral ventricle to allow for controlled drainage of CSF. Blood pressure is closely monitored. The goal is to maintain blood pressure low enough to prevent another stroke or hemorrhage without decreasing cerebral perfusion. The client may require continuous mechanical ventilation and hyperventilation to decrease ICP. Mannitol, an osmotic diuretic, helps in lowering increased ICP. Surgical evacuation of the intracerebral hematoma may be performed. Increasing ICP, central herniation, and brain stem hemorrhage can lead to death from depression of the vital centers in the medulla, that is, brain stem failure.

Blood Glucose Control. Severe hyperglycemia can lead to poor outcomes and reduced perfusion of the brain during thrombolysis. Even nondiabetic clients should not be given excessive glucose via intravenous fluids.

Stroke Recurrence. The incidence of stroke recurrence in the first 4 weeks after acute ischemic stroke ranges from 0.6% to 2.2% per week. The risks of anticoagulation include intracranial hemorrhage, systemic bleeding, and death. Therefore the general use of heparin in all clients with acute ischemic stroke is no longer recommended. Heparin is indicated to prevent stroke recurrence in clients at risk for cardiogenic emboli. Initially unfractionated heparin, dose based on body weight, is administered intravenously, and then warfarin is administered orally.

SAFETY ALERT

Intravenous heparin is delivered with an infusion pump for accurate and safe delivery. Monitoring of clotting times is important to detect over-anticoagulation, which increases the risk of bleeding. Activated partial thromboplastin time (aPTT) should be at 1.5 to 2.5 times control for anticoagulation to be effective.

After a therapeutic anticoagulant level has been achieved with heparin therapy, warfarin administration is begun. Because warfarin has a long half-life, the physician initiates the warfarin therapy while the client is still receiving intravenous heparin. Once the client has a therapeutic response to heparin, in about 24 to 48 hours, the physician discontinues the heparin and continues the warfarin therapy. The therapeutic International Normalized Ratio (INR) for prophylaxis against cardiogenic embolization is 2.0 to 3.0. Clients receiving anticoagulation therapy should be assessed for bruising, hematuria, blood in feces, bleeding from mucous membranes, and new-onset or worsening headaches.

The long-term risk for stroke recurrence is 4% to 14% per year. Antiplatelet agents, including aspirin, ticlopidine, extended-release dipyridamole plus aspirin, and clopidogrel, decrease the risk for secondary stroke. Antiplatelet agents inhibit platelet function to decrease the risk of thrombus formation. The selection of the specific antiplatelet agent is individualized according to the client's medical history.

Aspiration. Clients with stroke are at high risk for aspiration pneumonia, which is the direct cause of death in 6% of clients following stroke. Aspiration is most common in the early period and is related to loss of pharyngeal sensation, loss of oropharyngeal motor control, and decreased LOC. Oral food and fluids are generally withheld for 24 to 48 hours.

SAFETY ALERT

Feeding by mouth must proceed cautiously; check gag reflex to determine if the client can swallow fluids. Hold feeding if there is any sign of aspiration.

If the client cannot eat or drink after 48 hours, alternate feeding routes are used, such as tube-feeding or hyperalimentation. When the swallowing mechanism has returned, the client can be fed orally. Progressive feeding programs for dysphagia are based on the degree of swallowing ability.

Other Potential Complications. Other complications of stroke depend primarily on the location of the lesion or infarcted tissue. If the brain stem is affected, blood pressure fluctuations, altered respiratory patterns, and cardiac dysrhythmias are all possible. Physical injury related to the client's inability to realize his or her limitations can occur. Complications of immobility can also occur.

Coma can follow strokes of various causes. The blood supply to the brain stem or reticular activating system, which controls consciousness, may have been directly occluded. Similarly, the deep structures of the thalamus that relay information to the cerebral cortex may be involved. Vascular occlusion of the internal carotid artery or one of its major branches may also decrease LOC. Sometimes the cerebral edema that follows stroke may produce midline shifts, resulting in coma.

Hyperthermia is treated immediately with antipyretics. Temperature elevations lead to increased cerebral metabolic needs, which in turn cause cerebral edema and increased risk for cerebral ischemia. Antipyretics are given and, if needed, a hypothermia blanket or ice packs to reduce body temperature. Causing the client to shiver should be avoided, however, because shivering increases oxygen consumption and ICP. If seizures develop, phenytoin (Dilantin) may be used.

Strokes caused by occlusive disease (e.g., thrombus, embolus) rarely cause sudden death. When stroke is fatal, death may occur within 3 to 12 hours, but it occurs more often between 1 and 14 days after the original episode. Typically, with any type of fatal stroke, a rise in temperature, heart rate, and respiratory rate occurs along with deepening coma several hours or days before death. These manifestations result from damage to the vasomotor and heat-regulating centers. The Case Study on p. 1857, which is continued on the website, presents a scenario of a client at risk for stroke.

Rehabilitation After Stroke

From the onset of stroke, interventions are aimed at maximizing the client's physical and cognitive recovery. Early pre-mobilization efforts are aimed at preventing the complications of neurologic deficit and immobility. After the first few days of the acute event, cerebral edema has usually subsided and the residual deficits of stroke can be identified. Clients with stroke and their families face difficult adjustments as the acute stages pass and residual disabilities become obvious.

Previously it was thought that damage to the central nervous system (CNS) was irreversible. Now it has been shown that even in adults with significant brain injury relearning can take place. It is extremely important that relearning take place as soon as possible after the injury. Early rehabilitation makes this relearning possible. The severity of a client's stroke will impact the length of time it may take to recover function.

Meningioma, Fractured Hip, and Possible Stroke

Mrs. Olsen is a 72-year-old white woman who resides at Shady Oaks Care Center. She fell today and could not get up again because of the pain. An x-ray examination obtained at the nursing home showed a proximal femoral fracture near the right hip joint. She has been transferred to your hospital for a preoperative medical evaluation in preparation for possible surgical repair of her right hip fracture later today . . .

Case Study continued on the website and the CD-ROM with discussions, multiple-choice questions, and a nursing care plan.

An interdisciplinary rehabilitation team is necessary to assist and support clients and their families during this time. Assessing the functional abilities of the client and setting realistic goals are part of this approach. Because stroke is a common health care problem, many facilities have developed clinical pathways to guide care. (See the CareMap of the Clinical Pathway feature on Stroke on the website.)

INTERDISCIPLINARY MANAGEMENT

Several disciplines facilitate recovery of the client following a stroke. It is the coordinated effort of the entire team that best serves the client and family.

The recommended plan of care includes using interdisciplinary services to do the following:

- Document the client's condition and course fully, including deficits, status of other diseases, complications, changes in status, and functional status before stroke.
- Begin physical activity as soon as the client's medical condition is stable; use caution with early mobilization in clients with progressing neurologic deficit, subarachnoid or intracerebral hemorrhage, severe orthostatic hypotension, acute myocardial infarction, or acute deep vein thrombosis.
- Assist in managing general health functions throughout all stages of treatment, such as managing dysphagia, nutrition, hydration, bladder and bowel function, sleep and rest, co-morbid conditions, and acute illnesses.
- Prevent complications, including deep vein thrombosis and pulmonary embolism, aspiration, skin breakdown, urinary tract infections, falls, spasticity and contractures, shoulder injury, and seizures.

- Prevent recurrent strokes through control of modifiable risk factors, oral anticoagulation, antiplatelet therapy, or surgical intervention.
- Assess throughout acute and rehabilitation stages.
- Use reliable standardized instruments for evaluation.
- Evaluate for formal rehabilitation during the acute stage.
- Choose an individual or interdisciplinary program based on the client's and family's needs; success of the program requires full support and active participation of the client and family; families must be involved at the outset.
- Choose the local rehabilitation program that best meets the client's and family's needs.

Physical Therapy

Physical therapists work with the client to build strength and preserve range of motion (ROM) and tone in noninvolved muscles. Physical therapy also builds ROM and tone and retrains muscles affected by the stroke. The client also works on balance and proprioception skills. This may enable the client, with continued improvement, to sit on the edge of the bed and eventually to ambulate. Exercise and bed mobility skills are taught at the client's bedside, as are wheelchair mobility and transfers. Clients who would benefit from the use of an orthosis are identified and instructed on how to apply and remove it. A hemiplegic client is usually able to ambulate using a quad cane following gait training.

Occupational Therapy

Occupational therapists work with the client to relearn activities of daily living (ADL) and to use assistive devices that promote independence. For example, a client with hemiplegia may be able to dress if the clothing can be closed with self-fastening tape (Velcro) fasteners rather than buttons.

Many clients experience severe pain in the affected shoulder and hand after a stroke. This pain can be so severe that it results in lack of balance and loss of ROM, which further restricts mobility and self-care. Overstretching from turns and transfers can aggravate the problem. Some clients have experienced partial dislocation or subluxation of the shoulder both from having the shoulder pulled on and from the weight of the arm pulling it. Chronic subluxation results in shoulder-hand syndrome, characterized by a painful or frozen shoulder and hand edema. Occupational therapists assist in treating this problem and in instructing the client and caregivers in proper transfer and positioning techniques to prevent further injury.

Speech Therapy

Speech pathologists work with the client to foster the maximum amount of speech recovery possible through relearning, accentuation of speech sounds, or use of alternative communication devices. The speech pathologist also assesses the client's swallowing mechanism and makes recommendations for initiation and progression of foods and fluids to decrease the risk of aspiration.

Case Management

Case managers are often assigned to clients following stroke. Their role is to facilitate all care providers and to advocate for the client and family. (See Case Management feature on Stroke on the website.)

Nursing Management of the Medical Client

Assessment. Ongoing assessments of all body systems are needed. The use of a standardized neurologic assessment tool such as the GCS assists the nurse in documenting changes in the client's status and in monitoring progress. The NIH stroke scale (Table 70-3) is also commonly assessed. In addition to the neurologic assessment, the client's blood pressure, heart sounds, heart rate and rhythm, respiratory rate and rhythm, temperature, levels of nutrition, ability to swallow, bladder and bowel elimination, and communication need to be assessed. The client's and family's psychosocial and learning needs should be assessed daily.

Diagnosis, Outcomes, Interventions
Diagnosis: Ineffective Tissue Perfusion. Cerebral perfusion of the cerebrum is critical for survival and long-term outcome. Therefore it should be the first priority in the care of clients with acute stroke. Decreased cerebral blood flow may be secondary to thrombus, embolus, hemorrhage, edema, or spasm. Ongoing assessment and intervention are required beyond the critical stage. Data indicating that the risk for altered perfusion has become an actual problem are shown in the Critical Monitoring box above, right.

Outcomes. The client will have improved cerebral tissue perfusion as evidenced by ICP less than 15 mm Hg, cerebral perfusion pressure (CPP) greater than 65 mm Hg, no type A waves (when using intracranial monitors), no reports of headache, no decreases in LOC, and stable or improving GCS score.

Interventions. Serial assessments of these data may be required as often as every 15 minutes for unstable clients to every 2 to 4 hours for stable clients. Analyze data for trends, and if the client is deteriorating neurologically, notify the physician. Manifestations of progressive deterioration include decreasing LOC, changes in motor or sensory function, pupillary changes, respiratory difficulty, and development of visual or perceptual defects or aphasia.

CRITICAL MONITORING

Manifestations Indicating an Acute Change in Cerebral Perfusion

- Intracranial pressure greater than 15 mm Hg sustained for 15 to 30 seconds or longer
- Cerebral perfusion pressure less than 70 mm Hg
- Decrease in Glasgow Coma Scale score of 2 or more points from baseline
- Decreasing levels of consciousness
- Mean arterial pressure of less than 80 mm Hg or systolic blood pressure less than 100 mm Hg
- Bradycardia
- Altered pattern of breathing
- Loss of response to painful stimuli
- Change in pupil size or response to light
- Headache
- Vomiting
- Abnormal flexion or extension posturing

Maintain the client's blood pressure within the range prescribed by the physician to maintain perfusion without promoting cerebral edema. Maintain normothermia to reduce cerebral glucose and oxygen consumption. Cluster nursing interventions to reduce unneeded movement and stimulation. Elevate the head of the bed 30 degrees to reduce cerebral edema. Maintain the client's head in a neutral position to improve venous drainage.

Administer medications to improve cerebral tissue perfusion as prescribed. Anticoagulants or antiplatelet agents will be used to decrease risk of further thrombus formation. Nimodipine, a calcium-channel blocker, is used to treat vasospasm secondary to subarachnoid hemorrhage.

Delirium and restlessness should be controlled, with sedatives if necessary. Be certain, however, that restlessness is not the result of treatable causes, such as hypoxia, full bladder, bowel impaction, or pain. Restraints should be avoided because they often increase agitation and ICP.

Straining at stool or with excessive coughing, vomiting, lifting, or use of the arms to change position should be avoided, because the Valsalva maneuver increases ICP. Mild laxatives and stool softeners are often prescribed.

Collaborative Problem: Hemorrhage. Because of the increased risk for systemic bleeding secondary to the use of thrombolytic therapy or anticoagulation, monitoring for bleeding is an important collaborative problem. Write the collaborative problem as *Risk for Prolonged Bleeding Times related to use of thrombolytic agents or anticoagulation.*

Outcomes. The nurse will monitor for hemorrhage and, if present, will control bleeding and notify the physician.

Interventions

For the client who is receiving thrombolytic therapy, certain interventions can prevent systemic bleeding, including the following: do not perform arterial punctures or insertions of nasogastric tubes, rectal thermometers, or rectal medications for 24 hours after the infusion; monitor all puncture sites and body fluids for manifestations of bleeding for 24 hours; and maintain bed rest for 24 hours after completion of the infusion.

Gingival bleeding and oozing from intravenous sites have been associated with intracranial hemorrhage. Pressure may be applied to any compressible bleeding sites.

For the client who is receiving anticoagulation, monitor the aPTT and INR and adjust the client's dosage based on the physician's orders. Report any manifestations of bleeding to the physician immediately.

Diagnosis: Risk for Aspiration. The nursing diagnosis *Increased Risk for Aspiration* is listed here because of its importance in maintaining airway and oxygenation. Not all clients are at risk for aspiration after stroke, and the risk depends on the time since injury and the area of infarction. When considering this nursing diagnosis, use the following causes of aspiration to guide your analysis: impaired swallowing, depressed cough and gag reflexes, and decreased LOC.

Outcomes. The client will have a reduced risk of aspiration as evidenced by easily managing saliva, no choking or coughing while eating, no fever, and no crackles or rhonchi.

Interventions. Assess the client for clinical manifestations of aspiration, such as fever, dyspnea, crackles and rhonchi, confusion, and decreased Pao_2 in arterial blood gases. Use caution in feeding the client, either orally or enterally. If the client is receiving enteral feedings, add food coloring to the tube feeding to assist with identifying aspiration via suctioned aspirate. Monitor chest x-ray results, and report findings of pulmonary infiltrate.

Diagnosis: Impaired Physical Mobility. Almost all clients have some degree of immobility after a stroke. In the early phases of stroke recovery, the client may be completely immobile and need assistance just to turn over in bed. Later in recovery, mobility may be hampered in one extremity only. Various causes can be used to individualize this diagnosis. These include (1) loss of muscle tone secondary to flaccid paralysis or spasticity and (2) reluctance to move because of the fear of self-injury or prolonged disuse.

Outcomes. The client will achieve maximal physical mobility within the limitations imposed by the stroke as evidenced by more normal movement of the affected extremity, improved muscle strength, and effective use of adaptive devices. This outcome may require a long time frame; shorter outcomes may be indicated for acute care.

Interventions. Assess the client's degree of muscle strength to use as a baseline value and for determining and evaluating outcomes. A comprehensive assessment by a physical therapist helps to determine appropriate activity levels.

Encourage Bed Exercises. Encouraging clients with hemiplegia to exercise while on bed rest not only prepares them for later activities but also offers hope and a sense of optimism about recovery. A hemiplegic client can learn to move the weak leg by sliding the unaffected leg under it to lift and move the weak leg. The client can also use the unaffected arm to move the affected arm and hand. Keep in mind that clients may have difficulty crossing the midline.

Frequent gluteal and quadriceps muscle setting exercises during the day help to prepare the client for later ambulation. Begin with 5 repetitions, and increase gradually to 20 repetitions each time. Instruct the client as follows:

- *Gluteal setting:* "Pinch" or contract the buttocks together and count to five. Then relax and count to five. Repeat.
- *Quadriceps setting:* Contract the quadriceps muscles on the anterior portion of the thigh while raising the heel and trying to squash a rolled towel placed under the popliteal fossa against the mattress. While keeping the muscle contracted, count to five. Then relax and count to five. Repeat. Perform on both legs if possible. Start quadriceps setting exercise as soon as the client is conscious. The quadriceps muscle is the most important in giving knee joint stability in walking.

Help the Client Sit Up

Help the client out of bed as soon as the client's condition is medically stable. Remember, however, that hemiplegia can severely affect balance. Assistance is needed to provide security and safety. Raise the head of the bed slowly to reduce orthostatic hypotension.

Assist the client to sit up the first time and closely monitor for balance and safety awareness.

SAFETY

⚠

ALERT

When the client first sits up, support the affected side, especially the back and the head. Gradually the client will learn to sit alone with the head of the bed elevated and then to sit on the edge of the bed with the feet on a firm surface. Help the client maintain balance by extending the affected arm and placing the palm flat on the bed. Be patient and encouraging as the client regains balance. When the client is sitting in a chair, support the weak side with pillows.

Eventually the client will learn to raise the weak leg with the unaffected leg and to swing both legs laterally over the side of the bed onto the floor. It is safest to have the client pivot on the unaffected leg. Therefore position the chair at a right angle to the unaffected side.

Teach the Client How to Use a Wheelchair. A hemiplegic client needs to learn safe transfers from the bed to the chair, commode, or wheelchair. The Client Education Guide below shows one method of moving safely from the bed to a wheelchair. The client with hemiplegia can propel a wheelchair with the unaffected arm and leg; one-arm-drive wheelchairs also are available. Once in a wheelchair, the client's level of independence increases greatly. Deficits in spatial relations, decreased awareness, and unilateral neglect can result in problems such as falling and running into doors. Clients must not be allowed to perform wheelchair self-transfers until they have demonstrated competence.

Promote Walking. A tilt table may be used in physical therapy to help the client assume a standing position if difficulty with balance is a problem. The client can begin standing as soon as the quadriceps muscles on the unaffected side have normal strength. Have the client seated on the edge of the bed. Encourage the client to rise by using the muscle power of the unaffected leg. The client may tend to swing around toward the affected side. Gradually the client will learn to take increasing amounts of weight onto the weaker side.

Despite weakness in the affected limb, a hemiplegic client often develops an extensor reflex, which facilitates standing. Position yourself on the weaker side when helping the client to stand. To avoid pulling on the affected arm and increasing the risk for shoulder injury, provide support with ambulation by using a gait belt. A quad cane should be used on the unaffected side to allow walking with a three-point gait.

Most hemiplegic clients can be taught to walk. Remind them to keep the body weight forward over the feet. Practice is important for learning to walk correctly. Incorrect habits, once developed, may be difficult to overcome later. Supervise clients carefully until they can safely walk alone without fear of falling. When walking, the client should not show circumduction or toe scraping or stoop forward. Heel-toe walking with a reciprocal gait pattern is the goal of ambulation.

Teach Bracing. If bracing is used, teach the client and family how to apply and remove the brace, to observe skin for breakdown, to give proper skin care, and to care for the brace itself.

Diagnosis: Risk for Hyperthermia. Bleeding or edema of the hypothalamus can lead to ischemia of the thermoregulatory center of the brain.

Outcomes. The client will have a reduced risk of hyperthermia or will have a normal temperature.

Interventions. Treat fever with antipyretics. A hypothermia blanket may be used to bring down a high temperature quickly. When hypothermia blankets are used, assess the skin frequently for pressure points and cold injury. Shivering must be avoided because the muscle activity increases body temperature. Keeping the feet warm with blankets may decrease shivering. Phenothiazine agents may be used to help stabilize neuronal membranes if fever is related to damaged brain structures.

Diagnosis: Risk for Impaired Skin Integrity. The loss of protective sensation and decreased ability to move increase the risk for injury to the skin. In addition, skin damage may develop from friction and shearing or increased skin fragility from inadequate nutritional status or edema.

Outcomes. The client's skin will remain intact as evidenced by an absence of stage I pressure ulcer development and an absence of manifestations of redness from friction or shearing.

Interventions. Assess the skin every 2 hours. Turn the client with hemiplegia or decreased LOC every 2 hours. Develop a written turning schedule for other health care providers and family members to follow. When positioning the client on the affected side, make sure that body weight does not harm affected limbs. Support the affected arm and leg when turning and positioning.

CLIENT EDUCATION GUIDE

Transfer from Bed to Wheelchair by a Hemiplegic Client

- Lock the wheelchair for safety, and keep it beside the bed on your unaffected side.
- Use your unaffected arm and leg to move your affected arm and leg.
- As your legs drop over the edge of the bed, swing your torso up to a sitting position.
- Push yourself up to a standing position by using your unaffected arm and leg.
- Reach across the wheelchair to grasp the far arm of the chair, and turn to seat yourself.
- Shading on the right side of the client indicates the affected side.

a hemiplegic client. Complete shoulder and hip dislocation can occur if the flaccid extremity is not supported properly. Place a pillow between the client's legs to provide support. The client may be able to tolerate lying only for 30 minutes on the affected side because of the impaired circulation or pain.

Collaborative Problem: Risk for Contracture. Normally the brain inhibits spastic muscle contraction. Early in stroke recovery, flaccidity is usually present because of a loss of cerebral connections for afferent sensory and efferent motor nerves. During recovery affected muscles may be spastic because the injured brain cannot inhibit spastic muscle contraction. Therefore the collaborative problem *Risk for Contracture* is due to flaccid paralysis or spasticity.

Outcomes. The nurse will monitor for the development of contractures as evidenced by no muscle shortening and by maintaining normal ROM.

Interventions. Assess the client's ROM in both the involved and noninvolved joints. These findings can be used as a baseline and as an expected outcome.

Perform passive ROM exercises two times daily after the first 24 hours following a stroke unless otherwise prescribed. Motor impulses usually begin to return between 2 and 14 days after a stroke. The affected part (initially flaccid) becomes spastic as the spinal cord motor systems establish their autonomy, and the potential for contractures increases. Passive ROM exercises are more difficult to perform once affected muscles begin to tighten.

Do not force extremities beyond the point of initiating pain or continuous spasm. Always support the joint you are exercising, and move the extremity smoothly, without jerking movements. Frequent passive ROM exercises (1) prevent joint immobility, tendon contractures, and muscle atrophy; (2) stimulate circulation; and (3) help reestablish neuromuscular pathways. Performing these exercises before dressing and undressing the client may facilitate self-care.

Teach the client to use the unaffected hand to lift the weak arm and to put it through ROM exercises. Exercise each finger separately. While in bed, teach the client (1) to exercise the affected arm by grasping it at the wrist with the unaffected hand and raising it above the head and (2) to stretch and rub the fingers of the affected hand several times each day. Active ROM to the unaffected extremities assists in maintaining or increasing muscle strength.

Once some voluntary movement returns, encourage the client with assisted movements. As motor strength increases, resisted movements may strengthen weakened muscles and help restore muscle bulk. Shoulder slings are not recommended because they may increase the risk of contractures.

Several interventions are used to reduce the risk for joint contracture:

- Allow the client to sit upright for short periods only; sitting can contribute to hip and knee flexion deformities.
- When the client is on one side, do not flex the hip acutely.
- Do not place a pillow under the affected knee when the client is supine; this encourages flexion deformity and impedes circulation.
- If the client's knees tend to hyperextend, place a folded towel under the knee for short periods while the client is lying supine.

If the client can tolerate the prone position, place the client in this position for 15 to 30 minutes several times a day, with a small pillow placed under the pelvis (from the umbilicus to the upper third of the thigh) to hyperextend the hip joints.

Prevent footdrop, heel cord shortening, and plantiflexion by (1) avoiding pressure on the feet, (2) performing frequent passive ROM exercises, and (3) having the client sit in a chair as soon as possible with the feet flat on the floor. While the client is in bed, keep the foot flexed at 90 degrees by using high-top tennis shoes or orthotics.

A trochanter roll, extending from the crest of the ilium to mid thigh, prevents external hip rotation by wedging under the projection of the greater trochanter and stopping the femur from rolling. Because trochanter rolls increase the risk of skin impairment, assess the skin beneath the roll often.

When the client is in bed, prevent adduction of the affected shoulder by placing a pillow in the axilla, between the upper arm and the chest wall, to keep the arm abducted about 60 degrees. Keep the arm slightly flexed in a neutral position. Place the forearm on another pillow with the elbow above the shoulder and the wrist above the elbow. This position stretches the shoulder's internal rotators. Elevating the arm also helps to prevent edema and resultant fibrosis.

Place the affected hand in a position of function (i.e., slightly supinated with fingers slightly flexed and the thumb in opposition). Frequent passive ROM exercises are important. The use of splints to prevent flexion contractures is more effective if the splints are designed individually by occupational therapists and scheduled for on-and-off periods to allow for skin assessment and ROM. Squeezing a rubber ball is not recommended because it promotes flexion when extension is desired.

The weight of an immobile arm may cause pain and movement limitation (frozen shoulder) or subluxation of the shoulder joint. Prevent these manifestations by supporting a completely flaccid arm with a pillow when the client is in bed or seated in a chair.

Diagnosis: Self-Care Deficit. Self-care deficits may range from not being able to reach with a weak arm to full dependence on others. This diagnosis is applicable if an achievable outcome can be obtained. Clients with complete paralysis and cognitive deficits may not be able to perform self-care. Other nursing diagnoses may be more applicable, such as *Impaired Physical Mobility* and *Impaired Skin Integrity.* Several nursing diagnoses can be used to describe *Self-Care Deficit,* including *Impaired Physical Mobility, Disturbed Sensory Perception (Visual), Unilateral Neglect,* or *Disturbed Thought Processes.*

Outcomes. The client will perform as many ADL as possible within limitations as evidenced by use of adaptive devices and techniques.

Interventions. Initially a client who has had a stroke may need considerable help with all self-care activities, including washing, eating, and grooming. Encourage clients to perform as many self-care activities as possible and to use the affected arm to avoid the tendency to do everything with the unaffected arm. This activity helps to preserve independent self-care, prevents complications of immobility, and enhances self-esteem.

Remember that stroke clients are easily frustrated and may need a lot of encouragement. Self-care activities provide an excellent opportunity for family teaching. Family members find it difficult to watch a loved one struggle with a task, and they often perform the task for the client. Explain how it benefits the client to be as independent as possible.

In clients with diplopia, an eye patch over one eye removes the second image and promotes better vision. Alternating the patch daily helps to maintain the function and strength of the extraocular muscles in both eyes. Provide mouth care at least three or four times a day, giving special attention to the affected side of the tongue and mouth. Focus rehabilitation plans on self-care deficits and ADL.

Diagnosis: Risk for Injury. The *Risk for Injury* and trauma continues throughout recovery from stroke. It may also extend into the home environment, where clients attempt to perform former activities, such as cooking or driving. Factors that increase the risk for injury include decreased LOC, weakness, flaccidity, spasticity, impulsive behavior, altered thought processes, and motor, visual, and spatial-perceptual impairments.

Outcomes. The client will remain free from injury as evidenced by an absence of abrasions, burns, or falls. The client will also seek needed help to perform tasks that are beyond his or her capabilities.

Interventions. Keep the side rails of the bed raised for clients with recent hemiplegia to protect them from rolling out of bed. As recovery proceeds, the client may pull against side rails when sitting up or turning. Once the client can get out of bed unassisted, half side rails may be more useful. Full side rails hinder ambulation.

A client with impaired sensation is especially prone to injury. Frequent skin inspections for manifestations of injury are essential. Visual disturbances may also increase a hemiplegic client's potential for injury. Weakness on one side makes clients susceptible to falls.

Remind clients to walk slowly, rest adequately between intervals of walking, use effective lighting, and look where they are going. Be especially alert during toileting. Make sure that support staff and family members know not to leave these clients alone in the bathroom.

Diagnosis: Imbalanced Nutrition: Less Than Body Requirements. Use the nursing diagnosis *Imbalanced Nutrition: Less Than Body Requirements* if your client has an inability to swallow secondary to stroke. Support the diagnosis with data on intake and output, ability to swallow, caloric intake and weight change over the past 3 days, and levels of hemoglobin, hematocrit, albumin, prealbumin, and lymphocyte count over the past 3 days.

Outcomes. The client will demonstrate manifestations of adequate nutrition as evidenced by (1) maintenance of stable weight; (2) consumption of adequate calories for age, height, and weight; (3) intake equaling output; (4) hemoglobin and hematocrit levels within normal limits for age and gender; (5) lymphocyte count, prealbumin levels, and albumin levels within normal limits; and (6) healing of incisions and wounds within 12 to 14 days, as applicable.

Interventions. Carefully assess the client's diet to ensure adequate nutrition. Assess total intake. Feeding clients with partial paralysis of the tongue, mouth, and throat requires patience and care for prevention of choking and aspiration. Clients often fear choking and are embarrassed and frustrated by eating difficulties. Consequently, they may avoid eating and may not obtain adequate nutrition. Give supplemental meals as necessary. If the client cannot swallow at all, tube-feeding may be used. With help and encouragement, hemiplegic clients can usually learn to feed themselves. Many helpful orthotic devices are available through consultation with an occupational therapist. These might include utensils with built-up handles or scoop plates. Make mealtimes pleasant and unhurried. Serve food attractively and at an appropriate temperature.

Feeding can be very frustrating for a dysphagic client, especially if the caregiver is not familiar with the client's specific disabilities. Support personnel and family members need to be taught basic feeding techniques and also to be informed of each client's individual needs and limitations. To facilitate feeding, assess the following and intervene as necessary. The speech pathologist can recommend additional feeding techniques based on the client's specific deficits and needs.

Promote Head Control. If the client has limited or no voluntary head control, placing a hand on the forehead may help. The caregiver approaches the client from the midline rather than from the side so that the client does not have to turn the head to be fed. Remind the client not to throw the head back to propel food because this can lead to aspiration. The head should be midline and flexed slightly forward.

Assist in Positioning. Have the client in an upright position, as close to 90 degrees as possible, either in bed or in a chair. Support the client's head to counteract hyperextension.

Promote Mouth Opening. If the client does not open the mouth, lightly touch both lips with the tip of a spoon. If this does not work, apply light pressure with a finger to the chin just below the lower lip. Ask the client to open at the same time. Stroking the muscle under the chin (digastric muscle), without crossing the midline, also stimulates mouth opening.

Stimulate Mouth Closing. If a client does not close the lips, swallowing is more difficult. Stimulate lip closure by stroking the lips with a finger or ice or by applying gentle pressure just above the upper lip with your thumb or forefinger.

Help the Client with Swallowing. A dysphagic client must concentrate on swallowing. A quiet environment, free from distractions, is helpful. Feed the client slowly and offer small amounts. Begin feeding the client with foods that require no chewing and are easy to swallow (Table 70-4). Gradually progress to foods that require more chewing and swallowing effort as tolerated. Alternate liquids with solids whenever possible to prevent food from being left in the mouth. Avoid unthickened liquids. Place food in the unaffected side of the mouth. Encourage the client to chew each bite thoroughly. After clients have swallowed, teach them to check for food on the paralyzed side by turning the head to the unaffected side and sweeping the mouth with the tongue.

Diagnosis: Impaired Verbal Communication. The inability to speak is frustrating for clients. Early recognition of this problem decreases some of the frustration in meeting everyday needs. Loss of verbal communication is usually caused by ischemia of the dominant cerebral hemisphere, leading to loss of the function of muscles that produce speech.

Outcomes. The client will be able to communicate effectively, the client's needs will be understood and met, and the client will indicate understanding of the communication of others.

Interventions. Communication involves the dual processes of sending and receiving language. Although either can be affected, the expressive deficit is usually greater than the receptive deficit after initial recovery. Clients may understand more than they can respond to clearly.

Most aphasic clients regain some speech through spontaneous recovery or speech therapy. Speech therapy should be started early. Occasionally residual brain function is not adequate for an aphasic client to relearn the complicated processes of communication. A picture board may be helpful.

TABLE 70–4   Progressive Feeding Program for Clients with Dysphagia

	Stage I	Stage II	Stage III	Stage IV
Description	Severe swallowing difficulty	Chewing and swallowing difficulty with various textures	Less difficulty swallowing, beginning to control foods better in mouth, able to tolerate various food textures and consistencies	Able to swallow most foods very well
Meats	Puréed meat with gravy, baby food, egg yolks	Junior baby food meats with gravy; scrambled, soft, or poached eggs; cottage cheese	Ground meat with gravy, soft meats (tuna) in casseroles, macaroni and cheese, fish without bones, chopped meats	Soft diet
Starch	Mashed potatoes with gravy	Muffins (no seeds), pancakes, French toast, cooked cereal (thick)	Toast (no seeds), rice, soft baked potato	Soft foods
Vegetables	Puréed	Junior vegetables	Peas, squash, cooked carrots; avoid stringy foods (celery, spinach)	Soft foods
Fruits	Puréed	Cooked fruit, ripe banana, soft canned fruit	Grapefruit and orange sections; peeled ripe peaches, pears, and nectarines	Soft foods
Dessert	Custard, pudding	Cakes (no seeds, nuts)	Pies, cakes, sherbet, ice cream	Soft foods
Liquids	None	None	Thick liquids, nectars, strained cream soups, eggnog, liquid caloric supplements, milk shakes	May be able to have thickened liquids

Assessment of dysarthria usually includes examination of the peripheral muscles of speech, tests for specific speech skills, and assessment of the client's functional ability based on the clarity of speech in conversation. Speech therapy is beneficial for many dysarthric clients.

Reinforce the lessons that a speech therapist has initiated. Remember, the client may have a short attention span. Use every encounter to encourage and support communication, and yet be careful not to cause frustration and fatigue. In general, when working with an aphasic client, speak at a slower rate and give the client time to respond. Listen and watch carefully when an aphasic client attempts to communicate. Try hard to understand. This reduces the client's frustration. Anticipate an aphasic client's needs to reduce feelings of communication helplessness.

When a client *cannot identify objects by name,* give the client practice in receiving word images. For example, point to an object and clearly state its name. Then ask the client to repeat the word.

When a client *cannot understand spoken words or has receptive difficulty,* repeat simple directions until they are understood. Do not shout; the client can hear. Speak slowly and clearly. Talk without pressing for a response. Use nonverbal methods of communication to reinforce your words. Stand within 6 feet, and face the client directly. Gradually shift topics of conversation, and tell the client when you are going to change the topic.

When a client has *difficulty with verbal expression,* give the client practice in repeating words after you. Begin with simple words and then progress to simple sentences.

Help the family to communicate with the aphasic client. Act as a role model for such communication by being calm, patient, and gentle. Explain how damaging it can be to the client's self-image if others appear to be embarrassed or amused by the client's attempts to communicate. Likewise, the family should not do all of the speaking for the client.

Always try to put aphasic clients at ease. Reduce the feelings of panic that may occur when they first realize that they cannot communicate as before. The fact that others understand the problem is helpful. Offer calm reassurance. Demonstrate the use of the call light and allow the client to practice. Use gestures and one-step commands.

Collaborative Problem: Risk for Corneal Abrasion. Following stroke, clients may lose their ability to blink. Without a blink reflex, the cornea will dry and become abraded. The collaborative problem is *Risk for Corneal Abrasion.*

Outcomes. Monitor the client for risk factors for the development of corneal abrasion, including the absence of eye closure or blinking and lack of eye moisture.

Interventions. Protect the eye with an eye patch if no blinking is noted. Instill prescribed artificial tears or consult the physician for a prescription if none exists.

Diagnosis: Disturbed Thought Processes. Sometimes it is difficult to make a nursing diagnosis of *Disturbed Thought Processes* unless you spend time with the client. Asking simple or common questions may get fixed, yet correct, answers. Often, after spending a morning with a client, you may note difficulty with thought processing that was not evident on first assessment. Changes in behavior may be caused by alterations in body image, sensation, vision, mobility, and perception. Cerebral edema may also increase confusion.

Outcomes. The client will have improved thought processing as evidenced by recall of information, improved Mini-Mental State Examination scores, decreased agitation, cooperation with interventions, and appropriate responses to questions about recent and past events.

Interventions. Try to prevent disorientation by reorienting the client as LOC improves. Continually reorient a confused client. Glasses and hearing aids assist the client in maintaining awareness of the environment and thus improve thought processes. Activity such as sitting up in a chair for meals or at scheduled times throughout the day also improves LOC and orientation. Position a calendar and a clock where the client can see them. Stroke contributes to altered behavioral patterns, including confusion, memory loss, and emotional lability. To decrease agitation, explain all nursing activities before initiating them. Avoid sensory overload.

Diagnosis: Disturbed Sensory Perception: Visual. Ischemia of visual pathways can lead to altered vision. The client may not notice you when you approach from one side or may not eat food from one side of the food tray. A thorough assessment of visual fields is usually needed for this diagnosis.

Outcomes. The client will successfully compensate for altered visual perceptions as evidenced by safely performing ADL and safely compensating for visual deficit through scanning or other techniques.

Interventions. Approach the client from the side that is not visually impaired. Position the call light and telephone on that side. If possible, position the bed so that the client's side that is not visually impaired is toward the center of the room. Teach clients to position the head to increase the visual field. Warn hemiplegic clients to be careful when crossing streets because they may not see traffic approaching from the affected side. An eye patch over one eye in clients with diplopia removes the second image and assists vision.

A client with perceptual deficits benefits from simplicity A busy or noisy environment is difficult to interpret and may increase confusion. Reduce complexity and the need for decision-making. The following are examples:

- Obtain clothing that is simply designed and easy to put on.
- Give brief, simple directions.
- Prepare food trays with a minimum number of utensils, dishes, and foods.

Diagnosis: Unilateral Neglect. *Unilateral Neglect* is a pattern of lack of awareness of one side of the body. The client behaves as if that part is simply not there. He or she does not look for the paralyzed limb when moving about. It is caused by damage to portions of the nondominant cerebral hemisphere. Unilateral neglect creates an increased risk of injury. It is possible to relearn to look for and to move the limb.

Outcomes. The client will be able to compensate for unilateral neglect as evidenced by being free from injury and demonstrating an increased awareness of the neglected body side.

Interventions. Initially adapt the environment to the deficit by focusing on the client's unaffected side. Greet the client as you enter the room, especially if the entrance is toward the neglected side. Keep personal care items and a bedside chair and commode on the unaffected side. Set up the client's food tray toward the unaffected side. Position the client's extremities in correct alignment. Gradually begin to focus the client's attention to the affected side. Move the personal items, bedside chair, and commode to the affected side. Assist the client from the affected side. Have the client groom the affected side first. Cue the client to scan the entire environment and remind the client to keep track of the affected extremities.

Diagnosis: Ineffective Coping. Coping strategies are quite varied among people. Any major illness or change in the body challenges a client's or family's coping skills. This process is particularly true after a stroke because of the physiologic changes and frustrations associated with the resulting deficits. The term *coping* refers to the use of all forms of coping strategies: emotional, cognitive, support systems, and risk appraisal.

Outcomes. The client will develop effective coping strategies as evidenced by appropriate lifestyle modifications, use of the assistance of others, and appropriate social interactions.

Interventions. After a stroke, the client may experience grief over lost mobility, inability to communicate, alterations in sensation and vision, and loss of roles within society. Stroke clients express feelings of profound suffering related to the sudden, devastating changes that accompany stroke. Be understanding and kind. Supportive statements are often helpful, such as "I am sure it's hard for you not to be able to dress alone." The client needs to feel listened to and cared about.

Loss of independence is of particular concern for the stroke client. Care for clients in a way that encourages their independence. Arrange the environment and anticipate needs to reduce frustration. Praise all successes, however small. Break a long-term goal into several short-term goals so that the client can experience successes along the way. For example, a long-term goal may be to walk independently, but short-term goals such as sitting on the side of the bed and ambulating with a quad cane will allow the client to have successes and the long-term goal will seem more attainable. Inappropriate behavior may occur. When necessary, point out the behavior in a matter-of-fact manner and ask the client to stop. Significant others often need help to understand that these behaviors may be caused by damage to the inhibitory centers in the brain or they may be a part of the normal grief response. Provide support by helping the client and family understand this.

Aphasic clients often express their emotional state by irritability and "moodiness." These frustrated clients are often anxious, bewildered, and depressed. Emotional lability may also be present. Accept such behavior in a matter-of-fact but kind manner, without embarrassment. Help families by encouraging short visits by one or two people. If children are allowed to visit, ensure that they are adequately supervised.

Psychosocial Nursing Diagnoses. Various psychosocial nursing diagnoses may be appropriate for clients experiencing stroke, depending on the client and the circumstances. These include *Interrupted Family Processes, Deficient Diversional Activity, Anxiety, Fear, Powerlessness, Situational Low Self-Esteem,* and *Social Isolation.* Shift in spousal roles often occurs. The ways a couple copes will determine how satisfying their lives are after a stroke. Include significant others in the plan of care; let them help care for the client if they wish. Provide them with the information they need to understand the client's condition. Many clients with strokes are in ICUs during the acute phase. The complexity of equipment and activity within an ICU may be frightening to the client and to significant others. Explain carefully what is happening, and provide opportunities for questions and discussion. Give frequent reassurance and support.

Evaluation. Evaluate the degree of outcome attainment on an ongoing basis. After a stroke, some outcomes, such as cerebral perfusion, are achieved early; others, such as self-care deficit, may require long-term rehabilitation. Monitor progress toward outcomes, working with both the client and the family.

Surgical Management

Several criteria are used to identify candidates for rapid evacuation of the hematoma in hemorrhagic stroke. The clients most likely to benefit from surgery are those who are younger than 70 years of age, can open their eyes and follow commands, have elevated ICP (>30 mm Hg), or are rapidly deteriorating neurologically. Clients who have large blood clots removed often can recover a substantial portion of speech. Surgery is usually not performed in clients with bleeding in deep cerebral structures such as the basal ganglia or thalamus.

Most therapies are aimed at reducing increased ICP. Surgery is also performed on some intracranial aneurysms and on the carotid arteries to reduce the risk for stroke.

Modifications for Older Clients

Because stroke affects older people more than it affects others, the nursing care discussed here does not have to be significantly altered for older clients. Older people often have multiple medical problems that must be monitored and treated simultaneously.

Self-Care

Clients who have experienced a stroke often are transferred to a rehabilitation unit after they are medically stable. The client is evaluated for rehabilitation potential, and plans are made for ongoing therapy. The plan of care established during acute care can continue. The major nursing diagnoses and collaborative problems include *Impaired Physical Mobility, Self-Care Deficit, Impaired Verbal Communication, Risk for Contracture, Imbalanced Nutrition: Less Than Body Requirements,* and *Ineffective Coping.*

The following are adjuncts to discharge from rehabilitation settings to home:

- Self-medication
- Use of therapeutic passes
- Rehabilitation home visits

Self-medication means that clients can manage their own medications. Goals are to help the client learn about the medications, including dosage, action, and side effects. Provide a supervised trial to evaluate the client's knowledge and compliance and to enable clients to develop increased responsibility for their own care. A clear and accurate medication chart is helpful.

Therapeutic passes allow the client to return to home or family for short stays. They facilitate discharge planning and improve the transition into the community. Passes help the stroke survivor adjust to the home environment and to practice self-care activities at home, and help the family adjust to living with the stroke survivor and to any alterations in physical, cognitive, and emotional functioning. Clients and family members can practice problem solving and can perform some physical care skills needed after discharge from the facility. Much effort goes into planning for the passes and preparing the client and family. Passes are usually for 8 hours at first and then are increased to a weekend. When the client returns to the facility, the client and family discuss any difficulties they had during the pass interval. Team members intervene with information, retraining, or procurement of needed supplies.

For the *rehabilitation home visit,* team members, including the nurse, social worker, and physical and occupational therapists, visit the client's home.

The purpose is to evaluate the accessibility of the home and the safety of the home environment based on the client's level of functioning, specifically the client's ability (1) to get in and out of the house; (2) to perform specific tasks in each room; (3) to transfer onto and off of the toilet, bed, and chair; and (4) to move about from room to room. The client's ability to use the telephone and various appliances safely is also evaluated. On the basis of findings from the visit, the team recommends home modifications, further teaching, or adaptive equipment.

The family needs a clear understanding of the client's residual deficits. If spatial or perceptual deficits or unilateral neglect is present, emphasize the need for assistance with ADL and the need for adherence to safety precautions to prevent injury.

Writing lists of tasks or activities may help clients with impaired memory. Reinforce measures to improve mobility and the ability to perform ADL. The client should have a plan for exercises. Equally important, the family and client need to have realistic expectations about the client's abilities so that they can encourage independence when and where the client is able.

Provide written documentation of any anticoagulant schedule as well as a list of warning signs of bleeding. Reinforce the need for caution when the client is using sharp instruments and tools. If appropriate, contact sports must be curtailed while the client is receiving anticoagulants. The INR is closely monitored, and medications are adjusted as needed. The client should be taught to carry Medic-Alert identification.

Provide information about community resources that can assist the client and family with home management and adjustments to residual deficits. These resources include Meals-on-Wheels, the American Stroke Association (a division of the American Heart Association), the National Stroke Association, stroke support groups, social services, local service groups to assist with the purchase of equipment, and individual and family counselors.

At times the stroke client may not be able to tolerate the intensive therapy of a rehabilitation setting, and placement in an extended care facility may be necessary. This is usually very stressful for the client and family, particularly an older spouse. In some cases, care by nurses and allied health professionals in the home may prevent placement in an extended care facility. If both partners are older or in poor health, placement in an extended care facility may be the only option, which can create feelings of guilt and abandonment. Emotional support must be provided to both the client and family members. Education in how to choose a facility and how to monitor care can be helpful.

TRANSIENT ISCHEMIC ATTACKS

Transient ischemic attacks (TIAs) are sudden, brief episodes of neurologic dysfunction caused by temporary, focal cerebral ischemia. Recovery is complete. By definition, a TIA lasts less than 24 hours, and most TIAs last only 5 to 20 minutes. TIAs that last longer than 1 hour are often caused by small infarcts. TIAs often serve as warning signs of an impending stroke, especially in the first few days.

Etiology and Risk Factors

During a TIA, a transient decrease in blood supply to a focal area of the cerebrum or brain stem occurs. Many factors can cause this ischemia. Thromboembolism from ulcerated plaque on the carotid arteries is the most common cause of TIAs, accounting for 80% of cases. Thromboemboli may originate in the vertebrobasilar system. Other sources of emboli include blood clots forming on diseased or prosthetic heart valves, atrial fibrillation, or breakdown of plaque.

Pathophysiology

The pathophysiology of a TIA is similar to that of a stroke. The major differences are the short duration of ischemia and the lack of permanent deficits associated with TIAs.

Clinical Manifestations

Manifestations of TIAs vary, depending on which area of the brain is affected. Common manifestations of a TIA in the carotid artery circulation include a rapid onset of weakness or numbness in an arm or leg, aphasia, and visual-field cuts. Manifestations of a TIA in the vertebrobasilar circulation include two or more of the following: vertigo, diplopia, dysphagia, dysarthria, and ataxia.

Transient ischemic attacks are often recurrent; however, some clients have only one or two episodes before having a complete stroke. TIAs may occur for 1 to 6 years before cerebral infarction, or clusters of TIAs may first appear only a few hours or days before a cerebral infarction. Between episodes, neurologic assessment findings are normal.

The diagnosis of TIA is confirmed by the client's reported clinical manifestations. The causes of the TIA and the potential risk for stroke are diagnosed by the following examinations:

- Auscultation for a carotid bruit
- CT to rule out stroke or other causes of neurologic deficit
- Doppler, computed tomographic angiography (CTA), or magnetic resonance angiography (MRA) studies of the carotid arteries
- Cerebral angiogram
- ECG to assess for atrial fibrillation
- Transthoracic or transesophageal echocardiography (TTE and TEE, respectively) to rule out mural thrombosis and valvular disorders

The results of the noninvasive carotid artery studies, which include the Doppler, CTA, and MRA, determine whether the more invasive cerebral angiogram is performed. The TTE is often performed before the TEE because it is less invasive; however, the TEE may better visualize prosthetic valves and the left atrium.

Conditions that mimic a TIA include intracranial hemorrhage, seizures, hypoglycemia, migraine, and inner ear disorders.

OUTCOME MANAGEMENT

Medical Management

Preventing the progression of a TIA to a stroke is the goal of medical management. Every effort is made to determine the cause of the TIAs. If the TIA is not from the heart or from embolism, the client is placed on anti-platelet therapy. Common agents include aspirin and sustained-release dipyridamole. For clients with persistent or paroxysmal atrial fibrillation, anticoagulation is recommended to maintain an INR of 2.5. Another important medical intervention is to identify and decrease the client's modifiable risk factors for stroke. All smokers should be encouraged to stop smoking. Physical activity of at least 10 minutes of exercise daily should be encouraged. Lowering blood pressure and serum lipid levels is also advised. Diabetic clients should keep fasting blood glucose levels below 126 mg/dl.

Teach the client and family about the manifestations of stroke, risk factors for stroke, and emergency care if a stroke occurs at home. If the client is hospitalized, assess neurologic status frequently for progressive ischemia.

Clients experiencing TIAs are often afraid that they are having a stroke. They need emotional support and education during this stressful time. The diagnostic work-up as well as the manifestations themselves can produce anxiety. Thorough, simple explanations of upcoming events can help. Stress the importance of completing the work-up. Baseline neurologic status must be recorded for postoperative comparison.

Surgical Management

Clients who are considered for surgery are those who have a low risk for postoperative morbidity and mortality and one of the following: (1) asymptomatic carotid artery disease with 50% or greater stenosis or (2) symptomatic carotid artery disease with 70% or greater stenosis. In these clients, the incidence of stroke with surgical management is significantly reduced compared with those with medical management. Clients considered at increased risk for postoperative morbidity and mortality include those with coronary artery disease, pulmonary disease, and moderate to severe stroke on the ipsilateral side. Surgery is usually performed only on stenotic arteries, not on those that are totally occluded. A client may require bilateral endarterectomy. The interval between surgeries is determined by the client's tolerance of the procedure and the likelihood of symptom progression from the remaining stenotic vessel.

Cerebral angiography may be performed before carotid artery surgery to establish the degree of carotid stenosis. The risk for stroke from cerebral angiography is 1% to 3%. Because of the vast improvements in the technology of noninvasive carotid artery studies (carotid ultrasound, carotid duplex, and MRA), these studies may also be used to evaluate stenosis and guide the planning for surgery. Preoperative aspirin is often administered to decrease the formation of embolism at the carotid suture line. If the client is receiving heparin, it is usually stopped on arrival to the operating room.

Carotid Endarterectomy

Carotid endarterectomy is useful in preventing stroke. Carotid endarterectomy is the opening of the carotid artery to remove obstructing and embolizing plaque (Figure 70-5). An incision is made on the anterior border of the sternocleidomastoid muscle. The vessel is clamped, and the plaque or atheroma is removed. Some surgeons use intraoperative electroencephalogram (EEG) and transcranial Doppler monitoring to detect decreased cerebral perfusion while the carotid artery is clamped. In addition, some surgeons shunt blood from below the targeted carotid artery incision to above it to provide a temporary blood supply to the brain. Neurologic status is closely monitored following surgery and the client is usually discharged the following day.

Prognosis. Follow-up Doppler studies are performed at 3 months postoperatively to assess for artery patency

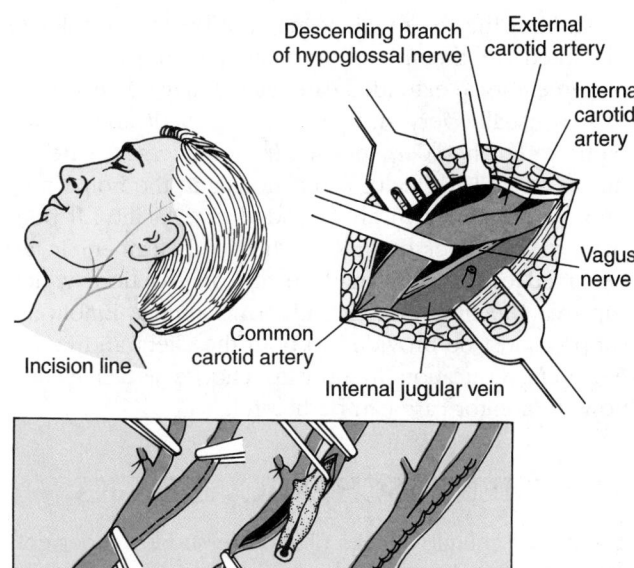

FIGURE 70-5 Carotid endarterectomy. **A,** The common carotid artery is clamped, and an incision is made along the carotid bifurcation. **B,** Plaque is removed. Sometimes portions of the artery are also removed and reconstructed with vein grafts or polyester, such as Dacron. **C,** The artery is sutured closed, and the clamps are removed.

and again at 6 months to 1 year to detect restenosis on the operated side and disease on the nonoperated side. Restenosis may occur in about 1% to 37% of clients after carotid endarterectomy.

Complications. Neurologic complications of carotid endarterectomy include the following:

- Embolization during surgery, causing cerebral vessel occlusion and ischemia
- Thrombosis of the artery at the endarterectomy site, causing cerebral ischemia
- Inadequate cerebral perfusion from intolerance of the temporary artery clamping during surgery

Other Techniques

Recent advances in microcatheter and microballoon technology have led to the investigational use of interventional neurovascular procedures to treat and prevent cerebrovascular disorders. Results of studies of the use of carotid angioplasty and stenting have been promising. The less invasive procedures would treat severe carotid stenosis in a less invasive way than traditional surgery.

Cerebral angioplasty is similar to coronary angioplasty. A balloon catheter is threaded through the arterial system via the femoral artery to the area of carotid stenosis. A small balloon is inflated to dilate the lesion. A stent catheter can also be used to further open the area of stenosis. The U.S. Food and Dru

Administration (FDA) considers both these procedures to be experimental. The complications and complication rate are comparable to those of carotid endarterectomy.

Nursing Management of the Surgical Client

Postoperative care after carotid endarterectomy includes neurologic assessments every 1 to 2 hours. Immediately report indications of deterioration of neurologic status. In addition, several cranial nerves (CNs) are close to the operative site. The function of the following CNs is assessed: facial (VII), vagus (X), spinal accessory (XI), and hypoglossal (XII). CN dysfunction is usually temporary but may last for months. The most common CN damage causes vocal cord paralysis, difficulty managing saliva, or tongue deviation.

Keep the client's head aligned in a straight position to help maintain airway patency and to minimize stress on the operative site. Antiplatelet agents are often administered. The client can lie supine or on the side, as long as the neck is not flexed. Elevate the head of the bed when vital signs are stable. Local applications of cold to the operative site may be prescribed.

Frequently assess the client's breathing pattern, pulse, and blood pressure. Maintain the client's blood pressure within 20 mm Hg of the preoperative normal values. Hypertension or hypotension may lead to hemorrhage, ischemia, or occlusion of the anastomosis. Labile blood pressure is a common postsurgical problem. Baroreceptors located in the lining of the carotid sinus are one of the primary mechanisms of maintaining normotension. Manipulation of the baroreceptors during surgery causes a short-term disruption in blood pressure regulation.

Observe the operative site. Airway obstruction can occur from excessive swelling of the neck or hematoma formation. Bleeding and hemorrhage are a concern because anticoagulation from intraoperative heparin is not yet reversed. Risk factor modification is essential to the long-term success of the surgery and the general health of the client.

🕯️ CLIENT AND PUBLIC EDUCATION

The general public has limited knowledge of the manifestations of stroke. In one study, only slightly more than half of the respondents could name at least one stroke manifestation. In addition, only 68% could name a risk factor for stroke. A public education campaign is under way to promote awareness of the manifestations of a stroke. In this campaign, stroke is referred to as a "brain attack" to indicate the need for emergency care with the same intensity as a heart attack. Prompt recognition allows for early treatment of a stroke, which may

---

lessen residual deficits and decrease disability. Recognition and modification of risk factors for stroke, shown in the Client Education Guide above, is the most effective prevention available.

CONCLUSIONS

Stroke is being managed today as a treatable problem if recognized early; however, because of the limited knowledge of the public about early warning signs, many clients still suffer the consequences of stroke. Treatment of the client with stroke is aimed at maximizing function and preventing disability.

THINKING CRITICALLY

1. A 70-year-old man had a left-side stroke 2 days ago. While obtaining his assessment, you note that his blood pressure is elevated at 200 mm Hg systolic; his usual systolic blood pressure is 140 to 160 mm Hg. He is receiving oxygen at 5 L, but his oxygen saturation has dropped from 95% to 88% in the last hour. The client was oriented to person, place, and time an hour ago but has become increasingly restless and slightly confused. The confusion has led him to pull out the nasogastric tube that had been placed for nutritional maintenance. What other neurologic assessments should you do? What is the first priority? Is the suddenness of this change significant?

Factors to Consider. How has the client's assessment changed from baseline values? Is there any relationship between the increased blood pressure and the hypoxia? Is the removal of the nasogastric tube an immediate problem?

2. A 78-year-old woman with a history of hypertension has a stroke. Her family reports that she has felt good and has refused to take her antihypertensive medication. She now has hemiparesis and is able to respond verbally. She does not recognize people or objects in her line of vision on the left side. Three days after her stroke, she is able to move her fingers and wiggle her toes on the affected side, and she is transferred to the rehabilitation unit. What are the most likely rehabilitation goals for this client? How should you proceed with teaching about the complications, motivation to comply with the prescribed therapies, and the importance of antihypertensive medications?

Factors to Consider. What types of rehabilitation will she require? How soon can teaching begin? How will you teach the client and family to provide her care after discharge?

3. A client is seen in the emergency department at 9 AM on Monday morning. His chief complaint is a severe headache. He states, "I am having the worst headache of my life. The pain awakened me around 5 AM and has gotten worse and worse." On examination, the client scores 15 on the Glasgow Coma Scale, complains of nausea, and has a stiff neck. The left-hand grip is slightly weaker than the right-hand grip, and there is a slight pronator drift of the left arm. In addition, there is flattening of the left nasolabial fold. A computed tomography scan of the brain reveals moderate hemorrhage on the right side with increased blood present in the right sylvian fissure. What tests would you expect to be ordered? What complications are important to assess for in this client?

Factors to Consider. What problem is probably in progress? Is the client a surgical candidate, either at the present time or in the future?

evolve   *Discussions for these questions can be found on the website.*

BIBLIOGRAPHY

Citations appearing in red refer to primary research.

Citations appearing in blue refer to evidence-based practice guidelines and protocols.

1. Adams, H.P., del Zoppa, G., Alberts, M.J., et al. (2007). Guidelines for the early management of adults with ischemic stroke. *Stroke, 38*(5), 1655-1711.
2. Ailawadi, G., et al. (2002). Carotid stenosis: Medical and surgical aspects. *Cardiology Clinics, 20*(4), 599-609.
3. American Heart Association. (2002). *Heart disease and stroke statistics—2003 update*. Dallas, Tex: American Heart Association.
4. Barch, C., et al., and the NINDS rt-PA Stroke Study Group. (1997). Nursing management of acute complications following rt-PA in acute ischemic stroke. *Journal of Neuroscience Nursing, 29*(6), 367-372.
5. Biller, J., & Love, B.B. (2000). Ischemic cerebrovascular disease. In W.G. Bradley (Ed.), *Neurology in clinical practice: Principles of diagnosis and management* (3rd ed.). Boston: Butterworth-Heinemann.
6. Biller, J., et al. (1998). Guidelines for carotid endarterectomy, a statement for healthcare professionals from a special writing group of the Stroke Council, American Heart Association. *Circulation, 97,* 501-509.
7. Broderick, J., et al. (1998). The greater Cincinnati/northern Kentucky stroke study: Preliminary first-ever and total incidence rates of stroke among blacks. *Stroke, 29*(2), 415-421.
8. Caplan, L.R. (1998). 10 most commonly asked questions about stroke. *The Neurologist, 4*(4), 227-231.
9. Cates, C. (2000). 10 most commonly asked questions about carotid angioplasty and stenting. *The Neurologist, 6*(1), 58-62.
10. Coombs, U.E. (2007). Spousal caregiving for stroke survivors. *Journal of Neuroscience Nursing, 39*(2), 112-119.
11. Kase, C.S. (2000). Intracerebral hemorrhage. In W.G. Bradley (Ed.), *Neurology in clinical practice: Principles of diagnosis and management* (3rd ed.). Boston: Butterworth-Heinemann.
12. Kasner, S.E. (2000). Stroke treatment-specific considerations. *Neurologic Clinics, 8*(2), 399-417.
13. King, R.B., Hartke, R.J., & Denby, F. (2007). Problem-solving early intervention: A pilot study of stroke caregivers. *Rehabilitation Nursing, 32*(2), 68-76, 84.
14. Hershey, L. (1999). 10 most commonly asked questions about stroke in women. *The Neurologist, 5*(3), 166-168.
15. Hinkle, J.L. (1998). Biological and behavioral correlates of stroke and depression. *Journal of Neuroscience Nursing, 30*(1), 25-31.
16. Johnson, S.C., Nguyen-Huynh, M.N., Schwarz, M.E., et al. (2007). *National Stroke Association Guidelines for the Management of TIA.* Accessed June 2007 from Stroke.org.
17. Lee, J., Soeken, K., & Picot, S.J. (2007). A meta-analysis of interventions for informal stroke caregivers. *Western Journal of Nursing Research, 29*(3), 344-356.
18. Manno, E.M., et al. (1999). The effects of mannitol on cerebral edema after large hemispheric cerebral infarct. *Neurology, 52,* 583-587.
19. Mayo, N.E., et al. (2000). There's no place like home: An evaluation of early supported discharge for stroke. *Stroke, 31*(5), 1016-1023.
20. Michael, K.M., & Shaughnessy, M. (2006). Stroke prevention and management in older adults. *Journal of Cardiovascular Nursing, 21*(5 Suppl), S21-26.
21. National Center for Health Statistics, Centers for Disease Control and Prevention. (2007). *Fast stats A to Z, stroke*. Retrieved June 2007 from www.cdc.gov/nchs/fastats/stroke.htm.
22. National Institute of Neurological Disorders and Stroke rt-PA Stroke Study Group. (1995). Tissue plasminogen activator for acute ischemic stroke. *New England Journal of Medicine, 333*(24), 1581-1587.
23. Pancioli, A., et al. (1998). Public perception of stroke warning signs and knowledge of potential risk factors. *Journal of the American Medical Association, 279*(16), 1288-1292.
24. Pilkington, F.B. (1999). A qualitative study of life after stroke. *Journal of Neuroscience Nursing, 31*(6), 336-347.
25. Post-stroke Rehabilitation Guideline Panel. (1995). *Post-stroke rehabilitation: Assessment, referral and patient management. Quick reference guide for clinicians* (Pub No. 95-0663). Rockville, Md: U.S. Department of Health and Human Services, Agency for Health Care Policy and Research.
26. Rapp, K., et al., and the NINDS rt-PA Stroke Study Group. (1997). Code stroke: Rapid transport, triage and treatment using rt-PA therapy. *Journal of Neuroscience Nursing, 29*(6), 361-366.
27. Reynolds, K., et al. (2003). Alcohol consumption and risk of stroke. A meta-analysis. *Journal of the American Medical Association, 289*(5), 579-588.
28. Siroky, M.B. (2003). Neurological disorders, cerebrovascular disease and parkinsonism. *Urologic Clinics of North America, 30*(1), 27-47.
29. Smith, G.R., & Mahoney, C. (1995). Coping and marital equilibrium after stroke. *Journal of Neuroscience Nursing, 27*(2), 83-89.
30. Suarez, J.L., et al. (1999). Predictors of clinical improvement, angiographic recanalization, and intracranial hemorrhage after intra-arterial thrombolysis for acute ischemic stroke. *Stroke, 30,* 2094-2100.

31. Swanson, R.A. (1999). Intravenous heparin for acute stroke: What can we learn from the megatrials? *Neurology, 52,* 1746-1750.

32. Tanne, D., et al. (2002). Markers of increased risk of intracerebral hemorrhage after intravenous recombinant tissue plasminogen activator therapy for acute ischemic stroke in clinical practice, The Multicenter rt-PA Acute Stroke Survey. *Circulation, 105,* 1679-1685.

33. Testani-Dufour, L., & Marano Morrison, C.A. (1997). Brain attack: Correlative anatomy. *Journal of Neuroscience Nursing, 29*(4), 213-222.

34. Wardlaw, J.M., Zoppo, G., Yamaguchi, T. & Berge, E. (2003). Thrombolysis for acute ischemic stroke. *Cochrane Data Base Systematic Review* (2), CD000213.

35. Williams, L.S., et al. (2002). Effects of admission hyperglycemia on mortality and costs in acute ischemic stroke. *Neurology, 59,* 67-71.

evolve *Did you remember to check out the bonus material on the Evolve website and the CD-ROM, including NCLEX®-Examination Style Review Questions, Open-Book Quizzes, and Chapter Review Audio Podcasts?*

http://evolve.elsevier.com/Black/medsurg

71

Management of Clients with Peripheral Nervous System Disorders

SHARON R. REDDING

The peripheral nervous system is that portion of the nervous system that exists outside of the brain and spinal cord itself. The peripheral nervous system is made up of three types of nerves:

- Motor nerves (responsible for voluntary movement)
- Sensory nerves (responsible for sensing temperature, pain, touch, and limb positioning)
- Autonomic nerves (responsible for involuntary functions, e.g., breathing, blood pressure, sexual function, digestion)

This chapter addresses problems with the spine and cranial nerves.

LOWER BACK PAIN

Lower back pain is the second most common reason for visits to health care providers (the most common reason being respiratory problems) and because of treatment and lost work hours it results in more health care costs than any other medical condition. The problem of lower back pain is a source of fascination, frustration, and often confusion by clinicians and scientists who attempt to study and treat this problem. The spine is the only organ that consists of bones, joints, ligaments, fatty tissue, multiple layers of muscles, peripheral nerves, sensory ganglia, autonomic ganglia, and the spinal cord. These structures are in turn fed by an intricate system of arteries and veins. Furthermore, the movement of the spine is complex and injury to the spine and other structures leads to unique patterns of pain.

Etiology

The spine is a mechanical organ that has been described as a crane with the ability to support weight, maintain balance, and counter numerous daily strains during normal work and recreational activities. Although it has tremendous ability to withstand most mechanical stresses, it can be stressed beyond its limits. Forces that exceed the capacity of the tissues to stretch can lead to injury and pain.

The origin of back pain is not well-known and has never been fully described. Many groups have given up trying to describe the cause of lower back pain and instead have listed several *red flag* conditions that are associated with the problem. Four groups of problems lead to back pain:

1. *Biomechanical and destructive* origins include compression of the disks, herniation of the disks, torsion injury, and vibration. These problems are seen when clients have occupations that require strenuous or repetitive lifting in a stooped position or jobs that require operating vibrating machinery.
2. *Destructive origins* include infection, tumors, and rheumatoid disorders. These conditions can place pressure on the spinal roots or cord, or alter the structure of the vertebrae.
3. *Degenerative* problems include osteoporosis and spinal stenosis. Osteoporosis can cause collapse of the vertebrae and lead to compression of the nerve roots. The spinal canal can narrow and compress the nerves, a condition called *spinal stenosis,*

evolve *Web Enhancements*

Client Education Guide   Lower Back Care (English Version and Spanish Translation)

Home Care After Cervical Laminectomy or Fusion (English Version and Spanish Translation)

Home Care After Carpal Tunnel Release (English Version and Spanish Translation)

Be sure to check out the bonus material on the Evolve website and the CD-ROM, including free self-assessment exercises. **http://evolve.elsevier. com/Black/medsurg**

usually occurring in older people. The severity ranges from entrapment of one nerve root to compression of the entire cord.

4. *Other disorders* include those that have no clear physiologic cause, yet lead to loss of income and pain. There is a growing body of data that show strong psychological influences on the response of clients to lower back pain. The primary determining factors for disability from lower back pain appear to be based on whether the client is depressed, is unhappy in a work setting, or involved in litigation. These psychosocial issues do not negate the presence of real pain. The manner in which the brain processes pain may be implicated. The psychosocial aspects may suppress the serotonergic pathways and limit the secretion of endorphins.

Specific Injuries to the Back

There are many causes of back pain (Figure 71-1). It is important to differentiate those conditions that are non-emergent from those that require surgery.

Back Strain

Back strain is an acute injury leading to lower back pain. Back strain occurs when the client flexes the back without bending the knees or makes rotating movements, creating significant stress on the intervertebral disks and muscles of the lower back.

Disk Herniation

Strenuous activity or degeneration of the disk or vertebrae can permit movement of the disk from its normal location. With aging, changes in disk cartilage and elasticity of the disk may cause the disk to prolapse. Displacement of intervertebral disk material may be referred to as *prolapse, herniation, rupture,* or *extrusion.* Ruptured intervertebral disks may occur at any level of the spine. Lumbar disks are more likely to rupture than cervical disks, because of the force of gravity, continual movement in this region, and improper movements of the spine as with lifting or turning. Thoracic disk disorders are the least common. More than half of people with clinical manifestations of a herniated disk give a history of a previous back injury. Heavy physical labor, strenuous exercise, and weak abdominal and back muscles all increase the risk of herniated disk. Repeated stress progressively weakens the disk, resulting in bulging and herniation.

Spinal Stenosis

Spinal stenosis is narrowing of the spinal canal, nerve root canals or foramen. It is due to excess bone growth from chronic stress on the bone. The excess bone produces pressure on the entire spinal cord. If compression remains untreated, weakness or paralysis of the innervated muscle groups may result.

Lordosis

Lordosis is an excessive backward concavity in the lumbar spine. It is commonly associated with sagging shoulders, medial rotation of the legs, and an exaggerated pelvic angle. Excessive lordosis may result in swayback and kyphosis. Back pain is common.

Spondylolisthesis

Spondylolisthesis is the forward slipping of one vertebra. It commonly occurs at L4–5, where the upper vertebra slips forward out of alignment. Spondylolisthesis is graded from 1 to 4. Grades 1 and 2 are managed conservatively. Grades 3 and 4 usually require surgery for stabilization (Figure 71-2).

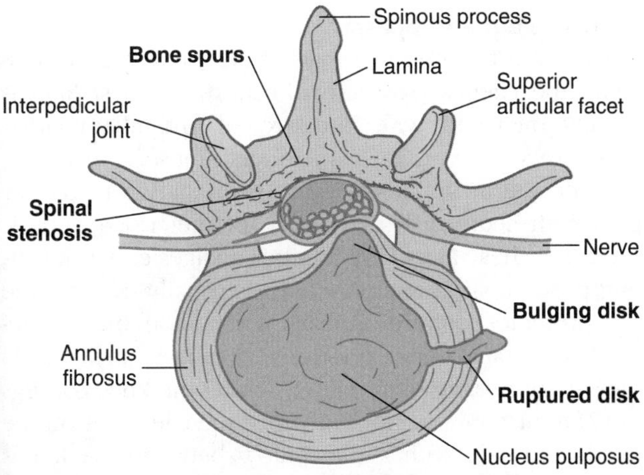

■ **FIGURE 71-1** The usual causes of lower back pain are disk herniation and spinal stenosis.

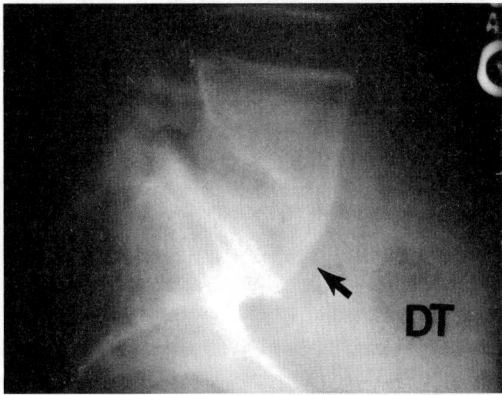

■ **FIGURE 71-2** Preoperative radiograph of spondylolisthesis. Note the slippage of the vertebrae. *(Courtesy James Manz, MD, Mayo Clinic, Eau Claire, Wis.)*

Spondylolysis

Spondylolysis is structural defect in which repeated microtrauma causes the vertebral arch to slip forward, resulting in stress fractures. The fifth lumbar vertebrae is most commonly involved.

Pathophysiology

Compressive loads have different effects on the intervertebral disk, body of the vertebrae, facets, and spinal ligaments. Under compressive loads, the annular fibers of the disks are stretched. The vertebrae are also compressed and may fracture at the end-plates. Spinal ligaments tend to buckle easily and the facet joints offer little resistance to compression.

The result is that the disk can herniate. When the disk only bulges, the annulus remains intact. With herniation, the annulus is usually torn, allowing extrusion of the nucleus pulposus (Figure 71-3). Compression of spinal nerve roots may result from herniation of the disk. The disks that separate and pad the vertebrae are innervated with fine nerve endings. When the disk impinges on the sciatic nerve, the condition and resulting pain is called *sciatica*. Sciatica is a severe, usually constant pain in the leg that occurs along the course of the sciatic nerve and its branches.

Clinical Manifestations

Rupture or herniation of a lumbar disk leads to lower back pain that radiates down the sciatic nerve into the posterior thigh as a result of compression of the spinal nerve roots. Typically, the pain of sciatica begins in the buttocks and extends down the back of the thigh and leg to the ankle. Disk herniation can result in groin pain. The client frequently has muscle spasms and hyperesthesia (numbness and tingling) in the area of distribution of affected nerve roots. The pain is aggravated by straining (coughing, sneezing, defecation, bending, lifting, and straight-leg raising) or prolonged sitting and is reduced by assuming the side-lying position with the knees flexed. Any movement of the lower extremities that stretches the nerve causes pain and involuntary resistance. Straight-leg raising on the affected side is

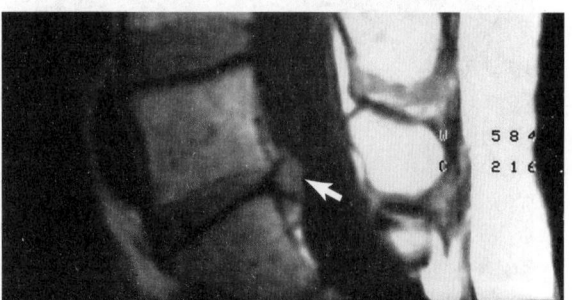

■ **FIGURE 71–3** Magnetic resonance imaging of the lumbar spine showing herniation of the disk between L5 and S1.

limited. Complete extension of the leg is not possible when the thigh is flexed on the abdomen (Lasègue's sign). There may be depression of deep tendon reflexes.

Manifestations of spinal stenosis usually begin slowly and are due to pressure placed on nerve roots as they exit the vertebrae. The most common manifestations are aching pain with standing and walking, paresthesias, and heaviness in the legs that progressively worsens with walking. There is rapid improvement in manifestations with trunk flexion, stooping, or sitting. The manifestations of spinal stenosis must be differentiated from claudication.

Diagnostic Findings

Computerized tomography (CT) and magnetic resonance imaging (MRI) scans provide precise images of the spine, disk, spinal cord, and paraspinal tissues (see Figure 71-3). Myelography and diskography are seldom used for initial evaluation.

OUTCOME MANAGEMENT

Medical Management

Goals of medical care include reducing pain and spasms, improving mobility, and repairing any structural problems in the spine or disks. Initial assessment of the client with lower back pain helps pinpoint the cause. The client's medical history is obtained to help determine whether a serious underlying condition is responsible for the pain, such as a fracture, tumor, or infection. The client's psychological and socioeconomic history is obtained, because these problems can complicate both assessment and management. The client is also asked to rate the pain. Physical examination determines whether lumbar nerve roots are involved by testing for reflexes, muscle strength, and the presence of neurologic deficits (Figure 71-4).

Control Pain and Spasms

Initial care of acute lower back pain is directed at managing the client's pain and directing activities. Pain is usually managed with nonsteroidal anti-inflammatory drugs (NSAIDs), COX-2 inhibitors, muscle relaxants, and short-term opioids. Ice has been shown to reduce pain with acute disk herniation for the first 48 hours. After that, heat is usually a better analgesic. A semi-sitting position (in a recliner chair) is usually comfortable and promotes forward lumbar spine flexion, thus reducing back strain. Other positions of comfort include (1) the supine position with pillows under the knees or legs or (2) the lateral position, in which the client lies on the unaffected side with a thin pillow between the knees and with the painful leg flexed to reduce tension on the sciatic nerve. Lying in a prone position and sleeping

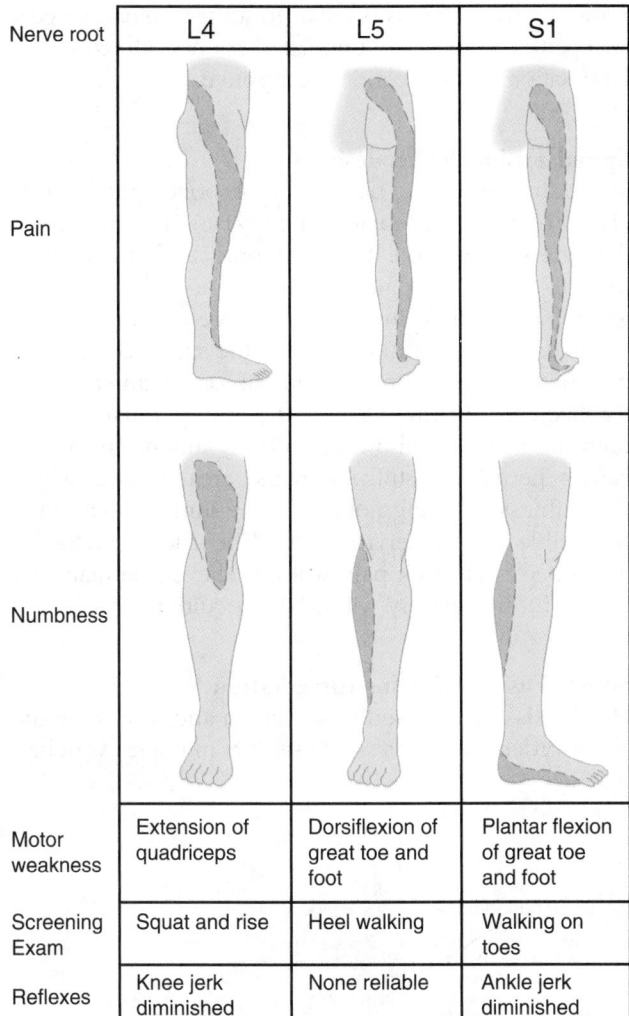

Nerve root	L4	L5	S1
Pain			
Numbness			
Motor weakness	Extension of quadriceps	Dorsiflexion of great toe and foot	Plantar flexion of great toe and foot
Screening Exam	Squat and rise	Heel walking	Walking on toes
Reflexes	Knee jerk diminished	None reliable	Ankle jerk diminished

■ **FIGURE 71–4** Assessment of lumbar nerve root compromise includes testing for motor weakness and reflexes, and eliciting pain (screening examination). *(Redrawn from Agency for Health Care Policy and Research. [1994]. Acute low back problems in adults: Assessment and treatment. Quick reference guide for clinicians (No. 14). Rockville, Md: Author.)*

with thick pillows under the head should be avoided. Physical therapists may be able to reduce pain and spasm with stretching exercises, massage, ultrasonic heat treatments, or transcutaneous electrical nerve stimulation (TENS). Work space or environmental modifications may also be necessary. Acupuncture and yoga exercises may be of therapeutic benefit.

For the client with nonspecific lower back pain, manipulation may be used by a physical therapist or chiropractor. *Spinal manipulation* is the use of the hands on the spine to stretch, mobilize, or manipulate the spine and paravertebral tissues. It is usually performed for clients with manifestations of back pain for more than 1 month's duration. There is no evidence that spinal traction with weights is effective in reducing lower back pain. Although unproven, deep ultrasonic heat treatment and moist local heat applications may

help reduce pain. Progressive muscle relaxation exercises, muscle stretching, and other stress reduction techniques can be helpful.

For severe lumbar disk problems with leg pain, conservative intervention involves 2 to 4 days of bed rest on a firm mattress. Bed rest reduces back pain by relieving the back muscles and vertebrae of the stresses. The forces of gravity (e.g., weight of the head with cervical problems) and motion can increase back pain during activity.

Improve Mobility

Activity modifications are prescribed to reduce back irritation and prevent debilitation from inactivity. Most clients do not require bed rest; in fact, more than 4 days of bed rest can be debilitating and slow recovery. The client is taught to minimize the stress of lifting by using good body mechanics, keeping objects close to the body, and to avoid twisting when lifting. Sitting may aggravate leg pain and clients who sit at work should change positions often. Aerobic activities should be prescribed to help avoid debilitation.

Walking, stationary bicycling, and even light jogging can be performed. Exercise should begin within the first 2 weeks after injury and each activity should be performed for 20 to 30 minutes, two or three times a week, for best aerobic conditioning.

Work activities need to be individualized for each client based on his or her job requirements. See the Client Education Guide feature on Lower Back Care on the website.

A back brace or corset is often prescribed for a client with a ruptured lumbar disk. Back supports are usually not recommended once clinical manifestations are relieved, because restricted back motion progressively weakens muscles and causes further degeneration of spinal structures. Strengthening the back and abdominal muscles helps prevent further problems when the exercises are done daily throughout life.

Nursing Care of the Medical Client

Nursing care focuses on assisting the client to adjust his or her lifestyle to reduce the risk of further back injuries. Many clients are frustrated with the lack of cure of their back pain. Clients have become accustomed to having a well-defined cause of a health problem and a well-researched approach for management. Many clients with lower back pain have pain for years without relief. This level of chronic pain can lead to depression and personality changes or relationship difficulties. Nurses should remain sensitive to the exasperation felt by the clients as well as the health care team. Clients reported higher satisfaction with treatment programs for low back pain when they received effective communication regarding treatment plans and care that was given.

Surgical Management

Surgery is indicated for spinal disk problems when (1) sciatica is severe and disabling, (2) manifestations of sciatica persist without improvement or worsen, and (3) physiologic evidence of specific nerve root dysfunction is present. Surgery is also used to stabilize spinal fractures and correct scoliosis and kyphoscoliosis. Some surgeons use other criteria.

Microdiskectomy

Microdiskectomy is the use of microsurgical instruments to remove the herniated fragment of disk. Use of this technique results in less trauma to the surgical site than standard diskectomy and more tissue integrity is preserved. Advantages of microsurgery include (1) minimal nerve root retraction, (2) preservation of an intact joint capsule (no bone is removed), (3) improved hemostasis, and (4) minimal stripping of the muscle and fascia from the spine.

Decompressive Laminectomy

The term *laminectomy* is confusing and is used loosely. The term *laminectomy* means complete removal of the bone between the spinous process and the facet. This much surgical removal is seldom necessary. The more correct term for what is done is *laminotomy,* which is the creation of a hole in the lamina. However, since the term is so common, it is used here.

Decompressive laminectomy is surgical removal of the posterior arch of a vertebra, exposing the spinal cord (Figure 71-5). This gives access to the spinal canal for (1) removing a spinal cord tumor, (2) removing portions of the facets, or (3) decompressing bony infringement on the spinal cord. Sometimes foraminotomy is performed to enlarge the intervertebral foramen if it is narrowed and osteophytic processes (overgrowth of bone) entrap the nerve root and impinge on neural structures.

Artificial Disk Replacement

Recent advances in research have developed replacement disks to provide spinal motion rather than fusion.

Postoperative care is similar to other spinal surgery except that clients are ambulated sooner. Outcomes of ambulation and recreation are positive.

Spinal Fusion/Arthrodesis

Spinal fusion is the placement of bone grafts (bone chips) between vertebrae (Figure 71-6). The new bone that grows fuses the two vertebrae and immobilizes them to reduce the pain. Usually no more than five vertebrae are fused; fusing more than five vertebrae causes considerable loss of movement in the spine. Bone grafts may be obtained from a bone bank or the anterosuperior iliac crest. During healing, the graft gradually grows onto the vertebrae and forms a bony union. This union causes permanent stiffness in the area. After a while, the stiffness is hardly noticed in the lumbar area but is noticeable in the cervical area. The client cannot be guaranteed that back pain will be relieved permanently or that further surgery will not be required.

Spinal Fusion with Instrumentation

Metal rods may be used to straighten and fuse the spine in disorders such as scoliosis or multiple vertebral

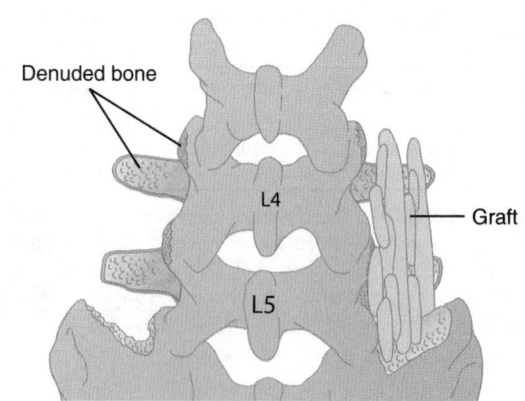

■ **FIGURE 71-6** Lumbar interbody spinal fusion. Bone grafts are taken from the iliac crest and inserted between the vertebrae. In this illustration, the "bed" of raw bone is shown on the left, and the graft material is shown in place on the right.

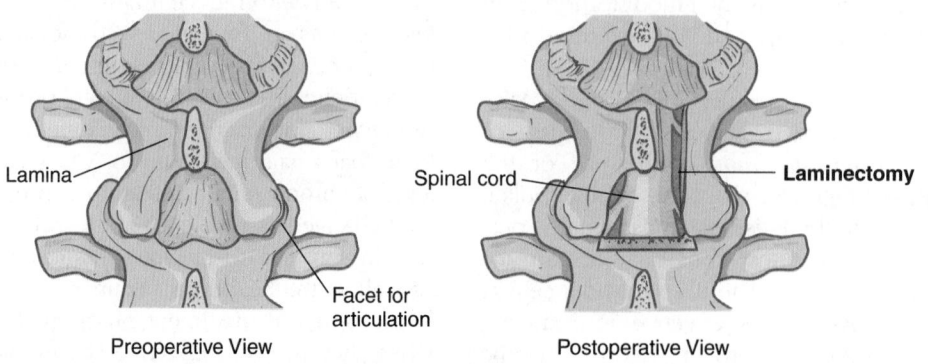

■ **FIGURE 71-5** Laminectomy for the interlaminal removal of a herniated disk.

fractures. Orthotic devices and braces can also be used to provide additional support while the bones heal in a fused manner (see Figure 27-4).

Complications

General potential complications following spinal disk surgery at any level include infection and inflammation, injury to nerve roots, dural tears, cauda equina syndrome, and hematoma. Non-union of the surgical area is also a risk and is associated with smoking. Some surgeons assess serum or salivary nicotine levels before surgery to reduce the risk of non-union and validate statements of smoking cessation.

Prognosis

The Agency for Healthcare Research and Quality (AHRQ) reviewed outcomes of surgery for lower back problems.[29] In general, lumbar diskectomy often relieved manifestations of pain in clients with severe and disabling leg pain faster than continued medical management. However, in individuals with no leg pain, there appeared to be little difference in outcome between diskectomy and conservative care. Most clients who had chymopapain injections required eventual diskectomy for permanent pain relief. More research is needed to determine who is best served by the various techniques; client preference also plays a big role in the technique chosen.

Nursing Management of the Surgical Client

The nursing care of clients having spinal surgery is shown in the Care Plan. (See Care Plan titled Management of the Client Undergoing Spinal Surgery, pp. 1878-1880.) Before surgery, encourage the client to become actively involved in their own care

Assessment. Following spinal surgery, assessment is similar to that performed for other surgical clients beginning with a head-to-toe assessment and evaluation of current pain level including response to analgesia. Assess neurologic function by asking the client to move his or her legs and comparing the results with those of the baseline evaluation. Question the client about the presence of numbness or tingling and changes in sensation or pain. New paresthesias may be a consequence of the edema from the surgery and the surgeon should be notified of them. If progressive weakness or paralysis of the lower extremities, loss of sphincter control, anal numbness, or urinary retention (called the *cauda equina syndrome*) occurs, notify the surgeon immediately. Emergency surgical decompression may be required.

Assess the wound for bulging or clear drainage, which may indicate cerebrospinal fluid (CSF) leakage. If the client had an anterior approach for surgery, usual care following abdominal surgery is required (e.g., assessment for atelectasis and ileus). Dressings and

drains are checked, including those at the donor site. Blood salvage during surgery is common and the client may return to the nursing unit with blood salvage equipment connected to incisional drains. Follow agency protocol and equipment guidelines to collect, filter, and reinfuse the client's salvaged blood.

Immediately following lumbar diskectomy, the client typically is not turned for an hour or so but remains flat to aid hemostasis. Begin side-to-side logrolling and repeat every 2 hours. If a dural tear was repaired, the surgeon may order the client to remain flat longer to minimize the risk of spinal headache, CSF leak, or a tear in the dural sutures.

After lumbar fusion, the bed is generally kept flat. The client logrolls from side to side, usually beginning about 4 hours after surgery and then every 2 to 4 hours thereafter; initially, extra assistance may be necessary (Figure 71-7, A-C on p. 1881). Spinal bone grafts are delicate and heal slowly. Eventually, turning is permitted without help, while keeping the spine rigid. Keep the bed linens loose at the foot of the bed to promote independent movement. If the client requires assistance to turn, or when turning to place a bedpan, turn the client in the logrolling manner. A fracture bedpan is used to reduce back arching and strain. Use of a trapeze over the bed is contraindicated because it promotes twisting. Usually the client is assisted to a chair the morning following surgery. Be sure to follow the physician's activity prescriptions.

Clients who have had fusions are on bed rest longer and thus are at greater risk for deep vein thrombosis (DVT). Compression devices on the legs may be used to improve venous return. Continuous compression stockings may be used, and the client is encouraged to move his or her legs and feet while on bed rest to promote venous return. If a client is supine following spinal surgery (e.g., using a bedpan), the lower back muscles may be relaxed somewhat if pillows are placed under the entire length of the legs. This may also prevent thrombophlebitis in the femoral vessels. Do not flex the client's knees by placing anything under the popliteal space, because the flexion increases the risk of DVT. Observe for and report any manifestations of DVT: redness or swelling in the one leg, Homans' sign (not a very specific sign, however), or sudden chest pain, dyspnea, and anxiety, which may indicate a pulmonary embolism.

After spinal surgery, a brace or corset may be required temporarily to support the spine. Clients who have lumbar or thoracic spinal fusions wear a fiberglass brace, which resembles a shell. Initially, back braces or corsets may be worn constantly, whether the client is in or out of bed. As the client's muscles strengthen, the use of braces or corsets is usually decreased. Again, follow the physician's activity prescriptions. Casts may be used for a while following any thoracic spinal surgery for clients with unstable thoracic spines (e.g., thoracic spinal cord trauma).

Management of the Client Undergoing Spinal Surgery

Nursing Diagnosis: Deficient knowledge related to client and family understanding of the preoperative, operative, and postoperative phases of spinal surgery.

Outcomes: Client and family will be able to explain the surgical procedure, preoperative preparations, and the postoperative precautions and needs. The client will demonstrate safe mobility, including logrolling, and transfer to and from the bed.

| NOC OUTCOMES | Knowledge: Treatment Regimen |

Interventions	NIC INTERVENTIONS	Rationales

1. Obtain baseline neurologic assessment:
  a. Motor and sensory function
  b. Psychological readiness
	Neurologic Monitoring	1. Establishes baseline motor and sensory function for later comparisons
		Determines level of ability and knowledge.

2. Explain logrolling.	Teaching: Preoperative	2. Protects back and enhances mobility.
3. Discuss activity limitations and avoidance of straining.	Teaching: Preoperative	3. Prevents damage (flexion, extension, twisting) to surgical site.
4. Explain need to seek assistance with ADL.	Teaching: Preoperative	4. Avoid stretching when reaching.
5. Explain use of stool softeners.	Teaching: Preoperative	5. Minimize straining with bowel movements.
6. Explain reason for non-ambulation.	Teaching: Preoperative	6. Clients with recent injury may exacerbate condition.
7. Encourage clients who smoke to stop smoking.	Teaching: Preoperative	7. Increases cardiovascular complications, risk of poor wound healing, and non-union if fusion is performed.
8. Evaluate for autologous blood donation.	Surgical Precautions	8. Two or three units should be donated at least 1 week before surgery. Older adults may require more time.
9. Review care of bone autograft donor site and pain management.	Teaching: Preoperative	9. Prepares client for additional pain.

10. Discuss changes in home environment:
  a. Bathroom facilities
  b. Shower/toilet use
  c. Ambulation devices
  d. Seat rises/grab bars
	Teaching: Preoperative	10. Anticipate home care needs.

Evaluation: Client and family will be knowledgeable of upcoming surgical procedure, understand postoperative nursing care, and have fears and concerns allayed. If questions arise about the operation, ask the surgeon to answer them. Do not attempt to provide information outside of your area of expertise.

Nursing Diagnosis: Fear and anxiety related to postoperative problems such as paralysis and chronic pain.

Outcomes: Client and family will express low level of fear or anxiety related to upcoming surgery and will use positive coping strategies to decrease fear or anxiety.

| NOC OUTCOMES | Fear Level, Anxiety Level |

Interventions	NIC INTERVENTIONS	Rationales
1. Encourage client and family to express fears and concerns.	Emotional Support	1. Allays concerns and fears.

Evaluation: Client and family will express fears and concerns, thus reducing anxiety level and improving compliance with surgical treatment regimen. For example, clients need to be aware that some edema is expected at the surgical site and therefore some of the preoperative deficit may still exist after surgery, but the client's condition should improve as the edema lessens.

Nursing Diagnosis: Acute Pain related to tissue trauma secondary to back (and/or abdominal) incision.

Outcomes: The client will express comfort, for example, a low level of tolerable pain, such as a 3 on a pain scale of 0 to 10.

| NOC OUTCOMES | Pain Level |

Interventions	NIC INTERVENTIONS	Rationales

1. Monitor pain:
  a. Incisional
  b. In extremity
	Pain Management	1. Incisional pain is expected, and leg pain is often significantly less after herniated disk surgery.

2. Administer pain medications:
  a. Basal (continuous) dose of opioid via IV pump and/or patient-controlled analgesia (PCA)
  b. PO
	Pain Management	2. Provide for client comfort. Provide PCA assistance. Avoid breakthrough pain. Combination strategy may be more effective.

Interventions	NIC INTERVENTIONS	Rationales
3. Teach client to ask for PO pain med before pain is too great.	Pain Management	3. Provide for client comfort.
4. Monitor epidural catheter for basal dose of analgesic.	Pain Management	4. Catheter to be maintained in position.
5. Avoid low-molecular-weight heparin injections.	Medication Safety	5. LMWH injections are associated with epidural hematoma when epidural catheters are in place.
6. Apply ice bag to incision using abdominal wrap to lumbar area and to bone graft donor site.	Pain Management: Cold Application	6. Provide for client comfort.

Evaluation: The client may have immediate relief from pain as many surgeons inject long-acting local anesthetics into disk spaces during surgery. This promotes a positive attitude toward the outcome of surgery. Often the pain recurs on the second postoperative day. This is due to both the increase in swelling and the fact that the local anesthetic is wearing off.

Nursing Diagnosis: Impaired Physical Mobility related to pain, leg weakness, prolonged immobility, or fear of pain and spasms. Choose the etiology that best fits your client.

Outcomes: The client will resume a maximal level of progressive activity, starting with logrolling on the day of surgery, progressing to independent movement from the bed to a standing position, followed by independent ambulation before discharge.

NOC OUTCOMES   Immobility Consequences: Physiologic, Mobility

Interventions	NIC INTERVENTIONS	Rationales
1. Use transfer device and ample people to assist with initial transfer to bed from surgery.	Body Mechanics Promotion	1. Support spine and maintain alignment. Transfer is smooth and gentle. Ensure safety.
2. Begin side-to-side logrolling every 2-4 hours; use extra help in turning.	Body Mechanics Promotion	2. Support spine and maintain alignment. Avoid twisting spine and hips. Ensure safety.
3. Administer analgesics before moving.	Pain Management	3. Lessens discomfort caused by spasms and pain with movement.
4. Tilt client back onto pillows; flex upper leg and place pillow between legs; place pillow to support upper arm; splint abdominal incision.	Body Mechanics Promotion Pain Management	4. Reduces pressure on donor site (iliac crest); keeps spine straight; prevents upper shoulder from sagging; reduces incisional pain.
5. Elevate head of bed as ordered.	Body Mechanics Promotion	5. Provides for client comfort and facilitates breathing and digestion.
6. Use pressure-redistribution mattress.	Pressure Management	6. Reduces risk of pressure ulcers.
7. Keep call light and PCA control so client can access them.	Body Mechanics Promotion	7. Avoid straining and twisting.
8. Instruct client about contraindicated positions and activities.	Body Mechanics Promotion	8. Avoid straining and twisting.
9. Assist client into chair; keep bed flat; have client roll onto side (see Fig. 71-7); have client then push torso from bed with arms to rise from the bed.	Body Mechanics Promotion	9. Lessen strain on spine Client may already be familiar with technique.
10. Anticipate spasms with turning and rising from the bed. Teach client to relax, deep breathe through spasm. Consider antispasmodics if prolonged or impaired movement.	Body Mechanics Promotion	10. Spasms are common with movement. Most spasms are transient. Prolonged or intense spasm will impair mobility.

Evaluation: Clients who have spinal surgery will have varying degrees of mobility limitations. Return to activity may depend upon the client's ability to manage pain, the extent of proper bone healing, muscle strength, and the use of proper body mechanics. Spasm control following surgery may be needed for some clients.

Nursing Diagnosis: Impaired Urinary Elimination related to pain and spasms with movement, inability to void in a supine position, and side effects from opioids.

Outcomes: The client will resume normal bladder emptying by the time the client is ambulating.

NOC OUTCOMES   Urinary Continence

Interventions	NIC INTERVENTIONS	Rationales
1. Assess for bladder distention and pain 8 hours after surgery.	Urinary Elimination Management	1. Urine is manufactured continuously by functional kidneys, even though the client has been NPO.
2. Try noninvasive methods to assist client to void	Urinary Elimination Management	2. Urinary catheterization increases the risk of urinary tract infection. Noninvasive measures do not carry this risk.

(Continued)

C A R E   P L A N   *evolve*

Management of the Client Undergoing Spinal Surgery—Cont'd

3. Straight catheterization is usually done twice.	Urinary Elimination Management	3. Straight catheterization empties the bladder, allowing time for resumption of normal voiding sensations.
4. Indwelling catheter is inserted if client still cannot void.	Urinary Elimination Management	4. Bladder or prostate problems may be present, preventing the client from voiding normally.
5. Maintain indwelling catheter until client is ambulating and using less pain medication.	Urinary Elimination Management	5. Pain and decreased activity hinder bladder function.
6. Assist client to urinate when standing or sitting.	Urinary Elimination Management	6. Lying supine can hinder sphincter function.
7. Straight catheterization is done to check for residual urine, if ordered.	Urinary Elimination Management	7. Promotes return of normal bladder function and prevents urinary tract infection.

Evaluation: Urinary retention occurs when the cauda equina is affected. Normal bladder function is dependent upon adequate pain management and resumption of ambulation and ADL.

Collaborative Problem: Risk for Paralytic Ileus is a common bowel problem after laminectomy and spinal fusion. Loss of bowel sounds and abdominal distention is due to lack of peristalsis from a sudden loss of parasympathetic function innervating the bowels and manipulation of the intestines in anterior approaches to spinal surgery.

Outcomes: The nurse will assess the client for return of normal bowel function, including normal bowel sound patterns, and evacuation without straining, by the time he or she is ambulating. This problem is expressed as a collaborative problem; therefore the outcome is written in terms of the nurse's actions. The nurse's actions cannot independently alter the outcome, as occurs with nursing diagnoses.

NOC OUTCOMES   Bowel Continence

Interventions	NIC INTERVENTIONS	Rationales
1. Assess abdominal status every 4 hours.	Bowel Management	1. Common findings include anorexia, nausea, vomiting, hard and possibly distended or tympanic abdomen, absence of bowel sounds.
2. Insert and maintain nasogastric tube to low intermittent suction.	Bowel Management	2. Reduce gastric distention and/or prevent paralytic ileus.
3. Maintain NPO status.	Bowel Management	3. Reduce gastric secretions.
4. Provide oral hygiene every 2 hours.	Oral Health Maintenance	4. Oral mucosa dries quickly when the client is NPO.
5. Resume clear liquid diet; advance diet as tolerated, when ordered.	Bowel Management	5. Hunger, bowel movement, or passing flatus indicates return of bowel function.
6. Encourage client to sit to defecate.	Bowel Management	6. Clients find it difficult or impossible to defecate when flat.

Evaluation: Expect bowel function to return within 12 to 24 hours after surgery; however, it may be longer if the client requires potent opioids. Return of hunger and reduced anorexia and nausea are the earliest signs that peristalsis has resumed. Ambulation is helpful in resuming peristalsis. The client should be able to eat before discharge.

Ileus is common for several days postoperatively. Inactivity and the use of opioid analgesia slow peristalsis. Fluids are forced as ordered; a regular time for bowel movements and bowel care is encouraged; fiber is provided in the diet (when allowed), and prescribed medications (e.g., stool softeners, mild bulk laxatives, or a suppository) and enemas are administered. Instruct the client not to strain for a bowel movement, because this increases pain and CSF pressure. Bowel movements are documented.

Disk problems often create fears and concerns related to pain, treatments, sexual activity, possible length of illness, and possible lifestyle changes. Provide psychosocial support to the client and family. Impaired mobility and altered urinary or bowel elimination are also common problems experienced after disk surgery. Smoking cessation is imperative because smoking delays the healing of bone. Considerations about employment and finances should be referred to a social worker.

Self-Care

Approximately 80% of the population experience lower back pain at some point in their lives. It is estimated that 10% of those who seek medical attention for back pain have herniated disks. Because of the frequency of herniated disk problems, health promotion is an essential activity for health care providers. See the Client Education Guide feature Lower Back Care on the website.

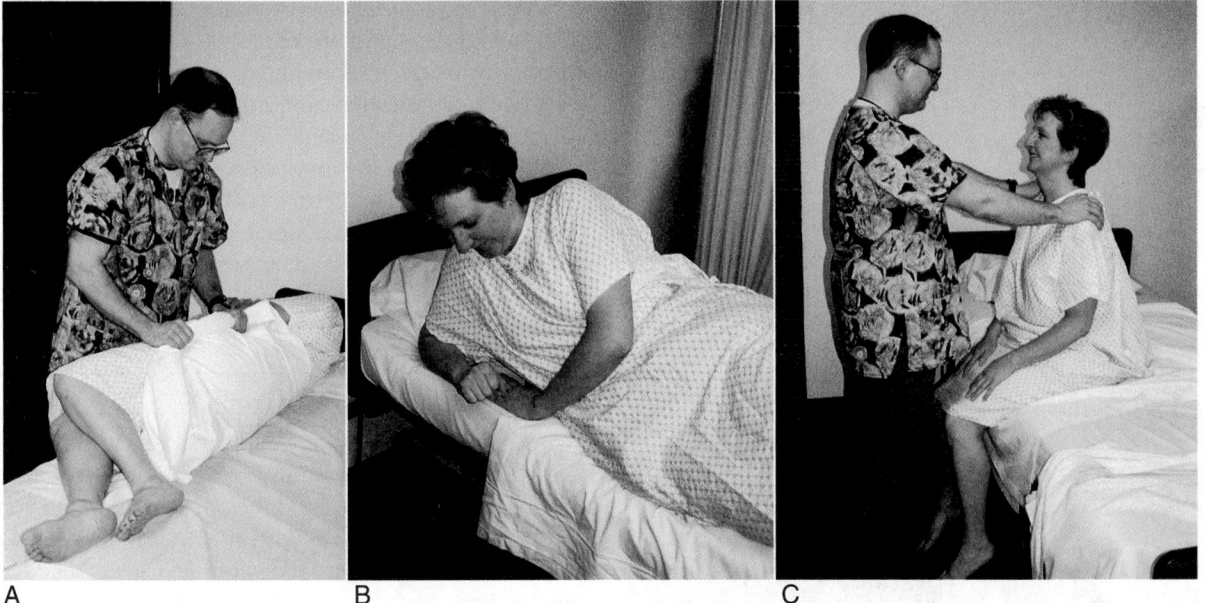

■ **FIGURE 71–7** Helping the client stand after lumbar fusion. **A,** Logroll the client to the edge of the bed using a turning sheet if needed. Leave the bed in that position. **B,** The client pushes off the bed with the hand and the other elbow to sit up without twisting. The client drops his or her legs off the side of the bed at the same time. **C,** With the client seated on the edge of the bed, the nurse assesses for orthostatic hypotension. The client stands from the bed without flexing the back.

CERVICAL DISK DISORDERS

Disks may become entrapped in the cervical spine. The process is much like that with herniated lumbar disks. Manifestations include arm pain, neck pain and spasms, and loss of function (grip strength) and changes in sensation in the hands.

OUTCOME MANAGEMENT

Initial treatment is with NSAIDs, muscle stretching, and teaching proper body mechanics. Opinions differ concerning the advisability of performing head and neck range-of-motion exercises in the presence of significant cervical disease. Tell the client to avoid activities that increase cervical disk pain. To prevent neck extension when in bed, only one flat pillow (to prevent neck flexion) is recommended. The neck should not be hyperextended. Intermittent traction may be applied for cervical disk herniation (5- to 8-lb weight) to reduce pain. The head of the bed may be slightly elevated with cervical traction. Otherwise, it is best kept flat when cervical pain is present.

A review of posture at work is important for clients who work at computer terminals. Keyboards, screens, and written materials should be kept at a height that reduces strain on the neck and shoulders. Stretching routinely also allows muscles to relax.

A soft cervical collar may be prescribed for mild to moderate cervical disk problems to keep the head slightly flexed. After fracture of a cervical vertebra, cervical disk rupture, or whiplash injury, the client may wear a neck brace (fitted so the chin rests on a cup and the neck is kept hyperextended), a hard collar (which extends up under the chin and prevents flexion of the neck), or a soft collar. Neck braces tend to limit vision, because people wearing them cannot look down at their feet.

> **Implement safety precautions when clients wear neck braces. Vision is impaired because they cannot turn the head or look down. Teach the client to climb stairs using a handrail.**

SAFETY

ALERT

Surgical Management

Sometimes conservative treatment does not work and clients require surgery. Surgery to stabilize bone fragments is necessary when a neck injury involves a bone fracture. Cervical fusion is most commonly performed through an anterior approach, so the incision will be on the front of the neck. Immediately after a posterior cervical diskectomy, a cervical collar is worn (Figure 71-8). A hard cervical collar is usually prescribed following fusion.

Treat any reports of nausea after cervical fusion. Vomiting can lead to aspiration because of difficulty in clearing the airway and not being able to turn the head or flex the neck.

Complications after posterior cervical surgery include soft tissue hematoma, air embolism, and subcutaneous wound dehiscence. Complications following anterior cervical surgeries include laryngeal nerve damage and injury to neck structures such as the carotid arteries, trachea, esophagus, and soft tissue.

After microdiskectomy, the client may have the head of the bed elevated to whatever position is comfortable. Following cervical spine fusion, the surgeon indicates

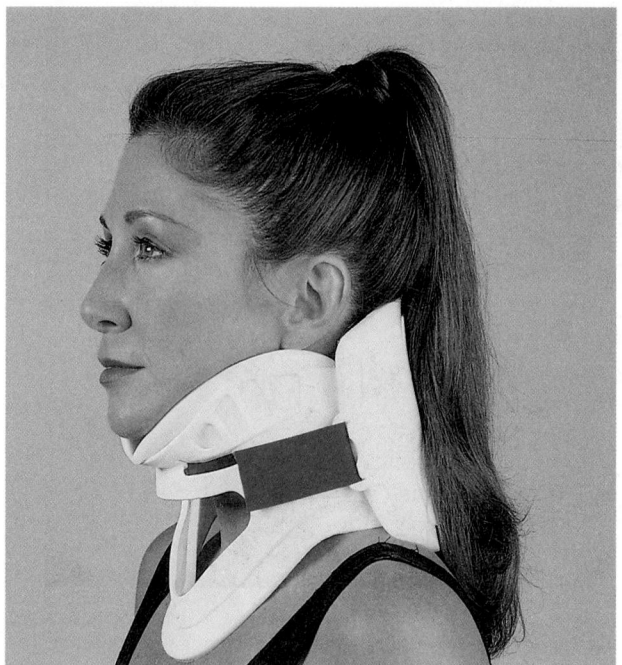

■ **FIGURE 71–8** A cervical collar with a chin piece. This orthosis provides additional support for the head and some restriction of cervical spine motion. *(Courtesy Zimmer, Inc., Dover, Ohio.)*

the degree of head elevation for comfort and to reduce edema. Make sure the spine is in anatomic alignment by keeping the head placed in neutral alignment. The client's head may be elevated and a folded small towel, bath blanket, or small pillow is placed under the head to maintain spinal alignment while the client lies supine or on the side.

Assess and document the client's neurologic status frequently.

SAFETY

ALERT

The development or worsening of a neurologic deficit must be promptly reported to the surgeon. During the first 24 hours after an anterior cervical diskectomy, assess the client's ability to breathe, check the operative site for excessive swelling, and changes in the client's voice. Laryngeal nerve damage during surgery may cause permanent vocal impairment, such as hoarseness. Watch for indications of respiratory paralysis resulting from spinal cord edema. Emergency tracheostomy equipment is kept at hand. If a spinal fusion was performed with the anterior cervical diskectomy, the surgeon is notified if upper extremity pain suddenly recurs. This could mean that the bone graft has moved out of place and surgery needs to be repeated.

Also assess the client for indications of postoperative improvement such as absence of paresthesias.

Tell the client that it is not unusual for preoperative manifestations to persist for a few days secondary to edema at the operative site, although these manifestations are usually less uncomfortable. Difficulty

swallowing and throat discomfort are usually present for several days and are commonly a result of local irritation from the endotracheal tube. A soft diet, throat lozenges, humidified air, minimal talking, and other comfort measures lessen the discomfort.

A wound drain may be present and is usually removed by the surgeon on the second postoperative day, after drainage has decreased. Bladder and bowel management are the same as for clients after lumbar surgery. Cervical surgery may affect the parasympathetic chain, causing urinary retention.

Self-Care

With shorter postoperative hospital stays, most clients are discharged before suture or staple removal. Instruction for care of the incision includes keeping the sutures or staples clean and dry and noting any increased redness or drainage from the wound. Clients need clear instructions on walking, lifting, driving, and returning to work. Most clients can resume regular activity 6 weeks after surgery. Specific physician instructions need to be followed.

Prolonged sitting or standing in one position strains the healing back. Contraindicated activities vary. The client is instructed to ask the surgeon when it will be safe to perform activities that could damage the back (climbing stairs, lifting a weight greater than 5 lb, prolonged travel, sexual activity, sports, exercise, and driving a car). Clients must not smoke. Smoking reduces blood supply to the tissues and delays healing. See the Client Education Guide feature on Home Care After Cervical Laminectomy or Fusion on the website.

POST-POLIO SYNDROME

Poliomyelitis is an acute form of paralysis characterized by destruction of motor cells in the spinal cord and brain stem. The disease has been controlled since the 1950s when mass immunization was used. However, post-polio syndrome can develop in polio survivors 30 years after the original disease. No form of prevention of post-polio syndrome has been identified.

Post-polio syndrome is a new onset of progressive weakness, fatigue, decreased temperature tolerance, emotional distress, dysphagia, pain in the joints and muscles, and respiratory problems. The onset is insidious, and weakness occasionally extends to muscles that were not involved during the initial illness. The prognosis is generally good; progression to further weakness is usually slow, with plateau periods that range from 1 to 10 years. The syndrome is thought to be due to progressive dysfunction and loss of motor neurons that compensated for the neurons lost during the original infection and not to persistent or reactivated poliovirus infection.

Management of post-polio syndrome has three components: energy conservation and lifestyle modification, medications, and measures to promote quality of life. Energy conservation includes pacing of activities, making the environment more ergonomic, sitting rather than standing, and use of electric mobility. Assistive devices to correct and minimize postural and gait abnormalities (e.g., canes, crutches, walkers) and braces designed to provide support to weakened muscles and joints can reduce pain, improve safety, and enhance energy conservation; they also help clients reduce fatigue, avoid overuse, and recover faster after activity. Occupational therapists can help clients assess their lifestyles and design appropriate changes. Despite the benefits of assistive devices, many polio survivors are reluctant to use them. They remember the intense rehabilitation efforts during their childhood and how they were encouraged to become independent and "like everyone else" again. It is important for a knowledgeable orthotist to fully explain the advantages of assistive devices and discuss the newer designs and materials.

Polio survivors may have also been instructed not to exercise, in order to avoid activity-induced muscle pain and "save" what muscle strength they have. This advice results in declining strength as a result of muscle deconditioning and increased long-term risk of cardiac deconditioning. Currently, several studies have demonstrated both the safety and the efficacy of nonfatiguing exercise for polio survivors. Progressive resistive strength training with reduced repetitive motion (e.g., 3 sets of 4 to 10 repetitions) done every other day demonstrated significant increases in static and dynamic strength without manifestations of injury or worsening manifestations.

Medications are used to reduce fatigue. Pyridostigmine (Mestinon) is commonly prescribed, but side effects of increased muscle twitching, nausea, diarrhea, and frequency are common. The weakness is treated with strengthening exercises, steroids to reduce inflammation, and electrical stimulation. Other manifestations are also treated symptomatically.

Symptomatic treatment of pain is important for optimizing both functional ability and quality of life. Polio survivors with pain can benefit from a multidisciplinary approach to pain management, which may include medication. The cause of the pain determines the choice of drug used to treat it. Primary post-polio muscle pain may have features of neuropathic pain. Additionally, primary neuropathic pain from nerve compression may be present. Neuropathic pain responds to NSAIDs, topical capsaicin, lidocaine (Xylocaine) preparations, and membrane-stabilizing agents. Biomechanical pain can be treated with steroids (oral or injectable), NSAIDs, or muscle relaxants, as well as with rehabilitation techniques, topical cold or heat, TENS, and relaxation/biofeedback. Overuse pain and cramps should not be casually medicated, because they are signs that changes in lifestyle and body mechanics are overdue.

Quality of life can be affected when post-polio syndrome develops in clients who have successfully adapted to their disease and disability. Respiratory distress may bring back memories of the initial infection and treatment in an iron lung (a very early form of a respirator in which the client's entire body was placed in a large metal cylinder).

Perceived barriers to health that furthered disablement in polio survivors have included fatigue, lack of money and time, lack of convenient resources, and lack of supportive health care providers. Additional restrictions are difficult to accept. Emotional support is vital. Teach the client to balance rest and activity.

SPINAL CORD DISORDERS

SPINAL TUMORS

Spinal tumors are similar in nature and origin to intracranial tumors but occur much less often. They are most common in young or middle-age adults and most often involve the thoracic region. Spinal tumors may occur outside of the spinal cord, such as in the meninges, nerve roots, or vertebrae (extramedullary), or within the substance of the spinal cord (intramedullary). Neurofibromas and meningiomas are the most common spinal cord tumors. Both are benign and operable and may not produce permanent damage if removed early.

Clinical manifestations of spinal tumors vary according to their location. Extramedullary tumors cause manifestations by compressing the spinal cord or some of its nerve roots or by occluding blood vessels supplying the cord. Early characteristics of spinal cord compression include pain, sensory loss, muscle weakness, and muscle wasting. Progressive cord compression is manifested by spastic weakness below the level of the lesion, decreased sensation, and increased reflexes. Severe cord compression at the cervical level destroys cord function and produces quadriplegia; compression at the thoracic or lumbar level results in paraplegia.

Intramedullary tumors produce more variable clinical manifestations. High cervical cord involvement causes spastic quadriplegia and sensory changes. Tumors in descending areas of the spinal cord produce motor and sensory changes appropriate to functions at that level.

Medical diagnosis is made after a complete general neurologic examination. Diagnostic testing includes CT scan or MRI scan.

Intervention for spinal tumors is usually surgery, radiation therapy, or both. Immediate surgery is indicated if compression of the cord or nerve roots is evident. Often, surgery results in marked improvement or even complete restoration of function, especially when the tumor is benign and encapsulated (e.g., meningioma or lipoma). However, functional improvement is less common when cord necrosis has developed. Complete surgical removal of an intramedullary tumor is rare. However, partial resection followed by radiation may improve the client's condition. Usually the course of the condition is gradually progressive.

SYRINGOMYELIA

Syringomyelia is often associated with Arnold-Chiari malformation (an abnormal protrusion of the medulla into the spinal canal) or spina bifida. Syringomyelia consists of abnormal cavities filled with dense, glue-like tissue in the spinal cord substance, especially the cervical cord. Scar tissue surrounds the cysts. Syringomyelia is characterized by (1) muscular weakness and wasting, (2) sensory defects, and (3) indications of injury to the long tracts of the spinal cord, such as hyperreflexia.

Early manifestations of cervical syringomyelia often include the following:

- Atrophy, weakness, and fibrillations of the small muscles of the hands
- Loss of pain sensation in the fingers or forearms
- Weakness and atrophy of the shoulder girdle muscles
- Horner syndrome, which is characterized by ptosis (droop) of the upper eyelid, constriction of the pupil, anhidrosis (absence of sweating), and flushing of the affected side of the face
- Nystagmus
- Vasomotor and trophic disturbances of the upper extremities

Although there is segmental loss or impairment of pain and temperature sensation, sensation for light touch remains. Segments of sensory loss may be separated by zones of normal sensation. Spasticity, ataxia, or paralysis of the lower extremities may occur, as may disturbed bladder control, if the lumbosacral region of the spinal cord is involved.

Cranial nerve involvement may produce additional problems such as impairment of facial pain and temperature sensation, loss of the corneal reflex (necessitating protection of the eye), dysphagia, dysarthria, laryngeal stridor (possibly necessitating tracheostomy), nystagmus, and atrophy and fibrillation of the tongue muscles.

Syringomyelia may progress rapidly at first and then become quiescent for many years. Some clients live 40 years after onset. Others become incapacitated (from paralysis or sensory defects) or die within a few years.

Treatment includes relieving increased pressure on the cord from the fluid content of the cavities within the spinal canal. The fluid buildup can be removed and CSF outflow restored by direct surgical drainage or by shunt placement.

NEUROSYPHILIS

Neurosyphilis is a chronic or late stage of syphilis involving infection of the brain or spinal cord. The oculomotor nerves may be affected, leading to an inability of the pupil to react to light, called an Argyll Robertson pupil. The posterior columns and nerve roots of the spinal cord may be affected, which is called *tabes dorsalis*. Because these are sensory nerves, the most common manifestation is pain. The pain can occur almost anywhere in the body, although abdominal pain is most common. The pain is severe enough to be confused with gastric ulcers and gallbladder disease. In addition to pain, areas of paresthesias may be noted. A common finding in tabes dorsalis is the loss of position sense in the feet and legs. As a result, clients walk with a slapping step. They are at increased risk of falls when walking in the dark because they must rely on visual cues for placement of their feet with each step. In addition, because the gait is abnormal, bone alignment with walking is altered. Eventually the foot is abnormally shaped (called *Charcot's joint*). This alteration in foot structure can lead to foot ulcerations, because the client bears the body weight on abnormal areas. The brain can also be involved in later stages of syphilis. A general deterioration of mental status can develop.

With improved case finding and the use of penicillin to treat syphilis in its early stages, the management of syphilis is improving. However, with development of resistant strains of organisms and a recent increase in the incidence of sexually transmitted diseases, problems may recur in the future.

UPPER/LOWER MOTOR NEURON LESIONS

Any lesion that destroys the UMNs initially results in contralateral paralysis, such as is seen with stroke. Initially, the involved area is flaccid and hyporeflexic. The flaccidity gradually recedes, and the reflex arc becomes hyperactive because of the lack of inhibition by the UMNs. Muscle tone is hypertonic and the extremity becomes spastic. Despite the spasms, the muscle becomes atrophied from disuse. The atrophy seen with UMN lesions occurs later than that seen with lower motor neuron (LMN) problems. The Babinski reflex is present.

When a lesion develops in lower motor neurons, the client develops flaccid muscle weakness or paralysis, loss of reflexes, loss of muscle tone, and atrophy of the involved muscles. The degree to which these clinical manifestations develop depends on the extent of the lesion. Each anterior horn cell innervates several separate muscle fibers, and because several anterior horn cells exist at each spinal level, a lesion confined to one spinal segment may not damage all of the anterior horn cells innervating an entire muscle. This type of lesion would cause muscle weakness rather than paralysis. Paralysis occurs when a lesion involves the column or anterior horn cells in several spinal segments. When all the peripheral motor nerves are involved, the entire muscle becomes flaccid. The muscles atrophy early from lack of innervation. LMN lesions are often associated with spinal cord injury or tumors and surgery on the aorta, which alters blood flow to the spinal cord.

DISORDERS OF THE CRANIAL NERVES

Cranial nerves can be affected in many ways by various nervous system disorders. For example, they may be secondarily affected by compression resulting from increased intracranial pressure or they may be directly damaged as a result of head injuries. In this section, only the two most common disorders specific to the cranial nerves, not those associated with other disorders, are discussed. Other cranial nerve disorders do exist. Regeneration of the cranial nerves can occur except for the first (olfactory) or second (optic) cranial nerve, because these nerves are actually part of the central nervous system (CNS).

TRIGEMINAL NEURALGIA

Chronic irritation of the fifth cranial nerve results in trigeminal neuralgia, also called *tic douloureux*. Although most commonly occurring in 50- to 70-year-old people, trigeminal neuralgia can occur in adults of any age. Approximately 60% of clients are women. The trigeminal nerve has three divisions: the ophthalmic, maxillary, and mandibular (Figure 71-9). Trigeminal neuralgia may occur in any one or more of these divisions.

Causes of trigeminal neuralgia can be divided into intrinsic and extrinsic lesions within the nerve itself, such as gross abnormalities of the axon or myelin, as may occur with multiple sclerosis. Extrinsic lesions are outside the trigeminal root and include mechanical compression by tumors, vascular anomalies, dental abscesses, or jaw malformation.

Trigeminal neuralgia is characterized by intermittent episodes of a sudden onset of intense pain. The pain is rarely relieved by analgesics. Tactile stimulation, such as touch and facial hygiene, and even talking, may trigger an attack. Trigeminal neuralgia is more prevalent in the maxillary and mandibular distributions and on the right side of the face. Bilateral trigeminal neuralgia is rare but does occur. The pain from trigeminal neuralgia can become so intense that the client ponders suicide.

None of the current diagnostic studies identify trigeminal neuralgia. Angiography, CT scan, and MRI can identify a causative lesion. The actual diagnosis is made on the

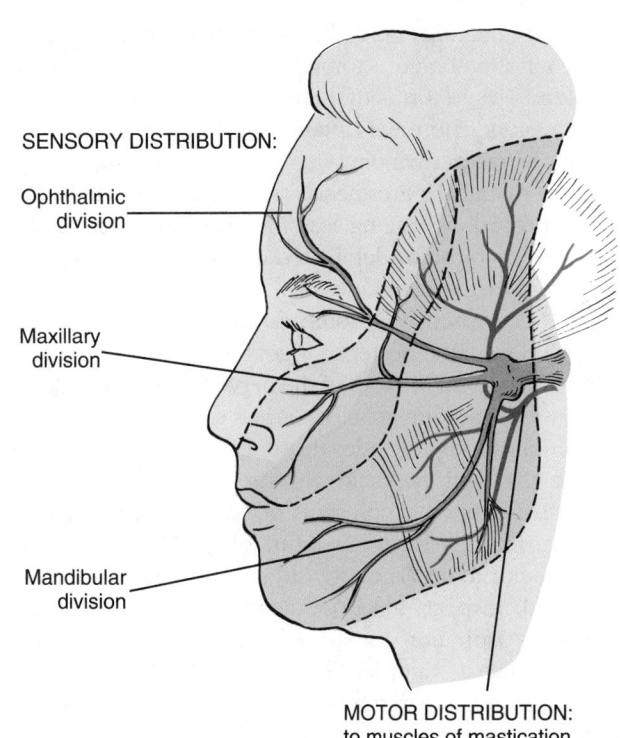

SENSORY DISTRIBUTION:

Ophthalmic division

Maxillary division

Mandibular division

MOTOR DISTRIBUTION: to muscles of mastication

■ **FIGURE 71–9** Distribution of the trigeminal nerve. Trigeminal neuralgia develops along the course of this nerve.

basis of an in-depth history with attention paid to triggering stimuli and the nature and site of the pain. A careful history is obtained from the client regarding stimuli that trigger an attack. This information is used to plan care so as to minimize triggering events. The client's dental hygiene and nutritional intake are evaluated. These clients often do not eat enough to meet their daily nutritional needs and neglect their teeth because of the pain.

OUTCOME MANAGEMENT

Anticonvulsants such as carbamazepine (Tegretol) and gabapentin (Neurontin) are often prescribed as the initial treatment of trigeminal neuralgia. These drugs may dampen the reactivity of the neurons within the trigeminal nerve. For some clients, these medications are all the treatment that is ever needed. Liver impairment may result from administration of both carbamazepine and phenytoin. Liver enzymes must be monitored before and during therapy. If the client cannot tolerate the dose needed for pain control, phenytoin can be used. These medications should be used cautiously in clients with a history of alcohol abuse. Baclofen (Lioresal) is an antispasmodic that may be used alone or in conjunction with anticonvulsants. Opioids are not particularly effective in relieving trigeminal neuralgia pain. Help clients use and improve any pain control strategies they have developed. Clients with trigeminal neuralgia need emotional support to help them deal with pain that has often been present for a long time.

Surgery includes nerve blocks with alcohol and glycerol, peripheral neurectomy, and percutaneous radiofrequency wave forms that create lesions that alter pain transmission. The relief obtained with these procedures is not always permanent. Complications include development of facial paresthesias and muscular weakness. These procedures, being less invasive, are often better tolerated by older or debilitated clients.

More invasive techniques include major surgical procedures. Microvascular decompression involves removing the vessel from the posterior trigeminal root. A rhizotomy is the resection of the root of the nerve. These procedures require a craniotomy to allow access to the nerve.

Complications include those of any surgical procedure, as well as facial weakness and paresthesias. If facial numbness is present following surgery, clients must learn to test the temperature of food before putting it into their mouth. They should chew on the unaffected side and inspect mucous membranes for irritation. Assess for aspiration and advance the diet slowly. Teach clients to use a water jet device instead of a toothbrush for dental hygiene and advise them to visit their dentist as soon as possible after surgery.

If the corneal reflex has been impaired, the client should be taught eye care. During the acute postoperative period, apply eye drops and a protective shield. The client assumes these tasks with supervision and then independently.

BELL'S PALSY

Bell's palsy affects the motor aspects of the facial nerve, the seventh cranial nerve (Figure 71-10). Bell's palsy is the most common type of peripheral facial paralysis. It affects both women and men in all age groups. However, it occurs most commonly between ages 20 and 40 years.

Bell's palsy results in a unilateral paralysis of the facial muscles of expression. There is no obvious pathologic cause although there is accumulating evidence that reactivation of herpesvirus (simplex type 1 or zoster) and Lyme disease may be implicated. Facial paralysis may be central or peripheral in origin. Central facial palsy is an upper motor neuron paralysis or paresis. Sometimes it produces dissociation of motor function. In this situation, the client cannot voluntarily show his or her teeth on the paralyzed side, but can show them with emotional stimulation such as that causing smiles or laughter. This phenomenon is called *voluntary emotional dissociation*.

Typical clinical manifestations include (1) upward movement of the eyeball on closing the eye (Bell's phenomenon), (2) drooping of the mouth, (3) flattening of the nasolabial fold, (4) widening of the palpebral fissure, and (5) a slight lag in closing the eye. Eating may be difficult.

There is no known cure for Bell's palsy. Care is palliative and includes analgesics if discomfort occurs from herpetic lesions, corticosteroids to decrease nerve tissue edema and often in combination with antiviral agents such as Acyclovir, physical therapy with moist heat, gentle massage, and stimulation of the facial nerve with faradic current. The cornea is protected with artificial tears, sunglasses, an eye patch at night, and periodic gentle closure of the eye.

Clients experiencing Bell's palsy often think they have had a stroke. Reassure the client that this is not the case. Most clients recover from Bell's palsy within a few weeks without residual manifestations. If permanent complete facial paralysis occurs, surgery may be necessary. Anastomosis of the peripheral end of the facial nerve with the spinal accessory or hypoglossal nerve allows closure of the eye during sleep and restores tone to the facial musculature.

DISORDERS OF THE PERIPHERAL NERVES

Peripheral neuropathy is a general term referring to disorders of peripheral nerves. Peripheral neuropathy can be associated with poor nutrition, a large number of diseases, and pressure or trauma. Many people suffer from the disorder without ever identifying the cause.

Peripheral neuropathy also can be classified by where it occurs in the body. Nerve damage that occurs in one area of the body is called *mononeuropathy;* that which occurs in many areas is called *polyneuropathy.* Radiculopathy is the term for neuropathy that affects nerve roots.

Neuropathy also can be categorized by cause, such as diabetic neuropathy and nutritional neuropathy. When a cause cannot be identified, the condition is called *idiopathic neuropathy.*

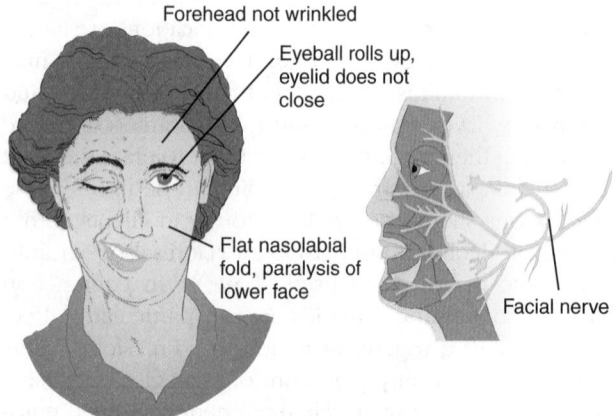

Forehead not wrinkled

Eyeball rolls up, eyelid does not close

Flat nasolabial fold, paralysis of lower face

Facial nerve

■ **FIGURE 71-10** Bell's palsy is paralysis of the facial muscles innervated by the seventh cranial nerve.

Peripheral neuropathy can be caused by disease; nerve compression, entrapment, or laceration; exposure to toxins; or inflammation. In many cases, especially in clients older than age 60 years, no cause can be determined. Several conditions are associated with neuropathy, including alcoholism, amyloidosis (metabolic disorder), autoimmune disorders (e.g., Guillain-Barré syndrome), Bell's palsy, cancer, carpal tunnel syndrome, renal failure, connective tissue diseases (rheumatoid arthritis), diabetes, Lyme disease, and vitamin deficiencies.

Clinical manifestations depend on the type of nerve affected (motor, sensory, autonomic) and where the nerve is located in the body. One or more types of nerve may be damaged.

Muscle weakness, cramps, and spasms are associated with motor nerve damage. In some cases, there may be loss of balance and coordination.

Sensory nerve damage can produce tingling, numbness, and pain. Pain associated with sensory nerve damage is variably described in the following manner:

- Sensation of wearing an invisible "glove" or "sock"
- Burning, freezing, or electric-like
- Extreme sensitivity to touch

If the autonomic nerves are damaged, involuntary functions may be affected. Orthostatic hypotension, bradycardia, reduced ability to perspire, constipation, bladder dysfunction, and sexual dysfunction may occur.

Because analgesics (e.g., aspirin, ibuprofen) are usually ineffective against pain caused by neuropathy, treatment often involves medications that target nerve cells. Anticonvulsants and antidepressants such as gabapentin (Neurontin) and amitriptyline (Elavil) are usually the first medications prescribed. Topical treatment with capsaicin cream (Zostrix) may be prescribed for focal neuropathy. The area surrounding the affected nerves may also be injected with lidocaine (Xylocaine) to temporarily reduce pain. Vitamin supplements may be used to treat nutritional neuropathy. Physical therapy (e.g., exercise, massage, heat) and acupuncture may be used to reduce manifestations.

CUMULATIVE TRAUMA DISORDERS

Cumulative trauma disorders (CTDs) include a group of overuse syndromes that predominantly affect the wrist and hand. They are also called *repetitive strain injuries* because some repetitive work activities seem to cause or exacerbate the manifestations. There are several forms (see Table 71-1). The client often describes fatigue in the extremity, and aching and tiredness during the activity. Rest generally relieves the manifestations in the first clinical stage. As the disorder progresses, manifestations persist despite rest. Finally, chronic aching, fatigue in the extremity, and weakness develop despite rest. To minimize the incidence and effects of CTDs, health specialists in business and industry have modified work tasks, workstations, work environment, tools, and equipment. Prevention focuses on exercises to reduce muscle strain and tension of the hands and wrist.

CARPAL TUNNEL SYNDROME

Carpal tunnel syndrome (CTS) is an entrapment neuropathy that occurs when the median nerve is compressed as it passes through the wrist along a pathway to the hand. The tunnel, called the *carpal tunnel,* is bordered by the flexor retinaculum, which is a band of fibrous tissue that prevents the wrist tendons from bowing when the wrist is flexed. Compression causes sensory and motor changes in the thumb, the index and middle fingers, and the radial aspect of the ring finger. CTS also leads to atrophy of the radial half of the thenar eminence.

CTS may develop spontaneously without a known cause or may result from disease or injury. The most commonly reported cause of CTS is repetitive motion of the wrist, with the wrist in constant flexion. A higher incidence of CTS is reported among homemakers, factory workers, bricklayers, cashiers, musicians, secretaries, and computer operators. Pregnancy, hypothyroidism, gout, and rheumatoid arthritis are other conditions associated with CTS.

Initially, the client may be awakened at night by pain and paresthesia. Although these initial manifestations are temporary and relieved by shaking the hand, later stages may be accompanied by motor loss (e.g., progressive weakness, inability to perform fine motor activities, and burning or numbness in the thumb, index finger, or middle finger) and daytime pain.

Assessment of the client begins with a thorough history, including occupational tasks. Diagnostic assessment for CTS includes assessing for Tinel's and Phalen's signs (Figure 71-11, *A* and *B*). Tinel's sign is the development of tingling in the hands and fingers when the wrist is tapped. Phalen's test is assessing for the development of numbness and tingling following forceful flexion of the wrists for 20 to 30 seconds (see Figure 71-11, *B*). Finally, the wrist compression test is done. The wrist compression test is manual application of 30 seconds of pressure over the flexor retinaculum (see Figure 71-11, *C*). If paresthesias develop after compression, the result is positive. The wrist compression test has been demonstrated to be 87% accurate in diagnosing CTS. Electromyography may also be used in differential diagnosis to rule out other possible causes.

OUTCOME MANAGEMENT

Initially the wrist is splinted in a neutral position to prevent mechanical irritation of the nerve. Injection of steroids into the flexor tendons is done less frequently than in the past because of reported problems with scarring, median nerve damage, and infection. In

TABLE 71–1 Repetitive Motion Injuries

Condition	Manifestations	People/Occupations at Risk	Usual Treatment
Neck			
Tension neck syndrome	Stiff, aching neck; headache	Typists, keypunch operators, cashiers, and others who must maintain a restricted posture	Prevention is key: (1) pause frequently when typing or keying to stretch about 30 sec every 30 min; (2) place screen directly in front of typist, avoid twisting; (3) place material to be typed at eye level if possible; avoid having materials to be typed consistently on one side of typist; conservative*
Cervical syndrome	Pain on flexion or extension of the neck with radiation down the arm	Common in people who assume awkward positions for a long time, such as painters, dentists	Conservative,* cervical collar, surgery
Shoulder			
Thoracic outlet syndrome	Numbness, pain, ischemia, and weakened pulse in upper extremity with hyperextension of shoulder	Overhead assembly workers, automobile repair mechanics, letter carriers	Conservative,* transcutaneous nerve stimulation, surgery
Supraspinatus tendinitis	Pain on elevating arm above 70 degrees at shoulder	People who must maintain abduction with elbow extended: painters, construction workers	Conservative,* physical therapy, steroid injections
Bicipital tendinitis	Pain over bicipital tendon in bicipital groove	Window washers, construction workers, shipping clerks	Conservative,* physical therapy, steroid injections
Elbow, Hand, and Wrist			
Lateral or medial epicondylitis (tennis elbow)	Local pain and pain on resisted hand motion	Repeated and forceful rotation of forearm with wrist bent; can be seen in bowlers, tennis players, and pitchers	Conservative,* steroid injections, surgery
de Quervain's tenosynovitis (inflammation of the extensor pollicis brevis tendons)	Gradual onset of pain, and sometimes swelling of radial styloid; popping sensation on extension of thumb	Middle-age women and those subject to repetitive stress of thumb	Conservative,* steroid injections, surgery
Carpal tunnel syndrome	Pain and paresthesias on percussion over median nerve at wrist (Tinel's sign) or with flexed wrists pressed together (positive Phalen's maneuver); night pain after 3-4 hr of sleep, morning stiffness, daytime numbness	Repetitive forced hand movements, keypunch operators, cashiers, typists, people with degenerative joint disease	Prevention is key: (1) while typing pause frequently, at least 30 sec every 30 min; (2) adjust keyboard so elbows are at 90-degree angle and wrists are straight; (3) do not rest wrists on a hard surface or restpad; wrists should "float" above keyboard; (4) use a light touch when striking keys; conservative,* steroid injections, surgery
Ulnar nerve entrapment	Pain and paresthesias on percussion of ulnar nerve over epicondyle (Tinel's sign); local swelling and tissue hypertrophy around elbow	Rheumatoid arthritis clients, occupational stress on elbow	Conservative,* surgery

*Conservative treatment consists of restriction of the harmful motion, splinting (if appropriate and only for short periods of time or at night), application of ice or heat, use of mild analgesics and nonsteroidal anti-inflammatory drugs, and performing gentle stretching exercises.

addition to rest, pyridoxine hydrochloride (vitamin B_6) has been reported to be helpful. For some clients, pain can be relieved by gently squeezing the distal metacarpal heads together with the affected hand palm up; in some instances, stretch of digits III and IV is also required. This maneuver may also help in the clinical diagnosis of CTS.

Surgery is indicated with (1) severe manifestations of long duration, (2) muscle atrophy, or (3) progressive sensory loss in the fingers and hand. Carpal tunnel release can be performed by opening the wrist or through an endoscope. General or regional anesthesia can be used. During the surgery, the transverse carpal ligament is divided to relieve pressure.

After surgery, blood flow is assessed hourly by checking the color, capillary refill, and warmth of the fingertips. When the anesthetic has worn off, assess the fingers for sensation.

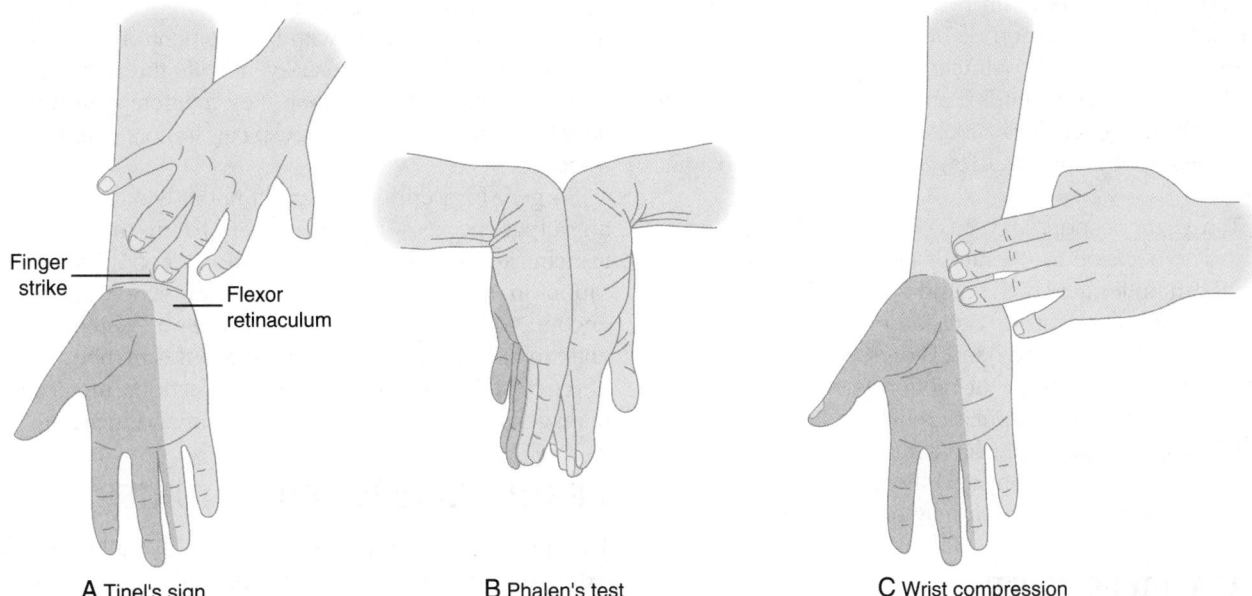

Finger strike
Flexor retinaculum

A Tinel's sign   **B** Phalen's test   **C** Wrist compression

■ **FIGURE 71–11**   Clinical examination for carpal tunnel syndrome includes tests for **(A)** Tinel's sign, **(B)** Phalen's sign, and **(C)** wrist compression. Each of these maneuvers elicits numbness and pain in the thumb, the index and middle fingers, and the radial aspect of the ring finger when carpal tunnel syndrome is present.

Initially, postoperative care centers on wrist immobilization using bulky dressings and a wrist splint. The arm is elevated on pillows to reduce edema. Encourage the client to try to move the fingers, even though they are splinted. Heavy gripping and pinching should be avoided for up to 6 weeks. These actions need to be avoided to keep the tendons from pushing out against the healing transverse ligament. After 6 weeks, the client should be safe to resume gripping and pinching without irritating the wrist. The client often returns to the same type of work, so recovery of strength and flexibility are imperative. Work site analysis should also be completed to avoid reinjury.

The client and family are the care providers beyond the immediate postoperative period. Because this surgery is usually performed on an outpatient basis, provide detailed instructions on home care. See the Client Education Guide feature on Home Care After Carpal Tunnel Release on the website.

CUBITAL TUNNEL SYNDROME

Cubital tunnel syndrome results from a combination of local pressure and stretching of the ulnar nerve at the elbow as it passes behind the medial epicondyle. The problem may arise following local trauma, but most often is spontaneous, with elbow position during sleep being the largest contributing factor. Problems include pain, numbness, altered sensation, and weakness, and may be permanent if nerve damage has occurred. Electrical nerve testing may be helpful in assessing nerve damage, but may be normal even in clients with symptomatic nerve compression. Nerve irritation at the neck may produce similar manifestations and may coexist with

this problem. Most mild cases can be treated with a splint or elbow pad and avoidance of flexion and direct pressure on the nerve. More advanced cases require surgery to decompress and transpose the nerve out of the cubital tunnel.

TARSAL TUNNEL SYNDROME

Tarsal tunnel syndrome is the counterpart of the CTS in the lower extremity. In this syndrome, the posterior tibial nerve is trapped beneath the flexor retinaculum and deep fascia along the foot's medial border. Entrapment compresses the nerve, causing pain, burning, and tingling on the sole of the foot; it usually worsens as the day progresses. This pain can usually be reduced by rest, elevation, or massage.

Conservative treatment, such as arch supports and wider shoes, may successfully relieve the discomfort of tarsal tunnel syndrome. If inflammation of the nerve is causing the compression, NSAIDs may be prescribed. Steroid injections may also be effective. If the problem is caused by flat feet, custom orthotics can help restore the foot's natural arch.

Surgery to release the laciniate ligament may be required to provide room for expansion of the nerve. If a cyst is impinging on the nerve, it can be removed.

DUPUYTREN'S CONTRACTURE

Dupuytren's contracture is permanent flexor contracture of the fourth and fifth fingers. Dupuytren's contracture is inherited as an autosomal dominant trait and is common in people of Northern European descent. It is also more common in alcoholic and diabetic clients.

In severe forms of contracture, a longitudinal fibrous cord forms, which extends from the fingers to the palm and pulls the fingers into a locked position. Milder forms have less contracture and fewer nodules in the palmar fascia.

Ten years or more may pass before surgery is necessary. The decision to operate is usually made when the client can no longer lay the hand outstretched on a table. The operation consists of excision of part of the palmar fascia. After surgery, the hand is dressed in a large compression dressing. Range of motion is encouraged. Frequent assessments of capillary refill and finger color are needed. Splints are often used at night to promote extension. Many months of physical therapy may be needed, and even then, full function may not be achievable.

GANGLION CYST

A ganglion can be described simply as a fluid-filled sac arising from an adjacent joint capsule or tendon sheath. A ganglion can form from almost any joint or tendon sheath in the wrist and hand. Trauma or degenerative changes in the fibrous joint capsule are thought to contribute to development of ganglia.

Ganglions may limit motion in the adjacent joints, or produce discomfort from compression or distention of local soft tissues. Large ganglions can be cosmetically unpleasant. Ganglion cysts of the distal interphalangeal (DIP) joint may produce deformities of the fingernail. Ganglion cysts arising from the flexor tendon sheath at the base of the finger may produce pain when grasping. On rare occasions, ganglion cysts (particularly those associated with the wrist) may cause changes in the bone. Ganglion cysts can frequently be diagnosed simply by their location and shape. They are usually not adherent to the overlying skin and are firmly attached to the underlying joint or tendon sheath. Large ganglions may permit the passage of light through their substance (transillumination). X-ray studies are sometimes helpful in diagnosing ganglion cysts, particularly around the DIP joint where associated degenerative arthritis is often found.

To relieve pain or numbness, the ganglion may be aspirated or surgically excised. The area may then be injected with a corticosteroid before a pressure dressing and splint are applied. NSAIDs are commonly used for pain. Wrist ganglions may recur in up to 30% of clients.

PERIPHERAL NERVE TUMORS

Although solitary tumors (generally neurofibromas) may develop on any peripheral nerve, multiple tumors most often occur and are part of a syndrome known as *neurofibromatosis* (von Recklinghausen's disease). This hereditary disorder is characterized by multiple tumors of the spinal and cranial nerves along with involvement of many other systems. The disease is usually not life-threatening, and lesions are excised only when they interfere with normal activity. Intracranial and intraspinal tumors are usually removed.

Surgery for peripheral nerve tumors is often done on an outpatient basis. In the recovery room, the dressings are checked for drainage; circulation, motion, and sensation in the extremity are also assessed. Clients are encouraged to perform range-of-motion exercises. Clients and family members are taught the manifestations of circulatory compromise and infection, medication management, and care of the dressing and incision.

PERIPHERAL NERVE INJURIES

The peripheral nerves most commonly subjected to external pressure are the median, radial, ulnar, sciatic, common peroneal, tibial, and long thoracic nerves. The common peroneal nerve (a terminal branch of the sciatic) is injured more frequently than any other nerve. Because of its course and distribution, the sciatic nerve is exposed to internal and external trauma and inflammation more than any other nerve. The sciatic nerve may also be injured directly during medication injections. The median nerve is most often injured by constriction from fascial bands. The axillary nerve may be injured as the result of an allergic reaction to serum injections or secondary to improper crutch walking. Any peripheral nerve can be injured by bone fractures or perforating wounds. Nerves can also be injured in common household accidents (cut on glass) or in motor-vehicle accidents.

Assessment includes a full examination of the injured area. Assessment findings with nerve damage depend on the type of nerve injured and the extent of damage. Damaged motor nerves cause clinical manifestations such as flaccid paralysis, and reflex loss in the muscle innervated by the injured nerve. Damaged mixed nerves or sensory nerves cause vasomotor and trophic disturbances following either partial or complete interruption of the nerve. Following partial injury or incomplete division of a nerve, the person may experience stabbing pains, paresthesias ("pins and needles" sensation), and, occasionally, the burning pains of causalgia. Damaged sensory nerves cause loss of sensation in the nerves' area of anatomic distribution. If the hand is injured, document the client's occupation and the dominant hand.

Conservative management may include splinting, ice, elevation of the limb, administration of anti-inflammatory and analgesic agents, or a combination of these modalities. If a peripheral nerve is traumatically severed, the ends should be surgically anastomosed to enable healing. The nearer the site of injury occurs to the CNS, the less chance of regeneration. When nerves are only slightly damaged, mild edema occurs at the injury site. This may cause temporary manifestations that recede in a few days or possibly weeks.

Postoperative care of clients having nerve repair or grafting includes elevation of the extremity. Elevation is critical to reduce edema and improve venous return. The procedure is usually performed with local anesthesia, so assessment of neurovascular status is not conclusive until the anesthesia has worn off. Color, warmth, movement, sensation, capillary refill, and strength are assessed. Some of these assessments can be hampered by dressings, but as many as possible should be performed. Monitor the fingertips for blood flow with Doppler laser or standard Doppler ultrasonography and temperature probes. The temperature of the hand is usually less than the core temperature and the surgeon indicates acceptable ranges of temperature. Physical therapy begins within a few days to promote movement after severe injuries.

If the injury is severe, the client may have recurring dreams about the accident and his or her injury. These dreams are generally normal, but if they are bothersome to the client, a psychiatric consultant may be helpful.

CONCLUSIONS

The physical and psychological impairments vary with the degree of damage as well as the client's response and ability to cope with the body changes. The coping response is not always related to the degree of physiologic damage. A client can have facial paralysis or trigeminal neuralgia and be more compromised psychologically than a client with spinal cord injury who has strong coping skills. It is imperative that nurses comprehend the severity of the client's dysfunction as it relates to quality of life, as well as the impact it has on family dynamics.

THINKING CRITICALLY

1. The client, a 34-year-old woman, had a lumbar laminectomy done earlier today. A prior assessment showed that movement and sensation of both lower extremities were intact. During the current postoperative assessment, she states that her right toes feel numb, and the dorsiflexion and plantiflexion of the right foot are weaker than earlier. She has requested an analgesic because she is starting to get a headache. What are the priorities for her care? What assessments and interventions might be used?

Factors to Consider. What assessment methods can be used to determine the extent of vascular insufficiency? What type of neurologic checks should be done?

A discussion for this question can be found on the website.

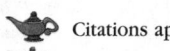

BIBLIOGRAPHY

Citations appearing in red refer to primary research.

Citations appearing in blue refer to evidence-based practice guidelines and protocols.

1. Ashkenazi, A., & Levin, M. (2004). Three common neuralgias. *Postgraduate Medicine, 116*(3), 16-32.
2. ASPAN pain and comfort clinical guideline. (2003). *Journal of Peri-Anesthesia Nursing, 18*(4), 232-236.
3. *Bell's palsy fact sheet*. National Institute of Neurological Disorders and Stroke website. Accessed 07/16/06 at www.ninds.nih.gov/disorders/bells/detail_bells.htm.
4. Boswell, M.V., Shah, R.V., Everett, C.R., et al. (2005). Interventional techniques in the management of chronic spinal pain: Evidence-based practice guidelines. *Pain Physician, 8*(1), 1-47.
5. Bridwell, K.H., Anderson, P.A., Boden, S.D., et al. (2005). What's new in spine surgery? *Journal of Bone and Joint Surgery, 87*(8), 1892-1901.
6. Brigham and Women's Hospital. (2003). *Upper extremity musculoskeletal disorders. A guide to prevention, diagnosis and treatment.* Boston, Mass: Brigham and Women's Hospital.
7. Cain, J.E. (2006). Gentle yoga effective for chronic low-back pain. *American Journal of Nursing, 106*(3), 22.
8. Canter, P. (2006). How effective is spinal manipulation? *General Practitioner, April 14*, 30-31.
9. Carlson, D. (2005). When your patient has acute facial paralysis. *Nursing, 35*(4), 54-55.
10. Childs, S.G. (2005). Dupuytren's disease. *Orthopaedic Nursing, 24* (2), 160-165.
11. Chronic pain relief. (2006). *British Journal of Community Nursing, 11*(4), 175.
12. D'Arcy, Y. (2006). Treatment strategies for low back pain relief. *Nurse Practitioner, 31*(4), 16-27.
13. Exercises for aching hands. (2005). *Harvard Women's Health Watch, 13*(3), 2-3.
14. Implant eases low back pain. (2006). *Nursing, 36*(2), 34-35.
15. Institute for Clinical Systems Improvement (ICSI). (2005). *Adult low back pain*. Bloomington, Minn: ICSI.
16. Institute for Clinical Systems Improvement (ICSI). (2005). *Assessment and management of chronic pain*. Bloomington, Minn: ICSI.
17. Kramasz, V.C., & Roman, L.M. (2005). Polio patients take a second. *RN, 68*(11), 33-37.
18. Kwon, B. (2006). A review of the 2001 Volvo Award winner in clinical studies: Lumbar fusion versus nonsurgical treatment for chronic low back pain: A multicenter randomized controlled trial from the Swedish Lumbar Spine Study Group. *Spine, 31*(2), 245-249.
19. Lively, M.W. (2005). Acute lumbar disk injuries in active patients: Making optimal management decisions. *Physician and Sportsmedicine, 33*(4), 21-27.
20. Low level heat wrap therapy helps low back pain. (2006). *Journal of Pain & Palliative Care Pharmacotherapy, 20*(1), 78-79.
21. Meadows, G.R. (2005). Microendoscopic lumbar diskectomy. *Operative Techniques in Sports Medicine, 13*(2), 122-124.
22. Mueller, D.M., & Oro, J.J. (2004). Prospective analysis of presenting symptoms among 265 patients with radiographic evidence of Chiari malformation type I with or without syringomyelia. *Journal of the American Academy of Nurse Practitioners, 16*(3), 134-138.
23. New concepts in Bell's palsy improve treatment options. (2005). *American Family Physician, 72*(1), 169-170.
24. National Institute of Dental and Craniofacial Research website. Accessed 10/12/05 at www.nidcr.nih.gov/.
25. Posture and back health. (2005). *Harvard Women's Health Watch, 12*(12), 6-7.
26. Shaw, W.S., Zaia, A., Pransky, G., et al. (2005). Perceptions of provider communication and patient satisfaction for treatment of acute low back pain. *Journal of Occupational and Environmental Medicine, 47*(10), 1036-1043.
27. Stevenson, K., Lewis, M., & Hay, E. (2006). Does physiotherapy management of low back pain change as a result of an evidence-based educational programme? *Journal of Evaluation in Clinical Practice, 12*(3), 365-375.

28. University of Michigan Health System. (2004). *Acute low back pain.* Ann Arbor, Mich: University of Michigan Health System.

29. U.S. Preventive Services Task Force (USPSTF). (2004). *Primary care interventions to prevent low back pain in adults: Recommendation statement.* Rockville, Md: Agency for Healthcare Research and Quality (AHRQ).

30. Schoen, D.C. (2005). Injuries of the wrist. *Orthopaedic Nursing, 24* (4), 304-307.

31. Washington State Department of Labor and Industries. (2005). *Antiepileptic drugs guideline for chronic pain.* Provider Bulletin (PB 05-10), 1-3.

32. Watkins, J. (2005). Independent nurse: Clinical—Diagnosis and care of Bell's palsy. *General Practitioner, June 6,* 119-120.

33. Work Loss Data Institute. (2006). *Carpal tunnel syndrome (acute & chronic).* Corpus Christi, Tex: Work Loss Data Institute.

34. Work Loss Data Institute. (2006). *Forearm, wrist & hand.* Corpus Christi, Tex: Work Loss Data Institute.

35. Work Loss Data Institute. (2006). *Low back—Lumbar & thoracic (acute & chronic).* Corpus Christi, Tex: Work Loss Data Institute.

36. Work Loss Data Institute. (2006). *Neck and upper back (acute & chronic).* Corpus Christi, Tex: Work Loss Data Institute.

evolve *Did you remember to check out the bonus material on the Evolve website and the CD-ROM, including NCLEX®-Examination Style Review Questions, Open-Book Quizzes, and Chapter Review Audio Podcasts?*

http://evolve.elsevier.com/Black/medsurg

CHAPTER 72

Management of Clients with Degenerative Neurologic Disorders

PATRICIA E. GRAHAM

Degenerative neurologic disorders pose a great challenge to the client, the family, and the caregiver, whether it is a nurse, a family member, or a significant other. By their very nature, these disorders cause progressive decline in neurologic function. Some progress relatively quickly (over months to 1 or 2 years), whereas others progress more gradually, sometimes over decades. Common nursing diagnoses for clients with these disorders are *Altered Thought Processes, Memory Deficit, Visual-Perceptual Alteration, Impaired Physical Mobility, Incontinence, Self-Care Deficit,* and *Impaired Individual and Family Coping.* A major goal of intervention is to help the client achieve an optimal level of functioning in light of chronic neurologic deficits. The family should also be taught what to expect, such as the usual areas of decline, how to provide care and support to the client, and how to manage stress and cope with the progressive nature of the disorder.

The diagnosis of degenerative neurologic disease is most often made in an outpatient setting; however, hospital admission may be necessary when acute relapses or life-threatening events occur. Many clients return to their homes and have regular follow-up in outpatient clinics; however, some may require rehabilitation, in either inpatient or outpatient settings, for newly acquired deficits. Other clients may require transfer to long-term care facilities because of a significant decline in their ability to provide self-care. Still other clients may not survive their acute illness.

ALZHEIMER'S DISEASE AND RELATED DEMENTIAS

The term *dementia* refers to the loss of memory, reasoning, judgment, and language to such an extent that it interferes with everyday life. The changes may occur gradually or quickly, and how they come about is key to determining whether the condition causing dementia is temporary.

Cognition is the act or process of thinking, perceiving, and learning. Cognitive activities that become impaired in dementia include decision-making, judgment, memory, spatial orientation, thinking, reasoning, calculation, personality, and verbal communication. A client with dementia may undergo behavioral and personality changes as well, depending on the area(s) of the brain affected. There are many causes of dementia. Because the brain is quickly injured from hypoxia, reduced blood flow, or drugs, the causes are numerous (Box 72-1).

Types of Dementia

Alzheimer's disease (AD) is the most common form of dementia among people over age 65. AD constitutes at least half of all dementias. Alzheimer's disease affects about 4 million Americans. Slightly more than half of these people receive care at home, and the remainder receive institutional nursing care. The prevalence of AD doubles every 5 years after the age of 65. In fact, some estimates indicate that nearly half of all people older than 85 have AD.

BOX 72-1 Causes of Dementia

- Alzheimer's disease
- Multi-infarct dementia (arteriosclerotic dementia)
- Parkinson's disease
- Lewy body disease
- Alcoholic dementia
- Binswanger's disease
- Creutzfeldt-Jakob disease
- Huntington's chorea
- AIDS-related dementia
- Normal pressure hydrocephalus
- Genetic or metabolic disease (e.g., thyroid)
- Toxic or traumatic injury
- Malignant disease: primary, metastatic, or iatrogenic from the treatment

---

Multi-infarct (multiple stroke) disease is the second most common cause of irreversible dementia. Blood clots block small blood vessels in the brain and destroy brain tissue. Typically multiple infarct dementias occur in men more than 50 years old. The effect of multiple infarcts (strokes) over time leads to the progressive decline in cognition.

Lewy body dementia is similar to Alzheimer's disease but may progress more rapidly. Abnormal brain cells called cortical Lewy bodies occur throughout the brain and produce manifestations. Lewy bodies are also associated with Parkinson's and Alzheimer's diseases, but it is not clear whether dementia with Lewy bodies is a distinct clinical entity or perhaps a variant of Alzheimer's or Parkinson's disease.

Pick's disease also is a form of dementia but differs from AD in several ways. First, the two diseases produce different abnormalities in the cells of the brain. Pick's disease is marked by "Pick bodies," rounded, microscopic structures found within affected cells. Neurons swell, taking on a "ballooned" appearance. Neither of these changes appears in Alzheimer's disease, and the pathology of Alzheimer's disease (plaques and tangles) is not found in Pick's disease. Second, Pick's disease is usually sharply confined to the front parts of the brain, particularly the frontal and anterior temporal lobes. This contrasts with Alzheimer's disease, which is more widely distributed.

Etiology and Risk Factors

The cause of AD has not been found, although several risk factors have been identified. Increasing age is a risk factor. Genetic factors are also linked to AD. At least five chromosomes (1, 12, 14, 19, and 21) are involved in some forms of familial AD. Four genetic loci have also been identified as contributing to AD, including the amyloid precursor gene, the presenilin 1 gene, the presenilin 2 gene, and the apolipoprotein E gene on chromosome 19. Research has also shown that the age of AD development is also

genetic. The Genetic Links feature on p. 1895 describes other genetic disorders in addition to AD.

Clinical situations associated with AD development include elevated homocysteine levels (also a risk factor for heart disease), inflammation, stroke, and oxidative damage from free radicals. (The Complementary and Alternative Therapy feature on p. 1896 summarizes promising research findings in using omega-3 fatty acids to lower the risk of Alzheimer's disease.) Research is active in these areas to find the pathophysiologic connections and prevent them.

Pathophysiology

Alzheimer's disease disrupts the three neuronal processes that keep neurons healthy: communication, metabolism, and repair. Alois Alzheimer first described presenile dementia in 1907. He used a new staining technique of human brain tissue to demonstrate the pathologic changes. The changes he noted are now termed *beta-amyloid plaques* and *neurofibrillary tangles* (Figure 72-1). *Plaque* is a cluster of beta-amyloid, a protein fragment snipped from a larger protein, called *amyloid precursor protein*. Plaques have been described as dense, mostly insoluble deposits of protein and cellular material outside and around the neuron. Plaques develop in the hippocampus, an area of the brain that helps encode memories. Degenerating nerve terminals, both dendritic and axonal, contain amyloid protein. Healthy neurons have an internal support structure, called *microtubules*. These tubules serve as tracts to guide nutrients to the end of the axon and back. The tubule is stable because of a protein called tau. In AD, the tau is changed chemically and becomes tangled. Once tangled, the tubules degenerate and so do the cells they support. The destruction leads to memory failure, personality changes, and problems carrying out activities of daily living (ADL).

Gross brain changes evident in clients with AD include thickening of the leptomeninges, shrunken gyri, widened sulci, enlarged ventricles, hippocampal shrinkage, and generalized atrophy (Figure 72-2). In addition to structural changes, neurotransmitter changes, for example acetylcholine, are evident in the brain of clients with AD. Acetylcholine decreases because there is a decline in cholinergic neurons in the basal nucleus that leads to loss of choline acetyltransferase in the neocortex and hippocampus.

Clinical Manifestations

Clinically, AD is characterized by a relentless impairment of decision-making that generally begins insidiously and can progress for a decade or so. Manifestations can vary depending on the portion of the brain involved and on genetic predisposition. The onset of AD typically occurs in late middle age (age 65 years and older), although some familial cases occur in a person's 40s and 50s.

GENETIC LINKS

Examples of Neurodegenerative Genetic Disorders

Disorder	Features	Inheritance	Gene Defect	Genetic Testing Available?
Huntington's disease (HD)	Progressive disorder of motor, cognitive, and psychiatric disturbance; onset 35-44 yr; median survival 15-18 yr after onset	AD	HD	Yes
Early-onset familial Alzheimer's disease (EOFAD)	Early onset of progressive impairment of memory, judgment, decision making, and language; mean onset under age 65 yr; comprise <2% of all AD cases	AD	PSEN1 APP PSEN2	Yes No Yes
Late-onset Alzheimer's disease (AD2)	Multiple affected family members, with onset of dementia after age 60-65 yr; estimated to account for ≈25% of Alzheimer's disease	Complex trait; one or more susceptibility genes	APOE	Yes*
Parkinson's disease (familial PD)	Progressive disorder characterized by resting tremor, akinesia, and rigidity; rare occurrence	AD	PARK1 PARK2 PARK3 PARK4 UCH-L1 PARK6 PARK7 PARK8	Yes No No No No No No No
Spinocerebellar ataxias, 21 types	Poor coordination of movement and wide-based uncoordinated, unsteady gait; poor coordination of limbs and speech often present; onset, frequency, and features vary and overlap	AD AR XL	SCA1 SCA2 SCA3 SCA6 SCA7 SCA8 SCA10 SCA12 SCA17	Yes Yes Yes Yes Yes Yes Yes Yes Yes
Friedreich's ataxia	Slowly progressive ataxia; onset age <25 yr; depressed tendon reflexes	AR	FRDA	Yes
Early-onset primary dystonia (DYT1)	Onset age <21 yr; involuntary sustained muscle contractions that cause posturing of limbs	AD	DYT1	Yes

AR, Autosomal recessive; *AD*, autosomal dominant; *XL*, X-linked.
*Presymptomatic testing is not routinely performed.

Preclinical Alzheimer's Disease

Alzheimer's disease begins near the hippocampus, a structure essential to the formation of both short- and long-term memories. Affected regions begin to shrink and in time (10 to 20 years perhaps) lead to memory loss.

Mild Alzheimer's Disease

As the cerebral cortex begins to shrink, other cognitive losses become apparent. *Memory disturbance* is usually noticed by family members or co-workers before the client does. The client may demonstrate poor judgment and problem-solving skills and become careless in work habits and household chores. Clients may become confused about where they are and they begin to get lost

easily. Routine activities such as bill paying and other daily tasks take longer. The client may do well in familiar surroundings and may be able to follow well-established routines but lacks the ability to adapt to new challenges. The person may become irritable, suspicious, or indifferent. Agitation, apathy, dysphoria, and aberrant motor behavior are associated with cognitive impairments.

Moderate Alzheimer's Disease

The client may demonstrate *language disturbance,* characterized by impaired word-finding and *circumlocution* (talking around a subject rather than about it directly). Later, spontaneous speech becomes increasingly empty, and *paraphasias* (words used in the wrong context)

COMPLEMENTARY AND ALTERNATIVE THERAPY

Omega-3 Fatty Acids from Fish and a Lower Risk of Alzheimer's Disease

A prospective study conducted from 1993 to 2000 followed 815 individuals (ages 65 to 94 years) in a community in the United States for an average of 3.9 years. These individuals completed a dietary questionnaire on average 2.3 years before clinical evaluation. A total of 131 individuals developed Alzheimer's disease in this study. Individuals who consumed fish once per week or more had 60% less risk of developing Alzheimer's disease compared with those who rarely or never ate fish.

REFERENCE

Morris, M., et al. (2003). Consumption of fish and omega-3 fatty acids and risk of incident Alzheimer disease. *Archives of Neurology, 60,* 940-946.

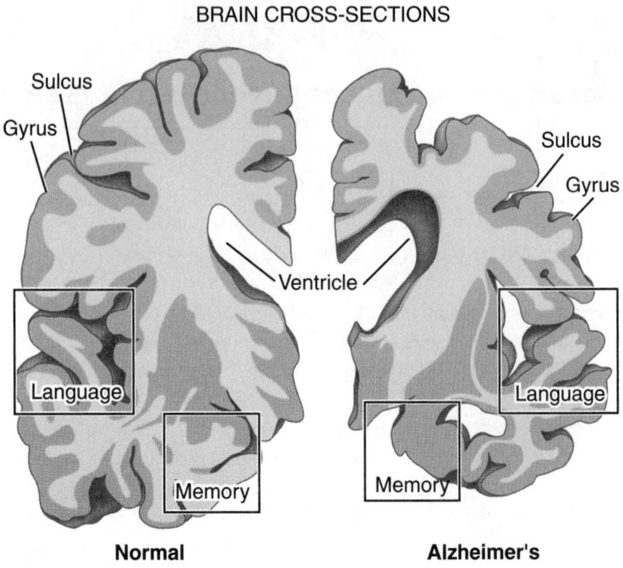

BRAIN CROSS-SECTIONS

FIGURE 72–2 Alzheimer's disease affects many portions of the brain, especially those required for memory and speech.

are used. Clients may repeat words and phrases just spoken by themselves *(palilalia)* or by others *(echolalia)*. Motor disturbance *(apraxia)* is characterized by difficulty in using everyday objects such as a toothbrush, comb, razor, and utensils. Apraxia combined with forgetfulness can create serious safety problems. The person may leave a stove burner on in the kitchen or forget to extinguish a cigarette. Indifference worsens, and restlessness with frequent pacing appears. *Hyperorality* (the desire to take everything into the mouth to suck, chew, or taste) may develop. Swallowing may become difficult.

Depression and irritability may worsen, and delusions and psychosis may appear. The person fears personal harm, theft of property, or infidelity of the spouse. Clients may see bugs crawling on the bed or throughout the house. Wandering at night is common. Occasional incontinence may occur.

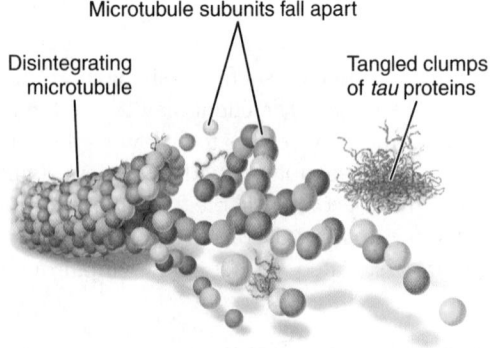

Microtubule subunits fall apart

Disintegrating microtubule

Tangled clumps of *tau* proteins

FIGURE 72–1 Neurofibrillary tangles. In clients with Alzheimer's disease and some other neurologic disorders, these tangles replace the normal neuronal cytoplasm. The tangles are often seen with senile plaques and appear throughout the cortex, hippocampus, and amygdala. The number of plaques and tangles correlates roughly with the severity of the dementia.

Severe Alzheimer's Disease

In the final stage, plaques and tangles are widespread throughout the brain. Clients cannot recognize family or friends and do not communicate in any way. Voluntary movement is minimal, and the limbs become rigid with flexor posturing. Urinary and fecal incontinence is frequent. Aspiration and aspiration pneumonia are frequent.

Diagnostic Findings

A diagnosis is best made by a multidisciplinary group that can assist the client and family to understand what is happening and what interventions or assistance will be needed. Because there is no definitive test for AD, the diagnosis is made by exclusion of known causes of dementia (e.g., toxic or metabolic alterations, drug side effects, cerebrovascular disease, cancer, infection). The diagnosis is confirmed with (1) the presence of dementia involving two or more areas of cognition, (2) insidious onset and steady progression, and (3) loss of normal alertness.

Computed tomography (CT) scan can be used to identify ventricular dilation and sulcal enlargement and cerebral atrophy of the portions of the brain most affected. Magnetic resonance imaging (MRI), single-positron emission computed tomography (SPECT), and positron emission tomography (PET) are also used to detect changes in brain function.

Finally, laboratory studies are performed to rule out metabolic and drug-related causes of dementia. These studies include urinalysis, complete blood count (CBC), erythrocyte sedimentation rate (ESR), electrolytes, blood urea nitrogen (BUN) and creatinine values, thyroid and liver function tests, calcium, serum B_{12} levels, syphilis serology, and human immunodeficiency virus (HIV) testing.

Manifestations of Other Dementias

Manifestations of multi-infarct dementia (MID) often develop in a stepwise manner and include confusion, problems with recent memory, wandering or getting lost in familiar places, incontinence, emotional lability such as laughing or crying inappropriately, difficulty following instructions, and problems handling money. Usually the damage is so slight that the change is noticeable only as a series of small steps. Over time, however, as more small vessels are blocked, gradual mental decline occurs. MID, which typically begins between the ages of 60 and 75, affects men more often than women.

Manifestations of Lewy body dementia can range from traditional parkinsonian effects, such as loss of spontaneous movement *(bradykinesia)*, rigidity (muscles feel stiff and resist movement), tremor, and shuffling gait, to effects similar to those of AD, such as acute confusion, loss of memory, and loss of or fluctuating cognition. Visual hallucinations may be one of the first manifestations noted, and clients may suffer from other psychiatric disturbances such as delusions and depression.

OUTCOME MANAGEMENT

No cure has been found for AD. Management of the client centers on helping maintain mental function and slowing the process of deterioration.

Medical Management

Maintain Mental Function

Several medications are used to retain ACh in the neurojunctions. Tacrine (Cognex), donepezil (Aricept), galanthamine (Reminyl), and rivastigmine (Exelon) are used to maintain memory. These drugs can have small but noticeable effects, depending on the stage of disease, differences in the way the drugs act in different clients, and other factors. At least temporarily, many clients taking these drugs experience improvements in their thinking abilities and are less likely to demonstrate common manifestations of advanced AD, such as wandering, agitation, and socially inappropriate behaviors. None of these drugs prevents AD from worsening over time.

In an effort to combat the effect of oxygen free radicals, alpha-tocopherol (vitamin E) and selegiline have been studied. Both agents have been reported to delay the development of the later stages of AD and show some improvement in levels of independent and behavioral manifestations. The Complementary and Alternative Therapy features here and on p. 1898 summarize research findings in the use of vitamin E supplements for Alzheimer's disease and in the use of ginkgo biloba to improve memory in healthy people. An extract of ginkgo biloba may improve cognitive function for 6 to 12 months. Propentofylline has been effective in the management of AD. See the Complementary and Alternative Therapy

feature Use It or Lose It: Reducing the Risk of Dementia on the website.

Over the short term, other medicines can somewhat relieve anxiety, agitation, depression, and psychotic or inappropriate behavior: anxiolytics for anxiety and agitation, neuroleptics for unusual or troublesome behavior, and antidepressants or mood stabilizers for mood disorders and specific problems such as spells of anger or rage. No specific drugs or dosages address the wide range of problems that clients with AD experience. Medications such as risperidone (Risperdal), olanzapine (Zyprexa), quetiapine (Seroquel), sertraline (Zoloft), or citalopram (Celexa) should be used as seldom as possible and at the lowest effective doses. This will help minimize side effects in frail

---

COMPLEMENTARY AND ALTERNATIVE THERAPY

Vitamin E Supplements for Clients with Alzheimer's Disease

The only agent that has been shown to slow the progression of Alzheimer's disease in a prospective study (in clients diagnosed with this condition) is vitamin E supplements. A multi-institutional, double-blind, placebo-controlled prospective study included 341 moderately impaired clients (Clinical Dementia Rating score of 2). Clients were randomly assigned to receive 2000 international units of vitamin E; 10 mg of selegiline; vitamin E and selegiline; or placebo for 2 years. The primary end-point was the time to progression to any of the following end-points: institutionalization, loss of any two of three basic activities of daily living (eating, dressing, and toileting), a rating of 3 on the Clinical Dementia Rating Scale, or death. Using an intention-to-treat analysis and after adjusting for differences among the groups in the baseline Mini-Mental State Examination score, the researchers observed a significant delay in the primary outcome among the treatment groups. There was an increase in median survival of 230 days for clients taking vitamin E alone, 215 days for clients taking selegiline, and 145 days for clients taking vitamin E and selegiline compared with clients receiving placebo.[2] The interpretation of this trial was somewhat controversial because of the need to include the baseline Mini-Mental State Examination score as a covariant in order to reveal a statistically significant difference between the treatment and placebo groups. Regardless, the American Academy of Neurology now recommends 2000 international units of vitamin E daily (1000 international units twice daily) as a standard care for the treatment of clients with Alzheimer's disease.[1]

REFERENCES

1. Doody, R., et al. (2001). Practice parameter: Management of dementia (an evidence-based review). Report of the Quality Standards Subcommittee of the American Academy of Neurology. *Neurology, 56,* 1154-1166.
2. Sano, M., et al. (1997). A controlled trial of selegiline, alpha-tocopherol, or both as treatment for Alzheimer's disease. The Alzheimer's Disease Cooperative Study. *New England Journal of Medicine, 336,* 1216-1222.

COMPLEMENTARY AND ALTERNATIVE THERAPY

Ginkgo Biloba in Healthy Individuals for Memory Enhancement

Extracts or compounds from ginkgo have shown some initial promise in enhancing memory in demented older individuals.[1] However, researchers wanted to test the potential claims of some manufacturers that ginkgo could, in general, enhance mental focus and improve memory and concentration. Community-dwelling, functionally independent individuals older than 60 years volunteered for this study of memory.[2] Participants were excluded if they scored less than 27 out of a possible 30 points on the Mini-Mental State Examination at baseline. Highly educated or intelligent participants with mild dementia may have been included in this study. Participants in this randomized controlled trial received 40 mg of ginkgo biloba three times daily (dose recommended by many manufacturers) or placebo for 6 weeks. This duration was 2 weeks longer than the manufacturer's suggested onset of action. A total of 230 participants were included. No statistically significant differences were observed between ginkgo and placebo on any of the scales measured. No significant changes from baseline to post-treatment and no adverse effects were noted in the groups. In other words, ginkgo, in standard doses for 6 weeks, was ineffective in improving memory, intelligence, and concentration in older clients without dementia.

REFERENCES

1. Le Bars, P., et al. (2002). Influence of the severity of cognitive impairment on the effect of the ginkgo biloba extract Egb 761 in Alzheimer's disease. *Neuropsychobiology, 45,* 19-26.
2. Solomon, P., et al. (2002). Ginkgo for memory enhancement: A randomized controlled trial. *Journal of the American Medical Association, 288,* 835-840.

older clients. The use of these medications to "control behavior problems" is avoided; rather, the behavior should be considered an attempt to communicate a specific need.

Nursing Management of Alzheimer's Disease

Assessment. When AD is suspected, a complete history should be taken to assess for other causes of dementia. Data should be obtained from the client, family, and co-workers (if possible). Secondary sources are used because the client is often unaware of a problem with thought processing and minimizes it. Ask specific questions about difficulties with ADL, increasing forgetfulness, and changes in personality. Assess past medical history for previous head injury or surgery, recent falls, headache, and a family history of AD. A Mini-Mental State examination may provide objective data for ongoing evaluation of the client (see Chapter 67). AD has a profound impact on psychosocial behaviors. Ask about the client's reactions to changes in routine or in the environment. It is not uncommon for a client with AD to become very agitated over small

changes, and apathy, social isolation, and irritability may be noted. As the brain continues to atrophy and the limbic system becomes dysfunctional, the client may become paranoid, use abusive language, and become suspicious of others.

Alzheimer's disease has a profound impact on the family. Assess the family for strengths and weaknesses, their ability to provide care for the client, and their financial concerns. In large centers, assessment of the client and family is performed through a team approach. The Client Education Guide website feature titled Caring for Family Members with Alzheimer's Disease provides instructions and resources for caregivers of people with AD.

> **The home environment should be evaluated for safety before the client is sent home from the hospital:**
>
> - Is the home on a busy street?
> - Can doors be secured so that the client cannot leave without supervision?
> - Are potentially dangerous appliances out of reach?

Diagnosis, Outcomes, Interventions

Diagnosis: Impaired Verbal Communication. Use the nursing diagnosis of *Impaired Verbal Communication related to loss of cognitive function* to describe the client with AD.

Outcomes. The client's needs will be communicated effectively, as evidenced by making her or his needs known and by interacting meaningfully with others. This outcome is only possible in the early stages. In later stages, a more appropriate outcome might be expressed as the client's needs are interpreted appropriately.

Interventions. In the initial stage of AD, the client's receptive and expressive language skills are relatively intact. The nurse must be prepared to adapt to the communication level of the client. If the client speaks only single words or short phrases, the nurse should do likewise. It is best to speak slowly and simply, with a firm volume and low pitch. The tone of voice should always be calm and reassuring and project control of the situation. When language becomes impaired in the second stage of the illness, be prepared to apply new techniques for communicating with the client.

Nonverbal behavior can provide clues about specific needs. Clients with AD often avert their eyes, look down, back away, and increase hand gesturing when they do not understand. If they are frustrated, angry, or hostile, they may increase motor activity by pacing, rattling doorknobs, waving their arms or shaking their fists, frowning, raising their voice volume and pitch, or tightening their facial muscles. These behaviors should signal staff to increase their alertness, search for the cause of the distress, and prepare to intervene.

The identification of pain or discomfort in clients with advanced AD is also difficult. Behavioral indicators of discomfort include noisy breathing, negative vocalization (constant muttering, making sounds with a negative quality), a sad or frightened facial expression, frowning, tense body language, and fidgeting.

Diagnosis: Impaired Memory. *Impaired Memory* is an ideal diagnosis for clients with AD. State this diagnosis as *Impaired Memory related to loss of short-term memory, inability to execute complex mental processes, or inability to concentrate or focus on specific tasks.*

Outcomes. The client will retain information to maximal capacity, maintain maximal orientation, and share meaningful life experiences.

Interventions. Because memory deficit occurs in all stages of AD, continually apply interventions to enhance memory. Reorient the client as necessary by placing a calendar and clock in obvious places. Because the client's long-term memory is retained longer than short-term memory, allow clients to reminisce. Become aware of a client's past experiences so that they can be shared meaningfully. Repetition is useful for ensuring maximal retention of information.

The client's memory loss can be an advantage in distracting him or her from the stressful situation. If removed from the situation and provided with calm, nonthreatening environment, clients may forget why they are upset. Elicit listening behavior by reaching out and touching, holding a hand, putting an arm around the waist, or in some way maintaining physical contact with the client. Dementia sufferers can perceive nonverbal behavior of others and can become agitated or upset if they sense negative nonverbal behavior from them. Having activities or interests, exercise periods, and opportunities to wander in a safe environment can do much to reduce anxiety and stress. The Management and Delegation feature at right discusses Communicating with Agitated Clients.

Diagnosis: Risk for Injury. Altered thought processes lead to impairments in judgment and forgetfulness. These changes increase risk for injury. State this common nursing diagnosis as *Risk for Injury related to impaired judgment, forgetfulness, and/or motor impairments.*

Outcomes. The client will be at reduced risk of injury by having the staff maintain a safe physical environment and the client having no physical injuries, near-falls, or falls.

Interventions

In the inpatient setting, ensure that clients cannot leave the premises without being noticed, that they wear an identification badge in case they become lost, and that doors and windows are secured. In the home, electrical devices, toxic substances, loose rugs, hot tap water, inadequate lighting, and unlocked doors can be sources of injury. Teach family members how to eliminate these safety hazards. Dangerous objects should be kept out of

reach, and potentially dangerous activities, such as cooking, should be supervised. The client's driving skill should be evaluated at regular intervals. The Bridge to Home Health Care feature on p. 1900 addresses additional safety considerations for clients with AD.

Diagnosis: Self-Care Deficit. Clients in the middle stage of AD require assistance to put clothes on properly, bathe, and toilet. State this diagnosis as *Self-Care Deficit related to loss of memory and motor impairments.*

Outcomes. Clients will maintain self-care ability as evidenced by completing the tasks they are capable of performing and receiving assistance with ADL that they are incapable of performing.

Interventions. Encourage the client with AD to do as much as possible, as long as it is safe and appropriate. Carefully balance helping the client with maintaining his or her autonomy; this can boost the client's confidence and self-respect, which can be very fragile during

---

MANAGEMENT AND DELEGATION

Communicating with Agitated Clients

Many aspects of client care are performed by unlicensed assistive personnel. Almost all of these activities, from taking vital signs to giving a bath, require communicating with the client. When clients are demented, they often cannot understand spoken directions and respond with aggressive or frightened behavior.

Communication with clients who have dementia is difficult. They do not always understand what you are saying and may respond differently each time you attempt to work with them. For clients who need help to put on clothes, bathe, and get to the bathroom, spoken words can usually be understood if the words are simplified and the caregiver is patient. Identify yourself and call the client by name. Be certain that the client is wearing a hearing aid and glasses, if necessary. Do not startle the client or speak to the client in a derogatory manner. Use simple, direct statements, speaking slowly and calmly. Look at the face of the client and have light shining on your face. For example, do not stand with your back toward the window; you will be in a shadow from the client's view.

If the client makes no attempts to speak, nonverbal forms of communication become more important. Avoid approaching the client from the side or from behind. Keep your facial expression positive, your body language open. You should continue to speak using a calm tone of voice. A person with dementia who feels threatened or confused by your communication may react in negative ways, such as striking out or crying. Try to use the same caregiver each day. Use nonverbal cues, such as moving your arms and hands, to indicate "Please come with me" or "Please take this pill." Do not give more than one instruction at a time.

BRIDGE TO HOME HEALTH CARE

Safety Solutions for People with Alzheimer's Disease

To live with damaged thinking and judgment is to live at risk. People with Alzheimer's disease cannot take responsibility for their own safety. They are unable to evaluate the potential consequences of their actions and they forget quickly. Verbal reminders and written notes have little value, but there are many other ways to promote safety.

Many older people love to live surrounded by their treasures. Although a neat home is always safer than a cluttered one, anticipate that only small changes can be made. Suggest moving knickknacks so that the edges of surfaces can be used for balance. Retain the existing furniture arrangements but consider removing or altering furniture with sharp corners, rocking chairs that tip easily, coffee tables, and fragile antiques. Block off unsafe areas by placing a sturdy chair in front of them. Eliminate hazards such as trailing wires, extension cords, or telephone cords. Caution caregivers to watch for paper or wooden objects that are tossed into gas fireplaces.

Most accidents happen in the kitchen and the bathroom. Therefore it is important to thoroughly assess how the person with Alzheimer's disease uses those areas. Disable stoves by removing knobs, installing a special switch behind the stove, removing a fuse, or turning the stove off at the breaker. Because people with AD may retain overlearned food preparation skills, they may be able to use sharp utensils and hot surfaces safely, but do need to be supervised. Encourage them to participate in meal preparation by doing single steps of a task, such as tearing lettuce for a salad or putting plates on the table.

Remove rugs and runners that tend to slide, especially those in the bathroom. Install grab bars to help prevent falls during transfers into or out of the tub or shower. Bars should be attached to structural supports rather than drywall or plaster. Consider using a raised toilet seat if rising is difficult and a bedside commode at night if urgency is a problem. Bath benches with nonskid feet are best, and hand-held showers minimize the need for the person to move about. Lower the temperature on the water heater to 120° F so that the water cannot become hot enough to scald anyone. If hot pipes are exposed, cover them with insulation.

While walking is good exercise and can reduce stress, wandering can become a safety issue. If the environment is secured with a fence, camouflaged doors, or locks, people with dementia may move freely within a relatively safe area, reducing the stress of caregivers who are afraid to let them out of sight. It is important to balance freedom, safety, and client rights. If wandering away from home is a potential hazard, the Alzheimer's Association has an excellent program called "safe return." More information about this low-cost program is available by calling 1-800-272-3900; website www.alz.org.

---

the early and middle stages of the disease. Give directions one at a time and plenty of time to complete a task.

Diagnosis: Urge Urinary and Fecal Incontinence. Clients in the middle stage of AD develop both urinary and bowel incontinence in the absence of pathology. State this nursing diagnosis as *Urge Urinary Incontinence or Self-Care Deficit: Toileting related to neuronal degeneration and forgetfulness.*

Outcomes. The client will have optimal bowel and bladder continence as evidenced by having dry, clean clothing and bedding as much as possible, having intact skin, and voiding appropriately in the bathroom.

Interventions. Anticipation of elimination needs and scheduled voiding and defecation times can help in the initial stages. The client may show nonverbal signs of needing to void or defecate, such as restlessness, grasping the genital area, or picking at clothing. Sometimes the client forgets where the bathroom is located. Having clear, bright signs indicating where the bathroom is and frequently taking the client there may help control

incontinence. Fluid intake after the dinner meal can be restricted to help maintain continence during the night.

Try to arrange a bowel program to coincide with the client's usual pattern. In the later stages of AD, clients may need to wear incontinence briefs during the day and external urinary drainage devices at night. Indwelling catheters should be avoided because of the risk of infection and injury. Several varieties of disposable and extra-absorbent washable underwear, bed pads, and mattress covers are available. If the client is male, choose undergarments that allow him to urinate through an opened fly.

Diagnosis: Caregiver Role Strain. Family members and especially caregivers (usually the spouse or adult children) of the client with AD face a great deal of emotional and physical burden. (See Translating Evidence into Practice feature on p. 1901.) State this nursing diagnosis as *Caregiver Role Strain related to grieving the loss of a family member to AD, a change in social role, and intense demands for time commitment and provision of care.*

TRANSLATING EVIDENCE INTO PRACTICE

Caregivers and Caregiver Role Strain

The annual direct and indirect cost of caring for the 4.5 million people with Alzheimer's disease in the United States is estimated to be at least $100 billion. By 2030, when the entire Baby Boomer generation is age 65 and older, the increased number of people with Alzheimer's disease could exceed the ability to absorb the added cost. Historically, most of the long-term care for functionally impaired older adults has been provided by informal caregivers. Family caregivers provide 80% of chronic illness home care services to clients age 50 and older by providing day to day services. It is noted that as AD progresses, caregivers spend as many as 70 hours per week primarily monitoring and managing the cognitive decline of AD clients.[1] In 1997 the National Family Caregiver Survey found that nearly 1 in 4 (23% or 22.4 million) U.S. households was involved in helping care for an individual 50 years old or older, at some point during the previous 12 months. In telephone interviews of 1002 households, the results showed only 20% of the informal caregivers received any assistance in providing care from the formal health care system. Further, 60% of the caregivers reported they had had no formal training in the care they were providing.[2]

The burden of providing care for clients with dementia is particularly troublesome. The degree of cognitive impairment, amount of help required with activities of daily living, personality changes, and presence of psychiatric symptoms and behavioral disturbances cause the greatest concern.[2,3] The relationship between the client and the caregiver can become strained and isolation from friends and activities creates additional social isolation. Caregivers often experience clinically significant changes in physical and mental health, particularly depression.[1,4]

In a series of interviews, family members reported that they coped in two styles. One style, emotion-focused, was seen as grieving, worrying, and self-accusation. They were also the only ones using wishful thinking and stoicism as strategies. Problem-based copers confronted the problem and sought information and social support. The problem-based copers also used the emotion-focused strategy of acceptance in combination with seeking information and social support.[2] Spirituality was identified as an important coping mechanism among wife caregivers of people with dementia. It was shown that caregivers of persons with AD relied on prayer and religious coping to help them through the caregiving experience. To mix approaches like these seems to be an effective choice of strategy.[5]

Interventions on the communication techniques, behavioral strategies, and environmental modifications improved the quality of life of primary caregivers while reducing the anxiety and depression levels.[6,7] Family caregivers can provide practical training to enable health care professionals to provide better care for their family member. In addition, family caregivers need information and support in self-care activities that promote their health and well-being. A community-based interventional study investigated the effectiveness of a comprehensive educational program exploring problems most likely to be experienced by caregivers of Alzheimer's clients. Results of this study indicate that problems among caregivers of Alzheimer's clients, especially in an environment with limited respite care options, were improved by participating in the comprehensive educational intervention program.[8]

REFERENCES

1. Burns, A. (2000). The burden of Alzheimer's disease. *International Journal of Neuropsychopharmacology, 3*(7), 31-38.
2. Navaie-Waliser, M., Feldman, P.H., Gould, D.A., et al. (2001). Long-term care provision: Striking a balance between informal and formal caregiving. *Abstracts from the Academy of Health Service Research and Health Policy Meeting, 18*, 97.
3. Almberg, B., Grafstrom, M., & Winblad, B. (1997). Major strain and coping strategies as reported by family members who care for aged demented relatives. *Journal of Advanced Nursing, 26*(4), 683-691.
4. Takano, M., & Arai, H. (2005). Gender difference and caregivers' burden in early-onset Alzheimer's disease. *Psychogeriatrics, 5*(3), 73-77.
5. Spurlock, W.R. (2005). Spiritual well-being and caregiver burden in Alzheimer's caregivers. *Geriatric Nursing, 26*(30), 154-161.
6. Yahas, N., McGowan, B., et al. (2006). Psychosocial interventions for disruptive symptoms of dementia. *Journal of Psychosocial Nursing and Mental Health Services, 44*(11), 34-42.
7. Perry, J. (2002). Wives giving care to husband's with Alzheimer's disease: A process of interpretive caring. *Research in Nursing and Health, 25*(4), 307-316.
8. Kuzu, N., Beser, N., Zencir, M., et al. (2005). Effects of a comprehensive educational program on quality of life and emotional issues of dementia patient caregivers. *Geriatric Nursing, 26*(6), 378-385.

Outcomes. The family will demonstrate reduced role strain as evidenced by voicing their emotional concern, seeking appropriate assistance, and providing adequate care for the client.

Interventions. AD is called a "long goodbye" because the client with AD remains alive for many months to years during which time the client cannot interact with the family. Family members grieve the loss of the person they used to know. Each decline in cognitive function becomes another source of grief. Two stages of grief in the family have been described. The process of grief begins during the caregiving stage and continues after the client's death. Normal family routines are lost, and the relationship between the family member and the dementia sufferer changes. Factors that have the most profound effect on the emotional well-being of caregivers include incontinence, overly demanding behavior, and the need for constant supervision.

Wives tend to experience a higher degree of emotional burden as caregivers than husbands do. Paradoxically, the closer the emotional bond between caregiver and dementia sufferer, the less the strain for the caregiver. Conversely, a low past level of intimacy is associated with an increased level of both perceived strain and depression in the spouse caregiver. According to the literature, caregivers tend to be women.

Support for Caregivers. Interview family members to determine their understanding of the diagnosis and prognosis of AD and to allow them to discuss their concerns about caring for the client:

- Do they know about community resources?
- Do they have someone to call when they can no longer cope with caregiving?

The Alzheimer's Disease and Related Disorders Association has local chapters that offer support groups in many major cities in the United States (Phone: 1-800-272-3900).

A variety of options are available to caregivers. Chore service workers can help with household chores and relieve the caregiver of these duties. Other paid help can provide in-home respite care by observing the dementia sufferer while the caregiver tends to business outside the home, seeks social interaction, or meets recreational needs.

Adult day care provides time away from home for the dementia sufferer. Day care usually offers a lunchtime meal as well as several hours of scheduled activities that are tailored to the client's abilities. These activities may include games, crafts, music, and exercise.

Respite care involves admission of the client to an extended care facility for a few days to a few weeks to allow the caregiver time to recover from the demands of providing 24-hour care (see the Bridge to Home Health Care website feature on Respite Care for Caregivers of People with Alzheimer's Disease). Assisted living facilities with dementia units can also be used. These settings are home-like and can provide needed supervision as long as the client is ambulatory.

Nursing home care is usually the final and most difficult and trying option for a caregiver. This decision creates guilt, self-doubt, and anxiety; however, it may be the only option when the caregiver suffers burnout and becomes unable to provide adequate care. Table 72-1 lists nursing guidelines for meeting family needs.

Diagnosis: Decisional Conflict. State this diagnosis as *Decision Conflict related to the need to make crucial decisions about life and death for a loved one.*

Outcomes. The family will experience comfort that the decisions that they have made meet the needs and wishes of the client with AD and will be acceptable to themselves and other family members.

Interventions. When the person with AD reaches the terminal stage of illness, the family needs to plan for the inevitable end-of-life issues. Questions about CPR and use of feeding tubes and antibiotics for the treatment of pneumonia and other infections will need answers. Ideally, decisions about these questions are raised and discussed with the client and family members before the person loses the capacity to make decisions.

Two forms of *advance directives* (means of expressing one's wishes about life-sustaining treatment after losing the mental capacity to make informed decisions) are available. One is the *living will,* a written document signed by the individual (while he or she is still mentally capable of making informed decisions) in the presence of a witness. The living will lists conditions under which the person wishes life-sustaining treatments to be withheld or withdrawn. The other advance directive is a *durable power of attorney for health care.* This is a legal document in which the person (while still mentally capable) assigns someone to act on his or her behalf in matters of health care decisions if the person loses decisional capacity (e.g., becomes demented). The family needs to be advised early to seek legal assistance to set up trusts, power of attorney documents for finances and for health care, and a living will.

The nurses' role during this time is to listen and facilitate discussion and comprehension of decisions. For example, if the family decides not to tube-feed the client, they may later ask "is she hungry?" for which the answer is "no, she has no sensation of hunger." The nurse may also have to guide the family through grieving over the finality of the decisions they made. Consultation with clergy is often beneficial.

PARKINSON'S DISEASE

Parkinson's disease (PD) is a chronic, progressive, neurologic disorder that results from the loss of the neurotransmitter dopamine in a group of brain structures that control movements. Its major manifestations are variable but can include hand tremor, slowness of movements, limb stiffness, and difficulties with gait and balance. For the vast majority of individuals, PD is not thought to be an inherited disease. Even when a second person within a family is diagnosed with PD, this is thought to be more of a coincidence than an emerging genetic pattern because PD is a fairly common disorder among the older population. Parkinson's disease develops most often in people in their 60s, although it can strike much younger people as well. It occurs worldwide. About 1% of people older than age 50 have PD.

Parkinsonian manifestations may also develop from other problems, such as long-term use of phenothiazines; poisoning from carbon monoxide, mercury, or manganese; or traumatic injury to the midbrain.

When PD occurs, degenerative changes are found in an area of the brain known as the *substantia nigra,* which produces *dopamine,* a chemical substance that enables people to move normally and smoothly. Once

TABLE 72–1 **Nursing Guidelines for Meeting the Needs of the Family of the Client with Dementia of the Alzheimer's Type**

Goals	Selected Interventions
Physical	
Monitor chronic health problems or physical limitations of family caregiver.	Obtain health history of family caregiver to identify past and new health problems.
	Support family in following through with routine health examinations.
	Refer family members to physician when health problems are observed.
Identify development of new health problems.	Assess family's understanding of medical management of own health problems.
	Teach family members to preserve own health in order to continue caring for client with Alzheimer's disease.
Identify cues for stress.	Emphasize family's need for adequate nutrition, hydration, exercise, and rest.
Examine somatic health problems.	Help family members to be alert to signs of caregiver stress.
Psychosocial	
Assist family in coping positively with stress.	Instruct family to get respite regularly for rest and relaxation.
	Teach stress management techniques (e.g., relaxation, supportive relationships, goal setting, time management, diversion).
Identify destructive methods of coping (e.g., alcohol, drugs, tobacco, overeating or under-eating, physical abuse of client).	Refer family to physician, therapist when stress remains unmanageable even with social or psychological resources.
Assess family dynamics.	Refer signs of physical abuse to adult protective services.
Assist family members in dealing with role change and conflict.	Recognize the family's role, discuss capacity to provide care, and give reinforcement for care provided.
	Counsel family in dealing with role conflicts, unmet expectations, or interpersonal conflicts.
	Teach family the need to maintain roles and social activities outside caregiving experience.
	Administer burden interview.
	Reinforce family's attempt to cope.
	Acknowledge family fears of being unable to continue with caregiving.
If need for support identified, direct family members to sources (e.g., in-home respite care or senior day services, nursing home).	Refer family to a support group to share with others in similar situations.
	Refer family to nearest office on aging or Alzheimer's Disease and Related Disorders Association, Inc. (ADRDA), to identify benefits in community available to Alzheimer's disease clients.
Identify family's mixed emotions (e.g., depression, anger, resentment, pity, embarrassment, guilt).	Listen to family and facilitate sharing of emotions and feelings in supportive, empathic environment.
Identify alternative plans for care if family members or social support systems become unable to provide care or are ineffective.	Counsel and support family if client placed in care of others; allay feelings of guilt.
	Facilitate family meeting to identify time for socialization.
Identify financial limitations.	Encourage family to be specific about financial limitations.
	Offer family referrals (legal, financial, or social service) for information on eligibility for private, county, state, or federal financial support for home services; advise and counsel regarding power of attorney or guardianship, trust or estate planning.
Assess family's ability to make funeral plans.	Help family anticipate and cope with grief process.
	Assist family in making prefuneral arrangements.
	Address family's fear regarding the possible role of heredity in development of Alzheimer's disease, and assist in making decision regarding autopsy.
Environmental	
Identify compatibility of environment with family and client.	Conduct a family meeting to discuss relationship of family, client, and environment.
Assess learning needs regarding client care tasks.	Teach management of concurrent physical health problems of the client with Alzheimer's disease.
	Include family in development of client care plan.
	Teach family to encourage the client to continue daily habits to extent possible.
	Complete behavior problems' checklist.
	Anticipate likely problems and teach how to manage them.
	Teach environmental modification (consistent, simple, calm routines) to maximize family endurance and enhance safety.
	Teach family to relate to client with creative connectedness (touch, humor, flexibility, reminiscence, music, planned activities).
Assess family's need and desire for information about Alzheimer's disease and how it affects the client's behavior.	Assist family in understanding symptoms related to memory loss, nature of the illness, symptoms, stages of disease progression, and behavior manifestations.
	Provide written material to reinforce education and understanding (e.g., *The 36-Hour Day, Coping and Caring: Living with Alzheimer's Disease;* literature from local, state, or national ADRDA chapters).
	Supply ADRDA 24-hour hotline number: 1-800-272-3900; website: www.alz.org.

odified from Stevenson, J.P. (1990). Family stress to home care of Alzheimer's disease patients and implications for support. *Journal of Neuroscience Nursing*, 22(3), 185.

cell loss in the substantia nigra reaches 80%, manifestations appear. The cause of nigral cell degeneration is not known. PD is characterized by a severe shortage of dopamine in relation to ACh in the basal ganglia, which leads to the clinical characteristics of PD.

Clinical Manifestations

The diagnosis of Parkinson's disease (PD) can be difficult. It is recommended that all people suspected of having PD be referred to a neurologist for diagnosis and initial planning of care. The manifestations do not appear until about 60% of the normal amount of dopamine is lost. The disease has six cardinal features: (1) tremor at rest on one side, the first manifestation in 70% of clients; (2) rigidity, increased tone, and stiffness in the muscles at rest; (3) bradykinesia (slow movement), fine movements become clumsy; (4) flexed posture of the neck, trunk, and limbs; (5) loss of postural reflexes; and (6) freezing movement.

Early in the disease, the client may notice a slight slowing in the ability to perform ADL *(bradykinesia)*. A general feeling of stiffness *(rigidity)* may be noticed, along with mild, diffuse muscular pain. *Tremor* is a common early manifestation that usually occurs in one of the upper limbs. It occurs at rest and involves a coarse "pill-rolling" movement of the thumb against the fingers that can vary in intensity and distribution. Voluntary movement stops or reduces the tremor in some people; however, others may have tremor during voluntary movement *(intention tremor)* as well.

Bradykinesia makes voluntary movements difficult to execute. When manifestations are severe, total lack of movement *(akinesia)* may occur and the client is literally frozen in one spot. Bradykinesia also affects gait. Initially there may be a slight stiffness of one leg while walking, and the ipsilateral arm may be held flexed at the elbow and abducted at the shoulder. The person may catch or drag one foot. Later, when both sides of the body are involved, the typical shuffling gait with short steps may develop. There is lack of associated swinging of the arms while walking. In advanced PD, the client stands with head, shoulders, and spine flexed forward, giving the appearance of a stooped posture (Figure 72-3).

The face of someone with advanced PD appears stiff, mask-like, and without expression. Speech is low in volume, monotonous in tone, and slow. Words are poorly articulated *(dysarthria)*. Saliva may flow involuntarily from the mouth because of the lack of spontaneous swallowing. PD clients may also exhibit *micrographia*—small, cramped handwriting.

Usually PD does not affect intellectual ability; however, a dementia similar to that of AD develops in 15% to 20% of clients with PD. Fatigue is a common occurrence; everyday tasks take longer and require more concentration. PD symptoms can disturb sleep. Immobility

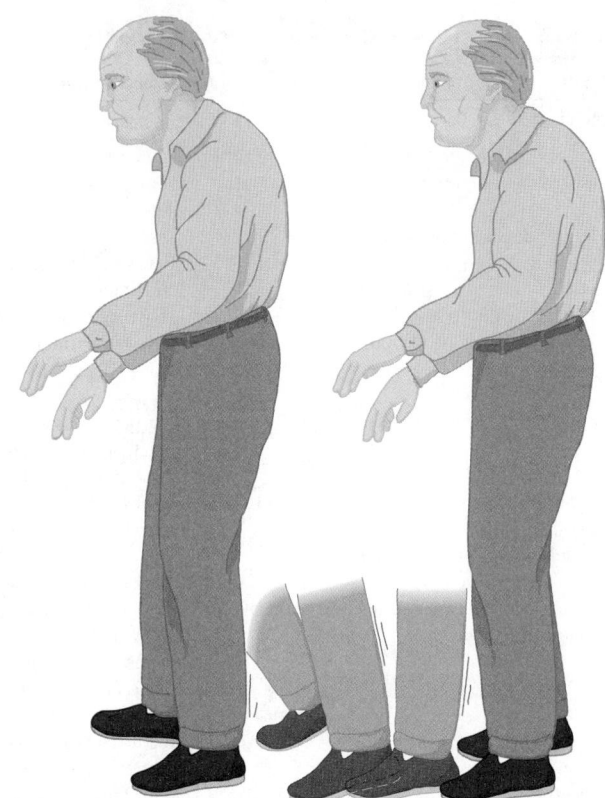

■ **FIGURE 72–3** Gait changes seen in Parkinson's disease. Some of the clinical manifestations of Parkinson's disease are stooped posture, bradykinesia, and a festinant gait.

slows gastric motility, and drug therapy contributes to constipation. Mood disturbance can occur, and emotional stress may intensify clinical manifestations. As many as 50% of PD clients have an episode of depression during this illness.

The course of the disease is slowly progressive. The person becomes more rigid and more disabled, eventually requiring full assistance with ADL.

OUTCOME MANAGEMENT

The goal of management of PD is to control the manifestations with the lowest possible dose of medication in order to avoid side effects. Medication selection and dosage are tailored to the client; factors considered are the severity of manifestations, the age of the client, and the presence of other medical conditions. Every client responds differently to a medication or dosage level, so this process involves experimentation, persistence, and patience.

Because clients with PD lack dopamine, it follows that a pharmacologic replacement of dopamine would be used. Dopamine does not cross the blood-brain barrier, but its precursor, L-dopa does. L-dopa is combined with carbidopa to prevent the breakdown of L-dopa so that smaller doses can be used. In general, most clients are treated with selegiline, a monoamine oxidase inhibitor, to block one pathway in the breakdown of dopamine. When manifestations become more pronounced, L-dopa/carbidopa (Sinemet) or a dopamine receptor agonist (pergolide) is used. Anticholinergics and antivirals are also used. These medications are gradually increased until the optimal therapeutic response is achieved. This process may take several months. When the daily dose of L-dopa approaches the desired level, the client often has involuntary *dyskinesias* (jerky, writhing movements), especially of the face, mouth, and tongue. Some clients prefer this stage to being severely bradykinetic because at least they can be mobile and perform voluntary movements more easily. Anticholinergics are used to reduce the tremor. The Complementary and Alternative Therapy feature below describes the possible benefits of coenzyme Q_{10} therapy.

Medical Management

Manage the Parkinsonian Crisis

Occasionally clients with PD experience a parkinsonian crisis as a result of emotional trauma or sudden or inadvertent withdrawal of anti-parkinsonian medication. Severe exacerbation of tremor, rigidity, and bradykinesia, accompanied by acute anxiety, sweating, tachycardia, and hyperpnea, occur. Intervention for parkinsonian crisis includes respiratory and cardiac support. The client should be placed in a quiet room with subdued lighting. Barbiturates may be prescribed in addition to anti-parkinsonian drugs.

Manage the On/Off Response

An *on/off response* (rapid fluctuation of clinical manifestations) may occur in clients with PD; the client may be mobile and active ("on") one moment and akinetic and rigid ("off") the next. This transition may happen quickly, within 1 to 2 minutes. Initially the off periods tend to occur 3 to 4 hours after a dose of anti-parkinsonian medication. Later the transition may happen any time and may be unrelated to medication ingestion. Apparently, off periods are due to dopamine deficit, but this factor is not clear. A person experiencing on/off response may be temporarily helped by shortening the interval between medication doses or by gradually increasing the total dosage.

Medications such as ropinirole may be given in addition to other PD medications to help stabilize the fluctuations.

Nursing Management of Parkinson's Disease

Nursing care of the PD client includes health assessment, medication instruction and monitoring, liaison with other members of the health care team, and client and family education. Case managers are often used to guide transitions from one facility to the next.

Advise the client to maintain fluid intake of 2 L every 24 hours and to increase the intake of dietary fiber. Stool softeners and mild laxatives can be used. A regular time for bowel movements should be established, usually ½ hour after the morning or evening meal.

Teach the client various techniques to enhance voluntary physical movement. Clients often need to try different strategies on their own to find what helps most. Some clients grasp coins in their pocket to reduce embarrassing hand tremor. Others grip the arms of a chair. Mental thoughts, such as walking over imaginary lines, can aid ambulation. One client may find that tossing small scraps of paper in front of him aids his walking, and another may find that rocking back and forth helps initiate movement. Encourage daily range-of-motion exercises to avoid rigidity and contractures. Remind the client to maintain good posture and to avoid flexion of the neck and shoulders. The client should sleep on a firm mattress. When resting, the client should avoid using a pillow to prevent flexion of the spine. Periodically lying prone also helps.

The benefits of regular daytime rest should be encouraged. The PD client should be encouraged to rest in bed laying flat for 30 minutes to 1 hour at the same

---

COMPLEMENTARY AND ALTERNATIVE THERAPY

Coenzyme Q_{10} Supplements and Parkinson's Disease

Parkinson's disease is a neurologic disorder that currently has no treatment that has demonstrated a reduction in the progression of this disease. Researchers conducted a multicenter, randomized, parallel-group, placebo-controlled, double-blind, dosing-ranging trial. The participants in this trial were 80 individuals with early Parkinson's disease that did not require treatment for their condition. Clients were randomly assigned to placebo or coenzyme Q_{10} at dosages of 300, 600, or 1200 mg/day. Clients were followed for 16 months or until disability requiring treatment with levodopa had developed. Researchers found that coenzyme Q_{10} supplements were safe and well tolerated at dosages of up to 1200 mg/day. Less overall disability developed in clients assigned to coenzyme Q_{10} than in those assigned to placebo, and the benefit was greatest in the clients consuming the highest dose. Coenzyme Q_{10} seemed to slow the progressive deterioration of function in Parkinson's disease. Clients taking the highest dosage (1200 mg/day) had deterioration slowed by 44%. The greatest benefit was observed for daily activities such as feeding, dressing, bathing, and walking. By the eighth month, clients taking the highest dose scored significantly better than the placebo group.

REFERENCE

Shults, C., et al. (2002). Effects of coenzyme Q10 in early Parkinson disease: Evidence of slowing of the functional decline. *Archives of Neurology, 59,* 1541-1550.

time every day. By resting during the day, the PD client will experience renewed energy for the rest of the day.

Because self-care activities are performed more slowly by the client with PD, extra time should be allowed for completion of tasks such as dressing, bathing, and eating. Warming trays can keep food hot. Recommend rest periods during meals to avoid aspiration. Activities of daily living (ADL) or exercise should be performed when drugs are working well to avoid injury to the client and caregiver.

As PD progresses, clients become rigid and unresponsive to verbal stimuli. During these stages, continue to treat clients with dignity, speaking to the clients rather than ignoring them.

Teach the client about home safety. Loose carpeting should be removed. Grab bars should be placed in the bathroom. An elevated toilet seat should be installed. Clients with severe tremor should avoid carrying hot liquids. Walking aids such as a cane or walker can provide added stability. The Client Education Guide below suggests additional interventions for clients with Parkinson's disease.

CLIENT EDUCATION GUIDE

Parkinson's Disease

Make sure that you understand how to take your medications on schedule and to not forget a dose. Know the importance of following the correct diet, and what side effects you can expect from your medications.

To avoid rigidity and the development of contractures:

- Exercise and stretch regularly.
- Perform the exercises recommended in your self-help booklets.
- Exercise first thing in the morning, when your energy levels are highest.
- Exercise in bed if getting to the floor is difficult.
- Get out of a chair by bending over slowly so that your head is over your toes; avoid soft, deep chairs.

If your health care provider has told you that you have bradykinesia (slow movements):

- Rock back and forth to get going.
- Imagine that you are stepping over an imaginary line when you walk.
- Throw small objects (e.g., small scraps of paper) in front of you to practice fine motor movements.
- Count to yourself while walking.
- Visualize your intended movement.
- Maintain a wide-based gait.
- Maintain upright posture and look up, not down, especially when walking.

If you have a tremor:

- Hold change in your pocket or squeeze a small rubber ball.
- Use both hands to accomplish tasks.
- Lie face down on the floor and relax your entire body.
- Sleep on the side that has the tremor.

If you have trouble getting dressed:

- Dress and undress in front of a mirror.
- Use adaptive devices such as long-handled shoehorns and button fasteners.
- Buy clothes with self-fasteners (e.g., Velcro) and slide-locking buckles.

To ensure safety:

- Wear good, sturdy shoes.
- Use a cane or walker.
- Concentrate on standing upright.
- Consciously pick up your feet to take steps.
- Remove all throw rugs, electrical cords, and clutter from the floor.
- Make sure that you have adequate lighting.
- Arrange essential items so that they are within easy reach.
- Use a bath chair and a hand-held shower nozzle.
- Have grab bars installed in the bathroom.
- Have a raised toilet seat installed.

To ensure good communication:

- Pause between every few words.
- Exaggerate the pronunciation of words.
- Finish saying the final consonant of a word before starting to say the next word.
- Express ideas in short, concise phrases.
- Plan what to say.
- Face the listener.

To ensure adequate swallowing and prevent aspiration:

- Think through the steps of swallowing:
  - Keep your lips closed.
  - Keep your teeth together.
  - Put food on your tongue.
  - Lift your tongue up and back.
  - Swallow.
- Eat slowly, taking small bites.
- Chew hard and move food around with your tongue.
- Finish one bite before taking another.
- Eat in an upright chair.
- Consume a high-fiber diet to prevent constipation.
- Avoid caffeine; caffeine increases PD symptoms.

To keep saliva from building up in your mouth:

- Make a conscious effort to swallow saliva often.
- Keep your head in an upright position so saliva will collect in the back of your throat and *stimulate automatic swallowing*.
- Swallow excess saliva before attempting to speak.

The client and family need emotional support. Support groups are available in most major cities. Refer the client and family to the American Parkinson Disease Association (1-800-223-APDA) or the website www.apdaparkinson.com.

Surgical Management

Surgical interventions are used for PD. Intractable tremor *(dyskinetic movement)* may be ameliorated by pallidotomy. Fetal tissue transplantation and genetically engineered cells that produce dopamine are in experimental stages. Deep brain stimulation is also used to treat uncontrollable movement. Deep brain stimulation involves electrodes implanted in the thalamus or globus pallidus. The device uses electrical currents to "jam" abnormal brain signals.

CREUTZFELDT-JAKOB DISEASE

Creutzfeldt-Jakob disease (CJD) is a rare, fatal brain disease that produces progressive dementia, myoclonus, and distinctive electroencephalographic (EEG) changes. CJD is a unique disease that apparently can arise from two separate mechanisms: genetic and infectious. People with the genetic form have a mutated gene. The infectious form does not develop from a known virus or other pathogen; therefore words such as *virion, slow virus,* and *prion* are sometimes used to describe the etiologic agent. Several reports document human-to-human spread of CJD from transplanted tissue from a person with CJD. Incubation periods have ranged from 4 to 21 years, which indicates the enormous difficulty of tracing the infection. In 1996 CJD was associated with ingestion of infected beef. This led to the popular term *mad cow disease.*

Clinical Manifestations

Manifestations include vague psychiatric or behavior changes suggesting a personality change. About one third of clients report weight loss, anorexia, insomnia, malaise, and dizziness for a period of weeks to months. In the early stages, there is progressive memory loss, visual impairment, and dysphagia. Within a few weeks or months, a relentlessly progressive dementia develops and marked deterioration is noted from week to week. *Myoclonus* (twitching) is usually present. Deterioration is rapid, with 90% of clients dying within 1 year.

A definitive diagnosis attempts to differentiate CJD from AD, which has a more protracted course and no myoclonus or EEG changes. Lithium toxicity can mimic the manifestations, but they clear within about 2 weeks after discontinuation of the drug. Brain biopsy during hospitalization or on autopsy is the usual method of establishing a definitive diagnosis. According to the World Health Organization, diagnostic criteria for CJD include progressive dementia and the presence of at least two of the following: myoclonus, extraocular or cerebellar disturbance, pyramidal/extrapyramidal dysfunction, and akinetic mutism. In addition there should be at least one of the following findings: electroencephalogram (EEG) typical for CJD regardless of the clinical duration of the disease; a positive 14-3-3 assay for cerebrospinal fluid. Laboratory values have been more helpful than EEGs in diagnosing CJD.

OUTCOME MANAGEMENT

No effective treatment is available, and CJD appears to be uniformly fatal. Nursing care is directed at supportive care—preventing skin breakdown, supplying nutrition, and providing emotional support to the client and family. Families require much support, care, and concern as they try to cope with the sudden onset of this debilitating disease and with managing the day-to-day care of the client.

Although CJD can be transmitted, the risk to health care workers and others having contact with the client is no more than that to the general population. Isolation of clients is not indicated, but personnel should wear gloves when handling tissues, blood, and spinal fluid. Accidental skin contact with possibly infected material should be followed by washing in 10% normal sodium hydroxide or a solution of 5% household chlorine bleach. The agent can be inactivated on surfaces by using a 10% bleach solution for 1 hour. Surgical and pathologic instruments should be steam-autoclaved for 1 hour at 132° C. No organs, tissue, or tissue products from clients with CJD or any other ill-defined neurologic disorders should be used for transplantation or replacement therapy.

HUNTINGTON'S DISEASE

Huntington's disease (HD), also known as *Huntington's chorea,* is an autosomal-dominant degenerative neurologic disease. It is characterized by abnormal movements *(chorea* has the same word root as *choreography),* intellectual decline, and emotional disturbance. Clinical manifestations usually begin in the 30s and 40s, although occasionally they begin in young adulthood or even in children. Women and men are equally affected. The disease is relentlessly progressive, leading to disability and death within 15 to 20 years. Death usually results from respiratory tract complications caused by aspiration. According to 1 report in the United States alone, about 30,000 people have HD and its prevalence is estimated to be about 1 in every 10,000 people. It is estimated that at least 150,000 others have a 50% risk of developing the disease and thousands more of their relatives live with the possibility that they may develop HD.

The disease is autosomal dominant; offspring of an affected person have a 50% chance of inheriting the disease. Because HD does not skip generations, offspring who have not inherited the disease will not pass it on to their offspring. The abnormal gene has been isolated on chromosome 4.

Pathophysiology

The pathologic changes of HD involve degeneration of the striatum (caudate and putamen) in the basal ganglia. Other subtle changes occur in the cortex and cerebellum, namely, loss of neurons and an increased number of glial cells (gliosis). The degeneration of the caudate nucleus leads to a reduction in several neurotransmitters, including gamma-aminobutyric acid, ACh, substance P, and metenkephalin, and their synthetic enzymes. This change leaves relatively higher concentrations of the other neurotransmitters—dopamine, and norepinephrine. The relative excess of dopamine in HD, a disorder of excessive movement, can be contrasted to the lack of dopamine in Parkinson's disease (PD), a disorder of lack of movement.

Clinical Manifestations

Emotional disturbances and mental deterioration may precede the abnormal movements. The person may become negative, suspicious, and irritable. This condition may progress to depression and psychosis. Temper outbursts and sexual promiscuity may also occur. Severe mood swings are common. Cognitive decline progresses, and eventually the person becomes demented, incontinent, and completely unable to provide self-care.

The abnormal movements in HD are subtle at first. The person may appear restless or fidgety. The person may be aware of these movements and try to mask them by making them seem to be parts of intentional movements, such as head scratching or leg crossing. As the disease progresses, the rapid, jerky choreiform movements become more pronounced and involve all muscles. The person is constantly in motion. Stress, emotional situations, and attempts to perform voluntary movement can aggravate the abnormal movements. During sleep the movements diminish or disappear.

The diagnosis of HD is made on the basis of clinical manifestations and family history because there is no specific diagnostic test for the disease itself. CT or MRI imaging of the brain may show atrophy of the head of the caudate, but this factor alone is not diagnostic of HD.

OUTCOME MANAGEMENT

Medical Management

There is no pharmacologic treatment for HD. Haloperidol, a dopamine blocker, can control the abnormal movements and some behavioral manifestations. Diazepam can be used to lower anxiety, thereby aiding in control of movements. Antidepressants can help depression.

The duration of HD ranges from 10 to 30 years. The most common causes of death are infection (most commonly pneumonia) and injuries related to a fall or other complications.

Nursing Management of Huntington's Disease

One of the most common and dangerous problems in the middle to late stages is dysphagia. Several interventions should be tried. Medications need to be evaluated for their anticholinergic and sedative effects, which may impair swallowing. Mealtimes should be free of stress and clutter and have an unhurried atmosphere. Use of adaptive eating utensils can encourage and extend independence in eating. The diet should include foods that are easy to swallow and form a bolus in the mouth (e.g., canned peaches, chopped meat in gravy and mashed potatoes, custards). Many clients with HD may require an intake of 5,000 calories a day without gaining weight because of their excessive movements. They should try eating frequent, small meals containing high-calorie foods. Vitamins or other nutritional supplements may be added to their diet. Clients should sit upright when eating. While swallowing, they should keep the chin down toward the chest. They can be trained to hold their breath before swallowing and cough after each mouthful is swallowed to clear the throat of any residual food. Clients with HD are at risk for dehydration and may require large quantities of fluids, especially during hot weather. In some cases water may be thickened with commercial additives to give it the consistency of syrup.

If the client continues to have difficulty eating and loses weight despite dietary and environmental modifications, a feeding tube may become necessary; however, artificial feeding methods often frighten families, and they pose ethical dilemmas about prolonging life. Nurses can help clients and their families make these difficult decisions by clarifying the issues and providing information on the types, risks, benefits, and long-term effects of artificial feeding methods.

Poor control of oral and respiratory muscles can make communication difficult. The nurse can assist the family in developing signals such as raising a hand or keeping the eyes open or closed for yes and no responses. If physical signals are not an option, cards with printed words may be helpful. Keep communication simple and unstrained. Repeat words that are understood to let the client know that communication has been successful.

Excessive movements and falls may cause physical injury and can restrict independence. Pads on wheelchairs and beds, shin guards, and walking belts can prevent injury. Aids for ambulation (e.g., walking behind a wheelchair) can extend independence. Clothing should be light and simple to put on and take off.

Huntington's disease has a major impact on the family, not only because of the burden of caregiving but also because of the risk to offspring of inheriting the disease. Many ethical dilemmas surrounding the issue of privacy can surface in cases of HD. Whether test results are positive or negative, the results are of interest to the spouse, other family members, employers, and insurers; however, principles of confidentiality forbid disclosure of medical information to anyone without the client's consent. Be sensitive to the client's desire for confidentiality, but use this opportunity to teach the client about the effect the disease may have on other family members. Because a blood test is now available to check for the presence of the abnormal gene, family members face difficult choices about whether to find out if they have the Huntington gene. Information is available for clients and families living with HD from the Huntington's Disease Society of America (telephone: 1-800-345-HDSA, website: www.hdsa.org).

MULTIPLE SCLEROSIS

Multiple sclerosis (MS) is a chronic demyelinating disease that affects the myelin sheath of neurons in the central nervous system (CNS). The myelin sheath is essential for normal conduction of nerve impulses. Patches of myelin deteriorate at irregular intervals along the nerve axon, causing slowing of nerve conduction. Axonal destruction also occurs in MS.

The onset of MS usually occurs between 20 and 40 years of age, and it affects women twice as often as men. Whites are affected more often than Hispanics, blacks, or Asians. The disease is most prevalent in the colder climates of North America and Europe. If someone is born in an area of high risk for MS and moves to an area of low risk after age 15, the person carries the risk of the area of origin.

Etiology and Risk Factors

The exact cause of MS is unknown. Most theories suggest that MS is an immunogenetic-viral disease, that is, an immune-mediated demyelination triggered by a viral infection, probably with the Epstein-Barr virus. A genetic susceptibility apparently alters the body's immune response to viral infection. Multiple genes are probably involved; however, the only consistently identified disease locus is on the human leukocyte antigen (HLA) gene complex on chromosome 6.

A variety of precipitating factors can precede the onset or an exacerbation of MS, such as infection, physical injury, emotional stress, pregnancy, and fatigue. Most pregnancy-related exacerbations occur 3 months postpartum and may relate more to the stress of labor and fatigue during the puerperium than to the pregnancy itself.

Pathophysiology

Myelin is a highly conductive fatty material that surrounds the axon and speeds conduction of nerve impulses along the axon. Myelin is made by oligodendrocytes. Both autoimmune processes and infectious agents have been implicated in the pathogenesis of multiple sclerosis. Activated T cells, which recognize self-antigens expressed in the CNS, and macrophages enter the brain from the peripheral circulation and initiate the inflammation. Through the production of inflammatory cytokines and reactive oxygen species, activated T lymphocytes and microglia/macrophages cause the demyelination and destruction of oligodendrocytes. Plaques form along the myelin sheath, eventually causing scarring and destruction (Figure 72-4). When edema and inflammation subside, some remyelination occurs but is often incomplete. Although plaques may occur anywhere in the white matter of the CNS, the areas most commonly involved are the optic nerves, cerebrum, and cervical spinal cord.

Clinical Manifestations

The wide variety of manifestations possible with MS and the unpredictable nature of the disease pose many challenges to the client and family. The course of illness varies from person to person. Four clinical patterns have been identified (Figure 72-5). The most common initial pattern is *relapsing-remitting* MS. Clients experience manifestations that eventually remit with little or no progression of disability.

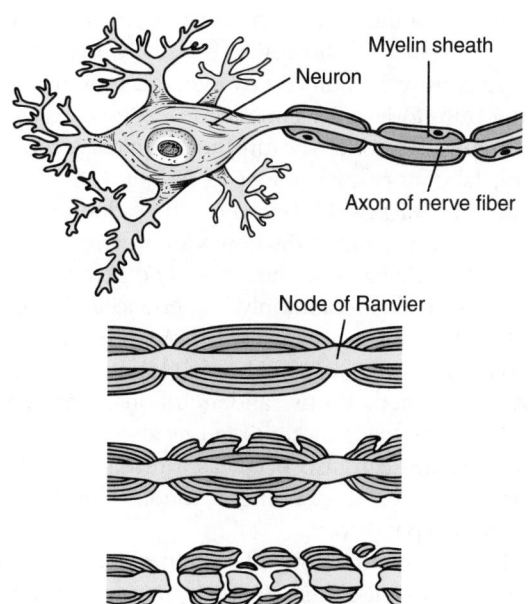

■ **FIGURE 72-4** Changes in the nerve sheath, as seen in multiple sclerosis. Myelin is made by oligodendrocytes and coats peripheral nerves, facilitating the nerve impulse. In clients with multiple sclerosis, the myelin degenerates in patches, causing nerve transmission to become erratic.

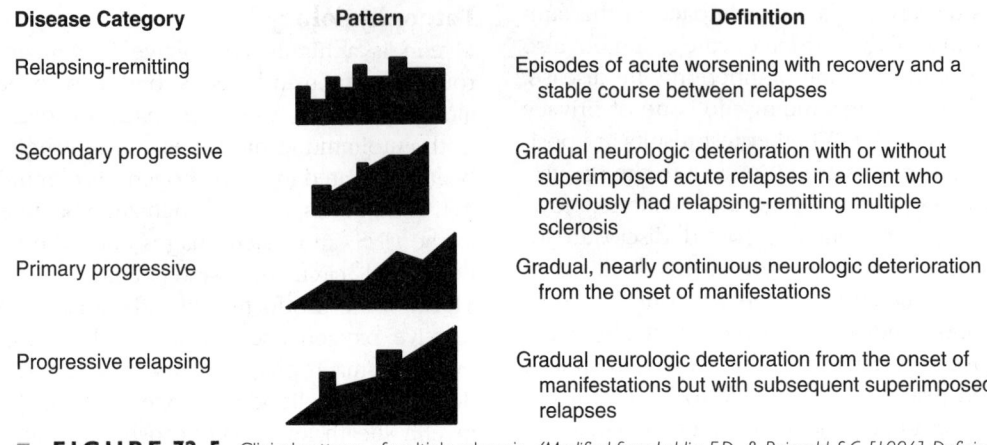

Disease Category	Pattern	Definition
Relapsing-remitting		Episodes of acute worsening with recovery and a stable course between relapses
Secondary progressive		Gradual neurologic deterioration with or without superimposed acute relapses in a client who previously had relapsing-remitting multiple sclerosis
Primary progressive		Gradual, nearly continuous neurologic deterioration from the onset of manifestations
Progressive relapsing		Gradual neurologic deterioration from the onset of manifestations but with subsequent superimposed relapses

■ **FIGURE 72–5** Clinical patterns of multiple sclerosis. *(Modified from Lublin, F.D., & Reingold, S.C. [1996]. Defining the clinical course of multiple sclerosis: Results of an international survey. Neurology, 46, 907-911.)*

The random distribution of MS plaques leads to several clinical manifestations:

- Weakness or tingling sensations (paresthesias) of one or more extremities caused by involvement of the cerebrum or spinal cord
- Vision loss from optic neuritis
- Incoordination that is due to cerebellar involvement
- Bowel and bladder dysfunction as a result of spinal cord involvement

Bladder dysfunction can take several forms, depending on which neural pathways are affected. Dysfunction may involve hesitancy, frequency, loss of sensation, incontinence, and retention. Increased or decreased detrusor muscle, bladder neck, or external sphincter tone, or a combination of these problems, may occur. The ultimate bladder dysfunction, however, is usually hyperreflexia in association with sphincter dyssynergia (sphincter contraction during detrusor contraction).[3] Proper diagnosis of the type of bladder dysfunction requires a thorough history, laboratory assessment of kidney function, and identification of possible infection. If bladder emptying is defective, further investigation with urography, cystoscopy, and urodynamic studies should be performed.

Constipation is commonly experienced by clients with MS. Dysfunction can result from one or more of the following factors: spinal cord lesion, immobility, dehydration, medications, and nutritional deficiencies. Fecal incontinence, although rarer, is also possible. Sexual dysfunction can also occur as a result of lesions in the ascending or descending autonomic and sensory fibers in the spinal cord.

Fatigue is a common manifestation of MS and usually one of the most disabling. Spasticity can reduce energy, inhibit motor control, and interfere with self-care, sexuality, vocational responsibilities, and recreation. Physical fatigue can be easily induced in MS by a short walk or other physical activity. For some reason, also not fully understood, the efficiency of demyelinated nerves deteriorates very rapidly with use. Almost everyone whose physical functioning has been disturbed through MS finds that their ability to perform an activity is reduced each time it is attempted.

Because MS strikes young adults during their years of establishing a family and an occupation, the impact of the disease can be devastating. Depression often occurs in clients, but it is not clear whether depression is a reaction to disability or a function of the disease itself. Others may experience euphoria, emotional instability, or apathy.

Because there is no definitive test for MS, clinicians rely on a detailed history, clinical findings, and a variety of diagnostic tests. The history often reveals several episodes of neurologic dysfunction, separated by time and by different locations in the CNS. Current research looking at clients who experience only one manifestation, such as optic neuritis, is changing the way clinicians diagnose MS.

Diagnostic tests include the following:

- Cerebrospinal fluid (CSF) evaluation for the presence of oligoclonal banding
- Evoked potentials of the optic pathways and auditory system to assess the presence of slowed nerve conduction
- MRI of the brain and spinal cord to determine the presence of MS plaques

OUTCOME MANAGEMENT

Medical Management of Multiple Sclerosis

The most important therapeutic aim of any disease modifying treatment of MS is to prevent or postpone long-term disability. Long-term disability in MS often evolves slowly over many years. Treatment generally falls into one of three categories: (1) treatment of acute relapses, (2) treatment aimed at disease management, and (3) symptomatic treatment.

Treat Acute Relapses

Treatment of acute relapses usually involves the use of intravenous (IV) or oral corticosteroids, which have both anti-inflammatory and immunosuppressive properties. They are often used to enhance recovery from an exacerbation. Methylprednisolone is standard therapy for acute exacerbations sometimes followed by an oral prednisone taper. Azathioprine (Imuran) and cyclophosphamide (Cytoxan), other immunosuppressive agents, may be used for more severe exacerbations or progressive MS.

Treat Exacerbations

Interferon-β_{1b} (Betaseron) is used for ambulatory clients with relapsing-remitting MS. Interferon-β_{1b} is a genetically engineered complex protein with both antiviral and immunoregulatory properties that can reduce the number of MS exacerbations. The drug is injected subcutaneously every other day. Interferon-β_{1a} (Avonex) is also available for the treatment of relapsing forms of MS. In addition to reducing the number and severity of relapses, interferon-β_{1a} has provided a delay in disability in placebo-controlled studies.

The third disease-modifying agent available for use in the United States is glatiramer acetate (Copaxone), a synthetic polypeptide approved for use in relapsing-remitting MS. It is not an interferon but is believed to work by mimicking myelin basic protein and interrupting the inflammatory cascade to prevent damage to myelin.

Side effects of the interferons include fever, fatigue, and flu-like manifestations. Clients taking interferon-β_{1a} have also reported increased depression and injection site reactions. Copaxone does not produce the interferon-type side effects of fever and flu-like manifestations, but rare episodes of face flushing, chest tightness, and shortness of breath lasting less than 15 minutes have been reported. Numerous other therapeutic agents are undergoing clinical trials.

Symptomatic Treatment

Several strategies are available for symptomatic management in MS. Pharmacologic interventions can be used for bladder dysfunction (oxybutynin, propantheline), constipation (psyllium hydrophilic mucilloid, bisacodyl pills or suppositories), fatigue (amantadine, modafinil), spasticity (baclofen, diazepam, dantrolene), tremor (propranolol, phenobarbital, clonazepam), and dysesthesias and trigeminal neuralgia (carbamazepine, phenytoin, amitriptyline).

Transcutaneous electrical nerve stimulation (TENS) is also helpful for dysesthesias. Areas of numbness should

be inspected regularly to prevent injury and development of pressure ulcers. Skin should be kept dry and free of urine and feces. A seat cushion that distributes pressure should be used for wheelchair-bound clients with insensate buttock skin. Blindness or severely impaired vision may occur. In this case, refer the client to Services for the Blind for rehabilitation. Cognitive and perceptual impairment necessitates psychometric and functional testing for accurate assessment and rehabilitation services.

Nursing Management of Multiple Sclerosis

Assessment. If the client is being assessed for possible MS, you should assess the client for clinical manifestations of the disorder. Ocular manifestations are very common. As a result of the fluctuations of clinical manifestations, the client may report a past history of similar findings that disappeared. The Care Plan on pp. 1912-1913 includes applicable nursing diagnoses and interventions for a client with multiple sclerosis.

If the client is being hospitalized for an exacerbation of MS, focus on the client's ability to perform ADL as well as other areas that require fine motor movements. Gross motor activities, such as walking, may also be impaired and may lead to problems with bowel and bladder continence.

Depression is commonly seen in clients with MS. It may be caused by the situation or stress. The potential for MS to progress to permanent disability can instigate depression. Likewise, MS may destroy the insulating myelin that surrounds nerves that transmit signals affecting mood, thus causing depression. Depression is also a side effect of some drugs used to treat MS, such as steroids or interferon.

Fatigue is common in clients with MS. Sleep disturbance is cited as one possible explanation; clients with MS are three times as likely to have disturbed sleep as the rest of the population. A number of factors contribute to this, including a reduction in sleep efficiency (demonstrated by polysomnographic studies), periodic involuntary leg movements, and urinary urgency.

The client with MS needs to have a clear understanding of the unpredictability of this disorder. The client may be free of manifestations for many weeks to months, even years, and then experience them. If the client can identify stressors that exacerbate the clinical manifestations, sometimes these stressors can be avoided. The National Multiple Sclerosis Society can be an excellent resource for education and support. For clients receiving one of the three disease-modifying pharmacologic agents, each pharmaceutical company has a support program to offer education, financial information, and support for clients with MS and their families.

Evaluate the client's social support system, which contributes to a sense of well-being. Grieving the loss

CARE PLAN *evolve*

Client with Multiple Sclerosis

Nursing Diagnosis: Impaired Urinary Elimination. Demyelination of the nerves supplying the bladder may result in altered bladder function (neurogenic bladder). This nursing diagnosis is stated as *Impaired Urinary Elimination related to bladder dysfunction.*

Outcomes: The client will maintain urinary continence and normal bladder filling as evidenced by residual volumes of less than 100 ml, application of appropriate bladder elimination procedures, and verbalization of personal satisfaction with urinary elimination status.

| NOC OUTCOMES | Urinary Elimination |

Interventions	NIC INTERVENTIONS	Rationales
1. Assess skin for incontinence-associated dermatitis with each voiding.	Urinary Incontinence Care	1. Urine in contact with skin causes injury to the skin and denudement.
2. Maintain fluid intake of 2000 ml/24 hr: a. 400-500 ml with each meal b. 200 ml tid between meals c. Limited fluid intake after 6 PM	Fluid Management	2. Adequate fluid intake promotes adequate urine production and improves urine volume at each voiding. Limited fluids after the evening meal reduces nighttime voiding/incontinence.
3. Toilet every 3 hr while awake.	Urinary Elimination Management	3. Bladder training with routine voiding reduces the risk of incontinence.
4. Scan bladder to confirm postvoid residual (PVR) volume.	Urinary Elimination Management	4. Urinary retention is determined by measuring the postvoid residual (PVR) urine volume 10-20 min after the person has voided.
5. If PVR is >100 ml, catheterize the bladder using sterile technique in the hospital.	Urinary Catheterization: Intermittent	5. A PVR volume >100 ml indicates incomplete bladder emptying. In older adult clients, a PVR of 150-200 ml or greater (measured on 2 separate occasions) indicates incomplete bladder emptying.
6. Instruct client on self-catheterization with a clean catheter.	Urinary Catheterization: Intermittent	6. Sterile equipment is not required for ongoing catheterization at home. A clean red rubber catheter can be reused for up to 1 week so long as it is washed thoroughly with soap and water and placed in a clean, tightly sealed plastic bag after every catheterization.

Nursing Diagnosis: Constipation. Immobility and demyelination lead to constipation. State this common nursing diagnosis as *Constipation related to immobility and demyelination.*

Outcomes: The client will have bowel movements of normal consistency and frequency.

| NOC OUTCOMES | Bowel Elimination, Bowel Continence |

Interventions	NIC INTERVENTIONS	Rationales
1. Assess normal bowel movement pattern.	Bowel Training Intervention	1. Daily BM is not everyone's pattern.
2. Develop a bowel program with suppositories or digital stimulation 45 min after breakfast.	Bowel Management Intervention	2. The gastrocolic reflex is most intense after breakfast.
3. Avoid routine use of enemas and laxatives.	Bowel Management Intervention	3. Routine use of laxatives and enemas leads to dependence for BMs.
4. Perform manual disimpaction if other methods do not work.	Bowel Management Intervention	4. Manual disimpaction is the last step of any bowel program.
5. Teach client to consume a high-fiber diet and 2000 ml of fluid.	Bowel Training Intervention	5. Fiber is not digested, so it adds to the bulk of BM, making it easier to pass. Fluid is absorbed from the large colon; so maintaining fluid intake softens stool.

Nursing Diagnosis: Fatigue. State this common nursing diagnosis as *Fatigue related to fatigue and muscle weakness.*
Outcomes: The client will demonstrate reduced fatigue as evidenced by (1) maintaining a balance between work, rest, and exercise and recreation; (2) performing ADL without excessive fatigue; (3) using energy-saving devices and techniques; (4) avoiding elevations in environmental and body temperatures; and (5) consuming a diet adequate in calories and protein for body size, frame, and age.

| NOC OUTCOMES | Activity Tolerance, Endurance, Energy Conservation |

Interventions	NIC INTERVENTIONS	Rationales
1. Keep the environment cool.	Energy Management	1. Mental fatigue can vary between mild and severely disabling and is usually exacerbated by exercise or increased body or ambient temperature.
2. Teach client to plan activities during peak energy periods.	Energy Management	2. Promotes optimal synchrony between the client's circadian rhythms and physical demands.
3. Plan for rest periods during the day.	Energy Management	3. Prevents some fatigue.
4. Facilitate sleep by reducing nighttime interruptions, noise, and light.	Energy Management	4. Sleep disturbance may lead to fatigue.

Nursing Diagnosis: Impaired Physical Mobility. Several aspects of MS lead to difficulties with mobility. State this common nursing diagnosis as *Impaired Physical Mobility related to weakness, contractures, spasticity, and ataxia.*
Outcomes: The client will demonstrate improved mobility as evidenced by performing ADL without excessive fatigue.

| NOC OUTCOMES | Ambulation: Walking, Joint Movement: Active, Mobility Level |

Interventions	NIC INTERVENTIONS	Rationales
1. Assess degree of muscle spasticity.	Exercise Therapy: Joint Mobility	1. Muscle spasticity can be painful and limit mobility. Some clients rely on muscle spasms to stabilize limbs for ambulation.
2. Stretch muscles and perform ROM on joints bid.	Exercise Promotion: Stretching	2. Muscle flexibility and joint mobility can be preserved with ROM exercises.
3. Administer antispasmodics as ordered.	Exercise Therapy: Muscle Control	3. Antispasmodics are often prescribed to control muscle spasm.
4. Position in neutral alignment.	Exercise Therapy: Joint Mobility	4. Maintaining body alignment prevents contractures.
5. Consult with physical therapists for mobility aids.	Exercise Therapy: Ambulation	5. Canes, walkers, and wheelchairs are used to promote mobility; they must be fit to the client and the client taught how to use them.
6. Consult with occupational therapists for utensils and splints.	Exercise Therapy: Joint Mobility	6. Splints help to maintain joint position and reduce contractures.
7. Avoid intense aerobic exercise.	Exercise Therapy: Joint Mobility	7. Exercise can exacerbate muscle fatigue in involved muscles because demyelinated nerve fatigues easily.

Nursing Diagnosis: Situational Self-Esteem. Because of the client's age, loss of independence and fear of disability or need for institutionalization can be devastating. State this diagnosis as *Situational Self-Esteem related to loss of independence and fear of disability.*
Outcomes: The client will achieve improved self-esteem as evidenced by verbalizing awareness that personal goals and body image will need to be adjusted, willingness to maintain appropriate independence, and positive thoughts and statements about self.

| NOC OUTCOMES | Self-Esteem |

Interventions	NIC INTERVENTIONS	Rationales
1. Assess for the presence of depression and any previous treatment for depression.	Coping Enhancement	1. Depression may be due to MS or caused by MS or the medications used for treatment.
2. Assess the client's problem-solving strategies.	Coping Enhancement	2. Identifies coping behavior strengths and defense mechanisms such as denial, avoidance, or intellectualization used to mask depression.
3. Evaluate the client's support systems.	Socialization Enhancement	3. The family and other people can be great assistance to the client, both physically and emotionally.
4. Provide experiences that increase the client's autotomy.	Self-Esteem Enhancement	4. Doing activities for oneself promotes a positive self-esteem.
5. Assist client to accept dependence on others.	Self-Esteem Enhancement	5. Accepting limitations resulting from disease and accepting help are crucial steps in being realistic about the disease and its impact.

Evaluation: The degree of expected outcome attainment for all of the above diagnoses should be evaluated on an ongoing basis. Most outcomes are long-term and may require weeks to months to attain.

of function in MS can lead to a reactive depression and require provision of support group therapy for both the client and the family. Some clients may not benefit from this type of therapy, however, because they may see people whose condition is much worse than their own and fear developing that level of disability. Online computer services for MS clients can provide a means of social support.

PARALYTIC DISEASES

Paralysis, the lost of both motor and sensory function, can occur from virus-like poliomyelitis or Guillain-Barré syndrome. Unfortunately, it can also develop from botulism. The Terrorism Alert feature below describes manifestations of and interventions for this rare paralytic condition.

GUILLAIN-BARRÉ SYNDROME

Guillain-Barré syndrome (GBS) is an inflammatory disease of unknown origin that involves degeneration of the myelin sheath of peripheral nerves. GBS is seen worldwide and affects people of all ages and races. Since the virtual elimination of poliomyelitis, GBS has become the most common cause of acute generalized paralysis, which affects between 1 and 4 per 100,000 of the population annually throughout the world. In one half to two thirds of cases, an upper respiratory or gastrointestinal tract infection precedes the onset of the syndrome by 1 to 4 weeks.

Although many organisms have been suspected, including cytomegalovirus and Epstein-Barr virus, *Campylobacter jejuni* is the organism most often implicated. This gram-negative rod is found in poultry, pets, raw milk, and contaminated water. *C. jejuni* targets the myelin

---

TERRORISM ALERT

Botulism

Botulism is a serious paralytic illness caused by a nerve toxin that is produced by the bacterium *Clostridium botulinum*. Botulinum is the most poisonous substance known. Two types of botulinum toxin are of concern in bioterrorism: food-borne and inhalational forms. Food-borne botulism can be especially dangerous because many people can be poisoned by eating a contaminated food. Food-borne botulism can occur from contaminated low-acid foods such as asparagus, green beans, beets, and corn. Outbreaks of botulism have been reported from chopped garlic in oil, chili peppers, tomatoes, improperly handled baked potatoes wrapped in aluminum foil, and home-canned or fermented fish. Inhalational botulism has been released intentionally via weapons.

The classic clinical manifestations of botulinum toxin exposure depend on the amount of toxin absorbed into the circulation. Manifestations include double vision, blurred vision, drooping eyelids, slurred speech, difficulty swallowing, dry mouth, and muscle weakness. All manifestations are due to muscle paralysis caused by the bacterial toxin. If untreated, these manifestations may progress to cause paralysis of the arms, legs, trunk, and respiratory muscles. In food-borne botulism, symptoms generally begin 18 to 36 hours after eating a contaminated food, but they can occur as early as 6 hours or as late as 10 days. Accordingly, food suspected of being contaminated should be refrigerated until it is retrieved by the public health department staff. The most direct way to confirm the diagnosis is to detect the botulinum toxin in the serum or stool.

Therapy for botulism is considered supportive with passive immunization with equine antitoxin. According to current reports, optimal use of botulism antitoxin requires early suspicion of botulism. Apparently, timely administration of

passive neutralizing antibody will help minimize nerve damage and the severity of the disease, but will not reverse existent paralysis. Supportive care may include enteral or parenteral nutrition, intensive care, and mechanical ventilation. The respiratory failure and paralysis that occur with severe botulism may require mechanical ventilation for weeks. After several weeks, the paralysis slowly improves. Because of the risk of respiratory failure and aspiration, the client should be frequently assessed for the gag and cough reflexes and control of oropharyngeal secretions and oxygen saturation.

If diagnosed early, food-borne and wound botulism can be treated with an antitoxin that blocks the action of the toxin. Contaminated food still in the gut can be partially removed by inducing vomiting or by using enemas. A careful travel and dietary history should be taken on any client suspected of botulism. Wounds should be treated, usually surgically, to remove the source of the toxin-producing bacteria. After exposure to suspected botulism, clothing and skin should be washed with soap and water. Contaminated surfaces should be cleaned with 0.1% hypochlorite solution.

Botulism is a rare disease. Intentional exposure should be considered if a large number of clients are seen with flaccid paralysis, if unusual types are found that are not seen in food poisoning, or if outbreaks are occurring in unusual settings (e.g., airports). Suspected outbreaks of botulism are quickly investigated. If they involve a commercial product, the appropriate control measures are coordinated among public health and regulatory agencies. Physicians should report suspected cases of botulism to the hospital epidemiologist or infection control practitioner and the state health department.

REFERENCE

Arnon, S., et al. (2002). *Bioterrorism: Guidelines for medical and public health management* (pp. 141-165). Chicago, Ill: American Medical Association.

sheath. Macrophages penetrate the basal lamina surrounding the axon, displace the Schwann cell from the myelin sheath, and phagocytose the myelin lamellae. An association between HIV and GBS has also been reported, and clients with GBS should be tested for HIV.

Clinical Manifestations

A characteristic feature is ascending weakness, usually beginning in the lower extremities and spreading, sometimes rapidly, to the trunk, upper extremities, and even the face. The weakness evolves over hours to days, with maximal deficit by 4 weeks in 90% of cases. Deep tendon reflexes are lost. Paresthesias (tingling sensation) in the limbs may occur early in the course of the illness.

This *initial phase* is usually followed by a *plateau phase* during which the disease no longer seems to progress, but the client does not recover functions initially lost. Deep, aching muscle pain in the shoulder girdle and thighs is common. The two most dangerous features of the disease are respiratory muscle weakness and autonomic neuropathy involving both the sympathetic and parasympathetic systems. The latter feature can involve orthostatic hypotension, hypertension, pupillary disturbances, sweating dysfunction, cardiac dysrhythmias, paralytic ileus, and urinary retention.

The third phase of the disease is the *recovery phase.* Improvement and recovery occur with remyelination. If nerve axons are damaged, however, some residual deficits may remain. Remyelination occurs in a descending pattern; the functions lost last are thus the first to be regained. Recovery is usually maximal at 6 months, although severe cases may take up to 2 years for maximal recovery. Fortunately, 85% to 90% of clients with GBS recover completely.

Diagnosis of GBS is based on history and physical examination, CSF examination, and electrophysiologic studies. The CSF contains increased protein, with few or no white blood cells. Nerve-conduction velocity is slowed, although it may be normal in the early stage of the illness. *Conduction block,* a diminution in amplitude or an absence of elicited muscle action potentials from stimulation of a peripheral nerve, also occurs.

OUTCOME MANAGEMENT

The focus of therapy is supportive care. Monitor respiratory or cardiovascular status carefully: vital signs, serial measurement of vital capacity, peripheral oxygen saturation, and electrocardiography. When vital capacity falls to 15 ml/kg of body weight, intubation and artificial ventilation are usually necessary.

Medical Management

Current practice guidelines for GBS include treatment with plasma exchange (PE) or IV immunoglobulin (IVIg), which hastens recovery from GBS. In addition, corticosteroids are not recommended for the treatment of GBS. Early treatment with (PE) may accelerate recovery, although the exact mechanism for this effect is not known. Hypotheses include the removal of circulating antibodies or other humoral myelinotoxic or immunopathogenic factors. IV immunoglobulin G (IVIG) therapy may prove to be the treatment of choice because it can be administered easily and can be given with other drugs simultaneously (PE removes co-medication jointly with adverse disease factors).

Nursing Management

During the first several days after hospital admission, it is crucial to assess the client's respiratory, swallowing, and autonomic function. The Critical Monitoring feature below summarizes nursing assessments for clients with Guillain-Barré syndrome who are in respiratory distress. Assess the following at least every 4 hours: vital signs, forced vital capacity, swallowing, strength in the extremities, and intake and output balance. If ascending weakness is noted, increase the frequency of assessment to every 2 hours or even more often. Cardiac monitoring and supplemental oxygen are often needed. Common complications include bladder infection, deep vein thrombosis, pulmonary emboli, pneumonia, and syndrome of inappropriate antidiuretic hormone (SIADH).

CRITICAL MONITORING

Respiratory Distress with Guillain-Barré Syndrome

Monitor the client for the following:
- Complaints of headache
- Myoclonic jerks
- Drowsiness
- Confusion
- Restlessness
- Reduced cough
- Decreased ability to move pulmonary secretions

Assess pulmonary function studies for the following:
- Decreased forced vital capacity (<15 ml/kg)
- Decreased tidal volume (<3-4 ml/kg)
- Decreased maximum inspiratory pressure (<10-20 cm H_2O)
- Decreased maximum expiratory pressure (<40 cm H_2O)

Assess arterial blood gases for the following:
- Decreased Pao_2 (<80 mm Hg on 50% Fio_2 with normal Pco_2)
- Alveolar-arterial gradient >300 on 50% Fio_2
- $Paco_2$ >50 mm Hg
- V_D/V_T >0.6

Fio$_2$, Fraction of inspired oxygen; *Paco$_2$,* partial pressure of arterial carbon dioxide; *Pao$_2$,* partial pressure of arterial oxygen; *V_D/V_T,* ratio of dead space volume to tidal volume.

Interventions to control infection and prevent complications of immobility are vital. Proper body alignment should be maintained to prevent deformities and injury to paralyzed limbs. Once the client's condition is stabilized, rehabilitative interventions can be implemented.

Assist the client in coping with the progressive nature of GBS. During the early stages, clients are frightened because their paralysis can ascend rapidly. They are often admitted to an acute care agency with progressive weakness and within days are completely paralyzed. Clients fear they will never recover. Help clients in verbalizing their fears, and offer support and encouragement that although the disorder is progressive, most clients gain full recovery. Encouragement is not hollow, however. The client is not taught to expect immediate resolution but is assisted to realize the usual time frames for recovery.

MYASTHENIA GRAVIS

Myasthenia gravis (MG) is an autoimmune disease that presents as muscular weakness and fatigue that worsens with exercise and improves with rest. The manifestations result from a loss of ACh receptors in the postsynaptic neurons of the neuromuscular junction. The cause of MG is unknown, but 80% of people with the generalized form of the disease have elevated titers of antibodies to the ACh receptor in their serum. MG may appear at any age, although there are two peaks of onset. In early-onset MG, at age 20 to 30 years, women are more often affected than men. In late-onset MG, after age 50, men are more often affected.

Clinical Manifestations

The primary feature of MG is increasing weakness with sustained muscle contraction. For instance, if the person is asked to hold the arms up, the power of muscle contraction diminishes and the arms gradually drift downward. After a period of rest, the muscles regain their strength. Muscle weakness is greatest after exertion or at the end of the day.

Ocular manifestations are most common, with *ptosis* (drooping of the upper eyelid) or *diplopia* (double vision) occurring in many clients. Ptosis is due to weakness of the levator palpebrae muscles of the eye. If not present at the examination, ptosis can be elicited by prolonged upward gaze, which creates fatigue of the muscle.

Diplopia is a result of weakness or fatigue of the extraocular muscles. Other manifestations are weakness of the orbicularis oculi muscles (which help close the eye), the facial muscles, the muscles of chewing and swallowing, and the limb muscles. Weakness of the facial and levator palpebrae muscles produces an expressionless face, with droopy eyelids, smoothed features, and a tendency for the mouth to hang open.

An attempt to smile often turns into a snarl because of the weakness. A person may hold a hand under the jaw to keep it closed. Dysphagia and a nasal quality to speech occur when the muscles of chewing and swallowing are involved. In severe cases, respiratory muscle weakness may occur, which may necessitate intubation and mechanical ventilation (see The Critical Monitoring Box on p. 1917).

The course of MG varies, and remissions and exacerbations may occur. Clinical manifestations may progress quickly or slowly and may fluctuate from day to day. The severity of the disease varies greatly from person to person.

Diagnostic Findings

The diagnosis of MG is based on the clinical presentation and can be confirmed by testing the client's response to anticholinesterase drugs. These drugs inhibit cholinesterase, an enzyme that breaks down ACh in the neuromuscular junction, thereby allowing more ACh to bind to the remaining ACh receptors. Edrophonium (Tensilon) is a short-acting drug that is given intravenously *(Tensilon test)*. A test dose of 2 mg (for adults) is injected first. If no untoward reaction occurs (such as increased weakness, change in heart rate or rhythm, nausea, or abdominal cramps), the remaining 8 mg is injected. The client is then observed for objective manifestations of improvement in muscle strength. The effect is transitory, wearing off after 3 to 5 minutes. Another drug, neostigmine methylsulfate (Prostigmin), may be used because of its longer duration of effect on muscle strength (1 to 2 hours), which allows better analysis of its effect.

When either drug is used, IV atropine sulfate should be available to inject as an antidote. This medication counteracts any severe cholinergic reactions (cardiac dysrhythmias or abdominal cramping). Electromyography (EMG) helps confirm the diagnosis. Repetitive stimulation of the nerve with recording from the involved muscle shows a characteristic decrementing response of the muscle action potential. Generally, after the initial diagnostic testing is performed by the practitioner, referral to a neurologist and/or pulmonologist may be necessary for long-term management.

OUTCOME MANAGEMENT

No cure for MG exists as yet. Pharmacologic intervention consists of two groups of medications: (1) short-acting anticholinesterase compounds and (2) corticosteroids. The most effective anticholinesterase drugs are pyridostigmine (Mestinon) and neostigmine (Prostigmin). Dosages are highly individualized, based on physiologic response to the medication. The goal is to achieve the maximum benefit (muscle strength and endurance) with the fewest side effects (excessive salivation, sweating, nausea, diarrhea, abdominal cramps, or tachycardia). Corticosteroids (usually prednisone) are directed toward reducing the level of serum ACh receptor antibodies. Corticosteroids may temporarily worsen manifestations; however, this is followed by gradual improvement in muscle strength.

After a peak of improvement is reached and maintained for several weeks, the dosage of both prednisone and anticholinesterase medication may be gradually decreased. A low maintenance dose of alternate-day prednisone may be effective for many months or years. Precautions with any steroid therapy are important, including potassium supplements if indicated and liberal use of antacids.

Potential complications of steroid use are cataracts, hypertension, diabetes, fluid retention, delayed wound healing, insomnia, and osteoporosis. Other treatments include azathioprine (Imuran) and cyclosporine (Sandimmune), which reduce the level of circulating ACh receptor antibodies, and plasmapheresis and IVIG.

Plasmapheresis

Plasmapheresis is an adjunctive therapy for clients with refractory MG. It is a process by which plasma is separated from formed elements of blood. The plasma is discarded and the packed red blood cells are joined with albumin, normal saline, and electrolytes and returned to the client. The purpose is to remove plasma proteins containing antibodies that are believed to cause MG. Plasmapheresis may produce transient improvement in clients who have actual or pending respiratory failure.

Usually, three to five treatments given once daily over 5 to 7 days are required. Potential complications include myasthenic or cholinergic crisis and, rarely, hypovolemia. Muscle strength should be assessed before and after the procedure, with particular attention paid to vital capacity, swallowing ability, diplopia, and ptosis to evaluate the effectiveness of the treatment.

Complications

Two major complications of MG may occur: *myasthenic crisis* and *cholinergic crisis*. The Critical Monitoring feature at right highlights clinical manifestations of these medical emergencies and outlines appropriate nursing interventions.

Myasthenic Crisis

Clients with moderate or severe generalized MG, especially those who have difficulty swallowing or breathing, may experience a sudden worsening of their condition. This is usually precipitated by an intercurrent infection or sudden withdrawal of anticholinesterase drugs, but it may occur spontaneously. If an increase in the dosage of the anticholinesterase drug does not improve the weakness, endotracheal intubation and mechanical ventilation may be required. In many instances, drug responsiveness returns in 24 to 48 hours, and weaning from the respirator can proceed.

CRITICAL MONITORING

Myasthenic and Cholinergic Crises in Clients with Myasthenia Gravis

MYASTHENIC CRISIS IS CAUSED BY UNDERMEDICATION

Clinical Manifestations
- Sudden marked rise in blood pressure because of hypoxia
- Increased heart rate
- Severe respiratory distress and cyanosis
- Absent cough and swallow reflexes
- Increased secretions, increased diaphoresis, and increased lacrimation
- Restlessness, dysarthria
- Bowel and bladder incontinence

Intervention
- Increased doses of cholinergic drugs as long as the client responds positively to edrophonium treatment
- Possible mechanical ventilation if respiratory muscle paralysis is acute

CHOLINERGIC CRISIS IS CAUSED BY DEPOLARIZATION BLOCK RESULTING FROM EXCESSIVE MEDICATIONS

Clinical Manifestations
- Weakness with difficulty swallowing, chewing, speaking, and breathing
- Apprehension, nausea, and vomiting
- Abdominal cramps and diarrhea
- Increased secretions and saliva
- Sweating, lacrimation, fasciculations, and blurred vision

Intervention
- Discontinue all cholinergic drugs until cholinergic effects decrease
- Provide adequate ventilatory support
- 1 mg intravenous atropine may be necessary to counteract severe cholinergic reactions

---

Cholinergic Crisis

Cholinergic crisis occurs as a result of overmedication. The muscarinic effect of a toxic level of anticholinesterase medication causes abdominal cramps, diarrhea, and excessive pulmonary secretions. The nicotinic effect paradoxically worsens weakness and can cause bronchial spasm. If respiratory status is compromised, the client may need intubation and mechanical ventilation.

Nursing Management of Myasthenia Gravis (MG)

Because MG may involve the muscles of respiration, the client may experience dyspnea and ineffective cough and swallow mechanisms, which may lead to aspiration and pneumonia. Encourage deep breathing and coughing. Have suction equipment available at the bedside, and instruct the client on how to use it. Instruct the client to sit upright when eating, to swallow only when the chin is tipped downward toward the chest, and never to speak while food is in the mouth. Oxygen and, in severe cases, mechanical ventilation may be required.

In MG, weakness is usually greatest following exertion and at the end of the day. Activities should be carefully planned to include rest periods so that energy is conserved and the muscles have a chance to regain their strength. Rearrangement of the home environment may help prevent unnecessary energy expenditure. Vocational retraining may be indicated for those who can no longer meet the physical demands of their jobs. Clients with severe disease or an acute exacerbation will be totally dependent on nursing care for ADL. This level of care requires that complications of immobility be avoided.

Provide the client and family with information about MG and its treatment. They should be aware of adverse reactions of both anticholinesterase drugs and steroids. Explain how to recognize myasthenic and cholinergic crises and how to have a plan to seek medical intervention, if necessary.

Surgical Management

Thymectomy can be used for treatment. The thymus gland, located in the superior mediastinum, is important during fetal growth for development of the immune system. It is usually atrophied and nonfunctioning in adulthood. The effect of thymectomy is not fully understood. It may alter some immunologic control mechanism that affects the production of antibodies to the ACh receptor, or it may eliminate a trigger to antibody production. Thymectomy is indicated for clients with thymoma, selected clients with generalized MG without thymoma, and selected clients with disabling ocular MG.[14] The procedure is recommended early in the course of the disease. Nursing management is similar to care following thoracic surgery.

AMYOTROPHIC LATERAL SCLEROSIS

Amyotrophic lateral sclerosis (ALS) is the most common of the motor neuron diseases. It is an age-dependent, fatal paralytic disorder also known as *Charcot's disease* and *Lou Gehrig's disease*. Onset is usually in middle age. Men are affected more often than women.

Amyotrophic lateral sclerosis involves degeneration of both the anterior horn cells and the corticospinal tracts. Consequently, both upper and lower motor neuron clinical manifestations are seen. Lower motor neuron clinical manifestations include weakness, atrophy, cramps, and fasciculations (irregular twitchings of muscle fibers or bundles). Upper motor neuron manifestations include spasticity and hyperreflexia. Involvement of the corticobulbar tracts causes dysphagia (difficulty swallowing)

and dysarthria (slurred speech). These clients are at risk for suboptimal caloric and fluid intake and a worsening of muscle atrophy, weakness, and fatigue. The sensory system is not involved, and cognition is not affected. The client remains alert and mentally intact throughout the course of the disease. The course of the disease is relentlessly progressive. Death usually results from pneumonia caused by respiratory compromise within 2 to 5 years.

Weakness typically begins in the upper extremities and progressively involves the upper arms and shoulders and then the muscles of the neck and throat. The trunk and lower extremities are usually not affected until late in the disease. When the intercostal muscles and diaphragm become involved, respirations are shallow and coughing is ineffective. Cognition, as well as bowel and bladder sphincters, remains intact, even when the client is totally debilitated. In some cases, weakness begins in the brain stem, causing problems with speech and swallowing. This is called *bulbar ALS*.

Diagnosis of ALS is made by the clinical presentation and EMG. The EMG criteria for the diagnosis of ALS include the presence of widespread anterior horn cell dysfunction with fibrillations, positive waves, fasciculations, and chronic neurogenic motor unit potential changes in multiple nerve root distribution in at least three limbs and the paraspinal muscles in the presence of normal sensory responses.

OUTCOME MANAGEMENT

Supportive therapy was the only intervention for ALS until riluzole (Rilutek) was approved in 1996. Its mechanism of action is unknown, but it is thought to have a neuroprotective effect. The drug extends the life of ALS clients by a few months. Clients with ALS are usually admitted to health care facilities only twice in their illness, first for diagnosis and later in the final stage of debilitation.

The antibiotic minocycline is being studied for ALS. Laboratory studies have linked inducible nitric oxide and caspase enzyme activation to motor nerve cell death in ALS. Minocycline is in the tetracycline group of antibiotics that penetrates barriers around the CNS when taken orally and helps to inhibit caspase enzymes, which are involved in cell death pathways. Genetic treatments are also being researched.

Supportive nursing care is an important aspect of managing the ALS client. In the outpatient arena, the nurse can provide ongoing assessment of daily living needs and make suggestions for modifications in activity level, clothing, and diet. Often just allowing the client or family to talk about problems reduces anxiety and helps them find solutions to problems.[19] Interventions should be aimed at conserving energy. Activities should be spaced during the day. Muscle stress, strenuous activity and extremes of hot and cold should be avoided. Leg braces, canes, and walkers can prolong independence in ambulation. Hand braces, special utensils, and adaptive devices such as buttonhooks can help with dressing and self-feeding. Pressure ulcers are not usually a problem because the sensory system remains intact and the client can feel when pressure on a body part is too great.

In the acute care setting, gather information from the client and family about communication needs and which positions are best for respiration, handling secretions, eating, and turning routines.

Encourage fluid intake regularly, when the client is not fatigued. Proper positioning is imperative. Providing a cup with a spout may prevent liquid from running out of the corners of the mouth. Give liquids by using a large syringe with short tubing on the tip. The tube is placed on the anterior portion of the tongue, and gentle force is used to deliver small amounts of liquid.

Encourage small, frequent, high-nutrient feedings. Tell the client to sit upright, with the head slightly flexed forward while eating. Papase tablets placed under the tongue 10 minutes before meals can make thick saliva less sticky. Plenty of time should be allowed for eating, and the client should not attempt to speak while food is in the mouth. Have suction equipment available during meals to reduce the risk of aspiration of food and secretions that become lodged in the mouth and pharynx. The head may need to be stabilized with a soft cervical collar. Consult the dietitian for special diet recommendations. As dysphagia progresses, percutaneous endoscopic gastrostomy (PEG) should be considered as an alternative or supplemental route for oral nutrition.

Although speech remains intelligible, the client can be trained to slow the rate of speech and exaggerate articulation. As manifestations progress, the client may need to repeat words or have an interpreter (usually the spouse). At this stage, it is important to eliminate extraneous noise, face the client when he or she is talking, and maintain eye contact. When the client's speech contains only one-word phrases or is no longer possible, writing can be an effective means of communicating and should be encouraged. When writing is no longer possible, a speech pathologist can provide communication devices such as alphabet boards and portable memo writers.[9]

If the client is a smoker, encourage him or her to stop. Exposure to people with respiratory tract infections should be avoided. Remind the client to use good posture. Pulmonary function tests should be performed regularly to assess ventilatory status. Clients generally experience respiratory fatigue when vital capacity is less than 1.5 L. Some clients can be taught to use their abdominal muscles to enhance respirations when the intercostal muscles and diaphragm become weak. A manifestation of pending respiratory insufficiency is shortness of breath while eating.

Encourage the client and family to talk about the losses they are experiencing and the feelings associated with them. Family members should be encouraged to take time for rest and activities away from the client. Refer the client and family to an ALS support group.

Eventually clients face the difficult choice of deciding whether they will accept artificial ventilation. Encourage them to discuss this with family and friends and to seek input from ALS support groups. Encourage clients to complete advance directives to indicate whether they desire life-sustaining treatments such as cardiopulmonary resuscitation, but this should be reassessed at regular intervals. Clients may change their minds on the basis of their experience with their illness, changes in their subjective appreciation of their quality of life, or changes in their evaluation of the benefits and burdens of life-sustaining measures as they come to terms with the imminence of death.[21]

CONCLUSIONS

Degenerative neurologic disorders have many causes, including viruses, autoimmune responses, and heredity. Some have no known cause. In general, they are relentlessly progressive, slowly taking away both physical and mental ability. Nurses should focus care on the management of clinical manifestations and prevention of complications. Family support throughout the process of care is essential.

THINKING CRITICALLY

1. A 52-year-old man with multiple sclerosis is wheelchair-bound and has a neurogenic bladder. He complains of a sudden onset of generalized weakness, fever, and chills and is admitted to the hospital. What priorities should be set for his care?

Factors to Consider. What do generalized weakness, fever, and chills suggest in *any* client? If your client has not been following good bladder management, how can you intervene?

2. A 70-year-old man with Parkinson's disease is admitted to the hospital after experiencing severe nightmares and periods of confusion. During lucid periods, he is very disturbed by these manifestations. At other times, he believes that his wife is participating in a conspiracy to harm him. What assessments and interventions should you consider?

Factors to Consider. Are hallucinations and paranoia typical manifestations of Parkinson's disease? Might the client's manifestations be related to treatment or to some cause other than Parkinson's disease?

3. A 41-year-old woman with myasthenia gravis is taking pyridostigmine and prednisone. She is complaining of increased fatigue and weakness and has difficulty breathing. What concerns should you have?

Factors to Consider. Might the client's difficulty breathing be related to her fatigue and weakness? Could these manifestations be related to myasthenia gravis or its treatment?

evolve   *Discussions for these questions can be found on the website.*

BIBLIOGRAPHY

Citations appearing in red refer to primary research.

Citations appearing in blue refer to evidence-based practice guidelines and protocols.

1. American Academy of Neurology Guideline Summary for Clinicians. (2006). *Manage ALS from the beginning: Care makes a difference* (pp. 1-2). St. Paul, Mn: American Academy of Neurology.
2. Andrews, K.L., & Husmann, D.A. (1997). Bladder dysfunction and management in multiple sclerosis. *Mayo Clinic Proceedings, 74,* 1176-1183.
3. Armstrong Mortenson, S., & Schumann, L. (2003). Myasthenia gravis: Diagnosis and treatment. *Clinical Practice, 15*(2), 72-78.
4. Brown, P. (1997). The risk of bovine spongiform encephalopathy ('mad cow disease') to human health. *Journal of the American Medical Association, 278*(12), 1008-1011.
5. Calne, S. (2005). Late-stage Parkinson's disease for the rehabilitation specialist: A nursing perspective. *Topics in Geriatric Rehabilitation, 21*(3), 233-246.
6. Friedlander, R. (2003). Apoptosis and caspases in neurodegenerative diseases. *New England Journal of Medicine, 348*(14), 1365-1375.
7. Goodwin, D.S., Frohman, E.M., & Garmany, G. (2002). Disease modifying therapies in multiple sclerosis. *Neurology, 58*(2), 169-178.
8. Gwyther, L.P. (2000). Family issues in dementia: Finding a new normal. *Neurology Clinics, 18*(4), 993-1010.
9. Haberman, B., & Davis, L.L. (2005). Caring for family with Alzheimer's disease and Parkinson's disease: Needs, challenges, and satisfaction. *Journal of Gerontological Nursing, 31*(6), 49-54.
10. Halper, J., et al. (2003). Rethinking cognitive function in multiple sclerosis: A nursing perspective. *Journal of Neuroscience Nursing, 35*(2), 70-81.
11. Handley, J. (2005). Using drugs to treat Parkinson's disease: A nurse's perspective. *Practice Nurse, July 8, 30*(1).
12. Hecht, M.J., et al. (2003). Burden of care in amyotrophic lateral sclerosis. *Palliative Medicine, 17*(4), 327-333.
13. Hogancamp, W.E., Rodriguez, M., & Weinshenker, B.G. (1997). The epidemiology of multiple sclerosis. *Mayo Clinic Proceedings, 74,* 871-878.
14. Hughes, R.A.C., Wijdicks, E.F.M., & Barohn, R. (2003). Practice parameters: Immunotherapy for Guillain-Barré syndrome. *Neurology, 61,* 736-740.
15. Jones, P.S., & Martinson, I.M. (1992). The experience of bereavement in care givers of family members with Alzheimer's disease. *Image—The Journal of Nursing Scholarship, 24*(3), 174-176.
16. Knopman, D.S., Boeve, B.F., & Petersen, R.C. (2003). Essentials of the proper diagnosis of mild cognitive impairment, dementia and major subtypes of dementia. *Mayo Clinic Proceedings, 78,* 1290-1308.
17. Lang, A.E., & Lozano, A.M. (1998). Parkinson's disease. *New England Journal of Medicine, 339*(16), 1130-1143.
18. Le Bars, P.L., et al. (1997). A placebo-controlled, double-blind, randomized trial of an extract of ginkgo biloba for dementia. *Journal of the American Medical Association, 278*(16), 1327-1332.
19. Levin, L.I., Munger, K., Ruberton, M., et al. (2003). Multiple sclerosis and Epstein Barr virus. *Journal of the American Medical Association, 289*(12), 1533-1536.
20. Lucchinetti, C.F., & Rodriguez, M. (1997). The controversy surrounding pathogenesis of the multiple sclerosis lesion. *Mayo Clinic Proceedings, 74,* 665-678.
21. Mayo Foundation for Medical Education and Research. (1996, Oct). Alzheimer's disease: Living with a 'long goodbye.' *Mayo Clinic Health Letter* (Suppl), 1-8.
22. McGonigal-Kenney, M.L., & Schultte, D.L. (2004). *Non-pharmacologic management of agitated behaviors in persons with Alzheimer's disease and other chronic dementing illnesses.* University of Iowa Gerontological Nursing Interventions Research Center, Research Dissemination Core.
23. Mezey, M., et al. (1996). Life-sustaining treatment decisions by spouses of patients with Alzheimer's disease. *Journal of the American Geriatrics Society, 44*(2), 144-150.
24. Miller, R.G., Rosenberg, J.A., Gelinas, D.F., and the ALS Practice Parameters Task Force. (2003). Practice Parameters: The care of the patient with amyotrophic lateral sclerosis (an evidence based review). *Report of the Quality Standards of Subcommittees of the American Academy of Neurology, 52*(7), 1311-1323.
25. National Institute of Neurological Disorders and Stroke Publication. (2006). *Huntington Disease: Hope through research* (NIH Pub No. 98-49). Bethesda, Md: NIH.
26. Nowotny, M.L. (1998). My journey with amyotrophic lateral sclerosis. *Journal of Neuroscience Nursing, 30*(1), 68-70.
27. Palmieri, R. (2005). Is it myasthenia gravis or Guillain-Barré syndrome? *Nursing, 35*(12), 1-4.
28. Perry, J. (2002). Wives giving care to husbands with Alzheimer's disease: A process of interpretive caring. *Research in Nursing and Health, 25*(4), 307-316.
29. Post, S.G., et al. (1997). The clinical introduction of genetic testing for Alzheimer disease: An ethical perspective. *Journal of the American Medical Association, 277*(10), 832-836.
30. Prusiner, S. (2001). Neurodegenerative diseases and prions. *New England Journal of Medicine, 344*(20), 1516-1524.
31. Robinson, L. (2003). The importance of touch for the patient with dementia. *Home HealthCare Nurse, 21*(1), 16-19.
32. Robinson, B.E. (1997). Guideline for initial evaluation of the patient with memory loss. *Geriatrics, 52*(12), 30-39.
33. Rodriguez, M. (1997). Multiple sclerosis: Insights into molecular pathogenesis and therapy. *Mayo Clinic Proceedings, 74,* 663-664.
34. Rudick, R.A., et al. (1997). Management of multiple sclerosis. *New England Journal of Medicine, 337*(22), 1604-1611.
35. Schechter, R., Inglesby, T.V., & Henderson, D.A. (2002). *Botulinum toxin as a biological weapon: Medical and public health management. (2) Botulinum toxin as a biological weapon. (Addendum)* (pp. 141-165). Chicago, Ill: American Medical Association.
36. Spurlock, W.R. (2005). Spiritual well-being and caregiver burden in Alzheimer's caregivers. *Geriatric Nursing, 26*(30), 154-161.
37. Vrabec, N.J. (1997). Literature review of social support and caregiver burden, 1980 to 1995. *Image—The Journal of Nursing Scholarship, 29*(4), 383-388.

evolve   **Did you remember to check out the bonus material on the Evolve website and the CD-ROM, including NCLEX®-Examination Style Review Questions, Open-Book Quizzes, and Chapter Review Audio Podcasts?**

http://evolve.elsevier.com/Black/medsurg

CHAPTER 73

Management of Clients with Neurologic Trauma

NORMA D. MCNAIR AND JUDI L. KURIC

The complexity of the central nervous system (CNS) allows the human organism to evaluate information about the outside world. Failure of the brain or the spinal cord to process information correctly prevents the affected person from accurately performing tasks and may impair interactions with others as well as self-appraisal.

Admission of a client with CNS trauma to the emergency department requires rapid mobilization of a trauma team. The team provides initial assessment and resuscitation of the trauma victim and performs triage to the appropriate radiologic studies and surgical service. Ultimately the management of a client with a head injury, spinal cord injury, or a combination of neurologic injuries is directed by the neurosurgical service. This chapter examines the needs of clients with CNS trauma, including head and spinal cord injuries.

The discussion will begin with crucial information in caring for any client with neurologic disease or trauma. Discussions about specific diseases will follow.

INCREASED INTRACRANIAL PRESSURE

The skull is a hard, bony vault filled with brain tissue, blood, and cerebrospinal fluid (CSF). A balance between these three components maintains the pressure within the cranium. The modified *Munro-Kellie hypothesis,* a theory for understanding intracranial pressure (ICP), states that because the bony skull cannot expand, when one of the three components expands, the other two must compensate by decreasing in volume for the total brain volume and pressure to remain constant.

Intracranial pressure is the pressure exerted in the cranium by its contents: the brain, blood, and CSF (Figure 73-1). ICP is measured with a monitor in the ventricle, the brain parenchyma, or the subarachnoid space. The normal ICP is 5 to 15 mm Hg. Pressures greater than 20 mm Hg are considered to represent *increased ICP,* which seriously impairs cerebral perfusion. Recognition of increased ICP is one of the most important assessments made by nurses caring for clients with neurologic disorders.

Cerebral perfusion pressure (CPP) is the amount of blood flow from the systemic circulation required to provide adequate oxygen and glucose for brain metabolism. *Mean arterial pressure* (MAP) represents the average pressure during the cardiac cycle. It is calculated by adding the systolic pressure to twice the diastolic pressure and dividing by 3. (Diastole is twice as long as systole.) The formula for calculating CPP is as follows:

$$CPP = MAP - ICP$$

When MAP and ICP are equal, there is no CPP and brain perfusion ceases. Therefore it is crucial to maintain control of both ICP and MAP.

Etiology and Risk Factors

Increased ICP is most often associated with a space-occupying lesion (such as a tumor, edema, or bleeding). However, a cerebral infarction, an obstruction to the outflow of CSF, an abscess, an ingested or accumulated toxin,

---

evolve Web Enhancements

Case Study Spinal Cord Injury

Client Education Guide Monitoring Family Members After Head Injury (English Version and Spanish Translation)

Use of a Halo Vest (English Version and Spanish Translation)

Ethical Issues in Nursing What is the Government's Obligation to Put Care for Its Citizens Above Care for Noncitizens, Given Scarce Resources?

Figure A Neurologic Observation Chart

Be sure to check out the bonus material on the Evolve website and the CD-ROM, including free self-assessment exercises. **http://evolve.elsevier.com/Black/medsurg**

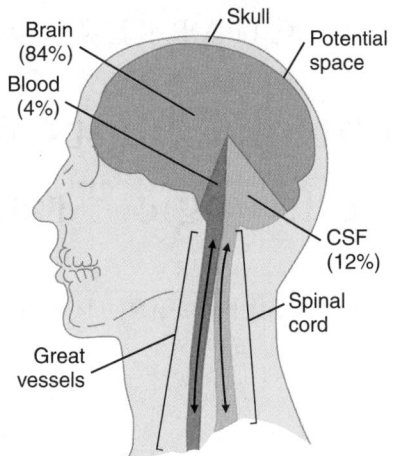

■ **FIGURE 73–1** Components of the intracranial vault. A balance between these three compartments maintains normal intracranial pressure.

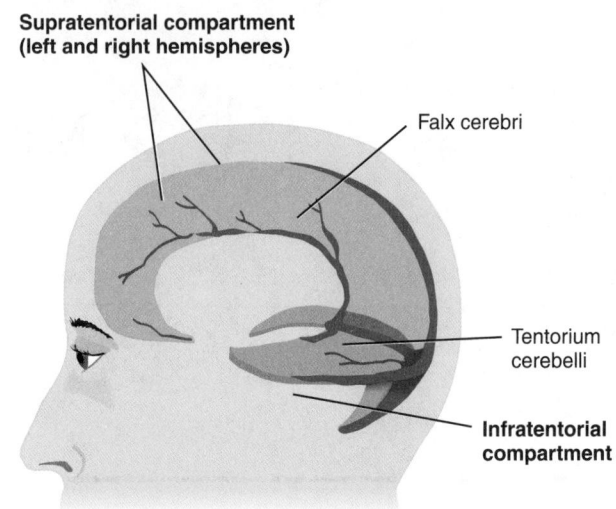

■ **FIGURE 73–2** The intracranial compartments are divided by inelastic fibers to provide support.

impaired blood flow to or from the brain, vasodilation from increased carbon dioxide ($PaCO_2$) or decreased partial pressure of oxygen (PaO_2), systemic hypertension, or increased intrathoracic pressure can also increase the pressure. Risk factors include head injury, brain tumors, cerebral bleeding, hydrocephalus, and edema from surgery or injury.

Pathophysiology

As an intracranial mass enlarges, initial compensation occurs through *displacement of CSF* into the spinal canal. The ability of the brain to adapt to increasing pressure without increasing ICP is called *compliance*. The movement of CSF out of the cranium is the first and major compensatory mechanism, but the cranial vault can accommodate increasing intracranial volume only to a point. When the compliance of the brain is exceeded, the ICP rises, clinical manifestations develop, and other compensatory efforts to reduce pressure begin.

The second form of compensation is *reduction of blood volume* in the brain. *Autoregulation* is the occurrence of compensatory changes in the diameter of intracranial blood vessels designed to maintain a constant blood flow during changes in CPP. Autoregulation is lost with increasing ICP. Small increases in brain volume can then cause dramatic increases in ICP, with a longer time required to return to baseline level. When ICP approaches systemic blood pressure, cerebral perfusion decreases and the brain suffers severe hypoxia and acidosis.

When blood flow is reduced by 40%, cerebral tissue becomes acidotic. When 60% of blood flow is lost, the electroencephalogram (EEG) begins to change. This stage of compensation alters cerebral metabolism, eventually leading to brain tissue hypoxia and areas of brain tissue ischemia.

The last stage of compensation and the most lethal is *displacement of brain tissue* across the dividing structures of the brain. The brain is supported within various intracranial compartments (Figure 73-2). The supratentorial compartment contains all the brain tissue from the top of the midbrain upward. This section is divided into right and left chambers by the tough, inelastic fibers of the falx cerebri. The supratentorial compartment is separated from the infratentorial compartment (containing the brain stem and cerebellum) by the tentorium cerebelli. The brain is capable of some movement within these compartments. Pressure increases in one compartment affect surrounding areas of lower pressure.

When swollen, the brain can bulge into the tentorium, under the falx cerebri, or through the foramen magnum into the spinal canal. This process is called *herniation* and often results in death from brain stem compression.

Cerebral Edema

The terms *cerebral edema, brain swelling,* and *increased ICP* are sometimes used interchangeably, but they are not the same. Cerebral edema and brain swelling are causes of increased ICP. An increase in brain bulk caused by an increase in cerebral blood volume is called *brain swelling.* *Brain edema,* in contrast, is an increase in the fluid surrounding the tissues of the brain, such as in the extracellular spaces or the white matter, or within the cells themselves. The distinction between these two conditions is important because the interventions differ.

After head injury, edema develops because of a disruption of the blood-brain barrier. This type of edema is similar to other forms of edema, such as that seen in a sprained ankle. The fluid contains electrolytes, proteins, and blood. Edema reaches its maximum within 48 to 72 hours after brain surgery or injury. The fluid returns to the systemic circulation via the CSF or the venous system. This form of edema is usually treated with osmotic diuretics.

Brain swelling is caused by increased blood volume resulting from dilated cerebral blood vessels. Brain swelling, in conjunction with cerebral edema, appears to be a major mechanism responsible for increasing ICP and for decreasing the size of the ventricles when compensation occurs. This form of swelling may be treated with therapeutic hyperventilation using mechanical ventilation to cause vasoconstriction.

Clinical Manifestations

Manifestations of increased ICP are caused by traction on the cerebral blood vessels from swelling tissues and by pressure on the pain-sensitive dura mater and various structures within the brain. The pathologic process of increased ICP actually comprises several entities that occur at the same time. No single set of clinical manifestations occurs in all clients. Indications of increased ICP relate to the location and cause of the raised pressure and to the speed and extent of its development.

Initial manifestations of increased ICP are subtle, and diligent observation for changes in the client's condition is necessary. Clinical manifestations include *any* alteration in level of consciousness (e.g., restlessness, irritability, confusion) and may include a decrease in the Glasgow Coma Scale (GCS) score. In addition, the client may have changes in speech, pupillary reactivity, motor or sensory ability, or cardiac rate and rhythm. Headache, nausea, vomiting, or blurred or double vision (diplopia) may be reported. The optic nerve is an extension of the brain, and increased tension in the skull is transmitted to the optic nerve to cause papilledema. *Papilledema* is swelling and hyperemia of the optic disc and can be observed only through an ophthalmoscope. Early detection of increased ICP (i.e., before clinical manifestations develop) by means of ICP monitoring in the critical care unit can greatly improve a client's outcome.

Cushing's triad—increased systolic blood pressure with widened pulse pressure and bradycardia—is a late response and indicates severe increased ICP with failure of autoregulation. Respiratory patterns progress from Cheyne-Stokes respiration to central neurogenic hyperventilation to apneustic breathing and ataxic breathing as ICP increases (see Chapter 68). These respiratory patterns will not be noticed in the client receiving mechanical ventilation, however. Hyperthermia is typically present when the hypothalamus is first affected by the increase in pressure, followed by hypothermia as ICP increases (Figure 73-3).

Common diagnostic studies performed to determine the source of increased ICP include skull radiography, computed tomography (CT) scanning, and magnetic resonance imaging (MRI). A lumbar puncture is not usually performed because of the risk of causing herniation of

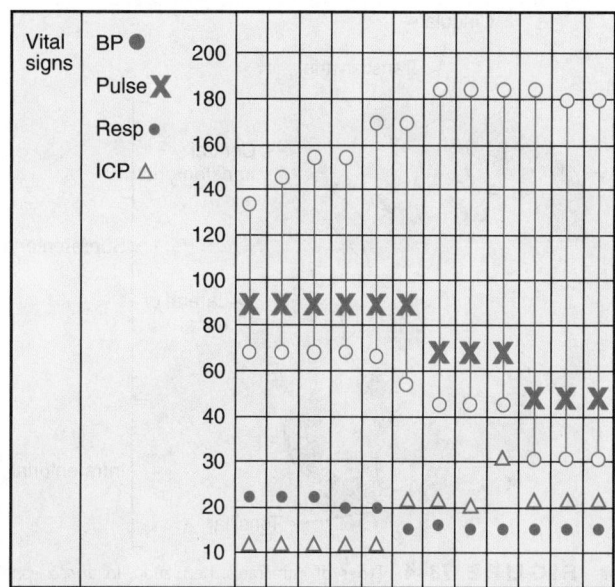

■ FIGURE 73–3 A late response to increased intracranial pressure is Cushing's triad (also called Cushing's response): bradycardia, systolic hypertension, and a wide pulse pressure, which result from pressure on the medulla. These manifestations can occur with intracranial hypertension or herniation. Alterations in the respiratory pattern also accompany Cushing's triad.

the brain stem when the pressure of the CSF in the spinal cord is lower than that in the cranium. In addition, the CSF pressure at the lumbar level is not always an accurate reflection of the intracranial CSF pressure.

Herniation Syndromes

Herniation syndromes have been classified into five types (Figure 73-4). These conditions occur late in the course of increased ICP and represent the body's last attempt to restore normal brain volume and pressure through displacement of blood, brain tissue, or CSF.

Herniation, regardless of the type, always constitutes an emergency. Notify the physician immediately of any manifestations that indicate a worsening of the client's condition as a result of increasing ICP.

Supratentorial Herniation Syndromes

Transcalvarial Herniation. Transcalvarial herniation occurs with open head injuries when brain tissue is extruded through an unstable skull fracture. Clinical manifestations vary greatly, depending on the location and extent of the open skull fracture.

Central Transtentorial Herniation. Central transtentorial herniation is the downward displacement of the diencephalon through the tentorial notch. It is caused by injuries or masses located in the cerebral tissue or on the outward perimeter of the cerebrum. An early indication of central transtentorial herniation is a rapid change in the level of consciousness. As the pressure increases,

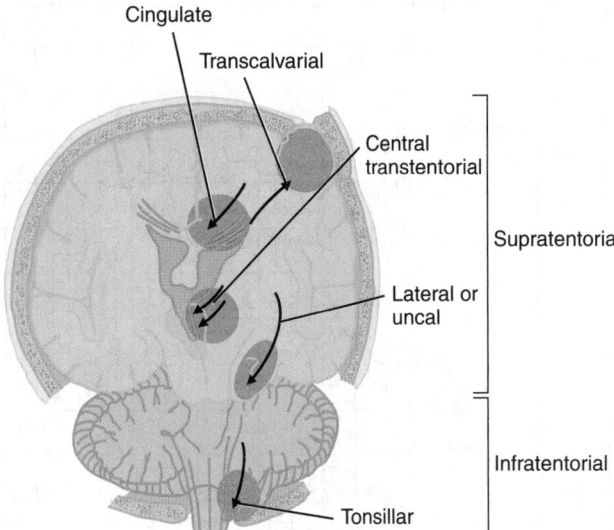

■ **FIGURE 73–4** Types of intracranial herniation. In *transcalvarial* herniation, edematous brain tissue is extruded through the skull. In *central transtentorial* herniation, the lesion is located centrally or superiorly in the cranium, and compression of central and midbrain structures may result. In *lateral* (or *uncal*) herniation, the lesion is located laterally within the cranium and can cause pressure on the midbrain. *Cingulate* herniation occurs between the two frontal lobes; the brain is pressed under the falx cerebri. In *tonsillar* herniation, the cerebellar tonsils are driven between the posterior arch of the atlas and the medulla and may be compressed.

changes in respiratory patterns are seen: first, Cheyne-Stokes respirations and then central neurogenic hyperventilation; later, apneustic breathing and also ataxic breathing (Biot's respiration); and, finally, apnea (see Chapter 68). Pupils become small but at first remain reactive, with progression to a dilated and fixed state. Pathologic reflexes begin with Babinski's sign (see Chapter 67) and then progress from abnormal flexion to abnormal extensor posturing. Doll's eye reflex and a positive response to caloric testing are noted when brain stem function is still intact but are absent if the brain stem dies (see Chapter 68). The Critical Monitoring feature on p. 1925 lists the specific areas of brain involvement that are correlated with pathologic manifestation.

Lateral Transtentorial Herniation. Lateral transtentorial herniation occurs from displacement by masses in or along the temporal lobe. It is also called *uncal herniation* because as the temporal lobe is compressed, the *uncus* (the anteromedial portion of the hippocampus) or the hippocampal gyrus shifts from the middle fossa through the tentorial notch into the posterior fossa. As the herniation progresses, the pupils first become sluggish in response to light and then become unresponsive; lack of response is seen first in the ipsilateral pupil and then in the contralateral pupil, as a result of third cranial nerve compression at the midbrain level. Other progressive clinical manifestations include a decreasing level of consciousness (stupor to coma), Cheyne-Stokes respirations

followed by central neurogenic hyperventilation, and abnormal flexor posturing that progresses to abnormal extensor posturing.

Cingulate Herniation. Cingulate herniation occurs when the frontal lobes of the cerebrum are compressed, resulting in compression of the cingulate gyrus (an arch-shaped convolution situated just above the corpus callosum) under the falx cerebri. Manifestations are related to cerebral artery compression resulting in ischemia and congestion, edema, and increasing ICP.

Infratentorial (Tonsillar) Herniation Syndrome

Tonsillar herniation, also known as *cerebellar herniation,* occurs when the cerebellar tonsil shifts through the foramen magnum, compressing the medulla and upper portion of the spinal cord. Increasing pressure in the posterior fossa, often secondary to cerebellar bleeding, is the usual underlying problem. Manifestations often progress rapidly and include erratic changes in blood pressure, pulse rate, and breathing; decreased level of consciousness; an arched, stiff neck; and quadriparesis.

OUTCOME MANAGEMENT OF HERNIATION SYNDROMES

Hyperventilation has been the standard treatment for herniation for many years. Based on the reduction in cerebral blood flow by vasoconstriction from "blowing off carbon dioxide," CPP is reduced in the brain. The tradeoff, however, is a serious reduction in arterial blood flow to the brain; therefore the routine practice of hyperventilation is questioned because the lack of arterial blood flow causes secondary brain injury. Today hyperventilation is used as a temporary measure for clients who exhibit manifestations of herniation.

Management of clients with head injury and increased intracranial pressure begins at the scene of injury and continues until the client reaches maximal function. This discussion begins in the emergent settings.

Medical Management

The goals of medical management are to maintain cerebral oxygenation, to decrease ICP, to maintain optimal neurologic function, and to ready the client for rehabilitation.

Maintain Cerebral Oxygenation

The swollen or bruised brain has an increased need for oxygen and glucose because of an increased metabolic rate. The Pao_2 must be kept between 90 and 100 mm Hg. Hypoxemia (apnea, cyanosis, oxygen saturation below 90%) is corrected immediately by opening the airway or intubating the client (cervical spine injury must be considered). Routine prophylactic hyperventilation

Manifestations of Changes in Neurologic Status

"Change" is the key word. Notify the physician whenever there is a change in the client's neurologic status. The following manifestations are listed in the order that indicates a *worsening* in the client's condition. Remember, a client may display a "transient" deterioration in neurologic responses that does not warrant calling a physician. For example, after you have just performed suctioning of the client's airway or have turned the client, you would anticipate a possible change in neurologic status. If you hyperoxygenate the client and ensure proper positioning for venous return from the jugular veins and airway maintenance, however, any manifestations of increased deficit should last only a few seconds or no more than 4 or 5 minutes. Worsening deficit that lasts longer than this increases the risk for irreversible brain injury and requires immediate attention.

NORMAL

- Alert, oriented to person, place, time
- Responds appropriately to verbal commands
- Eyes open spontaneously with any stimulus, unless in a deep sleep

ABNORMAL; CHANGES RESULTING FROM ALTERED PERFUSION OF THE CEREBRAL CORTEX

- Altered level of consciousness
- Altered perception of time, then place, and lastly person
- Motor deficits (e.g., hemiparesis, hemiplegia)
- Speech deficits (e.g., expressive or receptive speech or both)
- Memory deficits (e.g., recent, intermediate, remote)
- Hyperreflexia
- Babinski's sign
- Seizures
- Decorticate rigidity
- Emotional lability
- Altered sensory interpretation
- Cheyne-Stokes respiration
- Headache, nausea, vomiting, papilledema

ABNORMAL; CHANGES RESULTING FROM ALTERED PERFUSION JUST INFERIOR TO THE CORTEX

- Pupillary changes: asymmetry of size, shape, or time-responsiveness
- Loss of reaction to direct light
- Visual field changes (e.g., homonymous hemianopsia; see Chapter 70)

ABNORMAL; CHANGES RESULTING FROM ALTERED PERFUSION OF THE DIENCEPHALON

- Altered temperature; first high fevers, then hypothermia
- Cheyne-Stokes respiration

ABNORMAL; CHANGES RESULTING FROM ALTERED PERFUSION OF THE POSTERIOR PITUITARY GLAND

- Diabetes insipidus (decreased antidiuretic hormone)

ABNORMAL; CHANGES RESULTING FROM ALTERED PERFUSION OF THE MIDBRAIN

- Dysfunction of CN III (loss of reaction to indirect or consensual light, disconjugate eye movement)
- Dysfunction of CN IV (disconjugate eye movement)
- Central neurogenic hyperventilation

ABNORMAL; CHANGES RESULTING FROM ALTERED PERFUSION OF THE UPPER PONS

- Dysfunction of CN V (altered sensory function to cornea, nasal membranes, face, oral cavity, tongue, teeth, or altered mastication)
- Dysfunction of CN VI (altered lateral eye movement)
- Dysfunction of CN VII (altered facial expression, taste, and salivation)
- Central neurogenic hyperventilation
- Abnormal extension posture
- Pinpoint pupils

ABNORMAL; CHANGES RESULTING FROM ALTERED PERFUSION OF THE LOWER PONS

- Apneustic breathing
- Flaccidity

ABNORMAL; CHANGES RESULTING FROM ALTERED PERFUSION OF THE MEDULLA

- Dysfunction of CN VIII (altered equilibrium and hearing)
- Dysfunction of CN IX (altered taste, pharyngeal sensations, and cough and swallowing)
- Dysfunction of CN X (altered sensations in pharynx, larynx, external ear, and altered cough and swallowing; altered parasympathetic nervous system functions in thoracic and abdominal viscera)
- Dysfunction of CN XI (altered neck and shoulder movement)
- Dysfunction of CN XII (altered tongue movement)
- Projectile vomiting
- Cushing's triad (increased systolic blood pressure, wide pulse pressure, bradycardia)
- Ataxic (Biot's respiration)

CN, Cranial nerve.

---

s avoided unless the client shows evidence of cerebral herniation (see later discussion).

Steroids have been prescribed for decades to control cerebral edema, and their use was shown to improve outcomes over 30 years ago. Recent studies, however, have not shown improved client outcomes with steroids, and so their use is no longer recommended.

Decrease Intracranial Pressure

Emergency care of the client at high risk for development of increased ICP focuses on maintaining the airway, improving breathing, and promoting circulation. Hypoxemia and hypotension are often associated with poor outcomes in head injuries. Immediate interventions may include intubation followed by hyperventilation, administration of osmotic diuretics, and elevation of the head to promote venous drainage.

Cerebral Perfusion

Intravenous (IV) fluids are administered to avoid or limit hypotension and to prevent secondary brain injury. Vasoactive medication, given either to raise or to lower blood pressure, may be required to maintain CPP at a normal level. CPP is a result of the relationship between blood pressure and ICP. If the physician has not left orders to treat blood pressure changes, notification must occur if the blood pressure range is below 100 or above 150 mm Hg systolic. Several clinical studies suggest that a CPP of 70 to 80 mm Hg is the critical threshold, although some recommend maintaining CPP over 60 mm Hg. Often physician orders specify titration of medication to maintain the CPP at greater than 60 mm Hg. General reduction measures include elevating the head of the bed, preventing obstruction of the jugular veins, controlling body temperature, preventing seizures, and providing sedation and analgesia. Nurses often titrate several medications simultaneously to achieve ideal CPP.

Hyperventilation

Hyperventilation had been recommended as the primary treatment of head-injured clients because elevated carbon dioxide levels cause cerebral blood vessels to dilate. By manually hyperventilating or increasing the ventilator settings to cause hyperventilation, a hypocarbic (low carbon dioxide) blood level is created. A partial pressure of CO_2 ($Paco_2$) level between 30 and 35 mm Hg results in vasoconstriction of the cerebral blood vessels, leading to decreased blood flow and thus decreased ICP. In traumatic brain injury, however, cerebral blood flow is reduced by as much as two thirds of normal and hyperventilation can seriously compromise cerebral perfusion. Therefore routine hyperventilation is no longer recommended unless the client is manifesting herniation. If the client has extensor posturing or pupillary asymmetry or nonreactivity, the client should be hyperventilated at a rate of 20 breaths/min until blood gas analyses can provide guidelines for ventilation rates.[9]

Osmotic Diuresis

Mannitol, a hyperosmotic agent, is used to immediately expand the volume of plasma and increases cerebral blood flow and oxygen delivery. Mannitol has a delayed effect of creating an osmotic gradient that pulls fluid out of the cells, resulting in diuresis over the following hours. Mannitol may accumulate in the brain over time; so to reduce this risk, it is usually given in bolus doses rather than by continuous infusion. Renal function, levels of electrolytes, and serum osmolality need to be monitored when the client is receiving mannitol. Diuresis is

expected, and the client may become hypotensive and dehydrated with the excessive use of mannitol. Monitoring for dehydration is crucial; it is manifested by increased serum sodium and osmolality values.

Hypertonic Saline. Hypertonic saline is any saline solution that is at a concentration higher than 0.9%. Common concentrations are 3%, 5%, 7%, and 23% sodium chloride. Hypertonic saline causes osmotic diuresis because its concentration is higher than that of tissue. Administration of hypertonic saline leads to an increase in plasma osmolarity and establishes an osmotic gradient that moves excess water from the cerebral tissue into the vasculature. By decreasing the water content of brain tissue, hypertonic saline can decrease mass effect and decrease ICP.

Prevent Complications

Many complications are associated with head injury (Box 73-1). Antibiotics may be prescribed, especially with an open head injury, the placement of an ICP monitor, or an infection in another body system. Infections increase metabolism and thus raise ICP.

Antiseizure medications (e.g., phenytoin, carbamazepine) may be given prophylactically to reduce the risk of seizures. Seizures significantly increase metabolic requirements and cerebral blood flow and volume and thus increase ICP. Chapter 69 describes the care of the client with seizures.

Intravenous fluids are given by IV infusion pump to help monitor the amount of fluids given. The client is maintained in a state of euvolemia. Hypotonic IV solutions are avoided because of the risk of promoting cerebral edema.

Temperature reduction decreases metabolism and cerebral blood flow and thus ICP. Antipyretics should be the first intervention to reset the hypothalamic thermostat. Other cooling measures include hypothermic blankets, bathing with tepid water, or placement of ice packs. Muscle relaxants are given to prevent shivering.

BOX 73-1   Complications of Head Injury

- Cerebral edema
- Stress ulcers
- Seizures
- Infections
- Acute hydrocephalus
- Diabetes insipidus
- Syndrome of inappropriate secretion of antidiuretic hormone
- Cardiac dysrhythmias
- Neurogenic pulmonary edema
- Subarachnoid hemorrhage/aneurysms
- Altered behavior
- Post-trauma response

Malnutrition, with wasting of lean muscle mass, can develop quickly because of the metabolic response to severe head injury. Hypoglycemia must be avoided; glucose is the primary fuel for the brain. Hypoglycemia should be avoided by close monitoring. Furthermore, severe hypoglycemia can also result in seizures and coma. Nutritional support is provided with jejunal feeding to reduce the risk of gastric regurgitation and aspiration. Recommended calorie intake is 140% of resting metabolic expenditures in nonparalyzed clients and 100% of resting metabolic expenditures in paralyzed clients with 15% of caloric intake as protein. Nutritional support should begin no later than the seventh day after injury.

Monitor Intracranial Pressure

Continuous ICP monitoring is used for clients experiencing conditions associated with potentially elevated ICP (e.g., head trauma with GCS scores of 8 and lower), preoperative and postoperative aneurysms, tumors, and posterior fossa lesions. ICP monitoring aids in earlier detection of intracranial mass lesions; it can limit the use of indiscriminate therapies to control ICP, which themselves can be harmful; it can reduce ICP by draining CSF and thus improve cerebral perfusion; it helps to determine prognosis; and it may improve outcomes.

Several methods of ICP monitoring are available. The most common types measure CSF pressure in the ventricles, brain parenchyma, or subarachnoid space. Intraventricular catheters provide the most accurate results. All monitoring devices are invasive and carry a risk of infection/colonization, hemorrhage, and obstruction, especially when the device is left in place for over 5 days.[9] Most surgeons prescribe antibiotics, limit the length of time for which the ICP monitor remains in place, and monitor CSF samples on a regular basis. The Bridge to Critical Care feature on Intracranial Pressure Monitoring below describes the nurse's role in caring for clients with these devices.

Monitoring ICP also allows the measurement of intracranial compliance. Introducing a known volume of fluid

BRIDGE TO CRITICAL CARE

Intracranial Pressure Monitoring

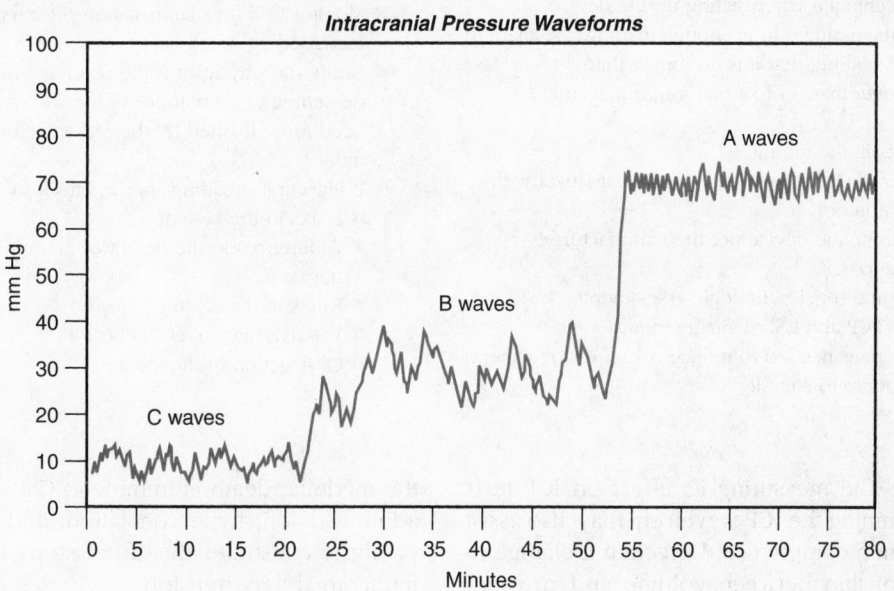

The shape of the waves is influenced by cardiac pulsations and respirations as well as by intracranial pressure (ICP).

C waves occur 4 to 8 times per minute and reflect fluctuations in arterial pressure. C waves are not considered significant.

B waves occur at intervals of 30 seconds to 2 minutes and represent increases in ICP to 50 mm Hg. They may be precursors to A waves and may indicate a decrease in compliance.

A waves are most pronounced when the amount of cranial contents is increased. Also called *plateau waves,* A waves represent recurrent ICP elevations to 100 mm Hg. An A wave may be caused by coughing or straining but, if recurrent or sustained, may indicate a reduced ability of the brain to compensate. The client may also show other manifestations of increasing ICP.

(Continued)

BRIDGE TO CRITICAL CARE

Intracranial Pressure Monitoring—Cont'd

To monitor   To monitor

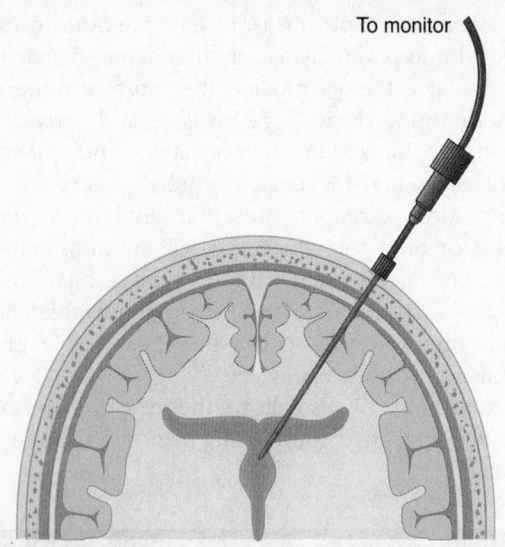

Ventricular catheter (ventriculostomy)

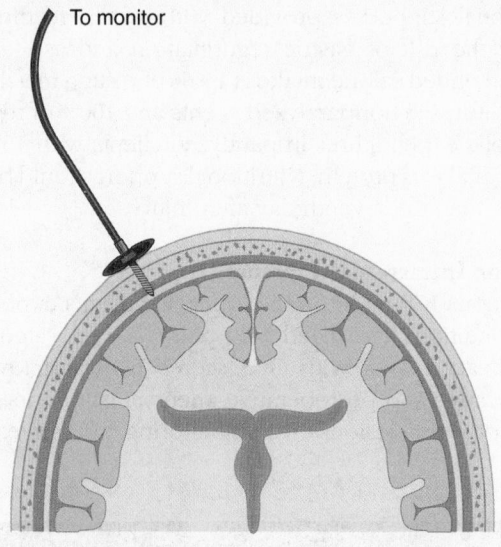

Subarachnoid screw (bolt) (ventriculostomy)

GENERAL INTERVENTIONS FOR MONITORING INTRACRANIAL PRESSURE AND VENTRICULOSTOMY DEVICES

- Use sterile technique when setting up the device.
- Ensure that the tubing is long enough to allow the client to be moved in bed but that it is no longer than 14 feet. Use of tubing longer than 14 feet may cause inaccurate readings.
- Prevent kinks in the tubing.
- Level the transducer at the tragus of the ear (level with foramen of Monroe).
- Zero or calibrate the device per the manufacturer's recommendations.
- Do baseline and serial neurologic assessments.
- Analyze ICP/PCP and CSF drainage trends.
- Medicate client as needed to reduce risk of dislodgement.
- Monitor response to stimuli.

- If head of bed is lowered, turn drainage device off to avoid draining the ventricles.
- Monitor insertion site for bleeding, drainage, CSF leakage.
- Monitor CSF for manifestations of infection (cloudy, increased volume).
- Notify the physician if the readings show damping (lessening of amplitude) of the waves. The catheter may need to be flushed by the physician or advanced practice nurse.
- If inaccurate readings occur, check for the following:
  - Leaks in the system
  - Differences in the height of the transducer and the device
  - Kinks in the tubing
  - Valsalva maneuver in client
  - Obstruction in the system

into the ventricle and measuring its effect on ICP tests compliance. Examining the ICP waveform may also assist in determining brain compliance. Detecting a change in the critical relationship between volume and pressure allows early treatment before the onset of clinical manifestations or sustained elevated ICP. Measurements of CPP can be made with ICP monitors. Ideally, CPP should be maintained at greater than 60 mm Hg.

Prevent Intracranial Hypertension

Intracranial hypertension is defined as an ICP greater than 20 to 25 mm Hg and can lead to a fatal herniation of the brain. When the herniation occurs at the level of

the medulla, death is imminent. CSF drainage, mannito administration, hyperventilation, and sedation/chemica paralysis constitute the usual steps in management o intracranial hypertension.

Sedation/Paralysis. Some clients have refractory intracra nial pressures and require very advanced methods to reduce cerebral metabolism. Methods can include seda tion and paralysis.

Barbiturates. High-dose barbiturates (pentobarbit or thiopental) induce coma, lower ICP, and decreas mortality in clients with uncontrollable ICP that refractory to all other medical and surgical treatments. These agents, however, can lead to hypotension, and their use is limited to clients with severe traumatic brain injury. Prophylactic use of barbiturates is not warranted. Barbiturate therapy requires sophisticated monitoring and special training. The client is intubated and placed on ventilatory support, and a pulmonary artery catheter is inserted. Additional monitoring modalities include jugular venous oxygenation ($Sjvo_2$) and brain tissue oxygenation (tbO_2).

Monitor serum drug levels daily; the dose should be reduced if serum levels exceed 5 mg/dl or if the burst suppression pattern on the EEG lasts longer than 10 seconds. Monitor temperature because barbiturates reduce metabolism, thereby cooling the body. If the temperature falls below 36° C, active warming is indicated. Propofol has been used instead of barbiturates to provide similar management of increased ICP but may not be as beneficial as barbiturates. The advantage of propofol is that it is short-acting, allowing for daily assessment of neurologic status. Similar monitoring of the EEG occurs as does care of the client.

Continue pupillary assessment. Even when a client is in a coma, the pupils dilate if the brain stem becomes compressed. Notify the physician of this change. Barbiturate therapy eliminates the client's normal protective functions. The client is completely dependent on nursing care for all basic needs (see Chapter 68). Wean clients slowly from barbiturate therapy/propofol to prevent rebound intracranial hypertension.

Neuromuscular Blocking Agents. Nondepolarizing neuromuscular blocking agents are sometimes used to induce skeletal muscle relaxation and to promote synchronous breathing during mechanical ventilation. Decreasing muscle activity may be necessary to control ICP. Nurses use a peripheral nerve stimulator to monitor for adequacy of drug dosage as well as for the risk of overdose (see Chapter 63). Pentobarbital and neuromuscular blocking agents usually are not given concomitantly. If the client is receiving a neuromuscular blocking agent, sedation and analgesia must be given because the neuromuscular blocking agents do not provide it. Other complications may result and are described in Box 73-1.

Nursing Management

Assessment. The Glasgow Coma Scale (GCS) is the most commonly used neurologic assessment tool in clinical care (Box 73-2). This scale provides objective measurement of three essential components of the neurologic examination: spontaneity of eye opening, best verbal response, and best motor response. The total score can range from 3 to 15. The client who is unresponsive

to painful stimuli, does not open the eyes, and has complete muscular flaccidity has a score of 3. The client who is oriented, opens the eyes spontaneously, and follows commands scores 15. A score of 8 or less indicates coma. Because the scoring of the GCS is based on the client's ability to respond and to communicate, the following criteria may render the GCS invalid:

- The client is intubated and cannot speak.
- Eyes are swollen closed.
- The client is unable to communicate in English.
- The client has a hearing loss.
- The client is blind.
- The client is aphasic.
- The client is paralyzed or hemiplegic.

The first GCS score recorded for the client becomes the baseline score. Subsequent scores allow assessment of trends or changes in neurologic status and provide a significant and reliable indicator of the severity of head injury. A single measurement cannot predict outcome; however, a decrease of 2 points in the GCS with a score of 9 or lower indicates serious injury. The use of consistent criteria for client assessment is more important than the specific tool used. Specific behaviors dictating a given score should be indicated. If variations occur in scoring criteria, the value of the scale is lost, and serious changes in the client's condition can be overlooked or treated unnecessarily (see the neurologic observation chart on the website). While the Glasgow Coma Scale is quick and easily repeated, more detailed neurologic assessments are conducted to identify specific trends in responses.

Level of Consciousness

The first change in a client who presents with altered cerebral tissue perfusion is a change in the level of consciousness (LOC). When decreased LOC is noted, serial and detailed assessments are required until the client has achieved maximum recovery. To eliminate the subjectivity associated with use of terms such as *lethargy, obtundation, semi-coma,* or *coma,* the GCS both objictifies the client's LOC and assists in identifying very subtle changes (see Box 73-2).

SAFETY

⚠

ALERT

Pupil Response. A pupil check includes assessing pupil appearance and physiologic response. The affected pupil is usually on the same (*ipsilateral*) side as the brain lesion, whereas the motor and sensory deficits are usually on the opposite (*contralateral*) side. Be careful not to mistake a prosthetic eye for a fixed pupil.

Pupil Equality. Document pupil equality, noting the relative size of each pupil.

BOX 73-2 Assessment of Clients Using the Glasgow Coma Scale

The Glasgow Coma Scale (GCS) is a numeric expression of cognition, behavior, and neurologic function. It is the most commonly used scale and was designed to measure level of consciousness and severity of injury through eye opening, verbal responsiveness, and motor response. The total of the three scores ranges from 3 to 15, with 3 being the most severe and 15 being normal. Assessments of abstract thought and problem solving should be combined with the GCS to give a more complete picture of neurologic status.

Documentation should contain specific descriptive terms. For example, instead of just indicating that the client is "stuporous," record the evidence of stupor that you observe: "no response to verbal commands, responded only to tracheal suctioning with abnormal flexor posturing." Words such as "lethargic," "stuporous," or "comatose" are open to individual interpretation, and a clear description of behavior is less likely to be misunderstood.

SCALE COMPONENTS

Eye Opening

Observe eye opening without speaking to the client. Does the client open the eyes and look around? If the eyes are closed, call the client's name. If no response is noted, raise your voice. If there is still no response, use a mildly painful stimulus, given in the central part of the body, such as squeezing the trapezius muscle or rubbing the sternum.

Avoid supraorbital pressure, as it can cause damage to the eyes. Pinching of the body can cause severe bruising and is unnecessary in a neurologic examination.

Motor Response

Asking the client to follow specific commands such as "Raise your right arm" or "Wiggle your toes" assesses motor responses. Do not ask the client to squeeze your hand, because grasp is a reflexive response that can occur with head injury. If agency protocol lists grasp as a neurologic assessment component, ask the client to "let go" after grasping to measure cognitive ability to control movement.

In a client who is unable to follow commands, observe the response to a painful stimulus. Responses may include (1) localizing (trying to remove the stimulus), (2) withdrawing, and (3) posturing. In addition, a response may not be elicited and the client may remain motionless.

Compare the right and left sides and the upper and lower extremities. Record the best response while also recording any abnormality that indicates decreased movement in a particular extremity.

Motor Activity

Motor activity assessment is the measure of strength of voluntary movement of the arms and legs. If a client cannot cooperate with testing, paralysis may be difficult to detect. Observe the client carefully. If a client is restless, paralysis may become obvious because the paralyzed part does not move as other body parts move. Additional information may be obtained in the following ways:

1. Comparing the tone of one side of the body with that of the other
2. Lifting the arms or legs on both sides, releasing them, and watching them drop to the bed
3. Observing the position of the limbs at rest

If a client can cooperate, assessing "drift" may demonstrate subtle tone and strength alterations. For this assessment, have the client hold both arms up in front of the body with the palms upward and the eyes closed. This position should be maintained for 10 seconds. Muscles are weak if one arm "drifts" (gradually moves) downward or if the hand pronates (turns over). This maneuver is often referred to as the *pronator drift test*. Drift can also be assessed in the lower extremities by having the patient raise one leg off the bed and hold it for five seconds with eyes closed. If the leg cannot be held up, it is weak and therefore has a drift.

Posturing

Review posturing in Chapter 68. As the client's intracranial pressure increases at the cortical level, abnormal flexor posturing occurs. As pressure reaches the pons level, abnormal extensor posturing occurs. When the pressure reaches further to the medullary level, flaccidity is noted, or a response is totally lacking—the gravest of all signs.

Verbal Response

Verbal responses assess the client's orientation to self, environment, and time. Ask appropriate questions such as the following: "What is your name? Where are you? What is the month, year, season, nearest holiday?" Avoid asking questions about the date or day of the week.

Being hospitalized can alter the accuracy of that response even in a person with normal cognitive function. Structure the conversation to elicit information that can be verified by family members, such as home address or employer's name. In many cases, a slight degree of confusion is not noticeable until some time is spent with the client. An apparently oriented client may ask the same question a few minutes after it was originally asked and answered, or the client may have "learned" the answers to common questions such as "What is your name?" and "What hospital are you in?" Therefore it is helpful to reassess the client regularly to check memory or to challenge cognitive integrity with various questions. If addition, observing the patient during the course of a normal conversation may provide evidence of confusion or disorientation.

SCORING

After obtaining the data for all three parts of the GCS, total the points for each part and compare the score obtained with the client's baseline score. If a decrease in the score of even 1 point occurs, complete a detailed neurologic assessment, including pupillary responses, cranial nerves, and motor/sensory examinations and notify the physician.

Pupil Size. Estimate the size of each pupil in millimeters (mm) before and after light stimulation. A penlight provides more accurate data than obtainable with a flashlight because of the smaller size of the light and the ability to focus the beam directly at the pupil.

Pupil Position. Note whether the pupil is positioned in the midline or deviated from midline.

Pupil Reaction to Light. Bring the penlight from the lateral aspect of the client's head toward the eye. Observe for constriction in that eye as well as in the opposite eye. Then test the opposite eye in the same way. The detection of subtle change may require four approaches with the penlight. Brisk and equal constriction of the pupils to direct and indirect light is a normal response. Sluggish or unequal direct or indirect *(consensual)* response is abnormal. *Anisocoria,* or unequal pupils, occurs normally in about 17% of the population, with one pupil being about 1 mm larger. It is important to ascertain information about pupil inequality from the client or family members so that an unnecessary procedure is not performed.

Pupil Shape. Normally, pupils are round. Describe abnormal shapes with a drawing. Pupils may be oddly shaped as a result of previous eye surgery. A pupil that looks oval may be early evidence of increasing ICP.

Pupil Accommodation. Normally, the size of the pupil and the lens (which is not visible to the naked eye) accommodates (adjusts) to varying focal lengths. Having the conscious client focus on a distant object and then quickly focus on a close object tests accommodation. Pupils should become smaller as the object is brought nearer the eye and should dilate when the object is moved away from the eye. Accommodation is often not tested in the acute care setting because of the client's inability to cooperate.

The acronym PERRLA is often used in practice and indicates that the *p*upils are *e*qual, *r*ound, and *r*eactive to *l*ight and *a*ccommodation. Notify the physician immediately if any change occurs in the pupillary response.

Eye Movement. Document any changes in eye movement. Observe the position of the eyes when assessing the pupils. The eyes should move together. If *disconjugate* (not together) movement is noted, the physician should be notified.

Vital Signs. Initially vital signs should be assessed continuously and recorded every 15 minutes until they are stable. Body temperature should be monitored every 2 hours. If hypothermia or hyperthermia occurs,

temperature should be monitored continuously; axillary thermometers or thermometers within urinary catheters are commonly used. Trends in vital signs and respiratory patterns should be analyzed. As ICP increases and herniation occurs at the level of the medulla, Cushing's response occurs (see Figure 73-3).

Vital sign changes are *late* changes. See the following discussion of altered cerebral tissue perfusion for care of a client with increasing ICP. Once the vital signs begin to deteriorate, many other changes have already occurred, such as a decrease in LOC. Ongoing monitoring for such changes is imperative; do not wait for vital signs to change because the delay may prove fatal for the client. Any changes in neurologic status may be significant and must be reported to the physician, no matter how minor they may seem.

Other assessments can also be made of the cranial nerves. Extraocular movements are tested on clients who are awake enough to follow directions. Ask the clients to follow your fingers with their eyes without moving the head. Move your fingers in a figure H, and observe both eyes as they move across, up, and down. Conjugate eye movements occur when both eyes move in a parallel motion. Disconjugate eye movements occur when the eyes do not move in a lateral direction together (one eye may move laterally while the other is fixed or moves in another direction). Tracking occurs when the client is consciously following someone's or something's movement around the room.

The *blink reflex* can be tested by lightly stroking the eyelashes. When the eyelids are closed, they will flutter slightly if the reflex is present. Observe for blinking in the conscious and alert client. The *gag reflex* is tested by asking the alert client to cough or swallow. If the client is unable or unconscious, stroke the back of the client's throat with a long cotton-tipped swab. The gag reflex should be swift; do not continue to test gagging once it is present because it will provoke vomiting.

Note the symmetry of the facial muscles. Note the ability of the eyelids to open spontaneously and equally. Ask the client to close the eyes as tightly as possible. Ask the client to smile, and note the corners of the mouth to identify symmetrical patterns. Ask the client to frown/wrinkle the forehead. Finally, note whether speech is clear, slurred, rambling, or aphasic.

Diagnosis, Outcomes, Interventions
Diagnosis: Ineffective Cerebral Tissue Perfusion. If the client is in a coma because of increased ICP, use this diagnosis to reflect the risk to cerebral tissue perfusion. Write the diagnosis as *Ineffective Tissue Perfusion: Cerebral related to increased ICP.* The term *patient* is used to refer to a person in a coma. The *client* in this case is the patient's family, who serves as his or her advocate.

Outcomes. The patient will maintain normal cerebral perfusion as evidenced by (1) stable or improving levels of consciousness; (2) stable or improving GCS score; (3) ICP of 15 mm Hg or less; (4) no restlessness, irritability, or headache; and (5) no pupillary changes, no seizures, no widening pulse pressure, no respiratory irregularity, and no hypertension or bradycardia.

Interventions. Administer the medications ordered to reduce cerebral edema (e.g., osmotic diuretics) and to decrease the risk of seizure (e.g., anticonvulsants), and monitor the patient's response to these medications. If the patient's baseline manifestations of increased ICP are not improving, if the patient's status deteriorates, or if seizures develop, notify the physician. Also, consult the physician for medication to promote bowel evacuation without straining because straining increases ICP. Disimpaction is not advised because of the vasovagal response that occurs.

Position the Patient. Place the patient supine with the head elevated 30 degrees unless contraindicated (e.g., with some spinal injuries, some aneurysms). Keep the patient's head in a neutral position to facilitate venous drainage from the brain. Avoid extreme rotation and flexion of the neck because these positions compress the jugular veins and increase ICP. Also avoid extreme hip flexion because this position increases intra-abdominal and intrathoracic pressures, which increase ICP. As the coma lightens, the patient may become disoriented and combative, making it difficult to maintain proper positioning. If restraints must be used, remember that they often increase agitation, which increases ICP.

If the patient's condition indicates that it will be considerable time before the neurologic condition will improve, consider placing the patient on a pressure-redistribution surface if turning from side to side cannot occur.

Maintain a Patent Airway. Patients need to maintain a patent airway even in the presence of increased ICP. Suctioning prevents the buildup of secretions, which results in elevations of CO_2 levels that lead to an increase of ICP. Adequately oxygenate intubated patients before initiating suctioning, between suctioning efforts, and after suctioning. Try to limit suctioning to three passes, and limit each pass to 10 seconds. Nasal drainage may indicate a dural tear; therefore suctioning of the nares is contraindicated because of the risk of injury to the dura and meningitis.

Balance Fluid Levels. In the past, only small amounts of fluids were administered to clients with head injury, in an effort to decrease cerebral edema. Current data indicate that fluid restriction may actually reduce blood volume and decrease cerebral circulation. The lack of volume causes the blood to be thick and sluggish and may decrease the mobilization of nutrition and toxins into and out of the circulation. Patients should be maintained in a euvolemic state rather than a fluid-restricted state. Fluid restriction may be appropriate for certain conditions (such as syndrome of inappropriate secretion of antidiuretic hormone [SIADH]) but otherwise is contraindicated. Strict intake and output measurement every 1 to 4 hours is necessary to assess fluid balance.

Control Body Temperature. Hyperthermia increases ICP because it increases metabolic demand. Therefore notify the physician immediately if hyperthermia occurs. If a patient's temperature is being managed with a hypothermia blanket, notify the physician if the patient's response is not within the prescribed parameters. Administer any ordered antipyretics. Observe for shivering because this phenomenon also increases metabolism and ICP. Assess for skin breakdown if cooling blankets are used for extended periods, especially in patients who are thin.

Monitor Intracranial Pressure. The ICP reading should be less than 15 mm Hg, the MAP reading 80 mm Hg or higher, and the CPP reading greater than 60 mm Hg.

Plateau waves (A waves) are noted when ICP is greater than 50 mm Hg and can be sustained for longer than 5 minutes. Whenever these sustained pressures are present, assess for contributing factors and intervene appropriately. For example, neck flexion, excessive hip flexion, airway secretions, excess water in the ventilator tubing, taping the endotracheal tube tightly over the jugular veins, and discussing the patient's condition at the bedside have all been known to increase ICP. Plan and space nursing interventions (e.g., turning the patient) for when the patient's ICP is not elevated to help prevent plateau waves. Plateau waves may not be obvious on the ICP monitor screen; a printout generated at a slow rate may be required for accurate observation of these waves. Whenever ICP is greater than 20 mm Hg, interventions to decrease ICP should begin. Use caution when adjusting the patient's position when intracranial monitoring systems are in use. If the system is open to the patient, changing position will quickly alter ventricular fluid levels.

Always close the stopcock on intracranial monitors before moving the patient or lowering the head of the bed.

Assessing the ICP monitor site for infection and leakage, using sterile technique for dressing and drainage bag changes, and maintaining a closed system are helpful in preventing infection or in promoting early intervention if infection occurs. If CSF drainage is required, most systems have a stopcock for attaching the tubing and drainage bag that maintains the closed system, decreasing the likelihood of infection. The system is opened only to change the drainage bag. The drainage bag is changed using strict sterile technique.

Evaluation. Evaluate the client's response to treatment as often as every 15 minutes, progressing to hourly, then every 2 to 4 hours, and every 8 hours as the client improves. Once the physician has determined that the client's clinical condition has been optimized, the frequency and extent of evaluation can diminish even further. In the immediate and acute stages, anticipate ongoing modification in the care plan to help the client reach maximum recovery.

Surgical Management

Various surgical techniques are used to treat increased ICP. Optimally, the cause of increased ICP is located and removed. Decompressive surgery removes some brain tissue (e.g., part of the temporal lobe) or a large portion of the skull to give the remaining structures room to expand. If brain compliance is low during surgery, the bone flap removed to gain access to the brain is not replaced, or the dura may not be closed. Subsequent surgery is then required to repair the defect. Postoperative care is the same as that required after craniotomy (see Chapter 69). If the bone flap remains unattached, special care is required to keep the patient off the side of the defect and a helmet may be required until the bone flap is replaced. Surgical placement of a ventriculoperitoneal shunt to allow drainage if CSF circulation is blocked can be done for chronic problems (Figure 73-5).

TRAUMATIC BRAIN INJURY

Traumatic brain injury is an insult to the brain that is capable of producing physical, intellectual, emotional, social, and vocational changes. In the United States, a head injury is experienced approximately every 15 seconds. Head injuries occur in about 7 million Americans every year. Among these head-injured people, more than 500,000 are hospitalized, 100,000 experience chronic disability, and about 2000 are left in a persistent vegetative state.

In more than 30% of cases, because of the seriousness of the injury, head injuries are fatal before the injured person arrives at the hospital. An additional 20% die later because of secondary brain injury. Secondary brain events include ischemia from hypoxia and hypotension, secondary hemorrhage, and cerebral edema.

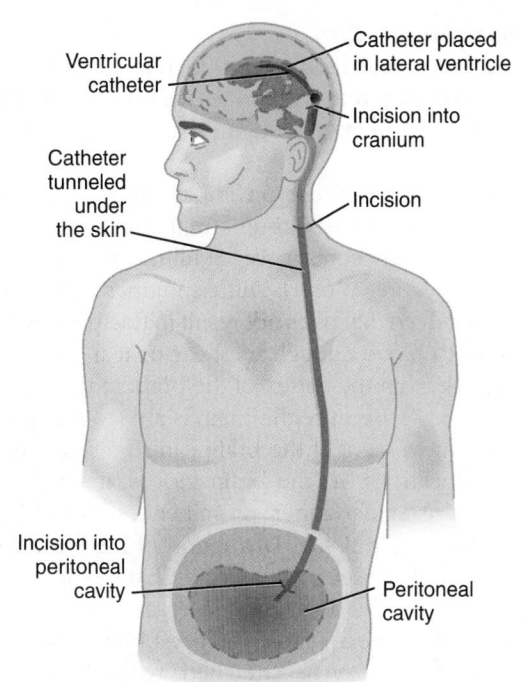

■ **FIGURE 73-5** Ventriculoperitoneal shunt placed for chronic hydrocephalus.

Clients with traumatic head injuries often have other major injuries, including injury to the facial structures, lungs, heart, cervical spine, abdomen, and bones. Facial fractures and lung injuries may contribute to respiratory insufficiency. Airway obstruction and decreased ability to breathe (e.g., from pulmonary contusion, flail chest, pneumothorax) contribute to respiratory insufficiency and poor oxygenation of the brain and other tissues. Ischemia of brain tissue may result.

Hemorrhagic shock in clients with multiple trauma is rarely caused by head injury alone. Frequently shock is due to ruptured abdominal organs or musculoskeletal injuries (e.g., fractured femur and pelvis). Circulation may be further compromised by cardiac contusion and associated dysrhythmias.

Etiology and Risk Factors

Motor-vehicle accidents are the leading cause of head injuries. Of clients admitted to the emergency department, most are males younger than 30 years and 50% have evidence of ingestion of alcohol or other substances of abuse. Alcohol slows the reflexes and alters cognitive processes and perception. These physiologic changes increase the chances of being involved in an accident or altercation. A second risk factor is driving without seat belts. Peak occurrence is during evenings, nights, and weekends. Other causes are assaults, falls, and sports-related injuries.

Mechanisms of Injury

Head injuries are caused by a sudden impact force to the head or inertial forces within the skull (Figure 73-6). The results are complex. Three mechanisms contribute to head trauma.

Primary injuries occur on impact and are the direct result of the impact resulting in injury to the area of the brain beneath the contact site. Skull fractures commonly occur (see Figure 73-6, A). Diffuse injuries occur when a blow is received that does not result in fracture but causes the brain to move enough to shear or tear some of the veins going from the cortex of the brain to the skull (see Figure 73-6, B). Because the brain is able to move within the skull, movement of the brain can result in injuries at different locations. As the brain moves, it scrapes over the skull's irregular inner prominences, which bruise and lacerate brain tissue. Disruption of the brain's small surface blood vessels may occur. Changes in capillary integrity lead to fluid shifts and petechial hemorrhages. Cranial nerves, nerve tracts, larger blood vessels, and other structures may be stretched, twisted, or rotated, and their functions disrupted. An example is an automobile accident in which the head hits the steering wheel.

Coup-Contrecoup Injuries.

A unique term can be used for this complex head injury: *coup-contrecoup injury*. From the French word *coup,* which means "blow," this diagnosis indicates that the client has sustained a combined injury at the point of impact and an injury on the side of the brain opposite from the movement of the brain within the skull. That is, a contrecoup injury (see Figure 73-6, *C*) from the French for "counterblow." Figure 73-7, *A* depicts a contrecoup injury as shown in an MRI scan.

Penetrating Trauma.

Penetrating injuries are a form of primary injury and include head wounds made by foreign bodies (e.g., knives or bullets) or those made by bone fragments from a skull fracture. The damage caused by a penetrating injury often relates to the velocity with which a penetrating object pierces the skull and brain. Bone fragments from a skull fracture may cause local brain injury by lacerating brain tissue and damaging other structures (e.g., nerves, blood vessels). If a major blood vessel is severed or ruptured, a large clot *(hematoma)* may form, with resultant damage to adjacent or remote structures (e.g., brain compression as in a herniation syndrome). Thus a hematoma itself can cause extensive brain tissue damage.

High-velocity objects (e.g., bullets) produce shock waves in the skull and brain. The shock waves may significantly damage brain structures beyond those in the object's path. Frequently penetrating wounds create an open communication between the external environment and the cranial cavity, and infection is thus a possible complication.[8]

Scalp Injuries.

Scalp injuries can cause lacerations, hematomas, and contusions or abrasions to the skin. These

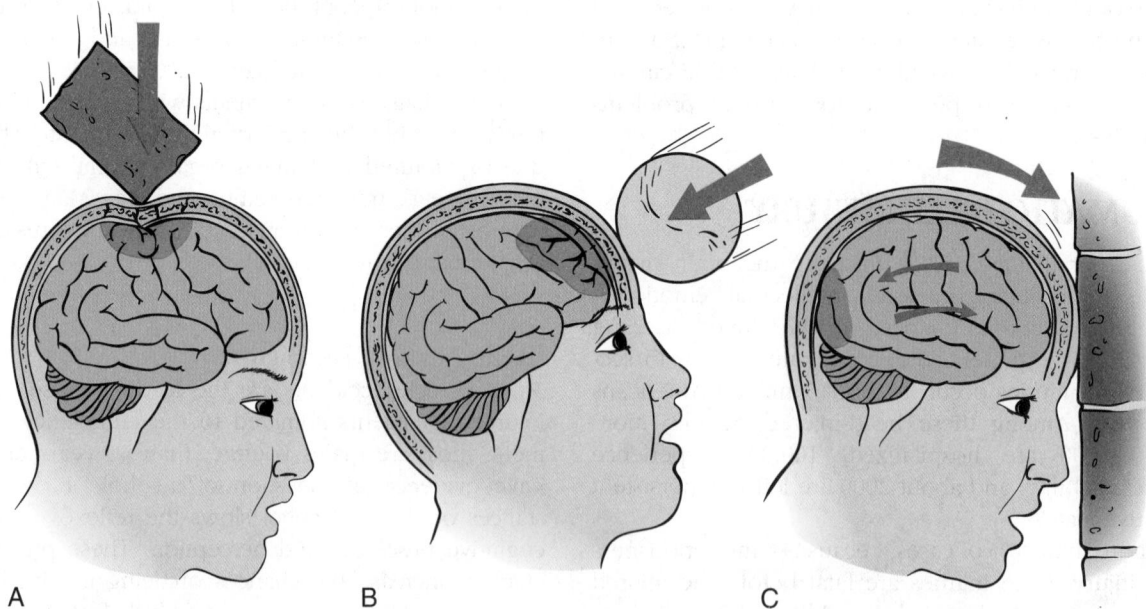

A   B   C

■ **FIGURE 73–6** Some mechanisms of head injury. **A,** Penetrating injury may fracture the skull. **B,** Diffuse injuries such as a blow to the skull do not result in fracture; they may cause the brain to move enough to tear some of the veins traversing from the cortical surface to the dura. Subdural hematoma may then develop. Note the areas of cerebral contusion (dark brown). **C,** Rebound of the cranial contents may result in an area of injury opposite the point of impact. Such an injury is called a *contrecoup* injury. In addition to the direct damage sustained in the three injuries depicted, additional brain damage may occur.

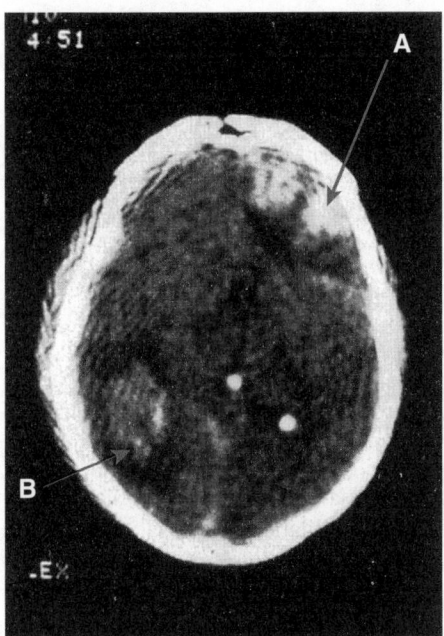

■ **FIGURE 73–7** A magnetic resonance imaging scan showing coup (A) contrecoup (B) injury after head injury.

injuries may be unsightly and may bleed profusely. Clients with minor scalp injuries not accompanied by damage to other areas do not require hospitalization. The care of these injuries is discussed in Chapter 82.

Skull Fractures. Skull fractures are often caused by a force sufficient to fracture the skull and cause brain injury. The fractures themselves do not signal that brain injury is also present; however, skull fractures often cause serious brain damage. Depressed skull fractures injure the brain by bruising it (resulting in a contusion) or by driving bone fragments into it (causing lacerations). The site of a fracture and the extent of brain injury may not correlate.

The three types of skull fractures are as follows:

- *Linear skull fractures* appear as thin lines on x-ray and do not require treatment; they are important only if there is significant underlying brain damage.
- *Depressed skull fractures* may be palpated and are seen on x-ray.
- *Basilar skull fractures* occur in bones over the base of the frontal and temporal lobes. These are not observable on plain x-ray but may be manifested as ecchymosis around the eyes or behind the ears or by blood or CSF leakage from the ear.

Brain Injuries

A single classification of brain injuries does not exist; however, the terms *open, closed, contusion,* and *concussion* are often applied to brain injuries. Open head injuries are those that penetrate the skull. Closed injuries are from blunt trauma.

Concussions. A *concussion* is head trauma that may result in loss of consciousness for 5 minutes or less and retrograde amnesia. There is no break in the skull or dura, and no damage is visible on CT or MRI scans.

Contusions. Contusions are associated with more extensive damage than that from concussions. With contusions the brain itself is damaged, often with multiple areas of small hemorrhage and bruised areas in brain tissue. Diffuse axonal injury resulting in anatomic disruption of the white matter may result from serious contusions. Microscopic nerve fiber lesions also occur. Abnormalities may be located primarily in one area of the brain, but other areas may also be injured. This is particularly true of brain stem contusions, which are a very serious type of lesion.

Diffuse Axonal Injury. Diffuse axonal injury is the most severe form of head injury because there is no focal lesion to remove. The injury involves the tissue of the entire brain and occurs at the microscopic level. Diffuse axonal injury is classified as mild, moderate, or severe. With *mild diffuse axonal injury,* loss of consciousness lasting 6 to 24 hours is characteristic, and short-term disability may be associated with it. With *moderate diffuse axonal injury,* coma lasting less than 24 hours is the predominant clinical feature, with incomplete recovery on awakening. *Severe diffuse axonal injury* also involves primary injury to the brain stem. The patient may present with abnormal posturing and in coma, but there may not be evidence of cerebral edema or increased ICP. Diffuse axonal injury begins with immediate loss of consciousness, prolonged coma, abnormal flexion or extensor posturing, hypertension, and fever.

Focal Injuries

Epidural Hematoma. An epidural hematoma, also called an *extradural hematoma,* forms between the skull and the dura mater (Figure 73–8). It occurs in about 10% of severe head injuries and is usually associated with a skull fracture. An epidural hematoma occurs from injury to the cerebral blood vessels, most often the middle meningeal artery. Bleeding is usually continuous, and a large clot forms, which separates the dura from the skull.

Manifestations are usually acute in onset because the bleeding is often arterial. With an epidural hematoma, the following sequence of events may occur:

1. The client is unconscious immediately after head trauma.
2. The client awakens and is quite lucid.
3. Loss of consciousness occurs and pupil dilation response rapidly deteriorates, with onset of eye movement paralysis, on the same side as that of the hematoma.
4. The client lapses into a coma.

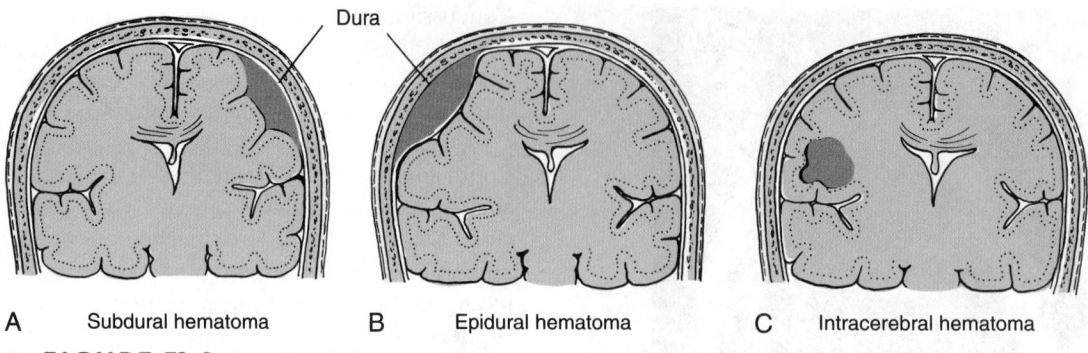

A   Subdural hematoma   B   Epidural hematoma   C   Intracerebral hematoma

■ **FIGURE 73–8** Formation of a hematoma after head injury. Note the shift of the brain structures.

Although these manifestations are often described as "classic" for an epidural hematoma, few clients present with such classic manifestations and astute assessment is necessary to prevent death.

Computed tomography scanning confirms the diagnosis. Rapid diagnosis and prompt intervention are essential with an epidural hematoma. Careful, ongoing assessment of neurologic status is also necessary.

Subdural Hematoma. Subdural hematoma is a collection of blood in the subdural space (i.e., between the dura mater and arachnoid mater). Tearing of the bridging veins over the brain causes most subdural hematomas.

Subdural hematomas may be classified as acute, subacute, or chronic, depending on how rapidly clinical manifestations develop. Another classification system recognizes only acute and chronic, combining the acute and subacute categories.

Acute and Subacute Subdural Hematoma. Acute subdural hematoma usually results from brain or blood vessel laceration. Acute subdural hematomas are a serious complication requiring prompt treatment because they compress and distort an already damaged, edematous brain. Acute subdural hematoma is symptomatic within 24 to 48 hours of injury and is seen in about 24% of clients with severe head injuries.

Clinical manifestations of acute subdural hematoma are similar to those of acute epidural hematoma. The onset and development of the clinical manifestations may be somewhat slower because the bleeding is more often venous rather than arterial. Recognition of clinical manifestations may be difficult because subdural hematoma is often associated with moderate or severe brain injury. A patient who develops an acute subdural hematoma may remain unconscious after injury or may have a variable LOC (depending on the extent of injury). A conscious client usually has a headache. The client may become irritable and confused and lapse into a coma or show a fluctuating LOC. Manifestations of increasing ICP appear. Subtle changes in LOC and development

of lateralizing changes (i.e., on one side) such as hemiparesis, pupillary dilation, or extraocular eye movement paralysis may be the only findings.

Chronic Subdural Hematoma. Chronic subdural hematoma is most common in older and alcoholic clients (Figure 73-9). These clients experience atrophy of the brain, which results in stretching of the bridging veins and an increase in the size of the subdural space. These stretched veins are easily ruptured in a fall, even if the fall does not result in other injuries. It develops several weeks or even months after injury because of a slow accumulation of fluid in a larger-than-normal space. Older or alcoholic clients may not even recall the mechanism of injury. The initial injury may have been relatively minor, and the client may not associate current

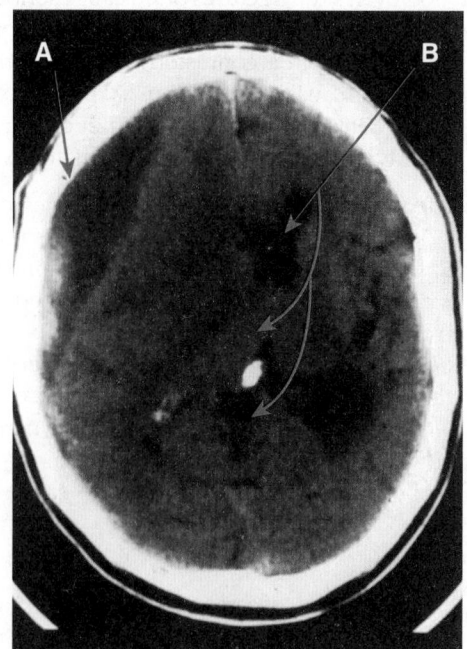

■ **FIGURE 73–9** A, Magnetic resonance image of a chronic subdural hematoma with an area of acute bleeding. B, Severe midline shift results.

clinical manifestations with the past injury. In addition, family members may not recognize the subtle neurologic changes or may not give credence to them because of the client's age or alcohol use.

Gradually the enlarging blood clot creates pressure on the brain. There is an interval during which the client appears to be recovering or seems completely recovered. Later, manifestations of neurologic deterioration develop. The client may become drowsy, inattentive, and incoherent and display personality changes. Headaches are another prominent symptom. These indications of chronic subdural hematoma may be overlooked until focal or lateralizing signs appear (e.g., hemiparesis, pupil signs). Changes in LOC continue, and LOC may fluctuate widely. Clinical assessment with subdural hematoma is similar to that with epidural hematomas. Surgical intervention usually consists of placing several burr holes or performing a craniotomy to remove the hematoma. Treatment results depend on the client's condition before surgery and the degree of primary brain tissue damage.

A client who has undergone evacuation of a chronic subdural hematoma usually has a drain placed in the cavity to prevent reaccumulation of the fluid and blood. These clients are typically kept flat during the immediate postoperative period, which allows the brain to reexpand to fill the cranial cavity.

Intracerebral Hematoma. Intracerebral hematomas occur less often than epidural or subdural hematomas. They are caused by bleeding directly into brain tissue and may occur at the area of injury, some distance away, or deep within the brain. These hematomas cause problems with increased ICP. Surgical resection may cause as much damage as the clot itself and is usually not performed unless the clot is easily accessible. Clinical manifestations are similar to those that occur with epidural or subdural hematomas, although hemiplegia is more common than hemiparesis. Many assessment findings relate to the lesion's mass effect. Various other clinical manifestations may also be present, depending on the location of the intracerebral hematoma. A diagnosis is established as with other types of hematomas. One form of hematoma, called *delayed traumatic intracerebral hematoma,* occurs after a few days. It is most common in people with disseminated intravascular coagulation, hypertension, a history of alcohol abuse, or hypoxia. It carries a poor prognosis.

Pathophysiology

Major head injuries cause direct damage to the parenchyma of the brain. Kinetic energy is transmitted to the brain, and bruising analogous to that seen in soft tissue injuries results. A blow to the surface of the brain results in rapid brain tissue displacement and disruption of blood vessels, leading to bleeding, tissue injury, and edema. Damage to the brain and skull includes the blow itself *(primary injury)* and continuing injury from edema, inflammation, and hemorrhage within the brain *(secondary injury)*. Secondary injury can result in more severe manifestations than those attributable to the impact itself. Inflammation leads to cerebral edema and increased ICP. Hemorrhage may be diffuse if it is due to tearing of several small vessels within the brain. Whenever pressure is increased within the brain, the brain can become hypoxic. The secondary problems occur hours to days after the initial impact.

A concussion usually causes injury to the brain that is reversible. Some biochemical and ultrastructural damage, such as depletion in mitochondrial adenosine triphosphate and changes in vascular permeability, also can occur.

Clients with diffuse axonal damage have microscopic injury to the axons in the cerebrum, the corpus callosum, and the brain stem. Widespread white-matter injury, white-matter degeneration, neuronal dysfunction, and global cerebral edema are characteristic features.

Studies have noted a significantly increased mortality in the client who experiences hypotension, especially early in the postinjury period. When autoregulation is disrupted, as in head injury, cerebral hypoperfusion leads to brain tissue ischemia. Hypoxia has a diminished effect on mortality so long as cerebral perfusion is adequate because the brain can extract extra oxygen for short periods. The combination of arterial hypotension and hypoxemia is significant in the progression of secondary injury. Other causes of secondary brain injury include increased ICP, respiratory problems, electrolyte imbalance, and infection.

Reperfusion injury occurs when ischemia is reversed and blood flow is reestablished; it also leads to secondary injury. Reperfusion injury is also recognized in myocardial infarction and stroke. Reperfusion injury is probably caused by oxygen free radicals, which are normal by-products of aerobic metabolism that usually break down into oxygen and water. In cell injury, breakdown of these radicals is impaired so that they accumulate, causing destruction of nucleic acids, proteins, carbohydrates, and lipids and, eventually, cell membranes in the brain tissue. Currently, research is targeted at developing neuroprotective agents that prevent delayed injury progression.[61]

Clinical Manifestations
Skull Fractures

Other than a history of skull fracture, clients may not have clear manifestations of the injury. Therefore they need careful ongoing assessment. They may develop other clinical signs, including the following:

- CSF or other fluid draining from the ear or nose
- Evidence of various cranial nerve injuries

- Blood behind the tympanic membrane
- Periorbital ecchymoses (bruises around the eyes)
- Later, a bruise over the mastoid process (Battle's sign)

Indications of cranial nerve and inner ear damage may be noted at the time of the initial injury or may not appear until later. They include the following:

- Vision changes from optic nerve damage
- Hearing loss from auditory nerve damage
- Loss of the sense of smell from olfactory nerve damage
- Squint or fixed, dilated pupil and loss of some eye movements from oculomotor nerve damage
- Facial paresis or paralysis (unilateral) from facial nerve damage
- Vertigo caused by damage from otoliths in the inner ear
- Nystagmus from damage to the vestibular system

Basilar skull fractures, depressed fractures, and other open (compound) fractures allow communication between the external environment and the brain. Infection is therefore a possible complication. See Chapter 69 for a discussion of brain abscess and meningitis. Increasing ICP with basilar skull fractures can be difficult to assess because the pressure is not exerted on the motor strip of the frontal lobes, which means that there will be no weakness in the contralateral extremities. Assess for subtle changes in vital signs, especially heart rate and rhythm and breathing patterns. Headache may be present if there is bleeding at the site of injury.

Concussions

After concussion, observers report loss of consciousness for 5 minutes or less. Retrograde amnesia, post-traumatic amnesia, or both may be present. The duration of amnesia may directly correlate with the severity of the concussion. The client usually has a headache and dizziness and may complain of nausea and vomiting. There is no break in the skull or dura, and no visible damage is seen on CT or MRI scans.

Contusions

The clinical manifestations of contusions are varied, partly because any area of the brain can suffer contusion. Contusions are often associated with other serious injuries, including cervical fractures. Secondary effects (e.g., brain swelling and edema) accompany serious contusions. Increased ICP and herniation syndromes may result. Contusions may be divided into cerebral contusions and brain stem contusions.

Cerebral Contusions. Manifestations of cerebral contusions vary, depending on which areas of the cerebral hemispheres are damaged. An agitated, confused head-injured client who remains alert may have a temporal lobe contusion. Hemiparesis in an alert head-injured client may indicate a frontal contusion. An aphasic head-injured client may have a frontotemporal contusion. Other findings indicate contusions in other areas. Although these findings correlate with cerebral contusion, they do not rule out other abnormalities, such as a developing mass lesion. Adverse changes in the client's condition require immediate medical attention. If treated early, these complications may be reversible.

Brain Stem Contusions. Brain stem contusions render a client immediately unresponsive or partially comatose because of significant brain stem disruption. Typically an altered LOC continues for at least several hours and usually days or weeks. The client may regain partial consciousness within hours or remain in a coma.

Damage to the reticular activating system may render the client permanently comatose. Other neurologic abnormalities are present and are usually symmetrical (i.e., evenly distributed on both sides of the body). Some may be lateralized (asymmetrical, or on one side of the body only), indicating development of a secondary event, such as a hematoma.

In addition to the altered LOC that is always present with brain stem contusion, respiratory, pupillary, eye movement, and motor abnormalities may occur.

- Respirations may be normal, periodic, very rapid, or ataxic.
- Pupils are usually small, equal, and reactive. Damage to the upper brain stem (third cranial nerve) may cause pupillary abnormalities.
- Loss of normal eye movements may occur because pathways controlling eye movements traverse the midbrain and pons.
- The client may respond to light or noxious stimuli by purposeful movements, such as pushing the stimulus away, or the client may have no response to stimuli (i.e., may be in a flaccid state). In the presence of profound alteration in LOC, flexor or extensor posturing may be elicited with or without noxious stimuli (see Chapter 68).

Brain stem contusions do not usually injure the brain stem alone. Localized swelling or direct injury to the hypothalamus may produce autonomic nervous system effects. The client may have a high temperature and a rapid pulse rate and respirations and may perspire profusely. These effects may wax and wane but, if sustained, can lead to serious complications.

These clinical manifestations often vary from one observation to another, whereas findings with a developing hematoma are more consistent. Careful documentation of assessment findings to identify patterns or trends in the client's condition is important.

Diagnostic assessments such as CT or MRI scanning may reveal fractures and areas of bleeding or brain shift (see Figure 73-9). Lumbar puncture can also be used to assess for bleeding within the subarachnoid space if any possibility of increased ICP has been ruled out. Currently, CT scans can identify blood in the subarachnoid space, and lumbar punctures are rarely done for this purpose.

OUTCOME MANAGEMENT

Major goals in the care of severely head-injured clients are as follows:

- Prompt recognition and treatment of hypoxia and acid-base disorders that can contribute to cerebral edema
- Control of increasing ICP resulting from factors such as cerebral edema or expanding hematoma
- Stabilization of other conditions.

Medical Management

The medical management of severely head-injured clients focuses on supporting all organ systems while recovery from the injuries takes place. This involves (1) ventilatory support, (2) management of fluid balance and elimination, and (3) management of nutrition and gastrointestinal function. Head trauma affects all systems of the body, and managing its effects requires a holistic perspective. The Translating Evidence into Practice feature on Management of Fever in Clients with Head Injury on p. 1940 describes assessments and interventions related to hyperpyrexia. Clinical manifestations may be the result of the initial head injury or may arise from a complicating process.

Initial Management

The initial management of clients with head injury is the same as for any other injured client: airway, breathing, and circulation. There is a high association of cervical fracture with head injury; therefore the client must be immobilized at the scene of the injury. Lateral cervical spine x-ray films are obtained before the client's head is moved, or the immobilization devices are removed. The client with head injury is protected from possible complications of cord injury by immobilizing the head and neck immediately, using a cervical collar or sandbags until a collar can be obtained.

If intubation is necessary, a jaw thrust maneuver must be used rather than neck flexion to open the airway without possible injury to the spine. A baseline assessment of the client's motor and sensory function is obtained at the scene of the accident. Interventions include achieving oxygenation and lowering the ICP with hyperventilation by mechanical ventilation or by manually hyperventilating the client with a bag-valve-mask device if the client has evidence of herniation.[9]

An IV line is placed and fluids are given to stabilize the blood pressure to systolic pressures over 90 mm Hg. Head injury alone does not cause major loss of blood. If substantial blood loss is suspected, look for other injuries (e.g., fractures, abdominal injury, and severe scalp laceration).

A complete history, including the mechanism of injury, is important. These data allow the physician to determine the probable extent of injury and allow emergency department personnel to prepare for the client's arrival. Open head wounds should be covered and pressure applied to control bleeding unless there appears to be an underlying depressed or compound skull fracture.

Do not attempt to remove foreign objects or any penetrating objects from the wound. Uncomplicated scalp wounds (that do not lie over depressed or compound skull fractures) are anesthetized with a local anesthetic agent, cleansed, and sutured. In the emergency department, primary and secondary surveys of the client's injuries are performed. Resuscitation continues with fluid administration.

Laboratory studies are performed, as are necessary radiologic studies. If any identified injuries require emergency surgery, the client is taken directly to the operating room (OR) before admission to the intensive care unit (ICU). Once the client is stabilized enough for transfer to the ICU, the neurosurgical and trauma teams and the nursing staff maintain ongoing care.

Ongoing Management

Ongoing care to maintain cerebral perfusion and reduce ICP is the focus of critical care. The cerebral metabolic rate is reduced with sedatives, paralytic agents, antipyretics, barbiturates, and hypothermia. Morphine is a commonly used opioid for the head-injured client. It reduces pain and can be given intravenously. Respiratory depression is controlled in the client who is intubated and ventilated. Paralytic agents may be used to promote adequate ventilation and should be administered in conjunction with a sedative and an analgesic because paralytic agents have no sedative or analgesic effect.

Prognosis

Few clients die instantly from head injury; however, many head-injured clients die within the first few minutes after injury from shock or impaired respiration. Early death may also result from brain stem damage. According to the results of several studies, coma duration is the best predictor of damage severity because it correlates highly with the probability of death, intellectual deficit, and social skill impairment. These studies classified a *mild* head injury as loss of consciousness

TRANSLATING EVIDENCE INTO PRACTICE

Management of Fever in Clients with Head Injury

Fever is defined as a core temperature greater than 38° C or 100.4° F. Other definitions of fever include two or more consecutive elevations greater than 38.3° C or 101° F.[5,6] Fever (hyperpyrexia) implies that the thermoregulatory response is intact but that the body temperature is maintained at a higher level. In the presence of fever, compensatory cooling responses occur. Hyperthermia is the loss of thermoregulatory ability, which can occur with injury to the hypothalamus or in malignant hyperthermia. Hyperthermia requires aggressive treatment to prevent cellular damage as the temperature approaches 40° C.

The management of fever in the head-injured patient can be complex because the etiology of fever is not always clear. Assessment of the fever is the first step in management. The nurse needs to evaluate the diagnosis of the patient, the disease processes that might be occurring in conjunction with the fever, and the pattern of the fever that the patient is experiencing. In addition, the presence of intravenous lines or other invasive devices (e.g., ICP monitor or indwelling bladder catheter) needs to be evaluated as causes of the fever.

Infectious causes of fever include ventilator-acquired or nosocomial pneumonia, bacteremia from central lines, and drug fever from antimicrobials, diuretics, or other medications. Noninfectious fever can occur as a result of neurologic events (stroke, head injury, seizure, or hemorrhage), malignancies, or acute myocardial infarction.

Whereas the literature suggests that fever can enhance the host defense by activating the body's physiologic adaptive response, in certain vulnerable populations (neurologic, cardiac, immune compromised, and older clients), evidence shows that fever is maladaptive and needs aggressive management.[2,4,6]

When fever is present, the physician is notified, and appropriate cultures are obtained. Antipyretics should be given as the first line of therapy for temperatures greater than 38.5° C. Acetaminophen, aspirin, or nonsteroidal anti-inflammatory drugs are given to "re-set" the hypothalamic thermoregulatory mechanism or "thermostat."[5,6]

Which cooling measures to use and when to use them have not been answered in the literature in scientifically rigorous studies. Cooling measures should be directed toward increasing heat loss. Examples of this include placing ice packs at the groin or axilla or sponging with alcohol and tepid water. It is important to prevent shivering, however, because shivering increases metabolic activity and the potential to increase rather than decrease the fever. Cooling measures that allow evaporation may be more effective than the use of cooling blankets.[1,4]

The use of cooling blankets should be reserved for clients whose core temperatures rise to 39° to 40° C (>103.5° F). The cooling blanket should be set at 23.9° C to prevent shivering episodes and clients should not be cooled at greater than 0.5° C every 30 minutes. The cooling blanket should be turned off once the patient temperature reaches a desirable level (<38° C).[1] Skin integrity should be assessed while on the cooling blanket because areas of "frost bite" can develop, especially if the skin is damp.

REFERENCES

1. Caruso, C.C., et al. (1992). Cooling effects and comfort of four cooling blanket temperatures in humans with fever. *Nursing Research, 41*(2), 68-72.
2. Henker, R. (1999). Evidence-based practice: Fever-related interventions. *American Journal of Critical Care, 8*(1), 481-489.
3. Kluger, M.J. (1986). Is fever beneficial? *Yale Journal of Biological Medicine, 58*, 89-95.
4. McIlvoy, L.H. (2005). The effect of hypothermia and hyperthermia on acute brain injury. *AACN Clinical Issues, 16*(4), 488-500.
5. O'Donnell, J., et al. (1997). Use and effectiveness of hypothermia blankets for febrile patients in the intensive care unit. *Clinical Infectious Diseases, 24*, 1208-1213.
6. Vaughn, L.K., Veale, W.L., & Cooper, K.E. (1980). Antipyresis: Its effect on mortality rate of bacterially infected rabbits. *Brain Research Bulletin, 5*, 69-73.
7. Wright, J.E. (2005). Therapeutic hypothermia in traumatic brain injury. *Critical Care Nursing Quarterly, 28*(2), 150-161.

---

for 20 minutes or less, a *moderate* head injury as 21 to 59 minutes of unconsciousness, and *severe* head injury as coma for 1 hour or longer.

Nursing Management

Assessment. A description of the mechanism of injury is helpful in understanding the nature of a head injury. Whenever there are witnesses to the accident, information obtained can be valuable in determining the extent of the injury. Information about the client's activity and LOC before and after the injury is also helpful. Also important is whether the client was conscious at all or unconscious after injury.

As soon as possible after head injury, assess and document the client's vital signs and neurologic status. This initial assessment and the data obtained from witnesses at the accident scene establish a baseline for later observations. Carefully document all assessment findings. Assessment data collection is described earlier in this chapter.

The physician should be notified promptly of any findings that indicate the possible development of complications. It is particularly difficult to accurately assess the condition of a head-injured client who has ingested large amounts of alcohol or other drugs before injury because the effects of these substances may obscure significant clinical abnormalities.

Diagnosis, Outcomes, Interventions. Many nursing and collaborative problems are present in the client with a head injury, such as risk for *Ineffective Airway Clearance, Ineffective Tissue Perfusion,* seizures, paralysis, infection, diabetes insipidus, and *Post-trauma Syndrome.* Othe problems that a client with a head injury may experience include the following:

- Risk for contractures
- Impaired skin integrity
- Impaired oral mucous membranes
- Imbalanced nutrition
- Risk for imbalanced fluid volume
- Risk for falls
- Risk for increased ICP
- Disturbed thought processes
- Interrupted family processes

Nursing diagnoses for these problems are discussed in Chapters 68 and 69. Investigation of the underlying causes of these problems and the interventions for them must be individualized according to the client's needs. A sample care plan for managing clients with traumatic injury appears on pp. 1942 to 1947.

Diagnosis: Risk for Ineffective Airway Clearance. The client with traumatic brain injury may have an altered state of consciousness and may not be able to expectorate secretions. The client is also at increased risk for aspiration.

Outcomes. The client will have effective airway clearance. The upper airway should be free of secretions. Respirations should be of a regular rate (16 to 22 breaths/min), rhythm, and depth. Breath sounds should be clear in both lungs, and the chest should have symmetrical movement. The trachea should be in a midline position, and no dyspnea or accessory muscle use should be noted. Aspiration should be prevented. The Pao_2 should be maintained greater than 90 mm Hg and the $Paco_2$ between 30 and 35 mm Hg initially. The chest film should be clear.

Interventions. Nursing actions aimed at maintaining adequate airway clearance include clearing the mouth and oral pharynx of foreign bodies (e.g., broken teeth) and suctioning the oropharynx and trachea every 1 or 2 hours and as needed. Avoid suctioning the nasopharynx until after a basilar fracture or meningeal tear is ruled out. A semiprone lateral position may facilitate drainage of secretions and prevent aspiration but is contraindicated with increased ICP or a cervical fracture. Humidified oxygen, endotracheal intubation, mechanical ventilation, or a tracheostomy may be required to maintain the client's Pao_2 and $Paco_2$ within set parameters.

Diagnosis: Ineffective Cerebral Tissue Perfusion. In clients who suffer from traumatic brain injuries, another appropriate nursing diagnosis is *Risk for Ineffective Cerebral Tissue Perfusion secondary to hypotension, hypertension, intracranial hemorrhage, hematoma, or other injuries.*

Outcomes. The client will have adequate cerebral tissue perfusion. The client will have a stable or improving LOC with a stable GCS score and an ICP of less than

15 mm Hg. Temperature will be maintained at less than 38.5° C. The client's blood pressure will be maintained within established parameters. Urine output will be a minimum of 0.5 ml/kg/hour and not greater than 200 ml/hour. Laboratory values will remain within normal limits.

Interventions. Although anticipatory, prudent monitoring is key to early detection of ineffective cerebral tissue perfusion, nursing interventions can actually prevent, delay, or minimize ineffective cerebral perfusion. These interventions are discussed earlier in this chapter. Briefly they include maintaining all physiologic parameters within normal limits, positioning the client for optimal venous return, and monitoring extracerebral systems for complications. Communicating a client's neurologic status accurately and completely through verbal reporting and documentation is essential to early identification of change and early intervention. ICP monitoring may be required (see earlier discussion).

Surgical Management

Conditions that may require surgery include subdural and epidural hematomas, depressed skull fractures, and penetrating foreign bodies. An epidural clot may be surgically evacuated through burr holes (Figure 73-10) or a craniotomy. During surgery the wound may be drained and bleeding vessels ligated. After surgery nursing care is the same as that for any client recovering from a craniotomy. Simple skull depressions are treated electively by surgically elevating the depressed bone tissue, removing fragments, and repairing lacerated dura. Compound depressed skull fractures are immediately treated surgically. The scalp, skull, and devitalized brain are debrided, and the wound is cleaned thoroughly. Unless all foreign material is removed, a brain abscess or seizures may develop. Debridement of a penetrating wound or depressed skull fracture frequently leaves a cranial

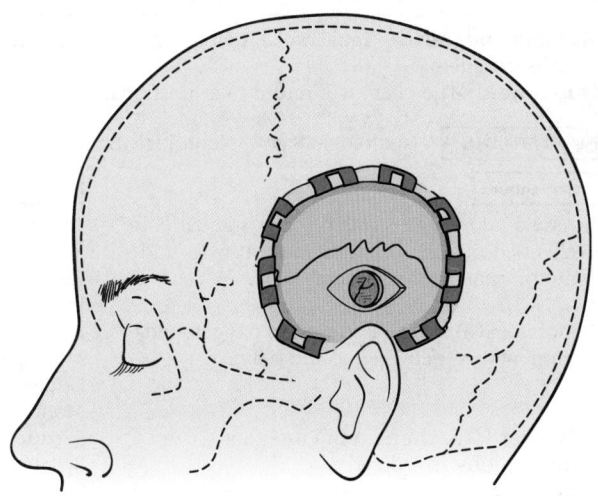

■ FIGURE 73-10 Placement of burr holes in the skull.

C A R E P L A N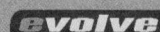

Management of the Client with Traumatic Brain Injury

Nursing Diagnosis: Airway Clearance, Ineffective (NANDA) related to decreased level of consciousness, loss of protection of airway and inability to maintain positioning.
Outcomes: Client will be free of respiratory distress or aspiration pneumonia.

NOC OUTCOMES Aspiration Prevention; Respiratory Status: Airway Patency; Respiratory Status: Ventilation

Interventions	NIC INTERVENTIONS	Rationales
1. Maintain patent airway using suctioning or coughing.	Airway Suctioning	1. A clear airway allows for adequate oxygenation and ventilation.
2. Position patient with HOB elevated 30 degrees.	Cough Management Aspiration Precautions: Positioning	2. Reduces risk of secretions from entering the lungs.
3. Assess client's ability to maintain own airway (cough, gag reflexes present).	Airway Management	3. Clients who are comatose may have lost reflexes needed to maintain airway.
4. Assess patency of artificial airway (ETT or tracheostomy).	Airway Management	4. Artificial airways can become plugged with mucus or from biting. Maintaining airway patency allows for effective oxygenation and ventilation.
5. Monitor oxygenation using pulse oximetry.	Respiratory Monitoring	5. Pulse oximetry provides information about oxygen status and should be >90%.
6. Provide oxygen support as needed.	Ventilation Assistance	6. Supplemental oxygen may be necessary to support the injured brain.

Evaluation: With interventions, client will be able to maintain/protect airway and oxygenate and ventilate without difficulty.

Nursing Diagnosis: Tissue Perfusion: Cerebral, Ineffective (NANDA) related to edema from traumatic brain injury.
Outcomes: The client will maintain cerebral perfusion.

NOC OUTCOMES Circulation Status; Cognition; Neurologic Status; Neurologic Status: Consciousness; Tissue Perfusion: Cerebral

Interventions	NIC INTERVENTIONS	Rationales
1. Maintain blood pressure within ordered range. Assess hemodynamic status to ensure appropriate cardiac output.	Cerebral Perfusion Promotion	1. Cerebral perfusion should be maintained to ensure oxygenation and nutrient delivery to brain tissue.
2. Monitor neurologic examination as per unit standard.	Neurologic Monitoring	2. Neurologic status is the most important indicator of the client's condition.
3. Maintain ICP <20 mm Hg. Treat ICP >25 mm Hg with diuresis, CSF drainage, mild hyperventilation.	Intracranial Pressure Monitoring	3. ICP monitoring provides an early warning system of possible changes within the cranial vault that could lead to a change in neurologic status.

Evaluation: The client will maintain a stable neurologic examination with ICP <20 mm Hg and CPP >60 mm Hg.

Nursing Diagnosis: Intracranial Adaptive Capacity, Decreased (NANDA) related to traumatic brain injury, increased ICP, and cerebral edema.
Outcomes: The client will return to a functional neurologic status and will be seizure-free.

NOC OUTCOMES Neurologic Status; Neurologic Status: Consciousness; Seizure Control; Tissue Perfusion: Cerebral

Interventions	NIC INTERVENTIONS	Rationales
1. Assess neurologic status per unit standard and client condition, including mental status and motor, sensory, and cranial nerves.	Cerebral Edema Management Cerebral Perfusion Promotion	1. Changes in neurologic status are the first indicators of problems developing within the cranial vault.
2. Monitor ICP and CPP to ensure oxygen and nutrients are delivered to the brain.	Intracranial Pressure Monitoring Neurologic Monitoring	2. ICP and CPP provide additional information about the status of the brain.
3. Monitor for seizures. Administer antiseizure medications as ordered.	Seizure Precautions Seizure Management	3. Seizures increase metabolic rate in the brain and lead to poor outcomes after TBI.

Evaluation: The client will maintain a stable neurologic examination.

Nursing Diagnosis: Confusion, Acute (NANDA) related to traumatic brain injury, hospitalization in an unfamiliar environment, effect of medications provided.

Outcomes: Client will be alert, oriented to person, place, and situation.

| NOC OUTCOMES | Cognitive Orientation; Neurologic Status: Consciousness |

Interventions	NIC INTERVENTIONS	Rationales
1. Evaluate the possible causes of delirium or delusion such as medications, environment, or lack of sleep.	Delirium Management Delusion Management	1. Determining the causes of changes in orientation will provide direction for management.
2. Attempt to modify those causes that can be modified.	Reality Orientation	2. When possible, a quiet environment with minimal stimulation will assist in calming and reorienting the client.
3. Orient the patient as much as is possible.		3. Reorienting the client may not be possible. It is important not to argue with the patient's current reality.
4. Provide medication that will decrease the delirium or delusion.		4. Use of sedative medications is a last resort, but should be used when the client indicates potential for self-harm or harm to others.
5. Ensure that a total assessment is completed by the medical team.		5. Ensuring that the change in orientation is not related to a structural change in the brain is a priority.
6. Determine the need for a psychiatric consultation.		6. Psychiatric consultation can assist with medication management for delirium/delusion.
7. Monitor neurologic status as required for area of care.	Neurologic Monitoring	7. Provides early identification of changes in level of consciousness.
8. Maintain ICP <20 mm Hg and CPP >60 mm Hg.	Cerebral Perfusion Promotion	8. Prevents secondary brain injury from edema or poor blood flow.

Evaluation: With interventions, client will show no evidence of delirium or delusion and will be aware of current situation. ICP and CPP will be maintained within normal limits.

Nursing Diagnosis: Fluid Volume Deficit or Excess (NANDA) related to need for fluid resuscitation after traumatic brain injury or need for diuresis.

Outcomes: Client will maintain fluids and electrolytes within normal limits and will maintain a regular diet.

| NOC OUTCOMES | Electrolyte and Acid-Base Balance; Fluid Balance; Hydration; Nutritional Status: Food and Fluid Intake |

Interventions	NIC INTERVENTIONS	Rationales
1. Monitor acid-base balance, fluid intake and output, and electrolyte results.	Acid-Base Management Fluid/Electrolyte Management	1. Values outside of normal range can cause changes in mentation and ability to participate in rehabilitation activities.
2. Assess fluid volume status.	Fluid Management Fluid Monitoring Hypovolemia Management Hypervolemia Management	2. Management of fluid volume will avoid hypovolemia and hypervolemia.
3. Provide fluid and electrolytes via IV access until client able to take liquids by mouth.	Intravenous Therapy	3. IV therapy provides hydration and electrolytes until the client can eat or be fed through a nasogastric tube.

Evaluation: The client will have stable fluid volume and electrolyte status.

Nursing Diagnosis: Hyperthermia (NANDA) related to traumatic brain injury or infection.

Outcomes: The client will be maintained without a fever.

| NOC OUTCOMES | Thermoregulation; Vital Signs |

Interventions	NIC INTERVENTIONS	Rationales
1. Monitor temperature per unit standard.	Temperature Regulation	1. Fever can occur from infection or from inability of the hypothalamus to regulate properly.
2. Initiate treatment of fever once >38.5° C.	Fever Treatment	2. Treatment of fever will reset the thermostat to decrease the event of further fever.

Evaluation: The client will maintain a temperature <38.5° C.

(Continued)

C A R E   P L A N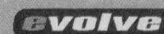

Management of the Client with Traumatic Brain Injury—Cont'd

Nursing Diagnosis: Pain, Acute or Chronic (NANDA) due to injuries sustained at the time of the traumatic brain injury.
Outcomes: The client will have pain control and will not become depressed as a result of pain.

NOC OUTCOMES	Comfort Level; Pain Control; Pain Level; Depression Level

Interventions	NIC INTERVENTIONS	Rationales
1. Educate client regarding medications, dosage, side effects.	Medication Management	1. Understanding of all medications allows for more appropriate choices.
2. Provide information about appropriate pain management and weaning from pain medication.	Pain Management	2. Excessive use of pain medication can lead to tolerance and may require additional support for weaning.
3. Assess the client's level of pain and if the client is not able to verbally express pain, use other pain assessment tools.	Pain Assessment Analgesic Administration	3. Pain management begins with assessment of level of pain.
4. Educate the client about analgesics and appropriate management of pain using various types of analgesia.	Sedation Management	4. Understanding all analgesia options helps the client in decision making for pain relief.
5. Provide information about the sedative effects of certain analgesics so that the client will not drive.		5. Sedation caused by medication can impair the ability to drive or perform complex tasks.

Evaluation: The client will have comfort at a tolerable level and will develop a self-management plan for pain control if needed.

Nursing Diagnosis: Skin Integrity, Impaired (NANDA) related to prolonged bed rest.
Outcomes: The client will have no evidence of skin breakdown or poor wound healing.

NOC OUTCOMES	Tissue Integrity: Skin and Mucous Membranes; Wound Healing: Primary/Secondary Intention

Interventions	NIC INTERVENTIONS	Rationales
1. Assess skin every shift to identify potential pressure areas and begin treatment if necessary.	Pressure Management	1. Clients who are on bed rest have increased risk of skin breakdown from pressure.
2. Turn the client q 2 hours.	Pressure Ulcer Care Skin Surveillance	2. Turning relieves pressure and decreases risk of skin breakdown.
3. Assess incision line to ensure that it remains clean, dry, and intact.	Incision Site Care	3. Incision line infection causes a delay in wound healing.
4. Provide appropriate care to incisions or pressure ulcers to promote healing.	Wound Care Pressure Ulcer Care Wound Care	4. Delay in wound healing leads to delays in mobility and rehabilitation.

Evaluation: The client's skin will remain intact and incisions will heal in a timely manner without evidence of infection.

Nursing Diagnosis: Nutrition: Imbalanced: Less Than or More Than Body Requirements (NANDA) related to inability to consume food or from eating too much food as a result of traumatic brain injury.
Outcomes: The client will maintain a normal weight and will consume a balanced diet.

NOC OUTCOMES	Appetite; Nutritional Status: Food, Fluid and Nutrient Intake; Weight Control

Interventions	NIC INTERVENTIONS	Rationales
1. Assess caloric consumption.	Nutrition Therapy Nutritional Monitoring	1. Too many calories or too few calories can inhibit healing and mobility.
2. Provide information about appropriate dietary intake.	Nutrition Management Weight Gain/Loss Assistance	2. Many clients need education about proper dietary intake, which will prevent future health care problems.
3. Educate regarding weight loss or gain as appropriate.		3. Weight gain or loss may affect strength and ability to regain independence.

Evaluation: The client will maintain an appropriate intake without excessive weight gain or loss.

Nursing Diagnosis: Self-Care Deficit: Bathing/Hygiene, Dressing/Grooming, Feeding, Oral Hygiene, Toileting (NANDA)

Outcomes: The client will have a satisfactory level of self-care as evidenced by independently performing as many activities of daily living as possible. The client will direct a caregiver to provide any needs not independently met.

NOC OUTCOMES   Self-Care Activities of Daily Living; Nutritional Status; Swallowing Status

Interventions	NIC INTERVENTIONS	Rationales
1. Assist the client in activities of daily living.	Self-Care Assistance: Bathing/Hygiene	1. Allowing the client to do as much as possible leads to increased independence.
2. Provide education regarding feeding and swallowing.	Oral Health Maintenance Self-Care Assistance: Dressing/Grooming	2. Careful monitoring of food intake and appropriate feeding/swallowing techniques will minimize aspiration.
3. Provide education about bowel management.	Self-Care Assistance: Feeding Swallowing Therapy Self-Care Assistance: Toileting Bowel Management	3. A regular bowel regimen will promote bowel continence and decrease constipation.

Evaluation: The client will become as independent as possible in all activities of daily living.

Nursing Diagnosis: Urinary Retention (NANDA) due to traumatic brain injury affecting neuronal control of the bladder.

Outcomes: The client will be continent and without bladder distention.

NOC OUTCOMES   Urinary Continence; Urinary Elimination

Interventions	NIC INTERVENTIONS	Rationales
1. Assess for bladder distention, particularly after urinary catheter is removed; use bladder scan if available.	Urinary Retention Care Urinary Catheterization	1. Bladder distention is a common problem after neurologic injury and can contribute to urinary tract infections.
2. Insert urinary catheter if client is unable to void, has history of urinary retention or prostatic hypertrophy, or has a post-void residual of >250 ml.		2. Catheterization removes excess urine and decreases the likelihood of infection from retention of urine. Good catheter care decreases the risk of infection from the catheter.
3. Assess for volume, color, odor of urine; frequency of urination; difficulty with urination; and overflow urination.	Urinary Elimination Management Urinary Retention Care	3. Voiding high volumes of urine could be related to diuresis or to diabetes insipidus. Clients with urinary retention may void frequently and in small amounts.

Evaluation: The client will be able to void or be able to notify caregivers of need to void.

Nursing Diagnosis: Sleep Deprivation (NANDA) due to traumatic brain injury, lack of sleep in the hospital, and changes in diurnal patterns from hospitalization.

Outcomes: The client will report a normal sleep pattern.

NOC OUTCOMES   Mood Equilibrium; Rest; Sleep; Symptom Severity

Interventions	NIC INTERVENTIONS	Rationales
1. Assess the client's mood and ability to tolerate stressful situations. Provide opportunities for sleep.	Mood Management Sleep Enhancement	1. Inability to sleep leads to intolerance of stressful situations, delays healing and recovery, and slows the rehabilitation process.
2. Assess medications provided to temper mood and promote sleep.	Medication Management	2. Medications may be necessary for the short-term to assist with stabilizing the sleep pattern.
3. Encourage increased activity during the day.	Energy Management	3. Increasing activity will promote sleep.
4. Avoid long naps during the day.	Sleep Enhancement	4. Naps during the day will prevent long periods of sleep at night.

Evaluation: After interventions, the client will return to a normal sleep schedule and will be able to tolerate stress and daily activities.

(Continued)

C A R E   P L A N   *evolve*

Management of the Client with Traumatic Brain Injury—Cont'd

Nursing Diagnosis: Communication, Impaired Verbal (NANDA) related to the results of traumatic brain injury.
Outcomes: Client will be able to communicate within limitations.

NOC OUTCOMES Communication: Expressive and Receptive; Information Processing

Interventions	NIC INTERVENTIONS	Rationales
1. Assess the client's ability to understand verbal and visual input and follow instructions, utilizing occupational therapists and speech/language pathologists.	Active Listening Communication Enhancement: Speech Deficit Communication Enhancement: Visual Deficit	1. Understanding communication deficits will assist in identifying alternate strategies for communication. The therapists will be able to provide opportunities for learning for the client and caregivers.
2. Identify anxiety that may be present in the client related to inability to communicate or remember.	Anxiety Reduction Memory Training	2. Providing strategies for dealing with communication and memory deficits will decrease the client's anxiety about functioning in society.

Evaluation: Client will develop strategies to enhance memory and communication.

Nursing Diagnosis: Mobility, Physical: Impaired (NANDA) related to prolonged bed rest, traumatic brain injury, and physical injuries from the cause of the brain injury.
Outcomes: The client will be able to ambulate and transfer to achieve independence.

NOC OUTCOMES Ambulation; Balance; Coordinated Movement; Mobility; Transfer Performance

Interventions	NIC INTERVENTIONS	Rationales
1. Provide early ambulation and out of bed activities.	Exercise Promotion: Strength Training Exercise Therapy: Ambulation	1. Increasing activity will lead to increased strength. Being able to ambulate out of the room improves the client's overall outlook.
2. Assist with balance activity when the client is out of bed.	Exercise Promotion: Strength Training Exercise Therapy: Balance	2. Reinforcing information taught by therapists will assist the client in improving balance.
3. Teach client and caregiver range-of-motion and isometric exercises that can be conducted in bed.	Exercise Therapy: Joint Mobility Exercise Therapy: Muscle Control	3. Exercises conducted in bed will improve client's strength and increase independence.
4. Provide opportunities for the client to transfer from bed to chair and back.	Self-Care Assistance: Transfer	4. Self-transfer allows the client to become more independent.

Evaluation: The client will increase strength and mobility within bed or be able to be placed in a wheelchair with tolerance for sitting and ability to propel self.

Nursing Diagnosis: Activity Intolerance (NANDA) related to prolonged bed rest, fluid and electrolyte imbalance, poor nutrition and physical deficits.
Outcomes: Client will feel rested with fewer complaints of fatigue and increasing tolerance for activities.

NOC OUTCOMES Activity Tolerance, Endurance; Self-Care: Activities of Daily Living (ADL)

Interventions	NIC INTERVENTIONS	Rationales
1. Alternate rest and activity.	Energy Management Activity Therapy	1. Conserves energy and reduces demands on musculoskeletal system. Increases activity tolerance and endurance.
2. Assist with activities.	Self-Care Assistance	2. Being assisted as needed with activity of daily living (ADL) conserves energy and reduces demands on musculoskeletal system.
3. Monitor fluids and electrolytes. Assist with treatment of abnormal results.	Fluid/Electrolyte Management	3. Allows detection and treatment of abnormal laboratory results.

Evaluation: Upon discharge from the intensive care unit (ICU), if interventions are successful, the client will have an increased tolerance to activity, perform more ADL, and experience fewer fluid/electrolyte changes. Fluid/electrolyte replacement will improve tolerance to activity. Activity therapy will result in an increase in activity endurance.

Nursing Diagnosis: Adjustment, Impaired (NANDA) related to body and cognitive changes due to traumatic brain injury.

Outcomes: Client will be able to adjust to changes in health status, cognitive and physical disabilities.

| NOC OUTCOMES | Acceptance: Health Status, Adaptation to Physical Disability, Coping, Motivation, Psychosocial Adjustment: Life Change |

Interventions	NIC INTERVENTIONS	Rationales
1. Assist with identifying strategies for adjusting to body and cognitive changes.	Anticipatory Guidance	1. Helps client begin to realistically accept changes that might be permanent.
2. Provide opportunities for client to express concerns	Coping Enhancement Emotional Support Counseling	2. Respects the client's concerns about changes in body and loss of cognitive function.
3. Provide resources and opportunities for venting of feelings, particularly social services or psychiatric consultation service.	Crisis Intervention	3. Assists the client during the early emotional period of adjustment after injury.

Evaluation: With interventions, the client will begin to accept changes that have occurred from the traumatic brain injury and will identify resources to assist with emotional recovery.

Nursing Diagnosis: Self-Esteem Disturbed (NANDA) related to changes in physical abilities, mental abilities, and appearance as a result of traumatic brain injury.

Outcomes: Client will be able to acknowledge changes in physical and cognitive abilities resulting from the brain injury. Client will cope with body image disturbance, avoid isolation, and initiate or reestablish support systems.

| NOC OUTCOMES | Adaptation to Physical Disability; Psychosocial Adjustment: Life Change; Self-Esteem |

Interventions	NIC INTERVENTIONS	Rationales
1. Assess the client's response to body changes.	Body Image Enhancement	1. Determines the extent of body image disturbance
2. Promote accepting and nonjudgmental attitude.	Active Listening Emotional Support Self-Esteem Enhancement	2. Respects the client's sensitivity to body image changes.
3. Listen and encourage ventilation of feelings.	Active Listening Emotional Support	3. Helps the client feel valued.
4. Provide information regarding adaptive equipment and/or techniques.	Anticipatory Guidance Coping Enhancement	4. Helps provide the client some control over the situation.

Evaluation: Some degree of change in body functioning may persist and the client will learn to accept the altered body image. In addition, it is expected that the client will maintain or establish new interpersonal relationships and activities.

Nursing Diagnosis: Caregiver Role Strain (NANDA) related to efforts to care for client, other family members and running of a household.

Outcomes: Caregiver will maintain an emotionally and physically stable relationship with the client by assuring that the caregiver achieves respite from care.

| NOC OUTCOMES | Caregiver Emotional Health; Caregiver Lifestyle Disruption; Caregiver-Patient Relationship; Caregiver Physical Health; Caregiver Well-Being |

Interventions	NIC INTERVENTIONS	Rationales
1. Assist primary caregiver in identifying resources to relieve the burden of caring for a brain-injured client.	Caregiver Support Coping Enhancement Respite Care	1. Helping the caregiver adjust to role changes enables caregiver to identify additional resources for support. Care of a client with TBI is demanding and draining and the caregiver will need breaks.
2. Allow the caregiver to express concerns about the role changes that the TBI has presented.	Coping Enhancement Presence Role Enhancement	2. When the caregiver can express concerns and begin to identify role changes, the caregiver is more prepared to care for the client.
3. Provide education to the caregiver regarding the need for rest, healthy eating, and exercise.	Energy Management Nutrition Management	3. Ensuring that the caregiver is rested and healthy will enable the caregiver to provide care without becoming ill.
4. Provide education to the caregiver regarding how to manage the day to day needs of the client.	Caregiver Support Respite Care Teaching: Individual	4. Providing the caregiver with information early in the recovery period will assist in identifying needs for learning.

Evaluation: Caregiver will recognize the additional demands of caring for a brain-injured individual and will develop strategies to minimize strain, provide respite, and maintain own activities and interests.

defect that is cosmetically unsightly. The defect may be surgically corrected by cranioplasty later.

Before surgery ICP is reduced as much as possible. Baseline neurologic data are documented. Informed consent needs to be obtained from the family if the patient is unconscious or confused. After surgery, provide nursing care for the client following the guidelines for craniotomy (see Chapter 69).

Self-Care

Clients with possible head injury or mild head injury were previously hospitalized for observation for a minimum of 6 hours (ideally for 48 hours) because of the risk of extradural hemorrhage. If the client is sent home, give clear instructions to help the client's caregiver assess for complications (see the Client Education Guide website feature on Monitoring Family Members After Head Injury).

Rehabilitation

Most clients hospitalized for more than 48 hours because of a head injury ultimately require some rehabilitation. Clients with mild head injury may be overlooked in the population of people who need follow-up care. Mild head injuries can cause headache, memory difficulties, difficulty performing simple tasks, and irritability. These clinical manifestations may persist for a month or longer.

Rehabilitation may take place in an inpatient or outpatient setting, depending on the client's condition. Rehabilitation may include physical, occupational, speech and cognitive therapy and is essential in returning the client to maximal function. Nurses play a major role in the rehabilitation of the head-injured client and in the education of significant others.

More severely injured clients may be sent to rehabilitation facilities with feeding tubes or tracheostomy tubes in place. Clients and families need assistance in choosing a new health care facility that can deliver the level of care needed. If recovery is unlikely, the client may need to be transferred to an extended-care facility. Because many head-injured clients are young, previously healthy people, placement in a nursing home may be a very difficult reality for family members to accept. Teaching and support can greatly improve coping. Involvement of disciplines such as social services, pastoral care, or discharge planning can increase the family members' understanding of the next phase of care.

The rehabilitation of clients with brain injuries is challenging. In some cases, community reintegration is unsuccessful. Studies have reported improvement in the client's ability to lead a productive life with the use of interdisciplinary techniques that include rehabilitation in cognition, compensatory techniques, social skills, emotional adjustment, leisure skills, physical fitness, and health maintenance. Most clients require at least 6 months in an ongoing program of rehabilitation both in-patient and out-patient. The ability of a client in a persistent vegetative state to respond to stimuli is constantly being reviewed. Hopefully, with continued research families will be given accurate and compassionate answers to their questions and concerns about the patient's ability to respond.

Modifications for Older Clients

Although most head injuries caused by motor-vehicle accidents do not occur in the older population, injury caused by falls is common. Diagnosis of a head injury is often more difficult in older adults because of an atypical presentation. These clients also experience more complications. An older client may be less able to tolerate respiratory problems or cardiac dysrhythmias. The presence of chronic diseases such as chronic obstructive pulmonary disease or heart failure can make managing ventilation and fluid balance more difficult. If any type of mental impairment was present before the injury, recovery to full independence is less likely. Poor stamina and medical complications may impede rehabilitation.

SPINAL CORD INJURY

Injury to the spinal cord can range in severity from mild flexion-extension "whiplash" injuries to complete transection of the cord with permanent quadriplegia. Trauma to the cord can occur at any level but most commonly occurs in the cervical and lower thoracic-upper lumbar vertebrae. These common cord injuries are due in part to the support given by the ribs to the thoracic spine and the flexibility of the cervical and lumbar spinal segments.

Although this discussion focuses on nursing management of *acute* spinal cord injury (SCI), it should be appreciated that about 200,000 people with spinal cord injury are living in the United States.

Etiology and Risk Factors

Trauma is the most common cause of SCI. Each year about 10,000 people sustain such injury. Most victims are males between the ages of 16 and 30 years; only 9% of injuries occur in people over the age of 60. Traumatic SCI is most often caused by automobile or motorcycle accidents, gunshot or knife wounds, falls, and sports mishaps. More than half of all SCIs involve the cervical spine, and the rest occur in the thoracic, lumbar, and sacral spinal segments.

The feeling of immortality often experienced by adolescents and young adults contributes strongly to their risk of SCI. Young people may believe they can engage in dangerous behavior without being injured. The use of alcohol and illicit drugs can reinforce this belief in immortality. A young person who has experienced the devastation of SCI may best deliver the message of primary prevention. In several nationwide programs, head-injured and spinal cord–injured people are available to speak at school-sponsored educational programs.

Nontraumatic disorders may also result in SCI. These problems include the following:

- Cervical spondylosis with myelopathy (spinal canal narrowing with progressive injury to the cord and roots)
- Myelitis (infective or noninfective)
- Osteoporosis causing vertebral compression fractures
- Syringomyelia (central cavitation of the cord)
- Tumors, both infiltrative and compressive
- Vascular diseases, usually infarction or hemorrhage

Whatever the cause, SCI produces distinctive and debilitating damage. Nowhere else in the body can a local insult produce such devastation in proportion to the extent of tissue involved.

Flexion-Rotation, Dislocation, and Fracture-Dislocation Injuries

By far the most common SCI is flexion injury. When the head strikes the steering wheel or windshield, the spine is forced into acute hyperflexion (Figure 73-11, *A*). Rupture of the posterior ligaments results in forward dislocation of the vertebrae. Nutrient blood vessels may be damaged, leading to ischemia of the spinal cord. The cervical spine, usually at the C5-6 level, is most commonly affected by a flexion injury. In the thoracic-lumbar spine, this type of injury is most frequently seen at the T12-L1 level.

Hyperextension Injuries

Hyperextension injuries result after a fall in which the chin hits an object and the head is thrown back (see Figure 73-11, *B*). The anterior ligament is ruptured, with fracture of the posterior elements of the vertebral body. Hyperextension of the spinal cord against the ligamentum flavum can lead to dorsal column contusion and posterior dislocation of the vertebrae. Complete transection of the cord can follow a hyperextension injury, although transection of the cord is rare. Clients who have complete lesions of the spinal cord do not necessarily have transection of the cord. Complete lesions of the cord result in loss of all voluntary movement and sensation below the lesion and loss of reflex function in isolated segments of the cord.

Compression Injuries

Compression injuries are often caused by falls or jumps in which the person lands directly on the head, sacrum, or feet (see Figure 73-11, *C*). The force of impact fractures the vertebrae and the fragments compress the cord. Disk and bone fragments may be propelled into the spinal cord on impact. The lumbar and the lower thoracic vertebrae are the most commonly injured regions after a compression impact when the person lands on the feet. If the person lands on the head (as in diving into shallow water), the injury is to the cervical spine. About 50% of these injuries result in incomplete lesions. Incomplete lesions occur when some of the spinal tracts remain intact.

Unique Cervical Injuries

Three types of fractures are unique to the cervical spine (Figure 73-12):

1. *Fractures of the odontoid process* (the superior projection on C2) may be intact, with no detectable movement, or may be displaced, with movement and entrapment of the spinal cord.
2. A *hangman's fracture* is a bilateral fracture through the pedicles of C2, separating the posterior elements from the body of the vertebra.
3. The *Jefferson fracture* involves bursting of the ring of C1. The spinal canal usually widens.

These injuries are usually associated with other spinal injuries. Clients with these cervical fractures either die of the injury immediately or are stable and may walk into the emergency department reporting only neck pain.

Pathophysiology

Most often SCIs occur as a result of injury to the vertebrae. The most common sites of injury are at the C1-2, C4-6, and T11-L2 vertebrae. These segments of the spine are the most mobile and therefore the most easily injured.

The cord is injured as the result of acceleration, deceleration, or another force (e.g., impact) applied to the spine. The forces injure the spinal cord by compressing, pulling, or tearing the tissues. Microscopic bleeding occurs immediately after injury, primarily in the gray matter of the cord. Within the first hour, edema develops and often spreads along segments of the spinal cord. Arachidonic acid and its metabolites (prostaglandins, thromboxanes, and leukotrienes) cause edema. Cord edema peaks within 2 to 3 days and subsides within the first 7 days after injury. Although the site of the initial injury has the most edema and bleeding, some edema and bleeding extend at least for two cord segments on either side of the injury. The edema of the cord leads to temporary loss of sensation and function. Spinal cord tissue injury is related to the initial insult, biochemical changes, and hemodynamic instability. Therefore immediately after injury, it is not easy to determine the ultimate degree of permanent impairment.

Further changes include fragmentation of the axonal covering and loss of myelin. Phagocytic cells can injure

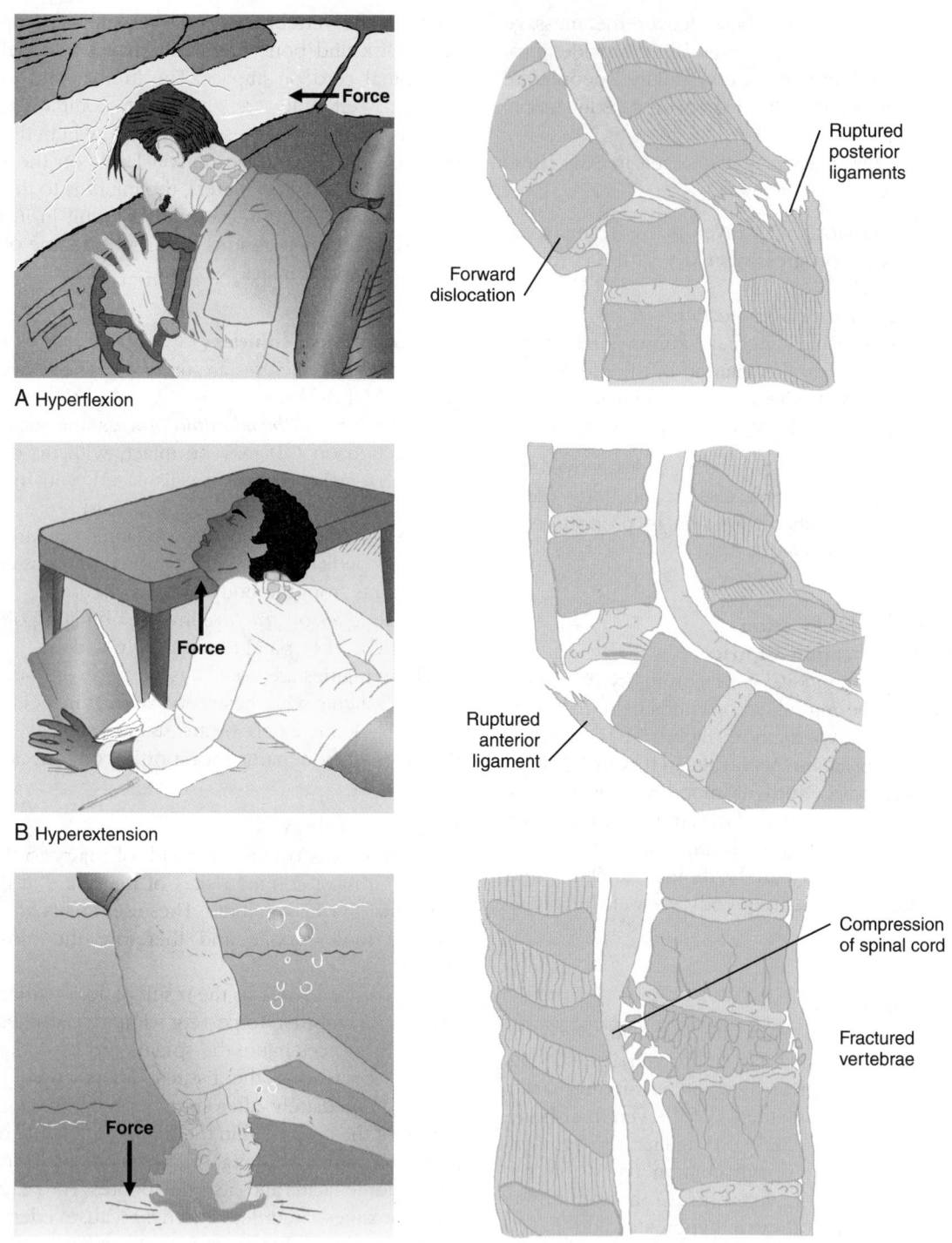

A Hyperflexion

Forward dislocation

Ruptured posterior ligaments

B Hyperextension

Ruptured anterior ligament

C Compression

Compression of spinal cord

Fractured vertebrae

■ **FIGURE 73–11**   Patterns of cervical spine injury. **A,** Hyperflexion injury of the cervical spine ruptures the posterior ligaments. **B,** Hyperextension injury of the cervical spine ruptures the anterior ligaments. **C,** Compression fractures crush the vertebrae and force bony fragments into the spinal canal.

surviving axons as they scavenge cellular debris. Chemotactic and inflammatory mediators further extend tissue necrosis. Macrophages engulf the spinal cord tissue and may cause a central cavity (called *post-traumatic syringomyelia*) to develop as early as 9 days after injury.

In addition, the oligodendroglial cells that support the cord are lost. Injury to the cord leads to rapid loss of axonal conduction from ion changes, such as very rapid increases in extracellular potassium and influx of calcium into the cell. Finally, free radicals are produced.

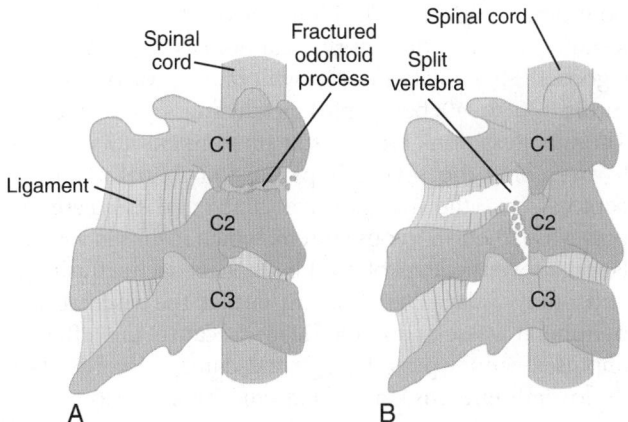

■ **FIGURE 73–12** Fractures of the cervical spine. **A,** Odontoid fractures are fractures of the superior projection of C2 that normally projects into C1. **B,** Hangman's fractures are of the pedicle of C2. The vertebra is split in half.

Free radicals are normally found in the body but are quickly controlled by antioxidant enzyme systems. When the antioxidant systems are overwhelmed, the free radicals damage tissues.

The physiologic response to SCI extends beyond changes within the spinal cord. For example, the sympathetic nervous system stress response results in reduced perfusion of the gastrointestinal tract and reduced production of gastric mucus to protect the lining. Ulceration and bleeding may develop.

Spasticity is the increased tone or contraction of muscles, producing stiff movements. Various CNS injuries or diseases such as SCI, strokes, and cerebral palsy may result in spasticity. After SCI, the brain can no longer influence reflex movements through the spinal cord. Eventually the lower part of the cord, using spinal reflex arcs, begins to work automatically. Spinal reflex activities include the flexor withdrawal reflex and reflex emptying of the bladder and bowel. These primitive spinal mechanisms, normally kept inactive by higher centers, are "released" when the normal inhibitions of the higher centers are destroyed. As recovery progresses, flexor responses are interspersed with extensor spasms. These movements ultimately develop into predominantly extensor activity. The client's limbs spasm into extension with movement. Spasticity may remain indefinitely or gradually decrease over time.

Clinical Manifestations
Level of Injury
The initial clinical manifestations of acute SCI depend on the level and extent of injury to the cord. Below the level of injury or lesion, the following functions are lost:

- Voluntary movement
- Sensation of pain, temperature, pressure, and *proprioception* (the ability to know where the body is in space)
- Bowel and bladder function
- Spinal and autonomic reflexes

The level of injury may be described in terms of (1) skeletal injury and (2) neurologic level of injury. Skeletal injury refers to the vertebral damage demonstrated by x-ray study. The criterion of the American Spinal Injury Association (ASIA) is useful in describing the level of spinal cord involvement: *The neurologic level of injury is the lowest segment of the spinal cord with bilateral intact sensory and motor function.* Sensory function is assessed according to dermatomes to identify the areas of skin with normal sensation. Motor function is measured by testing myotomes to identify muscles with active movement and full range of motion (ROM) against gravity. The ASIA Impairment Scale is as follows:

- Normal with sensory and motor function preserved
- Incomplete with the majority of motor function preserved
- Incomplete with nonfunctional motor function preserved
- Incomplete with only sensation preserved
- Complete with loss of sensation and motor function

Injury to the cervical cord produces quadriplegia. Injuries above the C4 level may be fatal because of loss of innervation to the diaphragm and intercostal muscles. Without immediate rescue breathing after the accident, the injured person will die of asphyxiation. Today, with the general public's knowledge of cardiopulmonary resuscitation, many people survive this injury to the cervical spine. Injuries to the remainder of the cervical spine create specific patterns of motor loss. Note that a person with a C7 injury is able to lift the shoulders, elbows, and wrists and has some hand function, but below C7 no motor function or sensation remains.

Injuries to the thoracic or lumbar spinal segment produce paraplegia. People with such injuries have function in their upper extremities and can be mobile in a wheelchair or with crutches and braces. People with L5 injury can extend the great toe and dorsiflex the ankle. They have no sensation in the perianal area, calf, heel, or small toe.

Changes in Reflexes
Reflexes, which normally cross the spinal cord and return to the stimulated limb, are absent in early SCI because of spinal shock. Blood pressure and temperature in denervated (without nervous function or innervation) areas fall markedly and respond poorly to reflex stimuli.

After spinal shock subsides, some body functions may return by reflex (e.g., control of the urinary bladder), but they lack integration with other visceral activities. Visceral activities may be initiated by atypical stimuli. For example, scratching the skin may cause vasodilation, sweating, and urination. Nervous system lesions may produce a type of defective urinary bladder function known as *neurogenic bladder.* For example, stimulation of the skin on the lower abdomen or thighs may cause reflex urination. This form of cord bladder is called a *reflex bladder.* Such stimulation may also cause reflex ejaculation and priapism (persistent abnormal penile erection without sexual desire) in paralyzed men.

Muscle Spasms

Intense and painful muscular spasms of the lower extremities occur following a traumatic complete transverse spinal cord lesion. In assisting the client and the family members to understand these movements, it should be explained that these muscle spasms are involuntary and do not mean that voluntary movement is returning. This information, although disappointing, is essential.

Muscle spasms range in intensity from mild muscular twitching to vigorous mass reflexogenic states. Extreme, involuntary muscle spasms can actually throw a client out of bed or wheelchair. Bed side rails are kept up and restraining straps are comfortably secured over the client lying on a stretcher. Muscle spasms, often aggravated by cold weather, prolonged periods of sitting, infections, or emotionally upsetting events, may become intolerable. Reflex spasms may be triggered by extrinsic or visceral stimuli, such as a distended bladder.

Emotion (e.g., anxiety, crying, anger, laughing) or cutaneous stimulation (e.g., tickling, stroking, pinching) may initiate spastic movements. By learning to recognize events that trigger such reflex spasms, the client may use these potentially annoying movements to achieve functional activities such as urination.

Autonomic Dysreflexia

Autonomic dysreflexia, also known as *autonomic hyperreflexia,* is a life-threatening syndrome. It is a cluster of clinical manifestations that results when multiple spinal cord autonomic responses discharge simultaneously. This syndrome, observed in as many as 85% of clients with cord injury above the T6 level, can occur anytime after spinal shock has resolved. Dysreflexia often lessens as time after injury passes, but it may recur. The manifestations of autonomic dysreflexia result from an exaggerated sympathetic response to a noxious stimulus below the level of the cord lesion. Common stimuli are bladder and bowel distention but may also include pressure ulcers, spasms, pain, pressure on the penis, excessive rectal stimulation, bladder stones, ingrown toenails, abdominal abnormalities, or uterine contractions.

Exaggerated sympathetic responses cause the blood vessels below the level of injury to constrict. As a result, the client develops hypertension (readings of 20 mm Hg above baseline are considered hypertensive), a pounding headache, flushing above the level of the lesion, nasal stuffiness, diaphoresis, piloerection ("gooseflesh"), dilated pupils with blurred vision, bradycardia (30 to 40 beats/min), restlessness, and nausea. The manifestations are a result of compensatory efforts to overcome the severe hypertension. Initially baroreceptors sense the hypertensive stimuli and stimulate the parasympathetic nervous system, which results in vasodilation above the level of cord injury (headache, flushing) and bradycardia. The problem is that the visceral and peripheral vessels do not dilate because the efferent impulses cannot pass through the damaged cord. Thus the overall effect is one of extreme hypertension (with pressures possibly as high as 300 mm Hg). Seizures and cerebral hemorrhage occur in about 10% to 15% of cases. See the later discussion on Risk for Autonomic Dysreflexia for interventions.

Clinical Syndromes Causing Partial Paralysis

Five spinal cord syndromes cause partial paralysis (Figure 73-13): central cord syndrome, anterior cord syndrome, Brown-Séquard syndrome, conus medullaris syndrome, and cauda equina syndrome. Each has distinctive neurologic features.

Central Cord Syndrome. Central cord syndrome (most common with hyperextension-hyperflexion injuries) produces more weakness in the upper extremities than in the lower extremities. This type of injury occurs most often in the older adult who has a pre-existing spinal stenosis. This injury may also occur in a person who lands on the head such as when diving into shallow water and hitting the bottom. The common mechanism of injury is a fall forward. The weakness is caused by edema and hemorrhage in the central area of the cord, which is predominantly occupied by nerve tracts to the hands and arms.

Anterior Cord Syndrome. A lesion in the anterior spinal cord causes anterior cord syndrome, with complete motor function loss and decreased pain sensation. Deep pressure, position sense, and two-point discrimination sensations remain intact. Often the anterior spinal artery is affected, causing an infarction of spinal cord tissue. Cervical cord concussion may produce various degrees of motor and sensory deficit, which completely resolve within hours. Occasionally cervical cord trauma produces only root injuries, which may paralyze isolated muscles or muscle groups in the arms and shoulders. These deficits are usually permanent.

Brown-Séquard Syndrome. Brown-Séquard syndrome is caused by lateral hemisection of the cord (i.e., when half the cord is cut or otherwise damaged, as in a bullet or knife wound). This injury results in ipsilateral (same

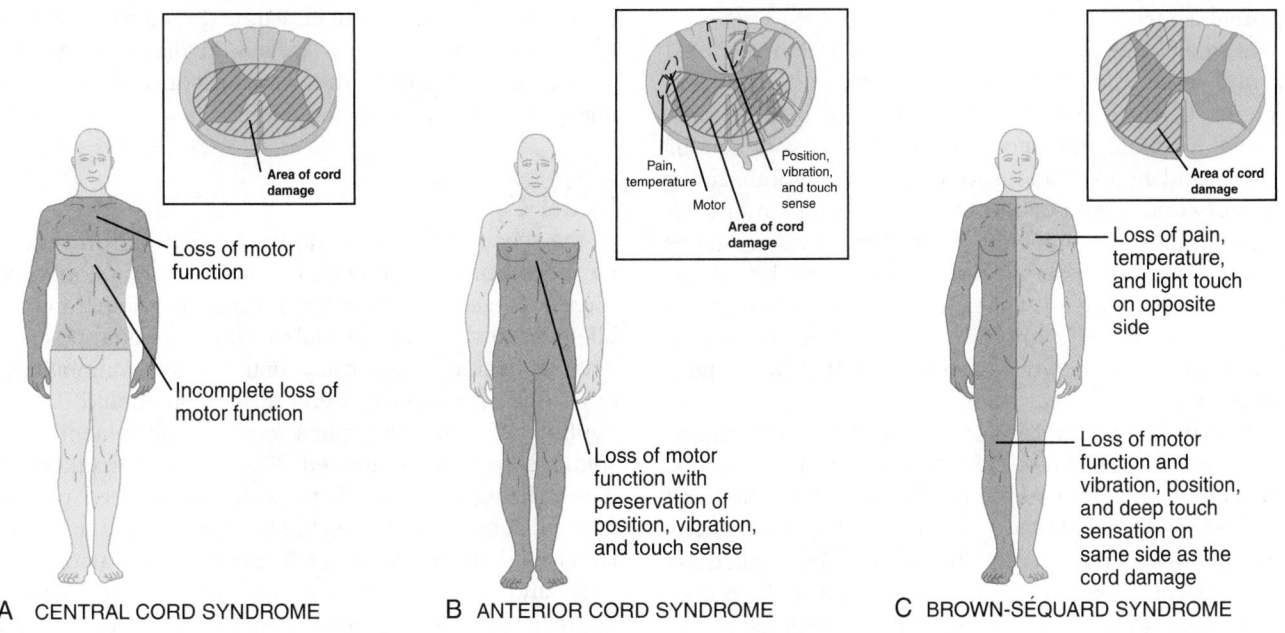

A   CENTRAL CORD SYNDROME

B   ANTERIOR CORD SYNDROME

C   BROWN-SÉQUARD SYNDROME

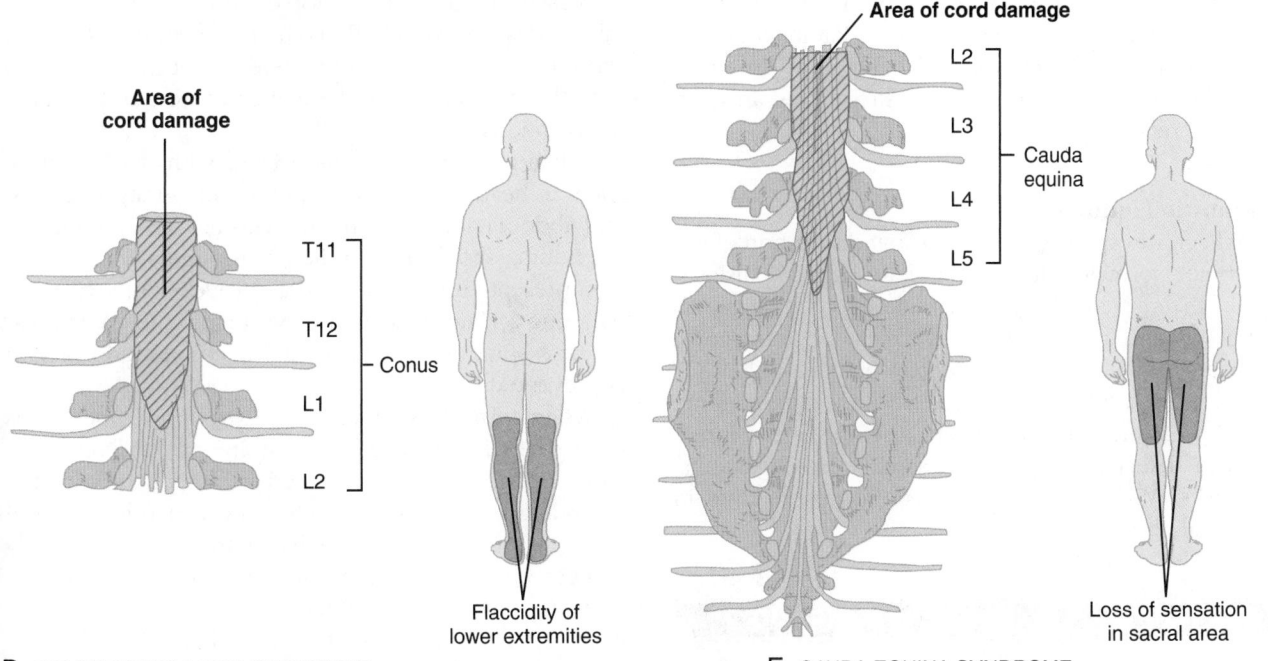

D   CONUS MEDULLARIS SYNDROME

E   CAUDA EQUINA SYNDROME

■ **FIGURE 73–13**   Patterns of injury leading to partial paralysis. **A,** Central cord syndrome. **B,** Anterior cord syndrome. **C,** Brown-Séquard syndrome. **D,** Conus medullaris syndrome. **E,** Cauda equina syndrome.

side) motor paralysis, loss of vibratory and position sense, and contralateral (opposite side) loss of pain and temperature sensation.

Conus Medullaris Syndrome. *Conus medullaris syndrome* follows damage to the lumbar nerve roots and the conus medullaris in the spinal cord. The client usually has bowel and bladder areflexia and flaccid lower

extremities. The bulbocavernosus penile (erection) and micturition reflexes may be preserved when damage is limited to the upper sacral segments of the spinal cord.

Cauda Equina Syndrome. Injury to the lumbosacral nerve roots below the conus medullaris results in the cauda equina syndrome. The client experiences areflexia of the bowel, bladder, and lower extremities.

Spinal Shock

The immediate response to cord transection is called *spinal shock*. The client with SCI experiences a complete loss of skeletal muscle function, bowel and bladder tone, sexual function, and autonomic reflexes. Loss of venous return and hypotension also occur. The hypothalamus cannot control temperature by vasoconstriction and increased metabolism; therefore the client's body assumes the environmental temperature. Spinal shock is most severe in clients with higher levels of SCI. Clients with thoracic or lumbar injuries are often unaffected because the sympathetic nervous system is spared with these levels of injury.

Spinal shock may last for 1 to 6 weeks. Indications that spinal shock is resolving include return of reflexes, development of hyperreflexia rather than flaccidity, and return of reflex emptying of the bladder. The earliest reflexes recovered are the flexor reflexes evoked by noxious cutaneous stimulation. The return of the bulbo-cavernosus reflex (anal sphincter contraction in response to squeezing the glans penis or tugging on the urinary catheter) in male patients is also an early indicator of recovery from spinal shock. Babinski's reflex (dorsiflexion of the great toe with fanning of the other toes when the sole of the foot is stroked) is an early returning reflex.

Diagnostic Findings

Lateral cervical spine x-rays may show dislocation of the vertebrae. Normally, the vertebrae are aligned. Dislocation of the vertebrae appears as one or more segments being offset. If present, there is likely also damage to the ligaments that connect one vertebra to another. CT scans are used to see in great detail how the vertebrae are aligned and whether other structures are injured. MRI can detect damage to the spinal cord, ligaments, and disks. MRI can also detect edema or bleeding in the spinal cord.

OUTCOME MANAGEMENT

Both initial (especially during the first hour after injury) and long-term interventions provided for a client who has sustained an SCI significantly influence the following:

- The extent of the injury and associated deficits
- How well the person survives the acute phase of injury
- The success of recovery and rehabilitation

People with SCI can lead productive and, in many cases, independent lives. As with head injury, information obtained from witnesses to the accident can assist in diagnosis and treatment. Information from witnesses or the client should include the mechanism of injury, the presence and duration of loss of consciousness, and impairment of motor function. It is also important to diagnose SCI correctly. Delays in diagnosis can be attributed to alcohol intoxication, concomitant head injury, or other multiple injuries.

Initial Care

At the scene of the accident, the injured person should be moved only when adequate numbers of people are present to accomplish while keeping the spinal immobile. The neck should be stabilized in a neutral position without flexion or extension until a fixed immobilizing device can be applied. Cervical traction should not be applied. Without x-ray films to guide movements, the spinal cord can be injured. The simplest method of immobilizing the spine is to place the affected person on a spine board and to secure the spine with a hard collar around the neck and self-fastening ties across the torso and legs. Transparent stiff collars have become popular because they allow visualization of the carotid arteries and trachea. Excellent on-the-scene care has increased the number of people who are neurologically intact despite vertebral column fractures. Accurate reporting of the person's baseline deficits is essential to help the physician plan the aggressiveness of treatment interventions.

Spinal trauma is often associated with other injuries, such as head injury, chest trauma, extremity fractures, and abdominal injury. Anyone who has sustained multiple trauma should be handled as though spinal injuries are present until assessment proves otherwise. In handling a client in whom cervical spine injury is present, the spine is kept in neutral alignment and flexion is prevented.

When turning is required, a *logrolling* maneuver is used. The client is placed in a supine position on a firm surface. The head is supported in alignment with the body and is immobilized with a firm, padded cervical collar. Some physicians use halter traction immediately to keep the cervical spine aligned and prevent movement. Clothing is cut off rather than removed. The client is transported on a flat, firm stretcher with the neck immobilized. SCI-trained personnel should remain with the client while x-ray studies are taken to ensure that the cervical spine is not moved.

Cervical spine injury may produce respiratory distress. When breathing difficulty is noted, immediate action is taken to maintain a patent airway and to provide adequate oxygenation. It is important that the client's neck not be hyperextended during intubation; therefore the jaw thrust technique is used. Suctioning is performed as necessary to maintain a patent airway. Mechanically assisted ventilation is required when definite loss or impairment of respiratory muscle function occurs. Respiratory parameters can be used to guide the decision of whether to ventilate the client mechanically. Serial decreases in vital capacity (less than 15 ml/kg), along with an increase in the partial pressure of arterial carbon dioxide ($Paco_2$), constitute a good predictor of impending pulmonary failure.

In the emergency department, a client who has sustained a severe cervical injury should be placed immediately in skeletal traction to immobilize the cervical spine and reduce the fracture and dislocation. Gardner-Wells tongs are inserted through the outer table of the skull (Figure 73-14). Traction is applied to the tongs via rope, pulleys, and weights. Traction weight is begun with 10 to 20 pounds (4.5 to 9.1 kg) and is gradually increased to accomplish bone reduction. When proper alignment is obtained and verified by x-ray examination, the traction weight may be lessened to maintain the reduction. Traction is not used to stabilize and immobilize thoracic or lumbar spinal fractures or fracture-dislocations because there is no effective way to provide it. Therefore the spine is kept in alignment, and logrolling is used as needed, until surgical stabilization can be performed.

A cross-table lateral x-ray film of the cervical spine is obtained before transport of the injured person. Lateral and anteroposterior x-ray studies are not usually sufficient. To visualize lower cervical fractures, it is necessary either to apply downward traction to the arms or have the arms in the swimmer's position during x-ray examination. If a high-level cervical lesion is suspected, a view of the odontoid bone through the open mouth may be required. CT and MRI are often used to establish the extent of the injury. A brief but thorough neurologic examination is made to assess the extent of injury and to establish a baseline of function and involvement for later comparison.

Common emergency interventions include insertion of an IV line and infusion of normal saline, insertion of an indwelling catheter, administration of high-dose steroids, administration of vasoactive medications to maintain systolic blood pressure, insertion of a nasogastric tube, and provision of oxygen if oxygen saturation is low.

Once orthopedic and medical stabilization of the fracture has been achieved, the client is transferred to an ICU or to an SCI center. It is important that the client be appropriately immobilized before transport.

Medical Management

Maintaining Vital Functions

Respiratory compromise may occur, and if the client develops diaphragmatic fatigue mechanical ventilation may be needed. Arterial blood gases are monitored closely. The client may be transferred to a kinetic treatment bed to reduce the risk of pressure ulcer development, improve pulmonary function, and minimize complications of immobility. These beds are shown in Figure 68-2 on p. 1801.

Vasoactive agents are commonly used to support blood pressure immediately after injury. Short-term high-dose methylprednisolone therapy is started in people with SCI less than 8 hours old. A bolus dose of 30 mg/kg infused over 1 hour followed by 5.4 mg/kg infused over 23 hours is usual. Other therapies may include the use of neuropeptides and thyrotropin-releasing hormone, which may induce some reversal of lesions by decreasing post-traumatic ischemia. Histamine-2 (H_2) receptor-blocking agents are often given to reduce the risk of gastric and intestinal bleeding. Long-term pharmacologic management may include urinary antiseptics, anticoagulants, laxatives, and antispasmodics.

Respiratory impairment, position, emotional status, or gastrointestinal function may compromise nutritional intake. Intubation eliminates the possibility of oral intake, whereas a tracheostomy does not. Clients with a tracheostomy require time to adjust to swallowing with the tube in place and must be carefully monitored to prevent aspiration.

Aspiration is also a risk for clients who must remain flat while in tongs and traction. Although these clients may be capable of swallowing, it is unlikely that they

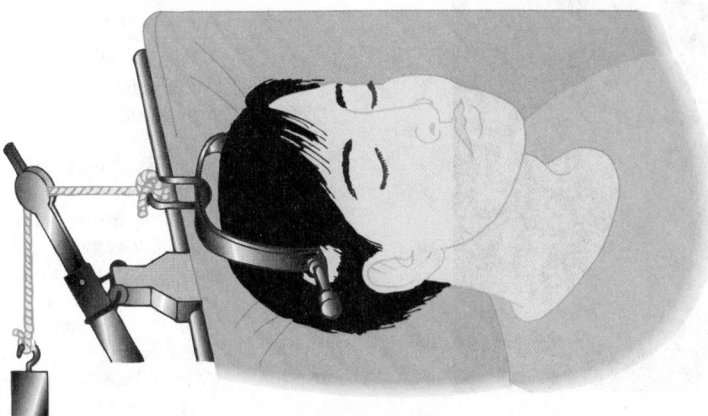

■ **FIGURE 73-14** Gardner-Wells tongs are used to provide skeletal traction on the cervical spine before operative stabilization.

will be able to consume safely enough food to meet their metabolic needs. Clients wearing a halo jacket (Figure 73-15) often experience difficulty eating because the halo jacket immobilizes the head. They should be encouraged to take small bites, eat slowly, and concentrate on swallowing.

Assessment of Other Injuries

Once the client's spine and emergency medical conditions have been stabilized, a complete neurologic assessment is performed. Several associated injuries are commonly seen with SCI. These include orthopedic injury to the spine, head injury, chest injury, abdominal injury, and genitourinary injury. Some of these injuries may not be immediately evident in the emergency department, and ongoing assessments are made until the problem is ruled out.

Monitoring for Complications

Potential complications include spinal shock, atelectasis, pneumonia, bradycardia, hypotension, deep vein thrombosis (DVT), gastrointestinal bleeding, pressure ulcers, joint contractures, and psychological dysfunction such as denial and depression. Depression is a common reaction to SCI and may be associated with inhibition of the appetite. Choosing when and what to eat may be one of the few areas of control left to the person with SCI.

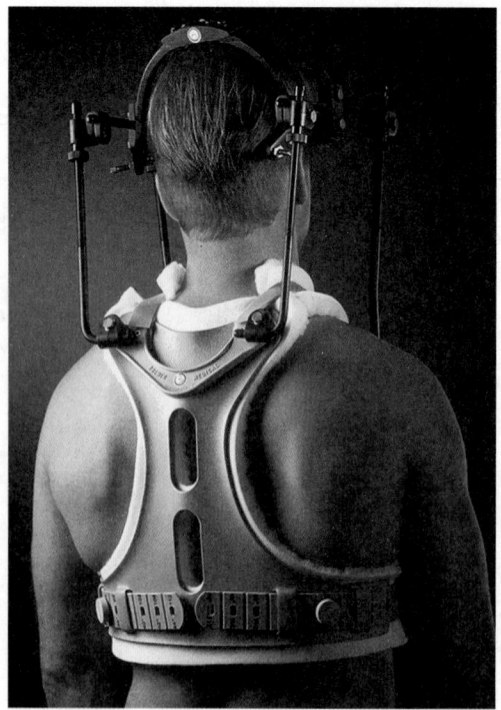

■ **FIGURE 73-15** Halo traction. This form of traction immobilizes the cervical spine so that the client can move without risk of further injury. *(Courtesy DePuy Spine, a Johnson & Johnson Company, Raynham, Mass.)*

As much free choice of dietary intake as is feasible should be encouraged. Any of these conditions can severely limit a spinal injury client's oral intake at a time when a high-calorie, high-protein diet is needed. Enteral feeding or total parenteral hyperalimentation is often prescribed until oral intake is sufficient to meet the body's needs.

Initial Nursing Management of the Client with Spinal Cord Injury

---

Assessment. A holistic assessment approach is essential in planning for nursing care of clients with SCI. Every system of the body is affected with these injuries. A complete baseline assessment is obtained initially. The results of subsequent assessments are then compared with the baseline results. Specific components in the assessment of the client with an SCI depend on the client's phase of treatment. Therefore assessment is addressed within the following sections.

Careful monitoring of hemodynamic parameters is essential. Heart rate, blood pressure, temperature, respirations, fluid balance, and peripheral oxygen saturation (by pulse oximetry) should be monitored continuously.

If the client is conscious, ask whether there is any pain. Sensation of touch and pinprick is assessed in the feet, legs, trunk, hands, and arms. Levels of sensation are documented according to dermatomes. To assess motor function, ask the client to wiggle toes, move ankles, flex knees, and move hands and arms. The location, symmetry, and strength of muscle movement are documented (Table 73-1). The major reflexes—that is, the Achilles, patellar, biceps, and triceps tendon reflexes—are briefly tested. Assessment for intact sensation in areas such as the perineum is also necessary. If the patient is

TABLE 73-1	Motor Assessment After Spinal Cord Injury
Spinal Nerve(s)	**Assessment Technique**
C4-5	Shoulders are shrugged against downward pressure of examiner's hands
C5-6	Arm is pulled up from resting position against resistance
C7	From flexed position, arm is straightened out against resistance
C7	Index finger is held firmly to thumb against resistance to pull it away
C8	Hand grasp strength is evaluated
L2-4	Leg is lifted from bed against resistance
L2-4	From flexed position, knee is extended against resistance
L5-S1	Knee is flexed against resistance
L5	Foot is pulled up toward nose against resistance
S1	Foot is pushed down (as in stepping on automobile gas pedal) against resistance

unresponsive, assessment is more limited. Assess respiratory status by observing for spontaneous movement and thorax expansion. Sensation and movement of extremities are assessed by watching the client for a few moments or by applying a painful stimulus (nail bed pressure) and observing for withdrawal.

Usually the client is awake and may be concerned about obtaining pain relief, the chances of survival, and the safety of any other people in the accident. Once these issues are addressed, the client may begin to appraise the severity of his or her own injury.

Rehabilitation begins when the client is admitted to the acute health care facility. During the acute stage, nursing and medical attention is appropriately focused on immediate needs. It is also imperative to remember that the client probably will have severe residual disabilities and must make major lifestyle changes. Care provided in the acute period can significantly affect the client's later life. Prevention of complications such as infection, pressure sores, and contractures facilitates rehabilitation and reduces suffering, disability, and expense. Challenges in caring for clients with SCI are presented in the Case Study below.

Diagnosis, Outcomes, Interventions

Collaborative Problem: Risk for Hypotension. Clients suffering from SCI are at risk for the development of hypotension. The collaborative problem of *Risk for Hypotension* is related to vasodilation and the inability to vasoconstrict attributable to loss of reflexes rather than to volume depletion.

Outcomes. The nurse will monitor for hypotension and pulmonary fluid overload as evidenced by systolic blood pressure greater than 90 mm Hg, heart rate more than 60 beats/min, and the client alert and oriented with an adequate urine output.

Interventions. Hypotension associated with spinal shock is initially treated with IV fluid. It is important to remember that fluid depletion is seldom the cause of hypotension; rather, lack of reflexes is the likely cause. Therefore fluid resuscitation should be carefully monitored to avoid fluid

---

CASE STUDY   *evolve*

Spinal Cord Injury

Ben Brown is a 21-year-old college junior who was admitted to the intensive care unit (ICU) via the emergency department for evaluation and treatment of a spinal cord injury (SCI) sustained in a diving accident. Consider the type of fracture most typical from this type of accident. He is accompanied by his fiancée and his parents....

Case Study continued on the website and the CD-ROM with discussions, multiple-choice questions, and a nursing care plan.

---

overload, which can lead to pulmonary edema. Vasopressor agents are often given in the acute phase of SCI to maintain blood pressure. Elevating the feet can aid venous return in acute situations.

Diagnosis: Impaired Spontaneous Ventilation, Ineffective Airway Clearance, Impaired Gas Exchange. Cervical-level SCI carries a high risk of respiratory compromise. Any or all three of these nursing diagnoses may be appropriate.

Outcomes. The client will show no manifestations of respiratory compromise as evidenced by clear lung sounds; Pao_2, Pco_2, pH, and oxygen saturation values within normal limits; unlabored respirations; and normal vital capacity.

Interventions. Chest physical therapy can help mobilize secretions and prevent pneumonia, as can suctioning and assisted coughing. When spinal cord edema has temporarily impaired respiratory function, mechanical ventilation is used to support respiration. Intubation and ventilation can be frightening to a person who has been able to breathe independently. Sedation is administered as needed after intubation. Provide reassurance that mechanical ventilation will probably not be permanent. Clients may also be placed on a kinetic bed to maximize pulmonary function.

For extended airway management, a tracheostomy may be required to allow for long-term controlled ventilation, to facilitate the removal of tracheobronchial secretions, and to seal off the esophagus from the trachea for the prevention of aspiration. An abdominal binder is often used to provide abdominal support, to facilitate diaphragmatic breathing, and to increase venous return.

Diagnosis: Risk for Aspiration. Clients without a tracheostomy or with ineffective airway clearance or in whom the gag reflex is absent are at higher risk for aspiration. Aspiration is a common cause of morbidity in SCI clients.

Outcomes. The client will exhibit no manifestations of aspiration as evidenced by clear lung sounds; absence of stridor and fever; minimal amounts of clear mucus upon suctioning; and Pao_2, $Paco_2$, pH, and oxygen saturation values within normal limits.

Interventions. Suctioning equipment should be kept available and breath sounds assessed every 1 or 2 hours in acutely ill clients. The results of arterial blood gas analysis and pulse oximetry are monitored to determine the degree of oxygenation provided with mechanical ventilation or supplemental oxygen administration. Tracheobronchial suctioning is performed frequently to prevent or reduce the accumulation of secretions from immobility, lack of a cough reflex, or pneumonia. Monitor the electrocardiogram for dysrhythmias (e.g., premature ventricular contractions) resulting from hypoxia during suctioning.

Diagnosis: Ineffective Thermoregulation. Thermoregulation may be altered because of loss of hypothalamic control of the sympathetic nervous system in clients with SCI above the T6 level.

Outcomes. The client will maintain normothermic status.

Interventions. Rectal or core temperature is monitored every 4 hours during the first 72 hours after injury. Skin surfaces are palpated for areas of warmth, coolness, and moisture. Control the environmental temperature by using bed linens as needed to warm the client, eliminating drafts in the room, and using hypothermia blankets cautiously.

Evaluation. The problems identified in the early period of SCI care may resolve within 72 hours, especially if no other serious injuries or medical problems are present. If the client remains in an ICU for a prolonged time, implement other aspects of SCI care as discussed later.

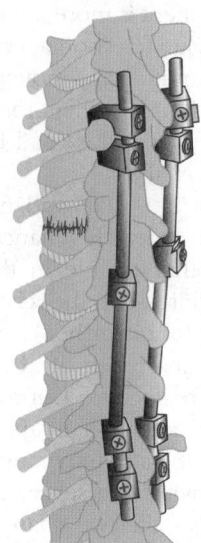

■ **FIGURE 73-16** Fractures of the spine are often stabilized with internal fixation devices.

Surgical Management

The goal of surgical intervention is to stabilize the spine. Decompressive laminectomy, in which the laminae of the vertebrae are removed to minimize pressure on the spinal cord, can be used for complete SCIs. Stabilization by surgical fusion can be done by insertion of metal plates and screws or the use of bone grafts alone or in combination.

Cervical fractures can also be allowed to heal with stabilization of bone fragments achieved by immobilization in a brace or halo jacket (see Figure 73-15). The halo jacket has a ring that is fixed to the skull with pins. This ring is then attached to the jacket by rods. This system provides the traction required to maintain cervical alignment. A halo jacket allows early mobilization and rehabilitation.

SAFETY
ALERT

The wrench that comes with the brace should always be taped to the front of the jacket to allow quick removal in case of emergency. If the client has some mobility remaining, always assist during the client's first attempt at any activity. The halo jacket changes the client's center of gravity, making falls a constant risk. Never grasp the rods to help reposition the client. Perform pin site care around the pin insertion sites daily. See your agency's policy manual for guidelines.

Burst fractures of the thoracic and lumbar spinal segments can be treated with body casts, Harrington rods, or other devices for spine stabilization. Spine stabilization devices are commonly inserted through a posterior incision (Figure 73-16). After the operation, perform the usual postoperative assessments, including an assessment of the neurovascular status of the legs. Chest tubes and nasogastric tubes are inserted during surgery. The client is logrolled to facilitate maintenance of respiration and skin perfusion. Pain is managed with continuous-infusion or injected opioids. The client usually is fitted for a body brace, and mobilization begins on the fourth day.

Complications of surgery include infection and poor wound healing as well as those related to anesthesia. Both infection and impaired wound healing are more likely to occur in a malnourished client.

Spinal Cord Injury Rehabilitation

Clients with all levels of injury and of all ages benefit from rehabilitation. The client and family are involved in all phases. In all phases of rehabilitation, it is imperative that a motivated client be given the opportunity to perform any skill, even if the nurse or the physician can accomplish it more quickly. Allowing the client to attempt a complex skill demonstrates support of the client's self-care abilities. The key to rehabilitation is a multidisciplinary team of physicians, nurses, and allied health care providers (physical therapists, occupational therapists, speech and language pathologists) to reduce morbidity, maximize functional recovery, and promote independence.

Establish Functional Goals
Prediction of functional ability after SCI can generally be guided by the degree of residual muscle function (Table 73-2). It is intended to be a guide and might not represent ability in all clients with various levels of injury.

Promote Mobility
Wheelchairs provide mobility, and having the proper wheelchair is crucial. The wheelchair design must provide the client with the ability to propel the chair and prevent development of spinal deformities and pressure

TABLE 73–2 Functional Goals in Rehabilitation After Spinal Cord Injury

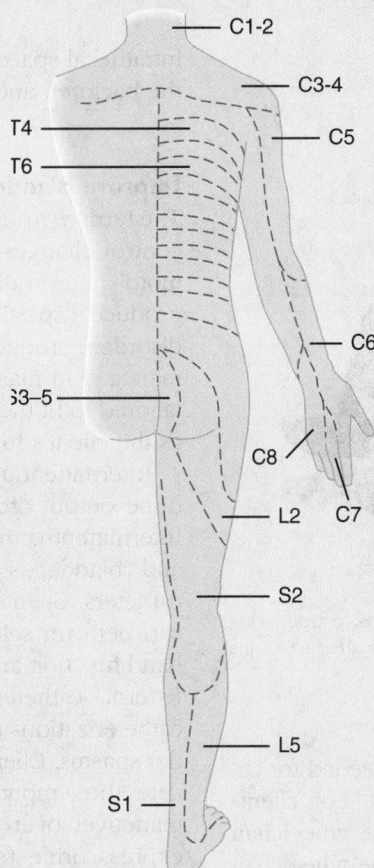

Spinal Cord Level	Muscle Function/Sensory Impairment	Functional Goals
C1-2	No phrenic nerve function; no sensation below neck	Respirations managed with phrenic pacemaker
C3-4	Neck control; scapular elevators; diaphragm function may be weak or absent	Manipulate electric wheelchair with breath control, chin control, or voice activation
C5	Fair to good shoulder control; functional deltoids/biceps; elbow flexion	Dress upper trunk; turn self in bed with or without arm slings
		Propel wheelchair with hand splints or after tenodesis
	No sensation below clavicles	Assist in getting into and out of bed; may learn to write or type
C6	Ability to lift shoulders, elbows, and wrists (partial)	Dress upper trunk; sometimes dress lower trunk
	Sensation as in C5 but more in arms and thumbs	Propel wheelchair with hand rim projections
		Self-feeding with hand splints
		Transfer from wheelchair to bed with or without minimal assistance (e.g., sliding board)
		Assist in getting to and from bedside commode; self-catheterization
C7	Ability to lift shoulders, elbows, wrists, and hands (partial)	Independent in transfer to bed, car, and toilet
	Sensation as in C6 level, with more in arms and middle fingers	Total dressing independence
		Propel wheelchair with standard hand rims
		Self-feeding with no assistive devices
C8	Ability to lift shoulders, elbows, wrists, and hands (partial)	Independent in transfer to bed, car, and toilet
	Sensation as in C7 level, with more in arms and little fingers	Total dressing independence
		Propel wheelchair with standard hand rims
		Self-feeding with no assistive devices
T1-4	Ability to use arms and hands normally	Independent in transfer to bed, car, and toilet
	No sensation below nipple line	Total dressing independence
	No trunk control	Propel wheelchair with standard hand rims
		Self-feeding with no assistive devices
		Transfer from wheelchair to floor and return
		Propel wheelchair up and down curb
		Transfer from wheelchair to tub and return
T5-L2	Partial to good trunk stability	Total wheelchair independence
	Able to use intercostal muscles	Limited ambulation with bilateral long leg braces and crutches (injury at T12 or below)
	No sensation below level of injury	
L3-4	All trunk-pelvic stabilizers intact; hip flexors, adductors, quadriceps	Ambulation with short leg braces with or without crutches depending on level of injury
L5-S3	Hip extensors, abductors; knee flexors; ankle control	No equipment needed if plantar flexion is strong enough for push-off at end of stance
	No sensation below midanterior thigh or in perianal area	

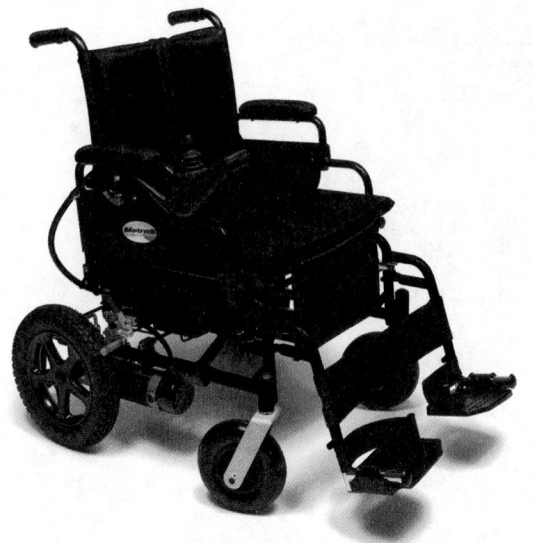

■ **FIGURE 73–17** A wheelchair with power hand controls for clients with C1-3 cervical spine injury. A respirator can be attached to the wheelchair. *(Courtesy Graham-Field Health Products, Atlanta, Ga.)*

ulcers. A high back and head support are needed for clients without arm function (Figure 73-17). For clients who can use their arms, the back of the wheelchair should be at the level of the scapula and the wheelchair should be lower than normal to facilitate transfers. Cushions help reduce pressure and the risk of pressure ulcers. Cushions, however, do not prevent pressure ulcers, and weight shifts are still needed every 10 to 15 minutes of time spent in the wheelchair. Physical therapists work with the client to teach how to transfer from bed to a wheelchair, from a wheelchair into and out of a car, and from the wheelchair onto a toilet.

Current emphasis is on strengthening muscles rather than using braces; however, back braces may be prescribed after lumbar spinal injury or for intervertebral disk problems. More frequently, a thoracolumbosacral orthosis is used. This device is a custom-made plastic brace with front and back pieces that attach together with self-fastening straps. This brace provides stability for the healing spine. The nurse is responsible for supervising the unlicensed professional whenever he or she is assisting with positioning transfers for a client with a spinal abnormality.

Reduce Spasticity

Spasticity often interferes with positioning and functional activities. However, spasticity also maintains muscle bulk, facilitates venous return, prevents DVT, and can aid in transfers. Treatment includes ROM exercises. Oral antispasmodic medications such as baclofen, dantrolene sodium, and clonidine are used only when the spasms cause discomfort or safety concerns. An implanted pump designed to deliver baclofen through a catheter into the intrathecal space can be used to increase the efficacy of the baclofen and decreasing dosages.

Improve Bladder and Bowel Control

The term *neurogenic bladder* is used to describe bladder control changes that occur with both upper and lower motor neuron disorders. Upper motor neuron disorders produce a spastic or reflex bladder. Lower motor neuron disorders produce a flaccid bladder. The bladder can be managed in many ways, and treatment options must be tailored to fit the client's preferences and lifestyle as well as the client's functional abilities.

Intermittent urinary catheterization is begun when the urine output drops to less than 600 ml in 4 to 6 hours. Intermittent catheterization reduces the risk of infection and bladder stone formation caused by indwelling catheters. Clients with injuries at the C6 level and lower can perform self-catheterization, if they have adequate hand function and can manage lower extremity clothing. External catheters are used for men who void between catheterizations or for those who leak urine during bladder spasms. Clients with arm function are taught to facilitate the emptying of their bladder using the Credé maneuver over the bladder to relax the sphincter and express urine (see Promote Bladder Retraining in the later nursing management section).

Urinary complications occur because of incomplete emptying of the bladder, necessitating catheterization. Catheterization may predispose the client to infection and vesicoureteral reflux, which may lead to kidney complications. Renal calculi, pyelonephritis, and hydronephrosis are major causes of considerable disability and even death in paralyzed clients.

Compared to indwelling catheters, suprapubic catheters seem to offer the advantages of less infection and urethral injury. Indwelling catheters are not ideal from a medical standpoint but are preferred by many clients because of the ease of management. Complications from catheters include infection, bladder stones, urethral damage, and a reported increased incidence of bladder cancer. A neurogenic bladder may also be managed pharmacologically with medications such as bethanechol (Urecholine) to stimulate bladder contraction or oxybutynin (Ditropan) to reduce bladder contraction. Urine-acidifying agents may also be prescribed to reduce the risk of infection.

A neurogenic bowel is similar to a neurogenic bladder in that the client cannot control defecation. The goal is to develop a bowel elimination method that is convenient, effective, and least expensive for the client. Sufficient fluid and fiber intake is essential. Consistent timing and position are important to a successful program. When fiber is added to or increased in the diet, it must be done slowly to avoid cramping and diarrhea. Stool softeners and bulk laxatives may also be used.

Bowel movements of clients with upper motor neuron damage are generally regulated with suppositories or digital stimulation every day or every other day to reduce the risk of autonomic dysreflexia. A lower motor neuron neurogenic bowel is more difficult to regulate, and often the client requires manual removal of impacted fecal material.

Prevent Pressure Ulcers

Numb skin is associated with an increased frequency of pressure ulcers. During the acute care period, the risk of pressure ulcer development is related to the level of injury, completeness of the injury, and duration of immobilization. Once the client is seated in a wheelchair, pressure ulcers can develop on the ischia as a result of prolonged sitting. Clients should be turned every 2 hours when in bed. If the client can reposition or turn without assistance in bed, an overlay mattress should be used and an alarm clock set to ring every two hours as a reminder during sleep.

A client with spinal fractures may be placed on a rotating bed (see Figure 68-2). It is equipped with supportive packs and straps that keep the body in neutral alignment while the bed continuously oscillates from side to side. If rotation is greater than 40 degrees, the continuous motion helps to prevent skin breakdown, reduce urinary stasis, and promote lung aeration. Skin inspection must be performed closely on the sacrum for signs of shearing. Unfortunately, the constant movement may also stimulate peristalsis, resulting in severe diarrhea. Some clients also experience disorientation from the constant movement and have reported fear of falling. Staff members should remain with the client initially to provide emotional support and reassurance. Also, it is important to pull window curtains at night because a client in a rotating bed who can see himself or herself "floating" in the window reflection can become disoriented or frightened.

Reduce Respiratory Dysfunction

Respiratory dysfunction is a significant cause of morbidity and mortality after SCI. Clients with injury to C3 have paralyzed diaphragms and will need phrenic pacing once they are weaned from a ventilator. In injuries lower than C3, the diaphragm may be the only functional muscle that is active in respiration because the intercostal and abdominal muscles are often paralyzed. Vital capacity and inspiratory reserve volume are markedly diminished. The client should be taught to use incentive spirometry and diaphragmatic breathing to enhance vital capacity. Glossopharyngeal breathing uses the tongue and muscles of the pharynx to force air into the lungs. This technique enhances vital capacity and promotes chest expansion.

Promote Expression of Sexuality

Sexual function in spinal cord–injured men depends on the location of the lesion (Box 73-3). Reflex erection is possible in some clients with upper motor neuron lesions and also with some lower motor neuron lesions. Ejaculation is possible with lower motor neuron lesions and if the lesion is more caudal. Fertility after SCI remains low but has been improved by electroejaculation, artificial insemination, and in vitro fertilization. Sexual dysfunction is approached from two avenues: psychological counseling and education about technological advances in the facilitation of sexual activity. Erection can be restored with external aids, an implantable penile prosthesis, or medications.

Female clients retain fertility after SCI. Problems with sexual function generally relate to positioning and the lack of vaginal lubrication. These problems can usually be addressed through client education.

Control Pain

Long-term pain occurs frequently in spinal cord–injured clients with intact sensation. Dysesthetic pain, which is distal to the site of injury, is extremely disabling. It is similar to the phantom sensation experienced after amputation. It is described as cutting, burning, piercing, radiating, or tightening. The usual treatment is with nonopioid analgesics and transcutaneous nerve stimulators. An "as-needed" approach to pain management is not recommended for chronic pain; however, routine analgesics may need to be supplemented with other

---

BOX 73-3 Sexual Function in Clients with Spinal Cord Injury

FEMALES

Lesions at C1-3: Reflex lubrication is probable; erogenous areas may develop above injury; libido is intact

Lesions at C4-6: Psychogenic lubrication is unlikely; nongenital orgasm may be experienced

Lesions at C7: Able to use hands for holding and caressing

Lesions at T12-L5: Psychogenic stimulation of the clitoris, lubrication, labial swelling, and skin flush are possible but unlikely

MALES

Lesions at C1-3: Reflex erection is caused by genital stimulation; psychogenic erection is not possible; erogenous zones above injury site may develop; libido is intact

Lesions at C4-6: Reflex erection is possible; nongenital orgasm may be experienced; no ejaculation; oral sex is possible; libido is intact

Lesions at C7: Able to use hands for holding

Lesions at T12-L6: Psychogenic stimulation and erection are possible; no reflex erection

Lesions at S2-4: Reflex erection is possible; ejaculation is possible but may be retrograde

pain-relieving medications given as needed during a client's pain peaks. Gabapentin (Neurontin) has been used successfully for patients with neuropathic pain.

Reduce Abnormal Bone Growth

Heterotopic ossification is the formation of bone in abnormal locations, occurring most often around the hips and knees after SCI. The client may develop swelling in the joint or loss of ROM. Heterotopic ossification is diagnosed by x-ray study or bone scan. Treatment includes the use of etidronate disodium (Didronel) and ROM exercises of the affected joints. Sometimes the bone is removed surgically.

Promote Psychological Adjustment

Psychological counseling is ongoing. Commonly, spinal cord–injured clients participate in peer group counseling sessions in which experiences and solutions are shared to help newly injured clients to cope better with their losses. Vocational rehabilitation may help clients reach their maximum rehabilitation potential.

Ongoing Nursing Management of the Client with Spinal Cord Injury

---

Assessment. The client usually is transferred to a rehabilitation setting when the acute illness is stable. Clients with high cervical injuries may remain on ventilators. The care of the ventilator-dependent client is discussed in Chapter 63. Some of the nursing diagnoses that applied in the acute care setting may still apply after transfer. The client remains at risk for skin impairment and may still have difficulty swallowing, with attendant risk for aspiration. A baseline assessment should be completed at transfer.

Diagnosis, Outcomes, Interventions
Diagnosis: Impaired Physical Mobility. Spinal cord injury that causes permanent impaired physical mobility produces problems with ambulation and potential complications arising from immobility. The relevant nursing diagnosis is *Impaired Physical Mobility related to inability to move upper and/or lower extremities secondary to paralysis.*

Outcomes. The client will have maximal physical mobility as evidenced by absence of tendon contractures, joint ankylosis, and muscle shortening and will demonstrate effective use of adaptive devices.

Interventions. Throughout the acute and rehabilitative phases of nursing care, make every effort to maximize functional abilities and independence by encouraging the client to perform independently any activities of daily living (ADL) for which capability remains.

Provide Positioning and Adaptive Equipment. Improper positioning of the client in the bed or chair and lack of joint movements (e.g., related to spasticity or immobility) lead to tendon contractures, joint ankylosis, and muscle shortening. Interventions to prevent such problems include the following:

- Frequent position changes
- Proper positioning of joints
- Use of splints and removable casts
- Intermittent turning to a prone position
- Positioning of upper extremities away from the body
- Draping of bed linen over frames to keep pressure off the feet
- Keeping knee joints flexed 15 degrees when the client is supine
- Use of active and passive conditioning exercises (see Risk for Contractures)

Wristdrop and footdrop are inevitable sequelae in paralyzed extremities unless specific preventive measures are used. Footdrop may be prevented by keeping the client's feet firmly supported in dorsiflexion at right angles to the hips to counteract the force of gravity on weakened muscles. Many devices are available to prevent footdrop; they are designed to stretch the Achilles tendons. Wearing shoes also helps prevent footdrop when the client lies down. Support a paralyzed arm in a sling when the client is out of bed and in a cock-up splint when the client is in bed. Usually the hand end of the splint is elevated 2 inches to support the wrist, and the fingers are maintained in a position of function. Posterior molded casts may be used instead of splints to support a paralyzed wrist while the client is in bed. For some clients, pillows and a hand roll are adequate. Skin must be frequently assessed under any braces or splints.

Assist with Transfers and Ambulation. Rehabilitative programs often require strength and endurance. To prepare a client for ambulation, the unaffected parts of the body must be strengthened and suitable exercises started early. Tolerance for activity gradually increases. Take care not to fatigue the client. Periods of planned rest and recreation are important.

Braces or corsets should be applied before the client is assisted to get out of bed. A thin, knitted undershirt is worn under the brace or corset to protect the skin and to keep the appliance clean. To apply the brace or corset, turn the client to one side, place the appliance against the back, and then roll the client back into it. The brace or corset is secured while the client lies supine. As recovery and rehabilitation progress, many clients learn to apply their own brace or corset while in bed. Others continue to need help. The degree of arm and hand function determines the client's ability to apply a brace.

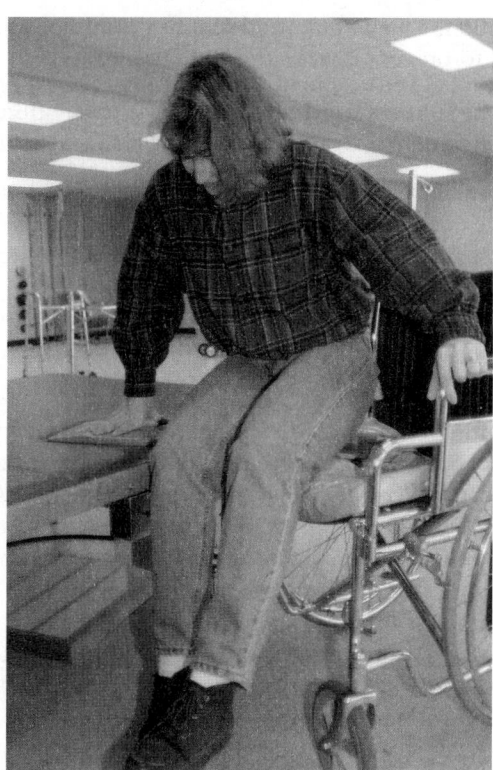

■ FIGURE 73–18 Bed-to-wheelchair lateral transfer using a sliding board.

Physical therapy is essential for all clients with SCI. Paraplegic clients need to learn various transfers to become self-sufficient. One transfer method is illustrated in Figure 73-18. Learning to sit up precedes learning to transfer. Take care in helping clients to stand or sit in a chair for the first time. Because of the loss of venous return from reflexes with movement, these clients are prone to orthostatic hypotension. Always check blood pressure before and after transfers. Syncope during a wheelchair transfer may be avoided in the quadriplegic client by using an abdominal binder, thigh-high support hose, and slowly elevating the head of the bed to 90 degrees. Using a recliner or a wheelchair with an adjustable back will help achieve gradual elevations.

Weight-bearing begins as early as possible after SCI. Weight-bearing stimulates osteoblastic (bone formation) activity and thus decreases demineralization of bone (osteoporosis) that develops with prolonged immobilization. Use of a standing board or tilt table assists the client to tolerate gradually a standing position. Having the client stand periodically each day also helps prevent contractures (e.g., hip contractures resulting from long periods of sitting).

Clients easily lose balance when wearing braces, particularly the halo brace, and must be careful to avoid falling. (See the Client Education Guide website feature on Use of a Halo Vest.) A brace feels surprisingly heavy at first, especially if the client is weak. For safety, shoes (rather than slippers or just stockings or socks) should be worn during ambulation. Shoes should tie or have self-fastening straps for firm support and have a low heel. High-top athletic shoes give added support. Slick soles, high or narrow heels, and stocking feet are hazardous.

The fit, comfort, and appearance of braces, corsets, and shoes are important to the client. Try to accommodate the preferences of clients who want to be as stylish as possible as well as benefit from therapeutic garments. Disabled clients are helped by being encouraged to express their feelings concerning their self-image and by having their desires taken into consideration when being fitted for therapeutic garments. Some garments can be painful when first worn. The pain worsens if the garments do not fit properly.

Diagnosis: Ineffective Airway Clearance. Airway clearance may be impaired because of paralysis of the abdominal and intercostal muscles. The relevant nursing diagnosis is *Ineffective Airway Clearance related to inability to cough.*

Outcomes. The client has adequate airway clearance as evidenced by participating in "quad-assisted" coughing, remaining afebrile, and having normal blood gas or pulse oximetry values and clear sputum.

Interventions. Use the "quad-assisted" cough maneuver to promote airway clearance. Quad-assisted coughing is accomplished by placing a fist or heel of the hand between the umbilicus and the xiphoid process. Press inward and upward during the client's cough (Figure 73-19). Other interventions, such as turning, hydration, and chest physical therapy, may also be used.

Collaborative Problem: Risk for Thrombophlebitis. Muscular activity is a major factor in venous circulation. A paralyzed client experiences slowed venous return and pooling of blood in dependent limbs. These phenomena constitute the basis for the collaborative problem *Risk for Thrombophlebitis.*

Outcomes. The nurse will monitor for thrombophlebitis as evidenced by unilateral leg edema, erythema, and warmth.

Interventions. In the acute phase of SCI, anti-embolism stockings, sequential compression devices, and subcutaneous heparin may be used prophylactically.

Education is vital to preventing vascular complications and minimizing their impact. Teach the client the importance of all preventive activities. During assessment of the legs for manifestations of clot formation (i.e., redness and unilateral swelling and warmth), explain the components of assessment and emphasize the importance of incorporating this activity into daily

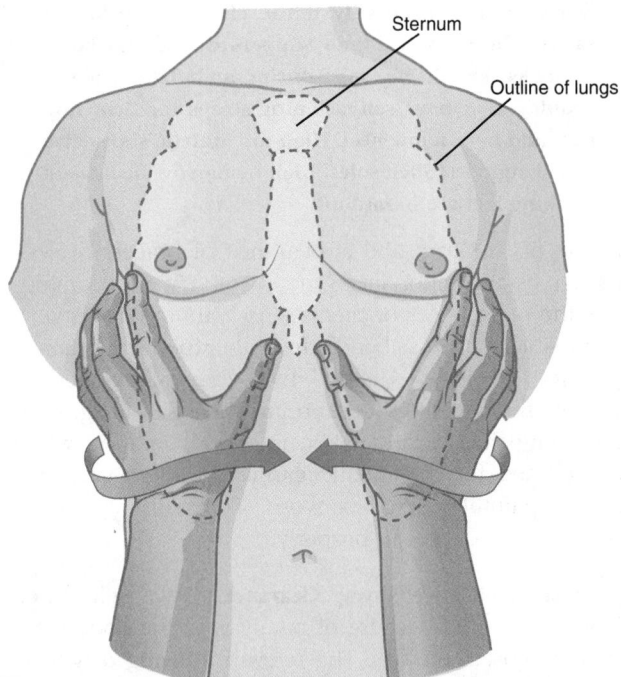

Sternum

Outline of lungs

■ **FIGURE 73–19** Cough assistance. In this technique, which can be performed with the client sitting in a wheelchair, the hands are placed on the midline of the upper abdomen. After the client inhales, pressure is directed inward and upward as the client attempts to cough. *(From AACN, & Carlson, K. [Eds.] [2008]. AACN advanced critical care nursing, St. Louis: Saunders.)*

routines. Measuring calf diameter on both legs daily to detect any changes is a more objective way of assessing swelling. Clients also learn not to cross their legs while sitting in a wheelchair.

Collaborative Problem: Risk for Contractures. Active ROM is severely limited or nonexistent in the upper extremities and nonexistent in the lower extremities in a client with cervical cord damage; it is also nonexistent in the lower extremities in a client with thoracic or lumbar cord damage. This deficit increases the risk for contractures. The collaborative problem is *Risk for Contractures related to inability to move purposefully secondary to spinal injury.*

Outcomes. The client will have reduced risk of contractures as evidenced by maintaining ROM present before the injury.

Interventions. Monitor the degree of ROM in all involved joints. Passive exercises prevent contractures and painful reflex dystrophies of the hand and shoulder. Such exercises may be prescribed as soon as 48 to 72 hours after injury. Active exercises, massage, and electrical stimulation may also be prescribed. Begin shoulder and arm exercises early. Strength in these areas and in the chest and back is essential for effective self-transfers and

ambulation. Clients may find that the prone position is helpful to prevent hip flexure contracture.

Diagnosis: Self-Care Deficit. The client who has suffered an SCI is often unable to perform many self-care activities.

Outcomes. The client will have a satisfactory level of self-care as evidenced by independently performing as many ADL tasks as possible. If unable to perform an activity independently, the client will be able to direct a caregiver's performance. These goals will be evaluated by observing successful performance of ADL by the client or under the client's direction.

Interventions. Self-care deficit can lead to a feeling of powerlessness. Assisting the client to maximize independence can lessen this feeling. The client is assisted with muscle-strengthening exercises and the use of adaptive devices. Clients with high cervical injuries are able to perform few activities independently. Allow them adequate time to accomplish whatever tasks they can. If help with ADL is needed, adapt nursing care to the client's routine. In collaborating to maintain intact oral mucous membranes, a schedule is established for brushing the teeth at least twice daily and cleaning the tongue, roof of the mouth, and gums with agents that do not contain lemon or alcohol.

Diagnosis: Risk for Imbalanced Nutrition: Less Than Body Requirements. After traumatic injury metabolic demand increases because of the response to stress and the body's requirements for healing. The relevant nursing diagnosis is written *Risk for Imbalanced Nutrition: Less Than Body Requirements related to increased metabolic demand and inability to access nutrients.* Anorexia related to depression may be another etiologic factor.

Outcomes. The client will have balanced nutrition as evidenced by maintaining a reasonable weight for height.

Interventions. The client should be weighed on admission to obtain a baseline measurement. Compare current weight to ideal body weight. Whereas weight loss is not encouraged during the healing phase of injury, once the client is stable, excess weight should be shed to promote activity and transferring. For clients below ideal body weight, nutrient supplementation should begin by 72 hours after injury if the client is not eating. Enteral feeding can be used if the client has bowel sounds. If the client still has paralytic ileus, hyperalimentation is commonly used. Weigh the client at least once a week to monitor progress. Laboratory values for albumin and prealbumin should also be monitored.

Diagnosis: Total Urinary Incontinence. Urinary bladder *atony* (absence of tone) may last several weeks or months after SCI. In clients with upper motor neuron lesions, when spinal shock subsides and the reflexes return, a reflex contraction may empty the bladder

Observe the client carefully for indications of problems with bladder control and infection, including incontinence, retention, urgency, dribbling, frequency, enuresis, and precipitate micturition. Document such observations and inform the physician. The relevant nursing diagnosis is written *Total Urinary Incontinence related to paralysis.*

Outcomes. The client will have improved bladder control as evidenced by absence of infection and by emptying of the bladder every 4 to 6 hours.

Interventions. Nursing intervention is planned to prevent urinary tract infection, to preserve existing bladder capacity and muscle tone, and to establish and maintain a routine pattern of elimination requiring minimal artificial assistance.

It is important to check a postvoid residual or to use an ultrasound to measure bladder volume to ensure near-complete bladder emptying. During the period of atony, a retention catheter may be inserted to prevent bladder distention and keep the client dry and comfortable.

> **Bladder overdistention causes stretching and fissure formation—a predisposing factor for infection—and may result in bladder rupture. When sensory pathways are damaged, the client does not feel the discomfort of bladder distention; however, prolonged catheter use also predisposes to infection. Therefore catheterization every 4 to 6 hours to keep urine volumes less than 600 ml is preferred over a retention catheter.**
>
> **Urinary complications may be avoided by periodically examining the client for bladder distention, accurately documenting fluid intake and output, using aseptic technique when handling urinary catheters, and observing for manifestations of bladder infection. Encourage the client to drink water to keep the urine diluted, which lessens the possibility of infection.**

Urine acidifiers may be prescribed. To prevent development of renal calculi, encourage the client to drink about 3000 ml of fluid per day, unless contraindicated by other medical conditions. This is sufficient to maintain a minimal urine output of 2000 ml/day. Drinking this much fluid may increase incontinence but is necessary to prevent renal calculi.

Self bladder care is discussed later, under Therapeutic Regimen Management.

Diagnosis: Bowel Incontinence or Constipation. Bowel dysfunction is a common but manageable problem in a client with SCI. This common nursing diagnosis is written as *Constipation related to paralysis.*

Outcomes. The client will have reduced risk of bowel incontinence or constipation as evidenced by a bowel movement every 1 to 2 days, no manifestations of fecal impaction, no incontinence, and no manifestations of hyperreflexia.

Interventions. Nursing intervention is planned to prevent constipation, distention, and impaction; to detect and treat these conditions if they occur; and to reestablish habitual, controlled bowel movements by conditioned reflex activity. Paralytic ileus is common after SCI. By frequently assessing bowel sounds and documenting the passage of stool, return of peristalsis can be determined and the client can resume oral intake. The client is observed carefully for indications of constipation, diarrhea, or *tenesmus* (straining at stool). If the bowel becomes impacted, a cleansing enema may be prescribed to initially empty the lower bowel. Enemas should be avoided for long-term bowel management, however. A paraplegic or quadriplegic client cannot retain an enema solution, nor can the degree of intestinal distention be felt. Therefore enemas must be administered carefully to avoid overdistending the intestine with excessive fluid; 500 ml or less is usually given.

Document the client's intake of fluid and food and elimination patterns. A bowel program should be established early. The program should occur at the same time every day (or every other day), after a meal or large snack with the patient as upright as possible. The use of water-based suppositories or digital stimulation provides a signal to the body for reflex evacuation.

A daily fluid intake of 3000 ml/day is important for proper bowel function as well as bladder function. Also, the diet must be high in bulk and roughage, such as bran, whole grains, fresh and dried fruits, and leafy green and raw vegetables. A stool softener such as docusate sodium (Colace) may be taken daily, but laxatives should be carefully administered. Bulk-forming medications (e.g., psyllium hydrophilic mucilloid [Metamucil]) are effective for spinal cord–injured clients so long as adequate hydration is maintained. Self bowel care is discussed later, under Therapeutic Regimen Management.

Diagnosis: Risk for Impaired Skin Integrity. Clients with SCI are at higher risk of impairment of skin integrity because of immobility and loss of protective functions.

Outcomes. The client will have intact skin as evidenced by no reddened areas over bony prominences and no areas or manifestations of skin irritation or dryness.

Interventions. The spinal cord–injured client cannot respond to the sensory cues to local tissue hypoxia resulting from being in one position for an extended period. Therefore, the development of pressure ulcers is frequent. Spinal cord–injured clients should be placed on pressure-redistributing beds or mattresses. Use of these special beds does not, however, eliminate the need to assess the skin every shift, turn the client every 2 hours, or eliminate the risk of pressure ulcers. In addition, the client's nutritional needs must be met to reduce the risk of pressure ulcers.

Wheelchairs need to be fitted with pressure reduction seating cushions that allow movement for transfers as well as pressure reduction. Because ischial pressure ulcers can develop quickly, clients should be taught to inspect their own skin with a long handled mirror or have their caregiver do so daily. The cushion also needs to be assessed; air columns should be full, foam should not be compressed, and gel cushions should not show wear. Seating evaluation for pressure areas is helpful to choose a chair cushion that provides pressure redistribution. Once an ulcer forms, complete bed rest may be needed to heal the ulcer; so prevention and early detection are crucial.

Once the client is seated, he or she should be taught to perform a daily systematic skin inspection. For example, at bedtime the client can use a long-handled mirror to see the buttocks before transferring to bed. Clothing should be worn that does not have seams, pockets, or rivets because these items cause unusual pressure points. Prevention of pressure ulcers should include use of pressure-relieving devices in both chair and bed. Wheelchairs should be fitted with gel cushions for those clients who transfer and with air column cushions for those who do not transfer. Pressure relief in wheelchairs is usually accomplished by pushing off the arms of the wheelchair or leaning forward every 15 to 30 minutes.

Diagnosis: Chronic Pain. Clients with SCI may experience pain at the level of the injury and radiating along spinal nerves originating in the area. Phantom sensation may also be experienced. The onset of pain is usually later than that for muscle spasms. Some paraplegic and quadriplegic clients experience both pain and spasm. Pain most often occurs in the lower extremities.

Outcomes. The client will experience adequate pain relief as evidenced by verbalization of improvement in comfort, ability to rest without interruption by pain, and ability to participate in therapies without hindrance by pain.

Interventions. Analgesics such as aspirin and nonsteroidal anti-inflammatory drugs (NSAIDs) may be prescribed. Opioids are seldom used after the initial injury and are contraindicated in clients with high cervical-level injuries because of the risk of respiratory depression.

Clients with thoracic pulmonary injuries tend to breathe more shallowly to avoid pain. Inadequate depth of respirations can lead to complications. Give prescribed pain medication and encourage deep breathing and coughing to aerate the lungs and remove secretions from the respiratory tract.

Antispasmodics, NSAIDs, and non-opioid analgesics are prescribed for pain associated with spasticity. Surgery (e.g., neurectomy, chordotomy) is sometimes required for pain relief.

Collaborative Problem: Risk for Autonomic Dysreflexia. Autonomic dysreflexia/hyperreflexia is a serious complication of SCI when injury is above the T6 level. This collaborative problem is documented as *Risk for Autonomic Dysreflexia related to spinal cord injury.*

Outcomes. The nurse will monitor for clinical manifestations of autonomic dysreflexia and respond to them quickly.

Interventions. Assess the client for sudden onset of severe hypertension, severe throbbing headache, profuse diaphoresis, flushing of the skin above the level of the lesion, nasal stuffiness, pilomotor spasm, blurred vision, nausea, and bradycardia. The Critical Monitoring feature below lists additional assessment findings related to this serious complication.

Educate the client about early warning signs and symptoms of autonomic dysreflexia and the importance of calling for a nurse immediately if any occur. Adaptive call lights are available to facilitate calling for assistance. If autonomic dysreflexia does occur, institute the following measures:

1. Elevate the head of the bed to a sitting position immediately.
2. Check blood pressure.
3. Check for possible sources of irritation (e.g., kinked or clogged catheter or distended bladder or lower bowel).
4. Remove the stimulus if it can be done quickly. Once the source of irritation is removed, manifestations of autonomic dysreflexia usually subside.
5. If blood pressure remains elevated, antihypertensive medication (nitrates, hydralazine, guanethidine, or diazoxide) may be administered according to prescription or procedural policy (intravenously, intranasally, or sublingually).
6. If there is no order or policy or if these measures do not correct the problem, notify the physician.

CRITICAL MONITORING

Features of Autonomic Dysreflexia

- Severe hypertension (up to 300 mm Hg)
- Pounding headache
- Flushing (above the level of the lesion)
- Piloerection
- Diaphoresis
- Dilated pupils, blurred vision
- Nasal stuffiness
- Bradycardia (pulse rate <60 beats/min)
- Restlessness
- Nausea

Once manifestations have subsided, observe the client's vital signs and neurologic status closely for 3 to 4 hours. If an antihypertensive medication has been given, the client may become hypotensive after the stimulus is removed. Autonomic dysreflexia may recur if the stimulus is not completely removed. If the identified source is bladder distention, use caution when emptying the bladder. Remove 500 ml every 5 to 15 minutes. If the identified source of irritation is bowel distention, be careful when removing the impacted material from the bowel. An anesthetic lubricant is used, and another nurse must monitor the client's blood pressure every few minutes. The stimulation of trying to remove the impacted material can increase the severity of the autonomic response.

When a quadriplegic client complains of a headache, *do not automatically give analgesics without first checking the blood pressure.*

Diagnosis: Risk for Injury. In clients with SCI, another appropriate nursing diagnosis is *Risk for Injury related to abnormal reflexes, spasms, and corneal drying.* Corneal abrasions may result unless proper interventions are instituted.

Outcomes. The client will sustain no injuries from spasms as evidenced by no abrasions or bruising. Corneal abrasions will not occur.

Interventions. Injections should be avoided whenever possible. Medications should be given orally or intravenously if needed. When injections must be given, inject them above the level of the cord lesion whenever possible. Absorption may be compromised in denervated areas of the body with impaired capillary and precapillary circulation. Moisten the cornea with natural tears every 4 hours for a client with altered blinking reflexes.

Clients can also be injured from involuntary spasms. Avoid unnecessary stimulation of areas that elicit reflex spinal automatisms. When such reactions do occur, an unembarrassed, accepting response helps relieve the client's anxiety and embarrassment. Gentle, slow hyperextension of a limb in spasm can often override the trigger points and interrupt the spasm. Abnormal spinal reflexes make clients respond to stimuli in ways that may be puzzling to both the client and others unless the origin of such responses is explained. For example, stimulation of the limbs (perhaps toe flexion while the person's foot is being dried) may cause mass flexion of the upper and lower extremities. Mass flexion reactions may be accompanied by massive contractions of the abdominal wall, evacuation of the urinary bladder and bowel, and automatic response such as sweating, flushing, penile erection, or pilomotor reactions below the level of the lesion.

Diagnosis: Ineffective Coping. When the reality of the injury and the permanent deficits are understood, coping skills may need to be taught. The nursing diagnosis can be written as *Ineffective Coping related to awareness of the permanent paralysis and its effect on life goals.*

Outcomes. The client will use adaptive coping strategies and resources appropriately.

Interventions. Clients need to find appropriate methods for coping with new approaches to performing ADL and managing bodily functions. The learning needs of spinal cord–injured clients and their family members are complex and ongoing. In the acute phase, education about spinal anatomy and physiology is needed. This teaching begins in the acute phase of hospitalization and should be incorporated into all aspects of care. Successful learning in this stage affects the client's entire life. Over time many SCI clients develop unique and resourceful adaptations to their living and work environments to facilitate independence.

Diagnosis: Anticipatory Grieving. Clients with SCI experience many changes (e.g., functional ability, role definition, body image, financial security). Grief is a normal response to these losses. Write the nursing diagnosis as *Anticipatory Grieving related to multiple losses.*

Outcomes. The client will progress through the grieving process and develop adaptive coping strategies as evidenced by verbalizing his or her feelings about the injury and the future, participating in community activities, and expressing positive thoughts about the future.

Interventions. Adjusting to paralysis is difficult physically and psychosocially for the client and family. Family members may experience the same reactions as those experienced by the disabled client and may need the same type of help. Sudden paralysis in a previously healthy, active person can be devastating. Typically the sudden lifestyle changes brought about by serious SCI produce a grief reaction. The reaction may involve initial shock and denial, leading to depression and anger. Crying and talking about the injury may be helpful. Social services or pastoral care may also be of assistance during this time of grief.

It takes time to adjust to disability and to develop ways of coping. Psychological adjustment occurs when the client can function appropriately in the real world. A client may use psychological defense mechanisms in adjusting to paralysis. When caring for such a client, assess the possible reasons for observed behavior. Hostility, depression, anger, or withdrawal may be upsetting to staff and family. These emotions and behaviors represent coping mechanisms and should not be taken personally.

Paralysis may cause complex changes in self-concept and body image. In the acute phase, immobilization can contribute to sensory deprivation and its consequences (e.g., hallucinations). Providing visual, auditory, and tactile stimulation as desired by the client may minimize the experience of deprivation.

Paralyzed clients are often helped initially by being with others who are experiencing similar problems. Clients should be allowed to wear their own clothing as soon as possible and encouraged to be out of bed and out of the hospital room. Planned social activities may reduce feelings of social isolation and may help clients regain self-confidence. Peer counseling, in which newly disabled clients are provided opportunities to talk with others who have adjusted to similar disabilities, may be helpful. Young clients may find enjoyment in sports designed for people in wheelchairs (Figure 73-20).

A sense of security is particularly important for a newly paralyzed client adjusting to enforced dependency. A paralyzed client should always have a means of summoning help and yet needs to learn that it is safe to be alone at times. Blow lights, minimal-pressure call lights, pads, and voice-activated call lights are now available in many settings.

Gradually the client develops trust in his or her abilities and resources and relinquishes some reliance on others. These feelings and attitudes develop slowly as the client experiences genuinely trustworthy relationships.

To avoid unnecessary frustrations, try to keep the client's environment comfortable, with necessary items conveniently placed. It is difficult and depressing for the client to have to ask for help repeatedly. Although recent advances have been made in the rehabilitation prognosis of paraplegic and quadriplegic clients, it is important to be realistic as well as optimistic. Nurses need to understand the tremendous lifestyle changes disabled clients must make. Some clients can be rehabilitated to a level of near-independence: walking (perhaps with braces or other appliances), driving a car, and coping with full-time employment outside the home. Quadriplegic clients usually rely on a wheelchair and other devices and appliances.

Most paralyzed clients can become productive and happy. After his devastating SCI, actor Christopher Reeve served as a positive role model regarding *abilities* that remain after SCI. Even if some clients are unable to be "productive," all disabled clients have a right to a satisfying, happy life. Although many paralyzed clients achieve complete rehabilitation, others lead lives that are difficult, frustrating, and psychophysiologically complex. At times, severe mental depression develops. Depression is assessed, and professional counseling is offered as indicated. Unfortunately, ideations of suicide are frequent.

Diagnosis: Disabled Family Coping. A family is a unit. A trauma as devastating as SCI to one of the members of the family unit affects the entire family. The relevant nursing diagnosis can be written *Disabled Family Coping: related to multiple changes in the family roles.*

Outcomes. The client and family members will use adaptive coping by identifying areas of significant or potential loss and changes in family roles, working together to overcome obstacles, seeking appropriate support services, and being able to restore a supportive family structure.

Interventions. The injury affects not only physical functioning but also the psychological, vocational, educational, and social aspects of life. An organized team approach is vital to helping the injured client and family cope with lifestyle changes. Nurses are often the first health care professionals to assess client and family coping. An open, empathetic manner can allow the people involved to express their grief and uncertainty and to ask questions. Educate the family about the normal grief response. Carefully probe into persistent denial of grief or lack of progression through grieving. Encouraging as much optimism as possible while remaining truthful and realistic may help SCI survivors to face the future.

Assess the previous roles of the client and other family members and how they have handled stressful situations or losses. Identify the family's sources of strength. Assess patterns of interaction between family members; their spiritual, social, and economic status; and their lifestyle. Cultural or ethnic influences should also be noted. These variables often influence how the family responds to grief. Sometimes the nurse can play a valuable role simply by giving family members permission to have a day off from visiting.

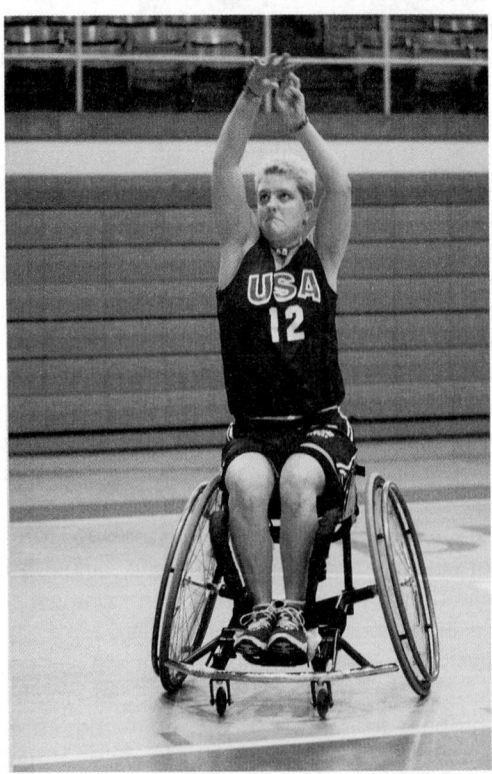

■ **FIGURE 73–20** The Paralympics offer young athletes opportunities to play sports.

Diagnosis: Ineffective Therapeutic Regimen Management. Clients with SCI have bladder and bowel function changes. Bladder emptying has to be learned using a different approach, and bowel retraining is often necessary. A common nursing diagnosis in this circumstance is *Ineffective Therapeutic Regimen Management.*

Outcomes. The client will be able to manage his or her bowel and bladder or instruct others how to do so.

Interventions. One of the most common stimuli for autonomic dysreflexia, a life-threatening complication in people with SCI, is bladder distention. Therefore intervention leading to bladder management is crucial.

Promote Bladder Retraining. When the initial indwelling catheter is removed, a program of intermittent catheterization is commonly prescribed to empty the bladder regularly every 4 to 6 hours for several weeks. During this time, the client may be taught methods of emptying the bladder without catheterization. Such methods promote urination by increasing intra-abdominal pressure on the bladder. For some clients with SCI, urinary flow can be initiated by using the Credé maneuver, the Valsalva maneuver, or the rectal stretch.

The *Credé maneuver* involves placing the fist or fingers directly over the bladder and pressing down toward the pubic bone with a kneading motion. This motion is continued until the bladder is empty.

The *Valsalva maneuver* involves inhaling deeply, holding the breath, and bearing down as hard as possible, as if for a bowel movement.

The *rectal stretch* involves inserting a lubricated, gloved finger into the rectum. When the anal sphincter is relaxed, the client maintains the relaxation by gently pulling on the sphincter. This relaxes the perineal floor. The Valsalva maneuver is performed at the same time.

Urination may also be prompted by reflex stimulation. The following stimuli may be successful: tapping the suprapubic area; stroking the glans penis, thigh, or vulva; tugging pubic hairs; or flexing the toes. The client or caregiver may apply the stimulation. As training continues, less stimulation is needed to initiate urination.

Catheterization may be required at home. Teach the client and caregiver clean, rather than sterile, technique. This technique has the same infection rate as for sterile insertion methods used for home catheterization. Suprapubic catheters may be inserted for long-term bladder management.

Occasionally a surgical procedure such as sphincterotomy is necessary. The bladder then empties continuously. An external, condom-type catheter connected to a closed drainage bag may be used to collect urine in men. External appliances for females are not consistently effective. The Mitrofanoff procedure is a surgical option that creates an opening from the bladder to the umbilicus. It allows for catheterization of the stoma and bladder emptying with less hand function and disrobing needed.

Teach Bowel Retraining. Bowel retraining is possible for most paraplegic and quadriplegic clients. It involves developing controlled bowel movements by conditioned reflex activity. Begin bowel retraining as soon as feasible. Ensure privacy during the daily bowel routine, and if possible, have the client sitting upright. When possible, include appropriate family members in the bowel retraining program because they may be involved in this aspect of long-term management. Always assess the family members' willingness to participate in such care. If the sexual partner is also responsible for hygiene and personal care, problems in role separation and intimacy may result. These issues should be openly discussed between partners.

With an effective bowel program, a client has a bowel movement once a day or every other day and is not incontinent at other times. Attaining continence may influence a paralyzed client's vocational future and positively affect ability to have satisfying social relationships. It can also give the client the confidence to cope with other problems.

Diagnosis: Sexual Dysfunction. Spinal cord–injured clients are often concerned about sexuality and their ability to achieve sexual fulfillment. They often worry about such concerns long before they express them to others. Nurses are often asked about sexuality issues before other professionals are approached, perhaps because nurses provide intimate care. Such care can promote a high degree of trust.

Outcomes. The client will develop personally satisfying and socially acceptable means of expressing sexuality as evidenced by interacting appropriately in social situations, verbalizing the effects of the injury on sexual function, discussing sexual issues with a health care team member, verbalizing methods of sexual expression, and verbalizing understanding of contraceptive implications.

Interventions. To be helpful, nurses need to be able to talk about sexuality without embarrassment. They also need accurate information about "normal" sexuality and how physiologic changes that occur because of the injury affect sexual function. Some clients discuss their own sexual potential directly. Others refer to it subtly or appear crude in the way they introduce the topic, such as making inappropriate sexual comments or gestures. Such behaviors are attempts to acknowledge sexuality. Try to look beyond the behavior to the underlying emotional concerns. Acknowledge the client's concerns and offer to open a discussion, by saying, for example, "You seem concerned about your sexuality, James. This is a common concern that others with spinal cord injury have had. Sometimes talking about it helps. If you like, we can talk about how this has affected you, and when you are ready, I can share with you interventions that have helped others who have had similar problems."

The client can be referred to another person or an agency if appropriate. Referral should not be made too hastily, however. If a client talks with a nurse about this subject, it is probably because the client feels most comfortable speaking with that nurse at that time. Allow the client to lead the conversation, which may be difficult. Professionals must be aware that they do not always know what a client needs and wants and should listen carefully to the client's voiced concerns.

In general, a physiologic sexual response requires an intact nervous system. For example, psychogenic erection requires an intact spinal cord with preservation of S2-4 nerve roots and spinal reflexes; ejaculation is a function of skeletal muscle controlled by the somatic center in the pudendal nerve originating in the S2-4 roots; and orgasm involves contraction of both smooth and skeletal muscle. It should be remembered, however, that there is more involved in sexual expression than physiologic response.

To some extent, sexual function can be predicted by the level of the spinal cord lesion (see Box 73-3). For example, psychogenic erection is often difficult or impossible after SCI. Although physical limitations certainly exist, every person is different. Many men do have reflex erections after SCI. Many disabled people enjoy *paraorgasm* (phantom orgasm) by developing alternative erogenous zones. The genitals are not the only body areas where sexual stimulation is possible, and intercourse is not the only means of sexual expression.

Some people find it disappointing, perhaps devastating, that they can no longer function sexually as they did before the injury; however, they can be helped to learn new ways of giving and receiving sexual pleasure. Sexual and relationship counseling is sometimes helpful. Some form of sexual expression is possible for anyone, regardless of disability. Before making specific suggestions for alternative expressions of sexuality, discussion with the client should occur to identify past sexual behavior and cultural taboos. Some clients may find some methods of giving and receiving sexual pleasure unacceptable. Lack of a sexual partner may be a deterrent but should not preclude discussion of sexuality. Society as a whole is becoming progressively more open about sexuality.

Increasingly, the parenting potential of disabled people is receiving societal attention. Physical assessment is needed to determine a client's ability to reproduce. Male infertility is a frequent complication of SCI because of testicular atrophy, decreased sperm formation, and infrequent ejaculation. Most men are unable to ejaculate after SCI. Women usually remain fertile and can conceive and deliver a child. Adoption is a viable option, and conception by artificial insemination is possible.

Disabled people may have contraception concerns. Little is known about the effects of various kinds of contraceptives on disabled people. Oral contraceptives may be contraindicated. Paralyzed women often have slowed circulation, increasing the potential circulatory complications of oral contraceptives. To use an intrauterine device, a woman must have feeling in her pelvis to be able to recognize early manifestations of pelvic inflammatory disease. Many paralyzed women do not have such sensation. Barrier devices, such as a diaphragm, a condom, or foam, may be used if at least one partner has enough manual dexterity to insert the diaphragm or foam or put on the condom.

Diagnosis: Risk for Injury. Sensory loss poses serious problems for paralyzed clients because they cannot feel the pain or pressure that normally warns of tissue damage.

Outcomes. The client will be free of injury as evidenced by absence of abrasions, reddened areas, ulcerations, or burns.

Interventions. Spinal cord–injured clients should not wear tight, restrictive clothing or ill-fitting shoes or braces. They need to develop the habit of preventive thinking to avoid potential danger.

> **Dangerous situations include getting too close to heaters, radiators, and fireplaces; using heating pads or hot-water bottles; and rubbing against shoes or parts of the wheelchair. Burns can be a serious problem because impaired circulation delays healing. External heat should not be applied if there is a loss of sensation, and the bath water should not be too hot.**

Regular foot and nail care is required to prevent overgrown nails from rubbing or cutting the skin and to prevent ingrown nails. Instruct the client not to cut corns or calluses; cutting too deep is easy to do and may lead to a foot infection. Cocoa butter or oils without alcohol may be used to soften calluses and reduce cracking.

Diagnosis: Ineffective Health Maintenance. Spinal cord injuries result in many alterations in physiologic functioning that place the client at risk for maintaining normal health status. A possible nursing diagnosis is *Ineffective Health Maintenance.*

Outcomes. The client and family members will be able to meet the client's needs as evidenced by intact skin, bowel and bladder continence, ability to transfer into and out of a wheelchair, absence of infection, maintenance of appropriate weight, and satisfaction with personal relationships.

Interventions. Teaching should be conducted in short sessions, using easily understood terms. For example, teach the caregiver the importance of providing good skin care on the hands and skin folds to prevent

Candida overgrowth. Complex tasks should be taught in steps, with return demonstrations provided by the client or caregiver.

Most spinal cord–injured people are transferred from an acute care hospital to a rehabilitation facility. After functional capabilities have been maximized, the person is then discharged from the rehabilitation facility. The Bridge to Home Health Care feature on Managing the Immobile Client in Chapter 27 on p. 534 provides suggestions for helping caregivers support the client with SCI who lives at home.

Evaluation. Spinal cord–injured clients are hospitalized for a long time. Therefore certain functions important to expected outcomes need to be evaluated frequently, such as respiratory and cardiac function. Other expected outcomes will not be achieved for months, such as independence in performing ADL. The plan of care must reflect these individual needs of the client.

Modifications for Older Clients

For older adults with SCI, the most important modification of the nursing care plan is increased vigilance. Older people are more prone to the complications of immobility. A person with heart failure may have difficulty breathing when lying flat. Before initiation of halo traction in this age group, some neurosurgeons perform a temporary prophylactic tracheostomy because the older client has difficulty swallowing oral secretions and eating. Older people are also more susceptible to sensory deprivation. The nurse must make sure the client has his or her eyeglasses and hearing aid. If a window or clock is not within the range of vision, the client should be reoriented as needed. Discharge plans for older clients may be complicated if the caregiver is also an older adult. The spouse of an older spinal cord–injured person may not have the physical strength to provide the needed care. Learning to provide home care may also be problematic.

Self-Care

The skills learned in a rehabilitation setting must be adapted to the home environment and community setting before hospital discharge. This process can be accomplished by the use of therapeutic weekend passes and participation in community activities as a part of the rehabilitation process. The client needs to learn how to delegate needed skills to another caregiver so that care can be provided at home.

Paraplegic clients can usually live independently. Most quadriplegic clients need assistance with ADL. Depending on the amount of assistance needed and the specific situation, this care may be provided by family members or by a part-time or full-time paid attendant. By using a wheelchair, clients may become completely independent in ADL, with minimal help of social services personnel, a home health aide, or family members. Many clients drive and hold outside jobs.

Ventilator-dependent people who cannot obtain in-home care and others who do not have the personal or financial resources for in-home care may have no option except institutional living. The problem of limited government resources for all clients requiring rehabilitative care remains an important ethical issue in nursing. Group-living situations, especially for young adults, are becoming more available, however.

  CONCLUSIONS

Brain and spinal cord injuries are some of the most complex injuries the human can endure. Nurses who work with the neurologically impaired must develop and maintain astute assessment skills to detect the subtle signs of neurologic deterioration quickly. The physical and psychological impairments vary with the degree of damage as well as the client's response to and ability to cope with the body changes. The coping response is not always related to the degree of physiologic damage. It is imperative that nurses comprehend the severity of the client's dysfunction as it relates to quality of life as well as the impact it has on family dynamics.

THINKING CRITICALLY

1. A 23-year-old man was admitted from the emergency department (ED) following a car accident in which he sustained a concussion and thoracic injuries with thoracic spinal cord involvement. The client's baseline data included loss of consciousness for 15 minutes, headache, nausea, and an inability to move or feel any sensation from his thorax down. One hour after this man arrived in the intensive care unit (ICU), additional assessment changes included an inability to move his fingers and hands and to flex or extend his arms. Shoulder movement was still intact. He was fully conscious, and his vital signs were stable. What critical interventions initiated in the ED need to be continued in the ICU? What do these changes in data indicate? What nursing interventions are appropriate both initially and as precautions?

Factors to Consider. What are the implications when a high thoracic injury occurs? What changes indicate ascending cord dysfunction?

2. A 22-year-old man was admitted 4 hours after sustaining a C6 spinal cord compression injury. No neurologic deficits were found, but his blood alcohol level was very high on admission. Initially, he kept falling asleep after you completed your assessments. Gardner-Wells tongs with 10 pounds of traction were placed. Now that the client is more awake, he has begun thrashing his arms and attempting to roll over in bed. What are the priorities for his care? What nursing interventions should be used?

Factors to Consider. What is the purpose of the Gardner-Wells tongs? How would edema and microscopic bleeding compromise recovery in this client?

Discussions for these questions can be found on the website.

BIBLIOGRAPHY

Citations appearing in red refer to primary research.

Citations appearing in blue refer to evidence-based practice guidelines and protocols.

1. Aito, S., Cariaggi, B., & Perazza, S. (2002). The use of high-dose methylprednisolone in acute spinal cord injuries: NASCIS review. National Acute Spinal Cord Injury Study. *Europa Medicophysica, 38*(2), 89-95.
2. American Association of Neuroscience Nurses. (2005). *AANN Reference Series for Clinical Practice: Guide to the care of the patient with intracranial pressure monitoring.* Chicago: Author.
3. American Spinal Injury Association (ASIA). (2002). *International standards for neurological classification of SCI.* Chicago: Author.
4. Anson, K., & Ponsford, J. (2006). Coping and emotional adjustment following traumatic brain injury. *Journal of Head Trauma Rehabilitation, 21*(5), 248-259.
5. Bader, M.K., Arbour, R., & Palmer, S. (2005). Refractory increased intracranial pressure in severe traumatic brain injury: Barbiturate coma and bispectral index monitoring. *AACN Clinical Issues, 16*(4), 526-541.
6. Bauman, W.A., & Spungen, A.M. (2000). Metabolic changes in persons after spinal cord injury. *Physical Medicine and Rehabilitation Clinics of North America, 11*(1), 109-140.
7. Bell, G.B. (1999). Spinal cord injury, pressure ulcers, support surfaces. *Ostomy and Wound Management, 45*(6), 48-50, 52–53.
8. Blank-Reid, C., & Reid, P.C. (2000). Penetrating trauma to the head. *Critical Care Nursing Clinics of North America, 12*(4), 477-487.
9. Bond, A.E., Draeger, C.R.L., Mandleco, B., Donnelly, M. (2003). Needs of family members of patients with severe traumatic brain injury: Implications for evidence-based practice. *Critical Care Nurse, 23*(4), 63-72.
10. Brain Trauma Foundation. (2000). *Management and prognosis of severe traumatic brain injury.* New York: Author.
11. Brewer, T., & Therrien, B. (2000). Minor brain injury: New insights for early nursing care. *Journal of Neuroscience Nursing, 32*(6), 311-317.
12. Bryce, T.N., & Ragnarsson, K.T. (2000). Pain after spinal cord injury. *Physical Medicine and Rehabilitation Clinics of North America, 11*(1), 157-168.
13. Chamberlain, D.J. (2006). The experience of surviving traumatic brain injury. *Journal of Advanced Nursing, 54*(4), 407-417.
14. Chaviano, A.H., et al. (2000). Mitrofanoff continent catheterizable stoma for pediatric patients with spinal cord injury. *Topics in Spinal Cord Injury Rehabilitation, Summer Suppl* (6), 30-35.
15. Chen, D., & Nussbaum, S.B. (2000). The gastrointestinal system and bowel management following spinal cord injury. *Physical Medicine and Rehabilitation Clinics of North America, 11*(1), 45-56, viii.
16. Christensen, M.A., Janson, S., & Seago, J.A. (2001). Alcohol, head injury and pulmonary complications. *Journal of Neuroscience Nursing, 33*(4), 184-189.
17. Clear, D., & Chadwick, D.W. (2000). Seizures provoked by blows to the head. *Epilepsia, 41*(2), 243-244.
18. Consortium for Spinal Cord Medicine. (2001). *Autonomic dysreflexia in individuals with spinal cord injury presenting to health care facilities* (2nd ed). Washington, DC: Paralyzed Veterans of America.
19. Consortium for Spinal Cord Medicine. (1999). *Neurogenic bowel management in adults with spinal cord injury.* Washington, DC: Paralyzed Veterans of America.
20. Consortium for Spinal Cord Medicine. (1999). *Outcomes following traumatic spinal cord injury.* Washington, DC: Paralyzed Veterans of America.
21. Consortium for Spinal Cord Medicine. (2000). *Pressure ulcer prevention and treatment following spinal cord injury.* Washington, DC: Paralyzed Veterans of America.
22. Consortium for Spinal Cord Medicine. (1999). *Prevention of thromboembolism in spinal cord injury.* Washington, DC: Paralyzed Veterans of America.
23. Davis, A.E. (2000). Mechanisms of traumatic brain injury: Biomechanical, structural and cellular considerations. *Critical Care Nursing Quarterly, 23*(3), 1-13.
24. Davis, A.E. (2000). Cognitive impairments following traumatic brain injury. *Critical Care Nursing Clinics of North America, 12*(4), 447-456.
25. Domeier, R.M., et al. (2002). Multicenter prospective validation of prehospital clinical spinal clearance criteria. *Journal of Trauma: Injury, Infection, and Critical Care, 53*(4), 744-750.
26. Dubendorf, P. (1999). Spinal cord injury pathophysiology. *Critical Care Nursing Quarterly, 22*(2), 31-35.
27. Ellenbogen, P.S., Meade, M.A., Jackson, M.N., et al. (2006). The impact of spinal cord injury on the employment of family caregivers. *Journal of Vocational Rehabilitation, 25*(1), 35-44.
28. Fan, J. (2004). Effect of backrest position on intracranial pressure and cerebral perfusion in individuals with brain injury: A systematic review. *Journal of Neuroscience Nursing, 36*(5), 278-288.
29. Flanagan, S.R., Hibbard, M.R., Riordan, B., et al. (2006). Traumatic brain injury in the elderly: Diagnostic and treatment challenges. *Clinics in Geriatric Medicine, 22*(2), 449-468.
30. Franzen, M.D. (2000). Neuropsychological assessment in traumatic brain injury. *Critical Care Nursing Quarterly, 23*(3), 58-64.
31. Goldstein, B. (2000). Musculoskeletal conditions after spinal cord injury. *Physical Medicine and Rehabilitation Clinics of North America, 11*(1), 91-108, viii-ix.
32. Hauber, R.P., & Testani-Dufour, L. (2000). Living in limbo: The low-level brain-injured patient and the patient's family. *Journal of Neuroscience Nursing, 32*(1), 22-26.
33. Henker, R. (2000). Use of blood cultures in the critically ill. *Critical Care Nurse, 20*(1), 45-50.
34. Henker, R. (1999). Evidence-based practice: Fever-related interventions. *American Journal of Critical Care, 8*(1), 481-489.
35. Hickey, J.V. (2003). Craniocerebral trauma. In J.V. Hickey (Ed.), *The clinical practice of neurological and neurosurgical nursing* (5th ed., pp. 373-406). Philadelphia: J.B. Lippincott.
36. Hickey, J.V. (2003). Vertebral and spinal cord injuries. In J.V. Hickey (Ed.), *The clinical practice of neurological and neurosurgical nursing* (5th ed., pp. 407-450). Philadelphia: J.B. Lippincott.
37. Hickey, J.V. (2003). Intracranial hypertension: Theory and management of increased intracranial pressure. In J.V. Hickey (Ed.), *The clinical practice of neurological and neurosurgical nursing* (5th ed., pp. 285-318). Philadelphia: J.B. Lippincott.
38. Iacono, L.A. (2000). Exploring the guidelines for the management of severe head injury. *Journal of Neuroscience Nursing, 32*(1), 54-60.
39. Iacono, L.A., & Lyons, K.A. (2005). Making GCS as easy as 1, 2, 3, 4, 5, 6. *Journal of Trauma Nursing, 12*(3), 77-81.
40. Johnson, M., Bulechek, G., Butcher, H., et al. (2006). *NANDA, NOC and NIC linkages* (2nd ed). St. Louis: Mosby.
41. Jumisko, E., Lexell, J., & Soderberg, S. (2005). The meaning of living with traumatic brain injury in people with moderate or severe traumatic brain injury. *Journal of Neuroscience Nursing, 37*(1), 42-50.
42. Karlet, M.C. (2001). Acute management of the patient with spinal cord injury. *International Journal of Trauma Nursing, 7*(2), 43-48.
43. Kavchak-Keyes, M.A. (2000). Autonomic hyperreflexia. *Rehabilitation Nursing, 25*(1), 31-35.
44. Kemp, B., & Thompson, L. (2002). Aging and spinal cord injury: Medical, functional, and psychosocial changes. *SCI Nursing, 19*(2), 51-60.
45. Kinder, R.A. (2005). Psychological hardiness in women with paraplegia. *Rehabilitation Nursing, 30*(2), 1-27.
46. Kirkness, C.J. (2005). Cerebral blood flow monitoring in clinical practice. *AACN Clinical Issues, 16*(4), 476-487.
47. Kirshblum, S.C., & O'Connor, K.C. (2000). Levels of spinal cord injury and predictors for neurologic recovery. *Physical Medicine and Rehabilitation Clinics of North America, 11*(1), 1-27, vii.

48. LeJeune, G., & Howard-Fain, T. (2002). Nursing assessment and management of patients with head injuries. *Dimensions of Critical Care Nursing, 27*(6), 226-229.

49. Lohne, V. (2001). Hope in patients with spinal cord injury: A literature review related to nursing. *Journal of Neuroscience Nursing, 82*(2), 173-187.

50. March, K. (2000). Intracranial pressure monitoring and assessing intracranial compliance in brain injury. *Critical Care Nursing Clinics of North America, 12*(4), 429-435.

51. Marion, D.W. (2004). Controlled normothermia in neurologic intensive care. *Critical Care Medicine, 32*(2, Suppl), S43-S45.

52. Marion, D.W., & Speigel, T.P. (2000). Changes in the management of severe traumatic brain injury: 1991-1997. *Critical Care Medicine, 28*(1), 16-18.

53. McIlvoy, L.H. (2005). The effect of hypothermia and hyperthermia on acute brain injury. *AACN Clinical Issues, 16*(4), 488-500.

54. McIlvoy, L., et al. (2001). Successful incorporation of the severe head injury guidelines into a phased-outcome clinical pathway. *Journal of Neuroscience Nursing, 33*(2), 72-78.

55. Mitchell, P.H., Ozuna, J., & Lipe, H. (1981). Moving the patient in bed: Effects on intracranial pressure. *Nursing Research, 30*(4), 212-218.

56. Moore, K.N., Burt, J., & Voaklander, D.C. (2006). Intermittent catheterization in the rehabilitation setting: A comparison of clean and sterile technique. *Clinical Rehabilitation, 20*(6), 461-468.

57. Mortimer, D.S., & Jancik, J. (2006). Administering hypertonic saline to patients with severe traumatic brain injury. *Journal of Neuroscience Nursing, 38*(3), 142-146.

58. Oertel, M., Kelly, D.F., Lee, J.H., et al. (2002). Metabolic suppression therapy as a treatment for intracranial hypertension: Why it works and when it fails. *Acta Neurochirurgica, 81*(Suppl), 69-70.

59. Olson, D.M., & Graffagnino, C. (2005). Consciousness, coma, and caring for the brain-injured patient. *AACN Clinical Issues, 16*(4), 441-455.

60. Pagni, C.A., & Zenga, F. (2005). Posttraumatic epilepsy with special emphasis on prophylaxis and prevention. *Acta Neurochirurgica, 93*(Suppl), 27-34.

61. Pryor, J. (2004). What environmental factors irritate people with acquired brain injury? *Disability and Rehabilitation, 26*(16), 974-980.

62. Pryor, J. (2006). What do nurses do in response to their predictions of aggression? *Journal of Neuroscience Nursing, 38*(3), 177-182.

63. Quint, D.J. (2000). Indications for emergent MRI of the central nervous system. *Journal of the American Medical Association, 283*(7), 853-855.

64. Ronne-Engstrom, E., & Winkler, T. (2006). Continuous EEG monitoring in patients with traumatic brain injury reveals a high incidence of epileptiform activity. *Acta Neurologica Scandinavica, 114*(1), 47-53.

65. Roth, P., & Farls, K. (2000). Pathophysiology of traumatic brain injury. *Critical Care Nursing Quarterly, 23*(3), 14-25.

66. Rovlias, A., & Kotson, S. (2000). The influence of hyperglycemia on neurologic outcome in patients with severe head injury. *Neurosurgery, 46*(2), 335-342.

67. Stempien, L., & Tsai, T. (2000). Intrathecal baclofen pump use for spasticity: A clinical survey. *American Journal of Physical Medicine & Rehabilitation, 79*(6), 536-541, 547-550, 564.

68. Sullivan, J. (2000). Positioning of patients with severe traumatic brain injury: Research based practice. *Journal of Neuroscience Nursing, 32*(4), 204-209.

69. Verhaeghe, S., Defloor, T., & Grypdonck, M. (2005). Stress and coping among families of patients with traumatic brain injury: A review of the literature. *Journal of Clinical Nursing, 14*(8), 1004-1012.

70. Wells, R., Dywan, J., & Dumas, J. (2005). Life satisfaction and distress in family caregivers as related to specific behavioural changes after traumatic brain injury. *Brain Injury, 19*(13), 1105-1115.

71. Wilensky, E.M., Bloom, S., Leichter, D., et al. (2005). Brain tissue oxygen practice guidelines using the LICOX CMP monitoring system. *Journal of Neuroscience Nursing, 37*(5), 278-288.

72. Winemuller, M.K., et al. (1999). Prevention of venous thromboembolism in patients with spinal cord injury: Effects of sequential pneumatic compression and heparin. *Journal of Spinal Cord Medicine, 23*(3), 182-191.

73. Winkelman, C. (2000). Effect of backrest position on intracranial and cerebral perfusion pressures in traumatically brain-injured adults. *American Journal of Critical Care, 9*(6), 373-380.

74. Winter, C.D., Adamides, A.A., & Rosenfeld, J.V. (2005). The role of decompressive craniectomy in the management of traumatic brain injury: A critical review. *Journal of Clinical Neuroscience, 12*(6), 619-623.

75. Wood, R.L.L., & Rutterford, N.A. (2006). Demographic and cognitive predictors of long-term psychological outcome following traumatic brain injury. *Journal of the International Neuropsychological Society, 12*(3), 350-358.

76. Wong, F.W.H. (2000). Prevention of secondary brain injury. *Critical Care Nurse, 20*(5), 18-27.

77. Wright, J.E. (2005). Therapeutic hypothermia in traumatic brain injury. *Critical Care Nursing Quarterly, 28*(2), 150-161.

78. Zuccarelli, L.A. (2000). Altered cellular anatomy of acute brain injury and spinal cord injury. *Critical Care Nursing Clinics of North America, 12*(4), 403-411.

evolve *Did you remember to check out the bonus material on the Evolve website and the CD-ROM, including NCLEX®-Examination Style Review Questions, Open-Book Quizzes, and Chapter Review Audio Podcasts?*

http://evolve.elsevier.com/Black/medsurg

UNIT 17

PROTECTIVE DISORDERS

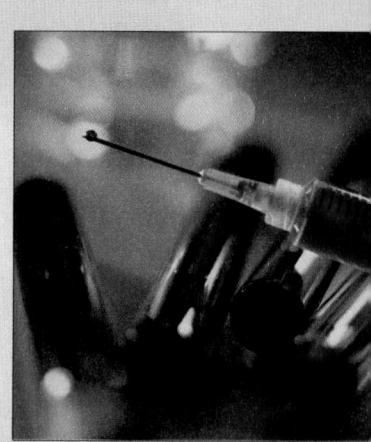

ANATOMY AND PHYSIOLOGY REVIEW:

The Hematopoietic System

Robert G. Carroll

Survival depends on maintaining a barrier separating the inside of the body from pathogens outside of the body and on employing effective defense mechanisms against those pathogens that break that barrier. The epithelium of the skin and of the gastrointestinal (GI), respiratory, urinary, and reproductive tracts provides the barrier. The body defends itself against attack by viruses, bacteria, and other parasites using two sets of separate but interrelated functions: (1) innate immunity and (2) adaptive immunity. Both of these systems must be present and operating properly in order to block establishment of infectious agents, to minimize damage caused by disease in progress, and to expel, destroy, or isolate infectious agents that gain access to inner tissues.

Together, the body is protected using both *surveillance* ("inside" threats) and *defense* ("outside" threats) functions. The importance of these mechanisms to our health and well-being becomes apparent when the defenses of a healthy body are compromised by infection or suppressed by medication or chemotherapy. Parts of the defense system in a healthy body may function inappropriately to reject organ and tissue transplants and may produce autoimmune disease or hypersensitivity states that cause pathologic changes and sometimes death.

RESISTANCE: A FORM OF NONSPECIFIC DEFENSE

The first line of defense in the body is the aspect of resistance that stops a threatening agent or condition. Defenses provide a form of resistance against disease by combating anything not recognized as *self*. Resistance components are usually the first to encounter infectious agents or parasites. Many of these functions operate independently of the immune system but, as shown later, some of the components and features participate in or amplify acquired immune responses.

SURFACE DEFENSES

Intact skin and mucous membranes, combined with surface-clearing mechanisms, are sufficient to provide barriers that prevent penetration to underlying tissues by many pathogens. Lysozyme in tears and bile in the gut inhibit gram-positive bacteria; hydrochloric acid in the stomach is lethal to many pathogens; and fatty acids help protect the skin from infectious agents.

The *reticuloendothelial system* (RES) includes mononuclear phagocytic cells (macrophages). Fixed (attached) macrophages in the sinusoids of the liver, spleen, and bone marrow monitor the circulating blood and remove all foreign particulates and any moribund self cells. Resident mobile macrophages in lymph nodes remove foreign particulate matter. Macrophages in the alveolar spaces are the most active of the RES cells and help remove inspired particulates that reach the lower recesses of the lung.

ORGANS OF THE IMMUNE AND HEMATOLOGIC SYSTEMS

The organs of the immune and hematologic systems are shown in Figure A&P17-1. There are both (1) peripheral sites for the production of the molecules and cells that serve as effector units of the immune response and (2) central organs that prepare antigens for recognition.

Lymph Nodes

Lymph nodes are mostly small organs (many are less than 5 mm in diameter) that are present throughout the body and interconnected by means of lymph vessels. Their structure is fairly complex and provides both RES and immune functions. The lymph node receives fluids, particulates, and solutes that are taken up by lymphatic capillaries from distal tissue sites. Resident macrophages within the node monitor the lymph fluid passing through the node for the presence of foreign particulates and remove them by phagocytic action. Antigenic substances, either particulates or solutes, are taken up by the macrophages or dendritic cells serving as antigen presenting cells (APCs). Immunocompetent cells in the lymph node can initiate either a humoral immune response or a cell-mediated immune response.

Lymph nodes are found in large numbers in the thoracic and abdominal cavities. Those lying close to the body surface are called *superficial nodes*. Cervical nodes lie alongside the neck, axillary nodes in the armpit, and inguinal nodes in the crease between the upper thigh and the trunk. When inflamed, these nodes become swollen and may be palpated, serving as diagnostic signs.

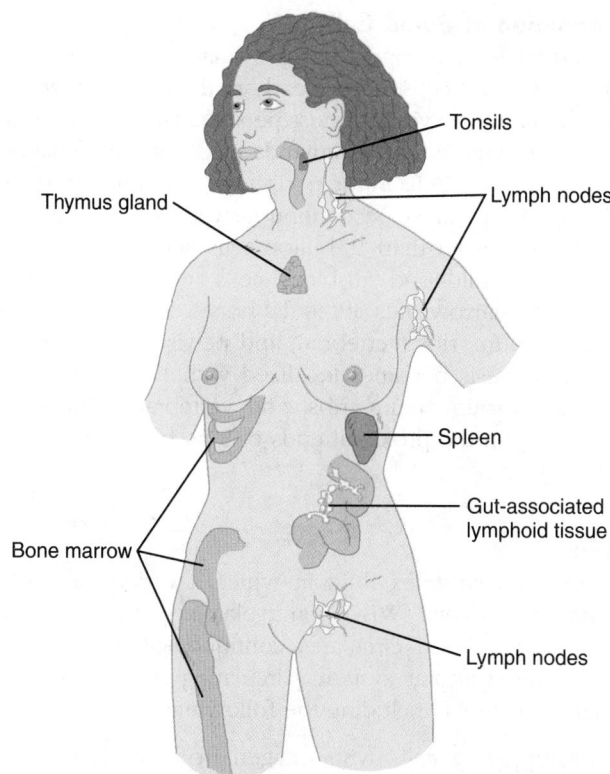

■ FIGURE A&P17–1 Organs of the immune system. The bone marrow, spleen, lymph nodes, tonsils, and gut-associated lymphoid tissue (GALT) function in both specific and nonspecific immunity, whereas the thymus functions primarily in specific immunity.

Lymph Nodules

The structure of the lymph nodules is much less organized than that of the lymph nodes. The nodules occur in the mucosal epithelium lining the respiratory, GI, and urogenital tracts. Antigenic materials are translocated across the epithelium through a special cell (M cell). The translocated material is deposited directly into the nodule structure where it is taken up by APCs. Immunocompetent B cells in lymph nodules produce either immunoglobulin E (IgE) or immunoglobulin A (IgA). These immunoglobulins provide for the development either of an allergic response of the immediate hypersensitivity type or, for IgA, of a mucosal immune response.

Spleen

The spleen is the largest lymphoid organ in the body. Its defensive functions include the blood-clearing process via fixed macrophages in sinusoids as well as serving as a major site of humoral immune responses to blood-borne antigens. The splenic pulp is divided into red zones and white zones. The white zones are accumulations of lymphocytes and APCs. Loss of the spleen or diminished function resulting from injury or infection greatly increases the risk of infection with extracellular bacteria.

Other functions of the spleen include (1) assisting in recycling iron by capturing hemoglobin released from destroyed red blood cells (RBCs) and (2) performing pitting (removal of particles from RBCs without destroying the cell itself).

Thymus

The thymus is located in the mediastinum, and reaches peak development during childhood. After puberty, it begins to atrophy but remnants persist into old age. The thymus is an endocrine organ that secretes hormones that contribute to the maintenance and function of peripheral T-cell populations.

A fundamental paradigm in immunology is the rearrangement of germ line genes during differentiation of lymphocytes in the central lymphoid tissues, leading to the production of molecules for the recognition of antigen. In both cell types, the antigen recognition unit is inserted into the membrane with the antigen-reactive ends extending out into the extracellular environment. The T cell uses the T-cell antigen receptor, and the B cell has a tetrapeptide monomer called *surface immunoglobulin* (SIg). The individual cells each have a unique receptor capable of reacting only with a single antigenic determinant (Figure A&P17-2). Each specifically reacting cell is called a *clonotype;* when properly stimulated by an antigen, the clonotype produces effector units (either antibody molecules or specially reactive cells) and a memory cell clone, both of which have the identical specificity of the original clonotype.

The positive and negative selection processes acting on cells in the thymus make it possible for the mechanism to discriminate between *self* and *non-self* in

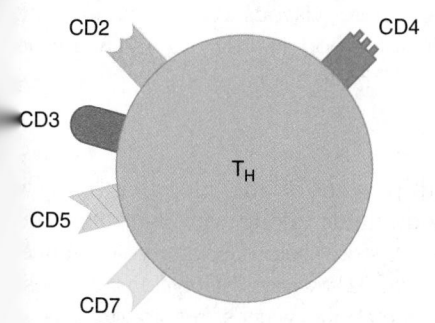

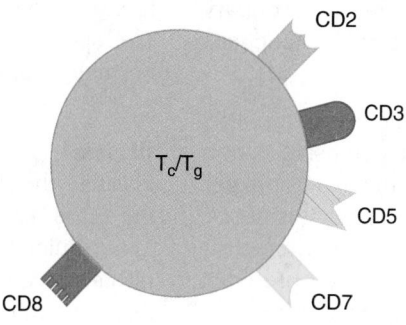

■ FIGURE A&P17–2 T cells can be distinguished by distinctive molecules located on their cell surfaces. They are called cluster designations (CDs). All mature T cells carry markers known as T2 (or CD2), T3 (or CD3), T5 (or CD5), and T7 (or CD7). T helper (T$_H$) cells carry a T4 (CD4) marker, and suppressor and cytotoxic T (T$_c$/T$_g$) cells carry a T8 (CD8) marker.

immune function. This distinction is accomplished by making antigen recognition absolutely dependent on the variable but individually unique composition of the transcription products of gene loci located in the major histocompatibility region of the genome.

The major histocompatibility complex (MHC) consists of integral cell membrane glycoproteins. Class I MHC molecules are found on nearly all nucleated cells in the body and represent a major antigenic distinction between individuals of a given species with different genotypes. This molecule is necessary for antigen recognition by cytotoxic T cells with CD8 surface markers. Class II MHC molecules are found on some APCs, on all B cells, and on antigen-activated T cells. This molecule is necessary for antigen recognition by helper T cells with CD4 surface markers. MHC antigens in humans were initially discovered on leukocyte membranes and are thus called *human leukocyte antigens* (HLAs). It is this recognition system that forms the basis for the rejection of foreign or transplanted tissue. The cells in the recipient's immune system recognize the surface HLA proteins of the donor's tissue as being non-self.

Bone Marrow

Bone marrow constitutes one of the largest organs in the body, with an aggregate weight in adults of about 3000 g (comparable in mass to the liver). Based on visual appearance, the marrow mass was originally described as being either red or yellow. *Red marrow* consists of a mass of supporting cells surrounding aggregates of hematopoietic cells and interspaced with sinusoidal capillaries. *Yellow marrow* is less active in hematopoiesis, with the light color resulting from adipose cells.

Function of Bone Marrow

Bone marrow provides for the following:

- Maintenance of a self-renewing pluripotent stem cell population from which all blood cells are derived
- An environment for the differentiation and maturation of blood cells
- A storage site for large numbers of neutrophils and erythrocytes
- Transformation of undifferentiated lymphocytes into mature B cells
- A site of antibody production in a secondary immune response to thymic-dependent antigens administered intravenously

Sinusoids bearing fixed macrophages serve an RES function in blood clearing. This is a defensive action based on the phagocytic activity of the macrophages attached to the luminal side of the marrow sinuses. These phagocytes, part of the RES or mononuclear phagocytic system, monitor the blood for the presence of foreign particulate matter, remove it, and destroy it.

Formation of Blood Cells

Hematopoiesis, the process of formation and development of blood cells, begins early in the development of the human embryo and must persist unabated throughout one's lifetime. The demands made on this function are enormous. Cells in the peripheral blood have a finite life span and must be continuously renewed at a rate probably greater than 10 billion cells per day.

During childhood, all blood cells are essentially produced in marrow sites of the flat bones of the skull, clavicle, sternum, ribs, vertebrae, and pelvis. After puberty, hematopoiesis becomes localized within the flat bones of the sternum, ilium, ribs, and vertebrae, sometimes occurring in the proximal ends of long bones (humerus and femur).

Blood

Blood is a complex fluid in which a variety of RBCs, white blood cells (WBCs), and platelets are suspended in plasma. Blood circulates continuously through the heart and vascular system. Circulating blood performs many functions, including the following:

- Supplying cells with oxygen from the lungs and absorbed nutrients from the GI tract
- Removing waste products from tissues to the kidney, skin, and lungs for excretion
- Transporting hormones from their origin in the endocrine glands to their targets in other parts of the body
- Protecting the body from dangerous microorganisms
- Promoting *hemostasis* (the arrest of bleeding)
- Regulating body temperature by heat transfer

Composition

About 8% of our total body weight is blood; for example, a healthy young female has 4 to 5 L and a male has about 5 to 6 L. Blood volume also varies by age and body composition. The less body fat, the more blood per kilogram of body weight is present.

Arterial blood is bright red because of the oxygen bound to the hemoglobin within RBCs. Venous blood is dark red because of the lower amount of oxygenated hemoglobin. Pulse oximetry uses this change in color to estimate the oxygen saturation in tissues. Blood is three to four times more viscous (thick) than water. The specific gravity of blood is 1.048 to 1.066. Blood normally has a pH of 7.35 to 7.45.

Plasma

Plasma, the liquid portion of the blood, is one of the three major body fluids (along with interstitial and intracellular fluids). A straw-colored, watery substance, plasma is composed of 92% water, 7% proteins, and less than 1% nutrients, metabolic wastes, respiratory gases enzymes, hormones, clotting factors, and inorganic salts. Serum albumin and gamma-globulin contribute to colloidal osmotic pressure (see the Anatomy and Physiology Review for Unit 12). Gamma-globulin also contains the antibody immunoglobulins IgM, IgG, IgA, IgD, and IgE, which are essential in the body's defense against microorganisms.

Plasma makes up about 55% of the blood, and solid suspended particles (blood cells and platelets) compose the other 45%. If a tube of blood is allowed to stand or is spun in a centrifuge, the cells separate. The term *packed cell volume* or *hematocrit* is used to express the volume or percent of the RBCs in the sample. Normal hematocrit levels are 35% to 45%. Hematocrit can be increased from loss of plasma (e.g., dehydration) or increased production of RBCs (polycythemia). Low hematocrit levels are seen in overhydration, during enhanced RBC loss, or during diminished RBC synthesis (Figure A&P17-3). The WBCs and platelets make up less than 1% of the blood volume. These cells form a buffy coat or white layer and are seen at the interface of the RBCs and plasma.

Hematopoiesis

Stem cells are poorly characterized, undifferentiated cells that exist within the red marrow. These totipotent, or pluripotent, stem cells are self-replicating and maintain a small population throughout the lifetime of the individual. Following stimulation by one or more signal

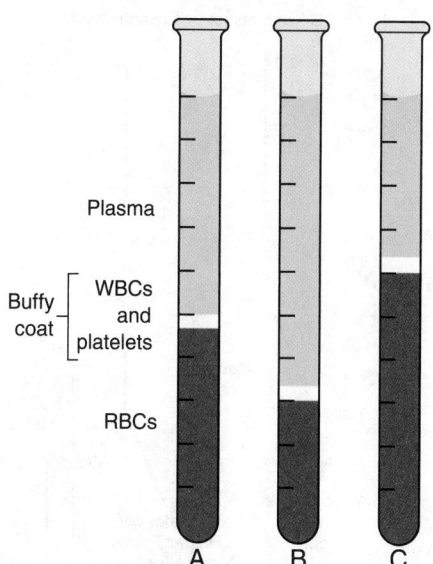

■ **FIGURE A&P17-3** Tubes showing hematocrit levels of normal blood, anemia, and polycythemia. Note the buffy coat located between the packed red blood cells (RBCs) and the plasma. **A,** A normal percentage of RBCs (45%). **B,** Anemia (a low percentage of RBCs, 30%). **C,** Polycythemia (a high percentage of RBCs, 60%). *WBCs,* White blood cells. *(Modified from Thibodeau, G., & Patton, K. [2007]. Anatomy and physiology [6th ed.]. St. Louis: Mosby.)*

molecules called *poietins,* the stem cells can undergo differentiation into erythrocytes (RBCs), megakaryocytes, and leukocytes. The steps of hematopoiesis and the divisions of each cell, once it takes a committed path, are shown in Figure A&P17-4.

Control of Hematopoiesis. Growth factors *(cytokines)* control blood cell growth, proliferation, and differentiation. Growth factors are usually identified by using acronyms that are a legacy from original studies of colony-forming cells. The suffix "-CSF" (colony-stimulating factor) describes the growth factor that stimulates or regulates the development of the corresponding cell type identified by the prefix "CFU-." For example, G-CSF is the growth factor for CFU-G (colony-forming unit–granulocytic series), and M-CSF is the growth factor regulating the development of monocytes (CFU-M). Other growth factors—interleukins (ILs)—are given numbers to distinguish between different molecules.

Red Blood Cells

RBCs (erythrocytes) carry oxygen to the cells and help transport carbon dioxide back to the lungs. RBCs also assist with acid-base balance. They contain carbonic anhydrase, an enzyme that joins carbon dioxide to water to form carbonic acid. The acid dissociates to form bicarbonate and hydrogen ions, which diffuse out of the RBC.

The mature RBC has no nucleus and is only 7.5 mm in diameter. Each RBC has a depression on the flat surface that provides a thin center and thicker edges. The unique structure of the RBC supplies a large surface area relative to its volume (to facilitate exchange by diffusion) and allows the cell to change shape passively as it flows through capillaries that are smaller than 7.5 mm in diameter. The average RBC count is 5,500,000 cells/mm^3 of blood.

Packed within each RBC are about 200 to 300 million molecules of hemoglobin. Each hemoglobin molecule is composed of four protein chains (globin). The globin is bound to a heme group that contains one iron atom. In healthy men, 100 ml of blood contains 14 to 16 g of hemoglobin. Women have slightly less, about 12 to 14 g. Anemia is present when hemoglobin levels decrease to less than 10 g per 100 ml of blood.

Erythrocyte Production. The production of erythrocytes is termed *erythropoiesis.* Normally, more than 100 million RBCs, or about 1% of the body's total, are formed to replace an equal number of destroyed cells. Erythropoietin increases the rate of RBC production when oxygen levels decrease or during pregnancy. Healthy bone marrow has the capacity to increase its production of erythrocytes six to eight times over the normal rate and is thus able to keep pace with increased destruction or

CELLS SEEN
IN BONE MARROW

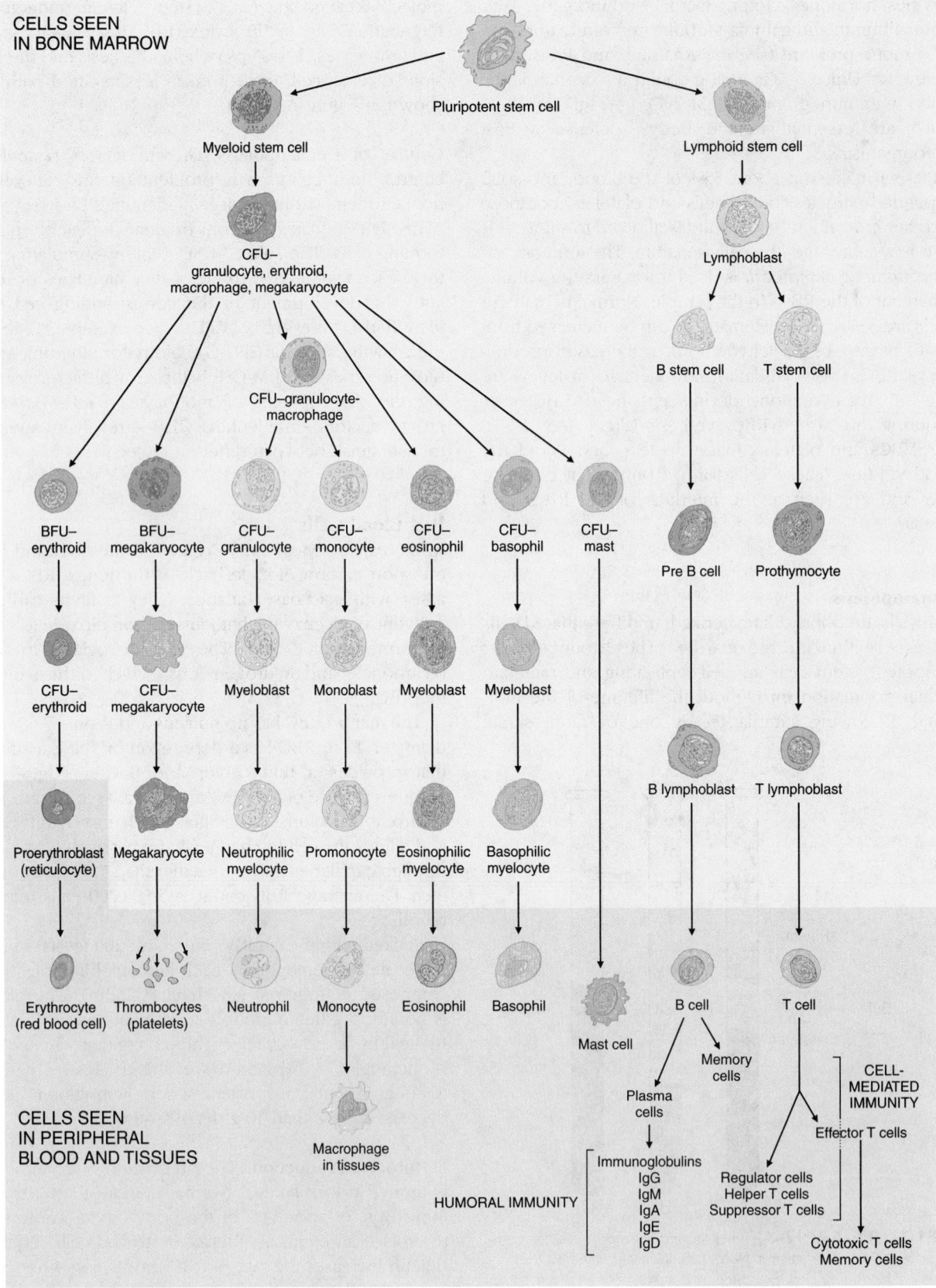

CELLS SEEN
IN PERIPHERAL
BLOOD AND TISSUES

■ **FIGURE A&PI7–4** Hematopoietic cascade. The pluripotent stem cell is the origin of all cells. Once a pathway is chosen, the cell is committed to the final cell type.

loss of RBCs. This response mechanism leads to a remarkably constant number of erythrocytes.

Erythrocytes are produced in the red bone marrow. Required for this process are (1) precursor cells, (2) a proper microenvironment, and (3) adequate supplies of iron, vitamin B_{12}, folic acid, protein, pyridoxine, and traces of copper. If any of these factors is missing, the resultant erythrocytes are fragile, misshapen, abnormally large or small, deficient in hemoglobin, or too few in number. Erythrocytes arise from nucleated cells called *hematopoietic stem cells*. *Stem cells* can maintain a constant population of newly differentiating cells. Differentiation takes about 7 days and involves about six stages (see Figure A&P17-4).

Immature erythrocytes leave the bone marrow via veins in the marrow and enter the general circulation as nucleated reticulocytes. After their release from the marrow sites, the reticulocytes travel to the spleen, where they undergo conditioning and evolve into mature erythrocytes before being released into the general circulation.

The life span of RBCs is about 105 to 120 days. As erythrocytes age, they become increasingly fragile and eventually rupture. The released hemoglobin and the empty membranes ("ghost cells") are taken up by macrophages within the liver, spleen, lymph nodes, and bone marrow. The hemoglobin is broken down into heme (iron and porphyrin) and globin (polypeptide chain) fractions. The iron of the heme fraction is returned to the liver, spleen, and bone marrow to be reused in making hemoglobin. The liver converts the porphyrin of the heme fraction into bilirubin, an orange pigment, and secretes it into the bile to be excreted from the body in the feces and urine (Figure A&P17-5). During periods of increased RBC destruction (e.g., in hemolytic anemia),

excessive amounts of bilirubin are formed and may accumulate in the body's tissues.

Nutritional Influences on Red Blood Cell Production. Vitamin B_{12} and folic acid are essential for normal RBC maturation and nervous system function. Because it is not synthesized in the body, vitamin B_{12} must be a component of the daily diet. Animal products such as meat and dairy products are primary sources of this vitamin. When released from food during digestion, vitamin B_{12} binds with *intrinsic factor,* and the complex is absorbed in the distal ileum. Folic acid, a B-group vitamin synthesized by many plants and bacteria, is also necessary for RBC formation and maturation.

Iron is essential to hemoglobin production. The adult human body contains about 50 mg of iron per 100 ml of blood. Total body iron ranges between 2 and 6 g, depending on the size of the person and the amount of hemoglobin sequestered within the cellular compartment. Hemoglobin accounts for about two thirds of the total iron (called *essential iron*). The other one third resides in the bone marrow, spleen, liver, and muscle. When an iron deficiency develops, the latter iron stores are depleted first, followed by a gradual loss of the iron contained in hemoglobin.

Megakaryocytes and Platelets

Platelets *(thrombocytes)* have two essential roles in hemostasis: (1) occlusion of small openings in blood vessels (a hemostatic function) and (2) provision of chemical components in the molecular cascade leading to coagulation (a thromboplastic function).

Individual platelets are produced by a fragmentation process from giant multinucleated cells in the red bone marrow called *megakaryocytes* (see Figure A&P17-4). The time required for the formation of human platelets is about 5 days. Cytoplasmic extensions from megakaryoblasts are extruded into sinusoids, and platelets are formed by fragmentation at the terminal ends of the filaments. Normal human marrow may have up to 6 million megakaryocytes per kilogram of body weight, with each megakaryocyte being able to produce 1000 or more individual platelets. Platelet production in a normal person appears to be under tight control by the hepatic hormone *thrombopoietin* and is remarkably consistent, with the numbers in a healthy person often remaining constant for years.

Hemostasis. Normal hemostasis is a process that repairs vascular breaks to reduce blood loss from blood vessels while maintaining the flow of blood through the vascular system. Hemostasis occurs in three stages: (1) *vasoconstriction* of the blood vessels, (2) formation of a platelet plug, and (3) coagulation or formation of a fibrin clot. Once the fibrin clot has served its purpose, further

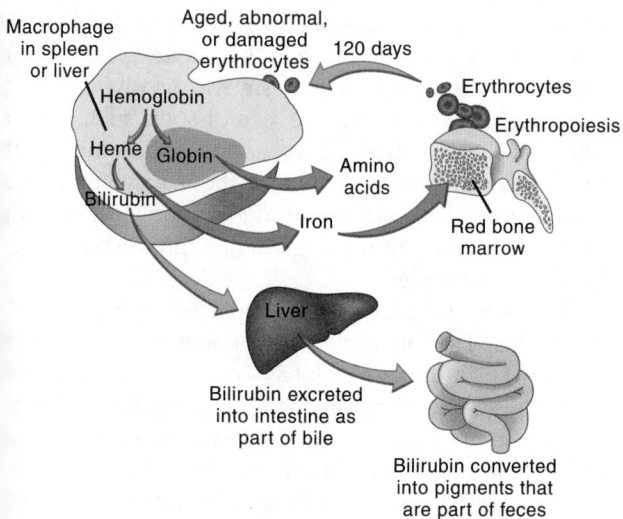

FIGURE A&P17-5 Destruction of red blood cells. *(From Thibodeau, G., & Patton, K. [2007]. Anatomy and physiology [6th ed.]. St. Louis: Mosby.)*

clot formation is balanced by anticoagulation and by *fibrinolysis* (clot dissolution).

Whenever bleeding results from injury or disease, the blood vessels that supply the damaged site constrict. Vasoconstriction slows the flow of blood to the injured area, decreasing blood loss. Vasoconstriction results from muscular tissue and reflex nervous system reactions. *Thromboxane A_2*, a potent local vasoconstrictor, is secreted by platelets and promotes constriction of small blood vessels following injury.

Adequate numbers of platelets (150,000 to 400,000/mm^3) are required in the peripheral blood for hemostasis. When platelets come into contact with an alteration of the endothelial cell lining of a blood vessel, they become sticky and adhere to one another, thus sealing the surface of the vessel lining. These platelet constituents can activate additional platelets that aggregate to form a *thrombus*.

Platelets control hemostasis unless large blood vessels have been damaged. If bleeding is severe, coagulation factors must join with platelets to form a permanent clot. The coagulation system consists of a series of interactions that result in the formation of a fibrin clot. The system consists of clotting proteins, most of which circulate in the plasma in an inactive state.

The formation of a fibrin clot can result from activation of one of two pathways: *intrinsic* or *extrinsic* (Figure A&P17-6). Various factors are needed by these two pathways for completion of a final common pathway that results in a fibrin clot. The *extrinsic pathway* is initiated when tissue injury occurs outside the vessels, such as a burn. The *intrinsic pathway* involves the blood itself (i.e., antigen-antibody reactions and endotoxins) or damage to the blood vessels. Blood in normal vessels that is stagnant for a long time can form clots.

Activated factor X is responsible for the conversion of prothrombin to thrombin and of soluble fibrinogen to an insoluble fibrin clot. The protein fibrin forms dense interlacing threads that entrap erythrocytes and platelets. The platelets then release a contractile protein, which causes shrinkage and retraction of the clot into a firm, insoluble fibrin mass. The process of retraction squeezes out the clear yellow serum. Serum differs from plasma in that it does not contain clotting factors.

In some cases, formation of a fibrin clot is unnecessary because hemostasis occurs at an early stage. Temporary clots are sometimes insufficient. For example, bleeding from a small pinprick can normally be ended by a platelet plug, whereas more serious cuts require the interaction of the various coagulation factors.

Fibrinolysis and Anticoagulants. The coagulation system is controlled by several mechanisms to maintain a flow of blood through the vascular space. The blood carries natural anticoagulants (e.g., heparin, antithrombin, antithromboplastin) that act continuously to inhibit

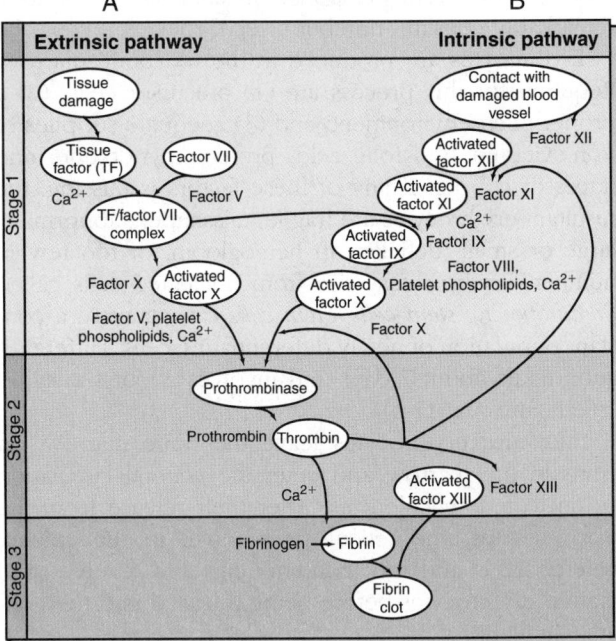

■ **FIGURE A&P17–6** Clot formation. **A,** Extrinsic clotting pathway. *Stage 1:* Damaged tissue releases tissue factor (TF), which with factor VII and calcium ions activate factor X. Activated factor X, factor V, phospholipids, and calcium ions form prothrombinase. *Stage 2:* Prothrombin is converted to thrombin by prothrombinase. *Stage 3:* Fibrinogen is converted to fibrin by thrombin. Fibrin forms a clot. **B,** Intrinsic clotting pathway. *Stage 1:* Damaged vessels cause activation of factor XII. Activated factor XII activates factor XI, which activates factor IX. Factor IX, along with factor VIII and platelet phospholipids, activates factor X. Activated factor X, factor V, phospholipids, and calcium ions form prothrombinase. *Stages 2 and 3* take the same course as in the extrinsic clotting pathway. *(From Thibodeau, G., & Patton, K. [2007]. Anatomy and physiology [6th ed.]. St. Louis: Mosby.)*

coagulation. The liver and RES also aid in controlling coagulation by removing activated clotting factors and fibrin.

In fibrinolysis, the fibrin clot is dissolved. The fibrinolytic mechanism activates in less than a day after clot formation. Formation of plasmin by *tissue plasminogen activator* is the major mechanism for dissolving a clot. Plasmin, a proteolytic enzyme, can dissolve such protein material as fibrin, fibrinogen, and factors V and VIII. Plasminogen, a serum globulin, is the inactive precursor of plasmin. Lysis of the clot produces formation of fibrin split products (or fibrin degradation products), which also act as anticoagulants.

Blood vessels break and are repaired continuously in the body. The multiple and complex interactions between clot formation, clot lysis, and anticoagulation allow normal vessel repair without precipitating a massive clot throughout the vascular system. Clots formed in the venous system often break free (embolus) and are transported to the lung capillaries, which have enhanced clot lysis properties. In contrast, emboli formed on the arterial system travel progressively through the arteriolar tree until they occlude an arteriole and block blood flow to areas distal to the occlusion. Clots lodging in the coronary circulation can cause a myocardial infarction, and clots lodging in the cerebral circulation can cause a stroke.

Roles of the Liver and Spleen

The spleen and liver both have important roles in the hematopoietic system. The spleen, lung, and liver sequester some of the peripheral blood erythrocytes, providing a ready reserve supply whenever the RBC count decreases significantly. The liver is also important in the blood-clearing process. Fixed macrophages (*Kupffer cells*) remove inanimate particulates and bacterial cells that appear in the peripheral blood. The roles of the liver in hematopoiesis are mostly indirect, related to the synthesis of plasma proteins and clotting factors, the decomposition of hemoglobin into bilirubin, and the storage of iron in the form of *ferritin*.

White Blood Cells (Leukocytes)

There are five types of WBCs, or *leukocytes*, classified according to the presence or absence of granules and the staining characteristics of their cytoplasm. As a group, the leukocytes appear brightly colored when stained. *Granulocytes* are derived from a myeloid stem cell that differentiates (see Figure A&P17-4). Granulocytes include three types of WBCs that have large granules in their cytoplasm. Their names are derived from the staining properties: (1) *neutrophils,* (2) *eosinophils,* and (3) *basophils*. There are two types of agranulocytes (WBCs without cytoplasmic granules): (1) *monocytes* and (2) *lymphocytes.*

Granulocytes

Neutrophils. Neutrophils stain very light pink-purple with neutral dyes. The granules in their cytoplasm make them appear "coarse," and they have nuclei with many lobes. Because of the appearance of their nuclei, they are also called polymorphonuclear leukocytes ("polys").

The neutrophil is the primary cell to respond during an acute inflammatory response (see Figure A&P17-4). About 90% of mature neutrophils remain in the bone marrow, a storage arrangement that enables the body to quickly release large numbers of these cells when inflammation occurs. The remaining 10% of neutrophils in the peripheral blood are subdivided, about half and half, into a circulating cell group and a cell group that adheres to endothelial linings in small blood vessels.

Thus a complete blood count (CBC) for a healthy person accounts for only about 5% of the total number of mature neutrophils actually present in the body at that time. The increases seen in peripheral WBC counts during episodes of inflammation are the result of large numbers of neutrophils being released from the bone marrow reserve. If the inflamed state is prolonged, the supply of mature cells with lobed nuclei becomes exhausted, and immature neutrophils with a banded nucleus appear in the circulating blood. The life span of the neutrophil is hours to 3 days.

Eosinophils. Eosinophils contain numerous large granules that stain orange. Under normal circumstances, mature eosinophils do not remain long in the marrow; they are present only in small numbers in the peripheral blood (less than 3% of the total WBC count in a healthy person). These cells exit the peripheral blood compartment and accumulate in extravascular sites near epithelial surfaces. From there, they can be recruited to protect against parasitic infections and to modulate IgE-mediated allergic responses. Their life span is hours to 3 days.

Basophils. The basophil stains purple and has large granules. Details of its normal role in body homeostasis are lacking. The intracytoplasmic granules (storage vesicles) include heparin, histamine, and a chemotactic factor for eosinophils. There is disagreement as to whether this cell is a precursor to a similar cell found in solid tissues: the mast cell. Vesicular contents in the mast cell are similar to those found in the basophil, and the human mast cell is known to bind IgE and to be a primary participant in the induction of IgE-mediated allergic cascades.

Agranulocytes

Monocytes. The monocyte is derived from a precursor cell that is indistinguishable from a myeloblast. Subsequent differentiation, however, leads to a cell structure that is markedly different from that of the granulocyte. The monocyte released from the bone marrow into the circulation is a hypoactive phagocytic cell. After becoming attached to sinusoidal endothelium in the spleen, bone marrow, and liver, or after emigrating from the blood into lung, connective, or lymphoid tissue, this cell becomes transformed into a *macrophage* with full phagocytic function. These cells constitute the RES and are responsible for removing all foreign particulate material that enters the body.

The macrophage is attracted secondarily to acute inflamed sites and is the characteristic cell in chronic and in many secretory T-cell–orchestrated inflammatory lesions. Some macrophages also have immune functions by serving as antigen-processing cells and APCs.

Lymphocytes. In their mature form, lymphocytes are assigned to one of three groups according to the presence of characteristic surface markers and cell function (see Figure A&P17-2): (1) Some lymphocytes are programmed in the thymus to become *T cells;* (2) others are programmed in the bone marrow to become *B cells;*

(3) some lymphocytes, not identifiable as either T cells or B cells, are *natural killer (NK) cells*. *B cells* function in antibody-mediated immune responses, helping to defend the body against invasive types of bacteria, bacterial toxins, and some viruses. *T cells* are the basis of cell-mediated immune functions that defend against facultative and obligate intracellular pathogens, fungi, and viruses. *NK cells* make up about 5% to 10% of the circulating lymphocytes. They are involved in killing some tumor cells and some virally infected cells. Their cytotoxicity can be enhanced by exposure to cytokines, which convert a naive NK cell into a lymphokine-activated cell. After binding to a target cell, the NK cell secretes *perforins,* which cause holes to form in the target cell membrane in a manner analogous to the membrane attack complex (MAC) of complement. Interestingly, people who have normal T-cell and B-cell populations but who are deficient in NK cells experience repetitive life-threatening infections by viruses such as varicella and cytomegalovirus.

Inflammation

Inflammation is a complex response to sublethal injury to a tissue, having both local and systemic consequences. The process can be initiated by products released from damaged cells, by components from microbial cells, and by the interaction of effector units and antigen. Within the injured tissue site, the first indication is a transient constriction followed by a sustained dilation of small blood vessels. Swelling at the site is caused by increased capillary permeability and the escape of plasma (with its solutes: complement, fibrinogen, immunoglobulins). At about the same time that the vessels are responding, WBCs begin to stick to the vascular endothelium, a process called *margination*. Neutrophils are the first to escape from the vessels *(diapedesis)* and, in response to a chemotactic gradient, accumulate at the site of injury.

After a few hours, monocytes from the local circulation and macrophages present in local connective tissues begin to infiltrate the site of injury. In a limited type of injury, the healing and resolution begin shortly afterward. Some cytokines produced by stimulated macrophages act locally to stimulate vascular changes and to activate fibroblasts and other cells. The same or other cytokines are distributed systemically and help to initiate the *acute phase response*. This systemic response accompanies a strong local inflammatory response. Many aspects of the acute phase response are initiated by the action of cytokines produced by stimulated macrophages. These stimulatory molecules include interleukin-1 (IL-1), tumor necrosis factor (TNF), and IL-6. The systemic responses of the host include (1) elevation of serum cortisol level, (2) induction of fever, (3) leukocytosis, (4) the de novo appearance of C-reactive protein, an opsonizing protein

that aids in phagocytosis, (5) increased production of complement components, and (6) increased production of siderophores (iron-binding proteins).

IMMUNITY

We can become immunized following *direct* (active) exposure to an antigen and generation of our own effector units or following *indirect* (passive) receipt of effector units produced by an animal, by another human, or by gene-engineering procedures. Indirect natural immunity occurs in utero via colostrum (topologic protection in humans) and across the placenta (systemic protection in humans). Artificial indirect immunity is produced through pooled gamma (immune)-globulin, $RH_o(D)$ immunoglobulin (RhoGAM), and genetically engineered human antibody.

ACQUIRED IMMUNITY

Four types (or compartments) of active immunity are identified based on the type and body location of the effector units:

1. *Humoral immunity.* The effector units are immunoglobulins (IgM, IgG, and IgA) present in the peripheral blood.
2. *Mucosal immunity.* The effector unit is an immunoglobulin (secretory IgA) present in mucous secretions of the respiratory tract, GI tract, and urogenital tract.
3. *Cell-mediated immunity.* The effector units are cytotoxic T cells that circulate in peripheral blood and are present in peripheral lymphoid tissues.
4. *Atopic hypersensitivity (type I hypersensitivity).* The effector unit is IgE, which is attached to surface receptors on mast cells found in connective tissues and subsurface tissues of the respiratory and GI tracts.

THE PRIMARY IMMUNE RESPONSE AND THE IMMUNE CASCADE

A primary immune response arguably occurs only once (Figure A&P17-7). The quality and quantity of the primary immune response depend on many factors, some of which are host-related whereas others depend on the composition of the antigen and how it is presented to the recipient. The primary immune response can be divided into three stages (the immune cascade).

Phase 1: Afferent Phase
Application or Exposure to the Antigen
Topical (skin) exposure is successful only with certain materials called *proantigens*. Examples of these substances include plant secretions (poison oak, poison ivy

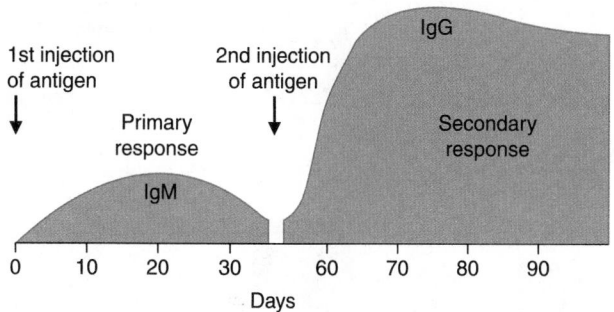

Antibody concentration in serum

1st injection of antigen

2nd injection of antigen

Primary response

Secondary response

IgG

IgM

Days

■ **FIGURE A&PI7–7** Primary and secondary antibody response. The second exposure of an antigen to the host causes a more rapid, stronger, and longer-acting response than the first exposure, owing to the presence of memory cells. Immunoglobulin M (IgM) is most often produced in the primary response, whereas IgG is more likely to be produced predominantly in the secondary response.

salts of nickel and chromium, and formaldehyde. Mucosal exposure, through epithelia in the respiratory, GI, or urogenital tract, is triggered by foods (strawberries, peanuts), drugs (aspirin), pollens, or house dust. Parenteral (subcutaneous, intradermal, intravenous) exposure is via vaccines or allergens for testing.

Transport of Antigen

Lymph nodules lie immediately under modified mucosal epithelium (M cells in the gut). No transport of antigen is required. Antigen deposited into solid tissues gains access to draining lymphatics and is then carried to the nearest regional lymph node. Antigen introduced intravenously localizes in the white pulp of the spleen. Proantigens applied to the skin are absorbed and, in conjunction with Langerhans cells in the subepithelial tissues, are coupled with an autogenous protein. The resultant complex is transported to a regional lymph node.

Arrival of Antigen

Arrival of antigen in peripheral lymphoid tissue is followed by its uptake by APCs. Any exogenous molecule or any cell that does not have the self-markers of the recipient can serve as an antigen. Antigens may be natural, artificial, or synthetic.

1. *Natural* antigens include unmodified bacteria, fungi, viruses, parasites, foreign tissue cells, and large individual molecules such as proteins.
2. *Artificial* antigens are natural antigens that have been altered, usually to produce a vaccine (e.g., killed or attenuated bacteria, inactivated viruses, and toxoids).
3. *Synthetic* antigens are not found in nature but are produced in the laboratory (e.g., molecules genetically engineered to improve current or proposed immunization protocols).

The reactive sites of antigens are called determinant sites (or *epitopes*) and consist of three to five monosaccharide or amino acid residues that act together as a unit. The determinant sites are complementary to the reactive sites of the T-cell antigen receptor (on T cells) and the serum immunoglobulin (on B cells). Each natural antigen has many different epitopes, each of which is capable of stimulating a specific B-cell or T-cell clonotype (Figure A&P17-8).

Phase 2: Central Phase

In phase 2, the central phase, antigen is taken up by or becomes affiliated with processing and presenting cells. Protein antigens are processed intracellularly by the APCs into peptide fragments. The fragments, in association with the major histocompatibility molecules, are placed on the surface of the APCs for presentation to T cells. B cells can react to antigen in solute form, or the antigen can be adsorbed to the surfaces of follicular dendritic cells. T and B lymphocytes become activated and produce effector units and memory clonotypes.

Phase 3: Efferent Phase

Effector units and memory clonotypes are exported to all body sites. If residual antigen remains in the tissues, effector units may combine with it, causing manifestations until the antigen is neutralized or removed. Residual antigen is most often seen with obligate or facultative intracellular parasites or pathogens. This condition is not likely to occur with an extracellular pathogen.

THE SECONDARY IMMUNE RESPONSE

The secondary immune response occurs when a person who has been previously immunized with an antigen is rechallenged later with the same substance. In this second (and any subsequent) response, effector units are generally produced in greater quantity for a longer

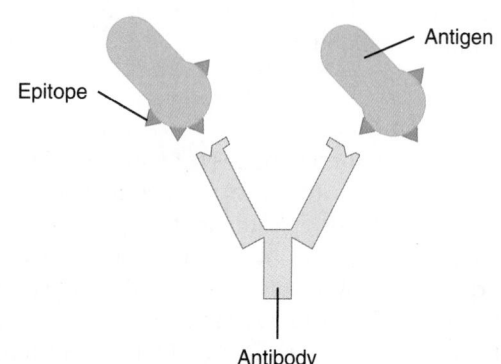

Antigen

Epitope

Antibody

■ **FIGURE A&PI7–8** Epitopes protrude from the surface of an antigen and combine with the appropriate receptor of an antibody, much as a key fits into a lock.

period, and antibody molecules may exhibit a higher affinity for antigen (see Figure A&P17-7).

Antigen Processing and Presentation

T-cell recognition of antigen is limited to peptide fragments presented by an APC in conjunction with an MHC molecule. The recognition process is assisted by CD4 or CD8 molecules on the T-cell surface. Class I MHC molecules are used to present peptides to CD8 cells, and class II molecules present peptides to CD4 cells. This recognition process is said to be self-MHC–restricted; that is, the APC and the T cell both must have the same MHC molecules (each must recognize the other as self). The cells that can function as APCs in peripheral lymphoid tissue sites are B cells, dendritic cells, and some macrophages. Other locations include endothelial cells in peripheral vasculature (in humans) and Langerhans cells in the skin.

B Cells and the Antibody Response

B cells recognize antigen in one of two forms:

1. When free, unprocessed antigen (characteristically carbohydrate) is encountered, the response is limited; only IgM is produced, and there are no memory B clonotypes developed.
2. When proteins or protein conjugates are used as antigens, the APCs must first process the molecules to produce peptide fragments, which are combined with MHC molecules and then presented to T helper cells (Figure A&P17-9).

The activated T cells secrete cytokines, which assist the B cell in responding to its own set of determinant sites present on the protein antigen. The cytokines stimulate growth and maturation in B cells, induce isotype switching, and make possible the development of memory clonotypes in both T and B cell lines.

After being activated by antigen and stimulated by cytokines, the B cell is transformed morphologically and physiologically into a distinct cell type: the *plasma cell*. Plasma cells are highly differentiated and specialized cells that are capable of producing large quantities of secreted immunoglobulin.

Immunoglobulins

Antibodies, or immunoglobulins (Ig), are a family of glycoprotein molecules that are present in the body as solutes in body fluids (plasma and mucous secretions) and attached to a group of cells in solid tissues. Once attached, they inactivate and bind to antigens to facilitate phagocytosis and initiate inflammation by activating the complement cascade (Figure A&P17-10). The terminal amino acid residues react with receptors on the surface of macrophages, neutrophils, B cells, and mast cells. There are five types (Table A&P17-1).

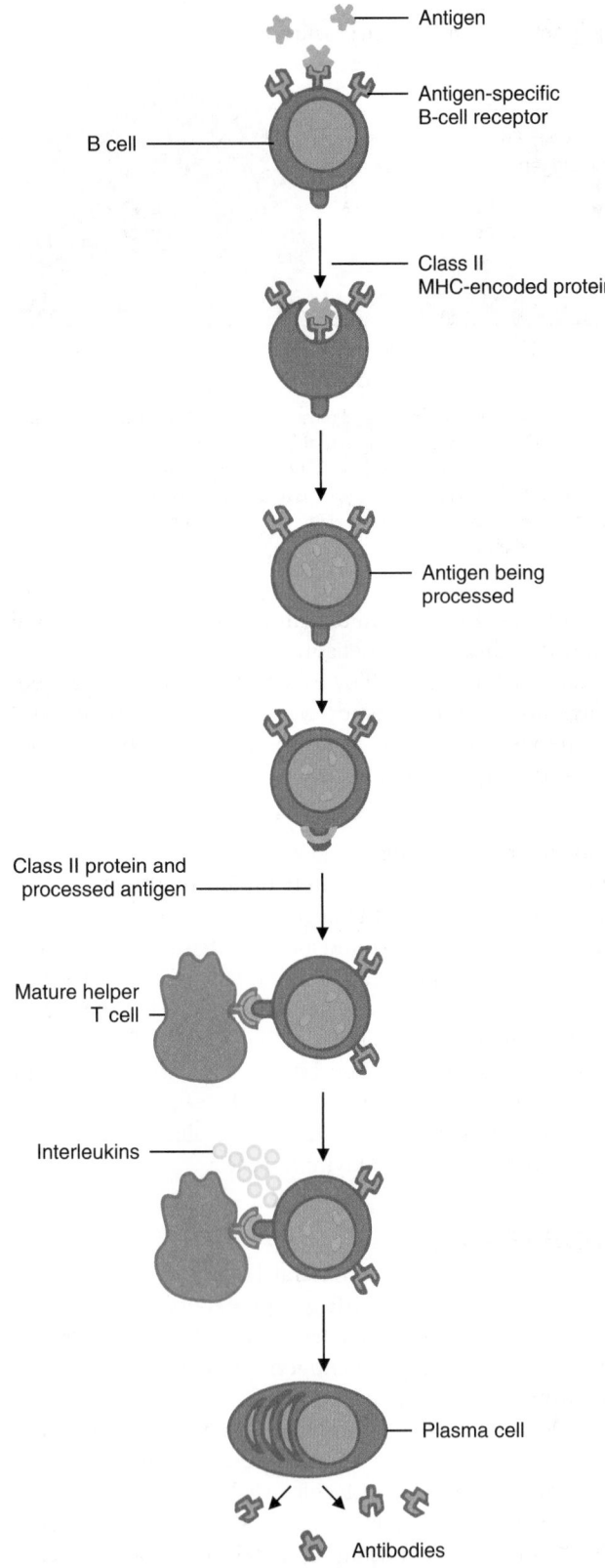

■ **FIGURE A&P17–9** Activation of B cells to make antibody. The B cell uses its receptor to bind matching antigen, which it engulfs and processes. The B cell then presents a piece of antigen, bound to class II protein on its surface. The complex binds to the mature T helper cell, which releases interleukins that transform the B cell into an antibody-secreting plasma cell. *(Redrawn from Schindler, L.W. [1991]. Understanding the immune system. Washington, DC: National Institutes of Health.)*

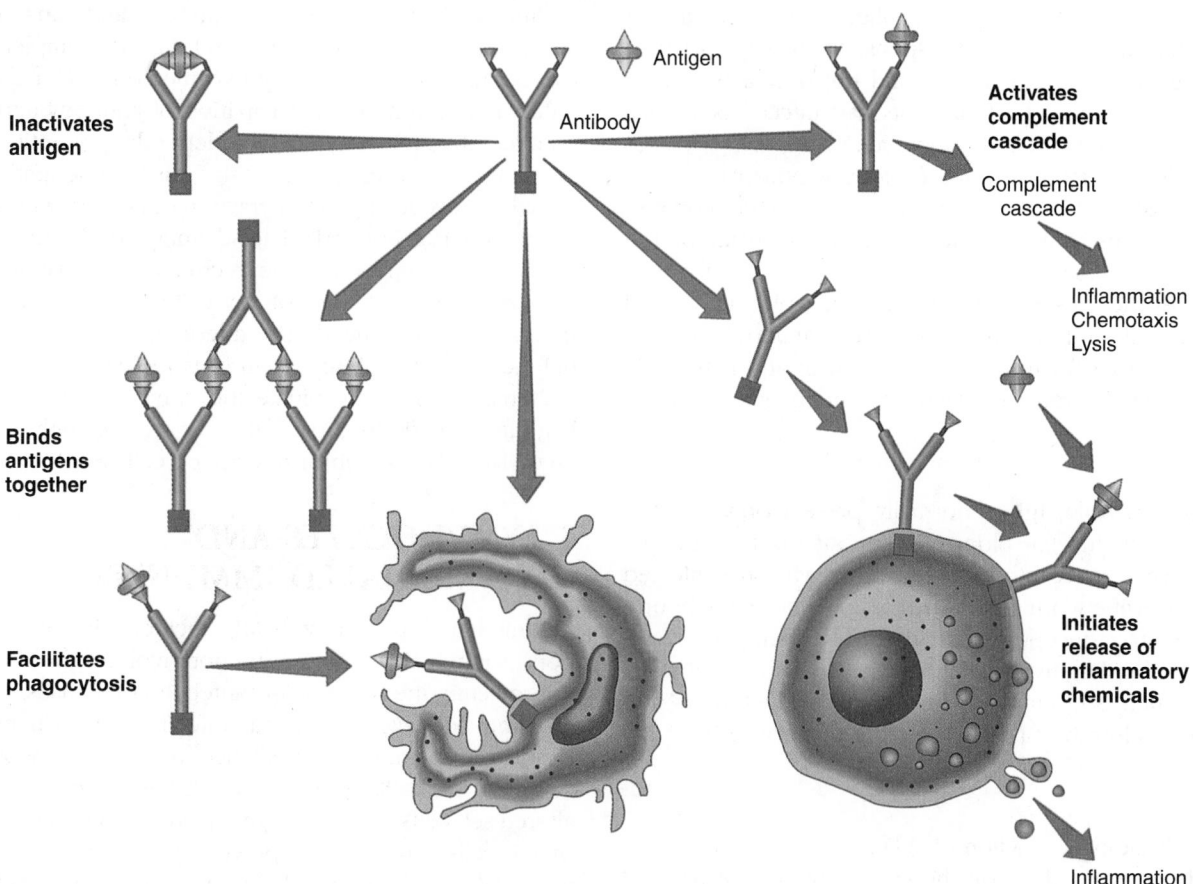

■ **FIGURE A&P17–10** Actions of antibodies. Antibodies act on antigens by inactivating and binding them together to facilitate phagocytosis and by initiating inflammation and activating the complement cascade. *(From Thibodeau, G., & Patton, K. [2007]. Anatomy and physiology [6th ed.]. St. Louis: Mosby.)*

TABLE A&P17–1 Classes and Characteristics of Immunoglobulins (Ig)

Class	% of Total	Characteristics
IgG	75	Present in circulation and tissue spaces Opsonizes antigen Activates complement Transferred transplacentally First Ig synthesized in secondary immune response
IgA	15	Present in circulation and seromucous secretions Prevents adherence of microorganisms to mucosal surface
IgM	10	Present primarily in circulation Powerful agglutinating antibody First Ig of primary immune response Activates complement
IgE	<1.0	Mediates hypersensitivity reactions Binds to mast cells and triggers mediator release
IgD	<1.0	Lymphocyte differentiation Full function unknown

IgG

IgG is available to react either by opsonizing antigens for accelerated uptake by RES cells or by activating complement via the classic pathway. When inflammation occurs in extravascular tissues, IgG is carried out of the vascular compartment to the septic site. There are four subclasses of IgG based on variation in amino acid composition in the heavy chain.

IgA

IgA is the predominant immunoglobulin in saliva, tears, colostrum, breast milk, and intestinal and bronchial secretions. The secretory (or mucosal) form of IgA prevents the adherence of microorganisms to mucosal epithelium and thus supplements resistance mechanisms against local infections in the respiratory, GI, and urogenital tracts.

IgM

IgM is normally present as a pentamer stabilized by a peptide J chain. It is the largest of the immunoglobulin molecules and is the class identified by the designation "natural." It is produced in response to challenge by bacteria in the normal gut flora and not only acts against these and similar bacteria that may infect tissue sites but also is the main immunoglobulin composing the iso-agglutinins reacting with blood group antigens.

IgM is more effective than IgG in activating complement, because only a single pentameric molecule bound to a cell is sufficient to initiate the cascade sequence (IgG requires the presence of two adjacent molecules bound to the cell surface). IgM is the early antibody seen in response to a thymic-dependent antigen and is the sole antibody produced against a thymic-independent antigen.

IgE

In most people, IgE is normally present only in trace amounts within the blood. Exceptions occur in people who have active atopic allergies or who are infected with parasitic worms. In humans, IgE is normally bound to a surface receptor on mast cells, where, following antigen binding, it triggers the release of chemical mediators such as histamine, which helps initiate the cascade of events leading to the expression of atopic allergy.

IgD

The physiologic function of IgD is unknown. It is present in large numbers on the cell membrane of naive B lymphocytes, and its only role is thought to be for antigen recognition.

MONOCLONAL ANTIBODIES

Monoclonal antibodies are immunoglobulins that can be synthesized by fusing a normal plasma cell (for antibody) with a myeloma cell (for longevity). The products of such a hybrid cell are immunoglobulins with an identical specificity. Current technology enables large quantities of immunoglobulins with almost any specificity to be produced at reasonable cost. Because they have a single specificity, they are widely used in research and for diagnostic and therapeutic regimens. Some of the applications include leukocyte identification, parasite and pathogen identification, quantitative estimation of peptide hormones, antitumor therapy, immunosuppression, and fertility control.

COMPLEMENT AND AMPLIFICATION OF ANTIBODY FUNCTION

Complement refers to a group of dissolved plasma proteins. When activated, the various components react in a cascade fashion. Complement activated by antibodies forms holes in the plasma membrane of the bacterium.

Sodium and water diffuse into the cell and cause it to swell and burst (Figure A&P17-11). Plasma complement can be activated by either of two methods: (1) a classic pathway requiring the participation of antibody and (2) an alternative pathway that is independent of antibody.

Activation of complement by the classic pathway must be preceded by the interaction of antigen with antibody (either IgG or IgM). The advantage of this pathway is that complement can be recruited to assist in the removal of any solute or of any cell against which antibody can be produced. The alternative pathway helps defend against pathogens. Surface molecules of many bacterial species can initiate the complement cascade, leading to the destruction of the bacterial cell either indirectly by opsonization or directly by cell lysis.

T LYMPHOCYTES AND CELL-MEDIATED IMMUNITY

Cell-mediated immunity (CMI) includes immune responses in which antibodies are not involved. CMI is vital in protecting the body against infection by viruses, slow-growing bacteria, and fungal infections. It also has a major role in immunosurveillance, reacting to abnormal clones of self cells, some of which are malignant. Such altered self cells can be destroyed in early stages by cytotoxic T cells or by NK cells, preventing them from becoming established tumors. Other CMI functions include primary rejection of allografts and development of delayed hypersensitivity reactions such as contact dermatitis (poison oak) and hypersensitivity to products of the tubercle bacillus. Many of the biologic actions of T lymphocytes are mediated through the secretion of factors called *lymphokines* (cytokines). Although humoral and

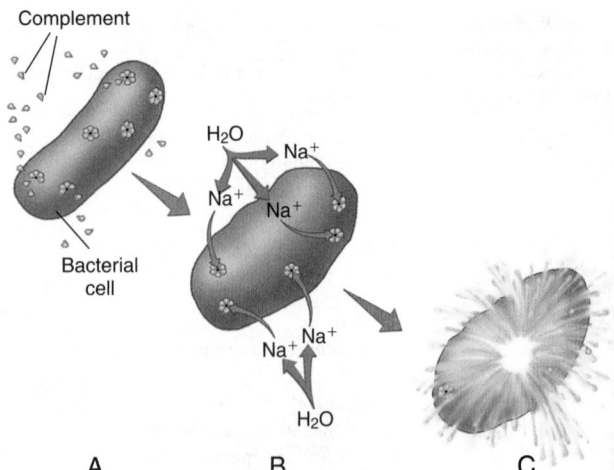

■ **FIGURE A&P17–11** Complement fixation. **A,** Complement molecules activated by antibodies form doughnut-shaped complexes in a bacterium's plasma membrane. **B,** Holes in the complement complex allow sodium (Na+) and then water (H2O) to diffuse into the bacterium. **C,** After enough water has entered, the swollen bacterium bursts. *(From Thibodeau, G., & Patton, K. [2007]. Anatomy and physiology [6th ed.]. St. Louis: Mosby.)*

cell-mediated responses are often discussed separately, these two arms of the immune system work together (Figure A&P17-12), sometimes inseparably, and failure or malfunction in one part of the system frequently alters the effectiveness of the other.

The T lymphocytes that play a predominant role in CMI belong to a variety of T-cell subsets. Some have a regulatory function and are designated as *T helper cells* or *T suppressor cells;* others act as effector cells. Cytokines from antigen-activated T helper cells assist B cells to mature and produce antibody and also modulate the maturation and function of cytotoxic T cells (see Figure A&P17-12). The importance of T helper cell function is reflected by the severe consequences seen when it is suppressed by physical or chemical means or depleted during infection with human immunodeficiency virus (HIV); the T helper cell is a primary target of HIV. The decline of T helper cells in infected people is almost inevitably followed by recurrent episodes of opportunistic infections and the development of malignancy in people with acquired immunodeficiency syndrome (AIDS).

The homeostatic reduction or suppression of B- and T-cell responses to antigen is no longer considered to be restricted to a single suppressor cell population (once thought to be a subset of T cells bearing the CD8 marker). It is currently hypothesized that this type of negative regulation may be a function of essentially all T cells. Whether a given cell will act to produce a positive immune response (produce effector units) or will mediate a negative response (tolerance) may be a function of the mechanism by which an individual T cell is activated by antigen.

The cytotoxic T lymphocyte reacts individually with target cells to establish a contact boundary that is required for target cell destruction. The intimate contact between the target cell and the cytotoxic T lymphocyte is mediated by an antigen-specific process and allows the cytotoxic T lymphocyte to release lytic molecules *(porins)* directly into the membrane of the target cell. Cytokines produced and released by the cytotoxic T lymphocyte during the cell contact phase enhance the action of porins. The cytotoxic T-lymphocyte function

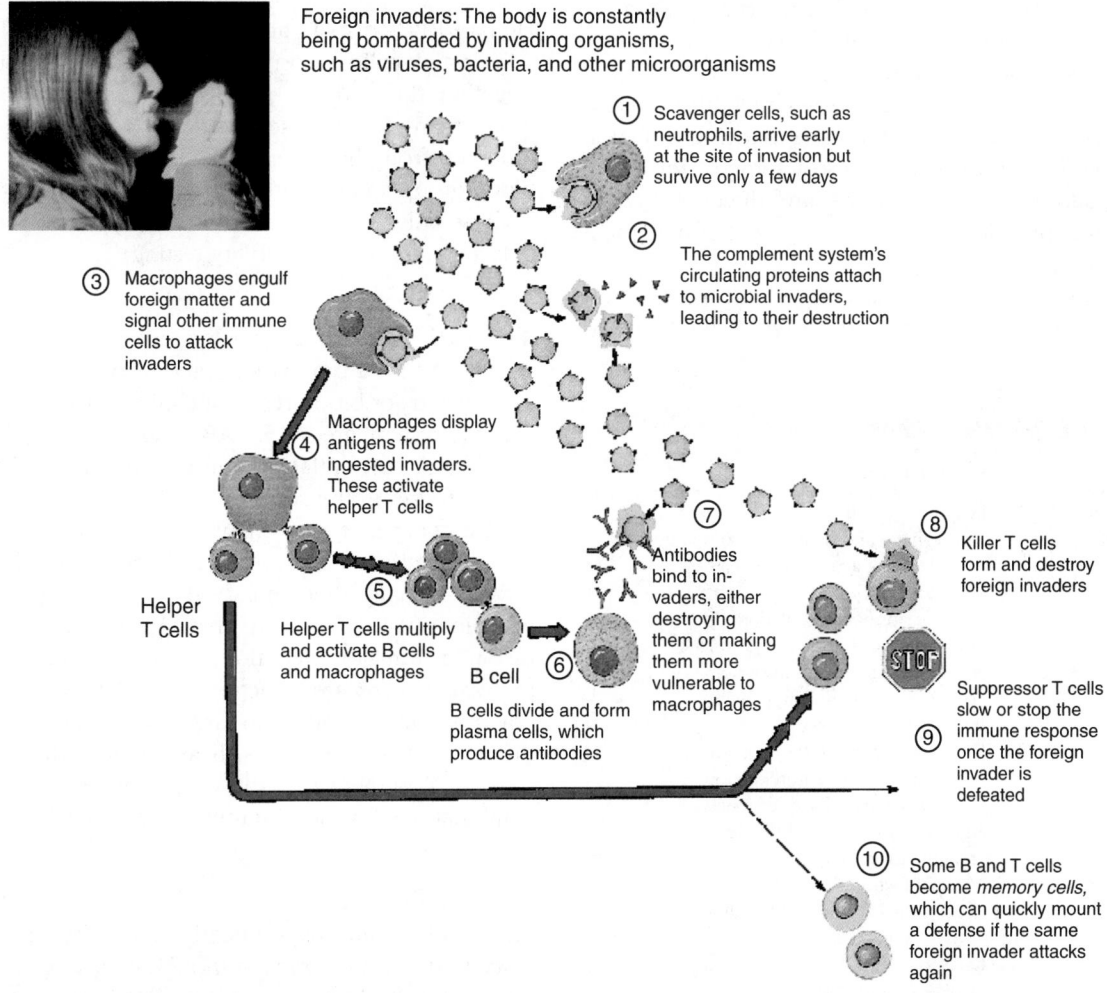

■ **FIGURE A&P17-12** The protective systems include both arms of defense. Sneezing decreases exposure to the virus. Humoral immunity is shown in steps *1* and *2,* cell-mediated immunity in steps *3* and *10.* *(From Thibodeau, G., & Patton, K. [2007]. Anatomy and physiology [6th ed.]. St. Louis: Mosby.)*

is to kill viral-infected host cells, malignant cells, and cells in allograft transplants.

CYTOKINES

The *cytokine* is a general term for cell-derived factors that mediate interactions between cells. Cytokines produced by lymphocytes are called *lymphokines;* those produced by monocyte-macrophage cells are called *monokines.* Some of these factors are called interleukins, indicating service as regulatory signals between various leukocytes (Table A&P17-2).

Cytokines are a diverse group of proteins with four areas of function:
1. Enhancement of mononuclear phagocytes
2. Regulation of lymphocyte growth, differentiation, maturation, and secretory activities
3. Inflammation
4. Systemic effects such as fever induction and induction of hemopoietic activity in the bone marrow

One of the best known cytokines is *IL-1,* originally described in the early 1960s. Produced by macrophages, IL-1 plays a role in induction of fever, acts as a coactivator of T cells, assists in activation of B cells and NK cells, and initiates the acute-phase response.

IL-2 is also well-known from its first identification as a T-cell growth factor. The growth-enhancing function was crucial in the original studies of some of the retroviruses. Current research efforts are directed toward finding an application for IL-2 for treatment of malignant conditions.

IL-3 and *IL-4* are necessary for inducing antigen-stimulated B cells to undergo isotype switching to change from synthesis and secretion of IgM to IgG (or IgA or IgE). IL-3 also stimulates bone marrow stem cells to differentiate into monocytic and granulocytic precursors.

Interferons (IFNs) are another group of molecules that serve as intercellular messengers. There are three major types: IFN-α, produced by many cells; IFN-β, produced by fibroblasts; and IFN-γ, produced by T lymphocytes. All interferons have antiviral activity and have a downregulating effect on proliferation of both normal and malignant cells.

Tumor necrosis factor acts as a growth factor for fibroblasts and has a necrotizing effect on tumor cells. TNF participates in inducing the acute-phase response and is apparently one of the major factors in inducing endotoxic shock (sometimes seen in infections with gram-negative bacteria). This cytokine is thought to be a major cause of infection-related cachexia.

BLOOD GROUPS AND BLOOD TYPING

Human RBCs display antigens that are either glycoproteins or glycolipids on the surface of the membrane. Together the various blood group systems contribute more than 400 characterized antigens. Antigens are inherited from the parents. Fewer than a dozen of these blood group antigens attract frequent clinical notice, and of these only the ABO and rhesus (Rh) systems are major determinants of compatibility testing.

The ABO Blood Group System
The ABO blood type is inherited as an autosomal trait. The four major blood types of clinical importance in this genetic system are A, B, AB, and O. Blood is typed according to the antigens found on the RBC and the antibodies found in the serum.

The two major antigens within the blood group system are antigens A and B. For the antibodies to be formed, usually there must be exposure to foreign or homologous RBC antigens through pregnancy or transfusion. The major exceptions are the A and B antigens, for which there are structurally similar proteins in the environment, resulting in antibody formation against the missing A or B, or both antigens by the age of 3 months. Table A&P17-3 shows the antigen and antibody combinations for the different blood groups.

The Rh System
The Rh blood groups are nearly equal in clinical importance to the ABO groups. Although Rh serology involves more than 20 different antigens, the D antigen has the most clinical significance because of the high risk of formation of an anti-D in an Rh-negative recipient. The

TABLE A&P17–2	Major Cytokines
Cytokine	**Principal Effects**
Interleukin-1 (IL-1)	Lymphocyte activation
	Macrophage and neutrophil stimulation
	Stimulation of acute-phase proteins
	Fever and sleep
	Pituitary hormone regulation
Interleukin-2 (IL-2)	Enhances T-cell growth and function
Interleukin-3 (IL-3)	Stimulates differentiation of hematopoietic cells (colony-stimulating factor)
Interleukin-4 (IL-4)	B-cell growth factor
Interleukin-5 (IL-5)	B-cell growth and differentiation
Interleukin-6 (IL-6)	B-cell growth and differentiation
	Stimulates acute-phase response
Colony-stimulating factor	Stimulates division and differentiation of bone marrow stem cells
Interferon	Antiviral factor
Tumor necrosis factor	Activates macrophages, granulocytes, and cytotoxic cells
	Cachexia
	Mediates septic shock
	Increases leukocyte adhesion
	Enhances antigen presentation

TABLE A&P17–3   The ABO Blood Group System

Blood Type	Agglutinogens on RBCs	Agglutinins in Plasma	Frequency in United States
A	A	Anti-B	41%
B	B	Anti-A	10%
AB	A and B	None	4%
O	None	Anti-A and anti-B	45%

RBCs, Red blood cells.

term *Rh-positive* means that the client has the D antigen; the *Rh-negative* client has no D antigen.

The most striking difference between the ABO and Rh systems is that, in the ABO system, there is spontaneous development of antibodies directed against A and B antigens not present on the RBC. In the Rh system, antibody formation is never spontaneous. Instead, a client must first be exposed to the Rh antigen, for example, through a blood transfusion or pregnancy. Thus clients with Rh-negative blood, transfused for the first time with Rh-positive blood, do not experience a reaction because their blood does not yet contain anti-Rh antibodies (anti-D). About 50% of people, however, develop sensitivity and form antibodies against the D antigen as a result of exposure to it from transfusion or pregnancy. If a sensitized client receives a second transfusion or has a second pregnancy with exposure to the D antigen, some degree of RBC destruction will occur. However, it is usually possible to prevent sensitization from occurring the first time by administering a single dose of anti-Rh antibodies in the form of Rh$_o$(D) immune globulin (RhoGAM) immediately following exposure to the D antigen.

THE HLA SYSTEM

HLAs are also called *histocompatibility antigens* because the antigens (glycoproteins) are found on the surface of most cells in the body except RBCs (including circulating and tissue cells). The HLA system is a series of closely linked genes located on the short arm of chromosome 6. The major function of the HLA antigen is regulation of the immune response, distinguishing self from non-self. This plays a major role in the rejection of transplanted tissues when donor and recipient HLA antigens do not match. There also is an association between HLA antigens and some diseases. For example, in ankylosing spondylitis, the association with HLA factor is so strong that HLA typing can be used diagnostically.

CONCLUSIONS

The immune system is extremely complex. It has evolved through the years to become a pervasive and highly structured group of complex functions that defend the body against pathogens and parasites from the outside and that are able to detect and attack altered self cells that pose threats to an individual's homeostasis.

BIBLIOGRAPHY

1. Goldsby, R.A., et al. (2000). *Kuby immunology* (4th ed.). Philadelphia: W.H. Freeman.
2. Thibodeau, G., & Patton, K. (2007). *Anatomy and physiology* (6th ed.). St. Louis: Mosby.
3. Travers, P., Walport, M., & Shlomchik, M. (2001). *Immunobiology* (5th ed.). New York: Garland.
4. Actor, J.K., DeBord, C. (2007). *Elsevier's integrated immunology and microbiology*. St. Louis: Mosby.

CHAPTER 74
Assessment of the Hematopoietic System

LINDA H. YODER

HISTORY

The nature of the presenting problem determines the focus of the health history for the hematopoietic and immune system. Clients may present with manifestations that suggest a hematologic or immunologic problem.

Biographical and Demographic Data

The immune response is diminished in both very young and older people. Some hematologic and immunologic disorders occur more frequently at certain ages, in women or men, and in those of a particular race or ethnic background. Collect family health history data because several hematologic and immunologic disorders are inherited. In addition, the normal values of some hematologic tests have age-specific and gender-specific norms. For example, hemoglobin and hematocrit levels are lower in women, particularly during the menstrual years, than in men. Hemoglobin values in African Americans are about 0.5 g/dl lower than those in whites.[14]

Current Health

Disorders of the protective system often affect all organs and tissues of the body, resulting in widespread pathophysiologic manifestations. Manifestations may be vague and nonspecific, such as fatigue, malaise, fever, anorexia, weight loss, and chronic diarrhea.

The body's defense against infectious or malignant disease occurs through the immune system. Two main functions of the immune system are to recognize substances that are foreign (non-self) and to eliminate these foreign substances with return to homeostasis. Factors that may affect immune responses are stress, aging, gonadal hormones (specifically estrogen, progesterone, and testosterone), nutrition, alcohol and other central nervous system acting drugs, physical exercise, and sleep.

Chief Complaint

It is important to note the timing; quality and quantity; severity and location; and precipitating, aggravating, and relieving factors associated with hemapoietic system manifestations. The chief complaint of the client may be fever, fatigue, or bleeding. Figure 74-1 provides an overview of the assessment of clinical manifestations related to the hematopoietic system.

Clinical Manifestations

In general, anemias often manifest with fatigue, paleness, and weakness; bleeding disorders with bruising, petechiae, epistaxis, and bleeding gums; and immunodeficiencies with recurrent infections and fever. Allergic manifestations may present as simple skin rashes, nasal stuffiness, and cough, or they may be more severe, such as wheezing and respiratory distress. Assess if different allergens trigger different responses and if the client ever experienced an anaphylactic reaction. Allergic manifestations range from mild to severe and can be systemic or organ specific, such as integumentary, respiratory, gastrointestinal, or cardiovascular reactions.

Fever. Clients with severe neutropenia or immunosuppression may be unable to mount the inflammatory

---

evolve Web Enhancements

Assessment Terms English and Spanish

Appendix B A Health History Format that Integrates the Assessment of Functional Health Patterns

Web Tables Sequence and Palpation Technique for Lymph Nodes

Lymphocyte Immunophenotyping

Immunoglobulin (Ig) Isotopes

Be sure to check out the bonus material on the Evolve website and the CD-ROM, including free self-assessment exercises. **http://evolve.elsevier.com/Black/medsurg**

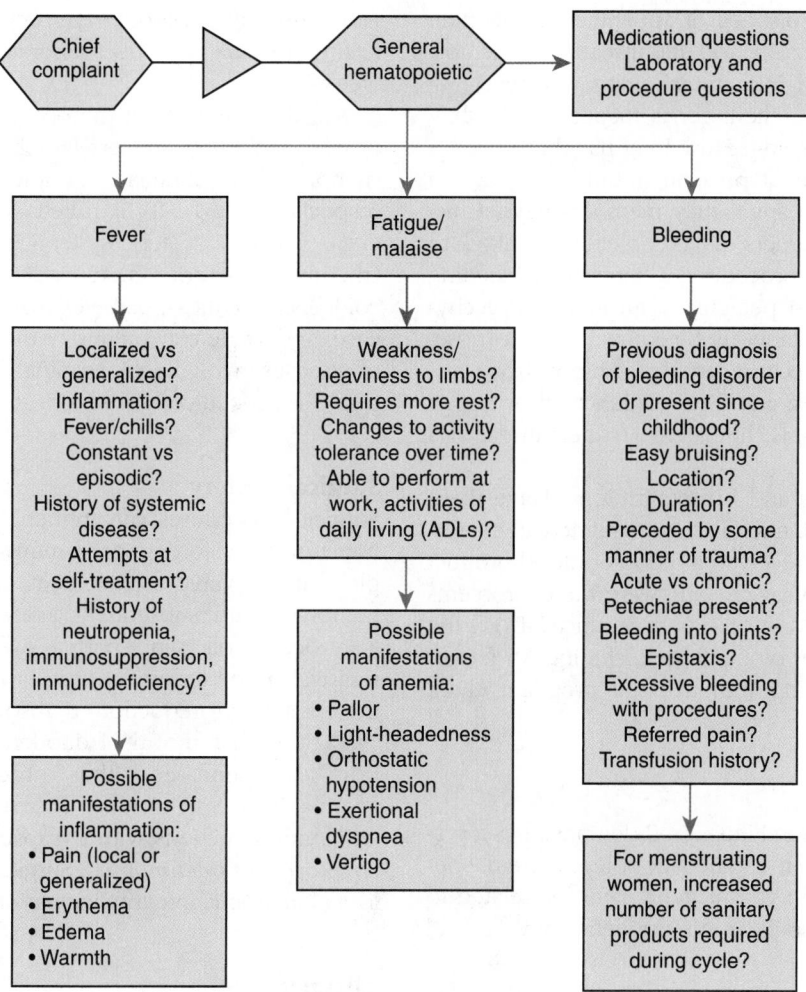

■ **FIGURE 74–1** Expanded hematopoietic assessment.

response of fever, redness, and pus formation. Assess for local inflammation (redness, heat, swelling, pain). Immunodeficiencies may be present at birth or may develop later in life, and they may be *iatrogenic* (a result of treatment with cytotoxic agents, corticosteroids or other immunosuppressants, or radiation). Immunodeficiencies also may result from protein-deficiency malnutrition, protein-losing enteropathy, nephrotic syndrome, or hypercatabolic states (major trauma, severe thermal injury). Immunodeficiencies may be related to loss of anatomic integrity from instrumentation (catheters), impaired dermatologic barrier function (burns, psoriasis, atopic dermatitis), mucosal inflammation (atopic diseases, irritants such as cigarette smoke), or mucociliary elevator dysfunction (cystic fibrosis or immotile cilia syndrome). Any episode of fever should be detailed as completely as possible, including any associated manifestations such as chills or night sweats.

Fatigue/Malaise. Anemia is characterized by pallor, weakness, and lightheadedness; severe anemia manifests with chronic severe fatigue, exertional dyspnea, headache, or vertigo. Does the client have sufficient energy to perform normal activities and occupational tasks? Do fatigue, dyspnea, or other manifestations interfere with a productive lifestyle? Has the client missed time from work or school, resulting in financial loss or other economic concerns, such as health or life insurance eligibility? Does the client feel rested after sleeping? The fatigue from anemia will not improve with increased amounts of sleep. The client should be questioned about a feeling of weakness or heaviness in the limbs.

Bleeding. Assess for bleeding disorders. Ask whether the disorder might be related to genetic factors, exposure to toxins, or liver disease. Cirrhosis, hepatitis, and other liver diseases can result in reduced production of clotting factors as well as reduced clearance of factors that inhibit clotting or promote fibrinolysis. Clients with hemophilia and other congenital coagulation disorders have a history of lifelong bleeding tendencies, such as excessive or prolonged bleeding after circumcision or dental extraction, repeated episodes of spontaneous bleeding into joints (hemarthrosis), and life-threatening hemorrhages (retroperitoneal, intracranial, or paratracheal).

When assessing the client for a suspected bleeding disorder, ask the following: How long has there been a bleeding problem? Was it present in childhood, or did it appear recently? Do any family members have a history of bleeding disorders? Is the bleeding linked to any specific event or procedure? Clients with bleeding disorders may manifest petechiae, purpura, and ecchymoses (bruises); spontaneous bleeding from the nose, gingiva, vagina, and rectum; oozing of blood from cuts and venipuncture sites; jaundice; conjunctival or retinal hemorrhage; hemoptysis, hematemesis, hematuria, and back and flank pain.

Ask about illnesses and hospitalizations. Have there been retroperitoneal, intracranial, or paratracheal hemorrhages? Has the client received a blood or blood product transfusion, and for what reason? Were there problems or reactions to the blood or blood products? Does the client know his or her blood type, including Rh factor? This information is important for the pregnant client who is Rh negative.

Review of Systems

The review of systems in Figure 74-2 demonstrates a systematic history relative to the hematopoietic system. Specific manifestations can vary if the disorder is related to allergy, anemia, bleeding, or immunodeficiency.

Past Medical History

Assess for hematologic disorders by asking whether there is a history of anemia, concurrent disorders (such as renal, liver, or autoimmune disease), cancer, or organ transplantation.

Clients with immunodeficiencies have a history of recurrent infections, especially of mucous membranes (such as the oral cavity, anorectal area, genitourinary tract, or respiratory tract). There may be a history of poor wound healing, diarrhea, or manifestations of systemic activation of the inflammatory response (fever, malaise, fatigue, anorexia, unexplained weight loss, headache, and irritability). There may be a history of unusually frequent bacterial infections, unusually severe viral infections, or development of an infection with an unusual microorganism (fungus or protozoa). When assessing lymphatic problems, inquire about trauma or other injury, especially to an extremity. Has the client had a recent infection or cancer?

Did the client experience an unusually severe course of measles, mumps, or other infectious diseases of childhood? Were there severe reactions to vaccinations, especially immunizations with live virus vaccines such as measles and mumps? Are vaccinations current? Has the client recently donated blood or blood components?

Donating whole blood, erythrocytes, leukocytes, platelets, or plasma can affect laboratory values for days or weeks.

Ask the client about the occurrence of any major illnesses, including cancer, lymphoproliferative diseases (lymphoma, leukemia, multiple myeloma), infection (especially HIV-1, HIV-2, rubella, cytomegalovirus, influenza, varicella zoster), systemic inflammatory diseases (rheumatoid arthritis, systemic lupus erythematosus, sarcoidosis, vasculitis), diabetes mellitus, renal or liver disease, and sickle cell anemia or disease. Is there a history of diseases involving the terminal ileum, Crohn's disease, tropical sprue, ulcers, or severe atrophic gastritis?

Surgical History

Surgical procedures can influence the development of hematologic disorders or immunodeficiency. For example, cardiac valve replacement may cause erythrocyte hemolysis and subsequent anemia. Anemia may also occur following partial or total gastrectomy or removal of the terminal portion of the ileum because of the consequent reduction in absorption of vitamin B_{12}. Surgical removal of duodenal tissue can decrease iron absorption and thus produce iron deficiency anemia. Splenectomy increases the risk of overwhelming infections with encapsulated bacteria such as *Streptococcus pneumoniae*. Surgical instrumentation and loss of anatomic integrity increase the risk of infection.

Allergies

If the client has a history of transfusions with blood or blood products, ask about complications. Reactions to blood products include fever, chills, back or flank pain, wheezing, headache, vomiting, urticaria (hives), and shock. Inquire about food and drug allergies or sensitivities. Has the client ever had an anaphylactic reaction or been hospitalized for an allergic reaction?

Clients with allergies may have rhinitis, sinusitis, urticaria, and pruritus. Ask whether allergic manifestations have been present since childhood. Can the client identify triggers? Is there a seasonal pattern associated with the manifestations? Has hospitalization or emergency treatment been necessary for a severe allergic reaction? Was desensitization therapy (allergy shots) undertaken, and if so was it effective?

Medications

Note the client's past and current use of both prescription and over-the-counter (OTC) drugs as well as herbal or complementary remedies and alcohol intake. Many medications can prolong bleeding; cause hemolysis of red blood cells; or, through selective or general bone marrow suppression, produce anemia, thrombocytopenia, or leukopenia. Medications also can inhibit folic acid

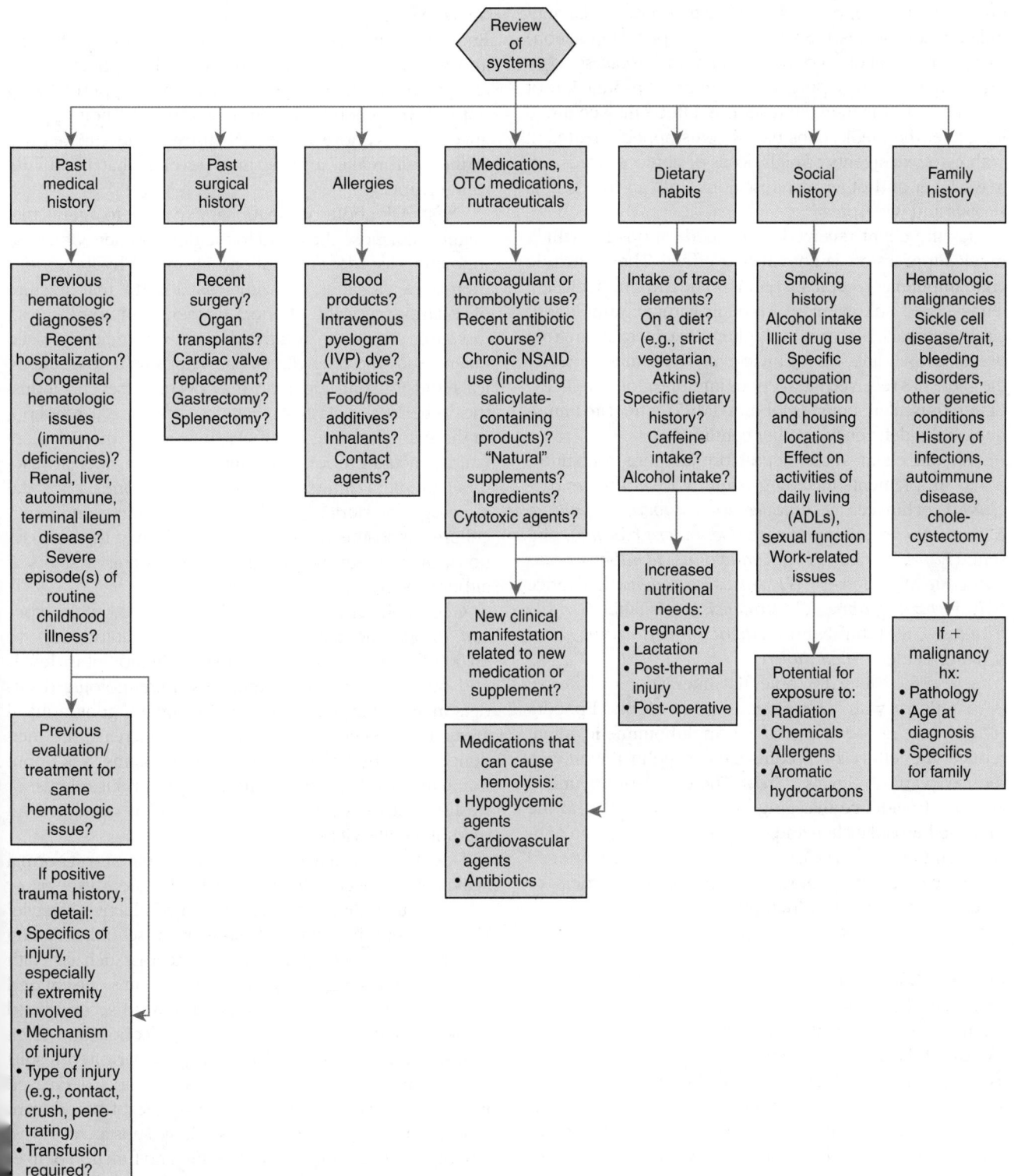

FIGURE 74–2 Expanded hematopoietic history.

absorption from the intestine, leading to folic acid deficiency and anemia.

Ask about current or recent anticoagulant therapy or thrombolytic treatment. The anticoagulants heparin and warfarin prolong bleeding, and heparin may also cause immune-mediated thrombocytopenia. The thrombolytic agents streptokinase, tissue plasminogen activator (t-PA), and urokinase also prolong bleeding.

Has the client taken corticosteroids, cytotoxic agents (cyclophosphamide, chlorambucil, cisplatin, etoposide), other immunosuppressants (gold salts, nonsteroidal anti-inflammatory drugs [NSAIDs]), or therapies (irradiation) for the treatment of cancer or autoimmune diseases? These agents may suppress bone marrow production of blood cells or the immune response. Effects may continue long after the medications have been stopped. Treatment with cytotoxic agents or high doses of corticosteroids can mask fever and other manifestations until an infection is serious and widespread.

Has the client received other medications for which myelosuppression is an adverse effect? These include chloramphenicol, cephalosporins, clindamycin, penicillin, tetracycline, sulfonamides, D-penicillamine, amphotericin B, antimalarials, captopril, phenothiazines, antithyroid drugs, zidovudine, and ganciclovir. Determine whether the client has received intravenous immune globulin (IVIG) or intramuscular immune globulin (IMIG) to treat an immunoglobulin deficiency or other conditions.

Ask the client about herbal preparations and nutritional supplements including comfrey *(Symphytum officinale),* echinacea *(Echinacea angustifolia, E. pallida, E. purpura),* evening primrose *(Oenothera biennis),* ginseng *(Panax ginseng, P. quinquefolius, Eleutherococcus senticosus),* goldenseal *(Hydrastis canadensis),* licorice *(Glycyrrhiza glabra, G. uralensis),* maitake *(Grifola frondosa),* St. John's wort *(Hypericum perforatum),* and stinging nettle *(Urtica dioica).*

Assess the client for potential interactions of herbal preparations with prescription medications. Ephedra *(Ma-huang, Ephedra sinica),* a sympathomimetic, might reduce the effect of prednisone. St. John's wort can reduce warfarin levels.[26] There is some limited anecdotal evidence that gingko, garlic, fish oil, and the Chinese herbs danshen and dong quai may exert an anti-coagulant effect.[26] The use of these products may need to be avoided in people with bleeding disorders or receiving anticoagulant therapy.

Dietary Habits

The hematopoietic and immune systems depend on the adequate intake of protein, calories, vitamins (A, B_{12}, folic acid), minerals, and trace elements such as iron and zinc. Inadequate intake of any of these substances can lead to anemia or immunodeficiency. Assess for conditions that increase nutritional needs, such as pregnancy, lactation, and hypercatabolic states that occur with thermal injuries. When assessing anemia, obtain a dietary history focusing on the intake of foods such as meat, fish, eggs, dairy products, whole grains, dark green vegetables, legumes, and nuts. Strict vegetarians who do not eat foods of animal origin may be at higher risk for a deficiency anemia, especially related to inadequate intake of vitamin B_{12} (see Chapter 28).

Social History

Encourage the client to discuss current levels of stress and whether they seem to relate to the appearance of allergic manifestations. Some clients may report breaking out in hives when under emotional stress. Their appearance triggers more emotional distress and can lead to further outbreaks; a cycle may develop that is difficult to interrupt.

Ask about occupational exposure to agents that might predispose the client to the development of hematopoietic disorders: radiation, aromatic hydrocarbons (kerosene, gasoline), benzene (used in the manufacture of pharmaceuticals, rubber, leather, and explosives), inorganic arsenics, trinitrotoluene, insecticides, weed killers, lead, and phenylbutazone. Exposure to toxic chemicals and ionizing radiation may occur in several industries (chemicals, plastics, ceramics, steel, metal refinery); in the manufacturing of rubber tires, shoes, incandescent lamps, vacuum tubes, glue, and varnish; in nuclear reactors, uranium mines, research laboratories, hospital radiology, or sterile supplies; and in farming and horticulture. Exposure to allergens at work may trigger reactions. Ask about the heating and cooling systems if airborne allergens are suspected.

Geographical location may be associated with exposure to possible health hazards. Living at altitudes above 10,000 feet may result in increased hemoglobin levels and other physiologic adaptations. Immunologic disorders may be more prevalent in certain geographical areas. High levels of air pollution can increase the incidence of allergy-related respiratory problems. Ask about home and work environments. Are pets, houseplants, or fresh-cut flowers present? What type of vegetation is in the immediate vicinity?

Does the client have sufficient energy to perform normal activities and occupational tasks? Do fatigue, dyspnea, or other manifestations interfere with a productive lifestyle? Has the client missed time from work or school, resulting in financial loss or other economic concerns, such as health or life insurance eligibility? Assess the client's current and past use of tobacco (including exposure to second-hand smoke that can aggravate allergies), alcohol, and illicit drugs. Excessive use of alcohol in particular often results in poor nutrition, folic acid deficiency, and decreased immunity as well as acute or chronic loss of blood from gastritis and esophageal varices. Many substances, most notably alcohol, damage the structure and function of liver cells, decreasing the production of clotting factors and reducing the clearance of factors that promote clot dissolution; the result is a bleeding tendency.

Family Health History

Explore the family history for common hematopoietic conditions, such as anemia, thrombocytopenia, bleeding disorders such as hemophilia or von Willebrand's disease, and congenital blood disorders such as sickle cell anemia. Inquire about a family history of jaundice; infections that were unusually frequent, unusually severe, or caused by an unusual organism; or a history of delayed healing. There may also be a history of cancer or autoimmune disease. A family history of neonatal jaundice or early cholecystectomy (gallbladder removal) may indicate a genetic hematologic disorder. Ask the client to identify allergies and sensitivities in family members, particularly atopic reactions. Hay fever tends to occur among family members.

PHYSICAL EXAMINATION

The physical examination of the hematopoietic system can entail both a complete head-to-toe examination and examinations of specific systems, depending on the nature of the client's problem. For example, anemia or fever can cause tachycardia and systolic ejection murmur; immunodeficiency manifested by repeated episodes of pulmonary infections may result in adventitious breath sounds. See Chapters 54 and 59, respectively, for discussions of cardiac and respiratory assessment. The Physical Assessment Findings in the Healthy Adult feature below outlines expected normal findings for the hematopoietic system.

The portions of the lymphatic system accessible for a physical examination are the superficial lymph nodes, liver, and spleen. Note the presence of a surgical splenectomy scar. For more specific information about physical assessment see the physical assessment texts provided in the references for this chapter. Table 74-1

describes possible abnormal physical findings related to the hematopoietic system and possible causes.

Inspection

Inspect surfaces overlying the lymph nodes for masses, scars, swelling, and redness. Note extremity swelling or edema. Look for symmetry and compare with the contralateral side.

Palpation

Use a methodical approach to examine the lymph nodes; do not overlook single nodes or chains of nodes. Palpate nodes for location, size, shape, consistency, symmetry, discreteness, mobility, tenderness, temperature, overlying edema, or red streaks.

Lymph nodes are generally nonpalpable; however, small (1 cm in diameter), single, round, soft, mobile, nontender nodes are common, particularly in the head, neck, and inguinal areas, and are usually not significant. Nodes that are inflamed, tender, large (>1 cm in diameter), hard, matted together, or fixed to underlying structures are abnormal. Describe their characteristics thoroughly. If you see a mass, palpate the area and compare with the contralateral side. The supraclavicular area is a frequent site of metastatic disease; investigate palpable nodes in this site.

The nodes of the head and neck and the clavicular and epitrochlear areas are most easily palpated while the client is sitting. Palpate the inguinal and popliteal nodes when the client is lying down. Axillary nodes may be palpated with the client sitting or lying. Specific guidelines for palpating the lymph nodes are presented in the website table Sequence and Palpation Technique *evolve* for Lymph Nodes.

DIAGNOSTIC TESTING

Diagnosis of hematologic, bleeding, or immunologic disorders depends primarily on laboratory analysis. No particular preprocedure or postprocedure care is associated with the simple blood tests involved in most hematopoietic assessments.

Although dozens of specific tests are used to diagnose individual disorders, all cases generally call for (1) a complete blood count (CBC) to determine the number of leukocytes, erythrocytes, and platelets; (2) a white blood cell (WBC) differential count to indicate the relative percentages of the different leukocytes; (3) coagulation studies such as prothrombin time (PT), partial thromboplastin time (PTT), and bleeding time; and (4) a peripheral blood smear for red blood cell (RBC) morphology to differentiate various anemias and blood dyscrasias.

Physical Assessment Findings in the Healthy Adult

The Hematopoietic System

INSPECTION

Alert and oriented; afebrile. Skin color even, without pallor, flushing, jaundice, bruises, or petechiae. Lumps or masses absent; no draining lesions. Sclerae white. Lingual papillae visible; oral lesions absent. Eupneic. Joints not swollen; full range of motion.

PALPATION

Lumps, masses absent. Lymph nodes, liver, and spleen nonpalpable and nontender. Joints nontender. Several round, small (0.5 cm), discrete, soft, mobile nodes palpable in submandibular area.

AUSCULTATION

Heart sounds regular, without murmurs or palpitations.

TABLE 74–1 Abnormal Assessment Findings

Anatomic Area	Manifestation	Possible Cause
Eyes	Visual disturbances	Anemia, polycythemia
	Blindness	Retinal hemorrhage related to thrombocytopenia or bleeding disorder
	Scleral jaundice	Hemolytic anemia
	Conjunctivitis, tearing, eye rubbing, styes, dark circles or "allergic shiners," "raccoon eyes"	Allergies
Ears	Vertigo or tinnitus	Severe anemia
	Blood in external auditory canal or bluish tympanic membrane, suggesting blood in middle ear	Bleeding disorders
	Chronic otitis media, mastoiditis	Immunodeficiencies or chronic infections and treatment with ototoxic drugs
	Hearing impairment related to eardrum rupture, scarring, perforated tympanic membrane	
Nose	Epistaxis	Thrombocytopenia and bleeding disorders
	Crusting around nares, sinopulmonary drainage, and indications of chronic sinusitis	Immunodeficiency
	Sneezing, sniffling, rhinitis, nasal polyps, nasal voice quality	Allergies
Mouth	Smooth, glossy, bright red, and sore tongue	Pernicious anemia, iron deficiency anemia
	Gingival bleeding	Thrombocytopenia, bleeding disorders
	Oral ulcers, candidiasis, gingivitis, periodontitis, dental caries, and tooth loss	Immunodeficiencies
	Tonsils may be enlarged, inflamed, or pustular; lip and tongue swelling, frequent throat clearing from postnasal drip, sore throat, itching of palate, throat, or neck, and hoarseness	Allergies
Respiratory tract	Dyspnea and orthopnea	Anemia, sickle cell crisis
	Wheezing, frequent cough, ineffective cough, and respiratory arrest	Allergies
Cardiovascular system	Tachycardia, palpitations, murmurs, particularly systolic and angina	Anemia
Gastrointestinal tract	Dysphagia	Mucous membrane atrophy related to iron deficiency anemia
	Abdominal pain	
	Hepatomegaly, splenomegaly	Sickle cell disease, retroperitoneal bleeding, acute hemolysis
	Hematemesis and melena	
	Vomiting, cramping, and diarrhea	Hemolytic anemia resulting in increased need for removal of erythrocytes
		Thrombocytopenia and bleeding disorders
		Allergies
Genitourinary tract	Hematuria	Hemolysis and bleeding disorders
	Amenorrhea and menorrhagia	Iron deficiency and bleeding disorders
	Decreased fertility	Severe anemia
Musculoskeletal system	Back pain	Hemolysis
	Sternal tenderness and excruciating bone pain, joint pain	Sickle cell crises
		Hemarthroses or bleeding into joints, often related to hemophilia
Nervous system	Headache and confusion	Anemia, polycythemia
	Brain hemorrhage	Thrombocytopenia or bleeding disorder
	Peripheral neuropathy, paresthesias, loss of balance	Pernicious anemia

The diagnosis of deficiency anemias may require measuring serum levels of iron, total iron-binding capacity (TIBC), transferrin saturation, ferritin, folic acid, and vitamin B_{12} (Table 74-2). Bone marrow aspiration and biopsy are performed to determine both the cellularity of the bone marrow and the morphology of the cells present. The diagnosis of particular hematologic disorders requires specialized blood tests, such as the Schilling test, hemoglobin electrophoresis, and measurement of levels of specific clotting factors. These specialized tests are discussed in Chapter 75. Table 74-3 and the website tables Lymphocyte Immunophenotyping and Immunoglobulin (Ig) Isotopes provide additional information concerning

TABLE 74–2 Laboratory Tests Used in the Diagnosis of Anemia

Test	Normal Value
Iron	50-150 mcg/dl
Total iron-binding capacity (TIBC)	250-350 mcg/dl
Transferrin	250-430 mg/dl
Transferrin saturation	20-55%
Ferritin	Men: 15-200 mcg/ml
	Women: 11-200 mcg/ml
Folate	7-20 mcg/ml
Vitamin B_{12}	200-800 pg/ml
Schilling test (vitamin B_{12} absorption)	8.5-28% excretion in 24-48 hr

dl, Deciliter; *mcg,* microgram; *ml,* milliliter; *pg,* picogram.

TABLE 74–3   Diagnostic Tests of the Hematopoietic System

Test Description	Purpose	Findings
Bone Marrow Aspiration and Biopsy		
Most commonly taken from posterior iliac crests; alternative site is sternum	Used to assess and identify most blood dyscrasias such as aplastic anemia, leukemias, pernicious anemia, thrombocytopenia	Reveals number, size, and shape of RBCs, WBCs, and platelet precursors
Lymphocyte Immunophenotyping		
Lymphocyte subpopulation analysis by flow cytometry	Measures total numbers and percentages of B lymphocytes, T lymphocytes, and T lymphocyte subsets (CD4, CD8) in a peripheral blood sample	See table on Lymphocyte Immunophenotyping on website Lists normal levels of T and B lymphocytes and conditions in which abnormal levels of T cells and B cells occur
Immunoglobulin isotypes	Measures serum level of various immunoglobulins: IgG, IgA, IgM, IgD, and IgE; subclasses of IgG may also be measured (IgG1, IgG2, IgG3, IgG4)	See table on Immunoglobulin (Ig) Isotopes on website
Radiography		
Chest x-ray	Assesses upper chest and lower part of the neck	Detects congenital absence of thymic tissue or tumor of thymus gland
Computed tomography (CT)	Assesses integrity of sinuses	See diagnostic testing textbook
Lymphangiography	Allows visualization of lymphatic system to assess malignancy, metastases, or obstruction	See diagnostic testing textbook
Skin Tests		
Skin tests confirm sensitivity to a specific allergen; antigens are applied by one of three methods:	A known antigen is placed on or directly beneath skin to detect presence of antibodies	
1. Patch tests		See Chapters 48 and 76
2. Scratch tests (tine tests or prick tests)		See Chapter 76
3. Delayed-type hypersensitivity skin testing		See Chapter 76

diagnostic tests that may be used with clients who have hemapoietic disorders.

Hematologic Tests
Complete Blood Cell Count (CBC)
The CBC includes the RBC count, hemoglobin, hematocrit, RBC indices, WBC count with or without differential, and platelet count. Table 74-4 presents the purpose for the various indices within a CBC and Table 74-5 presents reference values for the CBC. Table 74-6 reviews the effects of diseases, disorders, and conditions on the CBC and the RBC indices.

Peripheral Blood Smear
A peripheral blood smear is obtained to determine variations and abnormalities in erythrocytes, leukocytes, and platelets. Cells of normal size and shape are termed *normocytes;* cells of normal color are *normochromic.* Abnormalities of erythrocyte size, shape, and color usually indicate some form of anemia.

Antiglobulin Tests
The *direct* antiglobulin test (Coombs' test) is used to detect certain antigen-antibody reactions between serum antibodies and RBC antigens, differentiate between various forms of hemolytic anemia, determine unusual blood types, and identify hemolytic disease in newborns. This test examines erythrocytes for the presence of antibodies (agglutinins) that damage erythrocytes without causing clumping or hemolysis. It is used to crossmatch blood for blood transfusions, test umbilical cord blood for erythroblastosis fetalis, and diagnose acquired hemolytic anemia.

The *indirect* antiglobulin test identifies antibodies to erythrocyte antigens in the serum of clients who have a greater than normal chance of developing transfusion reactions. Both the direct and the indirect tests are agglutination procedures that use a suspension of RBCs.

Coagulation Screening Tests
Laboratory studies are the most crucial for pinpointing the type and cause of bleeding disorders. Initially, four basic laboratory tests are performed to discern whether the bleeding problem is related to a platelet, coagulation, or vascular defect: platelet count, PT, PTT, and bleeding time. Most bleeding disorders are diagnosed by the PT and PTT (Table 74-7).

Because the normal and therapeutic ranges for PT vary according to the type of reagent used in the assay, the PT is standardized by conversion to the International Normalized Ratio (INR). For most clinical

TABLE 74–4 Purpose of Complete Blood Cell Count Indices

Test Component	Purpose
Red blood cell count	Measures number of RBCs per cubic millimeter (mm³) of blood. Normal values vary with age and gender.
Hemoglobin level	Used to evaluate hemoglobin content (iron and oxygen-carrying capacity) of erythrocytes by measuring number of grams of hemoglobin per 100 ml of blood (dl).
Hematocrit level	Measure of volume of RBCs in whole blood expressed as a percentage. Normal values vary with age and gender.
Red blood cell indices	
Mean corpuscular volume (MCV)	Measures erythrocyte size and hemoglobin content. Normal value: 76-100 μm³. MCV <76 μm means abnormally small *(microcytic)* RBCs. MCV >100 μm means abnormally large *(macrocytic)* RBCs.
Mean corpuscular hemoglobin (MCH)	Measures hemoglobin content within one RBC of average size. Normal value: 27-33 pg. MCH <27 pg indicates hemoglobin deficiency, hypochromic RBCs. MCH >33 pg indicates macrocytic cells with abnormally large volume of hemoglobin.
Mean corpuscular hemoglobin concentration (MCHC)	Measures average hemoglobin concentration within 100 ml (1 dl) of packed RBCs. Normal value: 32-36 g/dl of packed RBCs. MCHC <32 g/dl indicates hemoglobin deficiency. MCHC remains normal when MCH >32 g/dl because cells are oversized (fewer cells can be packed together within 1 dl).
Platelet count	Platelets have a key role in blood clotting. Number of platelets (thrombocytes) per cubic millimeter (mm³) of blood.
White blood cell count	Number of WBCs in a cubic millimeter of blood.
White blood cell differential	Determines proportion of each of the 5 types of WBCs in a sample of 100 WBCs.
Reticulocyte count	A reflection of RBC production, reticulocyte count measures responsiveness of bone marrow to a decreased number of circulating erythrocytes. Specifically, this test measures number of reticulocytes released from bone marrow into blood.

dl, Deciliter; *pg*, picogram; *μm³*, cubic micrometer.

TABLE 74–5 Normal Values for Complete Blood Cell Counts in Adults

Measure	Value*
Erythrocytes	
RBC count (number of cells/mm³ of blood)	Women: 4.2-5.4 million/mm³ Men: 4.7-6.1 million/mm³
Hemoglobin (oxygen-carrying pigment of RBC)	Women: 12-16.0 g/dl Men: 13.5-18.0 g/dl
Hematocrit (% volume of RBCs in whole blood)	Women: 37%-47% (pregnancy >33%) Men: 42%-52%
Reticulocytes	0.5%-2% of total erythrocytes
Leukocytes	
WBC count (number of cells/mm³ of blood)	4000-9000/mm³
WBC differential	
Granulocytes	
Neutrophils	55%-70%
Eosinophils	1%-4%
Basophils	0.5%-1.0%
Agranulocytes	
Lymphocytes	20%-40%
Monocytes	2%-8%
Platelets	
Platelet (thrombocyte) count (number of cells/mm³ of blood)	150,000-450,000/mm³

g/dl, Grams per deciliter; *mm³*, cubic millimeter; *RBC*, red blood cell; *WBC*, white blood cell.
* Normal values may differ significantly among laboratories.

conditions that necessitate anticoagulation, the recommended INR is 2 to 3.0. Clients with mechanical prosthetic valves or recurrent systemic embolism may need higher INR levels.

Immunologic Status Tests

Most immunodeficiencies can be identified through three blood tests: (1) WBC and differential, (2) immunoglobulin levels, and (3) total serum complement.

TABLE 74–6 Diseases, Disorders, and Conditions Affecting the Complete Blood Cell Count and Red Blood Cell Indices

CBC, RBC Index	Increased by	Decreased by
RBC count	Polycythemia vera, cardiac and pulmonary disorders characterized by cyanosis, dehydration, acute poisoning	Anemia, fluid overload, recent hemorrhage, leukemia
Reticulocyte count	Hemolytic anemia, hemorrhage, following effective treatment for pernicious anemia	Bone marrow failure, pernicious anemia
Hemoglobin	Hemoconcentration from polycythemia or dehydration	Hemodilution (fluid overload), anemia, recent hemorrhage
Hematocrit	Hemoconcentration from loss of fluid, dehydration, polycythemia	Hemodilution, anemia, acute massive blood loss
Mean corpuscular volume	Pernicious anemia, macrocytic anemia, folic acid, or vitamin B_{12} deficiency anemias	Microcytic anemia, iron deficiency anemia, hypochromic anemia, thalassemia, lead poisoning
Mean corpuscular hemoglobin	Macrocytic anemia	Microcytic anemia
Mean corpuscular hemoglobin concentration	Spherocytosis	Microcytic anemia, hypochromic anemia, thalassemia, iron deficiency anemia
WBC count	Infection, leukemia, tissue necrosis	Bone marrow depression
Neutrophils	Inflammatory disease or response, tissue necrosis (burns, myocardial infarction), granulocytic leukemia and other malignancies, acute stress response, bacterial infection	Bone marrow depression, viral diseases, drugs (chemotherapy, some antibiotics, psychotropics)
Eosinophils	Allergic reactions, parasitic infections, skin diseases, cancers, pernicious anemia	Stress response, Cushing's syndrome
Basophils	Leukemia, some hemolytic anemias, polycythemia vera	Corticosteroids, allergic reactions, acute infections (*Note:* decline is unlikely to be detected because normal count is 0%-2%)
Lymphocytes	Infectious mononucleosis, chronic bacterial infections, tuberculosis, pertussis, lymphocytic leukemia	AIDS, corticosteroids, immunosuppressive drugs
Monocytes	Infections (tuberculosis, malaria, Rocky Mountain spotted fever), collagen-vascular diseases, monocytic leukemia	Drug therapy, prednisone
Platelet count	Malignancies, polycythemia vera, splenectomy (rebound thrombocytosis)	Idiopathic thrombocytopenia purpura, aplastic anemia, hemolytic disorders, chemotherapeutic drugs or radiation, hypersplenism or splenomegaly, infiltrative bone marrow disease, disseminated intravascular coagulation, viral infections, AIDS

AIDS, Acquired immunodeficiency syndrome; *RBC,* red blood cell; *WBC,* white blood cell.

TABLE 74-7 Laboratory Tests Used in the Diagnosis of Hemorrhagic Disorders

Name of Test	Purpose	Normal Values	Interpretation of Findings
Platelet count	Measures number of circulating platelets in venous or arterial blood	150,000-450,000/mm³	Low count results in prolonged bleeding time and impaired clot retraction; diagnostic of thrombocytopenia
Prothrombin time (PT)	Determines activity and interaction of factors V, VII, and X, prothrombin, and fibrinogen; determines dosages of oral anticoagulant drugs	11-15 sec (one-stage) INR: 2-3	Prolonged PT is seen in clients receiving anticoagulant therapy; with low levels or deficiencies of fibrinogen, clotting factors II, V, VII, and X; impaired prothrombin activity; in presence of circulating anticoagulants as seen in SLE
Partial thromboplastin time (PTT, aPTT)	Complex method for testing normalcy of intrinsic coagulation process; used to identify deficiencies of coagulation factors, prothrombin, and fibrinogen; used to monitor heparin therapy	25-38 sec	Prolongation of time indicates coagulation disorder that is related to deficiency of a coagulation factor; not diagnostic for platelet disorders
Thrombin time	Measures functional fibrinogen available, as shown by time needed to form fibrin clot after thrombin is added	10-15 sec	Prolonged time indicates DIC or hypofibrinogenemia; presence in blood of excess heparin or other anticoagulants
Thromboplastin generation test (TGT)	Measures generation of thromboplastin; if result abnormal, second stage is done to identify missing coagulation factor	<12 sec (100%)	Abnormal values found in hemophilia
Fibrinogen level	Measures level of fibrinogen	200-400 mg/dl	Abnormally low values may indicate DIC, liver disease, congenital or acquired afibrinogenemia
Fibrin split products (FSPs), fibrin degradation products (FDPs) test	Measures products that result from breakdown of fibrin	Less than 10 mcg/ml	Abnormally high levels are seen in DIC; helpful in monitoring fibrinolytic therapy
D-dimer	Measures a specific product resulting from breakdown of fibrin	Less than 0.5 mcg/ml	Abnormally high levels confirm diagnosis of DIC; screen for abruptio placentae (placental abruption)
Activated clotting time	Crude measure of coagulation process in venous blood; used to control heparin therapy; commonly used during cardiovascular surgery and in ICU	7-120 sec (depends on type of activator used)	Prolonged time occurs in severe coagulation problems and therapeutic administration of heparin
Bleeding time	Measures ability to stop bleeding after a small puncture wound	3-8 min in adults (varies with test method)	Prolonged bleeding time occurs in vascular maladies and after aspirin ingestion
Capillary fragility test (tourniquet test, Rumpel-Leede test)	Crude test of vascular resistance and platelet number and function; BP cuff is placed on arm and inflated to pressure midway between systolic and diastolic BP for 5 min; petechiae in area are counted	No petechiae	Petechiae (five or more) are seen in thrombocytopenia and vascular purpura
Clot retraction	Indicates function and number of platelets; measures time needed for contraction of an undisturbed clot	50%-100% in 24 hr	Clot retraction is retarded in thrombocytopenia; clot is small and soft in thrombasthenia (functional disturbance of platelets)

BP, Blood pressure; *DIC,* disseminated intravascular coagulation; *ICU,* intensive care unit; *INR,* International Normalized Ratio; *SLE,* systemic lupus erythematosus.

Additional immunodeficiencies can be determined through more complex tests, including lymphocyte immunophenotyping, measures of immunoglobulin subclasses, complement assays, and the presence of specific antibodies (after immunizations or exposure to antigens as with communicable diseases).

CONCLUSIONS

The hematopoietic and immune systems are extremely complex. Understanding the structure, function, and assessment of the protective system will help you care for clients with any of the wide variety of disorders that affect this highly complex system.

BIBLIOGRAPHY

 Citations appearing in red refer to primary research.

 Citations appearing in blue refer to evidence-based practice guidelines and protocols.

1. Abbott, M.B., & Levin, R.H. (2001). Anaphylactoid reactions to radiocontrast agents. *Pediatric Revue, 22*(10), 356.
2. Ahya, S., et al. (Eds.) (2001). *The Washington manual of medical therapeutics* (30th ed.). Philadelphia: Lippincott Williams & Wilkins.
3. Anderson, K.N. (Ed.) (2002). *Mosby's medical, nursing, & allied health dictionary* (6th ed.). St. Louis: Mosby.
4. Bickley, L.S., & Szilagyi, P.G. (2005). *Bates' guide to physical examination & history taking* (9th ed.). Philadelphia: Lippincott Williams & Wilkins.
5. Cavanaugh, B.M. (2003). *Nurse's manual of laboratory and diagnostic tests* (4th ed.). Philadelphia: F.A. Davis.
6. Chernecky, C.C., & Berger, B.J. (Eds.) (2003). *Laboratory tests and diagnostic procedures* (4th ed.). Philadelphia: Saunders.
7. Corbett, J.V. (2003). *Laboratory tests and diagnostic procedures with nursing diagnoses* (6th ed.). Upper Saddle River, NJ: Prentice Hall.
8. Doenges, M.E., et al. (2006). *Nurse's pocket guide: Diagnosis, prioritized interventions and rationales* (10th ed.). Philadelphia: F.A. Davis.
9. Etkin, S., et al. (Eds.) (2005). *Professional guide to diseases* (8th ed.). Philadelphia: Lippincott Williams & Wilkins.
10. Ferri, F.F. (2006). *Ferri's clinical advisor: Instant diagnosis and treatment*. Philadelphia: Saunders.
11. Fishbach, F.T. (2003). *A manual of laboratory and diagnostic tests* (7th ed.). Philadelphia: Lippincott Williams & Wilkins.
12. Goldman, L., & Ausiello, D.A. (Eds.) (2003). *Cecil's textbook of medicine* (22nd ed.). Philadelphia: Saunders.
13. Guyton, A.C., & Hall, J.E. (2005). *Textbook of medical physiology* (11th ed.). Philadelphia: Saunders.
14. Harmening, D. (Ed.) (2001). *Clinical hematology and fundamentals of hemostasis* (4th ed.). Philadelphia: F.A. Davis.
15. Healey, P.M., & Jacobson, E. (2006). *Common medical diagnoses: An algorithmic approach*. Philadelphia: Saunders.
16. Kasper, D.L., et al. (Eds.) (2004). *Harrison's principles of internal medicine* (16th ed.). New York: McGraw-Hill.
17. McPherson, R.A., & Pincus, M.R. (Eds.) (2006). *Henry's clinical diagnosis and management by laboratory methods* (21st ed.). Philadelphia: Saunders.
18. Jacobs, D.S., et al. (Eds.) (2001). *Jacobs & DeMott laboratory test handbook* (5th ed.). Cleveland: Lexi-Comp.
19. Jarvis, C. (2003). *Physical examination and health assessment* (4th ed.). Philadelphia: Saunders.
20. Kee, J.L. (2004). *Laboratory and diagnostic tests with nursing implications* (7th ed.). Upper Saddle River, NJ: Prentice Hall.
21. Mandell, G.L., et al. (Eds.) (2000). *Mandell, Douglas, and Bennett's principles & practice of infectious diseases* (5th ed.). Philadelphia: Churchill Livingstone.
22. Miller-Keane, B.F., & O'Toole, M.T. (Ed.) (2005). *Encyclopedia & dictionary of medicine, nursing, & allied health* (7th ed.). Philadelphia: Saunders.
23. Pagana, K.D., & Pagana, T.J. (2004). *Mosby's diagnostic and laboratory test reference* (7th ed.). St. Louis: Mosby.
24. Seidel, H.M., et al. (Eds.) (2006). *Mosby's guide to physical examination* (6th ed.). St. Louis: Mosby.
25. Shils, M.E., et al. (Eds.) (2006). *Modern nutrition in health & disease* (10th ed.). Philadelphia: Lippincott Williams & Wilkins.
26. Skidmore-Roth, L. (2005). *Mosby's handbook of herbs & natural supplements* (3rd ed.). St. Louis: Mosby.
27. Tierney, L.M., et al. (Eds.) (2006). *Current medical diagnosis and treatment* (45th ed.). New York: McGraw-Hill.
28. Turgeon, M.L. (2004). *Clinical hematology: Theory and procedures* (4th ed.). Philadelphia: Lippincott Williams & Wilkins.

evolve *Did you remember to check out the bonus material on the Evolve website and the CD-ROM, including NCLEX®-Examination Style Review Questions, Open-Book Quizzes, and Chapter Review Audio Podcasts?*

http://evolve.elsevier.com/Black/medsurg

CHAPTER 75

Management of Clients with Hematologic Disorders

LINDA H. YODER

This chapter provides information about disorders that affect red blood cells *(erythrocytes)*, white blood cells *(leukocytes)*, the spleen, platelets, and clotting factors. Priorities of nursing care center on the lack of oxygenated blood flow and risk of hemorrhage. Leukemia and lymphoma are discussed in Chapter 79.

DISORDERS AFFECTING RED BLOOD CELLS

THE ANEMIAS

Anemia is a clinical condition that results from an insufficient supply of healthy red blood cells (RBCs), the volume of packed RBCs, and/or the quantity of hemoglobin. Hypoxia results because the body's tissues are not adequately oxygenated. Not a disease in itself, anemia reflects a number of underlying pathologic processes leading to an abnormality in RBC number, structure, or function. When anemia is identified, further testing must be done to determine its cause.

Risk Factors, Etiology, and Classification

Anemia can arise from primary hematologic problems or can occur as a secondary consequence of defects in other body systems. Those at risk for developing anemia differ with the various etiologies. Because the prevalence of anemia increases with age, adults 65 and older are at particular risk; the estimated prevalence in this age-group is 20%. Aging cannot be assumed to be the cause of anemia, however, without excluding other reversible causes. Hereditary anemias have several cultural and ethnic considerations. The prevalence of sickle cell disease and thalassemia is high in African Americans. Thalassemia is also high in people of Mediterranean

origin. Pernicious anemia rates are high in Scandinavians and African Americans.

The anemias are classified by either the etiology or the morphology of the specific anemia. Anemia is caused in one of three ways: (1) decreased production of healthy RBCs, (2) increased RBC destruction *(hemolysis)*, or (3) loss of blood. A number of underlying problems lead to these conditions. Etiologic categories are listed in Box 75-1.

Morphologic classification is based on erythrocyte size, shape, and color. Normal RBCs are shown in Figure 75-1, *A*. Morphologic categories include normocytic/normochromic (normal size and color), macrocytic/normochromic (large size, normal color), and microcytic/hypochromic (small size, pale color). Some anemias are named for the abnormal shape of the RBCs. For instance, normal RBCs have a biconcave shape, and *sickle cell anemia* has sickle-shaped RBCs (Figure 75-1, *B*); spherocytosis, a hereditary disorder leading to hemolytic anemia, has spherical-shaped RBCs.

Table 75-1 gives a general overview of blood components, including composition, compatibility, special considerations, and outcomes. (See Table 74-6 on p. 2001 for other abnormalities of erythrocytes and their associated conditions.)

---

evolve Web Enhancements

Concept Map Understanding DIC and Its Treatment

Ethical Issues in Nursing Should Parents Who Are Jehovah's Witnesses Have the Right to Refuse a Life-Saving Transfusion for Their Child?

Be sure to check out the bonus material on the Evolve website and the CD-ROM, including free self-assessment exercises. **http://evolve.elsevier. com/Black/medsurg**

BOX 75-1 Etiologic Categories of Anemia

DECREASED RBC PRODUCTION

Defective DNA Synthesis
- Cobalamin/vitamin B_{12} deficiency
- Folic acid deficiency

Decreased Hemoglobin Synthesis
- Iron deficiency
- Thalassemia (decreased globin synthesis)
- Sideroblastic anemia (failure to completely form heme)

Decreased Number of Erythrocyte Precursors
- Aplastic anemia
- Anemia of leukemia and myelodysplasia
- Chronic diseases

INCREASED RBC DESTRUCTION (HEMOLYSIS)

Intrinsic
- Abnormal hemoglobin (sickle cell anemia)
- Enzyme deficiency
- Membrane abnormalities

Extrinsic
- Physical trauma
- Antibodies (autoimmune and isoimmune)
- Infectious agents
- Toxins (snake venom; chemotherapy)

BLOOD LOSS

Acute
- Trauma
- Blood vessel rupture

Chronic
- Gastritis
- Hemorrhoids
- Menstruation

Pathophysiology

Transport of oxygen is impaired with anemia. Hemoglobin is lacking or the number of RBCs is too low to carry adequate oxygen to tissues and hypoxia develops. The body attempts to compensate for tissue hypoxia by increasing the rate of RBC production, increasing cardiac output by increasing stroke volume or heart rate, redistributing blood from tissues of low oxygen needs to tissues with high oxygen needs, and shifting the oxygen-hemoglobin dissociation curve to the right to facilitate the removal of more oxygen by the tissues at the same partial pressure of oxygen.

Clinical Manifestations

Manifestations accompanying anemia are due primarily to the body's response to hypoxia. The manifestations differ depending on the severity and speed of blood loss, the chronicity of the anemia, the client's age, and the presence of other disorders. Hemoglobin (Hb) levels are used to determine the severity of anemia. Clients with mild anemia (Hb levels of 10 to 14 g/dl) are usually asymptomatic. If manifestations do occur, they typically follow strenuous exertion. Clients with moderate anemia (Hb levels of 6 to 10 g/dl) may suffer from *dyspnea* (shortness of breath), palpitations, *diaphoresis* (profuse perspiration) with exertion, and chronic fatigue. Some clients with severe anemia (Hb levels <6 g/dl), such as those with chronic renal failure, may be asymptomatic because their anemia develops gradually; others may have significant clinical manifestations involving multiple body systems. Additional manifestations are due to the underlying etiology; a careful work-up can provide clues to the etiology. Table 75-2 on p. 2009 lists typical manifestations of severe anemia by body system. ➤ The Translating Evidence into Practice feature on p. 2011 provides additional information on how anemia can cause fatigue and compromise quality of life.

The RBC count, hemoglobin level, and hematocrit value confirm the presence of anemia. A bone marrow specimen may be required to confirm the type of anemia. A peripheral blood smear (RBC indices) is needed to determine the size of the RBC. Table 75-3 on p. 2010 identifies laboratory study findings in various anemias.

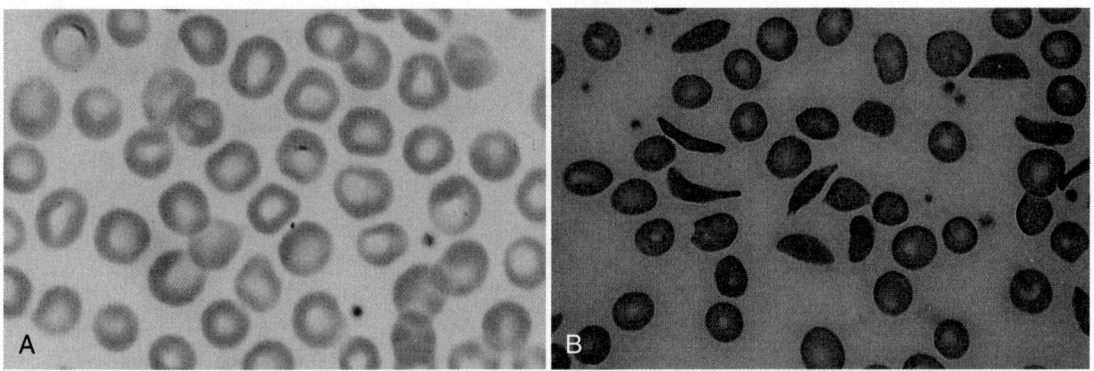

■ **FIGURE 75-1 A,** Normal red blood cells. **B,** Sickle cell anemia. (Magnification ×875.) Note the elongated and sickle-shaped cells. (*From Rodak, B. [2002]. Hematology: Clinical principles and applications [2nd ed.]. Philadelphia: Saunders.)*

TABLE 75–1 Blood Components

	Whole Blood	Red Blood Cells	Platelet Concentrates	Fresh Frozen Plasma	Cryoprecipitate	Granulocyte Concentrates	Plasma Derivatives	Coagulation Factor Concentrates
Composition	RBC, plasma, plasma proteins (globulins, antibodies), 63 ml of anticoagulant-preservative	RBC with CPDA-1 solution (anticoagulant-preservative only), final hematocrit no higher than 80% (80% RBC, 20% plasma) RBC with 100 ml of additive solution, final hematocrit about 55%-60%	Single-unit platelets contain minimum of 5.5×10^{10} (1 unit) platelets in 50-70 ml of plasma obtained by separating platelet-rich plasma from 1 unit of fresh whole blood; 6-10 units may be pooled for 1 transfusion Single-donor platelets contain minimum of 3.0×10^{11} platelets (6 units) obtained from single donor by use of automated cell separator during apheresis; recipient exposed to fewer donors, which decreases complications	91% water, 7% protein (globulin, antibodies, clotting factors), and 2% carbohydrates Freezing within 8 hr of collection preserves all clotting factors	Each unit contains 50% of antihemophilic factor VIII (80-120 units) and 20-30% of factor XIII originally present in a unit of whole blood, as well as vWF and 250 mg of fibrinogen suspended in 10-20 ml of plasma	Unit obtained by granulocytapheresis contains minimum of 1×10^{10} granulocytes, variable amounts of lymphocytes (usually <10%), 30-50 ml of RBC and 100-400 ml of plasma, and 6-10 units of platelets; platelets can be separated from the unit if granulocyte recipient is not thrombocytopenic	*Albumin:* 96% albumin, 4% globulin and other proteins extracted from plasma; available as a 5% solution, oncotically equivalent to plasma, and also concentrated 25% solution *Plasma protein fraction:* 83% albumin and 17% globulins extracted from plasma; less pure than albumin and has higher degree of contamination with other plasma proteins; in 5% solution only	*Factor VIII:* Lyophilized concentrate containing large quantities of factor VIII; prepared from large pools of donor plasma, but heat treatment during fractionation process significantly reduces risk of transmitting viral disease *Factor IX:* Lyophilized concentrate containing large quantities of factor IX; also contains factors II, VII, and X; product prepared from large pools of donor plasma, but heat treatment during fractionation process significantly reduces risk of transmitting viral disease
Volume	500 ml/unit	250-350 ml/unit 350-400 ml/unit	50-70 ml/unit 200-400 ml/unit	200-250 ml	5-10 ml/unit	200-400 ml with platelets 100-200 ml without platelets	Albumin: 250 and 500 ml (5%); 50 and 100 ml (25%)	Multiple-dose vial

ABO/Rh Compatibility							
ABO type of donor should be identical with recipient's Rh− blood can be given to an Rh− or Rh+ recipient	A can match with A or O; B can match with B or O; O can match only with O; AB can match with A, B, or O Rh− blood can be given to either Rh+ or Rh− recipient	Whereas platelets have no ABO or Rh antigens, they are suspended in 200-400 ml of plasma containing donor antibodies and a small number of RBC ABO and Rh compatibility is recommended	A can match with A or AB; B can match with B or AB; AB can match only with AB; O can match with A, B, or O Rh− and Rh+ blood can be given to either Rh+ or Rh− recipient	Cryoprecipitate contains no RBC and a small volume of plasma ABO crossmatching not needed, and plasma compatibility preferred but not required	Granulocytes contain a significant number of RBC and plasma; therefore ABO of donor should be identical with recipient's Rh− components may be transfused to Rh+ recipient	Antibodies destroyed during processing; therefore compatibility not a factor	Antibodies destroyed during processing, so compatibility not a factor
Special Considerations							
Whole blood transfusion is rarely indicated Treatment with specific blood components is usually recommended	RBC may be viscous; thus 0.9% saline may be added to achieve optimal flow rates For some clients, leukocyte depletion filter may be used to prevent complications	Because platelet concentrates contain few RBC, crossmatch testing is not required Plasma ABO and Rh compatibility is recommended, especially when total volume of transfusion exceeds 150-200 ml Only filters specially designed for platelet transfusion should be used	Plasma carries same risk of disease transmission as does whole blood If only volume expansion is required, products of choice are crystalloid or colloid solutions, such as saline or albumin Plasma contains no RBC, and Rh compatibility and crossmatching are not required ABO compatibility must be confirmed before administration	Single units of cryoprecipitate may be pooled into 1 container by blood collection center If individual bags are issued, products may need to be added to rinse residual cryoprecipitate from bags and tubing	Granulocytes have short survival (<24 hr); infuse as soon as possible Granulocyte concentrates contain significant number of RBC; pretransfusion testing recommended Increased incidence of febrile, nonhemolytic reactions with granulocyte transfusions; infuse slowly, observe client closely; premedication with antihistamine, acetaminophen, steroids advised	PPF and albumin cannot transmit hepatitis or HIV infection; pasteurization process used to prepare products destroys such viruses Hypotension has been associated with rapid infusion of PPF; 25% albumin can cause significantly increased blood pressure because of its ability to draw fluid into intravascular space	Factor VIII and factor IX assays should be performed at appropriate intervals to assess response Factor VIII concentration lacks vWF and should not be used in treatment of von Willebrand's disease

(Continued)

TABLE 75-1 Blood Components—Cont'd

	Whole Blood	Red Blood Cells	Platelet Concentrates	Fresh Frozen Plasma	Cryoprecipitate	Granulocyte Concentrates	Plasma Derivatives	Coagulation Factor Concentrates
Outcomes	Prevention or resolution of hypovolemic shock and anemia In a nonbleeding adult, 1 unit of whole blood should increase hematocrit by 3% and hemoglobin by 1 g/dl	Resolution of manifestations of anemia In a nonbleeding adult, 1 unit of RBC should increase hematocrit by 3% and hemoglobin by 1 g/dl	Prevention or resolution of bleeding caused by thrombocytopenia or platelet dysfunction 1 unit should raise peripheral platelet count 5000-10,000/mm³ if underlying cause is resolved or controlled Efficacy of platelet transfusion can be determined by obtaining platelet counts at 1 hr and 18-24 hr after infusion	Treatment effectiveness is assessed by monitoring coagulation function (specifically PT and PTT) or by specific factor assays	Correction of factor VIII, vWF, factor XIII, and fibrinogen deficiency; cessation of bleeding in uremic clients Laboratory values required to assess effectiveness of treatment	Do *not* administer amphotericin B within 4 hr of granulocyte transfusion to avoid pulmonary insufficiency Improvement in or resolution of infection Increase in peripheral WBC count not usually seen after granulocyte transfusion in adults, although increase may be seen in children An improvement in clinical condition because of resolving infection is only measure of treatment effectiveness	Client will acquire and maintain adequate blood pressure and volume support	Client will develop hemostasis because of increased levels of factor VIII and factor IX activity

CPDA-I, Citrate-phosphate-dextrose-adenine; *FFP*, fresh frozen plasma; *HIV*, human immunodeficiency virus; *IV*, intravenous; *PPF*, plasma protein fraction; *PT*, prothrombin time; *PTT*, partial thromboplastin time; *RBC*, red blood cells; *vWF*, von Willebrand's factor; *WBC*, white blood cells.

TABLE 75–2 Clinical Manifestations of Severe Anemia (Hb <6 g/dl)

Area	Clinical Manifestations
General	Pallor, severe fatigue, malaise, weakness, lightheadedness, fever, exertional dyspnea, headache, vertigo, sensitivity to cold, weight loss
Skin (integumentary)	Pallor (anemia); jaundice (HA); dry skin, brittle nails, spoon-shaped concave nails with longitudinal ridges (IDA)
Eyes	Blurred vision (anemia, PV); sclera jaundice and retinal hemorrhage (HA)
Ears	Vertigo, tinnitus
Mouth	Smooth, glossy, bright red, and sore tongue (PA, IDA)
Lungs	Dyspnea, orthopnea (anemia, HbS crisis)
Cardiovascular	Tachycardia, palpitations, murmurs (particularly systolic), angina, hypertension, cardiomegaly, intermittent claudication, heart failure, MI
Gastrointestinal	Anorexia; dysphagia (IDA); abdominal pain (HbS, HA); hematemesis (vomiting blood), tarry stools (HA); hepatomegaly, splenomegaly
Genitourinary	Amenorrhea and menorrhagia (IDA); decreased fertility (anemia); hematuria (HA)
Musculoskeletal	Back pain (HA); sternal tenderness and severe bone and joint pain (HbS)
Nervous system	Headache, confusion (anemia); peripheral neuropathy, paresthesias, and loss of balance (PA); mental depression, anxiety, coping difficulties (especially life-threatening conditions)

AP, Aplastic anemia; *HA*, hemolytic anemia; *HbS*, sickle cell anemia; *IDA*, iron deficiency anemia; *MI*, myocardial infarction; *PA*, pernicious anemia; *PV*, polycythemia vera.

OUTCOME MANAGEMENT

Medical Management

The goals of care for clients with anemia include (1) alleviating or controlling the causes, (2) relieving the manifestations, and (3) preventing complications. Treatment varies in intensity and duration because some anemias resolve after blood transfusion, others resolve within a few weeks or months, and still other forms require lifelong intervention.

Alleviate and Control the Causes

Depending on the etiology of the anemia, interventions may include (1) supplemental iron therapy, (2) nutritional therapy, (3) surgery to repair sites of hemorrhage, (4) splenectomy, (5) removal of toxic agents that cause aplasia, (6) stem cell or bone marrow transplantation, (7) corticosteroid therapy, and (8) immunosuppressive therapy.

Relieve Manifestations

Oxygen Therapy. Oxygen therapy may be prescribed for clients with severe anemia because their blood has a reduced capacity for oxygen. Oxygen helps to prevent tissue hypoxia and lessens the workload of the heart as it struggles to compensate for the lower Hb levels.

Erythropoietin. Subcutaneous injections of erythropoietin can be given to treat anemias of chronic disease because this drug increases the production of RBCs. For this drug to be effective, the client must have bone marrow capable of producing RBCs and sufficient nutrients for the production of RBCs.

Iron Replacement. Iron can be given to augment oral intake in cases where the need for iron is immediate or the demands are beyond dietary measures (e.g., pregnancy). The oral form of iron should be used because it is inexpensive and convenient. It is usually given for mild forms of anemia. The medications of choice are ferrous sulfate (Feosol) or ferrous gluconate (Fergon), 200 to 325 mg orally in three or four doses a day, with or after meals. Taking iron with vitamin C or orange juice aids in the absorption of iron. Clients usually receive iron supplements for at least 6 months for repletion of the body stores. Side effects may include nausea, vomiting, constipation or diarrhea, and blackened stools. The consequences of iron replacement therapy are outlined in the Integrating Pharmacology feature on p. 2012.

Blood Component Therapy

Traditionally the term *blood transfusion* has meant the administration of whole blood. The term now has a broader meaning because of the ability to administer specific blood components such as platelets or plasma. Blood component therapy is used to manage hematologic diseases and some surgical/therapeutic procedures depend on blood product support. Blood products obtained from another person are called homologous. Those reinfused from the client's own blood are called autologous.

Risks Associated with Homologous Blood Transfusions. Blood transfusions should not be used as a substitute for a specific therapy to treat the underlying cause of the anemia.

TABLE 75-3 Laboratory Study Findings in Erythrocytic Disorders

	Iron Deficiency	Thalassemia Major	Cobalamin B$_{12}$	Folic Acid Deficiency	Aplastic Anemia	Hemolytic Anemia	Sickle Cell Anemia	Polycythemia Vera	Hemachromatosis
RBC count	−	N to −	−	−	−	−	−	+	+
Hb/HcT	−	− (beta trait +)	−	−	−	−	−	+	+
RBC	Mic/H	Mic/H	Mac/N	Mac/N	N/N	N/N		Few cells	
Morphology	Target cells	Target cells	Hypersegmented Polymorphonuclear Leukocytes	Hypersegmented polymorphonuclear leukocytes		Fragmented Bizarre shape	Sickle cell Target cell	N/N	
Reticulocyte	N or −	—	—	−	−	+	+	+	
Platelets	N or −	—	+	+	−		+	+	
MCV	−	−	− to N	− to N	N				
MCH	−	−	+	+	N				
MCHC	−	−	−		N	+ with spherocytosis >36			
Serum iron	−	+	− with malabsorption			+	N or +	−	+
TIBC	+	+	−			−	N or −	−	+
Serum ferritin	−								+
Bilirubin	N or −	+				N or + Indirect bilirubinemia	+		
Marrow aspirate	Absence of hemosiderin		Megaloblasts	Megaloblasts	− Aplastic: remaining cells normal Myelodysplastic: remaining cells abnormal			Hyperplastic	
Other	− Transferrin saturation	Hb electrophoresis Amniocentesis	− Serum vitamin B$_{12}$ + Schilling	− Serum folate	− WBC	− Folate	+ HbS on Hb electrophoresis − Haptoglobin + Fibrinogen + Urobilinogen + Stercobilinogen Amniocentesis	− Serum erythropoietin + Serum B$_{12}$ + Fibrinogen + WBC (neutrophils)	+ Transferrin saturation Liver biopsy: +iron stores Genetic test to detect *HFE* gene mutation

+, Increase or positive; −, decrease or negative; *Hb*, hemoglobin; *Hb/HcT*, hemoglobin/hematocrit; *HbS*, sickle hemoglobin; *HFE*, hemachromatosis gene symbol; *Mac/N*, macrocytic/normochromic; *MCH*, mean corpuscular hemoglobin; *MCHC*, mean corpuscular hemoglobin concentration; *MCV*, mean corpuscular volume; *Mic/H*, microcytic/hypochromic; *N*, normal; *N/N*, normocytic/normochromic; *RBC*, red blood cell; *TIBC*, total iron-binding capacity; *WBC*, white blood cell.

TRANSLATING EVIDENCE INTO PRACTICE

Fatigue and Quality of Life

One of the most debilitating manifestations of anemia is profound fatigue that significantly affects the client's quality of life. A growing body of literature documents that fatigue not only is often overlooked and undertreated but also is considered an inevitable sequela of disease and treatment to be endured. Most of the research into fatigue and its management has occurred in the cancer model; however, manifestations accompanying fatigue in the ill client are endemic to all client populations. For example, clients with anemia experience classic clinical manifestations of profound fatigue, dyspnea, shortness of breath, pallor, weakness, and below normal Hb serum blood levels.[1,2]

Only recently have researchers found that fatigue is so far reaching that it is known to decrease the quality of life in the four domains of living: physical, psychological, social, and spiritual well-being. The correlation between fatigue and physical well-being is well-known but not always well understood. Clients most often report they cannot keep pace with their normal activities of functioning as a parent, work at their jobs, exercise, or have energy for pleasurable activities such as going to the movies or visiting friends.[1-4]

Psychological well-being is affected by emotional distress, fears of the unknown, the inability to concentrate, forgetfulness, and the notion that their disease is worsening. Cognitive dysfunction secondary to cancer treatment is only beginning to be explored.[4,5] Studies suggest that women with cancer who have been treated with adjuvant therapy show cognitive dysfunction 2 years after treatment.[6] The cognitive functions that appear to be affected by chemotherapy include verbal and short-term memory, verbal fluency, and concentration.[6] A randomized study about the effect of the use of epoetin alfa on cognitive function, fatigue, and quality of life in women with breast cancer who had received adjuvant or neoadjuvant chemotherapy found that less fatigue and better quality of life were seen in the epoetin alfa arm than in the placebo arm during chemotherapy.[7] However, in a longitudinal study of breast cancer clients, the strongest predictor for fatigue was poor mental health.[8]

Social well-being affected by fatigue is manifested in the client's reluctance to attend support groups or attend community activities because of the profound fatigue. Clients find themselves becoming isolated and often depressed because they must conserve their energy for the basic tasks of daily living.[1]

Finally, the spiritual well-being domain encompasses the client's concern for his or her mortality and often causes a shift in life priorities from the need to accumulate tangible goals (e.g., promotions at work, gaining more financial security) to focus on the small but joyous events of even one day (e.g., the change of seasons, gardening, or return to a religion that might have been abandoned for some years).

More research is required to understand fully the manifestations of fatigue and its enormous consequences for the client and the client's family. Although the impact of fatigue is well documented in its physical consequences, psychological, social, and spiritual consequences are only beginning to be researched. Similar to shifts in understanding and treating the manifestations of pain in a humanistic and nonjudgmental fashion, fatigue is emerging as an important manifestation to be managed by health care clinicians.[9]

Nursing research is emerging to document that all the domains of fatigue can be diminished by teaching clients and their families to practice certain behaviors.[10-12]

1. Treating anemia with erythropoietin colony-stimulating factors or RBC transfusion when appropriate
2. Promoting sleep and rest
   a. Take short naps instead of long ones.
3. Providing optimal nutritional support
   a. Eat low-fat, high-fiber meals.
4. Alternative therapies
   a. Use relaxation techniques, biofeedback, or massage therapy.
5. Energy conservation and body mechanics
   a. Wash hair in the shower, not in the tub or over a sink.
   b. Use a terry-cloth robe instead of a towel to dry off.
   c. Use a hand-held shower while sitting in the tub.
   d. Install a handrail.
6. Exercise
   a. Exercise moderately.
   b. Take walks.
7. Cognitive dysfunction
   a. Do crossword puzzles.
   b. Do jigsaw puzzles.

REFERENCES

1. Nail, L.M. (2004). Fatigue. In C.H. Yarbro, M.H. Frogge, & M. Goodman (Eds.), *Cancer symptom management* (3rd ed., pp. 47-60). Boston, Mass: Jones & Bartlett.
2. Fletchner, H., & Bottomley, A. (2003). Fatigue and quality of life: Lessons from the real world. *The Oncologist, 8*(Suppl 1), 5-9.
3. Ferrell, B.R., et al. (1996). "Bone tired": The experience of fatigue and impact on quality of life. *Oncology Nursing Forum, 23*, 1539-1547.
4. Fu, M.R., McDaniel, R.W., & Rhodes, V.A. (2005). Fatigue. In C.H. Yarbro, M.H. Frogge, & M. Goodman (Eds.), *Cancer nursing: Principles & practice* (6th ed., pp. 741-760). Boston, Mass: Jones & Bartlett.
5. Holzner, B., et al. (2002). The impact of hemoglobin levels on fatigue and quality of life in cancer patients. *Annals of Oncology, 13*, 965-973.
6. Schagen, S.B., et al. (1998). Impairment of cognitive function in women receiving adjuvant treatment for high-risk breast cancer; high dose versus standard-dose chemotherapy. *Journal of the National Cancer Institute, 90*, 210-218.
7. O'Shaughnessy, J., et al. (2002). *Impact of epoetin alfa on cognitive function, asthenia, and quality of life in women with breast cancer receiving adjuvant or neoadjuvant chemotherapy: Analysis of a 6-month follow-up data.* Presented at the 25th Annual San Antonio Breast Cancer Symposium, Dec 11-14, San Antonio, Tex.
8. Nieboer, P., et al. (2005). Fatigue and relating factors in high-risk breast cancer patients treated with adjuvant standard or high-dose chemotherapy: A longitudinal study. *Journal of Clinical Oncology, 23*(33), 8296-8304.
9. National Cancer Institute (NCI). Fatigue. Retrieved 04/18/07 from www.cancer.gov/cancertopics/pdq/supportivecare/fatigue/HealthProfessional/.
10. Crimpton, B. (1995). Symptom management: Loss of concentration. *Seminars in Oncology Nursing, 11*, 279-288.
11. Swartz, A. (1998). Patterns of exercise and fatigue in physically active cancer survivors. *Oncology Nursing Forum, 25*(3), 1-12.
12. Young-McCaughan, S. (2006). Exercise in the rehabilitation from cancer. *MEDSURG Nursing: The Journal of Adult Health, 15*(6), 384-388.

INTEGRATING P H A R M A C O L O G Y

Oral and Parenteral Iron Replacement Therapy

Iron deficiency anemia is often treated with oral ferrous sulfate and, more recently, with parenteral iron administration. Although oral iron is an over-the-counter medication, its frequent side effects often cause the client to discontinue the medication. Nurses can teach clients the nature of the side effects and how to manage them. You may teach your client to drink ginger tea or suck on ginger candy to avoid or minimize nausea and vomiting. Stool softeners to avoid constipation are also important. Conversely, IV iron replacements, long discouraged because of the danger of anaphylactic shock, are being replaced by newer preparations with fewer adverse effects. Because of the history of adverse events, fear of administering the IV iron agent warrants discussion of this new preparation.

Functional iron deficiency may develop in clients with normal ferritin levels but low transferrin saturation (<20%) because of the inability of the client to mobilize iron stores rapidly enough to support increased erythropoiesis. Some factors that influence the absorption of iron include the dose, iron stores, the degree of erythropoiesis, diet, and the route of administration. In iron deficient clients, the amount of iron absorbed can be 10% to 30% and as high as 60%. In healthy clients, about 5% to 10% of dietary iron is absorbed. In clients with iron deficiencies such

as iron deficiency anemia, oral or IV iron replacement may be needed.

Oral iron supplementation therapy is preferred, provided the client can adequately absorb iron and can tolerate oral therapy. If no blood is lost, the usual adult daily dose of elemental iron is in the range of 180 to 200 mg in divided doses preferably taken on an empty stomach. Oral iron supplementation is available as ferrous sulfate, ferrous gluconate, or ferrous fumarate. These iron salts are absorbed equally; however, they differ in the amount of elemental iron they contain. Ferrous gluconate, ferrous sulfate, and ferrous fumarate provide about 11%, 20%, and 33% of elemental iron, respectively. All three iron salts are known to be associated with GI side effects such as nausea and vomiting, constipation, diarrhea, or dark coloration of feces.

Some clients may inadequately respond to oral iron supplementation because of poor absorption, noncompliance, or intolerance of therapy.

Parenteral iron therapy does not induce GI side effects, thereby reducing client noncompliance, and it is convenient to take; however, parenteral iron preparations are also known to be associated with hypersensitivity reactions, including anaphylactic reactions and local adverse reactions. Three different IV iron preparations are currently available for iron deficiency anemia: (1) iron dextran, (2) sodium ferric gluconate, and (3) iron sucrose. All iron dextran products are indicated for use as a second-line therapy only after clients fail oral iron therapy.

SAFETY

⚠

ALERT

A homologous transfusion can have significant risks for the client. These risks include hemolytic transfusion reactions and the possibility of contracting infectious diseases such as human immunodeficiency virus (HIV)/acquired immunodeficiency syndrome (AIDS), hepatitis B or C, graft-versus-host disease (GVHD), cytomegalovirus (CMV), Epstein-Barr virus (EBV), and West Nile virus. Transfusions should be avoided in clients who might be candidates for bone marrow transplantation (BMT) (e.g., those with aplastic disorders or sickle cell disease) because transfusion decreases the probability of cure. In addition, clients who may have multiple antibodies against RBCs and those with autoimmune antibodies are at a higher risk for complications because of the complexities of obtaining crossmatched donor blood. Considering the potential risks, alternative interventions should be taken when possible to reduce the need for transfusion. The Joint Commission (TJC) requires that all blood transfusions be evaluated to confirm that clear medical indications for the transfusion exist and that the client responds as expected.

Because of the risks associated with blood transfusion, a client's informed consent is required. Blood is administered only after informed consent is obtained. Consent includes an explanation to the client or family member, if necessary, of medical indications for

homologous transfusion and its benefits, risks, and alternatives. Documentation of informed consent may consist of a form in the medical record stating that this information was presented in a manner understandable to the client or family member (e.g., the risks of and alternatives to blood transfusion were explained, and the client consented). If no family member is available or time does not allow, place a note to this effect in the chart.

Transfusion Reactions Associated with Homologous Blood Transfusions. A blood transfusion reaction is an adverse reaction to blood component therapy that can range from mild symptoms to a life-threatening condition. Complications can be acute or delayed, occurring days to years after a transfusion. Acute reactions may be immunogenic or nonimmunogenic. Immunogenic reactions include allergic, acute hemolytic, and anaphylactic reactions as well as fever; nonimmunogenic reactions include circulatory overload and septicemia. Table 75-4 details acute transfusion reactions.

Delayed reactions may include a delayed hemolytic reaction, hepatitis B, hepatitis C, HIV, GVHD, iron overload, and other infections and agents such as CMV, EBV, human T-cell leukemia virus type 1 (HTLV-1, the organism

TABLE 75–4 **Acute Transfusion Reactions**

Reaction	Cause	Clinical Manifestations	Management	Prevention
Immunogenic				
Allergic Incidence: 1%	Sensitivity to foreign proteins in plasma	Urticaria, flushing, itching (no fever)	Administer antihistamines as directed If manifestations mild and transient, transfusion may resume	Treat prophylactically with antihistamines
Febrile, nonhemolytic Incidence: 0.5-1%	Sensitization to donor white blood cells, platelets, or plasma proteins	Fever and/or pulmonary symptoms Sudden chills and fever (rise in temperature >1° C [1.8° F]), headache, flushing, anxiety, muscle pain	If fever and/or pulmonary manifestations occur, *do not* resume transfusion Give antipyretics as prescribed; avoid aspirin thrombocytopenic clients Treat shock	Consider leukocyte-poor blood products (filtered, washed, or frozen) if fever occurs more than once
Acute hemolytic Incidence: 1:25,000 Fatal: 2:1 × 10^6	Infusion of ABO-incompatible RBCs	Chills, fever, low back pain, flushing, tachycardia, tachypnea, hemoglobinuria, hemoglobinemia, hypotension, vascular collapse, bleeding, acute renal failure, shock, cardiac arrest, death	Send blood samples for serologic testing, and send urine samples to lab Maintain blood pressure Give diuretics as prescribed to maintain urine flow Insert indwelling catheter or measure hourly output Dialysis may be needed	Meticulously verify recipient from sample collection to transfusion
Anaphylactic Incidence: 1:150,000	Infusion of IgA proteins to IgA-deficient recipient who has developed anti-IgA antibodies	Anxiety, urticaria, wheezing progressing to cyanosis, shock, and possible cardiac arrest	Do not transfuse additional RBCs Initiate CPR if indicated Have epinephrine ready for injection (0.4 ml of a 1:1000 solution subcutaneously)	Give blood components from IgA-deficient donors or remove *all* plasma by washing
Nonimmunogenic				
Circulatory overload Estimated incidence: 1:10,000 (not usually reported to blood bank)	Infusion of blood at a rate too rapid for size, cardiac status, or clinical condition of recipient	Cough, dyspnea, pulmonary congestion (rales), headache, hypertension, tachycardia, distended neck veins	Place client in upright position with feet in dependent position Administer diuretics, oxygen, and morphine as prescribed Phlebotomy may be required	Adjust transfusion volume and flow rate on basis of client size and clinical status If slow transfusion will exceed 4 hr, request that unit be aliquoted into smaller volumes
Septicemia Incidence: very rare	Transfusion of component contaminated with microorganism	Rapid onset of chills, high fever, vomiting, diarrhea, marked hypotension, and shock	Treat manifestations and administer antibiotics, IV fluids, vasopressors, and steroids as directed Obtain culture of client and blood containers	Collect, process, store, and transfuse blood according to industry standards Infuse within 4 hr of starting time

CPR, Cardiopulmonary resuscitation; *Ig,* immunoglobulin; *IV,* intravenous; *RBC,* red blood cells.

that causes malaria), and West Nile virus. Table 75-5 provides details on delayed transfusion reactions.

Autologous Blood Transfusion. *Autologous* blood transfusion is the alternative to *homologous* (random) transfusion and should be considered. Clients who do not have leukemia or bacteremia should be offered the option of donating their own blood before a scheduled surgical procedure when there is a reasonable expectation that blood will be required. Although the risk-benefit ratio should be evaluated, experience to date indicates that even clients with heart disease and other high-risk conditions tolerate donating blood well. The elimination of disease transmission, alloimmunization, and other potential transfusion complications makes this a reasonable option for many surgical clients.

Autologous donations can be made every 3 days if the donor's Hb level remains at or above 11 g/dl. For the

blood to be maintained in a liquid state, donations should begin within 5 weeks of the transfusion date. Donations should cease at least 3 days before the date of transfusion.

Transfusion Procedures

Confirm Physician's Order. The physician's order for transfusion should specify blood component, volume, and rate of infusion.

Obtain Venous Access. The gauge of the needle used for transfusion varies with the product being infused.

When packed RBCs weighing less than 300 g are infused, a 19-gauge or larger needle is needed to achieve the maximal flow rate. If a smaller-gauge needle must be used, the RBCs can be diluted with 0.9% saline. To prevent hemolysis, add no solution other than normal saline to blood components.

TABLE 75–5 Delayed Transfusion Reactions

Reaction	Clinical Manifestations
Delayed hemolytic	Fever, mild jaundice, decreased hemoglobin and hematocrit
	Occurs as early as 3 days or as late as several months but usually 7 to 14 days posttransfusion as result of destruction of transfused RBCs by alloantibodies not detected during crossmatch
	Generally, no acute treatment is required, but hemolysis may be severe enough to warrant further transfusions
	Although uncommon, severe complications such as renal failure and DIC have been reported
Hepatitis B*	Elevated liver enzymes (AST and ALT), anorexia, malaise, nausea and vomiting, fever, dark urine, jaundice
	Incubation period is about 8-12 wk, although it may extend to 6 mo or longer
	Usually resolves spontaneously within 4-6 wk; chronic carrier state can develop and can result in permanent liver damage
	Treat symptomatically
Hepatitis C*	Similar to hepatitis B, but manifestations are usually less severe
	Approximately 20% of acute infections resolve
	Chronic liver disease and cirrhosis may develop
	Before introduction of anti-HCV test, accounted for 90%-95% of all posttransfusion hepatitis
	Treat symptomatically
Human immunodeficiency virus (HIV)	Can be asymptomatic for up to several years or may develop flu-like manifestations within 2-4 wk
	Later manifestations include weight loss, diarrhea, fever, lymphadenopathy, thrush, *Pneumocystis* pneumonia
Iron overload	Heart failure, dysrhythmias, impaired thyroid and gonadal function, diabetes mellitus, arthritis, cirrhosis
	Excess iron is deposited in heart, liver, pancreas, and joints, causing dysfunction
	Commonly occurs in clients receiving >100 units for chronic anemia over a period of time
	Prevented by iron chelation therapy [deferoxamine (Desferal)], which chelates and removes accumulated iron via kidneys, may be administered IV or subcutaneously
	Treat clinical manifestations
Graft-versus-host disease	Fever, rash, diarrhea, nausea, jaundice, hepatitis
	Result of replication of donor lymphocytes (graft) in transfusion recipient (host)
	Onset 3-30 days posttransfusion
	No effective therapy available
	To prevent, irradiate blood products before transfusion in at-risk recipient
	Some believe that irradiated blood products are indicated for first-degree family members' donations also
Other	Other infectious diseases and agents may be transmitted via transfusion, including cytomegalovirus, HTLV-1, and those causing malaria

ALT, Alanine aminotransferase; *AST*, aspartate aminotransferase; *HTLV-1*, human T-cell leukemia virus, type 1; *IV*, intravenous; *RBCs*, red blood cells.
*New cases of transfusion-related hepatitis B and C are not common.
From Blaney, K.D., & Howard, P.R. (2000). *Basic and applied concepts of immunohematology*. St. Louis: Mosby; and Hillyer, C.D., et al. (2003). *Blood banking and transfusion medicine: Basi principles and practice*. Philadelphia: Churchill Livingstone.

Components that contain a significant volume of plasma or other diluent can be safely infused at a rapid rate through smaller-gauge needles or catheters.

A central venous catheter is an acceptable access option for blood transfusion; however, a large volume of refrigerated blood infused rapidly into the ventricle of the heart may cause cardiac dysrhythmias. Warming the blood can reduce the risk of this complication.

Another issue of concern is the use of multilumen catheters, which may allow blood to mix with incompatible solutions and medications as they exit the catheter tips. Experience indicates that the circulation achieved through a blood vessel that is suitable for central line placement results in rapid mixing of fluids. As a result no harmful effects have been reported.

Preparation for the Infusion. Blood-bank regulations state that refrigerated components may not be returned to inventory if they have been warmed to more than 10° C (50° F). To meet this requirement, most transfusion medicine services consider 30 minutes to be the maximal allowable time out of monitored storage. To avoid wasting a scarce commodity, certain procedures should be performed before blood is requested: (1) An intravenous (IV) catheter appropriate for transfusing the requested component should be functional, flushed with normal saline, and maintained at a keep-vein-open (KVO) rate. (2) Vital signs should then be taken and recorded. (3) The existence of a fever may be a reason for delaying the transfusion. In addition to masking a possible manifestation of an acute transfusion reaction, fever can also compromise the efficacy of platelet transfusions. (4) Premedication may be required if the client has a history of adverse reactions. In many cases, febrile reactions can be prevented by administering acetaminophen. A history of allergic reactions may warrant prophylactic administration of antihistamines (e.g., diphenhydramine HCl). To ensure effectiveness, administer oral medication 30 minutes before the transfusion is started. IV medication may be given immediately before the transfusion is initiated.

Confirm Blood Acceptability

The most crucial phase of transfusion is confirming product compatibility and verifying the client's identity. The name and identification number of the recipient must be provided, and a permanent record of this information must be maintained in the blood bank. To avoid delivery to the wrong client, blood should be transported to only one client at a time.

An estimated 90% of transfusion reactions are due to improper product-to-client identification. Before going to the client's bedside, verify ABO and Rh compatibility, usually by comparing the bag label with the medical record and forms issued from the blood bank. Also check the bag label to ensure that the correct component has been issued, and check for the expiration date.

Inspect the unit for leaks, abnormal color, clots, excessive air, and bubbles. Check carefully for important labels (e.g., "autologous" or "directed") or instructions (e.g., "use a leukocyte-depleting filter"). Cellular components (whole blood, RBCs, and platelets) for an immunosuppressed client should be clearly marked "irradiated."

At the bedside compare the name and number on the identification bracelet with the tag on the blood bag. If applicable, check the secondary identification system. The American Association of Blood Banks recommends that two qualified people perform this critical step.

Infuse Blood. Most blood products should be infused through administration sets designed specifically for this use. The set usually contains a 170-micrometer filter designed to trap fibrin clots and other debris that accumulates during blood storage. Most standard filters can filter 4 units of blood. Tubing is available in two basic configurations: straight or Y-type. The use of Y-type tubing simplifies the process of adding normal saline to RBCs and provides ready access to a saline flush if the transfusion must be interrupted. Straight tubing usually has a medication injection site a few inches from the needle. If an adverse reaction develops, a KVO saline drip initiated at this site maintains patency of the IV line but avoids exposure to the 30 to 50 ml of blood remaining in the tubing and filter.

To reduce the risk of septicemia, change the administration set every 4 to 6 hours or according to institution policy.

Blood warmers may be used to prevent hypothermia, which can be induced by rapid infusion of large volumes of refrigerated blood.

Monitor During the Transfusion

The first 10 to 15 minutes of any transfusion are the most critical. If a major ABO incompatibility exists or a severe allergic reaction such as anaphylaxis occurs, it is usually evident within the first 50 ml of the transfusion. Therefore it is recommended that the transfusion begin slowly and that the client be closely monitored. If no evidence of a reaction is noted within the first 15 minutes, flow can be increased to the prescribed rate.

Before leaving the client unattended, instruct the client to report anything unusual immediately. Take and record vital signs before the transfusion begins, after the first 15 minutes, and every hour until 1 hour after the transfusion has been discontinued. Check vital signs immediately if the client displays any untoward manifestations.

The recommended rate of infusion varies with the blood component being transfused. Components such as platelets, plasma, and cryoprecipitate may be infused rapidly, but you must take care to avoid circulatory overload, especially with geriatric clients and clients with cardiac disease. To avoid the risk of septicemia, infusions should not exceed 4 hours. If the client's size or medical condition does not allow infusion within 4 hours, the unit may be split into smaller aliquots in the blood bank. Regulatory agencies require complete documentation of the transfusion, including identification of personnel starting and ending the transfusion, unique product number, and outcome (e.g., "no reaction noted").

Watch for Transfusion Reaction

SAFETY ALERT

Exposure to foreign blood elements may mediate immunologic and nonimmunologic reactions affecting all major body systems. Consider any unusual manifestation that occurs during or immediately after a transfusion a potential reaction. Monitor unconscious clients closely because manifestations of a reaction may be inhibited in the unconscious state. The acute reactions most frequently seen are described in Table 75-4.

Although treatment may vary depending on the manifestations, certain standard procedures must be followed when a reaction is suspected. It is important to know your institutional policies regarding management of transfusion reactions; however, the following steps are indicated:
1. Stop the transfusion.
2. Keep the IV line open with normal saline.
3. Contact the client's physician and the blood bank.
4. Recheck identifying tags and numbers on the blood and the client.
5. Monitor vital signs and urine output.
6. Treat symptoms per physician's orders.
7. Save blood bag and tubing and send it to the blood bank for examination with transfusion reaction report.
8. Complete transfusion reaction report.
9. Obtain blood and urine samples, in accordance with institutional policy.
10. Document client's condition and all actions taken in the client's record and transfusion reaction forms per hospital policy.

Nursing Management of the Medical Client

Assessment. The general nursing care of clients with anemia includes adequate assessment by the nurse to help identify the cause of the anemia and client education deficits relating to the underlying illness causing the anemia. You can help in the diagnosis by taking a complete health history focusing on the elements outlined in Chapter 74. Client and family teaching is extremely important in treating the anemias because most of the care takes place in an outpatient clinic or in the client's home. Help the client and family to become knowledgeable about self-care in both preventing and treating anemia.

Diagnosis, Outcomes, Interventions
Diagnosis: Activity Intolerance and/or Fatigue. Write the nursing diagnosis as *Activity Intolerance and/or fatigue related to decreased blood supply or low hemoglobin levels as evidenced by complaints of fatigue and lack of energy, dyspnea, pallor, tachycardia, and cognitive dysfunction.*

Outcomes. The client will tolerate activity as evidenced by being able to sit up without fatigue, dyspnea, pallor, or tachycardia; walking increasing distances; and participating in activities of daily living such as bathing, dressing, grooming, and feeding, to the greatest extent possible.

Interventions. Teach the client about the condition, self-care activities, lifestyle changes, nutritional needs, and medication information. Inform the client that iron salts are gastric irritants and should always be taken with or after meals. Liquid iron preparations should be well diluted and taken through a straw (undiluted liquid iron stains teeth). The client can avoid constipation, commonly seen during iron therapy, by eating a high-fiber diet and using stool softeners or laxatives as required. Avoid consumption of coffee and tea with iron; absorption is hampered by the tannates. See the discussion of transfusion therapy procedures earlier in the chapter if a blood transfusion is required.

Evaluation. Resolution of anemia requires time. When packed RBCs are used, anemia will be corrected immediately. When oral iron preparations are used, it takes weeks for anemia to resolve; the client will thus need assessments at intervals to monitor the progress of therapy. Ultimate prognosis depends on how well the underlying disease is resolved or controlled; progress in this regard should also be monitored.

Modifications for Older Clients

Older adults have an especially high prevalence of anemia, primarily attributable to poor nutrition with decreased intestinal absorption of iron, often resulting from debilitation or depression or both. Anemia in older clients is often asymptomatic or mistakenly diagnosed as normal aging changes. Such manifestations include fatigue, confusion, angina, ataxia, and heart failure. Special care should be taken to provide a thorough work-up of these clients to determine whether an etiology exists that might be reversible and thus treatable.

ANEMIA CAUSED BY DECREASED ERYTHROCYTE PRODUCTION

Normally the production and destruction of erythrocytes are in equilibrium in the body. In situations where the production of erythrocytes is decreased, anemia results. Decreased production may be due to (1) decreased synthesis of normal hemoglobin, as seen in iron deficiency anemia, thalassemia, and sideroblastic anemia; (2) defective DNA synthesis, as seen in megaloblastic anemia resulting from cobalamin (vitamin B$_{12}$) and folate deficiency; or (3) reduced availability of erythrocyte precursors, as seen in aplastic anemia and anemia of chronic disease.

IRON DEFICIENCY ANEMIA

Iron deficiency anemia (IDA) is a chronic, hypochromic, microcytic anemia resulting from an insufficient supply of iron in the body. Without iron, hemoglobin concentration in the RBCs is reduced and the cells are unable to oxygenate the body's tissues adequately, resulting in anemia.

Etiology and Risk Factors

The National Academy of Sciences recommends an iron intake of 15 mg daily for women and 10 mg daily for men. An average diet supplies the body with about 12 to 15 mg/day of iron, of which only 5% to 10% (0.6 to 1.5 mg) is absorbed. IDA is associated with either inadequate absorption or excessive loss of iron. Major risk factors for IDA include (1) insufficient dietary intake of iron, (2) blood loss, (3) impaired absorption of iron, and (4) excessive demands for RBC production as a result of hemolysis. It is important to know the population groups that have a higher association with these risk factors.

Populations in poor countries and people whose diets lack meat are at particular risk for iron deficiency anemia from insufficient dietary intake of iron, the most prevalent hematologic disorder worldwide. About 30% of the world's population has this anemia. It is an important international economic concern for two reasons: (1) the diminished capacity of individuals to perform physical labor and (2) the impact on the growth, development, and learning of infants and children. Alcoholics are also at increased risk because of poor diets.

Other populations may have increased requirements for iron intake at particular times in their lives. The amount of iron normally absorbed daily is sufficient for meeting the needs of healthy men and women past childbearing age, but it does not meet the additional needs of menstruating and pregnant women, infants, children, adolescent females, older adults (>65 years),

regular blood donors, and those on strict vegetarian diets. These groups are at a sufficiently high risk to warrant consideration of prophylactic iron therapy. In the United States women have twice the prevalence of IDA as men (8% versus 4%) because of the excess needs of women of childbearing age. An estimated 4% to 8% of premenopausal women are iron deficient. The most common etiologies of IDA for women are menstruation and pregnancy. Normal iron excretion is less than 1 mg daily. Iron is excreted in urine, sweat, bile, and feces and from the skin in desquamated cells. The average woman loses another 15 mg monthly during menses. About 500 mg of iron is lost during a normal pregnancy.

Older adults are a population at risk for IDA. An estimated 20% of adults more than 65 years of age suffer from this condition. Economic constraints, poor dentition, lack of interest in food preparation, malnutrition, and increased rates of chronic disease and cancers, particularly of the gastrointestinal (GI) tract, contribute to a higher prevalence rate in older adults.

Blood loss is the most common etiologic factor in men, and the GI tract is the most common site. Hemorrhage may result from peptic ulcers, hiatal hernia, gastritis, gastroesophageal reflux disease (GERD), cancer, hemorrhoids, diverticula, Crohn's disease, ulcerative colitis, or salicylate poisoning. It may also be related to gastritis from the use of aspirin, steroids, or nonsteroidal anti-inflammatory drugs (NSAIDs). Bleeding from the GI tract is usually chronic and occult (too small to be seen). A chronic blood loss of as little as 2 to 4 ml daily can result in iron deficiency anemia because every 2 ml of blood contains 1 mg of iron. The body can compensate for such losses to some degree by excreting less than 0.5 mg of iron daily rather than the normal 1 mg.

Malabsorption of iron may result from alterations in the mucosa of the duodenum and proximal jejunum (as in chronic diarrhea, malabsorption syndromes such as sprue and celiac disease, gastrectomy, and removal of the proximal small bowel), resulting in IDA. Tannates (in tea and coffee), carbonates, the chelating agent ethylenediaminetetraacetic acid (EDTA), and the medicinal antacid magnesium trisilicate all hinder nonheme iron absorption. Eating starch and clay, which occurs in some cultures, also leads to malabsorption.

Pathophysiology

Iron is present in all RBCs as heme in Hb; heme accounts for two thirds of the body's iron. Iron is also vital for the metabolic processes of DNA synthesis and electron transport. Iron concentration in the body is regulated by the absorptive cells in the proximal small intestine; these cells alter iron absorption to match body losses of iron intake. Errors in this balance also lead to anemia. Fortunately the GI tract can increase its absorption of iron from 10% daily to about 20% to 30% daily. In this way, the body often compensates for diminishing iron stores resulting from inadequate iron intake or excessive iron loss. The other one third of the body's iron (non-heme) is stored in the form of ferritin, an iron-phosphorus-protein complex that contains about 23% iron.

Clinical Manifestations

In mild cases of iron deficiency anemia, the client is asymptomatic; in more severe cases, assessment reveals the general manifestations of anemia, including fatigue; headache; dyspnea; palpitations; pallor in the face, palm of the hand, nail bed, and mucous membranes of the mouth and conjunctiva; *angular stomatitis* (inflammation of the mucosa of the mouth), *glossitis* (inflammation of the tongue), and *cheilitis* (inflammation of the lips); and brittle nails. Laboratory results characteristic of iron deficiency anemia are presented in Table 75-3. Once a diagnosis of iron deficiency anemia is confirmed, studies are conducted to find the cause. Radiographic studies (GI tract series), stool examination for occult blood, esophagoscopy, gastroscopy, and sigmoidoscopy are commonly done to identify the site of blood loss. Correction of the underlying problem (malnutrition, alcoholism, hemorrhage) must follow so that the deficiency does not recur.

OUTCOME MANAGEMENT

Management of IDA focuses on (1) diagnosis of and correction of the underlying cause and (2) treatment through diet and supplemental iron preparations. Supplemental iron is administered to increase iron available in the blood. Monitoring the client to ensure compliance is important. An increase in reticulocytes 5 to 10 days after initiation of iron therapy can document a positive response. Clients with increased daily needs should be given supplemental iron prophylactically (during pregnancy) (see the Integrating Pharmacology feature on Oral and Parenteral Iron Replacement Therapy, p. 2012).

Diets high in iron should be planned with the client and family members. The nurse plays a key role in this intervention. Clients and families may need to be taught the elements of high-iron diets, both in terms of the food to be consumed (Box 75-2) and with respect to how it should be prepared to increase (cooking in iron skillets) or prevent the loss of dietary iron.

THALASSEMIA

Thalassemia is an autosomal-recessive genetic disorder that results in inadequate normal Hb production. Whereas IDA affects heme synthesis, thalassemia disrupts the synthesis of globin.

Etiology and Risk Factors

Thalassemia is frequently found in people of Mediterranean, African, and Southeast Asian origin. Individuals

---

BOX 75-2 Foods High in Iron, Vitamin B$_{12}$, and Folic Acid

EXCELLENT SOURCE OF IRON

Almonds, asparagus, bran, beans, Boston brown bread, carrots, cauliflower, celery, chard, dandelions, egg yolk, graham bread, kale, kidney, lettuce, liver, oatmeal, oysters, soybeans, spinach, and whole wheat. (Cook foods in iron pans.)

GOOD SOURCE OF IRON

Apricots, beef, beets, cabbage, cornmeal, cucumbers, currants, dates, duck, goose, greens, lamb, molasses, mushrooms, oranges, parsnips, peanuts, peas, peppers, potatoes, prunes, radishes, raisins, rhubarb, pineapple, tomatoes, and turnips.

VITAMIN B$_{12}$

Red meats, especially liver, dairy products, and eggs.

FOLIC ACID

Asparagus, broccoli, spinach, lettuce, lemons, bananas, melons, green leafy vegetables, fish, legumes, whole grains, liver, organ meats, mushrooms, strawberries, milk, eggs, yeast, wheat germ, kidney beans, beef, potatoes, dried peas and beans, and nuts. (Foods should not be cooked with excessive heat or large amounts of water.)

---

who inherit an alpha-gene(s) have alpha-thalassemia, the most common of the thalassemias; the alpha-trait (*heterozygous* state) is asymptomatic in about 30% of African Americans. Those who inherit just one beta-gene (*heterozygotes*) have thalassemia minor, also called *thalassemia trait,* the carrier state of thalassemia major. Those who inherit both beta-genes (*homozygotes*) have thalassemia major, which results in a profound and life-threatening anemia.

Pathophysiology

In alpha-thalassemia, there is a mutation in the alpha-globin gene(s). In thalassemia minor, one beta-globin gene is mutated, leading to minor disruptions in beta-globin synthesis. In thalassemia major, a mutation exists in both beta-genes, resulting in significant impairment of beta-globin synthesis, marked reduction in hemoglobin production, and profound anemia. Hemolysis results from an imbalance in the alpha- and beta-globin chains, which are normally paired. The excess unpaired alpha- or beta-globin chains aggregate and form a precipitate that damages RBC membranes, leading to intravascular hemolysis.

Clinical Manifestations

Individuals with alpha-thalassemia may have very mild anemia and are typically asymptomatic. Those with thalassemia minor have clinical manifestations of mild to moderate anemia. These disorders may be undiagnosed for several years.

Individuals with thalassemia major are diagnosed early in life because the lack of Hb becomes quickly apparent. Affected children appear normal at birth because fetal Hb contains no beta-globin; however, in the first few months of life, as Hb synthesis switches from fetal to adult form, manifestations of severe anemia begin to appear. The children also have pain, failure to thrive, frequent infections, diarrhea, splenomegaly, hepatomegaly, jaundice from RBC hemolysis, and bone marrow hyperplasia.

Fetal diagnosis for a specific type of thalassemia can be made through amniocentesis. Molecular diagnostic tests can determine whether a mutation is present after 8 weeks of gestation.

OUTCOME MANAGEMENT

Thalassemia minor usually does not require treatment. For thalassemia major, the treatment goals are to provide adequate normal Hb for erythropoiesis and to alleviate the effects of iron overload. Chronic transfusions are administered to correct the anemia with the targeted Hb level at 9 to 10 g/dl. Iron chelation with deferoxamine is necessary to prevent iron overload. Iron supplementation should not be used. Because RBCs may be sequestered in the spleen, a splenectomy may be necessary to decrease transfusion requirements. Genetic counseling and testing for families should be encouraged.

MEGALOBLASTIC ANEMIAS

Megaloblastic anemias are a group of disorders caused by impaired DNA synthesis resulting in defective, large RBCs (megaloblasts). They are caused by deficiencies of vitamin B_{12} (cobalamin) and folic acid.

Cobalamin/B_{12} Deficiency (Pernicious Anemia)

Pernicious anemia is an autoimmune disorder characterized by the absence of intrinsic factor (IF) in gastric secretions, leading to malabsorption of cobalamin (vitamin B_{12}). Pernicious anemia has been incorrectly used to describe any cobalamin deficiency, but it is actually only one cause of inadequate cobalamin.

Etiology and Risk Factors

Pernicious anemia (PA) is the most prevalent form of vitamin B_{12} deficiency in the United States and Canada (Box 75-3). It is associated with gastric atrophy and loss of IF as well as a rare genetic autosomal-recessive disorder (congenital pernicious anemia) in which IF is lacking without gastric atrophy. Ninety percent of people with PA have antibodies that react specifically against the parietal gastric cells where IF is produced; 60% have anti-IF antibodies. It occurs more often in families of PA clients and is associated with human leukocyte

---

> **BOX 75-3   Causes of Cobalamin and Folate Deficiencies**
>
> - Insufficient dietary intake: Rare with cobalamin (Cbl) but common with folate
> - Drugs that impede absorption in the stomach: Purine analogs (azathioprine), pyrimidine analogs (5-fluorouracil [5-FU]), ribonucleotide reductase inhibitors (hydroxyurea), anticonvulsants (phenytoin), and oral contraceptives
> - Drugs that impair uptake in the ileum: Nitrous oxide, cholestyramine, *p*-aminosalicylic acid, neomycin, metformin, phenformin, and colchicine
> - Genetic disorders causing defects in the ileal receptors of intrinsic factor (IF): Imerslund-Graesbeck syndrome, hereditary transcobalamin II (TCII) deficiency
> - Impaired absorption resulting from medications, cancers, gastrointestinal (GI) diseases, or surgical resection of the terminal ileum
> - GI disorders: Gastric atrophy, gastrectomy, gastric stapling, bypass for pancreatic insufficiency of protease, which releases Cbl from R-protein binders so that Cbl can bind with IF
> - Zollinger-Ellison syndrome

---

antigen (HLA) types A2, A3, and B7 and in type A blood groups. PA typically arises in people between 40 and 70 years of age with peak incidence around 70 years of age. It is more prevalent in people of Celtic and Scandinavian ancestry.

Pathophysiology

Cobalamin (B_{12}) and folate deficiency is believed to lead to attenuated production of DNA. In normal metabolism cobalamin (extrinsic factor) is released from its ingested protein-bound state by gastric acid. It is bound to IF, a glycoprotein produced by parietal cells of the gastric lining, and absorbed in the terminal ileum. It is then bound to the protein transcobalamin II (TCII) and transported to storage sites in the liver. Problems with any of these steps can lead to deficiency. Without cobalamin, DNA synthesis and cell replication are impaired. RBC precursors (erythrocytes/reticulocytes) do not divide normally, and large, poorly functioning RBCs are created. Production of myelin on nerves is greatly affected, also resulting in neurologic deterioration.

Clinical Manifestations

The major manifestations of PA are low Hb, hematocrit (HcT), and RBC levels. The diagnosis is based on the presence of anemia, GI manifestations (weight loss, appetite loss, nausea, vomiting, abdominal distention, diarrhea, constipation, steatorrhea), and neurologic disorders (paresthesias of feet and hands, poor gate, memory loss, cognitive problems, depression). Laboratory studies include a complete blood count (CBC), peripheral smear, reticulocyte count, Hb and HcT levels, serum iron level, total iron-binding capacity, and serum ferritin levels (see Table 75-3). In addition the Schilling test is the definitive test for PA and is used to diagnose and determine the cobalamin deficiency. The Schilling test measures the absorption of orally administered radioactive vitamin B_{12} (tagged with cobalt 60) before and after parenteral administration of IF. Gastric secretion analysis to check for the presence of free HCl is another important test. Most clients with pernicious anemia have low-volume gastric secretions with high pH and free hydrochloric (HCl) acid levels. These findings do not change, even after the administration of histamine, which normally stimulates gastric secretion.

OUTCOME MANAGEMENT

Medical Management

Cobalamin/Vitamin B_{12} Therapy

Clients with PA need both immediate treatment and lifelong therapy with maintenance vitamin B_{12}. The standard treatment is parenteral administration of cobalamin (cyanocobalamin or hydroxocobalamin) at 1000 mcg daily for 2 weeks and then weekly until the HcT returns to normal. Once the HcT is normal, monthly injections for life are required. An intranasal form of cyanocobalamin (Nascobal) is available as a nasal gel that is self-applied weekly. The response to the injections is usually quick and dramatic, often occurring within 24 to 48 hours. Within 72 hours, reticulocytes begin to increase; by the end of the first week, the total RBC count rises significantly. Cardiovascular involvement usually lessens with improved erythropoiesis. Peripheral nerve function may improve, but long-term neuromuscular complications are rarely reversed with treatment.

Iron Supplements

Additionally the client may need oral or IV iron supplements if the Hb level fails to rise in proportion to an increased RBC count. Iron deficiency may be an etiologic factor in pernicious anemia and must be corrected if it is present. Iron deficiency anemia can also develop during treatment of pernicious anemia. Injections of vitamin B_{12} may cause a rapid regeneration of RBCs that depletes iron. As a result the Hb level remains low, although the total RBC count rises. Once the acute stage of the illness is past, the client with pernicious anemia must undertake a lifelong program of maintenance therapy. Monthly injections of vitamin B_{12} are needed to avoid relapse. Encourage the client to eat a diet high in folic acid and iron to supplement the medication used to treat the anemia (see Box 75-2).

If the cause involves altered absorption of vitamin B_{12}, nutritional supplements are useless. If the disease is related to decreased intake of the vitamin, a diet high in vitamin B_{12} is encouraged.

Digestants

Digestants may be given to enhance the metabolism of vitamins; for example, HCl acid may be diluted in water and given with meals during the first few weeks of vitamin B_{12} therapy.

Treat Neurologic Complications

Multidrug combinations of high doses of folate, cobalamin, and pyridoxine have been proposed to help prevent neurologic complications.

Nursing Management of the Medical Client

Because clients with PA must receive weekly or monthly treatment for life, the nurse plays an important role in monitoring client progress. Response to treatment should be carefully monitored with blood counts and clinical blood chemistry tests. The client must be educated about the importance of adherence to the treatment regimen on a lifelong basis if the anemia is to be controlled and about the life-threatening consequences of not doing so. The progress of neurologic complications should be continually assessed. Clients with existing neurologic problems should be monitored for and educated about the possibility of injuries attributable to diminished sensitivity to heat and pain from nerve damage. Because gastric carcinoma is commonly associated with PA, clients should be evaluated frequently for the presence of this cancer.

Folic Acid Deficiency Anemia

Etiology and Risk Factors

Anemia associated with folic acid deficiency is common. There are many causes, most of which are the same as those of vitamin B_{12} deficiency. Usually folic acid deficiency results from a diet lacking in such foods as green leafy vegetables, liver, citrus fruits, nuts, grains, and yeast. Clients with chronic alcoholism or eating disorders, such as anorexia, because of their typically inadequate diets, are particularly at risk. High levels of alcohol in the blood also partially block the response of the bone marrow to folic acid, which thereby interferes with RBC production. Hemodialysis clients have to be carefully watched for folic acid deficiency because folic acid is lost during dialysis.

Folic acid deficiency, like vitamin B_{12} deficiency, can develop with malabsorption syndromes (e.g., sprue, celiac disease, steatorrhea). Certain medications can also impede folic acid absorption and utilization.

For example, a serious anemia may develop under the following conditions:

- Long-term use of anticonvulsant medications (e.g., primidone, phenytoin, phenobarbital)
- Administration of antimetabolites (e.g., folic acid antagonists, purine, pyrimidine analogs) to clients with cancer and leukemia
- Use of certain oral contraceptives

Finally, folic acid deficiency may occur with increased demands for folate, such as during pregnancy and the growth spurts of childhood and adolescence.

Clinical Manifestations

Folic acid, like vitamin B_{12}, is necessary for DNA synthesis; unlike PA, however, folic acid deficiency does not cause neurologic manifestations. The presence of neurologic problems generally rules out folic acid deficiency as the etiology. Anemia resulting from folic acid deficiency has a slow and insidious onset. The client, often thin and emaciated, usually appears quite ill. The client's malnourished and debilitated state frequently leads to other deficiencies, for example, of iron, protein, minerals, and other vitamins. Some clients may also have an electrolyte imbalance, and neurologic manifestations may develop as a result of thiamine, calcium, or magnesium deficiency (commonly linked with alcoholism).

The megaloblastic anemia caused by folic acid deficiency is the same as that seen in pernicious anemia (see Table 75-3). The diagnosis is confirmed by blood smear and bone marrow examinations. With folic acid deficiency, the serum folate level is less than 4 ng/ml (normal: 7 to 20 ng/ml); the Schilling test finding is normal. HCl is probably present in the gastric juice. Neurologic manifestations are absent; and the client responds favorably to a therapeutic trial of 50 to 100 mg of folic acid administered intramuscularly (IM) daily for 10 days.

OUTCOME MANAGEMENT

For correction of anemia caused by folate deficiency, the client receives oral doses of folic acid 0.1 to 5 mg daily until the blood profile improves or the cause of intestinal malabsorption is corrected. Clients with malabsorption syndromes may need parenteral folic acid initially, followed by maintenance therapy with oral doses. Folic acid is administered IM in the form of folinic acid (leucovorin calcium injection). In addition, vitamin C is sometimes prescribed because it increases the role of folic acid in promoting erythropoiesis. Diets with foods rich in folic acid (see Box 75-2) and food preparation methods that ensure that folate is not destroyed are important. Lifelong monthly doses of folate may be necessary for clients with partial or total gastrectomies.

Multivitamins with folate are often prescribed for older clients. Nursing interventions are similar to those discussed for the client with PA.

ANEMIAS CAUSED BY INCREASED ERYTHROCYTE DESTRUCTION
HEMOLYTIC ANEMIA

Hemolytic anemia is an end result of conditions that lead to hemolysis. Hemolysis, the premature destruction of erythrocytes, can result from physical damage, intrinsic membrane defects, abnormal Hb, erythrocytic enzymatic defects, immune destruction of RBCs by macrophages, or hypersplenism. Anemia occurs when the bone marrow fails to replace RBCs at the rate they are destroyed.

Etiology and Risk Factors

Hemolytic anemias constitute about 5% of all anemias. Hemolysis can result from hereditary disorders or acquired hemolytic conditions. Hemolysis can happen because of problems intrinsic or extrinsic to the RBCs. Extrinsic hemolytic anemias are the most common type and are acquired. In this type of hemolytic anemia, the RBCs are normal, but damage is caused by external factors such as toxins, mechanical injury (prosthetic heart valves), or trapping of cells within the sinuses of the liver or spleen. Intrinsic hemolytic anemias are caused by defects in the RBCs themselves resulting from abnormal Hb (e.g., sickle cell disease), enzyme deficiencies that alter glycolysis (glucose-6-phosphate dehydrogenase deficiency [G-6-PD]), or RBC membrane abnormalities.

The two sites of hemolysis are either intravascular or extravascular. Intravascular destruction takes place in the circulation whereas extravascular hemolysis takes place in the liver, spleen, and bone marrow.

Clinical Manifestations

The clinical manifestations of hemolytic anemia are numerous and diverse and are due primarily to anemia, the extent of compensation, previous treatment, and the underlying cause. The client with hemolytic anemia may suffer from all the general manifestations of anemia discussed previously (weakness, fatigue). Manifestations of specific disorders may be present, such as *hemochromatosis* (bronze skin tone and diabetes), or *hemoglobinuria* (dark urine) caused by intravascular hemolysis. Renal failure may be caused by an increased load of RBC breakdown products. Jaundice is often present because of the increased destruction of RBCs, causing an elevation in bilirubin levels. The spleen and liver may enlarge because of hyperactivity.

Because of the large number of causes for hemolytic anemia, numerous laboratory tests are conducted to determine or rule out known etiologies. These include a CBC, peripheral smear and morphologic examination, RBC indices, increased red blood cell distribution width (RDW), reticulocyte count, lactic acid dehydrogenase level, serum haptoglobin level, indirect bilirubin level, and other studies suggested by the history or physical examination (see Table 75-3). Increased RBC fragility, shortened erythrocyte life span, increased fecal and urinary urobilinogen levels, and hemoglobinemia in cases of massive intravascular hemolysis are typically seen.

OUTCOME MANAGEMENT

Interventions are undertaken to counter the complications of the hemolysis and to treat the underlying disorder. Removal of the offending agent, if it is known, is key. Transfusion therapy may be necessary (packed RBCs should be administered slowly to avoid cardiac arrest). Adequate fluids are given to flush the kidneys. In addition, sodium bicarbonate or sodium lactate is administered to alkalize the urine, which decreases the likelihood of precipitation in the renal tubules. Folate acid may be given to offset the consumption of folate that results from active hemolysis. Corticosteroids (prednisone) may be indicated and iron replacement therapy may be needed for those with severe intravascular hemolysis to counter persistent hemoglobinuria. Erythropoietin is given for anemia that has resulted from renal failure. Finally, clients should be educated to recognize the manifestations of hemolysis and to seek immediate medical attention if they occur.

SICKLE CELL DISEASE

Sickle cell disease (SCD) is a group of inherited disorders of mutant hemoglobin (hemoglobin S [HbS]) that causes the characteristic sickling of RBCs. Sickling occurs only under conditions of low oxygenation. The abnormally shaped RBCs become trapped in capillaries, causing organ damage from infarcts and tissue hypoxia, or are damaged in transit, leading to severe anemia. The most common variant, *sickle cell anemia,* is an autosomal-recessive disorder in which the person is homozygous for HbS. The heterozygous form, known as *sickle cell trait,* is a much milder form of the disease and the carrier state of HbS. SCD is a lifelong condition that manifests in the first year of life and persists throughout one's life span.

Etiology and Risk Factors

Sickle cell disease is found in races of people from areas of the world where malaria is endemic, including Africa, the Mediterranean, the Middle East, and India. It is the most common form of anemia worldwide; there are more than 200 million carriers of sickle cell trait worldwide. In the United States, about 1 in 375 African Americans are affected, and 8% of African Americans carry the gene and have the sickle cell trait. It is also found, although rarely, in people of Mediterranean, Middle East, or East Indian descent. The prevalence rate is less than the incidence rate because of high early mortality. Whether an individual will have sickle cell anemia or sickle cell trait or will be free of the disorder depends on the Hb genes inherited from each parent. Figure 75-2 shows the distribution of the sickle cell gene and the inheritance pattern for the gene. Life expectancy is currently 42 years for males and 48 years for females. The leading cause of death is *acute chest syndrome.*

Pathophysiology

The genetics, molecular biology, and pathophysiology of SCD are well understood. The defective hemoglobin (HbS), when exposed to a decrease in oxygen, becomes viscous, has decreased solubility, and forms a gel-like substance containing hemoglobin crystals within the affected RBCs. These crystals clump together into long chains that form a parallel array of filaments, which disrupt the membrane, and the cell assumes a crescent or classic sickle shape (see Figure 75-1, *B*). The sickled cells become rigid, sticky, and fragile. These cells agglutinate and impede circulation in the capillaries, causing microinfarcts, tissue hypoxia, and further sickling. These responses to HbS

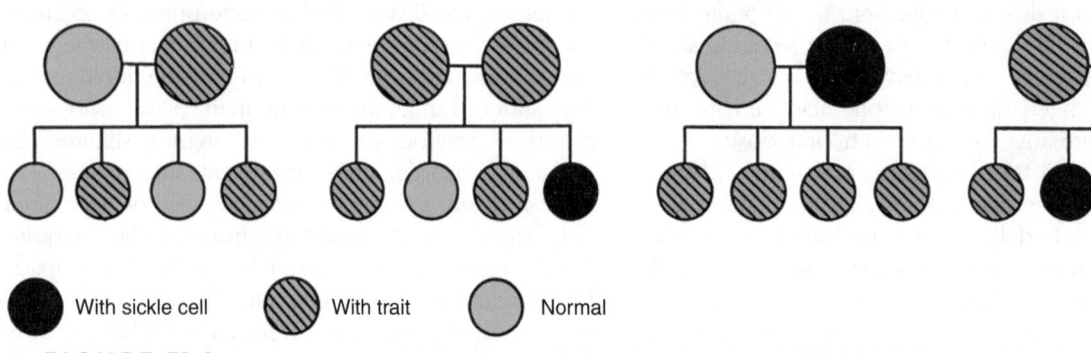

With sickle cell   With trait   Normal

■ **FIGURE 75–2** Inheritance pattern of sickle cell gene. (Redrawn from Page, J., et al. [1981]. *Blood: The river of life.* Washington, DC: Torstar Books.)

lead to the profound clinical manifestations of sickling disorders: hemolytic anemia, painful sickle cell crisis, and multiple organ system damage.

Sickle cell crisis is an acute, episodic exacerbation of the disorder instigated by reduced oxygen levels and associated crises. Exposure to low oxygen levels (low oxygen tension) triggers the process of sickling, such as living in high altitudes, flying in planes that are not pressurized, exercising strenuously (including military boot camp), acquiring respiratory tract infections, or undergoing anesthesia without receiving adequate oxygenation. A sickle cell crisis is most typically the result of vaso-occlusion in tissues and organs *(vaso-occlusive crisis)*. This crisis is the most common reason for seeking medical care. It may be induced by stress, exposure to cold water or temperature, hypoxia, or infection; most crises occur with no obvious cause.

Organ-damage syndromes are also a hallmark of SCD. Organ damage is due to increased fibrinogen levels and plasma-clotting factors (products of hemolysis) that contribute to the formation of microthrombi and the resultant microinfarcts and tissue necrosis of vital organs. The organs most vulnerable to infarction and necrosis are the brain, heart, lung, and kidneys because of their constant demand for oxygen and the bone marrow and spleen because of increased demands on these organs to replace damaged erythrocytes.

Clinical Manifestations

The typical clinical picture of SCD is associated with profound manifestations of chronic hemolytic anemia, painful sickle cell crisis, and manifestations of the various associated organ-damage syndromes. Many people with SCD are in good health and asymptomatic, except for the occasional but painful periods of vaso-occlusive crisis, the most common manifestation of SCD in adulthood.

Chronic hemolytic anemia is universally present but usually well tolerated. Clients often present with the classic manifestations of chronic anemia such as pallor of the mucosa, fatigue, and low tolerance for exercise. Jaundice is a common side effect of chronic hemolysis. Folate deficiency with resulting megaloblastic changes is also common because of increased demands for folate required for the replacement of destroyed cells.

Sickle cell crisis is predominantly a *vaso-occlusive crisis* (sometimes referred to as *pain crisis*), a serious manifestation that requires immediate medical attention. It has a sudden onset and results in severe pain in the long bones, joints, the chest, the back, and the abdomen (resembling an acute condition of the abdomen); the face may also be involved. The painful bone infarction of the *hand-foot syndrome* is often the first symptom of SCD. Fever, malaise, and leukocytosis may be present. The duration of crises is extremely variable from client to client and may range from six or more per year, to relatively few over a lifetime, to none. Individual clients

appear to have established frequency patterns. About 50% of individuals with homozygous HbS have vaso-occlusive crises.

Aplastic, hemolytic, and sequestration crises are seen much less frequently but also require immediate medical attention. *Aplastic crisis* is a serious complication caused by infection with the parvovirus B19. This virus infects red cell progenitors in the bone marrow, leading to cessation of erythropoiesis. Hb levels drop precipitously; however, this condition is self-limiting because bone marrow usually recovers in 7 to 10 days. Pain may be a presenting manifestation of this condition. *Hemolytic crisis,* resulting from the abnormal destruction of RBCs, also may be seen. This condition presents with manifestations of severe hemolytic anemia. The client is usually febrile. *Sequestration crisis* occurs when there is a sudden and massive trapping of destroyed RBC components by visceral organs; splenic sequestration is a common and painful complication.

Acute chest syndrome is the current most common cause of SCD-related mortality followed by cerebrovascular, cardiac, and pulmonary infarcts. This syndrome presents with chest pain, fever, cough, tachypnea, leukocytosis, and pulmonary infiltrates. Fat emboli resulting from bone marrow infarction are thought to be the major cause of this syndrome. It is a medical emergency and, if not treated immediately, can result in acute respiratory distress and death.

The involvement of multiple organ systems, caused primarily by microinfarcts and resulting tissue necrosis, is the basis for the complications most commonly seen in SCD. Nearly every major organ system is affected (Table 75-6). Cerebrovascular, myocardial, and pulmonary infarctions are serious complications. The most severe manifestation is stroke, typically of thrombotic origin. It is a life-threatening condition and often leads to brain-related deficits (e.g., sensory, motor, cognitive, affective) and paralysis. Heart involvement, caused by ischemia from chronic anemia and microinfarcts, usually includes hemosiderin deposits in the myocardium, systolic murmur, and dilation of the ventricles and left atrium, leading to heart failure. Pulmonary infarcts lead to pulmonary hypertension, heart failure, and eventually cor pulmonale.

Splenomegaly is evident by the latter part of the person's first year of life and may present as a sudden and painful splenic sequestration crisis. Impaired function follows, and eventually the spleen shrinks *(autosplenectomy)*. As a result immune deficiency develops, and infections are commonly seen, particularly with encapsulated microorganisms such as *Streptococcus pneumoniae*. Hepatomegaly- and infarction-related hepatopathy is often present, as are bile stones, as a result of chronic hemolysis with hyperbilirubinemia. Renal medullary ischemia may be present, resulting in a diminished capacity to concentrate urine; nephritic syndrome, although uncommon, may occur.

TABLE 75–6 Organ System Manifestations in Sickle Cell Anemia

Organ Systems	Clinical Manifestations
Central nervous system	Thrombosis- or hemorrhage-related paralysis, cerebral deficits, or death
Cardiac	Systolic murmur, cardiomegaly, heart failure
Pulmonary	Acute chest syndrome, hypertension, infiltrates, pneumonia, heart failure
Renal	Hematuria, renal failure
Spleen	Splenomegaly, splenic atrophy (autosplenectomy)
Hepatic	Hepatomegaly, gallstones
Skeletal	Hand-foot syndrome, osteonecrotic skeletal deformities, osteomyelitis, osteoporosis
Genital	Penile priapism
Optic	Hemorrhage, retinal detachment, retinopathy, blindness
Dermis	Stasis ulcers of extremities

Hyperactivity of the bone marrow can lead to spindly legs, a short trunk, and a tower-shaped skull. Skeletal manifestations of aseptic necrosis, especially on the heads of weight-bearing long bones, are due to repeated infarction of the bone, joints, and growth plates, and may lead to osteomyelitis, osteoporosis, and osteosclerosis. Related pain in the joints and long bones is common and usually severe; necrotic bone marrow with associated development of infection is often present. Skeletal and joint involvements are associated with chronic pain and disability and may require changes in lifestyle and employment. This is the single most important economic effect of the disease.

Impaired circulation leads to edema of the hands and feet and often results in leg and foot ulcers because of delayed healing and opportunistic infections. Leg ulcers are a chronic painful problem and are found in about 75% of older children and adults with the disease. Ophthalmologic manifestations may include ptosis from periorbital infarction, retinal vascular changes, and proliferative retinitis, which may result in a loss of vision. Diagnosis of HbS disease is suggested by findings of chronic hemolytic anemia and vaso-occlusive crisis and is confirmed by the existence of homozygous HbS. Typical laboratory study findings are shown in Table 75-3.

Four specific laboratory procedures demonstrate the presence of HbS in either homozygous or heterozygous clients. A stained blood smear is examined for the presence of sickle cells. A sickle slide preparation is used to detect the sickling phenomenon after deoxygenation of the blood. This test is accurate but time-consuming. The sickle-turbidity tube test is an excellent mass screening test to detect HbS. After a finger prick, blood is mixed with Sickledex solution in a test tube. Five minutes later, the specimen is observed for cloudiness, which indicates the presence of HbS. Solutions mixed

with normal Hb will remain clear. If the test demonstrates HbS, it does not however differentiate SCD from sickle cell trait and other variants. The final study, Hb electrophoresis, is the diagnostic test for HbS and also differentiates SCD from sickle cell trait.

Imaging studies are also frequently used. Skeletal x-rays may show deformities and flattening of the bones and joints and areas of infarction. Magnetic resonance imaging (MRI) can demonstrate areas of avascular necrosis and distinguish between osteomyelitis and bony infarction. An abdominal sonogram can document spleen size and the presence of bile stones. Transcranial Doppler ultrasonography can identify clients at risk for stroke.

Many African Americans are unaware that they carry the sickle cell trait and that they can transmit this trait to their future children. Consequently, researchers are perfecting mass screening tests for the detection of HbS among the African-American population. Clients who have only the sickle cell trait may never be detected unless they are exposed to extremely low oxygen tension, strenuous work or exercise, or pregnancy. When exposed to extreme stressors, the client with the trait may experience manifestations of SCD.

OUTCOME MANAGEMENT

Medical Management

No safe, effective treatment is currently available. Treatment strategies are aimed at control of manifestations and management of disease complications and include management of the following: (1) vaso-occlusive crisis; (2) acute and chronic pain; (3) chronic hemolytic anemia; (4) acute chest syndrome and organ-damage syndromes; and (5) infections. Vaso-occlusive crisis is typically treated with hydration and analgesics. Intravenous fluids (normal saline or 5% dextrose in saline) are administered to correct dehydration and to replace continuing loss.

Reduce Pain

Acute pain control is best accomplished by the administration of opioids, with morphine sulfate being the drug of choice. The drug is given IV, hourly at first, until an effective dose is established; then the dose is tapered off once pain control is achieved, usually in 24 to 48 hours. Often patient-controlled analgesia (PCA) pumps are used to provide the best pain control. When the client is discharged, sustained-release morphine is given with the dose gradually reduced over several days. Morphine elixir is most commonly used for breakthrough pain. Chronic pain control is achieved with acetaminophen and NSAIDs. The NSAIDs are best for treating deep bone pain, although the use of opioids may be required. If so, codeine and hydrocodone should be tried first; morphine should be used only for more severe cases. Tricyclic antidepressants may reduce the dose of opioids because of their ability to interfere with pain perception. Many clients are depressed, and lifting depression may have a positive effect on the pain. Non-pharmacologic measures, such as physical therapy, heat and cold applications, transcutaneous nerve stimulation (TENS), hypnosis, and acupuncture, may also be used.

Pharmacologic Agents

Hydroxyurea is the only drug currently approved by the Food and Drug Administrative (FDA) for the treatment of SCD. Hydroxyurea increases the production of HbF, which retards sickling, the Hb level increases, and vaso-occlusive crises become less frequent and less severe or totally eliminated. A decrease in chronic pain and a lowering of reticulocyte levels also occur; however, hydroxyurea has been identified as a potential leukemogenic and carcinogenic agent. Data on long-term use are currently not available. Candidates for this therapy should include only those who have frequent, painful crises (>6 per year), uncontrolled pain using conservative treatment, acute chest syndrome, or a history of or high risk for stroke. For clients receiving hydroxyurea, frequent blood tests to monitor for leukopenia or thrombocytopenia are necessary.

Sodium cromoglycate has shown promising results in significantly reducing the percentage of sickle cells in venous blood. This effect appears to be retained when the blood is deoxygenated. The drug is given by inhalation or the nasal route.

Folic acid supplementation is required because all clients have a folate deficiency. Iron supplementation may also be required for menstruating women.

Blood Transfusion

Blood transfusion is indicated only for special situations such as acute chest syndrome, stroke, aplastic crisis, pregnancy, and general anesthesia. The goal of the transfusion is to reduce the concentration of HbS to 30% or less. Those receiving repeated transfusions should be given iron-chelating agents.

Acute chest syndrome is treated with analgesics, oxygen, antibiotics, and transfusion. The goal of treatment is to reduce the level of HbS to 30% or less. If the HcT is 30% or higher, an exchange transfusion is required. This entails removing 1 unit of blood, transfusing 1 unit, and repeating the process or using a continuous-flow phoresis machine.

Prevent Infection

Prevention of infection greatly improves survival. In the past, infection was the leading cause of mortality. Penicillin prophylaxis, beginning in infancy, and pneumococcal vaccination at 2 years with a booster at 5 years, controls infections of pneumoniae origin. All infections must be treated promptly with broad-spectrum antibiotics until the causative organism is identified and appropriate antibiotic therapy instituted.

Nursing Management of the Medical Client

Assessment. Assess the client for the patterns that may indicate sickle cell crisis. Assess for the ability of the family and client to cope with the disorder and their understanding of the disease and triggers of crisis.

Diagnosis, Outcomes, Interventions
Diagnosis: Acute Pain. Because of the long bone pain, joint swelling, and abdominal pain secondary to sickling crisis, one nursing diagnosis is *Acute Pain related to sickle cell crisis.*

Outcomes. The client will experience diminished pain as evidenced by verbalization of pain reduction and reliance on fewer opiates for control of pain.

Interventions. Assess for the earliest manifestations of vaso-occlusive crisis and initiate analgesics as needed and ordered. Monitor for the effectiveness of analgesia. Apply heat to joints as ordered. Provide rest periods. Administer fluids to prevent dehydration and recurrence of pain crisis. Increase oral fluid intake, and monitor intake and output.

Diagnosis: Readiness for Enhanced Self-Care. Another nursing diagnosis is *Readiness for Enhanced Self-Care related to disease, treatment, and prevention of crises.*

Outcomes. The client and family will understand the disease, treatment, and prevention of crises as evidenced by the client's and the family's statements and the absence or lessened frequency of crises.

Interventions. When educating clients about sickle cell anemia or sickle cell trait, remember the following:
1. Explain the nature of the disease and answer any related questions the client or family may have.
2. Explain that because SCD is a lifelong condition, adherence to therapy and follow-up visits is critical for effective control of the disease.
3. Encourage African-American parents to have themselves and their children tested for the presence of HbS. Advise parents-to-be that sickle cell screening procedures for the fetus and newborn are available, as is genetic counseling.
4. Advise the client and family to have routine medical examinations that include an RBC count.
5. Encourage young adults who carry HbS to ask their physician for genetic counseling before marrying or having children.
6. Alert young women with sickle cell anemia that pregnancy carries a high risk for them.

7. Explain that multiple organ system complications, particularly pulmonary, cerebrovascular, cardiovascular or renal complications, may develop. The client and family should be taught the manifestations of these complications and be advised to seek prompt medical attention if any arise.

8. Explain how to prevent crises, such as (a) avoiding lower oxygen tension and (b) taking caution against becoming dehydrated. Instruct the client and family to call a physician if vomiting, diarrhea, high fever, or any other cause of water loss develops.

The nurse plays an important role in the lifelong management of this disease. The nurse should be aware that the risk for failure to maintain the treatment regimen might be high. Many clients may be of lower socioeconomic and education levels and without adequate health insurance coverage. These factors often lead to noncompliance with treatment regimens.

Evaluation. An appropriate outcome for the client with SCD is that the disease will remain in remission as long as possible. It is impossible to prevent every crisis; however, with education and an effort by the client and family, the number of attacks can be reduced and the severity lessened.

POLYCYTHEMIA VERA

Polycythemia vera (PV), the excessive production of erythrocytes, leukocytes, and platelets, is caused by excessive activation of pluripotent stem cells in the bone marrow. It is a chronic, life-shortening, pan-hyperplastic, malignant, neoplastic marrow disorder. The inordinate mass production of these three cell lines results in (1) an increase in blood viscosity; (2) an increase in the total blood volume, which may be twice or even three times greater than normal; and (3) severe blood congestion of all tissues and organs.

Etiology and Risk Factors

In the United States, PV is relatively rare; its prevalence is 0.6 to 1.6 per million population. Although it occurs in people of every age group, its peak incidence is in the group 50 to 70 years of age. All ethnic groups are affected, and predilection of people of Jewish descent may exist. No cure is currently available. With the advent of new therapeutic regimens for management of PV, survival is now between 10 and 20 years. The most common causes of mortality are thrombosis, particularly pulmonary emboli (up to 40%), and hemorrhagic complications, especially for those with myelofibrosis or pancytopenia (up to 30%).

Pathophysiology

Polycythemia vera is due to the excessive production of a single line of clonal stem cells present in the bone marrow. These cells interfere with or stimulate normal stem cell growth and maturation. Unregulated neoplastic proliferation is thought to be the etiology. The origin of the abnormal clonal cells is currently unknown; however, these cells have an increased sensitivity to growth factors for maturation, indicating the presence of a defect in the signal pathway common to different growth factors.

Clinical Manifestations

In its early stages polycythemia usually remains asymptomatic (an increased HcT level may be an incidental finding). Presenting manifestations are usually related to hypoxia from impairment of the microcirculation caused by blood hyperviscosity secondary to hypervolemia. Manifestations include dizziness, headache, vertigo, tinnitus, visual disturbances, and angina pectoris. Other manifestations can appear depending on the body system that is affected. The client may also have a ruddy complexion and dusky, red mucosa; cardiovascular hypertension and heart failure (shortness of breath, orthopnea); increased clotting leading to stroke, myocardial infarction, or peripheral gangrene; bleeding (hemorrhage in capillaries, venules, and arterioles), which causes rupture of vessels, GI peptic ulcers, and enlargement of liver and spleen; and skeletal gout (painful swollen joints, usually the big toe) characterized by an increased uric acid level.

Diagnostic findings (see Table 75-3) include (1) an RBC count as high as 8 to 12 million/mm^3; (2) Hb level of 18 to 25 g/dl; (3) HcT greater than 54% in men and 49% in women; (4) platelet count usually increased; (5) normal arterial blood gas (ABG) values; (6) hyperplastic bone marrow; and (7) a serum uric acid level three to four times normal.

OUTCOME MANAGEMENT

A permanent cure for PV is currently unavailable, but remission of many years can be achieved. The goals of care in PV are 2-fold: reduction of (1) blood volume and viscosity and (2) myeloproliferative activity. These decreases are accomplished through phlebotomy, administration of myelosuppressive agents, and radiation therapy. Emergency phlebotomy can be used to normalize red cell mass as quickly as possible (removal of 500 to 2000 ml of blood until the HcT reaches 45%). Clients with hematocrits of less than 70% may be bled twice a week. Clients who are older or who have cardiovascular compromise or cerebrovascular complications should receive volume replacement with saline solution to avoid postural hypotension. If platelet counts are elevated, a myelosuppressive agent should be used in combination with aspirin (300 mg three times a day) to avoid thrombotic or hemorrhagic complications. Women of childbearing age should be treated only with phlebotomy. Once normal HcT levels are reached, subsequent phlebotomies should be carried out as frequently (monthly) as necessary to maintain the HcT at about 45%. Iron deficiency will likely result, but as it supervenes, RBC production will be retarded so that clients managed by phlebotomy alone may require as few as two or three phlebotomies a year.

The myelosuppressive agent hydroxyurea is commonly used in clients older than 50 years of age. Radioactive phosphorus, chlorambucil, busulfan (Myleran), and melphalan (Alkeran) have also been tried but are not indicated for long-term use because of the increased incidence of acute leukemia (17%) after 15 years. Radioactive phosphorus, however, may be used for clients older than 80 years or for those with co-morbid conditions in which life expectancy is shorter than 5 to 10 years. Anagrelide may be used in younger clients (50 to 70 years) if hydroxyurea is contraindicated. In young males, myelosuppressive therapy can lead to aspermia; use of this treatment should be carefully evaluated for these clients.

Hyperuricemia is treated with allopurinol until remission is attained; acute gouty attacks are treated with colchicine or other anti-inflammatory agents.

HEMOCHROMATOSIS

Hemochromatosis (HH), also called *iron overload disease,* is the most common genetic disorder in the United States. It is an inherited metabolic disorder that causes increased absorption of iron that is deposited in the body tissues and organs, particularly the liver, heart, and pancreas. As iron levels increase, toxicity results and leads to damage of vital organs.

Etiology and Risk Factors
Hemochromatosis is associated with a defect in a gene (*HFE*) that helps regulate the amount of iron absorbed from food. The body's normal iron concentration is 2 to 6 g. Individuals with HH accumulate between 0.5 and 10 g/year and eventually may have in excess of 50 g. Individuals who inherit a defective gene from each parent (*homozygous*) may develop the disease. Those with only one defective gene from each parent (*heterozygous*) are carriers and rarely develop the disease. HH is present at birth, but manifestations seldom manifest before adulthood.

Hemochromatosis is the most common genetic disorder among Caucasians, with an incidence of 1 in 100 to 500 Caucasians of European heritage. About 0.5% (5 in 1000) of the American Caucasian population is homozygous for the disorder. About 1 person in 10 is a carrier. Men and women are equally at risk for HH, but men are five times more likely to be diagnosed than women and to have manifestations at a much younger age. Women seldom have manifestations before menopause.

Clinical Manifestations
Joint pain is the most common manifestation of HH. Other manifestations include fatigue, lack of energy, irritability, depression, loss of body hair, abdominal pain, loss of sex drive, and heart problems. Early diagnosis and treatment are critical to a positive outcome in HH. If the disease is not detected early and treated before the accumulation of iron in the body tissues, serious disorders such as arthritis, liver disease, pancreatic disease, heart complications, impotence, bronzing of the skin, and other problems can arise.

Hemochromatosis is one of the most underdiagnosed disorders. Certain blood tests can determine whether iron stores in the body are higher than normal. The transferring saturation test (TS) can calculate how much iron is bound to the protein that carries iron in the blood. The serum ferritin test shows the level of iron in the liver. If HH is suspected, a special blood test to detect the *HFE* mutation can be ordered as a definitive diagnosis. A liver biopsy is sometimes undertaken to determine how much damage the liver has sustained (see Table 75-3).

OUTCOME MANAGEMENT

Treatment is simple, inexpensive, and safe. The major goal of treatment is to rid the body of excess iron, which is accomplished with phlebotomy. Depending on the severity of iron overload, 500 ml of blood can be drawn each week for up to 2 or 3 years until iron levels return to normal limits. Then maintenance phlebotomy, usually once every 2 to 4 months for life, is initiated. Clients with HH should not take iron supplements, and dietary intake of iron may be limited. Those with liver damage should avoid alcoholic beverages. If tissue damage has occurred, specialists in the organ system involved usually treat the resulting organ system complications.

DISORDERS AFFECTING WHITE BLOOD CELLS

White blood cells (WBCs), also called *leukocytes,* are divided into two groups:

- *Granulocytes* (polymorphonuclear leukocytes)
- *Agranulocytes* (mononuclear cells)

Granulocytes, in turn, are divided into three groups: (1) neutrophils, (2) basophils, and (3) eosinophils. The names denote affinity for the dyes used in staining. Agranulocytes include lymphocytes (B and T) and monocytes.

Plasmacytes (plasma cells) are derived from B lymphocytes. Plasmacytes are formed within the bone marrow and lymph nodes and are active in producing immunoglobulins (antibodies). Leukemia and lymphoma are discussed in Chapter 79.

AGRANULOCYTOSIS

Agranulocytosis (granulocytopenia, malignant neutropenia) is an acute, potentially fatal blood dyscrasia characterized by profound *neutropenia* (a reduced number of circulating neutrophils). Because neutrophils make up roughly 93% of all granulocytes, the terms *neutropenia* and *agranulocytosis* are often used interchangeably.

Etiology and Risk Factors

Agranulocytosis is a fairly rare condition. For unknown reasons, females are much more susceptible to this condition than males, although even among females, agranulocytosis is relatively rare.

Agranulocytosis results from either inadequate neutrophil production or excessive destruction of neutrophils. The most common cause of agranulocytosis is drug or chemical toxicity or hypersensitivity. Any drug or chemical that leads to aplasia can also cause agranulocytosis. More than 75 drugs have been associated with development of agranulocytosis. Agents that also produce neutropenia, when given in sufficiently large does over time, include many cancer chemotherapeutic agents, ionizing radiation, and benzene. Agents that frequently produce neutropenia (usually only in clients sensitive to the drug) include tranquilizers (phenothiazine, chlorpromazine), antithyroid agents (thiouracil, propylthiouracil), anticonvulsants (phenytoin), antibiotics (chloramphenicol, sulfonamides), and analgesics (aminopyrine, phenylbutazone). Some of these agents (including valproic acid, carbamazepine, and beta-lactam antibiotics) inhibit myelopoiesis, whereas others induce the formation of antibodies that destroy granulocytes (antithyroid drugs, gold compounds, aminopyrine).

Additional causes include (1) anemias related to diminished erythropoiesis (aplastic and megaloblastic anemias); (2) certain diseases such as uremia, tuberculosis, typhoid fever, malaria, yellow fever, EBV, hepatitis B, CMV, and influenza; (3) ionizing radiation exposure; (4) autoimmune diseases such as systemic lupus erythematosus and rheumatoid arthritis; and (5) genetic aberrations, which may be suspected if a family history of recurrent infections beginning in childhood exists.

Pathophysiology

The exact mechanisms of neutropenia are not clearly understood. Bone marrow and the peripheral blood are the organ systems most affected in neutropenia. Neutrophils are the first blood cells to respond to an injury and constitute a swift and powerful defense against invading microorganisms through normal surveillance and phagocytosis. Failure to produce adequate numbers of neutrophils leads to a greater susceptibility to bacterial invasion, especially when the absolute neutrophil count (ANC) drops below 500/mm^3. In profound neutropenia (<100/mm^3), infection occurs in nearly 100% of cases.

Clinical Manifestations

The manifestations of agranulocytosis are a result of neutropenia. Typically the onset of this acute disease is rapid. For the first 2 or 3 days, severe fatigue and weakness occur, followed by a sore throat, ulcerations of the pharyngeal and buccal mucosa, dysphagia, high fever, weak and rapid pulse, and severe chills. The mucous membranes of the throat and mouth are particularly vulnerable. Without prompt antibiotic treatment, the disorder usually causes septicemia and death within a week.

OUTCOME MANAGEMENT

Treatment of clients with agranulocytosis involves eliminating potentially toxic agents that may be responsible for marrow suppression. Agranulocytosis caused by toxic substances is usually reversed within 2 to 3 weeks after their elimination. An allogenic bone marrow transplant (BMT) may be required for survival if agranulocytosis is not reversed when the cause is removed.

Surveillance cultures of blood, throat, sputum, urine, and stool should be taken at frequent intervals to monitor the status of infections. Broad-spectrum antibiotics are usually administered until the offending organism is identified and appropriate antibiotic therapy, along with rehydration, is initiated to treat the infection. Control of oral and gingival pain is performed with meticulous mouth care, saline rinses, and local anesthetic gels and gargles. Diet needs include soft or liquid foods until mouth and gum sores are diminished.

Treatment of agranulocytosis includes various *colony-stimulating factors,* such as granulocyte colony-stimulating factor (G-CSF), granulocyte macrophage colony-stimulating factor (GM-CSF), recombinant neutrophil cytokine filgrastim (Neupogen), and erythropoietin (EPO). These factors are given after the offending agent has been eliminated. If given before a serious infection is established, the duration of the infection is shortened and recovery hastened.

MULTIPLE MYELOMA

Multiple myeloma is a malignancy of the plasma B cell characterized by infiltration of the cells into the bone marrow, which leads to destruction of other marrow cells, destruction of the bone cortex, and the secretion by the cells of the monoclonal paraprotein (Bence-Jones).

Etiology and Risk Factors

The etiology of multiple myeloma is a neoplastic proliferation of the plasma B cells. Risk factors include an increased incidence in some families, ionizing radiation, and occupational chemical exposures. The incidence rate is 4 per 100,000 people. Men are affected twice as often as women and African Americans twice as often as Caucasians. It usually develops after the age of 40 and peaks in the sixth decade. It accounts for 1% of all malignancies and 10% of hematologic malignancies.

Pathophysiology

Multiple myeloma is characterized by an abnormal proliferation of plasma B cells. These cells infiltrate the bone marrow and produce abnormal and excessive amounts of immunoglobulin *(myeloma protein)*. Accumulation of these cells in the marrow disrupts RBC, leukocyte, and platelet production, which leads to anemia, increased vulnerability to infection, and bleeding tendencies, respectively. In addition, abnormal and excessive amounts of cytokine are produced, which plays an important role in bone destruction (lytic lesions and osteoporosis). Cell destruction leads to hypercalcemia, which can cause renal problems and failure (polyuria, hyperuricemia), GI problems (nausea, anorexia), and neurologic manifestations (confusion). Further complications include hematopoietic suppression, immunosuppression, chronic infections, proteinuria, and soft tissue masses.

Clinical Manifestations

Once manifestations appear, they typically involve the skeletal system, particularly the pelvis, spine, and ribs. The most common presenting complaint is bone pain (70%). The most common cause of the pain is pathologic fractures and bone lesions, which occur in 93% of clients over the course of the illness. Diffuse osteoporosis is common and manifests as multiple osteolytic lesions of the skull, sternum, rib cage, and spine (10% to 20% have spinal cord compression). Thirty percent of clients present with manifestations of hypercalcemia (confusion, somnolence, bone pain, constipation, nausea, and thirst); renal stones may be seen with this condition. Hyperuricemia is usually present and manifests as renal impairment/renal failure attributable to renal tubule obstruction and interstitial nephritis. Infections resulting from the high volume of monoclonal proteins, bleeding attributable to thrombocytopenia, and carpal tunnel syndrome may also be present.

A diagnosis of multiple myeloma is made with radiographic studies, bone marrow biopsy, and blood and urine examinations. Radiographic studies may reveal diffuse lesions in the bone, widespread demineralization, and osteoporosis. The CBC shows anemia, leukopenia, and thrombocytopenia. The bone marrow contains large numbers of immature plasma cells, which usually constitute 5% of the bone marrow cell population. Because of the abnormal number of plasma cells producing immunoglobulins, peripheral blood samples sent for plasma electrophoresis reveal a large amount of abnormal immunoglobulins. Another diagnostic manifestation of multiple myeloma is the appearance of Bence Jones paraprotein in a 24-hour urine test. A beta$_2$-microglobulin test is an important test because it is an overall marker of the total body tumor burden and (along with the level of renal damage) is a strong indicator of outcome. Median survival is 3 years.

OUTCOME MANAGEMENT

Currently no cure for multiple myeloma exists. Management is aimed at early recognition and treatment of complications of the disease. Clients may require hospitalization for pain management and treatment of bone-related complications. Not all clients with multiple myeloma should be treated initially. Clients who are asymptomatic are often carefully monitored until the disease progresses and then are treated with chemotherapy.

Medical Management

Suppress the Bone Marrow

If overt manifestations are present, chemotherapy is the preferred initial treatment. Some controversy exists over which chemotherapy regimen is most effective. The most commonly used regimen is melphalan and prednisone given orally for 4 to 7 days and repeated at 4- to 6-week intervals. It is well tolerated and has a 50% to 60% response rate. Other combinations of alkylating agents can also be effective. The VAD regimen of vincristine (Oncovin), doxorubicin (Adriamycin), and dexamethasone (Decadron) is used for clients who do not respond to alkylating agents and is well tolerated. Thalidomide has recently been shown to have positive results, with a 30% response rate. Leukocyte and platelet counts are monitored regularly and doses are adjusted until modest cytopenia occurs. Chemotherapy may continue for 1 to 2 years, but almost all cases recur when chemotherapy is discontinued. Interferon-alfa appears to be beneficial in prolonging the duration of remission.

Autologous bone marrow and peripheral blood stem cell transplantation in combination with high-dose chemotherapy has had a significantly higher response rate (80% versus 57%) and better 5-year event-free survival (28% versus 10%) than those treated with chemotherapy alone.

Reduce Serum Calcium Levels

Corticosteroids and hydration are used to reduce serum calcium levels. A new group of corticosteroid agents now exists for treating hypercalcemia. The most effective agent to date is pamidronate sodium (Aredia); etidronate disodium (Didronel) and gallium nitrate (Ganite) are also effective agents. Medications such as furosemide (Lasix), steroids, etidronate, gallium, or pamidronate are used to increase calcium excretion and to decrease calcium loss from bone. If the client is able, encourage activity that places stress on the long bones to increase calcium absorption.

Administer IV fluids in amounts adequate to maintain an output of 1.5 to 2 L daily. Clients with multiple myeloma usually require about 3 to 4 L of fluid per day. The client needs sufficient fluid not only to dilute the calcium overload, but also to prevent protein from precipitating in the renal tubules.

Treat Complications

Nursing care is focused primarily on management of the various complications caused by dissemination of the disease. Bone pain management can be obtained with palliative radiotherapy of localized myeloma lesions and with NSAIDs, acetaminophen, or an acetaminophen-opioid combination.

Antiemetics may be required for relief of nausea and vomiting. Small, frequent feedings may be better tolerated, and stool softeners may be routinely required. Closely monitor intake, output, and blood studies to determine the effectiveness of treatment. Weigh the client daily so that any significant loss can be noted and corrected. Measure the client's calcium level at regular intervals for assessment of the development of hypercalcemia.

Because of skeletal complications, care should be taken when moving the client because there is a high potential for pathologic fractures. Closely monitor the client's mental status. If disorientation or confusion occurs, remove sharp objects and other potentially hazardous items from the environment. The side rails should be raised, and light restraints may be required.

Teach the client and family about the manifestations of hypercalcemia and instruct them to report any manifestations immediately to the physician.

SAFETY ALERT

Instruct family members or significant others on how to institute safety measures to prevent falls and injuries. The client may need some assistive devices at home, such as a toilet riser and handhold bars in the bathroom.

Counseling may be needed for the client and family to deal with the eventual fatal outcome of multiple myeloma.

INFECTIOUS MONONUCLEOSIS

Infectious mononucleosis is an acute disorder that is self-limiting and usually is benign.

Etiology and Risk Factors

The cause of 85% of infectious mononucleosis-like cases is the EBV, a herpesvirus. Infectious mononucleosis should be suspected in clients 10 to 30 years of age and is most common in populations with many young adults such as college students and military personnel. The mode of transmission is primarily through saliva during close contact and the incubation period is 4 to 6 weeks.

Clinical Manifestations

The epithelial cells of the oropharynx, nasopharynx, and salivary glands are infected first before spreading to the lymphoid tissue via infected B lymphocytes. The infection is characterized by painful enlargement of the lymph nodes, numerous large lymphoblasts, lymphocytosis, sore throat, and fever. The onset of infectious mononucleosis follows an incubation period of 4 to 8 weeks. Before frank clinical manifestations occur, the person may experience fatigue, headaches, malaise, and myalgias.

Clients present with sore throat; palatal petechiae; posterior, cervical, or auricular adenopathy; or marked diffuse adenopathy and significant fatigue. Subsequently, assessment may reveal temperatures up to 39° C (102.2° F), pharyngitis, and lymphadenopathy that is more pronounced in the cervical regions. Splenic enlargement causes left upper quadrant pain. In rare cases, liver involvement may develop into a hepatitis-like syndrome. When infectious mononucleosis is severe, two complications may develop: (1) splenic rupture resulting from the infiltration of the spleen by massive numbers of lymphocytes and (2) streptococcal pharyngitis secondary to bacterial invasion of the throat.

The diagnosis of infectious mononucleosis is based on three criteria: (1) physical assessment, (2) laboratory tests (WBC with differential), and (3) tests specific for EBV antibodies (*Monospot;* heterophile antibody test). The WBC count usually ranges from 12,000 to 20,000/mm³, of which >50% are lymphocytes and 10% are atypical lymphoblasts.

OUTCOME MANAGEMENT

No specific intervention either mitigates or shortens the disease process. Because infectious mononucleosis must simply run its course, treatments are directed at control of manifestations. Symptomatic treatment is the focus of care, which includes adequate hydration, analgesics, antipyretics, and adequate rest. Bed rest should not be enforced; the client's energy level should guide appropriate activity. Aspirin is avoided in children because of the risk of Reye's syndrome; therefore nonsteroidal anti-inflammatory drugs (NSAIDs) are used to treat fever, headache, sore throat, and myalgias. Amoxicillin and ampicillin should be avoided because they may cause a morbilliform rash in clients with infectious mononucleosis. Cool sponge baths and a large fluid intake help control fever. Warm saline or 2% lidocaine solution throat gargles may relieve sore throat. Contact sports must be avoided for at least 4 weeks after the onset of clinical manifestations to reduce the risk of splenic rupture. Corticosteroids are recommended only in clients with significant pharyngeal edema that causes or threatens respiratory compromise.

Although complications sometimes develop, the prognosis for clients with infectious mononucleosis is generally excellent. During the long convalescence the client slowly regains strength and energy although between 9% and 22% of clients report persistent fatigue or hypersomnia 6 months after infectious mononucleosis.

SPLENIC RUPTURE AND HYPERSPLENISM

Rupture of the spleen, complicated by severe hemorrhage, is the most frequent indication for splenectomy. Hypersplenism is the second most important indication for splenectomy.

Etiology and Risk Factors

Causes of splenic rupture include the following:

- Trauma (e.g., automobile accidents, bullet or knife wounds, severe blows to the spleen)
- Accidental tearing of the splenic capsule during surgery on neighboring organs
- Disease of the spleen that causes softening or damage (e.g., infectious mononucleosis and malaria)

In hypersplenism the spleen destroys, in excessive numbers, one of the blood cell types (i.e., erythrocytes, leukocytes, or platelets). Primary hypersplenism occurs in idiopathic thrombocytopenic purpura and congenital spherocytosis. Some etiologic factors associated with secondary hypersplenism include lymphomas (including Hodgkin's disease), leukemia, polycythemia vera, acute infections (including infectious mononucleosis), chronic infections, malaria, syphilis, hemoglobinopathy, and cirrhosis of the liver.

Clinical Manifestations

Manifestations of hypersplenism include moderate to massive splenomegaly, anemia, leukopenia, or thrombocytopenia and a compensatory increase in the production of the affected blood cell line by the bone marrow. Overactivity of the spleen develops either as a primary condition of unknown origin or as a condition secondary to another disease.

OUTCOME MANAGEMENT

Primary hypersplenism can be alleviated by splenectomy. Splenectomy is palliative only for clients with secondary hypersplenism because the surgery has little or no effect on the course of the primary illness. When the diagnosis is confirmed, it is important to teach the client to prevent complications associated with the specific cytopenia.

The spleen has an important role in the phagocytosis of circulating opsonized organisms. Clients are at increased risk for infection, especially during the first 3 years after surgery. The splenectomized client should be advised to seek medical treatment at the earliest manifestations of infection.

The unique functions performed by the spleen are eventually assumed by other organs; however, loss of the spleen because of the cessation of function or splenectomy does require the client to be monitored for potentially serious complications. Nursing care of the client undergoing splenectomy is generally the same as that discussed in Chapter 14 for any client undergoing surgery.

DISORDERS OF PLATELETS AND CLOTTING FACTORS

Disorders of hemostasis that affect platelets and clotting factors include (1) purpura and (2) coagulation disorders (Box 75-4). They are classified with the hemorrhagic disorders. The Terrorism Alert feature on p. 2032 discusses viruses that can cause hemorrhage.

HEMORRHAGIC DISORDERS

Normal clot formation and lysis depend on (1) intact blood vessels, (2) an adequate number of functioning platelets, (3) sufficient amounts of the 12 clotting factors (I to XIII; VI is no longer used), and (4) a well-controlled fibrinolytic system. Consequently, the four basic problems underlying hemorrhagic (bleeding) disorders are as follows:

- Weak, damaged vessels that rupture easily or spontaneously
- Platelet deficiency (*thrombocytopenia*) resulting from hypoproliferation, excessive pooling of platelets in the spleen, or excessive platelet destruction
- Deficiency or total lack of one of the clotting factors
- Excessive or insufficient fibrinolysis

The diagnosis of a hemorrhagic disorder is based on a complete health and family history, physical examination, and laboratory tests for platelet and clotting defects. The

---

BOX 75-4   Classification of Disorders of Hemostasis

PURPURA

Vascular Defect Purpura
- Familial hemorrhagic telangiectasia
- Anaphylactoid purpura (allergic purpura)
- Toxic purpura

Platelet Disorder Purpura
- Idiopathic thrombocytopenic purpura
- Secondary thrombocytopenias

COAGULATION DISORDERS
- Hemophilia
- Hypoprothrombinemia
- Disseminated intravascular coagulation (DIC)

TERRORISM ALERT

Hemorrhagic Fever Viruses

HEMORRHAGIC FEVER VIRUSES

Historically, hemorrhagic fever viruses (HFVs) refer to a clinical illness associated with fever and a bleeding disorder caused by a virus belonging to one of four distinct families: Filoviridae, Arenaviridae, Bunyaviridae, and Flaviviridae. Ebola and Marburg are in the Filoviridae family; Lassa and New World Arenaviridae are in the Arenaviridae family; Rift Valley fever is in the Bunyaviridae family; and Dengue, Omsk hemorrhagic fever, Kyasanur Forest disease, and yellow fever are in the Flaviviridae family.

The HFVs are transmitted to humans via contact with infected animal reservoirs or arthropod vectors, although the reservoirs and vectors for Marburg and Ebola viruses are unknown. The Working Group on Civilian Biodefense previously established nine features that characterize biologic agents that pose serious risks if used as biologic weapons against civilian populations. Several HFVs exhibit a number of these features and pose serious risk as biologic weapons, including Ebola and Marburg viruses, Lassa fever and New World arenaviruses, Rift Valley fever, yellow fever, Omsk hemorrhage fever, and Kyasanur Forest disease. These viruses can be spread through unannounced aerosol attacks. The overall incubation period is 2 to 21 days.

A variety of clinical manifestations follow infection with HFVs, including fever, headache, hypotension, abdominal pain, diarrhea, myalgias, skin rash, encephalitis, and eventually manifestations of progressive hemorrhaging such as conjunctival hemorrhage, petechiae, hematuria, hematemesis, and melena. DIC and circulatory shock may ensue. Therefore in the event of a bioterrorist attack with one of these agents, infected clients may have a variety of clinical presentations, complicating early detection and management.

The mainstay of treatment of HFV is supportive, with careful maintenance of fluid and electrolyte balance, circulatory volume, and blood pressure. Vasopressor support is with hemodynamic monitoring as well as mechanical ventilation and renal dialysis. IM injections, aspirin, NSAIDs, and anticoagulant therapies are contraindicated. Steroids are not indicated. No antiviral drugs have been approved by the U.S. FDA for treatment of HFVs. Ribavirin (used for treatment of chronic hepatitis C) has some in vitro and in vivo activity against Arenaviridae and Bunyaviridae but no utility against Filoviridae or Flaviviridae.

Protective measures against nosocomial transmission of HFVs include double gloves, impermeable gowns, strict hand hygiene, N-95 masks or powered air-purifying respirators, a negative isolation room with 6 to 12 air changes per hour, leg and shoe coverings, face shields, goggles for eye protection, restricted access of nonessential staff and visitors, environmental disinfection with 1:100 dilution of household bleach, and placing all clients with HFVs in the same part of the hospital to minimize exposures to other clients and health care workers.

Data from Borio, L, et al. (2002). Hemorrhagic fever viruses as biological weapons: Medical and public health management. *Journal of the American Medical Association, 287*(18), 2391-2405.

history usually offers numerous clues to the type of bleeding problem and its cause. *Petechiae* (tiny hemorrhagic spots caused by intradermal or submucosal bleeding) are usually present in vascular and thrombocytopenic purpuras. The presence of *ecchymoses* (large, blotchy subcutaneous hemorrhagic areas), *hematomas* (subdermal hemorrhage), and *hemarthrosis* (blood within the joints) points to *hemophilia;* however, ecchymoses may develop in any hemorrhagic disorder. Clients who hemorrhage severely from several areas during childbirth or a major surgical procedure may have a fibrinogen deficiency. In addition to any evidence of bleeding, search for manifestations of hepatic cirrhosis (e.g., hepatomegaly, jaundice) and splenomegaly. Laboratory studies provide the most crucial evidence for pinpointing the type and cause of a bleeding disorder.

Clients with hemorrhagic disorders need to understand (1) why they are at risk for bleeding, (2) the manifestations of bleeding, and (3) preventive measures to avoid bleeding. Those who can be managed by home health care should be referred to appropriate health care agencies. Clients with bleeding disorders should carry an identification card at all times that indicates their diagnosis, name of their physician or health care agency, and blood type.

IMMUNE THROMBOCYTOPENIC PURPURA

Immune thrombocytopenic purpura (ITP) is the most common thrombocytopenic disorder. It was previously called idiopathic thrombocytopenic purpura because its cause was unknown, but it is now clearly considered to be a hemorrhagic autoimmune disease that results in the destruction of platelets.

Etiology and Risk Factors

ITP is an acquired disorder in which circulating platelets are destroyed because of autoantibodies that bind with antigens on the platelet membrane. Although the platelets perform normally in the bloodstream, they are recognized as foreign and are destroyed by the macrophages when they reach the spleen and liver. The decrease in the number of platelets results in bruising and spontaneous bleeding into the skin and mucous membranes (purpura). Platelets normally survive 8 to 10 days within the circulation; with ITP, however, platelet survival is as brief as 1 to 3 days or less. ITP may be acute or chronic; in most cases, the course is one of remissions and exacerbations that, if untreated, may continue for years. Chronic ITP occurs most commonly in women between 20 and 40 years of age.

Clinical Manifestations

Clinical manifestations include petechiae, ecchymosis, epistaxis, bleeding from the gums, and easy bruising. Women may have extremely heavy menses or bleeding between periods.

Diagnostic findings that confirm the presence of ITP include the following:

- A platelet count below 100,000/mm^3
- Prolonged bleeding time with normal coagulation time (all coagulation factors are present and normal)
- Increased capillary fragility as demonstrated by the tourniquet test
- Positive platelet antibody screening
- Bone marrow aspirate containing normal or increased numbers of megakaryocytes

Complications of ITP include (1) spontaneous cerebral hemorrhage, which proves fatal in 1% to 5% of clients with ITP; (2) severe hemorrhages from the nose, GI tract, and urinary system; (3) bleeding into the diaphragm, which can result in pulmonary complications; and (4) nerve pain, extremity anesthesia, or paralysis resulting from the pressure of hematomas on nerves or brain tissues.

OUTCOME MANAGEMENT

Idiopathic thrombocytopenic purpura is treated with high-dose corticosteroids to inhibit the macrophage ingestion of the antibody-coated platelets. Plasmapheresis is sometimes used as short-term therapy until the steroid therapy takes effect. If the client is actively bleeding or requires surgery, IV gamma-globulin can be used to increase the platelet count.

If the client does not have a sustained remission, splenectomy may be needed. In 60% to 80% of cases, removal of the spleen results in complete and permanent remission. Danazol (Danocrine) has been used with success in some clients. Immunosuppressive therapy used in refractory cases includes vincristine, vinblastine (Velban), azathioprine (Imuran), and cyclophosphamide.

Nursing care of clients at high risk for bleeding is discussed in Chapter 79.

COAGULATION DISORDERS

Coagulation disorders stem from a defect in the clotting mechanisms. One or more of the clotting factors (I-XIII) is depleted or absent. The important coagulation disorders discussed here are (1) disseminated intravascular coagulation (DIC) and (2) the hemophilias. See Figure A&P17-6 on p. 1982 for an explanation of the coagulation cascade.

DISSEMINATED INTRAVASCULAR COAGULATION

Disseminated intravascular coagulation is a complex syndrome of activated coagulation that results in bleeding and thrombosis. It is basically a loss of balance between the clotting and lysing systems in the body caused by the simultaneous presence of thrombin and plasmin. Too much thrombin tips the balance toward the prothrombic state, resulting in thrombosis; too much plasmin triggers excessive clot lysis *(fibrinolysis),* in which clotting factors are consumed to such an extent that generalized bleeding occurs. This concept is referred to as *consumptive coagulopathy.* In DIC these seemingly contradictory states of excessive thrombosis and excessive lysis occur simultaneously.

Etiology and Risk Factors

The causes of DIC are many. Four categories of causative factors are (1) infection, (2) tissue coagulation factors traveling into the circulation, (3) damage to the vascular endothelium, and (4) stagnant blood flow. Infection is the leading cause (e.g., gram-negative septicemia, typhoid fever, Rocky Mountain spotted fever, viremia, parasites). Conditions that may lead to DIC are listed in Box 75-5. The key to managing DIC is treatment of the underlying cause/disease.

Pathophysiology

Excessive clotting can be precipitated through extrinsic or intrinsic coagulation pathways (see Figure A&P17-6). The extrinsic pathway is a response to massive tissue damage (e.g., burns or trauma); the intrinsic pathway is a response to damaged blood vessels (endothelium). Both release substances that activate thrombin, which in turn activates fibrinogen. This results in deposition of fibrin throughout the microcirculation. The formation of fibrin is triggered by increased production of thrombin, the suppression of anticoagulation mechanisms, and delayed removal of fibrin because of impaired fibrinolysis.

Platelet aggregation or adhesiveness is increased, enabling fibrin clots and microthrombi to form in the brain, kidneys, heart, and other organs; microinfarcts and tissue necrosis ensue. RBCs become trapped in the fibrin strands and are destroyed (hemolysis). The resultant sluggish circulation of blood reduces the flow of nutrients and oxygen to the cells. Platelets, prothrombin, and other clotting factors are consumed in the process, which compromises coagulation and predisposes to bleeding.

Excessive clotting activates the fibrinolytic mechanism, which causes the production of fibrin degradation products. Fibrin degradation products act to inhibit platelet clotting functions, which causes further bleeding. Ultimately, with lysis of clots and depletion of clotting factors,

---

BOX 75-5 **Conditions That May Precipitate Disseminated Intravascular Coagulation**

- Shock
- Cirrhosis
- Purpura fulminans
- Glomerulonephritis
- Acute fulminant hepatitis
- Acute bacterial and viral infections (septicemia)

CONDITIONS THAT MAY CAUSE THE RELEASE OF PLATELET FACTOR III

- Fat emboli
- Snakebites

Hemolytic processes caused by

- Infection
- Transfusion reactions
- Immunologic disorders

Tissue damage caused by

- Trauma
- Heatstroke
- Extensive burns
- Transplant rejections
- Surgery—particularly if extracorporeal circulation was used
- Glomerulonephritis
- Acute anoxia
- Prosthetic devices

CONDITIONS THAT MAY CAUSE THE RELEASE OF THROMBOPLASTIN FROM TISSUES

- Neoplastic growths
- Adenocarcinomas
- Acute leukemias
- Prostatic cancer
- Bronchogenic cancer
- Giant cavernous hemangioma
- Obstetric conditions
- Abruptio placentae (placental abruption)
- Retained dead fetus
- Amniotic fluid embolism
- Septic abortion
- Eclampsia

---

the blood loses its ability to clot (Concept Map feature on Understanding DIC and Its Treatment, p. 2035).

Clinical Manifestations

Clinically, DIC is termed acute, subacute, or chronic. *Acute* DIC usually presents as a hemorrhagic condition associated with excess plasmin formation. The onset is usually within days to hours after an initial assault to the body system. *Subacute* DIC may not be apparent initially but may become fulminant as the clinical course progresses. *Chronic* cases of DIC are typically seen in clients with cancer or in women carrying a dead fetus.

Subacute and chronic cases usually present as thrombosis attributable to excessive formation of thrombin.

Manifestations of acute DIC (hemorrhagic) include (1) purpura, petechiae, and ecchymoses on the skin, mucous membranes, heart lining, and lungs; (2) prolonged bleeding from venipuncture; (3) severe, uncontrolled hemorrhage during surgery or childbirth; (4) excessive bleeding from gums and the nose; (5) intracerebral and GI bleeding; (6) renal hematuria; (7) tachycardia and hypotension; and (8) dyspnea, hemoptysis, and respiratory congestion. Manifestations of microvascular thrombosis include oliguria and acute renal failure; pulmonary emboli and acute respiratory distress; delirium, convulsions, and coma; hemorrhagic necrosis; and ischemia of the peripheral tissue (acral cyanosis) with the risk of gangrene.

The prognosis for clients with DIC varies. Associated mortality is quite high, primarily because of the underlying illness. Hemorrhage, organ damage (especially acute respiratory distress syndrome [ARDS]), or even death may occur within a matter of hours if associated with gram-negative sepsis. In severe cases the mortality reaches 80%.

Diagnostic tests include screening assays and confirmatory assays. Findings of the screening assays show prolonged prothrombin time (PT) and activated partial thromboplastin time (PTT), a very low (and falling) platelet count ($<100,000/mm^3$), reduced fibrinogen level, and prolonged clotting times. Confirmatory tests such as fibrinogen degradation product (FDP), D-dimer, and factor assays identify the presence of products of DIC pathology. Table 75-7 provides the laboratory tests used in the diagnosis of DIC.

OUTCOME MANAGEMENT

Medical Management

The treatment of DIC is controversial, and efforts are under way to determine the most suitable regimen for managing this syndrome. Goals of treatment include (1) identification and correction of the precipitating cause or problem (e.g., infection, delivery of a fetus, surgery, or irradiation for cancer); (2) reestablishing hemostasis by replacing missing blood components; and (3) supportive therapy to control manifestations of hemorrhage and thrombosis.

Appropriate treatment is determined when (and if) the underlying cause is identified; for instance, antibiotic therapy to control infections or surgery to control severe obstetric complications. In the meantime, manifestations of hemorrhage and thrombosis must be addressed. Replacement of missing blood components is an important first step, particularly if bleeding is present. Washed packed RBCs can be administered to replace blood volume lost through hemorrhage without introducing anticoagulant substances. The specific blood product to be transfused is determined by the deficiency. Platelet

CONCEPT MAP

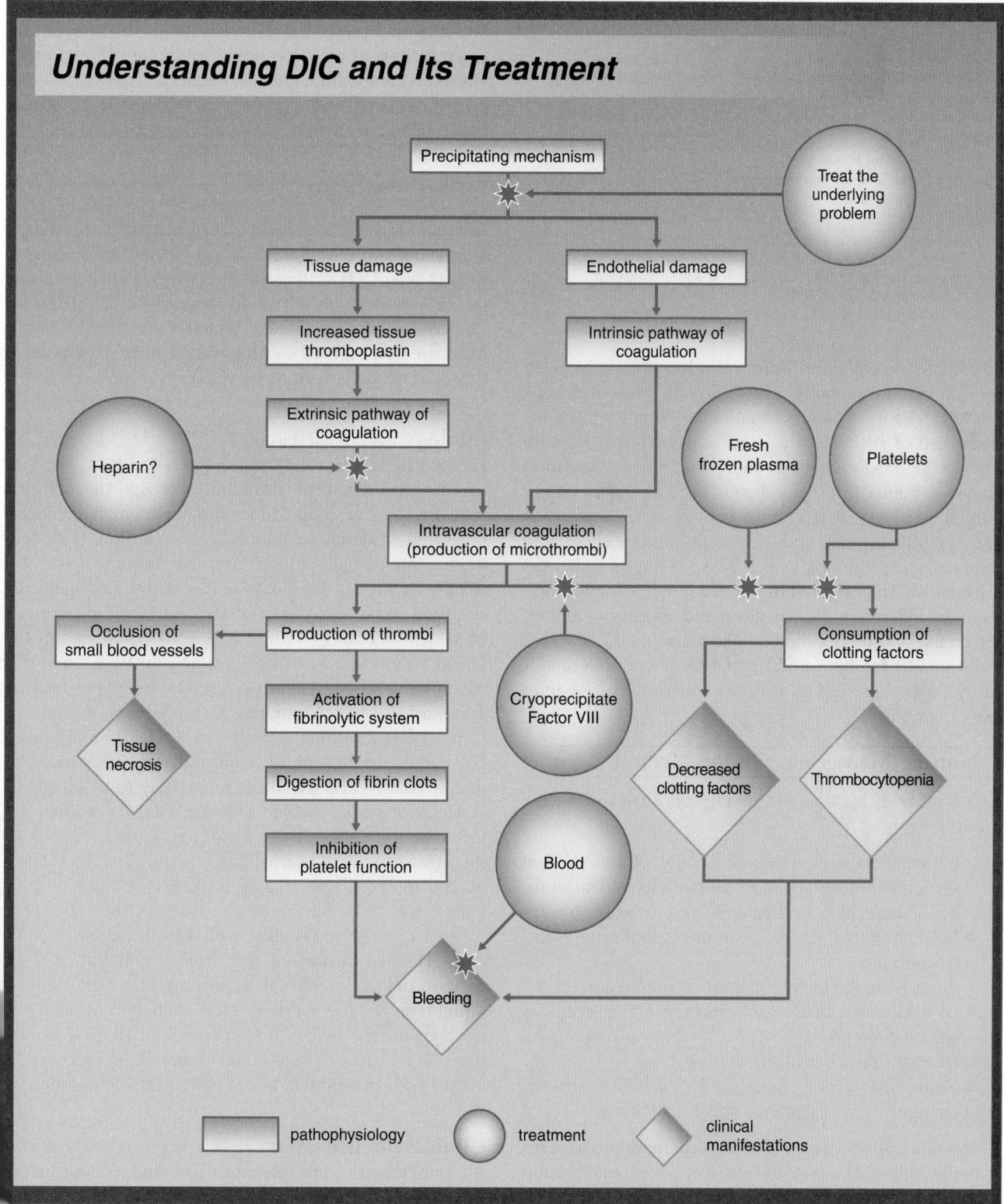

Understanding DIC and Its Treatment

Precipitating mechanism

Treat the underlying problem

Tissue damage

Endothelial damage

Increased tissue thromboplastin

Intrinsic pathway of coagulation

Extrinsic pathway of coagulation

Heparin?

Fresh frozen plasma

Platelets

Intravascular coagulation (production of microthrombi)

Occlusion of small blood vessels

Production of thrombi

Consumption of clotting factors

Tissue necrosis

Activation of fibrinolytic system

Cryoprecipitate Factor VIII

Decreased clotting factors

Thrombocytopenia

Digestion of fibrin clots

Inhibition of platelet function

Blood

Bleeding

pathophysiology   treatment   clinical manifestations

are given for thrombocytopenia. If fibrinogen levels are below 100 mg/dl, transfusions of cryoprecipitate are given until fibrinogen levels can be maintained at 100 to 150 mg/dl. Fresh frozen plasma is transfused if coagulation factors are decreased. Concerns that this may reaccelerate coagulation are unfounded because the plasma protease inhibitors in the plasma are sufficient to control such a reaction. 🪔 The protease

TABLE 75–7 Laboratory Tests Used in Diagnosis of Disseminated Intravascular Coagulation

Test	Results
Prothrombin time	Prolonged (75%)
Partial thromboplastin time	Usually prolonged
Thrombin time	Usually prolonged
Fibrinogen level	Usually depressed
Platelet count	Usually depressed
Fibrin degradation products	Elevated (75%-100%)
D-Dimer (cross-linked fibrin fragments)	Positive*
Protamine sulfate test	Strongly positive
Antithrombin III	Reduced (90%)
Factor assays II, V, VII, VIII, X, XIII	Reduced

*Important diagnostic test. Identifies presence of both thrombin and plasmin. More reliable than fibrin split products (FSP).

inhibitors gabexate and aprotinin (Trasylol) have been used in studies to control bleeding with some success.

The most controversial of the current treatments is the use of IV heparin to control thrombosis. Heparin inhibits the production of thrombin and other coagulation enzymes, but it can also accelerate bleeding. If heparin induces bleeding, ε-aminocaproic acid (Amicar) is given; cardiac, renal, and electrolyte studies should be followed closely during its use because Amicar enhances thrombosis. Antithrombin III (Desirudin), a natural coagulation inhibitor, may also be given and appears to shorten the course and reduce the complications of DIC. Hirudin, a thrombotic inhibitor and neutralizer is currently under study. Chronic DIC can be controlled by long-term use of heparin.

Nursing Management of the Medical Client

Assess all body systems for the effects of DIC, including the following:

- Integumentary bleeding or oozing of blood from venipuncture sites or mucosal surfaces and wounds, pallor, petechiae, ecchymoses, and hematomas
- Respiratory tachypnea, hemoptysis, orthopnea, and basilar rales
- Cardiovascular tachycardia and hypotension
- GI abdominal distention, guaiac-positive stools or gastric contents
- Genitourinary hematuria and oliguria
- Neurologic vision changes, dizziness, headache, changes in mental status, and irritability

Nursing care of clients with DIC is complex and requires extreme vigilance because the client must be treated simultaneously for the primary causative problem as well as the related manifestations of DIC. Generally the goal is to monitor and quantify blood loss and provide supportive therapy with blood components to resolve manifestations of hemorrhage and control further bleeding. Monitor appropriate laboratory values to determine treatment

effectiveness and observe for manifestations of thrombosis or transfusion reactions. To prevent further injury, avoid injections when possible, apply pressure to bleeding sites, and turn and reposition the client frequently and gently. Overt bleeding from body orifices and other clinical manifestations can be frightening to clients and their significant others, who all will require intense emotional support, especially if the client does not survive.

HEMOPHILIA

Hemophilia is an X-linked genetic disorder that results in a deficiency of coagulation factors. Two major forms are hemophilia A (HA), the classic form, which is due to a deficiency of factor VIII; and hemophilia B (HB), also known as Christmas disease, which is due to a deficiency of factor IX. Inherited clotting disorders are discussed in the Genetic Links feature on p. 2037.

Etiology and Risk Factors

Factor VIII and factor IX deficiencies result in an insufficient production of thrombin through the intrinsic pathway of the coagulation cascade, which creates a profound tendency for spontaneous bleeding. Both conditions are usually found only in males. Factor VIII (FVIII) deficiency also may be caused by a congenitally acquired molecular defect in the FVIII binding domain of von Willebrand factor (vWF). FVIII circulates in the blood bound to vWF. This disorder, von Willebrand disease, is the most common congenital bleeding disorder and may affect both genders. A comparison of the three forms of hemophilia appears in Table 75-8. Because HA makes up 80% of all hemophilia, the discussion of manifestations and treatment refers only to this form.

Hemophilia is classified as severe (<1% of normal factor level), moderate (1% to 5% of normal factor level), or mild (5% to 40% of normal factor level). The prevalence of HA in the United States is 20.6 cases per 100,000 males, with 60% having severe disease; the HB rate is 5.3 cases per 100,000 males, with 40% having severe disease. Female carriers of the disease will transmit the genetic defect to 50% of their sons and 50% of their daughters will be carriers. Men with hemophilia will not transmit the defect to their sons, but all their daughters will be carriers. Rare female hemophilia can occur if a man with hemophilia mates with a female carrier.

Clinical Manifestations

All manifestations are related to bleeding. Severe hemophilia often presents at circumcision or at the beginning of ambulation or primary dentition. The hallmark of this disorder is *hemarthrosis* (bleeding into the joints) in the knees, ankles, elbows, wrists, fingers, hips, and shoulders. Hemarthrosis is painful and leads to deterioration of the joints, which may become deformed and permanently

GENETIC LINKS

Examples of Inherited Clotting Disorders

Disorder	Features	Inheritance	Metabolic/Gene Defect	Genetic Testing vailable?
von Willebrand disease	Mucocutaneous bleeding; prolonged bleeding time	AD	Mutation in von Willebrand factor (VWF) gene on chromosome 12	Yes
Hemophilia A (factor VIII deficiency; classic hemophilia)	Easy bruising and hemorrhage into joints and muscles because of deficient clotting ability	XR	Mutation in factor VIII (FVIII) gene on chromosome 10	Yes
Hemophilia B (factor IX deficiency; Christmas disease)	Similar to hemophilia A	XR	Mutation in factor IX (FIX) gene on chromosome 10	Yes
Hemophilia C (factor XI deficiency)	Mild to moderate bleeding; mucocutaneous bleeding	AR	Mutation in factor XI (FXI) gene on chromosome 4; deficiency of plasma thromboplastin antecedent (PTA)	Yes

AD, Autosomal dominant; *AR*, autosomal recessive; *XR*, X-linked recessive.

crippled. Synovial hypertrophy, hemosiderin deposition, fibrosis, damage to the cartilage, and subchondral cyst formation are seen with this condition.

HA typically manifests in the following ways:

- Slow, persistent bleeding from cuts, scratches, and other minor traumas
- Delayed hemorrhage that follows minor injuries; bleeding may not start from a site until hours or even days after the traumatic event
- Severe hemorrhaging from the gums after dental extraction or even brushing the teeth with a hard toothbrush
- Severe, sometimes fatal, epistaxis after injury to the nose
- Overwhelming gastric hemorrhage, which may be linked to gastric disorders such as ulcers and gastritis
- Recurrent hematoma formation in the deep subcutaneous tissue in the intramuscular tissues (muscular atrophy sometimes results) and around the

peripheral nerves, causing compression that can result in severe pain, anesthesia of the innervated part, nerve damage, and paralysis
- Hematuria from genitourinary trauma
- Splenic rupture from falls or abdominal trauma
- Intracranial bleeding, which is the leading cause of hemorrhagic death

Life expectancy dramatically increased with the advent in the 1960s of antihemophilic factor (AHF) replacement therapy and prophylactic therapy with lyophilized concentrates that eliminate bleeding. Before this time, the life expectancy for clients with severe HA was 5 to 11 years; today it is 50 to 60 years. Intracranial hemorrhages currently account for about one third of HA-related deaths.

Platelet function, platelet count, bleeding time, and prothrombin time are normal. The activated partial thromboplastin time (aPTT) is prolonged. Quantitative assays for factor VIII determine the severity of the disease.

TABLE 75–8   **Comparison of the Three Forms of Hemophilia**

Form of Hemophilia	Etiology	Transmission	Major Laboratory Findings
Hemophilia A (classic hemophilia)	Inherited factor VIII (antihemophilic globulin) deficiency	Transmitted as sex-linked *recessive* trait; transmitted by females; occurs in males and, rarely, homozygous females	Coagulation time prolonged but bleeding time normal; factor VIII missing from plasma
Hemophilia B (Christmas disease)	Inherited factor IX (plasma thromboplastin component) deficiency	Transmitted as sex-linked *recessive* trait; transmitted by females; occurs in males and, rarely, homozygous females	Laboratory findings and symptoms same as in hemophilia A; factor IX missing
von Willebrand's disease	Inherited factor VIII deficiency and defective platelet dysfunction	Transmitted as autosomal *dominant* trait to both sexes; occurs in both males and females	Both coagulation time and bleeding time prolonged; low factor VIII levels; platelet adhesiveness decreased

OUTCOME MANAGEMENT

The goals of care for clients with hemophilia are as follows:

- Stop topical bleeding as quickly as possible.
- Supply the missing factor causing hemorrhage.
- Prevent complications leading to and caused by bleeding.

The nurse can control topical bleeding quickly by applying pressure or ice to the injured site, packing the area with fibrin foam, and applying topical hemostatic agents such as thrombin.

Primary factor replacement therapy should be initiated as ordered. This typically is the immediate transfusion of factor VIII (or IX) concentrate supplied as a lyophilized powder. One unit per kilogram of concentrate increases the plasma level of FVIII by 2%, with a reaction half-time of 8 to 12 hours. Because the procoagulant activity of AHF disappears rapidly, clients need transfusions every 12 hours until bleeding stops. For mild hemorrhage, an FVIII level of 30% should be maintained; for major hemorrhage, the level should be maintained at 50%; life-threatening bleeds require a level of 80% to 90%. Plasma levels must be maintained at higher than 50% for a minimum of 7 to 10 days. Prophylactic administration of FVIII to a level 50% above normal is recommended in cases of minor injury, surgery, and dental extractions. Transfusion of packed RBCs or WBCs is used only to replace blood volume when there has been severe loss.

With repeated transfusions and AHF therapy, some clients become sensitized to AHF and develop alloantibody inhibitors that can neutralize FVIII and complicate replacement therapy. These antibodies are seen in about 30% of clients with severe cases by the age of 10. In case of major and life-threatening hemorrhages, these clients are treated with massive doses of factor VIII from animal sources (bovine and porcine), inactivated prothrombin complex concentrates (Konyne 80, Proplex T), or activated prothrombin complex concentrates (Feiba VH Immuno, Autoplex T). Recent treatment with FVIIa for hemarthrosis has been effective for these clients. Clinicians are using various experimental treatments such as immunosuppressive therapy to combat this problem.

Hemarthrosis may be controlled if the client receives AHF in the early stages of bleeding. Joint immobilization and local chilling (such as packing ice around the joint) may bring relief. If pain is severe, it may be necessary to aspirate blood from the joint. Once bleeding stops and swelling subsides, the client should perform active range-of-motion exercises without weight-bearing to prevent further complications such as deformity and muscle atrophy.

Prophylactic home infusion of AHF can greatly reduce bleeding episodes and related complications. Training programs with strict guidelines for this regimen have been developed. As a result, clients with hemophilia lose less time from work or school and need fewer visits to the emergency department.

 Analgesics and corticosteroids often reduce joint pain and swelling and the pain of chronic arthritis. Avoid all aspirin products. In mild hemophilia, the use of IV desmopressin may eliminate the need for AHF. Desmopressin acts by causing an increase in plasma factor VIII activity.

Although most clients with hemophilia are successfully maintained with home health care, they may be seen in the hospital during acute bleeding episodes or for unrelated treatments. If even a minor invasive procedure is planned, it is crucial to assess the factor VIII level and to administer a sufficient quantity of factor concentrate before the procedure. During routine medical examinations, these clients should be assessed for the frequency of bleeding episodes and the effectiveness of home therapy. Examine joints for manifestations of bleeding and related atrophy.

Teach the client and family to recognize early manifestations of bleeding and why it is critical to intervene with treatment immediately. Effective and prompt administration of factors to reduce the incidence of bleeding episodes and resultant complications is a priority. The client and family will need to learn IV infusion administration techniques to control the bleeding. Discuss situations that require medical consultation. Discuss the need to curtail physical activities such as contact sports, minor invasive procedures, falls, and cuts that may precipitate a bleeding episode. If a client has HIV seroconversion, arrange for a referral for appropriate care.

CONCLUSIONS

Hematologic diseases are complex disorders that require the nurse to understand the hematopoietic system. The nurse is often involved in the administration of blood and blood products for treatment of these various disorders. Many of the blood disorders are life-threatening; others are easily controlled with proper nutrition or regular medication.

Because blood and blood product transfusions are widely used in the treatment of hematologic disorders, it is vital that you understand these procedures, the implications of these procedures, and the proper techniques of administration so the client will receive safe and effective care.

THINKING CRITICALLY

1. A 62-year-old client underwent a gastric resection for peptic ulcer disease 3 months ago at a hospital in another state. She comes to the nursing clinic complaining of shortness of breath and fatigue

with minimal physical exertion. She currently takes ranitidine (Zantac). What assessments should you make now?

Factors to Consider. What is the significance of the history of gastric resection? How might this contribute to the client's lethargy? What might be causing the shortness of breath and fatigue? What laboratory results would be appropriate to evaluate? What teaching should you consider with this client?

2. A 40-year-old client has recently been told that she has multiple myeloma. She has been admitted to the oncology inpatient unit for initial evaluation and treatment. On her fourth day after admission, she becomes confused and difficult to arouse. Bowel sounds are diminished, and she begins to vomit. What priority assessment should you make now?

Factors to Consider. What might predispose the client to this change in her level of consciousness? What additional assessments would you need to make? What interventions should you anticipate at this time?

Discussions for these questions can be found on the website.

BIBLIOGRAPHY

Citations appearing in red refer to primary research.

Citations appearing in blue refer to evidence-based practice guidelines and protocols.

1. Agaliotis, D. (2006). Hemophilia overview. *EMedicine.* Available: www.eMedicine.com/med/topic3528.htm.
2. Ahmed, S., Shahid, R.K., & Russo, L. (2005). Unusual causes of abdominal pain: Sickle cell anemia. *Best Practice & Research Clinical Gastroenterology, 19*(2), 297-310.
3. Auwaeter, P.G. (2004). Infectious mononucleosis: Return to play. *Clinics in Sports Medicine, 23,* 485-497.
4. Besa, E., & Woermann, U. (2003). Polycythemia vera. *eMedicine.* Available: www.emedicine.com/med/topic1864.htm.
5. Bryan, S. (2002). Hemolytic transfusion reaction: Safeguards for practice. *Journal of PeriAnesthesia Nursing, 17*(6), 399-403.
6. Busch, M., Kleinman, S., & Nemo, G. (2003). Current and emerging infectious risks of blood transfusions. *Journal of the American Medical Association, 289*(8), 959-961.
7. Conrad, M. (2006). Anemia. *EMedicine.* Available: www.emedicine. com/med/topic132.htm.
8. Conrad, M. (2006). Iron deficiency anemia. *EMedicine.* Available at www.emedicine.com/med/topic1188.htm.
9. Conrad, M. (2006). Pernicious anemia. *EMedicine.* Available at www.emedicine.com/med/topic132.htm.
10. De Franceschi, L., & Corrocher, R. (2004). Established and experimental treatments for sickle cell disease. *Haematologica, 89*(3), 348-356.
11. Distenfeld, A., & Woermann, U. (2005). Sickle cell anemia. *EMedicine.* Available at www.emedicine.com/med/topic12126.htm.
12. Distenfeld, A. (2006). Agranulocytosis. *EMedicine.* Available at www.emedicine.com/med/topic82.htm.
13. Doenges, M.E., et al. (2006). *Nurse's pocket guide:Diagnosis, prioritized interventions and rationales* (10th ed). Philadelphia, Pa: F.A. Davis.
14. Ebell, M.H. (2004). Epstein-Barr virus infectious mononucleosis. *American Family Physician, 70*(7), 1279-1287, 1289-1290.
15. Edwards, C.L., Scales, M.T., Loughlin, C., et al. (2005). A brief review of the pathophysiology, associated pain, and psychosocial issues in sickle cell disease. *International Journal of Behavioral Medicine, 12*(3), 171-179.
16. Epstein-Barr virus and infectious mononucleosis. Accessed 02/22/07 at www.cdc.gov/ncidod/diseases/ebv.htm.
17. Ferri, F.F. (2006). *Ferri's clinical advisor: Instant diagnosis and treatment.* Philadelphia: Saunders.
18. Gaines, K. (2003). Aminocaproic acid (Amicar): Potent antifibrolytic agent for treating hematuria. *Urologic Nursing, 23*(2), 156-158.
19. Gando, S., Iba, T., Eguchi, Y., et al. (2006). A multicenter, prospective validation of disseminated intravascular diagnostic criteria for critically ill patients: Comparing current criteria. *Critical Care Medicine, 34*(3), 625-631.
20. Grethlein, S. (2006). Multiple myeloma. *EMedicine.* Available at www.emedicine.com/med/topic1521.htm.
21. Hebert, P., et al. (2003). Clinical outcomes following institution of the Canadian universal leukoreduction program for red blood cell transfusions. *Journal of the American Medical Association, 289*(15), 1941-1949.
22. Hess, J.R., & Lawson, J.H. (2006). The coagulopathy of trauma versus disseminated intravascular coagulation. *Journal of Trauma, 60,* S12-S19.
23. Mehta, S.R., Afenyi-Annan, A., Byrns, P., et al. (2006). Opportunities to improve outcomes in sickle cell disease. *American Family Physician, 74,* 303-310, 313-314.
24. National Institute of Diabetes, Digestive, and Kidney Diseases. (2003). *Hemochromatosis.* National digestive diseases information clearinghouse. Available at www.niddk.nih.gov/health/digest/pubs/hemochrom/hemochromatosis.htm.
25. Rajkumar, S., et al. (2002). Current therapy for multiple myeloma. *Mayo Clinic Proceedings, 77,* 813-822.
26. Raphael, R.L., & Vichinsky, E.P. (2005). Pathophysiology and treatment of sickle cell disease. *Clinical Advances in Hematology & Oncology, 3*(6), 492-505.
27. Reed, W., & Vichinsky, E. (1999). Transfusion practice for patients with sickle cell disease. *Current Opinions in Hematology, 6*(6), 432-436.
28. Rosenfeld, S., et al. (2003). Antithymocyte globulin and cyclosporine for severe aplastic anemia: Association between hematologic response and long-term outcome. *Journal of the American Medical Association, 289*(9), 1130-1135.
29. Schick, P. (2005). Hemolytic anemia. *EMedicine.* Available at www.emedicine.com/med/topic979.htm.
30. Schick, P. (2005). Megaloblastic anemia. *EMedicine.* Available at www.emedicine.com/med/topic1420.htm.
31. Levi, M., & Schmaier, A. (2006). Disseminated intravascular coagulation. *EMedicine.* Available at www.emedicine.com/med/topic 557.htm.
32. Siddiqui, A.K., & Ahmed, S. (2003). Pulmonary manifestations of sickle cell disease. *Postgraduate Medicine Journal, 79,* 384-390.
33. Steinberg, M. (2006). Pathophysiologically based drug treatment of sickle cell disease. *Trends in Pharmacological Sciences, 27* (4), 204-210.
34. Steinberg, M., et al. (2003). Effect of hydroxyurea on mortality and morbidity in adult sickle cell anemia: Risks and benefits up to 9 years of treatment. *Journal of the American Medical Association, 289*(13), 1645-1651.
35. Takeshita, K. (2006). Thalassemia beta. *EMedicine.* Available at www.emedicine.com/med/topic2260.htm.
35a. The Joint Commission. (2008). National Patient Safety Goals Hospital Program. Available at www.JointCommission.org/Patient Safety/NationalPatientSafetyGoals/08_hap_npsgs.htm.
36. Weiner, D., & Brugnara, C. (2003). Hydroxyurea and sickle cell disease: A chance for every patient. *Journal of the American Medical Association, 289*(13), 1692-1695.

evolve **Did you remember to check out the bonus material on the Evolve website and the CD-ROM, including NCLEX®-Examination Style Review Questions, Open-Book Quizzes, and Chapter Review Audio Podcasts?**

http://evolve.elsevier.com/Black/medsurg

CHAPTER 76

Management of Clients with Immune Disorders

Linda M. Scott

The immune system constitutes the body's defense system against invading foreign substances. A functioning immune system must protect the body from potential pathogens. An immune system that is malfunctioning predisposes an individual to the development of a wide variety of diseases ranging from severe infection to autoimmune disease and the resultant tissue injury. The Unit 17 Anatomy and Physiology Review describes the normally functioning immune system; this chapter looks at alterations in the immune system and examines how these changes affect the human organism.

HYPERSENSITIVITY DISORDERS

As health care providers, nurses deal with allergic conditions far more often than might be suspected. Allergic rhinitis, asthma, and dermatitis are a few examples of these immunologic diseases.

The tendency to develop allergies for which there is a genetic predisposition and that involve immunoglobulin E (IgE) antibody formation is known as *atopy*. The terms *atopic, allergic,* and *hypersensitive* are frequently used interchangeably. *Allergy* (or, more appropriately, hypersensitivity) describes the increased immune response to the presence of an allergen, also known as an *antigen*. Between 20% and 30% of the population have allergies. We cannot predict who will have allergies; however, there is a higher incidence of allergies among children of allergic parents.

People must progress through a two-step process to become allergic. Step 1 starts with *sensitization*. Sensitization occurs when one develops IgE antibodies against a substance that is inhaled, ingested, or injected. Newly formed IgE antibodies stick to basophils and mast cells, which are found in the skin's mucosal surfaces and in the respiratory and gastrointestinal (GI) tracts. Hypersensitivity can be claimed only after IgE antibodies against a certain foreign substance have formed and are bound to the surface of tissue mast cells and circulating basophils.

Hypersensitivity does not produce any of the manifestations typically associated with allergic disease. It is not until step 2, *reexposure to the allergen,* that allergic manifestations such as sneezing, asthma, and anaphylaxis occur. Although the cellular events for all immediate allergic reactions tend to be similar, differences are found in the clinical sequelae that occur, based on the state of the individual's host defenses, the nature of the allergen, the concentration of the allergen, the route by which the allergen enters, the amount of allergen exposure received, and which organ is affected.

Etiology and Risk Factors
Host Defenses

Some people are more susceptible to hypersensitivity than others for reasons that are unclear (see the Complementary and Alternative Therapy feature on p. 2041). The increasing prevalence of allergic disease suggests that environmental factors acting either before or after birth contribute to the regulation of the development of Th_2 cells or their function. Th_2 cells play a triggering role in the activation and recruitment of IgE antibody–producing B cells, mast cells, and eosinophils—the cellular triad involved in allergy. The decrease in the number of reported childhood infectious

Allergies

Several studies have found a number of environmental factors that may be associated with a lower incidence of allergic disease. For example, taking oral supplements of a probiotic supplement such as *Lactobacillus ruminus*,[3] having a dog or other pet in the home,[5] attending a day care center or having siblings in the home,[1] and farm exposure[4] have all been found to decrease the incidence of allergic disease. However, exposure to tobacco smoke increased the production of allergen-specific IgE and exacerbated allergic responses in clients with allergies,[2] which suggests that clients with allergies should avoid tobacco smoke.

REFERENCES

1. Celedon, J., et al. (2002). Day care attendance, respiratory tract illnesses, wheezing, asthma, and total serum IgE level in early childhood. *Archives of Pediatric Adolescent Medicine, 156,* 241-245.
2. Diaz-Sanchez, D., et al. (2006). Challenge with environmental tobacco smoke exacerbates allergic airway disease in human beings. *The Journal of Allergy and Clinical Immunology, 118*(2), 441-446.
3. Kalliomaki, M., et al. (2001). Probiotics in primary prevention of atopic disease: A randomised placebo-controlled trial. *Lancet, 357,* 1076-1079.
4. Leynaert, B., et al. (2006). Association between farm exposure and atopy, according to the CD14 C-159T polymorphism. *The Journal of Allergy and Clinical Immunology, 118*(3), 658-665.
5. Reijonen, T., et al. (2000). Predictors of asthma three years after hospitalization admission for wheezing in infancy. *Pediatrics, 106,* 1406-1412.

diseases that has resulted from vast vaccination programs, antimicrobial therapy, and changing lifestyles are important influences on an individual's outcome in the Th response to an allergen. Specific IgE formation can be influenced by viral infections, especially those caused by cytomegalovirus (CMV) and mononucleosis. Factors such as air pollution, gender, age, and exposure to second-hand smoke can influence the manifestations of allergies.

Nature of the Allergen

Allergens are antigens that produce a clinical allergic reaction. In atopic diseases, allergens are capable of inducing IgE antibody, thus triggering an allergic response. Molecules that combine with proteins to produce antibodies are called *haptens*. Haptens, along with other environmental allergens, are carried on vectors that may become airborne (e.g., pollen, molds, dust particles, animal dander). Contact with these allergens causes sensitization and atopy and evokes the acute manifestations of allergy. Some haptens (e.g., penicillin) are highly antigenic.

Concentration of the Allergen

Higher concentrations usually result in hypersensitivity responses of greater intensity. Lower concentrations of the allergen may then cause severe manifestations when reexposure occurs.

Route of Entrance into the Body

Routes by which allergens enter the body include inhalation, injection, ingestion, and direct contact. Most allergens are inhaled.

Exposure to the Allergen

Sensitization to allergens is necessary for hypersensitivity to occur. A few factors that influence the likelihood of development of allergy are a person's age at the time of exposure (exposure early in life), the type of allergen (house dust mite, cockroach, various medications, and pollen), the allergen load (lower levels are capable of inducing specific IgE production), and the month of a person's birth (a greater affinity for allergies is seen in those born in the spring and fall).

Pathophysiology

The key intermediate in allergic disease is the IgE antibody. The production of IgE in response to an allergen renders an individual allergic. The two general categories of hypersensitivity reactions are (1) *immediate* (humoral or antigen-antibody) and (2) *delayed* (cell-mediated).

Immediate Reaction

The immediate (antigen-antibody) reaction occurs within minutes after exposure to the allergen. The resultant IgE production mediates the immediate response by activating mast cells and basophils, causing them to degranulate and release mediators such as histamine, leukotrienes from basophils and prostaglandins, and platelet-activating factor from eosinophils.

The mediators, whether preformed or newly formed after activation, are able to increase vascular permeability, dilate vessels, cause bronchospasm, contract smooth muscle, and ignite other inflammatory cells. Table 76-1 describes chemical mediators of the allergic reaction, their action, and the associated manifestations.

Manifestations of mediator release vary, depending on the organ where the mediators' receptors are found. For example, histamine is a preformed mast cell mediator that has receptors in various organs, including skin, oral and nasal mucosa, lungs, and the smooth muscle in the GI tract. Once histamine binds to its receptor, it can cause many reactions. Vasodilation causes edema; smooth muscle contraction results in dangerous airway narrowing; and glandular stimulation leads to increased mucus secretion in the nose, lungs, and GI tract.

TABLE 76–1   Chemical Mediators of the Allergic Reaction

Mediator	Action	Manifestations
Histamine	Dilates blood vessels and increases vascular permeability	Erythema, tissue swelling, and shock
	Constricts smooth muscles in bronchial airways	
	Stimulates nerve endings	Shortness of breath and wheezing
	Increases mucus production in airways and GI tract	Itching and painful skin
		Congestion, gastric reflux, and heartburn
Platelet-activating factor	Dilates blood vessels and constricts bronchial airways	Same as for histamine
	Aids in secretion and aggregation of platelets	Same as for histamine
Eosinophil chemotactic factor of anaphylaxis (ECF-A)	Increases eosinophil migration	Inflamed airways
Neutrophil chemotactic factor	Increases neutrophil migration	Inflamed airways
Heparin	Anticoagulation	Increased bleeding and bruising
Bradykinin	Slows smooth muscle contraction	Mucus plugging
	Increases vascular permeability	Swelling
	Increases mucus production	Congestion
Lipid Mediators or SRS-A		
Leukotrienes	Increase vascular permeability	Same as for histamine
	Increase smooth muscle contraction	
Prostaglandin D	Constricts bronchial airways	Wheezing, shortness of breath, and cough
	Vasodilation	Flushing and swelling
Cytokines (IL-4, IL-5, TNF-α)	Allow cells to influence activity and development of other unrelated cells	Inflammation, edema, and fibrosis
	Aid in eosinophil production	
	Increase vascular permeability	

GI, Gastrointestinal; *IL,* interleukin; *SRS,* slow-reacting substance of anaphylaxis; *TNF,* tumor necrosis factor.

Newly formed mediators, including lipid mediators and cytokines, are made after the mast cell has been activated and have similar actions to those of histamine, but their effects tend to last much longer. Once released into the blood and after binding to their receptors, these mediators cause more bronchial smooth muscle contraction, vasodilation in the skin, nasal congestion, and edema.

Delayed Reaction

The delayed (cell-mediated or late-phase) reaction is seen when there is a prolonged response to the initial allergen. T cells govern the delayed inflammatory response that occurs about 2 to 8 hours after mast cells have been activated by the initial allergen exposure.

Hypersensitivity reactions are divided into four main types (Table 76-2):

- Type 1, immediate or anaphylactic
- Type 2, cytolytic or cytotoxic
- Type 3, immune complex
- Type 4, cell-mediated or delayed

Type 1 (Anaphylactic) Hypersensitivity. The anaphylactic response (described previously) is a rapidly

TABLE 76–2   Types of Hypersensitivity Reactions

	Type	Causative Component	Pathologic Process	Reaction
1	Immediate/ anaphylactic	IgE	Mast cell degranulation ↓ Histamine and leukotriene release	Anaphylaxis Atopic diseases Skin reactions
2	Cytolytic/cytotoxic	IgG IgM Complement	Complement fixation ↓ Cell lysis	ABO incompatibility Drug-induced hemolytic anemia
3	Immune complex	Antigen-antibody complexes	Deposition in vessels and tissue walls ↓ Inflammation	Arthus reaction Serum sickness Systemic lupus erythematosus Acute glomerulonephritis
4	Cell-mediated/delayed	Sensitized T cells	Lymphokine release	Tuberculosis Contact dermatitis Transplant rejection

Ig, Immunoglobulin.

occurring reaction that is mediated by IgE antibodies. The allergen binds to IgE antibodies, which are attracted to the surface of mast cells and basophils, causing the release of mediators (see Table 76-1). Examples of type 1 hypersensitivity reactions include anaphylaxis, allergic rhinitis, asthma, and acute allergic drug reactions.

Type 2 (Cytolytic or Cytotoxic) Hypersensitivity. Cytolytic or cytotoxic reactions are complement dependent and thus involve IgG or IgM antibodies. The antigen-antibody binding results in activation of the complement system and destroys the cell on which the antigen is bound, usually a circulating blood cell, thus causing tissue injury. Examples of tissue injury caused by type 2 hypersensitivity include hemolytic anemia, Rh hemolytic disease in newborns, autoimmune hyperthyroidism, myasthenia gravis, and blood transfusion reactions.

During a blood transfusion, blood group incompatibility causes cell lysis, which results in a transfusion reaction. The antigen responsible for initiating the reaction is a part of the donor red blood cell membrane. Manifestations of a transfusion reaction result from intravascular hemolysis of red blood cells and include headache and back pain (flank), chest pain similar to angina, nausea and vomiting, tachycardia and hypotension, hematuria, and urticaria.

Transfusions of more than 100 ml of incompatible blood can result in severe, permanent renal damage, circulatory shock, and death. Therefore if manifestations develop, stop the transfusion at once, maintain an open intravenous (IV) line, check the client's vital signs, and notify the physician immediately. For detailed nursing interventions related to transfusion reactions, see Chapter 75.

Type 3 (Immune Complex) Hypersensitivity. Immune complex reactions result when antigens bind to antibodies, leading to tissue injury. The molecular size of the antigen-antibody complexes is an important feature in eliciting immune complex reactions. Larger complexes are rapidly cleared by phagocytic cells. The smaller complexes formed in antigen excess persist longer in the circulation because they are not so easily captured by phagocytic cells in the spleen and liver. Inflammation results and leads to acute or chronic disease of the organ system in which the immune complexes were deposited.

Immune complex–mediated inflammation is produced by IgG or IgM antibodies, antigen, and complement. The mediators of inflammatory injury include the complement cleavage peptides, which can activate mast cells, neutrophils, monocytes, and other cells. The release of lysosomal granules from white blood cells and macrophages causes further tissue injury.

The antigen may be tissue-fixed or released locally, as in Goodpasture's syndrome, in which circulating antibodies react with autologous antigens in the glomerular basement membranes of the kidneys, causing inflammation of the glomerulus.

Antigen-antibody complexes are formed in the bloodstream and get trapped in capillaries or deposited in vessel walls, causing urticaria, arthritis, arteritis, or glomerulonephritis. Alternatively, antigen-antibody complexes may form in the joint space, with resultant synovitis, as in rheumatoid arthritis and systemic lupus erythematous. The Arthus reaction is a localized area of tissue necrosis that results from immune complex hypersensitivity.

The antigen may also be circulating, as in serum sickness. Serum sickness develops 6 to 14 days after injection with a foreign serum. Deposition of complexes on vessel walls causes complement activation, with resultant edema, fever, inflammation of blood vessels and joints, and urticaria. Classic serum sickness is rare because large doses of heterologous sera (e.g., horse antisera to human lymphocytes) are seldom used.

A serum sickness–like reaction may occur, however, after administration of such medications as penicillin, sulfonamides, streptomycin, thiouracils, and hydantoin compounds. Rather than being dominated by cutaneous vasculitis, these reactions more often manifest with fever, arthralgias, lymphadenopathy, and urticaria. The illness is usually benign and self-limiting, and it resolves after discontinuation of the offending medication.

Nursing care of the client with serum sickness depends on the severity of the reaction. For a mild reaction, care includes control of fever and pain with aspirin and antihistamines. For a severe reaction, care may require steroids.

Serum sickness can be prevented by avoiding allergen exposure. Obtain an allergy history and information about any previous reactions to drugs or vaccines. Document findings in the client's chart, care plan, and medication record so that the risk of subsequent exposure is minimized.

Type 4 (Cell-Mediated, Late-Phase, or Delayed) Hypersensitivity. In cell-mediated hypersensitivity, sensitized T cells respond to antigens by releasing lymphokines, some of which direct phagocytic cell activity. This reaction occurs 24 to 72 hours after exposure to an allergen. Delayed hypersensitivity is induced by chronic infection (e.g., tuberculosis) or by contact sensitivities, as in contact dermatitis.

Type 4 reactions occur after the intradermal injection of tuberculosis antigen or purified protein derivative (PPD). If the client has been sensitized to tuberculosis, sensitized T cells react with the antigen at the injection site. The reaction leads to edema and fibrin deposits, which result in the induration characteristic of a positive tuberculosis reaction.

Graft-versus-host disease (GVHD) and transplant rejection are also type 4 reactions. In GVHD, immunocompetent donor bone marrow cells (the graft) react against various antigens in the bone marrow recipient (the host). Various clinical manifestations result, including skin, GI, and hepatic lesions. Transplant rejection is discussed in Chapter 80, and GVHD is discussed in Chapter 79.

Contact dermatitis is another type 4 reaction that occurs after sensitization to an allergen, commonly a cosmetic, adhesive, topical medication, drug additive (such as lanolin added to lotions), or plant toxin (such as poison ivy). With the first exposure, no reaction occurs, but antigens are formed. On subsequent exposures, hypersensitivity reactions are triggered, which lead to itching, erythema, and vesicular lesions.

Clinical Manifestations

During an allergic response, mast cell activation and the release of chemical mediators result in increased vascular permeability, edema, dilation of blood vessels, smooth muscle contraction, bronchospasm, and increased mucus secretion in the nose, lungs, and GI tract.

The diagnosis of an allergic disease is based on the client's history, manifestations experienced during or after allergen exposure, and the results from commonly used allergy tests. Common allergy tests include (1) skin testing; (2) radioallergosorbent test (RAST) or fluoroenzyme immunoassay test (ImmunoCAP FEIA), which are used to measure IgE levels to certain allergens in vitro; (3) pulmonary function tests (PFTs) to diagnose asthma; and (4) blood assays for IgE levels.

Skin Testing

Skin tests are the diagnostic test of choice for allergic diseases. In prick skin testing, the clinician introduces a small quantity of allergen into the skin by quickly pricking, scratching, or puncturing it. A wheal and flare reaction peaks in 15 to 20 minutes if the client is allergic. Skin testing is generally considered safe and is more specific, though less sensitive, than intradermal testing, but it always carries a risk of causing a systemic reaction such as anaphylaxis.

Intradermal testing is used if the prick skin test is negative. The allergen is injected directly below the skin by holding the skin taught and inserting the 26-gauge needle parallel to its surface, just far enough to cover the beveled portion and produce a bleb. There is a higher incidence of severe allergic reactions with this kind of testing. Therefore it should be used with extreme caution and under close supervision. A patch test can be used to evaluate contact allergies; the allergen is applied directly to the skin and then covered with a gauze dressing.

Nurses often administer skin tests and interpret test results. An *immediate* reaction (i.e., appearing within 10 to 20 minutes after the injection), marked by erythema and wheal formation greater than 3 mm of the positive control (usually histamine), denotes a positive reaction. *Positive* reactions indicate antibody response to previous exposure to this antigen and suggest that the client is allergic to the particular substance that causes the reaction. *Negative* reactions may be inconclusive, requiring further assessment. Negative results may indicate the following: (1) antibodies have not formed to this antigen, (2) the antigen was deposited too deeply into the skin (e.g., subcutaneously), (3) the client is immunosuppressed from disease or therapies (e.g., steroids, chemotherapy, radiation therapy), or (4) the client has taken antihistamines within the past 72 hours.

Problems that arise from skin testing range from minor itching to anaphylaxis. Itching and discomfort at the injection site are common and can be relieved by the application of cool compresses or topical steroid or antihistamine creams, and by the administration of oral antihistamines such as diphenhydramine (Benadryl). Ulceration of the injection site is best treated by keeping the area clean and dry. Anaphylactic shock is a rare but potentially lethal complication of skin testing. A client with a history of an anaphylactic reaction to a substance should never undergo skin testing for an allergy to that substance. This is especially true of allergens such as penicillin, which can produce lethal anaphylaxis in susceptible clients.

Radioallergosorbent Test

The RAST uses the principle of immunoabsorption and reveals elevated levels of allergen-specific IgE antibodies in the client's blood. The allergen of interest is first bound to some solid surface, usually a paper disk. The client's blood is then incubated with the disk. If the client has antibodies specific to the allergen being tested, they bind to that allergen. The unbound antibodies are washed away, and the level of antigen-specific IgE can be measured. This test is somewhat less sensitive than skin testing and is more time-consuming and costly. However, this may be indicated if the client is unable to omit certain medications, like antihistamines, before testing, has suffered from anaphylaxis to a known allergen, or has dermographism or a widespread skin disease.

ImmunoCAP FEIA (Fluoroenzyme Immunoassay Test)

This method uses as the solid phase a flexible, hydrophobic cellulosic disk to which an allergen has been linked. The advantage of this system compared to RAST testing is that it has a very high antigen-binding capacity and has minimal nonspecific binding with high total Ig output. This test is more readily used worldwide based on its increased sensitivity and equal specificity.

Pulmonary Function Test

The PFTs are done to confirm the diagnosis or to evaluate respiratory status in asthmatic disease, to assess the severity of lung obstruction, and to guide the medical treatment of asthma. The principal abnormality associated with asthma is reversible airway obstruction, reflected by a reduction in the forced expiratory volume measured in 1 second (FEV_1). Reversibility is noted if an increase of more than 15% in the FEV_1 is observed after giving a bronchodilator such as albuterol (Ventolin).

Blood Assays

Immunometric blood assays measure the total amount of IgE normally present in the circulation. Most studies have shown that blood concentrations of IgE are increased in the presence of allergic disease; however, a normal or even decreased level may occur in IgE-mediated sensitivities. Elevated serum eosinophil levels also may suggest hypersensitivities.

OUTCOME MANAGEMENT

Medical Management

Allergies are among the most common disorders seen in the medical community. The client often requires a combination of treatments, ranging from avoidance of known allergens to environmental control, immunotherapy, and follow-up.

Identify Allergen

It is imperative to obtain a detailed history that identifies any previous allergic problems in the client and also the presence of allergy in close family members, to perform a thorough assessment and examination, and to ensure that appropriate diagnostic tests are performed. The clinician must know the times of the year during which manifestations occur to determine a correct diagnosis on the basis of the offending allergen. If year-round manifestations are present, find out whether they are worse at any time. A careful search for environmental factors should be undertaken. The client should be questioned in detail regarding the home environment: location, type of heating, insulation, humidity, nature of the bedding, presence of carpeting, method of house cleaning, and so on.

Avoid Allergen

Avoidance of the allergen is often the easiest, cheapest, and safest way of dealing with allergies; however, identification of the specific allergen is sometimes difficult, especially if the client refuses, cannot afford, or cannot locate allergen-testing services. Even if the allergen can be identified, complete avoidance may not be possible, as with pollens and food additives.

Control Environment

Environmental control sometimes helps to eliminate airborne allergens. Figure 76-1 illustrates ways to desensitize a room. These environmental controls, combined with air filters that remove small particles from the air, can help to eliminate many allergens.

Administer Medications

Atopic clients benefit greatly from selected prescriptions and over-the-counter medications. Usually, clients self-administer these agents, although in some settings the nurse or a family member administers them. For more information on allergy medications, see the Integrating Pharmacology feature on p. 2047.

Promote Desensitization

Immunotherapy ("desensitization therapy") is designed for the treatment of type 1, IgE-mediated hypersensitivity reactions. Precise doses of allergens are injected at intervals over a prolonged period with the goal of altering the immune system's response to an allergen, thus reducing manifestations of rhinitis, sneezing, and generalized pruritus triggered by subsequent exposures. The doses are increased gradually over time, or injections may be given several times a day in increasing doses in "rush" protocols. Immunotherapy increases IgG antibody levels and may increase suppressor T-cell function. Specific IgG interferes with IgE binding to allergens and thus mitigates the hypersensitivity response. Immunotherapy is widely used in the treatment of allergic rhinitis (hay fever), for which its greatest success has been achieved because immunotherapy blunts the seasonal rise in specific IgE antibody levels. It also is used for Hymenoptera sensitivity (bee, yellow jacket, wasp, and hornet stings) with reportable success. There is some controversy regarding the efficacy of this treatment in the management of asthma.

Nurses often administer these injections and assess and treat side effects. Clients are asked to wait at least 30 to 40 minutes after receiving the injections so that immediate reactions can be treated. Side effects are similar to those seen in skin testing.

Nursing Management of the Medical Client

Assessment. As a nurse, you play a crucial role in obtaining a detailed medical history of the client and ensuring that appropriate diagnostic tests are performed. The most important part of evaluating the allergic client is the history. The history should elicit all the client's current manifestations. It is important for clinicians to know

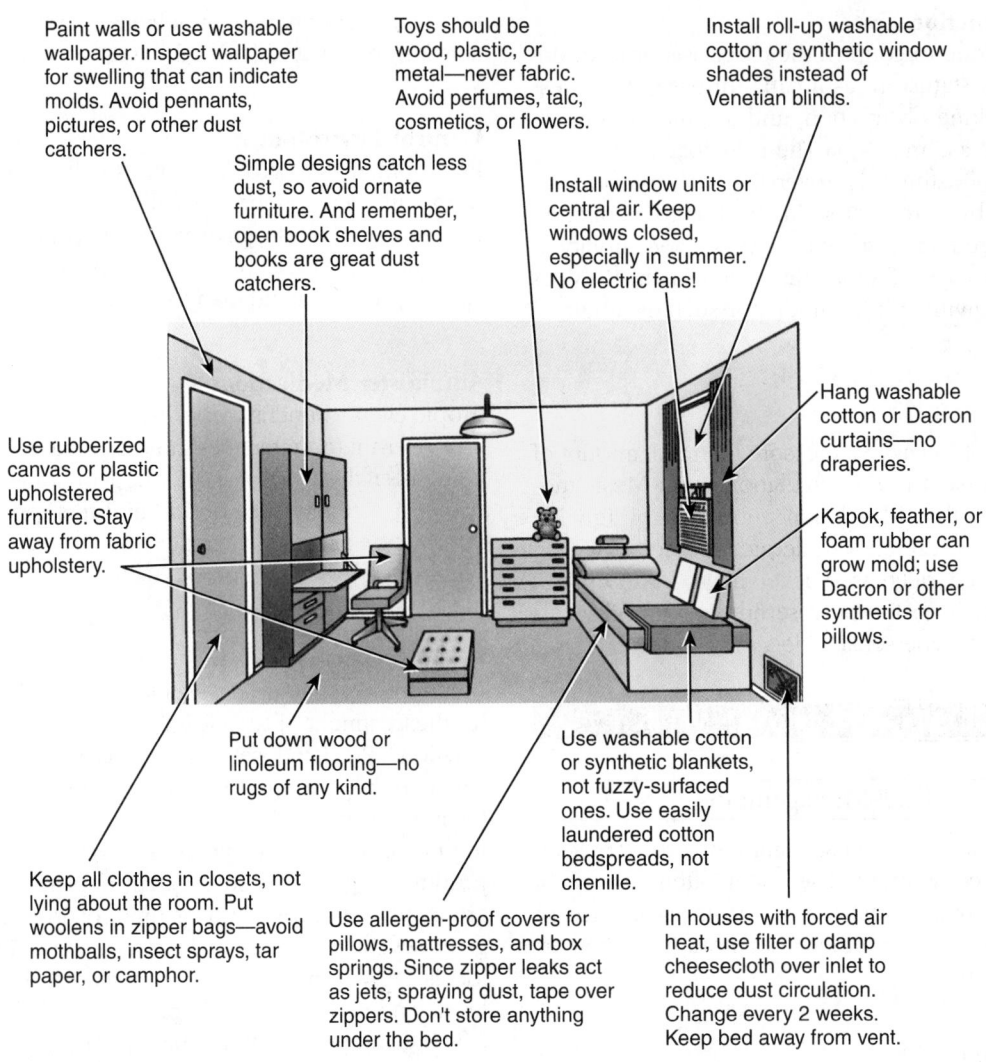

Paint walls or use washable wallpaper. Inspect wallpaper for swelling that can indicate molds. Avoid pennants, pictures, or other dust catchers.

Simple designs catch less dust, so avoid ornate furniture. And remember, open book shelves and books are great dust catchers.

Toys should be wood, plastic, or metal—never fabric. Avoid perfumes, talc, cosmetics, or flowers.

Install window units or central air. Keep windows closed, especially in summer. No electric fans!

Install roll-up washable cotton or synthetic window shades instead of Venetian blinds.

Use rubberized canvas or plastic upholstered furniture. Stay away from fabric upholstery.

Hang washable cotton or Dacron curtains—no draperies.

Kapok, feather, or foam rubber can grow mold; use Dacron or other synthetics for pillows.

Put down wood or linoleum flooring—no rugs of any kind.

Use washable cotton or synthetic blankets, not fuzzy-surfaced ones. Use easily laundered cotton bedspreads, not chenille.

Keep all clothes in closets, not lying about the room. Put woolens in zipper bags—avoid mothballs, insect sprays, tar paper, or camphor.

Use allergen-proof covers for pillows, mattresses, and box springs. Since zipper leaks act as jets, spraying dust, tape over zippers. Don't store anything under the bed.

In houses with forced air heat, use filter or damp cheesecloth over inlet to reduce dust circulation. Change every 2 weeks. Keep bed away from vent.

■ **FIGURE 76–1** Controlling the environment of a room. Dacron is a trade name for polyester. *(Courtesy A.H. Robins Co., Richmond, Va.)*

whether the manifestations are always present or what times of the year they worsen.

Indoor allergens are causing increasing amounts of distress. House dust mites and cockroach and animal allergens are problematic and are present year-round in many homes. Assess whether animals are present in the home and, if so, how many. Is the house filled with plants that could harbor mold spores? Is the client exposed to moist rooms, such as a basement, that is constantly damp?

Environmental factors such as smoke can exacerbate manifestations. Determining where these manifestations present is very important. Many occupations involve exposure to certain allergens such as smoke, latex, chemicals, and animals. Manifestations may be reported as worse during the workweek compared with the weekend. Inquiries such as these help to narrow down possible causes of manifestations.

Diagnosis, Outcomes, Interventions

Diagnosis: Health-Seeking Behaviors and Readiness for Enhanced Self-Care. The key nursing diagnoses for the client with hypersensitivity disorders is *Health-Seeking Behaviors* and *Readiness for Enhanced Self-Care related to the desire to learn about the disease process, treatment regimen, and risk control methods.*

Outcomes. The client will follow a mutually agreed on health maintenance plan that includes stated understanding of the disease process, treatment regimen, and control of risk factors.

Interventions

Provide Teaching. Although clients usually self-administer medications, as described under the medical management section, you are responsible for instructing clients and their significant others about these medications

Medications for Allergies

In addition to avoiding the allergen, several medications are available to minimize manifestations and decrease the inflammatory process.

Antihistamines are the major group of prescription and over-the-counter drugs used to alleviate the early phase allergic manifestations. These medications relieve sneezing, rhinitis, itching, and other manifestations of allergic rhinitis. They bind to the H_1 receptor. Traditional antihistamines such as diphenhydramine (Benadryl) pass the blood-brain barrier and can produce significant drowsiness. Because newer agents (cetirizine [Zyrtec], fexofenadine [Allegra], and loratadine [Claritin]) do not cross the blood-brain barrier (or do so poorly), they do not cause the drowsiness that limits the use of traditional medications.

Decongestants (oral sympathomimetics) such as pseudoephedrine and phenylephrine help relieve nasal congestion by stimulating the alpha-adrenergic receptors that control the capillary sphincters at the entrance to the venous plexuses of the turbinates. Nasal decongestants such as oxymetazoline hydrochloride and phenylephedrine sprays act primarily on turbinate swelling and are more effective and rapid in onset when used topically rather than orally. Because the prolonged use of topical nasal sprays can cause rhinitis medicamentosa (recurrence of congestion), however, it is advisable to limit their use to no more than 3 to 5 days. Practitioners are cautioned against the use of oral agents by clients with heart disease, hypertension, thyroid disease, diabetes, and urinary difficulties resulting from prostatic hypertrophy. These drugs can be combined with antihistamines to treat the multiple manifestations of allergy.

Corticosteroids, anti-inflammatory agents, and immunosuppressants can be used to treat allergic manifestations. Corticosteroids are the most effective drug for the treatment of rhinitis. Oral steroids are in general more effective and rapid in onset than topical forms, but their systemic effects can produce a myriad of complications. Topical steroid creams can be used to treat dermatitis. Beclomethasone dipropionate (Beconase), triamcinolone (Nasacort), flunisolide (Nasarel), budesonide (Rhinocort), and fluticasone (Flonase) are nasal sprays useful in treating allergic rhinitis, and they evoke few systemic side effects.

Cromolyn sodium is a topical or aerosol medication used to treat allergic rhinitis (Nasalcrom) and asthma (Intal). Its mechanism of action is not completely understood, but it helps prevent the release of chemical mediators (e.g., histamine and leukotrienes) by stabilizing mast cells during both immediate and late-phase reactions. Cromolyn sodium should be administered before allergen exposure. It should be started a week before allergy season to be most effective in the treatment of seasonal allergic rhinitis. It must be used on a regular basis and, unfortunately, dosing is required four to six times a day. Nasal steroids such as Flonase and Rhinocort are the mainstay of therapy for allergic rhinitis.

Inhaled steroids are fundamental to the treatment of asthma. New inhaled steroids with a greater topical potency ratio and fewer systemic effects allow greater control in asthma management. Fluticasone (Flovent), fluticasone and Serevent (Advair), triamcinolone (Azmacort), and beclomethasone (Vanceril) are examples of inhaled steroids.

Anticholinergics are used primarily to treat allergic rhinitis and rhinorrhea caused by the common cold. Ipratropium (Atrovent) was a major advance in the therapeutic regimen for asthma. It does not cross the blood-brain barrier and is relatively free of side effects. Anticholinergics inhibit the effects of acetylcholine by blocking its binding to receptors at neurotransmitter sites on glandular tissue, thereby decreasing the amount of watery discharge in clients with rhinitis. Anticholinergics are also available in oral forms in combination with antihistamines and decongestant preparations (Dura-Vent DA, Extendryl SR).

$Beta_2$ agonists are commonly used to control bronchospasm in asthma. Albuterol (Ventolin) and other short-acting bronchodilators have proved to be well tolerated. The drawback of the older bronchodilators is their short duration of action (only 4 to 6 hours), which limits their use for manifestations experienced at night. This problem has been addressed with the new generation of long-acting $beta_2$ agonists such as salmeterol (Serevent).

Anti-leukotrienes are used to treat manifestations of asthma and anaphylaxis. They block the synthesis or action of leukotriene mediators, which are known to contribute to airway edema, smooth muscle contraction, and the process of inflammation. These drugs include zafirlukast (Accolate), zileuton (Zyflo), and montelukast (Singulair).

The client needs to learn what the medication is, why it is being prescribed, how to take it, when to take it, and what the possible side effects might be. In addition, the client needs to know what to do during an anaphylactic reaction (see Anaphylaxis, Insect Sting Allergy, and Latex Allergy).

If an inhaler is prescribed, the client must be taught how to use it correctly (see Chapter 61). A spacer (an attachment added to the inhaler that holds the medication in the additional chamber or space until the client inhales) may be recommended to help the client obtain the maximal effect. Some clients are taught to perform desensitization injections themselves. In this case, teach clients the proper injection technique and the manifestations of any untoward reactions to the medications, such as shortness of breath, hoarseness, urticaria, and generalized flushing.

Clients may need to carry medications for anaphylaxis with them at all times. In such instances, clients should also wear a medical alert bracelet. Other nursing interventions are described in the following sections under specific disorders.

Evaluation. It is expected that the client will obtain relief from allergic manifestations when the treatment regimen is followed. The client will be able to avoid or control risk factors for allergic manifestations. Ideally, the client will be able to avoid anaphylactic events and obtain treatment before serious problems develop.

ALLERGIC DISORDERS

FOOD ALLERGY

Adverse food reactions can be classified in one of two ways: (1) *food allergies,* which occur by a specific IgE-mediated response to the offending food, such as food-induced anaphylaxis from peanuts; and (2) *food intolerances,* which do not result from an IgE-mediated response but cause manifestations such as diarrhea and vomiting. The prevalence of food intolerances is much higher than that of food allergies. Although food allergies can occur at any age, the condition is more common among infants and very young children, affecting about 8% of those under age 3.

A thorough history is the most important factor in the diagnosis of food allergy or intolerance. Eight foods account for nearly 90% of all food allergies: milk, eggs, peanuts, tree nuts, fish, shellfish, soybeans, and wheat. Fortunately, most food allergies are outgrown; however, allergies to peanuts, tree nuts, and shellfish are lifelong. Food allergies can be determined through skin testing. Food diaries (a record of events, including dietary intake for subsequent episodes) are used to provide insight for the correct diagnosis.

The standard of diagnosis in food allergy is the double-blind, placebo-controlled food challenge. The suspected food is eliminated from the diet for 10 to 14 days. Antihistamines are not to be taken for at least 24 hours before the challenge, and a fasting state should be maintained for 12 to 18 hours before testing. The challenge starts with the introduction of a very low dose of the suspected food, and the dose is gradually increased every 20 to 30 minutes until a reaction is noted or the amount of food present in a normal feeding is reached. *Elimination diets* are also used and consist of removing one food at a time until the adverse manifestations are relieved.

Measuring serum blood tryptase levels can also prove helpful because elevations in tryptase occur and are detectable in the blood for up to 2 hours after a severe systemic reaction. Negative results do not, however, rule out a positive reaction.

See the Bridge to Home Health Care website feature on Managing Immunosuppression and Nutrition.

ATOPIC DERMATITIS

Atopic dermatitis occurs in about 10% of the population. Clients typically have a history of or complaints about itchy skin, in addition to a history of rashes in the area of skin creases. Other common complaints are of generally dry skin initially experienced in children younger than 2 years of age, accompanied by manifestations of asthma, hay fever, or dermatitis. Lesions of atopic dermatitis are red and pruritic, contain exudates, and are maculopapular in younger clients, becoming drier and thicker as clients age (Figure 76-2). The lesions are typically found on the cheeks, scalp, and forehead; in later years, they may occur on the trunk and extremities.

Medical Management

Treatment is aimed at controlling and reducing the manifestations because there is no true cure. Antihistamines are used with good results to help alleviate the itch-scratch cycle that is common to atopic dermatitis.
The mainstay of therapy is topical corticosteroids, which control the inflammation in the skin lesions. Gels

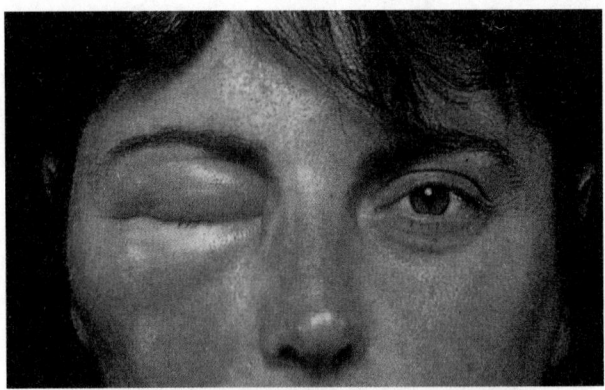

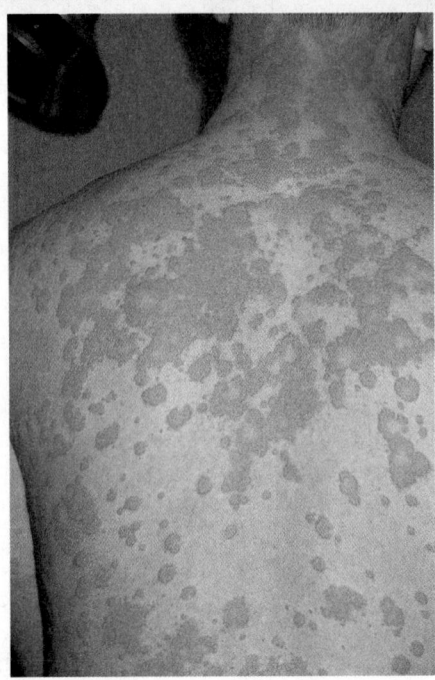

■ **FIGURE 76–2** Contact dermatitis.

penetrate more effectively but are drying. Ointments should be used in more severe cases because they promote hydration; however, some clients prefer not to use them because they are oily and become messy in the heat. Creams and lotions are the least penetrating but are preferred by most clients. They are absorbed quickly and promote comfort. Antibiotics may be needed to treat superficial skin infections caused by intense pruritus and scratching.

Nursing Management of the Medical Client

Teach clients the importance of environmental control. A key strategy is to minimize allergen exposure and physical stimuli that provoke pruritus. Explain that the client can reduce itching by avoiding severe changes in temperature, wearing loose cotton clothing, using gentle detergents, and rinsing clothing completely. Advise clients to avoid chemical irritants, emotional stress, aeroallergens such as dust and animal dander, and dietary allergens. Teach the client general skin care measures, such as how to perform the following:

1. Maintain good skin hydration by bathing in lukewarm water.
2. Use gentle soaps (e.g., Basis, Dove).
3. Apply a lubricant such as Alpha Keri, petroleum jelly, Eucerin, or Aquaphor to the skin immediately after bathing.
4. Avoid scratching.
5. Keep fingernails trimmed to avoid infection.

URTICARIA

Urticaria (or hives) is a cutaneous reaction associated with several different causes (Figure 76-3). It occurs in as many as 25% of all people at some time. Hives that are present daily or intermittently over a period of less than 6 weeks are termed *acute* urticaria. Hives present for more than 6 weeks are referred to as *chronic* urticaria.

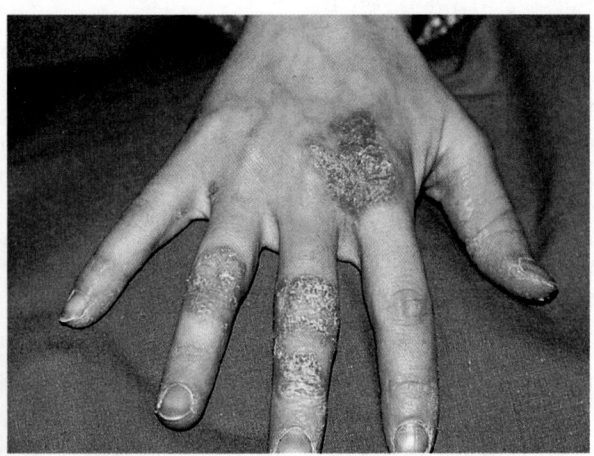

■ **FIGURE 76–3** Allergic urticaria.

Lesions of urticaria tend to be papules or plaques that fade within 24 hours. They do not leave areas of hyperpigmentation. Hives are round or oval and range in size from a few millimeters to several centimeters. Numerous agents can trigger the onset of urticaria: cold, heat, the sun, vibrations, rubbing, or pressure. Urticaria can also be caused by medications, foods, and infections.

Mast cells and their mediators may play a key role in urticaria, causing intense pruritus and vascular changes. A lesional skin biopsy to identify which types of inflammatory cells are present in the lesion is useful in structuring treatment. Some known provoking stimuli of urticaria are medications, foreign substances, foods and food additives, infections, insect bites and stings, contact irritants, inhalants, heat, cold, light, and pressure.

Medical Management

Although management focuses on identifying and eliminating any known causative factors, in about 80% of chronic cases no cause of urticaria is found. All clients with urticaria should be cautioned about aspirin and nonsteroidal anti-inflammatory drugs (NSAIDs), which may exacerbate existing hives. Opiates should be used cautiously as well because they are typically mast cell degranulators.

Antihistamines are the mainstay of therapy for urticaria. Nonsedating antihistamines are recommended during the day; more sedating antihistamines may be preferred at night. Doxepin (Sinequan), a tricyclic antidepressant, is sometimes used for treatment because of its actions on both H_1 and H_2 receptors. Corticosteroids should not be used except for short-term therapy.

Nursing Management of the Medical Client

Urticaria tends to evoke anxiety and frustration in both clients and clinicians. The most effective treatment is to eliminate any triggers. Help the client identify factors that may be suspect, and suggest elimination diets and challenges if foods or food additives are thought to provoke manifestations. Encourage clients to avoid initiating physical factors, such as pressure from tight clothing, heat, vibration, sunlight, and rubbing of the skin. Good skin hydration is mandatory; counsel the client to avoid harsh soaps and irritants and to apply moisturizing lotions after bathing while the skin is still damp.

ANAPHYLAXIS, INSECT STING ALLERGY, AND LATEX ALLERGY

The most common causes of anaphylaxis are drugs, foods, latex exposure, and insect bites and stings. Common food offenders in adults are peanuts, tree nuts, and shellfish (Box 76-1). Insect stings cause many deaths

BOX 76-1 Common Agents Causing Anaphylaxis

DRUGS
- Penicillins (most common)
- Cephalosporins
- Tetracyclines
- Streptomycin
- Kanamycin
- Neomycin
- Heparin
- Protamine
- Vancomycin
- Amphotericin B
- Polymyxin
- Bacitracin
- Aspirin, other anti-inflammatory agents
- Colchicine
- Tranquilizers

FOODS
- Peanuts
- Seafood
- Eggs
- Nuts
- Milk
- Citrus fruits
- Strawberries
- Legumes

INSECT VENOMS
- Hymenoptera (honeybees, wasps, yellow jackets, hornets, fire ants)

BIOLOGICALS
- Heterologous antisera (especially equine)
- Enzymes
- Hormones
- Vaccines (especially egg-cultured types)

BLOOD PRODUCTS
- Plasma
- Cryoprecipitate
- Whole blood
- Gamma-globulin

ALLERGEN EXTRACTS
- Skin-testing agents
- Desensitization

DIAGNOSTIC AGENTS
- Sulfobromophthalein
- Iodinated contrast media

tract obstruction, which can occur immediately and without other manifestations, are the primary cause of death from anaphylaxis. Although manifestations usually begin 5 to 30 minutes after the offending trigger has been encountered, there can be a delay of an hour or more. The more rapid the onset, the more severe the episode.

The incidence of anaphylaxis related to insect stings ranges from 0.3% to 3% in the general population. The sting insects are members of the order Hymenoptera. People may be allergic to one or all of the stinging insects, but the sting of the yellow jacket is the most common cause of allergy. Common reactions to an insect sting include pain, swelling, and redness that may be localized or may extend over a large area. The swelling usually peaks in 24 to 48 hours and may last for 7 to 10 days. There are no factors that identify those at potential risk for anaphylaxis from an insect sting other than a prior history. Those who have had severe anaphylaxis have an 80% chance of another reaction.

Health care workers are at particular risk for latex allergy. About 700,000 health care workers are affected. Workers with allergies to latex also have a high incidence of reactions to certain foods, such as chestnuts, bananas, kiwi, avocado, apricot, and papaya. Manifestations range from simple dermatitis to generalized itching, urticaria, sneezing, coughing, wheezing, hypotension, and shock on exposure. The diagnosis of type 1 hypersensitivity to latex is confirmed by in vivo skin testing with raw latex extracts or in vitro blood assays that measure specific IgE responses to latex.

Medical Management

Anaphylaxis is treated by (1) administering epinephrine, (2) removing or discontinuing the causative agent, (3) administering emergency oxygen, (4) maintaining an open airway, (5) placing the client in the Trendelenburg position, and (6) giving supportive IV fluids, such as 0.9% normal saline or lactated Ringer's solution as necessary.

Nursing Management of the Medical Client

The nursing diagnoses *Risk for Latex Allergy Response* and *Latex Allergy Response* are more specific nursing diagnoses for latex allergy reactions. Most of the interventions for these diagnoses have been described under the nursing diagnoses *Health-Seeking Behaviors* and *Readiness for Enhanced Self-Care*. In addition, the incidence and severity of anaphylactic reactions are decreased by both general and specific measures.

Take a thorough history for drug, food, insect, pollen, and animal allergies from every client. Counsel all clients with a history of anaphylaxis or anaphylactic-like reactions to carry epinephrine with them at all

in the United States every year. The incidence of anaphylaxis related to latex exposure, especially in health care workers, has dramatically increased since the 1990s with the increased use of latex gloves.

Anaphylactic events commonly present with hives and angioedema and often with dyspnea, wheezing, syncope, hypotension, nausea, vomiting, diarrhea, abdominal pain, flushing, headache, rhinitis, substernal pain, and itching. Cardiovascular collapse, shock, and respiratory

times in the form of an EpiPen or Ana-Kit for self-injection. Recommend that they carry a medical alert bracelet or necklace and an identification card in their wallet or purse and that they register with the proper authorities.

ALLERGIC RHINITIS

Manifestations of allergic rhinitis are persistent and show seasonal variation. Nasal manifestations are often accompanied by eye irritation, which causes pruritus, erythema, and excessive tearing. Numerous allergens may cause these manifestations, such as tree pollens (most common in the spring), grasses (summer), ragweed (fall), or dust mites and animal dander (year-round).

When the nasal mucosa is exposed to an allergen, a series of events is set in motion. Allergen exposure increases the production of IgE, which binds to the receptors on mast cells and basophils and eventually causes a release of mediators. The mediator release leads to increased swelling and congestion, watery discharge, sneezing, and nasal itching that persists for a period of at least 1 hour per day.

Medical Management

Avoidance therapy, symptomatic therapy, and immunotherapy are the three types of management for allergic rhinitis. Nasal glucocorticoid sprays are used with good results for the treatment of allergic rhinitis. The newer, nonsedating antihistamines are beneficial in maintaining control over allergic rhinitis and are a crucial component of therapy. Sympathomimetic agents such as pseudoephedrine help to vasoconstrict the nasal mucous membranes but should be used for short-term therapy only.

Nursing Management of the Medical Client

Educating the client is the most important component of therapy. Teach clients to avoid allergens and to use air filters and air conditioning. Emphasize that compliance with medication is essential. Explain the reasoning behind daily medication use as well as how to adjust the medication to control minor flare-ups and to prevent progression of the disease.

ASTHMA

Because the diagnosis and treatment of asthma account for a substantial number of outpatient visits in allergy clinics, a heightened awareness and thorough understanding of the disease are warranted. See Chapter 61 for a thorough discussion of asthma management.

CONCLUSIONS

The immune system is a complex, interrelated system that affects the whole body. As a nurse, you must understand immune responses to provide clients with complete and individualized care. Because the care of these clients requires multifaceted interventions, you must be able to develop and implement complex care plans to meet their needs.

THINKING CRITICALLY

1. L.S. is a 41-year-old woman admitted for surgery. After surgery, she was to receive prophylactic IV cephalosporin but received a dose of penicillin by mistake. She has a known allergy to penicillin. With a history of allergy to penicillin, what type of hypersensitivity reaction is L.S. most likely to experience? Using the concepts of hypersensitivity, explain this process.

Factors to Consider. What reactions might the nurse expect? What should be the nurse's first actions? What medications might the nurse expect the physician to prescribe to treat this reaction? How can such a reaction be prevented from occurring in the future?

2. A.W. is a 21-year-old college student admitted with an asthmatic attack that has not responded to his usual treatments. He is admitted for a course of IV medications and respiratory treatments. When you enter the room to start the IV line, his wheezing is audible. He is also anxious and gasping for air. What actions should you implement? What problems might you experience when you start the IV line?

Factors to Consider. After the acute phase is over, what might the nurse assess to determine the cause of the asthma attack and why the typical interventions were unsuccessful? What additional teaching might be required?

3. R.H. is a newly graduated registered nurse on an oncology unit. She has been wearing gloves more than ever during the past 2 weeks following orientation. A rash develops on her hands, and she complains of itching all over her body. What type of allergic reaction might be occurring? What actions to assess the allergy should be taken?

Factors to Consider. Can R.H. expect to continue in her new job? Does the organization have a responsibility to keep her employed?

Discussions for these questions can be found on the website. **evolve**

BIBLIOGRAPHY

Citations appearing in red refer to primary research.

Citations appearing in blue refer to evidence-based practice guidelines and protocols.

1. Brown, S. (2006). Anaphylaxis: Clinical concepts and research priorities. *Emergency Medicine Australasia, 18*(2), 155-169.

2. Casale, T., et al. (2001). Effect of omalizumab on symptoms of seasonal allergic rhinitis: A randomized controlled trial. *Journal of the American Medical Association, 286*(23), 2956-2968.

3. Craig, T.J. (2002). Allergic rhinitis remains an important disease. *Journal of the American Osteopathic Association, 102*(6 Suppl 2), S1-S2.

4. DiLorenzo, G. (2006). Is there a role for antileukotrienes in urticaria? *Clinical and Experimental Dermatology, 31*(Issue 3), 327-334.

5. Mohrenschlager, M. (2006). Atopic eczema: What's new? *Journal of the European Academy of Dermatology and Venereology, 20*(5), 503-513.

6. Price, D. (2006). International primary care respiratory group (IPCRG) guidelines: Management of allergic rhinitis. *Primary Care Respiratory Journal, 15*(1), 58-70.

7. Rote, N. (2006). Alterations in immunity and inflammation. In K. McCance & S. Huether (Eds.), *Pathophysiology: The biologic basis for disease in adults and children* (5th ed., pp. 249-291). St. Louis: Mosby.

8. Rote, N., & Trask, B. (2006). Adaptive immunity. In K. McCance & S. Huether (Eds.), *Pathophysiology: The biologic basis for disease in adults and children* (5th ed., pp. 211-248). St. Louis: Mosby.

9. Ryan, D. (2005). Management of allergic problems in primary care: Time for a rethink? *Primary Care Respiratory Journal, 14*(4), 195-203.

10. Solomon, W. (2003). Atopic dermatitis and urticaria. In S. Price & L. Wilson (Eds.), *Pathophysiology: Clinical concepts of disease processes* (6th ed., pp. 149-153). St. Louis: Mosby.

11. Solomon, W. (2003). Bronchial asthma: Allergic and otherwise. In S. Price & L. Wilson (Eds.), *Pathophysiology: Clinical concepts of disease processes* (6th ed., pp. 139-148). St. Louis: Mosby.

12. Solomon, W. (2003). Familiar (IgE-mediated) allergic disorders: Anaphylaxis and the atopic diseases. In S. Price & L. Wilson (Eds.), *Pathophysiology: Clinical concepts of disease processes* (6th ed., pp. 129-138). St. Louis: Mosby.

13. Sommers, M. (2003). Alterations in immunocompetence. In V. Carrieri-Kohlman, A. Lindsay, & C. West (Eds.), *Pathophysiological phenomena in nursing: Human responses to illness* (3rd ed., pp. 297-317). Philadelphia: Saunders.

14. Walker, S. (2005). Management of urticaria. *Primary Care Respiratory Journal, 14*(3), 166-168.

15. Willsie, S.K. (2002). Improved strategies and new treatment options for allergic rhinitis. *Journal of the American Osteopathic Association, 102*(6 Suppl 2), S7-S14.

CHAPTER 77

Management of Clients with Rheumatic Disorders

PATRICIA A. MACDONALD

Rheumatic disorders comprise autoimmune and inflammatory disorders, which have been called "the primary crippling diseases" of the developed world. The term arthritis literally means "inflammation of a joint" but arthritis is actually a collection of more than 100 related, but distinct, conditions. Approximately 49% of all Americans older than 65 feel that they have arthritis; this is 1 in every 7 Americans and 1 in every 3 families. The Centers for Disease Control and Prevention (CDC) reports that 70 million Americans currently suffer from arthritis and that by 2035 more than 20% of the U.S. population will be 65 years of age or older. Arthritis is the primary reason for work-related disability and is the leading cause of disability among people ages 65 or older.

Given the high prevalence and significant impact of rheumatic disorders in terms of economic, functional, social, and psychological consequences, these disorders should receive considerable attention from us all. The United Nations, the World Health Organization, and 37 countries have proclaimed the years 2000 to 2010 as the Bone and Joint Decade. This global initiative is intended to improve the lives of people with musculoskeletal disorders, such as arthritis, and to advance understanding and treatment of musculoskeletal disorders through prevention, education, and research. A consortium of national organizations produced the *National Arthritis Action Plan: A Public Health Strategy,* a comprehensive and ambitious plan for addressing the management of arthritis. In addition, autoimmunity was named a major priority women's health issue by the Office of Research on Women's Health, a unit of the National Institutes of Health, as these disorders target women 75% of the time. As the incidence of autoimmune and inflammatory disorders continues to rise, research efforts focus on the role of overuse, injury, obesity, gene defects, infection, immunosuppression, amino acids, interleukin, and environmental agents in both the development and the treatment of these life-altering diseases. The ultimate goals in managing rheumatic disorders are to relieve pain and clinical manifestations, assuage psychological distress, improve physical function, and generally aid in the well-being of the client. Equally important, however, are interventions to prevent and ameliorate socioeconomic problems. A majority of the costs, both economic and social, are due to lost function rather than direct medical costs. Until a cure for the many types of rheumatic disorders is found or far more effective therapies to prevent joint damage and physical disability are developed, people will continue to suffer severe, premature economic and social dislocations that will seriously affect their lives. As the population ages, society can expect that these impacts will mushroom.

Rheumatic disorders are characterized by chronic pain and progressive physical impairment of joints and soft tissues. They encompass more than 100 diseases and conditions including osteoarthritis (OA) (discussed in Chapter 26), rheumatoid arthritis (RA), psoriatic arthritis (PsA), systemic lupus erythematosus (SLE), fibromyalgia syndrome (FMS), systemic sclerosis (SSc), ankylosing spondylitis (AS), reactive arthritis, polymyositis (PM), dermatomyositis (DM), vasculitis, bursitis, polymyalgia rheumatica, and Lyme disease.

Because RA is the classic autoimmune and inflammatory disease, it is helpful to refer to the discussion of RA while studying the other disorders, which are outlined in

---

evolve **Web Enhancements**

Bridge to Home Health Care Increasing Independent Living with Rheumatoid Arthritis

Web Tables Extra-Articular Manifestations of Rheumatoid Arthritis

Common Diagnostic Studies Used in Rheumatic Disorders

Principles of Joint Protection and Associated Work Simplification Strategies

Be sure to check out the bonus material on the Evolve website and the CD-ROM, including free self-assessment exercises. **http://evolve.elsevier.com/Black/medsurg**

Chapter 26. Although the conditions have different clinical patterns, pain and impaired mobility are common problems among clients with these disorders.

Clinical trials and their results are used to support evidence-based practice (EBP). The American College of Rheumatology has set the standard for what is an acceptable indicator of disease improvement. The difficulty in evaluating the results of clinical trials is due to differences in designs (single agent vs. combination) and differences in client populations (early vs. late disease, rheumatoid factor positive vs. negative). Standardizing clinical trial designs ensures that the efficacy and safety of the treatments for rheumatic disorders is clearly demonstrated, subjectively as well as objectively, leading to the practice of evidence-based medicine. The treatment of RA is explored in the Translating Evidence into Practice feature on p. 2055.

AUTOIMMUNITY

Relationships between altered immune function and rheumatic disease are better understood as a result of continued research efforts. Autoimmune diseases are defined as conditions in which immunologic self-tolerance has been disrupted, with resultant damage to body tissues or cells normally recognized as self. Autoimmune disorders with muscle and joint involvement include SLE, RA, dermatomyositis (DM), scleroderma (SSc), Sjögren's syndrome, and mixed connective tissue disease.

To understand systemic, arthritic autoimmune diseases, it is important to briefly review key components of the immune system. Please see the anatomy and physiology review of the hematopoietic system at the beginning of Unit 17.

The ability of the immune system to distinguish self from non-self depends in large part on cell-surface antigens. These antigens (which are unique to every person) are encoded by a large cluster of genes called the *major histocompatibility complex* (MHC) located on the short end of chromosome 6. Histocompatibility antigens are also more typically referred to as *human leukocyte antigens* (HLAs) because they were first discovered on leukocytes. Seven closely related gene loci have been identified: HLA-A, HLA-B, HLA-C, HLA-D, HLA-DR, HLA-DQ, and HLA-DP. Each of these gene loci is occupied by multiple alleles (alternate genes) that code the development of each surface antigen. At least 23 gene products are associated with the HLA-A group, and 47 are associated with the HLA-B group.

HLAs have been categorized into two groups. Found on the surface of nucleated cells, class I antigens include HLA-A, HLA-B, and HLA-C. Class II antigens (D, DR, DQ, and DP) are found on macrophage and B cells, among others.

As a result of aberrations in HLA activity genetic coding, the body may lose some of its ability to recognize and differentiate self from non-self, resulting in autoimmune disorders. In other words, the body has decreased self-tolerance. Abnormalities of the HLA system, however, are but one key to the development of autoimmunity. Other factors involve abnormal T-cell or B-cell reactivity, resulting in altered recognition of foreign antigens and self by the immune system. For example, altered T-cell function has been implicated in the pathogenesis of arthritic diseases, such as RA. Research has begun to identify the specific roles of various T cells in these disease processes. For example, $CD4^+$ T cells have been shown to have a crucial role in the pathogenesis of arthritis, and $CD8^+$ T cells may play an immunoregulatory role. In addition, research suggests that B cells in the synovial membrane of joints expand as a result of local antigen stimulation. It is also likely that the immune system can be altered by interactions with chemical, environmental, viral, and bacterial agents.

Another important aspect of autoimmune disease is familial aggregation (or clustering), which suggests that there is a genetic predisposition to the development of specific disorders. This possibility is not surprising because an individual's HLA type is inherited. Indeed, some HLA types appear more frequently in certain disease conditions. For example, in Caucasians HLA-B27 appears in 80% to 90% of people with ankylosing spondylitis but in only 7% to 10% of the general population.

RHEUMATOID ARTHRITIS

Rheumatoid arthritis (RA) is a chronic, systemic autoimmune disorder whose major distinctive feature is chronic, symmetrical, and erosive inflammation of the synovial tissue of joints. The severity of the joint disease may fluctuate over time, but progressive development of various degrees of joint destruction, deformity, and disability is the most common outcome of established disease. Associated nonarticular manifestations may include subcutaneous nodules, vasculitis, pulmonary nodules or interstitial fibrosis, and pericarditis.

Rheumatoid arthritis occurs worldwide and affects all racial and ethnic groups. It can occur at any time of life, but its incidence tends to increase with age, peaking between the fourth and sixth decades. Women are affected two to three times more often than men. Clients with RA have a substantially reduced life expectancy, and mortality can be predicted, in most instances, by more severe clinical status.

The incidence of RA is estimated to range from 0.5% to 1.5% of the population. After age 55, the incidence rates for men and women are estimated to be 2% and 5%, respectively. Incidence rates for African Americans are similar to those for Caucasian Americans. RA appears to be a relatively "recent" disease. It was first described

TRANSLATING EVIDENCE INTO PRACTICE

Rheumatoid Arthritis Treatment

Have new pharmacologic treatments made a difference in treatment outcomes for rheumatoid arthritis (RA)? RA is a chronic, systemic autoimmune disorder whose major distinctive feature is exhibited primarily by chronic, symmetrical, and erosive inflammation of the synovial tissue of joints. Pharmacologic treatment of this disorder is one of the most thoroughly researched areas in the treatment of rheumatic disorders. However, this has not always been true. Many of the early treatments were based on anecdotal reports written by health care providers about clients treated within their own practice.

Careful review of the literature relating to new therapies as well as new evidence about older treatment standards is necessary. Recent studies that address the use of biologic response modifiers (BRMs) in addition to the more traditional disease-modifying antirheumatic drugs (DMARDs) have been reviewed. As a result of these studies, much more is known about RA, its progression, and the damage that occurs to joints without overt clinical manifestations.

All 10 of the studies used double-blind, controlled methods to evaluate the medications studied. Many measured ACR20 and Sharp Scores as recommended by the American College of Rheumatology.[2,3,5-7,9] Others used quality of life measurement instruments or radiographic findings.[1,4,5,7,8-10]

Methotrexate (MTX) and placebo were found to be less effective than methotrexate and infliximab combined[1] or MTX and abatacept combined.[4,10] Findings also found that combination therapy of MTX with adalimumab was superior to either MTX alone or adalimumab alone;[2] in addition, MTX with etanercept was superior to either MTX alone or etanercept alone.[8] Etanercept was also found to decrease fatigue for nearly 4 years in clients who received it.[7] Adalimumab was more effective than placebo at inhibiting the progression of structural joint damage, reducing the clinical manifestations of RA, and improving physical function in clients with active RA who had demonstrated an incomplete response to MTX.[6] Similarly, clients with an incomplete response to DMARDs showed improved responses when etanercept or infliximab was added to the treatment regimen.[3]

Dosages of 5 mg/day of prednisolone[9] or infliximab[3,5,9] in combination with DMARD therapy substantially decreased radiographic progression in early RA clients.[3,5,9] The use of more than one drug provided better outcomes than did single use of a drug.[1-5,8,9]

However, one study reported increased rates of serious adverse advents when abatacept was combined with DMARDs.[10]

Greater joint damage at baseline was associated with poorer physical function at baseline and less improvement in physical function after treatment, underlining the importance of early intervention to slow the progression of joint destruction.[1]

IMPLICATIONS

The most common finding was the improvement in clients who received more than one DMARD for the treatment of RA. Additional research is needed to determine whether continued long-term use of multiple agents will result in less progression of RA over time while also limiting adverse side effects. As more pharmacologic agents are introduced for treatment of RA, the nurse will need to monitor results of studies according to ACR20, Sharp, and other scores that measure client outcomes associated with treatment of rheumatoid arthritis. All of these agents have potential toxic side effects that need to be monitored closely by the nurse and the client.

REFERENCES

1. Breedveld, F., Han, C., et al. (2005). Association between baseline radiographic damage and improvement in physical function after treatment of patients with rheumatoid arthritis. *Annals of the Rheumatic Diseases, 64*(1), 52-55.
2. Breedveld, F., Weisman, M., et al. (2006). The PREMIER study: A multicenter, randomized, double-blind clinical trial of combination therapy with adalimumab plus methotrexate versus methotrexate alone or adalimumab alone in patients with early, aggressive rheumatoid arthritis who had not had previous methotrexate treatment. *Arthritis and Rheumatism, 54*(1), 26-27.
3. De Filippis, L., et al. (2006). Improving outcomes in tumor necrosis factor α treatment: Comparison of the efficacy of the tumor necrosis factor vs blocking agents etanercept and infliximab in patients with active rheumatoid arthritis. *PAN Minerva Medica, 48*(2), 129-135.
4. Emery, P., et al. (2006). Treatment of rheumatoid arthritis patients with abatacept and methotrexate significantly improved health-related quality of life. *The Journal of Rheumatology, 33*(4), 681-689.
5. Goekoop-Ruiterman, Y., et al. (2005). Clinical and radiographic outcomes of four different treatment strategies in patients with early rheumatoid arthritis (the BeSt study): A randomized, controlled trial. *Arthritis and Rheumatism, 52*(11), 3381-3390.
6. Keystone, E., et al. (2004). Radiographic, clinical, and functional outcomes of treatment with adalimumab (a human anti-tumor necrosis factor monoclonal antibody) in patients with active rheumatoid arthritis, receiving concomitant methotrexate therapy: A randomized, placebo-controlled, 52-week trial. *Arthritis and Rheumatism, 50*(5), 1400-1411.
7. Moreland, L., et al. (2006). Effect of etanercept on fatigue in patients with recent or established rheumatoid arthritis. *Arthritis and Rheumatism, 55*(2), 287-293.
8. Van der Heijde, D. (2006). Patient reported outcomes in a trial of combination therapy with etanercept and methotrexate for rheumatoid arthritis: The TEMPO trial. *Annals of the Rheumatic Diseases, 65*(3), 328-334.
9. Wassenberg, S., et al. (2005). Very low-dose prednisolone in early rheumatoid arthritis retards radiograph progression over two years: A multicenter, double-blind, placebo-controlled trial. *Arthritis and Rheumatism, 52*(11), 3371-3380.
10. Weinblatt, M., et al. (2006). Safety of the selective costimulation modulator abatacept in rheumatoid arthritis patients receiving background biologic and non biologic disease-modifying antirheumatic drugs: A one-year randomized, placebo-controlled study. *Arthritis and Rheumatism, 54*(9), 2807-2816.

in the mid-18th century and has not been found in skeletal remains from ancient European or Asian civilizations. However, erosive polyarthritis has been documented in the skeletons of prehistoric (3000 to 5000 years ago) Native Americans, which might indicate an infectious agent confined to a small geographic area before the 18th century.

Etiology and Risk Factors

RA is characterized by the presence of rheumatoid factor (RF), an autoantibody directed against immunoglobulin G (IgG), in more than 80% of those with the disease. In addition to RF, antibodies against collagen, Epstein-Barr virus, encoded nuclear antigen, and certain other antigens have been identified. The role of autoantibodies in RA is still unclear, but research has focused attention on pre-illness immunologic status. Antikeratin antibody (AKA) and anti-perinuclear factor (APF) appear to be markers that predict the development of RA in RF-positive clients. However, RA develops in only a proportion of cases. Other immunogenetic markers may aid in the identification of clients with early RA and those with more severe disease.

Genetic factors are important in the epidemiology of the disease. A genetic predisposition for RA is seen with a higher concordance rate of 32% in identical twins rather than the 9% rate observed in fraternal twins. Research suggests that the consistent reports by female RA clients that joint pain and swelling disappear during pregnancy, may be due to the genetic differences between mother and fetus. This is an exciting area for continuing research. The strongest genetic evidence, however, is seen in the association of RA with HLA-DR4, a genetically determined allele of the MHC on the short arm of chromosome 6.

Pathophysiology

The histologic changes in RA are not disease specific but largely depend on the organ involved. The primary joint lesion involves the synovium. Rheumatoid factor (RF) antibodies develop there against the immunoglobulin IgG, the largest of the five classes of immunoglobulins, to form immune complexes. Ironically, immunoglobulins (IgG) are natural human antibodies. It is not clear, however, why the body produces an antibody (RF) against its own antibody (IgG) and, in effect, transforms IgG to an antigen or foreign protein that must be destroyed. The products of macrophages and lymphocytes are thought to have critical roles in the pathogenesis of RA, as part of the immune response to an unidentified antigen. Moreover, it is the formation of these antibody-antigen immune complexes that leads to the activation of the complement system and the release of lysosomal enzymes from leukocytes. Both of these reactions cause inflammation. Initial research has demonstrated that interleukin-8, known as neutrophil-activating peptide 1 (NAP-1), has a definite role in the inflammatory process of RA and that circulating autoantibodies may provide a clinically useful marker for RA severity. With the initial formation of immune complexes, synovitis develops as the synovial membrane becomes swollen, irritated, and inflamed.

As the immune complexes are deposited onto the synovial membrane or the superficial layers of the articular cartilage, they are phagocytized by polymorphonuclear (PMN) leukocytes, monocytes, and lymphocytes. Unfortunately, phagocytosis deactivates the immune complexes and simultaneously produces additional enzymes (oxygen radicals, arachidonic acid) that lead to hyperemia, edema, swelling, and thickening of the synovial lining. The hypertrophied synovium literally invades the surrounding tissue, including cartilage, ligaments, joint capsule, and tendons. Eventually, granulation tissue forms to cover the entire articular cartilage, leading to the formation of *pannus,* a highly vascularized fibrous scar tissue composed of lymphocytes, macrophages, histiocytes, fibroblasts, and mast cells. Undoubtedly the most destructive element in RA, pannus can erode and destroy articular cartilage, eventually resulting in subchondral bone erosions, bone cysts, fissures, and development of bone spurs and osteophytes. Research has concluded that tumor necrosis factor (TNF) is produced by cells at the cartilage-pannus junction and may lead to cartilage destruction. Pannus can also scar and shorten tendons and ligaments, leading in turn to ligamentous laxity, subluxation, and contractures. The Concept Map on p. 2057 explores the pathophysiology and treatment of rheumatoid arthritis.

Clinical Manifestations

Rheumatoid arthritis may be mild and relapsing, involving a few joints for a brief period, or markedly progressive, with the development of deformities and severe systemic disease. Overall, RA is characterized by cycles of exacerbation and remission, the duration of which adds to the feelings of powerlessness and uncertainty that clients often experience, A small percentage of clients have severely progressive disease that does not respond to aggressive therapy.

Table 77-1 illustrates the seven criteria for the 1987 revised American College of Rheumatology (ACR) classification of RA. The 1987 criteria for the classification of RA serve as a framework for the clinical diagnosis. The classification system, however, is not intended to explicitly define diagnosis. It is important to remember that RA is a clinical diagnosis. Other findings, including the results of laboratory tests, radiologic examination, and synovial fluid analysis, help to confirm the diagnosis. The criteria highlight the symmetrical involvement of inflamed joints of the wrist, the metacarpophalangeal (MCP) joints, and the proximal interphalangeal (PIP)

CONCEPT MAP

Understanding Rheumatoid Arthritis and Its Treatment

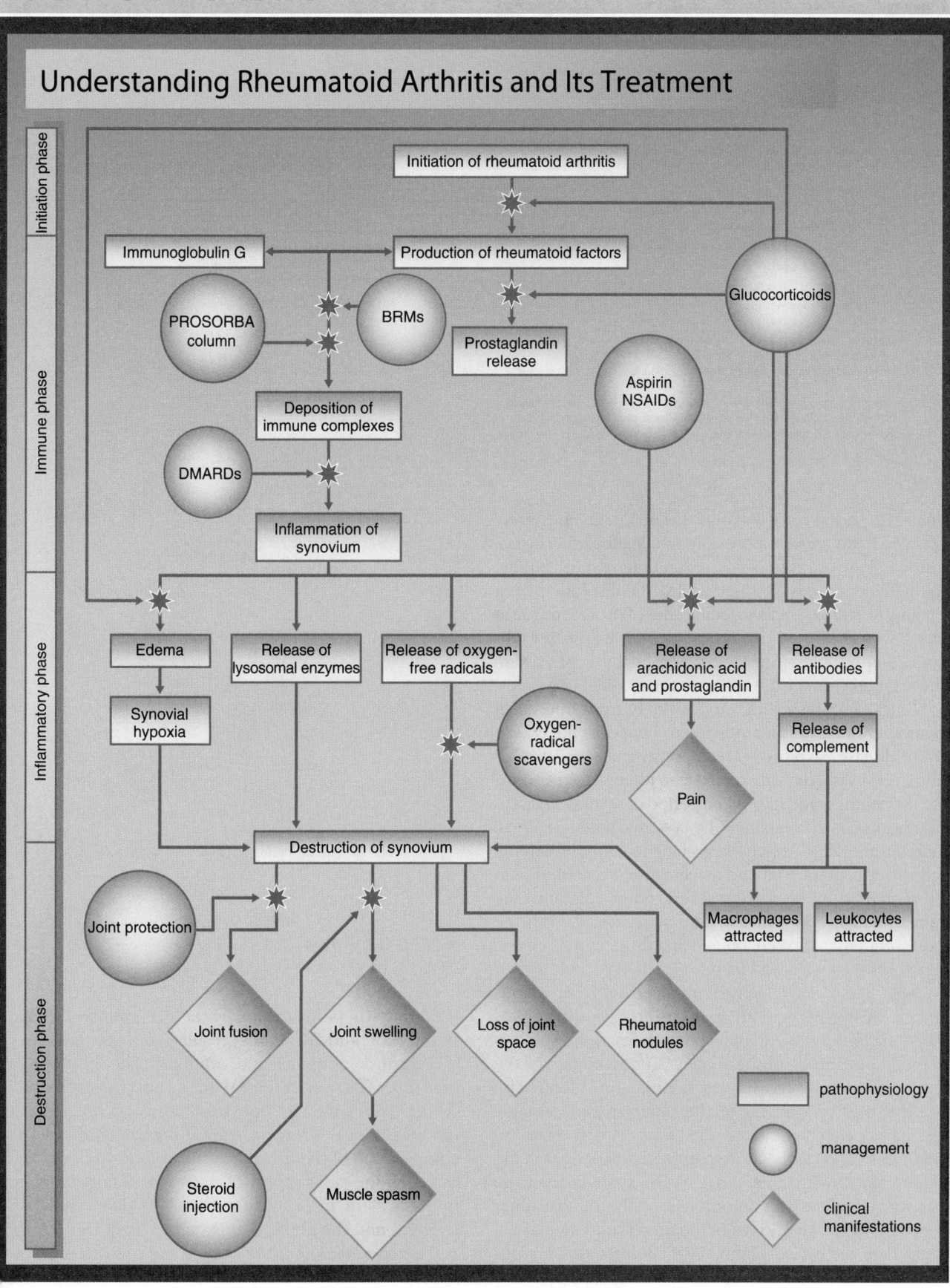

TABLE 77-1 1987 Revised Criteria of the American Rheumatism Association for the Classification of Rheumatoid Arthritis*

Criterion	Description
1	Morning stiffness in and around joints lasting at least 1 hr before maximal improvement
2	Soft tissue swelling (arthritis) of three or more joint areas (including right and left PIP,[†] MCP, wrist, elbow, knee, ankle, and MTP joints)
3	Swelling of at least one wrist, MCP, or PIP joint
4	Simultaneous symmetrical swelling in joints listed in criterion 2
5	Subcutaneous rheumatoid nodules
6	Presence of rheumatoid factor
7	Radiographic erosions or periarticular osteopenia in hand or wrist joints

* Note: Rheumatoid arthritis is defined by the presence of four or more criteria. Criteria 1 through 4 must have been present for at least 6 weeks. The American Rheumatism Association 1987 revised criteria for the classification of rheumatoid arthritis.
† MCP, Metacarpophalangeal; MTP, metatarsophalangeal; PIP, proximal interphalangeal.
Data from Arnett, F.C., et al. (1988). The American Rheumatism Association 1987 revised criteria for the classification of rheumatoid arthritis. *Arthritis and Rheumatism, 31*, 315-324.

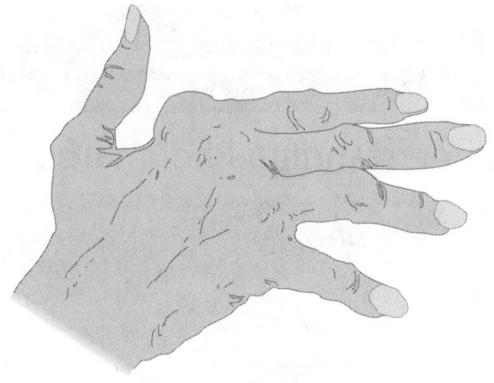

Ulnar drift

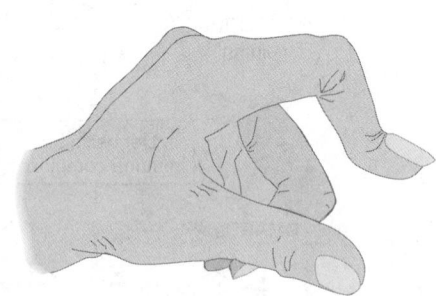

Boutonnière deformity

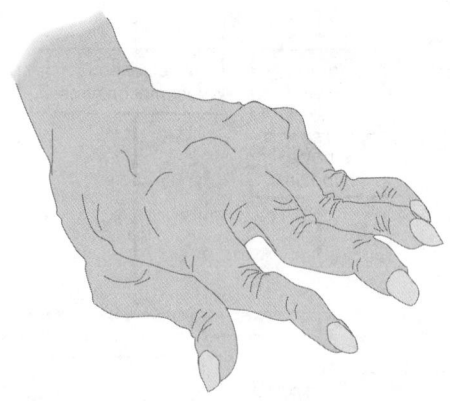

Swan-neck deformity

■ **FIGURE 77-1** Three types of hand deformity characteristic of clients with rheumatoid arthritis.

joints. The distal interphalangeal (DIP) joints are rarely involved in RA and are more commonly affected in osteo-arthritis. Four or more of the seven criteria must be met before the disease is classified as RA. The first four criteria relating to stiffness and swelling must be present for at least 6 weeks, and criteria 2 through 5 (swelling and sub-cutaneous nodules) must be observed by a physician. These criteria remain the hallmark for classification of RA.

Clinical features of RA vary not only from one client to another but also in an individual client over the course of the disease. Explosive acute polyarticular onset evolving over several days also can occur. Rheumatoid arthritis usually begins gradually, over a period of several weeks to months, and is accompanied by systemic manifestations, such as anorexia, weight loss, fatigue, muscle aching, and stiffness. Joint pain and swelling are associated with morning stiffness that can last several hours. Joint involvement is usually polyarticular and symmetrical, with the most frequently affected joints being those in the fingers, hands, wrists, knees, and feet.

Bilateral symmetrical involvement of the hands (wrists, MCP joints, and PIP joints) is characteristic of RA. Inflammation of the PIP joints contributes to the spindle-shaped appearance of the fingers. Tenosynovitis of the flexor tendons of the fingers is common, along with swelling and tenderness of the ulnar styloid process. Decreased dorsiflexion of the wrist occurs early in the disease and can be more painful than changes in the finger joints. With time, progressive synovial damage leads to characteristic deformities of the hands: ulnar deviation of the MCP joints of the fingers and medial deviation of the wrist. Figure 77-1 depicts three types of hand deformities characteristic of RA. A swan-neck deformity (hyperextension of the PIP joint with flexion of the MCP and DIP joints) results from contractures of the intrinsic muscles and tendons. The boutonnière deformity (flexion of the PIP joints and hyperextension of the DIP joints) is due to rupture of the extensor tendons over the fingers. Carpal tunnel syndrome, the compression of the median nerve as a result of tenosynovitis on the volar aspect of the wrist, is fairly common in RA. All of these changes lead to decreased hand strength and the ability to maintain a tight pinch.

The shoulders, elbows, and spine are also affected. Shoulder arthritis is seen with late disease, whereas the elbows can become flexed and contracted with early disease. Spinal involvement is usually limited to the cervical area. Atlantoaxial subluxation can lead to tenderness, muscle spasm, persistent head tilt, and occipital headache.

In the lower extremities, RA frequently affects the feet and knees. Cock-up toes result from plantar subluxation of the metatarsal heads. Walking can be difficult because of limited flexion and extension of the ankle. Active synovitis is often seen in swelling over the medial and lateral aspects of the patella. Popliteal cysts (Baker cysts) can develop behind the knee joint.

As a systemic disease, RA can affect almost every body system. Extra-articular manifestations of RA are summarized in the Extra-Articular Manifestations of Rheumatoid Arthritis table on the website. Three of these manifestations, however, are the most frequently seen in RA. These include rheumatoid nodules (Figure 77-2), Sjögren's syndrome, and Felty's syndrome. Rheumatoid nodules, granuloma-type lesions that develop around small blood vessels, can develop in up to 50% of clients with RA. Usually, those affected have high titers of RF. Generally firm, mobile, and painless, rheumatoid nodules appear over the extensor surfaces of joints, such as elbows and fingers, but may be found elsewhere in the body, including in the lungs. These nodules can easily break down or become infected.

Secondary Sjögren's syndrome, keratoconjunctivitis sicca, is seen in approximately 10% to 15% of clients. It may occur by itself or with other diseases, such as SLE or polymyositis. Clients with Sjögren's syndrome have diminished lacrimal and salivary gland secretion. They may complain of gritty, burning, or sandy eyes, with decreased tearing, itching, and photosensitivity.

Felty's syndrome was originally described as the combination of RA, splenomegaly, leukopenia, and leg ulcers. Subsequent observations have shown an association with lymphadenopathy, thrombocytopenia, and the HLA-DR4 haplotype. Felty's syndrome occurs most commonly in clients with severe, nodule-forming RA. Other extra-articular problems seen in RA include inflammatory eye disorders, infection, pulmonary disease, vasculitis, and cardiac abnormalities.

Diagnostic Testing

Laboratory Testing. The laboratory evaluation of clients with rheumatic disease is often informative but rarely definitive. Serum and urine chemistries are usually normal in RA. Anti-CCP (cyclic citrullinated protein antibodies) is a diagnostic marker and is predictive of the future development of rheumatoid arthritis. It is as sensitive as rheumatoid factor, but is more specific. Elevated erythrocyte sedimentation rates (ESRs) and C-reactive protein (CRP) levels are typical of active disease, with the CRP level being a more definitive indicator of inflammation. Hematologic studies often indicate a mild normocytic, hypochromic anemia along with thrombocytosis. An underlying iron deficiency anemia is usually present if the hemoglobin level is less than 10 g/ml and ferritin levels are low. Low eosinophil counts occur with increased disease activity, and granulocytopenia may indicate Felty's syndrome. Occasionally, proteinuria and microscopic hematuria are seen as a result of amyloid deposits in the kidney.

Serologic tests used to confirm the diagnosis of RA include antinuclear antibodies (ANAs) and RF. Antinuclear antibody titers are seen in 15% to 20% of clients, over half of who have Felty's syndrome. Rheumatoid factor, an autoantibody directed against the immunoglobulin IgM, is positive in only 80% of clients. Higher titers are seen in active disease. The presence of IgM RF, however, is not specific for RA. Increased levels can be seen in older adults or after infections or immunizations. Rheumatoid factor titers are also present in other rheumatic disorders, including SLE, dermatomyositis, and SSc, and in liver and pulmonary disease. The absence of a positive RF test does not exclude the diagnosis of RA in a client with typical clinical characteristics. Clients can convert from negative to positive with an exacerbation in their clinical manifestations. Clients with seronegative RA, however, have better outcomes and rarely have extra-articular involvement. Recent evidence points to recognition that seronegative and seropositive polyarthritis are separate entities. See the Common Diagnostic Studies Used in Rheumatic Disorders table on the website. **evolve**

Radiologic Studies. Radiologic findings help to confirm disease activity and monitor treatment results. In the early stages, soft tissue swelling is indicated by increased shadowing on the x-ray around the affected joint (Figure 77-3). Massive tissue swelling of the entire joint often precedes further destructive changes, such as periarticular osteoporosis. Subchondral cysts may develop from the invasion of granulation tissue. As the disease progresses, subchondral bone erosions develop, ultimately causing a narrowing of the joint space. In mild disease, erosions may not develop for 6 to 12 months. Initially

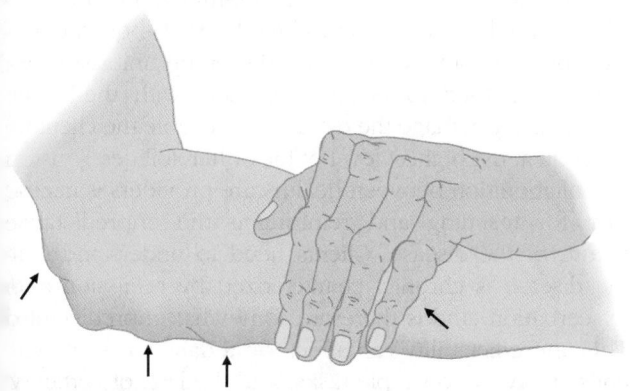

■ FIGURE 77–2   Rheumatoid nodules.

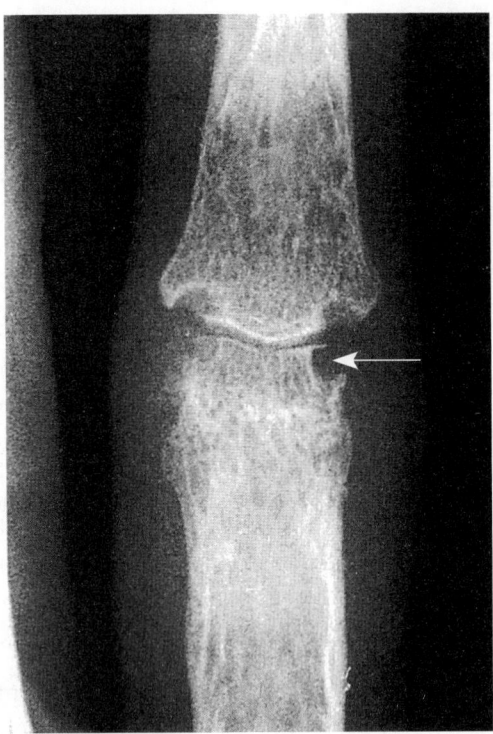

■ **FIGURE 77–3** Radiograph of an interphalangeal joint affected by rheumatoid arthritis. Pocket erosion is shown with the arrow. Pocket erosions can spread into trabecular bone and weaken the bone surface. There is also joint space narrowing and soft tissue swelling. *(From Resnick, D., Berthiaume, M.J., & Sartoris, D. [1993]. Imaging. In W.N. Kelley, et al. [Eds.], Textbook of rheumatology [4th ed., p. 600]. Philadelphia: Saunders.)*

occurring at the joint margins where the capsule is attached, erosions are first seen in the small joints of the hands and feet, where the bone is less dense. Subluxation and malalignment of the joints can be seen on x-ray, reflecting the destructive changes seen on physical examination. With advanced disease, subchondral bone destruction and diffuse osteoporosis appear.

Other Procedures. Synovial fluid analysis indicates a change from the normal transparent color to a milky, cloudy, or dark yellow fluid. Arthroscopic examinations typically show pale, thick, edematous synovial villi, cartilage destruction, and fibrous scar formation (pannus). Bone and joint scans can be used to detect early joint changes and more readily confirm the diagnosis.

OUTCOME MANAGEMENT

There has been considerable effort devoted to the development of outcome measures in RA. A proposed set of core RA measures includes pain measurement, disability, physician and client global assessment, number of tender and swollen joints, and acute-phase reactants. In addition, the American College of Rheumatology (ACR) developed a statistically powerful definition of improvement in

RA: 20% improvement in tender and swollen joint counts and 20% improvement in three of the five remaining ACR core set measures of client and physician global assessments, pain, disability, and an acute-phase reactant. These research advances continue to clarify effective and appropriate management strategies for RA clients. At the very least, the plan of care for clients with manifestations suggestive of RA should (1) establish a diagnosis of RA as early as possible, (2) determine the stage of disease (joint destruction) and disease activity (inflammation), (3) define relevant factors that will affect prognosis, (4) establish a plan for treatment as early as possible, (5) monitor disease activity and response to treatment, and (6) modify the treatment when client response is absent or inadequate.

Medical Management

Effective management of RA involves a combination of medications, rest, exercise, and methods of joint protection. The primary goals of RA treatment strategies are to provide pain relief, to decrease joint inflammation, to maintain or restore joint function, and to prevent bone and cartilage destruction. Proven treatments for arthritis must show in repeated, controlled scientific clinical trials that they are safe and provide benefit in one or more of the following areas:

- Pain reduction
- Reduction of inflammation
- Safe joint mobility
- Avoidance of stress damage to joints

The treatment and management of RA requires successful collaboration between the client and the entire health care team—health care provider (physician, physician's assistant, and nurse practitioner), nurse, and physical and/or occupational therapist. Other team members—orthopedic surgeon, nutritionist, social worker, and orthotist—may be required, as the client's needs change. The totally dependent RA client is uncommon today, in large part because of advances in joint replacement surgery and the advent of new therapies.

Education is critical in the successful treatment of RA. Clients and their families must be educated about the disease process and its impact on the entire unit. Families must be helped to become partners with the client to effectively manage the disease and enable the client to function at the highest level of his or her abilities.

Collaboration between health care providers is necessary for teaching and reinforcing the unpredictable nature of the disease. Clients need to understand that the disease is chronic, characterized by remission and exacerbation, and is therefore somewhat unpredictable. This unpredictability can affect, on a daily basis, the client's ability to do simple tasks, and the lack of certainty with which the client and family can plan ahead for outings and special activities can be frustrating for all involved. Individual and family stress can escalate to the point where family counseling is required. Reinforcing positive coping strategies and recommending stress-management techniques, however, can help to avoid feelings of powerlessness and helplessness.

Reduce Pain and Inflammation

Reduction of pain and inflammation is most often achieved with pharmacologic management, which usually combines a nonsteroidal anti-inflammatory drug (NSAID), a disease-modifying antirheumatic drug/biologic response modifier (DMARD/BRM), and short intermittent courses of oral glucocorticoids. Medications are changed in response to lack of efficacy or if the initial improvement fades. The use of single-drug therapy has been shown to be of limited benefit in the treatment of RA. The majority of clients who are prescribed a single agent are no longer on that agent 3 years later. Combination therapy is most effective if introduced within the first 2 years after diagnosis of RA. Methotrexate (MTX), in combination with the BRMs, has shown a synergistic effect, as well as with the immunodmodulator leflunomide. As explained in the Integrating Pharmacology feature on pp. 2062-2063, these medications reduce pain and inflammation as well as control systemic involvement. Also, see the Translating Evidence into Practice feature on p. 2055 for information related to pharmacologic management of RA.

PROSORBA Column

PROSORBA column, a medical device used in conjunction with apheresis, employs approximately 200 mg of protein A covalently bound to an inert silica matrix that is contained within a 300-ml polycarbonate housing. Each column contains 123 ± 2 g of this matrix. Protein A is a component of certain strains of the *Staphylococcus* bacterium, and it has the propensity to bind immunoglobulin G (IgG) and IgG bound to an antigen, i.e., circulating immune complex. The PROSORBA column is indicated for use in the therapeutic reduction of the clinical manifestations of severe RA in adult clients with long-standing disease who have failed to respond to or are intolerant of DMARDs. The procedure requires 12 weekly apheresis procedures. A plasma volume of 1250 ± 250 ml is passed through the column. Clients must have good intravenous access. The therapeutic effect is usually not noticed until completion of the 12 weeks.

Protect Articular Surfaces

One important interrelated area of medical management involves the principles of joint protection and work simplication. In a multidisciplinary setting, principles of joint protection and work simplification can be taught by the occupational therapist and reinforced by the nurse. Education in these areas can have a positive effect on increased energy levels and decreased fatigue, thereby improving the client's coping abilities and sense of control.

Specific suggestions or anticipatory guidance about self-care can be beneficial. For example, clients should select easy-to-grip combs and brushes with large handles. These devices are readily available at almost all stores. Using a long-handled bath brush to reach the feet and back during bathing is much less stressful on the joints. Selecting attractive, adaptable clothing is easier now that many stores and mail-order catalogs have included a home care section. Jogging suits with pull-on pants and large, easily zippered tops are comfortable and attractive. Adaptive equipment for dressing includes long-handled shoehorns, zipper pulls, and buttoners. Involvement of the feet, the metatarsalphalangeals (MTPs), can seriously affect the ability to ambulate and enjoy life. Referral to an orthotist for proper supportive shoes and/or orthotics is essential to reduce pain and prevent further joint damage. See the Principles of Joint Protection and Associated Work Simplification Strategies table on the website.

Maintain Function

Therapeutic exercise is another important modality in the initial and ongoing treatment of RA. Three types of exercises are typically used: range-of-motion (ROM), strengthening, and endurance. The purpose of ROM exercises is to improve joint motion. ROM exercises can be passive, assisted, or active. Carried out by the therapist, without any client effort, passive exercises are most often done when the client is totally unable to move the joint because of the lack of strength or voluntary control. The purpose of passive ROM is to ensure joint movement when there is a risk of developing contractures. Research has identified a safe role for progressive resistance exercise training in selected clients, leading to significant improvements in strength, pain, and fatigue without exacerbating disease activity or joint pain. Whatever form of exercise is prescribed, the client should not perform these exercises if joint inflammation or a flare-up exists. Although clients may be able to enjoy other therapeutic and recreational exercises, they need to understand that engaging in other activities or activities of daily living (ADL) is not a substitute for a ROM program.

Strengthening exercises are done to preserve or improve the muscle's ability to perform work. Two types of strengthening exercises are commonly used: isometric and isotonic. With isometric exercises, the muscle is contracted for 5 to 6 seconds, but the joint is not permitted to move. Common isometric techniques include gluteal folds and quadriceps-setting exercises. Isotonic exercises are used carefully in clients with RA because

INTEGRATING P H A R M A C O L O G Y

Medications Used in the Treatment of Rheumatoid Arthritis

Pharmacologic treatment of rheumatoid arthritis (RA) is directed at (1) relieving manifestations of pain, inflammation, and stiffness; (2) maintaining joint function and range of motion; (3) minimizing systemic involvement; and (4) delaying disease progression.

ANALGESICS

Acetaminophen (Tylenol) is given only for pain relief because it has analgesic and antipyretic properties equivalent to those of aspirin. However, acetaminophen does not have any anti-inflammatory or antirheumatic actions and is not helpful in reducing the inflammation and swelling of rheumatic arthritis.

NSAIDs

Nonselective nonsteroidal anti-inflammatory drugs (NSAIDs) such as aspirin, ibuprofen (Motrin, Advil), meloxicam (Mobic), nabumetone (Relafen), and diclofenac (Voltaren) are used to treat inflammation and swelling. They suppress inflammation by inhibiting the synthesis of prostaglandins, which play a major role in the process of inflammation. The most common side effects of NSAID therapy include nausea, GI irritation, and gastric and duodenal ulcers. NSAIDs do not alter the course of RA because they do not prevent joint damage or slow disease progression.

Cyclooxygenase is the key enzyme involved in the production of prostaglandins that is inhibited by NSAIDs. There are two forms of this enzyme—cyclooxygenase-1 (COX-1) and cyclooxygenase-2 (COX-2). COX-1 is present in all cells at all times and its purpose is to produce prostaglandins that regulate normal cellular processes; drugs that inhibit this enzyme are called nonselective NSAIDs. COX-2 is expressed almost completely in response to inflammation. COX-2 produces prostaglandins in the joints and synovium; drugs in this class are called selective NSAIDs. Celecoxib (Celebrex) is currently the only available COX-2 NSAID, and it is less likely to cause stomach ulcers and GI irritation than traditional NSAIDs.

The COX-2 NSAIDs and traditional NSAIDs have been shown to equally relieve arthritis pain and to share many of the same side effects, including the potential to cause fluid retention, high blood pressure, heart failure, and liver and kidney problems in some clients. As with all medications, clients are urged to use the lowest effect dose.

An additional important side effect of some of the COX-2 NSAIDs is an increase in the risk of heart attacks and strokes, especially when they are used at higher doses. Although all NSAIDs have the potential to cause high blood pressure and worsen congestive heart failure, present studies have not clearly shown traditional NSAIDs to cause an increase in heart attacks and strokes as was seen with some of the COX-2 NSAIDs pulled from the market (valdecoxib [Bextra] and rofecoxib [Vioxx]). More research is needed to understand if some or all of the traditional NSAIDs also increase the risk of these events.

DMARDs AND BRMs

Disease-modifying antirheumatic drugs (DMARDs) reduce joint destruction and retard disease progression, but they are more toxic than NSAIDs and require close monitoring. DMARDs are considered when the client does not show a decrease in pain, swelling, and stiffness or if x-rays show evidence of bony erosions within the first 30 to 60 days of onset. First-choice DMARDs include methotrexate (MTX), sulfasalazine (Azulfidine), and the antimalarial agent hydroxychloroquine (HCQ, Plaquenil). MTX is considered the first-choice drug among the DMARDs because of its efficacy, relative safety, low cost, and extensive use in RA. Other DMARDs include gold salts, penicillamine (Depen), azathioprine (Imuran), and cyclosporine (Sandimmune). Since 1998, seven new DMARDs, classified as biologic response modifiers (BRMs) and tumor necrosis factor (TNF) blockers, have been released in the United States: etanercept (Enbrel), infliximab (Remicade), anakinra (Kineret), adalimumab (Humira), rituximab (Rituxan), abatacept (Orencia), and leflunomide (Arava).

All of the DMARDs, including TNF blockers and BRMs, are toxic to multiple body organs including the liver, kidneys, GI tract, lungs, bone marrow, and eyes (HCQ), and must be monitored closely. These drugs suppress the bone marrow and place clients at risk for infection, anemia, and bleeding.

Many of the DMARDs may take days, weeks or months to begin controlling the manifestations of RA, which is why clients continue to receive, glucosteroids and/or NSAIDs while the DMARDs are initiated. MTX may result in a therapeutic effect in 3 to 6 weeks, but HCQ may require 3 to 6 months.

GLUCOCORTICOIDS

Glucocorticoids produce an immediate and profound anti-inflammatory response in clients with RA. At low doses, glucocorticoids demonstrate characteristics that are primarily anti-inflammatory rather than immunosuppressive. At higher doses, these agents are immunosuppressive by appearing to exert the greatest suppressive effect on T helper cells. Higher doses are reserved for rapid relief of acute manifestations seen with exacerbation of RA. Low-dose prednisone is used as a bridge, to carry clients from unsuccessful NSAID therapy until they experience the benefits of the slow-acting, disease-modifying agents. The bridge time has shortened considerably with the advent of the BMRs and TNFs. Long-term prednisone use is correlated with the development of several adverse effects, specifically serious infections, fractures and osteoporosis, increased urinary calcium excretion that can cause urolithiasis, and GI bleeding. Treatment guidelines have been published for treatment of steroid-induced osteoporosis. The defect in calcium absorption is treated with daily doses of 1500-mg calcium supplements and 800 units of vitamin D. Bisphosphonates (alendronate sodium and risedronate) are most frequently used for the treatment of osteoporosis.

Medications Used in the Treatment of Rheumatoid Arthritis—Cont'd

Determining if a surgical client is glucocorticoid dependent has important implications for those undergoing surgery. Taking a drug history of the client with RA requires exploration of the use of glucocorticoids: when they were initiated, dosage history, and date they were discontinued. Steroid-dependent clients are those currently taking glucocorticoids as well as those weaned from chronic glucocorticoid therapy within the last year. Other clients at risk of steroid dependency include those who received regular intra-articular injections of steroids, psoriasis clients who routinely used topical steroids on large areas of the skin, and clients with inflammatory bowel disease who routinely used steroid enemas. Steroid-dependent clients who undergo

general anesthesia must receive stress doses of glucocorticoids to prevent intraoperative shock. Three doses of intravenous hydrocortisone (100 mg each) are usually given before, during, and immediately after the surgical procedures.

COMBINATION THERAPIES

A combination of one or two medications may be used to provide relief of pain, swelling, and stiffness and to slow degeneration of a joint. The benefit of giving more than one medication is to maximize the therapeutic effect and minimize the side effects with smaller dosages of all medications prescribed. Common combinations include MTX + HCQ, MTX + Enbrel, or MTX + Arava.

INVESTIGATIONAL AGENTS

Rheumatoid arthritis research continues to focus on the pathogenesis of disease, halting disease progression and treating earlier in the course of the disease. For more information regarding clinical trials being conducting in RA and other rheumatic diseases, see the website www.clinicaltrials.gov.

---

they require repetitive joint motion. After joint pain and inflammation have been controlled, however, and the client has achieved increased isometric strength, dynamic, low-resistance exercises are appropriate. Appropriate low-resistance exercises for the client with RA include bike riding, swimming, golf, Ping-Pong, and dancing.

Other physical therapy modalities are also useful. For severely inflamed joints, splints appear to help resolve inflammation more quickly than does leaving the joint unsplinted. Heat therapy and cold therapy are important adjuncts to an exercise and rehabilitation program.

Superficial heat therapy can be given with hot packs, hydrotherapy, or paraffin baths. Deep heat is achieved through the use of diathermy or ultrasound. Superficial heat appears to cool joints by increasing the local blood flow, but deep heat actually raises the intra-articular joint temperature. As a result, superficial heat is generally preferred to deep heat. Heat seems to be more beneficial in the treatment of chronic conditions characterized by minimal swelling and inflammation. It also permits more effective stretching exercises.

Many clients find cold therapy provides relief of pain and stiffness. Cold packs, however, should not be used in clients with Raynaud's phenomenon, cold sensitivity, or cryoglobulinemia, or in anyone who finds it uncomfortable. The Arthritis Foundation has developed a wide selection of literature about RA. Support groups, self-help classes, and water-based or land-based exercises are available. To obtain this information from The Arthritis Foundation, call 1-800-283-7800. Requests for information can also be mailed to The Arthritis Foundation,

1414 Spring Street, NW, Atlanta, GA 30309, or visit their website at www.arthritis.org.

Nursing Management of the Medical Client

The goal of nursing care for clients with RA is to promote a healthy, positive life course adaptation. To achieve this goal, the nurse focuses on four domains of human response: comfort, self-care, control, and coping.

Adapting to a chronic illness is a demanding, complex process physically, emotionally, and socially. The energy required to achieve this adaptation can be easily exhausted, especially in the early stages of RA. Achieving normalcy, regulation, or adjustment can become a lifelong process, consuming increasing amounts of energy, unless clients learn to participate actively in modulating their responses to the illness. By working together, the nurse helps the client master adaptive strategies in each of the four domains so physical, psychological, and social energy is renewed.

The nurse's role is to assess, educate, and coordinate treatments, facilitate adaptations in the home, reevaluate periodically, and serve as client advocate. Providing information to help the client deal with chronic pain, comply with treatment, and cope with a chronic disease are some of the challenges faced in managing clients with RA. The nurse provides information and encourages the client's self-management by allowing choices about when to exercise, which adaptive equipment to use, and what other self-care techniques to use. Clients with RA appreciate caring and empathy by nurses. See the Bridge to Home Health Care feature on Increasing evolve

Independent Living with Rheumatoid Arthritis on the website.

Assessment. Nursing assessment begins by identifying the client's concerns and needs. The history should include information about the duration of clinical manifestations and ways the client has been managing those manifestations, particularly pain. The client's current understanding of RA and the coping strategies used for dealing with pain and fatigue are important. Determine the methods that the client is now using to reduce pain and the amount of pain the client considers tolerable. Find out what methods the client is using for joint protection.

Evaluate the amount of swelling and pain in each joint and the number of affected joints to obtain a "joint count." Determine physiologic measures of function such as a timed walk, measures of grip strength, and results of self-reported instruments that evaluate flexion and extension. Assess for clinical manifestations in the client's eyes, heart, lungs, and peripheral nerves. It is important to note new manifestations and marked changes in previous clinical manifestations.

Also evaluate the client's perception of his or her quality of life, usual role in the family, and social involvement. Physical changes in the body can lead to lower self-esteem. Clients may find it psychologically difficult to be seen in public and manage stares instigated by a hand deformity and other changes. Be sensitive to these issues and bring them into the discussion if the client or family hints at suicidal thoughts.

Diagnosis, Outcomes, Interventions
Diagnosis: Chronic Pain/Impaired Physical Mobility. The primary diagnosis of clients with RA is *Chronic Pain related to inflammation and swelling from pressure on surrounding tissues, joint deformity, and joint destruction.* Another common and related nursing diagnosis is *Impaired Physical Mobility related to pain, stiffness, and joint deformity.* The amount of pain these clients experience permeates all aspects of their lives including physical mobility.

Outcomes. The client's pain will be controlled at a level that permits the client to perform ADL. The client will maintain mobility at the highest level possible to carry out desired activities.

Interventions. Achieving a reasonable degree of comfort is a continuous challenge. Pain can be so pervasive and encompassing that it becomes a veil over daily activities, only to lift at unpredictable moments. Clients frequently use military terms, such as "struggle," "battle," "siege," "in the trenches," "attack," "fight," and "surrender," to describe their experiences with pain and discomfort. The importance of covering up the pain and keeping up with activities as a means of rejecting or disengaging from the disease has been emphasized. In fact, achieving some degree of comfort is the primary predictor of psychological well-being as well as maintaining mobility.

Teach About Medications. Numerous strategies can be used to help clients achieve pain relief and maintain mobility. Obviously, teaching clients about their medications and monitoring their response are important nursing responsibilities. Clients should receive information about the purpose, dose, frequency, and anticipated side effects of each medication. See the Integrating Pharmacology feature on Medications Used in the Treatment of Rheumatoid Arthritis, pp. 2062-2063. Clients need to understand clearly when they are to report adverse manifestations to the health care team and what to do if they miss a dose. Some of the new therapies include self-injectable medications, requiring that clients and their families be taught injection and preparation techniques. Preprinted or written instructions are essential to help clients recall the information. Appropriate educational materials on a variety of pharmacologic agents are available from The Arthritis Foundation and the pharmaceutical manufacturer.

Nurses play an important role in teaching clients to participate in their care by keeping a medication history. Clients can use a notebook or flow sheet to record essential medication information useful to themselves and other health care providers, such as dentists, other medical specialists, or emergency personnel. Initially, many clients find it helpful, as does the health care provider, to list the medications, date started, dosage, date discontinued, and reason for discontinuing the drug. This list should be reviewed and updated at each visit.

Promote Comfort with Nonpharmacologic Measures. Modulating the client's response to the experience of joint pain is another key principle of pain management. The uncertainty and unpredictability of the disease, with its concomitant impact on comfort, have been well documented. The following four interventions are used to help clients with the pain of RA: (1) making them comfortable, according to what has worked for them in the past; (2) listening to and learning from clients; (3) reducing anxiety; and (4) enlisting family and community support. Not all clients with RA have the same pain or the same experience with pain, so it is critical to understand the phenomenon from the individual client's perspective.

Other nonpharmacologic pain management strategies can be very useful. They not only can help to relieve pain but also can decrease anxiety and, thus, enhance overall comfort and a sense of control.

Positioning the client, ensuring that the limbs are correctly supported, and reinforcing the use of heat and cold are all important measures for promoting comfort. Some clients find that flannel nightwear, sleeping blankets, and thermal underwear are helpful means of retaining warmth while reducing pain and stiffness. A variety of relaxation techniques, including imagery, self-hypnosis, and controlled, rhythmic breathing, have been suggested. Progressive muscle relaxation techniques should be used with caution in clients with RA, however, because there is a danger that muscles could be tensed too tightly, thus exacerbating joint and muscle pain.

Manage Stiffness. Other comfort-promoting activities include the management of stiffness and the promotion of adequate sleep. If these areas are addressed through the nurse-client partnership, fatigue can also be significantly reduced. Clients need to be taught to distinguish between pain and stiffness and to understand why the nurse is interested in differentiating between the two manifestations. As one of the most important diagnostic criteria of RA (as well as several other arthritic diseases), *morning stiffness* can vary in duration or quality depending on disease activity. Typically, clients with morning stiffness wake up feeling comfortable until they begin to move. If the morning stiffness lasts longer than 1 hour or does not show evidence of decreasing, they may require additional rest and sleep plus changes in their medical regimen. Exercise can also decrease morning stiffness, pain, and fatigue. Clients may use pain medication before exercise to permit increased freedom of movement.

Occasionally, if stiffness is severe, family members may need to provide early morning assistance so the client is prepared for the day ahead. Another option is for clients to begin (or organize) as many tasks as possible the night before so they have enough time to complete ADL without rushing or undue anxiety. Clients might also be able to rearrange schedules so chores normally performed in the morning, when stiffness is most pronounced, are deferred until later in the day. Daytime stiffness can occur, but frequent position changes and pacing or alternating the types of activities usually alleviates it.

One unusual aspect of stiffness is that it is a disabling phenomenon that is not readily understood by other family members. Initially, family and co-workers may wonder if the client is feigning his or her inability to move rapidly or perform optimally in the morning. Helping the client and family understand the need for additional time to complete activities is an important measure in decreasing the family's frustration and the client's anxiety about moving slowly.

Promote Sleep and Rest. Disturbed sleep can significantly affect the client's level of comfort, especially when the client has a chronic illness. With RA, sleep is often interrupted because of joint pain, excessive fatigue, stiffness, or generalized musculoskeletal aching. Other important causes are anxiety and poor sleep hygiene. Before specific interventions are suggested, the nurse needs to determine how the sleep has been disturbed—for example, difficulty falling asleep, frequent periods of waking up during the night, or early morning awakening. Often the nurse's first interventions are to reinforce good sleep habits, such as maintaining a regular sleep schedule, avoiding caffeine or alcohol before bed, or engaging in soothing activities before retiring.

Other strategies address specific causes of impaired sleep in clients with RA. For example, warming the bed or taking a bath before bedtime can ease painful joints. Taking the prescribed NSAID (with a light snack of milk and crackers) half an hour before retiring can also promote sleep by relieving joint pain. If clients are awakened during the night because of pain or stiffness, they may need to use a smaller pillow, bed boards, or even lighter weight blankets. Those clients who have difficulty falling asleep because of worries or diffuse anxiety may benefit from using relaxation-imagery exercises. Avoidance of alcohol and caffeine before bed or engaging in soothing activities such as reading are also helpful.

Whole body rest can decrease joint inflammation and pain. Alternating rest and activity throughout the day may help with maintenance of mobility and management of pain. An afternoon nap also helps reduce fatigue.

Diagnosis: Readiness for Enhanced Self-Care. The nursing diagnosis is *Readiness for Enhanced Self-Care related to complex medication schedules, high risk of side effects of medications, health maintenance, and self-care.* Self-care includes taking medications as ordered, maintaining mobility with exercise and rest, and ensuring good nutrition. Self-care also includes all practices that clients undertake to promote their health and well-being despite having a chronic illness. Other modalities besides medications, such as heat, exercise, rest, positioning, or joint protection, are examples of these practices. Self-care practices must be taught and reinforced so the client does not develop self-care deficits.

Outcomes. The client will make informed decisions about the management of RA that will lead to a satisfactory quality of life despite the disease and will demonstrate ability to cope with the chronic illness.

Interventions. In general, clients with RA have a difficult time learning to live in partnership with the disease. RA clients may experience the fears of becoming crippled, being perceived as being old and nonproductive, and not being understood by loved ones. As with any chronic illness, clients need to maintain some degree of physical and psychological control over the disabling effects of their clinical manifestations. For some clients, however, the need to exercise control is so great that they can experience extreme powerlessness and helplessness during exacerbations of the illness. 🪔 Clients who can view their relationship with RA as an evolving partnership have better outcomes, both physically and psychosocially, than clients who perceive the disease to be the "enemy." This sense of partnership helps the client let go (i.e., rest and take care of himself or herself) during exacerbations of the disease yet respond actively by agreeing to engage in health-promoting, self-care practices. It can also help clients not to waste precious energy with anxiety, anger, and unresolved grief or guilt.

Promote Balanced Nutrition. Nutrition is an important aspect of self-care that is often misunderstood by the client with RA. This misunderstanding can occur because the popular press has promoted nutrition and unique diet therapies as instant cures for arthritis. Clients with RA may become overweight (because of decreased activity or mobility) or underweight (because of the anorexia of a chronic illness, the side effects of medications, or alterations in oral mucous membranes). In addition, diets may not provide sufficient iron to restore the deficit that results from the anemia of a chronic illness.

Clients need to understand that it is just as important to consume nutritionally sound diets as it is to achieve a reasonable body weight. Strategies to promote nutrition in anorectic clients include good oral hygiene before and after meals; small, frequent feedings; and high-calorie snacks. Clients with a dry mouth (xerostomia) benefit from moister foods and extra fluids with meals. Eliminating spicy or acidic foods, sitting upright to eat, and taking all medications with food and a full glass of water can ameliorate gastrointestinal distress. Clients with stiffness or hand deformities need assistive devices to feed themselves or require help to open cartons or packages.

Promote Decision Making. Exercising healthy control over the disease may include formulating causes of the illness. 🪔 Clients who reported causes for their arthritis (such as fate, personal habits, heredity, or the environment) were less anxious, depressed, and hostile than were those who did not report any cause. Most likely, clients who continue to ask "Why me?" and are unable to identify a specific cause of the illness have a more difficult time feeling in control.

Powerlessness can have physically and mentally detrimental effects on the client and can lead to anxiety, depression, and hopelessness. The key intervention for powerlessness is to increase the client's active participation in decision making by allowing the client as many choices as possible, for example, when to take medications or how to perform required ADL. Helping clients

to reframe their relationship with the disease to one of active partnership, as was previously mentioned, can also increase the sense of control.

Client education and hope are important to the client's perception of control. Arthritis education provides information that clients can use to make informed decisions about their care. Knowledge about the disease, its course, the appropriate treatment, and what clients can do to promote their well-being increases their mastery of the unknown. Client education in the safe environment of a support group can also decrease the uncertainties of the disease and thus enhance control.

Promote Hope. Having a sense of hopefulness about the future is a powerful ally against powerlessness. Everything clients do can be based on some level of hope. Nursing interventions to promote hope include avoiding false reassurance, helping clients to set realistic goals, praising them for all accomplishments (no matter how small), and active listening. Being sensitive to changes in mood and affect is important, particularly for clients receiving glucocorticoid therapy. When clients are taking steroids, views about the future often change from hopeful and positive to depressed, despairing expressions about their lives. If medication changes are not possible or if dosage adjustments do not relieve the depression, the nurse should consult the physician about the need for a psychiatric evaluation.

Promote Coping. Successful coping strategies help the client with RA to integrate the disease into the demands of daily living. Coping strategies can be viewed as either approach (positive or healthy) or avoidance strategies. Healthy approach strategies include seeking out information and assistance, finding strength through spiritual support, verbalizing feelings and concerns, setting goals, expressing positive thoughts, and maintaining realistic independence. The less adaptive, avoidance strategies include denial, excessive sleeping, other passive behaviors, and depression. Depression is often associated with increased levels of pain and functional impairment and increased use of health care services. As with clients who have other chronic illnesses, treatment with antidepressants may improve coping and pain control. In addition, the relationship between depression and pain may be influenced by the use of adaptive or maladaptive coping strategies and by clients' beliefs about their abilities to control their pain. Therefore the nurse's goal is clearly to help the client realize the benefits of the healthier approach strategies. Healthy coping strategies and the reframing of negative behaviors can be discussed, modeled, and safely tested in nurse-led client support groups.

For some clients, coping may be impaired because of changes in their body image and self-esteem. As the disease progresses, disfiguring joint changes or systemic alterations, such as rheumatoid nodules, may contribute to clients' sensitivity about their appearance and attractiveness. If changes occur in the performance of occupational, family, or social roles, self-esteem can be significantly affected. When clients with RA maintain employment with high levels of functional disability and exposure to stressful work, men and women, are at equal risk of experiencing emotional distress.

Evaluation. Rheumatoid arthritis is progressive and improvement can be slow. It may take several weeks to months for the expected outcomes to be achieved. Nevertheless, despite the many problems that people with RA face daily, many of these people courageously overcome these problems to maintain active, productive lives. There are multiple websites for arthritis that clients or health care providers can access, with the most comprehensive being The Arthritis Foundation at www.arthritis.org.

Surgical Management

Surgical procedures may be helpful for clients with arthritis. Surgery may be used to relieve pain, improve function, and correct deformities. When joints are already severely damaged and pain is uncontrollable, joint replacement may become an option. Previously, surgery was considered only late in the course of arthritis, often after severe joint destruction or deformity had developed. Now, however, early surgery is used to prevent deformities during the early phases or active stages of the disease.

Tendon Transfer and Osteotomy
Tendon transfers can prevent progressive deformity. During these procedures, nodules or benign bony tumors *(exostoses)* may be surgically removed and flexion contractures surgically relieved. *Osteotomies* (excising or cutting through bone) may improve the function of deformed joints or limbs. For example, a femoral head osteotomy may give symptomatic relief by changing the position of the head of the femur when it is being subjected to the stress of impact against the acetabulum. Postoperative care varies, depending on the joint treated. Postoperative physical therapy is critical.

Synovectomy
Synovectomy (surgical removal of synovia, as in the elbows, wrists, fingers, or knees) may be used in clients with RA to help maintain joint function. With RA, joint destruction begins in the synovial tissue and then proceeds to involve bone, cartilage, and other structures.

Short-term immobilization and physical therapy are needed after surgery.

Arthrodesis
Arthrodesis is an operation to produce bony fusion of a joint and is used for clients with bone loss after joint infection, tumors, musculoskeletal trauma, and paralysis. Arthrodesis may also help certain clients with RA or degenerative arthritis to regain some mobility. Although arthrodesis immobilizes the joint, the procedure may eliminate some of the discomfort of the arthritic process and improve functional mobility. The ankle is the joint most commonly treated with arthrodesis, usually to relieve post-traumatic arthritis. Arthrodesis often results in stiffness in adjacent joints and increases the energy required for ambulation. After surgery, the limb is casted. Nursing care is the same as for clients with casts (Chapter 27).

Joint Replacement
Arthroplasty (joint replacement) is the surgical replacement of diseased joints or joint components with artificial joints or joint components. The operation restores motion to a joint and function to the muscles, ligaments, and other soft tissue structures that control a joint. The selection of a prosthesis will require collaboration between the client and health care provider and will be dependent on the joint involved as well as the age and sex of the client. Joint prostheses can be a combination of a metal surface articulating with a polyethylene surface. The metal surfaces are made of strong, light-weight alloys such as cobalt-chromium and titanium-aluminum-vanadium. In some instances both surfaces of an arthritic joint may be replaced. Arthroplasties of the shoulder and hand are discussed next; hip and knee replacement is described in Chapter 26 following discussion of osteoarthritis.

Shoulder Arthroplasty. Disorders of the shoulder that require arthroplasty are much less common than those problems in weight-bearing joints. The shoulder relies on soft tissue and ligaments for stability, particularly the rotator cuff muscle-tendon unit. Shoulder arthroplasty is the replacement of the humeral head and glenoid articulating surface with a metal and polyethylene prosthesis (Figure 77-4). The primary indication for total shoulder replacement is pain and, secondarily, improvement in function and ROM.

Contraindications include infection and inability to comply with rehabilitation, such as clients with physiologic (e.g., neuropathy) or psychological problems. Complications include brachial nerve palsy, prosthetic loosening, joint dislocation or subluxation, and impingement syndrome.

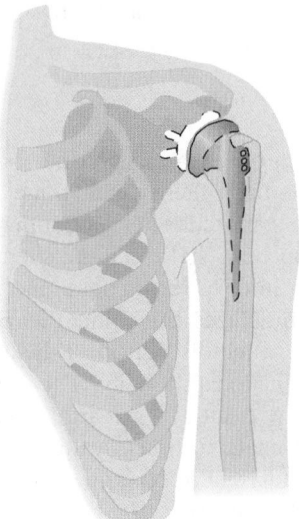

■ **FIGURE 77–4** Total shoulder arthroplasty.

Postoperative Care

SAFETY ALERT

Nursing assessment includes neurovascular examination of the operative arm at least every 4 hours. As shown in the Critical Monitoring feature at right, a possible complication is development of impingement syndrome because of the proximity of the brachial plexus.

Hemovac drainage should be less than 100 ml during the first 12 hours. Elevate the head of the bed 30 degrees to reduce swelling and improve comfort. Aggressive pain management is needed; shoulder arthroplasty usually causes more pain during the first 24 hours than the other joint replacements.

Patient-controlled analgesia (PCA) works well when supplemented with non-opioid anti-inflammatory agents. Ice is applied to the shoulder and the shoulder is positioned for comfort. Shoulder rehabilitation begins quickly after surgery and continues for about 6 weeks. For no other joint is rehabilitation as important as for the shoulder. The shoulder is placed through progressive external and internal ROM, hyperextension, and finally exercises with resistance once the rotator cuff has healed (approximately 6 weeks). Usually, the client can be taught how to use the nonoperative arm to move the operative arm through ROM.

Hand Arthroplasty. Various hand deformities develop from synovitis. Synovitis stretches the central portion of the extensor tendon, causing it to shift. Eventually, the tendons become shortened and fixed. Ulnar drift occurs when the imbalance of damaged extensor tendons and intact flexor tendons causes subluxation of the MCP joint. Other hand deformities develop from synovitis of the PIP joint: boutonnière deformity and swan-neck deformity.

Postoperative Brachial Plexus Compromise

- To assess median nerve status, have the client grasp your hand. Note the strength of the first and second fingers. A weak grip may indicate compromise of the median nerve.
- To assess radial nerve status, note the movement of the client's thumb toward the palm and then back to neutral. Problems with this motion may indicate compromise of the radial nerve.
- To assess ulnar nerve status, have the client spread all the fingers wide and resist pressure. Weakness against pressure may indicate compromise of the ulnar nerve.
- To assess cutaneous nerve status, assess for flexion of the biceps by having the client raise the forearm. Poor biceps flexion may indicate compromise of the cutaneous nerve.
- To assess axillary nerve status, have the client push the elbow outward against pressure. Hold the arm still while you palpate the deltoid for contraction. Weak contraction may indicate compromise of the axillary nerve.

A boutonnière deformity is flexion of the PIP joint and hyperextension of the DIP joint. There is no loss of MCP joint mobility. In the swan-neck deformity, the DIP joint is flexed and the PIP joint is hyperextended. Surgery includes tendon transfers to improve pinch grasp and arthrodesis for strength and position of the thumb for opposition. Hinge implants are placed to restore function to the fingers.

Postoperative Care. After surgery, neurovascular assessments are performed every hour for several hours. If the client has regional block anesthesia, the hand may be numb. The hand is elevated off the bed to prevent ulnar pressure. The hand is usually placed in a stockinette and suspended from the bed. An opening is made to assess the fingers. Encourage the client to exercise the fingers 10 times every hour, attempting full extension and flexion. Finger exercises reduce edema and pain. Place the client's personal items within easy reach of the nonoperative arm. If the opposite hand is equally deformed from RA, the client is often quite helpless and will require assistance with most components of ADL.

Encourage the client to use the nonoperative arm as much as possible. Some clients may express great concern about being dependent. Promote independence, and praise actions that foster self-care. Rehabilitation is a long process. Most clients are fitted with outrigger splints with rubber bands that allow exercise with resistance after 1 week. Therapy continues for several weeks to assist the client to regain strength and control.

Modifications for Older Clients

Older clients may have adapted to RA very well but often find any further dependency needed after surgery difficult to handle. They tend to be slower in their recovery from total joint replacement surgery. They may require prolonged hospitalization in an extended-care facility or subacute care setting until they regain adequate mobility to function independently or with some assistance and safety.

CONNECTIVE TISSUE DISORDERS

SYSTEMIC LUPUS ERYTHEMATOSUS

The term *lupus,* Latin for wolf, to describe various disfiguring cutaneous disorders, dates to the medieval period. The first clinical description of rashes that continue to be recognized as lupus was by Biett, in 1833. Credit is usually given to Kaposi for describing the systemic nature of the disease, including fever, weight loss, lymphadenopathy, and mental disturbances. Insights into the pathogenesis of systemic lupus erythematosus (SLE) were enhanced by the discovery of the lupus erythematosus (LE) cell phenomenon and the antinuclear factor.

SLE is a multisystem, inflammatory disorder associated with abnormalities of the immune system. It is a chronic condition characterized by various degrees of increased disease activity that are generally followed by a less active, remitting course. So many classic immunologic abnormalities can be present in SLE that it is considered the prototype of an autoimmune disease. Typically, multiple body organs and systems are affected at different times, thus producing widespread damage to connective tissues, blood vessels, and serous and mucous membranes.

SLE is primarily a disease of young women. Peak incidence occurs between the ages of 15 and 40 during the childbearing years, with a female to male ratio of 5:1. However, the onset can range from infancy to advanced age. In both pediatric and older-onset clients, the female to male ratio approximates 2:1. The 1982 revised criteria for the classification of SLE are listed in Table 77-2. The diagnosis of SLE is confirmed if a client has any 4 of the 11 criteria present, either serially or simultaneously, during any observation period.

Etiology and Risk Factors

In the general population, SLE affects approximately 1 in 2000 individuals. Incidence rates have increased over the past 40 years, most likely because of an increased availability of serologic tests and increased awareness of the disease. The disease has a predilection for women in

TABLE 77-2 1982 Revised Criteria for the Classification of Systemic Lupus Erythematosus

Criterion	Definition
Malar rash	Fixed erythema, flat or raised, over the malar eminences, tending to spare nasolabial folds
Discoid rash	Erythematous raised patches with adherent keratotic scaling and follicular plugging; atrophic scarring may occur in older lesions
Photosensitivity	Skin rash as a result of unusual reaction to sunlight, by client history or physician observation
Oral ulcers	Oral or nasopharyngeal ulceration, usually painless, observed by physician
Arthritis	Nonerosive arthritis involving two or more peripheral joints, characterized by tenderness, swelling, or effusion
Serositis	Pleuritis—convincing history of pleuritic pain or rub heard by a physician or evidence of pleural effusion *or* Pericarditis—documented by electrocardiogram or rub or evidence of pericardial effusion
Renal disorder	Persistent proteinuria greater than 0.5 g/day or greater than 3 g if quantification not performed *or* Cellular casts—may be red cell, hemoglobin, granular, tubular, or mixed
Neurologic disorder	Seizures—in the absence of offending drugs or known metabolic derangements, e.g., uremia, ketoacidosis, or electrolyte imbalance *or* Psychosis—in absence of offending drugs or known metabolic derangements, e.g., uremia, ketoacidosis, or electrolyte imbalance
Hematologic disorder	Hemolytic anemia—with reticulocytosis *or* Leukopenia—less than 4000/mm³ total on two or more occasions *or* Lymphopenia—less than 1500/mm³ on two or more occasions *or* Thrombocytopenia—less than 100,000/mm³ in absence of offending drugs
Immunologic disorder	Positive lupus erythematosus cell preparation *or* Anti-DNA—antibody to native DNA in abnormal titer *or* Anti-Sm—presence of antibody to Sm nuclear antigen *or* False-positive serologic test for syphilis known to be positive for at least 6 months and confirmed by *Treponema pallidum* immobilization or fluorescent treponemal antibody absorption test
Antinuclear antibody	Abnormal titer of antinuclear antibody by immunofluorescence or an equivalent assay at any point in time and in absence of drugs known to be associated with "drug-induced lupus" syndrome

Data from Tan, E., et al. (1982). The 1982 revised criteria for the classification of systemic lupus erythematosus (SLE). *Arthritis and Rheumatism, 25,* 1271-1277.

their childbearing years, with young African-American women the majority group affected. The prevalence of SLE varies with race, ethnicity, and socioeconomic status. The Lupus Foundation of America (www.lupus.org) estimates that 1,500,000 Americans have either systemic or limited forms of lupus. The female to male prevalence ratio is 10:1 for women in the childbearing years. However, men and African-American females have a worse renal outcome than women.

Once considered a fatal disease in young women, SLE now has improved outcomes. Over 85% of people with the disorder live longer than 15 years after diagnosis. Increased mortality, however, has been noted in African Americans, Asians, Puerto Ricans, and people of Hispanic descent living in the southwest United States. Poor survival has been associated with high serum creatinine levels, low hematocrit levels, proteinuria, and the source of medical care funding. The most common causes of death in SLE are active lupus nephritis, vascular events, and infections.

An underlying hormonal change may explain why the disease affects so many more women. Genetic factors may also be involved. Familial aggregation occurs in 10% of people having a first-degree relative with SLE, including its occurrence in identical twins.

Pathophysiology

The pathologic findings of SLE occur throughout the body and are manifested by inflammation, blood vessel abnormalities that encompass both bland vasculopathy and vasculitis, and immune complex deposition. SLE results from an abnormal reaction of the body against its own tissues, cells, and serum proteins. In other words, as an autoimmune disease, SLE is characterized by a decreased self-tolerance. In the North American Caucasian population, there is a positive association between SLE and two HLA antigens (DR2 and DR3) that are coded by the MHC. People with SLE have increased numbers of both self and non-self antigens, suggesting hyperactivity of the B cells. Interleukin-6 may have a role in B-cell hyperactivity. Another antibody, anti-DNA of the IgG type, may be responsible for the development of the engulfed LE bodies in the LE cells. The relationship between the serum LE factor and the pathologic changes that occur with SLE is not clear. The absence of the LE factor, however, is a strong indication that the disease is not present. Increased levels of anti–double-stranded DNA (anti-dsDNA) antibodies are associated with increased disease activity in clients with SLE.

Clinical Manifestations

SLE can be differentiated by the presence or development of glomerulonephritis, photosensitivity, characteristic skin rashes, central nervous system disease, and various cytopenias such as the Coombs' test positive hemolytic anemia, leukopenia, and thrombocytopenia. The clinical manifestations vary considerably, from general complaints of fever, fatigue, and malaise; to painful, swollen joints; to the psychological distress of a variety of skin lesions. The latter can include the classic butterfly rash over the bridge of the nose and cheeks, erythematous discoid lesions (which can result in permanent scars on the scalp, ears, face or neck), the temporary loss of hair on the scalp, painless mouth ulcers, and cutaneous vascular lesions. Sunlight may trigger a local dermatitis. Systemic manifestations (renal, cardiac, or pulmonary) as well as a variety of serum, immunologic, and antibody abnormalities may be present. Table 77-3 summarizes the changes in organ systems that occur in SLE.

The *most specific tests* for SLE are antibodies to double-stranded DNA and antibodies to Sm and ribosomal P proteins, which are seen exclusively in SLE. Measuring C-reactive protein levels can sometimes be a useful test for distinguishing between a lupus flare-up and infection. It usually remains normal in a flare-up but is elevated in infection.

The *most sensitive test* for SLE is the relatively nonspecific fluorescent anti-nuclear antibody (ANA) assay. Almost all clients with SLE have ANAs, but they also occur in many other situations, such as infections, advanced age, and RA, and with certain drug therapy regimens. Complements C3, C4, and CD 50 are useful measures of disease activity.

TABLE 77–3 System Changes with the Pathogenesis of Systemic Lupus Erythematosus

System	Pathogenesis with Systemic Lupus Erythematosus
Integumentary	Immune complex deposition, inflammation of dermal-epidermal junctions, vasculitis
Gastrointestinal	Collagen degeneration and vasculitis leading to mucous membrane ulcers; vasculitis leading to organ infarction and necrosis
Musculoskeletal	Increased fibrin deposits at synovial surfaces; inflammation of arterioles, venules, and tendon sheaths; eventual necrosis, degeneration, and fibrosis of muscle tissue
Pulmonary	Pleural inflammation, pneumonitis, pulmonary hypertension
Cardiovascular	Diffuse vasculitis; inflammation and scarring of atrioventricular and sinoatrial nodes; inflammation of pericardial sac
Renal	Deposition of immune complexes in glomerular basement membranes
Neurologic	Immune complex deposition; antineuronal antibody activity leading to cerebritis, seizures, organic brain syndrome, and peripheral neuropathies

OUTCOME MANAGEMENT

Medical Management

In general, the clinical pattern and prognosis of SLE are variable. The illness may develop rapidly with an acute fulminant course. More commonly, it develops insidiously and becomes chronic, with remissions and exacerbations. The course of the disorder is more severe when onset occurs at a young age. The survival rate has improved dramatically in recent years, although the disease is still potentially fatal. Improvements in early diagnosis and treatment allow clients the opportunity to live longer.

The primary management of SLE involves the use of drugs that suppress end-organ inflammation or interfere with immune function. Very few drug therapies have been subjected to randomized clinical trials. Treatment of acute SLE is based on the use of steroids, immunosuppressive agents, and experimental therapies. It is critical in the management of these clients to be aware of and to aggressively treat the co-morbid conditions that commonly occur in SLE—hypertension, infections, seizures, hyperlipidemia, and osteoporosis.

Reduce Inflammation and Minimize Complications

Only three drugs have been approved for the treatment of lupus, with the last approved more than 40 years ago. They are aspirin, glucocorticoids, and hydroxychloroquine. Off-label use includes NSAIDs, cyclophosphamide, and azathioprine. Medications used to treat lupus are reviewed in the Integrating Pharmacology feature on p. 2072.

Dialysis or Kidney Transplantation

Clients with end-stage lupus nephropathy are managed with dialysis or kidney transplantation. There is a tendency for decreased clinical and serologic lupus activity following the onset of end-stage renal disease. Survival rates of lupus clients and other end-stage renal clients are comparable. Most studies note an increased incidence of infections among SLE clients on dialysis. Kidney transplantation during an acute exacerbation of SLE is controversial and may increase the risk of poor outcome. Recurrence of lupus nephritis in transplanted allografts, often with the same histopathology as in the native kidney, develops in 2% to 4% of transplanted kidneys.

Promote Rest and Coping

Although drug therapy and the use of experimental treatments play a significant part in the management of SLE, perhaps the more important aspects of treatment are the supportive therapies of physical and emotional rest, diet and nutrition, and skin protection. Nurses have an important role in teaching clients how to manage the daily stress of coping with a chronic illness.

Nursing Management of the Medical Client

Obtain Nursing History

The nursing history of people with confirmed or suspected SLE must be sufficiently thorough to capture the range of possible manifestations that accompany an autoimmune disease. Clients need to be asked about general problems, such as fever, weight loss, and fatigue, and about changes in energy levels. A detailed medication history is essential in identifying the need for additional client teaching as well as in determining that the condition has not been drug induced. Clients should be asked about the names of their current medications, dosage, purpose, side effects, and length of time that they have been taking these drugs. Approximately 25 drugs have been implicated as causing a lupus-like syndrome, but only a few (hydralazine, procainamide, isoniazid) cause the disorder with any great frequency.

Questions about changes in skin should be elicited. The presence, location, and nature of rashes need to be explored as well as if the rashes are associated with exposure to sunlight or even fluorescent lighting. Clients should be asked about changes in their nails and nail beds, loss of hair on the scalp, and mouth or nasal sores.

Because SLE is occasionally characterized by generalized cerebritis, careful attention should be paid to the neuropsychiatric system. If seizure activity occurs, it is usually the generalized tonic-clonic type. The client should be asked about visual disturbances, vertigo, facial weakness, and presence of headaches. Changes in emotional status, including anxiety, insomnia, disorientation, and mood swings, are fairly common as a result of the disease and/or steroid therapy. The client may also complain of impaired cognition, such as mental dullness or a slow reaction time.

Complete Physical Assessment

The nursing assessment should begin with an examination of the integumentary and musculoskeletal systems because clients with SLE have a high percentage of physical changes involving the skin, muscles, and joints. Inspect the entire body carefully, noting the location, nature, and size of cutaneous and vascular lesions. Transient rashes can appear in any location, particularly after exposure to sunlight. Interestingly, the classic butterfly rash over the bridge of the nose and cheeks affects fewer than half of those with SLE. Discoid lesions, characterized by annular erythematous plaques, can appear as atrophied, scaling areas on the face, neck, and arms. Severe scarring is also possible. Fingers can be affected by erythema under the nail beds or by digital gangrene.

INTEGRATING PHARMACOLOGY

Medications Used to Treat Systemic Lupus Erythematosus

Systemic lupus erythematosus (SLE) is a chronic disease similar in many ways to rheumatoid arthritis (RA). However, with SLE, inflammation is not limited to joints; rather, it occurs throughout the body. Clinical manifestations include pleuritis, pericarditis, and nephritis and a severe episode can be fatal. Fortunately, the manifestations of SLE can usually be controlled with prompt and aggressive glucocorticoid therapy.

NSAIDs

Nonsteroidal antiinflammatory drugs (NSAIDs) are used to reduce musculoskeletal manifestations, mild serositis, and fever.

SAFETY
⚠
ALERT

Care must be taken when using NSAIDs in clients with SLE. NSAIDs inhibit prostaglandin synthesis within the kidney and impair renal blood flow. Clients with lupus nephritis are particularly susceptible because of a heightened dependency on prostaglandins to maintain renal function compromised by glomerular inflammation. Clients should be questioned about their nonprescription use of NSAIDs. Renal abnormalities produced by NSAIDs, particularly impaired renal function, are generally promptly reversible.

GLUCOCORTICOIDS

Glucocorticoids are required to control serious complications, such as thrombocytopenic purpura, hemolytic anemia, myocarditis, pericarditis, seizures, and nephritis. Prednisone is usually given orally in low doses (up to 15 mg/day), moderate doses (16 to 40 mg/day), or high doses (up to 120 mg/day). Divided doses are generally administered to ensure more sustained anti-inflammatory action and greater lupus-suppressing activity than the same amount of drug given as a single morning dose.

SAFETY
⚠
ALERT

Once the disease is under control, however, gradual reduction (tapering) is essential. Clients on a multiple daily dose regimen must first be converted to a single morning dose before attempting to reduce the actual drug dose. The length of time the client has been on the drug directly affects the length of drug taper. Many methods have been used with the most common being to decrease the dose by 10 mg in weekly increments.

See the discussion of surgery clients receiving glucocorticoid therapy in the Integrating Pharmacology feature on Medications Used in the Treatment of Rheumatoid Arthritis.

An alternative to the use of high-dose oral glucocorticoids is bolus intravenous steroid pulse therapy. Usually 1 to 1.5 g of methylprednisolone is given daily for 3 days to clients with severe disease, such as active nephritis, fulminating central nervous system disease, and hematologic crises. Generally, oral glucocorticoids (up to 60 mg/day of prednisone) are also given following this treatment period. Dysrhythmias and seizures have been associated with sudden death after administration of pulse therapy.

OTHER IMMUNOSUPPRESSANTS

The use of immunosuppressive agents has gradually become an accepted therapy for SLE. Methotrexate in low doses (7.5 to 15 mg/week) appears to be useful in managing arthritis, skin rashes, serositis, and other clinical manifestations. Treatment regimens, including azathioprine (Imuran) or cyclophosphamide (Cytoxan), have been able to halt the progression of glomerulonephritis or result in significantly less renal deterioration. Azathioprine, intravenous cyclophosphamide, and HCQ can also be given. See the Integrating Pharmacology feature on Medications used in the Treatment of Rheumatoid Arthritis for more information.

OTHER AGENTS

The attenuated androgen danazol has been shown to be useful in managing SLE thrombocytopenia. The mechanism of action has not been defined, but it is thought to involve endocrine influences such as the suppression of pituitary follicle-stimulating hormone and luteinizing hormone on immune or reticuloendothelial functions.

Intravenous immunoglobulin has been shown to be useful in managing severe SLE thrombocytopenia. The platelet count rises rapidly within hours of administration, occasionally peaking with extraordinarily high counts in which thrombotic events become a clinical concern. The rate of relapse following treatment is high. The primary role is to control acute bleeding associated with lupus thrombocytopenia or to rapidly increase the platelet count to allow for splenectomy or other surgery.

Dapsone, an antimicrobial agent used to treat leprosy (Hansen's disease), has been used to manage cutaneous manifestation of lupus, including discoid, subacute cutaneous lupus, bullous, and lupus profundus lesions. Hematologic side effects are common and require close monitoring.

There are several drugs in clinical trials for the treatment of lupus nephritis, including the use of mycophenolate mofetil (CellCept) and tolerogens that arrest the production of dsDNA antibodies. A placebo-controlled trial of dehydroepiandrosterone (DHEA) has reported benefits in clients with mild to moderate lupus activity. Stem cell transplant is also being aggressively explored.

Mild to moderate loss of scalp hair can occur when the disease is active. Vascular lesions can include petechiae, purpuric lesions, and Raynaud's phenomenon.

Joint manifestations, with or without active synovitis, occur in over 90% of those affected. Along with Raynaud's phenomenon, these findings are often the earliest features of the disease. Therefore the musculoskeletal examination should focus on a full assessment of the ROM of all joints, noting the location and presence of synovitis, diffuse swelling, joint and muscle pain, and stiffness. Joint involvement is symmetrical in SLE, but deformities are usually the result of soft tissue stresses rather than erosive changes. One of the more common deformities is Jaccoud's arthropathy, a rheumatoid-like deformity of the hands present in about 10% of clients with SLE. In this condition, the MCP joints are subluxed, ulnar deviation develops, and hyperextension of the PIP joints can be observed.

Manage Exacerbations

During exacerbations, clients may become acutely and seriously ill. Infectious complications can develop in about one half of clients with SLE, especially bacterial infections of the skin, respiratory tract, and urinary tract. Nursing care during this time is directed toward the assessment and management of acute confusional states, the prevention of seizures, the maintenance of skin integrity, the prevention of additional infection, the assessment of renal function, and the management of impaired gas exchange associated with lung disease and infection.

During this acute phase, increased fatigue, joint pain, and stiffness are often present as a result of inflammation and increased disease activity. Nursing activities to manage these acute flare-ups are similar to those used during exacerbations of RA. Self-care deficits are often exacerbated because of the increased disease activity. It is important to help clients maintain as much independence as possible during periods of acute flare-ups so both self-esteem and physical functions are enhanced. Clients may require considerably more time to complete even one task, so nursing interventions may need to help the client focus on conserving energy and prioritizing self-care actions.

Promote Orientation and Decision Making

Caring for a client with acutely impaired thought processes can be perplexing. Several factors can contribute to the cause of this nursing diagnosis, including increased inflammation of the central nervous system and psychosis from high doses of steroids. Clients typically have severe throbbing headaches that are sometimes accompanied by generalized tonic-clonic seizures. They may display impaired judgment, inappropriate speech and behavior, difficulty concentrating or comprehending simple instructions, or short-term memory deficits. As the disease progresses, they may have personality changes, with a decreased ability to carry out purposeful activity. Clients with impaired thought processes should be cared for in a quiet environment, particularly when headaches are severe. Clocks and calendars should be provided to help with orientation. Communication must be caring but clear and concise to decrease ambiguity and anxiety.

Provide Seizure Precautions

If clients are prone to seizures, they should be observed carefully for auras or specific activities that might trigger the seizure. During the seizure, the client should be protected from injury by removing dangerous objects, providing padding and blankets, and by turning the client to the side after muscle activity has stopped to prevent aspiration. Restraints should never be applied during the seizure because the intense muscular activity beneath the restraint could lead to fractures.

SAFETY

ALERT

Monitor Fluid Status

Another focus of nursing care during exacerbations of the disease is the management of excess fluid volume typically seen in peripheral edema. The goal is to maintain optimal renal function by assessing urinary output and urine specific gravity every 2 to 4 hours, monitoring fluid intake and electrolyte levels, and assessing changes in the level of consciousness.

Maintain Skin Integrity

The skin of a steroid-dependent client with SLE is characteristically tissue thin and fragile, so clients with peripheral edema must be moved and handled gently. The excess osmotic pressure beneath the skin surface can stress it easily so that minimal shearing forces can quickly denude the dermal layers.

SAFETY

ALERT

Promote Coping and Self-Esteem

During the chronic phase of the illness, clients can experience intense frustration because they often do not appear ill. The extreme weakness and fatigue they encounter during exacerbations of the disease, however, can lead to feelings of powerlessness and helplessness, ineffective coping, and a disturbance in self-concept. Helping clients with SLE develop a traditional support group is difficult. Lupus clients are often homebound because of extreme fatigue, impaired mobility, and commitment to their roles of spouse and parent. In these situations, the use of telephone support networks or Internet support networks for clients with SLE can be a powerful nursing strategy. At the same time that these networks provide social support and counseling for the homebound, they also encourage personal growth and development among other clients with SLE who have developed positive coping skills. Nurses can play an important role in helping to establish this type of network through the education and support of peer counselors.

Discuss Reproductive Issues

During remissions, clients often wonder about whether they can safely have children. This is a natural concern because most clients are women of childbearing age. Because fertility in clients with SLE is comparable to that of the general population, initiating and responding to clients' requests for health information are important functions of the nurse. Relapses of SLE can occur at any time during pregnancy but have not shown to result in an increase in the risk of fetal loss. The incidence of relapses during pregnancy has been reported to vary from 22% to 58%. However, most disease exacerbations can be reasonably well controlled with increasing doses of prednisone. Oral contraceptives containing low doses of estrogen are safe with mild lupus but should be used with caution by clients with severe lupus, as they can cause a flare-up. In addition, most studies report good neonatal outcomes in infants born to women with SLE, although a high incidence of prematurity has been observed.

SYSTEMIC SCLEROSIS

Systemic sclerosis (SSc), literally "hard" (scleros) "skin" (derma), encompasses both a disease restricted to the skin (localized scleroderma) and a disease with internal organ involvement (diffuse scleroderma or systemic sclerosis). One of the earliest definite descriptions of scleroderma was published by W.D. Chowne (1842, London), pertaining to a child, and in an adult by James Startin (1846, London). Maurice Raynaud (1862, Paris) described the vasospastic phenomenon that bears his name.

SSc is one of the least well understood of the rheumatic disorders. It occurs as a multisystem inflammatory disease characterized by skin thickening (scleroderma) and deposition of excessive quantities of connective tissue (particularly collagen), which eventually results in severe fibrosis. The skin, blood vessels, synovium, and skeletal muscles are affected along with the microvasculature of internal organs, such as the heart, lung, kidney, and gastrointestinal tract. Widespread vascular involvement, perhaps the earliest and most significant pathologic change, is also a prominent feature of SSc.

SSc is seen worldwide. The incidence for women is more than three times greater than that for men, especially for those between the ages of 14 and 40 years. The incidence has been calculated to be 10 per 100,000

people, with a total estimate of 250,000 to 300,000 cases in the United States.

SSc is considered one of the eight types of sclero derma, the classification of which depends on the degree and extent of skin thickening. The term "sclero derma" was first introduced in the mid-19th century to describe skin induration. Later, others used the term "progressive systemic sclerosis" to reflect its often generalized multisystem course. Currently, the term "systemic sclerosis" is preferred because many clients have limited skin and organ involvement.

Etiology and Risk Factors

Several risk factors have been associated with SSc. Over production of collagen and fibrous skin thickening have been associated with environmental factors (working with plastics, coal, or silica dust) and a high alcohol intake. Scleroderma-like conditions can also be present as a result of genetic factors (phenylketonuria), metabolic disorders (Hashimoto's thyroiditis), malignancies, postinfectious disorders, and neurologic conditions.

Pathophysiology

SSc is the result of an excessive production of collagen by fibroblasts. It seems likely that lymphocytes accumulate in the lower dermis. These cells, almost entirely T lymphocytes, generate lymphokines, which in turn stimulate fibroblasts to produce excessive amounts of procollagen. After the procollagen is secreted from the cell, it undergoes cross-linking in the extracellular environment to produce mature, relatively insoluble collagen. The skin undergoes fibrotic changes, leading to loss of elasticity and movement.

Vascular changes are also important in the development of SSc. When the vascular endothelium is injured, damaged blood vessels release vasoactive substances, which are stimulated to overproduce collagen and mucopolysaccharides. Proliferation of the subintimal connective tissue results, along with fibrous thickening and narrowing of the lumina, thus leading to tissue ischemia. A small number of clients with CREST (see Clinical Manifestations) develop pulmonary hypertension and intestinal malabsorption, which are the leading causes of death for these clients.

Clinical Manifestations

The two major types of SSc are classified according to the degree of their skin and systemic involvement. The first type, characterized by diffuse, cutaneous scleroderma, begins with symmetrical widespread thickening of the skin on the extremities, the face, and the trunk. In the early stages of the disease, bilateral symmetrical swelling of the fingers, face, and feet can be seen, and the skin has a tense, wrinkle-free appearance (Figure 77-5). A

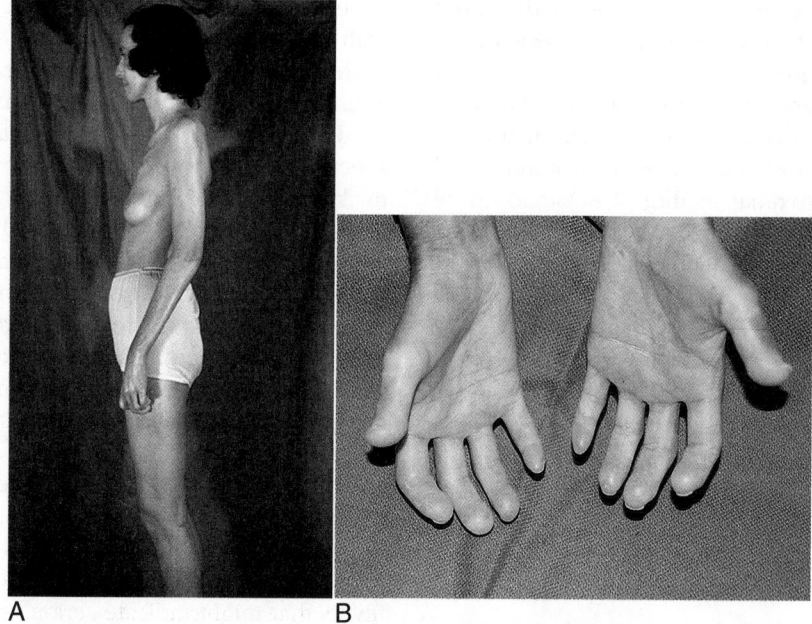

■ FIGURE 77–5 **A,** Long-term scleroderma. Note wrinkle-free appearance and shininess of the skin. **B,** Appearance of the hands in a client with scleroderma. Note thickening of the skin and swelling of the fingers.

the disease progresses, the skin becomes more thickened, hidebound, and shiny. Changes in pigmentation (both hypopigmentation and hyperpigmentation) are associated with the loss of normal skin folds. Distal thickening is always more severe than proximal thickening, so the extremities may show more changes than the face. Eventually, the face can become mask-like. The mouth is rigid, and the overall expression is blunted or immobile. Clients with this diffuse type have a tendency to develop early problems in the gastrointestinal tract, heart, lungs, and kidneys. The esophagus is particularly affected. Because of the early development of visceral changes, the pace, progression, and complications can be rapid.

The second type, limited cutaneous scleroderma, is characterized by skin changes that are usually confined to the fingers and distal portions of the extremities and face. In general, skin changes progress much more slowly than they do in the diffuse type of SSc. Truncal scleroderma is absent. Visceral changes (e.g., severe pulmonary arterial hypertension and biliary cirrhosis), if they do appear, are rare and are seen late in the course of the disease. Clients with limited scleroderma often develop "CREST":

- **C**alcinosis: Calcium deposits in the tissues
- **R**aynaud's phenomenon: Intermittent vasospasm of the finger tips
- **E**sophageal hardening: Sclerosis of the esophagus
- **S**clerodactyly: Scleroderma of the digits
- **T**elangiectasias: Capillary dilations that form vascular lesions on the face, lips, and fingers

The presence of the CREST manifestations is a poor prognostic indicator. The 10-year survival rate after diagnosis is approximately 65%.

Raynaud's phenomenon, a generally bilateral vasospastic condition, can be an especially important predictor of SSc. Tricolor changes affecting the fingers in Raynaud's disease consist of pallor (white) accompanying vasoconstriction, followed by cyanosis (blue) as capillary blood is desaturated of oxygen, followed by hyperemia (redness) secondary to vasodilation. Clients with the CREST syndrome often develop painful ulcers on the finger tips or in the areas of calcinosis because of chronic vascular insufficiency. Although not listed in the acronym CREST, there is evidence of pulmonary involvement in the majority of clients. An occasional client with limited cutaneous scleroderma will develop pulmonary artery hypertension.

Laboratory findings are relatively normal in clients with scleroderma. Mild hemolytic anemia is often present because of mechanical damage to red cells from diseased small vessels. Mild hypergammaglobulinemia (IgG) and rheumatoid factor are found in 30% of those affected. Slight elevation of the ESR is also common. Proteinuria is common with renal involvement. Most clients have positive titers for ANA. Anticentromere and anticentriole antibodies seem to be relatively specific for scleroderma. Clients with the serum anticentromere antibody have a more favorable prognosis. SCL-70, an antibody to topoisomerase, is found in about 35% of clients with diffuse SSc but is rarely seen in clients with limited cutaneous involvement and the CREST syndrome. The anticentromere ANA is seen in 80% of those with limited cutaneous involvement and in only 5% of those with diffuse cutaneous involvement.

A definite diagnosis of SSc requires the presence of one major or two minor criteria. The major criteria for proximal scleroderma are skin thickening and tightening of areas proximal to the MCP joints. These changes can affect the entire extremity, face, neck, thorax, and abdomen. The three minor criteria are (1) sclerodactyly (in which the skin changes are limited to the fingers); (2) digital pitting scars, with depressed areas at the tips of the fingers or loss of fingerpad tissue; and (3) bibasilar pulmonary fibrosis.

OUTCOME MANAGEMENT

Medical Management

The treatment of SSc involves the shared management of a chronic illness and pharmacologic support. Members of the health care team should educate the client about the nature, course, and treatment of SSc, the importance of avoiding cold, stress management techniques as a means to control Raynaud's phenomenon, the prevention of hand contractures and facial rigidity, the nutritional management of constipation and diarrhea and ideal body weight, and the prevention of injury. Protecting digits by using gloves or wearing warm socks, avoiding cold temperatures, and not smoking are important self-care measures that may require behavior modification to help the client have some control over the illness.

Reduce Inflammation, Sclerosis, and Vasospasm

Many medications are used in systemic sclerosis, but no single agent has been proved convincingly effective. Treatment and prevention of complications are the current goals of therapy. Three types of therapeutic agents have been used to treat SSc: (1) vasoactive agents, (2) anti-inflammatory medications, and (3) immunosuppressive drugs.

In Raynaud's disease, calcium-channel blockers have become widely prescribed. Nifedipine, 10 to 20 mg three times a day, was effective for Raynaud's disease in a controlled, double-blind trial. Digital ulcers and digital infarcts have been somewhat successfully treated with digital sympathectomies.

Glucocorticoids are the major anti-inflammatory agents used in SSc when clients have significant joint and muscle involvement or extensive skin disease. Low-dose steroid therapy (prednisone, 10 mg/day or every other day) is preferred. Overall, immunosuppressive agents (azathioprine, cyclophosphamide, cyclosporine, and methotrexate) have not consistently been proved effective in the

treatment of SSc. Cyclophosphamide is often used in client with progressive lung fibrosis.

Penicillamine, an immunomodulating agent that als interferes with the cross-linking of collagen, is a widel used drug in treating scleroderma. A large retrospective study showed significant improvement in ski thickening after 2 years of therapy and improved 5-yea survival compared with untreated clients Not all clin cians, however, accept penicillamine as established the apy for SSc. Initial doses should be low (125 mg/day and the dose should increase gradually. Reduction c skin thickness requires long-term therapy, so clien need considerable support and monitoring while the are taking penicillamine. In addition, numerous tox side effects can occur, including lupus-like syndrom myasthenia gravis, glomerulonephritis, pemphigu excessive skin wrinkling, and blood and liver dyscrasia Clients taking penicillamine must be carefully instructe to report skin rashes, burning, bleeding, sore throats, c fevers that might indicate serious side effects. The nurs and physician must explain the importance of period laboratory follow-up of liver, kidney, and renal functio to the client.

Various other agents are used to treat specif system problems. Minocycline has been effective in th treatment of diarrhea associated with malabsorption sy drome. This drug may reduce inflammation by blockir metalloproteases. A proton pump inhibitor should b administered to reduce the acidity of gastric reflux. Et nercept, a biologic response modifier (BMR), in an initi small (10 client), open-label pilot study was encou aging, as was the long-term extension, but furthe research is necessary to determine its effectiveness SSc management.

Reduce Renal Complications

Renal crisis and associated hypertension was the mc feared complication of systemic sclerosis. Th introduction of angiotensin-converting enzyme (AC inhibitors, which are capable of reversing underlyir hyperreninemia and controlling hypertension, h improved the outcome of renal crisis. Clients now ha an 80% 1-year survival and a 60% 5-year survival, in co trast to a 15% 1-year survival without the use of AC inhibitors.

Treat Pulmonary Arterial Hypertension

Pulmonary arterial hypertension (PAH) is a leading cau of mortality in SSc. Two-year survival of clients with PA has been 40% to 55%. Pulmonary vascular disease ca occur in isolation or in the setting of the later stages interstitial lung disease, complicating both diffuse a limited scleroderma. Initial endothelial cell injury resu in abnormal vascular reactivity, related to factors such local release of the vasoconstrictive mediator endothel and loss of the endothelial-derived vasodilators prostacyclin and nitric oxide (NO). Functional lesions progress to structural lesions of arteriolar fibrosis.

The newly approved pharmacologic treatments, epoprostenol (Flolan), bosentan (Tracleer), and terprostinil (Remodulin), are well matched to current understanding of the underlying pathophysiology. All three agents have been demonstrated in controlled clinical trials to have beneficial effects on exercise capacity and pulmonary hemodynamics. Factors affecting the use of these agents include the short half-life of the prostacyclin analogs (epoprostenol, 2 to 5 minutes; treprostinil, 3 hours), necessitating continuous infusion; the need for a central line for administration of epoprostenol; the potential teratogenicity (risk for congenital defects) of bosentan; and availability issues (e.g., bosentan is distributed only through centralized pharmacies).

Nursing Management of the Medical Client

Complete Nursing History

Clients should be interviewed with great sensitivity because of their possible fears about the disease and the changes in body image. The first manifestation of SSc is often puffiness of the fingers and toes and in limited scleroderma, Raynaud's phenomenon. Question clients carefully about their experiences. Ask them if they have had the sequence of blanching, cyanosis, and erythema that is associated with periodic vasospasm of the peripheral blood vessels. Ask which parts of the body have been affected. Although Raynaud's phenomenon is commonly seen in the hands and toes, it can affect the earlobes, nose, and tongue. It is also important to ask clients under what circumstances (i.e., cold or stress) they have experienced Raynaud's phenomenon.

Clients should be asked about changes in the texture, color, consistency, and moisture of their skin. Because skin changes can be widespread, it is usually helpful to tell clients you would like to review changes according to body location. Clients should be asked about subcutaneous nodules that they may have noticed under their finger tips.

Other systemic changes to be explored include those associated with the gastrointestinal tract. Clients should be asked about the ease with which they swallow food and the types of food they have had difficulty swallowing. The presence of diarrhea (related to bacterial overgrowth) or a malabsorption syndrome can occur; constipation (related to colonic hypomotility), nausea, vomiting, and abdominal distention should be explored within the framework of onset, severity, duration, aggravating factors, and relieving factors. The respiratory system can be affected, secondary to interstitial pulmonary fibrosis. Therefore ask clients if they have had any cough, shortness of breath, or dyspnea with activity.

Clients should be asked questions about their musculoskeletal health. The presence of bilateral symmetrical joint pain and swelling should be elicited. Changes in endurance and muscle strength, as indicated by the ability to perform ADL, should be explored.

Complete Physical Assessment

A careful assessment is required of the entire integumentary system, including the skin on the feet, trunk, and abdomen. The face and lips (as well as fingers, palms, and fingernails) may have telangiectasias, which are macular dilations of superficial blood vessels that collapse after firm palpation. The hands are inspected and palpated for edema, thickened or hardened skin, loss of skin folds, or wrinkles (see Figure 77-5, *B*). Fingers are also inspected and palpated for subcutaneous calcific nodules and dilated capillary loops or venules or ulcers on the tips of the fingernails. Nail beds are inspected for pitting, changes in contour, and the appearance of suppurative cuticles.

Changes in the skin over the forearms, face, legs, and trunk can occur in diffuse cutaneous scleroderma. Therefore each area should be carefully assessed for edema, thickening, or tightening. The face should be inspected for mobility of expression and ability to open the mouth. Clients with SSc are often unable to open the mouth fully as the disease progresses. Skin thickening is often accompanied by areas of hypopigmentation and hyperpigmentation, so these changes are most commonly observed on the extremities and chest.

The musculoskeletal assessment includes a thorough evaluation of ROM because reduced joint mobility and polyarthritis characterize SSc. Flexor and extensor tendons should be palpated for the presence of friction rubs. Often, coarse crepitus caused by fibrin deposits can be heard with tendon motion—a sign that is often considered specific for SSc. Eliciting Tinel's sign (see Figure 71-11, *A*, p. 1889) to rule out or confirm carpal tunnel syndrome is useful. Muscle strength should be assessed and graded because SSc may have a polymyositis-type myopathy affecting the proximal muscles.

Other body systems should be assessed to provide baseline data or to determine possible organ involvement. The respiratory system should be assessed for the ease and extent of thoracic excursion, presence of dyspnea, and presence of adventitious lung sounds. The heart is examined for changes in rhythm or signs of heart failure. Blood pressure must be monitored closely because sudden malignant hypertension associated with renal disease can occur in SSc.

Facilitate Muscle and Joint Movement

Most clients with SSc have significant muscle and joint involvement, including arthralgias, myalgia, and fibrosis of the tendons. When contractures develop, they are often due to the fibrotic changes in the skin. These muscle and joint changes lead to problems often encountered in clients with RA—joint pain, stiffness, fatigue, self-care deficits, and impaired physical mobility.

From the client's perspective, coping with an altered body image that accompanies extensive skin changes can be an overwhelming task. Nurses can help clients understand that successful coping often means assuming responsibility for self-care and the prevention of complications. Nursing interventions, therefore, are targeted at maintaining a full ROM of the mouth and hands as well as suggesting creative use of clothing and makeup to enhance the appearance.

Maintain Skin Integrity

Changes in skin integrity require meticulous nursing care. For the acutely ill client, all digits and extremities must be handled carefully and gently. If possible, the client should try to move or reposition himself or herself so minimal discomfort occurs. Debilitated or steroid-dependent clients or those undergoing orthopedic surgery should be placed on pressure-reducing beds or air mattresses to prevent the development of skin breakdown over bony prominences. Dressings must be removed carefully so that additional trauma does not occur. Although moist dressings are applied to injured areas, they should be dampened with sterile saline if they do not come off easily. Tape should be used only when absolutely essential, for example, to stabilize an intravenous catheter needle. Otherwise, all dressings should be secured with stretchable gauze.

Whenever possible, the administration of injections and intravenous therapy should be in sites free of fibrosis and sclerosis. Areas of tough, thickened skin and sclerotic veins cannot be easily punctured. It is possible, also, to cause additional damage (and a portal for infection) if needle punctures are not made successfully.

Provide Education

Client education is the cornerstone to effective nursing care of the client with Raynaud's phenomenon. Clients must be assisted to modify their dress and health practices so all controllable sources of vasospasm are eliminated. Newly diagnosed clients may need anticipatory guidance about how to dress protectively in cold weather and in air conditioning. They may readily recognize the need for gloves but not realize the importance of protecting the head, ears, nose, lips, and feet. Keeping a pair of gloves in a tote bag or pocket is helpful when in air-conditioned stores or when taking frozen items out of the grocery freezer. Clients must maintain their core temperature, always dressing warmly. Clients must often be helped to change their health practices so they eliminate the use of vasoconstrictive substances, such as alcohol and caffeine. Learning biofeedback or other stress management skills is indicated when clients identify stress as a cause of altered tissue perfusion.

Promote Adequate Nutrition

Clients with SSc often have difficulty maintaining their weight because of esophageal changes leading to dysphagia, esophagitis, and decreased intestinal motility. Consultation with the dietitian can help the nurse provide appropriate, easy-to-swallow, high-calorie snacks. The dietitian can plan meals to avoid foods contributing to esophagitis and gastric reflux. Remaining upright for 1 to 2 hours after eating also helps to prevent esophageal reflux. Avoiding heavy snacks close to retiring, using a large wedge pillow to elevate the head and shoulders, or elevating the head of the bed on shock blocks can prevent bedtime reflux. The client's ability to chew and swallow dry, compact foods, such as meat and bread, should be carefully evaluated. Often, these foods cause severe choking spells. Moistening them with gravies, sauces, or jellies helps them to be more easily tolerated. The achievement of nutritional goals is often affected by dental hygiene practices. Because of sclerotic skin changes, clients may have a difficult time completely opening the mouth. Mucous membranes may become inflamed or ulcerated because of lack of moisture or inadequate brushing and rinsing. Using a small angled toothbrush or Waterpik can help prevent these problems. Reinforcing the need to perform facial exercises to prevent rigidity of the face and mouth is a priority nursing intervention.

Promote Bowel Elimination

Chronic constipation and diarrhea are two other problems that are usually amenable to nursing intervention. Chronic constipation is associated with the decreased motility of the gastrointestinal tract that accompanies SSc. Nursing interventions include eating easy-to-swallow, high-fiber foods along with drinking more fluids and participating in exercise. The use of bulk stool softeners and suppositories may be needed as part of the bowel program. Diarrhea is associated with the malabsorption syndrome. Foods known to precipitate diarrhea should be eliminated from the diet, and natural antidiarrheal agents can be added to meals. When infectious organisms are present, antibiotic agents are prescribed, often tetracycline.

Monitor for Complications

Nursing care is also directed toward the monitoring and detecting of potential problems. The potential for impaired gas exchange exists when interstitial fibrosis of the lungs occurs. The presence of dyspnea, changes in activity tolerance, and an increased rate and depth of respirations may be noted. Auscultation of lung sounds may indicate fine crackles. Oxygen is usually administered as supportive therapy, and clients are educated about factors (pollen, smoking, humidity) that exacerbate the pulmonary condition.

SPONDYLOARTHROPATHIES

The *spondyloarthropathies* are a group of interrelated disorders that include psoriatic arthritis (PsA), reactive arthritis, arthritis-associated inflammatory bowel disease, and ankylosing spondylitis (AS). Spondyloarthropathies are distinguished from RA by the following three characteristics: (1) a negative test for RF, (2) the absence of rheumatoid nodules, and (3) an inflammatory peripheral arthritis that is typically asymmetrical. Three other features of the spondyloarthropathies have been noted. First, inflammation occurs where the ligament inserts into the bone (enthesis) rather than at the synovium. Extraskeletal changes can occur in the eye, skin, lung parenchyma, or aortic valve. Second, there is considerable overlap between the various spondyloarthropathies. For example, a person with PsA can develop the classic sacroiliitis seen in AS. Finally, there is a tendency toward familial aggregation in the development of the disease, with genes other than *B27* probably playing a role.

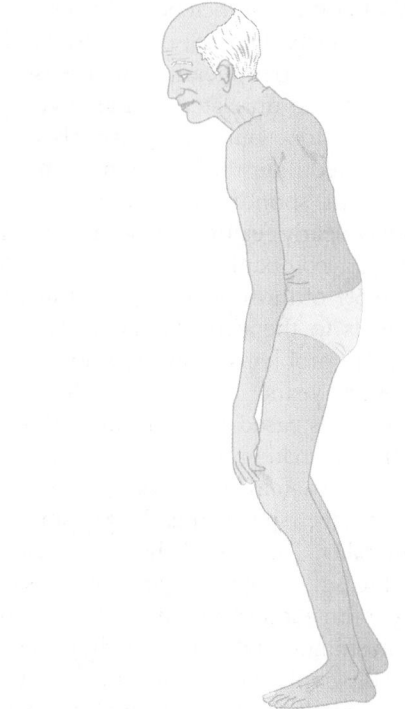

■ **FIGURE 77–6**   Ankylosing spondylitis.

ANKYLOSING SPONDYLITIS

Literally, ankylosing spondylitis (AS) refers to fusion (ankylosis) of inflamed vertebrae (spondylitis) (Figure 77-6). The disease typically begins in the spine of young men in their late teens or early twenties. The majority of clients have bilateral sacroiliitis that causes pain and some degree of restricted motion in the lumbar spine. Peripheral arthritis of the large joints, usually the hips and shoulders and more rarely the knees, occurs in 20% to 30% of people with AS. Small joint involvement is not usually seen. Chest expansion can also be decreased because of an associated costovertebral arthritis. By the time the client is 50 or 60, the fusion of the lumbar spine has proceeded to the cervical region. If AS is not treated, the disease tends to progress with remissions and exacerbations to a final stage of rigid lumbar and thoracic kyphosis that leaves the neck in a flexed position. Ankylosing spondylitis is associated with a shortening of the life span.

Etiology and Risk Factors

The average annual age-adjusted incidence rate of AS has been reported to be 6.6 per 100,000 population, with men affected three times as frequently as women. Although the usual age of onset has been established as between 15 and 35 years, the age group with the highest incidence rate is the 25- to 34-year-old group.

The overall incidence rate is estimated to be 129 per 100,000 population. Thus the overall incidence rate for the entire population has been estimated to fall between 1 and 2 per 1000 population.

Risk factors associated with AS include gender (with a 3:1 to 4:1 predominance of males over females), the young adult years of adolescence through adulthood (15 to 35 years old), and a genetic predisposition. A strong tendency toward familial aggregation has been seen and a sex-linked hormone may be important. The presence of HLA-B27 may also be a risk factor, as it appears frequently in the high-risk Indian population but is almost nonexistent in the low-risk U.S. African-American population. Although the disease is generally seen in men in the third decade of life, the condition may go undetected in women because of its milder course and the usual caution in performing pelvic x-rays in women of childbearing age.

Clinical Manifestations

Initially, morning backache and stiffness begin during young adulthood. The back pain and stiffness subside with movement but often return with inactivity. Back pain throughout the spinal column, difficulty sleeping, and neurologic changes such as bowel and bladder incontinence, paresthesia, and numbness may also occur.

Several other systemic manifestations of AS can be seen, such as uveitis, pulmonary fibrosis, inflammatory bowel disease, and aortic insufficiency. Uveitis occurs in up to 25% of all clients with AS, especially in HLA-B27-positive clients with peripheral joint disease, but its incidence seems to be unrelated to the severity of the spondylitis. Upper lobe pulmonary fibrosis is rare, but it has been reported. Intestinal inflammation is frequent in clients with spondylarthropathy, and one fourth of clients have early features of Crohn's disease. Aortic insufficiency, accompanied by a typical diastolic murmur, occurs in 5% of those with AS, and this problem frequently leads to the need for an aortic valve replacement. Cardiac problems, however, do not usually appear for several years.

The diagnosis of AS is based on the results of the history and physical examination and on radiologic findings. Positive physical examination findings include the presence of sacroiliitis, spinal muscle spasms, and decreased hip mobility. Decreased chest expansion is seen later in the disease. Along with symptomatic sacroiliitis, radiologic confirmation of sacroiliac joint changes is probably the most important finding early in the disease. Although radiographs taken early in the disease may show no abnormalities, later the typical changes of sacroiliitis develop, with patchy sclerosis at the joint margins. Early changes in AS include a squaring off of the anterior lumbar vertebral surfaces. This squaring is caused by erosion of the upper and lower margins of the vertebrae at the site of insertion of the annulus fibrosus. The intervertebral ligaments involved in the inflammatory process heal by ossification, leading to the formation of syndesmophytes in the outer layers of the annulus fibrosus. Eventually, the disk space becomes bridged by these bony syndesmophytes. In the end stage of the disease, complete spinal fusion (bamboo spine) and fusion of the sacroiliac joints occur along with ossification of all of the ligamentous structures.

Generally, laboratory studies are not helpful in diagnosing AS. Although the HLA-B27 antigen is seen in 90% of clients with AS, it is found in up to 10% of those without the disease, thus limiting its specificity in diagnosis. An elevated ESR is seen in most clients, but it may be normal in those with severe disease. Other findings may include elevated creatine kinase (CK) and alkaline phosphatase levels, but these are not confirming diagnostic tests.

OUTCOME MANAGEMENT

Medical Management

The treatment goals for AS are to maintain mobility, decrease inflammation, and control pain. As with other chronic conditions, treatment is more successful when clients are engaged in and assume responsibility for health promotion and other self-care activities.

Maintain Mobility

Instructing the client to perform appropriate exercises and engage in ADL is critical if the client is to maintain mobility with minimal spinal curvature. Good posture must be encouraged through exercises that promote stretching and extension of the spine. Swimming is an excellent general conditioner as well as an activity that promotes spinal extension without increased pain. The nurse may need to help the client solve problems about awkward furniture or equipment that reinforces spinal flexion. For example, the client who has a desk job may need to invest in a tilting artist's table so the neck and head are not forced into flexion with constant activity. Selecting ergonomic chairs or ensuring the correct placement of a computer workstation can also be beneficial for the client's comfort. Appropriate sleep posture must be reinforced, particularly in those with mild cervical flexion who are accustomed to sleeping with two pillows. Spinal extension is maximized during sleep if clients lie on a firm mattress, preferably with bed boards underneath, in a supine position, without a pillow. If the client insists on using a pillow, it should be as flat as possible.

Reduce Pain and Inflammation

As with many other chronic arthritic conditions, successful pain management depends on reducing inflammation and stiffness. NSAIDs are used to reduce inflammation, and the application of heat (or a warm shower or bath) helps to relieve morning pain and stiffness. Sulfasalazine and methotrexate have shown beneficial effects but their use is being supplanted by the approval of the "Tumor-Necrosis-Factor alpha (TNF-α) blockers," which have been shown to slow or even halt the progression of AS and to be highly effective in treating spinal arthritis. Etanercept and infliximab have been approved by the FDA for the treatment of AS.

Nursing Management of the Medical Client

Obtain Nursing History

Questions should focus on the typical clinical manifestations of pain, stiffness, and fatigue and their effects on performing ADL, as well as screening for extra-articular involvement. Question clients about the nature, onset, location, duration, and quality of their pain. Ask what self-care measures (e.g., use of heat or cold, showers or baths) they have used to cope with the pain-stiffness-fatigue cycle and which measures have been effective.

Determine whether the pain is in the lower back, thorax, or cervical area and if other large peripheral joints such as the knees, hips, or shoulders, cause discomfort. During the early phase of AS, clients complain of lumbosacral pain that radiates to the buttocks and thighs. Sleep for clients with AS is different from normal sleep

Therefore an assessment of sleep patterns should be completed. Ask clients if the pain is worse on rising, if it is associated with morning stiffness, and if it decreases with activity. Also determine the length of time that the client has been affected with back pain. These points are important because the following five features strongly suggest inflammatory spinal disease: (1) insidious onset of discomfort, (2) being younger than 40 years, (3) persistence of discomfort for more than 3 months, (4) association with morning stiffness, and (5) improvement with exercise.

Clients should also be questioned about fatigue, weight loss, and the presence of a low-grade fever. With advanced disease, cord compression can occur as a result of spinal fractures, so it is important to elicit information about neurologic changes, such as decreased motor activity, paresthesias, numbness, and bowel and bladder incontinence. Because of the possibility of extra-articular disease, it is important to ask clients about their eyes, respiratory status, and heart. The following are suggested screening parameters for each system:

Eyes: Presence of blurred vision, decreased vision, pain, excessive tearing, photophobia

Respiratory status: Presence and quality of cough, sputum production, dyspnea, shortness of breath, smoking history

Cardiovascular status: History of murmurs, tachycardia, and extra heart sounds

Complete Physical Assessment

The spinal assessment is often normal early in the disease, or there can be tenderness with deep palpation of the sacroiliac joint. As the disease progresses into the upper spinal segments, loss of the normal lumbar lordosis occurs, followed by decreased flexion, extension, and lateral movement. Asking the client to flex at the waist and observing the flattening of the lumbar spine can assess loss of lumbar lordosis. Tenderness along vertebral structures and marked paravertebral spasm can also be present with decreased lumbar lordosis.

A useful measure of lumbar flexion is the Schober's test. With the client standing erect, the nurse makes a mark at the L5-S1 area and another 10 cm above it. When the client bends forward in maximal flexion, the distance between the two marks normally should increase to 15 cm. In AS, however, this measurement does not significantly increase. The Schober's test is most useful in evaluating young clients because spinal flexion generally decreases with age. Alternatively, when screening for AS, measure the distance from fingers to floor when clients attempt to touch their toes. Clients with decreased flexion have a greater distance between their fingers and the floor. The tendency to develop a kyphotic posture in AS is reflected in diminished thoracic expansion. To assess chest expansion, place the tape measure at the nipples and then note the chest measurement with full lung expansion. A distance of less than 3 cm, along with other physical signs, is highly suggestive of AS.

As the disease progresses, loss of ROM in the neck leads to a fixed kyphosis that can seriously impair visual function. The serial tracking of measurements of the distance from the client's head to the wall can be used to detect the progression of cervical kyphosis. Positioning the client with the heels against the wall and instructing the client to extend the neck fully can obtain consistent results.

Clients with AS should also be assessed for two other musculoskeletal changes. The first change is the development of an inflammatory peripheral joint involvement, particularly of the hips, knees, and shoulders. Assess these joints bilaterally for changes in ROM, pain, tenderness, and synovitis. Also observe for signs of enthesitis, a problem commonly seen in juvenile AS and occasionally present in adults. Enthesitis can involve the plantar aspect of the foot (plantar fasciitis), the heel (Achilles tendinitis), and the knee. Other sites include the greater trochanters, superior anterior iliac crests, and ischial tuberosities. Attachment sites may or may not be swollen, but typically they are extremely painful to palpation. Because of the potential for developing extraskeletal problems with the eyes, lungs, and heart, these systems should be carefully assessed during the baseline screening.

Provide Education

The nurse plays a key role in educating the client about health promotion activities, exercise, and the management of pain. One of the most critical areas for skillful nursing intervention involves being attentive and providing positive, unconditional regard for those clients with changing appearances. If the disease progresses rapidly or if the client has not sought help until skeletal changes are noticeable, the client may be quite self-conscious and even depressed about the appearance. Businessmen may have found it increasingly more difficult to find clothing that fits. Some men have been known to avoid buying suits because of their embarrassment about being seen by salespersons or tailors. The client may be so concerned about appearance that he or she avoids social interaction outside of the job. Helping clients who have an altered body image or who are socially isolated is a significant challenge and an opportunity to establish a meaningful, therapeutic relationship. Although specific nursing interventions can be implemented that encourage group participation and interaction, it is often the nurse's positive, unconditional regard that helps the client work toward reintegration of self. Approximately one third of clients experience depression and women report more depression than men.

Promote Effective Breathing

Another important area for nursing intervention, especially as the disease progresses, is the maintenance of effective breathing patterns and adequate oxygenation. Ongoing assessment of chest wall expansion, instructions in deep-breathing exercises, and the avoidance of smoking and respiratory depressants can help the client to maintain optimal breathing. If dyspnea becomes a problem, instruct the client in pursed-lip breathing and the pacing of activities. For those clients with cervical involvement who become acutely ill or require surgery, notify the anesthesia department. Ankylosing spondylitis in the cervical area frequently causes problems with intubation.

REACTIVE ARTHRITIS

Reactive arthritis and Reiter's syndrome are both designations for a form of peripheral arthritis, often accompanied by one or more extra-articular manifestations, which appear shortly after certain infections of the genitourinary or gastrointestinal tracts. The majority of affected individuals, usually young men, have inherited the human leukocyte antigen HLA-B27. Reiter's syndrome originally referred to the clinical triad of nongonoccocal urethritis, conjunctivitis, and arthritis. Because of many overlapping clinical, epidemiologic, and genetic features, reactive arthritis is classified as a seronegative spondylarthropathy. Approximately 80% of clients experience chronic problems marked by periods of remission and exacerbation.

Etiology and Risk Factors

Reactive arthritis occurs following exposure to a bacterial gastrointestinal or genitourinary infection. Although the exact mechanism remains unclear, certain infective agents and a specific genetic background (presence of HLA-B27) are associated with reactive arthritis. Epidemic reactive arthritis has occurred in association with dysentery. Endemic or postvenereal reactive arthritis is the more common type found in the United States.

Endemic reactive arthritis occurs more frequently in young men (9:1) and is linked to the greater prevalence of HLA-B27 antigen in this population. Cases following food-borne enteric infections affect both genders equally. Caucasians are affected more commonly than African Americans or other racial groups who have a lower frequency of HLA-B27. Reactive arthritis is difficult to diagnose and probably occurs more frequently than reported.

Clinical Manifestations

Reactive arthritis demonstrates features in almost every system of the body. The most common features are polyarthritis, urethritis or cervicitis, and conjunctivitis. There is a link between the genitourinary system and reactive arthritis. Urethritis can occur symptomatically (discharge, slight burning on urination) or can be asymptomatic, which is a component in the difficulty in establishing a diagnosis. Reactive arthritis has been reported frequently in clients with human immunodeficiency virus (HIV) infection. There is a high incidence of prostatitis and acquired immunodeficiency syndrome (AIDS). The role of AIDS in the pathogenesis of reactive arthritis is still being investigated. Urethral infection is commonly accompanied by stomatitis, balanitis, and keratoderma blennorrhagicum. The keratodermal lesions are similar to psoriatic lesions and can appear on the soles of the feet, glans penis, and toes.

Conjunctivitis, considered a classic manifestation, is typically a transient, mild phenomenon. If a sterile discharge is present, it subsides within a few days. Uveitis can become a more significant clinical problem in this disorder.

Reactive arthritis is characteristically additive, asymmetrical, and oligoarticular, affecting an average of four joints. The arthritic process generally affects weight-bearing joints, especially of the knees and ankles. Large effusions can accompany it.

Diagnostic work-up includes radiography and laboratory examinations. Early in the disease, there are no radiographic changes. With disease progression, joint space narrowing and erosive changes can be seen. In advanced disease, the individual may develop sacroiliitis, as found in AS.

Laboratory findings may show an elevated erythrocyte sedimentation rate (ESR), but the ESR may be normal despite active joint involvement. Mild hypochromic or normochromic anemia may be present. Routine typing for HLA-B27 is considered unnecessary.

OUTCOME MANAGEMENT

Medical Management

Reactive arthritis usually runs a self-limited course of from 3 to 12 months in the majority of clients; however, some studies suggest that many clients continue to be plagued by minor musculoskeletal manifestations. Management of the client targets client education and management of clinical manifestations. There is a general recognition that reactive arthritis has a greater propensity for chronicity than previously appreciated, which should temper an overly optimistic prognosis. One study reported that at 1 year after diagnosis 40% of clients with post-genitourinary-acquired reactive arthritis and 20% of post-gastrointestinal-acquired reactive arthritis still had active disease, but almost all had recovered at 2-year follow-up.

Administer Medications

Pharmacologic management is similar to that used for AS. The attacks tend to be self-limiting, lasting 2 to 4 months, with a recurrence rate of 15% per year. The use of antibiotic therapy in the prevention or management of reactive arthritis remains controversial. For clients with ocular manifestations, steroid eye drops or subconjunctival preparations may be needed. Severe uveitis is relatively common and is a difficult clinical management problem.

Provide Physical Therapy

Joint pain and dysfunction are managed with a regimen of physical therapy. Splinting for joint protection along with a managed exercise and activity program are indicated.

Nursing Management of the Medical Client

Obtain Nursing History and Complete Physical Examination

The history should examine the pattern of orthopedic pain. Joint pain, back pain, heel pain, and a tendinitis-type pain can manifest in reactive arthritis. Clients with a nonspecific arthritis should be questioned about the presence of genitourinary and ocular manifestations. Ask the client if he or she has noted any atypical urethral discharge or slight pain or burning on urination for even a few days. An examination of past history of sexually transmitted diseases is important, as is the sexual history in relation to number and frequency of sexual partners. Question the client specifically about eye disease. Has the client experienced recent eye irritation and perhaps attributed it to smog or other chemical irritants? The client may have noted dermatologic lesions. Ask the client about any lesions for which he or she may have used a glucocorticosteroid cream. Has the client noticed any other vesicle-type lesions?

Physical examination targets the involved joints and inspects for dermatologic lesions and the presence of localized infections.

Provide Education

As with any chronic disease, client education plays a crucial role in helping the individual understand and manage the disease. Similar to RA (see prior discussion), clients and their families need information about the disease process and management. Because of the link to genitourinary pathology, education must target safe sexual practices. There is some evidence that use of a condom protects the client from postvenereal exacerbation of reactive arthritis. Clients are advised to avoid multiple sexual partners.

PSORIATIC ARTHRITIS

Psoriasis is a common skin disorder characterized by stippled nails, pruritus, and silvery scales on bright red plaques, usually on the elbows, knees, and scalp. It is a genetically determined disease associated with several histocompatibility antigens, including HLA-B14, HLA-Bw17, and HLA-Cw6. About 5% to 10% of those with psoriasis develop a distinctive inflammatory arthritis—psoriatic arthritis (PsA).

Three to five types of PsA have been proposed. In asymmetrical oligoarthropathy, there is asymmetrical involvement of both large and small joints, and sausage-shaped joints are common. With this type of arthritis, the asymmetrical pattern involves the interphalangeal and metatarsophalangeal joints of the feet and the DIP joints of the fingers. The second type, symmetrical polyarthropathy, closely resembles RA. Arthritis mutilans, a severe form of destructive arthritis, is characterized by telescoping digits also known as the "opera-glass hand." Psoriatic spondylitis is characterized by the sacroiliitis of AS. Clients with this last type, characterized by DIP involvement, often have nail changes, such as pitting, transverse depressions, and subungual hyperkeratosis, along with DIP joint disease.

The overall incidence of PsA is approximately 0.1% in the United States. Arthritis occurs in approximately 5% to 7% of clients with psoriasis but it may affect 40% of hospitalized clients with extensive skin involvement. Two percent of Caucasian North Americans and Europeans are believed to be affected with psoriasis but it is relatively uncommon in Asians. The male to female ratio is equal but varies in subsets of this disease. In contrast to psoriasis, where the peak age is between 5 and 15 years, the peak age of PsA is between 30 and 55 years, which is similar to RA.

Etiology and Risk Factors

The cause of PsA appears to be a complex combination of immunologic, genetic, and environmental factors. Immunologic changes seen in some clients include elevated titers of IgG and IgA and the presence of immune complexes. There is an increased prevalence of the disease among family members who have psoriatic arthritis. Possible environmental factors include group A streptococci and trauma.

Clinical Manifestations

The diagnosis of PsA is usually confirmed after a positive history of psoriasis and specific x-ray findings. It is important to realize that in some clients, particularly children, joint changes precede skin changes. Nevertheless, most rheumatologists agree that the diagnosis cannot be made without evidence of psoriatic skin or nail changes.

Some changes that appear on x-ray are suggestive of PsA. In early cases, soft tissue swelling can be seen in clients with psoriasis similar to that observed in RA. Periarticular demineralization of the bone, however, is less common in psoriatic arthritis. Radiologic findings indicative of the disease include erosions of the DIP joints (both hands and feet), which can lead to a whittled, "pencil-in-cup" appearance. Clients with spinal involvement have radiologic evidence of sacroiliitis, but the distribution of the joint changes is less predictable than it is in AS.

Laboratory tests often reveal a slightly elevated sedimentation rate and hypochromic anemia. Many clients have mild hyperuricemia, which is a confusing finding that could initially lead to the diagnosis of gout. Tests for RF are negative in 75% of clients; among the 25% with positive tests, many have coexisting psoriasis and RA.

OUTCOME MANAGEMENT

Medical Management

Although clients with PsA can have an explosive onset of polyarticular or monoarticular joint pain, erythema, and swelling, treatment goals are directed to the management of a chronic illness. Clients can be confused or discouraged when they first realize their diagnosis. They may perceive themselves as having not just one but two chronic diseases and thus feel increasingly powerless or helpless about their illness. Nurses and physicians, therefore, must work collaboratively to educate clients about the cause of the disease and the expected course of treatment. As with all other arthritic diseases, engaging the client's interest and partnership in actively managing the disease is essential for the best outcomes.

Nurses work with physicians to educate clients about key treatment strategies, many of which are similar to those implemented in RA and AS. During exacerbations of the disease, clients must avoid stressing inflamed joints, participate in active assistive ROM exercises to prevent joint contractures, and alternate periods of rest with activity. Those with foot and toenail involvement must be instructed to select appropriate footwear to protect swollen digits and keratotic nail beds.

Reduce Inflammation

The initial treatment for stable plaque psoriasis is topical. However, topical therapy may be impractical for clients with extensive psoriasis (more than 20% involvement) and systemic therapy may be indicated at the outset. Topical treatment includes emollients and keratolytic agents alone or in combination with anthralin, glucocorticoids, and vitamin D derivatives. Stress and certain drugs (beta-adrenergic blockers, angiotensin-converting enzyme inhibitors, lithium, and antimalarial

drugs) may exacerbate psoriasis and should be used with caution.

Unlike rheumatoid arthritis, which usually requires constant treatment, psoriatic arthritis may only require therapy when manifestations arise. When they subside, therapy can be stopped until further problems develop. Initial treatment usually consists of NSAIDs. If the arthritis does not respond, DMARDs may be used. These include sulfasalazine, methotrexate, and cyclosporine and the more recently available "anti-TNF agents" such as etanercept, infliximab, and adalimumab. The antimalarial drug hydroxychloroquine may be effective, but some people taking this will experience a flare-up of their psoriasis, so it is usually avoided. Azathioprine may benefit those with severe forms of PsA.

For severely swollen joints, glucocorticosteroid injections can be useful for controlling the inflammation. Surgery can be helpful to repair or replace badly damaged joints. Simultaneous joint and skin disease activity has been observed in up to one third of clients, particularly those with non–spondylitis disease.

For clients with intractable pain or loss of joint function, surgery may be indicated. Although several reports have raised concerns about a higher risk of infections, recurrent contracture or stiffness, or excessive bone formation after surgery, most of these fears seem ill founded and surgery should not be withheld.

Nursing Management of the Medical Client

Obtain Nursing History

The focus of the nursing history for clients with psoriatic arthritis is similar to that for clients with RA. Asymmetrical pauciarticular arthritis, however, often occurs in psoriatic arthritis, so clients should be questioned about the nature, onset, and location of any acutely occurring painful, swollen joints. Questions about back pain and stiffness can help to identify psoriatic spondylitis. In addition, clients should be asked about their psoriasis-associated skin changes—location, size, color, and degree of scaling of the plaques—as well as changes in the nail beds of the fingers and the toes. Because the disease seems to be caused by several other factors, ask clients if there is a family history of arthritis, psoriatic arthritis, or psoriasis. Determine whether the client has a history of severe infection before or after developing clinical manifestations of the disease or any episodes of local trauma to the hands, feet, or spine.

Complete Physical Assessment

Assessment of the client with psoriatic arthritis begins with a thorough assessment of the skin for evidence of psoriatic plaques or nail bed changes. Such completeness is essential because the disease cannot be confirmed, even with characteristic radiologic changes unless there is evidence of psoriasis. Usually located on extensor surfaces, psoriatic skin lesions are either macular or papular round scales that tend to bleed when they are removed. If clients deny that they have any skin involvement, examine all areas carefully, particularly the scalp, axillae, and umbilicus. Look carefully for pitting nails, which often precede skin rashes and are highly suggestive of psoriasis.

Defer the assessment of the musculoskeletal system until the examination of the integument is complete, so that subtle changes in either system are not overlooked. Because the range of joint involvement in psoriatic arthritis is extensive (e.g., asymmetrical or symmetrical, small or large, pauciarticular or monoarticular), each joint must be assessed for swelling, bogginess, and erythema. Pay particular attention to the small joints of the hands and feet, watching for swollen, sausage-shaped digits, which result from tenosynovitis of the flexor tendon sheath. Note whether any of the digits have assumed a spindle or telescopic shape.

Maintain Skin Integrity

Nursing interventions are especially important for the client with PsA experiencing impaired skin integrity. Clients with PsA may need basic instruction about how to care for their skin. If skin changes are severe, the client should be referred to a dermatologist, or the nurse (and physician) should collaborate with the dermatologist if the client has previously sought care from this specialist. The nurse should review skin care principles, such as the purpose and application techniques of emollients to keep the skin soft, patting the skin dry after bathing instead of vigorous towel drying, and the correct application of topical ointments with a thin layer, sparingly applied. If the client is hospitalized, it is important that he or she assume responsibility for skin care as soon as it is feasible.

Enhance Body Image

Because of the changes in both the skin and the joints, it is likely that the client has experienced a significant body image disturbance. Being sensitive to clients' expressions can help to assess the degree of integrity they perceive they have. It is not unusual for people to be so affected by their appearance that they wear long-sleeved shirts on the hottest days and buy only clothes with pockets to hide their altered fingers. The communication of positive unconditional regard by the nurse—and all members of the health care team—can be a powerful tool to help clients begin to feel comfortable exploring their feelings.

FIBROMYALGIA SYNDROME

Not all people complaining of musculoskeletal pain have arthritis. Fibromyalgia syndrome is an increasingly recognized chronic musculoskeletal pain disorder of unknown cause. It occurs in about 2% to 5% of the general population, predominantly in girls and young women. Active research is being conducted to find the cause. Clinical manifestations include fatigue, morning stiffness, non-refreshing sleep because of lack of stage 4 sleep, and postexertional muscle pain. About one third of clients have associated problems such as irritable bowel syndrome, tension headaches, premenstrual syndrome, numbness and tingling, and Raynaud's phenomenon. Fatigue is the most common clinical manifestation, and the most common cause of the fatigue is chronic depression.

OUTCOME MANAGEMENT

Management is symptomatic and includes L-tryptophan to increase sleep, tricyclic antidepressants to inhibit serotonin uptake, benzodiazepines for the treatment of anxiety associated with depression, and glucocorticoids and NSAIDs for pain control. Low-intensity exercise is also important and helps to decrease pain. Biofeedback, acupuncture, and hypnotherapy have also been used to help manage nonmuscular problems such as functional diarrhea, tension headache, and fatigue. The efficacy of these treatments is yet to be fully ascertained.

Many clients with fibromyalgia perceive themselves to be significantly disabled and have a reduced quality of life that rivals conditions such as RA and terminal emphysema. Clients with fibromyalgia have difficulty coping with "daily hassles" and this, in turn, increases the psychological stress. Cognitive behavioral therapy is often effective in providing these clients a sense of control over their lives.

IDIOPATHIC INFLAMMATORY MYOPATHY (POLYMYOSITIS AND DERMATOMYOSITIS)

Inflammatory diseases of muscle are a heterogeneous group of disorders characterized by proximal muscle weakness and nonsuppurative inflammation of skeletal muscle. Traditionally, the terms polymyositis and dermatomyositis have been used to represent these diseases. Today it is more appropriate to use the term *idiopathic inflammatory myopathy* to describe the entire group and reserve the terms polymyositis (PM) and dermatomyositis (DM) for more specific conditions or subsets.

The idiopathic myopathies are relatively rare diseases. Accurate estimates of their prevalence are difficult to obtain because the diseases are uncommon and lack universally accepted specific diagnostic criteria. Estimates of incidence range from 0.5 to 8.4 cases per million. The incidence appears to be increasing, although this may simply reflect increased awareness and more accurate diagnosis. Although polymyositis and dermatomyositis affect all age groups, there is a bimodal distribution of the age of onset with peaks at ages 10 and 15 years in children and between 45 and 60 years in adults. As with other rheumatic diseases, there is a 2:1 female to male predominance in PM-DM with the exception of inclusion body myositis, which affects men twice as often. Racial differences are apparent. In adults the lowest rates are reported in the Japanese and the highest in African Americans. Although no direct relationships have been established between an inflammatory myopathy and a specific genetic marker, several associations have been recognized. The strongest associations are for HLA-B8, HLA-DR3, and HLA-DRW52 phenotypes with polymyositis and dermatomyositis in all age groups.

Etiology and Risk Factors

The idiopathic myopathies are believed to be immune-mediated processes that are triggered by environmental factors in genetically susceptible individuals. This is supported by the following two observations: (1) there is a recognized association with other autoimmune and connective tissue diseases and (2) there is a high prevalence of circulating autoantibodies. The autoantibodies associated with PM-DM include the myositis-specific autoantibodies (MSAs) found almost exclusively in these diseases.

The triggering event of PM-DM is unknown, but viruses have been strongly implicated. The seasonal variation in the onset of disease is direct evidence that infectious agents play a role as well as the evidence found in animal models. Genetic factors play an important role. Individuals with HLA-DR3 are at increased risk for developing inflammatory muscle disease including polymyositis and juvenile dermatomyositis. All clients with the anti-Jo-1 antibodies have the HLA antigen DR52, and Caucasian clients also have a high prevalence of HLA-B8, HLA-DR3, and HLA-DR6. Inclusion body myositis is more likely associated with HLA-DR1, HLA-DR6, and HLA-DQ1.

A subset of clients with inflammatory myopathies develops muscle weakness with an underlying malignancy. Malignancy may precede or follow the onset of muscle weakness. The association is rare in children, but has occurred in clients of all ages in all subsets of disease, although associated malignancy may be more common with dermatomyositis. Subsequent studies seem to indicate that the types of tumors found roughly paralleled those found in the general population with the exception of ovarian cancer, which is over-represented in women with dermatomyositis.

Pathophysiology

The results of muscle biopsies, usually of the deltoid or quadriceps muscles, have provided useful information about the pathology of the disease. Several changes have been noted, including focal or extensive degeneration of muscle fibers caused by inflammatory infiltrates of lymphocytes and macrophages. In some cases, necrosis of parts or entire groups of muscle fibers can occur. Fibers, however, can also show evidence of regeneration.

Clinical Manifestations

The most frequently occurring idiopathic myopathies in adults, polymyositis and dermatomyositis are diffuse, systemic, inflammatory connective tissue diseases. Although these disorders can have an acute onset and progress rapidly, more typically there is a slower progression. Clients gradually develop significant weight loss, fatigue, and weakness over a period of months, sometimes not even being aware of when the changes began. Both diseases cause symmetrical progressive weakness of the proximal or limb-girdle muscles and occasionally atrophy of the muscles of the limbs, neck, and pharynx. Decreased muscle strength occurs in the pelvic girdle first, followed by weakness of the legs and shoulders and arms. Weakness of the flexor muscles of the neck occurs in about half of those affected with PM-DM. In acute disease, muscles can be tender or swollen and doughy. When classic skin changes are associated with polymyositis, the disease is classified as *dermatomyositis*. The classification of idiopathic inflammatory myopathies, to which polymyositis and dermatomyositis belong, includes the following seven groups: (1) polymyositis, (2) dermatomyositis, (3) amyopathic dermatomyositis, (4) juvenile dermatomyositis, (5) myositis associated with neoplasia, (6) myositis associated with collagen vascular disease, and (7) inclusion body myositis.

The criteria developed in 1975 for the diagnosis of PM and DM continue to be used: (1) proximal, symmetrical muscle weakness, with or without dysphagia or respiratory muscle weakness; (2) elevation of serum muscle enzyme levels; (3) characteristic electromyographic changes; (4) muscle biopsy evidence of myositis; and (5) the typical skin rash of DM. In addition, the diagnosis is confirmed after excluding other neuromuscular diseases, such as myasthenia gravis, amyotrophic lateral sclerosis, polymyalgia rheumatica, and Guillain-Barré syndrome. Research continues to refine the diagnostic criteria for PM-DM, and four additional criteria may become standard in the future.

The most important laboratory test is the measurement of the muscle enzyme creatine kinase (CK) (formerly creatine phosphokinase). An elevated CK level indicates muscle injury, but it is not specific to PM-DM. Elevated CK levels can be seen after intramuscular injections, muscle biopsies, or exercise, for example. The level of CK changes according to the activity of the disease. Other muscle enzymes are also elevated in most cases, including aldolase, ALT, AST, and LDH. The sedimentation rate is normal in 50% of clients.

Electromyographic (EMG) results often show bizarre, high-frequency discharges with spontaneous fibrillations and positive spikes at rest. Muscle biopsies are done if there is doubt about the diagnosis. The muscle chosen should be affected by the disease but not atrophied. The site should not be one where a previous EMG needle has been introduced. When biopsies are performed using general anesthesia, a permanent scar usually forms, and the area is sore for several weeks. For these reasons, physicians may prefer not to perform the biopsy unless it is essential to making the diagnosis. Muscle biopsy results, as was previously mentioned, show changes associated with necrosis and degeneration as well as evidence of regeneration. Fibrosis may be seen.

OUTCOME MANAGEMENT

Medical Management

The treatment of PM-DM usually begins with the daily administration of high doses of oral glucocorticosteroids. Prednisone (1 to 2 mg/kg/day) is given until elevated levels of muscle enzymes begin to decrease toward normal and clients show improvement in their ability to perform ADL. In severe cases, the daily dose can be divided or intravenous methylprednisolone may be used. Reduction in steroid dosages to alternate-day therapy may not be possible for several months. Some clients require long-term treatment with maintenance doses of steroids because the disease can recur when the steroids are withdrawn. Clients who do not respond to steroids or who cannot tolerate the high steroid doses usually require the addition of an immunosuppressive agent, such as daily azathioprine (50 to 150 mg/day) or weekly methotrexate therapy (7.5 mg/week PO or 0.5 to 0.8 mg/kg/week IV). Other immunosuppressive agents have been used in steroid-resistant clients. Cyclophosphamide, 6-mercaptopurine, chlorambucil, total-body (or total-nodal) irradiation, and intravenous immunoglobulins have also been used. Hydroxychloroquine can be used to treat the cutaneous lesions of dermatomyositis, although it has no recognized effect on the myositis.

Nursing Management of the Medical Client

Obtain Nursing History

Eliciting the history of a person with PM-DM begins with the client's perspective. The client seeks health care because of the nonspecific changes, usually occurring over several months, of increasing fatigue, weight loss, and malaise. When questioned about the nature of the fatigue and how it affects the ability to carry out activities of daily living, clients usually describe difficulty in performing tasks because of muscle weakness. Good screening questions include queries about the changes in ability to perform ADL that require the use of large muscle groups. Questions about the onset, duration, location, and quality of muscle pain should be asked. Muscle pain or tenderness may or may not be present in the early phases of the disease. Ask the client if he or she has had difficulty brushing the hair, reaching over the head for objects on a shelf or putting on clothes, or performing repetitive chores, such as mowing the lawn, hanging up laundry, or putting away groceries.

For a history of pelvic limb weakness, determine if the client has had difficulty rising from an armless chair, getting out of a car, climbing steps, or riding a bike. Ask if the client has had difficulties in raising the neck off the bed or pillow. Question the client about associated joint pains because arthritis and arthralgia occur in many clients who are in the overlap group V (i.e., they have both polymyositis and dermatomyositis and evidence of another collagen vascular disease, such as RA or SSc). Some clients may report a tendency to fall that is unrelated to balance, so explore changes in gait patterns with them. Because muscle weakness in the face and larynx is seen in PM-DM, determine if there has been any difficulty in chewing or swallowing, facial swelling, or hoarseness.

Because PM-DM is a systemic disease, questions must also be included about the integumentary, pulmonary, and cardiovascular systems. Determine whether the client has experienced any skin or nail changes—rash, reddened areas, scaling—typical of those seen in dermatomyositis. Common respiratory complications of PM-DM include aspiration pneumonia (because of a weakened cough, slow protective movements with vomiting, and pharyngeal muscle weakness) and interstitial lung disease. Questions about whether the clients had previous respiratory diseases, particularly pneumonia and influenza-like illnesses, and about how they recovered provide important information to surgical nurses for preoperative and postoperative pulmonary care. The client's cardiac history should be assessed via questions about dysrhythmias and the existence of a prolapsed mitral valve.

Complete Physical Assessment

The examination of the client with PM-DM requires a meticulous assessment of the skin and nail beds for the presence of erythema, macular-papular rashes, plaques, scaling, and nodules. Skin changes can help to direct this examination. To confirm the presence of a heliotrope rash on the client's face, hold the neck and head securely while it is lowered off the examination table or the side of the bed. This maneuver elicits increased suffusion to cause the distinctive color of the bluish red hue of the rash.

Initially test for muscle weakness by asking the client to walk, get up from a chair without arms, raise the neck off the bed or table, or lift a heavy book. Loss of hand strength is less noticeable, but it can be detected by a test of grip strength. Asking the client to shrug the shoulders upward against the nurse's hands can test proximal weakness of the shoulder girdle. Weakness of the masseter muscles (which can be seen in clients who have difficulty chewing) is assessed by palpating their strength when the client clenches the teeth. All muscle groups should be palpated for symmetry, atrophy, pain or tenderness, and the presence of contractures. Atrophy generally appears late in the disease, but contractures develop early if muscle weakness has been severe. As muscles are being assessed, large and small joints should be inspected for erythema, pain, presence of synovitis, and limitations in ROM.

Although the focus of the examination is on the integumentary and musculoskeletal systems, thorough assessment of the cardiopulmonary system is required because of the systemic nature of the disease. The bilateral assessment of chest expansion (diaphragmatic excursion) helps the nurse to know how compliant the muscles of respiration are. The quality of the breathing, the presence of dyspnea with simple activities, and the presence of a cough can indicate an acute or chronic respiratory problem with muscle disease. The quality of the lung sounds should be carefully assessed for fine rales (crackles) because aspiration pneumonia is a frequent complication of advanced PM-DM.

Provide Medication Teaching

The education of clients receiving high-dose steroid therapy focuses on teaching them about the potential side effects of long-term prednisone. Clients should be aware that they have an increased risk of infection, so they should monitor and report any manifestations, such as low-grade fevers, chills, or joint pain, to their primary caregivers. Other long-term effects include facial edema, increased appetite, and the development of diabetes mellitus, osteoporosis, and avascular necrosis.

SAFETY ALERT **Clients should also be instructed to wear a medical alert identification tag as long as they are receiving prednisone therapy. Clients must clearly understand that they should never change a dose of prednisone. Steroids must be tapered slowly after high-dose or long-term use because the body cannot respond quickly to changes in cortisol levels. During the period in which high doses of steroids have been administered, the hypothalamus-pituitary-adrenocortical axis has been suppressed, thus leading to negative feedback for the natural production of cortisol. Steroid-dependent clients who abruptly discontinue their therapy can experience an addisonian crisis (characterized by circulatory collapse, vomiting, and severe weakness) with minimal stress.**

Prevent Aspiration

Clients with involvement of the pharyngeal and respiratory muscles must be carefully monitored for the prevention of aspiration pneumonia. Helping clients maintain or regain effective swallowing can significantly reduce aspiration. Resting before meals, eating easily swallowed foods (such as those of a smooth, slippery consistency), and sitting upright during meals are measures that can enhance the client's ability to swallow.

Prevent Falls

Clients with PM-DM are also at risk of falling because of muscle weakness, gait changes, and the possibility of osteoporosis from high-dose prednisone therapy. Balancing a muscle-strengthening program with the use of assistive devices and instructions about safe ambulation helps to keep the client injury free.

BURSITIS

Bursitis is a painful inflammation of the bursae, those closed, minimally fluid-filled sacs that are lined with a synovium similar to the lining of joint spaces. The purpose of bursae is to reduce friction between adjacent tissues—tendon and bones or tendons and ligaments—by lubricating these enclosed structures with synovial fluid from the bursal sac. There are approximately 150 bursae in the body. They typically cover bony prominences, such as the olecranon, trochanter, or patella, and provide protection between the skin and other structures. They are usually quite thin, but with repeated stress, they can become thickened and fluid-filled secondary to inflammation. Bursitis can be either an acute or a chronic condition.

Approximately 3% of the adult population has been estimated to have painful, symptomatic bursitis. The problem peaks between the ages of 40 and 50, presumably as active adults first experience the beginning of degenerative changes in the joints. The shoulder joint is the most commonly affected, followed by the elbow, knee, and hip. When bursitis involves the upper extremities, the dominant arm is usually affected.

Risk factors associated with the development of bursitis include acute or chronic trauma, typically through participation in mechanical, highly repetitive activities. Other causes include such arthritic conditions as RA, gout, tumors, and degenerative changes associated with increasing age. Bursitis is considered a true inflammatory condition with the classic signs of inflammation, local redness, warmth, and swelling.

Typically, the client with acute bursitis complains of exquisite localized pain in the target area. Clients may experience point tenderness and can point specifically to the spot of greatest discomfort. They may also have diffuse soreness radiating to the tendons at the site. Depending on the location of the bursitis, clients may complain of interrupted sleep (e.g., with subacromial bursitis, calcaneal bursitis), difficulty walking (trochanteric bursitis, calcaneal bursitis), or difficulty performing ADL (subacromial or olecranon bursitis).

Occupational or avocational activities can also provide insight into the nature of the pain, for example, a woodcarver who has developed acute subacromial bursitis or a businesswoman who walks long distances in medium to high heels.

The diagnosis of bursitis is generally based on the results of the history and physical examination. Radiographs of the affected joint are usually normal in acute bursitis, whereas in chronic conditions calcium deposits may be present. Results of laboratory tests and synovial fluid analysis are normal unless the bursa has become infected.

OUTCOME MANAGEMENT

Acute bursitis is treated with rest and immobilization of the affected joint, non-opioid analgesics, and ROM exercises. In general, the pain of acute bursitis is controlled with NSAIDs. Client education focuses on the causes of bursitis, the prevention of additional attacks (by avoiding activities that cause constant friction or pressure), the correct application of moist heat, and medication and exercise instruction.

Relieve Pain

Helping clients obtain pain relief is the primary focus of nursing interventions. Without pain relief, joint mobility is impaired through frozen, protective measures. Nurses must instruct clients about the purpose of anti-inflammatory medications as well as the appropriate dose and untoward side effects.

Pain relief is also achieved by resting or immobilizing the joint or by elevating or compressing the involved area to control edema. Teaching clients about the correct application of ice and heat is important so they receive maximum pain relief. If clients receive intra-articular injections of cortisone, they should be informed about the possibility of a post-injection flare-up. They should also be reassured that the pain responds quickly to the application of ice packs.

Promote Self-Care

Self-care deficits are usually temporary in acute bursitis. If the condition becomes chronic, clients may experience more difficulties, particularly if the shoulder or elbow is involved. Dressing is easier if oversized garments are worn, especially those with long sleeves or wide pant legs. Shirts and tops that button in the front

are also helpful. Clients can be taught to minimize shoulder or elbow pain by putting clothing on the affected arm first and by taking it off the affected arm last.

VASCULITIS

Vasculitis comprises a group of disorders leading to inflammation and necrosis of blood vessel walls. Soluble immune complexes are deposited in blood vessel walls in areas where capillaries have increased permeability. After deposition, the immune system is activated and the complex is destroyed along with the blood vessel wall. These disorders include polyarteritis nodosa, systemic necrotizing vasculitis, and allergic granulomatous angiitis. Inflammation and damage to large and small vessels result in end-stage organ damage.

Specific manifestations vary, depending on the organs affected. Steroids are the treatment of choice for these disorders.

POLYMYALGIA RHEUMATICA

Polymyalgia rheumatica is a clinical syndrome occurring more commonly in women than in men. It is a disease of aging, rarely occurring before age 60 years. It is characterized by pain and stiffness in the neck, shoulder, back, and pelvic girdle, especially in the morning. Headaches or painful areas on the head may be present. The client also may have a low-grade fever or temporal arteritis. Laboratory findings include an elevated ESR, mild anemia, and possible elevation of immunoglobulins. Steroids usually produce symptomatic relief within days.

GIANT CELL ARTERITIS

Giant cell arteritis, also known as temporal or cranial arteritis, is also a disease of older people. The client often has manifestations of polymyalgia rheumatica for months, and then suddenly experiences the severe headaches associated with temporal arteritis. The onset of this disorder is usually sudden, with severe pain often appearing in the temporal area. The pain also may be felt in the occipital area, face, jaw, or side of the neck. It is usually associated with hyperesthesia, which makes any touch exquisitely painful. The client may experience visual changes, including sudden onset of blindness in one or both eyes.

It is very important to diagnose and treat this disorder before blindness occurs. Because older women are often affected, their complaints of decreased vision and headaches are sometimes ignored as normal aging. Treatment is with glucocorticoids, which are highly effective in controlling this disorder.

MIXED CONNECTIVE TISSUE DISEASE

Mixed connective tissue disease is a combination of several connective tissue diseases. Clients have manifestations that are not typical of any one disorder. Frequent combinations are SLE and SSc and RA. Mixed connective tissue diseases are managed according to their manifestations.

LYME DISEASE

Lyme disease is one form of rheumatic joint disease with a known cause. It is included as a connective tissue disorder because the skin, joints, nervous system, and heart are involved. This complex multisystem disease is caused by the tick-borne spirochete *Borrelia burgdorferi*. Clinical manifestations found from 3 to 32 days after the bite may include a red, flat rash that clears in the center, severe headache, stiff neck, fever, chills, myalgias, joint pain, severe malaise, and fatigue.

The disease can be treated with a course of antibiotic therapy. Doxycycline is the most common antibiotic used. Neurologic abnormalities may occur if treatment is ineffective. Intra-articular steroids and NSAIDs may be used to relieve joint inflammation and pain. Long-term effects include fatigue and arthralgia for many years after the initial infection.

CONCLUSIONS

Nursing clients with rheumatic disorders can prove to be challenging. Clients can experience acute exacerbations or crises with almost all of these diseases. Systemic manifestations can be as devastating as the musculoskeletal manifestations. Whether in remission or exacerbation these diseases are always present. This results in considerable uncertainty, which can lead to a cycle of ineffective coping, disturbed self-esteem, helplessness, and powerlessness. In many respects, the psychological and social problems that are associated with these chronic illnesses can be as disabling as the physical complaints.

Physiologically, clients with rheumatic disorders (autoimmune, spondylarthropathies, or inflammatory arthritis) experience many common problems. The triad of pain, fatigue, and stiffness must be controlled so that function is enhanced or maintained. Difficulty with self-care is usually accompanied by sleep disturbances, altered nutrition, and impaired mobility. These can adversely affect the individual's self-concept and self-esteem and lead to social isolation.

Because of the chronicity of these disorders, clients need skilled, knowledgeable nursing care that draws on the disciplines of rehabilitation, counseling, and self-care. The unique role of the nurse for these clients is one that assumes accountability and responsibility for guiding and directing the client through the health care maze. Clients with chronic, usually systemic illnesses require multiple therapies and follow-up appointments for pharmacologic management, nutritional counseling, lifestyle assessment, physical and occupational therapy, and psychological support. The personal and financial cost can exhaust the client's enthusiasm, job security, support systems, and sense of purpose in life. The nurse can provide a sense of consistency, hope, and reassurance that the client can learn to cope with, and positively adapt to, the demands of a chronic illness. Clients with arthritis need the nurse's expertise to teach them how to explore new self-care strategies so successful adaptation to the disease is a reality. Nurses help clients learn to become partners with the entire health care team as well as with themselves. When clients assume the role of partner, they exhibit greater control, greater accountability, and increased self-esteem as they learn self-management skills. This is nowhere more evident than clients giving themselves their bi-weekly or daily injections of some of the newer treatments.

THINKING CRITICALLY

1. You are working in an outpatient clinic and receive a call from a 66-year-old woman who is experiencing a flare-up of rheumatoid arthritis. She was seen 2 days ago in the clinic and was given a high dose of prednisone. Now she reports epigastric abdominal pain. She reports that her pain has a burning quality, is worse between meals, is relieved by food, and is aggravated by coffee. She has taken some over-the-counter ibuprofen for the pain but states, "It didn't help." What other information do you need to collect? What interventions would you advise?

Factors to Consider. Consider the side effects of glucocorticoids and NSAIDs.

2. A 55-year-old woman with a history of joint pain is scheduled for shoulder arthroplasty. She has experienced increasing pain while working as a waitress and handling orders that must be carried to tables of restaurant guests. She hopes to be able to work pain-free so she can resume her job as a waitress. What nursing assessments are pertinent to this type of condition and proposed surgery? How realistic is the client's desire to return to work as a waitress?

Factors to Consider. How will assessments help in the prevention of postoperative complications? Are clients able to return to an improved level of functioning after joint replacement surgery?

Discussions for these questions can be found on the website

BIBLIOGRAPHY

Citations appearing in red refer to primary research.

Citations appearing in blue refer to evidence-based practice guidelines and protocols.

1. Acorn, J., Joachim, G., & Wachs, J. (2003). Scleroderma: Living with unpredictability. *AAOHN Journal, 51*(8), 358-359.

2. American College of Rheumatology and Association of Rheumatology Health Professionals. (2007). *Rheumatoid arthritis.* Accessed 03/04/07 from www.rheumatology.org.

3. American College of Rheumatology, Subcommittee on Rheumatoid Arthritis Guidelines. (2002). Guidelines for the management of rheumatoid arthritis, 2002 update. *Arthritis and Rheumatism, 46*(2), 238-346. (Also available at www.rheumatology.org/research/guidelines.)

4. Arnett, F., et al. (1988). The American Rheumatism Association 1987 revised criteria for the classification of rheumatoid arthritis. *Arthritis and Rheumatism, 31,* 315-324.

5. Cooper, G., & Stroehla, B. (2003). The epidemiology of autoimmune diseases. *Autoimmune Review, 2*(3), 119-125.

6. Crowther, C., & McCance, K. (2006). Alterations of musculoskeletal function. In K. McCance & S. Huether (Eds.), *Pathophysiology: The biological basis for disease in adults and children* (5th ed., pp. 1497-1545). St. Louis: Mosby.

7. Egan, M., et al. (2006). Splints and orthosis for treating rheumatoid arthritis. *The Cochrane Library, 1,* CD004018.

8. Graham, D., et al. (2002). Ulcer prevention in long-term users of nonsteroidal anti-inflammatory drugs. *Archives of Internal Medicine, 162,* 169-175.

9. Hansen, A., Lipsky, P., & Dorner, T. (2003). New concepts in the pathogenesis of Sjögren's syndrome: Many questions, fewer answers. *Current Opinion in Rheumatology, 15*(5), 563-570.

10. Harris, E., et al. (2005). *Kelley's textbook of rheumatology* (7th ed.). Philadelphia: Saunders.

11. Koopman, E., & Moreland, L. (2005). *Arthritis and allied conditions: A textbook of rheumatology* (15th ed.). Philadelphia: Lippincott Williams & Wilkins

12. Marchesoni, A., et al. (2003). Radiographic progression in early rheumatoid arthritis: A 12-month randomized controlled study comparing the combination of cyclosporine and methotrexate with methotrexate alone. *Rheumatology, 42,* 1-5.

13. Mayes, M., et al. (2003). Prevalence, incidence, survival, and disease characteristics of systemic sclerosis in a large U.S. population. *Arthritis and Rheumatology, 48*(8), 2246-2255.

14. Meenan, R., Callahan, L., & Helmich, C. (1999). The Arthritis Action Plan: A public health strategy for a looming epidemic. *Arthritis Care and Research, 12,* 79-81.

15. National Center for Chronic Disease Prevention and Health Promotion. (1999). *National Arthritis Action Plan: A public health strategy.* Atlanta: Centers for Disease Control and Prevention.

16. Neumann, L., & Buskila, D. (2003). Epidemiology of fibromyalgia. *Current Pain and Headache Reports, 7*(5), 362-368.

17. Robinson, V., et al.. (2006). Thermotherapy for treating rheumatoid arthritis. *The Cochrane Library, 1,* CD002826.

18. Roth, S. (2004). Effects of Prosorba Column apheresis in patients with chronic refractory rheumatoid arthritis. *Journal of Rheumatology, 31*(11), 2131-2135.

19. Schneider, J., Matthews, J., & Graham, B. (2003). Reiter's syndrome. *Cutis, 71*(3), 198-200.

20. Tan, E., et al. (1982). The 1982 revised criteria for the Classification of Systemic Lupus Erythematosus (SLE). *Arthritis and Rheumatism, 25,* 1271-1277.

21. Turesson, C., O'Fallon, W., & Crowson, C. (2003). Extra-articular disease manifestations in rheumatoid arthritis: Incidence trends and risk factors over 46 years. *Annals of Rheumatic Diseases, 62*(8), 722-727.

22. Wolfe, F., et al. (2003). Predicting mortality in patients with rheumatoid arthritis. *Arthritis and Rheumatology, 48*(6), 1530-1542.

23. Wolfe, F., et al. (1990). The American College of Rheumatology 1990 Criteria for the classification of fibromyalgia: Report of the multicenter criteria committee. *Arthritis and Rheumatism, 33*(2), 160-172.

INTERNET RESOURCES

Arthritis Foundation: www.arthritis.org

Clinical Trial Information: www.Clinicaltrials.gov

Lupus Foundation of American: www.lfa.org

National Sjögren's Syndrome Association: www.sjogrens.org

Rheumatology Resources: www.rheumatology.org/resources.htm

Scleroderma Foundation: www.scleroderma.org

Sjögren's Syndrome and Anesthesia: www.sjogrens.org/ane.htm

Fibromyalgia: www.fibromyalgia.org

 Did you remember to check out the bonus material on the Evolve website and the CD-ROM, including NCLEX®-Examination Style Review Questions, Open-Book Quizzes, and Chapter Review Audio Podcasts?

http://evolve.elsevier.com/Black/medsurg

CHAPTER 78

Management of Clients with Acquired Immunodeficiency Syndrome

MEG BLAIR

HIV/AIDS

The year 2006 marked the 25th anniversary of the onset of HIV/AIDS. In June 1981 the first cases of what would come to be called HIV/AIDS were reported to the Centers for Disease Control (CDC). Currently, HIV/AIDS is one of the world's greatest public health crises. Globally, in 2006 more than 65 million people were living with HIV/AIDS. In 2005 there were 4.9 million people newly infected, and there were more than 3.1 million AIDS-related deaths. HIV kills more people than any other infectious disease and ranks fourth among the leading causes of death worldwide. In the United States, more than 944,000 cases have been recorded to date. The number of diagnosed cases continues to rise, with minority populations being among the hardest hit. African Americans comprise half of current HIV/AIDS cases, and AIDS was the leading cause of death for black women ages 25 to 44 years in 2002. Other groups heavily affected in the United States include men who have sex with other men, injecting drug users, women, older adults, and adolescents.

Infection with the human immunodeficiency virus (HIV) results in destruction of the body's host defenses and immune system. For many years, because of a lack of understanding and effective treatment, HIV was considered a rapidly progressing fatal disease. Today HIV infection is viewed more optimistically as a chronic disease that can be controlled with appropriate health care. The cost of such health care (which may top $28,000 per year, per person), however, limits its accessibility to developed, industrialized nations such as the United States. Because many parts of the world, such as Africa and Asia, lack adequate economic resources to treat this disease, HIV infection continues to be a rapidly progressing fatal illness in these areas.

From both a medical and a nursing perspective, clinical management parallels the HIV illness trajectory. Once infected with HIV, a person who receives appropriate treatment can live for many years and continue to function without major problems. In the latter stages of disease, for a variety of reasons to be discussed, the illness progresses, wearing out the immune system. The person is then given the diagnosis acquired immunodeficiency syndrome (AIDS). Because of this dual clinical picture, the material presented in this chapter is divided into (1) caring for the person with HIV disease and (2) caring for the person with AIDS.

Etiology and Risk Factors

Etiology

The etiologic agent associated with AIDS was first isolated by French scientists in 1983 and named the lymphadenopathy-associated virus. One year later, an American scientist claimed the discovery of the etiologic agent and named it the human T-cell lymphotropic virus type III. This led to much confusion, since both scientists actually identified the same virus. In 1986 the International Society on the Taxonomy of Viruses renamed the virus, calling it the human immunodeficiency virus (HIV). In that same year, a second and distinctly different strain of the

---

evolve Web Enhancements

Bridge to Home Health Care   Living with HIV/AIDS

Case Study   Human Immunodeficiency Virus

Diversity in Health Care   HIV and AIDS in Minority Populations

Ethical Issues in Nursing   Should a Client's Sexual Lifestyle Influence Nursing Care?

Boxes   HIV and AIDS Classification System for Adolescents and Adults

Common Nursing Diagnoses for Clients with HIV and AIDS

Be sure to check out the bonus material on the Evolve website and the CD-ROM, including free self-assessment exercises. **http://evolve.elsevier.com/Black/medsurg**

virus was discovered in Africa. Therefore since 1986 the scientific names use to distinguish the two viruses are HIV-1 and HIV-2.

This was a major—and alarming—discovery because it was the first clue that HIV could change its appearance, or mutate, rapidly. This capability is called genetic promiscuity, and it has become the hallmark of the virus, creating a monumental challenge for scientists and researchers alike. HIV-1 is distributed worldwide, but it is most prevalent in Europe and the United States. HIV-2 predominates in West African nations but has been isolated in other parts of the world. By 1996 scientists discovered that HIV-1 had also mutated several times. It has two major subtypes: (1) HIV-1 major (group M) viruses and (2) HIV-1 outlier (group O) viruses.

HIV-1 Group M

Group M viruses are assigned to 10 genetic subtypes, designated HIV-1, group M, subtypes A, B, C, D, E, F, G, H, I, and J, according to the phylogenetic analysis of their genes. The distribution of subtypes varies worldwide.

HIV-1 Group O

The designation O was deliberate because this mutation was an outlier and differed from the others. Group O was identified primarily in west and central Africa, with a few isolated cases found through special tests in France and the United States.

It is important to mention these complexities to illustrate the rapidly changing nature of HIV. The virus poses a considerable challenge to researchers investigating new drugs to treat the disease or developing vaccines because their work is usually limited to one specific subtype of HIV-1. Indeed, vaccine trials have shown that a vaccine for one subtype may not work for other subtypes.

Risk Factors

Modes of transmission have remained constant throughout the course of the HIV pandemic. The virus is spread through certain sexual practices, through exposure to blood and body fluids, and through perinatal (vertical) transmission. The patterns in the spread of HIV changed considerably during the first 19 years of the epidemic in the United States. Although most Americans infected with HIV continue to be men who have sex with men, significant increases have been noted in intravenous (IV) drug users, women, and heterosexuals. This decline, however, has been limited to white men; the number of new HIV infections among racial and ethnic minority men who have sex with men continues to increase, as outlined in the Diversity in Health Care website feature on HIV and AIDS in Minority Populations. In

young adults (ages 19 to 29), the number of new infections has been increasing, especially in the South and Midwest. Increased numbers of cases are also seen in rural areas and in smaller cities. HIV infection and AIDS are the second leading causes of death among adults ages 25 to 44.

Perhaps the most overlooked population in the HIV epidemic is adults ages 50 and older. Cumulatively they represent 12% of all known cases, but in 2004 they represented 16% of new infections. People in this age group may not be tested promptly for HIV because neither they nor their health care providers perceive them to be at risk for this disease. Women older than 50 acquire HIV infection primarily through heterosexual contact.

The principal mode of transmission of HIV throughout the world has been through sexual exposure. Except in Australia, Europe, and the United States, most HIV transmission has been through heterosexual activity. One important lesson health care professionals have learned from this epidemic is that sexual practices, not sexual preferences, place people at risk for sexually transmitted infections (STIs), including HIV/AIDS. Homosexual men who do not engage in unprotected sex or expose themselves to another person's body fluids are no more at risk for acquiring HIV infection than anyone else; similarly, heterosexual or homosexual couples in long-term, monogamous relationships are at low risk. Unsafe sexual encounters outside of these relationships do, however, pose a risk.

Sexual practices that are completely safe include (1) autosexual activities (such as masturbation), (2) mutually monogamous relationships between noninfected partners, and (3) abstinence. Very safe sexual practices include noninsertive activity. Insertive practices with a condom are considered probably safe so long as the condom is used correctly, does not break, and no contact with body fluids occurs. Everything else is considered risky. Other cofactors, such as engaging in sexual activities while under the influence of drugs or alcohol, having multiple sex partners, and the presence of sores in the genital area, increase the risk of acquiring HIV. Although the number of reported cases is small, oral sexual practices, whether performed on a man or a woman, have been implicated in transmission.

Transmission by exposure to blood is a broad category encompassing numerous possible routes, the most obvious being through transfusion of infected blood products and through transplantation of infected donated tissue or organs. Prevention of HIV infection by any of these means is possible by donor exclusion (excluding people from high-risk groups), routine serologic testing of donated tissues or fluids for HIV antibodies, and heat inactivation of certain blood products, such as factor VIII concentrate. Other means of preventing HIV infection related to blood products are adhering to autologous (self-donated) blood programs and limiting the administration of any blood product to situations in which it is absolutely necessary.

Use of injected drugs accounts for the largest number of HIV infections through exposure to contaminated blood. The only absolutely safe injecting drug use behavior is not to inject. Very safe practice is to use sterilized injection paraphernalia and never share needles and syringes. A probably safe practice is to clean injection paraphernalia with full-strength bleach before injecting, although disposable needles and syringes are difficult to clean. Anything else is considered risky. Other cofactors that increase the chances of acquiring HIV by drug injection include the seroprevalence of HIV in the geographical area of the drug user, the social setting of the drug use (e.g., "shooting galleries," where injection paraphernalia is shared), and the frequency of injection.

Needle exchange programs provide sterile injection equipment, latex condoms, counseling, and access to social and health programs, including drug treatment. Numerous studies have shown that needle exchange programs decrease the spread of HIV and hepatitis B and C and do not increase or promote injection drug use. Despite the proven success of this approach to disease prevention, state and federal legislators have been reluctant to appropriate funds to support this model of care. In the United States, needle exchange programs may operate as legal, illegal but tolerated, or illegal underground programs. In Europe, where this approach has more support, government studies have found that needle exchange programs not only reduce the incidence of HIV but also reduce health care spending for other diseases associated with IV drug injection.

HIV transmission to health care workers by clients is an ongoing concern for workers, employers, and public health officials. In the United States, the total number of health care workers with documented, occupationally acquired HIV or AIDS in 2002 was 57. The number with possible transmission was 139. Although most occupationally-related HIV infections are due to percutaneous exposure, other modes of transmission included mucocutaneous exposure and direct exposure to HIV in the laboratory setting. The actual average risk to a health care worker for exposure to HIV is extremely low (0.4% after a needle-stick or sharp instrument injury and 0.09% after a mucous membrane exposure). The risk is increased in situations in which a deep injury occurs, when there is visible blood on the device causing the injury, when the device involved was previously placed in a client's artery or vein, and when AIDS was diagnosed in the source client who died within 60 days after the health care worker's exposure.

SAFETY ALERT

Accidental needle-stick exposure poses the greatest hazard to health care workers. Nurses must learn and follow standard precautions when handling blood and body fluids and when performing

procedures that could lead to exposure to blood and body fluids. One of The Joint Commission's National Patient Safety Goals recommends following standard precautions and complying with the CDC guidelines. When any incident reflects potential exposure to blood-borne pathogens, seek medical treatment immediately. The CDC has guidelines for evaluating and possibly treating exposures to HIV.

In the United States, only one case of HIV transmission from a health care worker to clients has been documented. It was reported in 1990 and involved a Florida dentist. Six clients reportedly became infected with HIV after receiving dental care. The circumstances of this case implied inadequate disinfection and sterilization of instruments in the dental office. Since this incident, retrospective studies of possible HIV transmission from infected health care workers to clients have not identified any other cases in the United States. There have been two reported incidents of clients infected with HIV in France, one documented and one suspected.

Occupational exposure to blood and body fluids is a potential problem not only for health care workers but also for members of other occupations, such as police and corrections officers.

Perinatal HIV exposure can occur during pregnancy, during vaginal delivery, and post-partum through breast-feeding. In 2001 there were fewer than 200 neonatal cases of HIV in the United States; however, there were more than 700,000 new cases in sub-Saharan Africa alone. This is mostly because women in this resource-poor area do not have access to testing and treatment. Administration of zidovudine to pregnant women has been shown to reduce the rate of vertical HIV transmission from 23% to 8%. The CDC has published guidelines for the use of zidovudine and other antiretroviral therapies for pregnant women and their newborn infants.

The only absolute method of preventing perinatal exposure is to avoid pregnancy. Health care workers should discuss HIV infection as part of routine prenatal care with all clients because many mothers may be unaware that they are infected with HIV. Infected women who carry to term should be advised against breast-feeding because this is a mode of HIV transmission. However, a woman living where a reliable supply of clean, safe drinking water does not exist may expose her infant to more danger from other infectious illnesses with bottle feeding.

Primary prevention of HIV infection for exposed individuals is an emerging concept being applied not only to health care workers but also to the treatment of other accidental exposures. Post-exposure prophylaxis is being used as a health maintenance strategy by some clinicians for people who engage in some high-risk activities. Considerable controversy surrounds the use of post-exposure prophylaxis except in cases of rape, and the ethical aspects of providing such treatment continue to be discussed.

Vaccine research has been ongoing since 1987. However, the mainstay of disease prevention continues to be education and reduction of risky behaviors.

Pathophysiology

HIV-1 is a member of the lentivirus subfamily of human retroviruses. Diseases caused by lentiviruses are characterized by an insidious onset and progressive involvement of the central nervous system (CNS), and may result in disorders of the immune system. HIV-1 is one of five viruses in the lentivirus family (Figure 78-1). The others are HIV-2 and human T-lymphotropic virus (HTLV) types I, II, and IV.

A retrovirus belongs to the family Retroviridae and possesses ribonucleic acid (RNA)-dependent deoxyribonucleic acid (DNA) polymerase (reverse transcriptase). HIV infects T helper cells (T4 lymphocytes), macrophages, and B cells. HIV does not directly affect the CNS or peripheral neurons, astrocytes, or oligodendrocytes. HIV infection in the CNS is indirectly caused by neurotoxins produced by infected macrophages or chemical substances produced by the dysregulation of cytokines and chemokines.

T helper cells are infected more readily than other cells. The depletion of T helper cells occurs in the following steps:

1. Once inside the host, HIV attaches to the target cell membrane by way of its receptor molecule, CD4.
2. The virus is uncoated, and the RNA enters the cell.
3. The enzyme known as reverse transcriptase is released, and viral RNA is transcribed into DNA.
4. This newly created DNA moves into the nucleus and the DNA of the cell.
5. A provirus is created when the viral DNA integrates itself into the cellular DNA or genome of the cell.
6. Once the provirus is in place, its genetic material is no longer pure host DNA but is part viral DNA.
7. The cell may function abnormally.
8. The host cell dies, and viral budding occurs (Figure 78-2). The new virus now infects other cells.

The main target for HIV is the T4 helper cell; however, the "glue" to which HIV is attracted is the CD4 molecule, which acts as the receptor for HIV on the T4 helper cell. Even though the CD4 molecule is also found on other cells, such as macrophages and monocytes, clinicians usually refer to T4 helper cells as CD4$^+$ cells. Therefore in articles, research papers, or laboratory reports about HIV, the labels T4, T4 helper, CF4$^+$, and CD4$^+$ T helper cell are used synonymously. Another substance, chemokine, acts as a messenger to facilitate

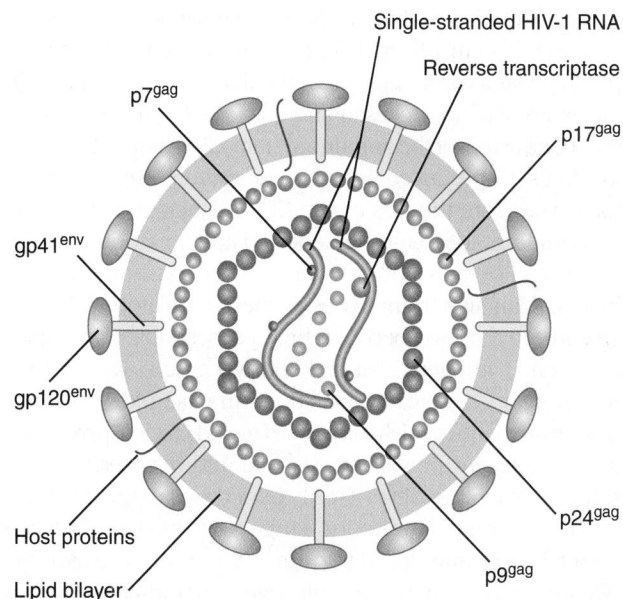

FIGURE 78–1 Schematic diagram of the human immunodeficiency virus-1 (HIV-1) virion. *RNA,* Ribonucleic acid. *(Redrawn from Sande, M., & Volberding, P. [1999]. The medical management of AIDS [6th ed.]. Philadelphia: Saunders.)*

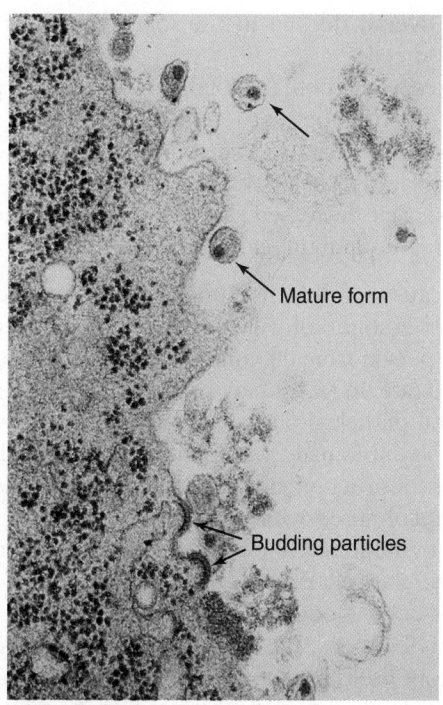

FIGURE 78–2 Human immunodeficiency virus. Electron micrograph of the virus budding from a T lymphocyte. *(From Friedman-Kien, A., & Cockerell, C. [1996]. Color atlas of AIDS [2nd ed., p. 11]. Philadelphia: Saunders.)*

HIV entry into cells. In 1996 scientists discovered that certain people have a genetic defect in a gene related to chemokines and, despite repeated exposure to HIV, never become infected.

The CD4$^+$ T helper cells are regulating cells in the immune system. They interact with monocytes, macrophages, cytotoxic T cells, natural killer cells, and B cells. In the analogy of an orchestra and a conductor, the T cells are the "conductor" of the immune system, directing all the activity ("music") produced by the other immune cells ("orchestra"). Therefore the loss of the CD4$^+$ T helper cells results in significant decreases in coordinated immune activity. The body loses its ability to maintain a consistent state of health. With significant losses of these regulatory cells, the HIV-infected person becomes highly susceptible to acquired infection. Pathogens that previously caused disease may reactivate and also cause infection. An example is the varicella zoster virus, which may have caused chickenpox when an HIV-infected person was a child and may reappear as shingles when the CD4$^+$ T-cell count drops to low levels.

The average laboratory range for the CD4$^+$ T-cell count is 500/mm^3 to 1600/mm^3. A gradual physiologic decline occurs in these cells over an individual's lifespan. In fact, CD4$^+$ T-cell counts in newborns are almost double those of an adult. In the adult, CD4$^+$ cell counts below 200/mm^3 are considered dangerously low and infection is likely to develop. Other laboratory changes that indicate immune dysfunction include the following:

- An overall decline in the total numbers of white blood cells
- Decreases in both the total number and the percentage of lymphocytes
- Significant changes in the CD4$^+$/CD8$^+$ ratio
- Decreased CD4$^+$ T-cell test findings
- Absent or decreased skin test reactivity (anergy)
- Increased immunoglobulin levels

The cause of this immune system damage is the extensive amount of HIV activity taking place in an infected person from the time of infection. HIV replicates at a rapid rate. In fact, it may produce 10 million new virions (viral particles) daily. Although a person with HIV may be asymptomatic with a normal CD4$^+$ cell count, insidious destruction of the immune system is taking place. Antiretroviral drugs interrupt the disease process by inhibiting the ability of the virus to replicate or to enter the cell, thus reducing the amount of circulating virus in the body and halting its destructive activity. Once this happens, the immune system begins to heal and restore itself, as noted by rising CD4$^+$ cell counts.

Sustaining the beneficial effects of antiretroviral therapy is challenging. The greatest problem is HIV's ability to mutate and become resistant to antiretroviral drugs. When this drug failure occurs, plasma viral load rises and the CD4$^+$ cell count decreases. The treatment regimen must then be changed. Because two to three drugs are usually used at the same time and the list of available approved drugs is still small, the number of combinations that can be prescribed is limited. Additionally, although the drugs can contain the disease in plasma, the virus can hide in many other cells in the body. Finally, because most antiretroviral agents do not cross the blood-brain barrier in the CNS, treatment of CNS problems caused by HIV infection can be very difficult.

The course of HIV illness varies from person to person. Several cofactors may accelerate immunodeficiency, including malnutrition, continued substance abuse, allergic conditions, genetics, age, pregnancy, gender, and presence of other infections. Factors that have been linked to increased mortality and morbidity include being of lower socioeconomic status, lacking access to adequate care, receiving care in a hospital with limited AIDS experience, and being treated by a physician with little experience in AIDS care.

Overall, survival among clients with AIDS has improved dramatically since the advent of highly active antiretroviral therapy (HAART) in 1996, which uses varying combinations of drugs from four different classes of antiretroviral medications. Since 2006, HAART has been called antiretroviral therapy (ART). Combined with prophylactic treatment for commonly occurring opportunistic infections, ART has led to HIV disease changing from a rapidly fatal disease to a chronic, mostly manageable condition (Figure 78-3).

To illustrate further the differences observed in HIV-infected people, scientists have reported that about 5% are perfectly healthy after many years and show no manifestations of disease progression. These long-term nonprogressors have the following:

- Documented evidence of HIV infection for more than 10 years
- Lack of manifestations
- Normal, stable immune profiles
- Never required any treatment for HIV disease

Long-term nonprogressors (LTNPs) appear to produce vigorous amounts of serum antibodies that keep HIV activity at extremely low levels, thus preventing damage to the immune system. LTNPs may have one part of a two-part genetic defect. People with both alleles on two genes cannot be infected with HIV. Do not confuse a long-term nonprogressor with a long-term survivor, defined as someone who has lived for more than 8 years after an AIDS diagnosis, who shows all clinical and laboratory manifestations of disease, and who continuously requires treatment.

Although the main target of HIV is the immune system, considerable damage occurs to other parts of the body as a result of HIV in body tissues. Examples of clinical conditions that can be directly attributed to HIV include cranial and peripheral neuropathies, uveitis, cardiomyopathy, pneumonitis, malabsorption in the small intestine, nephritis, cervicitis, arthritis, psoriasis, gonad dysfunction, and adrenalitis. Additionally, damage to the hematologic system—caused in part by impaired blood cell production—commonly results in anemia, granulocytopenia, and thrombocytopenia.

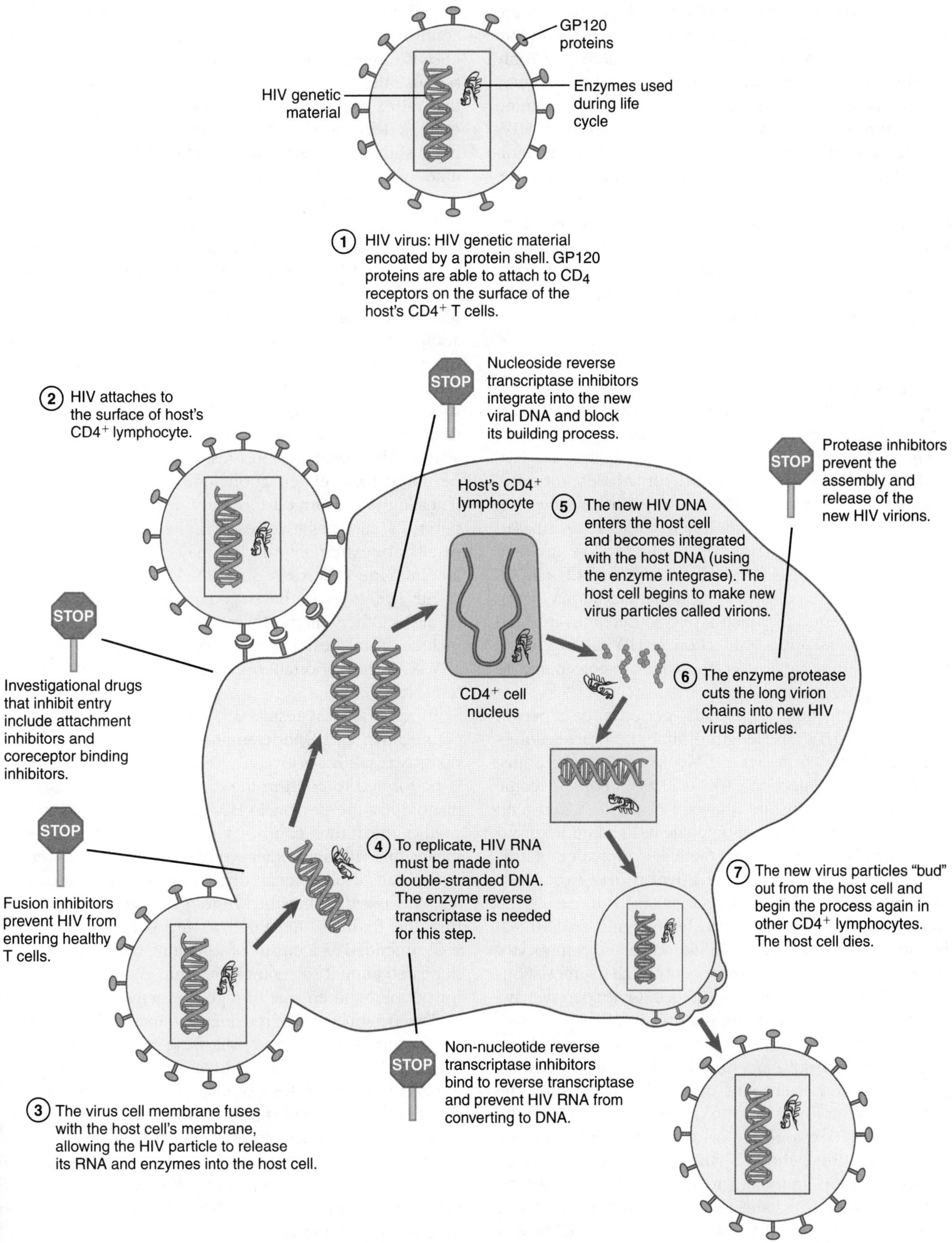

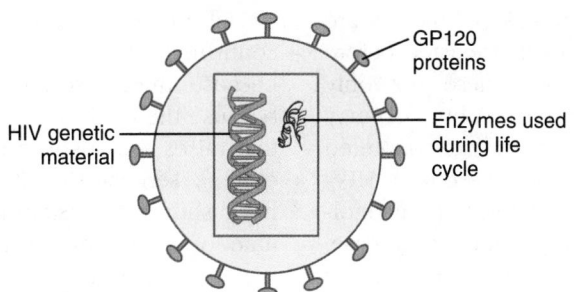

1 HIV virus: HIV genetic material encoated by a protein shell. GP120 proteins are able to attach to CD4 receptors on the surface of the host's CD4+ T cells.

GP120 proteins

Enzymes used during life cycle

HIV genetic material

2 HIV attaches to the surface of host's CD4+ lymphocyte.

STOP Nucleoside reverse transcriptase inhibitors integrate into the new viral DNA and block its building process.

STOP Protease inhibitors prevent the assembly and release of the new HIV virions.

Host's CD4+ lymphocyte

5 The new HIV DNA enters the host cell and becomes integrated with the host DNA (using the enzyme integrase). The host cell begins to make new virus particles called virions.

STOP Investigational drugs that inhibit entry include attachment inhibitors and coreceptor binding inhibitors.

CD4+ cell nucleus

6 The enzyme protease cuts the long virion chains into new HIV virus particles.

STOP Fusion inhibitors prevent HIV from entering healthy T cells.

4 To replicate, HIV RNA must be made into double-stranded DNA. The enzyme reverse transcriptase is needed for this step.

7 The new virus particles "bud" out from the host cell and begin the process again in other CD4+ lymphocytes. The host cell dies.

STOP Non-nucleotide reverse transcriptase inhibitors bind to reverse transcriptase and prevent HIV RNA from converting to DNA.

3 The virus cell membrane fuses with the host cell's membrane, allowing the HIV particle to release its RNA and enzymes into the host cell.

■ **FIGURE 78–3** The steps in the life cycle of the HIV virus with correlation to medications.

In addition to managing HIV disease, clinicians are challenged with addressing illnesses that existed before the person acquired HIV infection. These not only require continuing treatment and attention but also may complicate the course of illness. Frequently encountered pre-existing and co-morbid conditions seen in HIV-infected clients include, but are not limited to, alcoholism, drug dependence, liver disease, kidney disease, psychiatric illness, and a history of STIs. As therapy improves and people with HIV disease live longer, they will also require treatment for such illnesses as cancer, coronary artery disease, chronic obstructive lung disease, hypertension, and diabetes, all of which may occur in the aging population not infected with HIV.

Clinical Manifestations

As knowledge has evolved regarding the HIV disease process, the CDC has developed and revised numerous classification systems (see the box on HIV and AIDS Classification System for Adolescents and Adults on the website). The most recent classification system for HIV disease in adults and adolescents is based on two monitoring parameters used to follow a client: (1) laboratory data (CD4$^+$ cell counts) and (2) clinical presentation (the person's clinical manifestations of diseases). The period in which a person becomes infected is referred to as primary infection. If HIV is detected at the time of initial infection, the client is considered to be in category A.

Primary infection is the initial period after a person has acquired HIV. The length of time the primary infection lasts varies from several weeks to a few months. During primary infection, 50% to 70% of people become sick. Many clinicians are unaware of this fact and tend to think that primary infection is silent. In addition to systemic manifestations (fever, fatigue, lymphadenopathy, nausea, vomiting), the infected person may experience headache; truncal (torso and arms) rash; ulcers of the mouth, genitals, or both; thrush; pharyngitis; diarrhea; hepatomegaly; myalgia; arthralgia; anemia; thrombocytopenia; and leukopenia. In some people, the manifestations are mild and similar to mononucleosis. Other people have severe manifestations requiring hospitalization.

During primary infection, a sudden and intense burst of HIV activity results in a high viral load and a dramatic drop in the CD4$^+$ cell count. In fact, during this time, the CD4$^+$ cell count may drop to below 100/mm^3, with the concomitant development of an AIDS-defining illness. This is also the period in which most newly infected people develop antibodies to HIV, which can then be detected through enzyme immunoassay testing. There is a "window" period for seroconversion (the time it takes for a newly infected person to develop antibodies to HIV that can be detected in a laboratory specimen). On average, antibodies can be detected in 4 to 12 weeks.

Unfortunately, in most instances the diagnosis is not confirmed at the time of primary infection, either because the person does not seek medical care or because the clinician does not take an adequate history that raises the suspicion of HIV infection. This is quite a serious situation because preliminary studies have shown that starting antiretroviral therapy at the time of initial infection may prevent damage to the immune system and to other body systems.

Previously, the decision to seek an HIV test was left up to the individual, except in certain instances, such as when seeking a federal job or when donating blood or solid organs. However, in 2006, the CDC began recommending routine HIV screening for all adolescent, adult, and pregnant clients in all health care settings. Clients will be notified that testing will be done with other routine screening unless the client defers. This is a change from past practice in which clients had to be asked specifically and had to give consent. Testing also involves pre- and post-test counseling. Testing may be performed either anonymously or confidentially. If testing is performed too early in the initial infection period, a false-negative result may occur. False-positive results are extremely rare but may occur in clients with autoimmune disorders such as lupus erythematosus, or in clients who have taken part in HIV vaccine studies. Other methods for detecting HIV infection include home test kits, salivary tests, and urine tests. HIV/AIDS is reportable in all 50 states and in the territories.

In general, test results are reported as (1) positive, (2) negative, or (3) indeterminate. If the enzyme immunoassay result is positive, a second test, the Western blot, is performed to confirm the diagnosis. A positive result means that the person is HIV-infected, but it does not predict the future course of disease. A negative result means that HIV antibodies were not detected. Indeterminate results usually mean that the enzyme immunoassay test was positive, but the Western blot test did not confirm the findings. Repeated testing later is commonly recommended as a means of validating initial test results. Repeated annual screening is recommended by the CDC for people who engage in high-risk activities.

The person usually remains asymptomatic for many years during the period following primary infection; therefore clients with HIV disease are commonly categorized in group A for extended periods. Although the clients have no obvious major manifestations, they may start to notice recurrent infections of the sinuses or respiratory tract or may feel increasing fatigue. Although no significant disease is apparent, viral destruction takes place throughout the body. The majority of this destruction occurs in lymph tissue, resulting in a slowly declining CD4$^+$ cell count. The damage to lymphatic structures also has a negative effect on the quality of CD4$^+$ cells that continue to be produced. After a while, although the numbers may be adequate, $CD4^+$ cells lose their ability to contain the destructive nature of HIV.

Since the beginning of the HIV epidemic, clinical monitoring has focused on evaluating the quantity of $CD4^+$ cells. In essence, $CD4^+$ cell counts are an indirect measurement of the clinical course of HIV disease, showing the end result of HIV activity. In 1996 viral load testing became available to directly measure viral activity in a person with HIV. Viral load tests measure the amount of HIV RNA in plasma, quantify HIV activity, determine prognosis, indicate the need for treatment, evaluate the biologic response to treatment, and detect treatment failure. $CD4^+$ cell counts should not be a substitute for viral load testing because the correlation between the two is weak. High viral loads may not always correlate with clinical manifestations and a low $CD4^+$ cell count and vice versa. Viral load results may be reported in copies per milliliter (e.g., 10,000 copies/ml). The actual numbers may be reported as follows:

- Decimal numbers, as in 10,000 copies
- Exponents, as in 10^4, where the exponent 4 indicates the number of zeros after the 1
- A logarithm, in this case 4, which indicates 10^4 or 10,000

Thus a report that sets viral activity at 5 logs would be interpreted as 10^5 or 100,000 copies/ml.

As the disease progresses, manifestations such as thrush or vulvovaginal candidiasis usually appear, which are distinct manifestations of an underlying immunodeficiency. This development is what commonly causes people to seek HIV testing. Those who have symptomatic illness are then classified into group B (see the box on HIV and AIDS Classification System for Adolescents and Adults on the website). Eventually a client with HIV infection develops one or more AIDS-defining diseases and is finally classified into group C. Once again, this may be the first time that HIV infection is discovered.

OUTCOME MANAGEMENT FOR HIV INFECTION

The outcomes for medical and nursing management of the client infected with HIV are to maintain the person's health, initiate and maintain an effective antiretroviral regimen, and prevent infectious complications. This requires follow-up at specified intervals and an understanding that to achieve these outcomes the client has to make lifestyle changes.

Medical Management of the Client with HIV Infection

Maintain Health

Initiating a plan of care for any client infected with HIV requires a detailed laboratory and clinical assessment.

Initial and follow-up laboratory testing provides invaluable information on disease progression, serves as a guide for treatment decisions, and determines the efficacy of treatment. A complete blood count is needed to identify anemia, thrombocytopenia, leukopenia, and developing infections. Multichannel chemistry panels and urinalysis disclose renal, liver, metabolic, or nutritional disease. Both tests are repeated at 6- to 12-month intervals to detect any abnormalities from disease progression or treatment complications. These results are also needed to modify dosages of antiretroviral drugs for clients with impaired kidney or liver function.

An annual tuberculin skin test detects mycobacterial disease, and a chest x-ray identifies pulmonary problems. For women, a pregnancy test and Papanicolaou (Pap) smear are usually performed. Pap smears are performed twice during the first year after a diagnosis of HIV infection and then at least annually. Screening for STIs includes testing for syphilis, gonorrhea, and *Chlamydia*. These are repeated annually if the client is sexually active. Hepatitis antibody testing is performed to identify acute or prior infection and to determine the need for immunization. There is a high incidence of hepatitis C in people infected with HIV.

Testing for pathogens known to cause opportunistic infections in people infected with HIV includes serologic tests intended to detect previous exposure to toxoplasmosis, histoplasmosis, cryptococcosis, and cytomegalovirus. For seronegative clients, repeated testing may reveal a primary exposure. For seropositive clients, rising titers of antibodies to these pathogens indicate the need for prophylactic therapy.

Finally, $CD4^+$ cell counts, ratios, and percentages are performed to determine the degree of immunodeficiency, and viral load testing is ordered to calculate the amount of viral activity. Viral load test result interpretations are as follows:

- 10,000 copies/ml: poses a low risk for AIDS
- 10,000 to 100,000 copies/ml: doubles risk for AIDS
- >100,000 copies/ml: poses a high risk for AIDS

The initial test, without any treatment, may reveal viral loads of 80,000 to 1 million copies per milliliter or even higher. These same tests are repeated at intervals determined by the presence or absence of manifestations or disease in the client through the course of illness. Because several viral load tests have been approved for use, clinicians are advised to use the same viral load test when performing serial measurements to control variations in test results. Diseases such as influenza, herpes, or pneumonia, as well as testing immediately after the influenza vaccine is administered, can cause a temporary increase in test results. Therefore testing may be deferred in any of these situations.

Initiate and Maintain Antiretroviral Therapy

The decision to treat HIV disease should involve both the primary care provider and the client. Many clients, because of personal experience or preference, may refuse recommended antiretroviral therapy. Clinicians should, in a noncoercive manner, provide as much objective information as possible so that the person with HIV can make an informed choice about taking these drugs. Most clinicians recommend starting an antiretroviral combination therapy regimen early in the course of disease; however, this has become somewhat controversial. This debate is outlined in the Translating Evidence into Practice feature on p. 2101.

Current guidelines from the U.S. Department of Health and Human Services are as follows:

- Symptomatic clients: Treat
- Asymptomatic clients with a CD4 count <200/mm^3: Treat
- Asymptomatic clients with CD4 counts 200-350/ mm^3: Therapy should generally be offered
- Asymptomatic clients with CD4 counts >350/mm^3: Defer or consider therapy if viral load is high

The following classes of antiretroviral agents are most commonly used:

- Nucleoside/nucleotide reverse transcriptase inhibitors (NRTIs)
- Protease inhibitors (PIs)
- Non-nucleoside reverse transcriptase inhibitors (NNRTIs)
- Fusion inhibitors

Also called nucleoside/nucleotide analogs, NRTIs block HIV replication of HIV in newly infected cells. PIs attack infected cells and prevent the virus from maturing appropriately. NNRTIs work in a manner similar to that of NRTIs. Fusion inhibitors, the newest class of drugs for treatment of HIV, prevent HIV from entering healthy T cells in the body (see Figure 78-3 and the Integrating Pharmacology feature on p. 2102). The only approved entry inhibitor is enfuvirtide (Fuzeon). Enfuvirtide blocks HIV fusion with the cell membrane, thus preventing entry of the virus into the cell. Enfuvirtide is given by twice daily subcutaneous injection. Use of entry inhibitors is reserved for HIV-positive clients who have become resistant to PIs, NRTIs, and NNRTIs.

Combination pills are available that greatly decrease the number of pills needed daily and facilitate adherence to treatment (see the Translating Evidence into Practice feature on p. 2101). In ART, a combination of three drugs from two of the first three drug classes (NRTIs, PIs, and NNRTIs) is used. Atripla, a combination of an NNRTI and two NRTI drugs, was approved by the FDA in July 2006. This is the first once-a-day combination antiretroviral pill. Clinicians and clients strive to find combinations that are the least toxic and that produce the largest and most long-lasting viral response (lowest viral load) and the best immune response (highest CD4$^+$ cell counts). The goals of therapy are to inhibit the replication of HIV, reduce the viral load to undetectable levels, and stabilize the disease.

Perhaps the greatest challenge in treating HIV infection has been the genetic promiscuity of this virus. As stated earlier, HIV mutates rapidly. In the presence of an antiretroviral drug, it can develop resistance to the drug and continue to grow in the presence of the drug. Three types of drug resistance are of concern:

- Genotypic resistance, in which the virus mutates
- Phenotypic resistance, in which the virus shows a decrease in sensitivity to the drug
- Cross-resistance, in which the virus, having developed resistance to one drug, becomes resistant to other drugs in that class

Monotherapy (prescription of one antiretroviral agent at a time) is more likely to result in drug resistance than is combination therapy. Subtherapeutic levels of a drug also lead to drug resistance. Subtherapeutic levels can occur when the client does not take the prescribed dosage or does not take doses at specified intervals, or both, and can also occur when other prescribed drugs interact with the antiretroviral drug and cause lower blood levels.

Attempting to prevent drug resistance, clinicians order combination therapy, believing that combinations of drugs "confuse" the virus, thus interfering with its ability to develop resistance. Unfortunately, preliminary data show that even in combinations of three drugs at once, resistance may develop to one or more of the agents being taken over time. Evaluation of antiretroviral therapy is based on the client's clinical manifestations and on laboratory tests of viral load and CD4$^+$ cell counts. The most reliable objective determinant is viral load testing, which is performed 3 to 4 weeks after initiating or changing therapy. If the decrease in viral load is not at least three times the original laboratory reports, or decreased by at least 0.5 log, the therapy is usually changed. Repeated testing is usually performed at 3- to 4-month intervals.

Drug failure, in which the ordered combination is no longer effective, can occur after trying several standard combinations of antiretrovirals. The challenge to the clinician at that point is to try combinations of four to six drugs in an effort to suppress HIV activity once again. This approach to therapeutic intervention is commonly called salvage therapy. In many instances, salvage therapy fails because the HIV-infected person has developed drug resistance to most of the available drugs.

Studies are also being conducted to identify other chemotherapeutic strategies to control HIV infection. Scientists are looking at the use of HIV vaccines

Adherence to Antiretroviral Therapy (ART)

Adherence to prescribed medication is known to be problematic. Clients have difficulty fully complying with therapy, whether it is of short duration for an acute episode (for instance, antibiotics) or of long duration (as in the case of chronic illness). It is well documented that adherence declines as the urgency of treating the disease declines and as the duration of therapy lengthens.

The literature shows that overall medication adherence rates vary from 40% to 80%. Unfortunately, HIV presents a unique challenge. Among individuals taking ART (antiretroviral therapy), only 40% to 60% are 90% adherent. Nonadherence to therapy allows the viral load to increase as immune functioning decreases, and is the major contributing factor to the development of resistant strains of HIV, which can be transmitted to others. Compliance with anti-HIV medication must occur at an incredible 95% to prevent these sequelae.

People living with HIV (PLWH) undergoing treatment face a daunting challenge in remaining adherent to their regimen. ART requires that the person take multiple medications, at precise dosing intervals, and with specific restrictions regarding timing the medications with food and fluid. In addition, there may be particular dietary or storage requirements. PLWH may also be taking several drugs to combat or prevent opportunistic infections, nutritional supplements, drugs to counteract unpleasant side effects, and, as the population of PLWH ages, medications to control other chronic conditions.

Many research studies have attempted to shed light on this topic by investigating factors leading to nonadherence as well as factors promoting adherence to therapy. Nonadherence can be a result of personal factors or systems-level factors. Personal factors include such things as forgetfulness, unwillingness to suffer side effects, lack of knowledge, large pill burden, lack of social support, and unwillingness to make lifestyle changes required by the treatment regimen. Systems-level factors include client-health care provider relationship; having multiple services available at one location; ease of obtaining refills; and simplicity of arranging follow-up care, especially in light of new manifestations or side effects. Ongoing substance abuse and psychiatric conditions also are important considerations. Cultural factors also appear to play a role in adherence.

Medication nonadherence seems to be a multifactorial and unique experience to each client. It is incumbent on the nurse to assess this topic gently at every opportunity, attempting to learn, from the client's point of view, what barriers he or she is facing in remaining adherent to the medical regimen.

IMPLICATIONS

Several strategies to improving medication adherence seem to be beneficial. First and foremost is education. PLWH need detailed information about their medications and knowledge regarding the consequences of nonadherence. They also need ongoing information regarding their viral load and $CD4^+$ counts, which can be correlated with medication use. Motivate the client by including him or her in all decisions regarding drug treatment. Give the client information regarding dosing schedule, food and storage requirements, and side effects; then let the client decide whether that treatment is feasible. Some clinics let the PLWH "practice" the regimen with candy or jelly beans for several weeks before the client is asked to commit to the regimen.

Simplify the regimen as much as possible and use drugs that require the least amount of change in the client's lifestyle. Help the client schedule taking medications along with other daily routines. Anticipate unpleasant side effects and be prepared to deal with them promptly. Several "adherence-promoting devices" are available, including simple pill boxes, beepers and alarms, and computer-generated telephone reminder calls. PLWH may need specific skills-building sessions or assistance with problem-solving barriers to taking medications.

Clients with active substance abuse or untreated and undertreated psychiatric conditions (depression, anxiety) may not be able to adhere until these issues are under control. Likewise, a person must fulfill "survival needs" before managing a complex condition such as HIV. If a client is homeless, finding shelter will be a much higher priority than adhering to medications. For these types of clients, it probably is best to delay the start of therapy until these conditions have been stabilized.

Adherence to an HIV medication regimen is demanding and complex, and requires vigilance on the part of the client in maintaining his or her treatment schedule. It also requires the nurse to be vigilant, sensitive, creative, and a partner with the PLWH to design strategies to improve adherence. Adherence to therapy is the most significant determinant of its success. Nurses must be in the forefront to help their clients combat this disease.

REFERENCES

1. Acri, T., Coco, A., Lin, K., et al. (2005). Knowledge of structured treatment interruption and adherence to antiretroviral therapy. *AIDS Patient Care and STDs, 19,* 167-173.
2. Adamian, M.S., Golin, C.E., Shain, L.A., & DeVellis, B. (2004). Brief motivational interviewing to improve adherence to antiretroviral therapy: Development and qualitative pilot assessment of an intervention. *AIDS Patient Care and STDs, 18,* 229-238.
3. Corless, I.B., Nicholas, P.K., Davis, S.M., et al. (2005). Symptom status, medication adherence, and quality of life in HIV disease. *Journal of Hospice and Palliative Nursing, 7*(3), 129-138.
4. Deloria-Knoll, M., Chmiel, J.S., Moorman, A.C., et al. (2004). Factors related to and consequences of adherence to antiretroviral therapy in an ambulatory HIV-infected patient cohort. *AIDS Patient Care and STDs, 12,* 721-727.
5. Enriquez, M., Lackey, N.R., O'Connor, M.C., & McKensey, D.S. (2004). Successful adherence after multiple HIV treatment failures. *Journal of Advanced Nursing, 45,* 439-446.
6. Garcia, P.R., & Cote, J.K. (2003). Factors affecting adherence to antiretroviral therapy in people living with HIV/AIDS. *Journal of the Association of Nurses in AIDS Care, 14*(4), 37-45.
7. Kalichman, S., Cherry, J., & Cain, D. (2005). Nurse-delivered antiretroviral treatment adherence intervention for people with low literacy skills and living with HIV/AIDS. *Journal of the Association of Nurses in AIDS Care, 16*(5), 3-15.
8. Mills, E., Nachega, J., Buchan, I., et al. (2006). Adherence to antiretroviral therapy in sub-Saharan Africa and North America. *Journal of the American Medical Association, 296*(6), 679-690.
9. Oggins, J. (2003). Notions of HIV and medication among multiethnic people living with HIV. *Health and SocialWork, 28*(1), 53-62.
10. Piliero, P.J., & Colagreco, J.P. (2003). Simplified regimens for treating HIV infection and AIDS. *Journal of the American Academy of Nurse Practitioners, 15,* 305-312.
11. Russel, J., Krantz, S., & Neville, S. (2004). The patient-provider relationship and adherence to highly active antiretroviral therapy. *Journal of the Association of Nurses in AIDS Care, 15*(5), 40-47.
12. Trzynka, S.L., & Erlen, J.A. (2004). HIV disease susceptibility in women and the barriers adherence. *MEDSURG Nursing, 13*(2), 97-104.
13. Tugenberg, T., Ware, N.C., & Wyatt, M.A. (2006). Paradoxical effects of clinician emphasis on adherence to combination antiretroviral therapy for HIV/AIDS. *AIDS Patient Care and STDs, 20,* 269-274.

INTEGRATING P H A R M A C O L O G Y

Understanding Antiretroviral Therapy (ART)

Compared with the early days of the epidemic, many drugs now exist to treat HIV/AIDS and more are being developed. Treating HIV with monotherapy (using one drug) leads to rapid drug resistance. Combination therapy (ART, or antiretroviral therapy) consists of the simultaneous administration of drugs that have different mechanisms of action and without similar toxicities. ART drug combinations attack the HIV virus at different points necessary for its replication. Utilizing multiple drugs decreases the chance of developing resistance.

Since the advent of ART, dramatic declines in AIDS morbidity and mortality have occurred. Inhibiting viral replication allows for "reconstitution" (rebuilding) of the immune system and reducing clinical progression and the risk of death. Drugs to treat HIV/AIDS fall into categories based on where in the viral replication cycle they are effective.

REVERSE TRANSCRIPTASE INHIBITORS

To replicate, HIV's viral RNA must be converted into double-stranded DNA. The enzyme *reverse transcriptase* is responsible for this activity. The first drugs approved to treat HIV/AIDS were reverse transcriptase inhibitors, which prevent the enzyme from changing viral RNA into DNA.

Non-Nucleoside Reverse Transcriptase Inhibitors

Non-nucleoside reverse transcriptase inhibitors (NNRTIs) bind directly to the enzyme and prevent the conversion of RNA to DNA. Examples include the following:

- Rescriptor (delavirdine, DLV)
- Sustiva (efavirenz, EFV)
- Viramune (nevirapine, NVP)

Nucleoside/Nucleotide Reverse Transcriptase Inhibitors

Nucleoside/nucleotide reverse transcriptase inhibitors (NRTIs) incorporate themselves into viral DNA and cause its construction to be terminated. Examples include the following:

- Combivir (zidovudine/lamivudine, AZT + 3TC)
- Epivir (lamivudine, 3TC)
- Retrovir (zidovudine: ZDV or AZT)
- Zerit (stavudine or d4T)
- Ziagen (abacavir or ABC)
- Videx, Videx EC (didanosine, ddI)
- Viread (tenofovir disoproxil fumarate, DF)
- Trizivir (abacavir/lamivudine/zidovudine, ABC + AZT + 3TC)

PROTEASE INHIBITORS

These drugs work by preventing the successful assembly and release of new virus particles (virions). Problems with this class include intolerance, high "pill burden," and poor adherence to treatment. Examples include the following:

- Agenerase (amprenavir, APV)
- Crixivan (indinavir, IDV)
- Fortovase (saquinavir soft gels, SQV-SGC)
- Invirase (saquinavir capsules, SQV-HGC)
- Kaletra (lopinavir/ritonavir, LPV)
- Norvir (ritonavir, RTV)
- Viracept (nelfinavir, NFV)

The optimal time to start therapy has not been definitively determined by research studies. Most clinicians favor the "hit early and hard" approach; however, recent guidelines from the U.S. Department of Health and Human Services and the International AIDS Society—USA Panel delineate several factors to consider before initiating therapy: $CD4^+$ count, viral load, presence of manifestations or opportunistic infections, and the client's willingness to adhere to the regimen. Client willingness is key: nonadherence to this complex regimen leads to drug resistance (see the Translating Evidence into Practice feature on Adherence to ART on p. 2101). Other considerations include drug toxicity profile, "pill burden," dosing/storage/food requirements, and interactions with other drugs the client is taking.

There is no specific prescription for ART. Recommended combinations include the following:

- 2 NRTIs plus either 1 NNRTI or 1 PI or 2 PIs
- 3 NRTIs

In July 2006 the FDA approved Atripla, the first once-a-day combination antiretroviral pill. It is a combination of an NNRTI and two NRTI drugs.

ENTRY INHIBITORS

Entry inhibitors work by preventing HIV from entering healthy T cells. They work differently from the approved anti-HIV drugs described earlier that are active against HIV after it has infected a T cell. These drugs are recommended after initial regimens but before clients become multi-drug resistant. Entry inhibitors include *fusion inhibitors* such as enfuvirtide (Fuzeon, ENF). Fuzeon binds to the gp41 protein on the HIV's surface so that it cannot bind with T cells, thus preventing the virus from infecting healthy cells. Administration is more difficult because enfuvirtide cannot be taken by mouth and must be given as an injection twice a day every 12 hours. Other entry inhibitors are currently under investigation.

Other drugs that work to inhibit different phases of the HIV life cycle are currently being studied. Supervised drug interruptions are also being investigated as a way to boost the client's immune system and decrease the financial and emotional burden of such complex therapy.

as a therapeutic strategy to stimulate host responses and control viral replication. Research continues on immunomodulators—drugs designed to modulate or reconstitute the immune system, such as interleukin-2.

Other novel approaches to therapy include newer entry inhibitor agents, nonpeptidic protease inhibitors, second-generation NNRTIs, integrase inhibitors, and chemokine antagonists.

🪔 Prevent Infection

By 1986 surveillance data indicated that in more than 80% of people with HIV disease, *Pneumocystis (carinii) jiroveci* pneumonia occurred at least once before death. 🪔 Studies eventually showed that morbidity and mortality rates could be reduced significantly by giving a drug prophylactically for *P. jiroveci* pneumonia. Since 1989 the U.S. Public Health Service has recommended that all HIV-infected clients with a CD4$^+$ cell count below 200/mm^3 receive prophylaxis for *P. jiroveci* pneumonia. Drugs include trimethoprim-sulfamethoxazole (TMP-SMX); dapsone; dapsone, pyrimethamine, and folinic acid; aerosolized, intravenous, or intramuscular pentamidine; or atovaquone. TMP-SMX and dapsone also provide protection against toxoplasmosis.

Although surveillance data alone do not reflect the true incidence of infection with *Mycobacterium avium-intracellulare* complex, postmortem examinations revealed that more than 60% of HIV-infected people had an active infection. 🪔 Since 1993 the U.S. Public Health Service has recommended that all HIV-infected clients with a CD4$^+$ cell count below 50/mm^3 receive prophylaxis for *M. avium-intracellulare* complex. Recommended drugs include clarithromycin, azithromycin, and rifabutin. However, these drugs may interact with antiretrovirals.

All HIV-infected clients with a positive result to a tuberculin skin test who have no evidence of active tuberculosis should receive 9 months of preventive therapy with isoniazid. Pyridoxine should be added to reduce the potential for peripheral neuropathy. An alternative regimen is rifabutin and pyrazinamide for 2 months; however, these drugs may interact with antiretrovirals.

Other recommended prophylactic measures include prevention of respiratory tract infections by using pneumococcal vaccine and influenza vaccine and prevention of traveler's diarrhea when traveling to countries where diarrhea is common by using antimicrobials such as ciprofloxacin. Finally, prophylactic medication may be ordered to prevent cytomegalovirus infection, recurrent candidiasis, cryptococcosis, or histoplasmosis.

Nursing Management of the Client with HIV Infection

Assessment. To help a client with health maintenance behaviors, nurses should not restrict assessment to the client's immediate clinical status. Instead, focus on potential problems the client may encounter during the illness. For example, if the client has no health insurance or money to pay for follow-up visits, the nurse should initiate social work consultation. There are alternate sources for health care services, such as the federally funded AIDS Drug Assistance Program. If the client lives alone and has no one willing to assist, he or she may need to be placed in an institution when the illness progresses. As a coordinator of care, have information readily available to identify problems and plan ahead.

Before performing any teaching, evaluate the client's existing level of knowledge about HIV infection. Some clients may know little, whereas others may be knowledgeable. Instead of making any assumptions, try to assess exactly what the client does or does not know about transmission and health-promoting behaviors.

The psychological burden of HIV disease can be overwhelming. Crisis points at which the nurse can anticipate anxiety, fear, or depression include the following:

- Time of the initial HIV-positive diagnosis
- Time of the initial AIDS diagnosis
- Changes in treatment
- Development of new manifestations
- Recurrence of problems or relapse
- Terminal illness

Psychological conflicts that clients commonly experience include fear of transmitting HIV to others, constant worry about developing an infection, guilt about a previous lifestyle, and changes in personal relationships. Social stressors may include disclosure of one's HIV status, stigma related to that status, insecurity about employment and insurance, and loneliness and social isolation.

Diagnosis, Outcomes, Interventions

Diagnosis: Risk for Ineffective Therapeutic Regimen Management. The primary nursing diagnosis encountered with newly diagnosed HIV infection is *Risk for Ineffective Therapeutic Regimen Management related to complexity of health care regimen*. Although some clients may know about HIV disease, it is unlikely that they know all that can be done to improve their health.

Outcomes. The client will learn about HIV disease—how to prevent transmission, how to manage the disease, and how to prevent complications.

Interventions

Provide Education. Health teaching should be ongoing and repeated at frequent intervals. An HIV-infected person can adopt several behaviors that not only improve immune function but also increase a sense of well-being. The content outline for teaching health maintenance includes stress management, exercise, safer sex practices, pregnancy and HIV infection, nutrition (emphasizing a high-protein, high-calorie, low-fat diet), food and water safety, skin care, routine mouth care, proper hand-washing, environmental cleaning and safety, pet care, limiting alcohol consumption, use of injected drugs, travel safety and avoiding exposure to infectious pathogens, importance of health care follow-up, and understanding and interpreting viral load tests and CD4$^+$ cell counts.

SAFETY ALERT — **The Joint Commission (TJC) National Patient Safety Goals related to reducing the risk of infections and hand hygiene guidelines are an important part of promoting health maintenance and preventing infection in clients who are infected with HIV.**

Carefully explain viral load test results because many people misunderstand the results. When successful therapy begins, the viral load drops from high levels, such as 750,000 copies/ml, down to what are called "undetectable" levels; however, most laboratory tests can detect HIV copies down to only 50 copies/ml. Because anything lower cannot be measured, the laboratory report reads "undetectable levels." Although this is great news and indicates the success of the prescribed regimen, it does not mean that the person no longer has HIV infection. Some clients with HIV infection leave their primary care provider thinking that they are disease free and no longer at risk of spreading HIV. This must be clarified whenever you report laboratory results to a client; emphasize that the client must still practice safer sex, avoid sharing needles, and so on.

Encourage clients to tell their health care providers about any self-prescribed therapies they are taking because these therapies might have a positive or negative influence on the outcomes of care. Keep track of over-the-counter medications because they may interact with prescribed therapies. Some clients may also obtain drugs through buyers' clubs or underground pharmacies. This not only may be detrimental to the effectiveness of prescribed treatments but also may have an adverse effect on observations made during a drug trial.

Some clients may opt to try alternative or complementary treatments, including (1) spiritual or psychological interventions (e.g., guided imagery, meditation, faith healing), (2) nutritional alternatives (e.g., a macrobiotic diet), (3) drug and biologic therapies (e.g., homeopathy, oxygen, ozone therapy), and (4) physical forces (e.g., acupuncture, acupressure, massage therapy). In most cases, these choices can have a positive effect on the person's emotional well-being but may also have a negative effect. For example, a macrobiotic diet can lead to vitamin and mineral deficiencies as well as weight loss. Herbal remedies may cause nausea, vomiting, diarrhea, or CNS depression or interact with antiretrovirals. Despite these effects, some clients will continue to use these methods.

Initiate and Maintain Antiretroviral Therapy. One of the most important aspects of providing nursing care to the HIV-infected client is helping with the antiretroviral regimen. Studies suggest that clients with chronic diseases such as hypertension and diabetes mellitus take their prescribed drugs about 50% of the time. However,

to sustain the durability and efficacy of antiretroviral therapy, clients must maintain about a 95% compliance rate. This places high expectations on both the HIV-infected client and the physicians and nurses. Because therapy may last for many years, it is vital that the client understand the potential benefits and drawbacks of any regimen and the potential consequences of not adhering to therapy. Potential benefits of antiretroviral therapy include the following:

- Control of HIV replication and mutation, with reduction in viral load
- Prevention of destruction of the immune system and loss of CD4$^+$ T helper cells
- Delayed progression to AIDS-defining illnesses
- Decreased risk for development of HIV resistance to drugs
- Decreased risk of drug toxicity (drugs are started when the client is healthier)
- Increased survival with HIV disease (the most important benefit)

Potential risks of antiretroviral therapy include the following:

- Reduced quality of life from adverse drug effects and the inconvenience of a complex regimen
- Earlier development of drug resistance
- A limited number of drugs available to respond to drug resistance
- Unknown long-term toxicity of antiretroviral therapy
- Unknown duration of the effectiveness of current antiretroviral therapies

The decision of whether to take antiretrovirals is ultimately up to the client. The regimens ordered may be complex and require the client to take large numbers of pills daily (as many as 15 to 20), often at exactly spaced intervals and with differing requirements as to timing the pills related to food. Liquid preparations often taste horrible, and the client must try various strategies to mask the taste. All the drugs have side effects to which the person must learn to adjust and control, and they also interact with numerous other drugs. These drug-drug interactions are usually not life-threatening, but they may interfere with antiretroviral blood levels, causing subtherapeutic effects, drug resistance, and drug failure. Instruct all clients taking antiretrovirals as follows:

- Take the drug at specified intervals.
- Do not skip a dose.
- Do not increase or decrease the number of pills you take.
- Follow meal and fluid requirements.
- If side effects occur, tell your physician or nurse. If side effects are significant, ask your primary care provider for information or medication to help manage them.

■ Store all drugs as instructed.

■ If you do not want to take the drugs, tell your primary care provider.

■ If you take the drugs only periodically, it would be better not to take them at all. Discuss this with your physician or nurse.

■ Remember, the treatment plan is yours. If you do not agree with it, discuss it with your physician or nurse.

Because of concern over the development of drug resistance and drug failure, several studies have been conducted on methods to help people infected with HIV adhere to their drug regimens. Several strategies have proved very helpful, especially when used together (see the Translating Evidence into Practice feature on Adherence to ART on p. 2101). Primary care providers also need to incorporate cultural and religious beliefs when addressing drug adherence behaviors. Meal planning because of fat content requirements or dietary restrictions or preferences as well as the need to abstain from food and water on certain days because of religious practices may be necessary.

Prevent Infection. Nursing strategies to prevent infection include health teaching and helping the client take drugs properly to prevent opportunistic infections. Health teaching focuses on safer sex practices not only to prevent HIV transmission but also to keep clients from acquiring STIs. Practicing food and water safety can prevent such diseases as salmonellosis, cryptosporidiosis, and toxoplasmosis. Simple hand-washing is an effective technique for minimizing food-borne illnesses. Maintaining skin and mucous membrane integrity with good skin and mouth hygiene can reduce the incidence of candidiasis.

Evaluation. Evaluation includes the client's understanding of the teaching provided and the choices available. If a client chooses not to adopt a recommended behavior, it does not mean that the client is noncompliant. Health care providers can have a difficult time evaluating the outcomes of teaching and weighing them against the client's free choice. Remember that the ultimate decision about following a health care provider's advice belongs to the client. The client's decisions do not reflect failure on the part of the health care professional.

Evaluation of a client's ability to adhere to a prescribed drug regimen includes both subjective and objective techniques. Subjective evaluation is by self-report; clients and their care partner describe the client's ability to take all prescribed medications. Objective analysis of the success of the plan of care is by laboratory evaluation of CD4$^+$ cell counts and viral load.

A totally different situation exists when minimal learning takes place because of cognitive impairment. It is well documented that problems with thinking or memory may exist and go unidentified if they are not obvious. This is more likely to occur in clients with less than a 12th grade education and in clients older than 50 years of age. In such a situation, a care partner should be designated who receives all information when it is provided to the client. Whenever the care partner cannot make a clinic or office visit, provide telephone teaching and document that you accomplished this.

OUTCOME MANAGEMENT FOR AIDS

As both the quantity and the quality of CD4$^+$ cells diminish, "AIDS-indicator" diseases occur. The categories of AIDS-defining illnesses include opportunistic infections, cancers, and other conditions specific to HIV disease. The four main types of opportunistic infections are (1) bacterial, (2) fungal, (3) protozoal, and (4) viral (Table 78-1). Neoplasms associated with AIDS include Kaposi's sarcoma (KS), non-Hodgkin's lymphoma, and invasive cervical cancer. Two other conditions unique to AIDS are (1) HIV wasting syndrome and (2) HIV encephalopathy. Hepatitis C is now considered an AIDS-indicator disease. Since the introduction of ART in 1996, the onset of AIDS-defining illness has been delayed and treating these diseases has become easier.

Medical Management of the Client with AIDS

Prevent and Treat Opportunistic Infections

Most of the pathogens responsible for opportunistic infections are ubiquitous; that is, they are all around us. Most people do not become sick from the organisms that cause opportunistic infections because their immune systems are intact. Once the regulators of the immune system (CD4$^+$ cells) are destroyed by HIV, however, infection can occur. Most opportunistic infections result from secondary reactivation of previously acquired pathogens rather than from a new or primary infection. For example, most people are infected with *P. (carinii) jiroveci* in the early preschool years, when it causes respiratory manifestations and is probably dismissed as a common cold. The child's intact immune system brings the infection under control; however, the organism remains dormant in the person's body. The potential then exists for the organism to reactivate, causing disease again in an immunocompromised person. This concept applies to any person with an immunodeficiency, regardless of the cause. Single opportunistic infections are rare, and clients may have multiple infections. Many of these opportunistic infections are not curable. Because the immune system no longer has the strength to contain the infection, it becomes chronic and requires lifetime suppressive therapy. Helping the client comply with the antibiotic regimen to keep opportunistic infections under control is an essential part of the care planning process. Because the client must take antibiotics for extended periods, drug resistance may develop,

TABLE 78–1 Opportunistic Infections Seen in Clients with AIDS

Infection and Source	Manifestations	Treatment and Comments
Bacterial Infections		
Mycobacterium tuberculosis (airborne, droplets)	"Constitutional": fever, chills, weight loss, night sweats, lymphadenopathy, fatigue "Pulmonary": cough, dyspnea, chest pain, hemoptysis	Combination therapy including isoniazid, rifampin, pyrazinamide, ethambutol, or streptomycin. All clients with HIV-positive status should be tested for TB annually; multi-drug resistance is growing problem.
Mycobacterium avium (soil, water, eggs, unpasteurized diary products)	Fever, night sweats, fatigue, anorexia, weight loss, abdominal pain, diarrhea	Difficult to treat; may defer based on severity. Prophylaxis may be considered. Drugs include azithromycin, clarithromycin, ethambutol, ciprofloxacin, rifabutin, amikacin, ampicillin, chloramphenicol, TMP-SMX, ciprofloxacin, norfloxacin.
Salmonellosis (contaminated food and water, handling contaminated feces, sexual activity involving oral-anal contact; food handlers and pets may be source of exposure)	Fever, night sweats, fatigue, anorexia, weight loss, abdominal pain, diarrhea	Prevent and treat perianal skin breakdown. Antibiotic therapy based on culture and sensitivity.
Pneumonia, especially from *Streptococcus pneumoniae* and *Haemophilus influenzae* (airborne)	Cough, productive cough, fever, chills, chest pain, shortness of breath, fatigue	Especially common in IV drug injecting clients. Pneumococcal vaccination recommended every 5 years.
Fungal Infections		
Candida albicans (found in food, soil, on fomites, and normally found on skin and in mouth, vagina, and large intestine)	Related to site of infection: may include dysphagia with esophagitis, oral lesions with thrush, cutaneous lesions with intertrigo, vulvovaginal irritation and discharge, vaginitis; constitutional symptoms occur with disseminated disease	Various antifungals related to the site of infection. Oral: clotrimazole troches, nystatin suspension, fluconazole. Esophagitis: fluconazole, itraconazole, ketoconazole, amphotericin B. Intertrigo and vaginitis: clotrimazole, miconazole, ketoconazole, fluconazole, itraconazole. Disseminated disease: amphotericin B. Most infections are endogenous; that is, the person's own organism is the source of infection. Eating yogurt made with live cultures helps control recurrence.
Cryptococcus neoformans (found in pigeon droppings, nesting places, soil, fruit, and unpasteurized fruit juice; organism is aerosolized and inhaled)	Low-grade fever, fatigue, headache, nausea, vomiting, altered mental status, cough, dyspnea, pleuritic chest pain, cutaneous and oral lesions possible	Amphotericin B, with or without flucytosine, fluconazole, or itraconazole. Maintenance lifetime suppressive therapy may be required.
Histoplasma capsulatum: histoplasmosis (endemic to certain regions of United States, especially middle, central, southern states, and to Puerto Rico)	Fever; weight loss; enlarged lymph nodes, liver, and spleen; abdominal pain; oral and skin lesions; anemia; leukopenia; and thrombocytopenia	Amphotericin B, itraconazole, fluconazole. Maintenance lifetime suppressive therapy may be required.
Coccidioides immitis: coccidioidomycosis (fungus endemic to Southwestern United States; also called valley fever)	Fever, dyspnea, fatigue, weight loss, cough	Amphotericin B, ketoconazole, itraconazole, fluconazile. Lifetime suppressive therapy may be required.
Protozoal Infections		
Pneumocystis (carinii) jiroveci (airborne)	Presentation may be elusive; with pneumonia, cough may be first symptom Productive cough, fever, dyspnea Extrapulmonary infection can occur	TMP-SMX, pentamidine, atovaquone, TMP-dapsone, clindamycin-primaquine, trimetrexate. Lifetime suppressive therapy may be required.
Toxoplasma gondii: toxoplasmosis (contaminated meat, vegetables, eggs, unpasteurized dairy products, in utero transmission, contaminated cat feces)	Headache, impaired cognition, hemiparesis, aphasia, ataxia, vision loss, cranial nerve palsies, motor problems, seizures; infection can occur in other body systems	Pyrimethamine plus sulfadiazine, leukovorin, clindamycin plus pyrimethamine, clarithromycin, azithromycin. Lifetime suppressive therapy may be required. Fewer than 1% of domestic cats are infected and veterinarians can perform a simple blood test to determine if cat is infected.

TABLE 78–1   Opportunistic Infections Seen in Clients with AIDS—Cont'd

Infection and Source	Manifestations	Treatment and Comments
Cryptosporidium (mammals, birds, reptiles, fish; water and food-borne; contaminated swimming pools, anal-oral sexual contact)	Malabsorption, dehydration, malnutrition, profuse diarrhea (up to 25 L/day), steatorrhea, flatulence, abdominal cramping and pain, anorexia, nausea, vomiting, fever, fatigue, profound weight loss, myalgia, electrolyte imbalance	Chronic disease, may be fatal. No effective treatment exists; however, drugs that may be tried include paromomycin, azithromycin, clarithromycin, nitazoxanide, thalidomide, and symptomatic therapy to decrease peristalsis and control pain. Monitor for and treat perianal skin breakdown.
Isospora belli: isosporiasis (infected animals, human-to-human, contaminated water)	Diarrhea, anorexia, nausea, vomiting, weight loss, abdominal pain, fever	TMP-SMX, pyrimethamine plus folinic acid.
Viral Infections		
Cytomegalovirus (CMV) (blood and body fluids, including saliva; feces)	May be asymptomatic. May cause chorioretinitis, pneumonitis, encephalitis, adrenalitis, colitis, esophagitis, hepatitis, or cholangitis	Ganciclovir, foscarnet, cidofovir plus probenecid. Lifetime suppression may be required. Most healthy people eventually become infected with CMV.
Herpes simplex (direct contact with infectious lesions/secretions)	Painful vesicular lesions on the oral, genital, or perianal regions. May also cause encephalitis, esophagitis, bronchitis, keratitis, pericarditis, and hand infections	Acyclovir, foscarnet, famciclovir; topical acyclovir for skin lesions. Chronic disease requires lifetime suppressive therapy.
Progressive multifocal leukoencephalopathy; JC virus (common in nature; most healthy people infected)	Limb weakness, ataxia, cognitive impairment, vision loss, speech impairment, headache. May progress to dementia, blindness, paralysis, and death	No effective therapy, but may try acyclovir, foscarnet, adenine arabinoside, cytosine arabinoside, interferon alfa.
Hepatitis		The leading cause of death in AIDS clients remains liver failure, with hepatitis being the most common etiology. See Chapter 47 for a discussion of hepatitis.

and both physicians and nurses must constantly observe the client for recurrence of the infection.

Bacterial Infections. There are several important opportunistic infections caused by bacteria, including *Mycobacterium tuberculosis* (causing TB), *Mycobacterium-avium* complex, and *Salmonella.* Bacterial pneumonia is common and is usually caused by *Streptococcus pneumoniae* and *Haemophilus influenzae.* The risk of bacterial infection rises with low CD4$^+$ counts and often clients will take prophylactic antibiotics to prevent these diseases (see Table 78-1).

Fungal Infections. Fungal infections are a common source of illness in the client with AIDS. *Candida albicans* is a frequent culprit. *Cryptococcus neoformans, Histoplasma capsulatum,* and *Coccidioides immitis* are other fungi found in nature that cause disease when the immune system is severely compromised (see Table 78-1).

Protozoal Infections. *Pneumocystosis (carinii) jiroveci* causes a pneumonia that was once a leading cause of death in the AIDS client. Successful treatment and prophylaxis has greatly reduced the death rate from this protozoal infection. *Toxoplasma gondii, Cryptosporidium,* and *Isospora belli* are also ubiquitous in nature and cause problems in an immunocompromised state (see Table 78-1).

Viral Infections. Viral infections in the AIDS client are difficult to treat. Cytomegalovirus disease (CMV), herpes, progressive multifocal leukoencephalopathy, caused by the JC virus (initials of the first client in whom it was first discovered), and hepatitis are the most common viral illnesses seen in the AIDS client (see Table 78-1).

Treat Neoplasms

Kaposi's Sarcoma. Four types of KS may be encountered in clinical practice: (1) classic KS, which tends to occur in older men who are black, of Mediterranean descent, or from certain Jewish populations; (2) African KS, seen in Africa; (3) transplant KS, seen in people who receive organ transplants; and (4) HIV-related KS, which differs from the others in that it runs a fulminant course, is disseminated throughout the body, and results in shorter survival.

The only form associated with HIV disease is HIV-related KS. It has been diagnosed predominantly in men who have sex with men and is thought to be associated with a sexually transmitted pathogen that then predisposes the person to development. Researchers think it is caused by either human herpesvirus type 8 (HHV-8) or KS-associated herpesvirus (KSHV). KS differs from most AIDS-defining diseases in that it is unrelated to low $CD4^+$ cell counts and can occur early in HIV infection.

Clinical presentation typically starts with an initial "patch" that is flat and pink, looks like a bruise, and is symmetrical on both sides of the body. Later, it turns into dark violet or black plaques. Clinical presentation of the lesions can include the mouth, skin, mucous membranes, head, neck, torso, limbs (soles of feet), genitals, lung, brain, intestines, testes, liver, spleen, pancreas, adrenal gland, and lymph nodes. They can be painful.

Treatment depends on the extent of tumors (tumor burden), $CD4^+$ cell count, associated manifestations and diseases, and the client's functional ability. Local therapy includes radiation, localized chemotherapy, and cryotherapy. Systemic therapy includes doxorubicin, alpha interferon, bleomycin, paclitaxel, and daunorubicin. Experimental therapies under investigation include possible treatment of the underlying viral cause of KS with foscarnet or ganciclovir. Initially several therapies may be tried, which may be effective in suppressing the course of KS; eventually, however, the clinical decline in the client's condition makes continued treatment impossible.

Non-Hodgkin's Lymphoma. Non-Hodgkin's lymphoma tends to occur late in the course of HIV disease and is related to low $CD4^+$ cell counts. The primary sites of occurrence are the brain, gastrointestinal tract, bone marrow, and liver. The initial clinical presentation may be nonspecific and include fever, night sweats, and weight loss, all of which are associated with *M. avium* complex infection, TB, and CMV infection.

Treatment includes methotrexate, bleomycin, doxorubicin, cyclophosphamide, and vincristine. Despite aggressive treatment, the prognosis is poor except in clients on combination antiretroviral therapy, who tend to survive longer.

Invasive Cervical Cancer. Cervical intraepithelial neoplasia (CIN), the precursor to cervical cancer, occurs at a high rate in women infected with HIV and is related to low $CD4^+$ cell counts. In early stages of disease, the client is asymptomatic; however, it progresses rapidly. Cervical dysplasia is usually detected by Pap smear. Early clinical manifestations include postcoital bleeding, metrorrhagia, and a blood-tinged vaginal discharge. Manifestations of more extensive disease include back, pelvic, and leg pain; weight loss; vaginal bleeding; anemia; lymphadenopathy; and edema of the legs.

Treatment of CIN can include conization, laser therapy, cryosurgery, electrocautery, or hysterectomy. For invasive cancer, treatment may involve surgery, radiation, and chemotherapy with cisplatin, vincristine, bleomycin, or mitomycin. Follow-up care focuses on recurrent disease and control of manifestations and metastasis.

Treat Conditions Specific to AIDS

AIDS Dementia. HIV encephalopathy, also referred to as *AIDS dementia complex,* appears to affect the very young and older HIV-infected clients and clients with anemia and weight loss. In addition, HIV-infected people with less than a 12th grade education may be more likely to show clinical manifestations. Manifestations include cognitive dysfunction, motor problems, and behavioral changes. Cognitive manifestations include an inability to concentrate, decreased memory, impaired judgment, and slowed thinking. Motor impairment may be manifested as leg weakness, ataxia, and clumsiness. Behavioral changes can range from apathy, reduced spontaneity, and social withdrawal to irritability, hyperactivity, anxiety, mania, and delirium.

The staging system for AIDS dementia complex is as follows:

- Stage 1: Minimal manifestations, mild neurologic manifestations, no impairment of work or ability to perform activities of daily living (ADL)
- Stage 2: Obvious intellectual or motor impairment, still able to do all but the most demanding ADL
- Stage 3: Cannot work or perform demanding ADL, still capable of basic self-care, ambulatory but may need a single assistive device
- Stage 4: Major intellectual disability, cannot walk without assistance
- Stage 5: Nearly vegetative, paraplegic or quadriplegic, only rudimentary cognition remains

Some studies have shown a favorable response to combination antiretroviral therapy. Psychotropic drugs may be tried in small doses, but benzodiazepines, drugs with strong anticholinergic properties, and amitriptyline should be used with caution. Follow-up monitoring focuses on detecting the progression of AIDS dementia complex and on evaluating the client's ability to safely maintain independent living and comply with prescribed therapies.

HIV Wasting Syndrome. Weight loss occurs at some point in more than 90% of people with HIV infection. *HIV wasting* is defined as profound involuntary **weight loss** (>10% of total body baseline weight) with either chronic diarrhea or chronic weakness and fever. The primary causes of HIV wasting syndrome are reduced food intake, malabsorption of nutrients, and altered metabolism of nutrients. The evaluation of a client with HIV wasting syndrome includes determining and treating the cause. Reversing wasting syndrome is very difficult.

The goal of drug therapy in wasting syndrome is to stimulate appetite, produce weight gain, and increase lean muscle mass. Often weight gain is from water and body fat, which is not beneficial. Identified conditions that contribute to wasting should be treated first. Drugs used to treat HIV wasting syndrome include megestrol acetate, anabolic steroids, and dronabinol (the major psychoactive component of marijuana). The drug used most successfully to treat wasting syndrome is human growth hormone. Follow-up therapy includes constant assessment for factors that may interfere with the plan of care.

Nursing Management of the Client with AIDS

The goal of nursing care is to diagnose and treat human responses to actual or potential health problems related to the development of clinical manifestations and the diagnosis of AIDS. All efforts are directed at controlling manifestations. Actual or potential problems seen in people with AIDS include fever, fatigue, weight loss, nausea, diarrhea, dry and painful mouth, dry skin, skin lesions, pain, dyspnea, cough, impaired cognition, impaired vision, insomnia, and sexual dysfunction. Common nursing diagnoses associated with the diagnosis of AIDS are presented in the website box Common Nursing Diagnoses for Clients with HIV and AIDS. Four problems that affect most AIDS clients are described here, in the Case Study feature below, and in the Bridge to Home Health Care website feature on Living with HIV/AIDS.

Assessment. Assessment of clinical manifestations should include both subjective and objective data. All clinical manifestations should be quantified. The easiest way to measure the severity of a clinical manifestation is by asking the client to rate it on a scale from 0 to 10, with 0 being no problem at all and 10 being the worst

possible. This method works well for most manifestations, such as fatigue and pain. Fever assessment can be made easy if the client is willing to keep a fever diary (i.e., recording the temperature whenever it is measured). For clients who have no scale at home, the nurse will have to rely on client self-report to detect trends in weight.

Pain is a subjective experience. The single most reliable indicator of the existence and intensity of acute pain and any related discomfort or distress is the client's self-report. Neither behavior nor vital signs can substitute for self-report. A client may be in excruciating pain even while smiling or laughing in an attempt to cope with it.

Diagnosis, Outcomes, Interventions

Diagnosis: Hyperthermia. An important nursing diagnosis and collaborative problem for a client with AIDS is *Hyperthermia related to hypermetabolic state (secondary to chronic HIV infection), opportunistic infections, dehydration, side effects of medication, malnutrition, and sites for potential organism invasion, such as IV lines or Foley catheters.*

Outcomes. After discussing the assessment findings and the nursing diagnosis, select interventions in concert with the client, care partner, or both to control fever and replace fluid loss.

> **Involving the client in planning care and reducing the risk of infections are two of TJC's National Patient Safety Goals.**

SAFETY

ALERT

Interventions. Because of the underlying immunodeficiency and impaired inflammatory response, clinical manifestations of infection, including fever, may be greatly muted. Nonpharmacologic interventions include keeping the client in a warm room to avoid shivering and applying a sheet and a loosely woven blanket. Avoid fanning the bed covers, exposing skin, or rapidly removing clothing that might cause chilling.

Avoid tepid water sponge bathing, which causes defensive vasoconstriction and has not been shown to be an effective coolant in fever. Sponge baths can cause shivering and can be distressing. Avoid alcohol sponging as well, which also causes vasoconstriction, shivering, and toxic fumes. The alcohol also can be absorbed cutaneously, causing hypoglycemia.

Increase caloric and fluid intake by providing a plan for six feedings distributed over 24 hours and high-protein, high-calorie nutritional supplements, especially if the client has anorexia. Provide 2 to 2.5 L of fluid to drink daily.

Maintain comfort and safety by providing dry clothes and bed linens made out of cotton rather than synthetics. Use emollient creams for dry skin. Monitor mental status frequently, especially when the client has

---

a fever. Evaluate the client's need for assistance with all ADL. Teach the client how to manage chronic recurrent night fever and night sweats by doing the following:

- Take the antipyretic agent of choice before going to sleep.
- Have a change of bedclothes nearby in case a change is necessary.
- Keep a plastic cover on the pillow.
- Place a towel over the pillow in case of profuse diaphoresis.
- Keep liquids at the bedside to drink.

Pharmacologic treatment can include aspirin, nonsteroidal anti-inflammatory drugs (NSAIDs), or acetaminophen. Follow-up should include comparing patterns of use of these agents with laboratory evaluation of hepatic and hematologic abnormalities as well as interactions with other agents.

Diagnosis: Fatigue. Another common nursing diagnosis is *Fatigue related to hypermetabolic state secondary to viral infection, muscular weakness/wasting secondary to AIDS, anemia, dehydration, and psychological and situational factors.* Fatigue is the most common complaint both of clients with AIDS and of their caregivers.

Outcomes. After discussing and validating the findings of assessment and nursing diagnosis, select interventions in concert with the client, care partner, or both to increase self-awareness of fatigue, associated clinical manifestations, environmental factors affecting fatigue, and activity tolerance. Identify interventions to highlight the importance of resting when needed and accepting assistance when needed. Develop a plan for a lifestyle that keeps the client independent, socially active, and involved in activities of daily living.

Interventions. Promote self-care and self-awareness by having the client keep a daily fatigue diary for at least 1 week to identify sources of fatigue, appropriate interventions, and patterns of peak fitness. Advise the client to avoid coffee, tobacco, and alcohol, which may increase fatigue. Promote adequate sleep by increasing the amount of sleep each day. Reduce the amount of sleep-cycle interruptions by preparing for sleep and keeping needed items at the bedside.

Promote rest and activity by developing a written 24-hour schedule of daily activities that alternates short activities with rest periods. Identify activity priorities, such as eating breakfast and then resting before bathing in the morning, as opposed to the reverse. Evaluate the client's needs and point out ways to conserve energy, such as sitting down while dressing, shaving, or preparing food; sitting on a shower chair while bathing; or using disposable items for eating so that no cleanup is needed. Help the client write a plan for rest and activities. Encourage the client to always plan activities ahead of time.

Prepare an exercise schedule (immobilization may lead to decreased endurance and increased fatigue) and plan exercises at peak energy times (after a rest period). Follow the exercises with rest. Aerobic exercise, which increases endurance, can reduce fatigue. Additional natural techniques that may be of benefit include progressive muscle relaxation, acupressure, massage, reflexology, imagery and visualization, autogenic relaxation, reframing and positive affirmations, therapeutic touch, and social support and support groups.

Diagnosis: Imbalanced Nutrition: Less Than Body Requirements. A frequently encountered nursing diagnosis is *Imbalanced Nutrition: Less Than Body Requirements related to increased nutrient requirements and decreased food intake secondary to side effects of medications and infection, such as anorexia, nausea, vomiting, altered taste, impaired swallowing or chewing, diarrhea, fatigue, depression, or impaired cognition.*

Outcomes. After discussing and validating the findings of assessment and the nursing diagnosis, select interventions in concert with the client, care partner, or both to increase food intake, preserve lean body mass, and provide adequate levels of all nutrients.

Interventions

Minimize Anorexia. Minimize factors contributing to anorexia. For *hyperosmia* (increased sense of smell), avoid cooking odors by keeping windows open and the home well aerated. Encourage meals that include cold foods. For *hyposmia* (decreased sense of smell), use spices such as basil, oregano, rosemary, thyme, cloves, mint, cinnamon, or lemon juice to enhance the aroma. For alterations in sense of taste (especially related to distaste for red meat), marinate meat in a commercial marinade, wine, or vinegar before cooking it, and use substitutes for red meat, such as eggs, peanut butter, tofu, cheeses, poultry, and fish.

Prevent Weight Loss. Weight loss can be a significant problem for clients who live alone or who have fatigue or depression. Interventions include the following:

- Eating small meals frequently throughout the day
- Eating high-calorie snacks or commercially prepared supplements (liquids or bars)
- Indulging in favorite foods
- Consuming more nutrient-dense foods and beverages rather than filling up on low-calorie items
- Drinking liquids 30 minutes before eating instead of with meals
- Preparing meals (such as soups or casseroles) ahead of time so they can be divided into individual servings and frozen until ready to use
- Keeping easy-to-prepare foods on hand, such as frozen dinners, canned foods, and eggs

- Encouraging the client to dine with friends or family
- Getting family members and friends involved in meal preparation; the pleasant atmosphere they can provide may stimulate the client's appetite

Many communities have home food delivery service for people with AIDS as well.

Improve Food Intake. Minimize factors related to difficulty in chewing, dysphagia (difficulty in swallowing), or odynophagia (painful swallowing) by advising clients to avoid rough foods, such as (1) raw fruits and vegetables; spicy, acidic, or salty foods; (2) alcohol or tobacco; (3) excessively hot or cold foods; (4) sticky foods, such as peanut butter; and (5) slippery foods, such as gelatin, bologna, and elbow macaroni. Encourage the client to do the following:

- Eat foods at room temperature.
- Choose mild foods and drinks, such as apple juice rather than orange juice.
- Eat dry grain foods (such as breads, crackers, and cookies) after softening them in milk, tea, or another mild beverage.
- Eat nonabrasive foods that are easy to swallow, such as ice cream, pudding, well-cooked eggs, noodle dishes, baked fish, and soft cheese.
- Eat Popsicles (frozen dessert) to numb pain.
- Use a straw when drinking.
- Tilt the head forward or back to make swallowing easier.

Increase the Availability of Food. Minimize factors related to the client's inability to obtain food by evaluating the client's financial resources and the need for referral for Medicaid, food stamps, or other services. Evaluate the client's home and ability to prepare and obtain food. Look for problems such as an absence of cooking facilities and the need for alternative housing arrangements. Explore community resources that provide free meals.

Teach Nutritional Requirements. If the client has no metabolic condition that requires a special diet, the prescribed diet for people with HIV disease should include high-protein, high-calorie, low-fat foods. Help the client plan a 24-hour menu, and review the essential elements of a low-microbe diet and food safety and preparation. Nutritional teaching should follow the client's usual pattern of food intake as much as possible, rather than expecting the client to follow a totally new, unfamiliar prescription for meal planning.

Diagnosis: Acute Pain or Chronic Pain. A common nursing diagnosis is *Acute Pain or Chronic Pain related to arthralgia, myalgia, or neuropathy associated with HIV disease, mass lesions associated with opportunistic infection(s) or cancer, side effects of medications, co-morbid*

disease such as diabetic neuropathy, or interventions such as surgery.

Outcomes. After discussing and validating the findings of assessment, select interventions in concert with the client, care partner, or both to reduce the incidence and severity of pain, communicate effectively about pain experiences, and enhance comfort and satisfaction.

Interventions

Provide Comfort Measures. Help the client and/or care partner identify activities that increase pain. Provide comfort measures such as using a pressure-relieving mattress, positioning and supporting limbs comfortably when in bed or a chair, and using a "pull sheet" to move clients or help them change positions. For institutionalized clients, encourage family members or significant others to bring in familiar objects that will provide physical and/or emotional comfort. Encourage the client to groom as usual, including using make-up or after-shave lotion, to help maintain a sense of normalcy and dignity during illness.

Provide Physical Therapy. Physical therapy can be very helpful in managing pain. The physical therapist can provide the following:

- Exercise to maintain or increase physical activity levels and endurance
- Ultrasound and physical treatments, such as application of heat or cold, to reduce musculoskeletal pain
- Therapeutic massage
- Instruction and supervision in using a transcutaneous electrical nerve stimulation (TENS) device, commonly called a TENS unit

Administer Pain Medications. Pharmacologic treatments usually include (1) *non-opioid analgesics,* such as aspirin or acetaminophen for mild pain; (2) *weak opioids,* such as codeine and oxycodone for moderate pain; and (3) *strong opioids,* such as morphine for severe pain. For neuropathic pain (such as HIV-associated polyneuropathy, acute and postherpetic neuralgia, and nucleoside toxicity with some antiretroviral medications), adjuvants such as ibuprofen may be used as well as amitriptyline, desipramine, nortriptyline, doxepin, carbamazepine, divalproex, phenytoin, gabapentin, or mexiletine. Primary care providers should anticipate several changes in prescriptions for analgesics when starting the client on a pain-control regimen. A major error in initial pain management occurs when a clinician prescribes a 2-week supply of an analgesic, assumes that the prescription works, and has no further contact until the client returns 2 weeks later for follow-up. On the contrary, during the initial phase of pain control, the clinician should have daily contact with the client, even if by telephone, and should anticipate schedule changes. Dosage frequency should be adjusted to prevent pain from recurring once the duration of analgesic action is determined. Similarly, it is a waste of money to prescribe large amounts of an analgesic, such as a 30-day supply, knowing that the orders will change. Orders for opioid analgesics should include "rescue" doses for break-through pain when regularly scheduled doses are insufficient.

Orders for analgesics as needed result in delays in administration and intervals of inadequate pain control. Tell clients and their care partners that the client may sleep for extended periods and may appear very drowsy during the first few days of a pain control regimen. Although this may result in part from the initial effects of the drug, it probably also reflects exhaustion and the need for rest as a result of sleep deprivation caused by pain. This situation usually reverses itself within a few days after a scheduled pain management regimen is begun.

Clients may refuse an analgesic if they are not in pain or may forgo it when they are asleep. Explain that this decision may lower blood analgesia levels and cause a resurgence of pain and failure of the pain control plan. Although the anti-inflammatory effects of aspirin are highly effective as an analgesic adjuvant, because aspirin inhibits platelet function, it may be contraindicated if the client has a low platelet count.

Injecting drug users will experience pain as any other client would. Do not deny this client pain medication. Helpful guidelines for managing pain in these clients include (1) having a single practitioner prescribe medications, (2) refusing to refill lost prescriptions, (3) carefully rationing opioid prescriptions, and (4) limiting rescue doses of opioid analgesics on a monthly basis. Clients who are being treated with methadone maintenance for drug addiction probably will require higher and more frequent doses of analgesia than an opioid-naive client would. Some antiretroviral drugs, such as nevirapine and ritonavir, interfere with the half-life of methadone and may decrease its blood levels. The client will experience mild withdrawal manifestations. Increasing the daily dose of methadone usually resolves the problem.

Because diarrhea is common in clients with HIV disease, especially when protease inhibitors are prescribed, the constipating effects of analgesics may actually be beneficial. Evaluate each client's response to therapy instead of automatically using stool softeners when initiating the pain control plan.

Encourage Complementary Therapies. Complementary therapies that may be used include cognitive-behavioral interventions, such as education and instruction in pain control, relaxation exercises, imagery, music distraction, biofeedback, and therapeutic touch.

Evaluation. It is expected that the client will maintain or increase weight. It is expected that the client, care partner, or both will (1) identify factors related to anorexia, difficulty in chewing, dysphagia, or odynophagia; (2) identify sufficient resources to obtain and prepare food or make use of social work interventions employed to obtain food stamps or public assistance; (3) identify ways to increase protein and calorie intake; (4) identify key concepts in planning a low-microbial diet; and (5) select a balanced 24-hour menu. The client's weight will fluctuate during the course of HIV disease related to new disease processes and the side effects of prescribed medications.

It is expected that the client, care partner, or both will be able to (1) identify appropriate measures to take for a fever, (2) initiate and maintain adequate hydration and nutrition, and (3) demonstrate the ability to take and record the client's temperature accurately. Although infection-related fever can be controlled with appropriate antibiotic therapy, this problem can be expected to recur throughout the illness.

It is expected that the client, care partner, or both will be able to (1) identify causative factors that increase fatigue, (2) plan a schedule of paced activity for a 24-hour period, (3) demonstrate the ability to participate in a program of exercise, and (4) verbalize a decrease in the client's fatigue for a 24-hour period. Fatigue is a manifestation that can be expected to recur throughout HIV disease, especially because it is a side effect of some antiretroviral medications.

It is expected that the client, care partner, or both will (1) identify aggravating factors or precipitating factors related to the pain experienced, (2) identify measures to control pain, and (3) verbalize a decrease in the amount and type of pain experienced over 24 hours. Pain may be either chronic or acute, depending on the cause. In most instances, it can be managed effectively, as with any client with another diagnosis.

CONCLUSIONS

Human immunodeficiency virus is a major threat to human health worldwide. The nature of care is very complex, and the client's clinical needs are numerous. At one time or another, almost all nurses will care for a person with HIV infection or AIDS. To provide adequate care for a person with HIV infection, understanding the illness trajectory and the therapeutic interventions needed to maintain health will result in the ability to provide high-level care.

THINKING CRITICALLY

1. A 30-year-old woman presents with fever, fatigue, lymphadenopathy, thrush, diarrhea, and pain in her muscles and joints. She has

a rash on her torso and arms. What questions would you ask to determine her possible exposure to HIV? How will the client be evaluated and treated?

Factors to Consider. What tests confirm the diagnosis of AIDS? How is the CD4$^+$ cell count used? What is the purpose of the viral load test? What treatment should be used?

2. You are working in a homeless shelter and are scheduled to present a 20-minute program on AIDS prevention. A small class of four men and three women has gathered. They are all known to you, and you suspect that one couple may be infected with HIV. What should you plan to teach?

Factors to Consider. What main areas of HIV education should be addressed? What is an effective method of communicating this information?

3. Your HIV-infected female client leaves the physician's office and comes over to you and says, "I don't have HIV anymore. The doctor just told me that my viral load was undetectable." How would you respond?

Factors to Consider. What does an undetectable viral load test result mean? What would you tell this client about safer sex practices and becoming pregnant?

4. Your 40-year-old male client with AIDS and *P. carinii* pneumonia is about to be discharged from the hospital. His CD4$^+$ cell count is 35/mm^3. He asks you what he should do now. What teaching would you provide?

Factors to Consider. When does a person with HIV infection get an AIDS diagnosis? Does this client need any medication for his pneumonia? Given the fact that the CD4$^+$ cell count is 35/mm^3, does he need any medication to prevent any other opportunistic infections?

Discussions for these questions can be found on the website.

BIBLIOGRAPHY

🔥 Citations appearing in red refer to primary research.

🔥 Citations appearing in blue refer to evidence-based practice guidelines and protocols.

1. CNN.com. (2006). *CDC wants HIV test for everyone.* Available at www.cnn.com/2006/HEALTH/conditions/05/09/hiv.testing.ap/index. html
2. Barroso, J. (2002). HIV-related fatigue. *American Journal of Nursing, 102*(5), 83-86.
3. Centers for Disease Control and Prevention (CDC). (2006). A glance at the HIV/AIDS epidemic. Washington, DC: Author.
4. CDC. (2006). Revised recommendations for HIV testing of adults, adolescents, and pregnant women in health care settings. *Morbidity and Mortality Weekly Report, 55*(RR14), 1-17.
5. CDC. (2006). Rapid HIV test distribution—United States—2003-2005. *Morbidity and Mortality Weekly Report, 55*(24), 673-676.
6. CDC. (2006). *Twenty five years of HIV/AIDS—United States, 1981-2006.* Washington, DC: Author.
7. CDC. (2003). *Surveillance of healthcare personnel with HIV/AIDS as of December 2002.* Available at www.cdc.gov/ncidod/dhqp/bp_hiv_hp_with.html.

8. CDC. (1992). 1993 Revised classification system for HIV infection and expanded surveillance case definition for AIDS among adolescents and adults. *Morbidity and Mortality Weekly Report, 41* (RR-17), 1-19.
9. Charland, M.B. (2003). Management of adverse effects associated with the use of Interleukin-2 in patients with HIV infection. *Journal of the Association of Nurses in AIDS Care, 14*(6), 89-95.
10. Cibulka, N. (2006). Mother-to-child transmission of HIV in the United States. *American Journal of Nursing, 106*(7), 56-64.
11. Conrad, A. (2003). Interleukin-2: Where are we going? *Journal of the Association of Nurses in AIDS Care, 14*(6), 83-88.
12. Coyne-Meyers, K., & Trombley, L.E. (2004). A review of nutrition in human immunodeficiency virus infection in the era of highly active antiretroviral therapy. *Nutrition in Clinical Practice, 19* (8), 340-355.
13. Covington, L.W. (2005). Update on antiviral agents for HIV and AIDS. *Nursing Clinics of North America, 40*(1), 149-165.
14. Demmer, C. (2001). Dealing with AIDS-related loss and grief in a time of treatment advances. *American Journal of Hospice & Palliative Care, 18*(1), 35-41.
15. Foy, K., Bradley-Springer, L., Kempner, T., et al. (2005). Enfuvirtide nursing guidelines: A report from the Association of Nurses in AIDS Care Expert Panel on enfuvirtide. *Journal of the Association of Nurses in AIDS Care, 16*(2), 2-12.
16. Foy, K., & Juethner, S.N. (2004). Enfuvirtide (T-20): Potentials and challenges. *Journal of the Association of Nurses in AIDS Care, 15* (6), 65-71.
17. Garcia, P.R., & Cote, J.K. (2003). Factors affecting adherence to antiretroviral therapy in people living with HIV/AIDS. *Journal of the Association of Nurses in AIDS Care, 14*(4), 37-45.
18. Glutzer, E., & Lalezari, J.P. (2005). Enfuvirtide for nurses: Answering patient questions on activity, safety, and lifestyle impact. *Journal of the Association of Nurses in AIDS Care, 16*(5), 26-34.
19. Gostin, L.O. (2000). A proposed national policy on health care workers living with HIV/AIDS and other blood-borne pathogens. *Journal of the American Medical Association, 284*, 1965-1969.
20. Jaspan, H.B., & Garry, R.F. (2003). Preventing neonatal HIV: A review. *Current HIV Research, 1*, 321-327.
21. Kaiser Family Foundation. (2006). *HIV/AIDS policy fact sheet.* Washington, DC: Author.
22. Kaiser Family Foundation. (2006). *Survey of Americans on HIV/AIDS.* Washington, DC: Author.
23. Kenny, P.E. (2004). The changing face of AIDS. *Nursing 2004, 34* (8), 56-63.
24. Kirton, C.A., Talotta, D., & Zwolski, K. (2001). *Handbook of HIV/AIDS nursing.* St. Louis: Mosby.
25. Kotler, D.P. (2004). The biology of human immunodeficiency virus infection. *Nutrition in Clinical Practice, 19*, 324-329.
26. Manen, L.V., Laschinger, S.J., Stevenson, T., et al. (2005). The nature of multidisciplinary care in the ambulatory setting: A synthesis of the literature. *Journal of the Association of Nurses in AIDS Care, 16*(5), 49-57.
27. Matthews, W.C., Mar-Tang, M., Ballard, C., et al. (2002). Prevalence, predictors, and outcomes of early adherence after starting or changing antiretroviral therapy. *AIDS Patient Care and STDs, 16*(4), 157-172.
27a. McLean, J., Murray, C., Schreibman, F., & Rigsby, M. (2007). *Pneumocystis (carinii) jiroveci pneumonia.* Available at www.emedicine.com/med/topic1850.htm.
28. Moyle, G. (2002). Overcoming obstacles to the success of protease inhibitors in highly active antiretroviral therapy regimens. *AIDS Patient Care and STDs, 16*, 585-597.
29. Murphy, D.A., Lu, M.C., Martin, D., et al. (2002). Results of a pilot intervention trial to improve antiretroviral adherence among HIV-positive patients. *Journal of the Association of Nurses in AIDS Care, 13*(6), 57-69.
30. Nolan, M.L., Greenberg, A.E., & Fowler, M.G. (2002). A review of clinical trials to prevent mother-to-child HIV-1 transmission in Africa and inform rational intervention strategies. *AIDS, 16*, 1991-1999.
31. Peiperl, L. (2002). What are the causes of severe illness and death in individuals being treated for HIV? *HIV InSite.* Available at http://hivinsite.ucsf.edu/InSite?page=cf9croi02&ss=xsl/doc.

32. Piliero, P.J., & Colagreco, J.P. (2003). Simplified regimens for treating HIV infection and AIDS. *Journal of the American Academy of Nurse Practitioners, 15*, 305-312.

33. Powderly, W.G. (2002). Long-term exposure to lifelong therapies. *Journal of Acquired Immune Deficiency and Human Retrovirology, 29*(Suppl 1), S28-S40.

34. Raines, C., Radcliffe, O., & Treisman, G.J. (2005). Neurologic and psychiatric complications of antiretroviral agents. *Journal of the Association of Nurses in AIDS Care, 16*(5), 35-48.

35. Russel, J., Krantz, S., & Neville, S. (2004). The patient-provider relationship and adherence to highly active antiretroviral therapy. *Journal of the Association of Nurses in AIDS Care, 15*(5), 40-47.

36. Scarlotti, G. (2004). Mother-to-child transmission of HIV-1: Advances and controversies of the twentieth century. *AIDS Reviews, 6*, 67-78.

37. Sepkowitz, K.A., & Eisenberg, L. (2005). Occupational deaths among healthcare workers. *Emerging Infectious Diseases, 11*, 1003-1008.

38. Sobieszcyyk, M.E., Jones, J., Wilkin, T. & Hammer, S.M. (2006). Advances in antiretroviral therapy. *Topics in HIV Medicine, 14*(1), 1-42.

38a. The Joint Commission. (2008). *2008 National Patient Safety Goals Hospital Program*. Available at www.jointcommission.org/Patient Safety/NationalPatientSafetyGoals.

39. Young, T.P. (2003). Immune mechanisms in HIV infection. *Journal of the Association of Nurses in AIDS Care, 14*(6), 71-75.

40. UNIADS. (2006). *Report on the global AIDS epidemic: Executive summary*. Geneva, Switzerland: Author.

41. Verheggen, R. (2003). Immune restoration in patients with HIV infection: HAART and beyond. *Journal of the Association of Nurses in AIDS Care, 14*(6), 76-82.

42. Villarreal, H., & Fogg, C. (2006). Syringe-exchange programs and HIV prevention. *American Journal of Nursing, 106*(5), 58-64.

43. Wolf, S.A. (2004, Oct). State of AIDS care 2004: One world, multiple standards. *IAPAC Monthly*, 374-388.

44. World Health Organization. (2002). *AIDS epidemic update*. Available at www.unaids.org/worldaidsday/2002/press/update/epiupdate2002_en.doc.

45. Yenni, P.G., Hammer, S.M., Hirsch, M.S., et al. (2004). Treatment for adult HIV infection: 2004 recommendations of the International AIDS Society—USA Panel. *Journal of the American Medical Association, 292*, 251-265.

evolve   *Did you remember to check out the bonus material on the Evolve website and the CD-ROM, including NCLEX®-Examination Style Review Questions, Open-Book Quizzes, and Chapter Review Audio Podcasts?*

http://evolve.elsevier.com/Black/medsurg

CHAPTER 79

Management of Clients with Leukemia and Lymphoma

SUSAN NEWTON

Cancers of the hematopoietic system are disorders that result from the proliferation of malignant cells originating in the bone marrow, thymus, and lymphatic tissue. Blood cells that originate in bone marrow are called *hematopoietic cells;* cells that originate in the lymph are called *lymphoid cells. Leukemia* is cancer of the bone marrow, and *lymphoma* is cancer of the lymphoid tissue.

LEUKEMIA

Leukemia is a malignant disease of the blood-forming organs. The American Cancer Society estimated that in 2007 about 44,240 new cases of leukemia would be diagnosed, and about 21,790 deaths would be attributed to the disease.[2] Leukemia is the most common malignancy in children and young adults. Half of all leukemias are classified as *acute,* with rapid onset and progression of disease resulting in 100% mortality within days to months without appropriate therapy. The remaining leukemias, classified as *chronic,* have a more indolent course. In children 80% of leukemias are lymphocytic and 20% are nonlymphocytic. In adults the percentages are reversed, with 80% nonlymphocytic.

Etiology and Risk Factors

Although the cause of leukemia is unknown, several risk factors are associated with leukemia, including (1) genetic factors, (2) exposure to ionizing radiation and chemicals, (3) congenital abnormalities (e.g., Down syndrome), and (4) the presence of primary immunodeficiency and infection with the human T-cell leukemia virus type 1 (HTLV-1). Genetic factors increase the risk of leukemia. A high incidence of acute leukemias and *chronic lymphocytic leukemia* (CLL) is reported in certain families. Hereditary abnormalities associated with an increased incidence of leukemia are Down syndrome, Fanconi's aplastic anemia, Bloom syndrome, ataxia telangiectasia, trisomy 13

(Patau's syndrome), Wiskott-Aldrich syndrome, and congenital X-linked agammaglobulinemia. Identical twins, fraternal twins, and siblings of children with leukemia are also at increased risk. In *chronic myelogenous leukemia* (CML), more than 90% of clients have the Philadelphia chromosome, an abnormal chromosome (see Chronic Leukemia later in this chapter).

Overexposure to ionizing radiation is a major risk factor for development of leukemia, with the disease developing years after the initial exposure. Alkylating agents used to treat other cancers, especially in combination with radiation therapy, increase a person's risk of leukemia. Workers exposed to chemical agents, such as benzene (an aromatic hydrocarbon), are at a much higher risk.

Causal risk factors acting together with a genetic predisposition can alter nuclear deoxyribonucleic acid (DNA). The leukemic cell is then unable to mature and respond to normal regulatory mechanisms. Abnormal chromosomes are reported in 40% to 50% of clients with acute leukemia, and certain chromosomes are repeatedly more involved than others. A mutation in a single cell appears to give rise to some leukemias.

Pathophysiology

In normal bone marrow, efficient regulation ensures that cell proliferation and maturation are adequate to meet a person's needs. Pluripotent stem cells commit to differentiate along the myeloid, erythroid, or lymphoid pathway in the presence of growth factors. In leukemia, control is missing or abnormal. Leukemia is an uncontrolled proliferation of leukocytes. This lack of control

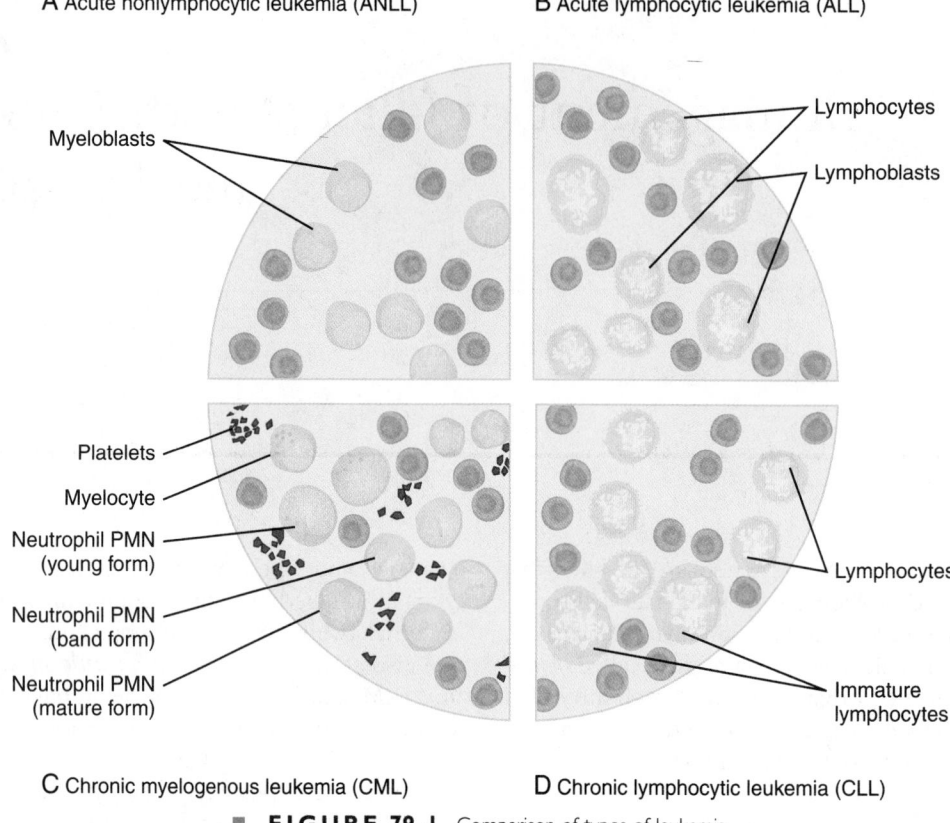

A Acute nonlymphocytic leukemia (ANLL)

B Acute lymphocytic leukemia (ALL)

Myeloblasts

Lymphocytes

Lymphoblasts

Platelets
Myelocyte
Neutrophil PMN
(young form)
Neutrophil PMN
(band form)
Neutrophil PMN
(mature form)

Lymphocytes

Immature
lymphocytes

C Chronic myelogenous leukemia (CML)

D Chronic lymphocytic leukemia (CLL)

■ **FIGURE 79–I** Comparison of types of leukemia.

causes normal bone marrow to be replaced by immature and undifferentiated leukocytes, or *blast cells* (Figure 79-1). Abnormal, immature leukocytes then circulate in the blood and infiltrate the blood-forming organs (liver, spleen, lymph nodes) and other sites throughout the body.

The French-American-British (FAB) Cooperative Group developed a classification system that is universally accepted. Under this system, acute leukemias are classified on the basis of morphologic characteristics and histochemical staining of blast cells, which indicates the percentage of immature cells in the bone marrow (Table 79-1).

Acute Leukemia

Acute leukemia is caused by a block in the differentiation of cells in the hematopoietic cell line. The result is a massive accumulation of immature, nonfunctional cells or blasts in the bone marrow or in other organs. *Acute lymphoblastic leukemia* (ALL) is most common in children (median age, 10 years). *Acute nonlymphocytic leukemia* (ANLL), also referred to as *acute myeloid leukemia* (AML), is more common in adults (median age, 65 years). Leukemias are considered clonal disorders in that a single cell undergoes transformation, and leukemic cells then proliferate. An interesting paradox is that leukemic cells apparently

TABLE 79–I French-American-British (FAB) Classification of Acute Leukemia

Acute Lymphocytic Leukemia

L1 Common childhood leukemia
L2 Adult acute lymphocytic leukemia
L3 Rare subtype, blasts resembling those in Burkitt's lymphoma

Acute Myeloblastic Leukemia

Granulocytic

M1 Myeloblastic leukemia without maturation
M2 Myeloblastic leukemia with maturation
M3 Hypergranular promyelocytic leukemia

Monocytic

M4 Myelomonocytic leukemia
M5 Monocytic

Erythroid

M6 Erythroleukemia

divide more slowly and take longer to synthesize DNA than do other blood precursors. Acute leukemia is not caused by rapid cellular proliferation but instead is caused by the blocking of blood cell precursors. Leukemic cells accumulate relentlessly in most affected individuals, and they compete with normal cellular proliferation. Acute leukemia has also been termed an *accumulation disorder* and *proliferation disorder.*

The development of leukemia occurs in the most primitive blood precursors, pluripotent stem cells, which give rise to all other blood cells (see the Unit 17 Anatomy and Physiology Review). The leukemia blasts, or precursor cells, literally "crowd out" the marrow and cause cellular proliferation of the other cell lines to cease. Normal granulocytic, monocytic, lymphocytic, erythrocytic, and megakaryocytic stem cells cease to function, causing *pancytopenia* (a reduction in all cellular components of the blood). Transformation also may occur, most often in the granulocyte-monocyte series, but transformation could also occur in the erythrocyte series.

Chronic Leukemia

Chronic leukemias are caused by unregulated proliferation of hematopoietic cells or disordered cell death *(apoptosis).* Chronic leukemia is classified as CML or CLL. CML originates in the pluripotent stem cell. Initially the marrow is hypercellular with most cells normal. Typically the peripheral blood smear reveals leukocytosis and thrombocytosis with an increased production of granulocytes. In 90% of cases examination of the bone marrow cells during metaphase shows a translocation of the long arms of chromosomes 9 and 22, called the *Philadelphia chromosome.* After a relatively slow course for a median period of 3 to 4 years, the client with CML invariably enters a *blast crisis* that resembles acute leukemia.

Blast crisis results in the death of more than 70% of clients with CML. During this phase increasing numbers of *blasts* (immature myeloid precursor cells, especially *myeloblasts,* the most primitive granulocyte precursors) proliferate in the blood and bone marrow. In blast crisis the blasts and *promyelocytes* (another myeloid cell precursor type) exceed 20% in the blood and 30% in the marrow. Increased fibrotic tissue in the marrow is another manifestation of blast crisis. Leukopenia, thrombocytopenia, and anemia also are evident. Without treatment death usually occurs within 6 months of onset of the blast crisis.

Chronic lymphocytic leukemia, which is characterized by the proliferation of early B lymphocytes, is an indolent leukemia that is seen most often in men older than 50 years of age. It is usually discovered when the complete blood count (CBC) is performed as part of a routine physical examination. A peripheral blood smear reveals increased numbers of mature and slightly immature lymphocytes. As the disease progresses, lymphocytes infiltrate the lymph nodes, liver, spleen, and ultimately the bone marrow. A staging system is based on the extent of lymphocyte infiltration. Progression of the disease may take up to 15 years, during which the client may not require therapy.

Clinical Manifestations

The manifestations of all types of leukemia are similar. The clinical history usually reveals anemia, thrombocytopenia, and leukopenia.

Clinical manifestations of bone marrow depression include fatigue caused by anemia, bleeding resulting from thrombocytopenia (reduced numbers of circulating platelets), fever caused by infection, anorexia, headaches, and papilledema. Bleeding can occur in the skin, gums, mucous membranes, and gastrointestinal (GI) and genitourinary tracts. Bleeding also is the underlying cause of petechiae and *ecchymosis* (discoloration visible through the skin).

Anorexia is associated with weight loss, diminished sensitivity to sour and sweet tastes, wasting away of muscle, and difficulty swallowing. Liver, spleen, and lymph node enlargement are more common in ALL than in ANLL. Splenomegaly and hepatomegaly usually occur together. The client with leukemia commonly experiences abdominal pain with tenderness and breast tenderness.

Headache, vomiting, and papilledema are associated with central nervous system (CNS) involvement. Facial nerve involvement causes facial palsy. Blurred vision, auditory disturbances, and meningeal irritation can occur if leukemic cells infiltrate the cerebral or spinal meninges. Intracranial hemorrhage and compression also can occur (Figure 79-2).

Complete Blood Cell Count

Complete blood cell count values vary greatly. The total white blood cell (WBC) count may be normal, abnormally low ($<1000/\text{mm}^3$), or extremely high ($>200,000/\text{mm}^3$). The differential may reveal that one type of leukocyte is overwhelmingly predominant. Abnormal leukocytes, including immature blast forms, may be noted on the peripheral smear. The platelet count and hemoglobin level usually are low.

Bone Marrow Aspiration

Bone marrow aspiration or biopsy is a key diagnostic tool for confirming the diagnosis and identifying the malignant cell type. Typical findings in the bone marrow aspirate and biopsy are an overall increase in the number of marrow cells and an increase in the proportion of earlier forms, suggesting immature cells.

Other Findings

Lumbar puncture determines the presence of blast cells in the CNS; 5% of clients have this abnormality at diagnosis. Lumbar puncture is rarely if ever performed during the acute phase of leukemia secondary to an increased risk of iatrogenic introduction of blast cells into the CNS. It is usually performed post-induction, especially in clients with ALL. Radiography of the chest

Severe infections (pneumonia, septicemia), ulcerations of the mouth and throat

Cause: High numbers of immature or abnormal leukocytes are unable to fight and destroy microorganisms

Headache, disorientation

Cause: Abnormal white cells infiltrating the central nervous system

Anemia accompanied by pallor, fatigue, malaise, hypoxia, and hemorrhage (gum bleeding, ecchymoses, petechiae, retinal hemorrhage)

Cause: Rapidly proliferating development of leukocytes inhibiting erythrocytes and thrombocytes

Enlarged organs (splenomegaly, hepatomegaly) exerting pressure on adjacent organs

Cause: High numbers of white cells accumulating within the liver and spleen, causing distention of tissues

Increased metabolic rate accompanied by weakness, pallor, and weight loss

Cause: Increased leukocyte production requiring large amounts of nutrients; cell destruction increases the amount of metabolic wastes

Hyperuricemia causing renal pain, obstruction (from stone formation), and infection; a late development is renal insufficiency with uremia

Cause: Large amounts of uric acid released as a result of destruction of great numbers of leukocytes; in late stages, abnormal leukocytes infiltrate the kidneys

Lymphadenopathy and bone pain

Cause: Excessive numbers of white cells accumulating in lymph nodes and bone marrow

■ **FIGURE 79–2** Clinical manifestations and pathophysiologic bases of leukemia.

and skeleton and magnetic resonance imaging (MRI) and computed tomography (CT) scans of the head and body detect lesions and sites of infection. Lymphangiography or lymph node biopsy may be performed to locate malignant lesions and classify the disease accurately.

OUTCOME MANAGEMENT

The treatment goals of all classifications of leukemia are targeted at destroying neoplastic cells and maintaining a sustained remission. During each phase of therapy, the medical treatment may vary, but the basic nursing principles are the same.

Medical Management

Acute Leukemia

The treatment plan for acute leukemia is determined by disease classification, the presence or absence of prognostic factors, and disease progression. The goal of treatment is complete remission with restoration of normal bone marrow function; this means a level of blast cells in the marrow less than 5%. About 70% to 80% of adults with ALL achieve complete remission, with 35% to 45% surviving 2 years. The cure rate remains low without bone marrow transplantation (BMT); however, of adults with ANLL, 60% to 70% achieve complete remission, and about 25% survive 5 years or longer.

Destruction of Neoplastic Cells

Chemotherapy. Chemotherapy is given to destroy the malignant cells of the bone marrow. The treatment protocol for acute leukemia may involve up to three phases: the induction phase, consolidation phase, and maintenance phase. The maintenance phase is usually only used in adult ALL. The three phases of the treatment protocol are as follows:

1. *Induction phase.* The client receives an intensive course of chemotherapy designed to induce complete remission. The usual criteria for complete

remission are blast cells less than 5% of the bone marrow cells and normal peripheral blood counts. Both conditions must be sustained for at least 1 month. Once remission is achieved, the consolidation phase begins.

2. *Consolidation phase.* Modified courses of intensive chemotherapy are given to eradicate any remaining disease. Usually a higher dose of one or more chemotherapeutic agents is administered.

3. *Maintenance phase.* Small doses of different combinations of chemotherapeutic agents are given every 3 to 4 weeks. This phase may continue for a year or longer and is structured to allow the client to live as normal a life as possible. This phase is used more commonly with ALL.

Radiation Therapy. Radiation therapy may be administered as an adjunct to chemotherapy when leukemic cells infiltrate the CNS, skin, rectum, and testes or when a large mediastinal mass is noted at diagnosis (as may occur in ALL).

Targeted Therapy. When AML relapses, treatment options are limited because of the associated toxicities and the health status of the client. Targeted therapies affect only the tumor cells and spare normal cells, hence decreasing the associated toxicities. Gemtuzumab ozogamicin (Mylotarg) is an anti-CD33 monoclonal antibody linked to calicheamicin, which is a potent cytotoxic agent. CD33 antigens are found on the surface of leukemic blast cells and myeloid precursors. This agent is approved for the treatment of CD33-positive AML in clients with first relapse who are 60 or older and who are not candidates for cytotoxic chemotherapy.

Treat or Prevent Tumor Lysis Syndrome. A potentially fatal complication resulting from the treatment of acute leukemia, *tumor lysis syndrome* is a group of metabolic complications associated with the rapid destruction of a large number of WBCs. If the WBC count is high when chemotherapy is initiated, rapid cell lysis can lead to (1) increased serum uric acid, phosphate, and potassium levels and (2) decreased serum calcium levels. Manifestations include confusion, weakness, bradycardia, electrocardiographic (ECG) changes, and dysrhythmias (hyperkalemia); numbness, tingling, muscle cramps, seizures, tetany, and ECG changes (hypocalcemia); and uric acid crystalluria, renal obstruction, and acute renal failure (hyperuricemia). Acute tumor lysis syndrome can be prevented by increasing intravenous (IV) hydration, alkalizing the urine, and administering allopurinol (Zyloprim). Rasburicase (Elitek) is a drug administered once a day for 5 days intravenously in pediatric clients with cancer to lower plasma uric acid concentrations and manage tumor lysis syndrome (TLS). This drug is also frequently given as a single larger dose in adult clients.[8] Often hemodialysis is necessary to decrease creatinine levels or leukapheresis is necessary to reduce the WBC count.

Replace Cells and Control Infection. Current treatment modalities for acute leukemia destroy normal and aberrant cells. Therapy is aimed at preventing and resolving the complications of acquired and induced pancytopenia: anemia, bleeding, and infection. Transfusions of red blood cells (RBCs) may be required until the marrow produces mature cells. All blood products should be human leukocyte antigen (HLA) matched, cytomegalovirus (CMV) negative, and irradiated. If the client requires IV infusions of RBCs and amphotericin B, an antifungal agent, they should be separated by at least 1 hour so that adverse (e.g., allergic) reactions can be detected.

Chronic Myelogenous Leukemia

Treatment of CML is usually divided into four areas: (1) stem cell transplantation (discussed later in this chapter), (2) interferon alfa therapy with or without chemotherapy, (3) single-agent chemotherapy (hydroxyurea), or (4) the use of specific tyrosine kinase inhibitors.

The goal of therapy in the chronic phase of CML is to control leukocytosis and thrombocytosis. When unwanted cells accumulate, apheresis is a method of blood collection in which blood is withdrawn from the client. The unwanted component is separated, and the remainder of the blood is returned to the client. *Apheresis* is usually performed with use of automated blood cell separators designed to remove selectively the desired blood element. *Leukapheresis* may be performed to lower an extremely high leukocyte count quickly and to prevent acute tumor lysis syndrome (Figure 79-3).

Leukapheresis is rarely performed in CML, however, unless peripheral blast count rises above $300,000/mm^3$ and the client is exhibiting abnormal clinical manifestations such as leukostasis. Leukapheresis can lower WBC counts rapidly and safely in clients with WBC counts greater than $300,000/mm^3$ and can alleviate acute manifestations of leukostasis, hyperviscosity, and tissue infiltration. This reduction is usually only temporary and often must be combined with chemotherapy and/or targeted therapy for more lasting effects. If painful splenomegaly develops, irradiating or removing the spleen may be recommended; however, splenectomy is considered an avenue of last resort secondary to high surgical mortality in this population.

The most widely used medications used to be interferon alfa administered IV or subcutaneously and hydroxyurea administered orally (PO). Clients with a

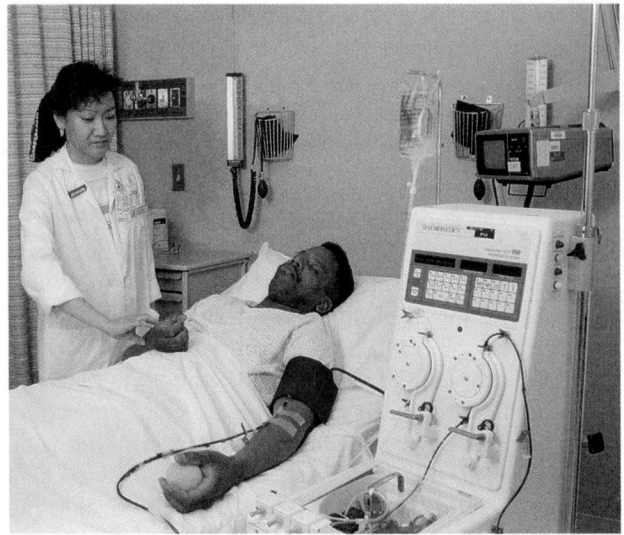

■ **FIGURE 79–3** The white blood cell (WBC) level can be temporarily lowered by leukapheresis. Several automated blood cell separators effectively remove large numbers of WBCs and return red blood cells and plasma to the client. The Haemonetics V50 cell separator is commonly used to perform this procedure.

leukemic cells in CML that are positive for the Philadelphia chromosome. 🪔 Data demonstrate 89% overall survival in after five years in patients that received imatinib as initial treatment for CML.

Dasatinib (Sprycel) is a newer drug in the class of tyrosine kinase inhibitors that often works to treat CML in clients when imatinib does not. While still in the class of tyrosine kinase inhibitors, dasatinib has the ability to bind to both the active and inactive conformation of the ABL kinase domain. Dasatinib is indicated for the treatment of adults with chronic, accelerated, or myeloid or lymphoid blast phase CML with resistance or intolerance to prior therapy including imatinib. It is also indicated for the treatment of adults with Ph+ ALL leukemia with resistance or intolerance to prior therapy.

The most recent kinase inhibitor was granted accelerated approval by the FDA in late 2007 is Nilotinib (Tasigna). This oral agent is indicated for use in the treatment of chronic phase (CP) and accelerated phase (AP) Philadelphia chromosome positive chronic myelogenous leukemia (CML) in adult patients resistant or intolerant to prior therapy that included imatinib.

blast crisis (Figure 79-4) require intensive chemotherapy with the same agents as used in acute leukemia. These drugs can destroy leukemic blast cells, transform them into normal granulocytes, or prevent leukemic cells from inhibiting formation of normal granulocytes. 🪔 Fortunately, the tyrosine kinase inhibitors have transformed the treatment of CML and are the standard of care today.

Targeted Therapy. 🪔 The class of tyrosine kinase inhibitors have revolutionized the treatment of CML. Imatinib mesylate (Gleevec) inhibits proliferation and induces apoptosis by inhibiting tyrosine kinase activity in cells positive for *bcr-abl*. This agent also targets new

Chronic Lymphocytic Leukemia

The goal of therapy in CLL is palliation or control of undesired manifestations. Local radiation to the spleen may be given as a palliative treatment to reduce complications. Two complications seen during the later stages are hemolytic anemia resulting from autoimmune disorder and hypogammaglobulinemia, which further increases susceptibility to infection. Antibiotics, transfusions of RBCs, and injections of gamma-globulin concentrates may be required for these clients. Leukapheresis is performed when the WBCs are enough to cause vascular thrombosis or embolism, especially in clients who are unresponsive to chemotherapy.

■ **FIGURE 79–4 A,** Microscopic view of a normal bone marrow specimen showing a normal distribution of blood cell types and fatty spaces. Blast cells appear as round, dark gray circles. **B,** During blast crisis the number of blast cells increases and fatty spaces shrink.

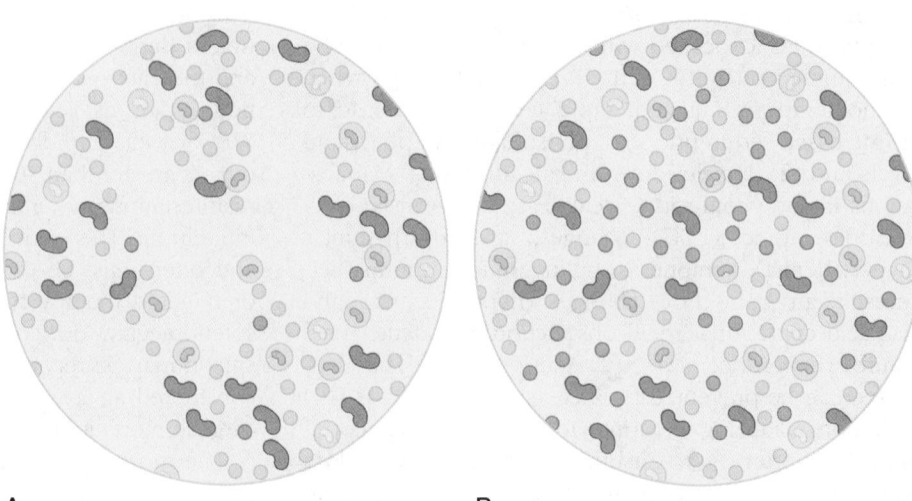

A   B

Chemotherapy. Chlorambucil (Leukeran) or cyclophosphamide (Cytoxan) may be given orally to reduce the manifestations of CLL. Chemotherapy generally is given for 2 weeks of every month. When anemia (stage III) and thrombocytopenia (stage IV) develop, daily oral prednisone is given as an adjunct to the alkylating agents. Prednisone has a marked lymphocytolytic effect and may stimulate the production of RBCs and platelets. Fludarabine (Fludara), classified as a nucleoside analog, is another chemotherapeutic agent that is used in treating CLL.

Targeted Therapy. Targeted therapies are now being used in the treatment of CLL. Alemtuzumab (Campath) is a monoclonal antibody approved by the FDA for the treatment of CLL in clients who have been treated with alkylating agents and for whom fludarabine therapy has not been successful. This agent is directed at the CD52 antigen of the lymphocytes, which slows their proliferation. Rituximab (Rituxan), which targets the CD20 antigen, also is effective as a second-line or third-line treatment and is frequently used in combination with IV Cytoxan and Fludarabine in a treatment known as FCR combination therapy.[5]

Nursing Management of the Medical Client

Assessment. Obtain a thorough health history from the client and family members to aid in diagnosis and treatment. The initial history and physical examination provide baseline data to facilitate assessment of complications of ablative chemotherapy and radiation therapy. The severity and longevity of the manifestations of leukemia are important facts to obtain and document.

Ask the client about risk factors and causative factors. Age is important to note because the incidence of leukemia increases with age. The client's occupational history and hobbies may also give hints about environmental exposures. Previous illnesses and medical history may indicate risk factors.

Because leukemia increases the risk of infection resulting from loss of WBC function, ask about the frequency and severity of infections, such as colds, pneumonia, bronchitis, and unexplained fever during the past 6 months. Leukemia reduces the production of RBCs. The client may report activity intolerance, shortness of breath, headache resulting from cerebral hypoxia, increased sleepiness, decreased attention span, anorexia, and weight loss.

The loss of platelet function increases the risk of bleeding. The client may report a tendency to bleed or bruise easily (e.g., nosebleeds), an inability to stop bleeding from small nicks, bleeding gums when brushing teeth, increased menstrual flow, or blood in the stool or urine.

Physical examination findings may include the manifestations shown in Figure 79-2. A complete head-to-toe assessment is performed. Clients with leukemia or blast crisis may have tachycardia, hypotension, tachypnea, murmurs or bruits, and increased capillary fill time resulting from low RBC counts. Skin and mucous membranes may show evidence of bruising and bleeding. *Petechiae* (small, raised red spots) may be present. Lymph node enlargement may be present. If the leukemic cells have infiltrated the spleen or liver, abdominal tenderness may be noted. If the leukemic cells have infiltrated the brain, the client may be confused, have seizures, or become comatose.

The therapeutic relationship initiated during assessment is used to support the psychosocial needs of clients and their families. Leukemia is a life-threatening illness, and working with the client and family as a team is beneficial. Educating the client is an ongoing process to increase understanding of the disease and may help in obtaining compliance with treatment.

The nursing role during the acute phases of leukemia is extremely challenging because the client has many physical and psychosocial needs. Modern therapies offer hope for remission and possibly cure for some clients, but leukemia is still a diagnosis equated with pain, expensive long-term therapy, and potential death.

Diagnosis, Outcomes, Interventions
Diagnosis: Ineffective Protection/Risk for Infection. The nursing diagnosis is written as *Ineffective Protection/Risk for Infection related to neutropenia or leukocytosis secondary to leukemia or treatment.*

Outcomes. Infection will be prevented or will be discovered early and treated effectively as evidenced by a neutrophil count greater than 1000/mm^3, an absence of fever, and no respiratory difficulty.

Interventions

In compliance with CDC hand hygiene guidelines and The Joint Commission (TJC) National Patient Safety Goals to reduce the risk of health-care–associated infections, it is necessary to institute required hand-washing for everyone coming in contact with the client. The client's risk for infection is estimated by calculating the absolute neutrophil count (ANC). The formula for calculating ANC and an example are given in the Critical Monitoring box on p. 2122. The client should be in protective isolation if the ANC count is below 500/mm^3. Visitors with possible communicable diseases should be screened for the presence of infection, and visitors or staff with colds or respiratory tract infections should not be allowed near the client. Avoid all live plants and flowers in the client's room.

SAFETY
ALERT

CRITICAL MONITORING

Determining the Absolute Neutrophil Count

A leading complication in oncology clients is infection. To recognize this risk, the absolute neutrophil count (ANC) is calculated daily. The ANC (or granulocyte count) provides a numerical estimate of the client's immune status, risk for bacterial infection, and need for reverse isolation. For example, a client with leukemia may have a high white blood cell (WBC) count or a normal count. On calculating the ANC, however, you may find that the client is at high risk for infection. For example, if a client has a WBC count of 9000/mm^3, composed of 10% segmented neutrophils (segs), 60% blast cells, and 30% other WBCs, the client would have an increased risk of infection because the functional neutrophils are only 900.

Three numbers are required:

- Banded neutrophil count
- Segmented neutrophil count
- Total WBC count

Obtain these numbers from the complete blood cell count and differential. The total WBC count is composed of five types of cells; the results from the laboratory show the total count and the percentage of each WBC type. For example, on the differential counts, the value next to monocytes represents the percentage of monocytes among the total number of WBCs.

Then use the following formula to calculate the ANC:

$$(\% \text{ Bands} + \% \text{ Segs}) \times \text{Total WBC count} = \text{ANC}$$

Example:

$$(2\% \text{ Bands} + 55\% \text{ Segs}) \times 1600 = 912$$

When the ANC is less than 1000, the client is at risk for bacterial infection.

When the ANC count is less than 500, the client is at high risk for bacterial infection.

SAFETY

ALERT

The client should be on a low-bacteria diet that excludes raw fruits and vegetables. Assist the client with a daily bath using antimicrobial soap. Encourage the client to perform meticulous oral hygiene several times a day. Female clients should not douche and should avoid the use of tampons. Daily stool softeners are ordered to reduce the risk of anal fissures. Perineal cleansing should occur after every bowel movement. Avoid insertion of rectal suppositories and rectal thermometers.

SAFETY

ALERT

Oral, axillary, or tympanic temperature should be taken every 4 hours, and the physician should be notified if a temperature is higher than 38° C (100.5° to 101° F) or lower than 36° C (97° to 97.5° F). Fever may be the only manifestation in a neutropenic client.

Assess the cause of fever before initiation of therapy by obtaining specimens of blood, sputum, urine, central line sites, and other potential sources of infection for culture.

Administer antibiotics as ordered. Therapy usually consists of multiple IV broad-spectrum antibiotics administered on alternating schedules. Administer analgesics as ordered for the relief of discomfort, avoiding aspirin if the client is thrombocytopenic. Aspirin, aspirin-containing products, and acetaminophen should be avoided because they may mask fever.

Invasive procedures should be avoided if possible. Provide meticulous skin decontamination before venipunctures. Maintain sterile occlusion of central venous catheters and perform routine dressing care according to institutional policy. Change IV tubing according to agency policy.

Monitor the client closely for manifestations of fungal or viral infections (i.e., increased respirations, rales, dyspnea, changed oral mucosa). Monitor the respiratory rate and auscultate breath sounds regularly. Viral and fungal pneumonia are common causes of death in the neutropenic client.

Diagnosis: Decreased Cardiac Output. The client eventually becomes thrombocytopenic because of the progression of the disease or because of chemotherapy treatment, leading to the nursing diagnosis of *Decreased Cardiac Output related to thrombocytopenia secondary to either leukemia or treatment.*

Outcomes. Bleeding as a result of injuries, such as falls, punctures, cuts, or other environmental hazards, will be prevented or will be diagnosed and treated successfully as evidenced by absence of bleeding and a platelet count greater than 20,000/mm^3.

Interventions

Institute bleeding precautions as follows:

- Provide a soft toothbrush for oral hygiene; avoid flossing, hard toothbrushes, and commercial mouthwashes containing alcohol.
- Instruct the client to avoid blowing or picking the nose, straining at bowel movements, douching or using tampons, or using razors. Men and women should use only electric shavers during the neutropenic phase.
- Do not give any intramuscular (IM) or subcutaneous injections.
- Do not insert rectal suppositories.
- Do not give medications containing aspirin, and instruct the client to avoid aspirin-containing medications.
- Avoid urinary catheters whenever possible. If a catheter must be inserted, use the smallest size possible, lubricate it well, and insert it gently.
- Avoid mucosal trauma during suctioning.

- Remove all potential hazards and sharp objects from the environment. Sharp corners or edges on furniture should be padded.
- Use a pressure-reducing mattress, and turn the client frequently to prevent pressure sores. Use bed cradles to protect extremities.
- Avoid overinflation of the blood pressure cuff, and rotate the cuff to different sites. Avoid prolonged use of tourniquets.
- Use only paper tape, and avoid strong adhesives that may cause skin adhesions.

Teach the client and significant others or family members to institute bleeding precautions during periods of thrombocytopenia. Monitor the client at least every 4 hours for manifestations of bleeding, such as ecchymosis, petechiae, epistaxis, gingival bleeding, hematuria, occult blood in stools, enlarged abdominal girth, disorientation, confusion, and changes in level of consciousness. All urine, stools, and emesis should be tested for blood. Take and record vital signs routinely, noting manifestations of altered tissue perfusion related to anemia (increased respirations and pulse rate, decreased blood pressure).

Check the platelet count, hemoglobin level, and hematocrit daily. Report a hemoglobin level of less than 10 g/dl and a platelet count of less than 20,000/mm³. Administer packed RBCs and platelets as ordered. Keep a current blood sample in the laboratory for crossmatching if needed in an emergency.

Diagnosis: Fatigue. Fatigue is a common complaint by clients. It may be cumulative, a gradually worsening response to treatments for cancer, low hematocrit and hemoglobin levels, altered blood glucose levels, decreased oxygen saturation levels, abnormal electrolyte levels, or unintentional weight loss. Fatigue is the greatest about 2 to 3 days after IV chemotherapy. The nursing diagnosis is written *Fatigue related to side effects of treatments, low hemoglobin levels, pain, lack of sleep, or other causes* as made evident by the client. A scale to rate fatigue numerically may be used, such as the Piper Fatigue Scale (see Evolve website), or, more simply, a 0 to 10 numerical scale (see Chapter 22).

Outcomes. The client will report less fatigue, plan adequate rest periods, and be able to do an increasing amount of usual activities with decreasing assistance from others.

Interventions. Assess for anemia and for the physical, psychological, and treatment-related causes of fatigue. Encourage exercise to maintain strength. Ask a physical therapist to assist with bed and strengthening exercises. An occupational therapist may be able to offer suggestions or devices to conserve energy. If the client has thrombocytopenia or fever or has just received chemotherapy (past 24 hours), exercise is not encouraged, in order to avoid injury. Advocate for adequate pain reduction, minimizing interruptions, and reducing visitors when rest is needed.

Diagnosis: Imbalanced Nutrition: Less Than Body Requirements. The client usually experiences decreased appetite and decreased nutritional intake as a result of the effects of radiation therapy and chemotherapy on the GI tract. Write the nursing diagnosis as *Imbalanced Nutrition: Less Than Body Requirements related to anorexia, pain, or fatigue.*

Outcomes. The client will maintain adequate nutrition and maintain body weight as evidenced by stable weight, adequate caloric intake, and maintenance of fluid and electrolyte balance.

Interventions. Administer antiemetics, as ordered, around the clock as necessary to prevent nausea and vomiting. Premedicate the client with sufficient antiemetics before meals to encourage food and fluid intake. Administer local and IV analgesics, as ordered, to reduce pain caused by mucositis.

Discuss daily dietary requirements with the client and provide high-carbohydrate meals and oral supplements. Allow the client to make food selections. Cold foods, shakes, and sandwiches are tolerated better than hot or spicy foods. Small, frequent feedings may be tolerated better than three large meals a day. Monitor weight daily. If the client cannot tolerate food for an extended period, begin total parenteral nutrition (TPN), as ordered, and monitor intake. The client's own digestive system should be used as long as possible, with TPN used as a last resort. Coordinate and plan rest periods and activities of daily living in increments as needed to minimize fatigue.

Diagnosis: Disturbed Body Image. Most clients experience body image disturbance. The nursing diagnosis is written as *Disturbed Body Image resulting from alopecia, weight loss, and fatigue.*

Outcomes. The client will be able to demonstrate and discuss understanding of the disease condition and the temporary nature of changes in body image and energy.

Interventions. Before treatment, inform the client about the potential for hair loss over the entire body. Encourage the use of scarves, hats, or wigs as desired. Explain the temporary nature of alopecia, although the hair may have a different color or texture when it returns. Alopecia may be permanent with whole-brain radiation therapy (WBXRT).

Encourage the client to balance rest with exercise and activities to maintain muscle tone without developing severe fatigue. Discuss daily dietary requirements with the client, and provide high-carbohydrate meals and oral supplements in an attempt to help clients maintain their body weight and an appearance that is acceptable to them.

Diagnosis: Risk for Sexual Dysfunction. Many clients experience reproductive or sexual dysfunction. The nursing diagnosis is written *Risk for Sexual Dysfunction related to the effects of chemotherapy or radiation therapy on reproductive organs.*

Outcomes. The client will be able to discuss the potential for sterility and decreased libido that may result from therapy.

Interventions. Describe the normal cellular destruction that might lead to temporary or permanent destruction of reproductive function in the client. Inform the client that sexual libido may be altered during and after the acute phase of the illness because of fatigue or other side effects of therapy. Provide the client with emotional support and references to support groups. Provide manuals for alternative sexual positioning and techniques. In appropriate cases, inform the client of reproductive alternatives, such as sperm banking, artificial insemination, and egg harvesting.

Diagnosis: Risk for Ineffective Therapeutic Regimen Management and Risk for Ineffective Family Therapeutic Regimen Management/Readiness for Enhanced Self-Care. Because hospital lengths of stay have become shorter and many oncology clients receive their care in outpatient settings, there is *Risk for Ineffective Therapeutic Regimen Management* and *Risk for Ineffective Family Therapeutic Regimen Management/Readiness for Enhanced Self-Care* related to the chronic nature of the disease process and the risk for complications.

Outcomes. The client and family will manage the therapeutic regimen as evidenced by effective medication administration, an absence of infections and hemorrhage, and the client's ability to remain independent at home.

Interventions. After the induction phase of therapy is completed successfully, the client frequently returns home to recover and to await subsequent courses of therapy that may be given on an outpatient basis if no serious complications arise. It is common for clients to return home with anemia and thrombocytopenia. They also may suffer from the residual effects of chemotherapy or radiation therapy, such as loss of appetite, nausea, and mucositis. Some clients find it difficult to leave the security of the hospital setting because of significantly altered body image, fatigue, and fear.

SAFETY
⚠
ALERT

Teach the client and the client's significant others how to recognize manifestations of complications as well as appropriate actions to take. Inform them of measures to ensure safety and to reduce risks of bleeding and infection. Provide clients with phone numbers of nursing personnel to call with questions and for suggestions for interventions. The client and

family should be referred to an oncology clinical nurse specialist or case manager as soon as possible after diagnosis. These nurses often educate the client and family about the disease process, the planned treatment, and strategies for successful transition from the hospital to home and outpatient care.

Evaluation. The desired outcome for the client with leukemia is that the disease will become a chronic condition that the client and family can cope with in a positive manner. If acute leukemia does not respond to therapy, the client's life expectancy is short.

Surgical Management

Bone Marrow Transplantation

To achieve cure with acute leukemia, bone marrow transplantation (BMT) is the most common current recommended treatment. Allogeneic BMT presents a treatment option for clients younger than 60 or 70 years of age, depending on the client's performance status, who have a suitable HLA-matched donor. Transplantation performed during the first remission has a higher success rate than transplantation performed during repeated remissions or in the blast phase of chronic leukemia. BMT is discussed later in this chapter.

Modifications for Older Clients

Older clients are at greater risk for chronic leukemia. The treatment of chronic leukemia in older clients is less vigorous. BMT is an option in older clients if they are otherwise fit and if their organ systems can endure the stress of the procedure. Some older adults with excellent physical and psychological functioning have done quite well with BMT.

LYMPHOMAS

Primary tumors originating from the lymphatic system were identified in 1932. Lymphoma is the most common tumor of the lymphoid system, with about 71,380 new cases diagnosed in 2007 and an estimated 19,730 deaths.[2] About 63,190 new cases of lymphoma will be non-Hodgkin's lymphoma (NHL) and about 8190 Hodgkin's lymphoma (Hodgkin's disease [HD]). *Lymphomas* are tumors of primary lymphoid tissue (thymus and bone marrow) or secondary tissue (lymph nodes, spleen, tonsils, and intestinal lymphoid tissue). Most lymphomas are cancers of secondary lymphoid tissue and involve mostly lymph nodes, the spleen, or both. Malignant lymphoid cells sometimes are found in circulating blood, indicating bone marrow involvement. The major subdivisions of malignant lymphomas are HD and NHL. Bone marrow involvement occurs more often in NHL than in HD.

HODGKIN'S DISEASE

In 1832 Hodgkin reported observations from autopsies showing unusually enlarged lymph nodes and biopsy tissue that showed a distinctive, large cell. Sixty years later Sternberg and Reed described the giant cells, which are called Reed-Sternberg cells of Hodgkin's lymphoma. Today the disease is called *Hodgkin's disease* and is known to be cancer of the lymph, or a lymphoma. Incidence rates differ with respect to age, gender, geographical locations, and socioeconomic class. In 2007 the American Cancer Society estimated the diagnosis of 8190 new cases of HD with 1070 related deaths in the United States.[2]

In economically advantaged countries, the incidence of HD is bimodal, with the first peak occurring in the mid-20s and the second peak occurring after age 50. In economically underdeveloped countries, the overall incidence of HD is lower than that in developed countries but the incidence of HD before age 15 is higher, with only a modest increase into young adulthood. The incidence in people older than age 60 is declining, probably because of improved diagnostic techniques that classify the disease more accurately.

Etiology and Risk Factors

The exact cause of HD is unknown, although indirect evidence indicates a viral cause. The Epstein-Barr virus (EBV) is believed to be a causative agent. EBV-associated lymphomas are well documented in clients who have received organ transplants or who have an immunodeficiency disease. A two-fold to three-fold increase in HD is seen among clients who have a history of mononucleosis, a disease caused by EBV. Researchers have shown that 30% to 50% of HD specimens contained EBV genome fragments in the diagnostic Reed-Sternberg cells.

Some studies indicate a genetic predisposition for HD. The disease occurs more frequently in Jews and among first-degree relatives. Siblings were shown to have a two-fold to five-fold increased risk, and same-sex siblings have a nine-fold increased risk. An increased risk was found among parent-child pairs but not among spouses, suggesting a genetic rather than an infectious cause. Research continues in an attempt to identify the genetic role in the development of HD.

Pathophysiology

Cancerous transformation occurs from a particular site in the lymph node. With continuing growth the entire node becomes replaced, with zones of necrosis obscuring the normal nodular pattern. The mechanism of growth and spread of HD remains unknown. Some have suggested that the disease progresses by extension to adjacent structures. It also may disseminate by the lymphatics because lymphoreticular cells inhabit all tissues of the body except the CNS. Hematologic spread also may occur, possibly by means of direct infiltration of blood vessels.

Clinical Manifestations

Clients often are asymptomatic and may have painless lymphadenopathy. Enlarged lymph nodes most commonly are found in the supraclavicular, cervical, and mediastinal regions (Figure 79-5). Local manifestations produced by lymphadenopathy usually are caused by pressure or obstruction. Involvement of the extremities can be manifested by pain, nerve irritation, and obliteration of the pulse. Clients may experience a nonproductive cough, with the chest radiograph revealing a mediastinal mass, which is present in about 50% of clients.

Pericardial involvement can occur by direct invasion from mediastinal lymph nodes. This involvement can cause pericardial friction rub, pericardial effusion, and engorgement of neck veins. Other manifestations arise when enlarged lymph nodes obstruct or compress an adjacent structure (e.g., edema of the face, neck, and right arm secondary to superior vena cava compression or renal failure secondary to urethral obstruction).

If the tumor infiltrates the spine and presses on the spinal cord, manifestations of spinal cord compression can develop. Manifestations range from early back pain with motor weakness and sensory loss to loss of motor function, urinary retention, constipation, and other manifestations of compression of the cord late in the disease.

Associated clinical manifestations of unexplained weight loss of more than 10% of body weight in 6 months, frequent drenching night sweats, and temperature above 38° C also may be present. Pruritus is a systemic manifestation that can be significant if it is recurrent. These additional manifestations are known as *B symptoms* for staging purposes; they occur in greater frequency in older clients and are negatively related to the prognosis.

The diagnosis is confirmed by lymph node and bone marrow biopsy. A chest radiograph to evaluate complaints of persistent cough or dyspnea may identify mediastinal involvement. The extent of disease is determined by CT scans of the thoracic, abdominal, and pelvic areas as well as gallium scan of mediastinal or hilar lymph nodes and lymphangiography of the lower extremities. If the extent of the disease cannot be determined by these diagnostic tests and confirmation of abdominal disease is necessary for determining treatment choice, a staging laparotomy may be performed.

Staging

Hodgkin's disease is divided into categories, or stages, according to the microscopic appearance of the involved

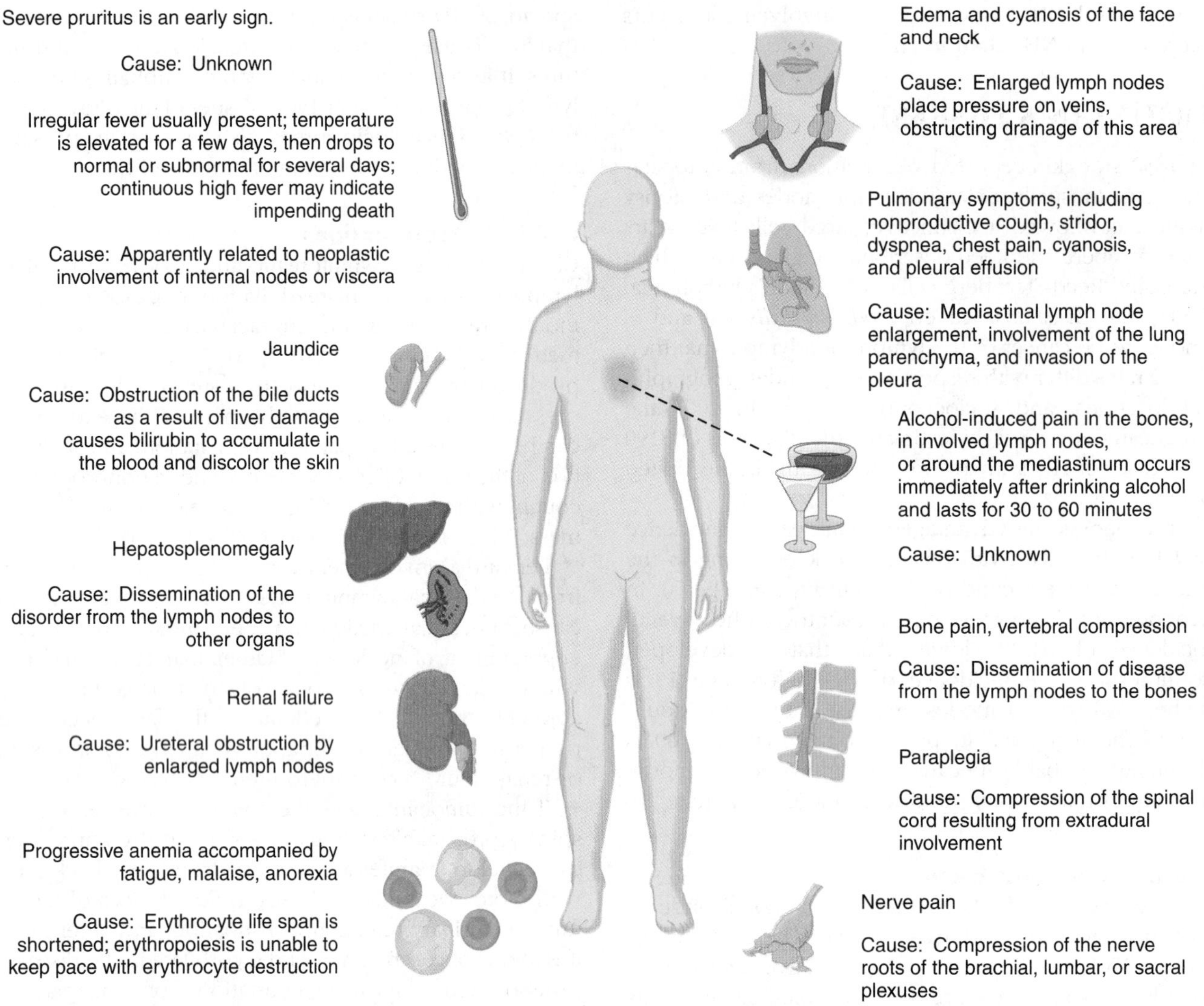

Severe pruritus is an early sign.

Cause: Unknown

Irregular fever usually present; temperature is elevated for a few days, then drops to normal or subnormal for several days; continuous high fever may indicate impending death

Cause: Apparently related to neoplastic involvement of internal nodes or viscera

Jaundice

Cause: Obstruction of the bile ducts as a result of liver damage causes bilirubin to accumulate in the blood and discolor the skin

Hepatosplenomegaly

Cause: Dissemination of the disorder from the lymph nodes to other organs

Renal failure

Cause: Ureteral obstruction by enlarged lymph nodes

Progressive anemia accompanied by fatigue, malaise, anorexia

Cause: Erythrocyte life span is shortened; erythropoiesis is unable to keep pace with erythrocyte destruction

Edema and cyanosis of the face and neck

Cause: Enlarged lymph nodes place pressure on veins, obstructing drainage of this area

Pulmonary symptoms, including nonproductive cough, stridor, dyspnea, chest pain, cyanosis, and pleural effusion

Cause: Mediastinal lymph node enlargement, involvement of the lung parenchyma, and invasion of the pleura

Alcohol-induced pain in the bones, in involved lymph nodes, or around the mediastinum occurs immediately after drinking alcohol and lasts for 30 to 60 minutes

Cause: Unknown

Bone pain, vertebral compression

Cause: Dissemination of disease from the lymph nodes to the bones

Paraplegia

Cause: Compression of the spinal cord resulting from extradural involvement

Nerve pain

Cause: Compression of the nerve roots of the brachial, lumbar, or sacral plexuses

■ **FIGURE 79–5** Clinical manifestations and pathophysiologic basis of Hodgkin's disease.

lymph nodes, the extent and severity of the disorder, and the prognosis. Accurate staging of HD is important for determining treatment options. Table 79-2 shows the Cotswold staging classification, which modified the Ann Arbor classification system primarily to incorporate the newer diagnostic tests and the evidence that bulky disease is an important prognostic indicator.

OUTCOME MANAGEMENT

Medical Management

Since the advent of combination chemotherapy, adult HD has become one of the most curable malignancies, resulting in a 5-year survival rate of 90% to 95% for stages I and II and 80% to 90% for stages III and IV. The goal of therapy for clients with stage I and II disease is to achieve long-term disease-free survival with minimal acute and long-term complications that affect quality of life. Treatment consists of radiation therapy alone or combined with chemotherapy.

Eradication of Tumor Cells

Radiation. Radiation treatment for HD involves three locations: the mantle, the para-aortic region, and the pelvis (Figure 79-6). The mantle field encompasses the submandibular, cervical, infraclavicular, axillary, mediastinal, subcarinal, and hilar lymph nodes. In clinical stages I and II disease, combined chemotherapy and radiation therapy are recommended for clients with unfavorable prognostic indicators. Most cancer centers classify B manifestations (fever, night sweats, and unexplained weight loss), high erythrocyte sedimentation rate (ESR), or large mediastinal adenopathy as poor prognostic factors. Some centers include large numbers of site involvement and older age as poor prognostic indicators.

TABLE 79–2   Cotswold Staging Classification for Hodgkin's Disease

Stage I	Involvement of a single lymph node region or a lymphoid structure (e.g., spleen, thymus, Waldeyer's ring)
Stage II	Involvement of two or more lymph node regions on same side of diaphragm (e.g., the mediastinum is a single site, hilar lymph nodes are lateralized); number of anatomic sites should be indicated by a subscript (e.g., II_2)
Stage III	Involvement of lymph node regions or structures on both sides of diaphragm: III_1: With or without involvement of splenic, hilar, celiac, or portal nodes III_2: With involvement of para-aortic, iliac, or mesenteric nodes
Stage IV	Involvement of extranodal site(s) beyond that designated as E

Designation Applicable to Any Disease Stage

A	No manifestations
B	Fever, drenching sweats, weight loss (B symptoms)
X	Bulky disease: $>\frac{1}{3}$ the width of mediastinum <10 cm maximal dimension of nodal mass
E	Involvement of a single extranodal site, contiguous or proximal to a known nodal site
CS	Clinical stage
PS	Pathologic stage

Data from Goldman, L., Krevans, J., & Ausiello, D. (2004). *Cecil textbook of medicine* (22nd ed.). Philadelphia: Saunders.

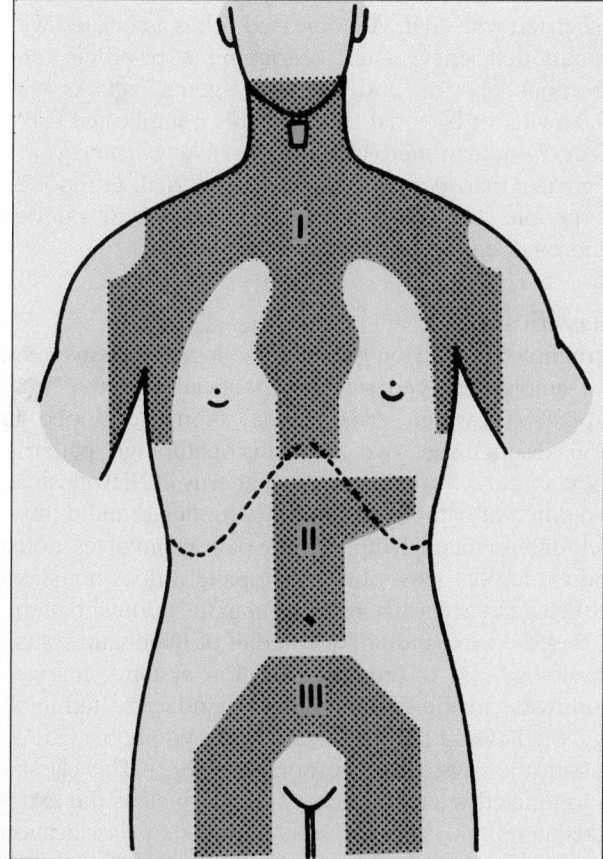

■ **FIGURE 79–6** Radiation fields in therapy for Hodgkin's disease. *Shaded areas* represent the three treatment fields. The *mantle field* is the uppermost field (I). Lungs and vocal cords are protected by lead blocks; the heart and thyroid gland are within the field. The *para-aortic field*, or middle field (II), extends from the diaphragm to just above the bifurcation of the aorta. When the spleen has not been removed, this field is extended to include the entire spleen and splenic hilum. The *pelvic* or *inverted Y field* is the lowest field (III). It encompasses the pelvic and inguinal nodes and includes a large area of bone marrow.

Chemotherapy. Chemotherapy has become the primary treatment strategy, with or without radiation therapy, in stages I and II disease with poor prognostic indicators and in clients with advanced HD. Numerous chemotherapy regimens are available for HD. For years, MOPP (mechlorethamine, vincristine [Oncovin], procarbazine, prednisone) was the gold standard of therapy; however, ABVD (doxorubicin [Adriamycin], bleomycin, vinblastine, and dacarbazine) has emerged as the best alternative to MOPP. Compared to MOPP, the primary advantages of ABVD are its ease of delivery in full doses, fewer side effects, and less risk of subsequent development of leukemia. With proper treatment, the 20-year disease-free survival rate of HD is 70% to 80%, and the overall survival rate, with salvage chemotherapy for clients who relapse, is 80% to 95%.

 Research has shown that clients with advanced disease (stages III and IV) may achieve better treatment results with MOPP plus ABVD than with MOPP alone. Other studies showed that ABVD alone could achieve results similar to MOPP plus ABVD. Many physicians recommend that ABVD alone be given for as many cycles as required to achieve a complete remission plus two consolidation cycles (usually six cycles total). The use of radiation therapy in advanced disease is individualized to the client, especially those with local-regional disease problems.

Clients who relapse after definitive HD therapy generally require some type of systemic therapy, which depends on the type of initial therapy used. Therapies range from chemotherapy and wide-field radiation to high-dose chemotherapy with autologous or allogeneic stem cell transplant. Of clients with stages I to II HD, 20% to 30% relapse within 5 years after radiation therapy. In these cases, the use of combination chemotherapy produces a 57% to 62% disease-free survival at 10 years. At the National Cancer Institute, a 93% second complete remission rate was seen in clients with initial remissions longer than 12 months after chemotherapy. The positive results of several studies investigating the use of stem cell transplant have provided the basis for recommending BMT and stem cell transplantation for all HD clients who relapsed or did not respond to any primary chemotherapy, regardless of the length of the initial remission.

Complications. The complications related to HD are numerous because they are a result of the disease itself or of radiation therapy, chemotherapy, or a combination of several of these factors (Table 79-3).

Nursing Management of the Medical Client

Obtain a thorough health history from the client and family members. The severity and longevity of the manifestations of the disease are important facts to obtain and document. Nurses play an essential role in symptom management associated with therapy. Because of the side effects of chemotherapy, clients may ask for a reduction of the dosage or may want to stop therapy completely. Provide clients with information about the effect of reducing or stopping therapy on long-term survival.

NON-HODGKIN'S LYMPHOMA

Non-Hodgkin's lymphoma comprises a group of malignancies with a common origin in the lymphoid cells. They are heterogeneous in cellular origin, morphologic

appearance, and clinical behavior. For 2007 the American Cancer Society estimated that in the United States about 63,190 new cases of NHL were diagnosed, with 18,660 related deaths.[2]

Between 1973 and 1991, the incidence of NHL increased by about 73%. Part of this increase was attributed to acquired immunodeficiency syndrome (AIDS). NHL is about 60 times more common in people with AIDS than in the general population of the United States. NHL is the eighth (male) and seventh (female) most common cause of cancer-related deaths in the United States. Men are affected more often than women, and the incidence is higher in whites than other races. NHL can occur in any age group, but an increase in incidence occurs in the 50s and 60s. Because the average age at diagnosis is in the 50s, the number of years of life lost to these malignancies ranks NHL fourth in economic impact among cancers in the United States.

Etiology and Risk Factors

No hereditary, ethnic, or dietary risk factors have been associated with NHL. An increased risk is associated with immunodeficiency states, autoimmune disorders, and infectious physical and chemical agents. As with HD, a viral or bacterial cause has been implicated (EBV, HTLV-1, human herpes virus 8, *Helicobacter pylori*). A greater than expected incidence of NHL is reported in people with ataxia-telangiectasia, Wiskott-Aldrich syndrome, and Chédiak-Higashi syndrome.

Classifications

Terminology describing NHL is complex, inconsistent, and ambiguous, and several classifications exist. Rappaport's widely used classification, developed in 1956, distinguishes two major histopathologic patterns: nodular and diffuse. These two patterns in NHL illustrate two different pathologic states. The nodular (and diffuse, well-differentiated lymphocytic) pattern involves nodal and extranodal sites. The diffuse pattern does not show the cell aggregates that are evident in the nodular pattern.

Based on expanding knowledge of lymphatic system physiology, six distinct classification systems emerged worldwide in the 1970s. To standardize terminology, the Revised European-American Lymphoma (REAL) classification system was proposed in 1994. This classification includes all lymphoma types as well as the extranodal lymphomas not included in the other classification systems.

Pathophysiology

In clients with NHL, an abnormal proliferation of neoplastic lymphocytes occurs. The cells remain fixed at one phase of development and continue to proliferate. Both T and B lymphocytes mature in the lymph nodes. Clinical manifestations are due to mechanical obstruction of the

---

TABLE 79–3 Complications of Hodgkin's Disease

Problem	Cause
Thyroid dysfunction Thymic hyperplasia	Underlying disease, therapy, or both
Hypothyroidism Thyroid cancer	Direct or indirect radiation exposure
Sexual dysfunction Male impotence Male and female infertility Female dyspareunia	Underlying disease, therapy, or both
Herpes zoster or varicella	Underlying disease, therapy, or both
Pulmonary dysfunction Pneumonitis (acute, chronic, or both)	Direct or indirect radiation exposure, bleomycin, nitrosoureas, radiation recall
Cardiac dysfunction Cardiomyopathy	Mediastinal radiation therapy, pericarditis (acute), doxorubicin, radiation recall
Pericarditis (chronic)	Mediastinal radiation therapy
Dental caries	Salivary changes related to radiation therapy
Myelodysplastic syndrome	Therapy, especially if age >40 yr or lymphocytic leukemia
Non-Hodgkin's lymphoma	Therapy
Solid tumors	Direct or indirect radiation exposure

enlarged lymph nodes. Lymphocytic infiltration of the abdomen or oropharynx also can occur.

Clinical Manifestations

Clients with NHL show localized or generalized lymphadenopathy. The cervical, axillary, inguinal, and femoral chains are the most frequent sites of lymph node enlargement. The swelling is generally painless, and the nodes have enlarged and transformed over months or years. Extranodal sites of involvement are the nasopharynx, GI tract, bone, thyroid, testes, and soft tissue. Some clients have retroperitoneal and abdominal masses with abdominal fullness, back pain, ascites (fluid in the peritoneal cavity), and leg swelling.

Several sites of involvement in NHL are not common in HD, such as Waldeyer's ring (lymphoid tissue that encircles the tonsils), the stomach, the small and large bowels, mesenteric lymph nodes, the thyroid, the skin, the pancreas, the kidneys, and the CNS. With diffuse NHL, clinical manifestations are variable and generally involve more systemic findings. Clients also may experience systemic B symptoms, including night sweats, fever, and weight loss. About one third of clients have hepatomegaly or splenomegaly.

Certain other clinical conditions mimic the malignant lymphomas, including tuberculosis, syphilis, systemic lupus erythematosus, lung cancer, and bone cancer. A thorough diagnostic evaluation is required.

Blood work includes a complete blood cell count (CBC), ESR, and peripheral smear to rule out other causes of lymphadenopathy, such as mononucleosis. Blood cultures and other serologic studies for viral and autoimmune diseases provide important differential information. Elevated lactate dehydrogenase (LDH) levels may be seen in advanced NHL.

A lymph node biopsy is an important diagnostic tool. The following are indications for biopsy:

- Adenopathy for longer than 3 weeks, which progresses in size or spreads to other areas
- B symptoms that cannot be attributed to other causes
- Abnormal blood test results indicative of lymphoma
- Radiographs that suggest possible extranodal involvement

Because of the aggressive nature of AIDS-related NHL, any symptomatic client at increased risk or known to be positive for human immunodeficiency virus (HIV) should have a biopsy to rule out high-grade lymphoma.

Just as in HD, once the diagnosis of NHL is made, disease staging should take place. Noninvasive imaging techniques, such as CT and MRI, are useful tools in the initial staging of NHL. Renal and liver function tests are performed to determine the presence of extranodal involvement. Bilateral bone marrow biopsies are important because metastasis to the bone marrow is common, especially in low-grade disease.

OUTCOME MANAGEMENT

Medical Management

Eradication of Tumor Cells

Many classification systems are used to differentiate NHL according to histologic type and cytologic characteristics. Treatment varies based on the histology and stage of the tumor. The treatment of a low-grade lymphoma is different from that for high-grade disease. Low-grade tumors tend to progress slowly and often are asymptomatic for long periods; the natural course of the disease may fluctuate considerably over 5 to 10 years, with or without treatment. Low-grade cells eventually transform into a more aggressive disease process, however, and may quickly cause the death of the client. Because of this process, indolent NHL is believed to be incurable, and many controversies exist concerning treatment standards, especially for clients who have disseminated disease.

Radiation and Chemotherapy. The progression of intermediate-grade and high-grade lymphomas is similar to that of other cancers. Because of their higher growth fraction, however, these tumors tend to be more sensitive to chemotherapy and radiation therapy; the response rate is higher when these tumors are treated. Combination chemotherapy is used to produce tumor shrinkage and remission. Cyclophosphamide and doxorubicin are active against lymphoma. Various combination drug regimens that include these two drugs are used in the treatment of NHL. Controversy regarding first-line standard of care therapy is ongoing. Studies comparing various treatment protocols affirmed the practice of using CHOP (cyclophosphamide, hydroxydaunorubicin [doxorubicin], vincristine [Oncovin], and prednisone) as first-line therapy in many academic and community settings.

For clients with low-grade NHL in stage I to II, radiation therapy alone may be curative, although there are reports of recurrence past 10 years. Depending on whether the disease is supradiaphragmatic or subdiaphragmatic, single-mode therapy includes mantle and inverted Y field irradiation (see Figure 79-6).

Clients with stage III to IV intermediate-grade lymphoma require combination chemotherapy as an immediate intervention. Clients who are older than age 60 and have elevated LDH levels, poor performance status, and stage III to IV intermediate disease are at higher risk and should be offered aggressive regimens that provide higher-dose intensities.

The diagnosis of a high-grade NHL warrants immediate and aggressive treatment. Clients may present with rapidly growing disease that has the potential to double in bulk in days or hours. Treatment includes dose-intense chemotherapy, with or without radiation therapy, and prophylactic CNS therapy. It is necessary to provide prophylaxis for the CNS because the blood-brain barrier prevents most chemotherapy drugs from getting into CNS spaces. Without such treatment, lymphoma cells may look for "sanctuary" in the CNS (CNS metastasis). High-grade NHL clients also are excellent candidates for BMT or stem cell transplantation because the tumors respond dramatically to high-dose chemotherapy, which is part of the preparative regimen of transplant.

Monoclonal Antibodies. Rituximab (Rituxan) is an unconjugated chimeric monoclonal antibody that binds to the CD20 antigen found on the surface of most B-cell lymphomas. This surface antigen is present in about 90% of B-cell lymphomas. This intravenous drug is FDA approved as a single agent in the treatment of relapsed low-grade follicular NHL, and also for first-line treatment of diffuse large B-cell, CD20+ NHL in combination with CHOP or other anthracycline-based chemotherapy regimens.

Targeted Therapy. Targeted therapy utilizing radiolabeled monoclonal antibodies is also available for the treatment of NHL. These radiolabeled agents recognize and react with specific antigens to target and kill specific tumor cells. Greater amounts of radiation are delivered to tumor cells than to normal cells, and critical organs that do not express the specific antigen are spared. There are two FDA-approved agents in this class of drugs for the treatment of clients with relapsed or refractory NHL: ibritumomab tiuxetan (Zevalin), which is labeled with yttrium 90, and tositumomab (Bexxar), which uses iodine 131.

Other Therapies. Experimental therapies are emerging in the treatment of NHL. Such therapies include vaccines, high-dose radioimmunotherapy and stem cell transplantation, and antisense anti-angiogenesis agents. These therapies are currently being investigated in clinical trials.

Nursing Management of the Medical Client

Assessment. Although the appearance of an enlarged lymph node in the absence of infection may cause worry, 56% of healthy adults may experience cervical adenopathy; however, any enlargement of lymph nodes warrants further evaluation.

The work-up for NHL begins with a thorough history and physical examination. On examination, lymph nodes involved in infectious processes may be tender or painful, whereas lymphomatous nodes tend to be firm and "rubbery" and are found in generalized patterns. Carcinomatous nodes often are hard and sometimes matted to one another or fixed to underlying structures in contiguous or regional patterns. Other hallmarks of

lymphoma, such as systemic B symptoms (fever, night sweats, unexplained weight loss), are seen in 20% to 30% of clients, but these manifestations also may be seen in other disease states, such as certain infections and connective tissue diseases.

The heterogeneous nature of NHL challenges nurses to meet a variety of physical and psychosocial needs for both clients and their families. The client and family members are confronted with managing a demanding diagnosis and treatment and coping with the effects of the disease on daily routines. Health care professionals often assume that clients with supportive families manage well, but family members share the strain of the illness, are deeply affected (psychologically, financially, and perhaps physically), and need ongoing support. It is crucial that nurses adapt their plans of care for these clients along the disease trajectory, which can wax and wane for many years.

Diagnosis, Outcomes, Interventions. The nursing diagnosis, outcomes, and interventions for HD and NHL are the same as those for the client with leukemia.

Nursing Diagnoses. These clients may have *Ineffective Protection/Risk for Infection* (related to neutropenia or the result of chemotherapy and radiation therapy), *Decreased Cardiac Output* (as a result of thrombocytopenia secondary to treatment), *Fatigue, Risk for Sexual Dysfunction, Imbalanced Nutrition: Less Than Body Requirements, Disturbed Body Image,* and *Risk for Ineffective Therapeutic Regimen Management* (Individuals and Families)/*Readiness for Enhanced Self-Care.*

Outcomes. The desired outcome for the client with lymphoma is that the disease will become a chronic condition that the client and family can cope with in a positive manner. If the disease becomes terminal, the outcome should include a death with dignity, in which comfort measures and psychological support are emphasized.

Interventions. Interventions for these problems were discussed previously for clients with leukemia.

Evaluation. Physiologic problems may resolve quickly with medication. Psychological diagnosis will require prolonged intervention.

BONE MARROW TRANSPLANTATION

Since the 1970s BMT has progressed from a treatment of last resort to a viable therapeutic modality for a variety of hematologic, malignant, and nonmalignant disorders. Peripheral stem cell transplantation and autologous transplants have further revolutionized the field. The status of the disease to be treated by BMT is an important determinant of the outcome for the client

Transplants for acute leukemias (ALL and AML) in remission at the time of transplant have survival rates of 55% to 68% if the donor is related and 26% to 50% if the donor is unrelated. High-dose chemotherapy and/or radiation therapy followed by bone marrow transplant is also used in the treatment of NHL. BMT has shown long-term survival of approximately 10% to 50% in clients with relapsed or refractory lymphoma.[15]

Indications

Bone marrow transplant may be considered as a treatment for clients with the following conditions:

- Aplastic anemia
- Malignant disorders, specifically myelodysplastic syndromes, leukemia (certain types of acute leukemic, chronic leukemic, and preleukemic states), lymphoma, multiple myeloma, neuroblastoma, and selected solid tumors (breast cancer, ovarian cancer, testicular cancer, poor-risk germ cell tumors)
- Nonmalignant hematologic disorders, such as Fanconi's anemia, thalassemia, and sickle cell anemia
- Immunodeficiency disorders, such as severe combined immunodeficiency disease and Wiskott-Aldrich syndrome

Bone Marrow Harvesting
Sources of Bone Marrow

The three types of bone marrow donors are (1) allogeneic, (2) syngeneic, and (3) autologous.

Allogeneic Bone Marrow. *Allogeneic* bone marrow is obtained from a relative or unrelated donor having a closely matched HLA type. This was the most common type of marrow transplant, but it carried the highest rate of morbidity and mortality because of complications of incompatibility such as graft-versus-host disease (GVHD). The rate of allogeneic transplants has dropped with the decreased birth rate and the increased use of autologous and peripheral stem cell transplants.

Syngeneic Bone Marrow. *Syngeneic* marrow is donated by an identical twin. Although syngeneic marrow is a perfect HLA match, which eliminates the risks of marrow rejection, the incidence of leukemic relapse is higher than when an allogeneic donor is used because GVHD is considered to have an antileukemic effect.

Autologous Bone Marrow. *Autologous* marrow is removed from the intended recipient during the remission phase to allow another course of ablative therapy to be given if a relapse occurs. Although autologous marrow eliminates the risk of adverse immunologic responses, such as GVHD and graft rejection, relapse after autologous BMT is a frequent occurrence. This relapse

may be due to contamination of the harvested bone marrow by malignant cells or the failure of pretransplant chemotherapy to eradicate completely the tumor cells from the body.

Histocompatibility Testing for Allogeneic and Syngeneic Transplantation

Immunologic recognition of the differences in HLA antigens is the first step in host transplant rejection. The HLA system antigens are a complex set of protein structures found on the surface membrane of all human nucleated cells, solid tissues, and circulating blood cells except RBCs. This genetically inherited mixture of antigens is considered representative of the tissue type of each person.

Siblings have a one in four chance of having identical sets of HLA antigens. This situation would provide the optimally matched allogeneic bone marrow donor. Because of the complexity of the HLA system, unrelated clients have less than a 1 in 5000 chance of having identical HLA types. The establishment of the National Bone Marrow Donor Program (NMDP) in 1986 has given hope to many clients who do not have a compatible relative donor. As of April 2007 the NMDP registry contained approximately 5.5 million potential donors and 40,000 cord blood units. This has increased the availability of unrelated donors for allogeneic transplants.

Allogeneic Donor Preparation

An extensive work-up is performed for ensuring compatibility and the mental and physical well-being of the prospective donor. This evaluation includes histocompatibility testing, medical history, physical examination, chest film, ECG, laboratory evaluation (CBC, chemistry profile, viral testing, rapid plasma reagin test [syphilis], ABO and Rh blood typing, coagulation studies), and psychological testing (may include psychiatric consultation).

Before marrow harvest, an informed consent, including potential donor complications (pain, fever, hematoma), must be obtained. In rare instances, the donor may experience serious adverse effects from general anesthesia. Spinal anesthesia is sometimes used instead of general anesthesia during the harvest. Because of the potential for significant blood loss during the harvesting process, syngeneic and allogeneic donors are advised to donate autologous blood for reinfusion before the procedure.

Newborns are currently being considered as potential donors through the use of their cord blood, which is rich in stem cells. Some parents are being encouraged to freeze their newborn's cord blood for potential future use, especially if there is a history of cancer in the family.

Marrow Collection

When collecting marrow, the client or donor is given general or spinal anesthesia in the operating room. The marrow is obtained in 5- to 10-ml aliquots from the marrow spaces of the pelvis or occasionally the anterior iliac crest and sternum. Numerous skin punctures may be required; the aspiration needle is redirected to various marrow spaces without being withdrawn. A total of 500 to 1000 ml of marrow usually is obtained. The blood is placed in heparinized tissue culture media and filtered for removal of fat and bone particles. Marrow can be infused immediately or frozen in a solution containing dimethyl sulfoxide (DMSO), which preserves stem cells in the frozen state.

Peripheral Stem Cell Collection

Peripheral stem (progenitor) cells are harvested by apheresis or leukapheresis, a process that removes blood through a large-bore catheter and runs it through a machine that removes the stem cells before returning the blood to the client. Because stem cell concentration is much lower in peripheral blood compared with bone marrow, a process to increase the concentration in the peripheral blood must be initiated first. To increase the number of circulating stem cells, a stimulus, such as a granulocyte colony-stimulating factor (GCSF), interleukins (ILs), fusion molecules (made from a combination of a CSF and IL-3), or some chemotherapeutic agents, may be given to the donor before the stem cell harvest. As mentioned earlier, the umbilical cord of newborns also is rich in stem cells.

Once the stem cells are harvested, they are preserved in the same manner as bone marrow. The engraftment of stem cells occurs at about the same rate as or slightly faster than with BMT.

Allogeneic Transplant
Recipient Preparation

The physical and psychological evaluation of the recipient is similar to that of the donor. Additional testing may be required to stage existing disease accurately. The recipient must undergo a preparative regimen before transplantation. Such a regimen serves three purposes:

1. Malignant cells are destroyed.
2. The immune system is inactivated, which reduces the risk of GVHD in allogeneic transplant clients.
3. The marrow cavities are emptied to provide space for implantation of the transfused stem cells.

Common protocols combine total body irradiation and high doses of a single chemotherapeutic agent (cyclophosphamide is one of the most common agents used) or fractionated/high doses of multiple agents. A multilumen central venous catheter is inserted to provide suitable access for marrow infusion as well as for antibiotics, blood products, hyperalimentation, and frequent blood sampling.

Bone Marrow Infusion

The infusion of the marrow is commonly anticlimactic after the client has undergone the rigorous preparatory chemotherapy and radiation therapy (often referred to as the *conditioning regimen*). The marrow is usually administered immediately after the conditioning regimen is complete. Before infusion, the client is premedicated with acetaminophen and diphenhydramine to prevent reaction. Marrow is administered from a large blood infusion bag by a multilumen catheter, using an infusion pump, or small volumes may be prefiltered and given by IV push by a physician.

The BMT client remains pancytopenic until the transplanted stem cells make their way to the medullary cavities, where subsequent growth and reconstitution of the marrow are confirmed. Indications of successful engraftment are an increase in platelets and RBCs in the peripheral blood count. This change may occur 14 days after marrow infusion. Each day that recovery is delayed places the client at added risk. Graft rejection is evident if the bone marrow fails to produce peripheral blood cells after several weeks.

Nursing Management

Nursing management of BMT clients follows the plan of care for any completely immunosuppressed client. Clients receiving allogeneic transplants must be observed closely for manifestations of GVHD. Potential immediate adverse reactions are allergic (urticaria, chills, fever), volume overload, and pulmonary complications secondary to fat emboli. Renal damage may occur from too many erythrocytes, or from the dimethyl sulfoxide (DMSO) preservative. The period immediately after transplant is crucial. Multisystem failure related to ablative therapy is common, as are immune reactions caused by the transplanted cells.

GRAFT-VERSUS-HOST DISEASE

The most common and potentially disastrous complication of allogeneic BMT is GVHD, which may occur 7 to 30 days after infusion of viable lymphocytes. The most important factor correlating with incidence and severity of GVHD is HLA disparity. The donor T lymphocytes form an immunologic reaction against the host cells. The clients at highest risk for development of GVHD are those who have had allogeneic BMT. Of those clients, risk is greatest when the donor mismatched two to three antigens and when the client is older than 3 years. With HLA-identical siblings used as bone marrow donors, incidence of moderate-to-severe acute GVHD ranges from less than 10% to 60%, depending on prophylaxis and other risk factors.

ACUTE GRAFT-VERSUS-HOST DISEASE

Acute GVHD is staged according to the organ system affected (Table 79-4). It usually affects the gut, skin, lungs, or liver. *Stage I* GVHD occurs in many allogeneic transplant clients. Skin manifestations may resolve without treatment. Systemic complications may be treated with immunosuppressive drug therapy.

Therapy for GVHD includes high doses of methylprednisolone, antithymocyte globulin, antilymphocyte globulin, cyclosporine, and anti–T-cell immunotoxins. These also leave the client immunosuppressed and vulnerable to infection. The prognosis and treatment depend on the severity of the syndrome. Acute GVHD that does not respond to treatment greatly increases the morbidity and mortality of BMT.

CHRONIC GRAFT-VERSUS-HOST DISEASE

Chronic GVHD, a long-term form of the disease with less acute manifestations, may occur even if the client has not experienced acute GVHD. Chronic GVHD appears about 100 days after transplantation; it may affect the liver, GI system, oral mucosa, and lungs as well as the skin. Chronic GVHD resembles autoimmune collagen-vascular disorders, such as systemic lupus erythematosus. It is characterized by scleroderma-like skin fibrosis and Sjögren's syndrome, in which the mucosa and lacrimal ducts are abnormally dry.

Diagnosis of chronic GVHD is confirmed by skin and oral mucosal biopsy. Although severe GVHD usually is fatal, researchers believe that a complete absence of this immune reaction increases the risk of leukemic relapse.

This situation may be due to a beneficial graft-versus-leukemic reaction that mild GVHD stimulates. In allogeneic BMT recipients with GVHD stages II through IV, the relapse rate is 2.5 times lower than in syngeneic recipients or allogeneic recipients without GVHD.

CONCLUSIONS

Leukemia and lymphoma are complex diseases affecting physiologic and psychological aspects of the client and the family. Nursing care focuses on protection of the client from infection resulting from loss of WBC function, protection from hemorrhage resulting from loss of platelet function, and protection from hypoxia resulting from loss of RBC function.

THINKING CRITICALLY

1. A 68-year-old woman is admitted with acute nonlymphocytic leukemia (ANLL). She is receiving chemotherapy. Her WBC count is 1000/mm³; 3% are banded neutrophils and 54% are segmented neutrophils. What, if any, precautions are needed?

Factors to Consider. How is her risk of sepsis determined? Why does body temperature serve as one marker of infection? What precautions are followed?

2. A 34-year-old man with acute myelogenous leukemia comes to the outpatient oncology facility for his second round of chemotherapy. Three days later the client calls the clinic nurse and is complaining of bleeding gums. What is the priority problem you should address? What instructions should you give the client at this time?

Factors to Consider. What pathologic process underlies the client's manifestations? Are there laboratory results you would want to check? What other precautions should you institute based on the client's other manifestations and the laboratory data? What other data are significant to collect at this time?

Discussions for these questions can be found on the website.

BIBLIOGRAPHY

 Citations appearing in red refer to primary research.

Citations appearing in blue refer to evidence-based practice guidelines and protocols.

1. Abraham, J., Allegra, C., & Gulley, J. (2005). *Bethesda handbook of clinical oncology*. Philadelphia: Lippincott Williams & Wilkins.
2. American Cancer Society. (2007). *Cancer facts and figures 2007.* Atlanta: American Cancer Society.
3. Burke, J.M. (2006). *Dx/Rx: Leukemia*. Sudbury: Jones and Bartlett.
4. Bush, S. (2002). Monoclonal antibodies conjugated with radioisotopes for the treatment of non-Hodgkin's lymphoma. *Seminars in Oncology Nursing, 18*(1 Suppl 1), 16-21.
5. Cheson, B.D. (2006). Monoclonal antibody therapy for B-cell malignancies. *Seminars in Oncology, 33*(2 Suppl 5), 2-14.
6. Copelan, E.A. (2006). Hematopoietic stem-cell transplantation. *New England Journal of Medicine, 354*(17), 1813-1826.
7. Gleevec Package Insert; accessed at www.gleevec.com on 11/23/3007.

TABLE 79–4 Stages of Acute Graft-Versus-Host Disease

Stage	Skin Manifestations	Liver Manifestations	Gastrointestinal Manifestations
1	Maculopapular rash <25% of body surface area	Bilirubin 2-3 mg/dl	Diarrhea 500-1000 ml/day
2	Maculopapular rash 25%-50% of body surface area	Bilirubin 3-6 mg/dl	Diarrhea 1000-1500 ml/day
3	Generalized erythroderma	Bilirubin 6-15 mg/dl	Diarrhea >1500 ml/day
4	Desquamation and bullae	Bilirubin >15 mg/dl	Abdominal pain or ileus

8. Leukemia and Lymphoma Society. (2007). *Leukemia and lymphoma latest news.* Available at www.leukemia-lymphoma.org.

9. McDonnell, A.M., Lenz, K.L., Frei-Lahr, D.A., et al. (2006). Single-dose rasburicase 6 mg in the management of tumor lysis syndrome in adults. *Pharmacotherapy, 26*(6), 806-812.

10. NCCN Practice Guidelines in Oncology v.2.2008; Chronic myelogenous leukemia. Available at www.NCCN.org.

11. Oncology Nursing Society. (2007). *Symptom management.* Available at www.ons.org/clinical/SymptomManagement.

12. Seeley, K.M., & DeMeyer, E. (2002). Nursing care of patients receiving Campath. *Clinical Journal of Oncology Nursing, 6*(3), 138-143.

13. Shannon-Dorcy, K. (2002). Nursing implications of Mylotarg: A novel antibody-targeted chemotherapy for CD33+ acute myeloid leukemia in first relapse. *Oncology Nursing Forum, 29*(4), 52-59.

14. Sprycel Package Insert; accessed at www.bms.com on 11/24/2007.

15. Steingass, S.K. (2006). Hematopoietic cell transplantation in non-Hodgkin's lymphoma. *Seminars in Oncology Nursing, 22*(2), 107-116.

16. Stolar, K. (1999). A graft versus host disease prevention and management tool: A mechanism for improving continuity of care. *Oncology Nursing Forum, 26*(6), 977-978.

17. Tasigna Package Insert; accessed at www.tasigna.com on 11/24/2007.

17a. The Joint Commission. (2008). *2008 National Patient Safety Goals Hospital Program.* Available at www.jointcommission.org/PatientSafety/NationalPatientSafetyGoals.

18. Yeager, K.A., et al. (2000). Implementation of an oral care standard for leukemia and transplantation patients. *Cancer Nursing, 23*(1), 40-47.

evolve *Did you remember to check out the bonus material on the Evolve website and the CD-ROM, including NCLEX®-Examination Style Review Questions, Open-Book Quizzes, and Chapter Review Audio Podcasts?*

http://evolve.elsevier.com/Black/medsurg

UNIT 18

MULTISYSTEM DISORDERS

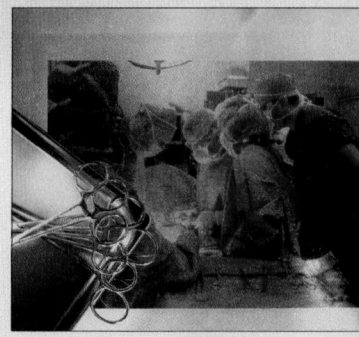

CHAPTER 80

Management of Clients Requiring Transplantation

CONNIE WHITE-WILLIAMS

The field of organ transplantation has evolved from the early beginnings of experimental kidney transplantation to the current practice of multiple organ transplantation. The advances made have been due largely to the increased knowledge in the areas of immunology and organ preservation, recipient and donor selection, and management of postoperative complications.

Organ transplantation is needed when an organ is irreversibly diseased or injured, leading to end-stage organ failure. Transplantation offers people with end-stage organ failure a chance to live longer and to overcome conditions that were once considered hopeless. Thus nurses have an increasing opportunity to care for clients with end-stage disease who are awaiting transplantation or who have undergone organ transplantation. In addition, nurses may also play a vital role in identification of potential donors and their management during the donor maintenance period.

HISTORICAL PERSPECTIVE

Transplantation had its beginnings in the 17th century with blood transfusions; however, the era of modern transplantation originated with a tooth replacement by John Hunter in the 18th century.[10] In 1912 Alexis Carrel developed the techniques for surgical suturing and vascular anastomosis that opened the pathway to solid organ transplantation.[9] Much of the work during the succeeding years focused on immunology, the importance of ABO and Rh blood group compatibility, and, later, the development of histocompatibility testing, all of which are crucial to organ transplantation today.[9,19] In 1945 Medawar[23] described the immune response of acute rejection, and by 1970 the relationship between donor and recipient histocompatibility in the role of acute rejection was recognized.[10]

Although many attempts at kidney transplantation were made in the early 1900s, it was not until 1954 that Merrell and Murray performed the first successful kidney transplantation between identical twin brothers.[10] Experimental heart transplantation took place in the early 1900s. In 1964 Hardy transplanted a chimpanzee heart (xenograft) into a 68-year-old man. In 1967 Barnard performed the first human-to-human heart transplantation.[5,10,16] The first lung transplantation was performed by Hardy in 1963.[10] Experimental liver transplantation began in the 1950s. The first human liver transplant was performed in 1963 by Starzl.[31] For a summary of the number of transplantation procedures reported by the United Network for Organ Sharing (UNOS), visit www.optn.org/data/annualreport.asp.[34]

With current success and survival statistics, these procedures are no longer deemed experimental. Organ transplantation is clearly an option for clients with end-stage organ disease. Much of the success is due to the availability of new immunosuppressive therapies, advances in organ preservation, improved surgical techniques, and the recognition of risk factors that affect survival after transplantation. Because transplant recipients

---

evolve Web Enhancements

Ethical Issues in Nursing Should Organ Procurement and Donation Be Discussed with the Dying and Their Families?

Do Clients with Transplants Have an Obligation to Comply with Their Post-Transplant Self-Care?

Are Health Care Workers Required to Continue Life- Supporting Interventions Until the Client's Body No Longer Responds?

Figures Transplantation Evaluation Summary Sheet

Tables Religious and Cultural Customs and Beliefs Related to Death and Organ Donation/Transplantation

Appendix A Religious Beliefs and Practices Affecting Health Care

Be sure to check out the bonus material on the Evolve website and the CD-ROM, including free self-assessment exercises. **http://evolve.elsevier. com/Black/medsurg**

now live longer, however, numerous social, economic, ethical, and quality of life (QOL) issues have arisen.

RELATED ISSUES

Cost

Average costs for the surgical procedure plus 5-year post-transplantation expenses are approximately $196,000 for kidney transplantation, $434,000 for heart transplantation, $361,000 for lung transplantation, and $394,000 for liver transplantation.[34] The Social Security Act was amended in 1972 to cover the cost of dialysis and transplantation for end-stage renal disease. Although coverage by private insurance companies, health maintenance organizations (HMOs), preferred provider organizations (PPOs), and Medicare/Medicaid has increased, the high cost remains a factor for clients who wish to undergo transplantation. In 1996 Medicare extended the coverage of immunosuppressive medications to 3 years after transplantation and then in 2001 to lifetime, which was a positive step toward helping clients financially.

Shortage of Organ Donors

The shortage of organ donors is the most significant limitation to transplantation. There are simply not enough organs for the thousands of clients waiting for transplantation. As of November 2007 the numbers of clients with end-stage disease waiting for an organ were as follows: 74,066 for a kidney, 2884 for a heart, 2841 for a lung, 17,471 for a liver, and 1767 for a pancreas.[27,34,35] (Because this information changes hourly, see www. unos.org/data/ for the most current data.[35]) Required request/referral and presumed consent programs are being implemented to increase organ donation. Also, the transplant community is investigating methods to increase donor organ supply. For example, redefining brain death to include cerebral death and anencephaly, use of xenotransplantation (transplanting organs from one species to another), and expanding the donor criteria to include older donors and living extrarenal donors (as in lobar transplantation of lung or liver) are all methods that increase donor organ supply.

Ethical Considerations

Many moral and ethical issues surround transplantation. Religious and cultural customs and beliefs related to death and organ donation and transplantation create challenges for health care professionals (see the website table on Religious and Cultural Customs and Beliefs *evolve* Related to Death and Organ Donation/Transplantation). As ways to increase the organ donor pool are explored, additional ethical dilemmas may be encountered. The future trends for transplantation include more living-related donation and new experimentation such as cell transplantation. It is important for nurses to be

knowledgeable about these issues and to communicate and discuss dilemmas with peers and professionals.

Definition of Death

Debate continues regarding the definition of death. The Uniform Determination of Death Act states that "an individual is considered dead if sustaining either (1) irreversible cessation of circulatory and respiratory function or (2) irreversible cessation of all functions of the entire brain, including the brain stem."[33] Different criteria are recognized for children and infants. In clients in chronic vegetative states or in anencephalic infants, brain stem function is intact but body and mental functions are not. Should death be redefined to include these people as donors? In transplantation, there will always be the dilemma of too few organs available in the face of the need to respect the life of people in a vegetative state who may be potential donors.

Buying and Selling of Organs

The National Organ Transplant Act of 1984 prohibits the sale of human organs and tissues. In addition, the Uniform Anatomical Gift Act of 1968 prohibits the sale or purchase of body parts or organs.[33] The conflict arises with respect to property rights. Supporters of organ sales believe that people own their bodies and have the right to do what they wish with their bodies—including the sale of their organs. The legal sale of blood plasma and sperm, which are body fluids, fuels the debate. The sale of organs in the United States is unlawful. A change in the law would alter the existing practice of free, altruistic donation.[15]

Prisoners as Donors or Recipients

A number of concerns arise in exploring solutions to the organ donor shortage. Once again, payment for organs enters the picture. Should prisoners be allowed to donate a kidney or bone marrow for a reduced sentence? This practice would not comply with current altruistic donation. In the same context, should a convicted criminal be allowed to be a transplant recipient? Some authorities believe that being a convicted criminal should not be an exclusion criterion, whereas others argue that it should be an exclusion criterion because of the prisoner's limited life expectancy outside prison.[15] Criminals may continue a life of crime outside of prison (drugs, guns, robberies), and therefore their chances of early death are greater.

Non–Heart-Beating Donors

Other potential organ donors are people who have experienced a respiratory or circulatory death. The hearts of these potential donors stop beating at the time of organ recovery. Ethical issues here involve the definition of brain death and determining when death occurs after asystole.

Xenotransplantation

Xenotransplantation—the transplantation of organs, tissues, or cells from one species to another (e.g., transplantation of a baboon heart into a human body)—has been proposed as one answer to the organ donor shortage. There are still many medical and ethical issues to consider with this concept. Medical issues include organ rejection, new modes of infection transmission, and incompatible immune system responses. Ethical considerations include informed consent, the use of animals as donors, potential benefits versus risks, and public health issues.[15]

OUTCOME MANAGEMENT

Clients with End-Stage Organ Disease
Referral and Recipient Selection

A primary responsibility of the transplant team is to transplant organs into clients who have the best chance for a long-term successful outcome. It is expected that the transplant recipient will experience an improvement in functional status, maintain long-term graft function, and enjoy improved QOL. This result is accomplished by the selection of an appropriate candidate. The transplant evaluation is a complex, multidisciplinary process that is usually initiated after a referral by the primary physician. The evaluation begins with an initial assessment of medical records and an examination of the client by the transplant team. On the basis of findings from the client's history and physical examination, the transplant team determines whether the client should undergo further evaluation for transplantation. Figure 80-1 shows the referral and evaluation process.

The goals of the evaluation process are to determine the following:

- The medical necessity for transplantation
- The surgical feasibility of the procedure
- Risk factors and the proper timing of transplantation
- Psychosocial suitability
- Immunologic status

The evaluation can be performed on either an inpatient or an outpatient basis and usually takes 3 to 5 days. During this period, extensive testing is completed, client education is provided, and the client and family members meet the members of the transplant team. Tests and procedures performed during the evaluation are listed in Box 80-1. These tests provide the transplant team with information regarding the status of all organ systems, infections, coexisting medical conditions, organ matching, and psychosocial issues that may affect the client and family. Psychosocial factors include

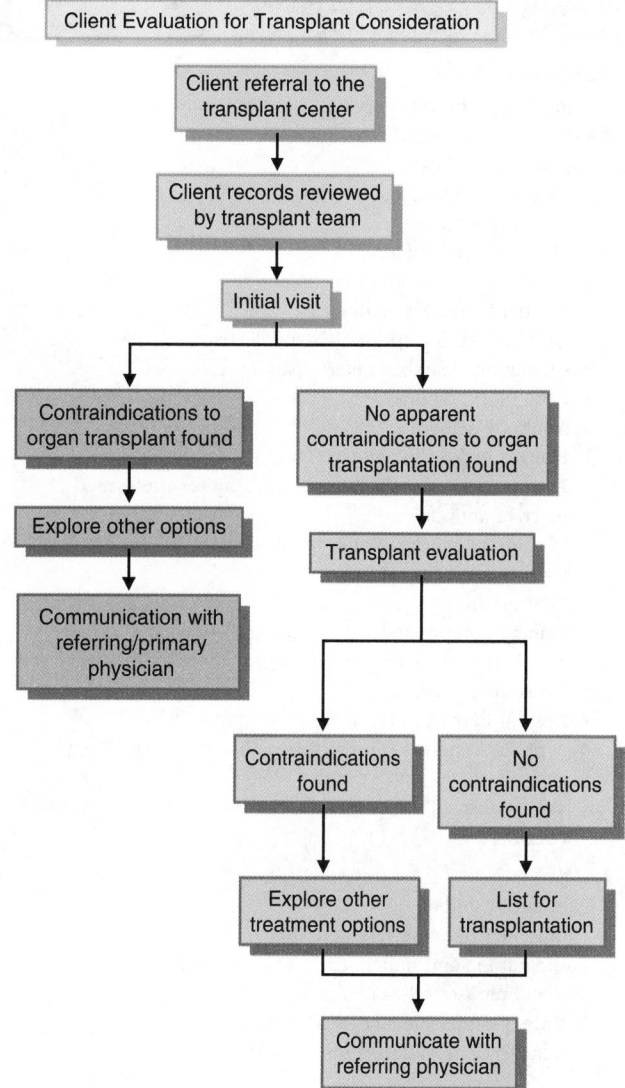

FIGURE 80–1 Client evaluation for transplantation.

neurocognitive status, coping skills, compliance history, availability of support systems, financial status, and extent of resources (Box 80-2). (See the website for an *evolve* example of an evaluation summary sheet to be completed for transplantation candidates.)

The details of the evaluation process may vary between transplant centers and with the organs being evaluated. It is important for you to understand the evaluation process and to know the indications for and contraindications to transplantation. In addition, preoperative education is an important responsibility of the nurse. The goal of education of the potential organ recipient is to provide the client and family with factual information regarding the waiting time for an organ, the surgical procedure, and the post-transplantation regimens, including diet, exercise, medication, routine follow-up, complications, and return to "normal" life expectations (return to work). Many centers provide this

---

BOX 80-1 **Evaluation for Organ Transplantation**

GENERAL
- Complete medical history and physical examination
- Psychiatric and social evaluation
- Laboratory studies
  - Electrolyte and metabolic profile
  - Liver function tests
  - Hematologic profile
  - Fasting cholesterol/lipid profile
  - Arterial blood gas analysis
  - Urinalysis, urine specific gravity determination
  - Creatinine clearance determination
  - ABO blood typing
  - Antibody screen
  - Human leukocyte antigen (HLA) tissue typing
  - Lymphocyte cytotoxicity screen (assay for preformed reactive antibodies)
- Virologic and microbiologic profile testing for the following:
  - Cytomegalovirus (CMV)
  - Toxoplasmosis
  - Human immunodeficiency virus (HIV)
- Hepatitis B surface antigen (HBsAg)
  - Hepatitis C antibody
  - Epstein-Barr virus (EBV)
  - Syphilis: Venereal Disease Research Laboratory (VDRL) assay
  - Tuberculosis: Purified protein derivative (PPD) testing with controls

KIDNEY
- Laboratory studies
- Glomerular filtration rate determination
- Radiographic and radionuclide scanning studies
  - Renal ultrasound examination
  - Kidney-ureter-bladder radiographic series
  - Renal radionuclide scanning

- Renal angiography
- Magnetic resonance imaging
- Renal biopsy
- Cystourethrography

HEART
- Radiographic and radionuclide scanning studies
  - Posteroanterior (PA) and lateral chest radiographs
  - Sinus and panoramic films
  - Resting radionuclide angiography
  - Pulmonary function tests
  - Ventilation-perfusion lung scan
  - Nuclear magnetic resonance imaging when indicated
  - Computed tomography (CT) studies when indicated
  - Resting and exercise gas exchange studies
- Cardiac catheterization
- Two-dimensional echocardiography
- Electrocardiography

LIVER
- Laboratory studies: additional blood work for diagnosis of specific liver disease may be indicated
- Radiographic and radionuclide scanning studies
  - Ultrasound examination of liver and biliary tree
  - CT scan of head
  - CT scan of abdomen with liver volumes
  - Endoscopic retrograde cholangiopancreatography
  - Percutaneous transhepatic cholangiogram
  - Pulmonary and cardiac evaluation

LUNG
- Radiographic and radionuclide scanning studies
  - CT scan of chest
  - Ventilation-perfusion scan
  - Pulmonary function tests
  - Cardiac evaluation

BOX 80-2 **Considerations in the Psychosocial Evaluation for Transplantation**

DEMOGRAPHICS
- Age
- Marital status
- Support systems

FINANCIAL
- Insurance
- Savings

SOCIAL HABITS
- Smoking
- Drinking

- Illicit drugs
- Coping skills

HEALTH MAINTENANCE
- Oxygen requirements
- Dialysis
- Compliance with medication regimen
- Compliance with clinical appointments

TRANSPORTATION
- Ability to get to clinic or hospital
- Travel time to transplantation center

HOME ENVIRONMENT
- Telephone
- Running water
- Trailer/home (e.g., financial? Steps? Cleanliness?)
- Heating and air-conditioning

---

education using several teaching skills, such as one-to-one teaching, group classes, and written information. The client uses this information to make an informed decision whether to undergo transplantation.

If contraindications are found during the transpla[n]t evaluation (Box 80-3), the transplant team reviews trea[t]ment options with the client and family. If no contrain[di]cations are found, the client can then be listed on th[e]

BOX 80-3   General Contraindications to Organ Transplantation

- Presence of active systemic infection (bacteremia, fungemia, viremia)
- HIV/AIDS
- Malignant disease (except skin cancer and some primary tumors of the diseased organ)
- Active peptic ulcer disease
- Active abuse of alcohol or other substances
- Severe damage to organ system(s) other than that to be transplanted (such as severe cardiovascular dysfunction in the potential liver transplant recipient)
- Severe psychiatric disease
- Demonstration of past or current inability to comply with a prescribed medical regimen
- Lack of a functional social support system
- Lack of sufficient financial resources to pay for surgery, hospitalization, medication, and follow-up care

---

national waiting list according to criteria established by UNOS, a nationwide system dedicated to the equitable sharing and distribution of donor organs.

Listing for Transplantation and Waiting for a Donor Organ

The criteria for listing a client for transplantation are governed by UNOS and vary according to the organ to be transplanted. These criteria include urgency, blood type, and recipient weight and height. Liver transplant candidates are assigned a MELD/PELD score, which is indicative of the severity of illness.[34] Likewise, lung transplant clients are assigned a lung allocation score (LAS), which assists in determining the order in which lung offers are made to transplant candidates. This score is a composite of diagnosis, pulmonary function test, and 6-minute walk results.[34]

Stable clients wait at home or near the transplant center. Many clients choose local housing, such as an apartment. A few centers provide hospital-owned housing dedicated to use by pretransplant and post-transplant clients and their families. Cellular telephones or beeper systems must be available to allow the transplant team to contact the client at any time. Usually, a client who lives at a distance from the transplant center requiring more than 2 hours' travel time must relocate or arrange air transportation to arrive at the center within an acceptable time.

Clients whose condition is unstable wait in the hospital, often in an intensive care unit. Some clients, particularly those awaiting heart transplantation, may live outside the hospital with continuous inotropic support. Intermittent hospitalization may be needed throughout the waiting period. Heart transplantation candidates who become hemodynamically unstable may need an intra-aortic balloon pump or a ventricular-assist device. Clients waiting for renal transplantation may be receiving dialysis, and those waiting for lung transplantation may require ventilator assistance. In liver transplantation candidates, mechanical assistance devices are not used during the wait for the transplant. Cardiac or pulmonary rehabilitation before transplantation is beneficial to optimize the client's strength and aerobic capacity.

Waiting for transplantation is perhaps the most stressful time for clients and families as they cope with terminal illness, altered lifestyles, financial strain, and impending surgery. Both the client and family members may experience feelings of anxiety, depression, and helplessness.[18,28,30] An often forgotten but important component of transplantation nursing is the care of clients with end-stage organ disease who are waiting for transplantation. The transplant nurse may care for clients while they wait in the hospital for a donor organ, in the clinic setting, or in the home. This wait may be days, months, or even years, and it is natural for the nurse to develop strong personal and professional relationships with these clients.

Along with the intense nursing that is involved in keeping the client alive during the waiting period, emotional stress may develop in nurses caring for these clients. It is important for nurses to have periodic meetings to discuss their feelings and difficult cases and to develop plans of care for the clients. More than 20 million people in the United States have chronic renal disease, whereas 400,000 have chronic kidney failure and receive dialysis each year.[25] Approximately 1.1 million Americans are expected to experience new or recurrent heart failure by the year 2010.[1] Cirrhosis is the fourth leading cause of death, accounting for 25,000 deaths yearly.[2] It is important for transplant nurses to understand that, although there may be many happy moments when an organ becomes available for the clients, there will also be tragedies when death occurs before an organ is located. Working with transplant clients can be both emotionally draining and frustrating during the waiting period for organ availability. Nurses can strive to provide excellent care for the client but they have little control over the availability of organs. It is important that emotional support be provided not only for transplant clients and their families but also for health care staff members and their families. Many centers have established support groups vital to the emotional well-being of the people involved.

During the waiting period, the nurse, as part of the transplant team, and the client with end-stage organ disease begin to establish a trusting relationship, participate in the client's education, and work together to grasp the realities of life after transplantation. Many clients and their families unrealistically expect that transplantation will cure all life's problems. The problems of end-stage organ disease may be resolved, but new problems associated with transplantation, including medication side effects, rejection, infections, and financial limitations, are frequently encountered. Help the client understand the post-transplantation regimen, and explain what to expect once the client is discharged from the hospital.

Organ Donation

The gifts of organ and tissue by donation are a vital part of transplantation. Without the gracious decision of the donor or donor family to give the "gift of life" by donation, there would be no post-transplantation miracles.

If the potential donor is a living relative, careful physical and psychosocial assessment is necessary. Potential donors must be psychologically evaluated as to their real desire to donate an organ, usually a kidney, and the ability to make a lifelong adjustment to having one kidney. To avoid conflict of interest, evaluation of the donor is commonly done by a team different from that caring for the recipient. Discussions with the donor should be held in strict confidence; if the potential donor decides not to donate, the medical team frequently cites a physical contraindication in order to allow continued acceptance of that person by the other family members.

Several legislative initiatives have advanced issues of donation and transplantation. In 1968 the Uniform Anatomical Gift Act, aimed at increasing volunteer organ donation, became law. Included in this law were the specifications for notifying legal next of kin of donation wishes, uniform donor cards, and designation of donation preference on the driver's license.[10] The National Transplant Act of 1984 addressed medical, legal, ethical, and social issues of donation such as requiring national scientific registries for assessment by the federal government and declaring it illegal to buy and sell human organs.[33] Also, the Organ Procurement and Transplant Network (OPTN) was established to create a national client registry and to coordinate organ allocation and distribution. UNOS is under contract from the U.S. Department of Health and Human Services to operate OPTN.[10]

The Omnibus Budget Reconciliation Act (OBRA) of 1986 requires hospitals to have written policies and procedures for identification and referral of potential donors. Under the 1987 Organ Donation Request Act, consideration of the donor's religious beliefs is mandated, and guidelines are set forth to guide the health care team's approach to next of kin for donor consent, attainment of consent, and notification of the organ procurement organization (OPO).

OBRA also requires transplant centers and OPOs to be members of OPTN. OPOs are nonprofit organ recovery services in the United States that constitute an integral link in the identification, acceptance, and management of the potential organ donor. In addition to the coordination of organ recovery, transplant procurement coordinators within the OPO provide professional and public education, assist hospitals during donor evaluation, and offer family counseling. Other responsibilities of the procurement coordinators are assisting in donor management, arranging transportation to and from the donor hospital, and assisting surgical personnel in the operating room. The procurement coordinator provides information to the clinical transplantation coordinator and the transplantation surgeon throughout the recovery process.[8,10]

OPOs are either hospital-based or independent. They must meet criteria mandated by the Health Care Finance Administration (HCFA), which includes (1) arranging for appropriate tissue typing, (2) demonstrating a working relationship with 75% of hospitals within the OPO area, (3) discussing accounting procedures, (4) providing a method of transport of donated organs, (5) submitting center-specific data, (6) cooperating with local tissue banks, and (7) having a governing board of directors.

Role of the Nurse in Organ Donation

The nurse plays an important role in organ donation and recovery with early identification of potential donors, making referrals to the OPO, and assisting in the medical management of the organ donor.[8] The nurse may act as a liaison with donor families or may be involved in the clinical management of the donor. This nursing role can be a very emotional experience. A nurse involved in this process must acknowledge the personal loss incurred when faced with the brain death of a donor client. The nurse then begins to focus on managing that client's vital systems until donation is completed.

The nurse's identification of a potential organ donor is a vital link to transplantation. To be a donor, a person must meet certain criteria, including sustaining an injury resulting in brain death.

The nurse may be the first to recognize the manifestations of brain death, including lack of responsiveness; absence of cough, gag, or corneal reflexes; and lack of response to painful stimuli. These findings should be reported to the physician. Refer all clients who meet brain death criteria to the local OPO.[8] It is most often a nurse who notifies the OPO of the potential donor. Notification should occur when brain death is imminent, to allow the procurement coordinator to become familiar with the potential donor's case. Figure 80-2 depicts the organ donor referral and triage procedure.

The first step in the donation process is awareness of potential organ donors. Organ donors are people who have suffered an injury leading to brain death

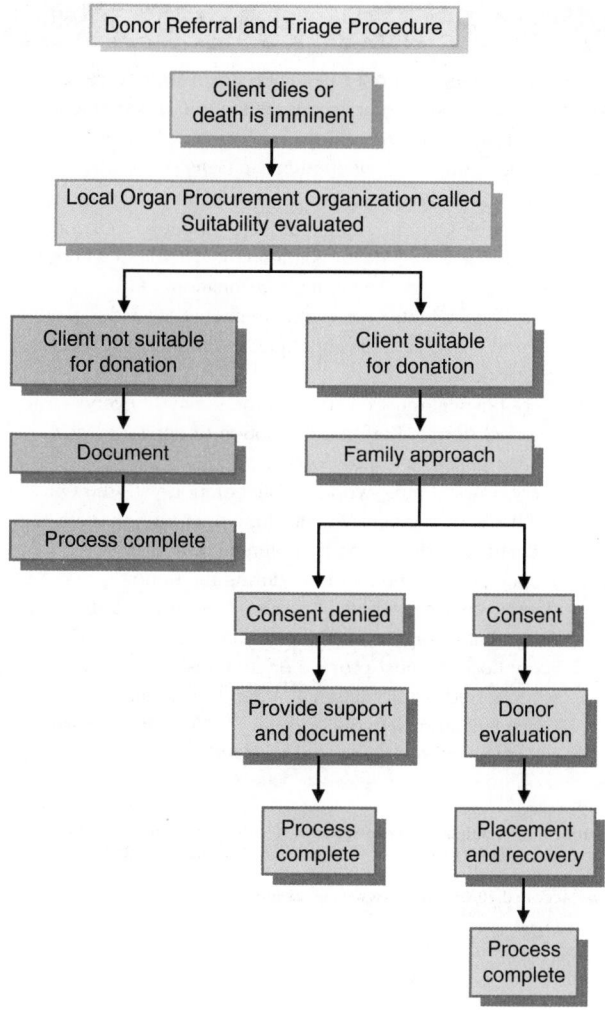

FIGURE 80–2   Organ recovery process.

thermoregulation. The ideal organ donor is a person whose fatal injury resulted in brain death but who was otherwise healthy and infection-free. Criteria for organ donation are listed in Box 80-4.

Initiation of the organ donor process should proceed according to hospital policy. Organ recovery occurs in the operating room only after (1) identifying a potential donor, (2) notifying an OPO, (3) diagnosing brain death, (4) obtaining family consent, and (5) managing the donor until organ removal is complete.

Organ Recovery

Multiple organ procurement, or recovery of more than one type of organ from a single donor, is standard practice. As many as four separate surgical teams may be present in the operating room, each focusing on recovery of one organ. Usually, a separate surgical team prepares the recipient for the new organ. After a midline incision is made, dissection of organs occurs. Once cross-clamping of the aorta is done and cardioplegia is begun, the heart is removed. Then lungs, liver, and finally kidneys are procured.

The organs are preserved in a cold storage solution selected by the transplant center. Examples of such solutions are University of Wisconsin solution (UW solution), Euro-Collins solution, Belzer's solution, and other, institution-specific solutions. Organs are preserved in a sterile storage solution, packed in ice, and transported in a cooler to the recipient.

Viability times for donated organs vary. Standard periods after organ recovery are as follows: for kidney, 48 to 72 hours; for heart, 4 to 5 hours; for lung, 4 to 6 hours; for liver, 24 to 30 hours; and for pancreas, 24 hours. For successful transplantation, the timing of organ removal, transport, and preparation of the recipient is essential. Surgical transplantation procedures for specific organs are discussed in their respective chapters.

Preparation of Recipient

While the procurement coordinator manages and coordinates the donor process, the clinical transplant coordinator manages and coordinates the preparation of the potential recipient. The potential recipient (or recipients—in many cases a second client is also told to come to the hospital in case the transplant team encounters a problem with use of the donated organ in the primary potential recipient) is admitted to the hospital and immediately prepared for surgery. Preparation involves obtaining blood work, administering preoperative medications, and performing other standard preoperative interventions such as shaving and skin preparation. Preparation of the recipient may become a race against the clock as the transplant team works within the time constraints of organ viability.

The most common causes of injury are head trauma, strokes, subarachnoid hemorrhage, and primary brain tumors. Once a potential donor is identified, the organ procurement agency should be notified. The next steps are documentation of brain death and family consent of donation.

Next, medical management of the potential donor begins. The goal of donor management is to maintain optimal conditions, ensuring functional and infection-free organs for transplantation. This goal is accomplished by the diligent management of hydration and tissue perfusion, oxygenation, infection control, diuresis, and temperature regulation. Guidelines that have been helpful in maintaining organ viability include the "rules of 100's," in which (1) systolic blood pressure is maintained at 100 mm Hg, (2) urine output at 100 ml/hour, (3) heart rate at 100 beats/min, and (4) Pao_2 at 100 mm Hg.[8] Common problems encountered in management of the potential donor are hypotension, shock, electrolyte imbalances, disseminated intravascular coagulation (DIC), and loss of

---

BOX 80-4   **Conditions of Participation for Organ Donation**

CONDITIONS OF PARTICIPATION

The Department of Health and Human Services (HHS), in an attempt to optimize donor potential and abate the critical shortage of organs for transplantation, issued the Hospital Conditions of Participation (COP) for Medicare and Medicaid on June 22, 1998. This rule took effect on August 21, 1998, and requires all U.S. hospitals to adopt a "routine notification" policy or mandates that hospitals have and implement written protocols to ensure that the organ procurement organization (OPO) is notified of all deaths. According to the COP, the hospital must, "in a timely fashion," notify the OPO of individuals who die or whose death is imminent," thus eliminating the need for hospital staff to identify a potential donor.* All patients who die should be considered a potential organ and/or tissue donor.

     Routine notification ensures that an individual who is most familiar with the current criteria on donation, specifically the OPO, evaluates every individual who dies to determine suitability for donation. If the policy were consistently followed, routine notification would make it virtually impossible for the hospital not to refer all potential organ donors. Thus routine notification places the decision making and determination of medical suitability for a person to be a donor in the hands of the procurement and transplant community, not in the hands of hospital staff.

This rule is designed not to exclude hospital professionals from the process but, rather, to ensure that the procurement professionals are included.

     Five stipulations are contained in the COP:

- A hospital must have an agreement with an OPO and must contact the OPO in a timely manner about all individuals who die or whose death is imminent. The OPO will then determine medical suitability for donation.
- Every hospital must have an agreement with a designated eye and tissue bank to cooperate in the recovery of eyes and tissues.
- Every hospital must ensure that the family of every potential donor is offered the option to donate organs and/or tissues or not to donate.
- Every hospital must work in collaboration with the OPO and tissue or eye bank in educating their staff, participating in death records to identify potential donors, and maintaining potential donors during the donor management period while necessary testing and the placement of organs and tissues take place.
- Every hospital must provide organ-transplant–related data, as requested by the national Organ Procurement and Transplantation Network and the U.S. Scientific Registry of Transplant Recipients and the OPOs.[†]

Source: United Network for Organ Sharing.
* Final Rule: *Federal Register,* Vol. 63, No. 119, June 22, 1998. 42 CFR Part 482.4.5. Department of Health and Human Services: Health Care Financing Administration. Medicare and Medicaid Programs; Hospital Conditions of Participation; Identification of Potential Organ, Tissue and Eye Donors and Transplant Hospitals, Provision of Transplant Related Data.
[†] From Chabalewski, F.L., et al. *Donation and transplantation: Into the new millennium.* Accessed 10/05/2000 at www.medscape.com.

Postoperative Transplant Clients

Management of the post-transplant client involves an intensive collaborative effort of the various members of the transplant team. The transplant team consists of transplant surgeons and other physicians, nurse coordinators, social workers, pharmacists, psychologists, nurse practitioners, nutritionists, members of the clergy, staff nurses, and consultants. Depending on which organ is transplanted, usually the same team members provide care to clients from initial referral throughout the client's lifetime. In many cases, kidney or liver transplant recipients return to their referring physicians for long-term care. Nursing care should be designed to recognize life-threatening clinical problems, to prevent complications, and to promote the client's return to normal activities with improved QOL. These goals are discussed in the Bridge to Critical Care feature on p. 2145.

Basic Immunology Related to Transplantation

To effectively care for the transplant client, you must understand basic immunology concepts related to transplantation (see Chapters 74 and 76). The immune response elicits mechanisms that direct the body to

recognize transplanted organs as foreign (non-self). Although this immune response is normal, it is the goal of immunosuppressive agents to alter this immune response in transplanted clients.

     The innate or nonspecific immune responses consist of natural mechanisms for the protection of the client against foreign antigens. These natural defenses are present at birth, lack memory, and do not need prior exposure for antigens to develop. Innate immunity mechanisms include physical barriers, chemical barriers, and leukocyte reactions, all of which play a role in the body's immune response.

     Acquired or specific immunity involves mechanisms elicited by the lymphoid system. Lymphoid cells include plasma cells and lymphocytes. Lymphocytes constitute 30% of the white blood cells (WBCs) and are responsible for the recognition of antigens. These lymphocyte defense mechanisms recognize foreign antigens and can elicit rejection of transplanted organs. Two types of lymphocytes can elicit a response: B lymphocytes, which mediate a humoral immune response through the production of antibodies; and T lymphocytes, which are derived from maturing stem cells in the thymus and act to defend the body by interaction with an antigen with

Solid Organ Transplantation

CORE BODY TEMPERATURE CHANGES

The client arrives at the intensive care unit directly from the operating room with the anesthetic agents unreversed. Postoperative hypothermia prolongs clearance of the anesthetic agents and can lead to other complications such as cardiac dysrhythmias, altered platelet function, and decreased oxygen delivery to the tissues. Nursing measures in the early postoperative phase are directed toward supporting and assisting the client while the core body temperature returns to normal. Warming blankets, heat lamps, commercially available rewarming devices, and head covers are important measures to expedite rewarming of the client. Frequent monitoring of arterial blood pressure, cardiac rhythm, central venous pressure, pulmonary artery pressures, and core body temperature is essential during this phase. Arterial blood pressure, systemic vascular resistance, and cardiac output are expected to decrease as core body temperature rises and vasodilation occurs; thus additional support measures often are required during this time of instability.

EARLY GRAFT DYSFUNCTION

The intensive care nurse must be aware of the manifestations of early graft dysfunction. During the first 24 hours, serologic laboratory findings, physical assessments, and objective hemodynamic measurements must be critically evaluated frequently for indications of graft function.

Organ	Indicators of Adequate Early Graft Function
Kidney	High-volume urine output
	Decreasing BUN and creatinine levels
	Normal serum potassium level
	Normal serum glucose level
	Nontender over graft (avoiding incision)
Heart	Normal cardiac output and cardiac index
	Decreasing to normal CVP
	Decreasing to normal PAP and PCWP
	Normal SVR
	Normal sinus rhythm with a ventricular rate of 90-100 beats/min
	Normal LVEF (>55%) by echocardiogram
	Normal S_1, S_2 heart sounds (pericardial rub may be present)
	Decreasing mediastinal drainage (<200 ml/hr in first 4 hr)
Lung	Normal Pao_2
	Normal CO_2 concentration
	Normal oxygen saturation
	Breath sounds clear and present in all allograft lung fields
	Decreasing pleural drainage
	Chest radiograph clear and well expanded
Liver	Adequate bile output
	Decreasing AST and ALT levels
	Increasing serum protein levels
	Normal to slightly elevated serum glucose level

ALT, Alanine aminotransferase; *AST,* aspartate aminotransferase; *CVP,* central venous pressure; *LVEF,* left ventricular ejection fraction; *PAP,* pulmonary artery pressure; *PCWP,* pulmonary capillary wedge pressure; *SVR,* systemic vascular resistance.

a sensitized T lymphocyte.[16,18,26,32,36] There are regulator (T helper and T suppressor) and effector (cytotoxic and memory) T lymphocytes.

In humans, the genetic factor used to determine specific antigen recognition is called the major histocompatibility complex (MHC). The MHC is the human leukocyte antigen (HLA) gene complex, located on chromosome 6. Antigens of the HLA complex are divided into two classes: class I comprises HLA types A, B, and C; class II consists of HLA types DR, DQ, and DP. Histocompatibility testing is used to minimize specific immune responses to the transplanted organ. The type of histocompatibility testing varies according to the organ transplanted and with time limitations.

Before transplantation, the potential recipient undergoes ABO typing, Rh typing, and HLA tissue typing. An assay for preformed reactive antibodies (PRAs) determines the presence of preformed antibodies to HLA antigens. Results range from 0% to 100%. If a potential recipient is found to have antibodies against specific HLA antigens, a donor organ with those antigens is not suitable for transplantation.

Several types of crossmatching procedures can be performed to identify the presence of antibodies in the potential recipient to antigens located on the lymphocytes of the potential donor. A positive result on crossmatching means that antibodies are present, and transplantation is usually inadvisable because of the associated higher risk of rejection. A negative result on crossmatching means that no antibodies are present, with a reduced risk of rejection.

Immunosuppression

The goal of immunosuppressive therapy involves the delicate balance of adequately suppressing the immune response to prevent organ rejection without developing complications from the therapy itself.

SAFETY
ALERT

This intricate balance of the immunosuppressive med-ication regimen is individualized for each client and is maintained throughout the client's lifetime. The trans-plant team aims to keep the dose of each drug within the therapeutic range. Management of the immuno-suppressive regimen is crucial to long-term outcomes in post-transplant clients; for example, excessive immunosuppression may lead to increased risk of infection, liver or kidney insufficiency, joint necrosis, cataracts, or malignancies, whereas inadequate immu-nosuppression may lead to rejection of the trans-planted organ. Although in many cases long-term graft acceptance can be maintained with less drug as time passes, most clients require immunosuppression for life to prevent rejection of the transplanted organ.[16]

Immunosuppressive agents are used in the post-transplant population in three categories of use: induction, maintenance, and antirejection. Specific agents and dosages vary according to category of use. Protocols are dependent on the type of organs trans-planted, transplant center–specific practices, and the client's history and current health status. See the Integ-rating Pharmacology feature on Immunosuppressive Agents Used in Transplantation. Most transplant centers use multiple-drug regimens containing agents that act on various functions of the immune system as well as minimize side effects. Many new immunosuppressant medications are being developed and tested in the United States and Europe.

Complications
Rejection

SAFETY
ALERT

Transplantation of allografts (organs transplanted between genetically different individuals in the same species) elicits an immune response in which the anti-gens in tissue of the transplanted organ are recog-nized as foreign; hence a series of events occurs, resulting in rejection of the organ. Rejection is classi-fied into three types: (1) hyperacute, (2) acute, and (3) chronic (Figure 80-3).[16,32]

Hyperacute Rejection. Hyperacute rejection can occur within minutes to hours of implantation of the organ. It is caused by the presence of antibodies. Usually, a destructive humoral or B-cell reaction to antigens on the vascular endothelium results in organ necrosis. Most hyperacute rejection episodes can be prevented by previous panel-reactive antibody (PRA) assay, histo-compatibility testing, and crossmatching. If hyper-acute rejection occurs, treatment options are limited. Clients who have received kidney or kidney-pancreas transplants may need to return to dialysis. Clients who have received other organ transplants may receive

INTEGRATING PHARMACOLOGY

Immunosuppressive Agents Used in Transplantation

Following transplantation, clients require continuous immunosuppression to prevent rejection of the transplanted organ. These immunosuppressive agents are often given in a combination of two to three agents that may vary from one transplant center to another. There are several classifications of immunosuppressive agents: (1) calcineurin inhibitors (also known as interleukin-2 [IL-2] inhibitors); (2) antiproliferatives; and (3) antibodies.

Calcineurin inhibitors are used to prevent and treat organ rejection and include agents such as cyclosporine (Sandimmune, Neoral, Gengraf), corticosteroids, tacrolimus (Prograf), and sirolimus (Rapamune). These drugs inhibit calcineurin and thereby suppress production of T lymphocytes, suppress T lymphocyte activity, and inhibit production of interleukin-2.

Antiproliferative agents are used to prevent organ rejection and include azathioprine (Imuran), mycophenolate mofetil (CellCept), methotrexate, and cyclophosphamide (Cytoxan). These drugs inhibit proliferation of T and B lymphocytes and interfere with DNA and RNA synthesis.

Antibodies are divided into monoclonal antibodies (muromonab-CD3 [Orthoclone OKT3], daclizumab [Zenapax], basiliximab [Simulect]) or polyclonal antibodies (Thymo-globulin, antithymocyte globulin [ATG]). These drugs inhibit T lymphocyte function, decrease the number of circulating lymphocytes, or block IL-2, which inhibits the activation of lymphocytes. They are used to prevent and treat organ rejection.

Because the client receiving immunosuppressive agents is at increased risk of infection, the client must be taught to recognize the clinical manifestations of infection as well as rejection. Many of the medications may cause serious side effects such as hypertension, fatigue, tremor, diabetes mellitus, renal dysfunction, cataracts, obesity, and various gastro-intestinal manifestations such as nausea, vomiting, bleeding, and diarrhea. These problems may also require medical or surgical management.

plasmapheresis, a procedure that removes circulating antibodies from the blood. If this measure fails, retrans-plantation is indicated.

Acute Rejection. Acute rejection usually occurs in the first 3 months after transplantation; however, it can occur at any time, particularly if the immunosuppression regi-men is altered or if an infection develops. Acute rejection can be a purely cellular immune response mediated by T cells or an antibody-mediated response, or a combina-tion of the two.[16,18,26,32] Diagnosis is based on clinical manifestations, laboratory data, or results of tests such

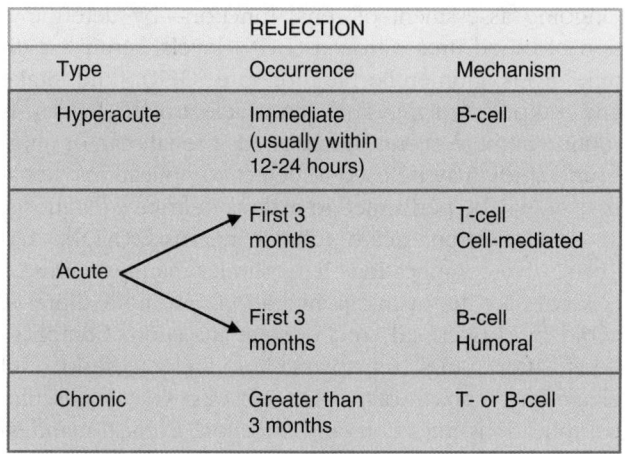

REJECTION		
Type	Occurrence	Mechanism
Hyperacute	Immediate (usually within 12-24 hours)	B-cell
Acute	First 3 months	T-cell Cell-mediated
	First 3 months	B-cell Humoral
Chronic	Greater than 3 months	T- or B-cell

■ **FIGURE 80–3**   Transplant rejection.

as organ biopsy. Clinical manifestations of rejection are listed in Box 80-5. Treatment usually consists of high-dose steroids; if recurrent episodes occur, muromonab-CD3 (Orthoclone OKT3) may be administered.

Chronic Rejection. Chronic rejection evolves gradually, usually after the first 3 months after transplantation. It may be the result of frequent episodes of acute rejection, increased ischemic time, or cytomegalovirus (CMV) infection. Chronic rejection results in progressive loss of graft function. The transplanted organ develops a persistent, perivascular inflammation associated with focal myocyte necrosis. Chronic rejection is treated in a similar fashion to test for acute rejection; however, retransplantation may be required as a result of the progressive deterioration of organ function.

Infection

Infection is the leading cause of morbidity and mortality after transplantation. Many factors contribute to the potential risk of infection, including the client's age, nutritional status, medical condition before transplantation, infection history and exposure, and the immunosuppressive regimen. Infections seen in transplant recipients are usually the result of immunosuppression or altered immune defenses.[18,26,36] During the first month after transplantation, nosocomial infections are common; then, between 1 and 6 months after transplantation, opportunistic infections such as *Pneumocystis (carinii) jiroveci* pneumonia, candidiasis, and CMV infection occur.[26,36] The lungs are the most common site for infection, followed by blood, urine, and the gastrointestinal tract. Common infections seen in transplant recipients are listed in Table 80-1. Infection is the most common indication for hospital readmission after transplantation.[13,36]

Malignancy

The development of post-transplantation malignancies caused by the immunodeficient state is well documented.[26,36] Types of malignancies seen in the post-transplantation population include basal cell and squamous cell carcinomas of the skin and lip, seen most commonly, followed by the lymphoproliferative disorders and cancers of the vulva, perineum, and lungs. Reduction in the level of immunosuppression, surgical resection, chemotherapy, and radiation therapy are treatment options.

SAFETY ALERT

All clients should be screened for development of cancer after transplantation. Routine gynecologic examinations, including mammography and cervical smear in women, annual prostate-specific antigen (PSA) testing in men, and regular physical examination of neck and groin lymph nodes, should be performed to detect any problems. Report any unusual lesions to the transplant team. In addition, monitor clients who are seronegative for Epstein-Barr virus for conversion to seropositivity, which may place them at higher risk for lymphoproliferative disease after transplantation. Clients need to be educated to use sunscreen products with a sun protection factor (SPF) of 15 or greater and to wear protective clothing to help prevent skin malignancies.

Clients Receiving a Specific Organ Transplant
Renal Transplantation

The potential renal transplant recipient has end-stage renal disease, most commonly the result of hypertension, diabetic nephropathy, or a hereditary or congenital disorder.[7,25] In most cases, the renal transplant candidate is anemic and fatigued and has been maintained by chronic hemodialysis (see Chapter 36). Contraindications to renal transplantation include seropositivity for the human immunodeficiency virus (HIV), active infection, severe coronary artery disease with left ventricular dysfunction, malignancy, severe peripheral vascular

TABLE 80-1 Common Infections After Transplantation

Infecting Organism	Site(s) Affected	Therapeutic Agent of Choice
Bacteria		
Gram-negative bacilli		Ticarcillin-clavulanate (Timentin)
Klebsiella	Lung	
Pseudomonas	Blood	
Escherichia coli	CNS	Gentamicin
Legionella	Lung	
Enterobacter		
Gram-positive cocci		Vancomycin
Enterococci		
Staphylococci		
Streptococci		
Viruses		
Cytomegalovirus	Lung	Ganciclovir
	Blood	
	GI tract	
Varicella-zoster virus	Skin	Acyclovir
	Blood	
Protozoa		
Toxoplasma gondii	Transplanted organ	Pyrimethamine Sulfadiazine
	Lung	Folinic acid
	Liver	
Pneumocystis jiroveci	Lung	Trimethoprim-sulfamethoxazole
Fungi		
Aspergillus	Lung	Amphotericin B
	CNS	
Candida	Oral mucosa	Nystatin Fluconazole Amphotericin B

CNS, Central nervous system; *GI,* gastrointestinal.

disease, severe carotid artery disease, and chronic active hepatitis.

Unlike the heart, lung, liver, or pancreas transplant candidate, the kidney transplant candidate has several potential donors: living related, living nonrelated, and cadaver. Eighty-five percent of all renal transplants are from cadaveric donors.

Extensive histocompatibility testing is completed for renal transplantation, because evidence indicates that six antigen matches are necessary for long-term graft survival. Six-antigen-matching means that six antigens recognized on recipient HLA tissue typing match six antigens found on donor HLA tissue typing. A negative result on crossmatching is required for transplantation to occur.

Nursing Care

Nursing care of the renal transplant recipient is focused on the recognition and prevention of complications.

Ongoing assessment of renal function—by determination of blood urea nitrogen (BUN) levels, serum creatinine levels, glomerular filtration rate (GFR), fluid intake and output, weight, and serum electrolyte levels—is routine in these clients. If indicated, a renal scan or ultrasound study may be used to detect complications. Renal biopsy may be performed to make a definitive diagnosis, in that rejection, acute tubular necrosis (ATN), and obstructive complications have similar manifestations.

Goals are to maintain hydration, promote diuresis, avoid fluid overload, and prevent infection. Complications after renal transplantation include fluid and electrolyte imbalances, ATN, obstructive or vascular complications, rejection, and infection. Clinical manifestations of potential complications in the renal transplant client are decreased urine output, graft tenderness or pain, increasing serum creatinine level, fever, and weight gain.

Pancreas and Pancreas-Kidney Transplantation

Pancreas transplantation is indicated for the client with type 1 diabetes mellitus to restore normal glucose metabolism.[11] Pancreas-kidney transplantation is performed in the diabetic client with end-stage renal disease (see Chapter 45).[11] Contraindications are the same as those for renal transplantation.

Nursing Care

Nursing care includes monitoring for fluid and electrolyte imbalances, especially BUN, serum creatinine, bicarbonate, and CO_2 levels. Urine amylase is also monitored to assess pancreatic function. With combined kidney-pancreas transplantation, clinical manifestations of graft thrombosis are a sudden increase in blood glucose concentration, severe graft pain, and increased serum creatinine level.

Heart Transplantation

Potential candidates for heart transplantation are usually New York Heart Association class III or class IV clients who are generally younger than age 65 years and have a life expectancy of less than 12 months. The most common diseases treated by heart transplantation are coronary artery disease and cardiomyopathy.[13,17] Contraindications to heart transplantation include malignancy; active infection; autoimmune disorders; irreversible kidney, lung, or liver disease; and severely elevated pulmonary vascular resistance. Relative contraindications, which vary between transplant centers, are peptic ulcer disease, stroke, peripheral vascular disease, diabetes mellitus, and obesity.[17]

When listed for transplantation, candidates are evaluated periodically, usually every 4 to 6 weeks, to monitor their overall condition. Clients whose condition is stable wait at home or near the hospital, and clients whose condition is hemodynamically unstable wait at the hospital. Clients who become critically ill may need continuous inotropic infusions or ventricular-assist devices.

Cardiac Transplantation Physiology Alterations

Unique to the cardiac transplant recipient is cardiac transplant denervation. Denervation occurs after orthotopic transplantation, in which the vagus nerve is severed. The lack of vagal nerve stimulation results in (1) a higher resting heart rate, (2) a gradual increase in heart rate with exercise and delayed return to baseline, (3) absence of angina, and (4) enhanced response to certain drugs (e.g., adrenaline, adenosine) and decreased response to other drugs (e.g., atropine, digoxin).[6,17] Finally, two P waves may be detected on the electrocardiogram resulting from the presence of both donor and recipient heart sinoatrial (SA) nodes. It is important to note that only the donor heart SA node regulates the electrical conduction of the heart.

Nursing Care

The nursing assessment is a vital component in the care of the cardiac transplant recipient. The physical assessment should include auscultation of heart and breath sounds and assessment of pedal pulses and of the jugular vein for distention. Ongoing assessment of renal and liver function and monitoring of immunosuppressant drug levels and the complete blood cell count (CBC) are important in the overall care of the client. Complications seen after heart transplantation include organ dysfunction, rejection, infection, coronary vasculopathy, and malignancy.[6,17] Chest radiography is used to monitor possible lung infection, whereas echocardiography and endomyocardial biopsy are used to detect rejection. Clinical manifestations of rejection include fever, shortness of breath, fatigue, presence of S_3 or S_4 heart sound, decreased blood pressure, decreased ejection fraction, and jugular vein distention.

Liver Transplantation

Indications for liver transplantation include chronic irreversible liver disease resulting from a number of underlying disorders. In adults, the most common indications are cirrhosis secondary to chronic hepatitis, cryptogenic cirrhosis, primary biliary cirrhosis, and primary sclerosing cholangitis (see Chapter 47).[20,21] Contraindications to liver transplantation are center-specific and may include portal vein thrombosis, active alcoholism, active infection, malignancy outside the hepatobiliary system, and advanced cardiopulmonary disease. The client evaluation takes into account technical feasibility and optimal timing of surgery in addition to the usual physical and psychosocial indications.

Nursing Care

The postoperative care of the liver transplant client is complex. Nursing care focuses on monitoring graft function, managing fluid and electrolyte imbalances, preventing problems with other organ systems, and assessing for manifestations of rejection or infection. Clinical manifestations of rejection include fever, elevation of liver enzymes, and change in color, amount, and consistency of bile drainage through the T tube.

Diagnosis of rejection is confirmed by liver biopsy. In addition, a sudden increase in the International Normalized Ratio (INR) (a system for reporting prothrombin values), serum bilirubin level, or levels of liver enzymes may indicate a complication such as hepatic artery thrombosis or biliary obstruction. If neurologic status is affected, serum ammonia levels may be monitored. Finally, as in all organ transplantation procedures, renal function, immunosuppressant drug levels, and white blood cell (WBC) counts should be closely monitored.

Lung Transplantation

The lung transplantation candidate has end-stage pulmonary disease and (1) is generally younger than 65 years of age for single-lung transplantation, 60 years for two-lung transplantation, or 55 years for heart-lung transplantation and (2) is able to participate in pulmonary rehabilitation (i.e., is not wheelchair-dependent).[3,6,37] The decision whether to perform a single-lung or double-lung procedure varies among transplant centers but is based on the likelihood of achieving the best outcome and most improvement in QOL.

Contraindications to lung transplantation are active malignancy, positive results on hepatitis B antigen assay, hepatitis C infection, autoimmune disorders, and dysfunction of organs other than the lungs. Risk factors that affect eligibility include symptomatic osteoporosis, the need for steroid therapy in doses greater than 20 mg/day, severe musculoskeletal disease, impaired nutritional status (malnutrition or obesity), the need for mechanical ventilation, and colonization with fungi or atypical mycobacteria.

Lung Transplantation Physiology Alterations

Removal of the native lung and lung replacement entail denervation of the transplanted lung. Denervation interferes with autonomic nervous system communication, resulting in dysfunctional ciliary movement, loss of cough reflex, and changes in mucus production, which lead to ineffective clearance of airway secretions. Health maintenance interventions to maintain patent airways are chest vibropercussion, postural drainage, and use of an incentive spirometer.

Nursing Care

The postoperative care of the lung transplant recipient is gratifying. It is a pleasure to watch an oxygen-dependent client who once gasped for breath become an active person requiring no oxygen after transplantation. Immunosuppressant drug levels, electrolyte determinations, liver function tests, CBC, chest radiography, and pulmonary function tests are important monitoring tests in this population.

Complications include surgical side effects, graft dysfunction, rejection, infection, and bronchiolitis obliterans or obliterating bronchiolitis (OB).[3,6,37] OB is the greatest limiting factor to long-term survival after lung transplantation. OB is progressive in nature, resulting in severe shortness of breath, and must be treated aggressively. Usual medical management may include administration of intravenous steroids, cytolytic therapy (with OKT3), administration of Thymoglobulin, photopheresis, and retransplantation. Goals in nursing management are to prevent and recognize complications and to promote return to a functional lifestyle.

Self-Care

Before discharge from the hospital, pertinent information is discussed with the client and family members. Postoperative education after transplantation can be challenging, because many clients are discharged between 1 and 2 weeks after surgery. Many institutions provide client education booklets. Information discussed with the client and family is presented in Box 80-6.

Of special importance are knowledge of the clinical manifestations of rejection and infection and indications for contacting the transplant team. A schedule of return appointments is usually given at discharge. Most clients reside close to the transplant center for 2 to 8 weeks before going home. This proximity allows for frequent medical visits, ongoing education, and familiarization of the client with the postoperative regimen. It also allows the client to become more independent and resume self-care responsibilities. Often it is the nurse who is best able to monitor compliance with the medical regimen and to identify difficulty coping with the post-transplantation regimen. Once the client returns home, it may be necessary for a home health nurse to provide wound care, perform intravenous infusions, or perform other nursing care measures. Findings on home visits are communicated to the transplant coordinator. Box 80-7 lists nursing diagnoses related to care of the post-transplant client.

Meticulous follow-up evaluation (assessing for manifestations of rejection, infection, or other complications)

BOX 80-7 Nursing Diagnoses for the Post-Transplant Client

- *Risk for Imbalanced Nutrition: More Than Body Requirements related to side effects of immunosuppressant agents/Less Than Body Requirements related to increased caloric needs after transplantation*
- *Ineffective Protection and Risk for Infection related to immunosuppression required after organ transplantation*
- *Readiness for Enhanced Self-Care and Deficient Knowledge related to post-transplantation regimen*
- *Pain related to transplantation surgery*
- *Risk for Ineffective Coping after transplantation related to increased stress, anxiety, fear, and lifestyle changes*
- *Risk for Injury: rejection of transplanted organ related to impaired immunocompetence; malignancy/diabetes mellitus/hypertension related to immunosuppression*

BOX 80-6 Client and Family Education After Transplantation

- Members of transplantation team
- When to call the transplant coordinator
- Immunosuppression
  - Administration of medications
  - Side effects of medications
- Rejection
  - Definition, manifestations, diagnosis, treatment
- Infection
  - Definition, manifestations, diagnosis, treatment
- Routine care
  - Temperature
  - Weight
  - Skin care
  - Incision care
  - Fluid intake and output

- Pedal pulses
- Incentive spirometry
- Clinic schedule
- Diet after transplantation
- Activities after transplantation
  - Precautions
  - Exercise
  - Physical therapy
- Self-care
  - Blood pressure
  - Blood glucose levels
  - Medical identification bracelet and card
  - Sun exposure
  - Sexual activity
  - Sending specimens for laboratory monitoring tests

- Vacations
- Over-the-counter medicines to be avoided
- Driving
- Birth control
- Psychosocial issues
  - Physical appearance
  - Family participation and support
  - Writing to the donor family
  - Cost of transplantation
- Health maintenance
  - Dental care
  - Ophthalmologic examinations
  - Gynecologic examinations
  - Yearly evaluations of transplant

is essential to the long-term well-being of the post-transplant client. Long-term care of the transplant recipient requires communication between the client and transplant team. Each client should be assessed for infection, rejection, malignancy, organ dysfunction, and adverse manifestations of immunosuppression such as diabetes mellitus, hypertension, hyperlipidemia, abnormalities on liver function testing, and gastrointestinal distress.

Psychosocial issues that should be investigated are financial status, family dynamics, and ability to return to work. The social worker at the transplant center can assist the client with insurance questions, medication assistance programs, and ways of dealing with the financial stresses of transplantation. Coping with QOL may also be an issue for the transplant client, as discussed in the Translating Evidence into Practice feature below.

Health maintenance areas to evaluate are screening by mammography and Papanicolaou (Pap) smears in women, colon cancer screening, and immunizations such as with the influenza vaccine and pneumococcal vaccine (Pneumovax). Routine dental and ophthalmologic examinations should be scheduled. Communication with the referring physician or the primary health care provider is also important. Constant relaying of information including laboratory findings, clinic visit results, and follow-up plans should occur between the transplant center and the client's primary health care provider.

TRANSLATING EVIDENCE INTO PRACTICE

Quality of Life After Transplantation

Quality of life (QOL) before and after transplantation, as well as how the client functions, copes, and lives after transplantation, is being investigated by nurses.[2-4,6,8-18,21,23-24] Other health care practitioners have completed similar studies of QOL.[1,5,7,19,20,22] Research studies may evaluate QOL at a specific period either before or after transplantation. Differences in the effects of drug treatment, device intervention, or medical therapy on QOL may be examined also. The diabetic client who is no longer insulin-dependent or the client who had end-stage renal disease who no longer requires dialysis has experienced a major change in lifestyle. Although there are challenges related to immunosuppressive therapy, most clients who undergo successful transplantation report improved QOL. Dew and colleagues reviewed 218 published studies using almost 15,000 total subjects from 1972 through 1996 and evaluated QOL in three areas: physical functioning, mental/cognitive health, and social functioning. Physical functioning was improved in all studies involving pancreas/kidney, pancreas, lung, and heart/lung clients.[1,4,8,22] Mental/cognitive and social improvement were reported in less than 80% of studies reviewed.[4] Of the studies reviewed by Dew and colleagues, few compared QOL ratings by transplant clients to QOL ratings by healthy people.[4]

Hathaway and colleagues and Johnson and colleagues reported improved QOL in renal transplant recipients regardless of race or gender of the client.[10,14] Hathaway and colleagues also completed a longitudinal study of 91 kidney transplant recipients who underwent QOL testing before transplantation and at 6 and 12 months after transplantation. The Sickness Impact Profile, the Adult Self-Image Scale, and the Personal Resource Questionnaire were used for this study. Variables that predicted post-transplantation QOL were employment status, the number of transplantation-related hospitalizations, and available social support.[11] White-Williams and colleagues found that males reported better QOL than females, both before heart transplantation and at 6 months after transplantation.[15,23]

Grady and colleagues reported on compliance at 1 year and at 2 years after heart transplantation in 120 recipients. Compliance was measured with the Heart Transplant Compliance Instrument developed for this study. The heart transplant recipients had no difficulty following medication regimens but did have difficulty with diet, exercise, and taking their vital signs.[8,9] De Geest and associates also examined compliance with taking medications in heart transplant recipients. They found that compliance with immunosuppressive medication was high; however, clients who were considered "moderate noncompliers" had a higher incidence of late acute rejection episodes. The findings in this study suggest that client compliance plays a pivotal role in long-term outcome after transplantation.[3]

Limbos and colleagues studied QOL in women before and after lung transplantation. Overall QOL improved after transplantation; however, the women reported impairments with sexuality and body satisfaction.[16] Manzetti reported that a health maintenance program of education and exercise improved QOL in clients awaiting lung transplantation.[18] Similarly, LoBiondo-Wood and colleagues reported improved QOL over time in 41 liver transplant recipients.[17] Post-transplant anxiety also reduced QOL in transplant recipients.[19,20,22]

IMPLICATIONS

QOL findings may vary from one type of transplant procedure to another, requiring nurses to be familiar with the QOL data for the type of transplant they encounter most frequently. Nurses working with a particular population of transplant clients may also share data about QOL that may be useful for transplant clients and families. It is important to remember that rating one's QOL may be relative because the experience of having a life-threatening illness changes how one thinks about life in general and about one's own particular life. Studies that compare QOL ratings by transplant recipients to QOL ratings by clients who have experienced near-death episodes, life-altering accidents, or medical treatment for severe illness should also be explored. Many studies were short term or asked clients about QOL only once or twice. This suggests that longitudinal studies of QOL are needed to enable nurses to understand and appreciate the impact of chronic illnesses and transplantation on clients and families.

(Continued)

TRANSLATING EVIDENCE INTO PRACTICE

Quality of Life After Transplantation—Cont'd

REFERENCES

1. Almenar-Pertejo, M., et al. (2006). Study on health-related quality of life in patients with advanced heart failure before and after transplantation. *Transplantation Proceedings, 38*(8), 2524-2526.
2. Cicutto, L., et al. (2004). Factors affecting attainment of paid employment after lung transplantation. *Journal of Heart and Lung Transplantation, 23*(4), 481-486.
3. De Geest, S., et al. (1998). Late acute rejection and subclinical noncompliance with cyclosporine therapy in heart transplant recipients. *Journal of Heart and Lung Transplantation, 17,* 854-863.
4. Dew, M., et al. (1997). Does transplantation produce quality of life benefits? A quantitative analysis. *Transplantation, 64,* 1261-1273.
5. Ekberg, H., et al. (2007). Increased prevalence of gastrointestinal symptoms associated with impaired quality of life in renal transplant recipients. *Transplantation, 83*(3), 282-289.
6. Forsberg, A. (2002). Liver transplant recipient's experienced meaning of health and quality of life one year after transplantation. *Theoria Journal of Nursing Theory, 11*(3), 4-14.
7. Girard, F., et al. (2006). Prevalence and impact of pain on the quality of life of lung transplant recipients: A prospective observational study. *Chest, 130*(5), 1535-1540.
8. Grady, K., et al. (1995). Predictors of quality of life in patients with advanced heart failure awaiting transplantation. *Journal of Heart and Lung Transplantation, 14,* 2-10.
9. Grady, K., et al. (1998). Patient compliance at one year and two years after heart transplantation. *Journal of Heart and Lung Transplantation, 17,* 383-394.
10. Hathaway, D., et al. (1996). Racial and gender differences in quality of life prior to and following kidney transplantation. *Proceedings of the Tenth Annual Southern Nursing Research Society Conference,* Feb 29, 2006, Miami, Fla.
11. Hathaway, D., et al. (1998). Post kidney transplantation quality of life prediction models. *Clinical Transplantation, 12,* 168-174.
12. Hilbrands, L., et al. (1995). The effect of immunosuppressive drugs on quality of life after renal transplantation. *Transplantation, 59,* 1263-1270.
13. Houle, N., et al. (2002). Health promoting behaviors, quality of life, and hospital resource utilization of patients receiving kidney transplants. *Nephrology Nursing Journal, 29,* 35-40.
14. Johnson, C., et al. (1998). Racial and gender differences in quality of life following kidney transplantation. *Image: Journal of Nursing Scholarship, 30,* 125-130.
15. Kirklin, J., & White-Williams, C. (2002). Quality of life after heart transplantation. In J. Kirklin, D. McGiffin, & J. Young (Eds.), *Heart transplantation.* New York: Churchill Livingstone.
16. Limbos, M., Chan, C., & Kesten, S. (1997). Quality of life in female lung transplant candidates and recipients. *Chest, 112,* 1165-1174.
17. LoBiondo-Wood, G., et al. (1997). Impact of liver transplantation on quality of life: A longitudinal perspective. *Applied Nursing Research, 10*(1), 27-32.
18. Manzetti, J., et al. (1994). Exercise, education and quality of life in lung transplant candidates. *Journal of Heart and Lung Transplantation, 13,* 297-305.
19. O'Reilly, F., et al. (2006). Baseline quality of life and anxiety in solid organ transplant recipients: A pilot study. *Dermatologic Surgery, 32*(11), 1480-1485.
20. Perez-San-Gregorio, M., et al. (2006). The influence of posttransplant anxiety on the long-term health of patients. *Transplantation Proceedings, 38*(8), 2406-2408.
21. Thomas, D. (1996). Returning to work after liver transplantation: Experiencing the roadblocks. *Journal of Transplantation Coordinators, 6,* 134-138.
22. Vermeulen, K., et al. (2007). Long-term health-related quality of life after lung transplantation: Different predictors for different dimensions. *Journal of Heart and Lung Transplantation, 26*(2), 177-193.
23. White-Williams, C., et al. (1997). Gender differences in quality of life outcomes before and 6 months after heart transplantation. *Journal of Heart and Lung Transplantation, 16,* 100.
24. Zarifian, A. (2006). Symptom occurrence, symptom distress, and quality of life in renal transplant recipients. *Nephrology Nursing Journal, 33*(6), 609-618.

CONCLUSIONS

Nursing care of the transplant client is both challenging and rewarding. With thorough understanding of the end-stage disease process and its manifestations, the organ donation and recovery process, and postoperative management, the nurse has the unique ability to work as a member of the interdisciplinary team caring for this group of clients. The nurse may serve as primary care provider, client advocate, and liaison with other team members. To maximize QOL, caring for the client and family must focus on both the physical and psychosocial aspects of transplantation, including not only medical treatments but also nursing interventions that address the client's specific QOL issues. If psychosocial issues are not fully explored, the client is likely to experience poorer satisfaction with the post-transplantation outcome. Performing meticulous medical care, providing long-term follow-up, and addressing physical and psychosocial QOL issues are all important components of management to improve both survival and QOL in the population of clients who have undergone organ transplantation.

THINKING CRITICALLY

1. A client has been receiving dialysis for several years while awaiting kidney transplantation. She is notified that a kidney donor has been found and that she should proceed to the hospital. What teaching will be completed before she goes to surgery? What psychosocial care should be offered?

Factors to Consider. What teaching and support will the family require? What are the ramifications if the donor kidney is found to be an unsuitable match for the client?

2. A client has recently undergone heart transplantation and is to be discharged from the hospital in 2 days. What client education should be completed? What education should be completed for the family

Factors to Consider. What living arrangements are required for the client after discharge? What are the long-term concerns related to financial factors, quality of life issues, and long-term immunosuppressive therapy?

3. At a pretransplantation support group, a client makes the following statement: "I think I may need to buy my new organ." How should the nurse react to this statement? What ethical issues are raised by this statement?

Factors to Consider. Of what other ethical considerations regarding organ donation should the transplant nurse be aware?

Discussions for these questions can be found on the website.

BIBLIOGRAPHY

Citations appearing in red refer to primary research.

Citations appearing in blue refer to evidence-based practice guidelines and protocols.

1. American Heart Association. (2007). *Heart transplant: Statistics.* Retrieved 03/01/07 from www.americanheart.org/presenter.jhtml?identifier=4588.
2. American Liver Foundation. (2007). *Liver transplant.* Retrieved 03/01/07 from www.liverfoundation.org/db/articles/1016.
3. American Lung Association. (2007). *Lung transplants fact sheet.* Retrieved 03/01/07 from www.lungusa.org/site/apps/s/content.asp?c=dvLUK9OE&b=34706&ct=3052341.
4. Banner, N., Polak, J., & Yacoub, M. (2003). *Lung transplantation.* Cambridge: Cambridge University Press.
5. Barnard, C.N. (1967). A human cardiac transplant. *South African Medical Journal, 41,* 1271-1274.
6. Baumgartner, W. (2002). *Heart and lung transplantation* (2nd ed.). Philadelphia: Saunders.
7. Danovitch, G. (2005). *Handbook of kidney transplantation* (4th ed.). Philadelphia: Lippincott Williams & Wilkins.
8. Ehrle, R., Shafer, T., & Nelson, K. (1999). Referral, request, and consent for organ donation: Best practice—a blueprint for success. *Critical Care Nurse, 19*(2), 21-33.
9. Guthrie, C (Ed.) (1912). Applications of blood vessel surgery. In *Blood vessel surgery.* New York: Longmans, Green.
10. Hakim, N., & Papalois, V. (2003). *History of organ and cell transplantation.* River Edge, NJ: Imperial College Press.
11. Hakim, N., Stratta, R., & Gray, D. (2002). *Pancreas and islet transplantation.* New York: Oxford University Press.
12. Hornick, P., & Rose, M. (2006). *Transplantation immunology: Methods and protocols.* Totowa, NJ: Humana Press.
13. International Society for Heart and Lung Transplantation. (2003). *Twenty-third annual meeting and scientific sessions,* April 9-12, 2003, Vienna, Austria.
14. Jonsen, A. (2005). *Bioethics beyond the headlines: Who lives? Who dies? Who decides?.* Lanham, Md: Rowman & Littlefield.
15. Kaserman, D., & Barnett, A. (2002). *The U.S. organ procurement system: A prescription for reform.* Washington, DC: AEI Press.
16. Kirklin, J., & George, J. (2002). Immunosuppressive modalities. In J. Kirklin, J. Young, & D. McGiffin (Eds.), *Heart transplantation* (pp. 390-463). New York: Churchill Livingstone.
17. Kirklin, J., Young, J., & McGiffin, D. (2002). *Heart transplantation.* New York: Churchill Livingstone.
18. Kuo, P., Schroeder, R., & Johnson, L. (2001). *Clinical management of the transplant patient.* New York: Arnold.
19. Landsteiner, K. (1928). Cell antigens and individual specificity. *Journal of Immunology, 15,* 589-600.
20. Lucey, M., Neuberger, J., & Shaked, A. (2003). *Liver transplantation.* Georgetown, Tex: Landes Bioscience.
21. Maddrey, W., Schiff, E., & Sorrell, M. (2001). *Transplantation of the liver* (3rd ed.). Philadelphia: Lippincott Williams & Wilkins.
22. Mancuso, D. (2006). *Progress in kidney transplantation.* New York: Nova Science.
23. Medawar, P.B. (1945). A second study of the behavior and fate of skin homografts in rabbits: A report to the War Wounds Committee of the Medical Research Council. *Journal of Anatomy,69,* 157-176.
24. Morris, P. (2001). *Kidney transplantation: Principles and practice* (5th ed.). Philadelphia: Saunders.
25. National Kidney Foundation. *Transplantation.* Retrieved 03/01/07 from www.kidney.org/atoz/atozTopic.cfm?topic=3.
26. Norman, D., & Turka, L. (2001). *Primer on transplantation* (2nd ed.). Mt. Laurel, NJ: American Society of Transplantation.
27. Organ Procurement and Transplantation Network (OPTN). (2007). *Data: Organ datasource: Kidney.* Retrieved 03/01/07 from www.optn.org/organdatasource/about.asp?display=kidney.
28. Palmer, R. (2006). Surgical innovations: Improving the quality of life. *Clinics in Geriatric Medicine, 22*(3), 499-734.
29. Parker, J., & Parker, P. (2004). *Heart transplant: A medical dictionary, bibliography and annotated research guide to internet references.* San Diego: ICON Health Publications.
30. Petty, M. (2003). Lung and heart-lung transplantation: Implications for nursing care when hospitalized outside the transplant center. *MEDSURG Nursing, 12*(4), 250-260.
31. Starzl, T.E., et al. (1963). Homotransplantation of the liver in humans. *Surgery, Gynecology and Obstetrics, 117,* 659-676.
32. Smith, S. (2002). Immunosuppressive therapies in organ transplantation. In S. Smith (Ed.), *Organ transplantation: Concepts, issues, practice, and outcomes.* Available at www.medscape.com.viewarticle/437182.
33. Task Force on Organ Transplantation. (1986). *Organ transplantation: Issues and recommendations* (HRP-0906976). Rockville, Md: Health Resources and Services Administration.
34. United Network of Organ Sharing (UNOS). (2006). *Annual Report of the U.S. Scientific Registry for Transplant Recipients and Organ Procurement and Transplantation Network—Transplant Data.* Richmond, Va: Author. Retrieved 11/20/07 from www.unos.org/data/annualReport.asp.
35. U.S. Department of Health and Human Services. (2006). *Annual Report of the U.S. Organ Procurement Transplantation Network and the Scientific Registry of Transplant Recipients: Transplant Data 1995-2005.* Rockville, Md: Health and Human Services Administration, Healthcare Systems Bureau, Division of Transplantation, United Network of Organ Sharing (UNOS) OPTN and Scientific Registry Data. Retrieved 03/01/07 from www.hrsa.gov/data/.
36. Urden, L., Stacy, K., & Lough, M. (2006). Transplantation. In L. Urden, K Stacey., & M. Lough (Eds.), *Thelan's critical care nursing: Diagnosis and management* (5th ed., pp. 1076-1127). St. Louis: Mosby.
37. White-Williams, C. (2002). Lung transplantation. In S. Smith (Ed.), *Organ transplantation: Concepts, issues, practice, and outcomes.* Available at www.medscape.com/viewpublication704.

evolve **Did you remember to check out the bonus material on the Evolve website and the CD-ROM, including NCLEX®-Examination Style Review Questions, Open-Book Quizzes, and Chapter Review Audio Podcasts?**

http://evolve.elsevier.com/Black/medsurg

CHAPTER 81

Management of Clients with Shock and Multisystem Disorders

LOUISE NELSON LAFRAMBOISE

SHOCK

Shock is a complex clinical syndrome that may occur at any time and in any place. It is a life-threatening condition often requiring team action by many health care providers, including nurses, physicians, laboratory technicians, pharmacists, and respiratory therapists. Shock causes thousands of deaths and unknown numbers of permanent injuries each year. The economic impact of shock is staggering, with annual health care costs for treatment of shock in the billions of dollars. Because shock is potentially lethal, debilitating, and costly, it is essential that nurses identify clients at risk for shock, recognize the early assessment findings indicating shock, and initiate appropriate interventions before shock ensues.

Shock is defined as failure of the circulatory system to maintain adequate perfusion of vital organs. Disorders leading to inadequate tissue perfusion result in decreased oxygenation at the cellular level. Inadequate oxygenation results in anaerobic cellular metabolism and accumulated waste products in cells. If this condition is untreated, cell death and organ death occur.

Classification

Shock is commonly divided into three major classifications:

- Hypovolemic
- Cardiogenic
- Distributive

Hypovolemic shock is due to inadequate circulating blood volume resulting from hemorrhage with actual blood loss, burns with massive shifts of fluids due to movement of plasma proteins into interstitial spaces, and fluid shifts or dehydration, with or without loss of fluid volume. Hypovolemic shock is the most common type of shock and develops when the intravascular volume decreases to the point where compensatory

mechanisms are unable to maintain organ and tissue perfusion.

Cardiogenic shock is due to inadequate pumping action of the heart. The heart muscle can be diseased as a result of primary cardiac muscle dysfunction or mechanical obstruction of blood flow caused by myocardial infarction (MI), valvular insufficiency caused by disease or trauma, cardiac dysrhythmias, or an obstructive condition such as pericardial tamponade or pulmonary embolus. The clinical definition of cardiogenic shock is decreased cardiac output and evidence of tissue hypoxia in the presence of adequate intravascular volume. Hemodynamic criteria for cardiogenic shock are sustained hypotension (systolic blood pressure <90 mm Hg for at least 30 min) and a reduced cardiac index (<2.2 L/min/m^2) in the presence of elevated pulmonary capillary occlusion pressure (>15 mm Hg). Other manifestations of tissue hypoperfusion include oliguria (<30 ml/hour), cool extremities, and altered mentation. Cardiogenic shock occurs in 10% to 15% of all clients after MI and carries an associated death rate of up to 80%. Cardiogenic shock after an MI usually occurs when 40% or more of the myocardium has been damaged.

The term *obstructive shock* is sometimes used to include conditions that lead to a sudden obstruction of blood flow (e.g., cardiac tamponade, tension

---

evolve **Web Enhancements**

Client Education Guide Shock (Spanish Translation)

Concept Map Understanding Septic Shock and Its Treatment

Ethical Issues in Nursing

Is There a Moral Difference Between Withholding and Withdrawing Treatments?

Be sure to check out the bonus material on the Evolve website and the CD-ROM, including free self-assessment exercises. **http://evolve.elsevier. com/Black/medsurg**

pneumothorax, pulmonary embolism). Obstructive causes are discussed under the topic of cardiogenic shock because the ability of the heart to pump effectively is the primary problem.

Distributive shock (also called *vasogenic shock*) is due to changes in blood vessel tone that increase the size of the vascular space without an increase in the circulating blood volume. The result is a relative hypovolemia (total fluid volume remains the same but is redistributed). Distributive shock is further divided into three types:

- *Anaphylactic shock* is a severe hypersensitivity reaction resulting in massive systemic vasodilation.
- *Neurogenic shock,* or interference with nervous system control of the blood vessels, can occur with conditions such as spinal cord injury (especially cervical spine injury), spinal anesthesia, or severe vaso-vagal reactions caused by pain or psychic trauma. Some amount of neurogenic shock is seen with all spinal cord injuries. More dramatic cases of neurogenic shock are seen with cervical spine injuries. The duration of neurogenic shock is usually 1 to 6 weeks as long as there is no irreparable cord injury, but recovery may take as long as 12 months.
- *Septic shock* is caused by a release of vasoactive substances. Current theories suggest there is a cascade of interactions between immune cells that happens rapidly and leads to microcirculatory alterations. Septic shock is the most common cause of mortality in intensive care units. Even with the best treatment, mortality ranges from 15% in clients with sepsis to 40% to 60% in clients with septic shock.

Etiology and Risk Factors

All causes of shock focus on some component of blood distribution throughout the body. There can be an insufficient quantity of blood (hypovolemic shock), an incompetent pump (cardiogenic shock), or an ineffective delivery of blood (distributive shock).

Hypovolemic Shock

The primary event precipitating hypovolemic shock is a large reduction in the circulating blood volume so that the body's metabolic needs cannot be met. Hypovolemic shock may be due to a loss of plasma or blood. Conditions that may cause a reduction in circulating blood volume include hemorrhage, burns, and dehydration.

Health promotion activities to prevent hypovolemic shock include client education to avoid injuries that would put someone at risk for hypovolemic shock. Health maintenance activities are the use of oxygen and maintenance of fluid and electrolyte balance. To restore health, monitor the client with telemetry and hemodynamic monitoring, and give vasoactive medications and blood and fluid replacements as ordered.

Hemorrhage. Hemorrhage is the loss of blood. Clinical manifestations may begin to appear with a blood volume deficit of 15% to 25%, or about 500 to 1500 ml in an adult with a normal circulating volume. Shock fully develops if a previously healthy client loses about one third of the normal circulating blood volume of 5 L. Wounds of the chest, abdomen, and thighs can lead to hemorrhagic shock.

The loss of smaller amounts of blood may cause shock in clients less able to compensate rapidly (e.g., older people with decreased vascular tone and impaired cardiac function). The extent to which shock develops after blood loss also depends on the length of time over which the blood loss occurs. Clients experiencing slow blood loss over a period of days or weeks tolerate their blood loss better than clients whose blood loss occurs rapidly over minutes or hours. Hypovolemic shock following trauma is typically the result of hemorrhage. The classes of hemorrhage and the associated assessment findings are listed in Table 81-1.

Burns. Hypovolemic shock produced by burns occurs most often in people with large partial-thickness or

TABLE 81-1   Assessment Findings and Classifications of Acute Hemorrhage*

Assessment Finding	Class I	Class II	Class III	Class IV
Blood loss (%)	<15	15-30	30-40	>40
Blood loss (ml)	<750	750-1500	1500-2000	>2000
Pulse rate (beats/min)	<100	>100	>120	>140
Respiratory rate (breaths/min)	Normal (14-20)	20-30	30-40	>35
Blood pressure	Normal	Normal	Decreased	Decreased
Pulse pressure	Normal or increased	Decreased	Decreased	Decreased
Central nervous system/mental status	Slightly anxious	Mildly anxious	Anxious, confused	Confused, lethargic
Urine output (ml/hr)	>30	20-30	5-15	Negligible
Intravenous fluid replacement	Crystalloid at 3 ml/1 ml of blood loss	Crystalloid at 3 ml/1 ml of blood loss	Crystalloid plus blood at 3 ml/1 ml of blood loss	Crystalloid plus blood at 3 ml/1 ml of blood loss

*Assumes a normal 70-kg man.
Data from American College of Surgeons Committee on Trauma. (1997). *Advanced trauma life support student manual* (p. 98). Chicago: Author.

full-thickness burns. It is caused primarily by a shift of plasma from the vascular space into the interstitial space. In addition to these fluid losses or shifts, the client may have cardiac dysfunction that is due to the presence of *myocardial depressant factor (MDF)*, a polypeptide (see Myocardial Deterioration). MDF affects the contractility of cardiac muscle by depressing myocardial muscle function. The result is impaired cardiac output, even in the presence of a normal circulating volume. Shock related to burns is discussed in Chapter 50.

Other causes of hypovolemic shock that may produce fluid shifts similar to those in burns include nephrotic syndrome, severe crush injuries, starvation, surgery, and conditions causing plasma fluids to accumulate in the abdominal cavity (e.g., cirrhosis of the liver, pancreatitis, bowel obstruction).

Dehydration. Shock may also occur either from reduced oral fluid intake or from significant fluid losses (e.g., rigorous exercise causing fluid loss from sweating and insensible fluid loss through the respiratory tract and in hot environments). Loss of fluid may occur in people with excessive urine output or prolonged vomiting or diarrhea, leading to dehydration-induced hypovolemic shock. Clients with chronic illnesses, especially older people, may be at increased risk because of impaired recognition of thirst, an inability to obtain fluids, inadequate maintenance of chronic conditions (e.g., increased blood glucose levels with diabetes), or inadequate monitoring of therapeutic regimens (e.g., diuretic-induced dehydration). With prolonged fluid deficit, all compartments—intravascular, interstitial, and intracellular—are depleted.

Cardiogenic Shock

Cardiogenic shock results primarily from an inability of heart muscle to function adequately or from mechanical obstructions of blood flow to or from the heart. The major cause of cardiogenic shock is ischemic heart disease of the right and left ventricle. As with other causes of shock, the lack of blood flow decreases tissue and organ perfusion.

Myocardial Infarction. Impaired heart muscle action is most often caused by MI (see Chapter 58). The area of dead or dying tissue that occurs with infarction impairs contractility of the myocardium, and cardiac output decreases. Impaired myocardial contractility may also occur with blunt cardiac trauma, cardiomyopathy, and heart failure.

Prevention of cardiogenic shock related to MI begins with health promotion activities directed at client education to decrease the risk factors associated with coronary artery disease (e.g., increasing exercise and modifying dietary intake). Supportive oxygenation and administration of inotropic agents and vasodilators are health maintenance activities. An intra-aortic balloon pump (IABP) (see Chapter 56) may be needed for health restoration.

Clients in cardiogenic shock may also develop some degree of hypovolemic shock. This is most often due to the therapeutic use of diuretics or to edema in the extremities or other dependent areas (caused by inadequate cardiac pumping activity and venous congestion). Clients in hypovolemic shock are also at risk for cardiogenic shock. The myocardium normally receives its blood supply during diastole. When the heart rate increases to compensate for the decreased blood volume to maintain cardiac output, diastole is shortened, sometimes leading to insufficient time for the coronary arteries to fill with blood. Because these arteries supply blood to the myocardium, the myocardial oxygen supply is impaired. The increased heart rate also increases the need of the myocardium for oxygen, predisposing the myocardium to injury because of the decreased blood flow and resultant decreased oxygen supply. In addition, the decreased venous return associated with hypovolemia results in decreased coronary artery perfusion and inadequate oxygenation of the myocardium.

Obstructive Conditions. Several types of mechanical obstructions of blood flow may cause cardiogenic shock:

1. *Large pulmonary embolism*. An *embolus* is usually the result of a blood clot that breaks loose in a person with deep vein thrombosis (DVT). This embolus travels through the venous system to the right side of the heart and into the pulmonary artery. The size of the embolus determines at what point it lodges in the pulmonary artery. A large embolus can inhibit perfusion of a major portion of the lung, resulting in an increased workload for the right ventricle.
2. *Pericardial tamponade* is an accumulation of blood or fluid in the pericardial space that compresses the myocardium and interferes with the ability of the myocardium to expand.
3. A *tension pneumothorax* is a significant amount of air in the pleural space that compresses the heart and great vessels, thus interfering with venous return to the heart.

Other Causes of Cardiogenic Shock. Most diseases of the heart have the potential to cause cardiogenic shock. They include (1) cardiac valvular insufficiency from trauma or disease, (2) myocardial aneurysms (usually resulting from previous MI or congenital abnormalities), (3) rupture of a valvular papillary muscle, (4) ventricular rupture, (5) aortic stenosis, (6) mitral regurgitation, (7) cardiac dysrhythmias, (8) infectious and inflammatory processes such as myocarditis and endocarditis, (9) pulmonary hypertension, and (10) toxic drugs.

Distributive (Vasogenic) Shock

Distributive shock results from inadequate vascular tone. Blood volume remains normal, but the size of the vascular space increases dramatically because of massive vasodilation. The result is maldistribution of the blood because of decreased blood pressure (BP) and lack of blood returning to the heart; this is why it is often referred to as "relative" hypovolemia. The volume of blood remains constant, but the blood has pooled because of increased capacity of the vascular system. After extensive vasodilation, the BP, return of venous blood to the heart, and cardiac output are decreased. As with other forms of shock, tissue anoxia and cell destruction result. The massive vasodilation present with distributive shock has several major causes.

Acute Allergic Reaction (Anaphylactic Shock). Anaphylactic shock occurs as a result of an acute allergic reaction from exposure to a substance to which the client has been sensitized. Common sensitizing agents are penicillin, penicillin derivatives, bee stings, chemotherapy, latex, chocolate, strawberries, peanuts, snake venom, iodine-based contrast for x-ray studies, seafood, and nonsteroidal anti-inflammatory drugs (NSAIDs).

Re-exposure to the foreign substance results in the offending antigen binding to previously synthesized immunoglobulins (i.e., IgE) on the mast cell. This binding causes the release of histamine (see Chapter 76). Manifestations include massive vasodilation, urticaria (hives), laryngeal edema, and bronchial constriction. Without prompt treatment, a person with anaphylactic shock will die from cardiovascular collapse and respiratory failure.

To help prevent the onset of anaphylactic shock, teach clients to avoid precipitators and to use an epinephrine injection (e.g., EpiPen). Encouraging clients to wear medical alert bracelets and to seek allergy desensitization also decreases their potential for anaphylactic shock.

Spinal Cord Injury (Neurogenic Shock). With injury to the cervical spine, commonly with injuries around the T6 level, the autonomic nervous system is affected. Below the level of injury there is blocking of sympathetic nervous stimulation, and the parasympathetic system acts unopposed. This unopposed stimulation causes vasodilation, decreased venous return, decreased cardiac output, and decreased tissue perfusion. Neurogenic shock is manifested by the triad of hypotension, bradycardia, and hypothermia.

Teaching clients safety measures may help prevent spinal cord injury and neurogenic shock. After injury, protect the client's spine, maintain the airway and breathing, provide circulatory support, and provide for thermoregulation. Health restoration involves rehabilitation when the client is stable.

Infection (Septic Shock). *Sepsis* is the presence of infection and activation of the inflammatory cascade. Systemic inflammatory response syndrome (SIRS) is a term used to define this clinical condition, and it is considered present if abnormalities exist in two of the following four clinical parameters: (1) body temperature, (2) heart rate, (3) respiratory rate, and (4) peripheral leukocyte count. Sepsis is defined as the presence of SIRS in the setting of infection. Severe sepsis is defined as sepsis with evidence of end-organ dysfunction as a result of hypoperfusion. Septic shock is defined as sepsis with persistent hypotension despite fluid resuscitation and resulting tissue hypoperfusion.

Bacteremia is defined as the presence of viable bacteria in blood. Bacteremia may be primary (without an identifiable focus of infection) or, more often, secondary (with a focus of infection). Sepsis is a disease seen most frequently in older adults and in those with co-morbid conditions that predispose them to infection. Clients who are immunocompromised are especially at high risk and include those with cancer who are receiving chemotherapeutic agents, those with end-stage renal or liver disease, those with advanced HIV, or those receiving steroids for chronic conditions. Clients with indwelling vascular catheters and urinary catheters are particularly at high risk. Although sepsis is commonly associated with bacterial infection, bacteremia does not need to be present to activate the massive inflammatory response that results in severe sepsis. In fact, fewer than 50% of cases of sepsis are associated with bacteremia.

Encouraging clients to treat infections immediately and completely may help reduce the incidence of septic shock. Older and immunocompromised clients should be monitored closely for infection, and treatment should begin immediately when infection is diagnosed. Identify high-risk clients and implement measures to prevent shock whenever possible.

Pathophysiology

Shock occurs when there is not adequate circulating volume to maintain aerobic metabolism in the cells. Adequate circulating volume is dependent on three interrelated components of the cardiovascular system: (1) the heart, (2) vascular tone, and (3) blood volume. Blood flows throughout the body because of its driving pressure as it leaves the left ventricle (LV). If there is a reduction in the volume of blood or if the heart muscle cannot pump effectively, cardiac output falls.

Vascular tone refers to the degree of constriction by the smooth muscle in the arteriole. The size of the body's larger blood vessels is regulated by the autonomic nervous system, but this is not true for the microcirculation. Arteriole and capillary sphincters are separate mechanisms governed by different controls. Typically, blood flow through the capillary bed is influenced by the varying needs of the cells located near the vessel. The capillaries open on demand of the cells adjacent to them.

A minor impairment in one component is compensated for by the other two, whereas prolonged or severe impairments lead to shock. Some of the problems with decreased organ and tissue perfusion in shock are due to failure of the normal mechanisms. If one of the three components of circulation fails, other parts of the system initiate compensatory mechanisms. For example, vasoconstriction and increased cardiac output may be used to compensate for decreased volume. As long as two of these factors can maintain a satisfactory compensatory action, adequate blood circulation can be maintained even though the third factor is not functioning normally. If compensatory mechanisms fail or if more than one of the three factors necessary for adequate circulation malfunctions, circulatory failure results and shock develops.

The systemic circulatory bed and the microcirculatory bed apparently do not have sensing devices that would allow a unified, coordinated response throughout the entire circulation. Thus events occurring within one bed do not influence events in the other. The relative autonomy of the microcirculation and the lack of coordination between it and the systemic circulation are important in determining the course of events in shock. Each type of shock progresses uniquely; the following sections discuss of the pathophysiology of each type.

Cardiogenic Shock

Cardiogenic shock is failure of the left ventricle to pump adequate blood volume. When cardiac output falls, the body compensates by releasing catecholamines (epinephrine and norepinephrine) to increase heart rate and systemic vascular resistance to increase venous return. However, these are only temporary measures to restore blood pressure and tissue blood flow to vital organs (heart and brain). The diseased heart cannot maintain its own myocardial tissue oxygenation, which results in a spiral of decreased cardiac output, hypotension, and further myocardial ischemia.

Anaphylactic Shock

Anaphylaxis is a systemic type I hypersensitivity reaction from the sudden release of inflammatory mediators from mast cells and basophils. When a sensitized client comes in contact with an antigen, IgE is stimulated and the mast cells and basophils release large amounts of histamine. Histamine leads to vasodilation, bronchial constriction, bronchorrhea, pruritus, laryngeal edema, and angioedema. Laryngeal edema obstructs the airway.

Septic Shock

Sepsis begins with the unchecked growth of organisms at a tissue site. About 50% of clients with septic shock have bacteremia, with gram-negative rods and gram-positive organisms being the most common agents. The organisms themselves start the disease. Endotoxins (also called lipopolysaccharides) are produced by gram-negative organisms. Gram-positive cocci also produce exotoxins. Host resistance and organism virulence are both factors that determine the body's response. Initially, there is an overwhelming inflammatory response to the microbes that is regulated by tumor necrosis factor (TNF), interferon, and the interleukins. In addition, complement is activated. These factors promote the systemic inflammatory response. As a result, mediators with vasodilatory and endotoxic properties are released systemically, including prostaglandins, thromboxane A_2, and nitric oxide. This results in vasodilation and endothelial damage, which leads to hypoperfusion and capillary leakage. In addition, cytokines activate the coagulation pathway, resulting in capillary microthrombi and end-organ ischemia.

Stages of Shock

Nonprogressive Stage. During the initial or nonprogressive stage of shock, cardiac output is slightly decreased because of the loss of actual or relative blood volume. During this stage, the body's compensatory mechanisms can maintain BP within a normal to low-normal range and can maintain perfusion to the vital organs. During the compensatory phase, the systemic circulation and microcirculation work together in a hyperdynamic state. This hyperdynamic state leads to an increase in lactic acid levels. Both levels of circulation undergo a major readjustment in which their activities are coordinated to preserve the entire system. Figure 81-1 illustrates these readjustments.

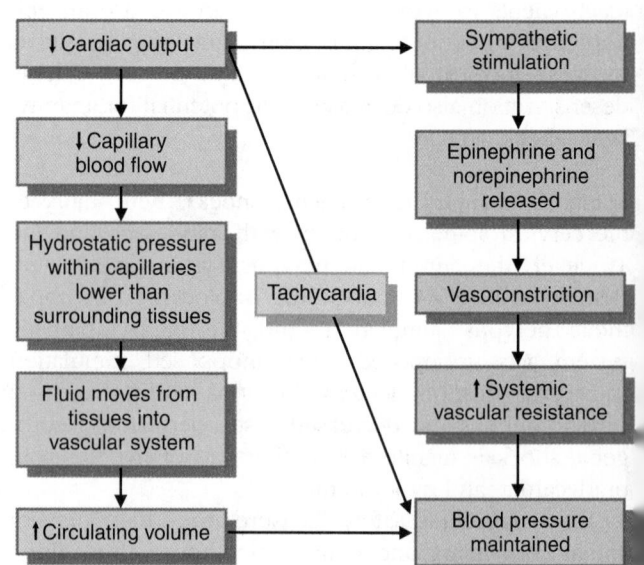

■ FIGURE 81-1   Nonprogressive stage of shock. Regardless of the cause, decreased cardiac output is generally the stimulus that precipitates the body's response to compensate for the hypovolemia (relative or actual) to maintain blood pressure.

Progressive Stage. If shock and the compensatory vasoconstriction persist, the body begins to decompensate and the systemic circulation and microcirculation no longer work in unison. As vasoconstriction continues, the supply of oxygenated blood to the tissues is reduced. This results in anaerobic metabolism and further lactic acidosis. Acidosis and the increasing $Paco_2$ cause the microcirculation to dilate. This dilation causes decreased venous return and decreased circulation of reoxygenated blood.

Lactic acidosis also causes increased capillary permeability and relaxation of the capillary sphincters. Relaxation of the sphincters allows increased blood in the capillaries and increased capillary pressure. This increased pressure along with the increased capillary permeability allows fluid to move out of the vascular space and back into the tissues. In doing so, the microcirculation reverses its pattern and tries to secure for itself (and the tissue it supplies) more of the limited supply of available blood. Thus the blood supply is progressively retained in the capillary bed, and blood pools in the microcirculation. Because the cells demand greater perfusion time, many or most of the capillaries remain open at any one time, increasing the vascular space in the microcirculation.

Increased vascular capacity, decreased blood volume, or decreased heart action reduces the mean arterial pressure (MAP). In turn, the pressure gradient for the venous return of blood decreases. This also contributes to venous pooling of blood, decreased venous return to the heart, and decreased cardiac output.

Because there are no feedback systems within the body to change this pattern, this cycle of events becomes progressively more severe. Eventually, the circulation is totally disrupted. Once the vascular space enlarges (because of vasodilation of the microcirculation), even normal blood volumes cannot fill all of these vessels. The result is a low central venous pressure (CVP) (except in cardiogenic shock) and inadequate venous return to the right side of the heart, with a further decrease in cardiac output.

This resultant decrease in circulating volume and capillary flow does not allow adequate perfusion and oxygenation of the vital organs. With the prolonged decrease in capillary blood flow, the tissues become hypoxic. This cycle of events is illustrated in Figure 81-2.

Irreversible Stage. The irreversible stage of shock occurs if the cycle of inadequate tissue perfusion is not interrupted. The shock state becomes progressively more severe, even though the initial cause of the shock is not itself becoming more severe. Cellular ischemia and necrosis lead to organ failure and death.

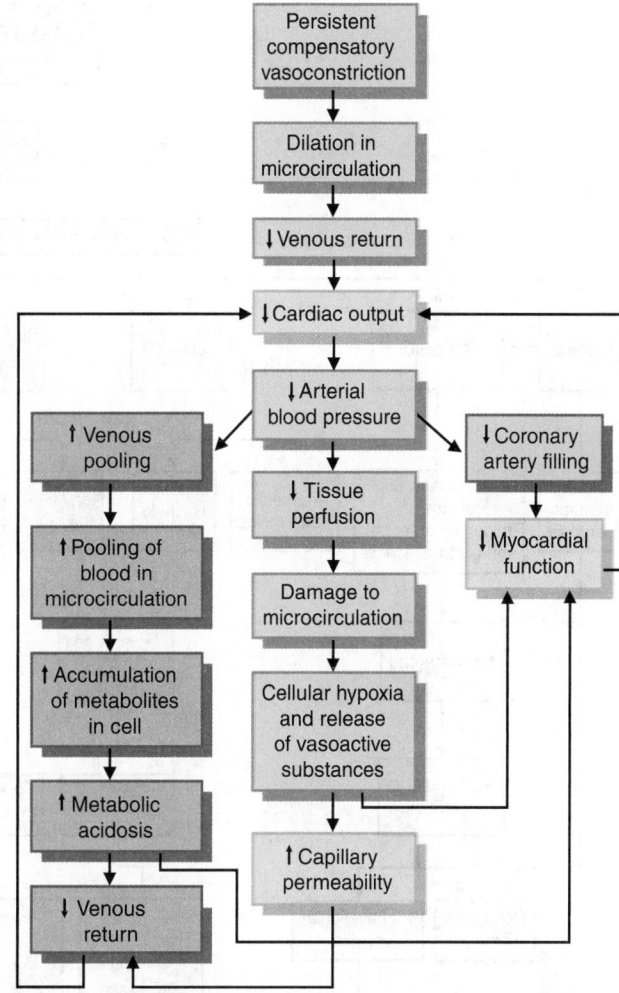

FIGURE 81–2   Vicious cycle of events occurring in the progressive stage of shock. The shock syndrome can be initiated anywhere in the cycle depending on the precipitating cause (e.g., impaired myocardial function because of myocardial infarction, blood loss caused by trauma, or the release of vasoactive toxins as a result of sepsis). Hypovolemic shock resulting from blood loss, for example, results in decreased arterial blood pressure, setting in motion a cascade of events that worsen the shock state.

Systemic Effects of Shock

Shock affects every system within the body. Equally important to understanding the cellular level of shock is understanding what happens to the various organs (Figure 81-3).

Respiratory System. Getting oxygen in *(ventilation)* and delivering oxygenated blood to the tissues *(perfusion)* are crucial for survival. Shock produces prolonged circulatory insufficiency that creates variable and inadequate perfusion of certain organs and tissues, particularly at the microcirculation level. Circulatory deprivation results in tissue hypoxia and anoxia. Hypoxia and anoxia can be tolerated for a short time. As the time lengthens, the chances of recovery diminish. A lack of oxygen appears to initiate the irreversible stage of shock. The greater the

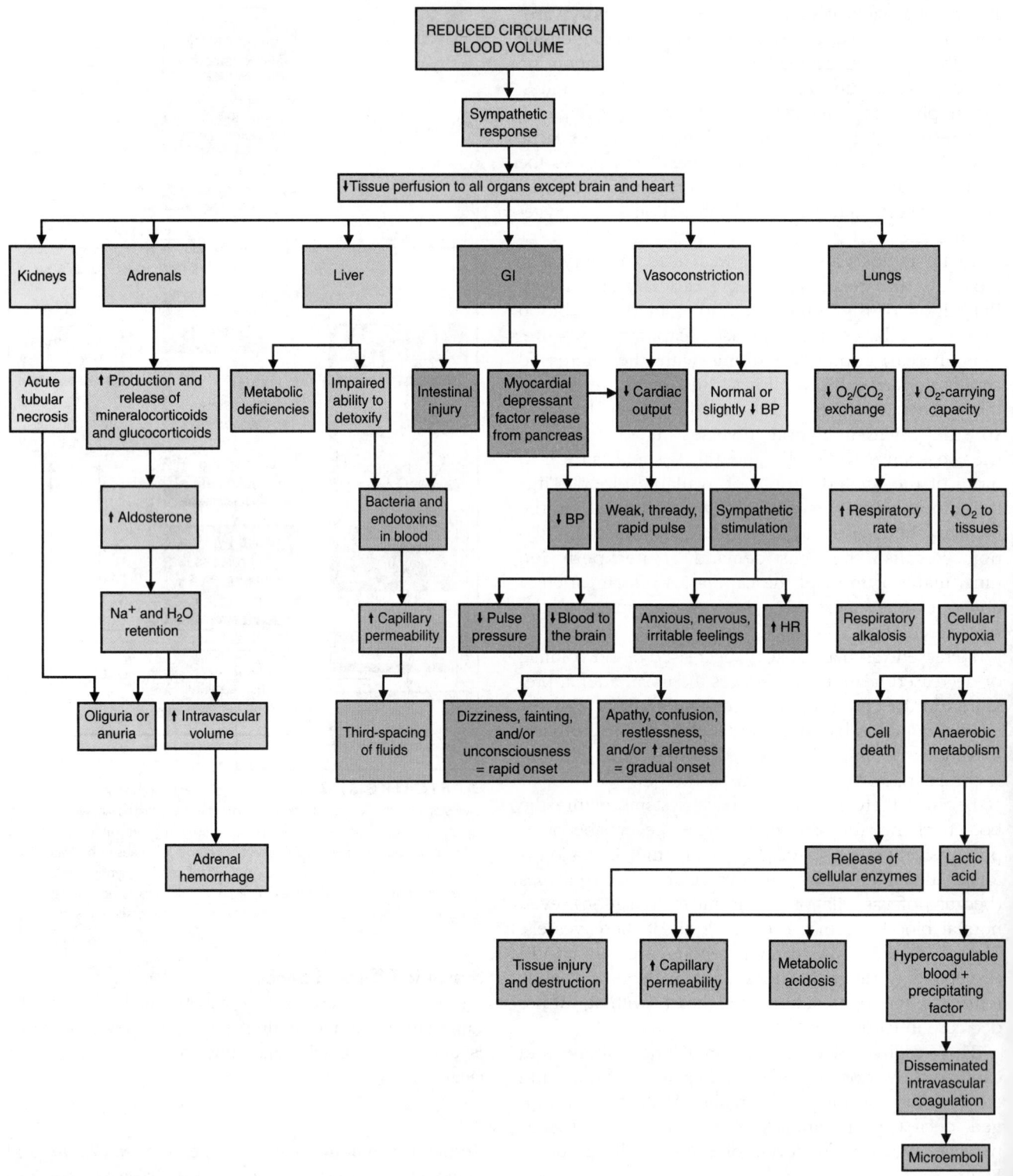

■ **FIGURE 81–3** Systemic effects of shock. The lack of blood flow is compensated by constricting flow to nonessential organs (all organs except the brain and heart).

difference between the amount of oxygen available and the amount needed, the more rapidly irreversible shock develops. If sufficient oxygen is available to the cells to meet the body's needs, irreversible shock is less likely to occur.

Respiratory failure continues to be a major cause of death in shock, despite many advances in shock prevention, early recognition, and management. The magnitude of this problem surfaced during the Vietnam War era when soldiers sustaining massive injuries and profound blood loss were successfully resuscitated, only to die several days later of acute respiratory distress syndrome (ARDS) (see Chapter 63). Although ARDS remains the greatest contributing factor to respiratory failure, other causes of respiratory failure during shock include aspiration and loss of neurologic control of breathing.

Acid-Base Balance. Oxygen and nutrients are essential to life because they synthesize adenosine triphosphate (ATP). ATP is the ultimate source of energy for life processes. When oxygen is not present, ATP is produced through *anaerobic metabolism*. Although production of ATP in this manner is a useful emergency measure, it is inefficient compared with the normal process of *aerobic (oxidative) metabolism*. Anaerobic metabolism produces anaerobic metabolites, such as lactic acid (which causes intracellular acidity with consequent cellular damage) and substrates of the adenylic acid system (which depress the heart) (see Figure 81-3).

In response to the chemoreceptors sensing decreased pH, the rate and depth of respirations are increased to "blow off" (exhale) CO_2 to compensate for the metabolic acidosis. This results in respiratory alkalosis. However, the cellular hypoxia is caused not by inadequate ventilation but rather by inadequate tissue perfusion. Therefore the increased respiratory effort does little to correct the problem.

Because lactic acid is not exhaled, it accumulates in tissue fluids, which become increasingly acidic. Metabolic acidosis is eventually produced. During metabolic acidosis, blood pH and bicarbonate levels decrease. Pyruvate, lactate, phosphate, and sulfate levels increase. Unless circulation is restored, the acidotic reaction resulting from metabolic acidosis ultimately kills the cells. The buildup of lactic acid causes such a severe local acidosis that cellular enzymes are inactivated. Cells soon die.

Respiratory alkalosis or *respiratory acidosis* (induced by pulmonary ventilatory or diffusion changes) may be superimposed on the metabolic acidosis. As perfusion and oxygen delivery to the tissues decrease, cellular energy production decreases. To compensate, cells increase anaerobic metabolism, which results in the buildup of lactic acid in the cell. As the pH of the cells decreases, lysosomes within the cell explode, releasing powerful, destructive enzymes. These enzymes destroy the cellular membrane and digest the cell contents. Once this process begins, the cellular changes are irreversible. The final result is cellular death (Figure 81-4).

Lysosomal Enzymes. Lysosomal enzymes are released from dead cells undergoing autolysis. They are also released from injured cells. Lysosomal enzymes become most active in an acid pH range. Thus as long as normal acid-base balance is maintained within the body, these enzymes are repressed within normal cells. During shock, however, the accompanying metabolic acidosis accelerates the activation of these enzymes in hypoxic tissues. The activation of lysosomal hydrolases within the cells and their release into the circulation markedly exacerbate the tissue injury that occurs during shock. The release of active lysosomal proteases and other enzymes from damaged tissue into the bloodstream and their action on extracellular and intracellular structures probably contribute to the progression of injury from cell to cell.

Cardiovascular System

Myocardial Deterioration. As shock progresses, the heart deteriorates. Cardiac deterioration is one of the major causes of death in shock. Although the exact cause of myocardial depression is unclear, much attention has been directed at MDF. MDF, a polypeptide with vasoactive properties, is released in response to ischemia of

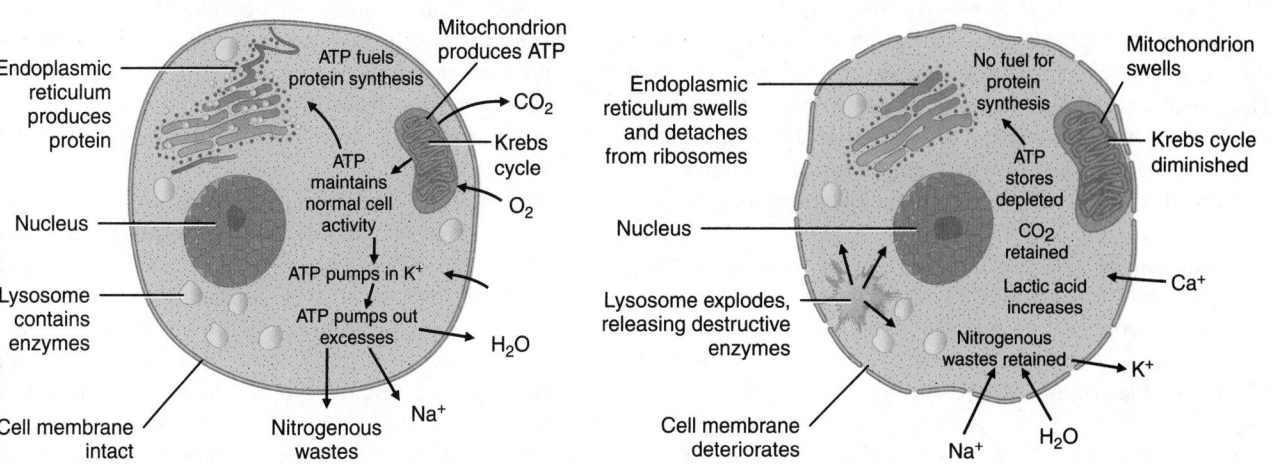

FIGURE 81-4 *Left,* Normal cell. *Right,* Alterations in cell function during late shock. *ATP,* Adenosine triphosphate; Ca^{++}, calcium; CO_2, carbon dioxide; H_2O, water; Na^+, sodium; O_2, oxygen.

the gastrointestinal (GI) tract. It causes a significant reduction in cardiac output, even in the presence of a normal circulating volume of blood. Another factor contributing to cardiac deterioration may be myocardial zonal lesions, which appear in the myocardium after ischemia or infarction. Cells in these areas do not fully repolarize and thus interfere with the usual efficient electrical conduction in the heart, which results in impaired contraction and possibly cardiac failure.

Cardiac depression is often compensated by the large cardiac reserve of a normal person. Because of this reserve, the heart can deteriorate to less than one third (sometimes less than one fifth) of its normal pumping strength without measurable evidence of cardiac failure.

Disseminated Intravascular Coagulation. During shock, tissue hypoxia results from the sluggish movement of blood in the capillaries. Anaerobic metabolism increases the production of lactic acid. The slow-moving acidic blood is hypercoagulable; however, it does not coagulate unless a clot-initiating factor is present. Such factors include bacterial endotoxins and thromboplastin of red blood cells (liberated by hemolysis). Hemolysis (destruction of red blood cells with the liberation of hemoglobin) accompanies trauma, especially when massive crushing injury occurs. When any of these factors is present along with the stagnant, acidic blood of shock, widespread intravascular clotting may occur in the vessels. This disorder is called *disseminated intravascular coagulation* (DIC) (see Chapter 75).

DIC is associated with multiple thrombi or emboli that are deposited in the microvascular circulation, with resultant organ obstruction and increased tissue ischemia. As blood attempts to flow through partially obstructed vessels, widespread hemolysis may occur. When red blood cells are destroyed, hemoglobin is again liberated. Anemia occurs because the liberated hemoglobin is excreted by the kidneys.

Because of the inappropriate clotting that occurs with DIC, the body attempts to reverse the process by breaking down clots. However, clots are destroyed throughout the body, not just the inappropriately formed clots. This results in bleeding in areas previously sealed by clots (e.g., venipuncture sites, vascular leaks in the brain). As DIC progresses, clotting factors are depleted, causing an inability to form normal clots in the presence of bleeding.

Treatment of the precipitating cause, anticoagulant therapy, and replacement of clotting factors must be started as soon as possible for maximal effectiveness. DIC is a serious complication that occurs in almost 40% of clients in septic shock and is often fatal.

Vasoconstriction. Sluggish circulation decreases the removal of CO_2 from the tissues. Increased levels of CO_2 dilate arterioles located in active tissues and constrict those in nonactive tissues. Because of the heart's increased activity, excessive CO_2 is produced in the myocardium. Increased concentration of CO_2 directly dilates the coronary arteries leading to the myocardium, which allows the myocardium to receive more arterial blood. CO_2 is also a powerful stimulant of the vasoconstrictor center in the sympathetic nervous system. With vasoconstriction of nonactive tissues, blood is shunted to the more active tissues, which have a greater immediate need.

Vasoactive Substances. Vasoactive substances (see below) are highly variable in promoting vasoconstriction or vasodilation in a person experiencing shock. The influence they exert may be altered by factors such as pH, the specific tissue (e.g., heart, lung), the presence of drugs or other substances, serum electrolyte levels, and sensitivity of the end organ.

Catecholamines. Catecholamines, such as epinephrine and norepinephrine, are present early in shock and are related to the fight-or-flight response. Their general effects are to increase blood flow to the brain, heart, and striated (skeletal) muscle and to decrease blood flow to the skin, kidneys, and splanchnic bed. Although the initial effect of vasoconstriction in the skin, kidneys, and splanchnic bed (GI tract) increases the intravascular volume, sustained vasoconstriction contributes to stagnant hypoxia and cellular death.

Vasoactive Polypeptides. Among the more important vasoactive polypeptides that appear to play significant roles in shock are the following:

1. *Histamine.* Histamine causes vasodilation, increased capillary permeability, bronchoconstriction, coronary vasodilation, and cutaneous reactions (flares, wheals). The effects of histamine are especially obvious in anaphylactic and septic shock.
2. *Bradykinin.* A kinin peptide, bradykinin produces vasodilation, increased capillary permeability, smooth muscle relaxation, pain, and infiltration of an area with leukocytes. Kinins appear to be most active in late shock. They may be a factor in the development of pulmonary insufficiency associated with shock.
3. *Angiotensin.* Angiotensin results from the action of renal renin on angiotensinogen. This potent substance causes vasoconstriction and increased vascular resistance. Although similar to norepinephrine in effect, angiotensin may produce fewer negative effects. Its role in sodium and water retention (through the stimulation of aldosterone secretion) is discussed under Adrenal Response.
4. *MDF.* MDF is a vasoactive polypeptide that contributes to cardiac failure in clients in shock by depressing cardiac muscle contraction.

Neuroendocrine System

General Adaptation Syndrome Response. Neuroendocrine responses during shock are defensive reactions that occur during the body's stage of resistance in the general adaptation syndrome (GAS). Because the length of the stage of resistance varies among people and is determined by the body's ability to compensate for its deficiencies, one person may be able to combat shock longer than another. For example, a previously healthy person may have a longer stage of resistance against shock compared with a person who is debilitated before shock develops. Various components of the sympathoadrenal (sympathetic part of the autonomic nervous system and adrenal medulla) response to a major stressor are shown in Figure 81-5.

Adrenal Response. Basic features of the neuroendocrine responses include (1) the release of epinephrine and norepinephrine from the adrenal medulla (which results in increased respiratory and heart rates, increased BP, increased blood flow to organs, decreased blood flow to peripheral tissues), and (2) the release of mineralocorticoids (which control fluid and electrolyte balance) and glucocorticoids (which increase blood glucose levels and reduce pain) from the adrenal cortex.

Increased production of adrenocortical mineralocorticoid hormones occurs. The main mineralocorticoids—aldosterone and desoxycorticosterone—help increase intravascular fluid volume by stimulating the kidneys to retain sodium and water. The renal tubular conservation of sodium occurs with any type of fluid loss or blood volume depletion. Aldosterone is essential to the conservation of sodium. Because water is retained in the body along with sodium, urine excretion is diminished during shock. This fluid is retained in the bloodstream to increase blood volume. Increasing the volume of blood in this way is aimed at increasing venous return, cardiac output, and BP.

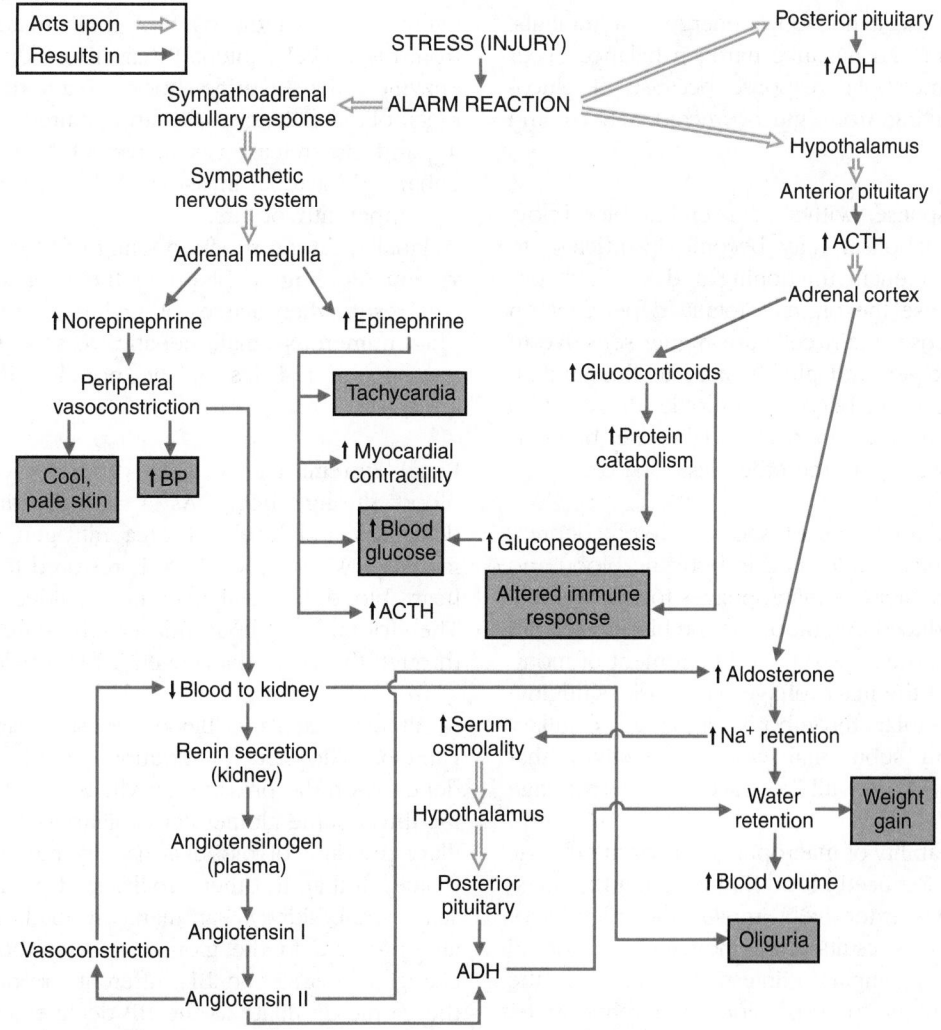

■ FIGURE 81–5 Components of the neuroendocrine response to a major stressor. Readily observed clinical manifestations as well as laboratory values are indicated by the boxes. *ACTH,* Adrenocorticotropic hormone; *ADH,* antidiuretic hormone; *BP,* blood pressure.

Pituitary Response. Of major importance in regulating water and sodium balance are aldosterone and ADH, also called *vasopressin*. ADH is produced by the posterior pituitary gland. The osmolality (osmotic concentration) of blood increases with dehydration. This stimulates osmoreceptors in the hypothalamus to release ADH from the posterior pituitary gland. ADH is carried via the blood to the kidneys, where it causes the body to retain water.

Metabolic Response. In general, the hormonal response to stress rapidly provides fuel for the body's various tissues, organs, and systems. These fuels (e.g., amino acids, fatty acids, glucose) are produced by the breakdown of food. These substances are then chemically converted into energy, resulting in the formation of ATP. ATP is the main source of energy produced and used inside the body's cells.

The glucocorticoids, particularly hydrocortisone, mobilize energy stores. During the initial phase of shock, the body's small stores of available carbohydrate are rapidly depleted. It then becomes necessary to mobilize protein and fat stores to meet the body's energy requirements. Protein catabolism and negative nitrogen balance occur as part of the metabolic response because of gluconeogenesis (resulting from glucocorticoid action) and starvation.

Neurologic Response. With shock, cerebral blood flow and cerebral metabolism may become insufficient to maintain normal mental functioning and level of consciousness. Because the brain is totally dependent on oxygen and glucose, brain cells are highly sensitive to a shortage of oxygen and glucose and to fluid imbalances. When the brain becomes hypoxic, the cerebral vessels dilate to restore blood flow. Likewise, blood is diverted to the brain from the other, less vital organs.

Immune System. All forms of shock severely depress macrophages, which are located in both the blood and the tissues. The capacity of macrophages to remove bacteria is greatly reduced. Alterations in the blood itself are partially due to tissue hypoxia and impairment of monitoring activities of the macrophage. The stasis, sludging, tendency for venular thrombosis, impaired capillary permeability, and subnormal vascular reactivity that occur during shock can all be traced to macrophage dysfunction.

The impaired ability of macrophages to ward off toxic agents is critical. Reduced blood flow through the intestines during shock extensively impairs the integrity of intestinal tissue. This results in the movement of normal GI flora across the impaired intestinal tissue into the bloodstream, leading to a possible bacteremic state. The person in a state of shock is more susceptible to bacterial products, particularly bacterial endotoxins, because of alterations in macrophage function.

Gastrointestinal System. Under sympathetic stimulation, vagal stimulation to the GI tract slows or stops, resulting in ileus with an absence of peristalsis. A lack of nutrient blood supply to the intestines increases the risk of tissue necrosis and sepsis. GI changes appear to have a more important role in the progression of shock than previously thought. The submucosa of the intestine becomes ischemic early in shock. If ischemia is prolonged, actual tissue necrosis of intestinal mucosa occurs. The intestinal arterioles and venules seem highly susceptible to the extensive vasoconstriction that occurs during shock. The massive amount of tissue destruction within the intestines that results from vasoconstriction and tissue anoxia is sufficient to cause tissue death even if bacteria are not present. Bacteria and their toxins contribute to shock by escaping into the systemic circulation following destruction of the intestinal mucosa barrier.

Shock causes serious changes in the functions of the liver, the major organ of detoxification. The liver suffers from this impaired circulation and appears to be a source of toxic materials. Normally, the liver protectively traps and disposes of toxic materials (released from the bowel contents) that are products of bacterial enzyme actions. During shock, the anoxic liver develops metabolic deficiencies, has an impaired ability to detoxify, and may release vasoactive substances. In addition, enhanced bacterial invasion of the liver from the intestine apparently occurs.

Finally, during shock, pooling of blood occurs in the viscera. Pooling of blood in the liver and portal bed may result when masses of agglutinated (clotted) blood plug numerous small hepatic vessels, sinusoids, and intrahepatic radicles of the portal vein and hepatic artery.

Renal System. The kidneys do not receive adequate blood during shock. As a result, urine production decreases and levels of urea nitrogen and creatinine increase. When blood flow is restored to the brain and heart, blood flow will again be provided to the kidneys. Therefore urine output indicates the status of circulation through the vital organs even if BP is below normal.

Altered Capillary Blood Pressure and Glomerular Filtration. Glomerular filtration within the kidneys depends on the pressure at which the blood is circulating through the glomerular capillaries. The average capillary pressure of blood is usually much higher in the glomeruli than in other capillaries. Under usual circumstances, the kidneys can maintain this heightened capillary pressure in the glomeruli even though there are changes in systemic BP. Afferent arterioles supplying the glomeruli dilate as the BP declines and constrict as it increases. However, this adaptive mechanism cannot protect the kidneys indefinitely against damage from a decreasing systemic BP.

When blood volume and BP decline steadily during shock, glomerular filtration is progressively reduced, which leads to an inability of the kidneys to excrete sodium and water. To compensate, the body excretes some sodium and water through the sweat glands. Damaged kidneys also lose their crucial ability to regulate electrolyte and acid-base balance.

Inadequate perfusion of renal capillaries is believed to be the cause of early prerenal failure in shock. The afferent and efferent arterioles constrict, shunting blood away from the glomeruli. If shock persists, actual renal shutdown occurs from focal tubular necrosis. Vasoconstriction in the kidneys may continue for a prolonged time after the systemic BP is restored to normal levels.

Renal Ischemia. During shock, the kidneys may experience renal ischemia. Because the kidneys have a high rate of metabolism, they are highly susceptible to injury of the tubule cells when the blood supply is deficient. When injury to the kidneys is extensive and renal failure ensues, acute tubular necrosis (ATN) occurs. With appropriate intervention, including careful fluid administration, the kidneys can heal. Normal kidney function usually returns after 10 to 14 days.

Clinical Manifestations
Systemic Manifestations of Shock

Because shock affects every system within the body, there are numerous clinical manifestations. Subjective complaints are usually nonspecific and may not be particularly helpful to the clinician attempting to diagnose shock and treat the client. The client may report feeling sick, weak, cold, hot, nauseated, dizzy, confused, frightened, thirsty, or short of breath. Observable and measurable manifestations are often conflicting (Figure 81-6). BP, cardiac output, and urine output are usually decreased. Respiratory rate is usually increased. Variable indicators of shock include alterations in heart rate, core body temperature, skin temperature, systemic vascular resistance, and skin color. Dyspnea, altered sensorium, and diaphoresis may be present. The manifestations discussed in the sections that follow are usually present in people with shock of any type.

Respiratory System. Rapid, shallow respirations (tachypnea) typically occur during shock because of decreased tissue perfusion. The respiratory rate increases as the oxygen-carrying capacity of the blood decreases. These changes may signal the development of hypoxemia and respiratory alkalosis.

Cardiovascular System

Tachycardia. Increased heart rate is the result of increased sympathetic stimulation. Tachycardia is an attempt to maintain adequate cardiac output and MAP when the blood's circulating volume declines. With increased rate, the pulse becomes typically weak and thready. At the onset of shock, the pulse rate does not

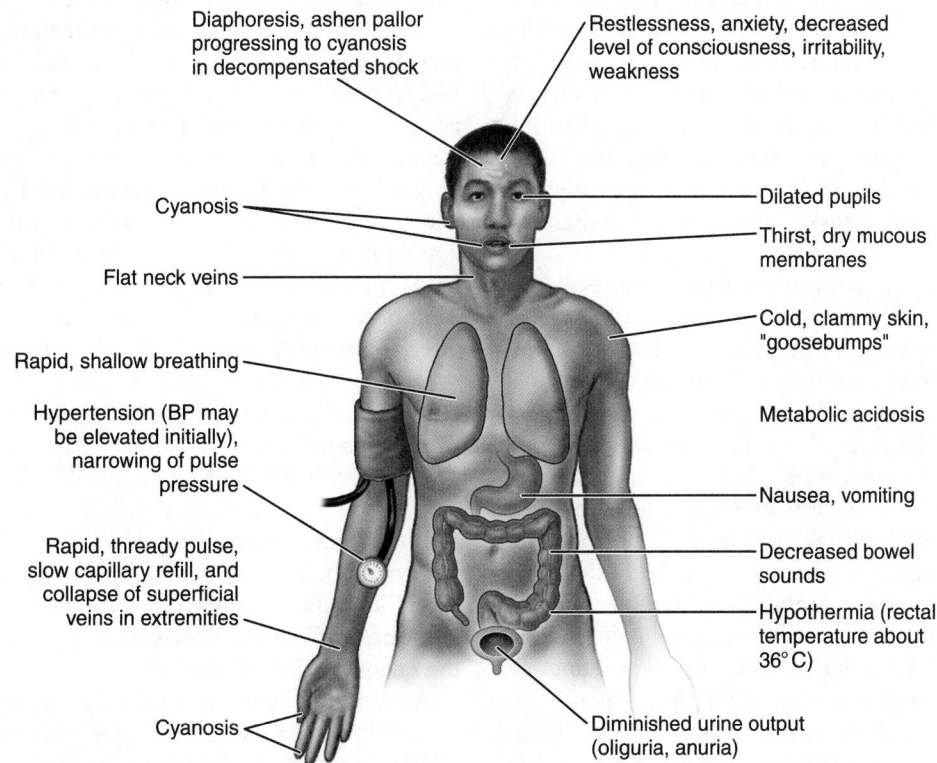

Diaphoresis, ashen pallor progressing to cyanosis in decompensated shock

Restlessness, anxiety, decreased level of consciousness, irritability, weakness

Cyanosis

Flat neck veins

Rapid, shallow breathing

Hypertension (BP may be elevated initially), narrowing of pulse pressure

Rapid, thready pulse, slow capillary refill, and collapse of superficial veins in extremities

Cyanosis

Dilated pupils

Thirst, dry mucous membranes

Cold, clammy skin, "goosebumps"

Metabolic acidosis

Nausea, vomiting

Decreased bowel sounds

Hypothermia (rectal temperature about 36° C)

Diminished urine output (oliguria, anuria)

FIGURE 81–6 Clinical manifestations of the client with hypovolemic shock.

relate as directly to the severity of shock as does BP, because in the early stage of shock, worry, excitement, and fear may influence the heart rate out of proportion to the underlying conditions. However, when emotional factors are no longer significant, serial observations of the pulse rate over a period of time are highly useful to assess the client's condition and the direction of the shock state and to evaluate the effectiveness of intervention.

Older clients (with and without various degrees of heart block) and clients taking beta-blocking medications, however, may show little change in heart rate despite the presence of conditions causing circulatory failure (e.g., hemorrhage). The pulse rate may become extremely slow in the terminal stages of shock and is usually slow in neurogenic shock.

Hypotension. The systolic BP indicates the integrity of the heart, arteries, and arterioles. The diastolic BP indicates the resistance (*systemic vascular resistance* [SVR] or *vasoconstriction*) of blood vessels. For example, an increasing diastolic BP indicates increasing systemic blood vessel resistance. Conversely, a declining diastolic BP indicates decreasing SVR. When the diastolic BP decreases significantly, vasoconstriction is being lost as a compensatory mechanism. When vasoconstriction is replaced by marked vasodilation, there is no resistance to blood flow and an adequate BP is difficult to maintain.

Usually, the BP begins to decrease when total blood volume is decreased by about 15% to 20%, although some clients may lose as much as 25% of the total blood volume without having a decline in BP. This is especially true in young adults; therefore in young adults, declining BP is a *very* late manifestation of shock. Typically, as shock progresses, both the systolic and the diastolic BPs drop, with the systolic pressure dropping more than the diastolic. The pulse pressure narrows because it is equal to the difference between the systolic and diastolic BPs.

During shock, pulse pressure is actually more significant than BP because it tends to parallel cardiac stroke volume. Pulse pressure is affected by stroke volume and by peripheral resistance. If stroke volume is decreased from a reduced circulating blood volume, pulse pressure decreases. In shock, pulse pressure may decrease even in the presence of an acceptable systolic BP. This may provide a clue to worsening shock. In shock, pulse pressure is often less than 20 mm Hg. The Critical Monitoring feature above, right, lists additional manifestations that require immediate intervention.

To maintain coronary circulation, a minimal systolic BP of 60 to 70 mm Hg is necessary. In interpreting BP readings, it is important to know what the client's BP has been. A systolic BP of 100 mm Hg or less is significant for clients whose systolic BP usually ranges from 110 to 140 mm Hg. When a client is supine, a decline

in BP may be a late finding. Hypotension by itself is not shock. Healthy clients often have BP readings lower than textbook normal values.

Additional problems need to be considered in assessment of BP that makes BP an unreliable criterion for assessing the presence and severity of shock. In the early, nonprogressive stage of shock, BP changes are generally unreliable because the arterial pressure may actually be normal or slightly elevated even though shock is present. In fact, blood volume deficits of 1 L or more may occur even though arterial and venous pressures are normal or elevated. When severe vasoconstriction is present, BP may be normal even though the circulation is actually highly inadequate. Conversely, the blood flow may be adequate even though BP is decreased (e.g., because of mechanisms such as vasodilation).

Valuable information about the level of arterial pressure in clients with vasoconstriction can be gained by assessing the strength of the femoral pulses. Doppler study may also be appropriate to obtain an accurate peripheral BP. Arterial lines are also used to monitor arterial pressures. With displaced or depleted blood volume, it is important to consider adequate venous filling. Hypovolemia, whether actual or relative, causes superficial veins to flatten. This change may hamper attempts to insert intravenous (IV) catheters for fluid replacement.

Neuroendocrine System. Early in shock, hyperactivity of the sympathetic nervous system with increased secretion of epinephrine usually causes the client to feel anxious, nervous, and irritable. Anxiety and worry are seen in the client's facial expressions.

Assessment findings associated with lack of blood flow to the brain are determined by the suddenness with which the shock develops and by its severity. With sudden, severe shock, the body may not have time to initiate its compensatory adjustment mechanisms. Consequently, the brain is deprived of its blood supply. The client may feel dizzy and faint on sitting up from a horizontal position because of postural hypotension. Fainting and unconsciousness may occur. If shock develops gradually over a period of hours, early assessment findings may include apathy and confusion or the opposite—restlessness and unusual alertness.

The systolic BP is important in maintaining blood flow to the brain. A cerebral perfusion pressure (CPP) of at least 50 mm Hg is required to deliver blood to the brain. Cerebral perfusion pressure can be computed by subtracting intracranial pressure from MAP (see Chapter 73 for measurement of intracranial pressure):

$$CPP = MAP - ICP$$

Usually, a decrease in systolic BP is accompanied by a reduced flow of blood to the brain. The vessels of the brain, like those of the heart, however, are not constricted by the vasoconstrictor center in the medulla oblongata. Thus blood from the peripheral vessels can be shifted to the brain as an emergency compensatory measure.

A client's level of consciousness decreases as circulation to brain tissue becomes increasingly impaired. Confusion, agitation, and restlessness may occur. In trauma situations, restlessness can be mistaken for pain. If opioids are given, the client's situation may be worsened or it may be difficult to detect worsening hypoxia. Drowsiness and stupor are more likely in shock related to severe infection than in shock caused by trauma and hemorrhage. As compensatory mechanisms fail, apathy may ensue. Ultimately, coma may develop.

Renal System. A decrease in urinary volume, often the earliest manifestation of developing shock, may occur even while arterial BP and pulse remain stable. Although urine output is one of the most sensitive indices in shock, any form of shock that develops rapidly shows other manifestations before decreased urine output is noticed.

Urine output should be kept greater than 0.5 ml/kg/hour. If the hourly output diminishes significantly, treatment must be instituted to prevent renal failure. Urinary flow of less than 0.5 ml/kg/hour can cause ATN from inadequate renal circulation.

Clinical Manifestations of Specific Types of Shock

Hypovolemic Shock. Initially, urine osmolality and specific gravity increase because of sodium and water reabsorption, which attempts to support circulating volume. As altered tissue perfusion and the hypovolemic shock progress, urine osmolality and specific gravity decrease because of the inability of the kidneys to reabsorb sodium and water. Sympathetic stimulation increases

pulse rate and respirations and decreases tissue perfusion to the skin, causing the skin to feel cool, clammy from diaphoresis, and to appear pale. Clients may sweat profusely, which increases insensible fluid loss, leading to further hypovolemia and temperature instability. Cyanosis may indicate either decreased tissue perfusion or decreased oxygenation, or both. Cyanosis is a late manifestation of decreased oxygenation.

Cardiogenic Shock. Because of the impaired muscle action or mechanical obstruction that caused the cardiogenic shock, blood is inadequately pumped through the heart. This results in a back-up of blood. When the shock is due to right-sided heart failure, this back-up is evidenced as jugular venous distention and increased CVP. (See Chapters 56 and 63 for discussions of cardiac tamponade and tension pneumothorax, respectively.) When the shock is due to left-sided failure, blood backs up into the pulmonary circulation, resulting in pulmonary edema, crackles in the lungs, and increased pulmonary capillary wedge pressure (PCWP). As in hypovolemic shock, there is stimulation of the sympathetic nervous system because of decreased cardiac output and decreased BP and all of the resultant clinical manifestations.

Distributive Shock

Anaphylactic Shock. Initially, the client may complain of a vague feeling of uneasiness or a feeling of impending doom. The massive vasodilation that occurs with anaphylaxis may cause complaints of headache as well. This may be followed by severe anxiety, dizziness, disorientation, and loss of consciousness.

The respiratory system develops many manifestations. The initial complaint may be a feeling of a lump in the throat, which is due to laryngeal edema and is followed by hoarseness, coughing, dyspnea, and stridor. Diffuse wheezes and a prolonged expiratory phase are heard on auscultation. If a pulse oximeter is in use, there may be a rapid decline in oxygen saturation. Additional complaints may include pruritus and urticaria. Direct observation may also demonstrate edema of the eyelids, lips, or tongue (angioedema).

Neurogenic Shock. Neurogenic shock may not present like the other forms of shock. The client often has bradycardia and hypotension (which cannot be corrected because of loss of the inability to vasoconstrict vessels). Below the level of injury, skin temperature takes on the same temperature as the room (poikilothermia). Skin is dry to the touch because of an inability to sweat.

Septic Shock. A person with severe sepsis develops the hypotension, coagulation disorders, and multisystem organ dysfunction of septic shock due, in part, to a dysregulated expression of the body's mediators of inflammation. The relationship between the outcomes of sepsis and the inflammatory response has led to a multitude of research.

Sepsis is diagnosed when two or more of these manifestations are present:

- Temperature greater than 38° C or less than 36° C
- Heart rate greater than 90 beats per minute
- Respiratory rate greater than 20 breaths per minute or a $Paco_2$ in arterial gas less than 32 mm Hg
- WBC count greater than 12,000 cells/ml, less than 4000 cells/ml, or greater than 10% band forms

In the early stages of septic shock, the body experiences massive vasodilation. Warm, dry, flushed skin is apparent during this hyperdynamic stage of septic shock. The compensatory increase in cardiac output and resultant increased perfusion of the skin give this stage the name "warm shock." During later stages, when compensatory mechanisms fail, the release of MDF and decreased venous return result in decreased perfusion and "cold shock," or the hypodynamic stage. At this point, the skin becomes pale, cold, clammy, and mottled. Body temperature decreases to subnormal levels. Auscultation of the lungs reveals crackles and wheezes, which develop secondary to pulmonary congestion as ARDS ensues. In addition to the clinical manifestations seen with shock in general, changes in the level of consciousness may include drowsiness and stupor progressing to coma. The Concept Map on p. 2169 illustrates the pathology, clinical manifestations, and related treatment interventions for the various stages of septic shock.

Diagnostic Assessment

Diagnostic assessments of clients in shock should include oxygenation, organ perfusion, and fluid balance. Assessment of respiratory status can be accomplished to some degree by noninvasive procedures such as spirometry, pulse oxymetry. Other noninvasive assessment and monitoring tools are the cardiac monitor and the 12-lead electrocardiogram (ECG). Laboratory studies include a complete blood cell count, blood chemistry, and blood and body fluid cultures for certain clients.

ABG analysis may also be done to determine whether the metabolic acidosis that occurs with shock is being effectively combated by hyperventilation. A low $Paco_2$, along with low pH and bicarbonate levels (metabolic acidosis), indicates that hyperventilation is trying to compensate. However, an increasing $Paco_2$ in the presence of a persistently low pH indicates that respiratory assistance is needed. It is also important to monitor Pao_2 levels to determine whether the client is being adequately oxygenated (see the Critical Monitoring feature on worsening shock on p. 2166).

CVP measurement is one of the first invasive assessments made in the presence of shock to estimate fluid

loss. A pulmonary artery or Swan-Ganz catheter may also be inserted to assist with assessments of fluid status, cardiac function, and tissue oxygen consumption (see Chapter 54).

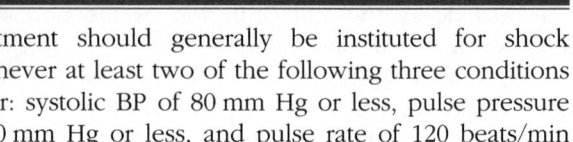

OUTCOME MANAGEMENT

Treatment should generally be instituted for shock whenever at least two of the following three conditions occur: systolic BP of 80 mm Hg or less, pulse pressure of 20 mm Hg or less, and pulse rate of 120 beats/min or more. Pulse pressure is calculated by subtracting diastolic BP from systolic BP and is normally between 30 and 50 mm Hg.

The therapeutic management of shock has changed markedly over recent years. Lowering the head, raising the feet, and administering potent vasoconstrictor drugs were once the foundation of treatment for a client in shock. Now, emphasis is placed on maintaining adequate circulating volume, using body positions that do not interfere with pulmonary ventilation, and the use of medications having both vasoconstrictor and vasodilator effects.

The following discussion addresses the general interventions for shock. Tables 81-2, 81-3, and 81-4 give specific interventions for hypovolemic, cardiogenic, and distributive shock, respectively.

Medical Management

Correct the Causative Factor

Assessment and an accurate differential medical diagnosis, which establish the specific cause of the shock state, form the basis for treatment. The differential medical diagnosis is usually readily made unless the shock is in an advanced stage, at which point several specific forms of shock may exist at the same time. Some forms of shock more easily recognized are hypovolemic shock that is due to extensive burns or trauma and cardiogenic shock with severe chest pain and acute MI. Septic shock is also treated initially with fluids because of ongoing capillary leakage. Of course, antibiotics are used and if the organisms are not known, antibiotics are prescribed empirically, based on what the suspected organisms might be. Blood cultures are drawn, allowing the antibiotics to be refined for specific bacteria.

Improve Oxygenation

Maintaining the client's airway is vital to the treatment of shock. In all types of shock, supplemental oxygen is administered to protect against hypoxemia. Oxygen can be delivered via a nasal cannula, a mask, a high-flow non-rebreathing mask, an endotracheal tube, or a tracheostomy tube.

Endotracheal intubation, or tracheostomy, may be performed to rest an exhausted client during severe or

Understanding Septic Shock and Its Treatment

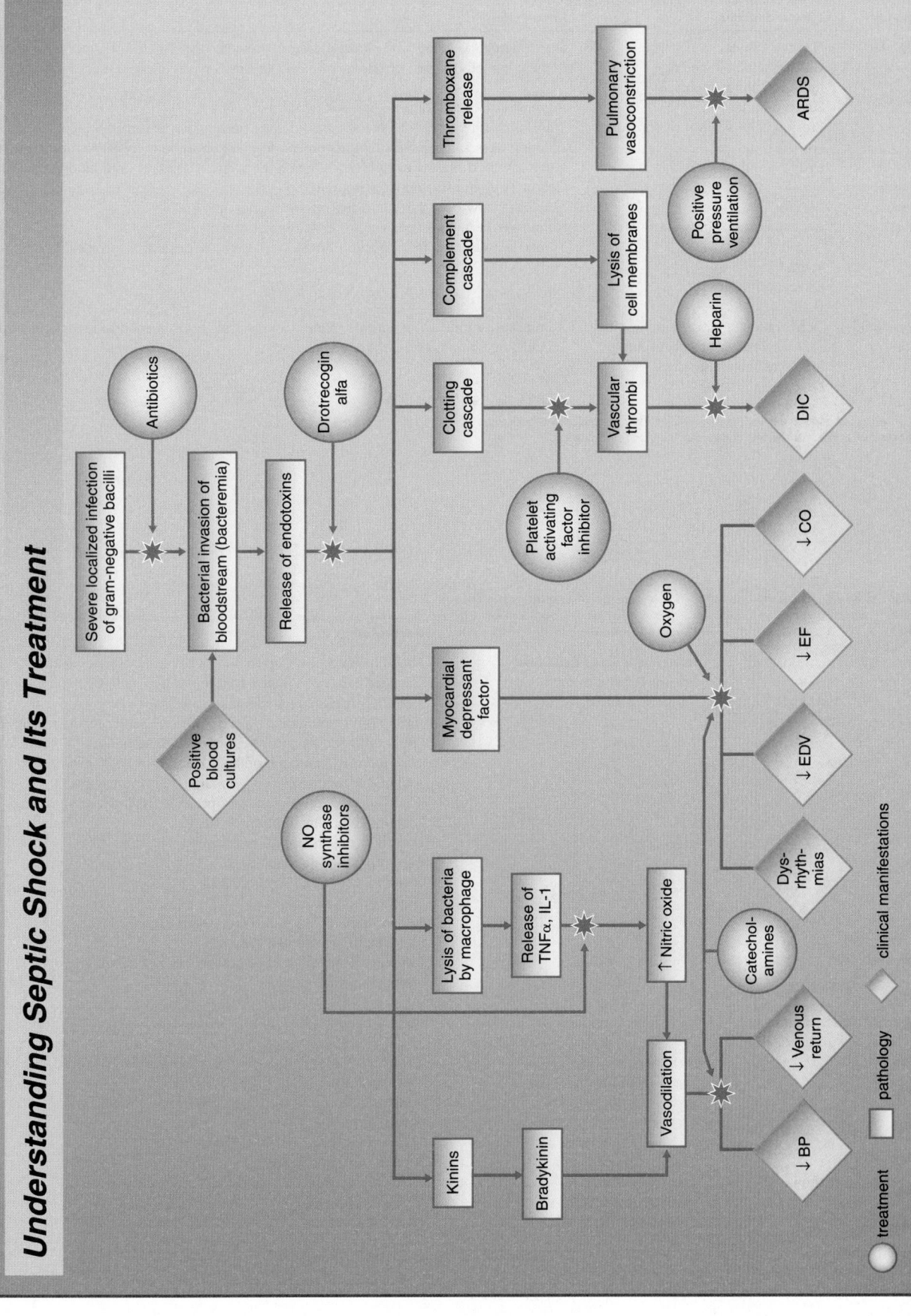

ARDS, Acute respiratory distress syndrome; *BP,* blood pressure; *CO,* cardiac output; *DIC,* disseminated intravascular coagulation; *EDV,* end-diastolic volume; *EF,* ejection fraction; *IL-1,* interleukin 1; *NO,* nitric oxide; *TNF,* tumor necrosis factor.

TABLE 81–2 Summary of the Management of Hypovolemic Shock

Etiology	Clinical Situation	Intervention*
Blood loss	Massive trauma	Stop external bleeding with direct pressure, pressure dressing, tourniquet (as last resort)
	Gastrointestinal bleeding	Reduce intra-abdominal or retroperitoneal bleeding or prepare for emergency surgery
	Ruptured aortic aneurysm	
	Surgery	Administer lactated Ringer's solution or normal saline
	Erosion of vessel from lesion, tubes, or other devices	Transfuse with fresh whole blood, packed cells, fresh frozen plasma, platelets, or other clotting factors, if significant improvement does not occur with crystalloid administration
	DIC	Use non-blood plasma expanders (albumin, hetastarch, dextran) until blood is available
		Conduct autotransfusion if appropriate
Plasma loss	Burns	Administer low-dose cardiotonics (dopamine, dobutamine)
	Accumulation of intra-abdominal fluid	Administer lactated Ringer's solution or normal saline
	Malnutrition	Administer albumin, fresh frozen plasma, hetastarch, or dextran if cardiac output is still low
	Severe dermatitis	
	DIC	
Crystalloid loss	Dehydration (e.g., diabetic ketoacidosis, heat exhaustion)	Administer isotonic or hypotonic saline with electrolytes as needed to maintain normal circulating volume and electrolyte balance
	Protracted vomiting, diarrhea	
	Nasogastric suction	

DIC, Disseminated intravascular coagulation; *MAST,* military or medical antishock trousers.
*Assumes that airway management and cardiac monitoring are ongoing.

TABLE 81–3 Summary of the Management of Cardiogenic Shock

Etiology	Clinical Situation	Intervention*
Myocardial disease or injury	Acute myocardial infarction	Fluid-challenge with up to 300 ml of normal saline solution or lactated Ringer's solution to rule out hypovolemia, unless heart failure or pulmonary edema is present
	Myocardial contusion	Insert CVP or pulmonary artery catheter; monitor cardiac output, pulmonary artery pressure, and PCWP; administer IV fluids to maintain left ventricular filling pressure of 15-20 mm Hg
	Cardiomyopathies	Administer inotropics (e.g., dopamine or dobutamine)
		Vasodilators (e.g., sodium nitroprusside, nitroglycerin, calcium-channel blockers, morphine)
		Diuretics (e.g., mannitol or furosemide)
		Cardiotonics (e.g., digitalis)
		Beta-blockers (e.g., propranolol)
		Glucocorticosteroids†
		Intra-aortic balloon pump or external counterpulsation device if unresponsive to other therapies
Valvular disease or injury	Ruptured aortic cusp	Same as above: if rapid response does not occur, prepare for prompt cardiac surgery
	Ruptured papillary muscle	
	Ball thrombus	
External pressure on heart interferes with heart filling or emptying	Pericardial tamponade caused by trauma, aneurysm, cardiac surgery, pericarditis	Relieve tamponade with ECG-assisted pericardiocentesis; repair surgically if it recurs
	Massive pulmonary embolus	Thrombolytic (streptokinase) or anticoagulant (heparin) therapy; surgery for removal of clot
	Tension pneumothorax	Relieve air accumulation with needle thoracostomy or chest tube insertion
	Ascites	
	Hemoperitoneum	Relieve fluid accumulation with paracentesis
	Mechanical ventilation	Reduce inspiratory pressure
Cardiac dysrhythmias	Tachydysrhythmias	Treat dysrhythmias; be prepared to initiate CPR, cardiac pacing
	Bradydysrhythmias	
	Pulseless electrical activity	

CPR, Cardiopulmonary resuscitation; *CVP,* central venous pressure; *ECG,* electrocardiogram; *IV,* intravenous; *PCWP,* pulmonary capillary wedge pressure.
*Assumes that airway management and cardiac monitoring are ongoing.
†Controversial.

TABLE 81–4 Summary of the Management of Distributive Shock

Etiology	Clinical Situation	Intervention*
Anaphylactic shock	Allergy to food, medicines, dyes, insect bites, stings, or latex	Prepare for surgical management of airway Decrease further absorption of antigen (e.g., stop IV fluid, place tourniquet between injection or sting site and heart if feasible) Epinephrine (1:100) 2 inhalations every 3 hr, *or* Epinephrine (1:1000) 0.2-0.5 ml every 5-15 min given subcutaneously, *or* Epinephrine (1:10,000) 0.5-1.0 ml every 5-15 min given at a rate of 1 mg/min IV fluid resuscitation with isotonic solution Diphenhydramine HCl or H_1-receptor antagonist IV Theophylline IV drip for bronchospasm Steroids IV Vasopressors (e.g., norepinephrine, metaraminol bitartrate, high-dose dopamine) Gastric lavage for ingested antigen Ice pack to injection or sting site Meat tenderizer paste to sting site
Septic shock	Often gram-negative septicemia but also caused by other organisms in debilitated, immunodeficient, or chronically ill clients	Identify origin of sepsis; culture all suspected sources Vigorous IV fluid resuscitation with normal saline Empirical antibiotic therapy until sensitivities are reported Administer cardiotonic agents (e.g., dopamine or dobutamine, norepinephrine, isoproterenol, digitalis, calcium) Naloxone (narcotic antagonist) Prostaglandins Monoclonal antibodies Drotrecogin alfa Temperature control (both hypothermia and hyperthermia are noted) Heparin, clotting factors, blood products if DIC develops
Neurogenic (spinal) shock	Spinal anesthesia Spinal cord injury	Normal saline to restore volume Treat bradycardia with atropine Vasopressors (e.g., norepinephrine, metaraminol bitartrate, high-dose dopamine, and phenylephrine) may be given Place client in modified Trendelenburg position
Vasovagal reaction	Severe pain Severe emotional stress	Place client in a head-down or recumbent position Give atropine if bradycardia and profound hypotension; eliminate pain

DIC, Disseminated intravascular coagulation; *IV,* intravenous.
*Assumes airway management and cardiac monitoring are ongoing.

prolonged shock and to correct respiratory failure. By increasing the rate of pulmonary ventilation (through spontaneous or mechanical hyperventilation), it is possible to compensate for minor degrees of metabolic acidosis. This increased "blowing off" of carbon dioxide with hyperventilation begins to compensate for acid-base imbalance. Positive end-expiratory pressure may be added when the client is being mechanically ventilated. This assists in preventing atelectasis and may provide a higher Pao_2 for the client at a lower oxygen concentration setting. The goal of therapy is to maintain a Pao_2 greater than 50 mm Hg and an Sao_2 greater than 90% to avoid anaerobic metabolism. If the chest is congested, chest physical therapy, including vibration, percussion, and postural drainage, may be required.

Sometimes the interventions discussed cannot establish optimal tissue oxygenation. In these instances, hyperbaric oxygenation (HBO) or extracorporeal membrane oxyge-

nation may be used. HBO involves the administration of 100% oxygen under 2 to 3 atmospheres of pressure. This raises tissue oxygen tension to normal or above-normal levels. HBO requires the use of special chambers, which usually are available only in highly specialized institutions.

Extracorporeal membrane oxygenation is most commonly used in adults as a temporary intervention for refractory ARDS. Arterial and venous catheters are inserted, and some of the client's blood is diverted through them into a machine that artificially oxygenates the blood. This is a relatively expensive form of therapy and is usually done only in large medical centers.

Restore and Maintain Adequate Perfusion

The primary aim in treating shock is to maintain an adequate circulating blood volume. Unless this is accomplished early, subsequent therapeutic measures are of no avail, and death can be anticipated. During shock intervention, all of the basic pathophysiologic changes associated with the development of shock must be corrected.

Some problems that must often be treated are (1) the vascular problem of vasoconstriction with the diminished tissue perfusion it causes, (2) the intravascular problem of coagulation and sludging of blood cells, and (3) the extravascular problem of extravasation of fluid into the extravascular space. The Integrating Pharmacology feature below discusses vasoactive medications commonly used to treat shock.

Nitric Oxide. Inducible nitric oxide synthase is a complex found in endothelial and vascular smooth muscle cells. Endothelial cells continually produce low levels of nitric oxide to maintain normal vascular tone. During inflammatory states, nitric oxide production is increased, resulting in hypotension and vasodilation.

Vasoconstrictors. Vasoconstrictors elevate the systemic BP by constricting peripheral arterioles. Vasoconstrictor

agents may be used briefly in shock if compensatory vasoconstriction is unable to maintain blood flow to vital organs. They may also be used to correct hypotension secondary to vasoconstrictor nerve paralysis, as in spinal anesthesia or conditions associated with massive vasodilation. However, vasoconstrictors should not be used exclusively but should be given concomitantly with IV fluids to restore adequate circulation and perfusion.

Perfusion of vital organs with blood is impossible when systolic BP is less than 50 mm Hg. Usually, the goal of using vasoconstrictors is to achieve and maintain a mean BP of 70 to 80 mm Hg, which is sufficient to perfuse tissues. Generally, attempts to increase the BP beyond this level are not advisable because vasoconstrictors increase the oxygen demand of the heart and may cause fatal dysrhythmias. Vasoconstrictors are used with extreme caution in cardiogenic shock. Other major adverse effects of vasoconstrictors include decreased renal and splanchnic blood flow, excessive or sudden increase in arterial BP (which may precipitate heart failure), pulmonary edema or left ventricular (LV) decompensation, and gangrene of the fingers and toes from prolonged vasoconstriction.

Although the use of vasoconstrictors during shock is being critically evaluated, they do favorably increase blood flow to the brain and heart in severely hypotensive clients. Reduced tissue perfusion when systolic pressures are less than 60 to 70 mm Hg may precipitate an MI or a stroke.

Vasodilators. Agents that induce vasodilation or inhibit vasoconstriction may promote recovery from shock in which intensive vasoconstriction is contributing to the problem. These include adrenergic blocking agents, ganglionic blocking agents, and direct-acting peripheral vasodilators.

Adrenergic blockade prevents harmful effects of prolonged vasoconstriction such as increased pressure in capillaries, promoting fluid loss from the vascular to the interstitial compartment, and altered blood flow, especially in the splanchnic area. These agents are also used to keep coronary arteries open. Prolonged vasoconstriction also impairs cellular nutrition and allows accumulation of waste products. Adrenergic blockade prevents these changes in circulation and may also induce opposite beneficial changes.

Vasodilators may be helpful during shock when vasoconstriction is severe and persists even though fluids have been infused in what should be adequate amounts for fluid replacement. Vasodilators may be administered to inhibit vasoconstriction of peripheral blood vessels (the result of norepinephrine from sympathetic stimulation) so that blood can be redistributed to enhance tissue perfusion and increase vascular volume. Vasodilator medications are sometimes given in combination with vasoconstrictor medications to offset the profound effects

INTEGRATING PHARMACOLOGY

Vasoactive Medications for Shock Management

It may seem contradictory to use medications that vasoconstrict and medications that vasodilate in caring for individuals in shock. However, both actions are needed at times during shock and many of the medications used have actions that are beneficial during each stage.

In the nonprogressive stage of shock, when the body is experiencing significant vasodilation, vasoconstrictors, such as high-dose dopamine, norepinephrine, and phenylephrine, help maintain blood pressure (BP). Adding medications that increase cardiac contractility, such as amrinone and dobutamine, further support BP by increasing cardiac output. As shock progresses and vasoconstriction ensues, these same drugs, with some changes in dosing, are still effective in supporting the client's hemodynamic stability. Low-dose dopamine causes vasodilation of the renal and mesenteric blood vessels, helping to support perfusion of the kidneys and gut. Amrinone and dobutamine contribute to vasodilation of blood vessels in the heart and skeletal muscle, ensuring adequate oxygenation to those organs and tissues. If significant systemic vasoconstriction continues, relaxation of the vascular smooth muscle may be necessary with drugs such as nitroglycerin and nitroprusside.

Titration and changing of medications are continued until the client's shock is clearly reversed. If the client progresses to the irreversible stage of shock despite the health care team's best efforts, these drugs will have little, if any, effectiveness.

that may occur with some vasoconstrictors and to provide the benefits both types of drugs have to offer.

When shock is caused by hypovolemia, rapid and adequate fluid replacement is essential before vasodilators are used. Vasodilators are dangerous because they lower arterial BP if they are given while circulating blood volume is deficient. When the circulating blood volume is inadequate, the body depends on vasoconstriction to maintain arterial pressure. However, when the vascular space is full and cardiac venous return is adequate, vasodilation should open arterioles in the lungs and elsewhere. This lets blood circulate, increasing cardiac output and capillary perfusion without lowering systemic BP. In fact, a vasodilator may produce a dramatic, sustained increase in the systemic arterial pressure.

Keep clients who are receiving vasodilators lying relatively flat. Elevation of the head can produce dangerous orthostatic hypotension. Older clients may have sclerotic blood vessels and may not tolerate the hypotension that may accompany administration of vasodilators. In this situation, a cardiotonic drug (such as dobutamine) may be given with the vasodilator to increase cardiac output.

Characteristically, impaired tissue perfusion is correctable during early shock. However, it may be fatal if treatment is not received or is inadequate. In the later stages of shock, impaired tissue perfusion becomes irreversible, leading to death despite treatment. However, treatment for irreversible shock is never abandoned while the client remains alive. Before a client's shock state is viewed as probably irreversible, identification and treatment of occult bleeding and restoration of circulating volume, correction of any factors interfering with cardiopulmonary function, and treatment of overwhelming infection must be attempted.

Assist Circulation

Mechanical devices that assist circulation or decrease the workload of the heart may be used as temporary measures in managing clients in shock.

Intra-Aortic Balloon Pump (IABP). An IABP is used primarily in clients with cardiogenic shock. The ability of the heart to adequately pump blood is augmented by a balloon-tipped catheter placed in the descending thoracic aorta. The catheter is attached to a unit that inflates during diastole and deflates just before systole. This counterpulsation displaces blood back into the aorta and improves coronary artery circulation. In cardiogenic shock, use of the IABP reduces afterload, allowing the heart to more efficiently empty, thereby increasing cardiac output. Details of the IABP are found in the Bridge to Critical Care feature on Intra-Aortic Balloon Pumping in Chapter 56.

Modified Trendelenburg Position. A client in shock is usually placed in a modified Trendelenburg position with the lower extremities elevated 30 to 45 degrees, the knees straight, the trunk horizontal or very slightly raised, and the neck comfortably positioned with the head level with the chest or slightly higher (Figure 81-7). This position promotes increased venous return from the lower extremities without compressing the abdominal organs against the diaphragm. The traditional Trendelenburg position (head down, with legs elevated at least 30 degrees above the head) was once the classic shock position but is no longer used for shock management because it compresses the abdominal contents against the diaphragm, interfering with pulmonary excursion, and promotes congestion of blood in the brain, possibly contributing to cerebral edema.

Elevating the legs mobilizes blood that has pooled in the lower extremities. As a result of gravity, the additional circulating blood increases venous return to the heart, thus improving cardiac output. The position is of temporary value in moderate hypovolemia. However, it does not help in severe hypovolemia, because the extremities have very little blood in them in such a state. Generally, the modified shock position is not used with cardiogenic shock, when there is already circulatory overload.

Replace Fluid Volume

The mainstay of hypovolemic shock therapy is expansion of circulating blood volume by IV administration of blood or other appropriate fluids. Fluid replacement should be administered through large-bore peripheral lines, central venous lines, or both. A sizable amount of fluid (about 4 L in moderately severe shock) leaves the interstitial space. This is in addition to fluid lost from the circulating volume. Thus fluid replacement therapy must replace both blood lost from the circulation and fluid lost from the interstitial space. Fluid replacement therapy must be closely monitored to prevent circulatory overload. Hypervolemia can be lethal; thus aggressive fluid replacement should be tapered off when urine output is at least 0.5 ml/kg/hour, systolic BP is greater than 100 mm Hg, or the heart rate is 60 to 100 beats/min.

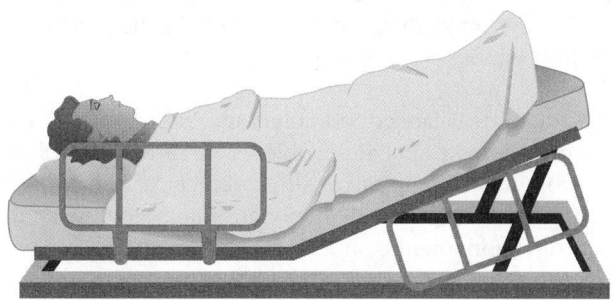

■ **FIGURE 81–7** Positioning of the person in shock. This position is a modification of Trendelenburg position and includes elevating the legs, leaving the trunk flat, and elevating the head and shoulders slightly.

In replacing fluids, enough volume must be administered to fill the capillaries and run through into the veins. Such fluid replacement maintains CVP and provides an adequate venous return to the heart. In addition, adequate fluid replacement decreases the sympathetic response and thus produces a vasodilation that promotes capillary flow. Adequate flow of fluids in the capillaries in turn perfuses tissues and prevents sludging and coagulation of blood within the vessels.

Blood. When hemorrhage is the primary cause of shock, the rapid administration of large volumes of packed cells or whole blood may be necessary. Type-specific, crossmatched blood is the most desirable form of blood replacement. However, if the client is hemorrhaging, it may be necessary to administer type-specific, un-crossmatched blood: O-negative blood or O-positive, low antibody titer blood. Women should receive Rh-negative blood.

When shock resulting from hemorrhage is treated, a crystalloid is usually given as an initial emergency treatment to sustain BP. Later, the acute anemia resulting from hemorrhage must be corrected by administration of packed cells for the prevention of hypoxemia.

During fluid replacement, a normal red blood cell mass should be maintained. Fluids given in excess of normal volume should be fluids other than blood so that they can be easily removed from the circulation by the kidneys once the shock is corrected. If the normal red blood cell mass is exceeded, it is difficult for the body to eliminate the excess red blood cells after the vascular volume returns to normal (after adequate perfusion of tissues with blood is achieved). Because dangers also are involved in blood transfusions, blood should not be used if another fluid can satisfactorily maintain an adequate oxygen-carrying capacity and can sufficiently increase blood volume. Blood can become so dilute that there are relatively few blood cells as the result of up to 8 to 12 L of fluid being administered in only a few hours.

Autotransfusion. Autotransfusion involves collecting and retransfusing blood into the same client. Autotransfusion is used to prevent or treat hypovolemic shock caused by hemorrhage. It is common in the treatment of chest injuries.

Crystalloid or Balanced Salt Solutions. Various fluids are given to correct specific problems, such as electrolyte or protein deficiencies or other defects of the blood, including acidosis and hyponatremia. However, in treating hypovolemic shock, the immediate results of therapy seem to depend less on the type of fluid administered for fluid replacement than on the amount of fluid administered. In general, enough fluid is given to exceed the normal blood volume. This "extra" fluid is required to replace intracellular fluid that was mobilized into the circulation as an early response to the hypovolemia. To assist with fluid administration, a three-to-one rule has been developed. For a client's estimated blood loss, three times as much crystalloid solution must be administered for adequate volume resuscitation. Crystalloid solutions that may be administered include normal saline, Ringer's lactate, or half-normal saline.

IV fluids used in shock management may include warmed crystalloids or balanced salt solutions, colloids, and blood. Dextrose and water should not be used to resuscitate a client; once the dextrose is metabolized, only hypotonic water remains, which leads to greater fluid shifts. Electrolyte solutions such as Ringer's lactate help expand extracellular volume, reduce viscosity, and prevent sludging. In a client with impaired liver function, a solution containing lactate could further compound the problem of lactic acidosis. In a normally functioning liver, lactate is converted to bicarbonate and does not accumulate. Because the liver is not an organ of primary perfusion during times of stress for the body and may not be functioning normally, other solutions should be considered before Ringer's lactate.

Abnormalities of electrolyte and acid-base balance are corrected with the specific substance needed rather than with a solution that administers multiple electrolytes and acid-base components. Therapy is gauged by serial ABG and electrolyte determinations.

Colloid Solutions. Colloid solutions contain proteins normally too large to exit at the capillary; thus they remain in the vascular compartment and increase osmotic pressure of the capillaries. This increased osmotic pressure helps pull fluid back into the vascular compartment and maintain circulating volume. These solutions may be used in conjunction with crystalloid solutions in treating hypovolemic shock to maintain an adequate circulating volume. The most commonly used colloid solutions include plasma and its components, plasma substitutes (e.g., dextran), oxygen-carrying solutions other than blood (e.g., perfluorocarbons and ultra-purified, stroma-free hemoglobin solutions), and hetastarch. (See discussions of blood and blood transfusions, Chapter 75.)

Colloid solutions cannot be used in clients with inflammatory conditions such as sepsis and burns. In these clients, capillary leakage is large enough that even the proteins escape.

Fresh frozen plasma (FFP) is the form commonly used to improve serum protein levels. FFP may be administered after massive transfusions to restore some clotting factors deficient in "banked" blood. Because FFP requires 15 to 30 minutes to thaw, it is not used in initial fluid resuscitation with shock.

Albumin may also be used to achieve adequate osmotic pressure. Occasionally, it is administered when sufficient amounts of other fluids fail to restore an adequate circulating volume. Use of albumin is controversial because it may move into the pulmonary interstitial space, drawing water along with it. Thus albumin may contribute to the development of ARDS.

Dextran may be used in both high- and low-molecular-weight forms. The advantage in using dextran is that it contains large molecules that should effectively and rapidly expand the intravascular volume. Dextran can interfere with blood type and crossmatch procedures and with clotting factors. It should therefore be used only after type and crossmatch have been done and until blood is available for transfusion. By initiating therapy with low-molecular-weight dextran and then progressing to high-molecular-weight forms, the incidence of hypersensitivity reactions to dextran can be lowered.

Blood Substitutes. Perfluorocarbons (e.g., Fluosol, Oxygent) are non-blood, oxygen-carrying solutions that remain in the circulation for about 12 to 24 hours. Major limitations associated with the use of perfluorochemicals relate to limited immediate availability (the product must be stored frozen), administration of 80% to 100% O_2 for the solution to be effective, and accumulation of the chemicals in the body. Advantages include the high solubility of perfluorocarbons, making them readily available to the tissues, and their acceptability to clients whose religious beliefs prohibit the use of blood products. Perfluorocarbons have been researched since the 1970s and are still in various stages of experimentation.

Hemoglobin-based oxygen carriers (e.g., stroma-free hemoglobin, PolyHeme, Hemopure, Hemolink) are made from hemoglobin that has been extracted from red blood cells and have been developed from bovine, recombinant, and human sources. Advantages are that no type and crossmatch is required for administration, so oxygen-carrying solutions are more readily available for situations in which major traumas occur or during periods of diminished blood availability. Concerns that still exist relate to the toxicity of the solutions, their short half-life, and their relatively high colloid oncotic pressure.

Hetastarch, a glycogen-like synthetic colloid, has been used to treat hypovolemic shock and may provide alternatives to blood administration. Its effects last between 3 and 24 hours. Pentastarch is also available as a volume expander.

🪔 Goal-Directed Therapy for Sepsis

Early goal-directed therapy (EGDT) is used for the treatment of sepsis. EGDT emphasizes early recognition of clients with potential sepsis in the ED and early use of broad-spectrum antibiotics and a rapid crystalloid fluid bolus, followed by goal-directed therapy for those clients who remain hypotensive or severely ill after this initial therapy (Box 81-1). EGDT is a three-step process aimed at optimizing tissue perfusion.

Step 1. Titrate crystalloid fluid administration to CVP, or administer 500-ml boluses of fluid until the CVP measures between 8 and 12 mm Hg. CVP is a surrogate for intravascular volume, as excess circulating blood volume is contained within the venous system. Only after the CVP is greater than 8 mm Hg should vasopressors be considered. A central venous catheter in the internal jugular or subclavian vein is placed to measure central venous pressure (CVP) and an arterial catheter to directly measure arterial blood pressure for those clients who did respond to fluids.

Step 2. If the client has not improved with fluid alone, vasopressors are administered to attain a mean arterial pressure (MAP) greater than 65 mm Hg.

Step 3. Evaluate the central venous oxygen saturation (Svo_2). The sample is obtained from the CV line, the blood from which is a surrogate for peripheral tissue oxygenation and cardiac output. An Svo_2 of less than 70% is considered abnormal and indicative of suboptimal therapy. In this case, the hematocrit is checked and blood transfused until a hematocrit greater than 30% is attained. Once this is attained and the Svo_2 is still low, dobutamine is initiated to increase cardiac output.

BOX 81-1   Sepsis Bundle

To improve quality and outcomes of care, a "sepsis bundle" was developed. For implementation of the bundle of care, a client must meet the following criteria:

1. Two or more of the following four items:
   a. Temperature >38.3° C or <36.0° C
   b. Heart rate >90 beats/min
   c. Respiration >20 breaths/min
   d. White blood cell count >12,000/mm³ or <4000/mm³, or >10% bandemia (banded leukocytes)
2. A suspected infection
3. SBP <90 mm Hg after 20 ml/kg fluid bolus or lactate >4 mmol/L

6-HOUR EMERGENCY DEPARTMENT SEVERE SEPSIS BUNDLE

1. Initiate CVP/Svo_2 monitoring within 2 hours of meeting bundle criteria.
2. Give broad-spectrum antibiotics within 4 hours (preferably 1 hour) of meeting bundle criteria.
3. Complete early goal-directed therapy (CVP ≥8 mm Hg, SBP ≥90 mm Hg, or MAP ≥65 mm Hg and Svo_2 ≥70%) at 6 hours of meeting bundle criteria.
4. Give steroid if client is receiving vasopressor or if adrenal insufficiency is suspected.
5. Monitor for lactate clearance.

From Nguyen, H.B., Corbett, S.W., Steele, R., et al. (2007). Implementation of a bundle of quality indicators for the early management of severe sepsis and septic shock is associated with decreased mortality. *Critical Care Medicine, 35* (4), 1105-1112.

Evaluate Fluid Replacement

Often, fluid replacement is the only treatment required for shock. However, it is difficult to evaluate whether fluid replacement is adequate. Internal losses of circulating fluid volume, including whole blood, into areas of traumatized tissue or into third spaces are difficult to estimate. If a vasoconstrictor drug has been administered or if prolonged vasoconstriction occurs, an additional considerable loss of circulating volume may also occur because of vasoconstriction. Large volumes of IV fluid may be administered either until systemic BP, urinary volume, and lactate levels become relatively normal or until central venous or pulmonary artery pressures, or both, stabilize or become elevated.

Infusion of blood or other fluids usually continues only as long as the CVP is low, that is, less than 4 cm H_2O or 2 mm Hg. When the CVP is higher than normal (e.g., greater than 15 cm H_2O or 11 mm Hg), benefit cannot be expected from the continued infusion of fluids or blood beyond maintenance amounts. When the CVP is low and the lungs are clear, with no indications of heart failure, fluids are administered to improve the return of blood to the heart. However, some clients have a normal or low CVP despite faulty LV function. They readily develop heart failure or pulmonary edema. Thus a low or normal CVP does not always mean that fluid administration is advisable.

If there is an adequate systemic response, IV fluid administration should be stopped before extremely high elevations of pulmonary artery pressures occur. An adequate volume of circulating fluid causes an ample venous return to the right side of the heart and increases the right-sided output. Pulmonary artery hypertension may develop if continued pulmonary obstruction is present because of coagulation in the microcirculation or vasoconstriction. This appears as increased pulmonary artery pressure. In the presence of right-sided heart failure, this increased pressure may back up through the right side of the heart, causing an abnormal elevation in CVP. Vasodilators may help open this partially blocked pulmonary microcirculation.

Prevent Complications

Prevent Renal Impairment. To prevent acute renal damage, the urine output is monitored, and diuretics (e.g., furosemide) may be given if fluid volume has been corrected. The normal rate of urinary excretion from the kidneys is 0.5 ml/kg. A client who becomes acutely hypovolemic or is experiencing a redistribution of circulating volume cannot maintain an hourly output of 40 to 60 ml of urine. Decreased urine output (oliguria) typically occurs in shock. Anuria may develop. When anuria is present, the client is said to be in renal shutdown or renal failure. Oliguria does not contraindicate the administration of large volumes of fluid in the treatment of

shock. In fact, restoring renal capillary perfusion along with that of other vital capillaries restores urine volume production as long as tubular necrosis is not already present. If acute tubular necrosis is present, peritoneal dialysis or hemodialysis may be needed until regeneration of functioning renal tubular epithelium occurs (see also Chapter 36).

Correcting metabolic acidosis (see Chapter 13) and using other measures to increase blood volume and improve cardiac output also benefit the kidney. If a large amount of tissue damage (e.g., crush injuries) is present, myoglobin may be released from damaged muscle tissue. Because the myoglobin molecule is large, a type of mechanical renal failure may result from attempts to excrete it. Increased fluids to flush the myoglobin through the kidney are important to decrease damage to the tubules; occasionally osmotic diuretics are used.

Prevent Gastrointestinal Bleeding. An early physiologic response to shock is a decrease in splanchnic circulation. This reduces the nutrient blood supply to the stomach and bowel, causing inadequate GI tissue perfusion and delayed gastric emptying; thus vomiting with aspiration of gastric contents into the lung may occur. For this reason and for diagnostic purposes, nasogastric (NG) suction is often used during treatment of shock. A double-lumen, 16F NG tube is usually used in adults. In addition, because of the ischemia, the gastric mucosa does not produce mucus and may quickly ulcerate. Proton pump inhibitors, sucralfate, or histamine-2 blockers are given prophylactically to reduce the risk of bleeding.

When shock is caused by GI bleeding, other NG tubes may be used. If the suspected cause of bleeding is a gastric ulcer, a 36F Ewald tube may be used. The many large holes in this tube facilitate saline lavage and removal of blood clots. If esophageal varices are suspected or present, a Sengstaken-Blakemore tube may be used. This triple-lumen tube exerts pressure on the lower portion of the esophagus and the upper portion of the stomach, where varices are most prominent. Pressure is created by esophageal and gastric balloons inflated with air. Gentle traction is applied to keep the balloons in proper position (see Chapter 31).

Provide Pharmacologic Management

Antibiotics. Antibiotics are essential for septic shock. Draw blood samples for culture and sensitivity. Cultures of urine, sputum, and fluid from draining wounds, sinuses, and so forth will provide information about the source of the sepsis.

Cultures should be drawn before antibiotics are initiated. However, it is imperative that intravenous antibiotic therapy be started as soon as possible after the recognition of sepsis, ideally within 1 hour.

Effective anti-infective administration within the first hour of documented hypotension is associated with increased survival in septic shock. Selection of the initial antibiotics depends on the probable site and presumed organisms of infection and local susceptibility patterns. Initially, empirical anti-infective therapy should include one or two agents with activity against the most highly suspected pathogens that can penetrate to the presumed site of infection. The potential for resistance of the pathogens should also be considered. For these reasons, vancomycin and/or aminoglycosides (e.g., gentamicin, amikacin) are common first-line choices for antibiotic therapy. Antibiotic therapy should be reevaluated within 48 to 72 hours based on culture and sensitivity results and client response to therapy. If resistant strains are found to be the cause of the infection and resultant sepsis, some of the newer antibiotics with activity against resistant strains (e.g., linezolid, daptomycin, telithromycin, tigecycline) may be initiated. Antibiotics may also be administered along with appropriate surgical management to clients with open or potentially contaminated wounds who are experiencing shock.

Drotrecogin Alfa. Drotrecogin alfa (Xigris) is used for severe sepsis and SIRS. Drotrecogin alfa is a recombinant form of human activated protein C and has the ability to inhibit inflammation, inhibit coagulation, and promote fibrinolysis. The main effect of protein C is to reduce the production of thrombin by inactivating factors Va and VIII. Thrombin is proinflammatory, procoagulant, and antifibrinolytic. In addition, protein C reduces the production of IL-1, IL-6, and TNF-α by monocytes and has profibrinolytic properties. Large clinical trials have shown significant benefit from the use of this medication in septic shock. Bleeding remains a significant side effect.

Heparin. The anticoagulant effect of heparin may help prevent complications or treat DIC. The dosage is usually initiated based on body weight and adjusted according to clotting studies. Heparin is also used because of the prolonged immobility often associated with shock. Immobility predisposes clients to venous thrombosis and pulmonary emboli. The treatment of DIC may include heparin administration to minimize consumption of clotting factors. Heparin also may be appropriate for clients with ARDS if the primary cause of the respiratory insufficiency is suspected to be DIC or massive microembolism.

Steroids. Steroids have several effects that may assist the client in neurogenic shock after spinal cord injury. They are given to reduce edema in the cord and have been shown to improve recovery. They assist in treatment by stabilizing lysosomal membrane and preventing intracellular release of enzymes. Complications from high-dose steroid therapy include acute GI bleeding, aggravation of diabetes, and immunosuppression.

In septic shock, low-dose steroid use for 5 to 7 days with tapering has demonstrated increases in survival rate and shock reversal in clients with vasopressor-dependent septic shock.

Naloxone. Naloxone (Narcan), an opiate antagonist, is commonly used to treat opioid and synthetic opioid overdosages. During stress, opiate-like substances known as *enkephalins* and *endorphins* are released from the brain. Although the mechanisms of action are not clear, endorphins may play a role in capillary bed vasodilation found in all forms of shock. Studies indicate that when naloxone is administered in the absence of shock, no significant cardiovascular effects are noted. However, when administered during shock, naloxone reverses the hypotension and decreases cardiac contractility, resulting in significant hemodynamic improvement and decreased mortality. It is believed that naloxone blocks the effects of endorphins and enkephalins.

Insulin. Recent research studies have indicated a significant reduction in mortality and morbidity in ICU clients when intensive insulin therapy is provided. Average blood glucose levels should be between 80 and 110 mg/dl. Tight regulation of blood glucose level does place clients at risk for hypoglycemic episodes, but studies show that hypoglycemia does not increase the risk of mortality whereas hyperglycemia does.

Epinephrine. Epinephrine is the drug of choice for emergency treatment of allergic reactions (anaphylaxis). Epinephrine inhibits histamine release and antagonizes its effects on end organs, resulting in reversal of the bronchial constriction, increased capillary permeability, and vasodilation that occur with acute anaphylactic reactions. The overall effect is improved respiratory status and cardiovascular stability. Antihistamines, like diphenhydramine (Benadryl), can be used to relieve clinical manifestations associated with anaphylaxis rather than to stop the release of histamine.

Proton Pump Inhibitors, Sucralfate, and Histamine H$_2$-Receptor Antagonists. These agents inhibit gastric acid secretion. Stress ulcers are often lethal complications of severe illness or injury produced by continuous shunting of blood from the GI tract due to extended sympathetic nervous system stimulation.

Opioids. The need for pain reduction may be obvious in clients experiencing different types of shock. However, the use of opioids for pain management may be dangerous. Opioids can lead to vasodilation that interferes with vasoconstriction, the only mechanism by which the client's BP is maintained. However, morphine sulfate may be helpful in cardiogenic shock because it causes pooling of blood in the extremities and contributes to a decrease in anxiety.

Cardiotonic Medications. Medications that improve myocardial contraction are basic in treating those forms of shock that decrease cardiac output (e.g., hypovolemic shock and cardiogenic shock):

- Rate-regulating medications such as beta-blockers and calcium-channel blockers can be used to reduce cardiac oxygen consumption. If digitalis is used, blood levels are monitored to assess for toxicity (e.g., bradydysrhythmias or tachydysrhythmias, ST-segment depression).
- Amiodarone, lidocaine, bretylium, quinidine, and procainamide may treat dysrhythmias that tend to reduce cardiac efficiency. However, these medications reduce myocardial contractility. Amiodarone is considered first-line therapy because of the significantly higher survival rate over lidocaine.
- Atropine may treat bradycardia, which predisposes clients to cardiogenic shock.

Calcium. The value and dosages of calcium in treating shock are not clear. However, calcium may be administered if impaired cardiac function is evident.

SAFETY ⚠ **ALERT**

Calcium chloride should be given intravenously only and through large veins.

Calcium gluconate requires greater doses for the same outcome but is less toxic to tissues if the IV infiltrates. Although calcium chloride and calcium gluconate are both available as 10% solutions, they are not identical in concentration. Do not substitute one for the other. Indications of hypocalcemia may be subtle. Careful assessment is essential. (See discussions of calcium disorders in Chapter 12.) Calcium may also precipitate toxic effects in a person who has received digitalis and should be given cautiously.

Nursing Management of the Medical Client

Nursing outcomes are similar to medical outcomes in that the overall goals of care are to correct the causative factor if possible, improve oxygenation, restore and maintain adequate tissue perfusion, and prevent complications. However, most of the interventions provided for clients in shock require a physician's order and are not independent nursing actions. The nurse's major responsibilities in shock include assessment of the client's condition and timely and accurate performance of dependent interventions.

Assessment. Because a client's condition can change rapidly in shock, frequent nursing assessment is essential. Documentation of the progress and response to interventions needs to be concise, yet convey the client's status minute by minute. Initiate a flow sheet containing all pertinent data in an easily read format. This flow sheet must contain the assessments essential in treating shock. Blood chemistries, blood gases, oxygen saturations, and electrolytes need to be determined frequently and reported promptly so therapy can be adjusted to the client's rapidly changing physiologic status.

The first step in assessing a person in shock is a general overview, giving attention to airway, breathing, and circulation (ABC).

Oxygenation Monitoring. Several assessments should be performed to determine that no airway or breathing problems exist. To determine airway patency, assess for the presence of noisy respirations and check for obstructions. Listen to lung sounds to determine adequate air movement. Assess the respiratory rate and effort to evaluate the adequacy of breathing. Evaluate chest wall expansion and assess for chest wall bulges or defects. Monitor for tracheal deviation, which could indicate tension pneumothorax.

When caring for clients experiencing shock, carefully differentiate nursing diagnoses concerning pain and impaired gas exchange. Restlessness is an assessment finding common to both and can thus be easily misinterpreted. Too often clients who are restless, especially trauma victims, are given opioids because their behavior is incorrectly interpreted as resulting from pain. However, the restlessness frequently is actually due to hypoxia, and opioids worsen the problem. The decision to administer opioids is often a nursing decision. It is important to assess the need for these medications carefully. Attention to positioning, splinting of injured areas, breathing techniques, and comfort measures may provide safer and more effective pain reduction than opioids. (Pain is discussed in detail in Chapter 20.)

Perfusion Monitoring. To complete the critical assessment of ABCs, circulation must be evaluated. Assess the client's pulse, BP, skin color, temperature, heart sounds, peripheral pulses, state of hydration, and skin perfusion (e.g., capillary refill time less than 3 seconds). Check the condition of the mucous membranes, sclera, and conjunctivae; the presence of pallor or cyanosis; and fullness of the neck veins (jugular venous distention, which may suggest right heart failure and cardiogenic shock).

It is imperative that the adequacy of blood volume be determined before administration of opioids to a client suffering from multiple trauma. Opioid administration causes vasodilation, which results in severe hypotension or shock. If an opioid is administered intramuscularly to a client in shock, it also may not be completely absorbed because of the vasoconstriction that is present. Because the client experiences little or no pain reduction, a second injection may be given. Once fluid resuscitation is complete and the circulating volume is restored, the client may absorb both doses of the opioid.

No one in shock should be given intramuscular medications when rapid onset of action of the drug is needed.

When opioids are appropriate for a client in shock, they are most effective if administered intravenously in small doses. When caring for trauma victims, especially those with massive injury, the extent of the injury does not necessarily coincide with the amount of pain being experienced. Careful assessment is necessary once opioid administration seems safe (in terms of the client's hemodynamic status). Assess the client's BP more closely after IV administration of opioids to watch for hypotension.

Even though a person in shock may feel cold and may be hypothermic, do not apply heat to the skin. Heat application dilates peripheral blood vessels and draws blood away from the vital organs (where it is life-sustaining) into the vessels of the skin. This interferes with the body's initial compensatory mechanism of peripheral vasoconstriction. Heat also increases the body's metabolism. In turn, this increases the need for oxygen and puts an added strain on the heart.

This approach does not mean that the person is kept in a cold environment. The environment is kept warm because it is important that the person not become chilled. Chilling and shivering expend energy needed to maintain vital functions. Chilling also contributes to sludging of blood in the microcirculation. Hypothermia slows the heart, increases the likelihood of ventricular fibrillation, and inhibits the body's reparative processes.

After potentially life-threatening problems are treated, obtain complete vital signs, with BP taken in both arms to rule out other causes of hypovolemic shock (i.e., thoracic dissection, aneurysm). It is important to take postural vital signs if applicable, and if it is safe to do so. Do not take postural vital signs (1) if the client has multiple traumatic injuries; (2) if there is evidence of vertebral, pelvic, or femoral fracture; or (3) if hypotension already exists. Clients with postural hypotension should not be sent to the x-ray department for upright films until they are adequately volume-resuscitated. If x-ray studies must be obtained, clients require constant attendance by a nurse, who monitors vital signs, administers IV fluids, and provides guidance to x-ray department personnel regarding movement, positioning, and timing of studies.

Measurement of postural vital signs is done when there is a history or presence of significant blood loss, unexplained tachycardia, a history of fluid loss (e.g., diarrhea, vomiting, diuretic therapy, or third-space loss), unexplained syncope, blunt chest or abdominal trauma, or abdominal pain.

Blood Pressure Monitoring. Often when a client is in shock, it is difficult to auscultate BP with a standard stethoscope. Two commonly used techniques to obtain BP measurements are palpation of the radial or brachial pulse during deflation of the BP cuff and use of a Doppler instrument. When palpation is used, the first palpable pulse noted during deflation of the cuff is the systolic BP. Document the BP as such (e.g., 90/palp). A Doppler instrument amplifies arterial and venous pulsations by ultrasonography. Various Doppler probes are available and are used instead of a stethoscope to measure BP. Systolic BP is easily heard by placing the probe over the brachial artery after applying transmission gel. The diastolic BP is not obtainable when the Doppler is used. Direct measurement of arterial BP by use of an arterial line often is done during shock. Discussion of arterial lines is found in Chapter 54.

For clarity and accuracy, document the method by which BP readings are taken (in addition to the readings themselves) and whether palpation or a Doppler monitor is used. This is important because these readings may be higher or lower than those obtained in the standard way with a cuff and stethoscope. Likewise, document whether readings are obtained by automatic BP machines even though readings from these machines may not differ from those taken in the standard way.

Once the airway is patent, air exchange is adequate, a pulse is present, and the cervical spine is immobilized (if it is a trauma situation), perform a rapid, cursory initial head-to-toe physical assessment. The initial assessment goal is to identify major problems and gross abnormalities. Give further detailed attention to specific injuries or problems after shock is stabilized.

Temperature Monitoring. An accurate core temperature measurement is important in assessing a client in shock. Sometimes an indwelling flexible rectal probe connected to a continuous display monitor is more accurate and less traumatic than intermittent rectal temperature measurements with a standard thermometer. Core temperature can also be measured with an indwelling urinary catheter that contains a thermometer. Tympanic temperatures are commonly used in critical care settings and provide core temperature measurements. Core temperature can also be obtained if the client has a thermodilution (Swan-Ganz) catheter in place.

Oral temperature measurement is neither accurate nor safe. During shock, the buccal mucosa is poorly perfused, and the client should be receiving oxygen by mask or nasal prongs. (Because clients in shock are hypoxemic, the procedure of removing the oxygen long enough to obtain an oral temperature is not routinely recommended.)

Cardiac Monitoring. For assessment and evaluation purposes, the electrocardiogram needs to be continuously monitored in all clients in shock, regardless of age. Nurses caring for clients experiencing shock need to be able to initiate cardiac monitoring, recognize cardiac dysrhythmias, and initiate treatment for any potentially lethal dysrhythmias that occur (see Chapter 57).

During the initial resuscitation period, it may be more appropriate to place the ECG monitor electrodes on the client's shoulders than on the chest. This placement does not interfere with chest film findings. It also allows better access to the chest for thoracic procedures such as insertion of chest tubes, pericardiocentesis, and CVP line placement. Once the client's condition is stabilized, the electrodes may be moved to the chest.

Hemodynamic Monitoring. Measurement of CVP is one hemodynamic technique that may be used in initial shock management, especially with hypovolemic shock. However, because CVP only provides information regarding preload, peripheral intra-arterial lines or a pulmonary artery catheter is inserted as soon as possible. Blood volume needs to be expanded as the vascular space enlarges, and CVP measurements are used to determine the amount of fluid needed to fill the enlarging vascular space. The rate of fluid replacement is adjusted to maintain the desired CVP. It is serious if the CVP continues to decrease despite fluid replacement. This means that the rate and volume of fluid replacement are not sufficient to meet the client's physiologic needs.

Peripheral arterial catheters are commonly used in shock to measure arterial BP and MAP and to obtain blood samples for chemical and blood gas analysis. These catheters are usually placed in the radial artery but may also be placed in the femoral or brachial arteries. Pulmonary artery and pulmonary capillary wedge pressure (PCWP) measurements are monitored to assess left-sided heart function and to guide fluid administration. These pressures are measured through a Swan-Ganz catheter. The PCWP reflects the LV end-diastolic pressure. This is the pressure in the LV just before contraction. An increase in this pressure in a client with cardiogenic shock may indicate left-sided heart failure. A low value in a client with hypovolemic shock may indicate that volume replacement is needed. In a client with septic shock, lower values would be expected during the warm phase and higher values during the cold phase.

Depending on the type of Swan-Ganz catheter used, additional measurements may be obtained. Some catheters have a fiberoptic tip that allows measurement of oxygen saturation of hemoglobin in the venous blood (Svo_2). Svo_2 is measured in the pulmonary artery, just before reoxygenation of the blood in the lungs. This reading gives an average of the tissue uptake or use of oxygen in the body. The normal range for Svo_2 is 60% to 80%. When the Svo_2 goes below 60%, it may indicate either decreased arterial oxygenation or increased tissue oxygen demand. If the Svo_2 is greater than 80%, the indication, in relation to shock, is that the oxygen is unable either to reach the tissues or to be extracted by the tissues.

Most Swan-Ganz catheters also have a thermistor bead just proximal to the balloon. This may be used to determine cardiac output by a thermodilution technique. A fourth lumen opens at the level of the right atrium, and CVP measurements (preload) can be obtained through this lumen.

Cardiac Output Monitoring. Cardiac output, measured in liters per minute, is the amount of blood pumped by the LV into the aorta each minute. During shock, cardiac output may be decreased because of myocardial damage resulting from an MI or, in hypovolemic shock, from inadequate volume replacement.

Because of the widespread use of Swan-Ganz catheters and the ease of obtaining measurements, cardiac output monitoring is used in managing all types of shock. These measurements assess overall cardiac function and the function of the LV. Factors that may alter cardiac output include heart rate, SVR, age, body size, exercise, and (in people with cardiac problems) decreased filling or emptying of the LV.

Cardiac index is the cardiac output divided by the body surface area. Cardiac output as a separate reading does not take into account the amount of tissue that needs to be perfused. By figuring body size into the calculation, a more accurate assessment is obtained.

SVR can be computed by dividing the cardiac output by the MAP (SVR = MAP/CO). SVR measures afterload and provides information regarding vasoconstriction or vasodilation. Decreased SVR indicates systemic vasodilation and may indicate the need for administration of vasoconstrictors. Increased SVR indicates systemic vasoconstriction and the potential need for vasodilators. Arterial BP and cardiac function should always be taken into consideration before administering vasoconstrictors or vasodilators.

Prevent Complications. Although it is important to begin assessments and interventions with the ABCs, additional assessments are necessary to evaluate the client's overall condition and prevent complications.

Additional assessments important in preventing complications include evaluation of the following:

- Level of consciousness and orientation × 3 (i.e., person, place, time)
- Ability to move extremities
- Sensation in all extremities
- Hand grasps
- Response to verbal and painful stimuli
- Pupil size and reaction to light
- Presence of abnormal posturing; presence, location, intensity, and duration of pain, and what reduces the pain
- Bowel sounds
- Abdominal distention or rigidity
- Circumference of abdomen or extremities
- Presence of lacerations, contusions, ecchymoses, petechiae, and purpura (also check for bruising over flank area)
- Bone deformities
- Presence of medical alert tags or bracelets

Prevent Renal Impairment. An indwelling urinary catheter is a simple means of monitoring a client during shock. Continuously measuring urinary flow provides important information about peripheral blood flow and kidney function. Because the amount of urine excreted during shock is often small, it is important to have an accurate, calibrated urine collector. In some settings, the catheter may be attached to a urinometer collector or to a more complex electric urinometer.

Urinary volume changes can be highly important as an index of the success or failure of therapy. Minimal (less than 0.5 ml/kg/hour) or absent urine output indicates treatment is not successful. Increasing urine output is a favorable sign. Assess the client's urine output routinely and record it at least every hour.

Prevent Gastric Ulceration. Assess gastric aspirate periodically for blood. Guaiac solution can be used to check for blood; litmus paper checks the pH to determine the acidity of the stomach. Promptly report new findings of blood or increases in the amount of blood.

Diagnosis, Outcomes, Interventions
Diagnosis: Ineffective Tissue Perfusion. The nursing diagnosis *Ineffective Tissue Perfusion* can be used to describe the reduced tissue perfusion and inadequate effective circulating intravascular blood volume. This diagnosis does not describe the oxygen-carrying capacity of the blood, but rather the volume of circulating blood and its ability to reach the tissues. The nursing diagnosis can be written *Ineffective Tissue Perfusion (specify type) related to actual or relative (specify type) hypovolemia secondary to shock (specify type).* Other potential nursing diagnoses for the client in shock are listed in Box 81-2.

BOX 81-2 Potential Nursing Diagnoses for the Client in Shock

- Activity Intolerance
- Acute Pain
- Anticipatory Grieving
- Anxiety
- Bathing/Hygiene, Dressing/Grooming, Toileting Self-Care Deficit
- Compromised Family Coping
- Constipation
- Decreased Cardiac Output
- Deficient Fluid Volume
- Disturbed Body Image
- Disturbed Personal Identity
- Disturbed Sleep Pattern
- Disturbed Sensory Perception: Visual, Auditory, Kinesthetic, Gustatory, Tactile, Olfactory
- Fear
- Imbalanced Nutrition: Less Than Body Requirements
- Impaired Gas Exchange
- Impaired Physical Mobility
- Impaired or Risk for Impaired Skin Integrity
- Impaired Tissue Integrity
- Impaired Verbal Communication
- Ineffective Airway Clearance
- Ineffective Breathing Pattern
- Ineffective Protection
- Ineffective Tissue Perfusion: Cerebral, Cardiopulmonary, Gastrointestinal, Renal, Peripheral
- Interrupted Family Processes
- Spiritual Distress

Outcomes. Nursing care of the client with shock is complex. Specific nursing and medical interventions vary according to individual needs and the setting in which care is delivered (e.g., emergency department versus intensive care unit). However, two major physiologic outcomes of care are desired:

1. Adequate blood flow (tissue perfusion) and cellular oxygenation are achieved to maintain the integrity of the tissue or organ.
2. The metabolic needs of the tissue or organ are reduced or maintained.

Interventions. Provide continuous assessment of the client. Keep equipment and supplies (e.g., suction, emergency drugs) available and in working order. Cardiovascular and respiratory changes can occur rapidly, and interventions must be adjusted promptly. Document observations clearly and concisely.

Help decrease tissue oxygen demand. Because shock states can double the body's O_2 consumption, promote factors that decrease tissue oxygen need. Interventions are aimed at decreasing total body work, pain, anxiety, and temperature to decrease tissue oxygen demand.

Implement appropriate, planned nursing interventions to prevent complications that can develop from enforced immobilization. Provide adequate pain reduction, because pain intensifies shock. Base this intervention on careful assessment.

Diagnosis: Interrupted Family Processes. Sudden changes in the family's communication and ability to problem-solve without the client and concerns about the cause of illness, or worry about the outcome, create a situational crisis. The appropriate nursing diagnosis is *Interrupted Family Processes.*

Outcomes. The goal is that the usual processes of coping for the family remain intact or that a new process be adopted to facilitate problem solving. Outcomes may include that the family members remain supportive of each other, cope reasonably well with the crisis, and participate in problem solving or decision making with the health care team. Another goal might be that the client and significant others understand the cause of the problem and modify their lifestyle to minimize or eliminate the causative factor.

Interventions. Facilitate expression of concerns and questions by the client and family. For example, try to reduce the client's fears and anxieties about what is happening and about the equipment being used.

A client in shock is extremely ill and may die. In addition, the stress of the situation is compounded by emergency medical treatment, with all the people, equipment, and movement this entails. During shock management, nurses attend to numerous delegated medical care activities. However, there must be sufficient nursing resources to provide psychosocial care (e.g., reassurance, emotional support) to the client and family.

Keep the client's family informed of what is happening. They need information on which to base decisions. Because of the family's anxiety, the nurse may need to calmly repeat information several times. The Client Education Guide at right highlights information to be conveyed to the families of clients with shock. Remember that the client and significant others may be experiencing "psychological shock." They often need, and greatly appreciate, opportunities to discuss with care providers their important concerns.

Help the client (and family) feel physically and emotionally comfortable. Do not keep loved ones away from the client unnecessarily. Because of limited space, there may be times when they must wait in another room for a period of time. However, they should not be kept away long and should be given a reasonable explanation of why it is necessary to leave their loved one.

A client experiencing shock requires emotional support. When caught up in the sudden drama of an emergency or critical care, health professionals sometimes forget that the experience and setting are often new and very frightening for the client. Unfortunately, "dehumanization" of the client may occasionally occur during the rush of emergency treatment. Whether a client appears to be conscious or not, always explain what is happening. Keep the atmosphere as quiet and orderly as possible. Eliminate unnecessary chatter. Commonly, recovered clients remember hearing what was said and were aware of what happened to them even though they appeared to be unconscious.

Provide care to the family. Among a nurse's greatest responsibilities are providing support, comfort, and advocacy to clients receiving care and to their significant others. All of the people involved may be frightened, anxious, confused, and dependent. The Translating Evidence into Practice feature on p. 2183 addresses how to help families best manage the multiple, often overwhelming concerns related to the sudden onset and complex condition of shock. This is very important for nursing clients who are critically ill and are experiencing shock.

Evaluation. It is expected that the client will achieve adequate tissue perfusion and make a full recovery without complications from the type of shock being experienced, be transferred to a medical unit, and eventually be dismissed to home. Recovery from the cause of the shock may be delayed because of the complications created from the shock episode (e.g., wound healing).

CLIENT EDUCATION GUIDE

Family Support for the Client with Shock

- It is difficult to prevent the occurrence of shock because the causes are often unpredictable. If your family member is in shock, obtain precise, consistent information about his or her current status and prognosis.
- Learn about the monitoring equipment in use.
- Learn how to communicate with the client who is intubated or unconscious.
- Learn how to demonstrate love and caring to someone surrounded by equipment.
- Participate in your family member's care during the hospital stay; this increases your ability to provide care at home.
- Learn how to prevent recurrence if the cause was avoidable.

Helping Family Members Deal with Life-Threatening Illnesses

The etiologies leading to the various types of shock usually have a sudden onset. Families and significant others have little warning or preparation for the life-threatening nature of their loved one's illness, and few have had experience with a family member being critically ill. The illness trajectory is often characterized by periods of stability and instability, and the critically ill client may move back and forth between the two states. All of this leads to a great deal of uncertainty for the families of individuals with shock.

Uncertainty as a concept has been described as having four components: (1) ambiguity concerning the state of the illness, (2) complexity concerning treatment and the system of care, (3) lack of information regarding diagnosis and the severity of illness, and (4) unpredictability of the course of illness and outcome.[2] All four of these components may be experienced by families of an individual shock.

Three studies were reviewed to determine the factors that lead to uncertainty and to identify those interventions most effective in alleviating the uncertainty for families of critically ill clients.

Uncertainty may stem from the tension between the capabilities of modern medicine (i.e., high-tech interventions) to maintain life and the philosophical perspective held by some of death with dignity and the obligation to honor their loved one's wishes related to extraordinary measures to sustain life. Contributors to uncertainty include (1) the client's current health status, (2) treatments necessary to save the loved one's life and the decisions families make about those treatments, (3) lack of information overall, (4) unfamiliarity with the setting, and (5) the need to be with and to be vigilant for their loved one. The experiences families have described resemble a vortex in which there is a downward spiral of prognoses, difficult decisions, feelings of inadequacy, potential for loss despite best efforts, and the possibility that the loved one may remain unconscious and die with no opportunity to say goodbye.

Despite the best efforts of the health care team, sometimes critically ill clients die. However, there are many opportunities during the care of a critically ill client to diminish the family's feelings of uncertainty. Families describe "living it one day at a time" and often need "just in time" information rather than the entire trajectory of information laid out before them. Family members may feel positive about what they have to offer their loved one if they are allowed to participate in the loved one's care.

Families remain vigilant for their loved one. It is unhelpful to provide false hope, but it is equally unhelpful to paint a bleak picture if the outcomes for the client are not yet certain. Families have also described "drawing on God's strength" as something that helps them cope with the uncertainty. Family members may find comfort in talking with someone from pastoral care if that service is available.

Implications for practice include allowing open visitation so that families can spend as much time as they need with their loved one. Families also need to have access to the physicians, nurses, and other health care providers who will listen to their concerns, provide information, and correct any misconceptions they may have. Contact pastoral care or other hospital personnel who can help families find comfort if the family requests it.

Implications for research include exploring the interventions most helpful to families of clients in shock. How much information can families take in at one time? How can the overwhelming nature of the technology be made more manageable for families? Considering the time constraints of health care professionals, how can families' questions and concerns be addressed in a timely manner?

REFERENCES

1. Kirchhoff, K.T., et al (2002). The vortex: Families' experiences with death in the intensive care unit. *American Journal of Critical Care, 11*(3), 200-209.
2. Mishel, M.H. (1981). The measurement of uncertainty. *Nursing Research, 30,* 258-263.
3. Pelletier-Hibbert, M., & Sohi, P. (2001). Sources of uncertainty and coping strategies used by family members of individuals living with end stage renal disease. *Nephrology Nursing Journal, 28*(4), 411-419.
4. Plowfield, L.A. (1999). Living a nightmare: Family experiences of waiting following neurological crisis. *Journal of Neuroscience Nursing, 31*(4), 231-238.

Surgical Management

Although surgical interventions that can help in shock states are limited, they may be very useful. In hypovolemic shock caused by trauma, surgery can be performed to control sources of bleeding. Once bleeding is controlled, interventions aimed at restoring adequate fluid volume are more effective. In septic shock, surgery may help manage the source of infection.

Self-Care

Shock must be fully resolved before a client is transferred or discharged (unless the client is being transported for the treatment of shock). Clients who survive shock find that recovery from the precipitating problem is delayed. They may also experience some feelings of confusion, depression, or grief when they realize that they lived through a very critical illness.

SYSTEMIC INFLAMMATORY RESPONSE SYNDROME (SIRS)

SIRS is an inflammatory clinical response of the whole body without a proven source of infection. SIRS is non-specific and can be caused by ischemia, inflammation, trauma, infection, or a combination of several insults. SIRS with a confirmed source of infection, through blood or tissue cultures, is called *sepsis* (Table 81-5). SIRS is defined as two or more of the following variables:

- Temperature of more than 38° C or less than 36° C
- Heart rate of more than 90 beats per minute
- Respiratory rate of more than 20 breaths per minute or a $Paco_2$ level of less than 32 mm Hg
- Abnormal white blood cell count (>12,000/µl or <4000/µl or >10% bands)

MULTIPLE ORGAN DYSFUNCTION SYNDROME

Single-organ failure (e.g., heart failure, renal failure) has long been recognized as a cause of morbidity and mortality in critically ill clients. *Multiple organ dysfunction syndrome* (MODS) is present when two or more organs fail. MODS is the presence of altered organ function in a client who is acutely ill such that homeostasis cannot be maintained without intervention.

Etiology and Risk Factors

Causes of MODS include dead tissue, injured tissue, infection, perfusion deficits, and persistent sources of inflammation such as pancreatitis or pneumonitis. Acute lung injury is usually present in some form. People known to be at high risk for developing MODS include those with impaired immune responses, such as older adults, clients with chronic illnesses, clients with malnutrition, and clients with cancer. In addition, clients with prolonged or exaggerated inflammatory responses are at risk, including victims of severe trauma and clients with sepsis.

Prevention is a primary direction of current therapy. Source control is a major emphasis. When possible, the potential source of sepsis or inflammation is excised or removed (e.g., infected central line or pressure ulcer).

TABLE 81–5 The Relationship of SIRS to Sepsis

Condition	Definition
SIRS	Inflammatory state of whole body without a proven source of infection
Sepsis	SIRS caused by known infection
Severe Sepsis	Sepsis with evidence of organ hypoperfusion
Septic Shock	Severe sepsis with hypotension despite adequate fluid resuscitation or requirement for vasopressor or inotropics to maintain blood pressure

In many cases, however, the source cannot be removed, such as pneumonia, pancreatitis, soft tissue injury, and hematoma. When the source cannot be removed, empirical antimicrobial agents are used to reduce risk.

It would be helpful to clinicians to be able to predict which clients are at the highest risk, but accurate prediction remains elusive. The most predictive variables appear to be the ratio of arterial oxygen tension (Pao_2) to the fraction of inspired oxygen (Fio_2) on day 1; the plasma lactate concentration on day 2; the serum bilirubin level on day 6; and the serum creatinine level on day 12 after injury. When nurses note these predictors, increased surveillance should begin.

Pathophysiology

In the healthy person, the normal integrated inflammatory response protects tissue from microbial invasion and rids the body of cellular debris and foreign material. This process of responses continues until the insult slows and the client's condition stabilizes. The inflammatory response also normally stops once it is no longer needed. SIRS is a case of unchecked inflammatory responses. MODS is the end result of the prolonged response.

Once the inflammatory response becomes systemic, it is controlled by chemical mediators of inflammation. Mediators include bradykinin, complement, histamine, interleukin-1, prekallikrein, prostaglandins, and tumor necrosis factor. These powerful mediators of inflammation induce a systemic response. Endothelial cells are a common target for some mediators. The endothelium is destroyed, and blood flow is reduced to the tissues. Endothelial damage is produced by endotoxins from bacteria, tumor necrosis factor, interleukin-1, platelet activating factors, and many others. When this inflammatory response is unchecked, it produces damage to organs and tissues by altering perfusion, disturbing oxygen supply or demand, or changing metabolic dysfunctions. Metabolism increases under the direction of mediators such as cortisol and the catecholamines.

Many organs are affected by MODS. The lungs are usually the first to malfunction, because of the large surface area of pulmonary epithelium combined with the presence of bacterial contamination from systemic blood return. The GI tract is generally the second system to malfunction, and it propagates conditions for further deterioration of other organs. Once the GI tract is malfunctioning, bacteria quickly relocate from the GI tract to other organs. Additionally, the hypermetabolic state increases gastric acid production, increasing the risk of ulceration and bleeding. The most serious metabolic problem is hypermetabolism. The hypermetabolic state is continued by cell-to-cell communication, and the sympathetic nervous system responds with its usual "fight-or-flight" response.

Classification

There are two types of MODS. *Primary* MODS results directly from a well-defined insult in which organ dysfunction occurs early and is directly attributed to the insult itself. The direct insult initially causes a localized inflammatory response that may or may not progress to SIRS. An example of primary MODS is a primary pulmonary injury, such as aspiration. Only a small percentage of clients develop primary MODS.

Secondary MODS is a consequence of widespread systemic inflammation, which develops after a variety of insults, and results in dysfunction of organs not involved in the initial insult. The client enters a hypermetabolic state that lasts for 14 to 21 days. During this time, the body catabolizes muscle and fat for energy, which causes profound changes in the body's metabolic processes. Unless the process can be stopped, the outcome for the client is death. Secondary MODS occurs with conditions such as septic shock and ARDS.

Clinical Manifestations

There is usually a precipitating event to MODS, including aspiration, ruptured aneurysm, or septic shock, which is associated with resultant hypotension. The client is resuscitated, the cause is treated, and the client appears to do well for a few days. The following possible sequence of events often develops.

The client experiences SIRS before MODS develops. Within a few days, there is an insidious onset of a low-grade fever, tachycardia, increased numbers of banded and segmented neutrophils on the differential count (called a left shift), and dyspnea with the appearance of diffuse patchy infiltrates on the chest x-ray film. The client often has some deterioration in mental status, with reasonably normal renal and hepatic laboratory results. Dyspnea progresses, and intubation and mechanical ventilation are required. Some evidence of consumptive coagulopathy (DIC) is usually present. The client is usually stable hemodynamically and has relative polyuria, an increased cardiac index (greater than 4.5 L/min), and systemic vascular resistance of less than 600 dynes cm^{-5}. Clients often have increased blood glucose levels in the absence of diabetes. Some physicians use the criteria presented in Box 81-3 to make the diagnosis of MODS.

Between days 7 and 10, the bilirubin level increases and continues to increase, followed by an increase in serum creatinine level. Blood glucose and lactate levels continue to increase because of the hypermetabolic state. Other progressive changes include excretion of urinary nitrogen and protein combined with decreased levels of serum albumin, prealbumin, and retinol binding protein. Bacteremia with enteric organisms is also common. In addition, infections from *Candida* and viruses such as herpes and cytomegalovirus are common. Surgical wounds fail to heal, and pressure ulcers may develop. During this time, the client needs increasing amounts of fluids and inotropic medications to keep blood volume and cardiac preload near normal and to replace fluids lost through polyuria.

BOX 81-3 Modified Apache II Criteria for Diagnosis of Multiple Organ Dysfunction Syndrome

CARDIOVASCULAR FAILURE (PRESENCE OF ONE OR MORE OF THE FOLLOWING)

- Heart rate <54 beats/min
- Mean arterial pressure ≤49 mm Hg (systolic pressure ≤60 mm Hg)
- Occurrence of ventricular tachycardia or ventricular fibrillation
- Serum pH ≤7.24 with a $Paco_2$ of ≤40 mm Hg

RESPIRATORY FAILURE (PRESENCE OF ONE OR MORE OF THE FOLLOWING)

- Respiratory rate ≤5 breaths/min or ≥49 breaths/min with a $Paco_2$ ≥50 mm Hg
- Alveolar – arterial oxygen difference ≥350 mm Hg (at sea level calculate as follows: [713 × % oxygen in inspired gas] – $Paco_2$ – Pao_2)
- Dependent on ventilator or CPAP on the second day

RENAL FAILURE (PRESENCE OF ONE OR MORE OF THE FOLLOWING)

- Urine output ≤479 ml/24 hr or ≤159 ml/8 hr
- Serum BUN ≥100 mg/dl (35.7 mmol/L)
- Serum creatinine ≥3.5 mg/dl (309 μmol/L)

HEMATOLOGIC FAILURE (PRESENCE OF ONE OR MORE OF THE FOLLOWING)

- WBC count ≤1000/μl (1 × 10^9/L)
- Platelets ≤20,000/μl (20 × 10^9/L)
- Hematocrit ≤20%

NEUROLOGIC FAILURE

- Glasgow Coma Scale score ≤6 (in absence of sedation)

HEPATIC FAILURE (PRESENCE OF BOTH OF THE FOLLOWING)

- Serum bilirubin ≥6 mg%
- Prothrombin time ≥4 sec over control in the absence of systemic anticoagulation

CPAP, Continuous positive airway pressure; *BUN*, blood urea nitrogen; *WBC*, white blood cell.
From Knaus, W.A., & Wagner, D.P. (1989). Multiple systems organ failure: Epidemiology and prognosis. *Critical Care Clinics*, 5(2), 221.

Between day 14 and day 21, the client is unstable and appears close to death. The client may lose consciousness. Renal failure worsens to the point of considering dialysis. Edema may be present because of low serum protein levels. Mixed venous oxygen levels may increase because of problems with tissue uptake of oxygen caused by mitochondrial dysfunction. Lactic acidosis worsens, liver enzymes continue to increase, and coagulation disorders become impossible to correct.

Prognosis

If the process of MODS is not reversed by day 21, it is usually evident that the client will die. Death usually occurs between days 21 and 28 after the injury or precipitating event. Not all clients with MODS die; however, MODS remains the leading cause of death in the intensive care unit, with mortality rates from 50% to 90%, despite the development of better antibiotics, better resuscitation, and more sophisticated means of organ support. For those clients who survive, the average duration of intensive care unit stay is about 21 days. The rehabilitation, which is directed at recovery of muscle mass and neuromuscular function, lasts about 10 months.

OUTCOME MANAGEMENT

Medical Management

Restrain the Activators

Manifestations of potential infection must be quickly treated to restrain the activators of MODS. If the agent is known, antibiotics to which the organism is sensitive should be administered. If the organism is not known, broad-spectrum empirical antibiotics are given. Early aggressive management of sources of infection should be carried out. For example, the client may need to have a large infected wound incised and drained or necrotic tissue excised.

SAFETY ALERT

Extreme caution must be taken to avoid infecting the client. These clients have many invasive monitors and may have open wounds. Unfortunately, clients in critical care units exist in a paradox. The ICU is the only environment with sophisticated equipment and health care professionals to provide safe care, yet it is an environment where the risk of infection is higher. In addition, there is a high prevalence of multiresistant organisms, such as *vancomycin-resistant enterococci* (VRE) and methicillin-resistant *Staphylococcus aureus* (MRSA).

If the severity of the sepsis is identified early and drotrecogin alfa (Xigris) (see earlier discussion) is administered, progression to MODS may be prevented. However, if there is progression, the lungs are often the first organs to fail and so require special attention. Aggressive pulmonary care is needed in all clients who are at risk of MODS. Interventions may be as simple as coughing and deep breathing or ambulation. The client's oxygen saturation should be monitored as well.

Because malnutrition develops from the hypermetabolism and the GI tract often seeds other areas with bacteria, some clinicians require the client to be fed enterally. They believe that feeding enhances perfusion and decreases the bacterial load and the effects of endotoxins. Nutrient intake is usually 30 to 35 kcal/kg/day of carbohydrates. Fats are restricted to 0.5 to 1 g/kg/day. Proteins are given to the client via modified amino acids. Some practitioners administer protein until an increase in plasma transferrin or prealbumin level is noted. Increases in these values indicate hepatic protein

synthesis rather than a breakdown of body stores. Decontamination of the GI tract and pharynx decreases infection but has shown no effect on the death rate from MODS.

Control the Mediators

Controlling the mediators of inflammation is directed at (1) general levels of care and (2) specific treatments targeted at the problem cells. Maintenance of a positive nitrogen balance via nutrition, promotion of sleep and rest, and management of pain are important general care areas. Specific treatments include monoclonal antibodies to control mediators such as interleukin-1, endotoxins, and tumor necrosis factors. These therapies are shown in Table 81-6. Outcomes from research in these treatments are conflicting, and it appears that there is no "magic bullet" to cure the problem.

Protect the Affected Organs

Care is directed toward maintaining the function of organs that fail with MODS. The client is intubated and mechanically ventilated to maintain adequate oxygenation. Oxygen is given to the client until blood levels of lactate decrease toward normal. Elevated serum lactate levels indicate the use of anaerobic metabolism. Nurses must recognize that certain clinical problems further increase the need for oxygen. Problems such as fever, seizures, and shivering increase oxygen demands. These problems should be controlled with medications or environmental changes (e.g., warming).

TABLE 81–6 Summary of Potentially Useful Therapies for Multiple Organ Dysfunction Syndrome

Rationale	Therapy
Treatment of infection	Monoclonal antibodies
	Passive antibody protection
	Gut decontamination regimens
Support of gut function	Mucosal trophic agents (e.g., glutamine, bombesin, ketone bodies)
	Early enteral feeding
	Regulation of gut microbial flora
Improved resuscitation	Hypertonic saline
	In-line sensors
	Tissue-specific sensors
	Noninvasive monitoring
Endothelial cell protection	PAF inhibitors
	WBC adherence inhibition
	Antioxidant therapy
	Eicosanoid modulation
Modulation of macrophage function	$n3$-Polyunsaturated fatty acids
	Signal transduction modulation
Stimulation of lymphocyte function	Arginine
	ω3-Polyunsaturated fatty acids

PAF, Platelet activating factor; *WBC*, white blood cell.
From Lekander, B.J., & Cerra, F.B. (1990). The syndrome of multiple organ failure. *Critical Care Clinics of North America, 2*(2), 338.

Fluids and inotropic drugs are used to support hemo-dynamic parameters. The client often becomes more unstable and needs continuous monitoring. Nutritional support is also critical to reduce the catabolism that accompanies hypermetabolism. Dialysis is often used to reduce azotemia from renal failure.

Nursing Management of the Medical Client

Care of the client with MODS is multifaceted, balancing the needs of one system against the needs of another while trying to maintain optimal functioning of each system. Nursing diagnoses appropriate for the client with MODS are determined by the system involved and the clinical manifestations identified.

The number of independent nursing interventions for the client with MODS is limited. The overall goal for nursing is effective client and family coping. This complex disorder taxes the client and family. Nurses must remain sensitive to the needs of the family. Caring for the family of critically ill clients is a challenge in that understanding, predicting, and intervening with families in crisis are less exact than the calculation of oxygen needs. There are no easy formulas to use to provide hope, courage, coping, and caring. Nurses must remain alert to the needs of the family as well as the client during this stressful time.

CONCLUSIONS

This chapter discussed shock under three major classifications: hypovolemic, cardiogenic, and distributive. The pathophysiology, clinical manifestations, and medical and nursing management are presented. Shock is a critical condition with a high death rate. Early diagnosis and intervention are necessary for the best possible outcomes. Multiple organ dysfunction syndrome is a syndrome of multiple organs progressively failing because of prolonged inflammatory responses. Again, early diagnosis and intervention are critical for positive outcomes.

THINKING CRITICALLY

1. The client is a 20-year-old man with a gunshot wound to the right chest and massive hemorrhage. His systolic BP is 60 mm Hg (palpated), heart rate is 130 beats/min, and respiratory rate is 36 breaths/min. The skin is pale, cold, and clammy; capillary refill time is greater than 3 seconds; pulses are weak and thready. What priority assessments should be done? What interventions might be performed?

Factors to Consider. What do his vital signs tell you? What injuries might have occurred with a major chest trauma? How can his need for fluid and blood replacement best be met?

2. A 69-year-old man was brought to the emergency department by a rescue squad. He had undergone a colon resection 2 weeks previously. His wife said that he was having increased difficulty breathing, and he could feel his heart beating in his chest. He also has seemed "slower" to her. He is not moving as fast as usual and gets very dizzy when he stands up. He almost passed out, which is why she called the rescue squad. What priority assessments should be done? What interventions might be performed?

Factors to Consider. What might be happening that could lead to all of the problems with breathing, dizziness, and confusion? What risk might be present as a result of the surgery?

3. A 65-year-old man in the coronary care unit had an acute MI 3 days ago. The monitor alarms and assessments reveal that his BP is 76/50 mm Hg, and his respiratory rate is 20 breaths/min. His pulse is rapid (128 beats/min) and thready. His skin is cool and diaphoretic, with a slight ashen color; the capillary refill time is greater than 3 seconds. The client is restless and confused. What priority assessments should be done? What interventions might be performed?

Factors to Consider. What form of shock can quickly develop in a client after an MI? Does he need fluid resuscitation to increase his blood pressure? Why or why not? What medications are commonly used to support a heart in distress? Are special forms of monitoring needed while these medications are used?

Discussions for the questions can be found on the website.

BIBLIOGRAPHY

 Citations appearing in red refer to primary research.

Citations appearing in blue refer to evidence-based practice guidelines and protocols.

1. Angstwurm, M.W., Engelmann, L., Zimmermann, T., et al (2007). Selenium in intensive care (SIC): Results of a prospective randomized, placebo-controlled, multiple-center study in patients with severe systemic inflammatory response syndrome, sepsis, and septic shock. *Critical Care Medicine, 35*(1), 118-126.
2. Bassi, G., Radermacher, P., & Calzia, E. (2006). Catecholamines and vasopressin during critical illness. *Endocrinology and Metabolism Clinics of North America, 35*(4), 839-857.
3. Bilbault, P., Lavaux, T., Launoy, A., et al (2007). Influence of drotrecogin alpha (activated) infusion on the variation of Bax/Bcl-2 and Bax/Bcl-xl ratios in circulating mononuclear cells: A cohort study in septic shock patients. *Critical Care Medicine, 35*(1), 69-75.
4. Boeuf, B., Poirier, V., Gauvin, F., et al (2003). Naloxone for shock. *Cochrane Database of Systematic Reviews,* (4), CD004443.
5. Boos, L., Szalai, A.J., & Barnum, S.R. (2005). C3a expressed in the central nervous system protects against LPS-induced shock. *Neuroscience Letters, 387*(2), 68-71.
6. Brasel, K.J., Guse, C., Gentilello, L.M., Nirula, R. Heart rate: Is it truly a vital sign? *Journal of Trauma, 62*(4), 812-817.
7. Brown, E.J. (2004). The molecular basis of streptococcal toxic shock syndrome. *New England Journal of Medicine, 350,* 2093-2094.
8. Bulger, E.M., Cuschieri, J., Warner, K., Maier, R.V. Hypertonic resuscitation modulates the inflammatory response in patients with traumatic hemorrhagic shock. *Annals of Surgery, 245*(4), 635-641.
9. Cohn, S.M., Nathens, A.B., Moore, F.A., et al (2007). Tissue oxygen saturation predicts the development of organ dysfunction during traumatic shock resuscitation. *Journal of Trauma, 62*(1), 44-54, discussion 54-55.
10. Dellinger, R.P., Carlet, J.M., Masur, H., et al (2004). Surviving Sepsis Campaign guidelines for management of severe sepsis and septic shock. *Critical Care Medicine, 32*(3), 858-873.

11. Dewachter, P., Jouan-Hureaux, V., Franck, P., et al (2005). Anaphylactic shock: A form of distributive shock without inhibition of oxygen consumption. *Anesthesiology, 103*(1), 40-49.

12. Fisher, C.G., Noonan, V.K., Smith, D.E., et al (2005). Motor recovery, functional status, and health-related quality of life in patients with complete spinal cord injuries. *Spine, 30*(19), 2200-2207.

13. Geppert, A., Dorninger, A., Delle-Karth, G., et al (2006). Plasma concentrations of interleukin-6, organ failure, vasopressor support, and successful coronary revascularization in predicting 30-day mortality of patients with cardiogenic shock complicating acute myocardial infarction. *Critical Care Medicine, 34*(8), 2035-2042.

14. Gross, P.A. (2006). Hypotension and mortality in septic shock: The "golden hour." *Critical Care Medicine, 34*(6), 1819-1820.

15. Habler, O.P., & Messmer, K.F. (2000). Tissue perfusion and oxygenation with blood substitutes. *Advanced Drug Delivery Reviews, 40*(3), 171-184.

16. Hekmat, K., Kroener, A., Stuetzer, H., et al (2005). Daily assessment of organ dysfunction and survival in intensive care unit cardiac surgical patients. *Annals of Thoracic Surgery, 79*(5), 1555-1562.

17. Hotchkiss, R.S., & Karl, I.E. (2003). The pathophysiology and treatment of sepsis. *New England Journal of Medicine, 348*, 138-150.

18. Huang, S.C., Chen, Y.S., Chi, N.H., et al (2006). Out-of-center extracorporeal membrane oxygenation for adult cardiogenic shock patients. *Artificial Organs, 30*(1), 24-28.

19. Kasperska-Zajac, A., & Rogala, B. (2006). Platelet function in anaphylaxis. *Journal of Investigative Allergology and Clinical Immunology, 16*(1), 1-4.

20. Kohsaka, S., Menon, V., Iwata, K., et al (2007). Microbiological profile of septic complication in patients with cardiogenic shock following acute myocardial infarction (from the SHOCK study). *American Journal of Cardiology, 99*(6), 802-804.

21. Kumar, A., Roberts, D., Wood, K.E., et al (2006). Duration of hypotension before initiation of effective antimicrobial therapy is the critical determinant of survival in human septic shock. *Critical Care Medicine, 34*(6), 1589-1596.

22. Lowenstein, C.J., & Michel, T. (2006). What's in a name? eNOS and anaphylactic shock. *Journal of Clinical Investigation, 116*(8), 2075-2078.

23. Mann, H.J., & Nolan, P.E., Jr. (2006). Update on the management of cardiogenic shock. *Current Opinions in Critical Care, 12*(5), 431-436.

24. Minneci, P.C., Deans, K.J., Banks, S.M., et al (2004). Meta-analysis: The effect of steroids on survival and shock during sepsis depends on the dose. *Annals of Internal Medicine, 141*(1), 47-56.

25. Nguyen, H.B., Corbett, S.W., Steele, R., et al (2007). Implementation of a bundle of quality indicators for the early management of severe sepsis and septic shock is associated with decreased mortality. *Critical Care Medicine, 35*(4), 1105-1112.

26. Nguyen, H.B., Rivers, E.P., Abrahamian, F.M., et al (2006). Severe sepsis and septic shock: Review of the literature and emergency department management guidelines. *Annals of Emergency Medicine, 48*(1), 28-54.

27. Poupko, J.M., Baskin, S.I., & Moore, E. (2007). The pharmacological properties of anisodamine. *Journal of Applied Toxicology, 27*(2), 116-121.

28. Powers, J., & Jacobi, J. (2006). Pharmacologic treatment related to severe sepsis. *AACN Advanced Critical Care, 17*(4), 423-432, quiz 434.

29. Revelly, J.P., Tappy, L., Martinez, A., et al (2005). Lactate and glucose metabolism in severe sepsis and cardiogenic shock. *Critical Care Medicine, 33*(10), 2235-2240.

30. Rudiger, A., Gasser, S., Fischler, M., et al (2006). Comparable increase of B-type natriuretic peptide and amino-terminal pro-B-type natriuretic peptide levels in patients with severe sepsis, septic shock and acute heart failure. *Critical Care Medicine, 34*(8), 2140-2144.

31. Schmidt, H., Muller-Werdan, U., Hoffmann, T., et al (2005). Autonomic dysfunction predicts mortality in patients with multiple organ dysfunction syndrome of different age groups. *Critical Care Medicine, 33*(9), 1994-2002.

32. Sheikh, A., ten Broek, V., Brown, S.G., Simons, F.E. H1-antihistamines for the treatment of anaphylaxis with and without shock. *Cochrane Database of Systematic Reviews,* (1), CD006160.

33. Stephens, C., & Fawcett, T.N. (2007). Nitric oxide and nursing: A review. *Journal of Clinical Nursing, 16*(1), 67-76.

34. Turgeon, A.F., Hutton, B., Fergusson, D.A., et al (2007). Meta-analysis: Intravenous immunoglobulin in critically ill adult patients with sepsis. *Annals of Internal Medicine, 146*(3), 193-203.

35. Zardi, E.M., Zardi, D.M., Dobrina, A., et al (2007). Prostacyclin in sepsis: A systematic review. *Prostaglandins & Other Lipid Mediators, 83*(1-2), 1-24.

evolve *Did you remember to check out the bonus material on the Evolve website and the CD-ROM, including NCLEX®-Examination Style Review Questions, Open-Book Quizzes, and Chapter Review Audio Podcasts?*

http://evolve.elsevier.com/Black/medsurg

CHAPTER 82

Management of Clients in the Emergency Department

JUDITH S. HALPERN AND PATRICIA A. MANION

During the mid-1960s, the need for specialization of emergency services throughout the United States was identified as a national priority to reduce the associated morbidity and mortality resulting from catastrophic illness or injury. Since then, the specialties of emergency medicine, emergency nursing, and prehospital care services have grown. In the United States, emergency department (ED) visits have increased by 18% (from 93.4 million to 110.2 million) during the years from 1994 to 2004. More than 100 million clients use EDs for health care services each year. The number of EDs throughout the United States has not increased over that same time period, however; in fact, they have decreased by about 12%. This equates to approximately 209 visits to U.S. EDs every minute during 2004. The age groups with the most frequent visits were 50 to 64 year olds (up 17%), 22 to 49 year olds (up 15%), and 65 years and older (up 8%). The scope of services provided in an ED range from treatment of acute conditions that threaten the loss of life, limb, or vision to management of non-urgent, chronic conditions. The types of clinical manifestations that accounted for the most frequent visits were general (e.g., fever, fatigue, pain), musculoskeletal, digestive, and respiratory.

EMERGENCY MEDICAL SERVICES

The emergency medical services (EMS) system encompasses all aspects of emergency care. Federal, state, and county EMS systems are designed to complement each other. The systems are responsible for establishing, regulating, coordinating, and monitoring the components involved in the provision of emergency care. These components include entities such as 911 telephone access systems, Emergency Medical Technician (EMT) and paramedical personnel scopes of practice, ground and air ambulance services, dispatch communication between points of incident and responding

personnel, and telecommunications between paramedical personnel and specialty-designated EDs known as *base station hospitals*. EMS systems are also instrumental in the coordination of activities for management of disaster situations.

Two goals of the EMS system are (1) to provide emergency care to a client as quickly as possible and (2) to ensure that the "right client arrives at the right hospital in the least amount of time." Consequently, EMS systems are involved with specialty-designated hospital departments and EDs such as local or state trauma centers, burn centers, and pediatric care centers.

EMERGENCY NURSING

Emergency nursing was officially recognized as a specialty in 1970. The national association representing these nurses is the Emergency Nurses Association (ENA). In 2006 the ENA was comprised of approximately 30,000 nurses who have chosen this area of professional nursing. Emergency nurses throughout the world have realized both their similarities and their differences through use of the World Wide Web and increasing international globalization.

According to the ENA, the definition of emergency nursing involves "the assessment, diagnosis, and treatment of perceived, actual or potential, sudden or urgent,

---

evolve Web Enhancements

Ethical Issues in Nursing Are Emergency Personnel Obliged to Honor Clients' Advance Directives?

Appendix A Religious Beliefs and Practices Affecting Health Care

Be sure to check out the bonus material on the Evolve website and the CD-ROM, including free self-assessment exercises. **http://evolve.elsevier.com/Black/medsurg**

physical or psychosocial problems that are primarily episodic or acute." These may require minimal care or life-support measures, education of client and significant others, appropriate referral, and knowledge of legal implications.

The ED of the future is being formulated today. Not only is technology changing, but also the day-to-day processes that support the ED infrastructure are being challenged and redesigned. These include concepts such as incorporating multiple triage stations and bedside or back-end client registration; using computerized protocols, guidelines, and electronic medical records; integrating nontraditional health care modalities; initiating wireless communication technology; and creating "virtual" EDs. In addition to the provision of direct client care, other multifaceted roles exist within emergency nursing. The emergency nurse is involved in the initial triaging of clients according to illness severity, may perform as a mobile intensive care nurse (MICN) by directing prehospital care personnel via telecommunication, and frequently provides client care in the prehospital environment. Community clinics use ED nurses, and many emergency nurses have become active in injury prevention programs at both national and local levels. Advanced practice roles such as clinical nurse specialists and nurse practitioners are integrated into many EDs throughout the United States. Nurses in these advanced practice roles often have a master's degree level of education or higher in addition to specialty certification.

Nurses working in an ED must be prepared to provide care to clients of all age-groups who have a myriad of possible illnesses or injuries. It is often cited that emergency nurses must have an understanding of almost all disease processes specific to any age-group. However, ED nursing is not usually addressed in depth in generic nursing programs. The education of ED nurses frequently occurs through hospital orientation programs, post-employment internship courses, and continuing education programs. ED nurses can obtain national specialty certification through an examination process. A certified ED nurse can use the credential of Certified Emergency Nurse (CEN).

LEGAL ISSUES

Nurses deal with a variety of legal issues in whatever specialty area they practice. The ED is no exception; however, certain issues are of paramount importance in this setting.

Federal Legislation

Past federal legislation has mandated that any client who presents to an ED seeking treatment must be rendered aid regardless of financial ability to pay for services. Since the mid-1980s, additional specific legislation

has been enacted requiring ED personnel to stabilize the condition of any client considered medically unstable before transfer to another health care facility—the Consolidated Omnibus Budget Reconciliation Act (COBRA) of 1986 and the Omnibus Budget Reconciliation Act (OBRA) of 1990. This stabilization must occur regardless of the client's financial ability to pay for services. ED personnel who transfer clients to another institution without first providing this initial stabilization can incur substantial fines and penalties, as can the hospital administration.

Clients have continued to seek health care services in the ED, even with the proliferation of managed health care plans and gate-keeping policies. The financial integrity of the ED has been challenged over the years because of the legal obligations of the ED to provide service. Retrospectively, financial reimbursement for rendered services has been denied to EDs from managed health care plans following a determination that the client's problem did not constitute a true emergency. Additional legislation was enacted (Emergency Medical Treatment and Active Labor Act [EMTALA] in 1988, 1989, 1990, and 1994) requiring that a medical screening examination be performed on all ED clients before solicitation of information about ability to pay. This medical screening examination must be inclusive enough to determine whether the client is experiencing an emergency medical condition requiring treatment or, in the case of a pregnant woman, is experiencing labor contractions. An emergency medical condition includes drug abuse, hemodynamic instability, psychiatric illness, intoxication, severe pain, and labor. If a client has an emergency medical condition, stabilization must be rendered. Stabilization is interpreted to mean that deterioration of the client is unlikely during possible transfer or discharge of the client. Continued interpretations of this act have expanded the facilities that come under EMTALA. These include not only EDs, but also hospital-owned urgent care centers, anywhere unscheduled clients appear for medical care, and off-site locations that are within a 250-yard zone of a main hospital that is covered under the 2001 outpatient prospective payment system. Violations of this legislation can again result in fines and penalties. Each congressional year, new legislation and interpretations of existing law are proposed for providing appropriate emergency medical treatment to the public while continuing to acknowledge cost-containment issues.

In 1996 the Health Insurance Portability and Accountability Act (HIPAA), Public Law 104–191, was passed to provide national standards for electronic health care transactions. Subsequently, the rule was further defined, and in 2002, it was extended to protect privacy of protected health information. The Privacy Rule covers information found in medical records, conversations with health care personnel, insurance records, billing information, and other health information that is collected. The rule restricts who can look at and receive a person's health information and stipulates that personal information cannot be used or shared without authorization.

Consent to Treat

Most adult clients seeking treatment in the ED give voluntary consent to the standard and usual treatment performed in this setting. In some instances, however, a client is deemed unable to give consent for treatment. This inability may be due to the critical nature of the client's illness or injury or to other conditions, such as an altered level of consciousness. In these instances, emergency care may be rendered to the client under the implied emergency doctrine. This doctrine assumes that the client would consent to treatment to prevent death or disability if the client were so able.

Children younger than the age of legal majority must have the consent of their parent or legal guardian for medical care to be rendered. Exceptions include (1) emancipated minors; (2) minors seeking treatment for communicable diseases, including sexually transmitted diseases, injuries from abuse, and alcohol or drug rehabilitation; and (3) minor-age females requesting treatment for pregnancy or pregnancy-related concerns. Some states also allow the adult caregiver with whom the child resides to give treatment authorization even though that caregiver may not be the parent.

The issue of informed consent in the ED is the same as that in any other health care setting. Adult clients must be informed about the necessity of required treatments, expected outcomes, and potential complications. Clients must also be mentally competent and understand the information being explained. As in any other setting, a mentally competent adult client always maintains the right to refuse treatment or withdraw previously given consent.

Restraints

Restraining a client while he or she is in the ED may at times be necessary. The need for restraints usually arises because the client is becoming agitated or potentially violent. Hard leather or chemical restraints are used in the ED if the client is in danger of injuring self or others and when nonphysical methods of controlling the client are not viable.

According to The Joint Commission (TJC) National Patient Safety Goals, restraints may not be used to control a client solely for convenience or because of staffing issues. When restraints are required, departmental and hospital guidelines that are in compliance with The Joint Commission and the Centers for Medicare & Medicaid Services (formerly the Health Care Financing Administration) must be followed. A physician's order for applying restraints as well as the client's behavior mandating the use of restraints must be documented. The client must be periodically reevaluated both for the continued need for restraints and for the integrity of distal circulation, motor movement, and sensory level of the restrained extremities. The findings must be documented. Offering water to the client and providing opportunities to urinate or relieve other body needs are required, as is documentation of this nursing care. No client may be kept in restraints against his or her will unless the client's behavior indicates the existence of safety issues. Behavior modification techniques used in an attempt to release the client from restraints must also be documented. The ED staff must receive appropriate education pertaining to dealing with clients requiring physical restraint.

Clients in the ED who have psychological conditions that render them a danger to themselves or to others, or who are unable to provide food or shelter for themselves, can be placed and held on a legal psychiatric restraining order. This order mandates that such clients be placed in a locked psychiatric facility for their protection for a maximum of 72 hours. Within that 72-hour period, the client must be evaluated by a psychiatrist to determine whether the legal hold needs to be extended or whether the client can be released. Clients who may be at risk for suicide must be identified according to TJC's National Patient Safety Goals.

Mandatory Reporting

Every state has mandatory reporting regulations that affect emergency nurses. Incidents and conditions may need to be reported to federal, state, or local authorities or to the Department of Public Health, Department of Motor Vehicles, coroner's offices, or animal control agencies. The types of incidents requiring reporting are suspected child, sexual, domestic, and older adult abuse; assaults; motor vehicle crashes; communicable diseases such as hepatitis, sexually transmitted diseases, chickenpox, measles, mumps, meningitis, tuberculosis, and food poisoning; first-time or recurrent seizure activity; death; and animal bites. Every ED has written policies regarding these mandatory reports.

According to TJC's National Patient Safety Goals, clients and their families must be told how to report concerns about safety and encouraged to report such incidents.

SAFETY
ALERT

Evidence Collection and Preservation

Recognition of unusual circumstances surrounding a client's injury or death is an important aspect of ED nursing because of the associated legal implications.

Not only must the legal authorities be notified, but also, in many instances, the ED nurse may be required to collect and preserve evidence taken from the client. This evidence can include bullets, weapons, clothing, and body fluid specimens. All collected evidence must be identified by the client's name, hospital identification number, date and time of evidence collection, type of evidence and source (e.g., venipuncture, hematoma aspiration, vomitus, swab), and the initials or signature of the person collecting the evidence. Once the evidence has been collected, its preservation and the maintenance of the "chain of custody" are extremely important. Table 82-1 and Boxes 82-1 and 82-2 relate to evidence collection.

Violence

In 2005 the United States Department of Labor, Bureau of Labor Statistics, identified 5702 fatal work injuries, of which 14% were attributed to assaults and violent acts.

Violence directed against ED personnel has become an issue of concern throughout the late 1990s and into the 21st century. The environment inherent in the ED, the emotional circumstances often surrounding the illness or injury that affect both clients and family members, and the increasingly violent trends in the United States all play a role in this phenomenon. Administrative changes have been made in some EDs to enhance both public and health care worker safety. These measures have included the installation of items such as metal detectors, "panic buttons," bullet-proof glass, and lock-down doors at public entrances; increasing the visibility of security guards; using patrol guard dogs; and instituting visitor control policies. Changing the perception of the ED from one of fear and isolation for both clients and family members is also occurring.

BOX 82-1 Tips for Preserving Evidence in the Emergency Department

1. Do not contaminate specimens or person—use gloves.
2. Minimally handle the body of a deceased person.
3. Place paper bags on the hands and feet and possibly over the head of a deceased person to protect trace evidence or residue.
4. Collect and place evidence on clean, white sheet until it can be packaged and labeled.
5. Do not place wet clothing in plastic bags as wet clothes can "sweat," thereby destroying evidence. Allow item to air-dry, and then place inside individual paper bags. If item is soaked and continues to leak fluid, place inside another bag and label to alert crime lab that it contains body fluids.
6. Photograph inflicted wounds or injury before cleansing or repair.
7. Do not insert invasive tubes through pre-existing wounds or holes (e.g., do not place chest tubes through chest wounds or intravenous catheters through needle track marks).
8. Do not cut clothing through evidence holes such as stab wounds or bullet wounds.
9. Collect the client's personal items, such as written notes, drugs or medications, and items from clothing pockets.
10. Do not allow family members, significant others, or friends to be alone with the client.

BOX 82-2 Maintaining "Chain of Custody" of Evidence in the Emergency Department

1. Seal evidence with tape and label with client information data, date and time of collection, signature of person collecting evidence.
2. Document all collected evidence on designated forms.
3. Document all transfers of evidence from one person to another, and include the reason for transfer of evidence.
4. Obtain signatures of the person releasing evidence and of the person receiving evidence.
5. *Never* leave collected evidence unattended. Call police or forensic nurse examiner immediately to retrieve evidence.
6. Air-dry evidence before placing it in a collection container or paper envelope.

Instituting family-centered practices that recognize the importance of family participation and addressing the emotional needs of clients and families is a trend in ED management.

However, education of ED personnel in violence prevention is also of paramount importance in reducing the toll of violence. The following areas are crucial to address:

- **Recognizing potentially violent clients and situations**

TABLE 82-1 Evidence Collection in the Emergency Department

Evidence	Collection/Container
Glass fragments, bullets, broken fingernails, paint chips, loose hair follicles, fibers, or trace evidence such as soil	Place each item in a paper envelope or specimen container.
Head or pubic hair samples	Collected samples from combings and cuttings are each placed in a paper envelope.
Blood (from both venipuncture and possible hematoma evacuation), urine, gastric washings, or vomitus	A 20-30-ml sample is placed in a sealed container.
Swabs from wounds, membranes, or orifices	Air-dry before placing in a collection container or paper envelope.

From Selfridge-Thomas, J. (1995). *Manual of emergency nursing* (p. 382). Philadelphia: Saunders.

■ **Identifying verbally and physically abusive cues from clients, family members, or friends**

■ **Understanding the importance of instinct or "gut reactions"**

■ **Using simple communication strategies to defuse potentially problematic situations**

■ **Requiring clients to completely undress before physical examination**

■ **Minimizing the presence of "potential weapons" in client care areas such as scalpels, needles, excess tubing attached to oxygen flow meters, scissors, stethoscopes worn around the neck, and personal jewelry**

■ **Restraining clients, when necessary, using a team approach**

■ **Avoiding becoming a hostage in a volatile situation**

■ **Having a safety committee track all reported assaults on clients and employees**

■ **Ensuring Occupational Safety and Health Administration violence guidelines are followed**

■ **Encouraging employees to report both verbal and physical assaults**

Once a violent situation has erupted, the protection of ED personnel and others in the department is of utmost concern. Any means necessary to ensure their safety must be undertaken.

ETHICAL ISSUES

The ethical issues confronting ED nurses usually deal with end-of-life concerns. Initial resuscitation and stabilization of clients in critical condition constitute universal standard practice in the ED. At times, however, the desired outcome of client survivability is not achievable.

Unexpected Death

When death occurs in the ED setting, it is usually sudden and unexpected, even if the client has had a prolonged illness. The unexpected nature of the death, or impending death, can present ethical dilemmas for both the family survivors and the ED personnel. One such issue deals with the length of time to which resuscitation is performed. This is usually a physician's decision; however, family members may at times have input. Allowing family members or significant others to be present during client resuscitation is becoming more common. This practice is not necessarily disruptive to the resuscitation process, and it can be of comfort to the survivors and the involved ED personnel.

When death does occur, the ED nurse and the ED physician have important roles in informing the family:

■ Inform the family of the client's death, and refer to the deceased client by name.

■ Provide the family with an explanation of the course of events related to the death; use simple explanations.

■ Offer the family an opportunity to view the body. If a child has died, allow the parent to hold the child. Providing the parent with a lock of the child's hair may be comforting.

■ Help the family to focus on decisions requiring immediate attention such as taking possession of the deceased person's valuables, arranging postmortem examination if desired or required, identifying possible organ or tissue donation, and selecting a funeral home.

■ Inform family members when they can leave the ED setting.

■ Provide community agency referral as needed.

Advance Directives

In 1991 Congress enacted the Patient Self-Determination Act (PSDA), which allows a client, or the client's health care proxy, to make determinations related to end-of-life measures. Emergency care personnel are obligated to abide by the client's advance directive decisions, if that information is available and provided in writing. When this written information is not available, ED personnel have a responsibility to stabilize or resuscitate any client according to standard treatment guidelines, regardless of a family member's expressed wishes.

Organ and Tissue Donation

Issues related to potential organ or tissue donation often arise in the ED setting. Once a potential donor is identified, the surviving family members need to be approached. A team approach involving a physician, a nurse, and possibly an organ procurement coordinator is optimal. Utmost dignity and professionalism must be maintained. (Chapter 80 reviews religious and cultural customs and beliefs related to death and organ transplantation. Also see the WebLinks for Chapter 80, *evolve* which include links to various agencies, organizations, and the latest medical information.) Whatever decision the family makes regarding organ or tissue donation, that decision must be supported by health care personnel.

Child Abandonment

States are beginning to pass child abandonment laws in response to the number of newborn infants being abandoned following birth. In general, the law allows mothers to bring their newborn child to the ED and abandon the child in the care of the ED personnel. The mother bears no criminal responsibility. Local Departments of Social Services are then contacted so the child can be placed in their custody.

COMPONENTS OF EMERGENCY CARE

Even though treatment decisions in the ED may at first appear to occur in a chaotic fashion, there is an inherent order in the timing and choice of interventions performed throughout a client's stay. The organizational flow of events involves client triage (prioritizing), in-depth nursing assessment of the client, diagnostic testing, formulation of diagnoses, outcome management, evaluation, disposition, and documentation.

Triage

Whether clients arrive in the ED via ambulance or are ambulatory, they are triaged at some point by either an ED physician or an ED nurse. The purpose of this triage process is to expediently determine the severity of a client's problem or condition in order to deliver emergency care in the most appropriate time frame. In other words, which clients need treatment immediately and which can wait is determined. The acuity level of the presenting problem is rated according to predetermined categories; the most frequently used ratings are *emergent* (must be treated immediately otherwise life/limb/vision is threatened), *urgent* (requires treatment but life/limb/vision is not threatened and care can be provided within 1 to 2 hours), and *non-urgent* (requires evaluation and possible treatment, but time is not a critical factor). However, the American College of Emergency Physicians and the Emergency Nurses Association have a joint position paper supporting the adoption of a reliable, valid five-level triage scale. The five-level rating approach is currently being incorporated into client triage in many emergency departments. The five-level rating systems are one of two types. In one type, the previous *urgent* and *non-urgent* categories may be further subdivided into unstable and stable clients. Another five-level rating system is the Emergency Severity Index (ESI). This system is based on the triage nurse identifying the critical clients and then predetermining the number of department resources most likely required to treat the non-urgent client. Figure 82-1 displays this algometric approach. Once an initial determination is made about the severity of the client's condition, a more in-depth nursing and medical assessment is completed. Appropriate diagnostic testing and specific interventions are performed using a team approach as emergency physicians and nurses work collaboratively to provide appropriate and expeditious management of the client's problem.

Nursing Assessment

The nursing assessment process for any client entering the ED is divided into *primary* and *secondary* assessments (Figure 82-2).

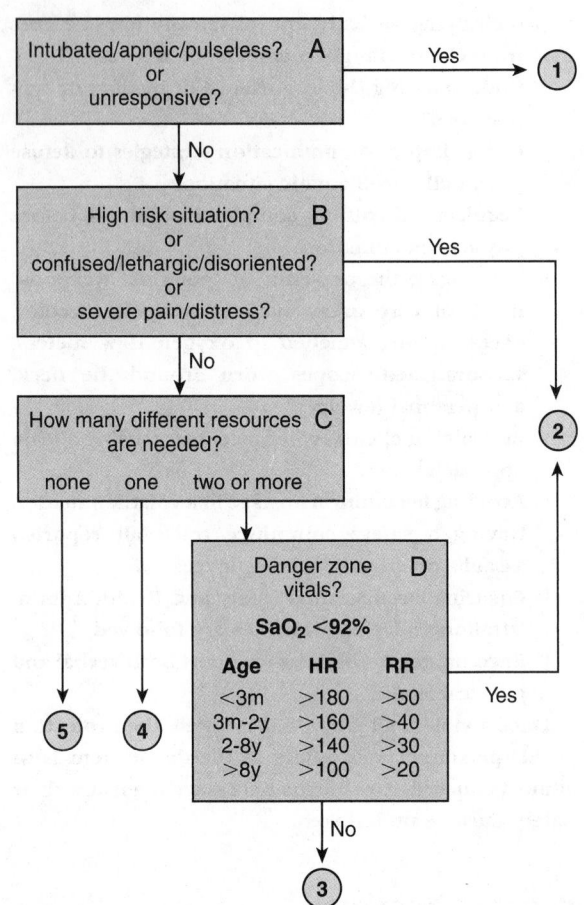

■ **FIGURE 82-1** Emergency Severity Index triage algorithm. *(From Wuerz, R.C., et al [2001]. Implementation and refinement of the Emergency Severity Index. Academic Emergency Medicine, 8, 170-176.)*

The purpose of the *primary assessment* is to immediately identify any client problem that poses a threat, immediate or potential, to life, limb, or vision. Information is gathered primarily through objective data, such as physical examination and vital signs. If any abnormalities are found during the primary assessment, immediate interventions such as Advanced Cardiac Life Support (ACLS) and Advanced Trauma Life Support (ATLS) must be instituted to aid in preserving the client's life, limb, or vision. The primary assessment uses the *ABC* mnemonic:

- *A* Airway patency
- *B* Breathing effectiveness
- *C* Circulation (both peripheral and organ-specific)

For any client arriving in the ED who has been involved in a major traumatic injury, the assessment of the airway also includes evaluation of the adequacy of the C-spine immobilization, and includes *D* for disability. This includes a brief evaluation of level of consciousness and pupil response to light.

Once it is determined that a client's ABC status is satisfactory, the *secondary assessment* is performed to

Primary Assessment

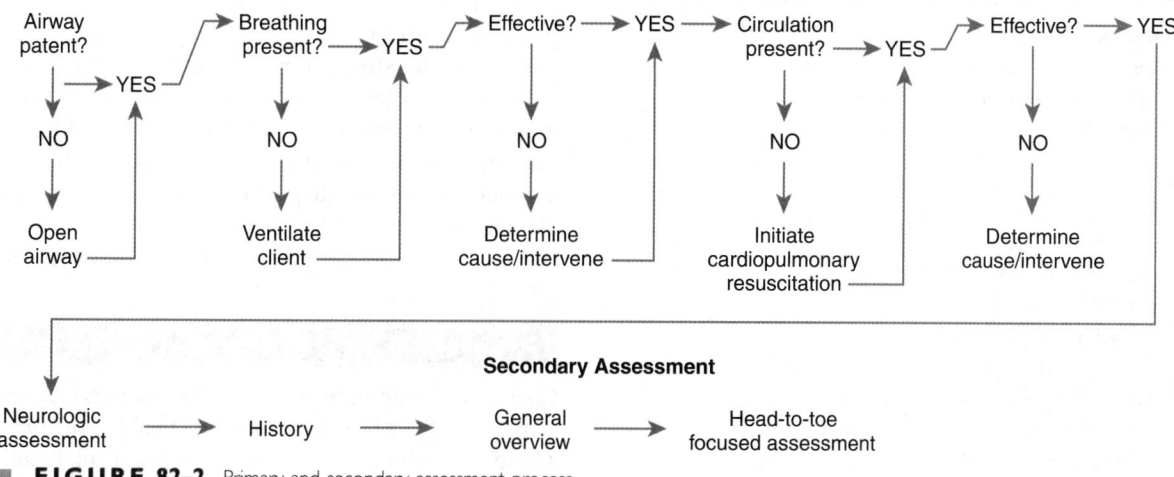

■ **FIGURE 82–2** Primary and secondary assessment process.

identify any other non–life-threatening problems the client may be experiencing. Both subjective information and objective data are obtained. The secondary assessment includes the following elements.

Neurologic Assessment

Determine the client's (1) level of consciousness; (2) orientation to person, place, time, and event; (3) Glasgow Coma Scale (GCS) score (Table 82-2); (4) pupillary size, equality, and reaction to light and accommodation; and (5) motor movement and strength of hand grips and pedal pushes. A brief neurologic assessment can also be determined using the *AVPU* mnemonic:

- *A* Alert (the client is awake and alert and needs no stimulus to respond to the environment)
- *V* Verbal (the client requires a verbal stimulus to elicit a response)
- *P* Pain (the client requires a painful stimulus to evoke a response)
- *U* Unresponsive (the client is unresponsive to any applied stimulus)

History

Elicit the nature of the client's chief complaint, duration of the problem, mechanism of injury from blunt or penetrating forces (Box 82-3), associated manifestations related to the primary problem, past pertinent medical history, current medications and compliance, use of over-the-counter (OTC) medications or herbs, routine use of alcohol or illicit drugs, known medication allergies, and immunization history. Women of childbearing age may need to be questioned about the date of the last normal menstrual period (LNMP) and the number of pregnancies and outcomes. Questions related to potential or actual child, sexual, domestic, or older adult abuse situations also must be addressed.

Pain

The most frequent complaint for which clients seek emergency care is related to both acute and chronic pain. Obtaining specific information regarding pain patterns can be extremely helpful. Asking questions according to the *PQRST* mnemonic often provides useful information:

- *P* Provokes: Are there any specific factors that cause the pain to increase or decrease?
- *Q* Quality: What descriptive terminology identifies the type of pain—dull, sharp, colicky, pressure?
- *R* Region/Radiation: Where is the pain located? Does it move to other areas?
- *S* Severity: Use a rating scale of 1 to 10, visual analogs, or word descriptors to describe pain severity.
- *T* Timing: How long has the pain been present? Are there cycles related to when the pain is present or absent?

TABLE 82–2	Glasgow Coma Scale	
Eye-opening response	Spontaneous	4
	To voice	3
	To pain	2
	None	1
Best verbal response	Oriented	5
	Confused	4
	Inappropriate words	3
	Incomprehensible sounds	2
	None	1
Best motor response	Obeys command	6
	Localizes pain	5
	Withdraws (to painful stimulus)	4
	Flexion (to painful stimulus)	3
	Extension (to painful stimulus)	2
	None	1
Total		3-15

BOX 82-3   History Questions Related to Injury

MOTOR VEHICLE CRASHES

- Do you remember the crash?
- Were you the driver or passenger?
- Were you wearing a seat belt?
- Did the airbag deploy?
- Did you hit the steering wheel or the dashboard? If so, with what part of your body?
- How fast was the vehicle going?
- What did the vehicle hit?
- Where is your pain?

BLUNT INJURY FROM FALLS

- How far did you fall?
- What precipitated the fall?
- What did you land on?
- Where is your pain?
- Self-reported loss of consciousness is not valid information.

GUNSHOT WOUNDS

- How long ago did the incident occur?
- What were you doing when you got shot?
- How many shots did you hear?
- What did the gun look like?
- Where is your pain?

PENETRATING WOUNDS OR STAB WOUNDS

- How long ago did the injury occur?
- How many times were you stabbed?
- What did the knife look like?
- Where is your pain?

Both adult and pediatric clients who rate their pain at a level of 7 or above, or use descriptive words denoting "severe" pain, need to be considered high risk and need to be evaluated by the ED physician as expediently as possible. Clients have a right to have their pain treated appropriately, in a timely manner, and effectively, without exception.

General Overview

Note the client's overall health condition, skin color, gait, posture, unusual skin markings or body odors, and mood and affect. Baseline measurements of blood pressure, heart rate, respiratory rate, pulse oximetry values, and temperature are important. Actual weight in a pediatric client and reported weight in an adult are also important.

Head-to-Toe (Focused) Assessment

Remove the client's clothing and examine the areas where the chief complaint and any other associated complaints are focused. The techniques of inspection, auscultation, percussion, and palpation are used to determine additional normal or abnormal findings.

Diagnosis

Upon completion of the medical and nursing assessment process, diagnostic tests (radiographic, cardiology, laboratory, special studies) may be initiated. Once all pertinent information has been collected, a working diagnosis is formulated. The physician provides a medical diagnosis; in addition, the ED nurse may incorporate a variety of nursing diagnoses. These diagnoses provide a framework on which to build a plan of appropriate client care and against which to measure outcomes.

OUTCOME MANAGEMENT

Client care interventions may be initiated by the ED nurse, the ED physician, or other health care providers. There is frequent collaboration among all health care providers involved, and interventions are assigned priority according to the severity of the client's condition.

Evaluation

The desired goal in client care is to achieve positive client outcomes after medical and nursing management. This is an integral component of ED nursing care. If the client's condition does not improve with initial interventions, the plan of care must be reexamined and additional interventions may be required.

Client Disposition

All clients entering the ED are eventually discharged from the ED. They may be transferred to another health care facility, admitted to the hospital, or released to home or another facility. Most clients are released to home following treatment. Before being discharged from the ED, a client or family members must be given both oral and written instructions concerning follow-up care. These instructions should identify the client's diagnosed problem, explain necessary continued treatments, describe potential complications, and specify time frames for rechecks and the name of the physician to whom the client is being referred. These instructions should be presented in both oral and written form in the client's primary language. At times, a hospital or family interpreter may be required to accomplish this outcome.

Nursing Documentation

Because ED nurses frequently are responsible for an assigned area, zone, or "pod" within the department and because clients enter and exit those areas on a continual basis, nursing documentation is of paramount importance. Documentation must include the recording of all assessment findings, diagnostic tests, interventions and management, responses to treatment, achieved outcomes, and client education. Documentation needs to be complete but concise, providing an ongoing record o the client's condition and responses. The format may be a flow sheet, narrative, computer-generated design, or a combination of these.

EMERGENCY CONDITIONS

INEFFECTIVE AIRWAY CLEARANCE

A compromised or ineffective airway may be due to either complete or partial airway obstruction. Common causes of airway compromise include the presence of a foreign object in the airway, airway edema, airway infection, facial or airway injury, and tongue obstruction.

Clinical Manifestations

The clinical manifestations of airway compromise include absence of breathing, drooling, stridor, intercostal or substernal retractions, alteration in skin color (pallor, gray, cyanotic), and agitation. A decreased level of consciousness may lead to airway compromise as a result of obstruction of the posterior pharynx by the relaxed tongue.

OUTCOME MANAGEMENT

Remove Obstruction

If an obstruction is present, the airway should be opened by a chin-lift or jaw-thrust maneuver (Figures 82-3 and 82-4, respectively). If either of these maneuvers opens the client's airway, patency is maintained via the insertion of a nasopharyngeal or oral airway device. If these maneuvers fail to relieve the obstruction, more aggressive interventions must be instituted, such as

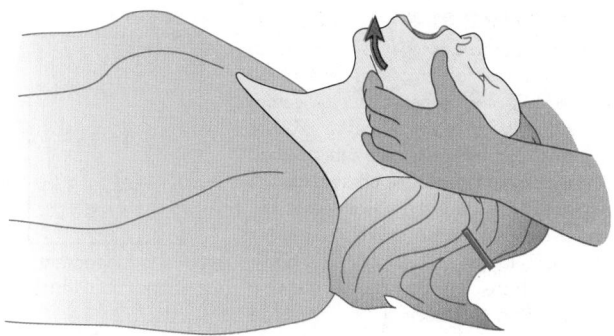

■ FIGURE 82–4   The jaw-thrust maneuver to open the airway is the preferred method for use in clients with head or cervical neck injury.

(1) performing abdominal or chest thrusts if an aspirated foreign object is the suspected cause (Figure 82-5), (2) suctioning the oral cavity to remove secretions or visible foreign objects, (3) intubating via the nasal or oral route, (4) using a laryngeal mask airway (LMA), or (5) assisting with creating a surgical airway via a cricothyroidotomy (Figure 82-6).

Intubate

In some cases, oral or nasal intubation may require the use of *rapid-sequence induction* (RSI). This procedure is used in awake clients who require intubation either to maintain the airway or as a mechanism to provide adequate ventilation. RSI is most frequently used in clients who have sustained a head or spinal injury and in clients who are rapidly tiring from the effort of maintaining effective breathing. RSI involves (1) establishing venous access, (2) hyperventilating the client with 100% oxygen, (3) administering intravenous (IV) lidocaine 1 mg/kg to blunt any transient increase in intracranial pressure from the actual intubation procedure, and (4) administering an IV general barbiturate or anesthetic medication such as thiopental 3 to 5 mg/kg, fentanyl (Sublimaze) 3 to 15 mcg/kg, ketamine (Ketalar) 1 to 2 mg/kg, etomidate (Amidate) 0.3 mg/kg, propofol (Diprivan) 2 mg/kg, or midazolam (Versed) 0.1 mg/kg followed immediately by the administration of an IV muscle-paralyzing agent such as succinylcholine (Anectine) 1.5 to 2 mg/kg, pancuronium (Pavulon) 0.04 to 0.1 mg/kg, or vecuronium (Norcuron) 0.08 to 0.1 mg/kg. Once the client loses consciousness and adequate muscle relaxation and paralysis have been obtained, intubation using equipment such as an intubating laryngeal mask airway, intubating fiberoptic bronchoscope, or nasal/endotracheal tubes is accomplished. The client is then ventilated using 100% oxygen via a bag until a ventilator is attached.

Verify Tube Placement

After an intubation procedure, there is immediate verification of tube placement by auscultation, verification

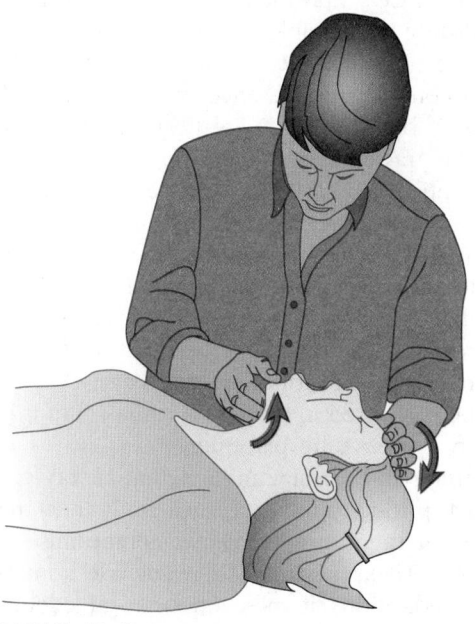

FIGURE 82–3   Chin-lift maneuver to open the airway.

■ **FIGURE 82–5** Abdominal-thrust maneuver (formerly known as the Heimlich maneuver) used for removal of foreign bodies blocking the upper airway. Vigorous upward chest or abdominal thrusts produce a rush of air that expels the foreign body. The abdominal thrust is the original Heimlich maneuver. The chest thrust is an adaptation that is useful for obese or pregnant victims. Use four quick thrusts in the positions shown. **A,** Hand placement. **B,** Maneuver for conscious victims. **C,** Maneuver for unconscious victims.

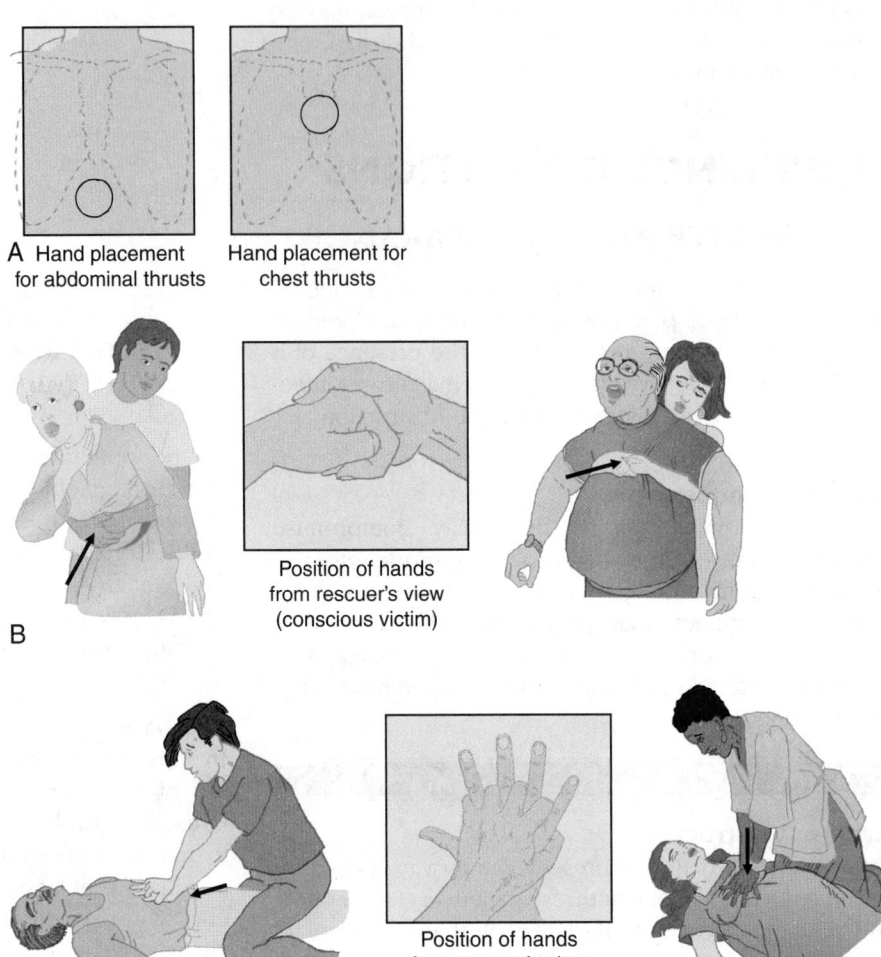

A Hand placement for abdominal thrusts

Hand placement for chest thrusts

Position of hands from rescuer's view (conscious victim)

B

Position of hands from rescuer's view (unconscious victim)

C

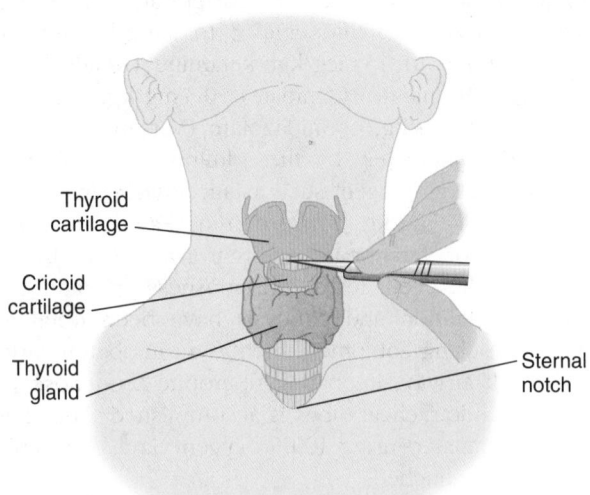

■ **FIGURE 82–6** A cricothyroidotomy procedure is performed to create a temporary airway. An opening is made into the trachea and is maintained with a small plastic tube.

Thyroid cartilage

Cricoid cartilage

Thyroid gland

Sternal notch

of end-tidal CO_2, and then chest x-ray. The ED nurse is immediately responsible for auscultation of the client's epigastric area and then chest during assisted ventilation to confirm the presence of equal bilateral breath sounds. If breath sounds are heard over the epigastric area, the tracheal tube must be removed, the client hyperventilated, and the procedure reattempted. Breath sounds heard more prominently over the upper right chest indicate that the tracheal tube has advanced too far into the right main bronchus. The tube needs to be pulled back and breath sounds reassessed. Once the presence of equal and bilateral breath sounds is confirmed and appropriate end-tidal CO_2 is present, the tube is secured in place and a chest film is obtained to verify correct tube placement.

Securing and maintaining a patent airway constitutes the first priority in any ED client. Other treatments directed at the cause of airway compromise are then instituted. These measures may include administration of IV medications if infection or local edema of the airway is present.

Immobilize the Spine

If the client with an actual or potential airway problem has also sustained a traumatic injury and arrives in the ED without C-spine immobilization, stabilization of the client's cervical, thoracic, and lumbar spine must be instituted and maintained until cleared by the physician. Stabilization is accomplished using a team approach and involves the following steps: (1) manually stabilizing the client's head and cervical spine, (2) applying an appropriate size hard cervical collar around the client's nuchal area, (3) placing the client on an ED stretcher, (4) logrolling as a unit until spine is cleared.

INEFFECTIVE BREATHING PATTERN

Effective breathing is affected if a client is either hyperventilating or hypoventilating. This may occur if the client is breathing too fast or too slowly. The normal respiratory rate for an adult is between 12 and 20 breaths/min; infant respiratory rates are between 30 and 40 breaths/min; and children have respiratory rates between 25 and 30 breaths/min until approximately the age of 10 years.

HYPERVENTILATION

Clinical Manifestations

Respiratory rates faster than normal constitute tachypnea and, in many cases, hyperventilation. Hyperventilation is defined as low arterial carbon dioxide level and may result in respiratory alkalosis. The client may report numbness and tingling sensations in the distal extremities or around the lips, along with carpal or pedal spasms. A sensation of chest pain may also be present. Frequently this condition is caused by client anxiety, but it is important to also investigate other possible causes, such as pain, aspirin toxicity, diabetic ketoacidosis, fluid loss, infection, central nervous system (CNS) lesions, and pulmonary embolism.

OUTCOME MANAGEMENT

The goals of treatment are to return the client's breathing pattern and rate to normal and to restore normal gas exchange. If anxiety is the cause of the hyperventilation, the client needs to be instructed to take slow, deep breaths through the nose and slowly exhale through the mouth. Having clients breathe into a paper bag and rebreathe their own carbon dioxide may be helpful. If another cause is identified as the reason for the client's altered breathing pattern, specific treatments such as administration of oxygen and inhaled, intravenous, or oral medications are initiated to reverse the process.

HYPOVENTILATION

Clinical Manifestations

Hypoventilation occurs when there is a decreased respiratory rate or inadequate exchange of gas at the alveolar level. This may occur when an adult client's respiratory rate falls below 12 breaths/min or, in the case of a child, the respiratory rate is below what is normal for the age group. At these rates, carbon dioxide accumulates in the alveoli, leading to respiratory acidosis. There may also not be enough oxygen available to maintain adequate tissue oxygenation. Clinical manifestations may include a decrease in the client's level of consciousness, pallor, cyanosis, and pulse oximetry readings of less than 96%. Causes of hypoventilation include brain stem lesions, head injury, drug-induced depression of the respiratory center, impaired respiratory muscle innervation from spinal cord injury, and the presence of neuromuscular diseases such as muscular dystrophy or Guillain-Barré syndrome.

OUTCOME MANAGEMENT

Improving ventilation via a bag-valve-mask device and, if necessary, endotracheal intubation is required to reduce carbon dioxide levels to near 38 to 42 mm Hg and to return oxygen levels to between 80 and 100 mm Hg. Recommendations for ventilating infants include using a pediatric size bag-valve-mask instead of an infant bag.

IMPAIRED GAS EXCHANGE

Etiology

Obstructions, infections, and injury within the pulmonary system can lead to the development of gas exchange abnormalities. Common causative disorders include asthma, other reactive airway diseases, chronic obstructive pulmonary disease, pulmonary embolism, pulmonary edema, bronchitis, pneumonia, tuberculosis, pneumothorax, and chest injuries such as a flail chest.

A less common cause of a gas exchange problem is noncardiac pulmonary edema, which results from acute damage to the alveolocapillary membrane. This damage can occur from inhalation injury, near-drowning, sepsis, trauma, and opioid overdose. As the alveolocapillary membrane permeability increases, fluid collects in the interstitial space, surfactant levels decrease, and the alveoli eventually collapse.

Clinical Manifestations

With constriction of the bronchi, accumulation of fluid, or lung consolidation occurs; abnormal lung sounds such as wheezes, rales (fine crackles), or rhonchi (coarse crackles) are often heard throughout the client's lung fields. With pulmonary infections, the client may have concurrent fever. If a pneumothorax is present, breath sounds are diminished or absent on the side of the pneumothorax. Asymmetrical chest wall movement suggests that there is something interfering with air entry or escape from that lung or that the client is splinting that side because of pain. Paradoxical chest wall movement with breathing should raise suspicion of a possible flail chest. In such cases, a chest film or spiral computed tomography (CT) scan provides valuable diagnostic information about the cause of the client's problem.

OUTCOME MANAGEMENT

Administer Oxygen

Oxygen therapy with a flow rate of between 2 and 10 L/min via nasal cannula for lower Fio_2 (fraction of inspired oxygen) or non-rebreather mask for 100% O_2 is the priority intervention for clients with an obstructive or infectious cause of ineffective gas exchange. Biphasic positive airway pressure (BiPAP) or continuous positive airway pressure (CPAP) are noninvasive ventilation masks used when the client requires assistance with ventilation and oxygenation.

Administer Medications to Open Lower Airways

Oxygen administration is frequently followed by administering aerosolized bronchodilator medications such as metaproterenol (Alupent) or albuterol (Ventolin) to open constricted upper or lower bronchi. Subcutaneous epinephrine 1:1000 may be administered to relax constricted bronchi and to reduce the degree of airway or bronchial edema. Administration of steroid medications, either intravenously or orally, is also frequently used as first-line therapy. A client with a pulmonary embolus or deep vein thrombosis may be given heparin or low molecular weight heparin.

Minimize Spread of Infection

Infectious diseases that are the cause of impaired gas exchange are treated with IV or oral antibiotic medications.

SAFETY ALERT **If the client has pneumonia, the IV antibiotic should be administered within 4 hours of arrival in the ED. This is part of The Joint Commission's (TJC) Core Measures.**

A client thought to have a highly contagious pulmonary disease such as tuberculosis must be isolated in a reverse or negative airflow room and will need to wear a high-efficiency particulate air (HEPA) filter mask placed over the nose and mouth when not in a reverse pressure room. Anyone entering the reverse pressure TB isolation room will need to wear a HEPA mask or particulate respirator (see Chapter 62).

TRAUMATIC PNEUMOTHORAX

A pneumothorax can be classified as a simple pneumothorax, open pneumothorax, or tension pneumothorax (see Figure 63-9). In a *simple pneumothorax,* air from the bronchus, bronchioles, or alveoli escapes into the pleural space and diminishes lung expansion capacity. With an *open pneumothorax,* a traumatically created opening in the client's chest wall may allow air to move freely into and out of the thoracic cavity during inspiration and exhalation. A tension pneumothorax occurs when air continues to become trapped in the pleural cavity with no mechanism of escape during the exhalation process. This type of pneumothorax is an emergent condition.

Clinical Manifestations

A simple pneumothorax can occur spontaneously but is frequently associated with penetrating injury to the chest or with blunt forces causing a rib fracture. An obvious chest wound is present with an open pneumothorax. If the wound is large enough, a sucking sound is heard as the client breathes. Pain with breathing is present, and diminished or absent breath sounds may be present on the side of the injury. The client may be tachypneic and may have decreased pulse oximetry readings.

A tension pneumothorax produces the clinical manifestations of extreme respiratory distress, distended jugular neck veins, and a mediastinal shift of the heart, trachea, esophagus, and great vessels to the side away from the tension pneumothorax. Hypotension and tachycardia are other findings. Pneumothorax is diagnosed by clinical manifestations, a chest radiograph, or a spiral CT.

OUTCOME MANAGEMENT

Administer Oxygen

Administration of 100% oxygen via a non-rebreather face mask is a priority treatment for a client who has sustained a pneumothorax.

Apply Occlusive Dressing

Any open chest wall wound should be covered with an occlusive gauze dressing, but this intervention may convert an open pneumothorax into the more dangerous tension pneumothorax because the gauze covering blocks the trapped air's escape route. If manifestations of a tension pneumothorax appear, the occlusive dressing must be immediately removed.

Release Trapped Air

If a tension pneumothorax is thought to be the cause of respiratory distress and if it has not been iatrogenically produced by covering an open chest wound, a 14- to 16-gauge catheter needle is immediately inserted into the client's anterior chest wall on the affected side at the second intercostal space, midclavicular line. This life-saving intervention allows the immediate release of trapped air and decompresses the pleural cavity.

Place Chest Tube

The simple, open, and tension varieties of pneumothorax are definitively treated with the insertion of a chest tube that is attached to a suction/collection device. This measure aids in reexpansion of the lung, leading to improvement in the client's gas exchange.

FLAIL CHEST

A flail chest involves serious rib fractures. It occurs when two or more ribs are fractured in two or more places on the same chest wall side or when the sternum is detached from the ribs. The fractured segment has no connection with the remaining rib cage. This segment then moves in a direction opposite that of the rest of the chest wall during the processes of inhalation and exhalation—so-called paradoxical chest wall movement (see Figure 63-8). The client may be tachypneic and in pain, and may complain of dyspnea.

Treatment often involves endotracheal intubation and mechanical ventilation. Pulmonary contusions are commonly present in conjunction with a flail chest, and within 24 to 48 hours, noncardiac pulmonary edema or adult (acute) respiratory distress syndrome (ARDS) may develop.

DEFICIENT FLUID VOLUME

A decrease in circulating blood volume leads to decreased tissue perfusion. Therefore any condition producing a profound volume deficit necessitates immediate intervention. The more common causes of volume loss include actual blood loss from the vascular compartment because of bleeding from solid organ injury, long bone fractures, vascular injuries, or GI bleeding. Illness leading to prolonged vomiting or diarrhea can also produce large fluid losses as can "third-spacing" volume loss or interstitial volume sequestering associated with major burn injury.

As volume loss occurs, various compensatory mechanisms produce vasoconstriction of the vasculature, retain fluid via the renal tubules, and increase cardiac output. These compensatory mechanisms—such as stimulation of the sympathetic nervous system; the release of renin, angiotensin, aldosterone, and antidiuretic hormones; and fluid shifts—continue in an effort to restore tissue perfusion, thus ensuring cell survival. However, these mechanisms are limited in scope, and if the lost volume is not restored, eventually cellular structures incur irreversible damage from the oxygen debt, and death ensues.

Clinical Manifestations

The client or prehospital personnel may provide a history of recent injury or illness with associated volume loss. Clinical manifestations may include agitation or decreasing level of consciousness, pale and diaphoretic skin, delayed capillary refill time of longer than 2 seconds, tachycardia, tachypnea, decreased urine output, and hypotension. Positive orthostatic vital signs (a decrease in systolic blood pressure by 20 mm Hg and an increase in pulse rate by 20 beats/min associated with the client changing from a lying to an upright position) may be present in clients with a mild to moderate volume loss. If blood has accumulated in the thoracic cavity (hemothorax) or abdominal cavity, percussion over the area elicits a dull sound. A collection of blood under the thoracic diaphragm or in the peritoneal cavity can produce Kehr's sign (referred shoulder pain unrelated to injury) or a rigid, hard abdomen with increased rebound tenderness upon palpation.

Diagnostic testing is directed at locating the source of any internal bleeding. Tests may include radiography, ultrasonography, and CT scans of the chest, pelvis, extremities, or abdomen. The laboratory tests of blood typing, complete blood count (CBC), hemoglobin concentration and hematocrit, and electrolyte panel are performed on collected blood samples. A urine specimen should be tested for specific gravity and the presence of blood and leukocytes and, in females, for pregnancy. If gastrointestinal bleeding is suspected, a nasogastric tube is passed and the aspirate tested for the presence of blood. Stool is tested for blood. Diagnostic testing not only helps in identifying the source and severity of volume loss but also aids in determining whether the client requires immediate surgery or hospital admission.

OUTCOME MANAGEMENT

Treatment is directed at preventing further volume loss and replacing fluid volume.

Maintain Blood Flow to Vital Organs

Oxygen (100%) is given via face mask to provide additional oxygen to tissues. The use of Trendelenburg positioning is not recommended.

Stop or Decrease Bleeding

If external bleeding is present, direct pressure should be applied to control further blood loss. The physician may suture or staple actively bleeding lacerations. If the bleeding source is the posterior nasal passages, the client needs to be seated and leaning forward in a high Fowler position. Nasal packing may be required.

Replace Fluids

Venous access must be obtained using a large-bore catheter (14 to 16 gauge). Usually two IV sites are required for fluid replacement. At the time of vein cannulation, blood samples should also be obtained for laboratory testing. If peripheral venous access is not possible, a central line may be inserted or an intraosseous procedure may be performed. This involves inserting an intraosseous needle into the proximal anterior tibia. Fluids, blood, and medications can then be infused into the bone marrow. This is a temporary lifeline and is removed once peripheral venous access can be obtained. The procedure is usually performed by a physician, but it may also be performed by educated personnel such as paramedics and ED nurses. In the past, this procedure was performed only on children younger than age 3 years, but this has recently been expanded so that the procedure can be performed on individuals of any age.

Crystalloids

Crystalloid fluids (normal saline, lactated Ringer's solution) are the replacement fluids of choice. They should be warmed and administered rapidly. If a client with actual loss of blood does not improve after 2 to 3 liters of crystalloid, then blood should be administered. In children, the infusion rate is 20 ml/kg administered as a bolus. This bolus may need to be repeated.

Colloids

Colloid fluids (e.g., blood, hetastarch, albumin) may also be given for fluid resuscitation. If the client has lost blood, then blood is the colloid of choice. These fluids contain proteins and are infused at a 1:1 ratio (1 unit of solution for every 1 unit of blood loss). Blood can be administered as whole blood or as packed red blood cells. It is best if the client's blood has been typed or, optimally, typed and crossmatched with the donor's blood, but universal type O Rh-negative blood can be used if speed is a vital consideration. Blood is usually warmed and can be infused quickly in an adult using a rapid infuser machine. In children, blood is infused at a rate of 40 ml/kg bolus.

Replace Fluids for Burns

Clients who have sustained major partial- or full-thickness burn injuries are at risk for associated fluid loss. Fluid replacement is calculated according to the client's weight in kilograms and the total body surface area (TBSA) involved, as determined by the *rule of 9s* (see Chapter 50). The usual formula is 2 to 4 ml of fluid × body weight in kilograms × TBSA. The calculated amount of fluid is used as the total fluid replacement volume required over the 24-hour period from the time of injury. One half of the total fluid amount is infused in the first 8-hour period, one fourth of the fluid amount in the second 8-hour period, and the remaining one fourth amount in the last 8-hour period.

Institute Other Measures

Once fluid resuscitation is begun, other interventions can be instituted. A nasogastric tube is passed to prevent vomiting and possible aspiration. In clients with gastrointestinal bleeding, gastric lavage is performed, instilling room-temperature normal saline; then, using a large syringe, the fluid is aspirated through the nasogastric tube. This procedure is repeated until there is a clearing of the bloody fluid aspirate. An indwelling urinary catheter is inserted to measure urine output. The client with volume loss is susceptible to the development of mild hypothermia. Keeping the client warm with blankets, warming lights, and infusion of warmed fluids aids in maintaining a normal body temperature. Continual monitoring of cardiac rate and rhythm, blood pressure, pulse oximetry readings, respiratory rate, level of consciousness, and temperature is indicated.

EXCESS FLUID VOLUME

Clients who have an excess of fluid volume can concurrently have pulmonary congestion, leading to respiratory distress. Although clients with renal failure experience fluid volume excess, the disorder most commonly associated with fluid overload in the ED is heart failure. Heart failure results in fluid excess because of the inability of the cardiac muscle to function effectively. Ejection fraction decreases, pressure in the left ventricle increases, and eventually pressure increases affect the left atrium and right ventricle and atrium. The client in heart failure also activates the renin-angiotensin-aldosterone axis and retains fluid.

Clinical Manifestations

The clinical manifestations of heart failure include agitation or restlessness, tachypnea and increased respiratory effort, respiratory rales, distended jugular neck veins, tachycardia, skin pallor, diaphoresis, ascites, and pitting-dependent edema. Pulse oximetry readings are often decreased on room air. The client may also cough up excessive, frothy sputum. Cardiac dysrhythmias, such as atrial fibrillation, may be noted with cardiac monitoring.

Because these clients often have a chronic history of heart failure, their daily medication regimen often includes digoxin, a diuretic, beta-blockers, angiotensin-converting enzyme (ACE) inhibitors, and potassium. Electrolyte imbalances are common, basic metabolic panel (BMP) levels are elevated, and serum levels of digoxin must be assessed via laboratory studies. Chest films provide information about the severity of the heart failure.

OUTCOME MANAGEMENT

Improve Oxygenation

Treatment is directed at improving the client's ability to breathe. Positioning the client in a high Fowler position facilitates the ability to breathe; 100% oxygen should be initiated via a non-rebreather mask although this intervention may be difficult for the client to tolerate. Noninvasive ventilatory assistance via BiPAP may be required. However, if respiratory fatigue develops, the client must be intubated to provide adequate ventilation. The use of RSI before intubation may be indicated.

Administer Medications

Establishing venous access for medication administration is necessary. If pharmacologic interventions with nitrates and diuretics are ineffective, recombinant human B-type natriuretic peptide nesiritide (Natrecor) may be administered to the client. The actions of this medication increase salt and water excretion in addition to producing vasodilation. The client must be monitored for urine output, hypotension, and respiratory improvement. Dobutamine, angiotensin-converting enzyme (ACE) inhibitor, and beta-blocker medications may be administered to reduce afterload. Dobutamine also has a positive inotropic effect.

Monitor Response to Treatment

Continual monitoring of the client's response to treatment is of paramount importance. Assessments should include level of consciousness, cardiac rhythm, blood pressure, respiratory rate and effort, pulse oximetry, and urine output.

DECREASED CARDIAC OUTPUT

Any illness or injury that has a direct effect on the heart can produce a decrease in cardiac output. Such disorders include cardiac dysrhythmias, acute myocardial infarction, cardiac injury, cardiac tamponade, and cardiac infection or myopathy.

When cardiac output decreases, tissue perfusion is adversely affected. Cardiac output (CO) is determined by stroke volume (SV) and heart rate (HR):

$$CO = SV \times HR$$

Therefore any disease process that produces a reduction in stroke volume or an alteration in heart rate has a direct effect on cardiac output. Entities such as cardiac dysrhythmias and acute myocardial infarction have a direct affect on heart rate. Acute myocardial infarction also reduces stroke volume as a result of the death of cardiac muscle. Cardiac tamponade results in compression of the cardiac muscle by the collection of blood or fluid in the pericardial sac. This effect produces a decrease in stroke volume. Infection and cardiac myopathy also affect the cardiac muscle structures, thereby reducing stroke volume.

Clinical Manifestations

Depending on the cause of the reduced cardiac output, clients may present with differing clinical manifestations.

Dysrhythmias are self-evident on cardiac monitoring. The most prominent manifestations associated with a decrease in cardiac output include chest pain, skin pallor, diaphoresis, hypotension, nausea, and agitation or a decrease in level of consciousness. External chest wall injury may be evident with blunt cardiac injury. Cardiac tamponade produces the additional findings of distended jugular neck veins and muffled heart sounds. Fever may be present with cardiac infections.

Diagnostic tests include cardiac monitoring, electrocardiography (ECG), chest radiography, ultrasonography, laboratory studies, noninvasive stress testing, two-dimensional echocardiography, myocardial perfusion imaging, CT scans, and invasive coronary angiography. Levels of the cardiac enzymes creatine kinase (CK) and the CK-MB fraction and of the cardiac markers myoglobin and troponin T (cTnT) and troponin I (cTnI) are especially important in diagnosing the occurrences of a myocardial infarction.

OUTCOME MANAGEMENT

Improve Cardiac Output

The goal of treatment is to improve cardiac output. High-flow oxygen should be administered via face mask, and venous access should be secured for the administration of medications. Supraventricular tachycardic dysrhythmias may be treated with IV adenosine (Adenocard), whereas bradycardic rhythms may be treated with IV atropine or with a pacemaker. Ventricular dysrhythmias may be suppressed by treating the cause if possible or by administering amiodarone or lidocaine. Clients who have sustained a blunt cardiac injury from traumatic injury may also develop cardiac dysrhythmias. For further discussion of dysrhythmia treatment, see Chapter 57.

Increase Coronary Artery Blood Flow

An acute myocardial infarction is often caused by an embolus or thrombus that occludes a coronary artery.

According to TJC Core Measures, all clients who arrive to the ED complaining of chest pain must be rapidly evaluated for acute myocardial infarction. An immediate dose of aspirin and a 12-lead ECG within 10 minutes will determine subsequent interventions. If the ECG indicates an ST-elevation MI (STEMI), the client will be transported to the cardiac catheterization laboratory for percutaneous intervention (PCI). If it is not possible to perform PCI within 90 minutes, administration of a fibrinolytic medication is the first-line choice for treatment. Fibrinolytic medication must be given within 30 minutes of arrival. If the ECG is indicative of a non–ST-elevation MI, treatment may then involve the administration of nitroglycerin, IV heparin, or IV enoxaparin

SAFETY

⚠️

ALERT

glycoprotein (GP) IIb/IIIa inhibitors, while further diagnostic testing occurs. Beta-blocker therapy is also instituted in clients who do not have concurrent heart failure or cardiogenic shock.

Clients who have received fibrinolytic medications must be continuously monitored for the presence of active bleeding. Other monitoring parameters include pain reduction, cardiac rate and rhythm, ST-segment patterns, blood pressure, pulse oximetry readings, and respiratory rate.

Remove Pericardial Fluid

Blunt or penetrating force injury, heart failure, and infections of heart structures can cause cardiac tamponade. If this condition is suspected or diagnosed, treatment involves pericardiocentesis (Figure 82-7). A long spinal needle attached to a 60-ml syringe is inserted beneath the xiphoid process and into the pericardial sac. The accumulated blood is removed, compression of the ventricles is relieved, and cardiac output is restored.

Treat Infectious Causes

Infections of the heart structures, such as pericarditis or endocarditis, may be treated with pain-reducing medications or antibiotics. Pericarditis is frequently caused by a viral organism, whereas endocarditis is of bacterial origin and requires antibiotic therapy.

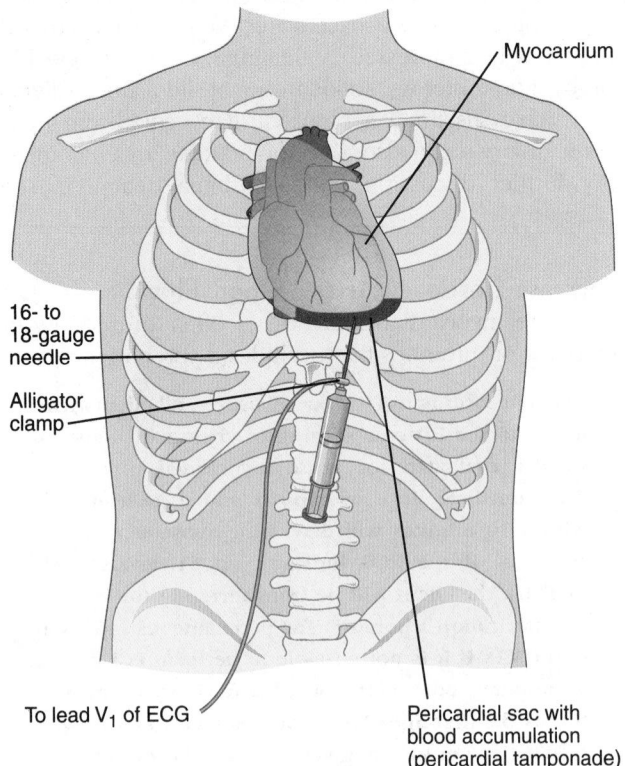

Myocardium

16- to 18-gauge needle

Alligator clamp

To lead V₁ of ECG

Pericardial sac with blood accumulation (pericardial tamponade)

■ **FIGURE 82–7** Pericardiocentesis procedure. *(Modified from Kosmos, C.A. [1995]. In S. Kitt, et al. [Eds.], Emergency nursing: A physiologic and clinical perspective [2nd ed., p. 66]. Philadelphia: Saunders.)*

ACUTE OR CHRONIC PAIN

Pain is one of the most common complaints of clients seeking emergency care. Pain can be caused by almost any entity; therefore identifying the source of pain is of paramount importance. The sensation of pain may be the only complaint, or pain may be associated with other clinical evidence of illness or injury. Pain is assessed as described earlier in the chapter.

OUTCOME MANAGEMENT

Promote Comfort

Pain reduction is the goal of treatment and may be provided by administering oral, intramuscular (IM), or IV analgesic or opioid medications. With isolated orthopedic injuries, such as digit injuries, pain reduction may be obtained by injecting affected nerves with anesthetizing medications. Client comfort measures should also be instituted. Measures may include client positioning to ease stress on painful areas, elevating injured extremities, applying ice or cool compresses to injured areas, and attempting to make the room environment comfortable for the client. Pain is to be assessed before and after each intervention, and the client's response should be documented.

Reduce Procedural Pain

Instituting conscious sedation before painful procedures is a routine practice in many EDs. This procedure involves controlled pharmacologic depression of the level of consciousness that nevertheless allows maintenance of the client's reflexes to protect the airway as well as maintain spontaneous ventilation. Conscious sedation is most commonly induced with medications such as midazolam (Versed), ketamine (Ketalar), or fentanyl (Sublimaze). Dose and route of administration vary with the agent used. It is not uncommon for a narcotic to be given along with a benzodiazepine for painful procedures. The ED nurse's responsibility is to continually monitor the client for airway patency, oxygen saturation levels, cardiac activity, and response to physical or verbal stimulation until recovery from the anesthesia has occurred.

ACUTE CONFUSION

Clients can have an altered level of consciousness from many causes. Underlying disorders such as stroke, metabolic abnormalities, seizure, intoxication, hemorrhage, or injury need to be considered. A helpful guide to use in attempting to determine the cause is the "vowels-TIPS" mnemonic: *A,* alcohol; *E,* epilepsy, encephalopathy, endocrine; *I,* insulin; *O,* overdose; *U,* underdose or uremia; *T,* trauma; *I,* infection; *P,* psychogenic; *S,* stroke or shock.

The normal state of wakefulness and consciousness is controlled by the reticular activating system (RAS) and the brain's cerebral hemispheres. Various factors can produce a decreased state of wakefulness. These include impairment of the central nervous system (CNS) from lesions, infection, or hemorrhage; a decreased supply of oxygen, blood, or glucose to cerebral tissues; and exposure to, ingestion of, or withdrawal from substances toxic to cerebral tissue.

Family members or prehospital personnel may be the only sources for obtaining historical information concerning the client's state of consciousness. It is extremely important to determine any known illnesses of the client, current medications, recent injury, known alcohol or drug use, and duration of the client's altered mental state.

Clinical Manifestations

Clinical manifestations vary according to the cause of the client's illness or injury. The Glasgow Coma Scale (GCS) score is less than 15 or different from baseline. The client may be disoriented or agitated. Pupil size and equality may be altered. Unequal pupil size and reaction may indicate compression of the third cranial nerve caused by increased intracranial pressure. Small, pinpoint pupils may signify opiate overdose, pontine hemorrhage, cholinesterase poisoning, or recent use of miotic eye drops. Cranial nerve abnormalities and unilateral decreased muscle strength may be present with a recent stroke. Tongue lacerations can indicate recent seizure activity. Pale, cool, clammy skin can occur with shock or hypoglycemia. Fresh needle marks on the skin indicate recent IV drug use. A petechial rash on the skin can be an indication of a lethal bacterial meningitis. Bruising of the face, eyes (raccoon eyes), or mastoid process (Battle's sign) or a bluish hue to the tympanic membrane can indicate recent head injury and an associated basilar skull fracture.

Diagnostic testing involves first obtaining a bedside blood glucose level. Other laboratory studies may be indicated, including serum levels of specific medications, serum and urine toxicology screening tests, CBC, blood cultures, electrolyte panel, arterial blood gas analysis, and urinalysis. Urine specimens should also be tested for the presence of myoglobin, because clients who have been comatose for a prolonged time can develop rhabdomyolysis, resulting from ischemia and damage to large muscle groups. Other diagnostic studies include ECG, chest film, and brain CT scan. Occasionally a lumbar puncture may need to be performed.

OUTCOME MANAGEMENT

Establish and Maintain Airway

The first treatment priority in a client with an altered level of consciousness is establishing and maintaining the airway. If the GCS is less than 9, then preparations for intubation should be undertaken. During interventions directed at maintaining airway patency, spinal immobilization should also be considered if there is any suspicion that a traumatic injury may have occurred. Also, 100% oxygen must be administered to provide supplemental oxygen to brain tissue.

Establish Vascular Access for Appropriate Medications

Venous access must be secured for possible IV fluid or medication administration. If a bedside glucose level reading is less than 45 mg/dl, 50% dextrose (D_{50}) is administered IV. If the bedside glucose level reading indicates a high level of glucose, therapy should be instituted for treatment of diabetic ketoacidosis or hyperglycemic hyperosmolar nonketotic coma (see Chapter 45).

Naloxone (Narcan) 2 to 4 mg IV may also be administered. If the cause of the alteration in consciousness is an opiate overdose, naloxone reverses the process.

If a stroke is considered to be the cause of the client's altered level of consciousness, rapid assessment of type of stroke by CT scan is vital to the process of determining the subsequent treatment of the client. Only clients with a nonhemorrhagic stroke, whose onset of clinical manifestations is clearly defined, and who have no contraindications to thrombolytic medication are eligible for thrombolytic therapy. And this is ONLY if the medication is given within 3 hours of the onset of clinical manifestations. If tonic-clonic seizure activity begins, the client is medicated with lorazepam (Ativan) 0.05 to 0.1 mg/kg IV to terminate the seizure. This intervention may need to be followed by IV administration of phenytoin (Dilantin). Phenytoin must be diluted in normal saline solution and infused at a rate of less than 50 mg/min.

IV antibiotic medications are administered in any client with known or suspected bacterial infection within the brain tissue or cerebrospinal fluid. In clients with bacterial meningitis, this can be a life-saving intervention.

Monitor Intoxicated Clients and Treat Toxicity States

Intoxicated clients with an altered level of consciousness must be monitored in the ED. Frequent vital signs and GCS scores must be obtained and documented. If the client sustained any traumatic event, then a brain CT should be obtained to rule out intracranial reasons for altered level of consciousness. Agitation may require RSI in order for CT to be obtained. Treatment involves IV fluid support and nutritional supplementation with thiamine, multivitamins, and occasionally folic acid.

Monitor Clients with Head Trauma and Treat the Injuries

Neurologic trauma can result in minor disturbances such as a concussion. Treatment for concussion varies according to clinical manifestations. A client with a GCS of 13 or higher is considered a mild head injury, a GCS of 9 to 13 is considered a moderate head injury, and a GCS of less than 9 is considered a severe head injury. If asymptomatic, a minor head-injury client is released to home without any definitive treatment. Before leaving the ED, the client or family members must be given instructions on manifestations that indicate worsening of the client's condition.

Other types of neurologic trauma, such as skull fractures, cerebral edema, subdural hematomas, epidural hematomas, and cerebral contusions, may require critical care management or operative intervention. The client must be closely monitored in the ED for any manifestations of increasing intracranial pressure. Mannitol may be administered IV to treat cerebral edema.

Prevent Injury

SAFETY ALERT

Safety is an important issue in a client with an altered level of consciousness. Medication and restraints to avoid dislodging of nasogastric and endotracheal tubes may be indicated. Seizure precautions may be necessary. If in place, spinal immobilization must be maintained and the client should be logrolled. Bed side rails must be up and locked in position at all times. Clients are monitored for changes in level of consciousness along with cardiac rate and rhythm, blood pressure, pulse oximetry, and respiratory rates.

DISTURBED SENSORY PERCEPTION

Sensory perceptions may be disturbed in any of the sensory organs, but an alteration in vision is one of the more common client complaints associated with sensory perceptual changes. Such alterations can be caused by infection, inflammation, or trauma.

Clinical Manifestations

The client may be able to provide information related to the visual changes and the circumstances surrounding the onset of the changes. The affected eye should be assessed for discharge from the eye, excessive tearing, redness of the conjunctiva, presence of a ciliary flush (a ring of inflammation surrounding the corneal-scleral junction), periorbital cellulitis, obvious foreign objects, presence of a cloudy cornea, extruded globe contents, and obvious ecchymosis, laceration, or trauma to the eye and surrounding structures. A baseline visual acuity test must be performed on all clients with a complaint related to the eye.

Changes in vision can be present with non-urgent conditions such as conjunctivitis. This infection of the conjunctival tissue is highly contagious. Foreign objects or chemicals in the eye, corneal abrasions, and deep

structure infections or injury are more significant problems, and the client usually presents with a complaint of pain as well as visual changes.

OUTCOME MANAGEMENT

Anesthetizing ophthalmic drops can be placed in the affected eye to diminish pain and allow for a more thorough examination of the eye. Superficial conjunctival infections are treated with topical ophthalmic antibiotic drops or ointments. Small superficial foreign objects are removed by the ED physician. For exposure to harmful chemicals, the eye must be irrigated with a minimum of 1 L of normal saline. After irrigation, the pH of the eye is checked; if it has not returned to a normal pH of 6 to 7, irrigation may need to be continued. If corneal abrasions are present, the client is given oral pain reduction medications and topical ophthalmic antibiotic medication. Patching of the affected eye is not recommended.

More serious problems associated with the eye necessitate an immediate consultation with, or referral to, an ophthalmologist. These problems include complaints of sudden changes in or loss of vision with or without pain, impaled foreign objects, extensive injury or infection, and globe rupture. Any client who receives treatment from the ED physician for an eye problem should be instructed to be rechecked within 24 hours by his or her primary physician or an ophthalmologist.

RISK FOR INFECTION

Clients frequently present to the ED because of an infectious process. The infection may be caused by either viral or bacterial organisms. The source of the infection may be localized, or the infection may have spread to surrounding tissues or be systemic. It also may be contagious. Hospital employees are frequently treated in the ED for needle-stick injury and prophylactically for hepatitis B and human immunodeficiency virus exposure.

Clinical Manifestations

Clinical manifestations depend on the organism causing the infection, the extent of the infection, and the location of the infection. Bacterial infections usually produce more obvious and severe manifestations than those seen in viral infections. With bacterial infections, the client may have a fever. However, older adults and neonates frequently have subnormal temperatures with an infectious process. The client may complain of pain at the site of the infection, such as in the ear, eye, throat, abdomen, genitourinary tract, or an area of skin. It is important to consider that airway, pharyngeal, and mouth infections can be associated with airway compromise. Meningeal infections can produce headache, vomiting, neck pain, and occasionally petechiae. Pulmonary infections are frequently accompanied by productive cough, nd sputum. Erythema, edema, lymphadenopathy, and observable discharge or pus may be present with ear, throat, or skin infections. A skin rash or abscess may also be the presenting problem of an underlying infection. Abdominal infections often present with pain and palpable abdominal tenderness. A systemic infectious process can lead to septic shock, in which endotoxins from bacterial organisms are released into the circulation. The client is acutely ill and may have clinical manifestations of fever, tachycardia, hypotension, and decreased urine output. In later stages of sepsis, the client may become hypothermic, the skin may have a mottled appearance, and the level of consciousness becomes diminished. These findings are usually associated with high death rate.

A primary decision must be made about whether the infection is considered contagious to other clients in the ED. If the infection is thought to be contagious, the client must be isolated as quickly as possible from other clients. This is in compliance with the TJC National Patient Safety Goal for reducing the risk of health care associated infections.

It then becomes important to identify the primary source of the infection. The ears, eyes, throat, lungs, skin, and genital and pelvic areas must be assessed for evidence of infection. A chest film is obtained, in addition to possible abdominal and pelvic ultrasound studies. Laboratory studies include a urinalysis, CBC, and culture of discharge and blood specimens. If the source of the infection is not identified, a lumbar puncture may be required.

OUTCOME MANAGEMENT

When dealing with clients with known or potential infections, it is important that the ED nurse be cognizant of the hospital-wide infection control policies and comply with the TJC National Patient Safety Goal related to reducing the risk of health care associated infections. Appropriate use of standard precautions at all times on all clients is the best protection for the nurse and for all ED clients.

Administer Medications

Treatment involves administering antibiotic or antiviral medications selected according to the identified or probable source of the infection. These agents may be administered orally, IM, or IV. The antipyretic medications acetaminophen (Tylenol) and ibuprofen can be administered orally or rectally (Tylenol) to reduce temperature. Other treatments to reduce temperature involve undressing the client and allowing heat to dissipate into the environment, but avoid shivering. Abscesses caused by skin infections may need to be incised, drained, and packed.

Hepatitis B prophylaxis treatment for unvaccinated employees exposed to a needle-stick consists of administering HBIG (hepatitis B immunoglobulin) and beginning the series of hepatitis B vaccinations. There is a risk of exposure to hepatitis C from needle-sticks, but to date there is no prophylactic treatment.

Monitor and Treat Sepsis

If sepsis is suspected, it is important to administer 100% oxygen to the client, infuse IV fluids of normal saline, and insert a nasogastric tube and an indwelling urinary catheter. Additional infused medications, after antibiotic administration, may include dopamine and corticosteroids. The client must be closely monitored for changes in blood pressure, heart rate, respiratory rate, oxygen saturation, cardiac rhythm, urine output, level of consciousness changes, and prolonged bleeding times. These clients are at risk for developing disseminated intravascular coagulopathy (DIC).

IMPAIRED PHYSICAL MOBILITY

Any injury to the musculoskeletal system can lead to a decrease in the client's mobility. Other causes of impaired mobility are injuries to the vertebral bodies and possibly the spinal cord. Sprains of ligaments, fractures to bones, dislocated joints, muscle strains, and amputated extremities or digits are the majority of problems for which clients seek emergency care related to mobility deficits.

Spinal cord injury can involve edema of the cord, with transitory or minimal deficits, or other cord injury, or the cord can actually be severed. With marked edema or cord severance, deficits are usually devastating and permanent. Neurogenic shock can develop with loss of the sympathetic component of the autonomic nervous system. With only the parasympathetic nervous system functioning, massive vasodilation occurs, and tissue perfusion is decreased.

Clinical Manifestations

Clinical manifestations in most musculoskeletal injuries include swelling around the injured area, presence of ecchymosis, obvious deformity of the area, palpable tenderness, and limited movement of the area. Amputations are self-evident, and depending upon whether a complete or partial amputation has occurred, active bleeding may be minimal or profuse. With a complete amputation, active bleeding is minimal as a result of constriction of the severed vessels. It is important that the ED nurse assess the effectiveness of circulation, motor movement, and presence and degree of sensation distal to any musculoskeletal injury.

An injury to the spinal cord produces a motor or sensory deficit, or both, below the level of injury. If the injury is in the upper thoracic or cervical area, the diaphragm and thoracic intercostal muscles can be affected, leading to respiratory compromise. A client with neurogenic shock has warm, dry skin caused by the massive vasodilation, hypotension, and bradycardia, with no movement or sensation below the level of injury.

Radiographic films of the injured area are obtained to aid in identifying fractures. Depending on the extent of the injury, additional laboratory tests or other diagnostic studies may be performed.

OUTCOME MANAGEMENT

Treat Sprains, Strains, and Fractures

Treatment of extremity sprains and fractures consists of immediately elevating the extremity above the level of the client's heart, applying ice to the area, and immobilizing the extremity with pillows or cardboard splints. Oral, IM, or IV pain-reducing medication may also need to be administered. More definitive immobilization of the area with the application of splints, molds, or immobilizers is accomplished before the client leaves the ED. Lower extremity injuries may require the client to use crutches. Detailed crutch-walking instructions must be provided, and the client should be able to demonstrate adequate use of the crutches to the ED nurse before his or her discharge from the department.

Pain-reducing medication is also administered to clients with muscle strains. Once clients achieve reduction of pain, they are usually discharged to home with instructions to rest and to apply alternating ice and heat to the injured area for the next 24 hours.

Reduce Dislocations

A joint dislocation requires reduction in the ED. This procedure is performed by the ED physician. Pain-reducing and muscle-relaxant medications may need to be administered before the reduction procedure. Once joint reduction has been achieved, a post-reduction radiographic film must be obtained. After successful reduction, the joint is immobilized with the required orthopedic device.

Treat Amputation

The goal in the management of a client who has sustained an amputation is to attempt to salvage the part so that possible replantation can occur or prevent further loss of tissue. Any profuse bleeding from the stump should be controlled with direct pressure. If the client has sustained significant blood loss, 100% oxygen is administered, venous access is established, and replacement fluids or blood are given.

The stump is then gently cleansed with normal saline. The amputated part is wrapped in sterile gauze moistened with normal saline. It is then placed in a plastic bag or container, and the plastic bag or container is placed o ice. The amputated part should *never* be place directly on ice, because the resultant freezing of the tissue makes replantation impossible. The client is give pain-reducing medications, antibiotic medications, an possible tetanus prophylaxis with tetanus and diphther toxoids (Td) 0.5 ml if more than 5 years have elapsed sinc the last tetanus immunization. The nurse should b prepared to transfer the client and the amputated part t a facility that performs reimplantations.

Treat Spinal Cord Injury

Clients with a spinal cord injury must be maintained i complete spinal immobilization. At a minimum, a cros table lateral cervical spine radiograph is required, an this study may be followed by more extensive spin films or a CT scan. When a high thoracic or cervic injury is present, the client may become fatigued wit the effort of maintaining respirations. The need for intu bation and assisted ventilation must be considere IV fluids are necessary to maintain perfusion. Administration of high-dose IV steroids such as methy prednisolone (Solu-Medrol) is controversial. IV admini tration of a vasopressor to counteract parasympathet nervous system effects is another treatment consideratio This therapy, however, must be instituted cautiousl because the vasoconstrictive effect of vasopressors m decrease perfusion to the injured cord. A nasogastric tul and indwelling urinary catheter are inserted.

The client must be kept warm with warmed fluid blankets, and heating lights as necessary, because ofte the ability to regulate internal body temperature h been lost. Stabilization of cervical fractures may invol applying Gardner-Wells tongs with traction, a halo tra tion device, or surgical repair. Monitoring of body ter perature, cardiac rate and rhythm, blood pressur respiratory rate and effort, pulse oximetry, urine outpu and changes in sensory and motor movement is vital.

IMPAIRED SKIN INTEGRITY

Skin and soft tissue injury is a common problem encou tered in ED clients. Injury to the skin and surroundir soft tissue can occur from sharp objects, blunt for injury, scraping mechanisms, or bites resulting in lacer tions, contusions, abrasions, avulsions, or punctu wounds.

Clinical Manifestations

Once the skin barrier is interrupted, the potential f infection is increased. Skin flora and other bacteria th have access to the underlying structures. After injury the skin, natural or secondary healing processes occ resulting in skin closure and scarring. Primary closu or suturing, of skin wounds also closes the skin a reduces the amount of scarring. Wounds caused by forces in which bacteria were deeply embedded in the tissues, or that are older than approximately 12 hours, are not routinely managed by primary closure because of the risk for developing infection. Diagnostic tests may involve radiographic films of the wound area. Such studies are important when a foreign object is suspected to be embedded in the wound or when gas in the wound may have developed.

OUTCOME MANAGEMENT

Skin and soft tissue wounds can occur anywhere on the body. Scalp and facial lacerations often bleed profusely because of the high vascularity of these areas. Direct pressure over the wound is usually sufficient to control bleeding.

Cleanse the Wound

Cleansing of wounds is best achieved using high-pressure irrigation and normal saline solution. Directing the stream flow from a 20- to 30-ml syringe directly into the wound adequately cleanses most wounds. A minimum of 100 ml of solution should be used. Shaving an area around a wound to remove hair is controversial. Clipping is the preferred method of removing hair, but any hair removal is controversial. In most instances, shaving is not necessary and should *never* be performed on a wound located in a client's eyebrow.

Open wounds often need to be anesthetized before cleansing and must be anesthetized before primary repair is attempted. A cotton ball can be saturated with a topical solution of tetracaine-adrenaline-cocaine (TAC) or lidocaine-epinephrine-tetracaine (LET) and then applied directly to a face or scalp wound, as long as it is not used near mucous membranes. Other anesthetic agents include lidocaine 1% or 2%, with or without epinephrine, and bupivacaine (Marcaine) 0.25% or 0.5%, with or without epinephrine. Anesthetic agents with epinephrine should never be injected into wounds located on the fingers, toes, ears, nose, or penis because of the vasoconstricting effects of epinephrine. Bupivacaine provides a longer anesthetic effect than that obtained with lidocaine. Sodium bicarbonate at a 1:10 ratio may be added to lidocaine or bupivacaine to reduce pain when the medication is injected into the wound.

Close the Wound

Small, superficial wounds may be closed with adhesive paper strips or Dermabond glue. It is important to evert and bring the wound edges close together and then apply the paper strips or glue.

Larger wounds that are gaping, that involve injury to deeper structures, that occur over joints, or that are

TABLE 82–3	Suture Material
Suture Size	**Indicated Use: Body Area(s)**
2-0, 3-0	Tissue subjected to strong tensile forces (e.g., knees, elbows, over joints)
3-0, 4-0	Epidermal and dermal layers, except for face
5-0, 6-0	Facial area

located in high-tension areas need to be sutured for optimal healing. The type of suture material required varies depending on the size and location of the open wound (Table 82-3).

Abrasion injuries are not sutured. Abrasion injuries need to be thoroughly cleansed in order to remove any particles or debris left in the wound. If particles remain in the wound, a tattooing effect results with the healing process. Human and animal bites are not routinely sutured because of the highly contaminated nature of the wound. The wound is thoroughly irrigated, and prophylactic antibiotic medications are frequently administered. Animal bites should be reported to the local animal control authorities.

Apply a Dressing

Protective dressings must be applied to wounds before the client leaves the ED. Most dressings involve first applying a thin layer of antibacterial ointment or gauze impregnated with petrolatum (Vaseline) or other occlusive substance. Then dry, sterile gauze is applied for padding, followed by a wrap of woven gauze (Kling or Kerlix). Adhesive tape is used to hold the dressing in place.

Administer Tetanus and Rabies Prophylaxis

Clients should be questioned about their tetanus immunization status. Because it is sound public health policy to take advantage of immunizing clients with combined vaccines whenever they are eligible, the CDC has specific recommendations for using vaccines that include protection against diphtheria and pertussis. Table 82-4 presents current recommendations for tetanus prophylaxis that take into consideration the appropriate doses for both children and adults. The vaccines used provide an active (acquired) immunity, but in select situations when immunity is questioned, the wound may be at a high risk for tetanus and the client may also be given passive antibodies in the form of human tetanus immune globulin (TIG) 250 units. If both preparations must be administered, they should be injected in separate sites in different extremities to avoid the globulin from potentially inactivating or inhibiting the immune response from the vaccine. In 2005 the United States licensed the use of a reduced

TABLE 82–4   Tetanus Prophylaxis in Wound Management*

History of Absorbed Tetanus Toxoid? (Doses)	Clean, Minor Wound; Tetanus Toxoid?	Clean, Minor Wound; Tetanus Immune Globulin (TIG)?	All Other Wounds; Tetanus Toxoid?	All Other Wounds; Tetanus Immune Globulin (TIG)?
Unknown or <3	Yes 1. For children <7 years, give DTP (pediatric form) or DT (pediatric form) if pertussis vaccine contraindicated 2. For people >7 years, Td (adult form) preferred 3. For people 11-18 years, give DTaP or Td (DTaP preferred for adolescents who have never received DTaP; Td preferred for adolescents who have received DTaP or if DTaP not available)	Not indicated	Yes 1. For children <7 years, give DTP (pediatric form) or DT (pediatric form) if pertussis vaccine contraindicated 2. For people >7 years, Td (adult form) preferred 3. For people 11-18 years, give DTaP or Td (DTaP preferred for adolescents who have never received DTaP; Td preferred for adolescents who have received DTaP or if DTaP not available)	Yes
+ history of 3 or more doses	If only 3 doses, then give 4th dose of absorbed toxoid Not indicated, unless >10 years since last dose	Not indicated	Yes if >5 years since last dose (more frequent boosters can increase incidence of adverse effects)	Not indicated

* Steps in tetanus prophylaxis include the following: (1) assess client's wound: (a) clean, minor (does not include descriptions listed in b); (b) includes (but is not limited to) wounds contaminated with dirt, feces, soil, saliva; puncture wounds; avulsions, wounds resulting from missiles, crushing injuries, burns, frostbite; (2) assess client's previous immunization history and age: (a) determine if client has received any previous tetanus vaccines (should have a history of receiving 3 doses as a primary series and then boosters as indicated); (b) client's age and wound will determine which vaccine(s) will be indicated.

DTaP, Reduced tetanus and diphtheria toxoid and acellular pertussis vaccine (use in adolescents 11 to 18 years of age); *DTP,* pediatric dose of diphtheria toxoid, tetanus toxoid, and pertussis vaccine (use only in children <7 years of age); *Td,* adult dose of diphtheria toxoid and tetanus toxoid (use only in children >6 years of age); *TIG,* tetanus immune globulin.

diphtheria toxoid and an acellular pertussis vaccine (DTaP) for use with people age 10 to 18 years. The newer vaccines help to reduce the risk of vaccination-related local and systemic reactions.

Rabies prophylaxis should be considered in clients who have been bitten by dogs, cats, skunks, raccoons, bats, squirrels, ferrets, or opossums. Prophylaxis is especially important if the animal cannot be located and placed under quarantine for an observation period.

Because a bat bite can be relatively minor in comparison to other animal bites, and bats are becoming a significant reservoir for the rabies virus, the Advisory Committee on Immunization Practices (ACIP) recommends that postexposure prophylaxis is appropriate for any bite, scratch, or mucous membrane exposure associated with bats.

The ACIP recommends two types of vaccine for people potentially exposed to rabies. These include rabies immune globulin (RIG), which provides rapid, passive immunity that persists for approximately 21 days; and rabies vaccine, which produces an active immune response that requires approximately 7 to 10 days to develop. The immunity lasts for approximately 2 years. The dose of human rabies immune globulin (RIG) for passive immunization is 20 units/kg. As much medication as possible should be injected into and around the wound site and the remainder of the dose injected intramuscularly in the buttocks. For active immunization with human diploid cell vaccine (HDCV), the dose is 1 ml

initially and again on days 0 (day 0 is date of exposure), 7, 14, and 28 following the bite incident.

Instruct on Wound Care

Instructions related to the care of the wound are given to the client or family members before they leave the ED. These instructions should identify the manifestations of infection and explain care of the wound. Timing for a follow-up appointment with the appropriate physician for a recheck of the wound and suture removal must also be included in the instructions.

ACCIDENTAL AND INTENTIONAL POISONINGS

Poisonings are either accidental or intentional. Accidental poisonings occur more commonly in the pediatric age group, whereas intentional poisonings are more frequent in the adolescent and adult population. Poisoning can also occur from injected venom, such as snake or insect bites.

Obtaining accurate information about the offending substance, amount, and time of ingestion or exposure can be difficult. Details may be available from family or friends. Other important information to obtain is whether the client has vomited since the exposure, whether the client has been depressed or had any previous episodes of intentional poisoning, if medication

ntainers or drug paraphernalia were found at scene,
d any other associated details.

linical Manifestations

Assessment must be directed toward the effective-
ss of the client's ABCs (airway, breathing, and circula-
n). There may be few outward clinical manifestations
at aid in determining the substance that was ingested,
haled, or injected.

Diagnostic tests may include electrocardiography and
ntinual cardiac monitoring. Blood and urine specimens
ed to be obtained for toxicology screening and testing.
many cases, the results of these tests are not rapidly
ailable. Chest films may aid in diagnosing possible
piration. If envenomation is the source of poisoning,
eeding and coagulation studies must be performed.

OUTCOME MANAGEMENT

aintain Airway

the client demonstrates a decrease in level of con-
iousness, initial interventions include establishing
d maintaining a patent airway, possibly with airway
ljunct devices. Oxygen should be administered, and
nous access should be obtained.

emove Offending Substance

eatment is directed at removing or absorbing the
fending substance. If the substance was injected, nal-
xone 2 to 4 mg IV may be administered. If the client's
vel of consciousness is decreased, a large nasogastric
wald) tube is passed either nasally or orally and gastric
vage performed if the ingestion was recent, potentially
xic, or considered significant. This procedure involves
stilling approximately 250 to 500 ml of normal saline
lution through the tube and then removing the solu-
n either with a syringe or by gravity drainage into
collection bag. This process is repeated until the
turned contents are clear of pill fragments. Then
quid-activated charcoal and a cathartic are instilled
rough the Ewald tube and allowed to remain in the
omach. The charcoal aids in adsorbing any other
maining particles of the toxic substance.

Awake and alert clients are given liquid-activated
arcoal to drink. This medication provides the greatest
nefit of adsorption if administered within 1 hour of
e ingestion. Occasionally, the charcoal slurry may
use the client to vomit, and an additional dose of the
arcoal may be required. The purpose of activated
arcoal is again to quickly adsorb the ingested toxic
bstance to minimize its harmful effects. Syrup
ipecac is not routinely administered. It is not effective
removing the toxic substance unless the ingestion
curred within the previous 30 minutes. Its emetic
fect prolongs the time until activated charcoal can be

administered. Clients who have ingested an alkaline-
based substance are not given syrup of ipecac, charcoal,
or any substance that can cause emesis.

If a specific toxic substance exposure is known and
an antidote is available, the antidote is administered.
Table 82-5 provides a list of the more common poisoning substances and antidotes. Dry chemicals that may
be present on the client's skin or external surfaces must
first be brushed off. Then the contaminated area is copi-
ously irrigated with water or normal saline.

Provide Psychiatric Evaluation as Needed

Any client who is in the ED because of an intentional poisoning must have a psychiatric evaluation
before discharge and release from the ED. This is a
TJC National Patient Safety Goal.

SAFETY ALERT

Many communities have psychiatric evaluation teams
(PETs) that provide this service.

SNAKE BITE

Snake antivenin is available for clients who have been
envenomed by a pit viper (a poisonous snake). The area
of the envenomation may be swollen and ecchymotic,

TABLE 82–5 Poisonings and Antidotes

Toxic Substance	Treatment
Beta-blocker medications	Treat hypotension initially with fluids; if unsuccessful, administer glucagons 100-150 mcg/kg IV followed by 2-5 mg/hr by infusion
Calcium-channel blocker medications	Calcium chloride 5-10 ml IV, or calcium gluconate 10-20 ml IV
Carbon monoxide	100% oxygen; possibly use of hyperbaric chamber
Iron	Deferoxamine (Desferal) 80 mg/kg IV or IM and repeated q 8 hr
Isoniazid (INH)	Pyridoxine (vitamin B_6) IV in dose equivalent to amount ingested (gram for gram); if ingested amount is unknown, administer 5 g IV over 3-5 min, then repeat q 3-5 min until seizures are controlled
Methanol, ethylene glycol	Fomepizole (Antizol) as an intravenous infusion, initially 15 mg/kg of body weight, followed by 10 mg/kg of body weight every 12 hr for 4 doses, then 15 mg/kg of body weight every 12 hr until ethylene glycol or methanol concentration decreases to less than 20 mg/dl
Phenothiazine medications	Diphenhydramine (Benadryl) 0.5-1 mg/kg IV or benztropine (Cogentin) 1-2 mg IM
Acetaminophen	N-Acetylcysteine (Mucomyst) 140 mg/kg PO, then 70 mg/kg every 4 hr for 17 doses

and pain may be present at the site. Pit viper venom produces both proteolytic and hemotoxic effects. Massive swelling producing a compartment syndrome may develop, and a coagulation disorder such as DIC may result. The wound area should be gently cleansed. Ice should not be applied to reduce swelling. Antivenin is administered intravenously, but skin or conjunctival testing must be performed before administering the antivenin.

HYPERTHERMIA

Hyperthermic emergencies are usually the result of environmental exposure. The pediatric and geriatric populations are at the greatest risk for developing hyperthermia. The types of hyperthermic problems are heat cramps, heat exhaustion, and heat stroke. Heat stroke is the most severe.

Clinical Manifestations
Muscle spasms of the arms and legs are evident with heat cramps. Often there is a depletion of sodium because the client has been perspiring excessively. Excessive sweating can lead to dehydration and heat exhaustion. The client may complain of headache, dizziness, nausea, and weakness. Mild hypotension can be present, and the skin is frequently cool and clammy to the touch.

Heat stroke is an emergent condition. The client is often comatose. Other clinical manifestations include hypotension, tachycardia, hot and flushed-appearing skin, and a core temperature of greater than 105 ° F (40.5 ° C).

OUTCOME MANAGEMENT

Administer Fluids and Electrolytes
For the client with mild heat cramps, administering oral fluids with electrolytes and removal from the hot environment are usually the only necessary treatments. Treatment of a client with heat exhaustion also involves removal from the hot environment and administering either oral or IV fluids to correct the problem.

Resolve Heat Stroke
Heat stroke treatment involves establishing and maintaining a patent airway, administering 100% oxygen, and establishing venous access. IV normal saline is administered to restore fluid volume. Cooling measures must be instituted quickly. These measures include removing all clothing from the client; spraying tepid mist over the client's body and using a fan to increase air flow; placing ice packs on the scalp and neck and in the axillae and groin; and using a cooling blanket. Gastric lavage with cool saline and peritoneal dialysis may be necessary. Cooling measures should continue until the client's body temperature is 101 ° F (38.4 ° C). As the temperature decreases, administering chlorprom azine (Thorazine) or diazepam (Valium) may required to reduce shivering. A nasogastric tube ar indwelling urinary catheter must be inserted. Continuo cardiac, pulse oximetry, blood pressure, respiratory ra level of consciousness, and temperature monitoring performed.

HYPOTHERMIA

Clinical Manifestations
A body temperature less than 94 ° F (34.4 ° C) indicat the condition of hypothermia. The development hypothermia is usually unintentional and involves ac dental and prolonged exposure to cold temperatures.

Hypothermia severity can be divided into stag depending on the client's core temperature. Differe clinical manifestations are present with each sta (Table 82-6).

OUTCOME MANAGEMENT

Rewarm the Client
After the establishment and maintenance of a patent a way, heated high-flow oxygen administration, ar venous access with warmed fluid replacement, treatme is then directed at rewarming the client. Rewarmi must be done slowly, because the hypothermic client especially susceptible to the development of ventricu fibrillation and cardiovascular collapse if warmed bloc is returned too rapidly to a cold heart. Rewarming met ods include the following:
1. Passive warming
   a. Removing wet clothing
   b. Covering the client with warm blankets
   c. Placing the client in a warm room
2. Active warming
   a. Immersing the client in a warm bath (104 ° [40 ° C])
   b. Placing the client on a warming blanket
   c. Placing radiant lamps over the client
3. Active core warming
   a. Infusing warmed IV fluids
   b. Providing heated, humidified supplemen oxygen
   c. Performing warm fluid lavage (peritoneal, g; tric, bladder, or colonic lavage)
   d. Performing continuous arteriovenous rewarr ing (CAVR), hemodialysis, or cardiopulmona bypass

Insertion of a nasogastric tube and indwelling urina catheter is an additional component of care. Continuo cardiac, pulse oximetry, blood pressure, respiratory ra level of consciousness, and temperature monitorii must be instituted.

TABLE 82–6	Stages of Hypothermia
Stage	**Clinical Manifestations**
Mild: 93-95 ° F (34.0-35 ° C)	Person conscious and alert but may have lethargy and confusion Shivering Bradycardia or tachycardia
Moderate: 86-93 ° F (30-34 ° C)	Decreased level of consciousness or coma Hypoventilation Bradycardia Atrial fibrillation Hypovolemia Cessation of shivering Possible hyperglycemia because of underutilization of glucose
Severe: <86 ° F (<30 ° C)	Coma Fixed and dilated pupils Bradycardia Apnea Hypotension Ventricular fibrillation Asystole

FROSTBITE

Hypothermia to the extremities can lead to frostbite injury. The feet, hands, nose, ears, and cheeks are most commonly affected. Damage to the tissues occurs, and peripheral blood flow is reduced. The area may appear red and swollen or may be pale in color. Formation of blisters containing either clear or purple bloody fluid may be seen. Rewarming of the frostbitten area should begin once the client is removed from the cold environment. The frostbitten part should be immersed in lukewarm water for 20 minutes. The frostbitten area needs to be handled gently so that blood-filled blisters remain intact. Loose, sterile, bulky dressings are then applied and changed daily. The rewarming process is painful; therefore pain-reducing medications must be administered.

INEFFECTIVE COPING

Clients present to the ED not only with medical and traumatically induced problems but also with psychological issues. Psychological disorders can range from mild anxiety to psychosis to deep depression. It is important that clients with psychological problems be taken as seriously as clients seeking treatment for medical problems.

A brief mental status examination needs to be conducted to assess the client's behavior, speech patterns, mood and affect, thought processes, and judgment and insight. Has the client recently experienced a crisis-producing situation? Is the client experiencing auditory or visual hallucinations? A physical examination must be performed to identify any concurrent medical condition or injury that may be compounding the problem.

It is important to communicate with the client in a calm, nonjudgmental, and accepting manner. Focusing the client on reality and explaining expected behaviors constitute part of the therapeutic communication process. In some cases, involuntary psychiatric hospitalization may be required. If the client is discharged from the ED, providing outside agency assistance and referral can be helpful.

DISASTER PLANNING/MASS CASUALTY INCIDENTS

After September 11, 2001 and subsequent national and international events, the U.S. health care system reassessed what constitutes a disaster and how to ensure an effective, unified response. Disasters are also referred to as mass casualty incidents (MCIs) and include such incidents as transportation crashes; forces of nature, such as hurricane, tornado, blizzard, earthquake, tsunami; or intentional events such as terrorist-related. As implied by the term, an MCI can suddenly overwhelm one department or hospital with a surge in clients.

Planning

The ED has typically been involved in both external (i.e., community) and internal (i.e., hospital) disaster planning. During a MCI, the ED serves as a central point for screening and the admission of critically ill or injured clients. They then institute a back-up plan to provide care to others. The entire hospital may be called into action to assist with providing care in the ED or expanding services throughout the institution. To help with emergency preparedness, the Centers for Disease Control and Prevention has developed a core set of competencies that include (1) understanding the necessary roles involved in responding to a disaster, (2) initiating and following the chain of command, and (3) activating the response plan. An ED nurse may help to coordinate responders and transfer clients; provide decontamination; deliver care for critically ill or injured clients admitted to ED; or be reassigned to other clinical areas that need additional nursing assistance.

Effective MCI care begins long before the first incident, and response agencies need a systematic approach to handling large numbers of clients. The United States Department of Homeland Security (USDHS) has worked with public health and acute care providers to develop the National Response Plan (NRP). This plan has several elements, including a standard incident management organizational structure, the National Incident Management System (NIMS), and an Incident Command Structure (ICS), that help individual agencies. In an MCI, an agency can divide their efforts into five functional areas—command, operations, planning, logistics, and finance/administration. The ICS structure can be used for any type of MCI that stresses an ED's ability to provide care, whether the incident is due to a sudden surge of clients from a one-time event or a more wide-spread incident.

All-Hazards Approach

The USDHS also encourages providers to plan for any type and level of MCI and to adopt an "all-hazards approach" to MCI care. The all-hazards approach encourages health care personnel to be aware of the potential for toxic exposure and to protect themselves before initiating care. Agencies involved in an MCI should provide different levels and types of personal protective equipment (PPE) for their staff. Depending on the suspected agents involved, PPE may range from changeable clothing; to protective eyewear and a mask; to full protective gear with self-contained air supply, gloves and boots, and impermeable coverall clothing. In some instances, health care providers may need to be pre-screened or eliminated from initial care if they are pregnant or cannot tolerate wearing PPE for a required time frame. EDs have created specific storage areas for PPE and provide orientation to help staff find what they should use for a given type of incident.

MCI Triage

During an MCI, the ED tends to be the portal through which injured clients are admitted to the hospital. The ED staff will be responsible for triage, decontamination for any suspected noxious substance (e.g., poisons, radiation), and isolation of any suspicious infectious cases. ED personnel may be the first to identify that a terrorist activity has occurred. For example, after a terrorist attack using biochemical weapons, clusters of otherwise healthy individuals may begin appearing at EDs requesting treatment for unknown illnesses (The Terrorism Alert feature above, right discusses staying alert for such patterns of illness.) These illnesses may be caused by the release of substances such as radiation, bacterial agents, toxic agents such as anthrax, nerve gas (see the Terrorism Alert feature on p. 2215 for details on sarin), or viral agents into the atmosphere, food supply, or other medium.

MCI triage is not the same as everyday triage in that clients are evaluated and categorized according to the institution's ability to provide care for the greatest number of victims. Instead of giving the most severely ill or injured person immediate and full attention, some clients receive no care and other lesser ill or injured clients may be sent away or asked to help care for others. The categories of MCI triage can be described as critical with a chance of survival, critical or close to death with minimal chance of survival, clients requiring hospital admission, clients with minor and treatable injuries, and clients with psychological injury. MCI triage allows the ED to rapidly determine which clients are to receive care.

TERRORISM ALERT

Being Alert to Patterns of Illness

All health care providers must remain alert for unusual illness patterns and clinical manifestations that might indicate an unusual infectious disease outbreak associated with intentional release of a biologic agent. The covert release of a biologic agent may not have an immediate impact because of the delay between exposure and illness onset, and outbreaks associated with intentional releases might closely resemble naturally occurring outbreaks. Indications of intentional release of a biologic agent include the following: (1) an unusual temporal or geographic clustering of illness (e.g., people who attended the same public event or gathering or development of a disease at an airport) or clients presenting with clinical manifestations that suggest an infectious disease outbreak (e.g., more than two clients presenting with an unexplained febrile illness associated with sepsis, pneumonia, respiratory failure, or rash or a botulism-like syndrome with flaccid muscle paralysis, especially if occurring in otherwise healthy people); (2) an unusual age distribution for common diseases (e.g., an increase in what appears to be a chickenpox-like illness among adults, but which might be smallpox); and (3) a large number of cases of acute flaccid paralysis with prominent bulbar palsies, suggestive of a release of *botulinum* toxin.

Clinical Manifestations

Each MCI disaster situation is unique in terms of the clients involved and the type of disaster that has occurred. Victims may have traumatic injuries, psychological manifestations, or a constellation of clinical manifestations indicating an exposure to a toxic substance.

Radiation Manifestations

The type and severity of clinical manifestations that clients demonstrate will be a direct result of the exposure to the blast itself and the type and dose of the thermal radiation. The effects may occur within hours of exposure or not appear until up to months afterward. Clinical manifestations of acute radiation exposure include nausea, diarrhea, malaise, development of immunocompromised infections, bleeding, shock, and death.

Chemical Agents

Nerve gas agents, such as sarin (see the Terrorism Alert feature on Sarin), enter the body via inhalation, skin contact, or ingestion. Depending on the route of exposure, clinical manifestations may begin to appear as soon as 20 to 30 minutes after exposure. These include respiratory arrest resulting from muscle paralysis, excessive salivation, diaphoresis, dyspnea, vomiting, incontinence, muscle weakness, and miosis.

Sarin

Sarin is one of the dangerous chemical weapons called nerve agents or nerve gases that have dominated chemical warfare since World War II. These gases are the most toxic and rapidly acting of the known chemical warfare agents. Sarin, a colorless and odorless gas, has a lethal dose of 0.5 mg for an adult and is 26 times more deadly than cyanide gas and 20 times more lethal than potassium cyanide. Just 0.01 mg/kg can kill a human. The vapor is slightly heavier than air, so it hovers close to the ground when released. Under cool, wet, and humid weather conditions, sarin degrades swiftly, but as the temperature increases, the lethal duration of the chemical increases despite high levels of humidity. Food and water may also be contaminated with sarin.

Nerve agents (e.g., sarin, tabun, soman, and VX) are potent acetylcholinesterase inhibitors. These agents alter cholinergic synaptic transmission at neuroeffector junctions (muscarinic effects), at skeletal myoneural junctions and autonomic ganglia (nicotinic effects), and in the central nervous system.

EXPOSURE

Following sarin gas release into air, people can be exposed through skin or eye contact or by breathing air that contains sarin. Small containers of sarin gas or liquid can be easily carried and released for an immediate, short-lived attack. Sarin mixes easily with water and can be used to poison water or food. Touching or drinking water that contains sarin or eating food contaminated with sarin may cause clinical manifestations such as those seen with sarin gas exposure.

PROTECTION

Chemical warfare suits that include body (skin and eye) and respiratory (mask) protection are available but are very hot when worn and are rarely available outside military or emergency rescue situations.

If exposure occurs without protection, people should leave the area where sarin was released and get into fresh air immediately, remove clothing, rapidly wash the entire body with soap and water, rinse eyes with plain water, and seek medical attention immediately. Contaminated clothing must be disposed of carefully with placement in plastic bags. Sarin is easily decontaminated with basic solutions.

CLINICAL MANIFESTATIONS

Exposure to large doses of sarin by any route results in loss of consciousness, convulsions, paralysis, and respiratory failure leading to death within seconds and minutes of the exposure if treatment is not initiated immediately. Other clinical manifestations are described below.

Exposure to small doses results in the following clinical manifestations within seconds to hours of exposure:

Muscarinic Effects

- Small, pinpoint pupils
- Blurred vision and eye pain
- Hypersecretion of salivary (drooling), lacrimal (watery eyes), sweat (diaphoresis), and bronchial (coughing) glands
- Runny nose
- Nausea and vomiting
- Diarrhea and abdominal cramps
- Urinary and fecal incontinence
- Slow heart rate

Nicotinic Effects

- Skeletal muscle twitching and weakness
- Convulsions
- Rapid heart rate and high blood pressure (which can mask muscarinic effects)

TREATMENT

Treatment consists of removing sarin from the body as soon as possible and providing supportive medical care. Emergency respondents must be trained and appropriately attired (skin and respiratory protection) before treating clients. Before transport to a hospital, all casualties must be decontaminated (clothing, skin, eyes). A patent airway must be ensured and antidotes, such as 2 mg of atropine IM and 600 mg of pralidoxime chloride (2-PAM Cl) IV, should be administered as soon as possible. These antidotes may be repeated at 5- to 10-minute intervals during transport and upon arrival to an ED. Emesis should not be induced if the client is alert and able to swallow a slurry of activated charcoal. Diazepam may be required to control convulsions. ALS guidelines are followed for clients with cardiac dysrhythmias or hypotension.

Data from CDC Fact Sheet on Chemical Emergencies, Department of Health and Human Services, Centers for Disease Control and Prevention. Retrieved 11/20/07 from www.bt.cdc.gov/agent/sarin/basics/facts.asp.

OUTCOME MANAGEMENT

Depending on the agent used to expose the population, client decontamination may or may not be required. If decontamination is necessary, specialized rooms and equipment must be used to prevent the spread of the agent to other clients or health care workers.

Managing a terrorist incident involves being able to recognize its occurrence and reacting quickly. In the effort to detect the occurrence of possible terrorist activities, emergency nurses must use epidemiologic clues to identify biochemical incidents, such as identifying (1) small or large outbreaks of a disease, (2) an increase in deaths of hospitalized clients within 72 hours of admission, (3) clusters of clients from a single location with the same illness, (4) childhood diseases in adults, (5) healthy people dying of flu, (6) unexplained blood disorders, and (7) unusual increases in complaints of fever, pulmonary, or gastrointestinal manifestations.

CONCLUSIONS

Providing care to clients in the ED setting can be challenging and rewarding. An understanding of the principles of emergency care is the cornerstone of the specialty of emergency nursing. Most clients present to the ED without a working diagnosis but only a cadre of clinical manifestations. Therefore assessing each client using an organized approach is paramount for the ED nurse in order to be able to establish care priorities and institute appropriate interventions. The nursing process from assessment to evaluation is continually used. The scope of ED nursing is constantly changing and expanding beyond the hospital walls into the areas of community practice and community education.

THINKING CRITICALLY

1. A 23-year-old man walks into the emergency department. He tells you that he was in a motor vehicle accident about 4 hours ago. The police were at the scene, but he refused to be transported to the emergency department because he felt fine; he went home. At home, however, the client started to experience worsening shoulder and posterior neck pain. His mother urged him to come to the emergency department. He tells you that he has "numbness" in his fingers and a "tingling" feeling in his right elbow. If you were the triage nurse, what potential problems would you consider that this client might have? Would you classify the client as emergent, urgent, or non-urgent? What measures should you take to ensure the client's safety?

Factors to Consider. What injuries sustained in a motor vehicle accident might account for the client's clinical manifestations?

2. A 35-year-old man is brought into the emergency department by the city police, who were arresting him for drunk and disorderly conduct. He had been involved in a barroom brawl, during which he acquired several small lacerations about the face and arms from broken glass, a hit to the head, and kicks to his ribs. He is conscious, verbally abusive, and threatening to fight his way out of the emergency department because he wants "to go home and be left alone." He has twice threatened you with bodily harm if you persist in preventing him from leaving. How would you proceed with this case?

Factors to Consider. Whom should you call? Would it be appropriate to sedate this client? What should you do if the client actually harms you physically?

3. A 60-year-old man has arrived at the emergency department with a complaint of headache. He states that he never had headaches until about 2 weeks ago, when he began awakening in the mornings with head pain. The headache would go away each day after he had been up and around for a few hours and had taken aspirin. In the last few days, however, neither aspirin nor acetaminophen has helped, and the headache has become nearly continuous. His wife states that his speech and balance have been "off" a little.

He wonders whether there can be any connection between his headaches and a recent fall or a recent elevation in blood pressure. Describe how you would proceed with an evaluation of this client. What further information should you elicit from him? What is your assessment priority? What triage classification would be best for this client? What interventions should you anticipate?

Factors to Consider. What diagnostic assessments should you anticipate? What should you include in your physical examination and nursing history?

4. The client, a 70-year-old man, has been brought to the emergency department by ambulance. His wife states that he has become increasingly confused over the past few months. Within the past few days, he has become worse, is difficult to awaken in the morning, and is "sleepy" all day. This situation progressed until today, when the client's wife could not keep him awake at all; she called an ambulance and had him brought in. The client has a long history of hypertension, coronary artery disease, diabetes mellitus, and depression. Ambulance records show evidence that the client is difficult to arouse, but upon aggressive stimulation, he "wakes up" and can follow basic commands. His vital signs are stable, but his pulse rate is slow and irregular. Blood pressure is lower than his "norm." His wife has brought his medications with her in a large paper bag. What is your priority assessment? What should you include in your physical assessment? What interventions should you anticipate?

Factors to Consider. What body systems should you assess? What diagnostic studies should you anticipate?

Discussions for these questions can be found on the website.

BIBLIOGRAPHY

🪔 Citations appearing in red refer to primary research.

🪔 Citations appearing in blue refer to evidence-based practice guidelines and protocols.

1. Agency for Healthcare Research, National Guideline Clearinghouse. (2003). *Use of physical restraints in the acute care setting.* Retrieved 10/09/06 from www.guideline.gov/summary/summary.aspx?ss=15&doc_id=3515&nbr=2741.
2. Agency for Healthcare Research, National Guideline Clearinghouse. (2006). *Assessment and management of acute pain.* Retrieved 10/09/06 from www.guidelines.gov/summary/summary.aspx?doc_id=9009&nbr=004884&string=pain.
3. Albers, G.W., Amarenco, P., Easton, J.D., et al. (2004). Antithrombotic and thrombolytic therapy for ischemic stroke: The Seventh ACCP Conference on Antithrombotic and Thrombolytic Therapy. *Chest,* 126(3 Suppl), 483S-512S.
4. American Academy of Emergency Medicine. (n.d.). EMTALA. Retrieved 10/09/06 from www.aaem.org/emtala/index.shtml.
5. American Heart Association, ECC Committee, Subcommittees and Task Forces of the American Heart Association. (2005a). 2005 American Heart Association Guidelines for Cardiopulmonary Resuscitation and Emergency Cardiovascular Care. Part 7.1. Adjuncts for airway control and ventilation. *Circulation,* 112(24 Suppl), IV 51-IV 57.
6. American Heart Association, ECC Committee, Subcommittees and Task Forces of the American Heart Association. (2005b). 2005 American Heart Association Guidelines for Cardiopulmonary Resuscitation and Emergency Cardiovascular Care. Part 11: Pediatric Basic Life Support. *Circulation,* 112(Suppl I), IV-156-IV-166.

7. Antman, E.M., Anbe, D.T., Armstrong, P.W., et al. (2004). ACC/AHA guidelines for the management of patients with ST-elevation myocardial infarction—Executive summary: A report of the American College of Cardiology/American Heart Association Task Force on Practice Guidelines (Writing Committee to Revise the 1999 Guidelines for the Management of Patients With Acute Myocardial Infarction). *Circulation, 110,* 588-636.

8. Bracken, M.B. (2006). Steroids for acute spinal cord injury. *The Cochrane Database of Systematic Reviews,* Issue 3. Available from www.cochrane.org/reviews/en/ab001046.html.

9. Bridges, N., & Jarquin-Valdivia, A.A. (2005). Use of the Trendelenburg position as the resuscitation position: To T or not to T? *American Journal of Critical Care, 14,* 364-368.

10. Broder, K.R., Cortese, M.M., Iskander, J.K., et al. (2006). Preventing tetanus, diphtheria, and pertussis among adolescents: Use of tetanus toxoid, reduced diphtheria toxoid, and acellular pertussis vaccines: Recommendations of the Advisory Committee on Immunization Practices (ACIP). *MMWR, 55*(RR03), 1-34.

11. Buller, H.R., Agnelli, G., Hull, R.D., et al.. (2004). Antithrombotic therapy for venous thromboembolic disease: The seventh ACCP conference on antithrombotic and thrombolytic therapy. *Chest, 126*(3 Suppl), 401S-428S.

12. Centers for Disease Control and Prevention. (1999). Human Rabies Prevention—United States, 1999. Recommendations of the Advisory Committee on Immunization Practices (ACIP). *MMWR, 48* (RR-1), 1-21.

13. Emergency Nurses Association. (2006a). *ENA history.* Retrieved 10/09/06 from www.ena.org/about/history.

14. Emergency Nurses Association. (2006b). *Violence in the emergency setting* (Position Statement). Retrieved 10/09/06 from www.ena.org/about/position.

15. Epifanio, P. (2000). Ocular emergencies. In K. Jordan (Ed.), *Emergency nursing core curriculum* (5th ed.). Philadelphia: Saunders.

16. Evans, M.M. (2003). Maintaining the chain of custody: Evidence handling in forensic-cases. *AORN Journal, 78,* 563-564, 566-567, 569.

17. Gebbie, K., & Qureshi, K. (2002). Emergency and disaster preparedness: Core competencies for nurses. *American Journal of Nursing, 102,* 46-51.

18. Gilboy, N., Tanabe, P., Travers, D.A., et al.. (2005). *Emergency Severity Index, Version 4: Implementation handbook* (AHRQ Pub No. 05-0046-2). Rockville, Md: Agency for Healthcare Research and Quality. Retrieved 10/09/06 from www.ahrq.gov/research/esi.

19. Heart Failure Society of America. (2006). HFSA 2006 Comprehensive Heart Failure Practice Guideline. *Journal of Cardiac Failure, 12,* e1-2.

20. Intracorp. (2005). Concussion, mild head injury. Retrieved 10/09/06 from www.guideline.gov/summary/summary.aspx?doc_id=7449&nbr=004395&string=concussion.

21. Killian, M. (Ed.) (1999). *Standards for emergency nursing practice* (4th ed.).Park Ridge, Ill: Emergency Nurses Association.

22. McCaig, L.F., & Nawar, E.W. (2006). National hospital ambulatory medical care survey: 2004 emergency department summary. *Advance Data for Vital and Health Statistics.* No. 372. Retrieved 10/09/06 from www.cdc.gov/nchs/data/ad/ad372.pdf.

23. National Heart, Lung, and Blood Institute (NHLBI), NAEPP Expert Panel Report. (2002). *Guidelines for the diagnosis and management of asthma—Update on selected topics 2002.* NIH Pub No. 02-5075.

24. National Institutes of Health. (2002). *Management of Hepatitis C: 2002.* Retrieved 10/09/06 from https://consensus.nih.gov/2002/2002HepatitisC2002116html.htm.

25. Schwartz, B., Weniger, B.G., Iskander, J.K., et al. (2002). General recommendations on immunization. Recommendations of the Advisory Committee on Immunization Practices (ACIP) and the American Academy of Family Physicians (AAFP). *MMWR, 51* (RR02), 1-36.

25a. The Joint Commission. (2008). *2008. National Patient Safety Goals Hospital Program.* Available at www.jointcommission.org/PatientSafety/NationalPatientSafetygoals.

26. The Leapfrog Group. *Quality measures: Pneumonia.* Retrieved 10/09/06 from https://leapfrog.medstat.com/hrp/references/Pneum.htm.

27. Trauma.Org. (2005). *Glasgow Coma Scale.* Retrieved 10/09/06 from www.trauma.org/scores/gcs.html.

28. Trauma.Org. (2005). *Steroids for spinal cord injury.* Retrieved 10/09/06 from www.trauma.org/spine/steroids.html.

29. Tucker, J. (2003). *Toxicity, acetaminophen.* Retrieved 10/09/06 from www.emedicine.com/ped/topic7.htm.

30. United States Department of Health and Human Services (USDHHS), Centers for Disease Control and Prevention. (n.d.), *Public Health Emergency Response Guide for State, Local, and Tribal Public Health Directors.* Retrieved 10/09/06 from www.bt.cdc.gov/planning/responseguide.asp.

31. United States Department of Health and Human Services (USDHHS), Office of Civil Rights. (2006). *Medical privacy—National standards to protect the privacy of personal health information.* Retrieved 10/09/06 from www.hhs.gov/ocr/hipaa/.

32. United States Department of Homeland Security (USDHHS). (2004). *National incident management system.* Available from www.dhs.gov/dhspublic/interapp/press_release/press_release_0367.xml.

33. United States Department of Homeland Security (USDHHS). (2006). *National response plan.* Retrieved 10/09/06 from www.dhs.gov/dhspublic/interapp/editorial/editorial_0566.xml.

34. United States Department of Labor (USDL), Bureau of Labor Statistics. (n.d.). Census of fatal occupational injuries charts, 1992-2005. *Census of Fatal Occupational Injuries (CFOI)—Current and Revised Data.* Retrieved 10/09/06 from www.bls.gov/iif/oshcfoi1.htm#charts.

35. United States General Accounting Office (USGAO). (2001). *Emergency care. EMTALA implementation and enforcement issues.* GAO-01-747.

36. Veenema, T., & Karam, P. (2003). Emergency: Radiation. *American Journal of Nursing, 103*(5), 32-50.

37. Wuerz, R.C., Travers, D., Gilboy, N., et al. (2001). Implementation and refinement of the emergency severity index. *Academic Emergency Medicine, 8,* 170-176.

38. Wyman, C. (n.d.). Conscious sedation a self-study guide. Retrieved 10/09/06 from www.gasnet.org/protocols/sedation/.

evolve **Did you remember to check out the bonus material on the Evolve website and the CD-ROM, including NCLEX®-Examination Style Review Questions, Open-Book Quizzes, and Chapter Review Audio Podcasts?**

http://evolve.elsevier.com/Black/medsurg

Index

NOTE: Page numbers followed by f indicate figures; those followed by t indicate tables; and those followed by b indicate boxed material.